Thyroid Function Test Reference Values

	Canine	Feline
T_4 (mcg/dl)	1.52-3.60	1.2-3.8
T_4 post-SH (mcg/dl)	>3- to 4-fold	>3- to 4-fold
T_3 (ng/dl)	48-154	–
T_3 post-TSH (ng/dl)	>10 ng increase	–
TSH (mIU/L)	0.14	0.37

Liver Function Test

Ammonia (mcg/dl)	45-120	
NH_3 post ATT (mcg/dl)	Minimal change from normal	No change from normal
Bile acids—fasting (μM)	<10	<2
Bile acids—2-hour postprandial (μM)	<15.5	<10

Normal Arterial Blood Gas Values and Ranges

	Human	Dog	Cat
pH	7.40 (7.35-7.45)	7.41 (7.35-7.46)	7.39 (7.31-7.46)
$PaCO_2$ (mm Hg)	40 (35-45)	37 (32-43)	31 (26-36)
Base deficit (mmol/L)	0 (–2 to +2)	–2 (+1 to –5)	–5 (–2 to –8)
Bicarbonate (mmol/L)	24 (22-26)	22 (18-26)	18 (14-22)
PaO_2 (mm Hg) (sea level)	95 (80-105)	92 (80-105)	107 (95-115)

Arterial vs. Venous Blood Gas Values for Normal Dogs

	Arterial	Mixed Venous	Jugular Venous	Cephalic Vein
pH	7.40 ± 0.03	7.36 ± 0.02	7.35 ± 0.02	7.36 ± 0.02
PCO_2 (mm Hg)	37 ± 3	43 ± 4	42 ± 5	43 ± 3
Base deficit (mmol/L)	–2 ± 2	–1 ± 1	–2 ± 2	–1 ± 1
Bicarbonate (mmol/L)	21 ± 2	23 ± 2	22 ± 2	23 ± 1
Total CO_2 (mmol/L)	22 ± 2	24 ± 2	23 ± 2	24 ± 2
PO_2 (mm Hg)	102 ± 7	53 ± 10	55 ± 10	58 ± 9

Coagulation Test Reference Ranges

	Canine	Feline
PT (sec)	6-11	6-12
PTT (sec)	10-25	10-25
FDP (mcg/ml)	<10	<10
D-dimer (ng/dl)	<250	<250
ACT (sec)	60-125	
BMBT (min)	1.7-4.2	1.4-2.4
Fibrinogen (mg/dl)	150-400	150-400

Urinalysis Reference Values

	Canine	Feline
Specific gravity		
Minimum	1.001	1.001
Maximum	1.060	1.080
Usual limits	1.018-1.050	1.018-1.050
Volume (ml/kg/day)	24-41	22-30
Osmolality (mOsm/kg)	500-1200	500-1200
Protein/creatinine ratio	<0.5 = normal 0.5-1.0 = gray zone >1.0 = abnormal	

Normal Adrenal Function Test Values

	Canine	Feline
Resting cortisol (mcg/dl)	1-5	6-18
Post-ACTH cortisol (mcg/dl)	0.5-5.5	6-12

Normal Fractional Electrolyte Clearance Values (%)

	Canine	Feline
Sodium	<1	<1
Chloride	<1	<1.3
Potassium	<20	<20
Phosphate	<40	<73

Cerebrospinal Fluid Analysis Reference for Dogs and Cats

Value	
Color	Colorless
Clarity	Transparent, clear
Refractive index	1.3347-1.3350
Protein concentration	Cisternal: <25 mg/dl Lumbar: <40 mg/dl
Total cell count	RBC: 0/μl WBC: <3/μl cisternal <5/μl lumbar
WBC differential count	Mononuclear cells Small mononuclear cells: 60%-70% Large mononuclear cells: 30%-40% Polymorphonuclear cells Neutrophils: <1% Eosinophils: <1% Others Ependymal lining cells: rare Nucleated RBC: rare in lumbar taps
Glucose (mg/dl)	61-116

RBC, Red blood cells; *WBC,* white blood cells.

Normal Synovial Fluid Values in Dogs and Cats

Value	
Amount	0.01-1 (ml)
Color	Clear/pale yellow
Viscosity	Very high
Mucin clot	Good
Spontaneous clot	None
White cells (mm^3)	<1000
Neutrophils	<5%
Mononuclear cells	>95%
Protein (g/dl)	2-2.5
Glucose (% of serum value)	>90

Categories of Effusions in Dogs and Cats

	Transudate	Modified Transudate	Exudate
Specific gravity	<1.017	1.017-1.025	>1.025
Total protein (g/dl)	<2.5	2.5-5.0	>3.0
Nucleated cell count (per μl)	<1000	500-10,000	>5,000
Predominant cell type	Mononuclear Mesothelial	Lymphocytes Monocytes Mesothelial RBCs Neutrophils	Neutrophils Mononuclear cells RBCs

SMALL ANIMAL CRITICAL CARE MEDICINE

SECOND EDITION

Deborah C. Silverstein, DVM, DACVECC
Associate Professor of Critical Care
Department of Clinical Studies
Matthew J. Ryan Veterinary Hospital
University of Pennsylvania
Philadelphia, Pennsylvania
Adjunct Professor
Temple University School of Pharmacy
Philadelphia, Pennsylvania

Kate Hopper, BVSc, PhD, DACVECC
Associate Professor of Small Animal Emergency & Critical Care
Department of Veterinary Surgical & Radiological Sciences
School of Veterinary Medicine
University of California–Davis
Davis, California

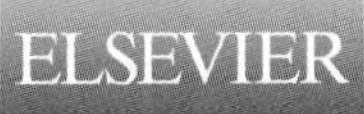

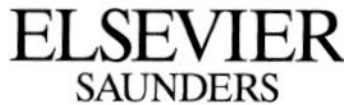

3251 Riverport Lane
St. Louis, Missouri 63043

SMALL ANIMAL CRITICAL CARE MEDICINE, SECOND EDITION ISBN: 978-1-4557-0306-7

International Standard Book Number: 978-1-4557-0306-7

Senior Vice President, Content: Loren Wilson
Content Strategy Director: Penny Rudolph
Content Development Specialist: Brandi Graham
Publishing Services Manager: Catherine Jackson
Senior Project Manager: David Stein
Design Direction: Ashley Eberts

Printed in Canada

Last digit is the print number: 9 8 7 6 5 4 3 2 1

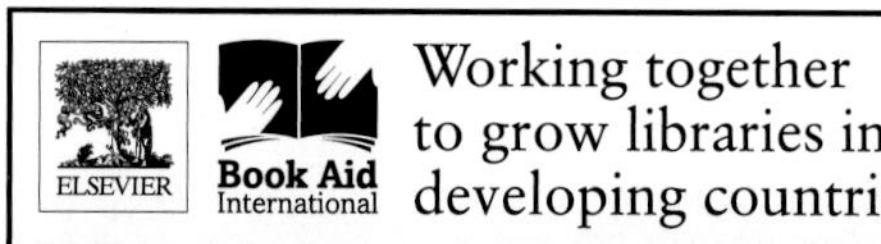

CONTRIBUTORS

Jonathan A. Abbott, DVM, DACVIM (Cardiology)
Associate Professor
Department of Small Animal Clinical Sciences
Virginia Maryland Regional College of Veterinary Medicine
Virginia Tech
Blacksburg, Virginia
Associate Professor
Department of Basic Sciences
Virginia Tech
Carilion School of Medicine
Roanoke, Virginia
Feline Cardiomyopathy

Sophie Adamantos, BVSc, CertVA, DACVECC, FHEA, MRCVS
Senior Lecturer in Emergency and Critical Care
Department of Veterinary Clinical Science
Royal Veterinary College
Hatfield, Hertfordshire, United Kingdom
Pulmonary Edema

Christopher A. Adin, DVM, DACVS
Associate Professor
Veterinary Clinical Sciences
The Ohio State University
Columbus, Ohio
Postthoracotomy Management

Ashley E. Allen-Durrance, DVM
Resident, EMCC
College of Veterinary Medicine
University of Florida
Gainsville, Florida
Magnesium and Phosphate Disorders

Robert A. Armentano, DVM, DACVIM
Small Animal Internist
Veterinary Medical Referral Services
Veterinary Specialty Center
Buffalo Grove, Illinois
Antitoxins and Antivenoms

Lillian R. Aronson, VMD, DACVS
Associate Professor of Surgery
Clinical Studies
University of Pennsylvania,
Philadelphia, Pennsylvania
Urosepsis
Kidney Transplantation

Anusha Balakrishnan, BVSc, AH
Resident, Emergency and Critical Care
Department of Clinical Studies–Philadelphia
School of Veterinary Medicine
University of Pennsylvania
Philadelphia, Pennsylvania
Shock Fluids and Fluid Challenge

Matthew W. Beal, DVM, DACVECC
Associate Professor, Emergency and Critical Care Medicine
Small Animal Clinical Sciences
Michigan State University
East Lansing, Michigan
Peritoneal Drainage Techniques

Allyson Berent, DVM, DACVIM (Internal Medicine)
Staff Doctor
Director of Interventional Endoscopy Services
Animal Medical Center
New York, New York
Hepatic Failure

Amanda K. Boag, MA, VetMB, DACVIM, DACVECC, MRCVS
Clinical Director
Vets Now
Dunfermline, Fife, United Kingdom
Aspiration Pneumonitis and Pneumonia
Pulmonary Contusions and Hemorrhage

Elise Mittleman Boller, DVM, DACVECC
Lecturer, Emergency and Critical Care
Faculty of Veterinary Sciences
University of Melbourne
Melbourne, Victoria, Australia
Sepsis and Septic Shock

Manuel Boller, DrMedVet, MTR, DACVECC
Senior Lecturer Emergency and Critical Care
Faculty of Veterinary Science
University of Melbourne
Melbourne, Victoria, Australia
Cardiopulmonary Resuscitation
Post–Cardiac Arrest Care

Dawn Merton Boothe, DVM, PhD, DACVIM (Internal Medicine), DACVCP
Professor, Director Clinical Pharmacology
Anatomy, Physiology, Pharmacology, and Department of Clinical Sciences
Auburn University
Montgomery, Alabama
Antimicrobial Use in the Critical Care Patient

Angela Borchers, DVM, DACVIM, DACVECC
Associate Veterinarian in Small Animal Emergency and Critical Care
William R. Pritchard Veterinary Medical Teaching Hospital
School of Veterinary Medicine
University of California, Davis,
Davis, California
Hemostatic Drugs

Søren R. Boysen, DVM, DACVECC
Associate Professor
Veterinary Clinical and Diagnostic Services
University of Calgary,
Calgary, Alberta, Canada
Gastrointestinal Hemorrhage
AFAST and TFAST in the Intensive Care Unit

Benjamin M. Brainard, VMD, DACVAA, DACVECC
Associate Professor, Critical Care
Small Animal Medicine and Surgery
College of Veterinary Medicine
University of Georgia
Athens, Georgia
Hypercoagulable States
Thrombocytopenia
Antiplatelet Drugs
Anticoagulants

Andrew J. Brown, MA, VetMB, MRCVS, DACVECC
Vets Now Referral Hospital
Glasgow, Scotland
Cardiogenic Shock
Rodenticides
Hemodynamic Monitoring

Scott Brown, VMD, PhD, DACVIM
Edward H. Gunst Professor of Small Animal Medicine
Department of Physiology and Pharmacology
College of Veterinary Medicine
The University of Georgia
Athens, Georgia
Hypertensive Crisis

Jamie M. Burkitt Creedon, DVM, DACVECC
Critical Consultations
Wichita Falls, Texas
Sodium Disorders
Critical Illness–Related Corticosteroid Insufficiency
Hypoadrenocorticism

Margret L. Casal, DrMedVet, PhD, DECAR
Associate Professor of Medical Genetics, Pediatrics, and Reproduction
Clinical Studies–Philadelphia
University of Pennsylvania,
Philadelphia, Pennsylvania
Mastitis

Ann M. Caulfield, VMD, CCRP, CVA
Director
Metropolitan Veterinary Associates
Rehabilitation Therapy
Norristown, Pennsylvania
Rehabilitation Therapy in the Critical Care Patient

Daniel L. Chan, DVM, DACVECC, DACVN, FHEA, MRCVS
Senior Lecturer in Emergency and Critical Care
Veterinary Clinical Sciences
The Royal Veterinary College,
North Mymms, Hertfordshire, Great Britain
Acute Lung Injury and Acute Respiratory Distress Syndrome
Nutritional Modulation of Critical Illness

Peter S. Chapman, BVetMed, DECVIM-CA, DACVIM (Internal Medicine), MRCVS
Staff Internist
Veterinary Specialty and Emergency Center
Levittown, Pennsylvania
Regurgitation and Vomiting

C.B. Chastain, DVM, MS, DACVIM (Internal Medicine)
Director of Undergraduate Biomedical Sciences
College of Veterinary Medicine
University of Missouri–Columbia
Columbia, Missouri
Syndrome of Inappropriate Antidiuretic Hormone

Dennis J. Chew, DVM, DACVIM (Internal Medicine)
Professor Emeritus
Veterinary Clinical Sciences
The Hospital for Companion Animals
Veterinary Clinical Sciences
College of Veterinary Medicine
The Ohio State University
Columbus, Ohio
Calcium Disorders

Dana L. Clarke, VMD, DACVECC
Lecturer in Interventional Radiology & Critical Care
Department of Small Animal Clinical Sciences
University of Pennsylvania
Philadelphia, Pennsylvania
Upper Airway Disease
Minimally Invasive Procedures

Melissa A. Claus, DVM, DACVECC
Lecturer
School of Veterinary and Biomedical Sciences
Murdoch University
Murdoch, Western Australia, Australia
Febrile Neutropenia

Leah A. Cohn, DVM, PhD, DACVIM (SAIM)
Professor
Department of Veterinary Medicine and Surgery
College of Veterinary Medicine
University of Missouri–Columbia
Columbia, Missouri
Acute Hemolytic Disorders

Edward Cooper, VMD, MS
Assistant Professor–Clinical
Veterinary Clinical Sciences
The Ohio State University
Columbus, Ohio
Hypotension

Etienne Côté, DVM, DACVIM (Cardiology, SAIM)
Associate Professor
Department of Companion Animals
Atlantic Veterinary College
University of Prince Edward Island
Charlottetown, Prince Edward Island, Canada
Pneumonia

M. Bronwyn Crane, DVM, MS, DACT
Assistant Professor
Health Management
Atlantic Veterinary College
University of Prince Edward Island
Charlottetown, Prince Edward Island, Canada
Pyometra

William T.N. Culp, VMD, DACVS
Assistant Professor
Department of Surgical and Radiological Sciences
University of California–Davis
Davis, California
Minimally Invasive Procedures
Thoracic and Abdominal Trauma

Meredith L. Daly, VMD, DACVECC
Director, Critical Care Service
Critical Care
Bluepearl Veterinary Partners
New York, New York
Hypoventilation
Fluoroquinolones

Emily Davis, DVM
Resident, Neurology
Department of Neurology and Neurosurgery
University of Pennsylvania
Philadelphia, Pennsylvania
Spinal Cord Injury

Harold Davis, BA, RVT, VTS (ECC) (Anesth)
Manager
Small Animal Emergency & Critical Care Service
William R. Pritchard Veterinary Medical Teaching Hospital
University of California–Davis
Davis, California
Peripheral Venous Catheterization
Central Venous Catheterization

Armelle de Laforcade, DVM, DACVECC
Associate Professor
Clinical Sciences
Tufts Cummings School of Veterinary Medicine
North Grafton, Massachusetts
Shock
Systemic Inflammatory Response Syndrome

Teresa DeFrancesco, DVM, DACVIM (CA), DACVECC
Professor of Cardiology and Critical Care
Department of Clinical Sciences
College of Veterinary Medicine
North Carolina State University
Raleigh, North Carolina
Temporary Cardiac Pacing

Amy Dixon-Jimenez, DVM
Cardiology Resident
Small Animal Medicine and Surgery
University of Georgia
Athens, Georgia
Anticoagulants

Suzanne Donahue, VMD, DACVECC
Veterinarian
Emergency/Critical Care
Hope Veterinary Specialists
Frazer, Pennsylvania
Chest Wall Disease

Patricia M. Dowling, DVM, MSc, DACVIM, DACVP
Professor
Veterinary Biomedical Sciences
Western College of Veterinary Medicine
Saskatoon, Saskatchewan, Canada
Motility Disorders
Anaphylaxis

Kenneth J. Drobatz, DVM, MSCE, DACVIM (Internal Medicine), DACVECC
Professor and Chief, Section of Critical Care
Department of Clinical Studies
Director, Emergency Service
Matthew J. Ryan Veterinary Hospital
School of Veterinary Medicine
University of Pennsylvania
Philadelphia, Pennsylvania
Acute Abdominal Pain
Heat Stroke

Adam E. Eatroff, DVM, DACVIM
Renal Medicine/Hemodialysis Unit
Animal Medical Center
New York, New York
Acute Kidney Injury
Chronic Kidney Disease

Melissa Edwards, DVM, DACVECC
Emergency and Critical Care Specialist
AVETS
Monroeville, Pennsylvania
Catheter-Related Bloodstream Infection

Laura Eirmann, DVM, DACVN
Nutritionist
Oradell Animal Hospital
Paramus, New Jersey
Veterinary Communications Manager
Nestle Purina Pet Care
St. Louis, Missouri
Enteral Nutrition
Parenteral Nutrition

Steven Epstein, DVM, DACVECC
Assistant Professor of Clinical Small Animal Emergency and Critical Care
Department of Surgical and Radiological Sciences
School of Veterinary Medicine
University of California–Davis
Davis, California
Care of the Ventilator Patient
Ventilator-Associated Pneumonia
Multidrug-Resistant Infections

Daniel J. Fletcher, PhD, DVM, DACVECC
Assistant Professor of Emergency and Critical Care
Clinical Sciences
College of Veterinary Medicine
Cornell University
Ithaca, New York
Cardiopulmonary Resuscitation
Post–Cardiac Arrest Care
Traumatic Brain Injury

Thierry Francey, DrMedVet, DACVIM
Diu Head, Small Animal Internal Medicine
Department of Clinical Veterinary Medicine
Vetsuisse Faculty University of Bern
Bern, Switzerland
Diuretics

Mack Fudge, DVM, MPVM, DACVECC
Colonel (ret)
U.S. Army Veterinary Corps
Helotes, Texas
Endotracheal Intubation and Tracheostomy

Caroline K. Garzotto, VMD, DACVS, CCRT
Owner, Surgeon
Veterinary Surgery of South Jersey, LLC
Haddonfield, New Jersey
Wound Management
Thermal Burn Injury

Alison R. Gaynor, DVM, DACVIM, DACVECC
Consultant
IDEXX Telemedicine
Portland, Oregon
Adjunct Assistant Professor
Department of Clinical Sciences
Cummings School of Veterinary Medicine
Tufts University
North Grafton, Massachusetts
Acute Pancreatitis

Urs Giger, PD, DrMedVet, MS, FVH, DACVIM, DECVIM-CA, DECVCP
Charlotte Newton Sheppard Professor of Medicine
Department of Clinical Studies
University of Pennsylvania
Philadelphia, Pennsylvania
Transfusion Therapy
Anemia

Massimo Giunti, DVM, PhD
Department of Veterinary Medical Science
University of Bologna
Bologna, Italy
Intraosseous Catheterization

Robert A.N. Goggs, BVSc, DACVECC, PhD, MRCVS
Lecturer, Emergency and Critical Care
Clinical Sciences
College of Veterinary Medicine
Cornell University
Ithaca, New York
Multiple Organ Dysfunction Syndrome
Aspiration Pneumonitis and Pneumonia

Richard E. Goldstein, DVM, DACVIM, DECVIM-CA
Chief Medical Officer
The Animal Medical Center
New York, New York
Diabetes Insipidus

Todd A. Green, DVM, MS, DACVIM (Internal Medicine)
Associate Professor
Small Animal Medicine and Surgery Program
School of Veterinary Medicine
St. George's University
Grenada, West Indies
Calcium Disorders

Reid P. Groman, DVM, DACVIM (Internal Medicine), DACVECC
Criticalist
Veterinary Specialty Center of Delaware
Castle, Delaware
Gram-Positive Infections
Gram-Negative Infections
Aminoglycosides
Miscellaneous Antibiotics

Julien Guillaumin, DrVet, DACVECC
Assistant Professor–Clinical–Emergency and Critical Care
Veterinary Clinical Sciences
The Ohio State University
Columbus, Ohio
Postthoracotomy Management

Tim B. Hackett, DVM, MS
Professor, Emergency and Critical Care Medicine
Clinical Sciences
Colorado State University
Fort Collins, Colorado
Physical Examination and Daily Assessment of the Critically Ill Patient

Susan G. Hackner, BVSc, MRCVS, DACVIM, DACVECC
Chief Medical Officer & Chief Operating Officer
Cornell University Veterinary Specialists
Stamford, Connecticut
Bleeding Disorders

Sarah Haldane, BVSc, BAnSc, MANZCVSc, DACVECC
Veterinary Science
University of Melbourne
Melbourne, Victoria, Australia
Nonsteroidal Antiinflammatory Drugs

Terry C. Hallowell, DVM, DACVECC
Critical Care Specialist
Critical Care
Allegheny Veterinary Emergency Trauma & Specialty
Monroeville, Pennsylvania
Urine Output

Ralph C. Harvey, DVM, MS, DACVAA
Associate Professor
Small Animal Clinical Sciences
College of Veterinary Medicine
University of Tennessee
Knoxville, Tennessee
Narcotic Agonists and Antagonists
Benzodiazepines

[†]Steve C. Haskins, DVM, MS, DACVAA, DACVECC
Professor Emeritus
Department of Surgery and Radiology
University of California–Davis
Davis, California
Hypoxemia
Catecholamines

Galina Hayes, BVSc, PhD, DACVECC
Department of Surgery
Valley Central Veterinary Referrals
Allentown, Pennsylvania
Illness Severity Scores in Veterinary Medicine

Rebecka S. Hess, DVM, DACVIM
Professor and Section Chief
Internal Medicine
University of Pennsylvania
Philadelphia, Pennsylvania
Diabetic Ketoacidosis
Hypothyroid Crisis in the Dog

Guillaume L. Hoareau, DrVet, DACVECC
Small Animal Emergency and Critical Care
William R. Pritchard Veterinary Medical Teaching Hospital
University of California–Davis
Davis, California
Brachycephalic Syndrome
Intraabdominal Pressure Monitoring

Daniel F. Hogan, DVM, DACVIM (Cardiology)
Associate Professor and Chief
Comparative Cardiovascular Medicine and Interventional Cardiology
Veterinary Clinical Sciences
Purdue University
West Lafayette, Indiana
Thrombolytic Agents

Steven R. Hollingsworth, DVM, DACVO
Associate Professor of Clinical Ophthalmology
Surgical and Radiological Sciences
University of California–Davis
Davis, California
Ocular Disease in the Intensive Care Unit

Bradford J. Holmberg, DVM, MS, PhD, DACVO
Animal Eye Center
Little Falls, New Jersey
Ocular Disease in the Intensive Care Unit

David Holt, BVSc, DACVS
Professor of Surgery
Department of Clinical Studies–Philadelphia
School of Veterinary Medicine
University of Pennsylvania
Philadelphia, Pennsylvania
Tracheal Trauma
Hepatic Encephalopathy

Kate Hopper, BVSc, PhD, DACVECC
Associate Professor of Small Animal Emergency & Critical Care
Department of Veterinary Surgical & Radiological Sciences
School of Veterinary Medicine
University of California–Davis
Davis, California
Hypertensive Crisis
Basic Mechanical Ventilation
Advanced Mechanical Ventilation
Discontinuing Mechanical Ventilation
Traditional Acid-Base Analysis
Nontraditional Acid-Base Analysis

Dez Hughes, BVSc, MRCVS, DACVECC
Associate Professor and Section Head, Emergency and Critical Care
Faculty of Veterinary Science
Associate Dean, eLearning
Faculty of Veterinary Science
University of Melbourne
Melbourne, Victoria, Australia
Pulmonary Edema
Hyperlactatemia

Daniel Z. Hume, DVM, DACVIM (Internal Medicine), DACVECC
Chief of Emergency and Critical Care
WestVet Animal Emergency and Specialty Center
Garden City, Idaho
Diarrhea

[†]Deceased.

Karen R. Humm, MA, VetMB, CertVA, DACVECC, MRCVS

Lecturer, Emergency and Critical Care
Department of Clinical Sciences & Services
The Royal Veterinary College, University of London
North Mymms, Hatfield, Hertfordshire
United Kingdom
Canine Parvovirus Infection

Karl E. Jandrey, DVM, MAS, DACVECC

Associate Professor of Clinical Small Animal Emergency and Critical Care
Department of Surgical and Radiological Sciences
University of California–Davis
Davis, California
Platelet Disorders
Abdominocentesis and Diagnostic Peritoneal Lavage

Shailen Jasani, MA, VetMB, MRCVS, DACVECC

Clinical Specialist
Vets Now Emergency Ltd.
Hertfordshire, United Kingdom
Smoke Inhalation

Lynelle R. Johnson, DVM, MS, PhD, DACVIM (SAIM)

Associate Professor
Medicine & Epidemiology
University of California–Davis
Davis, California
Pulmonary Thromboembolism

L. Ari Jutkowitz, VMD, DACVECC

Associate Professor
College of Veterinary Medicine
Michigan State University
East Lansing, Michigan
Massive Transfusion

Kayo Kanakubo, DVM

Resident, Clinical Nutrition
School of Veterinary Medicine
University of California–Davis
Davis, California
Blood Purification for Intoxications and Drug Overdose
Renal Replacement Therapies

Marie E. Kerl, DVM, MPH, DACVIM, DACVECC

Associate Teaching Professor
Department of Veterinary Medicine and Surgery
University of Missouri–Columbia
Columbia, Missouri
Fungal Infections
Antifungal Therapy

Lesley G. King, MVB, DACVECC, DACVIM (Internal Medicine)

Professor, Section of Critical Care
Department of Clinical Studies–Philadelphia
School of Veterinary Medicine
Director, Intensive Care Unit
Matthew J. Ryan Veterinary Hospital
University of Pennsylvania
Philadelphia, Pennsylvania
Calcium Channel Blocker and β-Blocker Drug Overdose
Management of the Intensive Care Unit

Marguerite F. Knipe, DVM, DACVIM (Neurology)

Health Sciences Assistant Clinical Professor, Neurology/Neurosurgery
Department of Surgical and Radiological Sciences
University of California–Davis
Davis, California
Deteriorating Mental Status

Amie Koenig, DVM, DACVIM (Internal Medicine), DACVECC

Associate Professor, Emergency and Critical Care
Department of Small Animal Medicine and Surgery
College of Veterinary Medicine
University of Georgia
Athens, Georgia
Hyperglycemic Hyperosmolar Syndrome
Hypoglycemia
Mycoplasma, Actinomyces, and Nocardia

Mary Anna Labato, DVM, DACVIM (Internal Medicine)

Clinical Professor, Department of Clinical Sciences
Section Head, Small Animal Medicine
Clinical Professor
Foster Hospital for Small Animals
Cummings School of Veterinary Medicine
Tufts University
North Grafton, Massachusetts
Antihypertensives

Catherine E. Langston, DVM, DACVIM (Internal Medicine)

Staff Doctor
Head of Renal Medicine and Hemodialysis
The Animal Medical Center
New York, New York
Acute Kidney Injury
Chronic Kidney Disease

Jennifer A. Larsen, DVM, PhD, DACVN

Assistant Professor of Clinical Nutrition
VM: Molecular Biosciences
University of California–Davis
Davis, California
Nutritional Assessment

Victoria S. Larson, BSc, DVM, MS, DACVIM (Oncology)
Adjunct Professor
Department of Clinical Sciences
University of Calgary
Calgary, Alberta, Canada
Staff Medical Oncologist
Oncology
Calgary Animal Referral and Emergency (Care) Centre
Calgary, Alberta, Canada
Complications of Chemotherapy Agents

Richard A. LeCouteur, BVSc, PhD, DACVIM (Neurology), DECVN
Professor of Neurology and Neurosurgery
Department of Surgical and Radiological Sciences
William R. Pritchard Veterinary Medical Teaching Hospital
School of Veterinary Medicine
University of California–Davis
Davis, California
Intracranial Hypertension

Justine A. Lee, DVM, DACVECC, DABT
CEO
VetGirl, LLC.
St. Paul, Minnesota
Nonrespiratory Look-Alikes
Approach to Drug Overdose
Analgesia and Constant Rate Infusions

Daniel Huw Lewis, MA, VetMB, CVA, DACVECC, MRCVS
Petmedics Veterinary Hospital
Petmedics (CVS) Ltd.
Manchester, Greater Manchester, United Kingdom
Multiple Organ Dysfunction Syndrome

Ronald Li, BSc, DVM, MVetMed, MRCVS
Senior Clinical Training Scholar in Emergency and Critical Care
Department of Veterinary Clinical Sciences
Queen Mother Hospital for Animals
The Royal Veterinary College
University of London
North Mymms, Hatfield, Hertfordshire, United Kingdom
Canine Parvovirus Infection

Debra T. Liu, DVM, DACVECC
Criticalist
Orange County Veterinary Specialists
Tustin, California
Veterinary Emergency Service
Fresno, California
Crystalloids, Colloids, and Hemoglobin-Based Oxygen-Carrying Solutions

Kristin A. MacDonald, DVM, PhD, DACVIM (Cardiology)
Veterinary Cardiologist
VCA–Animal Care Center of Sonoma
Rohnert Park, California
Infective Endocarditis

Maggie C. Machen
Resident, Cardiology
Ryan Hospital
School of Veterinary Medicine
University of Pennsylvania
Philadelphia, Pennsylvania
Ventricular Failure and Myocardial Infarction

Valerie Madden, DVM
Resident
College of Veterinary Medicine
Cornell University
Ithaca, New York
Complications of Chemotherapy Agents

Christina Maglaras, DVM
Resident, Small Animal Emergency and Critical Care
Department of Small Animal Medicine and Surgery
College of Veterinary Medicine
The University of Georgia
Athens, Georgia
Mycoplasma, Actinomyces, and Nocardia

Deborah C. Mandell, VMD, DACVECC
Staff Veterinarian, Emergency Service
Adjunct Associate Professor, Section of Critical Care
Emergency/Critical Care
Veterinary Hospital of the University of Pennsylvania
Philadelphia, Pennsylvania
Cardiogenic Shock
Pheochromocytoma
Methemoglobinemia
Pulmonary Artery Catheterization

F.A. (Tony) Mann, DVM, MS, DACVS, DACVECC
Professor
Veterinary Medicine and Surgery
University of Missouri–Columbia
Columbia, Missouri
Electrical and Lightning Injuries

Linda G. Martin, DVM, MS
Associate Professor, Emergency and Critical Care Medicine
Clinical Sciences
Auburn University
Auburn, Alabama
Magnesium and Phosphate Disorders

Christiane Massicotte, DVM, MS, PhD, DACVIM (Neurology)
Adjunct Faculty
Clinical Studies
University of Pennsylvania
Philadelphia, Pennsylvania
Neurologist
Animal Emergency and Referral Associates
Philadelphia, Pennsylvania
Diseases of the Motor Unit

Karol A. Mathews, DVM, DVSc, DACVECC
Professor Emerita
Clinical Studies
Ontario Veterinary College
University of Guelph
Guelph, Ontario, Canada
Illness Severity Scores in Veterinary Medicine

Elisa M. Mazzaferro, MS, DVM, PhD, DACVECC
Staff Criticalist
Cornell University Veterinary Specialist
Stamford, Connecticut
Oxygen Therapy
Perioperative Evaluation of the Critically Ill Patient
Arterial Catheterization

Robin L. McIntyre, DVM
Resident in Small Animal Emergency and Critical Care
Veterinary Medical Teaching Hospital
William R. Pritchard Veterinary Medical Teaching Hospital
University of California–Davis
Davis, California
Patient Suffering in the Intensive Care Unit
Cardiac Output Monitoring

Maureen McMichael, DVM, DACVECC
Associate Professor, Emergency & Critical Care Service Chief
Veterinary Clinical Medicine
Veterinary Teaching Hospital
University of Illinois
Urbana, Illinois
Prevention and Treatment of Transfusion Reactions
Critically Ill Neonatal and Pediatric Patients
Critically Ill Geriatric Patients

Margo Mehl, DVM, DACVS
VCA San Francisco Veterinary Specialists
Staff Surgeon
Surgery
San Francisco, California
Portosystemic Shunt Management

Matthew S. Mellema, DVM, PhD, DACVECC
Assistant Professor, Small Animal Emergency and Critical Care
Department of Veterinary Surgical and Radiological Sciences
University of California–Davis
Davis, California
Patient Suffering in the Intensive Care Unit
Brachycephalic Syndrome
Ventilator Waveforms
Cardiac Output Monitoring
Electrocardiogram Evaluation
Intraabdominal Pressure Monitoring

Kathryn E. Michel, DVM, MS, DACVN
Professor of Nutrition
Department of Clinical Studies
School of Veterinary Medicine
University of Pennsylvania
Philadelphia, Pennsylvania
Enteral Nutrition
Parenteral Nutrition

Carrie J. Miller, DVM, DACVIM (Internal Medicine)
Director of Internal Medicine
Virginia Veterinary Specialists
Charlottesville, Virginia
Allergic Airway Disease in Dogs and Cats and Feline Bronchopulmonary Disease
Inhaled Medications

James B. Miller, DVM, MS, DACVIM
Consultant
Antech Diagnostics
Stratford, Prince Edward Island, Canada
Hyperthermia and Fever

Adam Moeser, DVM, DACVIM (Neurology)
Veterinary Neurologist
Neurology/Neurosurgery
Animal Neurology and MRI Center
Commerce, Michigan
Anticonvulsants

Cynthia M. Otto, DVM, PhD, DACVECC
Associate Professor
Clinical Studies–Philadelphia
Executive Director
Penn Vet Working Dog Center
University of Pennsylvania
Philadelphia, Pennsylvania
Sepsis and Septic Shock
Intraosseous Catheterization

Trisha J. Oura, DVM, DACVR
Radiologist
Diagnostic Imaging
Tufts Veterinary Emergency Treatment & Specialties
Walpole, Massachusetts
Acute Lung Injury and Acute Respiratory Distress Syndrome

Mark A. Oyama, DVM, DACVIM (Cardiology)
Professor, Clinical Educator
Department of Clinical Studies–Philadelphia
University of Pennsylvania
Philadelphia, Pennsylvania
Mechanisms of Heart Failure

Carrie A. Palm, DVM, DACVIM
Assistant Professor of Clinical Small Animal Internal Medicine
Department of Medicine and Epidemiology
School of Veterinary Medicine
University of California–Davis
Davis, California
Blood Purification for Intoxications and Drug Overdose
Renal Replacement Therapies
Apheresis

Mark G. Papich, DVM, MS, DACVCP
Professor of Clinical Pharmacology
Veterinary Teaching Hospital
College of Veterinary Medicine
North Carolina State University
Raleigh, North Carolina
Strategies for Treating Infections in Critically Ill Patients

Romain Pariaut, DVM, DACVIM (Cardiology), DECVIM-CA (Cardiology)

Associate Professor of Cardiology
Veterinary Clinical Sciences
Louisiana State University
Baton Rouge, Louisiana
Bradyarrhythmias and Conduction Disturbances
Ventricular Tachyarrhythmias
Cardioversion and Defibrillation

Sandra Perkowski, VMD, PhD, DACVAA

Chief, Anesthesia Service
Clinical Studies–Philadelphia
School of Veterinary Medicine
University of Pennsylvania
Philadelphia, Pennsylvania
Pain and Sedation Assessment
Sedation of the Critically Ill Patient

Michele Pich, MA, MS

Veterinary Grief Counselor
Social Work
School of Veterinary Medicine
University of Pennsylvania
Philadelphia, Pennsylvania
Client Communication and Grief Counseling

Simon R. Platt, BVM&S, MRCVS, DACVIM (Neurology), DECVN

Professor of Neurology
Small Animal Medicine and Surgery
College of Veterinary Medicine
University of Georgia
Athens, Georgia
Coma Scales
Tetanus
Vestibular Disease

Lisa Leigh Powell, DVM, DACVECC

Veterinary Clinical Sciences
University of Minnesota
St. Paul, Minnesota
Drowning and Submersion Injury

Robert Prošek, DVM, MS, DACVIM (Cardiology), DECVIM-CA (Cardiology)

Adjunct Professor of Cardiology
Department of Small Animal Medicine and Surgery
University of Florida
Gainesville, Florida
President
Florida Veterinary Cardiology
Miami Beach; South Miami; Ocean Reef; Homestead; Key West, Florida
Canine Cardiomyopathy

Bruno H. Pypendop, DrMedVet, DrVetSci, DACVAA

Professor
Department of Surgical and Radiological Sciences
School of Veterinary Medicine
University of California–Davis
Davis, California
Jet Ventilation
α_2 Agonists and Antagonists
Capnography

Jane Quandt, BS, DVM, MS, DACVAA, DACVECC

Associate Professor–Comparative Anesthesia
Small Animal Medicine and Surgery
College of Veterinary Medicine
University of Georgia
Athens, Georgia
Anesthesia in the Critically Ill Patient
Analgesia and Constant Rate Infusions

Louisa J. Rahilly, DVM, DACVECC

Medical Director
Emergency and Critical Care
Cape Cod Veterinary Specialists
Buzzards Bay, Massachusetts
Methemoglobinemia

Alan G. Ralph, DVM, DACVECC

Resident in Emergency and Critical Care Medicine
Department of Small Animal Clinical Sciences
College of Veterinary Medicine
Michigan State University
East Lansing, Michigan
Hypercoagulable States

Shelley C. Rankin, BSc (Hons), PhD

Associate Professor Clinician Educator of Microbiology
School of Veterinary Medicine
University of Pennsylvania
Philadelphia, Pennsylvania
Nosocomial Infections and Zoonoses

Alan H. Rebar, DVM, PhD, DACVP

Senior Associate Vice President for Research
Professor of Veterinary Clinical Pathology
Department of Comparative Pathology
College of Veterinary Medicine
Purdue University
West Lafayette, Indiana
Blood Film Evaluation

Erica L. Reineke, VMD, DACVECC

Assistant Professor of Emergency and Critical Care Medicine
Clinical Studies–Philadelphia
School of Veterinary Medicine
University of Pennsylvania
Philadelphia, Pennsylvania
Evaluation and Triage of the Critically Ill Patient
Serotonin Syndrome

Adam J. Reiss, DVM, DACVECC

Staff Veterinarian
Southern Oregon Veterinary Specialty Center
Medford, Oregon
Myocardial Contusion

Caryn Reynolds, DVM, DACVIM (Cardiology)

Staff Cardiologist
Veterinary Emergency and Specialty Center of New Mexico
Albuquerque, New Mexico
Bradyarrhythmias and Conduction Disturbances

Laura L. Riordan, DVM, DACVIM

Florida Veterinary Referral Center
Estero, Florida
Potassium Disorders

Joris H. Robben, DVM, PhD, DECVIM-CA
Associate Professor, Emergency and Intensive Care Medicine
Department of Clinical Sciences of Companion Animals
Faculty of Veterinary Medicine
Utrecht University
Utrecht, the Netherlands
Intensive Care Unit Facility Design

Narda G. Robinson, DO, DVM, MS, FAAMA
Director, CSU Center for Comparative and Integrative Pain Medicine
Clinical Sciences
Colorado State University
Fort Collins, Colorado
Complementary and Alternative Medicine

Mark P. Rondeau, DVM, DACVIM (Internal Medicine)
Staff Veterinarian
Department of Clinical Studies–Philadelphia
School of Veterinary Medicine
University of Pennsylvania
Philadelphia, Pennsylvania
Acute Cholecystitis
Hepatitis and Cholangiohepatitis

Patricia G. Rosenstein, DVM
Emergency Veterinarian
Veterinary Hospital
The University of Melbourne
South Yarra, Victoria, Australia
Hyperlactatemia

Alexandre Rousseau, DVM, DACVIM (Internal Medicine), DACVECC
Cornell University Veterinary Specialists
Stamford, Connecticut
Bleeding Disorders

Elizabeth A. Rozanski, DVM, DACVIM, DACVECC
Associate Professor
Clinical Sciences
Tufts Cummings School of Veterinary Medicine
North Grafton, Massachusetts
Acute Lung Injury and Acute Respiratory Distress Syndrome

Elke Rudloff, DVM, DACVECC
Residency Training Supervisor
Lakeshore Veterinary Specialists
Glendale, Wisconsin
Assessment of Hydration
Necrotizing Soft Tissue Infections

Kari Santoro-Beer, DVM, DACVECC
Lecturer, Critical Care
Department of Clinical Studies–Philadelphia
Matthew J. Ryan Veterinary Hospital
University of Pennsylvania
Philadelphia, Pennsylvania
Daily Intravenous Fluid Therapy
Pheochromocytoma

Valérie Sauvé, DVM, DACVECC
Head of Critical Care
Emergency and Critical Care
Centre Vétérinaire DMV
Montreal, Quebec, Canada
Pleural Space Disease

Emily Savino, CVT, VTS (ECC)
ICU Nursing Supervisor
Matthew J. Ryan Veterinary Hospital
University of Pennsylvania
Philadelphia, Pennsylvania
Management of the Intensive Care Unit

Michael Schaer, DVM, DACVIM (Internal Medicine), DACVECC
Professor Emeritus
Small Animal Clinical Sciences; Section of Emergency and Critical Care
University of Florida
Gainesville, Florida
Potassium Disorders
Antitoxins and Antivenoms

Sergio Serrano, LV, DVM, DACVECC, MBA
Medical Director, Criticalist
Connecticut Veterinary Center
West Hartford, Connecticut
Pulmonary Contusions and Hemorrhage

Claire R. Sharp, BSc, BVMS (Hons), MS, DACVECC
Assistant Professor
Clinical Sciences
Tufts Cummings School of Veterinary Medicine
North Grafton, Massachusetts
Gastric Dilatation-Volvulus

Scott P. Shaw, DVM, DACVECC
Medical Director
New England Veterinary Center & Cancer Care
Windsor, Massachusetts
β-Lactam Antimicrobials
Macrolides

Nadja E. Sigrist, DrMedVet, FVH, DACVECC
VET ECC CE
Affoltern am Albis
Zürich, Switzerland
Thoracocentesis
Thoracostomy Tube Placement and Drainage

Deborah C. Silverstein, DVM, DACVECC

Associate Professor of Critical Care
Department of Clinical Studies
Matthew J. Ryan Veterinary Hospital
University of Pennsylvania
Philadelphia, Pennsylvania
Adjunct Professor
Temple University School of Pharmacy
Philadelphia, Pennsylvania
Shock
Chest Wall Disease
Crystalloids, Colloids, and Hemoglobin-Based Oxygen-Carrying Solutions
Daily Intravenous Fluid Therapy
Shock Fluids and Fluid Challenge
Thoracic and Abdominal Trauma
Vasopressin
Fluoroquinolones

Meg Sleeper, VMD, DACVIM (Cardiology)

Associate Professor of Cardiology
Clinical Studies–Philadelphia
University of Pennsylvania Veterinary School
Philadelphia, Pennsylvania
Ventricular Failure and Myocardial Infarction
Myocarditis

Sean Smarick, VMD, DACVECC

Hospital Director
AVETS
Monroeville, Pennsylvania
Catheter-Related Bloodstream Infection
Urine Output
Urinary Catheterization

Lisa Smart, BVSc (Hons), DACVECC

Senior Lecturer, Veterinary Emergency and Critical Care
School of Veterinary and Life Sciences, College of Veterinary Medicine
Murdoch University
Murdoch, Western Australia, Australia
Ventilator-Induced Lung Injury

Laurie Sorrell-Raschi, DVM, DACVAA, RRT

Anesthesiologist
Anesthesia/Pain Management and Complementary Therapy
Veterinary Specialty Center of Delaware
New Castle, Delaware
Blood Gas and Oximetry Monitoring

Sheldon A. Steinberg, VMD, DMSc, DACVIM (Neurology), DECVN

Emeritus Professor of Neurology/Neurosurgery
Clinical Studies–Philadelphia
School of Veterinary Medicine
University of Pennsylvania
Philadelphia, Pennsylvania
Anticonvulsants

Randolph H. Stewart, DVM, PhD

Clinical Associate Professor
Veterinary Physiology & Pharmacology
Texas A&M University
College Station, Texas
Interstitial Edema

Beverly K. Sturges, DVM, MS, DACVIM (Neurology)

Radiological & Surgical Sciences
University of California–Davis
Davis, California
Intracranial Hypertension
Intracranial Pressure Monitoring
Cerebrospinal Fluid Sampling

Jane E. Sykes, BVSc (Hons), PhD, DACVIM

Professor
Medicine and Epidemiology
University of California–Davis
Davis, California
Viral Infections

Rebecca S. Syring, DVM, DACVECC

Critical Care Specialist
Veterinary Specialty and Emergency Center
Levittown, Pennsylvania
Traumatic Brain Injury

Jeffrey M. Todd, DVM, DACVECC

Assistant Clinical Professor
Department of Veterinary Clinical Sciences
College of Veterinary Medicine
Veterinary Medical Center
University of Minnesota
St. Paul, Minnesota
Hypothermia

Tara K. Trotman, VMD, DACVIM (Internal Medicine)

Internal Medicine Consultant
Idexx Laboratories
Westbrook, Maine
Gastroenteritis

Karen M. Vernau, DVM, MAS, DACVIM (Neurology)

Associate Clinical Professor of Neurology/Neurosurgery
Surgical and Radiological Sciences
University of California–Davis
Davis, California
Seizures and Status Epilepticus

Cecilia Villaverde, BVSc, PhD, DACVN, DECVCN

Assistant Professor
Ciencia Animal i dels Aliments
Universitat Autònoma de Barcelona
Bellaterra, Barcelona, Spain
Chief of Service
Servei de Dietètica i Nutrició
Fundació Hospital Clínic Veterinari
Universitat Autònoma de Barcelona
Bellaterra, Barcelona, Spain
Nutritional Assessment

Charles H. Vite, DVM, PhD, DACVIM (Neurology)

Associate Professor, Neurology
Clinical Studies
School of Veterinary Medicine
University of Pennsylvania
Philadelphia, Pennsylvania
Spinal Cord Injury

Susan W. Volk, VMD, PhD, DACVS

Assistant Professor of Small Animal Surgery
Department of Clinical Studies–Philadelphia
School of Veterinary Medicine
University of Pennsylvania
Philadelphia, Pennsylvania
Peritonitis

Lori S. Waddell, DVM, DACVECC

Adjunct Assistant Professor, Critical Care
Department of Clinical Studies–Philadelphia
Matthew J. Ryan Veterinary Hospital
School of Veterinary Medicine
University of Pennsylvania
Philadelphia, Pennsylvania
Rodenticides
Hemodynamic Monitoring
Colloid Osmotic Pressure and Osmolality Monitoring

Andrea Wang, DVM, MA, DACVIM

Small Animal Internist, Board Certified
Advanced Veterinary Care
Salt Lake City, Utah
Thrombocytopenia

Cynthia R. Ward, VMD, PhD, DACVIM (Internal Medicine)

Professor, Small Animal Internal Medicine
Small Animal Medicine and Surgery
College of Veterinary Medicine
University of Georgia
Athens, Georgia
Thyroid Storm

Wendy A. Ware, DVM, MS, DACVIM (Cardiology)

Professor
Departments of Veterinary Clinical Sciences and Biomedical Sciences
Iowa State University
Ames, Iowa
Pericardial Diseases

Aaron C. Wey, DVM, DACVIM (Cardiology)

Owner
Cardiology
Upstate Veterinary Specialties, PLLC
Latham, New York
Valvular Heart Disease

Michael D. Willard, DVM, MS, DACVIM (Internal Medicine)

Professor
Department of Small Animal Clinical Sciences
Texas A&M University
College Station, Texas
Gastrointestinal Protectants
Antiemetics and Prokinetics

Kevin P. Winkler, DVM, DACVS

Surgeon
Georgia Veterinary Specialists
Atlanta, Georgia
Necrotizing Soft Tissue Infections

Annie Malouin Wright, DVM, DACVECC

Staff Criticalist
Critical Care
BluePearl Minnesota
Eden Prairie, Minnesota
Sedative, Muscle Relaxant, and Narcotic Overdose
Calcium Channel Blocker and β-Blocker Drug Overdose

Bonnie Wright, DVM, DACVAA

Associate
Fort Collins Veterinary Emergency & Rehabilitation Hospital
Fort Collins, Colorado
Air Embolism

Kathy N. Wright, DVM, DACVIM (Cardiology; Internal Medicine)

Lead Cardiologist, Cincinnati and Dayton locations
MedVet Medical and Cancer Center for Pets
Cincinnati and Dayton, Ohio
Supraventricular Tachyarrhythmias
Antiarrhythmic Agents

PREFACE

The field of critical care is an exciting one and rapidly growing in both human and veterinary medicine. New developments and recommendations are evolving faster than ever, making it especially important for veterinarians to have an up-to-date resource when caring for critically ill dogs and cats. The second edition of *Small Animal Critical Care Medicine* reflects the current knowledge of experts in the field, with extensive citations to the veterinary and medical literature at the end of each chapter. It builds upon the strong foundation of the first edition, focusing on a comprehensive approach to critical care medicine, from the pathophysiology of disease states to interpretation of diagnostic tests and descriptions of medical techniques that are unique to this specialty. In this edition, there is a greater focus on critical care medicine and fewer chapters devoted to routine care of emergent patients. There are 32 new chapters and all remaining chapters have been updated or completely rewritten. We are delighted to welcome many new contributors; this edition represents the work of over 150 authors from around the world. The scope of topics is broad and clinically oriented, helping practitioners provide the highest standard of care for their critically ill small animal patients. As with the first edition, this textbook is intended to be an essential, state-of-the-art resource for anyone working with critically ill patients in general practice settings, specialty veterinary practices, and university teaching hospitals.

An exciting feature of this new edition is its full-color layout, enabling effortless visibility of relevant color photographs throughout each chapter. The organization of this new edition has changed slightly, including a large section dedicated to intensive care unit procedures. All the chapters start with key points to quickly provide the reader with the most important take-home messages for each topic. The appendices provide an outstanding resource of useful information gathered together in one easy-to-access location, including lists of formulas, reference values, and constant rate infusion doses.

This text includes 23 major sections with 211 chapters that cover all aspects of critical care medicine. Several chapters of this new edition deserve to be highlighted. The chapter on cardiopulmonary resuscitation was rewritten and a new chapter on post-resuscitation care added, both authored by Daniel J. Fletcher and Manuel Boller, the current leaders of veterinary CPR and the RECOVER project. Another new chapter explores mechanisms of patient suffering in the intensive care unit, an immensely important but poorly recognized subject to date. The respiratory section has been broadened, with a stronger emphasis on the physiology of respiratory failure and new chapters on tracheobronchial injury and brachycephalic syndrome. In addition, the following chapters deserve special attention:

- The mechanical ventilation section has been expanded and represents the most thorough and advanced review of mechanical ventilation currently available for veterinary patients
- The acid-base and hyperlactatemia chapters have been completely rewritten and a new chapter reviewing nontraditional approaches to acid-base analysis has been added.
- The fluid therapy section has been completely rewritten and includes two new transfusion therapy chapters.
- There is a new section on therapeutic drug overdose, a well-recognized issue in the intensive care unit, that includes a new chapter on the role of blood purification in the treatment of toxins and drug overdose.
- There is a major emphasis on infectious diseases and antimicrobial therapy, including new chapters on approaches to multidrug-resistant infections and advanced antimicrobial strategies for critical patients.
- The focus on coagulation has been expanded, with outstanding chapters on antiplatelet drugs and hemostatic drugs.
- A new section focuses on intensive care unit design and management, areas unique to the field of critical care medicine that have not been addressed in previous veterinary publications.
- There are new chapters on such topics as noninvasive surgery and interventional radiology, AFAST/TFAST in the intensive care unit, and the pharmacology of antitoxins and antivenoms.

Critical care medicine poses a unique set of challenges and rewards, and the editors intend for this book to continue to fill the gap that exists between basic medical and surgical references and the available emergency-oriented manuals. Ultimately, we hope that this book will enable veterinarians, who have committed themselves to the knowledgeable and skillful care of their patients, to better deliver on that solemn promise and enhance both quality of life for pets and the ongoing relationship with those who love them.

ACKNOWLEDGMENTS

The editors are most appreciative to all of the Elsevier staff, especially Penny Rudolph, Brandi Graham, and David Stein, who made this textbook possible. We would also like to thank all of our contributors; it is their invaluable time and effort that have made this edition such an incredible resource for all veterinarians.

The second edition of this book would not have been possible without the love and support of my husband, Stefan, and precious boys, Maxwell and Henry. Thank you to all of our dedicated contributors, colleagues and mentors, as well as to my amazing co-editor, Kate. Although I am not convinced the second edition was any easier than the first, the "team" that made it possible is truly amazing! I feel honored to have worked with each and every one of you.

—Deb

For all the amazing mentors I have had from day one of my veterinary career. People such as Russell Mitten, Peter Irwin, Glen Edwards, Philip Hartney, Ava Firth, Steve Haskins, Janet Aldrich, Matt Mellema and Deb Silverstein. Each and every one of you showed me what being a clinician and a teacher really means. Thank you.

—Kate

In loving memory of all of our family and colleagues that have left this world prematurely and are missed so dearly every day, especially MaryLee Dombrowski, Sharon Drellich, and Dougie Macintire. You will never be forgotten. And last, but certainly not least, this book is in memory of Steve Haskins, who passed away shortly after contributing to this book. Neither of us would be where we are today if this amazing man had not touched our lives in such a positive and immeasurable way. To Steve and all of our loved ones, this book is for you.

—Deb and Kate

CONTENTS

Part V: Electrolyte and Acid-Base Disturbances

Part VI: Fluid Therapy

Part VII: Endocrine Disorders

Part VIII: Therapeutic Drug Overdose

Part IX: Neurologic Disorders

Part X: Infectious Disorders

Part XIX: Miscellaneous Disorders

Part XX: Pharmacology

Part XXI: Monitoring

Part XXII: Procedures

Part XXIII: ICU Design and Management

PART I KEY CRITICAL CARE CONCEPTS

CHAPTER 1

EVALUATION AND TRIAGE OF THE CRITICALLY ILL PATIENT

Erica L. Reineke, VMD, DACVECC

KEY POINTS

- *Triage* refers to the sorting of ill animals for treatment based on priority when resources are insufficient for all to be treated immediately.
- The use of triage lists may help to categorize patients based on treatment priority along with targeted waiting times.
- The triage examination consists of a *primary survey,* in which the cardiovascular, respiratory, neurologic, and urinary systems are evaluated to identify life-threatening abnormalities. It includes both subjective and objective assessments.
- Intravenous catheterization, emergency blood testing, and a FAST ultrasound evaluation can offer additional information to guide patient stabilization procedures.
- The *secondary survey,* or a more thorough physical examination, should be performed once the animal is stabilized.

INTRODUCTION

Triage, derived from the French word *trier,* refers to the sorting of patients for treatment priority when resources are insufficient for all to be treated immediately in an emergency setting. The roots of triage can be traced to the battlefields in the mid-1800s where the medical needs of military casualties were prioritized. Military triage was refined during subsequent wars and demonstrated that early triage assessment and prompt resuscitation significantly reduced mortality rates.[1] The utility of military triage captured the attention of hospital providers, and during the late 1970s emergency departments began to develop their own triage systems.[2]

In veterinary medicine the term *triage* is also used to describe the sorting of animals in an emergency department based on medical priority: the sickest are treated first. Rapid and accurate triage of the animal is also essential for a successful veterinary emergency department. An initial, brief assessment of the animal (described later) is performed by a trained veterinary technician and a veterinarian to identify those animals needing immediate, lifesaving interventions. If multiple emergent animals are presented at the same time, the veterinary medical team must determine how long the animals can safely wait.[3] Less urgent cases are typically treated on a "first come, first served" basis.

TRIAGE SYSTEMS

Triage systems have been developed for use in people to improve the acuity of triage because of the overcrowding of human emergency departments and prolonged waiting times.[3] These systems provide clear guidelines on how to assess the patient's clinical needs and priority for care. Many different triage systems, such as the Emergency Severity Index, Australasian Triage Scale, Canadian Triage & Acuity Scale, and Manchester Triage System, have been developed and validated for use in human emergency departments. These triage systems typically use a 5-level system to categorize patients (e.g., 1, resuscitation [red]; 2, emergent [orange]; 3, urgent [yellow]; 4, less urgent [blue]; 5, nonurgent [green]). Each level has an associated time required for physician assessment; all level 1 patients must be treated immediately.[4,5] The triage systems are generally based on vital signs (e.g., heart rate, respiratory rate) and, in some systems, on a presenting complaint algorithm.[6] In these systems, triage is generally performed by an emergency department nurse. However, in some recent studies, physician triage has been implemented in which a designated physician is used to intervene early in a patient's emergency department course to guide triage or accelerate the initial evaluation and treatment of patients. These studies have found that time to initial physician evaluation, length of stay, and number of patients leaving without being seen were reduced.[7-9]

The first veterinary triage scoring system was developed at the University of Pennsylvania for animals presented for treatment after acute trauma.[10] The Animal Trauma Triage (ATT) scoring system was devised to provide stratification of veterinary trauma patients. Although primarily developed for clinical research and outcome prediction, this scoring system may also be useful in identifying trauma patients requiring immediate medical or surgical intervention. In this system, physical examination findings in six categories (perfusion, cardiac, respiratory, eye/muscle/integument, skeletal, and neurologic) are scored on a 0 to 3 scale in which 0 indicates slight or no injury and 3 indicates severe injury. In this system, animals with higher ATT scores would receive treatment priority compared with animals with lower ATT scores. In several studies the ATT score has been shown to predict survival; animals with higher ATT scores are less likely to survive compared with animals with lower scores.[11-14]

More recently a veterinary triage list (VTL) based on a human 5-point scoring system was developed and evaluated for use in categorizing all emergency patients. In this triage system, animals are categorized into color-coded triage categories along with target waiting times: red, immediate; orange, 15 minutes; yellow, 30 to 60 minutes; green, 120 minutes. The VTL described in this study was developed by modifying the Manchester triage scale with common clinical conditions seen in veterinary medicine. For example, animals with severe decompensatory shock, exsanguinating hemorrhage, severe respiratory distress, or seizures would be triaged as red and require immediate treatment, whereas animals with mild respiratory distress, uncontrollable minor hemorrhage, and history of unconsciousness would be triaged to a yellow category. In this study, intuitive triage performed by trained veterinary technicians based on the medical history and a visual examination of the animal was compared with a retrospective evaluation of the VTL applied by a veterinary review team. The results of this study suggested that the use of the VTL was more effective at categorizing emergency patients with target waiting times as compared with intuitive triage performed by the veterinary technicians.[15] Although future prospective studies are needed to validate this veterinary triage list, this study raises awareness of the importance of triage and appropriate target waiting times in veterinary medicine, especially in a busy emergency service where resources may be limited.

INITIAL PATIENT TRIAGE

On arrival to the emergency service, an initial brief triage assessment of the animal should be performed. At the author's institution, experienced veterinary technicians who exclusively work in the emergency service and have specific training in veterinary triage typically perform this first assessment. The technician first obtains a brief medical history from the owner, including patient signalment, the reason for seeking medical care, and concurrent medical conditions. A brief visual inspection of the animal and a focused physical examination may be performed in the triage area. The brief focused physical examination includes an evaluation of the respiratory, cardiovascular, neurologic, and urinary systems.[16] Abnormalities in other organ systems, such as the gastrointestinal tract, may not be immediately life threatening but could result in significant intravascular fluid losses and hypotension, which are apparent during the cardiovascular evaluation. Patients with an abnormality in any of these four systems are brought quickly to the treatment area for a doctor assessment. Other conditions that warrant immediate evaluation by a veterinarian include severe pain, recent ingestion of a toxin or signs of intoxication, recent seizures, trauma, active bleeding, prolapsed organs, recent snake bites, hyperthermia or hypothermia, open wounds, fractures, burns, dystocia, and death.[17]

If the animal is triaged as needing immediate medical intervention, it should be brought quickly to the treatment area for assessment by a veterinarian. At this time, verbal permission or signed medical consent should be obtained from the owner that authorizes the veterinary hospital to initiate medical treatment or diagnostics and outlines the cost of this care. This approach allows for stabilizing treatments to be initiated immediately without removing the veterinarian from the treatment area. The triage area in the treatment room should be equipped with supplies to treat a critically ill animal, including an oxygen supply, supplies for intravenous or intraosseous catheterization, intravenous fluids, continuous electrocardiography (ECG), blood pressure measuring equipment, and a crash cart. The crash cart should be fully stocked with items needed for cardiopulmonary arrest, such as endotracheal tubes, laryngoscope, electrical defibrillator, and drugs for resuscitation (see Chapter 3). In-house laboratory equipment should be available for performing emergency blood testing, including but not limited to a minimum database (packed cell volume [PCV], total solids [TS], glucose, and blood urea nitrogen), blood gas evaluation, and lactate.

Primary Survey

The primary survey includes evaluation of the same physical parameters as performed during the technician triage, but it is much more detailed and may involve both subjective and objective evaluations (Figure 1-1). It should be performed quickly (<2 minutes) to allow for initiation of lifesaving therapies.

Respiratory system evaluation

Evaluation of the respiratory system is focused on determining the presence or absence of hypoxemia or hypoventilation (see Chapters 15 and 16). Prolonged hypoxemia and poor tissue oxygen delivery may result in multiple organ failure and therefore should be treated immediately. During evaluation of the respiratory system, the patency of the upper airway should be assessed first. If the patient is not breathing, immediate endotracheal intubation should be performed and positive pressure ventilation should be initiated (see Chapter 3). The presence of stertor or stridor, along with an increased inspiratory effort, may indicate an upper airway obstruction, and these animals should be brought immediately to the treatment area and administered supplemental oxygen (see Chapter 17).[18]

If the animal has a patent airway, the respiratory rate and effort (movement of the chest wall and abdomen and evaluation for paradoxical breathing efforts) along with mucous membrane color should be assessed; the trachea and thorax should also be auscultated. Cyanotic mucous membranes are considered to be a late and severe sign of hypoxemia. If significant abnormalities, such as dull lung sounds, pulmonary crackles, or wheezes, are auscultated along with an increased respiratory effort, the animal should be administered supplemental oxygen until more objective assessments can be made (see Chapter 15). Although tachypnea can indicate the presence of hypoxemia, it can also be associated with concurrent hypovolemia, pain, abdominal distention, and fear (see Chapter 29). Animals that have tachypnea secondary to respiratory compromise will also typically have an increased respiratory effort.

If tachypnea (respiratory rate > 40 breaths/min) or other abnormalities in the respiratory system are identified during the primary survey, a more objective noninvasive assessment of the blood oxygen content via pulse oximetry should be obtained. A pulse oximetry reading of at least 95% is normal; values less than 95% (corresponding to a $PaO_2 < 80$ mm Hg) indicate hypoxemia.[19] Arterial blood gas analysis, although more invasive than pulse oximetry, can also be useful in determining if hypoxemia is present (see Chapter 186).

If hypoxemia is suspected based on the animal's triage evaluation, supplemental oxygen therapy (either by mask, flow-by, or cage) should be instituted immediately and the clinical response to treatment should be evaluated. Definitive treatment for the cause of respiratory compromise (e.g., needle thoracocentesis if pleural space disease is suspected) should be provided as soon as possible.

There are unique considerations for the feline patient with clinical signs of respiratory distress. Generally, increased respiratory rate and effort along with open-mouth breathing indicate the presence of severe hypoxemia in cats. Even minor manipulations, such as performing a physical examination or placement of an intravenous catheter, can lead to respiratory and cardiac arrest. These cats often benefit from being placed immediately in an oxygen cage before performing a complete primary survey. The cat should be monitored closely for a brief period for improvement in the respiratory signs. Once the cat's respiratory signs have improved, the primary survey should be completed, or, if the size of the oxygen cage allows, the initial assessment of the cat can be performed within the oxygen cage itself.

Cardiovascular system evaluation

The evaluation of the cardiovascular system is done to identify poor tissue perfusion resulting in decreased tissue oxygen delivery. If inadequate tissue perfusion is not recognized and treated emergently, critical tissue hypoxia may result, triggering a cascade of events that could result in multiple organ dysfunction and death.[20] Conditions

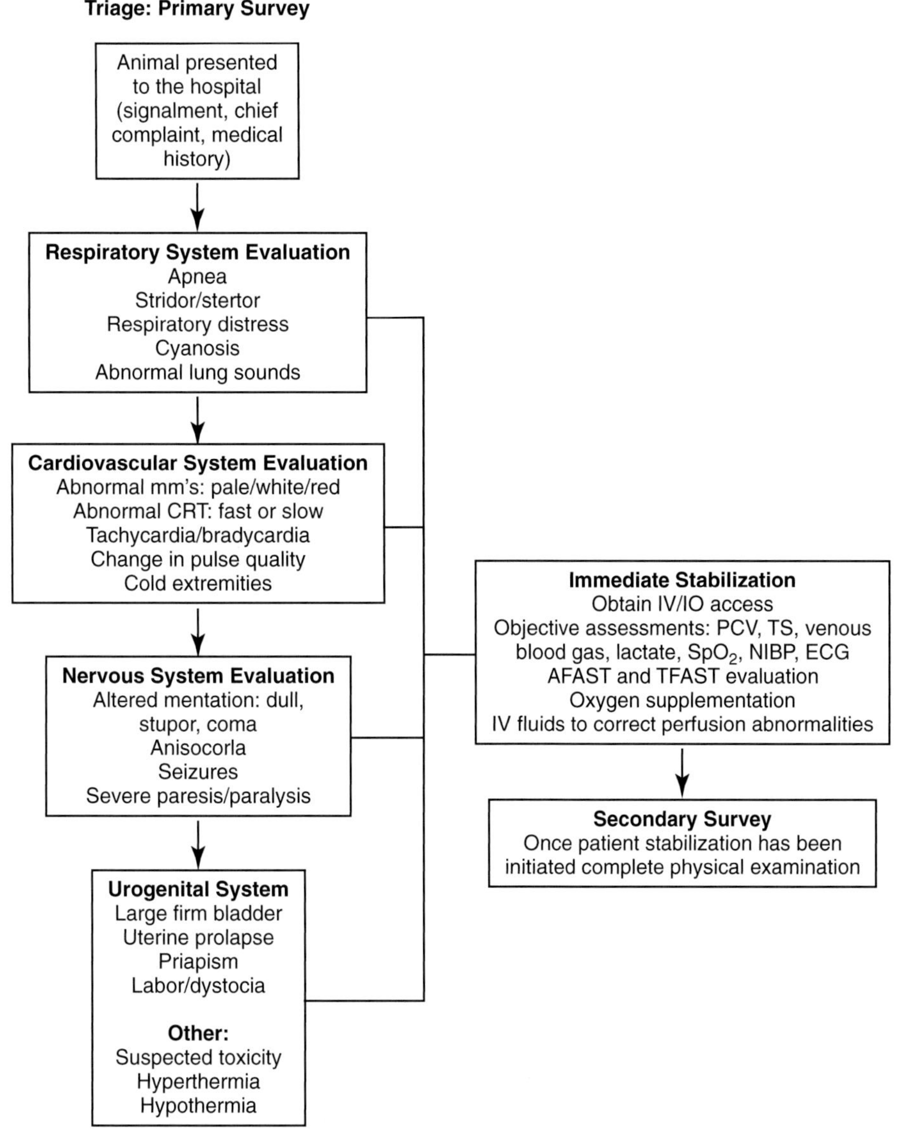

FIGURE 1-1 Triage algorithm for emergent small-animal patients that includes a primary survey and immediate stabilization.

that can result in poor tissue perfusion and clinical signs of shock include hypovolemia, cardiac disease, cardiac arrhythmias, and vasodilatory states such as sepsis or systemic inflammatory response syndrome (SIRS) (see Chapter 5). A thorough primary survey of the cardiovascular system includes evaluation of the mucous membrane color, capillary refill time, heart rate, and pulse quality (both femoral and dorsal metatarsal pulses) and auscultation of the heart. Physical examination findings consistent with poor tissue perfusion include pale mucous membranes, tachycardia (or bradycardia in cats), tall and narrow pulse profile, poor or absent pulses, and prolonged capillary refill time. Additionally, the animal may have a dull mentation, heart sounds may be quiet, the body temperature may be low, and the extremities may be cool to the touch (Table 1-1).[21]

It is important for the veterinarian performing the primary survey to keep in mind that animals in the early stages of compensatory shock may only have mild changes in their cardiovascular parameters (i.e., heart rate and pulse quality). It may not be until the late stages of shock (or decompensated shock) that marked changes (i.e., tachycardia, weak pulses) in these cardiovascular parameters are recognized. Those animals that are presented in the early stages of shock may be initially triaged as a lower priority and treatment

Table 1-1 Physical Examination and Diagnostic Parameters Consistent with Shock

Parameter	Value
Mentation	Depressed
Mucous membranes	Pale pink, white, injected
Capillary refill time	>2 sec
Heart rate	Cats: >220 beats/min, <160 beats/min Small-breed dogs: >160 beats/min Large-breed dogs: >100 beats/min
Respiratory rate	>40 breaths/min
Pulse quality	Absent or weak femoral or metatarsal pulse Narrow or wide pulse pressure
Systolic blood pressure	<90 mm Hg
Lactate	>2.5 mmol/L

thereby delayed; this could result in patient deterioration and subsequently a worse outcome. Therefore careful evaluation of the cardiovascular parameters in conjunction with the patient's clinical history should be performed to determine if shock might be present. If there is any concern during the primary survey that the patient may be in shock, more objective measurements of the cardiovascular system should be performed.

Objective assessments of the cardiovascular system during the primary survey may include an electrocardiographic tracing to evaluate for cardiac arrhythmias (both tachyarrhythmias and bradyarrhythmias) that may be affecting cardiac output and a noninvasive blood pressure measurement (see Chapter 183). A Doppler blood pressure measurement less than 90 mm Hg is considered low and may represent shock in both cats and dogs. A blood lactate measurement is another useful diagnostic test that can aid in assessing for the presence of poor perfusion to the tissues. Under conditions of hypoxia, cells switch to anaerobic metabolism and lactate will be produced. A blood lactate concentration greater than 2.5 mmol/L may be indicative of systemic hypoperfusion.[22,23]

Animals identified as having poor tissue perfusion should receive rapid therapy and the underlying cause for the shock identified as soon as possible (see Chapter 5). Additional tests, such as diagnostic imaging, may need to be delayed until the animal is stabilized.

Neurologic system evaluation

Evaluation of the animal's neurologic system should include an evaluation for brain or spinal cord injury. Problems affecting the neurologic system that require immediate stabilizing interventions include seizures, altered mental state (such as stupor or coma), and severe acute paralysis with loss of nociception. Seizures should be treated immediately because prolonged seizure activity can result in hyperthermia, cerebral edema, and irreversible brain injury, regardless of the underlying cause of the seizures.[24]

Increased intracranial pressure (e.g., secondary to traumatic brain injury or intracranial disease) should be suspected in any patient that is presented with a severely altered mental status. Prolonged elevations in intracranial pressure can lead to ischemia of the brain and herniation through the foramen magnum.[24] Therefore stabilizing therapies should be initiated immediately in these animals (see Chapter 84). Patients with suspected traumatic spinal cord injury should be immobilized on a backboard to prevent further injury, and movement of the animal should be minimized.

Urinary system evaluation

Acute kidney injury or urinary obstruction can lead to metabolic acidosis, hyperkalemia, cardiac arrhythmias, and death. In male cats, urethral obstruction is a common emergency condition accounting for approximately 9% of cat emergency visits at one veterinary teaching hospital.[25] Therefore all male cats that are presented on an emergency basis should have a bladder palpation performed to rule out the presence of a urethral obstruction. A large bladder (either in a cat or dog) that is not easily expressed, combined with the presence of bradycardia, warrants an electrocardiographic assessment to evaluate for cardiac arrhythmias that may result from hyperkalemia. These animals should have immediate stabilizing treatments performed, including urinary catheterization (see Chapter 208). Additionally, an animal with a history of decreased urination without a palpable bladder and concurrent bradycardia should be assessed for acute kidney injury and uroabdomen.

Additional considerations

Animals that are presented after ingestion of a toxin or possible intoxication should be triaged immediately to the treatment area. After completing the primary survey, decontamination procedures (emesis induction, activated charcoal administration, or intravenous fluid diuresis, if indicated) should be initiated as soon as possible because treatment delay could have life-threatening consequences. In addition, animals that are presented with a reproductive emergency, such as dystocia, priapism, or paraphimosis, should be immediately evaluated and treated. Animals with active bleeding or open wounds should have an occlusive bandage placed to help control hemorrhage and reduce additional contamination of the wound until definitive treatment can be performed. Finally, analgesics should be administered during the triage of animals that are in significant pain (e.g., animals with fractures). Ideally, these animals should have a complete neurologic examination performed before the administration of analgesics.

Triage Diagnostics: Vascular Access, Emergency Database, and Focused Ultrasound

Intravenous access should be obtained in any critically ill animal requiring immediate treatment for abnormalities that were noted during the primary survey. An intravenous catheter is typically placed in a peripheral vein, such as the cephalic or lateral saphenous vein, and can be used for administration of intravenous fluids or drugs (see Chapter 193). Central venous catheterization can also be considered; however, it should be avoided in animals if there is a suspicion of a coagulopathy or elevated intracranial pressure (see Chapter 195). Alternatively, an intraosseous catheter might prove lifesaving in neonates, very small animals, or animals in which intravascular access is difficult and require rapid resuscitation (see Chapter 194).

During placement of the intravenous catheter, blood should be drawn for clinical pathologic evaluation. A minimum database consisting of PCV, TS, AZO test strip, glucose, and a blood smear should be evaluated. Ideally a venous blood gas, electrolytes and lactate measurement should also be drawn during the initial evaluation of a critically ill animal. These blood values provide useful diagnostic information about the animal and help guide initial therapeutic interventions. For example, in an animal presenting for acute trauma, a normal PCV with low total solids and a lactate measurement of 6.0 mmol/L would be supportive of a diagnosis of acute hemorrhage. In a recent study, the admission base excess was found to be predictive of the need for a red blood cell transfusion in animals presenting with blunt trauma. In this study, a base excess of −6.6 was 88% sensitive and 73% specific for predicting animals that required a red blood cell transfusion.[11] This study provides evidence supporting the utility of a venous blood gas evaluation at admission in critically ill animals; it not only guides initial patient stabilization but also helps to predict the future medical needs of the animal.

An ultrasound evaluation, or the focused assessment with sonography (FAST), to assess for free abdominal, pleural, and pericardial fluid is another useful diagnostic tool in the hands of an emergency veterinarian during the triage evaluation.[26,27] In addition to the identification of free fluid, thoracic ultrasonography can also be useful in identification of pneumothorax, diaphragmatic hernia, and rib fractures.[27] In people, the use of thoracic ultrasound has proven to be faster and more accurate at detecting pleural effusion as compared with thoracic radiography.[28] Additionally, thoracic ultrasonography to evaluate cardiac contractility and left atrial size may be useful alongside the physical examination findings to help identify animals with congestive heart failure.

At the author's institution, both thoracic and abdominal FAST are routinely used during the primary survey. This can be done quickly, generally taking less than 5 minutes to perform. For example, both abdominal and thoracic FAST may be used to evaluate for free pericardial, pleural, or abdominal fluid during the triage evaluation of a dog or cat presenting with physical examination findings consistent with shock. Likewise, a FAST ultrasound examination would be performed on an animal with acute abdominal pain, abdominal distention, or a palpable abdominal fluid wave. A thoracic FAST evaluation is also routinely performed in animals with respiratory distress to evaluate for pleural effusion, pneumothorax, global cardiac contractility, and left atrial enlargement. The early identification of fluid during the triage evaluation expedites the diagnosis of the underlying cause of the animal's condition, guides diagnostic sampling of the fluid, and allows for prompt stabilization measures to be instituted (e.g., needle thoracocentesis in animals with pleural effusion or pericardiocentesis in animals with pericardial effusion).

Secondary Survey

After the primary survey has been completed and stabilizing treatments initiated (when indicated), a more thorough and complete physical examination should be performed. This is termed the secondary survey. During the secondary survey, a reevaluation of the respiratory, cardiovascular, neurologic, and urinary systems should be performed and a full "tip of the nose to the tip of the tail" physical examination should be completed.

SUMMARY

Animals that are presented on an emergency basis should be sorted according to treatment priority when resources are limited. High-priority animals—those in which abnormalities are identified during the primary survey—should receive immediate stabilizing interventions, and lower priority patients are treated in order of arrival to the hospital. Client consent should be obtained early in the triage process to determine the willingness and financial ability of the owner to treat the animal. In addition, decisions about cardiopulmonary resuscitation orders, such as whether resuscitation is desired, should be obtained from owners of unstable critically ill animals during or shortly after triage. Stabilizing treatments are aimed at correction of life-threatening abnormalities identified during the primary survey and generally involve treatment of shock, hypoxemia, and nervous system dysfunction. Once the animal has been stabilized, a complete secondary survey should be performed, which includes a reevaluation of the systems in the primary survey.

REFERENCES

1. Kennedy K, Aghababian R, Gans L, et al: Triage: technique and applications in decision making, Ann Emerg Med 28:136-144, 1996.
2. Fry M, Burr G: Review of the triage literature, Aust Emerg Nurs J 5(2):33-38, 2002.
3. Gilboy N, Tanabe T, Travers D, et al: Emergency severity index (ESI): a triage tool for emergency department care, Version 4. Implementation Handbook 2012 Edition. AHRQ Publication No. 12-0014. Rockville, MD, 2011, Agency for Healthcare Research and Quality.
4. Beveridge R, Clarke B, Janes L, et al: Canadian emergency department triage scale (CTAS) implementation guidelines, Can J Emerg Med 1 (suppl 3):S1-S24, 1999.
5. Fernandes CMB, Tanabe P, Golboy N, et al: Five-level triage: a report from the ACEP/ENA five level triage task force, J Emerg Nurs 31:39-50, 2005.
6. Barfod C, Lauritzen, MM, Danker JK, et al: Abnormal vital signs are strong predictors for intensive care unit admission and in-hospital mortality in adults triaged in the emergency department—a prospective cohort study, Scand J Trauma Resusc Emerg Med 20(28):1-9, 2012.
7. Chan TC, Killeen JP, Kelly D, et al: Impact of rapid entry and accelerated care at triage on reducing emergency department patient wait times, lengths of stay, and rate of left without being seen, Ann Emerg Med 46:491-497, 2005.
8. Han JH, France DJ, Levin SR, et al: The effect of physician triage on emergency department length of stay, J Emerg Med 2010;39:227-233, 2010.
9. Holroyd BR, Bullard MJ, Latoszek K, et al: Impact of a triage liaison physician on emergency department overcrowding and through-put: a randomized controlled trial, Acad Emerg Med 14:702-708, 2007.
10. Rockar RA, Drobatz KS, Shofer FS: Development of a scoring system for the veterinary trauma patient, J Vet Emerg Crit Care 4(2):77-83, 1994.
11. Stillion JR, Fletcher DJ: Admission base excess as a predictor of transfusion requirement and mortality in dogs with blunt trauma, J Vet Emerg Crit Care 22(5):588-594, 2012.
12. Simpson SA, Syring R, Otto CM: Severe blunt trauma in dogs: 235 cases (1997-2003), J Vet Emerg Crit Care 19(6):588-602, 2009.
13. Steeter EM, Rozanski EA, DeLaforcade-Burress AD, et al: Evaluation of vehicular trauma in dogs: 239 cases (January–December 2001), J Vet Emerg Crit Care 235(4):405-408, 2009.
14. Holowaychuk MK, Monteith G: Ionized hypocalcemia as a prognostic indicator in dogs following trauma, J Vet Emerg Crit Care 21(5):521-530, 2011.
15. Ruys LJ, Gunning M, Teske E, et al: Evaluation of a veterinary triage list modified from a human five-point triage system in 485 dogs and cats, J Vet Emerg Crit Care 22(3):303-312, 2012.
16. Aldrich J: Global assessment of the emergency patient, Vet Clinic Small Anim 35:281-305, 2005.
17. Drobatz KJ: Triage for the veterinary technician. 77th annual Western Veterinary Conference Proceedings, Las Vegas, Feb 20-24, 2005.
18. Sigrist NE, Adamik KN, Doherr MG, et al: Evaluation of respiratory parameters at presentation as clinical indicators of respiratory localization in dogs and cats with respiratory disease, J Vet Emerg Crit Care 21(1): 13-23, 2011.
19. Reeves RB, Park JS, Lapennas GN, et al: Oxygen affinity and Bohr coefficients of dog blood, J Appl Physiol 53(1):87-95, 1982.
20. Aldrich J: Shock fluids and fluid challenge. In Silverstein DC, Hopper K, editors: Small animal critical care medicine, St. Louis, 2009, Saunders Elsevier, pp 276-280.
21. Boag AK, Hughes D: Assessment and treatment of perfusion abnormalities in the emergency patient, Vet Clin Small Anim 35:319-342, 2005.
22. Hughes D, Rozanski ER, Shofer FS, et al: Effect of sampling site, repeated sampling, pH and PCO_2 on plasma lactate concentration in healthy dogs, Am J Vet Res 60:521-524, 1999.
23. Redavid LA, Sharp CR, Mitchell MA, et al: Plasma lactate measurements in healthy cats, J Vet Emerg Crit Care 22(5):580-587, 2012.
24. Syring RS: Assessment and treatment of central nervous system abnormalities in the emergency patient, Vet Clin Small Anim 35:343-358, 2005.
25. Lee JA, Drobatz KJ: Characterization of the clinical characteristics, electrolytes, acid-base, and renal parameters in male cats with urethral obstruction, J Vet Emerg Crit Care 13(4):227-233, 2003.
26. Boysen SR, Rozanski EA, Tidwell AS, et al: Evaluation of a focused assessment with sonography for trauma protocol to detect free abdominal fluid in dogs involved in motor vehicle accidents, J Am Vet Med Assoc 225(8):1198-1204, 2004.
27. Lisciandro GR, Lagutchik MS, Mann KA, et al: Evaluation of a thoracic focused assessment with sonography for trauma (TFAST) protocol to detect pneumothorax and concurrent thoracic injury in 145 traumatized dogs, J Vet Emerg Crit Care 18(3):258-269, 2008.
28. Zanobetti M, Poggioni C, Pini R: Can chest ultrasonography replace standard chest radiography for evaluation of acute dyspnea in the ED, Chest 139(5):1140-1147, 2011.

CHAPTER 2

PHYSICAL EXAMINATION AND DAILY ASSESSMENT OF THE CRITICALLY ILL PATIENT

Tim B. Hackett, DVM, MS, DACVECC

KEY POINTS

- Hands-on assessment of critically ill patients is essential to detect life-threatening changes in their condition.
- A careful physical examination should be used to evaluate the critically ill patient before performing blood tests, electrodiagnostic techniques, or imaging.
- Clinicians and other personnel should note and record both subjective and objective physical examination parameters as often as necessary, taking into consideration the patient's current problems and anticipated complications.
- The ideal monitoring plan allows for early detection of metabolic or physiologic derangements with minimal risks for iatrogenic insult, unnecessary expense to the client, and inappropriate use of intensive care unit resources.
- Use of checklists will enhance the critically ill patient's daily assessment.

Daily assessment of the critical patient begins with a thoughtful, history-guided physical examination. Physical examination is the core of critical care medicine. The goal of the intensivist is monitoring, recording, and interpreting physiologic variables in critically ill animals to detect problems with organ function and allow targeted, lifesaving intervention. Readers are also directed to Chapter 1 for further discussion of intensive care patient evaluation. Although monitoring is a vital component of intensive care unit (ICU) care, it is not the monitoring that is beneficial or protective but rather the clinician's interpretation of the data and actions based on changes in monitored parameters that are important. It is impossible for the presence of a monitoring device to alter outcome. A monitored variable is useful only if changes in that variable are linked to an intervention or therapy that affects outcome.[1] In addition to evaluating functions or parameters pertinent to the primary disease process, the daily assessment should include surveillance for new problems, because a common cause of ICU morbidity and mortality is progressive physiologic dysfunction in organ systems remote from the site of the primary disease process.

Arterial and venous blood gas analysis, blood pressure monitoring, pulse oximetry, ultrasonography, coagulation analysis, and other point-of-care tests have become commonplace in 24-hour emergency and critical care veterinary practices. Their appropriate use has improved our ability to provide the best care to our patients and is covered in detail in subsequent chapters. Despite this, one is reminded not to overlook the "art" of the physical examination. For example, to date there is no readily available technology that can measure perfusion or hydration. Although measurement of parameters such as blood pressure provides vital information, it can only be interpreted in light of the physical examination.

PHYSICAL EXAMINATION

The daily physical examination of the critically ill patient is approached much the same as the triage and primary survey of the emergency patient. With focus on the efficacy of oxygen delivery, the first priority is assessing the respiratory and cardiac systems. The ABCs (airway, breathing, and circulation) of resuscitation provide a simple systematic approach to the primary survey.[2]

Airway and Breathing

Patients adapt respirations to minimize the work of breathing. By noting abnormal breathing patterns, one is able to rank differential diagnoses and quickly arrive at an optimal treatment plan. Animals with upper airway obstruction, dynamic airway collapse, bronchitis, or other obstructions to airflow will often breathe slower and more deeply to minimize airway resistance. With laryngeal disease or extrathoracic tracheal collapse/obstruction, increased effort will be noted on inspiration. With collapse of the intrathoracic airways, there is greater effort on expiration. When there is a physical obstruction such as a mass or foreign body, the abnormal effort can be noticed on both inspiration and expiration. Auscultating the entire respiratory tract and finding the point of maximal intensity can help identify the location of the obstruction.

Animals with pulmonary parenchymal disease or pulmonary fibrosis may adopt a *restrictive breathing pattern* to overcome increased elastic forces of the pulmonary parenchyma. By minimizing the change in volume and increasing the respiratory rate, they can attempt to maintain alveolar minute ventilation despite decreased pulmonary compliance.

A very slow or apneustic respiratory pattern maybe indicative of impending respiratory arrest, and the patient should be rapidly assessed and stabilized as necessary.

Circulation

Alveolar ventilation is the first step in providing oxygen to the tissues. A normal cardiovascular system is then necessary to carry oxygenated blood from the lungs to the body. Physical assessment of the circulatory system relies on palpation of the arterial pulse (for synchrony, quality, and pulse rate), evaluation of venous distention, assessment of mucous membrane color and capillary refill time, and auscultation of the heart and lungs. Inadequate global perfusion is considered an indicator of circulatory shock and is a clinical diagnosis made from physical examination alone.[3]

Heart rate

A normal heart rate indicates that at least one component of cardiac output is normal. A heart rate of 70 to 120 beats/min is considered normal in small dogs, 60 to 120 beats/min in large dogs, and 140 to 200 beats/min in cats.

Bradycardia can result in decreased cardiac output and subsequent poor perfusion; cats often develop bradycardia (<120 beats/min) in shock, and this can be associated with imminent cardiac arrest. Bradycardia is an unusual finding in a critically ill patient and can result from electrolyte imbalances (hyperkalemia), neurologic disease (increased intracranial pressure), or conduction disturbances (atrioventricular block, sick sinus syndrome) or can be a side effect of analgesic or anesthetic drugs. An electrocardiogram (ECG) is indicated for full assessment of bradycardia.

Sinus tachycardia (dogs > 180 beats/min, cats > 220 beats/min) is the body's response to decreased blood volume, pain, anxiety, hypoxemia, and systemic inflammation. Increasing heart rate will temporarily increase cardiac output and oxygen delivery. However, there are some physiologic limitations to this response. When the heart rate becomes too fast, diastolic filling is compromised and stroke volume is inadequate. Sinus tachycardia often results from circulatory shock or pain. Tachycardia that is irregular or associated with pulse deficits usually indicates an arrhythmia, and an ECG is indicated.

Mucous membrane color

Evaluation of mucous membrane color is subjective but can give important information about peripheral capillary perfusion. Pale or white mucous membranes can be indicative of anemia or a vasoconstrictive response to shock. Red mucous membranes suggest vasodilation and are observed in systemic inflammatory states and hyperthermia. Cyanotic gums indicate severe hypoxemia in the face of a normal packed cell volume because cyanosis will not be clinically evident without adequate hemoglobin levels. A yellow hue (icterus) indicates increased serum bilirubin resulting from hepatic disease or hemolysis. A brown discoloration of the mucous membranes is observed with methemoglobinemia. During examination of the gums, petechiation or bleeding should be noted because petechiae and bruising are clinical signs of platelet deficiency or dysfunction and thrombocytopenia is an early finding in disseminated intravascular coagulation.

Capillary refill time

Evaluation of capillary refill time (CRT) provides further information on peripheral perfusion. Used in conjunction with pulse quality, respiratory effort, heart rate, and mucous membrane color, the CRT can help assess a patient's blood volume and peripheral perfusion and provide information on shock etiology. Normal CRT is 1 to 2 seconds. This is consistent with a normal blood volume and perfusion. A CRT longer than 2 seconds suggests poor perfusion due to peripheral vasoconstriction. Peripheral vasoconstriction is an appropriate response to low circulating blood volume and reduced oxygen delivery to vital tissues. Patients with hypovolemic and cardiogenic shock should be expected to have peripheral vasoconstriction. Peripheral vasoconstriction is also commonly associated with cool extremities, assessed by palpation of the distal limbs. Significant hypothermia will also cause vasoconstriction. A CRT of less than 1 second is suggestive of a hyperdynamic state and vasodilation. Hyperdynamic states can be associated with systemic inflammation, distributive shock, and heat stroke or hyperthermia.

Venous distention

Venous distention can be a sign of volume overload, right-sided congestive heart failure or increased right-sided filling pressure. Palpation of the jugular vein may demonstrate distention, although it may be easier to visualize by clipping hair over the lateral saphenous vein. The patient is positioned in lateral recumbency; if the lateral saphenous vein in the upper limb appears distended, the limb is slowly raised above the level of the heart. If the vein remains distended, it suggests an elevated central venous pressure. Potential causes of an elevated central venous pressure include volume overload, pericardial effusions, or right-sided congestive heart failure. A patient with pale mucous membranes and a prolonged CRT from vasoconstriction in response to hypovolemia would not be expected to have venous distention. In comparison, cardiogenic shock with biventricular failure is more likely to cause pale mucous membranes, prolonged CRT, and increased venous distention.

Pulse quality

The femoral pulse should be palpated while listening to the heart or palpating the cardiac apex beat. A strong pulse that is synchronous with each heartbeat is normal and consistent with adequate blood volume and cardiac output. Digital palpation of pulse quality is largely a reflection of pulse pressure. Pulse pressure equals the difference between the systolic and diastolic arterial blood pressures. A normal pulse pressure may be felt despite abnormal systolic and diastolic pressures. Global markers of anaerobic metabolism like base deficit and lactate along with low mixed venous oxygen saturation are more sensitive indicators of perfusion than blood pressure or physical examination parameters. If other indicators suggest inadequate perfusion, the patient should be evaluated for pathologic hyperdynamic conditions such as sepsis or causes of a low diastolic pressure. For example, the presence of a holosystolic murmur with normal to increased pulse pressure can indicate diastolic runoff through a patent ductus arteriosus. Both the femoral and dorsal pedal pulses should be palpated. It has been said that a palpable dorsal pedal arterial pulse indicates a systolic blood pressure of at least 80 mm Hg, although experienced clinicians will find they are able to feel these pulses in hypotensive patients. An irregular pulse or one that is asynchronous with cardiac auscultation is a sign of a significant cardiac arrhythmia. An ECG can confirm the arrhythmia and help determine the best treatment.

Weak pulses are a common finding in the critically ill and can be due to decreased cardiac output as a result of either low stroke volume or decreased contractility, peripheral vasoconstriction, or decreased pulse pressure. The simultaneous evaluation of pulse pressure and response to intravenous fluid therapy will help distinguish the common causes of shock.

Auscultation

Cardiac and pulmonary auscultation is an essential part of the physical examination. Clinicians and critical care nurses should perform serial auscultation throughout a patient's hospitalization. Nursing staff and clinicians should auscultate the heart and pulmonary sounds at least twice during a shift. Subtle changes in respiratory noise may identify potential fluid overload or early pulmonary dysfunction.

The respiratory system should be evaluated from the nasal cavity, larynx, and trachea to all lung fields. Stertor and wheezes in the upper airways and quiet crackles in the lungs may be an early sign of fluid overload.[4] Inspiratory stridor can be heard with laryngeal paralysis, whereas expiratory wheezes suggest small airway collapse and bronchitis. Crackles can be heard with pneumonia, pulmonary edema, pulmonary hemorrhage, and small airway disease. Aspiration pneumonia often affects the cranioventral lung fields, making them sound denser, with referred large airway sounds and minimal breath sounds. Pulmonary edema may begin in the perihilar lungs fields. Decreased lung sounds may be heard with pulmonary consolidation, pneumothorax, and pleural effusion. With pleural effusion, a fluid line may be detected by ausculting the patient's chest while the patient is standing or held in sternal recumbency. Changes in lung sounds may be an indication for further examination by thoracic radiography or ultrasound. Critically ill patients with evidence of pulmonary dysfunction should have their oxygenating ability evaluated with pulse oximetry or arterial blood gas measurement. Any change in respiratory character or sounds should prompt immediate reevaluation of oxygenation status.

Cardiac auscultation should be repeated at least once daily. As mentioned with pulse quality, the pulse should be palpated while listening to the heart. New murmurs or asynchronous pulses should be noted and investigated. Cardiac arrhythmias in the critically ill are an early sign of cardiac dysfunction. As with failure of any organ system, these abnormalities should be investigated and underlying metabolic or oxygen delivery problems corrected.

Level of Consciousness

The patient's level of consciousness and response to surroundings should be assessed frequently. If the patient appears normal, alert, and responsive, overall neurologic and metabolic status is likely normal. Patients that are obtunded or less responsive to visual and tactile stimuli may be suffering from a variety of complications and illnesses. Patients with stupor can be aroused only with painful stimuli. Stupor is a sign of severe neurologic or metabolic derangements. Coma and seizures are signs of abnormal cerebral electrical activity from either primary neurologic disease or severe metabolic derangements such as hepatic encephalopathy. One of the most concerning issues in the critically ill patient is any decrease in the gag reflex. This may be a result of a general decrease in the level of consciousness or a primary neurologic deficit. A decrease in the gag reflex places the animal at high risk of aspiration pneumonia, a potentially fatal complication. Oral intake should be withheld in animals with a compromised gag reflex, and if the gag reflex is absent, immediate endotracheal intubation to protect the airway is indicated.

Temperature

Body temperature should be monitored frequently, if not continuously, in the critically ill patient. Environmental hyperthermia should be differentiated from primary hyperthermia. Hospitalized animals may develop hyperthermia from cage heat or heating pads. Primary hyperthermia or true fever should be investigated quickly, because systemic inflammation and infectious complications are common complications of critical illness.

Hypothermia is also common in critically ill animals. Many have difficulty maintaining their body temperature and require external heat supplementation. Passive warming with a dry blanket is safer than active warming with external heat sources. Active warming should take care to prevent burns and iatrogenic hyperthermia. Circulating hot air systems are an excellent source for active rewarming. Heat may be supplied by circulating hot water blankets or by placing warm water-filled gloves or bottles in towels next to the animal. A warming waterbed can be made by placing a thick plastic bag over an appropriate-size container filled with warm water. A towel placed under the animal will prevent its nails from perforating the plastic. Blankets placed on top of the animal will prevent heat from escaping. Heating pads should be used with caution, using both a low temperature setting and insulating the animal with a blanket or fleece pad. Heat lamps should be used from a distance of more than 30 inches to prevent burns. Electric cage dryers or handheld blow dryers are useful if the animal is already wet. Intravenous fluids warmed to body temperature can be beneficial when rapid administration rates are used but are not effective at maintenance fluid rates.[5] To prevent overwarming, body temperature should be monitored at regular intervals and warming measures discontinued when the body temperature reaches 100° F. Animals should be monitored carefully to prevent iatrogenic hyperthermia and thermal burns.

Hydration

Whereas perfusion parameters such as mucous membrane color, CRT, and heart rate are a measure of intravascular volume, hydration status is a subjective measure of interstitial fluid content. It is important to assess intravascular and interstitial fluid compartments separately and individualize fluid plans according to needs in both spaces. Day-to-day changes in body weight reflect fluid balance; therefore, daily body weight is the most objective way to monitor hydration. A dehydrated patient should gain weight as fluid volumes are restored. Overhydration is associated with progressive increases in body weight. Evaluating skin turgor or skin elasticity is used to assess hydration. With dehydration, skin turgor is decreased and skin tenting becomes prolonged. With overhydration, skin turgor increases and the subcutaneous tissues gain a "jelly-like" consistency. Serous nasal discharge, peripheral edema, and chemosis are additional supporting signs of overhydration. Peripheral edema can also indicate vasculitis or decreased oncotic pressure such as that seen with hypoproteinemia. Skin turgor is affected by the amount of subcutaneous fat, making it difficult to assess in cachectic and obese animals.

Clinicians should be wary of third-space fluid accumulation. Third-space fluid loss is fluid collection within a body cavity that does not contribute to circulation. Pleural and abdominal effusions can lead to increases in body weight or maintenance of body weight in a patient that is becoming hypovolemic. Daily, or more often when appropriate, assessment of fluid balance is essential in critically ill animals. This requires accurate measurement of all fluid intake and output to include food and water consumption, urine, vomit, feces as well as any drain fluid production. Discrepancies in the volume of intake versus output require reevaluation of the patient and alteration of the fluid plan.

Abdominal Palpation and Gastrointestinal Assessment

The gastrointestinal (GI) tract may be difficult to evaluate on physical examination but not unimportant because GI problems are often seen with circulatory shock and critical illness. Thorough abdominal palpation is an important part of a complete physical examination. Clinicians and technicians should evaluate the patient's abdomen for effusion, organ size, and location and localize any discomfort. Contents of the intestinal tract can be evaluated by both gentle palpation and digital rectal examination. The frequency, character, and volume of GI losses should be monitored. If fresh or digested blood is observed, GI protectants and antibiotics may be indicated.

MONITORING AND LABORATORY DATA

The use of checklists has been promoted to enhance care for critically ill patients.[6] By combining aspects of the physical examination with the most essential diagnostic tests, patient status is reviewed in a systematic manner, minimizing the chance of missing significant changes in condition. Kirby's Rule of 20, a list of monitoring parameters for septic small-animal patients, predates much of the current human literature on the use of checklists.[7] Box 2-1 lists these 20 parameters and provides an excellent initial approach to monitoring most critically ill animals. This work provided the groundwork for critical care monitoring of the septic patient and has been adapted for most critical veterinary patients. Optimal care is provided when information collected by physical examination and clinical observation is integrated with the results of ancillary tests and technologically derived data. Fluid balance; oxygenation; mentation; perfusion and blood pressure; heart rate, rhythm, and contractility; GI motility;

BOX 2-1 *Kirby's Rule of 20 for Monitoring the Critically Ill Patient*[7]

- Fluid balance
- Oncotic pull
- Glucose
- Electrolyte and acid-base balance
- Oxygenation and ventilation
- Mentation
- Perfusion and blood pressure
- Heart rate, rhythm, and contractility
- Albumin levels
- Coagulation
- Red blood cell and hemoglobin concentration
- Renal function
- Immune status, antibiotic dosage and selection, WBC count
- GI motility and mucosal integrity
- Drug dosages and metabolism
- Nutrition
- Pain control
- Nursing care and patient mobilization
- Wound care and bandage change
- Tender loving care

GI, Gastrointestinal; *WBC,* white blood cell count.

mucosal integrity; and nursing care have all been discussed in the physical examination section of this chapter. The remainder of this checklist makes up the daily monitoring and laboratory assessment recommended for most critical patients.

Oncotic Pull, Total Protein, and Albumin

Hypoproteinemia is a common finding in critically ill patients. Total protein should be monitored at least daily, and serum albumin should be monitored every 24 to 48 hours. Hypoalbuminemic animals may require support with synthetic or natural colloids. Although albumin levels less than 2 mg/dl have been associated with increased mortality in human patients, albumin transfusions to increase serum levels have not resulted in increased survival.[8]

Colloid osmotic pressure (COP), the osmotic pressure exerted by large molecules, serves to hold water within the vascular space. It is normally the role of plasma proteins, primarily albumin, that stay within the vasculature. Inadequate COP can contribute to vascular volume loss and peripheral edema. The COP can be measured directly with a colloid osmometer; however, it is not commonly available, so most clinicians will base assessment of oncotic pressure on serum total protein (see Chapter 187). The limitation to the use of serum total protein is that the correlation between the refractive index of infused synthetic colloids and COP is not reliable.[9]

Glucose

Hypoglycemia can occur rapidly in critically ill patients. Blood glucose concentration should be monitored routinely. The frequency of measurement will depend on the severity of illness and the nature of the underlying disease. The development of hypoglycemia in a critically ill adult patient should prompt the consideration of sepsis. Studies of human ICU patients have demonstrated increased morbidity and mortality associated with hyperglycemia.[10] The 2012 Surviving Sepsis guidelines recommend targeting an upper blood glucose level of 180 mg/dl or less in patients with severe sepsis.[11] Although similar veterinary studies have not been performed, a similar goal would seem appropriate; however, it is important to avoid wide swings in blood glucose and hypoglycemia.

Electrolyte and Acid-Base Balance

Abnormalities in serum electrolytes are common in critically ill patients. Serum sodium, chloride, potassium, and calcium should be monitored and maintained within the normal ranges through appropriate supplementation and crystalloid fluid choices. Magnesium depletion has been identified as a common electrolyte abnormality in critically ill veterinary patients.[12]

Measurement of acid-base status has become routine, and both arterial and venous samples can be evaluated. Interpretation of acid-base abnormalities can be aided by measurement of lactate and electrolyte concentrations (see Chapter 54).

Oxygenation and Ventilation

In addition to the physical examination described for the respiratory system, additional monitoring is recommended to objectively assess respiratory function. Respiratory failure can be a failure of oxygenation, resulting in hypoxemia, or a failure of ventilation, resulting in hypercapnia (see Chapters 15 and 16). Pulse oximetry, end-tidal carbon dioxide measurement, and arterial and venous blood gases can all be used to assess oxygenation and ventilation.

Red Blood Cell and Hemoglobin Concentrations

The oxygen content of arterial blood is mostly bound to hemoglobin. Hemoglobin concentration should be monitored at least daily and optimized to ensure adequate oxygen delivery. The optimal hematocrit value for oxygen transport is from 27% to 33%. Human studies support a lower transfusion trigger of 7 g/dl of hemoglobin.[13] Transfusions of whole blood, packed red blood cells, or hemoglobin-containing solutions should be given as needed.

Blood Pressure

Blood pressure can be measured indirectly by Doppler or oscillometric techniques or directly via an indwelling arterial catheter. Blood pressure should be measured at least daily in critically ill patients. Continuous blood pressure monitoring maybe indicated for hemodynamically unstable patients (see Chapter 183).

Coagulation

Coagulation abnormalities often occur in critically ill patients. They can result from primary diseases such as vitamin K antagonist intoxication or hepatic disease, a coexisting problem such as von Willebrand disease or nonsteroidal anti-inflammatory drug administration, or because of an acquired problem such as dilutional coagulopathy or disseminated intravascular coagulation (DIC). The choice of coagulation test will depend on the patient's history, primary disease process, and tests available. Practices should be able to evaluate platelet number, function, and clotting factor function (see Section XI).

Renal Function and Urine Output

Urine output should be monitored in critically ill patients (see Chapter 192). Decreased urine output can reflect inadequate renal perfusion or acute renal failure. Patients who have experienced hypotension during anesthesia or secondary to their underlying disease are at risk of acute kidney injury. Critical patients often receive potentially nephrotoxic drugs. Normal urine output in a well-perfused, normally hydrated patient is 1 to 2 ml/kg/hr. In both oliguric and polyuric patients, measurement of fluid intake and GI and urinary losses can be used to facilitate fluid therapy. Indwelling urinary catheters are often used in the critically ill patient to maintain normal bladder size and prevent urine scald. By allowing frequent checks of urine output they should also be considered a simple monitoring technique. With careful attention to cleanliness, these can be very effective tools without significant risk of ascending urinary tract infection.[14]

Serum creatinine and blood urea nitrogen levels should be monitored daily during a crisis period. Urine should be evaluated daily for evidence of renal tubular casts or glucosuria.

Immune Status, Antibiotic Dosage and Selection, and White Blood Cell Count

Bacterial infection is a common complication in ICU admissions. Empiric broad-spectrum, parenteral antibiotic therapy is often initiated based on knowledge of common pathogens and results of Gram staining of appropriate specimens. Culture and sensitivity results should be reviewed when available and empiric antibiotic choices adjusted accordingly. White blood cell count and differential should be monitored frequently for evidence of new or nonresponsive infections.

Drug Dosages and Metabolism

Drug dosages should be reviewed daily. Animals with renal and hepatic dysfunction may have altered metabolism, and dosages may need to be adjusted. Interactions among drugs should be considered in animals receiving multiple therapies.

Nutrition

Caloric intake is an important variable to monitor daily. Nutrition is an essential yet commonly overlooked component of successful management of the critical patient. Patients that develop a negative energy and protein balance may develop a loss of host defenses, loss of muscle strength, visceral organ atrophy and dysfunction, gastrointestinal barrier breakdown, pneumonia, sepsis, and death. Enteral malnutrition is a predisposing factor in bacterial translocation and secondary sepsis, making enteral feeding the preferred route when possible (see Section XIV).

Nursing Care

Recumbent patients require attentive nursing care to prevent secondary complications. Patients should be turned every 4 to 6 hours and encouraged to take deep breaths to prevent pulmonary atelectasis. The skin should be assessed often. Pressure points over bony protuberances should be evaluated regularly to prevent decubitus ulcers. Moisture from urine, feces, or other draining fluids should be identified early to prevent scalding of the skin. Urine output and bladder size should be monitored frequently. This is especially true in animals at risk for renal failure or in patients with neurologic disease that prevents normal micturition.

Frequent assessment of patient comfort is subjective but important (see Chapter 141). Appropriate pain control should always be provided (see Chapter 144). Hands-on contact with the patient is invaluable in high-quality clinical assessment and monitoring. Mental health is as important as physical health. Comfortable, dry bedding, gentle handling by staff members, and visits from owners are important. If possible, normal circadian rhythms should be maintained, with lights out or dimmed at night. Owner visits may improve the attitude of the patient and provide insights that may not be appreciated with the physical examination alone.

REFERENCES

1. Prittie J: Optimal endpoints of resuscitation and early goal-directed therapy, J Vet Emerg Crit Care 16:329, 2006.
2. Aldrich J: Global assessment of the emergency patient, Vet Clin North Am Small Anim Pract 35:281, 2005.
3. Kittleson MD: Signalment, history and physical examination. In Kittleson MD, Kienle RD, editors: Small animal cardiovascular medicine, St. Louis, 1998, Mosby.
4. Kotlikoff MI, Gillespie JR: Lung sounds in veterinary medicine. Part I. Terminology and mechanisms of sound production, Comp Cont Educ Pract Vet 5:634, 1984.
5. Chiang V, Hopper K, Mellema MS: In vitro evaluation of the efficacy of a veterinary dry heat fluid warmer, J Vet Emerg Crit Care 21(6):639-647, 2011
6. Winters BD, Gurses AP, Lehmann H, Sexton, CJ, Pronovost PJ: Clinical review: checklists—translating evidence into practice, Crit Care 13:1, 2009.
7. Kirby R: Septic shock. In Bonagura JD, editor: Current veterinary therapy XII, Philadelphia, 1995, Saunders.
8. Mazzaferro EM, Rudloff E, Kirby R: The role of albumin replacement in the critically ill veterinary patient, J Vet Emerg Crit Care 12:113, 2002.
9. Bumpus SE, Haskins SC, Kass PH: Effect of synthetic colloids on refractometric readings of total solids, J Vet Emerg Crit Care 8:21-26, 1998.
10. Krinsley JS: Effect of an intensive glucose management protocol on the mortality of critically ill adult patient, Mayo Clin Proc 79:992, 2004.
11. Dellinger RP, Levy MM, Rhodes A, et al: Surviving Sepsis campaign: international guidelines for management of severe sepsis and septic shock, 2012, Intensive Care Med 39(2):165-228, 2013.
12. Martin LG, Matteson VL, Wingfield WE, et al: Abnormalities of serum magnesium in critically ill dogs: Incidence and implications, J Vet Emerg Crit Care 4:15, 1994.
13. Hebert PC, Wells G, Blajchman MA et al: A multicenter, randomized, controlled clinical trial of transfusion requirements in critical care, N Engl J Med 340:409, 1999.
14. Smarick SD, Haskins SC, Aldrich J, et al: Incidence of catheter-associated urinary tract infection among dogs in a small animal intensive care unit, J Am Vet Med Assoc 224:1936, 2004.

CHAPTER 3

CARDIOPULMONARY RESUSCITATION

Daniel J. Fletcher, PhD, DVM, DACVECC • Manuel Boller, DrMedVet, MTR, DACVECC

KEY POINTS

- Early recognition of cardiopulmonary arrest (CPA) and rapid initiation of cardiopulmonary resuscitation (CPR) are crucial for patient survival.
- Basic life support, consisting of high-quality chest compressions at a rate of 100 to 120 per minute and a depth of one third to one half the width of the chest, and delivered in uninterrupted cycles of 2 minutes, as well as ventilation at a rate of 10 breaths/min, is arguably the most important aspect of CPR.
- Monitoring priorities during CPR include electrocardiography to obtain a rhythm diagnosis and end-tidal carbon dioxide monitoring to evaluate the effectiveness of chest compressions and as an early indicator of return of spontaneous circulation.
- Advanced life support interventions for asystole and pulseless electrical activity include vasopressor therapy and parasympatholytic therapy, especially in cases of bradycardic arrest because of high vagal tone.
- The most effective advanced life support therapy for ventricular fibrillation is electrical defibrillation. Only a single shock should be delivered initially, followed by a full 2-minute cycle of basic life support before administering an additional shock in refractory ventricular fibrillation.

Cardiopulmonary arrest (CPA) in cats and dogs is a highly lethal condition, with rates of survival to discharge of only 6% to 7%.[1] Widespread training targeted at standardized cardiopulmonary resuscitation (CPR) guidelines in human medicine has led to substantial improvements in outcome after in-hospital CPA from 13.7% in 2000 to 22.3% in 2009.[2] An exhaustive literature review was recently completed by the Reassessment Campaign on Veterinary Resuscitation (RECOVER) initiative, the result of which was generation of the first evidence-based consensus veterinary CPR guidelines.[3] The evidence evaluation and guidelines were generated in five domains: Preparedness and Prevention,[4] Basic Life Support,[5] Advanced Life Support,[6] Monitoring[7], and Post–Cardiac Arrest Care.[8] The goal of this chapter is to summarize the most important treatment recommendations from the first four domains. Chapter 4 discusses the Post–Cardiac Arrest Care guidelines.

PREPAREDNESS AND PREVENTION

Early recognition of and response to CPA are critical if survival rates are to be improved. Including both didactic training targeted at establishing a baseline CPR knowledge base and hands-on practice for psychomotor skill development in training programs improves CPR performance and outcomes.[9,10] Once baseline training has been completed, refresher training at least every 6 months is recommended for personnel likely to be involved in CPR attempts to reduce decay of skills and knowledge.[11,12] A centrally located, routinely audited crash cart containing all necessary drugs and equipment should be maintained in the practice. Readily available cognitive aids, such as algorithm and dosing charts, improve adherence to guidelines as well as individual performance during CPR.[13-15] Staff should be trained in the use of these aids regularly. Even brief post-event debriefing sessions during which team performance is discussed and critically evaluated can help improve future performance and at the same time serve as refresher training.[16,17]

A standardized assessment leading to early recognition of CPA is crucial and should be applied immediately to any acutely unresponsive patient. In non-anesthetized patients, a diagnosis of CPA should be highly suspected in any unconscious patient that is not breathing. A brief assessment lasting no more than 10 to 15 seconds based on evaluation of airway, breathing, and circulation (ABCs) will efficiently identify CPA. If CPA cannot be definitively ruled out, CPR should be initiated immediately rather than pursuing further diagnostic assessment. The rationale for this aggressive approach includes the following: (a) Pulse palpation is an insensitive test for CPA in people, and this may also be the case in dogs and cats; (b) even short delays in starting CPR in pulseless patients reduce survival rates; and (c) starting CPR on a patient not in CPA carries minimal risks.[18,19] Therefore there should be no delay in starting CPR in any patient in which there is a suspicion of CPA.

BASIC LIFE SUPPORT

Basic life support (BLS) includes chest compressions to restore blood flow to the tissues and the pulmonary circulation and ventilation to provide oxygenation of the arterial blood and removal of carbon dioxide from the venous blood. BLS should be initiated as quickly as possible once a diagnosis of CPA has been made using the treatment mnemonic CAB (*c*irculation, *a*irway, *b*reathing). More than any other CPR intervention, high-quality BLS focused first on chest compressions followed by ventilation likely has the most significant impact on outcome.[18] However, given the higher incidence of primary respiratory arrest in dogs and cats than in people, early airway management and ventilation are strongly recommended. In multiple rescuer CPR, an airway should be established simultaneously with the initiation of chest compressions.

Circulation: Chest Compressions

Tissue hypoxia and ischemic injury occur rapidly in patients with untreated CPA, an immediate consequence of which is the exhaustion of cellular energy stores. Altered cellular membrane potentials and organ dysfunction follow rapidly, and longer duration of ischemia primes the system for more severe reperfusion injury when tissue blood flow resumes. Administration of high-quality chest compressions can provide vital blood flow to tissues, decreasing ischemic injury and blunting the reperfusion injury set in motion with return of spontaneous circulation (ROSC). Chest compressions are targeted at two main goals: (a) restoration of pulmonary CO_2 elimination and oxygen uptake by providing pulmonary blood flow, and (b) delivery of oxygen to tissues to restore organ function and metabolism by providing systemic arterial blood flow. Even well-executed chest compressions produce only approximately 30% of normal cardiac output; therefore meticulous attention to chest compression technique is essential. Any delay in starting high-quality chest compressions or excessive pauses in compressions reduce the likelihood of ROSC and survival to discharge.

During ventricular systole in the spontaneously beating heart, coronary blood flow is negligible and at times may be retrograde; several mechanisms have been proposed to explain this finding, including backward pressure waves, the intramyocardial pump theory, coronary systolic flow impediment, and cardiac compression.[20,21] This same phenomenon has been described during CPR using external chest compressions.[22,23] Therefore it is important to consider that the majority of myocardial perfusion during CPR occurs during the decompression phase of chest compressions and is determined predominantly by myocardial perfusion pressure (MPP, also known as coronary perfusion pressure [CPP]), defined as the difference between aortic diastolic pressure and right atrial diastolic pressure (MPP = ADP − RADP). There is strong evidence that higher MPP during CPR is associated with better success in both humans and dogs, leading to the use of MPP as a primary marker of CPR quality.[24,25]

Unfortunately, little experimental or clinical data are available to guide chest compression technique in dogs and cats, but anatomic principles suggest that chest compressions may be delivered with the patient in either left or right lateral recumbency,[26] with a compression depth of one third to one half the width of the chest and at a rate of 100 to 120 compressions per minute regardless of animal size or species. An experimental study in dogs showed that higher compression rates lead to higher MPP and coronary blood flow velocity, but because anterograde flow occurred only during chest decompression, net myocardial blood flow decreased at compression rates above 120 per minute, so faster rates should be avoided.[27] To ensure the correct compression frequency, the use of cues such as a metronome or a song with the correct tempo (e.g., the Bee Gee's "Staying Alive") is recommended. Leaning on the chest between compressions will reduce filling of the heart by preventing full elastic recoil of the chest and must be avoided. Compressions should be delivered without interruption in cycles of 2 minutes to optimize development of adequate MPP, because it takes approximately 60 seconds of continuous chest compressions before MPP reaches its maximum.[28] MPP is the primary determinant of myocardial blood flow, and higher MPP is associated with a higher likelihood of ROSC. Electrocardiography (ECG) analysis to diagnose the arrest rhythm and pulse palpation to identify ROSC require pauses in chest compressions and should be accomplished during a brief cessation (2 to 5 seconds) of compressions at the end of each 2-minute BLS cycle. To minimize compressor fatigue, a new team member should take over chest compressions during this planned pause.

The generation of blood flow to the tissues during CPR occurs in fundamentally different ways than in a patient with a spontaneously beating heart. There are two models explaining the mechanisms of forward flow during external chest compressions, and based on these models it is likely that the most effective technique for chest compressions will depend on patient size and chest geometry. The cardiac pump theory proposes that direct compression of the left and right ventricles increases ventricular pressure, opening the pulmonic and aortic valves and allowing blood flow to the lungs and the tissues, respectively.[29] Thoracic elastic properties allow the chest to recoil between compressions, creating a subatmospheric intrathoracic pressure that draws venous blood into the ventricles before the subsequent compression. In contrast, an increase in overall intrathoracic pressure during a chest compression forcing blood from the thorax into the systemic circulation is proposed in the thoracic pump theory. Rather than as a pump, the heart acts simply as a conduit for blood flow.[30] Taking into account these two theories and which is more likely to be most exploitable given an individual patient's thoracic shape and size, recommendations can be made for rescuer hand position during chest compressions.

Table 3-1 specifies the recommended approach to chest compressions in dogs and cats based upon size and thoracic conformation. It should be noted that although animals of the same breed tend to have similar chest conformations, each individual should be evaluated independently and the most appropriate technique applied regardless of breed. Medium to large dogs with round chest conformations (lateral width similar to dorsoventral height) are likely best compressed in lateral recumbency using the thoracic pump theory by placing the hands over the widest portion of the chest (the highest point when laying in lateral recumbency). In contrast, similarly sized dogs with deeper, keel-chested conformations (lateral width significantly smaller than dorsoventral height) are likely to be more

Table 3-1 Chest Compression Approaches

Conformation	Breed Examples	Predominant Theory	Technique
Medium- and large-breed round-chested dogs	• Labrador Retriever • Golden Retriever • Rottweiler • German Shepherd • American Pitbull Terrier	Thoracic pump	Lateral recumbency, two-hand technique, hands over the widest part of the chest (highest point in lateral recumbency)
Medium- and large-breed keel-chested dogs	• Greyhound • Doberman Pinscher	Cardiac pump	Lateral recumbency, two-hand technique, hands directly over the heart
Flat-chested dogs	• English Bulldog • French Bulldog	Cardiac pump	Dorsal recumbency, two-hand technique, hands directly over the sternum
Cats and small dogs in average body condition	• All cats • Chihuahua • Yorkshire Terrier • Maltese • Shih Tzu	Cardiac pump	Lateral recumbency; (1) one-hand technique, hand wrapped around sternum over heart; (2) two-hand technique, hands directly over the heart; take care not to overcompress the chest
Obese cats and small dogs		Cardiac pump or thoracic pump	Lateral recumbency, two-hand technique, hands over the heart (if chest is keel-shaped) or the widest part of the chest (if chest is round)

effectively compressed using a cardiac pump approach, with the hands placed directly over the heart. In markedly flat-chested dogs with dorsoventrally compressed chests similar to humans (lateral width significantly larger than dorsoventral depth), the cardiac pump theory may be maximally employed by positioning the hands over the sternum with the patient in dorsal recumbency. In medium to large dogs with low chest compliance, considerable compression force is necessary for CPR to be effective. The compressor's posture has a significant impact on efficacy; the compressor should lock the elbows with one hand on top of the other and position the shoulders directly above the hands. Engaging the core muscles rather than the biceps and triceps by using this posture will allow the compressor to maintain optimal compression force and reduce fatigue. The use of a stepstool is recommended if the patient is on a table and the elbows cannot be locked. Alternatively, the compressor can kneel over the patient by climbing onto the table or placing the patient on the floor.

Chest compressions should be done directly over the heart in most cats and small dogs. These patients tend to have highly compliant, predominantly keel-shaped chests that favor the cardiac pump mechanism. The same two-handed technique as described earlier for large dogs can be used or a single-handed technique with the hand wrapped around the sternum and compressions achieved by squeezing the chest. Circumferential compressions of the chest using both hands may also be considered.

Airway and Breathing—Ventilation

Dogs and cats in CPA should be ventilated as soon as possible after chest compressions are started. Patients should be intubated immediately if the equipment is available. Intubation should occur in lateral recumbency without interrupting chest compressions. In intubated patients, chest compressions and ventilation are done simultaneously. The inflated endotracheal tube cuff prevents gastric insufflation with air, allows pulmonary inflation during chest compressions, and minimizes interruptions in chest compressions. The following ventilation targets should be used during CPR: ventilation rate of 10 breaths/min, a short inspiratory time of approximately 1 second, and a tidal volume of approximately 10 ml/kg. This low minute ventilation is adequate during CPR because pulmonary blood flow is reduced. Because low arterial CO_2 tension causes cerebral vasoconstriction, leading to decreased cerebral blood flow and oxygen delivery, hyperventilation must be avoided. In addition, increased intrathoracic pressure caused by positive pressure ventilation will impede venous return to the chest, reducing effectiveness of chest compressions and reducing MPP. Therefore limiting the ventilation rate to reduce the mean intrathoracic pressure will improve cardiac output.

Mouth-to-snout ventilation is an alternative breathing strategy and will provide sufficient oxygenation and CO_2 removal but should only be used if endotracheal intubation is not possible. Firmly close the animal's mouth with one hand while extending the neck to align the snout with the spine. The rescuer should then make a seal over the patient's nares with his or her mouth and inflate the lungs by blowing firmly into the nares while visually inspecting the chest during the procedure, continuing the breath until a normal chest excursion is accomplished. An inspiratory time of approximately 1 second should be targeted.

Because ventilation cannot be accomplished simultaneously with chest compressions in nonintubated patients, rounds of 30 chest compressions should be delivered, immediately followed by two short breaths. Compressions and mouth-to-snout breaths at a ratio of 30:2 should be continued for 2-minute cycles and the rescuers rotated every cycle to prevent fatigue. This technique necessitates pauses in chest compressions and should only be employed when endotracheal intubation is impossible because of lack of equipment or trained personnel.

MONITORING

Because of motion artifact and the lack of adequate pulse quality during CPR, many monitoring devices are of limited use, including pulse oximeter and indirect blood pressure monitors such as Doppler and oscillometric devices. However, ECG and capnography are two useful monitoring modalities during CPR, and their use is recommended.

Electrocardiography

Many important decisions about ALS therapy are dependent on the ECG rhythm diagnosis. However, it is important to note that the ECG is highly susceptible to motion artifact and cannot be interpreted during ongoing chest compressions; therefore, to minimize pauses in chest compressions, the only time the ECG should be evaluated is between 2-minute cycles of BLS while compressors are being rotated. The team leader should clearly announce the rhythm diagnosis and invite other team members to express agreement or dissent to minimize misdiagnosis. In the event of differing opinions on the rhythm diagnosis, chest compressions should be resumed immediately and discussion should proceed into the next cycle. The three most common arrest rhythms leading to CPA in dogs and cats are asystole, pulseless electrical activity (PEA), and ventricular fibrillation (VF).[1,31,32]

Capnography

End-tidal CO_2 ($ETCO_2$) monitoring is safe and feasible during CPR and, regardless of technology, is resistant to motion artifact.[33,34] Detection of measurable $ETCO_2$ suggests (but is not definitive for) correct endotracheal tube placement; however, this may not be a reliable test of correct endotracheal tube placement in the CPA patient because of poor pulmonary blood flow.[35] $ETCO_2$ can also be used as an indicator of chest compression efficacy because when minute ventilation is held constant, $ETCO_2$ is proportional to pulmonary blood flow. A very low $ETCO_2$ value during CPR (e.g., <10 to 15 mm Hg) has been associated with a reduced likelihood of ROSC in dogs and humans.[1,36] $ETCO_2$ substantially increases upon ROSC and therefore is a valuable early indicator of ROSC during CPR.

ADVANCED LIFE SUPPORT

Advanced life support (ALS), including drug therapy and electrical defibrillation, is initiated once BLS procedures have been started. It should be emphasized that in the absence of high-quality BLS interventions, ALS procedures are unlikely to be successful; therefore all ALS interventions should be implemented so as to minimize any impact on BLS quality.

Drug Therapy

During CPR, drug therapy should be preferentially administered by the intravenous or intraosseous route, and early placement of a peripheral venous, central venous, or intraosseous catheter is recommended. Cutdown procedures to obtain peripheral venous access are commonly required. Note that BLS should not be paused during vascular access procedures. Vasopressors, parasympatholytics, and antiarrhythmics may be indicated in dogs and cats with CPA, depending on the underlying arrest rhythm. Depending on the type of arrest, the duration, and predisposing factors, other potentially useful ALS therapies may include reversal agents, intravenous fluids, and alkalinizing drugs. Table 3-2 summarizes the doses of drugs that may be of

Table 3-2 **CPR Drugs and Doses**

	Drug	Common Concentration	Dose/Route	Comments
Arrest	Epinephrine (low dose)	1 mg/ml (1:1000)	0.01 mg/kg IV/IO 0.02-0.1 mg/kg IT	Every other BLS cycle for asystole/PEA. Increase dose 2-10× and dilute for IT administration.
	Epinephrine (high dose)	1 mg/ml (1:1000)	0.1 mg/kg IV/IO/IT	Consider for prolonged (>10 minutes) CPR.
	Vasopressin	20 U/ml	0.8 U/kg IV/IO 1.2 U/kg IT	Every other BLS cycle. Increase dose for IT use.
	Atropine	0.54 mg/ml	0.04 mg/kg IV/IO 0.15-0.2 mg/kg IT	Every other BLS cycle during CPR. Recommended for bradycardic arrests and known or suspected high vagal tone. Increase dose for IT use.
	Bicarbonate	1 mEq/ml	1 mEq/kg IV/IO	For prolonged CPR / PCA phase when pH < 7.0. Do not use if hypoventilating.
Antiarrhythmic	Amiodarone	50 mg/ml	5 mg/kg IV/IO	For refractory VF/pulseless VT. Associated with anaphylaxis in dogs.
	Lidocaine	20 mg/ml	2 mg/kg slow IV/IO push (1-2 minutes)	For refractory VF/pulseless VT *only* if amiodarone is not available.
Reversals	Naloxone	0.4 mg/ml	0.04 mg/kg IV/IO	To reverse opioids.
	Flumazenil	0.1 mg/ml	0.01 mg/kg IV/IO	To reverse benzodiazepines.
	Atipamezole	5 mg/ml	50 μg/kg IV/IO	To reverse α2 agonists.
Electrical Defibrillation	Monophasic External		4-6 J/kg	May increase dose by 50% each cycle up to a maximum dose of 10 J/kg for refractory VF/pulseless VT.
	Monophasic Internal		0.5-1 J/kg	
	Biphasic External		2-4 J/kg	
	Biphasic Internal		0.2-0.4 J/kg	

BLS, Basic life support; *CPR*, cardiopulmonary resuscitation; *PCA*, postcardiac arrest; *PEA*, pulseless electrical activity; *IO*, intraosseous; *IT*, intrathecal; *IV*, intravenous; *VF*, ventricular fibrillation; *VT*, ventricular tachycardia.

use during CPR. As part of preparedness for CPR, a drug dose chart should be in plain view in the ready area of the hospital. CPR algorithms and drug dose charts produced as part of the RECOVER initiative are available at http://www.veccs.org.

Vasopressors

Because cardiac output during CPR is generally 30% of normal or less, increasing peripheral vascular resistance to redirect blood flow from the periphery to the core can be useful regardless of the arrest rhythm. The best-studied vasopressor during CPR is epinephrine, a catecholamine that causes peripheral vasoconstriction via stimulation of α_1 receptors but also acts on β_1 and β_2 receptors. The α_1 effects have been shown to be the most beneficial during CPR,[37] and these vasoconstrictive effects predominate in the periphery while sparing the myocardial and cerebral vasculature and preserving blood flow to these core organs.[38] A meta-analysis showed that low-dose epinephrine (0.01 mg/kg intravenously [IV]/intraosseously [IO] every other cycle of CPR) was associated with higher rates of survival to discharge in people, compared with high-dose epinephrine (0.1 mg/kg IV/IO every other cycle of CPR).[39] Therefore early in CPR low-dose epinephrine is recommended. However, after prolonged CPR, a higher dose (0.1 mg/kg IV/IO every other cycle of CPR) may be considered because of evidence that this dose is associated with a higher rate of ROSC. Endotracheal administration of epinephrine is also possible (0.02 mg/kg low dose; 0.2 mg/kg high dose) and should be accomplished by feeding a long catheter through the tube and diluting the epinephrine 1:1 with isotonic saline or sterile water.[40] Although still considered a mainstay of therapy for asystole and PEA, there is controversy regarding the utility of epinephrine during CPR. Despite evidence of increased ROSC rates with its use, no consistent long-term survival or functional outcome effect has been demonstrated.[41]

An alternative to epinephrine is vasopressin (0.8 U/kg IV/IO every other cycle of CPR), a vasopressor that acts via activation of peripheral V1 receptors. It may be used interchangeably or in combination with epinephrine during CPR. Unlike epinephrine, it is efficacious in acidic environments in which α_1 receptors may become unresponsive to epinephrine. It also lacks the inotropic and chronotropic β_1 effects that may worsen myocardial ischemia in patients that achieve ROSC.[42] Like epinephrine, vasopressin may be administered endotracheally as described earlier.

Parasympatholytics

Atropine is a parasympatholytic drug and has been extensively studied in CPR.[43-45] Its administration may be considered during CPR in all dogs and cats (0.04 mg/kg IV/IO every other cycle of CPR) and may be especially useful in patients with asystole or PEA associated with increased vagal tone, such as occurs with chronic and severe or acute gastrointestinal, respiratory, or ocular disease. Endotracheal administration is also possible (0.08 mg/kg).[46]

Antiarrhythmic drugs

Patients with VF refractory to electrical defibrillation (discussed in the next section) may benefit from treatment with the antiarrhythmic drug amiodarone at a dose of 2.5 to 5 mg/kg IV/IO.[47] There are reports of anaphylactic reactions in dogs, so close monitoring for signs of anaphylaxis is warranted once ROSC is achieved; if noted, they should be treated appropriately (see Chapter 152).

Lidocaine (2 mg/kg slow IV/IO push) is a less effective alternative to amiodarone for patients with refractory VF. Although lidocaine has been shown to increase the energy required for successful electrical defibrillation in dogs in one study, others have shown that this drug is beneficial.[48,49]

Reversal agents

If any reversible sedative drugs were administered to the patient before CPA, reversal agents may be beneficial and are unlikely to cause harm. Commonly available reversal agents include naloxone (0.04 mg/kg IV/IO) for opioids, flumazenil (0.01 mg/kg IV/IO) for benzodiazepines, and atipamezole (0.05 mg/kg IV/IO) or yohimbine (0.11 mg/kg IV/IO) for α_2 agonists.

Intravenous fluids

Administration of intravenous fluid boluses during CPR may be harmful to euvolemic or hypervolemic patients because they tend to increase central venous (and hence right atrial) pressure rather than arterial blood pressure in patients in CPA. This elevation in right atrial pressure can compromise perfusion of the brain and heart by decreasing MPP and cerebral perfusion pressure. Conversely, patients with documented or suspected hypovolemia will likely benefit from intravenous fluids, which will help to restore adequate preload and may increase the efficacy of chest compressions and improve arterial systolic and diastolic pressures, leading to increased cerebral perfusion pressure and MPP.

Corticosteroids

Most studies have shown no definitive evidence of benefit or harm from corticosteroid administration during CPR, although most were confounded by coadministration of other drugs.[50,51] One prospective observational study in dogs and cats showed an increased rate of ROSC in dogs and cats, but the type and dose of steroids administered were highly variable and a causative effect could not be inferred because of the study design.[1] It is well known that significant gastrointestinal ulceration can develop from a single high dose of corticosteroids.[52-54] In addition, immunosuppression and reduced renal perfusion because of decreased renal prostaglandin production are known side effects. Because of this nonadvantageous risk/benefit ratio, the routine use of corticosteroids is not recommended during CPR.

Alkalinizing agents

Severe metabolic acidosis can develop with prolonged CPA (>10 to 15 minutes), leading to inhibition of normal enzymatic and metabolic activity as well as severe vasodilation. Administration of sodium bicarbonate (1 mEq/kg, once, diluted IV) may be considered in these patients. It should be remembered that these metabolic disturbances may resolve rapidly after ROSC; therefore bicarbonate therapy in patients with prolonged CPA should be reserved for those with severe acidemia (pH < 7) of metabolic origin.

Electrical Defibrillation

Electrical defibrillation is the cornerstone of therapy for VF and pulseless ventricular tachycardia (VT). Guidelines for the approach to electrical defibrillation during CPR have recently been modified because of recent data suggesting a three-phase model of ischemia during VF in the absence of CPR. The initial electrical phase during the first 4 minutes is characterized by minimal ischemia and continued availability of cellular energy stores to maintain metabolic processes. The subsequent 6 minutes, constituting the circulatory phase, are characterized by reversible ischemic injury caused by depletion of cellular adenosine triphosphate (ATP) stores. After 10 minutes, the metabolic phase and potentially irreversible ischemic damage begin.

Based on this model, if the duration of VF is known or suspected to be 4 minutes or less, chest compressions should be continued only until the defibrillator is charged, and the patient should then be defibrillated immediately. However, one full cycle of CPR should be done before defibrillating if the patient has been in VF for more than 4 minutes. This allows blood flow and oxygen delivery to the myocardial cells, which can then generate ATP and restore normal membrane potentials, making the cells more likely to respond favorably to electrical defibrillation.[55]

Two types of defibrillators are available. Monophasic defibrillators deliver current in one direction between the paddles and across the patient's chest, whereas biphasic defibrillators deliver current in one direction before reversing polarity and delivering a current in the opposing direction. Biphasic defibrillators have been shown to successfully defibrillate patients at a lower energy output, leading to less myocardial damage, and are therefore recommended over monophasic devices. Dosing for monophasic defibrillators begins at 4 to 6 J/kg, whereas biphasic defibrillation dosing starts at 2 to 4 J/kg. The dose may be increased by 50% with each defibrillation attempt up to a maximum dose of 10 J/kg (see Chapter 204).

Regardless of the technology used, ALS algorithms no longer recommend three stacked shocks. Instead, chest compressions should be resumed immediately after a single defibrillation attempt without a pause for rhythm analysis. A full 2-minute cycle of BLS should then be administered before reassessing the ECG. If the patient is still in VF, defibrillation should be repeated at the end of this cycle of BLS.[56,57]

OPEN-CHEST CPR

The current International Liaison Committee on Resuscitation Consensus on Science does not currently provide any recommendations on open-chest CPR (OCCPR) because of the lack of controlled clinical trials.[58] However, a number of experimental studies in dogs and clinical studies in people indicate improvements in hemodynamic variables, MPP and cerebral perfusion pressure, and outcome when comparing OCCPR and closed-chest CPR.[59,60] There is also evidence that delays in starting OCCPR lead to poorer outcomes and that after 20 minutes of closed-chest CPR in dogs OCCPR is unlikely to be effective.[61] Although significantly more invasive and costly than closed-chest CPR, the prevailing evidence suggests that improved outcomes from CPA are likely with OCCPR compared with closed-chest CPR, and in cases in which owner consent has been obtained and no underlying diseases that would be contraindications to OCCPR are present (such as thrombocytopenia or coagulopathy), the procedure should be employed as soon as possible after diagnosis of CPA.

To perform OCCPR, a left lateral thoracotomy in the fourth to fifth intercostal space is performed with the animal in right lateral recumbency, and Finochietto retractors are used to open the chest for access to the heart. The pericardium may be removed in all cases to facilitate compressions but should always be removed in patients with pericardial effusion or other pericardial disease. The ventricles can then be directly compressed using either a two-hand technique with the right ventricle cupped in the left hand and the fingers of the right hand placed over the left ventricle or a one-hand technique with the fingers of the right hand placed over the left ventricle and the heart compressed against the sternum.[62] Care should be taken to compress the ventricles from apex to base to maximize forward blood flow. If ROSC is achieved, intensive post–cardiac arrest care will be required after the thoracotomy is closed and a chest tube placed to reduce the risk of pneumothorax.

Although OCCPR may be employed in any patient in CPA, for some conditions leading to CPA it is likely the only viable option. Conditions making external chest compressions futile include pleural space disease, pericardial effusion, and penetrating thoracic injuries. In addition, it is likely that closed-chest CPR will be ineffective in giant-breed dogs with round- or barrel-chested conformation and OCCPR is preferable. Finally, patients already in surgery that experience CPA should likely have OCCPR rather than closed-chest CPR. In patients undergoing abdominal surgery, the heart is easily accessible via an incision in the diaphragm, so thoracotomy is not required.

PROGNOSIS

There are limited data on prognosis in dogs and cats after CPA. It is likely, however, that the cause of the arrest is an important prognostic indicator, as evidenced by a retrospective study of dogs and cats with CPA. The authors found that of 15 dogs and 3 cats that survived to hospital discharge, only 3 of 18 had significant underlying chronic disease, whereas all other patients had acute disease leading to CPA.[31] It is likely that patients experiencing CPA as a consequence of severe, untreatable, or progressive chronic diseases are less likely to survive to hospital discharge, even though these outcomes are confounded by euthanasia. Patients that arrest in the perianesthetic period have a markedly better prognosis, as high as 47% survival to discharge in one recent prospective observational veterinary study, than patients that arrest because of other etiologies.[1] CPR efforts in the population of cats and dogs with acute, treatable disease are warranted and should be aggressive and persistent if the owner consents.

REFERENCES

1. Hofmeister EH, Brainard BM, Egger CM, et al: Prognostic indicators for dogs and cats with cardiopulmonary arrest treated by cardiopulmonary cerebral resuscitation at a university teaching hospital, J Am Vet Med Assoc 235(1):50-57, 2009.
2. Girotra S, Nallamothu BK, Spertus JA., et al: Trends in survival after in-hospital cardiac arrest, N Engl J Med 367(20):1912-1920, 2012.
3. Fletcher DJ, Boller M, Brainard BM, et al: RECOVER evidence and knowledge gap analysis on veterinary CPR. Part 7: Clinical guidelines, J Vet Emerg Criti Care (San Antonio, Tex.: 2001) 22 Suppl 1S102-131, 2012.
4. McMichael M, Herring J, Fletcher DJ, et al: RECOVER evidence and knowledge gap analysis on veterinary CPR. Part 2: Preparedness and prevention, J Vet Emerg Crit Care (San Antonio, Tex.: 2001) 22 Suppl 1S13-25, 2012.
5. Hopper K, Epstein SE, Fletcher DJ, et al: RECOVER evidence and knowledge gap analysis on veterinary CPR. Part 3: Basic life support, J Vet Emerg Crit Care (San Antonio, Tex.: 2001) 22 Suppl 1S26-43, 2012.
6. Rozanski EA, Rush JE, Buckley GJ, et al: RECOVER evidence and knowledge gap analysis on veterinary CPR. Part 4: Advanced life support, J Vet Emerg Crit Care (San Antonio, Tex.: 2001) 22 Suppl 1S44-64, 2012.
7. Brainard BM, Boller M, Fletcher DJ : RECOVER evidence and knowledge gap analysis on veterinary CPR. Part 5: Monitoring, J Vet Emerg Crit Care (San Antonio, Tex.: 2001) 22 Suppl 1S65-84, 2012.
8. Smarick SD, Haskins SC, Boller M, et al: RECOVER evidence and knowledge gap analysis on veterinary CPR. Part 6: Post-cardiac arrest care, J Vet Emerg Crit Care (San Antonio, Tex.: 2001) 22 Suppl 1S85-101, 2012.
9. Noordergraaf GJ, Gelder JM Van, Kesteren RG Van, et al: Learning cardiopulmonary resuscitation skills: does the type of mannequin make a difference? Eur J Emerg Med 4(4):204-209, 1997.
10. Cimrin AH, Topacoglu H, Karcioglu O, et al: A model of standardized training in basic life support skills of emergency medicine residents, Adv Ther 22(1):10-18, 2005.
11. Isbye DL, Meyhoff CS, Lippert FK, et al: Skill retention in adults and in children 3 months after basic life support training using a simple personal resuscitation manikin, Resuscitation 74(2):296-302, 2007.
12. Mpotos N, Lemoyne S, Wyler B, et al: Training to deeper compression depth reduces shallow compressions after six months in a manikin model, Resuscitation 82(10):1323-1327, 2011.
13. Royse AG: New resuscitation trolley: stages in development, Aust Clin Rev 9(3-4):107-114, 1989.
14. Schade J: An evaluation framework for code 99, QRB Qual Rev Bull 9(10):306-309, 1983.
15. Dyson E, Smith GB: Common faults in resuscitation equipment—guidelines for checking equipment and drugs used in adult cardiopulmonary resuscitation, Resuscitation 55(2):137-149, 2002.
16. Edelson DP, Litzinger B, Arora V, et al: Improving in-hospital cardiac arrest process and outcomes with performance debriefing, Arch Intern Med 168(10):1063-1069, 2008.
17. Dine CJ, Gersh RE, Leary M, et al: Improving cardiopulmonary resuscitation quality and resuscitation training by combining audiovisual feedback and debriefing, Crit Care Med 36(10):2817-2822, 2008.
18. Rittenberger JC, Menegazzi JJ, Callaway CW: Association of delay to first intervention with return of spontaneous circulation in a swine model of cardiac arrest, Resuscitation 73(1):154-160, 2007.
19. Dick WF, Eberle B, Wisser G, et al: The carotid pulse check revisited: what if there is no pulse? Criti Care Med 28(11 Suppl):N183-185, 2000.
20. Tyberg JV: Late-systolic retrograde coronary flow: an old observation finally explained by a novel mechanism, J Appl Physiol (Bethesda, Md: 1985) 108(3):479-480, 2010.
21. Khouri EM, Gregg DE, Rayford CR: Effect of exercise on cardiac output, left coronary flow and myocardial metabolism in the unanesthetized dog, Circ Res 17(5):427-437, 1965.
22. Kern KB, Hilwig R, Ewy GA: Retrograde coronary blood flow during cardiopulmonary resuscitation in swine: intracoronary Doppler evaluation, Am Heart J 128(3):490-499, 1994.
23. Andreka P, Frenneaux MP: Haemodynamics of cardiac arrest and resuscitation, Curr Opin Crit Care 12(3):198-203, 2006.
24. Kern KB, Ewy GA, Voorhees WD, et al: Myocardial perfusion pressure: a predictor of 24-hour survival during prolonged cardiac arrest in dogs, Resuscitation 16(4):241-250, 1988.
25. Paradis NA, Martin GB, Rivers EP, et al: Coronary perfusion pressure and the return of spontaneous circulation in human cardiopulmonary resuscitation, JAMA 263(8):1106-1113, 1990.
26. Maier GW, Tyson GS, Olsen CO, et al: The physiology of external cardiac massage: high-impulse cardiopulmonary resuscitation, Circulation 70(1):86-101, 1984.
27. Wolfe JA, Maier GW, Newton JR, et al: Physiologic determinants of coronary blood flow during external cardiac massage, J Thorac Cardiovasc Surg 95(3):523-532, 1988.
28. Kern K, Hilwig R, Berg R, et al: Importance of continuous chest compressions during cardiopulmonary resuscitation, Circulation 105(5):645-649, 2002.
29. Kouwenhoven WB, Jude JR, Knickerbocker GG: Closed-chest cardiac massage, JAMA 1731064-1731067, 1960.
30. Niemann JT, Rosborough J, Hausknecht M, et al: Blood flow without cardiac compression during closed chest CPR, Crit Care Med 9(5): 380-381, 1981.
31. Waldrop JE, Rozanski EA, Swanke ED, et al: Causes of cardiopulmonary arrest, resuscitation management, and functional outcome in dogs and cats surviving cardiopulmonary arrest, J Vet Emerg Crit Care 14(1): 22-29, 2004.
32. Plunkett SJ, McMichael M. Cardiopulmonary resuscitation in small animal medicine: an update, J Vet Intern Med 22(1):9-25, 2008.
33. Grmec S, Klemen P: Does the end-tidal carbon dioxide (EtCO2) concentration have prognostic value during out-of-hospital cardiac arrest? Eur J Emerg Med 8(4):263-269, 2001.
34. Pokorná M, Necas E, Kratochvíl J, et al: A sudden increase in partial pressure end-tidal carbon dioxide (P(ET)CO(2)) at the moment of return of spontaneous circulation, J Emerg Med 38(5):614-621, 2010.
35. Li J. Capnography alone is imperfect for endotracheal tube placement confirmation during emergency intubation, J Emerg Med 20(3):223-229, 2001.
36. Kolar M, Krizmaric M, Klemen P, et al: Partial pressure of end-tidal carbon dioxide successful predicts cardiopulmonary resuscitation in the field: a prospective observational study, Crit Care (London) 12(5):R115, 2008.
37. Bassiakou E, Xanthos T, Papadimitriou L: The potential beneficial effects of beta adrenergic blockade in the treatment of ventricular fibrillation, Eur J Pharmacol 616(1-3):1-6, 2009.
38. Koehler RC, Michael JR, Guerci AD, et al: Beneficial effect of epinephrine infusion on cerebral and myocardial blood flows during CPR, Ann Emerg Med 14(8):744-749, 1985.
39. Vandycke C, Martens P: High dose versus standard dose epinephrine in cardiac arrest - a meta-analysis, Resuscitation 45(3):161-166, 2000.
40. Manisterski Y, Vaknin Z, Ben-Abraham R, et al: Endotracheal epinephrine: a call for larger doses, Anesth Analg 95(4):1037-1041, table of contents, 2002.

41. Callaway CW: Epinephrine for cardiac arrest, Curr Opin Cardiol 28(1): 36-42, 2013.
42. Biondi-Zoccai GGL, Abbate A, Parisi Q, et al: Is vasopressin superior to adrenaline or placebo in the management of cardiac arrest? A meta-analysis, Resuscitation 59(2):221-224, 2003.
43. Blecic S, Chaskis C, Vincent JL: Atropine administration in experimental electromechanical dissociation, Am J Emerg Med 10(6):515-518, 1992.
44. DeBehnke DJ, Swart GL, Spreng D, et al: Standard and higher doses of atropine in a canine model of pulseless electrical activity, Acad Emerg Med 2(12):1034-1041, 1995.
45. Coon GA, Clinton JE, Ruiz E: Use of atropine for brady-asystolic prehospital cardiac arrest, Ann Emerg Med 10(9):462-467, 1981.
46. Paret G, Mazkereth R, Sella R, et al: Atropine pharmacokinetics and pharmacodynamics following endotracheal versus endobronchial administration in dogs, Resuscitation 41(1):57-62, 1999.
47. Anastasiou-Nana MI, Nanas JN, Nanas SN, et al: Effects of amiodarone on refractory ventricular fibrillation in acute myocardial infarction: experimental study, J Am Coll Cardiol 23(1):253-258, 1994.
48. Dorian P, Cass D, Schwartz B, et al: Amiodarone as compared with lidocaine for shock-resistant ventricular fibrillation, N Engl J Med 346(12):884-890, 2002.
49. Dorian P, Fain ES, Davy J-M, et al: Lidocaine causes a reversible, concentration-dependent increase in defibrillation energy requirements, J Am Coll Cardiol 8(2):327-332, 1986.
50. Mentzelopoulos SD, Zakynthinos SG, Tzoufi M, et al: Vasopressin, epinephrine, and corticosteroids for in-hospital cardiac arrest, Arch Intern Med 169(1):15-24, 2009.
51. Smithline H, Rivers E, Appleton T, et al: Corticosteroid supplementation during cardiac arrest in rats, Resuscitation 25(3):257-264, 1993.
52. Levine JM, Levine GJ, Boozer L, et al: Adverse effects and outcome associated with dexamethasone administration in dogs with acute thoracolumbar intervertebral disk herniation: 161 cases (2000-2006), J Am Vet Med Assoc 232(3):411-417, 2008.
53. Dillon AR, Sorjonen DC, Powers RD, et al: Effects of dexamethasone and surgical hypotension on hepatic morphologic features and enzymes of dogs, Am J Vet Res 44(11):1996-1999, 1983.
54. Rohrer CR, Hill RC, Fischer A, et al: Gastric hemorrhage in dogs given high doses of methylprednisolone sodium succinate, Am J Vet Res 1999;60(8):977-981, 1999.
55. Weisfeldt ML, Becker LB: Resuscitation after cardiac arrest: a 3-phase time-sensitive model, JAMA 288(23):3035-3038, 2002.
56. Cammarata G, Weil MH, Csapoczi P, et al: Challenging the rationale of three sequential shocks for defibrillation, Resuscitation 69(1):23-27, 2006.
57. Tang W, Snyder D, Wang J, et al: One-shock versus three-shock defibrillation protocol significantly improves outcome in a porcine model of prolonged ventricular fibrillation cardiac arrest, Circulation 113(23): 2683-2689, 2006.
58. Shuster M, Lim SH, Deakin CD, et al: Part 7: CPR techniques and devices: 2010 International Consensus on Cardiopulmonary Resuscitation and Emergency Cardiovascular Care Science with treatment recommendations, Circulation 122(16 Suppl 2):S338-344, 2010.
59. Alzaga-Fernandez AG, Varon J: Open-chest cardiopulmonary resuscitation: past, present and future, Resuscitation 64(2):149-156, 2005.
60. Benson DM, O'Neil B, Kakish E, et al: Open-chest CPR improves survival and neurologic outcome following cardiac arrest, Resuscitation 64(2):209-217, 2005.
61. Kern KB, Sanders AB, Ewy GA: Open-chest cardiac massage after closed-chest compression in a canine model: when to intervene, Resuscitation 15(1):51-57, 1987.
62. Barnett WM, Alifimoff JK, Paris PM, et al: Comparison of open-chest cardiac massage techniques in dogs, Ann Emerg Med 15(4):408-411, 1986.

CHAPTER 4
POST–CARDIAC ARREST CARE

Manuel Boller, DrMedVet, MTR, DACVECC • Daniel J. Fletcher, PhD, DVM, DACVECC

KEY POINTS

- The systemic response to ischemia and reperfusion, anoxic brain injury, postresuscitation myocardial dysfunction, and persistent precipitating pathologic conditions define post–cardiac arrest care measures needed for each individual patient.
- Immediate post–cardiac arrest care focuses on prevention of rearrest by ensuring optimal ventilation, oxygenation, and tissue perfusion, as well as identifying and correcting reversible causes of cardiopulmonary arrest.
- Hypoxemia and hyperoxemia early after return of spontaneous circulation (ROSC) should be prevented by controlled reoxygenation with a target SaO_2/SpO_2 of 94% to 98% or a PaO_2 of 80 to 100 mm Hg.
- Hemodynamic optimization measures after ROSC include administration of intravenous fluids, pressors, inotropes, and blood products to reach a mean arterial pressure (MAP) of 80 mm Hg or higher, an $ScvO_2$ of 70% or more, and a lactate of less than 2.5 mmol/L.
- Mild therapeutic hypothermia (32° to 34° C) for 24 to 48 hours is recommended in patients that remain comatose after ROSC if mechanical ventilation and advanced critical care capability is available.
- Additional neuroprotective strategies include permissive hypothermia, slow rewarming (0.25° to 0.5° C/hr), osmotic therapy, and seizure prophylaxis.
- Critically ill survivors should be referred to veterinary critical care centers for post–cardiac arrest care.

Ahead of his time, the Russian resuscitation scientist and physician Vladimir Negovsky stated in 1972 that "after the first step in resuscitation when heart function and respiration have been restored, the second step in resuscitation arises—the more complicated problems of treating the after-effects of a general hypoxia."[1] Since then, post–cardiac arrest (PCA) care has been increasingly emphasized as a key element of cardiopulmonary resuscitation (CPR). Current CPR guidelines in both human and veterinary medicine devote entire sections to the care of those patients that achieved return of spontaneous circulation (ROSC) after cardiopulmonary arrest (CPA).[2-5] The rationale behind this is twofold. First, epidemiologic studies in people show that two thirds of in-hospital cardiac arrest (IHCA) patients who achieve stable ROSC do not survive to hospital discharge.[6] In veterinary medicine 85% of dogs or cats with ROSC are euthanized or die before hospital discharge (Figure 4-1).[7] Thus optimization of PCA care has the potential to save many lives. Second, new opportunities for delivering complex therapies are now available. Foremost, clear evidence of the neuroprotective potential of mild therapeutic hypothermia (MTH) boosted the field of PCA care. The protective effect of cooling also demonstrated that PCA treatment, even if delayed after ROSC, can influence outcome dramatically. Recent human epidemiologic data suggest that the improvement in outcomes achieved after IHCA over the past 10 years in part is due to increased postresuscitation survival.[8] PCA arrest care is now considered the final essential link of a comprehensive treatment strategy to optimize outcomes from CPA (Figure 4-2).

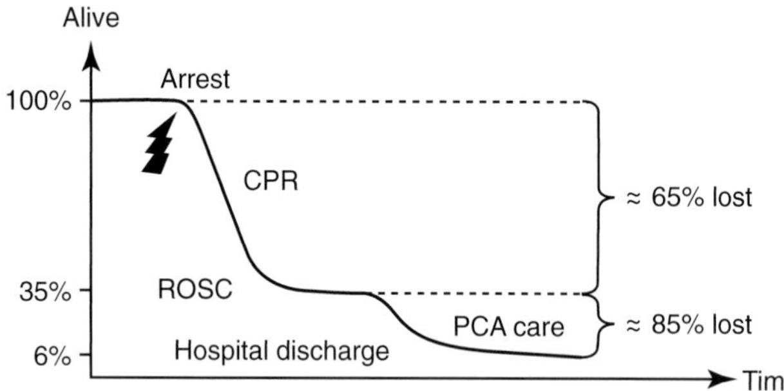

FIGURE 4-1 The epidemiology of veterinary CPR is characterized by two phases of patient losses. First, the two thirds of patients that do not reach ROSC despite initiation of CPR. Second, the large majority of patients that do not survive to hospital discharge, despite initial ROSC. Thus patient management during the PCA phase is as important as CPR to improve outcomes. *(Data from Hofmeister EH, Brainard BM, Egger CM, et al: Prognostic indicators for dogs and cats with cardiopulmonary arrest treated by cardiopulmonary cerebral resuscitation at a university teaching hospital, J Am Vet Med Assoc 235(1):50-57, 2009.)*

There are two paradigms of care during the PCA phase. One aims at pathophysiologic processes that occur in the postresuscitation phase, namely (1) ischemia and reperfusion (IR) injury, (2) PCA brain injury, (3) PCA myocardial dysfunction, and (4) persistent precipitating pathologic conditions (Figure 4-3). The other paradigm of care responds to a shift in treatment prioritization as time after ROSC progresses. Immediately after ROSC, the focus is on prevention of recurrence of cardiac arrest and limitation of organ injury. Later care emphasizes treatment of the underlying disease processes, prognostication, and rehabilitation.[2]

PROPAGATING SUSTAINED ROSC

The majority of dogs and cats that are initially successfully resuscitated die within the first few hours because of rearrest.[9] The goal immediately after ROSC is to sustain spontaneous circulation and perfusion of vital organs, such as the brain and the myocardium, attenuating further injury and preventing rearrest. Although patient monitoring options are limited during CPA (see Chapter 3), common monitoring such as noninvasive blood pressure measurement and pulse oximetry provide useful information after ROSC. Identification of any reversible cause of CPA needs to be proactively pursued. If not already addressed during advanced life support (ALS), it is important to assess for abnormalities in electrolytes, glucose, acid-base status, hematocrit, arterial oxygenation, and ventilation soon after ROSC. Abnormalities such as hypoxemia, severe anemia, hypotension, and hyperkalemia or hypocalcemia must be corrected aggressively. The incidence of rearrest rhythms has not been systematically reported in veterinary patients, but in people, shockable and nonshockable rhythms are equally prevalent, with ventricular fibrillation (VF) and pulseless ventricular tachycardia (VT) identified in 15% and 29%, respectively.[10] If VT persists, treatment with lidocaine (2 mg/kg intravenous [IV] bolus, followed by a 30 to 50 mcg/kg/min infusion) is recommended. Catecholamine administration may be necessary to maintain vascular tone and adequate blood pressure. Positive inotropic support can serve to attenuate postischemic left ventricular

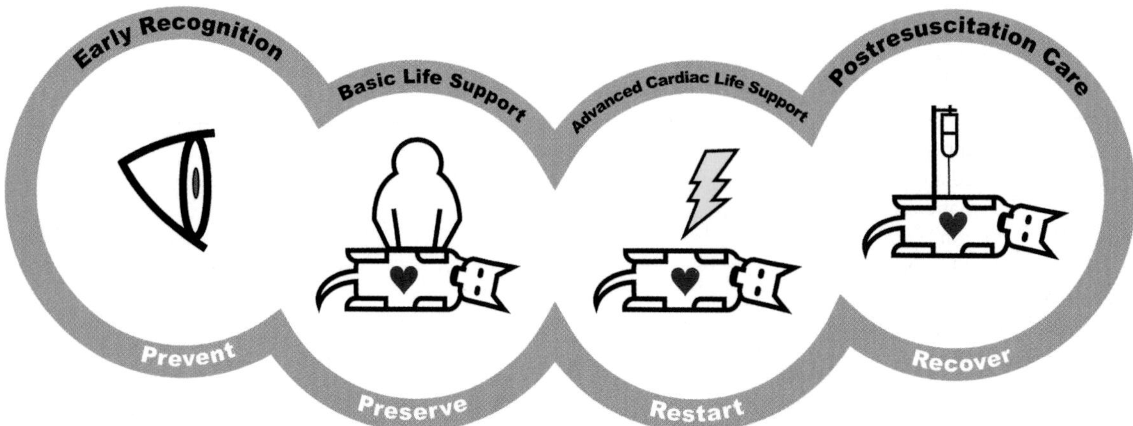

FIGURE 4-2 The chain of survival for dogs and cats symbolizing the continuum of care required to successfully manage CPA. *(From Boller M, Boller EM, Oodegard S, et al: Small animal cardiopulmonary resuscitation requires a continuum of care: proposal for a chain of survival for veterinary patients, J Am Vet Med Assoc 240(5):540-554, 2012.)*

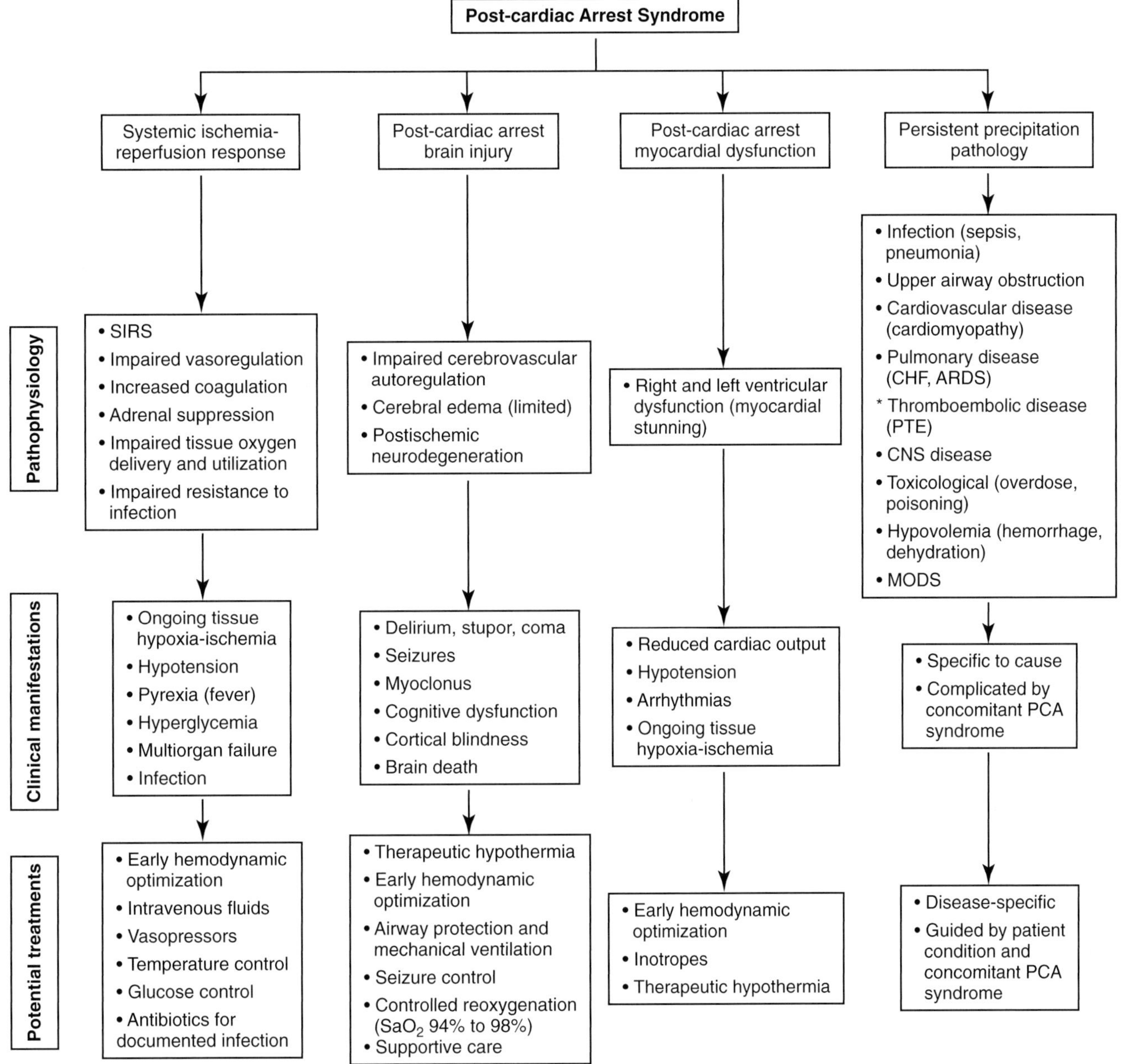

FIGURE 4-3 Flowchart summarizing pathophysiology, clinical manifestations, and potential treatments for the four major components of the post–cardiac arrest syndrome. *ARDS,* Acute respiratory distress syndrome; *CHF,* congestive heart failure; MODS, multiorgan dysfunction syndrome; *PCA,* Post–cardiac arrest; *PTE,* pulmonary thromboembolism; SIRS, systemic inflammatory response syndrome. *(Modified with permission from Boller M, Boller EM, Oodegard S, et al: Small animal cardiopulmonary resuscitation requires a continuum of care: proposal for a chain of survival for veterinary patients, J Am Vet Med Assoc 240(5):540-554, 2012.)*

systolic dysfunction.[11,12] Ventilatory assistance is almost invariably necessary during the immediate postresuscitation phase and needs to be delivered by either manual or mechanical ventilation with a target $PaCO_2$ of 32 to 43 mm Hg in dogs and 26 to 36 mm Hg in cats. Once sustained ROSC has been achieved for the first 20 to 40 minutes, the clinician's attention can be directed toward attenuation of the evolution of further organ injury that arises as a consequence of IR and to titrate supportive care to the needs of the patient.

SYSTEMIC RESPONSE TO ISCHEMIA AND REPERFUSION: SEPSIS-LIKE SYNDROME

ROSC after the global ischemic event of CPA leads to a whole-body IR syndrome that Negovsky characterized as "post-resuscitation disease" more than 40 years ago.[1] The syndrome shares many characteristics with severe sepsis, specifically in regard to inflammation, coagulation, and the endothelium.[1,13-28] After observing neutrophil and endothelial activation paired with high concentrations of circulating cytokines (tumor necrosis factor α [TNF-α], interleukin 6 [IL-6], IL-9, IL-10) in the postarrest phase in humans, Adrie et al coined the term *sepsis-like syndrome* to describe the phenotype of post–cardiac arrest abnormalities.[29] Thus the PCA patient may have characteristics that are similar to severe sepsis and multiorgan dysfunction syndrome. With that in mind, therapeutic considerations involving (1) early hemodynamic optimization, (2) glycemic control, and (3) critical illness–related corticosteroid insufficiency (CIRCI) are being examined in human medicine and have relevance to veterinary PCA care. Naturally, treatment is highly individualized, each element of care being carefully titrated to the patient's needs. This titration is guided by monitoring—that is, by assessment and reassessment of predefined treatment endpoints.

Hemodynamic Optimization

Early goal-directed therapy (EGDT) was studied by Rivers et al more than 10 years ago as a strategy of hemodynamic optimization in patients with severe sepsis and septic shock.[30] EGDT uses an algorithm in which single interventions are started or discontinued based on the achievement of predefined physiologic endpoints with an emphasis on early resuscitation. In human medicine, the EGDT approach has been implemented for PCA care as an early hemodynamic optimization protocol bundled together with mild therapeutic hypothermia.[31,32] Included interventions are those to optimize tissue oxygen delivery (fluid administration, vasopressors/inotropes, red blood cell transfusion, oxygen supplementation) and to decrease tissue oxygen demand (sedation, mechanical ventilation, neuromuscular blockade, temperature control). A veterinary PCA hemodynamic optimization algorithm has been published by the RECOVER initiative.[33] Resuscitation endpoints are central venous pressure (CVP; 0 mm Hg < CVP < 10 mm Hg), mean arterial blood pressure (MAP 80 to 120 mm Hg), and perfusion parameters (central venous oxygen saturation [$ScvO_2$] > 70 %; lactate < 2.5 mmol/L). Markers of vasodilation, such as injected mucous membranes or shortened capillary refill time, pulse quality, and echocardiographic determination of left ventricular function should also be included in a comprehensive hemodynamic assessment. Such monitoring will guide effective yet safe treatment with fluids, vasopressors, and inotropes (see Chapters 8 and 183). Although there are no veterinary studies validating this approach yet, goal-directed therapy is an excellent example for how monitoring interacts with treatment. There is considerable diversity of the PCA patient response to injury and treatment, and a "one-size-fits-all" therapeutic strategy is not appropriate.

Glycemic Control

Hyperglycemia commonly occurs after cardiac arrest in humans and has been associated with worse outcome.[34-37] Mild to moderate hyperglycemia combined with a total plasma insulin decrease of 60% was observed in experimental research in dogs early after ROSC.[38] Animal studies (including canine) have demonstrated that hyperglycemia worsens ischemic brain injury.[39-42] In humans, iatrogenic hypoglycemia occurred in 18% of PCA patients treated with tight glycemic control (4.4 to 6.1 mmol/L; 80 to 110 mg/dl). There is no evidence that tight glucose control provides additional benefits over a less stringent target, and moderate glycemic control targeting glucose levels less than 180 mg/dl is currently suggested for human PCA patients.[3,36,43] A similar strategy in dogs and cats after cardiac arrest may be considered. Implementation of glycemic control with intravenous insulin administration follows the recommendation for patients with severe sepsis (see Chapter 6).

Adrenal Dysfunction

Steroids are essential to the physiologic response to severe stress and are important for the regulation of vascular tone and endothelial permeability. CIRCI, or relative adrenal insufficiency (RAI), after ROSC was identified in several human clinical studies and has been associated with increased mortality.[44-49] Low-dose steroid administration for septic shock remains controversial,[50] and direct evidence supporting corticosteroid administration during PCA care is lacking. Because of this and the risk for infection, peptic ulcer, and exacerbation of postischemic neurologic injury associated with corticosteroid administration, routine administration of corticosteroids during PCA care is not recommended.[33] However, administration of low-dose hydrocortisone (1 mg/kg IV followed by either 1 mg/kg IV q6h or an intravenous infusion of 0.15 mg/kg/hr) in dogs and cats with vasopressor-dependent shock after CPA, with or without documented CIRCI, may be considered.[33]

POST–CARDIAC ARREST BRAIN INJURY

In humans, cerebral dysfunction after cardiac arrest is the single greatest concern and the most common single cause of death. In one study neurologic injury was the cause of death in two thirds of patients after out-of-hospital cardiac arrest (OHCA) and one fifth after IHCA.[51] In small animals, PCA brain injury has been described in experimental and clinical reports, but little is known about its epidemiology.[52-55] PCA brain injury results from global cerebral IR.[56] Although the process is complex and not understood in its entirety, some aspects of cerebral IR injury are clear:

1. Most of the injury is sustained during reperfusion and not during ischemia, affording the clinician the opportunity to intervene after ROSC is achieved.
2. Cytosolic and mitochondrial calcium overload leads to activation of proteases that may lead to neuronal death and production of reactive oxygen species (ROS).[57,58]
3. A burst of ROS occurs during reperfusion, leading to oxidative alterations of lipids, proteins, and nucleic acids propagating injury of neuronal cell components and limiting the cells' protective and repair mechanisms.[56]
4. Mild therapeutic hypothermia administered after ROSC is proven to reduce postresuscitation cerebral dysfunction.[59]

Brain Injury Sustained During Ischemia Versus During Reperfusion

Much of the injury sustained after CPA evolves during reperfusion rather than ischemia. By optimizing the reperfusion process, extended durations of ischemia can be tolerated.[60,61] Nevertheless, IR is a continuum that is initiated during cellular ischemia. A sudden decline in oxygen delivery occurs upon onset of CPA. Glycolysis allows for limited continued energy production, but cerebral adenosine triphosphate (ATP) stores are depleted within 2 to 4 minutes. In contrast, 20 to 40 minutes are required for the same to occur in the intestines and the myocardium.[62-64] Once ATP is depleted, cellular membrane potentials are rapidly lost. Clinically, any cardiac electrical activity as detected by electrocardiogram (ECG) provides evidence that the global myocardial membrane potential has not yet subsided, or, during reperfusion, has been reestablished once again. Large amounts of sodium, chloride, and calcium enter the cells, followed by cell swelling and membrane disruption. It is believed that the combined influences of increased exposure to calcium, oxidative stress, and energy depletion lead to mitochondrial injury, finally leading to more ROS production upon reperfusion and to apoptosis and necrosis.[56,65] Therefore, controlled reperfusion strategies include mild hypocalcemia and avoidance of hyperoxemia.[57,61,66] Recent experimental studies have demonstrated neurologically intact survival using these strategies even after 30 minutes of warm cerebral ischemia.[67,68]

Controlled Reoxygenation

Large amounts of ROS are generated after CPR.[69-71] Becker and Neumar summarized in detail the pathobiology of ROS because of IR in the PCA period.[72,73] Excessive production of ROS in the presence of exhausted protective mechanisms peaks in elaboration of highly reactive free radicals, namely hydroxyl radicals (•OH) and peroxynitrite (ONOO•), which in turn cause cell membrane damage, lipid peroxidation, DNA damage, and protein alterations.

Rapid reoxygenation following prolonged global ischemia is an implied goal of CPR and essential for saving lives from cardiac arrest. However, the absolute requirement of reintroducing oxygen conflicts with the toxic potential of oxygen as substrate for ROS.

Much evidence suggests that arterial hyperoxemia soon after ROSC increases oxidative brain injury, increases neurodegeneration, worsens functional neurologic outcome, and negatively affects overall survival.[72] Retrospective clinical studies in humans demonstrated an association between post-ROSC hyperoxemia and in-hospital mortality and documented a linear relationship between the degree of hyperoxemia and nonsurvival.[74,75] In a canine experimental study, titration of oxygen supplementation to an SpO_2 of 94% to 96% compared with a consistent FiO_2 of 1 lead to superior functional neurologic outcomes and a reduction in neuronal degeneration in vulnerable brain regions.[55] The inspired oxygen concentration, especially early after ROSC, should therefore be titrated to normoxemia (PaO_2 80 to 100 mm Hg; SpO_2 94% to 98%), avoiding both hypoxemia and hyperoxemia.[33]

Mild Therapeutic Hypothermia

Mild therapeutic hypothermia (MTH) is the only treatment proven in clinical trials to be effective in increasing neurologically intact survival after resuscitation from OHCA, whereas conclusive data are still awaited for IHCA.[3,76,77] MTH exerts its protective effects via a number of processes, including a reduction of mitochondrial injury and dysfunction, decrease in cerebral metabolism, reduction of calcium inflow into cells and neuronal excitotoxicity, reduced production of ROS and reduced apoptosis, and suppression of seizure activity.[59] MTH consists of reduction of the core body temperature to 32° to 34°C (89.6° to 93.2° F). A variety of cooling methods have been used in humans, including cooling blankets, simple icepacks, intravenous infusion of ice cold saline, and endovascular cooling devices.[78] Cooling to target temperature early after ROSC, or even during reperfusion, is likely more effective than a delay in cooling.[79] The optimal duration of MTH is unknown, and likely varies, with the more severely injured patients requiring a longer duration of cooling. MTH for 24 to 48 hours is recommended in dogs and cats that remain comatose after ROSC, followed by rewarming at a slow rate of 0.25° to 0.5° C (0.45° to 0.9° F) per hour.[33] Patient management and monitoring efforts may be considerable during MTH and are likely similar to that needed for mechanical ventilation. However, the use of hypothermia has been described in veterinary medicine indicating that implementation of MTH is feasible.[80,81] Clinical application of MTH requires managing the side effects. Cooling induces increased muscle tone and shivering, which in return leads to increased oxygen consumption, metabolic rate, and respiratory and heart rates and requires sedation, endotracheal intubation, and ventilation.[82] Cooling without sedation may abolish the protective effect of MTH.[59] Other physiologic disturbances can occur, including changes in metabolism, acid-base status, electrolytes, ECG, drug elimination, coagulation, and immune function, and the clinician should be familiar with those alterations when using PCA cooling.[59] However, adverse effects associated with PCA hypothermia in humans with OHCA were found to be on par with normothermic care and did not affect mortality.[83,84] Nevertheless, the side effects profile may be different in different species such as dogs and cats and after IHCA, where sepsis and coagulopathy is not uncommon. If either of these conditions is present, the benefit of MTH needs to be carefully weighed against the risk.

Many small animals are spontaneously hypothermic after CPA. Allowing the patient to slowly rewarm to normal core temperature over many hours after CPA without quick active rewarming (i.e., permissive hypothermia) offers an alternative to MTH. Even though the entire potential of MTH will not be realized with this approach, it may attenuate the harmful effects of a rapid increase in brain temperature after ischemia. It is reasonable to target a rewarming rate of 0.25° C to 0.5°C (0.45° to 0.9° F) per hour.[33] In addition, it is important to prevent fever or hyperthermia after CPA because it is associated with increased mortality.[3,37]

Other Neuroprotective Treatment Strategies

Although epidemiologic data are lacking, clinical experience suggests that post-CPA seizures can occur in dogs and cats. In humans, the occurrence of seizures during the first 3 days after CPA is associated with worse outcome. Nonconvulsive status epilepticus (i.e., only identified by electroencephalography) occurs commonly in humans who remain comatose after ROSC.[85] Seizure activity leads to a drastic increase in cerebral metabolism and oxygen demand, possibly outstripping oxygen supply. Thus patients should be monitored for seizures and treated accordingly if they occur (see Chapter 82). Prophylactic administration of barbiturates should also be considered.[33] This may be particularly relevant in animals that remain comatose or are sedated, because nonconvulsive seizure activity may be present and difficult to diagnose.

Cytotoxic and vasogenic cerebral edema have been described after CPA and are associated with poor neurologic outcome in people.[86] In contrast, intracranial hypertension (ICH) does not commonly occur,[87] but if it does it can compromise cerebral perfusion pressure and thus cerebral blood flow. In dogs, hypertonic fluid administration after 14 minutes of anoxic brain injury decreased cerebral edema but did not affect survival or functional neurologic outcome.[88] In general, the use of hypertonic solutions such as mannitol or hypertonic saline for reduction of cerebral edema after cardiac arrest has not been well examined, and the few studies available demonstrate neither benefit nor harm.[5] Thus the use of mannitol or hypertonic saline can be considered if the presence of cerebral edema is suggested by clinical signs, such as coma, stupor, or decerebrate posture.[33] Unfortunately the clinical signs of ICH overlap with the neurologic deficits often seen after CPA.

Induction of supranormal cerebral perfusion pressure during the PCA phase has been demonstrated to be beneficial, indicating that a clinically relevant increased intracranial pressure or resistance to blood flow exists. In dogs after 12.5 minutes of untreated ventricular fibrillation, more than 50% of the brain remained below baseline blood flow 1 to 4 hours after resuscitation but not in animals with hypertensive hemodilution with a hematocrit of 20% and a mean arterial pressure of 140 mm Hg.[89] Similar results were found in other animal studies of optimized brain perfusion after prolonged cardiac arrest.[68] In addition to an increased intracranial pressure, perivascular edema, intravascular coagulation, and a loss of blood flow autoregulation may also be responsible for the beneficial effect of supranormal cerebral perfusion pressures after prolonged cardiac arrest.[90-94] It is likely that these mechanisms are of less importance during shorter durations of CPA and thus a less aggressive perfusion pressure goal may be sufficient in most clinical veterinary cases.[33] Experimental evidence suggests that the CO_2 responsiveness of cerebral arteries is disturbed for the first several hours after prolonged ischemia such that arterial vasodilation in response to increasing $PaCO_2$ is abolished.[95-97] In contrast, with shorter durations of cerebral ischemia or later after reperfusion, CO_2 responsiveness was maintained or restored such that hyperventilation after ROSC reduced cerebral blood flow and worsened neurologic outcomes compared with normoventilation.[96,98-100] Similarly, the decreased tissue pH associated with hypoventilation could be harmful. It is therefore reasonable to avoid both hypoventilation and hyperventilation after ROSC and to control ventilation such that normoventilation is achieved (dog: $PaCO_2$ 32 to 42 mm Hg; cat: $PaCO_2$ 26 to 36 mm Hg).[33]

Neurologic Assessment and Prognostication

Assessing the patient's PCA neurologic status is relevant for treatment decisions and prognostication. Complete neurologic examinations should be undertaken directly after ROSC and initially every 2 to 4 hours. Care should be taken to interpret the findings in light of factors that confound the neurologic examination, such as sedation, neuromuscular blockade, seizures, and postictal status. Neurologic deficit scoring systems that include metrics of consciousness, motor and sensory function, and behavior have been used in clinical and experimental studies using dogs.[53,101] Alternatively, the Modified Glasgow Coma Scale (MGCS), originally developed for dogs with traumatic brain injury, can be used to systematically assess and track the patient's overall PCA neurologic status, although it has not been validated for this indication.[102] The MGCS assesses function of the brainstem (cranial nerve reflexes) and cerebral hemispheres (motor response) in conjunction with the level of consciousness.

In principle, any retention of normal neurologic function immediately after ROSC supports a favorable prognosis. Conversely, studies of comatose human survivors of CPA suggest that clinical neurologic examination is not a reliable predictor of poor outcome during the first 24 hours after ROSC.[103] Early absence of pupillary light response (PLR) in comatose patients led to a false-positive rate for prediction of irreversible unconsciousness of more than 30%.[104] Between 24 and 72 hours, presence of coma and absence of PLR significantly increased the likelihood of poor neurologic outcomes, but conscious survival is possible. It is not until 3 days after ROSC that lack of PLR and absence of motor response to a painful stimulus predict reliably that a human patient will fail to regain consciousness.[103] Sedation and MTH will further delay the ability for definitive prognostication.[105] Even though no comparable data are available for veterinary patients, the notion that early clinical prognostication of the final neurologic outcome is unreliable is likely true in dogs and cats also. Apart from clinical neurologic examinations, other prognostic tools have been examined. Electrophysiologic measurements, such as electroencephalography (EEG), somatosensory evoked potentials (SSEP) and brainstem auditory evoked response (BAER), were shown to aid in early detection of futility in humans.[103] Depending on the available veterinary expertise, electrophysiologic assessment may be useful in dogs and cats as an adjunct to neurologic examination. BAER has been well described in the veterinary literature for auditory assessment, although reports on its use in ischemic brain injury in dogs or cats are sparse.[106,107] Elevations of neuron-specific enolase (NSE) levels in cerebrospinal fluid (CSF) or plasma, a commonly used biomarker of neuronal injury after CPA, were found to imply poor neurologic outcome in experimental animal and clinical human studies, but the assay is not available for clinical veterinary use at this time.[103,108,109] Brain imaging modalities, such as computed tomography or magnetic resonance imaging, are currently insufficiently validated for prediction of neurologic outcomes.[103] Taken altogether, veterinary neurologic prognostication currently depends on clinical findings and in some instances BAER or EEG. Moreover, it is important to recognize that futility of care from a neurologic point of view is difficult to predict during the first 24 to 72 hours. One clinical implication of this is that costly PCA care in animals that remain comatose after ROSC has to be initiated in the absence of valid neurologic prognostication. In addition, it is important to recognize that there is significant potential for neurologic recovery, provided adequate supportive care is possible. Waldrop et al (2004) documented that neurologic abnormalities present after ROSC, such as dullness, ataxia, circling, seizures, and blindness, resolved in 90% of CPA survivors before hospital discharge.[110]

MYOCARDIAL DYSFUNCTION

Myocardial dysfunction (MD) is well described after cardiac arrest in experimental studies and in humans and has been the subject of one recent veterinary case report.[12,14,111] MD occurs even in cases free of coronary artery disease and, like brain injury, its extent is attenuated by hypothermia. PCA myocardial dysfunction is characterized by increased central venous and pulmonary capillary wedge pressure, reduced left- and right sided systolic and diastolic ventricular function with increased end-diastolic and end-systolic volume, and reduced left ventricular ejection fraction and cardiac output.[11,12,14,111,112] These changes may be further complicated by ventricular tachyarrhythmia, together leading to cardiogenic shock in severe cases. MD is reversible and typically resolves within 48 hours.[12,14] This reversibility in the absence of cell necrosis is the basis for the term *myocardial stunning.* Mechanisms of injury are not fully understood and are multifactorial. Myocyte dysfunction results from cellular processes associated with cellular IR comparable to those evolving in the nervous system.[113] Thus the severity of MD depends on the duration and extent of myocardial ischemia as well as the conditions under which reperfusion occurs (e.g., presence or absence of hypothermia). Second, a lack of capillary blood flow during PCA (myocardial no-reflow) may occur.[14,114] Microvascular obstruction or plugging may occur subsequent to endothelial cell activation and swelling, neutrophil–endothelial cell interactions, activation of coagulation, and platelet aggregation.[114] Pericapillary edema will further impede microvascular blood flow. With alterations in capillary permeability, the subsequent increase in microvascular hematocrit and total protein and the associated rheologic properties, tissue blood flow can be impaired. Moreover, postischemic red blood cells may have reduced deformability and have a tendency toward endothelial cell adhesion and to form erythrocyte plugs. Third, several factors were found to worsen MD, including intra-arrest administration of epinephrine and high energy and monophasic waveform defibrillation.[14] Diagnosis and monitoring of progression and resolution of MD during the PCA phase is best accomplished noninvasively via serial echocardiography.[12] However, therapeutic decision making demands additional monitoring of right-sided filling pressures, to limit the risk for hydrostatic pulmonary edema, and of perfusion parameters (e.g., lactate, $ScvO_2$). MTH attenuates MD.[115-117] No other treatments have been identified to be clinically effective in attenuating the occurrence of PCA MD at this time.[111] Dobutamine administration at typical clinical doses used in dogs and cats was shown to effectively improve left ventricular function and cardiac output. Cardiac arrhythmias should be addressed commensurate to their significance (see the Cardiac Disorders section).

PERSISTENT PRECIPITATING PATHOLOGY

IHCA, the most common CPA scenario confronting the small-animal clinician, is often triggered by preexisting disease processes, such as severe sepsis, trauma, or respiratory failure. These pathologic conditions will likely persist after ROSC. They will affect the specific PCA care provided and influence the prognosis. Precipitating processes and preexisting comorbidities add great variability to the PCA patient population. Limited information is available about what these factors are in small-animal patients. In one veterinary study including 204 dogs and cats, causes of CPA were identified as hypoxemia (36%), shock (18%), anemia (13%), arrhythmia (8%), MODS (6%), traumatic brain injury (5%), anaphylaxis (1%), or other causes (21%).[7] Another study suggests that trauma is a more common clinical feature in cats compared with dogs with CPA.[9] Meaney et al identified in 51,919 human patients with IHCA as cause of cardiac arrest: hypotension (39%); acute respiratory failure (37%); acute myocardial infarction (10%); and metabolic/electrolyte disturbances (10%).[118] In dogs, the first identified rhythm is by far more commonly asystole and PEA than pulseless VT/VF.[53] In humans, survival to hospital discharge after IHCA is markedly worse in patients with PEA/asystole compared with VT/VF.[8,118-120] Because nonshockable rhythms do more commonly occur as a result of severe systemic disease than VF/VT, this serves as indirect indicator of the importance of preexisting diseases on survival.[121] A recently published validated prognostic tool to be used in early survivors from IHCA included as predictors not only age, initial arrest rhythm, prearrest neurologic function, and duration of CPR but also scores for the presence of preexisting disease, including mechanical ventilation, renal and hepatic insufficiency, sepsis, malignancy, and hypotension.[122]

This information taken together indicates that the PCA population encountered after IHCA is influenced by a plethora of preexisting conditions. These demand an individualized patient approach using critical care principles to support oxygenation, ventilation, circulation, and metabolism in order to realize the animal's potential for a positive, meaningful outcome.

REFERENCES

1. Negovsky VA: The second step in resuscitation—the treatment of the 'post-resuscitation disease,' Resuscitation 1(1):1-7, 1972.
2. Neumar RW, Nolan JP, Adrie C, et al: Post-cardiac arrest syndrome: epidemiology, pathophysiology, treatment, and prognostication, Circulation 118(23):2452-2483, 2008.
3. Peberdy MA, Callaway CW, Neumar RW, et al: Part 9: post-cardiac arrest care: 2010 American Heart Association Guidelines for Cardiopulmonary Resuscitation and Emergency Cardiovascular Care, Circulation 122(18 Suppl 3):S768-786, 2010.
4. Boller M: Celebrating the 50th anniversary of cardiopulmonary resuscitation: from animals to humans…and back? J Vet Emerg Crit Care 20(6):553-557, 2010.
5. Smarick S, Haskins SC, Boller M, et al: RECOVER evidence and knowledge gap analysis on veterinary CPR. Part 6: Post-cardiac arrest care, J Vet Emerg Crit Care 22(S1):S85-101, 2012.
6. Goldberger ZD, Chan PS, Berg RA, et al: Duration of resuscitation efforts and survival after in-hospital cardiac arrest: an observational study, Lancet 380(9852):1473-1481, 2012.
7. Hofmeister EH, Brainard BM, Egger CM, et al: Prognostic indicators for dogs and cats with cardiopulmonary arrest treated by cardiopulmonary cerebral resuscitation at a university teaching hospital, J Am Vet Med Assoc 235(1):50-57, 2009.
8. Girotra S, Nallamothu BK, Spertus JA, et al: Trends in survival after in-hospital cardiac arrest, N Engl J Med 367(20):1912-1920, 2012.
9. Kass PH, Haskins SC: Survival following cardiopulmonary resuscitation in dogs and cats, J Vet Emerg Crit Care 2(2):57-65, 1992.
10. Salcido DD, Stephenson AM, Condle JP, et al: Incidence of rearrest after return of spontaneous circulation in out-of-hospital cardiac arrest, Prehosp Emerg Care 14(4):413-418, 2010.
11. Kern KB, Hilwig RW, Berg RA, et al: Postresuscitation left ventricular systolic and diastolic dysfunction. Treatment with dobutamine, Circulation 95(12):2610-2613, 1997.
12. Nakamura RK, Zuckerman IC, Yuhas DL, et al: Postresuscitation myocardial dysfunction in a dog, J Vet Emerg Crit Care 22(6):710-715, 2012.
13. Kern KB, Hilwig RW, Rhee KH, et al: Myocardial dysfunction after resuscitation from cardiac arrest: an example of global myocardial stunning, J Am Coll Cardiol 28(1):232-240, 1996.
14. Kern KB: Postresuscitation myocardial dysfunction, Cardiol Clin 20(1):89-101, 2002.
15. Ito T, Saitoh D, Takasu A, et al: Serum cortisol as a predictive marker of the outcome in patients resuscitated after cardiopulmonary arrest, Resuscitation 62(1):55-60, 2004.
16. Geppert A, Zorn G, Delle-Karth G, et al: Plasma concentrations of von Willebrand factor and intracellular adhesion molecule-1 for prediction of outcome after successful cardiopulmonary resuscitation, Crit Care Med 31(3):805-811, 2003.
17. Oppert M, Gleiter CH, Muller C, et al: Kinetics and characteristics of an acute phase response following cardiac arrest, Intensive Care Med 25(12):1386-1394, 1999.
18. Negovsky VA: Postresuscitation disease, Crit Care Med 16(10):942-946, 1988.
19. Adrie C, Monchi M, Laurent I, et al: Coagulopathy after successful cardiopulmonary resuscitation following cardiac arrest: implication of the protein C anticoagulant pathway, J Am Coll Cardiol 46(1):21-28, 2005.
20. Adrie C, Laurent I, Monchi M, et al: Postresuscitation disease after cardiac arrest: a sepsis-like syndrome? Curr Opin Crit Care 10(3):208-212, 2004.
21. Bottiger BW, Martin E: Thrombolytic therapy during cardiopulmonary resuscitation and the role of coagulation activation after cardiac arrest, Curr Opin Crit Care 7(3):176-183, 2001.
22. Fries M, Kunz D, Gressner AM, et al: Procalcitonin serum levels after out-of-hospital cardiac arrest, Resuscitation 59(1):105-109, 2003.
23. Gando S, Nanzaki S, Morimoto Y, et al: Alterations of soluble L- and P-selectins during cardiac arrest and CPR, Intensive Care Med 25(6):588-593, 1999.
24. Gando S, Nanzaki S, Morimoto Y, et al: Out-of-hospital cardiac arrest increases soluble vascular endothelial adhesion molecules and neutrophil elastase associated with endothelial injury, Intensive Care Med 26(1):38-44, 2000.
25. Mussack T, Biberthaler P, Kanz KG, et al: S-100b, sE-selectin, and sP-selectin for evaluation of hypoxic brain damage in patients after cardiopulmonary resuscitation: pilot study, World J Surg 25(5):539-543, 2001.
26. Gando S, Nanzaki S, Morimoto Y, et al: Tissue factor and tissue factor pathway inhibitor levels during and after cardiopulmonary resuscitation, Thromb Res 96(2):107-113, 1999.
27. Bottiger BW, Motsch J, Braun V, et al: Marked activation of complement and leukocytes and an increase in the concentrations of soluble endothelial adhesion molecules during cardiopulmonary resuscitation and early reperfusion after cardiac arrest in humans, Crit Care Med 30(11):2473-2480, 2002.
28. Geppert A, Zorn G, Karth GD, et al: Soluble selectins and the systemic inflammatory response syndrome after successful cardiopulmonary resuscitation, Crit Care Med 28(7):2360-2365, 2000.
29. Adrie C, Adib-Conquy M, Laurent I, et al: Successful cardiopulmonary resuscitation after cardiac arrest as a "sepsis-like" syndrome, Circulation 106(5):562-568, 2002.
30. Rivers E, Nguyen B, Havstad S, et al: Early goal-directed therapy in the treatment of severe sepsis and septic shock, N Engl J Med 345(19):1368-1377, 2001.
31. Gaieski DF, Band RA, Abella BS, et al: Early goal-directed hemodynamic optimization combined with therapeutic hypothermia in comatose survivors of out-of-hospital cardiac arrest, Resuscitation 80(4):418-424, 2009.
32. Sunde K, Pytte M, Jacobsen D, et al: Implementation of a standardised treatment protocol for post resuscitation care after out-of-hospital cardiac arrest, Resuscitation 73(1):29-39, 2007.
33. Fletcher DJ, Boller M, Brainard BM, et al: RECOVER evidence and knowledge gap analysis on veterinary CPR, Part 7: Clinical guidelines, J Vet Emerg Crit Care 22(S1):S102-131, 2012.
34. Mullner M, Sterz F, Binder M, et al: Blood glucose concentration after cardiopulmonary resuscitation influences functional neurological recovery in human cardiac arrest survivors, J Cerebral Blood Flow Metabol 17(4):430-436, 1997.
35. Longstreth WT, Inui TS: High blood-glucose level on hospital admission and poor neurological recovery after cardiac-arrest, Ann Neurol 15(1):59-63, 1984.
36. Losert H, Sterz F, Roine RO, et al: Strict normoglycaemic blood glucose levels in the therapeutic management of patients within 12 h after cardiac arrest might not be necessary, Resuscitation 76(2):214-220, 2008.
37. Nolan JP, Laver SR, Welch CA, et al: Outcome following admission to UK intensive care units after cardiac arrest: a secondary analysis of the ICNARC Case Mix Programme Database*, Anaesthesia 62(12):1207-1216, 2007.

38. Volkov A, Trubina I, Novoderzhkina I, et al: Changes in some hemodynamic, endocrine, and metabolic indexes in the early post-resuscitation period, Bull Exp Biol Med 87(1):1-4, 1979.
39. Siemkowicz E, Hansen AJ: Clinical restitution following cerebral ischemia in hypo-, normo- and hyperglycemic rats, Acta Neurol Scand 58(1):1-8, 1978.
40. Dalecy L, Lundy E, Barton K, Zelenock G: Dextrose containing intravenous fluid impairs outcome and increases death after 8 minutes of cardiac-arrest and resuscitation in dogs. Surgery 100(3):505-511, 1986.
41. Katz L, Wang Y, Ebmeyer U, et al: Glucose plus insulin infusion improves cerebral outcome after asphyxial cardiac arrest, Neuroreport 9(15):3363-3367, 1998.
42. Martin A, Rojas S, Chamorro A, et al: Why does acute hyperglycemia worsen the outcome of transient focal cerebral ischemia? Role of corticosteroids, inflammation, and protein O-glycosylation, Stroke 37(5):1288-1295, 2006.
43. Oksanen T, Skrifvars MB, Varpula T, et al: Strict versus moderate glucose control after resuscitation from ventricular fibrillation, Intensive Care Med 33(12):2093-2100, 2007.
44. Kim JJ, Hyun SY, Hwang SY, et al: Hormonal responses upon return of spontaneous circulation after cardiac arrest: a retrospective cohort study, Crit Care 15(1):R53, 2011.
45. de Jong MF, Beishuizen A, de Jong MJ, et al: The pituitary-adrenal axis is activated more in non-survivors than in survivors of cardiac arrest, irrespective of therapeutic hypothermia, Resuscitation 78(3):281-288, 2008.
46. Miller JB, Donnino MW, Rogan M, et al: Relative adrenal insufficiency in post-cardiac arrest shock is under-recognized, Resuscitation 76(2):221-225, 2008.
47. Kim JJ, Lim YS, Shin JH, et al: Relative adrenal insufficiency after cardiac arrest: Impact on postresuscitation disease outcome, Am J Emerg Med 24(6):684-688, 2006.
48. Pene F, Hyvernat H, Mallet V, et al: Prognostic value of relative adrenal insufficiency after out-of-hospital cardiac arrest, Intensive Care Med 31(5):627-633, 2005.
49. Hekimian G, Baugnon T, Thuong M, et al: Cortisol levels and adrenal reserve after successful cardiac arrest resuscitation, Shock 22(2):116-119, 2004.
50. Batzofin BM, Sprung CL, Weiss YG: The use of steroids in the treatment of severe sepsis and septic shock, Best Pract Res Clin Endocrinol Metab 25(5):735-743, 2011.
51. Laver S, Farrow C, Turner D, et al: Mode of death after admission to an intensive care unit following cardiac arrest. Intensive Care Med 30(11):2126-2128, 2004.
52. Palmer AC, Walker RG: The neuropathological effects of cardiac arrest in animals: a study of five cases, J Small Anim Pract 11(12):779-791, 1970.
53. Buckley GJ, Rozanski EA, Rush JE: Randomized blinded comparison of epinephrine and vasopressin for the treatment of naturally occurring cardiopulmonary arrest (CPA) in dogs, J Vet Intern Med 25(6):1334-1340, 2011.
54. Fukushima U, Sasaki S, Okano S, et al: Non-invasive diagnosis of ischemic brain damage after cardiopulmonary resuscitation in dogs by using transcranial Doppler ultrasonography, Vet Radiol Ultrasound 41(2): 172-177, 2000.
55. Balan IS, Fiskum G, Hazelton J, et al: Oximetry-guided reoxygenation improves neurological outcome after experimental cardiac arrest, Stroke 37(12):3008-3013, 2006.
56. O'Neil BJ, Koehler RC, Neumar RW, et al: Global brain ischemia and reperfusion. In Paradis NA, Halperin HR, Kern KB, Wenzel V, Chamberlain DA, editors: Cardiac arrest, ed 2. Cambridge, UK, 2007, Cambridge University Press, pp 236-281.
57. Starkov AA, Chinopoulos C, Fiskum G: Mitochondrial calcium and oxidative stress as mediators of ischemic brain injury, Cell Calcium 36(3-4):257-264, 2004.
58. White BC, Sullivan JM, DeGracia DJ, et al: Brain ischemia and reperfusion: molecular mechanisms of neuronal injury, J Neurol Sci 179(S 1-2): 1-33, 2000.
59. Polderman KH: Mechanisms of action, physiological effects, and complications of hypothermia, Crit Care Med 37(7 Suppl):S186-202, 2009.
60. Li D, Shao Z, Vanden Hoek TL, et al: Reperfusion accelerates acute neuronal death induced by simulated ischemia, Exp Neurol 206(2): 280-287, 2007.
61. Allen BS, Buckberg GD: Studies of isolated global brain ischaemia: I. overview of irreversible brain injury and evolution of a new concept—redefining the time of brain death, Eur J Cardiothor Surg 41(5):1132-1137, 2012.
62. Nishijima MK, Koehler RC, Hurn PD, et al: Postischemic recovery rate of cerebral ATP, phosphocreatine, pH, and evoked potentials, Am J Physiol Heart Circ Physiol 257(6):H1860-H1870, 1989.
63. Blum H, Summers JJ, Schnall MD, et al: Acute intestinal ischemia studies by phosphorus nuclear magnetic resonance spectroscopy, Ann Surg 204(1):83-88, 1986.
64. Jennings RB, Hawkins HK, Lowe JE, et al: Relation between high energy phosphate and lethal injury in myocardial ischemia in the dog, Am J Pathol 92(1):187-214, 1978.
65. Halestrap AP, McStay GP, Clarke SJ: The permeability transition pore complex: another view, Biochimie 84(2-3):153-166, 2002.
66. Hazelton JL, Balan I, Elmer GI, et al: Hyperoxic reperfusion after global cerebral ischemia promotes inflammation and long-term hippocampal neuronal death, J Neurotrauma 27(4):753-762, 2010.
67. Allen BS, Ko Y, Buckberg GD, et al: Studies of isolated global brain ischaemia: I. A new large animal model of global brain ischaemia and its baseline perfusion studies, Eur J Cardiothor Surg 41(5):1138-1146, 2012.
68. Allen BS, Ko Y, Buckberg GD, et al: Studies of isolated global brain ischaemia: II. Controlled reperfusion provides complete neurologic recovery following 30 min of warm ischaemia—the importance of perfusion pressure, Eur J Cardiothor Surg 41(5):1147-1154, 2012.
69. Idris AH, Roberts LJ 2nd, Caruso L, et al: Oxidant injury occurs rapidly after cardiac arrest, cardiopulmonary resuscitation, and reperfusion, Crit Care Med 33(9):2043-2048, 2005.
70. Basu S, Liu X, Nozari A, et al: Evidence for time-dependent maximum increase of free radical damage and eicosanoid formation in the brain as related to duration of cardiac arrest and cardio-pulmonary resuscitation, Free Radic Res 37(3):251-256, 2003.
71. Basu S, Nozari A, Liu XL, et al: Development of a novel biomarker of free radical damage in reperfusion injury after cardiac arrest, FEBS Lett 470(1):1-6, 2000.
72. Neumar RW: Optimal oxygenation during and after cardiopulmonary resuscitation, Curr Opin Crit Care 17(3):236-240, 2011.
73. Becker LB: New concepts in reactive oxygen species and cardiovascular reperfusion physiology, Cardiovasc Res 61(3):461-470, 2004.
74. Kilgannon JH, Jones AE, Shapiro NI, et al: Association between arterial hyperoxia following resuscitation from cardiac arrest and in-hospital mortality, JAMA 303(21):2165-2171, 2010.
75. Kilgannon JH, Jones AE, Parrillo JE, et al: Relationship between supranormal oxygen tension and outcome after resuscitation from cardiac arrest, Circulation 123(23):2717-2722, 2011.
76. Kory P, Fukunaga M, Mathew JP, et al: Outcomes of mild therapeutic hypothermia after in-hospital cardiac arrest, Neurocrit Care 16(3):406-412, 2012.
77. Nichol G, Huszti E, Kim F, et al: Does induction of hypothermia improve outcomes after in-hospital cardiac arrest? Resuscitation 84(5):620-625, 2013.
78. Sunde K, Soreide E: Therapeutic hypothermia after cardiac arrest: where are we now? Curr Opin Crit Care 17(3):247-253, 2011.
79. Nagao K, Kikushima K, Watanabe K, et al: Early induction of hypothermia during cardiac arrest improves neurological outcomes in patients with out-of-hospital cardiac arrest who undergo emergency cardiopulmonary bypass and percutaneous coronary intervention, Circ J 74(1):77-85, 2010.
80. Hayes GM: Severe seizures associated with traumatic brain injury managed by controlled hypothermia, pharmacologic coma, and mechanical ventilation in a dog, J Vet Emerg Crit Care 19(6):629-634, 2009.
81. Kanemoto I, Taguchi D, Yokoyama S, et al: Open heart surgery with deep hypothermia and cardiopulmonary bypass in small and toy dogs, Vet Surg 39(6):674-679, 2010.

82. Polderman KH, Herold I: Therapeutic hypothermia and controlled normothermia in the intensive care unit: practical considerations, side effects, and cooling methods, Crit Care Med 37(3):1101-1120, 2009.
83. Holzer M: Targeted temperature management for comatose survivors of cardiac arrest, N Engl J Med 363(13):1256-1264, 2010.
84. Nielsen N, Sunde K, Hovdenes J, et al: Adverse events and their relation to mortality in out-of-hospital cardiac arrest patients treated with therapeutic hypothermia, Crit Care Med 39(1):57-64, 2011.
85. Rittenberger JC, Popescu A, Brenner RP, et al: Frequency and timing of nonconvulsive status epilepticus in comatose post-cardiac arrest subjects treated with hypothermia, Neurocrit Care 16(1):114-122, 2012.
86. Xiao F: Bench to bedside: brain edema and cerebral resuscitation: the present and future, Acad Emerg Med 9(9):933-946, 2002.
87. Sakabe T, Tateishi A, Miyauchi Y, et al: Intracranial pressure following cardiopulmonary resuscitation, Intensive Care Med 13(4):256-259, 1987.
88. Kaupp HA, Jr, Lazarus RE, Wetzel N, et al: The role of cerebral edema in ischemic cerebral neuropathy after cardiac arrest in dogs and monkeys and its treatment with hypertonic urea, Surgery 48:404-410, 1960.
89. Leonov Y, Sterz F, Safar P, et al: Hypertension with hemodilution prevents multifocal cerebral hypoperfusion after cardiac arrest in dogs, Stroke 23(1):45-53, 1992.
90. Ames A 3rd, Wright RL, Kowada M, et al: Cerebral ischemia. II. The no-reflow phenomenon, Am J Pathol 52(2):437-453, 1968.
91. Fischer M, Hossmann KA: No-reflow after cardiac arrest, Intensive Care Med 21(2):132-141, 1995.
92. Fischer M, Hossmann KA: Volume expansion during cardiopulmonary resuscitation reduces cerebral no-reflow, Resuscitation 32(3):227-240, 1996.
93. Nishizawa H, Kudoh I: Cerebral autoregulation is impaired in patients resuscitated after cardiac arrest, Acta Anaesthesiol Scand 40(9):1149-1153, 1996.
94. Sundgreen C, Larsen FS, Herzog TM, et al: Autoregulation of cerebral blood flow in patients resuscitated from cardiac arrest, Stroke 32(1):128-132, 2001.
95. Nemoto EM, Snyder JV, Carroll RG, et al: Global ischemia in dogs: cerebrovascular CO2 reactivity and autoregulation, Stroke 6(4):425-431, 1975.
96. Koch KA, Jackson DL, Schmiedl M, et al: Total cerebral ischemia: effect of alterations in arterial PCO2 on cerebral microcirculation, J Cereb Blood Flow Metab 4(3):343-349, 1984.
97. Christopherson TJ, Milde JH, Michenfelder JD: Cerebral vascular autoregulation and CO2 reactivity following onset of the delayed postischemic hypoperfusion state in dogs, J Cereb Blood Flow Metab 13(2):260-268, 1993.
98. Buunk G, Van Der Hoeven JG, Meinders AE: Cerebrovascular reactivity in comatose patients resuscitated from a cardiac arrest, Stroke 28(8):1569-1573, 1997.
99. Bisschops LL, Hoedemaekers CW, Simons KS, et al: Preserved metabolic coupling and cerebrovascular reactivity during mild hypothermia after cardiac arrest, Crit Care Med 38(7):1542-1547, 2010.
100. Pynnonen L, Falkenbach P, Kamarainen A, et al: Therapeutic hypothermia after cardiac arrest—cerebral perfusion and metabolism during upper and lower threshold normocapnia, Resuscitation 82(9):1174-1179, 2011.
101. Safar P, Xiao F, Radovsky A, et al: Improved cerebral resuscitation from cardiac arrest in dogs with mild hypothermia plus blood flow promotion, Stroke 27(1):105-113, 1996.
102. Platt SR, Radaelli ST, McDonnell JJ: The prognostic value of the modified Glasgow Coma scale in head trauma in dogs, J Vet Intern Med15(6):581-584, 2001.
103. Morrison LJ, Deakin CD, Morley PT, et al: Part 8: Advanced life support: 2010 International Consensus on Cardiopulmonary Resuscitation and Emergency Cardiovascular Care Science with treatment recommendations, Circulation 122(16 Suppl 2):S345-421, 2010.
104. Geocadin RG, Eleff SM: Cardiac arrest resuscitation: neurologic prognostication and brain death, Curr Opin Crit Care 14(3):261-268, 2008.
105. Oddo M, Rossetti AO: Predicting neurological outcome after cardiac arrest, Curr Opin Crit Care 17(3):254-259, 2011.
106. Webb AA: Brainstem auditory evoked response (BAER) testing in animals, Can Vet J 50(3):313-318, 2009.
107. Cerchiari EL, Sclabassi RJ, Safar P, et al: Effects of combined superoxide dismutase and deferoxamine on recovery of brainstem auditory evoked potentials and EEG after asphyxial cardiac arrest in dogs, Resuscitation 19(1):25-40, 1990.
108. Usui A, Kato K, Murase M, et al: Neural tissue-related proteins (NSE, G0 alpha, 28-kDa calbindin-D, S100b and CK-BB) in serum and cerebrospinal fluid after cardiac arrest, J Neurol Sci 123(1-2):134-139, 1994.
109. Shinozaki K, Oda S, Sadahiro T, et al: S-100B and neuron-specific enolase as predictors of neurological outcome in patients after cardiac arrest and return of spontaneous circulation: a systematic review, Crit Care 13(4):R121, 2009.
110. Waldrop JE, Rozanski EA, Swanke ED, et al: Causes of cardiopulmonary arrest, resuscitation management, and functional outcome in dogs and cats surviving cardiopulmonary arrest, J Vet Emerg Crit Care 14(1):22-29, 2004.
111. Zia A, Kern KB: Management of postcardiac arrest myocardial dysfunction, Curr Opin Crit Care 17(3):241-246, 2011.
112. Meyer RJ, Kern KB, Berg RA, et al: Post-resuscitation right ventricular dysfunction: delineation and treatment with dobutamine, Resuscitation 55(2):187-191, 2002.
113. Frank A, Bonney M, Bonney S, et al: Myocardial ischemia reperfusion injury: from basic science to clinical bedside, Semin Cardiothorac Vasc Anesth 16(3):123-132, 2012.
114. Niccoli G, Burzotta F, Galiuto L, et al: Myocardial no-reflow in humans, J Am Coll Cardiol 54(4):281-292, 2009.
115. Hsu CY, Huang CH, Chang WT, et al: Cardioprotective effect of therapeutic hypothermia for postresuscitation myocardial dysfunction, Shock 32(2):210-216, 2009.
116. Tissier R, Ghaleh B, Cohen MV, et al: Myocardial protection with mild hypothermia, Cardiovasc Res 94(2):217-225, 2012.
117. Jacobshagen C, Pelster T, Pax A, et al: Effects of mild hypothermia on hemodynamics in cardiac arrest survivors and isolated failing human myocardium, Clin Res Cardiol 99(5):267-276, 2010.
118. Meaney PA, Nadkarni VM, Kern KB, et al: Rhythms and outcomes of adult in-hospital cardiac arrest, Crit Care Med 38(1):101-108, 2010.
119. Brindley PG, Markland DM, Mayers I, et al: Predictors of survival following in-hospital adult cardiopulmonary resuscitation, Can Med Assoc J 167(4):343-348, 2002.
120. Kutsogiannis DJ, Bagshaw SM, Laing B, et al: Predictors of survival after cardiac or respiratory arrest in critical care units, Can Med Assoc J 183(14):1589-1595, 2011.
121. Abella BS: Not all cardiac arrests are the same, Can Med Assoc J 183(14):1572-1573, 2011.
122. Chan PS, Spertus JA, Krumholz HM, et al: A validated prediction tool for initial survivors of in-hospital cardiac arrest, Arch Intern Med 172(12):947-953, 2012.

CHAPTER 5

SHOCK

Armelle de Laforcade, DVM, DACVECC • Deborah C. Silverstein, DVM, DACVECC

KEY POINTS

- *Shock* is defined as inadequate cellular energy production and most commonly occurs secondary to poor tissue perfusion from low or unevenly distributed blood flow. This leads to a critical decrease in oxygen delivery (DO_2) compared with oxygen consumption (VO_2) in the tissues.
- There are numerous ways to classify shock, and many patients suffer from more than one type of shock simultaneously. A common classification scheme includes hypovolemic, distributive, and cardiogenic etiologies, although metabolic and hypoxic causes of shock are also well recognized.
- For all forms of shock except cardiogenic, the mainstay of therapy involves rapid vascular access and administration of large volumes of isotonic crystalloid fluids. Studies have not shown a clear benefit of one type of fluid over another; however, failure to administer an adequate volume of fluids may contribute significantly to mortality.
- End points of resuscitation such as normalization of heart rate and blood pressure, improved pulse quality and mentation, and resolution of lactic acidosis are necessary to tailor therapy to the individual patient.
- Oxygen therapy and avoidance of stress are key components to the treatment of cardiogenic shock. Sedation and intubation may be required in dyspneic patients that fail to respond to diuretic and vasodilator therapy.

Shock is defined as inadequate cellular energy production. It most commonly occurs secondary to poor tissue perfusion from low or unevenly distributed blood flow that causes a critical decrease in oxygen delivery (DO_2) in relation to oxygen consumption (VO_2). Although metabolic disturbances (e.g., cytopathic hypoxia, hypoglycemia, toxic exposures) and hypoxemia (e.g., severe anemia, pulmonary dysfunction, methemoglobinemia) can lead to shock, it most commonly results from a reduction in DO_2 secondary to one of three major mechanisms: loss of intravascular volume (hypovolemic shock), maldistribution of vascular volume (distributive shock), or failure of the cardiac pump (cardiogenic shock). Box 5-1 lists all the functional classes of shock. An index of suspicion based on signalment and a brief history may help differentiate between these various causes of shock. Early recognition of cardiovascular instability, along with a combination of physical examination findings and point-of-care testing suggestive of reduced perfusion, are all that is necessary to initiate therapy. Rapid, aggressive therapy and appropriate monitoring, along with the removal of any underlying causes, are necessary to optimize the chance for a successful outcome.

CLINICAL PRESENTATION

Hypovolemic shock is commonly associated with internal or external blood loss or excessive loss of other body fluids (e.g., severe vomiting, diarrhea, polyuria, burns). In hypovolemic states, reduced cardiac output caused by diminished venous return triggers compensatory mechanisms that attempt to raise the circulating blood volume. An increase in sympathetic activity causes vasoconstriction, increased cardiac contractility, and tachycardia, with a resultant rise in cardiac output. Extreme vasoconstriction and microvascular alterations induce mobilization of fluid from the interstitial and extracellular spaces to the intravascular space. Additionally, a reduction in renal blood flow activates the renin-angiotensin-aldosterone system, which further upregulates the sympathetic nervous system and causes sodium and water retention via the production of both aldosterone and antidiuretic hormone, respectively. Because the net effect of these responses is to increase intravascular volume, clinical signs of shock may be subtle initially, characterized by mild to moderate mental depression, tachycardia with normal or prolonged capillary refill time, cool extremities, tachypnea, and a normal blood pressure. Pulse quality is often normal, and this stage is generally referred to as "compensated shock." With ongoing compromise of systemic perfusion, compensatory mechanisms are no longer adequate and often

BOX 5-1 ***Functional Classifications and Examples of Shock***

Hypovolemic: A Decrease in Circulating Blood Volume

Hemorrhage
Severe dehydration
Trauma

Cardiogenic: A Decrease in Forward Flow from the Heart

Congestive heart failure
Cardiac arrhythmia
Cardiac tamponade
Drug overdose (e.g., anesthetics, β-blockers, calcium channel blockers)

Distributive: A Marked Decrease or Increase in Systemic Vascular Resistance or Maldistribution of Blood

Sepsis
Obstruction (heartworm disease, saddle thrombosis)
Anaphylaxis
Catecholamine excess (pheochromocytoma, extreme fear)
Gastric dilatation-volvulus

Metabolic: Deranged Cellular Metabolic Machinery

Hypoglycemia
Cyanide toxicity
Mitochondrial dysfunction
Cytopathic hypoxia of sepsis

Hypoxemic: A Decrease in Oxygen Content in Arterial Blood

Anemia
Severe pulmonary disease
Carbon monoxide toxicity
Methemoglobinemia

begin to fail. Pale mucous membranes, poor peripheral pulse quality, depressed mentation, and a drop in blood pressure become apparent as the animal progresses to decompensated shock. Ultimately, if left untreated, reduced organ perfusion results in signs of end organ failure (e.g., oliguria) and ultimately death.

Rather than causing an absolute reduction in circulating blood volume/hypovolemia, diseases such as sepsis and gastric dilatation-volvulus lead to maldistribution of blood flow and result in distributive shock. Dogs with sepsis or a systemic inflammatory response syndrome (SIRS) may show clinical signs of hyperdynamic or hypodynamic shock (see Chapters 6 and 91). The initial hyperdynamic phase of sepsis or SIRS is characterized by tachycardia, fever, bounding peripheral pulse quality, and hyperemic mucous membranes secondary to cytokine (e.g., nitric oxide)–mediated peripheral vasodilation. This is often referred to as vasodilatory shock. If septic shock or SIRS progresses unchecked, a decreased cardiac output and signs of hypoperfusion often ensue as a result of cytokine effects on the myocardium or myocardial ischemia. Clinical changes may then include tachycardia, pale (and possibly icteric) mucous membranes with a prolonged capillary refill time, hypothermia, poor pulse quality, and a dull mentation. Hypodynamic septic shock is the decompensatory stage of sepsis and without intervention will result in organ damage and death (see Chapter 7). Lastly, the gastrointestinal tract is the shock organ in dogs, so shock often leads to ileus, diarrhea, hematochezia, and melena.

The hyperdynamic phase of shock is rarely recognized in cats. Also, in contrast to dogs, changes in heart rate in cats with shock are unpredictable; they may exhibit tachycardia or bradycardia. In general, cats typically present with pale mucous membranes (and possibly icterus), weak pulses, cool extremities, hypothermia, and generalized weakness or collapse. In cats the lungs are vulnerable to damage during shock or sepsis, and signs of respiratory dysfunction are common in this species.[1-3]

Dogs with gastric dilatation-volvulus may have normal circulating blood volume; however, compression of the major vessels secondary to severe gastric dilatation causes decreased venous return and reduced cardiac output. This is a form of relative hypovolemia. Although the classifications of shock are useful in understanding the underlying mechanism of cardiovascular instability, it is important to remember that different forms of shock can occur simultaneously in the same patient. A dog with gastric dilatation-volvulus, for example, will often have a component of hypovolemic shock secondary to blood loss associated with rupture of the short gastric vessels. Dogs with septic peritonitis may experience tissue hypoxia as a result of vasodilation and a relative hypovolemia but likely suffer from actual hypovolemia as well if severe cavitary effusions or protracted vomiting are present. In these dogs, metabolic changes leading to cytopathic hypoxia may also contribute to tissue/cellular hypoxia.

DIAGNOSTICS AND MONITORING

Some basic diagnostic tests should be completed for all shock patients in order to assess the extent of organ injury and identify the etiology of the shock state. A venous or arterial blood gas with lactate measurement, a complete blood cell count, blood chemistry panel, coagulation panel, blood typing, and urine analysis should be performed. Thoracic and abdominal radiographs, abdominal ultrasound, and echocardiography may be indicated once the patient is stabilized.

Additional monitoring techniques that are essential in the diagnosis and treatment of the shock patient include continuous electrocardiographic monitoring, blood pressure measurement, and pulse oximetry (see Monitoring section). Gradual resolution of tachycardia (and hypotension) often signals successful return of cardiovascular stability, whereas persistent tachycardia indicates ongoing cardiovascular instability. It is important to note that the best form of monitoring is a thorough physical examination, and frequent patient assessment will also provide important clues regarding response to therapy.

Monitoring Tissue Perfusion and Oxygen Delivery

The magnitude of the oxygen deficit is a key predictor of outcome in shock patients. Therefore optimizing oxygen delivery and tissue perfusion is the goal of treatment and sufficient monitoring tools are necessary to achieve this objective. A well-perfused patient possesses the following characteristics: central venous pressure between 0 and 5 cm H_2O; urine production of at least 1 ml/kg/hr; mean arterial pressure between 70 and 120 mm Hg; normal body temperature, heart rate, heart rhythm, and respiratory rate; and moist, pink mucous membranes with a capillary refill time of less than 2 seconds. Monitoring these parameters is the tenet of patient assessment. Additional monitoring tools that may prove beneficial include the measurement of blood lactate, indices of systemic oxygenation transport, and mixed venous oxygen saturation.

Blood Lactate Levels

Critically ill patients with inadequate oxygen delivery, oxygen uptake, or tissue perfusion often develop hyperlactatemia and acidemia that are reflective of the severity of cellular hypoxia. A lactic acidosis in human patients carries a greater risk for developing multiple organ failure, and these people demonstrate a higher mortality rate than those without an elevated lactate concentration.[4] High blood lactate levels may also aid in predicting mortality in dogs.[5-7] The normal lactate concentration in adult dogs and cats is less than 2.5 mmol/L; lactate concentrations greater than 7 mmol/L are severely elevated.[5] However, normal neonatal and pediatric patients may have higher lactate concentrations.[8] In addition, sample collection and handling procedures can affect lactate concentration.[9] Serial lactate measurements taken during the resuscitation period help to gauge response to treatment and evaluate resuscitation end points; the changes in lactate concentrations are a better predictor of survival than are single measurements (see Chapter 56 for further details).

Cardiac Output Monitoring and Indices of Oxygen Transport

The measurement of indices of systemic oxygen transport is a direct method of assessing the progress of resuscitation in shock patients. A right-sided cardiac catheter or pulmonary artery catheter (PAC, also termed Swan-Ganz catheter or balloon-directed thermodilution catheter) is typically used to monitor these parameters (see Chapters 184 and 202). The PAC enables the measurement of central venous and pulmonary arterial pressure, mixed venous blood gases (PvO_2 and SvO_2), pulmonary capillary wedge pressure (PCWP), and cardiac output. With this information, further parameters of circulatory and respiratory function can be derived (i.e., stroke volume, end-diastolic volume, systemic vascular resistance index, pulmonary vascular resistance index, arterial oxygen content, mixed-venous oxygen content, DO_2 index, VO_2 index, and oxygen extraction ratio). Although cardiac output is typically determined using thermodilution methods, other techniques are available (see Chapter 184).

A PAC allows the clinician to assess the cardiovascular and pulmonary function of shock patients. The response to treatment and titration of fluid therapy, vasopressors, and inotropic agents can also be monitored. Cardiac output and systemic DO_2 should be optimized using intravascular volume loading until the PCWP approaches 10 to 12 mm Hg. A high PCWP (>15 to 20 mm Hg) will promote the formation of pulmonary edema, further impairing oxygenation and overall oxygen transport. Despite potential benefits, the use of a PAC does not necessarily translate into reduced mortality in the critically ill shock patient; it is an invasive monitoring technique that is not without risk.[10] In addition, the accuracy of measurements provided by the PAC relies on catheter placement, calibration of transducers, coexisting cardiac or pericardial disease, and correct interpretation of waveforms and values.

Mixed Venous Oxygen Saturation (SvO_2) and Central Venous Oxygen Saturation ($ScvO_2$)

Changes in the global tissue oxygenation (oxygen supply to demand) can be assessed using SvO_2 measurements. Assuming VO_2 is constant, SvO_2 is determined by cardiac output, hemoglobin concentration, and SaO_2. SvO_2 is decreased if DO_2 decreases (i.e., low CO, hypoxia, severe anemia) or if VO_2 increases (i.e., fever, seizure activity). With conditions such as the hyperdynamic stages of sepsis and cytotoxic tissue hypoxia (e.g., cyanide poisoning), SvO_2 is increased. A reduction in SvO_2 may be an early indicator that the patient's clinical condition is deteriorating. In addition, SvO_2 may be an alternative to measuring cardiac index during resuscitative efforts.

Ideally, SvO_2 is measured in a blood sample from the pulmonary artery. However, in animals that do not have a PAC, venous oxygen saturation can be measured from the central circulation, using a central venous catheter in the cranial or proximal caudal vena cava. SvO_2 is then termed $ScvO_2$ (central venous oxygen saturation). Although the $ScvO_2$ values are generally higher than SvO_2 in critically ill patients with circulatory failure, the two measurements closely parallel each other. Therefore a pathologically low $ScvO_2$ likely indicates an even lower SvO_2. A recent prospective, randomized study comparing two algorithms for early goal-directed therapy in patients with severe sepsis and septic shock showed that maintenance of a continuously measured $ScvO_2$ above 70% (in addition to maintaining central venous pressure above 8 to 12 mm Hg, MAP pressure above 65 mm Hg and urine output above 0.5 ml/kg/hr) resulted in a 15% absolute reduction in mortality compared with the same treatment without $ScvO_2$ monitoring.[11] One study of dogs with severe sepsis and or septic shock evaluated changes in tissue perfusion parameters in response to goal-directed hemodynamic resuscitation.[12] In this study, resuscitation was aimed at restoring parameters related to tissue perfusion, including capillary refill time, central venous pressure, blood pressure, lactate, base deficit, and $ScvO_2$. A higher $ScvO_2$ was associated with a lower risk of death, highlighting the importance of microcirculatory and macrocirculatory dysfunction in severe sepsis and septic shock.[13] Until these parameters are more extensively studied in naturally occurring shock in dogs, early recognition of shock followed by aggressive goal-driven resuscitation is likely crucial to a successful outcome.

TREATMENT

Treatment of shock is based on early recognition of the condition and rapid restoration of the cardiovascular system so that DO_2 to the tissues is normalized as soon as possible. The mainstay of therapy for all forms of shock except cardiogenic shock is based on rapid administration of large volumes of intravenous fluids to restore an effective circulating volume and tissue perfusion.[14] Vascular access is essential for successful treatment of shock but can be difficult as a result of poor vascular filling and a collapsed cardiovascular state. Because speed of fluid administration is proportional to the diameter of the catheter lumen and inversely proportional to its length, short, large-bore catheters should be placed in a central or peripheral vein. When intravenous access is difficult or delayed because of cardiovascular collapse, a cutdown approach or intraosseous catheterization may be necessary (see Chapters 193 to 195).

The type of fluid selected for the treatment of shock may vary (see Chapter 60). Replacement isotonic crystalloids such as lactated Ringer's solution, 0.9% sodium chloride (NaCl), or Normosol R form the mainstay of therapy for shock, administered rapidly at doses up to 1 blood volume (90 ml/kg for the dog, 50 ml/kg for the cat). The administered fluid rapidly distributes into the extracellular fluid compartment so that only approximately 25% of the delivered volume remains in the intravascular space by 30 minutes after infusion,[15] and some animals will therefore require additional resuscitation at this time point. In patients that are bleeding, it may even be advantageous to perform hypotensive resuscitation (to a MAP of approximately 60 mm Hg) until the hemorrhage is controlled, because aggressive fluid therapy in this setting can worsen bleeding and outcome.[16] For animals with coexisting head trauma, the isotonic crystalloid of choice is 0.9% NaCl because it contains the highest concentration of sodium and is least likely to contribute to cerebral edema. The "shock doses" of crystalloids serve as useful guidelines for fluid resuscitation of the shock patient; however, the actual volume administered should be titrated according to the patient's clinical response in order to prevent volume overload. Excessive fluid administration is often evidenced by pulmonary or peripheral edema caused by any combination of increased hydrostatic pressure, hypoalbuminemia, and increases in vascular endothelial permeability (see Chapter 11). Animals with uncontrolled hemorrhage or deranged compensatory mechanisms may not respond adequately to crystalloid resuscitation and will require additional therapeutic, diagnostic, and monitoring strategies. Additional fluid therapy options in these patients include synthetic colloid solutions, hypertonic saline, blood products, and hemoglobin-based oxygen carrying (HBOC) solutions.

Synthetic colloids such as the hydroxyethyl starches are hyperoncotic to the normal animal and therefore pull fluid into the vascular space after intravenous administration (see Chapter 58). They therefore cause an increase in blood volume that is greater than that of the infused volume and help to retain this fluid in the intravascular space in animals with normal capillary permeability. They are appropriately used for shock therapy in acutely hypoproteinemic animals (total protein < 3.5 g/dl) with a decreased colloid osmotic pressure. They can also be used with isotonic or hypertonic crystalloids to maintain adequate plasma volume expansion with lower interstitial fluid volume expansion and to expand the intravascular space with smaller volumes over a shorter period. Because of the prevalence of occult cardiac disease in cats, hydroxyethyl starch solutions are typically administered more conservatively in this species, at doses ranging from 5 to 10 ml/kg compared with 10 to 20 ml/kg in dogs. With the exception of human trauma patients, studies have failed to support a survival benefit with the use of colloids compared with crystalloids in resuscitation from shock. In the specific population of human trauma patients, crystalloid use has been associated with reduced mortality compared with colloid therapy.[17] There are serious recent concerns in human medicine that hydroxyethyl starches contribute to acute kidney injury, especially in critically ill patients and those with sepsis, but there is no evidence to support this association in dogs and cats.

Human albumin, a natural hyperoncotic and hyperosmotic colloid solution with rising popularity in veterinary medicine, is another therapeutic option when crystalloid therapy alone has failed to restore or maintain an effective circulating blood volume. Preliminary studies in dogs found that albumin therapy increases circulating albumin concentrations, total solids, and colloid osmotic pressure, although the effect on mortality remains unknown. Potential complications are reportedly rare in critically ill animals and are similar to those for any blood product transfusion (i.e., fever, vomiting, increased respiratory effort), in addition to the potential for increasing clotting times. However, few studies have been published evaluating the safety of human albumin in animals. Recent reports of albumin administration to normal research dogs revealed potentially fatal reactions to the product, especially with repeated dosing.[18] Caution is therefore advised at this time. A commercial lyophilized canine albumin product is available for albumin replacement for those animals whose risk for complications or adverse outcome may be associated with profound albumin loss.

The use of 7% to 7.5% sodium chloride (hypertonic saline) can be lifesaving in the emergency setting (see Chapter 60). The long shelf life and affordability of this solution render it a necessity in the veterinary emergency hospital. After administration of hypertonic saline, there is a transient (<30 minutes) osmotic shift of water from the extravascular to the intravascular compartment. It is administered in small volumes (3 to 5 ml/kg) intravenously over 10 minutes. In addition to the fluid shift caused by hypertonic saline, there is evidence that it also reduces endothelial swelling, modulates inflammation, increases cardiac contractility, causes mild peripheral vasodilation, and decreases intracranial pressure. The effects of this solution are immediate, with a decrease in heart rate and improvement of pulse quality typically noted within 1 to 2 minutes of administration. Though short lived, this transient improvement in cardiovascular state may provide the necessary time for other therapies to take effect. Hypertonic saline should always be used in combination with other resuscitative fluids because of the osmotic diuresis and rapid sodium redistribution that occur after administration. A mixture of hypertonic saline and a synthetic colloid may further augment and prolong the rise in blood volume compared with hypertonic saline alone. Several studies in dogs suggest that the combination of hypertonic saline and dextran 70 is associated with more rapid improvement in hemodynamic status and with lower overall crystalloid requirements than when crystalloids are used alone.[19,20]

Blood component therapy is often used during resuscitation of the shock patient. Most fluid-responsive shock patients tolerate acute hemodilution to a hematocrit of less than 20%. In the dog, splenic contraction secondary to catecholamine release may mask the presence of anemia, and a reduced total protein concentration can be used to raise the index of suspicion for blood loss in this species. Both the dose of packed red blood cells and speed of administration may vary depending on the underlying condition and the hemodynamic state of the patient. In animals with acute blood loss that are unresponsive to fluid therapy alone, fresh whole blood or packed red blood cells and fresh frozen plasma should be used in an attempt to stabilize clinical signs of shock and maintain the hematocrit above 25% and the clotting times within the normal range (see Chapter 61). Packed red blood cells and fresh frozen plasma are administered at a dose of 10 to 20 ml/kg and fresh whole blood at a dose of 20 to 30 ml/kg. Although all blood products should be administered over at least 1 to 2 hours in order to monitor for a transfusion reaction and avoid volume overload, it may be necessary to administer these products in bolus doses in animals with severe internal or external blood loss. A blood type should be determined in all animals, especially cats, before transfusions are given. Packed red blood cells are given to increase oxygen content in animals with severe anemia or in conjunction with fresh frozen plasma in coagulopathic shock patients. Plasma products are most commonly used in animals with profound blood loss, a coagulopathy, or severe hypoalbuminemia (large volumes of intravenous fluids in a short period may also have a dilutional effect on circulating coagulation factors). Its ability to increase colloid osmotic pressure is limited compared with the hyperoncotic synthetic colloids, but it does supply albumin, an important carrier of certain drugs, hormones, metals, chemicals, toxins, and enzymes. Platelets are only present in fresh blood within 24 hours of collection, and their use is indicated in animals with thrombocytopenia/thrombocytopathia–induced bleeding disorders or massive hemorrhage.

Finally, HBOC solutions may be beneficial for the treatment of shock (see Chapter 58). In states of anemia, the HBOC solutions may increase oxygen delivery to tissues and increase perfusion of capillary beds affected by microvascular thrombosis because of the small size of the free hemoglobin. Despite these theoretical benefits and the long shelf life of this product, HBOC solutions are not widely used because of inconsistent supply, undesirable side effects, expense, and lack of clear benefit over other solutions available.

Shock patients that remain hypotensive despite intravascular volume resuscitation often require vasopressor or inotrope therapy. Because oxygen delivery to the tissue is dependent on both cardiac output and systemic vascular resistance, therapy for hypotensive patients includes maximizing cardiac output with fluid therapy, as discussed earlier, and inotropic drugs or modifying vascular tone with vasopressor agents (see Chapters 8, 157, and 158). Commonly used vasopressors include catecholamines (epinephrine, norepinephrine, dopamine), positive inotropic agents, and the sympathomimetic drug phenylephrine. In addition, vasopressin, corticosteroids, and glucagon have been used as adjunctive pressor agents.

Unlike hypovolemic or distributive shock, cardiogenic shock is characterized by a systolic or diastolic cardiac dysfunction resulting in hemodynamic abnormalities such as increased heart rate; decreased stroke volume; decreased cardiac output; decreased blood pressure; increased peripheral vascular resistance; and increases in the right atrial, pulmonary arterial, and pulmonary capillary wedge pressures (see Chapter 39). These pathologic changes result in diminished tissue perfusion and increased pulmonary venous pressures, resulting in pulmonary edema and dyspnea. Supplemental oxygen therapy and minimal handling are extremely important to avoid further decompensation in patients with cardiogenic shock. A brief physical examination consisting of thoracic auscultation alone may identify the presence of a cardiac murmur or gallop rhythm and pulmonary crackles. In cats, hypothermia secondary to reduced perfusion may be very helpful in differentiating heart failure from other causes of dyspnea.

Successful treatment of cardiogenic shock depends on rapid evaluation of signalment, a brief physical examination, and avoidance of stress. The diuretic furosemide (1 to 8 mg/kg) administered intravenously or intramuscularly is the mainstay of therapy for congestive heart failure. Animals that fail to show clinical signs of improvement after repeated doses of diuretics may require more specific therapy targeting the underlying cardiac abnormality (e.g., systolic dysfunction, diastolic failure, arrhythmias). Ultimately, the dyspneic patient in cardiogenic shock that fails to respond to therapy should be anesthetized, intubated, and positive pressure ventilated with 100% oxygen to stabilize the animal, remove the anxiety associated with shortness of breath, and allow the clinician to perform a thorough physical examination and pursue further diagnostics such as thoracic radiographs and echocardiography.

Early recognition and initiation of therapy are essential for successful treatment of the shock patient. Therapy for the shock patient is complicated by the need for rapid decision making in the absence of a complete medical history. In all forms of shock other than cardiogenic shock, intravenous fluid administration is the mainstay of therapy. Although underresuscitation or delayed onset of therapy could clearly contribute to a negative outcome, excessive or overaggressive resuscitation may also have undesirable consequences, including a dilutional coagulopathy and pulmonary edema. The combination of breed, signalment, and physical examination findings will help the emergency clinician identify the type of shock present, and serial evaluation with clearly defined end points of resuscitation are essential for successful management of the shock patient.

REFERENCES

1. Schutzer KM, Larsson A, Risberg B, et al: Lung protein leakage in feline septic shock, Am Rev Respir Dis 147:1380, 1993.
2. Brady CA, Otto CM, Van Winkle TJ, et al: Severe sepsis in cats: 29 cases (1986-1998), J Am Vet Med Assoc 217:531, 2000.
3. Costello MF, Drobatz KJ, Aronson LR, et al: Underlying cause, pathophysiologic abnormalities, and response to treatment in cats with septic peritonitis: 51 cases (1990-2001), J Am Vet Med Assoc 225:897, 2004.
4. Nguyen HB, Rivers EP, Knoblich BP, et al: Early lactate clearance is associated with improved outcome in severe sepsis and septic shock, Crit Care Med 32:1637, 2004.
5. Boag A, Hughes D: Assessment and treatment of perfusion abnormalities in the emergency patient, Vet Clin North Am Small Anim Pract 35:319, 2005.
6. dePapp E, Drobatz KJ, Hughes D, et al: Plasma lactate concentration as a predictor of gastric necrosis and survival among dogs with gastric volvulus: 102 cases (1995-1998), J Am Vet Med Assoc 215:49, 1999.
7. Nel M, Lobetti RG, Keller N, et al: Prognostic value of blood lactate, blood glucose and hematocrit in canine babesiosis, J Vet Intern Med 18:471, 2004.
8. McMichael MA, Lees GE, Hennessey J, et al: Serial plasma lactate concentration in 68 puppies aged 4 to 80 days, J Vet Emerg Crit Care 15:17, 2005.
9. Hughes D, Rozanski ER, Shofer FS, et al: Effect of sampling site, repeated sampling, pH and PCO2, on plasma lactate concentration in healthy dogs, Am J Vet Res 60:521, 1999.
10. Taylor RW: Pulmonary Artery Consensus Conference participants: Consensus statement, Crit Care Med 25:910, 1997.
11. Rivers E, Nguyen B, Havstad S, et al: Early goal-directed therapy in the treatment of severe sepsis and septic shock, N Engl J Med 345:1368, 2001.
12. Conti-Patara A, de Araujo Caldeira J, de Mattos-Junior E, et al: Changes in tissue perfusion parameters in dogs with severe sepsis/septic shock in response to goal-directed hemodynamic optimization at admission to ICU and the relation to outcome, J Vet Emerg Crit Care 22(4):409-418, 2012.
13. Trzeciak S, McCoy JV, Dellinger RP, et al. Early increases in microcirculatory perfusion during protocol-directed resuscitation are associated with reduced multi-organ failure at 24 h in patients with sepsis, Intensive Care Med 34(12):2210-2217, 2008.
14. Silverstein DC, Kleiner J, Drobatz KJ: Effectiveness of intravenous fluid resuscitation in the emergency room for treatment of hypotension in dogs: 35 cases (2000-2010), J Vet Emerg Crit Care 22(6):666-673, 2012.
15. Silverstein DC, Aldrich J, Haskins SC, et al: Assessment of changes in blood volume in response to resuscitative fluid administration in dog, J Vet Emerg Crit Care 15:185, 2005.
16. Stern SA, Wang S, Mertz M, et al: Under-resuscitation of near-lethal uncontrolled hemorrhage: effects on mortality and end-organ function at 72 hours, Shock 15:16, 2001.
17. Choi PT, Yip G, Quinonez LG, et al: Crystalloids vs. colloids in fluid resuscitation: A systematic review, Crit Care Med 27:200, 1999.
18. Cohn LA, Kerl ME, Dodam JR, et al: Clinical response to human albumin administration in healthy dogs, Am J Vet Res 68:657, 2007.
19. Shertel ER, Allen DA, Muir WW, et al: Evaluation of a hypertonic sodium chloride/dextran solution for treatment of traumatic shock in dogs, J Am Vet Med Assoc 208:366, 1996.
20. Fantoni DT, Auler JO Jr, Futema F, et al: Intravenous administration of hypertonic sodium chloride solution with dextran or isotonic sodium chloride solution for treatment of septic shock secondary to pyometra in dogs, J Am Vet Med Assoc 215:1283, 1999.

CHAPTER 6
SYSTEMIC INFLAMMATORY RESPONSE SYNDROME

Armelle de Laforcade, DVM, DACVECC

KEY POINTS

- Systemic inflammatory response syndrome (SIRS) is a widespread response to an infectious or a noninfectious insult and, if left untreated, can lead to multiple organ failure and death.
- Under normal conditions, the release of proinflammatory mediators and acute-phase proteins triggers a compensatory antiinflammatory response that leads to the restoration of a homeostatic state.
- Criteria used for the identification of SIRS are nonspecific and may lead to an overdiagnosis of this condition.
- Severe systemic inflammation often leads to vascular hyporesponsiveness, increased endothelial permeability, and a hypercoagulable state.
- Treatment of SIRS consists of supportive care and treatment of the underlying disease.

Systemic inflammatory response syndrome (SIRS) is a term introduced by the American College of Chest Physicians and Society of Critical Care Medicine (ACCM/SCCM) consensus conference in 1992 to acknowledge the importance of systemic activation of inflammation as a contributor to organ failure in sepsis.[1] The inherent heterogeneity of patients with sepsis and the observation of similar clinical courses in disease states lacking an infectious cause led to the breakdown of sepsis into a trigger (bacterial invasion) and a response to that trigger (the inflammatory response). From this emerged the concept of SIRS, or a systemic response to an insult that is infectious or noninfectious in origin.

Although SIRS is most commonly associated with sepsis, other disease states known to cause widespread release of proinflammatory endogenous mediators and subsequent systemic inflammation in people include trauma, burns, major surgery, and pancreatitis.[2] These insults can progress to multiple organ failure, shock, and death because of the magnitude of the inflammatory response alone (and

Table 6-1 Proposed Criteria for the Diagnosis of SIRS in Dogs and Cats

	Dogs (2/4 Changes Required)*	Cats (3/4 Changes Required)
Temperature (°C)	<100.6 or >102.6	<100 or > 104
HR (beats/min)	>120	<140 or >225
RR (breaths/min)	>20	>40
WBC ($\times 10^3/\mu l$); % bands	<6 or >16; >3%	>19 or <5

HR, Heart rate; *RR,* respiratory rate; *SIRS,* Systemic inflammatory response syndrome; *WBC,* white blood cells.

*Proposed criteria for the diagnosis of SIRS include at least two (in dogs) or three (in cats) of the changes listed. Criteria described for dogs were found to have a sensitivity of 97% and a specificity of 64% for the diagnosis of SIRS.[35]

in the absence of infection).[2,3] SIRS describes a clinical state rather than a disease entity. Proposed criteria for the diagnosis of SIRS consist of two out of the following four clinical signs: (1) hypothermia or hyperthermia, (2) leukocytosis or leukopenia, (3) tachycardia, and (4) tachypnea (Table 6-1).[1] Studies relating the magnitude of the inflammatory response to outcome highlight the importance of early recognition of systemic inflammation and treatment of the underlying disease process.[4]

SYSTEMIC INFLAMMATION

Systemic inflammation may be triggered by products of both gram-positive and gram-negative bacteria. Factors known to stimulate macrophages and monocytes include lipopolysaccharide (from gram-negative bacteria), lipoteichoic acid (gram-positive bacteria), peptidoglycan and flagellin (gram-positive and gram-negative bacteria), and mannan (fungi). Normally leukocyte activation resulting from exposure to these proteins, and subsequent release of tumor necrosis factor α (TNF-α), lead to an inflammatory response designed to protect the host. Excessive activation of inflammation, however, may contribute to the development of tissue damage, multiple organ failure, and death.

Although the release of mediators such as TNF-α, interleukin (IL)-1, IL-6, prekallikreins, bradykinin, platelet activating factor, and others in response to leukocyte activation has been well characterized, this proinflammatory response is accompanied by activation of antiinflammatory measures designed to counteract the proinflammatory state. This compensatory antiinflammatory response syndrome (CARS) is characterized by the release of antiinflammatory mediators (including IL-10, transforming growth factor β [TGF-β], and IL- 13); production of soluble receptors and receptor antagonists for cytokines such as TNF-α; and reduction of B and T lymphocyte production. Although clearly beneficial in its ability to control the proinflammatory state, excessive stimulation of the CARS may contribute to immunoparalysis and increased susceptibility to nosocomial infections seen in the late stages of sepsis.[5-7]

THE CONSEQUENCES OF SYSTEMIC INFLAMMATION

Disruptions in homeostasis caused by production of proinflammatory mediators include loss of vascular tone, disruption of the endothelial permeability barrier, and stimulation of coagulation (see Chapter 7). Loss of vascular tone is thought to occur secondary to excessive inducible nitric oxide synthase production, the precursor to nitric oxide release, and possibly a deficiency of vasopressin (a potent vasoconstrictor hormone) or cortisol. Disruption of the endothelial permeability barrier is a direct result of cytokine production.[8,9]

A hypercoagulable state, induced by cytokine-mediated tissue factor expression on the surface of leukocytes, leads to fibrin deposition in the microvasculature and is thought to contribute to organ failure in proinflammatory states. Endogenous anticoagulant systems such as antithrombin, protein C, and tissue factor pathway inhibitor are consumed and in some cases impaired in states of systemic inflammation.[10,11] Interestingly, studies have supported a close relationship between inflammation and coagulation.[12,13] Thrombin resulting from the activation coagulation stimulates leukocyte activation and further cytokine production.

TNF-α down regulates the activation of protein C, which is known to have antiinflammatory properties in addition to its role as an anticoagulant. Modulation of inflammation was thought to contribute to the apparent success of drotrecogin alpha (Xigris, or recombinant human activated protein C [rhAPC]) in improving survival in people with severe sepsis.[14,15] Ultimately, failure to show a survival benefit in human patients with septic shock led to discontinuation of all clinical trials related to Xigris and to its withdrawal from the market in 2011.[16]

SIRS AND SEPSIS

Although SIRS has been identified as an important component of sepsis, it can occur in the absence of infection yet have a clinic course resembling that of sepsis. Parameters such as body temperature, heart rate, and respiratory rate are useful to identify the presence of systemic inflammation, but they lack sensitivity and specificity for the diagnosis of sepsis. The time required to obtain culture and sensitivity results precludes their usefulness in differentiating non-septic SIRS from septic SIRS in most clinical situations. This need to differentiate sepsis from SIRS of noninfectious origin has led to the search for biological markers that would identify the presence (or lack of) bacterial infection in patients with clinical signs of SIRS. C-reactive protein (CRP) and procalcitonin (PCT) have both been studied extensively in people. Additionally, the use of the PIRO (*p*redisposition, *i*nsult/*i*nfection, *r*esponse, and *o*rgan *d*ysfunction) acronym was adopted following the 2001 Sepsis Definitions conference to more accurately stage sepsis and describe the clinical manifestations of the infection and the host response (see Chapter 91 for further details).

POTENTIAL MARKERS OF SEPSIS

CRP is an acute-phase protein produced by hepatocytes in response to inflammatory cytokine release, including TNF-α, and IL-1β. CRP release peaks 36 to 50 hours after secretion and it has a half-life of 19 hours. Although studies support a rise in CRP in humans with sepsis,[17] elevations have also been documented secondary to other inflammatory processes such as trauma, surgery, acute pancreatitis, and myocardial infarction.[18] Some studies have also suggested that CRP levels reflect the severity of the inflammatory process, but these levels have not been shown to differ between survivors and nonsurvivors.[19] Because of the prolonged half-life and lack of specificity, CRP is not considered the ideal marker for the diagnosis of sepsis.

Procalcitonin, the precursor molecule to calcitonin, has also been investigated as a potential marker of sepsis. Normally produced by the thyroid gland, PCT during sepsis is thought to originate from mononuclear leukocytes after endotoxin and cytokine stimulation.[20] PCT is released hours after endotoxin release, and peak levels persist for up to 24 hours. Although the exact role of PCT in patients with sepsis is still unknown, it has been shown to increase inducible nitric oxide synthase (iNOS)-mediated nitric oxide release and therefore may play a role in amplification of the inflammation.[21]

Studies have documented elevated PCT levels in people with bacterial infections complicated by systemic inflammation and little to no change in PCT in localized infections or in infections of viral etiology. These findings support the use of PCT to help differentiate between bacterial sepsis and SIRS of nonbacterial origin in humans and may be used as a guide to initiate antimicrobial therapy.[22-24] In some studies, PCT levels correlate with disease severity, and they may have prognostic value in people with sepsis and septic shock.[23,24] Overall, PCT is thought to represent a superior marker of sepsis than CRP in people.

TREATMENT OF SIRS IN HUMANS

Because systemic inflammation is a critical component of sepsis, studies investigating the benefit of therapeutic interventions for sepsis have focused on modulation of the inflammatory response. Cytokine blockade, in particular, has been investigated extensively as a means to control inflammation, prevent end-organ damage, and improve survival in severe sepsis and septic shock. TNF-α blockade using TNF antibody administration failed to improve survival in people with sepsis and was shown in some studies to have detrimental effects.[25,26] Similarly, the use of receptor antagonists to TNF, platelet activating factor, and IL-1 failed to improve 28-day survival in people with severe sepsis.[27,28]

The antiinflammatory benefits of ibuprofen were also studied in a prospective, randomized, double-blinded, placebo-controlled trial. A survival benefit was not shown in humans with sepsis.[29] High-dose corticosteroids, commonly used before the 1990s, were often administered to control the inflammatory response. This practice was discontinued because of failure to increase survival and, in some studies, increased mortality.[30] Human intravenous immunoglobulin was shown to increase survival in small study of humans with gram-negative sepsis.[31] The immune-modulating properties of statins, drugs commonly used to control cholesterol in humans, have led to recent studies investigating their effect in diseases known to be associated with systemic activation of inflammation. Their potential benefits in people with SIRS and sepsis have yet to be determined.[32] A recent multicenter, randomized, double-blind, placebo-controlled study of atorvastatin }in patients with severe sepsis did not show a difference in IL-6, mortality, or length of hospital stay between groups.[33] The promising results of the PROWESS study[14] led to the recommendation of rhAPC administration to patients with severe sepsis.[34] However, failure to show a survival benefit in subsequent studies led to its withdrawal from the market in 2011.[16]

SIRS IN SMALL ANIMALS

Knowledge relating to SIRS in animals is based on studies of animal models of sepsis and related diseases, and studies investigating the inflammatory response in naturally occurring animal diseases are lacking. Historically, studies of sepsis have often included both dogs and cats; however, increasing evidence supports significant differences in the manifestation of systemic inflammation in these species.

Common causes of SIRS in animals include sepsis, heat stroke, pancreatitis, immune disease, neoplasia, severe polytrauma, and burns. Criteria for SIRS have been extrapolated from human studies for dogs and cats, but few prospective studies have been performed to validate these criteria. In one study of 30 septic and 320 nonseptic dogs, criteria found to have the greatest sensitivity for the diagnosis of SIRS were determined; they are listed in Table 6-1.[35] In both animals and humans, the criteria used for identification of SIRS may lead to overdiagnosis of this condition. In cats, proposed criteria for SIRS were derived from a retrospective study in which severe sepsis was identified at necropsy. This study identified inappropriate (or relative) bradycardia (HR < 140 beats/min) in 66% of cats with severe sepsis.[36] Although the criteria for SIRS that were proposed as a result of this study have yet to be validated prospectively, relative bradycardia was also identified in 16% of cats with septic peritonitis.[37] This finding supports the fundamental difference between cats and dogs in the hemodynamic response to systemic inflammation.

Several studies have been performed investigating alterations in hemostasis in dogs with systemic inflammation. In one study, all nine dogs with parvoviral enteritis had evidence of hypercoagulability as determined using thromboelastography and a reduction in measured antithrombin activity.[38] Another study investigating the coagulation response in dogs with and without SIRS showed great variability in hemostatic alterations in both populations. When comparing dogs with and without SIRS to healthy controls, significant changes, including prolonged prothrombin time (PT) and activated partial thromboplastin time (aPTT), reduced antithrombin and protein C activities, and increased D-dimers, were seen both groups of sick dogs compared with controls.[39] Several studies documented reduced activities of PC and AT in dogs with naturally occurring sepsis, suggesting the tendency toward hypercoagulability in this disease process.[40-42] However, AT was also reduced in dogs with uncomplicated *Babesiosis* infection, although thromboelastography variables of infected dogs did not differ significantly from those of healthy controls.[43]

Potential uses of markers of inflammation in animals with SIRS include differentiation between infectious and noninfectious causes of systemic inflammation and determination of severity of disease and response to therapy. CRP is the acute-phase protein that has received the most attention in the veterinary literature to date. In one study of dogs with naturally occurring pancreatitis, serum CRP concentrations were elevated in all 16 dogs with acute pancreatitis compared with controls, and CRP concentration decreased in all dogs that were hospitalized for 5 days.[44] Increased CRP concentration has been documented in a variety of disease states, including immune-mediated hemolytic anemia, various neoplasias,[45] chronic valvular disease,[46] and other diseases known to cause acute inflammation. The usefulness of CRP measurements to differentiate infectious from noninfectious SIRS in animals with naturally disease has not yet been investigated.

Studies investigating the presence of inflammatory mediators in animals with naturally occurring disease are lacking. In one study of dogs with parvoviral enteritis, 7 of 17 dogs had measurable TNF activity.[47] Proinflammatory cytokines have also been documented in other disease states thought to have an inflammatory component (e.g., cranial cruciate rupture in the dog).[48] One study investigating inflammatory changes in 32 dogs with pyometra compared those with and without SIRS to healthy controls. In this study, CRP was elevated in dogs with pyometra both with and without SIRS. Among the cytokine changes identified in this study, IL-7 was significantly elevated in dogs with pyometra and SIRS compared with controls, and IL-10 was significantly elevated only in dogs with pyometra and SIRS.[49]

Clinical manifestations of SIRS are often nonspecific and may vary depending on the underlying disease process. In general, signs of SIRS often resemble those of sepsis and in most cases are managed similarly. Loss of appetite and depression are commonly reported in animals experiencing systemic inflammation. In addition to clinical signs listed in Table 6-1, animals may exhibit injected mucous membranes and bounding peripheral pulses, suggesting a compensated hyperdynamic state, or vomiting and diarrhea (even if the problem is not gastrointestinal in origin). A high index of suspicion for SIRS may also be based on complete blood cell count (CBC) changes such as a neutrophilic leukocytosis, with or without a left shift, and toxic cytologic changes to the neutrophils. Alterations often found on the biochemistry panel include hyperglycemia or hypoglycemia, hypoalbuminemia, elevated alanine aminotransferase and aspartate aminotransferase, and, in some cases, hyperbilirubinemia. Changes in blood glucose are thought to occur secondary to altered carbohydrate metabolism, with increased gluconeogenesis causing hyperglycemia in the early phase of infection/inflammation and hypoglycemia occurring late when glucose utilization exceeds production. Reduced albumin concentration occurs secondary to reduced manufacturing by the liver in favor of production of acute-phase proteins and also to loss induced by changes in endothelial permeability. Liver enzyme concentrations are likely altered as a result of changes in perfusion and decreased oxygen delivery to tissues. Finally, cholestasis may be the cause of elevated serum bilirubin, though it has also been suggested that immune-mediated hemolysis may play a role. The effect of acute inflammation on renal function is demonstrated by a study of urine protein excretion in dogs with SIRS. In this study, evidence of glomerular and tubular dysfunction was present with dogs with SIRS as demonstrated by changes in urinary protein to urinary creatinine ratio, urinary albumin to urinary creatinine ratio, and urinary retinol-binding protein to urinary creatinine ratio.[50]

It is important to note that cats and dogs differ in the manifestation of SIRS, with cats more likely to experience hypotension, hypoglycemia, and hyperbilirubinemia than dogs. Ultimately, clinical manifestation of SIRS resembles that of sepsis, with the finding of infection ultimately necessary to differentiate these two conditions.

The mainstay of treatment for SIRS consists of treatment of the underlying disease process and supportive care. If infection is found or suspected along with clinical signs of SIRS, then treatment for sepsis consisting of source control, antibiotic therapy, and cardiovascular support should be initiated. Although SIRS may not always be of infectious origin, antibiotics are often added when an infectious cause for SIRS is suspected but no specific infection is diagnosed. Until culture results are available, antibiotic therapy must be broad spectrum so that gram-positive, gram-negative, and anaerobic organisms are covered. Common combinations include a cephalosporin, enrofloxacin, and metronidazole, or ampicillin and enrofloxacin (see Chapters 91 and 175).

Once culture and susceptibility testing results are available, antimicrobial therapy may be tailored to target the identified pathogen. More aggressive antimicrobial therapy may be warranted if a hospital-acquired infection is suspected. Intravenous fluid therapy generally consists of replacement fluids such as lactated Ringer's solution or Normosol-R. Fluid therapy is aimed at resolving hypovolemia, maintaining daily requirements, and replacing any ongoing losses and must be tailored to the individual patient (see Chapter 59). It is important to note that inflammatory mediators associated with systemic inflammation also lead to changes in endothelial permeability; therefore excessive crystalloid administration may result in interstitial accumulation of fluids and clinical signs of peripheral edema.

Other therapies may include oxygen supplementation (see Chapter 14), nutritional support in the form of enteral or parenteral nutrition (see Chapters 129 and 130), and stress ulcer prophylaxis (see Chapter 161).

Monitoring the patient with SIRS consists of regular evaluation of volume and perfusion status through measurement of serum lactate concentration, central venous pressure measurements, central venous oxygen saturation, serial body weights and comparison of intake to output (see Chapter 183). Intermitted blood pressure measurements may be helpful, and vasopressor therapy is indicated if fluid therapy alone fails to resolve hypotension (see Chapters 157 and 158). Hematocrit and serum electrolyte, albumin, and glucose concentrations should be monitored regularly. Complications of SIRS include cardiovascular collapse, disseminated intravascular coagulation, and multiple organ dysfunction (see Chapter 7).

SUMMARY

Systemic inflammation has received widespread attention as a key component of sepsis in both people and animals. SIRS is classically associated with diseases such as pancreatitis and sepsis in dogs and cats but may be underrecognized as a contributor to cardiovascular collapse and organ failure in animals with other diseases (e.g., polytrauma, neoplasia). Cats in particular may be more susceptible to the development of noninfectious SIRS, a clinical state that may show similar signs as sepsis and result in organ failure and death.

Supportive care aimed at preserving organ function and treatment of the underlying disease process remain the mainstay of therapy. Low-dose glucocorticoid and intravenous immunoglobulin administration warrant further study in animals with naturally occurring disease.

REFERENCES

1. Bone RC, Balk RA, Cerra FB, et al: Definitions for sepsis and organ failure and guidelines for the use of innovative therapies in sepsis. ACCP/SCCM Consensus Conference Committee, Chest 101:1644, 1992.
2. Rangel-Frausto MS, Pittet D, Costigan M, et al: The natural history of the systemic inflammatory response syndrome (SIRS): a prospective study, J Am Med Assoc 273(2):117, 1995.
3. Beal AL, Cerra FB: Multiple organ failure syndrome in the 1990s. Systemic inflammatory response and organ dysfunction, J Am Med Assoc 271:226-233, 1994.
4. Jönsson B, Berglund J, Skau T, et al: Outcome of intra-abdominal infection in pigs depends more on host responses than on microbiology, Eur J Surg 159:571, 1993.
5. van der Poll T, van Deventer SJH: Cytokines and anticytokines in the pathogenesis of sepsis, Infect Dis Clin N Am 13:312, 1999.
6. van der Poll T: Immunotherapy of sepsis, Lancet Infect Dis 1:165, 2001.
7. Kox WJ, Volk T, Kox S, et al: Immunomodulatory therapies in sepsis, Int Care Med 26(S1):S124, 2000.
8. Trepels T, Zeiher AM, Fichtlscherer S: The endothelium and inflammation, Endothelium 13(6):423, 2006.
9. Harbrecht BG: Therapeutic use of nitric oxide scavengers in shock and sepsis, Curr Pharm Des 12(27):3543, 2006.
10. Mesters RM, Helterbrand J, Utterback BG, et al: Prognostic value of protein C concentrations in neutropenic patients at high risk of severe septic complications, Crit Care Med 28:2209, 2000.
11. Vary TC, Kimball SR: Regulation of hepatic protein synthesis in chronic inflammation and sepsis, Am J Physiol 262:C445, 1992.
12. Esmon CT, Fukudome K, Mather T, et al: Inflammation, sepsis, and coagulation, Haematologica 84:254, 1999.
13. Thijs LG, de Boer JP, de Groot M, et al: Coagulation disorders in septic shock, Int Care Med 19(Suppl 1):S1, 1993.
14. Bernard GR, Vincent JL, Laterre PF, et al: Efficacy and safety of recombinant human activated protein C for severe sepsis, N Engl J Med 344:699, 2001.
15. Rjewald M, Petrovan RJ, Donner Al, et al: Activated protein C signals through the thrombin receptor PAR1 in endothelial cells, J Endotoxin Res 9:317, 2003.

16. Ranieri VM, Thompson BT, Barie PS, et al: Drotecogin alpha (activated) in adults with septic shock, N Eng J Med 366(22):2055, 2012.
17. Povoa P, Almeida E, Moreira P, et al: C-reactive protein as an indicator of sepsis, Int Care Med 24:1052, 1998.
18. Pepys MB, Hirschfield GM: C-reactive protein: a critical update, J Clin Invest 111:1805, 2003.
19. Meisner M, Adina H, Schmidt J: Correlation of procalcitonin and C-reactive protein to inflammation, complications, and outcome during the intensive care unit course of multiple-trauma patients, Crit Care 10(1):R1, 2006.
20. Oberhoffer M, Stonans I, Russwurm S, et al: Procalcitonin expression in human peripheral blood mononuclear cells and its modulation by lipopolysaccharides and sepsis-related cytokines in vitro, J Lab Clin Med 134:49, 1999.
21. Hoffmann G, Totzke G, Smolny M, et al: In vitro modulation of inducible nitric oxide synthase gene expression and nitric oxide synthesis by procalcitonin, Crit Care Med 29(1):112, 2001.
22. Assicot M, Gendrel D, Carsin H, et al: High serum procalcitonin concentrations in patients with sepsis and infection, Lancet 341:515, 1993.
23. Jekarl DW, Lee SY, Lee J, et al. Procalcitonin as a diagnostic marker and IL-6 as a prognostic marker for sepsis, Diagn Microbiol Infect Dis http://dx.doi.org/10.1016/j.diagmicrobio.2012.12.011, 2013.
24. Georgopolous AP, Savva A, Giamarellos-Bourboulis EJ, et al: Early changes in procalcitonin may advise about prognosis and appropriateness of antimicrobial therapy in sepsis, J Crit Care 26(3):331e1, 2011.
25. Abraham E, Anzueto A, Gutierrez G, et al: Double-blind randomized controlled trial of monoclonal antibody to human tumour necrosis factor in treatment of septic shock, Lancet 351:929, 1998.
26. Panacek EA, Marshall J, Fischkoff S, et al: Neutralization of TNF by a monoclonal antibody improves survival and reduces organ dysfunction in human sepsis: results of the MONARCS trial, Chest 118:88S, 2000.
27. Opal S, Laterre PF, Abraham E: Recombinant human platelet-activating factor acetylhydrolase for treatment of severe sepsis: results of a phase III, multicenter, randomized, double-blind, placebo-controlled, clinical trial, Crit Care Med 32(2):332, 2004.
28. Opal SM, Fisher CJ Jr, Dhainaut JF, et al: Confirmatory interleukin-1 receptor antagonist trial in severe sepsis: a phase III, randomized, double-blind, placebo-controlled, multicenter trial, Crit Care Med 133:94, 1997.
29. Bernard GR, Wheeler AP, Russell JA, et al: The effects of ibuprofen on the physiology and survival of patients with sepsis. The Ibuprofen in Sepsis Study Group, N Engl J Med 336(13):912, 1997.
30. Luce JM, Montgomery AB, Marks JD, et al: Ineffectiveness of high-dose methylprednisolone in preventing parenchymal lung injury and improving survival in patients with septic shock, Am Rev Resp Dis 138:62, 1998.
31. Schedel I, Dreikhausen U, Nentwig B, et al: Treatment of gram-negative septic shock with an immunoglobulin preparation: a prospective, randomized clinical trial, Crit Care Med 19(9):1104, 1991.
32. Kruger P, Fitzsimmons K, Cook D, et al: Statin therapy is associated with fewer deaths in patients with bacteraemia, Int Care Med 32(1):75, 2006.
33. Kruger P, Bailey M, Bellomo R. A multicentre randomized trial of atorvastatin therapy in intensive care patients with severe sepsis, Am J Respir Crit Care Med doi:10.1164/rcm.201209-1718OC, 2013.
34. Dellinger RP, Carlet JM, Masur H, et al: Surviving Sepsis Campaign guidelines for management of severe sepsis and septic shock, Int Care Med 30(4):536, 2004.
35. Hauptman JG, Walshaw R, Olivier NB: Evaluation of the sensitivity and specificity of diagnostic criteria for sepsis in dogs, Vet Surg 26:393, 1997.
36. Brady CA, Otto CM, Van W, et al: Severe sepsis in cats: 29 cases (1986-1998), J Am Vet Med Assoc 217:531, 2000.
37. Costello MF, Drobatz KJ, Aronson L, et al: Underlying cause, pathophysiologic abnormalities, and response to treatment in cats with septic peritonitis: 51 cases (1990-2001), J Am Vet Med Assoc 225(6):897, 2004.
38. Otto CM, Rieser TM, Brooks MR, et al: Evidence of hypercoagulability in dogs with parvoviral enteritis, J Am Vet Med Assoc 217(10):1500, 2000.
39. Bauer N, Moritz A: Coagulation response in dogs with and without systemic inflammatory response syndrome—preliminary results, Res Vet Sci 94:122, 2013.
40. deLaforcade AM, Freeman LM, Shaw SP, et al: Hemostatic changes in dogs with naturally occurring sepsis, J Vet Intern Med 17:674, 2003.
41. Bentley AM, Mayhew PD, Culp WT, et al: Alterations in the hemostatic profiles of dogs with naturally occurring septic peritonitis, J Vet Emerg Crit Care 23(1):14, 2013.
42. DeLaforcade AM, Rozanski EA, Freeman LM, et al: Serial evaluation of protein C and antithrombin in dogs with sepsis, J Vet Intern Med 22(1):26, 2008.
43. Liebenberg C, Goddard A, Wiinberg B, et al: Hemostatic abnormalities in uncomplicated babesiosis (Babesia rossi) in dogs, J Vet Intern Med 27:150, 2013.
44. Holm J, Rozanski EA, Freeman LM, et al: C-reactive protein concentrations in canine acute pancreatitis, J Vet Emerg Crit Care 14(3):183, 2004.
45. Tecles F, Spiranelli E, Bonfanti U, et al: Preliminary studies of serum acute-phase protein concentrations in hematologic and neoplastic diseases of the dog, J Vet Intern Med 19(6):865, 2005.
46. Rush JE, Lee ND, Freeman LM, et al: C-reactive protein concentration in dogs with chronic valvular disease, J Vet Intern Med 20(3):635, 2006.
47. Otto CM, Drobatz KJ, Soter C: Endotoxemia and tumor necrosis factor activity in dogs with naturally occurring parvoviral enteritis, J Vet Int Med 11(2):65, 1997.
48. Fujita Y, Hara Y, Nezy Y, et al: Proinflammatory cytokine activities, matrix metalloproteinase-3 activity, and sulfated glycosaminoglycan content in synovial fluid of dogs with naturally acquired cranial cruciate ligament rupture, Vet Surg 35(4):369, 2006.
49. Karlsson I, Hagman R, Johannisoon A: Cytokines as immunological markers for systemic inflammation in dogs with pyometra, Reprod Dom Anim 47(suppl 6):337, 2012.
50. Schaefer H, Kohn B, Schweigert FJ, et al: Quantitative and qualitative urine protein excretion in dogs with severe inflammatory response syndrome, J Vet Intern Med 25:1292, 2011.

CHAPTER 7
MULTIPLE ORGAN DYSFUNCTION SYNDROME

Robert A.N. Goggs, BVSc, DACVECC, PhD, MRCVS • Daniel Huw Lewis, MA, VetMB, DACVECC, MRCVS

KEY POINTS

- Multiple organ dysfunction syndrome (MODS) is the potentially reversible abnormal function of at least two organ systems arising from a life-threatening physiologic insult such that homeostasis cannot be maintained without medical intervention.
- MODS most often develops secondary to severe systemic inflammation, trauma, or sepsis, and sustained organ failure is a leading cause of death in critically ill dogs and cats.
- Central to the pathogenesis of MODS is a dysregulated immune response. Interactions among systemic inflammation, the coagulation system, and the gastrointestinal tract promote MODS.
- Mortality increases with the severity of organ system dysfunction and number of organ systems involved.
- Numerous organ failure scoring systems have been developed for human patients. The most commonly used are the SOFA, MOD, and LODS scores, and of these the SOFA score is predictive of outcome in dogs.
- Every effort should be made to recognize patients at risk of MODS and intervene to prevent organ dysfunction from occurring secondary to other disease processes.
- Successful treatment of MODS requires aggressive support of organ function coupled with therapies directed at resolving the underlying cause.

The progression of critical illness to multiple organ failure and death has been recognized in human medicine since the 1950s,[1] and myriad terms have since been used to describe the development of multiple organ failure in the critically ill.[2] Improvements in acute trauma management and advances in intensive care over the past 60 years have created a population of patients who survive the initial life-threatening event but subsequently develop progressive organ dysfunction. Consequently, some have characterized this syndrome of secondary organ failure as a disease of medical progress—the unintended result of improvements in resuscitation and initial management of acute injury and illness.[3]

Growing recognition that systemic inflammation could develop from various acute physiologic insults,[4] that systemic inflammation might lead to development of dysfunction in initially unaffected organ systems, and that injury to one organ system might cause damage in others[5] paved the way for the 1991 American College of Chest Physicians and Society of Critical Care Medicine consensus conference on sepsis and organ failure. This conference proposed definitions for systemic inflammatory response syndrome (SIRS), sepsis, and MODS.[6] The 1991 conference defined MODS as "the presence of altered organ function in an acutely ill patient such that homeostasis cannot be maintained without intervention." This syndrome can be primary, where organ dysfunction arises from the primary insult, or secondary, where organ dysfunction arises from systemic inflammation.[7] The consensus definition is perhaps purposefully imprecise, and a more usable definition may be that proposed by Marshall[8]: "the development of potentially reversible physiologic derangement involving two or more organ systems not involved in the disorder that resulted in ICU admission, and arising in the wake of a potentially life-threatening physiologic insult."

EPIDEMIOLOGY

Most cases of MODS are secondary to shock, sepsis, and trauma, but multiple other conditions have been associated with MODS (Table 7-1). The reported incidence of MODS in human intensive care units (ICUs) varies with the patient population, the type of ICU, and the scoring system used to define organ dysfunction. Recent estimates for trauma patients suggest that up to 47% of adult trauma patients suffer organ failure while in ICU.[9,10] In surgical ICUs approximately 54% of patients develop MODS,[11] the most common cause of death in this population.[12] Longitudinal studies in people suggest the incidence and severity of MODS and the associated mortality rates are decreasing.[9,13] Nonetheless, MODS is still responsible for somewhere between 50% and 80% of surgical ICU deaths and is associated with a substantially greater mortality rate than that seen in patients without MODS.[12]

In trauma patients, the picture is complicated. Early reports suggested a bimodal distribution of organ failure in trauma patients, and this was linked to a "two-hit" theory of MODS.[14] Contemporaneous recognition of the potential for iatrogenic harm through interventions such as ventilation and fluid balance[15,16] led to institution of new treatment paradigms[17,18] to rapidly reverse physiologic abnormalities and reduce the risk of secondary insults.[19,20] These alterations to clinical practice may now be reducing the incidence of late events.[21]

Table 7-1 Conditions Associated with the Development of MODS

Risk Factor	Example(s)
Infection	Peritonitis Pneumonia Necrotizing wound infections
Inflammation (noninfectious)	Pancreatitis
Ischemia	GDV Mesenteric volvulus
Immune reactions	Autoimmune disease Transplant rejection Graft versus host disease
Iatrogenic injury	Surgical trauma Ventilator-induced lung injury
Intoxication	Pharmaceutical drug reactions Environmental agent toxicity
Endocrine	Adrenal crisis Pheochromocytoma

Adapted from Mizock BA: The multiple organ dysfunction syndrome, Disease-a-Month 55:476, 2009.
GDV, Gastric dilation-volvulus; *MODS,* multiple organ dysfunction syndrome.

Although advances in veterinary critical care have also resulted in increased numbers of patients with organ dysfunction secondary to critical illness, there remain relatively few primary reports of MODS in small animals. In part this may result from lack of a veterinary consensus definition of MODS.[22] Two recent studies have examined organ dysfunction in dogs with sepsis/systemic inflammatory response syndrome (SIRS); both studies clearly demonstrated a positive correlation between mortality and the degree of organ system dysfunction.[23,24] In dogs with septic peritonitis, single organ dysfunction complicated the primary disease in 78% of dogs, whereas MODS occurred in 50% cases, a prevalence similar to human surgical ICUs.[23] In the same study, mortality increased from 31% when one organ system was affected to 91% when four organ systems were dysfunctional; no dog with five affected organ systems survived.[23] In dogs with SIRS or sepsis, increased organ dysfunction severity as measured by modified sequential organ failure (SOFA) score was associated with increased mortality.[24]

PATHOPHYSIOLOGY

The pathogenesis of organ dysfunction secondary to severe physiologic insults such as sepsis is complex,[25] particularly because diverse primary causes incite dysfunction through distinct mechanisms in different organs. Our understanding remains incomplete, but central to the pathology of MODS is immune dysregulation that results in disordered systemic inflammatory processes (Figure 7-1; see Chapter 6). The degree of physiologic insult resulting from a primary event can be sufficient to create a massive inflammatory reaction, with consequent detrimental effects on the function of organs distant to the site of the initial injury—the "one-hit" theory of MODS.[26] There is also evidence that the initial immune dysfunction may be augmented by ongoing inflammation in the gastrointestinal tract (GIT),[27,28] the "sustained hit" theory, which can drive a patient to MODS.[27,28] Additional iatrogenic injuries, such as surgical trauma or drug reactions, or secondary insults, including ventilator-induced lung injury[29,30] and hospital-acquired infections,[31] have also been implicated in the pathogenesis of MODS through activation of previously primed inflammatory cells.[32] Irrespective of origin, the common biologic response to pathogen invasion, injury, severe localized inflammation, or autoimmunity is one of innate immune defense activation,[33] involving evolution of various soluble mediators and activation of immune effector cells.

Immune Dysregulation

Rather than simply an overproduction of proinflammatory mediators, the progression to MODS reflects dysregulation of the balance between proinflammatory and antiinflammatory agents. Initial host-defense responses induce proinflammatory cytokine release but also stimulate antiinflammatory mediator production, which should restore equilibrium in the system. A predominance of proinflammatory mediators gives rise to SIRS and its associated clinical signs, whereas an excess of antiinflammatory mediators can generate immunosuppression with a resultant predisposition to secondary infection—the compensatory antiinflammatory response syndrome (CARS). Although not diseases in themselves, both SIRS and CARS can result in MODS. These syndromes represent parts of a spectrum of inflammatory dysfunction and it should be recognized that both processes can occur at different times in an individual.

Activation of pattern recognition receptors (PRRs) on immune, epithelial, and endothelial cells initiates signaling cascades through nuclear factor kappa B (NFκB) that result in acute-phase protein secretion, inducible nitric oxide synthase (iNOS) expression, and the production of proinflammatory cytokines and chemokines. Pattern recognition receptors such as the Toll-like receptors (TLRs) are stimulated both by pathogen-associated molecular patterns (PAMPs) expressed by foreign organisms, and by danger-associated molecular patterns (DAMPs) that indicate host cell damage.

Key mediators in the proinflammatory response are tumor necrosis factor α (TNF-α) and interleukin (IL) 1, 6, 8 (CXCL8), and 12. Release of TNF-α and IL-1 are early events, whereas later production of IL-6 and IL-8 prolongs the inflammatory response. Many of the classical features of inflammation can be attributed to TNF-α through induction of iNOS and cyclooxygenase 2 (COX-2), leading to vasodilation, increased capillary permeability, and local slowing of blood flow.[34] Early inflammatory cytokines induce expression of tissue factor (TF) and adhesion molecules on endothelial surfaces and prime neutrophils. Activated neutrophils have upregulated adhesion molecule expression and once attached to the endothelium produce enzymes that enhance endothelial permeability. Overall, TNF-α and IL-1 activity leads to local conditions favoring the diapedesis of circulating defense cells and the extravasation of plasma. Extravasated, primed neutrophils have an increased capacity for generation of reactive oxygen species (ROS) and lipid mediators. Replication of this functional response on a body-wide scale leads to a reduction in effective circulating volume, diminished tissue perfusion, and unfavorable cellular energetics (shock),[35] as well as a propensity for local tissue injury by activated neutrophils.

Death of cells by necrosis, release of cytosolic and nuclear components, and degradation of proteoglycans in the extracellular matrix provide multiple new DAMPs, accelerating innate immune system activation and resulting in the production of yet more proinflammatory cytokines/chemokines. High-mobility group box 1 (HMGB1) protein is released by active innate immune cells as well as necrotic cells and acts to promote monocyte TF expression and inhibit protein C activation.[36] Such mediators then enter the circulation and travel to other organs where they exert their inflammatory influence, resulting in further cellular dysfunction and a vicious cycle of cell death and inflammation.

Complement activation through the classical, alternative, or lectin pathways is an important component of the innate host-defense system. Complement activation generates proinflammatory, biologically active peptides that, in the context of MODS, act as leukocyte chemoattractants, stimulate cytokine production, enhance adhesion molecule and TF expression, and increase vascular permeability. Central to these functions are the anaphylatoxins C3a and C5a.[37] Plasma concentrations of C3a are proportional to injury severity and mortality after trauma,[38] and treatment with anti-C5a antibodies attenuates MODS in a rodent model of sepsis.[39]

Coagulation

The development of MODS is propagated by the complex interplay between coagulation and inflammation, which leads to endothelial activation and injury and the generation of microvascular thromboses that ultimately causes organ systems to fail. The links between inflammation and coagulation pathways have been clearly established,[40] and the role of disordered coagulation in the pathogenesis of sepsis[41,42] and the subsequent development of disseminated intravascular coagulation (DIC) in small animals is well known.[43] Proinflammatory cytokines interact with the cellular regulators of thrombosis: endothelium, platelets, and leukocytes. The actions of TNF-α, IL-1, and IL-6 in particular lead to upregulation of reciprocal adhesion molecules on leukocytes and endothelial cells, promoting interactions designed to protect the host. In health, TF is concealed by the endothelium and coagulation activation is limited by various circulating proteins such as antithrombin, protein C, and tissue factor pathway inhibitor.[44] Abnormal TF expression by mononuclear phagocytes and tissue parenchymal cells is induced by inflammatory cytokines, C-reactive protein, and PAMPs such as lipopolysaccharide

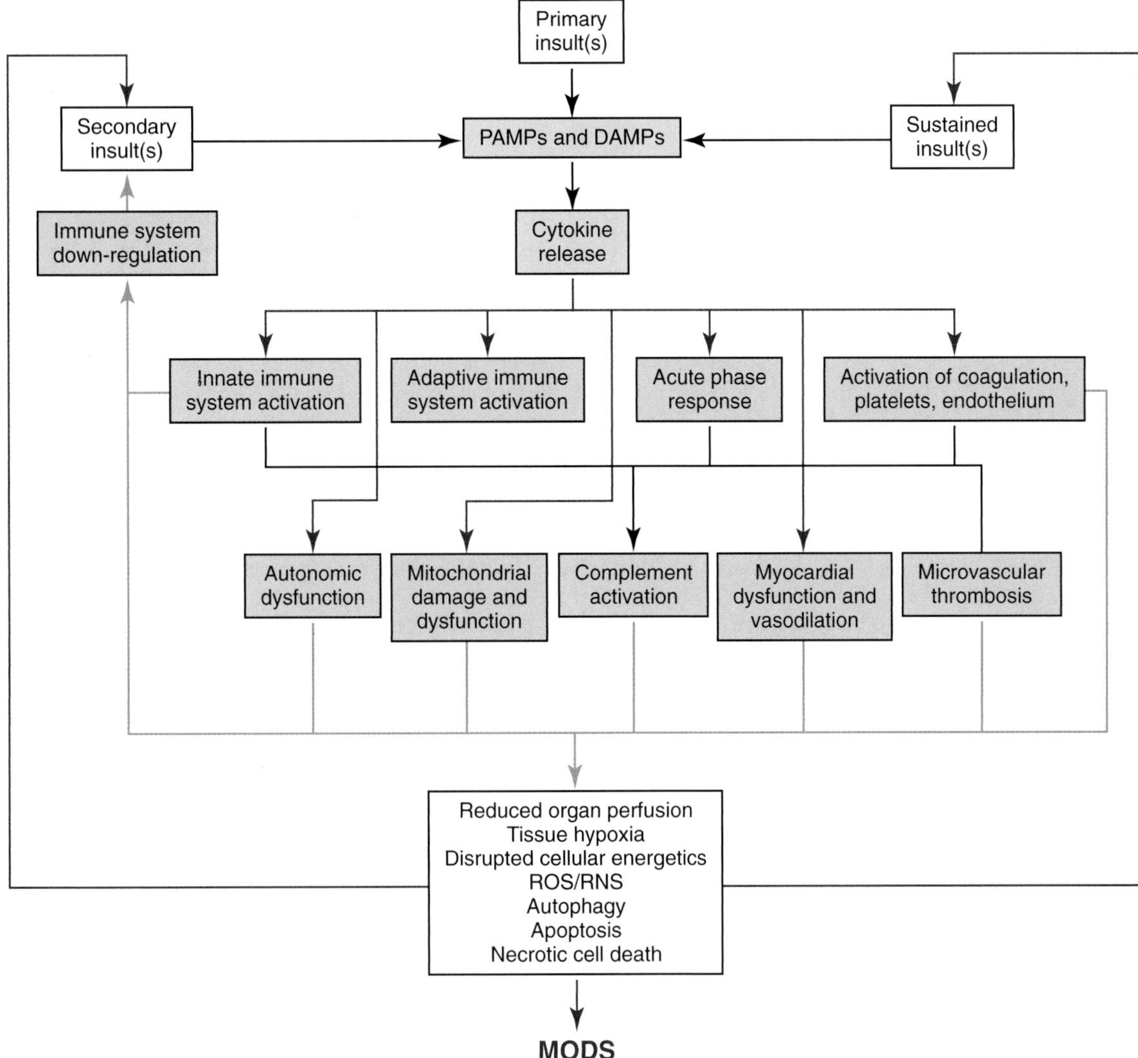

FIGURE 7-1 An overview of the pathogenesis of MODS. The most common primary insults leading to MODS are trauma, sepsis, and noninfectious SIRS; secondary insults that may contribute include opportunistic infections, ventilator-associated lung injury, surgical trauma, and anesthesia-related hypoperfusion. Sustained insults such as gut inflammation, crosstalk from other failing organs, or inadequate organ support can lead to the perpetuation of the physiologic insult. All these insults cause exposure of the immune system to pathogen-associated molecular patterns *(PAMPs)* such as LPS or peptidoglycans or to damage-associated molecular patterns *(DAMPs)* such as histones or high mobility group box 1 proteins. This triggers an immune response, activation of the innate and adaptive immune systems, and consequent increases in the plasma concentrations of both pro- and antiinflammatory cytokines. The effects of these increased circulating cytokine concentrations are myriad. Organ perfusion is adversely affected by autonomic and myocardial dysfunction and through the systemic vasodilation induced by inappropriate nitric oxide generation. Activation of the endothelium, platelets, and the coagulation and complement systems can lead to microvascular thrombosis and cellular injury. Mitochondrial damage may also ensue, which leads to derangement in cellular energy production and cell death by apoptosis or necrosis. *MODS,* Multiple organ dysfunction syndrome; *ROS,* reactive oxygen species; *RNS,* reactive nitrogen species.

(LPS)[45,46]; this triggers coagulation activation through binding of factor VII. In addition, proinflammatory cytokines reduce expression of antithrombotic proteins such as thrombomodulin, protein C, and the extracellular protein C receptor. These activities tip the balance away from anticoagulation and in favor of thrombin generation and the suppression of fibrinolysis. On a local level, such enhanced fibrin formation is protective because it limits hemorrhage and acts to contain pathogens. Activation of these processes on a systemic level, however, can lead to widespread microvascular thrombosis and endothelial injury. The combination of these phenomena impairs organ perfusion, limits reparative functions, and propagates organ dysfunction.[47]

Mitochondria

Although microcirculatory disturbances are clinically detectable in people and dogs with shock,[48,49] these abnormalities may be insufficient to explain the bioenergetic failure that accompanies many critical illnesses. It has been proposed that ineffective cellular oxygen utilization in intermediate metabolic processes leads to intracellular energy deficits that contribute to MODS development.[50] This cytopathic hypoxia[51] may be due to oxidative mitochondrial damage and subsequent loss by autophagy, which, coupled with a failure of mitochondrial biogenesis, leads to depletion of mitochondrial numbers.[52]

Although under normal circumstances, approximately 1% oxygen entering cells is converted to ROS by mitochondrial electron transport chains (ETC), several components of the inflammatory response disturb this activity, increasing ROS generation and resulting in deleterious effects on mitochondrial DNA and membrane integrity. In particular, iNOS-generated nitric oxide can directly interfere with ETC complexes IV and V and, via peroxynitrite, also inhibits ETC complex I.[53,54] TNF-α can directly inhibit ETC complex III. ROS and reactive nitrogen species (RNS) and certain cytokines activate poly-(ADP-ribose) polymerase, reducing availability of complex I substrates.[55] These effects combine to impair adenosine triphosphate (ATP) generation and increase oxidative stress. In addition to causing loss of mitochondria, the ROS/RNS-induced mitochondrial damage leads to release of cytochrome c into the cytosol, triggering apoptotic death and releasing mitochondrial DNA, which acts as a DAMP, triggering further cytokine generation via TLR-9.[56]

Gastrointestinal Tract

As demonstrated by the beneficial effects of selective gastrointestinal decontamination on respiratory tract and bloodstream infections in ICU patients,[57] the GIT clearly contributes to the pathology of critical illness. The precise role of the GIT in MODS pathogenesis remains contentious, however. At a panel discussion in 1985, Meakins and Marshall proposed that in septic ICU patients, commensal bacterial overgrowth coupled with a loss of mucosal barrier function might permit bacterial translocation, thus allowing the bowel to become a pathogen reservoir that drives the generation of MODS.[58] Others have since demonstrated increased GIT wall permeability in critically ill patients after splanchnic hypoperfusion, oxidative stress, and the action of inflammatory cytokines.[59] It has been shown that after ischemia-reperfusion injury, the GIT can generate sufficient proinflammatory cytokines to drive systemic inflammation into MODS[60] and that toxic GIT-derived substances entering mesenteric lymph are sufficient to cause acute respiratory distress syndrome (ARDS) and MODS (the GIT-lymph hypothesis).[61,62] However, others have argued that translocation of bacteria alone may be insufficient to generate SIRS, that such translocation may be a normal process important in creating an appropriate adaptive immune response, and that presence of bacteria in the blood may be a marker of host immunosuppression or colonization by a particularly virulent organism.[63] Ultimately, these discrepancies may relate to the patient population studied (abdominal surgery vs. trauma) or the endpoints of the study (lymph node bacterial culture vs. intestinal permeability measurements). Thus bacterial translocation may occur without GIT-derived sepsis, whereas GIT-derived sepsis can occur in the absence of bacterial translocation.[62]

Rather than examining each component or mechanism individually, the interplay of multiple components of the gastrointestinal system during critical illness may better explain the different roles played by the GIT in MODS pathogenesis in diverse patient populations.[27] In this model, the GIT comprises the intestinal epithelium, the mucosal immune system, and the commensal bacteria. In individual patients any or all of these components may be dysfunctional and the interplay between them gives rise to the clinical phenomena seen. For instance, diminished GIT barrier function caused by tight junction disruption[59] coupled with impaired local immunity may permit translocation of commensal bacteria. Alternatively, altered microbial flora secondary to antimicrobial administration[64] and inadequate epithelial nutrition impairs local immunity.[65] This allows for production of bacterial toxins or inflammatory mediators that are absorbed and transported in lymph to the lung.[66] This crosstalk hypothesis[27] posits that organ dysfunction is most likely to occur when reduced barrier function, impaired local immunity, and altered intestinal microflora all coexist, a scenario that may be a common occurrence in our sickest patients.

SPECIFIC ORGAN DYSFUNCTION

The temporal sequence of organ dysfunction in patients with MODS varies with inciting cause and host factors such as species, genetic propensity, age, comorbidities, and drug therapies. The pattern of organ failure in dogs with sepsis is unlikely to be identical to that in a traumatized cat. The pattern of failure in human surgical patients is first pulmonary, then liver, GIT, and kidney.[67] Likewise, pulmonary involvement is typically an early manifestation in human trauma and sepsis patients.[68,69] As mentioned previously, the pattern of organ failures may be changing with advances in therapy, and it seems probable that early organ failure and late organ failure represent different phenomena.[70] The manifestations of MODS in specific organ systems are briefly discussed next; additional information regarding treatment can be found in other chapters and are referenced later in this chapter.

Lung

The lungs are often affected in patients with MODS.[30] They may be injured primarily (e.g., pneumonia, contusions) or secondarily by systemic inflammation generated by a process elsewhere (e.g., trauma, septic peritonitis). The common pathogenesis of acute lung injury (ALI) and ARDS is now well described (see Chapter 24).[71] Lung injury is initiated by a local or systemic proinflammatory state that promotes the sequestration of primed neutrophils. Inflammatory mediator activity and the activities of sequestered neutrophils damage basement membranes and endothelial cells and disrupt tight junctions. Pulmonary capillary permeability increases, promoting formation of protein-rich pulmonary edema. The resultant alveolar flooding and surfactant inactivation cause collapse of alveoli and terminal airways, reducing lung compliance and leading to shunting, hypoxic pulmonary vasoconstriction, and hypoxemia. The changes in pulmonary blood flow result in pulmonary artery hypertension and increase right ventricular workload. The initial exudative phase may be followed by a proliferative phase characterized by type II pneumocyte recruitment and phenotypic change and the generation of fibrous tissue by fibroblasts. This phase should be restorative but can lead to pulmonary fibrosis.

Cardiac

Potentially reversible myocardial dysfunction in association with sepsis is well recognized in humans and is also documented in naturally occurring sepsis in dogs.[72-74] Sepsis cardiomyopathy is characterized by early contractile dysfunction leading to biventricular dilation, reduced ejection fraction and fractional shortening, as well as a reduced response to preload and catecholamines.[75] In experimental sepsis in dogs, decreased ejection fraction and increased preload accompany the myocardial depression. Assessment of oxygen transport variables in dogs with sepsis identified reduced oxygen delivery compared with healthy dogs.[76] However, nonseptic dogs with SIRS had significantly lower cardiac output and oxygen delivery compared with both healthy dogs and septic dogs, suggesting that myocardial depression in patients with sepsis and SIRS is not uniform. The mechanisms of this myocardial depression remain unclear but likely involve disrupted cellular energetics, altered calcium handling, effects of circulating proinflammatory cytokines, direct and indirect effects of nitric oxide, and induction of myocyte apoptosis.[77] Impaired autonomic function manifesting as inappropriate tachycardia and reduced heart rate variability has also been noted. This may reflect local effects on pacemaker cells or alterations to central nervous system function.

Liver

Normally, the liver helps to prevent systemic endotoxemia and bacteremia thanks to its substantial endogenous macrophage population

(Kupffer cells). These cells can also produce cytokines in response to inflammatory signals or changes in hepatic oxygenation and secrete proteins as part of the acute-phase response.[78] Initiation of liver dysfunction in patients with MODS may result from primary hepatic damage or, more commonly, secondary to inflammatory stimuli originating elsewhere. Liver dysfunction manifests as impaired gluconeogenesis and glycolysis, reduced synthetic and metabolic functions, and, most seriously, a coagulopathy (see Chapter 116).

Decreased hepatic perfusion during shock may cause temporary acute liver dysfunction. The liver normally receives around 75% of its blood supply from the GIT with the remainder coming from the hepatic arteries. Hypoperfusion secondary to trauma or sepsis alters this ratio, such that portal blood flow increases as hepatic arterial blood flow diminishes.[79] Consequently, the liver may become hypoxic, modulating the release, binding, and cytotoxicity of cytokines, including TNF-α. Increased hepatic and gastrointestinal inflammatory cytokine production during this period predisposes postsurgical patients to liver failure, despite the increased portal blood flow.[80] Glutamine depletion has been documented in dogs with experimental sepsis[81] and likely relates to liver dysfunction. Glutamine is necessary to maintain gastrointestinal enterocyte health and function and deficits may increase hepatic exposure to GIT-derived bacteria or bacterial toxins.[82] GIT-derived catecholamines may also contribute to hepatic dysfunction because Kupffer cell adrenoceptor activation enhances production of TNF-α, IL-6, and NO.[83]

Gastrointestinal

The GIT may be involved in the pathogenesis of MODS, but it is also clearly a target organ. Dysfunction typically manifests as ileus, gastrointestinal ulceration, intolerance of enteral feeding, vomiting, and diarrhea.[22] As discussed earlier, gastrointestinal disturbances may promote systemic inflammation and reduced mucosal barrier function may allow bacterial translocation. Increases in GIT wall permeability have been documented in dogs after trauma.[84] Endotoxemia also appears to reduce GIT motility in dogs.[85]

Kidneys

Renal dysfunction is a consistent yet discouraging development in the progression of MODS, linked to worsening mortality rates in sepsis.[69] Acute kidney injury (AKI) as recently defined by the Kidney Disease: Improving Global Outcomes work group,[86] represents a continuum of kidney damage that can be present before it is identifiable by standard laboratory tests (see Chapter 124). Recently the human RIFLE criteria[87] have been found to be predictive of outcome in dogs,[88] and specific scoring systems have been developed for veterinary patients but remain in their infancy.[89]

In patients with trauma and after hypovolemic or hemorrhagic shock, acute kidney injury likely results from renal hypoperfusion.[1] In the setting of acute ischemia, multiple pathologic mechanisms are induced, including adhesion molecule expression and cytokine release leading to leukocyte infiltration and endothelial injury. Reduced renal perfusion pressure activates intrarenal vasoconstrictive responses with associated ischemic necrosis, loss of tubular cell polarity, and sloughing of tubular cells into the tubular lumen.[90,91]

In AKI secondary to sepsis, however, injury may occur in the absence of renal hypoperfusion, with ischemic tubular damage of much lower significance. Rather, the renal circulation may participate in the vasodilatory processes that characterize hyperdynamic postresuscitation septic shock.[92] It has been demonstrated that sepsis-induced AKI can occur in the presence of normal renal blood flow[93,94] and that azotemia results from a loss of glomerular filtration pressure associated with afferent and efferent vasodilation.[95] The actual mechanism of AKI in sepsis remains unclear. Plausible hypotheses include direct nephrotoxicity from high levels of TNF-α[96] and renal cell apoptosis.[97] Pulmonary failure has been found to almost universally precede AKI in burn patients with MODS.[98] This suggests that organ crosstalk through soluble mediators, such as Fas ligand in plasma, may be damaging the kidney through apoptosis induction.[99]

Central Nervous System

Sepsis-associated encephalopathy is a well-recognized (although ill-defined) entity in people. To date it has not been definitively identified in small animals, although it seems probable that dogs may also suffer from central nervous system (CNS) complications of sepsis (see Chapter 80). Identification is hampered by a lack of sensitive or specific criteria. Encephalopathic patients suffering from sepsis, particularly those with gram-negative infections, have higher mortality rates than those with normal mentation. Pathologically, the cerebrum is most commonly involved. Typical lesions include leukoencephalopathy, hemorrhage, microabscessation, perivascular edema, and disruption of astrocyte foot processes. The pathophysiology of sepsis-associated encephalopathy is poorly understood and may involve microbial toxins, inflammatory mediators, metabolic and vascular abnormalities, mitochondrial dysfunction, oxidative stress, and apoptosis.[100]

Coagulation and the Endothelium

The interactions between inflammation and coagulation are complex and have been extensively reviewed elsewhere.[101-103] However, several new contributors to endothelial and coagulation dysfunction have recently been identified. Extracellular histones (H3 and H4 particularly) released from necrotic cells are known to mediate MODS pathogenesis and are toxic to endothelial cells in vitro.[104] Activated neutrophils can also be stimulated to release neutrophil extracellular traps (NETs) that contain histones, DNA, and granule proteins.[105] These structures may be designed to trap and kill microorganisms, but they are also capable of inducing thrombus formation,[106] potentially through platelet activation and polyphosphate release[107] and by impairing protein C activation.[108]

Activation of the endothelium is an early feature of systemic inflammation and sepsis that facilitates leukocyte transmigration and PAMP/DAMP recognition through TLR expression. Excessive endothelial activation is involved in the pathophysiology of MODS through links to disordered coagulation, excessive leukocyte recruitment, and the loss of microvascular barrier function, but it is also clear that the endothelium is a target organ in patients with MODS. Endothelial activation also leads to Weibel-Palade body degranulation and release of angiopoietins (Ang-) and von Willebrand factor (VWF). The angiopoietins are epithelial growth factors, of which Ang-1 and Ang-2 are best characterized but have opposing biologic effects. Ang-1 enhances endothelial cell survival and promotes barrier integrity, whereas Ang-2 is antagonistic to Ang-1 and promotes endothelial activation and dysfunction.[109] Correspondingly, plasma concentrations of these and other endothelial biomarkers appear to have prognostic value in sepsis.[110]

SCORING SYSTEMS

Scoring systems used for ICU patients may be designed to assess specific diseases or individual organ systems or be applicable to all critically ill patients irrespective of disease (see Chapter 13). These nonspecific illness severity scores are a means of assigning objective numerical values to individuals at ICU entry to predict outcome with an estimated probability. Such scoring systems account for comorbidities, patient demographics, and baseline characteristics in addition to recent physiologic information. The ideal system would be easy to generate using widely available data and provide consistent,

Table 7-2 **Comparison of SOFA, MOD, and LODS Scores for Organ Failure Assessment**[111,115]

	SOFA[118]	MOD[123]	LODS[124]
Score development	Consensus conference	Systematic literature review and logistic regression testing	Multiple logistic regression on multicenter dataset
Cardiovascular component	BP, vasopressor type and dose requirements	HR x (MAP/CVP)	HR and BP
Respiratory component	PaO_2/FiO_2 ratio	PaO_2/FiO_2 ratio	PaO_2/FiO_2 ratio
Neurologic component	Glasgow Coma Scale	Glasgow Coma Scale	Glasgow Coma Scale
Renal component	Serum creatinine and urine output	Serum creatinine	Serum urea, serum creatinine, urine output
Hepatic component	Serum bilirubin	Serum bilirubin	Serum bilirubin, prothrombin time
Hematologic component	Platelet count	Platelet count	WBC count, platelet count
Type of scale	No linear scale	Linear scale	Linear scale
Scoring	Each organ 0-4	Each organ 0-4	Organs weighted 0, 1, 3, or 5/organ
Data collection point	Worst value for last 24 hours	First value of day	Worst value for last 24 hours
Advantages	Simple, reliable, accurate Validated in various populations Reflects sequential organ dysfunction	Simple, reliable Reflects sequential dysfunction	Generated using large database Accounts for relative severity among organs systems Can be used as illness severity score
Disadvantages	Potential for variation in vasopressor use among clinicians/ centers	Need for central venous catheter for calculation of cardiovascular component	Complexity given weightings of various organ systems

BP, Blood pressure; *CVP,* central venous pressure; *HR,* heart rate; *MAP,* mean arterial pressure; *WBC,* white blood cell.

repeatable, and accurate prognostic information in a variety of patient populations in diverse ICU settings.

The most widely used illness severity scores in people are the Acute Physiology and Chronic Health Evaluation score, the Simplified Acute Physiology Score, and the Mortality Prediction Model.[111] These scores have been updated multiple times to encompass additional data and to maintain predictive accuracy and are now so complex that scores are typically generated by computer software. Scoring systems are underused in veterinary medicine, potentially because of the cumbersome nature of some scores and skepticism regarding the predictive ability of available systems. Two recently developed scores for use in dogs[112] and cats[113] have sought to improve this situation by providing species-specific systems and a categorical scoring approach.

In patient with MODS, as with other disease processes, care should be taken when applying population-based illness severity scores to individual patients. Such scores are not designed to predict outcome in individuals because clearly it is not possible to predict 80% mortality in a single patient, in whom the outcome is binary (patients either survive or they don't). Similarly, scores should not be used to provide prognostic information for clients; rather, they should only be used to guide therapy as part of overall patient assessment.[114] Most illness severity scores are used for research purposes to control for illness severity as a confounding variable, to provide objective context to single-center studies, or to assess the effectiveness of randomization in interventional clinical trials. Illness severity scores may be useful to monitor therapeutic interventions and to set therapeutic targets in ICU patients.

Organ failure scores for patients with MODS are typically diagnosis independent and use physiologic data to assess patient status. Organ failure scores are designed to be used repeatedly to serially evaluate changes occurring over time in individual patients. Although organ failure scores are primarily designed to describe the nature and extent of organ dysfunction rather than predict outcome, the number and magnitude of organ dysfunction in ICU patients is highly correlated with outcomes in people[115] and dogs.[23,24] At least 30 organ failure assessment scores have been described in the human literature.[2] Some, like the three described in Table 7-2, have been widely used, whereas others, such as the PELOD[116] or NEOMOD,[117] have been developed for specific patient populations. Although several disease-specific scores have been generated in veterinary species (e.g., for trauma, pancreatitis, and DIC), no specific veterinary MODS scoring systems have been developed to date. The application of human MODS scores to small animals is currently under investigation.

Sequential Organ Failure Assessment (SOFA)

The consensus-developed SOFA score is the least complex of the three commonly used systems.[118] Six organ systems are evaluated (cardiovascular, respiratory, neurologic, renal, hepatic, and hematologic) and the worst value of the day is used to calculate the score. Each organ system is equally weighted, with values from 0 to 4, such that the total score varies from 0 to 24 (Table 7-3). The cardiovascular score in SOFA is based on the need for, and dose of, vasopressor agents, which may not be ideal given the variation in clinical practice between locations. The simplicity of the SOFA score means it is reliable and accurate across clinicians and locations.[119] Initially validated in a mixed ICU population, it has since been successfully used in various patient populations.[120-122] Recently the SOFA score with minor modifications was applied to a population of dogs with sepsis and nonseptic SIRS.[24] In these dogs, both daily and cumulative SOFA scores over the first 3 days of hospitalization were significantly correlated with outcome. An increase in SOFA score was also strongly predictive of mortality in this study.

Multiple Organ Dysfunction (MOD) Score

The multiple organ dysfunction (MOD) score was developed from published characteristics of organ failure using an idealized set of

Table 7-3 **Sequential Organ Failure (SOFA) Score Criteria**[24,118]

	0	1	2	3	4
Cardiovascular					
MAP, or vasopressors*	≥60 mm Hg	<60 mm Hg	Dopamine <5 or dobutamine any dose	Dopamine >5 or epinephrine ≤0.1 or norepinephrine ≤1	Dopamine >15 or epinephrine >0.1 or norepinephrine >1
Respiratory					
PaO_2/FiO_2 (mm Hg)	>400	<400	<300	<200 (Ventilated)	<100 (Ventilated)
Neurologic					
Modified Glasgow Coma Scale†	>14	13-14	10-12	6-9	<6
Renal					
Creatinine mg/dl (Creatinine μmol/L)	<1.4 (<124)	1.4-1.9 (124-172)	2.0-3.4 (173-300)	3.5-4.9 (301-441)	>5 (442)
Hepatic					
Bilirubin mg/dl (Bilirubin μg/L)	<0.6 (<10)	0.6-1.4 (10-25)	1.5-5 (26-86)	5.1-11 (87-190)	>11.1 (>190)
Hematologic					
Platelet count $\times 10^3/\mu l$	>150	150-100	100-50	50-20	≤20

*Vasopressors given for at least 1-hour doses in μg/kg/min.
†We recommend using the modified Glasgow Coma Scale per Platt (see Chapter 81), 2001.[156]

criteria for an organ function score.[111] The score was then refined using logistic regression of data from one ICU and then tested against additional patients from the same location.[123] As for SOFA, each of the six organ systems are equally weighted, but for MOD the first measurements of the day are used. One peculiar and potentially problematic aspect of the MOD score is the use of a composite cardiovascular variable, the product of heart rate × (central venous pressure/mean arterial pressure). The MOD score is not designed to predict outcome but does correlate with it. As with biomarkers such as lactate, a change in MOD score over time may predict outcome more accurately.[123]

Logistic Organ Dysfunction System (LODS)

The logistic organ dysfunction system (LODS) score is a hybrid score with properties of a mortality prediction index and an organ failure score. The LODS was developed from a composite database of more than 13,000 patients from ICUs in 12 countries by multivariate logistic regression techniques.[124] In contrast to SOFA and the MOD score, the LODS is a weighted system in which failure of some organ systems (e.g., respiratory) contributes more to the final score than others (e.g., liver). The LODS score can also be converted to a mortality probability using the logistic regression equation. Although not originally intended for serial use, the LODS score has been shown to accurately chart the progression of patients during their stay in ICU.[125]

Predisposition Infection Response Organ (PIRO) Dysfunction

As sepsis is the most common underlying cause of MODS, we briefly discuss here a sepsis-specific approach to scoring organ failure. The 2001 sepsis definitions consensus conference[126] proposed stratifying patients based on their predisposing conditions, the nature and extent of both the infection and the host response, and the degree of resulting organ dysfunction (the predisposition infection response organ [PIRO] system). Although initially a conceptual framework, prognostic models have since been generated based on the PIRO system. These models have been evaluated by several groups using very large databases from randomized controlled trials and registries. The models correlate highly with mortality rates. These studies have each generated unique models, using different variables and weightings that preclude direct comparison but demonstrate the validity and value of the PIRO concept in evaluating septic patients with MODS.

Which Score To Use?

Despite considerable effort comparing the available systems, no one score performs perfectly. Although there are concerns with certain parameters for each of the scoring systems discussed here, the SOFA score may be easiest to apply. The commonly used scores (i.e., SOFA, MODS, LODS) generally have excellent discriminant ability, although in several studies the SOFA score was demonstrated to be superior.[111,115]

At this juncture, it is reasonable to question which system should be used in veterinary medicine. True illness severity scores have been developed for dogs and cats and should be applied whenever possible. For MODS scoring, some authors have adapted criteria from various sources to suit their needs,[23] whereas others have directly adopted human scoring systems.[24] Clearly the optimal way forward would be the application of a specific veterinary MODS score; until one is developed, however, the SOFA score might be a rational place to start (with minor modifications to facilitate ease of use).[24]

MANAGEMENT

As Arthur Baue sagely points out, the names and acronyms we give to the progressive organ dysfunction associated with critical illness are not diseases in their own right, but arbitrarily defined terms against which treatment cannot be specifically directed.[2] Rather, we must support organ function while the underlying cause is identified and specifically treated, to buy time to enable patients to repair and restore themselves. Marshall's 2001 definition of MODS as a "potentially reversible physiologic derangement" makes it clear that we can and should take all necessary steps to maximize the survival of these patients.

MODS should be viewed as a functional derangement rather than a structural defect. Ideally, early individualized therapeutic interventions in patients with severe physiologic insults will prevent the development of secondary organ dysfunction. The Surviving Sepsis campaign guidelines provide a suitable means by which to achieve this aim.[127] Clearly, however, prevention will not be uniformly possible and some patients will develop MODS in spite of, and occasionally as a result of, our best intentioned therapy. Indeed, the marked reductions in mortality associated with ARDS achieved between 1996 and 2005 are probably attributable to a reduction in iatrogenic harm, not improvements in therapy.[128]

Management strategies of patients with established MODS should address two principal aims: (1) Treat the source of the physiologic insult; (2) support organ function. Here we briefly discuss organ support strategies and mention some novel therapies under investigation. We refer readers to other chapters for more information where necessary.

Cardiovascular Support

Support of the cardiovascular system involves goal-directed therapy to optimize preload, restore effective circulating volume, and maintain perfusion pressure to brain, myocardium, kidneys, and GIT.[129] Although the specific parameters and interventions in the original early goal-directed therapy study[130] are currently being reevaluated,[131] the principles espoused by Rivers et al remain valid.[132] Regular monitoring of several upstream and downstream resuscitation parameters[133] and individualized therapy with fluids, vasopressors, and inotropic agents are the basis of goal-directed therapy. No single parameter represents the ideal resuscitation endpoint, and clinicians should use all available monitoring modalities to repeatedly assess the effectiveness of their interventions (see Chapter 183).[134]

Ventilatory Strategies

Mechanical ventilation is the principal means of support of the respiratory system in patients with MODS but has the potential to promote pulmonary damage through barotrauma, volutrauma, atelectrauma, and ventilator-associated pneumonia.[135] In addition to the well-recognized adverse pulmonary effects of ventilation, injurious mechanical ventilation is implicated in generating or sustaining dysfunction in distant organs (see Chapters 30 and 31).[29,30]

Multiple clinical trials have evaluated lung-protective strategies for ALI/ARDS patients, most of which demonstrated mortality benefits associated with low tidal volume, lung-protective strategies based on the baby-lung concept of ARDS.[136] Although attention has focused on a 6 ml/kg tidal volume, the protective value of these strategies may actually be due to lower plateau pressures. Other ARDS Network trials have also generated important recommendations about fluid management and catheter usage in ALI/ARDS patients.[16,137]

More recent ALI/ARDS studies have addressed lung recruitment and positive end-expiratory pressure (PEEP) optimization.[138] Several trials have been stopped for futility, and others are still ongoing. Meta-analysis of published studies suggests that higher PEEP values may be beneficial in patients with established ARDS.[139] Numerous pharmacologic interventions have been evaluated in ARDS patients, but none have been demonstrated to improve outcome. There is continued interest in alternative ventilation strategies (e.g., high-frequency oscillatory ventilation) and adjunctive therapies (e.g., extracorporeal membrane oxygenation), but few if any of these measures are currently applicable to veterinary medicine. Reports in the veterinary literature suggest that lung-protective ventilator strategies are safe in dogs[140] and that successful outcomes can be obtained even in severely affected patients.[141,142]

Renal Replacement Therapy

Evidence supporting the use of renal replacement therapy (RRT) in MODS patients is equivocal, and its interpretation is complicated by the myriad different technologies available (see Chapters 124 and 205).[143] Early reports supported the theory that plasma filtration by continuous RRT might limit the progression of sepsis to MODS by reducing blood inflammatory cytokine concentrations.[144] As discussed, however, the pathogenesis of MODS is more complex than simply the effects of a cytokine storm. As such, renal replacement therapy is currently only recommended when AKI exists.[127] There remains equipoise regarding the appropriate time to intervene with RRT and the dose to institute.[145] The current limited availability of these technologies in veterinary medicine requires that other means of renal function support must be employed. Hopefully, firmer recommendations in this area can be made in future.

Nutritional Support and Glucose Control (see Chapters 127 to 130)

Given the putative role for the gastrointestinal tract in the pathogenesis of MODS and the evidence that the GIT is itself a target organ, attempts have been made to support GIT health through early enteral nutrition and to examine the potential benefit of nutritional immunomodulation and supplementation (see Chapters 127 and 128).[146] Results of research examining specific nutritional supplements, such as arginine, glutamine, selenium, and omega-3 fatty acids, have been mixed. Current recommendations for septic patients from the European Society of Parenteral and Enteral Nutrition are that nutritional support should commence once patients are hemodynamically stable and that parenteral nutrition can be used if the enteral route is not tolerated (see Chapters 129 and 130). If parenteral nutrition is administered, supplementation with omega-3 and glutamine can be considered.[147]

Beginning with the original Leuven trial in 2001, which identified survival benefits attributed to lower levels of MODS in ICU patients treated with continuous insulin infusions,[148] considerable attention has been given to the potential benefits of insulin therapy/glucose control in ICU patient management. Multiple studies have since attempted to identify the optimal blood glucose concentration with varying success; few have been able to replicate the outcome benefits identified in the original study.[149,150] By comparison, all have documented higher frequencies of hypoglycemia in the more intensive insulin therapy arms. Current recommendations in people are that blood glucose be maintained at a more liberal level of 150 mg/dl (8.33 mmol/L).[127] In contrast, hyperglycemia requiring insulin therapy in critically ill veterinary patients is uncommon. As discussed, evidence for a benefit from insulin therapy is equivocal and the potential for life-threatening complications associated with hypoglycemia well recognized.[151] As such, administration of insulin to critically ill (nondiabetic) small animals for the purpose of tight glucose control is not recommended.

Corticosteroids

Glucocorticoids remain one of the most controversial therapies in critical care, and their role in MODS patients is no exception (see Chapter 72). Early animal models suggesting efficacy in endotoxemia have consistently failed to translate into benefits in human clinical trials. The associated adverse effects and lack of demonstrable benefit have rendered high-dose corticosteroids obsolete. Recent attention has been on identifying the subset of septic patients who might benefit from "low-dose" hydrocortisone therapy and whether drugs with mineralocorticoid properties are required in addition to glucocorticoids. Initial interest in this area centered on the concept of relative adrenal insufficiency (RAI), currently called critical illness–related corticosteroid insufficiency (CIRCI). Multiple clinical trials and meta-analyses later, the CORTICUS trial suggested no outcome benefit from universal low-dose steroid usage. The trial did indicate that hydrocortisone administration might hasten reversal of shock. As such, and for now, recommendations are that replacement levels of hydrocortisone be considered for patients with vasopressor-refractory septic shock.[127] Another large scale trial, the ADRENAL study (NCT01448109), is currently underway, specifically investigating hydrocortisone in vasopressor-dependent septic shock, with results expected in 2016.

Novel Therapeutic Approaches

Despite considerable progress in our understanding of the pathogenesis of MODS and conditions (e.g., sepsis) that most commonly give rise to organ failure, we have few (if any) effective novel pharmacologic interventions. Industry and taxpayers have poured huge amounts of money into a seemingly bottomless pit of false hopes and failed trials, including TNF-α antibodies, IL-1β receptor antagonists, protease inhibitors, and recombinant proteins such as tifacogin to name a few. There are many reasons why promising basic research has failed to translate into clinical benefit,[152,153] and even for drugs that are approved, open-label trials and meta-analyses can still sound the death knell for promising drugs such as drotrecogin alfa.[154] However, pathophysiologic insights, such as the roles of Toll-like receptors and the importance of DAMPs have provided novel avenues to explore and are yielding new drugs such as Toll-like receptor and CD28 antagonists.[155] Despite this, the complexity and multiple redundancies of the pathways linking systemic inflammation and MODS may mean that a single "magic bullet" for the treatment of the condition is unlikely to exist.[25] The development of therapeutic "bundles" incorporating multiple interventions may provide the best means of improving outcome.[17-20,127]

REFERENCES

1. Mizock BA: The multiple organ dysfunction syndrome, Disease-a-Month 55:476, 2009.
2. Baue AE: MOF, MODS, and SIRS, Shock 26:438, 2006.
3. Hackett TB: Introduction to multiple organ dysfunction and failure, Vet Clin North Am Small Anim Pract 41:703, 2011.
4. Goris RJ, te Boekhorst TP, Nuytinck JK, et al: Multiple-organ failure. Generalized autodestructive inflammation? Arch Surg 120:1109, 1985.
5. Baue AE: Multiple, progressive, or sequential systems failure. A syndrome of the 1970s, Arch Surg 110:779, 1975.
6. American College of Chest Physicians/Society of Critical Care Medicine Consensus Conference: Definitions for sepsis and organ failure and guidelines for the use of innovative therapies in sepsis, Crit Care Med 20:864, 1992.
7. Proulx F, Fayon M, Farrell CA, et al: Epidemiology of sepsis and multiple organ dysfunction syndrome in children, Chest 109:1033, 1996.
8. Marshall JC: The multiple organ dysfunction syndrome. In Holzheimer RG, Mannick JA, editors: Surgical treatment: evidence-based and problem-oriented. Munich: Zuckschwerdt Verlag, 2001, p 780.
9. Ciesla DJ, Moore EE, Johnson JL, et al: A 12-year prospective study of postinjury multiple organ failure: has anything changed? Arch Surg 140:432, 2005.
10. Ulvik A, Kvale R, Wentzel-Larsen T, et al: Multiple organ failure after trauma affects even long-term survival and functional status, Crit Care 11:R95, 2007.
11. Barie PS, Hydo LJ: Epidemiology of multiple organ dysfunction syndrome in critical surgical illness, Surg Infect (Larchmt) 1:173, 2000.
12. Barie PS, Hydo LJ, Pieracci FM, et al: Multiple organ dysfunction syndrome in critical surgical illness, Surg Infect (Larchmt) 10:369, 2009.
13. Barie PS, Hydo LJ, Shou J, et al: Decreasing magnitude of multiple organ dysfunction syndrome despite increasingly severe critical surgical illness: a 17-year longitudinal study, J Trauma 65:1227, 2008.
14. Moore FA, Sauaia A, Moore EE, et al: Postinjury multiple organ failure: a bimodal phenomenon, J Trauma 40:501, 1996.
15. Ventilation with lower tidal volumes as compared with traditional tidal volumes for acute lung injury and the acute respiratory distress syndrome. The Acute Respiratory Distress Syndrome Network, N Engl J Med 342:1301, 2000.
16. Wiedemann HP, Wheeler AP, Bernard GR, et al: Comparison of two fluid-management strategies in acute lung injury, N Engl J Med 354:2564, 2006.
17. Moore FA, McKinley BA, Moore EE, et al: Inflammation and the host response to injury. A large-scale collaborative project: patient-oriented research core—standard operating procedures for clinical care. III. Guidelines for shock resuscitation, J Trauma 61:82, 2006.
18. West MA, Shapiro MB, Nathens AB, et al: Inflammation and the host response to injury. A large-scale collaborative project: patient-oriented research core—standard operating procedures for clinical care. IV. Guidelines for transfusion in the trauma patient, J Trauma 61:436, 2006.
19. Nathens AB, Johnson JL, Minei JP, et al: Inflammation and the host response to injury. A large-scale collaborative project: patient-oriented research core—standard operating procedures for clinical care. I. Guidelines for mechanical ventilation of the trauma patient, J Trauma 59:764, 2005.
20. Minei JP, Nathens AB, West M, et al: Inflammation and the host response to injury. A large-scale collaborative project: patient-oriented research core—standard operating procedures for clinical care. II. Guidelines for prevention, diagnosis and treatment of ventilator-associated pneumonia (VAP) in the trauma patient, J Trauma 60:1106, 2006.
21. Minei JP, Cuschieri J, Sperry J, et al: The changing pattern and implications of multiple organ failure after blunt injury with hemorrhagic shock, Crit Care Med 40:1129, 2012.
22. Johnson V, Gaynor A, Chan DL, et al: Multiple organ dysfunction syndrome in humans and dogs, J Vet Emerg Crit Care 14:158, 2004.
23. Kenney EM, Rozanski EA, Rush JE, et al: Association between outcome and organ system dysfunction in dogs with sepsis: 114 cases (2003-2007), J Am Vet Med Assoc 236:83, 2010.
24. Ripanti D, Dino G, Piovano G, et al: Application of the Sequential Organ Failure Assessment Score to predict outcome in critically ill dogs: preliminary results, SAT Schweiz Arch Tierheilkunde 154:325, 2012.
25. Lewis DH, Chan DL, Pinheiro D, et al: The immunopathology of sepsis: pathogen recognition, systemic inflammation, the compensatory anti-inflammatory response, and regulatory T cells, J Vet Int Med 26:457, 2012.
26. Moore FA, Moore EE: Evolving concepts in the pathogenesis of postinjury multiple organ failure, Surg Clin North Am 75:257, 1995.
27. Clark JA, Coopersmith CM: Intestinal crosstalk: a new paradigm for understanding the gut as the "motor" of critical illness, Shock 28:384, 2007.
28. Puleo F, Arvanitakis M, Van Gossum A, et al: Gut failure in the ICU, Semin Respir Crit Care Med 32:626, 2011.
29. Slutsky AS, Tremblay LN: Multiple system organ failure. Is mechanical ventilation a contributing factor? Am J Respir Crit Care Med 157:1721, 1998.
30. Del Sorbo L, Slutsky AS: Acute respiratory distress syndrome and multiple organ failure, Curr Opin Crit Care 17:1, 2011.
31. Acosta JA, Yang JC, Winchell RJ, et al: Lethal injuries and time to death in a level I trauma center, J Am Coll Surg 186:528, 1998.
32. Saadia R, Schein M: Multiple organ failure. How valid is the "two hit" model? J Accid Emerg Med 16:163, 1999.
33. Tsukamoto T, Chanthaphavong RS, Pape H-C: Current theories on the pathophysiology of multiple organ failure after trauma, Injury 41:21, 2010.
34. Mark KS, Trickler WJ, Miller DW: Tumor necrosis factor-alpha induces cyclooxygenase-2 expression and prostaglandin release in brain microvessel endothelial cells, J Pharmacol Exp Ther 297:1051, 2001.
35. Kumar A, Parrillo JE. Shock: classification, pathophysiology, and approach to management. In Parrilo JE, Dellinger RP, editors: Critical care medicine: principles of diagnosis and management in the adult, ed 3, Philadelphia, 2008, Mosby Elsevier, p 379.
36. Sunden-Cullberg J, Norrby-Teglund A, Treutiger CJ: The role of high mobility group box-1 protein in severe sepsis, Curr Opin Infect Dis 19:231, 2006.
37. Rittirsch D, Flierl MA, Ward PA: Harmful molecular mechanisms in sepsis, Nat Rev Immunol 8:776, 2008.
38. Hecke F, Schmidt U, Kola A, et al: Circulating complement proteins in multiple trauma patients—correlation with injury severity, development of sepsis, and outcome, Crit Care Med 25:2015, 1997.

39. Huber-Lang MS, Sarma JV, McGuire SR, et al: Protective effects of anti-C5a peptide antibodies in experimental sepsis, FASEB J 15:568, 2001.
40. van der Poll T, de Boer JD, Levi M: The effect of inflammation on coagulation and vice versa, Curr Opin Infect Dis 24:273, 2011.
41. Hopper K, Bateman S: An updated view of hemostasis: mechanisms of hemostatic dysfunction associated with sepsis, J Vet Emerg Crit Care 15:83, 2005.
42. de Laforcade AM, Freeman LM, Shaw SP, et al: Hemostatic changes in dogs with naturally occurring sepsis, J Vet Int Med 17:674, 2003.
43. Estrin MA, Wehausen CE, Jessen CR, et al: Disseminated intravascular coagulation in cats, J Vet Int Med 20:1334, 2006.
44. Schouten M, Wiersinga WJ, Levi M, et al: Inflammation, endothelium, and coagulation in sepsis, J Leukoc Biol 83:536, 2008.
45. Pawlinski R, Mackman N: Cellular sources of tissue factor in endotoxemia and sepsis, Thromb Res 125(Suppl 1):S70, 2010.
46. Stokol T, Daddona JL, Choi B: Evaluation of tissue factor procoagulant activity on the surface of feline leukocytes in response to treatment with lipopolysaccharide and heat-inactivated fetal bovine serum, Am J Vet Res 71:623, 2010.
47. Gando S: Microvascular thrombosis and multiple organ dysfunction syndrome, Crit Care Med 38:S35, 2010.
48. Sakr Y, Dubois MJ, De Backer D, et al: Persistent microcirculatory alterations are associated with organ failure and death in patients with septic shock, Crit Care Med 32:1825, 2004.
49. Peruski AM, Cooper ES: Assessment of microcirculatory changes by use of sidestream dark field microscopy during hemorrhagic shock in dogs, Am J Vet Res 72:438, 2011.
50. Hotchkiss RS, Karl IE: Reevaluation of the role of cellular hypoxia and bioenergetic failure in sepsis, JAMA 267:1503, 1992.
51. Fink MP: Cytopathic hypoxia. Mitochondrial dysfunction as mechanism contributing to organ dysfunction in sepsis, Crit Care Clin 17:219, 2001.
52. Exline MC, Crouser ED: Mitochondrial mechanisms of sepsis-induced organ failure, Front Biosci 13:5030, 2008.
53. Wendel M, Heller AR: Mitochondrial function and dysfunction in sepsis, Wien Med Wochenschr 160:118, 2010.
54. Garrabou G, Moren C, Lopez S, et al: The effects of sepsis on mitochondria, J Infect Dis 205:392, 2011.
55. Pacher P, Beckman JS, Liaudet L: Nitric oxide and peroxynitrite in health and disease, Physiol Rev 87:315, 2007.
56. Zhang Q, Raoof M, Chen Y, et al: Circulating mitochondrial DAMPs cause inflammatory responses to injury, Nature 464:104, 2010.
57. Silvestri L, de la Cal MA, van Saene HK: Selective decontamination of the digestive tract: the mechanism of action is control of gut overgrowth, Intensive Care Med 38:1738, 2012.
58. Meakins J, Marshall J: The gastrointestinal tract: the "motor" of MOF, Arch Surg 121:197, 1986.
59. Fink MP, Delude RL: Epithelial barrier dysfunction: a unifying theme to explain the pathogenesis of multiple organ dysfunction at the cellular level, Crit Care Clin 21:177, 2005.
60. Hassoun HT, Kone BC, Mercer DW, et al: Post-injury multiple organ failure: the role of the gut, Shock 15:1, 2001.
61. Magnotti LJ, Xu DZ, Lu Q, et al: Gut-derived mesenteric lymph: a link between burn and lung injury, Arch Surg 134:1333, 1999.
62. Deitch EA: Gut-origin sepsis: Evolution of a concept, Surgeon 10:350, 2012.
63. Alverdy JC, Laughlin RS, Wu L: Influence of the critically ill state on host-pathogen interactions within the intestine: gut-derived sepsis redefined, Crit Care Med 31:598, 2003.
64. Shimizu K, Ogura H, Goto M, et al: Altered gut flora and environment in patients with severe SIRS, J Trauma 60:126, 2006.
65. Kang W, Kudsk KA: Is there evidence that the gut contributes to mucosal immunity in humans? JPEN J Parenter Enteral Nutr 31:246, 2007.
66. Jordan JR, Moore EE, Sarin EL, et al: Arachidonic acid in postshock mesenteric lymph induces pulmonary synthesis of leukotriene B4, J Appl Physiol 104:1161, 2008.
67. Cerra FB: The multiple organ failure syndrome, Hosp Pract (Off Ed) 25:169, 1990.
68. Ciesla DJ, Moore EE, Johnson JL, et al: The role of the lung in postinjury multiple organ failure, Surgery 138:749, 2005.
69. Russell JA, Singer J, Bernard GR, et al: Changing pattern of organ dysfunction in early human sepsis is related to mortality, Crit Care Med 28:3405, 2000.
70. Ciesla DJ, Moore EE, Johnson JL, et al: Multiple organ dysfunction during resuscitation is not postinjury multiple organ failure, Arch Surg 139:590, 2004.
71. Parent C, King LG, Walker LM, et al: Clinical and clinicopathologic findings in dogs with acute respiratory distress syndrome: 19 cases (1985-1993), J Am Vet Med Assoc 208:1419, 1996.
72. Nelson OL, Thompson PA: Cardiovascular dysfunction in dogs associated with critical illnesses, J Am Anim Hosp Assoc 42:344, 2006.
73. Dickinson AE, Rozanski EA, Rush JE: Reversible myocardial depression associated with sepsis in a dog, J Vet Int Med 21:1117, 2007.
74. Cavana P, Tomesello A, Ripanti D, et al: Multiple organ dysfunction syndrome in a dog with Klebsiella pneumoniae septicemia, Schweiz Arch Tierheilkd 151:69, 2009.
75. Flynn A, Chokkalingam Mani B, Mather PJ: Sepsis-induced cardiomyopathy: a review of pathophysiologic mechanisms, Heart Fail Rev 15:605, 2010.
76. Butler AL, Campbell VL: Assessment of oxygen transport and utilization in dogs with naturally occurring sepsis, J Am Vet Med Assoc 237:167, 2010.
77. Bulmer BJ: Cardiovascular dysfunction in sepsis and critical illness, Vet Clin North Am Small Anim Pract 41:717, 2011.
78. Matuschak GM: Lung-liver interactions in sepsis and multiple organ failure syndrome, Clin Chest Med 17:83, 1996.
79. Meier-Hellmann A, Specht M, Hannemann L, et al: Splanchnic blood flow is greater in septic shock treated with norepinephrine than in severe sepsis, Intensive Care Med 22:1354, 1996.
80. Poeze M, Ramsay G, Buurman WA, et al: Increased hepatosplanchnic inflammation precedes the development of organ dysfunction after elective high-risk surgery, Shock 17:451, 2002.
81. Karner J, Roth E, Ollenschlager G, et al: Glutamine-containing dipeptides as infusion substrates in the septic state, Surgery 106:893, 1989.
82. Novak F, Heyland DK, Avenell A, et al: Glutamine supplementation in serious illness: a systematic review of the evidence, Crit Care Med 30:2022, 2002.
83. Aninat C, Seguin P, Descheemaeker PN, et al: Catecholamines induce an inflammatory response in human hepatocytes, Crit Care Med 36:848, 2008.
84. Streeter EM, Zsombor-Murray E, Moore KE, et al: Intestinal permeability and absorption in dogs with traumatic injury, J Vet Intern Med 16:669, 2002.
85. Cullen JJ, Caropreso DK, Ephgrave KS, et al: The effect of endotoxin on canine jejunal motility and transit, J Surg Res 67:54, 1997.
86. Kidney Disease: Improving Global Outcomes (KDIGO) Acute Kidney Injury Work Group: Clinical practice guideline for acute kidney injury, Kidney Int Suppl 2:1, 2012.
87. Bellomo R, Ronco C, Kellum JA, et al: Acute renal failure—definition, outcome measures, animal models, fluid therapy and information technology needs: the Second International Consensus Conference of the Acute Dialysis Quality Initiative (ADQI) Group, Crit Care 8:R204, 2004.
88. Lee YJ, Chang CC, Chan JP, et al: Prognosis of acute kidney injury in dogs using RIFLE (Risk, Injury, Failure, Loss and End-stage renal failure)-like criteria, Vet Rec 168:264, 2011.
89. Thoen ME, Kerl ME: Characterization of acute kidney injury in hospitalized dogs and evaluation of a veterinary acute kidney injury staging system, J Vet Emerg Crit Care 21:648-657, 2011.
90. Lunn KF: The kidney in critically ill small animals, Vet Clin North Am Small Anim Pract 41:727, 2011.
91. Bellomo R, Kellum JA, Ronco C: Acute kidney injury, Lancet 380:756, 2012.
92. Wan L, Bagshaw SM, Langenberg C, et al: Pathophysiology of septic acute kidney injury: what do we really know? Crit Care Med 36:S198, 2008.
93. Langenberg C, Bellomo R, May C, et al: Renal blood flow in sepsis, Crit Care 9:R363, 2005.
94. Langenberg C, Bellomo R, May CN, et al: Renal vascular resistance in sepsis, Nephron Physiol 104:p1, 2006.

95. Langenberg C, Wan L, Egi M, et al: Renal blood flow and function during recovery from experimental septic acute kidney injury, Intensive Care Med 33:1614, 2007.
96. Cunningham PN, Dyanov HM, Park P, et al: Acute renal failure in endotoxemia is caused by TNF acting directly on TNF receptor-1 in kidney, J Immunol 168:5817, 2002.
97. Jo SK, Cha DR, Cho WY, et al: Inflammatory cytokines and lipopolysaccharide induce Fas-mediated apoptosis in renal tubular cells, Nephron 91:406, 2002.
98. Steinvall I, Bak Z, Sjoberg F: Acute kidney injury is common, parallels organ dysfunction or failure, and carries appreciable mortality in patients with major burns: a prospective exploratory cohort study, Crit Care 12:R124, 2008.
99. Imai Y, Parodo J, Kajikawa O, et al: Injurious mechanical ventilation and end-organ epithelial cell apoptosis and organ dysfunction in an experimental model of acute respiratory distress syndrome, JAMA 289:2104, 2003.
100. Consales G, De Gaudio AR: Sepsis associated encephalopathy, Minerva Anestesiol 71:39, 2005.
101. Brainard BM, Brown AJ: Defects in coagulation encountered in small animal critical care, Vet Clin of North Am Small Anim Pract 41:783, 2011.
102. O'Brien M: The reciprocal relationship between inflammation and coagulation, Top Companion Anim Med 27:46, 2012.
103. Cheng T, Mathews K, Abrams-Ogg A, et al: The link between inflammation and coagulation: influence on the interpretation of diagnostic laboratory tests, Compendium 33:E1, 2011.
104. Xu J, Zhang X, Pelayo R, et al: Extracellular histones are major mediators of death in sepsis, Nat Med 15:1318, 2009.
105. Papayannopoulos V, Metzler KD, Hakkim A, et al: Neutrophil elastase and myeloperoxidase regulate the formation of neutrophil extracellular traps, J Cell Biol 191:677, 2010.
106. Fuchs TA, Brill A, Duerschmied D, et al: Extracellular DNA traps promote thrombosis, Proc Natl Acad Sci U S A 107:15880, 2010.
107. Semeraro F, Ammollo CT, Morrissey JH, et al: Extracellular histones promote thrombin generation through platelet-dependent mechanisms: involvement of platelet TLR2 and TLR4, Blood 118:1952, 2011.
108. Ammollo CT, Semeraro F, Xu J, et al: Extracellular histones increase plasma thrombin generation by impairing thrombomodulin-dependent protein C activation, J Thromb Haemost 9:1795, 2011.
109. Lee WL, Liles WC: Endothelial activation, dysfunction and permeability during severe infections, Curr Opin Hematol 18:191, 2011.
110. Paulus P, Jennewein C, Zacharowski K: Biomarkers of endothelial dysfunction: can they help us deciphering systemic inflammation and sepsis? Biomarkers 16:S11, 2011.
111. Vincent JL, Moreno R: Clinical review: scoring systems in the critically ill, Crit Care 14:207, 2010.
112. Hayes G, Mathews K, Doig G, et al: The acute patient physiologic and laboratory evaluation (APPLE) score: a severity of illness stratification system for hospitalized dogs, J Vet Intern Med 24:1034, 2010.
113. Hayes G, Mathews K, Doig G, et al: The Feline Acute Patient Physiologic and Laboratory Evaluation (Feline APPLE) Score: a severity of illness stratification system for hospitalized cats, J Vet Intern Med 25:26, 2011.
114. Hayes G, Mathews K, Kruth S, et al: Illness severity scores in veterinary medicine: what can we learn? J Vet Intern Med 24:457, 2010.
115. Ferreira AM, Sakr Y: Organ dysfunction: general approach, epidemiology, and organ failure scores, Semin Respir Crit Care Med 32:543, 2011.
116. Leteurtre S, Martinot A, Duhamel A, et al: Validation of the paediatric logistic organ dysfunction (PELOD) score: prospective, observational, multicentre study, Lancet 362:192, 2003.
117. Janota J, Stranak Z, Statecna B, et al: Characterization of multiple organ dysfunction syndrome in very low birthweight infants: a new sequential scoring system, Shock 15:348, 2001.
118. Vincent JL, Moreno R, Takala J, et al: The SOFA (Sepsis-related Organ Failure Assessment) score to describe organ dysfunction/failure. On behalf of the Working Group on Sepsis-Related Problems of the European Society of Intensive Care Medicine, Intensive Care Med 22:707, 1996.
119. Arts DG, de Keizer NF, Vroom MB, et al: Reliability and accuracy of Sequential Organ Failure Assessment (SOFA) scoring, Crit Care Med 33:1988, 2005.
120. Ceriani R, Mazzoni M, Bortone F, et al: Application of the sequential organ failure assessment score to cardiac surgical patients, Chest 123:1229, 2003.
121. Tsai MH, Peng YS, Lien JM, et al: Multiple organ system failure in critically ill cirrhotic patients. A comparison of two multiple organ dysfunction/failure scoring systems, Digestion 69:190, 2004.
122. Lorente JA, Vallejo A, Galeiras R, et al: Organ dysfunction as estimated by the sequential organ failure assessment score is related to outcome in critically ill burn patients, Shock 31:125, 2009.
123. Marshall JC, Cook DJ, Christou NV, et al: Multiple organ dysfunction score: a reliable descriptor of a complex clinical outcome, Crit Care Med 23:1638, 1995.
124. Le Gall JR, Klar J, Lemeshow S, et al: The Logistic Organ Dysfunction system. A new way to assess organ dysfunction in the intensive care unit. ICU Scoring Group, JAMA 276:802, 1996.
125. Timsit JF, Fosse JP, Troche G, et al: Calibration and discrimination by daily Logistic Organ Dysfunction scoring comparatively with daily Sequential Organ Failure Assessment scoring for predicting hospital mortality in critically ill patients, Crit Care Med 30:2003, 2002.
126. Levy MM, Fink MP, Marshall JC, et al: 2001 SCCM/ESICM/ACCP/ATS/SIS International Sepsis Definitions Conference, Crit Care Med 31:1250, 2003.
127. Dellinger RP, Levy MM, Rhodes A, et al: Surviving Sepsis campaign: international guidelines for management of severe sepsis and septic shock: 2012, Intensive Care Med 39(2):165, 2013.
128. Mongardon N, Dyson A, Singer M: Is MOF an outcome parameter or a transient, adaptive state in critical illness? Curr Opin Crit Care 15:431, 2009.
129. Conti-Patara A, Caldeira JdA, de Mattos-Junior E, et al: Changes in tissue perfusion parameters in dogs with severe sepsis/septic shock in response to goal-directed hemodynamic optimization at admission to ICU and the relation to outcome, J Vet Emerg Crit Care 22:409, 2012.
130. Rivers E, Nguyen B, Havstad S, et al: Early goal-directed therapy in the treatment of severe sepsis and septic shock, N Engl J Med 345:1368, 2001.
131. Delaney A, Angus DC, Bellomo R, et al: Bench-to-bedside review: the evaluation of complex interventions in critical care, Crit Care 12:210, 2008.
132. Rivers EP, Coba V, Whitmill M: Early goal-directed therapy in severe sepsis and septic shock: a contemporary review of the literature, Curr Opin Anaesthesiol 21:128, 2008.
133. Trzeciak S, Rivers EP: Clinical manifestations of disordered microcirculatory perfusion in severe sepsis, Crit Care 9(Suppl 4):S20, 2005.
134. Butler AL: Goal-directed therapy in small animal critical illness, Vet Clin North Am Small Anim Pract 41:817, 2011.
135. Gattinoni L, Protti A, Caironi P, et al: Ventilator-induced lung injury: the anatomical and physiological framework, Crit Care Med 38:S539, 2010.
136. Cortes I, Penuelas O, Esteban A: Acute respiratory distress syndrome: evaluation and management, Minerva Anestesiol 78:343, 2012.
137. Wheeler AP, Bernard GR, Thompson BT, et al: Pulmonary-artery versus central venous catheter to guide treatment of acute lung injury, N Engl J Med 354:2213, 2006.
138. Matthay MA, Ware LB, Zimmerman GA: The acute respiratory distress syndrome, J Clin Invest 122:2731, 2012.
139. Briel M, Meade M, Mercat A, et al: Higher vs lower positive end-expiratory pressure in patients with acute lung injury and acute respiratory distress syndrome: systematic review and meta-analysis, JAMA 303:865, 2010.
140. Oura T, Rozanski EA, Buckley G, et al: Low tidal volume ventilation in healthy dogs, J Vet Emerg Crit Care 22:368, 2012.
141. Hopper K, Haskins SC, Kass PH, et al: Indications, management, and outcome of long-term positive-pressure ventilation in dogs and cats: 148 cases (1990-2001), J Am Vet Med Assoc 230:64, 2007.
142. Kelmer E, Love LC, Declue AE, et al: Successful treatment of acute respiratory distress syndrome in 2 dogs, Can Vet J 53:167, 2012.
143. Joannidis M: Continuous renal replacement therapy in sepsis and multisystem organ failure, Semin Dial 22:160, 2009.

144. Ronco C, Tetta C, Mariano F, et al: Interpreting the mechanisms of continuous renal replacement therapy in sepsis: the peak concentration hypothesis, Artif Organs 27:792, 2003.
145. Palevsky PM: Renal replacement therapy in acute kidney injury, Adv Chronic Kidney Dis 20:76, 2013.
146. Moore FA, Moore EE: The Evolving rationale for early enteral nutrition based on paradigms of multiple organ failure: a personal journey, Nutr Clin Pract 24:297, 2009.
147. Ortiz Leyba C, Montejo Gonzalez JC, Vaquerizo Alonso C: Guidelines for specialized nutritional and metabolic support in the critically-ill patient: update. Consensus SEMICYUC-SENPE: septic patient, Nutr Hosp 26(Suppl 2):67, 2011.
148. van den Berghe G, Wouters P, Weekers F, et al: Intensive insulin therapy in critically ill patients, N Engl J Med 345:1359, 2001.
149. Treggiari MM, Karir V, Yanez ND, et al: Intensive insulin therapy and mortality in critically ill patients, Crit Care 12:R29, 2008.
150. Finfer S, Chittock DR, Su SY, et al: Intensive versus conventional glucose control in critically ill patients, N Engl J Med 360:1283, 2009.
151. Finfer S, Liu B, Chittock DR, et al: Hypoglycemia and risk of death in critically ill patients, N Engl J Med 367:1108, 2012.
152. Kampmeier TG, Ertmer C, Rehberg S: Translational research in sepsis—an ultimate challenge? Exp Transl Stroke Med 3:14, 2011.
153. Hall TC, Bilku DK, Al-Leswas D, et al: The difficulties of clinical trials evaluating therapeutic agents in patients with severe sepsis, Irish J Med Sci 181:1, 2012.
154. Vincent JL: The rise and fall of drotrecogin alfa (activated), Lancet Infect Dis 12:649, 2012.
155. Artigas A, Niederman MS, Torres A, et al: What is next in sepsis: current trials in sepsis, Expert Rev Anti Infect Ther 10:859, 2012.
156. Platt SR, Radaelli ST, McDonnell JJ: The prognostic value of the modified Glasgow Coma Scale in head trauma in dogs, J Vet Intern Med Am Coll Vet Intern Med 15:581, 2001.

CHAPTER 8
HYPOTENSION

Edward Cooper, VMD

KEY POINTS

- Blood pressure is a combination of the effects of various elements. These include heart rate, stroke volume, and systemic vascular resistance.
- Hypotension occurs when at least one of the controls of blood pressure is overcome or neutralized.
- Treatment of hypotension involves treating the underlying cause and targeting the patient's normal control mechanisms.

Hypotension is a reduction in systemic arterial blood pressure, which results from disruption in normal cardiovascular homeostasis. Because numerous factors contribute to maintenance of normal blood pressure, hypotension only develops secondary to a disease process that has negatively affected this regulation. What follows is a review of the normal physiology and pathophysiology of blood pressure control as they relate to causes of hypotension in critically ill patients. Although covered elsewhere in greater detail, there is also consideration of various treatment options for these assorted disorders.

NORMAL DETERMINANTS OF BLOOD PRESSURE

Systemic arterial blood pressure provides the hydraulic force that drives blood flow and thereby significantly affects tissue perfusion. More specifically, it is the force exerted by blood against any unit area of the vessel wall.[1] Arterial blood pressure varies depending on the phase of the cardiac cycle (systolic vs. diastolic), but it is the mean arterial pressure (MAP) that plays the biggest role in tissue perfusion.[2] Understanding the main cardiovascular elements that determine MAP is essential to understanding the development of hypotension. These factors can be represented by the so-called tree of life (Figure 8-1).

True of any fluid that is pumped through a closed system, pressure (in this case MAP) is primarily determined by the product of flow (cardiac output [CO]) and resistance (systemic vascular resistance [SVR]). Cardiac output, in turn, is a function of the volume of blood ejected with each contraction of the heart (stroke volume [SV]) times the number of contractions per minute (heart rate [HR]). The determinants of SV are preload (stretching of the ventricle before contraction, largely a function of venous return), contractility (force of ventricular contraction), and afterload (the force needed to overcome

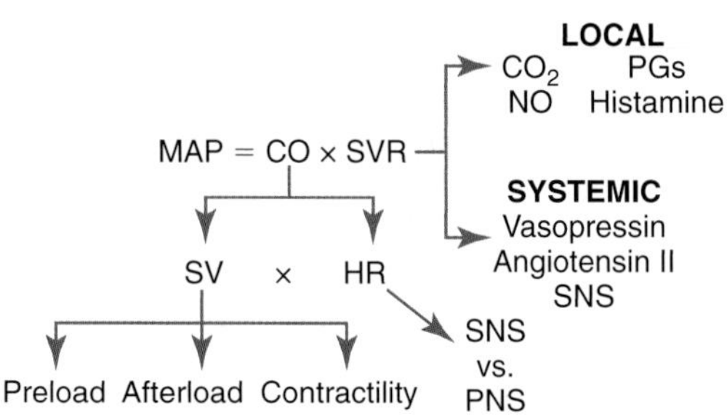

FIGURE 8-1 The "tree of life" representing the key physiologic factors that determine mean arterial pressure. *CO,* Cardiac output; *CO_2,* carbon dioxide; *HR,* heart rate; *PGs,* prostaglandins; *PNS,* parasympathetic nervous system; *MAP,* mean arterial pressure; *NO,* nitric oxide; *SNS,* sympathetic nervous system; *SV,* stroke volume; *SVR,* systemic vascular resistance.

aortic pressure and achieve left ventricular outflow). SV is directly related to preload and contractility, whereas it is inversely related to afterload. Heart rate, the other major contributor to CO, is dictated by the relative balance between input from the sympathetic nervous system (SNS) and parasympathetic nervous system (PNS).

Regulation of SVR is another major factor that serves to determine MAP. Vascular tone, and thereby SVR, is affected by both systemic and local mediators, which cause either vasoconstriction or vasodilation. Catecholamines released by the SNS are primarily responsible for basal systemic vascular tone, as well as minute-to-minute regulation of blood pressure.[1] Angiotensin II and vasopressin, also having vasoconstrictive effects, play more of a role in long-term regulation of vascular tone. In addition to these systemic mediators, local factors can also serve to affect blood flow in response to changes in metabolic demand, muscle activity, and vascular injury and to circumvent systemic vascular control. Examples include vasodilatory substances such as nitric oxide (NO), histamine, prostacyclin, and carbon dioxide, as well as vasoconstrictive agents such as endothelin, thromboxane, and thrombin.[1] Although their effects are to meant to alter local vascular tone, excessive/systemic release can result in significant changes to SVR.

POTENTIAL CAUSES OF HYPOTENSION

Significant alterations in any of the previously described components of the "tree of life" could result in a reduction in MAP and lead to the development of hypotension. A categorical approach to causes of hypotension can be helpful in recognizing the pathophysiology involved and thereby aid in recognition and treatment (Table 8-1).

Reduction in Preload

Reduction in preload is a common cause of hypotension and can result from a number of different disease processes. As a reflection of venous return, preload will be affected by any cause of significant fluid loss from the vascular space, including hemorrhage, gastrointestinal or urinary losses leading to severe dehydration, edema, or cavitary effusions (hypovolemic shock; see Chapter 5). For patients experiencing acute bleeding, it is typically necessary to have greater than 30% loss of vascular volume before hypotension will develop.[3] Another important (and sometimes overlooked) cause of relative hypovolemia and preload reduction is venodilation. Veins have a significant capacity for volume; relaxation results in pooling and diminished venous return (see Reduction in Systemic Vascular Resistance later in this chapter).

In addition to hypovolemia, any major obstruction in venous return will result in a preload reduction and the potential for hypotension to develop (obstructive shock). A classic example is gastric dilation/volvulus, whereby gastric distention results in compression of the vena cava and impedes return of blood from caudal circulation. Further, twisting of the stomach itself results in venous congestion and trapping of vascular volume away from effective circulation. Through similar mechanisms, caval or portal venous thrombosis, severe pneumothorax, mesenteric volvulus, and massive pulmonary thromboembolism could all be placed in this category. Another specific cause of obstruction is pericardial effusion with cardiac tamponade. Although there is sometimes a tendency to consider this a primary cardiogenic issue, the main pathogenesis involves collapse of the right atrium from increased pericardial pressure and failure of right-sided filling (i.e., preload). This becomes particularly important when considering therapeutic options, as will be discussed later.

Reduction in Cardiac Function

Diseases originating in the heart (primary) or externally affecting the heart (secondary) can also cause hypotension (cardiogenic shock; see Chapter 39). Myocardial dysfunction can occur as a primary disease with dilated cardiomyopathy, characterized by impaired myofibril contraction, decreased contractility, and progressive ventricular dilation (see Chapter 42). Secondary myocardial dysfunction can arise associated with severe acidosis or alkalosis, toxin exposure, drug administration, or systemic inflammatory response syndrome (SIRS)/sepsis. Numerous theories have been advanced to explain the occurrence of cardiomyopathy in patients with SIRS/sepsis, including

Table 8-1 **Causes of Hypotension and Recommended Treatment**

Cause	Sample Diseases	Treatments
Reduction in Preload		
Hypovolemia	Hemorrhage Severe dehydration Edema/cavitary effusions	Address underlying problem. Provide fluid resuscitation.
Obstructive	Gastric dilation-volvulus Mesenteric volvulus Caval/portal venous occlusion Pericardial effusion Severe pleural space disease Pulmonary thromboembolism	Relieve the obstruction if possible, with surgery, pericardiocentesis, or thoracentesis; administration of thrombolytics; or thrombectomy as needed. Provide fluid resuscitation.
Reduction in Cardiac Function		
Primary	Cardiomyopathy Valvular disease Tachyarrhythmia or bradyarrhythmia	Administer positive inotrope. Administer antiarrhythmics. Provide supportive measures for congestive heart failure
Secondary	Systemic inflammatory response syndrome/sepsis Electrolyte abnormalities Severe hypoxia Severe acidosis or alkalosis	Address the underlying cause. Administer positive inotrope.
Reduction in Systemic Vascular Resistance		
	SIRS/sepsis Electrolyte abnormalities Severe hypoxia Severe acidosis or alkalosis Drug or toxins	Address the underlying cause. Provide fluid resuscitation. Administer vasopressors.

myocardial ischemia, microcirculatory dysregulation, impact of various cytokines (tumor necrosis factor α [TNF-α], interleukin 1β [IL-1β], IL-6), impaired calcium transport, catecholamine insensitivity, and mitochondrial dysfunction function, among others.[4,5] No single mechanism has been identified; it is likely a combination of these factors.

Severe mitral regurgitation is another potential cause of cardiogenic hypotension. As the majority of the left ventricular volume moves backward into the atrium, rather than forward into arterial circulation, there is a significant reduction in effective stroke volume and thereby cardiac output (see Chapter 42). Severe tachyarrhythmias (ventricular or supraventricular) and bradyarrhythmias (third-degree AV block, sick sinus syndrome, hyperkalemia) are also potential causes of decreased cardiac output and hypotension (see Cardiac Disorders section below).

Reduction in Systemic Vascular Resistance

Diseases that cause hypotension through a decrease in SVR share a common mechanism of inappropriate vasodilation resulting in maldistribution of blood flow (maldistributive or vasodilatory shock). The cardiovascular changes brought about by SIRS and sepsis best exemplify this process (see Chapters 6 and 91). Vasodilation associated with SIRS/sepsis is related to excessive production of nitric oxide from upregulation of induced nitric oxide synthase by assorted cytokines (e.g., TNF-α, IL-1β, IL-6) and direct vasoactive properties of various other inflammatory mediators.[6] Additional factors implicated include upregulation of adenosine triphosphate (ATP)–sensitive potassium channels, depletion of vasopressin stores, and vascular insensitivity to catecholamines.[6] In the early stages of SIRS/sepsis, the afterload reduction brought about by arterial vasodilation actually results in an increase in CO and a hyperdynamic state during which blood pressure is sustained. However, progressive vasodilation, along with myocardial dysfunction, eventually leads to a hypodynamic state and hypotension. It is important to remember that concurrent venodilation and associated pooling of blood volume, especially in the splanchnic circulation, causes decreased venous return (preload) and further contributes to cardiovascular collapse.

Anaphylaxis represents another example of reduced SVR through systemic release of vasoactive substances (see Chapter 152). In susceptible patients, immunoglobulin E (IgE) produced in response to allergen exposure binds to mast cells and basophils. This binding triggers release of histamines, leukotrines, and other substances that promote vasodilation and increased vascular permeability.[7] Finally, disruption of sympathetic outflow, from either severe brain or spinal cord injury, can result in systemic vasodilation. Because of unchallenged vagal tone, bradycardia can also accompany and further potentiate the associated hypotension.

RESPONSE TO DECREASES IN BLOOD PRESSURE

Given the importance of MAP in tissue perfusion, especially to vital organ systems, all effort is made to preserve normal blood pressure and prevent the development of hypotension. To that end there are a number of mechanisms in place, both immediate and delayed, that respond to a decrease in blood pressure.

The main moment-to-moment regulator of blood pressure is the baroreceptor reflex system. With a fall in blood pressure, and thereby stretch of the baroreceptors (especially in the carotid sinus and aortic arch), stimulus to the vasomotor center of the medulla is decreased. The result is in an increase in sympathetic and a decrease in parasympathetic outflow. This shift in autonomic balance and release of catecholamines then leads to vasoconstriction (increase in SVR) and increased HR and contractility (and thereby CO), all functioning to raise blood pressure back to normal. Although most emphasis is placed on arterial vasoconstriction, a significant increase venous tone also occurs. This will cause decreased capacitance and promote venous return, thereby supporting preload. Another important contributor is the chemoreceptor reflex. This reflex, originating in chemoreceptor organs (such as the carotid and aortic bodies), responds to a decrease in tissue oxygen tension, increase in carbon dioxide, or decrease in pH. These changes reflect a decrease in blood flow or oxygen delivery rather than a change in blood pressure per se. Also unlike the baroreceptors, these changes cause increased signaling from the chemoreceptors and serve to excite the vasomotor center and promote sympathetic outflow.

Acute decreases in blood volume or pressure will also promote the movement of fluid from the interstitium into the vascular space. Associated decreases in capillary hydrostatic pressure cause a shift in the net balance of Starling's forces toward the vascular compartment. The resulting internal fluid resuscitation helps to maintain blood volume, preload, and MAP.

Through a number of mechanisms, decreased blood pressure and blood flow to the kidneys result in activation of the renin-angiotensin-aldosterone (RAA) system. Renin is released by juxtaglomerular cells in response to decreased baroreceptor activity, sympathetic activation, or decreased tubular chloride as sensed by the macula densa. The associated generation of angiotensin II exerts a number of effects to help return blood pressure to normal. Angiotensin II causes vasoconstriction by both direct (triggering vascular smooth muscle contraction) and indirect actions (stimulation of sympathetic activity and release of vasopressin). The RAA system also plays a major role in expanding blood volume. Angiotensin II promotes sodium and water retention in the proximal tubule and alters glomerular filtration rate through preferential constriction of the efferent arteriole. In addition, aldosterone release from the adrenal cortex drives sodium reabsorption and potassium excretion in the cortical collecting duct.

Release of vasopressin (also called antidiuretic hormone [ADH]) from the anterior pituitary is primarily regulated by changes in blood osmolarity. However, in the face of significant hypovolemia/hypotension (and with further input from the SNS and RAA system), release of vasopressin can increase significantly, independent of osmolarity (also known as nonosmotic stimulation of ADH). Through activation of V_1 receptors, vasopressin causes vasoconstriction and an increase in SVR. Further, ADH-mediated activation of V_2 receptors in the renal collecting duct promotes water retention to help support blood volume and preload.

These compensatory mechanisms are in place to maintain MAP at all costs, which is the reason for its central location in the "tree of life." It is only when these efforts are overwhelmed that blood pressure will significantly decrease. As such it is important to note that there can be significant disruption of the cardiovascular system before hypotension develops (as the patient is still in the compensated stages of shock). Once blood pressure drops, the patient has developed "decompensated shock" and the body can no longer keep up with the severity of the cardiovascular insult. If left unchecked, the compensatory mechanisms are not just overwhelmed but become exhausted. Tissue reserves and responsiveness to the various mediators become diminished, which, in conjunction with severe acidemia, leads to vasodilation, venous pooling, bradycardia, and ultimately complete cardiovascular collapse. Therefore early recognition and treatment are paramount in the management of impending or existing hypotension.

DIAGNOSIS OF HYPOTESION

Diagnosis of hypotension is largely related to the history, presenting clinical picture, and progression of signs through the course of treatment, including aspects of physical examination and blood pressure measurement.

Physical Examination

Indicators of hypotension found on physical examination are largely related to the systemic reflection of compensatory mechanisms and, for the most part, occur regardless of the underlying cause. These include clinical signs such as tachycardia (sympathetic stimulation of HR), as well as pale mucous membranes, prolonged capillary refill time (CRT), weak peripheral pulses, cool distal extremities, and altered mentation (all reflecting peripheral vasoconstriction or impaired perfusion). It is important to note that cats may also demonstrate bradycardia in shock states (especially cardiogenic and vasodilatory). As another exception to this, patients that are in the early (hyperdynamic) stages of vasodilatory shock may have bounding pulses, red mucous membranes, and shortened CRT to reflect the reduction in SVR and increase in peripheral perfusion. As described earlier, many of these signs will develop before a decrease in blood pressure (i.e., during compensation) but should definitely be present once the patient is hypotensive. Aside from disruption of these perfusion parameters, other clinical signs related to the specific underlying disease may be present (e.g., internal/external bleeding, abdominal distention, murmur/arrhythmias, and respiratory distress).

Measurement of Blood Pressure

By definition, a diagnosis of hypotension can only be made after obtaining a blood pressure measurement that is below the normal range (Table 8-2).[8] Because they are more reflective of tissue perfusion and less variable with peripheral measurement, MAP values are generally preferred.[2] In dogs and cats, hypotension could be considered when the MAP is below 80 mm Hg, although concern for impaired tissue perfusion, especially renal, generally does not occur until MAP gets below 60 to 65 mm Hg. Recognizing the limitations, in circumstances where MAP is not available (e.g., when using Doppler ultrasonography), a systolic blood pressure of less than 90 to 100 mm Hg could also be considered to reflect hypotension. Numerous methodologies can be used to measure blood pressure, including direct and indirect techniques (see Chapter 183).

Direct blood pressure monitoring

Direct measurement through use of an arterial catheter (typically dorsopedal or femoral) and pressure transducer is considered the gold standard for assessment of arterial blood pressure. In addition to being more accurate than indirect methods, direct measurement provides continuous reporting of systolic, diastolic, and mean pressures, as well as display of the arterial waveform. As such, this information can be used to detect and treat hypotension (e.g., with resuscitation fluid therapy, titration of vasopressors) on a minute-to-minute basis. Furthermore, the catheter can be used for arterial blood sampling to monitor acid-base status and blood gas parameters in critically ill patients.

Use of direct blood pressure is not without its drawbacks, risks, and complications. Obtaining arterial access can be challenging and invasive, the equipment can be very expensive, and there are potential complications from catheter placement (e.g., bleeding, infection, thrombosis). Despite these limitations, direct blood pressure monitoring is generally preferred in the management of a critically ill or hypotensive dog. Direct blood pressure monitoring is less commonly used in cats, except for temporary monitoring (e.g., during anesthesia) because secondary thrombosis and failure to establish collateral circulation are common in this species.

Table 8-2 Normal Arterial Blood Pressure Values in Dogs and Cats

	Dogs	Cats
Systolic arterial pressure	110 to 190 mm Hg	120 to 170 mm Hg
Diastolic arterial pressure	55 to 110 mm Hg	70 to 120 mm Hg
Mean arterial pressure	80 to 130 mm Hg	60 to 130 mm Hg

FromWadell LS: Direct blood pressure monitoring, Clin Tech Small Anim Pract 15(3):111, 2000.

Indirect blood pressure measurement

Indirect methods of blood pressure measurement (including Doppler ultrasonography and oscillometric sphygmomanometry) are generally less invasive, less expensive, less technically challenging, and more readily available when compared with direct. Therefore for practical considerations these methods are often used as the initial, if not only, means of obtaining a patient's blood pressure. In many clinical circumstances they can provide useful information to guide diagnosis and clinical decision making, but it is important to be aware of their limitations. The accuracy of indirect methods is less than direct measurement, with a general tendency to overestimate blood pressure in hypotension and underestimate in hypertension.[10] In addition, there are other limiting aspects related to either methodology that should be considered.

Doppler ultrasonography

Doppler blood pressure measurement is relatively sensitive in small patients (<10 kg) or patients in low-flow states and is readily available in most veterinary settings. However, there are a number of potential limitations. This method only provides a systolic pressure, although there is evidence that Doppler blood pressure may be more reflective of MAP in cats.[10] Accurate measurement can be affected by cuff size, which should be approximately 40% of the limb circumference. If the cuff is too large or too small, measurements may underestimate or overestimate the actual blood pressure, respectively. Doppler measurements also require patient handling, which may stimulate a stress response and "artificially" elevate the patient's blood pressure.

Oscillometric sphygmomanometry

Oscillometric methods carry the advantage of being more automated and providing information about systolic pressure, diastolic pressure, and MAP. Unlike Doppler ultrasonography, oscillometric readings do not require patient manipulation after cuff placement, and many devices are easily set to cycle for repeated pressure readings. Oscillometric measurements are affected by cuff size in a fashion similar to the Doppler technique. Other limitations that can affect accuracy include small patient size (especially cats), significant motion, low-perfusion states, and arrhythmias.

Additional Diagnostics

Diagnostic evaluation in the hypotensive patient is largely geared toward determining the underlying cause and assessing the extent of systemic compromise. Initial emphasis is placed on point-of-care diagnostics until the patient is stable for transport or a more involved workup. Preliminary laboratory analysis might include packed cell volume/total protein (PCV/TP), blood glucose, arterial or venous blood gas analysis, blood smear, and lactate measurement, with eventual submission of complete blood cell count, chemistry profile, and coagulation profile. The presence of fluid or air in the pleural or peritoneal cavity is easily assessed with ultrasound examination and can be performed at the bedside; thoracic/abdominal radiographs and complete abdominal ultrasound should be performed as indicated. Cardiac assessment can be achieved with electrocardiography

(ECG) and echocardiography. Bedside echocardiogram can be very useful for early detection of pericardial effusion, qualitative assessment of systolic function, and monitoring of relative volume status (cardiac underfilling or overfilling). Studies have demonstrated that some of these assessments can be performed accurately without extensive cardiology training.[11]

TREATMENT OF HYPOTENSION

The key to successful management of hypotension is early detection and swift therapeutic intervention. Whenever possible, therapy should be initiated at the earliest indication of cardiovascular instability (e.g., alteration of perfusion parameters), even if hypotension has not yet developed; once it does, the need to intervene becomes even more critical. Ultimately, addressing the underlying cause is the most essential aspect of treating hypotension. In the immediate sense, stabilization is largely geared toward supporting the affected components of the "tree of life"—preload, cardiac function, and SVR (see Table 8-1).

Fluid Resuscitation

Fluid administration is often the cornerstone of resuscitative efforts, especially if a reduction in preload is suspected. This includes causes of absolute (e.g., hemorrhage) or relative (e.g., obstruction or vasodilation) hypovolemia and typically not primary causes of cardiac dysfunction. A complete discussion of resuscitation fluid therapy is beyond the scope of this chapter (see Chapter 60, as well as suggested references), but a few points bear mentioning.

The classic approach to fluid resuscitation involves application of "shock doses" of crystalloids or colloids, titrated to effect based on resolution hypotension and abnormal perfusion parameters. However, there continues to be significant controversy regarding the optimal approach, especially with regard to volumes administered, use of synthetic colloids, and administration of blood products.[12-14] It is also important to recognize that once a "reasonable" amount has been administered but the hypotension has not resolved, additional fluids are unlikely to provide benefit and may be harmful. The challenge lies in determining what constitutes "reasonable." Measurement of central venous pressures or bedside echocardiography may provide some guidance but are not without limitations. Certainly if a full "shock dose" has been administered without improvement, measures to address cardiac dysfunction or vasodilatory processes should be considered.

Positive Inotropes

A positive inotrope should be used in cases of documented (through echocardiography) or highly suspected (based on clinical picture) myocardial/systolic dysfunction. This includes causes that are both primary (e.g., dilated cardiomyopathy) and secondary (e.g., sepsis associated). In these cases application of a β-adrenergic agonist is indicated, with dobutamine generally the preferred agent (see Chapter 157). Drawbacks to use of positive inotropes include increased myocardial oxygen demand and the potential to cause arrhythmias.

Vasopressor Agents

Patients with an inappropriate vasodilatory process may benefit from administration of a vasopressor agent. It is often challenging to make this determination. Signs consistent with early/hyperdynamic vasodilation (bounding pulses, red mucous membranes, shortened CRT) may be more obvious; however, once progressed to the hypodynamic stage it can be difficult to distinguish from other causes of hypotension. The associated clinical picture (e.g., sepsis, anesthesia, etc.) may also help guide the decision. Because fluid loading is often attempted first, failure to respond might suggest that vasoconstriction is needed. For this purpose an α_1 agonist or vasopressin may be used (see Chapters 157 and 158, respectively). Although dopamine has long been considered a first-line vasopressor, current human guidelines recommend use of norepinephrine with vasopressin added second, if needed, in septic patients.[12]

SUMMARY

Hypotension is a common and life-threatening occurrence in critically ill patients. Understanding the normal mechanisms of blood pressure regulation, the main factors that can result in disruption of cardiovascular hemostasis, and the body's compensatory responses are essential to timely recognition and appropriate therapy.

REFERENCES

1. Guyton AC, Hall JE, editors: The textbook of medical physiology, ed 12, Philadelphia, 2000, Saunders.
2. Marino PL: Arterial blood pressure. In Marino P, editor: The ICU book, ed 3, Philadelphia, 2006, Lippincott, Williams & Wilkins.
3. Garrioch MA: The body's response to blood loss, Vox Sanguinis 87(S1):S74, 2004.
4. Romero-Bermejo FJ, Ruiz-Bailen M, Gil-Cebrian J, Huertos-Ranchal MJ: Sepsis-induced cardiomyopathy, Curr Cardiol Rev 7(3):163, 2011.
5. Costello MF, Otto CM, Rubin LJ: The role of tumor necrosis factor-α (TNF-α) and the sphingosine pathway in sepsis-induced myocardial dysfunction, J Vet Emerg Crit Care 13:25, 2003.
6. Bridges EJ, Dukes S: Cardiovascular aspects of septic shock: pathophysiology, monitoring, and treatment, Crit Care Nurse 25(2):14, 2005.
7. Simons FE: Anaphylaxis, J Allergy Clin Immunol 125(Suppl 2):S161, 2010.
8. Wadell LS: Direct blood pressure monitoring, Clin Tech Small Anim Pract 15(3):111, 2000.
9. Reference deleted in pages.
10. Caulkett NA, Cantwell SL, Houston DM: A comparison of indirect blood pressure monitoring techniques in the anesthetized cat, Vet Surg 27:370, 1998.
11. Tse YC, Rush JE, Cunningham SM, et al: Evaluation of a training course in focused echocardiography for noncardiology house officers, J Vet Emerg Crit Care 23(3):268, 2013.
12. Driessen B, Brainard B: Fluid therapy for the traumatized patient, J Vet Emerg Crit Care 16(4):276, 2006.
13. Dellinger RP, Levy MM, Rhodes A, et al: Surviving sepsis campaign: international guidelines for management of severe sepsis and septic shock: 2012, Crit Care Med 41(2):580, 2013.
14. Kobayashi L, Costantini TW, Coimbra R: Hypovolemic shock resuscitation, Surg Clin North Am 92(6):1403, 2012.

CHAPTER 9
HYPERTENSIVE CRISIS

Kate Hopper, BVSc, PhD, DACVECC • Scott Brown, VMD, PhD, DACVIM

KEY POINTS

- An elevated arterial blood pressure is concerning because of its potential to cause target-organ damage.
- Target organs at risk of damage from hypertension include the eyes, brain, and kidneys.
- A hypertensive emergency is defined as a marked elevation in arterial blood pressure with evidence of new or progressive target-organ damage.
- Patients with a hypertensive emergency should have their mean arterial blood pressure decreased by no more than 25% within 1 hour.
- A hypertensive urgency is defined as a critically elevated arterial blood pressure with no evidence of target-organ damage and is an indication for a gradual reduction in blood pressure.

The definition of high arterial blood pressure (ABP) will vary among species and potentially genders, breeds, and ages of animals. An American College of Veterinary Internal Medicine (ACVIM) consensus statement released in 2007 defined hypertension for dogs and cats based on systolic ABP (Table 9-1).[1] Because the comparable accuracy of systolic versus mean ABP can vary between measurement technique, the use of systolic ABP may not always be ideal and clinicians should adjust the criteria for hypertension accordingly.

An elevated ABP is concerning because of its potential to cause target-organ damage (TOD). Organs vulnerable to hypertension-associated damage are listed in Table 9-2; ocular and brain injury are of greatest concern. Human medicine differentiates a hypertensive emergency as a patient with an elevated ABP with new or progressive TOD, whereas hypertensive urgency is a critically elevated ABP with no evidence of TOD. Patients with a hypertensive emergency require immediate lowering of blood pressure, whereas patients with a hypertensive urgency can have their ABP lowered over hours to days.[1,2]

Table 9-1 ACVIM System for Classification of Systolic Blood Pressure Levels in Dogs and Cats Based on Risk for Further Target Organ Damage[1]

Risk Category	Systolic Blood Pressure (mm Hg)	Diastolic Blood Pressure (mm Hg)	Risk of Further Target Organ Damage
AP0 (or I)	<150	<95	Minimal
AP1 (or II)	150 to 159	95-99	Mild
AP2 (or III)	160 to 179	100-119	Moderate
AP3 (or IV)	≥180	≥ 120	Severe

ACVIM, American College of Veterinary Internal Medicine.
When separate consideration of the systolic and diastolic blood pressure leads to different categorization, the patient should be assigned the higher risk category.
NOTE: Therapeutic target is generally a systolic ABP of 110 to 150 mm Hg (see text).

PATHOPHYSIOLOGY

Blood pressure is determined by both cardiac output and systemic vascular resistance. In health, blood pressure is tightly regulated such that mean arterial pressure varies minimally.[3] The autonomic nervous system serves to prevent acute changes in blood pressure while the renin-angiotensin-aldosterone system, stress relaxation responses of the vasculature, and fluid shifts between the vascular space and the interstitium respond within minutes to hours to correct abnormalities in blood pressure. Long-term blood pressure control is largely the responsibility of the kidneys through regulation of extracellular fluid volume.

Hypertension is the result of inappropriately high systemic vascular resistance with or without concurrent increases in blood volume. Uncontrolled vasoconstriction is due to local and systemic mediators, including catecholamines, angiotensin II, endothelin I, vasopressin, and thromboxane, in addition to inadequate local production of vasodilators such as nitric oxide and prostacyclin.[4] Increases in blood volume almost always are due to inadequate volume excretion by the kidneys. This may be due to intrinsic kidney disease or it can occur as a result of active renal reabsorption of salt and water, usually in response to a perceived lack of adequate effective circulating volume or hormonal influence (e.g., aldosterone or glucocorticoid excess).

Inflammation has been implicated both in the development of hypertension and as a consequence of hypertension. Oxidative stress has been demonstrated in both animal models of hypertension and human clinical patients. Oxidative stress is associated with endothelial dysfunction and has been suggested to cause hypertension through decreased nitric oxide bioavailability, although the exact role of reactive oxygen species in hypertension is an area of active investigation.[5] The vascular remodeling and endothelial injury that occur as a consequence of hypertension are associated with a proinflammatory response that includes cytokine production, white blood cell activation, and upregulation of endothelial adhesion molecules. In human patients with hypertensive emergencies, these inflammatory changes can lead to increased endothelial permeability and activation of coagulation cascades and may also contribute to the TOD seen in patients with chronic hypertension.[6] The vascular injury and associated inflammatory changes secondary to hypertension have not been studied in clinical veterinary patients, although the proteinuria that is often observed in these patients may be a marker of this injury.

BLOOD PRESSURE MEASUREMENT

Blood pressure can be measured via direct or indirect methods. Direct ABP is measured via an arterial catheter or needle, whereas indirect ABP methods use a compressive cuff that detects the presence or absence of a peripheral pulse.[7-16] Although direct ABP is considered the gold standard, indirect methods are far more commonly used in the clinical setting (see Chapters 183 and 201).

Table 9-2 **Hypertensive End-Organ Damage**

End Organ	Hypertensive Injury	Clinical Findings	Role for Emergency Antihypertensive Therapy?
Eye	Retinopathy	Acute blindness, retinal detachment, or hemorrhage	Yes
	Choroidopathy	Vitreal hemorrhage or hyphema	Yes
Brain	Encephalopathy Stroke	Central neurologic signs of acute onset	Yes
Kidney	Progression of chronic kidney disease	Serial increases in serum creatinine concentration Proteinuria	Not typically indicated
Heart and vessels	Cardiac failure	Left ventricular hypertrophy Systolic murmur Arrhythmias Evidence of cardiac failure	Not typically indicated

To obtain reliable values, it is important to follow a standard protocol for blood pressure measurement. The ABP may be affected by stress or anxiety associated with the measurement process,[17] and these changes may result in a false diagnosis of hypertension.[18] This anxiety-induced, artifactual elevation of ABP is often referred to as *white-coat hypertension,* a reference to the white coat of the medical professional measuring ABP. A measurement session consisting of three to seven consecutive indirect measurements, or possibly even at-home measurements, should be obtained before initiation of antihypertensive therapy. Although the general rule is to conduct at least two measurement sessions separated by 30 minutes or more before initiating therapy, the presence of ocular or neurologic end-organ damage constituting an emergency is an exception to this rule.

TARGET ORGAN DAMAGE

Ocular

Ocular lesions are observed in many animals with systemic hypertension; reported prevalence rates are as high as 100%.[19-24] The syndrome of hypertensive ocular injury is most often termed hypertensive retinopathy.[20,22,25,26] Sudden onset of blindness, intraocular hemorrhage, and retinal detachment are the most common indications for emergency lowering of ABP. Other ocular lesions associated with high ABP include retinal vessel tortuosity, edema, and retinal degeneration (Figures 9-1 and 9-2). Effective antihypertensive treatment can lead to retinal reattachment, although restoration of vision is not common and subsequent retinal degeneration leading to blindness may occur. Hypertensive ocular injury has been reported at systolic ABP as low as 168 mm Hg,[21] and there is a substantially elevated risk of occurrence with a systolic ABP that exceeds 180 mm Hg (particularly when this increase occurs suddenly).[24-26] In a retrospective study of 42 hypertensive dogs, 62% were found to have major ocular lesions. The median systolic ABP of dogs with major ocular lesions was 197 mm Hg (range 165 to 265 mm Hg) and was not significantly different from the median systolic ABP of hypertensive dogs without ocular lesions (189 mm Hg; range 165 to 210 mm Hg).[27]

Neurologic

Neurologic clinical signs are common in hypertensive dogs and cats. Signs include altered mentation, disorientation, lethargy, seizures, balance disturbances, head tilt, nystagmus, behavioral abnormalities, and focal neurologic defects. Hypertensive encephalopathy[1] is a complication justifying rapid lowering of ABP and has been reported in dogs[23] and cats,[22,25,28-30] occurring as a well-described entity in humans, characterized by white matter edema and vascular lesions.[31]

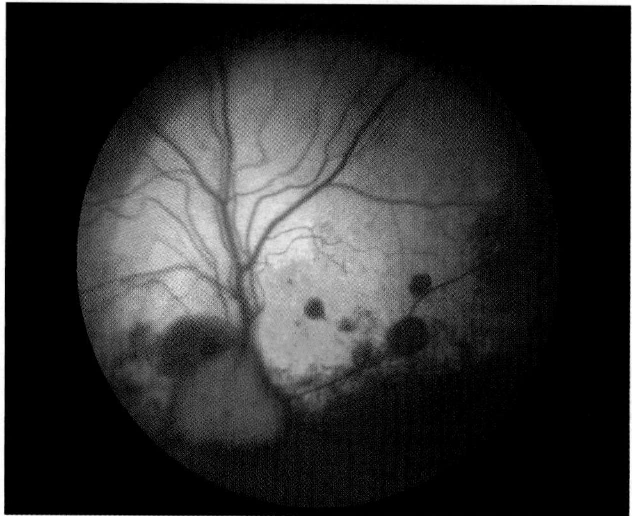

FIGURE 9-1 Retinal hemorrhage in a dog with hypertension. *(Image courtesy Dr. Steven Hollingsworth, Ophthalmology Service, Veterinary Medical Teaching Hospital, University of California, Davis.)*

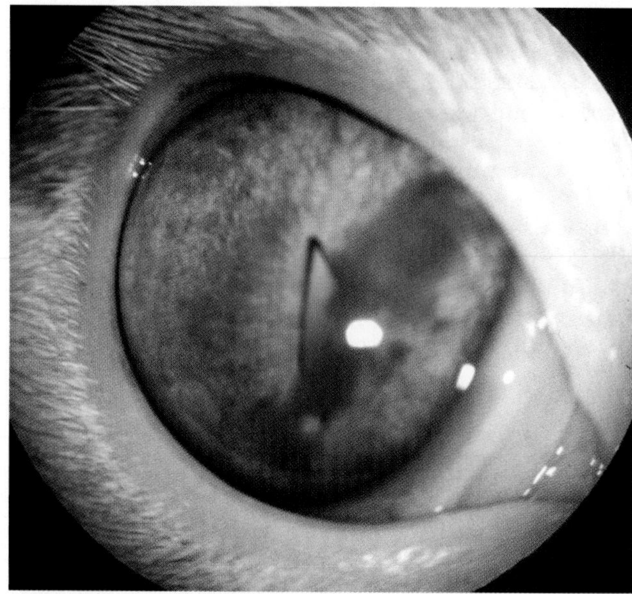

FIGURE 9-2 Hyphema in a cat with hypertension. *(Image courtesy Dr. Steven Hollingsworth, Ophthalmology Service, Veterinary Medical Teaching Hospital, University of California, Davis.)*

Hypertensive encephalopathy also occurs after renal transplantation in humans[32] and may be a cause of otherwise unexplained postoperative death in cats.[28] Hypertensive encephalopathy is more likely to occur with a sudden rise in ABP or a systolic ABP that exceeds 180 mm Hg.[33] This syndrome, in its early phases, is rapidly responsive to lowering of ABP.[28,33] Hemorrhagic and ischemic strokes are observed in dogs and cats, and these conditions may generally be distinguished from hypertensive encephalopathy by virtue of their slow and incomplete response to lowering ABP. Before treating hypertension in the patient with evidence of intracranial disease, Cushing's reflex (causing hypertension and bradycardia) in response to increased intracranial pressure must be distinguished from neurologic injury secondary to hypertension (see Chapter 191).

Renal

In the kidney, hypertensive injury generally manifests as an enhanced rate of decline of renal function, early renal death, and proteinuria. Proteinuria is a marker of hypertensive nephropathy in humans,[34] and severity was directly related to degree of elevation of ABP in an experimental study of chronic kidney disease in cats.[33] Further, treatment of hypertension in cats has been associated with a significant decrease in urine protein/creatinine ratio.[35] Malignant hypertension is a syndrome of severe, progressive elevations of ABP causing end-organ damage that is often associated with kidney disease and is a recognized cause of rapidly progressive renal injury in rats and people, necessitating quick reductions in ABP. However, hypertensive damage to the canine and feline kidneys is almost always a slow and insidious process, requiring weeks to years to fully manifest, and is thus rarely a rationale for emergency therapy in dogs and cats.

Cardiovascular

Cardiac changes in hypertensive animals may include systolic murmurs, cardiac gallops, and left ventricular hypertrophy.[19,22,36] Although cats with previously undiagnosed hypertension may unexpectedly develop signs of congestive heart failure after receiving fluid therapy, heart failure and other serious complications are infrequent[22,25,37] and slow to develop. While vascular injury within the eye or central nervous system is a rationale for emergent therapy, cardiac changes rarely mandate rapid reductions in ABP.

PATIENTS AT RISK FOR HYPERTENSION

Hypertension can occur as a primary, idiopathic disease process or may be secondary to an underlying disease. Although there have been reports of primary hypertension in dogs and cats, secondary hypertension is far more common in veterinary patients. Diseases associated with hypertension in dogs and cats are listed in Box 9-1, with kidney disease, diabetes mellitus, hyperadrenocorticism, and hyperthyroidism being most common. See Chapter 159 for further discussion on the causes of hypertension.

There are at least two primary indications for evaluating a patient with possible hypertension. First, ABP should be measured in patients with clinical abnormalities consistent with hypertensive TOD. This generally includes clinical signs of hypertensive retinopathy or hyphema, epistaxis, and unexplained intracranial neurologic signs (e.g., seizures, altered mentation, focal neurologic deficits). A second indication for ABP measurement is the presence of diseases or conditions commonly associated with secondary hypertension (see Box 9-1) or the use of therapy that may elevate ABP (e.g., sympathetic agonists). A thorough physical examination, including funduscopic evaluation, cardiac auscultation, and neurologic examination, should be performed concurrently in these at-risk patients to assess for TOD. Abnormalities of the urinary (e.g., microalbuminuria, proteinuria, azotemia, or structural changes in the kidney) and cardiovascular (e.g., unexplained left ventricular hypertrophy, gallop rhythm, arrhythmia, or systolic murmur) systems are also indications for ABP measurement.

BOX 9-1 ***Diseases Causing Hypertension in Dogs and Cats***

Common Causes

- Kidney disease
- Diabetes mellitus
- Hyperadrenocorticism
- Hyperthyroidism

Less Common Causes

- Pheochromocytoma
- Hyperaldosteronism
- Hepatic disease
- Polycythemia
- Chronic anemia
- Congestive heart failure
- Neoplasia
- Iatrogenic (drug induced)

HYPERTENSIVE URGENCY

Patients with a significant increase in blood pressure (systolic ABP ≥ 160 mm Hg) but no evidence of TOD are considered to have a hypertensive urgency. Epistaxis can occur as a consequence of hypertension. In the absence of TOD, epistaxis alone would be considered consistent with a hypertensive urgency. A gradual reduction in blood pressure over hours to days is important to prevent development of a hypertensive emergency such as organ damage or vascular accidents.[2]

HYPERTENSIVE EMERGENCY

A hypertensive emergency requires an immediate reduction in blood pressure. The current human recommendation is to reduce mean arterial blood pressure by no more than 25% within 1 hour, then to further reduce the blood pressure to 160/100 to 110 mm Hg within the next 2 to 6 hours. Excessive drops in blood pressure can precipitate organ ischemia and should be avoided.[2]

TREATMENT

Once a decision is made to treat an animal with high ABP, therapeutic interventions will generally involve a pharmacologic agent. Certain disease conditions identified during this evaluation may be best addressed with specific classes of agents, such as β-blockers for hypertension-associated hyperthyroidism or α-blockers and β-blockers or surgical excision for pheochromocytomas; aldosterone receptor blockers or surgical excision of adrenal tumors in animals with hypertension associated with hyperaldosteronism; or some combination of calcium channel blockers, angiotensin-converting enzyme inhibitors, angiotensin receptor blockers, and aldosterone receptor blockers for hypertension associated with kidney disease in dogs.[1,33,38-41] Chapter 159 discusses the pharmacologic management of hypertension in more detail.

Therapeutic Goals

The goal of antihypertensive therapy is to reduce the magnitude, severity, and likelihood of further TOD, generally to reduce systolic ABP to 110 to 150 mm Hg. Because end-organ damage is likely to be directly related to systolic ABP and adversely affected by wide fluctuations in ABP, it is preferable to achieve a stable reduction of ABP to the lower half of this range. Some severely hypertensive animals (i.e., systolic ABP > 250 mm Hg), and those with secondary vascular changes, may exhibit signs of hypotension (i.e., syncope, weakness, exercise intolerance, and prerenal azotemia) when ABP is lowered rapidly. This is uncommon if the systolic ABP is maintained above 120 mm Hg.

Follow-up

Measurement of ABP and assessment for changes related to end-organ damage should be performed at least every 8 to 12 hours initially. Patients receiving parenteral antihypertensive agents should be assessed more frequently, generally at 1- to 3-hour intervals. Choice of agents, drug dosage, and dosage interval should be adjusted according to ABP, with a goal of maintaining a stable systolic ABP between 110 and 150 mm Hg without evidence of effects of low ABP. It is important to carefully reevaluate any patient treated with emergency antihypertensive therapy before instituting further therapy. Follow-up evaluations should include measurement of ABP, funduscopic examination, and other assessments specific to the individual's end-organ damage and concurrent diseases. Once end-organ damage and ABP are stabilized, generally within 3 to 5 days, the transition to an oral antihypertensive regimen should be made gradually.

REFERENCES

1. Brown S, Atkins C, Bagley R, et al: Guidelines for the identification, evaluation, and management of systemic hypertension in dogs and cats, J Vet Intern Med 21:542, 2007.
2. Chobanian AV, Bakris GL, Black HR, et al: The seventh report of the Joint National Committee on Prevention, Detection, Evaluation and Treatment of High Blood Pressure, Hypertension 42:1206, 2003.
3. Guyton AC, Hall JE: Textbook of medical physiology, ed 12, Philadelphia, 2011, Saunders.
4. Donahoe M: Very high systemic arterial blood pressure. In Vincent JL, Abraham E, Moore FA, et al, editors: Textbook of critical care, ed 6, Philadelphia, 2011, Elsevier.
5. Briones AM, Touyz RM: Oxidative stress and hypertension: current concepts, Curr Hypertens Rep 12:135, 2010.
6. Verhaar MC, Beutler JJ, Gaillard CA, et al: Progressive vascular damage in hypertension is associated with increased levels of circulating P-selectin, J Hypertension 16:45, 1998.
7. Gordon DB, Goldblatt H: Direct percutaneous determination of systemic blood pressure and production of renal hypertension in the cat, Proc Soc Exp Biol Med 125:177, 1967.
8. Littman MP: Spontaneous systemic hypertension in 24 cats, J Vet Intern Med 8:79, 1994.
9. Egner B: Blood pressure measurement. In Egner B, Carr A, Brown S, editors: Essential facts of blood pressure in dogs and cats, ed 3, Babenhausen, Germany, 2003, Beate Egner Vet Verlag.
10. Stepien RL, Rapoport GS, Henik RA, et al: Comparative diagnostic test characteristics of oscillometric and Doppler ultrasonographic methods in the detection of systolic hypertension in dogs, J Vet Intern Med 17:65, 2003.
11. Bodey AR, Young LE, Bartram DH, et al: A comparison of direct and indirect (oscillometric) measurements of arterial blood pressure in anaesthetised dogs, using tail and limb cuffs, Res Vet Sci 57:265, 1994.
12. Haberman C, Morgan J, Kang C, et al: Evaluation of indirect blood pressure measurement techniques in cats, Int J Appl Res Vet Med 2:279, 2004.
13. Haberman C, Kang C, Morgan J, et al: Evaluation of indirect blood pressure measurement techniques in dogs, Can J Vet Res 70:211, 2006.
14. Binns SH, Sisson DD, Buoscio DA, et al: Doppler ultrasonographic, oscillometric sphygmomanometric, and photoplethysmographic techniques for noninvasive blood pressure measurement in anesthetized cats, J Vet Intern Med 9:405, 1995.
15. Mishina M, Watanabe T, Fujii K, et al: Noninvasive blood pressure measurements in cats: clinical significance of hypertension associated with chronic renal failure, J Vet Med Sci 60:805, 1998.
16. Stepien RL, Rapoport GS: Clinical comparison of three methods to measure blood pressure in nonsedated dogs, J Am Vet Med Assoc 215:1623, 1999.
17. Belew AM, Barlett T, Brown SA: Evaluation of the white-coat effect in cats, J Vet Intern Med 13:134, 1999.
18. Kallet AJ, Cowgill LD, Kass PH: Comparison of blood pressure measurements obtained in dogs by use of indirect oscillometry in a veterinary clinic versus at home, J Am Vet Med Assoc 210:651, 1997.
19. Elliott J, Barber PJ, Syme HM, et al: Feline hypertension: clinical findings and response to antihypertensive treatment in 30 cases, J Small Anim Pract 42:122, 2001.
20. Stiles J, Polzin DJ, Bistner SI: The prevalence of retinopathy in cats with systemic hypertension and chronic renal failure or hyperthyroidism, J Am Anim Hosp Assoc 30:564, 1994.
21. Sansom J, Rogers K, Wood JL: Blood pressure assessment in healthy cats and cats with hypertensive retinopathy, Am J Vet Res 65:245, 2004.
22. Maggio F, DeFrancesco TC, Atkins CE, et al: Ocular lesions associated with systemic hypertension in cats: 69 cases (1985-1998), J Am Vet Med Assoc 217:695, 2000.
23. Jacob F, Polzin DJ, Osborne CA, et al: Association between initial systolic blood pressure and risk of developing a uremic crisis or of dying in dogs with chronic renal failure, J Am Vet Med Assoc 222:322, 2003.
24. Littman MP, Robertson JL, Bovee KC: Spontaneous systemic hypertension in dogs: five cases (1981-1983), J Am Vet Med Assoc 193:486, 1988.
25. Littman MP: Spontaneous systemic hypertension in 24 cats, J Vet Intern Med 8:79, 1994.
26. Sansom J, Barnett K, Dunn K, et al: Ocular disease associated with hypertension in 16 cats, J Small Anim Pract 35:604, 1994.
27. Leblanc NL, Stepien RL, Bentley E: Oculate lesions associated with systemic hypertension in dogs: 65 cases (2005-2007), J Am Vet Med Assoc 238:915, 2011.
28. Kyles AE, Gregory CR, Wooldridge JD, et al: Management of hypertension controls postoperative neurologic disorders after renal transplantation in cats, Vet Surg 28:436, 1999.
29. Brown CA, Munday J, Mathur S, et al: Hypertensive encephalopathy in cats with reduced renal function, Vet Pathol 42:642, 2005.
30. O'neill J, Kent M, Glass EN, Platt SR. Clinicopathologic and MRI characteristics of presumptive hypertensive encephalopathy in two cats and two dogs, J Am Anim Hosp Assoc 49:412, 2013
31. Kletzmayr J, Uffmann M, Schmaldienst S: Severe but reversible hypertensive encephalopathy, Wien Klin Wochenschr 115:416, 2003.
32. Tejani A: Post-transplant hypertension and hypertensive encephalopathy in renal allograft recipients, Nephron 34:73, 1983.
33. Mathur S, Syme H, Brown CA, et al: Effects of the calcium channel antagonist amlodipine in cats with surgically induced hypertensive renal insufficiency, Am J Vet Res 63:833, 2002.
34. Palatini P: Microalbuminuria in hypertension, Curr Hypertens Rep 5:208, 2003.
35. Jepson RE, Elliott J, Brodbelt D, Syme HM: Effect of control of systolic blood pressure on survival in cats with systemic hypertension, J Vet Intern Med 21:402, 2007.
36. Lesser M, Fox PR, Bond BR: Assessment of hypertension in 40 cats with left ventricular hypertrophy by Doppler-shift sphygmomanometry, J Small Anim Pract 33:55, 1992.
37. Wey AC, Atkins CE: Aortic dissection and congestive heart failure associated with systemic hypertension in a cat, J Vet Intern Med 14:208, 2000.
38. Grauer G, Greco D, Gretzy D, et al: Effects of enalapril treatment versus placebo as a treatment for canine idiopathic glomerulonephritis, J Vet Intern Med 14:526, 2000.
39. Brown SA, Finco DR, Brown CA, et al: Evaluation of the effects of inhibition of angiotensin-converting enzyme with enalapril in dogs with induced chronic renal insufficiency, Am J Vet Res 64:321, 2003.
40. Brown SA, Walton CL, Crawford P, et al: Long-term effects of antihypertensive regimens on renal hemodynamics and proteinuria, Kidney Int 43:1210, 1993.
41. Gaber L, Walton C, Brown S, et al: Effects of different antihypertensive treatments on morphologic progression of diabetic nephropathy in uninephrectomized dogs, Kidney Int 46:161, 1994.

CHAPTER 10

HYPERTHERMIA AND FEVER

James B. Miller, DVM, MS, DACVIM

KEY POINTS

- Thermoregulation is controlled by the preoptic region of the hypothalamus. It responds to thermoreceptors in the brain and peripheral nervous system to maintain a narrow range of body temperature by increasing either heat production or loss.
- Hyperthermia describes any elevation in core body temperature above accepted normal values.
- A true fever is the body's normal response to infection, inflammation, or injury and is part of the acute-phase response. It is controlled by the thermoregulatory center in the hypothalamus.
- Other forms of hyperthermia are a result of an imbalance between heat production and heat loss. Hyperthermic patients are approached differently from those with a fever, both diagnostically and therapeutically.
- A fever may be beneficial to the host by decreasing bacterial growth and inhibiting viral replication. Most fevers are not a threat to life unless body temperature exceeds 107° F (41.6° C).
- A fever will increase water and caloric requirements, and this must be considered when treating the febrile patient.
- In most cases an accurate diagnosis should be obtained before initiating nonspecific therapy for a fever.
- Nonsteroidal antiinflammatory drugs and glucocorticoids will reduce a fever, but the latter will also block the acute-phase inflammatory response.
- Total body cooling may be counterproductive and usually is reserved for afebrile hyperthermia or when fevers approach 107° F (41.6° C).
- Antimicrobial therapy should not be used empirically for fever management unless there is a documented or strongly suspected indication of infection. Treatment should be based on culture and sensitivity testing, as indicated.

Obtaining a body temperature measurement is important in the evaluation of all patients, especially the critically ill patient. A rectal temperature higher than 102.5° F (39.2° C) is considered elevated in the unstressed dog or cat. The method of measurement must also be taken into account because ear, axillary, or toe web measurements will be lower than rectal temperatures. An intravascular thermistor is considered most accurate but is usually impractical in the clinical setting.

It is tempting for the veterinarian to associate any elevation in body temperature with true fever. The assumption is often made that the fever is caused by an infectious agent, even if there is no obvious cause. If the patient's fever resolves after antimicrobials are administered, the assumption is made that it was caused by a bacterial infection. A normal body temperature is often assumed to indicate the absence of infectious disease. This approach to fever, hyperthermia, or normothermia can be misleading and result in inaccurate diagnoses and inappropriate, or even lack of, therapy. In one French study almost half the 50 febrile dogs that were retrospectively examined had a noninfectious cause for the increased body temperature.[1]

THERMOREGULATION

Thermoregulation is the balance between heat loss and heat production. Metabolic, physiologic, and behavioral mechanisms are used by homeotherms to regulate heat loss and production. The thermoregulatory control center for the body is located in the central nervous system in the preoptic area of the anterior hypothalamus (AH).[2] Changes in ambient and core body temperatures are sensed by the peripheral and central thermoreceptors, and information is conveyed to the AH via the nervous system. The thermoreceptors sense that the body is below or above its normal temperature (set point) and subsequently cause the AH to stimulate the body to increase heat production and reduce heat loss through conservation if the body is too cold or to dissipate heat if the body is too warm (Figure 10-1). Through these mechanisms, the dog and cat can maintain a narrow core body temperature range in a wide variety of environmental conditions and activity levels. With normal ambient temperatures, most body heat is produced by muscular activity, even while at rest. Cachectic or anesthetized patients, or those with severe neurologic impairment, may not be able to maintain a normal set point or generate a normal response to changes in core body temperature.

HYPERTHERMIA

Hyperthermia is the term used to describe any elevation in core body temperature above the accepted normal range for that species. When heat is produced or stored in the body at a rate greater than it is lost, hyperthermia results.[3] The term *fever* is reserved for those hyperthermic animals in whom the set point in the AH has been reset to a higher temperature. In hyperthermic states other than fever, temperature elevation is not a result of the body attempting to raise its temperature but is due to the physiologic, pathologic, or pharmacologic changes that cause heat gain to exceed heat loss. Box 10-1 outlines the various classifications of hyperthermia.

TRUE FEVER

True fever is a normal response of the body to invasion or injury and is part of the acute-phase response.[4] Other parts of the acute-phase response include increased neutrophil numbers and phagocytic ability, enhanced T and B lymphocyte activity, increased acute-phase protein production by the liver, increased fibroblast activity, and increased sleep. Fever and other parts of the acute-phase response are initiated by exogenous pyrogens that lead to the release of endogenous pyrogens (Figure 10-2).[5]

Exogenous Pyrogens

True fever may be initiated by a variety of substances, including infectious agents or their products, immune complex formation, tissue inflammation or necrosis, and several pharmacologic agents. Collectively, these substances are called *exogenous pyrogens.* Their ability to directly affect the thermoregulatory center is probably minimal

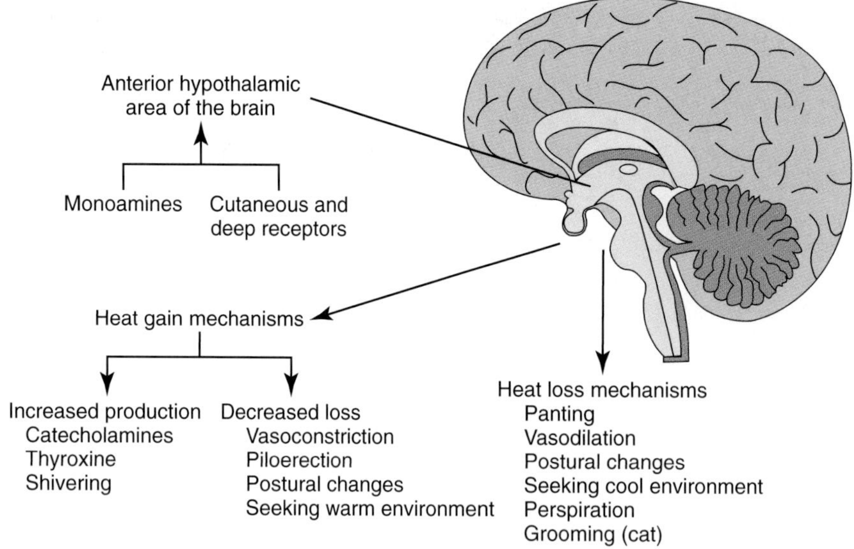

FIGURE 10-1 Schematic representation of normal thermoregulation. *(From Miller JB: Hyperthermia and fever of unknown origin. In Ettinger SJ, Feldman EC, editors: Textbook of veterinary internal medicine, ed 10, St Louis, 2010, Saunders.)*

BOX 10-1 *Classification of Hyperthermia*

True Fever

Production of endogenous pyrogens

Inadequate Heat Dissipation

Heat stroke
Hyperpyrexic syndromes

Exercise-Induced Hyperthermia

Normal exercise
Hypocalcemic tetany (eclampsia)
Seizure disorders

Pathologic or Pharmacologic Origin

Lesions in or around the anterior hypothalamus
Malignant hyperthermia
Hypermetabolic disorders
Monoamine metabolism disturbances

From Miller JB: Hyperthermia and fever of unknown origin. In Ettinger SJ, Feldman EC, editors: Textbook of veterinary internal medicine, ed 10, St Louis, 2010, Saunders.

and they primarily cause the release of endogenous pyrogens by the host. Box 10-2 lists some of the more important known exogenous pyrogens.

Endogenous Pyrogens

In response to stimulation by an exogenous pyrogen, proteins (cytokines) released from cells of the immune system trigger the febrile response. Macrophages are the primary immune cells involved, although T and B lymphocytes and other leukocytes may play significant roles. The proteins produced are called *endogenous pyrogens* or *fever-producing cytokines.* Although interleukin 1, interleukin 6, and tumor necrosis factor α are considered the most important fever-producing cytokines, at least 11 cytokines are capable of initiating a febrile response (Table 10-1).

Some neoplastic cells are also capable of producing cytokines that lead to a febrile response. The cytokines travel via the bloodstream to the AH, where they bind to the vascular endothelial cells within the AH and stimulate the release of prostaglandins (PGs), primarily PGE_2 and possibly $PGF_{2\alpha}$. The set point is raised and the core body temperature rises through increased heat production and conservation.

INADEQUATE HEAT DISSIPATION

Heat Stroke

Heat stroke is a common result of inadequate heat dissipation (see Chapter 149). Exposure to high ambient temperatures may increase heat load at a faster rate than it can be dissipated from the body. This is especially true in larger breeds of dogs and obese or brachycephalic animals. Heat stroke may occur rapidly, especially in closed environments with poor ventilation (e.g., inside a car with the windows closed on a moderately hot day). Environmental temperatures inside a closed car exposed to direct sun may exceed 120° F (48° C) in less than 20 minutes, even when the outside temperature is only 75° F (24° C). Death may occur in less than an hour, especially in the predisposed animal types described earlier.

Heat stroke will not respond to antipyretics used for the management of a true fever. The severely hyperthermic patient must undergo immediate total body cooling to prevent organ damage or death. Mechanisms of heat loss from the body include the following: radiation (electromagnetic or heat exchange between objects in the environment), conduction (between the body and environmental objects that are in direct contact with the skin, as determined by the relative temperatures and gradients), convection (the movement of fluid, air, or water over the surface of the body), and evaporation (disruption of heat by the energy required to convert the material from a liquid to a gas, as with panting). There are numerous strategies for cooling the hyperthermic patient (Box 10-3), and the techniques chosen should be based on the severity of the animal's condition, temperature, and response to therapy.

In most veterinary patients, total body cooling is best accomplished by administering intravenous fluid therapy (see Chapter 60), providing water baths and rinses using tepid water, and placing a fan near the animal. If the water applied to the animal is too cold, there is a tendency for peripheral vasoconstriction that will inhibit radiant heat loss and slow the cooling process. Cooling should be

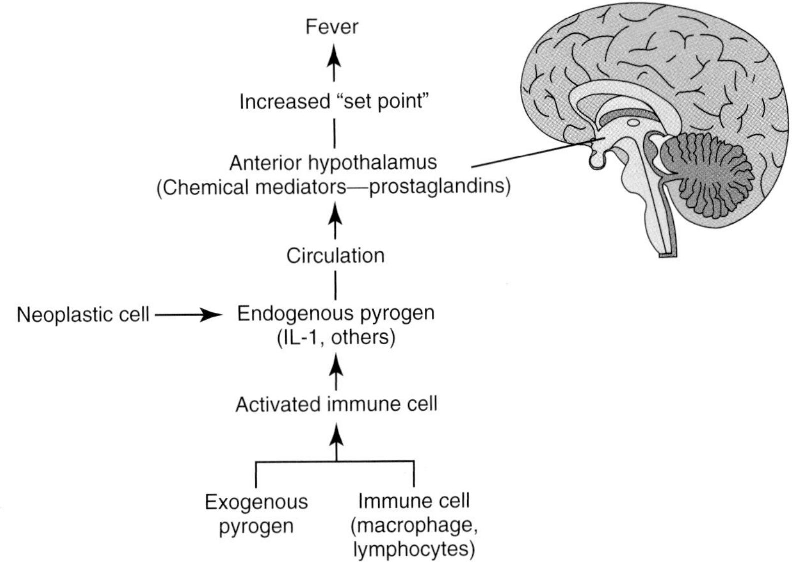

FIGURE 10-2 Schematic representation of the pathophysiology of fever. *(From Miller JB: Hyperthermia and fever of unknown origin. In Ettinger SJ, Feldman EC, editors: Textbook of veterinary internal medicine, ed 10, St Louis, 2010, Saunders.)*

BOX 10-2 ***Exogenous Pyrogens***

Infectious Agents

Bacteria (Live and Killed)

Gram positive

Gram negative

Bacterial Products

Lipopolysaccharides

Streptococcal exotoxin

Staphylococcal enterotoxin

Staphylococcal proteins

Fungi (Live and Killed)

Fungal products

Cryptococcal polysaccharide

Cryptococcal proteins

Viruses

Rickettsiae

Protozoa

Nonmicrobial Agents

Soluble Antigen-Antibody Complexes

Bile Acids

Pharmacologic Agents

Bleomycin

Colchicine

Tetracycline

Levamisole (cats)

Tissue Inflammation and Necrosis

From Miller JB: Hyperthermia and fever of unknown origin. In Ettinger SJ, Feldman EC, editors: Textbook of veterinary internal medicine, ed 7, St Louis, 2010, Saunders.

Table 10-1 Proteins with Pyrogenic Activity

Endogenous Pyrogen	Principal Source
Cachectin (TNF-α)	Macrophages
Lymphotoxin (TNF-β)	Lymphocytes (T and B)
IL-1α	Macrophages and many other cell types
IL-1β	Macrophages and many other cell types
Interferon α	Leukocytes (especially monocytes/macrophages)
Interferon β	Fibroblasts
Interferon γ	T lymphocytes
IL-6	Many cell types
Macrophage inflammatory protein 1α	Macrophages
Macrophage inflammatory protein 1β	Macrophages
IL-8	Macrophages

IL, Interleukin; *TNF*, tumor necrosis factor.

From Miller JB: Hyperthermia and fever of unknown origin. In Ettinger SJ, Feldman EC, editors: Textbook of veterinary internal medicine, ed 7, St Louis, 2010, Saunders. Adapted from Beutler B, Beutler SM: The pathogenesis of fever. In Bennett JC, Plum F, editors: Cecil textbook of medicine, ed 20, Philadelphia, 1996, Saunders.

discontinued when body temperature approaches normal (approximately 103° F [39.4° C]) to prevent iatrogenic hypothermia.

Hyperpyrexic Syndrome

Hyperpyrexic syndrome is associated with moderate to severe exercise in hot and humid climates. This syndrome may be more common in hunting dogs or dogs that "jog" with their owners. In humid environments, evaporative cooling via panting is minimal. In addition, heavy exercise may lead to vasodilation and increased blood flow to skeletal muscles but vasoconstriction of cutaneous vessels, thus compromising peripheral heat loss.

Many hunting dogs and dogs that run with their owners will continue to work or run until they become weak, stagger, and collapse. In suspected cases of hyperpyrexic syndrome, owners should measure the dog's rectal temperature at the first sign that the dog is becoming weak or does not want to continue. Owners should be instructed that rectal temperatures above 106° F (41° C) require immediate total body cooling and temperatures above 107° F (41.6° C) may lead to permanent organ damage or death.

Exercise-Induced Hyperthermia

The body temperature will rise with sustained exercise of even moderate intensity because of heat production associated with muscular activity. Even when extreme heat and humidity are not factors, dogs will occasionally reach temperatures that require total body cooling. This is especially true in dogs that do not exercise frequently, have thick undercoats, are overweight, or have respiratory disease.

BOX 10-3 ***Cooling Options for the Hyperthermic Patient***

Oxygen and Intravenous Isotonic Fluid Therapy

Surface Cooling Techniques

Clip fur if indicated
Tepid water applied to skin or whole body (manually or via bath)
Fan
Ice packs over areas with large vessels (neck, axilla, inguinal region)
Combination of above techniques

Internal Cooling Techniques

Rectal administration of cool isotonic fluids
Gastric lavage
Open body cavity
Peritoneal dialysis

Extracorporeal Techniques

Antipyretic Drugs

Antiprostaglandins
Dantrolene
Dipyrone
Aminopyrine
COX-2 inhibitors
Glucocorticoids
Additional NSAIDs

COX-2, Cyclooxygenase-2; *NSAIDs,* nonsteroidal antiinflammatory drugs.

Eclampsia results in extreme muscular activity that can lead to significant heat production and result in severe hyperthermia. Total body cooling should be initiated if the patient is hyperthermic, in conjunction with therapy for the eclampsia (see Chapter 52).

Seizure disorders from organic, metabolic, or idiopathic causes are encountered often in small animals (see Chapter 82). Hyperthermia associated with increased muscular activity can result, especially if the seizures are prolonged or occur in clusters. The initial concern of the clinician should be to stop the seizures, but when significant hyperthermia is present, total body cooling is also recommended.

Pathologic and Pharmacologic Hyperthermia

The pathologic and pharmacologic types of hyperthermia encompass several disorders that will impair the heat balance equation. Hypothalamic lesions may obliterate the thermoregulatory center, leading to impaired responses to both hot and cold environments. Malignant hyperthermia (MH) has been reported in dogs and cats. It leads to a myopathy and subsequent metabolic heat production secondary to disturbed calcium metabolism that is initiated by pharmacologic agents such as inhalation anesthetics (especially halothane) and muscle relaxants such as succinylcholine. Extreme muscle rigidity may or may not be present. Removal of the offending causative agent and total body cooling may prevent death. Dantrolene sodium, a muscle relaxant, is a specific and effective therapy for malignant hyperthermia and acts by binding to the ryanodine receptor to depress excitation-contraction coupling in skeletal muscle. It is dosed at 1 to 3 mg/kg IV or 1 to 5 mg/kg PO.

Hypermetabolic disorders may also lead to hyperthermic states. Endocrine disorders such as hyperthyroidism and pheochromocytoma can lead to an increased metabolic rate or vasoconstriction, resulting in excess heat production, decreased ability to dissipate heat, or both. These conditions rarely lead to severe hyperthermia that requires total body cooling.

BENEFITS AND DETRIMENTS OF FEVER

Benefits

Fever is part of the acute-phase response and is a normal response of the body. Even poikilotherms such as fish and reptiles will respond to a pyrogen by seeking higher environmental temperatures to raise their body temperatures.[6] It is logical to think that a true fever is beneficial to the host. Most studies have shown that a fever will reduce the duration of morbidity and decrease mortality from many infectious diseases. A fever decreases the ability of many bacteria to use iron, which is necessary for them to live and replicate.[6] Use of nonsteroidal antiinflammatory drugs (NSAIDs) to block fever in rabbits with *Pasteurella* infections significantly increases mortality rates. Many viruses are heat sensitive and cannot replicate in high temperatures. Raising the body temperature in neonatal dogs with herpesvirus infections significantly reduces the mortality rate.

Detriments

Hyperthermia increases tissue metabolism and oxygen consumption, thus raising both caloric and water requirements by approximately 7% for each degree Fahrenheit (0.6° C) above accepted normal values. In addition, hyperthermia leads to suppression of the appetite center in the hypothalamus but usually not the thirst center. Animals that have sustained head trauma or a cerebrovascular accident may suffer more severe brain damage if coexisting hyperthermia is present; total body cooling may be beneficial in these patients.

Body temperatures above 107° F (41.6° C) often lead to increases in cellular oxygen consumption that exceed oxygen delivery, resulting in deterioration of cellular function and integrity. This may lead to disseminated intravascular coagulation (DIC) (see Chapter 104), with thrombosis and bleeding, or cause serious damage to organ systems, including the brain (cerebral edema and subsequent confusion, delirium, obtundation, seizures, coma); heart (arrhythmias); liver (hypoglycemia, hyperbilirubinemia); gastrointestinal tract (epithelial desquamation, endotoxin absorption, bleeding); and kidneys (acute kidney injury). (For further details, see Chapters 7 and 149). Additional abnormalities might include hypoxemia, hyperkalemia, skeletal muscle cytolysis, tachypnea, metabolic acidosis, tachycardia, tachypnea, and hyperventilation.

Exertional heat stroke and malignant hyperthermia may lead to severe rhabdomyolysis, hyperkalemia, hypocalcemia, myoglobinemia, and myoglobinuria and elevated levels of creatine phosphokinase. Fortunately, true fevers rarely lead to body temperatures of this magnitude and are usually a result of other causes of hyperthermia that should be managed as medical emergencies.

CLINICAL APPROACH TO THE HYPERTHERMIC PATIENT

The evaluation of the hyperthermic patient should be approached in a logical manner to avoid making erroneous conclusions.[3] A complete history and physical examination should be performed unless the patient is critically ill or severely hyperthermic (temperature higher than 106° F [41° C]). In such cases, immediate total body cooling and supportive care should be initiated.

In stable patients, a thorough physical examination and specific questions concerning previous injuries or infections, exposure to other animals, disease in other household pets, previous geographic environment, and previous or current drug therapy are beneficial. This approach enables the clinician to decide if the elevated body temperature is a true fever. Temperatures less than 106° F (41° C), unless prolonged, are usually not life threatening, and antipyretic therapy should not be administered before performing a proper clinical evaluation.

NONSPECIFIC THERAPY FOR FEBRILE PATIENTS

Mild to moderate elevations in body temperature are rarely fatal and may be beneficial to the body. As stated before, hyperthermia may inhibit viral replication, increase leukocyte function, and decrease the uptake of iron by microbes (which is often necessary for their growth and replication). If a fever exceeds 107° F (41.6° C), there is a significant risk of permanent organ damage and DIC. The benefits of nonspecific therapy versus its potential negative effects should be considered before initiating such management.

Nonspecific therapy for true fever usually involves inhibitors of prostaglandin synthesis. The compounds most commonly used are the NSAIDs. These products inhibit the chemical mediators of fever production and allow normal thermoregulation. They do not block the production of endogenous pyrogens.[3] These products are relatively safe, although acetylsalicylic acid is potentially very toxic to the cat (cyclooxygenase-2 [COX-2] inhibitors are relatively safe) and animals with gastrointestinal ulceration or renal disease should not receive these drugs. Consensus guidelines have been published on the use on NSAIDS in cats.[7] Dipyrone, an injectable nonsteroidal antiinflammatory drug sometimes used in cats, may lead to bone marrow suppression, especially with prolonged use.

Total body cooling with water, fans, or both in a febrile patient will reduce body temperature; however, the thermoregulatory center in the hypothalamus will still be directing the body to increase the body temperature. This may result in a further increase in metabolic rate, oxygen consumption, and subsequent water and caloric requirements. Unless a fever is life threatening, this type of nonspecific therapy is counterproductive.

Glucocorticoids block the acute-phase response, fever, and most other parts of this (adaptive) response. In general, their use should be reserved for those patients in whom the cause of the fever is known to be noninfectious and blocking the rest of the acute-phase response will not be detrimental (and may prove beneficial). The most common indications include some immune-mediated diseases in which fever plays a significant role and glucocorticoid therapy is often part of the chemotherapeutic protocol (e.g., immune-mediated hemolytic anemia, immune-mediated polyarthritis).

Phenothiazines can be effective in alleviating a true fever by depressing normal thermoregulation and causing peripheral vasodilation. The sedative qualities of the phenothiazines and their potential for hypotension should be considered before administration to the febrile patient.

THE FEBRILE INTENSIVE CARE PATIENT

Fever is a common problem in critically ill veterinary patients. The clinician must attempt to exclude noninfectious causes and then determine the infection site and likely pathogens (see Chapter 175). Intensive care patients often have both infectious and noninfectious causes of fever, necessitating a systematic and comprehensive diagnostic approach. Altered immune function, indwelling catheter devices, and more invasive monitoring and treatment approaches put these patients at high risk for inflammation and nosocomial infections.

Noninfectious causes of fever in intensive care patients commonly include phlebitis or thrombophlebitis, postoperative inflammation, posttransfusion reactions, pancreatitis, hepatitis, cholecystitis, aspiration pneumonitis, acute respiratory distress syndrome, and neoplastic processes.

Nosocomial infection in critically ill patients is an important cause of new-onset fevers. Although incidence studies have not been performed in veterinary patients, the reported range in people is 3% to 31%. Commonly implicated sources include the lungs (aspiration or ventilator-associated pneumonia), the bloodstream, catheters, incisions, and the urinary tract. An initial diagnostic evaluation might include a complete blood cell count, thoracic and abdominal imaging, and close inspection of all catheter sites or incisions. Additional diagnostic tests that might be indicated include culture and sensitivity testing of blood, urine, airway fluid, pleural or peritoneal effusions, postoperative incisions, cerebrospinal fluid, joint fluid, nasal discharge, and diarrhea.

Antimicrobial therapy is indicated for the febrile patient only when a specific pathogen is known or strongly suspected.[3] The use of antimicrobials in these patients without knowledge that a microbial agent is causing the fever can lead to bacterial resistance (see Chapter 175). Dogs with evidence of a systemic inflammatory response syndrome have a higher mortality rate,[8] and the source should be rapidly identified and treated (see Chapter 6). However, if an infectious cause is not suspected and the patient is not deteriorating or neutropenic, antimicrobial additions or changes should be delayed until more definitive information is obtained.

REFERENCES

1. Chervier C, Chabanne L, Godde M, et al: Causes, diagnostic signs, and the utility of investigations of fever in dogs: 50 cases, Can Vet J 53(5):525, 2012.
2. Cunningham JG: Textbook of veterinary physiology, ed 2, St Louis, 1997, Saunders.
3. Mackowiac PA: Approach to the febrile patient. In Humes HD, editor: Kelley's textbook of internal medicine, ed 4, Philadelphia, 2000, Lippincott Williams & Wilkins.
4. Dinarella CA: The acute phase response. In Bennet JC, Plum F, editors: Cecil textbook of medicine, ed 20, Philadelphia, 1996, Saunders.
5. Beutler B, Buetler SM: The pathogenesis of fever. In Bennet JC, Plum F, editors: Cecil textbook of medicine, ed 20, Philadelphia, 1996, Saunders.
6. Berlin MT, Abeche AM: Evolutionary approach to medicine, South Med J 94:26, 2001.
7. Sparkes AH et al: ISFM and AAFP Consensus guidelines, long-term use of NSAIDs in cats, J Feline Med Surg 12(7):521, 2010.
8. DeClue AE: Biomarkers for sepsis in small animals. In Proceedings of the annual meeting of the ACVP/ASVCP, Seattle, WA, December 2012.

CHAPTER 11
INTERSTITIAL EDEMA

Randolph H. Stewart, DVM, PhD, DACVIM (Internal Medicine)

KEY POINTS

- Interstitial fluid is formed by filtration out of microvessels and removed via the lymphatic system or transudation across the serosal surface of a visceral organ.
- Interstitial edema and an increased interstitial fluid volume commonly form in response to increased microvascular pressure, increased microvascular permeability, and inflammatory-related changes in mechanical relationships within the interstitial space.
- Interstitial edema impairs tissue function by impeding oxygen diffusion to cells and altering the mechanical properties of the affected tissue.
- Management of interstitial edema requires an appreciation of the forces and tissue properties involved in interstitial fluid volume regulation.

Interstitial edema formation, an increase in interstitial fluid volume, is a common clinical condition observed in conjunction with heart failure, venous thrombosis, protein-losing disorders, excessive crystalloid administration, anaphylaxis, burns, and inflammatory disease/systemic inflammatory response syndrome (SIRS). Interstitial edema can negatively affect many organ systems, such as the skin, lung, intestine, brain, skeletal muscle, kidney, and heart. The presence of edema in these organs impairs proper oxygen delivery and cellular function in addition to altering the mechanical properties of the tissue (e.g., pulmonary compliance).

Because each organ system possesses a unique set of tissue properties, the specific manner in which each organ responds to an edemagenic challenge is necessarily organ specific. However, a common set of principles and mechanisms govern interstitial volume, pressure, and flow in all organs. Interstitial fluid volume is determined by the balance between filtration out of capillaries and venules into the interstitial space and lymphatic removal of that interstitial fluid. In organs located within body cavities—the heart, lungs, liver, and intestines—transudation of interstitial fluid across the organ's serosal surface into the surrounding space provides an additional avenue for interstitial fluid removal. The variable primarily responsible for mediating the balance between microvascular filtration and the two interstitial outflows is the interstitial fluid pressure.[1] An increase in interstitial pressure acts to inhibit filtration and simultaneously promote lymph flow and serosal transudation. The interstitial fluid volume depends on the interstitial fluid pressure and the current interstitial pressure–volume relationship.

MICROVASCULAR FILTRATION

The microvascular filtration rate is determined by forces and tissue properties modeled in the Starling-Landis equation:

Equation 1 $$J_V = L_pA[(P_{mv} - P_{int}) - \sigma_d(\Pi_p - \Pi_{int})]$$

where J_V is the microvascular filtration rate; L_p is the hydraulic conductivity (a measure of water permeability); A is the filtration surface area; P_{mv} and P_{int} are the hydrostatic pressures within the microvessels and interstitial space, respectively; σ_d is the osmotic reflection coefficient; and Π_p and Π_{int} are the colloid osmotic pressures exerted by plasma and interstitial fluid, respectively.[2]

Recent findings in some microvascular beds have resulted in a revision of the Starling-Landis principle based on two related ideas: (1) the endothelial glycocalyx is the primary barrier to microvascular filtration and (2) the colloid osmotic pressure of the fluid on the interstitial side of the glycocalyx and within the endothelial clefts has a more direct effect on filtration than that of the free interstitial fluid. The colloid osmotic pressure of this fluid can be substantially lower than that of the free interstitial fluid because of the combined effects of protein sieving by the endothelial glycocalyx and the convective flow of filtered fluid through the clefts.[2] Reversal of fluid flow across the microvascular barrier upsets this colloid osmotic pressure gradient and limits fluid reabsorption by the microvasculature.[2]

The Starling-Landis equation shows that the direction of microvascular filtration depends on the sum of the hydrostatic and colloid osmotic pressure gradients, whereas the magnitude of filtration is the product of the hydraulic conductivity, surface area, and net pressure gradient. P_{mv} in most organs is estimated between 7 and 17 mm Hg. That pressure is opposed by P_{int}, which in many tissues, such as subcutaneous tissue, lung, and resting skeletal muscle, is subatmospheric. This establishes a hydrostatic pressure gradient ($P_{mv} - P_{int}$) favoring filtration out of the microvessels into the interstitial space. The colloid osmotic pressure gradient, however, opposes filtration and favors retention of fluid within the microvasculature. Colloid osmotic pressure of plasma and interstitial fluid is a consequence of the concentration of proteins, particularly albumin, as well as the redistribution of permeable ions induced by the presence of the charges on those proteins. The colloid osmotic pressure of plasma is predictably higher than that of interstitial fluid; however, the interstitial fluid protein concentration and colloid osmotic pressure are not as low as commonly reported in textbooks. The protein concentration within the myocardial interstitial fluid is usually 70% to 80% that of plasma. It is similarly high in the interstitial fluid of the lung, skin, skeletal muscle, intestine, kidney, and liver.[3]

The colloid osmotic pressure gradient in Equation 1, $\Pi_p - \Pi_{int}$, is modified by σ_d. This coefficient is a function of the protein permeability of the microvascular barrier and possesses a value between 0 (indicating a membrane that is freely permeable to protein) and 1 (for a membrane that is impermeable to protein). The fraction of the colloid osmotic pressure gradient that is expressed across the microvascular barrier is represented by σ_d. Its value is close to 1 for the blood-brain barrier, and it approaches 0 for the sinusoids of the liver.

In most microvascular beds, there is a small net pressure gradient favoring filtration. The commonly reported view that filtration occurs at the arteriolar end of the capillary and reabsorption occurs at the venular end is not supported by experimental or theoretical analysis. Current evidence indicates that all the microvascular filtrate is removed by lymphatic drainage or transserosal flow and little or no microvascular reabsorption occurs under normal conditions in most tissues.[2]

LYMPHATIC DRAINAGE

The lymphatic system removes interstitial fluid and returns it to the venous blood. This system begins with terminal lymphatic vessels within the interstitial space, converges to progressively larger vessels through lymph nodes, and eventually terminates in the venous system. The determinants of lymph flow have been modeled on a modification of Ohm's law as given here:

Equation 2 $$Q_L = (P_{int} + P_{pump} - P_{sv})/R_L$$

where Q_L is lymph flow, P_{int} is the interstitial hydrostatic pressure, P_{pump} is the effective driving pressure generated by the cyclic intrinsic contraction and extrinsic compression of the lymphatic vessels working in concert with one-way valves, P_{sv} is systemic venous pressure, and R_L is the effective lymphatic resistance.[4]

Most lymphatic vessels possess intramural smooth muscle and contain one-way valves at regular intervals. Spontaneous phasic contraction and extrinsic compression of these vessels propel lymph antegrade. Lymphatic pumping explains why lymph is able flow from an interstitial space with subatmospheric pressure to the systemic venous blood where the pressure is 2 to 5 mm Hg.

Lymph flow is regulated by multiple factors. The strength and frequency of lymphatic contractions are modified by numerous vasoactive mediators, including prostaglandins, thromboxane, nitric oxide, epinephrine, acetylcholine, substance P, and bradykinin. In addition, increased stretch of lymphatic vessels stimulates increased strength and frequency of lymphatic contractions, and increased lymph flow results in a shear-mediated relaxation.[5,6] This shear-mediated response has a beneficial but counterintuitive effect. After edema-induced elevations in lymph flow, the reduction in lymphatic pumping further enhances flow because when lymphatic inlet pressure exceeds outlet pressure, passive flow can exceed the pumping capacity of the vessel.[7]

Pleural fluid and peritoneal fluid are removed by lymphatic drainage and returned to the venous circulation. This fluid exits these cavities through direct connections called lymphatic stomata into lymphatic vessels within the diaphragm and body wall.[8]

The lymphatic system drains into the great veins of the neck; therefore, systemic venous pressure is the downstream pressure against which lymph must flow (see Equation 2). Because of this arrangement, elevations in venous pressure can diminish lymph flow and therefore contribute to edema formation. This effect, however, is usually modest in unanesthetized animals. The lymphatic circulation is normally more sensitive to changes in interstitial pressure than it is to changes in systemic venous pressure. In other words, although lymph flow generally increases markedly in response to interstitial edema formation, it does not usually decrease markedly in response to venous hypertension. This is because lymphatic vessels respond to increased outflow pressure by increasing pumping activity via increases in the strength and frequency of contractions. However, in the presence of interstitial edema caused by increased microvascular filtration, increased neck vein pressure may significantly impede lymph flows and alter interstitial fluid balance.[9] In addition, many anesthetic agents significantly reduce lymphatic pumping and thus increase lymphatic sensitivity to venous hypertension. This means that the sensitivity to edemagenic challenges such as intravenous crystalloid administration is exaggerated in anesthetized patients.

SEROSAL TRANSUDATION

In organs suspended within potential spaces, such as the heart, lung, liver, and intestines, interstitial fluid may be removed, in part, via transudation across the serosal surface. This process is driven by the hydrostatic and colloid osmotic pressure gradients like those seen in Equation 1. Edema-induced increases in interstitial hydrostatic pressure will increase the rate of transudation and may result in effusion within the surrounding cavity.[10]

ANTIEDEMA MECHANISMS

When confronted with an edemagenic insult, interstitial edema formation is moderated by a set of antiedema mechanisms. These intrinsic interdependent mechanisms include (1) increased interstitial hydrostatic pressure, (2) increased lymph flow, (3) decreased interstitial colloid osmotic pressure, and (4) increased transserosal flow in organs within potential spaces. Interstitial pressure opposes microvascular filtration and promotes lymph flow and transserosal flow. In response to increased microvascular pressure, lymph flow can increase tenfold in many tissues. Increased microvascular filtration is characterized by an increase in water filtration that exceeds that of protein. This decrease in the protein concentration of the filtrate results in a fall in interstitial colloid osmotic pressure, which acts to reduce microvascular filtration (see Equation 1). Serosal transudation is enhanced by the combined effects of increased P_{int} and decreased Π_{int}.

These self-regulating mechanisms are efficient because they incur little energy cost and are effective because they respond rapidly to edema formation; however, their effectiveness diminishes in the presence of continued challenge. Therefore a patient that has responded to an edemagenic stress (e.g., hypoproteinemia) is at increased risk of edema development in response to additional challenge, such as crystalloid infusion.

MECHANISMS OF EDEMA FORMATION

The pathophysiology of interstitial edema formation involves changes in the factors responsible for interstitial fluid formation and removal (Table 11-1). However, edemagenic diseases commonly result

Table 11-1 Edemagenic Conditions with Related Mechanisms and Example Disease Processes

Condition	Mechanism	Relevant Disease Processes
Venous hypertension	Increased microvascular pressure and filtration	Heart disease, venous thrombosis
Hypoproteinemia	Decreased plasma colloid osmotic pressure, increased filtration	Protein-losing enteropathy and nephropathy
Increased microvascular permeability	Increased filtration, diminished influence of microvessel-interstitium colloid osmotic pressure gradient	Inflammation, infection
Impaired lymph flow	Vessel obstruction or damage, pharmacologic impairment of contractility	Trauma, surgical damage, systemic venous hypertension, anesthesia
Inflammatory edema	Shift in interstitial pressure–volume relationship, decreased interstitial pressure	Inflammation, anaphylaxis, burn injury, frostbite

in perturbations of more than one of these factors. In addition, therapeutic measures, such as intravenous fluid administration, may exacerbate these perturbations. In fact, because the pathogenesis of edemagenic disease processes may be quite complex, it is perhaps more beneficial clinically to emphasize the degree to which the sensitivity of the fluid balance system has been changed rather than the specific effects of changes in microvascular pressure, permeability, and so on. The degree to which the sensitivity of the system to edemagenic challenge, termed *edemagenic gain,* can be changed has been illustrated for histamine and endotoxin.[11]

Five basic edemagenic conditions are discussed next and shown in Table 11-1. It should also be noted that, although clinical assessment of interstitial edema is often limited to the lungs and subcutaneous tissue, other organs, such as the heart, liver, and intestines, may also be significantly affected.

Venous Hypertension

Elevations in venous pressure seen with heart failure, venous thrombosis, and cirrhotic liver disease reliably cause regional increases in microvascular pressure. The resulting increase in microvascular filtration (seen in Equation 1) expands interstitial fluid volume in the tissues drained by the affected veins. The severity of the edema is directly proportional to the magnitude of the venous pressure increase. In addition, hypertension affecting the central veins can retard lymph flow, particularly in anesthetized patients, because it increases lymphatic outflow pressure.

Hypoproteinemia

An acute decrease in plasma colloid osmotic pressure resulting from hypoproteinemia, particularly hypoalbuminemia, results in increased microvascular filtration (see Equation 1). The relationship between the degree of hypoproteinemia and the resulting edema formation is nonlinear such that mild to moderate protein deficits cause little edema formation. This nonlinearity is likely caused by the engagement of antiedema mechanisms that readily compensate for mild to moderate hypoproteinemia. However, because the protective mechanisms are already engaged, even moderate hypoproteinemia can make the patient particularly susceptible to further edemagenic challenge (e.g., crystalloid infusion).

Increased Microvascular Permeability

According to Equation 1, apparent changes in microvascular permeability may involve changes in water permeability (L_p), microvascular surface area (A), and protein permeability (σ_d). Experimentally, it is very difficult to differentiate between changes in L_p and changes in A. If L_p or A increase, the microvascular filtration rate will be greater for any given transmembrane pressure gradient. If protein permeability increases, the microvascular filtration rate increases because the effectiveness with which the plasma-to-interstitium colloid osmotic pressure gradient restrains water filtration is diminished. This increase in protein permeability also impairs the effectiveness of the fall in interstitial colloid osmotic pressure to serve as an antiedema mechanism.

Impaired Lymph Flow

In the short term, lymphatic obstruction or functional impairment generally results in only mild edema formation caused by the diminished interstitial fluid removal. However, the combination of impaired lymph flow with any additional edemagenic challenge can result in profound edema. This is true not only because increased lymph flow is a very important antiedema mechanism but because the effectiveness of the other antiedema mechanisms—decreased interstitial colloid osmotic pressure and increased transserosal flow—is dependent on adequate lymph flow. Recall that the inhibitory effect of systemic venous hypertension on lymph flow is increased in anesthetized patients and patients with preexisting interstitial edema.

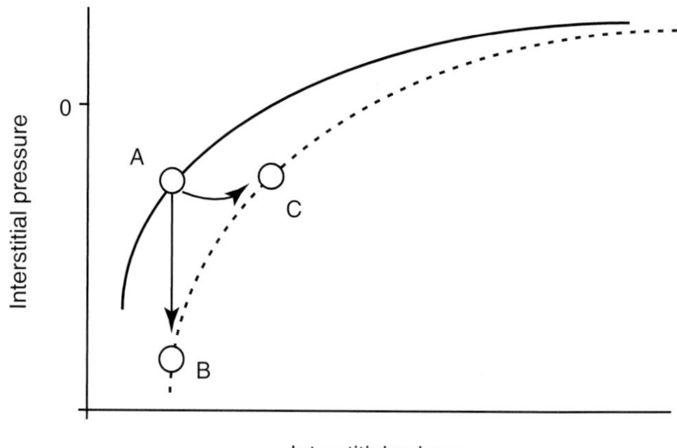

FIGURE 11-1 A proposed mechanism of inflammatory change in the interstitial pressure–volume relationship. Baseline interstitial pressure and volume values **(A)** lie along the normal pressure-volume relationship *(solid line).* With induction of inflammatory or immune-mediated disease, this relationship may change rapidly *(dashed line).* In experimental preparations in which microvascular filtration is hindered, interstitial pressure drops **(B).** More commonly, the fall in interstitial pressure promotes microvascular filtration, resulting in marked interstitial edema formation **(C).**

Inflammatory Edema

A greatly underappreciated mechanism of edema formation involves changes in the interstitial pressure–volume relationship. This phenomenon has been recently reviewed by the investigators primarily responsible for its elucidation.[12,13] Under normal conditions, interstitial pressure increases predictably with increases in interstitial volume. However, in response to inflammation, this mechanical relationship can shift markedly in a short period.[12-14] A consequence of this shift is a sudden fall in interstitial pressure and a consequent rapid increase in interstitial volume (Figure 11-1). This edema formation can occur with no significant changes in microvascular pressure or permeability. This phenomenon appears to be the result of a structural rearrangement of the extracellular matrix modulated by alterations in the attachment of collagen fibers to cells, particularly fibroblasts. Collagen fibers in the interstitial space act to restrain or compress interstitial volume. This effect is actuated by fibroblasts exerting tension on multiple collagen fibers via integrin-mediated connections, thus contracting the extracellular matrix.[12,13] Inflammation appears to disrupt this collagen-fibroblast bond.

This change in the interstitial pressure–volume relationship has been reported in skin and tracheal mucosa in select experimental models of inflammation, direct tissue damage of burns and freezing, ischemia-reperfusion, neurogenic inflammation induced by vagal nerve stimulation, and anaphylaxis.[12-15] This condition has been experimentally created by induction of mast cell degranulation, exposure to LPS, complement activation, and induction of asthma by antigen exposure as well as by introduction of inflammatory mediators, including tumor necrosis factor α (TNF-α), platelet activating factor, interleukin 1β (IL-1β), IL-6, and prostaglandins E_1, E_2, and I_2.[12,13] Several agents have been shown experimentally to prevent or reverse the fall in interstitial pressure, including prostaglandin $F_{2\alpha}$, corticotropin releasing factor, α-trinositol, platelet-derived growth factor BB, insulin, and vitamin C.[12,13]

CHRONIC EDEMAGENIC CONDITIONS

When evaluating chronic disease states, a difficulty arises when trying to ascribe the magnitude, persistence, or absence of edema to the mechanisms described earlier. Assessment of the mechanisms responsible for acute edema depends on parameters having relatively constant values (e.g., L_p and σ_d in Equation 1, P_{pump} and R_L in Equation 2) and variables with values that can change readily (e.g., P_{mv}, P_{int}, Π_p). However, the interstitial fluid balance system is not only complex but also adaptive. Chronic increases in interstitial volume, pressure, or flow induce adaptive changes in the values of those previously "constant" parameters.[16-18] These might include changes in microvascular permeability to water and protein, interstitial compliance, lymphatic contractile function, and serosal permeability as well as lymphangiogenesis, the growth of new lymphatic vessels. To add to the complexity, an adaptive change in one dimension, such as microvascular permeability, alters the signal for change in another dimension, such as lymphatic pumping. These multiple interdependent responses have the effect of changing both the magnitude of interstitial volume at equilibrium and the edemagenic gain, the sensitivity of the system to edemagenic challenge. These adaptive changes in fluid balance parameters make it difficult to predict the occurrence and severity of interstitial edema in chronic conditions.

CONCLUSION

Disease conditions characterized by interstitial edema development can best be understood via mechanisms responsible for interstitial fluid balance—increased venous and microvascular pressures, decreased plasma colloid osmotic pressure, increased microvascular permeability, impaired lymphatic function, and altered interstitial compliance. However, these cases can often be difficult to manage for two reasons. First, more than one mechanism of edema formation is often involved. For example, inflammatory disease may alter lymphatic pumping, microvascular permeability to water and protein, and the interstitial pressure–volume relationship simultaneously. Second, disease conditions that last for more than 1 to 2 days can induce adaptive responses in the interstitial fluid balance system that diminish clinical predictive accuracy.

Preliminary evidence exists for several therapeutic interventions specific to the treatment of interstitial edema. In a model of intestinal edema induced by mesenteric venous hypertension and crystalloid infusion, hypertonic saline treatment significantly reduced interstitial edema formation.[19] This effect appeared to be the result of fluid redistribution in that it concurrently increased urine production, intestinal luminal fluid volume, and peritoneal fluid volume.[19] In a model of anaphylaxis in albumin-sensitized rats, α-trinositol, an isomer of the intracellular messenger inositol trisphosphate, abolished the fall in tracheal interstitial fluid pressure induced by albumin administration, whereas hydrocortisone had no effect.[20] α-Trinositol also successfully prevented edema formation and the fall in interstitial pressure when used as a pretreatment in experimentally induced ischemia-reperfusion.[15] Perhaps more promising, platelet-derived growth factor BB was shown to be effective after treatment to speed resolution of the anaphylaxis-induced drop in dermal interstitial pressure.[21,22] Clinical trials demonstrating the effectiveness of these and related therapies remain to be performed.

REFERENCES

1. Dongaonkar RM, Laine GA, Stewart RH, Quick CM: Balance point characterization of interstitial fluid volume regulation, Am J Physiol Regul Integr Comp Physiol 297:R6, 2009.
2. Levick JR, Michel CC: Microvascular fluid exchange and the revised Starling principle, Cardiovasc Res 87:198, 2010.
3. Aukland K, Reed RK: Interstitial-lymphatic mechanisms in the control of extracellular fluid volume, Physiol Rev 73:1, 1993.
4. Drake RE, Laine GA, Allen SJ, et al: A model of the lung interstitial-lymphatic system, Microvasc Res 34:96, 1987.
5. Shirasawa Y, Benoit JN: Stretch-induced calcium sensitization of rat lymphatic smooth muscle, Am J Physiol Heart Circ Physiol 285:H2573, 2003.
6. Gashev AA, Davis MJ, Zawieja DC: Inhibition of the active lymph pump by flow in rat mesenteric lymphatics and thoracic duct, J Physiol (Lond) 540.3:1023, 2002.
7. Quick CM, Venugopal AM, Gashev AA, et al: Intrinsic pump-conduit behavior of lymphangions, Am J Physiol Regul Integr Comp Physiol 292:R1510, 2007.
8. Wang ZB, Li M, Li JC: Recent advances in the research of lymphatic stomata, Anat Rec 293:754, 2010.
9. Drake RE, Abbott RD: Effect of increased neck vein pressure on intestinal lymphatic pressure in awake sheep, Am J Physiol Regul Integr Comp Physiol 262:R892, 1992.
10. Stewart RH, Rohn DA, Allen SJ, Laine GA: Basic determinants of epicardial transudation, Am J Physiol Heart Circ Physiol 273:H1408, 1997.
11. Dongaonkar RM, Quick CM, Stewart RH, et al: Edemagenic gain and interstitial fluid volume regulation, Am J Physiol Regul Integr Comp Physiol 294:R651, 2008.
12. Reed RK, Liden A, Rubin K: Edema and fluid dynamics in connective tissue remodeling, J Mol Cell Cardiol 48:518, 2010.
13. Reed RK, Rubin K: Transcapillary exchange: role and importance of the interstitial fluid pressure and the extracellular matrix, Cardiovasc Res 87:211, 2010.
14. Wiig H, Rubin K, Reed RK: New and active role of the interstitium in control of interstitial fluid pressure: potential therapeutic consequences, Acta Anaesthesiol Scand 47:111, 2003.
15. Nedrebø T, Reed RK, Berg A: Effect of α-trinositol on interstitial fluid pressure, edema generation, and albumin extravasation after ischemia-reperfusion injury in rat hind limb, Shock 20:149, 2003.
16. Laine GA: Microvascular changes in the heart during chronic arterial hypertension, Circ Res 62:953, 1988.
17. Gashev AA, Delp MD, Zawieja DC: Inhibition of active lymph pump by simulated microgravity, Am J Physiol Heart Circ Physiol 290:H2295, 2006.
18. Desai KV, Laine GA, Stewart RH, et al: Mechanics of the left ventricular myocardial interstitium: effects of acute and chronic myocardial edema, Am J Physiol Heart Circ Physiol 294:H2428, 2008.
19. Radhakrishnan RS, Shah SK, Lance SH, et al: Hypertonic saline alters hydraulic conductivity and up-regulates mucosal/submucosal aquaporin 4 in resuscitation-induced intestinal edema, Crit Care Med 37:2946, 2009.
20. Woie K, Westerberg E, Reed RK: Lowering of interstitial fluid pressure will enhance edema in trachea of albumin-sensitized rats, Am J Respir Crit Care Med 153:1347, 1996.
21. Rodt S, Åhlén K, Berg A, et al: A novel physiologic function for platelet-derived growth factor-BB in rat dermis, J Physiol 495.1:193, 1996.
22. Lidén Å, Berg A, Nedrebø T, Reed RK, Rubin K: Platelet-derived growth factor BB-mediated normalization of dermal interstitial fluid pressure after mast cell degranulation depends on β3 but not β1 integrins, Circ Res 98:635, 2006.

CHAPTER 12
PATIENT SUFFERING IN THE INTENSIVE CARE UNIT

Matthew S. Mellema, DVM, PhD, DACVECC • Robin L. McIntyre, DVM

KEY POINTS

- Suffering is "an experience of unpleasantness and aversion associated with the perception of harm or threat of harm in an individual."
- Pain is far from the only unpleasant sensation critically ill animals are likely to experience.
- Relief of as many forms of patient suffering as possible is likely to lead to improved outcomes.

Patient suffering is a difficult topic to discuss in the clinical setting. A common perception is that the topic of animal suffering has been co-opted (some might say hijacked) by animal welfare advocates, including those perceived as extremist in their viewpoints. This perception seems to have led to a reactive pushback and reluctance to address the topic by many small animal clinicians. If this is the case, then it is unfortunate and also incompatible with the Veterinarian's Oath, which includes a mandate to use our training in "the prevention and relief of animal suffering." Another factor that may limit clinician consideration of patient suffering is the perception that if there are larger, more acutely life-threatening aspects of critical illness that require our attention, then patient suffering is a minor issue in the grander scheme of things and can underevaluated or undertreated.

Suffering in animals is challenging to define because of the inability of the patients to verbalize their perception of their sense of well being. One definition of suffering is that it is "the state of undergoing pain, distress, or hardship"; however, this definition is overly focused on pain and provides little guidance to clinicians. A more useful definition might be that suffering is "an experience of unpleasantness and aversion associated with the perception of harm or threat of harm in an individual." The authors prefer this definition because it can more easily be tied to the physiology of homeostasis in vertebrates. It captures the key concept that suffering is linked to the *perception* of both genuine harm and potential harm. It also offers the flexibility of treating harm as a multidimensional parameter rather than equating it to a single unpleasant sensation (e.g., pain). This definition also allows for consideration of forms of suffering that may be either physical or mental in nature and also allows for consideration of a continuous range in the intensity of suffering rather than just a binary process (e.g., mild, moderate, severe versus a present/absent model).

If one adopts the authors' preferred definition of suffering, then it can be put into a larger physiologic context that has relevance to critical illness and patient assessment. By focusing on patient perception of real or potential harm, one is led directly to consideration of how animals monitor their body systems for harm and how their behavior changes in response to harm surveillance signals. Vertebrates have a range of what some have called "primal alert signals" that appear to be highly conserved across species. These signals are linked to the fundamental needs required by animals to maintain homeostasis. Further, these signaling systems are designed to alert the animal to threats to these needs being met and drive both aversive and adaptive behaviors. The responses to these alarm signals can occur at the cortical and subcortical level. The best understood of these primal alert signals is pain. Pain is the alert signal tied to tissue integrity surveillance. Real or perceived threats to tissue integrity will be monitored by nociceptive fibers, conveyed by associated transmission pathways, and processed at brainstem and cortical centers. Activation of these receptors will lead to both aversive and adaptive behavioral responses. For example, if a child places his or her finger into a flame, then nociception will result in reflex withdrawal of the finger (aversive response) and hopefully from the pain perception the child will then learn not to repeat the process in the future (adaptive behavior). Although pain is an important alarm signal with great relevance to both animal suffering and clinical practice, there are several others and some evidence to suggest that pain is not the most unpleasant among them.

MASLOW'S HIERARCHY OF NEEDS AND PRIMAL ALERT SIGNALS

A consideration of animal suffering is inextricably linked to a consideration of their behavior as well. Indeed, ill animals have such a consistent clustering of disease manifestations when they are ill that the term *sickness behavior* has arisen to describe the four most common clinical signs associated with illness (i.e., fever, lethargy, anorexia, cachexia).[1] Psychologists have long sought to develop an understanding of what drives human behavior. One widely influential model was proposed by Abraham Maslow in 1934 and has come to be known as Maslow's hierarchy of needs model.[2] In Maslow's framework much of human (and perhaps animal) behavior is attributed to a perpetual drive to meet specific needs. These drives are akin to instincts. What was unique about Maslow's work was that he explicitly described a hierarchy and a continuum of dependencies. That is to say, Maslow considered not all needs to be of equal importance and proposed that humans will not exhibit behaviors designed to meet higher order needs (e.g., personal achievement) unless basic needs (e.g., food, water, shelter) are first adequately met. Maslow arranged the needs that may drive human behavior into a pyramid with the most important or essential needs at the bottom (Figure 12-1). The needs were arranged into several tiers (physiologic, safety, love/belonging, esteem, and self-actualization). Physiologic needs were assigned preeminence. Although sociology and psychology have moved on to embrace attachment theory as an alternative explanation of human behaviors, Maslow's hierarchy of needs remains better suited to application in veterinary clinical practice. Each of the physiologic needs may be linked to a primal alert signal that provides input regarding whether that need is being met or is under potential threat. Pain may be considered the alert signal linked to threats to tissue integrity. Dyspnea is considered the signal linked to alveolar ventilation adequacy. Thirst and hunger herald threats to water and nutrient

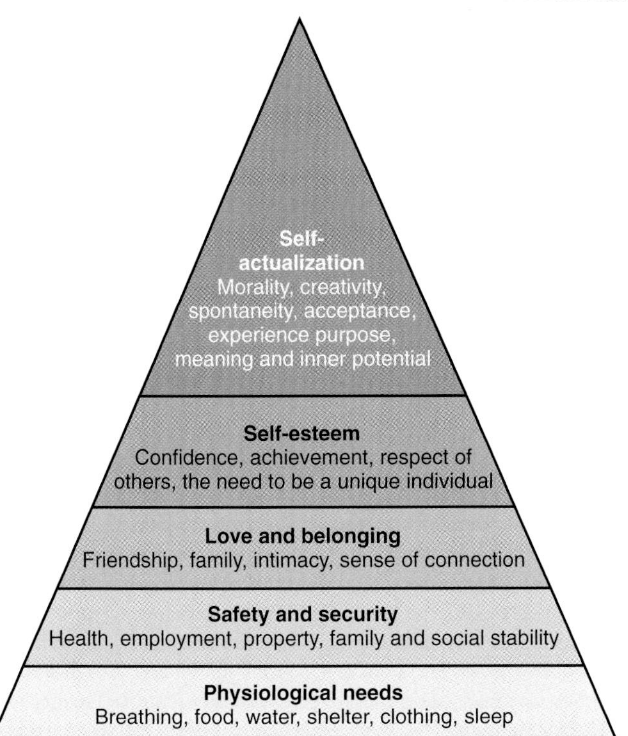

FIGURE 12-1 Maslow's original hierarchy of human needs. Highest priority needs are at the bottom of the pyramid. These needs must be met for needs in a tier lying above it to receive priority. Few would dispute that most of the highest priority needs are shared between humans and animals (excluding clothing, which in some cases may actually lead to patient suffering via humiliation; see also "dogs in sweaters").

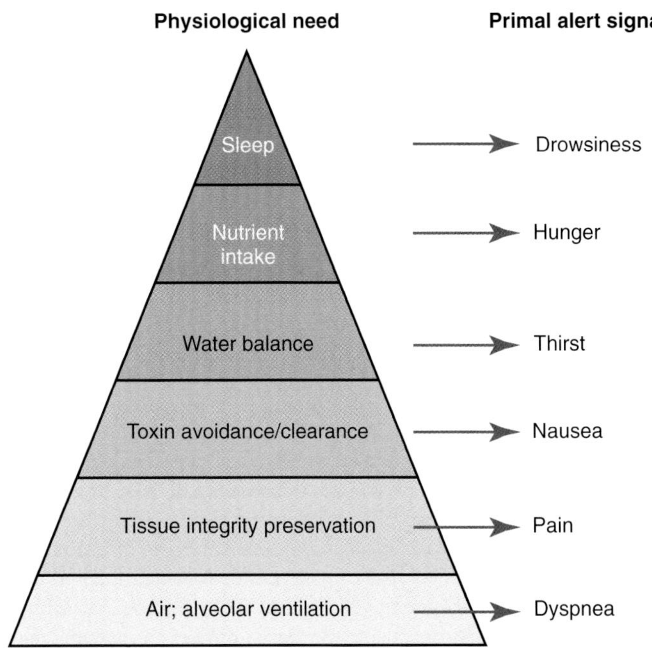

FIGURE 12-2 A second subhierarchy of the basic physiologic needs and the primal alert signals used to herald real or perceived threats to meeting those needs.

balance, respectively. Hunger may be a more nuanced signal that can be altered to drive behaviors geared toward meeting fairly specific nutrient requirements (e.g., cravings, pica). Nausea is likely tied to toxic threats or waste excretion and drives both aversive behaviors (vomiting) and adaptive behaviors (food aversion). Not all the primal alert signals are clearly evident as distinct or unique sensations, yet behavioral changes are still evident. Sleep is a fundamental need of vertebrate species and yet to date no specific, unique sensation linked to sleep inadequacy has been described. Feelings of drowsiness are nonspecific and may be elicited in subjects that have little or no sleep debt under some conditions (e.g., postprandial somnolence). Because primal alert signals linked to procreation have little or no relevance to critical care, the authors have elected to exclude them from this chapter.

Some researchers have expanded Maslow's hierarchy into subhierarchies. For example, physiologic needs are not all given equal priority (Figure 12-2). The available evidence indicates that the need for air is assigned the top priority. This proposed relationship comes from the finding that in human hospice patients with both pain and dyspnea these patients report that dyspnea is the more unpleasant sensation of the two.[3] In laboratory-induced models of pain and dyspnea, one finds that concurrent dyspnea makes pain less noticeable, whereas the converse is not true (i.e., pain does not make dyspnea less unpleasant). Animal studies have compared how unpleasant dyspnea is versus hunger and find that in most species animals will remain starved rather than seek out food that is made available in an environment that will result in sensations of dyspnea (e.g., argon-filled chamber).

Consideration of some, but perhaps not all, of these primal alert signals is a routine part of critically ill patient assessment. In the present era, it would be assumed by the authors that clinicians are frequently monitoring patients for evidence of pain. Signs of respiratory distress are often equated with sensations of dyspnea in veterinary practice. Periodic assessment of hunger, thirst, and nausea may be performed as well. Patients may be considered to have a significant sleep debt when microsleeps become apparent. Microsleeps are brief (1- to 60-second) periods of involuntary sleep that occur regardless of what the patient is doing (e.g., briefly falling asleep while sitting upright). Increases in the delta state effectively shut down the brain for a brief period in response to a large sleep debt. Surveillance for evidence of activation of these primal alert signals is a routine part of clinical practice whether it is done with a recognition of this conceptual framework or not. One entire specialty of medical practice (i.e., palliative care) is devoted to the recognition and alleviation of these symptoms/clinical signs, but all clinicians share a responsibility to monitor for these signs of basic needs not being met in their patients.

As described earlier, pain research has dominated the field of patient suffering research. This has clearly been to the patients' benefit, but much work remains to be done in expanding our understanding of other unpleasant sensations and how they may be alleviated. A growing body of evidence from human intensive care medicine suggests that even at the finest institutions symptom relief is far from optimal. In a study by Denise Li and colleagues out of the University of California at San Francisco, the prevalence of unaddressed symptoms (i.e., unpleasant sensations interfering with a sense of well-being) was 100%.[4] All patients reported some degree of dyspnea (i.e., shortness of breath). Prevalence rates were also quite high for most of the other symptoms that were evaluated (thirst, tiredness, anxiety, hunger, generalized discomfort, pain, dyspnea, depressed feelings, and nausea). Interestingly, this study found that there was a high degree of correlation between some symptoms and others (Figure 12-3). These associations may be of use in veterinary intensive care. For example, in Figure 12-3 one finds a high correlation among thirst, tiredness, general discomfort, and anxiety. This suggests that in patients that appear anxious and uncomfortable, providing greater opportunity for rest and meeting water intake needs may have a crossover benefit that translates to less sedative and

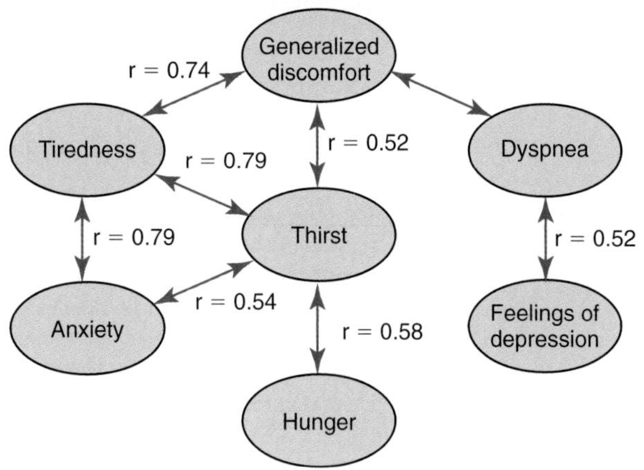

FIGURE 12-3 Correlation between symptoms in critically ill human patients.[4]

analgesic need. A similar study by Nelson et al, which focused on cancer patients in the intensive care unit (ICU) setting, identified prevalence rates of greater than 50% for six different symptoms (all at a moderate to severe level).[5] The six symptoms that had these high prevalence rates were discomfort, unsatisfied thirst, difficulty sleeping, anxiety, pain, and unsatisfied hunger. Depression and dyspnea were also identified in 34% to 39% of patients at moderate to severe levels. These same authors also investigated symptom burden in a population of chronically critically ill human patients, and in this group prevalence rates of greater than 50% were identified for all 16 symptoms assessed (weight loss, lack of energy, inappetence, pain, dry mouth, hunger, drowsiness, dyspnea in two settings, insomnia, nausea, difficulty communicating, thirst, worried, sad, and nervous).[6] Clearly some but not all of these symptoms may be relevant to small animal patients. For example, although human patients expressed distress over weight loss, it strains credibility to think that dogs are overly concerned with body image. However, this study does raise some interesting points. Human patients appeared to find dry mouth distressing and unpleasant. Although mucous membrane hydration is frequently assessed in small animal patients, the authors' impression is that little or no effort is made to maintain membrane moisture as a therapeutic goal.

Impact of Symptom Relief

Data would suggest that clinicians are far more likely to consider palliative relief as an important goal in and of itself when such measures can be tied to clinical outcomes. There is evidence that failure to address symptoms in humans and animal models can be linked to both outcomes and physiologic derangements. The ICU can be a noisy place and sleep patterns may be frequently disrupted by the chaos and commotion that can occur at unpredictable intervals. Studies in dogs in which their sleep was frequently disrupted by an alarm sounding have demonstrated that such sleep fragmentation leads to systemic hypertension. Considering the number of equipment alarms (e.g., ventilators, fluid pumps, syringe pumps) that may go off on a typical overnight shift in a busy veterinary ICU, it is not implausible to consider that this noise burden may contribute to cardiovascular instability in some cases. An industry-academia summit was convened recently to address "alarm fatigue" in the human ICU setting.[7] Addressing the human toll of alarm signals and hospital noise was the major focus of this meeting. Moreover, it has been shown that symptom experience is an independent predictor of important outcomes in human critically ill patients. Symptom distress has also been associated with unfavorable outcomes including higher mortality rates. Conversely, reduction of symptom burden may promote favorable outcomes such as physiologic stability and reduced resource expenditures. Taken together, the available evidence suggests that greater attention to relief of clinical signs may yield improved outcomes even when clinicians don't consider palliative measures to be their own reward.

Palliative Measures

Some aspects of palliative care may appear self-evident and represent current standard of care, whereas others might require a revision of patient care protocols. Addressing thirst, hunger, and pain in a proactive manner can be easily justified. Consideration should be given to offering small amounts of oral liquids to maintain membrane moisture (even when oral intake should be limited) and increase patient comfort. Providing adequate opportunity for uninterrupted sleep should also be a primary goal. Clustering treatments to minimize patient awakenings is advised. Providing quiet periods with reduced lighting overnight is recommended whenever feasible. Greater vigilance for signs of nausea and earlier intervention may be warranted based on the human ICU experience. Serial monitoring using validated pain scoring systems is advised as well. Nebulized furosemide may provide symptomatic relief from dyspnea, as may opioid administration. It is advised to encourage owner visitations and to make efforts to get patients outside for a portion of each day whenever such measures would not represent an undue risk. Providing opportunities for patients to express normal behaviors may enhance comfort and reduce anxiety.

In summary, pain is far from the only unpleasant sensation critically ill animals are likely to experience. The application of a broader definition of animal suffering in the hospital environment may lead to more comprehensive palliative care being provided and to improved outcomes. Increased patient comfort is likely to also lead to improved workplace safety and reduction in negative patient-caregiver interactions as patient tolerance of handling is enhanced.

REFERENCES

1. Tizard I: Sickness behavior, its mechanisms and significance, Anim Health Res Rev 9(1):87, 2008.
2. Zalenski RJ, Raspa R: Maslow's hierarchy of needs: a framework for achieving human potential in hospice, J Palliat Med 9(5):1120, 2006.
3. Banzett RB, Gracely RH, Lansing RW: When it's hard breathe, maybe pain doesn't matter, J Neurophysiol 97:959, 2007.
4. Li, DT, Puntillo K: A pilot study on coexisting symptoms in intensive care patients, Appl Nurs Res 19(4):216, 2006.
5. Nelson JE, Meier DE, Oei EJ, et al: Self-reported symptom experience of critically ill cancer patients receiving intensive care, Crit Care Med 29(2):277, 2001.
6. Nelson JE, Meier DE, Litke A, et al: The symptom burden of chronic critical illness, Crit Care Med 32(7):1527, 2004.
7. Improving clinical alarms: fall summit aims to develop action plan, Biomed Instrum Technol Suppl:7, 2011.

CHAPTER 13

ILLNESS SEVERITY SCORES IN VETERINARY MEDICINE

Galina Hayes, BVSc, PhD, DACVECC • Karol A. Mathews, DVM, DVSc, DACVECC

KEY POINTS

- Severity scores provide a quantitative and objective measure of patient illness.
- Multiple severity of disease scoring systems have been described and studied for use in dogs and cats.
- Severity scores are useful for guiding triage and analyzing clinical research groups.
- The use of severity of disease scores enables clinicians to assess the effectiveness of treatment while controlling for differences in illness severity between treatment groups. This can assist with interpretation of results in observational studies.
- The disease severity scores can be used to demonstrate effective randomization when group sizes are small in randomized controlled trials.

An illness severity score is a number assigned to a patient that correlates with a probability that a specific outcome will follow. This number is computed with varying degrees of complexity from several variables. Selection of an illness score or outcome model by the clinician or researcher is based on characteristics such as validated predictive accuracy, transferability to the intended patient population, and ease of application. The use of an illness score to manage individual patients or establish a prognosis has several limitations; however, illness severity scores provide a valuable and currently underused research tool. Although several diagnosis-specific and diagnosis-independent scores have been proposed in recent years and are being used clinically, scoring systems in general have achieved limited adoption in the veterinary clinical research setting. Potential reasons for this include lack of familiarity with score applications to research, the cumbersome or subjective nature of some of the models available, and lack of prospectively demonstrated association between model score and outcome.

APPLICATIONS OF ILLNES SEVERITY SCORES

Applications for the Individual Patient

Illness severity scores may be broadly considered as either diagnosis specific or diagnosis independent. Diagnosis-specific scores assess particular facets of a patient's primary problem, such as proteinuria in the feline renal International Renal Interest Society (IRIS) score[1] or stool frequency in the canine inflammatory bowel disease score.[2,3] Diagnosis-independent scores provide an objective assessment of a patient's global physiologic illness status, typically derived from variables such as blood pressure and temperature.[4-6] Severity scores can provide an objective tool for baseline assessment at admission or some other defined time point or can be calculated daily for patient trending.

Scores calculated for a specific patient often are presented as an outcome prediction score. Basing therapy on prediction of survival for the individual patient is not an appropriate use of scores. However, scores still can be useful in a clinical setting as an adjunctive tool for patient assessment, taken together with a traditional clinical assessment. Scores can provide the perspective of a database that may be larger than the experience of a single clinician[7,8] and help remove subjectivity from patient assessment.[9] Having to consider all data requirements of a particular scoring system may expand the clinician's knowledge on the topic. Also, inclusion of an objective validated score in the medical record may protect the clinician from accusations of false prognostication. When a clinician's assessment has included consideration of a score, accuracy of prediction has been shown to improve.[8] In human medicine, head-to-head comparisons between scores and clinicians have shown that experienced clinicians can accurately and consistently outperform even sophisticated models in predicting recovery of an individual from disease.[10,11] In agreement with this observation, when a veterinary score designed to predict the survival of critically ill foals was assessed, clinician prediction of outcome outperformed the score prediction by 83% to 81%. Combining the foal score with the clinician's assessment, however, improved the accuracy of survival prediction by an additional 12%.[8] Clinician assessments can be heavily swayed by recent case experience, and the inclusion of an objective score in the patient assessment process can help avoid this pitfall and ensure consistency.

Scoring various components of a patient's clinical presentation can also be used to scale severity of illness within a primary diagnostic category rather than to predict a mortality outcome. For instance, a symptom index was developed to predict the severity of benign prostatic hyperplasia (BPH) in a group of 373 dogs. In this study, a group of animals with BPH were graded as mildly, moderately, or severely affected and then a symptom grading system developed to predict category of severity.[12] In an alternate approach, components of ultrasonographic imaging findings were evaluated for prediction of a neoplastic diagnosis in dogs with prostatic disease. The presence of mineralization was found to be highly predictive of diagnosis.[13]

Inappropriate Score Use

Illness severity scores are not designed to be used in isolation to predict outcome for individuals; predictions should only be applied on a population basis. The confidence interval surrounding any prediction for an individual is substantially wider than for a group, and the introduction of this additional uncertainty into the estimate typically ensures that individual estimations are not clinically helpful. An additional issue, particularly for probability estimates, is that a probability likelihood intrinsically implies a population application. For instance, where a dichotomous outcome is being predicted (e.g., death, development of acute kidney injury/failure, remission failure), a score of 70% cannot predict a 70% chance of mortality for any one individual, but in a group of 100 similar patients, 70% may be expected to die or 30% will survive.[14] Where one can confidently predict a 40% mortality rate for canine intensive care unit (ICU) patients with a severity prediction index (SPI2) of 0.6, it is impossible to discriminate the survivors from the nonsurvivors within that group.[15] Similarly, the 10% of patients that survive in a 90% mortality prediction group will not have falsified the odds by surviving but instead confirmed the validity of the probabilities.[14]

These issues reflect the difficulty of attempting to apply a probability estimate ranging from 0 to 1 to an individual when the individual result will be 0 or 1.[9] Clinicians should be aware of this issue and take particular care if score results are quoted to clients. Scores should not be used for prognostication of individuals, and treatment decisions should not be made solely on the result of a score, particularly where the treatment decision could be deleterious to the misclassified patient.[14,16,17]

Applications in Triage and Clinician Performance Benchmarking

In human medicine, scores have been used to assist appropriate triage of patient groups—for example, triage of patients waiting for coronary artery bypass grafting[18] and transplant[18] and to guide appropriate site of care for pneumonia patients.[19] The authors of a veterinary score assessing illness severity in canine pancreatitis patients suggested that the score be used to assist prediction of requirement for intensive care unit (ICU) admission and appropriate triage.[20] Appropriate roles for the use of available scores in the management or triage of groups of veterinary patients have yet to be fully defined, particularly in companion animal medicine where the focus has been on individual recovery rather than the economic impact of group management. Table 13-1 details several diagnosis-specific and diagnosis-independent veterinary severity scores, together with some details of their construction and validation.

In general terms, use of a score as a component of the overall clinical assessment of the individual is appropriate, whereas use of the score as the sole means of justifying a treatment or euthanasia decision is not. Users of scores must take into consideration the issues

Table 13-1 Overview of Recent Veterinary Outcome Prediction Models

	Model Features						
Model	**Outcome Parameter**	**No. of Measured Parameters**	**Model Population**	**Model Format**	**Patient Numbers for Construction of Model**	**Validation Method**	**AUROC (If Reported)**
Clinical severity index for canine acute pancreatitis (2008)[18]	Mortality at discharge	4	Data collected over a 7-year period, primary and referral population	Table	61 dogs assessed, 14 deaths	Spearman rho correlation analysis on construction data set	None
Model estimating recovery from ARF in dogs requiring hemodialysis (2008)[40]	Alive and dialysis free at 30 days postdischarge	13-15	Presumed referral population, retrospective data collection, collection period not stated	Table	182 dogs assessed, 96 deaths	Model discrimination assessed on construction data set	0.91
Canine IBD activity index[2] (CIBDAI score, 2003)	Histologic grade of lesions, serum CRP, and haptoglobin	6	Presumed referral population, prospective data collection over 18 months	Table	58 dogs assessed	Spearman correlation analysis	None
Model estimating survival probability in hospitalized foals[13] (2006)	Mortality at discharge	6	Multicenter referral population, prospective data collection	Logistic regression equation	577 foals, 98 deaths	Validated prospectively on an independent data set	AUC not stated for construction or validation data set; 90% sensitivity and 46% specificity for survival at cut-point selected
Model estimating survival probability in canine ICU patients[8] (SPI2, 2001)	Mortality at 30 days postadmission	7	Multicenter referral population, prospective data collection	Logistic regression equation	624 dogs, 243 deaths	Validated on an independent data set	AUC on construction data = 0.76, on validation data = 0.68
Modified Glasgow Coma Scale for estimating survival in canine head trauma[49] (2001)	Mortality at 48 hours	Neurologic exam; 3 main categories of assessment	Referral population, retrospective data collection over a 9-year period	Table	38 dogs, 7 deaths	Logistic regression on construction data set *p* value in univariate analysis reported	None

ARF, Acute renal failure; *AUC,* area under the curve; *AUROC,* area under receiver operator characteristic; *CRP,* C-reactive protein; *IBD,* irritable bowel disease.

of score validation and transferability (discussed later) before applying them to patients.

Illness severity scores have been used as a performance measure in human medicine. Actual mortality rates are compared with those predicted by the score. Units achieving lower or higher mortality rates than those the scores predict can be designated as high or low achievers. The ratios of actual to predicted scores have been used to rank the performance of physicians (e.g., cardiac surgeons) or, more commonly, health care units.[6,21] This approach is an unexplored area in veterinary medicine; however, as subspecialization and treatment complexity increases, the use of these tools for the objective evaluation of both individual veterinarians and unit performance may become appropriate. Actual mortality is compared with mortality predicted by the score to calculate a mortality ratio. Before mortality ratios can be compared as a performance measure, similarities among patient groups must be carefully established.[16] Mortality ratios have been used to rank the performance of emergency doctors working shifts on a rolling patient population.[22] In conjunction with other performance measures, this approach may be a more ethical method by which to allocate clinician remuneration than a commission-oriented system.

RESEARCH APPLICATIONS

In veterinary medicine, the ability to select the most effective treatment, or form an accurate prognosis, is often hampered by lack of well-designed observational studies or randomized controlled trials for reference. Case series and retrospective descriptive studies make up a substantial proportion of the veterinary literature. These often are performed over several years and have many pitfalls, including lack of case homogeneity, lack of defined control groups, and change in management procedures over time. The findings of observational studies often are hampered by confounding, defined as the presence of an extraneous factor distorting the relationship between the outcome and the variable under study.[23] Control of confounders minimizes erroneous conclusions about the relationships between exposure (e.g., pancreatitis, trauma) and outcome. A common confounder of the relationship between treatment and outcome is illness severity. Objective quantification of illness severity facilitates analytical control of this variable and can improve the quality of observational studies.

Use of Illness Severity Scores in the Management of Confounding

The severity of a patient's illness or derangement of physiologic status can have a substantial impact on the association between treatment and outcome. Quantifying illness severity in an objective manner facilitates the use of design or analytical techniques to remove the confounding effects of illness variation among patient groups, allowing the true impact of the treatment to be identified. For instance, a minimum or maximum illness score can be set as a predefined criterion for study entry. Alternatively, illness severity can be entered as a covariable with treatment in a regression analysis of treatment effect on outcome. This approach will allow the effect of treatment on outcome to be estimated while controlling for illness severity. In this way, beneficial treatment effects can be identified that otherwise would be missed; conversely, treatments that may appear as risk factors in the initial analysis can have their true effect identified. This approach has been used in studies of human patients for many years. Several scoring systems for objectively quantifying illness severity that operate independent of primary diagnosis have been validated and are in common use in human medicine. These include the Acute Physiology and Chronic Health Evaluation (APACHE) score,[24] Mortality Probability Model (MPM) score,[25] Simplified Acute Physiology Score (SAPS),[26] and Intensive Care National Audit and Research Centre (ICNARC) model.[27] The APACHE score was first constructed in 1981 and is now in its fourth incarnation.[28] As an example of use, in a recent cohort study investigating administration of proton pump inhibitors (PPIs) as a risk factor for nosocomial pneumonia, measurement of illness severity across the cohort using the APACHE II score was pivotal in eliminating PPI administration as an independent risk factor for pneumonia, even though the initial analysis showed a weak positive association.[29] Because the initial analysis did not include illness severity, it failed to identify that PPIs generally are administered to the more critically ill and therefore to patients more prone to acquiring pneumonia.[29]

Several diagnosis-independent illness severity scores, including the Survival Prediction Index (SPI) and Acute Patient Physiologic and Laboratory Evaluation (APPLE) scores, have been constructed and validated for dogs and cats,[4,15,30,31] although adoption in veterinary research has been limited. The SPI score has been recalibrated in a multicenter study to give the SPI2 score, which is based on seven variables and is diagnosis independent and prospectively validated (Box 13-1). The authors are not aware of any veterinary studies in which illness severity has been objectively quantified and managed in the data analysis as a covariable with outcome. However, there has been a recent trend of documenting illness severity in patient groups, with several recent studies recording the SPI, SPI2, or APPLE scores of patient groups.[32-34] The Canine Inflammatory Bowel Disease Activity Index (CIBDAI) score has been used to objectively define treatment groups[35] and provide a benchmark for correlation of imaging findings in patients with clinical disease.[36] With the increasing availability of appropriately validated scores in veterinary medicine, research use is likely to increase.

Demonstration of Effective or Ineffective Randomization

The process of randomization in controlled trials is intended to equally distribute potential confounding factors, such as age or degree of illness severity, among treatment groups and thus eliminate

BOX 13-1 *SPI2 Score Calculation*

- Diagnosis-independent score designed to objectively stratify clinical canine ICU patients into groups according to severity of disease.
- Score predicts probability of survival based on seven variables.
- Variables used are the most abnormal values of the parameter identified within 24 hours of admission.

$$\begin{aligned}\text{Logit (P)} = {} & 0.3273 + (0.0108 \times \text{MAP [mm Hg]}) \\ & - (0.0102 \times \text{resp rate [bpm]}) - (0.2183 \times \text{creatinine [mg/dl]}) \\ & + (0.0164 \times \text{PCV [\%]}) + (0.3553 \times \text{albumin [g/dl]}) \\ & - (0.1184 \times \text{age [years]}) - (0.8069 \times \text{medical vs. surgical} \\ & \text{[medical} = 1\text{, surgical} = 0])\end{aligned}$$

Thus for a 6-year-old dog with mean arterial pressure 65 mm Hg, respiratory rate 40 beats/min, creatinine 2.82 mg/dl, packed cell volume 25%, albumin 2.5 g/dl, medical admission:

$$\begin{aligned}\text{Logit (P)} = {} & 0.3273 + (0.0108 \times 65) - (0.0102 \times 40) - (0.2183 \times 2.82) \\ & + (0.0164 \times 25) + (0.3553 \times 2.5) - (0.1184 \times 6) \\ & - (0.8069 \times 1) = -0.2134\end{aligned}$$

Logit P is then solved for P using $P = e^{\text{logit P}}/(1 + e^{\text{logit P}})$ $e^{-0.2134} = 0.8078$, so $P = 0.8078/1.8078 = 0.45$, or **survival probability = 45%**

Data from King LG, Wohl JS, Manning AM, et al: Evaluation of the survival prediction index as a model of risk stratification for clinical research in dogs admitted to intensive care units at four locations, Am J Vet Res 62:948-954, 2001.

the effects of confounding. However, when case numbers are small or confounding factors are numerous or variable, randomization may not be successful in achieving this goal and inaccurate estimates of a treatment effect can result. Delineating the severity of illness of animals assigned to treatment and control groups allows for both documentation and analytical control of ineffective randomization, decreasing the risk of an important treatment effect being missed or wrongly assessed.[9] Observational studies are typically undertaken when randomization is impractical or unethical. In this study type, scores can be used to objectively describe or stratify patient groups by illness severity.[22] Equivalent illness severity among treatment or exposure groups, despite lack of formal randomization, can then be demonstrated or disproved. In a recent study investigating the role of early hyperglycemia in survival from head trauma in human patients, blood glucose concentration was higher in the nonsurviving patients.[37] Illness severity was also worse in nonsurvivors, suggesting hyperglycemia to be an epiphenomenon only. However, when illness severity score was included as a covariable in the analysis, two levels of blood glucose were identified that were associated with increased mortality after controlling for the effect of illness severity. Thus blood glucose concentrations that might trigger therapeutic intervention were identified.[37]

Provision of Objective Context

Reporting a score that has a known and previously validated association with illness severity provides important contextual information in descriptive studies, giving observations greater interpretability and external validity.[14] High external validity allows study findings to be better generalized to the wider population. A retrospective veterinary study documenting use of human serum albumin used the veterinary SPI2 score in this manner.[32]

Reduction of Required Sample Sizes

Illness severity scores are an effective tool by which to improve power and therefore decrease the sample size required to detect a significant difference between treatment or exposure groups in clinical research. Stratifying patients by severity of illness to ensure patient group homogeneity can also decrease the sample size required to measure an effect.[16] This approach is of particular relevance to veterinary medicine where case numbers are often small. Multivariable regression can be thought of conceptually as the ultimate form of stratified analysis. In this context, the overall sample size required to identify a statistically significant measure of effect between a variable and outcome is decreased when an additional variable that explains a significant degree of the data variation is introduced.[38] In a hypothetical example, consider an observational study investigating the association between medication with an analgesic and comfort level after fracture repair. The relationship between analgesic administration and comfort level will be confounded by the severity of the fracture. Clinicians are more likely to give analgesics to patients with severe fractures, and patients with severe fractures are more likely to be in pain. An analysis that does not include a measure of fracture severity is likely to require a very large sample size to identify any association between analgesic administration and improved comfort in this situation, and a reverse association (i.e., analgesic administration associated with less comfort) may even be identified. However, if the variable "fracture severity" is introduced into a multivariable analysis, the data variation explained by this variable is effectively "subtracted" and any association between the analgesic and patient comfort will reach statistical significance with lower patient numbers.

Critical Evaluation of Illness Severity Scores

Appropriate selection and comparison of scores for clinical or research use requires some understanding of different score construction and validation methods. The approach to assessment of these factors is reviewed next.

Assessment of Model Validity

A scoring system has construct and content validity if it evaluates aspects of disease or illness known, by previous research or clinical experience, to correlate with severity across all aspects of the disease pathophysiology.[39] *Predictive validity* refers to the correlation between actual and predicted outcomes of patients to whom the score is applied.[39] It is this aspect of validity that is addressed in quantitative statistical score validation. The purpose of this process is to establish that the score predicts outcome reliably and to give a quantitative measure of score performance. The process of validation ideally involves prospectively comparing predicted with actual outcomes. This is an essential step in score assessment and is unfortunately lacking in several recent veterinary scores.

Some debate exists over the appropriate population on which to perform validation. All models will perform well if tested on the same data set used for model construction, and measures of model performance can be artificially inflated if this approach is used.[14] It is intuitive that evaluation of a score on the same set of patient data that generated the associations used to construct the score may result in a biased evaluation and an artificially inflated measure of performance. The area under receiver operator characteristic (AUROC) curve of 0.91 reported for the canine hemodialysis recovery prediction score (Figure 13-1) likely suffered from this issue. The authors of the original SPI score acknowledged the bias inherent in this method of validation and in response pursued validation of the SPI2 score on data collected prospectively at several centers.[15] Appropriate validation can also be performed by randomly dividing the original data set into separate score construction and validation groups.

These validation techniques, although important, only evaluate internal validity, defined as validity of inferences with respect to the population used for the study. Thus a model with excellent internal performance may still perform poorly if applied to a new and different population. A model constructed and validated in an ICU with a focus on management of oncologic patients may perform quite differently in an ICU with a focus on acute trauma. Furthermore, different management techniques and different resource availability (e.g., availability of mechanical ventilation) will have considerable

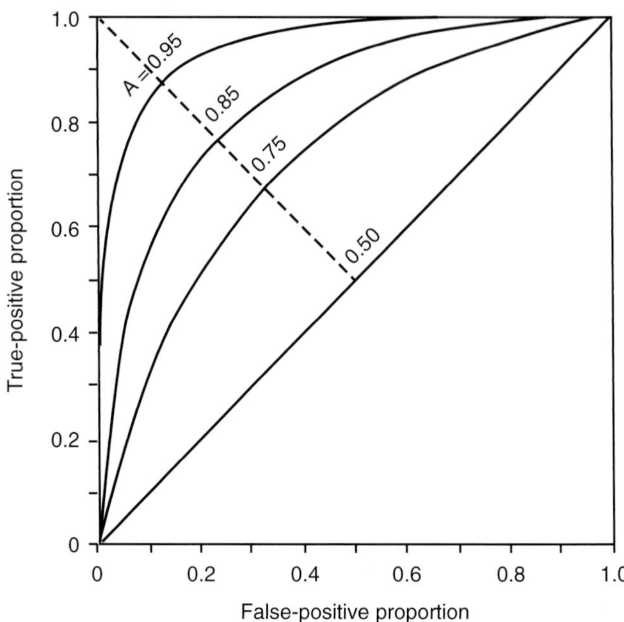

FIGURE 13-1 Area under the receiver operator characteristic curve.

impact on score transferability between centers. It is appropriate, when presenting a score, to provide considerable detail of the population characteristics used for score construction to allow the user to assess whether the score can appropriately be transferred to the intended patient group.

Discrimination and Calibration

Model calibration reflects the ability of a model to predict outcomes across the relevant outcome range in a population. For example, in a model predicting a 15% mortality rate in one group and 90% mortality in another group, the model is said to have good calibration if 15 of 100 patients in the first group and 90 of 100 patients in the second group do in fact die. The accuracy of a model reflects the degree to which model predictions reflect the true outcome and is closely related to model discrimination. Model discrimination measures the ability of the model to discriminate between those individuals expected to live and those expected to die (i.e., did the model identify the correct 15 and the correct 90 patients). The concepts of discrimination and calibration are not mutually exclusive. They measure different characteristics, but characterization of discrimination may only be truly appropriate if good calibration already has been demonstrated.[9]

Calibration is typically evaluated by the Hosmer-Lemeshow goodness-of-fit test,[16,42-44] whereas model discrimination is evaluated by a test of the AUROC curve, which is a plot of the true positive versus the false positive proportion predicted by the model at points throughout the predictive range.[45] An AUROC of 1.0 indicates perfect discrimination, whereas an AUROC of 0.5 indicates the model is no more predictive than a coin flip. The SPI2 score achieved an AUROC of 0.76 on the construction sample and 0.68 on the validation sample.[15] The canine and feline APPLE scores reported AUROCs of 0.93 and 0.91 for the canine model and 0.91 and 0.88 for the feline model.[30,31] An example of an AUROC curve with various values is shown in Figure 13-1.

Model Transferability

A model constructed on a particular case population and transferred to another may lose predictive accuracy. For instance, a severity score predicting survival in canine surgical patients[46] was constructed in 1994 on a population of referral patients undergoing laparotomy and subsequently managed in an ICU. This score might not transfer well to a population of patients undergoing exploratory laparotomy for foreign body removal at a general practice in 2009. Thus transferability depends heavily on the differences between the construction population and end-user population. All models constructed to date have been found to drift in accuracy both over time and when applied to new source populations.[47,49] The reasons for this drift, and potential methods to correct it in new populations,[15,46] have been the subject of much debate.

Clear and quantitative descriptions of the construction population can assist the end user in appropriate model selection. Geographic location, case mix, primary versus referral population mix, mortality rates, euthanasia rates, and other descriptive measures of the construction patient population may assist in establishing potential transferability. The commonly used models in humans are adjusted approximately every 5 years to account for changes in management of a specific illness over time.[46] External validity tends to be better when the construction data set is obtained from multiple locations.[15,24]

Intended model use is also an important factor. If a score is used to stratify, characterize, or demonstrate equivalence among patient groups, then drift in the quantitative predictive power of the model over time may be less of an issue. Describing two patient groups as having a similar average APACHE II score of 15 or two groups of canine acute pancreatitis patients as having dissimilar clinical severity indices of 4 and 6, respectively, has its own internal validity and adds contextual information. This holds true even when scores are no longer well correlated to a specific mortality outcome. At the time of score construction in 1985, an APACHE II score of 15 correlated to a 17% mortality risk.[50] Numerous studies since that time have demonstrated drift, with the APACHE II now consistently overpredicting mortality.[28] However, a Medline search identified approximately 265 studies of human patients in the last year that used the APACHE II score as a descriptive stratification term without reference to expected mortality. This is a valid technique employing a widely used and recognized clinical language to improve the power, relevance, and transferability of research findings. Use of a score in this manner loses validity when predicted mortality derived from an outdated model is compared with actual mortality as a measure of treatment effect.

Veterinary Models: Disease Specific and Disease Independent

Several of the more recent veterinary models available are detailed in Table 13-1. The main advantage of a disease-specific model is that model development has been performed on a relatively homogenous patient population where many of the clinical features specific to the disease process have been selected as variables. In this way, the end user of the model can expect reasonable fit and transferability of the model, often with the measurement of fewer variables than with diagnosis-independent models.[51] In addition, the selected outcome is often of particular relevance to the disease in question—for instance, development of systemic bacteremia after mastitis,[52] requirement for long-term hemodialysis after acute renal failure,[46] or likelihood of recovery from surgical colic.[53] Disadvantages of disease-specific models include lack of availability for rare diseases, difficulty selecting the primary disease in patients with multiple comorbidities, and lack of applicability in stratifying patient groups with multiple heterogeneous disease processes.

Models that operate independently of the primary diagnosis assume that across a wide and representative population, variables that do not make reference to the primary diagnosis, such as age and physiologic status, will suffice to model patient outcome.[4,27] Difficulties arise if the primary disease mix of the end user's population differs substantially from the population on which the model was developed. An important advantage to this model type is the applicability of the score to relatively heterogeneous patient groups, to individuals where a single primary diagnosis is difficult to assign, or before a diagnosis has been reached. Some models compromise between these two methodologies and assign a "primary diagnosis" coefficient as a component of the final score.[28]

FEATURES OF MODEL CONSTRUCTION

Selection of Predictive Variables

Variables used to determine outcome probabilities vary widely depending on the outcome being evaluated. They can be categorized into patient factors such as age, serum creatinine concentration,[15] and tumor histologic features,[54] or factors relating to treatments and other processes of care (e.g., whether the patient is admitted on a medical or surgical service).[15] Variables can be weighted with respect to their relative contribution to outcome prediction; for example, age was given a double weighting compared with heart rate in the first SAPS for human ICU patients.[5] Variables can be selected on the basis of expert opinion,[5] by multivariable logistic regression analysis of patient data in a population of patients in whom the outcome is known,[8] or by a combination of the two. In an example of the former, the canine modified Glasgow Coma Score for predicting outcome after head trauma was devised on neurologic markers selected by expert opinion as analogous to the human Glasgow Coma Scale,[55] whereas the variables in the foal survival score[8] were selected by optimal performance in regression analysis.

In multivariable logistic regression analysis, the variables that have a linear relationship and are most statistically predictive of the outcome are preferentially identified.[8] Ideally, selected variables should be independent of treatment or care process, because these factors are likely to vary among groups of clinicians and institutions. Inclusion of variables of this nature may decrease external validity and thus limit application of the model to the wider population.[16] Selection of variables that are infrequently measured or expensive to measure, however predictive, may also limit the wider applicability of the model.[9]

As a general rule, the more variables included in the model, the greater the estimated standard errors become and the more dependent the model becomes on the observed data. Using a large number of variables for score calculation may result in "overfitting" of the model to the construction data set and decrease model stability when it is used prospectively.[56,57]

Finally, variable selection is performed with the aim of minimizing the potential for interobserver variability, measurement error, and subjective bias. In a scoring system with a mortality outcome devised to reflect severity of injury in human burn patients, a precise definition of inhalation injury based on clinical and laboratory criteria was provided, with inhalation injury for the purposes of the score additionally defined as that requiring mechanical ventilation.[58] In this way, score miscalculation caused by clinician subjectivity or measurement error associated with a single test was minimized.

Outcome Selection

The degree to which the frequency of euthanasia outweighs "natural" death in veterinary medicine poses a unique challenge to models developed on a mortality outcome. The performance and timing of euthanasia reflects multiple factors, including severity of patient illness, owner financial and emotional status, diagnosis of a disease anticipated to be terminal at some future point, subjective assessments of degree of suffering, and individual clinician perspective. If all euthanized patients are excluded from the model development data set, available patient data may be limited and biased. If all patients are included regardless of euthanasia status, the significance of a particular variable as a risk factor for death may be masked by patients euthanized for financial reasons. Attempting to determine the exact reason for euthanasia, and discriminate among patient subsets on that basis, can be challenging because of lack of practicality or appropriateness of in-depth owner questioning at a time of emotional stress. Clinician subjectivity and clinician misconceptions can also be sources of error.[59] Handling of euthanized patients in veterinary models varies from complete exclusion[60] through exclusion of some subsets[46] to complete inclusion.[8]

The outcome selected as the endpoint of the model—for example, death,[15] survival from surgical colic,[53] or recovery of dogs from acute kidney injury/failure with hemodialysis,[46]—requires careful consideration. The outcome should be specific, easily and accurately determined, and an appropriate endpoint for all patients to which the model is applied. As an example, evaluation of time to tumor recurrence may seem useful as an outcome closely associated with tumor malignancy; however, in reality this outcome may be more closely associated with the type and frequency of performance of patient screening tests than tumor behavior. Equally, length of an animal's ICU stay may be more reflective of an owner's financial constraints than of the patient's requirement for hospital care, quality of care provided, or severity of underlying disease. The outcome should be clarified with a specific definition, such as "mortality at 30 days after hospital admission." If a more ambiguous outcome is used, such as "occurrence of melanoma metastasis," the means and methods by which this outcome is to be determined must be clearly stated.[16]

Examples of modeled outcomes include probability of survival to hospital discharge,[8] probability that a certain length of hospital stay will be exceeded,[6] probability of recurrence of a specific tumor type,[54] and probability that a septic focus is present.[60] The CIBDAI correlated historical and physical findings with bowel histology scores.[2] Outcome probabilities are calculated directly or indirectly

			Mentation score 0	*4* 1	*7* 2	*8* 3	*9* 4	
6 <36.1	*4* 36.1-37.0	*3* 37.1-38.5	**Temperature (C)** 38.6-39.4	*1* >39.4				
9 <61	*4* 61-100		**MAP (mm Hg)** 101-140	*1* >140				
			lactate (mg/dl) 0-17.1	*5* 17.2-36.0	*6* 36.1-63.1	*9* >63.1		
			PCV(%) <11	*11* 11-20	*16* 21-30	*14* 31-40	*13* 41-45	*17* >45
11 <14.9	*7* 14.9-21.3		**Urea (mg/dl)** 21.4-24.9	*12* 25.0-32.5	*7* 32.6-69.8	*6* >69.8		
12 <111	*9* 111-115	*11* 116-118	**Chloride (mEq/L)** 119-122	*11* 123-125	*7* >125			
			Body cavity fluid score 0	*3* 1	*6* 2			

Feline $APPLE_{full}$ score. The central cell in each figure represents the range of values for the variable for which 0 points would be assigned. The cells to either side show the appropriate score for the corresponding range of the variable. The final score for the patient is achieved by summing the scores for each variable. "Mentation score" is collected at admission; for all others use the most abnormal value identified over the 24-hour period following admission. If history and physical exam fail to prompt assessment of fluid score, assign zero.
MAP reflects the value recorded for MAP if direct or indirect manometry is used, or the pressure corresponding to first return of audible signal on cuff deflation if Doppler technique is used. The $APPLE_{full}$ score can be converted to a mortality risk probability (p) using the equation $p = \exp(R)/(1 + \exp[R])$ where $R = (0.213 \times APPLE_{full}) - 9.472$.

FIGURE 13-2 Conversion to mortality probability (p) using $APPLE_{full}$ equations in Figure 13-2.

through an intermediary score from the measured variables. The canine Glasgow Coma Scale[55] uses an intermediary score to model probability of survival after head trauma. With this score, a patient is assigned a number based on several components of a neurologic examination; these are summed, and the total score number is then correlated with a graph to obtain the percentage probability of survival. The more sophisticated and useful models allow calculation of percent outcome probability across the full range of the model, rather than only giving a selected cut-point at which death would be predicted.

MODEL-BUILDING PROCESS

When intensive care clinicians in human medicine were polled regarding desirable score properties, they requested a score that was simple, easy to calculate, and reflected the degree of physiologic derangement of the patient.[27] The challenge of model building is to balance simplicity in use and parsimony in the number of variables required against predictive power. Failure to achieve this balance is likely to result in poor model adoption.

BOX 13-2 ***Algorithm for Assignment of the Body Cavity Fluid Score and Mentation Score Used for Feline APPLE Score Calculation***

Mentation Score: Assessed at Admission Prior to Sedation/Analgesic Administration	Body Cavity Fluid Score (Ultrasonographic Evaluation, as Assessed by FAST or TFAST Technique*)
0 Normal	0 No abdominal, thoracic or pericardial free fluid identified
1 Able to stand unassisted, responsive but dull	1 Abdominal OR thoracic OR pericardial free fluid identified
2 Can stand only when assisted, responsive but dull	2 Two or more of abdominal, thoracic, or pericardial free fluid identified
3 Unable to stand, responsive	
4 Unable to stand, unresponsive	

*Boysen SR, Rozanski EA, Tidwell AS, et al: Evaluation of a FAST protocol to detect free abdominal fluid, J Am Vet Med Assoc 225:1198-1204, 2004.

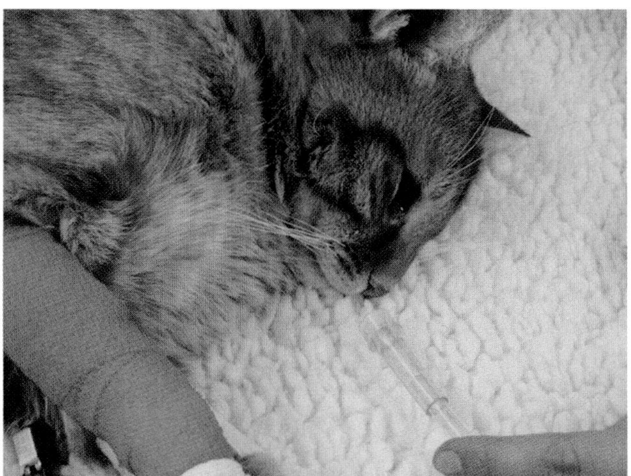

FIGURE 13-3 Example of patient $APPLE_{full}$ score calculation and conversion to mortality probability (*p*) for Rusty, a 6-year-old domestic short hair cat admitted to hospital with acute-onset dyspnea, maintained on oxygen support and intravenous fluids.

APPLE Scores

The diagnosis-independent APPLE scores were developed on ICU populations, with data from 598 dogs and 450 cats used for model construction and data from 212 dogs and 150 cats used for assessing model performance.[30,31] For the canine APPLE score, both 10 variable and 5 variable models were reported, whereas for the feline APPLE score the models contained 8 and 5 variables, $APPLE_{full}$ and $APPLE_{fast}$, respectively. The feline $APPLE_{full}$ calculation construct is shown in Figure 13-2 and Box 13-2. An example of $APPLE_{full}$ score calculation from clinical parameters is shown for a clinical patient in Figure 13-3 and Table 13-2. A feature of model construction was that the models allowed for nonlinear relationships between predictive variables; for example, the relationship between mortality risk and white blood cell counts for the canine score gave a higher risk when counts were either very low or high. The models showed good performance characteristics when validated, and the case populations used to evaluate model performance were maintained distinct from those used to construct the models. This reduced the risk of bias in overestimating good model performance. A recent study evaluating the performance characteristics of the SPI2 model and APPLE model in conjunction with cardiac troponins for mortality prediction in 42 dogs admitted to ICU with primary noncardiac disease found that the APPLE score showed better predictive capacity than the SPI2 (AUROC = 0.776 vs. 0.610) and that the addition of cardiac troponins improved model performance in that patient group.[62]

SUMMARY

What can we learn from illness severity scores? We can decrease bias and confounding and add important contextual information to our research. We can supplement our clinical judgment with objective measures of patient illness. We can benchmark performance and establish protocols for triage and therapeutic management based on objective measures. Many diagnosis-specific and diagnosis-independent veterinary scores have been presented in recent years. Score adoption may be maximized by the development of scores that

Table 13-2 **Example of Feline $APPLE_{full}$ Score Calculation**

Parameter	Most Abnormal Value Detected Over First 24 Hours of Admission	$APPLE_{full}$ Score
Rectal temperature (°C)	37	3
Mean arterial pressure (mm Hg) (Doppler)	80	4
Lactate (mmol/L)	3.2	5
PCV (%)	18	11
Urea (mmol/L)	15.2	7
Chloride (mmol/L)	121	0
Body cavity fluid score	Thoracic free fluid present	3

PCV, Packed cell volume.

Total $APPLE_{full}$ score = 8 + 3 + 4 + 5 + 11 + 7 + 0 + 3 = 41/80

Conversion to mortality probability (p) using $APPLE_{full}$ equations in Figure 13-2.

R = (0.213 x 41) − 9.472 = −0.739

p = exp(−0.739) / (1 + exp[−0.739]) = 0.32

Thus in the range 0 to 1 estimated mortality probability for this patient is 0.32 or 32% risk of nonsurvival to discharge.

Calculation mentation score at admission: Unable to stand, responsive—score 8.

can be calculated simply, are well validated, summarize a patient's physiologic condition, and reflect an accepted and trusted development methodology.[27] Clinician and researcher access to illness severity scores and score updates would be greatly assisted by the establishment of a central online score repository, perhaps associated with one of the specialty colleges. The prevalence of euthanasia in companion animal medicine poses a unique challenge to scores based on a mortality outcome.

REFERENCES

1. Syme HM, Markwell PJ, Pfeiffer D: Survival of cats with naturally occurring chronic renal failure is related to severity of proteinuria, J Vet Intern Med 20:528-535, 2006.
2. Jergens AE, Schreiner CA, Frank DE, Niyo Y: A scoring index for disease activity in canine inflammatory bowel disease, J Vet Intern Med 17:291-297, 2003.
3. Jergens AE: Clinical assessment of disease activity for canine inflammatory bowel disease, J Am Anim Hosp Assoc 40:437-445, 2004.
4. King LG, Stevens MT, Ostro EN: A model for prediction of survival in critically ill dogs, J Vet Emerg Crit Care 4:85-99, 1994.
5. Le Gall JR, Loirat P, Alperovitch A: A simplified acute physiology score for ICU patients, Crit Care Med 12:975-977, 1984.
6. Zimmerman JE, Kramer AA, McNair DS, et al: Intensive care unit length of stay: benchmarking based on APACHE IV, Crit Care Med 34:2517-2529, 2006.
7. Knaus WA, Wagner DP, Draper EA, et al: The APACHE III prognostic system: risk prediction of hospital mortality for critically ill hospitalized adults, Chest 100:1619-1636, 1991.
8. Rohrbach BW, Buchanan BR, Drake JM, et al: Use of a multivariable model to estimate the probability of discharge in hospitalised foals that are seven days of age or less, J Am Vet Med Assoc 228:1748-1756, 2006.
9. Higgins TL: Severity of illness indices and outcome prediction. In Fink MP, Abraham E, Vincent JL, Kochanek PM, editors: Textbook of critical care, Philadelphia, 2005, Elsevier Saunders, pp 2195-2206.
10. Sinuff T, Adhikari NK, Cook DJ, et al: Mortality predictions in the intensive care unit: comparing physicians with scoring systems, Crit Care Med 34:878-885, 2006.
11. Kruse JA, Thill-Baharozian MC, Carlson RW: Comparison of clinical assessment with APACHE II for predicting mortality risk in patients admitted to the intensive care unit, J Am Med Assoc 26:1739-1742, 1988.
12. Zambelli D, Cunto M, Gentilini F: Validation of a model to develop a symptom index for benign prostatic hyperplasia in dogs, Repro Dom Anim 47:229-231, 2012.
13. Bradbury CA, Westropp JL, Pollard RE: Relationship between prostatomegaly, prostatic mineralization, and cytologic diagnosis, Vet Radiol Ultrasound 50(2):167-171, 2009.
14. Le Gall JR: The use of severity scores in the intensive care unit, Intensive Care Med 31:1618-1623, 2005.
15. King LG, Wohl JS, Manning AM, et al: Evaluation of the survival prediction index as a model of risk stratification for clinical research in dogs admitted to intensive care units at four locations, Am J Vet Res 62:948-954, 2001.
16. Higgins TL: Quantifying risk and benchmarking performance in the adult intensive care unit, J Intensive Care Med 22:141-156, 2007.
17. Rogers J, Fuller HD: Use of daily APACHE II scores to predict individual patient survival rate, Crit Care Med 22:1402-1405, 1994.
18. Rexius H, Brandrup-Wognsen GB, et al: A simple score to assess mortality risk in patients waiting for coronary artery bypass grafting, Ann Thoracic Surg 81:577-582, 2006.
19. Valencia M, Badia J, et al: Pneumonia severity index class V patients, characteristics, outcomes, and value of severity scores, Chest 132:515-522, 2007.
20. Mansfield CS, James FE, Robertson ID: Development of a clinical severity index for dogs with acute pancreatitis, J Am Vet Med Assoc 233:936-944, 2008.
21. Rothen HU, Stricker K, et al: Variability in outcome and resource use in intensive care units, Intensive Care Med 33:1329-1336, 2006.
22. Lockrem JD Sirio CA: The use of intensive care unit severity scoring systems in reimbursement strategies, Crit Care Clin 10:145-146, 1994.
23. Dohoo I, Martin W, Stryhn H: Confounder bias: analytic control and matching, Charlottetown, Prince Edward Island, 2007, Veterinary Epidemiologic Research, pp 235-270.
24. Zimmerman JE, Kramer AA, et al: APACHE IV—hospital mortality assessment for today's critically ill patients, Crit Care Med 34:1297-1310, 2006.
25. Higgins TL, Teres D, Nathanson B: Outcome prediction in critical care: the Mortality Probability models, Curr Opin Crit Care 14:498-505, 2008.
26. Capuzzo M, Moreno R, LeGall JR: Outcome prediction in critical care: the Simplified Acute Physiology Score models, Curr Opin Crit Care 14:485-490, 2008.
27. Harrison DA, Parry GJ, Carpenter JR, et al: A new risk prediction model for critical care: the intensive care national audit and research centre (ICNARC) model, Crit Care Med 35:1091-1098, 2007.
28. Zimmerman JE, Kramer AA: Outcome prediction in critical care: the Acute Physiology and Chronic Health Evaluation models, Curr Opin Crit Care 14:491-497, 2008.
29. Beaulieu M, Williamson D, Sirois C: Do proton-pump inhibitors increase the risk for nosocomial pneumonia in a medical intensive care unit, J Crit Care 23:513-518, 2008.
30. Hayes G, Mathews K, Doig G, et al: The APPLE Score: a severity of illness stratification system for hospitalized dogs, J Vet Intern Med 24:1034-1047, 2010.
31. Hayes G, Mathews K, Doig G: The Feline APPLE Score: a severity of illness stratification system for hospitalized cats, J Vet Intern Med 25(1):26-38, 2011.
32. Trow A, Rozanski E, DeLaforcade A: Evaluation of use of human albumin in critically ill dogs: 73 cases (2003-2006), J Am Vet Med Assoc 233:607-612, 2008.
33. Chan DL, Rozanski EA, Freeman LM: Relationship among plasma amino acids, C reactive protein, illness severity and outcome in critically ill dogs, J Vet Intern Med 23:559-663, 2009.
34. Prittie JE, Barton LJ, Peterson ME, et al: Pituitary ACTH and adrenocortical secretion in critically ill dogs, J Am Vet Med Assoc 220:615-619, 2002.
35. Munster M, Horauf A, Bilzer T: Assessment of disease severity and outcome of dietary, antibiotic and immunosuppressive interventions by use of the canine IBD activity index in 21 dogs with chronic inflammatory bowel disease, Berl Munch Tierarztl Wochenschr 119:493-505, 2006 [German].
36. Gaschen L, Kircher P, Stussi A, et al: Comparison of ultrasonographic findings with clinical activity index (CIBDAI) and diagnosis in dogs with chronic enteropathies, Vet Radiol Ultrasound 49:56-64, 2008.
37. Liu-Deryk X, Collingridge DS, Orme J, et al: Clinical impact of early hyperglycemia during acute phase of traumatic brain injury, Neurocritical Care 11:151-157, 2009.
38. Greenland S: Introduction to regression models. In Rothman KJ, Greenland S, Lash TL, editors: Modern epidemiology, Philadelphia, 2008, Lippincott Williams, pp 381-417.
39. Kaplan RM, Sacuzzo DP: Validity. In Psychological testing, principles, applications and issues, Belmont, CA, 2008, Wadsworth Cengage Learning, pp 133-157.
40. Harrell FE: Regression modelling strategies with applications to linear models, logistic regression, and survival analysis, New York, 2001, Springer Verlag.
41. Reference deleted in pages.
42. Shapiro AR: The evaluation of clinical predictions, N Engl J Med 296:1509-1514, 1977.
43. Brier GW: Verification of forecasts expressed in terms of probability, Monthly Weather Rev 75:1-2, 1950.
44. Spieghalter DJ: Probabilistic prediction in patient management and clinical trials, Stat Med 1986;5:421-423.
45. Hanley JA, McNeil BJ: the meaning and use of the are under the receiver operating characteristics curve, Radiology 143:29-36, 1982.
46. Segev G, Kass PH, Francey T, Cowgill LD: A novel clinical scoring system for outcome prediction in dogs with acute kidney injury managed by hemodialysis, J Vet Intern Med 22:301-308, 2008.

47. Harrison DA, Brady AR, Parry GJ: Recalibration of risk prediction models in a large multicenter cohort of admissions to adult, general critical care units in the United Kingdom, Crit Care Med 34:1378-1388, 2006.
48. Reference deleted in pages.
49. Kramer A: Predictive mortality models are not like fine wine, Crit Care 9:636-637, 2005.
50. Knaus W, Draper E, Wagner D, et al: APACHE II A severity of disease classification system, Crit Care Med 13:818-825, 1985.
51. Rello J, Rodriguez A, Lisboa T, et al: PIRO score for community acquired pneumonia: a new prediction rule for assessment of severity in intensive care unit patients with community acquired pneumonia, Crit Care Med 37:456-462, 2009.
52. Wenz JR, Garry FB, Marrington GM: Comparison of disease severity scoring systems for dairy cattle with acute coliform mastitis, J Am Vet Med Assoc 229:259-262, 2006.
53. Grulke S, Olle E, et al: Determination of a gravity and shock score for prognosis in equine surgical colic, J Vet Med A 48:465-473, 2001.
54. Preziosi R, Sarli G, Paltrinieri M: Multivariate survival analysis of histological parameters and clinical presentation in canine cutaneous mast cell tumors, Vet Res Com 31:287-296, 2007.
55. Platt SR, Radaelli AT, McDonnell JJ: The prognostic value of the modified Glasgow Coma Scale in head trauma in dogs, J Vet Intern Med 15:581-584, 2001.
56. Hosmer DW, Lemeshow S: Variable selection. In Applied logistic regression, New York, 2000, Wiley and Sons, pp 92, 339-347.
57. Peduzzi PN, Concato J, Kemper E, Holford TR, Feinstein A: A simulation study for the number of events per variable in logistic regression analysis, J Clin Epidemiology 99:1373-1379, 1996.
58. The Belgian Outcome in Burn Injury Study Group: Development and validation of a model for prediction of mortality in patients with acute burn injury, Brit J Surg 96:111-117, 2009.
59. Rockar RA, Drobatz KS: Development of a scoring system for the veterinary trauma patient, J Vet Emerg Crit Care 4:77-82, 1994.
60. Brewer BD, Koterba AM: Development of a scoring system for the early diagnosis of equine neonatal sepsis, Equine Vet J 20:18-22, 1988.
61. Reference deleted in pages.
62. Langhorn R, Oyama M, King L, et al: Prognostic importance of myocardial injury in critically ill dogs with systemic inflammation, J Vet Intern Med [Epub ahead of print], 2013.

PART II RESPIRATORY DISORDERS

CHAPTER 14
OXYGEN THERAPY

Elisa M. Mazzaferro, MS, DVM, PhD, DACVECC

KEY POINTS

- Tissue hypoxia occurs in a variety of critical illnesses. Oxygen supplementation can improve oxygen delivery and decrease the incidence of lactic acidosis.
- Supplemental oxygen administration should be provided whenever a patient's PaO_2 is less than 70 mm Hg or oxygen saturation (SpO_2) is less than 93% on room air.
- Noninvasive means of oxygen supplementation, including flow-by, mask, hood, and oxygen cages, are simple means of providing an oxygen-enriched environment to a critical patient.
- Nasal and nasopharyngeal oxygen supplementation require minimal equipment and are well tolerated by many patients that are hypoxemic.
- Tracheal oxygen supplementation provides a higher FiO_2 than nasal or noninvasive means of oxygen therapy, but it is technically slightly more difficult and has greater inherent risks to the patient.

In clinical medicine the term *hypoxia* is defined as a decrease in the level of oxygen supply to the tissues, whereas *hypoxemia* strictly refers to inadequate oxygenation of arterial blood and is defined as a PaO_2 less than 80 mm Hg (at sea level) (see Chapter 15). Because hypoxemia reduces the oxygen content of the arterial blood (CaO_2), it may result in tissue hypoxia. Because oxygen delivery to the tissues (DO_2) is dependent on the product of cardiac output and CaO_2 (Box 14-1), increases in cardiac output can prevent tissue hypoxia in hypoxemic patients.

Hypoxemia can occur as a result of hypoventilation, ventilation-perfusion mismatch, diffusion impairment, decreased oxygen content of inspired air, and intrapulmonary shunt (see Chapter 15). Global oxygen delivery is often reduced in systemic illnesses such as sepsis, systemic inflammatory response syndrome, anemia, and acid-base imbalances.

ARTERIAL OXYGEN CONTENT

Arterial oxygen content depends on the concentration of hemoglobin and the binding affinity or degree of oxygen saturation (SaO_2) of the hemoglobin present. The majority of arterial oxygen is delivered to tissues while bound to hemoglobin. A small fraction is delivered dissolved (or unbound [$0.003 \times PaO_2$]) in plasma (see Box 14-1). Provision of supplemental oxygen by increasing the fraction of inspired oxygen over 21% is an effective means of increasing both bound and unbound oxygen in arterial blood, provided that a pulmonary parenchymal shunt is not present.[1]

INDICATIONS FOR OXYGEN THERAPY

Oxygen supplementation aims to increase CaO_2, which is of particular benefit to the hypoxemic animal but is considered of benefit to all patients at risk of tissue hypoxia. Supplemental oxygen administration is indicated in patients with a PaO_2 less than 70 mm Hg or oxygen saturation (SaO_2) less than 93% on room air.[1] Oxygen therapy can be divided into noninvasive and somewhat invasive administration techniques. The type of oxygen supplementation method of delivery is largely dependent on each patient's individual needs and tolerance, patient size, the degree of hypoxemia, the level of fraction of inspired oxygen (FiO_2) desired, the anticipated length of oxygen supplementation required, clinical experience and skill, and equipment and monitoring available.[2]

METHODS OF OXYGEN ADMINISTRATION

Humidification

A variety of methods of oxygen supplementation exist. All methods require some kind of humidification source in order to avoid drying and irritation of the nasal mucosa and airways if long-term oxygen therapy is required. The administration of nonhumidified oxygen for more than several hours will result in drying and dehydration of the nasal mucosa, respiratory epithelial degeneration, impaired mucociliary clearance, and increased risk of infection.[2] A supplemental oxygen source can easily be humidified by bubbling the delivered oxygen through a bottle of sterile saline or water.[2] As oxygen is bubbled through the liquid, it becomes humidified and accumulates above the surface of the solution. The gas that collects can then be delivered through a length of oxygen tubing to the patient's oxygen source, whether it is a mask or tube into some component of the respiratory tract. Commercial bubble humidifiers are readily available and can be a convenient way to provide humidified oxygen.

Noninvasive Methods

Flow-by oxygen

Flow-by oxygen supplementation is one of the simplest techniques to utilize in an emergent patient. Flow-by oxygen provides an increased concentration of oxygen to the patient when a length of oxygen tubing (ideally connected to a humidified oxygen source although not essential for short-term therapy) is held adjacent to or within 2 cm of a patient's nostril. An oxygen flow rate of 2 to 3 L/min generally provides an FiO_2 of 25% to 40%.[3] An advantage of this technique is that it is generally well tolerated by most patients and can be used while initial triage and assessment are being performed. Because this technique also delivers a large quantity of

BOX 14-1 *Equation of Oxygen Delivery (DO_2)*

$DO_2 = Q \times CaO_2$
Where Q = cardiac output and CaO_2 = arterial oxygen content and is calculated as:
$CaO_2 = [1.34 \text{ (ml } O_2\text{/g)} \times SaO_2 \text{ (\%)} \times \text{Hemoglobin (g/dl)}] + [PaO_2\text{(mm Hg)} \times 0.003 \text{ (ml } O_2\text{/dl/mm Hg)}]$

oxygen to the surrounding environment, it is thus wasteful and not appropriate or economical for long-term use.

Face mask

Short-term oxygen supplementation can be administered by placing a face mask over a patient's muzzle, then delivering humidified oxygen or tank oxygen in a circle rebreathing or a nonrebreathing circuit. With a tight-fitting face mask, flow rates of 8 to 12 L/min can provide an FiO_2 of up to 50% to 60%.[3] With loose-fitting face masks, higher flow rates of 2 to 5 L/min are recommended, depending on the size of the patient and degree of hypoxemia. With a tight-fitting face mask, rebreathing of carbon dioxide can occur. The face mask should be vented periodically or changed to a looser face mask or alternate means of oxygen supplementation as soon as possible. Awake and coherent patients often do not tolerate oxygen delivered by face mask for long periods. An attendant must be present to ensure that the mask does not become detached and that the patient does not struggle or damage its eyes with the edge of the mask.[4] Advantages of this technique are that minimal equipment is required and that the patient can be simultaneously treated and evaluated in emergent situations.

Oxygen hood

Several varieties of oxygen hoods are available from commercial manufacturers or can be easily made in hospital with cling film (e.g., Saran Wrap), tape, and a rigid Elizabethan collar. To create an oxygen hood, the front of a rigid Elizabethan collar is covered with lengths of cling film taped in place. A small portion of the front is left open to room air to allow the hood to vent. The collar is then placed over the patient's neck and secured snugly. A length of oxygen tubing is placed through the back of the collar and taped to the side of the collar so that it doesn't become dislodged with patient movement. Once the oxygen hood has been flooded with oxygen (1 to 2 L/min), oxygen flow rates of 0.5 to 1 L/min typically will deliver an FiO_2 of 30% to 40%,[5] depending on the size of the patient and how tightly fitted the collar is around the patient's neck. With extremely small patients, such as toy breeds or neonates, the entire patient can be placed into the collar for a homemade oxygen tent or mini-cage. Some patients will not tolerate the collar and can become hyperthermic. If left unvented, carbon dioxide and moisture can accumulate within the hood and contribute to patient distress. Overall, an oxygen hood is an economical and practical means of supplemental oxygen administration and is generally well tolerated by most patients.

Oxygen cage

Supplemental oxygen can be delivered into a Plexiglas box to administer higher FiO_2 concentrations than nasal, hood, or flow-by oxygen.[4] Oxygen cages that control oxygen concentration, humidity, and temperature are available from commercial sources. The cages are also vented to decrease buildup of expired CO_2. Oxygen cages can be manufactured from human pediatric incubator units into which humidified oxygen is supplied through a length of oxygen tubing. Fractions of inspired oxygen can reach up to 60%, depending on the size of cage and patient and oxygen flow rate but typically are maintained at 40% to 50%.[2,4] Oxygen cages are very useful but also are an expensive means of administering supplemental oxygen, because oxygen within the cage is let out into the external environment whenever the cage is opened. In some patients, hyperthermia can develop if the temperature within the cage is not maintained at 70° F (22° C).[4] Ice packs can be placed within an oxygen cage to decrease ambient temperature but should not be placed directly on the patient because peripheral vasoconstriction can potentially exacerbate hyperthermia. Although many authors describe lack of direct patient access as a disadvantage of this oxygen supplementation technique, the use of continuous monitoring of pulse oximetry, blood pressure, and electrocardiogram (ECG) allow patient monitoring through the Plexiglas cage doors.[4]

Table 14-1 Nasal Oxygen Flow Rates and Associated Tracheal FiO_2[7]

Total Oxygen Flow Rate (ml/kg/min)	Tracheal FiO_2 (%)
50	29.8 +/– 5.6
100	37.3 +/– 5.7
200*	57.9 +/– 12.7
400*	77.3 +/– 13.5

*Above flow rates of 100 ml/kg/min, patient discomfort is often noted. Note 400 ml/kg/min flow rate was achieved by bilateral nasal oxygen catheters each at 200 ml/kg/min.

Invasive Methods

Nasal prongs

Human nasal prongs can be used in medium and large dogs. They are easy to place, relatively inexpensive, and well tolerated by most dogs. The disadvantages include the ease with which the animal can dislodge the nasal prongs and the unknown FiO_2 they supply. It is likely that nasal prongs would provide an FiO_2 similar to or possibly higher than flow-by oxygen but less than that provided with a nasal oxygen catheter.

Nasal and nasopharyngeal oxygen

If supplemental oxygen is going to be required for more than 24 hours, placement of a nasal or nasopharyngeal oxygen catheter should be considered. Nasal oxygen catheters are fairly simple to place, require minimal equipment, and are generally well tolerated by most patients.[6] Oxygen insufflation catheters can be placed into the nasal cavity or directly into the nasopharyngeal region by a similar technique. To place a nasal oxygen catheter, the patient's nasal passage should be anesthetized first with topical 2% lidocaine or proparacaine. Next, the tip of a 5 to 10 French (depending on patient size) red rubber or polypropylene catheter should be premeasured. To approximate the distance to advance a nasal oxygen catheter, it should be premeasured from the nose to the level of the lateral canthus of the eye and the distance marked on the tube using a permanent marker. The tip of the tube is lubricated and the tube gently inserted into the ventral nasal meatus to the level of the mark on the tube. To enter the ventral meatus it may be necessary to angle the tube ventromedially when inserted. The tube can be secured adjacent to the nostril with suture or staples. The length of tube can then be secured to the lateral maxilla or between the patient's eyes with suture or staples. To help prevent patient intolerance of the tube, be sure to avoid securing the tube to the patient's whiskers. Oxygen should be provided from a humidified oxygen source to avoid drying and irritation of the nasal mucosa. A large range of FiO_2 can be provided by nasal catheters, depending on the size of the animal, respiratory rate, and panting or mouth-breathing.[4,7] Flow rates of 50 to 150 ml/kg/min can provide 30% to 70% FiO_2.[2,8,9] (Table 14-1).

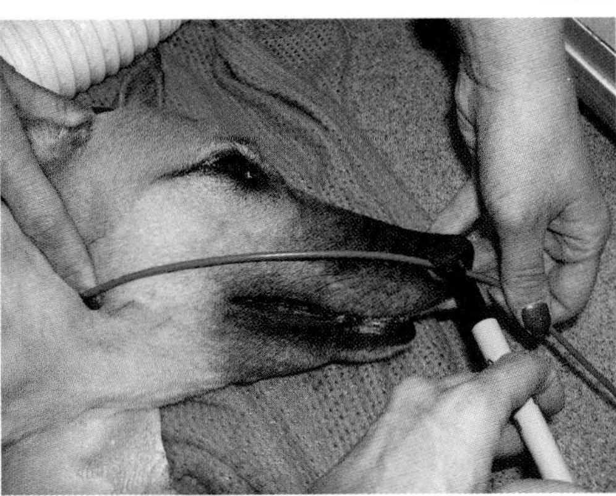

FIGURE 14-1 Measurement of a red rubber catheter to the ramus of the mandible in preparation for placement of a nasopharyngeal oxygen catheter.

Higher flow rates can be irritating to the patient and cause sneezing. Total oxygen flow rates provide similar tracheal FiO_2 when provided through one catheter or divided between two nasal catheters.[7] Sneezing and patient intolerance can be alleviated in most cases with reapplication of a topical anesthetic or advancement of the nasal catheter into the nasopharyngeal region.

The method to place a nasopharyngeal catheter is almost identical to placement of a catheter into the nasal meatus, with the exception of the anatomic landmark of where to premeasure the tube. After application of the topical anesthetic, the tip of the catheter is placed at the ramus of the mandible and marked at the tip of the nose (Figure 14-1). The lubricated tube is then placed ventromedially into the ventral nasal meatus. To facilitate passage of the tube ventrally and medially to the turbinates, the lateral aspect of the nostril should be pushed medially and the patient's nasal philtrum pushed dorsally as the tube is passed. Once the tube has been passed to the level of the mark on the tube, it can be secured to the patient's face in an identical manner as the nasal oxygen catheter. Overzealous pressure as either tube is placed can result in epistaxis. After placement of a nasal or nasopharyngeal catheter, an Elizabethan collar should be placed to help avoid iatrogenic tube dislodgement by the patient. A length of oxygen tubing attached to a humidified oxygen source can be attached to the proximal end of the nasal tube with a cut 1-ml syringe or Christmas tree adapter.

Transtracheal oxygen

Placement of a catheter directly into the trachea is an effective means of administering increased FiO_2 to patients that are intolerant of nasal or hood oxygen, are panting or displaying open-mouthed breathing, or have an upper airway obstruction. Although this technique is more labor intensive and requires a higher degree of skill than placement of a nasal catheter, higher FiO_2 with a degree of continuous airway pressure is provided[10] and can be beneficial for patients who require a higher degree of supplemental oxygen than that provided with a nasal catheter but who do not require mechanical ventilation, such as animals with severe bronchopneumonia.

Two methods of tracheal oxygen supplementation have been described. The first method uses a through-the needle large-bore catheter placed percutaneously through the skin and underlying tissues directly into the trachea.[4] The patient's ventral cervical region should be clipped just caudal to the larynx to the thoracic inlet and laterally off of midline. To avoid iatrogenic introduction of bacteria and debris into the tracheal lumen, aseptic technique must be followed at all times. The clipped area should be aseptically scrubbed. A small bleb of 2% lidocaine should be placed at the level of the third through fifth tracheal ring, infiltrating the subcutaneous tissues and skin as the needle is backed out. The area is aseptically scrubbed again. Wearing sterile gloves, the patient's trachea is gently palpated, then grasped in the operator's fingers for stabilization. A small nick incision can be made through the skin with a number 11 scalpel blade to decrease tissue drag as the catheter is inserted. The needle of the catheter is then inserted through the skin (with or without the nick incision), through the subcutaneous tissue and sternohyoideus muscle, and into the trachea. A pop will be felt as the needle enters the trachea. Once in place, the catheter with stylette is inserted through the needle into the tracheal lumen. The needle is then removed from the trachea once the catheter has been inserted to its hub. Depending on the size of the animal, the distal end of the catheter may run to the level of the carina. The catheter can be connected to a humidified oxygen source with a cut 1-ml syringe or Christmas tree adapter and oxygen run at a flow rate of 50 to 150 ml/kg/min.[10] The catheter should be secured to the neck with lengths of white tape. Caution must be exercised to monitor the patient carefully, because ventral flexion of the neck or excessive skin folds can cause kinking of the catheter and catheter occlusion. Excessive skin folds can be pulled dorsally and secured on dorsal cervical midline with several horizontal mattress sutures until the catheter is no longer required.

The second method of intratracheal oxygen supplementation is more invasive and requires heavy sedation or the administration of a short-acting anesthetic agent such as propofol or fentanyl/diazepam (see Chapters 142 and 143). The patient's ventral cervical region should be clipped and aseptically scrubbed in an identical manner as listed earlier. The area should be aseptically draped with sterile field towels and infiltrated with a local anesthetic (2% lidocaine, 1 to 2 mg/kg). A vertical skin incision should be made over the third through fifth tracheal rings. The subcutaneous tissues and sternohyoid muscle should be bluntly dissected with a curved hemostat or tips of a Metzenbaum scissors until the trachea is visible. A small incision is then made in between the fourth and fifth tracheal rings with a number 11 scalpel blade, taking care to avoid cutting more than 50% circumference of the trachea. A curved hemostat is used to open the hole between tracheal rings and a grooved director (from a spay pack) inserted into the tracheal lumen. A large-bore multifenestrated catheter with a stylette is then inserted into the tracheal lumen along the grooved director. Once the catheter is inserted, the grooved director and catheter stylette can be removed and the catheter secured in place. A 4-×-4 square of sterile gauze with antimicrobial ointment should be placed over the incision and the catheter secured with lengths of white tape. The cranial and caudal edges of large skin incisions should be sutured with nonabsorbable suture. The benefits of this technique is that larger catheters can be inserted and administer continuous airway pressure at higher oxygen flow rates than other methods of oxygen supplementation. Oxygen flow rates of 50 ml/kg/min are required to achieve 40% to 60% FiO_2.[10] This technique is well tolerated by many patients and is economical but has the inherent risks associated with sedation, general anesthesia, and introduction of bacteria directly into the tracheal lumen. Jet lesions and damage to the trachea with tracheitis can occur with this technique.[4]

HYPERBARIC OXYGEN

Hyperbaric oxygen administers 100% oxygen under supra-atmospheric pressures (>760 mm Hg) to increase the percent of dissolved oxygen in the patient's bloodstream by 10% to 20%.[1,9,11] Dissolved oxygen can diffuse readily into tissues that are damaged and may not have adequate circulation. Hyperbaric oxygen has been recommended for the treatment of severe soft tissue lesions, including burns, shearing injuries, and infection, and osteomyelitis.

Ruptured tympanum and pneumothorax have been associated with the use of hyperbaric oxygen therapy. Hyperbaric oxygen is rarely used in veterinary medicine, given the expense of the equipment and space required for a specialized "dive chamber" in which to place the patients during treatment. An additional disadvantage is that once the dive chamber has been pressurized to supra-atmospheric levels, the chamber cannot be opened to gain patient access should complications occur.

COMPLICATIONS OF OXYGEN THERAPY

The administration of supplemental oxygen is not an innocuous treatment. Hypercapnia is the primary stimulus for respiration in normal patients. In patients with chronic respiratory disease and hypercapnia, however, hypercapnic respiratory drive is diminished or lost and the patient becomes largely dependent on hypoxia as a respiratory stimulant. The administration of supplemental oxygen to a chronically hypercapnic patient depresses the hypoxic respiratory drive and can result in severe hypoventilation and respiratory failure. Mechanical ventilation may be necessary to treat the severe hypercapnia and hypoxia that develop.[1] This "blue bloater" syndrome is an uncommon occurrence in small animal medicine and is best described in human chronic obstructive pulmonary disease patients.

Oxygen Toxicity

Oxygen therapy can be directly toxic to the pulmonary epithelium. The severity and time of injury are dependent on the fraction of inspired oxygen and duration of therapy. Pulmonary oxygen toxicity can be divided into five distinct phases. During the initiation phase, oxygen-derived free radical species such as superoxide anion, peroxide, and hydroxyl radicals cause direct damage to pulmonary epithelial cells as cellular antioxidant stores become depleted.[1,9] The initiation phase occurs within 24 to 72 hours of exposure to 100% oxygen.[1] Next, destruction of the pulmonary epithelial lining causes airway inflammation and the recruitment of activated inflammatory cells to the site. During this inflammatory phase, massive release of inflammatory mediators results in increased tissue permeability and the development of pulmonary edema. Severe local destruction occurs and is most commonly associated with patient mortality. If the patient survives the destruction phase, type II pneumocytes and monocytes increase during a stage of proliferation. Finally, collagen deposition and interstitial fibrosis occur and can result in permanent damage to the lungs. An FiO_2 of more than 50% should not be administered for longer than 24 to 72 hours to avoid pulmonary oxygen toxicity.[9] Fortunately, without use of mechanical ventilation, FiO_2 greater than 50% is difficult to obtain, making the risk of pulmonary oxygen toxicity minimal with most methods of oxygen supplementation.

There is species variability in susceptibility to oxygen toxicity, and there is some concern that cats may be more sensitive than dogs. Minimizing exposure to high FiO_2 in cats is recommended. In neonates, oxygen toxicity may cause a retinal lesion called retrolental fibroplasia. Oxygen therapy should be titrated to the lowest possible concentration in neonatal patients.

REFERENCES

1. Tseng LW, Drobatz KJ: Oxygen supplementation and humidification. In King LG, editor: Textbook of respiratory disease in dogs and cats, St Louis, 2004, Elsevier, pp 205-213.
2. Camps-Palau MA, Marks SL, Cornick JL: Small animal oxygen therapy, Comp Contin Educ Pract Vet 21(7):587, 2000.
3. Loukopoulos P, Reynolds WW: Comparative evaluation of oxygen therapy techniques in anaesthetized dogs: face-mask and flow-by techniques, Aust Vet Practit 27(1):34, 1997.
4. Drobatz KJ, Hackner S, Powell S: Oxygen supplementation. In Bonagura JD, Kirk RW, editors: Current veterinary therapy XII: small animal practice, Philadelphia, 1995, WB Saunders.
5. Loukopoulos P, Reynolds W: Comparative evaluation of oxygen therapy techniques in anaesthetized dogs: intranasal catheter and Elizabethan collar canopy, Aust Vet Practit 26(4):199, 1996.
6. Marks SL: Nasal oxygen insufflation, JAAHA 35(5):366, 1999.
7. Dunphy ED, Mann FA, Dodam JR, et al: Comparison of unilateral versus bilateral catheters for oxygen administration in dogs, J Vet Emerg Crit Care 12(4):245, 2002.
8. Jackson RM. Pulmonary oxygen toxicity, Chest 86(6):900, 1985.
9. Mensack S, Murtaugh R: Oxygen toxicity, Compendium Continu Educ Pract Vet 21(4):341, 1999.
10. Mann FA, Wagner-Mann C, Allert JA, Smith J: Comparison of intranasal and intratracheal oxygen administration in healthy awake dogs, Am J Vet Res 53(5):856, 1992.
11. Braswell C, Crowe DT: Hyperbaric oxygen therapy, Compend Contin Educ Vet 34:E1-E5, 2012.

CHAPTER 15
HYPOXEMIA

†Steve C. Haskins, DVM, MS, DACVAA, DACVECC

KEY POINTS

- Hypoxemia is defined as a partial pressure of oxygen of less than 80 mm Hg or arterial blood hemoglobin saturation of less than 95%.
- When cyanosis is manifested as a sign of hypoxemia, it is always a late sign of severe hypoxemia.
- There are three causes of hypoxemia: low inspired oxygen concentration, hypoventilation, or venous admixture.
- There are four causes of venous admixture: low ventilation-perfusion regions; small airway and alveolar collapse (atelectasis); diffusion defects; and anatomic right-to-left shunts.

Hypoxemia is generally defined as an arterial partial pressure of oxygen (PaO_2) of less than 80 mm Hg or arterial blood hemoglobin saturation (SaO_2 or SpO_2) of less than 95%. Serious, potentially life-threatening hypoxemia is generally defined as a PaO_2 less than 60 mm Hg or an SaO_2 or SpO_2 of less than 90%. Atmospheric oxygen is normally ventilated into the alveoli; it then diffuses across the respiratory membrane along partial pressure gradients into the plasma. Anything that interferes with one or more of these processes will decrease the plasma PO_2. Oxygen diffuses from the plasma into the red blood cell and binds to hemoglobin. Both the PaO_2 and SaO_2 are affected by the same pulmonary processes, and SaO_2 or SpO_2 are often used as a surrogate marker of PaO_2. Blood oxygen can also be expressed as a concentration or content (milliliters of oxygen per 100 ml of whole blood), but this parameter is primarily determined by hemoglobin concentration and is not considered, per se, to be a marker of hypoxemia.

COLLECTION OF BLOOD SAMPLES FOR IN VITRO MEASUREMENT

Arterial blood must be used for an assessment of pulmonary function. Venous blood comes from the tissues and is more a reflection of tissue function than lung function. The details of blood sampling and storage before analysis have been detailed elsewhere.[1-3] The blood sample must be taken as anaerobically as possible (exposure to air will change the partial pressures of both oxygen and carbon dioxide) and analyzed as soon as possible. (In vitro metabolism and diffusion of gases into and through the plastic of the syringe will change the partial pressures of both oxygen and carbon dioxide.[4]) Excessive dilution with anticoagulant should be avoided.[5]

RECOGNITION OF HYPOXEMIA

PaO_2

The PaO_2 is the partial pressure (the vapor pressure) of oxygen dissolved in solution in the plasma of arterial blood and is measured with a blood gas analyzer, usually with a silver anode/platinum cathode system in an electrolyte solution (polarography) separated from the unknown solution (the blood) by a semipermeable (to oxygen) membrane. The arterial PO_2 (PaO_2) is a measure of the ability of the lungs to move oxygen from the atmosphere to the blood. The normal PaO_2 at sea level ranges between 80 and 110 mm Hg.

SpO_2

Hemoglobin saturation with oxygen (SaO_2) is the inevitable consequence of the increase in PaO_2 during the arterialization of venous blood as it traverses the lung; PaO_2 and SaO_2 are directionally (though not linearly) related. Hemoglobin saturation with oxygen can be measured with a bench-top oximeter (SaO_2) using many wavelengths of red to infrared light.

Pulse oximeters use only two wavelengths (660 and 940 nm) and are designed to measure only oxygenated hemoglobin (SpO_2) (see Chapters 109 and 186).[6,7]

SpO_2 is directionally, but not linearly, associated with PaO_2 (Figure 15-1) and therefore can be used as a surrogate marker of PaO_2 (Table 15-1). The SO_2/PO_2 relationship is described by a sigmoid curve, the oxygen-hemoglobin dissociation curve (see Figure 15-1 and Table 15-1). There are several important clinical implications of this relationship. Most importantly, the difference between normoxemia and hypoxemia is only a few saturation percentage points (see Table 15-1), and severe hypoxemia is only a few saturation percentage points below that. Small changes in SpO_2 represent large changes in PaO_2 in this region of the oxyhemoglobin dissociation curve. Second, severe hypoxemia is defined at a level when the hemoglobin is still 90% saturated. This may not seem fair, but it is the partial pressure of oxygen in the plasma, not hemoglobin saturation, that drives oxygen diffusion down to the mitochondria. PO_2 is the driving force; SO_2 (more specifically oxygen content) is the reservoir that prevents the rapid decrease in PO_2 that would otherwise occur when oxygen diffuses out of the blood. Third, saturation measurements cannot detect the difference between a PaO_2 of 100 and 500. This difference is important when monitoring and tracking the progress of animals breathing an enriched oxygen mixture. With these, and a few additional caveats, pulse oximeters noninvasively, continuously, and automatically monitor very well the parameter they were designed to measure—hypoxemia (see Chapter 186). Pulse oximeter readings are prone to error, and suspected hypoxemia should be corroborated with other clinical signs and an arterial blood gas analysis if necessary.

Cyanosis

Grayish to bluish discoloration of mucous membranes commonly signals the presence of deoxygenated hemoglobin in the observed tissues. The observation of cyanosis is dependent on the visual acuity of the observer (some individuals can see it earlier than others), lighting (it is more readily detected in a well-lit room than in the shadows of a cage), and the type of lighting used (it is more readily detectable with incandescent as opposed to fluorescent lighting).[12] In general, it requires an absolute concentration of deoxygenated hemoglobin to manifest sufficient cyanosis that everyone agrees to its

†Deceased.

existence; 5 gm/dl is the commonly cited figure.[13] This is important for two reasons. First, if a dog had a hemoglobin concentration of 15 gm/dl, cyanosis would manifest when the arterial blood saturation decreased to 67% (equivalent to a PaO_2 of about 37 mm Hg (see Figure 15-1). When cyanosis is manifested as a sign of hypoxemia, it is always a late sign of severe hypoxemia. Second, if an animal is anemic—for instance, having a hemoglobin concentration of 5 gm/dl—it would die of hypoxemia and the resultant tissue hypoxia long before manifesting cyanosis.

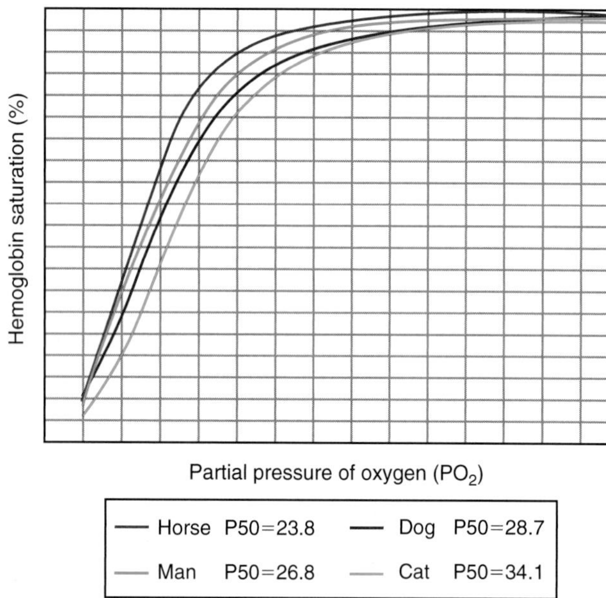

FIGURE 15-1 Oxyhemoglobin dissociation curves for the horse, man, dog, and cat.[8-11]

MECHANISMS OF HYPOXEMIA

There are three causes of hypoxemia: low inspired oxygen concentration, hypoventilation, and venous admixture (Figure 15-2; Tables 15-2 and 15-3). A fourth cause of hypoxemia can be a reduced venous oxygen content[14-18] secondary to low cardiac output or sluggish peripheral blood flow (shock) or high oxygen extraction by the tissues (seizures). When venous oxygen content is very low, it takes

Table 15-1 Correlation Between PaO_2 and SaO_2*

	PaO_2	SaO_2
Severe hyperoxemia	500	100
Hyperoxemia	125	99
Normoxemia	100	98
Hypoxemia	<80	<95
Severe hypoxemia	<60	<90
P50	29	50

*This chart represents rounded approximations of the relationship between PaO_2 and SaO_2 in people and dogs. Cats have a right-shifted curve, in comparison, and the corresponding SaO_2 values are lower (see Figure 15-1).

Table 15-2 Primary Physiologic Causes of Hypoxemia

Causes of Hypoxemia	Recognition and Examples	Treatment
Low inspired oxygen	Inspection of the apparatus Improper functioning apparatus to which the animal is attached Depleted oxygen supply; altitude	Oxygen supplementation if at altitude Disconnect patient from mechanical apparatus and repair/replace apparatus
Global hypoventilation	Elevated $PaCO_2$, end-tidal CO_2, or $PvCO_2$ Neuromuscular dysfunction; airway obstruction, abdominal distention, chest wall dysfunction, pleural space filling defect	Oxygen supplementation; positive pressure ventilation; remove/bypass obstruction; decompress abdomen; close or stabilize chest wall; provide thoracocentesis
Venous admixture	See Table 15-3	See Table 15-3.

CO_2, Carbon dioxide; *$PvCO_2$,* venous PCO_2.

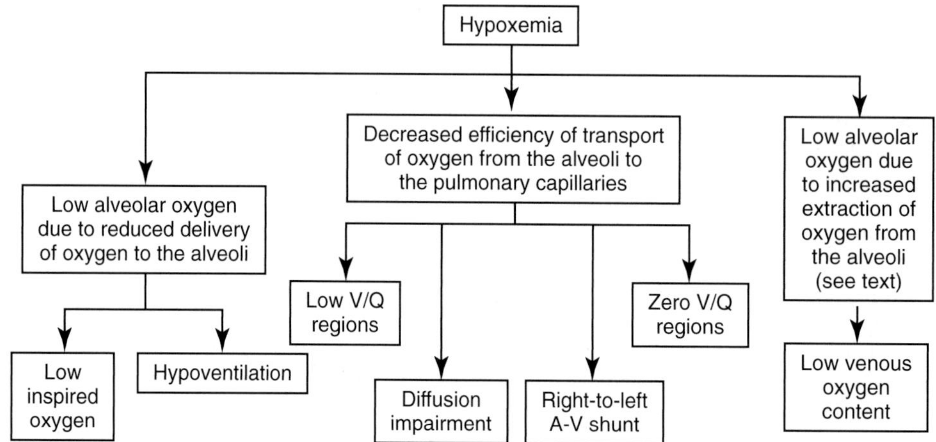

FIGURE 15-2 Categorical causes of hypoxemia.

Table 15-3 **Venous Admixture**

Mechanisms of Venous Admixture	Causes	Notes
Low V/Q regions	Moderate to severe diffuse lung disease (edema, pneumonia, hemorrhage)	Common; responsive to oxygen therapy
Atelectasis (No V/Q regions)	Severe to very severe diffuse lung disease (edema, pneumonia, hemorrhage)	Common; not responsive to oxygen but responsive to PPV
Diffusion defects	Moderate to severe, diffuse lung disease (oxygen toxicity, smoke inhalation, ARDS)	Uncommon; partially responsive to oxygen
Right-to-left shunts	Right-to-left PDA and VSD; intrapulmonary A-V anatomic shunts	Uncommon; not responsive to oxygen or PPV; surgery possible

A-V, Arterial to venous; *ARDS,* acute respiratory distress syndrome; *low V/Q ratio,* low ventilation compared with blood flow because of either low regional ventilation or high regional perfusion; *PDA,* patent ductus arteriosus; *PPV,* positive pressure ventilation; *Q,* perfusion; *V,* ventilation; *VSD,* ventricular septal defect.

more oxygen and more time for the capillary blood to be arterialized. This lowers alveolar PO_2 (P_AO_2) and therefore PaO_2 will be lowered. In practice, the impact of low venous oxygen and blood flow is often offset by a decrease in shunt fraction, which offsets the decrease in PaO_2.[14,19] Low venous oxygen is verified by measuring central or mixed venous oxygen.

Low Inspired Oxygen

Low inspired oxygen must be considered any time an animal is attached to mechanical apparatus such as a face mask, anesthetic circuit, or ventilator or is in an enclosed environment such as an oxygen cage. Inspired or ambient oxygen concentration can be measured with a variety of commercially available oxygen meters. The problem can often be identified by inspection and verification of the improper operation of the mechanical device and remedied by replacing the device with one that is operating properly. The decrease in inspired oxygen concentration decreases the alveolar oxygen concentration and subsequently arterial blood oxygenation.

High altitude is another cause of low inspired oxygen. Atmospheric oxygen concentration is 21% at any altitude, but as altitude increases, barometric pressure decreases and the partial pressure of oxygen in the atmosphere ($P_{atm}O_2$) represented by 21% also decreases. Normal individuals living at higher altitudes have lower PaO_2 values and compensate to some extent by hyperventilating.

Hypoventilation

Hypoventilation is defined by an elevated $PaCO_2$ (≥45 mm Hg) or one of its surrogate markers: end-tidal CO_2 (usually about 5 mm Hg lower than $PaCO_2$) or central venous PCO_2 (usually about 5 mm Hg higher than $PaCO_2$). See Chapter 16 for further discussion of this topic.

Alveolar oxygen is the balance between the amount of oxygen being delivered to the alveoli (inspired oxygen concentration and alveolar minute ventilation) and the amount of oxygen being removed from the alveoli by the arterialization of venous blood (ultimately, tissue metabolism). A decrease in alveolar minute ventilation (hypoventilation) decreases the delivery of oxygen to the alveoli and subsequently to the blood leading to hypoxemia. Increasing the inspired oxygen concentration is very effective in preventing hypoxemia secondary to hypoventilation.

There are only four gases of note in alveoli: oxygen, carbon dioxide, water vapor, and nitrogen. The partial pressure of alveolar oxygen (P_AO_2) can be determined by the alveolar air equation. The normal alveolar composition of gases when breathing room air at sea level is water vapor 50 mm Hg (fixed; alveolar gases are always 100% saturated at body temperature); carbon dioxide 40 mm Hg (regulated by the brainstem respiratory control center); oxygen 105 mm Hg; and nitrogen 560 mm Hg.[19] If an animal was to hypoventilate to a $PaCO_2$ of 80 mm Hg, the water vapor pressure and nitrogen levels would remain unchanged but the oxygen would fall to about 65 mm Hg and the patient would become hypoxemic. When breathing 100% oxygen for a time to allow the elimination of nitrogen from the readily mobilized stores (alveoli, blood, and vessel-rich tissues), the alveolar water vapor and carbon dioxide levels would not change but nitrogen would decrease to near 0 and oxygen would increase to near 665. If an animal were to severely hypoventilate while breathing 100% oxygen, the alveolar carbon dioxide could theoretically rise to about 550 mm Hg before the alveolar oxygen decreased to a level that would lead to hypoxemia ($PaO_2 < 80$ mm Hg). Hence hypoventilation is a cause of hypoxemia in patient's breathing room air but not in patients breathing enriched oxygen mixtures. Further hypoxemia as a result of hypoventilation is readily resolved with oxygen therapy.

Venous Admixture

Venous admixture is all the ways in which venous blood can get from the right side to the left side of the circulation without being properly oxygenated. Blood flowing through some regions of the lung may be suboptimally oxygenated or may not be oxygenated at all. When this "venous" blood admixes with optimally arterialized blood flowing from the more normally functioning regions of the lung, the net oxygen content and PaO_2 are reduced. There is typically a small amount of venous admixture in the normal lung (<5%).[20] An increase in venous admixture represents a reduced blood-oxygenating efficiency of the lung and implies the presence of intrinsic pulmonary parenchymal disease.

There are four causes of venous admixture (see Table 15-2): (1) low ventilation-perfusion regions, (2) small airway and alveolar collapse (atelectasis or zero ventilation but perfused lung units), (3) diffusion defects, and (4) anatomic right-to-left shunts. Most diffuse lung disease will have a variable combination of each of these mechanisms; however, one often predominates. These mechanisms have important therapeutic implications. It is also inappropriate to use the term *ventilation-perfusion (V/Q) mismatch* as a cause of hypoxemia without some adjective (i.e., "high" or "low") because not all types of V/Q mismatch contribute to hypoxemia (Table 15-4).

Regions of low ventilation-perfusion (V/Q) ratio

Alveoli with a low ventilation-perfusion (V/Q) ratio occur secondary to small airway narrowing, which impairs ventilation. Because it is a ratio, a low V/Q could also be caused by an increased Q, such as occurs in pulmonary thromboembolism. Small airway narrowing may be caused by bronchospasm, fluid accumulation along the walls of the lower airways, or epithelial edema. Like global hypoventilation, regional hypoventilation results in the reduced delivery of oxygen to alveoli (compared with that removed by the circulation) and a

Table 15-4 **Categories of Ventilation-Perfusion Mismatching and Their Contribution to PaO_2**

Category	Impact	Example
Ventilated but unperfused lung units	Alveolar dead space ventilation; no impact on net PaO_2 because there is no blood flow to or from these regions	Pulmonary thromboembolism
Higher than average ventilation/perfusion ratio lung units	Regional hyperventilation; tends to increase PaO_2	Hypovolemia; high tidal volumes
Average ventilation-perfusion ratio lung units	Normal situation; normal PaO_2	Normal
Lower than average ventilation-perfusion ratio lung units	Regional hypoventilation; tends to decrease PaO_2	Small airway narrowing secondary to lower airway disease; hypoxemia is oxygen responsive
No ventilation but perfused lung units	Physiologic shunt; tends to decrease PaO_2	Small airway and alveolar collapse; hypoxemia is not oxygen responsive but is responsive to PPV

PPV, Positive pressure ventilation.

reduction in alveolar and arterial PO_2. Poorly oxygenated blood from these capillary beds admixes with blood from more normally functioning regions of the lung, diluting and reducing the net oxygen concentration. This is a common mechanism of hypoxemia in moderate pulmonary disease. Like global hypoventilation, regional hypoventilation is very responsive to oxygen therapy.

Regions of zero V/Q

Small airway and alveolar collapse (regions of zero V/Q) occurs in diseases associated with the accumulation of airway fluids (transudate, exudates, or blood). Small airway and alveolar collapse is common in the dependent regions of the lung if animals are recumbent for prolonged periods of time (e.g., general anesthesia or coma) in the absence of an occasional deep (sigh) breath. Blood flowing through these areas will not be arterialized. This condition has been referred to as "physiologic shunt" (blood flowing past nonfunctional alveoli) to differentiate it from a "true or anatomic shunt," where blood completely bypasses all alveoli (be they functional or not). Hypoxemia due to zero V/Q regions is not responsive to oxygen therapy because oxygen cannot get to the gas exchange surface. Collapsed small airways and alveoli can only be "reactivated" by increasing airway or transpulmonary pressure, by taking a deep spontaneous breath, or by augmentation of airway pressure. This is a common mechanism of hypoxemia in severe pulmonary disease as proven by the fact that positive pressure ventilation and positive end-expiratory pressure (PEEP) are usually very effective at improving lung oxygenating efficiency.

Diffusion impairment

Diffusion impairment as a result of a thickened respiratory membrane is an uncommon cause of hypoxemia. Capillaries meander through the interstitial septae, between alveoli, bulging first into one alveolus and then into the adjacent alveolus. The interstitium between the endothelium and the epithelium on the "bulge side" or "thin side" of the capillary (encompassing two thirds to three fourths of the circumference of the capillary) is either nonexistent (the endothelial and epithelial basement membranes are one in the same) or is functionally nonexistent, and no fluid accumulates here. Transcapillary fluid leaks occur on the thick ("service") side of the capillary but do not accumulate here either. Fluid is forced (by the low compliance of the interstitial tissues and lymphatics) upward toward the loose interstitial tissues surrounding the medium-sized arterioles, venules, and bronchioles toward the hilus of the lung.[21] Eventually these interstitial fluids build up enough pressure that they break into the airways and distribute along the airway surfaces, causing first airway narrowing (low V/Q) and then small airway and alveolar collapse (0 V/Q), as discussed earlier and without a diffusion defect per se. In order for a diffusion defect to occur, the flat type I alveolar pneumocytes have to be damaged by inhalation or inflammatory injury. In the healing process, the thick, cuboidal type II alveolar pneumocytes proliferate across the surface of the gas exchange surface. This can occur with oxygen toxicity or during progression of the acute respiratory distress syndrome.[22] Such thickening of the gas exchange membrane represents a substantial diffusion defect until such time as the type II pneumocytes mature to type I pneumocytes. Diffusion defects are partially responsive to oxygen therapy.

Anatomic Shunts

Anatomic shunts that cause hypoxemia are vascular abnormalities where the blood flows from the right side to the left side of the circulation, bypassing all alveoli in the process. This is not a common mechanism of hypoxemia and most commonly found in young animals with congenital defects. This cause of hypoxemia is not responsive to either oxygen therapy or positive pressure ventilation. Some are amenable to surgical intervention.

ESTIMATING THE MAGNITUDE OF THE VENOUS ADMIXTURE

In pulmonary parenchymal disease, lungs often fail in their ability to get oxygen in before failing their ability to get carbon dioxide out. This is apparent from the rather common co-occurrence of hypocapnia and hypoxemia and is attributed to the fact that alveolar-capillary units that are working relatively well can easily compensate for those that are working relatively poorly with respect to carbon dioxide elimination but not for oxygen intake. It is for this reason that it is important to evaluate $PaCO_2$ and PaO_2 separately. $PaCO_2$ defines alveolar minute ventilation; PaO_2 defines blood oxygenation. Given the specifics of the situation, any combination of ventilation (normo-, hypo-, or hyper-) and oxygenation (normo-, hypo-, or hyper-) can coexist in a patient at a given time, and different combinations mandate different therapeutic strategies. Although PaO_2 defines the status of blood oxygenation, the clinical significance of the measurement (the status of lung function; the magnitude of the venous admixture) can only be fully appreciated when PaO_2 is referenced to the $PaCO_2$ and the inspired oxygen at the time of measurement.

Because factors including FiO_2 and the nature of ventilator settings can alter PaO_2, in general it is recommended to estimate venous admixture under some arbitrary conditions (such as "always while breathing room air" or "always while breathing 100% oxygen" or "always off ventilator support" or "always at a certain mean airway pressure"). Although the latter approach may provide a more consistent evaluation of the underlying pathophysiology, the former approach indexes therapeutic effectiveness and guides the withdrawal of such support.

$PaCO_2$ + PaO_2 Added Value ("The 120 rule")

When breathing 21% oxygen at sea level, the $PaCO_2$ + PaO_2 added value calculation will give the clinician some idea about lung function. A normal $PaCO_2$ of 40 mm Hg and a minimum PaO_2 value for normoxemia of 80 mm Hg add to 120. An added value of less than 120 mm Hg suggests the presence of venous admixture, and the greater the discrepancy, the worse the lung function. If $PaCO_2$ increases from 40 mm Hg to 60 mm Hg by hypoventilation, the PaO_2 should decrease from 80 mm Hg to about 60 mm Hg if the animal does not have lung disease, and the addition of the two values will still equal 120. The conclusion is that the cause of the hypoxemia in this situation was purely hypoventilation. If instead the animal has a $PaCO_2$ of 60 mm Hg and a PaO_2 of 40 mm Hg, the added value is 100 (less than 120) and it can be concluded that the animal has lung dysfunction in addition to hypoventilation. This added value rule or "120 rule" can only be used when the patient is breathing 21% oxygen at near-sea level conditions. At altitude, atmospheric and alveolar and arterial PO_2, and the "added value rule," need to be proportionately decreased.

Alveolar-Arterial PO_2 Gradient

The alveolar-arterial PO_2 gradient (A-a gradient) is the difference between the calculated alveolar partial pressure of oxygen (P_AO_2) and the measured arterial partial pressure of oxygen (PaO_2) and is described in further detail in Chapter 186. At sea level, breathing 21%, the alveolar air equation can be shortened to

$$P_AO_2 = 150 - PaCO_2$$

At different altitudes and inspired oxygen concentrations, the complete formula must be used. Once P_AO_2 has been calculated, the A-a gradient is calculated by subtracting the measured PaO_2 from the calculated P_AO_2. When breathing room air, the usual A-a gradient is less than 10 mm Hg; values above 20 mm Hg are considered to represent decreased oxygenating efficiency (venous admixture). Unfortunately the normal A-a gradient increases at higher inspired oxygen concentrations and may be as high as 100 to 150 mm Hg at an inspired oxygen concentration of 100%. As a result the A-a gradient is of most value when assessing room air blood gases.

PaO_2/FiO_2 Ratio

Many approaches have been suggested that could be used to compensate for the variation in A-a gradient associated with variation in inspired oxygen. The PaO_2/FiO_2 (or P/F) ratio is the easiest to calculate and is further described in Chapter 186.

The P/F ratio can be very misleading when used at 21% inspired oxygen concentrations if $PaCO_2$ values are elevated. $PaCO_2$ values have been ignored in this calculation, but when breathing room air, changes in $PaCO_2$ can have a significant impact on PaO_2. It is recommended to use the "120 rule" or A-a gradient when evaluating room air blood gases and to use the P/F ratio if evaluating arterial blood gases from patients on supplemental oxygen.

Venous Admixture (Shunt) Calculation

If a mixed venous blood sample (pulmonary artery) can be obtained, then venous admixture can be calculated as

$$Q_S/Q_T = (CcO_2 - CaO_2)/(CcO_2 - C\bar{v}O_2)$$

where Q_S is shunt fraction; Q_T, cardiac output; Q_S/Q_T, venous admixture expressed as a percent of cardiac output; CcO_2, oxygen content of end-capillary blood; CaO_2, oxygen content of arterial blood; and $C\bar{v}O_2$, oxygen content of mixed venous blood.

Jugular venous blood is sometimes used as a surrogate for pulmonary arterial blood. Arterial and mixed venous PO_2 is measured and oxygen content (ml/dl) is calculated as

$$(1.34 \times Hb \times SO_2) + (0.003 \times PO_2)$$

where SO_2 is percent hemoglobin saturation with oxygen. Capillary PO_2 is assumed to be equal to calculated P_AO_2 and is used to calculate capillary oxygen content. PO_2 is measured and SO_2 is either measured (accuracy mandates a bench-top oximeter) or extrapolated from a standard oxyhemoglobin dissociation curve (which is the value reported on the printout from some blood gas analyzers, or can be derived by hand from an oxyhemoglobin dissociation curve such as in Figure 15-1. Venous admixture is normally less than 5%.[20] Values greater than 10% are considered to be increased and may increase to more than 50% in severe, diffuse lung disease.

Although the equation shown earlier seems like a lot of math, it is considered to be the most accurate way to estimate venous admixture.[23] If blood samples are taken while the patient is breathing room air, all the previously discussed categorical mechanisms of venous admixture are assessed. If blood samples are taken while the patient is breathing 100% oxygen, the low V/Q mechanism of hypoxemia is eliminated from the assessment and diffusion defects are minimized. In this usage, the formula is referred to as the "shunt" formula because it assesses the magnitude of the remaining two causes of venous admixture: "physiologic" shunts secondary to atelectasis and true "anatomic" shunts. Intermediate inspired oxygen concentrations and particularly changes in inspired oxygen concentration will change the venous admixture calculated by this formula by virtue of the impact of the FiO_2 on the low V/Q regions.[24-26] Like P/F ratio, venous admixture will also be impacted by changes in mean airway pressure by virtue of its impact on the open/closed status of alveoli. It is usually recommended to determine the venous admixture at the current inspired oxygen and ventilator settings, whatever they might be, depending on the needs of the patient.[26]

REFERENCES

1. Haskins SC: Sampling and storage of blood for pH and blood gas analysis, J Am Vet Med Assoc 170:429-433, 1977.
2. Gray S, Powell LL: Blood gas analysis. In Burkitt-Creedon JM, Davis H: Advance monitoring and procedures for small animal emergency and critical care, Oxford, UK, 2012, John Wiley & Sons, Ch 22, pp 286-292.
3. Kennedy SA, Constable PD, Sen I, Couetil L: Effects of syringe type and storage conditions on results of equine blood gas and acid-base analysis, Am J Vet Res 73:979-987, 2012.
4. Rezende ML, Haskins SC, Hopper K: The effects of ice-water storage on blood gas and acid-base measurements, J Vet Emerg Crit Care 17:67-71, 2006.
5. Hopper K, Rezende ML, Haskins SC: Assessment of the effect of cilution of blood samples with sodium heparin on blood gas, electrolyte, and lactate measurements in dogs, Am J Vet Res 65:656-660, 2005.
6. Biebuyck JF: Pulse oximetry, Anesthesiology 70:98-108, 1989.
7. Ayres DA: Pulse oximetry and CO-oximetry. In Burkitt-Creedon JM, Davis H, editors: Advanced monitoring and procedures for small animal emergency and critical care, Oxford, UK, 2012, John Wiley & Sons, pp 274-285.
8. Smale K, Anderson LS, Butler PJ: An algorithm to describe the oxygen equilibrium curve for the Thoroughbred racehorse, Equine Vet J 26:500-502, 1994.
9. Kelman GR: Digital computer subroutine for the conversion of oxygen tension into saturation, J Appl Physiol 21:1375-1376, 1966.
10. Cambier C, Wierinckx M, Clerbaux T, Detry B, Liardet MP, Marville V, Frans A, Gustin P: Haemoglobin oxygen affinity and regulating factors of the blood oxygen transport in canine and feline blood, Res Vet Sci 77:83-88, 2004.

11. Clerbaux T, Gustin P, Detry B, Cao ML, Frans A: Comparative study of the oxyhaemoglobin dissociation curve of four mammals: man, dog, horse, and cattle, Comp Biochem Physiol 106:687-694, 1993.
12. Kelman GR, Nunn JF: Clinical recognition of hypoxaemia under fluorescent lamps, Lancet 1:1400-1403, 1966.
13. Martin L, Khalil H: How much reduced hemoglobin is necessary to generate central cyanosis? Chest 87:182-185, 1990.
14. Bishop MJ, Cheney FW: Effects of pulmonary blood flow and mixed venous O2 tension on gas exchange in dogs, Anesthesiology 58:130-135, 1983.
15. Giovannini I, Boldrini G, Sganga G, et al: Quantification of the determinants of arterial hypoxemia in critically ill patients, Crit Care Med 11:644-645, 1983.
16. Huttemeier PC, Ringsted C, Eliasen K, Mogensen T: Ventilation-perfusion inequality during endotoxin-induced pulmonary vasoconstriction in conscious sheep: mechanisms of hypoxia, Clin Physiol 8:351-358, 1988.
17. Santolicandro A, Prediletto R, Formai E, et al: Mechanisms of hypoxemia and hypocapnia in pulmonary embolism, Am J Respir Crit Care Med 152:336-347, 1995.
18. Cooper CB, Celli B: Venous admixture in COPD: pathophysiology and therapeutic approaches, J Clin Obst Pulm Dis 5:376-381, 2008.
19. Lumb AB: Nunn's applied respiratory physiology, ed 6, Oxford, 2005, Butterworth Heinemann.
20. Haskins SC, Pascoe PJ, Ilkiw JE, et al: Reference cardiopulmonary values in normal dogs, Comp Med 55:158-163, 2005.
21. Staub NC: The pathogenesis of pulmonary edema, Prog Cardiovasc Dis 23:53-80, 1980.
22. Ware LB, Matthay MA: The acute respiratory distress syndrome, N Engl J Med 342:1334-1349, 2000.
23. Wandrup JH: Quantifying pulmonary oxygen transfer deficits in critically ill patients, Act Anaesth Scand 107:37-44, 1996.
24. Gowda MS, Klocke RA: Variability of indices of hypoxemia in adult respiratory distress syndrome, Crit Care Med 25:41-45, 1997.
25. Whiteley JP, Gavaghan DJ, Hahn DEW: Variation of venous admixture, SF6 shunt, PaO2, and the PaO2/FIO2 ratio with FIO2, Brit J Anaesth 88:771-778, 2002.
26. Oliven A, Abinader E, Bursztein S: Influence of varying inspired oxygen tensions on the pulmonary venous admixture (shunt) of mechanically ventilated patients, Crit Care Med 8:99-101, 1980.

CHAPTER 16
HYPOVENTILATION

Meredith L. Daly, VMD, DACVECC

KEY POINTS

- Minute ventilation comprises alveolar ventilation and dead space ventilation and is calculated by multiplying the tidal volume by the respiratory rate.
- Hypercapnia results when alveolar ventilation is inadequate to remove the CO_2 produced in the body by aerobic metabolism.
- Hyperventilation is generally defined as a $PaCO_2$ less than 30 to 35 mm Hg.
- Hypoventilation is defined as a $PaCO_2$ greater than 40 to 45 mm Hg. Slight species-specific differences exist.
- Arterial CO_2 concentration is maintained within a narrow range by central and peripheral neuronal control, central and peripheral chemoreceptors, neuromuscular junctions, and respiratory mechanics.
- Clinical signs associated with hypoventilation may be the result of the systemic effects of hypercapnia, uncompensated respiratory acidosis, or secondary to the disease process causing the hypoventilation.
- The gold standard for assessment of arterial carbon dioxide ($PaCO_2$) levels is arterial blood gas analysis.
- Hypoventilation is treated by increasing alveolar ventilation through treatment of the underlying disease, chemical stimulation of breathing, and mechanical ventilation.

Carbon dioxide (CO_2) is the product of aerobic metabolism. It is produced primarily in the mitochondria and subsequently diffuses via a series of sequential partial pressure gradients into the cytoplasm, the extracellular space, the intravascular space, and the pulmonary capillaries. Upon reaching the pulmonary capillaries, CO_2 diffuses into the alveolus, where a balance between CO_2 production and alveolar ventilation determines its concentration. Therefore, in a patient with relatively constant CO_2 production, the arterial CO_2 concentration serves as a surrogate for alveolar ventilation. Increased blood CO_2 concentration, or hypercapnia, can be caused by hypoventilation or an increase in dead space ventilation, CO_2 production, or inspired CO_2 concentration. The most common cause of hypercapnia in clinical patients is hypoventilation because of decreased minute ventilation.

DEFINITIONS

Total ventilation, also called *minute ventilation*, is the total volume of gas exhaled per minute. It is equal to the tidal volume times the respiratory frequency. The volume of inhaled air is slightly greater than that exhaled because more oxygen is inhaled than carbon dioxide is exhaled; this difference is usually less than 1%. Tidal volume (V_t) comprises dead space volume (V_d), or the portion of tidal volume that does not actively participate in gas exchange, *and* the volume of fresh gas entering the alveoli (V_a).[1] Alveolar ventilation ($\dot{V}_A$) is the volume of fresh inspired air (non–dead space gas) available for gas exchange that enters the alveoli per minute, equivalent to the total amount of air breathed per minute ($\dot{V}_E$; minute ventilation) minus that air contained in the dead space per minute ($\dot{V}_D$). The alveolar ventilation also is measured theoretically during exhalation, but the inhaled and exhaled volumes are similar in health.

Alveolar ventilation ($\dot{V}_A$) can be derived from the following equations

$$V_t = V_d + V_a \quad \text{(equation 1)}$$

multiplying by respiratory rate,

$$\dot{V}_E = \dot{V}_A - \dot{V}_D \quad \text{(equation 2)}$$

which can be rearranged as

$$\dot{V}_A = \dot{V}_E - \dot{V}_D \quad \text{(equation 3)}$$

where $\dot{V}_E$ is the expired minute ventilation and $\dot{V}_D$ is the dead space ventilation.[1]

Dead space ventilation consists of the portion of tidal volume per minute that does not actively participate in gas exchange. Dead space can be subdivided into anatomic, alveolar, physiologic, and apparatus dead space. The volume of gas filling the upper airway, trachea, and lower airways to the level of the terminal bronchioles does not participate in gas exchange and therefore is considered anatomic dead space. Alveolar dead space is defined as the portion of inspired gas that passes through the anatomic dead space and mixes with gas in that alveoli but does not participate in gas exchange with the pulmonary capillaries.[1] Physiologic dead space comprises anatomic and alveolar dead space and is the sum of all portions of the tidal volume that do not participate in gas exchange. Physiologic dead space is approximately the same as anatomic dead space when the lung is normal. However, in the presence of ventilation-perfusion inequality (i.e., when a portion of tidal volume ventilates alveoli that are not perfused), physiologic dead space is increased, primarily because of the ventilated air that goes to lung units with abnormally high ventilation-perfusion ratios (increased alveolar dead space). Last, when patients are connected to a breathing device, the circuit may add dead space if any portion of tidal volume is rebreathed without fresh gas flow replacement. This is most important in patients that are small or have decreased ability to ventilate.

Dead space ventilation may be measured in several different ways; two of the most common include Fowler's method and Bohr's method. Fowler's method involves measuring the concentration of an exhaled tracer gas, typically nitrogen, over time and displaying its concentration graphically against the volume of gas exhaled. The anatomic dead space volume is subsequently derived from this graph; it is a function of the geometry of the airways.[2] Physiologic dead space can be measured via Bohr's method. This method uses the principle that all of the carbon dioxide in the exhaled gas originates from the alveolus. Therefore the concentration of CO_2 in the exhaled gas comprises alveolar CO_2 that is diluted by the CO_2-free air in the conducting airways and in the airways that are poorly perfused.[2] By measuring CO_2 in the exhaled gas, the clinician may calculate this dilution factor; it represents physiologic dead space as calculated by the Bohr equation

$$\dot{V}_D/\dot{V}_T = F_A - F_E/F_A \quad \text{(equation 5)}$$

The partial pressure of any gas is proportional to its concentration, therefore

$$\dot{V}_D/\dot{V}_T = P_ACO_2 - P_ECO_2/P_ACO_2 \quad \text{(equation 6)}$$

Assuming alveolar and arterial oxygen PCO_2 are equal, then

$$\dot{V}_D/\dot{V}_T = P_aCO_2 - P_ECO_2/P_aCO_2 \quad \text{(equation 7)}$$

Bohr's method is different from Fowler's method; it measures the volume of lung that does not eliminate carbon dioxide; therefore it is a measure of physiologic dead space rather than anatomic dead space. Once the corresponding dead space volume is measured, alveolar ventilation can be calculated by subtracting dead space ventilation from the total ventilation measured via spirometry. Alveolar ventilation is reduced by an increase in dead space ventilation, regardless of whether the dead space is of anatomic, alveolar, or apparatus origin. The corresponding changes in alveolar gas tensions are identical to those produced by a decreased minute ventilation of a different cause, such as a decreased respiratory rate.

Another way of measuring alveolar ventilation is to use the alveolar ventilation equation. The equation states that alveolar PCO_2 (P_ACO_2) is directly proportional to the amount of CO_2 produced by metabolism and delivered to the lungs ($\dot{V}CO_2$) and inversely proportional to the alveolar ventilation $\dot{V}_A$.[1]

$$P_ACO_2 \propto (\dot{V}CO_2/\dot{V}_A) \times K$$

Although the derivation of the equation is for alveolar PCO_2, its clinical usefulness stems from the fact that alveolar and arterial PCO_2 can be assumed to be equal in patients with normal lungs. Therefore

$$\dot{V}_A = (\dot{V}CO_2/PaCO_2) \times K$$

The constant 0.863 is necessary to equate dissimilar units for $\dot{V}CO_2$, $\dot{V}CO_2$ (ml/min), and $\dot{V}_A$ (L/min) to PCO_2 pressure units (mm Hg).[1] This means, for example, if the alveolar ventilation is halved, the $PaCO_2$ is doubled as long as CO_2 production remains unchanged. Even when alveolar and arterial PCO_2 are not equal (as in states of severe ventilation-perfusion imbalance), the relationship expressed by the equation remains valid: $PCO_2 \propto \dot{V}CO_2$ $\dot{V}_A$ because of the high solubility of this gas in the circulation. From the alveolar ventilation equation can be concluded that the only physiologic reason for increased $PaCO_2$ is a level of alveolar ventilation that is inadequate for the amount of CO_2 produced by aerobic metabolism and subsequently delivered to the lungs.[1]

Arterial PCO_2 is therefore a measure of the ventilatory status of a patient (see Chapter 186). Normal values vary, depending upon the analyzer used but generally fall within the range of 30 to 42 mm Hg in the dog and 25 to 36 mm Hg in the cat.[3] A $PaCO_2$ less than 30 to 35 mm Hg indicates hyperventilation, and a $PaCO_2$ greater than 40 to 45 mm Hg indicates hypoventilation. Venous CO_2 values represent a combination of arterial PCO_2, tissue metabolism, and blood flow. Venous CO_2 values are typically 3 to 6 mm Hg higher than the corresponding arterial values during steady state (33 to 42 mm Hg canine, 32 to 44 mm Hg feline) but can diverge significantly in disease states, particularly those associated with decreased tissue perfusion.[3]

CONTROL OF BREATHING

In the healthy patient, arterial CO_2 concentration is maintained within a narrow range through a complex interplay of several feedback mechanisms. Factors controlling alveolar minute ventilation include central and peripheral neuronal control, central and peripheral chemoreceptors, neuromuscular junctions, and respiratory mechanics/muscles. A disturbance in any one of these mechanisms can lead to altered alveolar minute ventilation and corresponding alterations in CO_2 concentrations. An understanding of the mechanisms of breath generation and execution is vital for the effective diagnosis and treatment of the patient with respiratory disease.

Central Neuronal Control of Breathing

The brainstem is the site of origin for automatic impulses that control breathing. The generation of the ventilatory pattern involves the integration of neural signals from three main groups of neurons located in the respiratory control centers in the medulla and pons: the medullary respiratory center, the apneustic center, and the pneumotaxic center. Respiratory neurons in the medulla are concentrated in two sites known as the ventral and dorsal respiratory groups. The dorsal respiratory group is located in the region of the nucleus tractus solitarius, where visceral afferents from cranial nerves IX and X terminate.[4] This area is responsible primarily for inspiration; neurons in this area are thought to have intrinsic periodic firing responsible for the basic rhythm of breathing.[5] The ventral respiratory group comprises four nuclei (nucleus retroambiguus, nucleus para-ambiguus, nucleus retrofacialis, and the pre-Bötzinger complex).[5] The ventral respiratory group controls voluntary forced exhalation and acts to increase the force of inspiration. The apneustic center, located in the lower pons, is responsible for coordinating the speed of inhalation and exhalation.[4] This center sends stimulatory impulses to the inspiratory area that activate and prolong inspiration. Impulses from this region can be overridden by signals from the pneumotaxic center to terminate inspiration. The pneumotaxic center, located in the upper pons, sends inhibitory impulses to the inspiratory center, terminating inspiration, and thereby regulating inspiratory volume and respiratory rate.[4] This center likely is involved in the fine-tuning of breathing. Breathing is also under voluntary control; the cerebral cortex can override impulses from the brainstem in certain situations (e.g., coughing and sniffing). These voluntary alterations are limited by changes in arterial blood gas tensions. In addition to these volitional changes in respiration, suprapontine reflex interference with respiration can occur during coughing, sneezing, and swallowing.[4]

The axons that project from the brainstem, cerebral cortex, and other suprapontine structures descend along the anterolateral white matter of the spinal cord to the phrenic, intercostal, and abdominal muscle motor neurons. Stimulation of these effector muscles leads to the generation of a breath. The descending automatic pathways most likely lie in the paramedian reticular formation of the medullary and pontine tegmentum and laterally in the high cervical cord in close proximity to the spinothalamic tract, whereas the descending pathways of the voluntary system are associated with the corticospinal tracts in the brainstem and upper cervical cord.[5] The nerve fibers mediating inspiration converge on the phrenic motor neurons in the ventral horns from C3 to C5 and the external intercostal motor neurons in the ventral horns throughout the thoracic spinal cord, typically from T2 to T12. The fibers responsible for active expiration converge primarily on the internal intercostal motor neurons in the thoracic spinal cord.[5]

Central and Peripheral Chemoreceptors

Regulation of breathing is a complex process involving multiple feedback loops. The process is centered in the brainstem (medulla), where information about respiratory rhythm is sent to the respiratory motoneurons in the spinal cord, based on feedback from various afferents. Afferent inputs include those from the central chemoreceptors within the medulla, peripheral chemoreceptors in the carotid and aortic bodies, and airway and lung receptors. These signals also reach higher areas of the central nervous system such as the pons, where they affect the patterning of breathing, and the cortex, where they may contribute to voluntary control of breathing.

Central chemoreceptors are responsible for approximately 85% of the respiratory response to carbon dioxide.[4] These receptors are located on the ventral surface of the medulla in close proximity to the dorsal and ventral respiratory neurons.[5] An increase in arterial CO_2 levels causes a corresponding increase in PCO_2 of the venous blood and cerebrospinal fluid (CSF). The PCO_2 value in the CSF and venous blood is approximately 10 mm Hg higher than that found in arterial blood. CO_2 readily penetrates membranes, including the blood-brain barrier. The CO_2 that diffuses across this barrier and into the brain and CSF becomes hydrated, forming carbonic acid. Carbonic acid promptly dissociates into H+ and HCO_3^-. The H+ concentration in the brain interstitium and the CSF therefore directly parallels changes in arterial PCO_2. The mechanism by which H+ concentration stimulates respiration is not completely understood; however, experimental studies have shown that if CSF PCO_2 concentrations are altered while H+ concentrations are held constant, respiration is minimally affected.[5] Alternatively, increases in CSF H+ concentrations result in proportional increases in ventilation. Therefore the CO_2 level in blood regulates ventilation primarily through its effect on the pH of the CSF.

Peripheral chemoreceptors are located in the carotid bodies at the bifurcation of the common carotid arteries and in the aortic bodies above and below the aortic arch.[4] The carotid bodies are responsible for the majority of the peripheral chemoreceptor control of ventilation, whereas the aortic bodies tend to have a greater role in the regulation of the circulation. The carotid bodies are highly perfused structures relative to their size, and as a result their arterial to venous PO_2 difference is small. Because of this, they are able to sense arterial blood gas tensions and respond rapidly, typically within 1 to 3 seconds. The peripheral chemoreceptors respond to a decrease in blood pH and partial pressure of oxygen, increased partial pressure of carbon dioxide, and hypoperfusion by stimulating an increase in ventilation.

The peripheral chemoreceptors are exclusively responsible for the increase in ventilation secondary to hypoxemia. In the absence of the carotid body receptors, hypoxemia depresses ventilation, likely through a direct effect on the respiratory center. The response of the peripheral chemoreceptors to arterial PCO_2 concentrations is substantially less important than that of the central chemoreceptors. However, their response is more rapid and therefore may be more important in adjusting ventilation in response to acute changes in PCO_2. Carotid body chemoreceptors stimulate ventilation in response to a decrease in arterial pH, regardless of whether this acidemia is respiratory or metabolic in origin.[2]

The automatic regulation of breathing relies upon the assimilation of central and peripheral chemoreceptor responses to blood levels of CO_2 and O_2. Therefore the integrated response to an increased arterial PCO_2 and decreased arterial PO_2 should be examined. In health, the most important factor in the control of breathing is the PCO_2 of the arterial blood. Feedback for CO_2 depends primarily on central chemoreceptors. Small increases of PCO_2 produce large increases in breathing, and vice versa. Central chemoreceptors sense changes in CO_2 and/or pH and provide a tonic drive to the network of respiratory neurons and a feedback on the blood levels of CO_2 and therefore the adequacy of ventilation for the metabolic needs.[2] Peripheral chemoreceptors also cause a minimal increase in ventilation secondary to increased arterial PCO_2 and decreased pH.

Hypoxemia stimulates ventilation primarily through its action on the peripheral chemoreceptors.[2] It has no action on the central chemoreceptors. The hypoxic stimulus for ventilation has a minimal role in health. In the face of a normal alveolar PCO_2, the alveolar PO_2 can be decreased to less than 50 mm Hg before any increase in ventilation is seen. However, in patients with increased PCO_2, increases in ventilation may be seen when alveolar PO_2 decreases below 100 mm Hg.[5] In patients with severe lung disease, the hypoxic drive for ventilation becomes more important. These patients have chronically increased CO_2 levels and thus have a diminished central and peripheral response to CO_2; arterial hypoxemia becomes the principal stimulus for ventilation in these patients.

Lung Receptors

Pulmonary stretch receptors present in the smooth muscle of the airways respond to excessive stretching of the lung during large inspirations. Once activated, they send action potentials through large myelinated fibers of the vagus nerve to the inspiratory area in the medulla and apneustic center of the pons. These impulses inhibit inspiratory discharge. The main effect of stimulating these receptors is a slowing of respiratory frequency by increasing expiratory time. This is known as the Hering-Breuer inflation reflex.[2]

Irritant receptors lie between airway epithelial cells and are stimulated by noxious gases, cold, and inhaled dusts. Once activated, they send action potentials via the vagus nerve leading to bronchoconstriction and increased respiratory rate. Juxtacapillary, or "J," receptors are located in the alveolar walls in close proximity to the capillaries. Because of their location, these receptors respond readily to chemicals in the pulmonary circulation, distention of the pulmonary capillary walls, and accumulation of interstitial fluid. Once stimulated, impulses travel via the vagus nerve in slow conducting fibers, leading to rapid, shallow breathing. Extreme stimulation may result in apnea. "J" receptors likely play a role in the apparent dyspnea seen in patients with left-sided congestive heart failure and interstitial lung disease.[4] Arterial baroreceptors function primarily to regulate the circulation but also play an important role in regulating ventilation in response to substantial fluctuations in blood pressure. A large decrease in arterial blood pressure causes hyperventilation, whereas a large increase in arterial blood pressure causes respiratory depression.[2]

Respiratory Mechanics and Muscular Control

Several different muscle groups are involved in creating a change in lung volume during a normal breath. These include the pharyngeal and laryngeal musculature, the diaphragm, rib cage, and spine and neck muscles, all of which play a role in inspiration, and the muscles of the abdominal wall, ribcage, and spine when active expiration is required.[4] The generation of an effective breath requires central neuronal impulses, modulated by chemical and physical stimuli, to trigger these muscle groups. As a result, the inspiratory muscles contract, expanding the thoracic wall and drawing the diaphragm caudally. The thoracic cavity expands, and because the lung is tethered to the thoracic wall by surface tension, the lung also expands. The strength of muscle contraction must be strong enough to overcome the two main sources of impedance to gas flow: the elastic recoil of the lungs and chest wall, and the resistance to gas flow, most prominent in the upper airways. Disease processes affecting respiratory muscle function, pulmonary compliance, airway resistance, or chest wall function interfere with the ability to generate a normal breath, and as a result lead to decreased alveolar ventilation.

DIFFERENTIAL DIAGNOSIS

Hypercapnia, defined as a PCO_2 in the arterial blood of greater than 36 mm Hg in a cat and 42 mm Hg in a dog,[3] can be caused by four possible abnormalities: hypoventilation, increased dead space ventilation, increased CO_2 production with a fixed minute ventilation, or increased inspired CO_2. The most common causes seen in clinical practice include hypoventilation, increased dead space ventilation, or a combination of the two. Hypoventilation can be caused by any process interfering with the ability to initiate or generate a normal tidal breath (Box 16-1). General categories include central neurologic disease, peripheral or central chemoreceptor dysfunction, lower motor neuron disease, neuromuscular disease, abnormal respiratory mechanics, or increased airway resistance.

CLINICAL SIGNS

Clinical signs associated with hypoventilation may be the result of the systemic effects of hypercapnia, uncompensated respiratory acidosis, or secondary to the disease process causing the hypoventilation. Patients with a decreased minute ventilation may present with shallow, rapid breathing or deep, slow breathing. Dyspnea may or may not be present, depending upon the condition causing hypoventilation. For example, patients with impaired central respiratory drive often do not appear to have difficulty breathing. However, in patients with acute mechanical failure of the respiratory system, such as a complete upper airway obstruction, dyspnea is readily apparent. In these situations, often hypoxemia, rather than hypercapnia, is the immediate threat to life. In patients with more chronic respiratory acidosis, clinical signs may be subtle. Although less common, patients may be hypercapnic despite an increased minute ventilation; that is, patients with increased physiologic dead space secondary to pulmonary thromboembolism may have CO_2 retention because of hypoperfusion of ventilated alveoli.

Hypercapnia and the accompanying respiratory acidosis can cause diffuse systemic effects; alterations in autonomic, cardiovascular, neurologic, and metabolic functions are common. Acute respiratory acidosis has variable effects on heart rate in canine patients. Hypercapnia and acidosis have been shown to directly decrease myocardial contractility and systemic vascular resistance.[4] However, these effects are offset commonly by the increased sympathetic nervous system stimulation and catecholamine release that occur secondary to acute hypercapnia and lead to an increased heart rate and systemic blood pressure. Tachyarrhythmias and prolongation of the QT interval have been reported rarely.[6]

Neurologic sequelae depend upon the magnitude and the duration of the hypercapnia, as well as the degree of concurrent hypoxemia. In general, cerebral blood flow is increased in response to increases in PCO_2 as a result of vasodilation of cerebral vasculature and increased systemic blood pressure. This increase in cerebral blood flow leads to increased intracranial pressure (ICP). Clinical signs of increased ICP are variable and include deteriorating level of consciousness, altered brainstem reflexes, and altered postural and motor responses. Carbon dioxide narcosis, seen when PCO_2 is greater than 90 mm Hg, is likely the result of alteration in intracellular pH and changes in cellular metabolism.[4]

Hypercapnia also may have metabolic and endocrine effects. At high levels of PCO_2, constriction of the renal afferent arteriole may cause acute kidney injury and a decrease in urine output. Hypercapnia may cause increased sodium and water retention, as well as hyperkalemia. The anterior pituitary may be stimulated by increased CO_2, leading to increased ACTH secretion.[4]

DIAGNOSIS

The gold standard for assessment of arterial carbon dioxide ($PaCO_2$) levels is arterial blood gas analysis. Arterial blood samples can be collected via percutaneous puncture of the femoral, dorsal pedal, coccygeal, sublingual, and dorsal auricular arteries in dogs. Obtaining an arterial sample in cats can be more difficult; the most accessible site is the femoral artery (see Chapter 186). If arterial blood cannot be obtained, a venous blood gas sample can be used. Central venous samples obtained from the jugular vein or vena cava, or mixed venous samples obtained from a pulmonary arterial catheter provide the most accurate results. If these are not available, peripheral venous samples can be used. In normal animals, the venous partial pressure of CO_2 is usually about 3 to 6 mm Hg higher than the arterial partial pressure of CO_2. This normal venous-arterial gradient occurs because CO_2 is removed from tissues and transported in venous blood back to the lungs as dissolved CO_2 in plasma (about 10%), and buffered within red blood cells as bicarbonate (about 90%).[4] However, the venous–arterial PCO_2 gradient ($P_{v-a}CO_2$) can increase significantly in states of decreased tissue perfusion. Venous CO_2 (P_VCo_2) is a reflection of arterial CO_2 inflow, de novo local tissue CO_2 production, and tissue blood flow. $PaCO_2$, as previously discussed, is most dependent on alveolar ventilation. During tissue hypoxia, tissue CO_2 production

BOX 16-1[14] ***Differential Diagnosis of Hypoventilation/Hypercarbia***

Decreased Respiratory Minute Ventilation

I. Central Neurological Disease
 1. Medulla, cerebrum, pons
  a. Drugs
   i. Opioids
   ii. General anesthetics
  b. Trauma
  c. Neoplasia
  d. Intracranial hemorrhage
  e. Cerebral edema
  f. Severe metabolic disturbances
  g. Severe hypothermia 80° F
 2. Cervical disease
  a. Trauma
   i. Spinal cord hemorrhage
   ii. Cervical fracture
  b. Tumor
  c. Surgery
  d. Infectious
  e. Intervertebral disk disease
  f. Inflammatory
  g. High epidural
  h. Anterior horn cell disease
II. Lower motor neuron disease/neuromuscular disease
 1. Myasthenia gravis
 2. Neuromuscular blockers
 3. Botulism
 4. Tick paralysis
 5. Demyelination
 6. Polyradiculoneuritis
 7. Toxoplasmosis
III. Chemoreceptor abnormalities
 1. Drugs
  a. Anesthetic agents
 2. Peripheral acidosis
  a. Metabolic derangements
 3. CSF acidosis
  a. Intracranial hemorrhage
  b. Metabolic derangements
IV. Abnormal respiratory mechanics
 1. Pulmonary fibrosis
 2. Respiratory fatigue from increased work of breathing
 3. Pickwickian syndrome
 4. Pleural space disease
  a. Pneumothorax
  b. Hemothorax
  c. Chylothorax
  d. Hydrothorax
  e. Malignant effusion
  f. Space-occupying mass
  g. Diaphragmatic hernia
 5. Loss of elasticity of chest wall/lungs
  a. Extrathoracic compression
  b. Fibrosis
 6. Loss of structural integrity of chest wall
  a. Flail chest
  b. Chest wound
 7. Decreased functional residual capacity
  a. Anesthetic agents
  b. Patient positioning (especially dorsal recumbency)
V. Increased airway resistance
 1. Upper airway obstruction
  a. Mucus plugs
  b. Neoplasia
  c. Foreign body
  d. Recurrent laryngeal nerve damage
  e. Laryngeal edema
  f. Inflammatory laryngitis
  g. Polyps
 2. Increased circuit resistance under anesthesia
 3. Tracheal or mainstem bronchus collapse
 4. Brachycephalic syndrome
 5. Bronchoconstriction
  a. Asthma
  b. Chronic bronchitis

Increased Dead Space Ventilation

I. Increased physiologic dead space (High V/Q)
 1. Poor cardiac output
 2. Shock
 3. Pulmonary emboli
 4. Pulmonary hypotension
 5. Pulmonary bulla
II. Increased anatomic dead space
 1. Excessive dead space in ventilator/anesthesia breathing circuit
 2. Excessively long endotracheal tube

Increased Carbon Dioxide Production with a Fixed Tidal Volume

I. Malignant hyperthermia
II. Reperfusion injury
III. Excessive nutritional support in a ventilated patient
IV. Fever
V. Iatrogenic hyperthermia

Increased Inspired Carbon Dioxide

I. Expired or old soda lime

is increased as a result of increased hydrogen ion production secondary to lactate formation and hydrolysis of ATP.[7] These protons are buffered by HCO_3^-, which subsequently leads to increased CO_2 production. In addition, CO_2 accumulates in tissues because of decreased blood flow. The net result is increased $PvCO_2$. The difference between venous and arterial PCO_2 ($P_{v\text{-}a}CO_2$) has been used to identify patients suffering from decreased tissue blood flow in a variety of disease states. $P_{v\text{-}a}CO_2$ has been correlated with decreased cardiac output in human and canine models of hemorrhagic and septic shock[8,9] and has been correlated with return of spontaneous circulation in animal models of cardiopulmonary arrest.[10] Therefore, although extremely useful, venous CO_2 values should be interpreted in conjunction with evaluation of measures of adequacy of oxygen delivery in clinical patients.

Direct measurement of $PaCO_2$ remains the gold standard for patient monitoring; however, blood gas analysis provides only a single measurement of what is often a rapidly changing clinical picture. In addition, arterial samples may be difficult to obtain or painful to the patient; a means of continuously monitoring $PaCO_2$ without the need for repeat blood gas analysis is desirable. Invasive continuous intraarterial blood gas monitoring systems are available in human medicine; however, they are costly and subject to technical difficulties related to the maintenance of arterial blood flow and motion artifact. These difficulties would likely restrict the use of these monitors in veterinary patients to those under general anesthesia or mechanical ventilation. Methods for the continuous noninvasive monitoring of $PaCO_2$ include end-tidal and transcutaneous devices.

End tidal capnography is a readily available, noninvasive surrogate for $PaCO_2$. Capnography analyzes the CO_2 concentration of the expiratory air stream, plotting CO_2 concentration against either time or exhaled volume. After anatomic dead space has been cleared, the CO_2 rises progressively to its maximal value at end-exhalation, a number that reflects the CO_2 tension of mixed alveolar gas. When ventilation and perfusion are distributed evenly, as they are in healthy subjects, end-tidal PCO_2 ($P_{ET}CO_2$) closely approximates $PaCO_2$. Normally $P_{ET}CO_2$ underestimates $PaCO_2$ by 2 to 6 mm Hg; this gradient is a function of dead space ventilation and cardiac output and has been shown to change in pathologic conditions that affect these physiologic variables.[4] In animals with severe lung disease, the PaO_2-$P_{ET}CO_2$ gradient is increased as a result of increased physiologic dead space. Low V/Q results when blood is delivered to regions of the lung with alveolar disease severe enough to affect CO_2 elimination, leading to a low end tidal CO_2 relative to $PaCO_2$. In portions of the lung that are hypoperfused, either because of decreased cardiac output or pulmonary embolism, less CO_2 is delivered to the lungs for elimination; this translates to a low $P_{ET}CO_2$ and an increased PaO_2-$P_{ET}CO_2$ gradient. The PaO_2-$P_{ET}CO_2$ difference is minimized when perfused alveoli are recruited maximally.

Transcutaneous CO_2 (TC-CO_2) monitors provide a second means of noninvasively monitoring $PaCO_2$. These monitors use heated electrodes to measure CO_2 in capillary beds. When compared with end tidal CO_2, TC-CO_2 monitoring has proven to be equally accurate in human patients with normal respiratory function and more accurate in patients with ventilation perfusion mismatching.[11] In addition, TC-CO_2 monitoring can be applied in situations that generally preclude end tidal CO_2 monitoring, such as high-frequency oscillatory ventilation and spontaneously breathing patients. It has been used to monitor acid-base balance in human patients with diabetic ketoacidosis.[11] Transcutaneous CO_2 monitors have been validated in veterinary patients but require frequent calibration and are often cost prohibitive.[12]

In addition to blood gas analysis and noninvasive CO_2 measurement, tests should be performed to help identify the underlying cause of hypoventilation. A baseline complete blood count, chemistry panel, and urinalysis are recommended. Additional tests include, but are not limited to, chest radiography, thoracic and abdominal ultrasound, cervical radiography, titers for infectious and neuromuscular disease, CT or MRI, electromyography, CSF analysis, endocrine function testing, and nerve and muscle biopsies. Test selection should be dictated by the clinical status of the patient and the suspected disease process(es).

TREATMENT

The only way to decrease arterial PCO_2 is to increase effective alveolar ventilation. This can be accomplished in several ways; typically therapy is approached in a stepwise fashion. Airway patency should be confirmed immediately, and if not present, supplemental oxygen should be administered while relief of airway obstruction, tracheostomy tube placement, or endotracheal intubation is performed. Once an airway has been secured, hemodynamic stability should be optimized to resolve hypercapnia secondary to poor pulmonary perfusion.

Additional therapies should be directed at treatment of the underlying cause of the hypoventilation. For example, patients receiving opioids, sedatives, or neuromuscular blockade should receive reversal medications if indicated; mechanical ventilation may be needed until the medications have been reversed or metabolized.

Provision of supplemental oxygen to the hypoventilating patient is controversial. The phenomenon of oxygen-induced hypercapnia in patients with chronic hypoventilation and acute hypoxemia may be observed. Sudden correction of arterial hypoxemia causes further hypercapnia by a combination of three mechanisms: (1) by depression of formerly hypoxic-driven peripheral chemoreceptors causing worsening hypoventilation, (2) relief of hypoxic pulmonary vasoconstriction in poorly ventilated lung regions that further reduces the ability of these units to eliminate CO_2 as local perfusion increases without concomitant increase in ventilation, and (3) significant correction of hypoxemia causes better saturation of hemoglobin so that previously buffered protons on deoxyhemoglobin are released with subsequent generation of new CO_2 from stores (Haldane effect).[13] Low-flow oxygen generally suffices to increase arterial PO_2 to satisfactory levels (~60 mm Hg and arterial oxygen saturation [SaO_2] ~ 90%); greater elevations are neither needed nor advisable in these patients.[13]

The next line of treatment is chemical stimulation of breathing. Several respiratory stimulants are currently available and include doxapram, aminophylline/theophylline, caffeine, and progesterone, among others. Doxapram stimulates respiration via activation of peripheral chemoreceptors; at higher doses, the medullary respiratory center is stimulated, causing an increase in tidal volume and respiratory rate. Side effects of doxapram result from systemic catecholamine release and central nervous system stimulation. In addition, this drug may increase the work of breathing, which can lead to increased oxygen consumption and carbon dioxide production.[14] Methylxanthine drugs, including aminophylline, theophylline, and caffeine, have been used as respiratory stimulants in veterinary patients. The mechanism by which the methylxanthines control breathing has not been fully elucidated, but they do cause central respiratory center stimulation leading to increased ventilation; improve skeletal muscle contraction, metabolic homeostasis, and oxygenation secondary to increased cardiac output; increase ventilation; and decrease hypoxic episodes.[15] Methylxanthines are believed to stimulate diaphragmatic contractility and prevent diaphragmatic fatigue in adult patients.[16] The specific effects appear to vary to some degree between methylxanthines. Caffeine is considered to be more effective in stimulating the central nervous and respiratory systems and appears to penetrate the cerebrospinal fluid more readily than theophylline.[17] Theophylline is considered a more potent cardiac stimulant and has greater diuretic and bronchodilator effects but is associated with a higher incidence of tachycardia.[17] Caffeine citrate is rapidly becoming the preferred drug in the management of apnea of prematurity because of more predictable pharmacokinetics and decreased adverse effects in comparison to theophylline. Studies evaluating safety and effectiveness of caffeine citrate in veterinary patients are warranted before this medication is routinely recommended.

Sodium bicarbonate administration is not indicated for the correction of acidemia secondary to respiratory acidosis. Hypercapnia may worsen after administration, and mechanical ventilation may become necessary. Acetazolamide is a diuretic that induces a metabolic acidosis via bicarbonate ion excretion. This acidosis may stimulate ventilation; however, caution should be exercised when using this drug in patients with a preexisting respiratory acidosis; severe systemic complications of acidemia may result.

The most effective treatment for hypoventilation is mechanical ventilation (see Chapter 30). Many patients with impaired respiratory drive or severe neuromuscular disease leading to hypoventilation require mechanical ventilation. Unfortunately this treatment modality is costly and labor intensive. Ventilated patients require 24-hour monitoring in an intensive care facility. Mechanical ventilation is lifesaving for patients with reversible causes causing hypoventilation and should be strongly considered in these patients when other therapeutic options are unsuccessful.

REFERENCES

1. Wagner PD, Powell FL, West JD: Ventilation, blood flow, and gas exchange. In Mason RJ, editor: Murray and Nadel's textbook of respiratory medicine, ed 5, Philadelphia, 2010, Saunders Elsevier.
2. West JB: Ventilation, control of ventilation. In West JB, editor: Respiratory physiology: the essentials, ed 6, Baltimore, 2000, Lippincott Williams & Wilkins.
3. Hopper K, Haskins SC: A case-based review of a simplified quantitative approach to acid-base analysis, J Vet Emerg Crit Care 18(5):467, 2008.
4. Lumb AJ: Control of breathing. In Lumb AJ, editor: Nunn's applied respiratory physiology, ed 6, Philadelphia, 2005, Elsevier Limited.
5. Nogués MA, Roncoroni AJ, Benarroch E: Breathing control in neurologic diseases, Clin Autonomic Res 12(6):440, 2002.
6. Johnson RA, Autran de Morais H: Respiratory acid-base disorders. In DiBartola SP, editor: Fluid, electrolyte, and acid-base disorders in small animal practice, ed 3, St Louis, 2006, Elsevier.
7. Boller MB: CO_2 in Low blood flow states. In Multidisciplinary systems review, 17th International VECC Symposium, 2011.
8. Bakker J, Vincent JL, Gris P, et al: Veno-arterial carbon dioxide gradient in human septic shock, Chest 101(2):509, 1992.
9. Van der Linden P, Rausin I, Deltell A, et al: Detection of tissue hypoxia by arteriovenous gradient for PCO_2 and pH in anesthetized dogs during progressive hemorrhage, Anesth Analg 80(2):269, 1995.
10. Grundler W, Weil MH, Rackow EC: Arterio-venous carbon dioxide and pH gradients during cardiac arrest, Circulation 74:1071, 1986.
11. Tobias JD: Transcutaneous carbon dioxide monitoring in infants and children, Paediatr Anaesth 19(5):434, 2009.
12. Vogt R, Rohling R, Kästner S: Evaluation of a combined transcutaneous carbon dioxide pressure and pulse oximetry sensor in adult sheep and dogs, Am J Vet Res 68(3):265, 2007.
13. McConville JF, Soloway J: Disorders of ventilation. In Longo DL, Fauci AS, Kasper DL, et al, editors: Harrison's principles of internal medicine, ed 18, New York, 2011, McGraw-Hill Professional.
14. Campbell VL, Perkowski S. Hypoventilation. In King LK, editor: Textbook of respiratory diseases in dogs and cats, St Louis, 2004, Elsevier.
15. Bhatia J: Current options in the management of apnea of prematurity, Clin Pediatr 39:327, 2000.
16. Randa JV, Gorman W, Bergsteinsson H, et al: Efficacy of caffeine in treatment of apnea in the low-birth-weight infant, J Pediatr 90:467, 1977.
17. Kriter KE, Blanchard J: Management of apnea in infants, Clin Pharmacy 8:577, 1989.

CHAPTER 17
UPPER AIRWAY DISEASE

Dana L. Clarke, VMD, DACVECC

KEY POINTS

- Upper airway obstruction is a common cause of respiratory distress in small animal emergency medicine requiring immediate recognition and treatment.
- Common diseases leading to upper airway obstruction include laryngeal paralysis, tracheal collapse, and brachycephalic airway disease.
- Patient stabilization, including oxygen, sedation, and anxiety control, should be a priority over diagnostics to avoid further patient distress.
- Complications of upper airway obstruction are common, including hyperthermia, aspiration pneumonia, and noncardiogenic pulmonary edema.

In veterinary medicine, upper airway disease causing airway obstruction and secondary respiratory distress is a common reason for emergency patient evaluation. Many underlying causes may result in respiratory compromise from upper airway obstruction, including brachycephalic airway syndrome, laryngeal paralysis, and tracheal collapse. Regardless of the cause, patients in distress often have exhausted their physiologic compensatory reserves for ventilation and oxygenation, and even small stresses such as restraint for examination can result in rapid decompensation. Prompt treatment with oxygen, anxiolytics, and for some patients, intubation or tracheostomy, may be necessary before the definitive cause is determined or diagnostics performed.

HISTORY AND CLINICAL SIGNS

Clinical signs noted by owners of patients with upper airway disease depend on the location, severity, chronicity, and species. Since cats breathe predominantly through their noses and only open-mouth breathe or pant with severe respiratory compromise, owners may not immediately recognize changes in respiratory comfort. The more sedentary lifestyle of cats also can delay diagnosis of respiratory disease because exercise intolerance is likely to be noticed only as a late change in cats. Dogs with upper airway disease often pant in response to respiratory difficulty. Because panting in dogs may not be recognized as abnormal, respiratory changes may not be obvious when panting is the only clinical sign.

The upper airway consists of the nasal passages and choanae, nasopharynx and oropharynx, larynx, and trachea. Clinical signs associated with disease along the upper respiratory tract can by dynamic or static. Dynamic signs occur during inspiration or expiration, depending on the location of the obstruction, or with stress, anxiety, and activity that alter airflow dynamics and precipitate obstruction. Static signs occur with fixed intraluminal or extraluminal obstructions. Disease in the rostral regions of the upper airway (nasal passages, choanae, and nasopharynx) can result in nasal discharge, sneezing, reverse sneezing, snoring, stertorous breathing, and inability to breathe comfortably when not panting. Stertorous respiration is characterized by low-pitched snoring like inspiratory and/or expiratory noise. Obstructive diseases of the larynx or trachea can result in coughing, gagging (particularly with eating or drinking), and respiratory stridor, which is a high-pitched noise associated with inspiration. Laryngeal and pharyngeal disease can lead to changes in vocalization (dysphonia).[1-4]

Coughing is a common clinical sign in animals with tracheal, mainstem, and laryngeal disease. Since it also commonly is associated with lower airway, pulmonary parenchymal, and cardiac disease, it is important to rule out other causes for coughing. Coughing that results from upper airway disease tends to be dry and nonproductive, whereas coughing of a lower airway or pulmonary parenchymal origin tends to result in a moist, productive cough.[5,6] However, many owners have difficulty appropriately determining the productivity of a cough because patients may quickly swallow sputum, or the cough may be associated with terminal, productive retching of gastrointestinal origin. Coughing upon exhalation is characteristic of intrathoracic tracheal and mainstem bronchial collapse. A classic "goose-honking" cough is common in many patients with tracheal collapse.

Many patients do not present for emergency examination when their respiratory signs are subtle; therefore most patients with upper airway disease are evaluated once there has been progression to obstruction and respiratory distress. In addition, because some clinical signs may have been present for long periods of time, such as coughing or snoring, or are attributed to aging (such as change in bark quality), owners may not recognize these signs as indicators of disease and instead perceive them as "normal" for their pet. For this reason, most upper airway obstruction patients have exhausted their physiologic respiratory reserves and are at risk of rapid decompensation with stress and handling by the time they present for emergency evaluation. In addition, upper airway obstruction and dyspnea can become a vicious self-perpetuating cycle, as continued work of breathing against an obstruction contributes to edema and inflammation, further airway narrowing, worsened obstruction, patient distress, and increased effort to breathe. Therefore initial examination of the patient may be limited, making observation and distant appreciation of audible sounds an important part of the triage assessment.

Laryngeal, tracheal, and thoracic auscultation often reveals loud, referred upper airway noise, which often can be localized to the point of maximal intensity with thorough auscultation of the entire respiratory tract. Patients with upper airway disease tend to have loud, noisy breathing and increased inspiratory time. Inspiratory noise and distress result from collapse of the upper airway rostral to the thoracic inlet trachea because generation of negative intrathoracic pressure upon inspiration collapses the weakened airway structure into the lumen. This collapse prolongs the inspiratory phase and creates noise from air and tissue reverberation in the lumen. Increased intrapleural pressure upon expiration collapses the upper airway caudal the thoracic inlet (intrathoracic trachea and mainstem bronchi) and results in prolonged expiration, expiratory dyspnea, and lower airway sounds (e.g., wheezes) on auscultation. In a retrospective evaluation of dogs and cats presenting for emergency evaluation of respiratory distress, inspiratory dyspnea in dogs and inspiratory noise in dogs and cats were significantly associated with disease localization to the upper airway. Too few cats in that study had disease isolated to the upper airway to fully characterize the nature of inspiratory dyspnea seen with upper airway disease.[7] The degree of upper airway noise often worsens with the severity of the obstruction.[1] Thorough auscultation of the pulmonary parenchyma can be difficult in the face of loud referred upper noise but is imperative because of parenchymal complications of upper airway obstruction such as noncardiogenic pulmonary edema and aspiration pneumonia.

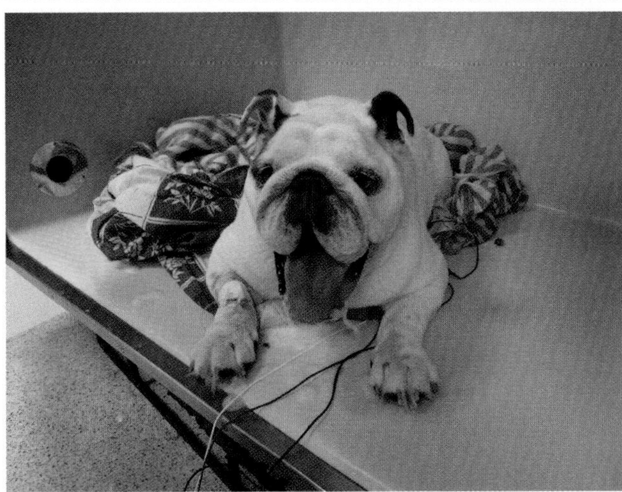

FIGURE 17-1 Bulldog in respiratory distress, demonstrating excessive panting, hypersalivation and orthopnea secondary to upper airway obstruction from brachycephalic airway syndrome (BAS).

Panting is a major method of thermoregulation, especially in dogs. Intolerance of warm and humid conditions is often seen in patients with upper airway disease resulting from decreased ability to efficiently increase minute ventilation to enhance heat dissipation and is a described risk factor for heat stroke.[8-11] Hyperthermia and heat stroke also can result from failure to effectively eliminate heat secondary to upper airway obstruction; these are common findings in patients with laryngeal paralysis and brachycephalic airway syndrome. Prompt recognition and treatment (see Chapter 149) of hyperthermia is essential to prevent secondary consequences such as renal, neurologic, cardiovascular, and coagulation disorders.[9-11] Since aspiration pneumonia is also a complication of upper airway obstruction, fever should be considered as a source of increased rectal temperature as well (see Chapter 10).

In addition to loud respiratory noise, marked respiratory distress, and hyperthermia, other clinical signs that can be recognized with severe upper airway obstruction include extension of the head and neck (orthopnea), cyanosis of the tongue and mucous membranes, and collapse (Figure 17-1). In such severe cases, immediate intubation or emergency tracheostomy (see Chapter 197) may be necessary life-saving interventions.

EMERGENCY STABILIZATION

The work of breathing against an upper airway obstruction can precipitate the cycle of edema and inflammation, patient distress, and progressive obstruction, so supplemental oxygen and techniques to minimize patient stress are universally recommended treatment strategies, regardless of the origin of the obstruction. For some patients, the restraint necessary for intravenous catheter placement, venipuncture, and other emergency diagnostics may exacerbate stress and oxygen demands, leading to further respiratory compromise or respiratory arrest. Therefore intramuscular (IM) administration of many emergency medications is necessary when catheter placement is not feasible.

Oxygen therapy can be provided in several different manners; the method selected depends on availability and patient tolerance (see Chapter 14). An oxygen cage is one of the best ways to provide high levels of inspired oxygen while minimizing patient stress and handling. However, enclosure within an oxygen cage prevents the clinicians and nurses from hearing upper airway noises that can indicate worsening obstruction, which can be dangerous in patients with upper airway disease.

Control of anxiety and discomfort is essential for patients with upper airway obstruction and respiratory distress (see Chapter 142). In cardiovascularly stable animals, acepromazine is an effective anxiolytic. Since it can be difficult to thoroughly assess cardiovascular stability in patients with upper airway obstruction, low doses (0.005 to 0.02 mg/kg IV and 0.01 to 0.05 mg/kg IM) should be used and repeated if needed, remembering that it can take approximately 15 minutes for full effect after intravenous administration.[12] Butorphanol provides sedation, cough suppression, and analgesia; the dose range is 0.1 to 0.5 mg/kg IM or IV. Other sedatives (dexmedetomidine, diazepam, midazolam, ketamine) and analgesics (methadone, fentanyl, hydromorphone) may be needed based on individual patient circumstances.

For patients in whom sedation and anxiety control do not relieve respiratory distress, or those at risk of imminent respiratory arrest, rapid induction for endotracheal intubation or tracheostomy is necessary (see Chapters 143 and 197). Propofol can be considered (0.05 to 1 mg/kg titrated to effect), with the acknowledgement of the risk of cardiopulmonary depression. It can be combined with diazepam for overall reduction of the propofol dose. Other options for rapid induction include ketamine combined with diazepam and etomidate.

Glucocorticoids (dexamethasone sodium phosphate 0.05 to 0.2 mg/kg IM, IV, SC) should be considered to reduce airway inflammation secondary to upper airway obstruction. Special consideration should be given to hypovolemic patients or those for whom perfusion is a concern because of risk of gastrointestinal ulceration, recent nonsteroidal antiinflammatory (NSAID) administration, and airway obstruction suspected to the secondary to neoplasia as steroid administration may interfere with diagnostic accuracy.

DIAGNOSTICS

Blood gas analysis is helpful in patients with upper airway obstruction to assess the degree of ventilatory dysfunction and/or hypoxemia. Although arterial blood gas analysis is the standard for assessing oxygenation and ventilation, collection of an arterial sample is often not possible upon presentation in patients with respiratory distress. With severe upper airway obstruction localized between the larynx and trachea, a respiratory acidosis characterized by increased partial pressure of carbon dioxide ($PvCO_2$) often is present. Animals with chronic airway obstructions and hypoventilation usually develop a compensatory retention of bicarbonate by the kidneys that contribute to improvement of the acidosis and negative base excess, but an increased $PvCO_2$ persists (see Chapters 16 and 186). Similar acid-base changes may be seen on an arterial sample with the same obstruction localization. An arterial sample provides objective determination of the partial pressure of oxygen in the sample to evaluate for hypoxemia. The alveolar-arterial (A-a) gradient must be calculated for all arterial samples to rule out hypoventilation as a contributor to hypoxemia, therefore determining if pulmonary dysfunction exits (see Chapters 15 and 186).

Thoracic radiographs are an important part of the diagnostic work-up in all patients with respiratory disease but must not be obtained at the risk of patient safety. Three view thoracic radiographs in the patient with upper airway disease are important to evaluate for noncardiogenic pulmonary edema, bronchopneumonia (aspiration or infectious), intrathoracic tracheal collapse, mainstem bronchial collapse, and airway or pulmonary neoplasia. Cervical radiographs are important to evaluate for laryngeal and pharyngeal masses, extrathoracic tracheal collapse, and radiolucent foreign bodies. Dynamic disease processes such as nasopharyngeal, tracheal, and mainstem bronchial collapse may not be seen or may be underestimated with radiography. Therefore fluoroscopy is preferable for a more thorough dynamic assessment of the entire upper respiratory tract throughout the respiratory cycle and while the patient is coughing to evaluate for collapse. Diagnostic imaging of the nasal passages, nasopharynx, and bulla generally is accomplished best with computed tomography (CT), although skull radiographs also may be considered. Heavy sedation or general anesthesia often is required for CT and skull radiography, so these diagnostics often are performed as second-tier diagnostics. In addition, dynamic disease processes such as nasopharyngeal, laryngeal, and tracheal collapse may not be seen on sedated or anesthetized CT examinations. More recent studies evaluating a clear plastic patient positioning device (Mouse-Trap) that contains the animal and restricts movement has shown promising results for dynamic CT evaluation of upper airway obstruction secondary to laryngeal, tracheal, and bronchial disease without the need for anesthesia or sedation.[13] Awake CT examination for cats with upper airway obstruction also has proven effective for diagnosing disease processes such as intramural airway masses, laryngeal paralysis, and laryngotracheitis.[14]

Sedated laryngeal examination is indicated in all patients with upper airway disease, even if laryngeal disease or dysfunction is not considered the primary pathology. Heavy sedation with medications that do not affect laryngeal function is essential for accurate assessment of laryngeal motion. Protocols proven to have minimal influence on laryngeal exam include intravenous propofol slowly titrated to effect, with or without the use of concurrent doxapram (1.1 to 2.2 mg/kg IV), or premedication with acepromazine (0.2 mg/kg IM) and butorphanol (0.4 mg/kg IM) 20 minutes before mask induction with isoflurane.[15-19] High-dose intramuscular acepromazine was recommended based on the results from normal dogs that did not permit mask induction when lower doses were used early in the trial, but caution is advised when using higher doses to avoid adverse effects.[17] Critically ill or compromised patients require lower doses of intramuscular acepromazine, and titration to effect starting with lower doses (0.01 to 0.05 mg/kg) should be considered for clinical patients (see Chapter 142). Regardless of the protocol used, it is important to have an assistant indicating the phases of respiration during laryngeal exam to confirm appropriate laryngeal motion and rule out paradoxical laryngeal motion, which can be confused as laryngeal function in dogs with laryngeal paralysis. Paradoxical laryngeal motion is defined as inward movement of the arytenoids secondary to negative pressure generated upon inspiration. A standard laryngoscope with blade and light source is used most commonly for direct visualization of the larynx, although rostral pulling of the tongue and pressure of the blade on the epiglottis may distort laryngeal and oropharyngeal examination. For this reason, some clinicians prefer transoral flexible endoscopy.[15,20,21] In addition to assessment of proper laryngeal function, the larynx also should be examined for collapse, inflammatory or proliferative abnormalities of the arytenoid cartilages, eversion of the laryngeal saccules, changes in the diameter of the rima glottis, and neoplasia. Epiglottic retroversion, or caudal displacement of the epiglottis into the rima glottis, also should be ruled out as an uncommon cause of upper airway obstruction and respiratory distress.[22] The length and appearance of the soft palate should be assessed, as should the tonsillar crypts and epiglottis. The caudal aspect of the soft palate should contact the epiglottis or extend no more than a few millimeters past it.[23] Palpation of the hard and soft palate for masses or defects also should be performed.

Rigid and flexible endoscopes are extremely helpful in the diagnosis of nasal, nasopharyngeal, oropharyngeal, and tracheal disease.

A rigid or flexible scope can be passed retrograde through the nasal passages to evaluate the nasal turbinates for proliferation, inflammation, plaques associated with fungal diseases, and masses. Biopsy and culture can be obtained with direct rigid scope visualization or blindly depending on the size of the patient and rigid scope used. Retroflexed flexible endoscopy allows for assessment of nasopharyngeal stenosis, polyps, nasopharyngeal turbinates, foreign bodies, and neoplasia. Dynamic nasopharyngeal collapse may be seen in nonintubated patients upon inspiration through their nose but may not be present with heavy sedation or with intubated patients who do not generate negative pressure through their nose. Flexible endoscopy also can be performed in the trachea to grade tracheal collapse; look for tracheal inflammation, foreign bodies, and masses; and assess for mainstem bronchial collapse. Tissue or fluid culture as well as biopsy can be performed through the working channel of the flexible endoscope using biopsy forceps.

Bronchopneumonia, whether secondary to aspiration, mucociliary dysfunction, or underlying chronic lower airway disease, is a common secondary complication to upper airway disease and obstruction (see Chapters 22 and 23). Sampling from the airway for cytology and culture is helpful to guide antimicrobial therapy, especially in patients with repeated episodes of pneumonia. However, in animals with severe respiratory distress, airway sampling may not be safe and a delay in antimicrobial therapy could hinder pulmonary parenchymal recovery. Therefore empiric antimicrobial therapy may be necessary. For patients stable enough to undergo airway sampling, transtracheal, endotracheal, and bronchoalveolar lavage can be considered for airway cytology and aerobic bacterial and *Mycoplasma* cultures (see Chapters 22 and 23).

DISEASES OF THE UPPER AIRWAY

Brachycephalic Airway Syndrome

Brachycephalic airway syndrome (BAS), brachycephalic syndrome (BS), and brachycephalic airway obstructive syndrome (BAOS) are synonymous terms used to describe the cluster of anatomic abnormalities seen in brachycephalic breeds, such as English bulldogs, Pugs, French bulldogs, and Boston terriers, that contribute to dysfunction of the upper airway. The classic primary anatomic components of BAS include stenotic nares and an elongated soft palate, although other commonly recognized components include tracheal hypoplasia and nasopharyngeal turbinates. Secondary complications from chronic increased resistance to airflow on inspiration include everted laryngeal saccules, tonsillar eversion, laryngeal collapse, tracheal collapse, chronic gastrointestinal signs, and even syncope.[24-30]

Approximately 80% of the resistance to airflow during inspiration is from the nose in normal dogs.[1,25,27,31,32] This is exaggerated in brachycephalic animals with stenotic nares, excessive pharyngeal tissues, elongated soft palate, and/or tracheal hypoplasia, which lead to turbulent airflow, edema, and increased inspiratory noise.[1,2,25,27] In addition to increased respiratory noise, other clinical signs seen in BAS patients include snoring, stertor, stridor, heat and exercise intolerance, hypersalivation, vomiting, and regurgitation.[24,25,28,29] It is most common in young adult dogs (2 to 3 years), although English Bulldogs have been reported to present at younger ages (i.e., 1 year).[33-35]

Diagnosis of BAS is made based on signalment, clinical signs, and examination of the nares, oropharynx, and larynx during a sedated oral examination using a laryngoscope or flexible endoscope. Oral examination should include assessment of the length of the soft palpate, size and shape of the rima glottis, and presence or absence of laryngeal saccule eversion or laryngeal collapse. Thoracic radiographs can be helpful to evaluate for tracheal hypoplasia, tracheal collapse, hiatal hernia, and pneumonia, although caution must be exercised when diagnosing tracheal hypoplasia when bronchopneumonia is present, because inflammation and edema of the trachea during an active airway infection may be deceiving.[36,37] Fluoroscopy can be helpful to evaluate for dynamic nasopharyngeal and tracheal collapse that may be secondary to BAS. Blood gas analysis may show signs of hypoxemia and/or hypoventilation, and brachycephalic breeds often have higher carbon dioxide levels and lower oxygen pressures than mesocephalic or dolicocephalic dogs.[38] Retroflexed endoscopy of the nasopharynx may show nasopharyngeal inflammation, collapse, or the presence of nasal turbinates protruding in the nasopharynx, which has been documented in approximately 20% of dogs symptomatic for BAS; 80% of those were Pugs in one study.[26] Bronchoscopic evaluation of dogs with BAS presenting for surgery showed that 87% of dogs had some degree of bronchoscopically detectable collapse or stenosis and that a worsened degree of bronchial collapse was associated with laryngeal collapse.[39] Upper gastrointestinal flexible endoscopy is helpful to evaluate for esophagitis, gastritis, reflux, hiatal hernia, and pyloric stenosis, which have been found in up to 80% of BAS patients, with worsened gastrointestinal signs correlated with worsened respiratory clinical signs.[29,30] Biomarker evaluation may show increased cardiac troponin I (cTnI), which may be secondary to myocardial injury from chronic hypoxemia. However, C-reactive protein and haptoglobin levels have not shown to be increased in dogs with upper airway obstruction secondary to BAS, indicating that there may be minimal systemic inflammation.[40]

First-line management of BAS includes weight loss, control of excitement and activity triggers, medical treatment for gastrointestinal signs, and treatment of underlying pulmonary parenchymal disease. However, surgical correction of BAS anatomic abnormalities often is required for successful management of most animals with clinical signs of upper airway obstruction. Since the nasal passage creates the most resistance to airflow, widening the nares is considered the most important aspect of surgery for BAS, especially because many of the other airway changes are considered to be secondary to stenotic nares. Therefore widening of the nares at a young age is proposed and shown to provide significant improvement in dogs postoperatively, regardless of the multiple techniques available.* Correction of other components of BAS, including soft palate resection, resection of everted laryngeal saccules, and tonsillectomy also may be needed and can be helpful even in advanced BAS cases with laryngeal collapse.[33,39,45] Tracheal hypoplasia and bronchial collapse has not been associated with outcome in dogs undergoing surgical intervention for BAS.[34,39] Cricoarytenoid lateralization combined with thyroarytenoid caudolateralization (arytenoid laryngoplasty) is a viable alternative for patients with advanced laryngeal collapse, a disease for which permanent tracheostomy was previously considered the only viable surgical intervention.[46] If tracheal collapse secondary to or concurrent with BAS continues to cause respiratory distress after surgical intervention for BAS, extraluminal rings or endotracheal stenting may be necessary.

Nasopharyngeal Polyps

Nasopharyngeal polyps are a common cause of upper airway obstruction in cats, accounting for 28% of cats with nasopharyngeal disease.[47] They also have been implicated in moderate to life-threatening upper airway obstruction in three dogs.[48-50] Nasopharyngeal polyps are benign inflammatory lesions that arise from the mucosa of the auditory tube or middle ear and grow into the nasopharynx or external ear canal. The exact cause is not known, and attempts to isolate and amplify feline herpes virus, feline calicivirus, *Mycoplasma* species,

*References 27, 30, 34, 39, 41-45.

Bartonella species, and *Chlamydophila felis* DNA or RNA from feline aural and nasopharyngeal polyps has been unsuccessful.[47,51-57] Clinical signs commonly seen in cats with nasopharyngeal polyps include respiratory noise or stertor, sneezing, nasal discharge, and dysphagia, which may contribute to weight loss.[51,52,54,56] Progression of the polyp can lead to dyspnea and signs consistent with upper airway obstruction. Diagnosis is usually made based on historical information, oropharyngeal examination with palpation of the soft palate, otoscopy, retroflexed rhinoscopy, radiographs, CT, and/or MRI[51,52,55,58] (Figure 17-2, *A*). Medical management is generally unrewarding; therefore surgical intervention is recommended. Traction-avulsion is the most simple method of removal but can be associated with a 40% to 50% chance of recurrence, especially if removed from the auditory canal[52,55,59,60] (Figure 17-2, *B*). For this reason, ventral bulla osteotomy (VBO) is recommended, especially for those patients with polyps in the auditory tube or evidence of middle ear disease.[52,56,60] VBO is associated with a higher incidence of postoperative Horner's syndrome (43% of cats treated with traction and 57% of cats treated with VBO), vestibular dysfunction, and facial and hypoglossal nerve paralysis.[52,56,60] In most cats, Horner's syndrome resolves postoperatively, although this can take up to 4 weeks.[59-61] Preoperative hearing deficits were not reversed in cats with polyps that had VBO performed.[62] Prolonged antimicrobial therapy is indicated for bacterial otitis media or interna; however, the role of postoperative steroids for nasopharyngeal polyps is unclear. However, one study showed decreased incidence of recurrence when prednisolone was administered postoperatively.[60] In general, the prognosis for cats treated surgically for inflammatory nasopharyngeal polyps is good.

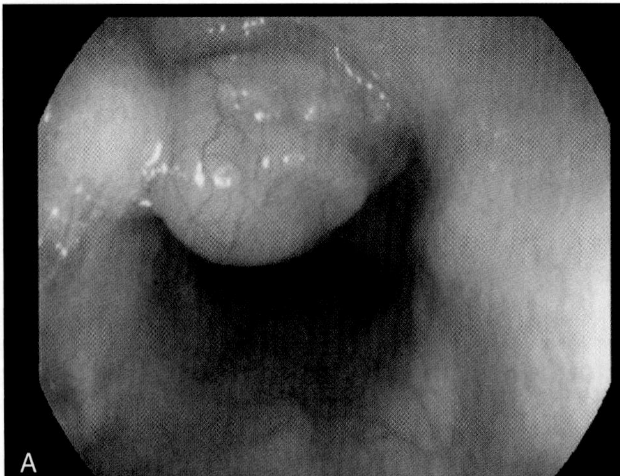

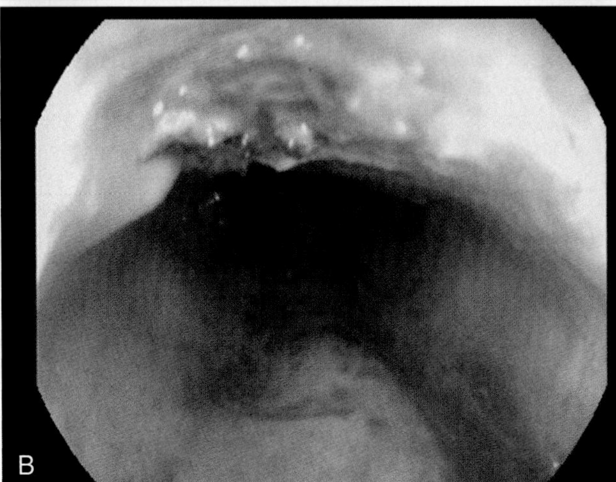

FIGURE 17-2 A, Retroflexed rhinoscopy of the caudal nasopharynx in an 11-year-old Shih Tzu showing the presence of a dorsal soft tissue mass. **B,** Appearance of the nasopharynx of the same dog after endoscopic electrocautery snare mass removal. Histopathology confirmed the mass was a benign inflammatory polyp.

Nasopharyngeal Stenosis

Nasopharyngeal stenosis (NPS) is reported uncommonly in dogs and cats.[63-67] Nasopharyngeal stenosis occurs when there is partial or complete narrowing of the nasopharynx by a membrane caudal to the choanae and rostral to the caudal aspect of the soft palate. It can overlie the hard or soft palate and may cover both if the membrane is thick enough. NPS can be a congenital lesion, or secondary to chronic inflammatory diseases such as rhinitis (infectious or aspiration), trauma, and neoplastic obstructions. Clinical signs, which often persist for months before diagnosis, include chronic nasal discharge, stertor, stridor, exercise intolerance, gagging, and in severe cases, dyspnea.[66-71] Diagnosis is generally made through computed tomography (CT) and retroflexed rhinoscopy, although barium contrast rhinography also has been described.[68] Surgical correction of the stenosis via surgical access through a midline incision in the soft palate has been described in cats.[72,73] When retroflexed flexible endoscopy is used to confirm or diagnose NPS, balloon dilation can be performed simultaneously to open the obstruction using minimally invasive techniques. An angioplasty balloon can be passed normograde through the ventral meatus of the nasal passage, or advanced retrograde through the oral cavity over a wire within a cut red rubber catheter that has been passed retrograde through the nose.[66,68-70] Balloon dilation is performed under constant retroflexed visualization, with or without concurrent fluoroscopy, once the balloon is positioned across the stenosis and confirming the balloon is not within the choanae. Re-stenosis over time is common, and repeated balloon dilations may be necessary depending on how clinically affected the patient is and the extent of re-stenosis.[66,67,69,70] In patients in whom balloon dilation has failed to resolve the NPS sufficiently, stent placement may be considered via surgical placement or using combined fluoroscopy and retroflexed rhinoscopy.[67,71] All animals had improvement in their respiratory signs post-stent placement. Complications include dysphagia and hair entrapment, tissue in-growth, and prolonged nasal discharge.[67] Stent erosion through the soft palpate in two dogs (4 and 20 months after placement of covered nasopharyngeal stents) has been described. It is a serious complication that should be considered before placement of nasopharyngeal stents, particularly over the soft palate.[74]

Congenital Choanal Atresia

Congenital choanal atresia also has been reported rarely in cats and in one dog and can cause similar clinical signs to NPS, including nasal discharge, stertor, exercise intolerance, and open-mouth breathing.[65,75-77] It results from abnormal bone or soft tissue obstructing the caudal nasal passage just rostral to the common nasopharynx and can be unilateral or bilateral. CT and retroflexed rhinoscopy can be used to make a diagnosis of choanal atresia. Treatment options include transnasal puncture with temporary stenting and surgical approach to the nasopharynx.[65,75-77]

Nasopharyngeal Foreign Bodies and Infection

Nasopharyngeal foreign bodies and infections occur infrequently in dogs and cats but can result in upper airway obstructive signs. Nasopharyngeal cryptococcosis, blastomycosis, and extensive bacterial infection and bony proliferation of the bulla are documented to result in nasopharyngeal obstruction.[78-80] Nasopharyngeal foreign bodies tend to cause acute-onset upper respiratory signs and also may result in sneezing. With chronicity, nasal discharge and halitosis can develop. Foreign bodies are presumed to become lodged in the nasopharynx secondary to inhalation, reflux during vomiting or regurgitation, or ingestion and secondary penetration through the soft palate. Foreign bodies can be removed via transoral removal via traction on the soft palate, retroflexed rhinoscopic basket retrieval, nasal flushing, and surgical excision via access through the soft palate. Nasopharyngeal foreign bodies found in dogs and cats include bones, foam, a premolar, a trichobezoar, plant material, a stone, sewing needles, and a pet fish.[81-87]

Laryngeal Paralysis

Laryngeal paralysis is the result of recurrent laryngeal nerve dysfunction that impairs arytenoid cartilage abduction during inspiration, leading to respiratory stridor and distress.[15,88-90] It is a common form of upper airway obstruction generally recognized in middle-age to older large and giant breed dogs.[90,91] Some studies suggest that Labrador Retrievers are overrepresented.[90-93] Congenital and acquired laryngeal paralysis have been described in dogs. The disease process also is recognized in cats, although not nearly as commonly.

In normal dogs, the larynx accounts for only 6% of resistance to airflow during nasal breathing because contraction of the dorsal cricoarytenoideus muscle, which is innervated by the recurrent laryngeal nerve, abducts the arytenoid cartilages and widens the glottis.[88] In cases of dysfunction of the recurrent laryngeal nerve, atrophy of one or both of the paired dorsal cricoarytenoideus muscles results, impairing abduction of the arytenoid cartilages and vocal folds. The net effect is narrowing of the glottis upon inspiration, causing increased velocity and turbulence of airflow, increased muscular effort for inspiration, dynamic collapse of the larynx, and ultimately, upper airway obstruction.[88] The cause of recurrent laryngeal nerve dysfunction can be congenital denervation, traumatic, iatrogenic, idiopathic, neoplastic, and associated with diffuse neuromuscular disease.[15,88,89] Congenital laryngeal paralysis has been described in Bouvier des Flandres, Rottweilers, Dalmatians, Siberian Huskies, and Husky mixed breeds, Bull Terriers, Pyrenean Mountain Dogs, and Leonbergers. Affected dogs were less than 1 year of age in all breeds except the Leonbergers.[94-100] Injury to the recurrent laryngeal nerve secondary to accidental cervical trauma, cervical, mediastinal or thoracic neoplasia, and iatrogenic injury during thyroidectomy and extraluminal tracheal ring prosthesis placement can result in acquired laryngeal paralysis.[15,88-90,101,102] Myasthenia gravis and hypothyroidism also have been implicated in cases of laryngeal paralysis, although the exact relationship is not understood completely.[90,101,103,104] However, an underlying cause is not confirmed for most cases of acquired laryngeal paralysis, resulting in many cases being labeled idiopathic, although evidence is growing that laryngeal paralysis is one component of generalized peripheral polyneuropathy.[90-93,102,105]

Clinical signs recognized in dogs with laryngeal paralysis depend on the severity of airway obstruction and can include inspiratory stridor, change in bark, exercise intolerance, coughing, and gagging. Most dogs do not develop significant clinical signs until bilateral laryngeal paralysis has developed.[90] Hypersalivation and vomiting or regurgitation may be seen in patients with laryngeal paralysis; however, the absence of gastrointestinal signs does not exclude the possibility of esophageal dysmotility.[91] In more severely affected animals respiratory distress, cyanosis, and collapse can result. Clinical signs can be exacerbated by exercise, stress, anxiety, and increased ambient temperature or humidity. Animals with profound airway obstruction and laryngeal edema may require emergency intubation or tracheostomy.

Before anesthesia for laryngeal examination or definitive surgery, thoracic radiographs are imperative to assess for evidence of pneumonia because resolving or subclinical aspiration pneumonia is common.[90,101] Other pulmonary pathology, such as noncardiogenic pulmonary edema, cardiomegaly, and intrathoracic or mediastinal neoplasia affecting the recurrent laryngeal nerve, hiatal hernia, and metastatic neoplasia should also be ruled out before anesthesia. Assessment of esophageal motility should be considered because dogs with esophageal dysmotility are at higher risk of aspiration pneumonia. Liquid-phase esophagram may better predict postoperative aspiration pneumonia compared with neurologic status.[91]

Laryngeal paralysis usually is confirmed via sedated, direct laryngeal examination or laryngoscopy. Care must be taken not to distort the oropharynx or larynx if a laryngoscope is used and to ensure paradoxical movement of the arytenoids during examination is not confused with proper, active arytenoid abduction.[15,20,21] Transoral flexible video endoscopy can be useful because it provides magnification and allows laryngeal examination without the need for manipulation of the tongue or epiglottis.[21] Transnasal flexible endoscopy for evaluation of the larynx also has been described in dogs weighing more than 20 kg and can be performed with lower doses of premedication and induction agents, especially if intranasal lidocaine is applied before the procedure.[106] Laryngeal ultrasound (echolaryngography) and computed tomography (CT) also has been used successfully for diagnosing unilateral and bilateral laryngeal paralysis.[13,107]

In dogs that are mildly affected by laryngeal paralysis, symptomatic medical care, including weight loss, avoidance of stressors, heat, and humidity, anxiolytic therapy, and medications for gastrointestinal supportive care (antacid therapy, promotility agents, antiemetic drugs) may ameliorate some clinical signs. Treatment of underlying disorders such as hypothyroidism and myasthenia gravis also may be beneficial. However, in more clinically affected dogs, especially those with upper airway obstruction, surgical intervention is needed to improve or resolve upper airway signs. Multiple surgical techniques are described, and the decision to perform unilateral or bilateral repair is debated in dogs that have bilateral laryngeal paralysis. The goal of surgical intervention is to widen the glottis to relieve the airway obstruction without deforming the laryngeal anatomy, to preserve the airway protective function of the larynx.[15,88] Surgical techniques are characterized into three main procedural outcome goal categories: widen the dorsal glottis (unilateral and bilateral arytenoid lateralization), widen the ventral glottis (vocal fold resection, partial laryngectomy, modified castellated laryngofissure), and widen the dorsal and ventral glottis (castellated laryngofissure combined with bilateral arytenoid lateralization).[88] Unilateral arytenoid lateralization (tie-back) is performed more commonly than bilateral lateralization, even in patients with bilateral laryngeal paralysis.[15,90,91,108,109] Bilateral arytenoid lateralization is associated with increased postoperative complications, including aspiration pneumonia and acute respiratory distress, and mortality as compared with unilateral lateralization and partial laryngectomy.[90] The most common postoperative complication is aspiration pneumonia, which is seen in 8% to 33% of patients.[90,108,110] Other reported complications include coughing and gagging, return of clinical signs, seroma formation, respiratory distress, and sudden death.[15,90,108,110] Despite complications, most animals (90%) experience improvement in their respiratory status and stridor postoperatively.[90,91,108] Arytenoid lateralization also has been described for small breed, nonbrachycephalic dogs with combined laryngeal paralysis and laryngeal collapse as a viable technique to improve upper airway obstructive symptoms.[111]

Even though laryngeal paralysis is uncommon in cats, the clinical signs are often similar to dogs.[112-114] Affected cats tend to be older, with median or mean ages reported from 8 to 16 years depending on the study.[112-114] Suspected congenital laryngeal paralysis also has been reported sporadically in young cats less than 2 years of age.[112,114] No clear guidelines exist regarding whether surgical intervention should be performed in cats with unilateral disease. Postoperative complications include transient Horner's syndrome, dyspnea, pulmonary edema, laryngeal edema, and obstructive laryngeal stenosis.[112-114] Immediate postoperative aspiration pneumonia is described in only two cats.[112]

Inflammatory Laryngeal Disease

Upper airway obstruction resulting from inflammatory or granulomatous laryngeal disease is uncommon in veterinary medicine and has been reported only sporadically in cats and dogs.[54,115-121] Little is known about the underlying cause, but potential causes include feline respiratory viruses, secondary bacterial infection, endotracheal intubation, previous foreign body, and secondary to laryngeal surgery.[115-117,120,121] Cervical radiography may show increased soft tissue opacity or laryngeal narrowing.[115,117-121] Sedated laryngeal examination reveals thickening and erythema of the larynx and vocal folds.[115,118] Nodules or mass-like lesions also may be seen on the arytenoid cartilages or within the rima glottis.[115,117-119] Since the gross appearance cannot differentiate inflammatory or granulomatous laryngitis from neoplasia, fine-needle aspirate, or preferably, biopsy and histopathology must be performed. Depending on the severity of clinical signs, temporary tracheostomy may be necessary, especially if significant inflammation develops secondary to biopsy.[115,116] Clinical outcome depends on response to treatment with corticosteroids, antibiotics, and surgical intervention, such as debulking of polypoid or mass-like inflammatory lesions.[54,115-118,120,121] Permanent tracheostomy may be necessary for refractory or nonresponsive cases.[115,117]

Tracheal Collapse

Tracheal collapse is a progressive, degenerative disease of the tracheal cartilages commonly seen in older toy and small breed dogs, particularly Yorkshire Terriers.[102] The disease has been reported in dogs of all ages, although the majority are middle age. It is rarely reported in cats. The exact cause of tracheal collapse is unknown; however, dorsal trachealis flaccidity and loss of rigidity of the tracheal cartilages resulting from decreased glycosaminoglycan, chondroitin, and calcium content are suspected.[122-124] The result is airway narrowing and an inability to withstand changing intraluminal airway pressures with respiration.

Tracheal collapse can affect the trachea along its length, and the location of collapse often determines clinical signs. Patients with cervical tracheal collapse tend to have inspiratory dyspnea resulting from the inability of the tracheal cartilages to withstand the negative airway pressure created by chest wall expansion and diaphragmatic contraction. Conversely, on expiration, increased intrapleural pressure collapses the intrathoracic trachea. Animals with collapse of the thoracic inlet trachea can have variable clinical signs.

Clinical signs can vary dramatically depending on the severity of collapse. Coughing, especially the classic "honking" cough, is a prominent feature that is often exacerbated by stress, activity, and excitement. Other clinical signs include stridor, gagging after eating or drinking, exercise intolerance, and respiratory distress.[102,123,125]

Thoracic radiographs are of modest benefit for diagnosing tracheal collapse because they rely on static images to document a dynamic process.[125] Paired inspiratory and expiratory thoracic radiographs improve their utility but can still underestimate severity and extent of disease.[126] Radiographs misdiagnosed the location of tracheal collapse in 44% of dogs and failed to diagnose tracheal collapse in 8% of dogs when compared with fluoroscopy.[126] However, thoracic radiographs are essential to assess for cardiomegaly, lower airway disease, bronchiectasis, and pulmonary parenchymal infiltrates such as pneumonia, which can be seen concurrently in patients with tracheal collapse.[102,125,127] Fluoroscopy allows for dynamic assessment of the entire length of trachea during the entire breath cycle and with coughing. Assessment for nasopharyngeal and mainstem bronchial collapse also can be performed during fluoroscopy. Tracheal ultrasound and computed tomography also have been shown to have adjunctive diagnostic benefit in tracheal collapse patients.[13,128] Bronchoscopy is helpful to grade the severity of tracheal collapse, rule out tracheal masses, and evaluate for bronchial collapse. One study showed that 83% of dogs with cervical tracheal collapse also had concurrent bronchial collapse.[125,129] However, because general anesthesia is required for tracheoscopy and bronchoscopy, recovery from this procedure can be complicated in patients with tracheal collapse and upper airway obstruction. If anesthesia is performed in patients with tracheal collapse, laryngeal examination also should be performed because laryngeal paralysis has been documented in 30% of patients with tracheal collapse in one study.[125] However, this may be an overestimation because other studies have not documented concurrent laryngeal paralysis with such frequency. Airway sampling via endotracheal wash or bronchoalveolar lavage for cytology and aerobic culture and susceptibility testing also should be performed in dogs with tracheal collapse but interpreted with caution because *Pasteurella, Staphylococcus, Streptococcus,* and *Klebsiella* spp. can be cultured from the airways of normal dogs.[130,131] Regardless, the mucociliary escalator is likely dysfunctional in dogs with tracheal collapse, and positive bacterial cultures with supportive cytologic findings of suppurative inflammation likely warrant appropriate antimicrobial treatment (see Chapters 22 and 23). The most commonly isolated bacterial species in dogs with tracheal collapse include *Pseudomonas* and *Pasteurella* spp., *E. coli,* and staphylococci.[131,132]

Complete blood count and serum chemistry evaluation should be performed in patients with tracheal collapse to look for inflammatory leukogram changes consistent with infection and evidence of liver dysfunction (elevated ALT and bile acids), which has been documented in dogs with tracheal collapse and is suspected to be secondary to hypoxemia.[133] Pulse oximetry and arterial blood gas analysis, if possible, should be performed for objective determination of oxygenation.

Aggressive cough control is the mainstay of medical management for dogs with tracheal collapse. Corticosteroids and bronchodilators may also be indicated if significant inflammation or bronchoconstriction is suspected to be contributing to clinical signs. The benefit of oral versus inhaled steroids and bronchodilators with tracheal collapse is yet to be determined. Use of a harness (rather than neck leads) and control of exacerbating factors, such as heat, stress, and excitement, are essential elements of conservative management. Gradual weight loss should be targeted for overweight patients. One study of 100 dogs with tracheal collapse showed that medical management was able to control clinical signs for more than 12 months in 71% of dogs.[102]

When medical management fails to control clinical signs of tracheal collapse, or the patient's quality of life is declining, surgical or interventional options should be considered. In dogs with cervical tracheal and/or proximal thoracic inlet collapse that have failed medical therapy, prosthetic extraluminal tracheal rings can be considered. Commercially made rings are available in four sizes from New Generation Devices (http://ngdvet.com) and also can be made by hand from polypropylene syringes or syringe cases. Extreme caution must be exercised during tracheal dissection and ring placement to avoid damaging the segmental tracheal blood supply and the recurrent laryngeal nerve. The success rate for prosthetic rings is reported to be 75% to 85%.[125,132] Postoperative complications include infection, laryngeal paralysis (10% to 21%), tracheal necrosis, and progressive tracheal collapse.[102,124,125,132,134] Patients typically are hospitalized for several days of intensive monitoring after ring placement. In dogs with cervical tracheal collapse treated with prosthetic ring placement, no survival difference was found between dogs with cervical collapse alone and those with concurrent intrathoracic tracheal collapse, indicating that even dogs with intrathoracic disease may benefit from ring placement if inspiratory dyspnea is severe enough to warrant intervention.[134]

In dogs with tracheal collapse at any point along the trachea or those deemed to be poor surgical candidates for ring placement, endoluminal tracheal stenting can be considered. Tracheal stenting is beneficial in tracheal collapse dogs that are presented in respiratory crisis that is nonresponsive to medical stabilization.[135,136] Initial experience with tracheal stenting when wall stents or balloon expandable stents were used was met with significant complications, such as foreshortening, migration, fracture, and excessive airway irritation.[137-142] Tracheal stents made for dogs (http://infinitimedical.com) have gone through multiple design iterations over the past several years, and engineering adjustments have improved their sizing and placement predictability, patient comfort, and fracture potential.[143] Complications seen with tracheal stenting, such as migration, foreshortening, and fracture, are greatly reduced when precise sizing is performed using positive pressure ventilation breath holds to determine maximal tracheal diameter along the length of the trachea. Fluoroscopy is used traditionally for stent placement, but bronchoscopic guidance has also been described.[144] Because measurements are performed under general anesthesia at the time of stenting, multiple sizes of tracheal stents should be readily available so that the appropriate size can be placed without having to attempt to recover a compromised patient. Tracheal stents are placed through an endotracheal tube, and when a bronchoscope adapter is used, the patient can continue to have oxygen insufflation during stent positioning and deployment. Patients often are discharged the day after stent placement. Long-term routine thoracic radiograph monitoring is important to detect migration, early fracture, or the development of inflammatory tissue. Currently, no long-term studies evaluating the outcome for dogs receiving later generation tracheal stents exist, although early information is positive.[144,145] Clinically significant tracheal stent fractures can be managed with placement of an additional tracheal stent within the original stent.[146]

Tracheal Stenosis/Stricture

Tracheal injury secondary to intraluminal trauma, as with endotracheal intubation, and extraluminal trauma, which is seen with bite wounds and vehicular trauma, is uncommonly reported in dogs and cats[147-151] (see Chapter 19). Injury and tearing of the dorsal tracheal membrane generally results from overinflation of the endotracheal tube cuff or repositioning of the head and neck during anesthesia without disconnecting the endotracheal tube from the tubing attached to the machine. Acute injury generally results in pneumomediastinum, pneumothorax, subcutaneous emphysema, and respiratory distress.[149] Less severe, full-thickness tracheal tears can result in circumferential tracheal stricture and ultimately tracheal narrowing, which, if severe enough, can result in upper airway obstruction. Tracheal stenosis also can be the result of scarring from prior surgery or tracheal avulsion.[147,148,152] Thoracic radiographs, computed tomography, and tracheoscopy can be used to confirm a diagnosis of tracheal stricture. Treatment options include surgical tracheal resection and anastomosis, bronchoscopic debridement of necrotic tissue, and intraluminal tracheal stenting.[147,148,150,152,153]

Tracheal narrowing leading to upper airway obstruction also has been reported secondary to intraluminal tracheal hemorrhage resulting from anticoagulant rodenticide toxicity and a tracheal hematoma in dogs.[154-156]

Tracheal Foreign Bodies

Aspiration of foreign material into the trachea can cause coughing, gagging, head and neck extension, and respiratory distress. The duration of clinical signs can vary depending on the type and extent of airway obstruction and the degree of associated inflammation. Retrieved tracheal materials in dogs and cats include grass awns, plant material, plastic material, stones and gravel, an owl tooth, and *Cuterebra* spp. in cats.[157-161] Cervical and thoracic radiographs can be helpful in the diagnosis of tracheal foreign material. Tracheoscopy allows for direct visualization and also can be used for removal of the foreign body using grasping forceps passed through the working channel of the bronchoscope (see Chapter 136).[157,159,160] One study reports an 86% success rate for bronchoscope assisted foreign body retrieval in dogs and 40% success in cats.[157] When bronchoscopic removal is not feasible or fails, surgical excision can be considered.[157,160,161] Retrieval using grasping forceps and fluoroscopic guidance also is described as a successful technique for tracheal foreign body removal in cats.[159] Novel retrieval techniques using the inflated balloon from a Foley catheter or fluoroscopic guided over-the-wire balloon angioplasty catheters also have been described.[158,162]

Upper Airway Neoplasia

Nasal and nasopharyngeal neoplasia are uncommon causes of upper airway obstructive signs, unless there is complete obstruction to nasal airflow, which can cause nasal discharge, inspiratory dyspnea, open-mouth breathing (cats), and inability to sleep (dogs). Canine nasal neoplasias are generally carcinomas (adenocarcinoma, squamous cell carcinoma, and undifferentiated carcinoma) or sarcomas (fibrosarcoma, osteosarcoma, and chondrosarcoma).[163] In cats, nasal lymphoma is most common, but sarcomas (fibrosarcoma, osteosarcoma, chondrosarcoma, and hemangiosarcoma), carcinomas (adenocarcinoma, undifferentiated carcinoma), and olfactory neuroblastomas are also reported.[163-165] Since achieving surgical margins is extremely difficult in the nasal passage, treatment usually involves systemic chemotherapy and radiation therapy. As experience with image guided interventional therapies for neoplasia grows, intraarterial chemotherapy delivery also likely will become an additional treatment modality for nasal neoplasia (see Chapter 136). Nasopharyngeal neoplasias reported in dogs include lymphoma, mast cell tumor, squamous cell carcinoma, undifferentiated carcinoma, adenocarcinoma, fibrosarcoma, osteosarcoma, and spindle cell tumor.[81] Nasopharyngeal neoplasias are less commonly reported in cats and include lymphoma and adenocarcinoma.[14,47,81,165] Surgical treatment may be possible for small or well-circumscribed nasopharyngeal neoplasias, although chemotherapy and radiation are more likely to be beneficial.

Primary laryngeal neoplasia is uncommon in dogs and cats and requires histopathology to differentiate from inflammatory/granulomatous laryngitis and benign lesions because they can have similar appearance on direct visual examination.[54,115,118] In general, animals with laryngeal tumors are older (median age of 8 years) and tend to have a history of coughing, choking, dyspnea, and voice change.[166] Most patients have significant disease progression by the time of presentation. In cats, reported laryngeal neoplasias include lymphoma, squamous cell carcinoma, poorly differentiated round cell tumor, carcinoma, and adenocarcinoma.[54,118,119,166,167] In dogs, confirmed laryngeal neoplasias include chondrosarcoma, extramedullary plasmacytoma, rhabdomyoma, carcinoma, mast cell tumor, squamous cell carcinoma, lymphoma, adenocarcinoma, melanoma, granular cell tumor, and chondroma.[166,168-171] Benign laryngeal lipomas and rhabdomyomas also are rarely seen in dogs.[166,167,172,173] Surgical resection is difficult and may require total laryngectomy and permanent tracheostomy for long-term management but can be successful for small or benign lesions.[166,172,173] Overall, prognosis for laryngeal tumors is guarded and depends on type, invasiveness, metastatic spread, and response to chemotherapy or radiation.[167]

Primary tracheal neoplasia is also uncommon in dogs and cats, and one study suggests it is less common than primary laryngeal neoplasia.[166] The most common tracheal tumor reported in dogs is osteochondroma; however, other reported types include chondrosarcoma, chondroma, adenocarcinoma, carcinoma, mast cell tumor, leiomyoma, extramedullary plasmacytoma, and osteosarcoma.[166,174] Lymphoma is the most common feline tracheal tumor; however, carcinoma, adenocarcinoma, adenoma, squamous cell carcinoma, neuroendocrine carcinoma, and basal cell carcinoma also have been reported[119,167,171,174-177] (Figure 17-3, *A*). The median age of dogs and cats with tracheal tumors is 9 years except for dogs with osteochondroma and enchondroma, which tend to be less than 2 years of age.[166,174] Coughing, wheezing, dyspnea, and stridor are common clinical signs in patients with tracheal tumors.[166,174] Cervical and thoracic radiographs can be helpful in the diagnosis of an intraluminal tracheal mass, which can be located at any point in the trachea from caudal to the larynx to the level of the carina. Computed tomography, which can even be performed in the awake, nonintubated patient, also can be helpful to more precisely determine extent of the mass and degree of luminal occlusion.[14] Tracheoscopy is valuable for direct visualization of the mass as well as obtaining biopsy or brush cytology samples but often requires extubation in small patients, which can be dangerous with obstructive lesions. Options for management of tracheal masses include surgical resection, endoscopic snaring, cryotherapy, radiation, chemotherapy, and palliative intraluminal stenting[119,174,175,152] (Figure 17-3, *B*). The prognosis varies and depends on extent of disease, mass type, and treatment response.

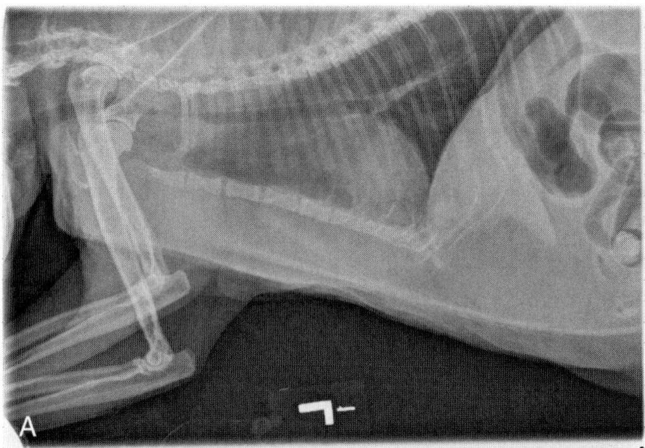

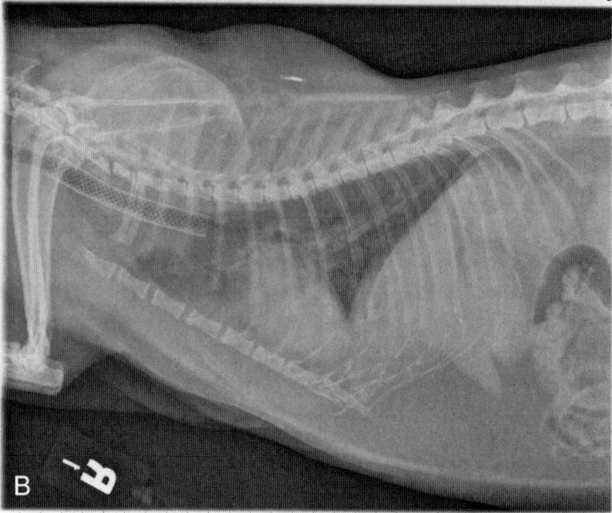

FIGURE 17-3 A, Intraluminal tracheal mass at the thoracic inlet of a 12-year-old cat with severe dyspnea, open-mouth breathing, and hypoventilation. **B,** Intraluminal tracheal stenting for palliation of the cat's tracheal mass, which quickly resolved his respiratory distress. Histopathology confirmed the tracheal mass was adenocarcinoma.

Complications of Upper Airway Obstruction

In addition to the respiratory distress, hypoxemia, and hypercarbia that can be associated with upper airway obstruction, there are numerous potential secondary complications that can result from obstructive upper airway disease, including hyperthermia (see Chapter 10), non-cardiogenic pulmonary edema (see Chapter 21), and aspiration pneumonia (see Chapter 23). Temperature should be monitored closely in all patients with upper airway disease, especially if there is concern for obstruction and failure to appropriately dissipate heat. Failure to actively cool a severely hyperthermic patient can result in respiratory, cardiovascular, neurologic, renal, and coagulation derangements that can progress to multiorgan dysfunction syndrome (MODS), multiorgan failure (MOF), and disseminated intravascular coagulation (DIC) (see Chapter 7). Identification of pulmonary pathology consistent with noncardiogenic edema (caudodorsal interstitial to alveolar infiltrates) and aspiration pneumonia (cranioventral interstitial to alveolar infiltrates) is important before any anesthetic procedure, and in the case of aspiration pneumonia, warrants consideration of airway sampling for cytology, culture and susceptibility testing, and institution of appropriate antimicrobial therapy. Treatment for noncardiogenic pulmonary edema is supportive and should include oxygen therapy and judicious crystalloid and colloid fluid therapy (see Chapters 57 through 60). The use of diuretics and β-agonists in noncardiogenic pulmonary edema is controversial because increased clearance of alveolar fluid has not been proven.[178-180]

REFERENCES

1. Holt DE: Upper airway obstruction, stertor, and stridor. In King LG, editor: Textbook of respiratory disease in dogs and cats, St Louis, 2004, Saunders.
2. Rozanski E, Chan DL: Approach to the patient with respiratory distress, Vet Clin North Am Small Anim Pract 35(2):307-317, 2005.
3. Miller CJ: Approach to the respiratory patient, Vet Clin North America Small Anim Pract 37(5):861-878, 2007.
4. Tseng LW, Waddell LS: Approach to the patient in respiratory distress, Clin Tech Small Anim Pract 15(2):53-62, 2000.
5. Corcoran B: Clinical evaluation of the patient with respiratory disease. In Ettinger SJ, Feldman EC, editors: Textbook of veterinary internal medicine, ed 5, St Louis, 2000, Saunders.
6. Harpster NK: Physical examination of the respiratory tract. In King LG, editor: Textbook of respiratory disease in dogs and cats, St Louis, 2004, Saunders.
7. Sigrist NE, Adamik KN, Doherr MG, et al: Evaluation of respiratory parameters at presentation as clinical indicators of the respiratory localization in dogs and cats with respiratory distress, J Vet Emerg Crit Care 21(1):13-23, 2011.
8. Hackner SG: Panting. In King LG, editor: Textbook of respiratory disease in dogs and cats, St Louis, 2004, Saunders.
9. Drobatz KJ, Macintire DK: Heat-induced illness in dogs: 42 cases (1976-1993), J Am Vet Med Assoc 209:1894-1899, 1996.
10. Johnson SI, McMichael M, White G: Heatstroke in small animal medicine: a clinical practice review, J Vet Emerg Crit 16(2):112-119, 2006.
11. Hemmelgarn C, Gannon K: Heatstroke: thermoregulation, pathophysiology, and predisposing factors, Compendium 35(7):E4-6, 2012.
12. Plumb DC: Plumb's veterinary drug handbook: desk, ed 7, Hoboken, NJ, 2011, Wiley.
13. Stadler K, Hartman S, Matheson J, et al: Computed tomography imaging of dogs with primary laryngeal or tracheal airway obstruction, Vet Rad Ultrasound 52(4):377-384, 2011.
14. Stadler K, O'Brien R: Computed tomography of nonanesthetized cats with upper airway obstruction, Vet Rad Ultrasound 54(3):231-236, 2013.
15. Millard RP, Tobias KM: Laryngeal paralysis in dogs, Compendium 31(5):212-219, 2009.

16. Tobias KM, Jackson AM, Harvey RC: Effects of doxapram HCl on laryngeal function of normal dogs and dogs with naturally occurring laryngeal paralysis, Vet Anaesth Analg 31(4):258-263, 2004.
17. Jackson AM, Tobias K, Long C, et al: Effects of various anesthetic agents on laryngeal motion during laryngoscopy in normal dogs, Vet Surg 33(2):102-106, 2004.
18. Gross ME, Dodam JR, Pope ER, et al: A comparison of thiopental, propofol, and diazepam-ketamine anesthesia for evaluation of laryngeal function in dogs premedicated with butorphanol-glycopyrrolate, J Am Anim Hosp Assoc 38(6):503-506, 2002.
19. Miller CJ, McKiernan BC, Pace J, et al: The effects of doxapram hydrochloride (dopram-V) on laryngeal function in healthy dogs, J Vet Intern Med 16(5):524-528, 2002.
20. Burbidge HM: A review of laryngeal paralysis in dogs, Br Vet J 151:71-82, 1995.
21. Creevy KE: Airway evaluation and flexible endoscopic procedures in dogs and cats: laryngoscopy, transtracheal wash, tracheobronchoscopy, and bronchoalveolar lavage, Vet Clin North Am Small Anim Pract 39(5):869-880, 2009.
22. Flanders JA, Thompson MS: Dyspnea caused by epiglottic retroversion in two dogs, J Am Vet Med Assoc 235(11):1330-1335, 2009.
23. MacPhail CM: Surgery of the upper airway. In Fossum TW, editor: Small animal surgery, ed 4, St Louis, 2013, Elsevier.
24. Hendricks JC: Brachycephalic airway syndrome. In King LG, editor: Textbook of respiratory disease in dogs and cats, St Louis, 2004, Saunders.
25. Lodato DL, Hedlund CS: Brachycephalic airway syndrome: pathophysiology and diagnosis, Compendium 34(7):E3-5, 2012.
26. Ginn JA, Kumar MSA, McKiernan BC, et al: Nasopharyngeal turbinates in brachycephalic dogs and cats, J Am Anim Hosp Assoc 4(5):243-249, 2008.
27. Koch DA, Arnold S, Hubler M, et al: Brachycephalic syndrome in dogs, Compend Contin Educ Pract Vet 25(1):48-55, 2003.
28. Trappler M, Moore K: Canine brachycephalic airway syndrome: pathophysiology, diagnosis, and nonsurgical management, Compendium 33(5):E1-4, 2011.
29. Poncet CM, Dupre GP, Freiche VG, et al: Prevalence of gastrointestinal tract lesions in 73 brachycephalic dogs with upper respiratory syndrome, J Small Anim Pract 46(6):273-279, 2005.
30. Poncet CM, Dupre GP, Freiche VG, et al: Long-term results of upper respiratory syndrome surgery and gastrointestinal tract medical treatment in 51 brachycephalic dogs, J Small Anim Pract 47(3):137-142, 2006.
31. Ohnishi T, Ogura JH: Partitioning of pulmonary resistance in the dog, Laryngoscope 79:1874, 1969.
32. Hoffman AM: Airway physiology and clinical function testing, Vet Clin North Am Small Anim Pract 37:829-843, 2007.
33. Torrez CV, Hunt GB: Results of surgical correction of abnormalities associated with brachycephalic airway obstruction syndrome in dogs in Australia, J Small Anim Pract 47(3):150-154, 2006.
34. Riecks TW, Birchard SJ, Stephens JA: Surgical correction of brachycephalic syndrome in dogs: 62 cases (1991-2004), J Am Vet Med Assoc 230(9):1324-1328, 2007.
35. Fasanella FJ, Shivley JM, Wardlaw JL, et al: Brachycephalic airway obstructive syndrome in dogs: 90 cases (1991-2008), J Am Vet Med Assoc 237(9):1048-1051, 2010.
36. Harvey CE, Fink EA: Tracheal diameter: analysis of radiographic measurements in brachycephalic and non-brachycephalic dogs, J Am Anim Hosp Assoc 18:570-576, 1982.
37. Clarke DL, Holt DE, King LG: Partial resolution of hypoplastic trachea in six English bulldog puppies with bronchopneumonia, J Am Anim Hosp Assoc 47(5):329-335, 2011.
38. Hoareau GL, Jourdan G, Mellema M, et al: Evaluation of arterial blood gases and arterial blood pressures in brachycephalic dogs, J Vet Intern Med 26(4):897-904, 2012.
39. De Lorenzi D, Bertoncello D, Drigo M: Bronchial abnormalities found in a consecutive series of 40 brachycephalic dogs, J Am Vet Med Assoc 235(7):835-840, 2009.
40. Planellas M, Cuenca R, Tabar M-D, et al: Evaluation of C-reactive protein, haptoglobin and cardiac troponin 1 levels in brachycephalic dogs with upper airway obstructive syndrome, BMC Vet Res 8:152-159, 2012.
41. Harvey CE: Stenotic nares surgery in brachycephalic dogs, J Am Anim Hosp Assoc 18:535-537, 1982.
42. Ellison GW: Alapexy: an alternative technique for repair of stenotic nares in dogs, J Am Anim Hosp Assoc 40:484-489, 2004.
43. Huck JL, Stanley BJ, Hauptman JG: Technique and outcome of nares amputation (Trader's technique) in immature shih tzus, J Am Anim Hosp Assoc 44(2):82-85, 2008.
44. Lodato DL, Hedlund CS: Brachycephalic airway syndrome: management, Compendium 34(8):E4-7, 2012.
45. Pink JJ, Doyle RS, Hughes JML, et al: Laryngeal collapse in seven brachycephalic puppies, J Small Anim Pract 47(3):131-135, 2006.
46. White RN: Surgical management of laryngeal collapse associated with brachycephalic airway obstruction syndrome in dogs, J Small Anim Pract 28;53(1):44-50, 2011.
47. Allen HS, Broussard J, Noone K: Nasopharyngeal diseases in cats: a retrospective study of 53 cases (1991-1998), J Am Anim Hosp Assoc 35(6):457-461, 1999.
48. Smart L, Jandrey KE: Upper airway obstruction caused by a nasopharyngeal polyp and brachycephalic airway syndrome in a Chinese Shar-Pei puppy, J Vet Emer Crit 18(4):393-398, 2008.
49. Fingland RB, Gratzek A, Vorhies MW, et al: Nasopharyngeal polyp in a dog, J Am Anim Hosp Assoc 29:311-314, 1993.
50. Pollock S: Nasopharyngeal polyp in a dog, a case study, Vet Med Small Anim Clin 66(7):705-706, 1971.
51. Holt DE: Nasopharyngeal polyps. In King LG, editor: Textbook of respiratory disease in dogs and cats, St Louis, 2004, Saunders.
52. Reed N, Gunn-Moore D: Nasopharyngeal disease in cats: 1. Diagnostic investigation, J Feline Med Surg 14(5):306-315, 2012.
53. Kudnig ST: Nasopharyngeal polyps in cats, Clin Tech Small Anim Pract 17(4):174-177, 2002.
54. Griffon DJ: Upper airway obstruction in cats: diagnosis and treatment, Compedium 22(10):897-909, 2000.
55. Muilenburg RK, Fry TR: Feline nasopharyngeal polyps, Vet Clin Small Anim Pract 32(4):839-849, 2002.
56. Tillson DM, Donnelly KE: Feline inflammatory polyps and ventral bulla osteotomy, Compendium 26(6):1-5, 2004.
57. Klose TC, Macphail CM, Schultheiss PC, et al: Prevalence of select infectious agents in inflammatory aural and nasopharyngeal polyps from client-owned cats, J Feline Med Surg 12(10):769-774, 2010.
58. Oliveira CR, O'Brien RT, Matheson JS, et al: Computed tomographic features of feline nasopharyngeal polyps, Vet Rad Ultrasound 53(4):406-411, 2012.
59. Kapatin AS, Mattheisen DT, Noone KE, et al: Results of surgery and long term follow up in 31 cats with nasopharyngeal polyps, J Am Anim Hosp Assoc 26:387-392, 1990.
60. Anderson DM, Robinson RK, White RA: Management of inflammatory polyps in 37 cats, Vet Rec 147(24):684-687, 2000.
61. Trevor PB, Martin RA: Tympanic bulla osteotomy for treatment of middle-ear disease in cats: 19 cases (1984-1991), J Am Vet Med Assoc 202(1):123-128, 1993.
62. Anders BB, Hoelzler MG, Scavelli TD, et al: Analysis of auditory and neurologic effects associated with ventral bulla osteotomy for removal of inflammatory polyps or nasopharyngeal masses in cats, J Am Vet Med Assoc 233(4):580-585, 2008.
63. Billen F, Day MJ, Clercx C: Diagnosis of pharyngeal disorders in dogs: a retrospective study of 67 cases, J Small Anim Pract 47(3):122-129, 2006.
64. Henderson SM, Bradley K, Day MJ, et al: Investigation of nasal disease in the cat—a retrospective study of 77 cases, J Feline Med Surg 6(4):245-257, 2004.
65. Coolman BR, Marretta SM, McKiernan BC, et al: Choanal atresia and secondary nasopharyngeal stenosis in a dog, J Am Anim Hosp Assoc 34(6):497-501, 1998.
66. Berent AC, Kinns J, Weisse C: Balloon dilatation of nasopharyngeal stenosis in a dog, J Am Vet Med Assoc 229(3):385-388, 2006.
67. Berent AC, Weisse C, Todd K, et al: Use of a balloon-expandable metallic stent for treatment of nasopharyngeal stenosis in dogs and cats: six cases (2005-2007), J Am Vet Med Assoc 233(9):1432-1440, 2008.

68. Boswood A, Lamb CR, Brockman DJ, et al: Balloon dilatation of nasopharyngeal stenosis in a cat, Vet Rad Ultrasound 44(1):53-55, 2003.
69. Glaus TM, Tomsa K, Reusch CE: Balloon dilation for the treatment of chronic recurrent nasopharyngeal stenosis in a cat, J Small Anim Pract 43(2):88-90, 2002.
70. Glaus TM, Gerber B, Tomsa K, et al: Reproducible and long-lasting success of balloon dilation of nasopharyngeal stenosis in cats, Vet Rec 157(9):257-259, 2005.
71. Novo RE, Kramek B: Surgical repair of nasopharyngeal stenosis in a cat using a stent, J Am Anim Hosp Assoc 35(3):251-256, 1999.
72. Mitten RW: Nasopharyngeal stenosis in four cats, J Small Anim Pract 29(6):341-345, 1988.
73. Griffon DJ, Tasker S: Use of a mucosal advancement flap for the treatment of nasopharyngeal stenosis in a cat, J Small Anim Pract 41(2):71-73, 2000.
74. Cook AK, Mankin KT, Saunders AB, et al: Palatal erosion and oronasal fistulation following covered nasopharyngeal stent placement in two dogs, Ir Vet J 66(1):8-14, 2013.
75. Khoo A, Marchevsky A, Barrs V, et al: Choanal atresia in a Himalayan cat—first reported case and successful treatment, J Feline Med Surg 9(4):346-349, 2007.
76. Azarpeykan S, Stickney A, Hill KE, et al: Choanal atresia in a cat, New Z Vet J 61(4):237-241, 2013.
77. Schafgans KE, Armstrong PJ, Kramek B, et al: Bilateral choanal atresia in a cat, J Feline Med Surg 14(10):759-763, 2012.
78. Wehner A, Crochik S, Howerth EW, et al: Diagnosis and treatment of blastomycosis affecting the nose and nasopharynx of a dog, J Am Vet Med Assoc 233(7):1112-1116, 2008.
79. Malik R, Martin P, Wigney DI, et al: Nasopharyngeal cryptococcosis, Aust Vet J 75(7):483-488, 1997.
80. Forster-van Hijfte MA, Groth AM, et al: Expansile, inflammatory middle ear disease causing nasopharyngeal obstruction in a cat, J Feline Med Surg 13(6):451-453, 2011.
81. Hunt GB, Perkins MC, Foster SF, et al: Nasopharyngeal disorders of dogs and cats: a review and retrospective study, Compendium 24(3):184-203, 2002.
82. Kang M-H, Lim C-Y, Park H-M: Nasopharyngeal tooth foreign body in a dog, J Vet Dent 28(1):26-29, 2011.
83. Haynes KJ, Anderson SE, Laszlo MP: Nasopharyngeal trichobezoar foreign body in a cat, J Feline Med Surg 12(11):878-881, 2010.
84. Riley P: Nasopharyngeal grass foreign body in eight cats, J Am Vet Med Assoc 202(2):299-300, 1993.
85. Ober CP, Barber D, Troy GC: What is your diagnosis? J Am Vet Med Assoc 231(8):1207-1208, 2007.
86. Papazoglau LG, Patsikas MN: What is your diagnosis? A radiopaque foreign body located in the nasopharynx, J Small Anim Prac 36(10):425, 434, 1995.
87. Simpson AM, Harkin KR, Hoskinson JJ: Radiographic diagnosis: nasopharyngeal foreign body in a dog, Vet Rad Ultrasound 41(4):326-328, 2000.
88. Holt DE, Brockman DJ: Laryngeal paralysis. In King LG, editor: Textbook of respiratory disease in dogs and cats, St Louis, 2004, Saunders.
89. Griffin J: Laryngeal paralysis: pathophysiology, diagnosis, and surgical repair, Compendium 7:1-13, 2005.
90. MacPhail CM, Monnet E: Outcome of and postoperative complications in dogs undergoing surgical treatment of laryngeal paralysis: 140 cases (1985-1998), J Am Vet Med Assoc 218(12):1949-1956, 2001.
91. Stanley BJ, Hauptman JG, Fritz MC, et al: Esophageal dysfunction in dogs with idiopathic laryngeal paralysis: a controlled cohort study, Vet Surg 39(2):139-149, 2010.
92. Thieman KM, Krahwinkel DJ, Shelton D, et al: Laryngeal paralysis: part of a generalized polyneuropathy syndrome in older dogs, Vet Surg 36:E26, 2007.
93. Thieman KM, Krahwinkel DJ, Sims MH, et al: Histopathological confirmation of polyneuropathy in 11 dogs with laryngeal paralysis, J Am Anim Hosp Assoc 46(3):161-167, 2010.
94. Venker-van Haagen AJ, Bouw J, et al: Hereditary transmission of laryngeal paralysis in Bouviers, J Am Anim Hosp Assoc 17:75-76, 1981.
95. Mahony OM, Knowles KE, Braund KG, et al: Laryngeal paralysis-polyneuropathy complex in young rottweilers, J Vet Intern Med 12:330-337, 1998.
96. Braund KG, Shores A, Cochrane S, et al: Laryngeal paralysis-polyneuropathy complex in young dalmatians, Am J Vet Res 55:534-542, 1994.
97. Polizopoulou ZS, Koutinas AF, Papadopoulos GC, et al: Juvenile laryngeal paralysis in three Siberian husky x Alaskan malamute puppies, Vet Rec 153:624-627, 2003.
98. O'Brien JA, Hendriks JC: Inherited laryngeal paralysis: analysis in the husky cross, Vet Q 8:301-302, 1986.
99. Gabriel A, Poncelet L, Van Ham L, et al: Laryngeal paralysis-polyneuropathy complex in young related Pyrenean mountain dogs, J Small Anim Pract 47(3):144-149, 2006.
100. Shelton GD, Podell M, Poncelet L, et al: Inherited polyneuropathy in Leonberger dogs: a mixed or intermediate form of Charcot-Marie-Tooth disease? Muscle & Nerve 27:471-477, 2003.
101. Klein MK, Powers BE, Withrow SJ, et al: Treatment of thyroid carcinoma in dogs by surgical resection alone: 20 cases (1981-1989), J AmVet Med Assoc 206:1007-1009, 1995.
102. White R, Williams JM: Tracheal collapse in the dog-is there really a role for surgery? A survey of 100 cases. J Small Anim Pract 35(4):191-196, 1994.
103. Jaggy A, Oliver JE, Ferguson DC, et al: Neurological manifestations of hypothyroidism: a retrospective study of 29 dogs, J Vet Intern Med 8:328-336, 1994.
104. Dewey CW, Bailey CS, Shelton GD, et al: Clinical forms of acquired myasthenia gravis in dogs: 25 cases (1988-1995), J Vet Intern Med 11:50-57, 1997.
105. Jeffery ND, Talbot CE, Smith PM, et al: Acquired idiopathic laryngeal paralysis as a prominent feature of generalised neuromuscular disease in 39 dogs, Vet Rec 158:17, 2006.
106. Radlinsky MG, Williams J, Frank PM, et al: Comparison of three clinical techniques for the diagnosis of laryngeal paralysis in dogs, Vet Surg 38(4):434-438, 2009.
107. Rudorf H, Barr FJ, Lane JG: The role of ultrasound in the assessment of laryngeal paralysis in the dog, Vet Rad Ultrasound 42(4):338-343, 2001.
108. Hammel SP, Hottinger HA, Novo RE: Postoperative results of unilateral arytenoid lateralization for treatment of idiopathic laryngeal paralysis in dogs: 39 cases (1996-2002), J Am Vet Med Assoc 228(8):1215-1220, 2006.
109. Snelling SR, Edwards GA: A retrospective study of unilateral arytenoid lateralisation in the treatment of laryngeal paralysis in 100 dogs (1992-2000), Aust Vet J 81(8):464-468, 2003.
110. Greenberg MJ, Reems MR, Monnet E: Use of perioperative metoclopramide in dogs undergoing surgical treatment of laryngeal parapysis: 43 cases, Vet Surg 36:E11, 2007.
111. Nelissen P, White RAS: Arytenoid lateralization for management of combined laryngeal paralysis and laryngeal collapse in small dogs, Vet Surg 21:261-265, 2011.
112. Hardie RJ, Gunby J, Bjorling DE: Arytenoid lateralization for treatment of laryngeal paralysis in 10 cats, Vet Surgery 38(4):445-451, 2009.
113. Thunberg B, Lantz GC: Evaluation of unilateral arytenoid lateralization for the treatment of laryngeal paralysis in 14 cats, J Am Anim Hosp Assoc 46(6):418-424, 2010.
114. Schachter S, Norris CR: Laryngeal paralysis in cats: 16 cases (1990-1999), J Am Vet Med Assoc 216(7):1100-1103, 2005.
115. Costello MF, Keith D, Hendrick M, et al: Acute upper airway obstruction due to inflammatory laryngeal disease in 5 cats, J Vet Emerg Crit Care 11(3):205-210, 2001.
116. Costello MF: Upper airway disease. In Silverstein DC, Hopper KA, editors: Small animal critical care medicine, St Louis, 2009, Elsevier.
117. Tasker S, Foster DJ, Corcoran BM, et al: Obstructive inflammatory laryngeal disease in three cats, J Fel Med Surg 1(1):53-59, 1999.
118. Taylor SS, Harvey AM, Barr FJ, et al: Laryngeal disease in cats: a retrospective study of 35 cases, J Fel Med Surg 11(12):954-962, 2009.
119. Jakubiak MJ, Siedlecki CT, Zenger E, et al: Laryngeal, laryngotracheal, and tracheal masses in cats: 27 cases (1998-2003), J Am Anim Hosp Assoc 41(5):310-316, 2005.

120. Oakes MG, McCarthy RJ: What is your diagnosis? [granulomatous laryngitis], J Am Vet Med Assoc 204:1891, 1994.
121. Harvey CE, O'Brien JA: Surgical treatment of miscellaneous laryngeal conditions in dogs and cats, J Am Anim Hosp Assoc 1982;18:557-562.
122. Dallman MJ, McClure RC, Brown EM: Histochemical study of normal and collapsed tracheas in dogs, Am J Vet Res 49(12):2117-2125, 1988.
123. Mason RA, Johnson LR: Tracheal collapse. In King LG, editor: Textbook of respiratory disease in dogs and cats, St Louis, 2004, Saunders.
124. Payne JD, Mehler SJ, Weisse C: Tracheal collapse, Compendium 28(5):373-383, 2006.
125. Tangner CH, Hobson H: A retrospective study of 20 surgically managed cases of collapsed trachea, Vet Surg 11(4):146-149, 1982.
126. Macready DM, Johnson LR, Pollard RE: Fluoroscopic and radiographic evaluation of tracheal collapse in dogs: 62 cases (2001-2006), J Am Vet Med Assoc 230(12):1870-1876, 2007.
127. Marolf A, Blaik M, Specht A: A retrospective study of the relationship between tracheal collapse and bronchiectasis in dogs, Vet Rad Ultrasound 48(3):199-203, 2007.
128. Eom K, Moon K, Seong Y, et al: Ultrasonographic evaluation of tracheal collapse in dogs, J Vet Sci 9(4):401-405, 2008.
129. Johnson LR, Pollard RE: Tracheal collapse and bronchomalacia in dogs: 58 cases (7/2001-1/2008), J Vet Intern Med 24(2):298-305, 2009.
130. McKiernan BC, Smith AR, Kissil M: Bacterial isolates from the lower trachea of clinically healthy dogs, J Am Anim Hosp Assoc 20:139-142, 1984.
131. Johnson LR, Fales WH: Clinical and microbiologic findings in dogs with bronchoscopically diagnosed tracheal collapse: 37 cases (1990-1995), J Am Vet Med Assoc 219(9):1247-1250, 2001.
132. Buback JL, Boothe HW, Hobson HP: Surgical treatment of tracheal collapse in dogs: 90 cases. J Am Vet Med Assoc 1996; 208:380-384.
133. Bauer NB, Schneider MA, Neiger R, et al: Liver disease in dogs with tracheal collapse, J Vet Intern Med 20(4):845-849, 2006.
134. Becker WM, Beal M, Stanley BJ, et al: Survival after surgery for tracheal collapse and the effect of intrathoracic collapse on survival, Vet Surg 41(4):501-506, 2012.
135. McGuire L, Winters C, Beal MW: Emergency tracheal stent placement for the relief of life-threatening airway obstruction in dogs with tracheal collapse, J Vet Emerg Crit Care 23(S1):S9, 2013.
136. Beal MW: Tracheal stent placement for the emergency management of tracheal collapse in dogs, Top Comp Anim Med 28(3):106-111, 2013.
137. Gellasch KL, Gomez TDC, McAnulty JF, et al: Use of intraluminal nitinol stents in the treatment of tracheal collapse in a dog, J Am Vet Med Assoc 221(12):1719-1723, 2002.
138. Radlinsky MG, Fossum TW, Walker MA, et al: Evaluation of the Palmaz stent in the trachea and mainstem bronchi of normal dogs, Vet Surg 26(2):99-107, 1997.
139. Sura PA, Krahwinkel DJ: Self-expanding nitinol stents for the treatment of tracheal collapse in dogs: 12 cases (2001-2004), J Am Vet Med Assoc 232(2):228-236, 2008.
140. Moritz A, Schneider M, Bauer N: Management of advanced tracheal collapse in dogs using intraluminal self-expanding biliary wallstents, J Vet Intern Med 18(1):31-42, 2004.
141. Sun F, Usón J, Ezquerra J, et al: Endotracheal stenting therapy in dogs with tracheal collapse, Vet J 175(2):186-193, 2008.
142. Mittleman E, Weisse C, Mehler SJ, et al: Fracture of an endoluminal nitinol stent used in the treatment of tracheal collapse in a dog, J Am Vet Med Assoc 225(8):1217-1221 2004.
143. Kim JY, Han HJ, Yun HY, et al: The safety and efficacy of a new self-expandable intratracheal nitinol stent for the tracheal collapse in dogs, J Vet Sci 9(1):91-93, 2008.
144. Durant AM, Sura P, Rohrbach B, et al: Use of nitinol stents for end-stage tracheal collapse in dogs, Vet Surg 41(7):807-817, 2012.
145. Clarke, DL, Tappin S, de Madron E, et al: Evaluation of a novel tracheal stent for the treatment of tracheal collapse in dogs. Accepted for research report presentation, ACVIM, June 2014.
146. Ouellet M, Dunn ME, Lussier B, et al: Noninvasive correction of a fractured endoluminal nitinol tracheal stent in a dog, J Am Anim Hosp Assoc 42(6):467-471, 2006.
147. Roach W, Krahwinkel DJ: Obstructive lesions and traumatic injuries of the canine and feline tracheas, Compendium 31(2):86-93, 2009.
148. Holt DE: Tracheal trauma. In King LG, editor: Textbook of respiratory disease in dogs and cats, St Louis, 2004, Saunders.
149. Mitchell SL, McCarthy R, Rudloff E, et al: Tracheal rupture associated with intubation in cats: 20 cases (1996-1998), J Am Vet Med Assoc 216(10):1592-1595, 2000.
150. Alderson B, Senior JM, Dugdale AHA: Tracheal necrosis following tracheal intubation in a dog, J Small Anim Pract 47(12):754-756, 2006.
151. Jordan CJ, Halfacree ZJ, Tivers MS: Airway injury associated with cervical bite wounds in dogs and cats: 56 cases, Vet Comp Ortho Trauma 26(2):89-93, 2013.
152. Culp WTN, Weisse C, Cole SG, et al: Intraluminal tracheal stenting for treatment of tracheal narrowing in three cats, Vet Surg 36(2):107-113, 2007.
153. White RN, Milner HR: Intrathoracic tracheal avulsion in three cats, J Amall Anim Pract. 36(8):343-347, 1995.
154. Blocker TL, Roberts BK: Acute tracheal obstruction associated with anticoagulant rodenticide intoxication in a dog, J Small Anim Pract 40(12):577-580, 1999.
155. Berry CR, Gallaway A, Thrall DE, et al: Thoracic radiographic features of anticoagulant rodenticide toxicity in fourteen dogs, Vet Rad Ultrasound 34:391-396, 1993.
156. Pink JJ: Intramural tracheal haematoma causing acute respiratory obstruction in a dog, J Small Anim Pract 47(3):161-164, 2006.
157. Tenwolde AC, Johnson LR, Hunt GB, et al: The role of bronchoscopy in foreign body removal in dogs and cats: 37 cases (2000-2008), J Vet Intern Med 24(5):1063-1068, 2010.
158. Goodnight ME, Scansen BA, Kidder AC, et al: Use of a unique method for removal of a foreign body from the trachea of a cat, J Am Vet Med Assoc 237(6):689-694, 2010.
159. Tivers MS, Moore AH: Tracheal foreign bodies in the cat and the use of fluoroscopy for removal: 12 cases, J Small Anim Pract 47(3):155-159, 2006.
160. Dvorak LD, Bay JD, Crouch DT, et al: Successful treatment of intratracheal cuterebrosis in two cats, J Am Anim Hosp Assoc 36(4):304-308, 2000.
161. Bordelon JT, Newcomb BT, Rochat MC: Surgical removal of a Cuterebra larva from the cervical trachea of a cat, J Am Anim Hosp Assoc 45(1):52-54, 2009.
162. Pratschke KM, Hughes JML, Guerin SR, et al: Foley catheter technique for removal of a tracheal foreign body in a cat, Vet Rec 144(7):181-182, 1999.
163. Malinowski C: Canine and feline nasal neoplasia, Clin Tech Small Anim Pract 21(2):89-94, 2006.
164. McEntee MC: Neoplasms of the nasal cavity. In King LG, editor: Textbook of respiratory disease in dogs and cats, St Louis, 2004, Saunders.
165. Little L, Patel R, Goldschmidt M: Nasal and nasopharyngeal lymphoma in cats: 50 cases (1989-2005), Vet Pathol 44(6):885-892, 2007.
166. Carlisle CH, Biery DN, Thrall DE: Tracheal and laryngeal tumors in the dog and cat: literature review and 13 additional patients, Vet Rad Ultrasound 32(5):229-235, 1991.
167. Saik JE, Toll SL, Diters RW, et al: Canine and feline laryngeal neoplasia: a 10-year survey, J Am Anim Hosp Assoc 22:359-365, 1986.
168. Muraro L, Aprea F, White RAS: Successful management of an arytenoid chondrosarcoma in a dog, J Small Anim Pract 54:33-35, 2013.
169. Witham AI, French AF, Hill KE: Extramedullary laryngeal plasmacytoma in a dog, New Zealand Vet J 60(1):61-64, 2012.
170. Hayes AM, Gregory SP, Murphy S, et al: Solitary extramedullary plasmacytoma of the canine larynx, J Small Anim Pract 48(5):288-291, 2007.
171. Rossi G, Magi GE, Tarantino C, et al: Tracheobronchial neuroendocrine carcinoma in a cat, J Comp Pathol 137(2-3):165-168, 2007.
172. O'Hara AJ, McConnell M, Wyatt K, et al: Laryngeal rhabdomyoma in a dog, Aust Vet J 79(12):817-821, 2001.
173. Brunnberg M, Cinquoncie S, Burger M, et al: Infiltrative laryngeal lipoma in a Yorkshire Terrier as cause of severe dyspnoea, Tierarztl Prax Ausg K Kleintiere Heimtiere 41(1):53-56, 2013.
174. Brown MR, Rogers KS: Primary tracheal tumors in dogs and cats, Compendium 25(11):854-860, 2003.

175. Drynan EA, Moles AD, Raisis AL: Anaesthetic and surgical management of an intra-tracheal mass in a cat, J Feline Med Surg 13(6):460-462, 2011.
176. Jelinek F, Vozkova D: Carcinoma of the trachea in a cat, J Comp Pathol 147(2-3):177-180, 2012.
177. Green ML, Smith J, Fineman L, et al: Diagnosis and treatment of tracheal basal cell carcinoma in a Maine Coon and long-term outcome, J Am Anim Hosp Assoc 48(4):273-277, 2012.
178. Bachmann M, Waldrop JE: Noncardiogenic pulmonary edema, Compendium 34(11):E1-E9, 2012.
179. Hughes D: Pulmonary edema. In Silverstein DC, Hopper KA, editors: Small animal critical care medicine, St Louis, 2009, Elsevier.
180. Boothe DM: Drugs affecting the respiratory system. In King LG, editor: Textbook of respiratory disease in dogs and cats, St Louis, 2004, Saunders.

CHAPTER 18
BRACHYCEPHALIC SYNDROME

Matthew S. Mellema, DVM PhD DACVECC • Guillaume L. Hoareau, DrVet, DACVECC

KEY POINTS

- The unique facial and tracheal conformations of brachycephalic dogs, when extreme, makes them prone to brachycephalic obstructive airway syndrome (BOAS).
- The main feature of BOAS is increased resistance to inspiratory flow. Although this is a chronic condition, patients might also be presented for acute decompensation.
- Management of upper airway obstructive crisis in patients suffering from BOAS is a common challenge for the critical care clinician.
- BOAS is associated with dysfunctions of other systems (e.g., pulmonary, cardiovascular, digestive, coagulation, immune) and should be regarded as a systemic disorder.
- Most of the systemic consequences of BOAS are similar to those of sleep apnea–hypopnea syndrome in humans.

Brachycephalic dogs (BD) are those belonging to a group of breeds characterized by "severe shortening of the muzzle, and therefore the underlying bones, and a more modest shortening and widening of the skull."[1] They are undoubtedly popular pets; the Bulldog and the Boxer are, respectively, the fifth and seventh most commonly registered breeds in the American Kennel Club canine registry. Because of their facial conformation, BD may suffer from disorders that represent a challenge for the intensive care clinician.

PATHOPHYSIOLOGY

As a result of their craniofacial and tracheal anatomy, BD often must overcome increased resistance to inspiratory (and to a lesser extent expiratory) air flow, especially when their brachycephalic features are accentuated. This is a multifactorial problem commonly referred to as brachycephalic obstructive airway syndrome (BOAS). Traditionally, BOAS has been characterized by narrowed nostrils (58% to 85% of BD[2,3]), an elongated and thickened soft palate (87% to 96%[2,3]), everted laryngeal saccules (55% to 58%[2,3]), and a hypoplastic trachea (46%[2-4]). Other anatomic structures may also contribute to the increased upper airway resistance to flow: Prominent nasopharyngeal turbinates have been reported,[5] and increased tongue base thickness may also be a significant contributor. In addition, one study reported that 53% of BD undergoing BOAS corrective surgery presented with laryngeal collapse,[6] which has been reported in patients as young as 4.5 months.[7] Finally, there are many reports of narrowed trachea compared with size-matched non-BD.[2,8] Of note, a single abstract described normalization of tracheal diameter in Bulldog puppies as they aged, suggesting that narrowing of tracheal lumen might improve over time in some young BD.[9]

In the authors' practice, not all brachycephalic breeds seem to be equally affected by BOAS. Bulldogs and French bulldogs are the breeds most often presented to critical care clinicians for BOAS or its systemic consequences. In one study, the Bulldog was the most common BD simultaneously affected by elongated soft palate (50% of BD), stenotic nares (39% of BD), everted saccules (56% of BD), hypoplastic trachea (54% of BD), and laryngeal collapse (40% of BD). Not surprisingly, the Bulldog has been used as a spontaneous model for human sleep apnea–hypopnea syndrome (SAHS).[10-13] SAHS is a common disorder in humans, affecting 2% to 4% of the middle-aged population.[14] It is characterized by repeat upper airway collapse during sleep. This can lead to edema, fibrosis, and ultimately weakness of the oropharyngeal inspiratory muscles, which are responsible for maintaining upper airway patency,[12,13] thus perpetuating further airway collapse during sleep. This progressive acquired oropharyngeal and laryngeal myopathy likely underlies the laryngeal collapse that is a common finding in BD,[6] sometimes at a young age.[7]

Patients suffering from SAHS are challenged by repeated hemoglobin desaturation episodes during their sleep. The number and severity of desaturation events are proportional to the severity of the disease itself. Sleep studies in a small group of BD confirmed nighttime desaturation in these dogs.[11] Five Bulldogs had pulse oximetry readings (SpO_2) below 90% during 32% of the time spent in rapid eye movement (REM) sleep, whereas no control dogs ever experience a drop in SpO_2 below 90%. Similarly, mean REM sleep SpO_2 values were significantly lower in Bulldogs (78 +/− 5%) than in control non-BD (95 +/− 2%).

The SAHS is associated with numerous systemic complications in humans (e.g., arrhythmia, thrombosis, systemic inflammation).[15-18] Although most of the literature regarding BD revolves around the upper airway, it might be prudent for veterinarians to begin to consider the BOAS as a systemic disorder.

RESPIRATORY CONSEQUENCES

Consequences of Chronic Upper Airway Obstruction

The consequences of chronic upper airway obstruction on the lower airways and pulmonary parenchyma are largely unknown.[19,20] It has been hypothesized that in order to overcome increased upper airway resistance, animals with BOAS generate greater subatmospheric pleural pressures on inspiration, thus creating more strain on intrathoracic tissues (humans with SAHS may generate pleural pressures as low as −65 mm Hg[21]).[6,22,23] BD have been shown to have significantly lower expiratory time–to–inspiratory time ratios, peak inspiratory flows, and higher peak expiratory flows when compared with a historical control group, further supporting the presence of more negative pleural pressures on inspiration.[24] Bronchial collapse has been reported in a cohort of BD, and the severity of the collapse was correlated with the presence of laryngeal collapse.[25] It was hypothesized that the repeated increases in subatmospheric pleural pressure may lead to degenerative weakening of the lower airways. However, an inflammatory rather than purely mechanical process may be responsible for airway weakening in this setting. Repetitive airway obstruction in an anesthetized dog model has been shown to result in pulmonary edema in this setting.[26] Moreover, markers of airway inflammation are increased in human sleep apnea patients.[27,28]

A group of BD, compared with non-BD controls, has been shown to have lower arterial partial pressures in oxygen (PaO_2) with a normal alveolar-to-arterial gradient and higher arterial partial pressures of carbon dioxide ($PaCO_2$).[23] BD may undergo a phenomenon called "habituation" by which they reset their chemoreceptor thresholds and tolerate lower PaO_2 and higher $PaCO_2$ without sensing the drive for increasing minute ventilation. Age may also play an important role in pulmonary function in BD because older dogs had lower PaO_2 than young and control dogs.[23] Like many others, this study could not control for the BOAS severity. Finally, measurements were taken in awake dogs; sleep values would be of great interest as well because they might explain occurrence of systemic complications of chronic upper airway obstruction.

In the intensive care setting, BD have been shown to be more likely to require mechanical ventilation than non-BD among dogs that were presented to an academic veterinary teaching hospital.[29] Aspiration pneumonia was the leading cause of respiratory failure in those same patients. It is proposed that chronic upper airway obstruction and greater subatmospheric pleural pressures may lead to disorders of the esophagus and stomach, making these patients more prone to regurgitation or vomiting, which are known risk factors for aspiration pneumonia. Also, BD with BOAS may prove challenging at the time of weaning from mechanical ventilation. Prolonged anesthesia promotes oropharyngeal inspiratory muscle weakness; oral, pharyngeal, and laryngeal edema are commonly seen in patients with prolonged transoral endotracheal intubation, further creating resistance to airflow. These complications place the brachycephalic patient at risk for airway obstruction on extubation. Temporary tracheotomy before weaning BD from mechanical ventilation might prove useful in select patients in order to bypass the oropharyngeal and laryngeal area if these appear inflamed. Of importance, outcomes for BD undergoing mechanical ventilation are similar to that of non-BD.[29,30]

Management of Upper Airway Obstructive Crises in BD

Upper airway obstructive crises are not uncommon in BD. Such acute deteriorations manifest as acute onset or progressive worsening of respiratory distress because of partial or complete upper airway occlusion. It can be a direct complication of BOAS or may also follow an anesthetic episode in which upper airway musculature is further weakened. Obstruction might be further worsened in this setting because of tissue swelling secondary to oropharyngeal surgery or prolonged intubation.

The management of upper airway disease is described elsewhere in this book (see Chapter 17). Patients should receive supplemental oxygen as soon as possible and remain in a cool and quiet environment. A recent retrospective study[31] evaluated the use of nasotracheal tube (NTT) placement in dogs after BOAS surgical correction. Humidified oxygen was delivered as needed via an NTT placed before recovery from anesthesia. Although deemed safe, NTT had to be removed in four dogs because it was perceived to be associated with vomiting, regurgitation, or coughing. In the postoperative period, five dogs without NTT experienced respiratory distress, whereas no dog with a NTT displayed similar signs. Fully gas-conditioned oxygen can also be delivered via a commercially available device (Precision-Flow, Vapotherm, Inc.), which provides high-flow (up to 40 L/min), humidified, and warmed supplemental oxygen. The inspired fraction of oxygen can also be precisely controlled with this device. High flow allows for creation of an "air-skeleton," maintaining airway patency in patients prone to upper airway collapse. To date, no study has critically evaluated the clinical utility of this device in BD in the postoperative period. Some patients might require orotracheal intubation or, rarely, emergent tracheotomy.

Sedation is an important step in the management of these patients because it decreases inspiratory efforts and reduces turbulent airflow. General anesthesia might be needed in some cases, and such patients should then be intubated.

Also, hyperthermia should be prevented because it creates a drive for panting that can promote airway collapse in some patients. The authors recommend active cooling for BD experiencing respiratory distress refractory to medical management if their temperature exceeds 103° F. Active warming of hypothermic brachycephalic patients (e.g., after anesthesia) should be discontinued once their temperature reaches 99° F.

Obese patients will benefit from weight loss. Some will also benefit from surgical therapy, which usually involves one or more of the following: wedge rhinoplasty, staphylectomy (soft palate resection), or ventriculectomy (sacculectomy). The role of tracheotomy tubes after BOAS surgical correction remains unclear. In the authors' practice, these are usually performed after long-term mechanical ventilation or if severe tissue swelling is observed after surgery. Favorable response to surgical therapy has been demonstrated,[2] but results are somewhat inconsistent and challenging to predict. Steroids can be used at antiinflammatory doses postoperatively, but no controlled study has evaluated their effects on outcome. Permanent tracheostomy is considered a surgical option of last resort because of the potential for severe complications such as recurrent lower airway infections. In some cases, the long-term prognosis remains poor, especially if laryngeal collapse is present.

Gastrointestinal Consequences

Upper digestive tract disorders have been recognized in BD. An endoscopy study[3] evaluated the esophagus and stomach of BD that were presented for upper airway disorders. Ninety-seven percent of the subjects had abnormalities in their esophagus (e.g., esophagitis, hiatal hernia, gastroesophageal reflux), stomach (e.g., pyloric hyperplasia, atresia, gastritis, duodenogastric reflux), or duodenum (duodenitis). Even patients without clinical evidence of upper gastrointestinal tract disorders had endoscopic abnormalities. Some with normal endoscopic examinations had histologic evidence of gastric or duodenal inflammation. There was an association between the severity of the respiratory signs and the upper digestive tract disorders' severity in the French bulldog. Another study by the same group[32] showed a favorable response of both the digestive and respiratory signs when medical therapy for the digestive problems was combined with BOAS corrective surgery.

Systemic Consequences

In humans, the SAHS is considered a systemic disease and not just a disease of the upper airway, and reports of systemic inflammation associated with SAHS are numerous and often reversible with therapy.[33,34] The most widely used therapeutic tool is the continuous positive airway pressure (CPAP) mask. With this device the patient wears a tightly fitted facial mask or nasal pillows, which allow for continuous air insufflation to promote upper airway patency. CPAP therapy is associated with improvement in the chronic inflammatory response and many other systemic markers of disease in SAHS.[35,36] There is a paucity of literature regarding the effect of chronic upper airway obstruction and BOAS on BD. Increased circulatory proinflammatory cytokines levels have been reported in a group of BD.[37] However, the chronic inflammatory state of SAHS in humans is not consistently characterized by increased inflammatory markers in a single "spot" blood sample, but rather by disruption and alteration of the normal diurnal variation in cytokine levels. In particular, an abnormal diurnal peak in TNF-α has been described and is felt to contribute to daytime somnolence.[16]

SUMMARY

BD are a popular group of dogs with unique conformational characteristics that when extreme make them prone to disorders that can represent a challenge for the critical care clinician. Further studies are required in order to better understand, diagnose, and treat BOAS.

REFERENCES

1. Bannasch D, Young A, Myers J, et al: Localization of canine brachycephaly using an across breed mapping approach, PLoS One 5:e9632, 2010.
2. Riecks TW, Birchard SJ, Stephens JA: Surgical correction of brachycephalic syndrome in dogs: 62 cases (1991-2004), J Am Vet Med Assoc 230:1324-1328, 2007.
3. Poncet CM, Dupre GP, Freiche VG, et al: Prevalence of gastrointestinal tract lesions in 73 brachycephalic dogs with upper respiratory syndrome, J Small Anim Pract 46:273-279, 2005.
4. Harvey CE, Fink EA: Tracheal diameter: analysis of radiographic measurements in brachycephalic and nonbrachycephalic dogs, J Am Anim Hosp Assoc 18:570-576, 1982.
5. Ginn JA, Kumar MS, McKiernan BC, et al: Nasopharyngeal turbinates in brachycephalic dogs and cats, J Am Anim Hosp Assoc 44:243-249, 2008.
6. Torrez CV, Hunt GB: Results of surgical correction of abnormalities associated with brachycephalic airway obstruction syndrome in dogs in Australia, J Small Anim Pract 47:150-154, 2006.
7. Pink JJ, Doyle RS, Hughes JML, et al: Laryngeal collapse in seven brachycephalic puppies, J Small Anim Pract 47:131-135, 2006.
8. Harvey CE: Inherited and congenital airway conditions, J Small Anim Pract 30:184-187, 1989.
9. Clarke DL, Otto MC: Resolution of severe hypoplastic trachea in six english bulldog puppies with bronchopneumonia, following growth to maturity. An abstract at a conference: International Veterinary Emergency & Critical Care Symposium, 2008; Phoenix, AZ.
10. Amis TC, Kurpershoek C: Pattern of breathing in brachycephalic dogs, Am J Vet Res 47:2200-2204, 1986.
11. Hendricks JC, Kline LR, Kovalski RJ, et al: The English bulldog: a natural model of sleep-disordered breathing, J App Physiol 63:1344-1350, 1987.
12. Petrof BJ, Pack AI, Kelly AM, et al: Pharyngeal myopathy of loaded upper airway in dogs with sleep apnea, J App Physiol 76:1746-1752, 1994.
13. Schotland HM, Insko EK, Panckeri KA, et al: Quantitative magnetic resonance imaging of upper airways musculature in an animal model of sleep apnea, J App Physiol 81:1339-1346, 1996.
14. Young T, Palta M, Dempsey J, et al: The occurrence of sleep-disordered breathing among middle-aged adults, N Engl J Med 1993;328:1230-1235, 1993.
15. Bounhoure JP, Galinier M, Didier A, et al: [Sleep apnea syndromes and cardiovascular disease], Bull Acad Natl Med 189:445-459; discussion 460-444, 2005.
16. Entzian P, Linnemann K, Schlaak M, et al: Obstructive sleep apnea syndrome and circadian rhythms of hormones and cytokines, Am J Respir Crit Care Med 153:1080-1086, 1996.
17. Carpagnano GE, Kharitonov SA, Resta O, et al: Increased 8-isoprostane and interleukin-6 in breath condensate of obstructive sleep apnea patients, Chest 122:1162-1167, 2002.
18. Hatipoglu U, Rubinstein I: Inflammation and obstructive sleep apnea syndrome pathogenesis: a working hypothesis, Respiration 70:665-671, 2003.
19. Ogura JH, Nelson JR, Suemitsu M, et al: Relationship between pulmonary resistance and changes in arterial blood gas tension in dogs with nasal obstruction, and partial laryngeal obstruction, Ann Otol Rhinol Laryngol 82:668-683, 1973.
20. Ogura JH: Effect of upper airway obstruction on the lower airway and cardiovascular system, Ann Otol Rhinol Laryngol 84:49, 1975.
21. Malone S, Liu PP, Holloway R, et al: Obstructive sleep apnoea in patients with dilated cardiomyopathy: effects of continuous positive airway pressure, Lancet 338:1480-1484, 1991.
22. Hoareau GL, Mellema MS, Silverstein DC: Indication, management, and outcome of brachycephalic dogs requiring mechanical ventilation, J Vet Emerg Crit Care 21(3): 226-235, 2011.
23. Hoareau GL, Jourdan G, Mellema M, et al: Evaluation of arterial blood gases and arterial blood pressures in brachycephalic dogs, J Vet Intern Med 26(4): 897-904, 2012.
24. Bernaerts F, Talavera J, Leemans J, et al: Description of original endoscopic findings and respiratory functional assessment using barometric whole-body plethysmography in dogs suffering from brachycephalic airway obstruction syndrome, Vet J 183(1):95-102, 2010.
25. De Lorenzi D, Bertoncello D, Drigo M: Bronchial abnormalities found in a consecutive series of 40 brachycephalic dogs, J Am Vet Med Assoc 235:835-840, 2009.
26. Fletcher EC, Proctor M, Yu J, et al: Pulmonary edema develops after recurrent obstructive apneas, Am J Respir Crit Care Med 160:1688-1696, 1999.
27. Aihara K, Oga T, Harada Y, et al: Comparison of biomarkers of subclinical lung injury in obstructive sleep apnea, Respir Med 105:939-945, 2011.
28. Aihara K, Oga T, Chihara Y, et al: Analysis of systemic and airway inflammation in obstructive sleep apnea, Sleep Breath 17:597-604, 2013.
29. Hoareau GL, Mellema MS, Silverstein DC: Indication, management, and outcome of brachycephalic dogs requiring mechanical ventilation, J Vet Emerg Crit Care (San Antonio) 21:226-235, 2011.
30. Hopper K, Haskins SC, Kass PH, et al: Indications, management, and outcome of long-term positive-pressure ventilation in dogs and cats: 148 cases (1990-2001), J Am Vet Med Assoc 230:64-75, 2007.
31. Senn D, Sigrist N, Forterre F, et al: Retrospective evaluation of postoperative nasotracheal tubes for oxygen supplementation in dogs following surgery for brachycephalic syndrome: 36 cases (2003-2007), J Vet Emerg Crit Care (San Antonio) 21:261-267, 2011.
32. Poncet CM, Dupre GP, Freiche VG, et al: Long-term results of upper respiratory syndrome surgery and gastrointestinal tract medical treatment in 51 brachycephalic dogs, J Small Anim Pract 47:137-142, 2006.
33. Akpinar ME, Yigit O, Altundag A, et al: Salivary and serum myeloperoxidase in obstructive sleep apnea, J Otolaryngol Head Neck Surg 41:215-221, 2012.
34. Aihara K, Oga T, Chihara Y, et al: Analysis of systemic and airway inflammation in obstructive sleep apnea, Sleep Breath 17(2):597-604, 2013.
35. Nural S, Gunay E, Halici B, et al: Inflammatory processes and effects of continuous positive airway pressure (CPAP) in overlap syndrome, Inflammation 36(1):66-74, 2013.
36. Guo Y, Pan L, Ren D, et al: Impact of continuous positive airway pressure on C-reactive protein in patients with obstructive sleep apnea: a meta-analysis, Sleep Breath 17(2):495-503, 2013.
37. Rancan L, Romussi S, Garcia P, et al: Assessment of circulating concentrations of proinflammatory and anti-inflammatory cytokines and nitric oxide in dogs with brachycephalic airway obstruction syndrome, Am J Vet Res 74:155-160, 2013.

CHAPTER 19
TRACHEAL TRAUMA

David Holt, BVSc, DACVS

KEY POINTS

- Cervical tracheal injury can result from bite wounds or overinflation of the endotracheal tube cuff.
- Cervical tracheal injury often results in subcutaneous emphysema.
- Tracheal tears caused by bite wounds or endotracheal tube cuff damage can often be managed conservatively but may require surgical exploration and repair.
- Intrathoracic tracheal tears can occur from blunt trauma and require careful anesthesia and intrathoracic surgical tracheal reconstruction.
- Tracheal strictures secondary to trauma or neoplasia can be treated with balloon dilation and stenting.

The trachea extends from the cricoid cartilage to the carina, dorsal to the heart base. The trachea, bronchi, and smaller airways conduct air to and from the lungs during respiration. The trachea is comprised of many C-shaped hyaline cartilages connected dorsally by the tracheal muscle and dorsal membrane. The cartilages are connected to each other by fibroelastic annular ligaments and lined with a ciliated mucosa and a submucosa containing elastic fibers, fat cells, and tubular seromucinous glands. Disruption of the trachea from external or iatrogenic trauma results in air leakage into the subcutaneous tissues and mediastinum as well as respiratory compromise of varying severity. Crushing injuries can result in subsequent stenosis. An accurate diagnosis can often be made based on the findings of physical examination and plain radiographs, but advanced imaging (e.g., computed tomography [CT], tracheoscopy) may be required.

Causes

Tracheal trauma can occur from projectile injuries, bite wounds, endotracheal tube damage, or blunt trauma. Projectiles can directly penetrate the trachea and damage tracheal cartilages and other structures adjacent to the perforation. The amount of damage depends on the size and mass of the projectile, its velocity, and the amount of kinetic energy transferred to the tissues. Bite wounds generate compressive and shearing forces that can easily damage the trachea. The teeth of the attacking animal may fracture or crush the tracheal cartilages, penetrate the interannular tracheal ligaments or cartilages, or completely transect the trachea. Blunt trauma can also result in segmental tracheal collapse. In cats specifically, intrathoracic tracheal disruption has been associated with blunt trauma.[1-8] The use of endotracheal tubes with low-volume, high-pressure cuffs has been linked with tearing of the dorsal tracheal membrane. This has been reported in cats and most likely results from overinflation of the cuff.

PATHOPHYSIOLOGY

Complete transection or avulsion of the cervical trachea results in severe respiratory compromise and often death. Crushing and fracture of cervical tracheal cartilages result in segmental tracheal collapse on inspiration. This causes variable degrees of inspiratory dyspnea and hypoxemia. Perforation of the cervical trachea also results in subcutaneous emphysema. Mild subcutaneous emphysema does not typically impair respiration. However, as air accumulates under the skin, cats in particular can become dyspneic and show signs of significant respiratory compromise. Air from the tracheal perforation can track into the cranial mediastinum and even retroperitoneal space, both of which communicate with the fascial planes of the cervical trachea. Pneumomediastinum rarely causes physiologic compromise unless the mediastinum ruptures, resulting in a pneumothorax.

Intrathoracic tracheal rupture in cats has been associated with blunt trauma episodes such as automobile accidents. It is theorized that hyperextension of the neck occurs and, because the carina is fixed, the trachea ruptures just cranial to this point as it is violently stretched.[1,9] Some of these injuries (and other concurrent injuries) are fatal. However, in some cats, the peritracheal adventitia and mediastinum maintain the continuity of the intrathoracic airway, allowing the animal to breathe. Initially, many cats do not have marked dyspnea.[1] It is speculated that dyspnea develops several days after the trauma because of stenosis or displacement of the proximal and distal tracheal segments.[9]

Tracheal tears secondary to intubation occur because of overinflation of the endotracheal tube cuff.[10] Other mechanisms of injury, including improper tube placement, injury from the use of a stylet, or failure to deflate the cuff before repositioning or removing the tube, have been suggested as additional causes for iatrogenic tracheal rupture. However, only overinflation of the cuff produced tracheal rupture in cadavers that was similar to what is seen in clinical cases.[10] Low-volume, high-pressure cuffs may be more likely to cause rupture than high-volume, low-pressure cuffs. In the majority of clinical cases reported, the tracheal rupture occurred after dental procedures.[10-12] Endotracheal tube cuffs may have been inflated excessively in these cases to prevent fluid or debris from leaking around the tube, or the animals may have been turned while the endotracheal tube was still connected to the anesthesia circuit.

Clinical Signs

Dogs and cats with tracheal perforation from a bite wound or projectile injury often present with subcutaneous emphysema. Subcutaneous emphysema is usually present in animals with relatively intact skin, thus creating the potential space for air accumulation. Occasionally the skin and soft tissue loss surrounding the tracheal perforation is large enough that air leaks directly from the perforation into the atmosphere and does not accumulate subcutaneously. Clinical signs of hypovolemia and shock are often associated with blood loss from the adjacent carotid arteries or jugular veins damaged by either a projectile or bite wounds, although coexisting injuries to distant areas of the body are also possible. Depending on the degree of bite wound trauma, coexisting injuries, and time from injury to presentation, animals may present with clinical signs associated with systemic inflammation and sepsis (see Chapters 6 and 91).

Animals with tracheal collapse or stenosis secondary to trauma can develop dyspnea over days to weeks.[7,13,14] The owner may or may not be aware of a history of trauma. Stridor on inspiration, indicative of upper airway obstruction, is often audible. Affected animals may not tolerate exertion and can become cyanotic when stressed.[7]

Cats with intrathoracic tracheal rupture can present with a known history of trauma (fall, motor vehicle accident), or return home after a variable period of absence. Clinical signs of shock, as well as neurologic and musculoskeletal injury, are often present after severe trauma and may mask signs of tracheal trauma. In animals with an uncertain history, finding avulsed or abraded nails or skin abrasions indicates possible trauma. Respiratory signs, including increased respiratory effort, dyspnea, exercise intolerance, open-mouthed breathing with exertion, and cyanosis, can be present immediately[2] or develop days to weeks after the trauma.[1] Other respiratory injuries, including rib fractures, pneumothorax, and pulmonary contusions, can also occur.[1]

Cats with tracheal rupture secondary to intubation invariably have moderate to marked subcutaneous emphysema that is usually apparent either during or immediately after the anesthetic episode. Other intermittent clinical signs include dyspnea, anorexia, coughing, and respiratory stridor.[10,11]

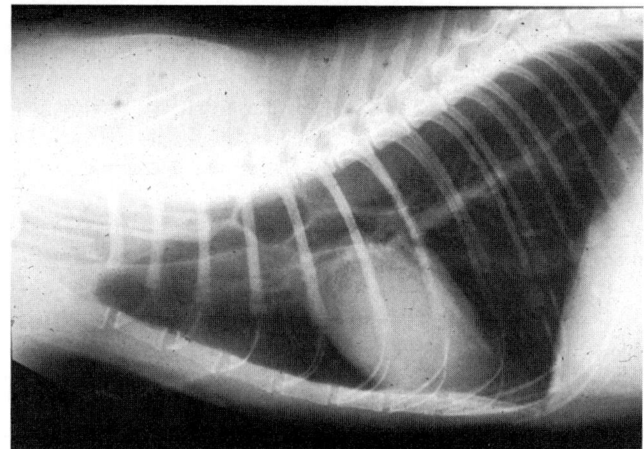

FIGURE 19-1 Avulsion of the intrathoracic portion of the trachea in a cat. *(Courtesy Dr. Daniel Brockman, Royal Veterinary College, London.)*

Differential Diagnosis and Diagnostic Testing

In addition to tracheal trauma, subcutaneous emphysema that develops after an anesthetic procedure can also be caused by barotrauma[9] that occurs when the machine pop-off valve is closed and markedly elevated intratracheal airway pressures develop in the anesthetized animal. Overinflation of the lungs causes marginal alveoli to rupture; air escapes through the base of marginal alveoli into perivascular or peribronchial connective tissue sheaths and migrates into the mediastinum and cervical tissue planes (and possibly the pleural space as well).[15] Other causes of subcutaneous emphysema include perforation of the larynx or esophagus, severe cervical bite wounds, and subcutaneous infections with gas-producing organisms. Cervical subcutaneous emphysema and dyspnea have also been reported in association with tracheoesophageal fistulas.[16]

The inspiratory stridor heard in some animals with tracheal stenosis secondary to trauma could also be associated with laryngeal diseases, including paralysis, trauma, or neoplasia; pharyngeal diseases, including injury, foreign body, or neoplasia; insect inhalation and perhaps other allergic reactions; and foreign body obstruction of the trachea or bronchi.

Animals with intrathoracic tracheal rupture usually present dyspneic with little stridor and no subcutaneous emphysema. Similar clinical signs might be seen in animals with airway foreign bodies[17]; laryngeal, tracheal, or bronchial tumors[18]; eosinophilic tracheal granuloma[19]; parasitic infestation of the trachea[20,21]; anticoagulant rodenticide intoxication[22]; tracheal polyps[23]; and tracheal cuterebriasis.[24] Conditions that might cause similar clinical signs include intrathoracic tracheal compression by esophageal foreign bodies or mediastinal tumors, abscesses, or hematomas; pneumothorax; pleural effusion; and diaphragmatic herniation.

In many cases, the diagnosis of tracheal damage is suspected from the history and physical examination findings. The tests used to confirm the diagnosis of tracheal trauma are often determined by the severity of the animal's respiratory distress. Plain lateral radiographs of the thorax and neck often provide a clear indication of tracheal disruption, particularly in cats with intrathoracic tracheal avulsion (Figure 19-1). In these animals either the interruption of the trachea or the bulging peritracheal or mediastinal tissues surrounding the rupture are clearly visible. However, in other cases the subcutaneous emphysema and pneumomediastinum associated with the tracheal damage make identifying the specific area of tracheal rupture extremely difficult. Fluoroscopy in the conscious animal may be useful to delineate areas of dynamic tracheal collapse. Recently, computerized tomography (CT) has been used to definitely diagnose laryngeal or tracheal diseases in dyspneic dogs. The majority of dogs were imaged without sedation or anesthesia, and the imaging accurately identified the cause of upper airway obstruction in all cases.[25]

Pharyngoscopy, laryngoscopy, esophagoscopy, and tracheobronchoscopy may be necessary to confirm a diagnosis of tracheal rupture and rule out other possible causes of the clinical signs. The larynx and laryngeal function must be rapidly inspected before intubation of dyspneic animals. Once the animal is intubated and breathing spontaneously, a gentle, thorough examination of the pharynx is performed, initially using a laryngoscope blade with a bright light source. The area dorsal to the soft palate can be inspected using either a dental mirror and a small spay hook to retract the palate rostrally or a flexible fiberoptic endoscope. Esophagoscopy is performed if a perforation of the esophagus is the suspected source of pneumomediastinum or an esophageal foreign body is suspected as a cause of tracheal compression.

In medium and large breed dogs, the trachea can be examined by passing an endoscope through the endotracheal tube. In small breed dogs and cats, the animal must be briefly extubated to allow passage of a small bronchoscope or cystoscope. Tracheal oxygen insufflation or high-frequency jet ventilation using a large-bore catheter can be used to prevent hypoxemia during extubation, although close monitoring for leakage of the supplemental oxygen is advised. Anesthesia must be maintained with injectable agents in these animals. The endoscope should be passed down the trachea carefully to avoid worsening a tracheal tear or creating or worsening a pneumothorax. Positive contrast tracheography has been performed during tracheoscopy to radiographically delineate a tracheal stricture.[7,26] More advanced imaging modalities, including computed tomography and magnetic resonance imaging, are now available in many hospitals to allow detailed imaging of the trachea and bronchi.

Treatment

Animals that are extremely dyspneic require general anesthesia and endotracheal intubation. The endotracheal tube should be substantially smaller than the tracheal lumen and extreme caution should be used during intubation if tracheal disruption is suspected. Passage of a large endotracheal tube in animals with cervical or cranial thoracic tracheal damage could cause complete disruption and separation of the tracheal ends, leaving the animal with no means of ventilating. The larynx and pharynx should be quickly inspected at the time of intubation for evidence of trauma, perforation, neoplasia, or laryngeal paralysis and the tube passed only into the larynx and proximal trachea. Ideally the plane of anesthesia should be light enough for the animal to maintain spontaneous respiration. Positive pressure ventilation should be avoided if possible, but if the animal is not spontaneously breathing, assisted breaths should be given with minimal pressure to provide adequate ventilation. In cats with complete intrathoracic tracheal disruption, positive pressure ventilation can "blow out" the tenuous membrane of mediastinum that has been maintaining airway continuity; thus effective ventilation of the lungs ceases and a rapidly worsening tension pneumothorax develops. Respiratory failure and death ensue.

High-frequency jet ventilation has been used to manage two cases of segmental tracheal stenosis,[6] but this technology is not widely available. If possible, animals with tracheal disruption confirmed before anesthesia should have the ventral cervical area and right thoracic wall clipped before induction of anesthesia. As soon as the animal is intubated, the anesthetist and surgeon should watch carefully for thoracic wall movement and spontaneous respiration. If the animal breathes spontaneously and pulse oximetry or arterial blood gas analysis indicates effective blood oxygenation, the tracheal tear can be approached as a more "elective" procedure. If, however, the animal is not spontaneously ventilating and the thoracic wall does not move with gentle positive pressure ventilation (peak inspiratory pressure ≤10 cm H_2O), the correct position of the endotracheal tube in the larynx should be quickly checked. If the endotracheal tube is correctly placed in the larynx but the animal is unable to ventilate effectively, an endotracheal tube must be surgically placed distal to the tracheal tear immediately.

If a confirmed cervical tear is present, the trachea is approached by a ventral midline cervical incision. In animals with intrathoracic tracheal avulsion, the trachea is approached via a right lateral third or fourth intercostal space thoracotomy. The distal end of the trachea is located; this is often difficult in patients with intrathoracic tears because the mediastinum obscures the trachea. A sterile endotracheal tube is placed in the distal trachea, connected to the anesthetic machine, and ventilation is reestablished.

Cervical tracheal tears are most often associated with bite wounds, penetrating missile injuries, or endotracheal tube cuff overinflation. In animals with bite wounds and penetrating missile injury, tracheal repair is combined with debridement, lavage, culture, and repair of the associated soft tissue injuries. During surgical exploration, vital cervical structures, including the recurrent laryngeal nerves, carotid arteries, and vagosympathetic trunks, must be identified and preserved. The trachea is carefully examined along its length. In animals with small tracheal lacerations, the endotracheal tube is passed beyond the damaged segment under direct surgical visualization and guidance. Small lacerations are debrided back to healthy, bleeding tissue and closed using 5/0 to 3/0 monofilament absorbable suture, depending on the animal's size.

If the animal has extensive cervical tracheal injury, a sterile endotracheal tube is placed into the trachea via a tracheostomy made at the (expected) distal site of tracheal resection. The tube is connected to the anesthetic machine using sterile tubing. The orally placed endotracheal tube is left in place for use during closure. The devitalized segment of trachea is resected, leaving the proximal and distal ends for anastomosis. Twenty percent of the trachea can be resected in a young dog and 25% to 50% can be resected in a mature dog. In medium and large breed dogs, a split cartilage technique should be used for anastomosis. The tracheal cartilage at the proximal and distal ends of the anastomosis is split circumferentially using a number 11 scalpel blade. The two remaining tracheal cartilage halves are apposed by preplacing 8 to 12 sutures of 4/0 to 3/0 monofilament absorbable material around the opposite cartilage halves and through the dorsal tracheal membrane on either side of the anastomosis. Experimentally, the split cartilage anastomosis technique results in better alignment and apposition of the tracheal ends and less long-term luminal stenosis than the annular ligament and cartilage technique.[27] However, in smaller dogs and cats the tracheal cartilages may not be wide enough to be split without fragmentation. In these animals, the trachea is resected by incising the annular ligament between the cartilage rings. Sutures are preplaced around the proximal and distal cartilage rings. The orally placed endotracheal tube is advanced across the anastomosis site if it is long enough, and the tracheostomy tube removed. If the orally placed tube is not long enough, the tracheostomy tube remains in place while the dorsal anastomosis sutures are tied. It is then removed and the ventral sutures are rapidly tied, reestablishing airway continuity and allowing effective ventilation through the orally placed endotracheal tube.

In cats with tracheal tears secondary to intubation, both surgical and conservative management strategies have been reported.[10-12] In one report, all cats (n = 7) treated conservatively with cage rest survived; clinical signs took 2 days to 5 weeks to resolve.[10] In the same report, 6 of the 9 cats treated surgically also survived.[10] Attempted surgical repairs of tears extending to the carina were unsuccessful. In a second report, 15 cats with moderate dyspnea were successfully treated with medical management,[11] including cage rest in all cats and supplemental oxygen (n = 3), sedatives (n = 2), and respiratory monitoring (n = 6) in some cats. Cats with severe respiratory distress, cyanosis unresponsive to oxygen supplementation, and worsening subcutaneous emphysema were treated surgically.[11] Surgical treatment was successful in 3 of 4 cats. All ruptures treated surgically in the second report were identified at the thoracic inlet on the dorsolateral aspect of the trachea at the junction of the tracheal rings and the trachealis muscle.[11] Definitive indications for surgical management of tracheal tears secondary to intubation have not been delineated. From these reports, however, surgery should be considered in animals with severe dyspnea or worsening dyspnea despite conservative management. The possibility of clinically significant tracheal stricture formation with conservative management is not known but seems minimal from the information available.[10,11]

Surgical repair of cervical tracheal tears is performed via a ventral midline cervical incision. Splitting the first several sternebrae may also be required for access.[10,11] Tears associated with intubation invariably involve the trachealis muscle. The trachea should be exposed and rotated so that the dorsal tracheal membrane is visible. The tissues are sutured using 5/0 or 4/0 monofilament absorbable suture.

Intrathoracic tracheal disruptions are approached via a right lateral thoracotomy. The third or fourth intercostal space is normally used; for more exposure, the third or fourth rib can be resected. Ideally, the animal should breathe spontaneously until the pleural space is opened, then positive pressure breaths should be provided using the minimum amount of positive pressure needed to maintain effective ventilation (peak inspiratory pressures ≤10 cm H_2O). The trachea lies dorsal to the cranial vena cava in the mediastinum. It may not be visible because of trauma-associated scarring and hemorrhage. Sterile endotracheal tubes of several appropriate sizes should be available on the surgery table before dissecting the mediastinum.

As soon the mediastinum is opened, the distal trachea must be located and intubated as quickly as possible. The thoracic endotracheal tube is connected to the anesthetic machine with sterile hoses. The ends of the trachea are debrided and apposed using single interrupted 4/0 or 5/0 monofilament absorbable sutures. The sutures should be preplaced and the medial sutures tied first. The thoracic endotracheal tube is removed and the lateral sutures rapidly tied. The orally placed endotracheal tube is used to assist ventilation. A chest tube is placed and the thoracotomy closed in a routine manner.

Tracheal strictures have been reported in the cervical,[2] thoracic inlet,[12] and intrathoracic[6,7,26,28,29] sections of the trachea. Stricture resection has been described; the approaches and anastomosis techniques are similar to those described previously for tracheal tears and avulsions. Tracheal resection and anastomosis is also described to treat traumatic tracheal collapse.[14] The length of the stenotic area should be carefully considered when planning a resection. As mentioned earlier, puppies and adult dogs can tolerate resection of 20% to 25% and 25% to 50% of the trachea, respectively.[30,31]

Successful balloon dilation of a tracheal stricture involving the carina of a cat has been described.[7] The balloon dilation catheter was passed through the lumen of the endotracheal tube and dilation was accomplished under direct visualization via a thoracotomy. Balloon dilation and stenting has also been performed using fluoroscopic or endoscopic guidance.[32] This should only be performed by clinicians with interventional radiology experience.

Outcome and Prognosis

The success of treating tracheal trauma depends largely on appropriate emergency and anesthetic case management. The majority of cases in which the trachea is successfully repaired recover well and breathe normally. Stenosis after resection and anastomosis is an infrequent complication.[13] The results of conservative versus surgical management of tracheal tears caused by overinflation of the endotracheal tube cuff were discussed earlier. Such injuries are far better prevented than treated. The use of an appropriately sized endotracheal tube; high-volume, low-pressure cuffs; and the minimum volume of air in the cuff necessary to create an airtight seal (0 to 3 ml in cats)[10] should prevent this iatrogenic injury. Cuff pressures can be readily measured using a pressure manometer connected to the endotracheal tube cuff (e.g., Posey Cufflator, Posey Co., Arcadia, CA). Pressures should be kept within 20 to 30 mm Hg to provide a sufficient seal without compromising tracheal mucosal perfusion.

REFERENCES

1. Lawrence DT, Lang J, Culvenor J, et al: Intrathoracic tracheal rupture, J Feline Med Surg 1:43, 1999.
2. White RN, Milner HR: Intrathoracic tracheal avulsion in three cats, J Small Anim Pract 36:343, 1995.
3. Jorger VK, Fluckiger M, Geret U: Ruptur der trachea bei drei katzen, Berl Munch Tierartzl Wschr 101:128, 1988.
4. Brouwer GJ, Burbidge HM, Jones DE: Tracheal rupture in a cat, J Small Anim Pract 25:71, 1984.
5. Kennedy RK: Traumatic tracheal separation with diverticuli in a cat, Vet Med Sm Anim Clin 71:1384, 1976.
6. Whitfield JB, Graves GM, Lappin MR, et al: Anesthetic and surgical management of intrathoracic segmental tracheal stenosis utilizing high-frequency jet ventilation, J Am Anim Hosp Assoc 25:443, 1989.
7. Berg J, Leveille CR, O'Callaghan MW: Treatment of posttraumatic carinal stenosis by balloon dilation during thoracotomy in a cat, J Am Vet Med Assoc 198:1025, 1991.
8. Corcoran BM: Posttraumatic tracheal stenosis in a cat, Vet Rec 124:342, 1989.
9. Nelson AW: Lower respiratory system. In Slatter DH, editor: Textbook of small animal surgery, ed 2, Philadelphia, 1993, WB Saunders, pp 777-804.
10. Hardie EM, Spodnick GJ, Gilson SD, et al: Tracheal rupture in cats: 16 cases, J Am Vet Med Assoc 214:508, 1999.
11. Mitchell SL, McCarthy R, Rudloff E, et al: Tracheal rupture associated with intubation in cats: 20 cases (1996-1998), J Am Vet Med Assoc 216:1592, 2000.
12. Wong WT, Brock KA: Tracheal laceration from endotracheal intubation in a cat, Vet Rec 134:622, 1994.
13. Smith MM Gourley IM, Amis TC, et al: Management of tracheal stenosis in a dog, J Am Vet Med Assoc 196:931, 1990.
14. Bradley RL, Schaaf JP. Tracheal resection and anastomosis for traumatic tracheal collapse in a dog, Comp Contin Educ Pract Vet 9:234, 1987.
15. Brown D, Holt DE: Subcutaneous emphysema, pneumothorax, pneumomediastinum and pneumopericardium in a cat. A case of barotrauma, J Am Vet Med Assoc 206:997, 1995.
16. Freeman LM, Rush JE, Schelling SH, et al: Tracheoesophageal fistula in two cats. J Am Anim Hosp Assoc 29:531, 1993.
17. Lotti U, Niebauer GW: Tracheobronchial foreign bodies of plant origin in 153 hunting dogs, Comp Cont Ed Pract Vet 14:7, 1992.
18. Carlisle CH, Biery DN, Thrall DE: Tracheal and laryngeal tumors of the dog and cat: literature review and 13 additional patients, Vet Radiol 32:229, 1991.
19. Brovida C, Castagnaro M: Tracheal obstruction due to an eosinophilic granuloma in a dog: surgical treatment and clinicopathological observations, J Am Anim Hosp Assoc 28:8, 1992.
20. Metcalfe SS. Filaroides osleri in a dog, Aust Vet Pract 27:65, 1997.
21. Cobb MA, Fischer MA. Crenosoma vulpis infection in a dog, Vet Rec 130:452, 1992.
22. Blocker TL, Roberts BK. Acute tracheal obstruction associated with anticoagulant rodenticide intoxication in a dog, J Small Anim Pract 40:577, 1999.
23. Sheaffer KA, Dillon AR: Obstructive tracheal mass due to an inflammatory polyp in a cat, J Am Anim Hosp Assoc 32:431, 1996.
24. Fitzgerald SD, Johnson CA, Peck EJ: A fatal case of intrathoracic cuterebriasis in a cat, J Am Anim Hosp Assoc 32:353, 1996.
25. Stadler K, Hartman S, Matheson J, O'Brien R: Computerized tomographic imaging of dogs with primary laryngeal or tracheal airway obstruction, Vet Radiol Ultrasound 52:377-384, 2011.
26. Hauptman J, White JV, Slocombe RF: Intrathoracic tracheal stricture management in a dog, J Am Anim Hosp Assoc 21:505, 1985.
27. Hedlund CS: Tracheal anastomosis in the dog. Comparison of two end-to-end techniques, Vet Surg 13:135, 1984.
28. McMillan FD: Iatrogenic tracheal stenosis in a cat, J Am Anim Hosp Assoc 21:747, 1985.
29. White RN, Burton CA: Surgical management of intrathoracic tracheal avulsion in cats; long term results in 9 consecutive cases, Vet Surg 29:430-435, 2000.
30. Maeda M, Grillo HC: Effect of tension on tracheal growth after resection and anastomosis in puppies, J Thoracic Cardiovasc Surg 65:658, 1973.
31. Cantrall JR, Folse JR: The repair of circumferential defects of the trachea by direct anastomosis: Experimental evaluation, J Thoracic Cardiovasc Surg 42:589, 1961.
32. Culp WTN, Weisse C, Cole SG, Solomon JA: Intraluminal tracheal stenting for treatment of tracheal narrowing in 3 cats, Vet Surg 36:107-113, 2007.

CHAPTER 20

ALLERGIC AIRWAY DISEASE IN DOGS AND CATS AND FELINE BRONCHOPULMONARY DISEASE

Carrie J. Miller, DVM, DACVIM (Internal Medicine)

KEY POINTS

- Allergic airway disease in dogs and cats encompasses a broad spectrum of diseases that are somewhat poorly defined, but the clinical signs and pathologic appearances are similar regardless of the cause.
- Diseases commonly included in this category include parasitic allergic airway disease, allergic bronchitis (eosinophilic bronchopneumopathy), feline asthma, and pulmonary infiltrates with eosinophils.
- Lower airway inflammation in response to either an extrinsic noxious stimulus or intrinsic hypersensitivity to antigenic stimulation is a known factor in the development of allergic respiratory disease in small animals. The airway inflammation causes mucosal edema, airway smooth muscle hypertrophy and constriction, and excessive production of airway secretions.
- Although the causes of canine and feline allergic airway disease are numerous, the medical treatment is similar because it is often difficult to remove the inciting cause (unless infectious in nature). The clinician therefore must attempt to control and dampen symptoms.
- Steroids, bronchodilators, and oxygen therapy are the mainstays of therapy for critical animals with severe allergic airway disease.

DEFINITION OF ALLERGIC AIRWAY DISEASE

Allergic airway disease in dogs and cats encompasses a broad spectrum of diseases that are somewhat poorly defined, but the clinical signs and pathologic appearances are similar regardless of the cause. Diseases commonly included in this category are parasitic allergic airway disease, allergic bronchitis (eosinophilic bronchopneumopathy), feline asthma, and pulmonary infiltrates with eosinophils (PIE). These diseases typically are characterized by bronchial or alveolar inflammatory changes, including submucosal wall edema, increased bronchial secretions, smooth muscle hypertrophy, and smooth muscle constriction of the bronchioles and small bronchi. Histologically, there is typically a predominance of eosinophils within the airways and submucosa of the bronchial tree. Clinical signs include labored breathing, rapid shallow breathing, increased expiratory effort, and coughing. Studies have shown variable degrees of inherent hypersensitivity in the bronchiolar smooth muscle in small animals with lower airway disease.[1,2] Animals may have an acute onset of respiratory signs with completely reversible changes or may develop chronic disease (defined as more than 2 months' duration) that is associated with irreversible bronchial wall alterations.[3] The pathogenesis of these diseases has not been investigated as thoroughly as has human asthma. Small animal allergic airway disease should not be named hastily as *asthma* because the pathogenesis and definition are much less clear than they are in humans.[4]

HUMAN ASTHMA

Human asthma is defined as a disease of the lower airways that makes affected individuals prone to inappropriate airway narrowing in response to a wide variety of provoking stimuli. The ease with which these airways narrow is termed *hyperreactivity*.[5] Human asthmatic patients develop large numbers of immunoglobulin E (IgE) antibodies in response to various inhaled allergens. These IgE antibodies then crosslink to mast cells in the submucosa of the bronchi and bronchioles of the lung, causing mast cell degranulation. Degranulation leads to the release of several inflammatory mediators (i.e., histamine, leukotrienes, eosinophilic chemotactic factor, bradykinin) that cause immediate airway constriction, as well as a late-phase inflammatory response that takes place several hours after initial release secondary to the effects of the leukotrienes.[5-7] These mediators are responsible for pulmonary mucosal edema, smooth muscle hypertrophy of the bronchi and bronchioles, accumulation of pulmonary secretions, and airway narrowing.[6] Because expiratory resistance and function is the primary breathing phase affected, there is air trapping within the lungs that leads to an increase in functional residual capacity (FRC) and appears radiographically as hyperinflation of the lungs.[6,8]

PATHOGENESIS OF SMALL ANIMAL ALLERGIC RESPIRATORY DISEASE

The pathophysiology of small animal allergic airway disease is less well understood than human asthma, but it is clear that these diseases in small animals are characterized clinically by coughing, a prominent increase in expiratory effort with or without appreciable wheezes, and a predictable response to glucocorticoids.[2,4,9] Allergic airway disease in small animals commonly causes increased numbers of eosinophils within the airways, hyperinflation of the lungs, and thickening of the bronchi and bronchioles. Lower airway inflammation, in response to either an extrinsic noxious stimulus or intrinsic hypersensitivity to antigenic stimulation, is a known component in animals with allergic respiratory disease. The airway inflammation causes mucosal edema, airway smooth muscle hypertrophy and constriction, and excessive production of airway secretions.[3,9] Although similar in clinical picture and treatment, diseases such as feline and canine bronchitis should not be termed *allergic* because they do not fit all of the above criteria (particularly overabundance of eosinophils in the airways). Diseases that should be included in small animal allergic airway disease include canine allergic bronchitis (also termed *eosinophilic bronchopneumopathy*), parasitic larval migration, PIE, and feline asthma.[10] Although the clinical picture and treatment of feline bronchopulmonary disease and feline asthma are similar, they may have separate causes because the cytopathologic features differ.

Table 20-1 Parasitic Diseases That May Cause an Inflammatory Pulmonary Reaction*

Parasite	Species	Location	Diagnosis	Management
Aelurostrongylus abstrusus	Cats	Southern United States and worldwide	Larvae in tracheal wash or fecal Baermann technique	Fenbendazole or ivermectin if clinical
Capillaria aerophila	Dogs and cats	Worldwide	Eggs in tracheal wash or fecal flotation	Fenbendazole or levamisole (dogs)
Filaroides hirthi	Dogs	North America, Japan, Europe	Zinc sulfate flotation or Baermann technique or larvae in tracheal wash	Albendazole or fenbendazole
Crenosoma vulpis	Dogs	Worldwide	Larvae in tracheal wash or fecal Baermann technique	Fenbendazole or levamisole
Paragonimus kellicotti	Dogs and cats	Great Lakes, Midwest, southern United States	Eggs in tracheal wash or fecal sedimentation	Praziquantel or fenbendazole
Intestinal parasite migration*: *Toxocara canis*	Dogs	Worldwide	Ova on fecal flotation	Pyrantel pamoate; for larval migration use either fenbendazole or ivermectin

*Clinical signs may include cough, respiratory distress, and often a peripheral eosinophilia. Other intestinal parasites to consider in animals with allergic lung disease include *Ancylostoma caninum* and *Strongyloides stercoralis.*

PARASITIC ALLERGIC AIRWAY DISEASE

Intestinal parasite migration as well as primary pulmonary parasitism can cause a parenchymal or lower airway allergic inflammatory response. The most common migratory parasite to cause an allergic response in the canine lungs is *Toxocara canis.* An inflammatory "allergic" reaction can take place in the lower airways and parenchyma of young dogs when this parasite migrates through the lungs as part of its normal development. Because of antigenic stimulation and the eosinophilic infiltrate induced by the larvae, these dogs may develop signs of respiratory disease that can vary in intensity.[11]

Other less common parasites known to migrate through the lungs include *Ancylostoma caninum* (dogs only) and *Strongyloides stercoralis* (dogs or cats). Primary lung parasites include *Paragonimus kellicotti, Aelurostrongylus abstrusus, Capillaria aerophila,* and *Filaroides hirthi* (Table 20-1). *Dirofilaria immitis* (heartworm infection) also can cause an allergic inflammatory response when large numbers of antimicrofilarial antibodies entrap microfilariae within the pulmonary capillaries.[12] All of these parasites elicit predominantly a type I hypersensitivity reaction in the lungs that leads to bronchoconstriction and inflammation within the airways and lung parenchyma.[11]

Clinical signs associated with larval migration or primary pulmonary parasitic infection vary markedly from asymptomatic to severe coughing, wheezing, and respiratory distress. A complete blood count may show eosinophilia or basophilia; however, this finding is not always present in animals suffering from parasitic allergic airway disease. Chest radiographs can show a variety of changes, including interstitial infiltrates, bronchial thickening, and even alveolar consolidation. *A. caninum* and *T. canis* can be seen using routine fecal flotation techniques.[10] *Strongyloides stercoralis* is more reliably found with the Baermann technique. However, negative fecal examination results do not rule out the possibility of migrating larval airway disease. Ova are often difficult to find on fecal examination because larvae typically begin to migrate through the lungs before shedding ova into the intestinal tract.[13]

Initially, a course of an appropriate antihelminthic medication (ivermectin or fenbendazole) can be used for treatment, particularly in mild to moderate clinical cases (see Table 20-1). Appropriate treatment for infection with *D. immitis* is discussed elsewhere.[14] In situations in which the clinical signs are severe, or fail to resolve completely, an antiinflammatory dosage of glucocorticoids (e.g., prednisone 0.5 to 1 mg/kg PO q24h) may be used to help control the inflammation associated with the infection.[10,11]

CANINE ALLERGIC BRONCHITIS OR EOSINOPHILIC BRONCHOPNEUMOPATHY

Canine allergic bronchitis (eosinophilic bronchopneumopathy) is characterized by pulmonary hypersensitivity with eosinophilic infiltration of lung and bronchial mucosa. The signalment of dogs with this disease tends to be different from that of either PIE or canine chronic bronchitis; these dogs tend to be younger (mean ± SD = 3.3 ± 2 years), and Siberian Huskies and Alaskan Malamutes are overrepresented. These dogs usually are in good physical condition but show clinical signs such as coughing, labored breathing, or nasal discharge that is mucopurulent or yellow-green.[12,15]

The most common radiographic finding in dogs with canine allergic bronchitis (eosinophilic bronchopneumopathy) is a diffuse, prominent, bronchointerstitial pattern. The bronchial inflammation, as well as mucous plugging, can sometimes create a nodular radiographic appearance as well. Forty percent of dogs have alveolar infiltrates (because of secondary pneumonia in some cases), and 26% have radiographic signs of bronchiectasis. A peripheral eosinophilia is present in about 60% of cases. Bronchoscopy typically reveals abundant yellow-green mucus or mucopurulent material, thickening with irregularities or polypoid changes to the mucosa, and exaggerated closure of the airways during expiration. Cytologic findings in fluid obtained from a bronchoalveolar lavage (BAL) or endotracheal wash (ETW) include more than 50% eosinophils in 87% of dogs and between 20% and 50% eosinophils in 13% of dogs.[15]

The mainstay of treatment for animals with this disease is glucocorticoids, with an induction dosage of prednisone of 1 mg/kg PO q12h, although larger dogs often require lower dosages. Most dogs relapse within months of discontinuing the steroids, but some dogs may remain disease free for years. A maintenance dosage of prednisone (0.25 to 0.5 mg/kg q48h) is suggested in an attempt to maintain remission. One study did demonstrate that the clinical signs of eosinophilic bronchopneumopathy could be controlled with chronic inhaled corticosteroids.[37] Other immunosuppressive drugs, as well as hyposensitization, are currently under investigation for the treatment of animals with this disease. Culture and susceptibility testing should be performed on the BAL or ETW fluid to rule out a secondary pneumonia. It is important to stress to the owner that this disease requires lifelong management, and the long-term use of steroids may have unwanted side effects.[12,15]

PULMONARY INFILTRATES WITH EOSINOPHILS

Pulmonary infiltrates with eosinophils (PIE) describes a spectrum of diseases that involve a type I hypersensitivity reaction occurring in the pulmonary parenchyma in response to various stimuli. PIE should be considered more of an "umbrella term" that encompasses several pulmonary diseases, all of which cause eosinophilic airway inflammation. The stimuli for this eosinophilic inflammation can include pulmonary or migrating parasites, heartworms, drugs, or inhaled allergens. One study showed that 65% of cases of PIE were caused by heartworm disease; however, this predominance may vary depending on the animal's geographic location.[16] The disease tends to occur in adult dogs, with no known sex or breed predilection.

Although PIE appears to be allergic in nature, based on the high numbers of eosinophils in the airways, it leads primarily to pulmonary parenchymal disease rather than airway disease. Affected dogs have classic symptoms of parenchymal disease, including respiratory distress with rapid, shallow breathing, coughing, and possibly cyanosis. Radiographically, a diffuse interstitial, bronchial, or alveolar pattern is apparent, and many dogs also have hilar lymphadenopathy. Bronchoscopy and BAL or ETW reveal a predominance of eosinophils within the airways. A peripheral eosinophilia is common, but its presence is dependent on the cause of the pulmonary eosinophilic inflammation. The morbidity and mortality in animals with PIE depends primarily on the underlying cause of PIE and whether the cause can be treated or removed. Given the heterogeneity of diseases represented by the term PIE, this classification should be avoided as an ultimate diagnosis and strive to uncover an underlying cause.[11,16]

FELINE BRONCHOPULMONARY DISEASE

Much like PIE, feline bronchopulmonary disease is a broad term that encompasses several disease processes. Although some cats may be truly allergic and asthmatic in nature, others may have chronic changes (chronic bronchitis) from prolonged and persistent irritation and inflammation to the lower airways related to nonallergenic stimuli.[2] Because these groups of cats look very similar clinically and the cause of feline bronchopulmonary disease is unknown, both diseases are presented here in detail. However, most clinical cases of feline bronchopulmonary disease do not fit the true definition of allergic airway disease.

Pathogenesis

The pathogenesis of the feline bronchopulmonary inflammatory response appears variable. The response is difficult to predict because it has been reported that up to 30% eosinophils may be seen in the BAL or ETW fluid of healthy cats.[17] The cellular inflammatory response is only partially responsible for feline bronchopulmonary disease. Another important factor is lower airway hyperreactivity, which is defined as the ease with which airways narrow in response to a nonspecific stimulus. Although some cats may have inherently reactive airways to truly allergic stimuli, others may have a degree of airway responsiveness to extrinsic noxious stimuli. Feline patients have been reported to have exacerbations of signs associated with exposure to scented hair sprays, clay-based litters, scented air fresheners, or cigarette smoke. In some cases, simply removing the noxious stimulus from the environment may noticeably improve a cat's symptoms.[2]

Clinical Signs

Respiratory distress, with increased expiratory effort and rapid, shallow breathing, is a common manifestation of feline bronchopulmonary disease. Cats often display open-mouth breathing, and excessive coughing with severe tracheal sensitivity is common. Although the inflammation within the airways is typically a chronic problem, the episode of respiratory distress may appear acute and severe in nature. Airway narrowing caused by inflammation and bronchoconstriction of the lower airways frequently causes wheezes and a forced abdominal push during exhalation.[1,18]

Feline bronchopulmonary disease appears to be the most common cause of coughing in cats, although 16% of cases had no coughing in the history or during physical examination.[2,12] In one study, 75% of cats coughed during examination, and many also exhibited wheezing or sneezing. The Siamese breed is overrepresented in cats with lower airway disease. There is no known sex or age predilection.[2,3]

Laboratory Diagnostic Tests

Once the cat is stabilized, a complete blood count, biochemical analysis, and urinalysis should be performed to help rule out systemic diseases that could be causing respiratory distress (see Chapter 1). These test results are typically normal in cats with feline bronchopulmonary disease, and it is a common misconception that they have a peripheral eosinophilia. In one study of cats with peripheral eosinophilia, only 9% were diagnosed with feline allergic airway disease.[2,3,19] A diagnosis of allergic airway disease in a cat with a peripheral eosinophilia should not be made without cytologic evidence demonstrating concurrent airway eosinophilia. A fecal examination helps rule in or rule out pulmonary parasites. A heartworm test is also important for any cat with labored breathing and evidence of bronchointerstitial disease. A bronchointerstitial pattern is the most persistent and chronic radiographic finding in feline heartworm disease, even without changes seen in the pulmonary vasculature.[12,20] Feline antibody and antigen heartworm tests should be performed because the amount of antigen can be extremely low or the antigen may be absent in some cats.[14]

Radiology

Thoracic radiographs are an essential diagnostic test in cats with respiratory distress; however, the cat should first be stabilized with oxygen, and other medications, if indicated. The radiographic appearance of feline bronchopulmonary disease can vary. The classic radiographic findings include an increase in bronchial densities, often described as *doughnuts, tram lines,* or *train tracks.* These terms describe the thickened bronchial walls viewed end-on or from the side. Other radiographic findings can include an increase in interstitial markings, an alveolar pattern, or hyperinflation of the lung fields with flattening of the diaphragm.[10-12] Alveolar infiltration and consolidation of the right middle lung lobe have been reported in 11% of cats with bronchopulmonary disease.[3] This radiographic appearance should not be mistaken for bronchopneumonia. Rare radiographic abnormalities that can be seen secondary to feline bronchopulmonary disease include pneumothorax, lung lobe torsion, or bronchiectasis.[34-36]

The severity of radiographic changes in cats with feline bronchopulmonary disease varies, ranging from mild to severe, and does not necessarily correlate with the severity of symptoms or diagnostic test results.[23] A prognosis therefore should not be made based solely on radiographic changes.

Bronchoscopy

Bronchoscopy allows direct visualization of the trachea and bronchial tree. Cats with feline bronchopulmonary disease often have thick mucus secretions in their lower airways, as well as hyperemic and edematous mucosa.[2,3] During bronchoscopy, a BAL should be performed. A BAL is preferred over a transtracheal wash because the BAL yields a cell population that is more representative of the lower airways and pulmonary interstitium. A BAL also has been shown to be more accurate than a transtracheal wash for the diagnosis of bacterial and mycotic infections of the lower airways.[21]

Fluid culture should be performed to rule out infectious causes of airway inflammation. A quantitative culture should be performed, with significant bacterial numbers indicating true bacterial infection. The bronchi of healthy cats are not considered sterile; thus a bacterial culture is generally considered significant only if the growth is greater than 2000 colony-forming units (CFU)/ml in cats. One study has shown that cats with feline bronchopulmonary disease have a significantly higher rate of mycoplasma colonization than that seen in cats with healthy airways.[2,3,17] The most predominant cell types found in bronchial washings of cats affected with bronchopulmonary disease are neutrophils and eosinophils. Dye and colleagues[2] reported that moderately and severely affected cats had statistically significantly higher percentages of eosinophils, neutrophils, and combined neutrophils and eosinophils than did healthy cats. However, mast cells were found infrequently and represented up to 8% of all the cell types.[2] Moise et al found that the predominant cell types in affected cats were eosinophils (24% of cats), neutrophils (33% of cats), macrophages (22% of cats), or a mixed cell population (21% of cats).[3] Clearly, cats with feline bronchopulmonary disease have variable cytologic findings, thus demonstrating why this disease is not routinely considered allergic in nature.

TREATMENT OF ALLERGIC AIRWAY DISEASE AND FELINE BRONCHOPULMONARY DISEASE

Glucocorticoids

Although the causes of canine and feline allergic airway disease are numerous, the medical treatment is similar because it is often difficult to remove the inciting cause (unless infectious in nature). The clinician must therefore attempt to control and dampen the clinical manifestations, which includes advising clients to remove inhalant irritants from the animal's environment, including such things as dusty litter, perfumes, aerosols, and cigarette smoke. Drug therapy and irritant avoidance are necessary in most animals with allergic airway disease. Several options exist for medical treatment of these patients. Steroids, bronchodilators, and oxygen therapy are the mainstay of emergency therapy.[22] Steroids are used in emergent patients and for long-term therapy to decrease inflammation and resistance in the lower airways (Table 20-2).[23] Airway inflammation can linger despite resolution of clinical signs in patients with feline bronchopulmonary disease. The clinician should be cautioned in tapering the glucocorticoids too rapidly. Although steroids are generally effective in decreasing airway resistance and inflammation, the common and often severe side effects of this class of drugs limit their feasibility for long-term control of allergic airway disease.[24] Some inhalant steroids (e.g., fluticasone and flunisolide) are used in the experimental setting to control airway inflammation without the systemic side effects[25,32] (see Chapter 172).

Bronchodilators

Two classes of bronchodilators can be used to manage allergic airway disease in veterinary patients. These include methylxanthines (theophylline, aminophylline) and selective β_2-receptor agonists (terbutaline or albuterol). Parenterally administered terbutaline has a rapid onset of action and is given most commonly to animals in acute, severe respiratory distress. Because β-agonist drugs may cause tachycardia or tachyarrhythmias in some animals, the clinician should attempt to rule out cardiac disease before administering these medications.[26] Inhaled β-agonist therapy is also an option for inpatient or outpatient therapy of allergic airway disease and may carry fewer side effects (see Chapter 172). Methylxanthine drugs may be preferable for long-term bronchodilation because tolerance to the β-agonist drugs may occur and subsequently decrease their efficacy in emergency situations. The brands of theophylline for which the pharmacokinetics were known to be therapeutic have unfortunately been taken off the market. The use and specific dose of theophylline recommended at this time is empiric.[27]

Antihelminthic medications are recommended routinely for animals with allergic airway disease. Although bronchoscopy and BAL washings offer the best chance of diagnosing parasitic allergic airway disease, migrating larvae and primary pulmonary parasites can be missed with these diagnostic tools.[11] Deworming protocols are generally very safe and can effectively cure animals with parasitic allergic airway disease.

Miscellaneous Drugs and Other Therapies

Because of the potent side effects of many steroids, other drugs have been used empirically for the treatment of allergic airway disease. No controlled, in vivo studies demonstrate the efficacy of these medications; however, they are sometimes prescribed when other medications appear unsuccessful. Cyclosporine is an immunosuppressant that specifically inhibits the T-helper cells of the immune system. Evidence suggests that the T-helper cells are a primary component of the allergic immune response.[24] Cyclosporine has been shown to block inflammatory changes associated with experimental asthma in

Table 20-2 Commonly Used Medications and Dosages for the Treatment of Allergic Airway Disease in the Dog and Cat

Drug	Class and Mechanism	Indication	Dosage Recommended
Dexamethasone sodium phosphate	Glucocorticoid: long-acting	Parenteral steroid for emergency use	0.2 to 0.5 mg/kg IV or IM
Prednisone or prednisolone	Glucocorticoid: short-acting	Appropriate for maintenance use and alternate-day therapy	1 to 2 mg/kg PO q12h for 2 weeks, then taper over 2 to 3 months
Methylprednisolone acetate	Glucocorticoid: long-acting	Appropriate only for cases with problems in compliance	20 mg per cat IM q4-6wk
Aminophylline	Bronchodilator: methylxanthine	Not recommended orally because of the short half-life in dogs and cats	5 to 10 mg/kg PO q8h or 5 to 10 mg/kg IV q6-8h
Theophylline	Bronchodilator: methylxanthine	Maintenance therapy: pharmacokinetics unknown	Cats: 5 mg/kg PO q8-12h Dogs: 5-10 mg/kg PO q12h
Terbutaline	Bronchodilator β_2-agonist	Parenteral or oral bronchodilator	0.01 mg/kg IV, SC, or IM q4-8h Cats: 1.25 mg PO q12h Dogs: 2.5 mg PO q8h

IM, Intramuscular; *IV,* intravenous; *PO,* per os; *SC,* subcutaneous.

cats; however, it has not been evaluated in naturally occurring cases of allergic airway disease.[28] Many humans with asthma are now treated with therapies such as leukotriene receptor blockers (montelukast and zafirlukast) or inhibitors of the enzyme 5-lipoxygenase (zileuton), which is responsible for the formation of leukotrienes themselves.[29] Cysteinyl leukotrienes do not appear to be important mediators of bronchoconstriction in cats, and the one veterinary study evaluating these medications did not show efficacy using a lipoxygenase blocker in a model of experimentally induced feline allergic airway disease.[30]

Cyproheptadine also has been suggested for use in cats with allergic airway disease. It is a serotonin receptor antagonist that inhibits feline airway smooth muscle contraction in vitro. Oral administration (2 mg q12h) was associated with a reduction in airway hyperreactivity in a subpopulation of cats with experimentally induced asthma, although some evidence suggests that higher dosages (i.e., 8 mg q8-12h) may be more appropriate.[30] It has yet to be determined whether cyproheptadine will work in vivo in cats with airway disease.[31]

Early research suggests that masitinib, a tyrosine kinase inhibitor, may help decrease airway eosinophilia and improve pulmonary mechanics in experimental cases of feline asthma.[33]

PROGNOSIS

The prognosis for small animals with allergic airway disease is variable and depends on the cause, chronicity, and continued exposure to irritants. The overall clinical picture can be exacerbated by concurrent underlying cardiac or other respiratory disease. Feline bronchopulmonary disease in cats is often a chronic disorder, one that manifests with either persistent signs or episodic flare-ups. Patient morbidity is high in affected cats because of the chronicity of the disease.

REFERENCES

1. Padrid PA: CVT update: Feline asthma. In Bonagura JD, editor: Kirk's current veterinary therapy XIII, St Louis, 2000, Saunders.
2. Dye JA, McKiernan BC, Rozanski EA, et al: Bronchopulmonary disease in the cat: historical, physical, radiographic, clinicopathologic, and pulmonary functional evaluation of 24 affected and 15 healthy cats, J Vet Intern Med 10:385, 1996.
3. Moise NS, Weidenkeller D, Yeager AE, et al: Clinical, radiographic, and bronchial cytologic features of cats with bronchial disease: 65 cases (1980-1986), J Am Vet Med Assoc 194:1467, 1989.
4. Johnson L: Diseases of the bronchus. In Ettinger SJ, Feldman EC, editors: Textbook of veterinary internal medicine, St Louis, 2000, Saunders.
5. Woolcock AJ: Asthma. In Murray JF, Nadel JA, editors: Murray and Nadel's textbook of respiratory medicine, ed 2, Philadelphia, 1994, Saunders.
6. Guyton AC, Hall JE, editors: The textbook of medical physiology, ed 9, Philadelphia, 1996, Saunders.
7. Felsburg PJ: Respiratory immunology. In Kirk RW, editor: Current veterinary therapy IX, St Louis, 1986, Saunders.
8. West JB: Respiratory physiology, ed 4, Baltimore, 1990, Williams & Wilkins.
9. Bauer T: Pulmonary hypersensitivity disorders. In Kirk RW, editor: Current veterinary therapy X, St Louis, 1989, Saunders.
10. Miller CJ, McKiernan BC: Allergic airway disease. In Wingfield WE, Raffe MR, editors: The veterinary ICU book, Jackson Hole, Wyo, 2002, Teton NewMedia.
11. Hawkins E: Pulmonary parenchymal diseases. In Ettinger S, Feldman E, editors: Textbook of veterinary internal medicine, St Louis, 2000, Saunders.
12. Norris CR, Mellema MS: Eosinophilic pneumonia. In King LG, editor: Textbook of respiratory disease in dogs and cats, St Louis, 2004, Saunders.
13. Urquhart GM, Armour J, Duncan JL, et al: Veterinary parasitology, New York, 1987, Churchill Livingstone.
14. Dillon R: Dirofilariasis in dogs and cats. In Ettinger SJ, Feldman EC, editors: Textbook of veterinary internal medicine, St Louis, 2000, Saunders.
15. Clercx C, Peeters D, Snaps F, et al: Eosinophilic bronchopneumopathy in dogs, J Vet Intern Med 14:282, 2000.
16. Calvert CA, Mahaffey MB, Lappin MR: Pulmonary and disseminated eosinophilic granulomatosis in dogs, J Am Anim Hosp Assoc 24:311, 1988.
17. Padrid PA, Feldman BF, Funk K, et al: Cytologic, microbiologic, and biochemical analysis of bronchoalveolar lavage fluid obtained from 24 healthy cats, Am J Vet Res 52:1300, 1991.
18. Corcoran BM, Foster DJ, Fuentes VL: Feline asthma syndrome: a retrospective study of the clinical presentation in 29 cats, J Small Anim Pract 36:481, 1995.
19. Center SA, Randolph JF, Erb HN, et al: Eosinophilia in the cat: a retrospective study of 312 cases (1975 to 1986), J Am Anim Hosp Assoc 26:349, 1990.
20. Selcer BA, Newell SM, Mansour AE, et al: Radiographic and 2-D echocardiographic findings in 18 cats experimentally exposed to *D. immitis* via mosquito bites, Vet Radiol Ultrasound 37:37, 1996.
21. Peeters DE, McKiernan BC, Weisiger RM: Quantitative bacterial cultures and cytological examination of bronchoalveolar lavage specimens in dogs, J Vet Intern Med 14:534, 2000.
22. Diehl KJ: Respiratory emergencies. In Wingfield WE, editor: Veterinary emergency medicine secrets, Philadelphia, 1997, Hanley & Belfus.
23. Schimmer B, Parker K: Adrenocorticotropic hormone: adrenocortical steroids and their synthetic analogs. In Goodman LS, Limbird LE, Milinoff PB, editors: Goodman & Gilman's the pharmacological basis of therapeutics, ed 9, New York, 1996, McGraw-Hill.
24. Boothe DM, Mealey KA: Glucocorticoid therapy in the dog and cat. In Boothe DM, editor: Small animal clinical pharmacology and therapeutics, St Louis, 2001, Saunders.
25. Padrid PA: Use of inhaled medications to treat respiratory diseases in dogs and cats, J Am Anim Hosp Assoc 42:165, 2006.
26. Plumb DC: Veterinary drug handbook, White Bear Lake, Minn, 1999, PharmaVet.
27. Bach JF, KuKanich B, Papich MG, et al: Evaluation of the bioavailability and pharmacokinetics of two extended release theophylline formulations in dogs, J Am Vet Med Assoc 224:1113, 2004.
28. Padrid PA, Cozzi D, Leff AR: Cyclosporine A inhibits airway reactivity and remodeling after chronic antigen challenge in cats, Am J Respir Crit Care Med 154:1812, 1996.
29. Villaran C, O'Neill SJ, Helbling A, et al: Montelukast versus salmeterol in patients with asthma and exercise-induced bronchoconstriction, J Allergy Clin Immunol 104:547, 1999.
30. Reinero CR, Decile KC, Byerly JR, et al: Effects of drug treatment on inflammation and hyperreactivity of airways and on immune variables in cats with experimentally induced asthma, Am J Vet Res 66:1121, 2005.
31. Padrid PA, Mitchell RW, Ndukwu IM, et al: Cyproheptadine-induced attenuation of type I immediate hypersensitivity reactions of airway smooth muscle from immune-sensitized cats, Am J Vet Res 56:109, 1995.
32. Cohn LA, DeClue AE, Cohen RL, et al: Effects of fluticasone propionate dosage in an experimental model of feline asthma, J Feline Med Surg 12(2):91-96, 2010.
33. Lee-Fowler TM, Guntur V, Dodam J, et al: The tyrosine kinase inhibitor masitinib blunts airway inflammation and improves associated lung mechanics in a feline model of chronic allergic asthma, Int Arch Allergy Immunol 158(4):369-374, 2012.
34. Mooney ET, Rozanski EA, King RG, et al: Spontaneous pneumothorax in 35 cats (2001-2010), J Feline Med Surg 14(6):384-391, 2012.
35. Dye TL, Teague HD, Poundstone ML: Lung lobe torsion in a cat with chronic feline asthma, J Am Anim Hosp Assoc 34(6):493-495, 1998.
36. Norris CR, Samii VF: Clinical, radiographic, and pathologic features of bronchiectasis in cats: 12 cases (1987-1999), J Am Vet Med Assoc 216(4):530-534, 2000.
37. Bexfield NH, Foale RD, Davison LJ, et al: Management of 13 cases of canine respiratory disease using inhaled corticosteroids, J Small Anim Practice 47(7):377-382, 2006.

CHAPTER 21

PULMONARY EDEMA

Sophie Adamantos, BVSc, CertVA, DACVECC, MRCVS, FHEA • Dez Hughes, BVSc, MRCVS, DACVECC

KEY POINTS

- Pulmonary edema is a common cause of respiratory distress in dogs and cats.
- Almost all parenchymal lung diseases have a component of edema.
- Two main pathophysiologic forms exist: high-pressure edema and increased permeability edema.
- Hydrostatic pressure is an important pathologic mechanism in both forms of edema.
- Cardiogenic edema is the most common form of high-pressure edema and the most common cause of pulmonary edema overall.
- Hypoproteinemia (decreased intravascular colloid osmotic pressure) is very rarely a sole cause of pulmonary edema.
- Pulmonary capillary pressure modification is important in treatment of both pathophysiologic forms.
- The prognosis for animals with pulmonary edema varies depending on the underlying cause.
- Cardiogenic pulmonary edema usually responds well to loop diuretic therapy, whereas most types of noncardiogenic pulmonary edema respond less readily to treatment.
- Fluid therapy should be administered with caution in patients with pulmonary edema.

Pulmonary edema is the accumulation of extravascular fluid within the pulmonary parenchyma or alveoli. The two main pathophysiologic forms are high-pressure edema (caused by increased pulmonary capillary hydrostatic pressure) and increased-permeability edema (caused by damage of the microvascular barrier and alveolar epithelium in more severe cases). Pulmonary edema is a relatively common disease process in veterinary patients that can rapidly become life threatening. The initial diagnostic approach is to differentiate cardiogenic (i.e., caused by left-sided, backward heart failure) from noncardiogenic edema (all causes other than left-sided heart failure).

PATHOPHYSIOLOGY

Transvascular fluid fluxes are determined by Starling's forces—that is, the balance among capillary hydrostatic pressure, interstitial hydrostatic pressure, capillary colloid osmotic pressure (COP), and interstitial COP. These factors also depend on the reflection and filtration coefficients of the tissues.[1] The reflection coefficient indicates the relative permeability of the membrane to protein (1 = 100% impermeable [i.e., 100% reflected]). The filtration coefficient is a measure of overall fluid flow from the vasculature of specific tissues and is dependent on the capillary surface area and the hydraulic conductivity. Tissue safety factors protect tissues against edema. In normal tissues, extravasation of low-protein fluid causes a fall in interstitial COP, which results in preservation of the net COP gradient, thereby protecting against further fluid extravasation.[2] Other safety factors that limit edema development in nondistensible tissues include increased interstitial hydrostatic pressure, which opposes further extravasation, and an increased driving pressure for lymphatic flow (which can increase up to 10 times normal).[3]

The pulmonary microvascular barrier (comprised of the endothelial cell and basement membrane) is relatively permeable to protein compared with other tissues. This means that the effective COP gradient that can be generated between the pulmonary intravascular space and pulmonary interstitium is lower.[3] Consequently, increased lymphatic flow is the main protection against edema in the lung[4] and hypoproteinemia (decreased COP) alone rarely causes pulmonary edema. Because of the lower COP gradient, hydrostatic pressure is the main determinant of fluid extravasation and edema formation in the lungs.[5] If interstitial fluid formation overwhelms the protective clearance mechanisms, edema occurs. The pulmonary ultrastructure protects and preserves gaseous diffusion. On one side of a pulmonary capillary the capillary endothelium is fused to the adjacent alveolar epithelial cell that is impermeable to fluids other than water and so that gas diffusion occurs directly through cells. On the other side, extravasated fluid can flow into the interstitium. The distensibility of the lung interstitium gradually increases toward the peribronchovascular region so that fluid drains into the more distensible peribronchovascular areas and not where gas exchange takes place.[6]

High-pressure edema forms because high pulmonary capillary pressures cause fluid extravasation that eventually overwhelms lymphatic removal. Fluid initially flows toward the peribronchovascular interstitium, then distends all parts of the pulmonary interstitium, finally spilling into the airspaces at the junction of the alveolar and airway epithelia.[5] In many dogs with cardiogenic edema, the increase in pressure occurs gradually and overt edema may take months to develop, but if there is an acute increase in hydrostatic pressure (e.g., chordae tendineae rupture), then edema can form peracutely.

Increased permeability edema happens when injury occurs to the microvascular barrier (and sometimes alveolar epithelium) allowing leakage of fluid with a high protein content.[5] The inciting cause may be hematogenous (to the capillary and then the alveolar epithelial cell), or aerogenous, where the alveolar cell is damaged and then the capillary. Because of the increased permeability (reduced reflection coefficient), the protective fall in interstitial COP is diminished so that hydrostatic pressure becomes the main determinant of edema formation. Interstitial fluid accumulation can then occur at lower hydrostatic pressures, and relatively small rises in pressure result in greater edema formation. In more severe cases, with concurrent endothelial and epithelial injury, there is a direct conduit between the intravascular space and the alveoli. Interstitial edema then progresses rapidly to alveolar flooding. This explains the greater severity and fulminant course of increased-permeability edema compared with hydrostatic edema.

Lymphatic drainage limits interstitial fluid accumulation, but pulmonary edema fluid is largely cleared via the bronchial circulation, probably because most fluid accumulates in the peribronchovascular areas.[7] The rate of edema clearance from the alveoli and interstitium depends on the fluid type, with pure water being reabsorbed in minutes whereas fluid containing macromolecules and cells takes many hours or days.

CLINICAL PRESENTATION

Pulmonary edema ultimately results in reduced oxygenation, so most animals have signs of hypoxemia and respiratory distress. Many are extremely fragile, so a risk-benefit assessment should be considered before even performing a physical examination. All respiratory distressed animals should be stabilized in a quiet, oxygen-enriched environment (see Chapter 14). Initial evaluation is to quantify the severity of respiratory distress and the region or regions of the respiratory tract affected using the respiratory rate, effort, pattern, noise, pulmonary auscultation, and presence or absence of paradoxical abdominal movement. Historical information sometimes raises the likelihood of a particular underlying cause. Smoke inhalation can cause increased permeability edema; vomiting predisposes a patient to aspiration pneumonia and increased permeability edema; if an animal has a previous diagnosis of congestive heart failure or a preexisting murmur or gallop, then left-sided heart failure and cardiogenic edema are most likely. Head trauma, seizures, or electric shock are all factors associated with neurogenic pulmonary edema.

Auscultation typically reveals pulmonary crackles or loud, coarse lung sounds. Crackles are difficult to hear with small tidal volumes or rapid respiratory rates. Careful auscultation may allow abnormal lung sounds to be localized to one region, and this may aid in the diagnosis, such as a cranioventral distribution with aspiration pneumonia and a perihilar distribution with cardiogenic pulmonary edema in the dog.

High-Pressure Edema

Cardiogenic edema

Cardiogenic pulmonary edema is probably the most common form of high-pressure edema in small animals. It occurs as a result of left-sided congestive heart failure. Cardiac disease is often chronic and in dogs there is usually a history of clinical signs consistent with heart disease: cough, orthopnea, exercise intolerance, and usually a heart murmur. An acute onset of signs may be seen, particularly if there has been a precipitating event such as stress. In contrast, cats often have no premonitory clinical signs before the onset of dyspnea, although again, there may be a precipitating stressful event. Most dogs with left-sided heart failure will have a heart murmur, and most cats have a murmur or gallop rhythm, although about 20% of cats with left-sided heart failure have been reported to have no auscultatory abnormalities.[8]

The chronic, compensatory mechanisms for heart failure result in fluid retention to maintain cardiac output, and, although beneficial in the short term, they eventually lead to signs of congestion, which in its most life-threatening form is pulmonary edema. In severe cases, blood vessel rupture may occur leading to a serosanguineous appearance of secretions, as evidenced by pink, frothy sputum.

Fortunately only a few common conditions cause cardiogenic pulmonary edema and signalment can be extremely useful in forming a differential diagnosis list. Middle-aged, large breed dogs tend to have dilated cardiomyopathy, whereas the smaller breeds tend to have mitral valve disease. Cats are more prone to myocardial disease, with hypertrophic and restrictive cardiomyopathies seen most commonly[8,9] (see Chapter 41).

Fluid therapy

Fluid therapy per se is a very uncommon cause of pulmonary edema without preexisting heart or lung disease because of the effective safety mechanisms within the lung. But fluid therapy may cause rapid increases in hydrostatic pressure in animals with preexisting (although asymptomatic) heart disease, leading to pulmonary edema. Experimental studies have demonstrated that healthy dogs are able to cope with large volumes: dosages of 360 ml/kg of crystalloid over 1 hour were given before severe fluid overload was seen.[10] Clinically, cats seem less able to cope with large volumes of intravenous fluid even if they appear otherwise healthy. This may be related to relative overdosing of fluid therapy because cats have a lower blood volume than dogs, a reduced capacity to cope with increased intravascular volume, or the high incidence of asymptomatic heart disease in cats.[11] Synthetic or natural colloid products and hemoglobin-based oxygen-carrying solutions cause much more volume expansion than crystalloids. Approximately 3 to 5 times the amount of colloid compared with isotonic crystalloid is retained within the intravascular space, so lower fluid rates and dosages should be used in cats. When there are other risk factors, such as systemic inflammation or pulmonary parenchymal disease, fluid therapy may be more likely to lead to pulmonary edema.

Increased-Permeability Edema

An increase in permeability is caused by direct injury to the microvascular barrier, alveolar epithelium or both. Increased permeability edema is synonymous with acute lung injury (ALI), which, in its more severe form, is referred to as acute respiratory distress syndrome (ARDS). Risk factors noted by the Dorothy Russell Havemeyer Working Group on ALI and ARDS in Veterinary Medicine were inflammation, infection, sepsis, systemic inflammatory response syndrome (SIRS), severe trauma (long bone fracture, head injury, and pulmonary contusion), multiple transfusions, smoke inhalation, submersion injury, aspiration of stomach contents, and ingestion of drugs and toxins.[12] ARDS is the most severe form of increased-permeability edema and is extremely difficult to manage. Furthermore, the early exudative, edematous stage of ALI/ARDS is a very different condition from the middle proliferative stage or the end-stage fibrotic phase. Clinical experience suggests that survival from ALI in veterinary patients is not uncommon but with ARDS the survival rate is low. Other causes of increased-permeability edema include pulmonary thromboembolism (see Chapter 26), ventilator-associated lung injury (see Chapter 36), and inhaled toxic insults such as volatile hydrocarbons.

Mixed-Cause Edema

There are other causes of pulmonary edema in which the pathophysiology is incompletely understood that probably are due to a combination of hydrostatic and increased-permeability edema. Neurogenic pulmonary edema (NPE) and negative pressure pulmonary edema (NPPE) are probably the commonest forms. NPE is seen acutely after an acute neurologic event—for example, head trauma, seizures, or electric cord bite. NPPE occurs after upper airway obstruction, such as strangulation or even a sharp pull on a lead.[13] These two forms of pulmonary edema are often combined and treated synonymously in veterinary medicine; however, there are subtle differences in their pathogenesis, although their clinical course and therapy are similar.

In NPE it is thought that massive, neuronal, sympathetic activity results in a sequence of events causing both hydrostatic and increased-permeability edema. This is known as the blast theory.[14,15] Initially, hydrostatic pressure edema occurs, but at very high pulmonary hydrostatic pressures, endothelial cell injury and vascular leak result in red blood cell and protein leakage into the alveolus. Sympathetic stimulation also causes vascular effects that can result in acute cardiac insufficiency.

NPPE is poorly described in veterinary patients but experimental models in dogs exist. The pathogenesis of NPPE is not clearly understood and is heavily debated. High pressure and increased permeability mechanisms have been suggested and both seem plausible.[16,17] During upper airway obstruction, extreme subatmospheric, intrathoracic pressures are generated that then causes pulmonary vascular pressure overload, an increase in vascular return, and preload. This is thought to be exacerbated by sympathetic stimulation associated with hypoxia causing an increase in afterload. As with NPE there is both hydrostatic pressure edema and resultant microvascular damage. Alternatively, endothelial cell injury and vascular leak cause the permeability edema.[13,16-18]

NPE and NPPE occur in cats and dogs but are more common in dogs. Clinical signs develop soon after the inciting cause and resolve within 24 to 48 hours. The prognosis for these conditions is good but depends on the underlying cause.

A relatively rare cause of pulmonary edema is reexpansion edema, which has been reported in dogs and cats after acute reexpansion of chronically collapsed lung lobes.[19] Suggested mechanisms include decreased surfactant levels in collapsed lung tissue, negative interstitial pressure, mechanical disruption of pulmonary parenchyma, oxygen free radical formation, and reperfusion injury.

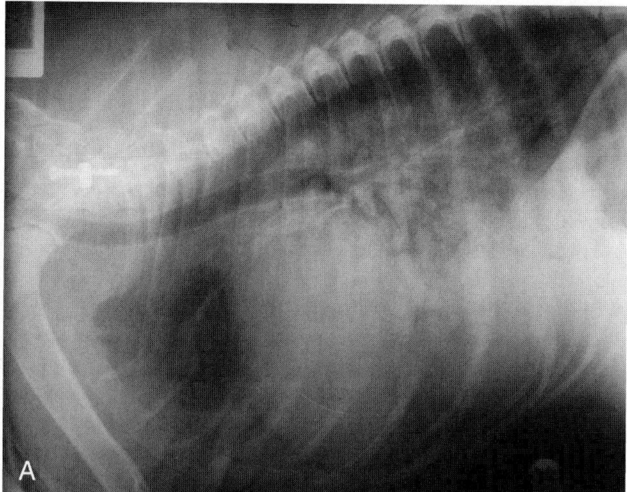

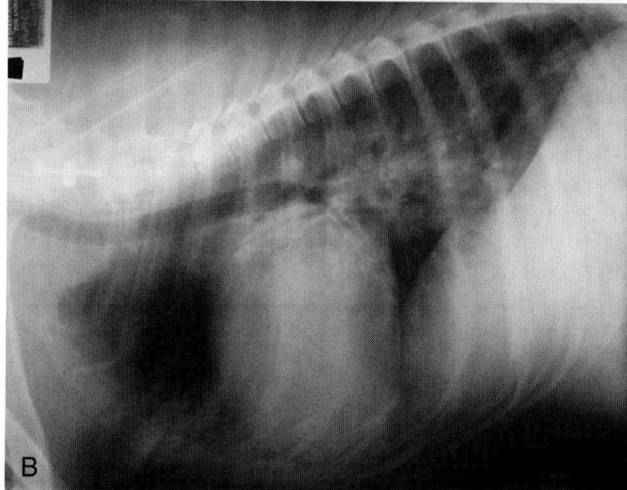

FIGURE 21-1 **A,** Lateral radiograph of a dog (Doberman Pinscher) showing marked perihilar alveolar infiltrates, an enlarged cardiac silhouette, and left atrial enlargement. This dog had severe congestive heart failure secondary to dilated cardiomyopathy. **B,** Lateral radiograph of the same dog 3 days later after intensive diuretic, positive inotropic, and vasodilator therapy (furosemide, dobutamine, pimobendan, and nitroprusside). There is marked improvement in the alveolar pattern, although mild perihilar infiltrates are still present.

DIAGNOSTIC TESTS

Practically all respiratory distress patients need nonstressful oxygen supplementation before performing diagnostic tests. A very quick ultrasound examination will confirm or rule out significant pleural effusion, and good ultrasonographers may get an estimate of left atrial size (almost always enlarged in left-sided heart failure). Thoracic radiographs are also useful to identify the cause of respiratory distress but can be highly stressful. In severely distressed patients they are best delayed until after initial empirical stabilization. All equipment necessary for radiographs should be organized in advance, including oxygen supplementation. The safest and most useful view in a dog is a quick lateral, and short exposure times should be used. Many distressed cats find lateral recumbency extremely stressful but most will tolerate sitting in sternal recumbency.

Pulmonary edema causes interstitial or alveolar infiltrates on a thoracic radiograph. In dogs, the distribution of the alveolar pattern can be helpful in discriminating between cardiogenic (Figure 21-1) and noncardiogenic (see Figure 24-1) edema, but nearly all causes of edema can produce a diffuse alveolar pattern. A dorsocaudal alveolar pattern suggests NPE or NPEE, whereas a cranioventral pattern is more suggestive of aspiration pneumonia.

Cardiogenic edema in dogs is typically seen in the perihilar region. In cats, however, there tends to be a mixed alveolar pattern that can be patchy and almost nodular (Figure 21-2). Pulmonary veins that are more distended than the pulmonary arteries may also be seen in some cases of left-sided heart failure. An enlarged left atrium seen on a brief echocardiogram raises the likelihood of congestive heart failure, but positioning may be challenging for echocardiography and respiratory distress animals should not be unduly stressed to obtain an echocardiogram.

Arterial blood gas analysis or pulse oximetry may be used to provide objective evidence of hypoxemia but are not essential for stabilization or diagnosis and maybe too stressful to be worthwhile in many animals (see Chapter 186). Some pulse oximeters are unreliable, especially in conscious patients that are moving or have darkly pigmented skin. Blood gas analyzers are becoming increasingly available and, with practice, arterial blood sampling is a relatively easy technique to master. Sampling from the dorsal metatarsal artery is less stressful than using the femoral artery and can even be performed in standing dogs. Arterial blood gas analysis will document severity of hypoxemia and allows monitoring of trends but is not specific for the type of lung disease.

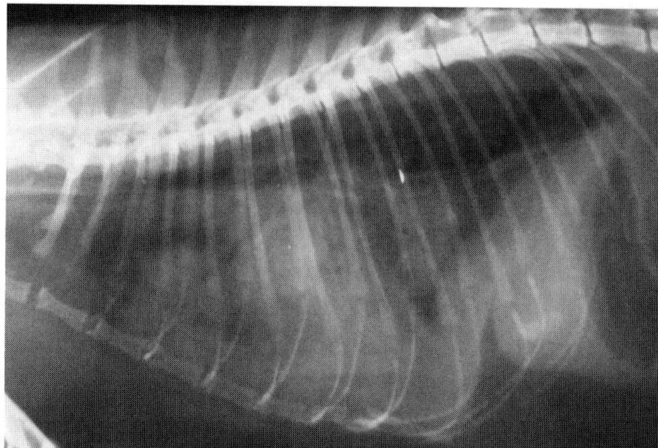

FIGURE 21-2 Lateral radiograph of a cat with congestive heart failure. Note the enlarged cardiac silhouette and widespread patchy alveolar infiltrates.

TREATMENT

Oxygen Therapy

Treatment of pulmonary edema depends on the underlying cause. No therapy is uniformly effective. Oxygen supplementation should be provided by the least stressful means to increase arterial oxygen content and tissue oxygen delivery. Patients should be subjected to minimal stress and movement should be limited to prevent increases in oxygen consumption. Animals in respiratory distress should never be forcibly restrained. A purpose-built oxygen cage is ideal, if available, but oxygen administration by flow-by, mask, or nasal cannula are also effective methods, if more stressful (see Chapter 14). Positive pressure ventilation (PPV) may be indicated in patients that cannot maintain a hemoglobin saturation greater than 90% or a partial pressure of arterial oxygen (PaO_2) greater than 60 mm Hg with noninvasive methods or in those with hypoventilation ($PaCO_2$ > 55 to 60 mm Hg) (see Chapter 30). If impending respiratory fatigue is a concern, PPV should be considered before there is significant deterioration. There is contradictory evidence regarding the effects of PPV on the resolution of pulmonary edema; PPV may help to resolve pulmonary edema in some situations but may slow it in others.[20,21]

Body position is also important to the patient with pulmonary parenchymal disease. If the animal will tolerate it, sternal recumbency aids with gas exchange, probably by reducing atelectasis and ventilation-perfusion (V/Q) mismatching.[22] In animals with unilateral disease, placing the affected lung on the uppermost side can be dangerous or even fatal, so sternal positioning or lateral recumbency with the diseased lung on the lower side is recommended.

Medical Therapy

The key to managing cardiogenic pulmonary edema is the reduction of pulmonary capillary pressures by reducing preload. Promotion of left-sided forward flow is also important in patients with large regurgitant fractions and likely in some with severe myocardial failure. The main drugs used are diuretics and vasodilators.

Furosemide, administered by bolus intravenous injection, is the mainstay of diuretic therapy for high-pressure edema because of its rapid onset of action (see Chapters 40 and 160). In addition to diuresis, furosemide also acts as a pulmonary venodilator and bronchodilator and causes an increase in COP secondary to hemoconcentration. These changes, in combination with the resultant reduction in pulmonary hydrostatic capillary pressure, may assist with alveolar fluid reabsorption.[23-25] Purported side effects of excessive use (hypovolemia and reduced mucociliary clearance because of dehydration) should not preclude furosemide use in life-threatening situations. In people, bolus injection and constant rate infusions are equally effective for management of heart failure[26,27] and the extrarenal effects seem to require bolus administration.

Because intravascular hydrostatic pressure promotes edema formation in patients with increased-permeability edema, hydrostatic pressure modification would seem logical, but most patients with increased-permeability edema do not respond as well. There is limited clinical evidence supporting furosemide use for increased-permeability edema and diuresis is not recommended in human patients, although experimental data support hydrostatic pressure modulation. The vasodilators used in acute high-pressure edema situations are the nitric oxide donors (nitroprusside, isosorbide dinitrate, and glycerol trinitrate/nitroglycerin). Nitroprusside causes arteriodilation and venodilation, whereas nitroglycerin is mainly a venodilator (see Chapters 40 and 159).

Other possible treatments for increased-permeability edema include α-adrenergic antagonists in experimental and human NPE[15,28] and β_2 agonism in toxic lung injury.[29,30] The latter act via cyclic adenosine monophosphate (cAMP) to increase fluid reabsorption by alveolar epithelial cells from the alveolar space,[29] so theoretically they could be beneficial. In people with respiratory failure and ARDS, intravenous and inhaled salbutamol were associated with a worse outcome,[30,31] likely because of increased cardiac output.

Fluid Therapy

Because the hydrostatic pressure gradient is so important in causing pulmonary edema, fluid restriction seems prudent but should be balanced against the risks of hypovolemia and compromised organ perfusion. The normal pulmonary microvascular barrier is relatively permeable to protein,[2] so natural or synthetic colloids (e.g., albumin and hydroxyethyl starches, respectively) may extravasate rapidly. If there is increased permeability such that more than half of the number of colloid molecules extravasate, colloid therapy may worsen pulmonary edema. Furthermore, macromolecular clearance from the alveoli is very slow compared with isotonic electrolyte solutions. Because vascular, interstitial, and epithelial permeability cannot be determined clinically, one has to rely on response to therapy. A trial dose of colloid may be administered cautiously in animals with suspected increased-permeability pulmonary edema, but the clinician should remain mindful that colloids could worsen some of these cases. The most recent Surviving Sepsis guidelines[33] recommend that, in patients with sepsis and septic shock, crystalloids be used for first-line resuscitation and that hydroxyethyl starches be avoided.

PROGNOSIS

Pulmonary edema has diverse causes that determine the prognosis. Usually, when there is no serious underlying disease, such as NPE in a puppy, the prognosis for resolution is relatively good. Severe increased permeability edema usually carries a poor prognosis. For cardiogenic edema the prognosis also depends on the severity of the underlying disease. Some dogs with left-sided heart failure from mitral valve disease may live for 2 or 3 years after diagnosis (median 276 days).[34] Dogs in forward failure with dilated cardiomyopathy have shorter survival times.[35] Few cats with congestive heart failure live beyond 1 to 1½ years from the time of diagnosis, with a median of 194 days.[7]

REFERENCES

1. Starling EH: On the absorption of fluid from connective tissue spaces, J Physiol (Lond) 19:312, 1896.
2. Parker JC, Perry MA, Taylor AE: Permeability of the microvascular barrier. In Staub NC, Taylor AE, editors: Edema, New York, 1984, Raven Press.
3. Taylor AE: The lymphatic safety factor: the role of edema-dependent lymphatic factors (EDLF), Lymphology 23:111, 1990.
4. Zarins CK, Rice CL, Smith DE, et al: Role of lymphatics in preventing hypooncotic pulmonary edema, Surg Forum 27:257, 1976.
5. Demling RH, LaLonde C, Ikegami K: Pulmonary edema: pathophysiology, methods of measurement, and clinical importance in acute respiratory failure, New Horiz 1:371, 1993.
6. Conhaim ROL, Lai-Fook SJ, Staub NC: Sequence of perivascular liquid accumulation in liquid-inflated dog lung lobes, J Appl Physiol 60:513, 1986.
7. Fukue M, Serikov VB, Jerome EH: Bronchial vascular reabsorption of low protein interstitial edema liquid perfused in sheep lungs, J Appl Physiol 81:810, 1996.
8. Payne J, Luis Fuentes V, Boswood A, et al: Population characteristics and survival in 127 referred cats with hypertrophic cardiomyopathy (1997 to 2005), J Small Anim Pract 51:540, 2010.
9. Ferasin L: Feline myocardial disease 1: classification, pathophysiology and clinical presentation, J Feline Med Surg 11:3, 2009.
10. Cornelius LM, Finco DR, Culver DH: Physiologic effects of rapid infusion of Ringers lactate solution into dogs, Am J Vet Res 39:1185, 1978.

11. Paige CF, Abbott JA, Elvinger F, et al: Prevalence of cardiomyopathy in apparently healthy cats, J Am Vet Med Assoc 234:1398, 2009.
12. Wilkins PA, Otto CM, Baumgardner JE, et al: Acute lung injury and acute respiratory distress syndromes in veterinary medicine: consensus definitions: The Dorothy Russell Havemeyer Working Group on ALI and ARDS in Veterinary Medicine, J Vet Emerg Crit Care 17:333, 2007.
13. O'Leary R, McKinlay J: Neurogenic pulmonary oedema, Contin Educ Anaesth Crit Care Pain 11:87, 2011.
14. Robin TJ: Speculations on neurogenic pulmonary edema (NPE), Am Rev Resp Dis 113:405, 1976.
15. Davison DL, Terek M, Chawla LS: Neurogenic pulmonary edema, Crit Care 16:212, 2012.
16. Krodel DJ, Bittner EA, Abdulnour R, et al: Case scenario: acute postoperative negative pressure pulmonary edema, Anesthesiology 113:200, 2010.
17. Al Ghofaily L, Simmons C, Chen L, et al: Negative pressure pulmonary edema after laryngospasm: a revisit with a case report, J Anesth Clin Res 3:10, 2012.
18. Udeshi A, Cantie SM, Pierre E: Postobstructive pulmonary edema, J Crit Care 25:508, 2010.
19. Fossum TW, Evering WN, Miller MW, et al: Severe bilateral pleuritis associated with chronic chylothorax in five cats and two dogs, J Am Vet Med Assoc 201:317, 1992.
20. Colmenero-Ruiz M, Fernandez-Mondejar E, Fernandez-Sacristan MA, et al: PEEP and low-tidal volume ventilation reduce lung water in porcine pulmonary edema, Am J Respir Crit Care Med 155:964, 1997.
21. Blomqvist H, Wickerts CJ, Berg B, et al: Does PEEP facilitate the resolution of extravascular lung water after experimental hydrostatic pulmonary oedema? Eur Respir J 4:1053, 1991.
22. McMillan MW, Whitaker KE, Hughes D, et al: Effect of body position on the arterial partial pressures of oxygen and carbon dioxide in spontaneously breathing, conscious dogs in an intensive care unit, J Vet Emerg Crit Care 19:564, 2009.
23. Luz da PL, Shubin H, Weil MH, et al: Pulmonary edema related to changes in colloid osmotic and pulmonary arterial wedge pressure in patients with acute myocardial infarction, Circulation 51:350, 1975.
24. Schuster CJ, Weil MH, Besso J, et al: Blood volume following diuresis induced by furosemide, Am J Med 76:585, 1984.
25. Ali J, Chernicki W, Wood LDH: Effect of furosemide in canine low-pressure edema, J Clin Invest 64:1494, 1979.
26. Amer M, Adomaityte J, Qayyum R: Continuous infusion versus intermittent bolus furosemide in ADHF: an updated meta-analysis of randomized control trials, J Hosp Med 7:270, 2012.
27. Felker GM, Lee KL, Bull DA, et al: Diuretic strategies in patients with acute decompensated heart failure, N Engl J Med 364:797, 2011.
28. Wohns RN, Tamas L, Pierce KR, Howe JF: Chlorpromazine treatment for neurogenic pulmonary edema, Crit Care Med 13:210, 1985.
29. McAuley DF, Frank JA, Fang X, et al: Clinically relevant concentrations of β_2-adrenergic agonists stimulate maximal cyclic adenosine monophosphate-dependent airspace fluid clearance and decrease pulmonary edema in experimental acid-induced lung injury, Crit Care Med 32:1470, 2004.
30. Sakuma T, Okaniwa G, Nakada T, et al: Alveolar fluid clearance in the resected human lung, Am J Respir Crit Care Med 150:305, 1994.
31 Matthay MA, Brower RG, Carson S, et al: Randomized, placebo-controlled clinical trial of an aerosolized beta-2 agonist for treatment of acute lung injury, Am J Respir Crit Care Med 342:1301, 2011.
32. Smith FG, Perkins GD, Gates S, et al: For the BALTI-2 study investigators: effect of intravenous β-2 agonist treatment on clinical outcomes in acute respiratory distress syndrome (BALTI-2): a multicentre, randomised controlled trial, Lancet 379:229, 2012.
33. Surviving Sepsis campaign: international guidelines for management of severe sepsis and septic shock: 2012, Crit Care Med 41:580, 2013.
34. Häggström J, Boswood A, O'Grady M, et al: Effect of pimobendan or benazepril hydrochloride on survival times in dogs with congestive heart failure caused by naturally occurring myxomatous mitral valve disease: the QUEST study, J Vet Intern Med 22:1124, 2008.
35. O'Grady MR, Minors SL, O'Sullivan ML, Horne R: Effect of pimobendan on case fatality rate in Doberman Pinschers with congestive heart failure caused by dilated cardiomyopathy, J Vet Intern Med 22:897, 2008.

CHAPTER 22
PNEUMONIA

Etienne Côté, DVM, DACVIM

KEY POINTS

- In dogs and cats with pneumonia, an underlying cause is almost always present. An essential part of managing these patients is to identify and correct any underlying causes in order to prevent persistence and recurrence of the disease.
- Complete blood count results are neither sensitive nor specific, and the white blood cell count cannot be used reliably to confirm or rule out pneumonia.
- More than half of dogs and cats with bacterial pneumonia are afebrile.
- In cats with pneumonia, coughing is usually absent but dyspnea is common.
- Obtaining three-view thoracic radiographs, avoiding radiographic overexposure or underexposure, and carefully examining all lung fields on all projections are important measures for detecting pneumonia radiographically.
- An endotracheal or transtracheal wash with bacterial culture and susceptibility testing is often useful for determining etiologic agents and optimal antibacterial drug selection.

Pneumonia is defined as inflammation of the lung parenchyma.[1,2] It commonly occurs in response to inhalation of infectious agents (bacteria, viruses, fungi, protozoa, helminths), either as a primary disorder or, more commonly, secondary to a predisposing disturbance. Noninfectious causes of pneumonia include idiopathic eosinophilic pneumonia, inflammation secondary to inhaled allergens or a hematogenous infection, and endogenous lipid infiltration.[1] For the criticalist, a patient with pneumonia presents at least three important possible challenges: respiratory system dysfunction, the emergence of systemic complications (e.g., multiple organ dysfunction), and the risk of contagion. Pneumonitis and pneumonia that occur as a result of inhalation of foreign substances or materials are described in Chapter 23. The focus of this chapter is infectious pneumonia.

CLINICAL PRESENTATION

Initial Evaluation

Critically ill animals with pneumonia require rapid identification and treatment because deterioration (hypoxemia, respiratory arrest) may occur quickly in fulminant cases. A soft cough, mild dyspnea, and nonspecific signs of lethargy and inappetence may be noted as the earliest manifestations in some dogs and cats. However, many patients with pneumonia show no respiratory signs (e.g., 36% of cats).[3] The spectrum of clinical signs ranges from none (the diagnosis is made incidentally on thoracic radiographs) to life-threatening dyspnea and impending cardiopulmonary arrest. Therefore pneumonia may become a consideration at one of at least three points in the evolution of a case: when clinical signs are noted by the owner, veterinarian, or both; when predisposing causes are identified; or when characteristic findings are apparent on thoracic radiographs.

History

Elements of a patient's history that should raise the clinician's index of suspicion for pneumonia are numerous. Broadly, historical clues include respiratory signs (cough, increased respiratory effort, purulent nasal discharge), systemic signs including lethargy and inappetence, and signs associated with predisposing or underlying causes (Table 22-1). Approximately 36% to 57% of dogs with pneumonia are found to have a concurrent predisposing disorder.[4,5] Geographic location and travel history may reveal important details to consider in patients suspected of having fungal or parasitic disease, and vaccination history may raise or lower the likelihood of specific infectious etiologies (e.g., canine distemper in puppies).

Physical Examination

Physical abnormalities in patients with pneumonia often are nonspecific beyond respiratory signs.[1,5] Demeanor may be normal, with some patients showing a bright and alert disposition despite having pneumonia, or abnormal, with lethargy, depression, or even obtundation predominating. Inappetence, weight loss, and signs attributable to the predisposing disorder are common. Respiratory signs are

Table 22-1 Factors Predisposing to or Associated with Pneumonia in Dogs and Cats

Factor	Comment
Impaired Patient Mobility	
Unconsciousness (natural or via general anesthesia)*	Attenuation, loss of reflexes (gag, cough)
Mechanical ventilation	Natural defense mechanisms of the upper airway bypassed by intubation and mechanical ventilation; normal movement and coughing prevented Regurgitation or aspiration of oropharyngeal bacteria may contribute
Weakness, paresis, paralysis*	—
Upper Airway Disorders	
Laryngeal mass or foreign body*	Successful laryngeal examination possible in many/most unsedated dogs using only a bright light source (Finnoff transilluminator), especially in dogs with marked dyspnea from upper airway obstruction
Laryngeal paralysis*	
Laryngeal or pharyngeal surgery*	Aspiration pneumonia (without overt clinical signs)—a common postoperative complication in animals with laryngeal paralysis (see Chapter 23)
Regurgitation Syndromes	
Esophageal motility disorder*	Dynamic esophagram (barium swallow) required for diagnosis Important if other tests do not identify an underlying cause for pneumonia
Esophageal obstruction*	Foreign body sometimes visible on thoracic radiographs Caution necessary with barium swallow procedures (barium aspiration risk); endoscopy may be preferable
Megaesophagus*	Often identifiable on plain thoracic radiographs
Other Factors	
Bronchoesophageal fistula	Usually acquired via trauma (e.g., perforating esophageal foreign body)
Cleft palate	Congenital abnormality that may cause ingesta to enter nasal cavity with subsequent aspiration
Crowded or unclean housing	Persistence and concentration of infectious organisms in environment contributors to risk
Forceful bottle feeding*	Aspiration possible when care provider squeezes the nursing bottle during suckling or if hole in nipple is too large
Gastric intubation*	—
Immune compromise	Specific conditions: anticancer or immunosuppressive chemotherapy; concurrent illness, including feline leukemia, feline infectious peritonitis, diabetes mellitus, or hyperadrenocorticism; primary ciliary dyskinesia; immunoglobulin or leukocyte defects or deficiencies
Inadequate vaccination	Viral, bacterial, or parasitic infection with secondary opportunistic bacterial pneumonia
Induced vomiting*	—
Seizures*	Must differentiate pneumonia radiographically from noncardiogenic pulmonary edema
Tracheostomy*	—

*Indicates predisposition to aspiration pneumonia.

rarely sensitive or specific. For example, dyspnea occurs with moderate or severe pneumonia but is absent in mild cases; 78% of puppies with pneumonia are tachypneic and 72% have an increased respiratory effort.[5] The cough of a patient with pneumonia may be moist or dry, and tracheal pressure may elicit a cough in some pneumonia patients and not in others. Most dogs with pneumonia (>90%) do have abnormally loud breath sounds, crackles, or wheezes on pulmonary auscultation[6]; however, these findings are nonspecific and do not allow differentiation from other causes of dyspnea (pulmonary edema, pulmonary hemorrhage). In contrast to dogs (47%),[6] cats with infectious pneumonia rarely cough (8%).[3] Mucopurulent nasal discharge may or may not be present in either species. Fever is a highly variable finding in both species, and pneumonia can be neither confirmed nor ruled out on the basis of body temperature. Animals with fungal, viral, parasitic, or protozoal pneumonia may have multisystem involvement (e.g., bone, intestinal tract, lymph nodes) and associated clinical signs. Overall, pneumonia is suspected in an animal when one or more compatible signs are noted in the history and physical examination, especially in a patient with a predisposing condition (see Table 22-1).

DIAGNOSTIC TESTING

Evaluation of patients suspected of having pneumonia is centered on diagnostic imaging and sampling respiratory secretions. Thoracic radiography remains the routine imaging test of choice. The characteristic finding is alveolar opacification. Air bronchograms, silhouetting of lung(s) with the heart, and consolidation, with or without interstitial patterns, typically are present with an asymmetric distribution (Figures 22-1 through 22-3). The alveolar pattern typical of pneumonia often is visualized more clearly in one radiographic view than in another. For example, a left lateral thoracic radiograph will allow optimal visualization of the right lung fields. Therefore, three-view thoracic radiography (a dorsoventral or ventrodorsal projection and both lateral projections) is recommended in all pneumonia suspects in order to minimize false-negative results and underdiagnosis. Computed tomography may be beneficial in animals with complicated pulmonary disease or those suspected of having foreign body–associated pneumonia; the results commonly assist in planning further surgical or diagnostic techniques.

Ancillary testing, including a complete blood count (CBC), serum biochemistry profile, and urinalysis, is important in all pneumonia suspects but rarely contributes directly to the diagnosis. Although many animals with pneumonia have unremarkable CBC results, abnormalities can include leukocytosis characterized by neutrophilia, left shift, and monocytosis.[6] Animals that are severely affected may be leukopenic, and dogs with idiopathic eosinophilic pneumonia may have a peripheral eosinophilia. Nonspecific biochemical abnormalities may be present, most commonly hypoalbuminemia secondary to inflammation or vascular leak syndromes.

A coagulation profile often is helpful in assessing critically ill patients that may have a bleeding disorder or pulmonary hemorrhage. Additional testing for hypercoagulability (e.g., thromboelastography, D-dimer, fibrin degradation product, and antithrombin levels) may be indicated in some patients, particularly if pulmonary thromboembolism is suspected.

Confirmation of bacterial lung infection requires demonstration of inflammation and infection in the lower respiratory tract. This information usually is obtained via transtracheal wash (TTW) or endotracheal wash (ETW), both of which can yield specimens for cytologic evaluation and bacterial or fungal culture and susceptibility testing. These tests are recommended when performing them is practical and safe. In all cases, a complete evaluation first must be made to identify other conditions, such as pulmonary hemorrhage (typically caused by anticoagulant ingestion) or cardiogenic pulmonary edema that would contraindicate such testing but could otherwise mimic pneumonia clinically.

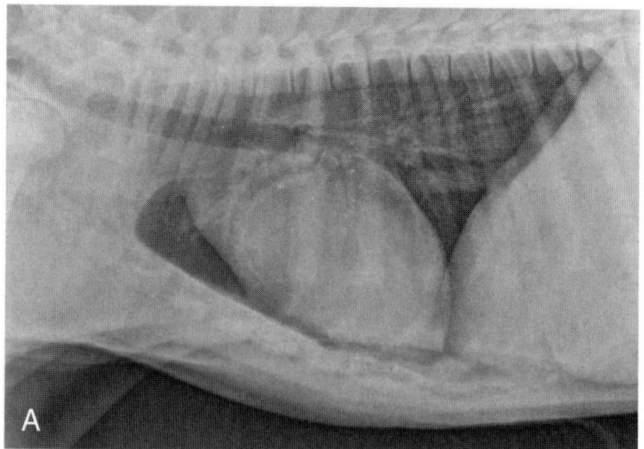

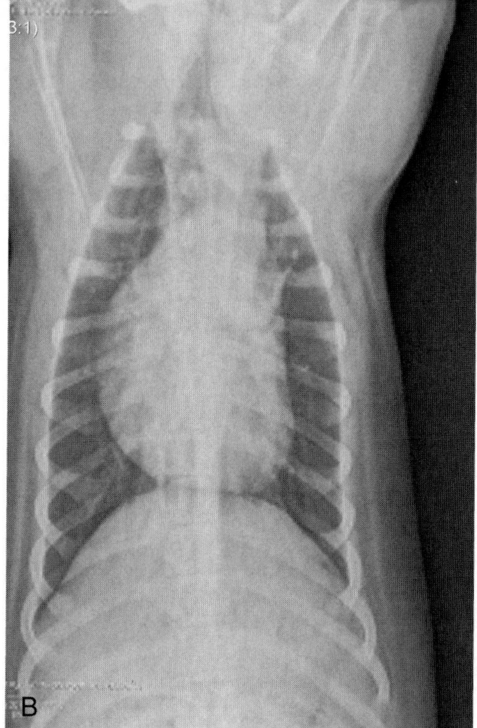

FIGURE 22-1 Thoracic radiographs (**A,** lateral projection; **B,** dorsoventral projection) of a dog with severe subaortic stenosis (SAS) and mild mitral valve dysplasia, taken at admission for surgery (cutting balloon valvuloplasty of SAS). On the lateral projection, there is a loss of the cranial cardiac waist consistent with poststenotic dilation of the ascending aorta and an enlarged dorsocaudal segment of the cardiac silhouette consistent with left atrial enlargement. The lung parenchyma is unremarkable.

Transcutaneous fine-needle aspiration of lung tissue in suspected cases of infectious pneumonia may be a low-yield, high-risk procedure, especially in dogs with diffuse pulmonary disease; a lower risk is expected if the patient is kept in lateral recumbency, aspirated side down, for 30 to 60 minutes after the procedure (15 to 20 minutes if anesthetized).[7] In cats with unexplained pulmonary parenchymal disease, fine-needle aspiration may provide a better yield than ETW.[8]

Additional diagnostic tests that may be indicated include fungal titers, serologic titers for heartworm disease and toxoplasmosis, viral testing, and fecal examination (flotation, Baermann sedimentation).

Blood gas evaluation (and pulse oximetry) can be valuable in all patients with dyspnea or respiratory distress, especially at baseline and for subsequent monitoring.[1] An arterial blood sample is

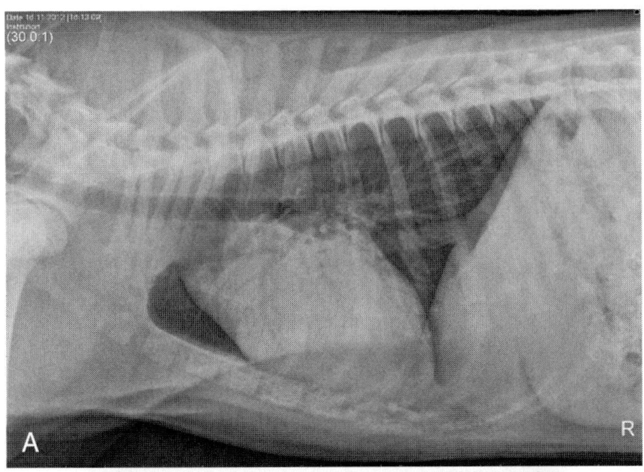

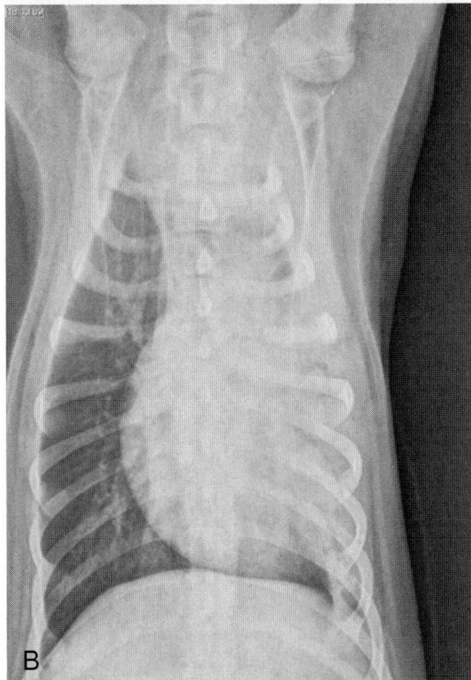

FIGURE 22-2 Thoracic radiographs (**A,** lateral projection; **B,** dorsoventral projection) from the same dog taken 24 hours later (6 hours postoperatively) because of new-onset severe dyspnea, fever, ataxia, and obtundation during anesthetic recovery. There is severe alveolar opacification of most of the left lung, consistent with pneumonia. Infiltrates are especially prominent over the cardiac silhouette in **A,** a finding that may be missed with a cursory evaluation of the radiographs. The peracute postoperative onset suggests the cause was aspiration of refluxed gastroesophageal contents; atelectasis caused by the patient's prolonged left-sided recumbency is less likely because the mediastinum has not shifted from midline.

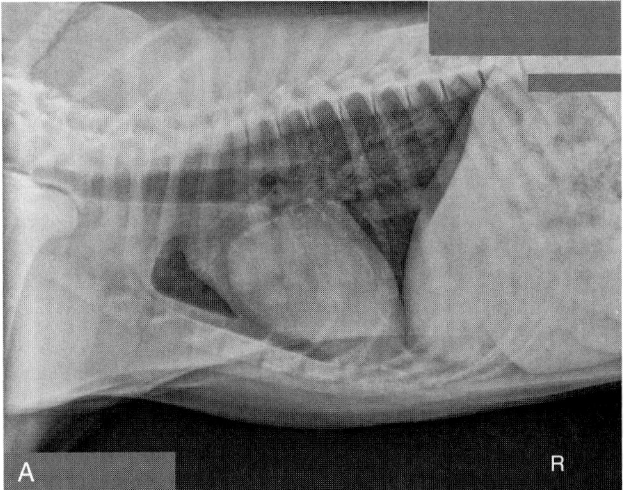

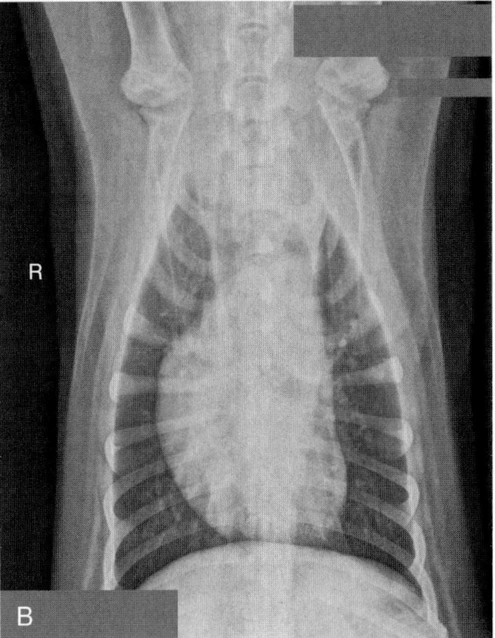

FIGURE 22-3 Thoracic radiographs (**A,** lateral projection; **B,** dorsoventral projection) from the same dog as seen in Figure 22-2 after treatment and discharge, 1 month postoperative recheck. The appearance of the lung parenchyma has returned to normal in all views.

necessary to accurately measure the partial pressure of oxygen (PaO_2) and oxygen saturation (normal: ≥80 mm Hg and ≥95%, respectively, when breathing room air at sea level). If hypoxemia is present, oxygen supplementation should be considered[1] (see Chapters 14 and 186). Abnormalities in dogs with pneumonia may include hypoxemia, decreased oxygen saturation, and increased alveolar-arterial oxygen gradient. Typically, hypercapnia is not present.[9]

PATHOPHYSIOLOGY

Mechanism

Infectious pneumonia represents an imbalance between natural defenses (upper airway mechanisms, airway barriers, humoral and cell-mediated immunity) and infectious agents. Pneumonia is characterized by bronchoalveolar inflammation. The bronchoalveolar junction is a major site of small particle (0.5 to 3 μm) deposition and is especially vulnerable to damage. Although large particles are cleared by the mucociliary apparatus, coughing, and the nasopharynx, particles smaller than 3 μm bypass the upper respiratory tract defenses and are deposited in the alveoli.[1] When large numbers of organisms, or those with high virulence, enter the lower airways, surfactant and alveolar macrophages are overwhelmed. An inflammatory response must ensue to effectively remove the offending organisms. Complex interactions between the cell-mediated and humoral immune systems, in conjunction with cytokines and chemokines, take place in an attempt to clear the offending agents.

Organisms and inflammatory exudates within the airways may lead to hypoxemia through several mechanisms. These include ventilation-perfusion mismatch, intrapulmonary shunting, and impaired diffusion. Severe or chronic pneumonia can lead to destruction of alveolar walls, damage to type II pneumocytes, and increases in pulmonary vascular permeability, all of which contribute to acute lung injury and acute respiratory distress syndrome (see Chapter 24).

If the infection and inflammation are not restricted to the lungs, a systemic inflammatory response syndrome, sepsis, and multiple organ dysfunction can occur (see Chapters 6 and 7). Animals with pneumonia may also develop bronchiectasis, pyothorax, polyarthritis, and/or glomerulonephritis.

Causes

Predisposing factors and disorders associated with pneumonia are listed in Table 22-1. Organisms commonly isolated via TTW from dogs with bacterial pneumonia include the gram-negative bacilli *Pasteurella* spp (22% to 28% of dogs with bacterial pneumonia) and Enterobacteriaceae such as *Escherichia coli* (17% to 46%), as well as gram-positive cocci such as *Staphylococcus* spp (10% to 16%) and *Streptococcus* spp (14% to 21%)[4,9,10]; in puppies with pneumonia, *Bordetella bronchiseptica* is most common (49%).[5] Anaerobic bacteria are isolated in 10% to 21% of cases,[4,9] and their presence warrants suspicion for pulmonary abscess formation. *Mycoplasma* spp commonly are detected, either as sole organisms (8%) or as coinfections with other bacteria in a large proportion of dogs with bacterial pneumonia (62%).[7,10]An emerging and poorly understood syndrome of acute, hemorrhagic, fatal pneumonia in dogs has been associated with *Streptococcus equi* subspecies *zooepidemicus* (Lancefield Group C); a unifying characteristic is housing in shelters, suggesting that contagion may play an important role.[11,12] Often, bacterial cultures from small animal patients with pneumonia reveal multiple species of bacteria (e.g., 43%,[4] 47%,[9] and 74% [including *Mycoplasma*][6] of dogs and 38% of cats[3]).

TREATMENT

Animals that are breathing comfortably and have mild pneumonia as an incidental finding should receive appropriate long-term antimicrobial therapy and supportive care, including management of underlying or predisposing factors. Immunocompromised animals should be monitored more frequently for worsening of clinical signs.

Oxygen supplementation should be provided to dyspneic and hypoxemic animals. Possible methods include flow-by delivery, intranasal cannula, oxygen cages, oxygen hoods, and oxygen tents, based on facilities and patient characteristics (see Chapter 14). The oxygen should be humidified and a sensor used for monitoring the inspired oxygen concentration. The approach to oxygen supplementation must be balanced against two important potential drawbacks: hyperthermia, especially for large breed or thick-coated dogs in an oxygen cage (even with air cooling settings) and reduced monitoring and handling because of the apparatus (oxygen cage, Elizabethan collar). Intranasal oxygen should be delivered at a flow rate of 50 to 100 ml/kg/min but never at a rate that causes discomfort or triggers the patient to actively close the nasopharynx (see Chapter 14).

Endotracheal intubation and positive pressure ventilation (see Chapter 30) are indicated if severe dyspnea leads to impending respiratory fatigue, if severe hypoxemia (partial pressure of arterial oxygen [PaO_2] < 60 mm Hg) is present, or if ventilatory failure (partial pressure of carbon dioxide [$PaCO_2$] > 60 mm Hg) occurs. An important consideration in decision making regarding mechanical ventilation in pneumonia patients is the long-term prognosis associated with the underlying cause that led to pneumonia. In some patients, pneumonia may be a surmountable obstacle and mechanical ventilation leads to a good outcome and long-term survival; such ideal candidates for mechanical ventilation have few or no preexisting illnesses and have a predisposing cause that is transient (e.g., trauma) or expected to respond to treatment. Conversely, in many patients pneumonia may be the final complication of longstanding or devastating illness, and implementation of mechanical ventilation is unlikely to lead to long-term resolution. Mechanical ventilation may still have value in such patients when owners want to try all reasonable options or when an initial response to treatment can be assessed as support for continuing treatment (good response to ventilation) versus euthanasia (poor response to ventilation). The decision to begin mechanical ventilation in a patient with pneumonia is therefore based on (1) respiratory status (respiratory rate and effort, thoracic radiographs, arterial oxygen content/pulse oximetry); (2) severity and reversibility of the inciting cause, which must be identified as completely as possible; and (3) the owner's opinion and abilities (financial, logistical, and emotional).

Empiric antimicrobial therapy is often appropriate in the initial stages of managing a patient with radiographically confirmed pneumonia, given the multiday turnaround time for bacterial culture and susceptibility testing results. Nevertheless, misuse of antimicrobial drugs can cause the patient harm. Therefore appropriate samples for bacterial culture (e.g., ETW or TTW fluid, sputum, blood, urine) should be collected before initiating antimicrobial treatment (Table 22-2). Empiric coverage should initially address gram-positive, gram-negative, and anaerobic bacteria. Animals with moderate to severe pneumonia (assessed based on respiratory signs, extent of pulmonary infiltrates on radiographs, appetite, and demeanor) should receive parenteral therapy.

For all these reasons, a common first choice approach is parenteral ampicillin and enrofloxacin, continued orally if bacterial culture results are positive and show susceptibility to these drugs. Preventive use of antimicrobials (e.g., patient hit by a car, has pulmonary contusions; antimicrobials given to prevent infection of contusions) is unsupported, selects for resistant bacteria, confers an unjustified sense of therapeutic effect, and is not recommended (see Chapter 175). Overall, antimicrobial drugs that penetrate lung tissue are preferable (such as chloramphenicol, doxycycline, enrofloxacin, trimethoprim-sulfamethoxazole, and clindamycin), although pulmonary inflammation may allow additional antimicrobials to penetrate during disease states. Such aminoglycosides as amikacin or gentamicin have the advantage of rapid onset of action and bactericidal activity. They are favored for treatment of euvolemic, normotensive, but rapidly deteriorating patients with fulminant pneumonia and sepsis that is considered likely to be of gram-negative bacterial origin, as seen in 33 of 65 puppies (51%) with bacterial pneumonia (see Figure 22-1).[5] Long-term oral therapy (6 weeks to 6 months) may be necessary after stabilization of the patient and marked improvement in oxygenating ability and radiographic infiltrates, but the exact duration must be adjusted to each patient because outcome depends on underlying cause, local immunity, nature of pathogenic organisms, and client factors. Generally, treatment is continued at least 2 weeks after radiographic resolution of pneumonia.

Animals diagnosed with idiopathic eosinophilic pneumonia or sterile inflammatory pneumonia should be treated with glucocorticoids and removal of potential allergens.

The use of bronchodilators in animals with pneumonia is controversial, but this class of drugs may be helpful in select cases by increasing airflow and mucokinetics by improving ciliary activity and increasing the serous nature of respiratory secretions. However, their use may suppress the cough reflex, worsen ventilation-perfusion mismatch, and allow exudates within the affected lung to spread to unaffected portions of the lung. β-Agonists may also have a direct antiinflammatory effect by decreasing mucosal edema and downregulating cytokine release. Methylxanthine bronchodilators may also increase mucociliary transport speed, inhibit degranulation of mast cells, and decrease microvascular permeability and leak. For example, aminophylline is a respiratory stimulant and it helps increase the strength of diaphragmatic contractility to assist animals with ventilatory fatigue. Intravenous caffeine has been used in place

Table 22-2 **Common Medications Used for Pneumonia**

Drug	Effect or Spectrum	Dosage	Formulation
Antibacterial Agents: Injectable			
Amikacin (Amiglyde-V)	G–	15 mg/kg (dog), 10 mg/kg (cat) IV q24h provided renal function and hydration are sufficient	50 mg/ml
Ampicillin (many names)	G+, some G– (certain *E. coli* and *Klebsiella* strains), some anaerobes *(Clostridia)*	22 mg/kg IV q6-8h	1-, 3-, 6-mg vials
Azithromycin	G+, G–, *Mycoplasma*	5-10 mg/kg IV q24h	500 mg/ml
Cefoxitin (Mefoxin)	Some G+, some anaerobes	30 mg/kg IV q6-8h	1-, 2-, 10-g vials
Clindamycin	G+, *Mycoplasma, Toxoplasma,* anaerobes	10 mg/kg IV q8-12h	150 mg/ml
Enrofloxacin (Baytril)	G–, *Mycoplasma*	5-10 mg/kg, dilute 1:1 in saline and give IV q12h or 12.5-20 mg/kg IV q24h (dog) or maximum 5 mg/kg q24h (cat)	22.7 mg/ml; IV is off label
Gentamicin (Gentocin)	G–	10 mg/kg (dog), 6 mg/kg (cat) IV q24h provided hydration and renal function are sufficient	50 mg/ml
Metronidazole (Flagyl)	Anaerobes	10 mg/kg slow IV infusion q12h	500 mg/100 ml
Ticarcillin-clavulanate (Timentin)	G+, G–, anaerobes	40-50 mg/kg slow IV infusion q6h	3-g vial
Trimethoprim-sulfamethoxazole	Some G+, some G–	15-30 mg/kg IV q12h	480 mg/ml
Antibacterial Agents: Oral			
Azithromycin (Zithromax)	G+, G–, *Mycoplasma*	5-10 mg/kg PO q24h	250-, 600-mg tablets; 20 or 40 mg/ml oral solution
Clindamycin (Antirobe)	G+, *Mycoplasma, Toxoplasma,* anaerobes	10 mg/kg PO q8-12h	25-, 75-, 150-mg capsules; 25 mg/ml oral solution
Metronidazole (Flagyl)	Anaerobes	10-15 mg/kg PO q12h	250 mg tablets
Trimethoprim-sulfamethoxazole (Ditrim, Tribrissen)	Some G+, some G–	15-30 mg/kg PO q12h	30, 120, 480, 960 mg tablets
Additional Therapeutic Agents			
Aminophylline	Bronchodilator and respiratory stimulant	5 mg/kg IV q8h (dilute and give over ≥30 minutes; up to 10 mg/kg in dog)	25 mg/ml
Caffeine	Bronchodilator, respiratory stimulant	5-10 mg/kg IV q6-8h (dilute and give over ≥30 minutes)	125 mg/ml
N-Acetylcysteine	Mucolytic	70 mg/kg IV q6h (dilute and give over ≥30 minutes)	20% solution
Terbutaline	Bronchodilator	0.01 mg/kg SC/IM/IV q4-6h	1 mg/ml

G–, Gram-negative; *G+*, gram-positive; *IM*, intramuscularly; *IV*, intravenously; *PO*, per os; *SC*, subcutaneously.

of aminophylline, although its benefit in veterinary medicine remains unproven.

Mucolytic therapy is used commonly in veterinary patients, but scientific proof of its benefit is lacking. *N*-acetylcysteine (NAC) leads to a breakdown of the disulfide bonds in thick airway mucus and is also a precursor to glutathione, a free radical scavenger. Aerosolized NAC may irritate the airways and cause a reflex bronchoconstriction, however, and is not recommended. Dilute intravenous NAC therapy has been used in small animals, but its effects on the respiratory system via this route are unknown.

Nebulization using 0.9% sodium chloride is an effective means of increasing particulate saline droplets in the inhaled airstream and to liquefy thick lower airway secretions in order to hydrate the mucociliary system and enhance productive clearing. Vaporizers and humidifiers are not effective because the particle size generated with these methods is greater than 3 μm in diameter.

Coupage of the chest refers to a rapid series of sharp percussions of the patient's chest using cupped hands and closed fingers. Compression of air between the cupped hand and the chest wall creates vibrational energy that is transmitted to the underlying lungs to loosen deep secretions and consolidated areas of the lung and stimulate the cough reflex. Although its effectiveness is contested in human medicine (see Chapter 23), coupage is typically performed for several minutes over affected areas of the lung. Nebulization with or without coupage should be performed every 4 to 6 hours (or continuously) in animals with pneumonia. Coupage is unnecessary in animals that are coughing spontaneously and frequently and may be contraindicated in animals that are coagulopathic, frequently regurgitating, show signs of pain in the chest region, or are fractious.

Because atelectasis can exacerbate respiratory insufficiency, hospitalized patients with pneumonia who are recumbent should be turned every 1 to 2 hours (with exceptions made to allow for restful sleep) and supported in an upright position at least every 12 hours. Short walks should be encouraged.

ADDITIONAL MANAGEMENT CONSIDERATIONS

Contagion and Zoonosis

In most cases, pneumonia-causing bacteria, as secondary invaders, are not contagious. However, contagion of the underlying process is possible by aerosol in dogs (e.g., canine distemper in the mucosal phase but not neurologic phase, infectious tracheobronchitis) and cats (e.g., feline herpesvirus, possibly calicivirus). Systemic mycoses are not contagious by aerosol from one animal directly to another.

Zoonotic concerns are minimal if the human is not immunocompromised, although *Mycobacteria* spp in dogs and cats, and the agents of plague *(Yersinia pestis)* and tularemia *(Francisella tularensis)* in cats have zoonotic potential even for immunocompetent human hosts (see Chapter 89).

MONITORING

The cornerstones of monitoring are observation and diagnostic testing. The two must occur jointly, and in the busy critical care environment it is essential to avoid managing and monitoring the patient's test results rather than the actual patient.

An attentive clinician can identify subtle changes in alertness, demeanor, appetite, respiratory effort, and other parameters that are not easily quantified but are highly valuable in assessing the patient's improvement or deterioration. More obvious changes in respiratory rate and effort, nasal flaring, cheek puffing, and orthopnea should be addressed immediately with diagnostic tests (e.g., repeated radiographs) or therapy (e.g., oxygen supplementation).

The interval between measurements of arterial blood gases and of pulse oximetry varies from minutes to days, depending on initial severity and clinical progression. Serial pulse oximetry measurements performed every 1 to 6 hours (or continuously) may reveal overall trends in arterial oxygen saturation that forewarn of positive or negative changes. However, single measurements should be interpreted with caution because erroneous readings may occur (see Chapter 186).

Thoracic radiographs may be used for monitoring progression of pulmonary disease, but for patients that are stable or improving, radiographic findings are unlikely to change during the first few days of treatment. Therefore retaking thoracic radiographs of a patient with pneumonia is not indicated during the first 3 to 5 days, except when the animal's condition is deteriorating or unexpected new clinical signs emerge. It is common for patients with severe pneumonia, especially puppies with *Bordetella* pneumonia, to show clinical and radiographic signs suggesting deterioration during the first few days of treatment, even when the subsequent outcome is excellent.[5]

PROGNOSIS AND OUTCOME

Response to antimicrobial therapy is observed in most dogs (69% to 88%) when pneumonia is managed appropriately[6,10]; acute, fulminant, hemorrhagic pneumonia of shelter dogs is an important exception.[11,12] Long-term outcome depends on the ability to resolve the inciting or associated cause, with a cure expected when reversal of the trigger is possible (e.g., surgical foreign body removal)[13] versus long-term management and frequent relapses expected when the predisposing cause lingers (e.g., idiopathic megaesophagus). Recurrent bouts of bacterial pneumonia should prompt the clinician to rule out bronchiectasis, an abscess or foreign body, other structural changes in the respiratory tract (e.g., ciliary dyskinesia), or inappropriate antimicrobial therapy (e.g., discontinuing therapy prematurely or antibiotic resistance) that may allow infection to persist or recur within the lungs. Surgical treatment (lung lobectomy) has led to resolution of pneumonia in 54% of dogs, with a higher percentage of success when a foreign body, or no bacterial isolates, were identified.[13] Anecdotal reports and observations suggest that certain bacteria, specific underlying disorders, and empiric antimicrobial treatment (instead of management based on culture and susceptibility) are associated with a worse prognosis.[6,10] Subjectively, the initial severity of clinical signs and response during intensive treatment also offer prognostic information. However, a comprehensive assessment of specific, evidence-based prognostic parameters is lacking for small animal bacterial pneumonia. Fungal, viral, parasitic, and protozoal pneumonias vary in their response to management, often depending on pathogenicity of the offending organism, degree of systemic involvement, immunnocompetence of the patient, and underlying risk factors.

REFERENCES

1. Brady CA: Bacterial pneumonia in dogs and cats. In King LG, editor: Textbook of respiratory disease in dogs and cats, St Louis, 2004, Saunders.
2. Cohn L: Pulmonary parenchymal diseases. In Ettinger SJ, Feldman EC, editors: Textbook of veterinary internal medicine, ed 7, St Louis, 2010, Elsevier.
3. Macdonald ES, Norris CR, Berghaus RB, Griffey SM: Clinicopathologic and radiographic features and etiologic agents in cats with histologically confirmed infectious pneumonia: 39 cases (1991-2000), J Am Vet Med Assoc 223:1142, 2003.
4. Angus JC, Jang SS, Hirsh DC: Microbiological study of transtracheal aspirates from dogs with suspected lower respiratory tract disease: 264 cases (1989-1995), J Am Vet Med Assoc 210:55, 1997.
5. Radhakrishnan A, Drobatz KJ, Culp WTN, et al: Community-acquired infectious pneumonia in puppies: 65 cases (1993-2002), J Am Vet Med Assoc 230:1493, 2007.
6. Thayer GW, Robinson SK: Bacterial bronchopneumonia in the dog: a review of 42 cases, J Am Anim Hosp Assoc 20:731, 1984.
7. Chandler JC, Lappin MR: Mycoplasmal respiratory infections in small animals: 17 cases (1988-1999), J Am Anim Hosp Assoc 38:111, 2002.
8. Sauve V, Drobatz KJ, Shokek AB, et al: Clinical course, diagnostic findings and necropsy diagnosis in dyspneic cats with primary pulmonary parenchymal disease: 15 cats (1996-2002), J Vet Emerg Crit Care 15:38, 2005.
9. Wingfield WE, Matteson VL, Hackett T, et al: Arterial blood gases in dogs with bacterial pneumonia, J Vet Emerg Crit Care 7:75, 1997.
10. Jameson PH, King LA, Lappin MR, Jones RL: Comparison of clinical signs, diagnostic findings, organisms isolated, and clinical outcome in dogs with bacterial pneumonia: 93 cases (1986-1991), J Am Vet Med Assoc 206:206, 1995.
11. Pesavento PA, Hurley KF, Bannasch MJ, Artiushin S, Timoney JF: A clonal outbreak of acute fatal hemorrhagic pneumonia in intensively housed (shelter) dogs caused by *Streptococcus equi* subsp. *zooepidemicus*, Vet Pathol 45:51, 2008.
12. Gower S, Payne R: Sudden deaths in greyhounds due to canine haemorrhagic pneumonia (letter), Vet Rec 170:630, 2012.
13. Murphy ST, Ellison GW, McKiernan BC, Mathews KG, Kubilis PS: Pulmonary lobectomy in the management of pneumonia in dogs: 59 cases (1972-1994), J Am Vet Med Assoc 210: 235, 1997.

CHAPTER 23

ASPIRATION PNEUMONITIS AND PNEUMONIA

Robert A.N. Goggs, BVSc, DACVECC, PhD, MRCVS • Amanda K. Boag, MA, VetMB, DACVIM, DACVECC, MRCVS

KEY POINTS

- Aspiration pneumonitis has a biphasic pathogenesis. Initial events are caused by direct chemical injury and are followed by localized inflammatory mediator cascades producing neutrophil chemotaxis, sequestration, and subsequent increased permeability edema.
- Aspiration pneumonia is an infectious process caused either by aspiration of contaminated material or by bacterial colonization of damaged lungs subsequent to a sterile aspiration episode. Acid-induced lung injury enhances bacterial adherence within the airways and reduces bacterial clearance from the lungs.
- Diagnosis is typically based on history, physical examination, and radiography. The severity of respiratory compromise is best assessed and monitored by arterial blood gas analysis.
- Treatment is principally supportive, consisting of airway management, cardiovascular support, oxygen therapy, and respiratory physiotherapy.
- Antimicrobial drug therapy should be directed by cytologic evaluation, Gram stain, and bacterial culture and susceptibility testing of samples collected by tracheal wash or bronchoalveolar lavage.
- The incidence of aspiration pneumonia can be reduced by recognizing the risk factors and attempting to control or minimize them.

Aspiration pneumonitis and pneumonia frequently coexist in veterinary patients and may cause significant morbidity and mortality. Both conditions share a common pathophysiology after direct pulmonary injury and the initiation of a localized inflammatory cascade that impairs respiratory function. Both conditions may incite development of acute lung injury (ALI) or acute respiratory distress syndrome (ARDS).[1] A number of risk factors exist for aspiration of gastric contents.[2,3] Clinicians should be aware of these risk factors and understand the subsequent pathogenesis of pulmonary damage to aid prevention, early recognition, and optimization of patient monitoring and treatment.

DEFINITIONS

Aspiration Pneumonitis

Aspiration pneumonitis is defined as acute lung injury caused by inhalation of chemical irritants. Inhalation of regurgitated gastric contents is the principal cause and is the focus of this chapter; other causes include inhalation of freshwater,[4] saltwater, and hydrocarbons.

Aspiration Pneumonia

Aspiration pneumonia is the pulmonary bacterial infection that develops after aspiration. Although pneumonitis and pneumonia are considered separate entities in people,[5] the distinction is poorly defined in veterinary species and the two syndromes are difficult to differentiate clinically. Aspiration pneumonia can result from bacterial colonization of lungs injured by acid aspiration or from aspiration of contaminated material. Because oropharyngeal colonization with pathogenic bacteria is extremely common in dogs and cats, both mechanisms likely occur. Inhalation of small quantities of oropharyngeal material contaminated by bacteria can occur in normal, healthy animals; bacterial colonization of the respiratory tree is prevented by rapid removal of this material by coughing and mucociliary clearance and infection prevented by robust humoral and cellular immunity. When the respiratory epithelium is damaged, the mucociliary clearance mechanisms impaired, or the immune system depleted or simply overwhelmed, pneumonia may ensue.

ASPIRATION PNEUMONITIS AND PNEUMONIA

Epidemiology

In veterinary medicine, between 5% and 26% cases of aspiration pneumonia are reported to be complications of anesthesia.[3] The incidence of aspiration pneumonitis is unknown but may be higher. In people, many instances of gastric aspiration are unwitnessed,[6] and silent gastric aspiration is a plausible cause of postoperative pulmonary complications in dogs.[7] Gastric aspiration complicates 1 in every 2000 to 3000 cases of general anesthesia in people[8]; a similar rate is plausible in veterinary medicine because large numbers of healthy animals are anesthetized for routine procedures.

Two recent studies have collectively reported information on more than 200 dogs with aspiration pneumonia.[2,3] These data suggest that gastrointestinal disorders are the most common risk factor, present in more than 60% cases, with megaesophagus the leading cause (26% of total cases). Neurologic disorders and laryngeal diseases occurred in 18% and 13% of the cases, respectively. Many dogs had multiple risk factors, including recent anesthesia. These risk factors closely parallel the situation in people.[9] Reported survival rates for aspiration pneumonia managed in academic referral institutions are 77% to 82%,[2,3] and outcome does not appear to be dependent on the type or number of underlying disorders. Dogs were typically hospitalized for 3 to 5 days at a cost of $2000 to $3000 in 2008. Few prognostic indicators have been identified in dogs, but it should be recognized that lung injury severity after gastric aspiration represents a continuum between subclinical pneumonitis and ARDS with respiratory failure. Disease progression to ARDS and the need for ventilation heralds a lower survival rate.

Pathophysiology

The magnitude of lung injury after gastric aspiration depends on the pH, volume, osmolality, and presence of particulate matter in the aspirate.[10] Severe histologic damage is caused by aspirates with a pH less than 1.5, but minimal damage is caused by aspirates with pH greater than 2.4 unless they contain particulate matter.[11,12] From these observations, three models of gastric aspiration have evolved: acid instillation, food particle injury, and combined acid-particle aspiration.[9]

Acid-induced lung injury, modeled by tracheal instillation of hydrochloric acid, has a biphasic pathogenesis.[13] Initially the direct caustic effects of the aspirate damage bronchial and alveolar epithelium and the pulmonary capillary endothelium. The acid aspirate also stimulates tracheobronchial substance P–immunoreactive neurons involved in control of bronchial smooth muscle tone and vascular permeability. Stimulation of these nerves induces tachykinin neuropeptide release, resulting in neurogenic inflammation, bronchoconstriction, vasodilation, and increased vascular permeability that peaks at 1 to 2 hours after aspiration.[14] In guinea pig models, tachykinin release in the lungs occurs after esophageal stimulation by gastric acid because of the presence of nonadrenergic, noncholinergic neural networks between the esophagus and the trachea.[15] Histologically, first-phase damage consists of epithelial and endothelial degeneration, necrosis of type I alveolar cells, and intraalveolar hemorrhage.

The second phase of acid-induced lung injury starts 4 to 6 hours after aspiration and is characterized by larger increases in pulmonary capillary permeability and protein extravasation. Extensive edema formation may ensue, compromising gas exchange and resulting in ventilation-perfusion mismatch and reduced lung compliance.[13] Chemotactic mediators released by alveolar macrophages, particularly interleukin 8,[16] tumor necrosis factor α,[17] and macrophage inflammatory protein 2,[18] attract neutrophils to the lung after the initial aspiration episode. Sequestration of activated neutrophils generates a localized proinflammatory state because of increased concentrations of reactive oxygen species,[19] proteinases[20] and complement proteins.[21] Complement activation by mast cell degranulation may lead to involvement of the contralateral lung even if the aspiration is unilateral.[22]

Particulate matter incites a neutrophilic response concomitant with increased inflammatory mediator concentrations but does not generate pulmonary edema.[12] Particulate matter may also cause small airway obstruction, prolong the inflammatory response, and act as a source of, and nidus for, bacterial infection.[23] Combination acid-particulate aspirates induce greater injury than either component alone,[24] characterized by larger and longer lasting tumor necrosis factor α expression, increased neutrophil sequestration, and greater levels of pulmonary capillary leak.[25]

Aspiration pneumonia may develop concomitantly with pneumonitis if the aspirated contents are contaminated with oropharyngeal bacteria. Alternatively, aspiration pneumonia may develop after pneumonitis by subsequent bacterial colonization of the damaged respiratory tract. Gastric aspiration increases the risk of subsequent pneumonia development through enhanced bacterial adherence to the respiratory epithelium[26] and reduced pulmonary clearance of bacteria.[27] Prior pneumonitis also increases the severity of subsequent pneumonia.[28] Bacteria reported in companion animals include enteric bacteria such as *Escherichia coli*, *Klebsiella* spp, and *Enterococcus* spp; oropharyngeal *Mycoplasma* spp; primary respiratory pathogens, including *Pasteurella* spp, *Pseudomonas* spp, and *Streptococcus* spp; and commensals such as *Staphylococcus* spp.[3,29] Polymicrobial infections are common. The development of pneumonia after gastric aspiration is a risk factor for subsequent development of both ARDS[1] and sepsis,[2,30] which substantially increase the risk of mortality.

Diagnosis

History

A full clinical history from the primary caregiver is essential in making a diagnosis of aspiration pneumonia. However, an index of suspicion must be maintained even in the absence of a clear history of aspiration, because aspiration episodes are rarely witnessed. Hospitalized patients perceived as at risk should have frequent respiratory system assessments; aspiration should be suspected if respiratory distress develops acutely.

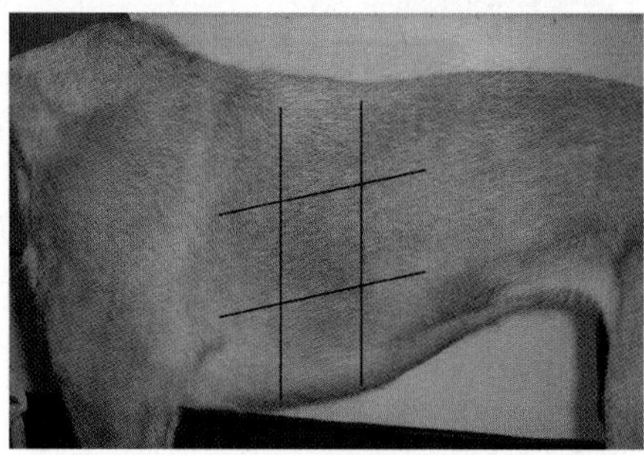

FIGURE 23-1 The "chessboard" analogy, wherein the lung fields are subdivided into smaller areas to enhance sensitivity of auscultation and to enable more accurate localization of abnormal lung sounds.

Physical examination

The clinical signs of aspiration include acute-onset respiratory distress, potentially accompanied by cough, lethargy, weakness, or collapse. Signs of associated disorders such as vomiting, regurgitation or neurologic abnormalities are often also present. Mucous membranes are typically normal, but hyperemic or cyanotic membranes may occur. Pyrexia is common (approximately 40% cases) and may be more frequent when aspiration events occur in hospital.[31] Respiratory pattern, rate, rhythm, effort, and depth should be observed. Most patients (70% to 75%)[3,31] with aspiration pneumonia have abnormal lung sounds on auscultation, but normal lung sounds do not preclude clinically relevant aspiration. Lung sounds in patients with aspiration pneumonia are often louder than normal; it is particularly important to consider whether the lung sounds are appropriate for the patient's respiratory rate and effort.[32] Fine crackles may be heard during inspiration, especially in the cranioventral areas. Rarely, lung sounds may be significantly decreased if a large bronchus becomes filled with exudates and cellular debris preventing the passage of air. Subdivision of the lung fields for auscultation may aid in lesion localization and improve detection rates (Figure 23-1).

Radiography and computed tomography

Thoracic radiography remains the mainstay for diagnosis of aspiration. Patients typically develop an alveolar lung pattern as a result of displacement of air from alveoli by fluid accumulation and cellular infiltration, although an interstitial pattern may also be seen.[31] In the dog and cat, aspiration pneumonia typically affects the right middle lung lobe and ventral parts of the other lobes (Figure 23-2). Lesion distribution may be affected by patient position at the time of aspiration.[33] History, clinical suspicion, and radiographic lesions are often sufficient to diagnose aspiration pneumonia. Radiologic differential diagnoses include infectious bronchopneumonia, pulmonary hemorrhage, neoplasia, and lobar collapse or torsion. Radiographic signs of aspiration pneumonia may change markedly over time, lag hours behind the onset of respiratory distress, or persist for several days despite clinical improvement. Correlations between radiographic severity and clinical signs, hypoxemia, or prognosis are generally poor, although involvement of multiple lobes was associated with reduced survival in a recent study.[3]

Radiography is also useful for identifying disorders that predispose to aspiration. Megaesophagus is identified readily on plain thoracic radiographs. Contrast studies may be needed to investigate and identify pharyngeal or esophageal motility disorders. However, they should be performed with caution because contrast media is aspirated easily by these patients (Figure 23-3).

Helical (spiral) thoracic computed tomography (CT) has not been widely used for evaluation of patients with aspiration

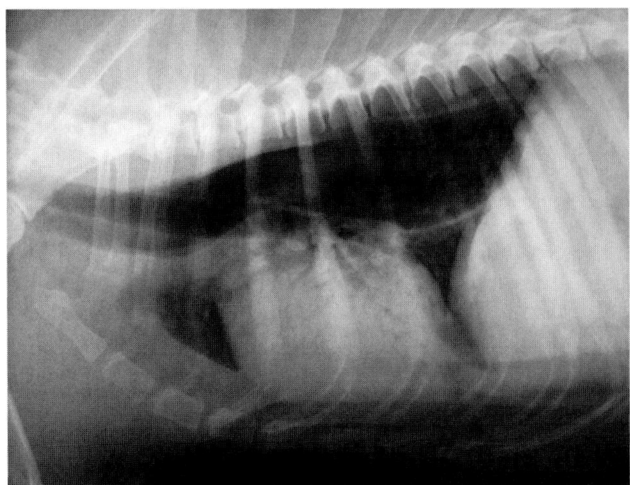

FIGURE 23-2 A right lateral thoracic radiograph of a dog with aspiration pneumonia secondary to megaesophagus. There is an alveolar pattern in the area of the right middle lung lobe and overlying the cardiac silhouette. Several air bronchograms can be seen.

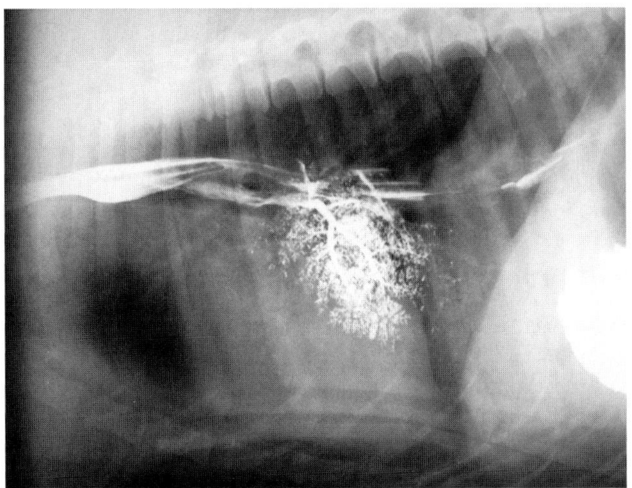

FIGURE 23-3 A right lateral thoracic radiograph of a dog with an esophageal motility disorder, showing contrast material within the esophagus, stomach, trachea, and right middle lung lobe.

pneumonia partly because of the accuracy of plain radiography for diagnosis of aspiration pneumonia. Limited access to this technology, potential risks associated with sedation for CT, and higher costs may also contribute. Typical CT findings in patients with aspiration pneumonia have been described,[33] and there is evidence to suggest CT may provide important additional information in select cases.[34]

Tracheal wash

Tracheal wash (TW) is a minimally invasive diagnostic test used in both dogs and cats to obtain airway samples for cytologic analysis and bacterial culture and susceptibility testing. TW can be performed via transtracheal (TTW) or endotracheal (ETW) wash techniques, depending on the size and stability of the patient. Both techniques are suitable for investigation of suspected aspiration pneumonia with ETW typically being preferred in smaller patients. In dogs, TTW may be as sensitive as transbronchial biopsy, lung aspirates, and bronchoalveolar lavage (BAL) for diagnosis of pneumonia,[35] although it may be less specific than other techniques. The use of TTW to diagnosis bacterial pneumonia has a sensitivity rate of 45% to 70%.[3,36,37] Oral swabs may be considered.[38]

Bronchoscopy and bronchoalveolar lavage

Bronchoscopy enables visualization of the respiratory tract lumen (typically to the tertiary bronchi level), assessment of airway injury, and collection of lavage samples. BAL retrieves larger volumes of fluid directly from visibly affected areas than TW, potentially providing greater sensitivity, specificity, and increased diagnostic yield. Guidelines for human adults recommend BAL for obtaining quantitative bacterial cultures and to differentiate pneumonitis from pneumonia.[39] In dogs and cats this distinction is less clear, however, and the procedure is not without risk in patients suffering from respiratory compromise. BAL is a more invasive diagnostic sampling technique than TW, necessitates anesthesia, and may cause bronchospasm and transient but potentially significant decreases in lung function. A blind BAL technique is described in which the sampling tube is inserted through the ET tube and advanced until resistance is met before the lavage fluid is injected. The technique is considered to be a valuable option in children.[40]

Complete blood cell count and serum biochemistry

Blood samples for complete blood cell count (CBC) and serum biochemistry values are indicated in all patients suspected of recently aspirating gastric contents. Common hematologic abnormalities include a neutrophilia or neutropenia with a left shift and lymphopenia.[3,31] These changes are nonspecific and labile reflecting the degree of inflammatory response. Both CBC and serum biochemistry analysis are useful for identifying and investigating comorbidities.

Oxygenation status

Patients with aspiration pneumonia often present with hypoxemia, which can be identified by pulse oximetry.[3] Arterial blood gas is, however, a more sensitive and reliable tool (see Chapter 15). Changes in arterial blood gas values have minimal lag time after aspiration. They provide an objective assessment of respiratory functional impairment, which can be measured serially to assess changes in lung function over time, as well as to guide and monitor therapeutic interventions. Typical changes include hypoxemia and hypocapnia, increased alveolar-arterial (A-a) gradient, and in some cases limited oxygen responsiveness. Hypercapnia is less common and suggests respiratory muscle fatigue, bronchoconstriction, or the presence of severe pulmonary parenchymal disease (see Chapter 186).

Biomarkers

Diagnosis of unwitnessed aspiration and differentiation of aspiration pneumonitis from pneumonia are diagnostic challenges. In animals with aspiration pneumonia, as elsewhere in medicine, biomarkers that might aid this process are avidly being sought. Single biomarkers such as procalcitonin,[41] sTREM-1, and C-reactive protein are not sufficiently specific to be of value, although procalcitonin may provide prognostic information.[42] Cytokine profiles in BAL fluid do correlate well with type and duration of injury but are yet to be validated in human studies.[43] Because cytokines have now been evaluated in various canine diseases, developments in this area may improve the clinician's diagnostic accuracy in the future.

Treatment

In veterinary patients, where the distinction between pneumonitis and pneumonia secondary to aspiration is often unclear, the principle aims of therapy are as follows:

1. Support respiratory function through airway management, oxygen supplementation, and mechanical ventilation if necessary. Other adjunctive respiratory therapies may be considered, but evidence for efficacy is limited.

2. Treat bacterial infections with appropriate antimicrobial therapy.
3. Manage underlying or predisposing conditions.

Airway management

After a witnessed aspiration event, airway patency should be established immediately; endotracheal intubation may be necessary. Foreign material obstructing the airway should be removed immediately. Aspirated liquid material will disperse quickly, but suctioning of the pharynx may reduce further aspiration and will facilitate intubation. Judicious airway suctioning may aid in fluid removal, but care should be taken not to cause atelectasis or mucosal damage. Therapeutic bronchoscopy is only indicated for atelectasis caused by mucous plugs, which are uncommon in animals after aspiration. Large-volume lavage of the affected areas is not recommended. Experimental work suggests that instillation of exogenous surfactant might be beneficial in canines with aspiration pneumonitis.[44] Although recent large-scale trials in human ALI/ARDS were not successful,[45] subgroup analyses suggested that patients with aspiration pneumonia might benefit.[46] Unfortunately a recent large scale trial investigating this treatment failed to confirm this; the future for surfactant therapy in aspiration is now uncertain.[47]

Oxygen therapy

Aspiration pneumonia results in severe hypoxemia as a result of V/Q mismatch, intrapulmonary shunting, and hypoventilation. Oxygen therapy is indicated in animals with respiratory distress, hypoxemia, or inadequate hemoglobin saturation. Numerous minimally invasive techniques are described, including nasal flow-by, masks, insufflation via nasopharyngeal catheters, oxygen hoods, and oxygen cages (see Chapter 14). Oxygen administration should be sufficient to alleviate respiratory distress and ensure adequate arterial partial pressure of oxygen (PaO_2). Oxygen toxicity has not been reported in the clinical veterinary literature, but experimental studies suggest prolonged, high inspired oxygen concentrations may have detrimental effects, including increased lung permeability, protein extravasation, and impaired compliance.[48] Oversupplementation should therefore be avoided.

Mechanical ventilation

Ventilatory support may be required in patients with progressive ventilatory failure (hypercarbia) or failure of pulmonary oxygen delivery or exchange (hypoxemia) when less invasive methods of oxygen support are inadequate (see Chapter 30). The decision to mechanically ventilate is typically made on the basis of serial arterial blood gas analyses and repeated patient examinations. Patients ventilated for pulmonary parenchymal diseases generally have a poorer prognosis than those ventilated for neuromuscular disease. This is likely because patients with pulmonary parenchymal disease have a much higher risk of complications of ventilation, including alveolar rupture, pneumothorax, capillary endothelial damage, impairment of venous return, and ventilator-associated pneumonia, compared with patients with hypercapnia and primary ventilatory failure. Use of lung-protective strategies has significantly improved survival rates in human with ARDS (see Chapter 31).[49] When possible, ventilation of these patients may be worthwhile because 30% are successfully discharged from the hospital.[50]

Antimicrobial therapy

Antimicrobial therapy is not indicated in the early stages of aspiration pneumonitis management. Early use of antimicrobials after aspiration may be more appropriate in patients with additional risk factors for pneumonia such as concurrent proton pump inhibitor use or gastrointestinal obstruction. Antimicrobials are, however, a vital part of treatment for patients with aspiration pneumonia. Antimicrobial selection should be based on culture and susceptibility testing results from samples obtained by TW or BAL. Cultures will not be possible in all cases and, regardless, results will not be available immediately. Cytologic analysis of airway washes, including Gram stain, should be used to guide antimicrobial choices while culture and susceptibility testing results are pending. The polymicrobial nature of many aspiration pneumonia infections supports the use of broad-spectrum antimicrobials or the use of several agents with overlapping spectra. Anaerobic coverage is unlikely to be necessary.[3,51] Empirical antimicrobial therapy should be chosen with consideration of local resistance profiles and should be deescalated or withdrawn if bacterial cultures are negative. Regardless of whether therapy is empirical or based on culture, it must be reevaluated based on clinical response; if patients are worsening, alternative therapy and repeated airway sampling and culture should be considered. In patients with worsening respiratory signs or failure, research suggests that the bacterial isolates may have different resistance profiles from those infecting patients with less severe disease.[51] The pharmacokinetics of antimicrobial agents should be considered during product selection (see Chapter 175). Polar drugs such as the cephalosporins and penicillins penetrate poorly, although they may achieve higher levels in inflamed tissues. Lipophilic molecules such as the fluoroquinolones penetrate natural body barriers readily and will reach therapeutic levels in bronchial secretions. Commonly used antimicrobials include β-lactamases in combination with fluoroquinolones.[2,3] Due consideration for prudent use of antimicrobials should be given before use of second- or third-line drugs.[52]

Bronchodilators

Bronchodilator drugs such as salbutamol and terbutaline may be of use in patients with acute aspiration pneumonitis if bronchoconstriction is part of the physiologic response to acid injury. Only when bronchospasm can be identified or is strongly suspected is bronchodilator therapy rational. Use of bronchodilators in animals with pneumonia is not recommended because the inotropic and vasodilator properties of these agents can increase perfusion of poorly ventilated lung units, thus worsening hypoxemia. Two recent human trials of inhaled albuterol in ALI/ARDS both suggest that this approach is unlikely to be beneficial and may worsen outcomes.[53,54]

Cardiovascular support

Fluid therapy should be used judiciously in patients with aspiration pneumonitis or pneumonia, because any increase in pulmonary capillary hydrostatic pressure will tend to exacerbate fluid extravasation into the alveoli. The patient's intravascular volume and hydration status should be assessed frequently and fluid therapy tailored to individual patient requirements, with due consideration for the degree of cardiovascular and respiratory compromise (see Chapters 57 and 59). In patients with sepsis secondary to aspiration pneumonia, optimization of hemodynamic parameters through use of goal-directed therapy should be undertaken (see Chapter 5 and the Surviving Sepsis guidelines).[55]

Chest physiotherapy

Respiratory physiotherapy is often employed to enhance clearance of airway secretions in patients with pneumonia. Systematic reviews report a lack of evidence to support this common practice,[56] although there is clearly equipoise among specialists regarding the use of physiotherapy in patients with pneumonia.[57] The evidence from children with community-acquired pneumonia does not support use of chest physiotherapy.[58] In contrast, two recent studies of ventilator-associated pneumonia have demonstrated reductions in pulmonary infection scores[59,60] and one of these publications suggested that twice daily chest physiotherapy may confer a survival benefit.[60]

Nebulization and coupage are the form of respiratory physiotherapy most often used in veterinary patients with aspiration pneumonia.[3] This therapy aims to humidify bronchial secretions and encourage their removal from the airways. No studies evaluating respiratory physiotherapy in veterinary patients have been performed. Respiratory physiotherapy may not be entirely benign because one study has documented a longer duration of pyrexia in those receiving this therapy.[61] The evidence suggests that ventilated patients are likely to benefit most from this practice, likely because anesthesia and intubation prevent the biological and behavioral mechanisms that aid in the clearance of airway secretions in the conscious patient. Airway humidification and coupage in ventilated patients may need to be coupled with careful airway suctioning in order to maximize the benefits.

Glucocorticoids

Few therapies in medicine cause more contention than the use of glucocorticoids; the situation is no different in pneumonia, where successive evidence reviews have reached opposing conclusions.[62-64] Glucocorticoids could theoretically be beneficial in suppressing the proinflammatory state that occurs in patients with aspiration pneumonitis, and some authors continue to consider steroid administration to these patients.[5] However, these agents suppress the immune system by decreasing levels of T-lymphocytes, inhibiting chemotaxis and phagocytosis, and antagonizing complement. The development of pneumonia is probable after gastric aspiration in veterinary patients; therefore glucocorticoid therapy may worsen the resulting infection and increase the associated mortality. In the absence of strong evidence of benefit, and in the face of risk of worsening outcome, routine use of glucocorticoid therapy in patients with pneumonia is not recommended. Only in the specific case of vasopressor-dependent septic shock secondary to pneumonia (or patients with previously diagnosed hypoadrenocorticism) should low-dose hydrocortisone be considered.[55]

Prevention

Preventing aspiration events is preferable to managing these patients once aspiration has already occurred. Clearly, this will not be possible in all patients, especially those with impaired airway reflexes or diseases that predispose to vomiting or regurgitation. Improved recognition of these patients and targeting preventive strategies towards them will be particularly beneficial. In addition, when our medical interventions place patients at risk,[65] we must attempt to minimize the impact through alterations in practice or by pharmacologic means when necessary.

Recently updated guidelines on perianesthetic fasting suggest that 6 hours is appropriate to minimize gastric volumes, although only 2 hours is necessary after liquid ingestion.[66] In dogs, fasting reliably increases gastric pH to a median 24-hour intragastric pH of 4.4.[67] The American Society of Anesthesiologists (ASA) recommendations may be excessive, however, and should not impede sedation or anesthesia in emergency situations.[68] Evacuation of the stomach via suction or using a nasogastric or orogastric tube in anesthetized, high-risk patients may be appropriate.[69]

For emergency anesthesia, short-term periprocedural gastric alkalinization to a pH higher than 2.5 may be appropriate to minimize the risk of acid-induced lung injury in patients considered to be at risk for aspiration.[69] Famotidine, pantoprazole, or omeprazole, but not ranitidine, would be suitable to achieve this in canine patients that have not fasted (see Chapter 161).[67] Conversely, long-term gastric alkalinization using histamine 2 (H_2) receptor antagonists or proton pump inhibitors may increase the risk of community- and hospital-acquired pneumonia in people, likely by promoting gastric bacterial colonization.[70-72] Similar veterinary studies are not available presenting evidence-based recommendations. However, these medications do increase intragastric pH in dogs; it is therefore probable that bacterial colonization may also occur in our patients. Patients on long-term gastric alkalinization therapy should be considered at increased risk of gastric bacterial colonization and aspiration pneumonia.

Prokinetic drugs such as metoclopramide enhance gastric emptying by increasing gastric contraction and small-intestine peristalsis. Metoclopramide is also an antidopaminergic antiemetic that, in combination with an H_2 receptor antagonist given 12 hours before and on the day of anesthesia, reliably reduces the risk of aspiration in humans. The periprocedural intravenous administration of metoclopramide and an H_2 receptor antagonist may be useful for emergency anesthesia in veterinary patients that have not been fasted.

Enteral feeding, whether it is esophageal, gastric, or postpyloric, predisposes patients to aspiration pneumonia.[73,74] Bacterial colonization of enteral feeding tubes occurs within 4 days of intensive care unit admission in human patients receiving gastric alkalinizing drugs.[75] Systemic antimicrobials will neither prevent nor manage this colonization. Because nutritional support of critical patients is important for recovery, the aspiration risk should be minimized using safe feeding protocols. Particular care should be taken when recumbent patients are fed enterally, and the residual gastric volume should be ascertained before administration of food if possible. Feeding should be stopped at any sign of patient discomfort or resistance and the tube position checked (see Chapter 129).

REFERENCES

1. Wilkins PA, Otto CM, Baumgardner JE, et al: Acute lung injury and acute respiratory distress syndromes in veterinary medicine: consensus definitions: The Dorothy Russell Havemeyer Working Group on ALI and ARDS in Veterinary Medicine, J Vet Emerg Crit Care 17:333, 2007.
2. Kogan DA, Johnson LR, Sturges BK, et al: Etiology and clinical outcome in dogs with aspiration pneumonia: 88 cases (2004-2006), J Am Vet Med Assoc 233:1748, 2008.
3. Tart KM, Babski DM, Lee JA: Potential risks, prognostic indicators, and diagnostic and treatment modalities affecting survival in dogs with presumptive aspiration pneumonia: 125 cases (2005-2008), J Vet Emerg Crit Care 20:319, 2010.
4. Heffner GG, Rozanski EA, Beal MW, et al: Evaluation of freshwater submersion in small animals: 28 cases (1996-2006), J Am Vet Med Assoc 232:244, 2008.
5. Marik PE: Pulmonary aspiration syndromes, Curr Opin Pulm Med 17:148, 2011.
6. Metheny NA, Clouse RE, Chang YH, et al: Tracheobronchial aspiration of gastric contents in critically ill tube-fed patients: frequency, outcomes, and risk factors, Crit Care Med 34:1007, 2006.
7. Alwood AJ, Brainard BM, LaFond E, et al: Postoperative pulmonary complications in dogs undergoing laparotomy: frequency, characterization and disease-related risk factors, J Vet Emerg Crit Care 16:176, 2006.
8. Olsson GL, Hallen B, Hambraeus-Jonzon K: Aspiration during anaesthesia: a computer-aided study of 185,358 anaesthetics, Acta Anaesthesiol Scand 30:84, 1986.
9. Raghavendran K, Nemzek J, Napolitano LM, et al: Aspiration-induced lung injury, Crit Care Med 39:818, 2011.
10. Exarhos ND, Logan WD, Jr., Abbott OA, et al: The importance of pH and volume in tracheobronchial aspiration, Dis Chest 47:167, 1965.
11. Schwartz DJ, Wynne JW, Gibbs CP, et al: The pulmonary consequences of aspiration of gastric contents at pH values greater than 2.5, Am Rev Respir Dis 121:119, 1980.
12. Knight PR, Rutter T, Tait AR, et al: Pathogenesis of gastric particulate lung injury: a comparison and interaction with acidic pneumonitis, Anesth Analg 77:754, 1993.
13. Kennedy TP, Johnson KJ, Kunkel RG, et al: Acute acid aspiration lung injury in the rat: biphasic pathogenesis, Anesth Analg 69:87, 1989.

14. Martling CR, Lundberg JM: Capsaicin sensitive afferents contribute to acute airway edema following tracheal instillation of hydrochloric acid or gastric juice in the rat, Anesthesiology 68:350, 1988.
15. Hamamoto J, Kohrogi H, Kawano O, et al: Esophageal stimulation by hydrochloric acid causes neurogenic inflammation in the airways in guinea pigs, J Appl Physiol 82:738, 1997.
16. Folkesson HG, Matthay MA, Hebert CA, et al: Acid aspiration-induced lung injury in rabbits is mediated by interleukin-8-dependent mechanisms, J Clin Invest 96:107, 1995.
17. Goldman G, Welbourn R, Kobzik L, et al: Tumor necrosis factor-alpha mediates acid aspiration-induced systemic organ injury, Ann Surg 212:513, 1990.
18. Shanley TP, Davidson BA, Nader ND, et al: Role of macrophage inflammatory protein-2 in aspiration-induced lung injury, Crit Care Med 28:2437, 2000.
19. Goldman G, Welbourn R, Kobzik L, et al: Reactive oxygen species and elastase mediate lung permeability after acid aspiration, J Appl Physiol 73:571, 1992.
20. Knight PR, Druskovich G, Tait AR, et al: The role of neutrophils, oxidants, and proteases in the pathogenesis of acid pulmonary injury, Anesthesiology 77:772, 1992.
21. Kyriakides C, Austen WG, Jr., Wang Y, et al: Mast cells mediate complement activation after acid aspiration, Shock 16:21, 2001.
22. Nishizawa H, Yamada H, Miyazaki H, et al: Soluble complement receptor type 1 inhibited the systemic organ injury caused by acid instillation into a lung, Anesthesiology 85:1120, 1996.
23. Britto J, Demling RH: Aspiration lung injury, New Horiz 1:435, 1993.
24. Knight PR, Davidson BA, Nader ND, et al: Progressive, severe lung injury secondary to the interaction of insults in gastric aspiration, Exp Lung Res 30:535, 2004.
25. Davidson BA, Knight PR, Helinski JD, et al: The role of tumor necrosis factor-alpha in the pathogenesis of aspiration pneumonitis in rats, Anesthesiology 91:486, 1999.
26. Ishizuka S, Yamaya M, Suzuki T, et al: Acid exposure stimulates the adherence of Streptococcus pneumoniae to cultured human airway epithelial cells: effects on platelet-activating factor receptor expression, Am J Respir Cell Mol Biol 24:459, 2001.
27. Rotta AT, Shiley KT, Davidson BA, et al: Gastric acid and particulate aspiration injury inhibits pulmonary bacterial clearance, Crit Care Med 32:747, 2004.
28. van Westerloo DJ, Knapp S, van't Veer C, et al: Aspiration pneumonitis primes the host for an exaggerated inflammatory response during pneumonia, Crit Care Med 33:1770, 2005.
29. Hoareau GL, Mellema MS, Silverstein DC: Indication, management, and outcome of brachycephalic dogs requiring mechanical ventilation, J Vet Emerg Crit Care 21:226, 2011.
30. Peyton JL, Burkitt JM: Critical illness-related corticosteroid insufficiency in a dog with septic shock, J Vet Emerg Crit Care 19:262, 2009.
31. Kogan DA, Johnson LR, Jandrey KE, et al: Clinical, clinicopathologic, and radiographic findings in dogs with aspiration pneumonia: 88 cases (2004-2006), J Am Vet Med Assoc 233:1742, 2008.
32. Sigrist NE, Adamik KN, Doherr MG, et al: Evaluation of respiratory parameters at presentation as clinical indicators of the respiratory localization in dogs and cats with respiratory distress, J Vet Emerg Crit Care 21:13, 2011.
33. Eom K, Seong Y, Park H, et al: Radiographic and computed tomographic evaluation of experimentally induced lung aspiration sites in dogs, J Vet Sci 7:397, 2006.
34. Prather AB, Berry CR, Thrall DE: Use of radiography in combination with computed tomography for the assessment of noncardiac thoracic disease in the dog and cat, Vet Radiol Ultrasound 46:114, 2005.
35. Moser KM, Maurer J, Jassy L, et al: Sensitivity, specificity, and risk of diagnostic procedures in a canine model of Streptococcus pneumoniae pneumonia, Am Rev Respir Dis 125:436, 1982.
36. Creighton SR, Wilkins RJ: Bacteriologic and cytologic evaluation of animals with lower respiratory tract disease using transtracheal aspiration biopsy, J Am Anim Hosp Assoc 10:227, 1974.
37. Angus JC, Jang SS, Hirsh DC: Microbiological study of transtracheal aspirates from dogs with suspected lower respiratory tract disease: 264 cases (1989-1995), J Am Vet Med Assoc 210:55, 1997.
38. Sumner CM, Rozanski EA, Sharp CR et al: The use of deep oral swabs as a surrogate for transoral tracheal wash to obtain bacterial cultures in dogs with pneumonia, J Vet Emerg Crit Care 21:515, 2011.
39. Woodhead M, Blasi F, Ewig S, et al: Guidelines for the management of adult lower respiratory tract infections—full version, Clin Microbiol Infect 17 Suppl 6:E1, 2011.
40. Sachdev A, Chugh K, Sethi M et al: Diagnosis of ventilator-associated pneumonia in children in resource-limited setting: a comparative study of bronchoscopic and nonbronchoscopic methods, Pediatr Crit Care Med 11:258, 2010.
41. El-Solh AA, Vora H, Knight PR 3rd, et al: Diagnostic use of serum procalcitonin levels in pulmonary aspiration syndromes, Crit Care Med 39:1251, 2011.
42. Berg P, Lindhardt BO: The role of procalcitonin in adult patients with community-acquired pneumonia—a systematic review, Dan Med J 59:A4357, 2012.
43. Jaoude PA, Knight PR, Ohtake P, et al: Biomarkers in the diagnosis of aspiration syndromes, Expert Rev Mol Diagn 10:309, 2010.
44. Zucker AR, Holm BA, Crawford GP, et al: PEEP is necessary for exogenous surfactant to reduce pulmonary edema in canine aspiration pneumonitis, J Appl Physiol 73:679, 1992.
45. Willson DF, Notter RH: The future of exogenous surfactant therapy, Respir Care 56:1369, 2011.
46. Taut FJ, Rippin G, Schenk P, et al: A Search for subgroups of patients with ARDS who may benefit from surfactant replacement therapy: a pooled analysis of five studies with recombinant surfactant protein-C surfactant (Venticute), Chest 134:724, 2008.
47. Spragg RG, Taut FJ, Lewis JF, et al: Recombinant surfactant protein C-based surfactant for patients with severe direct lung injury, Am J Respir Crit Care Med 183:1055, 2011.
48. Nader-Djalal N, Knight PR, Davidson BA, et al: Hyperoxia exacerbates microvascular lung injury following acid aspiration, Chest 112:1607, 1997.
49. Matthay MA, Ware LB, Zimmerman GA: The acute respiratory distress syndrome, J Clin Invest 122:2731, 2012.
50. Hopper K, Haskins SC, Kass PH, et al: Indications, management, and outcome of long-term positive-pressure ventilation in dogs and cats: 148 cases (1990-2001), J Am Vet Med Assoc 230:64, 2007.
51. Epstein SE, Mellema MS, Hopper K: Airway microbial culture and susceptibility patterns in dogs and cats with respiratory disease of varying severity, J Vet Emerg Crit Care 20:587, 2010.
52. Morley PS, Apley MD, Besser TE, et al: Antimicrobial drug use in veterinary medicine, J Vet Intern Med 19:617, 2005.
53. Matthay MA, Brower RG, Carson S, et al: Randomized, placebo-controlled clinical trial of an aerosolized beta(2)-agonist for treatment of acute lung injury, Am J Respir Crit Care Med 184:561, 2011.
54. Gao Smith F, Perkins GD, Gates S, et al: Effect of intravenous beta-2 agonist treatment on clinical outcomes in acute respiratory distress syndrome (BALTI-2): a multicentre, randomised controlled trial, Lancet 379:229, 2012.
55. Dellinger RP, Levy MM, Rhodes A, et al: Surviving Sepsis Campaign: international guidelines for management of severe sepsis and septic shock: 2012, Intensive Care Med 39:165, 2013.
56. Yang M, Yuping Y, Yin X, et al: Chest physiotherapy for pneumonia in adults, Cochrane Database Syst Rev CD006338, 2010.
57. Fleming S, Morgan G: Insufficient evidence to recommend routine adjunctive chest physiotherapy for adults with pneumonia, Evid Based Nurs 13:73, 2010.
58. Lukrafka JL, Fuchs SC, Fischer GB, et al: Chest physiotherapy in paediatric patients hospitalised with community-acquired pneumonia: a randomised clinical trial, Arch Dis Child, 2012.
59. Ntoumenopoulos G, Presneill JJ, McElholum M, et al: Chest physiotherapy for the prevention of ventilator-associated pneumonia, Intensive Care Med 28:850, 2002.
60. Pattanshetty RB, Gaude GS: Effect of multimodality chest physiotherapy in prevention of ventilator-associated pneumonia: A randomized clinical trial, Indian J Crit Care Med 14:70, 2010.
61. Britton S, Bejstedt M, Vedin L: Chest physiotherapy in primary pneumonia, Br Med J (Clin Res Ed) 290:1703, 1985.
62. Chen Y, Li K, Pu H, et al: Corticosteroids for pneumonia, Cochrane Database Syst Rev CD007720, 2011.

63. Salluh JI, Povoa P, Soares M, et al: The role of corticosteroids in severe community-acquired pneumonia: a systematic review, Crit Care 12:R76, 2008.
64. Povoa P, Salluh JI: What is the role of steroids in pneumonia therapy? Curr Opin Infect Dis 25:199, 2012.
65. Java MA, Drobatz KJ, Gilley RS, et al: Incidence of and risk factors for postoperative pneumonia in dogs anesthetized for diagnosis or treatment of intervertebral disk disease, J Am Vet Med Assoc 235:281, 2009.
66. ASA: Practice guidelines for preoperative fasting and the use of pharmacologic agents to reduce the risk of pulmonary aspiration: application to healthy patients undergoing elective procedures: an updated report by the American Society of Anesthesiologists Committee on Standards and Practice Parameters, Anesthesiology 114:495, 2011.
67. Bersenas AM, Mathews KA, Allen DG, et al: Effects of ranitidine, famotidine, pantoprazole, and omeprazole on intragastric pH in dogs, Am J Vet Res 66:425, 2005.
68. Thorpe RJ, Benger J: Pre-procedural fasting in emergency sedation, Emerg Med J 27:254, 2010.
69. Jensen AG, Callesen T, Hagemo JS, et al: Scandinavian clinical practice guidelines on general anaesthesia for emergency situations, Acta Anaesthesiol Scand 54:922, 2010.
70. Eom CS, Jeon CY, Lim JW, et al: Use of acid-suppressive drugs and risk of pneumonia: a systematic review and meta-analysis, CMAJ 183:310, 2011.
71. Yildizdas D, Yapicioglu H, Yilmaz HL: Occurrence of ventilator-associated pneumonia in mechanically ventilated pediatric intensive care patients during stress ulcer prophylaxis with sucralfate, ranitidine, and omeprazole, J Crit Care 17:240, 2002.
72. Lopriore E, Markhorst DG, Gemke RJ: Ventilator-associated pneumonia and upper airway colonisation with Gram negative bacilli: the role of stress ulcer prophylaxis in children, Intensive Care Med 28:763, 2002.
73. Kazi N, Mobarhan S: Enteral feeding associated gastroesophageal reflux and aspiration pneumonia: a review, Nutr Rev 54:324, 1996.
74. Marik PE, Zaloga GP: Gastric versus post-pyloric feeding: a systematic review, Crit Care 7:R46, 2003.
75. Garvey BM, McCambley JA, Tuxen DV: Effects of gastric alkalization on bacterial colonization in critically ill patients, Crit Care Med 17:211, 1989.

CHAPTER 24

ACUTE LUNG INJURY AND ACUTE RESPIRATORY DISTRESS SYNDROME

Elizabeth A. Rozanski, DVM, DACVIM, DACVECC • Trisha J. Oura, DVM, DACVR • Daniel L. Chan, DVM, DACVECC, DACVN, FHEA, MRCVS

KEY POINTS

- Acute lung injury may be a severe complication of critical illness or injury.
- Inflammation and alterations in the alveolar-capillary membrane lead to the influx of pulmonary edema, resulting in alveolar flooding with protein-rich fluid and loss of lung volume.
- Acute lung injury (ALI) and acute respiratory distress syndrome (ARDS) are clinical rather than histopathologic diagnoses.
- Computed tomography may provide valuable information in identification and treatment of patients with ALI/ARDS.
- Treatment is supportive; low tidal volume ventilation is appropriate in people and possibly dogs.
- Pharmacologic therapy, including glucocorticoids, has shown limited benefit to date.

Acute lung injury (ALI) and acute respiratory distress syndrome (ARDS) represent life-threatening complications of critical illness in people. The development of these complications actually reflects the advances in critical care that have occurred in human medicine in the last 50 years; patient survival beyond the initial injury or illness is considered a prerequisite for the development of any form of multiple organ failure.

Early pathologic and clinical reports from World War I describe findings consistent with the modern definitions of ALI, although this was not recognized as a clinical entity.[1] Concomitant with medical advances, and partly related to the influx of multitudes of young, previously healthy men injured in combat during the 1960s, physicians began to appreciate that although individuals could be resuscitated in the field, they would then die days to weeks later from progressive multiorgan failure. Ashbaugh and colleagues are credited with first modern description of 'adult respiratory distress syndrome' in 1967.[2] Since its recognition, ARDS has remained a devastating complication of critical illness, with survival rates now only slightly better than 40 years ago. Adult respiratory distress syndrome was reclassified as 'acute respiratory distress syndrome' in 1994 to include pediatric patients.[3]

THE HUMAN PERSPECTIVE

Criteria for the Diagnosis of ALI/ARDS

ALI/ARDS was initially defined by the American-European Consensus Conference in 1994 as severe respiratory failure after a catastrophic event.[3] The catastrophic event may be pulmonary (e.g., aspiration pneumonia or pulmonary contusion) or extrapulmonary (e.g., abdominal sepsis) in nature. More recently, other inciting events such as blood transfusions, have been recognized to result in

BOX 24-1 ***The Berlin Definition of Acute Respiratory Distress Syndrome***[5]

Timing

Within 1 week of a known clinical insult or new or worsening respiratory symptoms.

Chest Imaging*

Bilateral opacities—not fully explained by effusions, lobar/lung collapse, or nodules

Origin of Edema

Respiratory failure not fully explained by cardiac failure or fluid overload. Need objective assessment (e.g., echocardiography) to exclude hydrostatic edema if no risk factor present

Oxygenation†

Mild: 200 mm Hg < $PaO_2/FiO_2 \le 300$ mm Hg with PEEP or CPAP ≥ 5 cm H_2O

Moderate: 100 mm Hg < $PaO_2/FiO_2 \le 200$ mm Hg with PEEP $\ge$ 5 cm H_2O

Severe: $PaO_2/FiO_2 \le 100$ mm Hg with PEEP ≥ 5 cm H_2O

CPAP, Continuous positive airway pressure; *PEEP,* positive end-expiratory pressure.

*Chest radiograph or computed tomography.

†If at altitude higher than 1000 m, then correction factor should be calculated as follows: [$PaO_2/FiO_2 \times$ (barometric pressure/760)].

a specific form of ALI, which is termed transfusion-related acute lung injury or TRALI.[4] ALI/ARDS is further defined by the presence of a low oxygenation index (PaO_2/FiO_2 ratio) with an index of less than 200 being consistent with ARDS and an index of 201 to 300 being defined as ALI.[3] Additional criteria include bilateral pulmonary infiltrates on thoracic radiography, exclusion of cardiogenic pulmonary edema, and decreased lung compliance.

There are several limitations of this initial definition of ARDS, including the variability of the PaO_2/FiO_2 ratio with different ventilator settings and difficulties in determining the presence of high hydrostatic pressure. In an effort to improve the sensitivity of the diagnostic criteria, an updated definition for ARDS known as the Berlin definition was published in 2012 (Box 24-1).[5] This new definition was found to have a better predictive validity for mortality than the original 1994 definition.

Pathophysiology

The most consistent histologic pattern appreciated with ARDS is diffuse alveolar damage (DAD).[6,7] However, this pattern is considered nonspecific and may be associated with a variety of clinical syndromes in addition to ARDS, including other pulmonary conditions such as acute interstitial pneumonia, inhalation of toxic substances, and prior treatment with amiodarone.[8-10] In cases of suspected ARDS, stages of lung injury include exudative, proliferative, and, ultimately, fibrotic phases. During the initial insult, hemorrhage and protein-rich pulmonary edema accumulate within the alveoli. The exudative phase (days 0 to 6) is characterized by protein-rich edema and the presence of eosinophilic hyaline membranes in the walls of the alveolar ducts. The proliferative phase (days 4 to 10) is characterized by a decrease in edema and hyaline membranes and an increase in interstitial fibrosis. The final fibrotic phase (day 8 onward) is characterized by pronounced fibrosis that may ultimately obliterate areas of the lungs. Histopathologic criteria are useful in understanding the pathophysiology of and evaluating patients with ARDS, although this syndrome should be considered a clinical diagnosis, with a lung biopsy or autopsy/necropsy not required to reach the diagnosis.[5]

The underlying specific cause for ALI and ARDS is often unknown, although pneumonia, sepsis, and trauma are common precursors to systemic inflammation that results in multiple organ dysfunction syndrome (MODS). ALI/ARDS may occur independently or as a part of MODS.

Common features of lung injury in ALI/ARDS include pronounced microvascular permeability, leukocyte activation, and alterations in cytokine production. Inflammatory mediators are responsible at least in part for the development and propagation of ALI/ARDS. Overzealous response on the part of the host may magnify the initially appropriate inflammatory response and result in perpetuation of injury. Major humoral mediators of ALI/ARDS include the proinflammatory cytokines interleukin 1 and tumor necrosis factor α; cellular mediators include neutrophils and macrophages.[5]

The arterial hypoxemia observed in ALI/ARDS develops from a variety of factors, including low alveolar partial pressure of oxygen (PAO_2) ventilation-perfusion (V/Q) mismatch, and shunting of venous blood into the arterial circulation. Diffusion limitation is rarely a major contributor to hypoxemia in people with ARDS.

Decreased PAO_2 can occur as a result of hypoventilation associated with low pulmonary compliance; oxygen therapy or mechanical ventilation is useful to help overcome this problem. Ventilation-perfusion mismatch occurs as a result of poorly ventilated alveoli subsequent to fluid accumulation and perfusion abnormalities of ventilated lung regions. Physiologic shunt occurs when deoxygenated venous blood flows past collapsed or flooded alveoli, never participating in gas exchange. Further, venous oxygen desaturation magnifies abnormalities associated with shunting, and efforts to improve venous oxygenation by improving perfusion and decreasing oxygen consumption can improve arterial oxygenation in the presence of significant physiologic shunt. Sedation and anxiolytics may be effective for improving oxygenation in the presence of V/Q mismatch, although care must be taken in the use of these drugs in patients with severe respiratory compromise. Human patients with ARDS almost invariably require mechanical ventilation, which can improve V/Q matching and decrease physiologic shunt by recruiting collapsed alveoli. Mechanical ventilation also relieves the work of breathing, preventing fatigue and reducing oxygen consumption.[6]

In people with ALI/ARDS, pulmonary functional abnormalities noted in addition to hypoxemia include decreased functional residual capacity (FRC), mild to moderate reductions in the forced expiratory volume in 1 second (FEV_1) and forced vital capacity (FVC), decreased diffusing capacity (DLco), decreased compliance, and increased resistance. Lowered compliance is the hallmark finding in ARDS and is determined by the slope of a P-V curve.[11] Specifically, this means that higher pressures are required to generate adequate tidal volumes. Most critical care ventilators in clinical use will also calculate lung mechanics, which may be easily tracked over time. Decreased pulmonary compliance results in an increased work of breathing, and respiratory fatigue may develop.[12] Alterations in surfactant production and composition may also contribute to alveolar collapse, and pulmonary arterial hypertension may result from increased pulmonary vascular resistance.

Resolution of ARDS occurs in an orderly fashion, similar to repair in any other tissue. First, excessive fluid and proteins are removed from the airways and proteins (soluble and insoluble) from the alveoli. Next the type II alveolar epithelial cell must repopulate the epithelial lining and the abnormal interstitium must restore its normal matrix. Finally, the damaged endothelium must be repaired to restore blood flow and unnecessary or residual cellular components be removed.[7,13] If recovery in incomplete, persistent deficiencies in lung function may remain. The majority of the recovery occurs over the first 3 months after extubation, with some additional recovery over the first year.[14] Quality of life of survivors is typically good, although depending on the concurrent critical illness or injury, there may be persistent abnormalities.[14] Some long-term survivors of critical illness develop psychologic symptoms and may require ongoing therapy to resume their predisease state.[14]

Treatment

Therapy for ALI/ARDS is primarily supportive, with no specific pharmacologic therapy associated with an improved outcome. Inhaled nitric oxide and surfactant therapy have been shown to improve oxygenation, but positive survival benefits are not observed.[15,16] Surfactant therapy can be lifesaving in infants with respiratory distress syndrome, and modification of surfactant composition and administration technique trials are ongoing.[16,17] However, as of this writing there are no clear benefits of their use. Cytokine-blocking agents have not been shown to be effective despite initial early promise. Intravenous β_2 agonists were shown to effectively lower lung water in the BALTI-I trial; however, a larger, more recent study recommend against their use.[18,19] Furthermore, both a positive fluid balance and high tidal volumes have been associated with worse outcomes.[20] A major breakthrough in the treatment of ARDS patients included using lower tidal volumes in mechanical ventilation, which has been associated with decreased ventilator associated lung injury and improved patient outcomes.[21] Most current ventilation guidelines include limiting fluid balance to prevent overhydration, limiting tidal volumes, using appropriate positive end-expiratory pressure (PEEP), and avoiding other complications of critical illness.[22,23] Treatment with activated protein C was initially encouraging in sepsis, but more recent clinical trials have not supported its use across the board in sepsis or ARDS and has subsequently been withdrawn from the market. There is an the increasing appreciation of the role of bronchoalveolar hemostasis in lung injury and ARDS, which may lead to targeting the abnormal fibrin deposition.[24] A variety of other trials evaluating other pharmacologic and ventilatory maneuvers, including surfactant, inhaled nitric oxide, and granulocyte-macrophage colony-stimulating factor (GM-CSF) are currently recruiting patients, and further information can be found at www.clinicaltrials.gov. Vitamin D deficiency has been identified in some people with lung injury, and there may be a role for supplementation of Vitamin D in critically ill people.[25] There is also interest in the potential role of stem cells to modulate inflammation in ARDS/ALI and some evidence of a positive effect of therapy.[26]

THE CANINE PERSPECTIVE

ALI and ARDS are recognized with far less frequency in critically ill dogs than in people, and several case reports suggest a similar association with critical illnesses.[21-24] Parent and colleagues were the first to comprehensively describe the clinical characteristics and course of 19 dogs identified with ARDS on necropsy in 1996.[27,28] Risk factors identified for dogs included the presence of pneumonia, sepsis, and shock. Several other case reports have highlighted the histopathologic appearance of ARDS in dogs with a variety of critical illnesses.[29-32] Campbell and King described 10 dogs receiving mechanical ventilatory support for pulmonary contusions; many (if not all) of the dogs surviving the initial 24 hours likely had ARDS.[33] Other reviews on ventilatory management have also described dogs ventilated for respiratory failure that likely met the criteria for ARDS, although this was not definitively stated, as an underlying cause.[34,35] Finally, in 2005 Walker and colleagues described the recovery from ALI in a dog with anaphylaxis associated with multiple bee stings.[36] Since the last publication of this textbook, a case report of two dogs successfully treated for suspected ARDS has been published.[37] Dogs are widely used in experimental studies evaluating ARDS and ALI.[12]

Criteria for the Diagnosis of ALI/ARDS

The actual incidence of ALI/ARDS remains unclear in dogs because of potential overlap in sources or respiratory distress and in lack of universal recording mechanisms. In some instances, such as with severe pulmonary contusion, it may be easier to reach the diagnosis of ARDS to the patient still in respiratory distress 72 to 96 hours after the incidence, whereas in others, such as those with aspiration pneumonia, it may be difficult to ascertain if ALI has developed or if recurrent aspiration has occurred. A veterinary consensus statement on the definitions and diagnostic criteria of ALI/ARDS was published in 2007. These criteria are shown in Box 24-2. Criteria for defining canine ALI as proposed by these authors are listed in Box 24-3. As a summary, the criticalist should look to identify ARDS in dogs with an underlying disease or trauma, which demonstrate progressive severe respiratory failure sufficient to require oxygen support and likely mechanical ventilation with PEEP, without significant pleural space disease, localized infection, thrombotic disease, or volume overload.

Arterial blood gas should be evaluated for the presence of hypoxemia and for calculation of the alveolar-arterial (A-a) gradient or PaO_2/FiO_2 ratio (see Chapter 15). If the animal is extremely stressed or experiencing marked respiratory distress, sampling for an arterial blood gas should be postponed so as not to risk causing further compromise or even cardiopulmonary arrest. Similarly, a dog that is

BOX 24-2 *Definition of Veterinary Acute Lung Injury and Acute Respiratory Distress Syndrome*[38]

One of each of the following first four categories is necessary for diagnosis. The fifth category is an optional measure.

1. Acute onset (<72 hours) of tachypnea and labored breathing at rest
2. Known risk factors
3. Evidence of pulmonary capillary leak without increased pulmonary capillary pressure* (any one of the following):
   a. Bilateral/diffuse infiltrates on thoracic radiographs (more than 1 quadrant/lobe)
   b. Bilateral dependent density gradient on CT
   c. Proteinaceous fluid within the conducting airways
   d. Increased extravascular lung water
4. Evidence of inefficient gas exchange (any one or more of the following):
   a. Hypoxemia without PEEP or CPAP and known FiO_2
      i. PaO_2/FiO_2 ratio
         1. <300 mm Hg for VetALI
         2. <200 mm Hg for VetARDS
      ii. Increased alveolar-arterial oxygen gradient
      iii. Venous admixture (noncardiac shunt)
   b. Increased dead-space ventilation
5. Evidence of diffuse pulmonary inflammation
   a. Transtracheal wash/bronchoalveolar lavage sample neutrophilia
   b. Transtracheal wash/bronchoalveolar lavage biomarkers of inflammation
   c. Molecular imaging (PET)

CT, Computed tomography; *PEEP,* positive end-expiratory pressure; *CPAP,* continuous positive airway pressure; *FiO_2,* fraction of inspired oxygen; *PET,* positron emission tomography; *PAOP,* pulmonary artery occlusion pressure.

*No evidence of cardiogenic edema (one or more of the following): PAOP < 18 mm Hg; no clinical or diagnostic evidence supporting left-sided heart failure, including echocardiography.

BOX 24-3 *Proposed Criteria for Identification of Acute Lung Injury in Dogs*

1. Preexisting severe acute critical illness or injury (pulmonary or extrapulmonary in nature)
2. Increased respiratory rate and effort
3. Bilateral pulmonary infiltrates on thoracic radiographs or, preferably, high-resolution computed tomography
4. Hypoxemia on room air with $PaO_2 < 45$ mm Hg, $SpO_2 < 85\%$ on room air, or A-a gradient > 50; alternatively, in the presence of supplemental oxygen of a known concentration, $PaO_2/FiO_2 < 300$
5. No evidence of congestive heart failure/volume overload as assessed via either echocardiogram or pulmonary arterial catheterization

experiencing severe respiratory distress should not be removed from supplemental oxygen in order to make interpretation of blood gas more straightforward. Volume overload or congestive heart failure should be excluded by performing diagnostic imaging, such as echocardiography, or thoracic radiographs.

In people, the standard imaging method for evaluating acute lung injury and ventilator-induced lung injury is high-resolution computed tomography (HRCT) of the thorax. In dogs, traditionally, thoracic radiographs are used to document bilateral alveolar disease at the time of ALI/ARDS diagnosis and to monitor disease progression. Thoracic radiographs from a dog with ARDS are shown in Figure 24-1. Because of patient instability, these radiographs may be acquired with portable radiograph units or may be limited by incomplete studies or poor patient positioning. Although computed tomography has been used in several animal models of lung injury, there has been no prospective imaging study of these syndromes in clinically affected dogs. The computed tomography findings in dogs with ALI/ARDS are not well known, and it is unclear if, or to what extent, alveolar hyperinflation or ventilator-associated lung injury is present in dogs undergoing mechanical ventilation.

Increased availability of multidetector CT may allow incorporation of this modality into patient workup and monitoring of disease progression. The advantages of CT include rapid acquisition of data, tomographic information regarding severity and distribution of pulmonary disease, and assessment for comorbidities such as pulmonary thromboembolism. There are several disadvantages as well, including cost and difficulty transporting unstable patients. In a recent abstract, HRCT was used in addition to traditional thoracic radiographs and oxygenation indices to monitor dogs with ARDS undergoing mechanical ventilation and to quantify alveolar overdistention and recruitment/derecruitment during mechanical ventilation (Figure 24-2).[38,39]

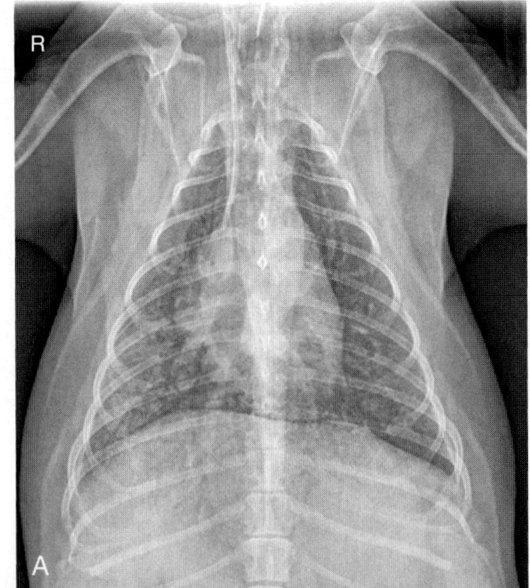

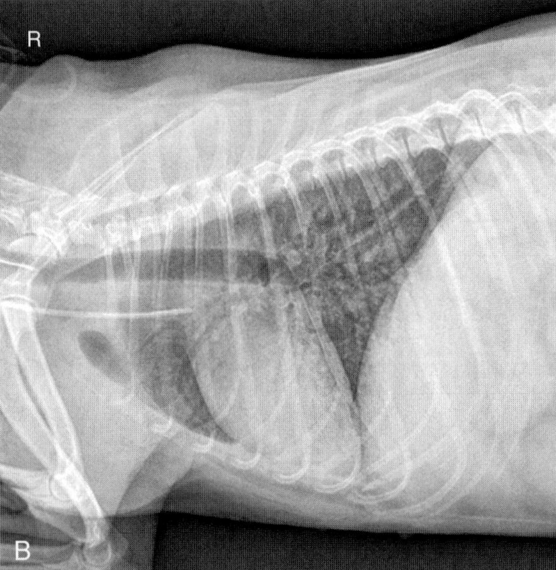

FIGURE 24-1 **A,** A ventral–dorsal thoracic radiograph from a dog with ARDS. **B,** A lateral thoracic radiograph from a dog with ARDS. Note the diffuse infiltrates and the lack of radiographically apparent left atrial enlargement.

Treatment

Recommendations for the treatment of potential ALI/ARDS in dogs focus on the elimination of other potentially more treatable causes. Thoracic radiographs should be evaluated for the presence of diffuse bilateral infiltrates. Bacterial pneumonia should be aggressively treated with antibiotics effective against hospital-acquired organisms. Pulmonary thromboembolism should be considered, and patients should be anticoagulated if clinically advisable and evaluated via echocardiogram or computed tomography.

Intermittent positive pressure ventilation with PEEP is the mainstay of support of the dog with ALI or ARDS (see Chapters 30 and 31). Suggested strategies for ventilatory management of animals with ARDS are largely derived from human data and have not been comprehensively evaluated in clinical veterinary patients.[40] Some less severely affected dogs may potentially be treated with cage rest and supplemental oxygen.

Recovery from lung injury is on the order of weeks; thus severe decreases in pulmonary compliance (or increases in inspiratory pressures) may suggest that prolonged mechanical ventilation will be required and owners need to be informed of the likely financial and emotional implications. No specific therapy for ALI/ARDS is available, and care is largely supportive. Ventilated dogs likely benefit from limiting tidal volume, but optimal tidal volumes for dogs with ARDS have not been established. One study did confirm that lower tidal volumes are well tolerated in healthy dogs.[41] Because of the substantial difference in thoracic cavity dimensions (e.g., Pug vs. an Irish Setter), it is possible that ultimately breed or body-type specific recommendations will be developed. Given the significant financial and emotional commitment required to support a critically ill dog undergoing mechanical ventilation, realistic and frequent client communications are recommended.

As we expand our understanding of the pathophysiology and our experience with ARDS/ALI in dogs, future therapies and

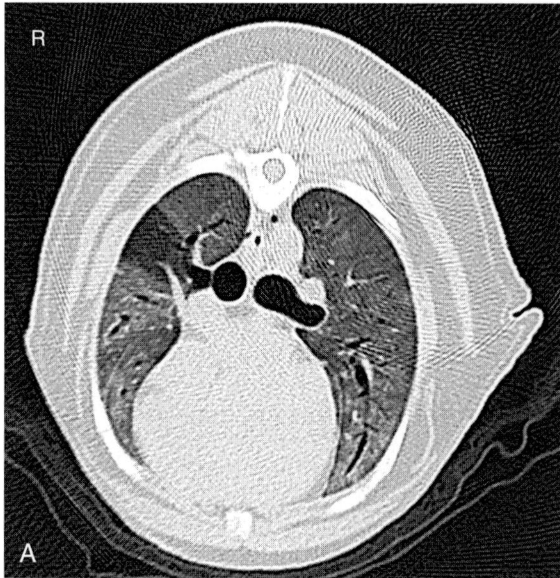

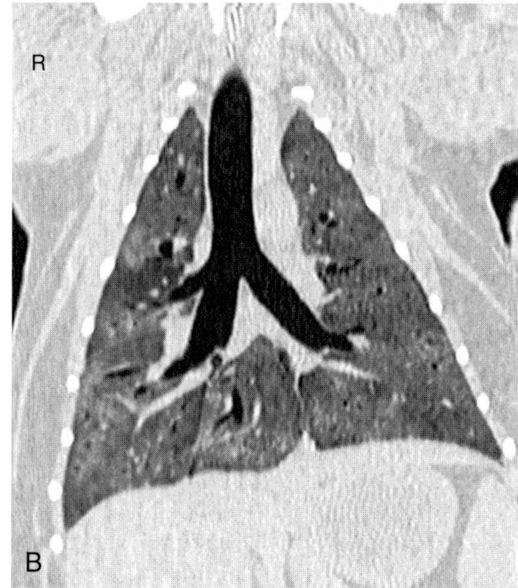

FIGURE 24-2 A, A computed tomography (CT) slice from the thorax of a dog with ARDS. Note the increased density consistent with noncardiogenic infiltrate. **B,** A CT reconstruction of a dog with ARDS. Note in particular that the entirety of the visible lung is affected; however, there is slightly heterogenous (patchy) distribution.

management strategies could be developed and tested to reduce morbidity and improve survival. An important first step involves increasing awareness and recognition of this disease entity in dogs. Efforts to better define this syndrome in dogs are warranted to allow us to compare any forthcoming case series and clinical trials.

REFERENCES

1. Simeone FA: Pulmonary complications of non-thoracic wounds: a historical perspective, J Trauma 8:625, 1968.
2. Ashbaugh DG, Bigelow DB, Petty TL, et al: Acute respiratory distress in adult, Lancet 2:319, 1967.
3. Bernard GR, Artigas A, Brigham KL, et al: Consensus Committee: The American-European Consensus Conference on ARDS: definitions, mechanisms, relevant outcomes, and clinical trial coordination, Am J Resp Crit Care 149:818, 1994.
4. Vlaar AP, Jeffermans NP: Transfusion-related acute lung injury: a clinical review, Lancet 382(9896):984, 2013.
5. Ferguson ND, Fan E, Camporota L, et al: The Berlin definition of ARDS: an expanded rationale, justification, and supplementary material, Intensive Care Med 38(10):1573, 2012.
6. Weinacker AB, Vaszar LT: Acute respiratory distress syndrome: physiology and new management strategies, Ann Rev Med 52:221, 2001.
7. Tomashefski JF: Pulmonary pathology of acute respiratory distress syndrome, Clin Chest Med 21:435, 2000.
8. Bouros D, Nicholson AC, Polychronopoulos V, et al: Acute interstitial pneumonia, Eur Respir J 15:412, 2000.
9. Erasmus JJ, McAdams HP, Rossi SE: Drug-induced lung injury, Semin Roentgenol 37:72, 2002.
10. Jirik FR, Henning H, Huckell VF, et al: Diffuse alveolar damage syndrome associated with amiodarone therapy, Can Med Assoc J 128:1192, 1983.
11. Kallet RH, Katz JA: Respiratory system mechanics in acute respiratory distress syndrome, Respir Care Clin N Am 9(3):297, 2003.
12. Zhang LF, Han LP, Wu XY, et al: Estimation of respiratory mechanics in dogs with acute lung injury, Adv Exp Med Biol 316:327, 1992.
13. Brower RG, Ware LB, Berthiaume Y, et al: Treatment of ARDS, Chest 120:1347, 2001.
14. Lee CM, Hudson LD: Long-term outcomes after ARDS, Semin Respir Crit Care Med 22:327, 2001.
15. Griffiths MJD, Evans TW: Inhaled nitric oxide therapy in adults, N Engl J Med 353:2683, 2005.
16. Willson DF, Thomas NJ, Markovitz BB, et al: Effect of exogenous surfactant (calfactant) in pediatric acute lung injury: a randomized controlled trial, JAMA 293:470, 2005.
17. Marraro GA: Perspectives for use of surfactant in children and adults, J Matern Fetal Neonatal Med 16(Suppl):29, 2004.
18. Perkins GD, McAuley DF, Thickett DR, et al: The Beta Agonist Lung Injury Trial (BALTI) a randomized placebo controlled clinical trial, Am J Resp Crit Care Med 173(3):281, 2006.
19. Smith G, Perkins GD, Gates S, et al. Effect of intravenous B-2 agonist treatment on clinical outcomes in acute respiratory distress syndrome (BALTI-2); a multicentre, randomized controlled trial, Lancet 379:229, 2012.
20. Sakr Y, Vincent JL, Reinhart K, et al: High tidal volume and positive fluid balance are associated with worse outcome in acute lung injury, Chest 128(5):3098, 2005.
21. The Acute Respiratory Distress Syndrome Network: Ventilation with lower tidal volumes as compared with traditional tidal volumes for acute lung injury and the acute respiratory distress syndrome, N Engl J Med 342:1301, 2000.
22. Lee WL, Detsky AS, Steward TE: Lung-protective mechanical ventilation strategies in ARDS, Int Care Med 26:1151, 2000.
23. Shuller D, Mitchell JP, Calandrino FS, et al: Fluid balance during pulmonary edema. Is fluid gain a marker or a cause of poor outcome? Chest 100:1068, 1991.
24. Glas GJ, van der Sluijs KF, Schultz M, et al: Bronchoalveolar hemostasis in lung injury and acute respiratory distress syndrome, Thromb Haemost 11:17, 2013. doi:10.1111/jth.12047
25. Parekh D, Thickett DR, Turner AM: Vitamin D deficiency and acute lung injury, Inflamm Allergy Drug Targets 12(4):253, 2013.
26. Curley GF, Laffey JG: Cell therapy demonstrates promise for acute respiratory distress syndrome—but which cell is best? Stem Cell Res Ther 4(2):29, 2013.
27. Parent C, King LG, Walker LM, et al: Clinical and clinicopathologic findings in dogs with acute respiratory distress syndrome: 19 cases (1985-1993), J Am Vet Med Assoc 208:1419-1427, 1996.
28. Parent C, King LG, Van Winkle TJ, et al: Respiratory function and treatment in dogs with acute respiratory distress syndrome: 19 cases (1985-1993), J Am Vet Med Assoc 208:1428, 1996.
29. Turk J, Miller M, Broen T, et al: Coliform septicemia and pulmonary disease associated with canine parvoviral enteritis: 88 cases (1987-1988), J Am Vet Med Assoc 196(5):771, 1990.
30. Frevert CW, Warner AE: Respiratory distress resulting from acute lung injury in the veterinary patient, J Vet Intern Med 6:154, 1992.
31. Lopez A, Lane IF, Hanna P: Adult respiratory distress syndrome in a dog with necrotizing pancreatitis, Can Vet J 36:240, 1995.
32. Jarvinen AK, Saario E, Andersen E, et al: Lung injury leading to respiratory distress syndrome in young Dalmatian dogs, J Vet Intern Med 9:162, 1995.

33. Campbell VL, King LG: Pulmonary function, ventilator management, and outcome of dogs with thoracic trauma and pulmonary contusions: 10 cases (1994-1998), J Am Vet Assoc 217(10):1505, 2000.
34. Orton CE, Wheeler SL: Continuous positive airway pressure therapy for aspiration pneumonia in a dog, J Am Vet Med Assoc 188:1437, 1986.
35. King LG, Hendricks JC: Use of positive-pressure ventilation in dogs and cats: 41 cases (1990-1992), J Am Vet Med Assoc 204(7):1045, 1994.
36. Walker T, Tidwell AS, Rozanski EA, et al: Imaging diagnosis: Acute lung injury following massive bee envenomation in a dog, Vet Radiol Ultrasound 46:300-303, 2005
37. Kelmer E, Love LC, DeClue A, et al: Successful treatment of acute respiratory distress syndrome in 2 dogs, Can Vet J 210:53:167, 2012.
38. Oura TJ, Hanel RM, Davies J, et al: Diagnostic Imaging enhances management of Acute respiratory distress syndrome, presented at 2012 ACVR Annual Scientific Meeting, Las Vegas, NV.
39. Wilkins PA, Otto CM, Baumgardner JE, et al: Acute lung injury and acute respiratory distress syndromes in veterinary medicine: consensus definitions: The Dorothy Russell Havemeyer Working Group on ALI and ARDS in Veterinary Medicine, J Vet Emerg Crit Care 17:333, 2007.
40. Mueller ER: Suggested strategies for ventilatory management of veterinary patients with acute respiratory distress syndrome, J Vet Emerg Crit Care 11:191, 2001.
41. Oura TJ, Rozanski EA, Buckley GJ, et al: Low tidal volume ventilation in healthy dogs, J Vet Emerg Crit Care 22(3):368, 2012.

CHAPTER 25
PULMONARY CONTUSIONS AND HEMORRHAGE

Sergio Serrano, LV, DVM, DACVECC • Amanda K. Boag, MA, VetMB, DACVIM, DACVECC, MRCVS

KEY POINTS

- Pulmonary contusions occur commonly in patients after blunt chest trauma. The contusions consist of interstitial and alveolar hemorrhage, accompanied by parenchymal destruction that starts immediately after the impact but can worsen for 24 to 48 hours after injury.
- The lesions typically resolve within 3 to 10 days, unless complications such as pneumonia or acute respiratory distress syndrome ensue.
- Clinical signs may be acute and severe or may develop progressively over several hours after trauma.
- The diagnosis of pulmonary contusions is based on a history of trauma and the presence of respiratory changes, ranging from tachypnea to severe respiratory distress, in conjunction with compatible blood gas abnormalities and characteristic changes seen on thoracic radiographs. Thoracic ultrasound and computed tomography (CT) scanning are becoming more widely used and may have diagnostic advantages compared with radiographs.
- Treatment of patients with pulmonary contusions is supportive and consists of oxygen therapy, judicious fluid administration, and analgesia for concurrent injuries. Ventilatory support may be necessary in severe cases.
- Less common causes of pulmonary hemorrhage include coagulopathies, thromboembolic disease, infectious disease (viral, bacterial, and parasitic), exercise-induced hemorrhage, and neoplasia.
- Treatment of atraumatic pulmonary hemorrhage is directed toward the underlying disease while providing respiratory and ventilatory support when needed.

Pulmonary contusions consist of pulmonary interstitial and alveolar hemorrhage and edema associated with blunt chest trauma, usually after a compression-decompression injury of the thoracic cage. Such injury in small animals is most commonly associated with motor vehicle trauma[1] and high-rise falls[2] in cats in urban areas. Thoracic bite trauma may also lead to severe contusions,[3] as may other animal interactions (e.g., horse kicks), human abuse, and shock waves from explosions.

Thoracic trauma has been reported in 34%,[4] 38.9%,[5] and 57%[6] of dogs and 17% of cats[5] that sustain limb fractures in road traffic accidents. Pulmonary contusions may also be present in traumatized animals without limb injuries; in one study, only 32% of dogs had concurrent fractures or luxations.[7] In general, pulmonary contusions are the most prevalent thoracic lesion after trauma and occur in roughly 50% of animals with thoracic injuries. They may occur as an isolated abnormality or in combination with other thoracic injuries, including pneumothorax, pleural effusion, rib fractures, diaphragmatic rupture, cardiac arrhythmias, and pericardial effusion.[5,8]

The clinical manifestations of pulmonary contusions can be acute and lead to immediate, severe respiratory distress or may develop progressively over several hours after the injury. Patients may display few clinical signs associated with the contusions initially; in one study, 79% of dogs with abnormal thoracic radiographic findings or low arterial partial pressure of oxygen (PaO_2) had no physical findings that were suggestive of thoracic injury on initial examination.[5] Another study found that American Society of Anesthesiologists (ASA) grade was significantly increased with the information provided by thoracic radiography.[9] However, radiographic changes may also be delayed. Because aggressive fluid therapy and general anesthesia have the potential to worsen contusions, the emergency clinician must not discount the possibility of their presence when evaluating more dramatic injuries, even if clinical signs of thoracic injury or respiratory distress are not apparent initially.

PATHOPHYSIOLOGY AND PATHOLOGY

Pulmonary contusions result from the release of direct or indirect energy within the lung. High-velocity missiles and blasts also lead to pulmonary contusions as shock waves pass through the parenchymal tissue and lead to bleeding into the alveolar spaces and disruption of normal lung structure and function. Several mechanisms have been postulated as important in the etiology of pulmonary contusion.[10]

Because of the compressible nature of the thoracic cage, acute compression and subsequent expansion lead to transmission of mechanical forces and energy to the pulmonary parenchyma. As a result, the lung is injured directly by the increased pressure in the so-called spalling effect, a shearing or bursting phenomenon that occurs at gas–liquid interfaces and may disrupt the alveolus at the point of initial contact with shock waves. The "inertial effect" that occurs when low-density alveolar tissue is stripped from heavier hilar structures as they accelerate at different rates results in both mechanical tearing and laceration of the lungs. Finally, an "implosion effect," resulting from rebound or overexpansion of gas bubbles after a pressure wave passes, can lead to tearing of the pulmonary parenchyma from excess distention.[11,12] The parenchyma may also be injured by the displacement of fractured ribs. Subsequent hemorrhage results in bronchospasm, increased mucus production, and alveolar collapse as a result of decreased production of surfactant.[13]

Damage to the lung leads to complex changes in respiratory function. The parenchymal damage causes ventilation-perfusion (V/Q) mismatch as the alveoli are flooded with blood and underventilated. In addition, an increase in lung water occurs as a result of the accumulation of protein-rich edema, subsequently decreasing lung compliance.[14] Recent experimental studies in pigs show that both true shunt and areas of low V/Q mismatch exist at both 2 and 6 hours after injury; true shunt appears to be the major cause of hypoxemia.[15,16] At the expense of blood flow to areas with normal ventilation-perfusion quotient, the shunt fraction and dead space ventilation increase. Both shunt (Q) and volume of poorly aerated and nonaerated lung tissue correlate independently with PaO_2.[15] There is also a variable vascular reaction in response to local hypoxia (hypoxic pulmonary vasoconstriction), which may be followed by a further decrease in local perfusion secondary to vascular congestion and thrombosis. In some patients, this leads to reduced perfusion to the unventilated lung, thus minimizing an increase in the shunt fraction.[17] Regardless, the patient subsequently displays dyspnea from hypoxemia. Either hypocarbia or hypercarbia may be present, depending on the severity of the contusions and the effects of concurrent injuries on ventilation.

In animals that survive the initial hours, the respiratory derangements associated with pulmonary contusions usually resolve in 3 to 7 days, but delayed deterioration may occur; this may be secondary to complications such as bacterial pneumonia or acute respiratory distress syndrome (ARDS) secondary to the local or systemic inflammatory response.[11] The frequency of these complications has not been well described in dogs and cats. In humans, pulmonary contusions cause severe immunodysfunction both locally and systemically, and this immunosuppression is associated with a decreased survival rate if a septic insult occurs.[18]

Histologic progression of pulmonary contusions has been demonstrated in a canine experimental model.[19] Immediate interstitial hemorrhage is followed by interstitial edema and infiltration of monocytes and neutrophils during the first few hours. Twenty-four hours after injury, the alveoli and smaller airways are full of protein, red blood cells, and inflammatory cells. At this stage, the normal architecture has been lost and edema is severe. Alveoli adjacent to the affected region remain normally perfused, but they are less compliant because of the edema and disruption of the surfactant layer. Thus they are poorly ventilated, which leads to an increase in ventilation-perfusion mismatch.[14,17,20,21] Furthermore, experimental studies in pigs have demonstrated that local pulmonary contusions may lead to generalized pulmonary dysfunction secondary to impaired surfactant activity and a subsequent decrease in alveolar diameter.[22] Forty-eight hours after injury, healing has started and the lymphatic vessels are dilated and filled with protein. The parenchyma and affected airways contain fibrin, cellular debris, granules from type II alveolar cells, neutrophils, and macrophages.[14] Another study found that within 7 to 10 days after trauma, canine lungs were almost completely healed with little scarring.[20]

Clinically there is not always a clear correlation between the apparent volume of affected lung and the clinical signs. At a mechanistic level, more recent studies on the pathophysiology of pulmonary contusions are focusing on the role of the acute inflammatory response and its impact on severity. Experimental studies highlight the potential importance of neutrophil activation, Toll-like receptors, and type II pneumocyte apoptosis in the progression of lung contusions.[23] Type II pneumocyte injury leading to generalized surfactant dysfunction may also play an important role and could be a therapeutic target.[24] Finally the interactions of lung contusion with other pulmonary injuries, such as silent aspiration of gastric contents, may exacerbate permeability changes and the inflammatory response, potentially contributing to the more severe forms of pulmonary contusions and their progression to acute lung injury (ALI)/ARDS and pneumonia.[24]

DIAGNOSIS

Physical Findings

Clinically patients have tachypnea or dyspnea, depending on the severity of the contusions and the time between injury and arrival at the veterinary hospital. Auscultation findings may be normal, or increased breath sounds and crackles can be present and may worsen over the initial 24-hour period. These abnormalities are often asymmetric and may be truly unilateral. Lung auscultation findings can be more difficult to interpret when concurrent conditions, such as pneumothorax, are present, and frequent monitoring of respiratory rate, effort, and pulmonary auscultation is warranted. Hemoptysis (the expectoration of blood from distal to the larynx) is present in a high proportion of human patients. It appears to be an uncommon finding in small animals but is usually associated with severe lesions.

Because there is a high incidence of thoracic trauma associated with skeletal injuries and respiratory symptoms may be absent or masked initially, the clinician should maintain a high index of suspicion for contusions in any traumatized patient.

Imaging: Radiology, Computed Tomography, and Ultrasound

Dyspneic patients should undergo stabilization before imaging is attempted. Animals that sustain thoracic trauma may have multiple thoracic injuries, making a precise diagnosis based on the physical examination alone challenging. Imaging studies may be helpful in identifying and defining all injuries; however, as with all dyspneic patients, the risk/benefit ratio of the imaging procedure should be considered carefully.

Radiographic changes in patients with pulmonary contusions consist of areas of patchy or diffuse interstitial or alveolar lung infiltrates that can be either localized or generalized (Figure 25-1). Radiographic changes may lag behind clinical signs by 12 to 24 hours and therefore "normal" radiographic findings may be seen in animals with pulmonary contusions. Patients with more severe radiographic changes initially may require a longer duration of oxygen supplementation and longer hospitalization times. However, the relationship between severity of the contusion based on radiographic changes and survival has not been established.[7]

Although computed tomography (CT) has been shown experimentally to be more sensitive for detecting initial lesions and accurately reflecting the extent of the lesion than standard radiographic techniques, lack of availability in veterinary hospitals and the need

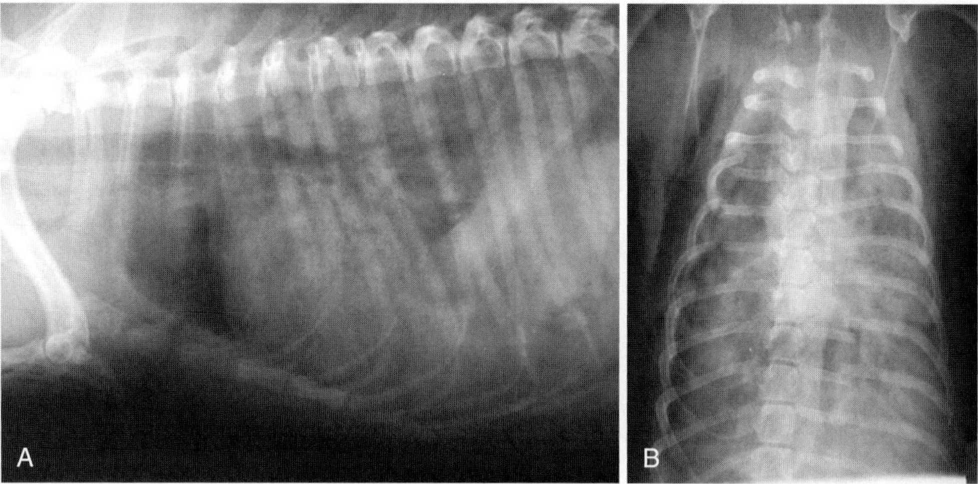

FIGURE 25-1 Lateral **(A)** and dorsoventral **(B)** radiographs showing the characteristic appearance of pulmonary contusions. Note the diffuse alveolar pattern. It is common to see additional radiographic abnormalities, such as multiple rib fractures, subcutaneous emphysema, pneumomediastinum, and pneumothorax, as seen in this case.

for sedation or anesthesia in a traumatized patient have so far limited its widespread use. An experimental canine model of pulmonary contusions found that a CT scan enabled detection of 100% of the pulmonary lesions, but initial thoracic radiographs failed to visualize them. In addition, 21% were still not visible radiographically after 6 hours. In this study, CT imaging underestimated the extent of the lesions in only 8% of the animals, whereas thoracic radiography underestimated the extent in 58% of the animals.[25]

In people, CT is considered the gold standard for the diagnosis of pulmonary contusions and may be predictive of progression and treatment needs. A contused volume of 20% or higher is highly predictive of the need for assisted ventilation (8% of patients with contused volume equal to or less than 20% compared with 40% of those patients with volumes higher than 20%).[26] The percentage of contused volume is also an independent predictive factor for the development of ARDS, with 21.5% being the best cutoff for severe pulmonary contusions.[27] Furthermore, in people with blunt pulmonary contusions, the absence of a blunt pulmonary contusion volume of 20% or more, more than four fractured ribs, or a Glasgow Coma Scale score higher than 14 precluded mechanical ventilation in 100% of the cases, while the presence of all three findings together predicted the need for mechanical ventilation in 100% of the cases.[28]

CT is undoubtedly a very sensitive tool and allows previously unrecognized injuries (occult injuries) to be identified. Patients with occult injury and those with no injury have similar ventilator needs and requirements; however, patients with occult injuries remain hospitalized longer. This has lead to the argument that occult injuries have minimal clinical consequences yet attract increased hospital resources.[29]

Thoracic ultrasound is gaining acceptance as a bedside test for the diagnosis of pulmonary contusions in people. Dependent on the ultrasonographic sign used (alveolointerstitial syndrome vs. the presence of a peripheral parenchymal lesion), sensitivity and specificity for the detection of contusions is high.[30] Other studies have shown thoracic ultrasonography to be a better diagnostic test than physical examination and thoracic radiographs when evaluating patients for pulmonary contusions or pneumothorax after chest trauma.[31] Utility of this technique has not been explored in small animal patients.

Blood Gas Analysis and Pulse Oximetry

Arterial blood gas analysis is the most objective method for assessing and monitoring the physiologic effects of thoracic trauma (see Chapter 186). Clinical data in dogs reveal a high incidence of hypoxemia; however, it is usually mild to moderate.[6,7] This may be because many of the most severe cases will die before arriving at the veterinary clinic. Either hypocarbia or hypercarbia may be seen, depending on the severity of the parenchymal injury, the nature of concurrent thoracic injuries, and other factors such as pain, distress, and the effect of concurrent metabolic acid-base derangements.

In humans, the arterial oxygen tension/fractional concentration of inspired oxygen ratio (PaO_2/FiO_2) is directly correlated with the volume of contused lung for the first 24 hours after injury, although this correlation is not consistent beyond 1 week.[32] Whether this association exists in small animal patients is unknown.

Although pulse oximetry has some limitations, it may be a useful quantitative assessment of oxygenation in cases in which an arterial blood gas analysis is not possible (e.g., cats). It is a less accurate indicator of impaired oxygenation, does not provide a measure of ventilation, and reliable measurements can be difficult to obtain in patients that are in shock. A pulse oximeter reading of less than 95% indicates hypoxemia and values less than 90% are consistent with severe hypoxemia.

MANAGEMENT

Initial Approach

Management of pulmonary contusions is supportive. Initial triage and major body system assessment should be done in any traumatized patient, and injuries should be ranked and managed based on their threat to patient life (see Chapter 1). Prehospital management rarely occurs. However, the animal should be transported to the clinic lying in its preferred posture or kept in sternal recumbency if possible.[33]

Oxygen therapy, judicious fluid therapy, and adequate analgesia are essential components of patient management.

Oxygen Therapy and Ventilation

Oxygen should be administered to all dyspneic patients (see Chapter 14). Noninvasive methods such as flow-by, nasal oxygen delivery, or oxygen cages and hoods are commonly used. In severely affected cases, intubation and ventilation may be necessary (see Chapters 30 and 31). This decision should be made based on the severity of the dyspnea and an assessment of arterial blood gas values, if possible.

In people, pressure-controlled ventilation with positive end-expiratory pressure is the preferred method of mechanical ventilation.[34] Improved ventilator strategies are being continuously evaluated. Recently the early use of high-frequency oscillatory ventilation (HFOV) has been deemed safe and efficacious,[35] and airway pressure release ventilation (a pressure-controlled mode consisting of a continuous positive airway pressure [CPAP] that at set intervals releases the pressure, effectively resulting in an inverted inspiration/expiration ratio) is associated with a reduced risk for ventilator-associated pneumonia, without changing either the need for ventilation days or the mortality rate.[36] One canine study examined 10 dogs with pulmonary contusions that required positive pressure ventilation and found that 50% of the dogs benefited from this intervention, and animals that weighed more than 25 kg were more likely to survive.[37] Alveolar recruitment strategies and the use of low tidal volumes have been shown to increase both oxygenation and lung aeration in humans with severe chest trauma,[38] although similar studies in dogs and cats are lacking.

Other advanced ventilatory techniques such as jet ventilation, selective bronchial intubation, dual-lung ventilation, and extracorporeal membrane oxygenation may prove useful but are not used routinely in the clinical setting for the management of pulmonary contusions in people or the veterinary field.

Fluid Therapy

Many patients with thoracic trauma will have some degree of concurrent hypovolemic shock. The debate regarding the optimal fluid therapy for use in trauma and shock patients has yet to be resolved; however, it seems that optimizing fluid therapy to maintain adequate perfusion while avoiding overzealous administration is likely to give the best results. In any patient with multiple trauma, the clinician must prioritize treatment decisions based on which major body system is most severely affected.

Many patients presenting with contusions also show some evidence of noncardiogenic shock. Several fluid options are available, and the fluid type and administration strategy chosen must take into account both the cardiovascular and pulmonary changes present (see Chapter 60). Regardless of the type of fluid chosen, increases in pulmonary capillary hydrostatic pressure may lead to increased fluid extravasation into the alveoli and worsening of pulmonary function. The clinician should aim to optimize tissue perfusion while avoiding excessive fluid administration that could worsen the pulmonary edema and hemorrhage. Careful monitoring and tailoring of the fluid protocol to the patient are preferable to administering preset volumes and rates. Replacement crystalloids are the most economical fluids and are at least as effective as colloids for resuscitation of the shock patient.[39,40] Evidence for the treatment of patients with pulmonary contusions is scarce, and papers yield conflicting results. Some have shown no benefits when using hypertonic saline over isotonic solutions in experimental porcine models of pulmonary contusions,[41] whereas others show less lung water retention and higher PaO_2 values with the use of hypertonic saline dextran versus Ringer's acetate.[42] Blood products and synthetic colloids may contribute to worsening pulmonary edema if they leak into the airways or interstitium. Hemoglobin-based oxygen carriers led to poorer oxygenation and more extensive pulmonary lesions compared with isotonic saline in a porcine model of pulmonary contusion and hemorrhage.[43]

Although clinical evidence is lacking, common sense dictates that although strict fluid restriction is not indicated, caution should be exercised when administering intravenous fluids to shock patients with suspected pulmonary contusions. Patients should be monitored carefully to detect any worsening of pulmonary function during fluid administration and fluid rates adjusted accordingly.

Analgesia

Hypoventilation caused by pain from concurrent injuries can be severe and should be managed proactively with analgesics (see Chapters 141 and 144). Ideally, drugs that cause minimal impairment of cardiac and respiratory functions should be used. Intercostal, intrapleural, and epidural analgesic administration can be used in conjunction with or as an alternative to systemic opioid administration. Further details can be found in Chapter 134.

Antimicrobial Therapy

Based on the reported low incidence of pneumonia after pulmonary contusions (1%),[7] indiscriminate use of antimicrobial agents should be avoided to limit bacterial resistance. In the small number of patients that do develop bacterial pneumonia, antibiotic therapy should be based on culture and susceptibility testing results of airway cytology (see Chapter 22).

Glucocorticoids

There are little supportive data for glucocorticoid use in the treatment of pulmonary contusions. Although some animal studies have shown a reduction in hypoxemia and lesion size after steroid administration,[44] others have shown no benefit.[45] Because of their potential deleterious effects, including increased susceptibility to infection and gastrointestinal ulceration, and the lack of positive effects on outcome, these agents are not recommended for the routine management of pulmonary contusions.

Other Therapies

Pulmonary contusion continues to be a significant cause of morbidity and mortality, despite the standard management strategies described earlier; work continues to identify improved treatment options. In people, the use of surfactant has been proven to improve both oxygenation and compliance in patients with severe pulmonary contusions.[46] Experimental studies suggest that dexmedetomidine improves hemodynamics, reduces the presence of inflammatory cells in the alveolar spaces, and modifies the inflammatory response by interfering with cytokine release.[47] The utility of these therapies in veterinary clinical patients is unknown.

PROGNOSIS AND OUTCOME

Outcome is related to the severity of pulmonary contusions as well as any coexisting thoracic and extrathoracic lesions. Survival rates of 82% have been described,[7] although the real survival rate may be lower because some of the most severely affected animals die before reaching a veterinary facility or before a diagnosis is made. Patients may require hospitalization for periods ranging from a few hours to several days, and oxygen supplementation can be required for several days to weeks.

In more severely affected patients, two retrospective studies have shown that approximately 30% of dogs requiring mechanical ventilation for contusions survived to discharge.[7,37] It is possible that newer lung-protective ventilatory strategies could improve outcomes (see Chapters 30 and 31).

Although the long-term prognosis for animals with pulmonary contusions has not been investigated, most animals that survive to discharge do not appear to have residual long-term sequelae. In people, even patients with severe injuries requiring ventilation show a substantial recovery, with postexercise oxygen saturations returning to normal values.[48]

ATRAUMATIC PULMONARY HEMORRHAGE

Atraumatic pulmonary hemorrhage may occur secondary to a diverse range of disease conditions (Table 25-1).

Although hemoptysis may occur in animals with pulmonary hemorrhage, it is an uncommon initial finding in small animals[49] and pulmonary hemorrhage cannot be ruled out based on the absence of

Table 25-1 Etiologies of Atraumatic Pulmonary Hemorrhage and Examples of Each

Infectious	Bacterial	Leptospirosis[53] *Escherichia coli*
	Fungal	—
	Mycoplasmal	—
	Parasitic	Heartworms (*Dirofilaria* spp) Lungworms (*Angiostrongylus vasorum*)
	Viral	—
Coagulation abnormalities	Defects of primary hemostasis	Thrombocytopathia Severe thrombocytopenia Uremia Hepatic failure
	Defects of secondary hemostasis	Anticoagulant rodenticide toxicity von Willebrand disease Hemophilia
	Thromboembolism	Cushing's disease Diabetes mellitus Nephrotic syndrome Glucocorticoid therapy
Cardiac	Heart failure Pulmonary hypertension	—
Neoplasia	Primary Metastatic	—
Anatomic	Lung lobe torsion	—
Environmental	Aspiration pneumonia Foreign bodies	—
Miscellaneous	Exercise-induced pulmonary hemorrhage in racing Greyhounds Post-seizure[54]	
Iatrogenic	Fine-needle aspiration Percutaneous biopsy	—

this symptom. In a population of cats undergoing airway cytologic analysis for a variety of disease conditions, pulmonary hemorrhage was identified in 63% of cases; the incidence of hemoptysis was not reported.[50]

DIAGNOSTIC EVALUATION

Pulmonary hemorrhage is identified by hemoptysis or hemorrhage on cytologic samples from tracheal, bronchial, or bronchoalveolar washes. The emergency clinician must be careful to distinguish true hemoptysis from hematemesis or bleeding from a source cranial to the larynx (nasal cavity, oropharynx). When using cytology specimens, acute hemorrhage is defined by presence of red blood cells and white blood cells in proportions similar to those in peripheral blood. Platelets may be present but tend to disappear within minutes after the hemorrhagic event. Within minutes to hours, erythrophagocytosis is present within the macrophages. Considering the diverse range of differential diagnoses, a thorough and careful diagnostic evaluation, including full history, diligent physical examination, and clinicopathologic testing and imaging, may be required to reach the correct diagnosis.

Historical information that suggests certain diagnoses may include exposure to toxins such as rodenticides or animals living in or having traveled to areas with a high incidence of certain infectious diseases (e.g., heartworms or lungworms). The influence of any concurrent drug therapy should be considered, such as high doses of glucocorticoids, especially in patients that are at risk for pulmonary thromboembolism. Historical information may also be suggestive of chronic medical conditions and may guide and inform further testing. The patient's signalment may suggest an increased possibility of certain coagulopathies, such as von Willebrand's disease in Doberman Pinschers.

The physical examination of animals with pulmonary hemorrhage may reveal clinical signs limited to the respiratory system, including hemoptysis, dyspnea, tachypnea, cough, and abnormal auscultation findings. Adventitious lung sounds are variable but may include focal or generalized harsh lung sounds progressing to crackles, focal muffled lung sounds corresponding to areas with consolidation or complete filling of the small airways, or wheezes. Heart murmurs or cardiac arrhythmias may also be noted and may suggest a cardiogenic cause for the pulmonary hemorrhage. However, because pulmonary hemorrhage may occur secondary to systemic disease, a full physical examination is mandatory. The presence of petechiae or ecchymoses should prompt the investigation of a bleeding disorder, whereas an elevated body temperature may suggest infectious or neoplastic disease.

Further diagnostic tests will be suggested by the patient's history and physical examination but may include a complete blood cell count (CBC), biochemical profile, coagulogram, urinalysis, and imaging techniques. An arterial blood gas analysis will provide the best evaluation of the functional impairment of the respiratory system and may reveal hypoxemia, hypocarbia (or hypercarbia in severe cases), and an increased alveolar–arterial gradient (see Chapter 186). However, in animals with suspected or confirmed pulmonary hemorrhage, arterial sampling should be avoided until clotting times and platelet numbers and function have been assessed. Animals with chronic diseases such as pulmonary neoplasia, chronic bronchitis, or pneumonia may have metabolic compensation for changes in arterial carbon dioxide tensions, whereas acutely affected animals often have uncompensated changes in acid-base status.

Thoracic radiographs may reveal an interstitial, alveolar, or mixed pattern, with a focal, patchy, or diffuse distribution. A peripheral interstitial and alveolar pattern in a young to middle-aged dog is a characteristic finding in *Angiostrongylus vasorum* infestation.[51] The cardiac silhouette may be enlarged and signs of pulmonary congestion may be evident in cases of congestive heart failure or *Dirofilaria* spp infestation. If cardiac disease is suspected, echocardiography is the test of choice for characterization of the disease.

Hematology findings may be unremarkable or may show changes suggestive of the underlying diagnosis, including normocytic normochromic anemia in case of chronic disease, eosinophilia with parasitic disease, and neutrophilia with or without a left shift in cases of inflammatory disease. Platelet numbers may be normal, mildly to moderately reduced (e.g., in disseminated intravascular coagulation, angiostrongylosis, and some cases of thromboembolism), or severely reduced (e.g., in immune-mediated thrombocytopenia). If platelet numbers are adequate but petechiae are present, thrombocytopathia may be present and a buccal mucosal bleeding time should be performed (see Chapter 105).

Clotting times (prothrombin time and activated partial thromboplastin time) are prolonged in animals with a coagulopathy. The prothrombin time is markedly prolonged in animals with anticoagulant rodenticide poisoning, although all clotting parameters may increase if bleeding has occurred. Increases in fibrin(ogen) degradation products or D-dimers may suggest pulmonary thromboembolism, although a CT scan with angiography is more definitive (see Chapter 104).[52] In recent years, thromboelastography (TEG) has emerged as a more comprehensive means to evaluate both the thrombotic and thrombolytic parts of hemostasis.

A fecal Baermann analysis should be performed if *A. vasorum* or other lungworm infections are suspected. Antigen or antibody detection tests for heartworm are indicated in dogs or cats living in, or traveling to, endemic areas.

TREATMENT

Treatment will ultimately need to be directed toward the underlying disease process. If the degree of respiratory compromise is marked, it may be necessary to use supportive or empiric therapy while the diagnosis is pursued. Oxygen should be administered to any dyspneic patient, and in particular to those animals showing hypoxemia on arterial blood gas analysis or low pulse oximetry readings. If noninvasive oxygen supplementation does not restore adequate oxygen levels, severe hypercarbia is present, or the patient displays significant dyspnea with impending fatigue, positive pressure ventilation may be required (see Chapter 30). Fluid therapy should be tailored to each animal's needs based on the cardiovascular and respiratory status, as with pulmonary contusions. Analgesia and sedation should also be used, as indicated by an animal's clinical status. It is often necessary to institute empiric antimicrobial therapy on the basis of a strong clinical suspicion while diagnostic test results are pending.

PROGNOSIS AND OUTCOME

Prognosis and long-term outcome will depend largely on the extent and severity of the process on admission, and on the etiology of the pathology. An overall mortality rate of up to 25%[49] in the 6 months after diagnosis has been reported, with patients dying as a result of the disease process or after humane euthanasia. It is difficult to predict whether any long-term impairment of function will ensue, but this likely depends on the underlying disease and its severity. Hence owners should be given a guarded to grave prognosis until a definitive diagnosis is reached.

REFERENCES

1. Spackman C, Caywood D: Management of thoracic trauma and chest wall reconstruction, Vet Clin North Am Small Anim Pract 17:431, 1987.
2. Vnuk D, Pirkic B, Maticic D, et al: Feline high-rise syndrome: 119 cases (1998-2001), J Feline Med Surg 6:305, 2004.
3. Scheepens ET, Peeters ME, Éplattenier HF, Kirpensteijn J: Thoracic bite trauma in dogs: a comparison of clinical and radiological parameters with surgical results, J Small Anim Pract 47(12):721, 2006.
4. Tamas P, Paddleford R, Krahwinkel D: Thoracic trauma in dogs and cats presented for limb fractures, J Am Anim Hosp Assoc 21:161, 1985.
5. Spackman C, Caywood D, Feeney D, et al: Thoracic wall and pulmonary trauma in dogs sustaining fractures as a result of motor vehicle accidents, J Am Vet Med Assoc 185:975, 1984.
6. Selcer B, Buttrick M, Barstad R, et al: The incidence of thoracic trauma in dogs with skeletal injury, J Small Anim Pract 28:21, 1987.
7. Powell L, Rozanski E, Tidwell A, et al: A retrospective analysis of pulmonary contusion secondary to motor vehicular accidents in 143 dogs: 1994-1997, J Vet Emerg Crit Care 9:127, 1999.
8. Sigrist N, Doherr M, Spreng D. Clinical findings and diagnostic value of post-traumatic thoracic radiographs in dogs and cats with blunt trauma, J Vet Emerg Crit Care 14:259, 2004.
9. Sigrist N, Mosing M, Iff I, et al: Influence of pre-anesthetic thoracic radiographs on ASA physical status classification and anaesthetic protocols in traumatized dogs and cats, Schweiz Arch Tierheilkd 150(10):507, 2008.
10. Clemedson C: Blast injury, Physiol Rev 36(3):336, 1956.
11. Huller T, Bazini Y: Blast injuries of the chest and abdomen, Arch Surg 100:24, 1970.
12. Cohn S: Pulmonary contusions: review of the clinical entity, J Trauma 45:973, 1997.
13. Demling R, Pomfret E: Blunt chest trauma, N Horizons 1:402, 1993.
14. Oppenheimer L, Craven K, Forkert L, et al: Pathophysiology of pulmonary contusion in dogs, J Appl Physiol 47:718, 1979.
15. Batchinsky AI, Weiss WB, Jordan BS, et al: Ventilation-perfusion relationships following experimental pulmonary contusion, J Appl Physiol 103(3):895, 2007.
16. Batchinsky AI, Jordan BS, Necsiou C, et al: Dynamic changes in shunt and ventilation-perfusion mismatch following experimental pulmonary contusion, Shock 33(4):419, 2010.
17. Wagner R, Slivko B, Jamieson P, et al: Effects of lung contusion on pulmonary haemodynamics, Ann Thorac Surg 52:51, 1991.
18. Perl M, Gebhard F, Bruckner U, et al: Pulmonary contusion causes impairment of macrophage and lymphocyte immune functions and increases mortality associated with a subsequent septic challenge, Crit Care Med 2005;33:1351, 2005.
19. Fulton R, Peter E: The progressive nature of pulmonary contusion, Surgery 67:499, 1970.
20. Moseley R, Vernick J, Doty D: Response to blunt chest injury: a new experimental model, J Trauma 101:673, 1970.
21. Hackner S: Emergency management of traumatic pulmonary contusions, Comp Cont Ed Pract Vet 17:677, 1995.
22. Hellinger A, Konerding M, Malkusch W, et al: Does lung contusion affect both the traumatized and the noninjured lung parenchyma? A morphological and morphometric study in the pig, J Trauma 39:712, 1995.
23. Raghavendran K, Notter RH, Davidson BA, et al: Lung contusion: inflammatory mechanisms and interaction with other injuries, Shock 32(2):122, 2009.
24. Raghavendran K, Davidson BA, Huebschmann JC, et al: Superimposed gastric aspiration increases the severity of inflammation and permeability injury in a rat model of lung contusion, J Surg Res 155(2):273, 2009.
25. Schild H, Strunk H, Weber W, et al: Pulmonary contusion: CT vs plain radiogram, J Comput Assist Tomogr 13:417, 1989.
26. Hamrick MC, Duhn RD, Ochsner MG: Critical evaluation of pulmonary contusion in the early post-traumatic period: risk of assisted ventilation, Am Surg 75(11):1054, 2009.
27. Wang S, Ruan Z, Zhang J, Jin W: The value of pulmonary contusion volume measurements with three-dimensional computed tomography in predicting acute respiratory distress syndrome development, Ann Thorac Surg 92(6):1977, 2011.
28. de Moya MA, Manolakaki D, Chang Y: Blunt pulmonary contusion: admission computed tomography scan predicts mechanical ventilation, J Trauma 71(6):1543, 2011.
29. Kaiser M, Wheaton M, Barrios C, et al: The clinical significance of occult thoracic injury in blunt trauma patients, Am Surg 76(10):1063, 2010.
30. Soldati G, Testa A, Silva FR, et al: Chest ultrasonography in lung contusion, Chest 130(2):533, 2006.
31. Hyacinthe AC, Broux C, Francony G, et al: Diagnostic accuracy of ultrasonography in the acute assessment of common thoracic lesions after trauma, Chest 141(5):1177, 2012.
32. Mizushima Y, Hiraide A, Shimazu T, et al: Changes in contused lung volume and oxygenation in patients with pulmonary parenchymal injury after blunt chest trauma, Am J Emerg Med 18:585, 2000.
33. MacMillan MW, Whitaker KE, Hughes D, Brodbelt DC, Boag AK: Effect of body position on the arterial partial pressures of oxygen in carbon dioxide in spontaneously breathing, conscious dogs in an intensive care unit, J Vet Emerg Crit Care 19(6):564, 2009.
34. Sharma S, Mullins R, Trunkey D: Ventilatory management of pulmonary contusion patients, Am J Surg 171:529, 1996.
35. Funk DJ, Lujan E, Moretti EW, et al: A brief report: the use of high-frequency oscillatory ventilation for severe pulmonary contusions, J Trauma 65(2):390, 2008.
36. Walkey AJ, Nair S, Papadopoulos S, et al: Use of airway pressure release ventilation is associated with a reduced incidence of ventilator-associated pneumonia in patients with pulmonary contusion, J Trauma 70(3):E42, 2011.

37. Campbell V, King L: Pulmonary function, ventilator management, and outcome of dogs with thoracic trauma and pulmonary contusions: 10 cases (1994-1998), J Am Vet Med Assoc 217:1505, 2000.
38. Schreiter D, Reske A, Stichert B, et al: Alveolar recruitment in combination with sufficient positive end-expiratory pressure increases oxygenation and lung aeration in patients with severe chest trauma, Crit Care Med 32:968, 2004.
39. Roberts I, Alderson P, Bunn F, et al: Colloids versus crystalloids for fluid resuscitation in critically ill patients (review), Cochrane Database Syst Rev (4):CD000567, 2004.
40. Investigators TSS: A comparison of albumin and saline for fluid resuscitation in the intensive care unit, N Engl J Med 350:2247, 2004.
41. Cohn S, Fisher B, Rosenfield A, et al: Resuscitation of pulmonary contusion: hypertonic saline is not beneficial, Shock 8:292, 1997.
42. Gryth D, Rocksen D, Drobin D, et al: Effects of fluid resuscitation with hypertonic saline dextran or Ringer's acetate after nonhemorrhagic shock caused by pulmonary contusions, J Trauma 69(4):741, 2010.
43. Cohn S, Zieg P, Rosenfield A, et al: Resuscitation of pulmonary contusion: effects of a red cell substitute, Crit Care Med 25:484, 1997.
44. Franz J, Richardson J, Grover F, et al: Effect of methylprednisolone sodium succinate on experimental pulmonary contusion, J Thor Cardiovasc Surg 68:842, 1974.
45. Shepard G, Ferguson J, Foster J. Pulmonary contusion, Ann Thorac Surg 7:110, 1969.
46. Tsangaris I, Galiatsou E, Kostanti E, Nakos G. The effect of exogenous surfactant in patients with lung contusions and acute lung injury, Intensive Care Med 33(5):851, 2007.
47. Wu X, Song X, Li N, et al: Protective effects of dexmedetomidine on blunt chest trauma-induced pulmonary contusions in rats, J Trauma Acute Care Surg 74(2):524, 2013.
48. Amital A, Shitrit D, Fox BD, et al: Long term pulmonary function after recovery from pulmonary contusion due to blunt chest trauma, Isr Med Assoc J 11(11):673, 2009.
49. Bailiff N, Norris C: Clinical signs, clinicopathological findings, etiology, and outcome associated with hemoptysis in dogs: 36 cases (1990-1999), J Am Anim Hosp Assoc 38:125, 2002.
50. DeHeer H, McManus P: Frequency and severity of tracheal wash hemosiderosis and association with underlying disease in 96 cats (2002-2003), Vet Clin Pathol 34:17, 2005.
51. Chapman P, Boag A, Guitian J, et al: Angiostrongylus vasorum infection in 23 dogs (1999-2002), J Small Anim Pract 45:435, 2004.
52. Nelson O: Use of the D-dimer assay for diagnosing thromboembolic disease in dogs, J Am Anim Hosp Assoc 41:145, 2005.
53. Klopfleisch R, Kohn B, Plog S, et al: An emerging pulmonary haemorrhagic syndrome in dogs: similar to the human leptospiral pulmonary haemorrhagic syndrome? Vet Med Int 2010:928541, 2010.
54. James FE, Johnson VS, Lenarz ZM, Mansfield CS: Severe haemoptysis associated with seizures in a dog, N Z Vet J 56(2):85, 2008.

CHAPTER 26
PULMONARY THROMBOEMBOLISM

Lynelle R. Johnson, DVM, MS, PhD, DACVIM

KEY POINTS

- Pulmonary thromboembolism (PTE) occurs as a secondary complication of diseases associated with hypercoagulability, endothelial damage, and stasis of blood flow.
- It is a challenging antemortem diagnosis and is associated with a guarded prognosis.
- Identification of risk factors and disease associations for PTE is important for clinical recognition of this complication.
- Clinical findings that support a diagnosis of PTE in a systemically ill patient include tachypnea, hypoxemia, echocardiographic detection of echogenic material in the pulmonary artery or evidence of acute right ventricular overload, and perfusion deficits on nuclear scintigraphy.
- Therapy for PTE relies primarily on treatment of the underlying disease process, support of oxygenation, and limitation of further growth of the clot through use of anticoagulants.
- Prophylaxis against thromboembolic complications should be considered in animals with serious disease syndromes that have been associated with PTE.

Obstruction of the pulmonary vascular bed can occur through blockage with fat, septic emboli, metastatic neoplasia, parasites (*Dirofilaria* or *Angiostrongylus*), or blood clots (pulmonary thromboembolism [PTE]). It is likely that PTE results most commonly from formation of clot material in the right side of the heart or at a distant site in the venous system that breaks free and lodges in the pulmonary vasculature. Thrombosis in situ may also occur in association with pulmonary hypertension, heartworm disease, or other disorders of the pulmonary vasculature. PTE is likely underdiagnosed in the veterinary population similar to the situation in human medicine. Thrombi undergo 50% reduction in clot volume in the first 3 hours postmortem because of fibrinolytic dissolution; with heparin administration, clot volume is further reduced as a result of inhibition of clot formation.[1] Thus necropsy confirmation of PTE can be difficult.

Clinical recognition of PTE antemortem is difficult because clinical signs and physical examination findings mimic those found in a variety of cardiopulmonary conditions. In an early report, PTE was a differential diagnosis for respiratory distress in less than 5% of dogs with PTE confirmed at necropsy.[2] In a later study,[3] PTE was suspected in 65% of dogs presenting with relevant respiratory signs and a recognized predisposing condition for thromboembolism, suggesting increased awareness of the condition. In dogs, immune-mediated hemolytic anemia, sepsis, neoplasia, amyloidosis, hyperadrenocorticism, and dilated cardiomyopathy are associated with increased risk for PTE, whereas neoplasia and cardiomyopathy are found most often in cats with PTE.[3-5] The majority of cases have comorbid conditions complicating the primary clinical disease and potentially

BOX 26-1 ***Disorders Associated with Pulmonary Thromboembolism***

Immune-mediated hemolytic anemia
Neoplasia
Sepsis
Protein-losing nephropathy/enteropathy
Cardiac disease
Hyperadrenocorticism
Central catheter use
  Hemodialysis
  Total parenteral nutrition
Hip replacement surgery (cemented)
Trauma

increasing the risk for thromboembolism. Because PTE is associated with nonspecific clinical signs such as tachypnea or respiratory distress, knowledge of predisposing conditions (Box 26-1) is important for appropriate diagnosis and treatment.

PATHOPHYSIOLOGY

Thromboembolism occurs in association with a hypercoagulable state. This is reviewed further in Chapter 104.

The key pathophysiologic responses to PTE include alterations in hemodynamics as a result of increased pulmonary vascular resistance, abnormalities in gas exchange, altered ventilatory control, and derangements in pulmonary mechanics. Rarely, pulmonary infarction contributes to the clinical presentation. Unlike the systemic circulation, the pulmonary circulation is able to accommodate substantial changes in blood flow without increases in pulmonary vascular pressure as a result of distention and recruitment of pulmonary vessels. Vascular obstruction from embolization results in both mechanical obstruction of the vasculature and reactive vasoconstriction because of the release of vasoactive mediators. The combination of these events causes a reduction in the cross-sectional area of the pulmonary circulatory bed, increases in vascular resistance, and, in moderate to severe cases, increases in pulmonary arterial pressure.

PTE results in hypoxemia primarily from low ventilation-perfusion (V/Q) areas of the lung, although physiologic shunting and reduced diffusion capacity also contribute to reduced arterial oxygen content. Hypoxemia can be present with as little as 13% obstruction of the vascular bed in humans,[6] suggesting that even minor embolic disease is physiologically relevant. The severity of hypoxemia will be impacted by the presence of underlying cardiopulmonary disease, reflex bronchoconstriction, and atelectasis. In the normal lung, most lung units have a V/Q ratio of approximately 1; however, PTE causes a redistribution of blood flow, resulting in a wide spectrum of high, normal, and low V/Q units. Low V/Q units are the most important contributors to hypoxemia. As the degree of vascular obstruction exceeds 50% of the surface area of the circulatory bed, intrapulmonary shunting (areas of no V/Q) occurs, leading to venous admixture.[7]

Ventilation is controlled by the interaction between the sensors, which are activated by elevated CO_2 in the central nervous system and decreased PaO_2 in the periphery, with the responders (respiratory muscles). PTE is associated with tachypnea and alveolar hyperventilation, although the mechanisms responsible for hyperventilation have not been fully defined. Hypoxemia could drive hyperventilation. Platelet aggregation with release of humoral mediators and cytokines could activate C fibers and irritant receptors to cause breathlessness. Embolization of additional organs often occurs with PTE,[3,8] and vascular obstruction in the central nervous system could also affect ventilatory control.

Changes in lung mechanics are likely important contributors to tachypnea because increased resistance and decreased compliance greatly affect the work of breathing. Experimental studies in dogs have documented increased airway resistance after PTE; 5-hydroxytryptamine (serotonin) likely mediates this bronchoconstriction.[9] Lung compliance is reduced in PTE because of pulmonary edema and atelectasis. Pulmonary edema appears to result from increased hydrostatic pressure associated with increased blood flow to nonembolized lung regions and from release of humoral factors that increase microvascular permeability.

HISTORY AND CLINICAL SIGNS

Historical features consistent with PTE included labored breathing, tachypnea, lethargy, and altered neurologic status. Additional clinical signs that can be observed include cough, syncope, and hemoptysis. Altered mental state is reported in 20% of human patients with PTE and might be related to transient hypoxemia or cerebral ischemia. In a report in dogs, abnormal neurologic status was recorded in more than one third of affected animals[3] and thus might be a common finding with PTE. Importantly, obvious respiratory distress and tachypnea can be absent in some dogs or cats that have pulmonary embolization documented at necropsy.

It is essential to obtain information regarding concurrent disease processes and treatment to determine the risk of embolization in hospitalized patients. In dogs with clinical syndromes associated with PTE, intravenous catheters had been placed in the majority of cases, exogenous glucocorticoid excess was reported in half, use of cytotoxic agents was found in more than one third, 21% had undergone recent surgical procedures, and 10% of dogs were given blood transfusions.[3]

PHYSICAL EXAMINATION

Dogs with pulmonary thromboembolism typically demonstrate tachypnea or hyperpnea. Physical examination findings potentially consistent with PTE include labored breathing, tachycardia, and harsh or abnormal lung sounds such as crackles or wheezes. Alternately, lung and heart sounds may be dampened because of pleural effusion. Cardiac murmurs are not uncommon in affected dogs or cats because of the presence of underlying cardiac pathology (particularly cardiomyopathy in cats) or development of pulmonary hypertension.

DIAGNOSTIC TESTING

The history of a disease association along with the acute onset of tachypnea and labored respirations is highly suspicious for pulmonary embolization; however, proving the presence of embolic disease antemortem is challenging. Routine laboratory work (complete blood cell count [CBC], chemistry profile, and urinalysis) is submitted to investigate the underlying disease. Hyperbilirubinemia and negative Coombs test were considered suggestive of PTE in dogs with immune-mediated hemolytic anemia (IMHA).[4] Hypoalbuminemia should prompt investigation of systemic protein loss, which could be associated with concurrent loss of antithrombin III. Antithrombin concentrations less than 50% to 75% of normal are suspicious for hypercoagulability and potentially increased risk of embolic complications. In animals with concurrent loss of albumin and globulin, a protein-losing enteropathy (PLE) should be considered. Low vitamin B_{12} serum levels are supportive of intestinal dysfunction, and hypercoagulability has been documented by thromboelastography (TEG) in dogs with PLE.[10] Thromboelastography is a newer diagnostic test that evaluates the kinetics and efficiency of clot formation. Although its role in diagnosis and management of PTE has not been established, this test provides a dynamic assessment of clot construction and strength and can identify both hypocoagulable and hypercoagulable states. In comparison, standard tests of coagulation (activated partial thromboplastin time [aPTT], prothrombin time [PT]) assess only the time required to form a clot.

Assessment of D-dimer concentration has been recommended as a way to exclude PTE when the test is negative or to increase the likelihood that embolization is present when a high titer is detected.[11] D-Dimer is a degradation product of fibrin that has undergone cross-linkage, and a positive test is more specific for fibrin formation than the fibrin degradation product test (FDP) because the FDP detects both fibrin and fibrinogen breakdown products. Unfortunately, many diseases in veterinary medicine result in elevation of D-dimer,[11] and a negative test does not exclusively rule out thromboembolism.[12] A study in human medicine evaluating the accuracy of D-dimer testing versus location of embolus reported that a negative D-dimer could be used to rule out the majority (93%) of large pulmonary emboli but only half of the subsegmental emboli.[13]

Arterial blood gas analysis reveals hypoxemia, hypocapnia, and a widened alveolar-arterial (A-a) gradient in most patients assessed. Calculation of the alveolar-arterial gradient corrects for the contribution of alveolar hypoventilation to arterial hypoxemia but does not differentiate V/Q mismatch from other causes of hypoxemia. The A-a gradient is measured by the following formula using data obtained from an arterial blood gas:

$$(A-a) = PAO_2 - PaO_2$$

$$(A-a) = [FiO_2(P_b - P_{H2O}) - PaCO_2/RQ] - PaO_2$$

where FIO_2 is fraction of inspired oxygen; P_b, barometric pressure (760 mm Hg at sea level); P_{H2O}, water vapor pressure at a given body temperature (50 mm Hg); and RQ, respiratory quotient (0.8 to 1.0). The normal A-a gradient is less than 10 to 15 mm Hg when breathing room air (see Chapter 15).

Arterial blood gas analysis during oxygen supplementation provides information on the potential mechanism underlying hypoxemia but does not help determine prognosis for recovery. A positive response to exogenous oxygen supplementation suggests that low V/Q regions are the primary pathophysiologic mechanism for hypoxemia. A negative response suggests that intrapulmonary shunting (zero V/Q regions) or pulmonary infarction could be present. Trends in oxygen responsiveness can be followed by calculating the partial pressure of oxygen/fraction of inspired oxygen (PF) ratio. This value is calculated by dividing the PaO_2 by the FiO_2. Normal values should exceed 450; the lower the PF ratio, the more severe the pulmonary abnormality. Although patients with PTE are classically described as being oxygen responsive, this is not always the case and response to oxygen therapy cannot be used as a definitive diagnostic test.

Thoracic radiographs can help elucidate the underlying disease responsible for embolization or can reveal abnormalities associated with vascular obstruction (Figure 26-1) Previously reported thoracic radiographic abnormalities associated with PTE in dogs include pleural effusion, loss of definition of the pulmonary artery, alveolar infiltrates, cardiomegaly, hyperlucent lung regions, and enlargement of the main pulmonary artery.[14] Interstitial or alveolar infiltrates can represent focal or diffuse edema associated with overperfusion or atelectasis. Normal thoracic radiographs do not rule out the possibility of pulmonary thromboembolization, and normal thoracic radiographs in a patient with dramatic tachypnea and respiratory distress should be considered highly suspicious for PTE.[3]

Echocardiography can be considered as a diagnostic modality for noninvasive assessment of major pulmonary vessels, and thrombi can occasionally be seen in pulmonary arteries or in the right atrium. Signs of acute right ventricular overload may be evident, such as right ventricular hypokinesis or dilation, abnormal septal motion, or tricuspid regurgitation. In human medicine, echocardiographic changes of right ventricular dilation, paradoxical septal motion, and increased velocity of tricuspid regurgitant jet are evident in the majority of patients with clinically relevant pulmonary embolization.[15]

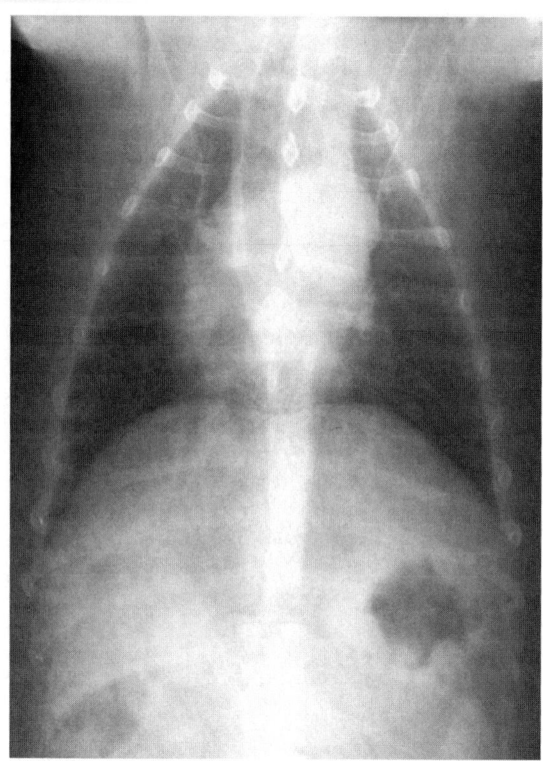

FIGURE 26-1 Dorsoventral thoracic radiograph of the dog displayed in Figure 26-2. Note the subtlety of the changes. The artery to the right caudal lung lobe appears to terminate abruptly at the eighth intercostal space. There is mild enlargement of the main pulmonary artery but the cardiac silhouette is unremarkable. Lung fields are essentially unremarkable with the exception of a focal area of interstitial opacity at the periphery of the right caudal lung lobe. *(Courtesy Dr. Narelle Brown, University of California, Davis.)*

Definitive diagnosis of pulmonary embolization in human medicine relies on selective pulmonary angiography, although contrast angiography during computed tomography is increasingly used. Neither technique has been embraced in veterinary patients because they require anesthesia. Ventilation-perfusion scans have compared favorably to angiography for diagnosis of PTE in human and veterinary patients[16]; however, the ventilation phase of the study requires anesthesia to ensure adequate deposition of radioactive gas throughout the airways. Perfusion scanning, using technetium-labeled macroaggregated albumin, is a less invasive tool that can be performed without anesthesia. This diagnostic test can reveal regions of absent radioactivity because of loss of pulmonary blood supply from embolization (Figure 26-2). In human medicine, a normal perfusion scan virtually excludes pulmonary embolization. An abnormal perfusion scan, however, can reflect PTE or a variety of pulmonary conditions, including pneumonia, atelectasis, edema, or contusions.

TREATMENT AND PROPHYLAXIS

Treatment and stabilization of the underlying condition should be initiated in order to limit further thrombus formation and subsequent embolization. Oxygen therapy is essential to reverse hypoxemia associated with V/Q mismatching and diffusion impairment. It is important to note that the degree of improvement in PaO_2 in

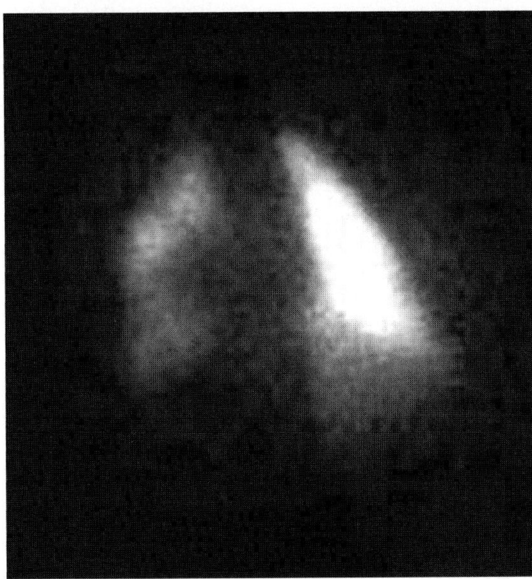

FIGURE 26-2 Nuclear scintigraphy using technetium-99m–labeled macroaggregated albumin. This ventral view reveals a large perfusion deficit in the region of the right caudal lung lobe. *(Courtesy Dr. Narelle Brown, University of California, Davis.)*

response to exogenous oxygen supplementation will depend on the percentage of the vascular bed that is obstructed, the concentration of inspired O_2 administered, the distribution of V/Q mismatching across the lung, and the degree of shunting that is present.

Thrombolysis offers the potential to resolve the embolus, but this benefit must be weighed against the concerns for hemorrhage. The current human guidelines recommend thrombolysis for massive pulmonary embolism, defined as pulmonary embolism with hypotension or cardiogenic shock. Thrombolysis is also recommended for pulmonary embolism associated with right ventricular enlargement or hypokinesis (submassive pulmonary embolism).[17] In less severe cases, the risk for hemorrhage is considered to outweigh the benefits. Thrombolysis is performed using tissue plasminogen activator (tPA) to cause direct fibrinolysis at the site of the clot. It can be delivered systemically or in a catheter-directed approach. Although the use of tPA has not been reported in clinical veterinary patients with PTE, it has been used extensively in canine experimental studies of thrombosis and anecdotally it has been used at the author's institution for treating PTE, with mixed results. Streptokinase is another thrombolytic drug that has been used successfully in canine patients, but the availability of this drug is currently limited. Further discussion of thrombolysis can be found in Chapter 169.

Anticoagulant therapy aims to reduce further growth of the embolus and prevent new embolic events. It is recommended for use in all human patients with PTE. The duration of anticoagulant therapy recommended depends on various underlying risk factors, with 3 months of therapy as a minimum in most scenarios.[17] Options for anticoagulant therapy include heparins, antiplatelet drugs, and novel anticoagulant drugs. These drugs are reviewed in Chapter 168. The efficacy of anticoagulant drugs in veterinary patients is poorly defined. Aspirin therapy has been associated with improved survival when combined with standard immunotherapy for management of immune-mediated hemolytic anemia,[18] although the effects specifically on PTE are difficult to determine.

SUMMARY

Pulmonary thromboembolism is often a devastating consequence of an already serious illness. Treatment of the primary condition and supportive care during recanalization of the clot can be successful; however, the possibility of further embolization exists. Prophylaxis for PTE should be considered in animals predisposed to the development of embolic complications.

REFERENCES

1. Moser KM, Guisan M, Bartimmo EE, et al: In vivo and post mortem dissolution rates of pulmonary emboli and venous thrombi in the dog, Circulation 48:170, 1973.
2. La Rue MG, Murtaugh RJ: Pulmonary thromboembolism in dogs: 47 cases (1986-1987), J Am Vet Med Assoc 197:1369, 1990.
3. Johnson LR, Lappin MR, Baker DC: Pulmonary thromboembolism in 29 dogs: 1985-1995, J Vet Intern Med 13:338, 1999.
4. Klein MK, Dow SW, Rosychuk RAW: Pulmonary thromboembolism associated with immune-mediated hemolytic anemia in dogs: ten cases (1982-1987), J Am Vet Med Assoc 195:146, 1989.
5. Norris CR, Griffey SM, Samii VF: Pulmonary thromboembolism in cats: 29 cases (1987-1997), J Am Vet Med Assoc 215:1650, 1999.
6. McIntyre KM, Sasahara AA: The hemodynamic response to pulmonary embolism in patients without prior cardiopulmonary disease, Am J Cardiol 28:288, 1971.
7. West JB: Pulmonary pathophysiology: the essentials, ed 5, Baltimore, 1998, Williams and Wilkins, pp 95-112.
8. Carr AP, Panciera DL, Kidd L: Prognostic factors for mortality and thromboembolism in canine immune-mediated hemolytic anemia: a retrospective of 72 cases, J Vet Intern Med 16:504, 2002
9. Thomas D, Steiz M, Rtanabe G, et al: Mechanism of bronchoconstriction produced by thromboemboil in dogs, Am J Phys 206:1207, 1964.
10. Goodwin LV, Goggs R, Chan DL, et al: Hypercoagulability in dogs with protein-losing enteropathy, J Vet Intern Med 25:273, 2012.
11. Nelson OL, Andreason C: The utility of plasma D-dimer to identify thromboembolic disease in the dog, J Vet Intern Med 17:830, 2003
12. Epstein SE, Hopper K, Mellema MS, et al: Diagnostic utility of D-Dimers in dogs with pulmonary embolism, J Vet Intern Med 27:1646, 2013.
13. Monye WDE, Sanson B, Mac Gillavry MR, et al: Embolus location affects the sensitivity of a rapid quantitative D-dimer assay in the diagnosis of pulmonary embolism, Am J Resp Crit Care Med 165:345, 2002.
14. Fluckiger MA, Gomez JA: Radiographic findings in dogs with spontaneous pulmonary thrombosis or embolism, Vet Rad 23:124, 1984
15. Nazeyrollas P, Metz D, Chapoutot L, et al: Diagnostic accuracy of echocardiography-Doppler in acute pulmonary embolism, Int J Cardiol 47:273, 1995.
16. Koblik PD, Hornoff W, Harnagel SH, et al: A comparison of pulmonary angiography, digital subtraction angiography, and ^{99m}Tc-DTPA/MAA ventilation-perfusion scintigraphy for detection of experimental pulmonary emboli in the dog, Vet Radiol Ultrasound 30:159, 1989.
17. Kearon C, Akl EA, Comerota AJ, et al: Antithrombotic therapy for VTE disease: Antithrombotic Therapy and Prevention of Thrombosis, 9th ed: American College of Chest Physicians evidence-based clinical practice guidelines, Chest 141:e419S, 2012.
18. Weinkle TK, Center SA, Randolph JF, et al: Evaluation of prognostic factors, survival rates, and treatment protocols for immune-mediated hemolytic anemia in dogs: 151 cases (1993-2002), J Am Vet Med Assoc 226:1869, 2005.

CHAPTER 27

CHEST WALL DISEASE

Suzanne Donahue, VMD, DACVECC • Deborah C. Silverstein, DVM, DACVECC

KEY POINTS

- The chest wall is necessary for respiration and protection of the thoracic cavity.
- Diseases of the chest wall include congenital anomalies, neoplasia, trauma-induced abnormalities (rib fractures, flail chest, penetrating wounds), cervical spine disease, and neuromuscular disease.
- The history and physical examination can usually establish a diagnosis of chest wall disease. Thoracic radiographs may also be informative.
- Initial treatment is aimed at stabilizing the patient and providing mechanical ventilatory assistance if indicated. Medical or surgical management of underlying diseases may be necessary.

Diseases of the chest wall are always a differential diagnosis for animals suffering from respiratory distress. A thorough history and physical examination will often help to confirm a diagnosis and ensure appropriate and timely therapy.

CHEST WALL ANATOMY AND FUNCTION

The chest wall has two main functions. The bones of the chest wall (13 pair of ribs, 13 vertebrae, and 9 sternebrae) serve to protect the internal structures of the thorax. The muscles of the chest wall (mainly the diaphragm and the external and internal intercostal muscles), and the nerves that innervate them, are necessary for normal respiration to occur.

When the diaphragm is stimulated, it contracts and moves caudally in animals. At the same time, the intercostal muscles move the ribcage cranially and outward. When the chest wall moves outward, the lungs are "pulled" with it as negative pressure is generated within the pleural space. As the intrathoracic volume increases during spontaneous inspiration, the pressure within the alveoli decreases slightly. Airway pressure becomes lower than atmospheric pressure, which causes air to flow into the lung. When the diaphragm and intercostal muscles relax during exhalation, the elastic recoil of the lungs and chest wall compresses the lungs and expels the air. During heavy breathing, the abdominal muscles also assist with exhalation.

DIAGNOSIS OF CHEST WALL DISEASE

Diagnosis of chest wall disease is based mainly on history and physical examination. A hallmark of chest wall disease is a paradoxical breathing pattern, especially in animals with respiratory muscle paralysis or weakness. This is characterized by decreased chest wall movement and inward movement of the abdominal wall during inspiration instead of the normal outward movement. Radiographs may be helpful when certain disease processes are suspected (e.g., rib fractures, congenital deformities, or neoplasia). Lastly, evidence of hypoventilation on arterial blood gas analysis is often present in animals with chest wall disease. In general, an arterial partial pressure of carbon dioxide ($PaCO_2$) greater than 50 mm Hg is consistent with hypoventilation that could be due to one of several disease processes, including chest wall disease.

DISEASES OF THE CHEST WALL

Congenital

Congenital disease of the chest wall is rare. The most common abnormality is pectus excavatum, an inward concavity of the sternum and costal cartilages. Animals with this disease are often asymptomatic; however, respiratory distress can occur via either "restrictive ventilation or paradoxical movement of the deformity during inspiration."[1] Surgical management is indicated only if there is significant respiratory impairment.

Neoplasia

Neoplasia of the chest wall, although fairly common, does not often lead to respiratory distress. A biopsy is needed to determine whether the mass is benign or malignant and to determine treatment options. Common masses of the chest wall include lipoma, chondrosarcoma, osteosarcoma, fibrosarcoma, mast cell tumor, and hemangiosarcoma.[1] Surgical management, including aggressive resection, movement of the diaphragm cranially, mesh placement, or flap procedures, may be necessary and could lead to respiratory difficulties postoperatively, especially in animals that require one or more concomitant lobectomies. Pain control is an important part of patient treatment in these cases (see Chapter 144).

Rib Fractures

Trauma

Rib fractures often cause significant pain. The patient may hypoventilate if severe discomfort is present during respiration. Although rib fractures do not routinely require surgical stabilization, their presence should alert the clinician to the possibility of underlying soft tissue thoracic injury, including pulmonary contusions, diaphragmatic hernia, hemothorax, or pneumothorax (see Chapters 25 and 28). If the rib fractures are very unstable, they can cause further trauma to the surrounding tissues and intrathoracic structures (i.e., lungs), thus necessitating surgical intervention.[2]

Flail chest and intercostal muscle damage

Flail chest is defined as a "fracture of several adjoining ribs resulting in a segment of thoracic wall that has lost continuity with the rest of the hemithorax."[2] This results in the fractured segment moving paradoxically throughout respiration. During inspiration, as the chest wall moves outward, the flail segment collapses inward because of negative intrapleural pressure, and vice versa.[2]

Respiratory distress often occurs in patients with flail chest for two main reasons: (1) Patients may hypoventilate purely because of pain, and (2) many animals with flail chest have other pulmonary injuries that cause hypoxemia, such as pneumothorax, hemothorax, pulmonary contusions, or a diaphragmatic hernia.

Management of flail chest can be only medical or a combination of medical and surgical approaches. Initially the patient should be laid down on the side with the flail segment, or the chest can be wrapped. This reduces bulging of the segment during exhalation to minimize pain and secondary trauma (although it will still be pulled inward with inhalation). If ventilation is severely impaired, intubation and manual ventilation may be lifesaving by ensuring that a tension pneumothorax is not present before positive pressure ventilation is initiated (see Chapter 30). Aggressive analgesia is often beneficial, although the animal must be monitored closely for respiratory depression and mechanical ventilation provided if necessary (see Chapters 141 and 144).

Time and cage rest are often the treatments of choice. An external stabilization splint, which covers the affected and unaffected surrounding areas and is sutured to the chest wall, has been used to provide chest wall support. Whether to surgically stabilize the flail chest segment is controversial. Often the actual flail segment contributes very little to dyspnea, hypoxemia, or hypoventilation, and pain or coexisting disease is the primary cause of these abnormalities. However, surgical stabilization of the segment reduces pain and improves thoracic wall excursion and ventilation and should be considered if anesthesia and surgery are required for other reasons. If the flail segment is displaced or adding to further lung dysfunction (laceration of the lung or vasculature by the flail segment), surgery is necessary (see Chapter 138).

Tearing of the intercostal muscles secondary to fractured ribs or a penetrating injury may cause a loss of chest wall rigidity and paradoxical movement of the affected area or flail segment. The degree of ventilatory impairment depends on the size of the destabilized area. This condition rarely causes direct respiratory impairment but rather leads to pain and may be a marker of additional injuries.

Penetrating wounds

If penetrating chest wall injuries allow air to enter into the pleural space, an open pneumothorax will develop. This should be closed manually to create an airtight seal and a chest tube placed, either at the site of the wound or a different location, in order to remove the air and reestablish negative pressure in the pleural space. A liberal amount of sterile ointment and an occlusive chest wrap can be used to cover the wound and maintain an airtight seal. As soon as the patient is stabilized, debridement and surgical repair should be performed. It is very important to monitor these patients closely because other internal organs are often damaged as well, leading to continued pneumothorax, hemothorax, diaphragmatic hernia, or pulmonary contusions (see Chapter 138).

Nontraumatic rib fractures

Some patients present with rib fractures and no history of trauma. In humans, this is most commonly seen secondary to excessive coughing or strenuous exercise. In cats, nontraumatic rib fractures have been seen secondary to chronic respiratory disease (i.e., asthma, pneumonia, and upper airway obstructions), chronic renal disease, and neoplasia.[3] This type of stress fracture is often seen mid-rib, in the caudal aspect of the ribcage.

Cervical Spine Disease

Cervical spinal diseases, such as cervical spine fractures or intervertebral disk disease, can cause significant hypoventilation (see Chapter 83). The exact mechanism is unknown, although there are many potential contributing factors. In dogs, the medullary respiratory center sends information via the reticulospinal tracts to the phrenic nerve and the segmental intercostal nerves. The phrenic nerve leaves the spinal cord between the fourth and sixth vertebral bodies and provides motor innervation to the diaphragm. The segmental intercostal nerves innervate the intercostal muscles and leave the spinal cord between C6 and T2. If these pathways are disrupted, ventilatory failure can ensue.[4] In cats, there is some evidence that afferent tracts to the respiratory center may be damaged during surgery on the cervical spine.[5]

Neuromuscular Disease *(see Chapter 85)*

Tick paralysis

Tick paralysis is induced when an engorged female tick secretes a neurotoxin into the patient that either inhibits depolarization of motor nerves or blocks the release of acetylcholine.[6] In the United States, the ticks most commonly involved are the American dog tick *(Dermacentor variabilis)* and the Rocky Mountain wood tick *(Dermacentor andersoni)*.[7] Signs typically develop 1 week after attachment of the tick. Patients often demonstrate marked ataxia of all four limbs, which progresses quickly to tetraparesis with generalized lower motor neuron symptoms. For an unknown reason, cranial nerve involvement is rare in the United States. If the tick is not found and removed, patients can progress to respiratory failure and ultimately death. Diagnosis is often made on cessation of signs after tick removal. This often occurs within 24 hours, with a complete recovery by 72 hours.[7] If tick paralysis is suspected but no ticks are found, rapid-acting insecticide solutions should be applied to the patient.

Tick paralysis in Australia occurs most commonly secondary neurotoxin secreted by the *Ixodes holocyclus* tick. Clinical signs are commonly severe and most affected animals require mechanical ventilation for a median duration of 23 hours[6] and hospitalization for 3 to 4 days. Animals requiring ventilation for hypoventilation alone had a good prognosis in one study, with more than 90% of animals surviving to discharge. Those with hypoxemia survived only 53% of the time.[6]

Acute idiopathic polyradiculoneuritis

Acute idiopathic polyradiculoneuritis, also known as Coonhound paralysis, is seen primarily in hunting dogs that presumably have been exposed to raccoons, but it also has been seen in dogs with no raccoon exposure.[7] One study has found an increased level of *Toxoplasma gondii* serum IgG antibody titers in affected dogs, but a definitive relationship has not been proven.[8] The disease occurs via immune-mediated demyelination and degeneration of axons of the ventral roots and spinal nerves.[7] This leads to an effective blockade of motor signals from the spinal cord to the muscles.

Clinical signs begin with pelvic limb paresis and hyporeflexia and can progress to tetraparesis within several days. The clinician will often detect diffuse hyperesthesia. If the disease is rapidly progressive, the patient may develop respiratory paralysis. Cranial nerve involvement is uncommon with coonhound paralysis. The clinical course tends to be approximately 3 to 6 weeks but can be significantly longer. Improvement usually begins by the third week.[7]

Diagnosis is based mainly on clinical suspicion. Coonhound paralysis is suspected after tick paralysis and botulism are ruled out. The diagnosis can be supported by electromyelographic evidence of diffuse denervation of affected muscles.[7] Management is supportive and may be prolonged in severe cases. The use of human intravenous immunoglobulin therapy was found to decrease the time until affected animals can ambulate without assistance in one study (75.5 days compared with 27.5 days in treated dogs).[9] The prognosis is typically good if complications are prevented, but recurrences have been described.

Botulism

Botulism is seen when the preformed *Clostridium botulinum* toxin is ingested. There are several types of botulism toxin, but all cases reported in dogs have been the result of type C toxin,[7] which is known to inhibit the release of acetylcholine from nerve terminals.

Clinical signs occur within 1 week of ingestion. These include mild generalized weakness or, in more severe cases, tetraparesis and possible respiratory failure. Unlike Coonhound paralysis, cranial nerve deficits can be seen with botulism. Duration of the disease is usually less than 2 weeks.[7]

Diagnosis is confirmed only by identification of the toxin in the serum, feces, or vomitus of the patient or in the food or carrion that the patient ingested. Electromyelography may help to differentiate botulism from Coonhound paralysis, but it is not definitive.

As with the other lower motor neuron diseases, management is largely supportive. There is an antitoxin available, but it needs to be administered before the toxin binds to receptors, which is not often possible.[7] Efficacy of antimicrobial therapy to manage *Clostridium* is unknown. Prognosis is generally good with aggressive supportive care and prevention of complications (e.g., aspiration pneumonia).

Fulminant myasthenia gravis

Myasthenia gravis occurs most commonly as a result of an autoimmune blockade, alteration, or destruction of the acetylcholine receptors at the neuromuscular junctions, but it can also be due to a congenital decrease in the number of these receptors on the postsynaptic membrane. Physical examination often reveals normal neurologic findings in the resting animal. Muscle weakness becomes apparent with exercise and worsens with continued exertion. The limbs are most grossly affected. Regurgitation (with or without aspiration pneumonia) secondary to megaesophagus is commonly present.

A presumptive diagnosis is made based on exercise-induced weakness, a decreasing response to repetitive nerve stimulation, or a positive response to acetylcholinesterase drugs such as edrophonium.[7] A definitive diagnosis is made when acetylcholine receptor antibodies are detected in the serum. Muscle biopsy with special staining is also used to diagnose congenital myasthenia gravis.

Management entails the use of an anticholinesterase agent like pyridostigmine and often glucocorticoids (see Chapter 85). Management with azathioprine and mycophenolate mofetil has also proven useful and may minimize side effects of steroid administration. Thymectomy has also been described for patients that respond poorly to medical management, because thymoma has been found to cause myasthenia gravis.[7]

Elapidae snake envenomation

Bites from Elapidae family of snakes (e.g., cobras, mambas, and tiger snakes), including the Eastern coral snake *(Micrurus fulvius fulvius)* in the southeastern United States and the Texas coral snake *(M. f. tenere)* in Texas, Louisiana and Arkansas, also lead to lower motor neuron disease. The venom from these snakes contains neurotoxic components, which leads to postsynaptic, nondepolarizing neuromuscular blockade. Clinical signs develop rapidly, and unfortunately there is usually minimal to no local tissue reaction as is seen with other snake bites. Signs range from peripheral weakness to tetraparesis. In severe cases, paralysis of respiratory muscles occurs. Patients may or may not have evidence of hemolysis and hemoglobinuria.[10]

Management is mostly supportive, although coral snake antivenom can be used early in the disease process. Unfortunately, once signs are evident, effectiveness of antivenom diminishes rapidly (see Chapter 174).[10] One study reported a 71% survival in dogs and cats treated with early antivenom.[11]

REFERENCES

1. Orton EC: Thoracic wall. In Slatter D, editor: Textbook of small animal surgery, ed 2, St Louis, 1993, Saunders.
2. MacPhail CM: Thoracic injuries. In Wingfield WE, Raffe MR, editors: The veterinary ICU book, Jackson Hole, WY, 2002, Teton NewMedia.
3. Adams C, Streeter EM, King R, Rozanski E: Cause and clinical characteristics of rib fractures in cats: 33 cases (2000-3009), J Vet Emerg Crit Care 20:4, 2010.
4. King AS: Autonomic components of the CNS. In King AS, editor: Physiological and clinical anatomy of the domestic mammal, Oxford, 1987, Oxford University Press.
5. Krieger AJ: Respiratory failure after ventral spinal surgery: a clinical and experimental study, J Surg Res 14:512, 1973.
6. Webster RA, Mills PC, Morton JM: Indications, durations and outcomes of mechanical ventilation in dogs and cats with tick paralysis caused by Ixodes holocyclus: 61 cases (2008-2011), Aust Vet J 91(6):233, 2013.
7. Oliver JE, Lorenz MD, Kornegay JN: Tetraparesis, hemiparesis, and ataxia. In Oliver JE, Lorenz MD, Kornegay JN, editors: Handbook of veterinary neurology, ed 3, St Louis, 1997, Saunders.
8. Holt N, Murray M, Cuddon PA, Lappin MR: Seroprevalence of various infectious agents in dogs with suspected acute canine polyradiculoneuritis, J Vet Intern Med 25(2):261, 2011.
9. Hirschvogel K, Jurina L, Steinberg T, et al: Fischer Polyradiculoneuritis Following Treatment with Human IV Immunoglobulin, J Am Anim Hosp Assoc 48(5):299, 2012.
10. Kremer KA, Schaer M: Coral snake (Micrurus fulvius fulvius) envenomation in five dogs: present and earlier findings, J Vet Emerg Crit Care 5:1, 1995.
11. Pérez M, Fox K, Schaer M: A retrospective evaluation of coral snake envenomation in dogs and cats: 20 cases (1996-2011), J Vet Emerg Crit Care 22(6):682, 2012.

CHAPTER 28

PLEURAL SPACE DISEASE

Valérie Sauvé, DVM, DACVECC

KEY POINTS

- Abnormalities within the pleural space may include pleural effusion, pneumothorax, or space-occupying soft tissue structures (diaphragmatic hernia, neoplasia).
- A diagnostic thoracocentesis may also prove therapeutic in severely affected patients.
- Fluid analysis and cytologic evaluation should always be performed on aspirates from a patient with newly diagnosed pleural effusion of unconfirmed etiology.
- Aerobic and anaerobic culture and susceptibility testing of suppurative effusions are imperative.
- Comparison of pleural fluid and serum triglyceride levels and cholesterol concentrations are necessary to confirm the diagnosis of chylothorax.
- Clinical evidence of cardiovascular shock often precedes dyspnea in patients with hemothorax.
- Tension pneumothorax, regardless of its origin, rapidly may be fatal. Immediate drainage via thoracocentesis or thoracostomy tube placement is required before taking thoracic radiographs.
- Clinical signs of a traumatic diaphragmatic hernia may be delayed; however, early detection and correction are important because perioperative outcome is worse in chronically affected patients.
- Tools such as ultrasonography, computed tomography (CT), and thoracoscopy are becoming increasingly available to aid in the diagnostic evaluation and treatment of pleural space disease.

PLEURAL SPACE

The pleural space is a potential space formed by the parietal and visceral pleura. It normally contains a minimal amount (few milliliters) of serous fluid to facilitate motion of the lungs in relation to the thoracic cavity and to each other, as well as force distribution during normal breathing.[1,2] The pleura is a thin epithelium formed of mesothelial cells overlying a thin basal membrane. The partition between the right and left hemithoraces is incomplete in small animals, but unilateral or unevenly distributed disease is common, especially when copious fibrin is present within the pleural space.[3]

Physiologic fluid flux in the pleural space is governed by Starling's law (Box 28-1), the degree of mesothelial and endothelial permeability, and the lymphatic drainage.[2] The visceral pleura assumes a larger role in determining the net pressure and favors reabsorption of fluid from the pleural space, where a greater vascular supply and lower hydrostatic pressure exist. Pleural lymphatic vessels are also an important component of fluid and cell reabsorption from the thorax.[2,3]

BOX 28-1 ***Modified Starling's Law Applied to the Pleural Cavity***[3]

$$\text{Net filtration} = K\{[(P_{c\,\text{parietal}} - P_{c\,\text{visceral}}) - P_{if}] - (\pi_c - \pi_{if})\}$$

P_c: capillary hydrostatic pressure of the visceral and parietal pleura
P_{if}: intrapleural hydrostatic pressure
π_c: plasma oncotic pressure
π_{if}: intrapleural oncotic pressure

There is an average pleural pressure of −5 cm H_2O, representing the difference between the elastic recoil properties of the lung and the thoracic cavity expanding forces at rest.[4] Air, fluid, or soft tissue within the pleural space can cause the lungs to collapse and the chest wall to expand outward by increasing the pressure within the thorax.[5] Pleural pathologic conditions such as these subsequently lead to a decrease in tidal volume, total vital capacity, and functional residual capacity.[6] The resulting atelectasis can lead to both hypoxemia and hypoventilation.

CLINICAL EVALUATION

Clinical signs of pleural disease may include tachypnea, open-mouth breathing, coughing, extended head and neck, crouched sternal recumbency with elbow abduction (orthopnea), cyanosis, and short, shallow breathing with an increased abdominal component. Paradoxical breathing has been strongly associated with pleural space disease, particularly in cats.[7] The degree of dyspnea varies depending on the amount of fluid/air/soft tissue, rate of fluid/air/soft tissue accumulation, and concurrent respiratory and metabolic disturbances. Auscultation reveals muffled breath sounds ventrally (fluid or tissue) or dorsally (air). The heart sounds may be muffled by fluid or tissue or abnormally loud or displaced with unilateral or focal disease.

Thoracic radiographs are extremely helpful in diagnosing and quantifying pleural space disease and other intrathoracic pathology. Repeat radiographs after thoracocentesis can be of diagnostic utility to assess improvement and better visualize intrathoracic structures (Figure 28-1). Horizontal beam thoracic radiographs have higher sensitivity for detection of small-volume pneumothorax and pleural effusion in human patients. It has been shown that the lateral recumbency horizontal beam (VD) thoracic radiograph with the standard left lateral view (vertical beam) have the highest detection rate for small volume pneumothorax and allows better severity assessment in traumatized pets or pets suspected of having a pneumothorax.[8]

Ultrasonographic examination is very helpful for rapid identification of pleural fluid in the emergency setting and guiding thoracocentesis. Furthermore, thoracic focused assessment with sonography for trauma (TFAST) ultrasound examination is becoming current practice in the emergency room to evaluate for presence and severity of pneumothoraces as well as other thoracic anomalies (see Chapter 189).[9,10] A pneumothorax is identified by the absence of "lung sliding" or "glide sign," which is the motion of the lung margins sliding against the chest wall surface during normal respiratory movement.[9,11] The transition zone (lung point) is the location where the lung sliding reappears, which helps determine grossly the quantity of

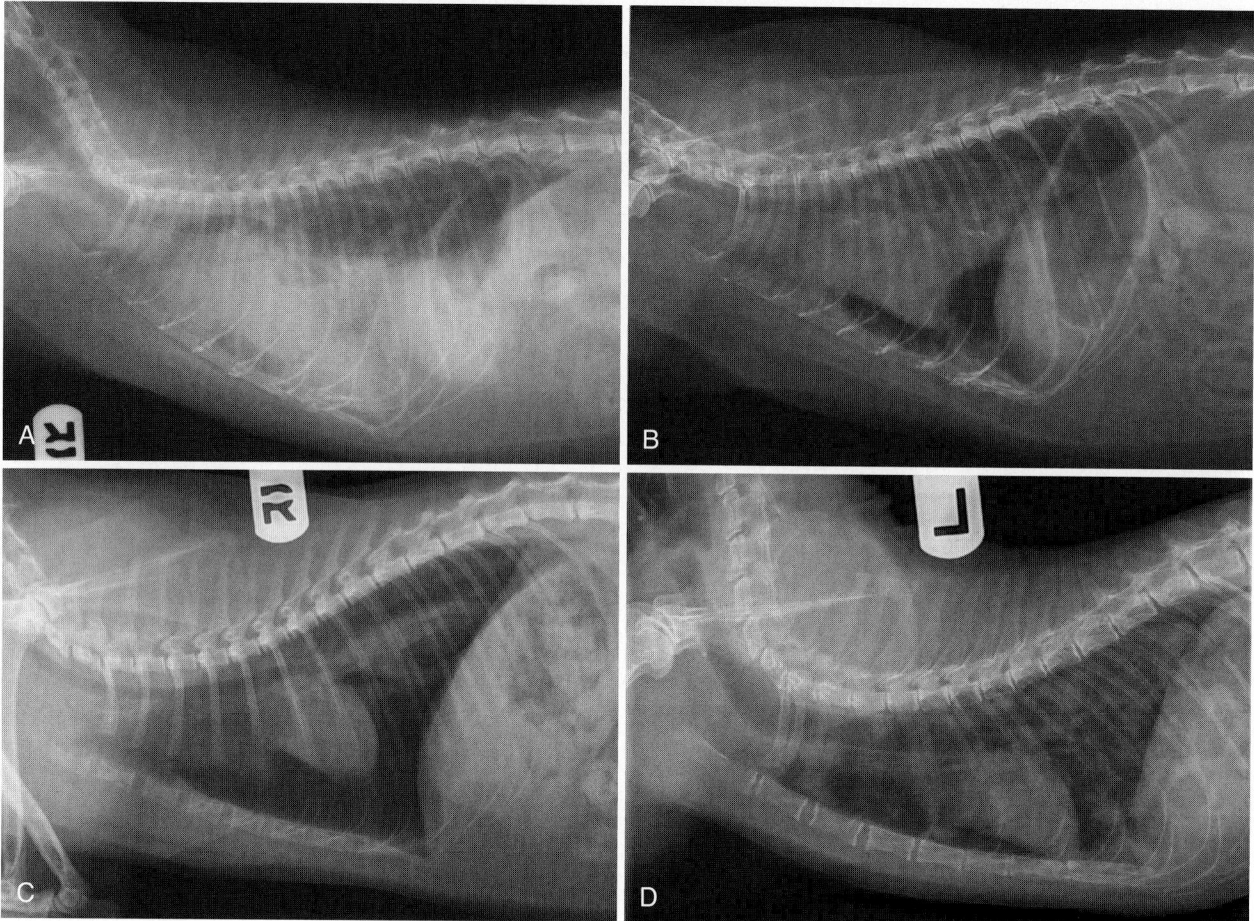

FIGURE 28-1 Cats with pleural space disease. **A,** Moderate volume of malignant effusion secondary to bronchogenic adenocarcinoma. **B,** Pneumothorax after thoracocentesis in the patient shown in **A. C,** Traumatic pneumothorax from high-rise syndrome. **D,** Spontaneous pneumothorax from diffuse pulmonary metastasis of salivary gland adenocarcinoma.

air present in the pleural space. Complete thoracic ultrasonography may reveal underlying pathology such as a diaphragmatic hernia, neoplastic process, thoracic wall disease, or lung lobe torsion.[12,13] Echocardiography will assist in the diagnosis of cardiac disease, heart base tumor, and pericardial disease.

Computed tomography is increasingly used to identify and characterize pleural and pulmonary lesions.[12,14] Thoracoscopy is another useful diagnostic and therapeutic tool in patients with pleural effusion and other intrathoracic pathology, allowing good visualization of the thoracic structures and acquisition of adequate biopsy samples.[15-18]

Thoracocentesis is an invaluable diagnostic, and often therapeutic, tool (see Chapter 198). Indications include (1) the presence of any undiagnosed pleural effusion and (2) therapeutic thoracocentesis to relieve respiratory signs caused by large amounts of air or fluid. However, if the cause of the effusion is known and the patient is not dyspneic, the procedure may be delayed and the clinical signs followed.[19,20] Fluid analysis has great diagnostic utility in patients with pleural effusion of an undetermined etiology.[19-21]

PLEURAL EFFUSION

Pure Transudates and Modified Transudates

Transudative pleural effusion, or hydrothorax, is the result of variations in the Starling forces that govern pleural fluid flux (see Box 28-1). Pure transudates are characterized by a low total protein and total nucleated cell count (Table 28-1) and generally develop secondary to decreased oncotic pressure (e.g., hypoalbuminemia) within the vasculature. It may also originate from presinusoidal or sinusoidal increased in hydrostatic pressure (e.g., portal hypertension, lymphatic obstruction). Modified transudates are associated with an increased posthepatic hydrostatic pressure (i.e., heart failure) or vascular permeability (e.g., vasculitis, lung lobe torsion, diaphragmatic hernia) causing leakage of a higher protein ultrafiltrate.[8,21] However, in animals with chronic effusion, irritation of the pleura may cause an increased nucleated cell count and water can be reabsorbed in

Table 28-1 **Fluid Type and Characteristics**[21,22]

Fluid Type	Classic Fluid Characteristics	New Proposed Criteria (Cats)
Pure transudate	TP < 2.5 g/dl TNCC <1500/μl	TP < 3.5 g/dl TPr < 0.56 TNCC < 5900/μl LDHp < 226 IU/L
Modified transudate	TP 2.5 to 7.5 g/dl TNCC 1000 to 7000/μl	
Exudate	TP >3.0 g/dl TNCC >7000/μl	TP > 3.5 g/dl TPr > 0.56 TNCC > 5900/μl LDHp > 226 IU/L

TP, Total protein; *TPr,* total protein ratio; *TNCC,* total nucleated cell count; *LDHp,* pleural lactate dehydrogenase.
Note that the new proposed criteria in cats do not differentiate between a pure transudate and a modified transudate.

excess of protein and cells, thus increasing the cell count and protein concentration.[6] Translocation of abdominal effusion, neoplastic effusion, and chylothorax are other causes of transudates or modified transudates.

Exudates

Exudative effusions are the result of alterations in the permeability of the capillaries.[22] Degenerate neutrophils usually will predominate with an infectious process (e.g., pyothorax).[21] Bacteria may originate from hematogenous or lymphatic spread, penetrating insults (iatrogenic, inhaled or external foreign body, bite wounds, trauma), or spread from infected organs (lung, gastrointestinal).[21] Aerobic and anaerobic cultures are recommended for all exudates. *Nocardia* spp, *Actinomyces* spp, and *Fusobacterium* spp are filamentous rods that are difficult to grow on culture media or identify with culture, cytologic, or histologic examination.[21,23] Other types of organisms, such as fungi, protozoa, and rickettsiae, may also cause septic pleural exudates.[21]

In aseptic exudates, the predominant cell type may vary to include nondegenerate neutrophils (inflammation), small lymphocytes (chylothorax), or neoplastic cells. Potential causes of an aseptic exudate include pneumonia and other well-circumscribed infections (e.g., abscess), generalized sepsis, pancreatitis, or necrosis of intracavitary neoplasia.[21]

Other fluid parameters are gaining interest in veterinary patients in order to classify effusions and help determine the etiology of pleural effusion. Among the markers studied in cats, pleural fluid lactate and total protein, as well as the ratio between the pleural and serum values, have higher capacity to distinguish between transudates and exudates[22] (see Table 28-1).

Feline Infectious Peritonitis

Feline infectious peritonitis (FIP), caused by a coronavirus (feline infectious peritonitis virus [FIPV] or feline coronavirus [FCoV]), is a common cause of aseptic pleural exudative effusion in cats, but it may also cause a modified transudate. Abdominal and pericardial effusion can be concomitant. The effusive form is a more acute disease process but may be present at the onset of the disease or terminally in animals with noneffusive FIP.[23,24] Deposition of infected macrophages forming pyogranulomas adjacent to small venules in the affected tissues and the inflammatory response associated with this cause a severe vasculitis associated with effusion formation.[23]

The diagnosis of FIP should be based on cumulative information rather than one diagnostic test. Pleural or peritoneal fluid typically will be viscous, straw-colored, and have a high protein concentration (>3.5 g/dl) with a relatively low nucleated cell count (<5000 cells/µl, although up to 25,000 cells/µl has been reported).[23,24] Nondegenerate neutrophils predominate in the fluid, with or without macrophages and lymphocytes.[23] A high serum antibody titer range (≥1 : 1600) is strongly suggestive of the disease.[25] Reverse transcriptase polymerase chain reaction (RT-PCR) on the effusion has shown good results at demonstrating the disease, although false positive results are possible.[24,25] Immunohistochemistry can be performed on the cells of the effusion; alternatively, examination of formalin fixed tissues for viral antigens will permit a definitive diagnosis.[24]

Pyothorax

A pyothorax is an accumulation of purulent exudate within the thoracic cavity. Bacterial infection within a feline thorax was previously attributed to bite wounds.[26] However, increasing evidence now suggests that the extension of pulmonary infections is a common cause, possibly secondary to aspiration of oropharyngeal flora.[27-29] Migrating inhaled foreign bodies and traumatic thoracic penetration are more common in dogs.[30-33] Other bacterial sources reported include pneumonia, pleuropneumonia, lung abscess, aberrant migration of *Cuterebra* larvae or grass awns, hematogenous or lymphatic dissemination, esophageal or tracheal perforations, lung parasites, diskospondylitis, neoplasia with abscess formation, and iatrogenic causes.[26,30,31] Septic suppurative effusion typically is diagnosed when intracellular organisms are present on cytologic examination and the presence of intracellular organisms. Culture and susceptibility testing should be performed on the fluid and antibiotic therapy initiated. Anaerobic bacteria are found commonly,[33-35] and infections with multiple organisms are highly prevalent.[26,34] In cats, nonenteric bacteria are most common and *Pasteurella* spp is most often isolated.[26,35] In dogs, *Escherichia coli* and other members of the family Enterobacteriaceae are isolated most often.[35,36] *Actinomyces* spp and *Nocardia* spp infections have been associated with intrathoracic pyogranulomatous infections in dogs.[37]

Hospitalization for appropriate supportive care and intravenous antibiotics is recommended. Pending culture and susceptibility testing results, broad-spectrum intravenous antibiotic therapy, such as enrofloxacin for gram-negative bacteria and ampicillin with sulbactam or ticarcillin with clavulanate for gram-positive and anaerobic infections,[38] should be instituted as soon as possible. However, an increasing resistance of *E. coli* to enrofloxacin has been documented and amikacin and ceftizoxime have shown to have better efficacy against this organism.[35] Clindamycin is also effective against many of the offending organisms in cats. Medical management with thoracostomy tubes (bilateral in most cases) is recommended, and sterile lavage with warm physiologic saline (10 to 20 ml/kg q6-12h daily) may be used initially if the effusion is thick and flocculent (see Chapter 199). Absorbed lavage solution by the inflamed pleura can lead to fluid overload, so close monitoring of fluid "ins and outs" is recommended. The use of pleural lavage with heparin may improve outcome in dogs with pyothorax treated with thoracostomy tubes by decreasing adhesion within the pleural space.[33] Intermittent thoracocentesis is not a recommended means of drainage and is associated with high mortality in both cats and dogs.[16,33] Tubes will often be necessary for 4 to 6 days [28,34,36] and removal is based on daily fluid reevaluation and the quantity of fluid produced (<2.2 ml/kg per tube q24h, although this can vary depending on the severity of pleuritis).[30] Thoracic radiographs or ultrasonographic examination should be used to monitor the efficacy of drainage. A thoracotomy with or without pneumonectomy should be performed if compartmentalized fluid, lung or pleural abscess, foreign body, perforated esophagus, thoracic wall lesion, or neoplasia is suspected or if medical management is failing.[33,39] Thoracoscopy is an alternative to thoracotomy in certain cases and should be consider as it is associated with lower morbidity and complication rate.[32]

Overall survival rate in small animals with pyothorax is good (63% to 66.1%).[26,33] In cats, success rates have been found to be up to 95% in cats treated with thoracostomy tubes.[28] Medical management is reported to fail in a minority of cats (5% to 9%),[26,28] but cats requiring thoracotomy maintain an excellent prognosis.[26,39,40] In dogs, surgical treatment has been associated with a better outcome.[36] In animals treated with thoracostomy tubes or thoracotomy, the prognosis was significantly better, 71% to 77.6%. The need for surgical exploration has not been associated with poorer outcome.[26,33]

Chylothorax

Chylous effusion is opaque and white or pink. Small lymphocytes usually predominate; however, nondegenerate neutrophils may become predominant after repeated thoracocenteses or with chronic disease.[21] The triglyceride concentration within the effusion is higher than the concentration in the serum, whereas the cholesterol level is equal to or lower than that of the serum. Causes of chylothorax include heart disease (e.g., cardiomyopathy, congestive heart failure, pericardial disease), thoracic duct obstruction (e.g., intraluminal or extraluminal neoplasia or granuloma), traumatic rupture of the thoracic duct, cranial mediastinal mass (e.g., thymoma, lymphosarcoma, aortic body tumor), lung lobe torsion, diaphragmatic or peritoneopericardial hernia, pacemaker implantation in cats, heartworm disease, congenital malformations, cranial vena caval thromboembolism, ligation of the left brachiocephalic vein, and idiopathic diseases.[41,42]

Idiopathic chylous effusion is diagnosed by exclusion in most animals with true chylothorax.[41,43] Medical management consists of intermittent thoracocentesis, a reduced-fat diet, medium-chain triglycerides, and rutin. Rutin is a benzopyrone nutraceutical that stimulates macrophage breakdown of protein in lymph, accelerating its reabsorption.[44] Thoracostomy tubes are indicated in animals with a traumatic chylothorax, if thoracocentesis is required several times weekly, or following surgery.[6] Surgical intervention is recommended if the medical management is unsuccessful at providing good quality of life to the animal. Multiple surgical interventions have been described; however, a combination of thoracic duct ligation with subphrenic pericardectomy has become the most successful procedure and is often performed via thoracotomy or thoracoscopy.[43,45,46] Long-term recovery rates vary from 73% to 100%.[45-47] The placement of pleural access ports at the time of surgery enable aspiration of pleural fluid by veterinary staff and owners after surgery and can allow animals with slowly resolving effusion to go home for continued postoperative care. Complications of chylous effusion and its drainage include weight loss, electrolyte abnormalities (pseudoaddisonian changes), lymphopenia, hypoproteinemia, dehydration, and fibrosing pleuritis.[41] Rarely, spontaneous resolution of idiopathic effusion occurs. This is expected in most animals suffering from traumatic thoracic duct rupture.

Hemothorax

A hemothorax is defined as a pleural space effusion with a hematocrit greater than 10%.[8] A lack of gross clotting and evidence of erythrophagocytosis and absence of platelets on cytologic examination differentiate iatrogenic hemorrhage from a true hemorrhagic effusion (unless peracute). Hemorrhage within the pleural cavity can be caused by a severe coagulopathy, often associated with ingestion of an anticoagulant rodenticide (see Chapter 111). Blunt or penetrating trauma, diaphragmatic hernia, hiatal hernia, thymic hemorrhage, neoplasia, pulmonary thromboembolism, lung lobe torsion, *Spirocerca lupi*, pancreatitis, and dirofilariasis are other reported causes. The most common cause of spontaneous hemothorax in dogs with a normal coagulation profile is neoplasia.[48] Finally, iatrogenic hemorrhage may be caused by venipuncture, jugular catheter placement, Swan-Ganz catheter placement, thoracocentesis, intrathoracic biopsy, and intrathoracic fine-needle aspiration, and may occur after thoracotomy or herniorrhaphy.

Cardiovascular shock often precedes respiratory compromise because as much as 30 to 60 ml/kg (dogs) or 20 ml/kg (cats) of pleural effusion is required to impair ventilation in those animals with normal lungs.[49,50] Therefore treatment includes appropriate fluid resuscitation and blood transfusions as needed. Only sufficient blood should be retrieved from the pleural space to relieve dyspnea and allow adequate oxygenation because the red blood cells that remain will be reabsorbed over the ensuing several days. Autotransfusion should be considered in trauma patients if more than 10 ml/kg of effusion is present.[49] Thoracostomy tube placement should be considered if the animal cannot be stabilized with thoracocentesis and the hemorrhage is ongoing (see Chapter 199). Surgery is rarely indicated in animals with a traumatic hemothorax unless a penetrating injury or uncontrollable hemorrhage is present but is often necessary for noncoagulopathic spontaneous hemothoraces.

Neoplastic Effusions and Pleural Neoplasia

Intrathoracic neoplasia may result in transudates or exudates by causing increased vascular permeability, obstruction of pleural and pulmonary lymphatic vessels or veins, shedding of necrotic material at the pleural surface (increasing oncotic pressure within pleural space), and obstruction or perforation of the thoracic duct.[51] Hemorrhage and pneumothorax may also result from neoplasia. Common primary thoracic cancers include mesothelioma, pulmonary carcinomas, and lymphosarcoma, but metastatic disease can also result in pleural abnormalities. Fluid analysis and cytologic studies are informative, but thoracic ultrasonography, computed tomography, thoracotomy, or thoracoscopy with fine-needle aspiration or biopsy will often be necessary to obtain a definitive diagnosis. In addition to treating the underlying neoplasia, long-term and palliative management of neoplastic effusions can be achieved in some patients by surgically creating a drainage system, such as placement of vascular access ports with intrathoracic drains or thoracic omentalization.[52,53] In human medicine, chemical pleurodesis is often also performed palliatively.[54] Intracavitary chemotherapy may also prove beneficial in some cases.

Fibrosing Pleuritis

Fibrosing pleuritis is a chronic condition in which the visceral pleura becomes thickened and restricts lung expansion as a result of inflammation within the thoracic cavity. Causes of this condition in humans include chylothorax, hemothorax, pleural infection, drugs, neoplasia, asbestosis, rheumatoid pleurisy, coronary bypass surgery, and uremia.[51] In veterinary medicine, this pathology is most often associated with chylous effusion.[55] Development of fibrosis depends on the degree of mesothelial cell and basement membrane damage and regeneration.[55] Radiographs show rounded, retracted lung lobes that will not expand after thoracocentesis. Pulmonary edema and interstitial fibrosis may contribute to dyspnea.[56] Decortication is the only successful therapy in humans and should be considered early for better outcome, while pulmonary changes are minimal. Pneumothorax is a common complication, and reexpansion pulmonary edema is also possible. The prognosis is guarded with diffuse disease.[56]

PNEUMOTHORAX

A pneumothorax is open if it results from an insult to the thoracic wall, such as a penetrating thoracic trauma. In patients with a closed pneumothorax, the thoracic cavity is intact and the air originates from a lesion within the lung parenchyma, trachea, airways, esophagus, mediastinum, or diaphragm. A tension pneumothorax develops if the site of air leakage creates a one-way valve during inspiration and results in a rapidly increasing pleural pressure that exceeds atmospheric pressure.

Traumatic pneumothorax is a common sequela of motor vehicular accidents and was found concurrently in 47% of dogs with pulmonary contusions.[57] It has also been reported in most (63%) cats with high-rise syndrome.[58] External wounds, such as a projectile injury, bite wounds, and penetrating sharp objects to the thorax and cervical spine, are also common causes. Iatrogenic pneumothorax after thoracocentesis is common, with an incidence of 3% to 20% in humans, with approximately 20% of those patients requiring thoracostomy tube placement.[20] Other common iatrogenic causes include leakage after lung lobectomy or respiratory tract surgery, thoracostomy tubes, fine-needle lung aspiration, barotrauma during positive pressure ventilation, and tracheal tears. Spontaneous pneumothorax is most often associated with pulmonary bullous emphysema in dogs, with the Siberian Husky being overrepresented.[59] Multiple other pathologic conditions can lead to a spontaneous pneumothorax:

neoplasia, feline asthma, pulmonary abscess, heartworm disease and other parasitic infections, foreign body migration, subpleural blebs, and pneumonia.[6] Finally, an infectious pneumothorax can be created by gas-forming bacteria within the thoracic cavity.

A tension pneumothorax can rapidly become life threatening, and immediate thoracocentesis is indicated in animals suspected to have this condition. If the pneumothorax is not easily relieved with thoracocentesis, an emergency mini-thoracotomy or rapid placement of a thoracostomy tube with intubation and mechanical ventilation may prove lifesaving. Decreased venous return to the thorax in animals with a tension pneumothorax can be associated with cardiovascular collapse and shock. The thorax may become barrel shaped, and limited chest expansion is noted despite significant respiratory effort. However, animals with subclinical air accumulation may not require thoracocentesis and the animal's progression should be followed closely because the air will be reabsorbed over days to weeks. A small amount of air in animals with severe pulmonary pathology may contribute significantly to dyspnea and should be relieved. Most patients with a closed traumatic or iatrogenic pneumothorax require thoracocentesis only once or twice.

Animals should be monitored closely after thoracocentesis for return of dyspnea, and cage rest is recommended for 2 weeks. The indications for a thoracostomy tube vary according to the clinical situation, but a tube should be placed in patients requiring more than two thoracocenteses within 6 to 12 hours (see Chapter 199). Other indications include patients with a tension pneumothorax and those with a pneumothorax that require mechanical ventilation.

Constant negative pressure applied within the pleural cavity is recommended using a two-chambered or three-chambered continuous suction device or commercially available Pleur-evac. Alternatively, a Heimlich valve may be used in medium and large breed dogs (although caution should be exercised if fluid accumulation is also present within the pleural space).

An exploratory thoracostomy is indicated if a closed traumatic pneumothorax does not resolve after 3 to 5 days of drainage. If an open pneumothorax is caused by a penetrating injury, the injury should be covered with an occlusive bandage and thoracocentesis performed; surgical repair is required as soon as the patient is stable. A spontaneous pneumothorax in dogs is best treated with surgical exploration, leading to a higher survival rate and decreased recurrence.[59] Thoracoscopic lobectomy has also been described in these patients.[60] Overall prognosis is good, with an 86% survival rate for treated dogs and cats with various causes of air accumulation.[61]

SPACE-OCCUPYING LESIONS

Space-occupying lesions within the pleural space may occur secondary to benign or malignant masses within the mediastinum or chest wall. These typically are diagnosed with thoracic radiographs or computed tomography. Further details on these diseases are beyond the scope of this chapter.

DIAPHRAGMATIC HERNIA

Acquired diaphragmatic hernias are usually the result of blunt trauma associated with vehicular trauma, high-rise syndrome, or dog fighting or attacks but may also be iatrogenic. Congenital diaphragmatic hernias are a result of aberrant embryogenesis and may be pleuroperitoneal, peritoneopericardial, or hiatal. These hernias are rare and beyond the scope of this chapter.

Clinical signs may occur immediately after the traumatic event but are considered chronic if present for more than 2 weeks.[62,63] Dyspnea varies from none to severe according to the organ herniated, resulting pleural effusion, and concomitant thoracic injuries. The organs most often involved are the liver, stomach, and small intestine; the omentum and spleen are also commonly herniated.[62-64] On physical examination, borborygmus over the chest or asymmetrically quiet heart or lung sounds may be ausculted. The abdomen may be further tucked in or palpated "empty," with failure to distinguish certain organs. Thoracic radiographs may reveal gas-filled abdominal organs within the thorax, an incomplete diaphragmatic border, pleural effusion, or cranially displaced abdominal organs. Additional radiographic views, ultrasonography, positive contrast celiography, and an upper gastrointestinal contrast study may aid in the diagnosis.

Thoracocentesis and gastrocentesis may relieve the dyspnea before surgery. Cardiovascular stabilization before surgery is also important. Indications for immediate surgical intervention include herniated stomach, strangulated bowel or organ, inability to oxygenate properly after medical intervention, and ruptured viscera. Most data suggest that early surgical intervention (within 24 hours of admission) provides an excellent prognosis for acute cases.[63]

Postoperative complications include pneumothorax, hemorrhage, aspiration pneumonia, sepsis, arrhythmias, and death.[62-64] Reexpansion pulmonary edema (RPE) is a rare complication after surgery. It results from release of endotoxins and oxygen free radicals, decreased surfactant concentrations, negative interstitial pressures, or chronic hypoxia causing increased vascular permeability and protein-rich pulmonary edema. Increased incidence of RPE has been associated with a longer duration of collapsed lung (≥72 hours). Care should be given to keep peak airway pressure below 20 cm H_2O to avoid positive end-expiratory pressure, and pleural air should be slowly evacuated postoperatively (>12 hours).[65] Prognosis for full recovery is excellent for acute cases (survival rate 94%).[63] Perioperative survival rate is lower (82% to 89%) when chronic acquired cases are included in the statistical analysis.[62-64] In some studies, dyspnea did not affect prognosis,[63] but older age, lower respiratory rate, and concurrent multiple injuries were associated with higher mortality in cats.[64]

REFERENCES

1. Dyce KM, Sack WO, Wensing CJC, editors: Textbook of veterinary anatomy, ed 3, St Louis, 2002, Saunders.
2. Dempsey SM, Ewing PJ: A review of the pathophysiology, classification and analysis of canine and feline cavitary effusions, J Am Anim Hosp Assoc 47:1, 2011.
3. Noone KE: Pleural effusion and diseases of the pleura, Vet Clin North Am Small Anim Pract 15:1069, 1985.
4. West JB: Respiratory physiology, ed 4, Baltimore, 1990, Williams & Wilkins.
5. West JB: Pulmonary pathophysiology: the essentials, ed 5, Philadelphia, 1995, Lippincott Williams & Wilkins.
6. King LG, editor: Textbook of respiratory disease in dogs and cats, St Louis, 2004, Saunders.
7. Le Boedec K, Arnaud C, Chetboul V: Relationship between paradoxical breathing and pleural diseases in dyspneic dogs and cats: 389 cases (2011-2009), J Am Vet Med Assoc 240(9):1095, 2012.
8. Lynch KC, Oliveira CR, Matheson JS, et al: Detection of pneumothorax and pleural effusion with horizontal beam radiography, Vet Radiol Ultrasound 53(1):38, 2012.
9. Lisciandro GR, Lagutchik MS, Mann KA: Evaluation of thoracic focused assessment for trauma (TFAST) protocols to detect pneumothorax and concurrent thoracic injury in 145 traumatized dogs, J Vet Emerg Crit Care 18(3):258, 2008.
10. Lischiandro GR: Abdominal and thoracic focused assessment with sonography for trauma, triage, and monitoring in small animals, J Vet Emerg Crit Care 21(2):104, 2011.
11. Lichtenstein DA, Menu Y: A bedside ultrasound sign ruling out pneumothorax in the critically ill. Lung sliding, Chest 108:1345, 1995.
12. Schwarz LA, Tidwell AS: Alternative imaging of the lung, Clin Tech Small Anim Pract 14:187, 1999.

13. Larson MM: Ultrasound of the thorax (noncardiac), Vet Clin North Am Small Anim Pract 39(4):733, 2009.
14. Reetz JA, Buza EL, Krick EL: CT features of pleural masses and nodules, Vet Radiol Ultrasound 53(2):121, 2012.
15. Kovak JR, Bergman PJ, Baer KE: Use of thoracoscopy to determine the etiology of pleural effusion in dogs and cats: 18 cases (1998-2001), J Am Vet Med Assoc 221(7):990, 2002.
16. Radslinsky MG: Complications and need for conversion from thoracoscopy to thoracotomy in small animals, Vet Clin North Am Small Anim Pract 39(5):977, 2009.
17. Schmiedt C: Small animal exploratory thoracoscopy, Vet Clin North Am Small Anim Pract 39(5):953, 2009.
18. Monet E: Interventional thoracoscopy in small animals, Vet Clin North Am Small Anim Pract 39(5): 965-975, 2009.
19. American Thoracic Society: Guidelines for thoracentesis and needle biopsy of the pleura, Am Rev Respir Dis 140:257, 1989.
20. Collins TR, Sahn SA: Thoracentesis: clinical value, complications, technical problems, and patient experience, Chest 121:178, 2002.
21. Cowell RL, Tyler RD, Meinkoth JH: Diagnostic cytology and hematology of the dog and cat, ed 2, St Louis, Mosby, 1999.
22. Zoia A, Slater LA, Heller J: A new approach to pleural effusion in cats: markers for distinguishing transudates from exudates, J Feline Med Surg 11(10):847, 2009.
23. Greene C: Infectious diseases of the dog and cat, ed 3, St Louis, 2006, Saunders.
24. Peterson NC: A review of feline infectious peritonitis virus infection: 1963-2008, J Feline Med Surg 11:225, 2009.
25. Hartmann K, Binder C, Hirschberger J: Comparison of different tests to diagnose feline infectious peritonitis, J Vet Intern Med 17:781, 2005.
26. Waddell LS, Brady CA, Drobatz KJ: Risk factors, prognostic indicators, and outcome of pyothorax in cats: 80 cases (1986-1999), J Am Vet Med Assoc 221:819, 2002.
27. Barrs VR, Beatty JA: Feline pyothorax—new insights into an old problem. Part 1. Aetiopathogenesis and diagnostic investigation, Vet J 179:163, 2009.
28. Barrs VR: Feline pyothorax: a retrospective study of 27 cases in Australia, J Feline Med Surg 7(4):211, 2005.
29. Anastasio J, Sharp C, Needle D: Histopathology of lung lobes in cats with pyothorax: 17 cases (1987-2010). In Small Animal IVECCS Abstracts 2012, presented at 18th International Veterinary Emergency & Critical Care Symposium, San Antonio, TX, Sept 8-12, 2012.
30. Demetriou JL, Foale RD, Ladlow J et al: Canine and feline pyothorax: a retrospective study of 50 cases in the UK and Ireland, J Small Anim Pract 43:388, 2002.
31. Scott JA, Macintire DK: Canine pyothorax: pleural anatomy and pathophysiology, Compendium 25:172, 2003.
32. Jimanez Pelaiez M, Jolliffe C: Thoracoscopic foreign body removal and right middle lung lobectomy to treat pyothorax in a dog, J Small Anim Pract 53(4):240, 2012.
33. Boothe HW, Howe LM, Boothe DM: Evaluation of outcomes in dogs treated for pyothorax: 46 cases (1983-2001), J Am Vet Med Assoc 236(6):657, 2010.
34. Scott JA, Macintire DK: Canine pyothorax: clinical presentation, diagnosis and treatment, Compendium 25:180, 2003.
35. Walker AL, Spencer JS, Hirsh DC: Bacteria associated with pyothorax of dogs and cats: 98 cases (1989-1998), J Am Vet Med Assoc 216:359, 2000.
36. Rooney MB, Monnet E: Medical and surgical treatment of pyothorax in dogs: 26 cases (1991-2001), J Am Vet Med Assoc 221:86, 2002.
37. Dovie JL, Kuipers RG, Worth AJ: Intra-thoracic pyogranulomatous disease in four working dogs, N Z Vet J 57(6):346, 2009.
38. Jang SS, Breher JE, Dabaco LA, et al: Organisms from dogs and cats with anaerobic infections and susceptibility to selected antimicrobial agents, J Vet Intern Med 210:1610, 1997.
39. Crawford AH, Halfacree ZJ, Lee KCL: Clinical outcome following pneumonectomy for management of chronic pyothorax in four cats, J Feline Med Surg 13(10):762, 2011.
40. Barrs VR, Beatty JA: Feline pyothorax—new insights into an old problem. Part 2. Treatment recommendations and prophylaxis, Vet J 179:171, 2009.
41. Birchard SJ, Smeak DD, McLoughlin MA: Treatment of idiopathic chylothorax in dogs and cats, J Am Vet Med Assoc 212:652, 1998.
42. Greenberg MJ, Weisse CW: Spontaneous resolution of chylothorax in a cat, J Am Vet Med Assoc 226:1667, 2005.
43. Fossum TW, Mertens MM, Miller MW: Thoracic duct ligation and pericardectomy for treatment of idiopathic chylothorax, J Vet Intern Med 18:307, 2004.
44. Thompson MS, Cohn LA, Jordan RC: Use of rutin for medical treatment of idiopathic chylothorax in four cats, J Am Vet Med Assoc 3:345, 1999.
45. Radlinsky MG, Mason DE, Biller DS, et al: Thoracoscopic visualization and ligation of the thoracic duct in dogs, Vet Surg 31:138, 2002.
46. Mayhew PD, Culp WTN, Mayhew KN: Minimally invasive treatment of idiopathic chylothorax in dogs by thoracoscopic thoracic duct ligation and subphrenic pericardectomy: 6 cases (2007-2010), J Am Vet Med Assoc 241(7):904, 2012.
47. da Silva CA, Monnet E: Long-term outcome of dogs treated surgically for idiopathic chylothorax: 11 cases (1995-2009), J Am Vet Med Assoc 239(1):107, 2011.
48. Nakamura RK, Rozanski EA, Rush JE: Non-coagulopathic spontaneous hemothorax in dogs, J Vet Emerg Crit Care 18(3):292, 2008.
49. Ludwig LL: Surgical emergencies of the respiratory system, Vet Clin North Am Small Anim Pract 30:531, 2000.
50. Cockshutt JR: Treatment of fracture-associated thoracic trauma, Vet Clin North Am Small Anim Pract 25:1031, 1995.
51. Taubert J: Treatment of malignant pleural effusion, Nurs Clin North Am 36:665, 2001.
52. Talavera J, Agut A, del Palacio JF: Thoracic omentalization for long-term management of neoplastic pleural effusion in a cat, J Am Vet Med Assoc 234(10):1299, 2009.
53. Cahalane AK, Flanders JA, Steffey MA: Use of vascular access ports with intrathoracic drains for treatment of pleural effusion in three dogs, J Am Vet Med Assoc 230(4):527, 2007.
54. American Thoracic Society: Management of malignant pleural effusion, Am J Respir Crit Care Med 162:1987, 2000.
55. Huggins JT, Sahn SA: Causes and treatment of pleural fibrosis, Respirology 9:441, 2004.
56. Fossum TW, Evering WN, Miller MW, et al: Severe bilateral fibrosing pleuritis associated with chronic chylothorax in five cats and two dogs, J Am Vet Med Assoc 201:317, 1992.
57. Powell LL, Rozanski EA, Tidwell AS, et al: A retrospective analysis of pulmonary contusion secondary to motor vehicular accidents in 143 dogs: 1994-1997, J Vet Emerg Crit Care 9:127, 1999.
58. Kapatkin AS, Matthiesen DT: Feline high-rise syndrome, Comp Cont Educ Vet Pract 13:1389, 1991.
59. Puerto DA, Brockman DJ, Lindquist C, et al: Surgical and nonsurgical treatment of and selected risk factors for spontaneous pneumothorax in dogs: 64 cases (1986-1999), J Am Vet Med Assoc 220:1670, 2002.
60. Brissot HN, Dupre GP, Bouvy MW et al: Thoracoscopic treatment of bullous emphysema in three dogs, Vet Surg 32:524, 2003.
61. Krahwinkel DJ, Rohrbach BW, Hollis BA: Factors associated with survival in dogs and cats with pneumothorax, J Vet Emerg Crit Care 9:7, 1999.
62. Minihan AC, Berg J, Evans KL: Chronic diaphragmatic hernia in 34 dogs and 16 cats, J Am Anim Hosp Assoc 40:51, 2004.
63. Gibson TWG, Brisson BA, Sears W: Perioperative survival rates after surgery for diaphragmatic hernia in dogs and cats: 92 cases (1990-2002), J Am Vet Med Assoc 227:105, 2005.
64. Schmiedt CW, Tobias KM, Stevenson MA: Traumatic diaphragmatic hernia in cats: 34 cases (1991-2001), J Am Vet Med Assoc 222:1237, 2003.
65. Stampley AR, Waldron DR: Reexpansion pulmonary edema after surgery to repair a diaphragmatic hernia in a cat, J Am Vet Med Assoc 203:1699, 1993.

CHAPTER 29

NONRESPIRATORY LOOK-ALIKES

Justine A. Lee, DVM, DACVECC, DABT

KEY POINTS

- Respiratory disease typically is defined as occurring within the following anatomic locations: upper and lower airways, pulmonary parenchyma, pulmonary circulation, pleural space, chest wall, or diaphragm.
- Patients presenting with clinical signs of respiratory distress, tachypnea, or dyspnea may have underlying cardiopulmonary disease or nonrespiratory look-alikes.
- Nonrespiratory look-alikes are those disease processes that result in increased respiratory effort as a result of noncardiopulmonary causes, such as respiratory compensation for metabolic acidosis, decreased oxygen content, hypovolemia, pain, anxiety, stress, hyperthermia, abdominal enlargement, metabolic derangements, drugs, and neurologic disease.
- Pulse oximetry can be used to simply and noninvasively differentiate nonrespiratory look-alikes from hypoxemia; alternatively, the gold standard of arterial blood gas analysis and evaluation of the alveolar-arterial (A-a) gradient is warranted.
- The respiratory system is unique in that it is the only vital function with both automatic and voluntary components.
- The compensatory response to a metabolic acidosis is hyperventilation; this results in a respiratory alkalosis in dogs, but has not been well studied in cats.
- Decreased oxygen delivery to chemoreceptors because of a decrease in oxygen content (e.g., anemia, dysfunctional hemoglobin, pericardial tamponade, or a decrease in the partial pressure of oxygen in the plasma) or decreased cardiac output (e.g., hypovolemia, hypotension) results in clinical signs of tachypnea.
- Pain, anxiety, and stress can affect the voluntary component of respiration, resulting in apparent tachypnea or dyspnea.
- When hyperthermia occurs, evaporative cooling via the respiratory tract results in tachypnea and a shallow breathing pattern.
- Severe abdominal distention (e.g., secondary to ascites, organomegaly, neoplasia) may cause pain, discomfort, decreased venous return to the heart, and metabolic acidosis, in addition to displacing the diaphragm cranially and inhibiting normal inspiratory movement.
- Metabolic diseases (e.g., hyperadrenocorticism, hyperthyroidism) and severe biochemical derangements (e.g., potassium, calcium, glucose) affect the respiratory pattern as a result of altered respiratory mechanics, input to respiratory sensors, and compromise of respiratory muscles.
- Drugs (e.g., opioids) or brain lesions affecting areas that are responsible for respiratory signaling (e.g., medulla, cerebral cortex) directly affect breathing rate and rhythm.
- Neuromuscular disease processes (e.g., affecting the nerves, muscles, or neuromuscular junctions to the intercostal muscles or diaphragm) may result in an abnormal respiratory pattern and an increase in the abdominal component of breathing.

The respiratory system is regulated by a complex system centered in the brain and helps adjust the delivery rate of oxygen to the lungs and the removal of carbon dioxide from the body. The respiratory system is unique in that it is the only vital function that has both an automatic (e.g., brainstem) and a voluntary (e.g., cortical) component.[1] Breathing is controlled by the medulla, which generates signals that are transmitted to both the upper airway and main and accessory respiratory muscles. Afferent feedback from mechanoreceptors in the lung, airway, diaphragm, and chest wall, as well as central and peripheral chemoreceptors (which monitor pH and partial pressures of carbon dioxide [PCO_2] and oxygen [PO_2]), allow for changes in the respiratory rate and pattern. Additionally, the cortex and supramedullary regions of the subcortex can affect the respiratory rate and pattern with volition, emotion, and onset of exercise.[2,3]

Traditionally, respiratory disease is anatomically located within the following locations: upper and lower airways, pulmonary parenchyma, pulmonary circulation, pleural space, chest wall, or diaphragm. However, because of the extensive network of input that can affect respiratory rate and pattern, patients with disease processes not directly related to the cardiopulmonary system may display a nonrespiratory "look-alike," presenting with clinical signs of tachypnea, apparent dyspnea, or even respiratory distress.

As a result, veterinarians must be able to appropriately evaluate patients presenting with respiratory signs and differentiate cardiopulmonary disease from nonrespiratory "look-alikes." Specific nonrespiratory look-alikes include respiratory compensation for a metabolic acidosis, a decrease in oxygen content (e.g., anemia, dysfunctional hemoglobin), hypovolemia, hypotension, pain, anxiety, stress, hyperthermia, abdominal enlargement, metabolic disease, drug therapy, and neurologic disease. A concise history from the owner, a thorough physical examination, and appropriate diagnostic techniques should all be used concurrently to differentiate cardiopulmonary system disease from these nonrespiratory look-alikes. Multiple concurrent disease processes are common, and the astute clinician must be able to differentiate between true hypoxemia versus nonrespiratory look-alikes.

PH AND PCO_2 RECEPTOR ACTIVATION

The most common acid-base abnormality in small animals is metabolic acidosis,[4] which is characterized by an increased hydrogen ion concentration, decreased pH, and decreased bicarbonate ion (HCO_3^-) concentration (see Chapter 54).[5] Metabolic acidosis most often results from a loss of bicarbonate-rich fluid from the body, increased hydrogen ion production, or decreased renal hydrogen ion excretion. In small animal medicine, the more common processes that cause metabolic acidoses are diabetic ketoacidosis (DKA), lactic acidosis, uremic acidosis, diarrhea-induced hyperchloremic acidosis,[5] and toxicoses (e.g., ethylene glycol, salicylates). The normal compensatory mechanism for metabolic acidosis is to expel additional carbon dioxide via hyperventilation, as evidenced by a decrease in the partial pressure of carbon dioxide in the peripheral arterial blood ($PaCO_2$). This compensatory mechanism is initiated as a result of the increased number of hydrogen ions stimulating peripheral and central chemoreceptors, which in turn increase alveolar ventilation (hyperventilation).[5]

Canine patients with disorders causing metabolic acidosis may demonstrate increased respiratory depth and rate in an attempt to normalize systemic pH (by blowing off carbon dioxide, an acid). The expected compensatory respiratory response is a decrement in $PaCO_2$ by 0.7 mm Hg per 1 mEq/L decrease in plasma bicarbonate concentration.[5] Although data are limited, this respiratory compensation is less commonly observed in cats.[6]

With certain metabolic diseases such as DKA, respiratory compensation may result in characteristic patterns such as Kussmaul respirations; this is clinically recognized as a deep, rhythmic breathing pattern.[5] Although this may not be classically seen in veterinary medicine, compensatory hypocapnia should be differentiated from underlying lung disease in these patients.

PO_2 RECEPTOR ACTIVATION

Inadequate oxygen delivery is sensed by receptors located in the carotid and aortic bodies and results in an increase in respiratory rate and depth. Under normal circumstances, central respiratory drive is modified primarily by changes in arterial PCO_2, which leads to an increase in the hydrogen ion concentration. However, hypoxemia becomes the primary stimulation for ventilation when the partial pressure of oxygen in the peripheral arterial blood (PaO_2) drops below 50 mm Hg.[7]

Recall that the formula to determine arterial oxygen content (CaO_2) is:

$$CaO_2 = (Hg \times SaO_2 \times 1.34) + 0.003 \times PaO_2$$

and for oxygen delivery (DO_2) is:

$$DO_2 = CaO_2 \times CO$$

where Hg is the hemoglobin concentration (g/dl), SaO_2 is the percent oxyhemoglobin saturation of arterial blood, PaO_2 is the partial pressure of oxygen in the arterial blood (mm Hg), and CO is cardiac output (dl/min).[7] See Chapter 15 for further details.

Patients with anemia, hypovolemia, pericardial tamponade, or other types of blood flow obstruction (e.g., intraabdominal hypertension) may appear tachypneic in an attempt to increase DO_2. A decrease in DO_2 to chemoreceptors in the carotid and aortic bodies will stimulate an increase in respiratory rate and depth in order to deliver more oxygen to the alveoli for gas exchange. Clinically this increase in respiratory rate and effort may result in a decrease in $PaCO_2$, even with coexisting pulmonary parenchymal disease. Primarily this is because the normal alveolar/arterial blood PCO_2 values are positioned on the steep, linear portion of the PCO_2/CO_2 content curve and an increase in alveolar ventilation causes a proportional decrease in CO_2 content. In addition, carbon dioxide is 20 times more diffusible than oxygen.[7] Anemia, whether from decreased production, blood loss, destruction, or sequestration, will significantly affect hemoglobin oxygen-carrying capacity and the delivery of oxygen to PO_2 chemoreceptors. In animals with acute blood loss, the heart rate (HR) will increase in an attempt to increase CO, with the goal of increasing oxygen delivery (e.g., CO = HR × SV, where SV is stroke volume); this is seen clinically as signs of hypovolemic shock (e.g., tachycardia). In chronically anemic patients, compensation occurs via increases in CO or changes in the affinity of hemoglobin for oxygen.[8]

Patients with altered hemoglobin-oxygen binding, including methemoglobinemia (e.g., acetaminophen toxicosis) or carboxyhemoglobinemia (e.g., carbon monoxide toxicosis secondary to smoke inhalation), will have a decreased SaO_2. It is important to recognize that pulse oximetry measurements are inaccurate with dysfunctional hemoglobin.

Finally, patients with underlying heart disease may have an increased respiratory rate and altered respiratory pattern caused by a decrease in cardiac output. Clinically this should be distinguished from primary respiratory disease, which may also be present.

In summary, patients with decreased DO_2 from either anemia or an absolute or relative hypovolemia may have a component of tachypnea or dyspnea from carotid and aortic receptor stimulation or simultaneous anatomic respiratory disease. Clinical evaluation includes serial physical examinations, blood pressure monitoring, volume resuscitation with fluid therapy (if cardiogenic shock has been ruled out), packed cell volume or hemoglobin measurement, and pulse oximetry.

CORTICAL MODIFICATION OF RESPIRATION

Dyspnea is defined as a subjective experience of breathing discomfort, which may have a cyclic component when related to pain, stress, or anxiety.[1] The voluntary (cortical) component of respiratory control can be altered in situations that cause pain, stress, or anxiety. Sympathetic stimulation (e.g., fight or flight) from pain, stress, or anxiety may result in hyperventilation and apparent dyspnea. The sympathetic response helps prepare the animal for immediate action by increasing oxygen delivery to the tissues and removing carbon dioxide generated with increased muscle activity.[9] When physical activity (e.g., fighting or escaping) does not occur, additional anxiety may result in hyperventilation.

Additionally, pain may limit chest expansion and cause anxiety, which may further increase respiratory distress (e.g., flail chest). Changes in the brain and spinal cord neurons result in central sensitization or a heightened perception of pain.[10] Subsequently, pain elicits the stress response, producing potentially detrimental physiologic effects such as increased sympathetic tone and vasoconstriction; this can lead to decreased oxygen delivery to tissues and compensatory increases in SV and HR (resulting in increased CO). As a result of the increased sympathetic tone and vasoconstriction, decreased venous blood flow can result in diminished pulmonary function, which can lead to atelectasis, hypoxemia, and ventilation-perfusion mismatch.[11]

Clinically pain, stress, and anxiety are seen most commonly as tachypnea and panting. This may worsen respiratory distress or even mask underlying lung pathology. For example, a dog with upper airway obstruction secondary to laryngeal paralysis may have exacerbated dyspnea as a result of both the anxiety of dyspnea and secondary laryngeal swelling. Although blood oxygenation may improve with oxygen supplementation, resolution of dyspnea typically requires immediate anxiolytic and/or analgesic therapy (e.g., sedation with acepromazine, butorphanol). (See Chapter 17 for further details.)

THERMAL RECEPTOR CHANGES

A small animal's primary method of thermoregulation is evaporative cooling from the respiratory tract through an increased respiratory rate. When body temperature is above the set point of the hypothalamic thermoregulatory center, the animal begins to pant. The set point of the thermoregulatory center is increased in disease (e.g., fever); as a result, normal cooling measures (e.g., panting) may not be stimulated with elevations in body temperature. Drugs such as μ opioids (e.g., morphine, fentanyl, meperidine, methadone, oxymorphone, hydromorphone) may falsely decrease the thermoregulatory center's set point; clinically, this may result in panting and tachypnea despite a normal body temperature.[12] Likewise, opioids may cause the opposite effect on the central respiratory center, resulting in respiratory depression. Hyperthermic patients or those treated with opioids may be tachypneic, and a thorough evaluation of the respiratory system should be conducted to ensure that underlying lung disease is not present. Clinically this may be important when considering analgesic therapy in an unstable patient. For example, in a hit-by-car patient, initial stabilization of airway, breathing, circulation, and dysfunction (e.g., ABCDs) is imperative; once the cardiopulmonary system is stabilized, the use of a reversible, quick-acting partial agonist-antagonist (e.g., butorphanol) may be beneficial initially, because less tachypnea is seen compared with a pure-μ opioid. Likewise, for a patient requiring sedation for abdominal ultrasonography, a μ opioid should be used cautiously to prevent excessive panting and decreased visualization during the procedure.

ELECTROLYTE IMBALANCES AND METABOLIC DISEASE

Electrolyte imbalances or metabolic disease may result in nonrespiratory causes of tachypnea. Significant alterations in potassium, glucose, or calcium concentrations may result in respiratory system muscle dysfunction (e.g., diaphragm, intercostal muscles, and accessory muscles). Metabolic disease, such as hyperadrenocorticism and hyperthyroidism, can affect respiratory patterns because of altered respiratory mechanics or changes in respiratory sensor input.

Severe hypokalemia (<2 mEq/L) may result in respiratory muscle weakness causing ineffective respiration, resulting in hypoventilation and hypoxemia. Such profound, severe hypokalemia is rarely seen in dogs and cats. Potential causes of hypokalemia include insulin administration, vomiting, chronic renal failure (cats), DKA, postobstructive diuresis, and diuretic administration (see Chapter 51).[13]

Hypoglycemia may alter respiratory muscle function and diminish proper signaling from the cortex and medulla to the respiratory system. Causes of hypoglycemia in dogs and cats include excess insulin (e.g., iatrogenic, insulinoma), severe liver disease (e.g., end-stage disease, portosystemic shunt, glycogen storage disease), insulinlike hormone–secreting tumors (e.g., hepatic carcinoma, hemangiosarcoma, leiomyoma), metabolic disease (e.g., hypoadrenocorticism, growth hormone deficiency), neonatal and juvenile hypoglycemia (e.g., in toy breed puppies), toxicosis (e.g., xylitol, ethanol), sepsis, and, less commonly, pregnancy toxemia, polycythemia, and hunting dog hypoglycemia.[14] (See Chapter 66 for further details.)

Hypocalcemia (or more specifically, a reduction in the biologically active form, ionized calcium) may also affect respiratory muscle function (see Chapter 52). Conditions most commonly associated with clinically significant decreases in ionized calcium include acute kidney injury, chronic renal failure, acute pancreatitis, and acute eclampsia (puerperal tetany) as seen in periparturient or nursing queens and bitches.[15]

Deficiencies in potassium, glucose, or calcium should be identified rapidly via diagnostic means such as venous blood gas analysis or glucometry in tachypneic patients to rule out nonrespiratory look-alikes. Appropriate, prompt therapy may lead to clinical improvement while the underlying disease process is identified and addressed.

Dogs with hyperadrenocorticism or those receiving glucocorticoid therapy often display tachypnea at rest, which may be a result of respiratory muscle weakness, muscle wasting, or fat deposition within the chest wall. Additionally, hepatomegaly and abdominal fat deposition may cause increased pressure on the diaphragm and contribute to the clinical signs.[16] Because these patients are predisposed to a hypercoagulable state and secondary pulmonary thromboembolism, advanced diagnostics may be necessary to differentiate primary respiratory disease from nonrespiratory look-alikes (see Chapter 104).

Hyperthyroid cats may be tachypneic because of increased carbon dioxide production (secondary to an increased metabolic rate, necessitating an increase in respiratory rate and minute ventilation), respiratory muscle weakness (from muscle wasting), or occasionally hypokalemia[16] resulting from a thyroid storm (see Chapter 69). Cats may exhibit open-mouth breathing or have clinical signs of respiratory distress while maintaining normal oxygen levels. Underlying thyroid-induced cardiomyopathy with secondary congestive heart failure may also occur and may result in primary cardiopulmonary disease (e.g., pulmonary edema, pleural effusion); this should be clinically distinguished from thyroid storm or other causes of nonrespiratory look-alikes.

PERIPHERAL NERVOUS SYSTEM DISEASE

Neuromuscular junction diseases such as myasthenia gravis, botulism, polyradiculoneuritis (e.g., coonhound paralysis), and tick paralysis can lead to hypoventilation and an abnormal respiratory pattern (see Chapters 16 and 85). Stimulation of the phrenic nerve results in contraction of the diaphragm, a subsequent increase in the thoracic cavity size, and expansion of the lungs to enable oxygen delivery to small airways and alveoli. With neuromuscular junction disease, signals from the phrenic nerve to the diaphragm are impaired, resulting in hypoventilation that may lead to hypercapnia and hypoxemia. Clinically, decreased expansion of the chest, increased abdominal effort, "cheek puffing," and short, shallow breaths may be observed. Similar clinical signs may be seen with spinal cord lesions at C_1 to C_5 or C_6 to T_2 (see Chapter 83). Although increasing the inspired oxygen concentration (FiO_2) with supplementation may mildly improve blood oxygen content, the patient will remain hypercarbic without ventilatory assistance. As a result, these patients often require positive pressure ventilation until correction of the primary abnormality is achieved (see Chapter 30).

Drugs and medications that affect the neuromuscular junction may also result in hypoventilation. As previously mentioned, opioids are a common cause of tachypnea (or less commonly, respiratory depression), and these drugs are often used in veterinary medicine. Less commonly used are paralytic agents (e.g., pancuronium, atracurium, vecuronium), which are nondepolarizing neuromuscular junction blockers that will cause respiratory paralysis. Pancuronium is used intraoperatively to help create muscle relaxation, particularly during orthopedic or ophthalmologic procedures. These patients must be manually or mechanically ventilated until the effect of the pancuronium is reversed or wears off (approximately 30 to 45 minutes). Reversal can be accomplished by administering an anticholinesterase agent (e.g., edrophonium, physostigmine, or neostigmine) with an anticholinergic agent (e.g., atropine or glycopyrrolate).

CENTRAL NERVOUS SYSTEM DISEASE

As previously described, the respiratory drive originates in the medulla (e.g., brainstem), whereas voluntary control of breathing occurs in the cerebral cortex. Additionally, chemoreceptors that monitor PCO_2 and pH are located centrally.[3] With central nervous system (CNS) disorders such as head trauma or a space-occupying lesion (e.g., brain tumor), patients may manifest abnormal respiratory patterns because of cerebral edema, bleeding, or increases in intracranial pressure affecting respiratory centers. Because respiratory system controllers are located throughout the CNS (e.g., medulla, cortex, chemoreceptors in various locations), a thorough cranial and peripheral nerve examination should be completed to locate additional abnormalities that may help the clinician localize the disease, formulate an appropriate diagnosis, and provide timely therapy.

CLINICAL EVALUATION

Arterial blood gas analysis is considered the gold standard in assessing oxygenation and ventilation (see Chapter 15). With arterial blood gas analysis, one can calculate the A-a gradient to evaluate the severity of lung disease. In veterinary medicine, the use of this formula is generally limited to assessment on room air (e.g., FiO_2 of 21%). The A-a gradient formula is as follows[17]:

$$[FiO_2 \times (P_{atm} - P_{H2O}) - (PaCO_2/0.8)] - PaO_2$$

Calculating the "Big A" (alveolar):

$$PAO_2 = FiO_2(760 - 47) - PaCO_2/0.8$$

At sea level, the barometric pressure (P_{atm}) is represented by 760 mm Hg and the water vapor pressure (P_{H2O}) is approximately 47 mm Hg. The respiratory quotient is represented as a denominator of 0.8 (or sometimes as a numerator of 1.2). When breathing room air at sea level, this can be simplified to: $PAO_2 = 150 - PaCO_2/0.8$. This value ("A") is then subtracted from the little "a" (arterial) PaO_2 (which is obtained from an arterial blood gas). A normal A-a gradient is 0 to 15 mm Hg. Values greater than 15 mm Hg are suggestive of underlying pulmonary parenchymal disease (from ventilation-perfusion [V/Q] mismatch or shunting), whereas normal values may be seen with hypoventilation (despite abnormal blood gas parameters). Chest radiographs should be performed in patients with an elevated A-a gradient to rule out underlying pulmonary disease.

The benefit of calculating an A-a gradient is that an arterial blood gas may look grossly acceptable when in fact there is severe lung disease and abnormal gas exchange within the alveoli. Alternatively, if the patient is hypoventilating (e.g., from excessive sedation), the arterial blood gas may appear very abnormal when in fact there is no underlying lung disease. For example, a dog with laryngeal paralysis that has an upper airway obstruction may be hypoventilating. On arterial blood gas analysis, the $PaCO_2$ may look very abnormal (e.g., 70 mm Hg; normal reference range 30 to 35 mm Hg) and the PaO_2 look very low (e.g., 60 mm Hg; normal reference range 80 to 110 mm Hg) as carbon dioxide is filling the alveolar space, leaving little room for oxygen. However, in this situation, the calculated A-a gradient is normal, indicating that the patient does not have lung disease or V/Q mismatch; rather, the patient is just hypoventilating because of a nonpulmonary parenchymal problem (e.g., laryngeal paralysis). Sedation and airway control will often resolve the clinical signs in this situation.

SUMMARY

In the emergency critical care setting, veterinarians are often presented with tachypneic, panting, or even apparently dyspneic patients. Approach to the patient with respiratory distress can be one of the most daunting tasks for a practicing veterinarian. Although there is no "cookbook" approach to the dyspneic patient, an appropriate diagnostic workup (including historical findings, clinical signs, a brief yet focused physical examination, clinicopathologic data, pulse oximetry, chest radiography, blood gas analysis, A-a gradient assessment, thoracic ultrasound, and so forth) is imperative. Although the goals of this chapter are not to discuss the approach to the dyspneic patient (see Chapter 1), it is imperative that the clinician be cognizant of a rapid, plausible differential list that includes nonrespiratory look-alikes. Primary respiratory system diseases should be ruled out from nonrespiratory look-alikes because the latter causes may mask underlying respiratory disease.

REFERENCES

1. American Thoracic Society: Mechanisms, assessment, and treatment: a consensus statement, Am J Respir Crit Care Med 159:321, 1999.
2. Moss IR: Canadian Association of Neuroscience Review: respiratory control and behavior in humans: lessons from imaging and experiments of nature, Can J Neurol Sci 32:287, 2005.
3. Corne S, Bshouty Z: Basic principles of control of breathing, Respir Care Clin N Am 11:147, 2005.
4. Cornelius LM, Rawlings CA: Arterial blood gas and acid–base values in dogs with various diseases and signs of disease, J Am Vet Med Assoc 178:992, 1981.
5. DiBartola SP: Metabolic acid–base disorders. In DiBartola SP, editor: Fluid therapy in small animal practice, St Louis, 2000, Saunders.
6. Lemieux G, Lemieux C, Duplessis S, Berkofsky J: Metabolic characteristics of cat kidney: failure to adapt to metabolic acidosis, Am J Physiol 259:R277, 1990.
7. West JB: Respiratory physiology: the essentials, ed 7, Baltimore, 2005, Lippincott Williams & Wilkins.
8. Pascoe PJ: Perioperative treatment of fluid therapy. In DiBartola SP, editor: Fluid therapy in small animal practice, St Louis, 2000, Saunders.
9. Wilhelm FH, Gevirtz R, Roth WT: Respiratory dysregulation in anxiety, functional cardiac, and pain disorders, Behav Modif 25:513, 2001.
10. Quandt JE, Lee JA, Powell LL: Analgesia in critically ill patients, Compend Contin Educ Vet Pract 27:433, 2005.
11. Crowe DT: Managing pain in the critically ill or injured animal, DVM Best Pract Aug:16, 2002.
12. Adler MW, Geller EB, Rosow CE: The opioids system and temperature regulation, Annu Rev Pharmacol Toxicol 28:429, 1988.
13. DiBartola SP, DeMorais HA: Disorders of potassium. In DiBartola SP, editor: Fluid therapy in small animal practice, St Louis, 2000, Saunders.
14. Grooters AM: Fluid therapy in endocrine and metabolic disorders. In Dibartola SP, editor: Fluid therapy in small animal practice, St Louis, 2000, Saunders.
15. Rosol TJ, Chew DJ, Nagode LA: Disorders of calcium. In DiBartola SP, editor: Fluid therapy in small animal practice, St Louis, 2000, Saunders.
16. Feldman EC, Nelson RW: Canine and feline endocrinology and reproduction, ed 2, St Louis, 1996, Saunders.
17. Haskins SC: Interpretation of blood gas measurements. In King LG, editor: Textbook of respiratory disease in dogs and cats, St Louis, 2004, Saunders.

PART III MECHANICAL VENTILATION

CHAPTER 30

BASIC MECHANICAL VENTILATION

Kate Hopper, BVSc, PhD, DACVECC

KEY POINTS

- Animals requiring mechanical ventilation most commonly suffer from lung disease, central neurologic system derangement, neuromuscular dysfunction, or combinations thereof.
- The three classic indications for mechanical ventilation are severe hypoxemia despite oxygen supplementation, severe hypoventilation despite therapy, and excessive respiratory effort.
- A fourth indication for mechanical ventilation is severe hemodynamic compromise that is unresponsive to conventional therapy.
- The goal of mechanical ventilation is to maintain adequate arterial blood gas parameters with the least aggressive ventilator settings.
- Animals with lung disease generally require more aggressive ventilator settings and may have a poorer prognosis than animals with neuromuscular diseases.
- The "ideal" ventilator settings for a given patient can be determined only by trial and error.
- Positive end-expiratory pressure (PEEP) increases the oxygenating efficiency of diseased lungs by preventing alveolar collapse and reducing ventilator-induced lung injury. PEEP is also used to prevent atelectasis in animals requiring prolonged anesthesia and mechanical ventilation.

Mechanical positive pressure ventilation (PPV) is of growing importance in veterinary critical care medicine. Mechanical ventilators use an increase in airway pressure to move gas into the lungs, in contrast to spontaneous breathing when airway pressure decreases below atmospheric pressure in order to generate the inspiratory phase of a breath.[1]

The respiratory function of the lungs is to oxygenate the arterial blood and remove carbon dioxide from the venous blood. *Oxygenation* refers to the movement of oxygen from the alveoli into the pulmonary capillaries and is primarily dependent on the surface area available for gas exchange and preservation of the delicate structure of the gas-exchange barrier.[2] *Ventilation* refers to the removal of carbon dioxide and is primarily dependent on fresh gas movement into the alveoli. When managing patients on mechanical ventilation it is useful to think of oxygenation and ventilation as two separate processes.

COMPLIANCE

Compliance is a measure of the distensibility of the lung and is defined as the change in lung volume for a given change in pressure.[2] A lung with high compliance will accept a large increase in volume for a small pressure change, whereas low compliance would be characterized as requiring a large pressure change to create a small increase in volume. The normal, healthy lung is very compliant and, as a result, requires relatively low airway pressures for adequate mechanical ventilation. In contrast, most pulmonary disease processes common to veterinary medicine will reduce pulmonary compliance and require higher airway pressures to adequately oxygenate and ventilate the patient.[1]

THE VENTILATOR BREATH

Ventilator breaths can be spontaneous, assisted, or controlled. Spontaneous breaths occur when the patient determines the respiratory rate and tidal volume. Assisted breaths occur when the patient determines the respiratory rate but the tidal volume is generated by the machine. During controlled ventilation the machine determines both the respiratory rate and the tidal volume.[3] Further definitions of breath types can be found in Chapter 31.

The ventilator can generate a breath in one of two basic ways. It can deliver a preset tidal volume over a given inspiratory time (volume controlled), or the machine can provide and maintain a preset airway pressure for a given inspiratory time (pressure controlled). When delivering a volume-controlled breath, the peak airway pressure generated will be dependent on the preset tidal volume chosen and the compliance of the respiratory system. When a pressure-controlled breath is delivered, the tidal volume will depend on the preset airway pressure chosen and the compliance of the respiratory system.[1,3] The more basic machines tend to be either volume-controlled ventilators or pressure-controlled ventilators. More modern, advanced machines have the capability to generate several different breath types.

VENTILATOR SETTINGS

Every ventilator model has a different range of settings. The more modern and advanced the machine, the more options it will provide for the operator to manipulate the ventilator breath. It is important to note that there is no standardization of ventilator terminology; the name of specific ventilator settings may vary between different brands of machine. Despite the apparent complexity of modern ventilators, a few important ventilator settings, available on almost all machines, allow the clinician to determine an effective ventilation protocol for each patient. These include respiratory rate, tidal volume, inspiratory pressure, inspiratory time, inspiratory-to-expiratory ratio (I:E ratio), trigger sensitivity, and positive end-expiratory pressure (PEEP; Table 30-1). The parameters that the operator can preset

Table 30-1 Important Characteristics of a Ventilator Breath

Parameter	Definition
Fraction of inspired oxygen (FiO_2)	Concentration of oxygen in the inhaled gas
Respiratory rate (RR)	Number of breaths per minute
Tidal volume (TV)	Volume of a single breath (ml)
Total minute ventilation (V_T)	Total volume of breaths in a minute (ml) (V_T = TV × RR)
Inspiratory time	Duration of inspiration (sec)
Inspiratory-to-expiratory (I:E) ratio	Duration of inspiration versus duration of expiration
Peak inspired pressure (PIP)	Peak pressure measured in the proximal airway (cm H_2O) during inspiration
Positive end-expiratory pressure (PEEP)	Positive airway pressure maintained during exhalation and the expiratory pause

Table 30-2 Suggested Initial Ventilator Settings

Ventilator Parameter	Pateint with Normal Lungs	Patient with Lung Disease
Fraction of inspired oxygen	100%	100%
Tidal volume (ml/kg)	8 to 12	6 to 8
Respiratory rate (breaths per minute)	10 to 20	15 to 30
Minute ventilation (ml/kg)	150 to 250	100 to 250
Pressure above PEEP (cm H_2O)	8 to 10	10 to 15
Positive end-expiratory pressure (cm H_2O)	0 to 4	4 to 8
Inspiratory flow rate (L/min)	40 to 60	40 to 60
Inspiratory time (seconds)	0.8 to 1	0.8 to 1
Rise time (seconds)	0.1 to 0.5	0.1 to 0.5
Inspiratory-to-expiratory ratio	1:2	1:1 to 1:2
Inspiratory trigger	1 to 2 cm H_2O or 1 to 2 L/min	1 to 2 cm H_2O or 1 to 2 L/min

will depend on the type of ventilation being used. With volume-controlled ventilation the tidal volume (or minute ventilation) is preset by the operator and peak airway pressure is a dependent variable. A peak airway pressure alarm limit is set to alert the operator of excessive airway pressures. If pressure-controlled ventilation is used, the airway pressure generated during inspiration is preset and tidal volume is a dependent variable. In some cases the parameters can be set directly, but in others they are indirectly determined by other settings. For example, the I:E ratio can be preset directly on some ventilators, but with some machines it is the consequence of the inspiratory time and respiratory rate that is chosen by the operator.[1,3]

The appropriate airway pressure and tidal volume for a given patient will depend on the patient's size and the nature of the underlying disease. The normal tidal volume for a healthy dog and cat is approximately 10 to 15 ml/kg. Patients with significant pulmonary disease may benefit from a lower tidal volume (e.g., 6 to 8 ml/kg is recommended for human patients with acute respiratory distress syndrome). Airway pressure is generally kept below 20 cm H_2O, often closer to 10 cm H_2O in patients with normal lungs. Animals with pulmonary disease have reduced pulmonary compliance and therefore require higher pressures in order to deliver an adequate tidal volume. As a result, airway pressures up to 30 cm H_2O may be necessary in animals with severe, diffuse lung disease.

When using volume-controlled ventilation on an intensive care unit (ICU) ventilator, the flow rate may need to be set in addition to the tidal volume. The flow rate will determine the inspiratory time and initial flow rates are set in the range of 40 to 60 L/min.[4] It can then be titrated as necessary. In pressure-controlled ventilation, some ventilators have a parameter called "rise time." This is the time in which the airway pressure increases from baseline to peak pressure. Faster rise times are indicated in patients with rapid respiratory rates, although caution is advised in animals with small endotracheal tubes because of increased resistance to flow (Table 30-2).

The trigger variable is the parameter that initiates inspiration; that is, how the ventilator determines when to deliver a breath. In animals that are not making respiratory efforts of their own, the trigger variable is time and is determined from the set respiratory rate. If the animal is making respiratory efforts, the trigger variable may be a change in airway pressure or gas flow in the circuit resulting from the patient attempting to initiate inspiration.[3,4] The trigger variable on most machines is set by the operator. An airway pressure drop of 1 to 2 cm H_2O or gas flow change of 1 to 2 L/min is an appropriate trigger variable in most patients. Lower settings are used in smaller patients. It is important to always set the trigger variable low enough that any genuine respiratory efforts made by the patient are detected by the machine and result in the delivery of an assisted breath. This will increase patient-ventilator synchrony and is important for patient safety. An increase in respiratory rate may be the only mechanism by which a ventilated patient is able to indicate there is a problem. However, the trigger variable can be too sensitive, such that nonrespiratory movement, such as patient handling, may initiate breaths. This should be avoided.

PEEP is available on many ventilators. If not provided by the machine, PEEP can be added by attaching a tube to the exhalation port of the ventilator. This can then be attached to a PEEP valve or the end of the tube can be submerged in the desired depth of water (depth in cm = cm H_2O pressure). PEEP, as the name suggests, maintains positive pressure in the airway during exhalation that prevents the lung from emptying completely. As a result the lung is "held" at a higher volume and pressure during exhalation.[1,3,5] PEEP is thought to increase the oxygenating efficiency of diseased lungs by recruiting previously collapsed alveoli, preventing further alveolar collapse and reducing ventilator-induced lung injury.[1,3,4] The appropriate magnitude of PEEP depends on the severity of the lung disease and the clinical response of the patient. Initially it may be set between 2 and 5 cm H_2O and then titrated appropriately.

INDICATIONS FOR MECHANICAL VENTILATION

There are three main indications for mechanical ventilation: (1) severe hypoxemia despite oxygen supplementation, (2) severe hypoventilation despite therapy, and (3) excessive respiratory effort with impending respiratory fatigue or failure.[1,4,6] Hypoxemia is defined as a partial pressure of arterial oxygen (PaO_2) of less than 80 mm Hg or a hemoglobin saturation (SpO_2) of less than 95%. A PaO_2 of less than 60 mm Hg or an SpO_2 of less than 90% is considered severe hypoxemia. (See Chapter 15 for further details.) It is important to note that venous values for PO_2 cannot be used to diagnose hypoxemia. A fourth indication for PPV is severe hemodynamic compromise that is refractory to therapy.[7] Anesthesia is often feasible in these patients with opioid and benzodiazepine drugs alone. Mechanical ventilation and anesthesia both serve to decrease oxygen consumption and may allow ongoing support of the patient while definitive measures to improve the hemodynamic state can be made (see Chapter 8).

When patients have severe hypoxemia despite oxygen therapy and specific treatment of the primary disease, mechanical ventilation is indicated. Most of these animals have primary lung disease.[2,5] Inspired oxygen concentrations of greater than 60% for a prolonged period (24 to 48 hours) can lead to oxygen toxicity and subsequent pulmonary damage.[5] Therefore animals that require high concentrations of inspired oxygen for longer than 24 hours in order to achieve adequate oxygenation may also benefit from mechanical ventilation.[1]

Hypoventilation is defined as an elevation in the partial pressure of carbon dioxide (PCO_2). (See Chapter 16 for further details.) In patients that are hemodynamically stable, venous PCO_2 is an accurate reflection of arterial PCO_2 and can be used to evaluate hypoventilation. Severe hypoventilation is defined as a $PaCO_2$ higher than 60 mm Hg and may be an indication for mechanical ventilation if the patient is unresponsive to therapy for the primary disease. Hypercapnia is a consequence of reduced effective alveolar ventilation. This may be due to increased dead space in a breathing circuit, upper airway obstruction, sedative overdose, or neurologic or neuromuscular diseases that impair respiratory rate or chest wall movement.[2,4] Most patients with increased apparatus dead space, upper airway obstruction, or sedative overdoses respond to appropriate therapy and do not require mechanical ventilation. Patients requiring ventilation in this category have neurologic, muscular, or neuromuscular disease processes such as brain disease, high cervical spinal cord disease, peripheral neuropathies, neuromuscular junction abnormalities, or primary myopathies. For simplicity, this group of disease processes will be referred to as neuromuscular diseases. Animals with brain disease may not tolerate small elevations in PCO_2, and mechanical ventilation may be beneficial in these patients if the $PaCO_2$ is higher than 45 mm Hg.[5] Another group of patients that may require PPV to prevent hypoventilation are those animals that require general anesthesia for reasons such as maintenance of an endotracheal tube or provision of effective analgesia. In such cases the anesthetic drugs invariably cause hypoventilation, and PPV during the anesthetized period is ideal.

Many post–cardiopulmonary arrest patients will require PPV for a time after return of spontaneous circulation. For short durations, manual ventilation may be sufficient, but animals with apnea, inadequate or unreliable ventilatory efforts, hypercapnia, or concerns for intracranial hypertension will benefit from mechanical ventilation as described in Chapter 4.

Animals with pulmonary disease may be able to maintain adequate oxygenation and ventilation by increasing their respiratory effort. If respiratory effort is marked, patients can become exhausted and respiratory arrest may occur despite acceptable blood gas values. Intervention before the arrest and initiation of mechanical ventilation may successfully stabilize these patients.[1,4] There are no objective measures of respiratory effort and impending fatigue; therefore this evaluation is one of clinical judgment.

APPROACH TO INITIATION OF MECHANICAL VENTILATION

Before initiating mechanical ventilation, appropriate machine setup and monitoring is required. If the patient is in a life-threatening state, it maybe necessary to anesthetize, intubate, and provide manual PPV while ventilator setup is performed. The "ideal" ventilator settings for a given patient can only be determined by a process of trial and error. The initial ventilator settings are based on guidelines such as those given in Table 30-2. The operator should anticipate that animals with primary lung disease may require more PEEP and higher inspired oxygen concentrations than patients with neuromuscular disease. Chapter 31 further describes ventilator protocols for animals with severe lung disease.

The machine should be turned on and tested with an artificial lung or rebreathing bag to ensure it is functioning properly. It is advisable to always start mechanical ventilation with 100% oxygen until appropriate machine function and patient stability can be confirmed. After initial stabilization, the FiO_2 can be tailored appropriately. A separate source of 100% oxygen with a means to provide manual ventilation should be available at all times in case of machine failure. Constant, intensive monitoring is essential for patients that are ventilated because they are completely dependent on their caregivers for survival. Anesthesia or the primary disease process may mask problems and the respiratory rate is no longer a reliable indicator of life; ventilators will easily ventilate a dead patient. Electrocardiography, core body temperature, arterial blood pressure, end-tidal carbon dioxide levels, and pulse oximetry monitoring should be used with every ventilator patient. Arterial blood gas measurements are of great benefit for evaluation of patients with pulmonary disease.

Patients require general anesthesia in order to start mechanical ventilation unless they have severe neurologic deficits. Anesthesia is required to enable intubation and allow the patient to tolerate positive pressure ventilation. Anesthesia induction should be rapid to allow immediate control of the airway and initiation of ventilation (see Chapters 143 and 197). All patients should receive high levels of inspired oxygen before and during induction. This is best provided by a tightly fitting face mask.

After induction, maintenance anesthesia is required. Inhalant anesthetics are not recommended because most ventilator patients require long-term anesthesia (hours to days) and these agents raise serious personnel safety concerns. In addition, most ICU style ventilators do not allow concurrent inhalant anesthesia; therefore this is generally not an option for long-term ventilation. The anesthetic protocol for maintaining ventilated patients depends somewhat on the animal's clinical state. The combination of a benzodiazepine infusion with one or two other injectable agents may offer the advantages of balanced anesthesia. Anesthetic drug options are discussed further in Chapters 34 and 143.

Animals that are immobile and unable to fight the ventilator, such as patients with respiratory paralysis, may benefit from placement of a temporary tracheostomy tube. This will allow the reduction (or even removal) of anesthetic agents and make neurologic evaluation and patient treatment simpler to interpret. Patients with normal neurologic function cannot be ventilated without general anesthesia, even with a temporary tracheostomy tube. Brachycephalic animals may benefit from the placement of a temporary tracheostomy tube for the weaning process (see Chapter 35).[8]

Immediately after the patient is connected to the ventilator, the chest should be observed for appropriate movements. The ventilator settings should be adjusted if the chest wall movements appear excessive or inadequate. Auscultation should then be performed to confirm the presence of breath sounds bilaterally. If breath sounds are not audible bilaterally, endobronchial intubation may have occurred and the endotracheal tube should be repositioned appropriately.

Auscultation over the larynx may help detect tracheal cuff leaks that can compromise the effectiveness of ventilation. Tracheal cuff pressures should not exceed 25 mm Hg; use of cuff pressure manometers help to prevent tracheal necrosis (e.g., Posey Cufflator).[9] Monitoring tools such as electrocardiography, pulse oximetry, end-tidal carbon dioxide, and arterial blood pressure should then be evaluated and significant abnormalities addressed immediately. Once the patient is considered stable, an arterial blood gas is evaluated while the animal is still receiving 100% oxygen, and the ventilator settings should be modified accordingly. In the absence of arterial blood gases, ventilator management is based on physical examination findings, venous PCO_2 levels, and pulse oximetry.

GOALS

The goal of mechanical ventilation is to maintain adequate arterial blood gas levels ($PaCO_2$ 35 to 50 mm Hg, PaO_2 80 to 120 mm Hg) with the least aggressive ventilator settings possible. If blood gas values are inadequate using the initial ventilator settings, the machine is first inspected to ensure that it is functioning correctly. The ventilator settings may then need to be adjusted to improve oxygenation or ventilation, as appropriate. It is always simpler to make one change at a time in the ventilator settings so that the effect of each change can be interpreted accurately. Careful recording of ventilator settings with the concurrent arterial blood gas value, end-tidal carbon dioxide level, and pulse oximetry reading is essential in evaluating and modifying the ventilator protocol.

Carbon Dioxide

Total minute ventilation (V_T) is equal to the product of the respiratory rate and the tidal volume. Carbon dioxide levels are controlled primarily by the alveolar minute ventilation ($V_A = V_T$ − dead-space volume). Dead space is any portion of the tidal volume that does not participate in gas exchange; increases in dead space result in decreases in effective alveolar ventilation and hypercapnia.[2,5] In small patients, excess tubing length between the breathing circuit Y-piece and the animal's mouth can cause significant increases in dead space. This maybe a consequence of excessive endotracheal tube length, extension pieces, or monitoring devices connected to the end of the endotracheal tube. Endotracheal tube obstruction caused by kinks or the accumulation of airway secretions may also reduce the volume of effective alveolar ventilation. In the absence of these equipment issues, hypercapnia is considered to be a result of inadequate V_A. Because minute ventilation is equal to the product of the respiratory rate and tidal volume, one or both of these ventilator settings can be increased and the PCO_2 concentration reevaluated to determine if the new ventilator protocol is adequate. Alternatively, if the PCO_2 is low, V_A should be decreased.

Oxygen

The initial arterial blood gas result is usually evaluated while the patient is breathing 100% oxygen. The first priority is to reduce the FiO_2 to less than or equal to 60% as soon as possible to reduce the risk of oxygen toxicity. The magnitude of reduction in the FiO_2 will be dictated by the measured PaO_2. After any reduction in oxygen concentration, the PaO_2 should be reevaluated. If SpO_2 correlates well with the PaO_2 (or arterial blood samples are unavailable), pulse oximetry can be used to help guide changes in ventilator settings as well.

Once the FiO_2 can be reduced to less than 60%, the focus then becomes reducing the magnitude of the ventilator settings, namely PEEP and the peak inspired airway pressure, in an attempt to minimize the likelihood of ventilator-induced lung injury (see Chapter 36).

In severe cases, hypoxemia will persist despite ventilation with 100% oxygen. In these animals, changes in the ventilator settings are required. Increases in PEEP, peak inspired airway pressure/tidal volume, or respiratory rate may help improve the oxygenating efficiency of the lung.[1] The following chapter on advanced mechanical ventilation discusses ventilator protocols in more detail. Prone positioning will maximize lung function in most patients, and animals with hypoxemia should be maintained in sternal recumbency until stabilized.

MAINTENANCE OF MECHANICAL VENTILATION

Short-term mechanical ventilation (less than 24 hours) requires appropriate monitoring and intensive nursing care but is feasible in many practice settings. Long-term mechanical ventilation is far more challenging and requires a well-staffed, 24-hour facility. Patient care issues such as cardiovascular support, nutritional support, airway care, and prevention of decubitus ulcers require continuous evaluation and treatment in order to prevent significant, life-threatening complications (see Chapter 34).

COMPLICATIONS

Mechanical ventilation is not benign; cardiovascular compromise, ventilator-induced lung injury, ventilator-induced pneumonia, and pneumothorax are all potential complications for ventilator patients.[1,2,10] Cardiovascular compromise as a result of impairment of intrathoracic blood flow is often an issue for patients with cardiovascular instability or when aggressive ventilator settings are necessary. Cardiovascular monitoring is recommended for all ventilator patients and is essential when high PEEP levels or more aggressive ventilator settings are used. Volutrauma and repetitive alveolar opening and collapse are believed to be the major causes of ventilator-induced lung injury and may be reduced with protective ventilation strategies (see Chapter 31).[11] Aseptic airway procedures, intensive oral care, and reducing the incidence of gastric regurgitation are all important in preventing ventilator-associated pneumonia (see Chapter 37).[1,2] Patients should be monitored continuously for evidence of a nosocomial infection and changes in pulmonary function. Routine sampling of airway fluid for cytology and culture and sensitivity testing may help to detect early ventilator-associated pneumonia.

Pneumothorax is a feared complication of PPV, but the contribution of ventilator settings in causing pneumothoraces is controversial. Pneumothorax has been shown to occur more often when very high airway pressures are used in human patients (plateau airway pressure > 35 cm H_2O).[12] When more conventional ventilator settings are used, there is no correlation among airway pressure, PEEP or other settings, and the occurrence of pneumothorax.[13,14] The development of a pneumothorax is more likely the result of underlying lung disease rather than the ventilator settings used. Minimizing the magnitude of ventilator settings should always be the goal of ventilator management. Pneumothorax should be a primary consideration when a patient has an acute decline in oxygenating ability, elevation in PCO_2, decreased chest wall movement and compliance, and patient–ventilator asynchrony. If not diagnosed and treated rapidly, a pneumothorax rapidly can prove fatal in animals receiving positive pressure ventilation. Unilateral or bilateral thoracostomy tubes with continuous drainage are indicated when managing these ventilated animals (see Chapter 199). If an acute, life-threatening pneumothorax develops in the ventilator patient, an emergency thoracotomy to create an open pneumothorax may be required to prevent cardiopulmonary arrest. After stabilization of cardiovascular parameters, thoracostomy tube(s) are then placed as mentioned earlier and the thoracotomy site is closed in a routine fashion.

TROUBLESHOOTING

Patient–ventilator asynchrony, called *bucking the ventilator,* occurs when the patient is breathing against the machine. This is a common

BOX 30-1 *Evaluation of Causes of Patient–Ventilator Aysnchrony*

- Hypoxemia*
- Hypercapnia†
- Pneumothorax
  - Pneumothorax is typified by a rapidly climbing PCO_2, falling PaO_2, and decreased compliance. Careful auscultation with or without thoracocentesis is needed to diagnose.
- Hyperthermia
  - Anesthetized animals often have relatively low temperatures, and even a rectal temperature of 102° F may cause dogs to pant while on the ventilator. Active cooling is required to control panting in hyperthermic ventilator patients.
- Inappropriate ventilator settings
  - Observe when the patient is trying to inhale and exhale; see if it is possible to match that pattern with your ventilator settings. (See Chapter 31 for further details.)
- Full urinary bladder or colon
  - Palpate the abdomen; consider placement of a urinary catheter and/or perform enema.
- Inadequate depth of anesthesia
  - Rely on the routine clinical signs of anesthetic depth. This may be the most common cause of bucking, but care should be taken not to blindly increase the anesthetic drug dose without fully assessing the patient when patient begins bucking the machine.

*See Box 30-2 for further details.
†See Box 30-3 for further details.
Information taken from Hopper K, Powell L: Basics of mechanical ventilation in dogs and cats, *Vet Clin North Am Small Anim Pract* 43:955, 2013.

BOX 30-2 *Causes of Decreases in Oxygenation in the PPV Patient*

- Loss of oxygen supply
- Machine or circuit malfunction
- Deterioration of the underlying pulmonary disease
- Development of new pulmonary disease
  - Pneumothorax, pneumonia, ventilator-induced lung injury, acute respiratory distress syndrome

issue; it can prevent effective ventilation and may lead to hypoxemia and hypercapnia. In addition, it increases the work of breathing and can increase patient morbidity.[4] A systematic approach to evaluation of patient–ventilator asynchrony is recommended. Box 30-1 provides a list of ruleouts for patient–ventilator asynchrony.

If a sudden decrease in oxygenation occurs, the oxygen supply to the machine should be checked as well as confirmation that the breathing circuit is intact and the ventilator is delivering breaths as prescribed. If the patient has become hypoxemic, the FiO_2 should be increased immediately to 100% and the animal placed in sternal recumbency until the condition is improved. See Box 30-2 for an outline of causes of decreases in oxygenating ability.

Sudden elevations in PCO_2 can occur as a consequence of equipment faults, patient problems (e.g., pneumothorax, airway obstruction), or inappropriate ventilator settings (Box 30-3). If no mechanical abnormalities are evident and patient disease such as pneumothorax is ruled out, the ventilator settings should then be changed to increase minute ventilation. Hypercapnia may be an acceptable consequence of some protective ventilation strategies (also known as permissive hypercapnia).[1,2,4,11]

BOX 30-3 *Causes of Hypercapnia in the PPV Patient*

- Pneumothorax
- Bronchoconstriction
- Obstruction of endotracheal or tracheostomy tube
- Increased apparatus dead space—excess tubing / connectors between the patient and the ventilator circuit Y-piece
- Incorrect assembly of the ventilator circuit, including large airway leaks, obstruction of the exhalation circuit, or any problem that would prevent effective generation or delivery of a tidal volume
- Increased pulmonary dead space, which may occur with overdistention of alveoli or large pulmonary embolism; classically causes increases in the $PaCO_2$—$ETCO_2$ gradient
- Inadequate ventilator settings.
  - In particular inadequate tidal volume, inadequate respiratory rate or both. Settings that can impair exhalation such as insufficient expiratory time can also cause hypercapnia. Hypercapnia may be an acceptable consequence of some protective ventilation strategies.

Data from Hopper K, Powell L: Basics of mechanical ventilation in dogs and cats, *Vet Clin North Am Small Anim Pract* 43:955, 2013.

PROGNOSIS

Prognosis for successful weaning from mechanical ventilation is largely dependent on the primary disease process. Human and veterinary clinical studies have repeatedly reported lower weaning rates for patients requiring ventilation for pulmonary parenchymal disease (inability to oxygenate) compared with patients with primary hypoventilation caused by intracranial or neuromuscular disease processes. Veterinary studies have reported that approximately 30% of dogs ventilated for pulmonary parenchymal disease are successfully weaned and about 20% leave the hospital; in comparison, 50% or more of dogs with intracranial or neuromuscular disease processes are weaned and approximately 40% survive to hospital discharge.[10] When compared with other breeds receiving mechanical ventilation, brachycephalic dogs do not appear to have a poorer prognosis for weaning or survival to hospital discharge.[8] Overall, cats tend to have a poorer prognosis than dogs for weaning, although like dogs, it varies with the underlying disease process (see Chapter 35).[9,15]

REFERENCES

1. Haskins SC, King LG: Positive pressure ventilation. In King LG, editor: Textbook of respiratory disease in dogs and cats, St Louis, 2004, Saunders.
2. West JB: Respiratory physiology: the essentials, ed 8, Baltimore, 2008, Lippincott Williams & Wilkins.
3. MacIntyre NR, Branson RD: Mechanical ventilation, ed 2, Philadelphia, 2009, Saunders.
4. Tobin MJ: Mechanical ventilation, New Engl J Med 330:1056, 1994.
5. Lumb AB: Nunn's applied respiratory physiology, ed 7, Oxford, 2010, Churchill Livingston.
6. Hess DR, Kacmarek RM. Essentials of mechanical ventilation, ed 2, New York, 2002, McGraw-Hill.
7. Rivers E, Nguyen B, Havstad S, et al: Early goal directed therapy in the treatment of severe sepsis and septic shock, N Engl J Med 345:1368, 2001.
8. Hoareau GL, Mellema MS, Silverstein DC: Indication, management and outcome of brachycephalic dogs requiring mechanical ventilation, J Vet Emer Crit Care 21:226, 2011.
9. Briganti A, Portela DA, Barsotti G, et al: Evaluation oft he endotracheal tube cuff pressure resulting from four different measures of inflation in dogs, Vet Anaesth Analg 39:488, 2012.

10. Hopper K, Haskins SC, Kass PH, et al: Indications, management and outcome of long-term positive-pressure ventilation in dogs and cats (1990-2001), J Am Vet Med Assoc 230:64, 2007.
11. Carney D, DiRocco J, Nieman G: Dynamic alveolar mechanics and ventilator-induced lung injury, Crit Care Med 33:S122, 2005.
12. Boussarsar M, Thierry G, Jaber S, et al: Relationship between ventilator settings and barotrauma in the acute respiratory distress syndrome, Intensive Care Med 28:406, 2002.
13. Weg MD, Anzueto A, Balk RA, et al: The relation of pneumothorax and other air leaks to mortality in the acute respiratory distress syndrome, N Engl J Med 338:341, 1998.
14. Anzueto A, Frutos-Vivar F, Esteban A, et al: Incidence, risk factors and outcome of barotrauma in mechanically ventilated patients, Intensive Care Med 30:612, 2004.
15. Lee JA, Drobatz KJ, Koch MW, King LG: Indications for and outcome of positive-pressure ventilation in cats: 53 cases (1993-2002), J Am Vet Med Assoc 226:924, 2005.

CHAPTER 31
ADVANCED MECHANICAL VENTILATION

Kate Hopper, BVSc, PhD, DACVECC

KEY POINTS

- The ventilator mode is defined by the control variable, breath pattern, and phase variables selected.
- Ventilator breaths can be volume controlled or pressure controlled. The three main breath patterns are continuous mandatory ventilation, continuous spontaneous ventilation, and intermittent mandatory ventilation.
- The goal of selection of the ventilator mode is to provide adequate gas exchange while preventing ventilator-induced lung injury.
- Lung-protective strategies may be important for treatment of severe, diffuse lung disease such as acute respiratory distress syndrome.
- Patient–ventilator asynchrony is a common, often unrecognized problem that can impair effective gas exchange, increase work of breathing, and create patient discomfort.

VENTILATOR CONCEPTS

An understanding of ventilator function requires an appreciation of how the machine is generating and controlling a given breath. This requires knowledge of what determines each phase of the breath and the source of energy for that breath (i.e., patient or ventilator).

Respiratory Cycle

The respiratory cycle can be divided into four phases: (1) inspiratory flow, (2) inspiratory pause, (3) expiratory flow, and (4) expiratory pause (Figure 31-1).[1,2] By defining how each respiratory phase is determined during a ventilator breath, the ventilator mode can be described. The respiratory phases also provide a context in which to define common ventilator parameters. For example, peak inspired pressure is the maximal airway pressure measured during the inspiratory flow phase. The plateau pressure is the airway pressure measured at the end of the inspiratory pause. The difference between the peak inspiratory pressure and plateau pressure is usually minimal in patients with normal lungs. Some pulmonary disease processes that increase airway resistance (e.g., asthma) can cause a significant difference between the peak and plateau pressure.

Equation of Motion

Patient–ventilator interactions can be described by the equation of motion. This equation is built into the ventilator software and is the basis for machine operation (Box 31-1).[2-4] The equation of motion states that the total pressure required to deliver a breath (includes patient effort and pressure generated by the machine) depends on the tidal volume and flow of the breath in addition to the resistance and compliance of the system. The resistance and compliance are determined largely by the characteristics of the patient and the ventilator circuit, whereas pressure, volume, and flow are the three interdependent variables that may be manipulated by the machine. To understand a ventilator breath, knowledge of changes in airway pressure, volume, and flow during each respiratory phase is required.

DEFINING THE VENTILATOR MODE

The ventilator mode is defined by the nature of the breath type and pattern, control variable, and phase variables used.

Breath Type

A ventilator breath is one of two major types: mandatory or spontaneous. During a spontaneous breath, the patient is responsible for both initiation and termination of inspiration, as well as generation of the entire inspiratory flow (tidal volume). A spontaneous breath in which the inspiratory flow is augmented by the machine is considered a supported breath. When the machine controls initiation and termination of inspiration as well as generating the entire inspiratory flow, it is considered a mandatory breath. When a mandatory breath is initiated by the patient, it is classified as an assisted breath (Table 31-1).[2-4]

Control Variable

The control variable is the primary variable manipulated by the machine to generate an inspiration.[2-4] Ventilator breaths can be flow, volume, or pressure controlled. In a pressure-controlled breath, the machine will maintain airway pressure at a constant, preset (by the operator) level, and inspiration ends when a preset inspiratory time is reached. The tidal volume and gas flow rate generated during this breath are dependent on the magnitude of the preset airway pressure and the resistance and compliance inherent to that system as per the equation of motion.

BOX 31-1 ***Equation of Motion***

Muscle pressure + Ventilator pressure =
(Tidal volume ÷ Compliance) + (Resistance × Flow)

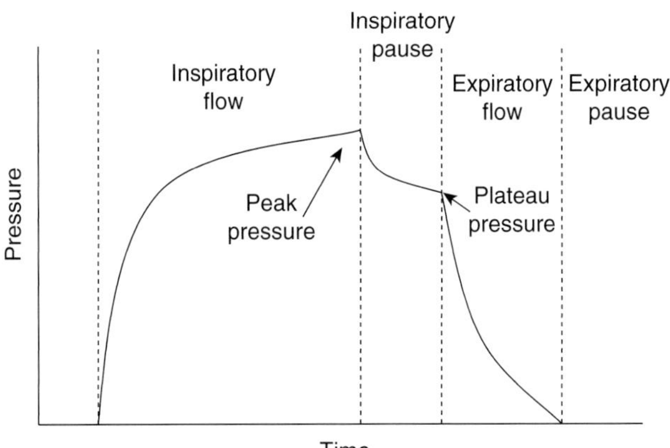

FIGURE 31-1 The respiratory cycle.

During a volume-controlled breath, the flow and tidal volume are fixed to a level preset by the operator; the machine will maintain a constant gas flow, and the inspiration ends when a preset tidal volume is delivered. As the equation of motion describes, airway pressure reached during these breaths is dependent on the magnitude of the preset tidal volume and the resistance and compliance of the patient's respiratory system.[2-4] The basic waveforms for a pressure-controlled and a volume-controlled breath are shown in Figure 31-2. Exhalation is passive, and it can be seen that it has an exponential character.

Phase Variables

The respiratory cycle helps define the four phases of a breath that can be controlled by the ventilator (see Figure 31-1): (1) the start of inspiration, (2) inspiration, (3) the end of inspiration, and (4) exhalation.[2,3]

Table 31-1 Categorization of Ventilator Breath Types

Breath Type	Initiation (Trigger)	Termination (Cycle)	Inspiratory Flow
Mandatory	Ventilator	Ventilator	Ventilator
Assisted	Patient	Ventilator	Ventilator
Spontaneous	Patient	Patient	Patient
Supported	Patient	Patient	Ventilator

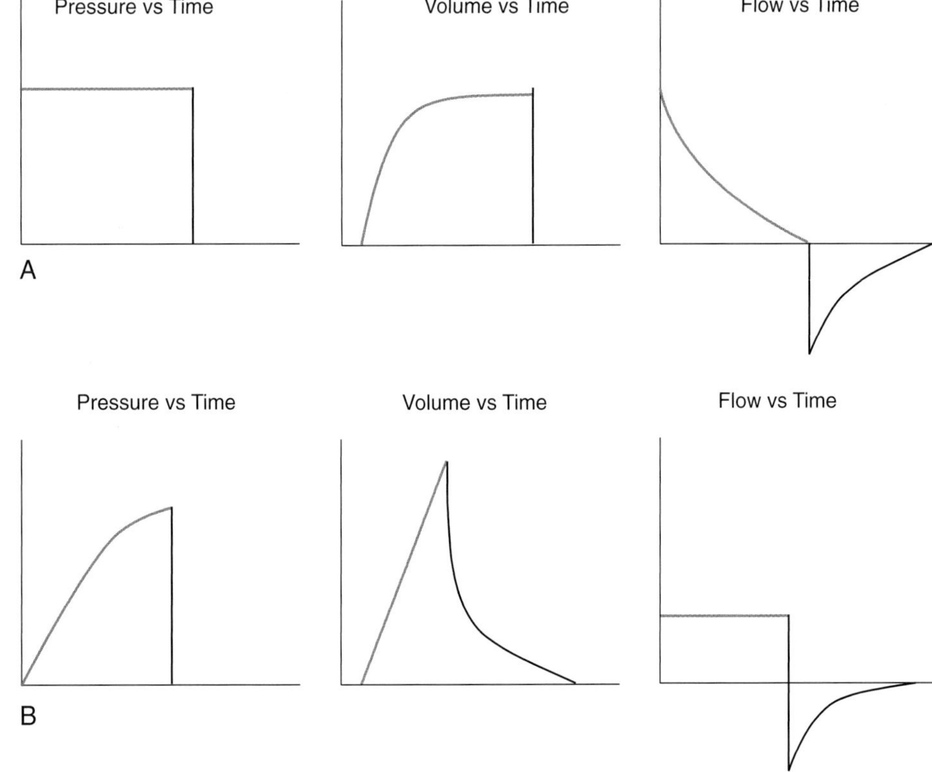

FIGURE 31-2 Pressure, volume, and flow time scalars for pressure-controlled and volume-controlled ventilation. (Note the inspiratory portion of each waveform is in *blue*.) **A,** In pressure-controlled ventilation, airway pressure is maintained at a constant level throughout the inspiration, volume increases with time, and the flow rate of the breath decelerates as the lungs fill with gas. **B,** In volume-controlled ventilation, the flow rate is held constant throughout inspiration but tidal volume and airway pressure both increase with time.

Trigger variable

The trigger variable is the parameter that initiates inspiration. It is how the ventilator determines when to deliver a breath.[2-4] In animals that are not making respiratory efforts of their own, the trigger variable will be time and is determined from the set respiratory rate. If the animal is making respiratory efforts, the trigger variable may be a change in airway pressure or gas flow in the circuit resulting from the patient's attempt to initiate inspiration. On most machines, the trigger sensitivity can be set by the operator. An airway pressure decrease of 2 cm H_2O or gas flow change of 2 L/min are usually effective initial trigger sensitivities, although lower settings may be necessary in small patients. Appropriate trigger sensitivity is essential to ensure that ventilator breaths are synchronized with genuine respiratory efforts made by the patient. This increases comfort and allows the patient to increase its respiratory rate as required. The trigger variable can be too sensitive, leading to the initiation of breaths after nonrespiratory movements such as patient handling. This should be prevented.

Cycle variable

The cycle variable is the parameter by which inspiration is terminated.[2-4] For example, to give a pressure-controlled breath, the ventilator maintains gas flow at a preset pressure for a given time. When that time has elapsed, inspiration is terminated and exhalation begins, so time is the cycle variable. Time is the most common cycle variable and will be determined by the preset respiratory rate and the inspiratory/expiratory (I:E) ratio. An inspiratory time of approximately 1 second is commonly recommended.

Limit variable

The limit variable is a parameter that the breath cannot exceed during inspiration, but it is different from the cycle variable because it does not terminate the breath.[2-4] This variable may be found on modern intensive care ventilators. For example, a volume-controlled, pressure-limited breath means that the ventilator will generate the breath by delivering a preset tidal volume, but it will not exceed the limit set for airway pressure at any time during the delivery.

Baseline variable

The baseline variable is controlled during exhalation; airway pressure is the most common baseline variable manipulated.[2-4] If airway pressure during exhalation is maintained above atmospheric pressure, this is referred to as *positive end-expiratory pressure (PEEP).*

Breath Pattern

Continuous mandatory ventilation

In the continuous mandatory mode of ventilation, the ventilator is responsible for all components of the breath. The operator sets the respiratory rate, and if the patient is unable to trigger breaths it is considered controlled ventilation. More commonly patients are allowed to trigger a respiratory rate higher than the preset value, and this is called assist-control ventilation. All the breaths delivered in assist-control ventilation are mandatory in nature. The terms *controlled* and *assist-control ventilation* are generally used interchangeably.[2-4] Assist-control ventilation provides maximal support of the respiratory system and is used in patients with severe pulmonary disease or those with no respiratory drive.

Continuous spontaneous ventilation

Every breath during continuous spontaneous ventilation is triggered and cycled by the patient; consequently this breath pattern can be used only in patients with a reliable, adequate respiratory drive. The inspiratory time and tidal volume are also determined by the patient. Continuous positive airway pressure (CPAP) and pressure support ventilation (PSV) are the two most common forms of continuous spontaneous ventilation.

CPAP provides a constant level of positive pressure (preset by the operator) throughout the respiratory cycle. CPAP increases functional residual capacity and compliance, enhancing gas exchange and oxygenation; it does not augment airflow during inspiration more than the baseline pressure provides. CPAP is commonly used in conjunction with PSV. CPAP alone is only suitable for use in patients with a strong respiratory drive and adequate ventilatory function. This is most commonly appropriate as part of a spontaneous breathing trial to determine a patient's suitability for weaning (see Chapter 35).

When using PSV, the ventilator augments inspiration during spontaneous breaths by increasing airway pressure, as set by the operator. As the names implies, these are *supported* breaths. This reduces the effort required to maintain spontaneous breathing in patients with adequate respiratory drive but inadequate ventilatory (inspiratory) strength. The degree of support provided will depend on the magnitude of preset pressure support. PSV can help overcome the resistance of breathing through the endotracheal tube and ventilator breathing circuit.[2-4] It can be used alone, in conjunction with CPAP, or to augment the spontaneous breaths during synchronized intermittent mandatory ventilation (see later).

The cycle variable in PSV is usually flow; the machine aims to detect when the patient is ready to exhale. This improves patient–ventilator synchrony and decreases the work of breathing.[4] There is some variation among machines regarding how the ventilator determines the end of inspiration in PSV. A common algorithm is the detection of a proportional drop in inspiratory flow such as a decrease to 5% to 25% of initial peak flow. Because these are spontaneous breaths, there are additional cycle variables for PSV built in to the software for safety reasons. These include inspiratory time and peak inspiratory pressure. Breaths are not allowed to be excessively long; they are commonly terminated if inspiratory time reaches 3 seconds. Breaths are also terminated on most machines if the airway pressure exceeds a preset pressure limit or the pressure alarm setting.[4]

PSV (usually with CPAP) is designed for use in patients with a normal respiratory drive but inadequate ventilatory ability. For example, a patient recovering from respiratory paralysis caused by a disease such as polyradiculoneuritis may benefit from the pressure support. PSV is particularly suited to patients that are awake and aware (and often have a tracheostomy) because it is designed to maximize patient comfort on the ventilator.

Intermittent mandatory ventilation

Intermittent mandatory ventilation is a combination of both mandatory and spontaneous breaths. A set number of mandatory breaths are delivered with either pressure or volume control. Between these breaths, patients can breathe spontaneously as often or as little as they choose.[2-4] The spontaneous breaths can be augmented with PSV on most machines. With most modern ventilators, the machine tries to synchronize the mandatory breaths with the patient's inspiratory efforts (assisted breaths), a pattern called *synchronized intermittent mandatory ventilation (SIMV).* If no breaths are detected by the machine during the period of synchronization, a mandatory breath will be given. The operator can control only the minimum respiratory rate and minimum minute ventilation; there is no control over the maximum rate or maximum minute ventilation.[2-4] SIMV is suitable for use in patients with an unreliable respiratory drive or patients that do not require maximal respiratory support.

Ventilator Mode

The basic definition of a ventilator mode requires identification of the control variable and the breath pattern (e.g., pressure-controlled, continuous mandatory ventilation). A more detailed definition would include a description of the nature of any phase variables that are used. For example, a patient may receive pressure assist-control, continuous mandatory, flow-triggered, time-cycled ventilation with PEEP.

RESPIRATORY RATE AND INSPIRATORY-TO-EXPIRATORY RATIO

The mandatory respiratory rate can be set on all ventilators. A normal respiratory rate of 15 to 30 breaths is usually selected when assisted ventilation is initiated. This can then be changed as appropriate. The I:E ratio may be preset by the operator, or in some older ventilators it is a default setting within the machine. Depending on the ventilator, the I:E ratio may be set directly or indirectly by manipulation of inspiratory time, percent inspiratory time, or inspiratory flow rate in conjunction with the respiratory rate. An I:E ratio of 1:2, with inspiratory times of approximately 1 second, is ideal to ensure that the patient has exhaled fully before the onset of the next breath. As respiratory rates are increased, the expiratory time will be sacrificed to "squeeze" in the necessary number of inspirations.

High respiratory rates can lead to a situation known as breath stacking, auto PEEP or intrinsic PEEP, because the animal is not able to exhale fully before the start of the next inspiration. Longer inspiratory times can be used in an effort to improve oxygenation. In some lung disease processes, a reverse I:E ratio (where inspiration is longer than exhalation) has been found beneficial, but this should be used with caution because associated intrinsic PEEP and hemodynamic compromise can have serious consequences.[2-4]

POSITIVE END-EXPIRATORY PRESSURE

PEEP is achieved by maintaining a pressure above atmospheric pressure during the expiratory phase of the breath, preventing complete emptying of the lungs on exhalation (increasing functional residual capacity). Extrinsic PEEP is a baseline phase variable that can be set on most modern ventilators. In addition, intrinsic PEEP can be developed as a consequence of inadequate time for exhalation or small airway collapse during exhalation. Physiologically, intrinsic PEEP has effects on pulmonary function and hemodynamics identical to those of extrinsic PEEP.[2-4]

Pulmonary parenchymal disease creates areas of low ventilation to perfusion matching (low V/Q) and areas of alveolar collapse (no V/Q), leading to decreased oxygenating ability. When pulmonary disease causes severe hypoxemia that will not resolve with oxygen therapy alone, positive pressure ventilation is indicated (see Chapter 30). In patients with pulmonary edema, loss of surfactant, and resultant alveolar collapse, PEEP can open or "recruit" collapsed alveoli and prevent further collapse of unstable alveoli, improving V/Q matching and hence improving oxygenation. Appropriate levels of PEEP can improve pulmonary compliance and reduce the work of breathing, although excessive PEEP can decrease compliance. Appropriate use of PEEP is also thought to reduce ventilator-induced lung injury by preventing injury associated with the cyclic reopening and collapse of alveoli with each breath (see Chapter 36).[5,6]

PEEP can also have detrimental effects; it can cause overdistention of healthier alveoli, which have a higher compliance, and lead to lung injury. Other adverse effects of PEEP may include increased alveolar dead space caused by obstruction of alveolar capillary flow, increased pulmonary vascular assistance, decreased left ventricular compliance, and reductions in cardiac output caused by impaired venous return during the expiratory phase. This latter effect is greatest when pulmonary compliance is high and preexisting cardiovascular compromise is present (e.g., in hypovolemic patients). Hemodynamic monitoring is recommended for all ventilated patients and is essential when high levels of PEEP or more aggressive ventilator settings are used (see Chapter 183).[2-5]

VENTILATOR ALARMS

Intensive care ventilators have numerous alarms built in for safety reasons. It is inevitable that ventilator alarms often will be activated for benign reasons (i.e., when moving the patient or if there is inadequate anesthetic depth). As a result, it is easy to ignore ventilator alarms, or it may be tempting to adjust the alarm settings to such extreme values that it is impossible for them to be triggered. These practices should be avoided because ventilator alarms can be lifesaving and are essential to the safety of the patient.[4]

Low Airway Pressure Alarm

The low airway pressure alarm should be set to approximately 5 to 10 cm H_2O below that of the patient's peak airway pressure. A low airway pressure alarm is suggestive of a leak or patient disconnection from the circuit and should be addressed immediately.[3]

High Airway Pressure Alarm

A high airway pressure alarm should always be set to a level that is above the current patient setting but not so high that it is irrelevant to the patient. A setting of approximately 10 cm H_2O above the patient's peak airway pressure is a reasonable guideline.[3] If the high airway pressure alarm is activated, immediate evaluation of the situation should be performed.

Potential causes of high airway pressures depend on the mode of ventilation being used. In volume control ventilation a high pressure alarm could be due to a sudden decrease in pulmonary compliance (e.g., endobronchial intubation, pneumothorax) or increased system resistance from an obstruction in the circuit or airways. Patient–ventilator asynchrony can generate high airway pressures in any mode of ventilation. If the high airway pressure alarm persistently sounds and the cause is not immediately obvious, it is advisable to disconnect the patient from the ventilator and manually ventilate until the issue can be resolved.

Low Tidal Volume Alarm

The low tidal volume alarm should be set at about 15% of the preset tidal volume.[3] A low tidal volume alarm should prompt the operator to look for leaks or disconnects in the circuit. If ventilating in a pressure control mode, a low tidal volume alarm could suggest a drop in compliance, an increase in resistance or an inadequate preset pressure.

High Tidal Volume Alarm

The high tidal volume alarm should be set at approximately 20% larger than the patient's tidal volume. A high tidal volume alarm may be due to the patient making spontaneous inspiratory efforts. In pressure-controlled ventilation, it could reflect an increase in compliance of the system.

LUNG-PROTECTIVE VENTILATION

It has been well demonstrated that overdistention of alveoli is injurious and should always be prevented.[6] In many patients this can be achieved by maintaining recommended tidal volumes when designing a ventilation protocol. In patients with severe lung disease such as acute respiratory distress syndrome (ARDS), lower tidal volumes should be targeted. ARDS causes collapse and consolidation of alveoli, leaving fewer aerated lung regions; these regions are especially vulnerable to overdistention if regular tidal volumes are delivered.

The ARDS Network reported a significant reduction in mortality of human patients with ARDS who were ventilated with a tidal volume of 6 ml/kg compared with 12 ml/kg. This lung-protective ventilation strategy included high PEEP levels and limited plateau pressures (no higher than 30 cm H_2O).[6] This finding was further supported by a Cochrane database review in 2007; it concluded that lower tidal volume ventilation in ARDS patients does reduce 28-day mortality.[7] The role of high levels of PEEP in protective lung ventilation remains controversial.[8] A likely consequence of low tidal volume ventilation is elevations in PCO_2. In human patients, high PCO_2 levels may be tolerated, a situation referred to as *permissive hypercapnia,* although heavier sedation or paralysis is often required to prevent patient–ventilator asynchrony.[4-6]

The ventilatory strategy of low tidal volumes and moderate to high PEEP, with or without permissive hypercapnia, is considered lung-protective ventilation. Given the evidence from experimental animal studies and human clinical trials, it would be reasonable to assume that lung-protective ventilation has a valid role in veterinary patients. It is important to appreciate that this ventilation strategy is designed for the lung with ARDS and should be applied with caution to those with other disease states. Potential adverse effects, including increases in intracranial pressure, acidemia, and PEEP-associated cardiovascular compromise, should to be considered before implementing a low tidal volume, moderate- to high-PEEP ventilator approach.

Setting Optimal PEEP

The method by which to select the ideal PEEP in patients with acute lung injury (ALI) or ARDS is a subject of great interest, but little consensus exists to date. It is unclear whether PEEP should be set to maximize pulmonary gas exchange or whether it would be safer to target the minimally acceptable PaO_2 to minimize adverse effects. Approaches include gradual increases in PEEP (e.g., use of the ARDS Network PEEP/FiO_2 titration tables), decremental PEEP titration, and choosing a PEEP 2 cm H_2O above the lower inflection point on the pressure-volume curve (Figure 31-3).[9-11] Tools by which to assess PEEP effectiveness have included the pressure-volume curve, monitoring changes in gas exchange (i.e., increases in PaO_2 and/or decreases in $PaCO_2$), and computed tomography. Three major clinical trials (the ALVEOLI, LOV, and ExPress trials) have evaluated PEEP selection, and a meta-analysis reviewed these trials in detail.[9,12-14] Although treatment with a higher PEEP was not associated with improved hospital survival overall, it was found to improve survival in the subgroup of patients with ARDS. The 2012 Surviving Sepsis guidelines state, "Strategies based on higher rather than lower levels of PEEP [should] be used for patients with sepsis-induced moderate or severe ARDS (grade 2C)."[15]

In veterinary clinical patients with ALI or ARDS, PEEP may be an effective option to improve lung oxygenating efficiency. In an effort to avoid adverse effects, patients should be monitored for hypotension, changes in alveolar dead space, and alveolar overdistention. Ventilator waveform analysis can be a valuable tool in helping to titrate PEEP (see Chapter 33).

Recruitment Maneuvers

A recruitment maneuver is a ventilator strategy used in the management of the ARDS lung by which the transpulmonary pressure (distending pressure of the lung) is increased transiently in an effort to open (recruit) collapsed alveoli. The role of recruitment maneuvers and the best way to perform them is another controversial topic in mechanical ventilation literature. Recruitment maneuvers have been associated with a varying degree of improvement on oxygenation; patients on lower PEEP and earlier in their disease process tend to show greater benefits.[16,17] Improvement is only sustained if the recruitment maneuver is followed by an adequate PEEP setting. The major adverse effects associated with recruitment maneuvers include hemodynamic compromise and alveolar overdistention, although these appear to be relatively uncommon in human patients.[17]

The method by which to perform a recruitment maneuver is also debated. Before starting, patients must be hemodynamically stable and placed on an FiO_2 of 1.0. Options include using a CPAP of 35 to 50 cm H_2O for 20 to 40 seconds; alternatively the patient can be placed on pressure control with a PEEP of 20 cm H_2O and pressure above PEEP of 20 cm H_2O for 1 to 3 minutes.[17,18] Patients must

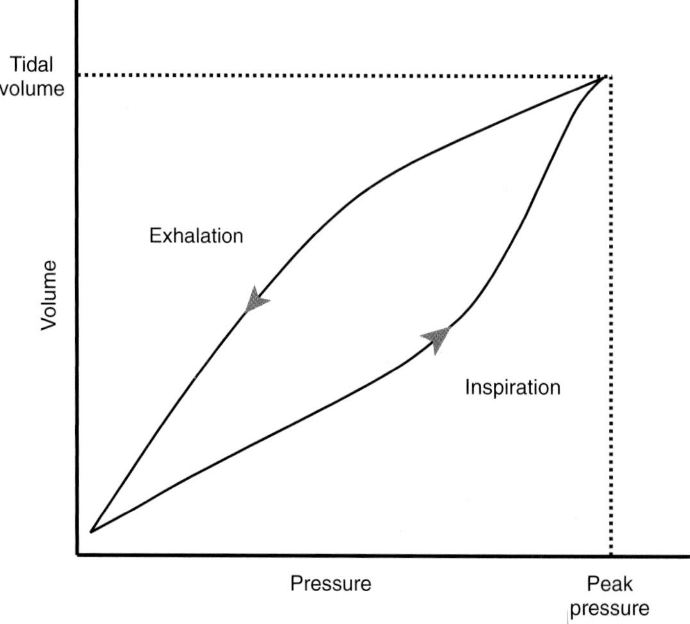

FIGURE 31-3 An idealized pressure-volume loop. Note that for a positive-pressure breath the loop flows in a counterclockwise direction, with inspiration represented by the lower limb and exhalation represented by the upper limb.

Table 31-2 **Common Causes of Patient–Ventilator Asynchrony***

Nature of Problem	Diagnostic Approach	Therapeutic Approach
Patient Related		
Hypoxemia	Obtain arterial blood gas analysis or monitor pulse oximetry	See Box 30-2
Hypercapnia	Obtain arterial or venous blood gas analysis	See Box 30-3
Hyperthermia	Monitor temperature	Provide active cooling Turn off heated humidifier for short periods
Pneumothorax	Auscultate Obtain blood gas analysis and radiographs Perform thoracocentesis	Perform thoracocentesis Thoracostomy tube placement
Drug-induced panting (opioids)	Assess respiratory pattern and concurrent drug administration	Consider change in anesthetic or sedation protocol
Inadequate anesthesia depth	Assess palpebral reflex, jaw tone, heart rate	Increase anesthetic depth
Equipment Related		
Disconnection or circuit leak	Evaluate circuit and endotracheal connection Auscultate neck for cuff leak Observe waveforms	Resolve disconnection or leak
Endotracheal tube kinked, obstructed, dislodged	Observe endotracheal tube position Auscultate chest Evaluate tidal volumes and waveforms Measure PCO_2	Reposition or replace endotracheal tube
Inappropriate trigger setting	Observe patient's respiratory efforts compared with ventilator responses Analyze ventilator waveforms	Change trigger setting accordingly
Insufficient tidal volume	Animal appears to try to increase inspiratory effort: observe waveforms	Consider increasing tidal volume (consider concerns for volutruma first)
Inspiratory time too long	Animal trying to exhale during inspiration: observe waveforms	Decrease inspiratory time and/or increase inspiratory flow rate

PCO_2, Partial pressure of carbon dioxide.
*NOTE: Patients may develop more than one problem concurrently.

be closely monitored through out the period of the recruitment maneuver. The 2012 Surviving Sepsis guidelines recommend recruitment maneuvers in septic patients with severe refractory hypoxemia caused by ARDS (grade 2C).[15] The role of recruitment maneuvers in veterinary ARDS patients is unknown.

PATIENT–VENTILATOR ASYNCHRONY

Patient–ventilator asynchrony occurs whenever there is a mismatch in the machine settings for the trigger sensitivity, gas delivery, or breath cycle determinants and the patient's respiratory drive.. Patient–ventilator asynchrony can impair gas exchange, increase the work of breathing, and create a sense of dyspnea for the patient.[2-4,19] Although there are no specific diagnostic criteria for the condition, it is commonly evidenced by animals fighting, or "bucking," the ventilator.

Less obvious signs of patient–ventilator asynchrony may be best observed by studying real-time ventilator waveforms and loops (see Chapter 33).[2,3,19,20] Studies report that patient–ventilator asynchrony is underestimated and often goes unrecognized in human patients, so it is likely that more subtle forms are poorly recognized in veterinary patients as well. To try and optimize the patient–ventilator interaction, the operator must continually attempt to match the trigger, gas flow, and cycling of breaths to the animal's needs.

Patient–ventilator asynchrony can have ventilator-related or patient-related causes. Because patient requirements can change constantly, continuous clinical assessment and physiologic monitoring is required, in conjunction with continuous manipulation of the machine settings or patient care in response to changes observed.[2-4,19] Table 31-2 lists common machine-related and patient-related causes of patient–ventilator asynchrony that should be evaluated when troubleshooting this problem. It is important to avoid the knee-jerk reaction of increasing anesthetic depth, because this may mask a significant underlying problem and increases the risk of anesthetic-related complications.

REFERENCES

1. Mushin M: Automatic ventilation of the lungs, Oxford, 1980, Blackwell.
2. Pilbeam SP, Cairo JM: Mechanical ventilation: physiological and clinical applications, ed 4, St Louis, 2006, Mosby.
3. Hess DR, Kacmarek RM: Essentials of mechanical ventilation, ed 2, New York, 2002, McGraw-Hill.
4. MacIntyre NR, Branson RD: Mechanical ventilation, ed 2, Philadelphia, 2009, WB Saunders.
5. Tobin MJ: Advances in mechanical ventilation, N Engl J Med 344:1986, 2001.
6. ARDS Network: Ventilation with lower tidal volumes as compared with traditional tidal volumes for acute lung injury and the acute respiratory distress syndrome, N Engl J Med 342:1301, 2000.
7. Petrucci N, Iacovelli W: Lung protective ventilation strategy for the acute respiratory distress syndrome, Cochrane Database Syst Rev 18:CD003844, 2007.
8. Briel M, Meade M, Mercat A, et al: Higher vs lower positive end expiratory pressure in patients with acute lung injury and acute respiratory distress syndrome, J Am Med Assoc 303:865, 2010.
9. Brower RG, Lanken PN, MacIntyre N, et al: National Heart, Lung, and Blood Institute ARDS Clinical Trials Network. Higher versus lower positive end expiratory pressures in patients with the acute respiratory distress syndrome, N Engl J Med 351(4):327, 2004.
10. Hodgson CL, Tuxen DV, Davies AR, et al. A randomized controlled trial of an open lung strategy with staircase recruitment, titrated PEEP and targeted low airway pressures in patients with acute respiratory distress syndrome, Crit Care 15:R133, 2011.

11. Lemaire F, Harf A, Simmonneau G, et al. Gas exchange, static pressure-volume curve and positive-pressure ventilation at the end of expiration. Study of 16 cases of acute respiratory insufficiency in adults, Ann Anesthesiol Fr 22:435, 1981.
12. Meade MO, Cook DJ, Guyatt GH, et al: Ventilation strategy using low tidal volumes, recruitment maneuvers, and high positive end-expiratory pressure for acute lung injury and acute respiratory distress syndrome: a randomized controlled trial, JAMA 299(6):637, 2008.
13. Mercat A, Richard JC, Vielle B, et al; Expiratory Pressure (Express) Study Group. Positive end expiratory pressure setting in adults with acute lung injury and acute respiratory distress syndrome: a randomized controlled trial, JAMA 299(6):646-655, 2008.
14. Briel M, Meade M, Mercat A, et al: Higher vs lower positive end-expiratory pressure in patients with acute lung injury and acute respiratory distress syndrome: systematic review and meta-analysis, JAMA 303(9):865, 2010.
15. Dellinger RP, Levy MM, Rhodes A, et al: Surviving Sepsis campaign: international guidelines for management of severe sepsis and septic shock, 2012, Intensive Care Med 39(2):165, 2013.
16. Grasso S, Mascia L, Del Turco M, et al: Effects of recruitment maneuvers in patients with acute respiratory distress syndrome ventilated with protective ventilatory strategy, Anesthesiology 96:795, 2002.
17. Kacmarek RM, Villar J: Lung recruitment maneuvers during acute respiratory distress syndrome: is it useful? Minerva Anesthesiol 77:85, 2011.
18. Lapinsky SE, Aubin M, Mehta S, et al: Safety and efficacy of a sustained inflation for alveolar recruitment in adults with respiratory failure, Intensive Care Med 25:1297, 1999.
19. Ranieri VM, Gregoretti C, Squadrone V: Patient–ventilator interaction. In Vincent JL, Abraham E, Moore FA, et al, editors: Textbook of critical care, ed 6, Philadelphia, 2011, Elsevier Saunders.
20. Waugh JB, Deshpande VM, Harwood RJ: Rapid interpretation of ventilator waveforms, Upper Saddle River, NJ, 1999, Prentice Hall.

CHAPTER 32
JET VENTILATION

Bruno H. Pypendop, DrMedVet, DrVetSci, DACVA

KEY POINTS

- Transtracheal jet ventilation can be used for emergency ventilation; high-frequency jet ventilation can be used to ventilate patients when tracheal intubation is not possible or practical.
- High-frequency ventilation can produce normoxemia and normocapnia with tidal volumes less than the volume of the dead space.
- High-frequency ventilation requires the use of very high minute volumes.
- During jet ventilation, distribution of ventilation and tidal volume depend more on airway resistance than on respiratory system compliance.
- Tidal volume and end-tidal carbon dioxide concentration cannot be measured accurately during jet ventilation.
- Adequacy of ventilation and oxygenation should be assessed using blood gas analysis, particularly if jet ventilation is used for extended periods.
- Interpretation of blood gas data should not be influenced by the mode of ventilation (spontaneous vs. conventional mechanical vs. jet).

High-frequency ventilation was first explored in the 1960s in an attempt to find a positive pressure ventilation technique that would have minimal impact on circulation.[1] It was assumed that insufflation of gas at a high frequency, directly in the airway, would enable a reduction in tidal volume and thereby in intrathoracic pressure.

Different strategies can be used to deliver high-frequency ventilation. These include high-frequency oscillation, high-frequency jet ventilation (or jet ventilation), high-frequency flow interruption, and high-frequency positive pressure ventilation.[2] This chapter focuses on jet ventilation.

Jet ventilation was first used during bronchoscopy.[1] A cannula was placed in an open-ended bronchoscope, and gas was delivered from a high-pressure source. Ambient air was entrained by the Venturi effect. The system was later adapted to deliver gas through a ventilating laryngoscope and through a catheter placed between the vocal cords. Percutaneous transtracheal jet ventilation was introduced during anesthesia in the early 1970s.

During jet ventilation, pulses of gas are delivered at high velocity through an orifice in a T-piece connected to a tracheal tube, through a narrow tube incorporated in the tracheal tube, or through a catheter placed in the upper airway.[3] Typical frequencies are in the range of 100 to 300 breaths/min.[4] The major advantage of jet ventilation resides in the flexibility of the patient interface, allowing ventilation in situations where tracheal intubation is not possible.

In addition to high-frequency jet ventilation, transtracheal jet ventilation can be used for emergency ventilation if a tracheal tube cannot be placed. Acceptable gas exchange can be achieved using a high-pressure oxygen source, a valve, a jet injector, a catheter, and noncompliant tubing. A jet injector can be made of a cut-off 1 ml syringe; the flush valve of an anesthesia machine can be used as valve.[5] Ventilation is then provided at a rate of 12 to 20 breaths/min.[6]

PHYSICS AND PHYSIOLOGY

High-frequency ventilation is based on the premises that transpulmonary pressure (i.e., the pressure that distends alveoli) can be divided into a steady and an oscillatory component. Eucapnia can then be maintained at low tidal volumes by an increase in the frequency of oscillation.[7] By decreasing tidal excursion (i.e., transpulmonary pressure excursion above and below its mean), high-frequency ventilation should also limit alveolar derecruitment caused by insufficient lung volume. Interestingly, panting in dogs may be considered to represent the physiologic counterpart to mechanical high-frequency, low tidal volume ventilation and has been used as a model to study gas exchange during conditions of high-frequency ventilation.[8]

The volume of gas delivered to the alveoli depends on the volume of gas passing through the jet, the volume of gas entrained into the tracheal tube or airway, and the volume of the dead space.[9] As frequency increases, tidal volume decreases, but dead-space ventilation increases and alveolar ventilation can therefore only be maintained with very high minute ventilation. At frequencies above 1 Hz (60 breaths/min), tidal volume is usually less than the volume of the dead space. It has been suggested that when tidal volume is less than 1.2 times the volume of the dead space, CO_2 elimination is greatly reduced, compared with conventional convective gas exchange, and that the length of the dead space has a larger influence than its volume on CO_2 elimination.[9] It may therefore be beneficial to administer jet ventilation as distally as possible or practical. However, it has been shown that the physical characteristics of a jet depend on the ratio of the jet diameter to tube or airway diameter, the ratio of jet diameter to tube length, the position of the jet entrance, and the driving pressure.[10] Injectors can be designed to maximize flow. With distal jet ventilation, optimization of the injector is not possible, potentially resulting in decreased efficiency and flow.

Although the gas volume of the jet after a single injection may not travel more than a few diameters, a continuing distal motion of previously injected gas occurs with the repetition of this jet injection, particularly at high frequencies.[11] High-frequency jet ventilation results in inhomogeneous ventilation.[12] Regional variation in gas concentration, air space volumes, and pressures are observed. Caudal lung lobes are usually ventilated better because of inertial factors. However, this lack of uniform ventilation is expected to have minimal impact on overall gas exchange.

The volume of the jet impulse (tidal volume) is influenced by the geometry of the injector, the amount of gas entrained, the pressure of the jet, the back pressure, and the impulse duration.[10] Effective injectors can entrain four to five times the jet flow during the early part of inspiration,[4,10] although some studies suggest that this effect is minimal.[13] The entrained volume, measured as a fraction of the tidal volume, is minimally affected by respiratory rate in the 12 to 200 breaths/min range.[14] Entrainment is optimized by positioning the jet entrance in the proximal part of the endotracheal tube.[10] Entrainment is due to a Venturi effect as a high-velocity gas stream exits the injector.[14] Entrainment is limited to the early part of inspiration (first 0.08 seconds, regardless of respiratory rate), because as the lungs begin to fill, the airway pressure increases, which opposes and eventually prevents entrainment of gas. For the remainder of inspiration, some of the jet gas comes out of the airway opening without entering the lungs.[14] The amount of gas lost this way (spilt volume) decreases as respiratory rate increases. During gas entrainment, there can be no spillage. As respiratory rate increases, inspiratory time decreases, but the time during which entrainment occurs remains fairly constant; therefore the time available for spillage decreases.[14] Because high frequencies are required, expiratory time is short and end-expiratory lung volume is increased. Therefore end-expiratory pressure is usually positive. This raises the pressure at the beginning of inspiration and may limit gas entrainment when high respiratory rates are used. Because of the high velocity of gas flow required to produce adequate ventilation at these high frequencies, changes in airway resistance will have a larger effect on tidal volume than respiratory system compliance, especially because volume changes are minimal. Similarly, distribution of ventilation will depend more on airway resistance than regional compliance, which may be beneficial in lung diseases that do not affect the airway.[7]

EQUIPMENT

Various devices to administer jet ventilation are commercially available. They are based on a high-pressure gas source and solenoid valves to admit/interrupt gas flow. Typical settings include peak airway pressure, respiratory rate, and inspiratory time or inspiratory/expiratory time ratio (I/E ratio). Some ventilators allow the control of mean airway pressure, positive end-expiratory pressure, minute volume, and driving pressure. Rates usually range from 30 to 150 breaths/min and sometimes may be as high as 600 breaths/min.

INDICATIONS

Jet ventilation is indicated in situations where mechanical ventilation is necessary or beneficial but traditional positive pressure ventilation cannot be delivered. These may include laryngeal and tracheal surgery, bronchial resection, laryngoscopy, and bronchoscopy and whenever limitation of movement associated with respiration is beneficial.[15] In addition, it has been suggested that jet ventilation in acute respiratory failure with circulatory shock resulted in higher cardiac output than traditional ventilation.[16] Finally, jet ventilation is indicated if ventilation is required in patients with a tracheal lesion secondary to tracheostomy or prolonged intubation.[15] Jet ventilation may also be used if the laryngeal opening is too small to allow intubation. It has been suggested that because of lower peak airway pressure than in traditional mechanical ventilation, jet ventilation may be preferable in airway leak situations.[17]

In dogs and cats, high-frequency jet ventilation has been used to maintain oxygenation and ventilation during resection and anastomosis of the intrathoracic trachea and during bronchoscopy.[18,19]

At the author's institution, jet ventilation is primarily used to maintain oxygenation and carbon dioxide elimination during bronchoscopy in small dogs and cats. Ventilation is delivered through a 14- or 16-gauge catheter positioned in the trachea. The bronchoscope can then be passed alongside that catheter (Figure 32-1).

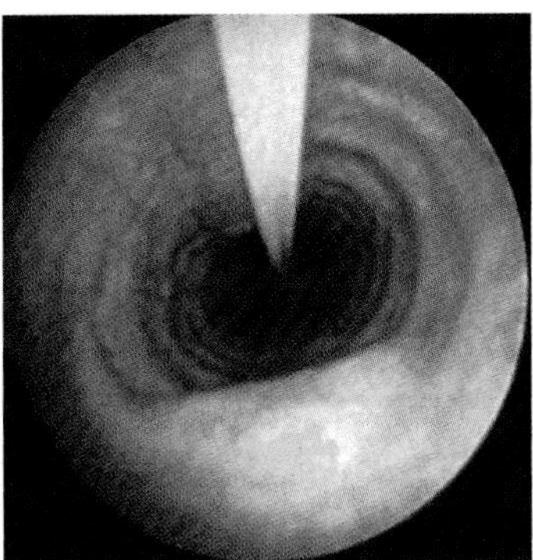

FIGURE 32-1 Endoscopic view showing the tip of a 13-gauge catheter used to deliver jet ventilation in a cat's trachea. *(From McCarthy TC: Veterinary endoscopy for the small animal practitioner, St Louis, 2005, Elsevier.)*

Transtracheal high-frequency jet ventilation can be used in emergency situations. A catheter is placed percutaneously through the cricothyroid membrane. The catheter is then secured to the neck of the patient. Migration of the catheter outside the trachea would result in severe subcutaneous emphysema.[17]

DISADVANTAGES

Tidal volume is very difficult to measure during jet ventilation. The high velocity of the jet and entrainment of additional gas make inspiratory volume measurement very difficult; spillage of gas out of the open airway and the common addition of a bias flow make measurement of expired volume inaccurate.[14] Similarly, end-tidal carbon dioxide concentration cannot be reliably measured during this mode of ventilation.[3] Therefore adequacy of ventilation should be confirmed by end-tidal carbon dioxide concentration measurement during intermittent ventilation with large tidal volume or by arterial blood gas analysis.

Jet ventilation may cause fluctuations in the amplitude of chest excursions and phasic changes in heart rate and systemic and pulmonary arterial pressures, resulting in fluctuations in blood flow.[20] The small tidal volumes and therefore low peak airway pressure and possibly mean airway pressure during jet ventilation are expected to limit the cardiovascular effects of this mode of ventilation. However, compared with conventional mechanical ventilation, high-frequency jet ventilation may result in similar, larger, or smaller cardiovascular effects.

Jet ventilation, particularly during severe bronchoconstriction or other forms of airway obstruction, may result in lung overinflation as gas accumulates because of short expiratory times. Lung hyperinflation may also result from steady alveolar pressure in excess of steady airway pressure.[7] This likely is due to unequal inspiratory and expiratory impedances, distribution of oscillatory flow, and expiratory flow limitation.[11,21] In addition, high-velocity gas streams as generated during high-frequency ventilation preferentially follow straight pathways. Because of the geometry of the central airway, this may result in regional differences, with an increased tendency of the lung base to be overinflated, compared with the apex.[7]

Prolonged use (i.e., hours) of high-frequency jet ventilation administered in the trachea via a catheter was shown to result in endoscopic evidence of tracheal injury characterized by hypervascularity, mucus accumulation, focal hemorrhage, linear epithelial loss, and diffuse erythema and epithelial loss.[22]

MONITORING OF GAS EXCHANGE DURING JET VENTILATION

Despite the technical difficulties limiting the ability to monitor the adequacy of ventilation during high-frequency jet ventilation, the same principles apply as for conventional mechanical ventilation.[23] Arterial blood gas analysis remains the "gold standard" to judge adequacy of oxygenation and ventilation and should be available if jet ventilation is used for extended periods. The same normal and abnormal PaO_2 and $PaCO_2$ values as during conventional mechanical ventilation should be used in the interpretation of blood gas data.

VENTILATOR SETTINGS

The goal of jet ventilation is to maintain adequate oxygenation and carbon dioxide elimination. However, because of the characteristics of jet ventilation, it is difficult to give guidelines for adjusting ventilatory parameters that will result in normal ventilation in different situations.[4] Our clinical experience suggests that at a frequency of 180 breaths/min, tidal volumes resulting in barely detectable chest excursions usually result in adequate oxygenation and normocapnia to moderate hypocapnia. One study in dogs and cats reported that with driving pressures of 0.33 kg/cm^2 and an I/E ratio of 1:2, cats were mildly hyperventilated at a frequency of 140 breaths/min; in dogs, a driving pressure of 1.3 to 1.8 kg/cm^2 and 120 to 150 breaths/min resulted in a similar degree of hyperventilation.[17]

REFERENCES

1. Bohn D: The history of high-frequency ventilation, Respir Care Clin N Am 7:535, 2001.
2. Cotten M, Clark RH: The science of neonatal high-frequency ventilation, Respir Care Clin N Am 7:611, 2001.
3. Sykes MK: High frequency ventilation, Br J Anaesth 62:475, 1989.
4. Mutz N, Baum M, Benzer H, et al: Clinical experience with several types of high frequency ventilation, Acta Anaesthesiol Scand Suppl 90:140, 1989.
5. Benumof JL, Scheller MS: The importance of transtracheal jet ventilation in the management of the difficult airway, Anesthesiology 71:769, 1989.
6. Hess DR, Gillette MA: Tracheal gas insufflation and related techniques to introduce gas flow into the trachea, Respir Care 46:119, 2001.
7. Fredberg JJ, Allen J, Tsuda A, et al: Mechanics of the respiratory system during high frequency ventilation, Acta Anaesthesiol Scand Suppl 90:39, 1989.
8. Meyer M, Hahn G, Piiper J: Pulmonary gas exchange in panting dogs: a model for high frequency ventilation, Acta Anaesthesiol Scand Suppl 90:22, 1989.
9. Sykes MK: Gas exchange during high frequency ventilation, Acta Anaesthesiol Scand Suppl 90:32, 1989.
10. Baum M, Mutz N: Physical characteristics of a jet in the airways, Acta Anaesthesiol Scand Suppl 90:46, 1989.
11. Scherer PW, Muller WJ, Raub JB, et al: Convective mixing mechanisms in high frequency intermittent jet ventilation, Acta Anaesthesiol Scand Suppl 90:58, 1989.
12. Wagner PD: HFV and pulmonary physiology, Acta Anaesthesiol Scand Suppl 90:172, 1989.
13. Tamsma TJ, Spoelstra AJ: Gas flow distribution and tidal volume during distal high frequency jet ventilation in dogs, Acta Anaesthesiol Scand Suppl 90:75, 1989.
14. Young JD: Gas movement during jet ventilation, Acta Anaesthesiol Scand Suppl 90:72, 1989.
15. Rouby JJ, Viars P: Clinical use of high frequency ventilation, Acta Anaesthesiol Scand Suppl 90:134, 1989.
16. Fusciardi J, Rouby JJ, Barakat T, et al: Hemodynamic effects of high-frequency jet ventilation in patients with and without circulatory shock, Anesthesiology 65:485, 1986.
17. Haskins SC, Orima H, Yamamoto Y, et al: High-frequency jet ventilation in anesthetized, paralyzed dogs and cats via transtracheal and endotracheal tube routes, J Vet Emerg Crit Care 1:55, 1991.
18. Whitfield JB, Graves GM, Lappin MR, et al: Anesthetic and surgical management of intrathoracic segmental tracheal stenosis utilizing high-frequency jet ventilation, J Am Anim Hosp Assoc 25:443, 1989.
19. Bjorling DE, Lappin MR, Whitfield JB: High-frequency jet ventilation during bronchoscopy in a dog, J Am Vet Med Assoc 187:1373, 1985.
20. Calkins JM: Physiologic consequences of high frequency jet ventilation, Med Instrum 19:203, 1985.
21. Simon BA, Weinmann GG, Mitzner W: Mean airway pressure and alveolar pressure during high-frequency ventilation, J Appl Physiol 57:1069, 1984.
22. Haskins SC, Orima H, Yamamoto Y, et al: Clinical tolerance and bronchoscopic changes associated with transtracheal high-frequency jet ventilation in dogs and cats, J Vet Emerg Crit Care 2:6, 1992.
23. Wagner PD: Interpretation of conventional measurement of gas exchange in high frequency ventilation (HFV), Acta Anaesthesiol Scand Suppl 90:158, 1989.

CHAPTER 33
VENTILATOR WAVEFORMS

Matthew S. Mellema, DVM, PhD, DACVECC

KEY POINTS

- Ventilator waveform analysis can be an invaluable tool in monitoring and troubleshooting the ventilator patient.
- Inspection of ventilator waveforms can be crucial in recognizing system leaks, the need for suctioning, and changes in respiratory mechanics.
- Ventilator waveforms should be inspected hourly in any patient on long-term mechanical ventilatory support.
- Ventilator waveforms should be inspected immediately whenever the patient appears to be "fighting" the ventilator.

Long-term (>24 hours) intermittent positive pressure ventilation (IPPV) can be a lifesaving therapy for patients with severe respiratory compromise.[1,2] It is also commonly employed as a short-term supportive measure for patients with transient respiratory dysfunction (e.g., depressed respiratory drive during anesthesia).[3,4] When choosing ventilator settings the operator must first choose a mode of ventilation and then select machine settings based on general guidelines, disease-specific guidelines, and presumed patient needs.[5] These initial settings may be adjusted based on an evolving understanding of the nature of the patient's respiratory disease and response to empiric trial. After initiation of mechanical ventilation, the ventilator settings are altered as necessary to achieve the targeted gas exchange levels. Inspection of ventilator waveforms, in combination with arterial blood gas values and inspection of the patient, often provides the most comprehensive overview of the appropriateness of the current settings, allows monitoring of disease status and ventilator troubleshooting, and may also help to identify sources of the patient-ventilator dyssynchrony (PVD).[6-11] Waveform interpretation can be challenging and this chapter is meant to serve as an introduction to the process for the interested reader.

WAVEFORM TYPES

General

Ventilator waveforms are typically divided into those wherein a single parameter is plotted over time (scalars) or two parameters are plotted simultaneously (loops). Scalar waveforms generally take on six characteristics shapes (Figure 33-1): square, ascending ramp, descending ramp, sine, exponential rise, and exponential decay.

Ramp and exponential waveforms are functionally similar enough that exponential waveforms are often lumped into the ramp category, leaving three characteristic shapes: square, ramp, and sine. Sine waveforms are characteristic of patient efforts such as are seen with spontaneous breaths in continuous positive airway pressure (CPAP) or synchronized intermittent mandatory ventilation (SIMV). Square waveforms indicate that the given parameter changes abruptly but is then held at a near constant value for a time. Ramp and exponential waveforms indicate that a parameter is changing gradually over time, with a rate of change that is either constant (ramp) or variable (exponential) (Figure 33-2).

Scalars are made up of a series of these waveforms plotted above and below the axis over time. Many modern ventilators can display multiple different scalars simultaneously (see Figure 33-2). Deflections below the axis either indicate values are lower than a reference point (e.g. pressure below baseline) or can indicate directionality (e.g., flow into or out of the patient). Determining which waveform to monitor most closely depends on the machine settings and clinician need. As a rule of thumb, the scalar that represents the dependent variable will have the information that most directly reflects the patient's respiratory mechanics. For example, if the patient is being ventilated in a pressure control mode, then the flow and volume scalars will contain useful information, whereas the pressure scalar should appear however the clinician set it to appear. This rule does not wholly apply to PVD, however, because patient effort in this setting often leads to subtle alterations in the plot of the independent variable.

Waveforms in Different Ventilation Modes

The scalar waveforms take on characteristic shapes depending on the mode of ventilation employed. Ventilator waveforms associated with commonly employed modes of ventilation are shown in Figure 33-2 and Figure 33-3. In Figure 33-2, the characteristic shape of the waveforms seen with volume control modes (V-ACV, SIMV-VC) are shown.[12] Two successive machine-delivered breaths are shown with no patient-triggering or spontaneous breaths. The pressure waveforms have the characteristic exponential rise shape ("shark fin"). The highlighted area denotes a period of inspiratory hold, which allows time for intrapulmonary redistribution of gas *("pendelluft")* with a resultant pressure decline from peak inspiratory pressure (PIP) to plateau pressure (Pplat).[13] If the inspiratory hold was removed, then this concavity would not be present and expiration would begin once the preset tidal volume had been achieved. Note that the flow profile in this setting is constant (square) throughout inspiration. The delivery of flow at a constant rate allows for meaningful assessment of airway resistance (Raw). However, some ventilators allow for delivery of flow during volume control modes with a descending ramp profile, which has several potential benefits. The inspiratory hold also results in a prominent plateau in the volume waveform as is shown (see Figure 33-3).

In Figure 33-3 the characteristic shape of the waveforms seen with pressure control modes (P-ACV, SIMV-PC) and support modes are shown. In pressure control modes the pressure waveform is now the one with the characteristic shape, whereas the flow waveform typically assumes the shape of an exponential decay.[14] The volume waveform may be indistinguishable from those observed with volume control modes. The series of waveforms to the right in Figure 33-3 show typical profiles for pressure support modes (e.g., SIMV with PSV). In this setting, inspiratory flow is not expected to reach zero before expiration begins. In these instances, the inspiratory flow is set to cycle off once a preset percentage of peak flow is achieved (e.g.,

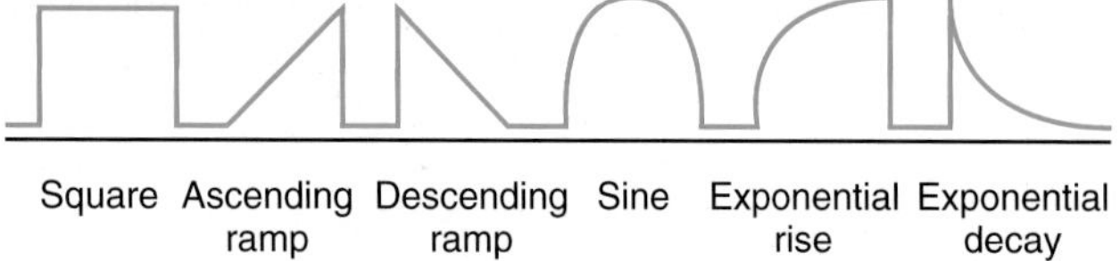

FIGURE 33-1 Characteristic shapes of ventilator waveforms. The six basic forms that make up standard ventilator scalar graphics are shown.

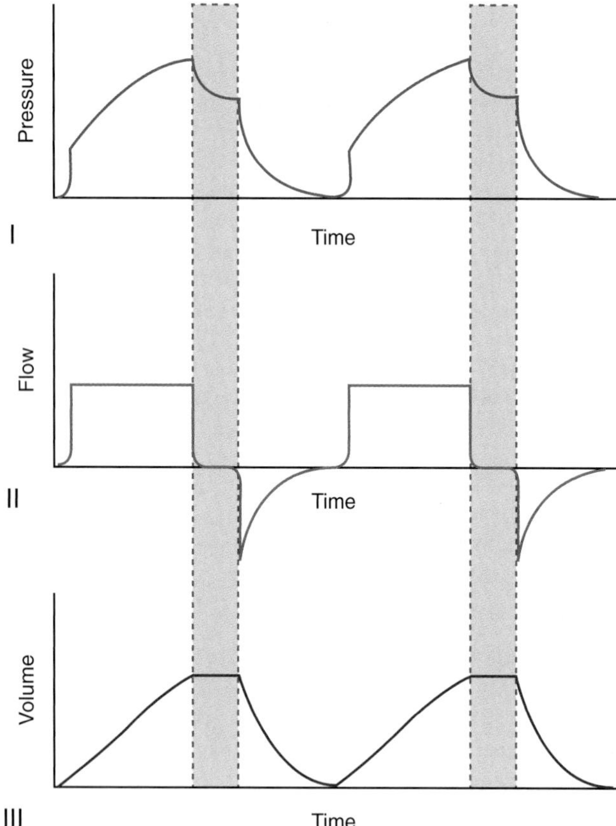

FIGURE 33-2 I-III, The pressure, flow, and volume scalars typical of volume control modes of ventilation are shown. An inspiratory hold is in place (shaded zones), which gives the pressure scalar (I) the classic appearance of a shark fin with a bite taken out of it.

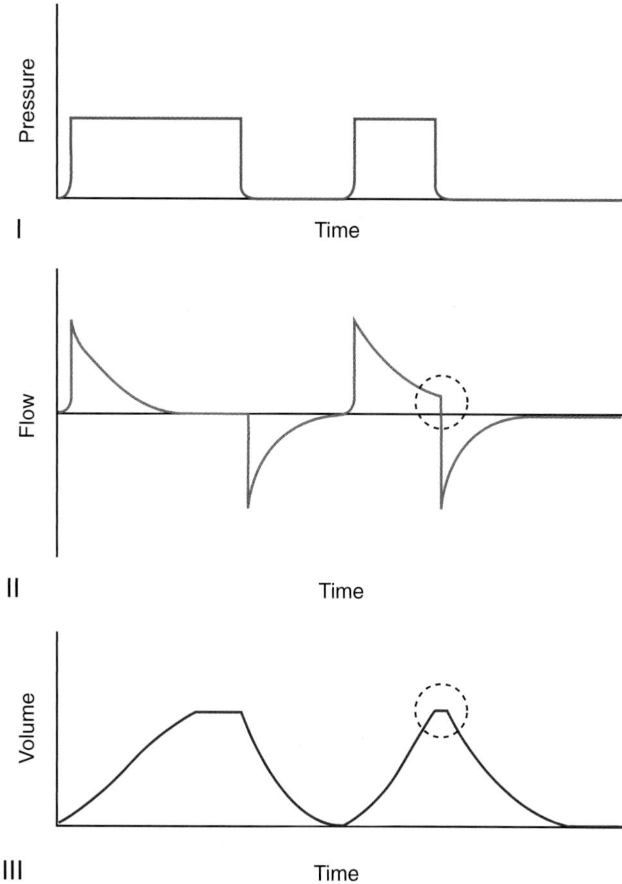

FIGURE 33-3 I-III, The pressure, flow, and volume scalars typical of pressure control modes of ventilation are shown. An inspiratory hold may still be prescribed (encircled), and this will result in plateau of the volume scalar (III). The scalars for the second breath are typical of pressure support modes of ventilation.

30% of peak). This point is reached within the upper dashed circle in the figure. Because the termination of inspiratory flow occurs when flow is low but not zero, the volume waveform shows a minimal plateau (lower dashed circle).

The use of SIMV as a mode of ventilation may be preferred in some clinical settings; however, it represents an additional level of complexity when it comes to ventilator waveform interpretation. In Figure 33-4 four archetypal sorts of SIMV breaths are displayed for comparison.[15] The vertical series labeled "A" depicts the typical waveforms associated with a mandatory breath in SIMV-VC. In this setting the shark fin pressure tracing and square wave flow tracing are evident. No inspiratory hold has been prescribed so expiration begins once the target tidal volume is achieved. Before the initiation of inspiratory flow there is no evidence of patient effort (triggering). The second breath (vertical series "B") is a spontaneous breath with characteristic sine wave appearance. Note that the negative portion of the pressure tracing is associated with inward flow because this is a spontaneous breath and not a positive pressure machine-delivered/assisted/supported breath. The tidal volume the patient achieves is lower than that seen with the preceding mandatory breath, which is what is typically observed (but not obligatory because it depends on

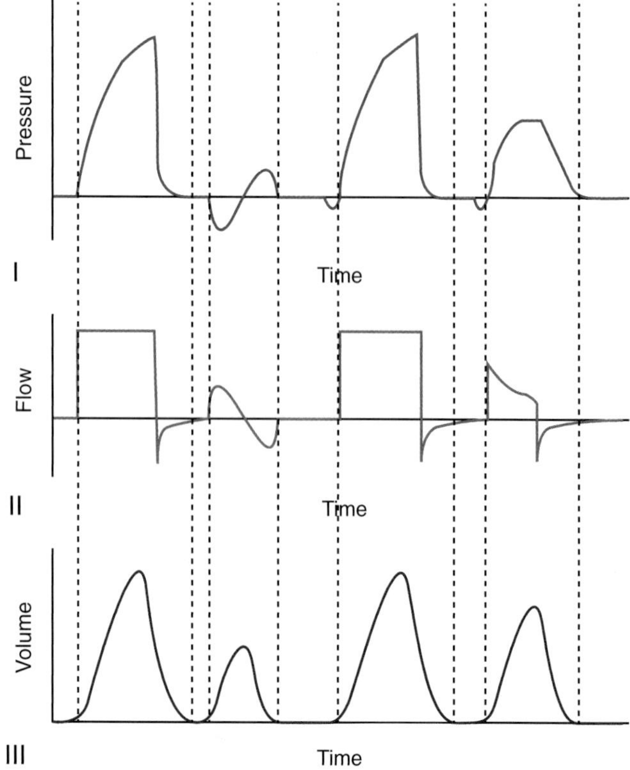

FIGURE 33-4 I-III, Scalar waveforms typical of SIMV breaths.

patient effort and capacity). The third breath (vertical series "C") represents a synchronized, patient-triggered but machine-delivered breath. In this instance the patient's inspiratory effort fell near to the time when the next mandatory breath was due. As such, the ventilator delivered a breath equivalent to the mandatory breath (series "A") but did so at a time synchronous with the patient's respiratory efforts. The tidal volume is identical to that achieved with the first breath. The patient's efforts only altered the timing of the breath, not its character. The nature of SIMV is such that there are preset periods immediately *after* a mandatory breath wherein the patient may breathe spontaneously and small time intervals *before* a mandatory breath during which patient efforts will trigger early delivery of the next ventilator-delivered breath (thus the *synchronized* nature of SIMV vs. IMV). The fourth breath (vertical series "D") represents the waveforms typical of SIMV with pressure support. Here the patient's inspiratory efforts for a spontaneous breath result in the ventilator delivering additional flow to supplement that achieved by the patient's own efforts. This pressure support is set to cease once a predetermined level of inspiratory flow is reached (e.g., 30% of peak flow). This is reflected in the flow waveform by the fact that inspiratory flow abruptly ceases at a level above zero. The tidal volume achieved is larger than the patient achieved with a spontaneous breath ("B") but smaller than the mandatory breaths ("A" and "C"). However, equivalent tidal volumes could be achieved by increasing the level of pressure support.

Pressure Waveform

The pressure waveform typically takes on an exponential rising (volume control modes with constant flow) or square waveform (pressure control) (Figure 33-5). In volume control modes with an exponential decay flow profile, the pressure scalar profile often appears as less square and more rounded. As mentioned earlier, when an inspiratory pause is in place the pressure waveform takes on the shape seen in Figure 33-5I, label B. Figure 33-5II shows that when positive end-expiratory pressure (PEEP) is being applied it is expected that pressure never returns to baseline, but rather remains at this preset level above atmospheric pressure between breaths (dashed line). Pressure decreases below this preset level indicate either patient effort, artifact, or circuit leaks.[16]

When an inspiratory pause is in place, inspection of the pressure waveform may reveal a great deal of information regarding the patient's lung mechanics. Figure 33-5III. In this setting PIP (denoted "a" on the figure) and Pplat (denoted "c" on the figure) can be determined. These pressures can be used to calculate dynamic and static compliances, respectively. For example, tidal volume/(PIP-PEEP) would estimate dynamic compliance and tidal volume/(Pplat-PEEP) would estimate static compliance. Dynamic compliance (Cdyn) is lower than static compliance (Cs) because of the increased pressure required overcoming circuit and airway resistance (Raw). This pressure would be reflected by the size of the region labeled "1" in Figure 33-5III. True static compliance can only be determined once bulk flow (gas delivery) and intrapulmonary flow (pendelluft) have ceased (point "c"). In many cases clinicians may be reluctant to design a breath with an inspiratory hold of the requisite length (~1.5 seconds) to truly measure static compliance and instead design application of a more brief inspiratory hold. In this case the pressure drops to the point labeled "b" and compliance measurements derived using these values are termed quasistatic (i.e., Cqs). In Figure 33-5III, the determinants of mean airway pressure (MAP) can be appreciated. The major influences on MAP values are the relative height and width of four distinct pressures: (1) pressure used to overcome circuit and airway resistances, (2) pressure used to deform the lung and expand the alveoli, (3) pressure throughout the expiratory flow phase, and (4) PEEP.[17] An increase in the surface area of any of these regions without an equivalent decrease in another will result in a higher MAP (Figure 33-6).

The PIP value on the pressure scalar can also be used in the estimation of Raw because resistance is equal to driving pressure divided by flow. An increase in Raw is seen as an increase in PIP without an accompanying increase in Pplat (see Figure 33-6I). Conversely, a decrease in compliance is evidenced by an increase in PIP and Pplat both with an unchanging difference between the two values (see Figure 33-6I).

Although an inspiratory hold can generate a wealth of information regarding pulmonary mechanics, an expiratory hold can also

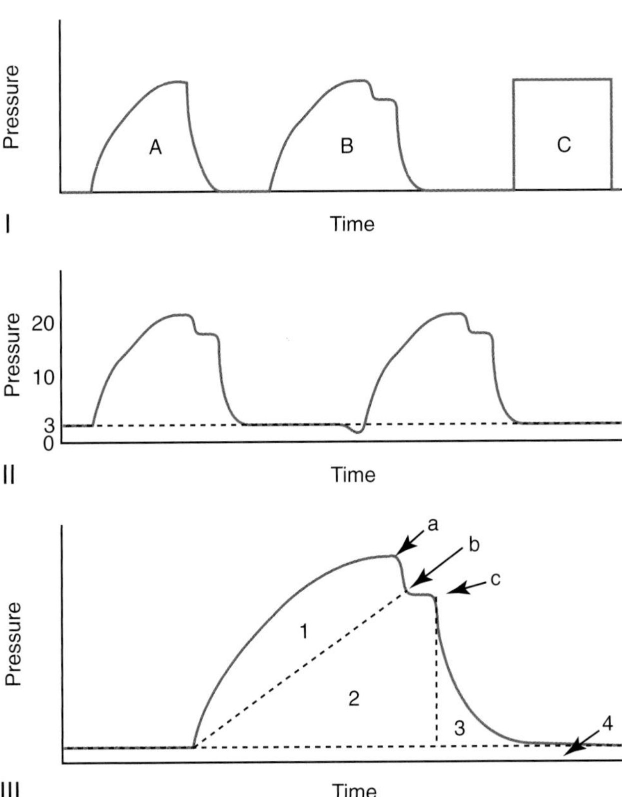

FIGURE 33-5 I-III, Pressure waveforms. Point (a) represents PIP and point (c) indicates Pplat.

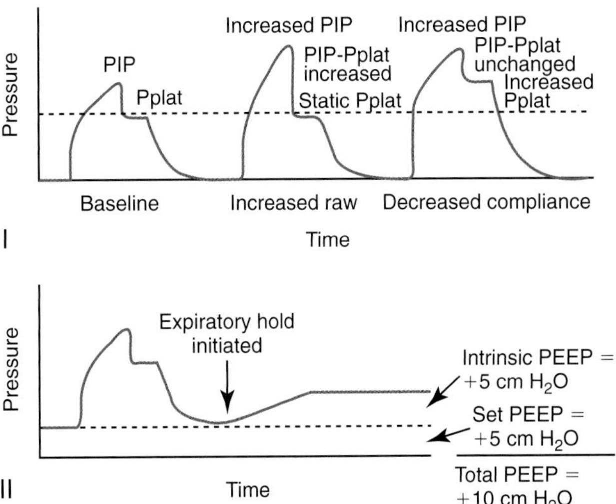

FIGURE 33-6 I-II, Using the pressure waveform to assess changes in lung mechanics.

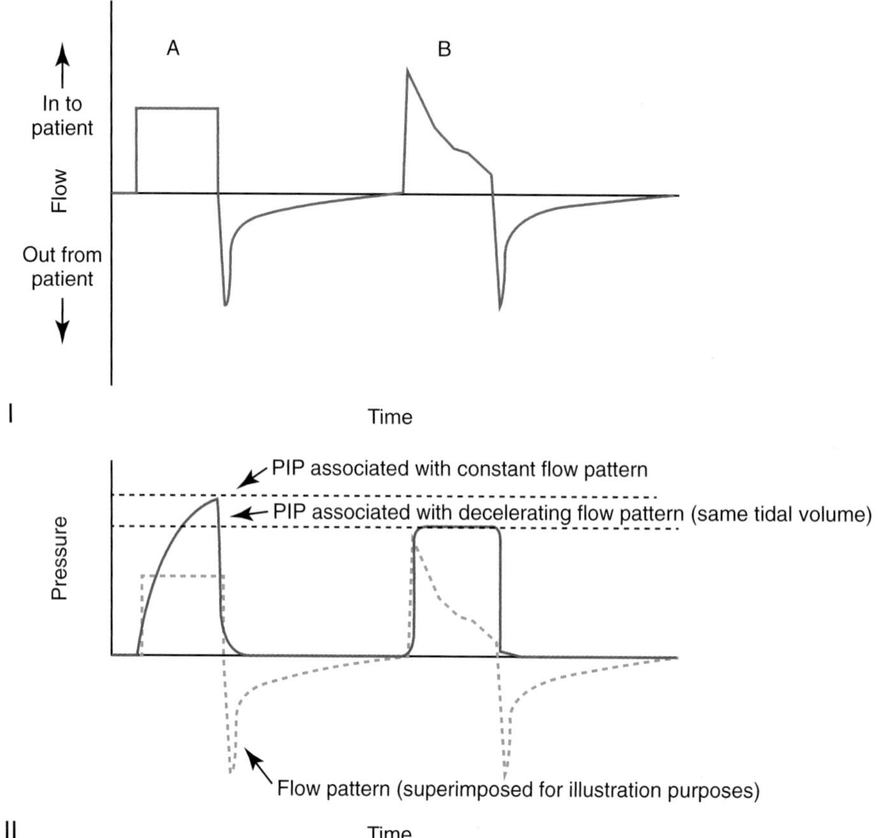

FIGURE 33-7 I-II, The flow waveforms typically seen when volume control modes of ventilation are employed. (I.A.)

yield useful information.[18] Many ventilators come equipped with an option for performing expiratory hold maneuvers. Performing this task allows one to quantify intrinsic PEEP caused by gas trapping (auto-PEEP) as long as auto-PEEP is of a value greater than set PEEP (see Figure 33-6II). In the example shown, set PEEP is +5 cm H_2O, but auto-PEEP is present and total PEEP is actually +10 cm H_2O. In these situations the auto-PEEP can have many adverse effects, including making patient triggering of the ventilator more challenging. In this instance, if the trigger value was set to −2 cm H_2O below PEEP, the patient would have to drop airway pressure to −7 cm H_2O instead of −2 cm H_2O before a breath would be triggered because of the additional airway pressure from auto-PEEP.

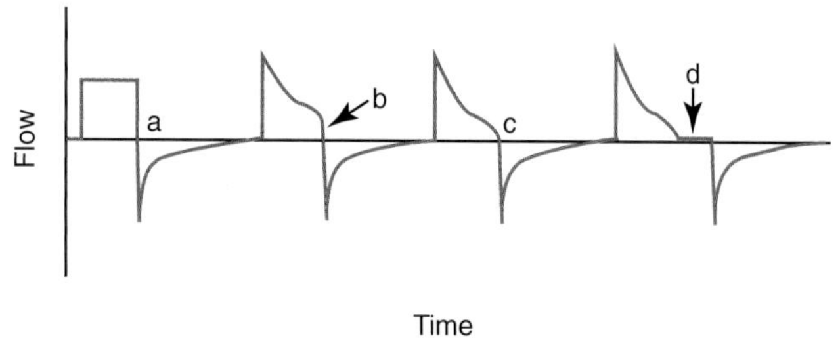

FIGURE 33-8 The flow waveform for four different volume control mandatory breaths with two different flow profiles are depicted.

Flow Waveform

The flow scalar takes on either a predictable, repeatable shape or a variable shape depending on the ventilation mode employed. In volume control modes of ventilation, the flow waveform will typically be square or descending ramp in conformation.[19] Many ventilators allow the operator to choose the flow profile in this setting. In spontaneous breathing, the flow profile will be sine wave in appearance. Lastly, in pressure control modes the flow waveform typically takes on an exponential decay appearance (see Figures 33-2 and 33-3).[20] Using a constant flow pattern (square wave) does allow for certain pulmonary mechanics measurements to be made because one can assign an absolute value to flow, next measure pressure differential, and then finally calculate resistance. However, the constant flow approach does have some drawbacks. For a given tidal volume delivered, using a constant flow delivery results in modestly higher peak inspiratory pressures (PIP) than if a decelerating ramp approach is taken, as illustrated in Figure 33-7I and II.[21-25] Moreover, the use of a decelerating ramp pattern allows for fine-tuning of inspiratory time (I-time) (Figures 33-7 and 33-8).

Figure 33-8 shows four different volume control mandatory breaths with two different flow profiles. For the breath to the far left (a), a constant (square) flow delivery was selected, whereas for the remaining three ("b" to "d") a decelerating ramp flow pattern was chosen. The third breath ("c") shows the appearance of the waveform when I-time is optimal. Flow returns all the way to zero before exhalation begins. In breath "b" the I-time is too short, and this may lead to flow asynchrony. In the case of breath "d," the I-time is too prolonged and there is a noticeable period of "zero-flow state" before exhalation. This zero-flow state puts the patient at risk for double triggering and other forms of PVD.[26] When one looks at breath "a," one can see that the constant flow rate option does not lend itself to the adjustment of I-time because the transition from inspiration to expiration is always abrupt when this flow pattern is selected unless an inspiratory hold is put in place. Thus, if the clinician opts for a volume control mode of ventilation, the selection of a decelerating ramp flow pattern may both allow for a lower PIP as well as allow one to optimize I-time using waveform inspection methods.

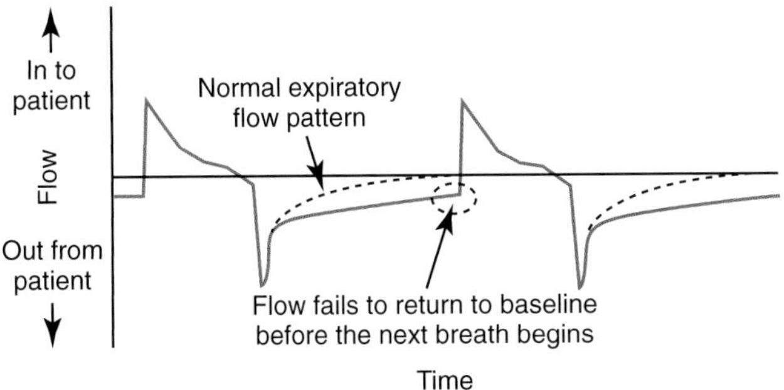

FIGURE 33-9 The pressure tracing from two successive breaths delivered in volume control mode with descending ramp flow patterns are depicted. In this example expiratory flow fails to return to zero before the next breath is delivered, indicating that auto-PEEP is present.

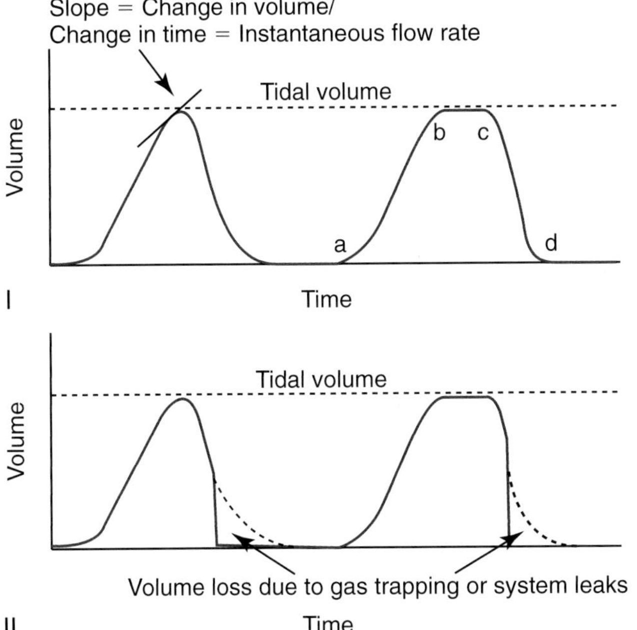

FIGURE 33-10 I-II, The volume waveforms from two successive breaths are represented.

The flow scalar is also a key tool in the detection of auto-PEEP without having to apply an expiratory hold. When auto-PEEP is present, the expiratory flow does not return to zero before the next breath is delivered (Figure 33-9). That is to say, the patient is not done exhaling the last breath when the next one is applied. In this way auto-PEEP can occur even in patients without intrathoracic airway dysfunction.

Volume Waveform

Of the three standard scalar waveforms (Figure 33-10), the volume tracing typically contains the least information that would lead a clinician to alter ventilator settings. This is because most ventilators that can display graphic outputs also provide numeric outputs as well. As such one often relies on numeric outputs of tidal volume and spends more time inspecting the other two scalars. However, there is some value to visual inspection of the volume scalar. In particular, it can provide a rapid qualitative picture of the relative size of spontaneous and mandatory breaths during SIMV or of patient effort during CPAP breathing. The volume waveform is the inextricably linked to the flow waveform. One parameter is generally derived from the other. In many modern ventilators, the circuit flow is determined (often via a flow disruptor and differential pressure transducer) and it is the flow signal over time that is used to calculate the delivered or exhaled volume. Thus when one looks at the volume tracing one can see that the slope of the curve at any point reflects the instantaneous flow rate ($\Delta V/\Delta t$), as shown in Figure 33-10I. In this same figure, one can see that between the points labeled "a" and "b" the slope is large and positive and thus the flow scalar should have a large positive deflection at this same point. Between "b" and "c" the slope of the volume waveform is zero, thus volume is unchanging, and thus a corresponding zero flow period is expected on the flow scalar. Lastly, between "c" and "d" one would expect to see a large negative deflection on the flow scalar to reflect the rapidly decreasing volume in the circuit. Tidal volume can also be determined from inspection of the volume scalar, as shown in this same figure. Lastly, the other major role for volume waveform inspection is in the identification of circuit leaks or gas trapping. As shown in Figure 33-10II, a volume waveform that takes a vertical plunge straight to baseline in the mid-to late-expiratory phase indicates that more volume came in across the flow sensor than ultimately came back. This can mean that there is a leak in the circuit or that a given volume of gas has unexpectedly remained within the patient (e.g., gas trapping or unidirectional flow into the pleural cavity).

Pressure-Volume Loops

Pressure-volume loops (PV loops) are graphic representations of the dynamic interconnection between changes in circuit pressure and circuit volume. Inspection of PV loops has long been used in the assessment of lung mechanics in ventilator patients.[27] In the last two decades PV loop assessment has also come to play an important role in designing protective lung strategies for the support of ARDS patients.[28] Figure 33-11I shows a typical PV loop for a mandatory, machine-delivered breath in a patient on a ventilator. Because the patient is receiving IPPV, inflation of the lungs corresponds with a rise in circuit pressure (inspiratory limb). Note that in a spontaneously breathing patient (or one in a negative pressure ventilator/iron lung), the addition of volume to the circuit would be associated with a decrease in circuit pressure and thus the tracing of the loop would proceed in a clockwise fashion instead (not shown). Several features of Figure 33-11I, are noteworthy. First, the loop does not begin at a pressure value of zero. This indicates the patient is on PEEP. Next, the pressure and volume values recorded at the highest value of the loop (upper right hand area of the plot) would correspond to PIP and tidal volume, respectively. Finally, a dashed line connecting the two points at which volume is not changing has been added. This line connects the starting and end-inspiratory points. Because no significant circuit flow is occurring at these points, the pressure value largely reflects that required to distend the lung to that volume and not the additional pressure required to overcome airway and circuit resistance. The bowing of the inspiratory limb away from this line reflects the additional pressure required to overcome these resistances. The slope of this line is a measure of pulmonary compliance. Because intrapulmonary flows have not been given enough time to cease, this form of compliance would be termed dynamic compliance (Cdyn) rather than static compliance (see Figure 33-11).

Figure 33-11II shows a patient-triggered PV loop for comparison. This "figure eight" type of loop is typical of patient effort.[29] In this case the patient effort is triggering/initiating activity and thus the small loop lies in the lower left aspect of the tracing (shaded area). Patient-ventilator dyssynchrony may result in small patient-generated loops at other points in the tracing (e.g., the expiratory limb). The dashed vertical line and arrow indicate the PEEP value, and one can note that the patient efforts bring airway pressure below this resting value. Once the triggering threshold is reached, a machine-delivered breath proceeds. The size of the shaded area of the patient effort loop indicates the work done by the patient to trigger the breath. If the

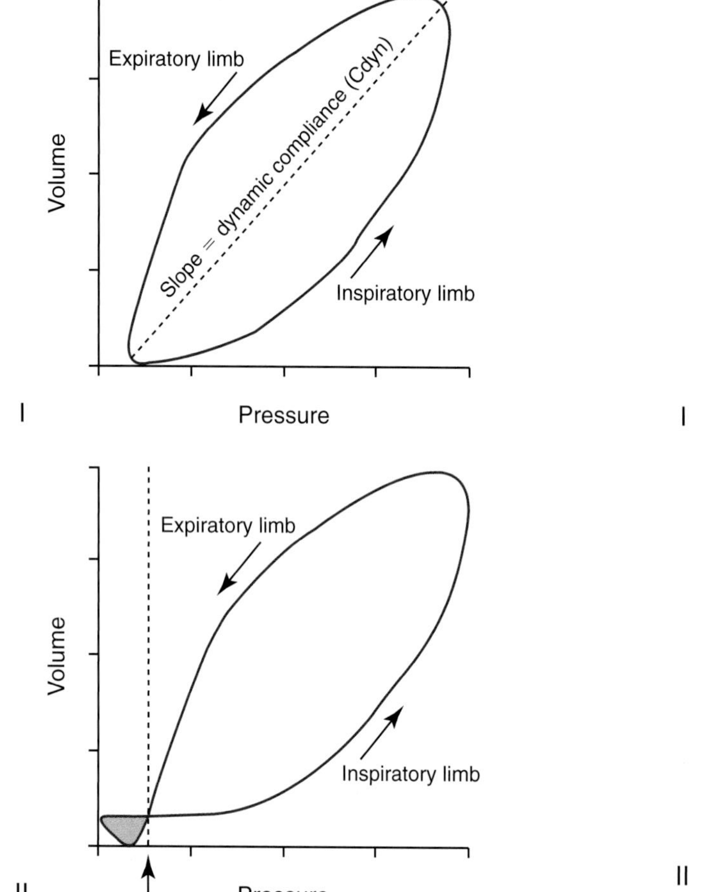

FIGURE 33-11 I-II, Typical PV loops for machine-triggered (I) and patient-triggered (II) breaths are depicted.

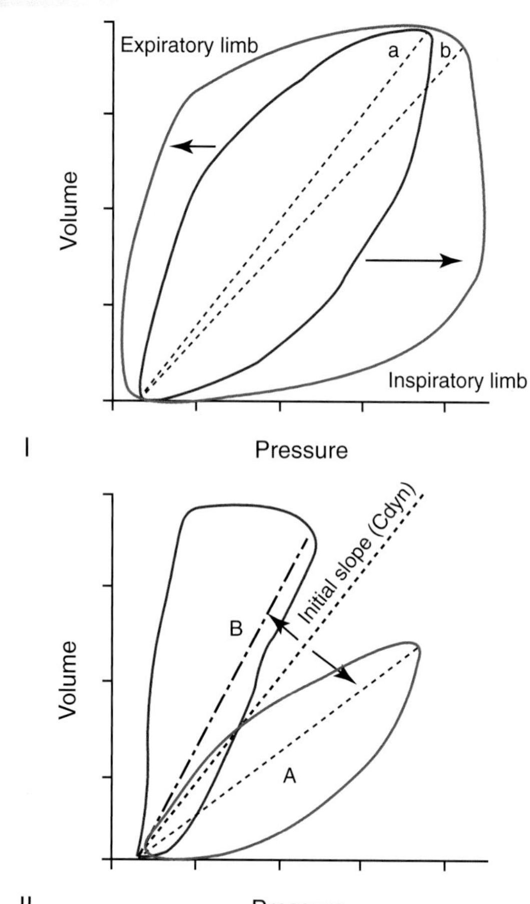

FIGURE 33-12 I-II, Pressure-volume loop changes seen with alterations in pulmonary mechanics.

trigger sensitivity is altered, then the patient will need to do more or less work to trigger the ventilator and the size of this area will change.

Changes in the orientation and area of PV loops can indicate alterations in the mechanical properties of the patient's lungs, the circuit, or both.[29] Figure 33-12I shows two loops from the same patient. The purple loop is the initial tracing, and the blue loop shows the changes expected to occur with an increase in airway or circuit resistances. The loop bows out farther from the dynamic compliance line, indicating that relatively greater applied pressure is required to overcome resistance and reach a given volume. Note that the Cdyn (as indicated by the slope of the line) has decreased. Unlike static compliance, the value of Cdyn is altered by changes in resistance because flow is not allowed to cease entirely. Increased bowing of the PV loop should prompt the clinician to investigate whether the endotracheal tube is kinked or obstructed, heat-moisture exchanger occlusion has occurred, or airway suctioning or bronchodilator administration is needed. Compliance changes also alter the shape and position of PV loops. As shown in Figure 33-12II, a reduction in compliance (e.g., pulmonary edema develops) causes the PV loop to rotate (labeled "A") as if its starting point was anchored and the loop rotated toward the x-axis. Conversely, if compliance increases (e.g., edema resolves) the loop moves as if its starting point was anchored and the loop rotated toward the y-axis (labeled "B"). The change in compliance can be appreciated by the significant alteration in the slopes of the Cdyn lines.

One must keep in mind that the shape of the PV loops is not entirely independent of the ventilator settings. Providing the same tidal volume with more rapid flow rates will result in increased bowing of the loop away from the compliance line. Moreover, in pressure control modes, the latter portion of the inspiratory limb can appear nearly vertical as constant inspiratory pressure is maintained (Figure 33-13I). Excessively large tidal volumes can lead to alveolar overdistention and "beaking" of the terminal portion of the inspiratory limb.[27] Beaking reflects further increases in circuit pressure with minimal additional volume increase. This shape is assumed once the alveoli have been expanded excessively and can only accept additional volume with large pressure increases (Figures 33-13 and 33-14).

The recognition of the mechanisms underlying ventilator-induced lung injury has lead to a greater role for PV loop inspection in optimizing ventilator settings. In this setting the clinician is advised to inspect the loop in search of two important inflection points (see Figure 33-14I). The lower inflection point (LIP) reflects a point at which pulmonary compliance significantly increases. This is thought to be the point at which a number of collapsed conducting and/or gas exchange units open. The cyclic opening and closing of these areas can lead to significant pulmonary damage (atelectrauma).[30] This atelectrauma can be minimized by increasing PEEP to a value greater or equal to the value at which the LIP is observed. In contrast, the upper inflection point (UIP) reflects the point at which pulmonary compliance significantly decreases because of alveolar overdistention and risk of alveolar injury (volutrauma) is increased.[31] It is generally advised to keep PIP below the pressure at which the UIP is noted. It must be noted that in small patients (<2 kg) the flow signal (and thus volume changes) may be difficult to acquire for all but the most sensitive equipment. When the monitoring equipment can't

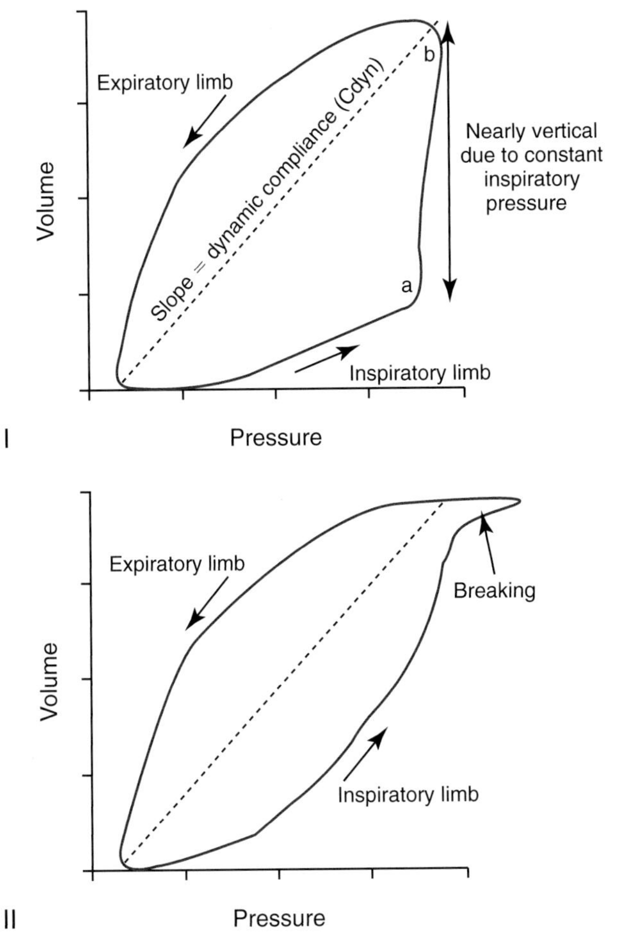

FIGURE 33-13 I-II, Pressure control and overdistention effects on PV loops.

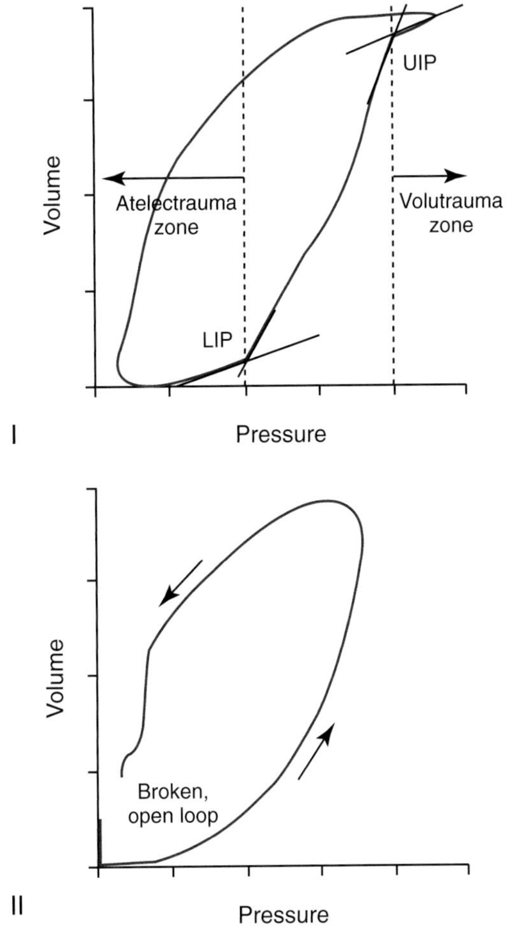

FIGURE 33-14 I-II, Upper inflection point (UIP), lower inflection point (LIP), and circuit leaks on PV loops.

acquire the signal, many models will continue to plot the last recorded value. The plot of a rising pressure with an absolutely constant volume will result in a sharp, narrow horizontal beak at end inspiration where flow is lowest. This signal acquisition artifact can mimic true beaking in these small patients. The clinician should remember that biologic processes rarely result in biophysical relationships that are absolutely linear in nature.

A leak in the ventilator circuit can also be reflected by changes in the PV loop. Figure 33-14II shows an open, broken, incomplete loop that is typical of a circuit leak. Monitoring for leaks is important for ensuring proper cuff inflation, ensuring delivery of targeted tidal volume, and alerting the clinician to the possibility of air leakage from the respiratory tract to the pleural space.

Flow-Volume Loops

Flow-volume loops are related to the flow scalar, and the inspiratory and expiratory limbs should roughly match the shape of the flow scalar portions (IA vs. IIA; IB vs. IIB) above and below the x-axis, respectively (Figure 33-15I and II).[29] The morphology of the waveforms will not match precisely because one is plotting flow against time and the other against volume, but the waveforms should be qualitatively similar. Flow-volume loops are particularly important in the assessment of excessive airway resistance and in alerting the clinician to the presence of copious airway secretions or circuit leaks. Flow asynchrony can also be detected via flow-volume loops, as is discussed in the Patient–Ventilator Dyssynchrony section later in this chapter (Figures 33-15 and 33-16).[10]

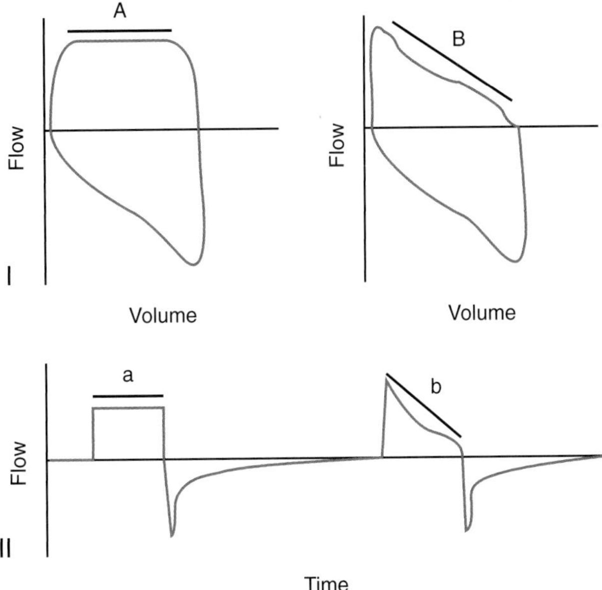

FIGURE 33-15 I-II, The flow-volume loop and corresponding flow scalars.

In ventilator waveform presentation the flow-volume loop is typically presented with the inspiratory limb above the x-axis (see Figure 33-16). In pulmonary function testing, the flow-volume loops are more typically presented with the expiratory limb above the x-axis and end-inspiration closest to the y-axis (i.e., upside down and inverted; picture the loop in Figure 33-16 rotated clockwise 180 degrees). In Figure 33-16, "a" denotes the start of inspiration. Inspiration continues to point "b" then ceases. The overall shape of the inspiratory limb is square, suggesting a constant flow volume control mode is being employed in this instance. The expiratory limb begins with the transition from point "b" to point "c." Peak expiratory flow is achieved early in exhalation and is patient effort dependent (usually not relevant in anesthetized patients on full assist-control ventilation). After peak flow is achieved, the expiratory limb tracing progresses to the effort-independent portion of the curve ("d"). The portion of the curve labeled "d" is the most relevant to the assessment of airway resistance (Raw) changes, although peak flow is also often altered as well. In the case of a significant increase in Raw, a "scooped out" appearance of the mid-to-late portion of the expiratory limb is noted with an accompanying reduction in peak expiratory flow (Figure 33-17I).[32] Such changes should prompt the clinician to investigate whether airway suctioning or bronchodilator administration is needed.

Circuit leaks can also be detected on flow-volume loops (see Figure 33-17II). In each case the key feature is that inspiratory and expiratory volumes are not equivalent. Much as was seen with the PV loop, the effect of a circuit leak on a flow-volume loop is to create a broken, incomplete appearance.[29]

Excessive airway secretions can also be detected via flow-volume loop inspection. Figure 33-17III shows an example of a flow-volume loop with a saw-tooth appearance to the effort-independent portion of the expiratory limb. This finding (along with auscultation of the trachea) is considered one of the most reliable indicators of the need for tracheal suction, whereas auscultation of crackles over the thorax is less predictive of suctioning need (see Figure 33-17).[32]

PATIENT–VENTILATOR DYSSYNCHRONY

Patient–ventilator dyssynchrony, or PVD (also called patient–ventilator interactions [PVI] or patient–ventilator asynchrony) is increasingly recognized as an important contributor to outcomes in patients requiring long-term mechanical ventilatory support.[6-11]

The ventilator patient's respiratory cycle can be divided into four distinct phases (Figure 33-18). Patient–ventilator dyssynchrony may occur during any of them, and more than one form of PVD may be detected concurrently. The first (phase 1) is the initiation of inspiration, which is also called the trigger mechanism. PVD during phase 1 is often referred to as *trigger asynchrony.* Trigger asynchrony has been shown to be by far the most common form of PVD in human patients.[11] The predominant types of trigger asynchrony include ineffective triggering, auto-triggering, and double triggering (Figure 33-19I, II, and III, respectively).[33] Ineffective triggering involves a patient-generated decrease in airway pressure with a simultaneous increase in airflow without triggering a machine-delivered breath. This form of PVD is often the result of an inappropriately set sensitivity setting on the ventilator. However, it has been shown that increasing levels of pressure support suppress respiratory drive and lead to increased frequency of ineffective triggering.[33-35] Triggering delay and ineffective triggering are often easier to identify on the flow scalar than on the pressure scalar because of the larger relative change in that parameter (i.e., bigger relative change in flow than pressure with ineffective efforts to trigger inspiration). When ineffective triggering is detected, the clinician should look for evidence of an improper triggering threshold, auto-PEEP (PEEPi), significant muscle weakness/fatigue, reduced respiratory drive, or an excessively deep level of anesthesia. Not all forms of trigger asynchrony may be corrected solely by adjusting the threshold.

Auto-triggering is another form of trigger asynchrony and occurs when a breath is delivered by the ventilator because of a change in airway pressure or flow not caused by patient effort. Most often auto-triggering is due to an inappropriately small threshold/sensitivity setting. Alternatively, flow or pressure distortions may be due to other factors, including circuit leaks, fluid/secretions within the circuit, or cardiac oscillations. Auto-triggering is more common when there are

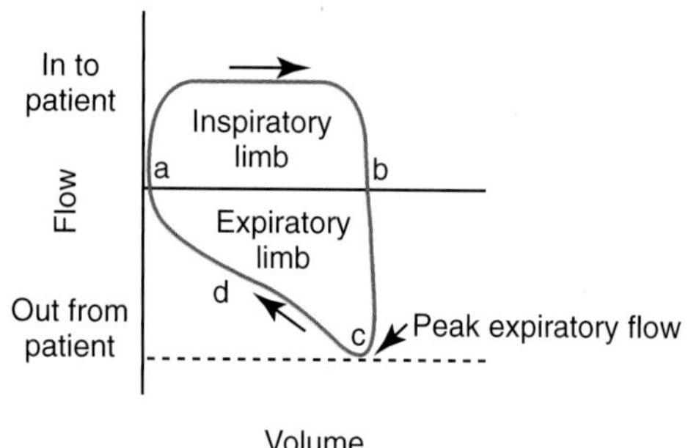

FIGURE 33-16 Typical appearance of a flow-volume loop.

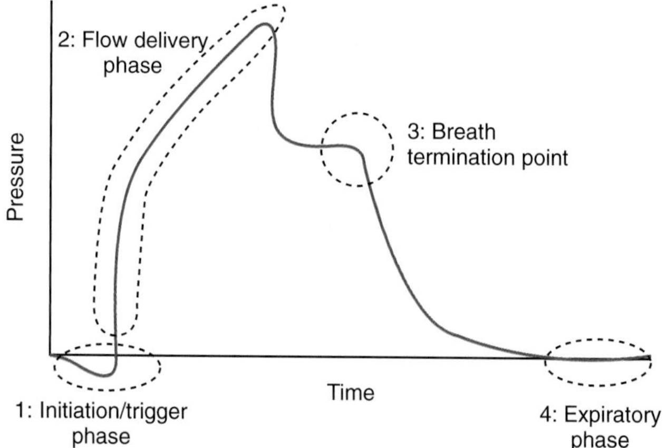

FIGURE 33-18 Phases of the machine-delivered breath. The four phases of a patient-triggered, machine-delivered breath are depicted and labeled on a pressure scalar waveform. The shape of the waveform is indicative that the breath was delivered in a volume control mode with an inspiratory hold.

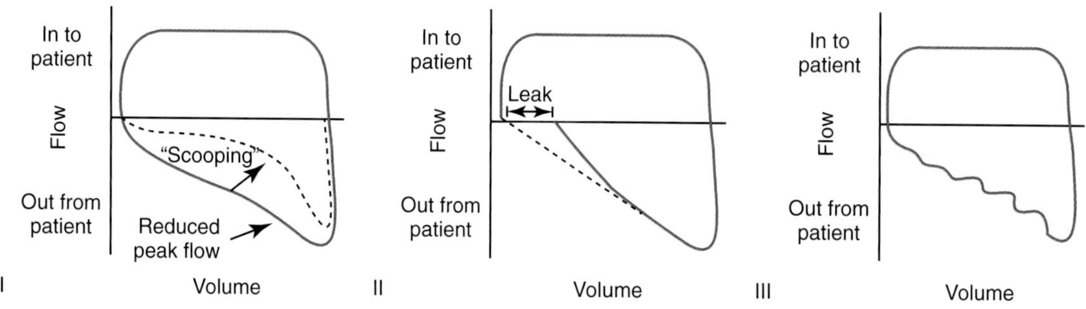

FIGURE 33-17 I-III, Flow-volume loops with increased Raw, circuit leaks, and excessive secretions.

prolonged periods of no expiratory flow between breaths. Double-triggering is defined as two delivered breaths separated by an expiratory time less than half the mean expiratory time. It occurs when a patient's inspiratory effort continues throughout the ventilator's preset I-time and thus remains present after the I-time has been completed. This prolonged effort triggers another breath. The end result is the patient receiving a tidal volume twice the desired or preset size. This carries with it risk of overdistention and alveolar trauma. This type of trigger asynchrony may be due to exceptionally high ventilatory demand on the part of the patient, low tidal volumes, an I-time that is too short, or a flow-cycle threshold set too high (see Figure 33-19).

Flow asynchrony is the result of ventilator supply of fresh gas to the inspiratory circuit that is either too fast or too slow for the individual patient. Flow asynchrony may be recognized using ventilator waveforms during either volume control or pressure control but manifests somewhat differently in each circumstance. In volume-controlled modes with constant inspiratory flow rates, it is easiest to detect flow asynchrony by comparing passive and patient-triggered breaths on both the pressure and flow scalars. In patients with flow asynchrony the triggered breaths will often have a "scooped out," concave appearance on the upswing of the pressure tracing (Figure 33-20I, labeled "A") and a saw-tooth appearance to the plateau phase of the flow tracing (see Figure 33-20II, labeled "B") relative to the convex mandatory breaths. Flow asynchrony may also be evident on flow volume and pressure-volume loops and manifest as irregular concavities of the inspiratory limbs (Figure 33-20III and 33-20IV, labeled "C" and "D"). Such findings should prompt the clinician to increase inspiratory flow until the two types of breaths have similar appearing waveforms. In pressure control (with variable inspiratory flow), one should look at the pressure-time scalar. When inspiratory flow is inadequate the pressure-time scalar will assume a "scooped out" appearance during the inspiratory plateau. When inspiratory flow is excessive one may see an early overshoot in the airway pressure waveform (Figure 33-21III). The clinician should adjust rise time in this setting until the pressure waveforms appear nearly square, have no plateau concavity, and show no evidence of overshoot.

Termination asynchrony is also termed cycling asynchrony. The two main types of termination asynchrony involve inspiration being terminated too early (premature cycling; Figure 33-21I) or too late (delayed cycling; see Figure 33-21II). In the first instance, the patient is continuing to make inspiratory efforts at the time the ventilator cycles off. In the latter circumstance, the patient initiates active expiratory efforts while the ventilator is continuing to deliver inspiratory flow. Premature cycling may be associated with double-triggering (see Figure 33-19III) if the inspiratory efforts are sufficient to trigger a second breath after the first has been terminated. On the ventilator waveforms, premature cycling may be detected by visualizing an abrupt initial reversal in the expiratory flow waveform (often with a concurrent concavity in the pressure waveform). Increasing I-time or tidal volume should address premature termination. On the ventilator waveforms, delayed termination manifests as a pressure spike on the pressure scalar during mid- to late inspiration (see Figure 33-21II). On the flow-scalar one sees an abrupt, rapid decline

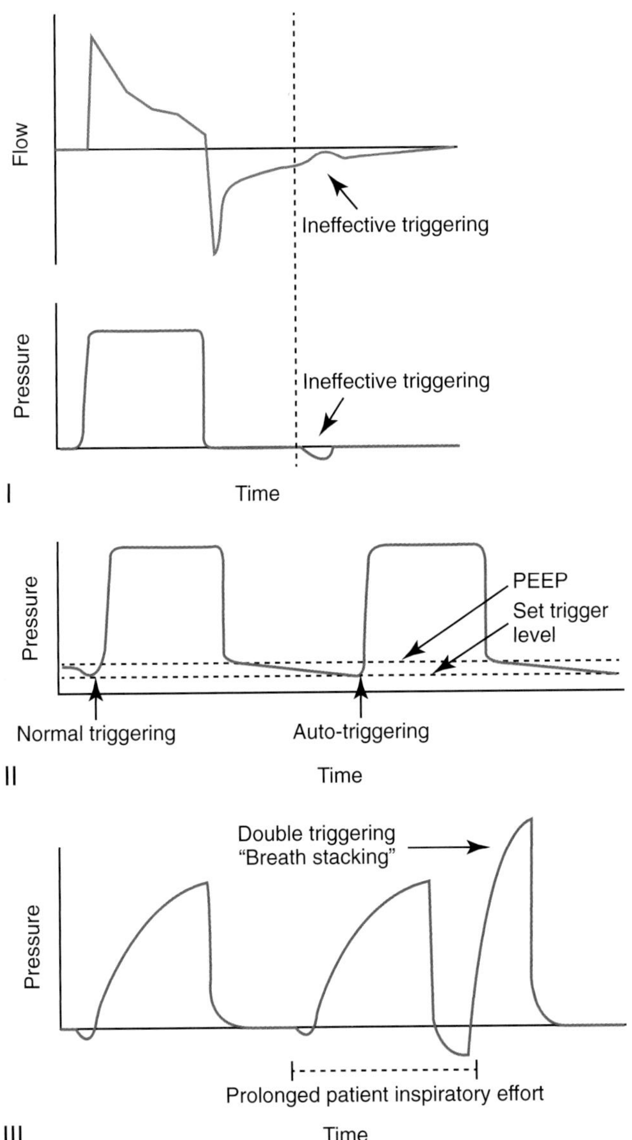

FIGURE 33-19 I-III, Evidence of various forms of trigger asynchrony on ventilator waveforms.

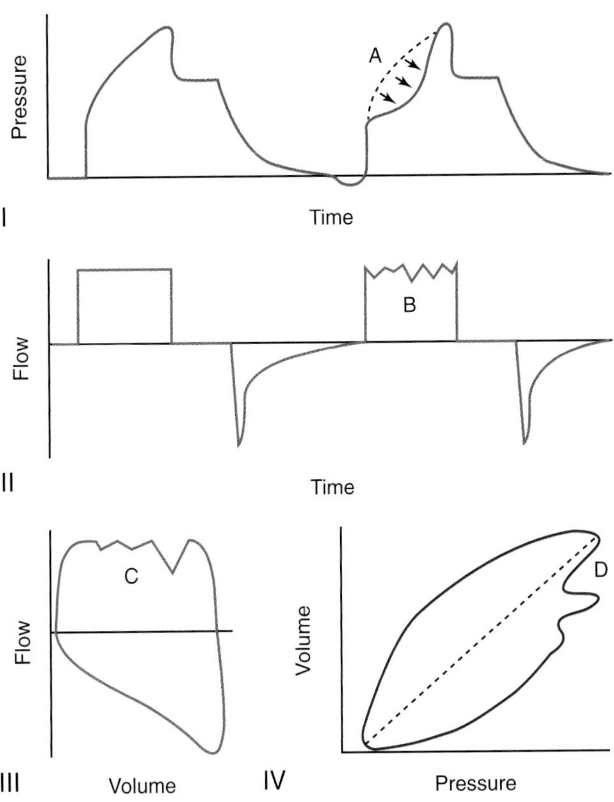

FIGURE 33-20 I-IV, Waveform appearance of flow asynchrony.

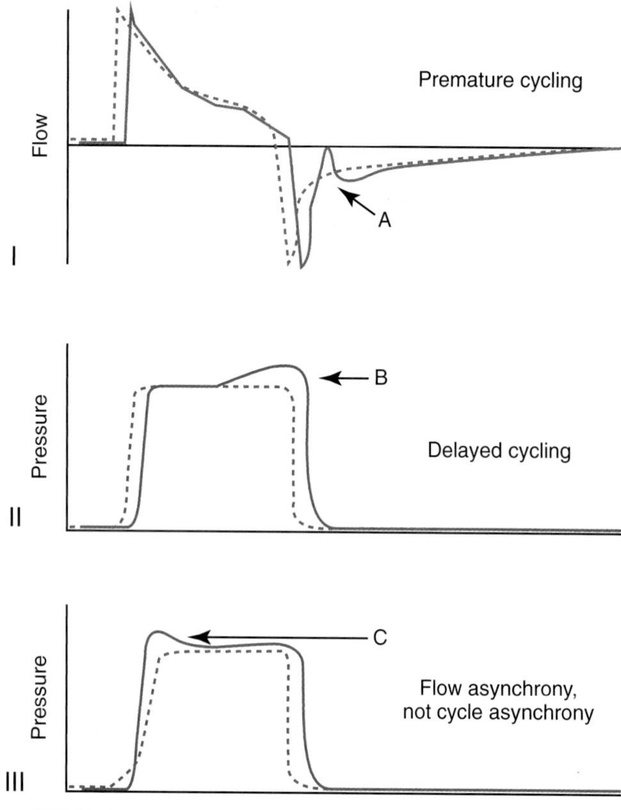

FIGURE 33-21 I-III, Waveform appearance of cycle asynchrony.

in inspiratory flow near end-inspiration. This type of asynchrony is managed by reducing I-time or tidal volumes. It is important not to confuse the early plateau change seen with flow asynchrony and the late plateau change seen with delayed cycling because the adjustments needed to address each of these are quite different. The waveforms for each of these forms of PVD are placed together in Figure 33-21 (II and III) to assist direct comparison.

Expiratory asynchrony typically manifests as auto-PEEP (gas-trapping), which has been described earlier in the section on the flow scalar (see Figure 33-9). If auto-PEEP is detected, then a number of parameters may be adjusted, nearly all of which serve to prolong expiratory time (e.g., trigger sensitivity, peak flow, flow pattern, rise time, I-time, cycle threshold, I/E ratio, and respiratory rate).[36] One major adverse aspect of auto-PEEP is the effect that it has on triggering (see also discussion of trigger asynchrony earlier). Auto-PEEP increases the difficulty the patient faces in reaching the triggering threshold. Increasing PEEP to account for auto-PEEP may improve triggering sensitivity and efficacy.

SUMMARY

In closing, ventilator waveforms should be inspected hourly in any patient on long-term mechanical ventilatory support and immediately whenever the patient appears to be "fighting" the ventilator. Ventilator waveforms can be crucial in recognizing system leaks, the need for suctioning, and changes in respiratory mechanics. The waveforms can also help place blood gas values into a more meaningful context and help with disease monitoring, in addition to evaluating the response to bronchodilators. The frequency with which PVD is recognized is largely dependent on how frequently one looks for it.[11] A systematic, step-wise approach evaluating all four phases can help the clinician to optimize ventilator settings and avoid over-anesthetizing patients with its associated adverse effects.

REFERENCES

1. Hopper K, Haskins SC, Kass PH, et al: Indications, management, and outcome of long-term positive-pressure ventilation in dogs and cats: 148 cases (1990-2001), J Am Vet Med Assoc 230(1):64, 2007.
2. Hopper K, Aldrich J, Haskins SC: Ivermectin toxicity in 17 collies, J Vet Intern Med 16(1):892, 2002.
3. Sedgwick CJ: Veterinary anesthesia ventilation, Mod Vet Pract 60(2):120, 1979.
4. Moens Y: Mechanical ventilation and respiratory mechanics during equine anesthesia, Vet Clin North Am Equine Pract 29(1):51, 2013.
5. ARDSnet authors: Ventilation with lower tidal volumes as compared with traditional tidal volumes for acute lung injury and the acute respiratory distress syndrome. The Acute Respiratory Distress Syndrome Network, N Engl J Med 342(18):1301, 2000.
6. MacIntyre NR: Patient-ventilator interactions: optimizing conventional ventilation modes, Respir Care 56(1):73, 2011.
7. Younes M, Brochard L, Grasso S, et al: (2007). A method for monitoring and improving patient: ventilator interaction, Intensive Care Med 33(8):1337, 2007.
8. Georgopoulos D, Prinianakis G, Kondili E, et al: Bedside waveforms interpretation as a tool to identify patient-ventilator asynchronies, Intensive Care Med 32(1):34, 2006.
9. Pierson DJ: Patient-ventilator interaction, Respir Care 56(2):214, 2011.
10. Nilsestuen JO, Hargett KD: Using ventilator graphics to identify patient-ventilator asynchrony, Respir Care 50(2):202; discussion 232-204, 2005.
11. de Wit M: Monitoring of patient-ventilator interaction at the bedside, Respir Care 56(1):61, 2011.
12. Waugh JB, Deshpande VM, et al: Waveforms for common ventilator modes. In Rapid interpretation of ventilator waveforms, Upper Saddle River, NJ, 2007, Pearson Education, 53-76.
13. Henderson WR, Sheel AW: Pulmonary mechanics during mechanical ventilation, Respir Physiol Neurobiol 180(2-3):162, 2012.
14. Hess DR: Ventilator waveforms and the physiology of pressure support ventilation, Respir Care 50(2):166; discussion 183-166, 2005.
15. Giuliani R, Mascia L, Recchia F, et al: Patient-ventilator interaction during synchronized intermittent mandatory ventilation. Effects of flow triggering, Am J Respir Crit Care Med 151(1):1, 1995.
16. Vignaux L, Vargas F, Roeseler J, et al: Patient-ventilator asynchrony during non-invasive ventilation for acute respiratory failure: a multicenter study, Intensive Care Med 35(5):840, 2009.
17. Marini JJ, Ravenscraft SA: Mean airway pressure: physiologic determinants and clinical importance. Part 1: Physiologic determinants and measurements, Crit Care Med 20(10):1461, 1992.
18. Blanch L, Bernabe F, Lucangelo U: Measurement of air trapping, intrinsic positive end-expiratory pressure, and dynamic hyperinflation in mechanically ventilated patients, Respir Care 50(1):110; discussion 123, 2005.
19. Koh SO: Mode of mechanical ventilation: volume controlled mode, Crit Care Clin 23(2):161, viii, 2007.
20. Singer BD, Corbridge TC: Pressure modes of invasive mechanical ventilation, South Med J 104(10):701, 2011.
21. Al-Saady N, Bennett ED: Decelerating inspiratory flow waveform improves lung mechanics and gas exchange in patients on intermittent positive-pressure ventilation, Intensive Care Med 11(2):68, 1985.
22. Wong PW, Nygard S, Sogoloff H, et al: The effect of varying inspiratory flow waveforms on pulmonary mechanics in critically ill patients, J Crit Care 15(4):133, 2000.
23. Bergman NA: Effect of different pressure breathing patterns on alveolar-arterial gradients in dogs, J Appl Physiol 18:1049, 1963.
24. Adams AP, Economides AP, Finlay WE, et al: The effects of variations of inspiratory flow waveform on cardiorespiratory function during controlled ventilation in normo-, hypo- and hypervolaemic dogs, Br J Anaesth 42(10):818, 1970.
25. Modell HI, Cheney FW: Effects of inspiratory flow pattern on gas exchange in normal and abnormal lungs, J Appl Physiol 46(6):1103, 1979.
26. de Wit M, Pedram S, Best AM, et al: Observational study of patient-ventilator asynchrony and relationship to sedation level, J Crit Care 24(1):74, 2009.

27. Harris RS: Pressure-volume curves of the respiratory system, Respir Care 50(1):78, discussion 98-79, 2005.
28. Terragni PP, Rosboch GL, Lisi A, et al: How respiratory system mechanics may help in minimising ventilator-induced lung injury in ARDS patients, Eur Respir J Suppl 42:15s-21s, 2003.
29. Waugh JB, Deshpande VM, et al: Pressure-volume and flow-volume loops. In Rapid interpretation of ventilator waveforms, Upper Saddle River, NJ, 2007, Pearson Education, 23-52.
30. Muscedere JG, Mullen JB, Gan K, et al: Tidal ventilation at low airway pressures can augment lung injury, Am J Respir Crit Care Med 149(5):1327,1994.
31. Dreyfuss D, Soler P, Basset G, et al: High inflation pressure pulmonary edema. Respective effects of high airway pressure, high tidal volume, and positive end-expiratory pressure, Am Rev Respir Dis 137(5):1159, 1988.
32. Guglielminotti J, Alzieu M, Maury E, et al: Bedside detection of retained tracheobronchial secretions in patients receiving mechanical ventilation: is it time for tracheal suctioning? Chest 118(4):1095, 2000.
33. Thille AW, Rodriguez P, Cabello B, et al: Patient-ventilator asynchrony during assisted mechanical ventilation, Intensive Care Med 32(10):1515, 2006.
34. Thille AW, Cabello B, Galia F, et al: Reduction of patient-ventilator asynchrony by reducing tidal volume during pressure-support ventilation, Intensive Care Med 34(8):1477, 2008.
35. Leung P, Jubran A, Tobin MJ: Comparison of assisted ventilator modes on triggering, patient effort, and dyspnea, Am J Respir Crit Care Med 155(6):1940, 1997.
36. Laghi F, Goyal A: Auto-PEEP in respiratory failure, Minerva Anestesiol 78(2):201, 2012.

CHAPTER 34
CARE OF THE VENTILATOR PATIENT

Steven Epstein, DVM DACVECC

KEY POINTS

- Long-term ventilation requires specialized equipment, 24-hour one-on-one nursing care, and intensive monitoring.
- Ventilator-associated pneumonia is a potentially fatal complication, and the risk of development can be reduced with detailed management strategies.
- Every body system should be evaluated on a daily basis to ensure that optimal care for each organ system is provided.

Mechanical ventilation, either short term (<24 hours), or long term (days to months), is becoming increasingly common in small animal practice. Much of the success or failure of these patients to survive is due to not only the respiratory effects of positive pressure ventilation but also the nursing care that goes along with it. Because most of these patients are anesthetized, many of the normal homeostatic functions of the body are compromised, creating potential complications for the patient. Care of the ventilator patient is aimed to minimize these complications. With short-term ventilation, care of the ventilated patient may not need to be as intense; however, long-term ventilation requires specialized care for optimal success.

It has been suggested that patients requiring short-term ventilation have better outcomes than patients requiring long-term ventilation.[1] Multiple complications associated with long-term ventilation have been documented, many of which relate to nursing care issues.[2] These include oral and corneal ulceration, tracheal tube occlusion or dislodgement, and gastric distention requiring decompression. The importance of nursing care for ventilator patients in human medicine is highlighted because the risk of late-onset, but not early-onset, ventilator-associated pneumonia (VAP) is affected by a lower nurse staffing level.[3] Ideally each patient on the ventilator will have a dedicated veterinary technician at all times. The focus of this chapter is to review the basic concepts of for care of the ventilator patient.

ANESTHESIA

Anesthetizing a patient for mechanical ventilation has two phases: induction and maintenance. A plan for both phases should be made before induction of anesthesia if the patient's condition allows for it. If injectable anesthesia is to be used for maintenance, adequate amounts for the first few hours should be drawn up and constant rate infusion (CRI) dosages calculated ahead of time. There is no optimal protocol for every patient, and the patient's comorbidities should be taken into account when creating a protocol. In general, a balanced approach minimizing cardiovascular adverse effects is recommended.

Before induction of anesthesia the patient should be preoxygenated if at all possible (see Chapter 143). Induction with ketamine, propofol, etomidate, or an opioid (all in combination with a benzodiazepine) may be appropriate. Although it may seem appealing because of the ability to deliver 100% FiO_2, mask induction with inhalant gasses should be avoided.[4]

Any anesthetic agent can be used for short-term ventilation; however, no agent is ideal for long-term ventilation (Table 34-1). If the patient requires ventilation for hypoxemic reasons, avoidance of the inhalant gasses is recommended because they inhibit hypoxic pulmonary vasoconstriction, which may worsen hypoxemia in the patient. As a result, a total intravenous anesthetic technique is typically used, ranging from a sole agent (propofol) to a multimodal approach of two to four agents. The choice of number of agents, and which agents are to be used, generally depends on the comorbidities of the patient as well as hemodynamic stability. A combination of an opioid and a benzodiazepine often can be used in a patient with more severe systemic illness, whereas the addition of either ketamine or

Table 34-1 Anesthetic Agents for Maintenance of the Ventilator Patient

Agent	Pros	Potential Problems
Benzodiazepines	Adjunct to reduce amount of other agent needed Minimal cardiovascular depression	Diazepam is hyperosmolar and may create phlebitis if given peripherally Propylene glycol toxicity as prolonged CRI
Etomidate	Minimal cardiovascular depression	Inhibits cortisol production Propylene glycol toxicity as prolonged CRI
Inhalants	Effective Familiarity with agent	Impair hypoxic pulmonary vasoconstriction Cardiovascular depression Environmental pollution without scavenging system
Ketamine	Useful adjunct Analgesia	Increases intracranial and intraocular pressure Muscle hypertonia
Opioids	Minimal cardiovascular depression Can be reversed with naloxone	Panting Hyperthermia
Dexmedetomidine	Useful adjunct Analgesia	Reduced cardiac output
Propofol	Rapid onset and recovery	Hypotension Lipemia Heinz body anemia in cats
Pentobarbital	Effective Good for intracranial disease	Prolonged recovery Can cause seizures on recovery with prolonged use Not currently available

propofol often is required to maintain an acceptable level of sedation in patients with less severe systemic illness. The addition of dexmedetomidine can be considered as well.

Various total intravenous anesthesia techniques for short-term ventilation have been studied in dogs and cats. A combination of a benzodiazepine (e.g., diazepam or midazolam) with morphine and medetomidine or a combination of a benzodiazepine with fentanyl and propofol has been shown to produce acceptable anesthesia and oxygen delivery to the tissues in dogs.[5] A study evaluating the administration of propofol versus ketamine versus propofol and ketamine (all three protocols also received fentanyl and midazolam) in cats reported that cats receiving propofol, fentanyl, and midazolam had a lower oxygen delivery and more hypotension than cats receiving ketamine, fentanyl, and midazolam.[6] This study documented prolonged recovery times in cats anesthetized for 24 hours with all three protocols (>18 hours to normal walking) and is consistent with the author's experience. Recovery times were statistically longer in the group that received ketamine compared with propofol and propofol with ketamine, although qualitatively there was no difference. Prolonged propofol administration (>24 hours) must be avoided in cats because of the development of Heinz body anemia. If propofol is chosen for maintenance, no more than 6 hours of medication should be kept in a syringe at time and it is recommended to change the administration line every 24 hours to help prevent bacterial contamination.

Whichever protocol is chosen for maintenance, the lowest possible dose should be used to achieve the desired effect. Evaluation of the depth of anesthesia should be performed every hour, with the minimal dosed titrated for immobilization and patient comfort. Adjunctive techniques such as cotton balls in the ears or covering of the eyes with a towel may be helpful to reduce stimulation. If the patient is being ventilated because of an inability to move (e.g., neuromuscular disease or cervical myelopathy), a tracheostomy tube can be considered because this will usually reduce or even remove the need for anesthetic agents. Caution should be exercised in choosing a tracheostomy tube in hypoxemic patients, because their need for sedation is often related to the need for mechanical ventilation to be performed and maintaining immobility, not the presence of an orotracheal tube.

MONITORING

Ventilator patients need intensive monitoring for optimal chances of success in weaning. Ideal monitoring includes continuous electrocardiography, placement of a rectal thermistor for continuous temperature, pulse oximetry, capnography, and serial blood pressure. Auscultation of the chest and a cardiovascular physical examination should be performed every 4 hours to detect abnormalities as early as possible. Blood pressure monitoring may be accomplished by indirect (Doppler or oscillometric) or direct (placement of an arterial catheter) means. The advantage of placing an arterial catheter is that it allows continuous blood pressure monitoring, in addition to ease in obtaining arterial blood gasses. At the author's institution the dorsal pedal artery or coccygeal artery are usually used with success, even in small (<5 kg) dogs. Caution must be exercised in cannulizing the dorsal pedal artery of a cat because they have poor collateral circulation to the distal limb and the risk of necrosis is higher than in dogs. As such it is recommended not to leave an arterial line in the dorsal pedal artery of a cat for longer than 6 to 8 hours.[4]

If an arterial catheter is in place, arterial blood gas analysis should be performed every 4 to 8 hours or more frequently if indicated. If an arterial catheter cannot be placed, then pulse oximetry may be used as a substitute for PaO_2 as an assessment of oxygenation status. The SpO_2/FiO_2 ratio has been used in adult humans with acute lung injury (ALI) or acute respiratory distress syndrome (ARDS) and in children with ALI and found to be an acceptable substitute for the PaO_2/FiO_2 ratio.[7,8] A pilot study in dogs demonstrated moderate correlation of the SpO_2/FiO_2 ratio to the PaO_2/FiO_2 ratio in a heterogeneous population of dogs spontaneously breathing room air.[9] Whether this relationship holds true in mechanically ventilated dogs and cats has yet to be determined. Even if an arterial catheter is placed, continuous pulse oximetry is recommended because it provides continuous feedback and may alert the clinician to a rapid change in oxygenation status. An arterial blood gas should be used to verify any large change in SpO_2 where possible. If indirect blood pressure monitoring is used, it should be monitored every 5 to 60 minutes depending on the hemodynamic stability of the patient.

Ventilator patients may suffer from either hyper- or hypothermia. Patients that develop asynchrony with the ventilator are prone to having elevations in body temperature because of increased heat production from muscular effort. This may be treated by improving ventilator–patient synchrony, using surface cooling methods (e.g., placement of a fan or use of a cold-water spray bottle), or turning off or removing the humidification system. Removal of airway humidification should only be performed for short periods because humidification is key to airway management (see later section). Hypothermia should be treated with circulating warm-water blankets or forced-air warming device or by covering the patient with a blanket to reduce heat loss, depending on the degree of hypothermia.

AIRWAY MANAGEMENT

Endotracheal Tube

Patients undergoing mechanical ventilation need intubation with either an endotracheal (ET) tube or a tracheostomy tube, with the majority of patients having intubation via the oral route (see Chapter 197). Ideally the ET tube should be sterile and have a low-pressure cuff and the intubation process performed with sterile gloves. Whenever the airway is being handled after intubation, hand hygiene should be performed first and examination gloves used. When low-volume, low-pressure (LVLP) tracheal tube cuffs were compared with high-volume, low-pressure cuffs (HVHP), the LVLP group reduced pulmonary aspiration in both a bench top and a group of anesthetized critically ill human patients.[10] This likely was due to the presence of longitudinal folds in the cuff in the HVHP group. The use of low-pressure cuffs is important because cuff pressure greater than 25 cm H_2O has been shown to reduce tracheal blood flow, which can lead to necrosis, and cuff pressures greater than 30 cm H_2O should be avoided.[11] The use of a cuff pressure monitoring device (commercially available or constructed in-house), which can directly measure cuff pressure, is recommended to help prevent tracheal damage.

To help prevent tracheal necrosis, it has been suggested to deflate the cuff and reposition it every 4 hours in veterinary medicine.[4] However, to help prevent VAP, the American Thoracic Society recommends that cuff pressure be maintained at more than 20 cm H_2O.[12] The risk of tracheal necrosis versus the risk of VAP should be weighed in each individual patient. The author recommends the following guidelines: If an HVLP or LVLP ET tube is used and the cuff pressure can be monitored, then the cuff should not be deflated and repositioned, but the cuff pressure should be checked every 4 hours. If a high-volume, high-pressure ET tube is used (e.g., for cats and small dogs) or if cuff pressure cannot be monitored, then the cuff should be deflated and repositioned every 4 hours. Before deflation and repositioning, oral care and suctioning must be performed.

The ET tube should be secured with a nonporous material such as plastic intravenous tubing. Gauze exposed to oral secretions provides a growth medium for bacteria. The ET tube tie should be retied every 4 hours to prevent damage to the lips. The tie used to secure the ET tube should be replaced every 24 hours to help prevent biofilm accumulation.

The decision to change the ET tube must be made on an individual patient basis. Reintubation has been shown to increase the risk of VAP in humans, whereas ET tube occlusion has been reported to occur in up to 14% of animals.[2] Patients with exudative pulmonary secretions and smaller diameter ET tubes put them at risk for occlusion and may benefit from an ET tube change every 24 to 48 hours. Patients being ventilated without significant pulmonary secretions or relatively large diameter ET tubes may only need ET tube changes on an as-needed basis.

Humidification

Patients undergoing long-term ventilation need humidification of the airways. Lack of humidification leads to increased mucus viscosity and inspissation, which can cause ET tube occlusion, tracheal inflammation, and depressed ciliary function. There are two major methods of humidification of the airways: heat and moisture exchangers (HME) and hot water humidifiers. Passive HMEs act as an "artificial nose," working by trapping the heat and moisture of exhaled air in the device and then returning them on the following inspiration. HMEs increase dead space and resistance to airflow. They also have the potential to become obstructed by airway secretions and are often avoided in patients that have copious or tenacious pulmonary secretions. HMEs should be changed every 24 to 48 hours or sooner if they become obstructed. Ventilator waveforms can be evaluated for increased resistance, indicating a partially occluded HME (see Chapter 33). Hot water humidifiers were traditionally considered the gold standard. Potential complications include overheating and condensation of water in the inspiratory limb, which contributes to bacterial colonization of the breathing circuit. The ideal type of humidifier is unknown, with each type having benefits and complications. The decision of which type to use should be made on availability, expected level of secretions, and concerns of increased dead space and resistance to the breathing circuit.

Airway Suctioning

Suctioning of the airway is of key importance to help prevent ET tube occlusion with airway secretions. In the awake patient, coughing helps clear secretions; however, the cough reflex is blunted or absent in the anesthetized patient. Suctioning can be performed by either an open or closed system suction method. It should be performed every 4 hours or more frequently on an as-needed basis.

The ideal catheter should be soft and flexible, have more than one distal opening, be sterile, and occlude no more than 50% of the internal diameter of the ET tube. Before suctioning, the patient should be preoxygenated with 100% oxygen for at least 5 minutes to help prevent hypoxemia during the process. With open suctioning, sterile gloves should be worn and the suction catheter inserted to the end of the ET tube. A second person wearing nonsterile gloves should disconnect the breathing circuit from the tube to facilitate sterile insertion of the catheter. Insertion of the catheter farther than the distal opening of the ET tube risks tracheal inflammation, induction of coughing, or vagal-mediated bradycardia. The process should be quick, with the catheter partially occluding the lumen of the ET tube for no more than 10 to 15 seconds per suctioning. The procedure should be repeated multiple times until secretions are no longer being aspirated. If an open system is used, then sterile saline should be poured into a sterile cup so the suction catheter can be cleansed between suction passes. A new cup is used each time to avoid bacterial contamination of the residual saline container. Closed-system suction catheters are available for use. These systems are kept in place between the breathing circuit and the patient between suctioning events. They have the advantage that the circuit does not have to be opened for suctioning, thereby reducing the risk of contamination. If either an open or closed system is used, the suction canister and tubing used should be replaced every 24 hours to minimize the chance of bacterial colonization.

The addition of saline to the airway to facilitate mucus recovery during suctioning remains controversial. Before suctioning, adding 0.1 to 0.2 ml/kg of 0.9% NaCl can be considered to help mobilize dry secretions. Concerns of saline instillation center around dislodging bacteria from the ET tube and promoting VAP as well as inducing hypoxemia. The benefit may be more effective removal of secretions, which may reduce the likelihood of VAP. In a group of human patients in an oncologic hospital, saline instillation decreased the risk of microbiologically proven ventilator-associated pneumonia.[13]

If the patient has a tracheostomy tube, all of these procedures apply, with the addition of routine care as discussed in Chapter 197. Suctioning either an ET tube or tracheostomy tube carry possible risks. These include iatrogenic hypoxemia, collapse of alveoli as a result of temporary lack of positive end-expiratory pressure, tracheal irritation, bradycardia, and hypotension. The patient should have continuous pulse oximetry during the procedure, and if hypoxemia develops, abort the suctioning process and reconnect the breathing circuit.

ORAL CARE

Patients anesthetized for prolonged periods can develop a significant number of complications involving the oral cavity.[14] These include oral ulceration, ranula formation, and reflux of gastric contents into the oral cavity. Anesthesia inhibits the swallowing reflex, which allows for pooling of secretions in the caudal oral and pharyngeal cavities. Swallowing normally helps prevent the accumulation of bacteria within the oral cavity and prevents desiccation of oral mucous membranes. To help prevent drying of the tongue, it is usually covered in an alternating dilute glycerin-soaked or saline-soaked gauze. Avoid wrapping the tongue circumferentially with gauze because this can lead to ranula formation. A lack of swallowing also allows for bacteria to proliferate and pool in secretions around the endotracheal tube, increasing the risk for VAP. Meticulous oral care focusing on subglottic suctioning and selective oral decontamination has been shown to decrease the incidence of VAP and oral lesions. The importance of oral care cannot be emphasized enough.

Whenever the oral cavity is to be handled, proper hand hygiene, including hand washing and wearing of examination gloves, is recommended. Oral care should be performed every 4 hours. During oral care the pulse oximeter should be repositioned within the oral cavity to help prevent ulceration. The tongue should be uncovered and the underside inspected for development of a ranula. If a ranula is forming, elevating the ET tube to avoid causing pressure on the base of the tongue may be helpful. Care to avoid placement of the tongue over the teeth, as well as a mouth gag, may help prevent ulceration. The entire oral cavity should be inspected for mucosal ulceration and any recorded in both depth and size.

In addition to the care just described, oral care consists of removing the pulse oximeter probe and any mouth gag and cleaning of them with a dilute 0.05% chlorhexidine solution. The entire oral cavity should then be cleansed with a 0.05% chlorhexidine solution. The oral cavity and caudal oropharynx should be gently suctioned, removing remaining chlorhexidine solution and oral secretions and avoiding excess stimulation, which may induce regurgitation. Brushing of the teeth twice daily can reduce the oral bacterial load and may be considered, but no beneficial effect over chlorhexidine antisepsis has been established. The mouth gag and pulse oximeter is then replaced.

EYE CARE

Ventilator patients are at increased risk of exposure keratopathy and microbial keratitis. Because they do not blink, the tear film cannot be spread over the cornea adequately, compromising the health of the eye. Additionally, many patients have lagophthalmos, predisposing them to exposure keratopathy. Despite eye care, up to 25% of children and 37.5% of adults on mechanical ventilation may develop ocular surface disorders.[15,16] The majority of ulceration develops within the first week; however, a significant proportion can develop within 48 hours of initiation of mechanical ventilation.

There are two major methods of providing lubrication to the eye: use of lubricating ointments or moisture chambers. A *moisture chamber* refers to a substance that completely seals off the eye from the environment, such as Doggles, swimmers' goggles, or polyethylene covers. The advantage of this method is that the cornea is protected even if the eye is open. Repetitive lubrication involves regular cleaning of the eye with sterile saline and replacement with a petroleum-based lubricant every 2 hours. A recent meta-analysis of human eye care in the intensive care unit (ICU) showed that use of the moisture chamber was superior in preventing exposure keratopathies compared with lubricating ointments.[17]

Because of the difficulty in obtaining a good seal from a moisture chamber with the various skull structures of dogs and cats, lubricating ointment is still considered the standard of care. Eye care should be performed every 2 hours. The eye should be lavaged with sterile saline and inspected for chemosis, corneal disease, and conjunctivitis. Fluorescein staining should be performed every 24 hours to evaluate for ulcer formation. If no ulceration is present, a petroleum-based lubricant should be reinstilled. If ulceration is present, a broad-spectrum antibiotic ointment should be used every 4 hours. For progressive or deep ulceration, refer to Chapter 154. For some patients with lagophthalmos or exophthalmos, a temporary tarsorrhaphy maybe been needed.

URINARY CARE

Patients undergoing short-term ventilation should have their bladders palpated and expressed every 4 to 6 hours. Voided urine can be collected in a diaper and weighed to track urinary volumes. If long-term ventilation is indicated, the patient may benefit from urinary catheterization. This avoids the repeated pressure and trauma of expressing the bladder and allows for more accurate documentation of urine volumes. Urinary catheterization can also be considered for any animal whose large size prohibits adequate bladder expression.

Urinary catheterization carries the risk of development of bacteriuria either from true urinary tract infection or colonization of the catheter. In dogs the incidence of urinary tract infections associated with indwelling catheterization in nonmyelopathic conditions ranges from 10% to 20%, with length of catheterization being a risk factor.[18,19] The incidence of urinary tract infections in dogs with a thoracolumbar myelopathy was not different with indwelling versus intermittent catheterization or manual expression.[20] Urinary catheter care should be performed every 8 hours as long as an indwelling catheter is in place to minimize the risk of urinary tract infections (see Chapter 208).

GASTROINTESTINAL TRACT

Gastrointestinal complications can occur because of mechanical ventilation, including esophagitis, gastrointestinal bleeding, diarrhea, ileus, constipation, or gastric distention and regurgitation. Splanchnic hypoperfusion plays an important role in the development of many of these complications because of diminished venous return from high levels of PEEP and increased levels of circulating catecholamines or proinflammatory cytokines.[21] The incidence of gastrointestinal bleeding in human patients can be as high as 47%, with clinically significant bleeding in 3.3% of patients ventilated for more than 48 hours.[22] A modifiable risk factor for bleeding identified was a peak inspiratory pressure 30 cm H_2O or greater. Using the minimal ventilator settings needed to provide adequate oxygenation and ventilation may improve gastrointestinal health.

The role of histamine-2 receptor antagonists (H_2RAs) in mechanical ventilation is controversial. The proposed benefit is to reduce stress-related mucosal disease and ulceration, whereas the proposed detriment is a higher rate of gastric colonization with bacteria. A meta-analysis comparing the use of H_2RA versus sucralfate showed no difference in effectiveness in the treatment of overt bleeding, but H_2RA use had higher rates of gastric colonization and VAP.[23] Although there was no difference in mortality identified in human patients, because of the increased incidence of VAP the routine use of H_2RAs cannot be recommended in veterinary patients.

Enteric nutrition in mechanical ventilation carries risks and benefits. It has been shown to decrease the incidence of gastrointestinal bleeding and prevent villous atrophy of the intestinal mucosa that may increase the risk of bacterial translocation. Enteric nutrition may increase the incidence of gastroesophageal reflux and aspiration pneumonia caused by ileus. The risks versus the benefits and the estimated length of ventilation should be considered before deciding to initiate enteric feeding. If enteric feeding is judged to be too risky or enteral feeding is not being tolerated and the expected length of ventilation exceeds a week, then parenteral nutrition can be considered.

Enteral feeding may be delivered via a nasogastric, gastrotomy, or jejunostomy tube. The use of an esophagostomy tube is not recommended for patients on mechanical ventilation. Post-pyloric feeding may be associated with a decreased risk of aspiration pneumonia. Feeding may be accomplished via continuous delivery or by intermittent bolus. The diet can be dyed with food coloring of a color not native to the body for detection of regurgitation during oral care. The role of monitoring of gastric residual volumes in ventilated human patients is controversial. Reignier et al[24] showed that in a group of mechanically ventilated people with early enteral feeding, the absence of gastric residual volume monitoring did not affect the incidence of patients that developed ventilator-associated pneumonia; however, there was an increased incidence of vomiting and regurgitation in that group. The role of gastric residual volume monitoring in mechanically ventilated dogs and cats is unclear at this time.

Ventilated patients may develop either diarrhea or constipation. If diarrhea develops, the perianal region should be kept clean and dry. To evaluate for constipation, the colon should be palpated daily. If constipation is noted, enemas may be needed to evacuate the colon.

RECUMBENT PATIENT CARE

Prolonged recumbency can induce decubital ulcers, tissue necrosis, atelectasis, muscle and ligament contracture, and regional dependent edema.[4] ICU-acquired weakness and critical illness neuromyopathy are also possible sequelae in long-term ventilation in humans but have not been documented in clinical veterinary medicine. ICU-acquired weakness starts to occur within hours and can result in prolonged disability. This condition is due to muscle and nerve dysfunction and can result in inability to wean a patient from the ventilator because of poor respiratory muscle strength. Both corticosteroids and neuromuscular blocking agents have been implicated in the development of this disease, and they should be avoided if possible. The diaphragm can start to atrophy within 18 hours of controlled ventilation; only short periods of intermittent spontaneous ventilation can minimize this dysfunction.[25]

To minimize these complications, patients should be kept well padded at all times and limbs should not be allowed to hang over the edge of the table. With giant breed dogs, ventilation on the floor should be considered if a large enough table is not accessible. Passive range of motion should be performed every 4 hours, including the flexion and extension of every joint in the limbs as distal as the phalanges. If patient conditions permit, a short (i.e., 5-minute), spontaneous breathing trial should be performed daily to "exercise" the respiratory muscles.

After passive range of motion is performed, the position of recumbency should also be changed every 4 hours, alternating between sternal and each lateral position, if the oxygenation status will tolerate it. If lateral recumbency is not possible, then the cranial half of the patient can be kept in sternal recumbency and the hips of the patient moved from right side down to left side down every 2 to 4 hours. Special attention for ulcer formation at the elbows or for development of dermal lesions in the antebrachium is needed if the cranial half of the patient is always in sternal recumbency.

For patients ventilated on a table that tilts, the ideal tilt for the table has yet to be determined. The current recommendation in human medicine is to elevate the torso 30 to 45 degrees. Ventilation with the trachea elevated above horizontal is thought to decrease gastroesophageal reflux, whereas ventilation with the trachea below horizontal may prevent aspiration of oropharyngeal secretions into the trachea. In a porcine model of sternal recumbency, all pigs with the trachea elevated 45 degrees above horizontal developed pneumonia, whereas none of the pigs with the trachea oriented 10 degrees below horizontal did.[26] At this time ventilation with the trachea elevated 45 degrees cannot be recommended in veterinary medicine. It seems reasonable to keep patients in a neutral horizontal position until further research is performed.

APPARATUS CARE

Part of caring for a patient on the ventilator also includes caring for the equipment. The ventilator circuit should be sterilized before use and put together wearing sterile gloves to minimize the chance of nosocomial infections. The ideal length of time for use of a single ventilator circuit has not been established. A meta-analysis showed an increased risk of pneumonia when circuits were changed every 2 days versus every 7 days, and no routine changing of the ventilator circuit did not increase the odds of VAP.[27] Based on this it is safe to not routinely change the ventilator circuit but to change the circuit if gross contamination is noted.

REFERENCES

1. Mellema MS, Haskins SC: Weaning from mechanical ventilation, Clin Tech Small Anim Pract 15:157, 2000.
2. Hopper K, Haskins SC, Kass PH, et al: Indication, management, and outcome of long-term positive-pressure ventilation in dogs and cats: 148 cases (1990-2001), J Am Vet Met Assoc 230:64 2007.
3. Hugonnet S, Uckay I, Pittet D: Staffing level: a determinant of late-onset ventilator-associated pneumonia, Crit Care 11:R80, 2007.
4. Haskins SC, King LG: Positive-pressure ventilation. In King LG, editor: Textbook of respiratory disease in dogs and cats, St Louis, 2004, Saunders.
5. Ethier MR, Mathews KA, Valverde AV, et al: Evaluation of the efficacy and safety for use of two sedation and analgesia protocols to facilitate assisted ventilation of healthy dogs, Am J Vet Res 69:1351, 2008.
6. Boudreau AE, Bersenas AME, Kerr CL, et al: A comparison of 3 anesthetic protocols for 24 hours of mechanical ventilation in cats, J Vet Emerg Crit Care 22:239, 2012.
7. Khemani RG, Thomas NJ, Venkatachalam V, et al: Comparison of SpO_2 to PaO_2 based markers of lung disease severity for children with acute lung injury, Crit Care Med 40:1309, 2012.
8. Rice TW, Wheeler AP, Bernard GR, et al: Comparison of the SpO_2/FiO_2 ratio and the PaO_2/FiO_2 ratio in patients with acute lung injury or ARDS, Chest 132:410, 2007.
9. Calabro JM, Prittie JE, Palma DA: Preliminary evaluation of the utility of comparing SpO_2/FiO_2 and PaO_2/FiO_2 ratios in dogs, J Vet Emerg Crit Care 23:280, 2005.

10. Young PJ, Pakeerathan S, Blunt MC, et al: A low-volume, low-pressure tracheal tube cuff reduces pulmonary aspiration, Crit Care Med 34:632, 2006.
11. Seegobin RD, van Hasselt GL: Endotracheal cuff pressure and tracheal mucosal blood flow: endoscopic study of the effects of four large volume cuffs, Br Med J 288:965, 1984.
12. American Thoracic Society, Infectious Diseases Society of America: Guidelines for the management of adults with hospital-acquired, ventilator-associated and healthcare-associated pneumonia, Am J Respir Crit Care Med 171:388, 2005.
13. Caruso P, Denari SAL, Ruiz S, et al: Saline instillation before tracheal suctioning decreases the incidence of ventilator-associated pneumonia, Crit Care Med 37:32, 2009.
14. Fudge M, Anderson JG, Aldrich J, et al: Oral lesions associated with orotracheal administered mechanical ventilation in critically ill dogs, J Vet Emerg Crit Care 7:79, 1997.
15. Dawson D: Development of a new eye care guideline for critically ill patients, Intensive Crit Care Nurs 21:119, 2005.
16. Germano EM, Mello MJG, Sena DF, et al: Incidence and risk factors for corneal epithelial defects in mechanically ventilated children: Crit Care Med 37:1097, 2009.
17. Rosenberg JB, Eisen LA: Eye care in the intensive care unit: narrative review and meta-analysis, Crit Care Med 36:3151 2008.
18. Smarick SD, Haskins SC, Aldrich J, et al: Incidence of catheter-associated urinary tract infection among dogs in a small animal intensive care unit, J Am Vet Med Assoc 224:1936, 2004.
19. Ogeer-Gyles J, Mathews K, Weese JS, et al: Evaluation of catheter-associated urinary tract infections and multi-drug-resistant Escherichia coli isolate from the urine of dogs with indwelling urinary catheters, J Am Vet Med Assoc 229:1584, 2006.
20. Bubenik L, Hosgood G: Urinary tract infection in dogs with thoracolumbar intervertebral disc herniation and urinary bladder dysfunction managed by manual expression, indwelling catheterization or intermittent catheterization, Vet Surg 37:791, 2008.
21. Mutlu GM, Mutlu EA, Factor P: GI complications in patients receiving mechanical ventilation, Chest 119:1222, 2001.
22. Chu Y, Jiang Y, Meng M, et al: Incidence and risk factors of gastrointestinal bleeding in mechanically ventilated patients, World J Emerg Med 1:32, 2010.
23. Huang J, Cao Y, Liao C, et al: Effect of histamine-2-receptor antagonists versus sucralfate on stress ulcer prophylaxis in mechanically ventilated patients: a meta-analysis of 10 randomized controlled trials, Crit Care 14:R194, 2010.
24. Reignier J, Mercier E, Le Gouge A, et al: Effect of not monitoring residual gastric volume on risk of ventilator-associated pneumonia in adults receiving mechanical ventilation and early enteral feeding, J Am Med Assoc 309:249, 2013.
25. Griffiths RD, Hall JB: Intensive care unit-acquired weakness, Crit Care Med 38:779, 2010.
26. Zanella A, Cressoni M, Epp M, et al: Effects of tracheal orientation on development of ventilator-associated pneumonia: an experimental study, Intensive Care Med 38:677, 2012
27. Han J, Liu Y: Effect of ventilator circuit changes on ventilator-associated pneumonia: a systematic review and meta-analysis, Respir Care 55:467, 2010.

CHAPTER 35
DISCONTINUING MECHANICAL VENTILATION

Kate Hopper, BVSc, PhD, DACVECC

KEY POINTS

- A patient must attain certain physiologic goals before successful weaning from mechanical ventilation.
- After short-term mechanical ventilation (<48 hours), an animal may be rapidly weaned without gradual reductions in ventilator settings.
- Weaning of animals after longer periods of mechanical ventilation involves a process of stepwise reduction in the level of ventilator support and the use of daily spontaneous breathing trials.
- Anesthetic management is a key aspect of successful weaning of the veterinary patient.
- Intensive monitoring is necessary after discontinuing mechanical ventilation. Weaning failures require immediate action to prevent complications and maximize future success.

Mechanical ventilation is a lifesaving intervention, but longer periods of ventilation have been associated with higher rates of morbidity and mortality in human patients.[1] It is clear that mechanical ventilation should be discontinued as soon as the patient is able to breathe adequately on its own. The challenge is accurately predicting when ventilation can be discontinued without putting the patient at risk of harm. The process of discontinuing ventilator support, otherwise known as *weaning,* has been the focus of a great deal of study in human medicine, although little information is available in the veterinary literature. In many patients receiving short-term ventilator support that have rapidly resolving disease processes, discontinuation is simply a matter of disconnecting the patient from the ventilator. Patients receiving mechanical ventilation for longer periods (greater than 2 to 3 days) and those with complex disease processes may require a true weaning process.

A patient must attain certain physiologic goals to be weaned from the ventilator. These include adequate gas exchange without the support of aggressive ventilator settings, an appropriate ventilatory drive, and recovery from significant systemic disease such as cardiovascular instability or organ failure. However, attaining these goals does not guarantee that the patient will be weaned successfully. Prolonged mechanical ventilation (longer than 48 hours) can cause inspiratory muscle weakness that is proportional to the duration of ventilation.[2] In addition, short-term controlled mechanical ventilation can cause decreased diaphragmatic force-generating capacity, also known as *ventilator-induced diaphragmatic dysfunction.*[3] As a result, sudden discontinuation of mechanical ventilation may be poorly tolerated despite adequate gas exchange. There is some

BOX 35-1 *Criteria for Readiness for a Spontaneous Breathing Trial*[5,6,13]

- Improvement in the primary disease process
- PaO_2:FiO_2 ratio > 150-200 with FiO_2 < 0.5
- PEEP ≤ 5 cm H_2O
- Adequate respiratory drive
- Hemodynamic stability
- Absence of major organ failure

FiO_2, Fraction of inspired oxygen (0.21-1.0); *PaO_2*, partial pressure of arterial oxygen (mm Hg); *PEEP*, positive end-expiratory pressure.

suggestion in the current human literature that direct monitoring of respiratory muscle function maybe of benefit in determining readiness to wean.[4] This is likely to be an area of future investigations.

In long-term ventilator patients, the weaning process must force the patient to assume some of the work of breathing to recondition the inspiratory muscles. Further, patients must be monitored closely subsequent to discontinuation of ventilation in case respiratory muscle fatigue develops.

Weaning from mechanical ventilation in human medicine is often protocol driven; the weaning process is started only after specific criteria of readiness are fulfilled, respiratory performance is tested regularly in an effort to predict the likelihood of successful weaning, and management of the ventilator settings during weaning follows preset guidelines. A recent meta-analysis of human studies concluded that protocol-driven weaning might result in shorter duration of ventilation compared with weaning without the use of protocols, but variability between studies made it difficult to make definitive recommendations.[1]

WHEN TO WEAN

Although weaning criteria are poorly defined in veterinary medicine, there is generally a time when the decision is made to significantly reduce the amount of ventilatory support provided. A set of criteria used in human patients to identify readiness to wean can be readily applied to veterinary patients (Box 35-1).[5,6] The original disease process necessitating mechanical ventilation should be stable or improving. The patient needs an adequate respiratory drive and should no longer be dependent on significant ventilator support for adequate gas exchange. Adequate oxygenation, as evidenced by a PaO_2:FiO_2 ratio of at least 150 to 200, is recommended before initiating weaning. A requirement for high inspired oxygen levels (>50%), high peak inspired airway pressures (>25 cm H_2O), and high positive end-expiratory pressure levels (>5 cm H_2O) to maintain oxygenation should preclude any weaning attempts. Weaning is not advised in animals that are hemodynamically unstable or have severe systemic disease such as organ dysfunction. It is recommended that patients are assessed daily for suitability for weaning (the "daily wean screen") using these criteria.[7] It should be noted that in human medicine the ability of a standardized screening process, similar to the one described here, to predict ability to wean decreases over time, and after 10 days of positive pressure ventilation (PPV) it was found to no longer be predictive.[8]

ANESTHETIC CONSIDERATIONS

When a patient is deemed ready for discontinuation of ventilation, disconnection of the machine and often extubation are desired as soon as possible but this requires the patient to be awake. Long-acting anesthetic agents such as pentobarbital are associated with prolonged recoveries (several hours to days). Discontinuing these agents 24 hours or more before weaning may occur is recommended to prevent undesirable prolongation of the anesthetic period. Changing the anesthetic protocol to that of short-acting agents, such as propofol or a benzodiazepine, or both, for the last 1 to 2 days of the ventilation period can provide effective control of anesthetic depth and may smooth out the rough recovery associated with prolonged infusions of agents such as ketamine or pentobarbital. Reversible drugs such as fentanyl and dexmedetomidine can be beneficial because they provide analgesia and contribute to a balanced anesthetic protocol but may be reversed during the weaning process as necessary. (See Chapter 34 for further discussion of anesthetic choices.)

Cats have extremely prolonged recovery times after long periods of injectable anesthesia, and this must be considered when managing feline patients on the ventilator.[9] Management strategies include reducing drug doses early based on predictions of when weaning will be possible and continuing mechanical ventilation until anesthetic recovery is achieved, even though the primary disease process may be resolved.

In human patients, spontaneous breathing trials (SBTs), described later in this chapter, are usually performed in awake patients, not under the influence of sedatives.[10] This is not feasible in most veterinary patients that require sedation or general anesthesia to maintain endotracheal intubation, control anxiety, and prevent excess mobility. This may be a limitation in translation of human ventilator weaning guidelines to veterinary patients. However, it is important to maximally reduce anesthetic depth when SBTs are performed.

WEANING PREDICTION

In human medicine many indexes have been evaluated as potential predictors of weaning success. The rapid shallow breathing index (f/V_T) has been shown to have some correlation with successful weaning in adults. It is calculated as the ratio of respiratory rate (f) and tidal volume (V_T). Those patients who develop increased rapid shallow breathing during a spontaneous breathing trial (marked by a higher f/V_T ratio) are more likely to fail the weaning trial. A ratio of less than 100 is used in human medicine to identify patients that can be weaned.[11] Unfortunately, even this ratio has not been a consistently reliable predictor of weaning outcome.[12,13] In veterinary medicine this ratio may be difficult to adapt to our patients given the variability in normal respiratory rates, but it is possible that a fast, shallow breathing pattern during an SBT may be a poor prognostic indicator. Measures of physiologic dead space (V_D/V_T) may be of some use in predicting successful weaning. Pediatric patients with a lower V_D/V_T measurement (≤0.5) were more likely to be extubated successfully than patients with higher V_D/V_T measurements (>0.65).[14] Overall no single index of weaning performs adequately enough to be relied on alone.

In veterinary medicine, no predictive indexes of weaning have been evaluated. Readiness to wean remains a clinical judgment. A retrospective study of brachycephalic dogs receiving PPV found that dogs with a higher PaO_2:FiO_2 ratio were more likely to be weaned compared with animals with lower PaO_2:FiO_2 ratios.[15] The interested reader is referred to MacIntyre (2012)[16] for further discussion of weaning prediction.

None of the proposed weaning predictors have been shown to perform adequately enough to be used alone for clinical decision making.[16] Currently, evaluation of physiologic parameters (Box 35-2) and clinical judgment of a patient during an SBT is recommended for assessment for readiness to wean in human patients.[7,16]

BOX 35-2 *Criteria for Failure of a Spontaneous Breathing Trial*

- Tachypnea (RR >50)
- $PaO_2 < 60$ mm Hg or $SpO_2 < 90\%$
- $PaCO_2 > 55$ mm Hg or $PvCO_2 > 60$ mm Hg or $ETCO_2 > 50$ mm Hg
- Tidal volume < 7 ml/kg
- Tachycardia
- Hypertension
- Hyperthermia or increase in temperature of > 1° C
- Anxiety
- Clinical judgment

$ETCO_2$, End-tidal carbon dioxide; *PaO_2,* partial pressure of arterial oxygen; *$PaCO_2$,* partial pressure of arterial carbon dioxide; *$PvCO_2$,* partial pressure of venous carbon dioxide; *RR,* respiratory rate; *SpO_2,* oxygen saturation.

WEANING A PATIENT FROM MECHANICAL VENTILATION

The process of weaning involves a reduction in the work of breathing performed by the machine with a proportional increase in the work performed by the patient. In veterinary medicine this sometimes is achieved with assist-control ventilation modes (such as volume assist control or pressure assist control) in which the magnitude of the ventilator settings is decreased. However, this approach is not recommended in patients receiving long-term ventilation. Because every breath in assist-control ventilation is generated by the machine, this approach does not increase the patient's work of breathing adequately.

The three main weaning techniques are SBT, pressure support ventilation (PSV), and synchronized intermittent mandatory ventilation (SIMV).[17]

Spontaneous Breathing Trials

An SBT involves removing most or all ventilator support and monitoring the patient's ability to breathe spontaneously. This can be achieved by disconnecting the animal from the machine and allowing it to breathe an enriched oxygen source (usually with an FiO_2 similar to or above the level the patient was receiving while ventilated) via a breathing circuit (such as a Bain circuit). An alternative approach is to leave the patient connected to the ventilator and switch to a low level (2 to 5 cm H_2O) of continuous positive airway pressure (CPAP). The advantage of using CPAP is that all monitoring and ventilator alarms can remain attached and if the patient fails the SBT, ventilatory support can be reestablished rapidly. Spontaneous breathing through the circuit and the ventilator machine itself increases the work of breathing compared with spontaneous breathing when disconnected from the circuit; a low level of CPAP may compensate for this effect and prevent unnecessary weaning failures.[18] Additionally, CPAP reduces the occurrence of atelectasis, which could also reduce the possibility of successful weaning. Atelectasis is likely in sedated patients, especially those with low chest wall compliance such as the obese patient.

The concept behind SBTs is to use them as training exercises once the patient is deemed sufficiently stable; there may be no expectation that the patient will be weaned with the initial trial. In human medicine it is commonly recommended to perform a 30- to 120-minute SBT daily from the time the patient attains adequate physiologic goals (see Box 35-1). SBTs may be a superior method of weaning from mechanical ventilation compared with PSV or SIMV in human patients.[16,19] In veterinary medicine, it is more common to perform an SBT when the patient is considered ready to be removed completely from ventilator support. Evidence from the human literatures suggests that daily SBTs to improve respiratory muscle strength as a prelude to successful weaning could be of benefit to many long-term ventilated small animal patients.

Pressure Support Ventilation

PSV is a pressure-limited spontaneous breathing mode; the breath is triggered and terminated by the patient. As such, it can be used only in patients with a normal respiratory drive. The inspiration is augmented by additional inspiratory pressure as preset by the operator, but the patient controls the respiratory rate, inspiratory flow, and tidal volume of each breath. The level of pressure support can be decreased gradually as the patient improves (see Chapter 31). When the patient is stable on a low level of pressure support (i.e., <5 cm H_2O), discontinuation of ventilation can be considered. This discontinuation essentially involves an SBT. If the patient fails the SBT, it is returned to PSV at the previous or higher settings as required.

Synchronized Intermittent Mandatory Ventilation

SIMV is another approach to reduce ventilator support gradually. During SIMV there are both mandatory and spontaneous breaths (see Chapter 31). The mandatory breaths are synchronized with the patient's inspiratory efforts, and the tidal volume of the mandatory breaths is generated totally by the ventilator (controlled ventilation). Between mandatory breaths the patient can breathe spontaneously (with or without PSV). Weaning generally is achieved by a gradual reduction in the mandatory breath rate, which demands a progressive increase in the respiratory work performed by the patient. When the patient can maintain adequate oxygenation and ventilation with minimal machine support, an SBT is performed.

If the patient fails the SBT, SIMV is resumed. Patients may require a higher level of machine support than previously needed while recovering from any deleterious effects of the SBT. When first introduced, SIMV was thought to reduce patient–ventilator asynchrony, reduce respiratory muscle fatigue, and expedite weaning. There is now evidence that SIMV may worsen respiratory muscle fatigue. Two well-conducted human trials found SIMV to be the least effective method of ventilator weaning.[18,19] Because no such trial has been performed in veterinary medicine, the role of SIMV for weaning small animal patients is unknown.

In summary, the weaning process for patients after longer periods of mechanical ventilation is generally a process of stepwise reduction in the level of ventilator support (using SIMV or PSV) and the initiation of daily SBTs once the animal meets the necessary criteria (see Box 35-1). Waiting to perform SBTs until the animal is ready to be completely removed from mechanical ventilation may delay successful weaning.

Tracheostomy and Weaning

There is ongoing discussion in the human literature regarding the role of tracheostomy in the long-term ventilator patient, commonly defined as longer than 3 days' duration. Potential benefits may include improved oral care, more effective airway suctioning, and reduced work of breathing (because of reduced dead space and resistance).[20] Other potential advantages in human patients include less laryngeal damage (not a problem recognized in small animal patients) and reduced sedation requirements. However, it is unlikely that tracheostomized animals will tolerate immobility and positive pressure ventilation without anesthetic agents. One exception may be patients with neurologic or neuromuscular diseases causing immobilility and respiratory paralysis; in these patients a tracheostomy tube may allow reduction or even complete withdrawal of anesthetic and sedative agents.

Human studies evaluating the impact of a tracheostomy on ventilator weaning and length of intensive care unit (ICU) stay have yet to reach a consensus.[20-23] A meta-analysis concluded that tracheostomy may shorten the duration of PPV.[21] The role of tracheostomy in veterinary patients receiving PPV is yet to be defined. Based on preliminary research and logical reasoning, a tracheostomy should be considered before weaning animals with upper airway disease (e.g., brachycephalic dogs).[15] The risk/benefit ratio of tracheostomy in neurologically normal animals with pulmonary disease but no evidence of upper airway disease must be determined on a case by case basis. Animals with tracheostomies are prone to complications such as circuit disconnections, increased tracheal secretions, and gas distention of the stomach. The presence of a tracheostomy may delay discharge from the hospital and will increase client costs. Clinicians must consider all these issues when determining how best to manage the airway of long-term ventilator patients.

MONITORING

Because it is impossible to predict how successful a given weaning attempt (SBT) will be, it is vital that patients are monitored closely to rapidly identify weaning failure and reinstate ventilatory support. Monitoring requires that a dedicated caregiver observe the patient for tachypnea, tachycardia, anxiety, or abnormal respiratory efforts such as paradoxical abdominal-thoracic movements and nasal flaring. In addition, oxygenation status ideally is monitored by continuous pulse oximetry and intermittent arterial blood gas measurements. Ventilatory status can be determined with arterial or venous blood gas measurements and continuous capnometry (see Chapters 186 and 190). A continuous electrocardiogram, for heart rate evaluation, and arterial blood pressure measurement are also recommended (see Chapter 183). Temperature monitoring is important because hyperthermia can occur as a consequence of increased respiratory effort and tends to further exacerbate any respiratory difficulties. Conducting weaning attempts with the patient still connected to the ventilator using CPAP allows monitoring of respiratory parameters such as minute volume and airway pressure.

FAILURE TO WEAN

Failure of a weaning attempt is identified by deterioration in certain physiologic parameters (see Box 35-2). Significant hypoxemia or hypercapnia is an obvious indication for reinstatement of ventilatory support. Tachycardia, hypertension, and tachypnea are all ominous signs and suggest that the patient cannot be weaned during that attempt. Significant anxiety or abnormal respiratory efforts are also indications to restore ventilatory support.[5,6] There is some clinical judgment involved in evaluating a weaning trial; strictly adhering to criteria such as those given in Box 35-2 may not always be appropriate (e.g., patients with severe anxiety, pain, or dysphoria may display similar signs). One author stresses the importance of preventing patient exhaustion during weaning trials because respiratory muscle fatigue is believed to delay successful weaning.[6]

Most commonly, unsuccessful weaning is a result of incomplete resolution of the underlying disease process, although a ventilator-associated complication or new disease process can develop.

EXTUBATION

Extubation is performed subsequent to a successful SBT once adequate recovery from anesthesia has occurred and the patient is actively swallowing. In patients ventilated via a temporary tracheostomy tube, it maybe prudent to leave the tube in place for 24 hours or more in case the patient relapses and requires reinstitution of ventilatory support.

PROGNOSIS

Prognosis for successful weaning from mechanical ventilation depends largely on the primary disease process. Human and veterinary clinical studies have repeatedly reported lower weaning rates for patients requiring ventilation for pulmonary parenchymal disease (inability to oxygenate) compared with patients with neuromuscular disease processes (inability to ventilate). One retrospective study of 34 dogs and 7 cats with heterogeneous lung disease reported an overall survival to hospital discharge rate of 20% compared with 57% for animals with neuromuscular disease.[24] In a retrospective study of 148 dogs and cats receiving long-term mechanical ventilation (>24 hours), 36% of cases with lung disease were weaned and 22% survived to hospital discharge. In comparison, 50% of the animals with hypoventilation were weaned and 39% survived to hospital discharge.[25] These statistics are similar to those reported in human medicine. A retrospective study of human intensive care patients treated longer than 24 hours with PPV reported a survival to discharge (from the intensive care unit) rate of 29.3% in the group with oxygenation impairment and 57.8% in the group with ventilatory insufficiency.[26]

These weaning and survival numbers may be somewhat misleading because outcome varies widely with the underlying disease process. For example, a group of dogs with aspiration pneumonia had a 50% weaning rate in one study, whereas only 8% of dogs with acute respiratory distress syndrome were weaned.[25]

REFERENCES

1. Blackwood B, Alderdice F, Burns K, et al: Use of weaning protocols for reducing duration of mechanical ventilation in critically ill adult patients, Cochrane systematic review and meta-analysis, BMJ 342:c7237, 2011.
2. Chang AT, Boots RJ, Brown MG, et al: Reduced inspiratory muscle endurance following successful weaning from prolonged mechanical ventilation, Chest 128:553, 2005.
3. Decramer M, Gayan-Ramirez G: Ventilator-induced diaphragmatic dysfunction: towards a better treatment? Am J Respir Crit Care Med 170:1141, 2004.
4. Doorduin J, van Hess HWH, van der Hoeven JG, Heunks LMA: Monitoring of the respiratory muscles in the critically ill, Am J Respir Crit Care Med 187:20, 2013.
5. MacIntyre NR, Branson RD: Mechanical ventilation, ed 2, Philadelphia, 2009, Saunders.
6. Hess DR, Kacmarek RM: Essentials of mechanical ventilation, ed 2, New York, 2002, McGraw-Hill.
7. Ely EW, Baker AM, Evans GW, Haponik EF. The prognostic significance of passing a daily screen of weaning parameters, Intensive Care Med 25:581, 1999.
8. Ely EW, Baker AM, Dunagan DP, et al: Effect on the duration of mechanical ventilation of identifying patients capable of breathing spontaneously, N Engl J Med 335:1864, 1996.
9. Boudreau AE, Bersensas AME, Kerr CL, et al: A comparison of 3 anesthetic protocols for 24 hours of mechanical ventilation in cats, J Vet Emerg and Crit Care 22:239, 2012.
10. MacIntyre NR, Cook DJ, Ely EW, et al: Evidence based guidelines for weaning and discontinuing ventilator support: a collective task force facilitated by the American College of Chest Physicians; the American Association for Respiratory Care; and the American College of Critical Care Medicine, Chest 120:375S, 2001.
11. Yang KL, Tobin MJ: A prospective study of indexes predicting the outcome of trials of weaning from mechanical ventilation, N Engl J Med 324:1445, 1991.

12. Epstein SK: Etiology of extubation failure and the predictive value of the rapid shallow breathing index, Am J Respir Crit Care Med 152:545, 1995.
13. Tanios MA, Nevins MI, Hendra KP, et al: A randomized controlled trial of the role of weaning predictors in clinical decision making, Crit Care Med 34:2530, 2006.
14. Hubble CL, Gentile MA, Tripp DS et al: Dead space-to-tidal volume ratio predicts successful extubation in infants and children, Crit Care Med 28:2034, 2000.
15. Hoareau GL, Mellema MS, Silverstein DC: Indication, management and outcome of brachycephalic dogs requiring mechanical ventilation, J Vet Emerg Crit Care 21:226, 2011.
16. MacIntyre NR: Evidence-based assessments in ventilator discontinuation process, Respir Care 57:1611, 2012.
17. Tobin MJ: Advances in mechanical ventilation, N Engl J Med 344:1986, 2001.
18. Brochard L, Rua F, Lorino H, et al: Inspiratory pressure support compensates for the additional work of breathing caused by the endotracheal tube, Anesthesiology 75:739, 1991.
19. Esteban A, Frutos F, Tobin MJ, et al: A comparison of four methods of weaning patients from mechanical ventilation, N Engl J Med 332:345, 1995.
20. Combes A, Luyt CE, Nieszkowska A, et al: Is tracheostomy associated with better outcomes for patients requiring long-term mechanical ventilation? Crit Care Med 35:802, 2007.
21. Griffiths J, Barber VS, Morgan L, Young JD: Systematic review and meta-analysis of studies of the timing of tracheostomy in adult patients undergoing artificial ventilation, BMJ 330:1243, 2005.
22. Clec'h C, Alberti C, Vincent F, et al: Tracheostomy does not improve the outcome of patients requiring prolonged mechanical ventilation: a propensity analysis, Crit Care Med 35:132, 2007.
23. Arabi YM, Alhashemi JA, Tamim HM, et al: The impact of time to tracheostomy on mechanical ventilation duration, length of stay and mortality in intensive care unit patients, J Crit Care 24:435, 2009.
24. King LG, Hendricks JC: Use of positive-pressure ventilation in dogs and cats: 41 cases (1990-1992), J Am Vet Med Assoc 204:1045, 1994.
25. Hopper K, Haskins SC, Kass PH, et al: Indications, management, and outcome of long-term positive-pressure ventilation in dogs and cats: 148 cases (1990-2001), J Am Vet Med Assoc 230:64, 2007.
26. Pesau B, Falger S, Berger E, et al: Influence of age on outcome of mechanically ventilated patients in an intensive care unit, Crit Care Med 20:489, 1992.

CHAPTER 36
VENTILATOR-INDUCED LUNG INJURY

Lisa Smart, BVSc, DACVECC

KEY POINTS

- The majority of ventilator-induced lung injury in experimental models is related to high end-inspiratory volume causing stretch injury.
- A second contributing factor is low end-expiratory volume, which can cause epithelial shear injury.
- Ventilator-associated lung injury can be a significant contributor to morbidity and mortality in patients on mechanical ventilation.
- Strategies to prevent ventilator-associated lung injury may decrease the duration of mechanical ventilation required and improve patient outcomes.

DEFINITIONS

For the purposes of this chapter the following definitions will be used. It is important to note that there is no consensus on the definition of these terms in the current literature and they are generally considered exchangeable.

Ventilator-induced lung injury (VILI): injury to the lung caused by mechanical ventilation in experimental models

Ventilator-associated lung injury: worsening of pulmonary function, or presence of lesions similar to acute respiratory distress syndrome, in clinical patients that is thought to be associated with the use of mechanical ventilation, with or without underlying lung disease

INTRODUCTION

Most criticalists will passionately debate that "putting a patient on the ventilator" is not a death sentence. But it is well documented that positive pressure ventilation (PPV) can cause significant pathology in the lung and can worsen lung dysfunction already present. Much research in the area, experimentally in animal models and clinically in people, has led to strategies designed to limit the amount of damage caused directly, or indirectly, by the ventilator. This chapter serves to review the pathophysiology and the clinical relevance of VILI and give an introduction to preventative measures. This chapter does not review effects of PPV on other organ systems, such as the cardiovascular system or neuroendocrine system, or other complications related to PPV such as ventilator-associated pneumonia (see Chapter 37).

EVIDENCE FROM EXPERIMENTAL MODELS

Ventilator-induced lung injury encompasses any pathologic lung condition associated with using positive pressure to create volume change within the lung. The term *volutrauma* has been used historically to describe injury associated with high-volume ventilation, and the term *barotrauma* has been used to describe extra-alveolar air related to high-pressure ventilation. In reality, VILI encompasses both these concepts, though as discussed later, high-volume ventilation causing stretch injury is likely more relevant.

Much of what is known about the pathophysiology of VILI is based on experimental animal models because there is inherent difficulty with relating the use of a ventilator in clinical patients with pathology arising in the lung. There is variation among the species in regards to their response to PPV, with rats developing VILI much more rapidly, within the hour, compared with larger animals.[1] In dog, sheep, and pig models it takes hours to days for moderate to severe VILI to develop.[2-4] Although there are no defined cutoffs for the point at which either pressure and volume creates injury, pathologic change tends to occur across species above peak inspiratory pressures of 30 cm H_2O or 40 ml/kg of tidal volume in experimental models.[2-6] In injured lungs it takes much less change in volume or pressure to exacerbate the injury already present[7,8] and VILI in combination with the original injury may have a synergistic effect in creating further damage.[9]

Stretch Injury

It appears that high volume is more injurious than high pressure, without a large increase in volume.[4,6,10,11] In one study, VILI was created in rats by high-volume/negative pressure ventilation, using an iron lung, but not with high-pressure/normal volume ventilation, via chest wall restriction.[10] Despite this, some positive pressure causes mild injury compared with negative pressure ventilation.[12] It has also been shown that even "normal" tidal volumes (7 ml/kg) in rats can be deleterious if combined with high positive end-expiratory pressure (PEEP), increasing functional residual capacity (FRC) and creating a high end-inspiratory volume.[13] These studies support the notion that an important component of VILI, and perhaps the most important, is stretch injury caused by high end-inspiratory volume.

Shear Injury

Repetitive opening and closing of small airways may cause shear injury and also contribute to VILI. This is also termed cyclic recruitment-derecruitment injury or atelectrauma. In the normal lung, inflated with physiologic tidal volume, it appears that inflation is mostly achieved by expansion of noncartilaginous airways/ducts and possibly additional alveoli "popping" open.[11,14-16] Alveoli size itself appears to change little, from start to end of inspiration, and, initially, small airways with functional surfactant seem tolerant of opening and closing. In injured lungs, alveoli become progressively unstable, changing shape during inflation and completely collapsing at the end of expiration.[11,16] Positive pressure ventilation, especially with high volume, shows a similar pattern in alveolar instability over time,[11] which may contribute to epithelial shear injury. Also, surface tension is increased as surfactant is inactivated or decreased by the effects of VILI,[2,17] which may explain why PPV can cause mild changes in normal lungs such as mildly decreased compliance, lower FRC, and progressive atelectasis.[12] Atelectasis may contribute to shear injury, as well as cause regional overdistention and associated stretch injury. These effects are even more pronounced in an open chest, because the lungs are able to completely collapse at the end of expiration as a result of lack of tethering to the chest wall.[18] Alveolar and airway flooding caused by development of increased vascular and epithelial permeability may worsen shear injury by washing out surfactant. The application of PEEP can mitigate, or even ameliorate, some of these problems.

Biotrauma

The effects of VILI are not just limited to the lung. Increased levels of circulating cytokines caused by VILI[19-23] may promote multiple organ dysfunction, and increased inflammatory cytokines worsening VILI in a circular fashion has been implicated as part of the pathophysiology of VILI.[9] This "two-hit" theory has also been described as "biotrauma," exacerbating the effects of "volutrauma" and "atelectrauma" described earlier. Another effect of PPV includes possibly increasing the risk of infection within the lung because it has been shown that PPV decreases mucociliary function in the trachea[24] and can help to disseminate bacteria within the lung and systemically.[25,26]

Histopathology

The histopathologic changes associated with VILI are hard to distinguish from changes associated with acute lung injury (ALI) or acute respiratory distress syndrome (ARDS) (see Chapter 24). These include decreased integrity of small airway epithelial cells, destruction of type 1 alveolar epithelial cells, alveolar and airway flooding, hyaline membrane formation, interstitial edema, and infiltration of inflammatory cells.[1] Lesions usually have an uneven distribution but tend to be worse in the dependent lung, likely because of worsened airway flooding and shear injury. However, experimentally in dogs this distribution of lesions disappears with prone, or sternally recumbent, positioning.[27]

Pneumothorax

Pneumothorax may also occur as a consequence of VILI and is commonly cited as caused by barotrauma, excessive pressure causing extra-alveolar air leaks, but is likely a combination of stretch injury and compromised lung integrity, with little relationship to the level of mean airway pressure. The occurrence of pneumothorax was one of the first indicators in clinical medicine that PPV could cause damage[28] and is one of the more extreme consequences of VILI. Evidence of extra-alveolar air or pneumothorax does not feature prominently in experimental studies; most of the damage is much more subtle. Pneumothorax is usually restricted to clinical patients with underlying lung pathology, as discussed later in the Clinical Relevance section of this chapter.

Oxygen Toxicity

Although oxygen toxicity is a separate entity from PPV, patients receiving PPV are invariably on supra-atmospheric levels of oxygen supplementation, up to 100% inspired oxygen concentration (FiO_2) (see Chapter 14). This may have an additive effect to the injury caused by VILI, especially if a high oxygen concentration is delivered for an extended period. Inspired oxygen concentration of 100%, in the short term, can cause absorption atelectasis and decrease oxygen diffusion capacity.[29] Beyond 24 hours, FiO_2 between 50% and 100% promotes the production of reactive oxygen and nitrogen species[30,31] and has been shown to cause pathologic change similar to ARDS and VILI, including interstitial edema, hyaline membrane formation, damage to the alveolar membrane, altered mucociliary function, and fibroproliferation.[29,30] The damage appears to be correlated to the level of FiO_2 and the length of time that oxygen was administered. Therefore, PPV needs to be a delicate balance among limiting volume change within the lung, applying appropriate PEEP, and limiting FiO_2 to whatever level the patient can tolerate.

CLINICAL RELEVANCE

Because of the growing evidence from experimental studies that high-volume/low-PEEP ventilation can cause harm and worsen lung injury already present, focus has shifted to the question of whether or not clinically acceptable forms of PPV can also cause harm in people. In the last decade, several studies have found evidence of an association between higher tidal volumes and development of ALI or respiratory failure in people.[32-36] Within the same time frame, various strategies for lung-protective ventilation have been developed, centering on volume limitation and the use of PEEP.

Volume limitation in patients with ALI and ARDS has shown the most dramatic results in outcome, with the landmark ARDSnet study showing a decrease in mortality when 6 ml/kg tidal volume was used versus 12 ml/kg.[37] The group receiving lower tidal volumes also, incidentally, received slightly higher PEEP and inspired oxygen concentration. Other studies focusing on volume limitation combined with PEEP strategies have shown minimal to no effects on mortality,[38,39] although some showed promise in regard to improving lung function, reducing days on the ventilator, and reducing organ failure.[40,41] Application of these strategies in people have also been associated with lower inflammatory cytokine production.[37,42-44]

More recently it has been shown that the benefits of volume limitation and higher PEEP may be conferred to people without ALI/ARDS at the start of ventilation. Two meta-analyses, one including people receiving primarily short-term intraoperative PPV[45] and a broader meta-analysis including people without ARDS receiving PPV,[46] both showed a decrease in lung injury development and lower incidence of pulmonary infection in the groups receiving lower tidal volume and higher PEEP.

There is little evidence in veterinary medicine that high-volume/low-PEEP ventilation is detrimental to clinical patients, specifically dogs and cats, or that lung-protective ventilation strategies affect outcome. There are some observational studies reporting the use of PPV for greater than 24 hours in dogs and cats[47-53]; use of tidal volume greater than 10 ml/kg appears common. One study included 14 dogs with cervical spinal disorders that had relatively normal lung function before PPV and reported two dogs euthanatized because of multiple organ dysfunction, including lung failure.[49] This study reported a mean tidal volume of 18 ± 5 ml/kg without a reference to PEEP. The incidence of pneumothorax, based on five different case series, varied from 0% to 28%,[48-52] with the largest cohort reporting an incidence of 7%,[48] which is fairly similar to the ARDSnet study.[37] The highest of these (28%), a case series of cats receiving PPV, did not find an association between peak inspiratory pressure above 25 cm H_2O, or presence of pulmonary parenchymal disease, and pneumothorax.[50] The mean tidal volume reported in this study was 23.7 ± 8.6 ml/kg, but an association between tidal volume and pneumothorax was not investigated. It is unknown whether any of the complications reported in these observational studies, including worsening lung function and pneumothorax, were associated with the ventilation strategy chosen. However, it is likely given the evidence from experimental data and clinical evidence from human medicine that lung-protective strategies will begin to surface in the veterinary medical literature.

PREVENTION

Conventional Mechanical Ventilation Strategies

See Box 36-1 for a summary of strategies for conventional mechanical ventilation.

BOX 36-1 *Preventative Strategies for Ventilator-Associated Lung Injury*

- Limit tidal volume to 6 to 10 ml/kg.
- Apply positive end-expiratory pressure (PEEP) at a minimum of 5 cm H_2O.
- Limit peak inspiratory pressure (PIP) to 30 cm H_2O.
  - Use subjective analysis of the PV loop to guide PEEP and PIP settings.
  - Avoid patient–ventilator asynchrony.
  - Consider recruitment maneuvers.
  - Maintain dogs in sternal recumbency most of the time.
  - Limit interstitial edema.
  - Allow permissive hypercapnia.
  - Allow permissive hypoxemia.

PV, Pressure-volume.

Low tidal volume

There is strong evidence for limiting tidal volume to 6 to 10 ml/kg, staying to the lower end of this range when the lungs are already compromised. Inflammation in the lung causes heterogeneous changes throughout, with regions of poorer compliance and atelectasis, which means more compliant regions become overdistended. Because it is difficult to know in any one patient which portions of the lung are being overdistended and which are not, it is prudent to limit tidal volume as much as possible. However, using low tidal volume also increases the risk of perpetuating atelectasis and creating further shear injury; therefore, application of PEEP is vital.

Positive end-expiratory pressure

It has been well established that some PEEP is better than no PEEP, or zero end-expiratory pressure; however, the minimum amount of PEEP in order to reduce VILI has not been established. Common levels of PEEP considered adequate in human medicine are in the range of 5 to 10 cm H_2O. Increasing PEEP above this level increases the risk of stretch injury, because total end-inspiratory volume increases; therefore, peak inspiratory pressure or plateau pressure needs to be monitored closely.

Limitation of plateau pressure

The combination of high PEEP, auto-PEEP (PEEP created by increased outflow resistance during expiration, asynchrony, or incomplete expiration), and tidal volume can lead to high end-inspiratory volume, which may be indicated by high plateau pressure. Peak inspiratory pressure may also be used as a surrogate for plateau pressure, and it is prudent to limit this pressure to less than 30 cm H_2O.

Using the Pressure-Volume Loop to Guide Settings

The pressure-volume (PV) loop often has two flatter portions, one at the start of inspiration and one at the end, called the lower inflection point (LIP) and the upper inflection point (UIP) (Figure 36-1). The LIP is the point at which compliance improves and there is much greater change in volume with change in pressure. This is thought to be due to overcoming the "opening" pressure of small airways and

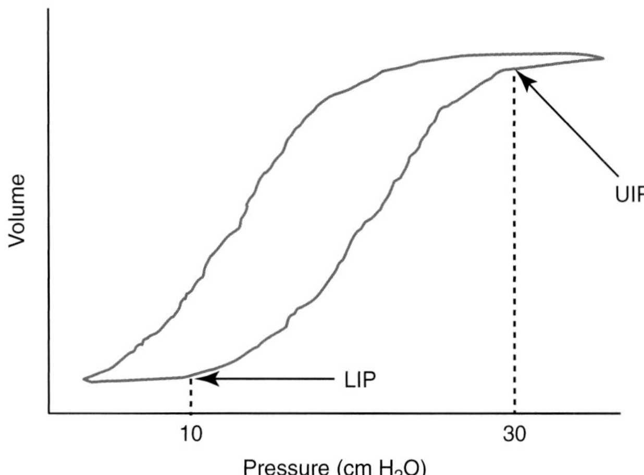

FIGURE 36-1 Subjectively interpreting a dynamic pressure-volume curve to identify the inflation pressure at which compliance increases (lower inflection point) and the point at which no further gain in volume is achieved (upper inflection point). Limiting peak or plateau pressure below the UIP may reduce the risk of stretch injury to the lung.

the point of lung recruitment. Changing the PEEP in order to stay above this level may reduce the degree of "opening-and-closing" injury or shear injury to small airways. The UIP is the point at which compliance is decreased dramatically so that there is little change in volume with increases in pressure. This is thought to be the point at which lung units become overdistended and may be at risk of high-volume injury; therefore, peak inspiratory pressure should be reduced to below this point. Correct measurement of the LIP and UIP is achieved by a static pressure-volume (PV) curve,[54] whereby a constant slow flow is injected and the plateau pressure is measured at set inflation volumes (see Figure 36-1). However, in order to achieve an accurate static pressure-volume curve, not only do you need the equipment but also a deeply anesthetized or paralyzed, stable patient that has respiratory efforts that are synchronous with the ventilator, as well as the ability to measure plateau pressure using esophageal pressure monitoring. The LIP and UIP can then be defined by various mathematical models.[54] Because of the technical difficulties of creating an accurate static PV curve, some clinicians use a subjective visual evaluation of the dynamic PV loop to estimate these points, as shown in Figure 36-1, and either raise PEEP or lower inspiratory pressure accordingly. However, chest wall compliance, patient–ventilator asynchrony, and even the particular mode of ventilation can interfere with inflection points, and this method may not be accurate or beneficial to the patient. Despite these limitations, small increases in PEEP and a reduction in inspiratory pressure are likely to benefit the patient rather than cause harm, depending on the individual. Use of the PV curve to guide ventilator settings in human medicine is controversial, and there is some debate still regarding what the LIP and UIP actually represent.

Avoid Patient–Ventilator Asynchrony

Patient–ventilator asynchrony can increase airway pressure or create auto-PEEP, depending on the type of asynchrony. This can contribute to regional overdistention and should be avoided if possible (see Chapter 31).

Other Strategies

The use of recruitment maneuvers, whereby the inspiratory pressure, or volume, and PEEP are increased for a short period (less than 1 minute), may recruit more lung that was previously atelectatic and improve oxygenation. However, these strategies can also cause overdistention and should only be used if absolutely necessary. The use of recruitment maneuvers is currently under debate in human medicine. See Chapter 31 for further discussion of recruitment maneuvers.

Other strategies to avoid regional atelectasis include maintaining the patient in sternal recumbency while periodically alternating the positioning of the pelvic limbs and limiting interstitial edema by keeping the patient with pulmonary disease on the "dry" side if the patient's cardiovascular system can tolerate it.

Permissive hypercapnia and permissive hypoxemia should also be considered in order to allow lower ventilator settings. Acid-base status needs to be monitored closely in regard to permissive hypercapnia. Regarding permissive hypoxemia, arterial hemoglobin saturation of 88% to 90% is often accepted as long as the physical examination, serum lactate concentration, and central venous saturation do not indicate a tissue oxygen deficit.

Advanced Pulmonary Support Techniques

Because of the risk of VILI using conventional mechanical ventilation in people with ARDS, advanced strategies such as partial liquid ventilation, high-frequency oscillatory ventilation, extracorporeal membrane oxygenation, and carbon dioxide removal are currently being researched.

REFERENCES

1. Dreyfuss D, Saumon G: Ventilator-induced lung injury: lessons from experimental studies, Am J Respir Crit Care Med 157:294, 1998.
2. Greenfield L, Ebert P, Benson D: Effect of positive pressure ventilation on surface tension properties of lung extracts, Anesthesiology 25:312, 1964.
3. Tsuno K, Prato P, Kolobow T: Acute lung injury from mechanical ventilation at moderately high airway pressures, J Appl Physiol 69:956, 1990.
4. Carlton D, Cummings J, Scheerer R, et al: Lung overexpansion increases pulmonary microvascular protein permeability in young lambs, J Appl Physiol 69:577, 1990.
5. Wilson M, Patel B, Takata M: Ventilation with "clinically relevant" high tidal volumes does not promote stretch-induced injury in the lungs of healthy mice, Crit Care Med 40:2850, 2012.
6. Hernandez L, Peevy K, Moise A, et al: Chest wall restriction limits high airway pressure-induced lung injury in young rabbits, J Appl Physiol 66:2364, 1989.
7. Hernandez L, Coker P, Thompson A, et al: Mechanical ventilation increases microvascular permeability in oleic acid-injured lungs, J Appl Physiol 69:2057, 1990.
8. Coker P, Hernandez L, Peevy K, et al: Increased sensitivity to mechanical ventilation after surfactant inactivation in young rabbit lungs, Crit Care Med 20:635, 1992.
9. de Prost N, Roux D, Dreyfuss D, et al: Alveolar edema dispersion and alveolar protein permeability during high volume ventialtion: effect of positive end-expiratory pressure, Intensive Care Med 33:711, 2007.
10. Dreyfuss D, Soler P, Basset G, et al: High inflation pressure pulmonary edema, Am Rev Respir Dis 137:1159, 1988.
11. Pavone L, Albert S, Carney D, et al: Injurious mechnical ventilation in the normal lung causes a progressive pathologic change in dynamic alveolar mechanics, Crit Care 11:1, 2007.
12. Grasso F, Engelberts D, Helm E, et al: Negative-pressure ventilation, Am J Respir Crit Care Med 177:412, 2008.
13. Dreyfuss D, Saumon G: Role of tidal volume, FRC, and end-inspiratory volume in the development of pulmonary edema following mechanical ventilation, Am Rev Respir Dis 148:1194, 1993.
14. Carney D, Bredenberg C, Schiller H, et al: The mechanism of lung volume change during mechnical ventilation, Am J Respir Crit Care Med 160:1697, 1999.
15. Prange H: LaPlace's law and the alveolus: a misconception of anatomy and a misapplication of physics, Adv Physiol Educ 27:34, 2003.
16. Schiller H, McCann II U, Carney D, et al: Altered alveolar mechanics in the acutely injured lung, Crit Care Med 29:1049, 2001.
17. Faridy E, Permutt S, Riley R. Effect of ventilation on surface forces in excised dogs' lungs, J Appl Physiol 21:1453, 1966.
18. Woo S, Hedley-Whyte J. Macrophage accumulation and pulmonary edema due to thoracotomy and lung overinflation, J Appl Physiol 33:14, 1972.
19. Tremblay L, Valenza F, Ribiero S, et al: Injurious ventilatory strategies increase cytokines and c-fos m-RNA expression in an isolated rat model, J Clin Invest 99:944, 1997.
20. Hegeman M, Hennus M, Heijnen C, et al: Ventilator-induced endothelial activation and inflammation in the lung and distal organs, Crit Care 13:1, 2009.
21. Imai Y, Parodo J, Kajikawa O, et al: Injurious mechanical ventilation and end-organ epithelial cell apoptosis and organ dysfunction in an experimental model of acute respiratory distress syndrome, JAMA 289:2104, 2003.
22. van Wessem K, Hennus M, van Wagenberg L, et al: Mechanical ventilation increases the inflammatory response induced by lung contusion, J Surg Res 183:377, 2013.
23. Hong C, Xu D, Lu Q, et al: Low tidal volume and high positive end-expiratory pressure mechanical ventilation results in increased inflammation and ventilator-associated lung injury in normal lungs, Anesth Analg 110:1652, 2010.
24. Piccin V, Calciolari C, Yoshizaki K, et al: Effects of different mechanical ventilation strategies on the mucociliary system, Intensive Care Med 37:132, 2011.
25. Schortgen F, Bouadma L, Joly-Guillou M, et al: Infectious and inflammatory dissemination are affected by ventilation strategy in rats with unilateral pneumonia, Intensive Care Med 30:693, 2004.

26. Nahum A, Hoyt J, Schmitz L, et al: Effect of mechanical ventilation strategy on dissemination of intratracheally instilled Escherichia coli in dogs, Crit Care Med 25:1733, 1997.
27. Broccard A, Shapiro R, Schmitz L, et al: Prone positioning attenuates and redistributes ventilator-induced lung injury in dogs, Crit Care Med 28:295, 2000.
28. de Prost N, Ricard J, Saumon G, et al: Ventilator-induced lung injury: historical perspectives and clinical implications, Ann Intensive Care 1:1, 2011.
29. Kafer E: Pulmonary oxygen toxicity, Br J Anaesth 43:687, 1971.
30. Fisher A, Forman H, Glass M: Mechanisms of pulmonary oxygen toxicity, Lung 162:255, 1984.
31. Demchenko I, Atochin D, Gutsaeva D, et al: Contributions of nitric oxide synthase isoforms to pulmonary oxygen toxicity, local vs. mediated effects, Am J Physiol Lung Cell Mol Physiol 294:L984, 2008.
32. Gajic O, Dara S, Mendez J, et al: Ventilator-associated lung injury in patients without acute lung injury at the onset of mechnical ventilation, Crit Care Med 32:1817, 2004.
33. Gajic O, Frutos-Vivar F, Esteban A, et al: Ventilator settings as a risk factor for acute respiratory distress syndrome in mechanically ventilated patients, Intensive Care Med 31:922, 2005.
34. Fernandez-Perez E, Keegan M, Brown D, et al: Intraoperative tidal volume as a risk factor for respiratory failure after pneumonectomy, Anesthesiology 105:14, 2006.
35. Mascia L, Zavala E, Bosma K, et al: High tidal volume is associated with the development of acute lung injury after severe brain injury: an international observational study, Crit Care Med 35:1815, 2007.
36. Determann R, Royakkers A, Wolthius E, et al: Ventilation with lower tidal volumes as compared with conventional tidal volumes for patients without acute lung injury: a preventative randomized controlled trial, Crit Care 14:1, 2010.
37. Network TARDS: Ventilation with lower tidal volumes as compared with traditional tidal volumes for acute lung injury and the acute respiratory distress syndrome, N Engl J Med 342:1301, 2000.
38. Brower R, Lanken P, MacIntyre N, et al: Higher versus lower positive end-expiratory pressures in patients with the acute respiratory distress syndrome, N Engl J Med 351:327, 2004.
39. Briel M, Meade M, Mercat A, et al: Higher vs lower positive end-expiratory pressure in patients with acute lung injury and acute respiratory distress syndrome: systematic review and meta-analysis, JAMA 303:865, 2010.
40. Meade M, Cook D, Guyatt G, et al: Ventilation strategy using low tidal volumes, recruitment maneuvers, and high positive end-expiratory pressure for acute lung injury and acute respiratory distress syndrome, JAMA 299:637, 2008.
41. Mercat A, Richard J, Vielle B, et al: Positive end-expiratory pressure setting in adults with acute lung injury and acute respiratory distress syndrome, JAMA 299:646, 2008.
42. Parsons P, Eisner M, Thompson B, et al: Lower tidal volume ventilation and plasma cytokine markers of inflammation in patients with acute lung injury, Crit Care Med 33, 2005.
43. Pinheiro de Oliviera R, Hetzel M, Silva M, et al: Mechanical ventilation with high tidal volume induces inflammation in patients without lung disease, Crit Care 14:1, 2010.
44. Ranieri V, Suter P, Tortorella C, et al: Effect of mechanical ventilation on inflammatory mediators in patients with acute respiratory distress syndrome: a randomized controlled trial, JAMA 282:54, 1999.
45. Hemmes S, Neto A, Schultz M: Intraoperative ventilatory strategies to prevent postoperative pulmonary complications: a meta-analysis, Curr Opin Anaesthesiol 26:126, 2013.
46. Neto A, Cardoso S, Manetta J, et al: Association between use of lung-protective ventilation with lower tidal volumes and clinical outcomes among patients without acute respiratory distress syndrome, JAMA 308:1651, 2012.
47. Kelmer E, Love L, DeClue A, et al: Successful treatment of acute respiratory distress syndrome in 2 dogs, Can Vet J 53:167, 2012.
48. Hopper K, Haskins S, Kass P, et al: Indications, management, and outcome of long-term positive-pressure ventilation in dogs and cats: 148 cases (1990-2001), J Am Vet Med Assoc 230:64, 2007.
49. Beal M, Paglia D, Griffin G, et al: Ventilatory failure, ventilator management, and outcome in dogs with cervical spinal disorders: 14 cases (1991-1999), J Am Vet Med Assoc 218:1598, 2001.
50. Lee J, Drobatz K, Koch M, et al: Indications for and outcome of positive-pressure ventilation in cats: 53 cases (1993-2002), J Am Vet Med Assoc 226:924, 2005.
51. Campbell V, King L. Pulmonary function, ventilator management, and outcome of dogs with thoracic trauma and pulmonary contusions: 10 cases (1994-1998), J Am Vet Med Assoc 217:1505, 2000.
52. Rutter C, Rozanski E, Sharp C, et al: Outcome and medical management in dogs with lower motor neuron disease undergoing mechanical ventilation: 14 cases (2003-2009), J Vet Emerg Crit Care 21:531, 2011.
53. Hoareau G, Mellema M, Silverstein D: Indication, management, and outcome of brachycephalic dogs requiring mechanical ventilation, J Vet Emerg Crit Care 21:226, 2011.
54. Gattinoni L, Eleonora C, Caironi P: Monitoring of pulmonary mechanics in acute respiratory distress syndrome to titrate therapy, Curr Opin Crit Care 11:252, 2005.

CHAPTER 37
VENTILATOR-ASSOCIATED PNEUMONIA

Steven Epstein, DVM, DACVECC

KEY POINTS

- Ventilator-associated pneumonia (VAP) is diagnosed clinically, based on the presence of systemic inflammation and new or progressive pulmonary infiltrates occurring after at least 48 hours of intubation.
- The main risk factor for the development of VAP is endotracheal intubation, and when VAP occurs, it is associated with high mortality rates.
- Prevention of VAP is most effective if preventative strategies are grouped in bundles and performed in every patient at risk.
- If VAP is suspected, early diagnostics included collection of lower airway samples should be performed and empiric therapy started with antimicrobial therapy altered when culture results are available.

Ventilator-associated pneumonia (VAP) refers to pneumonia that arises more than 48 hours after endotracheal intubation that was not present at the time of intubation.[1] In veterinary medicine, patients may be remain endotracheally intubated for prolonged periods without receiving mechanical ventilation. These patients are at risk for developing pneumonia from many of the same pathogenic factors as mechanically ventilated patients are. As such, all anesthetized dogs and cats with endotracheal intubation, regardless of mechanical ventilation status, are discussed together in this chapter.

In veterinary medicine the incidence of VAP has not been reported, but in human medicine it is a common complication of mechanical ventilation occurring in 8% to 28% of intubated human patients.[2] The incidence of VAP varies with study period, diagnostic criteria, and location, with current estimates of between 0 and 6 events per 1000 ventilator days reported to the Centers for Disease Control and Prevention by the National Healthcare Safety Network for 2010.[3] The risk for development of VAP varies with duration of ventilation with a daily hazard rate of 3.3% for the first 5 days, 2.3% for day 6 to 10, and 1.3% after.[4] Because most animals receive mechanical ventilation for less than a week, the majority of the cases of VAP would be expected to occur in the first few days of ventilation; however, the cumulative incidence will increase as number of days of intubation increases. Crude intensive care unit (ICU) mortality rates for VAP in humans have been reported to be between 24% to 76%.[2] The development of VAP also increases the length of time mechanical ventilation is necessary, which would contribute to mortality rates in veterinary medicine. With these high mortality rates, early diagnosis and prevention of the development of VAP are key to improving outcome.

PATHOGENESIS

One of the key factors in the pathogenesis of VAP is the introduction of a microbial pathogen into the airways. Once a pathogen gets past the cuff of the endotracheal tube there are several potential outcomes. The pathogen may be cleared by normal respiratory defenses, the lower airways may be colonized, the tracheobronchial tree may become infected (ventilator-associated tracheobronchitis [VAT]), or if the pulmonary parenchyma becomes infected, VAP occurs. Normal respiratory defenses to colonization or infection of the lower airways include cough, mucus clearance, and humoral and cellular immune responses. These normal defenses are compromised in an anesthetized critically ill animal, as there is a reduced ability to cough due to sedation and the presence of the endotracheal tube, inflation of a cuffed endotracheal tube depresses the mucociliary clearance rate,[5] and critical illness is associated with decreased immune system function and increased susceptibility to nosocomial infection.[6] In addition there is evidence for neutrophil dysfunction in VAP with a reduced phagocytic capability[7] and elevation in neutrophil proteases in the alveolar space.[8]

With these impaired respiratory defenses, the prime risk factor for the development of VAP is the presence of an endotracheal tube. In fact, the risk for the development of VAP in patients receiving noninvasive mechanical ventilation is lower than in patients with endotracheal intubation.[9] Reintubation after unsuccessful extubation is a risk factor for VAP as well.

Microaspiration past the cuff of the endotracheal tube and biofilm development within the endotracheal tube likely represent the two major pathologic mechanisms behind VAP. When the endotracheal cuff is inflated this allows for pooling of secretions beyond the vocal folds, but above the cuff (subglottic region). When high-volume, low-pressure cuffs are used to prevent tracheal injury, the longitudinal folds that develop are associated with microaspiration or macroaspiration of subglottic fluid with subsequent translocation of bacteria to the interior of the endotracheal tube or airways. Once bacteria are present on the internal surface of the endotracheal tube, in which most are made of polyvinyl chloride, these bacteria may easily adhere and produce a complex polysaccharide matrix known as biofilm. This biofilm is inaccessible to antimicrobials unless they are aerosolized. As the bacteria proliferate within the endotracheal tube, they may be dislodged into the lower airway because of airflow, suctioning, or bronchoscopic procedures. In a cohort of human patients with VAP, 70% had identical pathogens identified from endotracheal tube biofilm and tracheal secretions with antimicrobial susceptibility data showing greater antimicrobial resistance in the biofilm isolates.[10]

The bacteria associated with biofilm formation or VAP may come from either exogenous or endogenous source. Exogenous sources include contaminated respiratory equipment, the environment, or healthcare provider's hands. (See Chapter 34 for proper hand hygiene and apparatus care.) With proper hand hygiene the primary source of colonization is likely endogenous bacterial. Normal oral flora is typically a mixed population of bacteria, whereas in critical illness aerobic gram-negative bacteria predominate. This change in type and increased numbers of bacteria can be attributed to a lack oral hygiene seen with normal swallowing that results in the spread of saliva which contains proteases, immunoglobulins, and enzymes. Patients receiving antimicrobials may also see a change in population and increase in resistance of oral flora because of antimicrobial pressures. Dogs and cats with respiratory failure requiring mechanical ventilation also have a shift in bacterial flora and antimicrobial resistance compared to patients with less severe respiratory disease in one study. Lower respiratory cultures from the respiratory failure group had a larger population of aerobic gram-negative enterics and increased antimicrobial resistance rates compared to patients that did not need mechanical ventilation.[11]

Alternatively, the source of respiratory bacterial colonization may be gastric in origin. Critically ill patients receiving gastric antacid medications show greater rates of gastric colonization than those who do not.[12] The relationship between gastric colonization and VAP is currently controversial as there is evidence for and against their relationship.

A variety of pathogens can be isolated with VAP, with aerobic bacteria representing the majority of cases. Anaerobic bacteria, viruses, and fungus are rarely the cause of VAP. Infections may be monomicrobial or polymicrobial in origin. Polymicrobial infections can be as common as monomicrobial infections although mortality has not been shown to be different between groups.[13] Initially, early-onset VAP (first 5 days) was thought not to be associated with multidrug-resistant (MDR) bacteria; however, recent reports are challenging this initial belief.[14] It is difficult to define risk factors for the development of MDR VAP; however, previous antimicrobial use is implicated. Local epidemiologic data are important in determining the likely pathogens that may be identified with VAP.

DIAGNOSIS

Over the last 30 years many definitions have been used for VAP. Currently there is no "gold standard" that can be used for a diagnosis. This lack of standardized diagnosis reflects variable rates seen between hospitals and research settings. There is currently controversy in deciding what criteria should be used in the diagnosis of VAP.

The modified CDC National Healthcare Safety Network definition of pneumonia is listed in Box 37-1.[15] Patients must satisfy all three criteria (radiologic, systemic, and pulmonary) and have a tracheostomy or endotracheal tube in place for more than 48 hours before the diagnosis of infection to receive a diagnosis of VAP. Although definitions such as these can be useful for research purposes they are often subjective and may be limited for clinical decision making for individual patients. Recently more objective criteria have been proposed the diagnosis of VAP but they are not widely accepted yet.[16]

The clinical diagnosis of VAP in an individual patient usually requires two of the following three criteria: fever, either leukocytosis or leukopenia, and purulent airway secretions. VAT is an infection of the tracheobronchial tree of similar origin to VAP but does not affect the pulmonary parenchyma. VAT may produce the same clinical signs as VAP does, and if a patient fulfills the clinical criteria for VAT/VAP, thoracic imaging is indicated. To help differentiate VAT from VAP, a new or progressive pulmonary infiltrates on thoracic radiography or computed tomography is required to diagnosis VAP. A deteriorating oxygenation status or increased ventilatory demands would be supportive of VAP. Thoracic radiographs may difficult to interpret as pulmonary hemorrhage, atelectasis or ARDS may be mistaken as pneumonic infiltrates resulting in high sensitivity and low specificity of this test. Additionally the clinical criteria are not specific for pneumonia and may result from noninfectious pulmonary conditions.

If VAP/VAT is suspected clinically, then microbiological methods should be used to aid in the diagnosis. Clinicians may obtain respiratory samples from endotracheal aspirates, via bronchoscopic or nonbronchoscopic bronchoalveolar lavage (BAL), or by protected specimen brush (PSB). Once a sample is obtained, it can be submitted for quantitative (CFU/ml), semiquantitative (1+ to 4+ growth), or qualitative (growth, no growth) culture and susceptibility testing. A recent Cochrane database review showed no difference on outcomes, or antimicrobial use when either culture type was used.[17] In a meta-analysis of invasive cultures defined as either BAL or PSB samples, versus endotracheal aspirates, the decision to use invasive cultures did not affect mortality. Invasive testing however did result in a modification of antimicrobial usage more often.[18] De-escalation therapy rates were higher when a quantitative BAL culture was used over a quantitative endotracheal aspirate.[19] As the lower airways are not sterile in health quantitative or semiquantitative cultures help to distinguish infection from normal resident flora. Table 37-1 compares the quantitative threshold for various sampling techniques for the diagnosis of pneumonia based on CDC guidelines.[20] It is recommended that if VAP is suspected, a BAL or PSB specimen be obtained and submitted for quantitative culture and threshold values used to confirm infection.

Airway sampling for microbial culture has its limitations. Endotracheal aspirates may represent colonization of the endotracheal tube rather than true infections, or if a nonbronchoscopic technique is used, fluid from a noninfected part of the lung may be sampled.

BOX 37-1 *Modified Centers for Disease Control and Prevention Clinical Surveillance Definitions for Ventilator-Associated Pneumonia (PNU1)*[15]

Radiologic Criteria (Two or More Serial Radiographs with at Least One of The Following)

New or progressive and persistent infiltrate
Consolidation
Cavitation

Systemic Criteria (at Least One)

Fever
Leukopenia or leukocytosis

Pulmonary Criteria (at Least Two)

New onset of purulent sputum, or change in character of sputum, or increased respiratory secretions, or increased suctioning requirements
Worsening gas exchange (e.g., desaturation, increased oxygen requirements, or increased ventilator demands)
New-onset or worsening cough, or dyspnea or tachypnea
Crackles or bronchial breath sounds

Patients must fulfill all three (pulmonary, radiologic, and systemic) criteria.

Table 37-1 Threshold Values for Cultured Specimens Used in the Diagnosis of Pneumonia

Collection Technique	Quantitative Threshold
Bronchoscopic bronchoalveolar lavage	$\geq 10^4$ CFU/ml
Blind bronchoalveolar lavage	$\geq 10^4$ CFU/ml
Bronchoscopic protected specimen brush	$\geq 10^3$ CFU/ml
Blind protected specimen brush	$\geq 10^3$ CFU/ml
Endotracheal aspirate	$\geq 10^5$ CFU/ml

Additionally it may take up to 48 to 72 hours for culture results to return. Because of these limitations, search for an accurate biomarker to predict VAP is underway. Proposed benefits of biomarkers to aid in the diagnosis of VAP are that they may return in hours instead of days and may be noninvasively sampled by nursing staff. To date multiple biomarkers (C-reactive protein, procalcitonin, triggered receptor expressed on myeloid cells 1 [TREM-1]) have been evaluated, and none provide the sensitivity and specificity needed to be a good diagnostic test.

PREVENTION

Because VAP is associated with high mortality rates, much study has gone into how it can be prevented. There is no one modification or treatment that is effective against the development of VAP and preventative measures should be applied as a bundle for patients at risk. Implementation of preventative bundles from the Institute for Healthcare Improvement or the International Nosocomial Infection Control Consortium has been shown to decrease the incidence of VAP.[21,22] A summary of nonpharmacologic and pharmacologic prevention strategies applicable to veterinary medicine that can minimize the occurrence of VAP are presented in Box 37-2.

Nonpharmacologic Strategies

Training ICU personnel for the prevention of VAP can reduce incidence of this disease. Frequent evaluation of compliance with protocols and feedback to ICU nurses is needed to maintain a high level of care and has been shown to decrease the incidence of VAP and increase compliance with protocols.[23] If mechanical ventilation is not common, protocols should be reviewed at the initiation of each case to help ensure proper management.

The World Health Organization and the CDC state that hand hygiene is one of the most important strategies for prevention and spread of infections. Proper hand hygiene, including alcohol-based hand rubs, can reduce the risk of VAP. Before the patient is touched, hands should be washed or an alcohol-based hand rub should be used, then examination gloves worn. Immediately before ICU personnel touch the airway or oral cavity, proper hand hygiene should be performed. This includes, if other areas of the patient are examined, performing hand hygiene before returning to the airway or oral cavity.

Longer duration of intubation is associated with an increased cumulative risk for the duration of VAP.[4] When protocol driven weaning from mechanical ventilation is used, there is evidence of shorter duration of ventilation as well as lower incidence of VAP.[24]

BOX 37-2 *Preventative Measures That May Decrease the Incidence of VAP*

Nonpharmacologic

Provide educational program for caregivers and monitoring of compliance.
Use of strict alcohol-based hand hygiene.
Minimize time of intubation with weaning protocols.
Do not change ventilatory circuit unless contamination occurs.
Aspiration of subglottic secretions.
Maintain endotracheal tube cuff pressure ≥25 cm H_2O.

Pharmacologic

Perform oral care with dilute chlorhexidine.
Avoid increasing gastric pH prophylactically.

Once weaning protocols are in place, they may be nurse driven, which may decrease duration of mechanical ventilation compared with physician-driven protocols.[25] Tracheostomy has also been proposed as a method of reducing duration of mechanical ventilation. In a recent meta-analysis, the timing of tracheostomy did not affect mortality, duration of mechanical ventilation, or incidence of VAP.[26]

The ideal length of time for use of a single ventilator circuit has not been established. A meta-analysis showed an increased risk of pneumonia when circuits were changed every 2 days versus every 7 days; not routinely changing the ventilator circuit did not increase the odds of VAP.[27] Based on this, routine changing of the ventilator circuit should not occur unless contamination is noted.

As microaspiration and biofilm formation are two of the most important mechanisms in the development of VAP, much research into the ideal endotracheal tube has occurred. Novel shapes of cuffs, cuff material, and coating of the endotracheal tubes coated with silver have showed promise.[28] The North American Silver-Coated Endotracheal Tube (NASCENT) study showed a decrease in the VAP and in patients that developed VAP a decreased mortality when a silver-coated endotracheal tube was used.[29]

There is strong evidence that suctioning of subglottic secretions can help reduce the occurrence of VAP.[30] Tracheal tubes with a port that exits above the cuff for continuous suction exist, but their cost effectiveness is questionable. Intermittent suctioning of subglottic secretions is currently recommended. To help prevent micro aspiration, the cuff on the endotracheal tube should be maintained with a pressure 25 cm H_2O or greater. See Chapter 34 for a description of airway management to help prevent VAP.

Pharmacologic Strategies

Performing oral antisepsis with chlorhexidine can reduce the incidence of VAP. The ideal concentration of chlorhexidine to be used has not been determined; however, favorable effects have been seen from 0.12% to 2%.[31] Topical decontamination of the oral cavity with antimicrobials to reduce the load of gram-negative bacteria in the oral cavity has also shown some promise. Typically an aminoglycoside or other combinations of antimicrobials without anaerobic activity are used. In meta-analysis, topical oral antimicrobials have shown a reduction in VAP and have the potential to decrease all cause ICU-acquired infections.[31] Because of its comparative ease of use and noninferiority in preventing VAP, topical chlorhexidine is recommended for use in oral care. Selective digestive decontamination (SDD) involves the topical and parental use of antimicrobials to decrease the flora of the entire gastrointestinal tract. The main limitation of SDD is the higher emergence of resistant bacterial strains preventing its routine use.

The role of increasing gastric pH with histamine-2 receptor antagonists (H_2RA) and proton pump inhibitors in mechanical ventilation is controversial. The proposed benefit is to reduce stress-related mucosal disease and ulceration, whereas the proposed detriment is a higher rate of gastric colonization with bacteria. In a meta-analysis comparing the use of H_2RA versus sucralfate showed no difference in effectiveness in the treatment of overt bleeding, but H_2RA use had higher rates of gastric colonization and VAP.[32] Because gastric colonization has been linked to development of VAP, routine use of gastric antacid drugs is not recommended; they should be reserved for use in cases of demonstrated gastrointestinal ulceration.

A novel therapy investigated to reduce the incidence of VAP is probiotics. A recent meta-analysis of randomized controlled trials found 7 studies and included 1142 patients found no decrease in the incidence of VAP or any other end point.[33] However, the results should be interpreted with caution because there was significant heterogeneity among study designs and further research is needed.

TREATMENT

The initiation of antimicrobial therapy for VAP should commence as soon as there is clinical suspicion and airway microbiological samples have been taken. Delays in appropriate antimicrobial administration increase the already high mortality rates seen with VAP.[34,35] Changing antimicrobial therapy to an appropriate one based on culture results when they are available may not reduce the risk of death with VAP (i.e., getting it right the first time is important).

The American Thoracic Society (ATS) and Infectious Diseases Society of America (IDSA) guidelines for initial empiric selection of antimicrobial therapy[1] are based on "early" (<5 days of hospitalization) or "late" onset (≥5 days of hospitalization) of VAP and whether risk factors are present for MDR pathogens. Risk factors for MDR pathogens included recent antimicrobial therapy, prolonged duration of hospitalization (≥5 days), or an immunosuppressive disease or therapy. Recent evidence, however, suggests that the presence of MDR pathogens in "early onset" VAP is as common as "late onset" and that empiric choices should cover potential MDR pathogens regardless of timing of onset of VAP.[14,36]

In making empiric antimicrobial selections, locally derived (institution-specific) guidelines may provide better coverage than general recommendations for a larger population. In a recent study comparing local guidelines with ATS/IDSA recommendations showed that 49% to 83% of pneumonia would have been covered by the ATS/IDSA compared with 94% based local data.[36] If local guidelines are not available, then broad-spectrum antimicrobial coverage for MDR pathogens should be initiated. This includes the use of an antipseudomonal (ticarcillin-clavulanate, meropenem or ceftazidime) with a fluoroquinolone or aminoglycoside. (Refer to the antimicrobial section of this text for appropriate dose and frequency) If methicillin-resistant *Staphylococcus* is prevalent locally, and gram-positive cocci are seen on respiratory fluid cytology, vancomycin may be added empirically. Epstein et al. showed that in dogs and cats with respiratory failure and a positive lower respiratory tract culture, only amikacin and carbapenems had greater than 90% efficacy against all aerobic bacteria tested, making carbapenems a reasonable empiric option for dogs and cats.[11] Aminoglycosides, however, are not used as monotherapy because of their poor penetration into infected lung tissue. Choosing broad-spectrum empiric therapy mandates that, when culture and susceptibility results are available, de-escalation to an antimicrobial with a narrow, more focused spectrum should occur.

The majority of infections can be treated by a course of appropriate antimicrobial for 8 days. Chastre et al demonstrated that patients treated for 8 days had no difference in mortality, recurrent infections, or ventilator free days or length of ICU hospitalization compared with 15 days of antimicrobial therapy.[37] They did document that patients with VAP caused by gram-negative fermenting bacilli, such as *Pseudomonas aeruginosa* or *Acinetobacter sp.* had higher mortality if only 8 days of treatment were used. However, in patients with recurrent infections, MDR pathogens emerged less in the 8 day treatment group. If a fermenting gram-negative bacilli is cultured, a 14- to 21-day course of antimicrobial therapy should be considered.

Aerosolized antimicrobials have the potential advantage of achieving high drug concentrations in the lungs while avoiding systemic absorption and toxicities. Aminoglycosides or polymyxins are most commonly used, which both have concerns for nephrotoxicity. With mechanical ventilation, an ultrasonic or vibrating plate nebulizer should be used to maximize delivery to the site of infection. A recent study evaluated adjunctive aerosolized antimicrobial therapy for the treatment of *Pseudomonas aeruginosa* and *Acinetobacter baumannii* VAP. The researchers concluded that despite a greater of severity of illness and incidence of MDR bacteria, patients receiving adjunctive aerosolized therapy had similar outcomes to patients that did not.[38] For MDR gram-negative infections, aerosolized antimicrobials may be considered; however, the patient should be monitored for bronchoconstriction during the process and future nebulization with that antimicrobial avoided if bronchoconstriction occurs.

REFERENCES

1. ATS: Guidelines for the management of adults with hospital-acquired, ventilator-associated and healthcare-associated pneumonia, Am J Respir Crit Care Med 171:388, 2005.
2. Chastre J, Fagon J: Ventilator-associated Pneumonia, Am J Respir Crit Care Med 165:867, 2002.
3. Dudeck MA, Horan TC, Peterson KD, et al: National Healthcare Safety Network (NHSN) Report, data summary for 2010, device-associated module, Am J Infect Control 39:798, 2011.
4. Cook DJ, Walter SD, Cook RJ, et al: Incidence of and risk factors for ventilator-associated pneumonia in critically ill patients, Ann Intern Med 129:433, 1998.
5. Sackner MA, Hirsh J, Epstein S: Effect of cuffed endotracheal tubes on tracheal mucous velocity, Chest 68:774 1975.
6. Boomer JS, To K, Chang KC, et al: Immunosuppression in patients who die of sepsis and multiple organ failure, JAMA 306:2594, 2011.
7. Conway MA, Kefala K, Wilkinson TS, et al: C5a mediates peripheral blood neutrophil dysfunction in critically ill patients, Am J Respir Crit Care Med 180:19, 2009.
8. Wilkinson TS, Morris AC, Kefala K, et al: Ventilator-associated pneumonia is characterized by excessive release of neutrophil proteases in the lung, Chest 142:1425, 2012.
9. Hess DR: Noninvasive positive-pressure ventilation and ventilator-associated pneumonia, Respir Care 50:924, 2005.
10. Adair CG, Gorman SP, Feron BM, et al: Implications of endotracheal tube biofilm for ventilator-associated pneumonia, Intensive Care Med 25:1072, 1999.
11. Epstein SE, Mellema MS, Hopper K: Airway microbial culture and susceptibility patterns in dogs and cats with respiratory disease of varying severity, J Vet Emerg Crit Care 20:587, 2010.
12. Kantorova I, Svoboda P, Scheer P, et al: Stress ulcer prophylaxis in critically ill patients: a randomized controlled trial, Hepatogastroenterology 51:757, 2004.
13. Combes A, Figliolini C, Trouillet J, et al: Incidence and outcome of polymicrobial ventilator-associated pneumonia, Chest 121:1618, 2002.
14. Restrepo MI, Petereson J, Fernandez JF, et al: Comparison of the bacterial etiology of early-onset ventilator associated pneumonia and late-onset ventilator associated pneumonia in subjects enrolled in 2 large clinical studies, Respir Care E-pub January 9, 2013 doi: 10.4187/respcare.02173.
15. Horan TC, Andrus M, Dudeck MA: CDC/NHSN surveillance definition of health care-associated infection and criteria for specific types of infections in the acute care setting, Am J Infect Control 36:309, 2008.
16. Klompas M, Magill S, Robicsek A, et al: Objective surveillance definitions for ventilator-associated pneumonia, Crit Care Med 40:3154, 2012.
17. Berton DC, Kalil AC, Teixeira PJZ: Quantitative versus qualitative cultures of respiratory secretions for clinical outcomes in patients with ventilator associated pneumonia, Cochrane Database Syst Rev 1:CD006482. doi:10.1002/14651858.CD006482.pub3.
18. Shorr AF, Sherner JH, Jackson WL, et al: Invasive approaches to the diagnosis of ventilator-associated pneumonia: a meta-analysis, Crit Care Med 33:46, 2005.
19. Giantsou E, Liratzopoulos N, Efraimidou E, et al: De-escalation therapy rates are significantly higher by bronchoalveolar lavage than by tracheal aspirate, Intensive Care Med 33:1533, 2007.
20. Centers for Disease Control and Prevention: National Healthcare Safety Network manual, Device-associated module: ventilator-associated pneumonia event, Centers for disease control and prevention, Atlanta GA. www.cdc.gov/nhsn/pdfs/pscmanual/6pscvapcurrent.pdf. Accessed February 18, 2013.

21. Al-Tawfiq JA, Abed M: Decreasing ventilator-associated pneumonia in adult intensive care units using the institute for healthcare improvement bundle, Am J Infect Control 38:552, 2010.
22. Leblebicioglu H, Yalcin AN, Rosenthal VD, et al: Effectiveness of a multidimensional approach for prevention of ventilator-associated pneumonia in 11 adult intensive care units from 10 cities of Turkey: findings of the international nosocomial infection control consortium, Infection E-pub Januar 9, 2013 doi 10.1007/s15010-013-0407-1.
23. Sinuff T, Muscedere J, Cook DJ, et al: Implementation of clinical practice guidelines for ventilator-associated pneumonia: a multi-center prospective study, Crit Care Med, 41:15, 2013.
24. Dries DJ, McGonigal MD, Malian MS, et al: Protocol-driven ventilator weaning reduces use of mechanical ventilation, rate of early reintubation and ventilator-associated pneumonia, J Trauma 56:943, 2004.
25. Danckers M, Grosu H, Jean R, et al: Nurse-driven, protocol-directed weaning from mechanical ventilation improves clinical outcomes and is well accepted by intensive care unit physicians, J Crit Care E-pub Dec 19, 2012 doi 10.1016/j.jcrc.2012.10.012.
26. Wang F, Wu Y, Bo L, et al: The timing of tracheotomy in critically ill patients undergoing mechanical ventilation: a systematic review and meta-analysis of randomized controlled trials, Chest 140:1456 2011.
27. Han J, Liu Y: Effect of ventilator circuit changes on ventilator-associated pneumonia: a systematic review and meta-analysis, Respir Care 55:467, 2010.
28. Fernandez JF, Levine SM, Restrepo MI: Technological advances in endotracheal tubes for prevention of ventilator-associated pneumonia, Chest 142:231, 2012.
29. Afessa B, Shorr AF, Anzueto AR, et al: Association between silver-coated endotracheal tube and reduced mortality in patients with ventilator-associated pneumonia, Chest 137:1015, 2010.
30. Muscedere J, Rewa O, Mckechnie K, et al: Subglottic secretion drainage for the prevention of ventilator-associated pneumonia: a systematic review and meta-analysis, Crit Care Med 39:1985, 2011.
31. Pileggi C, Bianco A, Flotta D, et al: Prevention of ventilator-associated pneumonia, mortality and all intensive care unit acquired infections by topically applied antimicrobial or antiseptic agents: a meta-analysis of randomized controlled trials in intensive care units, Critical Care 15:R155, 2011.
32. Huang J, Cao Y, Liao C, et al: Effect of histamine-2-receptor antagonists versus sucralfate on stress ulcer prophylaxis in mechanically ventilated patients: a meta-analysis of 10 randomized controlled trials, Crit Care 14:R194, 2010.
33. Gu WJ, Wei CY, Yin RX: Lack of efficacy of probiotics in preventing ventilator-associated pneumonia, Chest 142:859, 2012.
34. Luna CM, Vujacich P, Niederman MS, et al: Impact of BAL data on the therapy and outcome of ventilator-associated pneumonia, Chest 111:676, 1997.
35. Iregui M, Ward S, Sherman G, et al: Clinical importance of delays in the initiation of appropriate antibiotic treatment for ventilator-associated pneumonia, Chest 122:262, 2002.
36. Becher RD, Hoth JJ, Rebo JJ, et al: Locally derived versus guideline-based approach to treatment of hospital-acquired pneumonia in the trauma intensive care unit, Surg Infect 13:352, 2012.
37. Chastre J, Wolff M, Fagon J, et al: Comparison of 8 vs 15 days of antibiotic therapy for ventilator-associated pneumonia in adults, JAMA 290:2588, 2003.
38. Arnold HM, Sawyer AM, Kollef MH: Use of adjunctive aerosolized antimicrobial therapy in the treatment of *Pseudomonas aeruginosa* and *Acinetobacter baumannii* ventilator-associated pneumonia, Respir Care 57:1226, 2012.

PART IV CARDIAC DISORDERS

CHAPTER 38
MECHANISMS OF HEART FAILURE

Mark A. Oyama, DVM, DACVIM (Cardiology)

KEY POINTS

- Neurohormonal activation is a key feature of heart failure.
- Myocardial tissue responds to disease through distinct patterns of hypertrophy.
- The relationship between preload and cardiac performance (Frank-Starling mechanism) provides insight into the genesis of congestive heart failure.
- Staging nomenclature has been developed to help describe the clinical progression of heart disease.

Heart failure is defined as the heart's inability to meet the metabolic needs of the peripheral tissues, or instances when the heart can only do so in the presence of increased venous filling pressures.[1] The specific mechanisms leading to heart failure are varied and complex, yet a basic understanding of the interplay between the heart and kidneys, as well as various neurohormonal systems such as the sympathetic nervous system (SNS) and renin-angiotensin-aldosterone system (RAAS), is needed for successful treatment of heart failure. Important mechanisms of cardiac injury also include alterations in intracellular calcium cycling, myocardial and vascular remodeling, and deficiencies in myocardial energy production, all of which perpetuate further neuroendocrine activation as part of a vicious cycle (Figure 38-1).

The clinical signs of heart failure include those relating to poor cardiac output (i.e., forward heart failure) and to congestion (i.e., backward heart failure). Typical signs of low cardiac output include weakness, activity intolerance, hypothermia, and depressed mentation. Inadequate tissue perfusion results in lactic acidosis, azotemia, and oliguria. In animals with congestive heart failure (CHF), elevated venous filling pressure causes exudation of fluid from pulmonary or systemic capillary beds, resulting in pulmonary edema, pleural effusion, or ascites. In reality, neither of these forms of heart failure occurs independent of the other and dysfunction always includes some combination of reduced cardiac output along with variably detected degrees of congestion.

The emergent heart failure patient requires acute manipulation of preload, afterload, contractility, atrioventricular synchrony, and heart rate so that forward cardiac output is improved and congestion alleviated. Chronic therapy for patients with heart failure concentrates on the heart as part of an integrated neuroendocrine system rather than an isolated muscular pump. Thus, with chronic therapy, targeting the neurohormonal pathways is of equal or greater importance than muscular pump function in the setting of the failing heart.

NEUROHORMONAL ASPECTS OF HEART FAILURE

The two classic neurohormonal pathways involved in the genesis of heart failure are the RAAS and the SNS. The natriuretic peptides, endothelin, and vasopressin systems also play a role. The importance of these and other neurohormonal systems is highlighted by the fact that many of the most effective drugs in treating heart failure are those that specifically target these systems.

Renin-Angiotensin-Aldosterone System

The primary trigger for activation of the RAAS is the heart's inability to provide normal renal perfusion. Decreased renal blood flow and sodium delivery to the distal portions of the nephron induces renin release from the macula densa. Renin converts angiotensinogen to angiotensin I, which is then rapidly converted to angiotensin II by angiotensin-converting enzyme (ACE) in the pulmonary vasculature. Angiotensin II is an important effector molecule for many of the maladaptive responses that promote further cardiac injury and heart failure, including renal sodium and water retention, production of aldosterone, myocardial apoptosis, cardiac and vascular remodeling and fibrosis, increased thirst, and vasoconstriction. Activation of the RAAS in dogs with heart failure has been well described.[2-4] The classic description of the RAAS involves circulating angiotensin II and aldosterone; local tissue RAAS is thought to significantly contribute to cardiac remodeling and injury. Moreover, angiotensin II can be generated from pathways independent of ACE and elevations of angiotensin II and aldosterone that can occur in spite of ACE inhibitor therapy. The end result of circulating and tissue RAAS activation is retention of fluid (which promotes development of CHF) and maladaptive myocardial and vascular remodeling (which cause further cardiac injury and depression of cardiac function).

Sympathetic Nervous System

The SNS is an evolutionary response to stress. In times of danger, the SNS, through its main effector molecules, norepinephrine and epinephrine, increase heart rate, cardiac output, and increase blood flow to important stress response organs such as skeletal muscle. The SNS is, however, a short-term response and chronic activation leads to adrenergic receptor downregulation, persistent tachycardia, increased myocardial oxygen demand, and myocyte necrosis. Thus when the acute response of the SNS becomes a chronic response, SNS activity ultimately leads to further cardiac damage. In humans with heart disease, increased norepinephrine concentrations are a significant risk factor for mortality. Increased SNS activity is likely one of the earliest systemic responses to cardiac injury. In the emergent patient

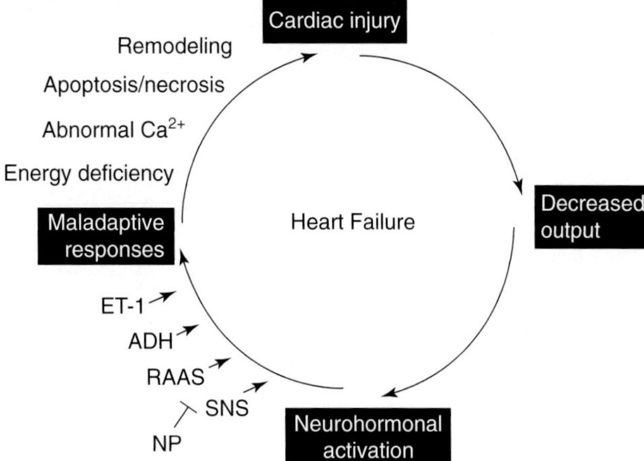

FIGURE 38-1 The vicious cycle of heart failure. Cardiac injury leads to decreased cardiac output and tissue perfusion and subsequent neurohormonal activation. Activity of the sympathetic nervous system (SNS), renin-angiotensin-aldosterone system (RAAS), vasopressin (antidiuretic hormone [ADH]) system, and endothelin-1 system (ET-1) is upregulated and triggers a host of maladaptive results. These responses include myocardiocyte energy depletion and deficiency, abnormal calcium ion transients, apoptosis/necrosis, and myocardial remodeling. The maladaptive responses contribute to ongoing cardiac injury, thus completing the vicious cycle of heart failure. The natriuretic peptide (NP) system counteracts activity of the SNS and RAAS but is not sufficiently potent to stop the cycle from continuing.

with low-output heart failure or CHF, temporary augmentation of already heightened SNS activity is occasionally needed to treat the acute event, but long-term stimulation of the SNS is not an objective of chronic heart failure therapy.

Natriuretic Peptide System

Myocardial tissue produces two main hormones that induce natriuresis, diuresis, and vasodilation. These so-called natriuretic peptides include atrial natriuretic peptide (ANP) and B-type natriuretic peptide (BNP), and both are produced primarily in response to stretch or stress of myocardial tissue. The natriuretic peptide system serves as a counterregulatory system to the RAAS and SNS. Circulating concentrations of ANP and BNP are increased in dogs and cats with heart disease, roughly in proportion to disease severity.[5-7] In the later stages of disease, the beneficial activity of the natriuretic peptide system is overwhelmed, resulting in the clinical appearance of CHF. The reasons for the loss of natriuretic peptide efficacy are complex but likely involve a combination of natriuretic peptide receptor downregulation, inappropriate or inadequate production or processing of the peptides, and increased peptide clearance or degradation. In humans with acute CHF, exogenous BNP helps alleviate the severity of dyspnea. Because of their important role in the pathophysiology of heart failure, both ANP and BNP are forming the basis for new diagnostic, staging, and prognostic assays in dogs and cats with heart disease.

Endothelin and Vasopressin Systems

Endothelin 1 is a potent vasoconstrictor produced by vascular endothelial cells in response to sheer stress, angiotensin II, and other various cytokines. Together with angiotensin II, endothelin 1 causes vasoconstriction and increased cardiac afterload. Endothelin 1 is elevated in dogs and cats with heart failure[8,9] and, in addition to its vascular effects, endothelin 1 alters normal calcium cycling within muscle cells and is directly toxic to myocardiocytes. There is a potential therapeutic role for endothelin 1 in cases of pulmonary hypertension, which is a serious complication in many patients with heart disease.

Arginine vasopressin or antidiuretic hormone increases reabsorption of free water within the renal collecting duct. Its pattern of activation closely resembles that of the RAAS and SNS, and in patients with advanced heart disease, excessive vasopressin contributes to development of fluid overload, CHF, and dilutional hyponatremia. Dilutional hyponatremia indicates heightened free water retention to the extent that serum sodium concentrations are decreased, despite an overall excess of body-wide sodium. In both humans and veterinary patients, dilutional hyponatremia is a marker of severe neurohormonal activation and is a poor prognostic sign.[10]

MYOCARDIAL REMODELING

The pathophysiology of heart failure and its resultant morbidity and mortality are closely related to progressive alterations in cardiac structure.[11] Angiotensin II, norepinephrine, aldosterone, and other related signaling molecules cause cardiac hypertrophy and alter cardiac architecture. These changes primarily consist of two different and distinct patterns of hypertrophy. Concentric hypertrophy is the response to conditions causing pressure overload (i.e., increased afterload), as in the case of systemic hypertension or subaortic stenosis. Increased afterload triggers replication of sarcomeres in parallel, resulting in an increase in the relative thickness of the ventricular walls. Conversely, in instances of volume overload, such as mitral regurgitation or dilated cardiomyopathy, sarcomeres replicate in series leading to elongation of myocytes and dilation of the ventricular chamber. Cardiac hypertrophy is not without consequence, and the limitations of concentric hypertrophy include increased myocardial oxygen demand, endocardial ischemia, fibrosis, collagen disruption, and injury to small coronary vessels. The limitations of concentric hypertrophy include increased myocardial wall stress, myocyte injury or necrosis, and myocyte slippage. The importance of myocardial remodeling to the pathophysiology of heart disease is highlighted by the fact that interventions that reduce or reverse remodeling are associated with improved survival.[11]

ABNORMAL CALCIUM ION HANDLING

Proper cardiac contraction relies on the influx and efflux of calcium ions within the myocardial cells (Figure 38-2). During systole, calcium ions enter the myocardial cell, which triggers release of additional calcium ions from the main storage area of calcium (sarcoplasmic reticulum [SR]). Calcium stored in the SRs flows through the ryanodine channel and then binds to troponin C located on the actin and myosin complex. The binding of calcium to troponin C begins the cascade of events that result in sarcomere contraction. As soon as contraction is complete, release of calcium from troponin C initiates the relaxation cycle, and calcium ions are quickly sequestered back into the SR through the sarcoplasmic/endoplasmic reticulum Ca^{2+}-ATPase (SERCA) channel. Other effector molecules in the cytosol, such as phospholamban, help regulate the reuptake of calcium. In patients with heart disease, there are a variety of abnormalities within this system that ultimately contribute to poor global systolic and diastolic function (see Figure 38-2). Inappropriate intracellular calcium distribution can predispose the cell to electrical abnormalities, apoptosis, or necrosis.

ABNORMAL MYOCARDIAL ENERGY PRODUCTION

Myocyte mitochondria provide high-energy phosphate molecules that fuel calcium and other ion pumps, sarcomere contraction and

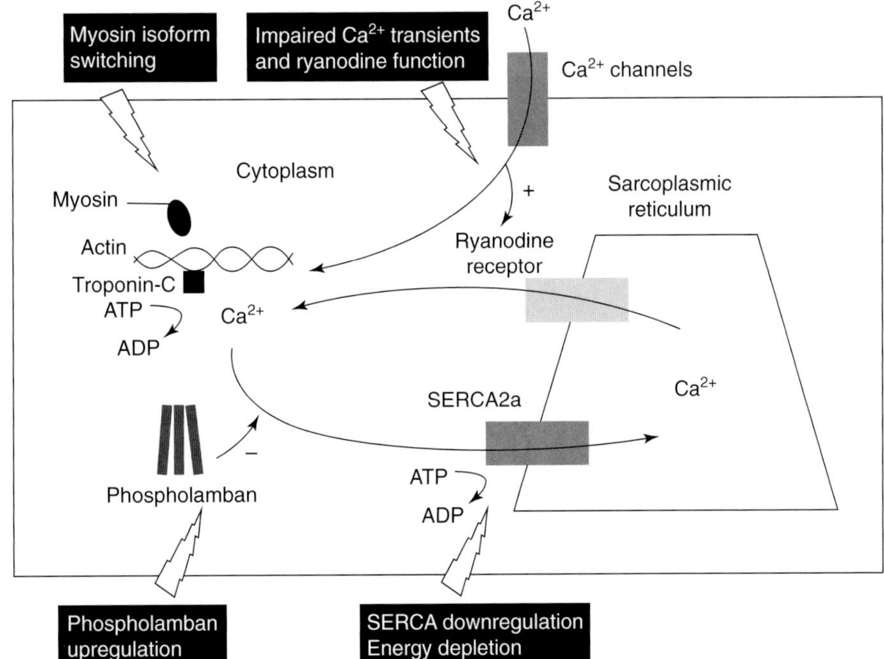

FIGURE 38-2 Myocyte calcium ion cycling in heart failure. Contraction of the actin-myosin sarcomere complex requires cytoplasmic calcium ions. These ions enter the cytoplasm partly through sarcolemmal calcium channels but mostly from intracellular calcium stores within the sarcoplasmic reticulum. Exit of calcium from the sarcoplasmic reticulum is mediated by the ryanodine receptor. Once released, the cytosolic calcium is then free to bind to troponin C located on the actin molecule. This binding initiates contraction of the sarcomere. Once contraction is complete, calcium is discharged from the troponin molecule and is taken back up into the sarcoplasmic reticulum by the ATP-dependent SERCA2a channel. Phospholamban is an intracellular calcium regulator of calcium and inhibits reuptake by SERCA2a. In animals with heart failure, numerous maladaptive changes within the calcium cycle lead to inappropriate distribution of intracellular calcium, poor sarcomeric contraction, cell injury, and apoptosis or necrosis. *SERCA,* Sarcoplasmic/endoplasmic reticulum Ca^{2+}-ATPase.

relaxation, maintenance of the resting cell membrane potential, and propagation of the cardiac action potential. In cases of severe heart disease, myocardial oxygen and substrate delivery may be decreased, resulting in ischemia and inefficient energy production via anaerobic metabolism. In dogs with myocardial disease, the oxidative phosphorylation chain located within mitochondria lack critical cytochromes and enzymes needed for energy production.[12] As its main substrate for energy production, the heart can utilize both glucose and free fatty acids. In cases of heart failure, the heart preferentially uses glucose, which requires less oxygen to metabolize than fatty acids.

GLOBAL CARDIAC FUNCTION

The Frank-Starling Mechanism as a Key to Understanding Heart Failure

The Frank-Starling mechanism describes a fundamental relationship between what is put into the heart (i.e., preload) and what comes out of the heart (i.e., cardiac output). The mechanism states that an increase in the initial volume or pressure within the ventricle increases the strength of the subsequent ventricular contraction. Thus, up to a physiologic limit, preload and contractility are positively associated. The Frank-Starling mechanism is a useful tool to describe the pathologic alternations to global cardiac function that occur in the setting of heart disease, as well as the rationale behind the use of many different cardiac medications.

In health, the heart operates within a range of preload conditions that acutely affect performance. In this way, the heart self-regulates its performance based on ventricular volume and pressure. During times of increased adrenergic drive, such as when exercising, the Frank-Starling relationship is shifted up and leftward, resulting in further improvement in cardiac performance, which is needed support the increased metabolic needs of the skeletal muscle and other organs (Figure 38-3, *A*). In conditions of disease, the Frank-Starling relationship is depressed downward and rightward so that despite fluid retention and increased preload, the subsequent contraction is less vigorous. Excessive amounts of preload produce CHF and its classic clinical signs such as shortness of breath or abdominal distention. The hearts of patients with CHF operate on a point to the far right of the disease curve (Figure 38-3, *B*). In patients with low-output heart failure, changes in preload produce an inadequate contractile response and clinical signs such as weakness, activity intolerance, or collapse predominate (Figure 38-3, *C*). In the direst of circumstances, clinical signs of both forward and backward heart failure exist simultaneously (Figure 38-3, *D*).

The Frank-Starling curve reveals why diuretics, vasodilators, and positive inotropes are used to acutely improve cardiac performance. Diuretics, by virtue of fluid loss, reduce preload and intravascular pressure, shifting the heart to the left along its curve (see Figure 38-3, *B*). This intervention alleviates signs of congestion without markedly affecting overall cardiac performance. Excessive diuresis could result in movement farther to the left and the potential to significantly reduce cardiac output. In the clinical situation this is unlikely to occur in the congested patient even with aggressive diuretic therapy. Positive inotropes, such as dobutamine, dopamine, and pimobendan, improve the contractility of the heart and shift the curve upward, resulting in improved cardiac output even as preload is reduced (see Figure 38-3, *C*). Finally, vasodilators act to either reduce afterload (arterial vasodilators) or preload (venous vasodilators). Arterial vasodilators such as amlodipine or hydralazine improve cardiac

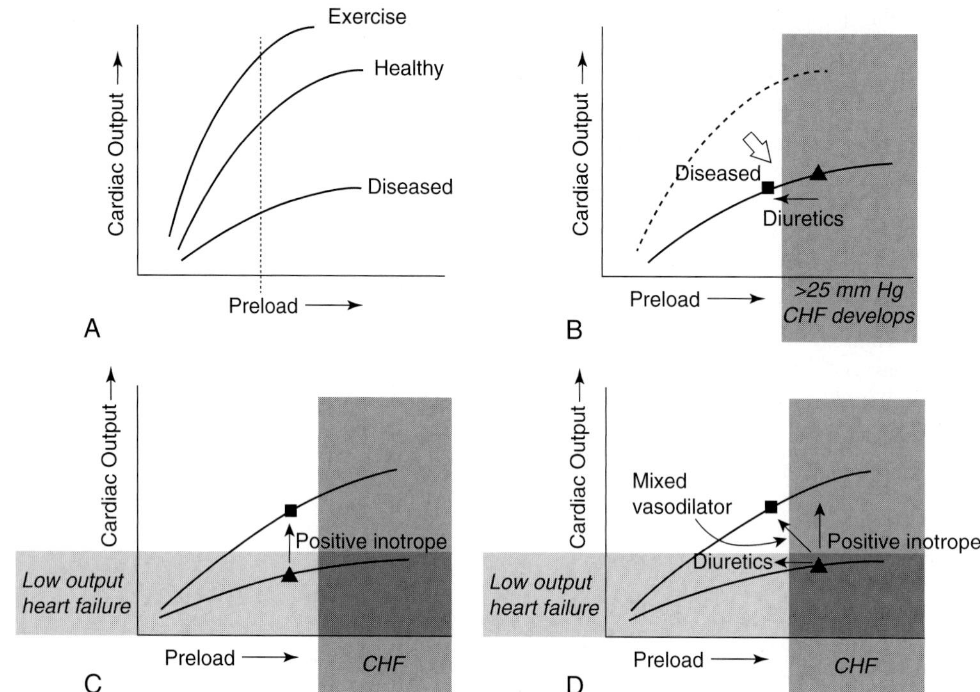

FIGURE 38-3 The Frank-Starling mechanism in health and disease. **A,** The Frank-Starling mechanism describes increased cardiac output in response to increased preload. During exercise, sympathetic tone present elevates the curve, whereas cardiac disease lowers the curve. The diseased state cardiac output at any given amount of preload is decreased. Additionally, in the diseased state, change in preload effects relatively little change in cardiac output because of the flat slope of the curve. **B,** Neurohormonal activation and excessive sodium and water retention leads to elevated intracardiac and venous pressure. Intravenous pressures greater than 25 mm Hg typically result in signs of congestion *(triangle)*. Diuretics, by reducing preload, move performance leftward along the curve and to a position below the threshold for congestion *(square)*. Because of the relatively flat slope of the curve, diuresis has relatively little detrimental effect on cardiac output. **C,** Cardiac injury can also result in low cardiac output *(triangle)*. Positive inotropic drugs shift the curve upward so that cardiac output at any given amount of preload is improved. **D,** Patients with severe heart failure can exhibit signs of both congestion and low output *(triangle)*. These patients require both diuretics and positive inotropes to improve function. Mixed vasodilators (those that provide both venous and arterial vasodilation) shift the curve both upward and leftward and are often used if systemic blood pressure will allow. CHF, Congestive heart failure.

performance by shifting the curve upward in a manner similar to a positive inotrope, whereas venous vasodilators such as nitrates reduce preload through an increase the capacitance of the venous system and shift the curve leftward, similar to diuretics. Mixed vasodilators such as ACE inhibitors result in a combination of both upward and leftward adjustment (see Figure 38-3, *D*).

Diastolic Heart Dysfunction

Many types of heart disease primarily are due to diastolic myocardial dysfunction, as opposed to systolic dysfunction. In veterinary medicine, the classic example of diastolic heart disease is hypertrophic cardiomyopathy in cats. Diastolic heart disease can be due to primary impairments of ventricular relaxation, filling, or compliance or secondary to disease of the pericardium. In the normal heart, the ventricle chamber expands readily in diastole because of high compliance (the ability of the ventricle to accommodate blood volume at a low hydrostatic filling pressure). Ventricular compliance is affected by the thickness of the ventricular wall (concentric hypertrophy decreases compliance), changes in the cytoskeleton and extracellular matrix (fibrosis decreases compliance), and function of the pericardium (pericardial disease or effusion reduces ventricular distensibility). In the early phase of diastole, relaxation requires energy as the movement of calcium ions back into the SR operates using ATP-driven pumps (see Figure 38-2). In circumstances of myocardial ischemia and energy deficit, active relaxation is delayed and early filling of the ventricle is diminished. The result of poor diastolic function is a reduction in cardiac output, which drives the same neurohormonal responses and clinical consequences that operate in systolic dysfunction. Treatment of diastolic dysfunction is targeted toward improving ventricular relaxation, increasing ventricular compliance, and alleviating any existing pericardial disease. In the absence of obvious pericardial disease, treatment focuses on increasing the time available for diastolic filling by decreasing heart rate, suppression of arrhythmias, and alleviation of congestion through the use of diuretics and vasodilators. Positive inotropes play little role in the management of diastolic dysfunction.

CLINICAL STAGING AND ASSESSMENT OF HEART FAILURE

Patients with heart disease are typically classified according to presence or absence of clinical signs and whether there is evidence of cardiac remodeling. A common veterinary staging system[13] involves four clinical classes, the first of which (Class A) describes overtly healthy animals that are at risk for developing heart disease. This class would contain, for instance, Doberman Pinschers over the age of 4 or adult Maine Coon cats. Animals in Class A have no detectable evidence of cardiac disease but might benefit from screening programs to detect the possible onset of disease as they age. Class B describes animals with diagnostic evidence of heart disease but without clinical signs, such as asymptomatic dogs with heart murmur or asymptomatic cats with an arrhythmia. Class B is further divided into Class B1, which describes patients with no radiographic or echocardiographic evidence of cardiac remodeling, and Class B2, which is the same as Class B1 but with radiographic or echocardiographic evidence of cardiac remodeling. Class C describes animals with cardiac remodeling, as well as current or historical clinical signs of heart failure, and Class D describes patients with severe and debilitating signs of heart failure even at rest. Thus the transition point between asymptomatic (preclinical) heart disease and symptomatic heart failure lies between Class B1 and Class C/D. It is important to note that not all animals in Class A will develop disease, nor will all animals in Class B suffer from sufficient severity of disease to cause clinical signs, and many animals will remain in Class A or B for the entirety of their life.

Clinical Manifestations of Heart Failure

Low output versus congestive failure

Most clinical signs of heart failure in the dog and cat involve CHF. Pulmonary venous pressures greater than 25 mm Hg and systemic venous pressures greater than 20 mm Hg are sufficient to produce congestion that manifests as pulmonary edema, pleural effusion, or ascites. Common owner complaints are increased respiratory effort and rate, coughing, activity intolerance, and abdominal distention. Peripheral edema of the limbs or subcutaneous tissues is rare in cases of CHF. In patients with severe myocardial dysfunction, cardiac performance is insufficient to provide adequate cardiac output and animals present with signs of low-output heart failure. Common clinical signs include weakness, depressed mentation, cardiac shock, and syncope. Diagnostic testing in these patients commonly reveals hypothermia, hypotension, azotemia, anuria or oliguria, and lactic acidosis. Patients with low-output heart failure require positive inotropes to improve contractility.

Left-sided versus right-sided heart failure

CHF presents as predominantly left- or right-sided failure or occasionally as biventricular failure. (See Chapters 39 to 43 for further details.) Common causes of left-sided heart failure in dogs include degenerative mitral valve disease, dilated cardiomyopathy, and patent ductus arteriosus. Common causes of left-sided heart failure in cats include hypertrophic and restrictive cardiomyopathy. In both dogs and cats pulmonary edema is exclusively a sign of left-sided heart failure. Common causes of right-sided heart failure in dogs include dilated cardiomyopathy, degenerative or congenital tricuspid valve disease, and pulmonary hypertension. In the dog, right-sided heart failure is manifest as pleural effusion or ascites, whereas in the cat, pleural effusion can occur as a result of either left- or right-sided heart failure. In the author's experience, right-sided heart failure is relatively rare in cats and most cases of cardiogenic pleural effusion in cats actually are due to left-sided disease. Ascites as a sign of right-sided heart failure in cats is relatively uncommon, and most cats with ascites are afflicted with noncardiac diseases.

REFERENCES

1. Givertz MM, Colucci WS, Braunwald E: Clinical aspects of heart failure; pulmonary edema, high-output failure. In Zipes DS, Libby P, Bonow RO, et al, editors: Heart disease: a textbook of cardiovascular medicine, ed 7, Philadelphia, 2005, Elsevier Saunders.
2. Tidholm A, Haggstrom J, Hansson K: Effects of dilated cardiomyopathy on the renin-angiotensin-aldosterone system, atrial natriuretic peptide activity, and thyroid hormone concentrations in dogs, Am J Vet Res 62:961, 2001.
3. Sisson DD: Neuroendocrine evaluation of cardiac disease, Vet Clin North Am Small Anim Pract 34:1105, 2004.
4. Haggstrom J, Hansson K, Kvart C, et al: Effects of naturally acquired decompensated mitral valve regurgitation on the renin-angiotensin-aldosterone system and atrial natriuretic peptide concentration in dogs, Am J Vet Res 58:77, 1997.
5. Fox PR, Rush JE, Reynolds CA, et al: Multicenter evaluation of plasma N-terminal probrain natriuretic peptide (NT-pro BNP) as a biochemical screening test for asymptomatic (occult) cardiomyopathy in cats, J Vet Intern Med 25:1010, 2011.
6. Oyama MA, Fox PR, Rush JE, et al: Clinical utility of serum N-terminal pro-B-type natriuretic peptide concentration for identifying cardiac disease in dogs and assessing disease severity, J Am Vet Med Assoc 232:1496, 2008.
7. Connolly DJ, Magalhaes RJ, Syme HM, et al: Circulating natriuretic peptides in cats with heart disease, J Vet Intern Med 22:96, 2008.
8. O'Sullivan ML, O'Grady MR, Minors SL: Plasma big endothelin-1, atrial natriuretic peptide, aldosterone, and norepinephrine concentrations in normal Doberman Pinschers and Doberman Pinschers with dilated cardiomyopathy, J Vet Intern Med 21:92, 2007.
9. Prosek R, Sisson DD, Oyama MA, et al: Measurements of plasma endothelin immunoreactivity in healthy cats and cats with cardiomyopathy, J Vet Intern Med 18:826, 2004.
10. Brady CA, Hughes D, Drobatz KJ: Association of hyponatremia and hyperglycemia with outcome in dogs with congestive heart failure, J Vet Emerg Crit Care 14:177, 2004.
11. Cohn JN, Ferrari R, Sharpe N: Cardiac remodeling—concepts and clinical implications: a consensus paper from an international forum on cardiac remodeling. Behalf of an International Forum on Cardiac Remodeling, J Am Coll Cardiol 35:569, 2000.
12. Lopes R, Solter PF, Sisson DD, et al: Characterization of canine mitochondrial protein expression in natural and induced forms of idiopathic dilated cardiomyopathy, Am J Vet Res 67:963, 2006.
13. Atkins C, Bonagura J, Ettinger S, et al: Guidelines for the diagnosis and treatment of canine chronic valvular heart disease, J Vet Intern Med 23:1142, 2009.

CHAPTER 39
CARDIOGENIC SHOCK

Andrew J. Brown, MA, VetMB, MRCVS, DACVECC • Deborah C. Mandell, VMD, DACVECC

KEY POINTS

- *Cardiogenic shock* is defined as inadequate cellular metabolism secondary to cardiac dysfunction, despite adequate intravascular volume.
- Clinical signs are consistent with global hypoperfusion. The aim of treatment is based on restoring cardiac output in order to normalize tissue perfusion and cellular metabolism.
- Systolic or diastolic dysfunction or arrhythmias can result in decreased stroke volume, forward flow failure, and cardiogenic shock.
- The most common cause of systolic dysfunction is dilated cardiomyopathy.
- Systolic dysfunction secondary to mechanical failure is less common. The causes include subaortic stenosis, hypertrophic obstructive cardiomyopathy, and acute mitral regurgitation secondary to ruptured chordae tendineae.
- Diastolic dysfunction can occur secondary to cardiac tamponade, hypertrophic cardiomyopathy, or tachyarrhythmias.
- Severe bradyarrhythmias such as third-degree atrioventricular block or sick sinus syndrome can lead to a severe decrease in cardiac output and thus cardiogenic shock.
- The prognosis for most forms of cardiogenic shock is guarded. A rapid diagnosis and appropriate therapeutic intervention(s) will enhance success.

Cardiogenic shock is defined as inadequate cellular metabolism secondary to cardiac dysfunction when there is adequate intravascular volume. It is a life-threatening emergency and must be recognized, diagnosed, and treated as soon as possible.

The etiology of cardiogenic shock is wide ranging and varied. Consequently diagnostic modalities, case management, and definitive therapy vary with the cause. Diagnosis is based on clinical demonstration of shock along with evidence of cardiac dysfunction. Ultimately, the aim of treatment is based on restoring cardiac output in order to normalize tissue perfusion and cellular metabolism.

PATHOPHYSIOLOGY

Shock is defined as inadequate cellular energy production. It can have multiple classifications, such as distributive, metabolic, hypoxic, or cardiogenic. Decreased tissue perfusion and subsequent inadequate metabolism and energy production at the cellular level will occur when cardiac output is reduced. This occurs most commonly as a result of inadequate intravascular volume or hypovolemic shock (classified under distributive shock; see Chapter 5). In the face of adequate intravascular volume, but reduced cardiac output from cardiac dysfunction, a patient has forward flow failure. When this forward flow failure is sufficient to cause inadequate tissue perfusion despite an adequate intravascular volume, the patient has cardiogenic shock. Heart failure can be classified as forward or backward ventricular failure. Backward flow failure occurs secondary to elevated venous pressures, and left ventricular failure (forward flow failure) occurs secondary to reduced forward flow into the aorta and systemic circulation (see Chapters 38 and 40).

Cardiac output is a product of stroke volume (SV) and heart rate (HR): SV × HR. A decrease in either stroke volume or heart rate can therefore lead to a reduction in cardiac output. The normal physiologic response to a decrease in stroke volume is a compensatory increase in heart rate (and systemic vascular resistance) to maintain cardiac output. This is due to a baroreceptor-mediated sympathetic stimulation to preserve blood pressure and tissue perfusion. A decrease in stroke volume that cannot be compensated for by a further increase in heart rate will lead to reduced cardiac output and forward flow failure. Similarly, forward failure may result from a severe decrease in heart rate without a primary decrease in stroke volume. Cardiogenic shock will ensue if the forward flow failure leads to decreased tissue perfusion that does not meet cellular energy demands.

Stroke volume is determined by preload, afterload, and contractility. Cardiogenic shock can ensue from alterations in any of these. For the purpose of this chapter, the cardiac cycle will be split into systole and diastole; compromise to either phase may result in a decreased stroke volume and cardiogenic shock.

In addition to the reflex increase in heart rate, strategies exist within the body to ensure normal tissue perfusion. In response to cardiac dysfunction–induced hypotension, neurohormonal mechanisms (e.g., renin-angiotensin-aldosterone system) increase the effective circulating volume (see Chapter 8). This increases preload, stroke volume, and therefore cardiac output and enables the animal to maintain a normal blood pressure. As a result, forward failure in patients with chronic cardiac conditions is rare. Most patients deteriorate secondary to the increase in preload and subsequent congestive (backward) heart failure and pulmonary edema. Examples of this include chronic valvular disease in dogs and hypertrophic cardiomyopathy in cats. Some patients may suffer from concurrent forward and backward failure (e.g., dogs with dilated cardiomyopathy).

Patients that demonstrate an acute decrease in cardiac output do not have time to compensate and, as a consequence, abruptly develop cardiogenic shock (e.g., acute pericardial effusion with cardiac tamponade). These animals commonly have signs consistent with cardiogenic shock (forward failure) but may also have evidence of right-sided backward failure (e.g., ascites).

A sustained decrease in cardiac output will eventually lead to organ dysfunction. Reduced coronary blood flow may result in arrhythmias or decreased contractility and will exacerbate existing cardiac dysfunction. Inadequate renal perfusion will lead to acute kidney injury, and decreased gastrointestinal perfusion may cause mucosal sloughing and hemorrhagic diarrhea.

CLINICAL SIGNS AND DIAGNOSIS

Cardiogenic shock is an extreme manifestation of forward failure, and clinical signs will reflect this state. Diagnosis is based on clinical evidence of shock and cardiac dysfunction. It is important to realize that there is overlap among the different classes of shock and that a definitive diagnosis can sometimes be difficult to ascertain.

Clinical signs are consistent with global hypoperfusion. A patient with cardiogenic shock will have a change in mentation manifested as depression, unresponsiveness, or disorientation. Peripheral extremities will be cold to the touch and the mucous membranes pale, with a prolonged capillary refill time caused by intense vasoconstriction (see Chapter 5). If the patient has backward failure and congestive heart failure, then parenchymal (pulmonary edema) or pleural space disease may result in tachypnea, dyspnea, and cyanosis. There may also be a compensatory respiratory alkalosis in response to a lactic acidosis.

The heart rate should be elevated in animals with cardiogenic shock unless a primary bradyarrhythmia is the cause of the cardiogenic shock or the patient is moribund. The tachycardia will be due either to an appropriate sympathetic response to hypotension or concurrent congestive heart failure (CHF) or may be a malignant arrhythmia (ventricular or supraventricular tachycardia) that is not allowing adequate diastolic filling and is the primary cause of cardiogenic shock. Correction of the malignant tachycardia in the latter case will likely improve stroke volume and cardiac output, whereas antiarrhythmic therapy for the compensatory tachycardia is contraindicated and the underlying cause should be addressed. This distinction can sometimes be difficult, and careful evaluation of the electrocardiogram and patient's volume status is necessary.

Careful auscultation of the heart and lungs should be performed. If the heart sounds are difficult to auscult, pericardial effusion should be considered, although the clinician should not forget other causes of quiet heart sounds (i.e., severe hypovolemia and obesity). If the patient has congestive heart failure, inspiratory crackles secondary to pulmonary edema may be heard on auscultation of the lungs or the lungs may be quiet ventrally as a result of pleural effusion. A murmur or gallop may also be ausculted, and although extracardiac ruleouts for a heart murmur should be considered, this may provide further evidence for cardiac disease. "Synchronous" peripheral pulse palpation and cardiac auscultation should be performed to detect pulse deficits or arrhythmias.

Renal blood flow will be reduced with cardiogenic shock and may result in azotemia, with or without oliguria or anuria. Gastrointestinal tract perfusion will also be reduced and may lead to vomiting and hemorrhagic diarrhea.

Venous blood gas analysis often reveals a metabolic acidosis. Inadequate cellular oxygenation may result in anaerobic metabolism and a lactic acidosis. Prerenal or renal azotemia may also contribute to the metabolic acidosis. The patient will usually have a compensatory respiratory alkalosis. If the patient has concurrent pulmonary edema, the alveolar-arteriolar (A-a) gradient will likely be increased on an arterial blood gas analysis (see Chapters 15 and 186).

An electrocardiogram should be performed on all patients that are in shock. Animals in cardiogenic shock may have a sinus tachycardia, bradyarrhythmia (e.g., atrioventricular [AV] block), or tachyarrhythmia such as atrial fibrillation or ventricular tachycardia. It is important to remember that patients with other causes of shock (e.g., distributive or hypoxic) can also have cardiac arrhythmias.

Chest radiographs should be performed when the patient is stable enough to withstand the stress of restraint and may help to rule out cardiac disease as the primary cause of shock. There may be an abnormality in the cardiac silhouette and evidence of congestive heart failure. Radiographic signs of CHF include enlarged pulmonary veins, an alveolar or interstitial pattern in the perihilar region (in dogs only; infiltrates are often patchy or diffuse in cats), and pleural effusion. However, it is important to remember that many animals in shock will have incidental cardiac disease that is not contributing to morbidity. Information derived from radiographs and the electrocardiogram will not enable the clinician to definitively diagnose cardiogenic shock; rather, it should be interpreted in conjunction with clinical findings and results of other diagnostic tests (i.e., radiographs and echocardiogram).

Echocardiographic findings will vary depending on the underlying cause of cardiogenic shock. Congenital or acquired structural abnormalities, along with changes in cardiac chamber size or myocardial thickness, may be described. Pressure gradients, blood flow, and an assessment of systolic and diastolic function can be obtained. A diagnosis of cardiogenic shock may be made if there is evidence of systolic dysfunction in the presence of adequate end-diastolic volume.

Even with advanced diagnostic imaging, the diagnosis of cardiogenic shock can still be difficult. A pulmonary arterial catheter (see Chapter 202) can be placed to aid in both diagnosis and monitoring. A patient with cardiogenic shock will have a decreased cardiac output with an increase in the preload parameters of central venous pressure, pulmonary arterial pressure, and pulmonary arterial occlusion (wedge) pressure. This catheter can be helpful for obtaining a diagnosis, guiding therapy, and monitoring the response to treatment.

SYSTOLIC DYSFUNCTION

Systolic dysfunction can result from a decrease in cardiac contractility or decreased flow through the left ventricular outflow tract (mechanical failure). The latter may be due to a functional obstruction (e.g., aortic stenosis or hypertrophic obstructive cardiomyopathy) or severe retrograde blood flow (e.g., chordae tendineae rupture and acute, severe mitral regurgitation; see Chapter 40).

Failure of Contractility

Dilated cardiomyopathy

The most common cause of cardiogenic shock resulting from systolic dysfunction is dilated cardiomyopathy (DCM) (see Chapter 42). This condition is most commonly seen in dogs (Doberman Pinscher, Boxer, Great Dane, Labrador Retriever, American Cocker Spaniel[1]) and is rarely seen in cats (except those with taurine deficiency). A progressive decrease in myocardial contractility that typically occurs over months to years results in a gradual decrease in stroke volume and forward failure. Activation of the renin-angiotensin system and sympathetic nervous system will stimulate renal retention of sodium and water. The increased intravascular volume results in increased end-diastolic volume. Eccentric hypertrophy occurs secondary to cardiac myocardial stretch. These compensatory mechanisms will maintain cardiac output until the myocardial failure becomes so severe that the cardiac chambers cannot sustain further enlargement. Any further increase in intravascular volume will result in an increased end-diastolic pressure, leading to an increase in pulmonary capillary hydrostatic pressure and cardiogenic pulmonary edema (with left-sided heart failure) or ascites (with right-sided heart failure).

Diagnosis of cardiogenic shock in dogs with DCM is made based on signs consistent with shock (see Clinical Signs and Diagnosis earlier in chapter) and cardiac dysfunction. Thoracic radiographs may reveal an enlarged heart along with evidence of CHF if present. An electrocardiogram may show a sinus tachycardia or arrhythmias such as atrial fibrillation or ventricular tachycardia.

An echocardiogram will demonstrate an enlarged and dilated heart with poor contractility. Valuable information can be gained from a pulmonary arterial catheter (see Chapters 202 and 184, Cardiac Output Monitoring). This catheter will enable the clinician to measure cardiac output, as well as determine preload parameters such as central venous pressure, pulmonary arterial pressure, and pulmonary arterial occlusion (wedge) pressure. This can help in the diagnosis, prognosis, and treatment of these patients.

The aim of treating patients with systolic dysfunction is to maximize cardiac output by increasing stroke volume. Preload parameters should be monitored closely and fluids given only if necessary, or diuretics administered if the dog has left-sided congestive heart failure (see Chapter 160). Positive inotropic agents such as the β_1-adrenergic receptor agonist dobutamine (see Chapter 157), phosphodiesterase inhibitors such as amrinone, pimobendan, or cardiac glycosides such as digoxin (see Chapters 40 and 42) can be titrated to optimize stroke volume. Optimal positive inotropic therapy has not been determined in human or veterinary medicine, and newer agents such as the calcium-sensitizing agent levosimendan are also being investigated.[2]

Sepsis

Studies in both humans and dogs have documented a dysfunctional myocardium in sepsis. Even during the hyperdynamic phase of septic shock (see Chapter 91) with increased cardiac output, a decrease in ejection fraction has been documented. A reduction in ventricular compliance, biventricular dilation, and decrease in contractile function all contribute to the decrease in ejection fraction.[3] In an experimental model of septic shock, dogs in the hyperdynamic phase (with an increased cardiac output) had decreased contractility and left ventricular dilation.[3] Myocardial dysfunction peaks within days of the onset of sepsis and has been shown to resolve within 7 to 10 days in patients who survive.[4] Low cardiac output is rare in patients with septic shock but often is due to end-stage decompensated myocardial depression.

Endomyocarditis

Endomyocarditis is a rare condition of cats that occurs several days after a routine procedure such as neutering (see Chapter 98). Cats have normal myocardial function before the anesthesia and the procedure is usually uneventful, but cardiac dysfunction, hypotension, pulmonary edema, and interstitial pneumonia rapidly develop. Although not well described, the endocardium is hyperechoic on echocardiography, and histopathology reveals neutrophilic inflammation and fibroplasia.[5] Supportive care is recommended, and even with positive pressure ventilation the prognosis is often poor.

Myocardial infarction

Myocardial infarction is the number one cause of cardiogenic shock in humans but is rarely seen (or recognized) in dogs and cats (see Chapter 40).

Mechanical Failure

Cardiogenic shock resulting from mechanical failure is rare in dogs and cats. Forward flow can be reduced by an obstruction to the left ventricular outflow tract (e.g., aortic stenosis or hypertrophic obstructive cardiomyopathy) or by severe acute retrograde blood flow as may occur with a chordae tendineae rupture.

Dogs with mitral endocardiosis and associated regurgitant flows typically have normal to increased myocardial contractility. However, chordae tendineae rupture leads to acute and extensive mitral regurgitation that commonly reduces forward flow sufficiently to result in cardiogenic shock and pulmonary edema.

DIASTOLIC FAILURE

Diastolic failure is due to inadequate ventricular filling. This can result from hypovolemia, a physical restriction (cardiac tamponade), inability of the myocardium to relax (hypertrophic cardiomyopathy), or inadequate time for filling (tachycardia). Diastolic failure will result in a decreased preload and therefore a reduced stroke volume. If the animal is unable to maintain cardiac output with an increase in heart rate, cardiogenic shock ensues.

The most common cause of a decreased preload resulting in an inadequate cardiac output is hypovolemia. This is corrected by restoration of intravascular volume and is therefore not truly cardiogenic shock (see Chapters 5 and 60).

Cardiac Tamponade

Diastolic ventricular filling will be impaired because of the physical restriction that occurs with cardiac tamponade. Cardiac tamponade occurs secondary to pericardial effusion (see Chapter 45). Effusions are most likely a result of neoplasia but can also be secondary to a coagulopathy, trauma, an atrial tear, or an idiopathic cause. The decreased diastolic ventricular filling will lead to a decrease in stroke volume and cardiac output. In an attempt to maintain normotension and tissue perfusion, a reflex tachycardia will ensue. Eventually the increase in heart rate will not be sufficient to maintain an adequate cardiac output and the patient will become hypotensive. Cardiac auscultation often reveals quiet or absent heart sounds, leading to a high index of suspicion of pericardial effusion; confirmation can be made quickly with ultrasonography. Despite the improved ability to visualize the heart in the presence of a pericardial effusion, a thorough echocardiogram should not be performed if a patient has cardiogenic shock. The reduced cardiac output will result in decreased tissue perfusion and a lactic acidosis. If the effusion is chronic, the patient may have decreased sodium and increased potassium concentrations from a reduced effective circulating volume–induced pseudohypoadrenocorticism. Because the systemic manifestations of this condition result from the decreased preload, increasing intravascular volume with a fluid bolus is warranted. However, emergency pericardiocentesis to allow for normal ventricular filling is also necessary to treat the cardiogenic shock. Pericardiocentesis in patients with coagulopathies or in dogs with a pericardial effusion secondary to an atrial tear is contraindicated, although the consequences of fulminant cardiogenic shock must be weighed against the risk of exsanguination.

Hypertrophic Cardiomyopathy

Failure of normal end-diastolic volume can occur secondary to an intrinsic inability of the myocardium to relax (e.g., hypertrophic cardiomyopathy). Hypertrophic cardiomyopathy (see Chapter 41) is the most commonly diagnosed feline cardiac disease and is characterized by concentric hypertrophy of the ventricular myocardium. Decreased end-diastolic ventricular volume (because of the inability of the myocardium to relax) leads to a decreased stroke volume and cardiac output. Activation of neurohormonal mechanisms will increase the intravascular volume to protect against hypotension and decreased tissue perfusion. Systolic function will normally remain adequate, and patients typically have backward (rather than forward) flow failure. However, cats with CHF that receive overzealous diuretic therapy can progress easily to hypovolemic (distributive) shock. In addition, cats with end-stage hypertrophic cardiomyopathy may also have severely impaired systolic function, leading to decreased stroke volume and cardiogenic shock. Treatment of cats with hypertrophic cardiomyopathy includes the use of β-blockers or calcium channel antagonists in an attempt to enhance lusitropy and diastolic filling (see Chapter 41).

Tachyarrhythmias

Inadequate ventricular filling occurs at elevated heart rates. End-diastolic volume is largely dependent on venous return, with atrial contraction contributing little to normal preload. When patients

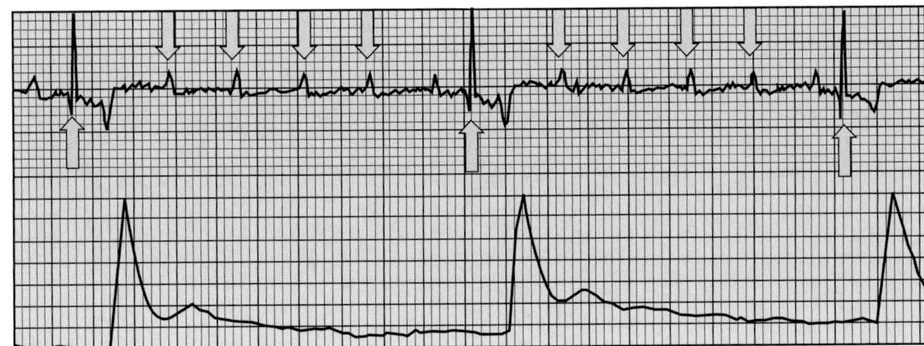

FIGURE 39-1 A lead II electrocardiogram at 25 mm/s with simultaneous arterial waveform of a patient with second-degree atrioventricular block. There are normal conducted QRS complexes *(up arrows)* with concurrent arterial pulses and nonconducted P waves *(down arrows)* with no associated cardiac output, as evidenced by an absence of an arterial pulse waveform.

become tachycardic (e.g., dogs with a heart rate over 200 beats/min), there is inadequate time for diastolic filling to occur before systole. As a result, end-diastolic volume and therefore stroke volume and cardiac output are reduced. The most common cause of this malignant tachycardia is a supraventricular tachycardia (see Chapter 47). This can be a result of primary cardiac disease or a cardiac manifestation of another systemic disease process. Therapy includes vagal maneuvers, calcium channel antagonists, and β-blockers to slow the heart rate, as well as management of the underlying condition (see Chapter 171).

BRADYARRHYTHMIAS

Severe bradycardia can lead to such a decrease in cardiac output that cardiogenic shock ensues. The most common cause of this is severe high-grade second-degree AV block (Figure 39-1) or third-degree AV block. Animals with severe sick sinus syndrome can also suffer from decreased tissue perfusion and shock. In patients with third-degree AV block, AV nodal conduction does not occur and escape complexes from the bundle of His, bundle branches, or Purkinje fibers induce cardiac contraction. Extranodal heart rates are much slower than normal, with the bundle of His producing 40 to 60 beats/min and ectopic beats from the bundle branches or distal Purkinje fibers producing 20 to 40 beats/min. Higher escape rates will be adequate for dogs at rest, but slower rates will result in a reduced cardiac output. An increase in stroke volume will occur secondary to an increased preload (because of the increased time for diastolic filling), but at low heart rates or during patient exertion, the cardiac output may be inadequate and cardiogenic shock will ensue. Cats with third-degree AV block typically have a higher ventricular escape rhythm of 100 to 140 beat/min and thus less commonly present for cardiogenic shock or syncope.[6]

Diagnosis can be made on the basis of the electrocardiographic evidence of severe second-degree or third-degree AV block or sick sinus syndrome and other signs consistent with shock (see Clinical Signs and Diagnosis earlier in this chapter). Blood pressure may be normal, but it is important to remember that blood pressure does not equal flow or perfusion. Second-degree AV block can be vagally mediated or secondary to sinoatrial or AV nodal pathology. An atropine response test (0.02 to 0.04 mg/kg intravenously [IV]) is warranted in all cases (lower doses generally suffice). A β agonist such as isoproterenol or dobutamine can be given as a constant rate infusion and will sometimes increase the heart rate sufficiently to treat the cardiogenic shock (see Chapter 157). If there is no response to medical therapy, the patient should have artificial cardiac pacing. This can be achieved by transthoracic pacing of the sedated patient or by placing an emergency temporary pacemaker. Intravenous fluids are contraindicated in these cases until a normal heart rate has been achieved, because preload is already increased and a further increase in left ventricular filling pressures may result in congestive (backward) heart failure.

REFERENCES

1. Kittleson MD, Kienle RD: Small animal cardiovascular medicine, ed 1, St Louis, 1998, Mosby.
2. Huang L, Weil MH, Tang W, et al: Comparison between dobutamine and levosimendan for treatment of postresuscitation myocardial dysfunction, Crit Care Med 33:487, 2005.
3. Natanson C, Fink MP, Ballantyne HK, et al: Gram-negative bacteremia produces both severe systolic and diastolic cardiac dysfunction in a canine model that simulates human septic shock, J Clin Invest 78:259, 1986.
4. Kumar A, Haery C, Parrillo JE: Myocardial dysfunction in septic shock: part I. Clinical manifestation of cardiovascular dysfunction, J Cardiothorac Vasc Anesth 15:364, 2001.
5. Stalis IH, Bossbaly MJ, Van Winkle TJ: Feline endomyocarditis and left ventricular endocardial fibrosis, Vet Pathol 32:122, 1995.
6. Kellum HB, Stepien RL: Third-degree atrioventricular block in 21 cats (1997-2004), J Vet Intern Med 20:97, 2006.

CHAPTER 40

VENTRICULAR FAILURE AND MYOCARDIAL INFARCTION

Maggie C. Machen, DVM • Meg Sleeper, VMD, DACVIM (Cardiology)

KEY POINTS

- Left ventricular failure can lead to decreased cardiac output and pulmonary edema and in many cases will be associated with arrhythmias.
- The primary aims of managing ventricular failure are to support contractility, relieve signs of congestion and suppress arrhythmias.
- Myocardial infarction is a rare occurrence in canine and feline patients.

BASIC TERMINOLOGY

The basic terminology of ventricular failure and myocardial infarction is summarized in the following list:

Heart failure: The pathophysiologic state in which the heart is unable to pump sufficient blood to meet the metabolic demands of the tissue while maintaining normal arterial and venous pressures.

Systolic heart failure: A defect in the pumping or contractile function of the heart.

Diastolic heart failure: A defect in the filling or relaxation function of the heart.

Congestive heart failure: The clinical syndrome that results when abnormal cardiac function causes accumulation and retention of fluid, resulting in signs of congestion and edema.

Forward heart failure: Decreased cardiac output results in inadequate delivery of blood to the arterial system, leading to diminished organ and muscle perfusion. As a result of reduced renal perfusion, plasma volume and extracellular fluid accumulate, leading to congestion of organs and tissues.[1] One example of a cause of forward failure is dilated cardiomyopathy.

Backward heart failure: Elevated filling pressure causes increased pressure within the left atrium and the pulmonary vasculature draining into the left atrium. This results in elevated capillary hydrostatic pressure, transudation of fluid into the interstitium, and pulmonary edema. If right-sided heart disease is present and right atrial pressure is increased, the same process can lead to elevated systemic venous pressure and ultimately ascites and subcutaneous edema.[1] One example of a cause of backward failure is degenerative valve disease.

Circulatory failure: When the delivery of oxygenated blood is insufficient to meet the metabolic demands of the body tissue.

CAUSES OF VENTRICULAR (SYSTOLIC) FAILURE

Primary Causes

Ventricular failure can be primary in origin, most commonly caused by dilated cardiomyopathy (DCM) affecting the left ventricle (LV) or by arrhythmogenic right ventricular cardiomyopathy (ARVC) affecting the right ventricle (Box 40-1). Clinical presentation depends on the stage of disease, and many animals with primary ventricular failure may remain asymptomatic for years. DCM and ARVC are discussed at length in Chapter 42.

BOX 40-1 ***Examples of Common Causes of Ventricular Failure***

Primary

- Left ventricular failure: dilated cardiomyopathy (DCM)
- Right ventricular failure: arrhythmogenic right ventricular cardiomyopathy (ARVC)

Secondary to Other Cardiac Disease

- Advanced degenerative valve disease with systolic dysfunction
- Tachycardia-induced cardiomyopathy

Extracardiac

- Sepsis
- Adriamycin toxicity
- Malnutrition

Secondary to Other Cardiac Disease

Ventricular failure can develop as a result of other cardiac diseases, either secondary to chronic pressure or volume overload. Untreated congenital diseases such as patent ductus arteriosus or ventricular septal defects result in chronic volume overload of the left side of the heart. The resultant eccentric hypertrophy, myocardial fibrosis, and decreased cardiac perfusion over time can lead to systolic dysfunction. Volume overload caused by acquired disease such as chronic degenerative valve disease (CVD) can also lead to systolic dysfunction. This sequela occurs more commonly in large breed dogs with CVD, for reasons that are not understood, and very rarely in small breeds (in which systolic function is often preserved until very late in the disease).

In cats, ventricular failure is most often seen with restrictive or unclassified cardiomyopathy. It is important to note that most cats presenting with congestive heart failure (CHF) do not have underlying systolic failure. For example, in a cat presenting with pleural effusion or pulmonary edema secondary to hypertrophic cardiomyopathy (HCM), congestive heart failure occurs because of elevated ventricular filling pressure caused by diastolic dysfunction. These cases rarely develop systolic dysfunction, and positive inotropes are actually contraindicated. In the rare feline cases of HCM that do develop systolic failure, a common cause is infarcted regions of myocardium that negatively affect regional myocardial function. For a full discussion of feline cardiomyopathy, refer to Chapter 41.

Chronic sustained tachycardia can also result in LV dysfunction and congestive heart failure. Tachycardia-induced cardiomyopathy is caused by persistent supraventricular or ventricular tachyarrhythmias and is characterized by systolic dysfunction and ventricular dilation.[2] In most instances, rate and rhythm control will result in improved myocardial function and associated clinical signs.

Extracardiac Causes

Systolic dysfunction can also develop secondary to several extracardiac disease processes. Sepsis can lead to myocardial depression, for reasons not completely understood. Myocardial depression occurs in almost 40% of septic human patients.[3] A circulating myocardial depressant in septic shock has long been proposed, and potential candidates include cytokines, prostanoids, and nitric oxide.[4] Other factors, such as decreased preload and systemic vasodilation, may contribute as well.

Certain drugs, such as anthracyclines (e.g., doxorubicin), are also known to be cardiotoxic and can result in left ventricular failure with chronic use (see Chapter 49 for a full discussion). Chronic severe nutritional deficiencies in taurine, L-carnitine, and vitamin E/selenium or vegan diets can result in systolic failure (see Chapter 42). Myocarditis, or inflammation affecting the heart, may cause ventricular dysfunction and is discussed in Chapter 49. Myocarditis may be infectious (e.g., viral, bacterial, tickborne) or secondary to cardiotoxic drugs (e.g., anthracyclines).

Myocardial Infarction

Although myocardial infarction (MI) is a leading cause of cardiovascular disease and death in humans, it is a relatively rare finding in small animal patients. Infarcts more commonly result secondary to systemic diseases that cause a hypercoagulable or hypofibrinolytic state.[5] The wide array of associated conditions includes neoplasia, disseminated intravascular coagulation, sepsis, hyperadrenocorticism, and glucocorticoid use.[5] Readers are directed to Chapter 104 for further discussion of hypercoagulable states. As mentioned earlier, MI can also be associated with end-stage feline or canine cardiomyopathies.

PHYSICAL EXAMINATION

Similar to the diagnostic tests discussed later, physical examination findings are highly dependent on the stage of disease, and animals in the occult phase of cardiac disease may have no obvious abnormalities. As left-sided occult disease progresses, subtle findings such as weak femoral pulse quality as a result of decreased cardiac output may be noted by the astute clinician. As LV dilation worsens and results in stretching of the mitral valve annulus, a soft left-apical murmur may develop because of mitral regurgitation. Ventricular ectopy with concurrent pulse deficits may also be noted with palpation of the pulses during auscultation. Once the patient has clinical signs of left-sided heart failure, there is respiratory compromise, varying from an occasional cough to tachypnea or dyspnea; in severe cases of fulminant edema, liquid or foam can be seen coming from the airway. Once in congestive heart failure, tachycardia caused by sympathetic drive can often help differentiate cardiogenic edema from other causes of respiratory distress. Some physical examination findings unique to right-sided congestion include development of jugular distention or pulsation and, possibly, signs of fluid accumulation either in the pleural space or the abdomen. All these physical examination findings should be evaluated in the greater context of the patient's presentation and history. For instance, a patient with suspected sepsis or myocarditis would also be expected to be lethargic and febrile.

DIAGNOSTIC TESTS

Although electrocardiography (ECG) is the gold standard for diagnosing arrhythmias or conduction disturbances, it provides no information regarding systolic function. Depending on the underlying cause of dysfunction and secondary compensatory changes, ECGs can give useful information regarding cardiac chamber enlargement should it be present. With ventricular hypertrophy the QRS may be prolonged, and with left-sided heart disease leads I, II, III and aVF often have tall R waves indicative of the increased LV mass. With right ventricular hypertrophy, the QRS complex is likely to have late negative deflections in leads I, II, III, and aVF, consistent with a rightward-shifted mean electrical axis. More importantly, many animals with ventricular failure may develop arrhythmias ranging from ventricular ectopy to conduction disturbances such as atrioventricular (AV) blocks or bundle branch blocks (depending on the underlying cause), ST segment changes, and so on. In severe cases, potentially life-threatening ventricular tachycardia may develop.

Thoracic radiographs (CXR) may be useful, depending on the phase of failure and the presenting complaint. Thoracic radiographs are the diagnostic tool of choice to confirm the presence of left-sided congestive heart failure (pulmonary edema). However, if a patient is in early systolic failure, the heart size and lungs may appear normal. This information may, in itself, be useful because cardiac disease would be unlikely to manifest in clinical signs with a normal vertebral heart size (VHS) (Figure 40-1) and clear lung fields.[6] This would not, of course, rule out an arrhythmia as a cause of clinical signs. Also, malignant arrhythmias may develop before the development of cardiomegaly or CHF. On the other hand, suspected dysfunction secondary to sepsis would be difficult to rule out based on normal thoracic radiographs given the acute nature of the dysfunction. (There is often insufficient time for cardiac dilation or hypertrophy, so heart size may be normal on CXR.)

Whatever the cause of dysfunction, as it progresses the appearance of CXR vary depending on whether the disease primarily affects the right or left side of the heart. With left-sided ventricular failure, classic cardiac findings include an increased VHS with dorsal elevation of the trachea caused by left atrial enlargement. Before or during an episode of CHF (as pulmonary venous pressure increases), pulmonary venous enlargement will develop, and eventually edema can be seen as an alveolar or interstitial pattern in the caudodorsal or

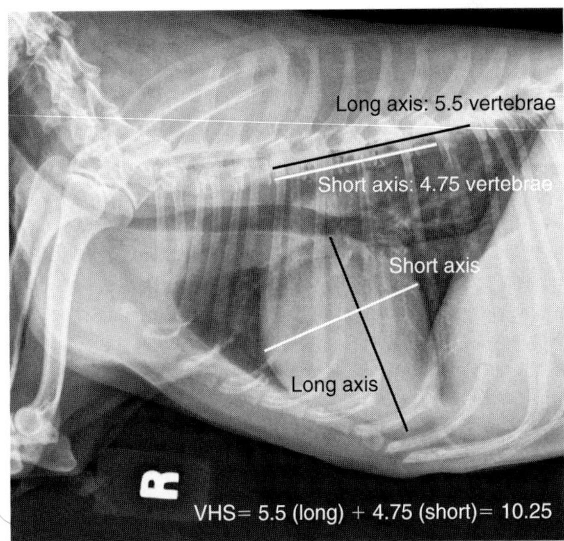

FIGURE 40-1 The vertebral heart size (VHS) calculation is determined by measuring the long axis and short axis of the heart as shown. These measurements are then evaluated as vertebral lengths, starting from the cranial border of the fourth thoracic vertebrae (as shown). The sum of the long axis and short axis, measured in vertebral lengths gives the VHS. For example, the VHS of the example shown is 5.5 + 4.75 = 10.25.
Normal VHS values:
Dog: <10.7 (for most breeds)
Cat: <8.0

perihilar lung fields. With right-sided disease such as ARVC, right-sided heart enlargement (which radiographically appears as a reverse-D cardiac silhouette on the DV or VD projection and increased sternal contact on the lateral projection) will develop before right-sided congestive signs such as enlargement of the caudal vena cava and ascites or pleural effusion.

The gold standard for diagnosis of systolic failure is echocardiography. Independent of disease stage or underlying cause, ventricular dilation and decreased systolic function (increase in ventricular end-systolic dimension) will be apparent. Decreased motion of the interventricular septum or free wall may also be seen. With concurrent congestive heart failure, atrial enlargement and dilation of the pulmonary veins would also be expected.

Biochemical screening abnormalities are highly dependent on the underlying cause. In regards to cardiac specific tests, biomarkers may be of some use for diagnosis of ventricular failure. B-type natriuretic peptide (BNP) is produced by myocardial tissue in response to increased pressure and wall stress and is a marker for cardiac dysfunction and heart failure. N-terminal–proBNP (NT-proBNP) may be useful to screen dogs with suspect occult systolic dysfunction.[7] Cardiac troponin (cTn) is a myofibrillar protein with two diagnostically relevant forms (cTnI and cTnT) that regulate contraction of the heart.[8] Blood concentrations of cTnI rise rapidly after cardiomyocyte damage, and assay of cTnI may be valuable in clinical diseases resulting in myocardial cell damage, such as myocarditis.[9]

PATHOPHYSIOLOGY

Once a patient develops forward heart failure with clinical signs of congestion and low cardiac output, treatment can be approached using Starling's curve (Figure 40-2). In a normal heart, as preload increases, cardiac performance also increases. However, at a certain point performance plateaus and then declines as preload continues to increase. In ventricular failure, the overall curve shifts downward, reflecting reduced cardiac performance at any given preload, and as preload increases, cardiac performance increases less. Moreover, as the heart dilates because of increased preload or the underlying cardiac disease, wall stress increases. As described by Laplace's law (wall stress = [pressure × radius] / 2 [wall thickness]), as the ventricle dilates, the resultant end-systolic and end-diastolic volumes cause increased wall stress throughout the entire cardiac cycle. Also, at any given left ventricular size (radius), the greater the developed pressure, the greater the wall stress. Increased wall stress caused by either of these mechanisms will increase the myocardial oxygen requirement and result in more myocardial energy expenditure.[10]

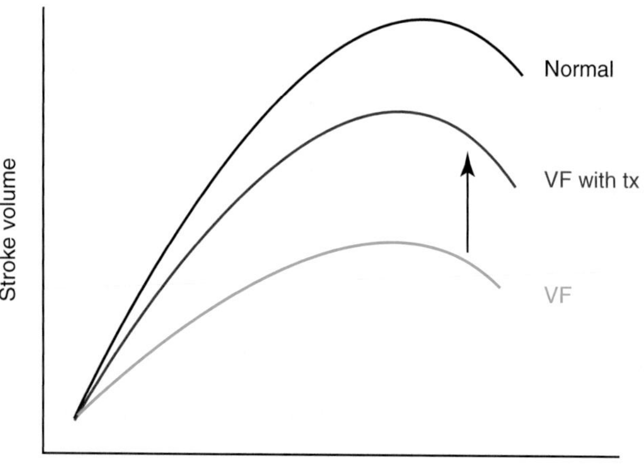

FIGURE 40-2 As described by the Frank-Starling mechanism, in a normal heart an increase in preload results in an increase in contractility, the result being a greater stroke volume *(normal curve)*. However, at a certain point performance plateaus, then declines. In ventricular failure (VF), the overall curve shifts downward, reflecting reduced contractility and stroke volume at any given preload. As preload increases, output increases less *(blue curve)*. With treatment (Tx), performance is improved, although not normalized *(red curve)*.

To summarize, the body's main compensatory mechanisms for cardiac dysfunction result in fluid retention to increase preload and sympathetic stimulation to increase heart rate and cardiac output. (See Chapter 38 for further discussion of the pathophysiology of heart failure.) Although these compensatory mechanisms are initially beneficial for increasing cardiac output, chronic sympathetic stimulation and fluid retention (increased blood volume) have deleterious results (e.g., increased myocardial energy usage, etc.). The goals of treatment in forward heart failure include supporting cardiac contractility and systemic blood pressure, relieving signs of congestion, and suppressing arrhythmias, collectively maximizing cardiac output. With treatment, cardiac performance is improved, although not normalized unless the underlying cause can be addressed directly. For all inotropic drugs discussed in the next section, specific drug information is listed in Table 40-1.

TREATMENT

Supporting Contractility and Maintaining Blood Pressure

Positive inotropic support is essential for ventricular (systolic) failure of any cause, and many animals that develop forward heart failure will have concurrent hypotension. In patients with hypotension but without clinical or radiographic evidence of congestion, it is crucial to rule out hypovolemia as the cause. In the absence of hypovolemia, positive inotropes such as dopamine or dobutamine can be used to raise systolic blood pressure in addition to increasing contractility.[10]

The most commonly used positive inotropes include dobutamine, dopamine, and pimobendan. Dobutamine is a potent nonselective β agonist (with greater effect on β1 receptors) that is administered as a constant rate infusion (CRI). Because of its nonselective β stimulation, the positive inotropic effects come with some degree of peripheral vasodilation, so blood pressure must be monitored. Dopamine (the precursor of norepinephrine), when given at low doses, has effects similar to dobutamine. However, when given at high doses, concurrent α receptor stimulation results in peripheral vasoconstriction. The combination of these effects makes dopamine and dobutamine attractive options for patients in cardiogenic shock. Careful monitoring is necessary when using these drugs with ventricular failure, because systemic hypertension and elevated afterload can cause cardiac output to plummet. Both these drugs also have positive chronotropic effects, which can result in decreased time for diastolic filling as the heart rate increases. Therefore concurrent ECG monitoring of heart rate and rhythm is necessary. Other less commonly used positive inotropic sympathomimetics include norepinephrine, epinephrine, and isoproterenol (see Table 40-1).

Pimobendan, an inodilator, is classified as both a calcium sensitizer and phosphodiesterase 3 inhibitor. It is a relatively new oral option for both acute and chronic inotropic support. Given its solely oral formulation, pimobendan may not be the ideal choice for an acute, severe episode of systolic failure; however, it has relatively rapid absorption and onset of effect. Pimobendan has also become widely available and may be a good option when CRIs are not feasible. Although not widely available in the veterinary setting, levosimendan and milrinone (both also phosphodiesterase 3 inhibitors) work similarly to pimobendan and are available in injectable formulations. (See

Table 40-1[10,11] **Positive Inotropes**

Drug	Mechanism of Action	Effect	Formulation	Suggested Dose†
Dobutamine HCl*	β-Adrenergic agonist; high dose weak α agonist $\beta_1 > \beta_2 > \alpha$	Positive inotropy Positive chronotropy Arteriolar vasodilation Vasoconstriction (high dose)	Injectable: 12.5 mg/ml	Dog: 2-20 mcg/kg/min Cat: 1-5 mcg/kg/min
Dopamine HCl*	Dopaminergic agonist, β-adrenergic agonist, high dose α agonist Dop > β High dose α	Positive inotropy Positive chronotropy, Peripheral vasodilation Vasoconstriction (high dose)	Injectable: 40, 80, 160 mg/ml	Dog: 2-10 mcg/kg/min Cat: 1-5 mcg/kg/min Titrate to desired effect: Low dose: inotropic support High dose: antihypertensive
Norepinephrine	β-Adrenergic agonist, α agonist $\beta_1 > \alpha > \beta_2$	Positive inotropy Positive chronotropy Vasoconstriction	Injectable: 1 mg/ml	0.01-3.0 mcg/kg/min
Epinephrine	β-Adrenergic agonist, α agonist $\beta_1 = \beta_2 > \alpha$	Positive inotropy Positive chronotropy Peripheral vasodilation Vasoconstriction HD	Injectable: 1 mg/ml, 0.1 mg/ml	0.01-0.1 mcg/kg/min
Isoproterenol	β-Adrenergic agonist $\beta_1 > \beta_2$	Positive inotropy Positive chronotropy Peripheral vasodilation	Injectable: 0.2mg/mL	Dog: 0.04-0.09 mcg/kg/min IV
Pimobendan*	Phosphodiesterase III inhibitor, Ca sensitizer	Positive inotropy Arteriolar vasodilation	Oral: 1.25, 5 mg chewable tablets	Dog: 0.25 mg/kg PO q12h Cat: 1.25 mg/cat PO q12h
Milrinone	Phosphodiesterase III inhibitor, Ca sensitizer	Positive inotropy Arteriolar vasodilation	Injectable: 1 mg/ml	0.375-0.75 mcg/kg/min

*Commonly used for inotropic support in veterinary medicine.
†Consult a pharmacology textbook for complete formulation and administration specifics.

Table 40-1 for specific drug information.) Digoxin (although historically widely used in veterinary medicine as a positive inotrope for chronic therapy) has very weak inotropic properties and has been largely supplanted by pimobendan. The exception is patients in which its negative chronotropic effect is indicated, in which case digoxin can be used in conjunction with pimobendan.

Relieving Signs of Congestion

Diuretics become critical should ventricular failure progress to clinical or radiographic signs of congestion, both in the acute stage and for chronic therapy. In many instances, the first knowledge of underlying ventricular failure comes when the patient develops signs of fluid overload and is presented for tachypnea, dyspnea, orthopnea, or coughing. Patients with biventricular or primarily right-sided failure may also develop ascites and abdominal distention. Furosemide is the most commonly used first-line diuretic choice (see Chapters 43 and Chapter 160 for doses). A potent loop diuretic, it works quickly to relieve life-threatening pulmonary edema, and can be given as a bolus (subcutaneously [SC], intramuscularly [IM], or intravenously [IV]) or as a CRI. With pulmonary edema, excess diuresis with overly aggressive preload reduction and relative volume depletion must be avoided.[10] If possible, baseline renal values should be obtained before diuretic therapy because patients with underlying renal insufficiency may require more conservative therapy. For animals with pleural or abdominal effusion causing respiratory distress, thoracocentesis or abdominocentesis should be performed at the time of presentation. Furosemide will decrease the rate of future fluid accumulation; however, it has very little effect on existing pleural or abdominal fluid. Secondary diuretics such as spironolactone, hydrochlorothiazide, and torsemide are important in chronic therapy for refractory failure; however, at this time they are only available in an oral formulation and have limited use in the emergency room setting. For information on chronic therapy for congestive heart failure, see Chapters 42 and 43.

Suppressing Arrhythmias

Despite variable underlying etiologies, many patients with ventricular failure will develop arrhythmias. All antiarrhythmic drugs can also be proarrhythmic, so it is important to note that prophylactic antiarrhythmic therapy is contraindicated in asymptomatic patients. For example, although it is common for patients to develop intermittent ventricular ectopy, only malignant arrhythmias warrant intervention. For a full discussion of antiarrhythmic therapy, see Chapters 47 and 48.

Treating the Underlying Cause

Although primary cardiac disease and myocardial infarctions are generally progressive and irreversible, some causes of heart failure can be treated primarily. For example, tachycardia-induced cardiomyopathy presents a unique situation for possible resolution. Depending on the severity and chronicity, successful rate control can often result in normal systolic function. Moreover, ventricular dysfunction secondary to some extracardiac causes (such as sepsis or nutritional deficiency) may improve or normalize with therapy. However, other causes, such as doxorubicin toxicity, are generally irreversible.

REFERENCES

1. Sisson D, Oyama M: Cardiovascular medicine of companion animals. Course outline for cardiovascular medicine, Champagne-Urbana, IL, 2003, University of Illinois School of Veterinary Medicine.
2. Umana E, Solares CA, Alpert MA: Tachycardia-induced cardiomyopathy, Am J Med 114:51, 2003.
3. Fernandes CJ Jr, de Assuncao MSC: Myocardial dysfunction in sepsis: a large, unsolved puzzle, Critical Care Res Pract 2012:896430, 2012.
4. Merx MW, Weber C: Sepsis and the heart, Circulation 116(7):793-802, 2007.
5. Driehuys S, Van Winkle TJ, Sammarco C, et al: Myocardial infarction in dogs and cats: 37 cases (1985-1994), J Am Vet Med Assoc 213(10):1444, 1998.

6. Buchanan JW: Vertebral scale system to measure heart size in radiographs, Vet Clin North Am Small Anim Pract 30:379, 2000.
7. Singletary GE, Morris NA, O'Sullivan L, et al: Prospective evaluation of NT-proBNP assay to detect occult dilated cardiomyopathy and predict survival in Doberman pinschers, J Vet Intern Med 26:1330, 2012.
8. Serra M, Papakonstantinou S, Adamcova M, et al: Veterinary and toxicological applications for the detection of cardiac injury using cardiac troponin, Vet J 185:50, 2010.
9. Sleeper MM, Clifford CA, Laster LL: Cardiac troponin I in the normal dog and cat, J Vet Intern Med 501, 2001.
10. Poole-Wilson PA, Opie LH: Acute and chronic heart failure: positive inotropes, vasodilators, and digoxin. In Opie LH, Gersh BJ, editors: Drugs for the heart, ed 7, Philadelphia, 2009, Saunders.
11. Smith FW, Tilley LP, Oyama MA, et al: Common cardiovascular drugs. In Tilley LP, Smith FW, Oyama MA, et al, editors: Manual of canine and feline cardiology, ed 7, St Louis, 2008, Saunders Elsevier.

CHAPTER 41
FELINE CARDIOMYOPATHY

Jonathan A. Abbott, DVM, DACVIM (Cardiology)

KEY POINTS

- Myocardial disease accounts for almost all acquired cardiac disorders in the cat.
- Cardiomyopathy, defined as a heart muscle disease that is associated with cardiac dysfunction, is an important cause of both morbidity and mortality in the cat.
- The most common forms of feline cardiomyopathy result in impaired ventricular filling.
- Clinical signs are associated with congestive heart failure (CHF) or systemic thromboembolism.
- Diagnostic imaging, through radiography and echocardiography, is vital to the diagnostic approach.
- Urgent medical management of CHF secondary to feline cardiomyopathy primarily consists of supportive care and interventions that decrease ventricular filling pressures.

Heart muscle disease is an important cause of morbidity and mortality in the cat. The various forms of myocardial disease account for virtually all acquired cardiac disorders in this species; disease that is primary to valvular structures, the pericardium, or specialized conduction system is uncommon. The nomenclature of myocardial disease is potentially problematic but evolving. Cardiomyopathy has been defined as a heart muscle disease that is associated with cardiac dysfunction.[1] Myocardial diseases generally are defined by morphopathologic features or, when it is known, cause. Based on this classification scheme, there are four basic types of cardiomyopathy: (1) dilated cardiomyopathy, (2) hypertrophic cardiomyopathy (HCM), (3) restrictive cardiomyopathy (RCM), and (4) arrhythmogenic right ventricular cardiomyopathy.[1] All these forms are observed in the cat.[2-6]

Heart muscle diseases that are associated with a known causal agent, hemodynamic abnormality, or metabolic derangement are known as specific cardiomyopathies.[1] In the cat, the most important disorders in this category are thyrotoxic cardiomyopathy and hypertensive HCM.[7] In general, these secondary cardiomyopathies seldom result in clinical signs and are reversible when the underlying disorder resolves.[8,9]

This chapter addresses the clinical picture and therapy of cardiomyopathy that develop as a result of abnormalities that are primary to the myocardium. HCM is the most common heart disease in the cat and therefore is emphasized.

ETIOPATHOGENESIS

HCM is a primary heart muscle disease in which ventricular hypertrophy develops in the absence of a hemodynamic or metabolic cause.[10] Although systolic dysfunction and wall thinning occasionally develop in patients with long-standing HCM, the disorder generally is characterized by hypertrophy of a nondilated ventricle.[10] It is accepted that HCM in humans is a genetic disease, and this disorder has been associated with hundreds of mutations of genes that encode sarcomeric proteins. The mutations responsible for familial HCM in Maine Coon cats and in Ragdoll cats have been identified.[11-13] This finding and the occurrence of HCM in related purebred and mixed breed cats support a genetic basis.[14-16]

Feline RCM is a disorder in which impaired ventricular filling occurs in the absence of myocardial hypertrophy or pericardial disease. The structural features of RCM are varied and diagnostic criteria are not rigidly defined. The term generally is applied when there is atrial enlargement associated with a ventricle that has a normal or nearly normal appearance.[7] The cause of feline RCM is not known. Endomyocardial fibrosis and myocardial functional deficits that impair relaxation are the presumed explanations for diastolic dysfunction and resultant atrial enlargement. It is possible that some examples of RCM represent the sequelae of endomyocardial inflammation.[4]

PATHOPHYSIOLOGY

Diastolic Dysfunction

The ability of the ventricle to fill at low diastolic pressures depends on the rate of the active, energy-requiring process known as *myocardial relaxation,* as well as on mechanical properties that determine chamber compliance.[17] Impaired myocardial relaxation and diminished chamber compliance alter the pressure-volume relationship so that diastolic pressures are high when ventricular volume is normal or small. High diastolic pressures are reflected upstream, potentially resulting in atrial enlargement and venous congestion. In cases in which the end-diastolic volume is diminished, stroke volume may also be reduced. Therefore diastolic dysfunction can explain subnormal cardiac output as well as venous congestion.

Diastolic dysfunction is the predominant pathophysiologic mechanism responsible for clinical signs in HCM and RCM.[7] With regard to HCM, intrinsic functional deficits of the cardiomyocytes and ischemia related to hypertrophy and abnormalities of the intramural coronary arteries are responsible for impaired myocardial relaxation. Hypertrophy and fibrosis stiffen the ventricle and explain diminished chamber compliance. The basis of cardiac dysfunction in feline RCM has been defined incompletely, although endomyocardial fibrosis likely plays an important role.

Systolic Anterior Motion of the Mitral Valve

Systolic anterior motion (SAM) of the mitral valve is echocardiographically detected in approximately 65% of cats with HCM.[3] The precise pathogenesis has been the subject of debate, but it is likely that abnormal drag forces are responsible for systolic movement of the valve leaflets toward the septum.[18] Abnormal papillary muscle orientation and dynamic systolic ventricular performance provide a structural and functional substrate that predisposes to SAM.[19] Movement of the mitral leaflets toward the septum results in dynamic—as opposed to fixed—left ventricular outflow tract obstruction and, usually, concurrent mitral valve regurgitation. SAM is a labile phenomenon; decreases in preload and afterload or increases in contractility may provoke or augment SAM, and this may explain the fact that the intensity of the associated murmur may vary from moment to moment.[20] The prognostic relevance of SAM in feline HCM has not been defined. Outflow tract obstruction caused by SAM has been associated with poor prognosis in humans with HCM.[21] Interestingly, the results of three retrospective studies of feline HCM suggest that SAM confers a more favorable prognosis than does its absence.[3,22,23] Possibly this finding reflects the limitations of retrospective evaluation of a referral population as the finding of SAM is associated with asymptomatic status. SAM is likely the most important cause of cardiac murmurs in cats with HCM.

Feline Arterial Thromboembolism (FATE)

Feline patients with myocardial disease are predisposed to the development of intracardiac thrombi. Intraventricular thrombi are occasionally observed, but the left atrium—specifically, its appendage—is more commonly the site of thrombus formation. If a portion of thrombus dislodges, it may embolize, the typical site of embolism being the aortic trifurcation. The causes of and risk factors for intracardiac thrombosis are incompletely defined. Left atrial enlargement, which presumably results in blood stasis, likely predisposes to thrombosis. Indeed, left atria of patients with feline arterial thromboembolism (FATE) are larger than those of patients with subclinical HCM or patients with heart failure caused by HCM.[22] However, systematic evaluation of risks and incidence of FATE has not been published and it is relevant that FATE occasionally occurs in patients in whom left atrial size is normal.[24] Left atrial enlargement is neither a sufficient nor necessary cause, but it is likely that left atrial enlargement is a risk factor for FATE as might be the echocardiographic findings of spontaneous contrast and systolic myocardial dysfunction.

The clinical syndrome of FATE does not result solely from arterial occlusion caused by the thrombus because experimental ligation of the distal feline aorta does not reproduce the clinical syndrome.[25] Available evidence suggests that vasoactive mediators, notably prostaglandins and serotonin, released from the thrombus decrease flow through collateral circulation, contributing importantly to the development of ischemia.[26-28]

CLINICAL PRESENTATION

Patient History and Physical Findings

Clinical manifestations of feline cardiomyopathy result from congestive heart failure (CHF) and FATE. When CHF is present, the observation of tachypnea or respiratory distress most commonly prompts the pet owner to seek veterinary evaluation. Cats with heart failure seldom cough. Nonspecific clinical signs such as lethargy, depression, and inappetence often are observed in patients with cardiomyopathy. Although the causative disorder is usually chronic, the onset of clinical signs associated with CHF is typically sudden.

Retrospectively evaluated case series have identified an association between the administration of glucocorticoids and the development of CHF in cats.[22,29] Some affected cats may have had preexisting but clinically silent HCM, but this has not been established. This association is relevant, because the long-term prognosis for cats with glucocorticoid-associated CHF may be better than for those with CHF from more typical causes.[29]

Patients with CHF often are depressed, and hypothermia commonly is observed. The heart rates of cats with heart failure differ little from those of healthy cats,[30] although bradycardia is occasionally evident. Many cats with HCM have a systolic murmur associated with SAM, but the prevalence of murmurs in cats with subclinical HCM is greater that in cats that have clinical signs of CHF.[23] The prevalence of murmurs in cats with other forms of cardiomyopathy is lower.[5] A gallop rhythm is a subtle but important auscultatory finding. The third and fourth heart sounds are seldom audible in healthy cats. In general, auscultation of a gallop sound signifies diminished ventricular compliance in association with high atrial pressures. A gallop sound more specifically identifies cats with heart disease than does a murmur. It is important to recognize that the prevalence of murmurs in echocardiographically normal cats is not inconsequential. Because of this, the finding of a cardiac murmur is sometimes incidental to a clinical picture that results from noncardiac disease.

Crackles are sometimes heard in feline patients with cardiogenic edema, but it is likely that the auscultation of adventitious pulmonary sounds has low sensitivity and specificity for pulmonary edema. Patients in which pleural effusions are responsible for respiratory distress generally have quiet heart sounds as well as diminished, dorsally displaced bronchial tones.

The anatomic site of embolism and time that has elapsed since the embolic event determines the clinical presentation of FATE. The distal aorta is embolized most commonly, but embolism of a brachial arterial, renal artery, mesenteric artery, or arteries of the central nervous system also occurs. Patients in which the clinical presentation is prompted by FATE of the aorta or brachial arteries have weak or absent arterial pulses. The resultant ischemic neuromyopathy causes variable degrees of pain, plegia, and nail bed cyanosis; when the distal aorta is affected, the gastrocnemius muscles often are firm.

Electrocardiography

In the absence of arrhythmias, the diagnostic utility of electrocardiography in the assessment of cats with cardiomyopathy generally is low. Electrocardiographic evaluation of cats with clinical signs resulting from feline cardiomyopathy generally reveals sinus rhythm, although pathologic tachyarrhythmias sometimes are observed. The heart rates of cats with heart failure seldom are higher than is normal, and bradycardia resulting from a slow sinus rate or AV conduction disturbances is occasionally evident.

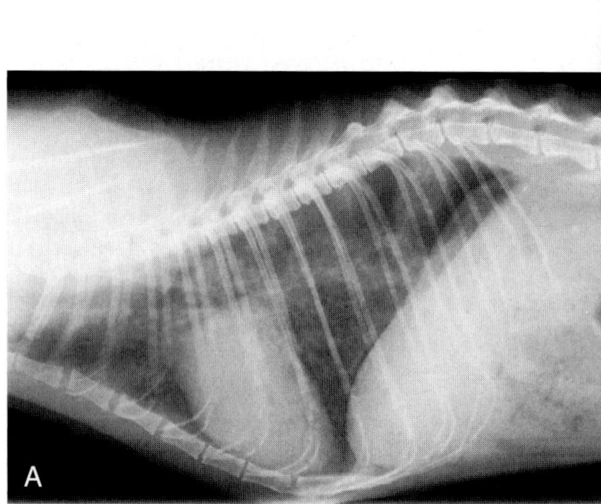

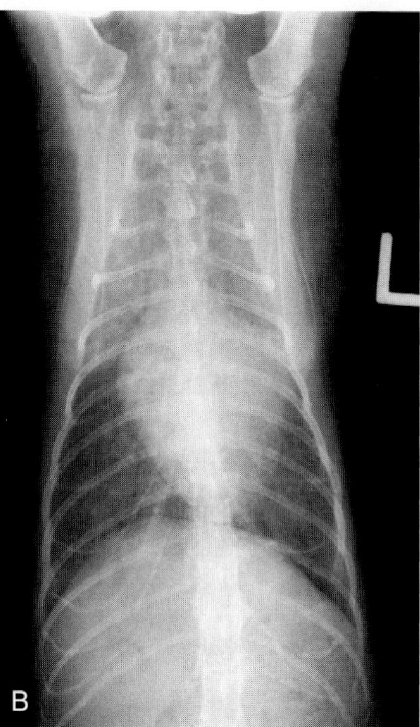

FIGURE 41-1 Lateral **(A)** and ventrodorsal **(B)** radiographic projections of the thorax of a cat with heart failure caused by hypertrophic cardiomyopathy. The cardiac silhouette is enlarged and there are patchy interstitial and alveolar densities distributed throughout the lung.

Radiography

In the cat, radiographic patterns associated with enlargement of specific chambers are relatively indistinct. Because of this, it is often impossible to draw conclusions regarding atrial or ventricular size, but rather, it is apparent only that the silhouette is enlarged. Radiographic cardiomegaly usually is evident when respiratory signs result from feline cardiomyopathy. Cardiogenic pulmonary edema in the cat typically is patchy but distributed diffusely through the lung (Figure 41-1). Fairly often the pulmonary arteries and veins are prominent if not obscured by infiltrates. Pulmonary edema is the most common manifestation of congestion in patients with HCM, but some cats develop large pleural effusions associated with HCM or other types of feline cardiomyopathy. Curiously, cats sometimes develop large pleural effusions as a result of cardiac diseases that affect primarily the left ventricle.

Echocardiography

Definitive antemortem diagnosis of feline cardiomyopathy requires echocardiographic evaluation. HCM is characterized echocardiographically by ventricular hypertrophy in the absence of chamber dilation. It is generally accepted that the end-diastolic thickness of the interventricular septum or left ventricular posterior wall is less than 6 mm in healthy cats, and measurements that exceed this figure suggest hypertrophy.[3] Left atrial enlargement resulting from diastolic dysfunction and sometimes concomitant mitral valve regurgitation is often present (Figure 41-2). This finding is clinically important because respiratory signs rarely result from cardiomyopathy in patients with normal atrial size.[31] It is important to know that echocardiographic pseudohypertrophy can result from hypovolemia.[32] When this is the case, atrial dimensions typically are small.

Systemic Blood Pressure

Systemic blood pressure is related to both tissue perfusion and vascular resistance. Serial evaluation of blood pressure is potentially useful in the treatment of critically ill patients with feline cardiomyopathy. Because abnormal ventricular loading conditions associated with systemic hypertension may result in compensatory hypertrophy, feline HCM is a diagnosis of exclusion. Systemic blood pressure can be measured by direct puncture of a peripheral artery but more often is estimated using indirect methods. In the cat, the Doppler technique is likely to be superior to the oscillometric method.[33] Accuracy of indirect blood pressure estimation is critically dependent on technique, and results must be interpreted in context of the inherent limitations of the method and the clinical scenario. Repeated measurements of systolic blood pressure in excess of 180 mm Hg are compatible with a diagnosis of hypertension.

Bloodborne Cardiac Biomarkers

Biomarkers are objectively determined characteristics that potentially have a role in diagnosis, risk stratification, evaluation of disease progression, and evaluation of response to therapy. Circulating B-type natriuretic peptide (BNP) concentration has a particular role in the diagnostic evaluation of patients suspected to have heart failure. This hormone is released by atrial and ventricular cardiomyocytes in response to increases in ventricular filling pressures; potentially therefore it is a bloodborne diagnostic marker of the heart failure state.[34]

Two separate studies have evaluated the diagnostic performance of N-terminal–BNP (NT-BNP) in populations of cats with respiratory distress.[35,36] Clinical findings including radiographic and echocardiographic data were used to define cardiac and non-cardiac causes of respiratory distress. The results of the two studies generally were concordant; NT-BNP concentration identified respiratory distress caused by feline cardiomyopathy with high sensitivity—near 90%—and a somewhat lower specificity that was in the high 80s.[35,36] A BNP assay is commercially available, but because of the time required for transport of samples to a central laboratory, it may be that the diagnostic potential for the evaluation of BNP concentrations will be fully realized only when BNP concentrations can be determined by a point-of-care assay.

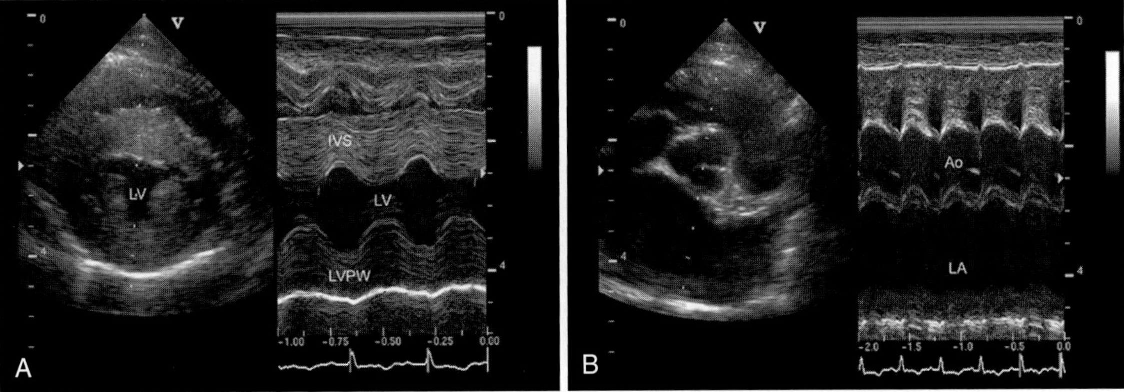

FIGURE 41-2 Echocardiographic images obtained from a cat with heart failure caused by hypertrophic cardiomyopathy. There is moderate left ventricular hypertrophy **(A)** and left atrial enlargement **(B).** Static two-dimensional, right parasternal short-axis images and related M-mode echocardiograms are shown for each image plane. *Ao,* Aorta; *IVS,* interventricular septum; *LA,* left atrium; *LV,* left ventricle; *LVPW,* left ventricular posterior wall.

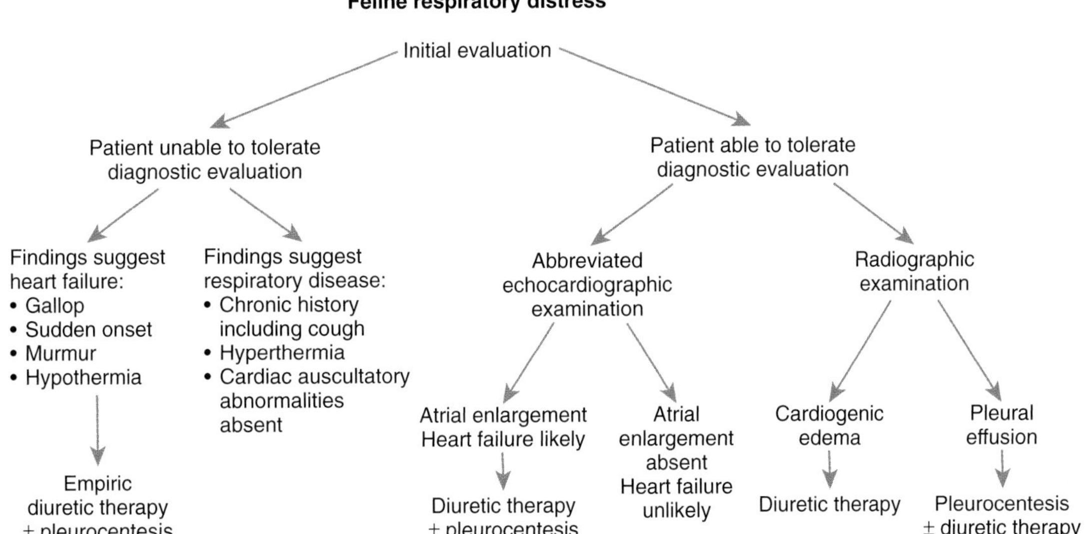

FIGURE 41-3 An algorithm that outlines one approach to the problem of feline respiratory distress; case management is determined by the tolerance of the patient and the availability of diagnostic modalities. When possible, the therapeutic approach is optimally determined by diagnostic data. It should be emphasized that these are only guidelines and that it can be difficult or impossible to distinguish cardiac and noncardiac causes of respiratory distress based on only patient history and physical findings (see text for details).

DIAGNOSTIC APPROACH

The therapeutic approach to feline cardiomyopathy is best formulated based on the results of diagnostic evaluation (Figure 41-3). When possible, clinical signs of tachypnea and respiratory distress should be investigated radiographically. The results of radiographic examination direct the therapeutic approach, and it is relevant that tachypnea was identified in 89% of patients with FATE in the absence of CHF.[37] When physical and radiographic findings suggest that cardiac disease is responsible for respiratory signs, echocardiographic evaluation is indicated. When the clinical picture is complicated by arrhythmias, the patient also should be evaluated electrocardiographically. However, it is important to recognize that feline patients in respiratory distress are fragile. Sometimes the risks associated with restraint for diagnostic evaluation cannot be justified, and empiric diuretic therapy should be considered. When empirical therapy is contemplated, it is important that the presumptive diagnosis is plausible based on signalment, history, and physical findings. Furthermore, an understanding of the expected response and a willingness to adapt to changing clinical circumstances is essential.

Sometimes it is possible to perform an abbreviated echocardiographic examination while the patient is sternally recumbent, minimally restrained, and receiving supplemental oxygen. In these circumstances, it is not always important to characterize definitively the nature of the myocardial disease. Documentation of left atrial enlargement provides indirect evidence of elevated filling pressures from which it can reasonably be surmised that the clinical signs result from congestion.[31] In most circumstances, the absence of left atrial enlargement suggests that respiratory signs are not the result of cardiac disease. It is important to note that patients who have suffered FATE often exhibit tachypnea that presumably is a manifestation of pain. In this patient population, tachypnea is inconsistently associated with congestion and it is therefore appropriate to obtain thoracic radiographs before administering diuretics to patients with FATE.

THERAPEUTIC APPROACH

Management of FATE

Urgent therapy of FATE is challenging and sometimes frustrating. In general, the syndrome is associated with a poor prognosis; mortality, not as a result of euthanasia, associated with FATE is close to 30% during initial hospitalization, and euthanasia is elected for approximately 30% of cases during the same period.[24,37,38] Survival is greater for patients in which only a single limb is affected.[24,37] Surgical thrombectomy, transcatheter thrombectomy, and the use of fibrinolytic drugs such as streptokinase and tissue plasminogen activator have been brought to bear, but none of these interventions is obviously superior to conservative medical therapy.[39-41] Narcotic analgesia is one of the few clear therapeutic indications in this clinical circumstance. Heparin is often administered in the 48 to 72 hours after an embolic event in the hopes that this treatment will prevent enlargement of the thrombus. The use of low-molecular-weight heparin (LMWH) has been suggested, but an advantage of LMWH over unfractionated heparin has not been demonstrated. Optimally, monitoring of the activated clotting time or prothrombin time is used to guide unfractionated heparin therapy. When this is impractical, the use of a relatively low dose of unfractionated heparin (60 to 100 IU/kg subcutaneously [SC] q8h) can be considered; this dose is seemingly associated with a low incidence of bleeding complications. (Chapter 168, provides further information on this topic.) Supportive care is important because many patients with FATE have concurrent CHF, and even when this is not the case, signs of low cardiac output such as azotemia and hypothermia are commonly observed.[24,37] Indeed, during the acute presentation, body temperature is of prognostic importance, with hypothermia being associated with reduced survival. A statistical model developed from retrospectively acquired data predicted 50% short-term survival for patients with a body temperature of 37.2°C.[37] For patients that survive the immediate aftermath of embolism, arterial pulses may become palpable within days but a return to normal limb function, if it occurs, may take weeks. As might be expected, some patients suffer the consequences of dermal or even muscular necrosis.

Prevention of future embolic events has received considerable attention, and the use of aspirin (acetylsalicylic acid [ASA]) and other antithrombotic medications, including clopidogrel, and LMWH is widespread despite lack of evidence of efficacy (see Chapters 167 and 168). Prophylaxis of FATE presents a particularly difficult problem because the risks for embolism are poorly defined; indeed, embolism is the first indication of cardiac disease in approximately 80% of affected patients.[24,37,38] Furthermore, the incidence of FATE in patients known to have cardiac disease is relatively low. Estimates from retrospective data vary, but FATE occurs in fewer than 20% of patients with previously identified cardiomyopathy.[24,37] These epidemiologic characteristics—most embolic events occur in patients not known to be at risk, together with the relatively low incidence of FATE in patients with presumed risk factors—present almost insurmountable difficulties. It is also important to consider the magnitude of effect of antithrombotic therapy. In a meta-analysis of trials that compared low-dose aspirin to placebo in human beings with stable cardiovascular disease, the absolute reduction in risk of adverse events—death, stroke, and myocardial infarction—associated with aspirin administration was 3.3%.[42] It is necessary to treat 30 human beings with aspirin to prevent a single adverse event. If the magnitude of effect is similar in cats, it is unlikely that an effect of aspirin will be evident in the clinical trials of the size generally performed in veterinary medicine. There is indirect evidence from retrospective data suggesting that low-dose aspirin is associated with fewer adverse effects than high-dose aspirin.[37] The author uses low-dose aspirin in selected cases—most often in those that have already suffered FATE or have a thrombus or spontaneous contrast that is echocardiographically visible in the left atrium.

Management of Acutely Decompensated Heart Failure

Heart failure is a syndrome that results from impaired filling or emptying of the heart. Clinical findings may reflect congestion, diminished cardiac output, or both. In veterinary patients it is necessary to use objective rather than subjective markers of disease, and therefore feline heart failure can be defined as pulmonary edema or pleural effusion that is caused by heart disease.

General supportive measures are indicated for feline heart failure. Indirect heat sources should be used when hypothermia is present. Supplemental oxygen can be administered by mask, by nasal insufflation, or via an oxygen administration cage. Most patients that respond to medical therapy for cardiogenic edema do so promptly, so mechanical ventilation generally is not required but can be considered for patients with marked respiratory distress. Thoracocentesis should be performed when physical or radiographic findings confirm that a large pleural effusion is responsible for respiratory distress. Intravenous fluids should be administered sparingly to patients with frank congestion and only if required as a vehicle for drug therapy. In animals with congestive failure, infusion of fluid further increases venous pressures but does not improve cardiac performance.

When cardiogenic pulmonary edema is present, diuretic therapy is indicated. Furosemide is a high-ceiling loop diuretic that increases urine production and therefore reduces intravascular volume and venous pressures. Furosemide can be administered intravenously, intramuscularly, or orally. During acute decompensation, the intravenous route is preferable, but intramuscular administration is appropriate when resistance to manual restraint or other factors make intravenous administration difficult or impossible. Generally the initial dosage is relatively high, perhaps 2 to 4 mg/kg.[43] The patient is then carefully observed for 40 to 60 minutes. If there is a decrease in respiratory rate or effort, a lower dose is administered. The dosage and interval for furosemide should be determined by clinical response. Frequent administration of low doses (0.5 to 1 mg/kg intravenously [IV] q1h) until respiratory signs resolve may provide a means to prevent excessive diuresis. Constant rate infusion of furosemide may accomplish the same objective, although the utility of furosemide infusion has not been specifically evaluated in the cat. If there is no change or if there is deterioration of clinical status after administration of two or three doses of parenteral furosemide, reevaluation of the presumptive diagnosis and therapeutic approach is indicated.

It is noteworthy that the clinical profile of heart failure resulting from feline cardiomyopathy is similar to that of feline endomyocarditis.[4] The latter is an idiopathic disorder that is associated with pneumonitis. Patients typically are brought for evaluation of respiratory distress that develops soon after a stressful event, such as surgical sterilization or onychectomy. Because respiratory signs associated with this disorder are apparently not cardiogenic, diuresis is unlikely to improve clinical status.

Nitroglycerin (NG) is an organic nitrate that is sometimes used with furosemide as an adjunctive therapy that may further reduce ventricular filling pressures.[43] NG causes venodilation as well as dilation of specific arteriolar beds, including those of the coronary circulation. In veterinary medicine, NG is used principally as a venodilator that increases venous capacitance, therefore causing a decrease in ventricular filling pressures. Thus the hemodynamic effect of NG is similar to that of diuretic therapy; it is primarily a preload-reducing intervention. The efficacy of NG in feline patients has not been established. NG is most commonly administered using a transdermal cream that is applied to the pinnae or inguinal area. In humans, absorption of transdermal NG depends on the surface area of the skin to which it is applied. The dosage in feline patients is based on anecdotal evidence, but ⅛ to ¼ inch of the transdermal cream has been suggested.

Preload reduction is used for heart failure because it may effectively eliminate clinical signs of congestion. However, preload reduction generally does not improve cardiac performance. Indeed, aggressive reduction in filling pressures can decrease stroke volume, potentially resulting in hypotension. This is particularly relevant in the discussion of feline cardiomyopathy because the disorders that most commonly cause heart failure in cats result in diastolic dysfunction. Patients with diastolic dysfunction develop congestion when ventricular volumes are normal or small. This may partly explain the sensitivity of feline patients to diuretic therapy.

Patient monitoring is an important aspect of critical care. In the management of feline cardiomyopathy, vital signs are perhaps the most important. It is useful to record body weight, body temperature, heart rate, and respiratory rate at frequent intervals. Other parameters including hematocrit, total serum protein values, blood urea nitrogen concentration, and systemic blood pressure may provide useful ancillary information.

Diastolic dysfunction resulting from HCM or RCM is the most common cause of feline heart failure. Other than furosemide, for which efficacy is assumed, no medical interventions have demonstrated efficacy for this syndrome. Based on this, the use of cardioactive ancillary therapy during acute decompensation is difficult to justify. An exception to this might be the use of antiarrhythmic agents for tachyarrhythmias that contribute to congestive signs. Primarily the management of acutely decompensated feline cardiomyopathy consists of supportive care and judicious lowering of ventricular filling pressures.

Management of Chronic Heart Failure

Long-term therapy for feline myocardial disease is best guided by echocardiographic findings. Management of diastolic dysfunction traditionally has been with drugs that slow heart rate or speed myocardial relaxation or both. β-Adrenergic antagonists such as atenolol are believed to indirectly improve ventricular filling by lowering heart rate. It is likely that slowing the heart rate is beneficial when tachycardia contributes to diastolic dysfunction. Furthermore, if diastolic function is markedly impaired, myocardial relaxation may be incomplete, even when the diastolic interval and heart rate are normal. Additionally, slowing the rate may improve coronary perfusion, which presumably is abnormal in cats with HCM. Still, elevated filling pressures resulting in congestion at rest are the most obvious cause of clinical signs in HCM, and it is likely that abnormal ventricular stiffness related to hypertrophy and fibrosis is at least partly responsible. It is therefore unclear whether heart rate reduction in patients in which heart rate initially is normal can decrease venous pressures. Relevant studies are lacking, and the optimal heart rate for patients with heart failure caused by feline HCM is not known. β-Adrenergic antagonists may have a particular role when dynamic left ventricular outflow tract obstruction is caused by SAM and when tachyarrhythmias complicate the clinical picture. Recently there has been interest in antagonists of the "funny" (I_f) sodium channel. Drugs such as ivabradine may have value as they slow heart rate but do not exert a negatively inotropic effect.[44]

Diltiazem is a benzothiazepine calcium channel antagonist. It has only a modest slowing effect on heart rate but is believed to speed myocardial relaxation. The latter effect may serve to reduce ventricular filling pressures. Additionally, diltiazem may dilate coronary arteries and improve diastolic function by improving coronary perfusion. In general, diltiazem has little effect on outflow tract obstruction caused by SAM.

Enalapril and benazepril, angiotensin-converting enzyme (ACE) inhibitors, also have been used in long-term management of feline HCM.[45,46] By interrupting the enzymatic conversion of angiotensin I to angiotensin II, these agents have diverse neuroendocrine effects. ACE inhibitors are vasodilators, although this effect is relatively weak. Most patients with HCM have normal or hyperdynamic systolic performance, and arteriolar dilation confers no obvious mechanical advantage. In contrast to patients with systolic dysfunction and chamber dilation, a reduction in afterload is unlikely to increase stroke volume simply because the ventricle empties almost completely in any case. Indeed, vasodilators generally are contraindicated in human HCM primarily because of the concern that vasodilation will provoke or worsen SAM.[47] The potential but theoretical benefits of ACE inhibition relate primarily to the neuroendocrine effects of these drugs. The resultant decrease in aldosterone activity might be beneficial by decreasing the renal retention of salt and water. Additionally, aldosterone and angiotensin II have been implicated as trophic factors that might be relevant to the development of hypertrophy and fibrosis.[48,49]

Although diastolic dysfunction is generally believed to be the dominant pathophysiologic mechanism responsible for clinical signs in HCM, recently published retrospective case series that included patients with HCM have evaluated the effect of pimobendan in feline myocardial disease.[50-52] It is possible that a lusitropic effect of pimobendan is beneficial, but studies to date have neither been prospective nor included a control group. Until more data are available, use of pimobendan should probably be reserved for feline patients with echocardiographically demonstrated systolic myocardial dysfunction, recognizing that any use of this drug in the feline species is "off-label."

Unfortunately, little is known of the efficacy of ancillary therapy for feline cardiomyopathy. In a small, open-label clinical trial, the effects of diltiazem, propranolol, and verapamil on cats with pulmonary edema caused by HCM were compared.[53] Diltiazem was the most efficacious of the three. However, this trial did not include a placebo group. A multicenter, randomized, placebo-controlled trial that was designed to evaluate the relative efficacy of atenolol, diltiazem, and enalapril in feline patients with CHF caused by HCM or RCM has been completed.[54] The results of this study have been presented but are not yet published. The primary endpoint of the trial was recurrence of congestive signs, and none of the agents were superior to placebo in this regard. Patients that received enalapril remained in the trial longer than those receiving the alternatives, although this result did not achieve statistical significance. Interestingly, patients receiving atenolol fared less well than did those in the placebo group. The finding that atenolol may harm cats with pulmonary edema was possibly unexpected but is consistent with the result of the only comparable study in which propranolol administration was associated with decreased survival.[31] Studies have not addressed the effect of multivalent therapy; it is possible that β-blockers or other agents are beneficial when used in combination with furosemide and an ACE inhibitor. Regardless, based on these as yet unpublished data, the use of enalapril with furosemide seems a reasonable initial approach to the long-term management of feline patients with CHF resulting from diastolic dysfunction.

REFERENCES

1. Richardson P, McKenna W, Bristow M, et al: Report of the 1995 World Health Organization/International Society and Federation of Cardiology

Task Force on the Definition and Classification of cardiomyopathies, Circulation 93:841, 1996.
2. Pion PD, Kittleson MD, Rogers QR, et al: Myocardial failure in cats associated with low plasma taurine: a reversible cardiomyopathy, Science 237:764, 1987.
3. Fox PR, Liu S-K, Maron BJ: Echocardiographic assessment of spontaneously occurring feline hypertrophic cardiomyopathy: an animal model of human disease, Circulation 92:2645, 1995.
4. Stalis IH, Bossbaly MJ, Van Winkle TJ: Feline endomyocarditis and left ventricular endocardial fibrosis, Vet Pathol 32:122, 1995.
5. Ferasin L, Sturgess CP, Cannon MJ, et al: Feline idiopathic cardiomyopathy: a retrospective study of 106 cats (1994-2001), J Fel Med Surg 5:151, 2003.
6. Fox PR, Maron BJ, Basso C, et al: Spontaneously occurring arrhythmogenic right ventricular cardiomyopathy in the domestic cat: a new animal model similar to the human disease, Circulation 102:1863, 2000.
7. Fox P: Feline cardiomyopathies. In Fox PR, Sisson DD, Moise NS, editors: Textbook of canine and feline cardiology: principles and clinical practice, ed 2, Philadelphia, 1999, Saunders, pp 621-678.
8. Nelson L, Reidesel E, Ware WA, et al: Echocardiographic and radiographic changes associated with systemic hypertension in cats, J Vet Intern Med 16:418, 2002.
9. Bond BR, Fox PR, Peterson ME, et al: Echocardiographic findings in 103 cats with hyperthyroidism, J Am Vet Med Assoc 192:1546, 1988.
10. Maron BJ: Hypertrophic cardiomyopathy: a systematic review, JAMA 287:1308,2002.
11. Meurs KM, Sanchez X, David RM, et al: A cardiac myosin binding protein C mutation in the Maine Coon cat with familial hypertrophic cardiomyopathy, Hum Mol Genet 14:3587, 2005.
12. Kittleson MD, Meurs KM, Munro MJ, et al: Familial hypertrophic cardiomyopathy in maine coon cats: an animal model of human disease, Circulation 99:3172, 1999.
13. Meurs KM, Norgard MM, Ederer MM, et al: A substitution mutation in the myosin binding protein C gene in ragdoll hypertrophic cardiomyopathy, Genomics 90:261, 2007.
14. Meurs KM, Kittleson MD, Towbin J, et al: Familial systolic anterior motion of the mitral valve and/or hypertrophic cardiomyopathy is apparently inherited as an autosomal dominant trait in a family of American shorthair cats, J Vet Intern Med 11:138, 1997.
15. Martin L, VandeWoude S, Boon J, et al: Left ventricular hypertrophy in a closed colony of Persian cats [abstract], J Vet Intern Med 8:143, 1994.
16. Kraus MS, Calvert CA, Jacobs GJ: Hypertrophic cardiomyopathy in a litter of five mixed-breed cats, J Am Anim Hosp Assoc 35:293, 1999.
17. Nishimura RA, Tajik J: Evaluation of diastolic filling of left ventricle in health and disease: Doppler echocardiography is the clinician's Rosetta stone, J Am Coll Cardiol 30:8, 1997.
18. Sherrid MV, Chaudhry FA, Swistel DG: Obstructive hypertrophic cardiomyopathy: echocardiography, pathophysiology, and the continuing evolution of surgery for obstruction, Ann Thorac Surg 75:620, 2003.
19. Levine RA, Vlahakes GJ, Lefebvre X, et al: Papillary muscle displacement causes systolic anterior motion of the mitral valve. Experimental validation and insights into the mechanism of subaortic obstruction, Circulation 91:1189, 1995.
20. Yoerger DM, Weyman AE: Hypertrophic obstructive cardiomyopathy: mechanism of obstruction and response to therapy, Rev Cardiovasc Med 4:199, 2003.
21. Maron MS, Olivotto I, Betocchi S, et al: Effect of left ventricular outflow tract obstruction on clinical outcome in hypertrophic cardiomyopathy, N Engl J Med 348:295, 2003.
22. Rush JE, Freeman LM, Fenollosa NK, et al: Population and survival characteristics of cats with hypertrophic cardiomyopathy: 260 cases (1990-1999), J Am Vet Med Assoc 220:202, 2002.
23. Payne J, Luis Fuentes V, Boswood A, et al: Population characteristics and survival in 127 referred cats with hypertrophic cardiomyopathy (1997 to 2005), J Small Anim Pract 51:540, 2010.
24. Laste NJ, Harpster NK: A retrospective study of 100 cases of feline distal aortic thromboembolism: 1977-1993, J Am Anim Hosp Assoc 31:492, 1995.
25. Imhoff RK: Production of aortic occlusion resembling acute aortic embolism syndrome in cats, Nature 192:979, 1961.
26. Butler HC: An investigation into the relationship of an aortic embolus to posterior paralysis in the cat, J Small Anim Pract 12:141, 1971.
27. Olmstead ML, Butler HC: Five-hydroxytryptamine antagonists and feline aortic embolism, J Small Anim Pract 18:247, 1977.
28. Schaub RG, Meyers KM, Sande RD, et al: Inhibition of feline collateral vessel development following experimental thrombolic occlusion, Circ Res 39:736, 1976.
29. Smith SA, Tobias AH, Fine DM, et al: Corticosteroid-associated congestive heart failure in 12 cats, J Appl Res Vet Med 2:159, 2004.
30. Hamlin RL: Heart rate of the cat, J Am Anim Hosp Assoc 25:284, 1989.
31. Smith S, Dukes-McEwan J: Clinical signs and left atrial size in cats with cardiovascular disease in general practice, J Small Anim Pract 53:27, 2012.
32. Campbell FE, Kittleson MD: The effect of hydration status on the echocardiographic measurements of normal cats, J Vet Intern Med 21:1008, 2007.
33. Binns SH, Sisson DD, Buoscio DA, et al: Doppler ultrasonographic, oscillometric sphygmomanometric, and photoplethysmographic techniques for noninvasive blood pressure measurement in anesthetized cats, J Vet Intern Med 9:405, 1995.
34. Sisson DD: Neuroendocrine evaluation of cardiac disease, Vet Clin North Am Small Anim Pract 34:1105, 2004.
35. Fox PR, Oyama MA, Reynolds C, et al: Utility of plasma N-terminal pro-brain natriuretic peptide (NT-proBNP) to distinguish between congestive heart failure and non-cardiac causes of acute dyspnea in cats, J Vet Cardiol 11:S51, 2009.
36. Connolly DJ, Soares Magalhaes RJ, Fuentes VL, et al: Assessment of the diagnostic accuracy of circulating natriuretic peptide concentrations to distinguish between cats with cardiac and non-cardiac causes of respiratory distress, J Vet Cardiol 11:S41, 2009.
37. Smith SA, Tobias AH, Jacob KA, et al: Arterial thromboembolism in cats: acute crisis in 127 cases (1992-2001) and long-term management with low-dose aspirin in 24 cases, J Vet Intern Med 17:73, 2003.
38. Schoeman JP: Feline distal aortic thromboembolism: a review of 44 cases (1990-1998), J Fel Med Surg 1:221, 1999.
39. Buchanan J, Baker G, Hill J: Aortic embolism in cats: prevalence, surgical treatment and electrocardiography, Vet Rec 79:496, 1966.
40. Reimer SB, Kittleson MD, Kyles AE: Use of rheolytic thrombectomy in the treatment of feline distal aortic thromboembolism, J Vet Intern Med 20:290, 2006.
41. Welch KM, Rozanski EA, Freeman LM, et al: Prospective evaluation of tissue plasminogen activator in 11 cats with arterial thromboembolism, J Fel Med Surg 12:122, 2010.
42. Berger JS, Brown DL, Becker RC: Low-dose aspirin in patients with stable cardiovascular disease: a meta-analysis, Am J Med 121:43, 2008.
43. Sisson DK: Management of heart failure: principles of treatment, therapeutic strategies, and pharmacology. In Fox PR, Sisson DD, Moise NS, editors: Textbook of canine and feline cardiology: principles and clinical practice, ed 2, Philadelphia, 1999, Saunders.
44. Riesen SC, Schober KE, Smith DN, et al: Effects of ivabradine on heart rate and left ventricular function in healthy cats and cats with hypertrophic cardiomyopathy, Am J Vet Res 73:202, 2012.
45. Amberger CN, Glardon O, Glaus T, et al: Effects of benazepril in the treatment of feline hypertrophic cardiomyopathy: results of a prospective, open-label, multicenter clinical trial, J Vet Cardiol 1:19, 1999.
46. Rush JE, Freeman LM, Brown DJ, et al: The use of enalapril in the treatment of feline hypertrophic cardiomyopathy, J Am Anim Hosp Assoc 34:38, 1998.
47. Maron BJ, McKenna WJ, Elliott P, et al: Hypertrophic cardiomyopathy, JAMA 282:2302, 1999.
48. Tsybouleva N, Zhang L, Chen S, et al: Aldosterone, through novel signaling proteins, is a fundamental molecular bridge between the genetic defect and the cardiac phenotype of hypertrophic cardiomyopathy, Circulation 109:1284, 2004.
49. Lim D-S, Lutucuta S, Bachireddy P, et al: Angiotensin II blockade reverses myocardial fibrosis in a transgenic mouse model of human hypertrophic cardiomyopathy, Circulation 103:789, 2001.
50. MacGregor JM, Rush JE, Laste NJ, et al: Use of pimobendan in 170 cats (2006-2010), J Vet Cardiol 13:251, 2011.

51. Gordon SG, Saunders AB, Roland RM, et al: Effect of oral administration of pimobendan in cats with heart failure, J Am Vet Med Assoc 241:89, 2012.
52. Hambrook LE, Bennett PF: Effect of pimobendan on the clinical outcome and survival of cats with non-taurine responsive dilated cardiomyopathy, J Fel Med Surg 14:233, 2012.
53. Bright JM, Golden AL, Gompf RE, et al: Evaluation of the calcium channel-blocking agents diltiazem and verapamil for treatment of feline hypertrophic cardiomyopathy, J Vet Intern Med 5:272, 1991.
54. Fox PR: Prospective, double-blinded, multicenter evaluation of chronic therapies for feline diastolic heart failure: interim analysis [abstract], J Vet Intern Med 17:398, 2003.

CHAPTER 42
CANINE CARDIOMYOPATHY

Robert Prošek, DVM, MS, DACVIM (Cardiology), DECVIM-CA (Cardiology)

KEY POINTS

- Primary cardiomyopathies, by definition, are idiopathic diseases that are not the result of an identifiable systemic disorder or any type of congenital or acquired heart disease.
- Myocardial diseases resulting from a well-defined disease process are appropriately referred to as *secondary myocardial diseases,* and these need to be considered before the diagnosis of a primary cardiomyopathy.
- Dilated (congestive) cardiomyopathy (DCM) is the most common form of primary myocardial disease in dogs and is characterized by chamber dilation and decreased contractility.
- Large and medium sized dogs are typically affected by DCM.
- Atrial fibrillation is common and often is one of the first abnormalities detected in giant breeds with DCM such as Great Danes, Irish Wolfhounds, and Newfoundlands.
- Breed variations in canine DCM should be considered in Cocker Spaniels, Dalmatians, Boxers, Doberman Pinschers, Portuguese Water Dogs, and the giant breeds.
- Boxers with arrhythmogenic right ventricular cardiomyopathy often have syncope and, as the name states, arrhythmias (ventricular).
- Myocardial failure that leads to congestion is an emergency that requires a low-stress environment, oxygen, diuretics, vasodilators, and inotropic support.

Primary myocardial diseases, or "true" cardiomyopathies, are those conditions that predominately affect the heart muscle; that are not the result of other congenital or acquired valvular, pericardial, vascular, or systemic diseases; and whose causes are unknown. The most common form of myocardial disease in the dog is dilated cardiomyopathy (DCM), but arrhythmogenic right ventricular cardiomyopathy (ARVC) (in Boxers) and hypertrophic cardiomyopathy (HCM) are also reported. There is increasing breed-specific information about canine DCM, especially in Doberman Pinschers, Dalmatians, Portuguese Water Dogs, Cocker Spaniels, and the giant breeds, which should be considered in diagnosis and treatment. Secondary myocardial diseases resulting from well-defined disease processes are listed in Box 42-1 and should be considered before making the diagnosis of a primary cardiomyopathy. Diagnostic and treatment techniques often are tailored to each patient and breed, with emphasis on control of a stable rhythm, prevention of congestive heart failure (CHF), and improvement in quality and length of life.

BOX 42-1 *Classification of Secondary Myocardial Diseases of Dogs***

Drugs and Toxins Anthracyclines (doxorubicin*) Catecholamines Ionophores **Canine X-Linked Muscular Dystrophy (Duchenne)*** **Infiltrative** Glycogen storage diseases Mucopolysaccharidosis **Neoplastic** **Ischemic** **Metabolic** Acromegaly Diabetes mellitus (see Chapter 64) Hyperthyroidism (see Chapter 70) Systemic hypertension (see Chapter 9) • Idiopathic • Renal disease	**Nutritional** L-Carnitine deficiency* Taurine deficiency* Vitamin E, selenium deficiency **Inflammatory** Myocarditis (see Chapter 49) **Infectious** Viral, bacterial, fungal, protozoal • Parvovirus, distemper • Lyme disease, trypanosomiasis

*Conditions discussed in this chapter.

DILATED CARDIOMYOPATHY

DCM is characterized by chamber dilation and impaired systolic and often diastolic function of one or both ventricles. It is an adult-onset disease, with the exception of the Portuguese Water Dog in which the young are affected (2 to 32 weeks old). Generally, it is a disease of large and medium sized dogs with increased incidence in the Doberman Pinscher, Great Dane, Irish Wolfhound, and American Cocker Spaniel in North American surveys, but European studies show an increased incidence in the Airedale Terrier, Newfoundland, English Cocker Spaniel, and Doberman Pinscher.[1]

Physical Examination

Often a soft, grade 1 to 3 of 6 systolic left or right apical murmur is noted and is a result of either mitral or tricuspid valve insufficiency, respectively. Auscultation may also reveal a chaotic rhythm of atrial fibrillation or an irregular rhythm caused by atrial or ventricular premature beats. With right-sided CHF the following may be noted: jugular pulses or distention or both, muffled heart and ventral lung sounds with pleural effusion (pleural fluid line), and hepatomegaly caused by congestion with or without ascites. With left-sided CHF, examination often reveals pulmonary crackles or rales, hypokinetic femoral pulses, pulse deficits with ventricular premature beats, or atrial fibrillation. Peripheral edema is rare. Finally, albeit rare, cardiogenic shock may be present as a result of decreased cardiac output (usually blood pressure is normal as a result of vasoconstriction and neurohormonal activation).

Thoracic Radiography

Thoracic radiographs should be examined for generalized cardiomegaly and signs of CHF. Signs of left-sided heart failure include interstitial or alveolar pulmonary edema and moderate to severe left atrial enlargement. Right-sided failure results in pleural effusion, enlarged caudal vena cava, hepatomegaly, and ascites (Figure 42-1).

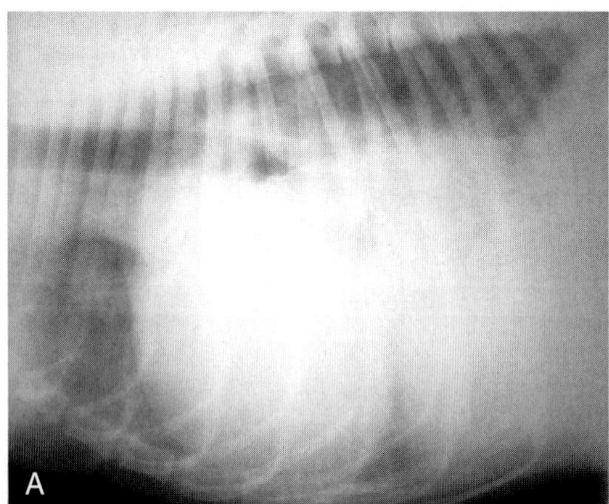

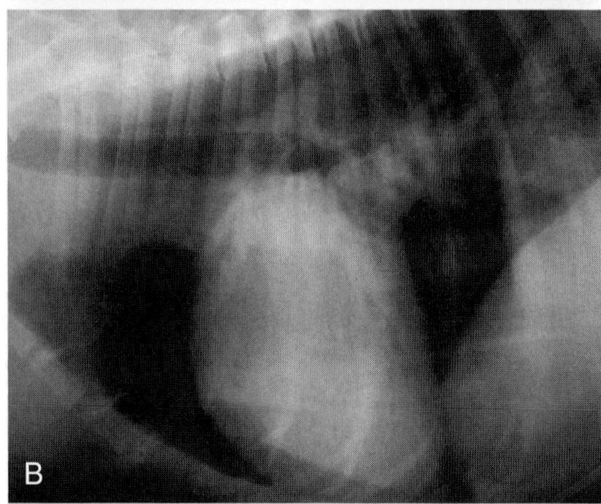

FIGURE 42-1 Lateral radiographs of a Doberman Pinscher with dilated cardiomyopathy. **A,** On presentation. **B,** Same patient after 36 hours of aggressive treatment of congestive heart failure (furosemide, O_2, nitroprusside, dobutamine).

Electrocardiography

The electrocardiogram (ECG) should be examined for sinus tachycardia, possibly with atrial or ventricular premature beats, atrial fibrillation, and ventricular tachycardia, especially in Boxers and Doberman Pinschers. Prolonged or increased voltage QRS complexes suggestive of left ventricular enlargement or low-voltage QRS complexes with pleural effusion may be noted.

Routine Blood Tests

Routine bloodwork findings are usually normal unless severe heart disease is present. Prerenal azotemia, high alanine aminotransferase levels, and electrolyte abnormalities may be evident in cases of severe heart disease. Hyponatremia and hypochloremia, if noted with CHF, are associated with a poorer prognosis. Hypokalemia, metabolic alkalosis, and prerenal azotemia may also be the result of diuretic therapy for heart disease.

Effusion Analysis

Peritoneal or pleural effusion in dogs with DCM is usually a modified transudate (nucleated cell count <2500/ml, total protein <4 g/dl), but on occasion a chylous effusion is found.

Echocardiography

Ventricular and atrial dilation are common with reduced myocardial systolic function (reduced left ventricular fractional shortening percentage [FS%] and ejection fraction). Increased E-point septal separation is also common with ventricular dilation.[2] Doppler studies confirm evidence of mitral and tricuspid regurgitation, low-velocity transaortic flow, diastolic ventricular dysfunction, and possible pulmonary hypertension (as a result of severe left-sided heart failure). Pleural effusion can also be noted along with mild pericardial effusion caused by CHF. Remember, most DCM cases with CHF should have moderate to severe atrial enlargement, and low FS% is not pathognomonic for DCM; many normal hearts contract more in apical-to-basilar direction, and this motion is not accounted for by the FS% (Figure 42-2).

ACUTE TREATMENT OF CONGESTIVE HEART FAILURE

Acute treatment of CHF is summarized in Box 42-2. CHF failure is discussed further in Chapter 40.

LONG-TERM TREATMENT OF DILATED CARDIOMYOPATHY

Pleurocentesis and abdominocentesis should be performed as needed to relieve clinical signs.

Diuretics

Diuretics are administered as needed to control edema. Furosemide is given at 1 to 4 mg/kg PO q8-24h, spironolactone at 1 to 2 mg/kg PO q12h, with or without hydrochlorothiazide 2 to 4 mg/kg PO q12h.The author often uses a combination of spironolactone-hydrochlorothiazide (Aldactazide) at 1 mg/kg PO q24h in refractory cases to decrease the number of drugs the owner has to administer (see Chapter 160).

Angiotensin-Converting Enzyme Inhibitors

Angiotensin-converting enzyme inhibitors are initiated early in the therapeutic regimen, and possible drug selection includes enalapril (0.5 mg/kg PO q12-24h), benazepril (0.25 to 0.5 mg/kg PO q12-24h), and lisinopril (0.5 mg/kg PO q24h).

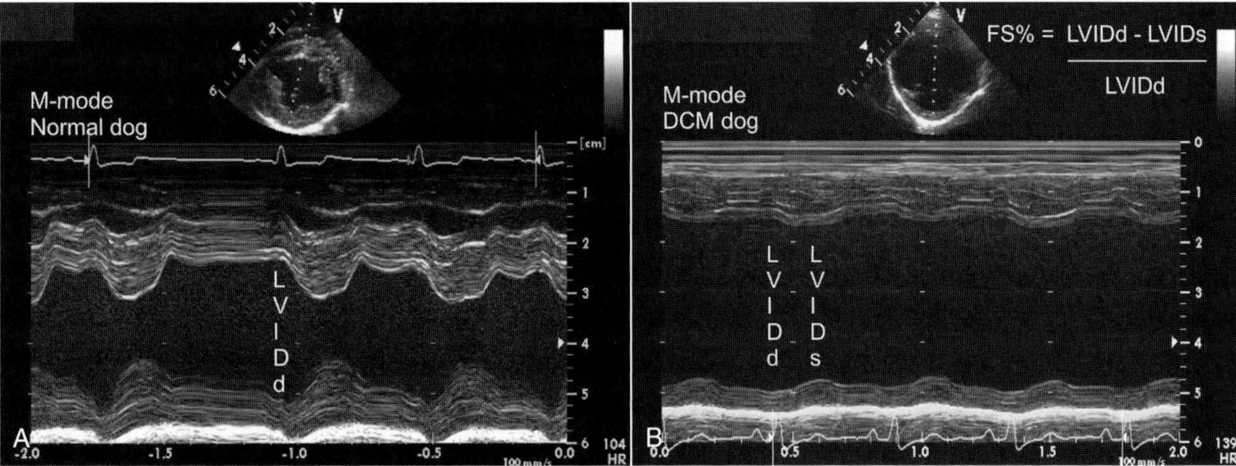

FIGURE 42-2 Example of a normal dog M-mode **(A)** and an M-mode from a dog with dilated cardiomyopathy **(B).** Dog in **B** would have a decreased fractional shortening percentage based on left ventricular internal dimension in diastole: left ventricular internal dimension in systole divided by left ventricular internal dimension in diastole = LVIDd – LVIDs/LVIDd.

BOX 42-2 ***Guidelines for Acute Management of Congestive Heart Failure***

- Minimize stress and ensure absolute rest.
- Perform thoracocentesis as needed for pleural effusion (therapeutic and diagnostic).
- Provide oxygen supplementation.
- If pulmonary edema: Administer furosemide 2 to 6 mg/kg IV or IM initial dose, then 1 to 2 mg/kg q2-3h as needed for resolution of pulmonary edema, then q8-12h for the first 3 days.
- Administer 2% topical nitroglycerin: 1 to 2 inches q8h.
- Treat life-threatening arrhythmias (see Chapters 47 and 48).
- Sodium nitroprusside: 2.0 μg/kg/min. If mean BP remains higher than 70 mm Hg, increase incrementally to 4 μg/kg/min until patient is stabilized or mean pressure falls below 70 mm Hg (rate >10 μg/kg/min rarely needed); extremely effective with furosemide in managing pulmonary edema.
- Dobutamine (if severe heart failure or cardiogenic shock; ECG monitoring needed): start at 2.5 to 5 μg/kg/min, increase q3-4h by 2.5 μg/kg/min until heart rate increases excessively (>180 beats/min or >10% rise from baseline); maximum infusion rate 15 μg/kg/min. If ventricular ectopy develops, reduce rate.
- Other options for positive inotropic support include amrinone, milrinone, and pimobendan.

NOTE: Management should be individually tailored, based on treatment history, clinical picture, complicating arrhythmias, and concurrent diseases. *BP,* Blood pressure; *ECG,* electrocardiogram; *IM,* intramuscularly; *IV,* intravenously.

Digoxin

Digoxin is administered to improve systolic function and to slow ventricular rate in animals with supraventricular tachyarrhythmias (0.003 mg/kg PO q12h, adjusting dosage based on blood levels) (see Chapter 171).

Pimobendan

Pimobendan (0.25 mg/kg PO q12h), a benzimidazole-pyridazinone drug, is classified as an inodilator because of its nonsympathomimetic, nonglycoside positive inotropic (through myocardial calcium sensitization) and vasodilator properties. It has become a mainstay in the treatment of patients with dilated cardiomyopathy. Pimobendan is approved for use in dogs to treat congestive heart failure originating from valvular insufficiency or dilated cardiomyopathy. However, a recent study (The PROTECT Study)[2a] has shown that administration of pimobendan to Doberman Pinschers with preclinical DCM prolongs the time to onset of clinical signs and extends survival, suggesting that pimobendan should be used earlier (preclinical phase) in Doberman Pinschers.

Novel Therapy

Novel therapies may be used after careful consideration of the benefits and risks involved; consultation with a cardiologist may be warranted. β-Blockers may be considered to blunt cardiotoxic effects of the sympathetic nervous system; however, heart failure must be well controlled and the dosage titrated slowly with careful monitoring. Carvedilol (0.5 mg/kg PO q12h; start with ¼ to ½ of a 3.125-mg tablet initially) or metoprolol (0.5 to 1 mg/kg PO q8h)can be used with caution.

Diet

It is important to keep patients eating an adequate level of protein, eliminate high salt–containing snacks, and in cats offer a sodium-restricted commercial diet (not at the expense of anorexia) such as Purina CV, Hills H/D, or Royal Canin Early Cardiac.

Supplements

Taurine (500 mg PO q12h) is started while waiting for taurine blood levels, especially in Cocker Spaniels. Omega-3 fatty acids may improve appetite and reduce cachexia (EPA 30 to 40 mg/kg PO q24h; DHA 20 to 25 mg/kg PO q24h). Consider L-carnitine (110 mg/kg PO q12h) in American Cocker Spaniels not responding to taurine and in Boxers.

TREATMENT OF ARRHYTHMIAS

Please see Chapters 47 and 48.

BREED VARIATIONS WITH DCM

Cocker Spaniels

DCM in some Cocker Spaniels is associated with low plasma taurine levels, and supplementation with taurine and L-carnitine (see earlier section for dosing) appears to improve myocardial function.[3] Normal plasma taurine levels should be more than 50 ng/ml. Additional measures should be used to address complications such as arrhythmias and CHF and might be withdrawn gradually pending response to taurine (usually 3 to 4 months).

Doberman Pinschers

Typically considered the poster child for DCM, the Doberman Pinscher does have some unique manifestations that are important for the clinician to recognize. On a molecular level, deficiency in calstabin-2 implicates this cytoskeletal protein abnormality as one of the possible causes of DCM in this breed. From the clinical perspective, 25% to 30% of Doberman Pinschers have ventricular arrhythmias without the classic ventricular dilation seen with DCM and CHF.[4] These patients are brought in most commonly for syncope or for arrhythmias noted on routine physical examinations. Sudden death is of great concern in this breed, and successful treatment of ventricular arrhythmias is imperative (see Chapter 48).

The author finds the most successful treatment consists of sotalol alone or in combination with mexiletine. A Holter monitor should be used on syncopal Doberman Pinschers to identify the causative arrhythmia (occasionally syncope caused by bradycardia in this breed)[5] and to monitor success of treatment. Doberman Pinschers with more than 50 ventricular premature complexes (VPCs) per 24 hours or with couplets or triplets are suspected for development of DCM. The rest of the Doberman Pinschers have left or biventricular failure, or both, and often have atrial fibrillation. Atrial fibrillation and bilateral CHF appear to be poor prognostic signs,[6] but outlook is also affected by treatment used and client and patient compliance.

Dalmatians

Male dogs appear to be overrepresented in Dalmatians with DCM. All dogs in one study had left-sided heart failure with no evidence of right-sided CHF or atrial fibrillation. Dalmatians fed a low-protein diet for prevention or treatment of urate stones that develop signs consistent with DCM should be switched to a balanced protein diet.[7] Otherwise, treatment is the same as for any dog with left-sided heart failure.

Great Danes and Irish Wolfhounds

Atrial fibrillation is the most common finding and in some cases develops before any other evidence of underlying myocardial disease.[8] Affected dogs commonly are presented for weight loss and loss of full exercise capacity, with occasional cough. Progression of the disease is relatively slow, especially in Irish Wolfhounds.[8] An X-linked pattern of inheritance is suspected in some families of Great Danes, with male dogs being overrepresented.[9]

Portuguese Water Dogs

A juvenile form of DCM has been reported in Portuguese Water Dogs. Affected puppies die from CHF at an average age of 13 weeks after rapid disease progression.[10]

ARRHYTHMOGENIC RIGHT VENTRICULAR CARDIOMYOPATHY IN BOXERS

In Boxer dogs affected with ARVC, approximately one third have predominately left-sided failure, another one third are brought in for syncope or collapse secondary to a rhythm disturbance, and the remaining one third are asymptomatic but have rhythm disturbances (primarily ventricular arrhythmias). Atrial fibrillation occurs less often in Boxers than in other breeds, and cardiomegaly usually is less marked on radiographic evaluation. The pathology of Boxer dog cardiomyopathy closely resembles that seen in humans with ARVC. Similarities between the populations include etiology, clinical picture, and histopathology of fibrous fatty infiltrate of the right ventricular free wall and septum.[11] ARVC appears as an autosomal dominant trait with variable penetrance in Boxers.[12]

Electrocardiography

Ventricular premature beats typically have a left bundle branch block morphology in leads I, II, III, and aVF, consistent with right ventricular origin. As in the Doberman Pinschers, a Holter monitor is helpful in quantifying the VPCs and diagnosing the cause of syncope or collapse (Figure 42-3). More than 100 VPCs in a 24-hour period, periods of couplets and triplets, and runs of ventricular tachycardia may be diagnostic in a symptomatic Boxer.

Treatment of Arrhythmogenic Right Ventricular Cardiomyopathy

Treatment of arrhythmias is based on clinical signs and generally is considered for animals that experience more than 500 to 1000 VPCs per 24 hours, runs of ventricular tachycardia, or evidence of R-on-T phenomenon. The author prefers sotalol (1.5 to 3 mg/kg PO q12h)

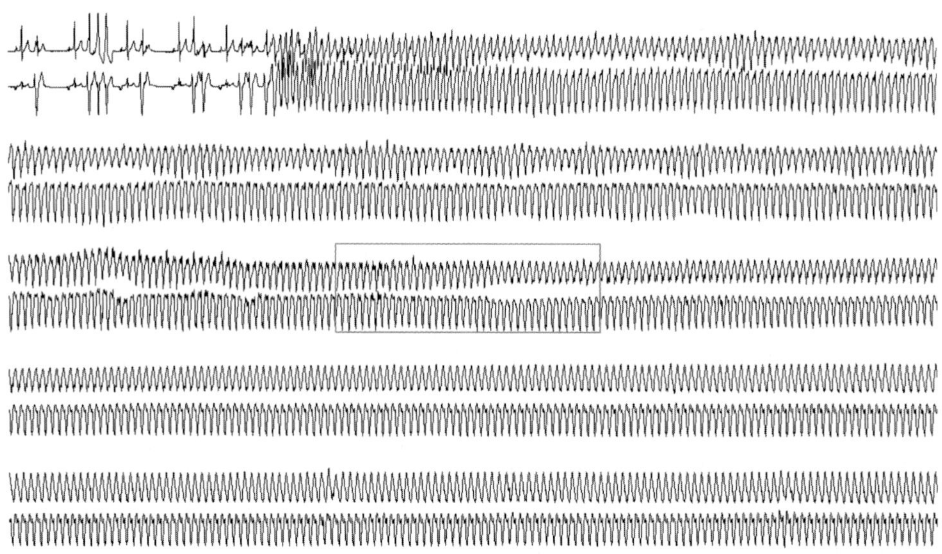

FIGURE 42-3 Sustained ventricular tachycardia in a Boxer dog wearing a Holter monitor (24-hour recorder).

with the combination of mexiletine (5 to 8 mg/kg PO q8h) in life-threatening ventricular arrhythmias in Boxers[13] (see Chapter 48). Another study found that treatment with sotalol or mexiletine-atenolol was well tolerated and efficacious in Boxer dogs with ventricular arrhythmias.[14] If CHF is present, or echocardiographic ventricular and atrial dilation are noted, treatment is the same as outlined earlier for other breeds. Additionally, supplementation with L-carnitine (110 mg/kg PO q12h) might be considered; a family of Boxers showed improvement in systolic function with this drug.[15]

HYPERTROPHIC CARDIOMYOPATHY IN DOGS

HCM is a condition characterized by idiopathic hypertrophy of the left ventricle. The term is applied appropriately only in circumstances in which a stimulus to hypertrophy cannot be identified. HCM has been recognized in only a small number of dogs and can be assumed to be an uncommon disorder.[16,17] A heritable form of hypertrophic obstructive cardiomyopathy has been described in Pointer dogs.[16] The cause of HCM in dogs is unknown. A genetic cause has been identified in most human patients,[18] but the precise pathogenic mechanism of hypertrophy remains a mystery. As with DCM, there may be more than one form (cause) of HCM.

Pathologic Features

The left ventricle is either symmetrically or asymmetrically hypertrophied (concentric hypertrophy), and the left atrium is dilated. Left ventricular mass is increased (heart weight/body weight ratio). When dynamic outflow tract obstruction is present, there is fibrosis of the anterior leaflet of the mitral valve, and a fibrous endocardial plaque on the ventricular septum opposite the mitral valve is noted. Myocardial fiber disarray, which characterizes the human form of this disease,[18] does not appear to be consistently present in affected dogs.

Important Differentials for Concentric Hypertrophy of the Left Ventricle

HCM and its variant hypertrophic obstructive cardiomyopathy are infrequent in dogs, and patients should be evaluated for other causes of concentric hypertrophy such as subvalvular or valvular aortic stenosis and systemic hypertension.

UNCOMMON MYOCARDIAL DISEASES OF DOGS

Duchenne Cardiomyopathy

Duchenne muscular dystrophy is an inherited neuromuscular disorder with an X-linked pattern of inheritance. Dystrophin, a cytoskeletal protein of the plasma membrane, is absent or defective in dogs and humans with Duchenne muscular dystrophy.[19,20] The disorder has been described best in Golden Retriever dogs.[19] Signs of skeletal muscle dysfunction predominate in most affected dogs. Some affected dogs develop deep and narrow Q waves in leads II, III, aVF, CV_6LU, and CV_6LL and may manifest a variety of ventricular arrhythmias. Echocardiography demonstrates hyperechoic areas (fibrosis and calcification) in the left ventricular myocardium as a sequela to myocardial necrosis.[19,20] Some affected dogs develop myocardial failure resembling DCM.

Atrioventricular Myopathy

Atrioventricular myopathy (silent atria, persistent atrial standstill) is a progressive idiopathic myocardial disease of dogs that may or may not be associated with a poorly characterized form of shoulder girdle skeletal muscular dystrophy. The unique features of this disorder include the marked degree of myocardial destruction and fibrosis and the characteristic bradyarrhythmias that result. Pathologic studies often reveal dilated, thin, almost transparent atria with little or no visible muscle. Involvement of the ventricles, especially the right ventricle, occurs somewhat later and is more variable. Histologic findings include variable amounts of mononuclear infiltration, myofiber necrosis and disappearance, and extensive replacement fibrosis. In dogs with muscular dystrophy, changes in skeletal muscle include muscle atrophy, hyalinized degenerated muscle fibers, and mild to moderate steatosis.[21,22] A similar cardiac disorder has been observed in human patients with Emery-Dreifuss (scapulohumeral) muscular dystrophy.

The most commonly affected dogs are English Springer Spaniels and Old English Sheepdogs. Affected dogs usually are brought in for weakness, collapse, or syncope caused by severe bradycardia. Less commonly, dogs have signs of right ventricular or biventricular CHF. Soft murmurs of atrioventricular valve insufficiency are audible in many cases. The most common ECG abnormality is persistent atrial standstill, but complete heart block and other rhythm and conduction disturbances may occur. Atrial enlargement is often found on thoracic radiographs, and generalized cardiomegaly is present in some dogs. Dilated, immobile atria can be identified by echocardiography or fluoroscopy. The clinical course usually is characterized by declining contractility, progressive ventricular dilation, and eventual heart failure. Management of the bradyarrhythmia by artificial pacemaker implantation usually results in immediate improvement in signs, but most dogs eventually develop refractory myocardial failure.[22]

Toxic Myocardial Disease

Doxorubicin (Adriamycin) and other anthracycline antibiotics can cause myocardial failure, typically after the administration of high cumulative doses (usually more than 200 to 300 mg/m^2 doxorubicin). Inasmuch as cardiac toxicity is irreversible, prevention is advised by avoiding high cumulative doses. Dexrazoxane, a cyclic derivative of ethylenediaminetetraacetic acid, protects against cardiomyopathy induced by doxorubicin and other anthracyclines, the main drawback for its use being expense.[23]

REFERENCES

1. Sisson DD, Thomas WP, Keene BW: Primary myocardial disease in the dog. In Ettinger SJ, Feldman EC, editors: Textbook of veterinary internal medicine, ed 5, St Louis, 2000, Saunders.
2. Bonagura JD, Luis Fuentes V: Echocardiography. In Ettinger SJ, Feldman EC, editors: Textbook of veterinary internal medicine, ed 5, St Louis, 2000, Saunders.

2a. Summerfield NJ, Boswood A, O'Grady MR, et al: Efficacy of pimobendan in the Prevention of Congestive Heart Failure or Sudden Death in Doberman Pinschers with Preclinical Dilated Cardiomyopathy (The PROTECT Study), J Vet Intern Med 26:1337, 2012.

3. Kittleson MD, Keene B, Pion P: Results of the multicenter spaniel trial (MUST): taurine-responsive and carnitine-responsive dilated cardiomyopathy in American Cocker Spaniels with decreased plasma taurine concentration, J Vet Intern Med 11:204, 1997.
4. Calvert CA, Meurs KM: CVT update: Doberman Pinscher occult cardiomyopathy. In Bonagura JD, editor: Kirk's current veterinary therapy XIII, St Louis, 2000, Saunders.
5. Calvert CA, Jacobs GJ, Pickus CW: Bradycardia-associated episodic weakness, syncope, and aborted sudden death in cardiomyopathic Doberman Pinschers, J Vet Intern Med 10:88, 1996.
6. Calvert CA, Pickus CW, Jacobs GJ, Brown J: Signalment, survival, and prognostic factors in Doberman Pinschers with end-stage cardiomyopathy, J Vet Intern Med 11:323, 1997.
7. Freeman LM, Michel KE, Brown DJ, et al: Idiopathic dilated cardiomyopathy in Dalmatians: nine cases (1990-1995), J Am Vet Med Assoc 209:1592, 1996.
8. Vollmar AC: The prevalence of cardiomyopathy in the Irish Wolfhound: a clinical study of 500 dogs, J Am Anim Hosp Assoc 36:125, 2000.

9. Meurs KM, Miller MW, Wright NA: Clinical features of dilated cardiomyopathy in Great Danes and results of a pedigree analysis: 17 cases (1990-2000), J Am Vet Med Assoc 218:729, 2001.
10. Dambach DM, Lannon A, Sleeper M, et al: Familial dilated cardiomyopathy of young Portugese Water Dogs, J Vet Intern Med 13:65, 1999.
11. Basso C, Fox PR, Meurs KM, et al: Arrhythmogenic right ventricular cardiomyopathy causing sudden cardiac death in Boxer dogs: a new animal model of human disease, Circulation 109:1180, 2004.
12. Meurs KM, Spier AW, Miller MW, et al: Familial ventricular arrhythmias in Boxers, J Vet Intern Med 13:437, 1999.
13. Prosek R, Estrada AH, Adin D: Comparison of sotalol and mexiletine versus stand-alone sotalol in treatment of Boxer dogs with ventricular arrhythmias, Proceedings of the American College of Veterinary Internal Medicine Forum, Louisville, KY, May 2006 (abstract).
14. Meurs KM, Spier AW, Wright NA, et al: Comparison of the effects of four antiarrhythmic treatments for familial ventricular arrhythmias in Boxers, J Am Vet Med Assoc 221:522, 2002.
15. Keene B, Panciera DP, Atkins CE, et al: Myocardial L-carnitine deficiency in a family of dogs with dilated cardiomyopathy, J Am Vet Med Assoc 198:647, 1991.
16. Sisson DD: Heritability of idiopathic myocardial hypertrophy and dynamic subaortic stenosis in Pointer dogs, J Vet Intern Med 9:118, 1995.
17. Thomas WP, Matthewson JW, Suter PF: Hypertrophic obstructive cardiomyopathy in a dog: clinical, hemodynamic, angiographic, and pathologic studies, J Am Anim Hosp Assoc 20:253, 1984.
18. Wynne J: The cardiomyopathies and myocarditis. In Braunwald E, editor: Heart disease, Philadelphia, 1992, Saunders.
19. Moise NS, Valentine BA, Brown CA, et al: Duchenne's cardiomyopathy in a canine model: electrocardiographic and echocardiographic studies, J Am Coll Cardiol 17:812, 1991.
20. Valentine BA, Winand NJ, Pradhan D, et al: Canine X-linked muscular dystrophy as an animal model of Duchenne muscular dystrophy: a review, Am J Med Genet 42:352, 1992.
21. Jeraj K, Ogburn PN, Edwards WD, Edwards JE: Atrial standstill, myocarditis and destruction of cardiac conduction system: clinicopathologic correlation in a dog, Am Heart J 99:185, 1980.
22. Miller MS, Tilley LP, Atkins CE, et al: Persistent atrial standstill (atrioventricular muscular dystrophy). In Kirk RW, Bonagura JD, editors: Kirk's current veterinary therapy XI, St Louis, 1992, Saunders.
23. Prošek R, Kitchell BE: Dexrazoxane pharm profile, Compendium 24:220, 2002.

CHAPTER 43
VALVULAR HEART DISEASE

Aaron C. Wey, DVM, DACVIM (Cardiology)

KEY POINTS

- Myxomatous valvular degeneration is the most common acquired cardiovascular disorder encountered in canine patients.
- The clinical picture of patients with valvular heart disease in the emergency setting is typically that of cardiogenic pulmonary edema (left-sided congestive heart failure).
- Virtually all patients with acquired degenerative valve disease that have congestive heart failure will have an audible cardiac murmur in the left apical position. If the patient does not have a murmur, other diagnoses should be considered.
- Radiographic and physical examination findings provide a working diagnosis for the management of most patients with valvular heart disease. Echocardiography is helpful but not essential for empiric emergency management.
- Goals of emergency therapy are to relieve signs of congestion, improve forward cardiac output, and improve tissue oxygenation and nutrient delivery.

Acquired degenerative valvular disease is the most common cardiovascular disorder identified in small animals, accounting for approximately 75% of cases of cardiovascular disease seen in dogs.[1] Its incidence (rate of occurrence over time) in older, small breed dogs approaches 100%.[2] The condition may also be referred to as *myxomatous valvular degeneration (MVD), mitral valve prolapse, acquired atrioventricular valvular degeneration,* or *valvular endocardiosis.* Because the mitral valve is most commonly affected, the condition is often referred to as *mitral valve disease.* This latter designation is technically incorrect, and the condition may affect all four cardiac valves.[2] For the purpose of this discussion, *myxomatous valvular degeneration* is used to describe the condition.

MVD most commonly affects canine patients, although it may occur in any mammalian species. Feline patients rarely are affected. In the dog, small breeds are overrepresented. Breeds commonly associated with the disease include the Poodle, Miniature Schnauzer, Chihuahua, Cocker Spaniel, Dachshund, Cavalier King Charles Spaniel, Miniature Pinscher, Lhasa Apso, Shih Tzu, Whippet, and Terrier breeds.[2,3] However, the differential should not be excluded in large breed dogs with a heart murmur in the left apical position. The disease typically is seen in elderly patients, but some breeds are known to develop MVD relatively early in life (e.g., Cavalier King Charles Spaniel).[4] A male predisposition has been suggested.[5]

PATHOLOGY

The exact cellular and hormonal mechanisms that result in MVD are unknown. It has been suggested for some time that collagen degeneration and synthesis are imbalanced, supported by the observation that chondrodystrophic breeds with other connective tissue disorders (collapsing trachea, intervertebral disk disease) often develop MVD. Histologic documentation of abnormal collagen distribution in MVD confirms this suspicion, and matrix metalloproteinases (MMPs) may play an important role in the turnover of collagen in the extracellular matrix of diseased valves.[6] Numerous neurohormonal factors have been implicated including serotonin, transforming growth factors α and β and I[2], insulin-like growth factor 1, angiotensin II, and nitric oxide, but the exact role of these hormonal messengers in the development and progression of the disease is unknown.[7-9] A common misconception is that vegetative endocarditis from periodontal disease contributes to MVD, but evidence to support this hypothesis is lacking, and inflammation does not appear to play a role in the development of the disease in dogs.[6]

Detailed descriptions of the histologic changes that accompany MVD are beyond the scope of this discussion, and readers are referred to other sources for this information.[3,10,11] Grossly the changes are evident as valve thickening and elongation, which subsequently alter the normal coaptation of valve leaflets and may result in valve prolapse. Histologically the valves are distorted and thickened by excessive accumulation of glycosaminoglycans and other extracellular matrix proteins.[7,10] The myxomatous changes have been characterized into classes of severity that are useful in a research setting, but these designations rarely are used clinically.[10]

If the degenerative changes or valve prolapse are significant, they result in a valve regurgitation that increases atrial pressure and decreases forward cardiac output (in the case of atrioventricular valve regurgitation). The degree of valvular insufficiency is dependent on the regurgitant orifice area, the pressure gradient across the valve, and the duration of systole (for the atrioventricular valves) or diastole (for the semilunar valves). In response to the decreased forward cardiac output and increased atrial pressure, several compensatory mechanisms are activated (see Pathophysiology) that result in eccentric hypertrophy (dilation) of the cardiac chambers on either side of the insufficient valve. The valve annulus then enlarges, causing further displacement of the leaflets and more regurgitation. In contrast to diseases with primary myocardial failure (i.e., dilated cardiomyopathy), ventricular function usually is maintained until late in the course of MVD, and patients often are symptomatic before severe myocardial failure develops. Large breed dogs may develop myocardial failure sooner during the course of the disease for reasons that are not completely understood, although increased wall stress as a result of a larger ventricular diameter may be a factor.[3] Many patients with MVD have a long asymptomatic phase before the onset of clinical signs. In these patients the murmur of valvular regurgitation often is identified during routine physical examination or when the patient is seen for an unrelated problem. The factors that result in progression from the asymptomatic stage to overt signs of heart failure in some dogs but not others are not completely understood.

PATHOPHYSIOLOGY

A detailed description of the pathophysiology of heart failure is presented elsewhere in this text (see Chapter 40), but a brief description is presented here. Decreased forward stroke volume and decreased mean arterial pressure result in neurohormonal activation: increased sympathetic tone, activation of the renin-angiotensin-aldosterone system, and a change in the concentration of numerous other neurohormones (endothelin 1, tumor necrosis factor α, nitric oxide).[12] The net result of these changes is vasoconstriction, sodium and water retention, and an increased forward cardiac output and blood pressure. This is accomplished through increased contractility (sympathetic stimulation), volume expansion, and eccentric hypertrophy. Other neurohormonal mechanisms may be activated to modulate this response (i.e., natriuretic peptide production secondary to increased atrial pressure and stretch), but these measures often are overwhelmed or downregulated with chronically altered cardiac output. Chronic activation of the renin-angiotensin-aldosterone system and sympathetic nervous system occurs at the expense of circulating volume and atrial pressure, which is ultimately transmitted to the pulmonary or systemic venous system. Capillary hydrostatic pressure eventually overcomes other forces in Starling's law (interstitial hydrostatic pressure and capillary oncotic pressure) that help to maintain a balance in movement of fluid across the capillary membrane, and fluid transudation results. Initially the pulmonary and systemic lymphatic systems accommodate the extra fluid transudation, but these systems eventually become overwhelmed and overt pulmonary edema or third-space fluid accumulation results (congestive heart failure). Additional complications particular to MVD such as rupture of chordae tendineae may also occur. This may be well tolerated with a minor chord but may result in a large increase in regurgitant orifice area and left atrial pressure with acute pulmonary edema.[10] Rarely, left atrial rupture occurs secondary to endothelial tearing at the site of impact of a high-velocity regurgitant jet. This complication may result in an acquired atrial septal defect but more commonly results in acute tamponade (see Chapter 45), collapse, and often death.[10,19]

HISTORY AND PHYSICAL EXAMINATION

Patients with MVD commonly have a history of a cardiac murmur that was identified during a routine physical examination. The murmur is often chronic, although it may be a new finding in the case of chordal rupture. The intensity of the murmur has been correlated with the severity of regurgitation.[13] The patient may be brought in for evaluation of a cough, dyspnea, exercise intolerance, syncope, or collapse. Physical examination findings with left-sided heart failure are attributable to pulmonary edema: dyspnea, orthopnea, cyanosis, and abnormal lung sounds. It should be noted that all patients with pulmonary crackles do not have cardiogenic pulmonary edema, and pulmonary edema can be present without crackles clearly evident on auscultation. Tachyarrhythmias (sinus tachycardia, premature contractions, or atrial fibrillation) may also be noted. Right-sided heart failure may result in the accumulation of pleural effusion or ascites, with decreased ventral lung sounds or abdominal distention, respectively. Jugular distention, pulsation, or a positive hepatojugular reflux test should be visible in patients with right-sided heart failure. An S_3 gallop sound may be detected with careful auscultation at the left sternal border in a patient with severe mitral regurgitation.[13] Femoral pulses usually are strong until late in the course of the disease unless acute chordal or left atrial rupture occurs. With left atrial rupture, patients demonstrate symptoms of cardiac tamponade (see Chapter 45).

LABORATORY EVALUATION

Laboratory findings for patients with MVD often are nonspecific. The complete blood cell count may be normal or may demonstrate a normochromic, normocytic nonregenerative anemia. A stress leukogram (neutrophilia, monocytosis, lymphopenia, eosinopenia) often is present in patients with congestive heart failure. The biochemical profile may demonstrate changes secondary to passive congestion of the liver (hepatopathy) or hyponatremia/hypochloridemia in chronic heart failure. Conversely, the biochemical panel may be normal or demonstrate abnormalities consistent with other diseases of aged patients (e.g., chronic renal failure, hepatopathies). Blood gas analysis may reveal varying degrees of hypoxemia with metabolic acidosis secondary to peripheral vasoconstriction and poor perfusion (lactic acidosis).

Research has identified several biochemical markers that may aid in the assessment of the patient with heart failure. The concentration of natriuretic peptides (ANP, BNP) is known to increase in congestive heart failure (CHF), although these peptides are difficult to measure in clinical samples because of their short half-life. Logistical difficulties associated with the stability of B-type natriuretic peptide have largely been overcome with the development of assays to evaluate the more stable amino terminal portion of the cleaved pro-hormone (NT-proBNP). These assays have been validated and demonstrate good sensitivity and specificity in differentiating patients with dyspnea secondary to cardiac disease versus primary respiratory disease.[14,15] Human "bedside" analyzers for B-type natriuretic peptide and NT-proBNP are available and may eventually be available in the veterinary emergency hospital laboratory. However, numerous other factors may influence NT-proBNP concentration in an emergency patient (e.g., pulmonary hypertension, renal dysfunction) and may confound interpretation of results of this assay.[16-18] Cardiac troponins (particularly cardiac troponin I, or cTnI) have also been investigated as blood-based biomarkers for heart disease in dogs and are sensitive but relatively nonspecific.[19,20]

ELECTROCARDIOGRAPHIC FINDINGS

The electrocardiogram is not a sensitive or specific diagnostic test for MVD. However, it should be performed in any patient with an arrhythmia or tachycardia. The most common rhythm changes seen in patients with MVD are sinus tachycardia, atrial premature contractions, and atrial fibrillation. Ventricular ectopy is unusual in the typical small breed dog with MVD but may occur with hypoxia, with other organ system failure, or in large breeds. Other abnormalities that may be identified in canine patients include P mitrale (P wave width >40 msec), P pulmonale (P wave height >0.5 mV), or evidence of left ventricular enlargement (R wave amplitude >2.5 mV or duration >60 msec). Severe cardiac disease may be present with normal electrocardiographic findings, and the absence of these electrocardiographic changes should not be interpreted by the clinician as an indicator of normal cardiac chamber size or function.

RADIOGRAPHIC FINDINGS

The radiographic findings in canine patients with MVD and congestive heart failure CHF are illustrated in Figure 43-1. Left-sided heart enlargement is apparent as loss of the caudal cardiac waist (left atrial enlargement) and a tall cardiac silhouette (left ventricular enlargement). These changes result in dorsal deviation of the trachea, carina, and mainstem bronchi. Pulmonary venous congestion may be evident in the cranial lobar veins on the lateral projection and the caudal lobar veins on the orthogonal projection. Dorsoventral positioning provides better visualization of the caudal pulmonary vasculature and is less stressful for the dyspneic patient than ventrodorsal positioning. Ventrodorsal positioning should be used in patients with pleural effusion for better visualization of the heart and accessory lung lobe.[22] In patients with significant tricuspid regurgitation, the heart may have changes consistent with right-sided heart enlargement (reverse D on dorsoventral films, increased sternal contact on lateral films). Often patients with advanced valvular disease will have global or generalized cardiomegaly. A vertebral scale system (vertebral heart score [VHS]) has been validated as an objective measure of assessing cardiac size in the dog and cat and may help substantiate a clinician's subjective impression of cardiomegaly.[23] Pulmonary edema in the dog initially is identified as a mild, perihilar, or central interstitial infiltrate. As the severity of the infiltrates increases in canine patients, they generally progress in a caudal and dorsal distribution but may be multifocal or asymmetric, particularly right caudal pulmonary interstitial infiltrates.[24] In cases with right-sided heart failure or biventricular disease, pleural fissure lines or overt effusion may be visible and there may be a loss of serosal detail in the abdomen.

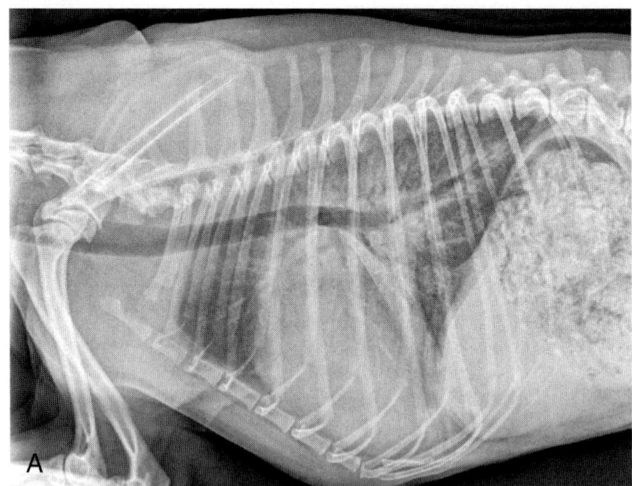

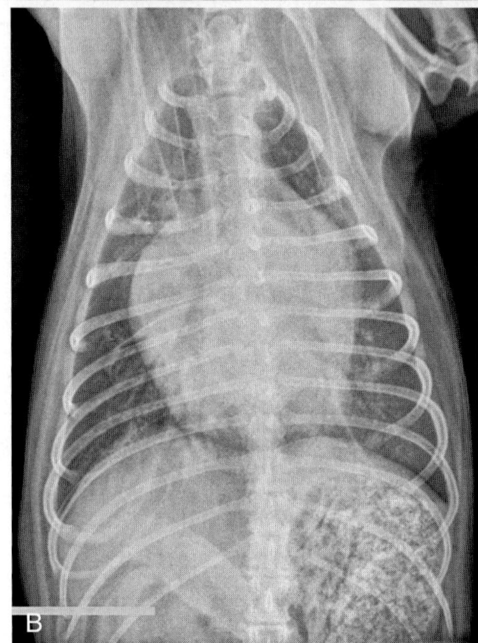

FIGURE 43-1 Right lateral **(A)** and dorsoventral **(B)** radiographs of a dog with myxomatous valvular degeneration and severe mitral regurgitation. **A,** Severe left-sided heart enlargement is visible as an increase in overall heart size (vertebral heart score 13.0) with a tall cardiac silhouette (left ventricular enlargement) and loss of the caudal cardiac waist (left atrial enlargement). The pulmonary vascular markings are difficult to evaluate because of a generalized pulmonary interstitial pattern that is more pronounced in the hilar and caudal lung fields. The liver is mildly enlarged. **B,** Severe generalized cardiomegaly is present with an enlarged left atrium. The pulmonary vasculature is difficult to evaluate. An interstitial pattern is visible in the caudal lung fields.

ECHOCARDIOGRAPHIC FINDINGS

Although echocardiography is not essential in generating an emergency medical treatment plan for patients with valvular disease, ultrasound machines commonly are used in the emergency setting. Echocardiography can help gauge disease severity, identify ruptured chordae tendineae, quantify pleural or pericardial effusion, confirm the diagnosis when radiographs are inconclusive, and guide therapy (e.g., thoracocentesis). The classic findings in a patient with MVD affecting the mitral valve include left ventricular and left atrial dilation, hyperdynamic left ventricular wall motion, and thickened mitral valve leaflets. For the emergency veterinarian, evaluation of left atrial size is the easiest assessment and has been reviewed

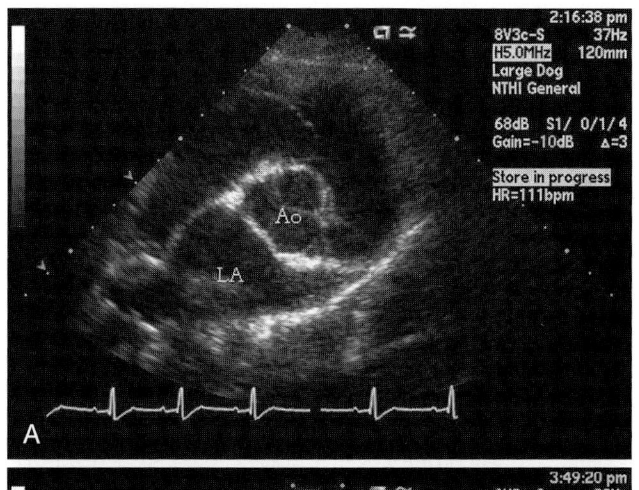

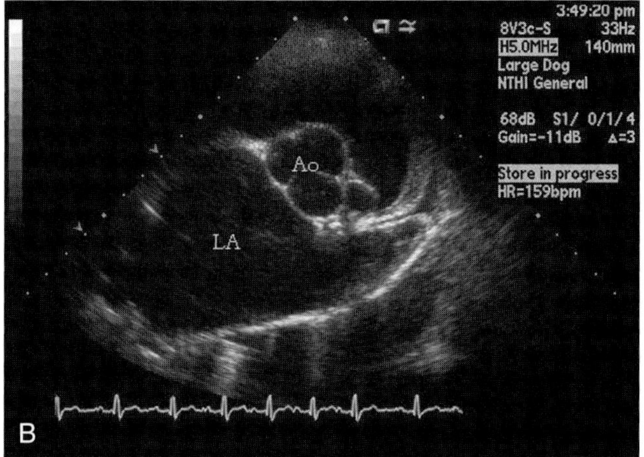

FIGURE 43-2 Right parasternal short-axis echocardiographic views of the aorta and left atrium in a normal dog **(A)** and a dog with myxomatous valve disease **(B).** The ratio of the cross-sectional dimensions of the left atrium and aorta *(LA/Ao)* should be less than 1.5 in normal dogs, as depicted in this example. In **B,** severe left atrial enlargement is present with an LA/Ao 2.0 or greater, suggestive of severe mitral regurgitation and elevated left atrial pressure. In the emergency setting this finding may be used to support a diagnosis of congestive heart failure.

elsewhere.[25,26] In general, patients in left-sided heart failure secondary to MVD will have a left atrium/aorta ratio of 2.0 or more (Figure 43-2). If this criterion is not met, other diagnoses should be considered for interstitial pulmonary infiltrates (e.g., pulmonary hypertension or thromboembolism, noncardiogenic edema, primary lung diseases, neoplasia). Other echocardiographic findings that may be identified include valve thickening or prolapse, leaflet flail (protrusion of the leaflet margin into the atrium during systole), and ruptured chordae tendineae. If available, color and spectral Doppler evaluation can confirm valve insufficiencies and offer subjective information regarding the severity of the regurgitant lesion. In patients with left atrial rupture, pericardial effusion and a pericardial thrombus may be identified. Although M-mode and spectral Doppler echocardiography offer many techniques for further evaluating cardiac function in patients with MVD, these techniques are highly dependent on sonographer experience and are beyond the scope of this text. The reader is referred to other sources for descriptions of these techniques.[26]

EMERGENCY MANAGEMENT

As with any cause of heart failure, ideal therapy would be to reverse or correct the underlying disease. Although this is not possible in the emergency setting for a patient with MVD, several hemodynamic variables can be manipulated to improve cardiovascular function and relieve clinical signs. The goals of emergency therapy for the patient in heart failure secondary to MVD are to relieve signs of congestion, improve forward cardiac output, and improve tissue oxygenation and nutrient delivery. An American College of Veterinary Internal Medicine panel has published a consensus statement outlining diagnostic and therapeutic guidelines for management of congestive heart failure secondary to MVD in dogs.[27] The reader is referred to this consensus statement for a more detailed discussion of treatment, but therapeutic recommendations are reviewed briefly here.

Congestive signs can be relieved by reducing the hydrostatic pressure in the pulmonary or systemic venous system or by removing third-space effusions. Reducing hydrostatic pressure can be accomplished by decreasing circulating volume or by venodilation. Relief of pulmonary edema usually is accomplished with diuretics to decrease intravascular volume. Furosemide is used most often (2 to 8 mg/kg in dogs or 1 to 4 mg/kg in cats intramuscularly [IM] or intravenously [IV]). A dosage-dependent venodilator effect has been observed with intravenous administration in humans.[28] A protocol for constant rate infusion (CRI) of furosemide has been investigated in normal dogs and is more effective than intermittent bolus injection.[29] Typical CRI dosing ranges from 0.5 to 1.0 mg/kg/hr after a bolus loading dose. Other loop diuretics (e.g., bumetanide, torsemide) may have greater potency and may be more useful in the future for management of canine patients.[30] Oral diuretics are not ideal because of the likelihood of impaired gastrointestinal absorption and a relatively slow onset of action. In patients with refractory edema, moderate restriction of fluid intake may also be helpful in reducing congestive signs. Side effects of diuretic therapy include prerenal azotemia, electrolyte disturbances (hypokalemia, hyponatremia, others), and acid-base derangements (metabolic alkalosis). Overzealous administration of diuretics or restriction of fluids can result in uremia, dangerous reductions in circulating plasma volume, and poor tissue perfusion.

Venodilators are not universally effective in veterinary patients, and their use should be considered adjunctive to diuretic therapy and oxygen administration. Topical nitroglycerin ointment (⅛ to ¼ inch q6h on the inner pinnae) is used most commonly. This modality increases venous capacitance in normal dogs,[31] but oral nitrates have minimal effect in normal dogs or dogs with CHF.[32]

Cardiac Output

Arterial vasodilators are helpful in reducing regurgitant fraction and increasing forward cardiac output. Hydralazine (0.5 to 2.5 mg/kg PO q12h) has been advocated in this setting for patients with refractory heart failure.[3] Side effects of this therapy include emesis and hypotension. Amlodipine (0.2 to 0.4 mg/kg PO q12h) may also be useful and generally has fewer side effects than hydralazine. Enalapril is not a potent vasodilator in dogs and cats and generally is not recommended for emergency management of CHF.[27] More aggressive approaches for improving forward cardiac output can be employed using an intravenous vasodilator in conjunction with a positive inotrope. This combination should be used only in settings where invasive blood pressure monitoring is available. Intravenous nitroprusside (1 to 2 mcg/kg/min titrated upward to a target blood pressure) can be administered alone or in conjunction with either dopamine or dobutamine (2.5 to 10 mcg/kg/min [dobutamine for cats: 1 to 5 mcg/kg/min]) to improve forward cardiac output and reduce capillary hydrostatic pressure. Mean arterial pressures should be maintained above 80 mm Hg with this regimen and can be adjusted quickly because of the short half-life of these medications. Potential complications of this therapy include severe hypotension and cyanide toxicity (with expired nitroprusside solutions or ≥3 days after mixing). With universal availability and increased experience with pimobendan, oral positive inotropic therapy with this agent is now recommended in the emergency setting.[27] Pimobendan is a phosphodiesterase inhibitor with both positive inotropic and vasodilatory properties that has significant benefits in the management of CHF.[35] This drug is now considered standard therapy in the emergency setting in patients able to tolerate oral administration, with a recommended oral dosage of 0.25 to 0.3 mg/kg PO q12h (see Chapter 40).[27] Digoxin and other digitalis glycosides have a long half-life that limits their usefulness for acute therapy. This can be overcome with intravenous administration or oral drug loading, but these approaches may result in toxicity.

Tissue Oxygenation

Oxygen therapy should be considered essential for the patient in heart failure from any cause. Increasing the fraction of inspired oxygen will help improve blood oxygen content, but the impaired pulmonary function caused by edema necessitates that oxygen be used in conjunction with the therapies described above. Detailed guidelines for administration of oxygen are given elsewhere in this text (see Chapter 14).

Arrhythmia Management and Adjunctive Therapy

Arrhythmias may be present in patients with MVD and complicate medical management. Isolated atrial or ventricular premature contractions rarely require therapy, but atrial fibrillation and ventricular or supraventricular tachycardia should be identified and addressed. These commonly result in a rapid heart rate that decreases diastolic filling and myocardial perfusion and affect forward cardiac output. Tachyarrhythmias may also decrease systolic function and result in myocardial failure if they are chronic (tachycardia-induced cardiomyopathy). Pharmacologic management of these arrhythmias is discussed elsewhere in this text (see Chapters 47 and 48). Direct current cardioversion may be employed for rhythms that are refractory to medical management (see Chapter 204).

Sedation is often helpful in managing anxiety associated with dyspnea in congestive heart failure patients, and opioid drugs such as morphine and butorphanol are often recommended for this purpose, although care and monitoring are necessary to minimize the risk of respiratory depression with these agents.[27] Control of ambient temperature and humidity should also be a priority, particularly when patients are confined to an oxygen cage.

Monitoring

Successful treatment of a patient with CHF from MVD requires monitoring of volume status, renal function, acid-base balance, and blood pressure. When patients are admitted in an emergency setting, a body weight, complete blood cell count, biochemical profile, urine specific gravity, blood pressure, and thoracic radiographs should be obtained before initiation of therapy (condition permitting). Twelve to 24 hours after initiation of therapy, a blood gas analysis, biochemical profile with electrolytes, and thoracic radiographs should be repeated. Frequent (every 12 hours) evaluation of patient weight is often helpful, with a target reduction of 5% to 7% of body weight on admission. If a patient develops significant azotemia (blood urea nitrogen >50 mg/dl, creatinine ≥2.5 mg/dl), dehydration, weight loss greater than 10% of weight on admission, alkalosis, or electrolyte disturbances, diuretic therapy should be modified and alternative modalities employed.

LONG-TERM THERAPY

In general, the goals of long-term therapy for MVD mirror those of the emergency setting but with orally administered medications, with additional emphasis on slowing disease progression, prolonging survival, and maintaining quality of life. The precise timing for initiation of therapy before the onset of CHF is a subject of much debate because clinical trials have demonstrated variable results with the early use of angiotensin-converting enzyme (ACE) inhibitors, and a consensus has still not been reached regarding the use of this drug class before the onset of clinical signs.[27,36] β-Blockers have also been evaluated in the preclinical phase of MVD, but recent data suggest that these drugs also do not slow progression of the disease or delay the onset of clinical symptoms.[37] Chronic treatment of patients with MVD and CHF should include a diuretic at the lowest effective dosage, pimobendan (0.25 to 0.3 mg/kg PO q12h), and an ACE inhibitor (enalapril, benazepril, or equivalent at 0.25 to 0.5 mg/kg PO q12h).[27] A balanced low-sodium diet should also play an integral role in the management of a patient's congestion and may reduce the dosage of diuretics required to control signs of edema but may be difficult to initiate at the onset of oral therapy because of poor palatability.[27,33] Spironolactone has gained recent recognition as an adjunctive agent that may be beneficial as an aldosterone antagonist rather than a diuretic, although a consensus has not been reached to date regarding initiation of therapy before or at the onset of heart failure.[27,34] As heart failure progresses or complications such as atrial arrhythmias or systolic dysfunction develop, digoxin is often added to this regimen. Adjunctive therapies (potassium gluconate and cough suppressants) are used on a case-by-case basis. When patients develop edema that is refractory to this therapy, additional diuretics (spironolactone, hydrochlorothiazide), positive inotropic agents (digoxin), vasodilators (amlodipine, hydralazine), cough suppressants (hydrocodone, dextromethorphan, butorphanol, tramadol) and bronchodilators (theophylline/aminophylline) are used in various combinations depending on the patient's coexisting disease states, ventricular function, and tolerance of therapy.[27,36] Sildenafil, a selective phosphodiesterase V inhibitor that causes nitric oxide–mediated vasodilation secondary to increases in cyclic GMP within the vascular endothelium, has been evaluated in the management of pulmonary hypertension secondary to congestive heart failure. This agent may become more important in the management of refractory heart failure as more prospective clinical trials are performed, but cost may also be a limiting factor. For patients whose disease is refractory to medical therapy, surgical intervention is a newer therapeutic modality that is offered at selected teaching institutions.[27,38-41]

PROGNOSIS

In general, MVD carries a more favorable prognosis than many other cardiovascular diseases. The condition has a long (1 to 3 years) preclinical phase when patients have an excellent quality of life with few clinical signs. When CHF signs develop, the prognosis worsens. Medical therapy may offer patients the possibility of approximately 6 to 18 months of good-quality life after the onset of CHF.[2] Patients with ruptured major chordae tendineae or a ruptured left atrium have a poor or grave prognosis. When patients decompensate while receiving long-term oral medications, aggressive parenteral therapy can still offer the possibility of temporary recovery and return to life at home with oral medication.

INFECTIOUS ENDOCARDITIS

This condition is mentioned here because of the similar hemodynamic changes that develop with valve regurgitation caused by vegetative lesions, but the condition is not typically associated with MVD. With the exception of one case report,[42] no published data are available that would suggest that MVD predisposes dogs to bacterial endocarditis. For detailed descriptions of this disease, the reader is referred to Chapter 98.[43,44]

REFERENCES

1. Detweiler DK, Patterson DF: The prevalence and types of cardiovascular disease in dogs, Ann N Y Acad Sci 127:481, 1965.
2. Borgarelli M, Buchanan JW: Historical review, epidemiology, and natural history of mitral valve disease, J Vet Card 14:93. 2012.
3. Kittleson MD: Myxomatous atrioventricular valvular degeneration. In Kittleson MD, Kienle RD: Small animal cardiovascular medicine, St Louis, 1998, Mosby.
4. Beardow AW, Buchanan JW: Chronic mitral valve disease in Cavalier King Charles Spaniels: 95 cases (1987-1991), J Am Vet Med Assoc 203:1023, 1993.
5. Swenson L, Häggström J, Kvart C, et al: Relationship between parental cardiac status in Cavalier King Charles Spaniels and prevalence and severity of chronic valvular disease in offspring, J Am Vet Med Assoc 208:2009, 1996.
6. Aupperle H, Disatian S: Pathology, protein expression and signaling in myxomatous mitral valve degeneration: Comparison of dogs and humans, J Vet Card 14:59, 2012.
7. Orton EC, Lacerda CMR, Maclea HB: Signaling pathways in mitral valve degeneration, J Vet Card 14:7, 2012.
8. Pedersen HD, Schutt T, Sondergaard R, et al: Decreased plasma concentration of nitric oxide metabolites in dogs with untreated mitral regurgitation, J Vet Intern Med 17:178, 2003.
9. Parker HG, Kilroy-Glynn P: Myxomatous mitral valve disease in dogs: does size matter? J Vet Card 14:19, 2012.
10. Fox PR: Pathology of myxomatous mitral valve disease in the dog, J Vet Card 14:103, 2012.
11. Sisson DK: Acquired valvular heart disease in dogs and cats. In Fox PR, Sisson DK, Moise NS, editors: Textbook of canine and feline cardiology, ed 2, St Louis, 1999, Saunders.
12. Martin MWS: Treatment of congestive heart failure, a neuroendocrine disorder, J Small Anim Pract 44:154, 2003.
13. Häggström J, Kvart C, Hansson K: Heart sounds and murmurs: changes related to severity of chronic valvular disease in the Cavalier King Charles Spaniel, J Vet Intern Med 9:75, 1995.
14. Prosek R, Sisson DD, Oyama MA, Solter PF: Distinguishing cardiac and non-cardiac dyspnea in 48 dogs using plasma atrial natriuretic factor, B-type natriuretic factor, endothelin, and cardiac troponin-I, J Vet Intern Med 21:238, 2007
15. Oyama MA, Rush JE, Rozanski EA, et al: Assessment of N-terminal pro-B-type natriuretic peptide concentration for differentiation of congestive heart failure from primary respiratory tract disease as the cause of respiratory signs in dogs, J Am Vet Med Assoc 235:1319, 2009.
16. Lee JA, Herndon WE, Rishniw M: The effect of noncardiac disease on plasma brain natriuretic peptide concentration in dogs, J Vet Emerg Crit Care 21:5, 2011.
17. Kellihan HB, MacKie BA, Stepien RA: NT-proBNP, NT-proANP and cTnI concentrations in dogs with pre-capillary pulmonary hypertension, J Vet Card 13:171, 2011.
18. Raffan E, Loureiro J, Dukes-McEwan J, et al: The cardiac biomarker NT-proBNP is increased in dogs with azotemia, J Vet Intern Med 23:1184, 2009.
19. Oyama MA, Sisson DD: Cardiac troponin-I concentration in dogs with cardiac disease, J Vet Intern Med 18:831, 2004.
20. Spratt DP, Mellanby RJ, Drury N, et al: Cardiac troponin I: evaluation of a biomarker for the diagnosis of heart disease in the dog, J Small Anim Pract 46:139, 2005.
21. Peddle GD, Buchanan JW: Acquired atrial septal defects secondary to rupture of the atrial septum in dogs with degenerative mitral valve disease, J Vet Card 12:129, 2010.
22. Saunders HM, Keith D: Thoracic imaging. In King LG, editor: Textbook of respiratory disease in dogs and cats, St Louis, 2004, Saunders.
23. Buchanan JW, Bucheler J: Vertebral scale system to measure canine heart size in radiographs, J Am Vet Med Assoc 206:194, 1995.
24. Diana A, Guglielmini C, Pivetta M, et al: Radiographic features of cardiogenic pulmonary edema in dogs with mitral regurgitation: 61 cases (1998-2007), J Am Vet Med Assoc 235:1058, 2009.
25. Rush JE: The use of echocardiography in the ICU and ER, Proceedings of the 23rd American College of Veterinary Internal Medicine Forum, Baltimore, June 2005.
26. Chetboul V, Tissier R: Echocardiographic assessment of canine degenerative mitral valve disease, J Vet Card, 14:127, 2012.
27. Atkins C, Bonagura J, Ettinger S, et al: Guidelines for the diagnosis and treatment of canine chronic valvular heart disease, J Vet Intern Med 23:1142, 2009.
28. Pickkers P, Dormans TP, Russel FG, et al: Direct vascular effects of furosemide in humans, Circulation 96:1847, 1997.
29. Adin DB, Taylor AW, Hill RC, et al: Intermittent bolus injection versus continuous infusion of furosemide in normal adult Greyhounds, J Vet Intern Med 17:632, 2003.
30. Peddle GD, Singletary GE, Reynolds CA, et al: Effect of torsemide and furosemide on clinical, laboratory, radiographic and quality of life variables in dogs with heart failure secondary to mitral valve disease, J Vet Card 14:253, 2012
31. Narayanan P, Hamlin RL, Nakayama T, et al: Increased splenic capacity in response to transdermal application of nitroglycerine in the dog, J Vet Intern Med 13:44, 1999.
32. Adin DB, Kittleson MD, Hornof WJ, et al: Efficacy of a single oral dose of isosorbide 5-mononitrate in normal dogs and in dogs with congestive heart failure, J Vet Intern Med 15:105, 2001.
33. Rush JE, Freeman LM, Brown DJ, et al: Clinical, echocardiographic, and neurohormonal effects of a sodium-restricted diet in dogs with heart failure, J Vet Intern Med 14:513, 2000.
34. Bernay F, Bland JM, Haggstrom J, et al: Efficacy of spironolactone on survival in dogs with naturally occurring mitral regurgitation caused by myxomatous mitral valve disease, J Vet Intern Med 24:331, 2010.
35. Boswood A: Current use of pimobendan in canine patients with heart disease. Vet Clin North Am Small Anim Pract 40:571, 2010.
36. Atkins CE, Haggstrom J: Pharmacologic management of myxomatous mitral valve disease in dogs, J Vet Card 14:165, 2012.
37. Keene BW, Fox PR, Hamlin RL, et al: Efficacy of BAY 41-9202 (bisoprolol oral solution) for the treatment of chronic valvular heart disease (CHVD) in dogs, Proceedings of the 24th American College of Veterinary Internal Medicine Forum, New Orleans, June 2012.
38. Buchanan JW, Sammarco CD: Circumferential suture of the mitral annulus for correction of mitral regurgitation in dogs, Vet Surg 27:182, 1998.
39. Griffiths LG, Orton EC, Boon JA: Evaluation of techniques and outcomes of mitral valve repair in dogs, J Am Vet Med Assoc 224:1941, 2004.
40. Orton EC, Hackett TB, Mama K, et al: Technique and outcome of mitral valve replacement in dogs, J Am Vet Med Assoc 226:1508, 2005.
41. Uechi M: Mitral valve repair in dogs, J Vet Card 14:185, 2012.
42. Tou SP, Adin DB, Castleman WL: Mitral valve endocarditis after dental prophylaxis in a dog, J Vet Intern Med 19:268, 2005.
43. Kittleson MD: Infective endocarditis (and annuloaortic ectasia). In Kittleson MD, Kienle RD: Small animal cardiovascular medicine, ed 1, St Louis, 1998, Mosby.
44. Miller MW, Sisson DK: Infectious endocarditis. In Fox PR, Sisson DK, Moise NS, editors: Textbook of canine and feline cardiology: principles and clinical practice, ed 2, St Louis, 1999, Saunders.

CHAPTER 44
MYOCARDIAL CONTUSION

Adam J. Reiss, DVM, DACVECC

KEY POINTS

- Myocardial injuries often are overlooked in the trauma patient.
- The most common physiologic consequence of myocardial injury in dogs and humans is arrhythmias.
- Arrhythmias associated with myocardial injury may be delayed in onset up to 48 hours.
- Holter monitoring or continuous electrocardiographic (ECG) monitoring should be considered in high-risk patients.
- Troponins, cardiac-specific proteins, are an effective biomarker of myocardial injury in dogs.
- Normal ECG findings and cardiac troponin I levels on admission in traumatized human patients are an efficient way to rule out myocardial injuries and arrhythmias associated with trauma.
- Management of myocardial injuries is aimed toward maintaining optimal cardiac output and suppressing life-threatening arrhythmias.
- The class I antiarrhythmic agents, including lidocaine and procainamide, are used commonly to manage ventricular ectopy associated with myocardial injury.

Traumatic myocarditis is a controversial subject. Much of the controversy in human studies revolves around a lack of consistent evidence that this injury has any effect on patient outcome and the expense associated with diagnostic testing, cardiac monitoring, and prolonged hospital stays.[1] Additional controversies associated with this injury revolve around its name, incidence, and how it is diagnosed. What appears to be agreed on consistently in the literature is the basic definition of this injury and that there is lack of an antemortem diagnostic gold standard. Direct visualization of the heart or histologic examination of damaged myocardium are considered the current diagnostic gold standard.[2]

The term *traumatic myocarditis* has been used often in veterinary literature to describe an assumed myocardial injury associated with arrhythmias in patients suffering from blunt thoracic trauma.[3] This term is used interchangeably with *myocardial injury* in this chapter.

INCIDENCE

Blunt thoracic trauma has been reported to result in myocardial injuries in 8% to 95% of human patients.[3-10] Reported variations in the frequency of myocardial injuries of dogs are similar to those described in humans. Several studies (three prospective, two retrospective) have examined the prevalence of traumatic myocarditis in the dog and report a range from 10% to 96%.[4,11-14] Variations in study design as well as disagreements regarding terminology, diagnostic modalities, and criteria used to identify myocardial injuries in humans and dogs contribute to the wide range in the reported frequency of this type of injury in both the human and veterinary literature.[2,3,7,13-21] The authors of these studies do agree, however, that myocardial injuries are easily overlooked.[18]

ETIOLOGY, MECHANISM OF INJURY, AND PATHOPHYSIOLOGY

Thoracic trauma is common in dogs injured by automobiles, animal attacks (bites, kicks), and falls from a height.* Because of the elastic nature of the thoracic cage, blunt trauma may subject the myocardium to compressive and concussive forces.[13,14,22-24] The most common mechanism of myocardial injury in the dog is that secondary to lateral chest compression.[22,24] In addition to potential concussive injury from forceful contact with the ribs, sternum, and vertebrae when rapid acceleration or deceleration occurs, it has been proposed that distortion of the thoracic cage results in a rise in intrathoracic and intracardiac pressures, causing shearing stresses within the myocardium powerful enough to result in contusions.[6]

In vivo studies performed in dogs to mimic blunt chest trauma have correlated histopathologic areas of myocardial injury with areas of injury found during echocardiographic examination. Experimental trauma delivered to the left side of the chest resulted in abnormalities that were located primarily in the craniolateral wall of the left ventricle, and right-sided chest trauma produced septal and right ventricular wall damage.[6]

Gross pathologic findings in the traumatized heart have been characterized by localized edema, ecchymosis, and intramyocardial hematoma formation. Myocardial injuries were often transmural, with the epicardial surface being more severely affected.[6]

Arrhythmias and conduction defects are the most commonly reported consequences of myocardial injuries in humans and dogs.[7,11,22-27] One proposed proarrhythmic mechanism of myocyte trauma is the lowering of the ratio of effective refractory period to action potential duration and an increase in the resting membrane potential (less negative) in damaged myocardial cells. Additionally it is proposed that myocyte injury results in alterations of sodium and calcium currents across cell membranes, increasing the availability of intracellular calcium, resulting in increased sensitivity to depolarization.[3] These proposed intracellular derangements secondary to trauma can potentiate arrhythmogenesis.[3] Arrhythmias become apparent when the injured myocardium becomes the site of the most rapid impulse formation, overcoming the sinus node as the dominant (overdrive) pacemaker. The injured myocardium becomes the new overdrive pacemaker, propagating the arrhythmia by depolarizing the sinus node before it has a chance to fire and recapture the cardiac rhythm.[3]

Isolated rabbit hearts have been subjected to injury during high-resolution mapping of epicardial excitation to identify the origin of arrhythmias in injured myocardium. The results of this study identified reentry as the mechanism of arrhythmia caused by myocardial contusion. The authors found that the site of impact became electrically silent (temporarily), resulting in a fixed and functional conduction block that caused reentry initiation.[28]

*References 2, 3, 11-13, 19-21.

Traumatized patients may also develop arrhythmias associated with metabolic acidosis, hypoxia, electrolyte imbalance, intracranial injuries, and catecholamine release.[23,25-27,29] These physiologic aberrations all promote alterations in membrane transport and permeability of cations (sodium, potassium, and calcium), which lead to a decrease in resting membrane potential, as described earlier, contributing to aberrant depolarization and arrhythmias.[3,23,25]

The most commonly reported arrhythmias secondary to canine myocardial injuries include premature ventricular contractions, ventricular tachycardia, and nonspecific ST segment elevation or depression.[6,22-27,29] Less commonly reported arrhythmias reported in dogs with chest trauma include atrial fibrillation, sinus arrest with ventricular or junctional escape complexes, and second-degree and third-degree atrioventricular block.[7,12,22,27]

DIAGNOSIS

Although uncommonly performed in the live patient, gross or histologic examination of the heart remains the diagnostic gold standard for myocardial contusions.[2,17,30] Because of the impracticality of visualizing the heart or performing myocardial biopsy, an understanding of the mechanism of injury, an awareness of associated injuries, and a high index of suspicion for myocardial injury are essential in making a diagnosis.[10] Emergency clinicians should consider myocardial injury in all traumatized dogs that have the following injuries: (1) fractures of extremities, spine, or pelvis, (2) external evidence of thoracic trauma, (3) radiographic evidence of chest trauma such as pulmonary contusions, pneumothorax, hemothorax, diaphragmatic rupture, and rib or scapular fractures, and (4) neurologic injury.*

Dogs with any of these injuries should have a lead II electrocardiograph (ECG) performed and, depending on the patient's condition and the clinician's index of suspicion, the ECG should be repeated intermittently (i.e., every 2 to 24 hours). ECG abnormalities commonly are delayed in onset for up to 48 hours after blunt chest trauma, so in cases in which there is a high index of suspicion for myocardial injury ECG monitoring should be considered for that time frame.[22,23,25] Holter monitoring is the most sensitive and least invasive indicator of arrhythmias in dogs with suspected myocardial injuries. However, the lack of immediate Holter interpretation (rapid turnaround time) may limit the practical application of this modality for veterinarians.[12] Other forms of continuous ECG monitoring, such as single patient monitors and telemetry, would likely provide a similar advantage over intermittent ECGs without the delays in interpretation encountered with Holter monitoring.[18]

An echocardiogram should be considered in severely traumatized dogs with a poor response to resuscitative efforts and evidence of thoracic injuries even if no ECG abnormalities are present. Transthoracic echocardiography in the dog can be used to identify and localize both structural and functional abnormalities of injured myocardium caused by blunt chest trauma. The echocardiographic features of myocardial injuries in the dog include (1) increased end-diastolic wall thickness; (2) impaired contractility, indicated by wall motion abnormalities and decreased fractional shortening; (3) increased echogenicity; and (4) localized areas of echolucency consistent with intramural hematomas.[6]

Serum myocardial isoenzyme analysis (cardiac troponins T and I [cTnT and cTnI]) has been used to diagnose myocardial injury in dogs and humans. The skeletal isoforms of the troponin proteins expressed are different from those in cardiac muscle.[19,31] The troponin structure is highly conserved across many differing species, allowing for veterinary application of tests currently in use at human care facilities.[32]

Troponin testing is based on immunologic detection of the cardiac-specific isoforms of troponin T and troponin I.[31] In both human and dogs, detectable levels appear in the circulation within 4 to 6 hours of cardiac myocyte injury and serum elevations may be present for up to 7 days.[7,19,32] In a comparison of multiple myocardial enzyme and protein markers and ECG to detect myocardial injury in traumatized dogs, cTnI was the most sensitive indicator of this type of injury.[2] One of the most important findings of the many human studies investigating the clinical use of cardiac troponins appears to be the negative predictive values for cardiac complications in trauma patients. In human trauma patients a normal cTnI level in combination with a normal ECG tracing on arrival has a negative predictive value of 100% for myocardial injuries, allowing these patients to avoid intensive cardiac monitoring and even be discharged safely in the absence of other significant injuries.[33] Because of the controversies and difficulty diagnosing myocardial injuries in dogs, veterinarians should consider using these two tests to rule out this disease in a quick and practical manner. Although there are no studies confirming this hypothesis in dogs, clinicians could consider performing a baseline ECG and cTnI measurement within 4 hours of injury. Extrapolating from human findings, dogs with a combination of normal ECG findings and cTnI levels (normal < 0.03 to 0.07 ng/ml[34]) would be less likely to develop arrhythmias and therefore would not require intensive cardiac monitoring. A positive finding on either test would suggest the possibility of myocardial injury and would indicate continuous ECG monitoring in those dogs.

TREATMENT

Treatment of myocardial injuries typically is aimed at suppressing potentially life-threatening arrhythmias and maintaining adequate tissue perfusion.[30] Antiarrhythmic therapy is not recommended if arterial pulse quality is good and synchronous on auscultation, mean arterial pressure is higher than 75 mm Hg, mucous membranes are pink, capillary refill time is 2 seconds or less, and the patient has no clinical signs of weakness or cardiopulmonary distress.[30] Antiarrhythmic therapy should be considered when properly stabilized patients (i.e., received adequate fluids, electrolytes, oxygen, pain control) develop arrhythmias such as multiform premature ventricular complexes, ventricular tachycardia, and the R-on-T phenomenon.[23,26,27,30] Treatment is imperative when arrhythmias are accompanied by clinical evidence of decreased cardiac output such as hypotension, weakness, pale mucous membranes, delayed capillary refill time, collapse, or syncope.[23,26,30] Additionally, treatment is indicated when an arrhythmia has a sustained (>15 to 30 seconds) ventricular rate that exceeds 140 to 180 beats/min in the dog.[12,23,26]

Lidocaine (2 mg/kg IV bolus) is the agent of choice for traumatized dogs suffering from ventricular ectopy fulfilling the criteria described in the previous paragraph.[30] Intravenous boluses of lidocaine may be repeated every 10 to 20 minutes until a cumulative dose of 8 mg/kg is given. A constant rate infusion (CRI) of 40 to 80 mcg/kg/min may be initiated to maintain a cardiac rate and rhythm that provides appropriate tissue perfusion.[23,30] Additional boluses of lidocaine are often required to suppress arrhythmias while steady-state blood levels are achieved by the CRI. The upper end of the recommended dosages of lidocaine may cause vomiting or seizures, so administration should be slowed or temporarily discontinued if these signs develop (see Chapter 48 for more information).[23,30,35]

If lidocaine does not resolve ventricular ectopy, procainamide may be administered intravenously or intramuscularly (6 to 15 mg/kg q4-6h).[23,30] If repeated boluses of procainamide are required to suppress arrhythmias, a CRI (10 to 40 mcg/kg/min) may be

*References 2, 12, 22, 25, 29, 30.

started. Oral procainamide (sustained release formulation 20 mg/kg q8h) may be initiated if continued management is required and oral medications can be tolerated. Potential side effects of procainamide administration include hypotension and atrioventricular conduction block.[23,35] Additional oral arrhythmia management options include tocainide (10 to 20 mg/kg PO q8-12h) and mexiletine (4 to 8 mg/kg PO q8h).[23] The reported side effects of tocainide include nausea, vomiting, and anorexia; although less commonly observed, complications associated with mexiletine include excitement or depression.[35]

β-Blockers (propranolol, metoprolol, atenolol, sotalol) should be considered cautiously when traumatized dogs with ventricular ectopy are unresponsive to class I antiarrhythmic agents, have been treated appropriately for shock and pain, and are not receiving positive inotropic medications.[30,35] An ultrashort-acting intravenous β-blocker, such as esmolol, may be used to test the efficacy of β-blockers in managing ventricular arrhythmias that have not responded to other medications.[26] The potential for serious side effects such as atrioventricular block, hypotension, bronchoconstriction, and decreased cardiac contractility must be considered when using β-blockers.[23,35]

Arrhythmias secondary to myocardial trauma that do not fulfill the stated guidelines for management are likely to be self-limiting and resolve within 3 to 10 days.[30] The end point of therapy is not necessarily complete resolution of the arrhythmia; appropriate therapeutic response includes reduction of the heart rate (<140 beats/min) and the return of adequate tissue perfusion.[30] In most cases antiarrhythmic therapy can be discontinued within 48 to 72 hours; however, it is recommended that intermittent ECG monitoring continue up to 1 week after discharge.[30] Medications being used to suppress arrhythmias should be discontinued a minimum of 24 hours before reexamination.[30] The most sensitive way to detect complete resolution of arrhythmias after discontinuing antiarrhythmic medications is continuous ECG (Holter) monitoring.[12] If some form of continuous monitoring is not available, intermittent lead II ECG monitoring can be performed to ensure that the arrhythmia has resolved and it is safe to discontinue therapy. If the arrhythmia persists, long-term oral therapy may be initiated.[30]

If a dog with a suspected myocardial injury must undergo anesthesia, agents that are least likely to induce arrhythmias, such as acepromazine, butorphanol, isoflurane, and glycopyrrolate, should be used.[3,23] Halothane, atropine sulfate, and the thiobarbiturates should be avoided because they are reported to exacerbate arrhythmias and to sensitize the heart to catecholamine-induced arrhythmias.[23,25]

SUMMARY

Although myocardial injuries may cause significant alterations in cardiac function in the traumatized dog, they are often overlooked in the face of severe trauma. Ventricular arrhythmias are the most common abnormalities caused by blunt myocardial injury. Although ECG monitoring traditionally has been used to diagnose myocardial injuries, the onset of arrhythmias associated with these injuries is often delayed, making recognition difficult. Arrhythmias may be secondary to alterations in transport of cations, such as calcium, potassium, and sodium, across the membranes of injured myocytes, resulting in a decrease of resting membrane potential, aberrant firing of injured cells, and loss of organized myocyte depolarization or reentry mechanisms.

The medical community has yet to provide a prospective study that investigates the need for therapeutic intervention of traumatic myocardial injuries in humans or dogs. Although newer noninvasive tests for myocardial injuries such as troponin levels may assist in diagnosing these injuries, they have not yet proven to be the single noninvasive diagnostic modality to detect myocardial injury.[18] In the real world of veterinary practice, continuous ECG monitoring has been shown to be a sensitive, noninvasive indicator of arrhythmias in traumatized dogs and should be considered in dogs with suspected myocardial injuries.[12]

A human study may have inadvertently stumbled upon an approach that makes more sense than those previously discussed: ruling out this disease rather than ruling it in. This study showed that in traumatized patients a combination of normal ECG and cTnI findings on admission had a 100% negative predictive value for cardiac complications, meaning that none of the patients with these test results developed arrhythmias requiring intervention.[33] These findings may be helpful in determining the need for continuous ECG monitoring in canine patients with suspected myocardial trauma and should be considered for further investigation in dogs.

REFERENCES

1. Beresky R, Klingler R, Peake J: Myocardial contusion: when does it have clinical significance? J Trauma 28:64, 1988.
2. Schober KE, Kirbach B, Oechtering G: Noninvasive assessment of myocardial cell injury in dogs with suspected cardiac contusion, J Vet Cardiol 1:17, 1999.
3. Paddleford RR: Anesthetic considerations for the high-risk patient requiring a short anesthetic procedure, AAHA Scientific Proceedings, Denver, March 1995.
4. Helling TS, Duke P, Beggs CW, et al: A prospective evaluation of 68 patients suffering blunt chest trauma for evidence of cardiac injury, J Trauma 29:961, 1989.
5. Feghali N, Prisant M: Blunt myocardial injury, Chest 108:1673, 1995.
6. Pandian N, Skorton DJ, Doty DB, et al: Immediate diagnosis of acute myocardial contusion by 2-dimensional echocardiography: studies in a canine model of blunt chest trauma, J Am Coll Cardiol 2:488, 1983.
7. Shorr RM, Crittenden M, Indeck M, et al: Blunt thoracic trauma, Ann Surg 206:200, 1988.
8. Maenza RL, Seaberg D, D'Amico F: A meta-analysis of blunt cardiac trauma: ending myocardial confusion, Am J Emerg Med 14:237, 1996.
9. Macdonald RC, O'Neill D, Hanning CD, et al: Myocardial contusion in blunt chest trauma: a 10-year review, Intensive Care Med 7:265, 1981.
10. Biffl WL, Moore FA, Moore EE, et al: Cardiac enzymes are irrelevant in the patient with suspected myocardial contusion, Am J Surg 168:523, 1994.
11. Selcer BA, Buttrick M, Barstad R, et al: The incidence of thoracic trauma in dogs with skeletal injury, J Small Anim Pract 28:21, 1987.
12. Snyder SS, Cooke KL, Murphy ST, et al: Electrocardiographic findings in dogs with motor vehicle-related trauma, J Am Anim Hosp Assoc 37:55, 2001.
13. Powell LL, Rozanski EA, Tidwell AS, et al: A retrospective analysis of pulmonary contusion secondary to motor vehicular accidents in 143 dogs: 1994-1997, J Vet Emerg Crit Care 9:127, 1999.
14. Campbell VL, King LG: Pulmonary function, ventilator treatment and outcome of dogs with thoracic trauma and pulmonary contusions: 10 cases (1994-1998), J Am Vet Med Assoc 217:1505, 2000.
15. Mucha P: Blunt myocardial injury (myocardial contusion). In Cameron JL, editor: Current surgical therapy, ed 8, St Louis, 2004, Mosby.
16. Ferjani M, Droc G, Dreux S, et al: Circulating cardiac troponin T in myocardial contusion, Chest 111:427, 1997.
17. Fulda GJ, Giberson F, Hailstone D, et al: An evaluation of serum troponin T and signal-averaged electrocardiographic abnormalities after blunt chest trauma, J Trauma 43:304, 1997.
18. Reiss AJ, McKiernan BC: Myocardial injury secondary to blunt thoracic trauma in dogs: diagnosis and treatment, Comp Cont Educ Pract Vet 24:944, 2002.
19. Kolata RJ: Trauma in dogs and cats: an overview, Vet Clin North Am Small Anim Pract 10:515, 1980.
20. Kolata RJ, Johnston DE: Motor vehicle accidents in urban dogs: a study of 600 cases, J Am Vet Med Assoc 167:938, 1975.
21. Kolata RJ, Kraut NH, Johnston DE: Patterns of trauma in urban dogs and cats: a study of 1000 cases, J Am Vet Med Assoc 164:499, 1974.

22. Alexander JW, Bolton GR, Koslow GL: Electrocardiographic changes in nonpenetrating trauma to the chest, J Am Anim Hosp Assoc 11:160, 1975.
23. Murtaugh RJ, Ross JN: Cardiac arrhythmias: pathogenesis and treatment in the trauma patient, Comp Cont Educ Pract 10:332, 1988.
24. Hunt C: Chest trauma: specific injuries, Comp Cont Educ Pract 1:624, 1979.
25. Macintire DK, Snider TG: Cardiac arrhythmias associated with multiple trauma in dogs, J Am Vet Med Assoc 184:541, 1984.
26. Abbott JA: Traumatic myocarditis. In Bonagura JD, editor: Kirk's current veterinary therapy XIII, St Louis, 2000, Saunders.
27. Wingfield WE, Henik RA: Treatment priorities in cases of multiple trauma, Semin Vet Med Surg (Small Anim) 3:193, 1988.
28. Robert E, Coussaye JE, Aya AG, et al: Mechanisms of ventricular arrhythmias induced by myocardial contusion: a high-resolution mapping study in the left ventricular rabbit heart, Anesthesiology 92:1132, 2000.
29. King JM, Roth L, Haschek WM: Myocardial necrosis secondary to neural lesions in domestic animals, J Am Vet Med Assoc 180:144, 1982.
30. Rush JE: Managing myocardial contusion and arrhythmias, Proceedings of the 22nd annual Waltham/OSU Symposium for the Treatment of Small Animal Diseases, Columbus, OH, October 10-11, 1998.
31. Adams JE: Utility of cardiac troponins in patients with suspected cardiac trauma or after cardiac surgery, Clin Lab Med 17:613, 1997.
32. O'Brien PJ, Dameron GW, Beck ML, et al: Cardiac troponin T is a sensitive biomarker of cardiac injury in laboratory animals, Lab Anim Sci 47:486, 1997.
33. Salim A, Velmahos GC, Jindal A, et al: Clinically significant blunt cardiac trauma: role of serum troponin levels combined with electrocardiographic findings, J Trauma 50:237, 2001.
34. Sleeper MM, Clifford CA, Laster LL: Cardiac troponin I in the normal dog and cat, J Vet Intern Med 15:501, 2001.
35. Muir WW, Sams RA, Moise NS: Pharmacology and pharmacokinetics of antiarrhythmic drugs. In Fox PR, Sisson DK, Moise NS, editors: Textbook of canine and feline cardiology: principles and clinical practice, ed 2, St Louis, 1999, Saunders.

CHAPTER 45
PERICARDIAL DISEASES

Wendy A. Ware, DVM, MS, DACVIM (Cardiology)

KEY POINTS

- Pericardial effusion is the most common pericardial disorder.
- Most pericardial effusions in dogs are hemorrhagic and of neoplastic or idiopathic origin.
- Hemangiosarcoma is by far the most common neoplasm causing pericardial effusion in dogs.
- Cardiac tamponade occurs when intrapericardial pressure rises to equal or greater than normal cardiac filling pressure.
- The rate of pericardial fluid accumulation influences how quickly cardiac tamponade develops; a large pericardial fluid volume implies a gradual process.
- Clinical signs usually reflect poor cardiac output and systemic venous congestion.
- Echocardiography is the main clinical tool for diagnosing pericardial effusion and cardiac masses.
- Right atrial collapse is a characteristic echocardiographic finding with cardiac tamponade.
- Immediate pericardiocentesis is indicated for cardiac tamponade.

The pericardium is a closed serosal sac that envelops the heart and is attached to the great vessels at the heart base. It provides a barrier to infection and inflammation from adjacent tissues and helps balance the output of the right and left ventricles. A small amount (approximately 0.25 ml/kg body weight) of clear, serous fluid normally serves as a lubricant between the visceral pericardium (epicardium), which is directly adhered to the heart, and the outer fibrous, parietal pericardial layer.[1]

The most common pericardial disorder involves excess or abnormal fluid accumulation within the pericardial sac (pericardial effusion). This occurs most often in dogs and can lead to signs of severe cardiac dysfunction. Other acquired and congenital pericardial diseases are seen infrequently. Acquired pericardial disease that causes clinical signs is uncommon in cats.[2]

PERICARDIAL EFFUSION

Hemorrhagic Pericardial Effusion

Most pericardial effusions in dogs are serosanguineous or sanguineous. The fluid usually appears dark red, with a packed cell volume (PCV) more than 7%, a specific gravity greater than 1.015, and a protein concentration greater than 3 g/dl. The underlying etiology usually is either neoplastic or idiopathic. Neoplastic effusions are more likely in dogs older than 7 years of age.[3]

Other, less common causes of intrapericardial hemorrhage include left atrial rupture secondary to severe mitral insufficiency, coagulopathy (especially from rodenticide toxicity or disseminated intravascular coagulation), and penetrating trauma.

Hemangiosarcoma

Hemangiosarcoma (HSA) is by far the most common neoplasm causing hemorrhagic pericardial effusion in dogs; it is rare in cats. Most HSAs arise in the right atrium or right auricle, but some also infiltrate the ventricular wall.[4,5] Occasionally, HSA occurs in the left ventricle, in the septum, or at the heart base. Metastases are common by the time of diagnosis.

Heart base tumors

The most common heart base tumor is the chemodectoma (aortic body tumor), which arises from chemoreceptor cells at the base of the aorta.[4] Thyroid, parathyroid, lymphoid, and connective tissue neoplasms also can occur at the heart base. Heart base tumors tend to be locally invasive around the root of the aorta and surrounding structures; however, metastases to other organs can occur.[6]

Other neoplasia

Hemorrhagic pericardial effusion also can occur with pericardial mesothelioma, malignant histiocytosis, some cases of cardiac lymphoma, and occasionally with metastatic carcinoma. Pericardial mesothelioma may cause mass lesions at the heart base or elsewhere but often has a diffuse distribution and may mimic idiopathic disease.[7,8] Lymphoma involving various parts of the heart is more common in cats than in dogs (and often causes a modified transudative effusion). Other primary tumors of the heart are rare but include myxoma, and various types of sarcoma.

Idiopathic (benign) pericardial effusion

Idiopathic pericardial effusion is also a relatively common cause of canine hemorrhagic pericardial effusion. It is reported most often in medium to large breed, middle-aged dogs. More cases have been reported in males than females. Its cause is still unknown; however, mild pericardial inflammation, with diffuse or perivascular fibrosis and focal hemorrhage, are common histopathologic findings.[9-11]

Transudative Pericardial Effusion

Transudates or modified transudates occasionally accumulate in the pericardial space of both dogs and cats. A chylous effusion occurs rarely. Pure transudates are clear, with a low cell count (usually <1000 cells/μl), specific gravity (<1.012), and protein content (<2.5 g/dl). Modified transudates may appear slightly cloudy or pink tinged. Their cellularity (approximately 1000 to 8000 cells/μl) is still low, but total protein concentration (approximately 2.5 to 5 g/dl) and specific gravity (1.015 to 1.030) are higher than those of a pure transudate.

Transudative effusions can develop with congestive heart failure (CHF), hypoalbuminemia, congenital pericardial malformations, and toxemias that increase vascular permeability (including uremia). These conditions usually are associated with relatively small-volume pericardial effusion, and cardiac tamponade is rare. In cats, pericardial effusion is most commonly associated with CHF from cardiomyopathy.[12] Effusion associated with cardiac lymphoma also often appears transudative.

Exudative Pericardial Effusion

Exudative effusions are cloudy to opaque or serofibrinous to serosanguineous. They typically have a high nucleated cell count (usually much higher than 3000 cells/μl), protein content (often much above 3 g/dl), and specific gravity (>1.015). Cytologic findings are related to the etiology. Exudative pericardial effusions are uncommon in small animals. However, they have occurred from plant awn migration, extension of a pleural or mediastinal infection, and bite wounds. Various bacteria (aerobic and anaerobic), actinomycosis, coccidioidomycosis, aspergillosis, disseminated tuberculosis, and, rarely, systemic protozoal infections have been identified. Feline infectious peritonitis is the most important cause of symptomatic pericardial effusion in cats. Exudative effusions also have occurred in association with leptospirosis, canine distemper, and idiopathic pericardial effusion in dogs. Chronic uremia occasionally causes a sterile, serofibrinous or hemorrhagic effusion.

CARDIAC TAMPONADE

The development of clinical signs from pericardial effusion is associated mainly with increased intrapericardial pressure. Because the fibrous pericardium is relatively noncompliant, increases in fluid volume can sharply raise intrapericardial pressure. *Cardiac tamponade* develops when intrapericardial pressure rises toward and exceeds normal cardiac diastolic pressures.[3,13] The external cardiac compression progressively limits right ventricular filling and, with increasing severity, also reduces left ventricular filling.[3,13] Systemic venous pressure increases and forward cardiac output falls. Eventually, diastolic pressures in all cardiac chambers and great veins equilibrate.[3,13]

The rate of pericardial fluid accumulation and the distensibility of the pericardial sac determine whether and how quickly cardiac tamponade develops. Rapid accumulation of a relatively small-volume effusion (e.g., 50 to 100 ml) can raise intrapericardial pressure markedly because pericardial tissue stretches slowly. Conversely, a slow rate of fluid accumulation may allow for enough pericardial distension to maintain low intrapericardial pressure until the effusion is quite large. A large volume of pericardial fluid implies a gradual process. So long as intrapericardial pressure is low, cardiac filling and output remain relatively normal and clinical signs are absent. Fibrosis and thickening further limit the compliance of pericardial tissue, and this can increase the likelihood of cardiac tamponade.

Neurohormonal compensatory mechanisms are activated as cardiac output falls.[14,15] These contribute to fluid retention and other clinical manifestations of tamponade. Signs of systemic venous congestion become especially prominent over time. Although pericardial effusion does not directly affect myocardial contractility, reduced coronary perfusion during tamponade can impair both systolic and diastolic function. Low cardiac output, arterial hypotension, and poor perfusion of other organs besides the heart can ultimately precipitate cardiogenic shock and death.

Cardiac tamponade also causes an exaggerated respiratory variation in arterial blood pressure known as *pulsus paradoxus.* Inspiration normally lowers intrapericardial and right atrial pressures slightly, which enhances right-sided heart filling and pulmonary blood flow. Left-sided heart filling diminishes as more blood is held in the lungs and the inspiratory increase in right ventricular filling pushes the interventricular septum leftward. Thus left-ventricular output and systemic arterial pressure normally decrease slightly during inspiration. Pulsus paradoxus is an exaggeration of this normal pressure difference with respirations; patients with pulsus paradoxus exhibit a fall in arterial pressure during inspiration of 10 mm Hg or more.[16,17]

CLINICAL PRESENTATION

Cardiac tamponade is relatively common in dogs but rare in cats. Clinical findings reflect poor cardiac output and usually systemic venous congestion as well. The typical history includes exercise intolerance, abdominal enlargement, tachypnea, weakness, collapse or syncope, and sometimes cough. Collapse is more common in dogs with cardiac neoplasia than in those with idiopathic disease.[18] Nonspecific signs such as lethargy, inappetence, or other gastrointestinal maladies can develop before obvious ascites does. Cases with pericardial effusion but without cardiac tamponade may show signs of the underlying disease process or be asymptomatic.

Physical Findings with Tamponade

Jugular venous distention or a positive hepatojugular reflux,* hepatomegaly, ascites, labored respiration, and weakened femoral pulses

*The hepatojugular reflux is assessed by applying firm pressure to the cranial abdomen while the animal stands quietly with head in a normal position. This pressure transiently increases venous return, but normally there is little to no change in jugular vein appearance. Jugular distention that persists while abdominal pressure is applied constitutes a positive (abnormal) test result.

are common physical findings.[3,13,18-21] Pulsus paradoxus is detected occasionally by femoral pulse palpation. High sympathetic tone commonly produces sinus tachycardia, pale mucous membranes, and prolonged capillary refill time. The precordial impulse is palpably weak with a large pericardial fluid volume, and heart sounds are muffled by moderate to large pericardial effusions.[3,18,19] In addition, lung sounds can be muffled ventrally with pleural effusion. Pericardial effusion alone does not cause a murmur, but concurrent cardiac disease may do so. Reduced lean body mass (cachexia) is apparent in some chronic cases.

Although right-sided congestion predominates, signs of biventricular failure can occur. Rapid pericardial fluid accumulation can cause acute tamponade, shock, and death without signs of pleural effusion, ascites, or radiographic cardiomegaly. Pulmonary edema, jugular venous distention, and hypotension may be evident in such cases.

DIAGNOSIS

Cardiac tamponade is often suspected from the history and physical examination, but thoracic radiographs and especially echocardiography are important for diagnosis. The electrocardiogram (ECG) may suggest pericardial disease in some cases.

Thoracic Radiographs

The appearance of the cardiac silhouette depends on the volume of pericardial fluid as well as any underlying cardiomegaly.[3,13,22,23] Massive pericardial effusion causes the classic globoid-shaped cardiac shadow ("basketball heart") seen on both views. But other causes of a large, rounded heart shadow include dilated cardiomyopathy or marked tricuspid (with or without mitral) insufficiency. Smaller volumes of pericardial fluid allow some cardiac contours to be identified, especially those of the atria.

Other radiographic findings associated with tamponade include pleural effusion, caudal vena cava distention, hepatomegaly, and ascites. Pulmonary infiltrates of edema or distended pulmonary veins are noted only occasionally. Tracheal deviation, a soft tissue mass effect, or metastatic lung lesions are seen in some cases of heart base tumors. Metastatic lung lesions are common in dogs with hemangiosarcoma.

Advanced imaging techniques such as cardiac computed tomography (CT) and magnetic resonance imaging (MRI) are sometimes used to further characterize structures involving or near the heart. These may be most useful in helping define the extent and location of a mass lesion; however, their ability to diagnose the presence of a cardiac mass has not yet been shown superior to echocardiography.[24]

Echocardiography

Because echocardiography is highly sensitive for detecting even small-volume pericardial effusion, it is the diagnostic test of choice.[3,13,25,26] The effusion appears as an echo-free space between the bright parietal pericardium and the epicardium. Abnormal cardiac wall motion and chamber shape and intrapericardial or intracardiac mass lesions can also be visualized.[22,25-28] Identification of the parietal pericardium in relation to the echo-free fluid helps differentiate pleural from pericardial effusion. Evidence of collapsed lung lobes or pleural folds can often be seen within pleural effusion.

Cardiac tamponade is characterized by diastolic (and early systolic) compression or collapse of the right atrium and sometimes right ventricle (Figure 45-1).[3,13,27] The left ventricular chamber often appears small, with walls that look hypertrophied (pseudohypertrophy), because of the poor cardiac filling.

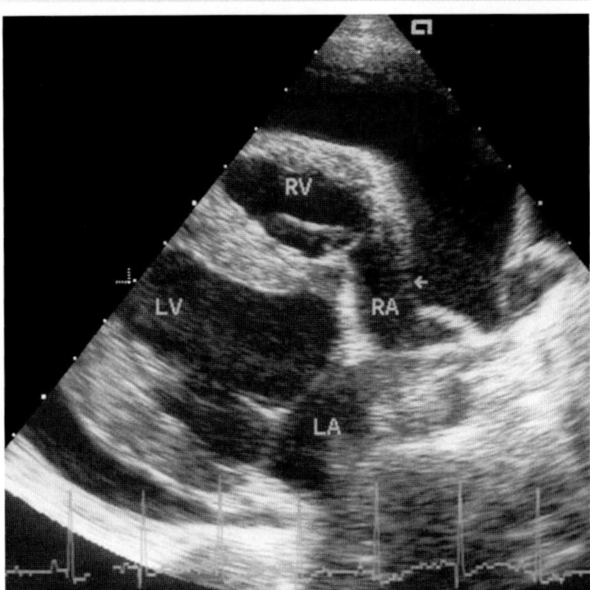

FIGURE 45-1 Right parasternal four-chamber echocardiographic image from a dog with cardiac tamponade. Pericardial fluid is seen surrounding the heart. Note the characteristic collapse of the right atrial wall *(arrow)* caused by elevated intrapericardial pressure. Electrocardiographic tracing along the bottom. *LA*, Left atrium; *LV*, left ventricle; *RA*, right atrium; *RV*, right ventricle.

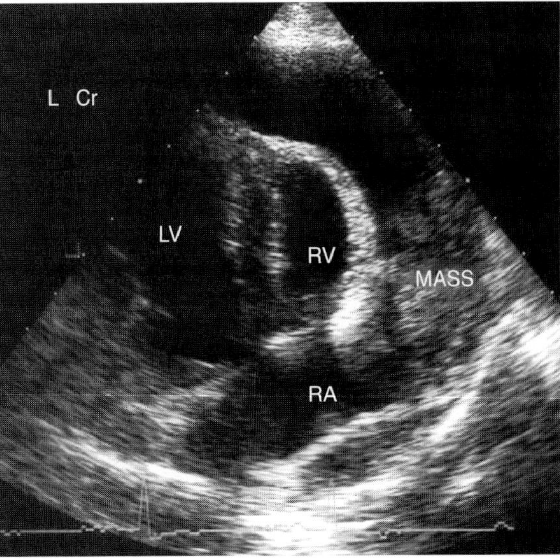

FIGURE 45-2 Left cranial long-axis echocardiographic image, optimized for right ventricular inflow tract and right auricle, from a dog with cardiac hemangiosarcoma. Pericardial effusion enhanced visualization of the tumor (MASS). This echo view confirmed the presence of the tumor and its origin from the tip of the right auricle. *LV*, Left ventricle; *RA*, right atrium; *RV*, right ventricle.

Visualization of structures at the heart base and mass lesions is usually better before pericardiocentesis is performed. It is important to carefully evaluate all portions of the heart, (especially the right atrium and auricle and right ventricle), ascending aorta, and the pericardium itself to screen for neoplasia. The left cranial parasternal (and transesophageal) transducer positions are especially useful (Figure 45-2). Some mass lesions are difficult to visualize. Mesothelioma may not cause discrete mass lesions and therefore may be indistinguishable from idiopathic pericardial effusion.

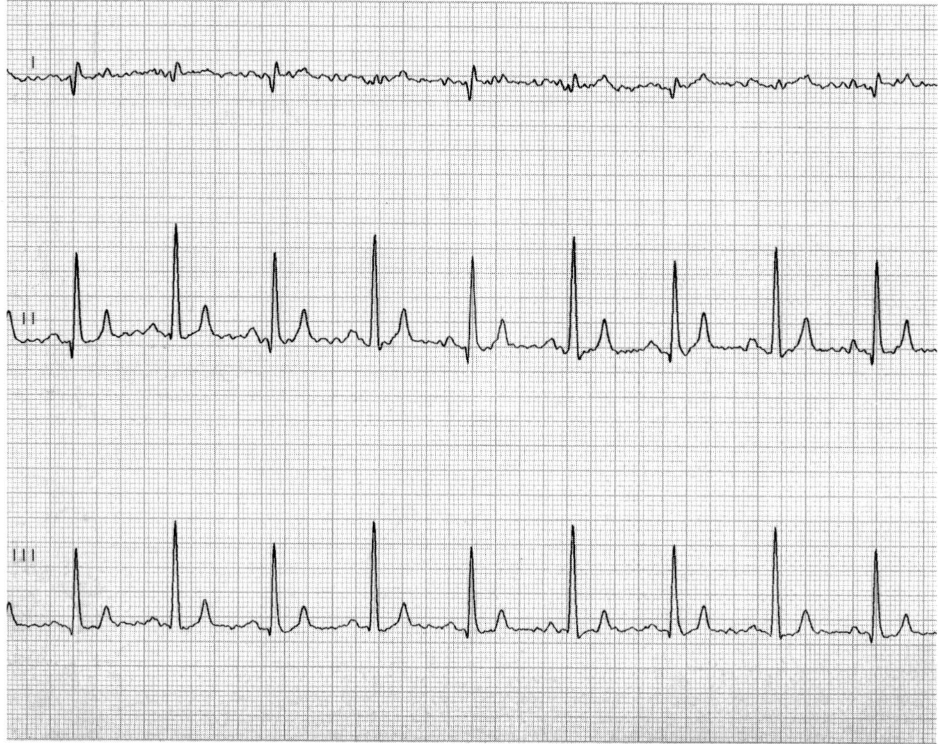

FIGURE 45-3 Electrocardiogram showing sinus rhythm with electrical alternans, from a dog with large-volume pericardial effusion. Note the every-other-beat change in QRS complex size and configuration in each lead. See text for further information. Leads I, II, III: 50 mm/sec, 1 cm = 1 mV.

Electrocardiography

Although not specific for tamponade, ECG findings associated with large-volume pericardial effusion include reduced amplitude QRS complexes (less than 1 mV in dogs) and electrical alternans. The latter is a recurring, beat-to-beat alteration in the size or configuration of the QRS complex (and sometimes T wave) that results from the heart swinging back and forth within the pericardium (Figure 45-3).[29] Electrical alternans may be more evident at heart rates between 90 and 140 beats/min or in certain body positions (e.g., standing). ST segment elevation, suggesting an epicardial injury current, also is seen in some cases of pericardial effusion.[19,29] Sinus tachycardia is common with cardiac tamponade; atrial and ventricular tachyarrhythmias occur in some cases.

Central Venous Pressure

Central venous pressure (CVP) measurement may be useful in identifying tamponade, especially if it is difficult to assess jugular veins or it is unclear whether right-sided heart filling pressure is elevated. Normal CVP is in the range of 0 to 8 cm H_2O. Cardiac tamponade commonly produces CVP measurements of 10 to 12 cm H_2O or higher.[3]

Clinicopathologic Findings

Routine laboratory findings may reflect underlying disease or tamponade-induced prerenal azotemia or hepatic congestion but are often otherwise nonspecific.[3,26] HSA may be associated with a regenerative anemia, increased number of nucleated red blood cells and schistocytes (with or without acanthocytes), leukocytosis, and thrombocytopenia. Pleural and peritoneal effusions associated with cardiac tamponade are usually modified transudates. Circulating cardiac troponin (cTn) concentrations or enzyme activities may be increased as a result of ischemia or myocardial invasion. Elevated plasma cTnI concentrations have been documented in dogs with cardiac HSA.[30]

Pericardial Fluid Analysis

Pericardial effusion samples (see Pericardiocentesis section later in this chapter) should be submitted for cytologic analysis and saved for possible bacterial (or fungal) culture. Nevertheless, differentiation of neoplastic effusions from benign hemorrhagic pericarditis is usually not possible on the basis of cytology alone.[31] Reactive mesothelial cells within the effusion may closely resemble neoplastic cells; furthermore, chemodectomas and HSAs may not shed cells into the effusion. Effusions associated with lymphoma typically are consistent with a modified transudate, and neoplastic cells usually are easily identified. Many neoplastic (and other noninflammatory) effusions have a pH of 7.0 or greater, whereas inflammatory effusions generally have lower pH. However, there is too much overlap for pericardial effusion pH to be a reliable discriminator.[32] Pericardial fluid culture is performed if cytology and pH suggest an infectious or inflammatory cause. It is currently unclear whether analysis of pericardial fluid for cardiac troponins or other substances will allow better differentiation of the underlying etiology.

MANAGEMENT OF CARDIAC TAMPONADE

It is important to differentiate cardiac tamponade from other diseases that cause right-sided congestive signs because its management is unique. The compressed ventricles require high venous pressure to fill. By reducing cardiac filling pressure, diuretics and vasodilators further decrease cardiac output and exacerbate hypotension. Positive inotropic drugs do not improve cardiac output or ameliorate the signs of tamponade because the underlying pathophysiology is impaired cardiac filling, not poor contractility.

Immediate pericardiocentesis is indicated for cardiac tamponade. This sometimes also provides diagnostic information. Congestive signs should resolve after intrapericardial pressure is reduced by fluid removal. A modest dose of diuretic can be given after pericardiocentesis, but this is not essential. Subsequent management is guided by the underlying cause of the pericardial effusion and other clinical circumstances.

PERICARDIOCENTESIS

Preparation and Positioning

Pericardiocentesis is a relatively safe procedure when performed carefully. Depending on the clinical status and temperament of the animal, sedation may be helpful. ECG monitoring is recommended during the procedure; needle or catheter contact with the heart commonly induces ventricular arrhythmias. Although cardiac tamponade is uncommonly caused by coagulopathy, verifying that coagulation parameters are normal is helpful, if patient status allows time for this. Pericardiocentesis usually is performed from the right side of the chest. This minimizes the risk of trauma to the lung (via the cardiac notch) and major coronary vessels, most of which are located on the left. The patient usually is placed in left lateral recumbency to allow more stable restraint; sometimes sternal recumbency is used if the dog is cooperative. Alternatively, the author has had good success using an elevated echocardiography table with a large cutout; the animal is placed in right lateral recumbency and the tap is performed from underneath (Figure 45-4). The advantage of this method is that gravity draws fluid down toward the collection site. But if adequate space is not available for wide sterile skin preparation or for needle or catheter manipulation, this approach is not advised. Echocardiographic guidance can be used but is not necessary unless the effusion is of very small volume or appears compartmentalized. Sometimes pericardiocentesis can be performed successfully on the standing animal, but the risk of injury is increased if the patient moves suddenly.

Several methods can be used for pericardiocentesis. An over-the-needle catheter system (e.g., 16 to 18 gauge, 1.5 inch to 2 inches long) can be used for most cases. Larger over-the-needle catheter systems (e.g., 12 to 14 gauge, 4 to 6 inches) allow for faster fluid removal in large dogs; a few extra small side holes can be cut (smoothly) near the tip of the catheter to facilitate flow, but care should be taken that the end of the catheter does not break off inside the patient. During initial catheter placement the extension tubing is attached to the needle stylet; after the catheter is advanced into the pericardial space and the stylet removed, the extension tubing is attached directly to the catheter. In emergency situations or when an over-the-needle catheter is unavailable, an appropriately long hypodermic or spinal needle attached to extension tubing is adequate. A butterfly needle (18 to 21 gauge) is generally used in cats. For all methods a three-way stopcock is placed between the extension tubing and a collection syringe.

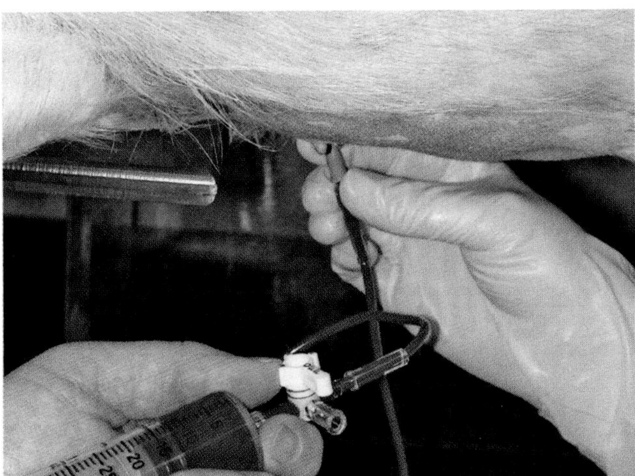

FIGURE 45-4 Alternative position for pericardiocentesis using an elevated table with side cutout designed for echocardiography (see text). The animal lies in right lateral recumbency and the puncture is performed from the dependent *(right)* side.

Pericardiocentesis Procedure

The skin is shaved and surgically prepared over the right precordium, from about the third to seventh intercostal spaces and from sternum to costochondral junction. Sterile gloves and aseptic technique should be used. The puncture site is identified by palpating for the cardiac impulse (usually between the fourth and sixth ribs just lateral to the sternum); the optimal site must be estimated if no precordial impulse is felt. Local anesthesia is recommended and is essential with use of a larger catheter. Two percent lidocaine is infiltrated (with sterile technique) at the skin puncture site, underlying intercostal muscle, and into the pleura. A small stab incision is made in the skin when using a larger catheter system.

The puncture site should be just cranial to a rib to avoid the intercostal vessels located caudal to each rib. Once the needle has penetrated the skin, an assistant should apply gentle negative pressure to the attached syringe, three-way stopcock (turned "off" to air), and extension tubing assembly as the operator slowly advances the needle toward the heart. In this way, any fluid will be detected as soon as it is encountered. Pleural fluid (usually straw colored) may enter the tubing first. It is helpful to aim the needle tip toward the patient's opposite shoulder. The pericardium causes increased resistance to needle advancement and may produce a subtle scratching sensation when contacted. The needle is advanced with gentle pressure through the pericardium; a loss of resistance may be noted with needle penetration, and pericardial fluid (usually dark red) will appear in the tubing. With a catheter system, the needle-catheter unit must be advanced far enough into the pericardial space that the catheter is not deflected by the pericardium as the needle stylet is removed. After the catheter is advanced into the pericardial space and the stylet removed, the extension tubing is attached to the catheter. Initial pericardial fluid samples are saved in sterile ethylenediaminetetraacetic acid (EDTA) and clot tubes for evaluation; then as much fluid as possible is drained.

A scratching or tapping sensation usually is felt if the needle or catheter contacts the heart; also, the device may move with the heartbeat, and ventricular premature complexes are often provoked. If this occurs the needle or catheter should be retracted slightly to avoid cardiac trauma. Care should be taken to minimize extraneous needle movement within the chest. If it is unclear whether pericardial fluid or intracardiac blood (from cardiac penetration) is being aspirated, a few drops can be placed on the table or into a clot tube and a sample spun in a hematocrit tube. Pericardial fluid does not clot (unless associated with very recent hemorrhage). The packed cell volume is usually lower than that of peripheral blood, and the supernatant appears yellow-tinged (xanthochromic). Furthermore, as pericardial fluid is drained, the patient's ECG complexes usually increase in amplitude, tachycardia diminishes, and the animal often breathes more deeply and appears more comfortable.

Complications of Pericardiocentesis

Ventricular premature beats occur commonly from direct myocardial injury or puncture. These are usually self-limited, resolving when the needle is withdrawn. Coronary artery laceration with myocardial infarction or further bleeding into the pericardial space can occur but is uncommon, especially when pericardiocentesis is done from the right side. Lung laceration causing pneumothorax or hemorrhage or both is also a potential complication during the procedure. In some cases, dissemination of infection or neoplastic cells into the pleural space may result.

ANCILLARY TREATMENT

Idiopathic Pericardial Effusion

Dogs with idiopathic pericardial effusion are initially treated conservatively by pericardiocentesis. After excluding an infectious cause by pericardial fluid culture or cytologic analysis, a glucocorticoid is often used (e.g., oral prednisone, 1 mg/kg/day, tapered over 2 to 4 weeks); however, its efficacy in preventing recurrent idiopathic pericardial effusion is unknown. Sometimes a 1- to 2-week course of a broad-spectrum antibiotic is used concurrently. Periodic radiographic or echocardiographic reevaluation is advised to screen for recurrence. Cardiac tamponade can recur after a variable time span (days to years). Nevertheless, extended survival times are possible in dogs with idiopathic pericardial effusion, even in those requiring more than three pericardiocenteses.[18,33] However, recurrent effusions can be caused by mesothelioma or other neoplasia, which sometimes becomes evident on repeated echocardiographic examination.[7,8]

Recurrent effusion that does not respond to repeated pericardiocenteses and antiinflammatory therapy is usually treated by subtotal pericardiectomy.[34] Removal of the pericardium ventral to the phrenic nerves allows pericardial fluid drainage to the larger absorptive surface of the pleural space. The less invasive techniques of thoracoscopic partial pericardiectomy or percutaneous balloon pericardiotomy are also used successfully to treat idiopathic and some cases of neoplastic pericardial effusion.[35-37] Biopsy samples of a mass (if identified) or even resection of a small right auricular mass can be accomplished through thoracoscopy.

Neoplastic Pericardial Effusion

Pericardiocentesis is done as needed to relieve cardiac tamponade. Attempted surgical resection (depending on tumor size and location) or surgical biopsy, and a trial of chemotherapy (based on biopsy or clinicopathologic findings) can be done; or conservative therapy can be pursued until episodes of cardiac tamponade become unmanageable. Surgical resection of HSA is often not possible because of the tumor's size and extent. Small masses involving only the tip of the right auricle have been successfully removed. Use of a pericardial patch graft may allow resection of larger masses.[38,39] However, this alone rarely results in prolonged long-term survival. Partial pericardiectomy may prevent the recurrence of tamponade.

Chemotherapy has allowed survival times of 4 to 8 months in some dogs with atrial HSA. Survival time in dogs with mesothelioma may be slightly longer than in those with HSA, but the overall prognosis is poor. Current chemotherapeutic recommendations should be consulted.

Heart base tumors (e.g., chemodectoma) tend to be slow growing and locally invasive and have a low metastatic potential. Partial pericardiectomy may prolong survival for years.

Infectious Pericarditis

Infectious pericarditis should be treated aggressively with appropriate antimicrobial drugs, based on culture and susceptibility testing, and pericardiocentesis as needed. Infusion of an appropriate antimicrobial agent directly into the pericardium after pericardiocentesis may be helpful. If a foreign body is suspected or intermittent pericardiocentesis is ineffective, continuous drainage with an indwelling pericardial catheter or surgical debridement should be pursued. Surgical therapy allows for removal of penetrating foreign bodies, more complete flushing of exudates, and management of pericardial constrictive disease. Even with successful elimination of infection, epicardial and pericardial fibrosis can lead to constrictive pericardial disease.

CONSTRICTIVE PERICARDIAL DISEASE

Constrictive pericardial disease is recognized occasionally in dogs but only rarely in cats. It occurs when scarring and thickening of the visceral or parietal pericardium restrict ventricular diastolic expansion and prevent normal cardiac filling. Usually the entire pericardium is involved symmetrically. In some cases fusion of parietal and visceral pericardial layers obliterates the pericardial space. In others the visceral layer (epicardium) alone is involved. A small amount of pericardial effusion (constrictive-effusive pericarditis) may be present.

Some cases are secondary to recurrent idiopathic hemorrhagic effusion, infectious pericarditis (especially from coccidioidomycosis but potentially also from other fungal or bacterial infections), a pericardial foreign body, tumors, or idiopathic osseous metaplasia or fibrosis of the pericardium.[3,13]

Compromised filling reduces cardiac output, and compensatory neurohormonal mechanisms cause fluid retention, tachycardia, and vasoconstriction.

Clinical Features

Middle-aged, medium to large breed dogs are most often affected. Males may be at higher risk. Some dogs have a history of pericardial effusion. Clinical signs of right-sided CHF predominate. These signs may develop over weeks to months. Ascites and jugular venous distention are the most consistent clinical findings, as in dogs with cardiac tamponade.

Diagnosis

The diagnosis of constrictive pericardial disease can be challenging. Typical radiographic findings include mild to moderate cardiomegaly, pleural effusion, and caudal vena cava distention. Echocardiographic changes in dogs with constrictive pericardial disease may be subtle; suggestive findings include mid- and late diastolic flattening of the left ventricular free wall, abnormal diastolic septal motion, and other findings secondary to abnormal hemodynamics. The pericardium may appear thickened and intensely echogenic, but differentiating this from normal pericardial echogenicity may be impossible. Mild pericardial effusion, without diastolic right atrial collapse, is seen in some cases. Serologic testing for Coccidioides (or other fungal agents) is advisable in endemic regions.

A CVP greater than 15 cm H_2O is common. Intracardiac pressure measurements are most useful diagnostically. Besides high mean atrial and diastolic ventricular pressures, the atrial pressure waveform shows a prominent y descent (during ventricular relaxation) because ventricular filling pressure is low only in early diastole. This is in contrast to cardiac tamponade, wherein the y descent is diminished. Another classic finding with constrictive pericardial disease is an early diastolic dip in ventricular pressure, followed by a mid-diastolic plateau, but this is not seen consistently. An angiocardiogram may appear normal or may show atrial and vena caval enlargement with increased endocardial-pericardial distance.

Treatment

Therapy for constrictive pericardial disease involves surgical pericardiectomy. If the visceral pericardial layer is affected, epicardial stripping is required, which increases the surgical difficulty and associated complications. Pulmonary thrombosis reportedly is a common and potentially life-threatening postoperative complication. Tachyarrhythmias are another complication.

CONGENITAL PERICARDIAL DISEASE

Peritoneopericardial diaphragmatic hernia (PPDH) is the most common pericardial malformation in dogs and cats. Abnormal embryonic development (probably of the septum transversum) allows persistent communication between the pericardial and peritoneal cavities at the ventral midline. The pleural space is not involved. Abdominal structures can herniate into the pericardial space, which may cause associated clinical signs.

Clinical Features

Most cases are diagnosed during the first several years of life, usually after gastrointestinal or respiratory signs develop. Vomiting, diarrhea, anorexia, weight loss, abdominal pain, cough, dyspnea, and wheezing are common signs. Physical examination findings can include muffled heart sounds on one or both sides of the chest, a weak or displaced cardiac precordial impulse, an "empty" feel on abdominal palpation (with herniation of many organs), and, rarely, signs of cardiac tamponade. However, some animals never develop clinical signs.

Diagnosis

Thoracic radiographs are often diagnostic or highly suggestive of PPDH. An enlarged cardiac silhouette, dorsal tracheal displacement, overlap of the diaphragmatic and caudal heart borders, and abnormal fat or gas densities within the cardiac silhouette are characteristic findings. Echocardiography may confirm the diagnosis when radiographic findings are equivocal. Other imaging techniques can also be used.

Treatment

Therapy involves surgical closure of the peritoneal-pericardial defect after viable abdominal structures are returned to their normal position. The presence of other congenital abnormalities and the animal's clinical signs influence the decision to operate. In uncomplicated cases prognosis is excellent; however, perioperative complications are common and, although often mild, can include death. Older animals without clinical signs may do well without surgery.

REFERENCES

1. Dyce KM, Sack WO, Wensing CJG: Textbook of veterinary anatomy, Philadelphia, 1996, WB Saunders, pp 219-220.
2. Hall DJ, Shofer F, Meier CK, et al: Pericardial effusion in cats: a retrospective study of clinical findings and outcome in 146 cats, J Vet Intern Med 21:1002, 2007.
3. Ware WA: Pericardial diseases. In Cardiovascular disease in small animal medicine, London, 2011, Manson Publishing, pp 320-339.
4. Ware WA, Hopper DL: Cardiac tumors in dogs: 1982-1995, J Vet Intern Med 13:95, 1999.
5. Boston SE, Higginson G, et al: Concurrent splenic and right atrial mass at presentation in dogs with HSA: a retrospective study, J Am Anim Hosp Assoc 47:336, 2011.
6. Vicari ED, et al: Survival times of and prognostic indicators for dogs with heart base masses: 25 cases (1986-1999), J Am Vet Med Assoc 219:485, 2001.
7. Machida N, Tanaka R, Takemura N, et al: Development of pericardial mesothelioma in Golden Retrievers with a long-term history of idiopathic haemorrhagic pericardial effusion, J Comp Path 131:166, 2004.
8. Stepien RL, Whitley NT, Dubielzig RR: Idiopathic or mesothelioma-related pericardial effusion: clinical findings and survival in 17 dogs studied retrospectively, J Small Anim Pract 41:342, 2000.
9. Day MJ, Martin MWS: Immunohistochemical characterization of the lesions of canine idiopathic pericarditis, J Small Anim Pract 43:382, 2002.
10. Martin MW, Green MJ, et al: Idiopathic pericarditis in dogs: no evidence for an immune-mediated aetiology, J Small Anim Pract 47:387, 2006.
11. Zini E, Glaus TM, et al: Evaluation of the presence of selected viral and bacterial nucleic acids in pericardial samples from dogs with or without idiopathic pericardial effusion, Vet J 179:225, 2009.
12. Davidson BJ, Paling AC, Lahmers SL, et al: Disease association and clinical assessment of feline pericardial effusion, J Am Anim Hosp Assoc 44:5, 2008.
13. Tobias AH: Pericardial diseases. In Ettinger SJ, Feldman EC, editors: Textbook of veterinary internal medicine, ed 7, Philadelphia, 2010, WB Saunders, pp 1342-1352.
14. Kaszaki J, Nagy S, Tarnoky K, et al: Humoral changes in shock induced by cardiac tamponade, Circ Shock 29:143, 1989.
15. Stokhof AA, Overduin LM, Mol JA, et al: Effect of pericardiocentesis on circulating concentrations of atrial natriuretic hormone and arginine vasopressin in dogs with spontaneous pericardial effusion, Eur J Endocrinology 130:357, 1994.
16. Fitchett DH, Sniderman AD: Inspiratory reduction in left heart filling as a mechanism of pulsus paradoxus in cardiac tamponade, Can J Cardiol 6:348-354, 1990.
17. Savitt MA, Tyson GS, Elbeery JR, et al: Physiology of cardiac tamponade and paradoxical pulse in conscious dogs, Am J Physiol 265:H1996, 1993.
18. Stafford Johnson M, Martin M, Binns S, et al: A retrospective study of clinical findings, treatment and outcome in 143 dogs with pericardial effusion, J Small Anim Pract 45:546, 2004.
19. Berg RJ: Pericardial effusion in the dog: a review of 42 cases, J Am Anim Hosp Assoc 20:721, 1984.
20. Gibbs C, Gaskell CJ, Darke PGG, et al: Idiopathic pericardial haemorrhage in dogs: a review of fourteen cases, J Small Anim Pract 23:483, 1982.
21. Vogtli T, Gaschen F, Vogtli-Burger R, et al: Hemorrhagic pericardial effusion in dogs. A retrospective study of 10 cases (1989-1994) with a review of the literature, Schweiz Arch Tierheilkd 139:217, 1997.
22. Bouvy BM, Bjorling DE: Pericardial effusion in dogs and cats. Part II. Diagnostic approach and treatment, Compend Contin Educ 13:633, 1991.
23. Guglielmini C, Diana A, Santarelli G, et al: Accuracy of radiographic veterbral heart score and sphericity index in the detection of pericardial effusion in dogs, J Am Vet Med Assoc 241:1048, 2012.
24. Boddy KN, Sleeper MM, Sammarco CD, et al: Cardiac magnetic resonance in the differentiation of neoplastic and nonneoplastic pericardial effusion, J Vet Intern Med 25:1003, 2011.
25. Thomas WP, Sisson D, Bauer TG, et al: Detection of cardiac masses in dogs by two-dimensional echocardiography, Vet Radiol 25:65, 1984.
26. MacDonald KA, Cagney O, Magne ML: Echocardiographic and clinicopathologic characterization of pericardial effusion in dogs: 107 cases (1985-2006), J Am Vet Med Assoc 235:1456, 2009.
27. Berry CR, Lombarde CW, Hager DA, et al: Echocardiographic evaluation of cardiac tamponade in dogs before and after pericardiocentesis: four cases (1984-1986), J Am Vet Med Assoc 192:1597, 1988.
28. Cobb MA, Brownlie SE: Intrapericardial neoplasia in 14 dogs, J Small Anim Pract 33:309, 1992.
29. Bonagura JD: Electrical alternans associated with pericardial effusion in the dog, J Am Vet Med Assoc 178:574, 1981.
30. Chun RHB, Kellihan HB, Henik RA, et al: Comparison of plasma cardiac troponin I concentrations among dogs with cardiac hemangiosarcoma, noncardiac hemangiosarcoma, other neoplasms, and pericardial effusion of nonhemangiosarcoma origin, J Am Vet Med Assoc 237:806, 2010.
31. De Laforcade AM, Freeman LM, Rozanski EA, et al: Biochemical analysis of pericardial fluid and whole blood in dogs with pericardial effusion, J Vet Intern Med 19:833, 2005.
32. Fine DM, Tobias AH, Jacob KA: Use of pericardial fluid pH to distinguish between idiopathic and neoplastic effusions, J Vet Intern Med 17:525, 2003.
33. Mellanby RJ, Herrtage ME: Long-term survival of 23 dogs with pericardial effusions, Vet Rec 156:568, 2005.
34. Aronsohn MG, Carpenter JL: Surgical treatment of idiopathic pericardial effusion in the dog: 25 cases (1978-1993), J Am Anim Hosp Assoc 35:521, 1999.

35. Mayhew KN, Mayhew PD, Sorrell-Raschi L, Brown DC: Thoracoscopic subphrenic pericardectomy using double-lumen endobronchial intubation for alternating one-lung ventilation, Vet Surg 38:961, 2009.
36. Monnet E: Interventional thoracoscopy in small animals, Vet Clin North Am Small Anim Pract 39:965, 2009.
37. Sidley JA, Atkins CE, Keene BW, et al: Percutaneous balloon pericardiotomy as a treatment for recurrent pericardial effusion in 6 dogs, J Vet Intern Med 16:541, 2002.
38. Crumbaker DM, Rooney MB, Case JB: Thoracoscopic subtotal pericardiectomy and right atrial mass resection in a dog, J Am Vet Med Assoc 237:551, 2010.
39. Morges M, Worley DR, Withrow SJ, et al: Pericardial free patch grafting as a rescue technique in surgical management of right atrial HSA, J Am Anim Hosp Assoc 47(3):224, 2011.

CHAPTER 46

BRADYARRHYTHMIAS AND CONDUCTION DISTURBANCES

Romain Pariaut, DVM, DACVIM (Cardiology), DECVIM-CA (Cardiology) •
Caryn Reynolds, DVM, DACVIM (Cardiology)

KEY POINTS

- Sinus bradycardia is usually secondary to a systemic disease causing high vagal tone.
- Bradyarrhythmias are more common in dogs than cats.
- Third-degree atrioventricular block and sick sinus syndrome account for the majority of bradyarrhythmias that require treatment.
- In the presence of atrial standstill, rule out hyperkalemia.
- Medical management of bradyarrhythmias is rarely successful.

DEFINITION

Bradyarrhythmias are defined as bradycardias (heart rate below than 60 beats/min in dogs, 100 beats/min in cats) associated with clinical signs, such as lethargy, decreased appetite, exercise intolerance, congestive heart failure, and syncope. During the diagnostic workup of a bradycardic animal, it is important to determine whether the arrhythmia results from an extracardiac disease and is therefore likely to resolve when the primary problem is corrected; no specific treatment to address the slow heart rate is usually necessary. In rare instances, immediate therapeutic action is needed when the animal is hemodynamically unstable or experiences syncopal episodes.

More commonly, bradyarrhythmias result from alterations in the conduction system, resulting in inadequate impulse formation or propagation. The normal cardiac impulse originates in the sinus node. A decrease in impulse discharge rate from nodal cells results in sinus bradycardia. Other abnormalities of impulse formation include sinus block and sinus arrest, resulting in asystolic pauses. These pauses may extend beyond 6 to 8 seconds and lead to syncopal episodes when atrioventricular or ventricular pacemaker cells fail to initiate an escape rhythm. Conduction disturbances include bundle branch blocks and first-, second-, and third-degree atrioventricular (AV) blocks. However, bundle branch blocks and first-degree AV blocks are not associated with clinical signs.

DIFFERENTIAL DIAGNOSIS

Bradyarrhythmias can result from alterations in autonomic tone, drug exposure, electrolyte abnormalities, trauma, hypoxia, inflammation or infiltration of the myocardium, and degenerative disease of the conduction system. Although the underlying pathologic condition cannot always be definitively determined, the clinician needs to decide (1) whether extracardiac factors are the cause for the arrhythmia, (2) if treatment is needed, and (3) how to choose between medical and pacemaker therapy. Determining the rhythm diagnosis from the electrocardiogram (ECG) is the essential first step (Figure 46-1). The common types of bradyarrhythmias in small animal patients are outlined next.

Sinus Bradycardia

Sinus bradycardia (or slow sinus arrhythmia) is rarely a primary disorder or a cause of clinical signs in the small animal patient. Rather, it is much more likely secondary to systemic disease causing increased vagal tone, particularly gastrointestinal, respiratory, neurologic, and ocular diseases. In these cases resolution of the primary disease results in an increased heart rate with no need for medical or pacemaker therapy. On the surface ECG, P waves, and QRS complexes are associated. The P waves are typically positive in leads II, III and aVF. When marked vagotonia is the cause for the bradycardia, a wandering pacemaker, which corresponds to a variation in the amplitude of the P wave in relation to the respiratory cycle, is usually present. The QRS complexes are usually narrow (60 msec in dogs; 40 msec in cats).

The presence of sinus bradycardia in an animal with impaired consciousness should raise the suspicion of increased intracranial pressure. Systemic hypertension and an abnormal breathing pattern complete the clinical picture of this physiologic response known as

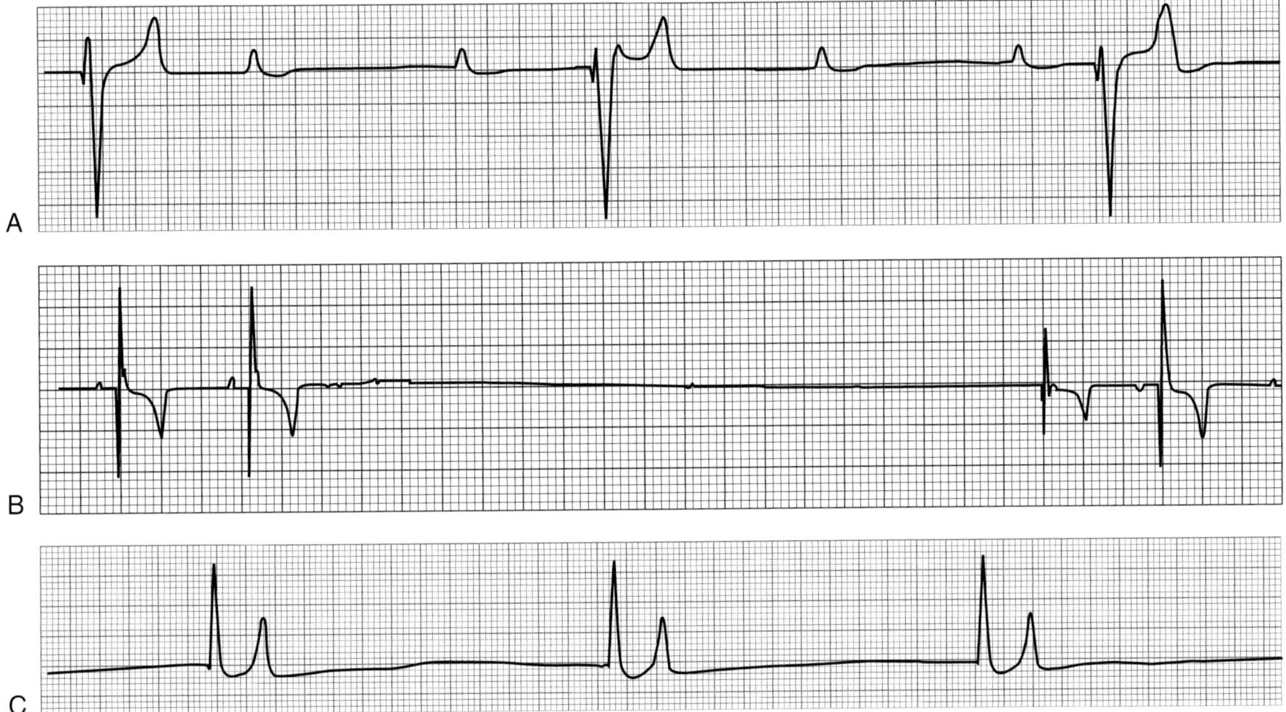

FIGURE 46-1 Electrocardiographic characteristics of bradyarrhythmias. **A,** Third-degree atrioventricular block. PP and RR intervals are regular but the P waves bear no constant relation to the R waves. Ventricular escape rhythm at a rate of 37 beats/min (recording speed: 50 mm/sec; amplitude: 10 mm/mV). **B,** Sick sinus syndrome. Two sinus beats are followed by a period of sinus arrest (3.9 seconds), which is terminated by an escape beat originating from the atrioventricular junction or the ventricles. The last beat is originating in the atrium. Its negative P wave is consistent with a wandering pacemaker or an impulse initiated at the bottom of the atrium. **C,** Acquired atrial standstill secondary to hyperkalemia. Note the bradycardia (38 beats/min), the tall and peaked T waves, and the absence of P waves (recording speed: 50 mm/sec; amplitude: 10 mm/mV).

Cushing's reflex. Measures to lower intracranial pressure should be rapidly initiated. Anticholinergic agents or pacing therapy are warranted if bradycardia is severe.[1]

Sinus Node Dysfunction

Sinus arrest is identified as a prolonged pause with no atrial activation or P wave on the ECG. Sinus block, which describes the failure of an impulse to exit the sinus node, cannot be differentiated from sinus arrest on a surface ECG. The lack of cardiac output resulting from a pause of approximately 6 to 8 seconds results in syncope. Sick sinus syndrome is a disease of the conduction system characterized by periods of normal sinus rhythm or sinus bradycardia, interspersed with long sinus arrest that can last up to 10 or 12 seconds because junctional and ventricular pacemakers fail to initiate escape beats. The use of opioids as sedatives often results in a prolongation of the periods of asystole. It is not uncommon that dogs that were asymptomatic while awake become hemodynamically unstable after sedation or under anesthesia. A variant of the disease, sometimes called bradycardia-tachycardia syndrome, is characterized by periods of paroxysmal atrial tachycardia followed by a temporary failure of the sinus rhythm to resume when the tachycardia abruptly terminates. It corresponds to an exaggeration of a normal physiologic response of the sinus node to the effect of a tachyarrhythmia, a mechanism known as overdrive suppression. Older Miniature Schnauzers and Terrier breeds are more commonly affected with sick sinus syndrome.

Atrioventricular Block

With first-degree AV block all the atrial impulses are conducted to the ventricles, but the PR interval is prolonged on the ECG (PR >130 msec in dogs, PR >90 msec in cats). It results from AV node fibrosis, increased vagal tone, or drugs that delay AV node conduction, including digoxin, calcium channel blockers, and β-blockers. Second-degree AV block is diagnosed when some P waves are not followed by a QRS complex on the surface ECG. The hemodynamic effect of this rhythm depends on the frequency of ventricular contraction. Second-degree AV block is said to be high grade when more atrial impulses fail to be conducted to the ventricles than are conducted. This can result in syncope or other signs of low cardiac output. Alternatively, a single P wave that does not get conducted can occur in normal dogs or those with increased vagal tone; it does not require treatment. Two types of second-degree AV blocks are recognized. Mobitz type I second-degree AV block is characterized by a progressive increase in the PR interval duration ending by a blocked P wave. It is known as Wenckebach's phenomenon. It usually results from a combination of AV node fibrosis and a progressive increase in vagal tone. This form of AV block is usually benign and does not require specific treatment. Mobitz type II second-degree AV block is characterized by the unexpected occurrence of blocked P waves. PR intervals before and after the blocked P waves are identical. The QRS complexes of conducted beats are usually wide because the area of block is below the His bundle, causing bundle branch blocks and intraventricular conduction delays. This form of block is more likely to worsen and result in clinical signs. Administration of atropine (0.04 mg/kg intravenously [IV]) can help the clinician to differentiate between the two forms of block. Type I usually improves after atropine and type II is unchanged or worsens.

Third-degree, or complete, AV block is typified by an absence of conducted P waves to the ventricles. The ECG displays independent atrial and ventricular activities. Cardiac output is dramatically reduced. In response, the atrial rate, which is under control of the adrenergic tone, is elevated. Electrical activation of the ventricles is dependent on an escape rhythm beyond the site of block. The QRS complexes are generally wide and bizarre at rates around 20 to 60 beats/min in dogs and 60 to 120 beats/min in cats. In addition, the ventricular rate is regular unless ventricular premature beats originating from an ischemic myocardium are present.

Causes of AV block include myocardial fibrosis, inflammation or infiltration, and potentially drug toxicity (calcium channel blockers, β-blockers, or digoxin). Age-related fibrodegenerative disease is the most common cause of AV block in dogs. An echocardiogram is indicated to identify concomitant structural cardiac disease. Although a mild elevation of plasma cardiac troponin I level is common in dogs with complete AV block, marked increase in concentration suggests myocarditis as the cause for the bradyarrhythmia.[2,3] Third-degree AV block in cats is often associated with structural heart disease.[4]

Clinical signs depend on the rate of ventricular contraction. Cats, and occasionally dogs, may show no apparent signs, and bradycardia is detected on physical examination. More commonly, animals present with signs of low cardiac output such as syncope, congestive heart failure, or weakness.

Atrial Standstill

Atrial standstill is defined by a lack of visible atrial electrical activity on the surface ECG. It can be temporary or persistent. Persistent atrial standstill is a rare disease that seems more prevalent in English Springer Spaniels, which also are predisposed to developing AV block.[5] It usually affects young dogs, and a genetic etiology is likely. Generally a significant myocardial pathologic condition is present and the long-term prognosis is guarded. The ECG is characterized by lack of P waves with a regular ventricular or AV nodal escape rhythm, at rates of 20 to 60 beats/min in dogs.

Hyperkalemia is a common cause of temporary atrial standstill. As plasma potassium concentration increases above 5.5 to 6 mmol/L, the initial change on the surface ECG is a narrowing of the T wave and an increase in its amplitude. As potassium concentration continues to rise, it leads to a decrease in heart rate associated with reduced P wave amplitude and a widening of the QRS complexes. P waves then become invisible, consistent with a diagnosis of atrial standstill.

TREATMENT

Medical Treatment

Vagally induced bradyarrhythmias and sick sinus syndrome may respond to the administration of parasympatholytic medications. An increase in heart rate after intravenous administration of atropine (0.04 mg/kg IV) or glycopyrrolate (0.01 mg/kg IV) confirms the contribution of vagal tone to the bradyarrhythmia. Side effects resulting from repeated injections limit their chronic use. They include mydriasis, dry mouth, constipation, urinary retention, and on occasion neurologic signs.

Sympathomimetic inotropes increase heart rate by β-adrenergic stimulation. Agents with β_2 effects cause systemic vasodilation, whereas drugs with associated α stimulation cause vasoconstriction. Dopamine (5 to 10 mcg/kg/min IV) and dobutamine (dog: 2 to 20 mcg/kg/min IV; cat: 1 to 5 mcg/kg/min IV) may contribute to an increase in heart rate and systolic function. They are usually administered as a constant rate infusion and the dose is increased to effect. They are indicated in the management of β-blocker overdose. Isoproterenol, a pure β agonist, improves conduction in the AV node and the His-Purkinje system, which may result in the partial or complete resolution of AV block. It may also increase the rate of a ventricular escape rhythm in complete AV block, but usually with limited success. It is administered as a constant rate infusion and its dose adjusted to effect. However, it causes a significant decrease in diastolic blood pressure via β_2 stimulation. Finally, respiratory and metabolic acidosis decrease its effectiveness.[6]

Terbutaline (0.2 mg/kg orally q8-12h, 0.01 mg/kg IV) is a selective β_2 agonist commonly used as a bronchodilator. Aminophylline (10 mg/kg twice orally q12h, or 10 mg/kg IV) is a phosphodiesterase inhibitor and bronchodilator with mild chronotropic effect. These drugs may temporarily increase heart rate in dogs with sick sinus syndrome.

Pacemaker Therapy

Transcutaneous pacing

Transcutaneous pacing is a quick and effective means of increasing the heart rate in an emergency situation. Many external defibrillators are multifunction devices that have this capability. Pacing electrodes are within adhesive pads that are available in adult or pediatric sizes. The pads are applied to clipped skin at the level of the third to fifth costrochondral junction (or over the palpable apex beat) on either side of the thorax.[7] The thorax can be bandaged to ensure good contact if the patient is not anesthetized or patient manipulation is anticipated. The ECG is recorded by the pads or via standard limb leads. The pacing rate is programmed, and the pads sense the intrinsic cardiac rhythm and deliver an impulse if necessary. The sensitivity can be adjusted until intrinsic QRS complexes are sensed. The current (in mA) should be gradually increased until ventricular capture is achieved. This is recognized by the appearance of wide QRS complexes on the ECG in addition to palpation of associated femoral pulses (see Chapter 203).

Transcutaneous pacing has been reported to be safe and effective in two reports of 42 and 27 dogs.[8,9] The major drawback of this method is that stimulation of the local skeletal muscles can be painful; therefore, this method is generally used only in anesthetized patients. Also, pacing of skeletal muscles can cause movement to the thorax and forelimbs. Despite this, temporary cutaneous pacing can be invaluable in severely unstable patients while more definitive therapy is prepared.

Temporary transvenous pacing

Temporary transvenous pacemakers involve a lead placed in the right side of the heart, generally the right ventricle, and connected to a generator external to the patient (Figure 46-2). Leads are usually

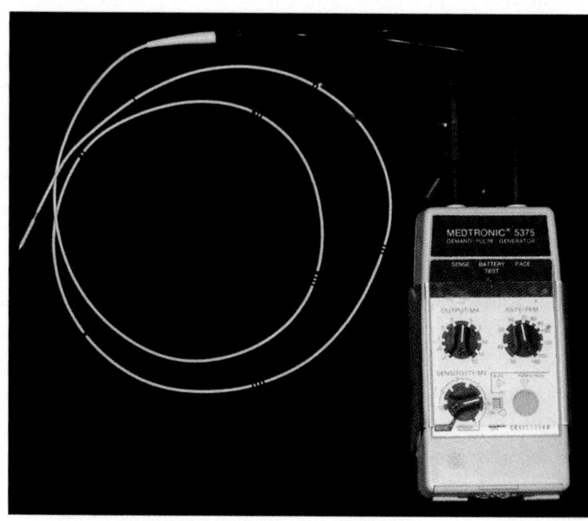

FIGURE 46-2 Temporary transvenous pacemaker.

bipolar, 100 to 110 cm in length and 4 to 6 Fr in diameter. Their tip is slightly curved, smooth, and not attached to the endocardium. Some leads are designed with a small balloon at their tip; once it is inflated with 1 ml of air, it helps the electrode to get "floated" along by blood flow through the cardiac chambers. The inflated balloon also prevents the risk of perforation when the lead is pushed against the walls of the right atrium or the ventricular apex. The jugular, saphenous, or femoral vein can be used, depending on the size of the patient. A vascular introducer sheath that is large enough to accommodate the pacing lead is secured in the vein, either percutaneously via Seldinger's technique or via a cutdown. The lead is then advanced into the right ventricular apex and attached to the generator. Fluoroscopic guidance is recommended to facilitate passage into the right ventricle; however, if this is not available, the distance from the introducer to the apex can be estimated and the lead gently advanced blindly. The electrode is connected to the external pacing generator, the heart rate is programmed at 80 to 100 pulses/min, and the highest output current is selected. As the lead progresses closer to the cardiac chamber, pacing spikes can be seen on the surface ECG until wide QRS complexes appear when the catheter reaches the right ventricle. Alternatively, ultrasound imaging could be used to identify the position of the lead in the cardiac chambers.[10] The team should be prepared for movement of the lead tip within the heart, causing loss of capture. If pacing is lost, the lead should be slightly adjusted until capture is regained. Because of this, the lead can be held in place with tape or sutured to the patient but should remain accessible in case adjustment is needed.

The external pacing generator is usually battery operated. When it is connected to the electrode positioned in the ventricle, it paces in the VVI mode (ventricle paced, ventricle sensed, inhibition of pacing when spontaneous ventricular activation sensed). This mode requires the selection of the appropriate current delivered to the endocardium to consistently activate ventricular contraction and sensitivity. The sensitivity is the minimum voltage of an electrical potential that the pacemaker will detect. The sensitivity value needs to be low enough to recognize spontaneous QRS complexes but high enough to prevent detection of other electrical potentials, such as T waves. A sensitivity of 1.5 mV is usually adequate. If T waves are detected by the pacemaker and inhibit pacing, sensitivity is decreased—that is, the number is increased (e.g., from 1.5 to 3 mV). A surface ECG is monitored to confirm control of the ventricles with the pacemaker. The paced QRS complexes are wide and sometimes preceded by a pacing spike. The output can usually be selected between 0.1 and 20 mA. A starting current of 2 mA is usually sufficient. The rate of the pacemaker is based on the disease process and needs of the patient. It is usually programmed between 70 and 130 beats/min (see Chapter 203).

Because this can be performed percutaneously in all but very small dogs or cats, this technique can be performed with the patient awake or only mildly sedated in most cases. This technique is easily performed and can rapidly improve cardiac output. For patients undergoing permanent pacemaker implantation, temporary transvenous pacemaker placement before induction of anesthesia can improve patient stability and does not cause stimulation of skeletal muscles, which can be a complication of transcutaneous pacing. This technique can also be used to support patients with transient bradycardia, as has been reported in a case of diltiazem toxicity in a dog.[11] The patient must remain sedated or be allowed limited mobility in order to keep the generator in close proximity and minimize lead dislodgement until decision to proceed with more permanent therapy is made.

REFERENCES

1. Agrawal A, Timothy J, Cincu R, et al: Bradycardia in neurosurgery, Clin Neurol Neurosurg 110:321, 2008.
2. Trafney DJ, Oyama MA, Wormser C, et al: Cardiac troponin-I concentrations in dogs with bradyarrhythmias before and after artificial pacing, J Vet Cardiol 12:183, 2010.
3. Church WM, Sisson DD, Oyama MA, et al: Third degree atrioventricular block and sudden death secondary to acute myocarditis in a dog, J Vet Cardiol 9:53, 2007.
4. Kellum, H, Stepien, R: Third-degree atrioventricular block in 21 cats (1997-2004), J Vet Intern Med 20:97, 2006.
5. Fonfara S, Loureiro JF, Swift S, et al: English springer spaniels with significant bradyarrhythmias—presentation, troponin I and follow-up after pacemaker implantation, J Small Anim Pract 51:155, 2010.
6. Guzman SV, Deleon AC, West JW, et al: Cardiac effects of isoproterenol, norepinephrine and epinephrine in complete AV heart block during experimental acidosis and hyperkalemia, Circulation Res 7:666, 1959.
7. Seungkeun L, Nam SJ, Hyun C: The optimal size and placement of transdermal electrodes are critical for the efficacy of a transcutaneous pacemaker in dogs, Vet J 183:196, 2010.
8. DeFrancesco TC, Hansen BD, Atkins CE, et al: Noninvasive transthoracic temporary cardiac pacing in dogs, J Vet Intern Med 17:663, 2003.
9. Noomanova N, Perego M, Perini A, Santilli RA: Use of transcutaneous external pacing during transvenous pacemaker implantation in dogs, Vet Rec 167:241, 2010.
10. Harrigan RA, Chan TC, Moonblatt S, et al: Temporary transvenous pacemaker placement in the emergency department, J Emerg Med 32:105, 2007.
11. Syring RS, Costello MF, Poppenga RH: Temporary transvenous cardiac pacing in a dog with diltiazem intoxication, J Vet Emerg Crit Care 18:75, 2008.

CHAPTER 47
SUPRAVENTRICULAR TACHYARRHYTHMIAS

Kathy N. Wright, DVM, DACVIM

KEY POINTS

- Supraventricular tachyarrhythmias (SVTs) are rapid rhythms originating from or dependent on tissues above the ventricles.
- Once thought relatively benign, SVTs are actually an important cause of morbidity, and even mortality, in small animals.
- Recognition of underlying structural heart disease and the contribution of SVTs to myocardial dysfunction are critical for accurate patient treatment.
- Acute termination of SVTs should be accomplished by medical means, based on the likely mechanism of the tachyarrhythmia.
- Long-term management can include antiarrhythmic therapy or procedures to eliminate an abnormal electrical circuit (such as an accessory pathway).

Supraventricular tachyarrhythmias (SVTs) are defined as rapid cardiac rhythms that (1) originate in the atria or atrioventricular (AV) junction (above the bundle of His) or (2) involve the atria or AV junction as a critical component of a tachyarrhythmia circuit.[1] The most clinically useful classification system broadly groups SVTs into atrial tachyarrhythmias or AV node–dependent tachyarrhythmias.[2] Such classification helps us to guide therapy of these abnormal heart rhythms and is discussed in detail later in this chapter.

The importance of managing SVTs has become clearer in recent years. Not only can these abnormal rhythms result from structural heart disease, but they can be the cause of structural heart disease as well. Pacing studies and clinical cases have demonstrated that sustained or frequently occurring SVTs can result in a poorly functioning, dilated heart.[3-8] This is known as *tachycardiomyopathy* or *tachycardia-induced cardiomyopathy* and cannot be distinguished initially from idiopathic dilated cardiomyopathy (DCM). Any young to middle-aged dog presenting with a clinical picture of DCM should have tachycardiomyopathy on the differential diagnosis list. Tachycardiomyopathy, unlike DCM, can be partially or completely reversible with adequate rhythm control. It is the most commonly unrecognized curable cause of heart failure in human (and likely veterinary) patients.[4] SVTs can also result in sudden death, although less often than does sustained ventricular tachycardia. Sudden death has occurred in several dogs with sustained tachyarrhythmias secondary to accessory pathways. The presumed mechanism is myocardial ischemia that gives rise to ventricular tachycardia and fibrillation, although the sudden onset of electromechanical dissociation has been seen in two dogs.

HISTORICAL DATA

Careful questioning of owners should be pursued to try to determine clinical signs that may be related to an SVT or structural heart disease. Those commonly reported include decreased exercise tolerance, weakness, signs of congestive heart failure, gastrointestinal (GI) signs (particularly vomiting and inappetence), collapse, noticeably rapid heart rate (most evident when the animal is in lateral recumbency), and pulsing of the ears or bobbing of the head with each heart beat. Several animals were diagnosed initially as having primary GI disease, only to find later that their GI signs were related to an SVT. Signs reported by owners whose animals have developed congestive heart failure include dyspnea, tachypnea, and abdominal distention. Some owners believe that their dogs are asymptomatic, only to realize how affected they have been once the tachyarrhythmias is controlled.

PHYSICAL EXAMINATION FINDINGS

It is important to remember that at the time an animal with SVT is presented to the veterinarian, the physical examination findings may be normal if the SVT was paroxysmal. On the other hand, a tachyarrhythmia may be detected at the time of arrival or while the animal is hospitalized. Decreased systemic arterial pulse quality, mucous membrane pallor, a peritoneal fluid wave, tachypnea or dyspnea with auscultable pulmonary abnormalities, murmurs of mitral or tricuspid regurgitation secondary to tachycardiomyopathy, and murmurs associated with a primary underlying heart disease are all potential physical examination findings.

EXAMINING THE ELECTROCARDIOGRAM

Distinguishing Supraventricular from Ventricular Tachyarrhythmias

It is most important to distinguish ventricular tachyarrhythmias from SVTs because the treatment and differential diagnoses for each will differ. A narrow QRS complex tachyarrhythmia will almost always be an SVT. The vast majority of wide complex tachyarrhythmias are ventricular tachyarrhythmias. Up to 80% of wide complex tachyarrhythmias in human case series are ventricular in origin.[9] If the patient has prior ECGs when in sinus rhythm or exhibits conversion, even briefly, to sinus rhythm during the tachyarrhythmia, the QRS complexes can be compared with those during tachyarrhythmia. Preexisting bundle branch block or ventricular preexcitation can thus be identified.[10] Distinguishing ventricular arrhythmias from SVTs with bundle branch aberration that develops during SVT or antegrade conduction of a tachycardia over an accessory pathway (rare that an accessory pathway can conduct antegrade at a very rapid rate in companion animals) is the most difficult task for the clinician. No criteria are absolute; however, the following rules are helpful[9,11]:

1. Identification of P′ waves (representing atrial depolarization that originates outside the sinoatrial node) with a consistent relationship to the QRS is indicative of an SVT with aberration. In dogs undergoing electrophysiologic studies, retrograde AV nodal conduction is noted in approximately 17% and most commonly has a long effective refractory period when it does occur. As many leads as possible should be run to identify P′ waves. Lewis leads, using the right and left arm electrodes of the standard ECG placed

on various positions over the precordium while monitoring the lead I channel, are very helpful in identifying P′ waves.

2. QRS fusion complexes are a hallmark of ventricular tachyarrhythmia.
3. If the tachycardia terminates in response to a vagal maneuver, this indicates that the tachycardia is supraventricular in origin. If the tachycardia does not terminate with a vagal maneuver, it may be of either supraventricular or ventricular origin.
4. If the tachycardia terminates with the administration of intravenous lidocaine, this diagnostic and therapeutic procedure indicates that the wide complex tachyarrhythmia is most likely ventricular in origin. Rarely, however, an atrial tachycardia will convert with lidocaine therapy, and some accessory pathways are lidocaine sensitive.

Diagnosing Atrial Versus Atrioventricular Node–Dependent Tachyarrhythmias

Once an SVT has been identified, it is helpful to determine if it is atrial or AV node–dependent. If the SVT is irregularly irregular and no organized atrial activity is identifiable, then atrial fibrillation is the diagnosis. Differentiation of regular SVTs involves several steps. Initiation and termination of the SVT are important diagnostic features. If an SVT continues despite AV block, it is atrial in origin. If a premature ventricular contraction terminates the SVT, it is far more likely that it is an AV node–dependent tachyarrhythmia. If a vagal maneuver terminates the SVT, it is also far more likely an AV node–dependent tachyarrhythmia.

Identification of P′ waves is an important diagnostic step, but it can be difficult in a rapid SVT. Precordial and Lewis leads help with their identification. The relationship of the P′ wave to the preceding QRS complex relative to the total RR interval identifies an SVT as either a short RP′ (RP′ interval ≤ 50% of the RR interval) or a long RP′ (RP′ interval > 50% of the RR interval) SVT.[1] Important identifying characteristics and mechanisms of the more common SVTs are reviewed in Table 47-1 and Figure 47-1. The most commonly occurring SVTs in small animals appear to be atrial fibrillation, intraatrial reentrant tachycardia, orthodromic AV reciprocating tachycardia (a macroreentrant circuit in which an impulse is carried from the atria to the AV node–His-Purkinje system to the ventricles to a retrograde-conducting accessory pathway to the atria), and automatic atrial tachycardia. Because the retrograde conduction properties of the canine AV node are typically poor and the antegrade fast pathway has a short effective refractory period, AV nodal reentrant tachycardia has not been identified in dogs undergoing electrophysiologic study for clinical tachyarrhythmias.

TREATMENT OF SUPRAVENTRICULAR TACHYARRHYTHMIAS

It is essential to identify predisposing factors that are contributing to the initiation or perpetuation of SVT in a given patient. Acid-base abnormalities, electrolyte disturbances, significant anemia, and hypoxemia should be corrected. AV node–dependent tachyarrhythmias are treated in some cases by single-agent therapy aimed at slowing conduction through the AV node. Most AV node–dependent SVTs, however, require that an additional drug be added to suppress another site in the circuit. Atrial tachyarrhythmias are best addressed by dual therapy: one drug to slow AV nodal conduction and a second drug to inhibit the atrial automatic focus or interrupt conduction in an atrial reentrant circuit. Sites of antiarrhythmic drug action in SVT are shown in Figure 47-2.

Emergent Therapy

Animals in incessant, rapid SVT require emergent interruption of the tachyarrhythmia. Vagal maneuvers may be tried first and may terminate the SVT if it is AV node dependent. Subjectively, the most effective vagal maneuver in small animals is carotid sinus massage. Sustained, gentle compression is applied for 5 to 10 seconds over the carotid sinus, which is located immediately caudal to the dorsal aspect of the larynx. The ECG needs to be monitored continuously throughout the procedure. Most often, however, the SVT does not terminate with such maneuvers and drug therapy must be initiated.

Parenteral negative dromotropic agents can be used to interrupt a tachyarrhythmic circuit that uses the AV node and is causing

Table 47-1 Characteristics of Common Supraventricular Tachyarrhythmias

SVT Mechanism	P′ Waves Visible?	P′ Wave Morphology	RP′ vs. RR Interval	Initiation and Termination	Response to AV Block
Atrial					
Automatic atrial	Yes	Variable, differs from sinus P	Varies with SVT rate, often long	Gradual rate acceleration and deceleration	SVT continues
Intraatrial reentry	Yes	Variable, differs from sinus P (may be subtle)	Varies with SVT rate, often long	Abrupt onset and offset at SVT rate	SVT continues
Atrial flutter	Flutter (F) waves	Identical saw-toothed F waves	Not applicable	Abrupt onset and offset at SVT rate	SVT continues
Atrial fibrillation	No, *f* waves may be seen	No visible P waves; *f* waves may be seen	Not applicable	Abrupt onset and offset at SVT rate, often incessant	SVT continues
AV Node–dependent					
OAVRT	Often visible within ST-T segment	Retrograde: (–) in II, III, avF	Typically short	Abrupt onset and offset	SVT terminates
Automatic junctional	Generally yes; AV dissociation common	Variable	Variable	Gradual rate acceleration and deceleration	SVT continues with AV dissociation
Typical AV nodal reentry	Generally no	Retrograde: (–) in II, III, avF	Short	Abrupt onset and offset	SVT terminates
PJRT	Typically visible in the T-P segment	Retrograde: (–) in II, III, avF	Long	Often incessant. Abrupt onset and offset.	SVT terminates

AV, Atrioventricular; *OAVRT*, orthodromic atrioventricular reciprocated tachycardia; *PJRT*, permanent junctional reciprocating tachycardia; *SVT*, supraventricular tachycardia.

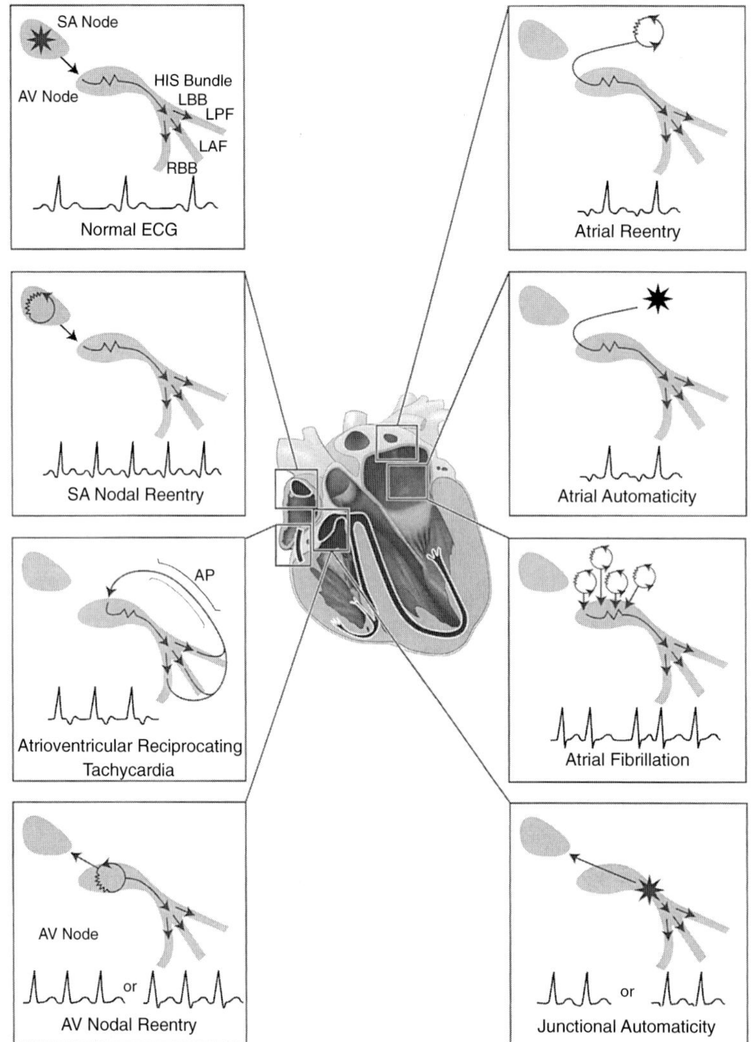

FIGURE 47-1 Representation of the mechanisms and electrocardiographic characteristics of the more common supraventricular tachyarrhythmias. *AP,* Accessory pathway; *AV,* atrioventricular; ECG, electrocardiogram; *LAF,* left anterior fascicle; *LBB,* left bundle branch; *LPF,* left posterior fascicle; *RBB,* right bundle branch; *SA,* sinoatrial. *(From Bonagura JD:* Kirk's current veterinary therapy XIII, *ed 13, Philadelphia, 2000, Saunders.)*

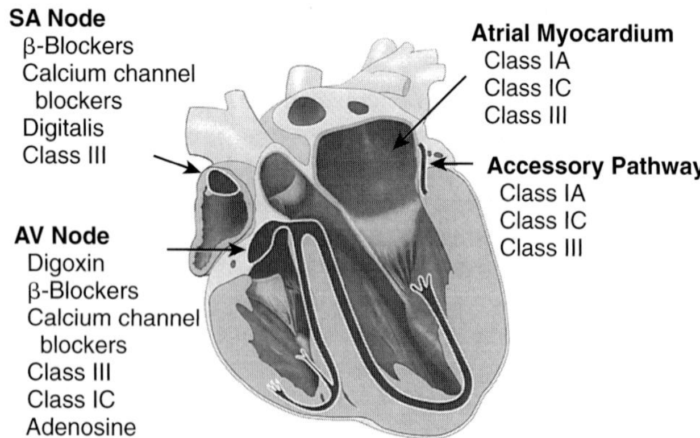

FIGURE 47-2 Sites of action for various antiarrhythmic drugs, highlighting their utility for specific supraventricular tachyarrhythmias. *AV,* Atrioventricular; *SA,* sinoatrial. *(From Bonagura JD:* Kirk's current veterinary therapy XIII, *ed 13, Philadelphia, 2000, Saunders.)*

hemodynamic compromise. In atrial tachyarrhythmias, such agents will not terminate the arrhythmia but will slow conduction to the ventricles. Intravenous calcium channel blockers, β-blockers, or adenosine have been used for this purpose. Blood pressure and ECG should be monitored before and throughout the procedure.

A comparison of the electrophysiologic and hemodynamic responses of intravenous diltiazem, esmolol, and adenosine in normal dogs demonstrated the superior efficacy of intravenous diltiazem in slowing AV nodal conduction while maintaining a favorable hemodynamic profile.[11] Esmolol was a significantly less effective negative dromotrope than diltiazem and caused a severe drop in left ventricular contractility measurements at dosages that did prolong AV nodal conduction. Adenosine, even at dosages of 2 mg/kg, was ineffective in slowing canine AV nodal conduction. A similar study has not been performed in cats. Diltiazem is administered at dosages of 0.125 to 0.35 mg/kg intravenously (IV) slowly over 2 to 3 minutes in dogs (Box 47-1).[1,12] A constant rate infusion (CRI) (0.125 to 0.35 mg/kg/hr) can be used if frequent recurrence of the arrhythmia occurs before the onset of efficacious oral antiarrhythmic therapy. Esmolol is an ultrashort-acting β_1-selective blocker that typically is administered at 0.5 mg/kg IV over 1 to 2 minutes.[1] Its brief half-life

BOX 47-1 *Emergency Therapy for Supraventricular Tachycardia in Dogs*

Diltiazem
- Intermittent Dosing: 0.125 to 0.35 mg/kg slowly IV over 2 to 3 minutes
- CRI: 0.125 to 0.35 mg/kg/hr if frequent reoccurrence

compared with that of propranolol makes esmolol the preferred parenteral β-blocker. It should nonetheless be used very cautiously in animals with impaired ventricular systolic function, because it will markedly depress ventricular contractility.

The calcium ion is critical for a number of cardiovascular functions. These include impulse formation within the sinoatrial node, conduction through the AV node, and excitation-contraction coupling in cardiac and vascular smooth muscles. Overdosage of calcium channel blockers can therefore result in hypotension, negative chronotropy caused by impaired discharge from the sinus node, negative dromotropy as a result of impaired AV nodal conduction, negative inotropy (decreased contractility), and impaired insulin release. The latter will cause blood glucose concentrations to rise while depleting intracellular calcium stores. The effects on the peripheral vasculature, cardiac muscle, and pancreatic β cells all can lead to hemodynamic collapse with high doses of calcium channel blockers.

There are two types of β receptors, β_1 and β_2. β_1 Receptors are located primarily within the heart and adipose tissue. The effects of β_1-receptor stimulation occur through coupling of β_1 receptors with adenyl cyclase, resulting in enhanced cyclic AMP production. This results in (1) increased heart rate secondary to stimulation of the funny current (I_f) and L-type calcium current; (2) enhanced myocardial contractility through L-type calcium current influx stimulating increased sarcoplasmic reticular calcium release; (3) improved myocardial relaxation through phosphorylation of phospholamban; and (4) enhanced automaticity of subsidiary pacemakers.[13] β_2 receptors are found primarily in bronchial and smooth muscles, where they produce relaxation. Overdosage of β-blocking drugs therefore can produce severe bradyarrhythmias, impaired atrial and ventricular contractility, bronchospasm, and decreased glycogenolysis, lipolysis, and gluconeogenesis.

Other agents can prolong the effective refractory period or slow conduction within the myocardium, including an accessory pathway or atrial myocardium. These agents can terminate both atrial and AV node–dependent tachyarrhythmias. Of these, procainamide is the agent most commonly used in veterinary medicine. A sodium and potassium channel blocker, procainamide decreases abnormal automaticity, slows conduction, and prolongs the effective refractory period in atrial (and ventricular), accessory pathway, and retrograde fast AV nodal tissue. In atrial tachyarrhythmias, other agents are used first to slow AV nodal conduction before administration of procainamide. Parenteral procainamide is administered in dosages of 6 to 8 mg/kg IV over 5 to 10 minutes or 6 to 20 mg/kg intramuscularly (IM) in dogs. A CRI of 20 to 40 mcg/kg/min can be used once a therapeutic response is obtained with bolus administration. Parenteral procainamide in cats is used cautiously at dosages of 1 to 2 mg/kg IV or 3 to 8 mg/kg IM and a CRI of 10 to 20 mcg/kg/min.

A precordial thump is a simple, brief procedure that has a low rate of success but has been used to successfully convert an SVT to sinus rhythm.[10,14] A sharp, concussive blow is delivered to the left precordium with the animal in right lateral recumbency. This will result in myocardial depolarization that could disrupt a reentrant tachycardia circuit. In addition to being a therapeutic procedure, it can be a diagnostic one in the case of wide complex tachycardias by allowing the clinician to see the morphology of the QRS complex during sinus rhythm. Unfortunately, often sinus rhythm will only last for a short time, so drug therapy or other intervention must be at the ready. Direct current (DC) cardioversion or overdrive pacing can be used to terminate certain hemodynamically unstable, sustained SVTs.[12] DC cardioversion in a proper critical care environment with appropriate hemodynamic and electrocardiographic monitoring offers certain distinct advantages over emergency drug therapy. The need to distinguish between supraventricular and ventricular tachyarrhythmias to design appropriate drug therapy is less important when DC cardioversion is employed. Sinus rhythm may be restored immediately with successful DC cardioversion, avoiding the slower titration and potential side effects seen with parenteral drug administration. The need for general anesthesia (albeit brief) is a risk factor for DC cardioversion but should not preclude its use in patients who would benefit from it. Biphasic cardioversion is more effective than using monophasic waveforms.

DC cardioversion and overdrive pacing are effective in terminating SVTs caused by reentry rather than abnormal automaticity. Overdrive pacing can be performed without general anesthesia if the patient is depressed or moribund. The jugular furrow can be locally anesthetized with lidocaine, a catheter introducer placed in the external jugular vein, and a multipolar catheter guided fluoroscopically into the right atrium (for intraatrial reentry) or ventricle (more effective for terminating orthodromic AV reciprocating tachycardia). The distal and second poles of this catheter are then attached to a programmable pacemaker. An electrophysiologic recorder (ideal but not necessary) or multilead surface ECG is used to continuously record cardiac electrical activity. Once the myocardium is captured, the pacing rate is increased to 10 to 20 beats/min faster than the tachyarrhythmia rate. One-to-one capture is ensured for a brief period, and then pacing is stopped once intracardiac electrograms confirm termination of the SVT. If only the surface ECG is recorded, pacing is stopped after a brief period to determine if the tachyarrhythmia terminated. If not, a longer period or slightly faster pacing rate is used. Failure to terminate or rapid resumption of the tachyarrhythmia can indicate either an SVT caused by an automatic mechanism or successful termination but then rapid reinitiation of a reentrant SVT.

Long-Term Therapy

Medical treatment

Long-term antiarrhythmic drug therapy must be tailored to each patient based on the type of SVT, the presence or absence of congestive heart failure or significant structural heart disease, comorbid conditions (particularly hepatic or renal dysfunction, acid-base disturbances, or endocrine diseases that alter the metabolism of specific antiarrhythmic drugs), and concurrent drug administration. Atrial tachyarrhythmias typically are managed by dual antiarrhythmic therapy, one drug to slow AV nodal conduction and a second to terminate the atrial tachyarrhythmia itself. This general rule is violated when persistent atrial fibrillation is present, when rate control typically becomes the goal. The other option with atrial fibrillation, however, is to cardiovert it to sinus rhythm using a biphasic defibrillator and use antiarrhythmic drug therapy to try to maintain sinus rhythm.[15] AV node–dependent tachyarrhythmias occasionally will respond to single- agent therapy aimed at slowing AV nodal conduction. In reality, however, these tachyarrhythmias most often require combination therapy as well. For instance, with orthodromic AV reciprocating tachycardia, one agent is used to slow AV nodal conduction and a second agent is used to block conduction or prolong the effective refractory period within an accessory pathway.

Drugs that slow AV nodal conduction include the classes that were discussed under emergent therapy. The three major classes include: digitalis glycosides, calcium channel blockers, and β-blockers.

Animals with systolic dysfunction classically are placed on digoxin as a first-line negative dromotrope (0.005 to 0.01 mg/kg PO q12h in a normokalemic dog with normal renal function; 0.0312 mg PO q24-48h in a normokalemic cat with normal renal function). The ventricular rate is almost never slowed adequately with digoxin as a single agent, however, and other drugs must be added. The calcium channel blocker diltiazem is effective in prolonging the effective and functional refractory periods of the AV node. This effect is most notable at faster stimulation rates (use dependence) and in depolarized fibers (voltage dependence).[16] Diltiazem has gained preference over verapamil because of its more favorable hemodynamic profile (i.e., minimal negative inotropic effect) at effective antiarrhythmic dosages. Standard diltiazem is administered three times a day, which can be difficult from a compliance standpoint. Sustained release preparations appear to have more variable absorption in companion animals, with resultant poorer arrhythmia control. Dilacor XR has been used successfully in dogs at 2 to 5 mg/kg PO q12h. These preparations can have a higher incidence of side effects in cats, including vomiting, inappetence, and hepatopathies.[12] A randomized, crossover study in 18 clinical dogs showed that the combination of digoxin and diltiazem produced better ventricular rate control in atrial fibrillation than either agent alone.[17]

Atenolol is a relatively β_1-selective blocker that competitively inhibits the effects of catecholamines on cardiac β receptors. Thus underlying sympathetic tone plays an important role in determining the effectiveness of atenolol in prolonging AV nodal conduction and refractoriness or suppressing abnormal atrial foci.[16,18] Because of its negative inotropic effects, the dosages required to significantly affect AV nodal conduction are often not well tolerated by animals with ventricular systolic dysfunction. The beneficial effects of β-adrenergic blockade in the face of impaired ventricular systolic function have been well demonstrated in human patients; therapy must begin at very low dosages and up-titration performed very slowly.[16] Patients with rapid SVTs do not have the luxury of this prolonged time for control of their ventricular rate. One must remember that the rapid ventricular rate is either worsening or may be the sole cause for their myocardial dysfunction. Atenolol is particularly useful in cats with hypertrophic cardiomyopathy and SVTs. Because of its renal clearance, the dosage of atenolol should be decreased in the face of concurrent renal failure.

Class I antiarrhythmic drugs block fast sodium channels and thus suppress abnormal automaticity and slow myocardial conduction velocity. Oral procainamide typically was used as an extended release preparation. Such preparations are no longer available, however, thus removing them from our armamentarium of effective antiarrhythmic drugs. The need for 2-hour to 6-hour dosing of formulations that are not extended release makes compliance nearly impossible. GI side effects can be prominent, and proarrhythmia is a definite concern with long-term procainamide therapy. Mexiletine, a class IB agent, can be useful as a component of multidrug therapy for some canine SVTs (some accessory pathways are sensitive to class IB agents, as are rare atrial tachyarrhythmias). It is used at 4 to 8 mg/kg PO q8h with food in dogs. Because of its side effect profile, it is not used in cats.

Class III antiarrhythmic agents are used to prolong the effective refractory period of atrial myocardium and accessory pathways. Sotalol and amiodarone, the two agents used in small animals, have additional antiarrhythmic actions, including slowing of AV nodal conduction. Sotalol typically is administered at 1 to 3 mg/kg PO q12h on an empty stomach for SVTs, but amiodarone dosing varies and typically includes a loading period.[12] The author uses 15 mg/kg q24h for 7 to 10 days, then 10 mg/kg q24h for 7 to 10 days, then 5 to 8 mg/kg q24h for maintenance. Serum amiodarone levels can be measured but may not correlate with tissue concentrations. The high incidence of reported extracardiac side effects in dogs receiving long-term amiodarone therapy has limited its widespread use.[12,19] Amiodarone has not been used in cats.

Catheter ablation

Certain SVTs can be cured, rather than simply controlled, with transvenous radiofrequency catheter ablation.[8,20-23] The tachyarrhythmia circuit is first mapped with numerous multielectrode catheters. Once, for example, an accessory pathway is identified, detailed mapping is used to locate precisely the atrial and ventricular insertions of the pathway along the AV groove. The distal electrode (4 mm to 5 mm) of a specialized catheter is positioned at the critical site, and radiofrequency energy is delivered to the tip electrode, causing thermal dessication of a small volume of tissue to permanently interrupt the tachycardia circuit. This technique has successfully been used by this author and others in a large number of canine cases, with long-term follow-up documenting that these dogs are, in fact, cured.

REFERENCES

1. Wright KN: Assessment and treatment of supraventricular tachyarrhythmias. In Bonagura JD, editor: Kirk's current veterinary therapy XIV, St Louis, 2009, Saunders Elsevier.
2. Wathen MS, Klein GJ, Yee R, et al: Classification and terminology of supraventricular tachycardia, Cardiol Clin 11:109, 1993.
3. Walker NL, Cobbe SM, Birnie DH: Tachycardiomyopathy: a diagnosis not to be missed, Heart 90:e7, 2004.
4. Salemi VM, Arteaga E, Mady C: Recovery of systolic and diastolic function after ablation of incessant supraventricular tachycardia, Eur J Heart Fail 7:1117, 2005.
5. Houmsse M, Tyler J, Kalbfleisch S: Supraventricular tachycardia causing heart failure, Curr Opin Cardiol 26:261, 2011.
6. Lishmanov A, Chockalingam P, Senthilkumar A, et al: Tachycardia-induced cardiomyopathy: evaluation and therapeutic options, Cong Heart Fail 16:122, 2010.
7. Knight BP, Jacobsen JT: Assessing patients for catheter ablation during hospitalization for acute heart failure, Heart Fail Rev 16:467, 2011.
8. Wright KN, Mehdirad AA, Giacobe P, et al: Radiofrequency catheter ablation of atrioventricular accessory pathways in three dogs with subsequent resolution of tachycardia-induced cardiomyopathy, J Vet Intern Med 13:361, 1999.
9. Miller JM, Hsia HH, Das M: Differential diagnosis for wide QRS complex tachycardia. In Zipes DP, Jaliffe J, editors: Cardiac electrophysiology: from cell to bedside, ed 5, Philadelphia, 2009, Saunders Elsevier.
10. Santilli RA, Diana A, Baron Toaldo M: Orthodromic atrioventricular reciprocating tachycardia conducted with intraventricular conduction disturbance mimicking ventricular tachycardia in an English Bulldog, J Vet Cardiol 14:363, 2012.
11. Wright KN, Schwartz DS, Hamlin R: Electrophysiologic and hemodynamic responses to adenosine, diltiazem, and esmolol in dogs, J Vet Intern Med 12:201, 1998.
12. Côté E: Electrocardiography and cardiac arrhythmias. In Ettinger S, Feldman B, editors: Textbook of veterinary medicine, ed 7, St Louis, 2010, Elsevier.
13. Opie LH, Horowitz JD: Beta-blocking agents. In Opie LH, Gersch BJ, editors: Drugs for the heart, ed 7, Philadelphia, 2009, Elsevier.
14. Jan SL, Fu YC, Lin MC, et al: Precordial thump in a newborn with refractory supraventricular tachycardia and cardiovascular collapse after amiodarone administration, Eur J Emerg Med 19:128, 2012.
15. Bright JM, zumBrunnen J: Chronicity of atrial fibrillation affects duration of sinus rhythm after transthoracic cardioversion of atrial fibrillation to sinus rhythm, J Vet Intern Med 22:114, 2008.
16. Miller JM, Zipes DP: Therapy of cardiac arrhythmias. In Braunwald E, Zipes DP, Libby P, Bonow RO, editors: Braunwald's heart disease: a textbook of cardiovascular medicine, ed 7, Philadelphia, 2005, Saunders.
17. Gelzer AR, Kraus MS, Rishniw M, et al: Combination therapy with digoxin and ditiazem controls ventricular rate in chronic atrial fibrillation in dogs better than digoxin or diltiazem monotherapy: a randomized, crossover study in 18 dogs, J Vet Intern Med 23:499, 2009.

18. Opie LH, Poole-Wilson PA: β-Blocking agents. In Opie LH, Gersch BJ, editors: Drugs for the heart, ed 7, Philadelphia, 2009, Elsevier.
19. Kraus MS, Ridge LG, Gelzer ARM, et al: Toxicity in Doberman Pinscher dogs with ventricular arrhythmias treated with amiodarone, Proceedings of the 23rd American College of Veterinary Internal Medicine Forum, Baltimore, June 2005.
20. Wright KN: Interventional catheterization for tachyarrhythmias, Vet Clin North Am Small Anim Pract 34:1171, 2004.
21. Wright KN, Knilans TK, Irvin HM: When, why, and how to perform radiofrequency catheter ablation, J Vet Cardiol 8:95, 2006.
22. Santilli RA, Spadacini G, Moretti P, et al: Anatomic distribution and electrophysiologic properties of accessory pathways in dogs, J Am Vet Med Assoc 231:393, 2007.
23. Santilli RA, Perego M, Perini A, et al: Electrophysiologic characteristics and topographical distribution of focal atrial tachycardia in dogs, J Vet Intern Med 24:539, 2009.

CHAPTER 48
VENTRICULAR TACHYARRHYTHMIAS

Romain Pariaut, DVM, DACVIM (Cardiology), DECVIM-CA (Cardiology)

KEY POINTS

- Wide QRS complex tachycardia with atrioventricular dissociation, fusion beats, and capture beats are electrocardiographic features diagnostic of ventricular tachycardia (VT).
- Clinical signs secondary to VT are determined by its rate and duration.
- The most common noncardiac causes of VT are hypoxemia, electrolyte imbalances (hypokalemia), acid-base disorders, and drugs.
- The most common cardiac diseases associated with clinical VT are arrhythmogenic cardiomyopathy in boxers and dilated cardiomyopathy in Doberman Pinschers.
- Antiarrhythmic medications do not prevent sudden death.
- Antiarrhythmic therapy is initiated if clinical signs associated with VT are present.
- When the origin (supraventricular or ventricular) of a wide QRS tachycardia cannot be determined, it must be managed as if it were VT.
- Lidocaine is the first-choice parenteral antiarrhythmic drug for treatment of VT in dogs.

INTRODUCTION

Physiologically, specialized ventricular cells known as *Purkinje fibers* may work as a pacemaker when the sinus and atrioventricular nodes fail to function appropriately, resulting in a ventricular escape rhythm or idioventricular rhythm at a rate of about 30 to 40 beats/min in dogs and 60 to 130 beats/min in cats.[1,2] Three arrhythmogenic mechanisms known as *enhanced automaticity, triggered activity,* and *reentry* (Box 48-1) may affect Purkinje cells or any excitable ventricular myocyte and result in ventricular tachycardia (VT).[3] They result in a ventricular rhythm faster than the physiologic idioventricular rhythm. Most human cardiologists define VT as three or more consecutive ventricular beats occurring at a rate faster than 100 beats/min, the conventional upper limit for normal sinus rhythm. In our patients, normal sinus rhythm can probably reach 150 to 180 beats/min in dogs and 220 beats/min in cats. These rates define the lower limit for VT. If a ventricular rhythm is faster than the physiologic idioventricular rhythm and slower than VT, it is called *accelerated idioventricular rhythm (AIVR).* The rate of an AIVR is within the range of the underlying sinus rhythm. Therefore both rhythms are seen competing on a surface electrocardiogram (ECG) because the faster pacemaker inhibits the slower one, a property known as *overdrive suppression.*[2] Besides rate, an important feature of VT is duration because both determine the clinical consequences of the arrhythmia. VT is described as nonsustained if it lasts less than 30 seconds and sustained if it lasts longer. Nonsustained VT is usually asymptomatic because of its short duration. The terms

BOX 48-1 *Electrophysiologic Mechanisms of Ventricular Tachycardia*

Reentry: Requires an impulse to leave a point of departure and return to its starting point with a sufficient delay that the cardiac tissue has recovered its excitability. It usually circles around an area of nonconductive tissue (fibrosis, vessel). Shortening of the refractory period and slow conduction favor this self-perpetuating mechanism.

Enhanced automaticity: Any myocardial cell can acquire the property of spontaneous depolarization when its environment is altered. Its membrane potential becomes less negative, which gives it the ability to generate an action potential similar to that of the sinus node.

Triggered activity: Results from small membrane depolarizations that appear after and are dependent on the upstroke of the action potential. They trigger an action potential when they reach the threshold potential. When they occur during the process of repolarization they are called *early afterdepolarizations (EADs),* and when they occur after full repolarization they are called *delayed afterdepolarizations (DADs).* Hypokalemia and drug-induced prolongation of the QT segment increase the risk of EADs. DADs occur secondary to intracellular calcium overload associated with sustained tachycardia and digoxin toxicity.

incessant VT and *VT storm* are used to describe recurrent episodes of sustained VT during a 24-hour period. VT storm is a life-threatening emergency.

ELECTROCARDIOGRAPHIC DIAGNOSIS

In the intensive care unit, VT is first suspected on physical examination or detected on a continuous ECG monitor. Confirmation of VT relies on a good-quality 6-lead surface ECG recording with the patient placed in right lateral recumbency.

Ventricular tachycardia is identified as a broad QRS tachycardia with complexes wider than 0.06 second in dogs and 0.04 second in cats. Each QRS complex is followed by a large T wave, directed opposite to the QRS deflection.

The challenge of ECG interpretation is to differentiate VT from supraventricular tachycardias (SVTs) with broad QRS complexes because of aberrant conduction of the electrical impulse within the ventricles. Aberrant ventricular conduction results from a structural bundle branch block, a functional or rate-related bundle branch block, or finally an accessory atrioventricular pathway causing preexcitation.[4] However, it is important to remember that VT is much more common than broad QRS complex SVT in dogs and cats.

The three most reliable diagnostic criteria of VT are atrioventricular dissociation, fusion beats, and capture beats (Figure 48-1). Atrioventricular dissociation is demonstrated when P waves are occasionally seen on the ECG tracing but are not related to ventricular complexes. These P waves reflect atrial activity independently from the ventricle. On occasion apparent atrioventricular association may be seen, or ventricular beats can conduct in a retrograde fashion to the atrium in a 1 : 1 ratio. Therefore signs of atrioventricular association do not rule out VT. Fusion beats and capture beats are seen with paroxysmal VT and AIVR. Fusion beats result from the summation of a ventricular impulse and a simultaneous supraventricular impulse resulting in a QRS complex of intermediate morphology and preceeded by a P wave (unless there is concurrent atrial fibrillation). A capture beat is a supraventricular impulse conducting through the normal conduction pathways to the ventricle during an episode of VT or AIVR. This complex occurs earlier than expected and is narrow if the conduction system is intact.[4]

Regularity of the rhythm is a less accurate criterion because VT can be slightly irregular. When the RR interval varies by 100 msec or more, it is suggestive of atrial fibrillation with aberrant ventricular conduction. Other criteria have been suggested by human cardiologists to make the correct diagnosis; for example, QRS complexes are usually wider with VT than with SVT.[4] Although rarely effective, vagal maneuvers can be done to slow the atrioventricular conduction, revealing P waves associated to the QRS complexes in case of SVT. It is also important to consider the overall clinical picture. For example, Boxers and Doberman Pinschers usually have VT. Finally, it is accepted that managing SVT as VT is usually less dangerous than the opposite, because drugs used to stop SVT or to slow the ventricular response rate to rapid atrial impulses (i.e., calcium channel blockers and β-blockers) do not interrupt VT and worsen hypotension with their vasodilatory or negative inotropic effects.

If doubt persists, a wide complex tachycardia should be treated as if it were VT.

APPROACH TO THE PATIENT WITH VENTRICULAR TACHYCARDIA

Once VT is confirmed on a surface ECG, the possible causes for the initiation and maintenance of the arrhythmia must be identified. The knowledge will help in planning an effective treatment protocol and predicting the short-term and long-term prognoses. It is useful to differentiate cardiac from noncardiac causes of VT.

Noncardiac Causes of Ventricular Tachycardia

Ventricular cells are sensitive to hypoxemia, electrolyte and acid-base imbalances, sympathetic stimulation, and various drugs. These changes typically affect the passive and energy-dependent ion exchanges across the cellular membrane of the myocyte during the initiation and propagation of the action potential.

Hypokalemia is the most commonly reported electrolyte disturbance responsible for or contributing to VT. It increases phase 4

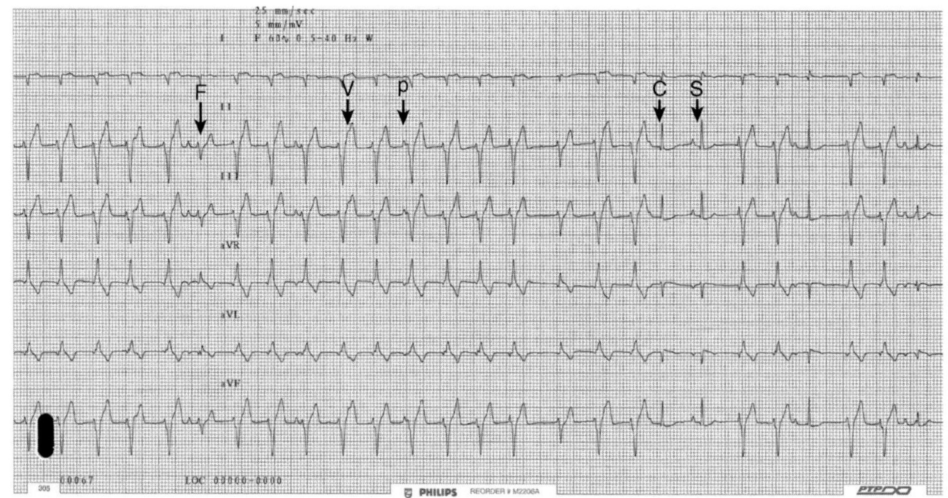

FIGURE 48-1 Electrocardiographic recording from a dog; paper speed is 25 mm/sec. There is ventricular tachycardia *(V)* at a rate of 150 beats/min. P waves *(p)* not related to the wide QRS complexes *(V)* indicate atrioventricular (AV) dissociation. There are fusion beats *(F)* with an intermediate morphology and capture beats *(C)*. Note that the PR interval of the capture beat is prolonged compared with a normal sinus beat *(S)*. It results from retrograde depolarization of the AV node by the preceding ventricular impulse and secondary slowing of the propagation of the sinus impulse in a partially refractory node, a phenomenon known as *concealed AV conduction.*

depolarization, increasing spontaneous automaticity, and prolongs the action potential duration, which promotes arrhythmias from triggered activity.[5] Because digoxin competes with potassium on its receptors, hypokalemia increases the risk of digoxin toxicity. Similar arrhythmias result from hypomagnesemia, because magnesium is necessary for proper functioning of the sodium-potassium ATP pump, which maintains normal intracellular potassium concentration. Hypocalcemia and hypercalcemia are also responsible for ventricular arrhythmias.

Increased adrenergic tone potentiates arrhythmias through various mechanisms. In the intensive care unit, drugs with sympathetic or sympatholytic activity are used commonly and should be stopped when possible to assess their role in the perpetuation of VT.

It is also important to evaluate the potential proarrhythmic effects of all the medications given to a patient with VT. There are many publications on drug-induced prolongation of the QT segment. Prolongation of the QT segment reflects prolongation of the cardiac cell membrane repolarization and indicates a risk of ventricular arrhythmia from triggered activity. Antiarrhythmic drugs such as procainamide and sotalol, but also domperidone, cisapride, chlorpromazine, and erythromycin, are known to prolong the QT segment. Bradycardia and hypokalemia contribute to this effect on repolarization and increase the risk of VT.[6]

Oxygen therapy, identification and correction of all electrolyte disturbances, and discontinuation of proarrhythmic medications are the initial and necessary first steps in the treatment of all patients with VT.

Cardiac Causes of Ventricular Tachycardia

In most patients with VT an echocardiogram is indicated as soon as possible to identify an underlying cardiac disease as the cause for the arrhythmia. In humans the association of sustained VT and heart failure is a marker of increased risk of sudden death from arrhythmia, and this is probably true in our patients as well.[7] Identification of cardiac disease may help to elaborate an effective treatment strategy, to know what to expect from the intervention, and to give the most accurate prognosis to the owner. Today there is valuable information on some breed-specific VTs.

VT is on occasion observed in patients with cardiac tumors (with or without associated tamponade), myocarditis, endocarditis, and ischemia.

VT is an important part of the clinical picture of dilated cardiomyopathy in some breeds. The prevalence of ventricular arrhythmias was 21% in a pool of breeds with dilated cardiomyopathy, 16% in Newfoundlands, and 92% in Doberman Pinschers. The natural history of the disease has been studied extensively in Doberman Pinschers. There is an occult stage of the disease with no clinical signs but with echocardiographic indicators of left ventricular dysfunction and a risk of sudden death of approximately 30%. It can last 2 to 4 years. In the overt stage of the disease, congestive heart failure is present and the risk of sudden death is about 30% to 50%. In Doberman Pinschers, most ventricular ectopies have a right bundle branch block morphology in lead II of the surface ECG, indicating their origin in the left ventricle.[8]

Cardiomyopathy of Boxers is known as *arrhythmogenic right ventricular cardiomyopathy (ARVC)*. It is an adult-onset disease with a concealed form characterized by occasional ventricular ectopies only, followed by an overt form with VT associated with exercise intolerance and collapse. On occasion myocardial failure is observed. In ARVC, ventricular ectopies typically have a left bundle branch block morphology, indicating their right-sided origin.[9] Recently it was shown that the disease not only affects the right ventricle but also the left ventricle and the atria. It is therefore not unusual to observe VT originating from the left side and supraventricular arrhythmias in these dogs.[10,11]

An inherited ventricular arrhythmia has been identified in some German Shepherds. In the most severe form of the disease these dogs have a propensity for sudden death until 18 months of age. The form of VT responsible for sudden death is polymorphic, rapid (>300 beats/min), nonsustained, and usually preceded by a pause.[12]

Dogs with severe subaortic stenosis and pulmonic stenosis are prone to syncope and sudden death. VT progressing to ventricular fibrillation may contribute to some of these episodes.

In cats, VT may be seen in association with idiopathic hypertrophic cardiomyopathy and with concentric hypertrophy secondary to hypertension and hyperthyroidism.

ANTIARRHYTHMIC TREATMENT

Decision to Treat

Antiarrhythmic agents are indicated to treat symptomatic VT and prevent its recurrence. Despite many large-scale randomized studies in humans and a few publications in veterinary medicine, there is no indication that antiarrhythmic agents can prevent sudden death and on some occasions they may precipitate it.[7]

Hemodynamic compromise usually is associated with rapid (>200 beats/min) and sustained VT in a patient with concurrent cardiac disease. Slower nonsustained VT and AIVR are usually auscultatory or ECG findings in patients with motor vehicle–related trauma, gastric dilation-volvulus, or metabolic imbalances and resolve spontaneously, with no antiarrhythmic medications, within 4 days.[13]

Some ECG characteristics of VT are viewed as indicators of an increased risk for sudden death and may influence the decision of the clinician toward treatment. Hemodynamic collapse is more likely to result from polymorphic VT, which is characterized by a continuously changing QRS complex pattern, than monomorphic VT. Antiarrhythmic agents are generally considered for sustained VT with rates greater than 180 to 200 beats/min. The presence of polymorphic VT may encourage treatment at the lower rate range. *R-on-T phenomenon* describes the superimposition of an ectopic beat on the T wave of the preceding beat, also known as the "vulnerable period." Some observations suggest that it may represent an increased risk for VT and sudden death from ventricular fibrillation. In an experimental study in dogs, ventricular fibrillation could be reliably induced by delivering an electrical impulse on the peak of T wave seen from lead II on the surface ECG.[14] However, ECG recordings collected from implantable cardiac defibrillators in human patients showed that ventricular tachycardia was as likely to be initiated by a late-occuring ventricular premature complex because it was from one originating on the T wave.[15] In veterinary patients, strong evidence is lacking and this finding by itself cannot justify treatment.

Regardless of its cause, rate, duration, or morphology, the decision to treat VT with antiarrhythmic medications must be dictated primarily by the clinical signs related to it.

Antiarrhythmic Drugs

A few antiarrhythmic agents will manage most VTs. Because studies in veterinary medicine are lacking and antiarrhythmic medications are complex drugs with many side effects, including proarrhythmic effects, it is important to gain experience with only a few commonly used drugs.

Lidocaine

Lidocaine is the first-choice intravenous agent to control VT. It works better on rapid VTs and in normokalemic animals. In dogs, boluses of 2 mg/kg can be repeated every 10 to 15 minutes. A maximum dose of 8 mg/kg/hr is recommended to avoid neurotoxic effects. The arrhythmia can be controlled over time with a continuous infusion of lidocaine at a rate between 25 and 80 mcg/kg/min. In cats, the safety margin is smaller and lower dosages of lidocaine can be used but β-blockers usually are preferred. Mexiletine has properties similar to those of lidocaine and is available as an oral medication. Mexiletine, 4 to 8 mg/kg q8h, combined with atenolol, 0.5 to 1 mg/kg q12-24h PO, has been shown to control VT in boxers with ARVC.[9,14]

Procainamide

Procainamide is used intravenously for VTs that do not respond to lidocaine. A bolus of 10 to 15 mg/kg over 1 to 2 minutes can be followed by a constant rate infusion at 25 to 50 mcg/kg/min. Rapid intravenous injection can cause hypotension. Long-term management of VT can be attempted with oral procainamide at 10 to 20 mg/kg q6h (or q8h if the sustained-release form is used).[14]

β-Blockers

Sympathetic activation has been implicated in the pathogenesis of ventricular arrhythmia. Alternatively, sustained VT causing hemodynamic instability increases circulating cathecolamine concentration. β-Blockers provide adrenergic system blockade and may help control arrhythmias. Esmolol is a short-acting β-blocker that can help control sympathetically driven VTs such as those associated with pheochromocytoma or thyrotoxic disease in cats, but its negative inotropic effects may be too pronounced in some patients and cause cardiovascular collapse. Esmolol should be injected slowly (0.2 to 0.5 mg/kg IV over 1 minute) because its effects dissipate within minutes after administration. Propranolol, a nonselective β-blocker, is the preferred β-blocker for the treatment of VT storm in human patients.[16] It is administered intravenously at a dose of 0.02 mg/kg.

Sotalol

Sotalol is an oral medication that is very effective at controlling VT. It is the main antiarrhythmic drug for long-term management of VT, especially in Boxers with arrhythmogenic cardiomyopathy.[9,17] In addition, the author often administers sotalol at 1 to 2 mg/kg PO to restore sinus rhythm in dogs with VT refractory to lidocaine and procainamide. Many dogs respond successfully within a few hours of oral sotalol administration.

Amiodarone

The author has only limited experience with intravenous amiodarone at a slow intravenous bolus of 5 mg/kg over 10 minutes in the setting of ventricular arrhythmias. When administering amiodarone intravenously, it is common that anaphylaxis-like reactions (urticaria, facial edema) occur; careful monitoring is required. These side effects can be treated with antihistamine and steroid injections.[18]

Magnesium sulfate

There are anecdotal accounts of the use of intravenous magnesium sulfate as an adjunct to other antiarrhythmic therapy in dogs with ventricular tachycardia. Although some experimental dog studies have evaluated magnesium therapy in prolonged QT syndrome,[19] there are no studies evaluating the efficacy of magnesium therapy in dogs with spontaneously occurring ventricular tachycardia. Currently in human medicine there are reports of magnesium sulfate therapy aiding the treatment of ventricular tachycardia caused by various therapeutic drug overdoses, but it is not considered mainstream antiarrhythmic therapy. The role of magnesium therapy in veterinary clinical patients remains to be defined.

Other Treatments

Anesthesia

Sedation and anesthesia may be used to decrease high sympathetic output contributing to VT maintenance. Sedation is recommended for the management of VT storm in human patients. Benzodiazepines and short-acting anesthetics such as propofol have been used.[16]

Electrical therapies

Rapid pacing is indicated to overdrive suppress some ventricular arrhythmias. In German Shepherds with inherited ventricular arrhythmias, bradycardia and pauses increase the risk of polymorphic VT. Therefore, atrial or ventricular pacing can be used to maintain a regular and faster heart rate, which prevents periods of slower rate and initiation of VT.

Finally, when antiarrhythmics fail to control ventricular tachycardia, the arrhythmia can be terminated via synchronized electrical cardioversion or defibrillation. Electrical therapies for the management of ventricular tachyarrhythmias are detailed in Chapter 204 of this book.

POSTINTERVENTION MONITORING

Because the response to antiarrhythmic agents cannot be predicted, continuous ECG monitoring is essential after the medication is started and for a minimum of 24 hours. It will give valuable information on the control of the arrhythmia and the possible proarrhythmic effects of the drugs. Twenty-four-hour Holter recording is more adapted to long-term management of the arrhythmia.

REFERENCES

1. Opie LH: Pacemakers, conduction system and electrocardiogram. In Opie LH, editor: The heart physiology, from cell to circulation, ed 3, Philadelphia, 1998, Lippincott-Raven.
2. Kittleson MD: Diagnosis and treatment of arrhythmias (dysrhythmias). In Kittleson MD, Kienle RD: Small animal cardiovascular medicine, ed 1, St Louis, 1998, Mosby.
3. Marriott HJL, Boudreau Conover M: Arrhythmogenic mechanisms and their modulation. In Marriott HJL, Boudreau Conover M, editors: Advanced concepts in arrhythmias, ed 3, St Louis, 1998, Mosby.
4. Brady WJ, Skiles J: Wide QRS complex tachycardia: ECG differential diagnosis, Am J Emerg Med 17:376, 1999.
5. Opie LH: Ventricular arrhythmias. In Opie LH, editor: The heart physiology, from cell to circulation, ed 3, Philadelphia, 1998, Lippincott-Raven.
6. Finley MR, Lillich JD, Gilmour RF Jr et al: Structural and functional basis for the long QT syndrome, J Vet Intern Med 17:473, 2003.
7. Huikuri HV, Castellanos A, Myerburg RJ: Sudden death due to cardiac arrhythmias, N Engl J Med 345:1473, 2001.
8. O'Grady MR, O'Sullivan ML: Dilated cardiomyopathy: an update, Vet Clin North Am Small Anim Pract 34(5):1187-207, 2004.
9. Meurs KM: Boxer dog cardiomyopathy: an update, Vet Clin North Am Small Anim Pract 34(5):1235-1244, 2004.
10. Oxford EM, Danko CG, Kornreich BG, et al: Ultrastructural changes in cardiac myocytes from Boxer dogs with arrhythmogenic right ventricular cardiomyopathy, J Vet Cardiol 13:101, 2011.
11. Vila J, Oxford EM, Saelinger C, et al: Structural and molecular pathology of the atrium of boxer arrhythmogenic cardiomyopathy. Research abstract, J Vet Intern Med 26:714, 2012.
12. Moise NS, Gilmour RF Jr, Riccio ML, et al: Diagnosis of inherited ventricular tachycardia in German Shepherd dogs, J Am Vet Med Assoc 210:403, 1997.
13. Snyder PS, Cooke KL, Murphy ST, et al: Electrocardiographic findings in dogs with motor vehicle-related trauma, J Am Anim Hosp Assoc 37:55, 2001.
14. Pariaut R, Saelinger C, Vila J, et al: Evaluation of shock waveform configuration on the defibrillation capacity of implantable cardioverter defibrillators in dogs, J Vet Cardiol 14:389, 2012.

15. Fries R, Steuer M, Schafers HJ, et al: The R-on-T phenomenon in patients with implantable Cardioverter-defibrillators, Am J Cardiol 91:752, 2003.
16. Eifling M, Razavi M, Massumi A: The evaluation and management of electrical storm, Tex Heart Inst J 38:111, 2011.
17. Moise NS: Diagnosis and management of canine arrhythmias. In Fox PR, Sisson DK, Moise NS, editors: Textbook of canine and feline cardiology: principles and clinical practice, ed 2, St Louis, 1999, WB Saunders.
18. Pedro B, Lopez-Alvarez J, Fonfara S, et al: Retrospective evaluation of the use of amiodarone in dogs with arrhythmias (from 2003 to 2010), J Small Anim Pract 53:19, 2012.
19. Chinushi M, Izumi D, Komura S, et al: Role of autonomic nervous activity in the antiarrhythmic effects of magnesium sulfate in a canine model of polymorphic ventricular tachyarrhythmia associated with prolonged QT interval, J Cardiovasc Pharmacol 48:121, 2006.

CHAPTER 49
MYOCARDITIS

Meg Sleeper, VMD, DACVIM (Cardiology)

KEY POINTS

- Myocarditis is an inflammatory process involving the heart. Inflammation may involve the myocytes, interstitium, or vascular tree.
- Myocarditis has been associated with a wide variety of diseases. Infectious agents (viral, bacterial, protozoal) may cause myocardial damage by myocardial invasion, production of myocardial toxins, or activation of immune-mediated disease.
- Myocarditis can also be associated with physical agents (doxorubicin), underlying metabolic disorders (uremia), toxins (heavy metals), or physical agents (heat stroke).

Myocarditis is a rare cause of heart failure in dogs and cats. Clinical features vary, including those of asymptomatic patients who may have electrocardiographic abnormalities and patients with or without heart enlargement, systolic dysfunction, or even full-blown congestive heart failure (CHF). The patient's history (i.e., environment and exposure) is often critical in determining likely risk and suggesting appropriate diagnostic tests. Clinical reports of canine myocarditis are most common in immunocompromised or immunonaïve patients.

INFECTIOUS MYOCARDITIS

Viral Myocarditis

Numerous viruses have been associated with myocarditis in humans. In dogs, viral myocarditis appears most commonly in immunonaïve patients, and the virus most commonly associated with the disease is parvovirus. However, at this time the entity appears to be very rare. In the late 1970s and early 1980s, when the parvovirus pandemic first was recognized, puppies did not receive maternal antibodies and very young puppies developed a fulminant infection with acute death as a result of pulmonary edema when exposed to the virus. Older puppies (2 to 4 months) often died subacutely from CHF, but others developed a milder myocarditis and later developed dilated cardiomyopathy (DCM), usually as young adults. Basophilic intranuclear inclusion bodies are found in the myocardium of acutely affected younger puppies but may be absent in older puppies.[1] Older dogs typically have gross myocardial scarring. Rare cases of parvovirus-induced myocarditis have been reported since the early to mid-1980s.

Rarely other viruses have been associated with myocarditis in dogs. In 2001 Maxson and others evaluated myocardial tissue from 18 dogs with an antemortem diagnosis of DCM and 9 dogs with a histopathologic diagnosis of myocarditis based on a polymerase chain reaction analysis to screen for canine parvovirus, adenovirus types 1 and 2, and herpesvirus. Canine adenovirus type 1 was amplified from myocardium of only one dog with DCM and none of the dogs with myocarditis, suggesting these pathogens are not commonly associated with DCM or active myocarditis in the dog.[2] Distemper virus–associated cardiomyopathy with a mild inflammatory infiltrate has been produced by experimental infection of immunonaïve puppies.[3] Natural infection with West Nile virus was associated with myocarditis in a wolf and a dog in 2002, the third season of the West Nile virus epidemic in the United States.[4] Viral genomic deoxyribonucleic acid has also been identified in feline myocardial tissue from patients with hypertrophic cardiomyopathy, DCM, and restrictive cardiomyopathy, suggesting that viral myocarditis may be a factor in these feline-acquired diseases.[1]

Protozoal Myocarditis

Chagas' disease

Chagas' disease is caused by *Trypanosoma cruzi,* a protozoal parasite. Chagas' disease is the leading cause of DCM in humans of Latin America, but it is rare in North America. In North American dogs, Chagas' disease occurs most commonly in Texas and Louisiana. There have been no reported feline cases in North America. The organism is transmitted by an insect vector (Reduviidae), and reservoir hosts include rodents, raccoons, opossums, dogs, cats, and humans. The trypomastigote is the infective stage, but on entering host cells the organism enters the reproductive stage and becomes an amastigote. Amastigotes multiply until the host cell ruptures.[1,5]

Dogs with clinical Chagas' disease have an acute or a chronic syndrome. In the acute stage, circulating trypomastigotes may be seen in a thick blood smear, and most dogs are brought for treatment

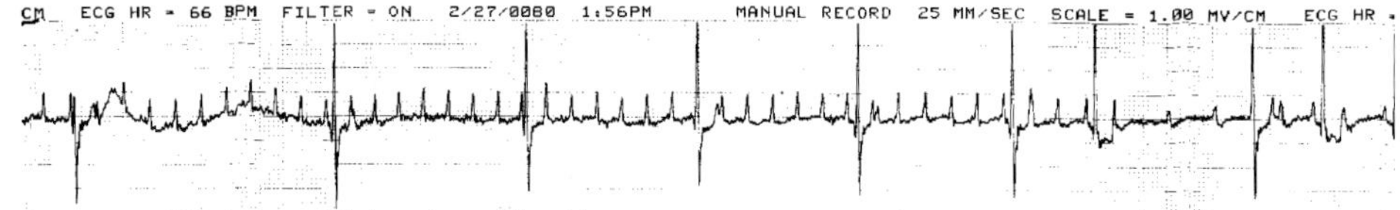

FIGURE 49-1 Electrocardiogram from a mixed breed dog with trichinosis involving the heart. The dog was brought in for collapse caused by complex arrhythmias. Note the ventricular escape beats. An underlying supraventricular tachycardia is likely as well.

because of sudden development of signs of right-sided heart failure (ascites, tachycardia, lethargy). Dogs with chronic Chagas' disease may enter a quiescent stage free of clinical signs for months or even years. Nervous system damage often causes ataxia and weakness in these patients.[1,5]

Bacterial and Other Causes of Myocarditis

Bacterial myocarditis is possible whenever bacteremia or sepsis is present, with the most common agents being staphylococcal and streptococcal species.[1] Myocarditis associated with *Citrobacter koseri,* an opportunistic pathogen of immunosuppressed human patients, has been described in two 12-week-old sibling Boxer puppies.[6] Tyzzer's disease (infection with *Bacillus piliformis*) was associated with severe necrotizing myocarditis in a wolf-dog hybrid puppy.[7] Two cases of feline *Streptococcus canis* myocarditis have been reported.[8,9]

Myocarditis has also been recognized secondary to rickettsial organisms such as *Rickettsia rickettsii, Ehrlichia canis,* and various *Bartonella* species.[1] Myocarditis has been noted in 2 of 12 dogs diagnosed with endocarditis, 11 of which were seroreactive to *Bartonella vinsonii* subspecies.[10] Lymphoplasmacytic myocarditis was observed in 8 cats experimentally infected with *Bartonella*; however, clinical signs consistent with heart disease were not observed.[11] *Bartonellae* have been implicated as an important cause of endocarditis in humans and dogs. Recently the organism has also been linked to endocarditis in the cat, and a few case reports suggest cats may develop myocarditis associated with *Bartonellae* as well.[12,13] Lyme disease (secondary to infection by the spirochete *Borrelia burgdorferi*) has been implicated as a cause of myocarditis in dogs, but documented cases are rare. Clinical signs are often vague and nonspecific, and serologic testing is not a reliable method to determine active infection.[1] In humans, Lyme myocarditis may be due to direct toxic effects or immunomediated mechanisms, and the disease is usually self-limiting.[14] Fungal infections of the myocardium are extremely rare but have occurred in immunocompromised patients.[1]

A group of cats was described with transient fever and depression that appeared to be infectious in nature. Postmortem examination revealed microscopic lesions consistent with myonecrosis and an inflammatory cell infiltrate. A viral etiology was suspected, but no organism was identified.[8] In a retrospective study reviewing 1472 feline necropsies over a 7-year period, 37 cases were diagnosed with endomyocarditis. The cats with endomyocarditis had a mean age at death of 3.4 years, and 62% of them had a history of a stressful event 5 to 10 days before being brought for treatment. Interstitial pneumonia was present in 77% of the cats at postmortem examination. Special stains for bacteria and fungi were negative.[15]

Parasitic agents can also lead to myocarditis. *Toxoplasma gondii* bradyzoites can encyst in the myocardium, resulting in chronic infection. Eventually the cysts rupture, leading to myocardial necrosis and hypersensitivity reactions.[1] Toxoplasmosis has been reported to be a cause of myocarditis in cats.[16] *Neospora caninum* can infect multiple tissues, including the heart, peripheral muscles, and central nervous system. Clinical signs associated with noncardiac tissues typically predominate; however, collapse and sudden death has been reported in affected dogs.[1] Infestation with *Trichinella spiralis* is a common cause of mild myocarditis in humans.[14] The parasite has been associated with at least one case of canine myocarditis complicated by arrhythmias (Figure 49-1).[17]

BOX 49-1 ***Characteristics Suggestive of Myocarditis***

- History suggests it is possible (e.g., oncology patient receiving doxorubicin, dog lives in Texas)
- Unusual signalment for heart disease (e.g., Irish Setter, German Shepherd)
- Supportive electrocardiographic findings include conduction abnormalities or arrhythmias
- Supportive echocardiographic findings include myocardial dysfunction (which may be regional) with or without heart enlargement
- Supportive clinical laboratory findings include leukocytosis, eosinophilia, elevated cardiac troponin I levels

NONINFECTIOUS MYOCARDITIS

Doxorubicin Toxicity

Doxorubicin cardiotoxicity may be manifested as arrhythmias, myocardial failure, or both. Cardiotoxicity is dosage dependent and irreversible and is more common at cumulative doses exceeding 250 mg/m^2; however, in one study in which only two doses of 30 mg/m^2 were administered, 3% of dogs developed cardiomyopathy.[1,8] The time to onset of CHF in affected dogs is highly variable. Although pathologic changes have been seen in the feline myocardium after administration, no antemortem echocardiographic or electrocardiographic changes associated with doxorubicin toxicity have been reported.

Other causes of noninfectious myocarditis, although rarely recognized in veterinary medicine, include allergic reactions, systemic diseases such as vasculitis, and physical agents such as radiation or heat stroke.[14] Numerous chemicals and drugs may lead to cardiac damage and dysfunction. A severe reversible DCM has been observed in humans with pheochromocytoma,[14] and similar findings have been observed in experimental animals receiving prolonged infusions of norepinephrine.[14] Myocardial coagulative necrosis was found in a dog that died suddenly after an episode of severe aggression, restraint, and sedation for grooming.[18] Myocardial lesions were presumed to be caused by catecholamine toxicity. A canine case of immune-mediated polymyositis with cardiac involvement has also been reported.[19]

DIAGNOSIS

Definitive diagnosis, unless the history clearly suggests myocarditis (e.g., doxorubicin toxicity), is elusive (Box 49-1). Supportive clinical laboratory tests include leukocytosis or eosinophilia, particularly in parasitic or allergic myocarditis. Elevated cardiac troponin I levels provide evidence of myocardial cell damage in patients suspected of having myocarditis. If a high suspicion for Chagas' disease is present,

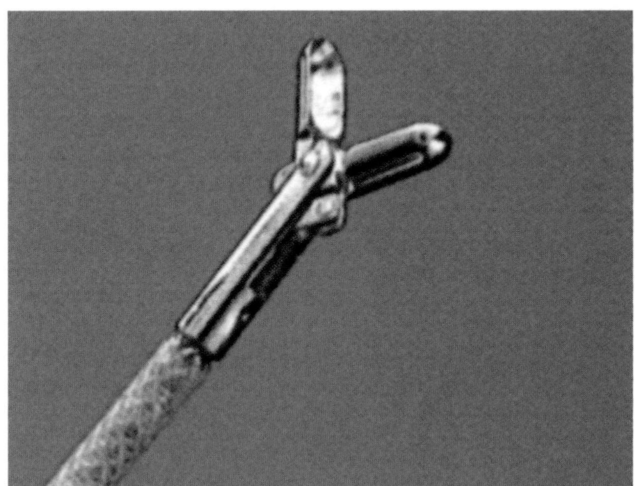

FIGURE 49-2 Photograph showing a bioptome used for endomyocardial biopsies via intravascular access.

serologic examination for *T. cruzi* is diagnostic. Demonstration of a rising titer is also helpful to establish the diagnosis of myocarditis associated with *T. gondii* or *N. caninum*. Viral and rickettsial testing should be performed if indicated. Blood cultures should be performed if a bacterial cause is suspected. Thoracic radiographs may show normal heart size or heart enlargement with or without evidence of CHF. The electrocardiographic findings may also be varied, and ventricular arrhythmias or conduction disturbances are common. Echocardiography most often demonstrates systolic dysfunction, either global or regional, and cardiac chambers may be normal or increased in size.

Endomyocardial biopsy (the gold standard for diagnosis of myocarditis in humans[20]) may allow definitive antemortem diagnosis (Figure 49-2). However, a focal myocarditis can still be missed because the sample size is small. At postmortem examination, immunohistochemistry or electron microscopy can confirm the diagnosis of *N. caninum* infection.[21] Gross pathology findings may be insignificant, or they may reveal cardiac dilation or ventricular hypertrophy, focal petechiae, and myocardial abscesses.[1] Specific findings depend on the underlying etiology. Focal or diffuse myocarditis is definitively diagnosed by histopathology when myocyte necrosis, degeneration, or both are associated with an inflammatory infiltrate.[1]

TREATMENT

Most recommendations for managing myocarditis in dogs and cats are extrapolated from human medicine or research with models of viral myocarditis. Supportive care is the first line of therapy for patients with myocarditis. In those patients with signs of CHF, typical therapy should include preload reduction with diuretics and afterload reduction with angiotensin-converting enzyme inhibitors (see Chapter 40). Digoxin increased expression of proinflammatory cytokines and increased mortality in experimental myocarditis, so it is recommended to be used with caution and at low dosages.[20] Intravenous inotropic therapy in the form of dobutamine can be useful if significant systolic dysfunction is present. Alternatively, pimobendan may be beneficial to address systolic dysfunction and reduce afterload.

Eliminating unnecessary medications may help reduce the possibility of allergic myocarditis. Results of recent studies suggest that immunosuppression is not routinely helpful in myocarditis patients, but it may have an important role in patients with myocardial dysfunction caused by systemic autoimmune disease.[20] Nonsteroidal antiinflammatory agents are contraindicated during the acute phase of myocarditis in humans (during the first 2 weeks) because they increase myocardial damage. However, they appear to be safe later in the course of disease.[14] In a murine model of viral myocarditis, angiotensin-converting enzyme inhibition (with captopril) was beneficial. Similarly, interferon therapy is beneficial in the experimental model of myocarditis and may be useful clinically.[14]

When diagnosis of acute Chagas' disease is possible, several agents appear to inhibit *T. cruzi*; however, by the time a diagnosis is made it is often too late for this approach. Patients with chronic Chagas' disease are treated symptomatically for CHF. Similarly, successful treatment has been reported using several agents in dogs affected with *N. caninum* myocarditis, but severely ill dogs often die.[1] Clindamycin is the drug of choice for treating clinical toxoplasmosis in dogs and cats; however, significant damage to the heart is irreversible.[21] In one report of a cat with presumed toxoplasmosis, signs of heart disease did resolve with clindamycin treatment.[22]

Dogs with evidence of bacteremia should be treated with antibiotics pending culture and susceptibility results. Empiric treatment should be effective against staphylococcal and streptococcal species (see Chapter 93). Animals with suspected rickettsial disease should be treated with doxycycline (5 to 10 mg/kg PO or IV q12-24h) pending titer results.

REFERENCES

1. Fox PR, Sisson DK, Moise NS, editors: Textbook of canine and feline cardiology: principles and clinical practice, ed 2, St Louis, 1999, WB Saunders.
2. Maxson TR, Meurs KM, Lehmkuhl LB, et al: Polymerase chain reaction analysis for viruses in paraffin-embedded myocardium from dogs with dilated cardiomyopathy or myocarditis, Am J Vet Res 62:130, 2001.
3. Higgins RJ, Krakowka S, Metzler AE, et al: Canine distemper virus-associated cardiac necrosis in the dog, Vet Pathol 18:472, 1981.
4. Lichtensteiger CA, Heinz-Taheny K, Osborne TS, et al: West Nile virus encephalitis and myocarditis in a wolf and dog, Emerg Infect Dis 9:1303, 2003.
5. Kittleson MD: Primary myocardial disease leading to chronic myocardial (dilated cardiomyopathy) and other related diseases. In Kittleson MD, Kienle RD: Small animal cardiovascular medicine, ed 1, St Louis, 1998, Mosby.
6. Cassidey JP, Callanan JJ, McCarthy G, et al: Myocarditis in sibling Boxer puppies associated with Citrobacter koseri infection, Vet Pathol 39:393, 2002.
7. Young JK, Baker DC, Burney DP: Naturally occurring Tyzzer's disease in a puppy, Vet Pathol 32:63, 1995.
8. Sura R, Hinckley LS, Risatti GR, et al: Fatal necrotizing fasciitis and myositis in cat associated with Streptococcus canis, Vet Rec 162:450, 2008.
9. Matsuu A, Kanda T, Sugiyama A, et al: Mitral stenosis with bacterial myocarditis in a cat, J Vet Med Sci 69:1171, 2007.
10. Breitschwerdt EB, Atkins CE, Brown TT, et al: Bartonella vinsonii subsp berkhoffii and related members of the alpha subdivision of the proteobacteria in dogs with cardiac arrhythmias, endocarditis or myocarditis, J Clin Microbiol 37:3618, 1999.
11. Kordick DL, Brown TT, Shin K, et al: Clinical and pathologic evaluation of chronic Bartonella henselae or Bartonella clarridgeiae infection in cats, J Clin Microbiol 37:1536, 1999.
12. Nakamura RK, Zimmerman SA, Lesser MB: Suspected Bartonella-associated myocarditis and supraventricular tachycardia in a cat, J Vet Cardiol 13:277, 2011.
13. Varanat M, Broadhurst J, Linder KE, et al: Identification of Bartonella henselae in 2 cats with pyogranulomatous myocarditis and diaphragmatic myositis. Vet Pathology 2012;49:608-61.
14. Wynne JA, Braunwald E: The cardiomyopathies and myocarditides. In Braunwald E, Zipes DP, Libby P, Bonow RO, editors: Braunwald's heart disease: a textbook of cardiovascular medicine, ed 7, Philadelphia, 2005, Saunders.
15. Stalis IH, Bossbaly MJ, Van Winkle TJ: Feline endomyocarditis and left ventricular endocardial fibrosis, Vet Pathol 32:122, 1999.

16. Dubey JP, Carpenter JL: Histologically confirmed clinical toxoplasmosis in cats: 100 cases (1952-1990), J Am Vet Med Assoc 203:1556, 1993.
17. Sleeper MM, Bissett S, Craig L: Canine trichinosis presenting with high grade second degree AV block, J Vet Intern Med 20:1228, 2006.
18. Pinson DM: Myocardial necrosis and sudden death after an episode of aggressive behavior in a dog, J Am Vet Med Assoc 211:1371, 1997.
19. Warman S, Pearson G, Barret E, et al: Dilation of the right atrium in a dog with polymyositis and myocarditis, J Small Anim Pract 49:302, 2008.
20. Feldman AM, McNamara D: Myocarditis, N Engl J Med 343:1388, 2000.
21. Dubey JP, Lappin MR: Toxoplasmosis and neosporosis. In Green CE, editor: Infectious diseases of the dog and cat, ed 3, St Louis, 2006, WB Saunders.
22. Simpson KE, Devine BC, Funn-Moore D: Suspected toxoplasmosis-associated myocarditis in a cat, J Fel Med Surg 7:203, 2005.

CHAPTER 50
SODIUM DISORDERS

Jamie M. Burkitt Creedon, DVM, DACVECC

KEY POINTS

- Most disorders of plasma sodium concentration result from abnormalities in the handling of water rather than sodium.
- Plasma sodium concentration is the major determinant of plasma osmolality.
- Hypernatremia or hyponatremia can cause central nervous system (CNS) disturbance resulting from changes in neuronal cell volume and function.
- Overly rapid correction of hypernatremia or hyponatremia can cause severe CNS dysfunction.
- Patients with hypernatremia or hyponatremia that require intravascular volume expansion should be treated with intravenous fluids that contain a similar sodium concentration as the patient's plasma.

Sodium concentration is important. Alterations in sodium concentration are associated with poor outcome in critically ill people[1,2]; even sodium concentration changes within the reference interval have been associated with increased mortality risk.[1] It is unclear whether small fluctuations in sodium concentration are themselves detrimental to outcome or if they portend a poorer prognosis because they indicate more severe disease.

Sodium concentration is expressed as milliequivalents (mEq) or millimoles (mmol) of sodium per liter of serum or plasma. In the vast majority of cases, disorders of sodium concentration in dogs and cats result from abnormalities in water handling rather than an increased or decreased number of sodium molecules. To understand what determines plasma sodium concentration and how changes in plasma sodium concentration alter cellular function, one must understand the distribution of body water and the concept and determinants of osmolality.

Distribution of Total Body Water

Water makes up approximately 60% of an adult animal's body weight; two thirds is intracellular and one third is extracellular. Extracellular water is distributed between the interstitial and intravascular compartments, which contain approximately 75% and 25% of the extracellular water, respectively (see Figure 59-1). The endothelium, which separates the intravascular fluid compartment from the interstitial space, and the cell membrane, which separates the interstitial and intracellular compartments, are freely permeable to water molecules. Therefore, in a closed system (no urinary or gastrointestinal [GI] output), when 1 L of free water (water containing no other molecules) is added to the animal, approximately 666 ml will be distributed to the intracellular space and 333 ml to the extracellular space. Of the 333 ml added to the extracellular space, approximately 250 ml (75% of 333 ml) will remain in the interstitial fluid space and 83 ml (25% of 333 ml) will be distributed to the intravascular compartment.

Osmolality and Osmotic Pressure

An osmole is 1 mole of any fully dissociated substance dissolved in water. Osmolality is the concentration of osmoles in a mass of solvent. In biologic systems, osmolality is expressed as mOsm/kg of water and can be measured using an osmometer. Osmolarity is the concentration of osmoles in a volume of solvent and in biologic systems is expressed as mOsm/L of water. In physiologic systems there is no appreciable difference between osmolality and osmolarity, so the term *osmolality* will be used for the rest of this discussion for simplicity. Every molecule dissolved in the total body water contributes to osmolality, regardless of size, weight, charge, or composition.[3] The most abundant osmoles in the extracellular fluid are sodium (and the accompanying anions chloride and bicarbonate), glucose, and urea. Because they are the most plentiful, these molecules are the main determinants of plasma osmolality in healthy dogs and cats.

Plasma osmolality (mOsm/kg) in healthy animals can be calculated by the equation shown in Box 50-1.[4,5] As this equation shows, plasma sodium concentration is the major determinant of plasma osmolality.

Osmoles that do not cross the cell membrane freely are considered *effective osmoles,* whereas those that do cross freely are termed *ineffective osmoles.* The water-permeable cell membrane is functionally impermeable to sodium and potassium. As a result, sodium and potassium molecules are effective osmoles and they exert osmotic pressure across the cell membrane. The net movement of water into or out of cells is dictated by the osmotic pressure gradient. Osmotic pressure causes water molecules from an area of lower osmolality (higher water concentration) to move to an area of higher osmolality (lower water concentration) until the osmolalities of the compartments are equal.

When sodium is added to the extracellular space at a concentration greater than that in the extracellular fluid, intracellular volume decreases (the cell shrinks) as water leaves the cell along its osmotic pressure gradient. Conversely, cells swell when free water is added to the interstitial space and water moves intracellularly along its osmotic pressure gradient.

Regulation of Plasma Osmolality

Hypothalamic osmoreceptors sense changes in plasma osmolality, and changes of only 2 to 3 mOsm/kg induce compensatory

BOX 50-1 Calculation of Serum Osmolality

Osmolality (mOsm/kg)

$$= 2([Na^+]) + (BUN\,[mg/dl] \div 2.8) + (glucose\,[mg/dl] \div 18)$$

Where $[Na^+]$ = sodium concentration and BUN is the concentration of blood urea nitrogen.

The BUN and glucose concentrations are divided by 2.8 and 18, respectively, to convert them from mg/dl to mmol/L.

mechanisms to return the plasma osmolality to its hypothalamic setpoint.[6] The two major physiologic mechanisms for controlling plasma osmolality are the antidiuretic hormone (ADH) system and thirst.

Antidiuretic hormone

ADH is a small peptide secreted by the posterior pituitary gland. There are two major stimuli for ADH release: elevated plasma osmolality and decreased effective circulating volume. Increased plasma osmolality causes shrinkage of a specialized group of cells in the hypothalamus called *osmoreceptors*. When their cell volume decreases, these hypothalamic osmoreceptors send impulses via neural afferents to the posterior pituitary, leading to ADH release.[7] When effective circulating volume is low, baroreceptor cells in the aortic arch and carotid bodies send neural impulses to the pituitary gland that stimulate ADH release.

In the absence of ADH, renal tubular collecting cells are relatively impermeable to water. When ADH activates the V2 receptor on the renal collecting tubular cell, aquaporin-2 molecules are inserted into the cell's luminal membrane. Aquaporins are channels that allow the movement of water into the renal tubular cell. Water molecules cross through these aquaporins into the hyperosmolar renal medulla down their osmotic gradient. If the kidney is unable to generate a hyperosmolar renal medulla because of disease or diuretic administration, water will not be reabsorbed, even with high concentrations of ADH. Circulating ADH concentration and ADH's effect on the normal kidney are the primary physiologic determinants of free water retention and excretion.

Thirst

Hyperosmolality and decreased effective circulating volume also stimulate thirst. The mechanisms by which hyperosmolality and hypovolemia stimulate thirst are similar to those that stimulate ADH release. Thirst and the resultant water consumption are the main physiologic determinants of free water intake.

Prioritization of Osmolality and Effective Circulating Volume

Under normal physiologic conditions, the renin-angiotensin-aldosterone system monitors and fine tunes effective circulating volume, and the ADH system maintains normal plasma osmolality. However, maintenance of effective circulating volume is always prioritized over maintenance of normal plasma osmolality. Therefore patients with poor effective circulating volume will have increased thirst and ADH release regardless of their osmolality. The resultant increased free water intake (from drinking) and water retention (from ADH action at the level of the kidney) can lead to hyponatremia (and thus hypoosmolality) in patients with poor effective circulating volume. An example of the defense of effective circulating volume at the expense of normal plasma osmolality is seen in patients with chronic congestive heart failure that present with hyponatremia.[8]

Total Body Sodium Content Versus Plasma Sodium Concentration

Plasma sodium concentration is different than, and independent of, total body sodium content. *Total body sodium content* refers to the total number of sodium molecules in the body, regardless of the ratio of sodium to water. Sodium content determines the *hydration status* of the animal. As it is used clinically, *hydration* is a misnomer, because findings such as skin tenting and moistness of the mucous membranes and conjunctival sac are determined by both the sodium content and the water that those sodium molecules hold in an animal's interstitial space.

When patients have increased total body sodium, an increased quantity of fluid is held within the interstitial space and the animal appears overhydrated, regardless of the plasma sodium concentration. Overhydrated patients may manifest a gelatinous subcutis; peripheral or ventral pitting edema; chemosis; or excessive serous nasal discharge.

When patients have decreased total body sodium, a decreased quantity of fluid is held within the interstitial space and the animal appears dehydrated, regardless of the plasma sodium concentration. Once a patient has lost 5% or more of its body weight in isotonic fluid (≥5% "dehydrated"), it may manifest decreased skin turgor, tacky or dry mucous membranes, decreased fluid in the conjunctival sac, or sunken eye position. Patients that are less than 5% dehydrated appear clinically normal. Patients with dehydration can become hypovolemic as fluid shifts from the intravascular space into the interstitial space as a result of decreased interstitial hydrostatic pressure.

The sodium/water ratio is independent of the total body sodium content: Patients may be normally hydrated, dehydrated, or overhydrated (normal, decreased, or increased total body sodium content) and have a normal plasma sodium concentration, hypernatremia, or hyponatremia.

HYPERNATREMIA

Hypernatremia is defined as plasma or serum sodium concentration above the reference interval. Hypernatremia is common in critically ill dogs and cats.

Etiology

Most dogs and cats with hypernatremia have excessive free water loss rather than increased sodium intake or retention.

Free water deficit

Normal animals can become severely hypernatremic if denied access to water for extended periods. Animals with vomiting, diarrhea, or polyuria of low-sodium urine may also develop hypernatremia. Hypernatremia can occur after administration of activated charcoal suspension containing a cathartic because the hypertonic cathartic draws electrolyte-free water into the GI tract. Osmotic diuresis with mannitol also causes an electrolyte-free water loss and thus can cause hypernatremia. Diabetes insipidus (DI), a syndrome of inadequate release of or response to ADH, can cause hypernatremia (see Chapter 67). Animals with DI become severely hypernatremic when they do not drink water, because they cannot reabsorb free water in the renal collecting duct. Acute or critical illness can unmask previously undiagnosed DI.[9] A syndrome of hypodipsic hypernatremia has been reported in Miniature Schnauzers,[10-12] one of which was diagnosed with congenital holoprosencephaly.[10] This syndrome most likely is due to impaired osmoreceptor or thirst center function. In other dog breeds and cats, hypodipsic hypernatremia has been associated with hypothalamic granulomatous meningoencephalitis, hydrocephalus, and other central nervous system (CNS) deformities and CNS lymphoma.[13-17]

Diagnostic differentiation between central DI, nephrogenic DI, and hypodipsic hypernatremia can be complex and is outside the scope of this chapter. The reader is referred to more detailed texts for further information.[18-20]

Sodium excess

Severe hypernatremia can also occur with the introduction of large quantities of sodium in the form of hypertonic saline, sodium bicarbonate, sodium phosphate enemas,[21] seawater, beef jerky, and salt-flour dough mixtures.[22]

Clinical Signs

Hypernatremia causes no specific clinical signs in many cases. If it is severe (usually >180 mEq/L) or occurs rapidly, it may be associated with CNS signs such as obtundation, head pressing, seizures, coma, and death. All cells that have Na^+/K^+-ATPase pumps shrink as a result of hypernatremia as water moves out of the cell down its osmotic gradient to the relatively hyperosmolar extracellular compartment, but neurons are clinically the least tolerant of this change in cell volume. Thus, neurologic signs are seen most commonly in patients with clinically significant hypernatremia. Patients that develop hypernatremia slowly are often asymptomatic for reasons explained later in Physiologic Adaptation to Hypernatremia.

An experimental study found decreased myocardial contractility during injection of hypernatremic or hyperosmolar solutions in dogs.[23] Hypernatremia has also been associated with hyperlipidemia, possibly a result of the inhibition of lipoprotein lipase.[13] Artifactual hemogram changes in the blood of two hypernatremic cats have been reported with a specific hematology analyzer.[24]

Physiologic Adaptation to Hypernatremia

Hypernatremia causes free water to move out of the relatively hypoosmolar intracellular space into the hyperosmolar extracellular space, leading to decreased cell volume. The brain has multiple ways to protect against and reverse neuronal water loss in cases of hypernatremia. In the early minutes to hours of a hyperosmolal state, as neuronal water is lost to the hypernatremic circulation, lowered interstitial hydraulic pressure draws fluid from the cerebrospinal fluid (CSF) into the brain interstitium.[19] As plasma osmolality rises, sodium and chloride also appear to move rapidly from the CSF into cerebral tissue, which helps minimize brain volume loss by increasing neuronal osmolality and thus drawing water back to the intracellular space.[25] These early fluid and ionic shifts appear to protect the brain from the magnitude of volume loss that would be expected for a given hyperosmolal state. Additionally, within 24 hours, neurons begin to accumulate organic solutes to increase intracellular osmolality and help shift lost water back to the intracellular space. Accumulated organic solutes are called idiogenic osmoles, or osmolytes, and include molecules such as inositol, glutamine, and glutamate.[19] Generation of these idiogenic osmoles begins within a few hours of cell volume loss, but full compensation may take as long as 2 to 7 days.[25] Restoration of neuronal cell volume is important for cellular function and is an important consideration during treatment of hypernatremia, as discussed later.

Treatment of the Normovolemic, Hypernatremic Patient

Hypernatremia should be treated, even if no clinical signs are apparent. Patients with hypernatremia have a free water deficit, so free water is replaced in the form of fluid with a lower effective osmolality than that of the patient. Treatment must be cautious, and close monitoring of plasma or serum sodium concentration and CNS signs is imperative.

In patients with mild to moderate hypernatremia ($[Na^+]_p$ < 180 mEq/L), sodium concentration should be decreased no more rapidly than 1 mEq/L/hr. In those with severe hypernatremia ($[Na^+]_p$ ≥ 180 mEq/L), it should be decreased no more rapidly than 0.5 to 1 mEq/L/hr. This slow decrease in plasma sodium concentration ($[Na^+]_p$) is important to prevent cellular swelling. Idiogenic osmoles are broken down slowly, so rapid drops in plasma sodium concentration (and thus plasma osmolality) cause free water to move back into the relatively hyperosmolar intracellular space and can lead to neuronal edema. Free water deficit can be calculated by the free water deficit equation[7] listed in Box 50-2. This formula gives the total volume of free water that needs to be replaced. This volume of free water, usually given as 5% dextrose in water, is infused over the number of hours calculated for safe reestablishment of normal plasma sodium concentration. This rate of free water replacement may be inadequate in cases of ongoing free water loss, as seen with diuresis of electrolyte-free water in patients with DI or unregulated diabetes mellitus, but it is a safe starting point in most cases.

BOX 50-2 *Calculation of Free Water Deficit*

Free water deficit

$$= ([\text{current}\,[Na^+]_p \div \text{normal}\,[Na^+]_p] - 1) \times (0.6 \times \text{body weight in kg})$$

where [current$[Na^+]_p$ is the patient's current plasma sodium concentration and normal $[Na^+]_p$ is the patient's normal plasma sodium concentration.

Plasma sodium concentration should be monitored no less often than every 4 hours to assess the adequacy of treatment, and CNS status should be monitored continuously for signs of obtundation, seizures, or other abnormalities. The rate of free water supplementation should be adjusted as needed to ensure an appropriate drop in plasma sodium concentration, the goal being a drop of no more than 1 mEq/hr and no clinical signs of cerebral edema. Water may be supplemented intravenously (as 5% dextrose in water) or orally on an hourly schedule in animals that are alert, willing to drink, and not vomiting. Free water replacement alone will not correct clinical dehydration or hypovolemia, because free water replacement does not provide the sodium required to correct these problems (see Total Body Sodium Content Versus Plasma Sodium Concentration). Free water replacement in the hypernatremic patient is relatively safe, even in animals with cardiac or renal disease, because two thirds of the volume administered will enter the cells.

Complications of Therapy for Hypernatremia

Cerebral edema is the primary complication of therapy for hypernatremia. Clinical signs of cerebral edema include obtundation, head pressing, coma, seizures, and other disorders of behavior or movement. If these signs develop during the treatment of hypernatremia, immediately stop the administration of any fluid that has a lower sodium concentration than the patient and disallow drinking. The patient's plasma sodium concentration should be measured to confirm that it is lower than it was when treatment was instituted. This is an important step because signs of worsening hypernatremia may be similar to those seen with cerebral edema. If the plasma sodium concentration has decreased, even if it has dropped at less than 1 mEq/L/hr, cerebral edema should be considered.

Cerebral edema is treated with a dose of mannitol at 0.5 to 1 g/kg intravenously (IV) over 20 to 30 minutes. Mannitol should be administered via a central vein if possible, but it may be diluted 1:1 in sterile water and given through a peripheral vein in an emergency situation. If mannitol is not available, or if a single dose does not improve signs, consider a dose of 7.2% sodium chloride at 3 to 5 ml/kg over 20 minutes. The administration method is similar to that used for mannitol. Hypertonic saline should not be administered as a rapid bolus because it can cause vasodilation.

HYPONATREMIA

Hyponatremia is defined as plasma or serum sodium concentration below the reference interval. Clinically detrimental hyponatremia is uncommon in critically ill dogs and cats.

Etiology

Dogs and cats with hyponatremia almost always have free water retention in excess of sodium retention; they may have sodium loss as well. Generation of hyponatremia usually requires water intake in addition to decreased water excretion.

Decreased effective circulating volume

A common cause of hyponatremia in dogs and cats is decreased effective circulating volume, which causes ADH release and water intake in defense of intravascular volume and thus decreases plasma sodium concentration. Possible causes include congestive heart failure,[8] excessive gastrointestinal losses,[26,27] excessive urinary losses, body cavity effusions,[28,29] and edematous states. Note that in the case of congestive heart failure, the patient has increased total body sodium (is "overhydrated") because of activation of the renin-angiotensin-aldosterone system, yet is hyponatremic because of increased water retention in excess of sodium retention. In the case of excessive salt and water losses from the GI or urinary tract, the patient is total body sodium depleted (is "dehydrated") and is hyponatremic as a result of compensatory water drinking and retention to maintain effective circulating volume.

Hypoadrenocorticism

Hypoadrenocorticism leads to hyponatremia through decreased sodium retention (caused by hypoaldosteronism) combined with increased water drinking and retention in defense of inadequate circulating volume. Animals with atypical hypoadrenocorticism, whose aldosterone production and release are normal, may also develop hyponatremia, because low circulating cortisol concentration leads to increased ADH release and resultant water retention regardless of intravascular volume status.[30]

Diuretics

Thiazide or loop diuretic administration can lead to hyponatremia by induction of hypovolemia, hypokalemia that causes an intracellular shift of sodium in exchange for potassium, and the inability to dilute urine.[30] Renal failure can cause hyponatremia by similar mechanisms.

Syndrome of inappropriate antidiuretic hormone secretion

Syndrome of inappropriate ADH secretion (SIADH) causes hyponatremia through water retention in response to improperly high circulating concentrations of ADH. The syndrome has been reported in dogs[31-34] and a cat[35] and has many known causes in humans[30] (see Chapter 68).

Other causes of hyponatremia

Hyponatremia has been reported in animals with GI parasitism,[26] infectious and inflammatory diseases,[36-39] psychogenic polydipsia, and pregnancy.[40] It has also been reported in a puppy fed a low-sodium, home-prepared diet.[41] A syndrome of cerebral salt wasting (CSW) has been described in humans with CNS disease but has not been reported clinically in dogs or cats. Patients with CSW have increased urinary sodium excretion in the face of intravascular volume depletion, which is inappropriate because a volume-depleted animal's kidney should avidly conserve sodium. The mechanisms—and even the syndrome's actual existence—are unclear, but both brain natriuretic peptide (too much) and aldosterone (not enough) have been implicated.[30] Cerebral salt wasting is differentiated from SIADH by evaluation of hydration status: patients with CSW are clinically dehydrated because of a decrease in total body sodium content, and those with SIADH are usually adequately hydrated with excessive free water retention.[42]

Clinical Signs

Mild to moderate hyponatremia usually causes no specific clinical signs. If hyponatremia is severe (usually <120 mEq/L) or occurs rapidly, it may be associated with CNS signs such as obtundation, head pressing, seizures, coma, and death. All cells that have Na^+/K^+-ATPase pumps swell as a result of hyponatremia as water moves into the relatively hyperosmolar cell from the hypoosmolar extracellular space, but brain cells are clinically the least tolerant of this change in cell volume.

An experimental study found increased myocardial contractility during injection of hyponatremic or hypoosmolar solutions in dogs.[23] Hyponatremia decreases renal concentrating ability in dogs.[43] There is one report of artifactual hemogram changes in canine blood secondary to hyponatremia using a specific hematology analyzer.[24]

Physiologic Adaptation to Hyponatremia

Hyponatremia causes free water to move into the relatively hyperosmolar cell from the hypoosmolar extracellular space, leading to increased cell volume. Interstitial and intracellular CNS edema increases intracranial tissue hydrostatic pressure. This pressure enhances fluid movement into the cerebrospinal fluid, which flows out of the cranium, through the subarachnoid space and central canal of the spinal cord, and back into venous circulation. Swollen neurons also expel solutes such as sodium, potassium, and organic osmolytes to decrease intracellular osmolality and encourage water loss to the extracellular fluid (ECF), returning cell volume toward normal. Ion expulsion occurs rapidly, but loss of organic osmolytes requires hours to days.[25] Therefore clinical signs associated with hyponatremia, and potential complications of management, are associated with both the magnitude and rate of sodium concentration change.

Treatment of the Normovolemic, Hyponatremic Patient

Patients asymptomatic for hyponatremia

Hyponatremia caused by decreased effective circulating volume is most often mild ($[Na^+]_p \geq 130$ mEq/L) and usually self-corrects with appropriate treatment of the underlying disease. Fluids with a sodium concentration less than that of the patient should be avoided. The plasma sodium concentration and the patient's CNS status should be monitored regularly, but complications of hyponatremia or its treatment are unlikely to occur in these situations. Patients with hyponatremia caused by congestive heart failure will likely remain hyponatremic as a result of diuretic administration, the resultant polydipsia, and ingestion of a low-sodium diet. Asymptomatic patients that are edematous may be treated with water restriction alone, and those that are asymptomatic and normally hydrated or dehydrated may be treated with administration of fluids containing a higher sodium concentration than that of the patient.

Patients symptomatic for hyponatremia

Symptomatic hyponatremia (acute or chronic) requires emergency therapy, although the best management approach is controversial. These patients usually have a plasma sodium concentration of 120 mEq/L or lower. The aim is to raise the patient's sodium concentration enough to resolve the clinical signs without causing complications (see later). One proactive method to achieve free water excretion is through administration of mannitol (0.5 to 1 g/kg IV over 20 to 30 minutes) along with furosemide (0.5 to 1 mg/kg IV) to ensure that electrolyte-free water is excreted along with the mannitol. Fluid loss should be replaced with standard replacement intravenous fluids, unless the patient is overhydrated and the fluid loss desired. Further explanation of this technique is available for review elsewhere.[44] The goal is to raise the plasma sodium concentration by no more than 10 mEq/L during the first 24 hours and by no more than 18 mEq/L during the first 48 hours of treatment, never to exceed the low end of the reference interval. The limit of 10 mEq/L during the first day of treatment is more important than the rate over a specific period within that day.[30]

When the patient's sodium concentration cannot be raised adequately with diuretics, or if a different approach is desired, hypertonic saline can be administered. In human medicine a common recommendation is to raise the symptomatic hyponatremic patient's sodium concentration by 10% to 15% in the first day of treatment. The rate of correction may be as high as 2 mEq/L/hr initially with a maximal increase of no more than 15 mEq/L in the first 24 hours. The sodium deficit should first be calculated using the formula in Box 50-3, using a target plasma sodium concentration of no more than 10% to 15% higher than the patient's current sodium concentration. The calculated sodium deficit determines the amount of hypertonic saline to be infused to raise plasma sodium no faster than 2 mEq/L/hr. The hypertonic saline is usually administered as a 3% solution. Co-administration of loop diuretics can further aid in excretion of free water and may be necessary in patients with concentrated urine.

Complications of Therapy for Hyponatremia

The major complication of treatment for hyponatremia is myelinolysis. Myelinolysis is a result of neuronal shrinking away from the myelin sheath as water moves out of the neuron during correction of hyponatremia. Clinical signs of myelinolysis usually manifest many days after intervention, so the clinician cannot assume that a rapid change in plasma sodium concentration has been well tolerated simply because no CNS signs are present during initial treatment. Overzealous correction of severe hyponatremia has led to paresis, ataxia, dysphagia, obtundation, and other neurologic signs in dogs.[45-48] All these dogs had initial plasma sodium concentrations of less than 110 mEq/L, and all had sodium concentration corrections that exceeded the above-recommended rate. Myelinolysis lesions in dogs are commonly seen in the thalamus, rather than the pons as in humans. Patients with myelinolysis may recover with intensive supportive treatment, although some do not.

Because the signs of myelinolysis are delayed, it is rare for a patient to develop abnormal CNS signs during initial treatment of hyponatremia. However, if new neurologic signs develop during treatment, administration of any fluid that is hyperosmolar to the patient (mannitol, hypertonic or isotonic fluids) should be stopped. The patient's plasma sodium concentration is checked to confirm that it has increased. This is an important step, because signs of worsening hyponatremia may be similar to those seen with treatment. If the plasma sodium concentration is higher than it was at the initiation of treatment, even if the concentration has increased slowly, CNS damage should be considered. Treatment of CNS signs caused by overly rapid correction of hyponatremia requires administration of free water. Precise guidelines for dropping plasma sodium concentration in case of overzealous correction are not available, but attempting to drop the sodium concentration to achieve no more than 10 mEq/L total correction during the first 24 hours and no more than 18 mEq/L total correction during the first 48 hours seems appropriate.[30] The free water volume to administer can be calculated using the free water deficit equation in Box 50-2, inserting the desired plasma sodium concentration in place of "normal $[Na^+]_p$." Decreasing sodium concentration in an already hyponatremic animal can be difficult unless the patient is treated with a loop diuretic such as furosemide to clamp urine osmolality, and water is replaced simultaneously.

BOX 50-3 *Calculation of Sodium Deficit*

Sodium Deficit =

$$(\text{target } [Na^+]_p - \text{patient } [Na^+]_p) \times (0.6 \times \text{lean body weight in kg})$$

where target $[Na^+]_p$ is the desired plasma sodium concentration and patient $[Na^+]_p$ is the patient's current plasma sodium concentration.

PSEUDOHYPONATREMIA

Pseudohyponatremia is the term used to describe hyponatremia in a patient with normal or elevated plasma osmolality. The most common cause of pseudohyponatremia in dogs and cats is hyperglycemia. Glucose is an effective osmole, so when hyperglycemia is present, the excess glucose molecules cause an increase in ECF water, diluting sodium to a lower concentration. For each 100 mg/dl increase in blood glucose, sodium concentration drops by approximately 1.6 mEq/L.[30] This effect is nonlinear, however; mild hyperglycemia leads to smaller changes in plasma sodium concentration than more severe hyperglycemia (see Chapter 64 for more information about this condition in diabetes mellitus). Pseudohyponatremia does not require specific treatment, and the sodium concentration will increase as the hyperglycemia resolves and water moves back into the cells. The other common cause of pseudohyponatremia in dogs and cats is mannitol infusion with retention (rather than renal excretion) of mannitol molecules.

VOLUME EXPANSION IN THE HYPOVOLEMIC, HYPONATREMIC, OR HYPERNATREMIC PATIENT

Patients with moderate to severe abnormalities in sodium concentration ($[Na^+]_p < 130$ or > 170) that require intravascular volume expansion should be resuscitated with a fluid that has a sodium concentration that matches that of the patient (±6 mEq/L). Hyponatremic animals may be resuscitated with a balanced electrolyte solution containing 130 mEq/L sodium if appropriate, or with a maintenance solution that has sodium chloride added to bring the sodium concentration of the solution up to that of the patient. Hypernatremic animals should be resuscitated with a balanced electrolyte solution with NaCl added in a quantity sufficient to bring the solution's sodium concentration up to that of the animal. The simplest way to add sodium to a bag of commercially available fluid is to add 23.4% NaCl to the bag. This product contains 4 mEq NaCl/ml solution, so it adds a significant quantity of sodium in a small volume.

REFERENCES

1. Sakr Y, Rother S, Ferreira AM, et al: Fluctuations in serum sodium level are associated with an increased risk of death in surgical ICU patients, Crit Care Med 41:133, 2013.

2. Hoorn EJ, Betjes MG, Weigel J, et al: Hypernatraemia in critically ill patients: too little water and too much salt, Nephrol Dial Transplant 23:1562, 2008.
3. Rose BD, Post TW: Introduction to renal function. In Rose BD,Post TW, editors. Clinical physiology of acid-base and electrolyte disorders, ed 5, New York, 2001, McGraw-Hill, pp 3-20.
4. Dugger DT, Mellema MS, Hopper K, et al: Comparitive accuracy of several published formulae for the estimation of serum omolality in cats, J Small Anim Pract 54(4):184, 2013.
5. Dugger DT, Mellema MS, Hopper K, et al: Estimated osmolality of canine serum: A comparison of the clinical ultility of several published formulae, J Vet Emerg Crit Care (In Press).
6. Giebisch G, Windhager E: Integration of salt and water balance. In Boron WF, Boulpaep EL, editors: Medical physiology, Philadelphia, 2003, Saunders, pp 861-876.
7. Rose BD, Post TW: Effects of hormones on renal function. In Rose BD, Post TW, eds. Clinical physiology of acid-base and electrolyte disorders, ed 5, New York, 2001, McGraw-Hill, pp 163-238.
8. Brady CA, Hughes D, Drobatz KJ: Association of hyponatremia and hyperglycemia with outcome in dogs with congestive heart failure, J Vet Emerg Crit Care 14:177, 2004.
9. Edwards DF, Richardson DC, Russell RG: Hypernatremic, hypertonic dehydration in a dog with diabetes insipidus and gastric dilation-volvulus, J Am Vet Med Assoc 182:973, 1983.
10. Sullivan SA, Harmon BG, Purinton PT, et al: Lobar holoprosencephaly in a Miniature Schnauzer with hypodipsic hypernatremia, J Am Vet Med Assoc 223:1783, 1778, 2003.
11. Van Heerden J, Geel J, Moore DJ: Hypodipsic hypernatraemia in a miniature schnauzer, J S Afr Vet Assoc 63:39, 1992.
12. Crawford MA, Kittleson MD, Fink GD: Hypernatremia and adipsia in a dog, J Am Vet Med Assoc 184:818, 1984.
13. Hanselman B, Kruth S, Poma R, et al: Hypernatremia and hyperlipidemia in a dog with central nervous system lymphosarcoma, J Vet Intern Med 20:1029, 2006.
14. Mackay BM, Curtis N. Adipsia and hypernatraemia in a dog with focal hypothalamic granulomatous meningoencephalitis, Aust Vet J 77:14, 1999.
15. DiBartola SP, Johnson SE, Johnson GC, et al: Hypodipsic hypernatremia in a dog with defective osmoregulation of antidiuretic hormone, J Am Vet Med Assoc 204:922, 1994.
16. Morrison JA, Fales-Williams A: Hypernatremia associated with intracranial B-cell lymphoma in a cat, Vet Clin Pathol 35:362, 2006.
17. Dow SW, Fettman MJ, LeCouteur RA, et al: Hypodipsic hypernatremia and associated myopathy in a hydrocephalic cat with transient hypopituitarism, J Am Vet Med Assoc 191:217, 1987.
18. DiBartola SP: Disorders of sodium and water: hypernatremia and hyponatremia. In DiBartola SP, editor: Fluid, electrolyte, and acid-base disorders in small animal practice, ed 3, St Louis, 2006, Saunders Elsevier, pp 47-79.
19. Rose BD, Post TW: Hyperosmolal states—hypernatremia. In Rose BD, Post TW, editors: Clinical physiology of acid-base and electrolyte disorders, New York, 2001, McGraw-Hill, pp 746-793.
20. Feldman EC, Nelson RW: Water metabolism and diabetes insipidus. In Feldman EC, Nelson RW, editors: Canine and feline endocrinology and reproduction, ed 3, St Louis, 2004, Saunders, pp 2-44.
21. Atkins CE, Tyler R, Greenlee P: Clinical, biochemical, acid-base, and electrolyte abnormalities in cats after hypertonic sodium phosphate enema administration, Am J Vet Res 46:980, 1985.
22. Barr JM, Khan SA, McCullough SM, et al: Hypernatremia secondary to homemade play dough ingestion in dogs: a review of 14 cases from 1998 to 2001, J Vet Emerg Crit Care 14:196, 2004.
23. Kozeny GA, Murdock DK, Euler DE, et al: In vivo effects of acute changes in osmolality and sodium concentration on myocardial contractility, Am Heart J 109:290, 1985.
24. Boisvert AM, Tvedten HW, Scott MA: Artifactual effects of hypernatremia and hyponatremia on red cell analytes measured by the Bayer H*1 analyzer, Vet Clin Pathol 28:91, 1999.
25. Verbalis JG: Brain volume regulation in response to changes in osmolality, Neuroscience 168:862, 2010.
26. DiBartola SP, Johnson SE, Davenport DJ, et al: Clinicopathologic findings resembling hypoadrenocorticism in dogs with primary gastrointestinal disease, J Am Vet Med Assoc 187:60, 1985.
27. Boag AK, Coe RJ, Martinez TA, et al: Acid-base and electrolyte abnormalities in dogs with gastrointestinal foreign bodies, J Vet Intern Med 19:816, 2005.
28. Willard MD, Fossum TW, Torrance A, et al: Hyponatremia and hyperkalemia associated with idiopathic or experimentally induced chylothorax in four dogs, J Am Vet Med Assoc 199:353, 1991.
29. Bissett SA, Lamb M, Ward CR: Hyponatremia and hyperkalemia associated with peritoneal effusion in four cats, J Am Vet Med Assoc 218:1580, 1590-1592, 2001.
30. Rose BD, Post TW: Hypoosmolal states—hyponatremia. In Rose BD, Post TW, editors. Clinical physiology of acid-base and electrolyte disorders, ed 5, New York, 2001 McGraw-Hill, pp 696-745.
31. Rijnberk A, Biewenga WJ, Mol JA: Inappropriate vasopressin secretion in two dogs, Acta Endocrinol (Copenh) 117:59, 1988.
32. Breitschwerdt EB, Root CR: Inappropriate secretion of antidiuretic hormone in a dog, J Am Vet Med Assoc 175:181, 1979.
33. Kang MH, Park HM: Syndrome of inappropriate antidiuretic hormone secretion concurrent with liver disease in a dog, J Vet Med Sci 74:645, 2012.
34. Shiel RE, Pinilla M, Mooney CT: Syndrome of inappropriate antidiuretic hormone secretion associated with congenital hydrocephalus in a dog, J Am Anim Hosp Assoc 45:249, 2009.
35. Cameron K, Gallagher A: Syndrome of inappropriate antidiuretic hormone secretion in a cat, J Am Anim Hosp Assoc 46:425, 2010.
36. Lobetti RG, Jacobson LS: Renal involvement in dogs with babesiosis, J S Afr Vet Assoc 72:23, 2001.
37. Keenan KP, Buhles WC, Jr., Huxsoll DL, et al: Studies on the pathogenesis of Rickettsia rickettsii in the dog: clinical and clinicopathologic changes of experimental infection, Am J Vet Res 38:851, 1977.
38. Son TT, Thompson L, Serrano S, et al: Surgical intervention in the management of severe acute pancreatitis in cats: 8 cases (2003-2007), J Vet Emerg Crit Care (San Antonio) 20:426, 2010.
39. Declue AE, Delgado C, Chang CH, et al: Clinical and immunologic assessment of sepsis and the systemic inflammatory response syndrome in cats, J Am Vet Med Assoc 238:890, 2011.
40. Schaer M, Halling KB, Collins KE, et al: Combined hyponatremia and hyperkalemia mimicking acute hypoadrenocorticism in three pregnant dogs, J Am Vet Med Assoc 218:897, 2001.
41. Hutchinson D, Freeman LM, McCarthy R, et al: Seizures and severe nutrient deficiencies in a puppy fed a homemade diet, J Am Vet Med Assoc 241:477, 2012.
42. Palmer BF: Hyponatremia in patients with central nervous system disease: SIADH versus CSW, Trends Endocrinol Metab 14:182-187, 2003.
43. Tyler RD, Qualls CW, Jr., Heald RD, et al: Renal concentrating ability in dehydrated hyponatremic dogs, J Am Vet Med Assoc 191:1095, 1987.
44. Porzio P, Halberthal M, Bohn D, et al: Treatment of acute hyponatremia: ensuring the excretion of a predictable amount of electrolyte-free water, Crit Care Med 28:1905, 2000.
45. MacMillan KL: Neurologic complications following treatment of canine hypoadrenocorticism, Can Vet J 44:490, 2003.
46. Churcher RK, Watson AD, Eaton A: Suspected myelinolysis following rapid correction of hyponatremia in a dog, J Am Anim Hosp Assoc 35:493, 1999.
47. Brady CA, Vite CH, Drobatz KJ: Severe neurologic sequelae in a dog after treatment of hypoadrenal crisis, J Am Vet Med Assoc 215:210, 222-225, 1999.
48. O'Brien DP, Kroll RA, Johnson GC, et al: Myelinolysis after correction of hyponatremia in two dogs, J Vet Intern Med 8:40, 1994.

CHAPTER 51

POTASSIUM DISORDERS

Laura L. Riordan, DVM, DACVIM • Michael Schaer, DVM, DACVIM, DACVECC

KEY POINTS

- A normal serum potassium concentration is essential for normal neuromuscular function.
- Common predisposing conditions for hypokalemia include diabetes mellitus, chronic renal disease (especially in cats), prolonged anorexia, diarrhea, hyperaldosteronism, and metabolic alkalosis.
- The main clinical manifestation in the dog and cat is hypokalemic myopathy.
- Rate of potassium infusion rather than total amount infused is of major therapeutic importance.
- Mild to moderate hypokalemia (serum potassium 2.5 to 3.5 mEq/L) can be corrected at a rate up to 0.5 mEq/kg/hr.
- Decreased renal excretion is the most common cause of hyperkalemia in small animal patients.
- Before determination of serum potassium level in any hyperkalemic patient or in any animal with urinary tract obstruction, an electrocardiogram (ECG) should be evaluated to detect bradycardia, atrial standstill, or ventricular arrhythmias.
- Renal failure, hypoadrenocorticism, and gastrointestinal disease are the most common causes of sodium/potassium ratios less than 27:1.
- When serum potassium exceeds 8 mEq/L or severe ECG changes are present, immediate therapy directed toward reducing and antagonizing the effects of serum potassium is warranted (i.e., 10% calcium gluconate, 10% calcium chloride, sodium bicarbonate, dextrose with or without insulin, β_2 agonists).
- Hemodialysis and hemoperfusion can effectively and rapidly lower serum potassium levels.

Few of the disturbances in fluid and electrolyte metabolism are as commonly encountered or as immediately life threatening as disturbances in potassium balance. Many clinicians are already sensitized to the detrimental effects of potassium disorders, especially hyperkalemia, but sometimes the adverse effects of hypokalemia are nearly as harmful. This chapter discusses the clinical essentials of hypokalemia and hyperkalemia in the critically ill dog and cat and shows why both are important to patient care.

Normal Distribution of Potassium in the Body

Potassium is the most abundant intracellular cation, with 98% to 99% located in the intracellular compartment. Most intracellular potassium lies in the skeletal muscle cells. The average potassium concentration in the intracellular space of dogs and cats is 140 mEq/L, and that in the plasma space averages 4 mEq/L.[1,2] Serum potassium levels therefore do not reflect whole body content or tissue concentrations.

HYPOKALEMIA

Definition and Causes

Hypokalemia occurs when the serum potassium concentration is less than 3.5 mEq/L (normal range 3.5 to 5.5 mEq/L). The general causes of hypokalemia are (1) disorders of internal balance and (2) disorders of external balance. The clinical conditions most commonly associated with each of these are provided in Box 51-1. Recently there has been a heightened recognition of feline hyperaldosteronism as the cause of marked hypokalemia, usually secondary to either an aldosteronoma or adrenocortical hyperplasia. It has also been associated with an adrenocortical adenoma in ferrets.[3]

Consequences

Abnormalities resulting from hypokalemia are divided into four categories: metabolic, neuromuscular, renal, and cardiovascular. Glucose intolerance is the most notable adverse metabolic effect of hypokalemia. Experiments have shown that release of insulin from the pancreatic β cells is impaired when total body potassium levels are decreased.[4]

Potassium is necessary for maintenance of normal resting membrane potential. Subsequently the most significant neuromuscular abnormality induced by hypokalemia in dogs and cats is skeletal muscle weakness from hyperpolarized (less excitable) myocyte plasma membranes that may progress to hypopolarized membranes.[5-7] Ventroflexion of the head and neck; a stiff, stilted gait; and a plantigrade stance may also be evident. In cats, hypokalemic myopathy typically is associated with chronic renal disease and poorly regulated diabetes mellitus.[2,8] It can also result from a potassium-deficient diet or prolonged anorexia.[14] More recently feline hyperaldosteronism as a result of aldosteronoma and adrenocortical hyperplasia has been described, although a diagnostic workup for these conditions is only indicated if the more common etiologies are not present. These cats can present with clinical signs

BOX 51-1 *Causes of Hypokalemia*[3,11,31-34]

Disorders of Internal Balance (Redistribution)

Metabolic alkalosis
Insulin administration
Increased levels of catecholamines
β-Adrenergic agonist therapy or intoxication
Refeeding syndrome

Disorders of External Balance (Depletion)

Renal potassium wasting
Prolonged inadequate intake
Diuretic drugs
Osmotic or postobstructive diuresis
Chronic liver disease
Inadequate parenteral fluid supplementation
Aldosterone-secreting tumor or any cause of hyperaldosteronism
Prolonged vomiting associated with pyloric outflow obstruction
Diabetic ketoacidosis
Renal tubular acidosis
Severe diarrhea

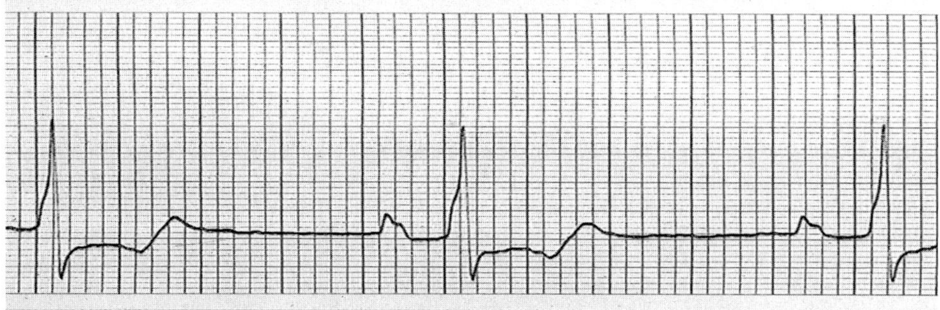

FIGURE 51-1 Lead II electrocardiogram at 50 mm/s taken from a dog with a serum potassium measuring 2.1 mEq/L. Note the increased P wave amplitude, the depressed ST segment, and the depressed T waves.

ranging from retinal hemorrhage caused by hypertension to profound muscle weakness with or without rhabdomyolysis.[9] Frank paralysis and death as a result of diaphragmatic failure and respiratory muscle failure can occur in severe cases.[10] Hypokalemia can also cause rhabdomyolysis, which may have a toxic effect on the renal tubules in some speciaes.[5,6]Smooth muscle impairment can also occur, leaving the patient with paralytic ileus and gastric atony.[11] These neuromuscular signs are seldom present until serum potassium levels fall below 2.5 mEq/L. Cats with chronic renal disease can become markedly potassium depleted, and the resulting hypokalemia may impair renal tubular function.[2,8,12]

In the myocardial cell, a high intracellular/extracellular potassium concentration ratio induces a state of electrical hyperpolarization leading to prolongation of the action potential. This may predispose the patient to atrial and ventricular tachyarrhythmias, atrioventricular dissociation and ventricular fibrillation. Abnormal electrocardiogram (ECG) findings in animals with hypokalemia are less reliable than in those with hyperkalemia.[13] Canine ECG abnormalities include depression of the ST segment and prolongation of the QT interval (Figure 51-1).[14] Increased P wave amplitude, prolongation of the PR interval, and widening of the QRS complex may also occur. In addition, hypokalemia predisposes to digitalis-induced cardiac arrhythmias and causes the myocardium to become refractory to the effects of class I antiarrhythmic agents (i.e., lidocaine, quinidine, and procainamide).

Management of Hypokalemia

The main management objectives include replacing potassium deficits and correcting the primary disease process. Treatment of moderate (2.5 to 3.4 mEq/L) to severe (<2.5 mEq/L) hypokalemia in the anorectic or vomiting patient requires parenteral administration of potassium chloride solution (or potassium phosphate in hypophosphatemic patients; Table 51-1). The rate of potassium infusion should seldom exceed 0.5 mEq/kg/hr for mild to moderate hypokalemia.[15] In profoundly hypokalemic patients with normal or increased urine output (serum potassium < 2.5 mEq/L) the rate can be increased cautiously to 1 to 1.5 mEq/kg/hr along with close ECG monitoring.[15] Adding 20 mEq potassium chloride solution to one liter of isotonic lactated Ringer's, 0.9% sodium chloride, and Plasma-Lyte A solutions will change the osmolality of those solutions to 312, 348, and 334 mEq/L, respectively.[16] Conditions that may predispose an animal to adverse effects of a potassium infusion include oliguria and anuria, hypoaldosteronism (Addison's disease), and coadministration of potassium-sparing drugs (spironolactone, triamterine). In patients with a primary metabolic acidosis, potassium chloride can be added to the buffer-containing intravenous fluids (lactated, acetated Ringer's or Plasma-Lyte A solutions), whereas potassium chloride is added preferentially to normal saline solution for the patient with metabolic alkalosis.

Table 51-1 **Guidelines for Routine Intravenous Supplementation of Potassium in Dogs and Cats[30]**

Serum Potassium Concentration (mEq/L)	mEq KCl to Add to 250 ml Fluid*	mEq KCl to Add to 1 L Fluid	Maximal Fluid Infusion Rate† (ml/kg/hr)
<2.0	20	80	6
2.1 to 2.5	15	60	8
2.6 to 3.0	10	40	12
3.1 to 3.5	7	28	18
3.6 to 5.0	5	20	25

*It is essential to shut off the flow valve to the patient and that the fluid container contents are thoroughly mixed during and after adding potassium to the parenteral fluids.
†So as not to exceed 0.5 mEq/kg/hr.

It is important to remember that these values are only ranges that must be adjusted to each patient's pathophysiologic needs. This is exemplified by the severely oliguric or anuric animal requiring minimal maintenance amounts of parenteral potassium chloride, in contrast with the polyuric ketoacidotic diabetic patient receiving regular crystalline insulin that will require much higher amounts. Animals with fluid-responsive shock states should be resuscitated with an isotonic crystalloid solution before adding potassium chloride to the crystalloid fluid infusion. In the severely hypokalemic patient (serum potassium < 2 mEq), it is prudent to begin potassium treatment during the rehydration period, either as a separate infusion or at a lower fluid rate in order to stay within acceptable guidelines for potassium infusion (0.5 to 1.5 mEq/kg/hr). Administration of sodium bicarbonate or insulin to hypokalemic diabetic patients should be postponed for the first 4 to 8 hours, or until the serum potassium level is greater than 3.5 mEq/L. Failure to do so can lead to marked, life-threatening hypokalemia secondary to translocation into the intracellular space.

Potassium gluconate powder$_{a,b}$ is a convenient form of dietary supplementation for stable dogs and cats with mild hypokalemia. It is given orally in food twice daily at a recommended dosage of ¼ teaspoonful (2 mEq) per 4.5 kg body weight. The maintenance dose should be titrated to effect. Its use is limited to animals that can be fed by mouth or by gastroenteral feeding tubes.

Anticipated Complications

Hyperkalemia can occur from excessive potassium supplementation. This is covered in the next section. Hypokalemic neuromuscular dysfunction is worsened and refractoriness to therapy may be evident when metabolic alkalosis, hypomagnesemia and hypocalcemia coexist.[17] It is important to correct all acid-base disorders and serum electrolyte deficiencies to attain normal neuromuscular function (see Chapter 53).

HYPERKALEMIA

Definition and Causes

Hyperkalemia occurs when the serum potassium concentration exceeds 5.5 mEq/L and is considered life threatening at serum concentrations greater than 7.5 mEq/L.[15,18]Hyperkalemia can result from four basic disturbances: increased intake or administration, translocation from the intracellular to the extracellular fluid space, decreased renal excretion, or an artifactual or pseudohyperkalemia (Box 51-2).

Excessive potassium supplementation (potassium chloride or potassium phosphate) in the intravenous fluids or overly rapid rates of administration can lead to hyperkalemia. To avoid cardiotoxicity, the intravenous rate generally should not exceed 0.5 mEq/kg/hr. Hyperkalemia can also occur from the administration of packed red blood cells that are past the expiration date or from angiotensin-converting enzyme inhibitors, potassium-sparing diuretics (e.g., spironolactone), or nonselective β-blocking drugs (e.g., propranolol) combined with potassium supplementation. Accidental overdose with the aforementioned medications can also lead to hyperkalemia.

An increased movement of potassium out of cells can lead to hyperkalemia, as seen with a mineral acidosis (uremic, respiratory, or induced by ammonium chloride, hydrogen chloride, or calcium chloride infusions) causing potassium to move out of the intracellular space in exchange for hydrogen ions. This extracellular translocation of potassium can also occur with heat stroke, crushing injuries, or tumor lysis syndrome associated with chemotherapy and after radiation therapy in dogs with lymphosarcoma.[19,20] Hyperkalemia has also been reported in cats treated with thrombolytic agents for aortic thromboembolism as a result of reperfusion of the affected limbs.[21]

BOX 51-2 *Causes of Hyperkalemia*

Increased Intake or Supplementation

Intravenous potassium-containing fluids
Expired RBC transfusion
Translocation from ICF to ECF
Mineral acidosis (NH_4Cl, HCl)
Diabetes mellitus with ketoacidosis or hyperosmolality
Acute tumor lysis syndrome
Extremity reperfusion following therapy for thromboembolism

Decreased Urinary Excretion

Anuric or oliguric renal failure
Urethral obstruction
Ruptured urinary bladder
Hypoadrenocorticism
Gastrointestinal disease (trichuriasis, salmonellosis, perforated duodenum)
Chylothorax with mechanical drainage
Drugs (ACE inhibitors, potassium-sparing diuretics, nonspecific β-blockers)

Pseudohyperkalemia

Thrombocytosis or leukocytosis
Akita dog and other dogs of Japanese origin

ACE, Angiotensin-converting enzyme; *ECF,* extracellular fluid; *HCl,* hydrogen chloride; *ICF,* intracellular fluid; *NH_4Cl,* ammonium chloride; *RBC,* red blood cell.

Although an osmotic diuresis decreases the total body potassium concentration in diabetic ketoacidosis, hyperkalemia may occur as a result of decreased cellular uptake of potassium secondary to insulin deficiency, extracellular translocation of potassium with water caused by serum hyperosmolality ("solute drag"), increased protein catabolism, prerenal azotemia, and any coexisting renal impairment. Insulin therapy normalizes the serum potassium concentration by correcting the insulin deficiency and hyperosmolality, enabling relocation of the potassium to the intracellular space and decreasing the need for protein catabolism.

Decreased urinary excretion secondary to prerenal, renal, or postrenal disease is the most common cause of hyperkalemia in small animal patients. In animals with complete urinary obstruction or uroabdomen, an ECG should be evaluated for evidence of changes secondary to hyperkalemia while the serum potassium concentration is determined. Blood pressure monitoring is also recommended. Intravenous, potassium-free fluids such as 0.9% saline should be administered as indicated, and further steps to reduce serum potassium or reduce the cardiotoxic effects of hyperkalemia should be taken if cardiac arrhythmias or hypotension are present (see Treatment of Hyperkalemia section).

Oliguria and anuria are most commonly associated with acute tubular damage, however oliguria can also occur with end-stage chronic renal failure. The distal tubule is dependent on both adequate glomerular filtration rate and urine flow to excrete potassium effectively. The severe reduction in both of these determinants with acute kidney injury significantly impairs the ability of the distal tubule to excrete sufficient potassium. Attempts to restore a normal effective circulating volume are essential to improving urine output and urinary potassium excretion. If no urine is produced after fluid therapy, additional measures should be taken (e.g., furosemide, mannitol, and/or diltiazem CRI), in attempts to convert the oliguric or anuric patient to a nonoliguric state (see Chapters 124 and 160). Chronic kidney disease can also be associated with hyperkalemia in dogs. This may be due to dietary potassium intake exceeding renal excretion as well as angiotensin-converting enzyme (ACE) inhibitor therapy that may be used in select patients with chronic kidney disease. It has been demonstrated that feeding a potassium-reduced diet can resolve hyperkalemia in these animals.[22]

Patients with classic, severe hypoadrenocorticism typically have hyperkalemia and hyponatremia and a sodium/potassium ratio less than 27:1. A resting cortisol or adrenocorticotropic hormone (ACTH) stimulation test is essential to differentiate this disease from acute renal failure because these patients might also be azotemic. Natriuresis in the absence of aldosterone leads to a reduced effective circulating volume, which further impairs distal tubule potassium excretion. This volume depletion also leads to reduced renal perfusion, prerenal azotemia, and further potassium retention. Initial therapy should include restoration of the effective circulating volume with potassium-free or potassium-deficient fluids (see Chapter 73). A case of hyporeninemic hypoaldosteronism has been reported in the dog. This condition results in low baseline and post-ACTH concentrations of aldosterone, but normal baseline and post-ACTH concentrations of cortisol. Hyporeninemic hypoaldosteronism should be considered in patients with persistent hyperkalemia in which other more common causes have been ruled out.[23]

Gastrointestinal disease, especially that associated with trichuriasis, salmonellosis, or duodenal perforation, can be associated with hyperkalemia and a reduced sodium/potassium ratio (<27:1).[24,25] Chronic chylothorax managed by intermittent or continual drainage can also result in hyperkalemia and hyponatremia.[26]In addition, these abnormalities were reported in a dog with a lung lobe torsion, another with a neoplastic pleural effusion, and three at-term pregnant Greyhounds.[27-29] Although the mechanism of hyperkalemia in such patients is unclear, a reduction in effective circulating volume and subsequent reduced distal renal tubular flow could lead to deficient urinary potassium excretion.

Consequences

Muscle weakness can occur when the serum potassium concentration exceeds 7.5 mEq/L. Hyperkalemia may cause bradycardia or atrial standstill due to prolonged depolarization and repolarization of the myocardial conduction system. ECG findings do not correlate precisely with serum potassium concentrations since the rate of increase or decrease also plays a role; however, generalizations can be made as to the progression of waveform and conduction changes (Table 51-2). Tachyarrhythmias may also occur secondary to hyperkalemia.[18]

Table 51-2 Electrocardiographic Changes Secondary to Hyperkalemia[14]

Serum Potassium Concentration	Electrocardiographic Change
>5.5 mEq/L	Peaked, narrow T wave
>6.5 mEq/L	Prolonged QRS complex and PR interval Depressed R wave amplitude Depressed ST segment
>7 mEq/L	Depressed P wave amplitude
>8.5 mEq/L	Atrial standstill Sinoventricular rhythm
>10 mEq/L	Biphasic QRS complex Ventricular flutter Ventricular fibrillation Ventricular asystole

PSEUDOHYPERKALEMIA

Potassium can be released from increased numbers of circulating blood cells, especially platelets and white blood cells, causing an artifactual increase in potassium termed *pseudohyperkalemia*. This is seen primarily in animals with severe thrombocytosis or leukocytosis. Pseudohyperkalemia can also be seen in Akita dogs (or other dogs of Japanese origin) secondary to in vitro hemolysis, because their erythrocytes have a functional sodium-potassium adenosine triphosphatase and, as such, have high intracellular potassium concentrations. This potassium is released and causes an artifactual hyperkalemia if hemolysis occurs in the serum blood tube. Confirmation of pseudohyperkalemia can be made by determining the plasma potassium concentration (blood collected in a heparinized tube) because this should not be affected by changes in platelet or white blood cell numbers (unless the patient suffers from leukemia).

Treatment of Hyperkalemia

An ECG should be performed in any patient with suspected or confirmed hyperkalemia. In asymptomatic animals with normal urine output, serum potassium concentrations between 5.5 and 6.5 mEq/L rarely warrant immediate therapy; however, the cause of the hyperkalemia should be investigated. In all hyperkalemic patients, exogenous potassium administration should be discontinued. Intravenous potassium-free or potassium-deficient isotonic crystalloids can be administered to promote diuresis, and this alone may be sufficient to correct mild hyperkalemia (≤6 mEq/L). Loop (furosemide 1 to 4 mg/kg intravenously [IV]) or thiazide (chlorothiazide 20 to 40 mg/kg PO) diuretics can increase urinary potassium excretion; however, their use must follow rehydration. Drugs that promote hyperkalemia, such as ACE inhibitors, β-adrenergic antagonists, and potassium-sparing diuretics, should be discontinued. In patients with chronic renal failure, a potassium-reduced diet should also be considered. Immediate therapy is directed toward reducing and antagonizing serum potassium in patients with severe ECG changes or when the serum potassium concentration exceeds 8 mEq/L. Ten percent calcium gluconate or calcium chloride can be administered to antagonize the cardiotoxic effects of hyperkalemia, but this has no effect on serum potassium concentrations. β-Adrenergic agonists, sodium bicarbonate, and dextrose with or without insulin can be administered to reduce serum potassium concentrations as described in Table 51-3. Peritoneal dialysis, hemodialysis, or continuous renal replacement therapy will effectively treat hyperkalemia that is not responsive to the previously mentioned interventions.

Table 51-3 Treatment of Life-Threatening Hyperkalemia

Drug	Dosage	Mechanism of Action	Onset of Action
10% Calcium gluconate	0.5 to 1.5 ml/kg IV slowly over 5 to 10 minutes with ECG monitoring	Increases threshold voltage but will not lower serum potassium	3 to 5 minutes
Sodium bicarbonate	1 to 2 mEq/kg IV slowly over 15 minutes	Increases extracellular pH, allowing for potassium to move intracellularly	15 minutes or longer
25% Dextrose	0.7 to 1 g/kg IV over 3 to 5 minutes	Allows for translocation of potassium into the intracellular space	<1 hour
25% Dextrose with insulin	Regular insulin at 0.5 U/kg* IV with IV dextrose at 2 g/U of insulin administered	As above	15 to 30 minutes
Terbutaline	0.01 mg/kg IV slowly	Stimulates Na^+/K^+-ATPase to cause translocation of potassium into the cell	20 to 40 minutes

*With hypoadrenocorticism the insulin dosage should be reduced to 0.25 U/kg IV because of the patient's predisposition to hypoglycemia.
ECG, Electrocardiogram; *IV*, intravenously; *Na^+/K^+-ATPase*, sodium-potassium adenosine triphosphatase.

REFERENCES

1. Faubel S, Topf J: The fluid, electrolyte and acid-base companion, San Diego, 1999, Alert and Oriented Publishers.
2. Wellman ML, DiBartola SP, Kohn: Applied physiology of body fluids in dogs and cats. In DiBartola SP, editor: Fluid therapy, electrolyte, and acid-base disorders in small animal practice, ed 4, St Louis, 2012, Saunders Elsevier.
3. Desmarchelier M, Lair S, Dunn M, et al: Primary hyperaldosteronism in a domestic ferret with an adrenocortical adenoma, J Am Vet Med Assoc 233:1297, 2008.
4. Rowe JW, Tobin JD, Rosa RM, et al: Effect of experimental potassium deficiency on glucose and insulin metabolism, Metabolism 29:498, 1980.
5. Gennari JF: Hypokalemia, N Engl J Med 339:451, 1998.
6. Dow SW, LeCouteur RA, Fettman MJ, et al: Potassium depletion in cats: hypokalemic polymyopathy, J Am Vet Med Assoc 191:1563, 1987.
7. Harrington ML, Bagley RS, Braund KG: Suspect hypokalemic myopathy in a dog, Prog Vet Neurol 7:130, 1996.
8. Dow SW, Fettman MJ, LeCouteur RA, et al: Potassium depletion in cats: renal and dietary influences, J Am Vet Med Assoc 191:1569, 1987.
9. Shiel R, Mooney C: Diagnosis and management of primary hyperaldosteronism in cats, In Pract 29:194, 2007.
10. Hammond TN, Holm JL: Successful use of short-term mechanical ventilation to manage respiratory failure secondary to profound hypokalemia in a cat with hyperaldosteronism. J Vet Emerg Crit Care 18(5):1476, 2008.
11. Brown RS: Potassium homeostasis and clinical implications, Am J Med 77:3, 1984.
12. Theisen SK, DiBartola SP, Radin MJ, et al: Muscle potassium content and potassium gluconate supplementation in normokalemic cats with naturally occurring chronic renal failure, J Vet Intern Med 11:212, 1997.
13. Diercks DB, Shumaik GM, Harrigan RA, et al: Electrocardiographic manifestations: electrolyte abnormalities, J Emerg Med 27:153, 2004.
14. Tilley LP: Essentials of canine and feline electrocardiography, ed 2, Philadelphia, 1985, Lea and Febiger.
15. DiBartola SP, DeMorais HA: Disorders of potassium: hypokalemia and hyperkalemia. In DiBartola SP, editor: Fluid, electrolyte, and acid-base disorders in small animal practice, ed 4, St Louis, 2012, Saunders Elsevier.
16. Bond D: Fluids and electrolytes in children. In Vincent JL, Abraham E, Moore FA, Kochanek PM, Fink MP, editors: Textbook of critical care, ed 6, Philadelphia, 2011, Elsevier.
17. Mcnutt MK, Kozar RA: Disorders of calcium and magnesium metabolism. In Vincent JL, Abraham E, Moore FA, Kochanek PM, Fink MP, editors: Textbook of critical care, ed 6, Philadelphia, 2011, Elsevier.
18. Fox PR, Sisson D, Moise NS: Textbook of canine and feline cardiology, Philadelphia, 1999, WB Saunders.
19. Laing EJ, Carter RF: Acute tumor lysis syndrome following therapy treatment of canine lymphoma, J Am Anim Hosp Assoc 24:691, 1988.
20. Laing EJ, Fitzpatrick PJ, Binnington AG, et al: Half-body radiotherapy in the treatment of canine lymphoma, J Vet Intern Med 3:102, 1989.
21. Rodriquez DB, Harpster N: Aortic thromboembolism associated with feline hypertrophic cardiomyopathy, Compend Contin Educ Pract Vet 24:478, 2002.
22. Segev G, Fascetti AJ, Weeth LP, et al: Correction of hyperkalemia in dogs with chronic kidney disease consuming commercial renal therapeutic diets—a potassium reduced home-prepared diet, J Vet Intern Med 24:546, 2010.
23. Kreissler JJ Langston CE: A case of hyporeninemic hypoaldosteronism in the dog, J Vet Inter Med 25:944, 2011.
24. DiBartola SP, Johnson SE, Davenport DJ, et al: Clinicopathologic findings resembling hypoadrenocorticism in dogs with primary gastrointestinal disease, J Am Vet Med Assoc 187:60, 1985.
25. Malik R, Hunt GB, Hinchliffe JM, et al: Severe whipworm infection in the dog, J Small Anim Pract 31:185, 1990.
26. Willard MD, Fossum TW, Torrance A, et al: Hyponatremia and hyperkalemia associated with idiopathic or experimentally induced chylothorax in four dogs, J Am Vet Med Assoc 199:353, 1991.
27. Zenger E: Persistent hyperkalemia associated with nonchylous pleural effusion in a dog, J Am Anim Hosp Assoc 28:411, 1992.
28. Lamb WA, Muir P: Lymphangiosarcoma associated with hyponatremia and hyperkalemia in a dog, J Small Anim Pract 35:374, 1994.
29. Schaer M, Halling KB, Collins KB, et al: Combined hyponatremia and hyperkalemia mimicking acute hypoadrenocorticism in three pregnant dogs, J Am Vet Med Assoc 218:897, 2001.
30. Greene RW, Scott RC: Lower urinary tract disease. In Ettinger SJ, editor: Textbook of veterinary internal medicine, Philadelphia, 1975, Saunders.
31. Thier SO: Potassium physiology, Am J Med 80(Suppl 4A):3, 1986.
32. Minaker KL, Meneilly GS, Flier JS, et al: Insulin-mediated hypokalemia and paralysis in familial hypokalemic periodic paralysis, Am J Med 84:101, 1988.
33. Halperin ML, Goldstein MB: Fluid, electrolyte and acid-base emergencies, Philadelphia, 1988, WB Saunders.
34. Adrogué HJ, Madias NE: Changes in plasma potassium concentration during acute acid-base disturbances, Am J Med 71:456, 1981.

CHAPTER 52

CALCIUM DISORDERS

Todd A. Green, DVM, MS, DACVIM • Dennis J. Chew, DVM, DACVIM

KEY POINTS

- Severe hypercalcemia or hypocalcemia can be lethal in dogs and cats, especially if rapid changes in serum calcium concentration occur.
- Disorders of hypocalcemia are encountered more commonly than those of hypercalcemia.
- Hypocalcemia based on total serum calcium is often mild and less often requires calcium-specific treatment than does hypercalcemia.
- Toxicity from hypercalcemia is greatly magnified if the serum phosphorus concentration is also increased.
- No calcium-specific treatment is indicated if the ionized calcium level is normal, despite an increase or decrease in the total serum calcium.
- No calcium-specific treatment is indicated when the total serum calcium is decreased but the ionized calcium level is normal.
- Hypercalcemic crisis is most likely to occur when there is toxicity from excess vitamin D metabolites circulating in the body.
- Acute treatment of moderate to severe ionized hypercalcemia involves intravenous saline, furosemide, calcitonin, and glucocorticoids.
- Severe hypercalcemia that is unlikely to resolve quickly may benefit from intermittent intravenous doses of bisphosphonates to decrease osteoclast function. Pamidronate is the first-choice bisphosphonate in veterinary medicine, but zoledronate is more potent and gaining popularity among small animal oncologists.
- In many instances, treatment of severe and symptomatic hypocalcemia involves the administration of immediate intravenous boluses of calcium salts followed by a constant rate infusion to maintain normal serum ionized calcium levels.
- Ionized hypocalcemia occurs more often than predicted when only the total serum calcium is measured, especially in the critical care setting.

CALCIUM HOMEOSTASIS

Calcium is an important electrolyte that is crucial for numerous intracellular functions, extracellular functions, and skeletal bone support. Calcium is necessary for muscle contraction because ionized calcium mediates acetylcholine release during neuromuscular transmission. Calcium also stabilizes nerve cell membranes by decreasing membrane permeability to sodium. Because of the complexity of its functions, normal homeostatic control mechanisms attempt to keep serum calcium within a narrow range, but only the circulating ionized component of total calcium is regulated. When these homeostatic mechanisms are disrupted or overwhelmed, conditions of hypocalcemia or hypercalcemia can occur. Three forms of circulating calcium exist in serum and plasma: ionized (free), protein bound, and complexed (calcium bound to phosphate, bicarbonate, lactate, citrate, oxalate).[1] Total calcium routinely measured on serum automated biochemical analyzers measures all three of these components. The ionized form of calcium is the biologically active form in the body and is considered the most important indicator of functional calcium levels.

Calcium regulation is a complex process involving primarily parathyroid hormone (PTH), vitamin D metabolites, and calcitonin. These calcium regulatory hormones exert most of their effects on the intestine, kidney, and bone. PTH is synthesized and secreted by the chief cells of the parathyroid gland in response to hypocalcemia or low calcitriol levels (also known as $1{,}25(OH)_2D_3$, the principal active vitamin D metabolite). PTH is synthesized and secreted constantly at low rates to maintain serum ionized calcium levels within a narrow range in healthy animals. PTH secretion is normally inhibited by increased serum ionized calcium levels, as well as by increased concentrations of circulating calcitriol. The principal action of PTH is to increase blood calcium levels through increased tubular reabsorption of calcium, increased osteoclastic bone resorption, and increased production of calcitriol.

Vitamin D and its metabolites also play a central role in calcium homeostasis. Dogs and cats, unlike humans, photosynthesize vitamin D inefficiently in their skin and therefore depend on vitamin D in their diet.[2] After ingestion and uptake, vitamin D is first hydroxylated in the liver to $25(OH)D_3$ (calcidiol), and then it is further hydroxylated to calcitriol by the proximal tubular cells of the kidney. This final hydroxylation by the 1α-hydroxylase enzyme system to form active calcitriol is under tight regulation and is influenced primarily by serum PTH, calcitriol, phosphorus, ionized calcium, and fibroblast growth factor 23 (FGF-23) concentrations. Decreased levels of phosphorus, calcitriol, and calcium promote calcitriol synthesis, and increased levels of these substances all cause a decrease in calcitriol synthesis. Increased PTH has a potent effect to enhance calcitriol synthesis, whereas FGF-23 inhibits the synthesis of calcitriol.[3]

With regard to calcium homeostasis, calcitriol primarily acts on the intestine, bone, kidney, and parathyroid gland. In the intestine, calcitriol enhances the absorption of calcium and phosphate at the level of the enterocyte. In the bone, calcitriol promotes bone formation and mineralization by regulation of proteins produced by osteoblasts. In addition, calcitriol is also necessary for normal bone resorption because of its effect on osteoclast differentiation. In the kidney, calcitriol acts to inhibit the 1α-hydroxylase enzyme system, as well as promote calcium and phosphorus reabsorption from the glomerular filtrate. In the parathyroid gland, calcitriol acts to inhibit the synthesis of PTH.

Although minor when compared with the effects of PTH and vitamin D metabolites, calcitonin also plays a role in calcium homeostasis. It is produced by the parafollicular C cells in the thyroid gland in response to an increased concentration of calcium after a calcium-rich meal and also during hypercalcemia. Calcitonin acts mostly on the bone to inhibit osteoclastic bone resorption activity but also decreases renal tubular reabsorption of calcium.

CALCIUM MEASUREMENT

Sample Handling Techniques

When collecting blood samples from patients for calcium measurements, the patient should be fasted before collection if possible to minimize postprandial increases in calcium. Both serum and heparinized plasma samples can be used. When plasma samples are used, certain anticoagulants such as oxalate, citrate, and ethylenediaminetetraacetic acid should not be used because they can dramatically lower calcium levels when measured in the laboratory. When measuring ionized calcium, serum is preferred over whole or heparinized blood because of less variation in results. In addition, anaerobic samples are preferred for ionized calcium measurement because pH can alter the concentration. In aerobic conditions, carbon dioxide can be lost, thus raising the pH in the sample. An alkalotic pH may increase the binding of calcium to protein, especially albumin, in the sample and therefore artificially decrease the amount of ionized calcium in the sample. Aerobic samples can be used with reasonable diagnostic accuracy for ionized calcium measurement when sent to a referral laboratory, but species-specific correction formulas are needed that correct the sample pH to 7.40. Handheld point-of-care analyzers consistently report ionized calcium values that are less than those from bench machines; this error increases with the magnitude of the calcium being measured.[4]

Ionized Versus Total Calcium

The calcium status of most animals is usually obtained first via measurement of total calcium. However, this parameter often does not reflect the ionized calcium concentration of the diseased patient,[5,6] especially in critically ill animals. When attempts are made to predict ionized calcium concentrations in the cat based on total calcium measurements, hypercalcemia and normocalcemia are often underestimated, whereas hypocalcemia is often overestimated.[6] In dogs, the opposite appears to be true; the frequency of hypercalcemia and normocalcemia is overestimated and hypocalcemia underestimated.[6] In dogs with chronic renal failure the magnitude of error greatly increases, with hypercalcemia being overdiagnosed.[6] Therefore for accurate assessment of patient calcium status, measurement of ionized calcium is recommended. So-called correction formulas that are used to predict ionized calcium status from total serum calcium are quite inaccurate.[5]

HYPERCALCEMIA

Hypercalcemia can be caused by numerous disease processes (Box 52-1) and may exert toxic systemic effects in multiple organs when ionized hypercalcemia is present.

Clinical Signs and Diagnosis

Clinical signs associated with hypercalcemia loosely parallel the severity of the calcium elevation. Common signs include polyuria and polydipsia (dogs, not cats), anorexia, constipation, lethargy, and weakness. Severely affected animals may display ataxia, obtundation, listlessness, muscle twitching, seizures, or coma. Bradycardia may be detected on physical examination, and electrocardiographic (ECG) monitoring may reveal a prolonged PR interval, widened QRS complex, shortened QT interval, shortened or absent ST segment, and a widened T wave. Bradyarrhythmias may progress to complete heart block, asystole, and cardiac arrest in severely affected animals. Other abnormalities may also be secondary to the underlying disease process causing the hypercalcemia.

Usually hypercalcemia is documented when total serum calcium is measured as part of the animal's diagnostic workup for clinical signs. Normal calcium values for dogs and cats can have a wide range and differ from laboratory to laboratory, so reference values should be used from the laboratory to which the sample was submitted. In general, normal total calcium values are approximately 10 mg/dl for dogs and 9 mg/dl for cats. These values are for mature animals because growing animals (dogs especially) can have higher total

BOX 52-1[1] *Differential Diagnoses for Hypercalcemia*

Nonpathologic

Postprandial
Juvenile, growing animal
Laboratory error
Lipemia

Transient or Inconsequential

Hemoconcentration
Hyperproteinemia
Hypoadrenocorticism

Pathologic or Persistent/Consequential

Parathyroid dependent

Primary hyperparathyroidism
- Adenoma
- Adenocarcinoma
- Hyperplasia
- Overdose of recombinant PTH

Parathyroid independent

Malignancy
Humoral hypercalcemia of malignancy
- Lymphosarcoma
- Anal sac apocrine gland adenocarcinoma
- Carcinoma (e.g., thyroid, prostate, mammary)
- Thymoma

Hematologic malignancies (bone marrow osteolysis, local osteolytic disease)
- Lymphosarcoma
- Multiple myeloma
- Leukemia
- Myeloproliferative disorders

Bone neoplasia (primary or metastatic)
Idiopathic hypercalcemia (cats)
Chronic renal failure
Calcinosis cutis—during recovery, especially after DMSO
Hypervitaminosis D
- Iatrogenic
- Plants (calcitriol glycosides)
- Rodenticide (cholecalciferol)
- Antipsoriasis creams (calcipotriene or calcipotriol)

Granulomatous disease (calcitriol synthesis)
- Fungal
- Injection site reaction
- Sterile dermatitis

Acute kidney injury
Skeletal lesions
- Osteomyelitis
- Hypertrophic osteodystrophy
- Disuse osteoporosis
- Bone infarction

Excessive oral or injectable calcium administration
- Calcium-containing intestinal phosphate binders
- Calcium supplementation (calcium carbonate, calcium gluconate, calcium chloride)

Hypervitaminosis A
Raisin/grape toxicity

DMSO, Dimethyl sulfoxide.

calcium values, likely secondary to normal bone growth. Once a diagnosis of hypercalcemia is suspected based on the total calcium value (>12 mg/dl in the dog and >11 mg/dl in the cat), an ionized calcium measurement should be performed to confirm the diagnosis.

A diagnosis of hypercalcemia is confirmed with an ionized calcium measurement greater than 6 mg/dl or 1.5 mmol/L in the dog or greater than 5.7 mg/dl or 1.4 mmol/L in the cat. The increase in ionized calcium typically parallels the increase in total serum calcium except in animals with renal failure, in which the increase in total calcium is caused by calcium binding with citrate, phosphate, or bicarbonate. In cats, hypercalcemia is more commonly discovered when ionized calcium is measured compared with the total calcium measurement in the same cat.[6]

Once the hypercalcemia is confirmed, a thorough physical examination should be repeated. The clinician should palpate the anal sacs (dogs) and peripheral lymph nodes for any enlargement, perform a fundic examination (e.g., systemic disease, mycoses, neoplasia), and do a thorough evaluation for any masses that may have been missed on initial examination (e.g., mammary tumors). Further diagnostic maneuvers should be tailored to the individual patient based on clinical signs, physical examination findings, initial laboratory testing, and suspected etiology, but may include a complete blood cell count, chemistry panel, urinalysis, imaging (thoracic radiographs, abdominal radiographs, abdominal ultrasonography, parathyroid ultrasonography), fine-needle aspiration with cytologic evaluation of any masses found, PTH measurement, PTH-related protein measurement, calcidiol measurement, calcitriol measurement, bone biopsy, and bone marrow aspiration.

Differential Diagnoses

A list of differential diagnoses for hypercalcemia is presented in Box 52-1, with neoplasia-associated hypercalcemia (specifically lymphoma) being the most common cause in dogs, followed by renal failure, hyperparathyroidism, and hypoadrenocorticism.[7] In cats, neoplasia is thought to be the third most common cause of hypercalcemia behind idiopathic hypercalcemia and renal failure. Serum phosphorus levels tend to be normal or low in animals with primary hyperparathyroidism or malignancies with an elevated PTH-related protein. Dogs with neoplasia-associated ionized hypercalcemia (specifically lymphoma and anal sac adenocarcinoma) often have higher serum ionized calcium concentrations than those with renal failure, hypoadrenocorticism, and other types of neoplasia.[7] However, the magnitude of ionized hypercalcemia alone does not predict specific disease states.[7] A thorough discussion of the pathophysiology of hypercalcemia in various disease processes is beyond the scope of this chapter; however, a thorough understanding of these principles is important because they serve as a guide for diagnosis and treatment.[1]

Treatment of Hypercalcemia

The consequences of hypercalcemia can be severe and affect multiple body systems including the central nervous system (CNS), gastrointestinal tract, heart, and kidneys. Therefore a timely diagnosis and rapid intervention can be vital, especially in animals with acute development of severe hypercalcemia. However, there is no absolute calcium value that should serve as a guide for initiating aggressive treatment. Rather, intervention should be guided by multiple factors, including the magnitude of hypercalcemia, rate of development, stable or progressive disease, clinical signs associated with hypercalcemia, organ dysfunction (renal, cardiac, CNS), clinical condition of the patient, and suspected etiology of the hypercalcemia (Figure 52-1). In addition, evaluation of phosphorus concentrations may help in guiding therapy, because a calcium-phosphorus product greater than 60 represents increased risk for soft tissue mineralization.

Definitive treatment for hypercalcemia involves removing the underlying cause. However, in many cases the cause is not readily apparent, and sometimes palliative therapy must be instituted before treating the primary disease (Table 52-1).

Acute therapy often involves the use of one or more of the following: intravenous fluids, diuretics (furosemide), glucocorticoids, and calcitonin (Figure 52-2). The therapeutic fluid of choice for animals with hypercalcemia is 0.9% sodium chloride because the additional sodium ions provide competition for renal tubular calcium reabsorption, resulting in enhanced calciuria. In addition, 0.9% sodium chloride is calcium free, thus decreasing the calcium load on the body. Intravenous fluid therapy should be used to correct dehydration over 4 to 6 hours (if stable) and then given at rates of at least 1.5 to 2 times maintenance (see Chapter 59). Potassium supplementation is often needed with this fluid protocol (potassium 5 to 40 mEq/L) depending on serum potassium concentrations (see Chapter 51). Judicious fluid therapy should be used in patients with

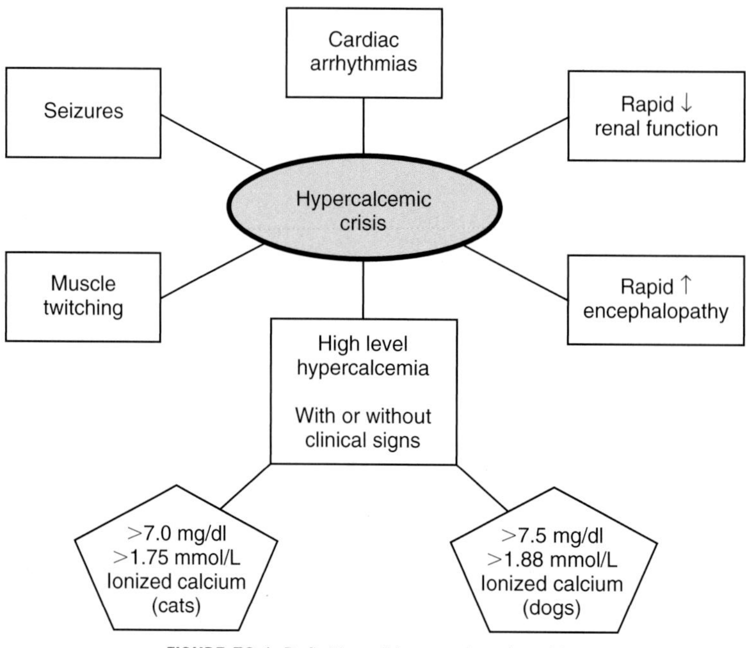

FIGURE 52-1 Definition of hypercalcemic crisis.

Table 52-1 **Treatment of Hypercalcemia**[1]

Treatment	Dosage	Indications	Comments
0.9% NaCl	4-6 ml/kg/hr IV CRI	Moderate to severe hypercalcemia	Contraindicated in congestive heart failure and hypertension
Furosemide	1 to 2 mg/kg IV, SC, PO q6-12h CRI 0.2 to 1 mg/kg/hr	Moderate to severe hypercalcemia	Volume expansion necessary before administration Rapid onset
Dexamethasone	0.1 to 0.22 mg/kg SC, IV q12h	Moderate to severe hypercalcemia	Use before identification of etiology may make definitive diagnosis difficult or impossible
Prednisone	1 to 2.2 mg/kg PO, SC, IV q12h	Moderate to severe hypercalcemia	Use prior to identification of etiology may make definitive diagnosis difficult or impossible
Calcitonin-salmon	4 to 6 IU/kg SC q8-12h	Hypervitaminosis D	Response may be short lived Vomiting may occur after multiple doses Rapid onset
Sodium bicarbonate	1 mEq/kg slowly IV bolus (may give up to 4 mEq/kg total dosage)	Severe, life-threatening hypercalcemia	Requires close monitoring Rapid onset
Pamidronate (Bisphosphonate)	1.3 to 2.0 mg/kg in 150 ml 0.9% NaCl IV over 2 to 4 hr	Moderate to severe hypercalcemia	Expensive Delayed onset
Cinacalcet (Calcimimetic)	No veterinary dosing published	Tertiary hyperparathyroidism Malignant primary hyperparathyroidism	Calcimimetic drug May have future uses in veterinary medicine

CRI, Constant rate infusion; *IV*, intravenous; *NaCl*, sodium chloride; *PO*, per os; *SC*, subcutaneous.

cardiac disease or hypertension, because volume overload and pulmonary congestion may easily occur. Furosemide enhances urinary calcium loss but should not be used in volume-depleted animals. Suggested dosages of furosemide are 1 to 2 mg/kg intravenously [IV], subcutaneously [SC], or orally [PO] q6-12h. A constant rate infusion (CRI) of 0.2 to 1 mg/kg/hr may occasionally be needed for several hours during a hypercalcemic crisis. Meticulous attention to fluid balance is essential when this method is used to avoid serious volume contraction. It is beneficial to place a urinary catheter in order to match the amount of fluid administered with the amount of urinary losses and ensure adequate volume replacement during aggressive diuresis.

Glucocorticoids can cause a reduction in serum calcium concentration in many animals with hypercalcemia. Glucocorticoids lead to reduced bone resorption, decreased intestinal calcium absorption, and increased renal calcium excretion. The magnitude of decline with therapy depends on the cause of the hypercalcemia. Dexamethasone often is given at dosages of 0.1 to 0.22 mg/kg SC or IV q12h, or prednisone at dosages of 1 to 2.2 mg/kg PO, SC, or IV q12h. However, in patients that have no definitive diagnosis for the hypercalcemia, calcitonin therapy should be considered instead of glucocorticosteroids because glucocorticosteroids may interfere with obtaining an accurate cytologic or histopathologic diagnosis as a result of cytolytic effects on lymphoid and plasma cells (e.g., lymphosarcoma, myeloma).

Calcitonin acts to decrease serum calcium concentrations mostly by reducing the activity and formation of osteoclasts. Calcitonin-salmon can be used at a dosage of 4 to 6 IU/kg SC q8-12h. Vomiting may occur after several days of administration in dogs. Sodium bicarbonate can also be considered for crisis therapy because it decreases the ionized and total calcium; effects on the bound fractions of calcium have not been examined in this situation.[8] Sodium bicarbonate is given at a dosage of 1 mEq/kg IV as a slow bolus (up to 4 mEq/kg total dose) when patients are at risk for death (see Table 52-1). Acid-base status should be monitored closely to avoid inducing alkalemia or other complications of bicarbonate therapy (i.e., paradoxical cerebral acidosis, hypernatremia, hypokalemia). Peritoneal or hemodialysis using calcium-free dialysate can be considered in cases refractory to traditional therapy. Fluid therapy should always be considered as the first treatment option and other modalities added based on response to therapy and the status of the patient.

Subacute or long-term treatment to decrease calcium levels may be needed in some cases, rather than acute rescue therapy. Glucocorticoids and furosemide can be used for long-term therapy and are usually administered orally. In addition, subcutaneous fluids (0.9% sodium chloride) can be given at dosages of 75 to 100 ml/kg q24h as needed.

Bisphosphonates are a class of drugs that have been used in human and veterinary medicine for management of hypercalcemia.[9] These drugs decrease osteoclastic activity, thus decreasing bone resorption. Bisphosphonates can take 1 to 3 days to maximally inhibit bone resorption, so they are not considered drugs of choice for acute or crisis therapy.[10] Pamidronate has been the most commonly used bisphosphonate in veterinary medicine for management of hypercalcemia; zoledronate is more potent than pamidronate and can be considered for use in selected patients. Pamidronate can be given intravenously at dosages of 1.3 to 2 mg/kg in 150 ml 0.9% saline as a 2-hour to 4-hour infusion.[9] This dose can be repeated in 1 week, if needed, but the salutary effect may last for 1 month in some instances. Crisis management for idiopathic hypercalcemia in cats is almost never needed because of the insidious development of hypercalcemia. Oral alendronate starting at 1 to 3 mg/kg/wk has been used for the chronic treatment of idiopathic hypercalcemia in cats.[11] This medication may provide more long-term control of idiopathic hypercalcemia in cats compared with other proposed treatments (author's unpublished observations). However, it should be noted that oral alendronate is not as effective as intravenous bisphosphonate therapy in the acute setting. Oral bisphosphonates can cause esophageal irritation and have been reported to cause abdominal discomfort, nausea, and vomiting in humans,[12] so standard precautionary measures should be taken to decrease esophageal transit time in patients receiving these medications. This may include giving several milliliters of water orally after the administration of these pills

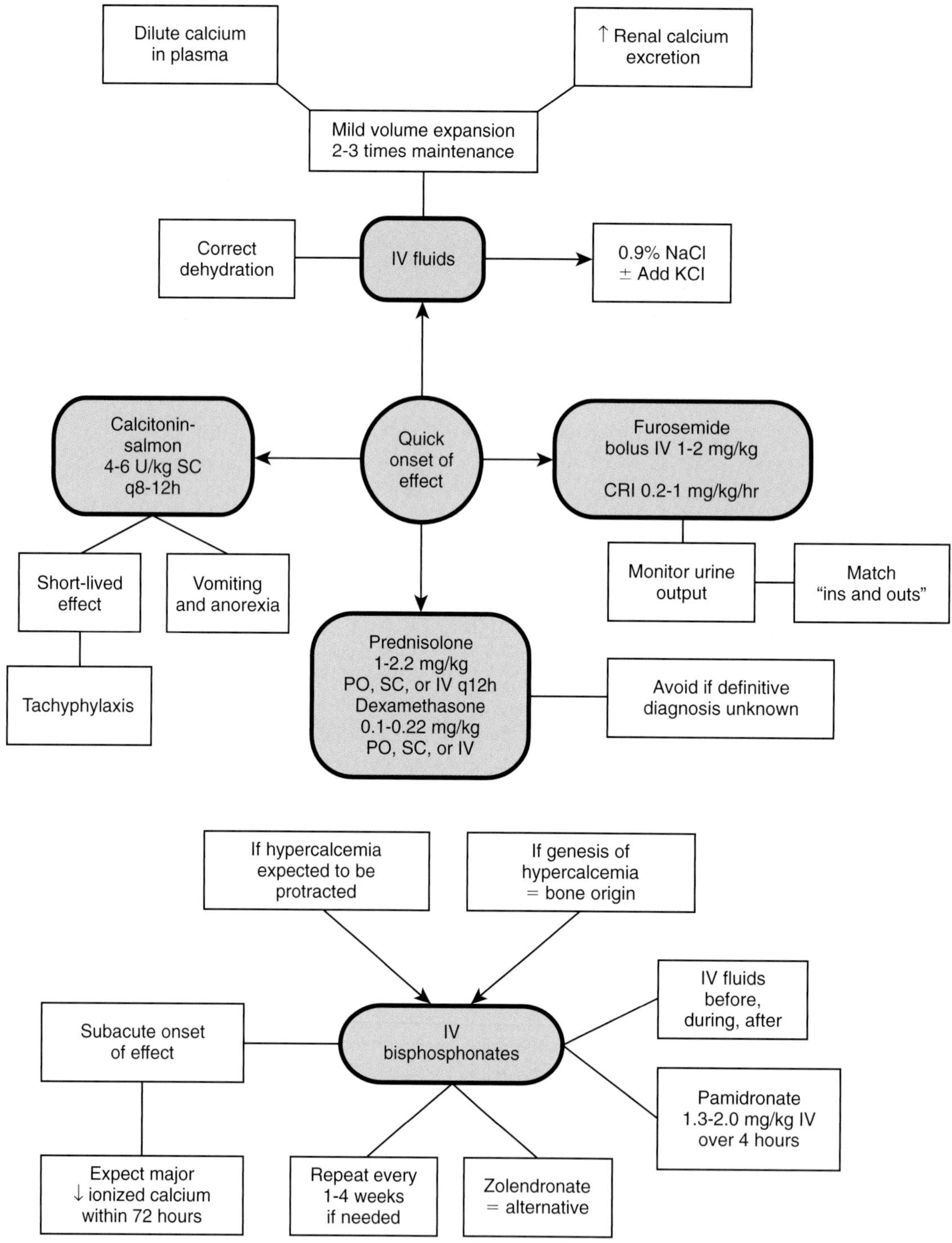

FIGURE 52-2 Treatment of critically ill patients with ionized hypercalcemia. *CRI,* Constant rate infusion; *IV,* intravenous; *PO,* per os; *SC,* subcutaneous.

and also "buttering" of the lips to encourage salivation and to decrease transit time of the pills into the stomach. Splitting of tablets is not recommended because of the potential for more severe corrosive effects.

Calcimimetics belong to a new class of drugs that will likely have future use in veterinary medicine to treat some cases of hypercalcemia in which the underlying cause cannot be treated adequately by other means (tertiary hyperparathyroidism, primary hyperparathyroidism caused by carcinoma). These drugs activate the calcium sensing receptor and thus decrease PTH secretion. Cinacalcet has been marketed for use in humans to treat renal secondary hyperparathyroidism and nonsurgical primary hyperparathyroidism.

HYPOCALCEMIA

Decreased total serum calcium is a relatively common electrolyte disturbance in critically ill dogs and cats. In two separate previous studies, the prevalence of ionized hypocalcemia was 31% in sick dogs and 27% in cats.[5,6]

Clinical Signs and Diagnosis

A list of clinical signs that occur with hypocalcemia is presented in Box 52-2. Signs of hypocalcemia are often not seen until serum total calcium concentrations are less than 6.5 mg/dl (<4 mg/dl or <1 mmol/L ionized calcium), and many animals show few signs even

BOX 52-2[1] *Clinical Signs Associated with Hypocalcemia*

Common	Occasional
None	Seizures
Muscle tremors or fasciculations	Panting
Facial rubbing	Pyrexia
Muscle cramping	Lethargy
Stiff gait	Anorexia
Behavioral change	Prolapse of third eyelid (cats)
• Restlessness or excitation	Posterior lenticular cataracts
• Aggression	Tachycardia or ECG alterations (i.e., prolonged QT interval)
• Hypersensitivity to stimuli	
• Disorientation	**Uncommon**
	Polyuria or polydipsia
	Hypotension
	Respiratory arrest or death

ECG, Electrocardiographic.

BOX 52-3 *Differential Diagnoses for Hypocalcemia*

- Hypoalbuminemia
- Chronic renal failure
- Eclampsia
- Acute kidney injury
- Pancreatitis
- Soft tissue trauma or rhabdomyolysis
- Hypoparathyroidism
  - Primary hypoparathyroidism
    Idiopathic
    Iatrogenic (postoperative bilateral thyroidectomy)
  - After sudden reversal of chronic hypercalcemia
  - Secondary to magnesium depletion, retention
- Ethylene glycol
- Phosphate enema
- Bicarbonate administration
- Improper sample anticoagulant (EDTA)
- Infarction of parathyroid gland adenoma
- Rapid IV infusion of phosphates
- Acute calcium-free IV infusion
- Intestinal malabsorption, PLE, starvation
- Hypovitaminosis D
- Blood transfusion (with citrate-containing anticoagulant)
- Hypomagnesemia (PTH secretion and receptor effects)
- Nutritional secondary hyperparathyroidism
- Acute tumor lysis syndrome
- Chelating agents
  - CaEDTA, dimercaprol (British anti-Lewisite), D-penicillamine, and meso-2,3-dimercaptosuccinic acid (succimer, IV radiocontrast)
- Excessive bisphosphonate treatment

Modified from Schenck PA, Chew DJ, Nagode LA, Rosol TJ: Disorders of calcium: hypercalcemia and hypocalcemia. In DiBartola SP, editor: *Fluid, electrolyte, and acid-base disorders in small animal practice*, ed 4, St Louis, 2012, Saunders Elsevier, pp 120-194.

EDTA, Ethylenediaminetetraacetic acid; *PLE*, protein-losing enteropathy; *PTH*, parathyroid hormone.

with lower calcium levels. Most animals with rapid development of hypocalcemia show clinical signs. Severely affected animals may have decreased inotropy and chronotropy (bradycardia), and ECG abnormalities may include a prolonged QT interval (because of prolonged ST segment), deep, wide T waves, or atrioventricular block.

Hypocalcemia is often discovered fortuitously after routine measurement of serum total calcium concentration. Hypocalcemia is defined as a total calcium concentration less than 8 mg/dl in dogs and less than 7 mg/dl in cats. When hypocalcemia is diagnosed via total calcium concentrations, it should always be confirmed with an ionized calcium measurement. Using ionized calcium concentrations, hypocalcemia is defined as less than 5 mg/dl (1.25 mmol/L) in dogs and less than 4.5 mg/dl (1.1 mmol/L) in cats.

After hypocalcemia is confirmed, other diagnostic strategies such as a complete blood cell count, chemistry panel, urinalysis, PTH measurement, and vitamin D metabolite measurements should be considered.

Differential Diagnoses

A list of differential diagnoses for hypocalcemia is presented in Box 52-3. The most common cause of a total serum hypocalcemia is hypoalbuminemia. However, the hypocalcemia associated with this is usually mild and typically no clinical signs result. Correction formulas have been advocated in the past to correct calcium levels for a low albumin, but these formulas do not accurately predict ionized or total calcium concentrations and are therefore not recommended.[5,6]

Renal dysfunction appears to be the second most common cause of hypocalcemia in dogs. Primary hypoparathyroidism is the one condition that will require long-term calcium-specific treatment. If the serum phosphorus level is above the reference range at the same time that hypocalcemia is discovered, the most likely diagnoses to rule out include renal dysfunction, pancreatitis (with or without prerenal azotemia), excessive phosphorous intake, and primary hypoparathyroidism.

Treatment

The consequences of untreated severe ionized hypocalcemia can be life threatening because of myocardial failure and respiratory arrest. This may be particularly important in dogs with sepsis because the presence of ionized hypocalcemia has been shown to be a negative prognostic indicator.[13] Septic cats also have a high prevalence of ionized hypocalcemia; failure to normalize during hospitalization is associated with a longer length of hospitalization and intensive care unit (ICU) stay. The decision to treat hypocalcemia should be based on multiple factors, including severity of clinical signs, rate of development of hypocalcemia, and etiology of the primary disease. Hypermagnesemia and hypomagnesemia can impair the secretion of PTH, and PTH actions on its receptor, so measurement of serum magnesium (preferably ionized magnesium) is important, especially in animals with refractory hypocalcemia.

Ionized hypocalcemia, low serum 25-hydroxyvitamin D (25[OH]D) concentrations, and elevated PTH serum concentrations have been reported in dogs with protein-losing enteropathies.[14] Many of these animals often undergo anesthetic procedures for diagnostic purposes (e.g., intestinal biopsy); therefore it may be warranted to treat ionized hypocalcemia, if present, because tachycardia, ECG alterations (i.e., prolonged QT interval), refractory hypotension, and respiratory arrest are all possible complications of ionized hypocalcemia.

Patients with decreased total calcium concentrations but normal ionized calcium concentrations require no treatment. If a decreased ionized calcium concentration is found, the clinician must decide if therapy is warranted. If the patient is stable, no clinical signs referable to hypocalcemia are documented, and the ionized calcium is not progressively decreasing, then it is reasonable to consider not treating these patients. Patients with a severe decrease in ionized calcium concentration warrant calcium-specific treatment regardless of clinical signs.[15,16] Therapy may also be initiated in an asymptomatic patient with moderate progressive ionized hypocalcemia to prevent the development of signs. Patients with clinical signs attributed to hypocalcemia clearly should receive calcium-specific rescue therapy.

Treatment of hypocalcemia can be divided into acute and subacute to long term. As with all cases of hypocalcemia, attempts should always be made to treat the primary disease causing the disorder. Most cases of hypocalcemia do not require long-term therapy, with hypoparathyroidism being the exception. Many cases will require acute treatment, especially those with tetany, seizures, or muscle fasciculations. Therapy typically involves the administration of calcium salts, as well as vitamin D metabolites.

For acute therapy, calcium should be administered intravenously to effect over a 10- to 20-minute period. Calcium gluconate and calcium chloride are both available for treatment, but calcium gluconate is preferred because it is not irritating if injected perivascularly (unlike calcium chloride). Calcium salts should **NEVER** be given subcutaneously because they can cause skin necrosis and abscess formation severe enough to warrant euthanasia, even when diluted calcium preparations are administered. Calcium gluconate (10% solution, calcium 9.3 mg/ml) can be given at dosages of 0.5 to 1.5 ml/kg IV slowly to effect. Heart rate and ECG should be monitored closely during administration to look for bradycardia; prolonged PR interval; widened QRS complex; shortened QT interval; elevated, shortened, or absent ST segment; and widened T wave, all of which may indicate cardiac toxicity. It is important to note that it may take up to 30 to 60 minutes for all clinical signs to resolve after correction of hypocalcemia, and some behavioral changes and panting may persist during this time.

For subacute management, the initial bolus of calcium salts often needs to be followed with a CRI of calcium, especially if the hypocalcemia is expected to persist. A CRI of elemental calcium can be delivered at a rate of 1 to 3 mg/kg/hr IV based on the severity of hypocalcemia to maintain normal calcium levels until oral calcium administration and or vitamin D metabolites can be used to control serum calcium concentrations. Vitamin D metabolites should also be started early if the hypocalcemia is expected to persist, because it may take several days for intestinal calcium transport to be maximized. Calcitriol is the preferred active vitamin D metabolite because it has a quick onset of action, short plasma half-life, and relatively short biologic effect half-life (important if overshoot hypercalcemia occurs). Calcitriol is dosed at 20 to 30 ng/kg q24h PO divided twice a day for 3 to 4 days for induction, then 5 to 15 ng/kg q24h divided twice a day for maintenance therapy, and titrated to the desired level of serum calcium concentration.

For long-term therapy (e.g., primary hypoparathyroidism), oral calcium usually is needed to control serum calcium levels. It should be noted, however, that the goal of therapy with hypoparathyroidism is not to return calcium levels completely to normal, because this can have deleterious effects (hypercalciuria despite normocalcemia in the absence of basal effects that PTH normally has on renal tubules). One should aim to control signs and correct calcium levels to just below normal. Many forms of oral calcium are available (calcium carbonate, calcium lactate, calcium chloride, calcium gluconate) and all are dosed at 25 to 50 mg/kg q24h (divided and given twice a day). Calcium carbonate is the most common form of calcium used and is generally well tolerated. Calcitriol can also be used at the previously mentioned dosages.

Calcilytics are a relatively new class of drugs that antagonize the calcium-sensing receptor and thus stimulate PTH secretion. They may have future use in veterinary medicine to treat some cases of hypocalcemia that are refractory to current therapies. Calcilytics are currently being investigated for their use in humans to treat osteoporosis and autosomal dominant hypocalcemia (familial hypercalciuric hypocalcemia).[17,18]

REFERENCES

1. Schenck PA, Chew DJ, Nagode LA, et al: Disorders of calcium. In DiBartola SP, editor: Fluid, electrolyte, and acid-base disorders in small animal practice, ed 4, St Louis, 2012, Saunders-Elsevier, pp 120-194.
2. How KL, Hazewinkel AW, Mol JA: Dietary vitamin D dependence of cat and dog due to inadequate cutaneous synthesis of vitamin D, Gen Comp Endocrinol 96:12, 1994.
3. de Brito Galvao JF, Nagode LA, Schenck PA, et al: Calcitriol, calcidiol, PTH, and FGF-23 interactions in chronic kidney disease (CKD), J Vet Emerg Crit Care 23(2):134-162, 2013.
4. Grosenbaugh DA, Gadawski JE, Muir WW: Evaluation of a portable clinical analyzer in a veterinary hospital setting, J Am Vet Med Assoc 213:691, 1998.
5. Schenck PA, Chew DJ: Prediction of serum ionized calcium concentration by serum total calcium measurement in dogs, Am J Vet Res 66:1330, 2005.
6. Schenck PA, Chew DJ: Prediction of serum ionized calcium concentration by serum total calcium measurement in cats, Can J Vet Res 74(3):209-213, 2010.
7. Messinger JS, Windham WR, Ward CR: Ionized hypercalcemia in dogs: a retrospective study of 109 cases (1998-2003), J Vet Intern Med 23(3):514-519, 2009.
8. Chew DJ, Leonard M, Muir W III: Effect of sodium bicarbonate infusions on ionized calcium and total calcium concentrations in serum of clinically normal cats, Am J Vet Res 50:145, 1989.
9. Hostutler RA, Chew DJ, Jaeger JQ, et al: Uses and effectiveness of pamidronate disodium for treatment of dogs and cats with hypercalcemia, J Vet Intern Med 19:29, 2005.
10. Guay DR: Ibandronate, an experimental intravenous bisphosphonate for osteoporosis, bone metastases, and hypercalcemia of malignancy, Pharmacotherapy 26:655, 2006.
11. Whitney JL, Barrs VR, Wilkinson MR, et al: Use of bisphosphonates to treat severe idiopathic hypercalcaemia in a young Ragdoll cat, J Feline Med Surg 13(2):129-134, 2011.
12. Twiss IM, van den Berk AH, de Kam ML, et al: A comparison of the gastrointestinal effects of the nitrogen-containing bisphosphonates pamidronate, alendronate, and olpadronate in humans, J Clin Pharmacol 46:483, 2006.
13. Luschini MA, Fletcher DJ, Schoeffler GL: Incidence of ionized hypocalcemia in septic dogs and its association with morbidity and mortality: 58 cases (2006-2007), J Vet Emerg Crit Care (San Antonio) 20(4):406-412, 2010.
14. Mellanby RJ, Mellor PJ, Roulois, et al: Hypocalcaemia associated with low serum vitamin D metabolite concentrations in two dogs with protein-losing enteropathies, J Small Anim Pract 46(7):345-351, 2005.
15. Drobatz KJ, Casey KK: Eclampsia in dogs: 31 cases (1995-1998), J Am Vet Med Assoc 217:216, 2000.
16. Drobatz KJ, Hughes D: Concentration of ionized calcium in plasma from cats with urethral obstruction, J Am Vet Med Assoc 211:1392, 1997.
17. Widler L, Altmann E, Beerli R, et al: 1-Alkyl-4-phenyl-6-alkoxy-1H-quinazolin-2-ones: a novel series of potent calcium-sensing receptor antagonists, J Med Chem 53(5):2250-2263, 2010.
18. Park SY, Mun HC, Eom YS, et al: Identification and characterization of D410E, a novel mutation in the loop 3 domain of CASR, in autosomal dominant hypocalcemia and a therapeutic approach using a novel calcilytic, AXT914, Clin Endocrinol (Oxf) 53(5):2250-2263, 2010.

CHAPTER 53

MAGNESIUM AND PHOSPHATE DISORDERS

Linda G. Martin, DVM, MS, DACVECC • Ashley E. Allen-Durrance, DVM

KEY POINTS

- Hypomagnesemia is a common electrolyte disorder in critically ill veterinary patients.
- Given that less than 1% of total body magnesium is located in the serum, serum magnesium concentrations do not always reflect total body magnesium stores. Consequently a normal serum magnesium concentration can occur when there is a total body magnesium deficiency.
- Magnesium homeostasis is primarily a function of intestinal absorption and urinary excretion; therefore hypomagnesemia is almost always caused by disturbances in one or both of these organ systems. Most cases of hypermagnesemia involve a component of renal insufficiency.
- Severe hypomagnesemia and hypermagnesemia cause clinical signs associated with the cardiovascular and neuromuscular systems.
- Phosphate is a key component of many physiologic processes, such as cellular energy regulation, synthesis of cell membranes and nucleic acids, bone mineralization, acid-base regulation, and cell signaling.
- Hypophosphatemia is common in critically ill patients and most often associated with transcellular shifts. Severe hypophosphatemia with depletion of total body stores can cause detrimental clinical consequences including hemolytic anemia, impaired platelet function, immune suppression, myocardial dysfunction, and neurologic signs.
- Hyperphosphatemia is most often associated with acute or chronic kidney disease, and clinical signs are typically a consequence of hypocalcemia and metastatic soft tissue mineralization.

MAGNESIUM

For more than a decade, there has been a growing interest in the clinical effects and therapeutic role of magnesium in veterinary medicine. Magnesium disorders are common in both feline and canine critically ill patients. Increased morbidity, mortality, and prevalence of concurrent electrolyte disorders occur in critically ill animals with altered total serum magnesium concentrations when compared with normomagnesemic critically ill animals.[1-3]

Magnesium is the second most abundant intracellular cation, exceeded only by potassium. The vast majority of magnesium is found in bone and muscle. Sixty percent of the total body magnesium content is present in bone, incorporated into the crystal mineral lattice or in the surface-limited exchangeable pool. This pool consists of magnesium that is in equilibrium with the magnesium ions in the extracellular fluid and serves as a reservoir for maintenance of the extracellular magnesium concentration. Twenty percent is located in skeletal muscle and the remainder is located in other tissues, primarily the heart and liver. Less than 1% of total body magnesium is present in the serum.[4,5] In the serum, magnesium exists in three distinct forms: ionized, anion-complexed, and protein-bound fractions. The ionized fraction is thought to be the physiologically active component and accounts for approximately 66% and 63% of the total serum magnesium concentration in cats and dogs, respectively. Approximately 4% and 6% are complexed to compounds such as phosphate, bicarbonate, sulfate, citrate, and lactate in cats and dogs, respectively. The remaining 30% and 31% of total serum magnesium are bound to protein (primarily albumin) in cats and dogs, respectively.[6,7]

Magnesium is required for many metabolic functions, most notably those involved in the production and use of adenosine triphosphate (ATP). This electrolyte is a coenzyme for the membrane-bound sodium-potassium ATPase pump and functions to maintain the sodium-potassium gradient across all membranes. Calcium ATPase and proton pumps also require magnesium. Magnesium is also essential for protein and nucleic acid synthesis, regulation of vascular smooth muscle tone, cellular second messenger systems, and signal transduction. In addition, there are data to suggest that magnesium exerts an important influence on lymphocyte activation, cytokine production, and systemic inflammation.[8-10]

Magnesium homeostasis is achieved through intestinal absorption and renal excretion. Absorption occurs primarily in the small intestine (jejunum and ileum) with little or none occurring in the large intestine. The loop of Henle is the main site of magnesium reabsorption in the kidney. The kidney appears to be the main regulator of serum magnesium concentration and total body magnesium content.[8] This is achieved by both glomerular filtration and tubular reabsorption.[5] Renal magnesium excretion will increase in proportion to the load presented to the kidney; conversely, the kidney conserves magnesium in response to a deficiency.[8]

Lactation appears to play a role in gastrointestinal (GI) and renal handling of magnesium. Increased concentrations of parathyroid hormone, in addition to calcium concentration, most likely participate in magnesium conservation during lactation to supply the mammary glands with a sufficient amount.[11] No primary regulatory hormone has been identified for magnesium homeostasis, although the parathyroid, thyroid, and adrenal glands are likely involved.[12]

Hypomagnesemia

Most magnesium-related disorders are caused by conditions that lead to the depletion of total body stores. Hypomagnesemia is a common electrolyte abnormality in both canine and feline intensive care unit patients.[1-3] However, this electrolyte disorder appears to be less common in the general canine hospital population.[13] Ionized hypomagnesemia has been documented in perioperative feline renal transplant recipients, as well as cats with diabetes mellitus and diabetic ketoacidosis.[14,15] Other evidence suggests that animals on peritoneal dialysis, dogs with congestive heart failure receiving furosemide therapy, dogs with protein-losing enteropathy, and lactating dogs are also at risk for hypomagnesemia.[16-19]

Causes

Causes of magnesium deficiency are both numerous and complex. Three general categories are involved: decreased intake (or absorption), increased losses, and alterations in distribution. Potential

BOX 53-1 ***Causes of Hypomagnesemia***

I. Decreased Intake
  A. Inadequate nutritional intake
  B. Prolonged intravenous fluid therapy or parenteral nutrition without magnesium replacement
II. Increased Losses
  A. Gastrointestinal
    1. Malabsorption syndromes
    2. Extensive small bowel resection
    3. Chronic diarrhea
    4. Inflammatory bowel disease
    5. Cholestatic liver disease
  B. Renal
    1. Intrinsic tubular disorders
      a. Glomerulonephritis
      b. Acute tubular necrosis
      c. Postobstructive diuresis
      d. Drug-induced tubular injury
        (1) Aminoglycosides
        (2) Amphotericin B
        (3) Cisplatin
        (4) Cyclosporine
    2. Extrarenal factors influencing renal magnesium handling
      a. Diuretic-induced states
        (1) Furosemide
        (2) Thiazides
        (3) Mannitol
      b. Digitalis administration
      c. Diabetic ketoacidosis
      d. Hyperthyroidism
      e. Primary hyperparathyroidism
  C. Lactation
III. Alterations in Distribution
  A. Extracellular to intracellular shifts
    1. Glucose, insulin, or amino acid administration
  B. Chelation
    1. Elevation in circulating catecholamines
      a. Sepsis or shock
      b. Trauma
      c. Hypothermia
    2. Massive blood transfusion
  C. Sequestration
    1. Pancreatitis

causes are listed in Box 53-1. Decreased dietary intake, if sustained for several weeks, can lead to significant magnesium depletion. In addition, catabolic illness and prolonged intravenous fluid therapy or parenteral nutrition without sufficient magnesium supplementation can contribute to depletion.[4,8,16]

Magnesium losses can occur through the GI tract, kidneys, or both. Because magnesium balance is primarily a function of intestinal absorption and urinary excretion, depletion is almost always caused by disturbances in one or both organ systems. Increased GI losses can result from inflammatory bowel disease, malabsorptive syndromes, cholestatic liver disease, or other diseases that cause prolonged diarrhea. Fluid from the intestinal tract contains a high concentration of magnesium. For this reason, patients with protracted episodes of large-volume diarrhea are prone to significant magnesium depletion.[4,9]

Because the kidney is the primary pathway of magnesium excretion, it often serves as a focal point for the development of hypomagnesemia through urinary loss. Acute renal dysfunction as a consequence of glomerulonephritis or the nonoliguric phase of acute tubular necrosis is often associated with a rise in the fractional excretion of magnesium. A number of endocrinopathies are also associated with an increase in the fractional excretion of magnesium, including diabetic ketoacidosis and hyperthyroidism.[9,15]

Numerous drugs that are commonly administered to critically ill patients can increase renal magnesium loss. Most of the commonly administered diuretic agents (furosemide, thiazides, mannitol) and cardiac glycosides induce hypomagnesemia by increasing urinary excretion. Other drugs, such as aminoglycosides, amphotericin B, cisplatin, and cyclosporine, predispose to renal tubular injury and excessive magnesium loss.[4,8]

Disease states or therapeutic modalities can cause the redistribution of circulating magnesium by producing extracellular to intracellular shifts, chelation, or sequestration. Administration of glucose, insulin, or amino acids causes magnesium to shift intracellularly. Also, catecholamine elevations in animals with sepsis, trauma, or hypothermia may cause ionized hypomagnesemia. It appears that β-adrenergic stimulation of lipolysis generates free fatty acids that chelate magnesium, thereby producing insoluble salts. In addition, citrated blood products can avidly chelate magnesium ions when administered in large quantities. In animals with acute pancreatitis, magnesium can form insoluble soaps, and magnesium sequestration may occur in areas of fat necrosis surrounding the pancreas.[4,8]

Clinical signs

Clinical signs of magnesium depletion are often related to its effects on the cell membrane that result in changes in resting membrane potential, signal transduction, and smooth muscle tone. The effects of magnesium on the myocardium are linked to its role as a regulator of other electrolytes, primarily calcium and potassium. For this reason, one of the most dramatic clinical signs associated with hypomagnesemia is cardiac arrhythmias, including atrial fibrillation, supraventricular tachycardia, ventricular tachycardia, and ventricular fibrillation. Hypomagnesemia also predisposes patients to digoxin-induced arrhythmias. Magnesium depletion not only enhances digoxin uptake by the myocardium but also inhibits the myocardial sodium-potassium ATPase pump, as does digoxin. Before overt arrhythmia development, subtle electrocardiographic (ECG) changes may be seen. These include prolongation of the PR interval, widening of the QRS complex, depression of the ST segment, and peaking of the T wave. In addition to these changes, hypomagnesemia can cause hypertension, coronary artery vasospasm, and platelet aggregation.[9,20]

Hypomagnesemia can cause various nonspecific neuromuscular signs. Concurrent hypocalcemia and hypokalemia may also contribute. Magnesium deficiency increases acetylcholine release from nerve terminals and enhances the excitability of nerve and muscle membranes. It also increases the intracellular calcium content in skeletal muscle. Clinical manifestations of magnesium deficiency can include generalized muscle weakness, muscle fasciculations, ataxia, and seizures. Esophageal or respiratory muscle weakness can be manifested as dysphagia or dyspnea, respectively.[4,9]

Because magnesium is necessary for the movement of sodium, potassium, and calcium into and out of cells, other manifestations of hypomagnesemia include metabolic abnormalities such as concurrent hypokalemia, hyponatremia, and hypocalcemia. Concurrent hypokalemia that is refractory to aggressive potassium supplementation may be due to magnesium deficiency causing excessive potassium loss through the kidneys. When hypokalemia is refractory to potassium supplementation, assessment of magnesium status and subsequent magnesium supplementation are recommended. Hypocalcemia is another manifestation of magnesium deficiency. Because hypomagnesemia impairs parathyroid hormone release and enhances calcium movement from extracellular fluid to bone, total and ionized hypocalcemia often accompanies magnesium depletion. Therefore clinical signs of hypocalcemia are often observed in patients with magnesium deficiency.[4,9]

Diagnosis

Magnesium deficiency should be suspected in patients predisposed to its development (disease processes or therapeutic modalities that can lead to hypomagnesemia) and exhibiting clinical signs and laboratory features consistent with magnesium depletion. Determination of total serum magnesium concentration is usually the most readily available technique for estimation of magnesium status. However, the precise clinical diagnosis of hypomagnesemia can be difficult. Because more than 99% of total body magnesium is located in the intracellular compartment, total serum concentrations do not always reflect total body stores. Therefore a normal total serum magnesium concentration can occur in an animal with a total body magnesium deficiency.[4,5] However, a low total serum concentration in a patient at risk for deficiency is usually significant. The reported reference range for total serum magnesium is 1.89 to 2.51 mg/dl in dogs, and 1.75 to 2.99 mg/dl in cats.[3,15]

The ionized magnesium concentration is thought to provide a more accurate reflection of intracellular ionized magnesium status and represents the "active" component. Ionized magnesium appears to equilibrate rapidly across the cell membrane; thus extracellular ionized magnesium values may be more reflective of intracellular stores. The canine reference range for ionized magnesium is 0.43 to 0.6 mmol/L, and the feline reference range is 0.43 to 0.7 mmol/L.[7]

Therapy

The amount and route of magnesium replacement depends on both the degree of hypomagnesemia and the patient's clinical condition. Mild hypomagnesemia may resolve with management of the underlying disorder and modification of intravenous fluid therapy. Animals receiving long-term diuretic or digoxin therapy may benefit from oral magnesium supplementation. Supplementation should be considered if total serum magnesium concentrations are lower than 1.5 mg/dl and at any concentration if clinical signs (cardiac arrhythmias, muscle tremors, refractory hypokalemia) are present. Renal function and cardiac conduction must be assessed before magnesium administration. Because magnesium is excreted primarily by the kidneys, the dosage should be reduced by 50% in azotemic patients and serum concentrations should be monitored frequently to prevent hypermagnesemia. Magnesium prolongs conduction through the atrioventricular (AV) node. Therefore any patient with cardiac conduction disturbances should have judicious supplementation and continuous ECG monitoring.

Both sulfate and chloride salts are available for parenteral supplementation. The intravenous route is preferred for rapid repletion of magnesium concentrations because the intramuscular route is generally painful. An initial dosage of 0.5 to 1 mEq/kg q24h can be administered by continuous rate infusion in 0.9% sodium chloride or 5% dextrose in water. A lower dosage of 0.25 to 0.5 mEq/kg q24h can be used for an additional 3 to 5 days. For management of life-threatening ventricular arrhythmias, a dose of 0.15 to 0.3 mEq/kg of magnesium diluted in normal saline or 5% dextrose in water can be administered slowly over 5 to 15 minutes.[21] Parenteral administration of magnesium sulfate may result in hypocalcemia because of chelation of calcium with sulfate. Therefore magnesium chloride should be given if hypocalcemia is also present. Other side effects of magnesium therapy include hypotension, atrioventricular block, and bundle branch blocks. Adverse effects usually are associated with intravenous boluses rather than continuous rate infusions.

Chloride, gluconate, oxide, and hydroxide magnesium salts are available for oral administration. The suggested dosage is 1 to 2 mEq/kg q24h. The main side effect of oral administration is diarrhea.[21]

It is important to recognize that many veterinary critical care diets contain low concentrations of magnesium (0.1 to 0.22 mg/kcal).[22] Given that many critically ill patients are fed at or below their resting energy requirement, the actual intake of magnesium may be well below the concentration needed to replete a magnesium deficient animal.[22] Additionally, magnesium supplementation in standard total parenteral nutrition formulations (0.13 to 0.22 mEq/kg/day) is also below the concentration recommended to treat hypomagnesemia (0.3 to 1.0 mEq/kg/day).[22] Based on the low concentrations of magnesium in critical care diets and total parenteral nutrition formulations, animals with moderate to severe hypomagnesemia will likely require intravenous or oral magnesium supplementation to normalize serum magnesium concentrations, especially if they have diseases resulting in continued loss of magnesium from the gastrointestinal tract or kidneys.

Hypermagnesemia

Hypermagnesemia appears to be a less common and simpler clinical entity than hypomagnesemia. Because large quantities of magnesium can be eliminated easily by the kidneys, it is unusual to encounter hypermagnesemia in the absence of azotemia. Unlike magnesium depletion, normal serum concentrations cannot hide increased body stores.

Causes

Conditions in which hypermagnesemia has been noted include renal failure, endocrinopathies, and iatrogenic overdose, especially in patients with impaired renal function. It appears that absolute magnesium excretion falls as the glomerular filtration rate declines, so it is not surprising that most patients with hypermagnesemia have some degree of renal insufficiency. In general the degree of hypermagnesemia parallels the degree of renal failure. Acute renal failure is more likely to be associated with clinically significant hypermagnesemia than chronic renal failure, but it may occur in the latter.[5]

Several endocrinopathies may be associated with hypermagnesemia, although the mechanisms are not well understood. These diseases include hypoadrenocorticism, hyperparathyroidism, and hypothyroidism. In comparison with renal failure, these diseases cause hypermagnesemia less often and to a milder degree. The prerenal azotemic state present in most patients with hypoadrenocorticism may contribute to hypermagnesemia.[22]

Improper dosing of magnesium replacement therapy or lack of consideration of the underlying renal function generally plays a role in iatrogenic hypermagnesemia.[23] Many cathartics, laxatives, and antacids contain magnesium, so care should be exercised if multiple doses are given to a patient with underlying renal disease. Sorbitol-containing cathartics are advised when patients have renal disease or require multiple doses to detoxify the GI tract.[5,20]

Clinical signs

Nonspecific clinical signs of hypermagnesemia include lethargy, depression, and weakness. Other clinical signs reflect the electrolyte's action on the nervous and cardiovascular systems. Hypermagnesemia usually results in varying degrees of neuromuscular blockade. One of the earliest clinical signs of magnesium toxicity is hyporeflexia. Profound magnesium toxicity has been associated with respiratory depression secondary to respiratory muscle paralysis. Severe respiratory depression can result in hypoventilation and subsequent hypoxemia. An absent menace and palpebral reflex have been reported in one dog and one cat that developed acute hypermagnesemia secondary to iatrogenic overdose.[24] Hypermagnesemia can also lead to blockade of the autonomic nervous system and vascular collapse.[20,22]

Cardiovascular effects of hypermagnesemia result in ECG changes, including prolongation of the PR interval and widening of the QRS complex. This is due to delayed atrioventricular and interventricular conduction. Bradycardia can occur in hypermagnesemic patients. At severely high serum magnesium concentrations, complete heart block and asystole can occur. Ectopy does not appear to be enhanced by elevated serum magnesium concentrations. Hypermagnesemia has also been reported to produce hypotension secondary to relaxation of vascular resistance vessels. Additionally, hypermagnesemia may impair platelet function and coagulation.[22]

Diagnosis

Unlike magnesium deficiency, normal serum concentrations cannot hide increased magnesium stores. Total serum magnesium concentrations greater than 2.99 mg/dl in cats and 2.51 mg/dl in dogs are considered indicative of hypermagnesemia.[3,15] Ionized magnesium concentrations above 0.7 mmol/L in cats and 0.6 mmol/L in dogs are considered ionized hypermagnesemia.[7]

Therapy

Therapy consists first and foremost of stopping all exogenous magnesium administration. Further treatment is based on the degree of hypermagnesemia, clinical signs, and renal function. A patient with mild clinical signs such as depression and hyporeflexia can be treated with supportive care and observation, provided that renal function is normal. More severe cases that involve unresponsiveness, respiratory depression, and any degree of hemodynamic instability should be treated with intravenous calcium. Calcium is a direct antagonist of magnesium at the neuromuscular junction and may be beneficial in reversing the cardiovascular effects of hypermagnesemia. Calcium gluconate (10%) can be given at 0.5 to 1.5 ml/kg as a slow intravenous bolus over 15 to 30 minutes. Saline diuresis and furosemide can also be used to accelerate renal magnesium excretion. Furosemide should not be given to a dehydrated or hypovolemic patient. Hypermagnesemic patients with severely impaired renal function may require peritoneal- or hemodialysis.

In patients with severe clinical signs, anticholinesterase treatment may be administered to offset the neurotoxic effects of hypermagnesemia. Physostigmine can be given at 0.02 mg/kg intravenously [IV] q12h until clinical signs subside. In severe cases complicated by cardiopulmonary arrest, intubation and mechanical ventilation are recommended. Hypermagnesemic shock may be refractory to epinephrine, norepinephrine, and other vasopressors, making resuscitation efforts extremely difficult.[5,22]

PHOSPHATE

Phosphorous is essential in numerous biologic processes and forms the body's major intracellular anion, phosphate. It is required in the production of ATP, guanosine triphosphate, cyclic adenosine monophosphate, and phosphocreatine, which function to maintain cellular membrane integrity, energy stores, metabolic processes, and biochemical messenger systems.[25,26] A major role of phosphate is maintenance of normal bone and teeth matrix in the form of hydroxyapatite.[25,27] Other roles include regulation of tissue oxygenation by way of 2,3-di-phosphoglycerate (2,3-DPG), which decreases the affinity of oxygen to hemoglobin, support of cellular membrane structure and ionic charge via phospholipids, mitochondrial production of ATP through the electron transport system by phosphoproteins, and buffering acidotic conditions in the body.[21,22]

Technically, phosphorus is an element and phosphate is a molecular anion (e.g., HPO_4^{2-}); however, the terms are often used interchangeably. For simplicity, *phosphate* will be used in this chapter to refer to either phosphorus or phosphate.[25] Distribution of whole body phosphate is as follows: 80% to 85% in the bone and teeth as inorganic hydroxyapatite, 14% to 15% in soft tissues, and less than 1% in the extracellular space.[25,26] Phosphorus is present in the body as organic and inorganic phosphates. Organic phosphate is mostly intracellular and inorganic phosphate is mostly extracellular.[25,28] Organic phosphates are components of phospholipids, phosphoproteins, nucleic acids, enzymes, cofactors, and biochemical intermediates.[28] Approximately two thirds of organic phosphate is in the form of phospholipids. Inorganic phosphate is further divided into orthophosphates and pyrophosphates. The quantity of pyrophosphates is insignificant; therefore most extracellular inorganic phosphate is in the form of orthophosphates. Approximately 85% of orthophosphates are free in circulation as monohydrogen phosphate (HPO_4^{2-}) or dihydrogen phosphate ($H_2PO_4^-$) with a ratio of 4:1 (HPO_4^{2-}:$H_2PO_4^-$) at a normal blood pH of 7.4. Alkalosis increases and acidosis decreases the ratio of divalent to monovalent phosphates.[25] The remaining 15% is either protein bound (10%) or complexed (5%) to magnesium, calcium, or sodium.[25,26] Inorganic phosphate in the form of 2,3-DPG accounts for 70% to 80% of phosphate in red blood cells.[29]

In plasma, both organic and inorganic phosphates are present. Organic phosphates include phosphate esters and phospholipids. Inorganic phosphates are composed primarily of the orthophosphates (free, protein bound, and complexed). It is important to note that only the inorganic phosphates are measured during blood chemistry analysis. Units are usually expressed as mmol/L or mEq/L. Conversion of units results in a normal plasma phosphate concentration of 3.1 mg/dl = 1 mmol/L phosphate = 1.8 mEq/L phosphate.[25] Serum or heparinized plasma, separated from cells within 1 hour, can be used to measure inorganic phosphate. Serum phosphate transiently peaks 6 to 8 hours after meals; therefore blood samples ideally should be collected after a 12-hour fast.[30] Spurious hyperphosphatemia can occur secondary to in vitro hemolysis or rupture of other blood cells, hypertriglyceridemia, and the presence of a monoclonal gammopathy.[27,31]

Phosphate balance is a complex interaction between phosphate intake and phosphate excretion. Intestinal absorption is linearly related to intake, and 60% to 70% of ingested phosphate is absorbed in the duodenum, jejunum, and ileum. In states of phosphate deficiency, calcitriol (1,25-dihydroxycholecalciferol) can increase active transport of inorganic phosphate.[25,26] Serum phosphate balance is dependent on glomerular filtration rate and tubular reabsorption, which occurs primarily in the proximal convoluted tubule.[26] Normally, 60% to 90% of filtered phosphate is reabsorbed in the proximal convoluted tubule.[25,27] The amount of phosphate reabsorbed is dependent on dietary intake, with maximal reabsorption occurring in animals consuming phosphate-deficient diets.[26] Parathyroid hormone (PTH) is considered a phosphaturic hormone because it decreases the tubular transport maximum for phosphate reabsorption. Growth hormone, insulin, insulinlike growth factor 1, and thyroxine increase tubular phosphate reabsorption.[25,26] Growth hormone partially accounts for the expected hyperphosphatemia in young, growing animals.[32] Phosphatonins, calcitonin, atrial natriuretic peptide, supraphysiologic doses of vasopressin, high doses of dexamethasone, and ACTH increase urinary phosphate excretion.[25,26] Phosphatonins are relatively new in the understanding of phosphate physiology; they are circulating substances that increase phosphate excretion in the kidneys, and it is believed intestinal phosphatonins exist as well. Fibroblast growth factor 23 is a phosphatonin thought to be heavily involved in the regulation of phosphate and vitamin D homeostasis.[26,27] The skeleton is the body's phosphate reservoir and provides a readily available source of phosphate during periods of hypophosphatemia under the regulation of PTH and calcitonin. PTH-mediated osteolysis is rapid and accounts for the acute changes (minutes to hours) in calcium and phosphate, whereas PTH-mediated activation of osteoclasts is a slower process (days to weeks). Hyperphosphatemia does not occur during this process because of the phosphaturic effects of PTH discussed earlier.[25,26]

Hypophosphatemia

Serum concentrations of phosphate measured by blood chemistry analyzers do not necessarily reflect whole-body phosphate balance. Phosphate is the predominant intracellular anion; therefore rapids shifts from the extracellular to intracellular space, or vice versa, can occur.[25] Blood chemistry analyzers measure serum phosphate (normal range 2.9 to 5.3 mg/dl depending on the age of the patient and chemistry analyzer).[27,32] Mild to moderate hypophosphatemia (1.0 to 2.5 mg/dl) may or may not be clinically significant and typically is not associated with phosphate depletion.[27,28,33] Severe hypophosphatemia (<1 mg/dl) is generally clinically significant and associated with total body phosphate depletion. However, a patient can suffer from phosphorous depletion despite a normal serum phosphate.[28] The decision to treat should be based on clinical assessment of the individual patient and measured serum phosphate concentration.

Causes

In general, hypophosphatemia can be caused by decreased intestinal absorption, transcellular shifts, or increased urinary excretion, with the most common cause being transcellular shifts.[26,28] In many clinical situations of hypophosphatemia, the etiology is often multifactorial. Potential causes of hypophosphatemia are listed in Box 53-2.

Decreased intestinal absorption is associated with chronic malnourishment, malabsorptive conditions (severe infiltrative disease), steatorrhea, vitamin D (1,25-dihydroxychcolecalciferol) deficiency, and administration of phosphate binding antacids.[27,28,34] Steatorrhea (increased fat content in feces) and diseases causing chronic diarrhea result in decreased intestinal phosphate absorption and secondary hyperparathyroidism due to vitamin D deficiency. Both mechanisms contribute to hypophosphatemia in this subset of patients. Iatrogenic hypophosphatemia can occur as a result of increased fecal excretion associated with phosphate-binding drugs such as aluminum hydroxide or lanthanum carbonate.[35]

Transcellular shifting of phosphate is associated with alkalemia, hyperventilation, refeeding syndrome, parenteral nutrition, insulin administration, glucose administration, catecholamine administration or release, and salicylate toxicity.[25,28,36] In critical care medicine, hypophosphatemia can occur as a result of hyperventilation caused by pain, anxiety, sepsis, heat stroke, and central nervous system disorders. Hyperventilation causes respiratory alkalosis, leading to rapid diffusion of carbon dioxide from the intracellular space to the extracellular space. The increase in intracellular pH activates phosphofructokinase and glycolysis, causing phosphate to rapidly shift into cells.[37] Hypophosphatemia is the most common and critical electrolyte disturbance associated with refeeding syndrome. During chronic malnutrition, phosphate depletion can occur and may not be reflected by a decrease in serum phosphate concentration. Administration of enteral or parental nutrition to a patient with chronic malnutrition stimulates insulin release, which promotes intracellular uptake of phosphate and glucose for glycolysis; this transcellular shift may result in severe hypophosphatemia.[38] Insulin and glucose administration can cause severe hypophosphatemia in a patient with total body phosphate depletion, such as patients being treated for diabetic ketoacidosis or hyperglycemic hyperosmolar nonketotic syndrome. Insulin and glucose stimulate glycolysis, promoting the synthesis of phosphorylated glucose compounds and intracellular shifts of phosphate.[27,33] Catecholamines (endogenous or exogenous) such as epinephrine or norepinephrine and β-receptor agonists such as terbutaline may cause hypophosphatemia as a result of β-adrenergic receptor–mediated cellular uptake of phosphate.[35,36] Salicylate toxicity causes uncoupling of oxidative phosphorylation and inhibition of the Kreb's cycle. Initially it causes hyperphosphatemia, which is thought to be a result of transcellular shifts from the intracellular to the extracellular compartment; however, this is rapidly (30 to 60 minutes) followed by hypophosphatemia caused by excessive urinary excretion.[39]

Excessive loss of phosphate through the kidneys can cause hypophosphatemia and phosphate depletion. This is more severe in patients with multifactorial causes of hypophosphatemia. For example, patients with diabetes mellitus have a high risk for phosphate depletion because of osmotic diuresis promoting phosphate excretion, loss of muscle mass, and impaired tissue phosphate utilization as a result of insulin deficiency. The severity of hypophosphatemia often worsens after treatment with insulin and intravenous fluid therapy because of transcellular shifts.[40] PTH is a phosphaturic hormone; therefore primary or nutritional secondary hyperparathyroidism may result in hypophosphatemia.[26] Primary hyperaldosteronism causes renal loss of calcium, resulting in hypocalcemia, which stimulates secretion of PTH and may result in normal or low serum phosphate. Hyperadrenocorticism is a reported cause of hypophosphatemia in humans; however, controversy exists in the veterinary

BOX 53-2 *Causes of Hypophosphatemia*

I. Decreased Gastrointestinal Absorption
  A. Chronic malnutrition
  B. Malabsorptive syndromes
  C. Steatorrhea
  D. Chronic vomiting and/or diarrhea
  E. Vitamin D deficiency
  F. Phosphate-binding antacids
II. Transcellular Shifts
  A. Alkalosis (respiratory or metabolic)
  B. Intravenous dextrose administration
  C. Insulin therapy
  D. Refeeding syndrome
  E. Catecholamines (endogenous or exogenous)
  F. Salicylate poisoning
  G. Eclampsia
  H. Hypercalcemia of malignancy
III. Increased Urinary Loss
  A. Diuresis
    1. Osmotic
      a. Diabetes mellitus/diabetic ketoacidosis
      b. Hyperosmolar hyperglycemic nonketotic syndrome
      c. Recovery phase of third-degree burns
    2. Drug induced
      a. Carbonic anhydrase inhibitors
      b. Mannitol
    3. Postobstructive
    4. Hypothermia induced
    5. Parenteral fluid therapy
  B. Hyperparathyroidism
    1. Primary
    2. Nutritional secondary
  C. Hyperaldosteronism
  D. Glucocorticoid therapy with or without hyperadrenocorticism
IV. Spurious or Laboratory Error
  A. Monoclonal gammopathy
  B. Hemolysis
  C. Hyperbilirubinemia
  D. Mannitol (blood levels >25 mmol/L)

literature. Initially it was thought that glucocorticoids decrease intestinal calcium absorption, leading to secondary hyperparathyroidism, and increase urinary excretion of phosphate, causing subsequent hypophosphatemia. However, in a prospective study, dogs with hyperadrenocorticism were found to have increased PTH concentrations and normal serum phosphate concentrations that were higher than the control group.[41] In humans, induction of therapeutic hypothermia for treatment of head trauma has resulted in severe electrolyte abnormalities, including depletion of magnesium, phosphate, potassium, and calcium. Increased urinary loss of electrolytes associated with hypothermia-induced diuresis is one possible mechanism of electrolyte depletion.[42] Hypophosphatemia occurs in patients with third-degree burns and is more significant in patients with higher total body surface area burns. The mechanism for hypophosphatemia is thought to be multifactorial; increased loss through the skin and increased urinary excretion during the recovery phase are likely mechanisms.[43]

Mannitol administration may cause spurious hypophosphatemia depending on the method used to measure serum phosphate. Mannitol, in concentrations as low as 25 mmol/L, interferes with the DuPont automatic clinical analyzer (ACA) colorimetric test by interfering with the formation of phosphomolybdate. This compound absorbs light and is proportional to serum phosphate concentrations. This has not been reported in the veterinary literature; however, it is feasible if the DuPont ACA endpoint method is used to measure serum phosphate.[35] Mannitol administration could theoretically also be associated with phosphate wasting because of its diuretic effects.

Sepsis has been associated with hypophosphatemia in people and may be attributable to increased circulation of inflammatory cytokines, especially interleukin-6 and tumor necrosis factor α.[44] Currently the mechanism by which cytokines cause hypophosphatemia is unknown. Acute respiratory alkalosis stimulates phosphofructokinase and glycolysis, which may play a role in the transcellular shift of phosphate during sepsis. Septic human patients with severe hypophosphatemia (serum phosphate concentration <1 mg/dl) are reported to have an eightfold increase in mortality.[45]

Clinical signs

Mild to moderate hypophosphatemia is typically asymptomatic; however, severe hypophosphatemia and total body phosphate depletion can result in widespread cellular dysfunction.[27,28] Depletion of ATP and 2,3-DPG is responsible for most of the severe clinical signs and can affect most cells in the body. Intracellular inorganic phosphate concentration is the critical determinant of cellular injury because it is necessary for the synthesis of ATP from adenosine diphosphate. Hemolysis can occur with severe hypophosphatemia because of decreased concentrations of red blood cell ATP and 2,3-DPG, spherocytosis, red cell membrane rigidity, and shorted red blood cell survival in some cats and dogs.[29,46-48] Decreased intracellular 2,3-DPG impairs release of oxygen by hemoglobin to tissues, leading to tissue hypoxia.[46] Severe hypophosphatemia causes impaired chemotaxis, phagocytosis, and bactericidal activity of leukocytes, which increases the risk of infection in critically ill animals.[49] Additionally, platelets have a shortened survival time with impaired clot retraction, which increases the risk of hemorrhage. Reversible myocardial dysfunction occurs with phosphate depletion and is a proposed mechanism for cardiac dysrhythmias associated with induction of therapeutic hypothermia in humans.[42] Clinical signs of severe hypophosphatemia-induced skeletal muscle changes include generalized weakness, tremors, and muscle pain (which can manifest as difficulty in weaning patients from mechanical ventilation). Rhabdomyolysis secondary to acute hypophosphatemia may occur during refeeding syndrome.[37] Neurologic signs may include ataxia, seizures, and coma associated with metabolic encephalopathy. Gastrointestinal signs can include anorexia, nausea, functional ileus, vomiting, and diarrhea.[28]

Diagnosis

Ideally the clinician should differentiate hypophosphatemia (decreased serum phosphate) from phosphate depletion (decreased total body phosphate). Unfortunately, differentiation may be difficult because phosphate is predominately intracellular, a fluid compartment that cannot easily be sampled for analysis. *Hypophosphatemia* refers to a decreased serum phosphate below the lower limit of the reference range and may occur with low, normal, or high total body phosphate. Mild to moderate hypophosphatemia correlates with a serum phosphate concentration of 1 to 2.5 mg/dl, and severe hypophosphatemia correlates with a serum phosphate of less than 1 mg/dl.[26,27] Phosphate depletion is a reduction in total body phosphate, usually resulting from decreased intake or increased loss through the kidneys, and can be compounded by transcellular shifts. Phosphate depletion can occur in the face of normal or high measured serum phosphate; therefore, phosphate depletion should be suspected in patients with predisposing causes and associated clinical signs.[27,33]

Therapy

The decision to treat a patient with hypophosphatemia will depend on the severity of the phosphate deficit, whether total body phosphate depletion is suspected or impending, anticipated duration of illness, clinical signs of the patient, and presence of concurrent illnesses associated with decreased intake or increased loss of phosphate. The focus should be on treating the primary disease and many cases of mild to moderate hypophosphatemia will subsequently resolve in this manner. For example, hypophosphatemia associated with respiratory alkalosis typically resolves when the patient's ventilatory and acid-base status normalizes.[28] Phosphate replacement can be administered orally or intravenously. Oral replacement is indicated in asymptomatic patients with mild to moderate (1 to 2.5 mg/dl) hypophosphatemia and the amount supplemented is often empirical. Bovine milk contains 0.032 mmol/ml of elemental phosphorous and can be used as an oral phosphate supplement.[33] Parenteral replacement is indicated in patients with severe hypophosphatemia (<1 mg/dl) that are at high risk of phosphate depletion. Commercially available hypertonic sodium and potassium phosphate solutions are available for parenteral use; they require dilution, typically in 0.9% saline, before administration. Dilution of phosphate salts in lactated Ringer's solution should be avoided because of potential for precipitation with calcium.[27] Sodium phosphate (Na_2HPO_4) contains 3 mmol/ml (93 mg/ml) phosphate and 4 mEq/L sodium. Potassium phosphate (KH_2PO_4) contains 3 mmol/ml (99.1 mg/ml) phosphate and 4.36 mEq/L potassium. When using potassium phosphate, it is important to account for the total amount of potassium supplementation in the patient's fluid therapy plan to avoid iatrogenic hyperkalemia. Reported dose ranges for intravenous phosphate therapy are 0.01 to 0.12 mmol/kg/hr.[27,28,40] Serum phosphate, ionized calcium, and serum potassium concentrations should initially be rechecked every 4 to 6 hours after starting parenteral phosphate replacement therapy. Potential adverse effects of overzealous supplementation include hyperphosphatemia, hypocalcemia with associated tetany, metastatic calcification, and renal failure. If potassium phosphate is oversupplemented, hyperkalemia may also occur.[27,33]

Hyperphosphatemia

The definition of hyperphosphatemia should vary depending on the age of the patient. A baseline normal serum phosphate range is 2.9 to 5.3 mg/dl; however, concentrations of 10 mg/dl have been reported in healthy puppies.[32]

Causes

Hyperphosphatemia can be caused by decreased renal excretion, increased intake or iatrogenic administration, and transcellular shifts. The most common cause in veterinary medicine is decreased renal excretion associated with acute kidney injury (AKI) or chronic kidney disease (CKD).[27,50] Hyperphosphatemia inhibits 1α-hydroxylase activity and stimulates secretion of PTH. Conversion of vitamin D to its active metabolite, calcitriol, is catalyzed by 1α-hydroxylase. Decreased calcitriol reduces intestinal absorption of phosphate; however, increased PTH enhances intestinal absorption and urinary excretion of phosphate, resulting in a small net effect of increased phosphate excretion. Calcitriol concentrations are subsequently restored by increased PTH. Initially, this restores serum phosphate; however, when PTH decreases, serum phosphate increases because of a decreased glomerular filtration rate and the cycle continues to preserve phosphate balance. Eventually, as CKD progresses, maximal inhibition of phosphate tubular reabsorption is surpassed, causing persistent hyperphosphatemia. As the number of functional tubular cells decrease, renal calcitriol synthesis tapers, and the magnitude of hyperphosphatemia progresses in spite of increased PTH. Renal secondary hyperparathyroidism occurs in 47% to 100% of dogs and cats with CKD, with a higher incidence in patients with more severe CKD (IRIS stage 3 and 4).[50] In the critical care setting, other common causes of hyperphosphatemia as a result of decreased excretion are AKI, acute-on-chronic kidney disease, urethral obstruction, and uroabdomen. Because of insufficient time for physiologic compensatory mechanisms to develop, AKI is often associated with significant hyperphosphatemia.

The most notable causes of transcellular shifts of phosphate resulting in hyperphosphatemia occur with tumor lysis syndrome, rhabdomyolysis, and hemolysis. Tumor lysis syndrome is the clinical manifestation and laboratory sequelae of acute death of tumor cells that release potassium, phosphate, and nucleic acids into circulation and may cause AKI. Renal tubular mineralization is thought to play a role in the pathogenesis of AKI associated with tumor lysis syndrome. Patients with a high tumor cell burden that respond rapidly to chemotherapy or radiation, such as stage IV and V lymphoma, are thought to be at higher risk for tumor lysis syndrome because these cells contain up to four times as much phosphate as normal cells.[26,27] Rhabdomyolysis is a syndrome of massive skeletal muscle tissue injury and can cause hyperphosphatemia directly from release of intracellular contents and indirectly by decreased renal excretion from resulting myoglobin-induced AKI (although this has never been reported in dogs or cats). Release of intracellular phosphate is the mechanism by which hemolysis is thought to cause hyperphosphatemia.[26,37]

Iatrogenic overdose and toxicities are conditions related to increased intake of phosphate. As mentioned in the previous section, parenteral administration of phosphate is not without risk and supplementation requires close monitoring to avoid iatrogenic overdose. Acute administration of large doses of parenteral phosphate can cause not only hyerphosphatemia but also hypomagnesemia, hypocalcemia, and hypotension.[33] Phosphate-containing enemas can cause severe hyperphosphatemia with the associated clinical consequences and can be fatal.[51] Ingestion of cholecalciferol rodenticides and vitamin D3 skin creams (e.g., calcipotriene) can rapidly increase serum phosphate concentration by increased intestinal absorption and release from bones.[52]

Hypoparathyroidism is rare in veterinary medicine but should be suspected in a patient presenting on emergency with acute tetany, muscle fasciculations, seizures, hypocalcemia, and normal kidney function (normal kidney values with appropriate urine specific gravity). In this disease, hyperphosphatemia may or may not be present.[27] Hyperthyroidism has also been associated with hyperphosphatemia because thyroxine increases renal tubular reabsorption of phosphate.[26]

Clinical signs

Clinical signs of hyperphosphatemia include anorexia, nausea, vomiting, weakness, tetany, seizures, and dysrhythmias. Hyperphosphatemia is often associated with hypocalcemia, hypomagnesemia, hypernatremia, and metabolic acidosis.[26,33] Clinical manifestations of hyperphosphatemia predominantly are due to hypocalcemia and metastatic soft tissue calcification. Tetany and seizures can develop in patients with severe hypocalcemia. Soft tissue calcium phosphate deposition occurs when the calcium phosphate product is greater than 58 to 70 mg^2/dl^2 and represents one mechanism for hypocalcemia. Tissues primarily affected by ectopic calcification include cardiac, vasculature, renal tubules, pulmonary, articular, periarticular, conjunctival, skeletal muscle, and skin.[26,27] Arrhythmias, such as polymorphic ventricular tachycardia or torsades de pointes caused by prolongation of the Q-T interval, are also associated with subsequent hypocalcemia and hypomagnesemia.[26]

Diagnosis

Diagnosis of hyperphosphatemia is based on a serum phosphate greater than 5.3 to 6 mg/dl in an adult dog or cat. Age of the patient should be considered when interpreting serum phosphate concentrations. Puppies and kittens less than 8 weeks of age have the highest plasma phosphate concentrations; this value steadily decrease as the animal ages, with normal adult values expected at 1 year of age.[26,27,32]

Treatment

A thorough investigation for the underlying cause should be sought to most effectively treat hyperphosphatemia. If rapid correction of hyperphosphatemia is needed, treatment includes crystalloid fluid therapy and dextrose administration with a goal of correcting azotemia (if present) and increasing intracellular uptake of phosphate. For patients with hyperphosphatemia caused by oliguric or anuric AKI, continuous renal replacement therapy or hemodialysis likely will be necessary. Continuous renal replacement therapy has been reported to be effective in a single case report for treatment of AKI and multiple electrolyte disturbances, including hyperphosphatemia, that was associated with acute tumor lysis syndrome and did not respond to conventional therapy.[53] Feeding a low-phosphate diet and administering phosphate binders such as aluminum hydroxide, ipakitine, lanthanum carbonate, or sevelamer should be considered when treating animals with hyperphosphatemia caused by chronic kidney disease.[27,54]

REFERENCES

1. Dhupa N: Serum magnesium abnormalities in a small animal intensive care population, J Vet Intern Med 8:156, 1994.
2. Toll J, Erb H, Birnbaum N, et al: Prevalence and incidence of serum magnesium abnormalities in hospitalized cats, J Vet Intern Med 16:217, 2002.
3. Martin LG, Matteson VL, Wingfield WE, et al: Abnormalities of serum magnesium in critically ill dogs: incidence and implications, J Vet Emerg Crit Care 4:15, 1994.
4. Berkelhammer C, Bear RA: A clinical approach to common electrolyte problems: 4. Hypomagnesemia, CMA J 132:360, 1985.
5. Sachter JJ: Magnesium in the 1990s: Implications for acute care, Top Emerg Med 14:23, 1992.
6. Schenck PA: Fractionation of canine serum magnesium, Vet Clin Pathol 34:137, 2005.
7. Schenck PA, Chew DJ: Understanding recent developments in hypocalcemia and hypomagnesemia, Proceedings of the 23rd American College of Veterinary Internal Medicine Forum, Baltimore, June 2005.

8. Friday BA, Reinhart RA: Magnesium metabolism: a case report and literature review, Crit Care Nurse 11:62, 1990.
9. Tong GM, Rude RK: Magnesium deficiency in critical illness, J Intensive Care Med 20:3, 2005.
10. King DE, Mainous AG, Geesey ME, et al: Dietary magnesium and C-reactive protein levels, J Am Coll Nutr 24:166, 2005.
11. Bateman S: Disorders of magnesium: Magnesium deficit and excess. In DiBartola SP, editor: Fluid, electrolyte, and acid-base disorders in small animal practice, ed 4, St Louis, 2012, Elsevier Saunders.
12. Dhupa N, Proulx J: Hypocalcemia and hypomagnesemia, Vet Clin North Am Small Anim Pract 28:587, 1998.
13. Khanna C, Lund EM, Raffe M, et al: Hypomagnesemia in 188 dogs: a hospital population-based prevalence study, J Vet Intern Med 12:304, 1998.
14. Wooldridge JD, Gregory CR: Ionized and total serum magnesium concentrations in feline renal transplant recipients, Vet Surg 28:31, 1999.
15. Norris CR, Nelson RW, Christopher MM: Serum total and ionized magnesium concentrations and urinary fractional excretion of magnesium in cats with diabetes mellitus and diabetic ketoacidosis, J Am Vet Med Assoc 215:1455, 1999.
16. Crisp MS, Chew DJ, DiBartola SP, et al: Peritoneal dialysis in dogs and cats: 27 cases (1976-1987), J Am Vet Med Assoc 195:1262, 1989.
17. Cobb M, Michell AR: Plasma electrolyte concentrations in dogs receiving diuretic therapy for cardiac failure, J Small Anim Pract 33:526, 1992.
18. Kimmel SE, Waddell LS, Michel KE: Hypomagnesemia and hypocalcemia associated with protein-losing enteropathy in Yorkshire Terriers: five cases (1992-1998), J Am Vet Med Assoc 217:703, 2000.
19. Aroch I, Ohad DG, Baneth G: Paresis and unusual electrocardiographic signs is a severely hypomagnesemic, hypocalcemic lactating bitch, J Small Anim Pract 39:299, 1998.
20. Arsenian M: Magnesium and cardiovascular disease, Prog Cardiovasc Dis 35:271, 1993.
21. Dhupa N: Magnesium therapy. In Bonagura JD, editor: Kirk's current veterinary therapy XII, ed 12, Philadelphia, 1995, Saunders.
22. Fascetti AJ: Magnesium: pathophysiological, clinical, and therapeutic aspects, Proceedings of the 21st American College of Veterinary Internal Medicine Forum, Charlotte, NC, June 2003.
23. Jackson CB, Drobatz KJ: Iatrogenic magnesium overdose: 2 case reports, J Vet Emerg Crit Care 14:115, 2004.
24. Van Hook JW: Hypermagnesemia, Crit Care Clin 7:215, 1991.
25. Yanagawa N, Nakhoul F, Kurokawa K, et al: Physiology of phosphorus metabolism. In Narins RG, editor: Maxwell & Kleeman's clinical disorders of fluid and electrolyte metabolism, ed 5, New York, 1994, McGraw-Hill.
26. DiBartola SP, Willard MD: Disorders of phosphorus: hypophosphatemia and hyperphosphatemia. In Dibartola SP, editor: Fluid, electrolyte, and acid-base disorders in small animal practice, ed 4, St Louis, 2012, Elsevier Saunders.
27. Schropp DM, Kovacic J: Phosphorous and phosphate metabolism in veterinary patients, J Vet Emerg Crit Care 17:127, 2007.
28. Forrester DS, Moreland KJ: Hypophosphatemia: causes and clinical consequences, J Vet Intern Med 3:149, 1989.
29. Yawata Y, Hebbel RP, Silvis S, et al: Blood cell abnormalities complicating the hypophosphatemia of hyperalimentation: erythrocyte and platelet ATP deficiency associated with hemolytic anemia and bleeding in hyperalimented dogs, J Lab Clin Med 84:643, 1974.
30. Lopez E, Aguilera-Tejero E, Estepa JC, et al: Diurnal variations in the plasma concentration of parathyroid hormone in dogs, Vet Rec 157:344, 2005.
31. Kristensen AT, Klausner JS, Weiss DJ, et al: Spurious hyperphosphatemia in a dog with chronic lymphocytic leukemia and an IgM monoclonal gammopathy, Vet Clin Pathol 20:45, 1991.
32. Harper EJ, Hackett RM, Wilkinson J: Age-related variations in hematologic and plasma biochemical test results in Beagles and Labrador Retrievers, J Am Vet Med Assoc 223:1436, 2003.
33. Geerse DA, Bindels AJ, Kuiper MA, et al: Treatment of hypophosphatemia in the intensive care unit: a review, Crit Care 14:R147, 2010.
34. Jergens AE, Crandel JM, Evans R, et al: A clinical index for disease activity in cats with chronic enteropathy, J Vet Intern Med 24:1027, 2010.
35. Liamia G, Milionis HJ, Elisaf M: Medication-induced hypophosphatemia: a review, Q J Med 103:449, 2010.
36. Kjeldsen SE, Moan A, Petrin J, et al: Effects of increased arterial epinephrine on insulin, glucose and phosphate, Blood Press 5:27, 1996.
37. Knochel JP, Barcenas C, Cotton JR, et al: Hypophosphatemia and rhabdomyoloysis, J Clin Invest 62:1240, 1978.
38. Justin RB, Hohenhaus AE: Hypophosphatemia associated with enteral alimentation in cats, J Vet Intern Med 9:228, 1995.
39. Quintanilla A, Kessler RH: Direct effects of salicylate on renal function in the dog, J Clin Invest 52:3143, 1973.
40. Adams LG, Hardy RM, Weiss DJ, et al: Hypophosphatemia and hemolytic anemia associated with diabetes mellitus and hepatic lipidosis in cats, J Vet Intern Med 7:266, 1993.
41. Ramsey IK, Tebb A, Harris, et al: Hyperparathyroidism in dogs with hyperadrenocorticism, J Small Anim Pract 46:531, 2005.
42. Polderman KH, Peerdeman SM, Girbes ARJ: Hypophosphatemia and hypomagnesemia induced by cooling in patients with severe head injury, J Neurosurg 94:697, 2001.
43. Loghmani S, Maracy MR, Kheirmand R: Serum phosphate level in burn patients, Burns 36:1112, 2010.
44. Barak V, Schwartz A, Kalickman I, et al: Prevalence of hypophosphatemia in sepsis and infection: the role of cytokines, Am J Med 104:40, 1998.
45. Shor R, Halabe A, Rishver S, et al: Severe hypophosphatemia in sepsis as a mortality predictor, Ann Clin Lab Sci 36:67, 2006.
46. Jacob HS, Amsden T: Acute hemolytic anemia with rigid red cells in hypophosphatemia, N Engl J Med 285:1446, 1971.
47. Chan PC, Calabrese V, Theil L: Species differences in the effect of sodium and potassium ions on the ATPase of erythrocyte membranes, Biochim Biophys Acta 79:424, 1964.
48. Fujise H, Higa K, Nakayama T, et al: Incidence of Dogs Possessing Red Blood Cells with High K in Japan and East Asia, J Vet Med Sci 59(6):495, 1997.
49. Craddock PR, Yawata Y, VanSanten L, et al: Acquired phagocyte dysfunction: a complication of the hypophosphatemia of parenteral hyperalimentation, N Engl J Med 290:1403, 1974.
50. Cortadellas O, Fernandez del Palacio MJ, Talavera J, et al: Calcium and phosphorus homeostasis in dogs with spontaneous chronic kidney disease at different stages of severity, J Vet Intern Med 24:73, 2010.
51. Schaer M: Iatrogenic hyperphosphatemia, hypocalcemia and hypernatremia in a cat (adverse reaction to phosphate enema), J Am Anim Hosp Assoc 13:39, 1977.
52. Pesillo SA, Khan SA, Rozanski EA, et al: Calcipotriene toxicosis in a dog successfully treated with pamidonate disodium, J Vet Emerg Crit Care 12:177, 2002.
53. Martin A, Acierno MJ: Continuous renal replacement therapy in the treatment of acute kidney injury and electrolyte disturbances associated with acute tumor lysis syndrome, J Vet Intern Med 24:986, 2010.
54. Kidder A, Chew D: Treatment options for hyperphosphatemia in feline CKD: what's out there? J Fel Med Surg 11:913, 2009.

CHAPTER 54

TRADITIONAL ACID-BASE ANALYSIS

Kate Hopper, BVSc, PhD, DACVECC

KEY POINTS

- Traditional acid-base analysis uses the Henderson-Hasselbalch equation to evaluate the blood pH as a direct consequence of the PCO_2, bicarbonate, and base excess.
- Blood pH is a measure of hydrogen ion concentration and is dependent on the ratio of bicarbonate to PCO_2.
- PCO_2 behaves as an acid in the body and represents the respiratory contribution to acid-base balance.
- Bicarbonate, base excess, and TCO_2 are all representations of the metabolic contribution to acid-base balance.
- The anion gap is a diagnostic tool that may help identify the cause of a metabolic acidosis.
- The treatment of most acid-base disorders is focused on resolution of the underlying disease.
- Sodium bicarbonate therapy is primarily indicated for the treatment of metabolic acidoses associated with kidney disease and diarrhea-associated loss of bicarbonate.

Regulation of hydrogen ion concentration within physiologically acceptable limits is essential. The evaluation of acid-base balance is an integral aspect of managing critically ill and injured patients. Clinically, adequate assessment of acid-base abnormalities requires an understanding of the etiology and magnitude of changes in order to guide further diagnostic and therapeutic interventions. Acid-base balance has been a focus of research and discussion in the medical literature since the beginning of the twentieth century.[1-5]

The normal concentration of hydrogen ions is very small (40 nanomoles/L) compared with other ions in the body, such as sodium (145 million nanomoles/L in the dog).[6] By convention, the concentration of hydrogen ions is described as pH, a dimensionless measure that is calculated as the negative logarithm of the hydrogen ion activity and allows the representation of a wide range of hydrogen ion concentrations in a simplified manner. The pH scale ranges from 0 for a 1 molar solution of hydrogen ion to 14 for a 10^{-14} molar solution.[4] The hydrogen ion concentration considered compatible with life for a mammalian system ranges from 10 to 160 nanomoles/L, which correlates with a pH from 8 to 6.8, respectively.[7] A blood pH below the normal range for the species is considered an acidemia and an elevated blood pH is considered an alkalemia. An individual process in the system that tends to decrease or increase pH is referred to as an acidosis or an alkalosis, respectively.

Clinical assessment of acid-base balance first evaluates the pH: normal, acidemia or alkalemia. The system is then partitioned into the respiratory and metabolic components and each is evaluated separately. PCO_2 represents the respiratory component universally, but there are numerous measures available for assessment of the metabolic component. These include the Henderson-Hasselbalch, or traditional, approach; the Stewart approach; and a semi-quantitative approach that combines aspects of both the traditional and Stewart approaches. This chapter will review traditional acid-base analysis and Chapter 55 will discuss the nontraditional approaches.

SAMPLE COLLECTION AND HANDLING

Before further discussion of acid-base analysis, it is important to appreciate the potential for preanalytical error if inappropriate sample collection or handling occurs. The site of sample collection affects acid-base variables. In healthy research dogs there was a statistically significant difference in pH, PCO_2, PO_2, and bicarbonate concentration when arterial values were compared with venous values. pH and PCO_2 were also different between jugular and cephalic venous samples (see Appendix 1).[8] These differences are relatively small, and for the purpose of acid-base analysis, venous samples have been found to be an adequate replacement for arterial values in critically ill human patients.[9,10] In states of poor peripheral perfusion, peripheral venous samples can have elevations in PCO_2 and lactate concentration, which will contribute to lower pH values that may not be representative of central venous or arterial values.[10]

Other sources of preanalytical error for acid-base analysis include time delays between sample collection and sample analysis; exposure to air, which will allow PCO_2 to equilibrate to a lower value; and inappropriate dilution of the blood sample with liquid anticoagulant such as sodium heparin.[11] Any bubbles in the sample should be immediately removed. If a delay of greater than 15 minutes between sample collection and analysis is anticipated, the sample should be maintained under airtight conditions and immersed in ice water.[12,13]

TRADITIONAL APPROACH

The traditional approach is based on the Henderson-Hasselbalch equation (Box 54-1) for carbonic acid (H_2CO_3) and uses pH, the partial pressure of carbon dioxide (PCO_2), and bicarbonate concentration (HCO_3^-). From this equation it is clear that pH has a direct relationship with bicarbonate concentration and an inverse relationship with PCO_2. Modern blood gas machines measure the hydrogen ion activity and PCO_2 of a blood or plasma sample and use the Henderson-Hasselbalch (HH) equation to derive the concentration of bicarbonate. The base excess (BE) and anion gap (AG) parameters have been added to the traditional approach to improve its diagnostic utility.

The body relies on three major processes to maintain acid-base balance: regulation of PCO_2 by alveolar ventilation, buffering of acids by bicarbonate and nonbicarbonate buffer systems, and changes in renal excretion of acid or base. As mentioned previously, PCO_2

BOX 54-1 ***Henderson-Hasselbalch Equation***

$$pH = 6.1 + \log([HCO_3^-] \div [0.03 \times PCO_2])$$

where 6.1 is the pKa in body fluids; HCO_3^- is the concentration of bicarbonate measured in mEq/L or mmol/L; 0.03 is the solubility coefficient for carbon dioxide in plasma; and PCO_2 is the partial pressure of carbon dioxide in mm Hg.

represents the respiratory component, and in the traditional approach changes in bicarbonate concentration (or BE) represent the metabolic component (influenced by both buffering systems and renal handling of acid). As the HH equation describes, pH is not dependent on having a specific PCO_2 and bicarbonate concentration. Rather, pH is the consequence of the ratio of bicarbonate to PCO_2. For example, a patient can have a high bicarbonate concentration, but as long as the PCO_2 has increased by a similar magnitude, the $HCO_3^-:PCO_2$ ratio will remain normal and hence pH will remain in the normal range. Because maintenance of an acceptable pH is optimal to maintain physiologic processes, it is no surprise that when an abnormality in one system (respiratory or metabolic) occurs, changes are made in the opposing system in an attempt to return the ratio of bicarbonate to PCO_2 toward normal; hence pH is driven back toward a more normal value. This process is known as compensation and tends to return pH toward normal, but it is generally accepted that compensation will not be complete. This means compensation will rarely result in a pH within the normal range and will not overcompensate. See later in this chapter for further discussion of compensation.

PCO_2

Carbon dioxide acts as an acid in the body because of its ability to react with water to produce carbonic acid. With increases in PCO_2, the ratio of bicarbonate to PCO_2 is decreased, hence pH falls. Another way to consider this process is that with an increase in PCO_2 the carbonic acid equation (shown below) will be driven to the right, increasing the hydrogen ion concentration.

$$CO_2 + H_2O \longleftrightarrow H_2CO_3 \longleftrightarrow H^+ + HCO_3^-$$

Because carbon dioxide is a gas and its concentration in the blood is controlled by pulmonary ventilation, the lung plays an important role in controlling acid-base status. Changes in alveolar ventilation occur rapidly and can alter blood pH within minutes. An increased PCO_2 has an acidotic influence (a respiratory acidosis) and a decreased PCO_2 represents a respiratory alkalosis.

Bicarbonate

Bicarbonate is a parameter calculated by blood gas machines, although some clinical laboratories do measure it directly. Elevations in bicarbonate are consistent with a metabolic alkalosis, whereas decreases in bicarbonate concentration represent a metabolic acidosis. One of the major criticisms of using bicarbonate as the measure of the metabolic component is that it is not independent of changes in PCO_2.[14-16] As discussed earlier, changes in PCO_2 will alter the equilibration of the carbonic acid equation. Elevations of PCO_2 will lead to elevations of bicarbonate, whereas decreases in PCO_2 will lead to a decrease in bicarbonate. As such it is important that changes in bicarbonate concentration are always evaluated in terms of the pH and PCO_2.

Base Excess

Base excess (BE) is the titratable acidity (or base) of the blood sample. It is defined as the amount of acid or base that must be added to a sample of oxygenated whole blood to restore the pH to 7.4 at 37° C and at a PCO_2 of 40 mm Hg.[17] Theoretically a normal individual should not have an excess or deficit of acid or base and hence BE would equal 0. An increased BE (more positive value) is consistent with an alkalotic process (either gain of bicarbonate or loss of acid). A decreased BE (more negative value), also known as a base deficit, represents an acidotic process. The BE is a parameter calculated by an algorithm programmed into blood gas machines. These machines use human algorithms with normal human blood having a BE of approximately 0 mmol/L. Unfortunately veterinary species do not have the same acid-base balance as humans. Herbivores tend to have a more positive "normal" BE than people, whereas carnivores tend to have a more negative "normal" BE than people. See Appendix 1 for a reported normal range of acid-base values for dogs and cats.

The major advantage of using BE over bicarbonate concentration is that it is independent of changes in the respiratory system. When there are minimal changes in PCO_2 present, the BE and bicarbonate should correlate well. The BE can be estimated by the measured bicarbonate concentration minus the normal bicarbonate concentration. In the face of substantial abnormalities in PCO_2, the BE is a more reliable measure of the metabolic component.[14,15,18]

Total Carbon Dioxide

Many blood gas machines and most diagnostic laboratories will provide a parameter called total carbon dioxide (TCO_2). This is a misleading name because this represents the metabolic acid-base component, not the respiratory system component. The TCO_2 is a measure of all the carbon dioxide in a blood sample, and the majority of carbon dioxide is carried as bicarbonate in the blood. In general, TCO_2 will be 1 to 2 mmol/L higher than the true bicarbonate concentration.[6]

Anion Gap

The anion gap (AG) was developed to better define the cause of a metabolic acidosis. Electroneutrality requires there to be an equal number of anions and cations in physiologic systems. In reality there is no actual AG; the apparent AG exists because more cations in the system are readily measured than anions. The AG is a reflection of unmeasured cations and unmeasured anions and is calculated according to the equation in Box 54-2. The AG of a normal individual is primarily composed of negatively charged plasma proteins, mostly albumin.[19]

There are two common mechanisms of metabolic acidosis. The first is the loss of bicarbonate from the body via the gastrointestinal tract or kidneys; this bicarbonate is produced by cells and involves the exchange of bicarbonate and chloride. The result is a rise in serum chloride as bicarbonate is lost, a hyperchloremic metabolic acidosis. No change in AG would be expected. The other common clinical cause of metabolic acidosis is the gain of acid. When there is excess acid in the system, hydrogen ions will titrate (combine) with bicarbonate, leading to a fall in bicarbonate concentration; the anion that accompanied the hydrogen ion (the conjugate base) will accumulate, maintaining electroneutrality and increasing the AG. Common acids associated with an increased AG include lactate, ketone bodies, sulfate, phosphate, and toxins such as ethylene glycol.[20] A useful mnemonic for increased AG metabolic acidosis in small animals is DUEL, standing for **d**iabetic ketoacidosis, **u**remic acids (sulfates, phosphates), **e**thylene glycol, and **l**actic acidosis (Box 54-3).

It is important to note that hypoalbuminemia can mask the presence of unmeasured anions. Albumin and phosphorus are the major contributors to the AG in the normal animal. In states of hypoalbuminemia, abnormal unmeasured anions (e.g., lactate or ketones) may be present but the calculated anion gap may still remain within the reported reference range. As a result the AG is not reliable in hypoalbuminemic patients.[21,22]

BOX 54-2 ***Anion Gap Equation***

$$\text{Anion gap}^* = ([Na^+] + [K^+]) - ([HCO_3^-] + [Cl^-])$$

*Physiologically there is no actual anion gap; rather, this is a measure of unmeasured anions and cations in the system. An increase in the anion gap usually reflects an increase in unmeasured anions.

BOX 54-3 ***Possible Causes for Metabolic Acidosis***

Increased Anion Gap Metabolic Acidosis

DUEL

- **D**iabetic ketoacidosis
- **U**remia
- **E**thylene glycol intoxication
- **L**-Lactic acidosis

Other Less Common Causes

- D-Lactic acidosis
- Salicylate ingestion
- Methanol intoxication

Normal (or Low) Anion Gap Metabolic Acidosis

- Renal bicarbonate loss
- Gastrointestinal bicarbonate loss
- Dilutional acidosis
- Hypoadrenocorticism
- Hypoalbuminemia

Table 54-1 Simple Acid-Base Disturbances Identified with the Traditional Acid-Base Approach

Acid-base Disturbance	pH	Primary Disorder	Compensation
Respiratory acidosis	Decreased	Increased PCO_2	Increased HCO_3^-
Respiratory alkalosis	Increased	Decreased PCO_2	Decreased HCO_3^-
Metabolic acidosis	Decreased	Decreased HCO_3^-	Decreased PCO_2
Metabolic alkalosis	Increased	Increased HCO_3^-	Increased PCO_2

HCO_3^-, Bicarbonate concentration measured in mEq/L or mmol/L; *PCO_2*, partial pressure of carbon dioxide measured in mm Hg.

Compensation

Traditional acid-base analysis can identify primary (or simple) acid-base disorders in which there is an abnormality of one system (respiratory or metabolic) and any changes evident in the opposing system are considered consistent with normal compensation (Table 54-1). For example, a primary metabolic acidosis should have respiratory compensation. The respiratory response to a primary metabolic abnormality is rapid in onset and complete within hours (assuming a stable level of the metabolic abnormality).[23,24] In comparison, the metabolic compensatory response to a primary respiratory disorder takes hours to begin and 2 to 5 days to complete.[24,25] The degree of expected compensation in dogs is commonly estimated from guidelines derived from healthy experimental animals (Table 54-2).[24] If the change observed in the secondary system is similar in magnitude to the calculated, expected response, it is consistent with compensation and the assessment is a simple acid-base disorder. In other words, the change in the secondary system is completely attributed to compensation and no other acid-base abnormality is suspected. A mixed acid-base disorder is diagnosed when the changes in the secondary system are not within a range compatible with expected compensation for the primary disorder. The assumption is that there is some disturbance of the secondary system preventing appropriate compensation from occurring or causing the appearance of "overcompensation" (which does not occur).

Some caution is necessary when interpreting the appropriateness of metabolic compensation to a primary respiratory disorder because it will depend on the chronicity of the respiratory abnormality, which may or may not be accurately determined. There are no published guidelines for the compensatory responses of cats. Cats may demonstrate similar metabolic compensation for respiratory disorders as dogs, although two of the three studies on this topic were performed in anesthetized cats.[26-28] There is a single study in the literature reporting that cats do not develop respiratory compensation in response to a metabolic acidosis and there are no studies evaluating the respiratory response of adult cats to a metabolic alkalosis.[29] Consequently extrapolation of the canine calculations of expected metabolic compensation to respiratory disorders should be performed with caution in cats. Extrapolation of the canine calculations of expected respiratory compensation to metabolic disorders cannot be recommended in cats.

Table 54-2 Expected Compensatory Changes to Primary Acid-Base Disorders

Primary Disorder	Expected Compensation
Metabolic acidosis	↓ PCO_2 of 0.7 mm Hg per 1 mEq/L decrease in $[HCO_3^-]$ ±3
Metabolic alkalosis	↑ PCO_2 of 0.7 mm Hg per 1 mEq/L decrease in $[HCO_3^-]$ ±3
Respiratory acidosis—acute	↑ $[HCO_3^-]$ of 0.15 mEq/L per 1 mm Hg ↑ PCO_2 ±2
Respiratory acidosis—chronic	↑ $[HCO^-_3]$ of 0.35 mEq/L per 1 mm Hg ↑ PCO_2 ±2
Respiratory alkalosis—acute	↓ $[HCO^-_3]$ of 0.25 mEq/L per 1 mm Hg ↓ PCO_2 ±2
Respiratory alkalosis—chronic	↓ $[HCO^-_3]$ of 0.55 mEq/L per 1 mm Hg ↓ PCO_2 ±2

$[HCO_3^-]$, Bicarbonate concentration measured in mEq/L or mmol/L; *PCO_2*, partial pressure of carbon dioxide measured in mm Hg, ↑ increased; ↓, decreased.

Acid-Base Analysis

Traditional acid-base analysis can identify four simple disorders, defined as a single acid-base abnormality, where any changes in the opposing system are attributed solely to compensation (see Table 54-1). In addition, mixed disorders can be diagnosed; these are any situation where there is an abnormality in both the metabolic and respiratory components. Mixed disorders are evident when both the respiratory and metabolic components have the same influence on acid-base balance (i.e., metabolic acidosis and respiratory acidosis or metabolic alkalosis and respiratory alkalosis). A mixed disorder is also present when there are abnormalities evident in both the metabolic and respiratory components but the pH is in the normal range. In this situation it is important to recall the rule that compensation does not return pH all the way back to normal. Lastly a mixed disorder may be identified when the change in the opposing system is not consistent with expected compensation.

There are numerous possible approaches to diagnosing an acid-base disturbance using the traditional approach. One such approach is provided in Box 54-4. In this method the pH is assessed as representing acidemia or alkalemia for that species. Then the respiratory component and the metabolic component are both assessed for their influence on the acid-base balance as acidosis, alkalosis, or normal. The process that is influencing acid-base in the same direction as the pH abnormality is the primary disorder. For example:

pH	7.26	(7.35 to 7.42)	= Acidemia
$PvCO_2$	30	(38 to 42 mm Hg)	= Respiratory alkalosis
HCO_3	12	(18 to 22 mmol/L)	= Metabolic acidosis

In this example, the only process that can be considered responsible for the change in pH is the metabolic system; the primary disturbance is therefore a metabolic acidosis. The next step is to determine if the opposing system (in this example the respiratory

BOX 54-4 ***Approach to Blood Gas Analysis***

1. Confirm the sample collection and handling was appropriate
2. Evaluate the pH (select one):
   In the normal range
   Acidemia
   Alkalemia
3. Evaluate the respiratory component, PCO_2 (select one):
   In the normal range
   Process (increased CO_2)
   Alkalotic process (decreased CO_2)
4. Evaluate the metabolic component, HCO_3 or SBE (select one):
   In the normal range
   Acidotic process (decreased HCO_3, negative SBE)
   Alkalotic process (increased HCO_3, positive SBE)
5. Define the primary process, either respiratory or metabolic—that is, which process is causing a change in the same direction as the pH change?
6. Evaluate if compensation is as expected
7. Determine the overall acid-base analysis
8. Is a primary metabolic acidosis present?
   If yes, calculate the anion gap.

system) is consistent with expected compensation. First the direction of the change in the opposing system needs to be evaluated to see if it is appropriate for compensation (see Table 54-1), keeping in mind the time required for metabolic compensation to occur. In many cases the presence of a change in the opposing system in the direction expected for compensation is sufficient to diagnose a simple disorder. In dogs the expected compensatory change can be calculated using Table 54-2 and, if the change in the opposing system is similar to that calculated, a simple disorder is then diagnosed. If the change in the opposing system is not similar to that expected (calculated), a mixed disorder is diagnosed. In this example the predicted respiratory compensation for a bicarbonate concentration of 12 mmol/L would be a PCO_2 in the range of ~31 ± 3 mm Hg. The patient has a PCO_2 of 30 mm Hg, consistent with compensation and a simple metabolic acidosis is the diagnosis. Lastly, if a metabolic acidosis has been identified, the AG can be calculated in an effort to help determine the underlying cause of the abnormality, assuming the patient is not hypoalbuminemic.

The advantage of the traditional approach to acid-base analysis is its relative simplicity and adherence to sound chemical principles. It has been tried and tested for the best part of a century in both the experimental and clinical environment and has been proven to be reliable and accurate. The major criticism of the traditional approach to metabolic acid-base disorders is its failure to identify individual disease processes that are contributing to the acid-base abnormality. Although the AG may help to determine causes of a metabolic acidosis, it is prone to error and only narrows the possible diagnoses but does not provide a definitive diagnosis.

CAUSES OF ACID-BASE ABNORMALITIES

Respiratory Acidosis

Elevations in PCO_2 can represent a primary respiratory acidosis or can occur in an attempt to compensate for a primary metabolic alkalosis. Respiratory acidosis results from an imbalance in CO_2 production via metabolism and alveolar minute ventilation in the lung. This is best described by the equation

$$PaCO_2 \sim \dot{V}CO_2/\dot{V}_A$$

where $\dot{V}CO_2$ is the production of CO_2 by the tissues and $\dot{V}_A$ is alveolar minute ventilation.[30]

A respiratory acidosis is the consequence of increased CO_2 production or decreased $\dot{V}_A$. Clinically the most common causes of changes in PCO_2 are a result of changes in $\dot{V}_A$. When primary metabolic acid-base abnormalities alter pH, it is sensed by both central and peripheral chemoreceptors and there is a resultant alteration in $\dot{V}_A$ to change PCO_2 in a manner to reduce the magnitude of pH change (respiratory compensation).

Because minute ventilation is the product of respiratory rate and tidal volume, common causes of a respiratory acidosis are diseases that reduce respiratory rate, tidal volume, or both. Airway obstruction can impair tidal volume. Depression of the respiratory center of the brainstem as a consequence of drugs (e.g., many anesthetics and sedatives), brain injury, mass lesion, and other conditions can lead to lack of stimulus for $\dot{V}_A$. Diseases that prevent transmission of impulses from the respiratory center to the respiratory muscles, such as cervical spinal cord disease, peripheral neuropathies, and diseases of the neuromuscular junction, can all cause respiratory paralysis and respiratory acidosis. Myopathies or muscular fatigue can also occur, impairing respiratory muscle function. Increases in CO_2 production can occur in patients with hyperthermia, seizures, fever, and malignant hyperthermia. However, the awake, neurologically intact animal should increase $\dot{V}_A$ to compensate for an increase in $\dot{V}CO_2$, so generally these abnormalities cause respiratory acidosis in the compromised or anesthetized animal. See Chapter 16 further discussion of this topic.

The ideal treatment for respiratory acidosis is resolution of the underlying disease when possible. In severe cases of hypoventilation that persists despite therapy, mechanical ventilation is indicated (see Chapter 30). Elevated levels of CO_2 can cause hypoxemia in patients breathing room air, and all animals with significant hypercapnia (>60 mm Hg) should receive oxygen therapy. It is important to note that bicarbonate therapy is contraindicated in patients with a respiratory acidosis.

Respiratory Alkalosis

From the previous discussion it is evident that a decreased PCO_2 is the result of an increase in $\dot{V}_A$ (decreased CO_2 production is not a clinically relevant issue). A low PCO_2 may occur as an appropriate compensatory response to a metabolic acidosis. Primary disease processes that may stimulate an increased respiratory rate or tidal volume include significant hypoxemia, pulmonary parenchymal disease (causing stimulation of stretch receptors or nociceptors), and airway inflammation.[31] In addition, central stimulation of respiratory rate and effort by the respiratory center can occur. This can be a pathologic process resulting from brain injury or it could be behavioral as a result of pain or anxiety. An animal's respiratory rate cannot be used to determine if it is hyper- or hypoventilating. Dead space ventilation, as occurs with panting, can allow a very rapid rate without change to PCO_2 while slow respiratory rates can be associated with hyperventilation if larger tidal volumes are generated. Ventilatory status can only be accurately determined by measurement of PCO_2.

Treatment of respiratory alkalosis is focused on therapy for the underlying disease; specific therapy for the respiratory alkalosis itself is rarely attempted.

Metabolic Acidosis

Metabolic acidosis occurs relatively commonly in small animal patients, identified in 43% of dogs and cats that had blood gas analysis at a university teaching hospital.[32] As described previously, metabolic acidosis can result from the loss of bicarbonate or the gain of acid, and the calculation of the AG may aid in determining which of these processes is present. Metabolic acidosis caused by bicarbonate loss, typified by hyperchloremia and a normal anion gap, can occur through the intestinal tract via diarrhea or can be due to renal losses. Hyperchloremic metabolic acidosis in association with small bowel diarrhea has been well reported in human patients and large animal species but is an infrequent occurrence in dogs and cats. Renal loss of bicarbonate can be an appropriate response to a persistent respiratory alkalosis (metabolic compensation). When it occurs as a primary disease process, it is known as renal tubular acidosis (RTA). It can be broadly categorized as proximal or distal tubular dysfunction. In animals with proximal RTA there is inadequate reabsorption of bicarbonate in the proximal nephron. Reported causes in dogs and cats include congenital abnormalities (e.g., Fanconi syndrome), as well as acquired abnormalities secondary to toxins, drugs, and various diseases (e.g., hypoparathyroidism and multiple myeloma). Distal RTA is a disorder involving inadequate hydrogen ion secretion in the distal tubule that prevents maximal acidification of the urine; it is often accompanied by hypokalemia and is more rarely reported in the veterinary literature than proximal RTA. Potential causes include pyelonephritis and immune mediated hemolytic anemia. The interested reader is directed to reference 33 for further reading on RTA. Hypoadrenocorticism not only leads to hypovolemia and a lactic acidosis but also impairs urine acidification, leading to metabolic acidosis.

Treatment of metabolic acidoses caused by bicarbonate loss is primarily based on therapy of underlying diseases. In addition, intravenous (IV) fluid therapy may speed the resolution of this disorder. Fluids containing a "buffer" such as lactated Ringer's solution will aid in the metabolism of hydrogen ions. When treating patients with a hyperchloremic metabolic acidosis, use of lower chloride containing fluids (i.e., avoiding 0.9% NaCl) will also be of benefit. When the acidosis is severe or the compensatory respiratory alkalosis is considered detrimental to the patient, bicarbonate administration is indicated (see Bicarbonate Therapy later in the chapter).

Metabolic acidosis caused by a gain in acid is typified by normochloremia and an elevated AG. The common causes in dogs and cats were mentioned previously—diabetic ketoacidosis (DKA), uremia, lactic acidosis, and ethylene glycol intoxication. Less common causes include D-lactic acidosis and various additional intoxications, including salicylates and methanol.[20]

Treatment of metabolic acidosis caused by an acid gain is primarily focused on resolution of the underlying cause and appropriate selection of IV fluid therapy, as described earlier. Bicarbonate administration may be beneficial in some uremic patients, but is not typically indicated for treatment of other acidoses (see Bicarbonate Therapy later in this chapter).

It is interesting to note that in a retrospective study of metabolic acidosis in dogs and cats, 25% of dogs and 34% of cats had neither an elevated AG nor hyperchloremia, suggesting there are limitations to this categorization of metabolic acidosis.[32]

Metabolic Alkalosis

Metabolic alkalosis appears to be less common in small animal patients, evident in 15% of a population of dogs and cats compared with the occurrence of metabolic acidosis in 43% of these animals.[33] Metabolic alkalosis broadly can be considered to occur because of either acid loss or bicarbonate gain. Causes of acid loss include selective gastric acid loss such as can occur with gastrointestinal obstructive processes (leading to sequestration or vomiting) and nasogastric tube suctioning. Renal acid loss can occur as a result of loop diuretic administration, mineralocorticoid excess, and the presence of nonreabsorbable anions such as carbenicillins.[34,35] Acid loss invariably occurs along with chloride in the gastrointestinal tract and renal system and as a result many animals with metabolic alkalosis will also be hypochloremic.

Increases in bicarbonate concentration can occur as an appropriate renal compensation to a respiratory acidosis. Pathologic increases in bicarbonate concentration can also occur with contraction alkaloses, iatrogenic administration of an alkalinizing therapy (e.g., sodium bicarbonate), or metabolism of organic anions such as lactate, ketones, acetate, and citrate. Hypokalemia can play a significant role in the generation and maintenance of metabolic alkalosis. Intracellular shifts of hydrogen ions in exchange for potassium ions leaving the cells will increase the pH of the extracellular fluid. Further, hypokalemia promotes renal acid loss.[35,36]

The kidney has the ability to excrete large quantities of bicarbonate, such that metabolic alkalosis should be rectified rapidly. When metabolic alkalosis is persistent, there must be factors limiting renal bicarbonate excretion. Decreased effective circulating volume and hypochloremia can both limit renal bicarbonate excretion. Hypokalemia and aldosterone excess further impair renal bicarbonate excretion.

There are three important aspects to treatment of metabolic alkalosis: (1) Ensure there is adequate effective circulating volume, (2) normalize electrolytes, and, (3) when possible, correct the primary disease.[36]

BICARBONATE THERAPY

There are many potential adverse effects of metabolic acidosis, including decreased myocardial contractility, arterial vasodilation, impaired coagulation, decreased renal and hepatic blood flow, insulin resistance, and altered central nervous function.[37-39] It is no surprise that clinicians are eager to resolve a metabolic acidosis by treatment of the primary disease, IV fluid administration, and, in some instances, alkalinizing therapy.

Sodium bicarbonate is the most common alkali therapy used in veterinary medicine. Alternative alkalinizing therapies include tris-hydoxymethyl aminomethane (also known as tromethamine [THAM]) and Carbicarb, an equimolar mixture of sodium bicarbonate and sodium carbonate. These alternative buffer therapies may have the advantage of having no (THAM) or less (Carbicarb) associated CO_2 production than sodium bicarbonate. The interested reader is directed to reference 38 for further reading on this topic.[38]

The indications for sodium bicarbonate administration have been somewhat controversial over the years, although some consensus has been reached in recent time. There are several concerns with bicarbonate therapy (Box 54-5). The first is that its use is based on the premise that acidemia has substantial negative consequences to the patient. Numerous human studies have demonstrated that a low pH is well tolerated; this includes patients subjected to permissive hypercapnia and patients with DKA.[40,41] One of the most commonly cited

BOX 54-5 ***Potential Adverse Effects Associated with Sodium Bicarbonate Administration***[48]

- Increased hemoglobin affinity for oxygen
- Increased blood lactate concentration
- Paradoxical intracellular acidosis
- Hypercapnia
- Hypervolemia
- Hyperosmolality
- Hypernatremia
- Hypocalcemia (ionized)
- Hypokalemia
- Phlebitis

adverse effects of acidemia is decreased myocardial contractility and vascular tone. Investigations have not been able to consistently demonstrate these negative hemodynamic effects; in addition, studies have failed to demonstrate that bicarbonate administration will improve hemodynamic performance in the face of acidemia (in some studies hemodynamic performance actually deteriorates after bicarbonate administration).[42-44] Another concern is that sodium bicarbonate therapy does not reliably increase pH. After administration, the bicarbonate binds hydrogen ions (hence the alkalinizing effect) to form carbonic acid; this rapidly dissociates to CO_2 and water. If ventilation does not increase appropriately, an elevated PCO_2 will cause a decrease in pH. For this reason, sodium bicarbonate therapy is strictly contraindicated in patients with evidence of hypoventilation.

Of greater concern is the paradoxical intracellular acidosis that has been shown to occur after sodium bicarbonate administration. Bicarbonate cannot freely cross cell membranes, but the CO_2 produced as bicarbonate is metabolized can freely enter cells. Once intracellular, the CO_2 combines with water, leading to hydrogen ion release and causing intracellular acidosis. Many animal studies have demonstrated decreases in cellular and cerebrospinal fluid pH after bicarbonate therapy.[45-48] Bicarbonate therapy has also been associated with increases in blood lactate concentration in studies of lactic acidosis, hemorrhagic shock, and DKA.[43,46,49,50] The exact mechanism for this response is not known, but left shifting of the oxygen-hemoglobin dissociation curve because of increases in blood pH may play a role.

Sodium bicarbonate therapy can be associated with other adverse effects, including hypervolemia, hyperosmolality, hypernatremia, hypocalcemia (ionized), hypokalemia, and decreases in PaO_2 (see Box 54-5). The many potential negative consequences of sodium bicarbonate therapy must be weighed against the potential benefits when considering its use in the clinical setting. If a specific therapy exists for the underlying cause of a metabolic acidosis, this in combination with appropriate IV fluid therapy should be the focus of treatment and bicarbonate therapy is not indicated. This is particularly relevant to animals with lactic acidosis or DKA, where bicarbonate therapy has been associated with no improvement in outcome or clinical deterioration despite severe acidemia.[44,48] It is likely that bicarbonate therapy will be beneficial in the treatment of diseases causing bicarbonate loss, such as chronic kidney disease and diarrhea (an uncommon cause of metabolic acidosis in small animal patients).[51,52] The role of bicarbonate therapy in the management of patients with acute kidney injury (AKI) is less well defined.[53] Because renal replacement therapy is rarely available for veterinary patients, the use of bicarbonate for management of metabolic acidosis and hyperkalemia is a reasonable option, although caution must be used to avoid volume overload in the oliguric or anuric patient.

Dose and Administration

There is no exact method by which to determine a sodium bicarbonate dose. An approximate dose can be calculated from the following formula:

$$\text{Sodium Bicarbonate Dose (mmol)} = 0.3 \times \text{BW (kg)} \times \text{Base Deficit}$$

where 0.3 is an approximate value for the distribution of bicarbonate, BW(kg) is the patient body weight in kilograms, and base deficit (mmol/L) is a calculated value provided by the blood gas machine (or can be approximated by patient's measured bicarbonate concentration minus the normal bicarbonate concentration).

This dose would theoretically return the blood bicarbonate concentration back to normal. It is common practice to only give a portion of this calculated dose (50% to 80%) in order to avoid causing an iatrogenic metabolic alkalosis. This is of particular concern when other simultaneous therapies may contribute to resolution of the metabolic acidosis. Because there is no way to accurately determine an appropriate bicarbonate dose, bicarbonate therapy should be guided by frequent reevaluation of acid-base status.

Hypertonic sodium bicarbonate should never be administered rapidly (other than in the cardiopulmonary resuscitation setting) because it can cause vasodilation and increases in intracranial pressure, which can be fatal.[54] The clinician has the choice of giving the dose slowly (over 30 minutes or longer) or diluting it with sterile water to make it an isotonic solution. Dilution usually results in a significant volume for administration; the rate of infusion should then be governed by the perceived fluid tolerance of the patient. If the hypertonic sodium bicarbonate solution is not diluted to an osmolality of less than 600 mOsm/L, it should be given via a central catheter to avoid phlebitis.[55] The commercially available 8.4% sodium bicarbonate solution has an osmolality of approximately 2000 mOsm/L, so a dilution of 1 part sodium bicarbonate to 3 parts diluent (e.g., sterile water for injection) would be appropriate for peripheral venous administration.

Before giving sodium bicarbonate, clinicians should consider their level of concern for the increase in intravascular volume and the potential for hypernatremia, hyperosmolality, hypercapnia, hypokalemia, and hypocalcemia (ionized) in the patient. These concerns may necessitate initiating other therapy before bicarbonate administration, a very slow bicarbonate administration rate, or even withholding the therapy if the level of concern outweighs the proposed benefit of the drug.

REFERENCES

1. Arrhenius SA: On the dissociation of substances dissociated in water, Z Phys Chem 1:631, 1887.
2. Brønsted JN: Some remarks on the concept of acids and bases, Recueil des Travaux Chimiques des Pays-Bas 42:718, 1923.
3. Henderson JL: Das Gleichgewicht zwischen Basen Und Sauren im Tierischen Organismus, Ergebn Physiol 8:254, 1909.
4. Sørenson SPL: Uber die Messung und Beeutung der Wasserstoffionen-konzentration bei biologischen Prozessen, Ergebn Physiol 12:393, 1912.
5. Van Slyke DD: Studies of acidosis, J Biol Chem 495-498, 1922.
6. DiBartola SP: Introduction to acid-base disorders. In DiBartola SP, editor: Fluid, electrolyte and acid-base disorders, ed 4, St Louis, 2012, Saunders Elsevier, pp 231-252.
7. Masoro EJ, Siegel PD: Acid-base regulation: its physiology, pathophysiology and the interpretation of blood-gas analysis, ed 2, Philadelphia, 1977, WB Saunders, pp 1-25.
8. Ilkiw JE, Rose RJ, Martin ICA: A comparison of simultaneously collected arterial, mixed venous, jugular venous and cephalic venous blood samples and the assessment of blood-gas and acid-base status in the dog, J Vet Intern Med 5:294, 1991.
9. Yildizdas D, Yapicioglu H, Yilmaz HL, et al: Correlation of simultaneously obtained capillary, venous, and arterial blood gases of patients in a paediatric intensive care unit, Arch Dis Child 89:176, 2004.
10. Treger R, Pirouz S, Kamangar N, et al: Agreement between central venous and arterial blood gas measurements in the intensive care unit, Clin J Am Soc Nephrol 5:390, 2010.
11. Hopper K, Rezende ML, Haskins SC: The effect of dilution of blood samples with sodium heparin on blood gas, electrolyte and lactate measurements in dogs, A J Vet Res 66:656, 2006.
12. Rezende ML, Haskins SC, Hopper K: The effects of ice water storage on blood gas and acid-base measurements, J Vet Emerg Crit Care 17:67, 2007.
13. Picandet V, Jeanneret S, Lavoie JP: Effects of syringe type and storage temperature on results of blood gas analysis in arterial blood of horses, J Vet Intern Med 21:476, 2007.
14. Corey HE: Stewart and beyond: New models of acid-base balance, Kid Int 64:777, 2003.

15. Kellum JA: Determinants of plasma acid-base balance, Crit Care Clin 21:329, 2005.
16. Stewart PA: Modern quantitative acid base chemistry, Can J Physiol Pharmacol 61:1444, 1983.
17. Siggaard Andersen O: The acid-base status of the blood, Scand J Clin Lab Invest 15:1, 1963.
18. Constable PD: Clinical assessment of acid-base status: comparison of the Henderson-Hasselbalch and strong ion approaches, Vet Clin Pathol 29:115, 2000.
19. Figge J, Rossing TH, Fencl V: The role of serum proteins in acid-base equilibria, J Lab Clin Med 117:453, 1991.
20. Oh MS, Carroll HJ: The anion gap, N Engl J Med 297(15):814, 1977.
21. Feldman M, Soni N, Dickson B: Influence of hypoalbuminemia or hyperalbuminemia on the serum anion gap, J Lab Clin Med 146:317, 2005.
22. Corey HE: The anion gap (AG): studies in the nephrotic syndrome and diabetic ketoacidosis (DKA), J Lab Clin Med 147:121, 2006.
23. Pierce NF, Fedson DS, Brigham KL, et al: The ventilatory response to acute base deficit in humans. The time course during development and correction of metabolic acidosis, Ann Intern Med 72:633, 1970.
24. de Morais HSA, DiBartola SP: Ventilatory and metabolic compensation in dogs with acid-base disturbances, J Vet Emerg Crit Care 1:39, 1991.
25. Polak A, Haynie GD, Hays RM, et al: Effects of chronic hypercapnia on electrolyte and acid base equilibrium. I. Adaptation, J Clin Invest 40:1223, 1961.
26. Szlyk PC, Jennings DB: Effects of hypercapnia on variability of normal respiratory behavior in awake cats, Am J Physiol 21:R538, 1987.
27. Lemieux G, Lemieux C, Duplessis S, et al: Metabolic characteristics of cat kidney: failure to adapt to metabolic acidosis, Am J Physiol 28:R277, 1990.
28. Hampson NB, Jobsis-VanderVliet FF, Piantadosi CA: Skeletal muscle oxygen availability during respiratory acid-base disturbances in cats, Resp Physiol 70:143, 1987.
29. Ching SV, Fettman MJ, Hamar DW, et al: The effect of chronic dietary acidification using ammonium chloride on acid-base and mineral metabolism in the adult cat, J Nutr 119:902, 1989.
30. Lumb AB: Carbon dioxide. In Nunn's applied respiratory physiology, ed 7, Philadelphia, 2010, Churchill Livingston, p 159.
31. Lumb AB: Control of breathing. In Nunn's applied respiratory physiology, ed 7, Philadelphia, 2010, Churchill Livingston, pp 61-82.
32. Hopper K, Epstein SE: Incidence, nature and etiology of metabolic acidosis in dogs and cats, J Vet Intern Med 26:1107, 2012.
33. Ha YS, Hopper K, Epstein SE: Incidence, nature and etiology of metabolic alkalosis in dogs and cats, J Vet Intern Med 27(4):847-853,2013.
34. DiBartola SP: Metabolic acid-base disorders. In DiBartola SP, editor: Fluid, electrolyte and acid-base disorders, ed 4, St Louis, 2012, Saunders Elsevier, pp 253-286.
35. Galla JH: Metabolic alkalosis, J Am Soc Nephrol 11:369, 2000.
36. Rose BD, Post TW: Metabolic alkalosis. In Clinical physiology of acid-base and electrolyte disorders, ed 5, New York, 2001, McGraw-Hill, pp 551-577.
37. Gauthier PM, Szerlip HM: Metabolic acidosis in the intensive care unit, Crit Care Clin 18:289, 2002.
38. Gehlbach BK, Schmidt GA: Bench-to-bedside review: treating acid-base abnormalities in the intensive care unit—the role of buffers, Crit Care 8:259, 2004.
39. Thorsen K, Ringdal KG, Strand K, et al: Clinical and cellular effects of hypothermia, acidosis and coagulopathy in major injury, Br J Surg 98:894, 2011.
40. Thorens JB, Jolliet P, Ritz M, et al: Effects of rapid permissive hypercapnia on hemodynamics, gas exchange, and oxygen transport and consumption during mechanical ventilation for the acute respiratory distress syndrome, Intensive Care Med 22:182, 1996.
41. Viallon A, Zeni F, Lafond P, et al: Does bicarbonate therapy improve the management of severe diabetic ketoacidosis? Crit Care Med 27:2690, 1999.
42. Graf H, Leach W, Arieff AI: Evidence for a detrimental effect of bicarbonate therapy in hypoxic lactic acidosis, Science 227(4688):754, 1985.
43. Rhee KH, Toro LO, McDonald GG, et al: Carbicarb, sodium bicarbonate, and sodium chloride in hypoxic lactic acidosis. Effect on arterial blood gases, lactate concentrations, hemodynamic variables, and myocardial intracellular pH, Chest 104(3):913, 1993.
44. Cooper DJ, Walley KR, Wiggs BR, et al: Bicarbonate does not improve hemodynamics in critically ill patients who have lactic acidosis. A prospective, controlled clinical study, Ann Intern Med 112:492, 1990.
45. Bureau MA, Bégin R, Berthiaume Y, et al: Cerebral hypoxia from bicarbonate infusion in diabetic acidosis, J Pediatr 96:968, 1980.
46. Arieff AI, Leach W, Park R, et al: Systemic effects of $NaHCO_3$ in experimental lactic acidosis in dogs, Am J Physiol 242:F586, 1982.
47. Kucera RR, Shapiro JI, Whalen MA, et al: Brain pH effects of NaHCO3 and Carbicarb in lactic acidosis. Crit Care Med 17(12):1320, 1989.
48. Chua HR, Schneider A, Bellomo R: Bicarbonate in diabetic ketoacidosis—a systematic review, Ann Intensive Care 1:23, 2011.
49. Graf H, Leach W, Arieff AI: Metabolic effects of sodium bicarbonate in hypoxic lactic acidosis in dogs, Am J Physiol 249(5 Pt 2):F630, 1985.
50. Beech JS, Williams SC, Iles RA, et al: Haemodynamic and metabolic effects in diabetic ketoacidosis in rats of treatment with sodium bicarbonate or a mixture of sodium bicarbonate and sodium carbonate, Diabetologia 38(8):889, 1995.
51. Trefz FM, Lorch A, Feist M, et al: Construction and validation of a decision tree for treating metabolic acidosis in calves with neonatal diarrhea, BMC Vet Res 8:238, 2012.
52. Kraut JA, Madias NE: Consequences and therapy of the metabolic acidosis of chronic kidney disease, Pediatr Nephrol 26(1):19, 2011.
53. Hewitt J, Uniacke M, Hansi NK, et al: Sodium bicarbonate supplements for treating acute kidney injury, Cochrane Database Syst Rev 6:CD009204, 2012.
54. Huseby JS, Gumprecht DG: Hemodynamic effects of rapid bolus hypertonic sodium bicarbonate, Chest 79(5):552, 1981.
55. Kuwahara T, Asanami S, Kubo S: Experimental infusion phlebitis: tolerance osmolality of peripheral venous endothelial cell, Nutrition 14:496, 1988.

CHAPTER 55

NONTRADITIONAL ACID-BASE ANALYSIS

Kate Hopper, BVSc, PhD, DACVECC

KEY POINTS

- The nontraditional approaches to acid-base analysis may provide greater insight to the underlying mechanisms of metabolic acid-base abnormalities.
- The Stewart approach identifies three independent determinants of acid-base balance: partial pressure of carbon dioxide (PCO_2), strong ion difference (SID), and total weak acids (A_{TOT}).
- Strong ion gap (SIG) is the Stewart measure of unmeasured anions or cations and is not affected by changes in albumin concentration.
- The semi-quantitative approach to acid-base analysis calculates the effects of five parameters on base excess: free water (marked by sodium concentration), changes in chloride concentration, albumin, phosphate, and lactate.
- The parameter XA is the semi-quantitative evaluation of unmeasured anions or cations.

Acid-base analysis involves evaluation of both the respiratory and metabolic contributions to blood pH. Evaluation of respiratory acid-base balance is similar across all diagnostic approaches (see Chapter 54). The nontraditional or quantitative approaches to acid-base analysis provide alternative methods to evaluate the metabolic contribution. The major criticism of the traditional approach to metabolic acid-base disorders is its failure to identify individual disease processes that contribute to a metabolic acid-base abnormality. The nontraditional approaches may provide greater insight to underlying causes of metabolic acid-base abnormalities.

THE STEWART APPROACH

According to the Stewart approach there are three independent determinants of acid-base balance: partial pressure of carbon dioxide (PCO_2); the difference between strong cations and strong anions, known as the strong ion difference (SID); and total weak acids (A_{TOT}).[1] The quantity of hydrogen (or bicarbonate) ions added to, or removed from, the system is not considered relevant to the final pH because hydrogen ion concentration is not an "independent" variable. SID and A_{TOT} are proposed to affect hydrogen ion concentration directly by altering the dissociation of water via electrochemical forces. Ultimately the Stewart approach is able to identify five metabolic acid-base abnormalities (Box 55-1).[2]

Strong Ion Difference

Strong ions are ions that are fully dissociated at physiologic pH. The major strong ions include sodium, potassium, calcium, magnesium, and chloride. Some authors include other anions as strong ions, such as lactate and ketoacids. The formula used to calculate SID is based on the total quantity of strong cations minus the quantity of strong anions. The exact formula used varies depending on the ions included in the calculation.[2,3] Quantitatively, sodium and chloride are the most important strong ions in the body and SID is commonly simplified as the difference between serum sodium and chloride concentrations. It is important to note that changes in SID will reflect changes in bicarbonate concentration if A_{TOT} remains constant (Figure 55-1).

A decreased SID metabolic acidosis can be due to hyponatremia, hyperchloremia, or a combination of the two. Conversely, an increased SID metabolic alkalosis may be due to hypernatremia, hypochloremia, or both. Treatment of abnormalities in SID generally focuses on fluid therapy to restore SID to normal. The SID of intravenous fluids can be determined as it is for plasma. This value can help guide fluid selection for patients with SID abnormalities. For example, a patient with an increased SID alkalosis may benefit from a fluid with a low SID such as 0.9% saline (SID = 0). In contrast, a patient with a decreased SID acidosis may be best treated with an IV fluid with a higher SID such as lactated Ringer's with an effective SID of approximately 28 mmol/L (after the lactate is metabolized).[4] Sodium bicarbonate is a fluid with a very high SID because bicarbonate is not counted as having any effect. As a result, sodium bicarbonate with a concentration of 2000 mmol/L has a SID of approximately 2000 mmol/L and is therefore considered an effective treatment of

BOX 55-1 *Metabolic Acid-Base Abnormalities Identified by the Stewart Approach*

- Increased SID metabolic alkalosis
- Decreased SID metabolic acidosis
- Increased A_{TOT} metabolic acidosis
- Decreased A_{TOT} metabolic alkalosis
- Increased SIG metabolic acidosis

SID, Strong ion difference; *A_{TOT},* total weak acids; *SIG,* strong ion gap.

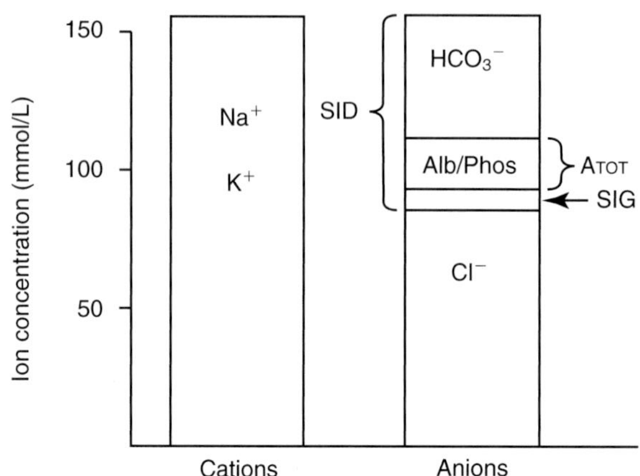

FIGURE 55-1 Gamblegram of normal plasma ion concentration. *Alb/Phos,* Albumin and phosphate concentration; *A_{TOT},* total weak acid concentration; *Cl^-,* chloride concentration; *K^+,* potassium concentration; *Na^+,* sodium concentration; *SID,* strong ion difference; *SIG,* strong ion gap.

patients with a low-SID metabolic acidosis. Further details regarding its use can be found later in this chapter.

Total Weak Acids (A_{TOT})

Weak acids are only partially dissociated at physiologic pH. The major contributors to A_{TOT} are albumin and phosphate. Because the dissociation of these substances varies with pH, there are complex formulas to calculate A_{TOT}.[2,3,5] Constable and colleagues have also developed simplified equations to estimate the plasma protein contribution to A_{TOT} using a species-specific dissociation constant (K_a), for dogs and cats. For dogs the net protein charge is 0.25 mEq/g for total protein or 0.42 mEq/g for albumin. The net protein charge for cats is 0.19 mEq/g of total protein or 0.41 mEq/g of albumin.[6,7] Because A_{TOT} represents a value for weak acids, increases in A_{TOT} indicate a metabolic acidosis and decreases in A_{TOT} (primarily from decreased albumin) indicate a metabolic alkalosis.

Treatment of abnormalities of A_{TOT} aim to normalize the levels of albumin and phosphate when possible.

Strong Ion Gap

The strong ion gap (SIG) is the Stewart evaluation of unmeasured anions in a manner similar to the use of anion gap (AG) in traditional acid-base analysis. Readers are directed to Chapter 54 for an explanation of AG. The SIG can be calculated from the SID minus the contribution of bicarbonate and A_{TOT}. As the Gamblegram in Figure 55-1 demonstrates, if there are no unmeasured anions (SIG = 0) in the system, the SID should equal the sum of the contributions of bicarbonate and A_{TOT}. If unmeasured cations are present in the system, this reduces the value determined for SIG. A simplified formula for the calculation of SIG has been developed by Constable for dogs as $SIG_{simplified} = ([alb] \times 4.9) - AG$; for cats it is $SIG_{simplified} = ([alb] \times 7.4) - AG$.[6,7] This simplified approach does not account for changes in phosphate concentration; in the presence of hyperphosphatemia the $SIG_{simplified}$ is determined by first modifying the AG equation with the following formula[6-8]:

$$AG_{\text{phosphate adjusted}} = AG + (2.52 - 0.58 \times [\text{phosphate}])$$

Increases in SIG, like increases in AG, reflect the presence of unmeasured anions (e.g., lactate, sulfates, ethylene glycol, ketones, etc.), which are assumed to have an acidifying influence on the system. There are many different formulas for determination of SIG in the literature, some of which include additional anions, such as lactate, and therefore affect interpretation of the SIG. A major advantage of SIG over AG is that it is independent of changes in albumin concentration. As a result, SIG is more sensitive to the presence of unmeasured anions in hypoalbuminemic patients.

A full explanation of the Stewart approach is beyond the scope of this chapter, and the interested reader is directed to references 2 and 3 for further discussion of the topic.

SEMI-QUANTITATIVE APPROACH

Several researchers have developed a clinical approach to acid-base analysis that is a combination of the traditional and Stewart methods.[9-12] This approach has been variably called the Stewart-Fencl approach, the Stewart-Figge approach, semi-quantitative analysis, and base excess partitioning. In this chapter the term *semi-quantitative metabolic acid-base analysis* is used.

This approach uses equations to estimate the magnitude of effect of individual acid-base processes on base excess (BE); each acid-base process is represented by one of five parameters. These parameters are as follows: (1) a free water effect (marked by sodium concentration), (2) an effect represented by changes in chloride concentration, (3) an albumin effect, (4) a phosphate effect, and (5) a lactate effect. Differences between the sum total of all these known, calculated effects and the BE are attributed to the presence of unmeasured (unknown) acids or bases. The formulas used to determine these effects are provided in Table 55-1.[12,13] A simplified or shorthand version of these formulas is provided in Table 55-2. These can be used to make a rough estimate of these parameters and allow clinical application of this approach without use of a computer spreadsheet. Semi-quantitative acid-base analysis as presented here requires measurement of pH and PCO_2, determination of BE, and measurement of as many of the following parameters as possible: sodium, chloride, albumin, lactate, and phosphate. From these measured parameters, 10 metabolic acid-base influences can be identified and the magnitude of their contribution to the overall BE estimated. Negative contributions indicate an acidotic influence on BE, whereas a positive calculated effect indicates an alkalotic influence.

Table 55-1 Formulas for Calculation of Semi-quantitative Acid-Base Parameters

Parameter	Formula
Free water effect	
Dogs	0.25([Na^+] − mid-normal [Na^+])
Cats	0.22([Na^+] − mid-normal [Na^+])
Corrected chloride	Measured [Cl^-] × (mid-normal [Na^+]/ measured [Na^+])
Chloride effect	Mid-normal [Cl^-] − corrected [Cl^-]
Phosphate effect	0.58 (mid-normal [phosphate] − measured [phosphate])
Albumin effect	3.7(mid-normal [albumin] − measured [albumin])
Lactate effect	−1 × [lactate]
Sum of effects	Free water effect + chloride effect + phosphate effect + albumin effect + lactate effect
Unmeasured ion effect	Base excess − sum of effects

[albumin], Albumin concentration in g/dl; Base excess in mmol/L; *[Cl^-],* chloride concentration in mmol/L; *[K^+],* potassium concentration in mmol/L; *[lactate],* lactate concentration in mmol/L; *[Na^+],* sodium concentration in mmol/L; *[phosphate],* phosphate concentration in mg/dl.

Table 55-2 Suggested Shorthand Formulas for Estimation of Semi-quantitative Acid-Base Effects

Effect	Shorthand Formula
Free water effect	(Measured sodium − Normal sodium) / 4
Corrected chloride	Measured chloride × (Normal sodium / Measured sodium)
Chloride effect	Normal chloride − Corrected chloride
Albumin effect	(Normal albumin − Measured albumin) × 4
Phosphate effect	(Normal phosphate − Measured phosphate) / 2
Lactate effect	Measured lactate × −1
Sum	Free water effect + Chloride effect + Albumin effect + Phosphate effect + Lactate effect
XA (Unmeasured)	Base Excess − Sum

Free Water Effect

The free water effect on BE is due to changes in the water balance. Clinically, the free water concentration is marked by sodium concentration; a deficit of free water causing hypernatremia and an excess of free water causing hyponatremia. An excess of free water (hyponatremia) will be evident by a negative free water effect indicating an acidotic effect—a dilutional acidosis. A deficit of free water (hypernatremia) will be evident by a positive free water effect indicating an alkalotic effect—a contraction alkalosis.[14]

Chloride Effect

In many processes within the body, chloride and bicarbonate are reciprocally linked (i.e., when a chloride ion is excreted, a bicarbonate ion is retained and vice versa). Such processes include gastric acid secretion, intestinal bicarbonate secretion, renal acid-base handling, and transcellular ion exchange. Evaluation of the change in chloride concentration can therefore be used to estimate the contribution to BE made by these processes. Because chloride concentration will also be altered by changes in free water concentration, it needs to be corrected before calculation of the chloride effect. The formula for determining the corrected chloride value (that is the value of chloride for the patient if there is no change in free water balance) is provided in Table 55-2. The difference between this corrected chloride concentration and the patient's normal chloride concentration (the mid-normal value for chloride for that species is usually used) estimates the contribution to BE by processes associated with the change in chloride concentration (see Table 55-1).

An increased (positive) chloride effect is associated with a process that increases bicarbonate concentration and is indicative of an alkalotic process; a decreased chloride effect (negative) marks an acidotic process (see Table 55-2).

Albumin Effect

Albumin acts as a weak acid. It has many H^+ binding sites associated with the imidazole group of the amino acid histidine. Hypoalbuminemia is equivalent to the removal of a weak acid from the system; it is evident as a positive effect and indicates an alkalotic effect. Conversely, hyperalbuminemia will be evident as a negative effect, indicating an acidotic influence.[6,11]

Phosphate Effect

Phosphoric and sulfuric acids are products of protein metabolism and are normally excreted by the kidneys. Patients with acute kidney injury or failure retain these acids, resulting in a metabolic acidosis. The phosphoric acid contribution toward BE, from a given inorganic phosphorus concentration, is determined by use of the equation in Table 55-1. Elevated phosphorus will cause a negative effect and indicates an acidotic influence on BE. Because serum phosphorus concentration is normally low, hypophosphatemia does not cause a clinically significant alkalosis. Sulfate is not usually measured and is therefore one of the unmeasured anions.

Lactate Effect

In acute clinical scenarios of lactic acidosis caused by anaerobic metabolism, lactate has an equimolar effect on BE (see Table 55-1). Elevations in lactate concentration will be evident as a negative calculated effect—an acidotic influence on BE. There are causes of hyperlactatemia that are associated with little or no acidosis, such as cytokine or catecholamine stimulation of glycolytic rate.[15] In addition, blood samples contaminated with sodium lactate (e.g., from lactated Ringer's) will also show an increase in lactate with no acidosis.[16] As a result, some clinical judgment is required when including the lactate value in the calculations.

Unmeasured Ions (XA)

The quantitative approach identifies many of the relevant contributors to the metabolic acid-base component. The difference between the sum of these identified effects and the patient's BE represents unidentified acids or bases contributing to the acid-base equilibrium (see Table 55-1). Unmeasured acids include ketoacids, sulfuric acid, ethylene glycol, salicylic acid, propylene glycol, and metaldehyde. As with the SIG value, the parameter XA is not affected by changes in albumin concentration, making it a more sensitive measure of unmeasured anions.

CONCLUSION

The major advantage of the Stewart and semi-quantitative approaches is the ability to recognize underlying mechanisms of acid-base disorders, in particular the effect of changes in albumin concentration. Although the nontraditional approaches cannot recognize compensatory changes to primary respiratory acid-base disorders, all changes in the metabolic system will be identified as pathologic. The Stewart approach is far more confusing and intimidating than the traditional approach for clinicians to use; it requires measurement of albumin and phosphorus concentration and really is best used with a computer spreadsheet. It is unknown if the increase in cost and complexity of this approach has sufficient clinical benefit to warrant its routine use. The semi-quantitative approach is also more complex than the traditional approach, although use of the simplified formulas may allow it to be more readily applied in the clinical setting. Another limitation of the Stewart approach is that SID and A_{TOT} are aggregate indices, much like anion gap. They will reflect general acid-base abnormalities, but unfortunately they are not specific. The semi-quantitative approach may provide a more useful clinical approach to acid-base analysis because it attempts to recognize the individual role of specific disease mechanisms. The semi-quantitative approach calculates small acid-base effects for each parameter. It is important to recognize that the inherent degree of error for each laboratory value could contribute to variability in these results. The semi-quantitative approach has not been validated in dogs and cats.

CLINICAL EXAMPLES

Case 1

A 13-year-old female spayed Terrier cross dog is presented with the history of vomiting and collapse. The bloodwork provided in Table 55-3 was obtained at presentation.

The traditional acid-base diagnosis of this case is a mixed disorder with a concurrent respiratory alkalosis and a metabolic acidosis resulting in a normal pH. The anion gap is slightly lower than the reference range. The Stewart approach reveals little more than the traditional approach in this case with essentially normal values for SID, A_{TOT}, and SIG. The abnormalities in chloride and sodium concentration lead to a mildly decreased SID, suggesting an acidotic process. It is interesting to note that the alkalotic influence of the hypoalbuminemia is counteracted by the acidotic influence of the hyperphosphatemia, resulting in an almost normal value for A_{TOT}.

In comparison, the semi-quantitative approach reveals a mild alkalotic effect attributable to a small free water deficit, an acidosis associated with bicarbonate-chloride exchange, and an acidosis caused by hyperphosphatemia. The hypoalbuminemia is exerting a strong alkalotic influence, which is reducing the severity of the metabolic acidosis. The sum of effects accounts for the majority of the BE with little suggestion of the presence of unmeasured ions. The semi-quantitative approach identified several contributors of acid-base abnormalities in this example, whereas the Stewart approach

Table 55-3 Clinical Examples of Acid-Base Abnormalities

Parameter	Case 1: Dog	Case 2: Cat
Sodium mmol/L	152 (144-152)	194 (148-156)
Potassium mmol/L	3 (3.6-4.7)	4.2 (3.4-4.7)
Chloride mmol/L	125 (111-121)	156 (115-126)
Albumin g/dl	1.1 (3.4-4.3)	4.2 (2.2-4.6)
Phosphorus* mg/dl	12.1 (2.6-5.2)	5.9 (3.2-6.3)
pH	7.383 (7.32-7.43)	7.241 (7.34-7.43)
$PvCO_2$ mmHg	28 (37-45)	45.5 (34-39)
Bicarbonate mmol/L	16 (18-26)	18.6 (20-23)
BE mmol/L	−7.8 (−4 to −1)	−7.3 (−5 to 0)
Lactate mmol/L	1.1 (<2)	1.2 (< 2)
Calculated Acid-Base Values (mmol/L)		
Corrected chloride	122	122
Anion gap	14 (8-16)	24 (16-20)
SID	30 (32-45)	42 (40-44)
A_{TOT}	9.8 (10-11)	14.3 (8-17)
SIG	6 (0-8)	14.3 (6-9)
Free water effect	1	9.4
Chloride effect	−6	2
Lactate effect	−1.1	−1.2
Albumin effect	7.2	−2.1
Phosphorus effect	−3.6	−0.6
Sum	−5.1	7.5
XA	−2.7	−14.8

A_{TOT}, Quantity of weak acids, was calculated as (measured albumin × [(0.123 × pH) − 0.631] × 10) + (measured phosphorus × 0.323 × [(0.309 × pH) − 0.469]). *SID*, strong ion difference, calculated as (Na^+ + K^+) − (Cl^-); *SIG*, strong ion gap, calculated as [SID − ([HCO_3^-] + A_{TOT})]; *XA*, unmeasured ion effect. Calculation of semi-quantitative parameters were based on formulas shown in Table 55-1.
*Phosphorus is interchangeable with phosphate.

suggested an essentially normal metabolic acid-base balance. This dog was ultimately diagnosed with pancreatitis and pyelonephritis.

Case 2

An 8-year-old female spayed cat with a 1-year history of diabetes mellitus is presented for ataxia and inappetence. The initial bloodwork is provided in Table 55-3.

The traditional approach reveals a mixed disorder of both respiratory acidosis and metabolic acidosis with an elevated anion gap. The Stewart approach shows an increased SID metabolic alkalosis, a normal A_{TOT}, and an increased SIG metabolic acidosis. The high SID is attributable to a hypernatremia of greater magnitude than the hyperchloremia, suggestive of a contraction alkalosis. The elevation in SIG suggests unmeasured anions such as lactate, sulfate, or ketoacids. Because lactate concentration is normal in this case, it is not a possible unmeasured anion.

The semi-quantitative approach shows a substantial alkalotic effect on BE from free water loss, a small acidotic effect from albumin, and a large unmeasured anion quantity. This case is a good example of the value of correcting the chloride concentration for changes in free water balance. At first glance the measured hyperchloremia of this cat might suggest a hyperchloremic metabolic acidosis, but once the influence of free water loss is accounted for, there is little abnormality in the patient's chloride concentration. This animal would clearly benefit from free water administration and, given the history of diabetes mellitus, further evaluation for ketoacids would be recommended given the large quantity of unmeasured anions evident. This cat was found to have diabetic ketoacidosis.

REFERENCES

1. Stewart PA: Modern quantitative acid-base chemistry, Can J Physiol Pharmacol 61:1444, 1983.
2. Kellum JA: Determinants of plasma acid-base balance, Crit Care Clin 21:329, 2005.
3. Constable PD: Clinical assessment of acid-base status: comparison of the Henderson-Hasselbalch and strong ion approaches, Vet Clin Pathol 29:115, 2000.
4. Morgan TJ, Balasubramanian V, Hall J: Crystalloid strong ion difference determines metabolic acid-base change during in vitro hemodilution, Crit Care Med 30:157, 2002.
5. Figge J, Mydosh T, Fencl V: Serum proteins and acid-base equilibria: a follow-up, J Lab Clin Med 120:713, 1992.
6. Constable PD, Stampfli HR: Experimental determination of net protein charge and Atot and Ka of nonvolatile buffers in canine plasma, J Vet Intern Med 19:507, 2005.
7. McCullough SM, Constable PD: Calculation of the total plasma concentration of nonvolatile weak acids and the effective dissociation constant of nonvolatile buffers in plasma for use in the strong ion approach to acid-base balance in cats, Am J Vet Res 64:1047, 2003.
8. Kaae J, de Morais HA: Anion gap and strong ion gap: a quick reference, Vet Clin Small Anim 38:443, 2008.
9. Fencl V, Rossing TH: Acid-base disorders in critical care medicine, Annu Rev Med 40:17, 1989.
10. Fencl V, Jabor A, Kazda A, et al: Diagnosis of metabolic acid-base disturbances in critically ill patients, Am J Respir Crit Care Med 162:2246, 2000.
11. Figge J, Rossing TH, Fencl V: The role of serum proteins in acid-base equilibria, J Lab Clin Med 117:453, 1991.
12. Leith DE: The new acid-base; power and simplicity, Proceedings of the 9th ACVIM Forum, New Orleans, 1991, pp 611-617.
13. de Morais HAS: A nontraditional approach to acid-base disorders. In DiBartola SP, editor: Fluid therapy in small animal practice, ed 1, Philadelphia, 1992, WB Saunders, pp 297-320.
14. Haskins SC, Hopper K, Rezende ML: The acid-base impact of free water removal from, and addition to, plasma, J Lab Clin Med 147:114, 2006.
15. Mizock BA: Controversies in lactic acidosis: implications in critically ill patients, J Am Med Assoc 258:497-501, 1987.
16. Jackson EV, Wiese J, Sigal B, et al: Effects of crystalloid solutions on circulating lactate concentrations. Part 1: Implications for the proper handling of blood specimens obtained from critically ill patients, Crit Care Med 25:1840-1846, 1997.

CHAPTER 56
HYPERLACTATEMIA

Patricia G. Rosenstein, DVM • Dez Hughes, BVSc, MRCVS, DACVECC

KEY POINTS

- Plasma lactate is a late but quantitative indicator of tissue hypoperfusion and can be used as a prognostic indicator and a treatment guide.
- Lactate is an intermediary metabolite of glucose oxidation that serves as a carbohydrate energy substrate reservoir.
- Lactate production is an adaptive and protective response to cellular energy deficiency that allows rapid or continued energy production when cellular energy requirements exceed the capacity of cellular aerobic respiration.

INTRODUCTION

The main use of plasma lactate concentration in clinical practice is as an adjunct to a shrewd physical examination to detect and monitor hypoperfusion. The clinical utility of lactate was first recognized after the First World War and reported definitively in 1964.[1] Its use became widespread in human and veterinary medicine in the 1990s with the advent of cheaper and simpler assays. Once considered a dead-end waste product of anaerobiosis, lactate is now recognized as an integral part of the cellular energy shuttle and as a metabolic regulator.

BIOCHEMISTRY

Lactate and lactic acid are not synonymous. Lactic acid, $CH_3CH(OH)COOH$, is a strong acid that at physiologic pH is almost completely dissociated to the lactate anion, $CH_3CH(OH)COO^-$ and H^+. Increased plasma lactate concentration is termed hyperlactatemia, which may or may not be associated with a net acidemia depending on the cause of the increased lactate, concurrent acid/base disturbances, and buffer reserves.

Glycolysis is the cytosolic process by which 1 mole of glucose is oxidized to 2 moles of pyruvate, adenosine triphosphate (ATP), and reduced nicotinamide adenine dinucleotide (NADH). Pyruvate enters the mitochondria and is converted into acetyl CoA, which then proceeds through the tricarboxylic acid (TCA) cycle, the electron transport chain, and oxidative phosphorylation to produce 36 moles of ATP (Figure 56-1). Under normal aerobic conditions only a small quantity of pyruvate is converted into lactate, catalyzed by lactate dehydrogenase (LDH) (see Figure 56-1). Lactate may then be either transported out of the cell or used within the same cell. Ultimately lactate is either converted back into pyruvate in local or distant tissues and oxidized to produce energy or converted back into glucose by gluconeogenesis.

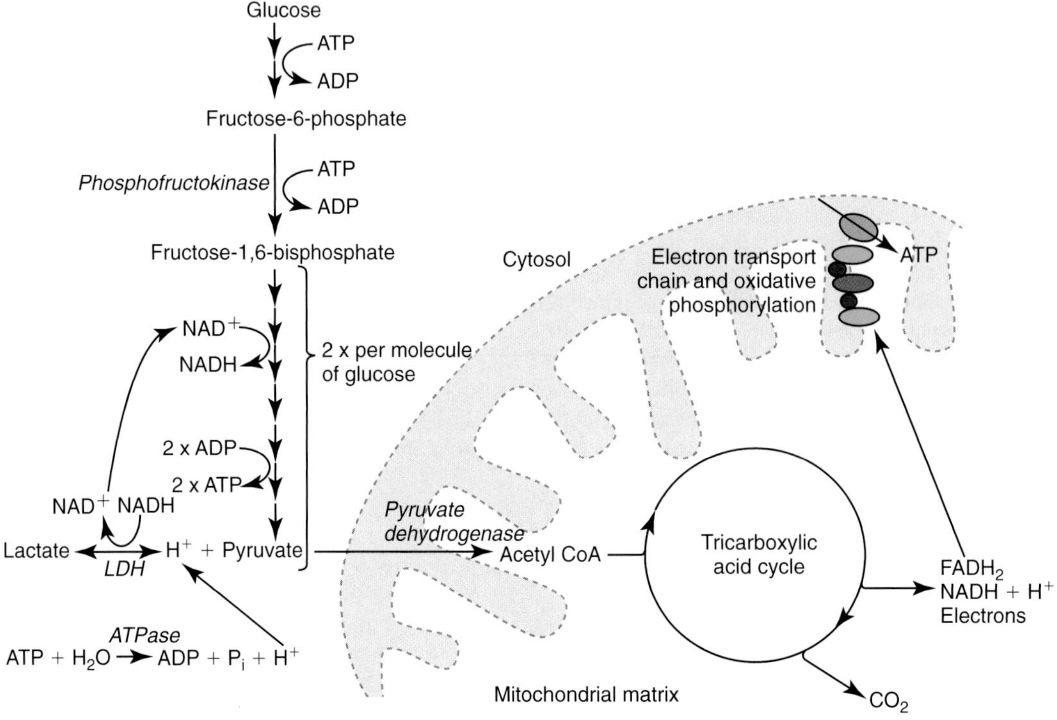

FIGURE 56-1 The biochemical pathways of cellular energy production: glycolysis, lactate production, the tricarboxylic acid cycle, oxidative phosphorylation, and the electron transport chain.

Glycolysis consumes NAD^+ and produces NADH and pyruvate. If there is a cellular oxygen deficiency, the TCA cycle and oxidative phosphorylation are slowed so NAD^+ falls and pyruvate and NADH build up, thereby hindering ongoing glycolysis. To allow glycolysis to continue, NAD^+ is replenished and pyruvate and H^+ ions are removed by conversion of pyruvate to lactate. Although glycolysis produces only 2 moles of ATP, it is very fast and so can temporarily satisfy energy demands.

Contrary to popular belief, the metabolic acidosis associated with lactate production is due to ATP use, not lactate production.[2] Glycolysis produces the lactate ion rather than lactic acid.[3] When the ATP made by glycolysis is utilized, H^+ is released into the cytosol. This proton would usually enter the mitochondrion and be used to maintain the proton gradient required for the electron transport chain and oxidative phosphorylation. When oxygen supplies are insufficient this cannot happen and H^+ ions accumulate and are then transported out of the cell. Hence, the acidosis from increased lactate production mostly is due to reduced H^+ consumption, not increased lactate production per se. Nevertheless, stoichiometrically, in acute anaerobic states, 1 mmol/L of lactate is associated with an equimolar production of H^+ ions and a concomitant reduction of the standardized base excess of 1 mmol/L. There are clinical states in which increased lactate production occurs while H^+ consumption by the mitochondria in maintained. The result will be hyperlactatemia without concurrent acidosis. This is discussed further later in this chapter.

PHYSIOLOGY

Lactate Pharmacokinetics in Health

Lactate is produced in the cytosol and then either converted back to pyruvate to proceed through local aerobic cellular metabolism or exported out of the cell and transported to distant tissues in the bloodstream. Although all tissues are capable of producing lactate, in resting conditions the majority of lactate production occurs in skeletal muscle, skin, brain, and erythrocytes by virtue of their inherent production capacities and mass relative to body weight.[4] Under conditions of health and aerobiosis, the liver and renal cortex are the predominant lactate-consuming organs. Hepatic metabolism accounts for 50% to 70% of lactate consumption, and the liver is capable of metabolizing markedly increased lactate loads.[5-7] The renal cortex metabolizes 25% to 30% of circulating lactate.[8-10] In keeping with its role as a carbohydrate energy substrate (essentially half a glucose molecule), lactate is not excreted in the urine until its plasma concentration is high. It is reabsorbed by the proximal convoluted tubule, and the renal threshold is 6 to 10 mmol/L.[11,12]

Lactate Pharmacokinetics in Disease

Tissue lactate production, distribution, metabolism, consumption, and excretion are different in disease states compared with normal homeostasis in healthy animals. During global hypoperfusion, lactate production in tissue beds depends on whether the blood flow is reduced or selectively preserved. In dogs with hypovolemia the splanchnic circulation, skin, subcutaneous tissue, and skeletal muscle produce the majority of lactate. Local disease can also affect tissue lactate production, for example, in acute lung injury the lungs increase lactate production.[13-15] During hyperlactatemia, some tissues, such as skeletal muscle, cardiac muscle, and brain tissue, increase their lactate uptake.[11,12,16-18] The liver continues to extract lactate until hepatic blood flow is less than 30% of normal,[19] but it can actually become a net lactate producer with poor perfusion, severe hypoxia, or hepatic failure.[16,19-21]

Lactate produced by tissues is exported by the cell into the interstitium, then passes into plasma. Once in plasma it then equilibrates with the intracellular space of erythrocytes. *Whole blood lactate* refers to the sum of intraerythrocytic and plasma lactate. Almost all analyzers measure lactate from plasma even though whole blood is aspirated by the machine.

ETIOLOGY OF HYPERLACTATEMIA

Hyperlactatemia is one of the most common conditions associated with metabolic acidosis in the dog and cat and occurs when lactate production exceeds consumption. "Lactic acidosis" has been defined as hyperlactatemia with a concurrent metabolic acidosis.

In 1961 Huckabee divided hyperlactatemia into type I, in which increased lactate occurred without an associated metabolic acidosis, and type II, defined as increased lactate with a concurrent metabolic acidosis.[22] Type II hyperlactatemia (lactic acidosis) was further classified into two categories: type A and type B. Type A (the most common) occurs with clinical evidence of a relative or absolute tissue oxygen deficiency. Type B occurs in the absence of clinical evidence of decreased oxygen delivery (Table 56-1).[23] Type A and B may exist concurrently. Clinical experience suggests that type B usually results in a mild to moderate increase in lactate (3 to 6 mmol/L). Conversely, severe hyperlactatemia (>6 mmol/L) usually is due to global hypoperfusion.

Type A Hyperlactatemia

Increased oxygen demand

Common causes of increased oxygen demand relate to muscle activity such as exercise, struggling, shivering, trembling, tremors, and seizures. Exercise-related hyperlactatemia ranges from 4.5 mmol/L in dogs after agility testing[24] to more than 30 mmol/L in racing Greyhounds.[25,26] Physiologic hyperlactatemia should resolve uneventfully once muscle activity ceases, with an elimination half-life of 30 to 60 minutes.[24,25,27] If resolution does not occur in a clinical patient within this time frame, a concurrent disease process is likely.

Decreased oxygen delivery

Hyperlactatemia is most commonly associated with decreased oxygen delivery secondary to systemic hypoperfusion (i.e., hypovolemic, maldistributive, cardiogenic, or obstructive shock). In dogs, progressively worsening hypoperfusion appears to demonstrate a fairly linear relationship with plasma lactate concentration. Mild hypoperfusion is associated with lactate concentrations of 3 to 4 mmol/L, moderate with 4 to 6 mmol/L, and severe with a plasma lactate concentration greater than 6 mmol/L. Anecdotal clinical experience suggest that cats demonstrate an exponential increase with a lesser increase in mild and moderate hypoperfusion, then a rapid rise when it is severe.

As would be expected, hyperlactatemia is a late indicator of hypoperfusion because lactate production does not occur until oxygen extraction has been maximized. Just as we recognize that falling blood pressure is a late indicator of hypovolemia, so is hyperlactatemia, a corollary being that subclinical hypoperfusion may exist with a normal blood lactate concentration.

Hyperlactatemia in normotensive, normovolemic patients caused by decreased oxygen content and oxygen delivery as a result of anemic or hypoxic hypoxia is rare. Anemia-related hyperlactatemia is highly dependent on intravascular volume status and chronicity. In experimental, acute, severe, euvolemic anemia, hyperlactatemia does not develop until the packed cell volume (PCV) drops below 15%.[28] Dogs and cats with chronic, euvolemic anemia may remain eulactatemic with a PCV of 10% or less. Dogs with anemia from hemolysis caused by immune-mediated hemolytic anemia (IMHA) have been reported to have hyperlactatemia, although this could also have been secondary to concurrent hypoperfusion.[29,30] Similarly, hypoxemia must also be severe (PaO_2 25 to 40 mm Hg) before pure hypoxemia-related hyperlactatemia develops.[23,28] Hence, hypoxia

Table 56-1 **Causes of Hyperlactatemia**

Type A Hyperlactatemia	
Increased Oxygen Demand*	**Decreased Oxygen Delivery**
Exercise	Systemic hypoperfusion*
Trembling/shivering	Local hypoperfusion
Muscle tremors	Severe anemia
Seizure activity	Severe hypoxemia
Struggling	Carbon monoxide poisoning

Type B Hyperlactatemia			
B_1: Associated with Underlying Disease	**B_2: Associated with Drugs or Toxins**		**B_3: Inborn Errors in Metabolism**
Sepsis/SIRS*	Acetaminophen	Halothane	Mitochondrial myopathies
Neoplasia	Activated charcoal	Insulin	Enzymatic deficiencies
Diabetes mellitus	β_2 Agonists	Lactulose	MELAS
Severe liver disease	Bicarbonate	Methanol	(mitochondrial encephalomyopathy,
Thiamine deficiency	Catecholamines	Morphine	lactic acidosis, and strokelike
Pheochromocytoma	Corticosteroids*	Nitroprusside	episodes)
	Cyanide	Salicylates	Miscellaneous
	Ethanol	Strychnine	D-lactic acidosis
	Ethylene glycol	Terbutaline	
	Propofol	Theophylline	
	Propylene glycol	TPN	
	Glucose	Xylitol	

SIRS, Systemic inflammatory response syndrome; *TPN,* total parenteral nutrition.
*Most commonly recognized.

should only rarely be considered as a sole diagnosis for increased lactate.

Local hypoperfusion, such as occurs with aortic thromboembolism or organ volvulus, causes local increases in lactate concentration in the veins draining that tissue. However, the effect on systemic plasma lactate concentration varies according to the remaining blood flow through the ischemic tissue and therefore how much lactate is washed into circulation. If there is little washout, then systemic lactate may not increase appreciably. Clinical experience suggests that organ torsion such as lung lobes, liver lobes, or spleens do not release much lactate and the systemic lactate concentration actually reflects the global perfusion status.

Type B Hyperlactatemia

Type B hyperlactatemia has conventionally been divided into three subcategories (see Table 56-1). Type B_1 is associated with underlying disease, B_2 with drugs or toxins, and B_3 with congenital or hereditary metabolic defects.

Type B_1

Hyperlactatemia occurs commonly in sepsis, systemic inflammatory response syndrome (SIRS), and septic shock and may persist despite aggressive correction of hypoperfusion, anemia, and hypoxemia.[31]

The pathophysiology of sepsis-associated hyperlactatemia is complex and multifactorial. Suggested mechanisms include skeletal muscle Na^+/K^+-ATPase upregulation[32]; mitochondrial dysfunction, including direct cytochrome inhibition[33]; increased hepatic lactate production; reduced hepatic lactate extraction[34]; impaired tissue oxygen extraction[35]; and capillary shunting.[35] Enhanced nitric oxide production, altered neurohormonal control of endothelial smooth muscle, reduced erythrocyte flexibility, increased leukocyte activation, and pyruvate dehydrogenase (PDH) inhibition[36,37] have also been implicated.

Hyperlactatemia associated with neoplasia may be due to hypoperfusion in some cases, but malignant cells are known to exhibit atypical carbohydrate metabolism by preferentially utilizing glycolytic pathways for energy production despite oxygen availability (Warburg's effect).[38,39] Rare cases of lymphoma and hemangiosarcoma may exhibit hyperlactatemia despite apparently normal perfusion. Some dogs with diabetes mellitus may have higher lactate than normal dogs, but this could also be due to concurrent type A causes.[40] Hepatic disease resulting in hyperlactatemia probably only occurs with severe hepatic dysfunction or failure or concurrent hypoperfusion.[41]

Type B_2

Many drugs and toxins can cause hyperlactatemia, and these are being increasingly reported in dogs (see Table 56-1). Both antiinflammatory and immunosuppressive doses of prednisone cause mild to moderate increases in lactate in clinically normal dogs.[42]

Metabolism of ethylene glycol (EG), ethanol, and methanol increases the $NADH/NAD^+$ ratio, which drives the LDH reaction toward lactate production.[43] But the severe metabolic acidosis and anion gap associated with EG toxicity is predominantly from acidic EG metabolites.[43,44] Propylene glycol, found in food items, chemical agents, and drugs, is metabolized to L-lactate, D-lactate, and pyruvate and can result in hyperlactatemia when ingested or administered in excess.[45] Some formulations of activated charcoal contain propylene glycol as well as the lactate precursor, glycerol, and can cause increased lactate concentrations.[46]

Catecholamines have been linked to increased Na^+/K^+-ATPase activity and increased glycogenolysis resulting in hyperlactatemia.[47] Not surprisingly, conditions resulting in excess endogenous catecholamine release, such as pheochromocytoma, have also been associated with hyperlactatemia.[48,49]

Type B_3

Congenital errors in metabolism that cause hyperlactatemia in people include glucose-6-phosphatase deficiency, pyruvate dehydrogenase deficiency and MELAS (mitochondrial encephalopathy, lactic acidosis, and stroke-like syndrome).[2] Mitochondrial myopathies have been reported in the Jack Russell Terrier, German Shepherd, and Old

English Sheepdog.[50-52] Pyruvate dehydrogenase deficiency has been recognized in the Clumber Spaniel and Sussex Spaniel.[53]

Hyperlactatemia Without Metabolic Acidosis

As previously mentioned, lactate production occurs independently of H^+ production in the cell and not all causes of hyperlactatemia are associated with a metabolic acidosis. Cytokine or catecholamine stimulation of glycolytic rate can lead to elevated pyruvate and subsequently lactate levels, while mitochondrial function remains normal and H^+ metabolism can continue.[54] Blood samples contaminated with sodium lactate (e.g., from lactated Ringer's) will also show an increase in lactate with no acidosis.[55]

D-Lactate

Lactate exists in levorotatory and dextrorotatory stereoisomeric forms: L-lactate and D-lactate. L-Lactate is the predominant form produced by mammalian cells. It is also the only stereoisomer measured by common clinical technology. D-Lactate is not detected by routine lactate analyzers and can only be measured by specialist laboratories. In health, D-Lactate is present at 1% to 5% of the concentration of L-lactate.[56] Both D- and L-lactate are produced by some bacteria under anaerobic conditions.[57] In people, D-hyperlactatemia associated with short bowel syndrome and exocrine pancreatic disease is thought to cause encephalopathy.[58-60]

D-Hyperlactatemia has been reported in cats with diabetic ketoacidosis,[61] propylene glycol intoxication,[62] and exocrine pancreatic insufficiency with bacterial dysbioisis.[63] Cats with gastrointestinal disease also have significantly higher D-lactate than cats without gastrointestinal disease.[64] In ruminants, hyperlactatemia caused by D-lactate is well documented with conditions such as grain overload.[65] D-Hyperlactatemia should be considered as a rare but possible cause of a high anion gap metabolic acidosis in dogs and cats.

CLINICAL USE

Because increased muscle activity causes hyperlactatemia, venipuncture should be performed with minimal struggling or trembling. If there is muscle activity, then this should be considered when interpreting results. Mild to moderate struggling seems to have minor effects on plasma lactate concentration,[66] but higher levels of muscle activity can significantly increase lactate (e.g., lots of struggling, trembling, tremors, marked exercise, and seizures).

Lactate measured in pulmonary arterial or peripheral arterial blood essentially reflects the mixture of all venous effluents in the body. In contrast, a venous sample reflects the net balance of the lactate entering that specific tissue in arterial blood and what happens in the tissue bed. If blood flow is normal and the animal is clinically healthy, cephalic vein lactate is slightly higher than arterial, but the difference is very small and clinically irrelevant.[67] If tissue blood flow is low and the tissue is producing lactate (e.g., a limb in an animal with global hypoperfusion), then venous lactate exceeds arterial by a larger amount. Hence, repeat lactate measurements should be taken from the same site. There is usually no clinical reason to need arterial blood samples for lactate measurement, but they could have better prognostic value than peripheral or central venous samples.

There are now a variety of handheld and bench-top lactate analyzers. Accuracy, precision, bias, and linearity differ among machines, and bench-top analyzers are superior to handhelds. Importantly, handheld analyzers may be inaccurate and imprecise at lactate concentrations within and just above the reference range. This means that a lactate concentration of approximately 3 mmol/L measured using a handheld may be artifactually high or a true high value. The reference ranges for plasma lactate concentration for dogs between 6 months and 12 years of age is 0.3 to 2.5 mmol/L.[67] Puppies may have higher blood lactate levels than adults during the 2 to 3 months of life.[68] Reference ranges in cats from two small studies vary from 0.3 to 1.7[69] and 0.3 to 2.9 mmol/L.[66] Lactate is only produced after tissue oxygen extraction is maximized, which means it is a late (i.e., insensitive) indicator of tissue hypoperfusion. Even a small rise is therefore very significant once other causes of hyperlactatemia have been ruled out.

Prognostic Use

Lactate is a useful prognostic indicator provided it is interpreted cautiously and appropriately. Low values make survival more likely and very high values make it less likely. Importantly, this depends on the underlying condition. If the process causing hyperlactatemia has a high mortality, then lactate is more likely to be prognostically useful (e.g., sepsis) but less helpful if the cause is easily correctable (e.g., simple hemorrhage that can be easily arrested). With hypoperfusion, a high initial lactate reflects the degree of hypoperfusion but not necessarily the reversibility. It has long been recognized that a decrease in lactate concentration with treatment is a much more reliable prognostic indicator. In general, with severe disease processes, if plasma lactate concentration does not fall back to normal within 24 to 48 hours, survival is less likely.

In people, lactate has shown prognostic value in trauma, sepsis, septic shock, SIRS, cardiac arrest, carbon monoxide toxicity, head trauma, malaria, and liver failure.[70-72] The addition of treatment targeted toward lactate clearance to the Surviving Sepsis campaign resuscitation bundle reduced mortality risk twofold in people with severe sepsis.[9]

Some degree of prognostic utility has been reported for ill and injured dogs[73]; systemically ill dogs[74]; and dogs with SIRS,[75] IMHA,[30] gastric dilation-volvulus,[76] severe soft tissue infections,[77] heartworm-associated caval syndrome,[78] babesiosis,[79,80] and abdominal evisceration.[81] Lactate has also been demonstrated to have some limited prognostic value in cats with hypertrophic cardiomyopathy[82] and septic peritonitis.[83,84] The APPLE (acute patient physiologic and laboratory evaluation) for dogs and cats found lactate to be one of the most significant variables associated with mortality and included lactate in both the full and fast scoring systems for both species.[85,86]

Diagnostic Use

Lactate can be used as an adjunctive diagnostic tool for certain conditions, especially septic peritonitis and other intraabdominal conditions requiring surgical intervention. It can be measured on abdominal fluid and used in conjunction with glucose, pH, PO_2, and PCO_2. Abdominal fluid from some severe cases of septic peritonitis may have a low glucose (<50 mg/dl; 2.8 mmol/L), PO_2, and pH (<7.0) and high PCO_2 and lactate. Intraabdominal values for glucose, PO_2, and pH will also often be lower than peripheral venous blood and PCO_2 and lactate will be higher.[87] Many noninfectious causes of abdominal effusion will not show these changes. The only studies of septic peritonitis published to date had such low numbers of patients that these diagnostic guidelines should not be used as a sole method for diagnosis of septic peritonitis.

Increased peritoneal lactate concentration or peritoneal fluid-to-blood gradients occur with aseptic abdominal crises such as small bowel strangulation,[88] mesenteric vascular thrombosis,[89] or abdominal neoplasia,[90] but these are also likely to be surgical conditions. The cause of high peritoneal fluid lactate concentrations with septic peritonitis has not been definitively confirmed. It is likely due to a combination of production by leukocytes, red blood cells (RBCs), and bacteria, as well as tissue anaerobiosis.

Lactate as a Therapeutic Endpoint

The most common clinical cause of hyperlactatemia is thought to be hypovolemia, and there is mounting evidence that lactate clearance can be used as a therapeutic endpoint to guide goal-directed fluid therapy. The underlying cause of hypoperfusion must be identified and treated, and therapy should be tailored to each patient. In certain cases, other interventions may be indicated to increase oxygen content (RBC transfusions, oxygen supplementation) and oxygen delivery (inotropes and sometimes pressors). If hyperlactatemia is the result of hypoperfusion secondary to cardiac dysfunction, specific cardiovascular therapeutics may be needed to restore perfusion and volume resuscitation may be contraindicated.

Plasma lactate concentration should rapidly decrease with ongoing volume resuscitation. As an approximate guideline, plasma lactate concentration should decrease by half every 1 to 2 hours. If this does not occur, this raises the suspicion for another source of lactate such as ongoing hypovolemia, maldistributive shock, obstructive shock, or an internal focus of ischemia or neoplasia.

Physiologic hyperlactatemia, such as after exercise or an uncomplicated seizure, does not require treatment. Hyperlactatemia is self-correcting without an ongoing cause, so treatment with sodium bicarbonate is not usually recommended. As thiamine pyrophosphate is a coenzyme associated with pyruvate dehydrogenase, thiamine supplementation may have theoretical benefits and can be considered as an adjunctive treatment.[13]

REFERENCES

1. Broder G, Weil MH: Excess lactate: an index of reversibility of shock in human patients, Science 143:1457, 1964.
2. Fall PJ: Lactic acidosis: from sour milk to septic shock, J Intensive Care Med 20:255, 2005.
3. Robergs RA, Ghiasvand F, Parker D. Biochemistry of exercise-induced metabolic acidosis, Am J Physiol Regul Integr Comp Physiol 287:R502, 2004.
4. Levy B: Lactate and shock state: the metabolic view, Curr Opin Crit Care 12:315, 2006.
5. Rowell LB, Kraning KK, Evans TO, et al: Splanchnic removal of lactate and pyruvate during prolonged exercise in man, J Appl Physiol 21:1773, 1966.
6. Arieff AI, Gertz EW, Park R, et al: Lactic acidosis and the cardiovascular system in the dog, Clin Sci 64:573, 1983.
7. Madias NE: Lactic acidosis, Kidney Int 29:752, 1986.
8. Bellomo R: Bench-to-bedside review: lactate and the kidney, Crit Care 6:322, 2002.
9. Nguyen HB, Kuan Sen W, Batech M, et al: Outcome effectiveness of the severe sepsis resuscitation bundle with addition of lactate clearance as a bundle item: a multi-national evaluation, Crit Care 15:R229, 2011.
10. Yudkin J, Cohen RD: The contribution of the kidney to the removal of a lactic acid load under normal and acidotic conditions in the conscious rat, Clin Sci Mol Med 48:121, 1975.
11. Miller AT, Miller JO: Renal excretion of lactic acid in exercise, J Appl Physiol 1:614, 1949.
12. Craig FN: Renal tubular reabsorption, metabolic utilization and isomeric fractionation of lactic acid in the dog, Am J Physiol 146:146, 1946.
13. Chadda K, Raynard B, Antoun S, et al: Acute lactic acidosis with Wernicke's encephalopathy due to acute thiamine deficiency, Intensive Care Med 28:1499, 2002.
14. Kellum JA, Kramer DJ, Lee K, et al: Release of lactate by the lung in acute lung injury, Chest 111:1301, 1997.
15. De Backer D, Creteur J, Zhang H, et al: Lactate production by the lungs in acute lung injury, Am J Respir Crit Care Med 156:1099, 1997.
16. Gladden LB: Net lactate uptake during progressive steady-level contractions in canine skeletal muscle, J Appl Physiol 71:514, 1991.
17. van Hall G, Strømstad M, Rasmussen P, et al: Blood lactate is an important energy source for the human brain, J Cereb Blood Flow Metab 29:1121, 2009.
18. Spitzer JJ, Spitzer JA: Myocardial metabolism in dogs during hemorrhagic shock, Am J Physiol 222:101, 1972.
19. Tashkin DP, Goldstein PJ, Simmons DH: Hepatic lactate uptake during decreased liver perfusion and hyposemia, Am J Physiol 223:968, 1972.
20. Samsel RW, Cherqui D, Pietrabissa A, et al: Hepatic oxygen and lactate extraction during stagnant hypoxia, J Appl Physiol 70:186, 1991.
21. Jeppesen JB, Mortensen C, Bendtsen F, et al: Lactate metabolism in chronic liver disease, Scand J Clin Lab Invest March 20, 2013 [Epub ahead of print].
22. Huckabee WE: Abnormal resting blood lactate: II. Lactic acidosis, Am J Med 30:840, 1961.
23. Cohen RD, Woods HF, Krebs HA: Clinical and biochemical aspects of lactic acidosis, Boston, 1976, Blackwell Scientific Publications.
24. Rovira S, Muñoz A, Benito M: Fluid and electrolyte shifts during and after agility competitions in dogs, J Vet Med Sci 69:31, 2007.
25. Pieschl RL, Toll PW, Leith DE, et al: Acid-base changes in the running greyhound: contributing variables, J Appl Physiol 73:2297, 1992.
26. Toll PW, Gaehtgens P, Neuhaus D, et al: Fluid, electrolyte, and packed cell volume shifts in racing greyhounds, Am J Vet Res 56:227, 1995.
27. Vincent JL, Dufaye P, Berré J, et al: Vincent, Dufaye, et al: Serial lactate determinations during circulatory shock, Crit Care Med 11:449, 1983.
28. Cain SM: Oxygen delivery and uptake in dogs during anemic and hypoxic hypoxia, J Appl Physiol 42:228, 1977.
29. Allen SE, Holm JL: Lactate: physiology and clinical utility, J Vet Emerg Crit Care (San Antonio) 18:123, 2008.
30. Holahan ML, Brown AJ, Drobatz KJ: The association of blood lactate concentration with outcome in dogs with idiopathic immune-mediated hemolytic anemia: 173 cases (2003-2006), J Vet Emerg Crit Care (San Antonio) 20:413, 2010.
31. James JH, Luchette FA, McCarter FD, et al: Lactate is an unreliable indicator of tissue hypoxia in injury or sepsis, Lancet 354:505, 1999.
32. Luchette FA, Friend LA, Brown CC, et al: Increased skeletal muscle Na+, K+-ATPase activity as a cause of increased lactate production after hemorrhagic shock, J Trauma 44:796, 1998.
33. Fink MP: Cytopathic hypoxia. Mitochondrial dysfunction as mechanism contributing to organ dysfunction in sepsis, Crit Care Clinics 17:219, 2001.
34. Chrusch C, Bands C, Bose D, et al: Impaired hepatic extraction and increased splanchnic production contribute to lactic acidosis in canine sepsis, Am J Respir Crit Care Med 161:517, 2000.
35. Elbers PWG, Ince C: Mechanisms of critical illness—classifying microcirculatory flow abnormalities in distributive shock, Crit Care 10:221, 2006.
36. Alamdari N, Constantin-Teodosiu D, Murton AJ, et al: Temporal changes in the involvement of pyruvate dehydrogenase complex in muscle lactate accumulation during lipopolysaccharide infusion in rats, J Physiol 586:1767, 2008.
37. Ince C: The microcirculation is the motor of sepsis, Crit Care 9(Suppl 4):S13, 2005.
38. Walenta S, Mueller-Klieser WF: Lactate: mirror and motor of tumor malignancy, Semin Radiat Oncol 14:267, 2004.
39. Touret M, Boysen SR, Nadeau M-E: Retrospective evaluation of potential causes associated with clinically relevant hyperlactatemia in dogs with lymphoma, Can Vet J 53:511, 2012.
40. Durocher LL, Hinchcliff KW, DiBartola SP, et al: Acid-base and hormonal abnormalities in dogs with naturally occurring diabetes mellitus, J Am Vet Med Assoc 232:1310, 2008.
41. Kruse JA, Zaidi SA, Carlson RW: Significance of blood lactate levels in critically ill patients with liver disease, Am J Med 83:77, 1987.
42. Boysen SR, Bozzetti M, Rose L, et al: Effects of prednisone on blood lactate concentrations in healthy dogs, J Vet Intern Med 23:1123, 2009.
43. Meng QH, Adeli K, Zello GA, et al: Elevated lactate in ethylene glycol poisoning: true or false? Clinica Chimica Acta 411:601, 2010.
44. Verelst S, Vermeersch P, Desmet K: Ethylene glycol poisoning presenting with a falsely elevated lactate level, Clin Toxicol 47:236, 2009.
45. Claus MA, Jandrey KE, Poppenga RH: Propylene glycol intoxication in a dog, J Vet Emerg Crit Care (San Antonio) 21:679–683, 2011.
46. Burkitt JM, Haskins SC, Aldrich J, et al: Effects of oral administration of a commercial activated charcoal suspension on serum osmolality and lactate concentration in the dog, J Vet Intern Med 19:683, 2005.
47. Levy B, Mansart A, Bollaert P-E, et al: Effects of epinephrine and norepinephrine on hemodynamics, oxidative metabolism, and organ energetics in endotoxemic rats, Intensive Care Med 29:292, 2003.
48. Radhi S, Nugent K, Alalawi R: Pheochromocytoma presenting as systemic inflammatory response syndrome and lactic acidosis, ICU Director 1:257, 2010.

49. Bornemann M, Hill SC, Kidd GS: Lactic acidosis in pheochromocytoma, Ann Intern Med 105:880, 1986.
50. Breitschwerdt EB, Kornegay JN, Wheeler SJ, et al: Episodic weakness associated with exertional lactic acidosis and myopathy in Old English sheepdog littermates, J Am Vet Med Assoc 201:731, 1992.
51. Vijayasarathy C, Giger U, Prociuk U, et al: Canine mitochondrial myopathy associated with reduced mitochondrial mRNA and altered cytochrome c oxidase activities in fibroblasts and skeletal muscle, Comp Biochem Physiol 109:887, 1994.
52. Olby NJ, Chan KK, Targett MP, et al: Suspected mitochondrial myopathy in a Jack Russell terrier, J Small Anim Pract 38:213, 1997.
53. Cameron JM, Maj MC, Levandovskiy V, et al: Identification of a canine model of pyruvate dehydrogenase phosphatase 1 deficiency, Mol Genet Metab 90:15, 2007.
54. Mizock BA: Controversies in lactic acidosis: implications in critically ill patients, JAMA 258:497, 1987.
55. Jackson EV, Wiese J, Sigal B, et al: Effects of crystalloid solutions on circulating lactate concentrations: Part 1. Implications for the proper handling of blood specimens obtained from critically ill patients, Crit Care Med 25:1840, 1997.
56. McLellan AC, Phillips SA, Thornalley PJ: Fluorimetric assay of D-lactate, Anal Biochem 1992:206;12, 1992.
57. Nielsen C, Mortensen FV, Erlandsen EJ, et al: L- and D-lactate as biomarkers of arterial-induced intestinal ischemia: an experimental study in pigs, Int J Surg 10:296, 2012.
58. Uribarri J, Oh MS, Carroll HJ: D-lactic acidosis. A review of clinical presentation, biochemical features, and pathophysiologic mechanisms, Medicine 77:73, 1998.
59. Zhang DL: D-lactic acidosis secondary to short bowel syndrome, Postgrad Med J 79:110, 2003.
60. Hove H, Mortensen PB: Colonic lactate metabolism and D-lactic acidosis, Dig Dis Sci 40:320, 1995.
61. Christopher MM, Broussard JD, Fallin CW, et al: Increased serum D-lactate associated with diabetic ketoacidosis, Metabolism 44:287, 1995.
62. Christopher MM, Eckfeldt JH, Eaton JW: Propylene glycol ingestion causes D-lactic acidosis, Lab Invest 62:114, 1990.
63. Packer RA, Cohn LA, Wohlstadter DR, et al: D-lactic acidosis secondary to exocrine pancreatic insufficiency in a cat, J Vet Intern Med 19:106, 2005.
64. Packer RA, Moore GE, Chang C-Y, et al: Serum D-lactate concentrations in cats with gastrointestinal disease, J Vet Intern Med 26:905, 2012.
65. Gentile A, Sconza S, Lorenz I, et al: D-Lactic acidosis in calves as a consequence of experimentally induced ruminal acidosis, J Vet Med A Physiol Pathol Clin Med 51:64, 2004.
66. Redavid LA, Sharp CR, Mitchell MA, et al: Plasma lactate measurements in healthy cats, J Vet Emerg Crit Care (San Antonio) 22:580, 2012.
67. Hughes D, Rozanski ER, Shofer FS, et al: Effect of sampling site, repeated sampling, pH, and PCO2 on plasma lactate concentration in healthy dogs, Am J Vet Res 60:521, 1999.
68. McMichael MA, Lees GE, Hennessey J, et al: Serial plasma lactate concentrations in 68 puppies aged 4 to 80 days, J Vet Emerg Crit Care (San Antonio) 15:17, 2005.
69. Rand JS, Kinnaird E, Baglioni A, et al: Acute stress hyperglycemia in cats is associated with struggling and increased concentrations of lactate and norepinephrine, J Vet Intern Med 16:123, 2002.
70. Blow O, Magliore L, Claridge JA, et al: The golden hour and the silver day: detection and correction of occult hypoperfusion within 24 hours improves outcome from major trauma, J Trauma Acute Care Surg 47:964, 1999.
71. Moon JM, Shin MH, Chun BJ: The value of initial lactate in patients with carbon monoxide intoxication: in the emergency department, Hum Exp Toxicol 30:836, 2011.
72. Okorie ON, Dellinger P: Lactate: biomarker and potential therapeutic target, Crit Care Clin 27:299, 2011.
73. Lagutchik MS, Ogilvie GK, Hackett TB, et al: Increased lactate concentrations in Ill and injured dogs, J Vet Emerg Crit Care (San Antonio) 8:117, 1998.
74. Stevenson CK, Kidney BA, Duke T, et al: Serial blood lactate concentrations in systemically ill dogs, Vet Clin Pathol 36:234-239, 2007.
75. Butler AL, Campbell VL, Wagner AE, et al: Lithium dilution cardiac output and oxygen delivery in conscious dogs with systemic inflammatory response syndrome, J Vet Emerg Crit Care 18:246, 2008.
76. Beer KAS, Syring RS, Drobatz KJ: Evaluation of plasma lactate concentration and base excess at the time of hospital admission as predictors of gastric necrosis and outcome and correlation between those variables in dogs with gastric dilatation-volvulus: 78 cases (2004-2009), J Am Vet Med Assoc 242:54, 2013.
77. Buriko Y, Van Winkle TJ, Drobatz KJ, et al: Severe soft tissue infections in dogs: 47 cases (1996-2006), J Vet Emerg Crit Care (San Antonio) 18:608, 2008.
78. Kitagawa H, Yasuda K, Kitoh K, et al: Blood gas analysis in dogs with heartworm caval syndrome, J Vet Med Sci 56:861, 1994.
79. Jacobson LS, Lobetti RG: Glucose, lactate, and pyruvate concentrations in dogs with babesiosis, Am J Vet Res 66:244, 2005.
80. Nel M, Lobetti RG, Keller N, et al: Prognostic value of blood lactate, blood glucose, and hematocrit in canine babesiosis, J Vet Intern Med 18:471, 2004.
81. Gower SB, Weisse CW, Brown DC: Major abdominal evisceration injuries in dogs and cats: 12 cases (1998-2008), J Am Vet Med Assoc 234:1566, 2009.
82. Bright JM, Golden AL, Gompf RE, et al: Evaluation of the calcium channel-blocking agents diltiazem and verapamil for treatment of feline hypertrophic cardiomyopathy, J Vet Intern Med 5:272, 1991.
83. Parsons KJ, Owen LJ, Lee K, et al: A retrospective study of surgically treated cases of septic peritonitis in the cat (2000-2007), J Small Anim Prac 50:518, 2009.
84. Costello MF, Drobatz KJ, Aronson LR, et al: Underlying cause, pathophysiologic abnormalities, and response to treatment in cats with septic peritonitis: 51 cases (1990-2001), J Am Vet Med Assoc 225:897, 2004.
85. Hayes G, Mathews K, Doig G, et al: The acute patient physiologic and laboratory evaluation (APPLE) score: a severity of illness stratification system for hospitalized dogs, J Vet Intern Med 24:1034, 2010.
86. Hayes G, Mathews K, Doig G, et al: The Feline Acute Patient Physiologic and Laboratory Evaluation (Feline APPLE) Score: a severity of illness stratification system for hospitalized cats, J Vet Intern Med 25:26, 2011.
87. Levin GM, Bonczynski JJ, Ludwig LL, et al: Lactate as a diagnostic test for septic peritoneal effusions in dogs and cats, J Am Anim Hosp Assoc 40:364, 2004.
88. DeLaurier GA, Cannon RM, Johnson RH Jr, et al: Increased peritoneal fluid lactic acid values and progressive bowel strangulation in dogs, Am J Surg 158:32, 1989.
89. Currao RL, Buote NJ, Flory AB, et al: Mesenteric vascular thrombosis associated with disseminated abdominal visceral hemangiosarcoma in a cat, J Am Anim Hosp Assoc 47:e168, 2011.
90. Nestor DD, McCullough SM, Schaeffer DJ: Biochemical analysis of neoplastic versus nonneoplastic abdominal effusions in dogs, J Am Anim Hosp Assoc 40:372, 2004.

PART VI FLUID THERAPY

CHAPTER 57

ASSESSMENT OF HYDRATION

Elke Rudloff, DVM, DACVECC

KEY POINTS

- Water is an essential component of organ homeostasis, and alterations in body water composition can affect patient outcome.
- Clinical factors such as physical examination parameters, plasma osmolality, urine osmolality, urine specific gravity, packed cell volume, total protein, and serum sodium concentration are used in the overall assessment of hydration status.
- There is no single index that accurately and easily measures hydration and individual fluid compartment water in the critical patient.
- A change in body weight may be the most practical method for estimating changes in total body water over a short period.
- Physical examination can only detect changes in extracellular fluid volume.
- The minimal degree of dehydration detectable on physical examination is 5% of body weight (kg).

INTRODUCTION

Water is the single most important medium for sustaining life. It is the medium that provides form to every organ and cell in the body, transports oxygen-carrying red blood cells and electrolytes as well as nutrients in plasma, carries substrates across membranes, evaporates to cool the body, is a solvent for organic and inorganic molecules, and is essential for most metabolic functions. Water imbalances can contribute to morbidity and mortality and need to be rapidly identified and corrected in the critically ill.

Water deficits affect body temperature regulation and neurologic function; severe deficits can result in electrolyte imbalances and hypovolemia resulting in reduced oxygen delivery, acute kidney injury, and death.[1,2] Excess water can result in altered ventilation and lung function, gastrointestinal dysfunction, and electrolyte imbalances.[3]

Physiologic Definitions

Although there are common terms used to identify hydration parameters in patients, uniformity in defining the physiologic definitions is necessary for consistency and accuracy.[4,5]

The definitions associated with the following terms are meant to be a resource for reference of terms used in this chapter.

Hydration: The taking in of water. A patient's total volume of body water (TBW) is reflected in its hydration status.

Euhydration: A condition of normal water content and a state of being within the range of minimal and maximal urine osmolality.

Hypohydration: A condition of reduced water content and a state of being over the maximal range of urine osmolality.

Dehydration: A dynamic state of reducing water content. It occurs as a result of a decreased water intake (water, food) in relation to water lost (in feces, urine, sweat, respiratory vapor). The term is used interchangeably with the term *hypohydration*. Clinically, this term represents a water deficit in the *interstitial and intracellular* fluid compartments and *not* a water deficit in the intravascular space.

Hypovolemia: A condition of reduced *intravascular* volume which occurs with plasma water or whole blood loss.

Hyperhydration: A condition of excess water content. It refers to the time the TBW increases above basal levels, between the ingestion of water and the renal excretion of water. It may result in a reduction in urine osmolality. It is used interchangeably with the term *overhydration*.

Rehydration: Dynamic state of replacing water lost. This term is *not* to be used synonymously with *intravascular volume resuscitation*.

VARIABILITY IN ASSESSING HYDRATION

The TBW is continuously in flux because it is being lost through evaporation, elimination, and metabolic processes and gained from food and water intake. An individual's overall body condition and illness will also affect water retention and losses, globally and in local fluid compartments. There is no single index that accurately and easily measures hydration and individual fluid compartment water in the critical patient. Although extracellular volume can be determined through a number of tests, the continuum of fluid movement from one moment to the next makes it impossible for a static moment in time to be reflected in any single measurement taken to assess TBW.[5] The veterinarian has to be familiar with the distribution and control of body water in order to understand how examination skills and point-of-care laboratory indices can be used to make an estimation of a patient's TBW and individual compartment hydration status and fluid needs.

DISTRIBUTION AND CONTROL OF TOTAL BODY WATER

The TBW that occupies the intra- and extracellular compartments is approximately 0.6 L/kg or 60% of body mass.[6] The TBW increases in the very young and decreases in overweight subjects. The intracellular fluid (ICF) compartment contains approximately 0.4 L/kg or 66% of TBW, and the extracellular fluid (ECF) compartment approximately 0.2 L/kg or approximately 33% of TBW (Figure 57-1). The

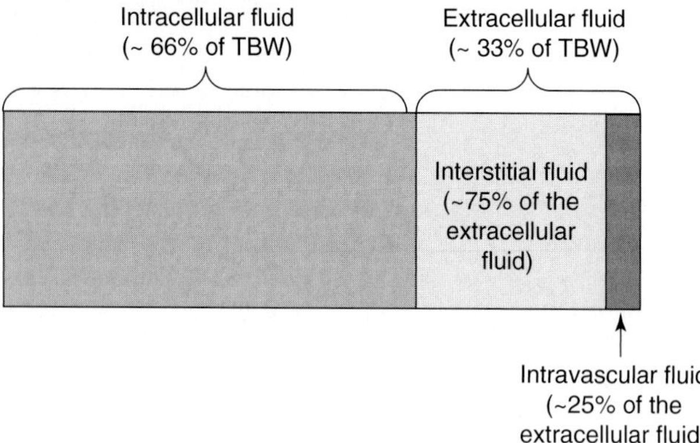

FIGURE 57-1 Graphical representation of the division of total body water in the body, also known as the Yannet-Darrow diagram. The intracellular and extracellular fluid compartments are separated by the cell membrane, and water movement across this barrier is dictated by osmotic gradients. The intravascular and interstitial compartments are separated by the capillary wall; water movement across this barrier is dictated by Starling's forces and is not determined by osmotic gradients.

ECF is further compartmentalized into the intravascular portion, which is approximately 25% of ECF volume (8% of TBW), and the remaining 75% of ECF volume (25% TBW) is interstitial fluid. Pregnancy, increased salt intake, exercise, and malnutrition as well as acute and chronic conditions will affect TBW and the division of water between the compartments.[7]

Body water is distributed across two compartmentalizing membranes, the endothelial cell lining of capillaries separating the intravascular from the interstitial space and the cell membranes separating the ICF from the ECF. The forces that dictate water movement across these two barriers differ. Water moves without restriction across the cell membranes under the influence of osmosis. The osmotic gradient across the cell membrane is dictated by the concentration of osmotically active particles on either side of the membrane and in the normal state is primarily the product of the relative sodium and potassium concentrations, which is controlled by the Na^+/K^+-ATPase pump on the cell membrane. In contrast, water movement across the capillary wall is dictated by Starling's forces (see Chapter 11).[8] It is important to note that osmolality does not affect distribution between the interstitial and intravascular space because the capillary wall is freely permeable to small solutes such as sodium and glucose.

The volume and distribution of TBW is under the control of hormonal mechanisms that maintain water and sodium balance by regulating renal water and salt excretion and reabsorption, whereas thirst mechanisms influence water intake.[9-12]

A hypotonic fluid loss (water with little or no solute content) will increase plasma solutes per kilogram water (osmolality). An increase in the plasma osmolality is detected by the supraoptic and paraventricular nuclei in the hypothalamus and causes the release of antidiuretic hormone (ADH; arginine vasopressin), an increase in water reabsorption by the renal collecting ducts, and more concentrated urine.[13,14] An increase in plasma osmolality and a reduction in baroreceptor stretch will also stimulate the thirst center, located near the supraoptic and preoptic nuclei in the anteroventral region of the third ventricle in the brain, and produce the sensation of thirst resulting in water intake.[15]

Hypovolemia stimulates baroreceptors that cause the hypothalamic-pituitary-adrenal axis to produce and release ADH, aldosterone, renin, and cortisol, which act in concert to cause renal conservation of water and sodium.[13] An overexpansion of the cardiovascular system causes stretch of the atria and release of atrial natriuretic peptide (ANP), which increases renal water and sodium excretion.[16,17]

MEASURING TOTAL BODY WATER

Most experiments investigating changes in TBW and hydration status are performed on athletes and normal subjects. The most accurate method of determining TBW is under controlled experimental conditions, when body water compartment volumes have equilibrated and are stable. Some consider that the "gold standard" of assessing hydration is by determination of TBW using isotope dilution and neutron activation analysis techniques.[5] This particular technique has not been investigated in the critically ill patient.

Multifrequency bioelectrical impedance analysis (MF-BIA) is a method that has be used to identify acute fluid shifts in critically ill people[18-20] and racing horses.[21] Bioelectrical impedance analysis measures the bioelectrical properties of tissue and dispersement of an electrical current to determine body water content. Controversies exist on its reliability, and specific studies in veterinary emergency and critical care medicine have not yet been performed using MF-BIA.[22] Until such time that sophisticated measurement techniques make their way to the intensive care unit (ICU) cage, the veterinarian must rely on using a combination of physical examination findings and point-of-care laboratory indices to make an estimation of a patient's hydration status.

Ninety percent of acute changes in body mass can be attributed to a change in total body water. This makes body weight measurements the most practical clinical way to monitor changes in TBW and estimating volumes gained or lost, where 1 kg change in TBW may be equivalent to 1 L change in TBW.[23-27] However, changes in body weight may not reliably correspond to clinical parameters of hydration in the small animal ICU population.[28] For example, the critical patient with abdominal effusion and peritonitis associated with acute pancreatitis may have a simultaneous collection of fluid in third space fluid compartments and reduction in interstitial and intravascular water. Although the body weight may not have changed, individual fluid compartment water has. Therefore, because they may not correlate with physical examination findings of hydration, body weight changes should not be used alone in determining a patient's level of hydration.

CLINICAL ASSESSMENT OF HYDRATION STATUS

Distinguishing among intravascular, interstitial, and intracellular water deficits is necessary for determining the fluid type to use for replenishment (see Chapter 59).

Interstitial Volume Changes

The interstitial fluid compartment is clinically evaluated by examining mucous membrane moisture, skin tent response, eye position, and corneal moisture as well as other parameters (Table 57-1).[29-34] Loss of interstitial volume causes mucous membranes to become "sticky" when touched (tacky); causes decreased subcutaneous fluidity, identified by decreased skin turgor (decreased skin elasticity evidenced by increased skin tent); and, when severe, results in dry corneas and retraction of the eye within the orbit. The clinician must estimate the degree of dehydration as a percentage of body weight in kilograms based on these parameters. As a general guideline the minimum degree of interstitial dehydration that can be detected in the average patient is approximately 5% of body weight.[34] Interstitial dehydration greater than 12% is likely to be fatal, so the clinician estimates dehydration in the range of 5% to 12% of body weight (see Table 57-1). It is important to note that there is substantial clinical variation in the correlation between clinical signs and degree of dehydration, so this is an estimate only.

Table 57-1 **Physical Examination Findings Used to Estimate Percent Interstitial Dehydration**[34]

Estimated % Dehydration	Physical Examination Findings
<5	Not detectable
5-6	Tacky mucous membranes
6-8	Decreased skin turgor Dry mucous membranes
8-10	Retracted globes within orbits
10-12	Persistent skin tent due to complete loss of skin elasticity Dull corneas Evidence of hypovolemia
>12	Hypovolemic shock Death

NOTE: There is substantial clinical variation in the correlation between clinical signs and degree of dehydration, so this is an estimate only.

As changes to the fluid volume of the interstitial space equilibrate with the intravascular space, all patients with evidence of interstitial dehydration will also have a degree of hypovolemia, although interstitial dehydration has to be severe (>10% to 12%) before clinically detectable changes in perfusion are likely to occur.[35]

Interstitial overhydration causes increased turgor of the skin and subcutaneous tissue, giving it a gelatinous nature; peripheral or ventral pitting edema can also occur. Chemosis and clear nasal discharge may also be evident. As fluid volumes are equilibrated between the interstitial space and the intravascular space, interstitial overhydration is associated with hypervolemia and dilution of the packed cell volume (PCV) and total protein (TP); in severe cases, pulmonary and other organ edema may occur.

Factors unrelated to hydration status that can alter parameters used to assess interstitial hydration include atropine administration (which reduces mucous membrane [MM] moisture), hypersalivation from nausea or pain, advanced age (which reduces skin elasticity), and changes in body fat content. It may be more challenging to appreciate dehydration in obese animals, whereas emaciated animals may appear to have decreased skin turgor even when euhydrated. Young puppies and kittens can also be difficult to assess because they have very elastic skin, so changes in skin turgor maybe harder to detect. Frequent reassessment and reevaluation are required to monitor response to treatment and adjust therapy accordingly.

Intravascular Volume Changes

Clinically, intravascular volume is assessed through the examination of perfusion parameters (mucous membrane color, capillary refill time, heart rate, and pulse quality) and determination of jugular venous distensibility (see Chapters 5 and 60). Although intravascular and interstitial water content equilibrates easily, rapid intravascular losses such as hemorrhage can cause hypovolemia without causing clinically detectable changes in the interstitial fluid compartment.

Excessive intravascular volume will manifest in increased jugular venous distention, in addition to increased central venous pressure. The most obvious and concerning clinical consequence of hypervolemia is pulmonary edema (see Chapter 21).

Intracellular Volume Changes

Intracellular volume changes cannot be identified on physical examination. The clinician must rely on changes in the effective osmolality of ECF (primarily changes in sodium concentration) to mark changes in cell volume. With decreases in ECF effective osmolality there will be an associated movement of water into the ICF compartment and a subsequent increase in intracellular volume. With increases in ECF effective osmolality there will be decreases in intracellular volume. Readers are directed to Chapters 50 and 187 for further discussion of this topic.

Table 57-2 **Laboratory and Clinical Parameters Used During the Assessment of a Patient's Extracellular Hydration Status and Expected Changes from Baseline with Hypohydration and Hyperhydration**

Parameter	Hypohydration	Hyperhydration
Skin turgor	↓	↑
Mucous membrane moisture	↓	↑
Packed cell volume	↑	↓
Total protein	↑	↓
Blood urea nitrogen	↑	↓
Urine osmolality	↑	↓
Urine specific gravity	↑	↓

HYPOTONIC FLUID LOSS

If TBW loss is due to loss of a fluid with little or no salt content (compared with ECF), the clinical consequences are different than the loss of isotonic fluid from the body (the more common clinical scenario). Hypotonic fluid losses will result in increases in ECF osmolality, reflected by increases in serum sodium concentration. As a consequence, water will move from the ICF compartment to the ECF compartment until osmolality is equalized. The loss of ICF volume has the greatest impact on the central nervous system, and if the degree of solute-free water loss is severe and acute it can result in neurologic abnormalities and possibly death as a result of neuronal cell shrinkage. In cases of substantial hypotonic fluid losses, as might happen with uncontrolled diabetes insipidus, the neurologic consequences will be fatal before there is sufficient ECF volume depletion for it to be clinically identified (i.e., less than approximately 5%).

ISOTONIC FLUID LOSS

The net loss or gain of fluid with a salt concentration similar to that of the ECF will cause changes in the ECF volume with little change in ECF osmolality, and hence there will be no change in the ICF volume. Isotonic fluid loss will lead to interstitial dehydration, causing the clinical signs listed in Table 57-2; isotonic fluid gain would cause interstitial overhydration. There will be minimal change in serum sodium concentration with isotonic fluid gain or loss. Isotonic fluid losses are a common cause of fluid imbalance in clinical medicine (often the product of hypotonic fluid loss combined with oral water intake) and are associated with gastrointestinal fluid loss, renal fluid loss, and third space translocation of fluid.

Changes in the ECF volume affect both the interstitial and intravascular volumes and manifest in changes in PCV and TP measurements. Measurements of PCV and TP may not reflect the ECF hydration status if the patient is anemic, polycythemic, or hypoproteinemic unless a baseline sample can be used for comparison. If the decrease in ECF volume is significant, it can be associated with elevations in kidney enzymes (prerenal azotemia).

Urine osmolality and specific gravity (SG) may also provide valuable information regarding ECF hydration status.[36,37] Urine osmolality reflects the total number of solutes per kilogram of urine[39] whereas urine SG is a measurement of the density (mass) of urine compared with water (which has a specific gravity of 1.000).[40] Urine osmolality and urine SG measured by refractometer show linear changes when urine water content changes.[29,38-40] Urine osmolality and SG will increase as water is reabsorbed from the urine filtrate in states of ECF dehydration and decrease as water is excreted from the urine in states of ECF hyperhydration. Evaluation of urine concentration will be limited if the patient has received intravenous (IV) fluid therapy or diuretic administration before urinalysis. Urine output can also reflect fluctuations in ECF volume, although it is a late marker for changes in the body fluid compartment,[41] particularly in situations of rapid volume turnover.

In the critically ill patient, comparing the volume of fluids taken in (e.g., IV fluid therapy, enteral support, voluntary ingestion) with the volume of fluid lost (e.g., in the urine, vomitus, stool, and drain production) can identify a potential state of ECF hyperhydration or hypohydration. Should the volume of fluid lost greatly exceed the volume taken in, the patient is assessed for signs of hyperhydration or causes of polyuria. Should the volume of fluid taken in greatly exceed the volume of fluid lost, the patient is assessed for signs of persistent hypohydration, third space fluid compartment sequestration, or oliguric renal failure.

SPECIAL CHALLENGES

Although the intravascular and interstitial compartments interact in a dynamic and continuous manner, alterations in any component of Starling's forces can result in an imbalance, making interpretation of physical examination findings challenging. For example, a patient with severe systemic inflammation may have increased capillary permeability leading to hypovolemia in conjunction with interstitial overhydration. A congestive heart failure patient can have local increases in pulmonary vascular volume leading to local interstitial hyperhydration (pulmonary edema) yet have reduced total circulating volume and global interstitial hypohydration because of chronic treatment with diuretics and afterload reducers. Other conditions that may require special considerations in assessing individual fluid compartments are listed in Box 57-1. They pose a challenge in both assessment of hydration as well as therapeutic manipulation in moving toward reestablishing euhydration.

CONCLUSION

Assessment of hydration is primarily dependent on the evaluation of physical and laboratory parameters that represent the water content of a dynamic medium involving interconnected fluid compartments. No single parameter should be used to estimate the hydration status of a patient. Changes in the clinical parameters of hydration (skin turgor, mucous membrane moistness, and eye position) all reflect changes in interstitial volume and can only occur with a combination of both salt and water losses. Changes in ICF volume cannot be detected on physical examination.

BOX 57-1 ***Conditions That May Result in Hydration Imbalances of Local Fluid Compartments***

Systemic inflammatory response syndrome
Diuretic or afterload reducer therapy
Noncardiogenic pulmonary edema
Uncontrolled hyperglycemia
Trauma of any organ
Hypoalbuminemia
Fluid therapy
Burns

REFERENCES

1. Armstrong LE, Maresh CM, Gabaree CV, et al: Thermal and circulatory responses during exercise: effects of hypohydration, dehydration, and water intake, J Appl Physiol 82:2028, 1997.
2. Leaf A: Regulation of intracellular fluid volume and disease, Am J Med 49:291, 1970.
3. Lee JY, Rozanski E, Anastasio M, et al: Iatrogenic water intoxication in two cats, J Vet Emerg Crit Care 23:53, 2013.
4. Mange K, Matasuura D, Cizman B, et al: Language guiding therapy: the case of dehydration versus volume depletion, Ann Intern Med 127:848, 1997.
5. Armstrong LE: Assessing hydration status: the elusive gold standard, J Amer College Nutr 26:575S, 2007.
6. Wamburg S, Sandgaard NCF, Bie P: Simultaneous determination of total body water and plasma volume in conscious dogs by the indicator dilution principle, J Nutr 132:1711S, 2002.
7. Armstrong LE, Kenefick RW, Castellani JW, et al: Bioimpedance spectroscopy technique: intra-, extracellular, and total body water, Med Sci Sports Exerc 29:1657, 1997.
8. Woodcock TE, Woodcock TM: Revised Starling equation and the glycocalyx model of transvascular fluid exchange: an improved paradigm for prescribing intravenous fluid therapy, Br J Anaesth 108:384, 2012.
9. Schrier RW, Berl T, Anderson RJ: Osmotic and non osmotic control of vasopressin release, Am J Physiol 236:F321, 1979.
10. Stachenfeld NS, Gleim GW, Zabetakis PM, et al: Fluid balance and renal response following dehydrating exercise in well-trained men and women, Eur J Appl Physiol Occup Physiol 72:468, 1996.
11. Robertson GL, Athar S: The interaction of blood osmolality and blood volume in regulating plasma vasopressin in man, J Clin Endocrinol Metab 42:613, 1976.
12. Robertson GL, Shelton RL, Athar S: The osmoregulation of vasopressin, Kidney Int 10:25, 1976.
13. Zucker A, Gleason SD, Schneider EG: Renal and endocrine response to water deprivation in dog, Am J Physiol 242:R296, 1982.
14. Metzler GH, Thrasher TN, Keil LC, et al: Endocrine mechanisms regulating sodium excretion during water deprivation in dogs, Am J Physiol 251:R560, 1986.
15. Fitzsimons JT: The physiological basis of thirst, Kidney Int 10:3, 1976.
16. Ackermann U, Irizawa TG, Milojevic S, et al: Cardiovascular effects of atrial extracts in anesthetized rats, Can J Physiol Pharmacol 62:819, 1984.
17. Genest J, Cantin M: Atrial natriuretic factor, Circulation 75:118, 1987.
18. Baldwin CE, Paratz JD, Bersten AD: Body composition analysis in critically ill survivors: a comparison of bioelectrical impedance spectroscopy devices, J Parenter Enteral Nutr 36:306, 2012.
19. Savalle M, Gillaizeau F, Maruani G, et al: Assessment of body cell mass at bedside in critically ill patients, Am J Physiol Endocrinol Metab 333:E389, 2012.
20. Baldwin CE, Paratz JD, Bersten AD: Body composition analysis in critically ill survivors: a comparison of bioelectrical impedance spectroscopy devices, J Parenter Enteral Nutr 36:306, 2012.
21. Waller A, Lindinger MI: Hydration of exercised Standardbred racehorses assessed noninvasively using multi-frequency bioelectrical impedance analysis, Equine Vet J 36:285, 2006.
22. Bordelon DJ, Wingfield W. Monitoring acute fluid shifts with bioelectrical impedance analysis: a review, J Vet Emerg Crit Care 12:153, 2002.
23. Cheuvront, SN, Ely BR, Kenefick RW, Sawka MN: Biological variation and diagnostic accuracy of dehydration assessment markers, Am J Clin Nutr 92:565, 2010.
24. Shirreffs SM: Markers of hydration status, Eur J Clin Nutr 57:S6, 2003.
25. Kavouras S: Assessing hydration status, Cur Opin Clin Nutr Metab Care 5:519, 2002.
26. Opplinger RA, Bartok C: Hydration testing of athletes, Sports Med 32:959, 2002.
27. Armstrong LE: Hydration assessment techniques, Nutr Rev 63:S40, 2005.
28. Hansen B, DeFrancesco T: Relationship between hydration estimate and body weight change after fluid therapy in critically ill dogs and cats, J Vet Emerg Crit Care 12:235, 2002.
29. Armstrong LE, Soto JA, Hacker Jr FT, et al: Urinary indices during dehydration, exercise, and rehydration, Int J Sport Nutr 8:345, 1998.

30. Hardy RM, Osborne CA: Water deprivation test in the dog: maximum normal values, J Am Vet Med Assoc 174:479, 1979.
31. Finco DR: Fluid therapy—detecting deviations from normal, J Am Anim Hosp Assoc 8:155, 1972.
32. Harrison JB, Sussman HH, Peckering DE: Fluid and electrolyte therapy in small animals, J Am Vet Med Assoc 137:637, 1960.
33. Cornelius LM: Fluid therapy in small animal practice, J Am Vet Med Assoc 176:110, 1980.
34. Langston C: Managing fluid and electrolyte disorders in renal failure. In DiBartola SP, editor: Fluid, electrolyte, and acid-base disorders in small animal practice, ed 4, St Louis, 2012, Saunders Elsevier, pp 545-556.
35. Francesconi RP, Hubbard RW, Szlyk PC, et al: Urinary and hematological indexes of hydration, J Appl Physiol 62:1271, 1987.
36. Popowski LA, Oppliger RA, Lambert GP, et al: Blood and urinary measures of hydration status during progressive acute dehydration, Med Sci Sports Exerc 33:747, 2001.
37. Shirreffs SM, Maughan RJ: Urine osmolality and conductivity as indices of hydration status in athletes in the heat, Med Sci Sport Exerc 30:1598, 1998.
38. Bovee KC: Urine osmolarity as a definitive indicator of renal concentrating ability, J Am Vet Med Assoc 155:30, 1969.
39. George JW: The usefulness and limitations of hand-held refractometers in veterinary laboratory medicine: an historical and technical review, Vet Clin Pathol 30:201, 2001.
40. Dossin O, Germain C, Braun JP: Comparison of the techniques of evaluation of urine dilution/concentration in the dog, J Vet Med A Physiol Pathol Clin Med 50:322, 2003.
41. Popowski LA, Oppliger RA, Lambert GP, et al: Blood and urinary measures of hydration status during progressive acute dehydration, Med Sci Sports Exerc 33:747, 2001.

CHAPTER 58

CRYSTALLOIDS, COLLOIDS, AND HEMOGLOBIN-BASED OXYGEN-CARRYING SOLUTIONS

Debra T. Liu, DVM, DACVECC • Deborah C. Silverstein, DVM, DACVECC

KEY POINTS

- The tonicity of a fluid is determined by the concentration of effective osmoles (osmoles not freely permeable through cell membranes between intracellular and extracellular space). However, small effective osmoles, such as sodium and other electrolytes, may diffuse across the capillary endothelium between cell junctions readily.
- The volume distribution of a crystalloid solution in the body depends on its tonicity relative to the extracellular fluid. The lower the tonicity of a crystalloid solution, the higher proportion of the fluid volume administered that will move into the intracellular space as a result of osmotic pressure differences. The osmolarity and tonicity of intracellular versus extracellular fluid compartments are equal during homeostasis.
- Colloidal solutions contain large molecules capable of increasing intravascular colloid osmotic pressure. Thereby the balance of Starling's forces is tilted to decrease transcapillary fluid flux into the interstitium and favors intravascular volume retention.
- Hemoglobin-based oxygen-carrying solutions (HBOCs) are colloidal solutions with oxygen-carrying capacity. Although the oxygen content of the blood is improved, tissue oxygenation and the hemodynamic effects of HBOCs are unpredictable because of its strong vasopressor effect.
- Fluid therapy is invaluable in treating hemodynamic, electrolyte, and acid-base derangements. Potential serious complications of fluid therapy include organ edema, cavitary effusion, electrolyte disturbances, and central pontine or thalamic myelinolysis that may be life threatening. Individualized treatment and close monitoring for potential side effects are the essence of safe fluid therapy.

Since the advent of intravenous fluid therapy in the early 1900s, many humans and animals have benefited from this life-saving treatment. Understanding the physiologic implications of different fluid losses from the body is equally important to having familiarity with the various solutions available commercially. This chapter describes the characteristics of common crystalloids, colloids, and hemoglobin-based oxygen-carrying solutions (HBOCs) and provides the foundation for fluid prescription. In addition to individual patient factors, fluid composition, osmolarity, tonicity, oncotic property, and acid-base effects of a given fluid must be considered before administration. Different volumes of distribution, rheologic properties (viscosity), oxygen-carrying abilities, and metabolism of the respective fluids also influence the hemodynamics in concert. Readers are directed to Chapters 59 and 60 for suggested dosages and administration options for these fluids.

Fundamentally, the osmolar gradient between fluid compartments dictates fluid shifts. During periods of homeostasis, the osmolarity and tonicity of the intracellular compartment are equal to that of the extracellular compartment. *Osmolarity* includes all osmoles in solution, whereas *tonicity* refers solely to effective osmoles, which do not freely permeate most cell membranes. It is changes in tonicity that will drive fluid movement in or out of cells. Sodium and its associated anions are the predominant extracellular effective osmoles, whereas potassium and its associated anions are the predominant intracellular effective osmoles. The Na^+/K^+-ATPase pumps on the cell membrane are the primary regulators of cell volume by maintaining an appropriate distribution of intracellular potassium and extracellular sodium. Most sodium ions of the body stay extracellular because of these Na^+/K^+-ATPase pumps.[1]

Starling's forces (i.e., hydrostatic and colloid osmotic pressures [COP] in the intravascular and interstitial spaces), as well as vascular endothelial permeability, govern the magnitude of fluid filtration through the capillary into the interstitial compartment. Normally, plasma albumin accounts for 80% of plasma COP, which is essential for minimizing fluid loss from the intravascular compartment into the interstitial space.[2] Readers are directed to Chapter 59 for further discussion of the physiology of fluid distribution in the body.

Potential adverse effects of fluid therapy include volume overload (e.g., pulmonary, peripheral tissue and other organ edema), inappropriate fluid shifts (e.g., cerebral edema as an example of intracellular overhydration), and electrolyte and acid-base derangements. Large volumes of fluid therapy may lead to a coagulopathy secondary to hemodilution and functional disturbances of primary hemostasis (e.g., synthetic colloidal fluids).[3] Aggressive volume resuscitation may exacerbate hemorrhage in bleeding patients. The clinical impacts of various fluids on the immune system and the causal relationship of synthetic starch colloids to kidney injury remain obscure and unproven in veterinary medicine.[4,5] Therefore a judicious approach to fluid therapy is necessary to minimize occurrences of these side effects.

CRYSTALLOIDS

Crystalloids are fluids containing small solutes with molecular weights less than 500 g/mole (1 g/mole = 1 dalton [Da]). The majority of solutes are electrolytes (<50 g/mole), which readily cross the capillary endothelium and equilibrate throughout the extracellular fluid compartment. There is a lag time of 20 to 30 minutes for electrolytes to distribute evenly in the extracellular fluid compartments (i.e., intravascular and interstitial fluid compartments). The net result of fluid shifts (i.e., osmosis) is dictated by the relative tonicity between different fluid compartments. Sodium and its respective anions (i.e., chloride mostly) are the most abundant effective osmoles in most crystalloids. Other small solutes such as glucose and lactate are readily metabolized; hence 5% dextrose in water is considered "free water" because it does not contain an effective osmole.

The lack of large molecules precludes crystalloids from exerting a colloidal effect. Less than one third of the volume of crystalloids administered remains in the intravascular space 30 minutes after administration.[6] The lower the fluid tonicity, the greater the extracellular fluid tonicity will be "diluted," resulting in an osmotic gradient favoring free water movement into the intracellular space and leaving less of the administered fluid volume in the extracellular space (i.e., intravascular and interstitial spaces).

Crystalloids are the most widely used fluids for treating clinical patients suffering from dehydration, cardiovascular shock, free water deficits, and electrolyte and acid-base imbalances. Crystalloids are often classified according to their tonicity. Features of isotonic, hypotonic, hypertonic solutions are discussed later in the chapter.

Isotonic Fluids

The osmolarity and sodium concentration of isotonic fluids are similar to that of plasma and extracellular fluid. Normal plasma osmolarity is 290 to 310 mOsm/L for dogs and 311 to 322 mOsm/L for cats, and isotonic fluids generally have an osmolality in the range of 270 to 310 mOsm/L.[7,8] These fluids are therefore useful for treatment of hypovolemic shock when rapid intravascular volume expansion is desired. Strictly speaking, isotonic fluid does not cause significant fluid shifts between intracellular and extracellular fluid compartments in normal animals (tonicities of the intracellular and extracellular fluids are unchanged; therefore there is no net osmotic shift).

Isotonic fluids are also commonly used for treating interstitial dehydration. Normal or abnormal body fluid losses are generally hypotonic or isotonic in nature. Although isotonic crystalloids are best suited for the treatment of dehydration secondary to isotonic fluid loss, they are commonly used to replace hypotonic loss as well. Although excess electrolytes are typically excreted by the kidneys, patients with compromised renal function should have their electrolytes closely monitored. Examples of isotonic fluids include Plasma-Lyte 148, Plasma-Lyte A, Normosol-R, lactated Ringer's solution, and 0.9% saline. Of note, 0.9% saline contains a much higher chloride concentration (154 mmol/L) than canine or feline plasma (see Table 59-2). It is useful for treating animals with a hypochloremic metabolic alkalosis, as in the case of pyloric obstruction. Conversely, patients with normal chloride concentration may develop a hyperchloremic metabolic acidosis when 0.9% saline is administered in large volumes.

Hypotonic Fluids

In comparison to extracellular fluid and plasma, the osmolarity and sodium concentration of hypotonic fluids are much lower (e.g., 0.45% saline has an osmolarity of 154 mOsm/L with a sodium [and chloride] concentration of 77 mEq/L). Five percent dextrose in free water is a unique isoosmotic solution (250 mOsm/L) with hypotonic effects because dextrose is rapidly metabolized and free water remains (tonicity of 0 mOsm/L). Sterile water with an osmolarity of 0 mOsm/L should never be administered directly into the vascular system because of the risk of intravascular hemolysis and endothelial damage.

Hypotonic fluids replenish free water deficits and are useful for treating animals with hypernatremia secondary to hypotonic fluid loss (although bolus therapy is contraindicated [see later in chapter]). Hypotonic fluids distribute throughout both intracellular and extracellular fluid compartments, with less remaining extracellularly (i.e., intravascular and interstitial space) in comparison to isotonic fluids. The large volume of distribution and free water content make hypotonic fluid a safer choice for slowly treating animals that have a decreased ability to excrete excess sodium or tolerate an elevated intravascular volume (e.g., kidney and heart diseases, respectively). Additionally, the low chloride content minimizes bromide loss in animals receiving potassium bromide therapy for seizure control.[9,10]

Hypotonic fluids should *never* be used as bolus therapy for intravascular volume resuscitation. Not only are these fluids ineffective at expanding the intravascular volume, they may also lead to life-threatening cerebral edema. A rapid intravenous administration of hypotonic fluids drops plasma and extracellular fluid osmolarity (mainly determined by sodium level) quickly; as a consequence, water shifts from the extracellular fluid space to the intracellular space. Frequent sodium level monitoring during hypotonic fluids administration is recommended.

Hypertonic Fluids

In contrast to hypotonic solutions, the high osmolarity and sodium concentration of hypertonic solutions, such as 7.5% saline, causes a free water shift (i.e., osmosis) from the intracellular space to the extracellular space, expanding the extracellular fluid volume by 3 to 5 times the volume administered. Osmotic fluid shifts from the interstitial space into the intravascular space start immediately after intravenous administration of hypertonic solution, even sooner than the uniform distribution of the electrolytes throughout the extracellular space. Free water from the intracellular fluid compartment then moves into the extracellular fluid compartment as the interstitial fluid osmolarity rises.

Hypertonic saline ranging from 3% to 7.5% is used for the therapy of hypovolemic shock, intracranial hypertension, and severe hyponatremia (see Chapter 50). It is often administered for patients with both hypovolemic shock and concerns for intracranial hypertension such as the head trauma patient. Similar to isotonic and hypotonic crystalloids, the intravascular volume expansion effect of hypertonic saline is transient (<30 minutes) because of the redistribution of electrolytes (i.e., sodium and its associated anions) throughout the extravascular space.[6] The ensuing osmotic diuresis also facilitates excess sodium excretion. To prolong the intravascular volume–expanding effect of hypertonic saline, it is often combined with a colloidal solution. A common preparation is made by mixing a stock solution of 23.4% hypertonic saline with 6% hetastarch or pentastarch in a 1:2 ratio to arrive at a total volume of 3 to 5 ml/kg.

Hypertonic saline has several beneficial effects on the cardiovascular system beyond increasing vascular volume. It transiently improves cardiac output and tissue perfusion via arteriolar vasodilation (decreased afterload), volume loading (increased preload), reduced endothelial swelling, and a weak positive inotropic effect.[11-13] It is important that administration rates do not exceed 1 ml/kg/min because hypotension may result from central vasomotor center inhibition or peripheral vasomotor effects mediated by the acute hyperosmolarity (bradycardia and vasodilation).[11] Hypertonic saline also has immune-modulatory effects including suppression of neutrophil respiratory burst activity and cytotoxic effects. The antiinflammatory effects of hypertonic saline may be especially advantageous in trauma patients.[13,14] Additionally, hypertonic saline improves cerebral perfusion pressure in head trauma patients by augmenting mean arterial blood pressure and decreasing intracranial pressure. At equal osmolar dosages, similar osmotic effects are achieved with either hypertonic saline or mannitol to reduce cerebral edema.[13,15] Hypernatremia is a potential side effect that prevents the safe use of repeated doses of hypertonic saline. A dose of 4 ml/kg of 7.5% saline will expand intravascular volume by 12 to16 ml/kg (a fraction of total shock dose), but the effect is transient secondary to the fluid redistribution to the interstitial space and osmotic diuresis that follows. Therefore additional volumes of isotonic crystalloids, colloids, or blood products are required to stabilize a patient suffering from hypovolemic or distributive shock (see Chapter 60 for details). Repeated administration of hyperosmotic solutions may lead to hemolysis and phlebitis if given into small peripheral veins.[16]

Acid-Base Effects of Crystalloids

The pH of intravenous fluids is usually acidic; largely this is due to dissolved carbon dioxide and the acidic nature of dextrose solutions. This low pH does not influence the acid-base balance of patients because of the lack of titratable acidity. Essentially the total quantity of free hydrogen ions in an intravenous fluid is small and easily buffered in the body and should not be considered as relevant to the acid-base effects of fluid therapy.

The acid-base effects of crystalloid administration depend largely on the buffer content of the fluid. Further discussion of the effects of various fluids on the pH of the blood is beyond the scope of this chapter but can be found in Chapters 54 and 55.

Acetate, gluconate, and lactate are weak buffers included in some crystalloids such as Normosol-R, lactated Ringer's solution, and Plasma-Lyte 148. Metabolism of these buffers consumes hydrogen ions, yielding an alkalinizing effect.[17] As such they are considered beneficial when treating patients with a metabolic acidosis. These fluids may not be as ideal for animals with a hypochloremic metabolic alkalosis, for which 0.9% saline is considered the fluid of choice. In hypovolemic shock, lactic acidosis is expected to be present. Although treatment with a buffered fluid may allow resolution of this metabolic acidosis slightly faster than treatment with an unbuffered fluid such as 0.9% saline, the greatest benefit to the patient is restoring adequate perfusion and the type of isotonic crystalloid utilized to achieve this is of less importance.[18-20]

The metabolism of lactate occurs mainly in the liver; therefore its use in animals with significant liver dysfunction is not recommended. Lactated Ringer's solution may be the ideal fluid for neonates because lactate is the preferred metabolic fuel in early life. The lactate anion found in crystalloids such as lactated Ringer's solution does not contribute to metabolic acidosis; it can, however, cause falsely elevated lactate meter readings if it is not yet metabolized. Clinically this concern is minimal unless the blood sample is contaminated. Acetate is metabolized primarily in the skeletal muscle and most cells in the body metabolize gluconate. Hypotension due to vasodilation is associated with rapid infusion of acetate and has been reported in humans and experimental dogs.[21,22,22a,22b] This has led to concerns of use of acetate containing crystalloids for shock resuscitation. Anecdotally, these fluids are used commonly for resuscitation, but further investigations of the hemodynamic effects of rapid administration of acetate containing fluids to hypovolemic animals are needed.

COLLOIDS

Colloidal solutions contain large molecules (>10,000 Da) that tend to remain in the intravascular space after intravenous administration and serve to increase blood viscosity and COP. This feature makes colloids attractive for intravascular volume resuscitation, particularly in patients with hypoalbuminemia and/or increased vascular permeability. Synthetic colloidal solutions contain colloidal particles that are suspended in isotonic crystalloids.

Normal COP is 15.3 to 26.3 mm Hg in dogs and 17.6 to 33.1 mm Hg in cats (whole blood).[23] Daily monitoring of COP is recommended for animals requiring oncotic support, with a target COP of 16 mm Hg (or lower in animals with chronic hypoproteinemia). Refractometer measurements of total protein do not correlate well with COP (or albumin and globulin concentration) after the administration of starch colloids.[24]

Available colloids are categorized to synthetic starch colloids, allogeneic blood products, and human albumin, as discussed next.

Synthetic Starch Colloids

Most synthetic starch colloid solutions are hyperoncotic relative to plasma and polydiverse (i.e., contain a wide spectrum of molecular weights). These solutions effectively increase and maintain intravascular COP; fluids are pulled into the vascular space because of the increased intravascular/ interstitial COP ratio. An increase in intravascular volume up to 1.4 to 1.5 times the volume administered was reported after the administration of either 6% hetastarch or Dextran 70 to normal dogs.[6] Hydroxyethyl starch molecules are branched polymers of glucose derived from hydrolysis of amylopectin. They are characterized by their concentration in the solution, molecular weight, degree of hydroxyl substitutions by hydroxyethyl groups, and ratio of hydroxyethyl group substitutions at the C2 versus C6 position. Each of the following are associated with a longer half-life (not higher oncotic pressure): larger molecular weight, higher degree of substitutions, and higher C2:C6 ratio.[25] For example, VetStarch, a veterinary formulation of Voluven, is a 6% tetrastarch solution with a weight average molecular weight of 130,000 Da, 4 hydroxyethyl group substitutions per 10 glucose molecules (designated as 130/0.4), and a C2:C6 ratio of 9:1. The molecular weight range of VetStarch and Voluven is 110,000 to 150,000 Da. The reported weight average molecular weight is weight based and is more representative of the larger hetastarch molecules. A number average molecular weight accounts for the relative distribution of various sized particles. In comparison to Hextend (670/0.75, 4:1), the half-life of VetStarch and

Voluven is shorter (38 hours vs. 10 hours in healthy humans). A high cumulative dosage can also prolong the half-life of synthetic starch colloids because of a saturable degradation process.[26,27]

Dextrans are another example of synthetic starch colloid solutions that are structured as linear polysaccharides. Purified bacterial dextran sucrase is used to digest sucrose to various sizes of dextran molecules to make these products.[25] Despite ample research available, dextran products are currently off the market, primarily because of their propensity to cause acute kidney injury and allergic reactions in humans.

The oncotic effect of synthetic colloids depends on the number of colloidal molecules. Small starch colloid molecules (e.g., hetastarch < 50,000 Da) are filtered through the glomeruli and rapidly excreted, causing a transient osmotic diuresis.[28,29] Colloidal molecules in the urine increase urine viscosity and specific gravity measurement by the refractometer. Urine osmolality is a more accurate measure of urine concentration in animals receiving colloidal fluids.[30] Larger starch molecules are metabolized slowly to smaller molecules. Synthetic starch molecules are degraded by the reticuloendothelial system (i.e., liver, spleen, and lymph nodes). Also, amylase in the blood metabolizes hydroxyethyl starches. If colloid molecules leak into the interstitial space, especially in patients with increased vascular permeability, they are returned to the circulation by the lymphatics or engulfed by macrophages. Kidneys are the main route for excretion of synthetic starch colloids.[25]

Synthetic starch colloids interfere with the function of platelets, von Willebrand's factor, and factor VIII, leading to a primary hemostatic coagulopathy and prolonged activated partial thromboplastin time, all of which are dose dependent. Hetastarch solutions typically prolong bleeding times when administered at doses greater than 20 ml/kg/day. The same characteristics of hydroxyethyl starches that enable a longer half-life also confer the greatest coagulopathic effects (higher molecular weight, degree of hydroxyethyl group substitution, and C2:C6 ratio of hydroxyethyl group substitution).[25] Clinical bleeding is not typically observed with the available commercial hydroxyethyl starch solutions in stable, noncoagulopathic animals, even with doses greater than 40 ml/kg/day; however, caution is advised when using higher doses in critically ill or coagulopathic animals. Lower-molecular-weight hydroxyethyl starch solutions may be preferable in patients with a higher risk of bleeding (e.g., surgical or coagulopathic patients) because of their decreased coagulopathic effects.[25] Allergic reaction to the synthetic starches is a possible side effect of synthetic colloids in humans but has not been reported in veterinary medicine.[25] Evidence for the increasing concern regarding acute kidney injury secondary to synthetic starch colloid use in the critically ill humans is accumulating and has led to their withdrawal from the market in some countries.[5] Decreased glomerular filtration, hypertonicity of glomerular filtrate, and direct hydroxyethyl starch deposits are thought to contribute to the renal toxicity of these products.[31,32] A direct association between hydroxyethyl starches and the occurrence of acute kidney injury has not been reported in veterinary medicine; however, similar risks are possible in the critically ill animals.

Allogenic Blood Products

Natural blood products provide either allogeneic albumin (i.e., canine or feline) or pooled human albumin (see next section). As mentioned earlier, albumin contributes to a large portion of COP in animals. Other essential physiologic functions of albumin involve wound healing, coagulation, and scavenging of free radicals. Albumin serves as a carrier for multiple substrates, including hormones, bilirubin, fatty acids, divalent cations, toxins, and drugs. Additionally, albumin also exerts a weak buffer effect via binding of hydrogen ions.[2]

Several colloidal blood products are derived from canine or feline donors (see Chapter 61 for further details). Fresh frozen plasma provides all the clotting factors and plasma protein. Plasma that remains at room temperature for more than 8 hours or is stored frozen for more than 1 year loses the labile clotting factors and is then considered frozen plasma. Frozen plasma provides plasma proteins and clotting factors II, VII, IX, and X. Cryosupernatant is the top portion of partially thawed fresh plasma after a hard spin (5000× g for 7 minutes) and contains albumin, globulin, antithrombin, protein C, protein S, and clotting factors II, VII, IX, X, XI and XII. The remaining portion is cryoprecipitate, which is rich in fibrinogen, fibronectin, factor VIII, and von Willebrand's factor. Fresh whole blood transfusion provides platelets and red blood cells in addition to plasma proteins and clotting factors.[33,34]

For colloid osmotic support, iso-oncotic plasma is less effective than hyperoncotic synthetic starch solutions. In order to raise the recipient's plasma albumin by 1g/dl, approximately 40 to 50 ml/kg of plasma from a normal dog is required.[35,36] In critically ill animals with an accelerated loss of albumin (e.g., septic peritonitis or large area skin burns), plasma transfusion therapy may not keep up with the rate of albumin loss. Circulatory overload is another concern when administering large volumes of plasma transfusion. Plasma transfusions to provide clotting factors and albumin are often used in addition to synthetic starch colloids to provide colloid osmotic support in coagulopathic and hypoalbuminemic animals. For animals with both clinical anemia and hypoproteinemia, whole blood transfusions are another option. All blood products carry some risks for transfusion reactions, in addition to immunomodulatory properties. Slow administration over 2 to 4 hours is recommended in stable patients in order to closely monitor for signs of a transfusion reaction or volume overload.

More recently, lyophilized pooled canine albumin became available, but the supply is intermittent (Animal Blood Resources International, Dixon, CA). Logically it seems that concentrated canine albumin administration would decrease the risk of circulatory overload associated with plasma transfusions and the hypersensitivity reactions associated with human albumin administration in small animals. There are currently two abstracts documenting the use of canine albumin in nine dogs with septic peritonitis.[37,38] More evidence is needed to support its purported benefit and clinical safety.

Human Albumin

Pooled human albumin has been administered to critically ill dogs to raise serum albumin and COP. Five percent (5 g/dl) human albumin is iso-osmolar and isooncotic, whereas the most commonly used 25% (25 g/dl) human albumin exerts 5 times the osmolar and oncotic effects of 5% human albumin. As expected, the high oncotic pressure of 25% albumin expands intravascular volume much more than the volume administered. Therefore judicious dosing and close monitoring for volume overload are crucial for patient safety. Although albumin is a well-conserved molecule across species, human and canine albumin molecules share only 79% homology.[39] The xenogenic transfusion of human albumin comes with the potential life-threatening risk of an immediate or delayed hypersensitivity reaction. Naturally occurring antibodies against human albumin have also been documented in healthy dogs with no prior human albumin transfusion.[40] Fortunately, several retrospective studies have found that the rate of severe adverse reaction is rare when used once in critically ill animals.[40,41] It is hypothesized that the immune system is compromised in severely ill animals and therefore unable to mount an immune response to the antigenic human albumin. Therefore human serum albumin is reserved only for critically ill animals with severe hypoalbuminemia, after carefully weighing the benefit and risks of human albumin administration. Extra-label use and potential risk must be clearly communicated to the pet owner before human albumin administration. Because immunoglobulin G (IgG) formation is well documented in dogs after exposure to human albumin, repeated administration within the lifetime of a given animal is not advised.[40] Although hypoalbuminemia is associated with poor clinical outcomes,[42] the effect of human albumin on mortality in small animals is currently unknown.

HEMOGLOBIN-BASED OXYGEN-CARRYING SOLUTIONS

Oxyglobin is the only veterinary FDA-approved HBOC for the treatment of canine anemia, although its supply has been intermittent; it was not available from the manufacturer in the United States at the time of the writing of this chapter, although it is currently available in Europe. It contains 13 g/dl of polymerized bovine hemoglobin that is ultrapurified and free of antigenic red blood cell stroma and is suspended in a modified lactated Ringer's solution. Bovine hemoglobin depends on chloride instead of 2,3-diphosphoglycerate in the red blood cells to regulate its oxygen affinity; readily available chloride in the extracellular fluid aids in the excellent oxygen transport ability of bovine hemoglobin.[43] Bovine hemoglobin has a P_{50} of 34 mm Hg, similar to that of canine and feline hemoglobin (P_{50} of canine and feline hemoglobin in red blood cells are 31.5 and 35.6 mm Hg, respectively).[44,45] Polymerization of bovine hemoglobin tetramers creates a more stable, larger molecule, which prolongs its half-life and eliminates renal toxicity associated with hemoglobin dimers (derived from rapid breakdown of individual hemoglobin tetramers).[43]

Oxyglobin is a polydiverse colloidal solution with an average weight molecular weight of 200 kDa (molecular weight range of 64 to 500 kDa). It is isoosmotic (300 mOsm/kg) and hyperoncotic (COP of 43 mm Hg). Free of cells, the viscosity of Oxyglobin is low (<2 cP). Increased preload, stroke volume, and cardiac output are observed after Oxyglobin administration. However, the hemodynamic effect of Oxyglobin is complicated by its nitric oxide scavenging effect. Normally, nitric oxide has a vasodilatory effect. Peripheral vasoconstriction subsequent to the decrease in nitric oxide with Oxyglobin therapy may ironically compromise tissue perfusion and oxygen delivery. In addition, the local regulatory response to improved tissue oxygenation may also lead to peripheral vasoconstriction after Oxyglobin administration.[46-48]

Blood typing and cross-matching are not necessary before Oxyglobin administration. Improvements in clinical signs of anemia mirror the increase of hemoglobin level. Hematocrit is no longer a useful measure of blood carrying capacity and may actually decrease after Oxyglobin administration because of its dilutional effect. The most concerning side effect of Oxyglobin is volume overload. Judicious dosing and close monitoring is imperative. The half-life of Oxyglobin is dose dependent and ranges from 18 to 43 hours after infusion of 10 to 30 ml/kg of Oxyglobin. Oxyglobin has a labeled shelf-life of 36 months at room temperature and does not require blood typing or cross-match before administration. Transient yellow-orange discoloration of the skin, mucous membranes, and sclera and orange- to brown-colored urine are increasingly obvious with higher dosages of Oxyglobin. Some serum chemistry and urine dipstick parameters will be invalidated because of serum discoloration.

CONCLUSION

Fluid therapy is versatile and plays a major role in the supportive care of hospitalized veterinary patients. In order to maximize the benefits and minimize side effects, treatment goals should be clearly delineated while formulating a fluid prescription. Familiarity with different fluid products, rational fluid prescription, and close patient monitoring (via physical examination and bloodwork) are the three major elements of proper fluid therapy.

REFERENCES

1. DiBartola SP, de Morais HA: Disorders of potassium: hypokalemia and hyperkalemia. In DiBartola SP, editor: Fluid, electrolyte, and acid-base disorders in small animal practice, ed 3, St Louis, 2006, Elsevier.
2. Mazzaferro EM, Rudloff E, Kirby R: The role of albumin replacement in the critically ill veterinary patient, J Vet Emerg Crit Care 12(2):113, 2002.
3. Kozek-Langenecker SA: Influence of fluid therapy on the haemostatic system of intensive care patients, Best Pract Res Clin Anaesthesiol 23:225, 2009.
4. Alam HB, Stanton K, Koustova E, et al: Effect of different resuscitation strategies on neutrophil activation in a swine model of hemorrhagic shock, Resuscitation 60:91, 2004.
5. Perner A, Haase N, Guttormsen AB, et al: Hydroxyethyl starch 130/0.42 versus Ringer's acetate in severe sepsis, N Engl J Med 367:124, 2012.
6. Silverstein DC, Aldrich J, Haskins SC, et al: Assessment of changes in blood volume in response to resuscitative fluid administration in dogs, J Vet Emerg Crit Care 15(3):185, 2005.
7. DiBartola SP: Disorders of sodium and water: hypernatremia and hyponatremia. In DiBartola SP, editor: Fluid, electrolyte, and acid-base disorders in small animal practice, ed 3, St Louis, 2006, Elsevier.
8. Dugger DT, Mellema MS, Hopper K, et al: Comparative accuracy of several published formulae for the estimation of serum osmolality in cats, J Small Anim Pract 54:184, 2013.
9. Shaw N, Trepanier LA, Center SA, et al: High dietary chloride content associated with loss of therapeutic serum bromide concentrations in an epileptic dog, J Am Vet Med Assoc 208:234, 1996.
10. Nichols ES, Trepanier LA, Linn K: Bromide toxicosis secondary to renal insufficiency in an epileptic dog, J Am Vet Med Assoc 208:231, 1996.
11. Kien ND, Kramer GC, White DA: Acute hypotension caused by rapid hypertonic saline infusion in anesthetized dogs, Anesth Analg 73:597, 1991.
12. Kien ND, Reitan JA, White DA, et al: Cardiac contractility and blood flow distribution following resuscitation with 7.5% hypertonic saline in anesthetized dogs, Circ Shock 35:109, 1991.
13. Bulger EM, Hoyt DB: Hypertonic resuscitation after severe injury: is it of benefit? Adv Surg 46:73, 2012.
14. Rizoli SB, Rhind SG, Shek PN, et al: The immunomodulatory effects of hypertonic saline resuscitation in patients sustaining traumatic hemorrhagic shock: a randomized, controlled, double-blinded trial, Ann Surg 243:47, 2006.
15. Cottenceau V, Masson F, Mahamid E, et al: Comparison of effects of equiosmolar doses of mannitol and hypertonic saline on cerebral blood flow and metabolism in traumatic brain injury, J Neurotrauma 28:2003, 2011.
16. Rocha e Silva M, Velasco IT, Porfirio MF: Hypertonic saline resuscitation: saturated salt-dextran solutions are equally effective, but induce hemolysis in dogs, Crit Care Med 18:203, 1990.
17. DiBartola SP, Bateman S: Introduction to fluid therapy. In DiBartola SP, editor: Fluid, electrolyte, and acid-base disorders in small animal practice, ed 3, St Louis, 2006, Elsevier.
18. Silverstein DC, Kleiner J, Drobatz KJ: Effectiveness of intravenous fluid resuscitation in the emergency room for treatment of hypotension in dogs: 35 cases (2000-2010), J Vet Emerg Crit Care (San Antonio) 22:666, 2012.
19. Driessen B, Brainard B: Fluid therapy for the traumatized patient, J Vet Emerg Crit Care 16:276, 2006.
20. Drobatz KJ, Cole SG: The influence of crystalloid type on acid-base and electrolyte status of cats with urethral obstruction, J Vet Emerg Crit Care 18:355, 2008.
21. Daugirdas JT, Nawab ZM, Ing TS: Acute hypotension during acetate-buffered dialysis in chemically sympathectomized dogs, Trans Am Soc Artif Intern Organs 31:517, 1985.
22. Noris M, Todeschini M, Casiraghi F, et al: Effect of acetate, bicarbonate dialysis, and acetate-free biofiltration on nitric oxide synthesis: implications for dialysis hypotension, Am J Kidney Dis 32:115, 1998.

22a. Saragoça MA, Bessa AM, Mulinari RA, et al: Sodium acetate, an arterial vasodilator: Haemodynamic characterisation in normal dogs, Proc Eur Dial Transplant Assoc Eur Ren Assoc 21:221-224, 1985.

22b. Saragoça MA, Mulinari RA, Bessa AM, et al: Comparison of the hemodynamic effects of sodium acetate in euvolemic dogs and in dogs submitted to hemorrhagic shock, Braz J Med Biol Res 19:455-458, 1986.

23. Mathews K: Monitoring fluid therapy and complications of fluid therapy. In DiBartola SP, editor: Fluid, electrolyte, and acid-base disorders in small animal practice, ed 3, St Louis, 2006, Elsevier.

24. Bumpus SE, Haskins SC, Kass PH: Effect of synthetic colloids on refractometric readings of total solids, J Vet Emerg Crit Care 8(1):21, 1998.

25. Mizzi A, Tran T, Karlnoski R, et al: Voluven, a new colloid solution, Anesthesiol Clin 29:547, 2011.

26. Jungheinrich C, Neff TA: Pharmacokinetics of hydroxyethyl starch, Clin Pharmacokinet 44:681, 2005.

27. Wilkes NJ, Woolf RL, Powanda MC, et al: Hydroxyethyl starch in balanced electrolyte solution (Hextend)—pharmacokinetic and pharmacodynamic profiles in healthy volunteers, Anesth Analg 94:538, 2002.

28. Plumb D: Hetastarch. In Plumb D, editor: Plumb's veterinary drug handbook, ed 6, Stockholm, 2008, Pharma Vet.

29. Klotz U, Kroemer H: Clinical pharmacokinetic considerations in the use of plasma expanders, Clin Pharmacokinet 12:123, 1987.

30. Smart L, Hopper K, Aldrich J, et al: The effect of hetastarch (670/0.75) on urine specific gravity and osmolality in the dog, J Vet Intern Med 23:388, 2009.

31. Dickenmann M, Oettl T, Mihatsch MJ: Osmotic nephrosis: acute kidney injury with accumulation of proximal tubular lysosomes due to administration of exogenous solutes, Am J Kidney Dis 51:491, 2008.

32. Schortgen F, Brochard L: Colloid-induced kidney injury: experimental evidence may help to understand mechanisms, Crit Care 13:130, 2009.

33. Abrams-Ogg ACG, Ann S: Principles of canine and feline blood collection, processing, and storage. In Weiss DJ, Wardrop KJ, editors: Schalm's Veterinary Hematology, ed 6, Ames, IA, 2010, Blackwell Publishing Ltd.

34. Benjamin RJ, McLaughlin LS: Plasma components: properties, differences, and uses, Transfusion 52(Suppl 1):9S, 2012.

35. Hughes D, Boag AK: Fluid therapy with macromolecular plasma volume expanders. In DiBartola SP, editor: Fluid, electrolyte, and acid-base disorders in small animal practice, ed 3, St Louis, 2006, Elsevier.

36. Wingfield WE: Fluid and electrolyte therapy. In Wingfield Weraffe MR, editors: The veterinary ICU book, Jackson,WY, 2002, Teton NewMedia.

37. Craft EM, de Laforcade AM, Rozanski EA, et al: The effect of transfusion with canine specific albumin in dogs with septic peritonitis. Abstract from the international veterinary emergency and critical symposium, J Vet Emerg Crit Care 2010.

38. Craft EM, Powell LL: Evaluation of the use of lyophilized canine specific albumin in dogs with septic peritonitis. Abstract from the international veterinary emergency and critical symposium, J Vet Emerg Crit Care 2010.

39. Gentilini F, Dondi F, Mastrorilli C, et al: Validation of a human immunoturbidimetric assay to measure canine albumin in urine and cerebrospinal fluid, J Vet Diagn Invest 17:179, 2005.

40. Martin LG, Luther TY, Alperin DC, et al: Serum antibodies against human albumin in critically ill and healthy dogs, J Am Vet Med Assoc 232:1004, 2008.

41. Mathews KA, Barry M: The use of 25% human serum albumin: outcome and efficacy in raising serum albumin and systemic blood pressure in critically ill dogs and cats, J Vet Emerg Crit Care 15(2):110, 2005.

42. Michel KE: Prognostic value of clinical nutritional assessment in canine patients, J Vet Emerg Crit Care 3(2):96, 1993.

43. Eike JH, Palmer AF: Effect of Cl- and H+ on the oxygen binding properties of glutaraldehyde-polymerized bovine hemoglobin-based blood substitutes, Biotechnol Prog 20:1543, 2004.

44. Rossing R, Cain S: A nomogram relating pO2, pH, temperature, and hemoglobin saturation in the dog, J Appl Physiol 21(1):195, 1966.

45. Herrmann K, Haskins S: Determination of P_{50} for feline hemoglobin, J Vet Emerg Crit Care 15:26, 2005.

46. Malhotra AK, Schweitzer JB, Fox JL, et al: Cerebral perfusion pressure elevation with oxygen-carrying pressor after traumatic brain injury and hypotension in swine, J Trauma 56:1049, 2004.

47. Knudson MM, Lee S, Erickson V, et al: Tissue oxygen monitoring during hemorrhagic shock and resuscitation: a comparison of lactated Ringer's solution, hypertonic saline Dextran, and HBOC-201, J Trauma 54:242, 2003.

48. Elmer J, Alam HB, Wilcox SR: Hemoglobin-based oxygen carriers for hemorrhagic shock, Resuscitation 83:285, 2012.

CHAPTER 59

DAILY INTRAVENOUS FLUID THERAPY

Deborah C. Silverstein, DVM, DACVECC • Kari Santoro-Beer, DVM, DACVECC

KEY POINTS

- Daily intravenous fluid therapy is used to correct dehydration, provide maintenance fluid and electrolyte needs, and replace ongoing losses.
- The movement of fluid within the body is determined by hydrostatic pressure, colloid osmotic pressure, vascular endothelial permeability, and osmolality.
- Total body water is distributed in the intracellular and extracellular (plasma and interstitium) fluid compartments. The intracellular space is much larger than the extracellular space.
- The most common types of daily intravenous fluids include isotonic crystalloids, hypotonic crystalloids, free water solutions, and synthetic colloids.
- The fluid type and rate should be tailored to the individual patient's needs.
- Potential complications of fluid therapy include pulmonary edema, subcutaneous edema, organ edema, and electrolyte imbalances.

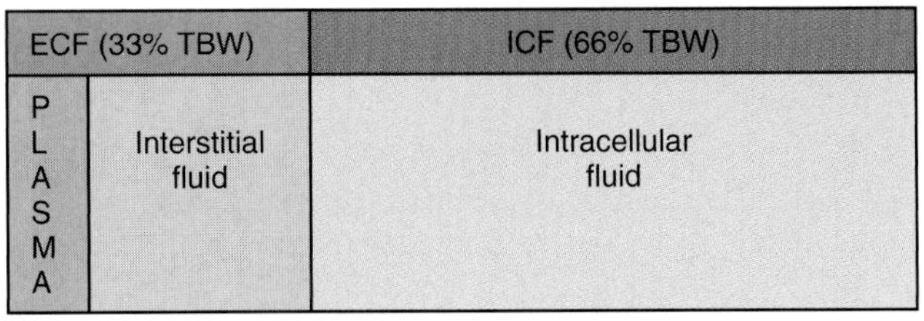

ECF (33% TBW)		ICF (66% TBW)
P L A S M A	Interstitial fluid	Intracellular fluid

FIGURE 59-1 The distribution of total body water *(TBW). ECF,* Extracellular fluid; *ICF,* intracellular fluid.

Intravenous fluid therapy is vital for the management of cardiovascular shock, interstitial dehydration, and daily maintenance fluid needs in critically ill animals (see Chapters 58, 60, and 193 to 195). This chapter focuses primarily on the distribution of total body water, patient assessment, and the delivery of synthetic intravenous fluids to maintain normal water, electrolyte, and acid-base status in critically ill dogs and cats that are hemodynamically stable. Because critically ill animals often have fluid and electrolyte balance derangements, overall recovery often depends on recognition and appropriate treatment of these disorders, in addition to diagnosing and treating the primary disease process.

TOTAL BODY WATER

Living organisms are predominantly composed of water. Total body water content is approximately 60% of body weight in a nonobese adult dog or cat. Total body water is distributed between two main compartments: intracellular fluid (ICF) and extracellular fluid (ECF) (Figure 59-1). Each compartment consists of solutes, primarily electrolytes, dissolved in water. The most important determinant of the size of each body fluid compartment is the quantity of solutes contained in that compartment.[1,2]

The ICF compartment is the larger of the two and comprises 66% of the total body water (40% of body weight). It is separated from the ECF compartment by the cell membrane, which is very permeable to water but impermeable to most solutes. Cell membranes contain numerous proteins, including ion channels and active solute pumps. The most important active pump is the Na^+/K^+-ATPase pump, which extrudes three sodium ions from the cell in exchange for two potassium ions into the cell. This pump is responsible for generation of the electrochemical gradient across cell membranes, typified by a high intracellular potassium concentration, high extracellular sodium concentration, and negative resting membrane potential. Therefore the most prevalent cation in the ICF is potassium, with much smaller contributions made by magnesium and sodium. The most prevalent anions in the ICF are phosphate and the polyanionic charges of the intracellular proteins.[1,2]

The ECF comprises the remaining 33% of the total body water and 20% of body weight. The ECF is subdivided into the plasma (25% of ECF) and interstitial (75% of ECF) fluid compartments. The interstitial fluid bathes all cells and includes lymph. The primary cation in the ECF is sodium and the most prevalent anions are Cl^- and HCO_3^- The proteins in plasma and the interstitial space also contribute to the negative charges. The oncotic pressure gradient between the intravascular and interstitial spaces is determined by the ratio of proteins in these two compartments.[1,2]

MOVEMENT OF FLUIDS WITHIN THE BODY

Water moves freely within most compartments in the body. Small particles such as electrolytes move freely between the intravascular and interstitial compartment but cannot enter or leave the cellular compartment without a transport system. Larger molecules (>20,000 Daltons) do not easily cross the vascular endothelial membrane and may attract small, charged particles, thus creating the *colloid osmotic pressure* (COP). There are three main natural colloid particles: albumin, globulins, and fibrinogen. An increase in the pressure of fluid within a compartment that pushes against a membrane is known as *hydrostatic pressure.*

In health, fluid distribution within the ECF is determined by the balance between forces that favor reabsorption of fluid into the vascular compartment (increased COP or decreased hydrostatic pressure) and those that favor filtration out of the vascular space (decreased COP or increased hydrostatic pressure).[1] Changes in the osmolality between any of the fluid compartments within the body will cause free water movement across the respective membrane.

In disease states, both increased fluid losses and decreased intake may lead to dehydration. The nature of the fluid loss (hypotonic, isotonic, or hypertonic) will determine the subsequent changes in osmolality. This will in turn dictate the relative effect of fluid loss on the ICF and ECF compartments.

Isotonic Fluid Loss

Isotonic fluid losses, as seen in animals with polyuric renal failure, vomiting, diarrhea, or bleeding, will lead to depletion of the ECF compartment and dehydration. If severe ECF losses are not replaced, hypovolemia may become clinically apparent. Because isotonic losses will not alter ECF osmolality, there will be no movement of water across the cell membrane and ICF volume will remain unchanged. In order to replace the ECF deficit, isotonic crystalloids should be administered (see Fluid Deficit). However, if the animal has been drinking water to replace the isotonic fluid losses, hyponatremia may result.

Hypotonic Fluid Loss

Hypotonic fluid losses, as seen with diabetes insipidus or excessive panting, will cause hypernatremia and an increase in ECF osmolality. This leads to movement of water out of the ICF space. Consequently, there is a depletion of both the ICF and ECF compartments. Isotonic fluid therapy may be sufficient if the hypernatremia is not severe, but in animals with significant hypotonic fluid losses, free water administration is indicated. Care must be taken to lower serum sodium slowly to avoid causing potentially life-threatening cerebral edema (see Chapter 50).

Hypertonic Fluid Loss

Loss of hypertonic fluid occurs infrequently in small animals. Excessive loss of solutes in the urine may occur with diseases such as hypoadrenocorticism but more commonly hyponatremia results from excessive free water intake or retention. Hyponatremia caused by hypertonic fluid loss is often exacerbated by electrolyte losses combined with hypotonic fluid replacement (i.e., oral water intake). If a hypertonic fluid loss does occur, a drop in ECF osmolality results and provides a gradient for water to move into the ICF compartment, leading to cell swelling. Significant hyponatremia or hypoosmolality requires careful fluid therapy to avoid rapid (>0.5 mEq/L increase per hour) changes in sodium concentration and subsequent central pontine myelinolysis (also known as osmotic demyelination syndrome).

Increased Vascular Permeability

Disease processes that cause an increase in vascular permeability may lead to high-protein fluid extravasation from the intravascular space. This can lead to a decrease in intravascular volume, possibly associated with interstitial edema. Because this will not alter the osmolality of the ECF compartment, increased vascular permeability alone is not expected to alter the ICF volume.

Patient history, physical examination, and laboratory data can provide useful information concerning the route of fluid losses, timeline of these losses, food and water consumption, and current clinical status. This will guide formulation of an appropriate fluid therapy plan.

FLUID THERAPY PLAN

The fluid type and rate of administration chosen depend primarily on the clinical status of the animal based on the physical examination and laboratory parameters. For animals with evidence of chronic dehydration on physical examination but stable cardiovascular parameters, fluid deficits should be replaced over 4 to 24 hours. Isotonic replacement fluids are administered according to the patient's estimated dehydration, maintenance needs, and anticipated ongoing losses.

To determine the quantity of fluid necessary for the stable patient with evidence of dehydration, the following formula is used:

$$\begin{aligned}&[\text{Body weight (kg)} \times 1000] \times [\text{percentage dehydration}/100]\\&\quad = \text{deficit (ml)}\\&\qquad + \text{estimated ongoing losses (ml)}\\&\qquad + \text{maintenance (ml)}\\&\quad = \text{amount to be given over next 4 to 24 hours}\end{aligned}$$

Fluid Deficit

Volume deficiencies in each of the body fluid compartments exhibit different clinical signs or laboratory abnormalities. ICF deficits lead to cerebral obtundation, hypernatremia, and hyperosmolality. ICF deficits alone will not cause clinical evidence of dehydration. In contrast, interstitial volume deficits are typically associated with a decrease in skin turgor (increased skin tenting) and dry mucous membranes. Skin turgor provides only a rough estimate of dehydration, and severe emaciation or obesity can make this assessment difficult. Serial body weight measurements may also be a useful and more objective indicator of dehydration (see Chapter 57). Intravascular volume deficits are commonly associated with compensatory vasoconstriction, pale mucous membranes, poor pulse quality, tachycardia, prolonged capillary refill time, and cold extremities. These symptoms are suggestive of poor tissue perfusion and require rapid intervention. Physical examination findings in animals with evidence of dehydration can be found in Chapter 57, Table 57-2.

Maintenance Fluid Therapy

Maintenance fluid therapy is administered either in conjunction with or after replacing the patient's fluid deficit. Maintenance fluid needs take into account the sensible and insensible ongoing fluid losses (feces, urine, panting, sweating). Despite extensive research examining the maintenance fluid needs of dogs and cats, results vary greatly with species, breed, body size and lean body weight, exercise level, season, gestation, and lactation, among other factors. Critical illness can also affect daily fluid requirements substantially. Because of these variations, it is especially important to reexamine animals receiving intravenous fluids several times per day.

Daily maintenance fluid volume requirements have been shown to parallel resting energy requirements; thus, calculations of resting energy requirements are often used to estimate fluid requirements (1 kcal of energy = 1ml of water). The resting energy requirement (RER) is the amount of energy (or water) needed to maintain homeostasis in the fed state in a thermoneutral environment and is equal to $70(BW_{kg})^{0.75}$. Additional commonly used formulas for calculating daily fluid needs are as follows:

Formula 1: $30(BW_{kg}) + 70$/day
Formula 2: $60(BW_{kg}) + 140$/day
Formula 3: 40-60 ml/kg/day
Formula 4: 2-4 ml/kg/hr

However, these estimates may not be as accurate for animals weighing less than 2 kg or more than 40 kg because of extreme alterations in body surface area and lean body mass changes; therefore the RER formula given earlier may be more appropriate in these patients ($70[BW_{kg}]^{0.75}$). In addition, because there is less water in fat than in muscle, most calculations overestimate the maintenance needs of overweight patients.[3-6] It is imperative to recognize that these maintenance calculations are variable and may not reflect the needs of critically ill patients in a hospital environment. Serial assessments of the patient's hydration status are required, and ongoing losses must be taken into account.

Ongoing Losses

Ongoing fluid losses are estimated from an understanding of the underlying disease process and historical data. For example, when treating animals with gastrointestinal losses, the approximate volume and frequency of vomiting and diarrhea is estimated. Obviously this predicted volume may be inaccurate; it allows calculation of an initial fluid therapy plan, but close patient monitoring and reevaluation are imperative. If the estimate of ongoing fluid losses is significantly inaccurate, the fluid plan should be altered accordingly.

Route of Administration

Although subcutaneous fluid administration can be effective in the management of fluid deficits, it is not adequate for the critically ill patient. Fluid therapy should be administered via an intravenous or intraosseous catheter that is assessed regularly for evidence of phlebitis (if venous) or inadvertent subcutaneous fluid administration. In general, fluids with an osmolality less than 600 mOsm/L can be given safely through a peripheral venous catheter; those with an osmolality greater than 700 mOsm/L should be given through a central catheter to decrease the risk of phlebitis or thrombosis.

FLUID TYPE

The type of fluid that should be administered depends on the individual patient. Options for the critically ill patient include replacement fluids, maintenance fluids, free water solutions, and synthetic colloids.

Replacement Fluids

Replacement fluids, also known as *isotonic crystalloids*, are electrolyte-containing fluids with a composition similar to that of the ECF. They have a similar osmolality as plasma (290 to 310 mOsm/L).[7,8] They may also contain buffer compounds and dextrose. Isotonic crystalloids are commonly used to expand the intravascular and interstitial spaces and maintain hydration. The constituents of commonly used isotonic fluids can be found in Table 59-1. Additional electrolytes, such as potassium, may be added to maintenance or replacement fluids as needed for an individual patient (see Part V, Electrolyte and Acid-Base Disturbances).

After infusion of isotonic crystalloids into the vascular space, the small electrolytes and water pass freely across the capillary vascular endothelium. These are extracellular-expanding fluids; 75% redistributes to the interstitial space, and only 25% remains in the vascular space after 30 minutes.[9] Although so-called *replacement fluids* are used commonly for maintenance of hydration, most animals are able to easily excrete the electrolyte constituents that are in excess of the body's needs. This practice is common because most hospitalized animals have ongoing electrolyte losses and poor enteral intake, and it is much easier to hang one bag of isotonic crystalloids than two separate bags (one for replacement and one for maintenance). The

Table 59-1 Isotonic Crystalloid Compositions

Fluid Type	Osmolality (mOsm/L)	$[Na^+]$ (mEq/L)	$[K^+]$ (mEq/L)	$[Cl^-]$ (mEq/L)	$[Mg^{2+}]$ (mEq/L)	$[Ca^{2+}]$ (mEq/L)	Lactate (mEq/L)	Acetate (mEq/L)	Gluconate (mEq/L)
0.9% NaCl	308	154	—	154	—	—	—	—	—
Lactated Ringer's solution	273	130	4	109	—	3	28	—	—
Plasmalyte 148	295	140	5	98	3	—	—	27	23
Normosol-R	295	140	5	98	3	—	—	27	23

Table 59-2 Maintenance and Free Water Solution Compositions

Fluid Type	Osmolality (mOsm/L)	[Na+] (mEq/L)	$[K^+]$ (mEq/L)	$[Cl^-]$ (mEq/L)	$[Mg^{2+}]$ (mEq/L)	$[Ca^{2+}]$ (mEq/L)	Lactate (mEq/L)	Acetate (mEq/L)	Dextrose
0.45% NaCl	150	77	0	77	—	—	—	—	—
0.45% NaCl with 2.5% dextrose	203	77	—	77	—	—	—	—	2.5%
Plasmalyte 56	110	40	13	40	3	—	—	16	—
Normosol-M	110	40	13	40	3	—	—	16	—
1/2 LRS with 2.5% dextrose	265	130	4	109	—	3	28	—	2.5%
D5W	252	—	—	—	—	—	—	—	5%

D5W, 5% Dextrose in water; *LRS*, lactated Ringer's solution.

rate of fluid replacement is determined as outlined earlier in this chapter.

Not all isotonic fluids are created equal, as seen in Table 59-1. Isotonic saline solution (0.9% NaCl) contains a higher concentration of sodium and chloride (154 mEq/L of each) than does normal blood and will cause proportional changes (increases) in the recipient electrolytes. Therefore large amounts of 0.9% NaCl will cause a mild increase in serum sodium, a marked increase in chloride, and a moderate decrease in bicarbonate and potassium. The kidneys typically will compensate, if possible, by excreting the excess electrolytes and conserving potassium.

Isotonic crystalloids can cause harm, especially in critically ill animals. The interstitial fluid gain can lead to interstitial edema, pulmonary edema, and cerebral edema. Patients with a low COP, pulmonary contusions, cerebral trauma, fluid-unresponsive renal disease, or cardiac disease/failure are at highest risk for complications. In addition, substantial hemodilution of blood constituents that are not found in the crystalloids can occur. Anemia, hypoproteinemia, electrolyte derangements, and hypocoagulability can occur after large-volume crystalloid administration.

Although all isotonic crystalloids have a similar composition, there are situations in which one specific fluid type may be preferable over another. Specifically, animals with diabetic ketoacidosis or liver disease should not receive lactate-containing fluids because of their decreased ability to convert the lactate to bicarbonate in the liver. However, lactated Ringer's solution may be preferred in very young animals because lactate is the preferred metabolic fuel in neonates with hypoglycemia. Patients with a hypochloremic metabolic alkalosis will benefit from 0.9% sodium chloride because this is the highest chloride-containing fluid, but animals with a severe acidosis may benefit from an alkalinizing fluid containing lactate, acetate, or gluconate (see Table 59-1). Animals with head trauma or increased intracranial pressure may benefit from 0.9% sodium chloride because this isotonic crystalloid is least likely to cause a decrease in osmolality that might promote water movement into the brain interstitium.

Maintenance Fluids

Maintenance fluids refers to the volume of fluid and amount of electrolytes that must be consumed on a daily basis to keep the volume of total body water and electrolyte content within the normal range. Obligate fluid losses are hypotonic and low in sodium but contain relatively more potassium than does the ECF.[10] Maintenance fluids are therefore hypotonic crystalloids that are low in sodium, chloride, and osmolality but high in potassium compared with normal plasma concentrations (Table 59-2). The inclusion of dextrose may make the fluid iso-osmotic to plasma, but the dextrose is metabolized rapidly to carbon dioxide and water, so these fluids are still hypotonic in nature. Maintenance-type fluids are distributed into all body fluid compartments and should never be administered as a rapid bolus because cerebral edema may result.

Free Water Administration

In order to give free water (fluids with no electrolytes or buffers) intravenously without using a dangerously hypotonic fluid, sterile water is combined with 5% dextrose to yield an osmolality of 252 mOsm/kg (safe for intravenous administration). This fluid is indicated in animals with a free water deficit (i.e., hypernatremia) or severe ongoing free water losses (e.g., diabetes insipidus). In order to safely lower the sodium concentration by 1 mEq/hr, a rate of 3.7 ml/kg/hr of free water is a good starting point and can be adjusted based on the patient's response. Alternatively, the patient's free water deficit can be calculated by the formula:

$$\text{Free water deficit} = ([\text{current}\,[Na^+] \div \text{normal}\,[Na^+]] - 1) \times (0.6 \times \text{body weight in kg})$$

This formula will provide the total volume of free water to be replaced and can be administered as 5% dextrose in water over the number of hours calculated for safe reestablishment of normal plasma sodium concentration (Na^+ change of no greater than 0.5 – 1.0 mEq/L/hr). Close monitoring of electrolyte status is advised. Dextrose 5% in water should never be administered as a rapid bolus because acute decreases in osmolality will cause potentially fatal cerebral edema (see Chapter 50 for further discussion of this topic).

Synthetic Colloids

The most commonly used synthetic colloid solutions are made from hydroxyethyl starch (hetastarch and tetrastarch products). Colloidal solutions contain large molecules (molecular weight > 10,000 Daltons) that do not readily sieve across the vascular membrane. The base solution is an isotonic crystalloid (e.g., 0.9% NaCl), and the colloidal particles are suspended within the crystalloid. These fluids are polydisperse (they contain molecules with a variety of molecular weights) and hyperoncotic to the normal animal and therefore cause the movement of fluid from the extravascular to the intravascular space. Synthetic colloids lead to an increase in blood volume that is greater than that of the infused volume and also aid in the retention of this fluid in the vascular space (in animals with normal capillary permeability). Hetastarch is a 6% hydroxyethyl starch solution, with particles ranging from 10,000 to 1,000,000 Daltons in molecular weight, a number average molecular weight of 69,000 Daltons, a mean average molecular weight of 450,000 Daltons, and a COP of 34 mm Hg in vitro. Excessive volumes can lead to volume overload, coagulopathies, and hemodilution. The use of synthetic colloids in critically ill humans has recently received a *Boxed Warning* from the U.S. Food and Drug Administration over concerns that it may increase mortality and the need for renal replacement therapy in this patient population (http://www.fda.gov/biologicsbloodvaccines/safetyavailability/ucm358271.htm). Still, there is no evidence to support this adverse effect in small animals. However, at volumes greater than 40 ml/kg/day, an increase in incisional bleeding has been reported with hetastarch solutions, which may be due to increased blood pressure and microcirculatory flow as well as dilutional and direct effects of hetastarch on coagulation. Hetastarch affects von Willebrand's factor, platelet function, and factor VIII function. Clinical evidence of bleeding has not been reported in animals receiving doses up to 20 ml/kg/day. An increase in the activated partial thromboplastin time (aPTT) may develop in animals that receive large amounts of synthetic colloid therapy, although the quantitative aPTT change is not predictive of clinical bleeding. Coagulation times should be monitored and transfusion therapy initiated as needed. VetStarch is a 6% tetrastarch solution, with particles ranging from 110,000 to 150,000 Daltons, a mean average molecular weight of 130,000 Daltons, and a COP of 40 mm Hg (observational data). Because of its lower average molecular weight and low molar substitution, VetStarch may be less likely to cause adverse renal and coagulation side effects but may also require higher doses to achieve similar effects to that of hetastarch. Synthetic colloids are typically used in combination with isotonic crystalloids to maintain adequate plasma volume expansion and colloid osmotic pressure with lower interstitial fluid volume expansion. Constant rate infusions are commonly used at a rate of 0.5 to 2 ml/kg/hr in animals with acute decreases in COP or total protein levels.[10,11]

The use of fresh or stored whole blood, packed red blood cells, or plasma products is often necessary in critically ill animals. A thorough discussion of transfusion medicine can be found in Chapter 61.

MONITORING

Animals receiving intravenous fluids should be monitored closely. Body weight should be monitored daily (or more often if indicated), and a physical examination should be performed at least twice daily to assess the animal's mental status, skin turgor, heart rate and pulse quality, mucous membrane color, capillary refill time, extremity temperature, and respiratory rate and effort. Serial lung auscultation should be performed to monitor for increased breath sounds, crackles, or wheezes. Clinical signs in animals receiving too much fluid include serous nasal discharge, chemosis, jugular venous distention, and interstitial pitting edema. In the early stages of pulmonary edema, an increase in the respiratory rate will occur, followed by inspiratory crackles, wheezes, and dyspnea. It is therefore of utmost importance to monitor the respiratory rate and effort of all patients receiving fluid therapy.

If an indwelling urinary catheter is present, urine output can be compared with fluid administered to help guide fluid therapy and prevent the administration of too much or too little fluid. Serum blood urea nitrogen and creatinine levels can be evaluated in conjunction with the urine specific gravity to determine whether there is prerenal or renal azotemia (or a combination of both). An increase in blood urea nitrogen and creatinine with an increase in urine specific gravity would suggest that the animal is receiving insufficient fluid volume. Inadequate tissue perfusion may result in an increase in blood lactate levels secondary to anaerobic metabolism. Serial lactate measurements may help guide fluid therapy as an indicator of tissue perfusion. Moderate to severely elevated lactate levels should alert the clinician that more aggressive treatment may be required.

If a central venous catheter is in place, central venous pressure monitoring may be used to help guide fluid therapy. Although this is a measurement of the pressure in the vena cava, it is used commonly to evaluate volume because changes in CVP may be reflective of changes in blood volume; there is normally a direct relationship between the two parameters (see Chapter 183). Additional monitoring techniques that might be helpful include arterial blood pressure; electrocardiogram; and repeated measurements of packed cell volume, total solids, blood glucose, electrolytes, lactate, and acid-base status. Pulmonary capillary wedge pressure monitoring, cardiac output monitoring, and mixed (or central) venous oxygen saturation measurements may be helpful in select patients.

DISCONTINUATION OF FLUID THERAPY

In most animals, fluid therapy should not be discontinued abruptly, especially if high flow rates are being administered. These animals may have renal medullary washout and therefore the urine-concentrating ability will be impaired for several days. This can lead to severe dehydration and hypovolemia in animals that are not drinking large amounts of water. Ideally, intravenous fluid therapy should be decreased gradually over a 24-hour period. Some animals may require slower weaning protocols, especially those receiving high flow rates. Owners should be informed that the animal may have increased water requirements for a few days after the discontinuation of intravenous fluid therapy.

In conclusion, intravenous fluid therapy should be used to maintain normal water, electrolyte, and acid-base status in dogs and cats that are hemodynamically stable. The fluid plan should be tailored to the animal's state of hydration, continued maintenance needs, coexisting diseases, laboratory abnormalities, and anticipated ongoing losses. Critically ill animals commonly require intravenous fluid therapy, and an understanding of body fluid compartments and the distribution of various fluid types is essential when formulating a treatment strategy. Judicious monitoring is vital, and a gradual weaning from fluid therapy is recommended.

REFERENCES

1. Greco DS: The distribution of body water and general approach to the patient, Vet Clin North Am Small Anim Pract 28:473, 1998.
2. Guyton AC, Hall JE: Functional organization of the human body and control of the "internal environment." In Guyton AC, Hall JE, editors: Textbook of medical physiology, ed 11, Philadelphia, 2005, Saunders.

3. National Research Council (NRC): Nutrient requirements of dogs and cats, Washington, DC, 2006, National Academies Press.
4. Mensack S: Fluid therapy: options and rational administration, Vet Clin Small Anim 38:575, 2008.
5. Abrams JT: The nutrition of the dog. In Rechcigl M, editor: CRC handbook series in nutrition and food. Section G: diets, culture media and food supplements, Boca Raton, FL, 1977, CRC Press, p 1.
6. Haskins SC: A simple fluid therapy planning guide, Semin Vet Med Surg (Small Anim) 3:227, 1988.
7. DiBartola SP: Fluid, electrolyte and acid-base disorders in small animal practice, ed 3, Philadelphia, 2006, WB Saunders.
8. Mathews KA: The various types of parenteral fluids and their indications, Vet Clin North Am Small Anim Pract 28:483, 1998.
9. Griffel MI, Kaufman BS: Pharmacology of colloids and crystalloids, Crit Care Clin 8:235, 1992.
10. Rudloff E, Kirby R: Fluid therapy. Crystalloids and colloids, Vet Clin North Am Small Anim Pract 28:297, 1998.
11. Kirby R, Rudloff E: The critical need for colloids: maintaining fluid balance, Comp Cont Educ Pract Vet 19:705, 1997.

CHAPTER 60
SHOCK FLUIDS AND FLUID CHALLENGE

Anusha Balakrishnan, BVSc, AH • Deborah C. Silverstein, DVM, DACVECC

KEY POINTS

- Several options are available for rapid reversal of hypovolemic shock, including crystalloids, synthetic colloids, albumin, hypertonic saline, and blood products.
- Shock fluids are best administered by intravenous or intraosseous routes.
- Isotonic crystalloids are typically the first choice for shock resuscitation but can cause interstitial and pulmonary volume overload.
- Synthetic colloids are excellent choices in hypo-oncotic states but can cause coagulopathies and potentially acute kidney injury in higher doses.
- Albumin and blood products (packed red blood cells and fresh frozen plasma) are other options available for shock resuscitation in certain conditions.
- Performing a fluid challenge is a useful tool to help guide therapeutic decisions regarding fluid therapy in hemodynamically unstable patients.

Fluid therapy is one of the mainstays of treatment in emergency and critical care medicine. Shock is a condition commonly seen in patients presenting to the emergency room as well in a large proportion of critically ill patients. Shock is defined as an inadequate production of energy at the cellular level (see Chapter 5). This usually occurs secondary to decreased delivery of oxygen and nutrients to tissues. Cardiovascular shock can occur secondary to an absolute decrease in the intravascular circulating volume (hypovolemic shock), a severe decrease in oxygen content in the blood (e.g., severe anemia or hypoxemia), maldistribution of the intravascular circulating volume secondary to widespread vasoconstriction or vasodilation (causing a relative hypovolemia, e.g., anaphylaxis or systemic inflammatory response syndrome [SIRS]), or because of failure of the cardiac pump (cardiogenic shock). A variety of metabolic causes for shock have also been identified, including hypoglycemia, various toxin exposures, and cytopathic hypoxia.

The treatment of shock aims to improve tissue perfusion and restore optimal oxygen and nutrient delivery to tissues. In animals with shock secondary to an absolute or relative decrease in the effective circulating intravascular volume, such as in hypovolemic or distributive shock, intravenous (IV) fluid therapy is the cornerstone of management. Various factors should be taken into consideration while administering IV fluid therapy for the treatment of shock, including timing; volume and rate of fluid administration; and safety, efficacy, and cost-effectiveness of the fluids. In recent years there has been an ongoing debate in the medical field regarding the optimal type of fluid for shock therapy, with a growing body of evidence suggesting that certain types of fluids may influence outcome in specific conditions such as trauma, severe sepsis, or septic shock. Regardless, it has been shown that rapid normalization of blood pressure in hypotensive, emergent dogs is associated with a greater survival-to-discharge rate.[1]

ADMINISTRATION OF SHOCK FLUIDS

Shock fluids are best administered intravenously, when possible. This is easily accomplished in patients that are already hospitalized and have adequate vascular access. However, patients that present to the emergency room in a shock state typically lack vascular access. Under these circumstances, establishing venous access can be extremely challenging. When possible, cephalic or saphenous venous access is quickly obtained by placement of the largest gauge, shortest length IV catheter that is appropriate for that particular patient (see Chapter 193). If rapid, large-volume shock fluid administration is necessary (e.g., dogs with severe hypovolemic shock secondary to acute gastric dilation-volvulus), multiple peripheral IV catheters can be placed. When peripheral venous access is difficult to achieve because of severe intravascular volume depletion, jugular venous access can be attempted with a large-bore, short IV catheter. These are typically secured by suturing them in place. Longer catheters can later be placed through the short catheter if long-term jugular venous access is desired after initial resuscitation. Occasionally, extremely unstable patients may be presented in cardiopulmonary arrest and a vascular cutdown procedure is necessary to achieve venous access. Alternatively, an intraosseous catheter can be placed for shock fluid administration. This can be achieved with a regular hypodermic needle in pediatric or neonatal animals. In older animals a commercially available intraosseous access device is usually necessary (see Chapter 194). Other fluid administration routes such as subcutaneous or intraperitoneal are generally not recommended for shock fluid administration because of longer absorption times.

RESUSCITATION ENDPOINTS AND MONITORING

Fluid therapy for the treatment of shock is performed under extremely close monitoring and should continue until various resuscitation endpoints have been reached (see Chapter 183). These endpoints include physical examination parameters such as improvement in heart rate, pulse quality, capillary refill time, temperature of extremities, and brighter mentation. Normalization of arterial blood pressure is another clinical parameter that is often used to guide shock fluid therapy.[1] Bloodwork parameters such as lactate levels and central venous oxygen saturation, when available, can be serially monitored to ensure improvement with fluid therapy. More recently, evaluation of the microcirculation has been considered as a potential endpoint for resuscitation in humans, particularly in septic patients. This is because there is growing evidence to suggest that normalization of conventional macrohemodynamic parameters does not necessarily reflect improved oxygen delivery and perfusion at the tissue level.[2-4] The concept of early goal-directed therapy for treatment of septic shock has received widespread acceptance in human medicine and uses targeted therapies that are instituted within the first 3 and 6 hours of presentation.[5] The 2012 Surviving Sepsis guidelines now mandate the use of this resuscitation strategy. The concept of goal-directed therapy for managing critically ill dogs and cats has also been gaining ground in recent years.[6] A recent veterinary study evaluating canine patients with septic shock also emphasized the importance of goal-directed hemodynamic optimization in improving outcomes.[7] Regardless, both human and veterinary medicine prioritize the use of fluid therapy for the rapid treatment of shock.

SHOCK FLUIDS

The various types of fluids available for shock resuscitation include isotonic and hypertonic crystalloids, synthetic colloids, hemoglobin-based oxygen carriers, albumin, and other blood products (fresh whole blood, fresh frozen plasma, and packed red blood cells).

Isotonic Crystalloids

Isotonic crystalloids are fluids that have a composition similar to that of the extracellular fluid (see Chapter 58). The principal component of crystalloid fluids is the inorganic salt sodium chloride (NaCl), with 0.9% NaCl being the prototype isotonic crystalloid. Sodium is the most abundant solute in the extracellular fluid, and it is distributed uniformly throughout the extracellular space. Because 75% of the extracellular fluids are located in the extravascular (interstitial) space, a similar proportion of the total body sodium is in the interstitial fluids. Exogenously administered sodium follows the same distribution, so 75% of the volume of sodium-based IV fluids is rapidly redistributed within the interstitium. This means that to increase plasma volume by a given amount, four times the desired volume needs to be administered to take into account the interstitial redistribution. However, when administered rapidly as a bolus, isotonic crystalloids can effectively expand plasma volume. A 2005 study showed that a rapid infusion of 80 ml/kg of 0.9% saline to four healthy dogs caused a 76.4% increase in intravascular volume. While rapid redistribution did occur, leaving a net intravascular volume increase of only 35% at 30 minutes and 18% at 4 hours post-infusion,[8] it is possible that a similar volume of infusion to hypovolemic animals may have resulted in a greater, more prolonged expansion of the vascular volume.

Isotonic crystalloids are inexpensive and readily available and as such are typically the first choice for shock resuscitation in most cases.[9] When used for shock resuscitation, the classic "shock dose" is approximately 60 to 90 ml/kg in dogs and approximately 45 to 60 ml/kg in cats, which reflects the approximate blood volumes in each species (Table 60-1). The actual dose used to treat patients with evidence of shock varies widely and is influenced by the species, individual patient, severity of shock, chronicity of disease, and any other co-morbidities (e.g., cardiac disease). A common recommendation is to begin shock treatment using a bolus of 10 to 20 ml/kg administered over 15 to 30 minutes. The patient should be closely monitored during delivery of the bolus, and it should be slowed or discontinued if any adverse effects are seen or if perfusion parameters improve before the end of the predetermined amount.

Adverse effects

Aggressive crystalloid-based resuscitation strategies can lead to several adverse effects, especially in patients predisposed to volume overload (e.g., patients with severe hypoproteinemia or cardiac disease). Because these fluids redistribute into the interstitium, organ edema can occur and may be life threatening (see Chapter 11). Pulmonary edema and acute lung injury are among the most commonly seen adverse effects of shock resuscitation, particularly in patients with increased vascular permeability secondary to systemic inflammation or sepsis.[10]

Other consequences of aggressive and overzealous crystalloid administration include changes to the gastrointestinal (GI) tract resulting in decreased motility, increased intestinal permeability predisposing the patient to bacterial translocation, and increased risk for abdominal compartment syndrome. Cardiac effects of crystalloid therapy have also been documented and include an increased risk of ventricular arrhythmias, disruption of cardiac contractility, and decreased cardiac output. This can be demonstrated by Starling's myocardial performance curve; when beyond a designated point on the curve, further increases in end-diastolic volume cause a decrease in cardiac output. Coagulation disturbances can also occur as a result of dilution of coagulation factors and decreased blood viscosity; however, these effects are significantly less than changes caused by synthetic colloids.[10,11]

Isotonic crystalloids, particularly lactated Ringer's solution, have been associated with alterations of the inflammatory cascade. Many formulations of this crystalloid contain racemic mixtures of both the L- and D-lactate stereoisomers. The D-lactate has been associated with an increase in neutrophil stimulation, whereas the L-lactate is rapidly metabolized by the liver.[12,13] Administration of lactated Ringer's solution that contains only the L-isomer may even decrease inflammation in humans with pancreatitis.[14] Even mild decreases in osmolality can lead to cellular swelling and subsequent activation of phospholipase A2, resulting in an increased production of prostaglandins, lipoxygenases, leukotrienes, and epoxyeicosatrienoic acids. Acute increases in cellular volume also stimulate production and release of tumor necrosis factor α (TNF-α) from macrophages. Increased levels of proinflammatory cytokines (e.g., interleukins such as IL-6, IL-8, and IL-10) may also occur; this can have deleterious effects on an already compromised microcirculation and further increase the risk of edema and fluid overload.[10,11,15,16]

Table 60-1 **Suggested Doses for Shock Fluid Resuscitation**

Shock Fluid	Dose	Comments	Examples of Products
Isotonic crystalloids	Typical bolus dose: 10-20 ml/kg IV over 15-30 minutes Total "shock" dose: 60-90 ml/kg in dogs, 45-60 ml/kg in cats	Rapid redistribution with short-lived intravascular volume expansion effect. Caution with use in patients with decreased colloid osmotic pressure or increased vascular permeability because of increased risk of pulmonary and interstitial edema.	0.9% NaCl, lactated Ringer's solution, Normosol-R, Plasmalyte-148
Synthetic colloids	Typical bolus dose: 2-5 ml/kg IV over 10-30 minutes Total "shock" dose: 10-20 ml/kg in dogs, 5-10 ml/kg in cats	Sustained intravascular volume expansion. Increased risk of coagulation disturbances with use of large doses. May potentially cause or exacerbate preexisting acute kidney injury.	Hespan (6% hetastarch in 0.9% NaCl) Hextend (6% hetastarch in lactated electrolyte solution) Pentaspan (10% pentastarch in 0.9% NaCl) Vetstarch, Voluven (6% tetrastarch in 0.9% NaCl)
Hypertonic solutions	Typical dose: 3-5 ml/kg of 7%-7.5% NaCl solution Can be combined in a 1:2 ratio of 23.4% NaCl to a synthetic colloid for sustained intravascular volume expansion	Monitor electrolytes, particularly sodium. Use with caution in chronic hyponatremia. Can exacerbate interstitial volume depletion in dehydrated patients. Good for small-volume resuscitation, particularly in septic shock, hemorrhagic shock, and traumatic brain injury.	Commercially available in concentrations ranging from 3%-23.4% NaCl
Albumin	Typical dose: 2 ml/kg of 25% human serum albumin IV over 2 hours followed by 0.1-0.2 ml/kg/hr IV for 10 hours for a total dose of 2 g/kg Alternatively, albumin deficit can be calculated and replaced over 6-12 hours (see text for calculation)	Ideal for critically ill hypoalbuminemic patients with severe sepsis, septic shock, or trauma. Monitor for anaphylactoid or delayed hypersensitivity reactions. Repeated use is NOT recommended due to sensitization and risk of anaphylactic reactions	Commercially available as 25% human serum albumin solution Lyophilized canine albumin previously marketed for use in dogs but is no longer commercially available in United States
Blood products	Typical dose: pRBCs and fresh frozen plasma: 10-20ml/kg given IV over 2-4 hours (can be given faster in rapidly decompensating patients up to a rate of 1.5ml/kg/min over 15-20 minutes) Fresh whole blood: 20-30 ml/kg over 2-4 hours	Check blood type before administration and crossmatch if necessary. Monitor for transfusion reactions throughout duration of administration. Ideal for patients presenting in acute hemorrhagic shock.	Canine and feline pRBCs Canine and feline FFP Canine and feline fresh whole blood (where donors available)
Oxyglobin	Typical dose: 10 to 30 ml/kg IV	No crossmatch or blood typing required. Hyperoncotic solution, so monitor for fluid overload. Increases systemic vascular resistance. Can cause yellow-orange discoloration of serum, tissues, and urine. Very expensive.	N/A

FFP, Fresh frozen plasma; *pRBCs,* packed red blood cells.

SYNTHETIC COLLOIDS

Colloids are large molecules (>10,000 Daltons) of varying sizes that do not readily cross diffusion barriers across normal blood vessels as crystalloids do. Colloids that are infused into the vascular space therefore tend to remain in the vascular space rather than redistribute to the interstitial space. This leads to a more sustained intravascular expansion effect. These fluids increase the colloid osmotic pressure of serum, creating a force that opposes the hydrostatic pressure in the vasculature and helps retain fluid in the vascular space.

Commercially available synthetic colloids typically contain large colloid molecules suspended in an isotonic crystalloid solution. Some of the more commonly available synthetic colloids are derivatives of hydroxyethyl starches (HESs) (see Chapter 58).

Hetastarch

Hetastarch is a synthetic colloid available as a 6% solution suspended in an isotonic crystalloid solution such as 0.9% saline (Hespan) or a lactated electrolyte solution (Hextend). The colloid particles are composed of amylopectin molecules that vary in size from a few hundred to more than a million Daltons. The clearance of hetastarch molecules from the intravascular space depends on the rate of their absorption by tissues (liver, spleen, kidney, and heart), uptake by the reticuloendothelial system, clearance through urine and bile, and enzymatic degradation to small particles by serum amylase. α-Amylase-mediated hydrolysis can reduce the molecular weight of these particles to less than 72 kDA. The degree of hydroxyl substitution in these starches is the primary determinant of how long they survive in the blood. In a study in healthy dogs, infusion of

20 ml/kg of hetastarch solution produced a 27.2% increase in blood volume immediately after infusion, an increase to 36.8% at 30 minutes, and maintenance of 26.6% at 4 hours post-infusion.[8]

Tetrastarch

Tetrastarch has particles with a slightly lower weight average molecular weight and a higher number of hydroxyl residues (lower substitution with hydroxyethyl groups) than the previously discussed hetastarch. These properties are likely responsible for causing fewer effects on coagulation than hetastarch solutions.[17,18] This product has recently been approved for use in small animals (Vetstarch). More studies in veterinary medicine evaluating the effects of this particular synthetic colloid are necessary to assess its effectiveness and safety as a volume expander.

Pentastarch

Pentastarch is a low-molecular-weight derivative of hetastarch that is available as a 6% or 10% solution in isotonic saline. Although it is not currently approved for clinical use in the United States, it has been used in other parts of the world as an effective volume expander. Pentastarch contains smaller but more numerous starch molecules than hetastarch and thus has a higher colloid osmotic pressure. It is a slightly more effective volume expander than hetastarch and can increase plasma volume by up to 1.5 times the infusion volume.[19]

Because colloids are retained in the vascular space longer than crystalloid solutions and can have adverse coagulation effects, the recommended rates and volumes of administration of these fluids are typically much lower than that of crystalloids. When synthetic colloids are used for the treatment of shock, the typical dose is 10 to 20 ml/kg in the dog and 5 to 10 ml/kg in the cat (see Table 60-1). This is commonly administered to effect in incremental boluses of 2 to 5 ml/kg over 10 to 20 minutes.

Adverse effects

Much emphasis has been placed in recent years on the various potential adverse effects of synthetic colloids, especially in people. There has been recent evidence in several human trials and meta-analyses that high molecular-weight starches (HES 200/0.6 and >200) may cause acute kidney injury in patients with severe sepsis, although HES 130/0.4 is considered to be less harmful.[9,19-24] However, a recently published study did not support this hypothesis and showed that even 6% HES 130/0.4 can cause more impairment of renal function than resuscitation with crystalloids alone in patients with severe sepsis.[24]

Another concern with the use of synthetic colloids is their effect on coagulation. All colloidal plasma substitutes are known to interfere with the physiologic mechanisms of hemostasis either through a nonspecific effect correlated to the degree of hemodilution or through specific actions of these macromolecules on platelet function, coagulation proteins, and the fibrinolytic system. High molecular-weight starches can cause decreases in the activity of von Willebrand's factor and its associated factor VIII and ristocetin cofactor activities, as well as some degree of platelet dysfunction.[25,26]

Studies have shown that the administration of more than 20 ml/kg/day of hetastarch in animals can cause coagulation derangements. This maximal limit is often exceeded in practice, but the potential for coagulopathic sequelae should be recognized. Because tetrastarch is purported to have fewer adverse effects on coagulation, higher doses can potentially be administered (up to 40 ml/kg/day).

HYPERTONIC SOLUTIONS

A hypertonic crystalloid solution is any saline solution that has an effective osmolarity exceeding that of normal plasma. Hypertonic saline solutions are available commercially in variable concentrations of 3% to 23.4%. Hypertonic saline has several beneficial properties that make it an excellent choice for rapid, small-volume resuscitation in shock patients. A 2005 study evaluating the changes in blood volume after a bolus of 4 ml/kg of 7.5% sodium chloride showed that the post-infusion plasma volume change was only about 17% despite a brief increase in blood volume about three times the volume of fluid administered.[8] Its ability to cause intravascular volume expansion in excess of the volume infused is due to the osmotic gradient generated by the sudden, dramatic increase in plasma osmolarity after administration, thus making it a good option for small-volume resuscitation.

In addition to its volume expansion ability, hypertonic saline has numerous other properties that make it an attractive choice for shock resuscitation, particularly in animals with septic shock, hemorrhagic shock, and traumatic brain injury. These properties include immunomodulatory effects, such as decreased neutrophil activation and adherence, stimulation of lymphocyte proliferation, and inhibition of proinflammatory cytokine production by macrophages. It also improves the rheologic properties of circulating blood, reduces endothelial cell swelling, and helps reduce intracranial pressure in patients with traumatic brain injury.[27-30] There is evidence to suggest that hypertonic saline administration improves myocardial function and causes coronary vasodilation, thereby improving overall cardiac function.[31] However, the clinical effect on cardiac contractility in dogs and cats requires further evaluation.

Hypertonic saline most commonly is used as either a 3% or 7.0% to 7.5% solution. Typically a 3 to 5 ml/kg dose of 7% to 7.5% solution is used for small-volume resuscitation (see Table 60-1). Because hypertonic saline rapidly redistributes into the interstitium within 30 minutes after administration and also causes an osmotic diuresis, its volume expansion effect is short lived. For this reason, it is often combined with a synthetic colloid such as hetastarch or pentastarch. This combined solution, sometimes referred to as "turbostarch," is administered at a dose of 3 to 5 ml/kg and is prepared by mixing a stock solution of 23.4% hypertonic saline with 6% hetastarch in a 1:2 ratio to arrive at a total volume of 3 to 5 ml/kg. For example, a 5 ml/kg dose for a 12-kg dog would be 60 ml. Therefore 1 part 23.4% hypertonic saline (20 ml) with 2 parts (40 ml) 6% hetastarch would create an approximately 7.5% hypertonic saline solution.

Adverse effects

The primary adverse effect of hypertonic saline is hypernatremia. This is seen immediately after administration but is usually transient. There is a risk for hypernatremia-induced central pontine myelinolysis when administered to patients with preexisting chronic hyponatremia; however, this has rarely been reported. Most critical patients have frequent monitoring of electrolytes, and the risk of transient hypernatremia does not outweigh the potential benefits hypertonic saline therapy.

Hypertonic saline should be used cautiously in patients with preexisting cardiac or pulmonary abnormalities because the increase in intravascular volume and hydrostatic pressure may lead to volume overload or pulmonary edema. It can also cause significant interstitial (and intravascular) volume depletion, particularly in patients that are already dehydrated. Therefore hypertonic fluid administration should be followed by additional fluid therapy as indicated.

ALBUMIN

Albumin is one of the most important plasma proteins because of its many physiologic effects in the body, including maintenance of colloid osmotic pressure and endothelial integrity, wound healing, metabolic and acid-base functions, coagulation, and free radical scavenging. Albumin levels are often low in critically ill patients (especially those with septic or hemorrhagic shock) because of loss, vascular leak, third-spacing, and decreased production as a result of shifting of hepatic production toward acute-phase proteins.

Hypoalbuminemic patients that require fluid resuscitation may be at increased risk for interstitial edema after large-volume crystalloid administration. Natural or synthetic colloid therapy should be considered. Albumin, a natural colloid, confers various additional advantages, as outlined earlier that are not provided by synthetic colloids, particularly in patients with systemic inflammatory syndromes and vascular leak disorders.

The use of albumin as a resuscitation fluid in human patients with severe sepsis and septic shock has been widely debated and remains controversial.[32-35] The landmark SAFE study showed no decrease in 28-day mortality in a heterogeneous population of critically ill patients who were administered either 4% human serum albumin (HSA) or 0.9% saline.[35] Trials in patients with traumatic brain injury have documented higher mortality rates when patients were resuscitated with albumin versus saline.[36] A large randomized controlled trial (the PRECISE RCT) evaluating the effectiveness of 5% HSA versus 0.9% saline in septic shock patients is currently underway and is expected to publish results over the next few months.[37]

The use of albumin in dogs is typically reserved for dogs with clinically severe hypoalbuminemia (usually <1 g/dl) secondary to severe sepsis, septic shock, or trauma or those with prolonged critical illness, especially after major surgery. Administration of albumin in dogs is associated with various logistical problems, including availability of species-specific albumin products. Concentrated canine albumin solutions have been only intermittently available; therefore 25% HSA is the most commonly used albumin solution.[38]

Several dosing regimens have been proposed for 25% human serum albumin therapy, including calculation of the patient's albumin deficit and administration over 6 to 12 hours (see Table 60-1).[38,39]

$$\text{Albumin deficit (gms)} = 10 \times (\text{desired albumin} - \text{patient albumin}) \times \text{weight (kg)} \times 0.3$$

Alternatively, 2 ml/kg 25% HSA over 2 hours IV followed by 0.1 to 0.2 ml/kg/hr for 10 hours for a total dose of 2 g/kg.[38,39]

Several veterinary studies in the past 10 years have evaluated the effects of 25% HSA in healthy and critically ill dogs.[39-43] When HSA was administered to healthy dogs, adverse effects, including life-threatening anaphylactoid reactions, were observed in three of nine dogs receiving a single infusion and in two of two dogs that received a second transfusion.[39] A study performed in 2008 found the use of 25% HSA in critically ill dogs significantly raised serum albumin and total protein concentrations, as well colloid osmotic pressure, particularly in survivors.[43] Although studies evaluating the use of HSA in critically ill dogs have observed increases in serum immunoglobulin G (IgG), acute type I hypersensitivity reactions have not been reported.[40-43] Therefore although the use of HSA in critically ill dogs appears to be safer than in healthy dogs, caution should be exercised and close monitoring is warranted.

BLOOD PRODUCTS

The use of blood products (whole blood, fresh frozen plasma [FFP], or packed red blood cells [pRBCs]) is of significant value in shock resuscitation, particularly in animals that present with signs of hemorrhagic shock secondary to trauma, nontraumatic hemoabdomen, gastrointestinal bleeding, rodenticide intoxication, or other primary or secondary coagulopathies.

Severe hemorrhagic shock results in an acute, dramatic drop in intravascular volume and a resultant decrease in oxygen delivery to tissues. These patients may require massive volume replacement within a very short time. Although traditional fluid therapy with crystalloids and synthetic colloids can be employed in the short term to replace circulating intravascular volume, blood products are often necessary to provide the hemoglobin necessary for oxygen-carrying capacity and to replace the coagulation factors that are lost and consumed during massive hemorrhage. Crystalloid and colloid therapy can also cause dilution of already depleted clotting factors, and colloids may interfere with clot formation and stability, all of which can worsen preexisting bleeding.

The use of fresh whole blood has been documented to be of greatest benefit in several human trauma studies. Fresh whole blood transfusions carry the benefit of increased levels of clotting factors, fibrinogen, and platelets compared with component therapy. Current recommendations in trauma resuscitation advocate minimizing or altogether avoiding crystalloid use in these patients. Aggressive use of fresh frozen plasma is recommended in situations where whole blood is not easily available with FFP/pRBCs given in the ratio of 1:1.[44,45]

Typical management of the patient presenting in acute hemorrhagic shock includes pRBCs and FFP at a dose of 10 to 20 ml/kg (see Chapter 61). Although transfusions are usually administered over a period of 2 to 4 hours, rapidly decompensating patients may require faster infusion rates (i.e., 1.5 ml/kg/min over 15 to 20 minutes) (see Table 60-1). The term *massive transfusion* has come into widespread use, defined as the replacement of a volume of whole blood or blood components that is greater than the patient's estimated blood volume. Massive transfusions carry a much higher risk of adverse transfusion related effects (e.g., electrolyte imbalances, acute lung injury, and immunologic reactions); they can be extremely cost prohibitive but lifesaving in certain patients.[46]

HYPOTENSIVE RESUSCITATION

Traditional fluid resuscitation for patients with hemorrhagic shock involves resuscitation until a normal systolic blood pressure is achieved. However, in recent years literature has pointed toward an improved survival (particularly in trauma patients) when a more conservative resuscitation strategy is employed in the acute setting during active hemorrhage, also known as hypotensive resuscitation.[47-49] Restoration of a lower-than-normal systolic blood pressure (approximately 80 to 90 mm Hg) helps facilitate control of hemorrhage and reduces the risk of rebleeding but at the same time ensures preserved blood flow to vital organs such as the kidney and GI tract. A classic example of the use of hypotensive resuscitation in veterinary medicine is the treatment of dogs with a nontraumatic hemoabdomen secondary to an actively bleeding intra-abdominal neoplasm. In these dogs, relative hemodynamic stability can be achieved with crystalloid, colloid, and blood product transfusions; however, overaggressive resuscitation is usually avoided, especially in the more stable patients, to avoid dislodging recently formed clots and helping to control active hemorrhage.

It is important to emphasize, however, that hypotensive resuscitation is a temporary solution and is only meant to bridge the gap between presentation and definitive hemostatic control (usually via surgical intervention). Hypotensive resuscitation should not be used as a long-term or permanent treatment approach because this puts the patient at risk for complications resulting from impairment of tissue perfusion.

FLUID CHALLENGE

A fluid challenge is defined as administration of fluids to patients that are hemodynamically unstable in order to assess their response to fluid therapy and guide further treatment decisions. This is usually reserved for critically ill patients and allows for subjective and objective assessment of the cardiovascular response during fluid infusion and rapid expansion of intravascular volume. It also helps guide therapy while minimizing the risk of volume overload that can occur as a result of overzealous or unnecessary fluid therapy. Performing a fluid challenge with specific targets helps provide a more objective method of guiding fluid therapy decisions.[50]

While performing a fluid challenge, the following factors should be considered:

- Type of fluid: Crystalloids or synthetic colloids are typically used to perform a fluid challenge. Because colloids are retained in the intravascular space longer than crystalloids, smaller volumes are required to complete a fluid challenge (e.g., a typical crystalloid volume for fluid challenge in a dog might be 10 to 20 ml/kg, whereas a synthetic colloid dose would be 3 to 5 ml/kg).
- Rate of fluid administration: Fluid challenges are typically performed over a period of 10 to 30 minutes.
- End points: Identify the parameters that are abnormal and indicative of hemodynamic instability, and aim to assess changes in these parameters after a fluid challenge. For example, hypotension, weak pulse quality, prolonged capillary refill time, tachycardia, or oliguria might be identified. Assess for reversal or improvement in these abnormalities after completion of a fluid challenge with specific endpoints. Lactate and central venous oxygen saturation ($ScVO_2$) monitoring, if available, can also be serially evaluated. (See Chapters 183 and 186 for further details.)
- Safety of the fluid challenge: Patients must be watched closely for signs of volume overload, particularly pulmonary edema, during any fluid challenge. Respiratory rate and effort, pulse oximetry, central venous pressures, and arterial blood gases should all be monitored.

REFERENCES

1. Silverstein DC, Kleiner J, Drobatz KJ: Effectiveness of intravenous fluid resuscitation in the emergency room for treatment of hypotension in dogs, J Vet Emerg Crit Care 22:666, 2012.
2. Ince C: The microcirculation is the motor of sepsis, Crit Care 9(4):S13, 2005.
3. Trzeciak S, McCoy JV, Dellinger RP, et al: Early increases in microcirculatory perfusion during protocol-directed resuscitation are associated with reduced multi-organ failure at 24h in patients with sepsis, Int Care Med 34:2210, 2008.
4. Vincent J, De Backer D: Microvascular dysfunction as a cause of organ dysfunction in severe sepsis, Crit Care 9(4):S9, 2005.
5. Rivers E, Nguyen B, Havstad S, et al: Early goal directed therapy in the treatment of severe sepsis and septic shock, N Engl J Med 345(19):1368, 2001.
6. Butler AL: Goal-directed therapy in small animal critical illness, Vet Clin N Am 41:817, 2011.
7. Conti-Patara A, de Araújo Caldeira J, de Mattos-Junior E, et al: Changes in tissue perfusion parameters in dogs with severe sepsis/septic shock in response to goal-directed hemodynamic optimization at admission to ICU and the relation to outcome, J Vet Emerg Crit Care 22:409, 2012.
8. Silverstein DC, Aldrich J, Haskins SC, et al: Assessment of changes in blood volume in response to resuscitative fluid administration in dogs, J Vet Emerg Crit Care 15(3):185, 2005.
9. Perel P, Roberts I: Colloids versus crystalloids for fluid resuscitation in critically ill patients, Cochrane Database Syst Rev 2012:6, 2012.
10. Cotton BA, Guy JS, Morris JA, et al: The cellular, metabolic and systemic consequences of aggressive fluid resuscitation strategies, Shock 26(2):115, 2006.
11. Shoemaker WC, Hauser CJ: Critique of crystalloid versus colloid therapy in shock and shock lung, Crit Care Med 7:117, 1979.
12. Rhee P, Burris D, Kaufmann C, et al: Lactated Ringer's solution causes neutrophil activation after hemorrhagic shock, J Trauma Inj Infect Crit Care 44(2):313, 1998.
13. Alam HB, Stanton K, Koustova E, et al: Effect of different resuscitation strategies on neutrophil activation in a swine model of hemorrhagic shock, Resuscitation 60:91, 2004.
14. Wu BU, Hwang JQ, Gardner TH, et al: Lactated Ringer's solution reduces systemic inflammation compared with saline in patients with acute pancreatitis, Clin Gastroen Hepatol 9(8):710, 2011.
15. Ng KF, Lam CK, Chan LC. In vivo effect of hemodilution with saline on coagulation: a randomized controlled trial, Br J Anaesth 88:475, 2002.
16. Lang F, Busch GL, Ritter M, et al: Functional significance of cell volume regulatory mechanisms, Physiol Rev 78:248, 1998.
17. Baron JF: A new hydroxyethyl starch: HES 130/0.4 Voluven®, Transfusion Altern Transfusion Med 2(2):13, 2000.
18. Langeron O, Doelberg M, Ang ET, et al: Voluven®, a lower substituted novel hydroxyethyl starch (HES 130/0.4), causes fewer effects on coagulation in major orthopedic surgery than HES 200/0.5, Anesthesia Analgesia 92(4):855, 2001.
19. Strauss RG, Pennell BJ, Stump DC. A randomized, blinded trial comparing the hemostatic effects of pentastarch versus hetastarch, Transfusion 42(1):27, 2002.
20. Bunn F, Trivedi D, Ashraf S: Colloid solutions for fluid resuscitation, Cochrane Database Syst Rev 2011:3, 2011.
21. Roberts I, Alderson P, Bunn F, et al: Colloids versus crystalloids for fluid resuscitation in critically ill patients, Cochrane Database Syst Rev 2004:4, 2004.
22. Perner A, Haase N, Wetterslev J, et al: Comparing the effect of hydroxyethyl starch 130/0.4 with balanced crystalloid solution on mortality and kidney failure in patients with severe sepsis (6S-Scandinavian Starch for Severe Sepsis/Septic Shock trial): study protocol, design and rationale for a double-blinded, randomized clinical trial, Trials 12(1):24, 2011.
23. Schortgen F, Girou E, Deye N, et al: The risk associated with hyperoncotic colloids in patients with shock, Int Care Med 34(12):2157, 2008.
24. Bayer O, Reinhart K, Sakr Y, et al: Renal effects of synthetic colloids and crystalloids in patients with severe sepsis: a prospective sequential comparison, Crit Care Med 39(6):1335, 2012.
25. Ekseth K, Abildgaard L, Vegfors M, et al: The in vitro effects of crystalloids and colloids on coagulation, Anaesthesia 57(11):1102, 2002.
26. Mortier E, Ongenae M, De Baerdemaeker L, et al: In vitro evaluation of the effect of profound hemodilution with hydroxyethyl starch 6%, modified fluid gelatin 4% and dextran 40 10% on coagulation profile measured by thromboelastography, Anaesthesia 52(11):1061, 2005.
27. Rizoli SB, Rhind SG, Shek PN, et al: The immunomodulatory effects of hypertonic saline resuscitation in patients sustaining traumatic hemorrhagic shock, Ann Surg 243(1):47, 2006.
28. Bulger EM, Jurkovich GJ, Nathens AB, et al: Hypertonic resuscitation of hypovolemic shock after blunt trauma: a randomized controlled trial, Arch Surg 143(2):139, 2008.
29. Mortazavi MM, Romeo AK, Deep A, et al: Hypertonic saline for treating raised intracranial pressure: literature review with meta-analyses, J Neurosurg 116:210, 2012.
30. Balbino M, Neto AC, Prist R, et al: Fluid resuscitation with isotonic or hypertonic saline solution avoids intraneural calcium influx after traumatic brain injury associated with hemorrhagic shock, J Trauma Inj Infect Crit Care 68:859, 2010.
31. Mouren S, Delayance S, Mion G, et al: Mechanisms of increased myocardial contractility with hypertonic saline solutions in isolated blood perfused rabbit hearts, Anesth Analg 81:777, 1995.
32. Delaney AP, Dan A, McCaffrey J, et al: The role of albumin as a resuscitation fluid for patients with sepsis: a systematic review and meta-analyses, Crit Care Med 39:386, 2011.
33. Friedman G, Jankowski S, Shahla M, et al: Hemodynamic effects of 6% and 10% hydroxyethyl starch solutions versus 4% albumin solution in septic patients, J Clin Anesth 20:528, 2008.
34. Boldt J, Heesen M, Muller M, et al: The effects of albumin versus hydroxyethyl starch solution on cardiorespiratory and circulatory variables in critically ill patients, Anesth Analg 83:254, 1996.
35. The SAFE Study Investigators: A comparison of albumin and saline for fluid resuscitation in the intensive care unit, N Engl J Med 350:2247, 2004.
36. Myburgh J, Cooper DJ, Finfer S, et al: Saline or albumin for fluid resuscitation in patients with traumatic brain injury, N Engl J Med 357:874, 2007.
37. McIntyre L, Fergusson DA, Rowe B, et al: The PRECISE RCT: evolution of an early septic shock fluid resuscitation trial, Transfus Med Rev 26:333, 2012.

38. Mazzaferro EM, Rudloff E, Kirby R: The role of albumin replacement in the critically ill veterinary patient, J Vet Emerg Crit Care 12:113, 2002.
39. Cohn LA, Kerl ME, Lenox CE, et al: Response of healthy dogs to infusions of human serum albumin, Am J Vet Res 2007;68:65, 2007.
40. Martin LG, Luther TY, Alperin DC, et al: Serum antibodies against human albumin in critically ill and healthy dogs, J Am Vet Med Assoc 232:1004, 2008.
41. Matthews KA, Barry M: The use of 25% human serum albumin: outcome and efficacy in raising serum albumin and blood pressure in critically ill dogs and cats, J Vet Emerg Crit Care 5(2):110, 2005.
42. Viganó F, Perissinotto L, Bosco VRF: Administration of 5% human serum albumin in critically ill small animal patients with hypoalbuminemia: 418 dogs and 170 cats (1994-2008), J Vet Emerg Crit Care 20:237, 2012.
43. Trow AV, Rozanski EA, deLaforcade AM, et al: Evaluation of use of human albumin in critically ill dogs: 73 cases (2003-2006), J Am Vet Med Assoc 233:607, 2008.
44. Como JJ, Dutton RP, Scalea TM, Edelman BB, Hess JR: Blood transfusion rates in the care of acute trauma, Transfusion 44:809, 2004.
45. Repine TB, Perkins JG, Kauvar DS, et al: The use of fresh whole blood in massive transfusion, J Trauma 60(Suppl):S59, 2006.
46. Jutkowitz AL, Rozanski EA, Moreau JA, et al: Massive transfusion in dogs: 15 cases (1997-2001), J Am Vet Med Assoc 220:1664, 2002.
47. Holcomb JB, Jenkins D, Rhee P, et al: Damage control resuscitation: directly addressing the coagulopathy of trauma, J Trauma 62:307, 2007.
48. Duchesne JC, McSwain NE, Cotton BA, et al: Damage control resuscitation: the new face of damage control, J Trauma Inj Infect Crit Care 69:976, 2010.
49. Morrison AC, Carrick MM, Normal MA, et al: Hypotensive resuscitation strategy reduces transfusion requirements and severe postoperative coagulopathy in trauma patients with hemorrhagic shock: preliminary results of a randomized controlled trial, J Trauma Inj Infect Crit Care 70:652, 2011.
50. Vincent JL, Weil MH: Fluid challenge revisited, Crit Care Med 34:1333, 2006.

CHAPTER 61
TRANSFUSION THERAPY

Urs Giger, PD, DrMedVet, MS, FVH, DACVIM-SA, DECVIM-CA, DECVCP

KEY POINTS

- *Transfusion therapy* refers to the safe and effective replacement of blood or one of its components, thereby offering support for critically ill anemic or bleeding patients.
- The indications for transfusions need to be clearly determined, and ideally only the deficient blood components are replaced using appropriate dosages.
- Although red blood cells and plasma clotting factors are crucial, the indications and efficacy of transfusing platelets, leukocytes, and other plasma proteins are limited.
- Blood products represent a limited resource; hence they should be given only when indicated, using the minimal dosage required and after carefully considering possible alternatives.
- All canine and feline donor blood must be typed for the dog erythrocyte antigen (DEA) 1 and the feline AB blood groups, respectively, and all donors must have regular health examinations including blood and infectious disease screening.
- All canine and feline recipient blood should be typed for the DEA 1 and AB blood group, respectively. Blood from animals previously transfused (>4 days after first transfusion ever received) should also be crossmatched before receiving another red blood cell transfusion (cats may be crossmatched even prior to the first transfusion because of possible anti-mik antibodies).
- Although acute hemolytic transfusion reactions are feared most, they can be avoided by prior compatibility testing; other transfusion reactions cannot be predicted by compatibility testing.
- The effectiveness and survival of transfused blood cells and plasma proteins should be monitored during and after transfusion using appropriate clinical and laboratory parameters.
- Lyophylized canine platelets and specific plasma components such as albumin and cryoprecipitate have recently become available, although no hemoglobin solutions are currently commercially available for veterinary use.

Critically ill animals or those undergoing surgical procedures often benefit from the administration of blood products. However, blood products are obtained from donor animals and thus represent a limited resource that is not available in all practice settings. Because they are biologic products, they bear the inherent risks of transmitting infectious diseases or causing other adverse reactions. Clinicians in the critical care setting play a key role in providing safe and effective transfusion therapy and therefore should be aware of the principles of transfusion medicine. The interested reader is referred at the end of the chapter to more comprehensive reviews and books on veterinary transfusion medicine.

INDICATIONS FOR TRANSFUSION THERAPY

Blood transfusions are indicated for management of anemia, coagulopathy, and, rarely, for other conditions such as thrombocytopenia, thrombopathia, and hypoproteinemia (Table 61-1). The disorders that lead to these medical problems and their detailed management are described in separate chapters. Fresh whole blood (FWB, kept at room temperature for <8 hours) contains all cellular and plasma components of blood, but specific blood component therapy provides the most effective and safest support and allows for optimal use of every blood donation. The decision to transfuse is based on the overall clinical assessment of a patient's history and clinical signs, routine laboratory test results, underlying cause, and sound clinical judgment. Although the optimal packed cell volume (PCV) is more than 30%, oxygen delivery in a normovolemic, resting animal can be maintained down to a PCV of 10% (although this is completely inadequate under most disease conditions). Thus there is no specific

Table 61-1 Blood Products, Storage Guidelines, and Indications

Blood Product	Storage	Temperature in Celsius	Indications
Fresh whole blood (FWB)	<8 hours	2 to 24	Combined red blood cell and plasma deficiency with need for platelets
FWB	<24 hours	4	Combined red blood cell and plasma deficiency without need for platelets
Stored whole blood (SWB)	28 days	4	Anemia Hypoproteinemia
pRBC	28 days	4	Anemia
Platelet rich plasma (PRP) or platelet concentrates	24 hours*	20-24	Thrombocytopenia with life-threatening bleeding
Fresh frozen plasma (FFP)	1 year	<–20 to –40	Any coagulation factor deficiencies; hypoproteinemia
Stored plasma	1 to 2 years	<–20 to –40	Hypoproteinemia
Cryoprecipitate (cryo)	1 year	<–20 to –40	von Willebrand's disease Hemophilia A (but not B) Hypofibrinogenemia
Cryoprecipitate-poor plasma (cryo-poor)	1 year	<–20 to –40	Hypoproteinemia Some coagulopathies (factors II, VII, IX, XI)

*If constantly mixed gently.

transfusion trigger in any patient (i.e., certain PCV or coagulation times). However, because transfusion carries inherent risks, blood should never be given without a clear indication or before exhausting alternative therapies. Furthermore, blood components represent a scarce resource and should not be used without a proper indication and assessment of the prognosis.

Red Blood Cell Transfusions

The most common indication for transfusions in dogs and cats is anemia (see Chapter 108). Transfusions are generally required after major loss of the blood's oxygen-carrying capacity (i.e., loss of hemoglobin) and subsequent tissue/organ ischemia but not as a simple volume expander. Depending on the type, degree, rapidity, and course of the anemia, a transfusion with blood products, such as stored packed red blood cells (pRBCs), FWB, or stored whole blood, may be warranted. Animals with rapidly progressive anemia should be transfused when the PCV is approximately 20% to 25%, but a patient with chronic anemia may not require a transfusion despite having a much lower PCV.

Healthy animals can readily tolerate a loss of up to 20% of blood volume (canine blood donors regularly give 20 ml/kg body weight while cats give 10 ml/kg q6-12wk) without any ill effects. However, animals with acute hemorrhage exceeding 20% of the blood volume may require a blood transfusion in addition to the initial shock fluid replacement therapy (see Chapter 60). It should be noted that animals with peracute blood loss will not show a drop in PCV for several hours after hemorrhage, until intercompartmental fluid shifts occur or fluid therapy is instituted. Hence other parameters are used to decide if transfusion therapy is indicated, such as mucous membrane color, capillary refill time, heart rate, blood pressure, venous oxygen saturation, and possibly blood lactate levels (see Chapter 183 for further details). Arterial blood gas values as well as respiratory rate and effort should be normal in uncomplicated anemia but are useful to evaluate animals with coexisting respiratory disease. In most animals with anemia secondary to acute blood loss, fluid therapy alone will restore vital organ perfusion, although pRBCs should be considered in any animal with evidence of anemia-related tissue hypoxia. A falling PCV is not a contraindication for fluid administration, although excessive blood collection for diagnostic tests may necessitate blood replacement in a sick animal and thus should be avoided. Animals that require anesthesia and surgery should have a PCV of at least 20% to ensure adequate oxygen-carrying capacity during anesthesia.

In animals with immune-mediated hemolytic anemia (see Chapter 110), red blood cell transfusions have proven lifesaving. There is no evidence that transfused red blood cells "add fuel to the fire" or are destroyed more rapidly than the patient's own erythrocytes. However, mismatched, incompatible transfusions must be avoided and older pRBCs may be less beneficial and safe than fresher pRBCs (<7 days), particularly in dogs with immune-mediated hemolytic anemia. The administration of a bovine hemoglobin solution (Oxyglobin) has also shown beneficial effects but is currently not available in the United States (see Chapter 58 for further details).

Fresh Frozen Plasma

Fresh frozen plasma (FFP) is used most commonly in veterinary practice to treat coagulopathies causing serious bleeding, because this product contains all coagulation factors. FFP is commonly used in animals with hemorrhage secondary to acquired coagulopathies (e.g., liver disease and anticoagulant rodenticide intoxications) or patients with hereditary coagulopathies and subsequent bleeding. Sudden hemorrhage caused by therapeutically used heparin (including accidental use of undiluted heparin flushes) or warfarin to counter thrombosis can also be corrected with FFP, although protamine and vitamin K can also rapidly reverse the heparin- and warfarin-induced effects, respectively. The use of FFP (with or without the administration of heparin) to replace deficient coagulation factors and antithrombin in patients with immune-mediated hemolytic anemia or disseminated intravascular coagulation is controversial. There are no studies documenting a definitive beneficial effect in animals or humans, except in a small study using high doses and strict anticoagulant monitoring. Similarly, evidence for the use of FFP in animals with acute pancreatitis (to replace α-macroglobulins and antiproteases) or in parvovirosis (to provide antiparvovirus antibodies and additional immunoglobulins and to stop gastrointestinal hemorrhage) is lacking. FFP is also commonly used to correct hypoproteinemias in animals with protein-losing nephropathies and enteropathies, but its effect on oncotic pressure in these animals is minimal at clinically used dosages, especially when compared with synthetic hyperoncotic agents such as the hydroxyethyl starch products. Critically ill animals with albumin concentrations less than 1.5 g/dl may benefit from plasma therapy because this protein is an important carrier of certain drugs, hormones, metals, chemicals, toxins, and enzymes. A canine albumin product is intermittently commercially available (see Chapter 58 for further details).

Other Blood Products

Other blood products are used less commonly in dogs and are generally not available for cats. Cryoprecipitate is rich in fibrinogen, fibronectin, factor VIII, and von Willebrand's factor and is the preferred treatment for bleeding dogs with these plasma protein deficiencies. In addition to frozen or freshly made cryoprecipitate from FFP, a lyophilized canine platelet product is now commercially available. Also cryoprecipitate-poor plasma may be administered to many coagulopathic and hypoproteinemic dogs when synthetic plasma expanders are of limited use or have undesirable side effects (e.g., exaggerate bleeding tendency). Because platelets are relatively short lived (1 week) and cannot readily be stored for any length of time (<8 hours at room temperature with agitation), they are rarely transfused. Life-threatening hemorrhage caused by thrombocytopenia in anemic dogs could be treated with FWB but generally requires only pRBCs to correct the anemia. Rarely, platelet-rich plasma (PRP) and platelet concentrates are required to control life-threatening bleeding (see Chapter 106). Furthermore, in dogs with immune-mediated thrombocytopenia, transfused platelets have a very short half-life (hours) and will not result in any appreciable platelet rise but may transiently stop severe hemorrhage. Cryopreserved platelets are short lived and lose their function and are no longer available, but lyophilized platelets have been intermittently available and may provide adequate hemostasis. Because of the very short half-life of granulocytes (hours), leukocyte transfusions are not generally performed in human or veterinary medicine.[1]

BLOOD TYPING

To ensure effective and safe transfusions, blood from both donor and recipient should be typed and, if previously transfused, a crossmatch also performed. Blood types are genetic markers on erythrocyte surfaces that are species-specific and antigenic in individuals that lack the same markers. This antigenicity results in the development of alloantibodies, so that the administration of a small volume (as little as 1 ml) of incompatible blood can result in life-threatening immune reactions. Blood typing is therefore clinically important to ensure blood compatibility and is recommended for any animal in need of a transfusion, any animal becoming a blood donor, and before breeding type B queens to avoid neonatal isoerythrolysis (NI). Unless blood compatibility tests are performed regularly, it is best to send ethylenediaminetetraacetic acid (EDTA) blood to a reputable laboratory for typing and crossmatching.[2,3]

Canine Blood Types

Dogs have more than a dozen blood group systems known as DEAs. Canine erythrocytes are either positive or negative for a blood type (e.g., DEA 4 positive or negative), and these blood types are thought to be codominantly inherited. In the DEA 1 system, various types (DEA 1.1, 1.2, and 1.3) have been postulated based on serology, but recent studies with monoclonal antibodies have shown that dogs can be either DEA 1 negative or to various degrees DEA 1 positive, similar to the Rh factor in humans.[3a] Fortunately, there are no clinically important alloantibodies present before sensitization of a dog with a transfusion (pregnancy has never been reported to cause sensitization).[2,4,5]

The most important canine blood type is DEA 1. DEA 1 elicits a strong alloantibody response after sensitization of a DEA 1–negative dog by a DEA 1–positive transfusion. This can lead to an acute hemolytic transfusion reaction in a DEA 1–negative dog previously transfused with DEA 1–positive blood. It is currently unknown if weakly DEA 1–positive blood elicits an alloantibody response in a DEA 1–negative dog or if weakly DEA 1–positive patients will react to strongly DEA 1–positive blood after being sensitized. Transfusion reactions against other blood types in previously transfused dogs have been described rarely. They include reactions against the DEA 4, Dal in Dalmatians and likely few other breeds, and another common red blood cell antigen in a Whippet. Additional clinically important blood types may yet be discovered.[6,7]

Simple blood typing cards using anticoagulated blood and a DEA 1 monoclonal antibody are available for DEA 1 typing of dogs (DMS Laboratories, Flemington, NJ), but there is some concern that weak agglutination reactions may be overlooked or autoagglutination may give false positive results (despite the control well). The reliable gel column technique is no longer available for animals, but an immunochromatographic strip-based method for in-clinic use has been documented to be very reliable (Alvedia, Lyon, France).[3a,8] A cartridge method with automatic reader has also been introduced but is apparently not as accurate and is more time consuming (Abaxis/DMS). Dogs that are DEA 1 negative are considered universal blood donors for a dog that has never been transfused. Canine blood typing sera for DEA 3, 4, and 7 and limited typing services are available (Animal Blood Resources International, Dixon, CA), but other blood group incompatibilites of clinical importance can be identified by crossmatching previously transfused dogs. Typing for the common red cell antigen Dal is currently hampered by the limited availability of antisera. Persistent autoagglutination after saline washing of the recipient's blood negates any typing and crossmatch testing except for the immunochromatographic method. Unless a bitch has been transfused previously with mismatched blood, there is no concern for NI.

Feline Blood Types

The main blood group system recognized in cats is known as the *AB blood group system* and consists of three types: type A, type B, and the extremely rare type AB. Type A is dominant over B.[9–11] Thus cats with type A blood have the genotype *a/a* or *a/b*, and only homozygous *b/b* cats express the type B antigen on their erythrocytes. In the extremely rare AB cat, a third allele recessive to *a* or codominant to *b* (or both) leads to the expression of both A (glycyl) and B (allyl) substances. Cats with type AB blood are not produced by mating of a cat with type A to a cat with type B unless the cat with type A carries a rare AB allele. Cats with type AB blood have been seen in many breeds, including domestic shorthaired cats but particularly in Ragdolls. The frequency of feline A and B blood types varies geographically and among breeds. For instance, all Siamese cats have type A blood, and Turkish Vans and Angoras have equal numbers of type A and B blood. Most domestic shorthaired cats have type A blood, but the proportion of cats with type B blood can be substantially different in certain geographic areas. Thus all donor blood must be typed. Most blood donors have type A blood, but some clinics also keep cats with the rare type B blood as donors.[2]

Cats have naturally occurring alloantibodies.[9] All cats with type B have very strong naturally occurring anti-A alloantibodies. Kittens receive anti-A alloantibodies through the colostrum from type B queens, and type B kittens develop high alloantibody titers (>1:32 to 1:2048) after a few weeks of age. Anti-A alloantibodies are responsible for serious transfusion reactions and NI in kittens with type A and AB blood born to type B queens. Cats with type A blood have weak anti-B alloantibodies, and their alloantibody titer is usually very low (1:2). Nevertheless, cats with type A blood can also develop hemolytic transfusion reactions when given B blood (in part due to the anti-A antibody in the type B donor blood), but no type A or AB queen has had a litter with NI caused by A-B incompatibility. Cats with type AB blood have no alloantibodies, although it is recommended that these cats receive type A pRBCs (mostly devoid of plasma with anti-B antibodies) if type AB blood is not available. Furthermore, additional blood group systems are being identified, such as the Mik RBC antigen in some domestic shorthaired cats. It is thought that Mik-negative cats may have naturally occurring alloantibodies or produce them, leading to blood incompatibility reactions beyond the AB blood group system.[12]

Simple AB blood typing cards are available for use in practice (DMS Laboratories, Flemington, NJ), but there are occasionally concerns that cats with type AB are not being recognized and misclassified as type A or B cats. Since withdrawal of the laboratory gel column AB-typing test, in-clinic immunochromatographic strip typing kits have become available, and one has been found to be very reliable (Alvedia, Lyon, France), although the other (DMS Laboratories, Flemington, NJ) has not yet been formally evaluated and seems to have off-center banding reactions.[13] Type B and AB should be confirmed by a laboratory and with back-typing; any type B cat older than 3 months has very strong anti-A alloantibodies, while AB cats have no alloantibodies.

BLOOD CROSSMATCHING

The blood crossmatch detects the serologic compatibility between the anemic recipient and potential donor and must be performed in cats if blood typing is not available and in dogs or cats that have previously received transfusion therapy.[1,2,10] This test looks for the presence or absence of alloantibodies in dogs or cats without determining the blood type; it does not replace blood typing. Crossmatching is done with anticoagulated blood from the recipient and the potential donor and requires some technical expertise but may be performed in private practice along with blood typing. Although laboratories use assays in tubes, microgel columns, or microtiter plates, a tube gel method (DMS Laboratories, Flemington, NJ) and strip (Alvedia, Lyon, France) crossmatch method have been recently introduced for clinical practice. The major crossmatch tests for alloantibodies in the recipient's plasma against donor cells. The minor crossmatch tests for alloantibodies in the donor's plasma against recipient's RBCs and is of lesser importance because the donor's plasma is mostly removed in pRBCs and will be diluted in the recipient patient (except if a type B cat is used as donor). It is also of lesser importance if all donors' types are known and if the donors, as generally recommended, have never received transfusions (i.e., have no prior sensitization). Persistent autoagglutination or severe hemoglobinemia (secondary to fragile red blood cells) may preclude testing at least by some methods. Washing the RBCs three times with physiologic saline (1 part blood and 5 to 9 parts saline) may resolve autoagglutination and rouleaux formation.

Because dogs do not have naturally occurring alloantibodies, the initial crossmatch of a dog that has not previously been transfused should be compatible.[4] However, a compatible crossmatch in a dog does not prevent sensitization against donor cells within 1 to 2 weeks. Thus a dog that was previously given a compatible transfusion from a donor dog may become incompatible with blood from the same donor 1 to 2 weeks later. Because cats have naturally occurring alloantibodies, a blood crossmatch test can detect an A-B mismatch as well as other incompatibilities (e.g., Mik). Mixing a drop of donor blood with recipient plasma (or vice versa) will detect the strong A-B incompatibilities. The practice of administering a small amount of blood (e.g., 1 ml) to the recipient animal to test for compatibility should be abandoned because it may result in fatal transfusion reactions. Transfusion of canine blood to feline patients should be avoided.

BLOOD DONORS AND SOURCES

Many larger veterinary specialty hospitals have few permanent canine and feline blood donors to cover their transfusion requirements or in case FWB or PRP (platelet concentrates) are needed. Several voluntary blood donor programs have emerged with client-owned or staff-owned dogs. More than a dozen commercial canine blood banks have been established in the United States that deliver blood products overnight; however, there may be a blood shortage at any time. Some blood banks are also providing feline products. If blood collection is only occasionally performed, it is advisable to get blood from a commercial resource with expertise in blood banking.

Autologous (self-) transfusion refers to the donation of blood by a patient from 4 weeks to a few days before a surgical procedure with the potential for substantial surgical blood loss. Blood can also be collected immediately before surgery. The patient's blood is diluted with crystalloid (and colloid) solutions, and the previously drawn blood is replaced when excessive bleeding occurs during or after surgery. Autotransfusion is another autologous transfusion technique in which shed blood salvaged intraoperatively or after intracavitary hemorrhage is reinfused intravenously after careful filtering. However, blood from longstanding (>1 hour), contaminated, or malignant hemorrhagic effusions should never be reinfused intravenously.

Blood donors should be young adult, lean, and good-tempered animals; dogs should weigh at least 23 kg to donate 450 ml (smaller dogs could be used if proportionally less blood is collected), and cats should weigh at least 4 kg to donate 40 ml of blood. They must have no history of transfusion and receive necessary vaccinations. In addition, blood donors must be healthy as determined by history, physical examination, and laboratory tests (complete blood cell count, chemistry screen, and fecal parasite examination every 6 to 12 months), as well as free of infectious diseases. Testing depends on species, breed, and geographic area but may include regular microfilaria, *Brucella, Babesia, Ehrlichia, Anaplasma, Borrelia, Bartonella, Mycoplasma*, and *Leishmania* spp testing in dogs and feline leukemia virus, feline immunodeficiency virus, feline infectious peritonitis, *Bartonella* and *Mycoplasma* spp testing in cats. Donors should receive a well-balanced, high-performance diet that may be supplemented twice weekly with oral ferrous sulfate (Feosol, 10 mg/kg q24h) if the donor is bled every 4 to 6 weeks. PCV or hemoglobin concentration should be more than 40% and more than 13 g/dl, respectively, in canine donors and more than 30% and more than 10 g/dl, respectively, in cats.[14]

BLOOD COLLECTION

Canine donors generally are not sedated, but cats regularly require sedation. Some sedatives, such as acepromazine, interfere with platelet function and induce hypotension and therefore should not be used. Blood is collected aseptically by gravity flow or blood bank vacuum pump from the jugular vein over a 5- to 10-minute period. Plastic blood bags (e.g., ABRI, Dixon, CA) containing citrate-phosphate-dextrose-adenine (CPD-A1), with or without satellite bags for blood component separation, are optimal. These commercial blood bags represent a closed collection system in which the blood does not come into contact with the environment at any time during collection or separation into blood components, thus minimizing the risk of bacterial contamination and allowing for rapid storage of the blood products. Large plastic syringes containing 1 ml CPD-A1 or 3.8% citrate per 9 ml blood and connected via three-way stopcock to a 19-gauge butterfly needle (and blood bag) are used commonly for blood collection in cats or toy breed dogs (ABRI, Dixon, CA). This represents an open collection system in which connections allow exposure of blood to the environment and potential contamination.[15] Because of the risk of bacterial contamination, blood collected via an open system should not be stored for more than 48 hours. A closed collection system for cats using small collection bags has been introduced but requires a tube welder to add the anticoagulant and connect to a pediatric apheresis catheter. Vacuum glass bottles containing acid-citrate-dextrose allow rapid collection but are not recommended because blood components are readily damaged and cannot be separated and stored for long periods. The maximal donated blood volume is 20 ml blood/kg or one regular blood bag unit of 450 ± 50 ml per 25-kg or larger dog and 10 ml blood/kg or 40 ml blood (one typical feline unit) per 4-kg or larger cat. Fluid replacement is generally not needed but can be considered in cats. Feeding donors should be limited to small amounts immediately post blood collection.

Blood components are prepared from a single donation of blood by simple physical separation methods, such as centrifugation, within 8 hours of blood collection; thereby, FWB can be separated into pRBCs, PRP or platelet concentrates, FFP, cryoprecipitate, and cryopoor plasma according to the *Technical Manual of the American Association of Blood Banking,* but this does require some expertise and equipment such as a large-volume cooled centrifuge. Blood component preparation is best accomplished by using plastic blood bags with satellite transfer containers to ensure sterility. Fluctuations in storage temperature significantly alter the length of storage; thus FWB and pRBCs should be kept at 4 ± 2° C (39 ± 3° F) and all plasma products at less than −20° C (−4° F) using blood bank refrigerators and freezers with alarms, if possible. Alternative refrigerator-freezer devices may be used as long as the temperature is monitored and the unit is not opened frequently. The bottom and top shelf in regular refrigerators may not hold the required temperature and may lead to freeze-induced hemolysis or bacterial growth, respectively. Storage of canine pRBCs will result in a gradual reduction of erythrocytic 2,3-diphosphoglyceride and accumulation of potentially large amounts of ammonia, but these metabolites are rapidly regenerated or eliminated, respectively, and do not typically affect pRBC efficacy or safety. Fresher pRBC units may be safer and have longer survival in vivo than older units, but using only FWB or fresh pRBCs is logistically impractical. Caution must be exercised, however, in animals that have severe liver insufficiency; these patients may also develop hypocalcemia when given large volumes of anticoagulated plasma products. Blood components that have been warmed to room or body temperature should not be recooled or stored again because of safety concerns (it affects product quality). Similarly, partially used or opened blood bags should be used within 24 hours because of the risk of contamination and product damage. Stored blood products should be rotated regularly and inspected; discolored units should be discarded.

ADMINISTRATION OF BLOOD PRODUCTS

For routine transfusion therapy in anemic patients, it is not necessary to warm blood after removal from the refrigerator. Warming may accelerate the deterioration of RBCs and permit rapid growth of contaminating microorganisms. However, there are specific clinical situations (such as transfusion of neonates or resuscitation of trauma patients) that necessitate the administration of rapid, massive transfusions such that warming of the blood products is indicated to prevent complications associated with hypothermia (e.g., cardiac arrhythmias). A temperature-controlled waterbath or bowl (≤39° C [<102° F]) is used to warm the blood products; a microwave should never be used because of the risk of regional overheating. Care should be taken to maintain absolute sterility and not to overheat any part of the blood products.

Blood bags are connected to infusion sets that have an in-line microfilter. Long (85 cm) blood infusion sets with a drip chamber for medium to large dogs and short infusion sets that can be attached to a syringe for small dogs and cats are available. A latex-free infusion set should be used for platelet administration to prevent aggregation. Microfilters with 170-µm pores are used commonly to remove clots and larger red blood cell and platelet aggregates. Finer filters with 40-µm pores will remove most platelets and microaggregates, but these commonly clog or become dysfunctional after filtering 50 to 100 ml of blood. Leukocyte reduction filters may be used at the time of blood collection to decrease febrile adverse reactions to white blood cell components, but they are expensive. Sterility must be maintained when connecting the blood component bag to the infusion set and the tubing to the catheter.

Blood components are best administered intravenously, although an intramedullary (intraosseous) catheter may be used when venous access cannot be obtained (see Chapter 194). Intraperitoneal administration is not generally recommended because absorption time is delayed and RBCs get damaged in the peritoneal cavity. Concurrent administration of drugs or fluids other than physiologic saline should be avoided to prevent lysis of erythrocytes or coagulation. Thus fluids containing calcium or glucose or those that are hypotonic or hypertonic should not be administered through the same intravenous line during the transfusion. Similarly no food should be given during a transfusion. Dripping blood via gravitational flow is preferred; most infusion pumps are not safe for the administration of RBC and platelet transfusions.

The rate of transfusion depends on the cardiovascular status, hydration status, degree of anemia, comorbidities and general condition of the recipient. The initial rate should be slow, starting with 1 to 3 ml over the first 5 minutes to observe for any transfusion reactions, even with blood-typed or crossmatched transfusions. In animals with cardiac disease, the transfusion should be given more slowly (i.e., 4 ml/kg/hr), and close monitoring is of utmost importance. Transfusion of a single bag should be completed within 4 hours to prevent functional loss or bacterial growth. The volume of the blood component needed depends on the type of deficiency and size of the animal. For treatment of anemia:

$$\text{Volume (ml) of whole blood} = 2 \times \text{PCV rise desired (\%)} \times \text{body weight (kg)}$$

In other words, administration of 2 ml whole blood/kg body weight raises the PCV by 1%. If pRBCs are used without prior resuspension in a RBC preservative, ½ to ¾ the volume should be administered, because non-resuspended pRBCs have a PCV of 70% to 80%.

In the absence of bleeding and hemolysis, at least 70% to 80% of transfused erythrocytes survive 24 hours (required blood bank standard) and transfused erythrocytes may thereafter be expected to have a near normal life span (up to 70 days in cats, 110 days in dogs). The response to the transfusion is monitored by obtaining a PCV and total protein reading before, during, and 6 and 24 hours after transfusion, and the clinician must consider continued blood loss and hemolysis when interpreting values.

In animals with thrombocytopenia or thrombopathia, one unit of platelet concentrate (~50 ml), PRP (~200 ml), or FWB (~450 ml) will increase the platelet count by approximately 10,000/µl in a recipient weighing 30 kg. In animals with serious or life-threatening bleeding, the platelet count should be increased to greater than 20,000 to 50,000/µl. Platelet counts should be monitored before and 1 hour and 24 hours after platelet transfusion.

In bleeding animals with coagulopathies or von Willebrand's disease, FFP is initially administered at a dosage of approximately 10 ml/kg to stop bleeding or prevent excessive bleeding during surgery. In some cases, larger volumes may be needed to control bleeding and, depending on the etiology of the coagulopathy, repeated administration of FFP may be required. Because of the short half-life of factors VII, VIII, and von Willebrand's factor, deficient animals may need treatment 2 to 4 times daily. Animals with other, less severe coagulopathies may be treated daily. Plasma support should be provided for an additional 1 to 3 days after the bleeding has been controlled to prevent rebleeding.

Cryoprecipitate at a dosage of 1 cryo unit (~50 ml)/10 kg or 1 to 2 ml/kg body weight twice daily is ideal to treat a bleeding animal with hemophilia A or von Willebrand's disease.

In contrast, cryo-poor plasma (6 to 10 ml/kg) is ideal for the treatment of bleeding induced by anticoagulant rodenticide poisoning because it contains the vitamin K–dependent coagulation factors.

ADVERSE TRANSFUSION REACTIONS

Although transfusion of blood and its components is usually a safe and temporarily effective form of therapy, there is always some risk involved. Adverse reactions usually occur during or shortly after the transfusion and can be caused by any component of the infused blood product. Most transfusion reactions can be avoided by carefully selecting only healthy donors; using appropriate collection, storage, and administration techniques; performing blood-typing and crossmatching; and administering only necessary blood components (see Chapter 62). The most common clinical sign of a transfusion reaction is fever, followed by vomiting and hemolysis; any reaction should lead to immediate cessation of the transfusion. Hemolytic transfusion reactions can be fatal and are therefore most concerning, whereas fever and vomiting are usually self-limiting. Adverse effects of transfusions can be divided into nonimmunologic reactions (transmission of infectious agents, vomiting, mechanical hemolysis, congestive heart failure, hypothermia, citrate toxicity, and pulmonary complications) and immunologic reactions (febrile nonhemolytic transfusion reactions, acute and delayed hemolytic transfusion reactions, manifestations ranging from urticaria to anaphylaxis, and graft-versus-host disease). Note that some clinical signs may be caused by both mechanisms.

Treatment of a suspected transfusion reaction initially involves stopping the transfusion, at least temporarily. Diphenhydramine, glucocorticoids, epinephrine, and isotonic crystalloid fluid administration are most commonly used to treat these reactions. Further details on these and other treatments can be found in Chapter 62.

ALTERNATIVES

Because blood is a scarce resource and may cause serious transfusion reactions, alternatives should be considered. In many animals, treatment of the underlying disease and other supportive measures are all that is needed. Crystalloid or synthetic colloidal fluids are appropriate when hypovolemia and low oncotic pressure are the main concerns. There are currently no alternative oxygen-carrier products, such as free hemoglobin, available for veterinary use. Placing a critically ill animal in an oxygen cage with an inspired oxygen concentration greater than 21% adds little to the oxygen content in a severely anemic patient (because of a lack of hemoglobin); it will increase the oxygen content only slightly, but it does allow the animal to rest away from the hustle of a busy treatment room. Furthermore, anemic animals with concomitant pulmonary disease (as often occurs with immune-mediated hemolytic anemia caused by pulmonary thromboemboli or pneumonia) will benefit from oxygen supplementation. Although human recombinant erythropoietin has a role in the treatment of anemia caused by chronic renal failure and a few other types of anemia, its effect is delayed. Therefore it is not effective for short-term treatment of anemia in the critical care patient (and does carry the risk of causing crossreacting antierythropoietin antibodies).

Although various recombinant human products are available as alternatives for supplementation of plasma proteins in human medicine, these treatment options have not been evaluated completely in small animals and may not be safe or cost effective. Human albumin concentrates have been used in dogs and cats with severe hypoalbuminemia, but serious concerns have arisen regarding its safety and effectiveness (lack of impact on survival in humans). Recombinant coagulation factors have drastically reduced the use of FFP in human patients. For instance, recombinant human FVIIa has been evaluated in dogs with factor VII deficiency (showing efficacy with minor bleeding) and other hemostatic diatheses. Similarly, there is no commercial product of a canine or feline immunoglobulin concentrate, and thus human intravenous immunoglobulin has been used successfully in the acute treatment of dermal and systemic toxic drug reactions, as well as the treatment of severe immune-mediated diseases. Again, these are human products that bear the risk of potentially fatal reactions, especially with repeated use. In conclusion, a good understanding of transfusion medicine and its benefits and risks is crucial for today's criticalist.

REFERENCES

1. Cotter SM, editor: Comparative transfusion medicine, San Diego, 1991, Academic Press.
2. Giger U: Blood typing and cross-matching to ensure compatible transfusions. In Bonagura JD, editor: Kirk's current veterinary therapy XIII, Philadelphia, 2000, WB Saunders.
3. Hohenhaus AE: Importance of blood groups and blood group antibodies in companion animals, Transfus Med Rev 18:117, 2004.

3a. Acierno MA, Raj K, Giger U: DEA 1 expression on dog erythrocytes analyzed by immunochromatographic and flow cytometric techniques, J Vet Intern Med (in press).

4. Giger U, Gelens J, Callan MB, et al: An acute hemolytic transfusion reaction caused by dog erythrocyte antigen 1:1 incompatibility in a previously sensitized dog, J Am Vet Med Assoc 206:1358, 1995.
5. Giger U, Blais MC: Ensuring blood compatibility: update on canine typing and cross-matching, Proc Am Coll Vet Intern Med Forum, 2005.
6. Melzer KJ, Wardrop KJ, Hale AS, Wong VM: A hemolytic transfusion reaction due to DEA 4 alloantibodies in a dog, J Vet Intern Med 17:931-33, 2003.
7. Blais MC, Berman L, Oakley DA, et al: Canine Dal blood type: a red cell antigen lacking in some Dalmatians, J Vet Intern Med 21:281, 2007.
8. Giger U, Palos H, Stieger K: Comparison of various canine blood typing methods, Am J Vet Res 66:1386, 2005.
9. Giger U, Bücheler J: Transfusion of type A and type B blood to cats, J Am Vet Med Assoc 198:411, 1991.
10. Griot-Wenk ME, Giger U: Feline transfusion medicine: feline blood types and their clinical importance, Vet Clin North Am Small Anim Pract 25:1305, 1995.
11. Griot-Wenk ME, Callan MB, Casal ML, et al: Blood type AB in the feline AB blood group system, Am J Vet Res 57:1438, 1996.
12. Weinstein NM, Blais MC, Harris K, et al: A newly recognized blood group in domestic shorthair cats: the Mik red cell antigen, J Vet Intern Med 21:287, 2007.
13. Stieger K, Palos H, Giger U: Comparison of various blood typing methods for the feline AB blood group system, Am J Vet Res 66:1393, 2005.
14. Wardrop KJ, Reine N, Birkenheuer A, et al: Canine and feline blood donor screening for infectious disease, J Vet Intern Med 19:135, 2005.
15. Brecher M, editor: AABB technical manual, ed 17, Bethesda, MD, 2013, American Association of Blood Banks.

CHAPTER 62

PREVENTION AND TREATMENT OF TRANSFUSION REACTIONS

Maureen McMichael, DVM, DACVECC

KEY POINTS

- *Transfusion therapy* refers to the safe and effective replacement of blood or one of its components, thereby offering support for many critically ill anemic or bleeding patients.
- The indications for transfusions need to be clearly determined, and ideally only the deficient blood component is replaced at the appropriate dosage.
- Although red blood cells and plasma clotting factors are crucial, the indications and efficacy of transfusing platelets, leukocytes, and other plasma proteins are limited.
- Blood products represent a limited resource; hence they should be given only when indicated, using the minimal dosage required and after carefully considering all alternatives.
- All canine and feline donor blood must be typed for the dog erythrocyte antigen (DEA) 1.1 and the feline AB blood groups, respectively, and all donors must have regular health examinations, including blood and infectious disease screening.
- All canine and feline recipient blood should be typed for DEA 1.1 and feline AB blood groups, respectively. Blood from any previously transfused (more than 4 days before) animal should also be crossmatched before receiving another red blood cell transfusion.
- Although acute hemolytic transfusion reactions are feared most, they can be avoided by prior compatibility testing; other transfusion reactions may not be predictable.
- The efficacy and survival of transfused blood cells and plasma proteins should be monitored during and after transfusion using appropriate clinical and laboratory parameters.

The transfusion of blood products, although necessary and often lifesaving, is associated with a significant and growing list of adverse effects. In addition to the known immunologic reactions, there are numerous effects related to antigenically compatible blood transfusions. Several studies support a relationship between transfusion of stored packed red blood cells (pRBCs) and deleterious clinical effects in humans, particularly with use of aged red cells (>2 weeks of storage). This chapter highlights some of the known adverse effects of transfusion as well as some of the more recently recognized factors, monitoring and treatment of transfusion related reactions, methods for elimination of reactants, and novel ways researchers are investigating to improve the safety of transfusion medicine.

COMPLICATIONS OF BLOOD PRODUCTS TRANSFUSIONS

Although blood product transfusion is an essential part of the treatment of many of the critical illnesses encountered in companion animals, a multitude of potential adverse effects are associated with the administration of blood products. Most studies report relatively infrequent percentages of overt transfusion reactions in dogs, with incidence rates of 3.0%, 3.3%, 4.2%, and 13%.[1-4] However, because many of our critically ill patients exhibit signs that are similar to the clinical signs of a transfusion reaction (fever, weakness, tachycardia, tachypnea) it is possible that some percentage of transfusion reactions are overlooked with the clinical signs attributed to the original illness.

Transfusion reactions are traditionally separated into immunologic and nonimmunologic reactions. The most common immunologic reactions seen in veterinary medicine include febrile nonhemolytic transfusion reactions (FNHTR) and urticaria.[2,3] Less common immune reactions reported in veterinary patients include hemolytic transfusion reactions, immune suppression, and decreased platelet counts.[2,3] The most common nonimmunologic transfusion reactions include infectious disease transmission (e.g., *Leishmania*), sepsis from bacterial contamination of the unit (e.g., *Serratia marcescens*), citrate toxicity leading to hypocalcemia (in patients receiving massive transfusions), and circulatory overload.

Febrile nonhemolytic reactions are the most commonly reported reactions in both human and veterinary medicine.[2,3,5] The cause is thought to be related to white blood cells (WBCs) present in transfused products. Residual WBCs in transfused products can have numerous deleterious effects, including production of cytokines in the unit and immune suppression, thrombocytopenia, and acute lung injury in the recipient.[5,6] Cytokine production has been shown to increase with storage time in both dogs and humans and contributes to the inflammatory response to transfusion.[7,8] Immune suppression has been documented in blood transfusion recipients and is thought to occur as a result of aberrant phagocytosis in natural killer cells and downregulation of both activity and production of T cells in the recipient.[9] Thrombocytopenia can occur as a result of nonimmune factors (splenic sequestration, sepsis, disseminated intravascular coagulation [DIC]) or immune factors. Immune-mediated platelet reactions can occur as a result of antibodies against human leukocyte antigen (HLA) or human platelet antigens (HPA).[10] Transfusion-associated acute lung injury (TRALI) is a significant concern in humans, and the HLA antibody in donor plasma (especially female donors) appears to be causative agent in most cases.[5,6] The clinical signs are caused by WBC aggregates in the pulmonary circulation leading to hypoxemia, respiratory distress, and often death. Hemolytic transfusion reactions occur when antibodies in the recipient react with the RBC surface antigen of the donor. The immunoglobulin G or M (IgG or IgM) antibodies then activate the complement system, which leads to formation of the membrane attack complex, which can damage the lipid bilayer of the RBC membrane leading to intravascular hemolysis. In addition, antibody or complement fragments adhering to the RBC surface increase RBC phagocytosis. If leukocytes recognize opsonized RBCs in circulation, the result is intravascular hemolysis, whereas extravascular recognition is termed extravascular hemolysis. Severity of the reaction is dependent on the amount of blood transfused, whether the antibody is cold or warm reacting, whether the immunoglobulin is IgG or IgM, and the concentration of the alloantibody in the recipient.[11]

Because many of our critically ill transfusion recipients have concomitant clinical signs similar to transfusion reactions, it is possible that we are underestimating a more common reaction. The mortality rates of dogs receiving a transfusion has been reported to range from 39% to 53%, with most deaths assumed to be due to the underlying disease process.[2,4] However, there are no published veterinary studies evaluating the effect of blood transfusion on morbidity and mortality in animals as a consequence of transfusion. Many critical patients have inflammatory conditions associated with their primary illness, and it is possible that a clinically silent inflammatory response to blood transfusion might be overlooked. Blood transfusion in humans and dogs has also been shown to be associated with an inflammatory response.[12-14] During storage of whole blood or pRBCs, contaminating leukocytes undergo lysis, which releases immunomodulators such as histamine, myeloperoxidase, plasminogen activator inhibitor 1, and eosinophilic cationic protein.[9] These mediators contribute significantly to an inflammatory response, potentially leading to the clinical signs of systemic inflammatory response syndrome (SIRS).

Detecting a transfusion reaction would be very difficult in specific disease populations because of the overlapping of some of the clinical signs of transfusion reaction with the illness itself. An example would be a dog with immune-mediated hemolytic anemia (IMHA) that develops sudden respiratory distress after a transfusion. This could be "assumed" to be due to a pulmonary thromboembolism, but without somewhat sophisticated diagnostics to verify this, TRALI would be overlooked. It is possible that TRALI is underappreciated in veterinary medicine because an acute onset of tachypnea in some animals receiving transfusions could be attributed to other disease processes. Further diagnostics may be discouraged because of the poor prognosis.

Monitoring

Although academically transfusion reactions are separated into immunologic and nonimmunologic categories, clinically this separation is not intuitive. For clinicians, separating the categories into mild, moderate, and severe make it much easier to diagnose and treat transfusion reactions in a timely manner. Before the transfusion begins, baseline recordings of the patient's temperature, pulse, and respiratory rate (TPR); pulse quality; heart and lung sounds; mentation; mucous membrane color; capillary refill time; and, ideally, blood pressure and pulse oximetry measurement should be recorded. An intensive care unit (ICU) transfusion form that includes space to record blood type and amount given, expiration date of unit, donor identification, recipient information, and start time of the transfusion as well as the previously listed baseline parameters can streamline the process. It is recommended that baseline parameters be recorded before and 5 minutes after the transfusion begins. They should then be evaluated every 15 minutes for the first hour, then hourly until the end of the transfusion. The same parameters are also recorded 1 hour after the transfusion ends. Additional monitoring is tailored to the specific patient (see later section).

Treatment for any suspected transfusion reaction begins with stopping the transfusion. Mild transfusion reactions are likely to include hypersensitivity reactions to plasma proteins and mild febrile, nonhemolytic reactions. Mild transfusion reactions are manifested by signs such as fever, urticarial, facial edema, and so on. In most of these cases the transfusion can usually be restarted in approximately 15 to 30 minutes at a slower rate. If there is evidence of a hypersensitivity reaction (cutaneous signs), diphenhydramine treatment (1 to 4 mg/kg subcutaneously [SC], intramuscularly [IM], or intravenously [IV]) can be considered. Antihistamines are more likely to benefit pets experiencing hypersensitivity reactions, which tend to occur in response to nonautologous plasma protein exposure and are more likely to occur with plasma transfusions. There is little evidence to suggest that prophylactic diphenhydramine or steroid therapy is of benefit in the treatment of febrile nonhemolytic transfusion reactions in humans and it is therefore unlikely to be helpful in pets.[15]

Moderate transfusion reactions can occur in response to both hemolytic and nonhemolytic transfusion reactions. Signs of a moderate transfusion reaction may include fever, tachycardia, tachypnea, weakness, vomiting, and so on. Supportive therapy may include one third to one half of a shock fluid bolus of isotonic crystalloids if the animal does not have signs of volume overload or a disease that would be worsened by fluids (e.g., congestive heart failure). Further fluid therapy guidelines can be found in Chapter 60. Because histamine release is not a feature of hemolytic or febrile, nonhemolytic transfusion reactions, diphenhydramine administration is unlikely to be of benefit, although, given the relative safety of diphenhydramine, it is unlikely to cause harm if administered. Glucocorticoids have long been considered a mainstay of therapy in the treatment of anaphylaxis and transfusion reactions. There is little evidence that prophylactic glucocorticoids are of benefit in the acute disease process; however, they may prevent the development of delayed immunologic reactions (occurring days later), which have been rarely reported in veterinary patients.[15] Because glucocorticoids have well-recognized adverse effects, the clinician must consider the risk/benefit ratio of these drugs for a given patient. The baseline parameters should be monitored closely for the next 30 to 60 minutes and further supportive care provided as necessary. Unless signs of a transfusion reaction resolve quickly, the transfusion should not be restarted, and the remaining blood product should not be administered to another patient.

Severe transfusion reactions or anaphylactic shock, although rare, affect dogs and cats differently. The most common presentation for cats is tachypnea (the lungs are the shock organ for cats) and for dogs it is hypotensive collapse (due to vasodilation of the splanchnic circulation). Epinephrine is given for its bronchodilator (cats) and vasoconstrictive (dogs) properties (0.01 mg/kg IV). In this chapter discussions of severe reactions are separated into canine and feline sections for streamlined reading.

Severe Transfusion Reactions in the Canine

If the transfusion reaction is severe (collapse, tachycardia or bradycardia, tachypnea, hypotension, fever, or hypothermia) and the dog is in shock, an airway should be secured immediately and ventilation provided as needed. Epinephrine (0.01 mg/kg IV) should be given along with half a shock bolus of isotonic crystalloids. Synthetic colloids should also be considered (see Chapter 60). The reader is also directed to Chapter 152 for further discussion of appropriate therapy. Repeat baseline parameter monitoring should be done every 5 minutes until the reaction has ceased. In addition, the blood product bag and recipient blood should be evaluated for evidence of hemolysis. A baseline chemistry panel and urinalysis should be assessed for renal function, along with a complete blood cell count (CBC) if there is not one from just before the transfusion (to assess for trends suggestive of sepsis).

Severe Transfusion Reactions in Felines

A severe transfusion reaction in felines may present as tachypnea, collapse, tachycardia or bradycardia, hypotension, fever, or hypothermia and most likely is due to an acute hemolytic transfusion reaction. These are most commonly seen with type B cats (having strong anti-A antibodies) inadvertently getting type A blood. Epinephrine

(0.01 mg/kg IV) or albuterol (albuterol inhaler attached to an Aerokat chamber and given as 2 actuations) should be given and the cat immediately provided with supplemental oxygen. The albuterol or epinephrine can be repeated if there is no improvement within 10 minutes. Because of the rapid, severe hemolysis that often accompanies these reactions, isotonic crystalloid fluids should be started immediately after the cat is stable, or sooner if necessary to aid resuscitation. In an acute hemolytic crisis, there is often no volume loss and fluid therapy should be used judiciously to prevent volume overload. Repeat baseline parameter monitoring should be done every 5 minutes until the cat is stable. In addition to checking the bag and recipient for hemolysis, a baseline chemistry panel and urinalysis should be assessed for renal function along with a CBC if there is not one from just before the transfusion (to assess for trends suggestive of sepsis). Renal function may decline because of hemolysis and should be monitored closely for several days.

Additional Diagnostics

Other diagnostics that should be performed for all patients suffering from a moderate to severe transfusion reaction include the recipient packed cell volume (PCV) (hemolysis) and urine (hemoglobinuria). Samples of the unit should be collected for PCV (hemolysis), gram stain (bacteria), and culture and susceptibility (C&S) testing and then placed in the refrigerator marked "Do Not Use" if a moderate to severe reaction is suspected. If there is any indication of contamination of the unit, the recipient should immediately begin broad-spectrum bactericidal antimicrobial therapy while awaiting C&S results.

Transfusion reactions can be delayed up to weeks or months, and the clinician should maintain an index of suspicion if an animal that has had a transfusion recently appears icteric, anorexic, or febrile. These reactions are usually mild and self-limiting but are commonly underestimated and unsuspected. For example, if a dog with IMHA begins to hemolyze red blood cells weeks after receiving a transfusion, the natural assumption would be that the dog is having a relapse of the IMHA and not necessarily a delayed transfusion reaction.

STORAGE LESIONS

Several studies have documented an association between storage time of pRBC units and adverse effects in critically ill patients,[16] septic patients,[17]and trauma patients.[18] Storage of pRBCs has been documented to lead to multiple deleterious changes in the RBC units, referred to as the storage lesion. During storage, RBCs undergo a series of physiologic, biochemical, and structural alterations leading to decreased viability and aggregation and increasing the risk for oxidative damage.[19] There are reports of significant disturbances in energy metabolism, rheologic properties, and oxidative damage to erythrocytes.[19] Several of the deleterious effects seen in stored RBCs, such as hemolysis and microparticle accumulation, are associated with an increased risk of adverse reactions in the recipients following the transfusion.[20]

Changes to the microenvironment of the pRBC unit occur as well. A decrease in the pH, accumulation of proinflammatory substances, release of free iron, and microparticles containing large amounts of free hemoglobin (Hb) have all been reported.[21-23] The formation of membrane vesicles (microparticles) causes increased cell density along with loss of surface area and has been associated with the induction of hypercoagulability.[24] Markers of hemolysis, such as potassium, arginase-1, and free Hb, increase with storage time in pRBC units. [21-23]

Free Hb is a potent scavenger of the essential endogenous vasodilator, nitric oxide (NO).[25] Decreased bioavailability of NO in capillaries may lead to decreased organ perfusion and contribute to multiple organ dysfunction syndrome (MODS).[25-27] Recent studies have documented hypertension after transfusion of free Hb in rats.[28] Prolonged storage has been shown to significantly increase free Hb and NO consumption within the pRBC storage medium.[29] In a human study, patients who received 2 units of pRBCs had a significantly higher level of free Hb and greater NO consumption than patients who received only 1 unit.[29] In canine pRBC units, both microparticles and cytokines have been documented to increase with storage time.[7,30] Free iron as a result of extravascular hemolysis has been reported in healthy human volunteers after transfusion of red blood cells.[22] The authors speculate that free iron may enhance transfusion-related complications and infection.[22] In a healthy human, approximately 1 ml of endogenous erythrocytes are cleared each hour, yielding approximately 1 mg of iron, which is either bound to transferrin in plasma or stored intracellularly.[22] If approximately 25% of a unit of pRBCs are cleared within 24 hours, this would amount to approximately 60 mg of iron. If most of this clearance occurs within the first hour, it would overwhelm the binding capacities of transferrin and ferritin, releasing free iron into the circulation and potentially enhancing oxidative stress and infection.[22]

Cytokines, regulatory polypeptides with numerous effects on immune cells, are essential to the modulation of inflammatory responses. They have been shown to accumulate in stored pRBC units, and this accumulation increases with storage time.[8,31] Transfusion of older units (>14 days of storage) has been described as giving a "cytokine soup" to the recipient because the older units promote systemic inflammation and may stimulate transfusion reactions. The accumulation of cytokines in stored blood is significantly decreased by prestorage leukoreduction of the unit.[31] A significant increase in ammonia concentration was documented in canine red cell units from day 1 (73 +/– 15 mmol/L) to day 35 (800 +/– 275 mmol/L).[32] In the same study, no increase in ammonia concentrations was noted in five anemic dogs receiving stored blood that contained elevated ammonia levels. However, all the dogs had normal hepatic function, which may not be indicative of the typical critical care patient. It might be prudent to avoid older (>14 days) blood in animals with hepatic dysfunction.

LEUKOREDUCTION

Leukoreduction (LR) attenuates or eliminates the inflammatory response to red blood cell transfusion in humans.[20,33] Leukoreduction has been shown to lower the incidence of virus transmission, alloimmunization, immunosuppression, and inflammation, all of which can contribute to morbidity and mortality in humans.[20,33] A decreased incidence of FNHTRs has been documented in patients receiving multiple transfusions with LR blood compared with NLR blood (61% in NLR group vs. 2.5% in LR group).[34] Leukoreduction exhibits a beneficial effect on the RBC storage lesion by improving both the incidence of hemolysis and the posttransfusion recovery of LR pRBCs.[33] One study documented a significant decrease in hemolysis, oxidative stress, loss of membrane integrity, and microparticle formation in LR units compared with non-LR units over time.[19] Seven randomized controlled trials showed that LR prevented HLA alloimmunization.[35] A multicenter, randomized, controlled trial (603 patients) in 1997 reported double the rate of platelet alloimmunization in the group without LR compared with the group that received LR blood.[35] Recently LR has been shown to abrogate the detrimental effects of aged pRBC units on trauma patients during transfusion.[36]

In dogs, LR has been shown to eliminate the inflammatory response to transfusion,[13] decrease microparticle formation compared with non-LR units,[30] and decrease cytokine production compared with non-LR units.[7] Leukoreduction is now standard veterinary practice in Canada and most of Europe because of the abundance of evidence supporting a reduced incidence of transfusion reactions and inflammatory responses in the recipients.[13]

Multiple techniques, including washing, apheresis, centrifugation, and filtration, are accepted approaches to perform LR. Filtration has been reported to remove the vast majority of WBCs from the blood via direct adhesion of WBCs to the filter, mechanical sieving, and indirect adhesion of aggregates (WBC and platelets) to the filter.[37] Filtration performed at collection for both human and dog blood has been shown to remove the majority of WBCs and platelets.[13,37] Human blood is generally submitted to LR before storage in order to prevent production of inflammatory mediators during storage. In humans, use of bedside LR filters (after storage) has been associated with hypotension in some populations and is therefore rarely used clinically.

Leukoreduction collection sets are only slightly more expensive than standard blood collection sets when purchased in bulk (they may add $35 to each unit), making them feasible for use in canine blood banks. A recent study documented successful LR in cats using specially designed filters to avoid significant blood loss through the larger filters for humans and dogs.[38]

FUTURE DIRECTIONS

In vitro–generated red blood cells could represent a very attractive alternative to current transfusion methodology. The specific production of blood products of a particular phenotype in a sterile environment has the potential to significantly reduce immunologic and infectious transfusion reactions. In vitro–generated RBCs would have to be able to appropriately bind oxygen in a reversible manner to reduce glutathione, maintain adenosine triphosphate (ATP), prevent accumulation of 2,3-diphosphoglycerate (2,3-DPG), and maintain satisfactory rheologic properties. Recently, in vitro–generated RBCs were documented to be functional with regard to all these properties, with a slightly diminished deformability in mice (comparable to stored RBCs).[39] During the first 5 days the RBCs showed approximately 94% to 100% survivability, but this dropped to 41% to 63% at 26 days. [39] Researchers have since gone on to transfuse these cells into one human with good results.[39] These RBCs did not show additional expression of blood group antigens. If this research continues to prove safe and successful, we could eventually see blood banks filled with blood phenotypes specifically chosen to match alloimmunized patients as well as patients with rare blood types.[39]

Other recent strategies to create safer blood transfusions include bioengineering coagulation factors to extend their half-life.[40] Chemical modification of therapeutic proteins with polyethylene glycol derivatives (PEGylation) is an established technology to increase the half- life of protein therapeutics.[41] Studies in hemophiliac mice demonstrated a significantly longer half-life of diPEGylated factor VIII molecules that maintained excellent hemostatic efficacy.[42] Albumin, with a circulating half-life of 20 days, can be fused with coagulation factors to extend the half-life of the transfused product.[43]

Transfusion medicine, although associated with significant adverse effects, is often lifesaving and necessary. The combined knowledge from clinical medicine and laboratory research on storage lesions and their effects on the recipient will aid in the development of improved blood products and preservative solutions. Future therapies focusing on specific cellular products, such as synthetic or bioengineered blood products and novel stem cell therapies, show great promise but are currently only feasible on a small scale. Until these therapies are available, maintaining strict quality control and the introduction of LR should improve the safety of veterinary transfusion medicine significantly.

REFERENCES

1. Assaraskakorn S, Niwetpathomwat A: A retrospective study of blood transfusion in dogs from a veterinary hospital in Bangkok, Thailand, Comp Clin Pathol 15:191, 2006.
2. Callan MB, Oakley DA, Shofer FS, et al: Canine red blood cell transfusion practice, J Am Anim Hosp Assoc 32:303, 1996.
3. Harrell K, Parrow J, Kristensen A: Canine transfusion reactions, part II. Prevention and treatment, Compend Contin Educ Pract Vet 19:193, 1997
4. Kerl ME, Hohenhaus AE. Packed red blood cell transfusion in dogs: 131 cases (1989), J Am Vet Med Assoc 202:1495, 1993.
5. Eder AF, Chambers LA: Noninfectious complications of blood transfusion, Arch Pathol Lab Med 131:708, 2007.
6. Sheppard CA, Logdberg LE, Zimring JC, et al: Transfusion-related acute lung injury, Hematol Oncol Clin North Am 21:63, 2007.
7. Corsi R, McMichael M, Smith SA, et al: Cytokines in stored canine erythrocyte concentrates, J Vet Emerg Crit Care, in review; abstract J Vet Intern Med 25(6):1502, 2011.
8. Snyder EL: The role of cytokines and adhesive molecules in febrile nonhemolytic transfusion reactions, Immunol Invest 24:333, 1995.
9. Neilsen HJ, Reimert C, Pedersen AN, et al: Leucocyte-derived bioactive substances in fresh frozen plasma, Br J Anaesth 78:548, 1997.
10. Pavenski K, Freedman J, Semple JW: HLA alloimmunization against platelet transfusions: pathophysiology, significance, prevention and management, Tissue Antigens 79:237, 2012.
11. Larison PJ, Cook LO: Adverse effects of blood transfusion. In Harmening D, editor: Modern blood banking and transfusion practices, ed 3, Philadelphia, 1995, FA Davis, pp 351-374.
12. Izbicki G, Rudensky B, Na'amad M, et al: Transfusion-related leukocytosis in critically ill patients, Crit Care Med 32:439, 2004.
13. McMichael M, Smith SA, Galligan A, et al: Effect of leukoreduction on transfusion-induced inflammation in dogs, J Vet Intern Med 24(5):1131, 2010.
14. McFaul SJ, Corley JB, Mester CW, et al: Packed blood cells stored in AS-5 become pro-inflammatory during storage, Transfusion 49:1451, 2009.
15. Marti-Carvajal AJ, Sola I, Gonzalez LE, et al: Pharmacological interventions for the prevention of allergic and febrile non-haemolytic transfusion reactions, Cochrane Database Syst Rev (6):CD007539, 2010. doi:10.1002/14651858.CD007539.pub2
16. Offner PJ, Moore EE, Biffl WL, et al: Increased rate of infection associated with transfusion of old blood after severe injury, Arch Surg 137:711, 2002.
17. Purdy FR, Tweeddale MG, Merrick PM. Association of mortality with age of blood transfused in septic ICU patients, Can J Anaesth 44:1256, 1997.
18. Zallen G. Offner PJ, Moore EE, et al: Age of transfused blood is an independent risk factor for post injury multiple organ failure, Am J Surg 178:570, 1999.
19. Antonelou MH, Tzounakas VL, Velentzas AD, et al: Effects of pre-storage leukoreduction on stored red blood cells signaling: a time-course evaluation from shape to proteome, J Proteomics 76(Spec No):220, 2012. doi:10.1016/j.jprot.2012.06.032
20. Zimrin AB, Hess JR: Current issues relating to transfusion of stored red blood cells, Vox Sang 96:93, 2009.
21. Gladwin MT, Kim-Shapiro DB: Storage lesion in banked blood due to hemolysis dependent disruption of nitric oxide homeostasis, Curr Opin Hematol 16:515, 2009.
22. Hod EA, Spitalnik SL: Harmful effects of transfusion of older stored red blood cells: iron and inflammation, Transfusion 51:881, 2011.
23. Zubair AC: Clinical impact of blood storage lesions, Am J Hematol 85:117, 2010.
24. Ho J, Sibbald WJ, Chin-Yee IH: Effects of storage on efficacy of red cell transfusion: when is it not safe? Crit Care Med 31:S687, 2003.
25. Reiter CD, Wang X, Tanus-Santos JE, et al: Cell free hemoglobin limits nitric oxide bioavailability in sickle cell disease, Nat Med 8(12):1383, 2002.
26. Minneci PC, Deans KJ, Zhi H, et al: Hemolysis associated endothelial dysfunction mediated by accelerated NO inactivation by decompartmentalized oxyhemoglobin, J Clin Invest 115:3409, 2005.
27. Vermeulen Windsant IC, Snoeijs MG, Hanssen SJ, et al: Hemolysis is associated with acute kidney injury during major aortic surgery, Kidney Int 77:913, 2010.

28. Donadee C, Raat NJ, Kanias T, et al: Nitric oxide scavenging by red blood cell microparticles and cell-free hemoglobin as a mechanism for the red cell storage lesion, Circulation 26:465, 2011.
29. Vermeulen Windsant IC, de Wit CJ, Sertorio JTC, et al: Blood transfusions increase circulating plasma free hemoglobin levels and plasma nitric oxide consumption: a prospective observational pilot study, Crit Care 16:R95, 2012.
30. Herring JM, Smith SA, McMichael M, et al: Procoagulant microparticles in stored canine erythrocyte concentrates, J Vet Emerg Crit Care 21(S1):S5, 2011.
31. Shanwell A, Kristoansson M: Generation of cytokines in red cell concentrates during storage is prevented by prestorage white cell reduction, Transfusion 35(3):199, 1995.
32. Waddell, LS, Holt DE, Hughes D, et al: The effect of storage on ammonia concentration in canine packed red blood cells, J Vet Emerg Crit Care 11(1):23, 2001.
33. Hess JR, Sparrow RL, van der Meer PF, et al: Red blood cell hemolysis during blood bank storage: using national quality management data to answer basic scientific questions, Transfusion 49:2599, 2009.
34. Blajchman MA: Landmark studies that have changed the practice of transfusion medicine, Transfusion 45:1523, 2005.
35. The Trial to Reduce Alloimmunization to Platelets study group: Leukocyte reduction and ultraviolet B irradiation of platelets to prevent alloimmunization and refractoriness to platelet transfusions, N Engl J Med 337:1861, 1997.
36. Phelan HA, Eastman AL, Aldy K, et al: Prestorage leukoreduction abrogates the detrimental effect of aging on packed red cells transfused after trauma: a prospective cohort study, Am J Surg 203:198, 2012.
37. Van Der Meer PF, Pietersz RN, Nelis JT, et al: Six filters for the removal of white cells from red cell concentrates, evaluated at 4 degrees C and/or at room temperature, Transfusion 39:265, 1999.
38. Schavone J, Rozanksi E, Schaeffer J, et al: Leukoreduction of feline whole blood using a neonatal leukocyte reduction filter: a pilot evaluation, J Vet Intern Med 26(3):777, 2012.
39. Giarratana MC, Rouard H, Dumont A, et al: Proof of principle for transfusion of in vitro-generated red blood cells, Blood 118(19):5071, 2011.
40. Sauna ZE, Pandey GS, Jain N, et al: Plasma derivatives: new products and new approaches, Biologicals 40:191, 2012.
41. Bailon P, Won CY: PEGylated biopharmaceuticals, Expert Opin Drug Deliv 6:1, 2009.
42. Rostin J, Smeds AL, Akerblom E: B-domain deleted recombinant coagulation factor VIII modified with monomethoxy polyethylene glycol, Bioconj Chem 11:387, 2000.
43. Mei B, Pan C, Jiang H, et al: Rational design of a fully active, long acting PEGylated factor VIII for hemophila A treatment, Blood 116:270, 2010.

CHAPTER 63
MASSIVE TRANSFUSION

L. Ari Jutkowitz, VMD, DACVECC

KEY POINTS

- Massive transfusion is traditionally defined as the transfusion of 1 or more blood volumes within a 24-hour period.
- Electrolyte abnormalities such as hypocalcemia, hypomagnesemia, and hyperkalemia are common after massive transfusion.
- Hemostatic defects often develop as a result of dilution, consumption of platelets and clotting factors, accelerated fibrinolysis, and release of anticoagulation factors such as activated protein C.
- Hypothermia and acidosis may exacerbate hemostatic defects.

Patients sustaining exsanguinating injuries as a result of trauma, coagulopathy, neoplasia, or surgery often require massive volume replacement during the resuscitation and perioperative periods. *Massive transfusion,* the term coined for this clinical entity, has traditionally been defined as the transfusion of a volume of whole blood or blood components that is greater than the patient's estimated blood volume (90 ml/kg in dogs and 66 ml/kg in cats) within a 24-hour period. Other definitions for massive transfusion have included the replacement of half the estimated blood volume in 3 to 4 hours or the administration of 1.5 ml/kg/min of blood products over a period of 20 minutes, reflecting a greater risk of adverse effects with rapid administration of blood products, as well as an increased injury severity in patients requiring more rapid administration.[1-4] Using the term *massive transfusion* has a number of limitations, including defining the entity by its treatment rather than its cause, the assignment of an arbitrary cutoff to a continuous variable (the volume of blood product transfused), and the fostering of retrospective analysis. Although there is still some value in discussing the common sequelae of massive transfusion, it may be more appropriate to focus future investigations on the early identification of patients in specific populations (such as acute traumatic coagulopathy) at risk for severe hemorrhage and to reserve the use of the term *massive transfusion* merely as a descriptor of the outcome of significant bleeding.

Massive transfusion imposes an incredible drain on blood banking resources. In veterinary clinics where blood products often are stored in limited quantities, a massively transfused patient may deplete most or all of the hospital's blood supply, making this commodity unavailable to other patients in need. This type of expenditure is also associated with significant cost to pet owners.

Given the severity of injuries that cause near exsanguination, it should not be surprising that massive transfusion has been associated with a high mortality rate, and this has led some to question whether massive transfusion may be futile or wasteful in veterinary patients.

BOX 63-1 *Abnormalities Associated with Massive Transfusion*

Electrolyte abnormalities • Hypocalcemia • Hypomagnesemia • Hyperkalemia Hemostatic defects • Thrombocytopenia • Secondary coagulopathy	Hypothermia Metabolic acidosis Immunosuppression Transfusion-related acute lung injury Other transfusion reactions

However, reports in the human literature have identified survival rates of between 25% to 84% after massive transfusion, and in one study of massively transfused dogs, 4 of 15 (27%) survived to discharge.[1,5-11] Complications associated with massive bleeding and resultant transfusion are numerous, however, and may include electrolyte disturbances, coagulation defects, hypothermia, alterations in acid-base status, immunosuppression, acute lung injury, other immunologic transfusion reactions, and transmission of infectious diseases (Box 63-1).

ELECTROLYTE DISTURBANCES

Stored blood undergoes changes in both the concentration and availability of various electrolytes. Recipients of massive transfusions may therefore develop electrolyte disturbances, with hypocalcemia, hypomagnesemia, and hyperkalemia most commonly reported.[9,12,13] Hypocalcemia and hypomagnesemia result from the citrate that is added to blood products as an anticoagulant. After transfusion, citrate binds rapidly to both calcium and magnesium with equal affinity, resulting in decreases in ionized calcium and magnesium levels. In one veterinary study, ionized hypocalcemia was documented in 100% of cases after massive transfusion, with severe hypocalcemia (<0.7 mmol/L) noted in 20%.[11] Changes in ionized magnesium concentration in this study tended to parallel those of ionized calcium. Ionized hypocalcemia has been reported to resolve quickly once perfusion is restored because citrate is metabolized rapidly by the liver.[14] Treatment with calcium gluconate is indicated in cases of severe hypocalcemia or when clinical signs such as hypotension, muscle tremors, arrhythmias, or prolonged QT interval manifest.

Potassium levels in stored (human) blood rise over time because of inactivation of the sodium-potassium ATPase pump by the cold storage temperatures. Humans receiving large volumes of stored blood products may therefore be at greater risk for the development of hyperkalemia. Most dogs, with the exception of Akitas and Shiba Inus, lack significant intracellular quantities of potassium in their red blood cells and, as a result, increased potassium levels are not observed in stored canine blood.[15,16] Although this would suggest that hyperkalemia in massively transfused canine patients should theoretically be less of a concern, hyperkalemia was identified in 20% of dogs in one study, a prevalence similar to that historically reported in human patients.[11] More recently, hyperkalemia was reported in fewer than 5% of traumatized human patients receiving massive transfusion, with preoperative potassium levels and postoperative pH accounting for the majority of cases.[17] It is likely that the hyperkalemia observed in canine cases resulted from similar causes, including potassium leakage into the bloodstream from damaged tissues, extracellular potassium shift secondary to acidosis, and reduced potassium excretion associated with oliguria.

HEMOSTATIC DEFECTS

Hemostatic defects are commonly seen in the massively transfused patient, with thrombocytopenia, hypofibrinogenemia, and dilutional coagulopathy most commonly reported. Thrombocytopenia after massive transfusion is believed to result primarily from blood loss and dilution. Blood products become devoid of platelets after 2 days of storage because the cold storage temperatures cause cell oxidation and death. Administering large volumes of these platelet-free blood products, especially after aggressive fluid resuscitation, can result in a dilutional thrombocytopenia. Thrombocytopenia resulting from dilution is generally less severe than the level that would have been predicted by the degree of dilution (i.e., the loss and replacement of 50% of a patients blood volume does not result in a 50% decrease in platelet count) because platelets are released from stores in the lungs and spleen.[18]

In studies of human patients wounded in war, nonhemostatic platelet counts of less than 50,000 cells/ml were noted only after transfusion of more than 2 blood volumes.[19] Similarly, in 15 massively transfused dogs, moderate thrombocytopenia developed in all dogs for which posttransfusion platelet counts were available, but none developed platelet counts below 50,000 cells/ml.[11]

Dilution alone, however, does not account for all the clinical observations regarding platelet counts. Blunt trauma, shock, sepsis, or systemic inflammation associated with the underlying injuries may also result in consumption of platelets and clotting factors. Platelet dysfunction resulting from acidosis or hypothermia is another well-documented phenomenon after massive transfusion and may be as important as platelet numbers in determining likelihood of bleeding.[20]

When large quantities of intravenous fluids and packed red blood cells are administered to replace massive blood loss, the dilutional effects may result in prolongation of prothrombin time (PT) and activated partial thromboplastin time (aPTT). Clotting factor consumption secondary to tissue injury may further exacerbate dilutional coagulopathy. Hemostasis is generally maintained as long as clotting factors are at least 30% of normal, and PT and aPTT values are not prolonged above 1.5 times normal.[21] Exchange transfusion models predict that loss and replacement of 1 blood volume removes slightly less than 70% of circulating factors in the plasma, so theoretically transfusions of up to 1 blood volume should not be associated with abnormal bleeding tendencies.[21] In human patients with war wounds, coagulopathy developed only after transfusion of more than 2 blood volumes.[19] Coagulopathy was identified in 70% of dogs after massive transfusion, although a correlation with transfused volumes could not be made because of the retrospective nature of the study.[11]

More recently, a subset of human trauma patients has been recognized with early evidence of coagulopathy that is mechanistically distinct from that mentioned earlier. This acute coagulopathy of trauma (ATC) is believed to result from altered coagulation enzyme activity, hyperfibrinolysis, and release of activated protein C secondary to tissue injury, hypoperfusion, and acidosis.[22] ATC has been documented before fluid resuscitation and has been associated with increased transfusion requirements, hospital stays, and mortality.[23] Coagulopathy after trauma has also been documented in dogs and has similarly been associated with injury severity, transfusion requirements, and outcome.[24]

Human trauma centers have traditionally employed empiric formulas for plasma and platelet replacement (e.g., giving 10 units of platelet concentrates and 5 units of plasma per 10 units of packed red blood cells administered) in an effort to correct coagulopathy, control bleeding, reduce transfusion requirements, and improve outcome. Increased fresh frozen plasma (FFP) and platelet/red blood cells (RBC) ratios (at least 2:1 and up to 1:1) appear to be associated with decreased mortality in human patients, but the optimum ratio of packed red blood cells, fresh frozen plasma, and platelet concentrates is still under investigation.[1,5,25,26]

HYPOTHERMIA

Hypothermia is a common complication of massive transfusion in human patients and was observed in 69% of massively transfused dogs.[11] Hypothermia results from shock secondary to the underlying illness or injury and the subsequent administration of large volumes of refrigerated blood products. Hypothermia can have profound effects on the coagulation system. Several studies have demonstrated a strong association between severity of hypothermia and the likelihood of developing microvascular bleeding.[10,27-29] Although hypothermia has little effect on clotting factor levels, it has been shown to inactivate the enzymes that initiate the intrinsic and extrinsic coagulation cascades and to enhance fibrinolysis.[4,27,28,30] Severe hypothermia can also result in decreased platelet activity.[20,28] Unfortunately, the contribution of hypothermia to coagulopathy is often overlooked in clinical patients because coagulation testing typically is performed at 37° C in the laboratory rather than at the patient's body temperature.[27]

METABOLIC ACIDOSIS

Another complication reported in the massively transfused patient is severe metabolic acidosis.[8,9,29] When blood is stored, glucose metabolism leads to an increase in lactic and pyruvic acids. Thus the pH of stored blood may be as low as 6.4 to 6.6.[9] When a patient is transfused with 1 or more blood volumes, severe acidosis can result. This is often compounded by lactic acidosis secondary to shock. The "bloody vicious cycle" of progressive hypothermia, persistent acidosis, and inability to establish hemostasis has been recognized increasingly in human medicine as a leading cause of death after blunt trauma.[29] The use of rapid infusers capable of quickly administering warmed blood and fluids, the increased use of warm air blankets, and the staging of laparotomy procedures to avoid prolonged hypotension secondary to anesthesia are measures that can significantly reduce the impact of hypothermia and acidosis on the coagulation system.[7,29]

IMMUNOSUPPRESSION AND WOUND HEALING

Immunosuppression has been well documented in human medicine after transfusion of large blood volumes. In one study of massively transfused human patients, the incidence of wound complications in the patients who survived for at least 1 week was 29.5%, 6 times the hospital average.[9] Similar findings of increased infection rates after transfusion have been documented in patients undergoing surgery for trauma, burns, fracture repair, gastrointestinal cancer, cardiac bypass, spinal surgery, and hip replacement.[31-39]

The mechanism by which blood transfusions reduce immune responsiveness is unclear, but donor white blood cells within the transfused blood have been implicated. These leukocytes are believed to exert immunosuppressive effects through alloimmunization, induction of tolerance in recipient lymphocytes, and release of humoral factors that suppress immune cell function. Experimental studies have identified decreased phagocytic cell function, decreased natural killer cell activity, decreased macrophage antigen presentation, and suppression of erythroid, myeloid, and lymphoid hematopoiesis as some of the changes seen after blood transfusion.[40] Leukoreduction, the use of filters to remove white blood cells before storage, has been shown in clinical studies to attenuate some of these changes.[34]

ACUTE LUNG INJURY

Massive transfusions have also been associated with transfusion-related acute lung injury. Blood stored under standard blood bank conditions develops microaggregates of platelets, white blood cells, and fibrin that may be removed only partially when transfused through a commercial (170-micron) blood filter. Embolization to the alveolar capillary beds has been shown experimentally to occur in dogs and may lead to acute lung injury.[41] In human medicine, antileukocyte antibodies in the donor blood have been implicated as one of the primary causes of in vivo agglutination and subsequent embolization of recipient neutrophils to the pulmonary vasculature, although this mechanism has not yet been identified in dogs.[42]

OTHER IMMUNOLOGIC TRANSFUSION REACTIONS

Because large volumes of blood are administered from a variety of donors, and because there is often insufficient time for crossmatching, massively transfused patients may be at greater risk for other immunologic transfusion reactions such as hemolytic reactions, type I hypersensitivity reactions, febrile nonhemolytic transfusion reactions, and posttransfusion purpura (thrombocytopenia). In massively transfused dogs, transfusion reactions consisting of fever, vomiting, facial swelling, and delayed hemolysis were noted in 40% of cases, well in excess of the hospital average.[11]

NONIMMUNOLOGIC TRANSFUSION REACTIONS

Other potential nonimmunologic complications of massive transfusions include bacterial contamination of stored blood, infectious disease transmission, and hyperammonemia. Blood is an excellent bacterial growth medium, and contamination may result from improper collection or handling techniques. Transfusion of contaminated blood can cause signs that may be difficult to distinguish from transfusion reactions, including fever, vomiting, hypotension, hemolysis, and death. Infectious disease transmission after transfusion is of major concern in human medicine because of human immunodeficiency virus, hepatitis, and other viral infections. The incidence of disease transmission in veterinary patients is not known, but the transmission of bloodborne pathogens like *Ehrlichia, Babesia,* and *Leishmania* is possible after transfusions in dogs.[43,44] Ammonia levels in stored blood rise significantly with time, so patients who receive large volumes may theoretically be at risk for hyperammonemia. Although this has not been a problem in healthy patients, those with severe liver disease or hypoperfusion secondary to shock may not be able to metabolize or excrete this ammonia and may consequently be at greater risk.[45]

RECOMMENDATIONS FOR MANAGEMENT

Hypothermia, metabolic acidosis, and coagulopathy have all been associated with increased mortality in human patients. Thus one of the priorities in management of massively transfused patients should be the recognition and arrest of this vicious cycle. Rapid resuscitation, measures to prevent cooling, and aggressive rewarming techniques should be employed to minimize hypothermia and acidosis. Useful techniques for temperature control include fluid warmers, warm air blankets, administration of warmed blood products, and admixture of blood products with warmed saline in a 1:1 ratio.

Surgical management of hemorrhage is critical, but initial surgical procedures should be aimed at "damage control," rather than definitive repair, to minimize the impact of hypothermia and acidosis associated with prolonged anesthesia. Using a staged laparotomy approach, sources of hemorrhage or contamination are initially controlled or packed off and the patient is then recovered. Completion of surgical procedures may be performed once cardiovascular status and coagulation have returned to acceptable levels.

To facilitate rapid identification and treatment of coagulation abnormalities, coagulation testing both before and during massive transfusion is recommended. Point-of-care testing for coagulation and electrolyte and acid-base status is a useful tool in these patients because samples sent to a laboratory rarely provide timely information. Formulaic administration of fresh frozen plasma and platelets should be considered, particularly in those patients with prolonged PT and aPTT or platelet counts of less than 50,000 cells/μl.

Abnormalities in electrolyte concentrations are nearly universal after massive transfusion, so careful monitoring is recommended, particularly if muscle tremors, hypotension, or arrhythmias are detected. Clinical signs of hypocalcemia and hypomagnesemia may be difficult to recognize in an anesthetized patient, and a prolonged QT interval on an electrocardiogram or unexplained hypotension may be the first warning of a problem. Treatment with 0.5 to 1.5 ml/kg intravenous [IV] calcium gluconate (10%) is recommended if ionized calcium levels are less than 0.8 mmol/L or when clinical signs are present.

OUTCOME

Despite the expectation that injuries necessitating massive transfusion are likely to be associated with a poor outcome, and despite the many associated risks, human and veterinary studies demonstrate that patients with exsanguinating injuries can be treated successfully. Survival rates of 25% to 84% in the veterinary and human literature, and a good functional outcome in most survivors, justify the high cost of acute care in these patients.

REFERENCES

1. Bhangu A, Nepogodiev D, Doughty H, et al: Meta-analysis of plasma to red blood cell ratios and mortality in massive blood transfusions for trauma, Injury 44:1693, 2013. doi: 10.1016/j.injury.2012.07.193
2. Mitra B, Cameron PA, Gruen RL, et al: The definition of massive transfusion in trauma: a critical variable in examining evidence for resuscitation, Eur J Emerg Med 18(3):137-42, 2011.
3. Blahut B. Indications for prothrombin complex concentrates in massive transfusions. Thromb Res 95:S63–S69, 1999.
4. Hardy JF, de Moerloose P, Samana CM: The coagulopathy of massive transfusion, Vox Sang 89:123-127, 2005.
5. Pidcoke, HF, Aden JK, Mora AG, et al: Ten-year analysis of transfusion in Operation Iraqi Freedom and Operation Enduring Freedom: increased plasma and platelet use correlates with improved survival, J Trauma Acute Care Surg 73: S445-S452, 2012.
6. Wudell JH, Morris JA, Yates K, et al: Massive transfusion: Outcome in blunt trauma patients, J Trauma 31:1-7, 1991.
7. Cinat ME, Wallace WC, Nastanski F, et al: Improved survival following massive transfusion in patients who have undergone trauma, Arch Surg 134:964-969, 1999.
8. Hakala P, Hiipala S, Syrjala, et al: Massive blood transfusion exceeding 50 units of plasma poor red cells or whole blood: the survival rate and the occurrence of leukopenia and acidosis, Injury Int J Care Injured 30:619, 1999.
9. Wilson RF, Mammen E, Walt AJ: Eight years of experience with massive transfusion, J Trauma 11:275, 1971.
10. Harvey MP, Greenfield TP, Sugrue ME, et al: Massive blood transfusion in a tertiary referral hospital: clinical outcomes and haemostatic complications, Med J Aust 163:356, 1995.
11. Jutkowitz LA, Rozanski EA, Moreau J, et al: Massive transfusion in dogs: 15 cases (1997-2002), J Am Vet Med Assoc 220:1664, 2002.
12. Meikle A, Milne B. Management of prolonged QT interval during a massive transfusion: calcium, magnesium, or both? Can J Anesth 47:792, 2000.
13. Ho KM, Leonard A: Risk factors and outcome associated with hypomagnesemia in massive transfusion, Transfusion 51:270, 2011.
14. Perkowski SZ, Callan MB, Oakley D, et al: Serum ionized calcium changes after infusion of citrated blood products in dogs (abstract), Vet Surg 25:186, 1996.
15. Degen M: Pseudohyperkalemia in Akitas, J Am Vet Med Assoc 190:541, 1987.
16. Fujise H, Nakayama T, Wada K, et al: Incidence of dogs possessing red blood cells with high K in Japan and East Asia, J Vet Med Sci 59:495, 1997.
17. Au BK, Dutton WD, Zaydfudim V, et al: Hyperkalemia following massive transfusion in trauma, J Surg Res 157:284, 2009.
18. Reed RL, Ciavarella D, Heimbach DM, et al: Prophylactic platelet administration during massive transfusion. A prospective, randomized, double-blind clinical study, Ann Surg 203:40, 1986.
19. Miller RD, Robbins TO, Barton SL: Coagulation defects associated with massive transfusions, Ann Surg 174:794, 1971.
20. Harrigan C, Lucas CE, Ledgerwood AM, et al: Serial changes in primary hemostasis after massive transfusion, Surgery 98:836-844, 1985.
21. Reiss RF: Hemostatic defects in massive transfusion: rapid diagnosis and management, Am J Crit Care 9:158, 2000.
22. Maegele M, Spinella PC, Schochl H: The acute coagulopathy of trauma: mechanisms and tools for risk stratification, Shock 38:450, 2012.
23. Brohi K, Singh J, Heron M, et al: Acute traumatic coagulopathy. J Trauma 54:1127, 2003.
24. Holowaychuk M, Hanel R, O'Keefe K, et al: Prognostic value of coagulation parameters in dogs following trauma (abstract). J Vet Emerg Crit Care 21:S6, 2011.
25. Brown JB, Cohen MJ, Minei JP, et al: Debunking the survival bias myth: characterization of mortality during the initial 24 hours for patients requiring massive transfusion, J Trauma Acute Care Surg 73:358, 2012.
26. Cap AP, Spinella PC, Borgman MA, et al: Timing and location of blood product transfusion and outcomes in massively transfused combat casualties, J Trauma Acute Care Surg 73:S89, 2012.
27. Gubler KD, Gentilello LM, Hassantash SA, et al: The impact of hypothermia on dilutional coagulopathy, J Trauma 36:847, 1994.
28. Watts DD, Trask A, Soeken K, et al: Hypothermic coagulopathy in trauma: Effect of varying levels of hypothermia on enzyme speed, platelet function, and fibrinolytic activity, J Trauma 44:846, 1998.
29. Cosgriff N, Moore EE, Sauaia A, et al: Predicting life-threatening coagulopathy in the massively transfused trauma patient: hypothermia and acidosis revisited, J Trauma 42:857, 1997.
30. Wolberg AS, Meng ZH, Monroe DM, et al: A systematic evaluation of the effect of temperature on coagulation enzyme activity and platelet function, J Trauma 56:1221, 2004.
31. Taylor RW, Manganaro L, O'Brien J, et al: Impact of allogenic packed red blood cell transfusion on nosocomial infection rates in the critically ill patient. Crit Care Med 30:2249, 2002.
32. Agarwal N, Murphy JG, Cayten CG, et al: Blood transfusion increases the risk of infection after trauma, Arch Surg 128:171, 1993.
33. Ford CD, VanMoorleghem G, Menlove RL: Blood transfusions and post-operative wound infection, Surgery 113:603, 1993.
34. Wheatley TJ, Veitch PS, Horsburgh T, et al: Transfusion induced immunosuppression: Abrogation by leucodepletion, Trans Proc 29:2962, 1997.
35. Jensen LS, Kissmeyer-Nelson P, Wolff B, et al: Randomized comparison of leucocyte-depleted versus buffy-coat-poor blood transfusions and complications after colorectal surgery, Lancet 348:841-845, 1996.
36. Houbiers JGA, Brand A, van de Watering LMG, et al: Randomized controlled trial comparing transfusion of leucocyte-depleted or buffy-coat-depleted blood in surgery for colorectal cancer, Lancet 344:573, 1994.
37. Murphy PJ, Connery C, Hicks GL, et al: Homologous blood transfusion as a risk factor for postoperative infection after coronary artery bypass graft operations, J Thorac Cardiovasc Surg 104:1092, 1992.

38. Triulzi DJ, Vanek K, Ryan DH, et al: A clinical and immunologic study of blood transfusion and postoperative bacterial infection in spinal surgery, Transfusion 32:517, 1992.
39. Murphy P, Heal JM, Blumberg N: Infection or suspected infection after hip replacement surgery with autologous or homologous blood transfusions, Transfusion 31:212-217, 1991.
40. Grzelak I, Zaleska M, Olszewski WL: Blood transfusions downregulate hematopoiesis and subsequently downregulate the immune response, Transfusion 38:1104-1114, 1998.
41. Barrett J, Dawidson I, Dhurandhar HN, et al: Pulmonary microembolism associated with massive transfusion: the basic pathophysiology of its pulmonary effects, Ann Surg 182:56, 1975.
42. Fung YL, Goodison KA, Wong JKL, et al: Investigating transfusion-related acute lung injury (TRALI), Int Med J 33:286, 2003.
43. Stegman JR, Birkenheuer AJ, Kruger JM, et al: Transfusion-associated Babesia gibsoni infection in a dog, J Am Vet Med Assoc 222:959, 2003.
44. Owens S, Oakley D, Marryott K, et al: Transmission of visceral leishmaniasis through blood transfusions from infected English Foxhounds to anemic dogs, J Am Vet Med Assoc 219:1081, 2001.
45. Waddell LS, Holt DE, Hughes D, et al: The effect of storage on ammonia concentration in canine packed red blood cells, J Vet Emerg Crit Care 11:23, 2001.

CHAPTER 64

DIABETIC KETOACIDOSIS

Rebecka S. Hess, DVM, DACVIM

KEY POINTS

- Diabetic ketoacidosis (DKA) is a severe form of complicated diabetes mellitus that requires emergency care.
- Acidosis and electrolyte abnormalities can be life threatening.
- Fluid therapy and correction of electrolyte abnormalities are the two most important components of therapy.
- Concurrent disease increases the risk for DKA and must be addressed as part of the diagnostic and therapeutic plan.
- Bicarbonate therapy usually is not needed, and its use is controversial.
- About 70% of treated dogs and cats are discharged from the hospital after 5 to 6 days of hospitalization.
- The degree of base deficit is associated with outcome in dogs with DKA. Additionally, dogs that have concurrent hyperadrenocorticism are less likely to be discharged from the hospital.

Diabetic ketoacidosis (DKA) is a severe form of complicated diabetes mellitus that requires emergency care. Ketones are synthesized from fatty acids as a substitute form of energy because glucose is not transported into the cells. Excess ketoacids results in acidosis and severe electrolyte abnormalities, which can be life threatening.

PATHOPHYSIOLOGY

Ketone bodies are synthesized as an alternative source of energy when intracellular glucose concentration cannot meet metabolic demands. Ketone bodies are synthesized from acetyl-coenzyme A (acetyl-CoA), which is a product of mitochondrial β-oxidation of fatty acids. This adenosine triphosphate (ATP)–dependent catabolism of fatty acids is associated with breakdown of two carbon fragments at a time and results in formation of acetyl-CoA. Synthesis of acetyl-CoA is facilitated by decreased insulin concentration and increased glucagon concentration. The anabolic effects of insulin include conversion of glucose to glycogen, storage of amino acids as protein, and storage of fatty acids in adipose tissue. Similarly, the catabolic effects of glucagon include glycogenolysis, proteolysis, and lipolysis. Therefore a low insulin concentration and increased glucagon concentration contribute to decreased mobilization of fatty acids into adipose tissue and increased lipolysis, resulting in increased acetyl-CoA concentration. In nondiabetics, acetyl-CoA and pyruvate enter the citric acid cycle to form ATP. However, in diabetic patients, glucose does not enter the cells in adequate amounts and production of pyruvate by glycolysis is decreased. The activity of the citric acid cycle is therefore diminished, resulting in decreased utilization of acetyl-CoA. The net effect of increased production and decreased utilization of acetyl-CoA is an increase in the concentration of acetyl-CoA, which is the precursor of ketone body synthesis.[1]

The three ketone bodies synthesized in the liver from acetyl-CoA are acetoacetate, β-hydroxybutyrate, and acetone. Acetyl-CoA is converted to acetoacetate by two metabolic pathways, and acetoacetate is then metabolized to β-hydroxybutyrate or acetone. One of the pathways for acetoacetate synthesis involves condensation of two acetyl-CoA units and the other utilizes three units of acetyl-CoA.[1]

Acetoacetate and β-hydroxybutyrate are anions of moderately strong acids. Therefore accumulation of these ketone bodies results in ketotic acidosis. Metabolic acidosis may be worsened by vomiting, dehydration, and renal hypoperfusion (see Chapter 54).[1] Metabolic acidosis and the electrolyte abnormalities that ensue are important determinants in the outcome of patients with DKA.[2]

It was previously believed that DKA patients have zero or undetectable endogenous insulin. However, in a study that included 7 dogs with DKA, 5 had detectable endogenous serum insulin concentrations, and 2 of these dogs had endogenous serum insulin concentration within the normal range.[3] Similarly, a study documenting resolution of diabetes mellitus in 7 of 12 cats with DKA suggested that in some cats, DKA can develop despite residual and ultimately adequate insulin concentrations.[4] Therefore it is possible that other factors, such as an increased glucagon, cortisol, or catecholamine concentrations, contribute to DKA. The concentration of these hormones may be increased because of concurrent disease.

Cytokine dysregulation is likely also involved in the pathophysiology of DKA. A recent study in dogs found that interleukin 18 (IL-18), resistin, and granulocyte-monocyte colony-stimulating factor concentrations were significantly higher in dogs with DKA before treatment compared with after resolution of ketoacidosis, and keratinocyte chemoattractant was significantly higher in dogs with DKA compared with dogs with uncomplicated diabetes. Additionally, IL-8 and monocyte chemoattractant protein 1 were significantly higher in dogs with uncomplicated diabetes compared with healthy controls. It is not yet known whether the cytokine dysregulation observed in patients with DKA is due to presence of concurrent disorders or other reasons. Interestingly, in this study the changes in cytokine concentrations were more pronounced than the changes noted in glucagon concentration.[5]

RISK FACTORS

The median age of dogs with DKA is 8 years (range 8 months to 16 years).[2] The mean age of cats with DKA is 9 years (range 2 to

16 years).[6] Breed or sex has not been shown to increase the risk of DKA in dogs or cats.[2,6,7]

Concurrent disease has been documented in about 70% of dogs with DKA and 90% of cats with DKA. The most common concurrent diseases noted in dogs with DKA are acute pancreatitis, bacterial urinary tract infection, and hyperadrenocorticism.[2] The most common concurrent diseases noted in cats with DKA are hepatic lipidosis, chronic renal failure, acute pancreatitis, bacterial or viral infections, and neoplasia.[6] It is possible that concurrent disease results in increased glucagon, cortisol, or catecholamine concentration and increased risk of DKA. Most dogs and cats with DKA are newly diagnosed diabetics. Insulin treatment may reduce the risk of DKA in dogs and cats.[2,6]

CLINICAL SIGNS AND PHYSICAL EXAMINATION FINDINGS

Clinical signs and physical examination findings may be attributed to chronic unmanaged diabetes mellitus, concurrent disease, or the acute onset of DKA. The most common clinical signs in dogs or cats with DKA are polyuria and polydipsia, lethargy, inappetence or anorexia, vomiting, and weight loss.[2,6,8] Common abnormalities noted on physical examination of dogs with DKA are subjectively overweight or underweight body condition, dehydration, cranial organomegaly, abdominal pain, cardiac murmur, mental dullness, dermatologic abnormalities, dyspnea, coughing, abnormal lung sounds, and cataracts.[2] Common abnormalities noted in cats with DKA are subjectively underweight body condition, dehydration, icterus, and hepatomegaly.[6]

CLINICAL PATHOLOGY

Approximately 50% of dogs with DKA have a nonregenerative anemia (which is not associated with hypophosphatemia), neutrophilia with a left shift, or thrombocytosis.[2] Anemia and neutrophilia with a left shift are also common features of feline DKA.[6] Cats with DKA also have significantly more red blood cell Heinz body formation than do normal cats, and the degree of Heinz body formation is correlated with plasma β-hydroxybutyrate concentration.[9]

Persistent hyperglycemia is apparent in all dogs and cats diagnosed with DKA unless they have received insulin.[2,6] Alkaline phosphatase activity is increased in almost all dogs with DKA.[2] Alanine aminotransferase activity, aspartate aminotransferase activity, and cholesterol concentration are increased in about half of dogs with DKA.[2] Increases in alanine aminotransferase activity and cholesterol concentration are also commonly observed in cats with DKA.[6] Azotemia is reported more commonly in cats than in dogs with DKA.[2,6,8]

Electrolyte abnormalities are common in both dogs and cats with DKA.[2,6,8] Initially an animal with DKA may appear to have extracellular hyperkalemia caused by dehydration, decreased renal excretion, hypoinsulinemia, decreased insulin function, hyperglycemia, and acidemia (leading to movement of hydrogen ions into the cells and potassium ions out to maintain cellular electronegativity). However, with rehydration, potassium ions are lost from the extracellular fluid and a true hypokalemia from depletion of total body potassium stores often becomes apparent. Hypokalemia may be exacerbated by binding of potassium to ketoacids, vomiting, anorexia, and osmotic diuresis. Insulin therapy may worsen extracellular hypokalemia as insulin shifts potassium into cells.[10] The most important clinical manifestation of hypokalemia in patients with DKA is profound muscle weakness, which can result in respiratory paralysis in extreme cases.

A total body phosphorous depletion often develops when phosphate shifts from the intracellular space to the extracellular space as a result of hyperglycemia, acidosis, and hypoinsulinemia; the phosphorous is then excreted as a result of the osmotic diuresis. Dehydration and decreased phosphorus excretion in the later stages of the disease may cause the serum phosphorous concentration to be normal or increased. Once fluid therapy is initiated, along with insulin therapy, a rapid decline in phosphorous often occurs secondary to extracellular and whole body phosphate depletion.[10] Hypophosphatemia related to DKA has been associated with hemolysis (in a cat) and seizures (in a dog).[11] Additional clinical signs that may develop because of hypophosphatemia include weakness, myocardial depression, and arrhythmias.

Decreased plasma ionized magnesium (iMg) concentration has been documented in four of seven cats with DKA and may be due to increased urinary excretion of magnesium.[12] The clinical significance of hypomagnesemia in cats is unknown. The clinical consequence of hypomagnesemia in humans with diabetes includes insulin resistance, hypertension, hyperlipidemia, and increased platelet aggregation. Dogs with DKA usually do not have low iMg concentrations at the time of initial examination.[2,13] In one study of 78 dogs with uncomplicated diabetes mellitus, 32 dogs with DKA, and 22 control dogs, plasma iMg concentration at the time of initial examination was significantly higher in dogs with DKA than in dogs with uncomplicated diabetes mellitus and control dogs.[13] Hyponatremia, hypochloremia, and decreased ionized calcium concentration have also been documented in about 50% of dogs with DKA. Low sodium concentration may develop secondary to hyperglycemia as intracellular fluid shifts to the extracellular compartment because of hyperglycemia (this is also known as *pseudohyponatremia).* Other explanations for hyponatremia, proposed in humans and experimental models of rodents, include ingestion of large amounts of water or retention of free water as a result of increased antidiuretic hormone secretion. In humans it is suggested that there is a decrease of 1 mEq/L in sodium concentration for every 62 mg/dl increase in glucose concentration. Venous pH is less than 7.35 in all dogs and cats with DKA. Lactate concentration is increased in about one third of dogs with DKA and is not correlated with the degree of acidosis.[2]

Urinalysis is usually indicative of glucosuria. Proteinuria or ketonuria may also be apparent. However, ketonuria may not be detected because the nitroprusside reagent in the urine dipstick reacts with acetoacetate and not with β-hydroxybutyrate, which is the dominant ketone body in DKA. Measurement of serum β-hydroxybutyrate is more sensitive than measurement of urine ketones.[14,15] The number of white blood cells per high-power field is usually 5 or fewer in the urine sediment, although 20% of dogs with DKA have aerobic bacterial growth on culture of urine obtained by cystocentesis.[2] This is likely a result of diabetic immunosuppression and decreased ability to mobilize white blood cells to the site of infection.

Results of additional clinicopathologic or imaging tests such as urine culture, abdominal ultrasonography, thoracic radiographs, adrenal or thyroid axis testing, pancreatic lipase immunoreactivity, liver function tests, or liver biopsy depend on concurrent disorders.

DIFFERENTIAL DIAGNOSIS

Differential diagnoses for ketonemia include DKA, acute pancreatitis, starvation, low-carbohydrate diet, persistent hypoglycemia, persistent fever, or pregnancy. Differential diagnoses for a primary metabolic acidosis include DKA, renal failure, lactic acidosis, toxin exposure, severe tissue destruction, renal tubular acidosis, and hyperchloremia.

TREATMENT

Administration and careful monitoring of intravenous (IV) fluid therapy is the most important component of treatment (see Chapters

59 and 60). Any commercially available isotonic crystalloid solution may be used. The use of 0.9% saline has been advocated because of its relatively high sodium concentration[10]; however, it may be contraindicated in hyperosmolar diabetics. Additionally, 0.9% saline may contribute further to the acidosis because of the high chloride concentration and lack of a buffer. Lactate (contained in lactated Ringer's solution) and acetate/gluconate (contained in Plasma-Lyte and Normosol-R) are converted to bicarbonate and may contribute to management of acidosis. Another advantage of these buffer-containing crystalloids is that they contain a small amount of potassium, which may blunt the acute decline in potassium concentration that the animal could suffer with initiation of fluid and insulin treatment. As long as the patient is monitored carefully, particularly in regard to hydration, mental status, and electrolyte concentrations, any of the above crystalloids can be used. Fluid therapy alone (with no insulin) significantly decreases blood glucose concentration in dogs with DKA.[16] Although the mechanism by which fluid therapy alone decreases blood glucose concentration is incompletely understood, one possible explanation is that improving renal perfusion decreases the concentration of counter regulatory hormones, most importantly glucagon.[17]

Correction and monitoring of electrolyte abnormalities is the second most important component of therapy. Electrolyte supplementation must be monitored frequently because frequent adjustments may be required. An animal that appears hyperkalemic at the time of initial examination may become hypokalemic shortly after fluid therapy has begun. Hypokalemia should be treated by administering potassium as an IV constant rate infusion (CRI) at a rate that should generally not exceed 0.5 mEq/kg/hr (Table 64-1). The potassium supplementation protocol described in Table 64-1 is based on the clinical experience and has not been scientifically validated. If higher dosages are required, continuous electrocardiographic monitoring should be performed simultaneously.

Hypophosphatemia is corrected with an IV CRI of potassium phosphate (solution contains 4.4 mEq/ml of potassium and 3 mM/ml of phosphate) at a rate of 0.03 to 0.12 mM/kg/hr. Serum potassium concentration must be taken into account when giving potassium phosphate for correction of hypophosphatemia. A magnesium sulfate solution (containing 4 mEq/ml of magnesium) given intravenously as a CRI of 0.5 to 1 mEq/kg q24h has been used successfully for correction of hypomagnesemia. Toxicity from erroneously administered intravenous magnesium has been reported in one diabetic cat and one dog with acute renal disease.[18] Signs of magnesium toxicity in these animals included vomiting, weakness, generalized flaccid muscle tone, mental dullness, bradycardia, respiratory depression, and hypotension.[18] Care must be taken to administer intravenous magnesium only to patients that have documented decreased iMg or total magnesium concentrations. As the hyperglycemia resolves, the sodium concentration is expected to increase secondary to the decrease in osmolality and subsequent movement of free water from the intravascular space (even without a change in sodium content). If hyponatremia and hypochloremia persist, they can be corrected by administering a 0.9% saline solution.

Hyperglycemia is corrected with insulin therapy after an average of 6 hours of fluid therapy with no insulin.[16] Because fluid therapy alone decreases blood glucose concentration significantly during the first few hours of treatment, administration of insulin at the onset of fluid therapy might decrease the blood glucose (and electrolyte) concentrations too rapidly, resulting in potentially harmful osmotic shifts.[16] Regular insulin (Humulin R, Novolin R) is used most commonly for treatment of DKA. Regular insulin is administered as an intravenous CRI (Table 64-2)[19] or intramuscularly.[20] When intravenous regular insulin is administered as a CRI, blood glucose is measured every 2 hours. When insulin is administered intramuscularly (IM), it is given every hour, and blood glucose is measured every hour. The initial dose of intramuscular therapy is 0.2 U/kg regular insulin, followed by 0.1 U/kg regular insulin IM 1 hour later. Treatment with intramuscular regular insulin is continued with 0.05 U/kg/hr, 0.1 U/kg/hr, or 0.2 U/kg/hr if blood glucose concentration drops by more than 75 mg/dl/hr, by 50 to 75 mg/dl/hr, or by less than 50 mg/dl/hr, respectively.[10] Monitoring of blood glucose concentration may be performed by use of a glucometer or a continuous interstitial glucose monitoring system, which provides a glucose measurement every 5 minutes.[21] Although a recent report of 15 cats with DKA documented a combination of intramuscular and subcutaneous glargine insulin treatment, it is difficult to recommend this treatment regimen because a specific protocol was not strictly adhered to throughout the study and electrolyte imbalances were common and severe, resulting in the need for a red blood cell transfusion in 2 cats with hypophosphatemia.[22]

The availability of genetically engineered rapidly acting insulin preparations has prompted investigations into their utility for treatment of DKA. A study of 12 dogs randomized to lispro or regular insulin treatment found that the median time to biochemical resolution of DKA in dogs treated with lispro insulin is significantly shorter than in dogs treated with regular insulin.[16] The clinical significance of this finding remains to be determined. Similarly, preliminary findings suggest that aspart insulin is safe and effective for treatment of DKA in dogs.[23] A study of 29 cats treated with a CRI of regular insulin has also determined that the published canine dose of insulin CRI (2.2 U/kg/day) does not increase the frequency of adverse neurologic or biochemical effects compared with the previously suggested insulin CRI dose of 1.1 U/kg/day.[8]

Table 64-1 Potassium Supplementation for Hypokalemic Animals with Diabetic Ketoacidosis

K Concentration (mmol/L)	Rate of Potassium Supplementation (mEq/kg/hr)*
<2	0.5
2 to 2.4	0.4
2.5 to 2.9	0.3
3.0 to 3.4	0.2
3.5 to 5	0.1

*Serum potassium concentration must be measured every 4 to 6 hours. If potassium concentration does not increase despite supplementation, the rate of supplementation can be increased, not to exceed 0.5 mEq/kg/hr without electrocardiographic monitoring.

Table 64-2 Administration of IV Insulin to Patients with DKA*

Blood Glucose Concentration (mg/dl)	Fluid Composition	Rate of Administration (ml/hr)
>250	0.9% NaCl	10
200 to 250	0.9% NaCl + 2.5% dextrose	7
150 to 200	0.9% NaCl + 2.5% dextrose	5
100 to 150	0.9% NaCl + 5% dextrose	5
<100	0.9% NaCl + 5% dextrose	Stop insulin administration

DKA, Diabetic ketoacidosis; *IV*, intravenous; *NaCl*, sodium chloride.
*2.2 U/kg of regular crystalline insulin added to 250 ml of 0.9% NaCl solution. The administration set must be flushed with 50 ml of the mixture before administering the solution to the animal.

Acidosis is usually corrected with intravenous fluid administration and insulin therapy alone.[2,6,16,17] Bicarbonate administration for correction of acidosis in humans with DKA is controversial.[17,24-26] The American Diabetes Association recommends bicarbonate supplementation only in patients with DKA in whom arterial pH remains less than 7.0 after 1 hour of fluid therapy.[24] Risks associated with bicarbonate treatment in humans with DKA include cerebral edema, exacerbation of hypokalemia, increased hepatic production of ketones, and paradoxical cerebral acidosis (as a result of increased carbon dioxide production in animals that are not adequately ventilating).[17,25,26] Bicarbonate treatment is not needed in most dogs and cats with DKA.[2,6,16] However, a retrospective study of 127 dogs with DKA reported that the degree of acidosis was associated with poor outcome.[2] The same study reported that intravenous sodium bicarbonate therapy was also associated with poor outcome.[2] It is not known if bicarbonate therapy in itself, or the severe degree of acidosis that prompted such therapy, caused the poor outcome in dogs treated with bicarbonate.

One bicarbonate treatment protocol is to administer sodium bicarbonate at ½ to ⅓ of (0.3 × body weight × negative base excess) over a 20-minute interval every hour, while monitoring bicarbonate and venous pH every hour. However, there are no studies to support this or any other bicarbonate treatment protocol in dogs and cats with DKA. The American Diabetes Association recommends treating pediatric patients with DKA who maintain a pH of less than 7.0 after 1 hour of fluid therapy with 2 mEq/kg sodium bicarbonate added to 0.9% sodium chloride, in a solution that does not exceed 155 mEq/L of sodium, over 1 hour.[24] The pH is monitored every hour and treatment is repeated until pH is 7.0 or greater.[25] See Chapter 54 for further details regarding bicarbonate therapy.

Concurrent disease is believed to contribute to DKA. Therefore identification and treatment of concurrent disease are indicated. It is possible that the latter decreases glucagon and cytokine secretion and contributes to improved diabetic regulation and resolution of DKA.

Long-term treatment of diabetes mellitus involves a fat-restricted diet containing high levels of insoluble fiber and complex carbohydrates for dogs and a high-protein, restricted-carbohydrate diet for cats. However, during episodes of diabetic ketoacidosis it is more important that patients eat than that they eat a specific diet aimed at long-term treatment goals. Dogs with an adequate body conditions score can be fasted for several days if they have vomiting or anorexia. However, dogs that have been fasted for more than 3 days and cats with any duration of anorexia must be treated with enteral or parenteral nutrition (see Chapters 129 and 130). The presence of concurrent disease (such as acute pancreatitis) may affect the choice of nutritional support.

OUTCOME

Most dogs and cats (70%) treated for DKA survive to discharge from the hospital.[2,6,8] Median hospitalization time for dogs and cats with DKA is 6 and 5 days, respectively.[2,6] At least 7% of dogs and up to 40% of cats experience recurring episodes of DKA.[2,6] Dogs with coexisting hyperadrenocorticism are less likely to be discharged from the hospital, and the degree of base deficit in dogs is associated with outcome.[2]

REFERENCES

1. Ganong WF: Review of medical physiology, ed 18, Stamford, CT, 1997, Appleton & Lange.
2. Hume DZ, Drobatz KJ, Hess RS: Outcome of dogs with diabetic ketoacidosis: 127 dogs (1993-2003), J Vet Intern Med 20:547, 2006.
3. Parsons SE, Drobatz KJ, Lamb SV, et al: Endogenous serum insulin concentration in dogs with diabetic ketoacidosis, J Vet Emerg Crit Care 12:147, 2002.
4. Sieber-Ruckstuhl NS, Kley S, Tschuor F, et al: Remission of diabetes mellitus in cats with diabetic ketoacidosis, Vet Intern Med 22:1326–1332, 2008.
5. O'Neill S, Drobatz K, Satyaraj E, et al: Evaluation of cytokines and hormones in dogs before and after treatment of diabetic ketoacidosis and in uncomplicated diabetes mellitus, Vet Immunol Immunopathol 148:276, 2012.
6. Bruskiewicz KA, Nelson RW, Feldman EC, et al: Diabetic ketosis and ketoacidosis in cats: 42 cases (1980-1995), J Am Vet Med Assoc 211:188, 1997.
7. Crenshaw KL, Peterson ME: Pretreatment clinical and laboratory evaluation of cats with diabetes mellitus: 104 cases (1992-1994), J Am Vet Med Assoc 209:943, 1996.
8. Claus MA, Silverstein DC, Shofer FS, et al: Comparison of regular insulin infusion doses in critically ill diabetic cats: 29 cases (1999-2007), J Vet Emerg Crit Care 20:509, 2010.
9. Christopher MM, Broussard JD, Peterson ME: Heinz body formation associated with ketoacidosis in diabetic cats, J Am Vet Med Assoc 9:24, 1995.
10. Feldman EC, Nelson RW: Diabetic ketoacidosis. In Feldman EC, Nelson RW: Canine and feline endocrinology and reproduction, ed 3, St Louis, 2004, WB Saunders.
11. Willard MD, Zerbe CA, Schall WD et al: Severe hypophosphatemia associated with diabetes mellitus in six dogs and one cat, J Am Vet Med Assoc 190:1007, 1987.
12. Norris CR, Nelson RW, Christopher MM: Serum total and ionized magnesium concentrations and urinary fractional excretion of magnesium in cats with diabetes mellitus and diabetic ketoacidosis, J Am Vet Med Assoc 215:1455, 1999.
13. Fincham SC, Drobatz KJ, Gillespie TN, et al: Evaluation of plasma ionized magnesium concentration in 122 dogs with diabetes mellitus: a retrospective study, J Vet Intern Med 18:612, 2004.
14. Tommaso MD, Aste G, Rocconi F, et al: Evaluation of a portable meter to measure ketonemia and comparison with ketonuria for the diagnosis of canine diabetic ketoacidosis, J Vet Intern Med 23:466, 2009.
15. Zeugswetter FK, Rebuzzi L: Point-of-care β-hydroxybutyrate measurement for the diagnosis of feline diabetic ketoacidaemia, J Small Anim Pract 53:328, 2012.
16. Sears KW, Drobatz KJ, Hess RS: Use of lispro insulin for treatment of diabetic ketoacidosis in dogs., J Vet Emerg Crit Care 22:211-218, 2012.
17. Glaser N, Kuppermann N: The evaluation and management of children with diabetic ketoacidosis in the emergency department, Pediatr Emerg Care 20:477, 2004.
18. Jackson CB, Drobatz KJ: Iatrogenic magnesium overdose: two case reports, J Vet Emerg Crit Care 14:115, 2004.
19. McIntire DK: Treatment of diabetic ketoacidosis in dogs by continuous low-dose intravenous infusion of insulin, J Am Vet Med Assoc 202:1266, 1993.
20. Chastain CB, Nichols CE: Low-dose intramuscular insulin therapy for diabetic ketoacidosis in dogs, J Am Vet Med Assoc 178:561, 1981.
21. Reineke EL, Fletcher DJ, King LG, et al: Accuracy of a continuous glucose monitoring system in dogs and cats with diabetic ketoacidosis, J Vet Emerg Crit Care 20: 303-312, 2010.
22. Marshall RD, Rand JS, Gunew MN, et al: Intramuscular glargine with or without concurrent subcutaneous administration for treatment of feline diabetic ketoacidosis, J Vet Emerg Crit Care 23:286-290, 2013.
23. Walsh ES, Drobatz KJ, Hess RS: Aspart insulin constant rate infusion for treatment of dogs with diabetic ketoacidosis, J Vet Intern Med 26:755, 2012 (abstract).
24. American Diabetes Association: Hyperglycemic crises in patients with diabetes mellitus, Diabetes Care 26:S109, 2003.
25. Chiasson JL, Aris-Jilwan N, Belanger R, et al: Diagnosis and treatment of diabetic ketoacidosis and the hyperglycemic hyperosmolar state, CMAJ 168:859, 2003.
26. Okuda Y, Adrogue HJ, Field JB: Counterproductive effects of sodium bicarbonate in diabetic ketoacidosis, J Clin Endocrinol Metab 81:314, 1996.

CHAPTER 65

HYPERGLYCEMIC HYPEROSMOLAR SYNDROME

Amie Koenig, DVM, DACVIM (Internal Medicine), DACVECC

KEY POINTS

- Hyperglycemic hyperosmolar syndrome (HHS) is a form of diabetic crisis marked by severe hyperglycemia (>600 mg/dl) and hyperosmolality with no or minimal urine ketones.
- Absence or resistance to insulin and increases in diabetogenic hormone levels stimulate glycogenolysis, and gluconeogenesis, hyperglycemia, osmotic diuresis, and dehydration result.
- Reduction of glomerular filtration rate (GFR) is essential to attain the severe, progressive hyperglycemia associated with HHS.
- Renal failure and congestive heart failure are common concurrent diseases that likely contribute to HHS via reduction of GFR.
- The most important goals of therapy are to replace fluid deficits and then slowly decrease the glucose concentration, thereby avoiding rapid intracranial shifts in osmolality and preventing cerebral edema. Fluid therapy will start to reduce blood glucose levels via dilution and by increasing GFR and subsequent urinary glucose excretion.
- Prognosis for feline HHS patients is poor (12% long-term survival), primarily as a result of concurrent disease. Dogs have a better prognosis (62% discharged from hospital).

Nonketotic hyperglycemic hyperosmolar syndrome (HHS) is an uncommon form of diabetic crisis marked by severe hyperglycemia (>600 mg/dl), minimal or absent urine ketones, and serum osmolality more than 350 mOsm/kg.[1] Other names for this syndrome include *hyperosmolar hyperglycemic nonketotic state* and *hyperosmolar nonketotic coma.* These terms have been replaced by *hyperglycemic hyperosmolar syndrome* in human medicine to better reflect the variable degrees of ketosis and inconsistent incidence of coma that occur with this syndrome.[2,3] Coma appears to be an uncommon form of this syndrome in animals.

HHS is an infrequent, albeit well-documented, complication of diabetes mellitus.[4-8] The incidence in humans with diabetes has been estimated to represent less than 1% of all adult human diabetic hospital admissions,[3,9,10] but incidence has been on the rise among diabetic children over the last decade [11,12] and has also been documented as a consequence of methadone toxicity in toddlers.[13] In comparison, HHS accounted for 6.4% of total emergency room visits by diabetic cats [4] and HHS, with or without ketosis, was identified in 5% of dogs with diabetes mellitus.[5]

This chapter reviews the pathogenesis, clinical findings, diagnostic evaluation, and treatment of HHS.

PATHOGENESIS

Pathogenesis of HHS involves hormonal alterations, reduction of glomerular filtration rate (GFR), and contributions from concurrent disease.

Hormonal Alterations

HHS begins with a relative or absolute lack of insulin coupled with increases in circulating levels of counterregulatory hormones including glucagon, epinephrine, cortisol, and growth hormone. These counterregulatory hormones are elevated in response to an additional stressor, such as concurrent disease. Epinephrine and glucagon inhibit insulin-mediated glucose uptake in muscle and stimulate hepatic glycogenolysis and gluconeogenesis, increasing circulating glucose concentration. Cortisol and growth hormone inhibit insulin activity and potentiate the effects of glucagon and epinephrine on hepatic glycogenolysis and gluconeogenesis. In conjunction with insulin deficiency, increases in the diabetogenic hormones increase protein catabolism, which in turn impairs insulin activity in muscle and provides amino acids for hepatic gluconeogenesis.[13] Pathogenesis of HHS is very similar to that of diabetic ketoacidosis, except that in HHS it is believed that small amounts of insulin and hepatic glucagon resistance inhibit lipolysis, thereby preventing ketosis[3,15,16] and instead promoting HHS. Lower levels of growth hormone have also been documented in patients with HHS.[16,17]

Hyperglycemia is the primary result of these hormonal alterations. It promotes osmotic diuresis, and osmotic diuresis increases the magnitude of the hyperglycemia, thus leading to a vicious circle of progressive diuresis, dehydration, and hyperosmolality. Neurologic signs are thought to develop secondary to cerebral dehydration induced by the severe hyperosmolality. In humans, elevated blood urea nitrogen (BUN) levels, acidemia, elevated sodium concentration, and osmolality, but not glucose concentration, are correlated with the severity of neurologic signs.[18]

Reduction of Glomerular Filtration Rate

Osmotic diuresis, additional losses such as via vomiting, and decreased water intake contribute to progressive dehydration, hypovolemia, and ultimately a reduction in the GFR as the syndrome progresses. Severe hyperglycemia can occur only in the presence of reduced GFR, because there is no maximum rate of glucose loss via the kidney.[19,20] That is, all glucose that enters the kidney in excess of the renal threshold will be excreted in the urine. An inverse correlation exists between GFR and serum glucose in diabetic humans.[19] Reductions in GFR increase the magnitude of hyperglycemia, which exacerbates glucosuria and osmotic diuresis. Human HHS survivors have also shown a reduced thirst response to rising vasopressin levels, which may also contribute to dehydration[21] and decreased GFR.

Influence of Concurrent Disease

Concurrent disease is important for initiating the hormonal changes associated with HHS and can also be important for exacerbating hyperglycemia. Diseases that are thought to predispose previously stable diabetics to a diabetic crisis include renal failure, congestive heart failure (CHF), infection, neoplasia, and other endocrinopathies,[1,22] although any disease can occur. Pancreatitis and hepatic disease appear to be uncommon concurrent diseases in cats with HHS,[4] while pancreatitis was more common in dogs, identified in approximately one third of all canine HHS patients.[5]

Renal failure and CHF also exacerbate the hyperglycemia associated with HHS because of their effects on GFR. Decreased GFR is inherent to renal failure. Inability to concentrate urine provides another source for obligatory diuresis. Myocardial failure, diuretic use, and third spacing of fluids associated with CHF may decrease GFR. Cardiac medications such as β-blockers and diuretics are also known to alter carbohydrate metabolism, thus predisposing to diabetic crisis.[3]

HISTORY AND CLINICAL SIGNS

Animals diagnosed with HHS may be previously diagnosed diabetics receiving insulin or may be newly diagnosed at the time HHS is recognized. The most common client complaints are fairly nonspecific and include decreased appetite, lethargy, vomiting, behavior changes, and weakness. Owners may report polyuria, polydipsia, and polyphagia consistent with diabetes, although these clinical signs may have gone unrecognized. History may also reveal recent onset of neurologic signs including circling, pacing, mentation changes, or seizure. Weight loss is an inconsistent finding. Recent steroid administration was seen in approximately 18% of dogs with HHS.[5]

PHYSICAL EXAMINATION

Vital parameters (temperature, pulse, and respiration) and body weight vary considerably with severity of the syndrome and presence and chronicity of comorbid diseases. Hypothermia is not uncommon as the syndrome progresses. Dehydration, marked by decreased skin turgor, dry or tacky mucous membranes, sunken eyes, and possibly prolonged capillary refill time, are common findings on physical examination in both dogs and cats. Mentation changes are also common. Most animals are reported as being depressed, but severely affected patients may be obtunded, stuporous, or comatose. Additional neurologic abnormalities including weakness or ataxia, abnormal pupillary light reflexes or other cranial nerve abnormalities, twitching, or seizure activity may be noted. Plantigrade stance, especially in cats, may be present subsequent to unregulated diabetes mellitus.

Other findings in patients with HHS are dependent on coexisting diseases. Animals should be examined closely for signs of heart disease, which may include any of the following: heart murmur, gallop, bradycardia, tachycardia or other arrhythmias, dull lung sounds, crackles, increased respiratory rate and effort, pallor, prolonged capillary refill time, and decreased blood pressure. Increased respiratory rate and effort may suggest cardiac failure but could also be secondary to infection, hyperosmolality, acidosis, asthma, or neoplasia. Animals with renal failure may have kidneys of abnormal size, oral ulceration, and pallor from anemia and may smell of uremia. Dogs with pancreatitis may have abdominal pain and vomiting.

DIAGNOSTIC CRITERIA

The criteria for diagnosis of HHS in veterinary medicine are a serum glucose concentration greater than 600 mg/dl, absence of urine ketones, and serum osmolality greater than 350 mOsm/kg.[1] In humans the criteria for diagnosis of HHS require a serum glucose greater than 600 mg/dl, arterial pH greater than 7.3, serum bicarbonate greater than 15 mmol/L, effective serum osmolality greater than 320 mOsm/kg, and anion gap less than 12 mmol/L. In addition, humans with HHS may have small quantities of urine and serum ketones, measured by the nitroprusside method.[2,3] Dogs with HHS have been classified as being ketotic or nonketotic at the time of the hyperosmolar event.[5]

Glucose concentrations can reach 1600 mg/dl in severely affected animals.[1] Blood glucose concentration may exceed the readable range on patient-side analyzers. Clinical suspicion for HHS should remain high in this situation, and additional diagnostic methods should be instituted to better define the severity of hyperglycemia, state of diabetes, and presence of coexisting diseases. Measuring glucose is also vital to rule out hypoglycemia as a cause of neurologic signs.

BOX 65-1 ***Important Calculations***

Dehydration deficit:
Fluid deficit (ml) = body wt (kg) × % dehydration (as decimal) × 1000 (ml/L)

Osmolality:
$\text{Serum osm}_{(calc)} = 2(Na^+) + (BUN \div 2.8) + (glucose \div 18)$

Effective osmolality:
$\text{Effective osm} = 2(Na^+) + (glucose \div 18)$

Corrected sodium:
$Na^+_{(corr)} = Na^+_{(meas)} + 1.6([\text{measured glucose} - \text{normal glucose}] \div 100)$

BUN, Blood urea nitrogen; *K*⁺, potassium; *Na*⁺, sodium; *osm,* osmolality; $Na^+_{(meas)}$, measured sodium concentration.
NOTE: BUN and glucose measured in mg/dl, electrolytes in mEq/L.

Osmolality measured by freezing point depression is not a commonly available patient-side test. Estimated serum osmolality can be calculated for dogs and cats using the following formula[23,24]:

$$\text{Serum osm}_{(calc)} = 2(Na^+) + (BUN \div 2.8) + (glucose \div 18)$$

BUN and glucose are measured in mg/dl and Na^+ is measured in mEq/L.

Because BUN equilibrates readily across cell membranes and effects of potassium on osmolality are small, calculating effective osmolality may be a better estimate[20]:

$$\text{Effective osm} = 2(Na^+) + (glucose \div 18)$$

Glucose is measured in mg/dl and Na^+ is measured in mEq/L.

Normal serum osmolality is 290 to 310 mOsm/kg. Neurologic signs have been documented in animals when osmolality exceeds 340 mOsm/kg (Box 65-1).[25]

Urine ketones can be assessed quickly using urine dipsticks. If urine is not available, serum ketones may be assessed by placing a few drops of serum on urine dipsticks[26] or using a blood ketone meter.[27-28]

Additional Diagnostic Evaluation

Additional diagnostic parameters, including serum chemistry analysis (with precise glucose measurement), complete blood cell count, urinalysis, urine culture, and (venous) blood gas, should be pursued in patients with confirmed or suspected HHS. Blood cell count abnormalities are varied and nonspecific. The packed cell volume and total solids level may be high secondary to dehydration. Chemistry abnormalities are dependent on degree of dehydration and presence of underlying disease. The most common biochemical abnormalities in cats with HHS include azotemia, hyperphosphatemia, elevated aspartate transaminase, acidosis, elevated lactate concentration, and hypochloremia.[4] Azotemia may be prerenal or renal in origin. Dogs with HHS and ketosis were less likely to be azotemic than their nonketotic counterparts.[5]

Venous blood gas analysis should be used to assess the degree of acidemia. It is not possible to differentiate HHS from DKA in cats based on the degree of metabolic acidosis.[4] In dogs, low pH has been associated with poorer outcome.[5] In HHS, metabolic acidosis is caused by accumulation of uremic acids and lactic acid, rather than ketones. Lactic acidosis is an indicator of poor tissue perfusion secondary to dehydration and hypovolemia.

Serum electrolytes should be monitored to help in choosing fluid therapy and to calculate the osmolality. Sodium concentration is the prime determinate of serum osmolality. In HHS the true magnitude of sodium concentration will be masked by the hyperglycemia. Measured serum sodium is reduced by hyperglycemia-induced osmotic pull of water into the vasculature.[29]

Sodium level should be expected to rise as glucose levels return to normal. Calculating the corrected serum sodium value can give a better indication of severity of free water loss (see Box 65-1). For every 100 mg/dl increase in glucose above normal, the measured serum sodium decreases by 1.6 mEq/dl.[29] A corrected serum sodium level can be calculated using the following formula:

$$Na^{+}_{(corr)} = Na^{+}_{(measured)} + 1.6\,([\text{measured glucose} - \text{normal glucose}]/100)$$

Sodium is measured in mEq/L and glucose is measured in mg/dl. This effect is nonlinear, however; mild hyperglycemia leads to smaller changes in plasma sodium concentration than more severe hyperglycemia

Animals in diabetic crisis are classically expected to have low total body potassium concentrations,[1] although cats with HHS tend to have a normal serum potassium concentration.[4] Dogs with nonketotic HHS had average potassium concentrations that were higher than dogs with HHS and ketotis.[5] Potassium losses are expected via diuresis, vomiting, and decreased intake; increases in potassium may occur secondary to acidosis, severe hyperosmolality,[30] insulin deficiency, and poor renal perfusion. Potassium levels are expected to decrease as acidosis improves and with insulin-induced cotransport of glucose and potassium into cells.

A thorough search for underlying disease should be undertaken in all patients with HHS. Additional diagnostic techniques, including thoracic and abdominal radiographs, abdominal ultrasonography, echocardiogram, retroviral testing (cats), and endocrine testing (thyroid hormone in cats and adrenal axis testing for dogs), may be indicated based on historical or physical findings or results of preliminary diagnostic results.

TREATMENT

Goals of therapy for patients with HHS include replacing the fluid deficit, slowly reducing serum glucose levels, addressing electrolyte abnormalities, and treating concurrent disease.[2]

Fluids

The fluid therapy plan should include resuscitation, dehydration deficit, ongoing losses and maintenance fluid needs (see Box 65-1). To prevent exacerbation of neurologic signs, it is important not to lower the serum glucose or sodium too rapidly. Hyperosmolality induces formation of osmotically active idiogenic osmoles in the brain. These idiogenic osmoles protect against cerebral dehydration by preventing movement of water from the brain into the hyperosmolar blood. Because idiogenic osmoles are eliminated slowly, rapid reduction of serum osmolality establishes an osmotic gradient across the blood-brain barrier, leading to cerebral edema and neurologic signs.[31]

In humans, fluid losses in HHS are estimated to be double that of a DKA patient and vascular volume is anticipated to decrease when water moves to the interstitium and intracellular space as intravascular glucose and osmolality decline. Insufficient fluid resuscitation can contribute to cardiovascular collapse and death.[3,32-36]

The first goal of therapy is to replace vascular volume in those patients with signs of hypovolemia or hypovolemic shock. An initial 20 ml/kg (cat) to 30 ml/kg (dog) bolus of an isotonic replacement crystalloid is recommended, after which the patient is reevaluated and the need for more boluses assessed. Isotonic saline (0.9% saline) is typically the initial fluid of choice because it both addresses the fluid deficits and replaces glucose with sodium in the extracellular space, thus preventing a rapid shift in osmolality. On its own, fluid therapy will start to reduce blood glucose levels via dilution and by increasing GFR and subsequent urinary glucose excretion.[37]

After vascular volume has been restored, dehydration deficits should be replaced more slowly using crystalloid solutions of varying sodium concentrations as needed to correct hypernatremia. Hypernatremia should be corrected slowly with a decrease of no more than 1 mEq/L/hr.[38] While lower sodium-containing fluids, such as 0.75% or 0.5% NaCl, may be needed to reduce the serum sodium, it may be necessary to switch back to isotonic saline if the sodium is dropping to quickly or if there are problems maintaining vascular volume as the hyperglycemia is corrected and water moves out of the vascular space.[39] Chapter 50 provides further discussion of the treatment of hypernatremia. Dehydration deficit (in milliters) should be calculated with the following formula:

$$\text{Body wt (kg)} \times \%\ \text{Dehydration (expressed as decimal)} \times 1000\ (\text{ml/L})$$

In humans the fluid deficit is assumed to be 12% to 15% of body weight,[3,33-35] and this massive dehydration deficit is often best replaced over 24 to 48 hours. Treating a patient with HHS and concurrent CHF presents a dilemma. Even maintenance amounts of parenteral fluids could be detrimental, so rehydration must be done more slowly and with care. Forced enteral fluid supplementation, as via a nasoesophageal tube, may be a viable option to aid in rehydration of some patients with CHF that are not vomiting.

Insulin

Unlike in DKA where insulin therapy is vital because of its role in reducing ketogenesis, insulin therapy is not as critical for reversal of HHS because much of the syndrome can be improved just by correcting fluid deficit. In the nonketotic HHS patient, insulin should not be given until the hypovolemia has resolved, the dehydration has improved, and the glucose concentrations are no longer adequately declining (<50 mg/dl/hr) with appropriate fluid therapy alone.[39] In the ketotic HHS patient, insulin may be needed somewhat sooner to reverse ketogenesis. Regardless, insulin therapy should be instituted only after several hours of fluid therapy and only if any potassium, magnesium, and phosphorus deficiencies have been corrected. Mechanics of insulin therapy for HHS are similar to those used in DKA, with protocol changes designed to lower the glucose levels more slowly. The ideal protocol for treating HHS in cats and dogs is unknown. Using intramuscular or intravenous protocols of regular insulin at dosages 50% of those used for DKA should reduce the risk of a too rapid decline of serum glucose.[1] Recommendations for children include an initial intravenous constant rate infusion of regular insulin of 0.025 to 0.05 U/kg/hr.[39] An intravenous protocol using lispro insulin has been reported for treating veterinary DKA patients but has yet to be reported for treating HHS patients.[40] For the intramuscular protocol, 0.1 U/kg of regular insulin can be given, followed by 0.05 U/kg q1-2h until the glucose is less than 300 mg/dl, then q4-6h. Initially, glucose should be monitored every 1 to 2 hours to ensure it is dropping at the optimal rate. (See Tables 65-1 and 65-2 for insulin protocols.) With both protocols the goal is to decrease the glucose levels by no more than 50 to 75 mg/dl/hr.[2,39,41] If the glucose is dropping too rapidly, the insulin dosage should be decreased by 25% to 50%.

Electrolytes

Electrolyte abnormalities may be present at admission or may develop upon treatment of HHS. Potassium, phosphorus, and

Table 65-1 Insulin Protocols for Use in Treating HHS

Insulin Protocol	Starting Dose	Subsequent Management
Intermittent intramuscular (IM)	Administer 0.1 U/kg of regular insulin, then 0.05 U/kg q2-4h.	Check blood glucose q4h. Goal is to reduce blood glucose by 50-75 mg/dl/hr. Subsequent insulin doses are increased or decreased by ~25% to meet this goal. Add dextrose to fluids when glucose <250 mg/dl.
Intravenous constant rate infusion (IV CRI)	Dilute 1 U/kg of regular insulin in 250 ml 0.9% NaCl. Start this solution at 10 ml/hr.	Check blood glucose q2h and adjust CRI rate as necessary (see Table 65-2).

Table 65-2 Insulin CRI Chart*

Blood Glucose (mg/dl)	Regular Insulin CRI Rate (ml/hr)	Maintenance/Replacement Fluid Composition
>250	10	As is
200-250	7	Plus 2.5% dextrose
150-199	5	Plus 2.5% dextrose
100-149	5	Plus 5% dextrose
<100	0	Plus 5% dextrose

CRI, Constant rate infusion.
*Example of an insulin CRI chart. These rates are guidelines only; the goal is to have the blood glucose concentration decline by no more than 50 to 75 mg/dl/hr.

Table 65-3 Electrolyte Supplementation

Electrolyte	Form	Dose for supplementation
Potassium (K)	Potassium chloride (KCl)	20-80 mEq K per liter of fluids (dependent on serum K concentration and fluid administration rate) up to a maximum rate of potassium 0.5 mEq/kg/hr
Phosphorus	Potassium phosphate (KPhos)	0.01-0.2 mmol/kg/hr *or* give 25% of potassium supplementation (see KCl) as KPhos and 75% as KCl
Magnesium	Magnesium sulfate	0.75-1 mEq/kg given as CRI over 24 hours

CRI, Constant rate infusion.

magnesium levels should initially be measured two to four times daily and supplemented in fluids as needed (Table 65-3). The concentrations of these three electrolytes may rapidly decrease once insulin is begun, so it is imperative that deficiencies are treated before initiating insulin therapy. Monitoring sodium is also critical in HHS because the presence of severe hypernatremia may be masked by a hyperglycemia-induced pseudohyponatremia.

Treating Concurrent Disease

Additional supportive and symptomatic therapies such as antibiotics for infection, antacids and phosphate binders for animals with renal failure, cardiac drugs for animals with heart failure, and antiemetics and analgesics for dogs with pancreatitis should be tailored to specific patient needs.

MONITORING

In addition to vigilant electrolyte monitoring, serial evaluations of physical and other biochemical parameters are vital to a successful outcome. Serial neurologic examinations should be performed to monitor for signs of cerebral edema that could develop if hyperosmolality is corrected too quickly. A subjective assessment of hydration status can be obtained by using skin turgor, serial body weight measurements (multiple times per day), intake and output calculations, packed cell volume/total protein (PCV/TP) measurements, and, possibly, urine specific gravity and renal parameters. Blood pressure and central venous pressure monitoring may be helpful in monitoring patients for evidence of hypovolemia. Electrocardiogram may be useful as a signs-of-life monitor and to assess for rhythm abnormalities in patients with electrolyte abnormalities or heart disease. Multilumen central venous catheters will facilitate glucose and electrolyte monitoring, central venous pressure measurements, and administration of multiple infusions. Ketones should be checked daily or as indicated to ensure an HHS patient is not developing DKA. Additional monitoring may be indicated based on presence of any concurrent diseases. Human HHS patients have been found to have an increased risk for venous thromboembolism, although this propensity has not been documented in animals with HHS.[42]

POSTCRISIS THERAPY

Attentive fluid and electrolyte therapy and regular insulin should be continued until the animal is no longer hyperosmolar and, ideally, is eating. Dextrose may need to be added to the fluids if the glucose drops less than 250 to 300 mg/dl and the animal is not yet eating. Once the animal is eating and drinking, long-acting insulin therapy, dietary management, and monitoring should be started as for a standard diabetic. Vigilant therapy and careful monitoring of the diabetes and any concurrent diseases are essential.

PROGNOSIS

The mortality rate for patients with HHS is high because of the severity of the syndrome as well as presence of concurrent disease. In humans, the mortality rate is consistently 15% to 17% of adult HHS admissions and has been documented as high as 72% in children.[18,43-46] Many outcome predictors have been identified in humans, including lower Glasgow Coma Scale score, higher plasma glucose level, and mild acidosis.[18,44-47] There are no clear predictors of survival from HHS for animals. In one feline study, in-hospital mortality was 64.7% and long-term (>2 month) survival was only 12%.[4] Outcome was not predicted by presence of neurologic signs, serum glucose concentration, measured serum sodium concentration, corrected serum sodium concentration, or total and effective serum osmolality. Long-term survivors had curable concurrent diseases. In one canine study, 38% of dogs with HHS died or were euthanized in-hospital and there was not a significant difference in survival if the HHS was documented with or without ketosis. Poor outome was associated with abnormal mental status and low venous pH.[5]

REFERENCES

1. Feldman EC, Nelson RW: Canine and feline endocrinology and reproduction, ed 3, St Louis, 2004, WB Saunders.
2. American Diabetes Association: Position statement: hyperglycemic crises in patients with diabetes mellitus, Diabetes Care 24:154, 2001.
3. Kitabchi AE, Umpierrez GE, Murphy MB, et al: Management of hyperglycemic crises in patients with diabetes, Diabetes Care 24:131, 2001.
4. Koenig A, Drobatz K, Beale AB, King L: Hyperglycemic, hyperosmolar syndrome in feline diabetics: 17 cases (1995-2001), J Vet Emerg Crit Care 14:30, 2004.
5. Trotman TK, Drobatz KJ, Hess RS: Retrospective evaluation of hyperosmolar hyperglycemia in 66 dogs (1993-2008), J Vet Emerg Crit Care 23(5):557-564, 2013.
6. Crenshaw KL, Peterson M: Pretreatment clinical and laboratory evaluation of cats with diabetes mellitus, J Am Vet Med Assoc 209:943, 1996.
7. Schaer M: Diabetic hyperosmolar nonketotic syndrome in a cat, J Am Anim Hosp Assoc 11:42, 1975.
8. Schaer M, Scott R, Wilkins R, et al: Hyperosmolar syndrome in the nonketoacidotic diabetic dog, J Am Anim Hosp Assoc 10:357, 1974.
9. Umpierrez GE, Kelly JP, Navarrete JE, et al: Hyperglycemic crises in urban blacks, Arch Intern Med 157:669, 1997.
10. Fishbein H, Palumbo PJ: Acute metabolic complications in diabetes. In Diabetes Data Group: Diabetes in America, Bethesda, MD, 1995, National Institutes of Health.
11. Bagdure D, Rewers A, Campagna E, Sills MR: Epidemiology of hyperglycemic hyperosmolar syndrome in children hospitalized in USA, Pediatr Diabetes 14:1, 2013.
12. Chen HF, Wang CY, Lee HY, See TT, et al: Short-term case fatality rate and associated factors among inpatients with diabetic ketoacidosis and hyperglycemic hyperosmolar state: a hospital-based analysis over a 15-year period, Intern Med 49:8, 2010.
13. Tiras S, Haas V, Chevret L, Decobert M, et al: Nonketotic hyperglycemic coma in toddlers after unintentional methadone ingestion, Ann Emerg Med 48:4, 2006.
14. Larsen PR, Kronenberg HM, Melmed S, Polonsky KS: Williams textbook of endocrinology, ed 10, Philadelphia, 2003, WB Saunders.
15. McGarry JD, Woeltje KF, Kuwajima M, Foster DW: Regulation of ketogenesis and the renaissance of carnitine palmitoyltransferase, Diabetes Metab Rev 5:271, 1989.
16. Chupin M, Charbonnel B, Chupin F: C-peptide blood levels in ketoacidosis and in hyperosmolar nonketotic diabetic coma, Acta Diabetolol Lat 18:123, 1981.
17. Gerich JE, Martin MM, Recant L: Clinical and metabolic characteristics of hyperosmolar nonketotic coma, Diabetes 20:228, 1971.
18. Pinies, JA, Cairo G, Gaztambide S, Vazquez JA: Course and prognosis of 132 patients with diabetic nonketotic hyperosmolar state, Diabetes Metab 20:43, 1994.
19. Kandel G, Aberman A: Selected developments in understanding of diabetic ketoacidosis, Can Med Assoc J 128:392, 1983.
20. Owen OE, Licht JH, Sapir DG: Renal function and effects of partial rehydration during diabetic ketoacidosis, Diabetes 30:510, 1981.
21. McKenna K, Morris AD, Azam H, et al: Exaggerated vasopressin secretion and attenuated osmoregulated thirst in human survivors of hyperosmolar coma, Diabetologia 42:534, 1999.
22. Bruskiewicz KA, Nelson RW, Feldman EC, Griffey SM: Diabetic ketosis and ketoacidosis in cats: 42 cases (1980-1995), J Am Vet Med Assoc 211:188, 1997.
23. Dugger DT, Mellema MS, Hopper K, Epstein SE: Estimated osmolality of canine serum a comparison of the clinical utility of several published formulae, J Vet Emerg Crit Care (in press).
24. Dugger DT, Epstein SE, Hopper K, Mellema MS: Comparative accuracy of several published formulae for the estimation of serum osmolality in cats, J Small Anim Pract 54:184, 2013.
25. Chrisman C: Problems in small animal neurology, ed 2, Philadelphia, 1991, Lea & Febiger.
26. Zeugswetter F, Pagitz ML: Ketone measurements using dipstick methodology in cats with diabetes mellitus, J Small Anim Pract 50:1, 2009.
27. Hoenig M, Dorfman M, Koenig A: Use of a hand-held meter for the measurement of blood beta-hydroxybutyrate in dogs and cats, J Vet Emerg Crit Care 18:1, 2008.
28. Tommaso M, Aste G, Rocconi F, et al: Evaluation of a portable meter to measure ketonemia and comparison with ketonuria for the diagnosis of canine diabetic ketoacidosis, J Vet Intern Med 23:3, 2009.
29. Katz MA: Hyperglycemia-induced hyponatremia: calculation of expected serum sodium depression, N Engl J Med 289:843, 1973.
30. Montolieu J, Revert L: Lethal hyperkalemia associated with severe hyperglycemia in diabetic patients with renal failure, Am J Kidney Dis 5:47, 1985.
31. Arieff AI, Kleeman CR: Studies on mechanisms of cerebral edema in diabetic comas. Effects of hyperglycemia and rapid lowering of plasma glucose in normal rabbits, J Clin Invest 52:571, 1973.
32. Delaney MF, Zisman A, Kettyle WM: Diabetic ketoacidosis and hyperglycemic hyperosmolar nonketotic syndrome, Endocrinol Metab Clin North Am 29:4, 2000.
33. Nugent BW: Hyperosmolar hyperglycemic state, Emerg Med Clin North Am 23:3, 2005.
34. Kitabchi AE, Umpierrez GE, Fisher JN, Murphy MB, Stentz FB: Thirty years of personal experience in hyperglycemic crises: diabetic ketoacidosis and hyperglycemic hyperosmolar state, J Clin Endocrinol Metab 93:5, 2008.
35. Kitabchi AE, Nyenwe EA: Hyperglycemic crises in diabetes mellitus: diabetic ketoacidosis and hyperglycemic hyperosmolar state, Endocrinol Metabol Clin North Am 35:4, 2006.
36. Ellis EN: Concepts of fluid therapy in diabetic ketoacidosis and hyperosmolar hyperglycemic nonketotic coma, Pediatr Clin North Am 37:2, 1990.
37. West ML, Marsden PA, Singer GG, Halperin ML: Quantitative analysis of glucose loss during acute therapy for hyperglycemic, hyperosmolar syndrome, Diabetes Care 9:465, 1986.
38. Kahn A, Brachet E, Blum D: Controlled fall in natremia and risk of seizures in hypertonic dehydration, Intensive Care Med 5:27, 1979.
39. Zeitler P, Haqq A, Rosenbloom A, Glaser N: Hyperglycemic hyperosmolar syndrome in children: pathophysiological considerations and suggested guidelines for treatment, J Pediatrics 158:1, 2011.
40. Sears KW, Drobatz K, Hess R: Use of lispro insulin for treatment of diabetic ketoacidosis in dogs, J Vet Emerg Crit Care 22(2):211, 2012.
41. Wagner A, Risse A, Brill H, et al: Therapy of severe diabetic ketoacidosis zero mortality under very-low-dose insulin application, Diabetes Care 22:674, 1999.
42. Keenan CR, Murin S, White RH: High risk for venous thromboembolism in diabetics with hyperosmolar state: comparison with other acute medical illnesses, J Thromb Haemost 5:6, 2007.
43. Cochran JB, Walters S, Losek JD: Pediatric hyperglycemic hyperosmolar syndrome: diagnostic difficulties and high mortality rate, Am J Emerg Med 24:3, 2006.
44. MacIsaac RJ, Lee LY, McNeil KJ, et al: Influence of age on the presentation and outcome of acidotic and hyperosmolar diabetic emergencies, Intern Med J 32:379, 2002.
45. Watchtel TJ, Silliman RA, Lamberton O: Prognostic factors in the diabetic hyperosmolar state, J Am Geriatr Soc 35:737, 1987.
46. Hamblin PS, Topliss DJ, Chosich N, et al: Deaths associated with diabetic ketoacidosis and hyperosmolar coma: 1973-1988, Med J Aust 151:439, 1989.
47. Fadini GP, de Kreutzenberg SV, Rigato M, et al: Characteristics and outcomes of the hyperglycemic hyperosmolar non-ketotic syndrome in a cohort of 51 consecutive cases at a single center, Diabetes Res Clin Pract 94:2, 2011.

CHAPTER 66

HYPOGLYCEMIA

Amie Koenig, DVM, DACVIM (Internal Medicine), DACVECC

KEY POINTS

- Normoglycemia is maintained by a balance between the glucose-lowering hormone insulin and glucose-elevating hormones glucagon, cortisol, epinephrine, and growth hormone.
- Hypoglycemia occurs via one of several mechanisms: excess insulin or insulin analogs, excessive glucose utilization, and decreased glucose production.
- The most common specific causes of hypoglycemia include exogenous insulin overdose, insulinoma and other insulin analog–secreting tumors, hypoglycemia of puppies and toy breeds, sepsis, hypoadrenocorticism, and severe liver disease.
- Neuroglycopenia causes alterations in mentation, seizures, blindness or alterations in vision, somnolence, and weakness or ataxia.
- Adrenergic stimulation in response to declining blood glucose accounts for other common clinical signs associated with hypoglycemia, including restlessness, anxiety, tachypnea, vomiting or diarrhea, and trembling.
- In hypoglycemic crises, parenteral dextrose administration is the most effective therapy. Food should be offered as soon as possible. Glucagon infusion may be used for cases of intractable hypoglycemia secondary to insulinoma or insulin analog–secreting neoplasms.

Euglycemia is maintained by a balance of glucose production, storage, and release from storage forms. Many disease processes can interfere with normal glucose homeostasis and lead to hypoglycemia. This chapter reviews normal glucose homeostatic mechanisms, clinical signs and causes of hypoglycemia, and treatment of a hypoglycemic crisis.

NORMAL GLUCOSE HOMEOSTASIS

Glucose comes from three sources: (1) intestinal absorption of glucose from digestion of carbohydrates; (2) breakdown of the storage form of glucose (glycogen) via glycogenolysis; and (3) production of glucose from precursors lactate, pyruvate, amino acids, and glycerol via gluconeogenesis. Glucose homeostasis is maintained by a balance between the glucose-lowering hormone insulin and glucose-elevating hormones, primarily glucagon, epinephrine, cortisol, and growth hormone.

Insulin is secreted by β cells of the pancreas in response to the rising concentrations of glucose, amino acids, and gastrointestinal (GI) hormones (gastrin, secretin, cholecystokinin, and gastric inhibitory peptide) present after a meal.[1] Insulin inhibits gluconeogenesis and glycogenolysis, promotes glycogen storage, stimulates glucose uptake and utilization by insulin-sensitive cells, and decreases glucagon secretion. Insulin also promotes triglyceride formation in adipose tissue and the synthesis of protein and glycogen in muscle. Decreased levels of insulin stimulate gluconeogenesis and reduce glucose used by peripheral tissues.

As blood glucose concentrations fall, the counterregulatory hormones glucagon, epinephrine, cortisol, and growth hormone are released. Both glucagon and epinephrine levels rise within minutes of hypoglycemia and have a transient effect on increasing glucose production; they subsequently support basal rates of glucose production.[2] Cortisol and growth hormone are released after a few hours, but their effects are also longer lasting.

Glucagon is secreted from pancreatic α cells. It acts on the liver to stimulate glycogenolysis and, to a lesser extent, gluconeogenesis, thereby increasing hepatic glucose production. This is transient, however, and glucose production quickly declines toward basal rates as increasing levels of insulin counteract the effects of glucagon. Glucagon directly stimulates hepatic glycogenolysis and gluconeogenesis, mobilizes gluconeogenic precursors, and reduces peripheral glucose utilization. Epinephrine limits insulin secretion and increases glucagon secretion. Cortisol increases glucose-facilitating lipolysis and release of amino acids from muscle for gluconeogenesis in the liver. Growth hormone antagonizes effects of insulin by decreasing peripheral glucose utilization and promoting lipolysis.

Hypoglycemia results when glucose utilization exceeds glucose entry into circulation. General mechanisms of hypoglycemia include (1) inadequate dietary intake, (2) excessive glucose utilization, (3) dysfunctional glycogenolytic or gluconeogenic pathways or inadequate precursors for these pathways, and (4) endocrine abnormalities. On its own accord, inadequate dietary intake is unlikely to cause hypoglycemia because gluconeogenic and glycolytic pathways dominate during periods of fast. In most animals a concurrent defect in one of the other mechanisms is required.

CLINICAL SIGNS AND CONSEQUENCES OF HYPOGLYCEMIA

Glucose is an obligate energy source for the brain. The brain has limited ability to use other substrates, can store minimal amounts of glycogen, and cannot manufacture glucose; therefore the brain relies on a constant stream of glucose for its energy needs.[3] Glucose enters the brain by facilitated diffusion. Adequate arterial glucose concentration is essential to maintaining a diffusion gradient. Because brain cells rely so heavily on glucose for energy, hypoglycemia results in neuroglycopenia (hypoglycemia of the central nervous system) and its neurologic manifestations. The degree, rate of decline, and duration of hypoglycemia all contribute to type and severity of symptoms.

Neuroglycopenic signs include altered mentation or dullness, sleepiness, weakness or recumbency, ataxia, blindness or altered vision, and seizures.[2,4] Prolonged neuroglycopenia can lead to permanent brain injury and neurologic signs, especially blindness, that persist beyond resolution of the hypoglycemia. Neurogenic signs result from activation of the adrenergic system in response to the hypoglycemia. Humans describe being hungry, a tingling sensation, tremors or shakiness, a pounding heart, and anxiety or nervousness.[2] Similar signs noted in hypoglycemic dogs and cats include pacing, vocalizing, restlessness, shaking, and trembling.[4] Vomiting, anorexia, panting or tachypnea, diarrhea, and urination have been noted in hypoglycemic dogs and cats. Bradycardia and circulatory collapse have also been documented.[5] Signs may be episodic. Some animals, especially those with prolonged hypoglycemia, demonstrate no associated signs.[4] This hypoglycemia unawareness may occur in patients whose brains are induced by chronic or recurrent hypoglycemia to upregulate cerebral glucose uptake, thereby decreasing the perception of peripheral hypoglycemia by the brain.[3]

DIAGNOSIS OF HYPOGLYCEMIA

By definition, hypoglycemia is diagnosed by a blood glucose level of 60 mg/dl or less, although clinical signs often do not develop until the level is less than 50 mg/dl. Whipple's triad provides guidelines for identifying hypoglycemia: clinical signs consistent with hypoglycemia, a low blood glucose level, and abatement of signs with correction of the hypoglycemia.[2]

Handheld glucometers may underestimate or overestimate serum glucose,[6,7] so glucose values obtained on a handheld glucometer should be confirmed via other methods. Falsely low glucose values, or pseudohypoglycemia, can be obtained if the serum is not separated from the red blood cells within 30 minutes of collection, because the red blood cells continue to consume glucose for glycolysis.[8] If centrifugation and serum separation must be delayed longer than 30 minutes, collection in a sodium fluoride tube will arrest glycolysis.

Once hypoglycemia is confirmed, additional diagnostic modalities may be indicated to identify its etiology. Complete blood cell count, serum chemistry analysis, urinalysis, imaging, insulin levels, and other endocrine testing may be indicated.

CAUSES OF HYPOGLYCEMIA

Many causes of hypoglycemia (Box 66-1) fall into the categories of excess insulin or insulin analog, inadequate glucose production, and excess cellular glucose consumption.

Excess Insulin or Insulin Analogs

Exogenous insulin overdose

Exogenous insulin overdose is possible in any animal receiving insulin therapy, whether for diabetes mellitus or for treatment of other disorders such as hyperkalemia or calcium channel blocker overdose. Insulin overdoses in diabetic animals occur more commonly in cats than dogs, in obese animals, and in cats receiving more than 6 units of insulin per injection.[4]

Anorexic or hyporexic diabetics receiving insulin are also at risk. Clinical signs are consistent with hypoglycemia. Treatment includes discontinuation of insulin therapy, feeding the animal as soon as possible, and administration of intravenous dextrose if the animal is too severely affected to eat. Duration of the hypoglycemia varies and is not necessarily dependent on the amount and type of insulin that caused the overdose.[4] Once the animal is stabilized and eating, the dextrose infusion can be tapered off while blood glucose levels continue to be monitored.

Some diabetic animals may not need insulin for several days, and others will become hyperglycemic more quickly. The animal should be monitored for onset of polyuria and polydipsia and hyperglycemia to verify need for insulin. Remission in transiently diabetic cats may be marked by a hypoglycemic episode. Once the need to restart insulin is confirmed, it is prudent to reduce the dosage by 25% to 50% initially and follow up with normal diabetic monitoring to attempt regulation.[9,10] There may be another underlying problem that predisposed the animal to hypoglycemia, and additional workup is warranted if hypoglycemia is ongoing or if the animal has additional history or signs unrelated to hypoglycemia.

BOX 66-1 *Causes of Hypoglycemia*

Artifact*

Pseudohypoglycemia*
Handheld glucometer*
- Hemoconcentration

Excess Insulin or Insulin Analogs

Exogenous insulin overdose
Insulinoma
Paraneoplastic syndrome
- Hepatomas, hepatocellular carcinoma
- Leiomyomas, leiomyosarcomas
- Pulmonary, mammary, and salivary carcinoma
- Lymphoma, plasmacytoid tumors
- Oral melanoma, hemangiosarcoma

Toxins and medications
- Sulfonylureas
- Xylitol

Excess Glucose Utilization

Infection
- Sepsis
- Babesiosis

Exercise-induced (hunting dog) hypoglycemia
Paraneoplastic
Polycythemia
Leukocytosis
Pregnancy

Decreased Glucose Production

Neonatal hypoglycemia
Hepatic dysfunction
- Portosystemic shunt
- Inflammatory or infectious hepatitis
- Hepatic lipidosis
- Cirrhosis
- Neoplasia
- Glycogen storage disease

Hypocortisolism
Counterregulatory hormone deficiencies
- Glucagon, growth hormone
- Thyroid hormone, catecholamines
- Hypopituitarism

Glycogenic or gluconeogenic enzyme deficiencies
β-Blockers

*Cause of apparent, not true, hypoglycemia.

Insulinoma

Insulinomas are insulin-secreting, usually malignant tumors of the pancreas. They are described more commonly in middle-aged to older dogs but have also been seen in cats.[10-19] Patients often exhibit weakness or collapse, and severe hypoglycemia is an isolated finding. Other clinical pathology data are generally unremarkable, although elevated liver enzyme activities and hypokalemia may be seen.[12,13,15,20]

Diagnosis is made by evaluating blood insulin concentration on a sample taken during an episode of hypoglycemia. High or normal insulin levels in the face of hypoglycemia are indicative of insulinoma. Some animals will have intermittent episodes of hypoglycemia and hyperinsulinemia that may require a supervised fast or multiple samples to identify.[20] Also, results may vary significantly between laboratories and this fact may prompt retesting those patients suspected of having insulinoma that do not have confirmatory endocrine testing.[14] If insulin levels are equivocal, an amended insulin/glucose ratio (AIGR) can be calculated:

$$\text{AIGR} = (\text{insulin} \times 100) \div (\text{plasma glucose} - 30)$$

A denominator of 1 is used if the plasma glucose is less than 30 mg/dl. An AIGR higher than 30 suggests insulinoma,[21] although is not definitive.[10] Performing the ratio on at least four samples may improve the sensitivity of the test.[20] Use of the ratio has fallen out of favor because patients with other causes of hypoglycemia can also have an abnormal ratio.[22,23] Low fructosamine values may also lend support to a diagnosis.[22-24] Provocative testing such as the glucagon tolerance test, oral glucose tolerance test, tolbutamide tolerance test, and epinephrine stimulation test have been tried but are no more sensitive than other tests and may precipitate hypoglycemia.[12]

Abdominal ultrasonography may or may not reveal a mass or nodule in the pancreas. Computed tomography (CT), magnetic resonance imaging (MRI) scintigraphy, and surgical exploration are other options for attempted identification of the insulinoma.[10,25-28] Thoracic radiographs are indicated to look for evidence of metastatic disease.

Emergency treatment for symptomatic hypoglycemia is outlined later in this chapter. A combination of surgical excision and medical management has resulted in the longest survival times for patients with insulinoma and surgical excision of the primary tumor and any obvious metastases is considered the treatment of choice.[29] Surgery is still considered palliative because approximately 50% of patients have metastatic disease evident at surgery and the majority of the others have occult metastases.[12,15,20] Medical options for animals not undergoing surgery or for those with metastatic disease and persistent hypoglycemia include dietary management (small, frequent feedings of a food low in simple sugars) and glucocorticoids (prednisone 0.5 to 1 mg/kg in divided doses PO q12h[30]). Higher doses of glucocorticoids and diazoxide (10 mg/kg initially, up to 60 mg/kg, divided q12h[30]), which directly inhibits pancreatic insulin secretion, can be used in patients with refractory disease. Other adjunctive therapies include streptozocin[31] (which selectively destroys pancreatic β cells), somatostatin analogs such as octreotide[32,33] (which suppresses synthesis and secretion of insulin), or alloxan (a β-cell cytotoxin).[10] Recent identification of growth hormone (GH), GH receptor, and insulinlike growth factor 1 (IGF-1) expression in the primary tumor and metastases suggests a potential future method to antagonize tumor growth.[34]

Survival times vary and depend on the extent of disease and therapeutic regimen. In one study, median survival time was 74 days for dogs with medical treatment only and 381 days for dogs undergoing surgery.[35] In another study, median survival time was 18 months for dogs with disease confined to the pancreas and local lymph nodes and less than 6 months for dogs with distant metastases.[15] Another reported that 10% to 15% of dogs undergoing surgery died or were euthanized within 1 month of surgery, 25% died within 6 months, and 60% to 70% lived more than 6 months, with many living longer than 1 year and some even longer than 2 years.[10] The longest survival times have been reported in dogs undergoing surgery followed by medical management upon recurrence of clinical signs.[29] The median survival time was 196 days for dogs undergoing only medical management, 785 days for those undergoing only surgery, and 1316 days for dogs undergoing surgery followed by prednisone upon relapse of clinical signs.[29] The biomarker Ki67 index shows promise for predicting disease-free intervals and survival time in clinical patients.[36]

Paraneoplastic hypoglycemia

Although any tumor can be associated with hypoglycemia, the most commonly described non–β-cell neoplasms associated with hypoglycemia include hepatomas and hepatocellular carcinoma, leiomyomas and leiomyosarcomas, and other carcinomas or adenocarcinomas (especially those of pulmonary, mammary, and salivary origin),[37] lymphoma, plasmacytoid tumors, oral melanoma, and hemangiosarcoma. Neoplasia can cause hypoglycemia via secretion of insulin or insulinlike peptides, accelerated consumption of glucose by the tumor cells, or by failure of glycogenolysis or gluconeogenesis by the liver. Historical and clinical findings and treatment are consistent with the specific tumor.

Toxins and medications

Certain toxins have been associated with hypoglycemia in dogs and cats. Excessive dosages of oral glucose-lowering agents such as the sulfonylurea drugs chlorpropamide and glipizide may cause hypoglycemia. These drugs are thought to stimulate insulin secretion from the pancreas, enhance tissue sensitivity to insulin, and decrease basal hepatic glucose production.[30] Xylitol-sweetened products, such as sugar-free gum, can cause hypoglycemia in dogs via its stimulation of insulin release from β cells.[38] Xylitol can also cause hepatic necrosis and failure, which can also cause hypoglycemia[39] β-Blockers such as atenolol are also thought to contribute to hypoglycemia via interference with adrenergic counterregulatory mechanisms.

A history of exposure or known ingestion coupled with consistent signs of low blood glucose levels would substantiate the diagnosis. In addition to treating hypoglycemia, induced emesis and activated charcoal administration may be indicated if the ingestion is identified early and the patient is not clinically impaired by hypoglycemia (see Chapter 74).

Inadequate Glucose Production

Hypoglycemia of neonates and toy breed dogs

Most commonly, hypoglycemia of neonatal and pediatric animals stems from inadequate substrate for glycolysis or gluconeogenesis. Glycogen stores are small and easily depleted in the face of inadequate food intake in these animals. Hepatic enzyme systems may also be immature.[40] Additionally, the brain accounts for most of the basal metabolic rate in the neonate, thus contributing to the common development of hypoglycemia in the young. In the nursing animal, factors predisposing to hypoglycemia include premature birth, debilitation of the bitch or queen at parturition, being the runt of the litter, and diabetes in the bitch.[40] Although seen most commonly in neonates, adult toy and small breed dogs are also at risk for hypoglycemia. In the weaned puppy or kitten, factors predisposing to hypoglycemia include concurrent infection, vaccinations, vigorous exercise, GI upset, hypothermia, poor nutrition, and extended fast.[40] Most affected animals respond readily to supplementation and increased feeding frequency. Recurrent or persistent hypoglycemia warrants further investigation. Other differentials for hypoglycemia that must be considered in a hypoglycemic puppy or kitten include portosystemic shunt or other hepatic disease, sepsis, glycogen storage disease, and counterregulatory hormone deficiency.

Hepatic disease

Portosystemic shunt, glycogen storage disease, severe inflammatory or infectious hepatitis, hepatic lipidosis, cirrhosis, hepatic neoplasia, and toxicity are specific etiologies of hepatic failure that can lead to hypoglycemia via dysfunctional glycogen storage, glycogenolytic, and gluconeogenic capabilities. Euglycemia usually is maintained until late in the course of hepatic disease until approximately 70% of hepatic function is lost.[8] Patients with portosystemic shunt and glycogen storage disease are usually young and may be small or unthrifty. Evaluation of an animal with severe liver disease may reveal a poor body condition score, microhepatica or enlarged liver, icterus, ascites, melena, vomiting, diarrhea, anorexia, or signs of hepatic encephalopathy such as depression or seizures. Clinical pathology data may show hypoalbuminemia, low blood urea nitrogen, hypocholesterolemia, hyperbilirubinemia, elevated liver enzyme activities, and low urine specific gravity (see Chapters 115, 116, and 132).

Hypocortisolism and other counterregulatory hormone deficiencies

Hypoadrenocorticism, specifically hypocortisolism, may lead to hypoglycemia via loss of cortisol-induced counterregulatory mechanisms. History may include anorexia, vomiting, diarrhea, melena or hematochezia, weakness, and possibly polyuria and polydipsia. Physical examination may reveal dehydration, bradycardia, muffled heart sounds, poor pulse quality, hypotension, and shock. Clinical pathology evaluation may reveal lack of stress leukogram, azotemia, hypercalcemia, hyponatremia, hypochloremia, and hyperkalemia. Confirmation of hypocortisolism is via the adrenocorticotropic hormone stimulation test. Treatment includes physiologic doses of glucocorticoids, and either fludrocortisone acetate (Florinef) or desoxycorticosterone pivalate if mineralocorticoids are also deficient. Fluid therapy is required in Addisonian crisis (see Chapter 73).

Deficiencies in other hormones such as glucagon, growth hormone, thyroid hormone, and catecholamines can all lead to hypoglycemia as a result of interference with counterregulatory mechanisms designed to prevent hypoglycemia.

Excess Glucose Utilization

Infection, extreme exercise, polycythemia or leukocytosis, and pregnancy can all lead to excessive cellular glucose consumption.

Infection

Sepsis is a common cause of hypoglycemia. Decreased intake, decreased hepatic function, and, most significantly, non–insulin-mediated increased consumption play a role in sepsis-induced hypoglycemia. Increased glucose consumption is believed to be induced by inflammatory mediators, such as tumor necrosis factor, especially in macrophage-rich tissues such as the spleen, liver, and lungs.[41] Hypotension or hypoxemia may also induce excess glucose consumption via increases in anaerobic glycolysis.

Patients with sepsis will be critically ill. Vasodilatory shock may be evidenced by injected mucous membranes and hypotension. Other clinical signs will depend on the type and location of infection. A complete workup and appropriate cultures are indicated (see Chapter 91). Canine babesiosis is an infection specifically associated with hypoglycemia, and hypoglycemia at admission is a poor prognostic indicator in canine babesiosis and may occur secondary to the same mechanisms as bacterial sepsis or by consumption of glucose by the parasites.[42-44]

Exercise-induced hypoglycemia

Exercise-induced hypoglycemia, also called *hunting dog hypoglycemia,* is generally seen in lean hunting or working dogs engaging in vigorous exercise. Glucose utilization by muscle markedly increases during exercise and endogenous glucose production, via glycolysis and gluconeogenesis, increases to meet this demand.[2] This form of hypoglycemia is believed to occur secondary to glycogen depletion in the face of increased glucose utilization. Affected animals should be fed small amounts frequently during exercise or should discontinue working if hypoglycemia continues.

Polycythemia and leukocytosis

Hypoglycemia in polycythemia occurs secondary to increased metabolism of glucose by the large red blood cell mass or because of reduced plasma volume.[7,8,45] Massive leukocytosis can have the same effect. Rapid processing of the blood sample is necessary to minimize in vitro glucose utilization by the cells. This measured reduction in blood glucose concentration is primarily an artifactual change and does not usually result in clinical signs of hypoglycemia.

TREATMENT OF HYPOGLYCEMIC CRISIS

Initial treatment for a symptomatic hypoglycemic patient, regardless of etiology, is usually intravenous dextrose. A bolus of 0.5 to 1 ml/kg of 50% dextrose (0.25 to 0.5 g/kg) can be diluted 1:2 to 1:4 and is then given intravenously over 5 minutes. This solution is hypertonic and can cause phlebitis. While acquiring or in the absence of intravenous access, such as in the home setting, Karo syrup, pancake syrup, or honey can be applied to the oral mucous membranes, and this may or may not significantly increase the glucose unless part of the dose is eventually swallowed.[46-48]

The goal of emergent therapy is to eliminate clinical signs; it may not be necessary to return the glucose to normal range. Marked improvements in neuroglycopenic signs usually are seen within 1 to 2 minutes of supplementation, although prolonged, severe neuroglycopenia can cause irreparable neuronal damage. If the patient is alert and it is not contraindicated, the recovering animal should be offered small, frequent meals that are low in simple sugars. Otherwise, a constant rate infusion (CRI) of 2.5% to 5% dextrose should be administered until the cause of the hypoglycemia is identified and resolved. Dextrose infusions should be formulated by adding the appropriate amount of 50% dextrose to an isotonic fluid such as lactated Ringer's solution or 0.9% saline (Table 66-1). Dextrose 5% in water (D_5W) should not be used as the sole fluid for treatment because it can result in severe, possibly life-threatening hyponatremia. Blood glucose should be monitored frequently to ensure adequate and not excessive supplementation is provided. Dextrose infusions may need to be continued for hours to days, depending on the underlying cause of the hypoglycemia. If a solution containing greater than 5% dextrose is needed to maintain blood glucose concentrations, ideally it should be administered via a central line to prevent vascular irritation.

Care should be taken using intravenous dextrose in animals with suspected insulinoma or other tumors secreting insulinlike analogs. In these patients, a bolus of intravenous dextrose can stimulate release of even more insulin from the tumor, leading to a vicious cycle of dextrose infusion followed by rebound hypoglycemia. Additionally, hyperinsulinemia has been shown to depress glucagon secretion in humans, thus removing one of the counterregulatory mechanisms vital to maintaining euglycemia.[49] Glucagon CRI is another option for treating animals with insulin or insulin like peptide–secreting tumors that are in a refractory hypoglycemic crisis.[50] Glucagon is reconstituted according the manufacturer's instructions and diluted in 0.9% saline. This resulting 1000 ng/ml solution is first administered as a bolus of 50 ng/kg followed by a CRI of 5 to 40 ng/kg/min,[30] the lowest rate necessary to eliminate clinical signs and maintain low normal euglycemia. Finally, glucocorticoids such as prednisone or dexamethasone antagonize insulin effects and stimulate gluconeogenesis, which may help stabilize blood glucose concentration in patients with paraneoplastic or endocrine-induced hypoglycemia, including hypoadrenocorticism and insulinoma.

Table 66-1 Emergency Management of Hypoglycemia

Drug	Dose/Route	Comments
Dextrose	Bolus: • 0.5-1 ml/kg (0.25-0.5 g/kg) of 50% dextrose (diluted at least 1:2) CRI: • 2.5%-5% dextrose (or more) as needed in fluids	• Avoid large dextrose bolus in patients with suspected insulinoma. • For 2.5% solution: add 50 ml of 50% dextrose to 950 ml crystalloid to make 1 L. • For 5% solution, add 100 ml of 50% dextrose to 900 ml crystalloid.
Frequent small meals	Oral feeding with diet low in simple sugars (higher in complex carbohydrates, proteins)	Institute when patient is alert enough to eat and swallow.
Glucagon	Bolus 50 ng/kg IV followed by CRI of 5-10 ng/kg/min (up to 40 ng/kg/min) to effect	Reconstitute based on manufacturer's instructions to a 1000 ng/ml solution.
Corticosteroids	Dexamethasone: 0.1-0.2 mg/kg IV as initial dose, then 0.05-0.1 mg/kg IV q12h Prednisone/prednisolone: • For hypoadrenocorticism: 0.1-0.22 mg/kg, then taper to lowest dose needed to control signs • For insulinoma: 0.25-0.5 mg/kg PO q12h	• Corticosteroids are for treating paraneoplastic or endocrine-induced hypoglycemia but are contraindicated for infection-induced hypoglycemia. • Dexamethasone is preferred form for patients with suspected hypoadrenocorticism before ACTH stimulation test because it will not be measured by the cortisol assay. • Prednisolone is preferred over prednisone in cats.

ACTH, Adrenocorticotropic hormone; *IV,* intravenously; *CRI,* constant rate infusion; *ng,* nanograms.

REFERENCES

1. Klein BG: Cunningham's textbook of veterinary physiology, ed 5, Philadelphia, 2012, Saunders.
2. Cryer PE: Hypoglycemia. In Melmed S, Polonsky KS, Larsen PR, Kronenberg HM, editors: Williams textbook of endocrinology, ed 12, Philadelphia, 2012, Saunders.
3. Boyle PJ: Alteration in brain glucose metabolism induced by hypoglycemia in man, Diabetologia 40:S69, 1997.
4. Whitley N, Drobatz K, Panciera D: Insulin overdose in dogs and cats: 28 cases (1986-1993), J Am Vet Med Assoc 211:326, 1997.
5. Little CJ: Hypoglycaemic bradycardia and circulatory collapse in a dog and a cat, J Soc Adm Pharm 46:445, 2005.
6. Wess G, Reusch C: Evaluation of five portable blood glucose meters for use in dogs, J Am Vet Med Assoc 216:203, 2000.
7. Paul A, Shiel RE, Juvet F, et al: Effect of hematocrit on accuracy of two point-of-care glucometers for use in dogs, Am J Vet Res 72(9):1204, 2011.
8. Latimer KS: Duncan and Prasse's veterinary laboratory medicine clinical pathology, ed 5, Hoboken, NJ, 2011, Wiley-Blackwell.
9. McIntire DK: Diabetic crises: insulin overdose, diabetic ketoacidosis, and hyperosmolar coma, Vet Clin North Am Small Anim Pract 25:639, 1995.
10. Feldman EC, Nelson RW: Canine and feline endocrinology and reproduction, ed 3, St Louis, 2004, Elsevier.
11. Dunn JK, Bostock DE, Herrtage ME, et al: Insulin-secreting tumors of the canine pancreas: clinical and pathological features of 11 cases, J Small Anim Pract 34:325, 1993.
12. Kruth SA, Feldman EC, Kennedy PC: Insulin-secreting islet cell tumors: establishing a diagnosis and the clinical course for 25 dogs, J Am Vet Med Assoc 181(1):54, 1982.
13. Leifer CE, Peterson ME, Matus RE: Insulin-secreting tumor: diagnosis and medical and surgical management in 55 dogs, J Am Vet Med Assoc 188(1):60, 1986.
14. Madarame H, Kayanuma H, Shida T, et al: Retrospective study of canine insulinomas: eight cases (2005-2008), J Vet Med Sci (7):905, 2009.
15. Caywood DD, Klausner JS, O'Leary TP, et al: Pancreatic insulin-secreting neoplasms: clinical, diagnostic, and prognostic features in 73 dogs, J Am Anim Hosp Assoc 24:577, 1988.
16. Trifonidou MA, Kirpensteijn J, Robben JH: A retrospective evaluation of 51 dogs with insulinoma, Vet Q 20:S114, 1998.
17. O'Brien, TD, Norton F, Turner TM, et al: Pancreatic endocrine tumor in a cat: clinical, pathological, and immunohistochemical evaluation, J Am Anim Hosp Assoc 26:453, 1990.
18. Hawks D, Peterson ME, Hawkins KL, et al: Insulin-secreting pancreatic (islet cell) carcinoma in a cat, J Vet Intern Med 6:193, 1992.
19. Kraje AC: Hypoglycemia and irreversible neurologic complications in a cat with insulinoma, J Am Vet Med Assoc 223:812, 2003.
20. Siliart B, Stambouli F: Laboratory diagnosis of insulinoma in the dog: a retrospective study and a new diagnostic procedure, J Small Anim Pract 37:367, 1996.
21. Thompson JC, Jones BR, Hickson PC: The amended insulin-to-glucose ratio and diagnosis of insulinoma in dogs, N Z Vet J 43:240, 1995.
22. Mellanby RJ, Herrtage ME: Insulinoma in a normoglycaemic dog with low serum fructosamine, J Small Anim Pract 43(11):506, 2002.
23. Loste A, Marca MC, Pérez M, et al: Clinical value of fructosamine measurements in non-healthy dogs, Vet Res Commun 25(2):109, 2001.
24. Thoresen SI, Aleksandersen M, Lonaas L, et al: Pancreatic insulin-secreting carcinoma in a dog: fructosamine for determining persistent hypoglycaemia, J Small Anim Pract 36:282, 1995.
25. Lester NV, Newell SM, Hill RC, Lanz OI: Scintigraphic diagnosis of insulinoma in a dog, Vet Radiol Ultrasound 40:174, 1999.
26. Robben JH, Pollak Y, Kirpensteijn J, et al: Comparison of ultrasonography, computed tomography, and single-photon emission computed tomography for the detection and localization of canine insulinoma, J Vet Intern Med 19:15, 2005.
27. Fukazawa K, Kayanuma H, Kanai E, et al: Insulinoma with basal ganglion involvement detected by magnetic resonance imaging in a dog, J Vet Med Sci 71(5):689, 2009.
28. Garden OA, Reubi JC, Dykes NL, et al: Somatostatin receptor imaging in vivo by planar scintigraphy facilitates the diagnosis of canine insulinomas, J Vet Intern Med 19:168, 2005.
29. Polton GA, White RN, Brearley MJ, et al: Improved survival in a retrospective cohort of 28 dogs with insulinoma, J Small Anim Pract 48(3):151, 2007.
30. Plumb DC: Veterinary drug handbook, ed 7, Stockholm, WI, 2011, Pharma Vet.
31. Moore AS, Nelson RW, Henry CJ, et al: Streptozocin for treatment of pancreatic islet cell tumors in dogs: 17 cases (1989-1999), J Am Vet Med Assoc 221:811, 2002.
32. Robben JH, Visser-Wisselaar HA, Rutteman GR, et al: In vitro and in vivo detection of functional somatostatin receptors in canine insulinomas, J Nucl Med 38:1036, 1997.
33. Robben JH, van den Brom WE, Mol JA, et al: Effect of octreotide on plasma concentrations of glucose, insulin, glucagon, growth hormone, and cortisol in healthy dogs and dogs with insulinoma, Res Vet Sci 80:25, 2006.

34. Buishand FO, van Erp MGM, Groenveld HA, et al: Expression of insulin-like growth factor-1 by canine insulinomas and their metastases, Vet J 191(3):334, 2012.
35. Tobin RL, Nelson RW, Lucroy MD, et al: Outcome of surgical versus medical treatment of dogs with β-cell neoplasia: 39 cases (1990-1997), J Am Vet Med Assoc 215:226, 1999.
36. Buishand FO, Kik M, Kirpensteijn J: Evaluation of clinico-pathological criteria and the Ki67 index as prognostic indicators in canine insulinoma, Vet J 185(1):62, 2010.
37. Bergman PJ: Paraneoplastic syndromes. In Withrow SJ, Vail DM, Page RL, editors: Withrow and MacEwen's small animal clinical oncology, ed 5, St Louis, 2013, Saunders.
38. Dunayer EK: Hypoglycemia following canine ingestion of xylitol-containing gum, Vet Hum Toxicol 46:87, 2004.
39. Dunaye EK, Gwaltney-Brant SM: Acute hepatic failure and coagulopathy associated with xylitol ingestion in eight dogs, J Am Vet Med Assoc 229(7):1113, 2006.
40. Chastain CB: The metabolic system. In Hoskins JD, editor: Veterinary pediatrics: dogs and cats from birth to six months, ed 3, Philadelphia, 2001, WB Saunders.
41. Meszaros K, Lang CH, Bagby GJ, et al: TNF increases in vivo glucose utilization of macrophage-rich tissues, Biochem Biophys Res Commun 149:1, 1987.
42. Nel M, Lobetti RG, Keller N, et al: Prognostic value of blood lactate, blood glucose, and hematocrit in canine babesiosis, J Vet Intern Med 18:471, 2004.
43. Jacobson LS, Lobetti RG: Glucose, lactate, and pyruvate concentrations in dogs with babesiosis, Am J Vet Res 66:244, 2005.
44. Keller N, Jacobson LS, Nel M, et al: Prevalence and risk factors of hypoglycemia in virulent canine babesiosis, J Vet Intern Med 18(3):265, 2004.
45. Rosenkrantz TS, Philipps AF, Skrzypczak PS, et al: Cerebral metabolism in the newborn lamb with polycythemia, Ped Res 23:3, 1988.
46. Chlup R, Zapletalova J, Peterson K, et al: Impact of buccal glucose spray, liquid sugars and dextrose tablets on the evolution of plasma glucose concentration in healthy persons, Biomed Pap Med Fac Univ Palacky Olomouc Czech Repub 153(3):205, 2009.
47. Gunning RR, Garber AJ: Bioactivity of instant glucose. Failure of absorption through oral mucosa, JAMA 240(15):1611, 1978.
48. Manning AS, Evered DF: The absorption of sugars from the human buccal cavity, Clin Sci Mol Med 51(2):127, 1976.
49. Banerer S, McGregor VP, Cryer PE: Intraislet hyperinsulinemia prevents the glucagon response to hypoglycemia despite an intact autonomic response, Diabetes 51:958, 2002.
50. Fischer JR, Smith SA, Harkin KR: Glucagon constant rate infusion: a novel strategy for the management of hyperinsulinemic-hypoglycemic crisis in the dog, J Am Anim Hosp Assoc 36:27, 2000.

CHAPTER 67
DIABETES INSIPIDUS

Richard E. Goldstein, DVM, DACVIM, DECVIM-CA

KEY POINTS

- Diabetes insipidus results from a lack of secretion of or a lack of an appropriate renal response to a hormone known as *vasopressin* or *antidiuretic hormone*.
- Primary diabetes insipidus is most commonly acquired and central in origin. Common causes include trauma and intracranial masses.
- Secondary diabetes insipidus is usually renal in origin. Common causes include hypercalcemia, gram-negative sepsis, and severe hypokalemia.
- The manifestation of diabetes insipidus that requires emergency intervention is severe hypernatremia and dehydration caused by urinary free water losses without appropriate intake.
- The water deprivation test does provide valuable diagnostic information and can be dangerous, resulting in severe dehydration and hypernatremia.

By definition diabetes *insipidus* is the tasteless or nonsweet diabetes. This differentiates it, of course, from the sweet diabetes, the better known diabetes *mellitus*. Diabetes insipidus is caused by a lack of the hormone vasopressin (otherwise known as *antidiuretic hormone* or *ADH*), a lack of renal receptors to vasopressin, or an inability of those receptors to respond to vasopressin. The presence of vasopressin and its ability to activate renal receptors are crucial to the kidneys' urine concentration capabilities. Vasopressin is a nonapeptide (nine amino acids) composed of six amino acids in a disulfide ring and three amino acids in a tail. In small animals the eighth amino acid in vasopressin is arginine, sometimes also called *AVP* or *arginine vasopressin*.[1]

Urine Concentration Mechanism

In a normally functioning kidney, as the solute within the tubule travels through the thick ascending loop of Henle, sodium (and subsequently chloride) is extracted by an energy-requiring ion pump from the solute in an area that is impermeable to water. This unusual feat renders the remaining solute hyposthenuric, or of lower osmolality than serum. The final urine concentration then depends on the presence and function of vasopressin. When the presence or function of vasopressin is lacking (diabetes insipidus), the final urine concentration can remain hyposthenuric or can be isosthenuric or even mildly hypersthenuric with partial disease.

Vasopressin Secretion and Sodium Homeostasis

Whole body water and sodium concentrations are kept constant despite a huge variability in dietary sodium intake and hydration status. A key factor of this control is the rate of vasopressin release from the neurohypothesis. The neurohypothesis consists of hypothalamic nuclei that secrete oxytocin and vasopressin. After the nuclear synthesis of these hormones they are transported in their axons and finally secreted from the termini in the posterior lobe of the pituitary gland. Several mechanisms regulate the release of vasopressin. Increases in extracellular fluid osmolality are detected by osmoreceptors of the hypothalamus and lead to a rapid increase in vasopressin release. Cardiovascular reflexes in response to changes in effective circulating volume also alter vasopressin release. Low-pressure baroreceptors of the cardiac atria and high-pressure baroreceptors of the aortic arch and carotid sinus stimulate vasopressin release in response to a decrease in blood pressure or blood volume. In addition, angiotensin II receptors in the hypothalamus increase vasopressin release in response to angiotensin II. The release of vasopressin is more sensitive to changes in osmolality than changes in effective circulating volume. An increase of only 1% in plasma osmolality will stimulate vasopressin release, whereas a drop in blood volume of approximately 10% is needed to stimulate vasopressin release.[2,3]

Antidiuretic Effects of Vasopressin

The antidiuretic effects of vasopressin occur in response to the binding of vasopressin to its receptor on the cells of the distal tubule and collecting duct. These are V_2 cyclic adenosine monophosphate–dependent receptors, which when activated cause an increase in water permeability of the luminal membrane by the insertion of aquaporin-2 water channels in the apical membrane of the renal epithelial cells. This allows a more rapid passive flow of water from the lumen through the epithelial cells and into the solute-rich, concentrated interstitium, causing a rapid and marked increase in osmolality within the tubular lumen.[4] Theoretically the maximum urine concentration of a given animal would be equal to the maximum solute concentration of the medullary interstitium. Thus in times of hypernatremia caused by excess salt intake or, more commonly, free water loss, resulting in a free water deficit or a hyperosmolar contraction of the extracellular space, the secretion of vasopressin causes an increase of water reabsorption from the kidney, a decrease in water excretion, and the normalization of sodium concentration in the body, while excreting heavily concentrated urine.

CENTRAL DIABETES INSIPIDUS

Central diabetes insipidus (CDI) is the most common primary form of diabetes insipidus. It is caused by a complete or partial lack of secretion of vasopressin from the axon termini in the anterior lobe of the pituitary gland. Documented causes of CDI in small animals include neoplastic, traumatic, inflammatory, congenital, and idiopathic conditions.[5,6] Glucocorticoid administration is thought to decrease vasopressin release in dogs and therefore can be included in the causes of canine acquired CDI.[1]

In humans CDI is associated most commonly with brain surgery, trauma, and immune-mediated disease. Neoplasia, infectious disease, and hereditary disorders are also relatively common in this population.[7] After brain trauma, at least 25% of long-term survivors suffer from what is defined in humans as *posttraumatic hypopituitarism.*[8] This syndrome most often includes suppression of hormone release from the anterior pituitary gland but can also include decreased vasopressin secretion from the posterior pituitary gland. Posttraumatic CDI is thought to resolve within a few days in most human cases[9] but may also be a sign of permanent or late brain damage. Postsurgical CDI may be the most common cause in humans. As intracranial surgery, including hypophysectomies, and better care of head trauma become more and more common in small animal practice, veterinary intensive care units will likely experience more of these cases as well. In humans pituitary gland radiation therapy can cause long-lasting pituitary gland damage with hormonal deficiencies. Interestingly, these rarely, if ever, include CDI. In dogs there are no large case series reporting the most common causes of CDI. Documented causes have included traumatic,[10] neoplastic, and idiopathic conditions[4] and have occurred secondary to iatrogenic steroid administration or hyperadrenocorticism.[1]

BOX 67-1 *Common Causes of Secondary Nephrogenic Diabetes Insipidus in Dogs and Cats*

- Hypercalcemia
- Hypokalemia
- Pyelonephritis
- Pyometra and gram-negative sepsis
- Portal systemic shunts
- Liver insufficiency
- Hypoadrenocorticism (more common in dogs)
- Hyperthyroidism (more common in cats)

NEPHROGENIC DIABETES INSIPIDUS

Nephrogenic diabetes insipidus (NDI) is caused by the failure of the kidney to respond to vasopressin. It is commonly divided into primary and secondary causes. Although primary NDI is uncommon and often congenital, secondary NDI is extremely common and likely the most common cause of diabetes insipidus seen in veterinary practice and intensive care units.

Primary NDI is most often considered to be hereditary in humans. Early diagnosis of this condition in humans through genetic screening has allowed for better care and increased survival. Most humans with congenital NDI have the X-linked form, causing the disease to manifest almost exclusively in male children.[11] In small animal patients primary or congenital NDI has been documented in a few rare reports in young dogs, never in cats. The canine reports included a Miniature Poodle, a German Shepherd, and a family of Huskies.[1]

By far the more common form of NDI in human[12] and veterinary patients is the acquired form. A partial list of causes of acquired NDI is included in Box 67-1. This syndrome is commonly seen in the emergency or critical care setting, caused by conditions such as pyometra or other causes of gram-negative sepsis, hypercalcemia, hypokalemia, liver failure, and hypoadrenocorticism. Each of these conditions causes an inability of the vasopressin to effectively bind and activate its receptor. In gram-negative sepsis bacterial endotoxins, especially from *Escherichia coli,* are thought to compete with vasopressin for binding sites on the tubular cell membranes, resulting in marked polyuria and polydipsia and possibly hypernatremia if water intake is insufficient. Similarly, hypercalcemia and severe hypokalemia are thought to interfere with vasopressin binding and subsequent activation of the V_2 receptor.

Another common mechanism of secondary NDI is the abolition of the medullary hypertonicity gradient. As mentioned previously the presence and proper function of vasopressin and its receptors allow water channels to be open in the tubular cells of the collecting duct. The passage of water, then, from the tubular lumen into the interstitium is still passive and based on the hypertonicity of the renal medulla, enabled by the renal counter-current mechanism. If this hypertonicity, a condition referred to as *medullary washout,* is absent, the urine will not become concentrated; it will be isosthenuric or even hyposthenuric. Medullary washout occurs in small animal patients for two common reasons:

1. Washout results from large amounts of urine passing through the tubules. This can occur in severely polyuric and polydipsic

animals, such as dogs with hyperadrenocorticism or dogs and cats receiving high volumes of intravenous fluids for extended periods.

2. The solutes necessary to produce the medullary hypertonicity gradient are lacking, such as insufficient urea in dogs and cats with hepatic insufficiency or insufficient sodium in dogs with hypoadrenocorticism. In both instances these animals may be severely polyuric and have a functional secondary NDI, despite absolutely normal renal function and normal vasopressin concentrations.

DIAGNOSING DIABETES INSIPIDUS

Diabetes insipidus should be high on the differential diagnosis list for any dog or cat with severe polyuria and polydipsia, especially when the urine is hyposthenuric. The first step in the diagnosis of primary diabetes insipidus is to exclude most other common causes of polyuria and polydipsia. This can be accomplished by evaluating the signalment and complaint, a complete history, physical examination, a serum biochemistry profile, and a complete urinalysis and urine culture.

Normal serum biochemistry results would rule out many causes of secondary NDI, including hypercalcemia, severe hypokalemia, low serum urea concentrations associated with liver disease, and low sodium concentrations associated with Addison's disease. Normoglycemia would rule out diabetes mellitus and a cause of polyuria and polydipsia. Normal urinalysis results and negative urine culture findings would exclude diabetes mellitus and primary renal glycosuria and would make pyelonephritis much less likely (Figure 67-1).

Additional testing may also be necessary when appropriate, including preprandial and postprandial serum bile acid concentrations to further exclude liver disease, serum thyroxine (T_4) concentrations to exclude hyperthyroidism, and imaging. Chronic kidney disease as a cause of polyuria and polydipsia is unlikely if the urine is hyposthenuric. If the urine is consistently isosthenuric, with normal or high-normal serum concentrations of blood urea nitrogen

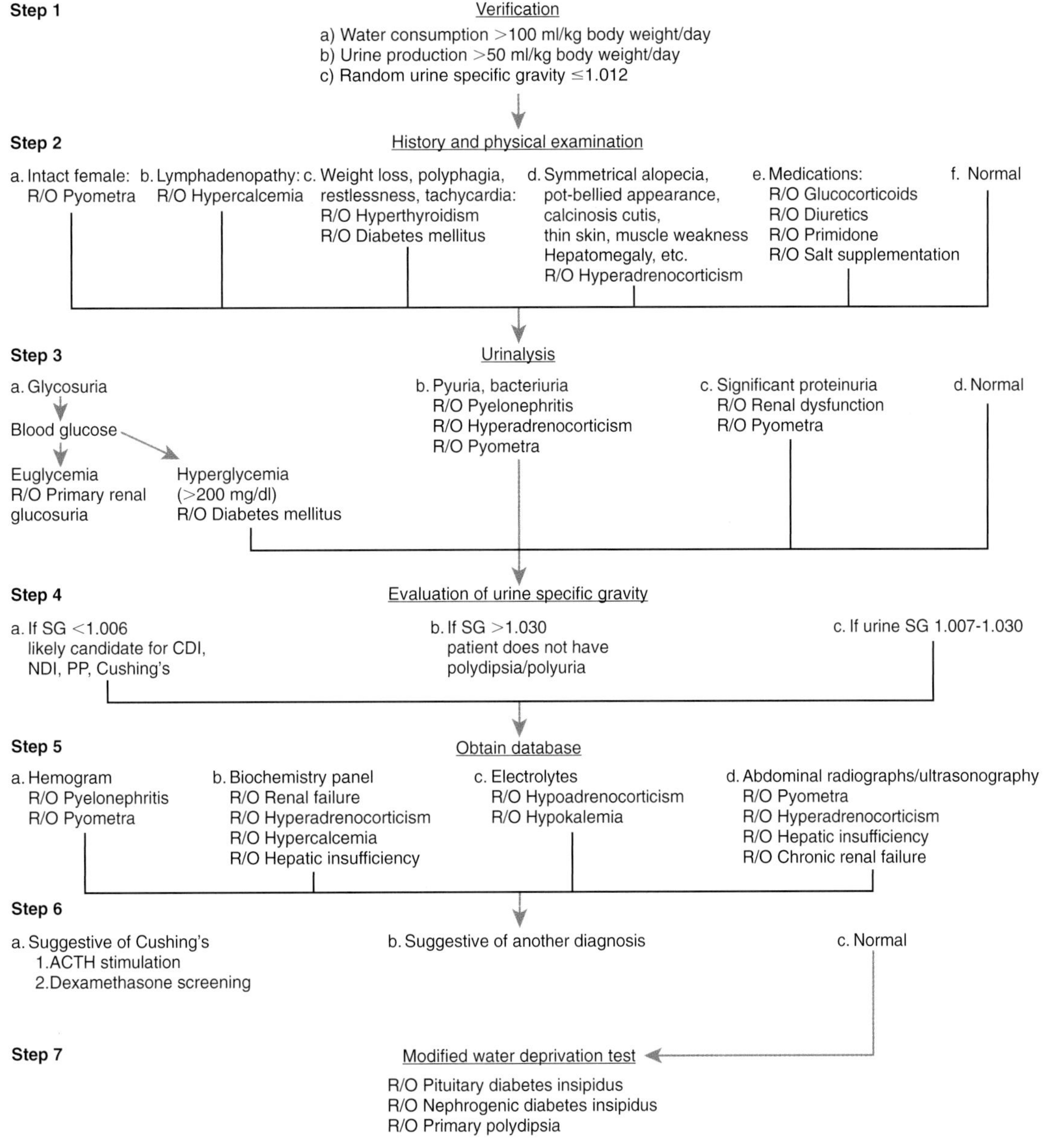

FIGURE 67-1 The diagnostic plan in a dog or cat with severe polydipsia and polyuria. *ACTH,* Adrenocorticotropic hormone; *CDI,* central diabetes insipidus; *NDI,* nephrogenic diabetes insipidus; *PP,* primary (psychogenic) polydipsia; *R/O,* rule out (a diagnosis); *SG,* specific gravity.

and creatinine, then a glomerular filtration study may be necessary to definitively rule out chronic kidney disease.

A relatively common scenario we are faced with is an older dog with severe polyuria, polydipsia, and hyposthenuric urine and no abnormal findings on physical examination, complete blood count, serum biochemistry profile, urinalysis (except the hyposthenuria), urine culture, and abdominal radiographs or ultrasonography. At this point in our diagnostic workup, the most likely remaining causes of the severe polyuria and polydipsia in this dog are hyperadrenocorticism, CDI or NDI, and primary or psychogenic polydipsia. The latter is a condition that is sometimes referred to as *psychogenic diabetes insipidus,* in which a dog drinks excessively for no apparent physiologic reason. Often these dogs are thought to drink this way because they are bored, stressed, or perhaps just enjoy drinking water.

The next step in the diagnosis is to attempt to exclude hyperadrenocorticism and psychogenic polydipsia. The first can be deemed much less likely based on a urine cortisol/creatinine ratio within the reference range or a low-dose dexamethasone suppression test with results within the reference range. An adrenocorticotropic hormone stimulation test is a less advisable option for this purpose because in many dogs with hyperadrenocorticism the results of an adrenocorticotropic hormone stimulation test lie within the normal reference range. It is absolutely essential to make every effort to exclude hyperadrenocorticism in these cases. If this step is missed and a water deprivation test or desmopressin acetate trial is used to confirm CDI, a misdiagnosis may occur. Dogs with hyperadrenocorticism may appear to have CDI per results of these tests and therefore will be mistakenly treated with desmopressin acetate instead of the proper diagnosis and treatment of their hyperadrenocorticism.

A random serum osmolality test may be used to attempt to diagnose psychogenic polydipsia. In this case dogs drink excessively as their primary disturbance and as a consequence are also polyuric. This is in contrast to diabetes insipidus, hyperadrenocorticism, and other causes or polyuria and polydipsia in which the primary disturbance is excessive urination. The polydipsia then, in these dogs, is an attempt to remain hydrated or to "catch up" with their urination. Theoretically the dogs with primary or psychogenic polydipsia should always be slightly overhydrated (with a low serum sodium concentration and low serum osmolality), and dogs with other causes of polyuria and polydipsia including diabetes insipidus should be slightly dehydrated (with a relatively high serum sodium concentration and serum osmolality).

On a random serum osmolality assay a result of less than 280 mOsm/L would be most consistent with psychogenic polydipsia. A result greater than 280 mOsm/L is hard to interpret because even if the dog did have psychogenic polydipsia, if it did not drink excessively that day (possibly because of the visit to the veterinarian), the osmolality could be more than 280 mOsm/L. If the random serum osmolality was indeed more than 280 mOsm/L, an additional test to confirm the diagnosis of primary diabetes insipidus and to differentiate between the more common CDI and the rare primary NDI is warranted. Two options are available to achieve these goals, a modified water deprivation test and a desmopressin acetate (synthetic vasopressin) trial.

Modified Water Deprivation Test

A modified water deprivation test is based on the premise that a dog that truly suffers from diabetes insipidus will not be able to concentrate its urine even under conditions of moderate dehydration. This is because of either a lack of vasopressin (CDI) or lack of an appropriate renal response to vasopressin (NDI). An appropriate rise in urine specific gravity while dehydrated would be suggestive of psychogenic polydipsia. Once dehydration has been achieved without an appropriate rise in urine concentration, desmopressin is given intramuscularly. A marked increase in urine specific gravity at that time would be diagnostic for CDI, and a complete lack of response to desmopressin would be suggestive of NDI. Although in many cases this test does provide a definitive diagnosis of diabetes insipidus, we do not recommend its routine use. This is because many problems and possible misdiagnoses are associated with the analysis of the test results and, more importantly, grave risks can be associated with this test, including severe dehydration, hypernatremia, and even death.[1]

Problems and risks

Causes of misdiagnoses

1. Medullary washout may occur. If the medullary interstitium has been "washed out" of solutes because of chronic severe polyuria and polydipsia for any reason, no urine concentration will occur despite the presence of endogenous vasopressin, desmopressin, and intact renal V_2 receptors. These dogs are then mistakenly diagnosed as suffering from NDI. The modified water deprivation test protocol attempts to eliminate this problem by recommending mild water restriction for a number of days before the test. Although helpful, this does not always eliminate the problem, is not always possible, and can be dangerous if dehydration is induced at home without proper monitoring.
2. Partial CDI, or a relative lack of vasopressin, can be very hard to diagnose, because a rise in urine specific gravity will be induced by dehydration. This rise, though, will be of inappropriately low magnitude and a very subjective value, and these dogs can be misdiagnosed as having psychogenic polydipsia. An additional rise in urine specific gravity should occur after desmopressin is given. Their response should be more dramatic, though, than in dogs with psychogenic polydipsia. This is a subjective value, making a definitive diagnosis of partial CDI very difficult.
3. Dogs with hyperadrenocorticism may appear to have CDI or partial CDI per a water deprivation test, leading to a misdiagnosis. This underlines the importance of establishing or excluding a diagnosis of hyperadrenocorticism in dogs before administering this test.

Associated risks

The main and most important risk, and the reason why we do not recommend the routine use of this test, is that severe dehydration can be associated with acute severe hypernatremia. This occurs in cases of CDI or NDI when dehydration continues past 5% of body weight because of a lack of intensive monitoring. In cases of complete diabetes insipidus this could happen in a very short time (a few hours). This may be accompanied by a rapid rise in serum sodium concentrations, resulting in neurologic symptoms. Despite aggressive fluid therapy, normal sodium concentrations may be difficult to restore. Desmopressin therapy is warranted in this case to slow the free water loss associated with the marked polyuria and to allow normalization of serum sodium concentrations.

Prevention of this complication includes only mild water deprivation at home during the days before the test, as well as aggressive, frequent monitoring of body weight, serum sodium, urea nitrogen, and creatinine (at least hourly) during the test. The test should be stopped at 5% loss of body weight or any marked increase in the above serum values. Water, intravenous fluids (an intravenous catheter should be preplaced), and desmopressin should be available for immediate use.

Desmopressin Acetate Trial

The other option available for the diagnosis of diabetes insipidus is the desmopressin acetate trial. Although this test does not yield immediate results, it is a much safer option for most dogs than the modified water deprivation test. This test is performed at home by the owner. The owner is instructed to collect urine, first thing in the morning, for a few days; to slightly limit access to water, if possible, for a few days; and then to begin therapy with desmopressin.

On days 5, 6, and 7 of this therapy urine is again collected first thing in the morning. All urine should be refrigerated after collection. At the end of the trial the urine samples are brought to the veterinarian for specific gravity measurement or, ideally, osmolality assays. The owners are encouraged to measure water intake during the trial if possible.

The theory behind this therapeutic trial is that given mild water deprivation and desmopressin, the dog's urine concentration will steadily increase over the trial period. Medullary washout will be eliminated slowly if it was present initially, and a dog with CDI should have a marked increase in urine concentration. No increase in urine concentration by the end of the trial would be consistent with NDI or psychogenic polydipsia. Because primary NDI is so uncommon in adult dogs, usually this is not a big problem. A definitive differentiation between those two conditions would require a modified water deprivation test.

Imaging After a Diagnosis of CDI

An extremely high percentage of adult dogs with acquired CDI appear to have intracranial mass lesions identifiable with magnetic resonance or computed tomographic imaging.[5] Such imaging is therefore recommended after the diagnosis of CDI, and radiation therapy is recommended if a lesion is identified.

TREATMENT OF DIABETES INSIPIDUS

A list of treatment options for CDI and NDI is included in Box 67-2. Most commonly CDI (partial or complete) is treated with desmopressin (oral or human nasal preparation given as eyedrops). This treatment is extremely effective and when given consistently will enable the dog to concentrate urine normally. Other therapies can also be used in those with CDI as well as those with NDI. These include therapies aimed at lowering total body sodium and commonly include thiazide diuretics and salt-restricted diets. These therapies typically have minimal success in those with NDI.

Another option for owners of pets suffering from CDI or NDI is not to treat. Theoretically, as long as these animals are allowed free access to water, are allowed to urinate outside, and are kept in conditions that help prevent dehydration through additional fluid loss (shade, no strenuous exercise in warm conditions), they will remain hydrated and may exhibit no clinical signs. This is especially important because of the high cost of desmopressin therapy for dogs with CDI and the lack of effective therapy for dogs with NDI.

BOX 67-2 *Therapies Available for Polydipsic/Polyuric Dogs with CDI, NDI, or Primary (Psychogenic) Polydipsia*[1]

A. Central diabetes insipidus (severe)
  1. DDAVP (desmopressin acetate)
    a. Effective
    b. Expensive
    c. May require drops in conjunctival sac if oral is ineffective
  2. LVP (lypressin [Diapid])
    a. Short duration of action; less potent than DDAVP
    b. Expensive
    c. Requires drops into nose or conjunctival sac
  3. No treatment—provide continuous source of water
B. Central diabetes insipidus (partial)
  1. DDAVP
  2. LVP
  3. Chlorpropamide
    a. 30% to 70% effective
    b. Inexpensive
    c. Pill form
    d. Takes 1 to 2 weeks to obtain effect of drug
    e. May cause hypoglycemia
  4. Clofibrate—untested in veterinary medicine
  5. Thiazides
    a. Mildly effective
    b. Inexpensive
    c. Pill form
    d. Should be used with low-sodium diet
  6. Low-sodium diet
  7. No treatment—provide continuous source of water
C. Nephrogenic diabetes insipidus
  1. Thiazides—as above
  2. Low-sodium diet
  3. No treatment—provide continuous source of water
D. Primary (psychogenic) polydipsia
  1. Water restriction at times
  2. Water limitation
  3. Behavior modification
    a. Exercise
    b. Another pet
    c. Larger living environment

Emergency Treatment

The most challenging aspect of this condition to an emergency or critical care clinician is the treatment of the severe dehydration, ongoing free water losses, and marked hypernatremia associated with small animals suffering from diabetes insipidus (primary or secondary) that for some reason have not had adequate access to water. This can be a result of vomiting or adipsia from an additional disease process, water deprivation by the owner (because of a belief that this will prevent urination in the house, or accidentally), the pet being lost without water, and animals that have sustained trauma (e.g., dog with diabetes insipidus that has been hit by a car and is presented for veterinary care hours or days later). In these instances the clinician is presented with a patient with inappropriately high free water losses, dehydration, and high sodium concentrations. The first challenge is recognition of this state by the clinician, and then aggressive medical therapy. Aggressive therapy includes fluids, therapy for acute or chronic hypernatremia, and possibly desmopressin. Desmopressin therapy (injectable or eyedrops) should be considered when dehydration and hypernatremia persist despite appropriate fluid therapy, urine volumes are high, and urine concentration is inappropriately low for the degree of clinical dehydration (see Chapter 50).

PROGNOSIS

The prognosis for dogs with CDI is good if they respond to therapy. Unfortunately, because of an apparently high incidence of intracranial masses in these dogs, the prognosis must remain guarded until advanced imaging can be pursued. The prognosis for dogs with primary NDI is guarded because of the lack of therapy for this condition. The prognosis for dogs with severe dehydration and hypernatremia is guarded as well, especially if the condition is chronic. Proper medical therapy can often induce complete resolution of these complications and allow long-term medical treatment of CDI or the primary cause of secondary NDI.

REFERENCES

1. Feldman EC, Nelson RW: Water metabolism and diabetes insipidus. In Feldman EC, Nelson RW, editors: Canine and feline endocrine and reproduction, St Louis, 2004, Elsevier Science.

2. Robertson GL: Physiology of ADH secretion, Kidney Int 21:S20, 1987.
3. Hall JE: Urine concentration and dilution; Regulation of extracellular fluid osmolarity and sodium concentration. In Guyton and Hall textbook of medical physiology, ed 12, Philadelphia, 2010, Saunders, pp 345-360.
4. Frokiaer J, Marples D, Knepper MA, et al: Pathophysiology of aquaporin-2 in water balance disorders, Am J Med Sci 316:291, 1998.
5. Harb MF, Nelson RW, Feldman EC, et al: Central diabetes insipidus in dogs: 20 cases (1986-1995), J Am Vet Med Assoc 209:1884, 1996.
6. Aroch I, Mazaki-Tovi M, Shemesh O, et al: Central diabetes insipidus in five cats: clinical presentation, diagnosis and oral desmopressin therapy, J Feline Med Surg 7:333, 2005.
7. Ghirardello S, Malattia C, Scagnelli P, et al: Current perspective on the pathogenesis of central diabetes insipidus, J Pediatr Endocrinol Metab 18:631, 2005.
8. Agha A, Thompson CJ: Anterior pituitary dysfunction following traumatic brain injury (TBI), Clin Endocrinol (Oxf) 64:481, 2006.
9. Ober PO: Endocrine emergencies. In Grenvik A, Ayres AM, Holbrook PH, et al, editors: Textbook of critical care, Philadelphia, 2000, WB Saunders.
10. Authement JM, Boudrieau RJ, Kaplan PM: Transient, traumatically induced, central diabetes insipidus in a dog, J Am Vet Med Assoc 194:683, 1989.
11. Sands JM, Bichet DG: Nephrogenic diabetes insipidus, Ann Intern Med 144:186, 2006.
12. Garofeanu CG, Weir M, Rosas-Arellano MP, et al: Causes of reversible nephrogenic diabetes insipidus: a systematic review, Am J Kidney Dis 45:626, 2005.

CHAPTER 68

SYNDROME OF INAPPROPRIATE ANTIDIURETIC HORMONE

C.B. Chastain, DVM, MS, DACVIM (Internal Medicine)

KEY POINTS

- Hyponatremia is the cardinal finding of the symptomatic syndrome of inappropriate antidiuretic hormone (SIADH).
- SIADH can be caused by cerebral disorders, pulmonary disease, or adverse effects of medications.
- Hyponatremia of SIADH is characterized by hypoosmolality and inappropriately concentrated urine and urine sodium excretion.
- Renal, adrenal, and thyroid functions are normal, and neither edema, dehydration, nor azotemia is typically present in animals with SIADH.

One of the most common electrolyte abnormalities in small animal veterinary patients is hyponatremia. Most cases are temporary and without clinical signs. One cause of hyponatremia that can be associated with clinical signs and may be fatal is the syndrome of inappropriate antidiuretic hormone (SIADH).

Antidiuretic hormone (ADH) deficiency is relatively well known and is referred to as central diabetes insipidus. The antithesis of diabetes insipidus, an excess of ADH, remains an obscure rarity in animals based on the frequency of case reports,[1-6] but its true incidence may be more common than diabetes insipidus. SIADH, also called Schwartz-Bartter's syndrome, is characterized by excessive release of ADH from the neurohypophysis or ectopically from another source. Signs of SIADH in humans are depression and confusion. Affected animals may have central nervous system disease, pulmonary disease, or conditions requiring drugs that can cause SIADH.

The failure to recognize the true incidence of SIADH may be caused by lack of clinical suspicion, transient nature of some forms of SIADH, insufficient monitoring, rapid demise of the patient, or clinician distraction from investigating and treating concurrent diseases. Recognition of SIADH is important for many reasons, including causes that can be iatrogenic and remedied by drug withdrawal and patient death that can be iatrogenic if SIADH is treated too aggressively.

CAUSES

ADH, also known as vasopressin, is normally secreted in response to an increase in serum osmolality (serum sodium concentration) or to maintain normal blood pressure and intravascular volume (see Chapter 158). ADH actions are achieved by the promotion of free water resorption by the kidneys, specifically the distal convoluted tubules and collecting ducts. Serum osmolality is monitored by the anterior portion of the hypothalamus. If blood pressure is normal or elevated, ADH secretion is inhibited by pressure receptors in the atria and great veins. A rise in serum osmolality is a more sensitive monitor (1% rise) and typical stimulus for ADH secretion than a decrease in blood pressure (9% decrease).[7,8] SIADH is defined as an excess of ADH in the absence of hypovolemia or hyperosmolality.

SIADH can be caused by cerebral disorders, pulmonary disease, or adverse effects of medications (Box 68-1).[7] The cause in some cases remains idiopathic. Three cases of idiopathic SIADH have been reported in dogs.[2,3] Cerebral causes of SIADH in humans include hypothalamic tumors, head trauma, meningitis, encephalitis, cerebrovascular accidents, and hydrocephalus. Hypothalamic tumors, granulomatous meningoencephalitis, congenital hydrocephalus, suspected immune-mediated hepatitis, and probable distemper encephalitis have been reported to cause SIADH in dogs.[5-8] SIADH has been reported in a cat after the administration of anesthetic drugs to

BOX 68-1 ***Selected Causes of the Syndrome of Inappropriate Secretion of ADH***[10]

Central Nervous System Disorders	Malignancies
Head trauma	Pancreatic carcinoma
Hydrocephalus	Prostatic carcinoma
Cerebrovascular accidents	Thymoma
Brain tumor	Osteosarcoma
Meningitis	**Drugs**
Encephalitis	Antidepressants
Pulmonary Lesions	Neuroleptics
Bacterial pneumonia	Antineoplastics
Aspergillosis	Nonsteroidal antiinflammatory drugs
Lung tumors	Opioids
Positive pressure ventilation	**Others**
Dirofilariasis	Pain
	Nausea
	Psychologic stress

ADH, Antidiuretic hormone.

perform a laparotomy to investigate the etiology of apparent liver disease.[9] Intracranial disease may directly stimulate the supraoptic or paraventricular nuclei to secrete ADH or may alter the osmoreceptors to inappropriately stimulate ADH secretion. Other cerebral causes of SIADH are perception of nausea, pain, and psychologic stress.[10]

Pulmonary diseases causing SIADH include tumors that ectopically produce ADH and diseases that interrupt the inhibitory impulses in vagal afferents from stretch receptors in the atria and great veins. Examples in humans have included tuberculosis pneumonia, aspergillosis, and lung abscesses. A dog had SIADH associated putatively with dirofilariasis.[1] Rarely, SIADH in humans has been caused by malignant tumors outside the thorax that have ectopically produced ADH.[10] In addition, positive pressure ventilation may inhibit low-pressure baroreceptors and stimulate the release of ADH.

Drugs may either increase ADH secretion or potentiate its action.[10,11] Drugs that are known to increase ADH secretion in humans include antidepressants (especially tricyclic antidepressants and monoamine oxidase inhibitors), anticancer drugs (intravenous cyclophosphamide and vinca alkaloids), opioids, and neuroleptics. Drugs that potentiate ADH action include cyclophosphamide and nonsteroidal antiinflammatory drugs.

The thirst center in the hypothalamus monitors plasma osmolality and extracellular fluid volume. If the patient is conscious, psychologically normal, and has a normal thirst center, water intake will subside to compensate for the reduction in plasma osmolality and expanded extracellular fluid volume of SIADH. Patients receiving fluid therapy, under sedation or anesthesia, that are psychologically deranged, or with central nervous system disease affecting the thirst center have an impaired ability to compensate for SIADH.

CLINICAL SIGNS

The clinical signs found in patients with SIADH depend on the cause of the syndrome and on the concentration of serum sodium. Signs of a central nervous system disease, pulmonary disorder, surgical or traumatic stress, or drug intoxication may overshadow signs of SIADH. This may account, in part, for its rare recognition in companion animals. Regardless of its cause, if the serum sodium is severely decreased (<120 mEq/L), signs of hyponatremia may prevail. Possible clinical signs of hyponatremia include nausea, anorexia, vomiting, irritable behavior, confusion, head pressing, seizures, cardiac arrhythmias, and coma. Neither hypertension nor edema will be present.

LABORATORY FINDINGS

The outstanding initial abnormal laboratory finding in patients with clinical manifestations of SIADH is hyponatremia secondary to renal retention of free water and ongoing urinary sodium losses. Sodium is lost in the urine despite hyponatremia because the secretion of renin and aldosterone is inhibited by normovolemia with expanding extracellular fluid caused by water retention. Serum osmolality is less than 280 mOsm/kg, whereas urine osmolality is more than 150 mOsm/kg and urine sodium usually more than 20 mEq/L. Atrial natriuretic peptide is secreted in response to expanding extracellular fluid volume, which further inhibits renin and aldosterone and promotes natriuresis. Even though water is retained, edema usually does not develop because of continuing natriuresis. The degree of natriuresis is quite variable and is dependent on the quantity of ingested dietary sodium.[10]

Other serum constituent concentrations, such as potassium and chloride, may also be diluted. Hypochloridemia may be severe enough to cause metabolic alkalosis. Blood urea nitrogen (BUN) and uric acid concentrations are decreased by dilution and increased glomerular clearance.[10] An increased BUN concentration typically excludes a diagnosis of SIADH.

DIAGNOSTIC IMAGING FINDINGS

If non–drug-induced SIADH is suspected, evidence for possible intrathoracic or intracranial lesions should be sought by routine radiographs and, in some cases, special imaging procedures such as computed tomography (CT) or magnetic resonance imaging (MRI).

DIAGNOSIS

A clinical diagnosis can be based on finding the characteristic clinical features of SIADH and the exclusion of other causes of hyponatremia. Plasma ADH determination is unreliable and unnecessary for diagnosis. Most cases of hyponatremia, hyposmolality, and hypovolemia are associated with an elevated ADH concentration, regardless of the cause. The water loading test can aggravate water intoxication of SIADH and is unnecessarily hazardous.

The clinical features of SIADH are most easily confused with those of primary hypoadrenocorticism. It differs from primary hypoadrenocorticism by having normal to low levels of BUN and serum potassium concentrations. Primary hypoadrenocorticism is associated with azotemia and hyperkalemia. Other differential diagnoses for hyponatremia include congestive heart failure, nephrosis, severe liver disease, hyperglycemia, and hyperlipidemia. In patients with SIADH without unrelated disease, renal, adrenal, cardiac, and liver functions are normal and blood glucose concentration is normal.

TREATMENT

Whenever possible, the cause for SIADH should be determined and corrected. The treatment of choice is discontinued fluid administration and restricted access to water. However, this may be insufficient in severe cases.

In acute severe cases, emergency treatment may include hypertonic (3%) saline, which should be given slowly in an intravenous dose over 2 to 4 hours if neurologic signs are thought to be secondary to acute hyponatremia and resulting cerebral edema. Isotonic saline infusion is unsuitable because of its low concentration of sodium, which will be excreted in the urine while the water will be retained, worsening the hyponatremia. When hyponatremia may have been present for more than 24 to 48 hours, care must be taken to prevent central pontine myelinolysis, an osmotically induced demyelination.[12] Serum sodium should not increase with treatment by more than 12 mEq/L/day (0.5 mEq/L/hr). The initial goal should be to increase serum sodium concentration to 125 to 130 mEq/L in a carefully controlled manner. When hypertonic saline is used, furosemide may also be beneficial to inhibit resorption of water in the renal tubules and reduce the risk of volume overload. Potassium should be supplemented as needed.

Demeclocycline, a tetracycline antibiotic, inhibits the action of ADH on the renal tubules. It has been effective in treating humans with SIADH caused by excessive secretion from hypothalamic nuclei or by the secretion of ectopic ADH. However, it is potentially nephrotoxic and renal function must be monitored closely. Improvement from demeclocycline treatment may take 1 to 2 weeks. A safe and effective dosage of demeclocycline in dogs has not been established. Lithium will also inhibit the action of ADH on the renal tubules, but its use is precluded by its toxicity, which is greater than that of demeclocycline.

PROGNOSIS

The prognosis for patients with SIADH depends on the cause. If caused by infection or drugs, successful treatment of the infection and withdrawal of the drug will lead to a cure. If caused by a malignant tumor that cannot be excised completely or destroyed by radiation, SIADH usually is incurable, although it can be controlled with water restriction and sodium supplementation.

REFERENCES

1. Breitschwerdt EB, Root CR: Inappropriate secretion of antidiuretic hormone in a dog, J Am Vet Med Assoc 175:181, 1979.
2. Biewenga WJ, Rijnberk A, Mol JA: Inappropriate vasopressin secretion in dogs, Tijdschr Diergeneeskd 113:104, 1988.
3. Rijnberk A, Biewenga WJ, Mol JA: Inappropriate vasopressin secretion in two dogs, Acta Endocrinol 117:59, 1988.
4. Houston DM, Allen DG, Kruth SA, et al: Syndrome of inappropriate antidiuretic hormone secretion in a dog, Can Vet J 30:423, 1989.
5. Fleeman LM, Irwin PJ, Phillips PA, et al: Effects of an oral vasopressin receptor antagonist (OPC-31260) in a dog with syndrome of inappropriate secretion of antidiuretic hormone, Aust Vet J 78:825, 2000.
6. Brofman PJ, Knostman KAB, DiBartola SP: Granulomatous amebic meningoencephalitis causing the syndrome of inappropriate secretion of antidiuretic hormone in a dog, J Vet Intern Med 17:230, 2003.
7. Kang MH, Park HM: Syndrome of inappropriate antidiuretic hormone secretion concurrent with liver disease in a dog, J Vet Med Sci 74:645, 2012.
8. Shiel RE, Pinilla M, Mooney CT: Syndrome of inappropriate antidiuretic hormone secretion associated with congenital hydrocephalus in a dog, J Am Anim Hosp Assoc 45:249, 2009.
9. Cameron K, Gallagher A: Syndrome of inappropriate antidiuretic hormone secretion in a cat, J Am Anim Hosp Assoc 46:425, 2010.
10. Cho KC: Electrolyte & acid-base disorders. In Papadakis MA, McPhee SJ, Rabow MW, editors: 2013 Current medical diagnosis & treatment, ed 52, New York, 2013, Lange Medical Books/McGraw-Hill.
11. Hauptman JG, Richter MA, Wood SL, et al: Effects of anesthesia, surgery, and intravenous administration of fluids on plasma antidiuretic hormone concentrations in healthy dogs, Am J Vet Res 61:1273, 2000.
12. O'Brien DP, Kroll RA, Johnson GC, et al: Myelinolysis after correction of hyponatremia in two dogs, J Vet Intern Med 8:40, 1994.

CHAPTER 69
THYROID STORM

Cynthia R. Ward, VMD, PhD, DACVIM (Internal Medicine)

KEY POINTS

- Thyroid storm is a syndrome of acute thyrotoxicosis that occurs primarily in hyperthyroid cats.
- The pathogenesis is unknown but probably results from rapid increases in serum thyroid hormone levels coupled with activation of the sympathetic nervous system.
- An event often triggers thyroid storm in previously diagnosed or undiagnosed hyperthyroid cats, although the event may not be readily apparent.
- Clinical signs include central nervous system disturbances, hyperthermia, acute or severe vomiting and diarrhea, abdominal pain, icterus, cardiac murmurs with or without arrhythmias, pleural effusion, pulmonary edema, tachypnea, hypertension, retinopathies, extreme muscle weakness and cervical ventroflexion, thromboembolic disease, and sudden death.
- Diagnosis is based on clinical signs and evidence of elevated serum thyroid hormones.
- Treatment is aimed at reducing production and secretion of thyroid hormones, blocking peripheral actions of thyroid hormones, systemic support, and elimination of the precipitating event.
- Successful outcome depends on rapid recognition of the clinical syndrome and aggressive therapy.

Thyroid storm is a syndrome described in human medicine to define a multisystem disorder resulting from organ exposure to excessive amounts of thyroid hormone. This form of acute thyrotoxicosis can be life threatening and is a significant cause of mortality in human patients treated in emergency rooms. Thyrotoxicosis describes any condition in which there is an excessive amount of circulating thyroid hormone, whether from excess production and secretion from an overactive thyroid gland, because of leakage from a damaged thyroid gland, or from an exogenous source. In contrast, hyperthyroidism describes thyroid gland hyperfunction. Therefore acute thyrotoxicosis may occur in the absence of thyroid gland hyperfunction, although this is rare in veterinary medicine.

In humans, thyroid storm can occur at any age. It can be present in euthyroid patients who have been oversupplemented with thyroid hormone, as well as undiagnosed, treated, and partially treated hyperthyroid patients. Hyperthyroidism is common in older feline patients. It is also seen rarely in dogs with thyroid carcinoma or extreme oversupplementation of thyroid replacement hormone to hypothyroid dogs. Hyperthyroid cats that experience an acute accentuation of thyrotoxicosis may be diagnosed with thyroid storm. This chapter discusses the human syndrome and compares it to that seen in hyperthyroid veterinary patients. The clinical signs of and treatment modalities for feline patients suffering from thyroid storm will also be presented.

PATHOGENESIS

Although the exact pathogenesis of thyroid storm remains to be elucidated, several factors appear to be involved, including high levels of circulating thyroid hormones, rapid increases in circulating thyroid hormones, hyperactivity of the sympathetic nervous system, and an increased cellular response to thyroid hormone.

High Levels of Circulating Thyroid Hormones

Although one would expect circulating thyroid hormones to be increased in patients with thyroid storm, there is no difference between serum thyroid hormone levels in human patients and in more stable hyperthyroid patients. The diagnosis therefore is made primarily based on clinical signs.[1]

Rapid, Acute Increases in Circulating Thyroid Hormones

The magnitude of change in serum thyroid hormone levels may be more important than the actual levels themselves. This would explain the occurrence of thyroid storm after radioactive iodine therapy and thyroid surgery that damage the thyroid gland and cause release of hormone or after abrupt cessation of antithyroid medication resulting in a rapid rise in serum thyroid hormone levels.[2] Certainly, nonthyroidal illness, known to be a precipitating factor in human medicine, has been shown to alter binding of thyroid hormones to their carriers and could also be responsible for rapid alterations in circulating thyroid hormone as well.

Hyperactivity of the Sympathetic Nervous System

Activation of the sympathetic nervous system has been implicated in the onset of thyroid storm.[3] Many of the clinical signs and physiologic signs are similar to those seen during catecholamine excess. Serum and urine catecholamine levels in humans are within normal limits during thyroid storm. However, thyroid hormones can alter tissue sensitivity to catecholamines at the cell surface receptor as well as the intracellular signaling levels, and this increased sensitivity may result in the clinical signs seen during thyroid storm. In addition, many of these clinical signs are controlled by β-adrenergic blockade.

Increased Cellular Response to Thyroid Hormones

This effect has been implicated in cases of thyroid storm resulting from infection, sepsis, hypoxemia, hypovolemia, and lactic acidosis or ketoacidosis.[4]

BOX 69-1 ***Potential Precipitating Events for Feline Thyroid Storm***

- Radioactive iodine therapy
- Thyroidal or parathyroidal surgery
- Abrupt withdrawal of antithyroid medications
- Stress
- Nonthyroidal illness
- Administration of iodinated contrast dyes
- Administration of stable iodine compounds
- Vigorous palpation of the thyroid

PRECIPITATING EVENTS

In most cases of thyroid storm in humans, a precipitating event can be identified, although no known cause is found in up to 2% of cases.[5] The most common precipitating events are infection, thyroidal and nonthyroidal surgery, radioactive iodine therapy, administration of iodinated contrast dyes, administration of stable iodine, withdrawal of antithyroid medication, amiodarone therapy, ingestion of excessive amounts of exogenous thyroid hormone, vigorous palpation of the thyroid gland, severe emotional stress, and a variety of acute nonthyroidal illnesses. Common events that precipitate thyroid storm in feline hyperthyroid patients include radioactive iodine therapy, abrupt withdrawal of antithyroid medication, thyroid surgery, vigorous thyroid palpation, stress, and administration of stable iodine compounds, as well as any of the other precipitating factors found in humans (Box 69-1).

CLINICAL SIGNS

Thyroid storm is the acute exacerbation of clinical signs of thyrotoxicosis; however, the diagnosis of thyroid storm in human medicine is based on the prevalence of four major clinical signs. These include (1) fever, (2) central nervous system (CNS) effects from mild agitation to seizures or coma, (3) gastrointestinal (GI) and hepatic dysfunction ranging from vomiting, diarrhea, and abdominal pain to unexplained jaundice, and (4) cardiovascular effects including sinus tachycardia, heart block, atrial fibrillation, ventricular tachycardia, and congestive heart failure. The combination of these clinical signs along with identification of a precipitating event allows for the diagnosis of thyroid storm.[5] In cats with presumed thyroid storm, many of these clinical signs also occur (Box 69-2).

In cats suffering from thyroid storm, hyperthermia is less common than in human patients. Central neurologic abnormalities, including severe obtundation and seizures, are common in cats with thyroid storm and often lead to the suspicion of the condition. Auscultation may reveal a cardiac murmur or arrhythmia (most often a gallop rhythm). Inspiratory crackles or dullness in the lung fields may be heard if pulmonary edema or pleural effusion is present, respectively.[6] Mild to severe hypertension may also be present during thyroid storm in cats.[7] Retinopathies, including hemorrhage, edema, degeneration, or even retinal detachment, may be found, especially in hypertensive thyrotoxic cats.[8] Tachypnea and hyperthermia may be present, and absent limb motor function may be detected as a result of thromboembolic disease occurring from acute thyrotoxicosis.[9] Sudden death may also occur. Severe, acute muscle weakness and ventroflexion of the neck may be seen in acutely thyrotoxic cats, often associated with hypokalemia.

DIAGNOSIS

The diagnosis of thyroid storm is based on identification of thyrotoxicosis, clinical signs, and evidence of a precipitating event.[5]

BOX 69-2 *Clinical Signs Associated with Feline Thyroid Storm*

Constitutional Signs

Hyperthermia
Dehydration

Cardiovascular Signs

Arrhythmias
Atrial fibrillation, ventricular tachycardia
Gallop rhythm
Sinus tachycardia
Congestive heart failure
Cardiomegaly
Pleural effusion
Pulmonary edema
Hypertension
Thromboembolic disease

Respiratory Signs

Tachypnea

Neuromuscular Signs

Behavior changes
Mental dullness/obtundation
Seizures
Muscle weakness
Cervical ventroflexion

Gastrointestinal and Hepatic Signs

Abdominal discomfort or pain
Vomiting
Diarrhea
Icterus

Ocular Signs

Hyphema
Retinal lesions
Retinal detachment

Thyrotoxicosis in hyperthyroid cats is demonstrated by an elevated total thyroxine (T_4) level, or a total T_4 level in the high-normal range combined with an elevated free T_4 level. The total T_4 level may be in the normal range in a hyperthyroid cat, but it is expected that in animals suffering from thyroid storm, the total T_4 and free T_4 levels will be above the normal range. In human medicine, thyroid storm is diagnosed based on a point system assigned to each of the main clinical components: fever, CNS signs, GI signs, and cardiovascular signs, as well as presence or absence of a precipitating event.[5] In hyperthyroid feline patients, thyroid storm may be diagnosed based on clinical signs of acute thyrotoxicosis. A precipitating event is identified in many cases.

LABORATORY ABNORMALITIES

Laboratory abnormalities result from uncomplicated thyrotoxicosis[10]; there is no distinguishing laboratory value for feline thyroid storm. In the hyperthyroid cat, hematologic abnormalities may include a mild erythrocytosis, macrocytosis, and Heinz body formation. In humans with thyroid storm, a leukocytosis with left shift in the absence of active infection or inflammation has been identified.[11] In hyperthyroid cats a mature neutrophilia, lymphopenia, and eosinopenia are more commonly identified as a stress response. Biochemical abnormalities seen in people with thyroid storm include a mild hyperglycemia and hypercalcemia. Elevated liver enzyme values are often seen as well, and hyperbilirubinemia may occur in severe cases; this finding carries a poor prognosis. In hyperthyroid cats, elevated liver enzyme levels, mild hyperglycemia, and severe hypokalemia may be seen in patients with acute thyrotoxicosis. Unexplained mild hyperbilirubinemia can occur, which leads to suspicion of thyroid storm. A decreased sodium/potassium ratio may be seen in thyrotoxic cats that experience heart failure and pleural effusion.[12] Radiographs may reveal cardiomegaly or evidence of congestive heart failure.

TREATMENT

Treatment of thyroid storm is aimed at controlling the four major problematic areas: (1) to reduce the production and/or secretion of thyroid hormones, (2) to counteract the peripheral effects of thyroid hormones, (3) to provide systemic support, and (4) to identify and eliminate the precipitating factor.[13]

Reduction in Production or Secretion of New Thyroid Hormones

The thioimidazole compound methimazole inhibits iodine incorporation into tyrosyl residues of thyroglobulin and thus prevents the synthesis of active thyroid hormone. In this way, methimazole should be the first line of defense against thyroid storm. However, it does not prevent the secretion of already formed thyroid hormones. Methimazole may be given orally, transdermally, or even rectally in cats. The dosage should be at the high end in cats that have normal renal function (5 mg per cat PO q12h). If there is suspected renal insufficiency or failure, the dosage of methimazole should be reduced by half to prevent a rapid decrease in renal blood flow.

Methimazole will block the formation of new, active thyroid hormone, but other measures must be instituted to prevent further secretion of formed hormone, which is stored in high concentrations in the thyroid gland. This can be done with stable iodine compounds such as potassium iodide. These compounds, in large dosages, can also decrease the synthesis rate of thyroid hormone. They must be given 1 hour after methimazole administration because a large load of iodine will initially stimulate thyroid hormone production. Potassium iodide may be given at 25 mg PO q8h. Instead of potassium iodide, lipid-soluble radiographic contrast agents, such as iopanoic acid, may be given at 100 mg per cat PO q12h.[14] Although iopanoic acid is available in parenteral form, oral administration is safer because it is a very hyperosmolar drug. This compound has the additional advantages of blocking peripheral conversion of thyroxine (T_4) to triiodothyronine (T_3), blocking T_3 from binding to its receptor, and inhibiting thyroid hormone synthesis. Dexamethasone at a dose of 0.1 to 0.2 mg/kg PO or IV may be used to inhibit the release of thyroid hormone from the thyroid gland and to block the peripheral conversion of T_4 to T_3.[15] This works synergistically with organic iodine compounds.

Inhibition of Peripheral Effects of Thyroid Hormone

The most rapid relief of signs caused by thyroid storm is accomplished with medications that block the β-adrenergic receptors, such as propranolol and atenolol. Propranolol, a nonselective β-adrenergic blocker, is used most commonly as a sympatholytic agent in human medicine, but it is inherently difficult to use in cats because of its poor oral bioavailability and short half-life, requiring administration every 8 hours in this species. The use of propranolol has been largely superseded by atenolol because of its selectivity and once-daily administration. However, propranolol inhibits the peripheral conversion of T_4 to T_3, although this effect happens slowly.[16] Therefore propranolol may be advantageous in severely thyrotoxic cats. High-end dosages of propranolol should be used to ensure β-adrenergic blockade at 5 mg PO q8h or 0.02 mg/kg intravenously (IV) over 1 minute. Alternatively, atenolol, a selective β_1-adrenergic blocker that has better oral bioavailability, may be prescribed at 1 mg/kg PO q12-24h. In emergent situations, a constant rate infusion (CRI) of the short-acting β_1-blocker esmolol may be given with a loading dose of 0.1 to 0.5 mg/kg IV over 1 minute, followed by a CRI of 10 to 200 mcg/kg/min.

An extreme method to counteract the peripheral actions of excess thyroid hormones is to reduce the systemic levels that are already present. Peritoneal dialysis, plasmapheresis, and hemodialysis have been used in human medicine, as has cholestyramine, which binds to thyroid hormone in the GI tract, and inhibits enterohepatic circulation. These methods rarely are used in human patients and probably have limited use in veterinary patients with thyroid storm.

Systemic Support

The third arm of treatment for patients with thyroid storm involves reversing the effects of thyroid hormones on the body. Hyperthermia should be treated with judicious use of parenteral fluids and fans. Volume depletion is another common systemic effect of thyroid storm and should be treated with intravenous isotonic crystalloid fluid replacement. Colloid fluid therapy generally is not indicated unless severe GI disease or another syndrome resulting in low oncotic pressure is present. Potassium supplementation should be added as necessary (some patients with thyroid storm become acutely hypokalemic). Dextrose supplementation of 5% to 10% should be considered, if needed, and B vitamin supplementation may prevent thiamine deficiency in hyperthyroid cats.

Cardiac disturbances are common in humans with thyroid storm, and it is not uncommon for cats with thyroid storm to arrive in cardiac failure. β-Adrenergic blockade therapy, as described earlier, may be also be helpful for managing cardiac failure because of its effects in reducing the elevated heart rate caused by thyrotoxicosis. Furosemide (1 to 4 mg/kg IV or intramuscularly [IM] q1-6h as needed; 0.5 to 2 mg/kg PO q6-24h), angiotensin-converting enzyme inhibitors (enalapril or benazepril at 0.5 to 2 mg/kg PO q12h), isosorbide dinitrate (0.5 to 2 mg/kg PO q8-12h), nitroglycerin (0.25 to 1.5 inch q6-12h topically), or hydralazine (0.5 to 1 mg/kg IV; 0.5 to 2 mg/kg PO, subcutaneously [SC], or IV q8-12h) may be useful to manage feline heart failure but must be used with care in patients with renal compromise (see Chapters 41, 159, and 160). In all cases, medications should be started at the lowest dosages and titrated upward to effect with close blood pressure monitoring.

Supraventricular arrhythmias are common in humans with thyroid storm, most commonly atrial fibrillation. Atrial fibrillation or ventricular tachycardias can also occur in thyrotoxic feline patients. β-adrenergic receptor blockade, as described earlier, is a first-line defense in treating these arrhythmias. A possible sequela in feline patients with heart failure or atrial fibrillation is thromboembolic disease. Anticoagulation should be considered using low-dose aspirin (5 mg/cat PO q72h), unfractionated heparin (200 to 400 U/kg SC q6-8h until activated partial thromboplastin time is 1.5 to 2 times prolonged), or low-molecular-weight heparin (with factor Xa monitoring). See Chapters 167 and 168 for further details.

Hypertension is often a complication of thyroid storm in cats. Blood pressure should be checked and antihypertensive therapy instituted with amlodipine (0.625 to 1.25 mg PO or rectally q12-24h) or β—adrenergic blockade, as discussed previously. In acute cases of hypertension, nitroprusside may be used as an intravenous CRI at 0.5 to 5 mcg/kg/min or nicardipine at 0.5 to 5 mcg/kg/min.

Eradication of the Precipitating Factor

In human patients with thyroid storm, a precipitating factor is one of the criteria that defines the disease. Precipitating factors should also be investigated thoroughly in cats with thyroid storm. A full workup, including hematology, and thyroid assays, biochemical analysis, urinalysis, retroviral testing, blood pressure measurement, and imaging studies should be performed. Abnormal findings should be further examined by culturing potentially infected fluids, detailed imaging studies, endoscopy, or other specialized testing. If another abnormality is identified, it should be treated in order to prevent recurrence of thyroid storm.

OUTCOME

Although thyroid storm is an uncommon finding in human emergency rooms, the mortality rate in patients with this syndrome is significant. Rapid recognition of the problem and aggressive treatment are necessary for a successful outcome. Thyroid storm is not as well defined in feline medicine, although acute manifestations of thyrotoxicosis result in a syndrome that can be considered a feline thyroid storm. Veterinary recognition of this syndrome may be lacking, so it is unknown what the true incidence and mortality from thyroid storm may be in cats. However, it is certainly recognized that death may arise from untreated, acute thyrotoxicosis. As in humans, it is anticipated that early recognition and aggressive treatment of feline thyroid storm will improve veterinary patient survival.

REFERENCES

1. Tietgens ST, Leinung MC: Thyroid storm, Med Clin North Am 79:169, 1995.
2. Maussier ML, D'Errico G, Putignano P, et al: Thyrotoxicosis: clinical and laboratory assessment, Rays 24:263, 1999.
3. Silva JE: Catecholamines and the sympathoadrenal system in thyrotoxicosis. In Braverman LE, Utiger RD, editors: Werner and Ingbar's the thyroid: a fundamental and clinical text, Philadelphia, 2000, Lippincott Williams & Wilkins.
4. Boelaert K, Franklyn JA: Thyroid hormone in health and disease, J Endocrinol 187:1, 2005.
5. Burch HB, Wartofsky L: Life-threatening thyrotoxicosis. Thyroid storm, Endocrinol Metab Clin North Am 22:263, 1993.
6. Kienle RD, Bruyette D, Pion PD: Effects of thyroid hormone and thyroid dysfunction on the cardiovascular system, Vet Clin North Am Small Anim Pract 24:495, 1994.
7. Elliott J, Barber PJ, Syme HM, et al: Feline hypertension: clinical findings and response to antihypertensive treatment in 30 cases, J Small Anim Pract 42:122, 2001.
8. Maggio F, DeFrancesco TC, Atkins CE, et al: Ocular lesions associated with systemic hypertension in cats: 69 cases (1985-1998), J Am Vet Med Assoc 217:695, 2000.
9. Smith SA, Tobias AH, Jacob KA, et al: Arterial thromboembolism in cats: acute crisis in 127 cases (1992-2001) and long-term management with low-dose aspirin in 24 cases, J Vet Intern Med 17:73, 2003.
10. Mooney CT: Hyperthyroidism. In Ettinger SJ, Feldman EC, editors: Textbook of veterinary internal medicine, ed 6, St Louis, 2005, Saunders.
11. Pimentel L, Hansen KN: Thyroid disease in the emergency department: a clinical and laboratory review, J Emerg Med 28:201, 2005.
12. Bell R, Mellor DJ, Ramsey I et al: Decreased sodium:potassium ratios in cats: 49 cases, Vet Clin Pathol 34:110, 2005.
13. Sarlis NJ, Gourgiotis L: Thyroid emergencies, Rev Endocr Metab Disord 4:129, 2003.
14. Bogazzi F, Miccoli, P, Berti P, et al: Preparation with iopanoic acid rapidly controls thyrotoxicosis in patients with aniodarone-induced thyrotoxicosis before thyroidectomy, Surgery 132:1114, 2002.
15. Mechanik JI, Davies TF: Medical management of hyperthyroidism theoretical and practical aspects. In Falk SA, editor: Thyroid disease: endocrinology, surgery, nuclear medicine, and radiotherapy, ed 2, New York, 1997, Lippincott Raven, p 253.
16. Geffner DL, Hershman JM: β-Adrenergic blockade for the treatment of hyperthyroidism, Am J Med 93:61, 1992.

CHAPTER 70

HYPOTHYROID CRISIS IN THE DOG

Rebecka S. Hess, DVM, DACVIM (Internal Medicine)

KEY POINTS

- Although *myxedema coma* is commonly used to describe a hypothyroid crisis, this is a misnomer. Many patients in a hypothyroid crisis are not comatose and do not have myxedema.
- A hypothyroid crisis is difficult to diagnose because it is rare and the clinical and clinicopathologic abnormalities may be nonspecific.
- Rottweiler dogs are at increased risk for a hypothyroid crisis.
- Concurrent disease, most commonly infection (pneumonia), may increase the risk for a hypothyroid crisis. Treatment with steroids, nonsteroidal medication, or surgery may also increase the risk for a hypothyroid crisis.
- Myxedema, obesity, mental dullness, hypercholesterolemia, and nonregenerative anemia are observed in many, but not all, dogs in a hypothyroid crisis.
- Intravenous (IV) administration of levothyroxine at a dosage of 5 mcg/kg q12h is a safe and effective treatment for dogs suffering from a hypothyroid crisis.
- Subjective improvement in mentation or ambulation occurs within 24 to 30 hours of IV levothyroxine administration in most dogs.
- When treated appropriately with supportive care and IV levothyroxine, most dogs with a hypothyroid crisis respond well and are discharged from the hospital.

Canine myxedema coma is a rare, life-threatening complication of hypothyroidism.[1-7] In human beings the name *myxedema coma* is considered a misnomer because human patients with this condition are rarely comatose and do not usually have myxedema.[8,9] Diagnosis of myxedema coma is difficult because it is rare, and therefore little is known of the condition.[1] Diagnosis is further complicated by nonspecific clinical signs. Recognition of an acute hypothyroid crisis in dogs that do not have coma or myxedema may advance the understanding and improve the outcome of dogs with a suspected hypothyroid crisis.[1]

PATHOPHYSIOLOGY

The pathophysiology of myxedema coma is incompletely understood. Thyroid hormones regulate cell function in many organs by binding intranuclear receptors and promoting expression of various enzymes.[10] Thyroid hormones exert chronotropic and inotropic effects in the heart, as well as catabolic, metabolic, calorigenic, and developmental effects in other organs.[10] Therefore decreased thyroid hormone concentrations have a profound effect on many body systems. The clinical hallmarks of myxedema coma in human beings are altered mental status, inadequate thermoregulation, decreased respiratory and cardiovascular function, and concurrent disease.[9,11]

In human beings, altered mental status may be limited to disorientation, confusion, or lethargy.[9] Coma is unusual.[8,9] In dogs, clinical signs such as disorientation and confusion may be difficult to appreciate. Although most dogs in a hypothyroid crisis have mental dullness, coma upon initial examination is uncommon.[1,2,4-6] The pathophysiology of altered mental status is multifactorial and may be a result of decreased blood flow and oxygen delivery to the brain, hyponatremia, lack of a direct effect of thyroid hormone on the brain, or disruption of the integrity of the blood-brain barrier.[9,12]

The pathophysiology of altered thermoregulation resulting in hypothermia likely is also multifactorial. Inadequate thyroid hormone function in the hypothalamus may result in inability to regulate body temperature.[9] Additionally, a decrease in the calorigenic effect of thyroid hormones contributes to hypothermia.[9] It is possible that hypoperfusion and hypotension also contribute to a low rectal temperature. The body temperature of some individuals with myxedema coma may appear to be normal because of a concurrent infection and fever.[9]

Hypoventilation develops secondary to decreased respiratory system responsiveness to hypoxia and hypercapnia and may be complicated by obese body condition, muscle weakness, pneumonia, pericardial or pleural effusion, and ascites.[11] In the heart, thyroid hormones increase the number of β-adrenergic receptors and their affinity to catecholamines, thereby increasing the inotropic and chronotropic effects of catecholamines.[10] Hypothyroid cardiomyopathy is also caused by an increase in α-myosin heavy chains (MHC), which have decreased adenosine triphosphatase (ATPase) activity, and a decrease in β-MHCs, which have more adenosine triphosphatase activity.[10] These changes result in hypothyroid cardiomyopathy typified by impaired left ventricular function or atrial fibrillation.[13,14] During a hypothyroid crisis, cardiovascular dysfunction is characterized by bradycardia, decreased cardiac contractility, cardiac enlargement, and hypotension, although diastolic hypertension has also been documented.[11]

Systolic hypotension is reported commonly in humans with myxedema coma and is thought to develop secondary to bradycardia, decreased cardiac output, and hypovolemia.[8,11] Blood pressure was not measured in most reports of canine myxedema coma.[4-6,15] Systolic hypotension was documented in four of five dogs in which the blood pressure was measured.[1,2] Diastolic hypertension is also recognized in humans with myxedema coma and is believed to develop because of peripheral vasoconstriction and central shunting of blood that occurs as a result of hypothermia and low oxygen consumption.[11]

Concurrent disease may prevent normal compensatory mechanisms from responding appropriately to a hypothyroid crisis and may therefore be involved in the pathophysiology of myxedema coma.[9] Absence of concurrent disease in most cases of hypothyroidism may explain why myxedema coma remains rare.

When myxedema does occur, it is thought to develop secondary to accumulation of the glycosaminoglycan hyaluronic acid in the dermis.[6,15] Impaired renal perfusion secondary to decreased cardiovascular function results in inability to excrete water and contributes to development of edema.[11] Excessive secretion of antidiuretic hormone may also contribute to hyponatremia, fluid retention, and edema in some patients.[16]

RISK FACTORS

Rottweiler dogs are at increased risk for myxedema coma.[1] Most dogs with a hypothyroid crisis are of middle age (median 6 years, range 4 to 10 years).[1] The age of dogs with a hypothyroid crisis is not significantly different from the age of other hypothyroid dogs. Female dogs do not appear to be at increased risk compared with other hypothyroid dogs, although myxedema coma is more common in women than men.[1,8,11] Dogs with untreated hypothyroidism are at increased risk.[1-6]

Most dogs with myxedema coma have a concurrent disorder, most commonly an infection. In a report of seven dogs with a hypothyroid crisis, concurrent disease was diagnosed in five.[1] Infection was diagnosed in four of the seven dogs. Three of the four dogs with infection had aspiration pneumonia. Additional infections included foreign body keratoconjunctivitis, pyometra, severe bilateral otitis, and pyoderma. The most commonly observed concurrent infections in humans with myxedema coma are pneumonia, influenza virus, urinary tract infection, and sepsis.[8]

Glucocorticoids were administered to three dogs with myxedema coma within 1 month of a hypothyroid crisis.[1,5] Oral prednisone at a dosage of 0.55 mg/kg q12h lowers the concentration of thyroid hormones in dogs.[17] Nonsteroidal antiinflammatory medications (carprofen and flunixin meglumine) were used in conjunction with glucocorticoids in one dog in a hypothyroid crisis.[1] Nonsteroidal antiinflammatory drugs (NSAIDs) may cause suppression of thyroid-stimulating hormone (TSH) secretion.[18] It is therefore possible that administration of glucocorticoids to dogs with untreated hypothyroidism may increase the risk of myxedema coma. An association between NSAIDs, or other thyroid hormone synthesis–altering drugs, and canine myxedema coma may become apparent in the future.

Surgery increases the risk of a hypothyroid crisis in human beings and has been reported in three dogs with myxedema coma.[1,6] It is possible that surgery compromises the ability of normal cardiovascular and pulmonary compensatory mechanisms to respond to a hypothyroid state and therefore increases the risk for a hypothyroid crisis.[8]

Other factors that increase the risk of myxedema coma in human beings include burns, carbon dioxide retention, gastrointestinal hemorrhage, hypoglycemia, infection, hypothermia (most cases are diagnosed during the winter), stroke, trauma, and various medications, including anesthetics, barbiturates, β-blockers, diuretics, narcotics, phenothiazines, and tranquilizers.[8]

CLINICAL SIGNS AND PHYSICAL EXAMINATION FINDINGS

Clinical signs and physical examination findings may be attributed to chronic untreated hypothyroidism, an acute hypothyroid crisis, or concurrent disease. Clinical signs commonly observed in dogs with chronic untreated hypothyroidism include weight gain or obese body condition, lethargy, mental dullness, weakness, and dermatologic abnormalities such as hyperkeratosis, alopecia, or thin hair coat.[7] In a study of seven dogs in a hypothyroid crisis, physical examination abnormalities included overweight or obese body condition (noted in five of seven dogs), nonpitting facial, jaw, or other edema (four of seven), tachypnea (four of seven), alopecia (three of seven), dehydration (two of seven), dermatitis (two of seven), otitis (one of seven), elevated or decreased body temperature (one dog each), heart murmur (one of seven), bradycardia (one dog), or tachycardia (one dog).[1] Neurologic findings included mental dullness (observed in five of seven dogs) and stupor (two of seven). None of the dogs was comatose.[1] In a literature review of five previously published manuscripts describing seven other dogs with myxedema coma, one dog was in a coma on initial examination,[3] although ultimately four of seven dogs developed coma.[2,4-6] Stupor was noted in six of these dogs.[2,4-6]

Most dogs in a hypothyroid crisis do not have all the classic physical hallmarks, including myxedema, hypothermia, bradycardia, hypoventilation, hypotension, and coma.[1,5,6]

CLINICAL PATHOLOGY

The most common abnormalities noted on complete blood cell count and serum chemistry screen are a mild nonregenerative anemia, hypercholesterolemia, lipemia, and increased alkaline phosphatase activity.[1] However, not all dogs with severe unregulated hypothyroidism have all these clinicopathologic abnormalities, and normal cholesterol concentration or hematocrit has been documented in dogs with myxedema coma.[1,5,6] Although hyponatremia and hypoglycemia are well recognized in humans with myxedema coma and have been noted anecdotally in dogs, they were not noted in any of seven dogs in a hypothyroid crisis.[1] Urinalysis and urine culture results are usually normal.[1]

Nonregenerative anemia is associated with hypothyroidism for at least a couple of reasons. Thyroid hormones bind thyroid hormone receptors on erythroid progenitors and act directly to increase erythroid proliferation.[19] Thyroid hormones also increase expression of the erythropoietin gene, further contributing to red blood cell formation.[19]

The mechanisms by which decreased thyroid hormone function induces dyslipidemia are widely studied and not fully understood. Alterations in both synthesis and transport of lipids are involved in the pathogenesis of hypothyroid dyslipidemia.[20] Decreased messenger ribonucleic acid (mRNA) expression of hepatic low-density lipoprotein (LDL) receptors results in fewer LDL receptors, decreased clearance of LDL by the liver, and elevated plasma LDL concentration.[20] High-density lipoprotein (HDL) subfraction concentration is also altered, with an increase in the subfraction HDL_2, attributed mainly to decreased hepatic lipase activity.[20]

Many possible explanations for hyponatremia have been investigated. These include increased renal reabsorption of sodium, impaired water clearance, increased antidiuretic hormone concentration, low plasma renin activity, and a low aldosterone concentration.[16] Hypoglycemia can develop in humans secondary to reduced insulin clearance or may be observed in patients with concurrent hypoadrenocorticism.[8,21] However, dogs with experimentally induced hypothyroidism have been shown to have decreased insulin sensitivity, which may lead to hyperglycemia.[22] Sepsis should also be considered in these cases.

Hypoxia and hypercarbia are reported in humans with myxedema coma. Venous blood gas analysis has been reported in seven dogs suffering from a hypothyroid crisis.[1,2] Hypercarbia was documented in one of these dogs,[2] and the arterial partial pressure of carbon dioxide ($PaCO_2$) was at the high end of normal in two other dogs[1] and normal in the remaining four dogs.[1] Lactate concentration was increased in five of the six dogs in which it was measured.[1]

Thyroid axis testing is performed to confirm the diagnosis of hypothyroidism. However, results often are not available immediately and treatment of a hypothyroid crisis must begin before confirmation of a diagnosis. Serum should be stored for future analysis before thyroid hormone supplementation is begun. Severe lipemia can interfere with hormone measurement, further complicating the diagnosis.[1] Hypothyroidism is confirmed based on low thyroxine and high TSH concentrations, although some hypothyroid dogs do not have elevated TSH concentrations. Endogenous TSH concentration was normal in 63% of measurements in dogs with spontaneous hypothyroidism.[23]

Several drugs can cause low thyroxine with or without high TSH concentrations and must be taken into account when confirming a diagnosis. These drugs include glucocorticoids, nonsteroidal antiinflammatory agents, trimethoprim-sulfonamide antibiotics, anticonvulsants (carbamazepine, valproate, and phenobarbital, potassium bromide), antituberculosis drugs (paraaminosalicylic acid, ethionamide, and prothionamide), propranolol, and lithium. Changes in thyroxine and TSH concentrations may be reversible with discontinuation of these medications.[24,25]

DIFFERENTIAL DIAGNOSIS

Many of the clinical and clinicopathologic abnormalities observed in dogs with myxedema coma are nonspecific. Differential diagnosis for obesity, lethargy, mental dullness, weakness, dermatologic abnormalities, and nonregenerative anemia are discussed elsewhere. Some nonspecific differentials might include chronic inflammatory disease, cardiac disease, metabolic disease (i.e., hypoadrenocorticism), intracranial disease, hypothermia, and sepsis.

Differential diagnoses for edema can be divided into those caused by increased hydrostatic pressure, decreased oncotic pressure, lymphatic obstruction, sodium retention, and vascular endothelial leak syndromes. Such differential diagnoses include heart failure, constrictive pericarditis, ascites, venous obstruction or compression, heat-induced illness, hormonal imbalance, protein-losing nephropathy or enteropathy, liver disease, malnutrition, neoplasia, renal hypoperfusion, sepsis, and excess secretion of renin, angiotensin, or aldosterone.

Differential diagnoses for hypercholesterolemia include hypothyroidism, diabetes mellitus, hyperadrenocorticism, protein-losing glomerulopathy, cholestatic disease, postprandial hyperlipidemia, primary hyperlipidemia (Miniature Schnauzers, Shetland Sheepdogs), lipoprotein lipase deficiency (cats), idiopathic causes (Doberman Pinschers, Rottweilers), and iatrogenic causes (glucocorticoids).

TREATMENT

Treatment is divided into supportive care, thyroid hormone supplementation, and treatment of concurrent conditions. Hypotension can be treated cautiously with fluids and vasopressors (see Chapters 60 and 157).[11] Dogs must be observed carefully for signs of fluid overload, which may exacerbate underlying cardiac disease or dysfunction. Hypothermia is treated by wrapping the dog with blankets and maintaining a warm ambient temperature.[11] Heating pads should be avoided because they can lead to vasodilation and worsening hypotension.[11] If respiratory depression is profound, mechanical ventilatory support is needed (see Chapter 30).[1,2] Hyponatremia can be corrected slowly (no more than 0.5 mEq/hr change in sodium concentration) with 0.9% saline solution.[11]

Ultimately, clinical signs resolve with thyroid hormone supplementation. Thyroid hormone is usually administered before results of thyroid axis testing are available and before the diagnosis of a hypothyroid crisis is confirmed. IV levothyroxine has a higher bioavailability than does oral levothyroxine, resulting in a more rapid clinical response. IV levothyroxine at a dosage of 5 mcg/kg administered q12h is safe and effective in dogs in a hypothyroid crisis.[1] Adverse side effects of IV thyroid hormone supplementation in humans may be reduced with thyroxine (T_4) rather than with intravenous triiodothyronine (T_3).[26,27] Such adverse side effects include cardiac arrhythmias, angina pectoris, and pneumonia.[26] Mortality of humans with myxedema coma is increased with high dosages of IV levothyroxine (>500 mcg/24 hours, which is equivalent to about 7 mcg/kg/24 hours).[28] Dogs should be monitored closely for these complications. Administration of IV levothyroxine may have led to the development of pneumonia in two dogs.[1] When the hypothyroid crisis is resolved, the oral route can be used (0.1 mg/5 to 7 kg PO q12h).[7]

Treatment of concurrent disease such as pneumonia, other infections, cardiac disease, concurrent endocrinopathy, or any other illness will facilitate recovery. Discontinuation of any medication that may have exacerbated the hypothyroid crisis is also recommended.

OUTCOME

Most dogs with myxedema coma respond well to therapy when given IV levothyroxine.[1,3] Seven of eight reported dogs that received IV levothyroxine were discharged from the hospital (87%).[1,3] Subjective improvement in mentation or ambulation occurs within 24 to 30 hours of administration of IV levothyroxine in most dogs.[1] Severity of concurrent disease, persistent hypothermia, advanced age, and degree of mental alteration (coma) is associated with a poor prognosis in humans.[29]

REFERENCES

1. Pullen WH, Hess RS: Hypothyroid dogs treated with intravenous levothyroxine, J Vet Intern Med 20:32, 2006.
2. Atkinson K, Aubert I: Myxedema coma leading to respiratory depression in a dog, Can Vet J 45:318, 2004.
3. Henik RA, Dixon RM: Intravenous administration of levothyroxine for treatment of suspected myxedema coma complicated by severe hypothermia in a dog, J Am Vet Med Assoc 216:713, 2000.
4. Kelly MJ, Hill JR: Canine myxedema stupor and coma, Compend Contin Educ Vet Pract 6:1049, 1984.
5. Chastain CB, Graham CL, Riley MG: Myxedema coma in two dogs, Canine Pract 9:20, 1982.
6. Johnson JA, Patterson JM: Multifocal myxedema and mixed thyroid neoplasm in a dog, Vet Pathol 18:13, 1981.
7. Feldman EC, Nelson RW: Hypothyroidism. In Feldman EC, Nelson RW: Canine and feline endocrinology and reproduction, ed 3, St Louis, 2004, WB Saunders.
8. Wall CR: Myxedema coma: diagnosis and treatment, Am Fam Physician 62:2485, 2000.
9. Fliers E, Wiersinga WM: Myxedema coma, Rev Endocr Metab Disord 4:137, 2003.
10. Ganong WF: Review of medical physiology, ed 18, Stamford, 1997, Appleton & Lange.
11. Sarlis NJ, Gourgiotis L: Thyroid emergencies, Rev Endocr Metab Disord 4:129, 2003.
12. Pancotto T, Rossmeisl JH Jr, Panciera DL: Blood-brain-barrier disruption in chronic canine hypothyroidism, Vet Clin Pathol 39(4):485, 2010.
13. Panciera DL: An echocardiographic and electrocardiographic study of cardiovascular function in hypothyroid dogs, J Am Vet Med Assoc 205:996, 1994.
14. Gerritsen RJ, van den Brom WE, Stokhof AA: Relationship between atrial fibrillation and primary hypothyroidism in the dog, Vet Q 18:49, 1996.
15. Doliger S, Delverdier M, More J, et al: Histochemical study of cutaneous mucins in hypothyroid dogs, Vet Pathol 32:628, 1995.
16. Park CW, Shin YS, Ahn SJ, et al: Thyroxine treatment induces upregulation of renin-angiotensin-aldosterone system due to decreasing effective plasma volume in patients with primary myxoedema, Nephrol Dial Transplant 16:1799, 2001.
17. Kaptein EM, Moore GM, Ferguson DE, et al: Effects of prednisone on thyroxine and 3.5.3'-triiodothyronine metabolism in normal dogs, Endocrinology 130:1669, 1992.
18. Surks MI: Drugs and thyroid function, N Engl J Med 333:1688, 1995.
19. Ma Y, Freitag P, Zhou J, et al: Thyroid hormone induces erythropoietin gene expression through augmented accumulation of hypoxia-inducible factor-1, Am J Physiol Regul Integr Comp Physiol 287:R600, 2004.
20. Tan KC, Shiu SW, Kung AW: Effect of thyroid dysfunction on high-density lipoprotein subfraction metabolism: roles of hepatic lipase and cholesteryl ester transfer protein, J Clin Endocrinol Metab 83:2921, 1998.

21. Kurtoglu S, Tutus A, Aydin K, et al: Persistent neonatal hypoglycemia: an unusual finding of congenital hypothyroidism, J Pediatr Endocrinol 11:277, 1998.
22. Hofer-Inteeworn N, Panciera DL, Monroe WE, et al. Effect of hypothyroidism on insulin sensitivity and glucose tolerance in dogs, Am J Vet Res 73(4):529, 2012.
23. Bruner JM, Scott-Moncrieff CR, Williams DA: Effect of time of sample collection on serum thyroid-stimulating hormone concentrations in euthyroid and hypothyroid dogs, J Am Vet Med Assoc 212:1572, 1998.
24. Daminet S, Ferguson DC: Influence of drugs on thyroid function in dogs, J Vet Intern Med 17:463, 2003.
25. Brenner K, Harkin K, Schermerhorn T: Iatrogenic, sulfonamide-induced hypothyroid crisis in a Labrador Retriever, Aust Vet J 87:503, 2009.
26. Ringel MD: Management of hypothyroidism and hyperthyroidism in the intensive care unit, Crit Care Clin 17:59, 2001.
27. Hylander B, Rosenqvist U: Treatment of myxoedema coma—factors associated with fatal outcome, Acta Endocrinol (Copenh) 108:65, 1985.
28. Yamamoto T, Fukuyama J, Fujiyoshi A: Factors associated with mortality of myxedema coma: report of eight cases and literature survey, Thyroid 9:1167, 1999.
29. Rodriguez I, Fluiters E, Perez-Mendez LF, et al: Factors associated with mortality of patients with myxoedema coma: prospective study in 11 cases treated in a single institution, J Endocrinol 180:347, 2004.

CHAPTER 71
PHEOCHROMOCYTOMA

Kari Santoro-Beer, DVM, DACVECC • Deborah C. Mandell, VMD, DACVECC

KEY POINTS

- Pheochromocytoma is a tumor of the chromaffin cells of the adrenal medulla.
- Clinical signs may include hypertension and manifestations of the elevated blood pressure, weakness, syncope, lethargy, vomiting, diarrhea, tachypnea, abdominal distention, tachyarrhythmias, bradyarrhythmias, and abdominal pain.
- Most pheochromocytomas in small animals are diagnosed either by abdominal imaging or during postmortem examination.
- Definitive treatment for a pheochromocytoma is surgical excision.
- Preoperative, perioperative, and postoperative management may be challenging.
- With complete surgical resection and an uneventful postoperative course, even dogs with vena caval thrombi may experience a significant survival time of 18 months to greater than 4 years.

Pheochromocytoma is a tumor of the chromaffin cells of the adrenal medulla. These cells synthesize, store, and secrete catecholamines in response to sympathetic stimulation (Figures 71-1 and 71-2).[1] Chromaffin cells are also termed APUD cells, because they are responsible for amine precursor uptake and decarboxylation. Pheochromocytoma may occur alone, or as part of a multiple endocrine neoplasia syndrome. In humans this is a heritable constellation of two or more endocrine neoplasias (or hyperplasia), usually involving the parathyroid and thyroid glands in addition to the adrenal glands.[2] Extra-adrenal pheochromocytomas (paragangliomas) occur rarely. Most (48% to 80%) pheochromocytomas in small animals and 30% to 76% in humans are diagnosed on postmortem examination. Others are incidental findings discovered during abdominal ultrasonography, despite the absence of clinical signs.[1,3-5] It is thought that pheochromocytomas represent between 0.01% and 0.13% of all canine tumors; however, these numbers may be low because the tumor may be benign or nonfunctional and thus not suspected or diagnosed.[6] These tumors may be both locally invasive and metastatic.[3,5] Most pheochromocytomas in humans secrete norepinephrine (NE) (versus epinephrine), but this has not been studied in dogs or cats.[2] It is thought that negative feedback of NE on tyrosine hydroxylase (which converts tyrosine to dopa, leading to synthesis of more NE) does not work normally in the tumor cells, or that the tumor metabolizes NE so quickly that the levels required for negative feedback are never reached.[2]

CLINICAL SIGNS

In dogs with pheochromocytomas, approximately 30% to 50% have clinical signs attributable to the tumor. Dogs tend to be older (10 to

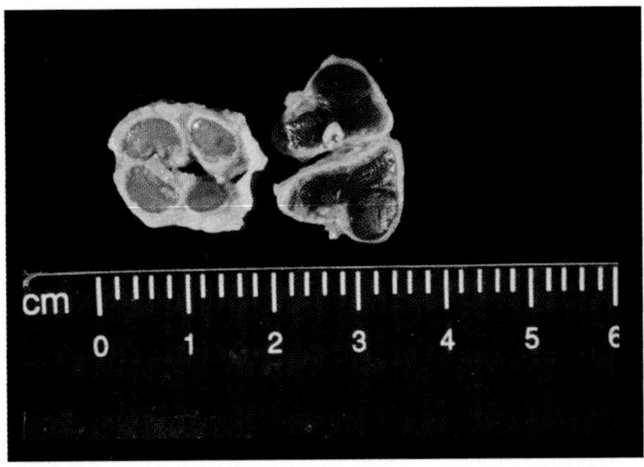

FIGURE 71-1 A normal adrenal gland on the left compared with a pheochromocytoma on the right. The pheochromocytoma was stained with potassium dichromate solution, which oxidizes catecholamines and produces a dark brown color.

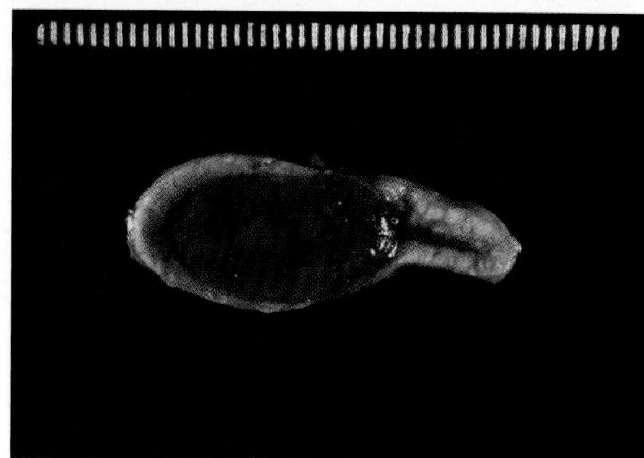

FIGURE 71-2 A large pheochromocytoma of the adrenal gland discovered as an incidental finding during necropsy. The pheochromocytoma is stained with potassium dichromate solution.

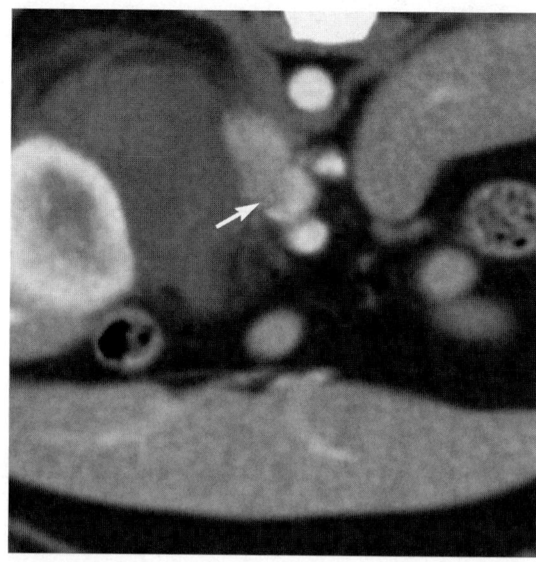

FIGURE 71-3 Transverse helical postcontrast computed tomography image at the level of the cranial pole of the right kidney. A right adrenal mass is seen, and a large filling defect is present in the caudal vena cava at that level *(arrow)*. This mass was determined to be a pheochromocytoma by histopathology.

12 years), and most retrospective studies have found no gender predilection although a recent paper reported that males were overrepresented.[1,5,7-9] Clinical signs may include hypertension, manifestations of the elevated blood pressure (e.g., blindness from retinal detachment), weakness, collapse, lethargy, vomiting, diarrhea, polyuria, polydipsia, tachypnea, abdominal distention, syncope, tachyarrhythmias, bradyarrhythmias, and abdominal pain.[5,8,10] These signs may be sustained or paroxysmal. Because the pheochromocytoma is not innervated like a normal adrenal gland, it is unclear what stimuli cause secretion of catecholamines from the tumor. A Budd-Chiari–like syndrome resulting from tumor invasion and extension up the caudal vena cava has been reported in a dog.[11] Approximately 15% to 38% of dogs with pheochromocytomas have neoplastic invasion of the caudal vena cava; however, clinical signs are not reliably associated with the extent or presence of vena caval invasion.[6,12,13]

Concurrent pheochromocytoma and hyperadrenocorticism have been reported in dogs, and some clinical signs may overlap.[14] Rupture of pheochromocytomas may result in hemoperitoneum or hemoretroperitoneum.[15-17] Dogs may exhibit neurologic deficits or paraparesis secondary to metastatic tumor in the spinal canal or secondary to aortic thromboembolic disease.[5,6,8] Cardiac arrhythmias may include third-degree atrioventricular block, second-degree atrioventricular block secondary to hypertension, supraventricular tachycardia, paroxysmal tachycardias, or ventricular ectopy.[10]

Of the few cats in the literature with an antemortem diagnoses of a pheochromocytoma, clinical signs consisted of lethargy, vomiting, polyuria, polydipsia, aggression, and weight gain or were associated with systemic hypertension (congestive heart failure and retinal detachment).[18-20]

DIAGNOSIS

As in humans, most pheochromocytomas in small animals are incidental findings, diagnosed by abdominal imaging or postmortem examination. In some dogs, an abdominal mass may be palpated.[5,8]

Abdominal radiography may show mineralization in the area of the adrenal glands or may demonstrate retroperitoneal effusion or an abdominal mass effect associated with the tumor (30% to 50% of cases).[5,21] Chest radiographs may show cardiomegaly and pulmonary venous congestion or pulmonary edema secondary to chronic hypertension or tachycardia.[1,5] These findings may be confirmed via echocardiography.[7] Rarely, metastatic disease may be seen on thoracic radiographs.[7,8]

In dogs 65% to 83% of pheochromocytomas are detected via abdominal ultrasonography, making it a useful first-line imaging modality.[2] The origin and architecture of the mass, as well as blood flow within the mass and invasion into adjacent structures, may be determined. Pheochromocytomas seem to have a higher likelihood for vena caval invasion than do adrenocortical tumors,[22] but ultrasonographically they appear similar to adrenocortical tumors.[23] It is difficult to determine the cellular origin of an adrenal mass based on ultrasonography, and some masses may be too small for detection by this means.[1,2] Invasive pheochromocytomas have been reported to invade not only the vena cava but also the aorta, renal veins, and hepatic veins.[12] Ultrasound-guided biopsies may be obtained, if indicated, but caution should be exercised.

Advanced imaging techniques such as computed tomography (CT) or magnetic resonance imaging (MRI) are very helpful for determining the size of the tumor and the extent of tumor invasion, although these require general anesthesia in the veterinary patient. Nonionic, low-osmolar contrast media is recommended for CT studies to minimize adverse reactions.[24] Gadolinium contrast for MRI studies is not contraindicated in patients with a suspected pheochromocytoma.[24] CT findings in dogs with pheochromocytoma show a lobulated, irregularly shaped mass associated with the adrenal gland. Areas of decreased intensity are interspersed with highly vascular areas with increased intensity (Figures 71-3 and 71-4).[24] CT is both sensitive and specific for identifying surrounding adrenal tumor invasion.[25] MRI may be used to differentiate between histologic types of adrenal tumors.[2] Scintigraphy using ^{123}iodinemetaiodobenzylguanidine (an NE analog) or ^{99m}technetium-methylene diphosphonate has been used in the dog to identify a pheochromocytoma.[26,27] One group used p-[^{18}F]fluorobenzylguani-dine to identify tumors in dogs using positron emission tomography.[28] These techniques are useful for identifying metastatic tumors as well.

Laboratory test results in animals with a pheochromocytoma are generally unremarkable. In dogs, a mild nonregenerative anemia may be present secondary to chronic disease or an increased mean cell volume or packed cell volume may be seen as a result of catecholamine or erythropoetin-like stimulation of the bone marrow.[1] A regenerative anemia may reflect hemorrhage from the tumor.[3] Leukocytosis or a stress leukogram may be found secondary to catecholamine release or inflammatory changes associated with the tumor.[2,3] If there has been hemorrhage or intravascular coagulation from the tumor, a consumptive thrombocytopenia may occur. Evidence of

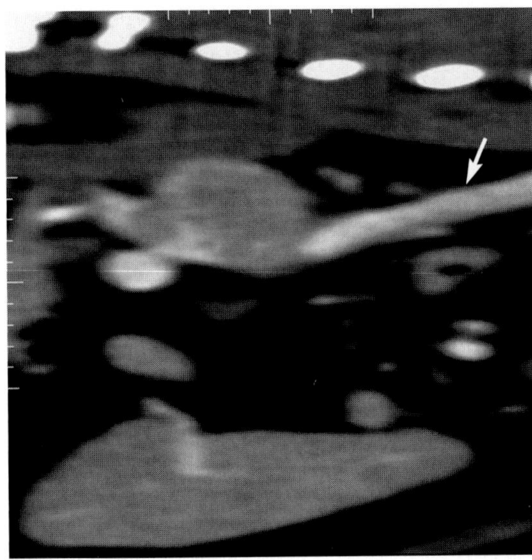

FIGURE 71-4 Sagittal reconstruction of the helical computed tomography scan in Figure 71-1 showing invasion of the caudal vena cava along the length (4 cm) of the mass. Irregular filling of the cava is present cranial and caudal to the mass, likely representing thrombus formation. The cranial aspect of the caudal vena cava is denoted with an *arrow.*

hypercoagulability may be present, but this has not been investigated in veterinary medicine (see Chapter 104).

Serum chemistry profiles may be normal or show elevations in liver enzymes (unrelated to liver metastasis).[3,7] Dogs with multiple endocrine neoplasia syndrome may be hypercalcemic as a result of elevated parathyroid hormone or parathyroid hormone–related peptide (PTH or PTH-rp). Dogs may be hyperglycemic from catecholamine stimulation of hepatic glucose production and decreased insulin release from α-receptor stimulation.[1] Pheochromocytomas may also secrete hormones such as vasoactive intestinal peptide, which can contribute to clinical signs such as diarrhea. In two retrospective reports of dogs with pheochromocytoma, hypercholesterolemia was present in 25% of dogs, possibly secondary to increased fat mobilization from catecholamine secretion or because of concurrent hyperadrenocorticism.[7,8]

In 20 dogs with a pheochromocytoma but without concurrent disease, 50% showed proteinuria, likely caused by a hypertensive glomerulopathy.[2] Measurement of urinary catecholamine concentrations (metanephrine, normetanephrine, vanillylmandelic acid) as a spot check referenced to urine creatinine, or over a 24-hour period, is performed in humans with suspected pheochromocytomas and has been investigated in dogs.[7, 29] One study showed that dogs with hyperadrenocorticism had increased concentrations of urinary catecholamines and normetanephine compared with normal dogs, and a high (four times normal) concentration of urinary normetanephrine was highly suggestive of pheochromocytoma.[29] Secondary factors, such as excitement, exercise, vanilla-containing foods, phenoxybenzamine therapy, and radiographic contrast agents may result in false-positive elevations.[2] Plasma metanephrine level measurements have recently been described in cats, including one cat with a suspected pheochromocytoma. In this study, sick cats with nonadrenal illness had significantly higher normetanephrine levels than healthy cats, and the cat with suspected pheochromocytoma had markedly higher normetanephrine levels.[30]

Because of the similarity in clinical signs and ultrasonographic appearance of pheochromocytomas and adrenocortical tumors, and reports of the coexistence of hyperadrenocorticism and pheochromocytoma, hyperadrenocorticism should be ruled out at the time of medical workup.[8]

Other tests reported in humans include the clonidine suppression test, which should decrease serum catecholamine levels in normal patients but not in patients with a functional pheochromocytoma (because catecholamine release from the tumor is not neurally mediated). The administration of intravenous phentolamine, an α-adrenergic antagonist, to hypertensive patients will cause a decrease in blood pressure if the hypertension is catecholamine mediated (close monitoring is vital). These tests have varying sensitivity and specificity, especially in the context of paroxysmal hypertension, and have not been evaluated thoroughly in veterinary patients.[2]

Provocation tests using metoclopramide, histamine, tyramine, and glucagon, all of which cause increased secretion of catecholamines from the tumor, are not recommended because of the potential for inducing acute hypertensive crises.[2] For this reason, the use of metoclopramide as an antiemetic in patients with suspected pheochromocytoma may be contraindicated.

Because hypertension and tachycardia may be paroxysmal, blood pressure and electrocardiogram (ECG) monitoring should be performed, but results may be low yield. Holter or continuous ECG monitoring may be necessary for the diagnosis of intermittent tachyarrhythmias.

The results of a biopsy or fine-needle aspiration of adrenal tumor masses are not discussed at length in the literature. This partially may be due to the difficulty of safely obtaining samples or because excisional biopsy is preferred. Gilson and others note a similarity in cytologic appearance between lymphosarcoma and pheochromocytoma when diagnosed from ascitic fluid in three dogs, so an adequate index of suspicion is necessary to prevent misdiagnosis.[7] Impression smears of a pheochromocytoma may also appear similar to a round cell tumor.[5] In addition, it is difficult to characterize relative malignancy on the basis of histopathologic evaluation, so it may be difficult to accurately predict tumor behavior on the basis of biopsy specimens.[7] Any tumor that demonstrates invasion of adjacent structures should be considered malignant.

TREATMENT

Definitive treatment for patients with a pheochromocytoma is surgical excision. Because of the systemic effects of pheochromocytomas, preoperative prophylactic treatment, careful anesthesia, and intensive perioperative monitoring and management are important. If which surgical excision is not possible or desired by the owner, medical management can be attempted.

Preoperative Treatment

Noncompetitive α-adrenergic blockade with phenoxybenzamine (0.5 to 2.5 mg/kg PO q12h) should be instituted at least 1 week before anesthesia for surgical resection of the tumor. This may help to blunt hypertensive episodes during anesthesia, although high dosages may be necessary.[31-33] In humans, preoperative α-adrenergic blockade decreased perioperative mortality associated with resection of pheochromocytoma from 13% to 45% to 0% to 3%.[34] In a recent retrospective study of dogs with pheochromocytoma undergoing adrenalectomy, those pretreated with phenoxybenzamine had a significantly decreased mortality rate compared with untreated patients.[9] α-Methylparatyrosine competitively inhibits tyrosine hydroxylase, interfering with catecholamine biosynthesis.[32] Some reports advocate the use of α-methylparatyrosine in conjunction with phenoxybenzamine, but it is associated with significant side effects and has not been studied in veterinary patients with pheochromocytoma.

Chronic sympathetic stimulation and vasoconstriction may result in intravascular volume depletion, which should be assessed and corrected before the induction of anesthesia.

Anesthesia and Monitoring

Anticholinergic drugs that may cause tachycardia and barbiturate agents that may lead to ventricular arrhythmias in the presence of excess catecholamines should be avoided during anesthetic premedication and induction. Long-lasting α-adrenergic antagonists such as acepromazine may complicate intraoperative or postoperative treatment and should be avoided, especially if the animal has been pretreated with phenoxybenzamine. A safe induction protocol might include an opioid, such as oxymorphone, hydromorphone, or fentanyl (minimal histamine release), combined with a benzodiazepine and propofol or etomidate to facilitate endotracheal intubation. Inhalant agents such as isoflurane or sevoflurane are preferred to halothane, which sensitizes the myocardium to catecholamine-induced arrhythmias. Desflurane can cause sympathetic stimulation and should be avoided. There are no contraindications to the use of nitrous oxide in humans undergoing surgery for pheochromocytoma.[32] Inhalant agents may be supplemented with balanced anesthetic techniques using potent opioids such as fentanyl, administered as a constant rate infusion (0.1 to 1.0 mcg/kg/min).

Intraoperative monitoring must include ECG and arterial blood pressure (preferably direct), as well as central venous pressure to estimate intravascular volume. Pulmonary arterial catheterization will give information about cardiac output and systemic vascular resistance that may help to tailor fluid and drug therapy during and after surgery; however, placement of these catheters may be associated with increased morbidity (see Chapter 202).[32] In one recent study of 60 dogs undergoing adrenalectomy, intraoperative complications included hypotension, hypertension, tachycardia, ventricular arrhythmias, and hemorrhage.[13]

During anesthesia, treatment with short-acting β-blocking drugs such as esmolol (0.05 to 0.5 mg/kg intravenously [IV] followed by 10 to 200 mcg/kg/min IV), or vasodilators such as nitroprusside (0.5 to 5 mcg/kg/min IV), may be necessary to maintain normal hemodynamics (see Chapters 47 and 159). Some human reports advocate magnesium sulfate for vasodilation during surgery for pheochromocytoma, although this has not been investigated in dogs.[33] Supraventricular tachycardia (SVT) is a common arrhythmia during surgery, although bradycardia with atrioventricular block and ventricular premature complexes have also been reported. Lidocaine may be used to treat ventricular arrhythmias (see Chapter 171). Before surgery, blood type and crossmatch to multiple units of packed red blood cells or fresh whole blood should be performed in case of severe intraoperative hemorrhage. Blood pressure during anesthesia in the hypertensive animal should be maintained at levels close to its resting blood pressure to prevent renal hypoperfusion, and urine output should be measured intraoperatively. If a venotomy is anticipated for removal of a thrombus, external cooling of the patient may be of benefit to protect tissues during intraoperative interruption of blood flow and ischemia.[22] Surgical manipulation of the tumor may cause catecholamine release. Alternatively, removal of the tumor may result in cardiovascular collapse from lack of catecholamines, requiring supplementation with sympathomimetic drugs such as phenylephrine (0.5 to 5 mcg/kg/min IV) or norepinephrine (0.1 to 2 mcg/kg/min IV) (see Chapter 157).

Surgical Excision

Surgery is often complicated and may necessitate vena caval venotomy or nephrectomy to fully remove or debulk the tumor. A recent study of 60 dogs with adrenal tumors found perioperative mortality rates of 6% for dogs undergoing elective adrenalectomy and 50% for dogs undergoing emergency adrenalectomy because of acute adrenal hemorrhage.[13] Adrenal tumor size and acute hemorrhage were predictive of perioperative mortality.[13] In another study of 41 dogs undergoing adrenalectomy, intraoperative mortality was 4.8% and preoperative hypokalemia or elevation in BUN along with concurrent nephrectomy were associated with shorter survival times.[30] A thorough abdominal exploration is recommended during surgery to identify gross metastatic disease. In a study of 61 dogs, 15% showed metastasis and 39% had locally invasive tumors.[8] In this study, concurrent neoplasia of various cellular origins was identified in 54% of the dogs.

Postoperative Monitoring and Complications

Many dogs experience significant complications during the first 24 to 72 hours postoperatively.[13,22,35] In a study of 60 dogs with adrenal tumors, 30% developed postoperative complications including hypotension, bradycardia, ventricular arrhythmias, tachypnea, vomiting, and cardiopulmonary arrest.[13] In another study of dogs with adrenal tumors, 51% (20 of 39) experienced postoperative complications after resection. These included ventricular tachyarrhythmias, dyspnea, disseminated intravascular coagulopathy, abdominal incisional dehiscence, internal hemorrhage, and vomiting.[22] One dog in this group experienced refractory hypertension after removal of the pheochromocytoma. Tumor type (adrenocortical versus pheochromocytoma) or presence of caval thrombi was not related to complications. Of the 11 dogs with pheochromocytomas in this study, seven experienced perioperative morbidity after resection of the tumor.[22] In another study of 52 dogs with adrenalectomy, 15% (8 of 30) died in the first 10 days after surgery from complications including refractory hypotension, pulmonary thromboembolism, acute kidney injury, acute pancreatitis, and cardiac arrest.[31,35]

Postoperatively, hypertension may or may not resolve, even with full excision of the tumor.[7] If bilateral adrenalectomy has been performed, supplementation with glucocorticoids and mineralocorticoids will be necessary. Postoperative hypotension or cardiovascular collapse is possible, and a decreased sensitivity to catecholamines from chronic stimulation may require noncatecholamine pressors such as vasopressin to maintain adequate blood pressure (see Chapter 158).[34] Blood glucose should be monitored postoperatively because removal of sympathetic stimulation may cause hypoglycemia.

Functional adrenocortical tumors may be associated with pulmonary thromboembolic disease; however, the association with pheochromocytomas is unclear. If an animal is suspected to be hypercoagulable, postoperative anticoagulation (i.e., heparin) may be indicated. See Chapter 168 for further details.

Medical Treatment

Symptomatic animals with pheochromocytomas that are nonresectable or metastatic may benefit from medical treatment with phenoxybenzamine, oral β-blockers, or other antiarrhythmic agents. β-Blockers should not be administered without concurrent α-blockade, because the loss of β_2 receptor–mediated vasodilation may exacerbate hypertension. Other therapy directed more specifically toward the clinical signs (e.g., diuretics to treat ascites) may also be indicated. Chemotherapeutic or radiotherapeutic treatment of pheochromocytoma in small animals has not been reported; however, they have been unrewarding in human medicine.[5]

PROGNOSIS

As more information regarding pheochromocytoma and its treatment becomes available in veterinary medicine, advances in diagnosis and treatment suggest that prognosis is guarded, although patients that survive surgery and the immediate postoperative period can have good survival times. In one study, factors associated with improved 10-day survival postoperatively included younger age, lack of intraoperative arrhythmias, shorter surgical time, and preoperative treatment with phenoxybenzamine.[9] Multiple studies suggest that factors associated with a poorer prognosis in dogs may include neurologic deficits, weight loss, abdominal distention, acute hemorrhage caused by tumor rupture, adrenal gland tumors with major axis length 5 cm or larger, larger tumors with invasion of neighboring structures, documented metastasis, and venous thrombosis.[13,25,31,35] In humans, histopathologic analysis that shows multiploidy (e.g., aneuploidy or tetraploidy) in the nuclear DNA of the tumor cells has been associated with a poorer prognosis.[36]

With complete resection and uneventful recovery from surgery, even dogs with vena caval thrombi may experience significant survival times, reported from 18 months to 4 years.[2,8,13, 22,35, 37] Recurrence of clinical signs or tumor-related death was not reported in the nine dogs that survived surgical resection of pheochromocytomas in the study by Kyles et al (median follow-up time was 9 months; range 1 to 36 months).[22] In the two most recent studies of all adrenal tumors in dogs, median survival times after adrenalectomy were 492 days for dogs that survived the postoperative period and 375 days overall (Lang, 60 cases) and 953 days (Massari, 52 cases), respectively.[13,35] Therefore recurrence of primary tumor or of metastatic disease appears to be rare in the limited studies currently available.[8]

REFERENCES

1. In Feldman EC, Nelson RW: Canine and feline endocrinology and reproduction, ed 3, St Louis, 2004, WB Saunders.
2. Maher ER Jr, McNeil EA: Pheochromocytoma in dogs and cats, Vet Clin North Am Small Anim Pract 27:359, 1997.
3. Barthez PY, Nyland TG, Feldman EC: Ultrasonographic evaluation of the adrenal glands in dogs, J Am Vet Med Assoc 207:1180, 1995.
4. Mansmann G, Lau J, Balk E: The clinically inapparent adrenal mass: update in diagnosis and management, Endocr Rev 25:309, 2004.
5. Platt SR, Sheppard BJ, Graham J, et al: Pheochromocytoma in the vertebral canal of two dogs, J Am Anim Hosp Assoc 34:365, 1998.
6. Santamarina G, Espino L, Vila M, et al: Aortic thromboembolism and retroperitoneal hemorrhage associated with a pheochromocytoma in a dog, J Vet Intern Med 17:917, 2003.
7. Gilson SD, Withrow SF, Wheeler SL, et al: Pheochromocytoma in 50 dogs, J Vet Intern Med 8:228, 1994.
8. Barthez PY, Marks SL, Woo J, et al: Pheochromocytoma in dogs: 61 cases (1984-1995), J Vet Intern Med 11:272, 1997.
9. Herrera MA, Mehl ML, Kass PH, et al: Predictive factors and the effect of phenoxybenzamine on outcome in dogs undergoing adrenalectomy for pheochromocytoma. J Vet Emerg Crit Care 2008; 22:1333.
10. Brown AJ, Alwood AJ, Cole SG: Malignant pheochromocytoma presenting as a bradyarrhythmia in a dog, J Vet Emerg Crit Care 17:164, 2007.
11. Schoeman JP, Stidworthy MF: Budd-Chiari–like syndrome associated with an adrenal pheochromocytoma in a dog, J Small Anim Pract 42:191, 2001.
12. Bouayad H, Feeney DA, Caywood DD, et al: Pheochromocytoma in dogs: 13 cases (1980-1985), J Am Vet Med Assoc 191:1610, 1987.
13. Lang JM, Schertel E, Kennedy S: Elective and emergency surgical management of adrenal gland tumors: 60 cases (1999-2006), J Am Anim Hosp Assoc 47:428, 2011.
14. vonDehn BJ, Nelson RW, Feldman EC, et al: Pheochromocytoma and hyperadrenocorticism in dogs: six cases (1982-1992), J Am Vet Med Assoc 207:322, 1995.
15. Whittemore JC, Preston CA, Kyles AE, et al: Nontraumatic rupture of an adrenal gland tumor causing intraabdominal or retroperitoneal hemorrhage in four dogs, J Am Vet Med Assoc 219:329, 2001.
16. Williams JE, Hackner SG: Pheochromocytoma presenting as acute retroperitoneal hemorrhage in a dog, J Vet Emerg Crit Care 11(3):221, 2001.
17. Evans K, Hosgood G, Boon GD, et al: Hemoperitoneum secondary to traumatic rupture of an adrenal tumor in a dog, J Am Vet Med Assoc 198:278, 1991.
18. Patnaik AK, Erlandson RA, Lieberman PH, et al: Extraadrenal pheochromocytoma (paraganglioma) in a cat, J Am Vet Med Assoc 197:104, 1990.
19. Gunn-Moore D: Feline endocrinopathies, Vet Clin North Am Small Anim Pract 35:171, 2005.
20. Calsyn J, Green RA, Davis GJ, et al: Adrenal pheochromocytoma with contralateral adrenocortical adenoma in a cat, J Am Anim Hosp Assoc 46:36, 2010.
21. Rosenstein DS: Diagnostic imaging in canine pheochromocytoma, Vet Radiol Ultrasound 41:499, 2000.
22. Kyles A, Feldman E, De Cock H, et al: Surgical management of adrenal gland tumor with and without associated tumor thrombi in 40 dogs (1994-2001), J Am Vet Med Assoc 223:654, 2003.
23. Besso JG, Penninck DG, Gliatto JM: Retrospective ultrasonographic evaluation of adrenal lesions in 26 dogs, Vet Radiol Ultrasound 38:448, 1997.
24. Prager G, Heinz-Peer G, Passler C, et al: Can dynamic gadolinium-enhanced magnetic resonance imaging with chemical shift studies predict the status of adrenal masses? World J Surg 26:958, 2002.
25. Schultz RM, Wisner ER, Johnson EG, et al: Contrast-enhanced computed tomography as a preoperative indicator of vascular invasion from adrenal masses in dogs, Vet Radiol Ultrasound 2009;50:625.
26. Wright KN, Breitschwerdt EB, Feldman JM, et al: Diagnostic and therapeutic considerations in a hypercalcemic dog with multiple endocrine neoplasia, J Am Anim Hosp Assoc 31:156, 1995.
27. Head LL, Daniel GB: Scintigraphic diagnosis: an unusual presentation of metastatic pheochromocytoma in a dog, Vet Radiol Ultrasound 45:574, 2004.
28. Berry CR, DeGrado TR, Nutter F, et al: Imaging of pheochromocytoma in 2 dogs using p-[18F] fluorobenzylguanidine, Vet Radiol Ultrasound 43:183, 2002.
29. Quante S, Boretti FS, Kook Ph, et al: Urinary catecholamine and metanephrine to creatinine ratios in dogs with hyperadrenocorticism or pheochromocytoma, and in healthy dogs, J Vet Intern Med 24:1093, 2010.
30. Wimpole JA, Adagra CF, Billson MF, et al: Plasma free metanephrines in healthy cats, cats with non-adrenal disease and a cat with suspected phaeochromocytoma, J Fel Med Surg 12:435, 2010.
31. Schwartz P, Kovak JR, Koprowski A, et al: Evaluation of prognostic factors in the surgical treatment of adrenal gland tumors in dogs: 41 cases (1999-2005), J Am Vet Med Assoc 232:77, 2008.
32. Kinney MAO, Narr BJ, Warner MA: Perioperative management of pheochromocytoma, J Cardiothorac Vasc Anesth 16:359, 2002.
33. James MF, Cronje L: Pheochromocytoma crisis: the use of magnesium sulfate, Anesth Analg 99:680, 2004.
34. Augoustides JG, Abrams M, Berkowitz D, et al: Vasopressin for hemodynamic rescue in catecholamine-resistant vasoplegic shock after resection of massive pheochromocytoma, Anesthesiology 101:1022, 2004.
35. Massari F, Nicoli S, Romanelli G, et al: Adrenalectomy in dogs with adrenal gland tumors: 52 cases (2002-2008), J Am Vet Med Assoc 239:216, 2011.
36. Nativ O, Grant CS, Sheps SG, et al: The clinical significance of nuclear DNA ploidy pattern in 184 patients with pheochromocytoma, Cancer 69:2683, 1992.
37. Guillaumot PJ, Heripret D, Bouvy BM, et al: 49-month survival following caval venectomy without nephrectomy in a dog with a pheochromocytoma, J Am Anim Hosp Assoc 2012;48:352.

CHAPTER 72

CRITICAL ILLNESS–RELATED CORTICOSTEROID INSUFFICIENCY

Jamie M. Burkitt Creedon, DVM, DACVECC

KEY POINTS

- Cortisol is involved in modulation of inflammation and regulation of vascular tone.
- Critical illness–related corticosteroid insufficiency (CIRCI) occurs in some individuals with severe sepsis, septic shock, and other types of critical illness.
- Critically ill human patients with poor hypothalamic-pituitary-adrenal (HPA) axis function have decreased survival compared with those with normal HPA axis function.
- Low dosages of hydrocortisone improve pressor responsiveness and may improve survival in human patients with pressor-resistant septic shock.
- The best method for diagnosing CIRCI is unknown.
- CIRCI likely occurs in a subpopulation of critically ill dogs and cats.
- Appropriate methods for the diagnosis and management of CIRCI in dogs and cats are unknown.

A syndrome of critical illness–related corticosteroid insufficiency (CIRCI) has been described in critically ill human beings. It is probably best described at this time as the improved pressor responsiveness and more rapid pressor weaning seen in some human patients with septic shock who are treated with low doses of hydrocortisone (usually 200 mg/day/adult human). The syndrome was formerly called relative adrenal insufficiency (RAI). *Critical illness–related corticosteroid insufficiency* is probably a more appropriate term because some studies suggest that some critically ill people benefit from corticosteroid therapy even if they are not adrenally "insufficient" based on plasma hormone tests; because there is no standard describing what constitutes adrenal insufficiency in this setting; and because many patients with CIRCI appear to have impaired cellular response to cortisol rather than inadequate production of it. Critical illness–related corticosteroid insufficiency has been reported most commonly and investigated most thoroughly in humans with septic shock,[1-5] which is defined as hypotension despite adequate fluid loading that is due to systemic inflammation from an infectious underlying cause.[6] CIRCI has also been described in patients with nonseptic critical illnesses including acute myocardial infarction,[7] hepatic failure,[8] severe pancreatitis,[9,10] burns,[11] and others.[12,13] Despite more than two decades of investigation of corticosteroid insufficiency in critical illness, significant debate in the human critical care community remains regarding CIRCI's underlying pathophysiology, identification, and treatment.[14-16] Currently, most prominent experts in the human critical care world seem to agree that *something* is going on with endogenous corticosteroid production or responsiveness in many human patients with septic shock and other severe illness. Accordingly, the most recent Surviving Sepsis Campaign guidelines recommend the use of low-dose hydrocortisone in septic shock patients who remain hypotensive despite pressor therapy,[17] even if the community still doesn't fully understand the pathophysiology of CIRCI or how to identify patients with it.

BACKGROUND

Modern investigations of CIRCI were prompted when several different researchers documented associations between altered hypothalamic-pituitary-adrenal (HPA) axis function and adverse events in critically ill patients.[4,18-20] Interest in the topic increased as some groups demonstrated improved pressor responsiveness or shock reversal in septic shock patients treated with low-dose hydrocortisone,[21,22] particularly in those with blunted cortisol response to corticotropin.[23-25] In 2002, Annane et al reported results from an investigation of 300 people with septic shock ("the French study"). In this study, people with blunted response to corticotropin treated with a combination of low-dose hydrocortisone (200 mg/day) and fludrocortisone (50 mcg/day) had improved survival, whereas those with an adequate response to corticotropin did not benefit from steroids.[1] In 2008, results of the Corticosteroid Therapy of Septic Shock (CORTICUS) trial were published. With 499 human septic shock patients included, CORTICUS is to date the largest published investigation regarding the use of hydrocortisone in the treatment of septic shock.[5] The CORTICUS trial found more rapid shock reversal in patients treated with hydrocortisone than in those treated with placebo, regardless of ACTH stimulation test results. There was no survival difference between patients treated with hydrocortisone and those treated with placebo, regardless of corticotropin responsiveness, and the steroid-treated group experienced more episodes of superinfection.

There has been much speculation in the critical care community attempting to explain the differences between the French study's results and those of CORTICUS, and authors are critical of many aspects of both studies. Differences between the French study and CORTICUS that have been implicated for poor agreement include differences in illness severity, timing of subject enrollment, percent of subjects receiving etomidate, and hydrocortisone treatment regimen.[14,26-32] Additionally, CORTICUS likely suffered from selection bias, failed to meet its enrollment target of 800 subjects, and is thus underpowered—the suggestion being that clinicians were reluctant to enroll subjects in CORTICUS to ensure that their septic shock patients received corticosteroids.[14,33,34]

Since 2008, relatively little new information has been published regarding CIRCI in people. The results of a preplanned analysis of secondary outcome data from the CORTICUS trial were published in 2011 and showed a decrease in Sequential Organ Failure Assessment (SOFA) score in patients treated with low-dose hydrocortisone compared with placebo, primarily because of improvements in cardiovascular and hepatic scores for those treated with steroids.[35]

Comments and editorials still appear in the human critical care literature regarding the most appropriate way to interpret CORTICUS and other available data regarding CIRCI.[14,36] At this time, there are many more questions than answers regarding specific underlying pathophysiology, appropriate nomenclature, diagnosis, and treatment of the syndrome.

SUSPECTED PATHOPHYSIOLOGY

Cortisol is a hormone released by the adrenal glands in small amounts in a circadian rhythm and in larger amounts during times of physiologic stress. It has many important homeostatic functions including regulation of carbohydrate, lipid, and protein metabolism; immune system modulation; ensuring proper production of catecholamines and function of adrenergic receptors; and stabilizing cell membranes. Serum cortisol concentration is determined by the hormonal cascade and negative feedback mechanisms of the hypothalamic-pituitary-adrenal (HPA) axis. The hypothalamus produces corticotropin-releasing hormone (CRH), which stimulates the anterior pituitary to release adrenocorticotropic hormone (ACTH). ACTH in circulation stimulates the zona fasciculata and zona reticularis of the adrenal gland to produce and release cortisol. Cortisol has negative feedback action on both the hypothalamic release of CRH and the pituitary release of ACTH. Thus, when circulating cortisol concentration is low, CRH and ACTH will increase, stimulating the adrenal glands to produce more cortisol. The increased serum cortisol concentration inhibits the release of more CRH and ACTH.

Once in circulation, most cortisol is bound to corticosteroid-binding globulin (CBG). Cortisol not CBG-bound is called "free cortisol," which is the biologically active cortisol fraction. Free cortisol enters target cells and binds the glucocorticoid receptor (GR) in the cytoplasm. The GR-cortisol complex translocates into the nucleus, where it affects gene transcription and ultimately cell function.

The underlying pathophysiology of CIRCI is unknown and is likely a complex combination of altered hypothalamic, pituitary, adrenal, hormonal, enzymatic, and receptor function.[15,37] Trauma, infarction, or medications can impair hypothalamic or pituitary function, thus preventing adequate CRH or ACTH production. Infarction, medications (e.g., etomidate or ketoconazole), hemorrhage from coagulopathy, or cytokines can impair adrenal synthesis of cortisol. Systemic inflammation causes decreased CBG concentration and causes dissociation of cortisol from CBG, increasing the percentage of circulating cortisol that is biologically active. Intracellular enzymes and the GR are also affected by cytokines, which can lead to a nonlinear relationship between plasma cortisol concentration and cortisol's tissue activity in critical illness. The combination of abnormalities in corticosteroid production and function may differ from individual to individual, complicating recognition of patients that may benefit from corticosteroid treatment. For instance, a patient could appear corticosteroid sufficient with standard plasma tests and still have inadequate tissue cortisol activity because of cytokines' effects on the GR.

CLINICAL MANIFESTATIONS

The most common clinical abnormality associated with CIRCI in humans with septic shock is pressor-resistant hypotension. Critically ill dogs with poor response to exogenous ACTH appear more likely to be hypotensive than those with more robust response.[38,39] Studies have shown that CIRCI is associated with poor pressor responsiveness in human patients that is restored with glucocorticoid administration.[5,23] There is one report each of a dog and a cat in septic shock in which pressors could be discontinued after addition of hydrocortisone to the treatment plan.[40,41] In vitro studies have shown that smooth muscle adrenergic receptor expression is modulated by glucocorticoids.[42,43] One human clinical study showed that myocardial adrenergic receptor downregulation in shock could be reversed by glucocorticoids.[44] Another study investigating the phenylephrine–mean arterial pressure relationship in humans with septic shock showed that physiologic dosages of hydrocortisone normalized vasomotor response to the drug,[45] underscoring the clinical importance of glucocorticoids in smooth muscle response to catecholamines.

Human patients with CIRCI may be more likely to die than those with similar illness severity and an intact HPA axis.[18,20,46] One study in septic dogs suggests that those with CIRCI are more likely to die than those with normal HPA function.[38]

DIAGNOSIS OF CIRCI

There is uncertainty in the human medical community regarding the definitive identification of patients with CIRCI. Continued uncertainty probably persists because pathophysiologic mechanisms likely differ by individual. At this time, the standard 250 mcg ACTH stimulation test is the method recommended to diagnose HPA axis abnormality in critically ill humans,[47] but it fails to identify patients whose corticosteroid insufficiency stems from tissue cortisol activity problems. The largest study on CIRCI in humans found no relationship between plasma cortisol testing and benefit from hydrocortisone therapy in pressor-resistant septic shock.[5] Thus the 2013 Surviving Sepsis Campaign guidelines suggest not using ACTH stimulation testing to identify which patients should be treated with hydrocortisone.[17] Nevertheless, some authors still believe that ACTH stimulation testing should be used to identify patients that would benefit from corticosteroid replacement.[48] The current recommendation in humans is to treat any pressor-resistant septic shock patient with low-dose hydrocortisone and monitor for decreased pressor requirements[17,47]; if improvement is seen, the implication seems to be that the patient has CIRCI, regardless of plasma hormone concentrations.

Moreover, the best way to identify critically ill patients who would benefit from corticosteroid replacement therapy is unclear. It is unknown for any individual exactly how much cortisol is needed or optimal for a given severity of illness, and the relationship between plasma cortisol and tissue cortisol activity is murky, particularly in critical illness.

Veterinary Data

No clinical veterinary studies have been performed to determine how best to identify CIRCI in dogs and cats. We performed a study to determine whether CIRCI occurs in dogs with sepsis using a standard 1-hour 250-mcg ACTH stimulation test.[38] Dogs with delta-cortisol 3 mcg/dl or less were significantly more likely to be hypotensive and had significantly decreased survival compared with dogs with delta-cortisol greater than 3 mcg/dl. Martin et al investigated HPA axis function in dogs with sepsis, severe trauma, or gastric dilation-volvulus.[39] The investigators performed 1-hour ACTH stimulation tests using 5 mcg/kg cosyntropin and found that dogs with delta-cortisol 3 mcg/dl or less were significantly more likely to receive vasopressors than dogs with delta-cortisol greater than 3 mcg/dl. Further study of larger populations of critically ill dogs is required to determine the best way to diagnose CIRCI in this population.

The studies performed in cats have used basal cortisol concentrations, stimulated cortisol concentrations, and delta-cortisol values. The ACTH stimulation test was performed using 125 mcg synthetic ACTH injected intravenously with samples collected 1 hour later for determination of poststimulated cortisol concentration.[49,50] A cutoff value for CIRCI was not proposed in either study, but Costello and colleagues found that septic cats had a mean delta-cortisol value of

2.3 mcg/dl (standard deviation [SD] ± 2.5 mcg/dl), whereas the mean delta-cortisol concentration in normal cats was 6.5 mcg/dl (SD ± 4.6).[50] Note that although the mean delta-cortisol value in septic cats was significantly lower than that in normal cats, the ranges likely overlap. There is a report of a critically ill cat with pressor-dependent hypotension in which hypotension resolved within 24 hours of glucocorticoid administration; this cat had an ACTH-stimulated delta-cortisol of 3.2 mcg/dl.[41] Although CIRCI appears to occur in cats, precise diagnostic criteria are undetermined.

For all species, it is unclear whether plasma hormone concentrations or HPA axis testing are related to the improved pressor responsiveness seen when some individuals are treated with hydrocortisone. It is possible, for example, that altered HPA axis function is a marker of disease severity and that the improved blood pressure seen with corticosteroid therapy is unrelated to HPA axis function. These remain hotly contested issues that may be resolved in the next decade. For now, CIRCI seems to be a diagnosis made by gauging response to therapy.

TREATMENT OF CIRCI

There are currently two consensus statements available regarding the treatment of human patients with CIRCI.[17,47] Both statements recommend against the use of hydrocortisone in septic shock patients unless they are poorly responsive to fluid therapy and vasopressor treatment, and both statements recommend hydrocortisone use in this patient set *regardless of basal or stimulated plasma hormone concentrations.* Marik et al recommend hydrocortisone be given either as four divided doses daily (50 mg/adult human every 6 hours, to total 200 mg/adult human/day), or as a dose of 100 mg hydrocortisone followed by 10 mg/hr as a continuous intravenous infusion (240 mg/adult human/day).[47] The 2013 Surviving Sepsis Campaign guidelines recommend 200 mg hydrocortisone/adult human/day as a continuous intravenous infusion.[17] Both groups recommend tapering the hydrocortisone over a few days rather than stopping abruptly.

Veterinary Data

There is little clinical evidence to determine whether dogs and cats with CIRCI would benefit from low-dosage steroid supplementation. One small study found no difference in survival of dogs with septic shock treated with hydrocortisone versus placebo,[51] though cases have been published that report pressor weaning in septic shock after administration of hydrocortisone.[40,41] At the author's hospital, dogs and cats with fluid-loaded, pressor-refractory septic shock are treated at the clinician's discretion with 2.5 to 3 mg/kg/day of hydrocortisone as a constant rate intravenous infusion, after undergoing a standard 1-hour ACTH stimulation test. It seems reasonable to continue steroid therapy only in patients that show significant improvement in cardiovascular status within 24 hours of starting the drug. We have poor clinical evidence to support the use of steroids in dogs and cats. Figure 72-1 provides an algorithm for clinical decision making in pressor-refractory septic shock.

PROGNOSIS

Human patients with CIRCI have a worse prognosis than those without corticosteroid insufficiency. However, with supplemental hydrocortisone therapy, patients with CIRCI may have the same prognosis as those with normal HPA axis function and the same severity of illness.[1] If the patient survives the primary underlying illness, prognosis for return of normal HPA axis function is good.[52]

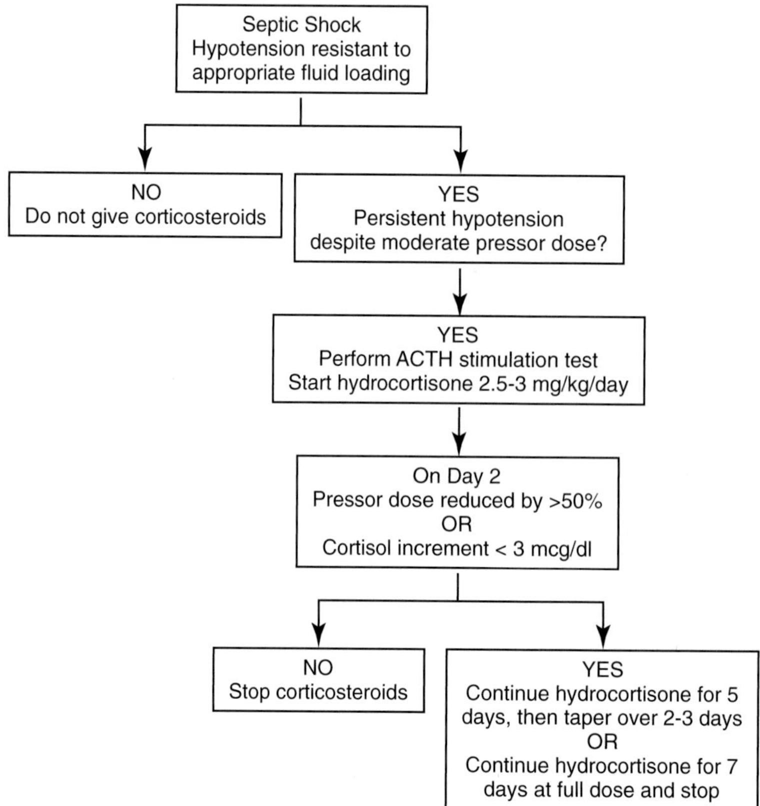

FIGURE 72-1 Decision tree for practical use of corticosteroids in dogs and cats with septic shock. *(Adapted from Annane D: Corticosteroids for severe sepsis: an evidence-based guide for physicians, Ann Intensive Care 1:7, 2011).*

REFERENCES

1. Annane D, Sebille V, Charpentier C, et al: Effect of treatment with low doses of hydrocortisone and fludrocortisone on mortality in patients with septic shock, JAMA 288:862, 2002.
2. Marik PE, Zaloga GP: Adrenal insufficiency during septic shock, Crit Care Med 31:141, 2003.
3. Manglik S, Flores E, Lubarsky L, et al: Glucocorticoid insufficiency in patients who present to the hospital with severe sepsis: a prospective clinical trial, Crit Care Med 31:1668, 2003.
4. Soni A, Pepper GM, Wyrwinski PM, et al: Adrenal insufficiency occurring during septic shock: incidence, outcome, and relationship to peripheral cytokine levels, Am J Med 98:266, 1995.
5. Sprung CL, Annane D, Keh D, et al: Hydrocortisone therapy for patients with septic shock, N Engl J Med 358:111, 2008.
6. Bone RC, Balk RA, Cerra FB, et al: American College of Chest Physicians/Society of Critical Care Medicine Consensus Conference: definitions for sepsis and organ failure and guidelines for the use of innovative therapies in sepsis, Crit Care Med 20:864, 1992.
7. Chang SS, Liaw SJ, Bullard MJ, et al: Adrenal insufficiency in critically ill emergency department patients: a Taiwan preliminary study, Acad Emerg Med 8:761, 2001.
8. Marik PE, Gayowski T, Starzl TE: The hepatoadrenal syndrome: a common yet unrecognized clinical condition, Crit Care Med 33:1254, 2005.
9. De Waele JJ, Hoste E, Decruyenaere J, et al: Adrenal insufficiency in severe acute pancreatitis, Pancreas 27:244, 2003.
10. De Waele JJ, Hoste EA, Baert D, et al: Relative adrenal insufficiency in patients with severe acute pancreatitis, Intensive Care Med 33:1754, 2007.
11. Graves KK, Faraklas I, Cochran A: Identification of risk factors associated with critical illness related corticosteroid insufficiency in burn patients, J Burn Care Res 33:330, 2012.
12. Bruno JJ, Hernandez M, Ghosh S, et al: Critical illness-related corticosteroid insufficiency in cancer patients, Support Care Cancer 20:1159, 2012.
13. Ho HC, Chapital AD, Yu M: Hypothyroidism and adrenal insufficiency in sepsis and hemorrhagic shock, Arch Surg 139:1199, 2004.
14. Marik PE: Glucocorticoids in sepsis: dissecting facts from fiction, Crit Care 15:158, 2011.
15. Venkatesh B, Cohen J: Adrenocortical (dys)function in septic shock—a sick euadrenal state, Best Pract Res Clin Endocrinol Metab 25:719, 2011.
16. Hsu JL, Liu V, Patterson AJ, et al: Potential for overuse of corticosteroids and vasopressin in septic shock, Crit Care 16:447, 2012.
17. Dellinger RP, Levy MM, Rhodes A, et al: Surviving Sepsis Campaign: international guidelines for management of severe sepsis and septic shock, 2012, Intensive Care Med 39:165, 2013.
18. Rothwell PM, Udwadia ZF, Lawler PG: Cortisol response to corticotropin and survival in septic shock, Lancet 337:582, 1991.
19. Span LF, Hermus AR, Bartelink AK, et al: Adrenocortical function: an indicator of severity of disease and survival in chronic critically ill patients, Intensive Care Med 18:93, 1992.
20. Annane D, Sebille V, Troche G, et al: A 3-level prognostic classification in septic shock based on cortisol levels and cortisol response to corticotrophin, JAMA 283:1038, 2000.
21. Bollaert PE, Charpentier C, Levy B, et al: Reversal of late septic shock with supraphysiologic doses of hydrocortisone, Crit Care Med 26:645, 1998.
22. Briegel J, Forst H, Haller M, et al: Stress doses of hydrocortisone reverse hyperdynamic septic shock: a prospective, randomized, double-blind, single-center study, Crit Care Med 27:723, 1999.
23. Annane D, Bellissant E, Sebille V, et al: Impaired pressor sensitivity to noradrenaline in septic shock patients with and without impaired adrenal function reserve, Br J Clin Pharmacol 46:589, 1998.
24. Oppert M, Reinicke A, Graf KJ, et al: Plasma cortisol levels before and during "low-dose" hydrocortisone therapy and their relationship to hemodynamic improvement in patients with septic shock, Intensive Care Med 26:1747, 2000.
25. Rivers EP, Gaspari M, Saad GA, et al: Adrenal insufficiency in high-risk surgical ICU patients, Chest 119:889, 2001.
26. Daley MR: Corticosteroids for septic shock, N Engl J Med 358:2068; author reply 2070, 2008.
27. Seam N: Corticosteroids for septic shock, N Engl J Med 358:2068; author reply 2070, 2008.
28. Luboshitzky R, Qupti G: Corticosteroids for septic shock, N Engl J Med 358:2069; author reply 2070, 2008.
29. Bollaert PE: Corticosteroids for septic shock, N Engl J Med 358:2069; author reply 2070, 2008.
30. Marik PE, Pastores SM, Kavanagh BP: Corticosteroids for septic shock, N Engl J Med 358:2069; author reply 2070, 2008.
31. Manoach S: Corticosteroids for septic shock, N Engl J Med 358:2070; author reply 2070, 2008.
32. Dellinger RP: Steroid therapy of septic shock: the decision is in the eye of the beholder, Crit Care Med 36:1987, 2008.
33. Chaudhury P, Marshall JC, Solomkin JS: CAGS and ACS evidence based reviews in surgery. 35: Efficacy and safety of low-dose hydrocortisone therapy in the treatment of septic shock, Can J Surg 53:415, 2010.
34. Lamontagne F, Meade MO: Low-dose hydrocortisone did not improve survival in patients with septic shock but reversed shock earlier, ACP J Club 148:6, 2008.
35. Moreno R, Sprung CL, Annane D, et al: Time course of organ failure in patients with septic shock treated with hydrocortisone: results of the Corticus study, Intensive Care Med 37:1765, 2011.
36. Sprung CL, Annane D, Singer M, et al: Glucocorticoids in sepsis: dissecting facts from fiction, Crit Care 15:446, 2011.
37. Cooper MS, Stewart PM: Corticosteroid insufficiency in acutely ill patients, N Engl J Med 348:727, 2003.
38. Burkitt JM, Haskins SC, Nelson RW, et al: Relative adrenal insufficiency in dogs with sepsis, J Vet Intern Med 21:226, 2007.
39. Martin LG, Groman RP, Fletcher DJ, et al: Pituitary-adrenal function in dogs with acute critical illness, J Am Vet Med Assoc 233:87, 2008.
40. Peyton JL, Burkitt JM: Critical illness-related corticosteroid insufficiency in a dog with septic shock, J Vet Emerg Crit Care (San Antonio) 19:262, 2009.
41. Durkan S, de Laforcade A, Rozanski E, et al: Suspected relative adrenal insufficiency in a critically ill cat, J Vet Emerg Crit Care 17:197, 2007.
42. Sakaue M, Hoffman BB: Glucocorticoids induce transcription and expression of the alpha 1B adrenergic receptor gene in DTT1 MF-2 smooth muscle cells, J Clin Invest 88:385, 1991.
43. Collins S, Caron MG, Lefkowitz RJ: Beta-adrenergic receptors in hamster smooth muscle cells are transcriptionally regulated by glucocorticoids, J Biol Chem 263:9067, 1988.
44. Saito T, Takanashi M, Gallagher E, et al: Corticosteroid effect on early beta-adrenergic down-regulation during circulatory shock: hemodynamic study and beta-adrenergic receptor assay, Intensive Care Med 21:204, 1995.
45. Bellissant E, Annane D: Effect of hydrocortisone on phenylephrine—mean arterial pressure dose-response relationship in septic shock, Clin Pharmacol Ther 68:293, 2000.
46. Schroeder S, Wichers M, Klingmuller D, et al: The hypothalamic-pituitary-adrenal axis of patients with severe sepsis: altered response to corticotropin-releasing hormone, Crit Care Med 29:310, 2001.
47. Marik PE, Pastores SM, Annane D, et al: Recommendations for the diagnosis and management of corticosteroid insufficiency in critically ill adult patients: consensus statements from an international task force by the American College of Critical Care Medicine, Crit Care Med 36:1937, 2008.
48. Annane D: Corticosteroids for severe sepsis: an evidence-based guide for physicians, Ann Intensive Care 1:7, 2011.
49. Prittie JE, Barton LJ, Peterson ME, et al: Hypothalamo-pituitary-adrenal (HPA) axis function in critically ill cats, J Vet Emerg Crit Care 13:165, 2003.
50. Costello MF, Fletcher DJ, Silverstein DC, et al: Adrenal insufficiency in feline sepsis. In: ACVECC postgraduate course 2006: sepsis in veterinary medicine, 2006, p 41.
51. Burkitt Creedon JM, Hopper K: Low-dose hydrocortisone in dogs with septic shock In 17th International Veterinary Emergency and Critical Care Symposium 2011, p 736.
52. Briegel J, Schelling G, Haller M, et al: A comparison of the adrenocortical response during septic shock and after complete recovery, Intensive Care Med 22:894, 1996.

CHAPTER 73

HYPOADRENOCORTICISM

Jamie M. Burkitt Creedon, DVM, DACVECC

KEY POINTS

- Hypoadrenocorticism (Addison's disease) is uncommon in dogs and rare in cats.
- Primary hypoadrenocorticism is due to failure of the adrenal glands, whereas secondary hypoadrenocorticism is due to pituitary or hypothalamic malfunction.
- Young to middle-aged female dogs are predisposed.
- Certain breeds are overrepresented, but most dogs with Addison's disease are of mixed breeding.
- Diagnosis is challenging because signs and clinicopathologic findings of hypoadrenocorticism mimic many other disease processes.
- Definitive diagnosis is by adrenocorticotropic hormone (ACTH) stimulation test, ideally coupled with an endogenous ACTH concentration.
- Treatment of the animal in crisis consists of aggressive, appropriate fluid resuscitation followed by hormone replacement.
- Hyperkalemia leading to electrocardiographic (ECG) changes can be life threatening and must be treated promptly and appropriately.
- Cats may require 3 to 5 days for a good clinical response to therapy.
- Long-term prognosis is very good with lifelong hormone supplementation.

The adrenal cortex is responsible for secreting many important hormones, including cortisol and aldosterone. Cortisol is a glucocorticoid released in small amounts in a circadian rhythm and in larger amounts during times of physiologic stress. It has many important homeostatic functions, including regulation of carbohydrate, lipid, and protein metabolism; modulation of immune system function; and ensuring proper production of catecholamines and function of adrenergic receptors. Serum cortisol concentration is determined by the hormonal cascade and negative feedback mechanisms of the hypothalamic-pituitary-adrenal axis. The hypothalamus produces corticotropin-releasing hormone (CRH), which stimulates the anterior pituitary to release adrenocorticotropic hormone (ACTH). ACTH in circulation stimulates the zona fasciculata and zona reticularis of the adrenal cortex to produce and release cortisol. Cortisol has negative feedback action on both the hypothalamic release of CRH and the pituitary release of ACTH. Thus, when circulating cortisol concentration is low, CRH and ACTH will increase, stimulating the adrenal glands to produce more cortisol. The increased serum cortisol concentration inhibits the release of more CRH and ACTH.

Aldosterone is a mineralocorticoid released from the zona glomerulosa of the adrenal cortex under the influence of a complex hormonal cascade that starts in the kidney. Its main purposes are to maintain normovolemia and enhance potassium excretion. When effective circulating volume is depleted, glomerular filtration decreases. The macula densa, a group of specialized cells in the distal portion of the thick ascending loop of Henle, senses decreased filtrate (specifically chloride) delivery. The macula densa then induces renin release from the nearby juxtaglomerular cells of the afferent arteriole serving that nephron. Renin cleaves the circulating hormone angiotensinogen into angiotensin I. Angiotensin I is then converted to angiotensin II by angiotensin-converting enzyme located in the lung, on endothelial cells throughout the body, and in many other organs. Angiotensin II stimulates the zona glomerulosa to release aldosterone, which stimulates cells of the renal collecting duct to reabsorb sodium and excrete potassium. Sodium reabsorption leads to water retention and thus augmentation of effective circulating volume. The adrenal cortex also releases a significant amount of aldosterone in response to hyperkalemia and a minimal amount in response to ACTH.

Hypoadrenocorticism, also called *Addison's disease,* is an uncommon disease in dogs and is rare in cats. Primary hypoadrenocorticism is caused by adrenal gland dysfunction, whereas secondary hypoadrenocorticism occurs when hypothalamic or pituitary malfunction prevents the release of CRH or ACTH, respectively. In most cases, patients with primary hypoadrenocorticism have both glucocorticoid and mineralocorticoid insufficiency. However, there are many reports of dogs with atypical primary hypoadrenocorticism who have only glucocorticoid insufficiency.[1-5] Dogs with atypical primary hypoadrenocorticism may develop mineralocorticoid deficiency within months of initial diagnosis.[1,2,4] Very rarely, mineralocorticoid deficiency may occur before glucocorticoid deficiency.[6] Because aldosterone release is mediated primarily by the renin-angiotensin cascade and serum potassium concentration, patients with secondary hypoadrenocorticism do not usually have the classic electrolyte abnormalities seen in patients with typical primary hypoadrenocorticism (see Clinicopathologic Findings).

WHO IS AFFECTED?

Hypoadrenocorticism usually occurs in young to middle-aged dogs, and females are reported to be more commonly affected than males.[2,4,7-11] Although the average age of onset is approximately 4 years,[4,5,7-11] naturally occurring hypoadrenocorticism has been documented in dogs as young as 2 months,[10] as well as in geriatric dogs. Dogs with only glucocorticoid deficiency may be older at time of onset than those with classic hypoadrenocorticism.[5] The most commonly affected pure breeds vary somewhat by report and include the Portuguese Water Dog, Great Dane, West Highland White Terrier, Standard Poodle, Wheaton Terrier, and Rottweiler.[7] It is important to note that mixed breed dogs are more commonly affected than any individual breed.[4,12] Primary hypoadrenocorticism is rare in cats. There appears to be no sex predilection in this species, and most are domestic shorthaired or longhaired cats.[4,13-19] Most cats are young to middle aged, with ages ranging from 1 to 14 years.[16,18] There is a single report of glucocorticoid-only hypoadrenocorticism in a cat.[18]

ETIOLOGY

The cause of naturally occurring primary hypoadrenocorticism in dogs and cats is unknown, but the most widely accepted theory is one of immune-mediated destruction of the adrenal cortices.[4,8] In support of this theory, young to middle-aged female dogs are most commonly affected by both Addison's disease and established immune-mediated diseases, and naturally occurring primary hypoadrenocorticism in humans is caused by immune-mediated destruction of the adrenal cortices. On necropsy, adrenal glands of affected animals are atrophied and fibrosed, consistent with prior immune-mediated destruction.[4,8,14,16] Other documented causes of primary hypoadrenocorticism in dogs and cats include adrenal neoplastic infiltration,[20,21] trauma,[22] suspected hemorrhage or hypoperfusion,[23] and iatrogenic destruction caused by mitotane[24] or trilostane[25-28] therapy for hyperadrenocorticism. Adrenal infiltration with infectious organisms has also been implicated.[4]

Secondary hypoadrenocorticism is due to hypothalamic or pituitary malfunction; decreased CRH or ACTH secretion causes decreased adrenal cortisol production. The most common cause of secondary hypoadrenocorticism is steroid withdrawal after long-term glucocorticoid therapy.[4,29] Long-term steroid administration causes negative feedback on the hypothalamus and pituitary, significantly decreasing ACTH production, which leads to adrenal cortical atrophy. Other documented causes of secondary hypoadrenocorticism in dogs and cats include hypothalamic or pituitary neoplasia,[30] trauma,[31,32] and iatrogenesis (surgical).

CLINICAL PRESENTATION

The clinical picture of hypoadrenocorticism is often vague and mimics other disease processes, most of which are significantly more common than Addison's disease. The classic signs and basic diagnostic test results in the hypoadrenal patient are generally nonspecific, and the vast majority of Addisonian patients will not have all the classic signs. Therefore the clinician must remember to place hypoadrenocorticism on the rule-out list for the patient that has any of these clinical signs.

History

The history for patients with Addison's disease is often vague and nonspecific and usually includes decreased appetite, lethargy, gastrointestinal (GI) disturbance, and weight loss. GI bleeding manifested by hematemesis, hematochezia, or melena may be present.[1,3,4,9,33] Other historical findings may include polyuria, polydipsia, weakness, shaking, pain, muscle cramps, and other nonspecific problems.[1,4,7,8,34] Because the clinical signs are often vague, patients may be brought for treatment in acute crisis without specific prior clinical signs. Thus the absence of such signs does not exclude hypoadrenocorticism as a diagnosis.

Physical Examination

Physical examination findings can vary significantly, depending on whether the hypoadrenocorticism involves hypoaldosteronism and on the severity and duration of illness. The most common physical examination findings include lethargy, weakness, poor body or coat condition, and dehydration. Collapse, hypovolemic shock, GI bleeding, abdominal pain, bradycardia, and hypothermia are common (particularly in emergency and critical care practice), although not all these abnormalities should be expected concurrently in any individual.[1,4,7-9,16] Patients with secondary hypoadrenocorticism or atypical primary hypoadrenocorticism may be less likely to arrive in crisis because these patients have adequate aldosterone to maintain intravascular volume and normal electrolyte concentrations.[1,3-5]

Clinicopathologic Findings

The most common clinicopathologic findings are a decrease in the sodium/potassium ratio, azotemia with an inappropriately low urine specific gravity, anemia, and a leukogram inconsistent with the patient's degree of illness. The normal sodium/potassium ratio is 27:1 to 40:1. Patients with typical primary hypoadrenocorticism (i.e., with aldosterone insufficiency) usually have a pretreatment sodium/potassium ratio (Na:K) of less than 28:1.[10] Note that these patients need not have both hyponatremia and hyperkalemia; rather, some have only one of these abnormalities, and the ratio of these cations can still be less than 28:1. Patients with only glucocorticoid insufficiency are unlikely to have these electrolyte changes.[1-5] Though hypoadrenocorticism appears to be the disease most commonly associated with low Na:K,[28] many other diseases and conditions occasionally are associated with low sodium/potassium ratios. Such diseases include renal failure or postrenal obstruction,[28,35,36] severe GI disease,[4,28,36,37] parasitic infestation,[35,37,38] pregnancy,[39] body cavity effusions,[36] and others.[4,36,40] Moreover, although a low sodium/potassium ratio is the classic electrolyte abnormality of Addison's disease, not all patients with hypoadrenocorticism have this change, which may be present with other conditions.

Most Addisonian patients are azotemic and hyperphosphatemic on arrival.[4,7-9,16] These changes are generally attributed to hypovolemia and are therefore prerenal in origin. However, most dogs and cats with hypoadrenocorticism have inappropriately low urine specific gravity (i.e., <1.030). Inability to appropriately concentrate urine has been attributed to lack of sodium retention and resultant renal medullary washout.[4,41] Renal concentrating ability returns with mineralocorticoid supplementation.

The complete blood cell count (CBC) usually reveals a mild to moderate nonregenerative anemia caused by lack of cortisol tropism at the level of the bone marrow. Patients with significant concomitant GI bleeding can have severe anemia that may be nonregenerative.[33] The degree of anemia may be masked initially by dehydration and resultant hemoconcentration. The CBC may reveal a "reverse stress leukogram," with relative or absolute neutropenia, lymphocytosis, and eosinophilia; however, the Addisonian patient can also have the neutrophilia and lymphopenia commonly seen with severe illness. Addisonian patients often have very normal-appearing CBC findings. It is important to interpret CBC values in light of the severity of disease; a normal CBC result or the "reverse stress leukogram" in an ill patient should raise the clinician's suspicion for hypoadrenocorticism. One recent study recommends using the lymphocyte count in combination with the Na:K ratio to screen for patients that should undergo definitive testing for hypoadrenocorticism (see later).[42]

Other blood work may reveal hypoglycemia, hypercalcemia, metabolic acidosis, hypoalbuminemia, and hypocholesterolemia. Hypoglycemia has been reported in up to 38% of dogs with hypoadrenocorticism.[1,4,7-9] Cortisol promotes glycogenolysis and gluconeogenesis, and lack of these processes may cause the hypoglycemia seen in some Addisonian patients. Seizures have been reported as a result of severe hypoglycemia in hypoadrenocorticism.[43,44] It is important to note that hyperglycemia has also been reported in dogs with hypoadrenocorticism,[4,7-9] so its presence does not exclude the diagnosis. Both total and ionized hypercalcemia have been reported in dogs and cats with hypoadrenocorticism*; the mechanism is unclear. Metabolic acidosis is seen commonly in dogs with hypoadrenocorticism. The acidosis is attributed to hypovolemia, with its resultant lactic acidosis, and decreased renal tubular hydrogen ion excretion, which is enhanced by aldosterone. Hypoalbuminemia has been reported in dogs with hypoadrenocorticism; the mechanism is unclear, but it may be related to GI bleeding, protein-losing enteropathy, or decreased hepatic synthesis.[4,48] Lastly, hypocholesterolemia has been reported in association with hypoadrenocorticism.[1,4,7,9]

*References 1, 4, 7-9, 16, 29, 45-47.

Elevated cholesterol concentration has also been reported in these patients; thus its importance in the diagnosis is equivocal. The most important feature of the basic clinicopathologic data in the hypoadrenal patient is its highly variable nature. One should not expect to find all the classic clinicopathologic changes in one animal.

Electrocardiographic Findings

An electrocardiogram (ECG) should be performed in all patients with clinical signs of hypovolemia or established hyperkalemia. Hypoadrenal patients may have bradycardia, which can be seen with or without hyperkalemia.[1,4,9] Those with hyperkalemia may have bradycardia, diminished or absent P waves, "tented" T waves, wide or bizarre QRS complexes, ventricular fibrillation, or asystole. Ventricular fibrillation and asystole require immediate cardiopulmonary resuscitation (see Chapter 3). Hyperkalemia-related ECG changes are of immediate life-threatening importance and should be treated promptly and appropriately (see Chapter 51). Before using insulin to treat hyperkalemic ECG abnormalities, make sure the patient is not already hypoglycemic and that glucose supplementation is adequate. There has been one report of atrial fibrillation in association with Addison's disease in a dog.[49]

Diagnostic Imaging

Radiographic findings in patients with hypoadrenocorticism may include microcardia, decreased size of pulmonary vasculature, small caudal vena cava, and microhepatica.[7,9,16,50] Although one study found that approximately 80% of dogs in Addisonian crisis had at least one of these radiographic abnormalities,[50] many hypoadrenal patients have normal radiographic findings. Abdominal ultrasonographic findings may reveal small adrenal glands bilaterally.[51,52] Because of the difficulty in locating normal adrenal glands in many animals, size interpretations should be made only by people highly trained and experienced in veterinary abdominal ultrasonography.

DIAGNOSIS

Although this clinical picture should increase the clinician's suspicion of hypoadrenocorticism, a definitive diagnosis is generally made using the ACTH stimulation test. A standard ACTH stimulation test can be performed using 250 mcg cosyntropin per dog or 125 mcg cosyntropin per cat; the drug can be given intramuscularly (IM) or intravenously (IV) in dogs and is recommended IM in cats. Blood is collected for serum cortisol measurement before ACTH administration and after 60 minutes in dogs, and after both 30 and 60 minutes in cats.[4] A recent study found a low-dose ACTH stimulation test using 5 mcg/kg of cosyntropin intravenously in dogs equally as effective as the standard ACTH stimulation test to diagnose hypoadrenocorticism.[53] If cosyntropin is not available, ACTH gel can be used. The protocol is 2.2 IU/kg ACTH gel IM in dogs and cats. Cortisol measurements are made before and 2 hours after ACTH administration in dogs and before and 1 and 2 hours after administration in cats.[4] Contact a veterinary reference laboratory for appropriate sample handling techniques, which can alter the results. A single basal plasma or serum cortisol concentration of 1 mcg/dl or less appears to have excellent sensitivity and very good specificity for hypoadrenocorticism.[54] The same study suggests that patients with a single basal plasma or serum cortisol concentration greater than 2 mcg/dl are highly unlikely to have hypoadrenocorticism, as long as they are not receiving medications that may alter the HPA axis.

Endogenous ACTH concentration is useful in differentiating primary from secondary hypoadrenocorticism. The distinction is particularly important in Addisonian patients with normal electrolyte values: If they have low endogenous ACTH concentration, they have secondary hypoadrenocorticism (hypothalamic or pituitary malfunction) and are unlikely to develop mineralocorticoid deficiency. However, the hypoadrenal patient with normal electrolyte values and an elevated endogenous ACTH concentration (atypical primary hypoadrenocorticism) may develop mineralocorticoid deficiency over time and therefore requires close monitoring. The sample for endogenous ACTH concentration should be taken along with the sample for baseline cortisol, before exogenous ACTH administration. Contact a veterinary reference laboratory for appropriate sample handling techniques, which can alter the results.

A recent study showed that a dog's cortisol/ACTH ratio, calculated from measured baseline cortisol and endogenous ACTH, could be used to diagnose primary hypoadrenocorticism.[11] All dogs in the study with a cortisol/ACTH ratio of 0.17 or less had hypoadrenocorticism, whereas all those with ratios 0.79 or greater were healthy (reference interval 1.1 to 26). The same study also suggests that a dog's ratio of plasma aldosterone concentration/plasma renin activity may be used to distinguish between typical and atypical primary hypoadrenocorticism. All dogs in the study with primary hypoadrenocorticism had a plasma aldosterone concentration/plasma renin activity ratio of 0.08 or less, whereas healthy dogs all had a ratio of 0.09 or more (reference interval 0.1 to 1.5).

Most exogenously administered glucocorticoids will interfere with adrenal function testing, affecting baseline cortisol, stimulated cortisol, and endogenous ACTH concentrations. Therefore, if the patient has a history of recent steroid administration, the tests should be delayed while glucocorticoids are withheld and the patient is treated symptomatically. The patient in crisis requires fluid resuscitation first and foremost; it is appropriate to collect an endogenous ACTH sample and complete the ACTH stimulation test before administration of supplemental steroids.

TREATMENT

By far the most important treatment for patients with hypoadrenocorticism is adequate and appropriate IV fluid therapy. Patients presenting to the emergency or intensive care setting are likely to be in crisis. Patients should be treated for shock as their physical examination and intensive monitoring results dictate (see Chapters 5 and 60).

Fluid Therapy

Traditionally, 0.9% saline has been recommended for initial fluid treatment of Addisonian patients because it has fluid and sodium to replace fluid and electrolyte deficits and no potassium to exacerbate hyperkalemia.[4] However, it is important to remember that patients with significant hyponatremia can suffer severe neurologic consequences if their serum sodium concentration is raised too rapidly; such complications have been reported in dogs treated for hypoadrenocorticism[55,56] (see Chapter 50). Because of the risks of rapidly increasing serum sodium concentration, a more appropriate therapy may be a balanced electrolyte solution with a lower sodium concentration (130 to 140 mEq/L), even though these solutions have 4 or 5 mEq potassium per liter. Restoration of effective circulating volume and resultant increase in glomerular filtration rate alone will help generate a kaliuresis, even if the fluid administered has potassium in it. Such decisions must be made on an individual basis. Frequent serum electrolyte measurements and neurologic examinations will help guide therapy.

Initial Hormonal Replacement

After endogenous ACTH measurement and ACTH stimulation testing, mineralocorticoid treatment should begin promptly. Mineralocorticoid supplementation should be provided for patients with confirmed aldosterone deficiency or those with low Na:K in the form of desoxycorticosterone pivalate at a dosage of 2.2 mg/kg IM or subcutaneously (SC) once every 25 days for the life of the patient.[4,57] Fludrocortisone can also be used, but it is available only in oral form and often is not tolerated during the initial crisis event because of GI disturbance. Glucocorticoid supplementation during the adrenal crisis is appropriate and is usually also required long term. Hydrocortisone, prednisolone, and dexamethasone are all available in injectable form; hydrocortisone is closest to endogenous cortisol, but any of these is adequate. Hydrocortisone is recommended at an initial dosage of 1.25 mg/kg IV once, and 0.5 to 1 mg/kg IV q6h on a tapering schedule. Prednisolone can be given at an initial dosage of 1 to 2 mg/kg IV followed by 0.5 to 1 mg/kg IV q8h on a tapering schedule. A reasonable initial dosage of dexamethasone is 0.1 mg/kg IV, with subsequent doses of 0.05 mg/kg q12h on a tapering schedule.

Supportive Therapies

Other therapy includes supportive care measures. Hypoglycemia should be corrected as required. Patients with GI disturbance may be treated with gastric protectants, and those with protracted vomiting may require antiemetic therapy. Patients with abdominal pain may require analgesia. Opiate medications are suitable for this purpose. Nonsteroidal antiinflammatory drugs should be avoided in patients with GI disturbance or azotemia and as such are almost always contraindicated in the hypoadrenal crisis. Concurrent disease such as aspiration pneumonia or sepsis should be treated appropriately.

Timeline for Clinical Improvement

Cats respond to therapy more slowly than dogs. Although a clinical response can be seen within hours in dogs, it may take 3 to 5 days for cats to show significant clinical improvement.[4,16]

ASSOCIATED DISORDERS

There are reports of Addisonian dogs concurrently diagnosed with immune-mediated diseases, including hemolytic anemia,[1,58] hypothyroidism,[1,7,59,60] myasthenia gravis,[1] keratoconjunctivitis sicca,[43] and bicytopenia.[61] These findings support an immune-mediated etiology for primary hypoaldosteronism in dogs.

Megaesophagus has been reported occasionally in dogs with uncontrolled hypoadrenocorticism.* The connection between the two problems is unclear. It has been reported in dogs with typical hypoadrenocorticism, as well as those deficient only in glucocorticoids. Megaesophagus resolves with treatment of the hypoadrenocorticism.

PROGNOSIS

If animals survive the initial crisis, long-term prognosis for both dogs and cats with naturally occurring Addison's disease is very good with appropriate, lifelong therapy. Patients with primary hypoadrenocorticism sometimes can be controlled with mineralocorticoid therapy alone, although most require glucocorticoid supplementation as well. Many patients with atypical primary hypoadrenocorticism (adrenal failure with normal electrolytes and normal pituitary function) will become mineralocorticoid deficient. These patients require frequent reexamination, electrolyte evaluation, and vigilant monitoring by the owner so that the development of a hypoaldosterone state does not lead to life-threatening crisis. Those with secondary hypoadrenocorticism are well controlled on lifelong glucocorticoid therapy.

*References 1, 4, 7, 9, 62, 63.

REFERENCES

1. Lifton SJ, King LG, Zerbe CA: Glucocorticoid deficient hypoadrenocorticism in dogs: 18 cases (1986-1995), J Am Vet Med Assoc 209:2076, 1996.
2. Sadek D, Schaer M: Atypical Addison's disease in the dog: a retrospective survey of 14 cases, J Am Anim Hosp Assoc 32:159, 1996.
3. Rogers W, Straus J, Chew D: Atypical hypoadrenocorticism in three dogs, J Am Vet Med Assoc 179:155, 1981.
4. Feldman EC, Nelson RW: Hypoadrenocorticism (Addison's disease). In Feldman EC, Nelson RW, editors: Canine and feline endocrinology and reproduction, ed 3, St Louis, 2004, Saunders, pp 394-439.
5. Thompson AL, Scott-Moncrieff JC, Anderson JD: Comparison of classic hypoadrenocorticism with glucocorticoid-deficient hypoadrenocorticism in dogs: 46 cases (1985-2005), J Am Vet Med Assoc 230:1190, 2007.
6. McGonigle KM, Randolph JF, Center SA, et al: Mineralocorticoid before glucocorticoid deficiency in a dog with primary hypoadrenocorticism and hypothyroidism, J Am Anim Hosp Assoc 49:54, 2013.
7. Peterson ME, Kintzer PP, Kass PH: Pretreatment clinical and laboratory findings in dogs with hypoadrenocorticism: 225 cases (1979-1993), J Am Vet Med Assoc 208:85, 1996.
8. Willard MD, Schall WD, McCaw DE, et al: Canine hypoadrenocorticism: report of 37 cases and review of 39 previously reported cases, J Am Vet Med Assoc 180:59, 1982.
9. Melian C, Peterson ME: Diagnosis and treatment of naturally occurring hypoadrenocorticism in 42 dogs, J Small Anim Pract 37:268, 1996.
10. Adler JA, Drobatz KJ, Hess RS: Abnormalities of serum electrolyte concentrations in dogs with hypoadrenocorticism, J Vet Intern Med 21:1168, 2007.
11. Javadi S, Galac S, Boer P, et al: Aldosterone-to-renin and cortisol-to-adrenocorticotropic hormone ratios in healthy dogs and dogs with primary hypoadrenocorticism, J Vet Intern Med 20:556, 2006.
12. Duesberg C, Peterson ME: Adrenal disorders in cats, Vet Clin North Am Small Anim Pract 27:321, 1997.
13. Stonehewer J, Tasker S: Hypoadrenocorticism in a cat, J Small Anim Pract 42:186, 2001.
14. Johnessee JS, Peterson ME, Gilbertson SR: Primary hypoadrenocorticism in a cat, J Am Vet Med Assoc 183:881, 1983.
15. Tasker S, MacKay AD, Sparkes AH: A case of feline primary hypoadrenocorticism, J Feline Med Surg 1:257, 1999.
16. Peterson ME, Greco DS, Orth DN: Primary hypoadrenocorticism in ten cats, J Vet Intern Med 3:55, 1989.
17. Mawhinney AD, Rahaley RS, Belford CJ: Primary hypoadrenocorticism in a cat, Aust Vet Pract 19:46, 1989.
18. Hock CE: Atypical hypoadrenocorticism in a Birman cat, Can Vet J 52:893, 2011.
19. Kasabalis D, Bodina E, Saridomichelakis MN: Severe hypoglycaemia in a cat with primary hypoadrenocorticism, J Feline Med Surg 14:755, 2012.
20. Labelle P, De Cock HE: Metastatic tumors to the adrenal glands in domestic animals, Vet Pathol 42:52, 2005.
21. Parnell NK, Powell LL, Hohenhaus AE, et al: Hypoadrenocorticism as the primary manifestation of lymphoma in two cats, J Am Vet Med Assoc 214:1208, 1200, 1999.
22. Berger SL, Reed JR: Traumatically induced hypoadrenocorticism in a cat, J Am Anim Hosp Assoc 29:337, 1993.
23. Rockwell JL, Monroe WE, Tromblee TC: Spontaneous hypoadrenocorticism in a dog after a diagnosis of hyperadrenocorticism, J Vet Intern Med 19:255, 2005.
24. Willard MD, Schall WD, Nachreiner RF, et al: Hypoadrenocorticism following therapy with o,p-DDD for hyperadrenocorticism in four dogs, J Am Vet Med Assoc 180:638, 1982.
25. Braddock JA, Church DB, Robertson ID, et al: Trilostane treatment in dogs with pituitary-dependent hyperadrenocorticism, Aust Vet J 81:600, 2003.
26. Cho KD, Kang JH, Chang D, et al: Efficacy of low- and high-dose trilostane treatment in dogs (<5 kg) with pituitary-dependent hyperadrenocorticism, J Vet Intern Med 27:91, 2013.
27. Ramsey IK, Richardson J, Lenard Z, et al: Persistent isolated hypocortisolism following brief treatment with trilostane, Aust Vet J 86:491, 2008.
28. Nielsen L, Bell R, Zoia A, et al: Low ratios of sodium to potassium in the serum of 238 dogs, Vet Rec 162:431, 2008.

29. Smith SA, Freeman LC, Bagladi-Swanson M: Hypercalcemia due to latrogenic secondary hypoadrenocorticism and diabetes mellitus in a cat, J Am Anim Hosp Assoc 38:41, 2002.
30. Eckersley GN, Bastianello S, Van Heerden J, et al: An expansile secondary hypophyseal mastocytoma in a dog, J S Afr Vet Assoc 60:113, 1989.
31. Platt SR, Chrisman CL, Graham J, et al: Secondary hypoadrenocorticism associated with craniocerebral trauma in a dog, J Am Anim Hosp Assoc 35:117, 1999.
32. Foley C, Bracker K, Drellich S: Hypothalamic-pituitary axis deficiency following traumatic brain injury in a dog, J Vet Emerg Crit Care (San Antonio) 19:269, 2009.
33. Medinger TL, Williams DA, Bruyette DS: Severe gastrointestinal tract hemorrhage in three dogs with hypoadrenocorticism, J Am Vet Med Assoc 202:1869, 1993.
34. Saito M, Olby NJ, Obledo L, et al: Muscle cramps in two standard poodles with hypoadrenocorticism, J Am Anim Hosp Assoc 38:437, 2002.
35. Pak SI: The clinical implication of sodium-potassium ratios in dogs, J Vet Sci 1:61, 2000.
36. Bell R, Mellor DJ, Ramsey I, et al: Decreased sodium:potassium ratios in cats: 49 cases, Vet Clin Pathol 34:110, 2005.
37. DiBartola SP, Johnson SE, Davenport DJ, et al: Clinicopathologic findings resembling hypoadrenocorticism in dogs with primary gastrointestinal disease, J Am Vet Med Assoc 187:60, 1985.
38. Graves TK, Schall WD, Refsal K, et al: Basal and ACTH-stimulated plasma aldosterone concentrations are normal or increased in dogs with trichuriasis-associated pseudohypoadrenocorticism, J Vet Intern Med 8:287, 1994.
39. Schaer M, Halling KB, Collins KE, et al: Combined hyponatremia and hyperkalemia mimicking acute hypoadrenocorticism in three pregnant dogs, J Am Vet Med Assoc 218:897, 2001.
40. Campbell VL, Butler AL, Lunn KF: Use of a point-of-care urine drug test in a dog to assist in diagnosing barbiturate toxicosis secondary to ingestion of a euthanized carcass, J Vet Emerg Crit Care (San Antonio) 19:286, 2009.
41. Tyler RD, Qualls CW Jr, Heald RD, et al: Renal concentrating ability in dehydrated hyponatremic dogs, J Am Vet Med Assoc 191:1095, 1987.
42. Seth M, Drobatz KJ, Church DB, et al: White blood cell count and the sodium to potassium ratio to screen for hypoadrenocorticism in dogs, J Vet Intern Med 25:1351, 2011.
43. Syme HM, Scott-Moncrieff JC: Chronic hypoglycaemia in a hunting dog due to secondary hypoadrenocorticism, J Small Anim Pract 39:348, 1998.
44. Levy JK: Hypoglycemic seizures attributable to hypoadrenocorticism in a dog, J Am Vet Med Assoc 204:526; discussion 528-530, 1994.
45. Peterson ME, Feinman JM: Hypercalcemia associated with hypoadrenocorticism in sixteen dogs, J Am Vet Med Assoc 181:802, 1982.
46. Messinger JS, Windham WR, Ward CR: Ionized hypercalcemia in dogs: a retrospective study of 109 cases (1998-2003), J Vet Intern Med 23:514, 2009.
47. Adamantos S, Boag A: Total and ionised calcium concentrations in dogs with hypoadrenocorticism, Vet Rec 163:25, 2008.
48. Langlais-Burgess L, Lumsden JH, Mackin A: Concurrent hypoadrenocorticism and hypoalbuminemia in dogs: a retrospective study, J Am Anim Hosp Assoc 31:307, 1995.
49. Riesen SC, Lombard CW: ECG of the month. Atrial fibrillation secondary to hypoadrenocorticism, J Am Vet Med Assoc 229:1890, 2006.
50. Melian C, Stefanacci J, Peterson ME, et al: Radiographic findings in dogs with naturally-occurring primary hypoadrenocorticism, J Am Anim Hosp Assoc 35:208, 1999.
51. Hoerauf A, Reusch C: Ultrasonographic evaluation of the adrenal glands in six dogs with hypoadrenocorticism, J Am Anim Hosp Assoc 35:214, 1999.
52. Wenger M, Mueller C, Kook PH, et al: Ultrasonographic evaluation of adrenal glands in dogs with primary hypoadrenocorticism or mimicking diseases, Vet Rec 167:207, 2010.
53. Lathan P, Moore GE, Zambon S, et al: Use of a low-dose ACTH stimulation test for diagnosis of hypoadrenocorticism in dogs, J Vet Intern Med 22:1070, 2008.
54. Lennon EM, Boyle TE, Hutchins RG, et al: Use of basal serum or plasma cortisol concentrations to rule out a diagnosis of hypoadrenocorticism in dogs: 123 cases (2000-2005), J Am Vet Med Assoc 231:413, 2007.
55. MacMillan KL: Neurologic complications following treatment of canine hypoadrenocorticism, Can Vet J 44:490, 2003.
56. Brady CA, Vite CH, Drobatz KJ: Severe neurologic sequelae in a dog after treatment of hypoadrenal crisis, J Am Vet Med Assoc 215:222, 210, 1999.
57. McCabe MD, Feldman EC, Lynn RC, et al: Subcutaneous administration of desoxycorticosterone pivalate for the treatment of canine hypoadrenocorticism, J Am Anim Hosp Assoc 31:151, 1995.
58. Willard MD: An unusual case of hypoadrenocorticism in a dog, Mod Vet Pract 61:830, 1980.
59. Smallwood LJ, Barsanti JA: Hypoadrenocorticism in a family of leonbergers, J Am Anim Hosp Assoc 31:301, 1995.
60. Blois SL, Dickie E, Kruth SA, et al: Multiple endocrine diseases in dogs: 35 cases (1996-2009), J Am Vet Med Assoc 238:1616, 2011.
61. Snead E, Vargo C, Myers S: Glucocorticoid-dependent hypoadrenocorticism with thrombocytopenia and neutropenia mimicking sepsis in a Labrador retriever dog, Can Vet J 52:1129, 2011.
62. Whitley NT: Megaoesophagus and glucocorticoid-deficient hypoadrenocorticism in a dog, J Small Anim Pract 36:132, 1995.
63. Bartges JW, Nielson DL: Reversible megaesophagus associated with atypical primary hypoadrenocorticism in a dog, J Am Vet Med Assoc 201:889, 1992.

PART VIII THERAPEUTIC DRUG OVERDOSE

CHAPTER 74

APPROACH TO DRUG OVERDOSE

Justine A. Lee, DVM, DACVECC, DABT

KEY POINTS

- When presented the poisoned patient, obtaining an appropriate toxicologic history is imperative.
- Triage—both on the phone *before* seeing the patient and upon presentation—is key with the poisoned patient.
- Confirmed identification of the active ingredients, milligram strength, and type of drug (e.g., immediate release, long-acting, extended-release) must be determined because this may alter the toxicologic management of the case.
- Toxicologic calculations should be performed to correctly identify (a) if the dose is toxic, (b) if it affects development of clinical signs (e.g., gastrointestinal vs. nephrotoxic toxic doses), and (c) if it approaches the LD_{50}.
- Appropriate decontamination (e.g., emesis induction, gastric lavage, administration of activated charcoal) is warranted in cases of drug overdose, if appropriate, because it is still the mainstay therapy for treatment of the poisoned patient in veterinary medicine.
- Antidote therapy should be used if available; however, for the vast majority of toxicants there is none. Therefore treatment of the poisoned patient is based on appropriate decontamination and symptomatic supportive care until clinical signs resolve or until risks for potential complications have passed.
- The four most common human drug toxicoses seen in veterinary medicine typically include selective serotonin reuptake inhibitor (SSRI) antidepressants, amphetamines, nonsteroidal antiinflammatory drugs (NSAIDs), and acetaminophen.
- The use of intravenous lipid emulsion (ILE) can be considered as a potentially lifesaving antidote for fat-soluble drug toxicosis (e.g., macrocyclic lactones, baclofen, calcium channel blockers, cholecalciferol). However, appropriate considerations such as lipophilicity of the drug, adverse effects from extra-label use, and potential drug interaction with other therapeutic interventions must be considered before its use in the poisoned patient.

According to the American Association of Poison Control Centers Toxic Exposure Surveillance System, the use of activated charcoal in human medicine has continued to steadily decline, dropping from 7.7% to 5.9% in 2003.[1] Although human medicine has moved away from decontamination (including emesis induction, gastric lavage, and administration of activated charcoal) with poisoned patients, the aggressive use of decontamination in veterinary medicine is still warranted. Certain modalities of therapy (e.g., antidotes [such as fomepizole, 2-PAM, digoxin-specific antibody fragments], plasmaparesis, hemodialysis, mechanical ventilation) that are less readily available in veterinary medicine, along with financial limitations of pet owners, often limit our ability to treat poisoned pets aggressively; as a result, the continued use of decontamination in veterinary medicine is still warranted as a first line of defense in treating the poisoned patient.

In veterinary medicine, with any poisoned patient the primary treatment for toxicant exposure should be decontamination and detoxification, along with symptomatic and supportive care of the patient. Initial steps when presented a poisoned patient should include obtaining an appropriate history, immediate stabilization and triage, performing a thorough physical examination, and initiating treatment (including decontamination and stabilization).

OBTAINING AN APPROPRIATE HISTORY

Often pet owners will call veterinary staff to determine if a product ingested is poisonous. Before recommending immediate decontamination, the veterinary professional (e.g., front desk staff, veterinary technician, and ultimately the veterinarian) must determine if the ingested product is toxic. More importantly, time must be taken to obtain an appropriate toxicologic history *before* recommendations for emesis induction. A toxicologic history differs somewhat from the standard history taking in veterinary medicine. Some key additional history questions to ask a pet owner include the following:

- What was the specific name of the product ingested? Do you know the active ingredient (AI)?
- How many total tablets could have been ingested? What was the minimum and maximum amount that your pet could have been exposed to?
- Was this an extended-release (XR), long-acting (LA), or sustained-release (SR) product? These initials will follow the name of the drug on the prescription vial.
- Was there an extra "letter" behind the brand name (e.g., Claritin vs. Claritin-D, Advil vs. Advil-PM)?
- What time did your pet get into this?
- Has your pet shown any clinical signs yet?
- Did you give your pet anything at home (e.g., hydrogen peroxide, milk, salt) when you found out he was poisoned?

TRIAGE

Once these key historical questions have been asked, the pet owner should be instructed to do the following:

- Safely remove their pet from the area of poisoning so additional ingestion does not occur
- Avoid the use of any home remedies found circulating on the Internet (e.g., milk, peanut butter, oil, grease, salt)
- Avoid emesis induction without consultation from a veterinarian or an animal poison control center (APCC) first

BOX 74-1 *Animal Poison Control Center Resources*

- ASPCA Animal Poison Control Center, 501(c)(3), Urbana, Illinois: (888) 426-4435. A $65 fee/call applies.
- Pet Poison Helpline, a division of SafetyCall International, Bloomington, Minnesota: (855) 213-6680. A $39 fee/call applies.
- Washington Poison Center Vet Pets, 501(c)(3), Seattle, Washington: (800) 572-5842. A $45 fee/call applies.

- Bring the original box/container/pill vial in to the veterinarian so they can assess the product for verification of the product name or active ingredient
- Call the original pharmacy to confirm the active ingredient, to identify how many total pills were prescribed, and to attempt to back-count how many were taken/ingested
- Call an APCC for medical assistance and toxicology advice if needed (Box 74-1)
- Seek immediate veterinary attention, if deemed toxic

Once the patient is presented to the veterinary professional, reconfirmation of the toxicologic history and immediate triage should be performed. The patient should be stabilized, with a focus on airway, breathing, circulation, and dysfunction (ABCD); preliminary temperature; heart rate; and pulse rate (TPR). Readers are referred to Chapter 1 for additional information. Once the patient is stabilized, a complete physical examination should be performed before decontamination.

WHEN TO DECONTAMINATE

The goal of decontamination is to inhibit or minimize further toxicant absorption and to promote excretion or elimination of the toxicant from the body.[2] Decontamination can only be performed within a narrow window of time for most substances (i.e., generally <1 to 2 hours); therefore it is important to obtain a thorough history and time since exposure to identify whether decontamination would be beneficial for the patient and if so would it be safe for the patient. Decontamination techniques may include ocular, dermal, inhalation, injection, gastrointestinal (GI), forced diuresis, and surgical removal to prevent absorption or enhance elimination of the toxicant.[2,3]

One of the most common ways of decontaminating veterinary patients is via emesis induction. Although gastric lavage is often more clinically effective at removing gastric contents, it is less often performed in veterinary medicine because it is more labor intensive. Veterinarians should be aware of which circumstances are appropriate or contraindicated for either emesis induction or gastric lavage to be performed.

Likewise, before counseling pet owners on performing "at-home" emesis induction, veterinarians should evaluate if it is medically appropriate. First, there is no safe emetic agent for pet owners to use at home in cats and immediate veterinary treatment is warranted. For dogs, the use of hydrogen peroxide can be considered at home, but only when appropriate: in asymptomatic patients with recent ingestion (i.e., generally <1 to 2 hours). Contraindications for at-home emesis induction are similar to those contraindications for emesis induction by veterinarians. For example, at-home emesis should never be performed with corrosive agents, hydrocarbons, in symptomatic patients, or those patients at risk for aspiration pneumonia. See Box 74-2 for more detailed indications and contraindications for emesis.

Gastric lavage, which is more labor intensive compared with emesis induction, requires intravenous (IV) catheter placement, sedation, intubation with a cuffed endotracheal tube (ETT), orogastric tube placement, multiple gavage cycles (followed by administration of activated charcoal, if appropriate), postanesthesia management, and supportive care.[3] As a result, many veterinarians often feel hesitant to perform it because of the time commitment and labor-intensiveness. Typically, gastric lavage is indicated for toxicants that remain in the stomach for a long time or that form large bezoars (e.g., bone meal, blood meal, large wads of aspirin, prenatal iron tablets).[3] Gastric lavage is also indicated in certain situations where emesis is contraindicated. In symptomatic patients at risk for aspiration (e.g., comatosed, seizuring, tremoring, hyperthermic), the use of gastric lavage may be beneficial to protect the airway while simultaneously removing any further toxicant within the stomach. Gastric lavage is also warranted with certain toxicants that have a very narrow margin of safety, result in severe clinical signs, or that approach 50% of the lethal dose (LD_{50}).[3] Some examples of toxicants that warrant gastric lavage include the following:

- Metaldehyde
- Strychnine
- Calcium channel blockers
- Baclofen
- β-Blockers
- Macrocyclic lactones (e.g., ivermectin, moxidectin)
- Organophosphates/carbamates

BOX 74-2 *Appropriate Indications and Contraindications to Inducing Emesis*

Emesis induction is appropriate in the following situations[3]:
- With recent ingestion (<1 to 2 hours) in an asymptomatic patient
- With unknown time of ingestion in an asymptomatic patient
- When ingestion of a product known to stay in the stomach for a long time is ingested by an asymptomatic patient (e.g., grapes, raisins, chocolate, xylitol gum, massive ingestions)

Emesis should *not* be induced in the following situations[3]:
- With corrosive toxicant ingestion (e.g., lye, ultra-bleach, batteries, oven cleaning chemicals)
- With hydrocarbon toxicant ingestion (e.g., tiki-torch oil, gasoline, kerosene)
- In symptomatic patients (e.g., tremoring, agitated, seizuring, hyperthermic, weak, collapsed)
- In patients with underlying disease predisposing them to aspiration pneumonia or complications associated with emesis induction (e.g., megaesophagus, history of aspiration pneumonia, laryngeal paralysis)

ACTIVATED CHARCOAL (AC)

After an appropriate history, triage, physical examination, and initial decontamination procedures have been performed in the poisoned pet, the next step is the administration of activated charcoal (AC), if appropriate. Activated charcoal should only be administered to the poisoned patient when the toxicant reliably binds to AC. Certain toxicants such as heavy metals (e.g., iron, zinc), xylitol, and alcohols (e.g., ethylene glycol, ethanol, methanol) do not reliably bind to AC, and administration of AC is contraindicated with these specific toxicants.[3] Likewise, symptomatic patients who are at risk for aspiration pneumonia should not be administered AC orally. Finally, the administration of AC with a cathartic should be used cautiously in dehydrated patients (e.g., vomiting, diarrhea) or those with excessive free water loss (e.g., diabetes mellitus, renal disease, diabetes insipidus); rarely, hypernatremia may be observed as a result of free water loss into the gastrointestinal tract (GIT).[3]

The beneficial effects of AC are dependent on timing of administration (to allow rapid binding to the toxicant within the GIT) and surface area of the AC (e.g., administering the appropriate volume of AC to bind with the toxicant). When administering AC, it should ideally be given within 5 minutes or less of ingestion to be most effective.[1] In veterinary medicine this is almost impossible because of driving time (to the clinic), lapsed time since ingestion, time to triage, and the amount of time it takes to physically deliver AC (e.g., syringe feeding, orogastric tube). As a result, administration of AC is often delayed up to an hour or more. Because time since ingestion is often unknown (e.g., pet owner coming home from work to find their pet poisoned), decontamination (including emesis and administration of AC) is often a relatively benign course of action, provided the patient is not already symptomatic. As always, when administering *any* drug, it is important that benefits outweigh the risks and that complications be prevented when possible. In veterinary medicine, administration of AC with a cathartic as long as 6 hours out may still be beneficial with certain types of toxicosis, particularly if the product has delayed release (e.g., XR, SR, LA) or undergoes enterohepatic recirculation (see Multidose Activated Charcoal later).

Current recommended dosing for single-dose AC is 1 to 5 g of AC/kg with a cathartic (e.g., sorbitol) to promote GIT transit time.[3] Several brands of AC exist (e.g., Toxiban, Universal Animal Antidote [UAA]), both with a cathartic or without. Care must be taken to administer the appropriate dose (not necessarily what is labeled); rather, calculating 1 to 5 g of AC/kg is appropriate.

Multidose Activated Charcoal

The use of multidose AC has been found to significantly decrease the serum half-life of certain drugs in humans, including antidepressants, theophylline, digitoxin, and phenobarbital.[1] Although veterinary studies are lacking, there is likely an added benefit from using multidose AC, provided the patient is well hydrated and monitored appropriately. Certain situations or toxicities, including drugs that undergo enterohepatic recirculation; drugs that diffuse from the systemic circulation back into the GIT down the concentration gradient; and ingestion of SR, XR, or LA products, will require multidose administration of AC.[3] Keep in mind that multidose AC should *not* contain a cathartic with additional doses because of increased risks for dehydration and secondary hypernatremia via fluid losses from the GIT. Current recommended dosing for multiple doses of AC is 1 to 2 g AC *without a cathartic* per kilogram of body weight PO q4-6h for 24 hours.[3]

Contraindications and Complications of Activated Charcoal Administration

Contraindications for AC include endoscopy (which would obscure visualization), gastric or intestinal obstruction, GI hemorrhage or perforation, recent surgery, late-stage presentation with clinical signs already present, dehydration, lack of borborgymi, ileus, hypovolemic shock, compromised airway (risk for aspiration pneumonia), and ingestion of a caustic substance or hydrocarbons.[3] In patients that have an unprotected airway that are at risk for aspiration pneumonia (e.g., a depressed state of consciousness, excessive sedation, laryngeal paralysis), the use of AC is contraindicated without ETT intubation (e.g., via gastric lavage).

Additional complications from AC administration include the risk for a transient increase in osmolality and potential risks of hypernatremia (typically secondary to cathartic administration or use of multidose AC). A study evaluating a commercial AC, Actidose-Aqua, in healthy dogs reported increases in serum osmolality, osmolal gap, and lactate after administration.[4] This raised the concern that the use of AC could confuse the diagnosis of intoxication of substances that can increase the osmolal gap such as ethylene glycol. Because this particular AC is not commonly used and does not contain sorbitol or a cathartic, the relevance to current clinical practice is unclear and further studies are needed.

Burkitt et al evaluated the use of a commercial AC, Actidose-Aqua, in a prospective, clinical trial in six dogs to determine if AC suspension containing propylene glycol (PG) and glycerol had any effects on serum osmolality, osmolal gap, and lactate.[4] Samples were also evaluated for acid-base status and concentrations of sodium, potassium, blood urea nitrogen (BUN), and glucose. In this study, dogs (n = 6) were given 4 g/kg of AC and samples were taken before and 1, 4, 6, 8, 12, and 24 hours post-AC.[4] In this study, mean serum osmolality, osmolal gap, and lactate concentration were significantly increased after suspension administration compared with baseline, typically increasing at 1 hour after AC administration, peaking at 4 hours, and returning to baseline by 24 hours. Hypernatremia was not detected in any of the study dogs; however, mild hypokalemia was seen ($p < .05$). Serum osmolality increased from 311 mOsm/kg at baseline to 353 mOsm/kg, osmolal gap increased from 5 to 52 mOsm/kg, and lactate concentration increased from 1.9 to 4.5 mmol/L after suspension administration ($p < .01$).[4] All six dogs drank frequently after AC administration, but water intake or urine output was not recorded. In addition, three of the dogs vomited within 1 to 3 hours of administration of AC, and four were lethargic.[4] Although this study was important in evaluating complications from AC, this particular AC did not contain sorbitol or a cathartic (Actidose with Sorbitol). A prospective study evaluating the use of a cathartic with AC would be important to evaluate the prevalence of hypernatremia seen with AC and cathartic administration.

CATHARTICS

The use of cathartics in the poisoned patient is designed to increase the speed and transit time of the GIT, promote fecal excretion of the toxin (ideally bound to AC), and decrease the time allowed for toxin absorption through the GIT. Typical cathartics used in veterinary medicine include osmotic cathartics such as saccharide (e.g., sorbitol) and saline cathartics (e.g., sodium sulfate, magnesium citrate, or magnesium sulfate). Sorbitol is most commonly used because it aids in the expulsion of the poison from the GIT while also masking the grittiness and poor palatability of AC with its sweet taste. Side effects of sorbitol administration include vomiting, dehydration, secondary hypernatremia (because of free water loss into the GIT), abdominal cramping or pain, and possible hypotension. The contraindications for cathartics are similar to those that exist for AC. Another important consideration in veterinary medicine is that mineral oil is no longer recommended as a cathartic because of the high risks of secondary aspiration. In general, if AC does not contain a preexisting cathartic (for the first dose administered), one can potentially add in sorbitol (70% solution) for single-dose dosing at 1 to 2 ml/kg PO given within 60 minutes of toxin ingestion. The use of a cathartic with additional doses (e.g., multidose) of AC is not warranted.

TREATMENT

Once the patient has been appropriately decontaminated, the focus of treatment should be based on symptomatic and supportive care. As previously mentioned, there are very few toxicants in veterinary medicine that have a readily available or specific antidote (e.g., fomepizole, 2-PAM, Vitamin K_1). As a result, symptomatic supportive care is imperative and considered the mainstay therapy once decontamination has been performed. Six broad categories of treatment for the poisoned patient are discussed here[3]:

1. Fluid therapy
2. Gastrointestinal support
3. Neurologic support

4. Sedatives/reversal agents
5. Hepatoprotectants
6. Miscellaneous

Fluid Therapy

Fluid therapy plays a key role in the poisoned patient and is indicated for several reasons: to aid in excretion of the drug (if it undergoes urinary excretion); to aid in perfusion (with toxicants resulting in hypotension or with vasoactive properties); to prevent dehydration; to encourage diuresis of nephrotoxins (e.g., grapes, lilies, ethylene glycol); to treat underlying azotemia or electrolyte abnormalities; and to vasodilate the renal vessels (particularly NSAID toxicosis). In general, a balanced, isotonic crystalloid (e.g., LRS, Norm-R) can be used at 1.5 to 4 times a normal maintenance rate. The exception to this would be with any toxicosis resulting in hypercalcemia (e.g., cholecalciferol, vitamin D_3, calcipotriene), where 0.9% NaCl would be the crystalloid of choice to promote calciuresis. While administering fluid therapy, frequent assessment of the poisoned patient should be performed to ensure appropriate hemodilution (e.g., evidence of appropriate weight gain, isosthenuria, packed cell volume/total solids [PCV/TS], physical examination parameters) and to ensure that volume overload does not occur (particularly if the patient has underlying cardiopulmonary disease).

On occasion, the use of colloids or transfusion of blood products may be warranted in the poisoned patient. The use of colloids should be reserved for patients with a low colloid osmotic pressure or profound hypoproteinemia; this may be seen after blood loss or acute hepatic insult. Blood products may be indicated for patients with clinical signs of anemia or coagulopathy secondary to anticoagulants or hepatotoxicants (e.g., xylitol, blue-green algae, sago palm, acetaminophen) resulting in secondary anemia and or coagulopathy. The reader is directed to Chapters 61 and 63 for further information.

Gastrointestinal Support

The use of antiemetics (e.g., maropitant, metoclopramide, ondansetron, dolasetron), antacids, antiulcer drugs, and gastric pH–altering medications is often indicated in the poisoned patient. In the author's opinion, the routine use of antiemetic therapy after emesis induction not only allows more rapid return to oral intake of water (thereby preventing hypernatremia) but also prevents the potential vomition of AC. In a recent study comparing the efficacy apomorphine and hydrogen peroxide, ongoing clinical adverse effects (e.g., nausea, vomiting) of these two emetic agents lasted anywhere from 27 to 42 minutes,[5] supporting the use of antiemetics to counter this prolonged vomition. Finally, certain toxicants result in gastric irritation, gastric distention, and other effects that may cause vomition. In those toxicants predisposing the patient to gastric ulceration (e.g., veterinary NSAIDs, human NSAIDs, corrosive toxicants), the use of antacids, antiulcer medication, and gastric pH–altering medications is also indicated.

Neurologic Support

Central nervous system (CNS) stimulatory (e.g., agitation, tremors, seizures) or sedatory (e.g., drowsiness, severe sedation, coma) clinical signs are often seen with certain toxicants. Toxicants that often result in CNS stimulation include amphetamines, SSRI antidepressants, sleep aids, tremorgenc mycotoxins, rodenticides (e.g., strychnine, bromethalin), methylxanthines, 5-fluorouracil (5-FU), and insecticides (e.g., pyrethrins, metaldehyde). CNS depression or sedatory effects may be seen with toxicants such as muscle relaxants (e.g., baclofen), sedatives (e.g., opioids), sleep aids, illicit drugs (e.g., marijuana), and macrocylic lactones (e.g., ivermectin, moxidectin). This list is not complete, and readers are referred to a toxicology resource for additional information.

With CNS stimulatory signs, the use of sedatives may be indicated (see later). The use of parenteral muscle relaxants (e.g., methocarbamol 40 to 110 mg/kg intravenously [IV] slow to effect) should be used for tremors. Appropriate anticonvulsant therapy (e.g., phenobarbital 4 to 16 mg/kg IV) should be used for grand mal or petit mal seizures.

Rarely, cerebral edema may be seen in the poisoned patient. This may be due to the primary toxicant (e.g., bromethalin, zinc phosphide) or secondary to uncontrolled, untreated seizures (e.g., 5-FU, caffeine). Appropriate therapy for cerebral edema includes hypertonic therapy such as mannitol or hypertonic saline and interventions for decreasing intracranial pressure. See Chapter 84 for more information.

Sedatives and Reversal Agents

With many of the CNS stimulatory toxicants, treatment includes the use of anxiolytics or sedatives such as acepromazine (e.g., 0.05 to 0.1 mg/kg, IV or intramuscularly [IM] prn, not to exceed 3 mg total per dog). The use of butorphanol (0.1 to 0.8 mg/kg, IV or IM prn) may also be used concurrently, depending on the severity of the anxiety, hypertension, and tachycardiac evident. With opioid toxicosis (e.g., fentanyl patch ingestion), the use of the opioid reversal agent, naloxone, is indicated (0.01 to 0.04 mg/kg, IV, IM, or subcutaneously [SC] prn); if not readily available, the use of butorphanol (an opiate agonist-antagonist) may also be considered. With severe sleep aid toxicosis, the use of flumazenil (0.01 to 0.02 mg/kg IV prn) can be considered, although is rarely necessary because of the wide margin of safety of this nonbenzodiazepine hypnotic. Finally, toxicants with α-agonist activity (such as imidazole decongestants found in nasal sprays and eyedrops or amitraz collars) can be reversed with the use of α-adrenergic antagonists such as yohimbine (0.1 mg/kg IV prn) or atipamezole (50 mcg/kg, IV or IM prn).

Hepatoprotectants

The use of hepatoprotectants such as S-adenosyl-methionine (SAMe) are benign nutraceuticals that are potentially beneficial for hepatotoxicants such as xylitol, blue-green algae, NSAIDs, *Amanita* mushrooms, acetaminophen, sago palm, and so on.[4,6-8] SAMe acts as a methyl donor and generates sulfur-containing compounds that are important for conjugation reactions used in detoxification and as a precursor to glutathione.[6] N-acetylcysteine (NAC) is commonly used to limit formation of the toxic metabolite NAPQI by providing alternate glutathione substrate with acetaminophen toxicosis[7] and has been anecdotally used for severe hepatotoxicity with sago palm and xylitol also.[8] With hepatotoxicants, the routine use of SAMe (18 mg/kg PO for 2 to 4 weeks) can be considered and adjusted based on routine monitoring of liver enzymes.

Miscellaneous

Other miscellaneous therapies are often used for the treatment of the poisoned patient, including β-blockers (for severe tachycardia associated with SSRI, amphetamine, chocolate toxicosis, and so forth); vitamin K_1 therapy (for anticoagulant rodenticide toxicosis), and so on. Readers are referred to a toxicology resource for additional information on these topics.

Intravenous Lipid Emulsion

Intravenous lipid emulsion (ILE), also called intravenous fat emulsion (IFE), has been used in both human and veterinary medicine for decades. Originally used as part of total parenteral nutrition (TPN), partial parenteral nutrition (PPN), or as a vehicle for drug delivery (e.g., propofol), ILE is now more recently used as a potential antidote for lipophilic drug toxicosis. Current theories on how ILE works in the poisoned patient include the following:

- Acting as a *lipid sink* by sequestration of lipophilic compounds into the newly created intravascular lipid compartment (a lipid or pharmacologic sink). With this lipid sink hypothesis, compartmentalization of the drug into the lipid phase results in a decreased free drug concentration available to tissues.
- Providing myocytes with energy substrates, thereby augmenting cardiac performance.
- Restoring myocardial function by increasing intracellular calcium concentration.
- Increasing the overall fatty acid pool, which overcomes inhibition of mitochondrial fatty acid metabolism (e.g., bupivacaine toxicosis).

Currently, the most supported hypotheses are that ILE improves cardiac performance and provides a lipid sink effect in the vascular compartment.

In veterinary medicine, the use of ILE has been advocated for toxicoses such as macrocyclic lactones (e.g., moxidectin, ivermectin), lidocaine, pyrethrins, and calcium channel blockers.[9-14] Recently, a state-of-the-art review by Fernandez et al[9] discussed the recommendations on the use of ILE in veterinary medicine; in this paper, dosage recommendations in veterinary medicine were based on extrapolation from human dosing and the dose used for TPN and PPN administration in veterinary medicine: administration of an initial 20% ILE bolus in the range between 1.5 ml/kg and 4 ml/kg (between 0.3 g/kg and 0.8 g/kg IV over 1 minute), followed by a constant rate infusion (CRI) of 0.25 ml/kg/min (0.05 g/kg/min IV over 30 to 60 minutes) as a generally conservative start in dogs. In patients that are nonresponsive after this traditional dosing, the authors recommended intermittent bolusing at 1.5 ml/kg q4-6h for 24 hours with anecdotal success. In addition, follow-up CRI doses of 0.5 ml/kg/hr (0.1 g/kg/hr) can be continued until clinical signs improve (not to exceed 24 hours) or until serum is lipemic. That said, there have been no safety studies evaluating the use of ILE in the clinically poisoned veterinary patient, and careful monitoring and risk assessment is imperative.

The author has had experienced anecdotal success with the use of ILE for certain additional medications with a narrow margin of safety (e.g., baclofen, cholecalciferol, β-blockers). However, there are reports—in both human and veterinary medicine—where ILE has not been beneficial. In general, the use of ILE should be limited to life-threatening ingestions, severely symptomatic patients, and those that fail to respond to traditional therapy. Keep in mind that rare adverse effects of this extra-label drug include fat embolism, fat overload syndrome, pancreatitis, worsening of acute respiratory distress syndrome (ARDS), and even coagulopathy. More importantly, the use of ILE is generally reserved until late-stage or late-treatment in human medicine (e.g., once cardiopulmonary arrest has occurred) because of the risk of drug interaction (e.g., cardiopulmonary resuscitation drug therapy, anticonvulsants, muscle relaxants, sedatives) with ILE.

The administration of ILE for the treatment of local anesthetic or other lipophilic drug toxicosis in veterinary medicine is still in its infancy and the true potential benefit is currently unknown. The judicious use of this new potential antidote should be considered based on the lipophilic nature of the drug. Readers are directed to the most recent resources on ILE for further information.

CONCLUSION

When the clinician is presented the poisoned patient, the use of appropriate history, triage, decontamination, and overall therapy is necessary to ensure an optimal outcome. Knowledge of the underlying mechanism of action, the pharmacokinetics (including absorption, distribution, metabolism, and excretion), and the toxic dose of the toxicant are imperative in determining appropriate decontamination and therapy for the patient.

REFERENCES

1. American Academy of Clinical Toxicology: Position Paper: single-dose activated charcoal, Clin Toxic 43:61, 2005.
2. Peterson ME, Talcott PA: Small animal toxicology, St. Louis, 2013, Elsevier.
3. Osweiler G, Hovda, L, Brutlag A, et al: The five-minute veterinary consult clinical companion: small animal toxicology, Ames, IA, 2011, Wiley-Blackwell.
4. Burkitt JM, Haskins SC, Jandrey KE, et al: The effect of oral administration of a commercial activated charcoal suspension on serum osmolality and lactate concentration in the dog, J Vet Int Med 19(5):683, 2005.
5. Khan SA, Mclean MK, Slater M, et al: Effectiveness and adverse effects of the use of apomorphine and 3% hydrogen peroxide solution to induce emesis in dogs, J Am Vet Med Assoc 241(9):1179, 2012.
6. Plumb DC: Plumb's veterinary drug handbook, ed 7, Stockholm, WI, 2011, PharmaVet.
7. Babski DM, Koenig A: Acetaminophen. In Osweiler G, Hovda L, Brutlag A, Lee JA, editors: Blackwell's five-minute veterinary consult clinical companion: small animal toxicology, ed 1, Iowa City, IA, 2010, Wiley-Blackwell, pp 687-695.
8. Ferguson D, Crowe M, McLaughlin L, et al: Survival and prognostic indicators for Cycad intoxication in dogs, J Vet Int Med 25(4):831, 2011.
9. Fernandez AL, Lee JA, Rahilly LJ, et al: The use of intravenous lipid emulsion as an antidote in veterinary toxicology, J Vet Emerg Crit Care 21(4):309, 2011.
10. Jamaty C, Bailey B, La Rocque A, et al: Lipid emulsions in the treatment of acute poisoning: a systematic review of human and animal studies, ClinTox 48:1, 2010.
11. Crandell DE, Weinberg GL: Moxidectin toxicosis in a puppy successfully treated with intravenous lipids, J Vet Emerg Crit Care (2):181, 2009.
12. Clarke DL, Lee JA, Murphy LA, et al: Use of intravenous lipid emulsion to treat ivermectin toxicosis in a Border collie, J Am Vet Med Assoc 239(10):1328, 2011.
13. O'Brien TQ, Clark-Price SC, Evans EE, et al: Infusion of a lipid emulsion to treat lidocaine intoxication in a cat, J Am Vet Med Assoc 237:1455, 2010.
14. Gwaltney-Brant S, Meadows I: Use of intravenous lipid emulsions for treating certain poisoning cases in small animals, Vet Clin Small Anim 42:251, 2012.

CHAPTER 75

BLOOD PURIFICATION FOR INTOXICATIONS AND DRUG OVERDOSE

Carrie A. Palm, DVM, DACVIM • Kayo Kanakubo, DVM

KEY POINTS

- Extracorporeal therapies can provide lifesaving treatments for patients with intoxications and drug overdoses.
- The use of extracorporeal therapies should be considered when they can significantly enhance toxin removal.
- Extracorporeal therapies should be combined with appropriate traditional medical management to maximize toxin and drug removal.

Extracorporeal therapies (ECTs) provide advanced treatment options for acute intoxications and drug overdoses in veterinary patients. Extracorporeal therapies are modalities whereby blood is removed from patient circulation and treated or processed before being returned to the patient. In human medicine, ECTs are used in the treatment of severe intoxications and poisonings, primarily when other methods of efficient elimination are lacking. These therapies are used when patients are diagnosed with or suspected to have exposure to lethal intoxications, with or without outward clinical signs evident at the time of diagnosis, especially when exposure poses a high risk of morbidity and mortality, as well as a high probability of success.[1]

Intervention with ECTs and peritoneal dialysis (PD) is most effective when the total body clearance of the exogenous toxin is increased significantly from its normal endogenous clearance; however, this information is often unavailable, especially in veterinary patients. In veterinary medicine the majority of intoxications are due to indiscriminate ingestion by the animal, making quantification and timing of exposure difficult to accurately assess in many cases. Therefore there are limited evidenced-based studies to accurately confirm or recommend the use of ECT for specific poisonings or drug overdoses. Based on human studies and published case series and reports in veterinary medicine, the use of ECT can be justified and on some occasions recommended as the treatment of choice for intoxications and drug overdoses.

METHODS

Successful application of renal replacement therapy (RRT) (intermittent hemodialysis [IHD], continuous renal replacement therapy [CRRT]), hemoperfusion (HF), and total plasma exchange (TPE) in the treatment of intoxications is dependent on the characteristics of the treatment modality and the characteristics of the toxin, including toxin pharmacokinetics and pharmacodynamics, dose and timing of exposure, exposure route, and the existence of comorbidities.

The two main mechanisms of solute removal in RRT are diffusion and convection. Diffusion is the movement of solute across a semipermeable membrane and is driven by the transmembrane concentration gradient. Convection across a permeable membrane, also known as ultrafiltration, is the movement of water and the resultant solvent drag that occurs due to the transmembrane pressure gradient playing a role in solute removal. In IHD, the continuous venovenous hemodialysis (CVVHD) mode of CRRT and PD, removal of solute is mainly by diffusion. On the other hand, with the continuous venovenous hemofiltration (CVVH) mode of CRRT, solute removal is mainly achieved by convection. The continuous venovenous hemodiafiltration (CVVHDF) mode of CRRT and application of ultrafiltration during IHD and PD combine diffusive and convective modalities. Efficiency of solute removal is dependent on the permeability of the membrane and the solute characteristics. The permeability of a dialyzer membrane is determined by pore size, membrane surface area, membrane thickness, and membrane material. Smaller molecules are better removed by diffusion, and larger molecules are better removed by convection.

ECT should be considered for intoxicated animals that develop severe adverse clinical signs (such as coma secondary to barbiturate ingestion), for animals with significant acid-base and electrolyte abnormalities, and for animals in which the intoxicant can lead to significant morbidity and mortality. In animals with concurrent disease (primary or secondary to the intoxication), such as altered renal function that might decrease intoxicant elimination, ECT should be considered. One benefit of IHD over CRRT in the treatment of poisoning is the rapid and efficient solute removal that can occur with the high dialysate and blood flow rates associated with IHD. Smaller molecular weight water-soluble intoxicants are removed most efficiently by diffusion in IHD. Continuous renal replacement therapy provides slow and continuous solute removal, which has been reported to be better tolerated than IHD in hemodynamically unstable human patients; however, rapid toxin removal is almost always more ideal, and when performed by an experienced RRT team, IHD rarely leads to hemodynamic instability.[2,3] Application of both diffusive and convective properties in CRRT allows for more efficient removal of larger molecular weight solutes than in IHD.[4] In addition, the membranes used in CRRT are often more permeable than IHD membranes, allowing better clearance of larger molecular weight solutes than IHD. Because of the slow and continuous clearance in CRRT, solutes with a large volume of distribution (Vd) that are redistributed into the intravascular compartment have better clearance with CRRT compared with shorter IHD treatments. It is important to note, however, that IHD treatments can be prolonged or repeated to allow for removal of toxins as they re-equilibrate into the intravascular space, and the combination of IHD and charcoal hemoperfusion (CH) allows for removal of large solutes. Peritoneal dialysis is the most inefficient ECT for treatment of intoxications but can be considered when other modalities are not available.

Charcoal hemoperfusion (CH) is another ECT whereby a sorbent, typically activated charcoal, is used to selectively or nonselectively (as with activated charcoal) adsorb a toxin after contact with the blood.

This modality is useful for removal of non–readily dialyzable intoxications, such as toxins with high protein-binding capacity or a large molecular weight ([MW]; up to 40,000 Da).[5] In human medicine, the use of CH for toxin removal has declined over the last several years because of the potential complications, high cost, and short storage life of charcoal cartridges and the improved efficiency of IHD and CRRT modalities.[6-8] The use of CH in veterinary medicine is still applicable and is often combined with other RRT modalities. There are technical complications that limit the use of this modality for every patient. In theory the nonselective adsorptive property of activated charcoal can cause hypocalcemia, hypoglycemia, and thrombocytopenia and can compromise coagulation. Therefore CH is performed in tandem with HD to decrease or eliminate these potential side effects, as the blood passes through the dialyzer after contact with the HF cartridge, allowing for normalization of electrolyte abnormalities. In addition, coating of the activated charcoal increases the biocompatibility of the charcoal. The extracorporeal blood volume (priming volume) of commercially available CH cartridges ranges from 150 ml to 240 ml; the total extracorporeal circuit blood volume can lead to development of hemodynamic instability in small animals (body weight [BW] < 10 kg),sometimes limiting this treatment modality to larger dogs, especially when used in combination with the HD dialyzer. Newer cartridges with small priming volumes are becoming available, allowing for combination HD/CH to be performed in smaller patients; however, smaller priming volumes correlate with smaller volumes of charcoal, and therefore fewer binding sites and more rapid saturation of the CH cartridge. In addition, specialized techniques, such as priming the extracorporeal circuit with blood, can be considered when treating smaller patients with ECT.

Total plasma exchange (TPE) or plasmapheresis is an extracorporeal procedure in which the blood is removed from a patient and passed through a medical device that separates the blood into its various components (either by centrifugation or filtration). With this modality the plasma component of the blood is removed and replaced with a replacement solution, such as a colloid (e.g., albumin, Hetastarch, or plasma) or a combination of crystalloid and colloid.[9] The efficiency of toxin removal with TPE is independent of the toxin size and protein binding, allowing for efficient and rapid removal of toxins that are not readily dialyzable.[10] In addition to removal of the inciting toxin, removal of toxic byproducts, such as circulating mediators of inflammation and other endogenous substances, may also reduce toxin-induced complications.[11] This treatment modality is generally most effective for treatment of intoxications shortly after ingestion and for those toxins that have a small volume of distribution (Vd), because only the blood compartment is being treated and procedures are performed over a shorter period, so there is less time for redistribution of toxin into the intravascular space. The exchanged plasma volume, solute intercompartment equilibration, and endogenous clearances also affect treatment efficiency.[12,13] Because reports on the use of TPE for the treatment of intoxications in veterinary patients are lacking, the recommendations and clinical application of this modality are based mostly on human literature, the clinician's experience, and characteristics of the ingested toxin.

TOXIN OVERVIEW

The MW and toxicokinetics (e.g., Vd, protein binding capacity, lipid solubility) of the intoxicant will affect treatment efficacy, as does the ECT modality prescribed.

When using IHD, CRRT, or PD, the toxicant must cross the permeable dialysis membrane from the blood compartment and into the dialysate compartment for effective clearance to occur from the body. Low MW toxins such as ethylene glycol (EG), with a MW of 62 Da, readily diffuse through dialyzer membranes, similar to urea (MW 66 Da). As the MW of the toxin increases, conventional IHD dialyzer clearances become less efficient compared with convective modality dialyzers for CRRT or the natural peritoneal membrane used in PD. This concept is also applied for protein-bound toxins, which are primarily bound to albumin (MW 69,000 Da). The protein-toxin complex will not cross the dialyzer membranes; however, other techniques such as plasmapheresis and hemoperfusion are not affected by this protein binding.

Volume of distribution of a toxic substance is the sum of all compartmental volumes that account for the total toxin distribution at an equilibrated state. For maximal clearance, the ideal solute Vd is less than or equal to the blood volume because toxin removal occurs directly from the intravascular compartment. For toxins with a large Vd, concentration within the intravascular compartment decreases as the solute distributes between the body fluid compartments (intercompartmental equilibration). The speed of equilibration depends on the characteristics of the toxin as well as the Vd. For example, a highly lipid-soluble, large-MW toxin with large Vd is likely to have a slower compartmental equilibration time. This can lead to a posttreatment "rebound," which refers to an increase in plasma toxin concentration after cessation of toxin removal via ECT, as the toxin redistributes from the other compartments into the intravascular space.[3] It is critical to recognize that initial resolution of clinical signs does not necessarily indicate adequate reduction of whole-body toxin concentration to an acceptable level, and plasma concentration of the intoxicant may return to a toxic level as intercompartmental equilibration occurs (Figure 75-1).

With IHD, CRRT, and PD, as the unbound solute (pharmacologically and toxicologically active form) is cleared, the rate of solute separation from the protein-bound state will affect the clearance rate. Highly protein bound toxins, depending on the affinity to the charcoal, in CH will competitively separate from the protein and adsorb to the charcoal for removal. In humans, for drugs and toxins with high affinity to albumin, albumin-supplemented dialysate has been used in CRRT. In this modality, as the free toxin crosses the membrane to bind with albumin in the dialysate, the concentration gradient will change and more toxin will dissociate from the albumin in the blood and will contribute to a greater clearance of toxin.[14]

In veterinary medicine the pharmacokinetics and toxicokinetics of many drugs and toxins are unknown, and this can make it difficult

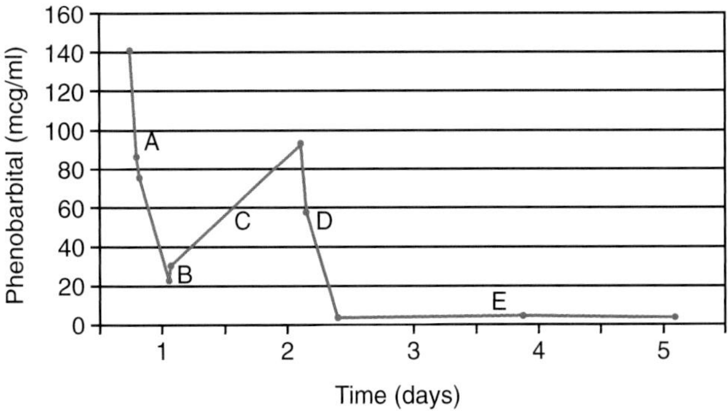

FIGURE 75-1 Representative graph for a patient undergoing blood purification (HD/CH) for treatment of phenobarbital overdose. **A,** The concentration of phenobarbital is decreasing secondary to removal during treatment 1. **B,** Rebound of phenobarbital into the intravascular space has occurred immediately after cessation of treatment. **C,** Rebound of phenobarbital into the intravascular space in the 24 hours after cessation of treatment 1. **D,** The concentration of phenobarbital is decreasing secondary to removal during treatment 2. **E,** Posttreatment phenobarbital concentrations. Note the lack of significant rebound into the intravascular space during this period.

to predict the efficacy of ECT for treatment of intoxications. In addition, the established pharmacokinetics and toxicokinetics of substances may vary when overdose occurs or when comorbidities are present. For example, uremia will alter the tissue binding capacity of some solutes, resulting in a decreased Vd.[15] In settings of low plasma protein concentrations and highly protein-bound drugs, the free fraction of drug increases but can re-equilibrate in tissue compartments and result in a higher Vd. Drug overdose can lead to saturation of protein binding sites in the plasma, and this may potentially decrease the protein binding ratio of the drug and lead to increased removal by HD.

CONSIDERATIONS

Considerations for treatment of toxicities with ECT include factors such as the associated morbidity and mortality of intoxication, treatment outcome with traditional therapies, patient characteristics (comorbidities, patient size, dose of intoxication, time of exposure), endogenous clearance, and characteristics of the toxin (MW, Vd, protein binding capacity, solubility, half-life).[10,16]

Ethylene Glycol

Ethylene glycol, a sweet and odorless glycol that is commonly used in automobile antifreeze products, is a common intoxication seen in dogs. The inherent toxicity of EG is very low, but significant morbidity and mortality results from generated metabolites, such as glycolic acid and oxalic acid. Calcium oxalate crystal formation develops in multiple organs, including the renal tubules, and can result in severe acute kidney injury and ultimately multiple organ failure.[17] The MW of EG is 62 Da with no protein binding capacity and a Vd of 0.5 to 0.8 L/kg of body weight (in humans). The absorption rate from the gastrointestinal tract is rapid (1 to 4 hours), and the plasma half-life in humans is about 3 to 9 hours. Because of its similar characteristics to urea, EG and its toxic metabolites are readily dialyzed with RRT.[18] The aim of the treatment is to readily remove EG and its metabolites (targeting 90% to 100% reduction) before there is significant conversion into oxalic acid. During the treatment, dialysate is formulated to correct and modify patient electrolyte, acid-base, and/or hemodynamic disorders. In addition, ethanol is added to the dialysate concentrate to inhibit ongoing metabolism of EG to its more toxic metabolites.[19] It is important to note that with the use of RRT, both EG and toxic metabolites are removed, while ethanol prevents further development of these toxic metabolites. This is in contrast to traditional medical management, where toxic metabolites are not removed. Current indications for use of HD in humans with EG toxicity include significant metabolic acidosis (pH < 7.25 to 7.30), acute kidney injury, and electrolyte abnormalities unresponsive to conventional therapy.[18] In veterinary medicine the definitive recommendations for initiation of HD for treatment of EG intoxication are not well defined; however, there is no question that early intervention is critical to prevent the development of life-threatening acute kidney injury. In our hospital, any patient with a recent history of exposure, as well as clinical evidence of EG exposure, is offered ECT as a treatment option. It is crucial that traditional medical intervention be employed immediately, pending the decision to pursue ECT.

Acetaminophen

According to the American Society for the Prevention of Cruelty to Animals (ASPCA) Animal Poison Control Center (APCC) data collected from 2002 to 2010, almost 25% of intoxication cases in dogs and cats in the United States were due to ingestion of human medications. The most common exposure reported in 2009 was acetaminophen (5.1%), followed by ibuprofen (2.1%).[24]

There are two main pathways for acetaminophen metabolism: conjugation with sulfate and glucuronide (accounting for 90% of the ingested dose) and metabolism by the cytochrome P-450 oxidase enzyme system (accounting for 5% of ingested dose). When acetaminophen is consumed in excess, the sulfation and glucuronidation pathways become saturated and formation of toxic substances increases.[25] N-acetyl-p-benzoquinone imine (NAPQI) has a direct toxic effect on the liver and on erythrocytes. In dogs and cats, acetaminophen toxicosis is usually associated with a single acute ingestion and liver and red blood cells are most commonly affected. In dogs, clinical signs are seen with 100 mg/kg of ingested dose, with peak plasma concentrations occurring at 2 to 4 hours postingestion. In cats, because of their reduced glucuronide metabolism and relative deficiency of glutathione, clinical signs can be seen from 10 mg/kg of ingestion, with peak plasma concentrations occurring at 0.5 hours postingestion. Plasma half-life (range 0.6 to 4.8 hours postingestion) is prolonged as the ingested dose increases.[26] Acetaminophen is a small (151 Da), non–protein bound, highly water-soluble compound with a small Vd. Although acetaminophen was shown to be readily dialyzed, the liver metabolism exceeded the clearance of the drug in normal dosages in uremic patients on maintenance hemodialysis.[27] In humans, HD and CH have been shown to reduce plasma half-life compared with conventional therapies.[28] In a human case report, where CVVHD was applied in combination with N-acetylcysteine administration, there was no significant change in the elimination half-life during dialysis or after dialysis had been stopped.[29] The author concluded that ongoing absorption of the drug from the gastrointestinal tract might have masked the true clearance rate of the drug by CVVHD. This highlights the importance of using medical therapy to bind drug from the intestinal tract, in conjunction with ECT. There are no reports in veterinary medicine on the application of ECT in acetaminophen intoxication; however, clinical experience at our institution has shown promising results in intoxicated patients with significant neurologic abnormalities at the time of presentation. ECT should be considered as a treatment option for animals with severe life-threatening complications and in animals with a history of recent (within 6 to 24 hours) ingestion, where decontamination is not possible or time of exposure makes decontamination unlikely to be successful.

Nonsteroidal Antiinflammatory Drugs

Nonsteroidal antiinflammatory drugs (NSAIDs) are cyclooxygenase-inhibiting medications that are prescribed often for acute and chronic orthopedic and surgical pain management. The pharmacokinetics of most drugs in this class are similar: small in size, highly protein bound (90% to 95%; mostly to albumin), and small Vd. As drug intoxication doses increase, protein binding sites become saturated, leading to an increase in the unbound fraction.[16] Most NSAIDs are absorbed efficiently after oral administration and are subsequently metabolized by the liver and then excreted in the urine. Some of these drugs undergo extensive enterohepatic recirculation, which may change the drug elimination rate (e.g., diclofenac, indomethacin, sulindac, etodolac, ibuprofen, naproxen, piroxicam, meloxicam, carprofen). Salicylate drug Vd can change with changes in blood pH, whereby a decrease in blood pH will increase the Vd as the drug diffuses out of the intravascular space.[30] Regardless of the specific NSAID ingested, initial treatment is directed to prevent further absorption of the drug from the gastrointestinal tract and at forced diuresis with fluid therapy. As with EG intoxication, it is critical to ensure that medical management is combined with ECT, especially during initial evaluation before ECT can be started. When making the decision to recommend ECT, it is critical to consider timing of exposure, the actual exposed dose, the presence of symptoms associated with the toxicity, and patient-specific characteristics. Detailed recommendations regarding the use of ECT in NSAID toxicity are not well defined. The high protein binding property of the drug favors the use of CH over conventional HD. In salicylate poisoning, patients can develop severe acid-base abnormalities, and in these cases, HD is considered a better treatment modality because it can modify acid-base status and prevent respiratory collapse.[31-33] As mentioned previously, in veterinary medicine, hemoperfusion is almost always performed simultaneously with HD to prevent the potential complications associated with CH. The large extracorporeal volume needed to perform combined HD/HP limits the application for this modality to larger patients. Efficient clearance of the unbound fraction of toxin may result in resolution of clinical signs as the patient is being dialyzed; however, as redistribution of the drug occurs, clinical signs may reappear. Online measurement of drug levels is not possible in veterinary medicine, so appropriate treatment times may be difficult to determine. Likewise, it is difficult to determine when a HP cartridge is saturated, although in the author's experience this typically occurs 4 to 6 hours after the start of therapy. If large quantities of residual drug remain in the gastrointestinal tract, leading to continued absorption, or if significant enterohepatic recirculation occurs, plasma concentrations may not decrease as anticipated. ECT should be continued until life-threatening symptoms associated with the drug resolve, and treatment should be combined with conventional medical therapy. TPE can also be utilized as a treatment for NSAID intoxication, given the high protein binding and low volume of distribution; however, evidence-based reports are lacking in both human and veterinary medicine.[9]

Mushrooms

Mushroom poisoning in animals and humans is associated with high morbidity and mortality. *Amanita phalloides*, also known as Death Cap, is found throughout North America, and associated toxins (amatoxins) are rapidly absorbed from the gastrointestinal tract.[34] These toxins target hepatocytes, crypt cells, and proximal convoluted tubules of the kidney via inhibition of protein synthesis. The plasma half-life is 25 to 50 minutes, and it is not detectable in plasma after 24 hours of exposure.[35] The amatoxin is water-soluble and non–protein bound with a molecular weight range of 373 to 990 Da. The Vd is small, 0.3 L/kg in humans, and it is 80% to 90% excreted in urine with 7% excretion in bile.[36] Alpha-amanitin, one of the most deadly amatoxins, is 60% excreted in the bile and returned to the liver via enterohepatic circulation.

Various methods have been recommended for treatment of Amanita poisoning. The characteristics of amatoxin make it an ideal toxin to be removed effectively by ECT; however, the rapid absorption and short plasma half-life limit the beneficial effect of the treatment. The high affinity of amatoxin to activated charcoal makes HP a more effective treatment compared with HD alone.[37] The use of TPE has been suggested to be useful for removal of the amatoxin itself, the toxic endogenous metabolites, and for removal of amatoxin-induced inflammatory mediators.[10,38] In humans it is recommended that TPE or CH be initiated within 24 to 48 hours of ingestion and that it be used in conjunction with other therapies. Studies in humans have shown decreased mortality with the use of these methods.[1,39,40] In veterinary medicine the limited diagnostics and lack of early detection of ingestion limit the therapeutic efficacy of ECT for treatment of many Amanita poisonings, but the use of TPE and hemoperfusion should be considered if early ingestion is identified.

Barbiturates

The long-acting barbiturate phenobarbital is used commonly in veterinary medicine, and in the author's experience is one of the most common barbiturate poisonings encountered. In human medicine, ECT is used to treat long-acting barbiturate intoxications when prolonged hypotension is present and when severe respiratory depression requiring ventilatory support is present.[41] Phenobarbital is absorbed slowly from the gastrointestinal tract of dogs and has a bioavailability of up to 90% after ingestion. Volume of distribution is 0.75 L/kg in dogs and metabolism occurs largely via conjugation in the liver. Human studies have shown that both hemoperfusion and HD can enhance elimination of barbiturates, but the overall benefit of this enhanced elimination is controversial. In veterinary medicine, when severe intoxication with long-acting barbiturates occurs, ECTs can be used to decrease hospital stay and to avoid complications such as aspiration pneumonia that can occur in severely obtunded or comatose patients. Given the large Vd, rebound of drug into the intravascular space is likely to occur after treatment with HD/HP, with resultant recurrence of clinical signs. In these situations, multiple or prolonged ECT sessions may be indicated. In addition, given the prolonged absorption of drug from the intestinal tract, as well as the presence of enterohepatic recirculation, medical therapy should be used in conjunction with ECT.

Lily Ingestion

Lilium and *Hemerocallis* plant species ingestion causes acute kidney injury in cats. According to the ASPCA, APCC, cases of lily toxicosis have increased since 2006.[42] The main toxin responsible for acute tubular necrosis in cats is still unknown. Rumbeiha et al demonstrated that toxic substances are present in the aqueous fraction of leaves and flowers.[43] In their report, cats showed clinical signs of vomiting and lethargy within 12 hours of ingestion and showed blood biochemistry and urine abnormalities within 24 hours after administration. The species-specific toxicity in cats is hypothesized to be due to a different metabolism of the toxin compared with other species.[44] Whether or not ECT provides additional clearance of toxins associated with lily ingestion is unknown. Currently in veterinary medicine, ECT is recommended only in cats with significant acute kidney injury but not for prevention of acute kidney injury secondary to lily intoxication.[45,46]

SUMMARY

The use of ECTs can aid in the treatment of poisonings and can improve outcomes for veterinary patients. When prescribing an ECT for treatment of intoxication, it is critical to have a solid understanding of the risks and benefits of treatment, as well as an understanding of drug toxicokinetics and of the EC modality chosen. It is also crucial that traditional medical management be used periprocedurally to allow for the best possible outcomes.

REFERENCES

1. Nenov VD, Marinov P, Sabeva J, et al: Current applications of plasmapheresis in clinical toxicology, Nephrol Dial Transplant 18(Suppl 5):56, 2003.
2. Tyagi PK, Winchester JF, Feinfeld DA: Extracorporeal removal of toxins, Kidney Int 74:1231, 2008.
3. Goodman JW, Goldfarb DS: The role of continuous renal replacement therapy in the treatment of poisoning, Semin Dial 19:402, 2006.
4. Messer J, Mulcahy B, Fissell WH: Middle-molecule clearance in CRRT: in vitro convection, diffusion and dialyzer area, ASAIO J 55:224, 2009.
5. Cutler RE, Forland SC, Hammond PG, et al: Extracorporeal removal of drugs and poisons by hemodialysis and hemoperfusion, Ann Rev Pharmacol Toxicol 27:169, 1987.
6. Ram Prabahar M, Raja Karthik K, Singh M, et al: Successful treatment of carbamazepine poisoning with hemodialysis: a case report and review of the literature, Hemodial Int 15:407, 2011.
7. Pilapil M, Petersen J: Efficacy of hemodialysis and charcoal hemoperfusion in carbamazepine overdose, Clin Toxicol (Phila) 46:342, 2008.

8. Tapolyai M, Campbell M, Dailey K, et al: Hemodialysis is as effective as hemoperfusion for drug removal in carbamazepine poisoning, Nephron 90:213, 2002.
9. Szczepiorkowski ZM, Winters JL, Bandarenko N, et al: Guidelines on the use of therapeutic apheresis in clinical practice—evidence-based approach from the Apheresis Applications Committee of the American Society for Apheresis, J Clin Apher 25:83, 2010.
10. Schutt RC, Ronco C, Rosner MH: The role of therapeutic plasma exchange in poisonings and intoxications, Semin Dial 25:201, 2012.
11. St Nenov D, Sv Nenov K: Therapeutic apheresis in exogenous poisoning and in myeloma, Nephrol Dial Transplant 16(Suppl 6):101, 2001.
12. Ezidiegwu C, Spektor Z, Nasr MR, et al: A case report on the role of plasma exchange in the management of a massive amlodipine besylate intoxication, Ther Apher Dial 12:180, 2008.
13. Ibrahim RB, Liu C, Cronin SM, et al: Drug removal by plasmapheresis: an evidence-based review, Pharmacotherapy 2007;27:1529, 2007.
14. Churchwell MD, Pasko DA, Smoyer WE, et al: Enhanced clearance of highly protein-bound drugs by albumin-supplemented dialysate during modeled continuous hemodialysis, Nephrol Dial Transplant 24:231, 2009.
15. Awdishu L, Bouchard J: How to optimize drug delivery in renal replacement therapy, Semin Dialysis 24:176, 2011.
16. Fertel BS, Nelson LS, Goldfarb DS: Extracorporeal removal techniques for the poisoned patient: a review for the intensivist, J Intensive Care Med 25:139, 2010.
17. McMartin K: Are calcium oxalate crystals involved in the mechanism of acute renal failure in ethylene glycol poisoning? Clin Toxicol (Phila) 47:859, 2009.
18. Barceloux DG, Krenzelok EP, Olson K, et al: American Academy of Clinical Toxicology practice guidelines on the treatment of ethylene glycol poisoning. Ad hoc committee, J Toxicol Clin Toxicol 37:537, 1999.
19. Cowgill LD: Urea kinetics and intermittent dialysis prescription in small animals, Vet Clin North Am Small Anim Pract 41:193, 2011.
20. Reference deleted in pages.
21. Reference deleted in pages.
22. Reference deleted in pages.
23. Reference deleted in pages.
24. McLean MK, Hansen SR: An overview of trends in animal poisoning cases in the United States: 2002-2010, Vet Clin North Am Small Anim Pract 42:219, v, 2012.
25. Bartlett D: Acetaminophen toxicity, J Emerg Nurs 30:281, 2004.
26. Savides MC, Oehme FW, Nash SL, et al: The toxicity and biotransformation of single doses of acetaminophen in dogs and cats, Toxicol Appl Pharmacol 1984;74:26, 1984.
27. Lee CS, Wang LH, Marbury TC, et al: Hemodialysis for acetaminophen detoxification, Clin Toxicol 18:431, 1981.
28. Higgins RM, Goldsmith DJ, MacDiarmid-Gordon A, et al: Treating paracetamol overdose by charcoal haemoperfusion and long-hours high-flux dialysis, QJM 89:297, 1996.
29. Wiegand TJ, Margaretten M, Olson KR: Massive acetaminophen ingestion with early metabolic acidosis and coma: treatment with IV NAC and continuous venovenous hemodiafiltration, Clin Toxicol (Phila) 48:156, 2010.
30. Hill JB: Salicylate intoxication, N Engl J Med 288:1110, 1973.
31. Winchester JF, Gelfand MC, Helliwell M, et al: Extracorporeal treatment of salicylate or acetaminophen poisoning—is there a role? Arch Intern Med 141:370, 1981.
32. Cohen DL, Post J, Ferroggiaro AA, et al: Chronic salicylism resulting in noncardiogenic pulmonary edema requiring hemodialysis, Am J Kidney Dis 36:E20, 2000.
33. Dargan PI, Wallace CI, Jones AL: An evidence based flowchart to guide the management of acute salicylate (aspirin) overdose, Emerg Med J 19:206, 2002.
34. Puschner B, Wegenast C: Mushroom poisoning cases in dogs and cats: diagnosis and treatment of hepatotoxic, neurotoxic, gastroenterotoxic, nephrotoxic, and muscarinic mushrooms, Vet Clin North Am Small Anim Pract 42:375, viii, 2012.
35. Faulstich H, Talas A, Wellhoner HH: Toxicokinetics of labeled amatoxins in the dog, Arch Toxicol 56:190, 1985.
36. Feinfeld DA, Rosenberg JW, Winchester JF: Three controversial issues in extracorporeal toxin removal, Semin Dial 19:358, 2006.
37. Paydas S, Kocak R, Erturk F, et al: Poisoning due to amatoxin-containing Lepiota species, Br J Clin Pract 44:450, 1990.
38. Jander S, Bischoff J, Woodcock BG: Plasmapheresis in the treatment of Amanita phalloides poisoning: II. A review and recommendations, Ther Apher 4:308, 2000.
39. Jander S, Bischoff J: Treatment of Amanita phalloides poisoning: I. Retrospective evaluation of plasmapheresis in 21 patients, Ther Apher 4:303, 2000.
40. Aji DY, Caliskan S, Nayir A, et al: Haemoperfusion in Amanita phalloides poisoning, J Trop Ped 41:371, 1995.
41. Roberts DM, Buckley NA: Enhanced elimination in acute barbiturate poisoning—a systematic review, Clin Toxicol 2011;49:2, 2011.
42. Slater MR, Gwaltney-Brant S: Exposure circumstances and outcomes of 48 households with 57 cats exposed to toxic lily species, J Am Anim Hosp Assoc 47:386, 2011.
43. Rumbeiha WK, Francis JA, Fitzgerald SD, et al: A comprehensive study of Easter lily poisoning in cats, J Vet Diagnost Invest 16:527, 2004.
44. Hall J: Lilies. In Peterson M, editor: Small animal toxicology, ed 3, St Louis, 2013, Elsevier, p 617.
45. Berg RI, Francey T, Segev G: Resolution of acute kidney injury in a cat after lily (Lilium lancifolium) intoxication, J Vet Intern Med 21:857, 2007.
46. Langston CE: Acute renal failure caused by lily ingestion in six cats, J Am Vet Med Assoc 220:49, 36, 2002.

CHAPTER 76
NONSTEROIDAL ANTIINFLAMMATORY DRUGS

Sarah Haldane, BVSc, BAnSc, MANZCVSc, DACVECC

KEY POINTS

- The incidence of adverse drug events caused by NSAIDs is high.
- Despite their increased safety margin, adverse gastrointestinal effects are still the most common side effects of COX-2–selective NSAIDs.
- The toxic dose of an NSAID can vary with the chronicity of administration as well as the patient's age, comorbidity, and concurrent medications.
- Overdose of NSAIDs should be treated as an emergency even if the patient is not yet showing clinical signs of toxicity.
- Client education plays a key role in reducing the risk and improving the outcome of NSAID toxicity.

Nonsteroidal antiinflammatory drugs (NSAIDs) are among the most commonly used medications in human and veterinary medicine. The potential for small animals to develop toxicoses is enormous because the drugs are encountered frequently in household medicine cabinets, and many of the NSAIDs have a small therapeutic margin for safety. The incidence of adverse drug events associated with NSAIDs is high in veterinary patients; they are among the most common medication-related calls to poison control centers and to the U.S. Federal Drug Administration's Center for Veterinary Medicine.[1,2]

COX-1, COX-2, AND PROSTAGLANDINS

After a tissue has been damaged, arachidonic acid is released from cell membranes, precipitating a chain of events known as the arachidonic acid cascade. Two enzyme groups metabolize arachidonic acid: the lipoxygenases (LOX) and the cyclooxygenases (COX). Products from the LOX cascade include leukotrienes and chemotactic factors. Products of the COX cascade include prostacyclin, thromboxanes, and prostaglandins.

Prostaglandins have diverse effects in many organ systems. They are often important in maintaining local blood supply to tissues. Continuously produced (constitutive) prostaglandins are required for the normal function of the brain, kidneys, gastrointestinal tract, primary hemostatic system, and reproductive system. Inducible prostaglandins are produced in response to tissue injury. They escalate the inflammatory response and increase peripheral nerve sensitization; they also have protective actions and play a role in tissue repair.[3,4]

The two main COX enzymes are known as COX-1 and COX-2. Although most COX-1–induced prostaglandins are constitutive and have homeostatic effects, some are also produced in response to tissue injury. Similarly, although many prostaglandins produced by COX-2 are inducible, there are constitutive COX-2 prostaglandins found in the brain, intestine, and kidneys in many species.[4-7]

NSAIDs are potent inhibitors of prostaglandin production. They are described as being nonspecific or dual acting if they inhibit both COX-1 and COX-2. Aspirin is the classic example of a dual-acting NSAID. Other examples in the veterinary market include ketoprofen and tepoxalin. COX-2–selective drugs have also been produced. The purpose of these drugs is to reduce inflammatory prostaglandin production via COX-2 inhibition with relatively less suppression of COX-1. However, all COX-2 inhibitors still inhibit COX-1 to some degree. A number of veterinary COX-2–selective NSAIDs are available, including carprofen, meloxicam, deracoxib, and firocoxib.

A COX variant, known as COX-3, has been isolated in the dog's brain and has similar inflammatory and pyretic effects to COX-1 and COX-2. Acetaminophen has been shown to specifically inhibit COX-3, so it has antiinflammatory and antipyretic effects in the brain. COX-3 in other species does not have the same inflammatory effects as in dogs.[8,9]

Older-generation NSAIDs, such as ibuprofen and naproxen, are far more likely to cause adverse effects than the newer formulations; however, the potential for complications still exists with chronic use or overdose of COX-2–selective NSAIDs. NSAID administration can have significant detrimental effects in animals with fluid deficits, gastrointestinal, renal, or hepatic disease or with disorders of primary coagulation.

POTENTIAL ADVERSE EFFECTS

Gastrointestinal Effects

Gastric ulceration is a common side effect of NSAID administration with prolonged use, high doses, or administration to hypovolemic or inappetent animals.[10,11] COX-1–induced prostaglandins in the gastric mucosa have protective effects: they increase gastric mucous production and enhance local blood flow. COX-2 is stimulated once damage has occurred to the intestinal mucosa and produces prostaglandins that play an important role in mucosal healing.[3,6,11-13] This means that NSAID administration can cause gastric ulceration and inhibit the ability of ulcers to heal. Some NSAIDs, such as aspirin, can cause direct injury to the gastric mucosa by disrupting surface phospholipids, allowing gastric acid to penetrate directly to the cells in the wall of the stomach.[6,14] In addition to their mucosal effects, COX-1– and COX-2–induced prostaglandins are important in the regulation of gastrointestinal motility.[15,16]

Despite their increased safety margin, adverse gastrointestinal effects are still the most common side effects of COX-2–selective NSAIDs.[10,11] NSAIDs are weak acids that become lipid soluble in the highly acidic environment in the stomach. This allows them to penetrate easily into gastric cells, where they become trapped in the relatively more alkaline environment. This leads to a high local concentration of NSAIDs in the gastric mucosa and may be an explanation for adverse effects occurring in the gastrointestinal system at lower doses than in other organ systems.[2] In one experimental study assessing long-term NSAID use in dogs, carprofen had the lowest incidence of gastrointestinal side effects when compared with meloxicam, ketoprofen, flunixin meglumine, and etodolac.[17] Multiple endoscopic and mucosal permeability studies have been performed evaluating the effects of short-term NSAID use, and no significant adverse effects have been found. However, because of the nature of these studies, only a few dogs were assessed in each, making it difficult to evaluate the importance of their findings.[14,18-22]

Deracoxib, meloxicam, and carprofen have been associated with gastrointestinal perforation. In most of these cases the drugs were administered at higher-than-recommended dosages or were administered concurrently with a corticosteroid or another NSAID.[23-28]

Renal Effects

When perfusion to the kidney declines, glomerular filtration rate (GFR) decreases accordingly. The juxtaglomerular apparatus (JGA) in the kidney releases prostaglandins that vasodilate the afferent renal arteriole to maintain renal blood flow and GFR. They also stimulate the release of renin from the JGA. This effect is mediated by the COX-1 and COX-2 enzymes.[29] When NSAIDs are administered to a hypovolemic patient, the prostaglandin-mediated effect of local vasodilation is diminished or lost. Significant damage to the kidneys can result and this can lead to acute renal failure.[7] Also, COX-2–selective medications can increase the relative production of thromboxanes, which have local vasoconstrictive effects and can exacerbate renal damage. Ketoprofen, carprofen, and tepoxalin at therapeutic doses have been shown to have little effect on renal perfusion in healthy anesthetized dogs. However, overdose or accidental ingestion of large doses of NSAIDs can potentially lead to acute renal failure despite normal blood volume.[7,10]

Hepatic Effects

NSAIDs are metabolized in the liver, primarily by conjugation with glycin or glucuronic acid. NSAID use has been associated with an increase in liver enzymes and hepatocellular injury in some patients. This toxicity does not depend on dose or duration of treatment and therefore is classified as an idiosyncratic reaction. In one report describing hepatoxicity secondary to carprofen administration, there was a marked similarity in the course of disease among Labrador Retrievers, which may indicate a possible underlying genetic basis in this breed. However, this result may have been influenced by the large number of Labradors that require NSAID administration for degenerative joint disease.[30] Because of the risk of hepatic toxicity, NSAID administration is not recommended for animals with concurrent liver disease.

Coagulation Effects

Prostacyclin (PGI_2) is produced from epithelial cells via COX-2 synthesis and inhibits platelet aggregation and causes vasodilation. COX-1 mediates production of thromboxane A_2 (TXA_2) from platelets, which increases platelet aggregation and causes vasoconstriction.[31] The balance between TXA_2 and PGI_2 is important in maintaining a functional coagulation system.

Aspirin is the most effective NSAID for reducing platelet aggregation because it binds permanently and decreases TXA_2 production for the life of the platelet. Conversely the COX-2–selective coxib class of drugs has been associated with increased risk of thrombosis-related cardiac events in humans.[32] In veterinary medicine, ketoprofen, carprofen, tepoxalin, meloxicam, and deracoxib have been studied to assess their affects on primary hemostasis. Ketoprofen and carprofen have been associated with decreased platelet function and deracoxib with potential for increased thrombosis in experimental trials; however, there are no published reports of clinically relevant hemostatic complications in dogs or cats.[17,31,33,34]

Bone and Cartilage Effects

Studies in animal models have shown that aspirin, indomethacin, and naproxen can have a deleterious effect on cartilage formation, which is significant because NSAIDs are often the primary therapeutic agents used to manage osteoarthritis in dogs and cats.[35-37] In contrast, *in vitro* studies have been performed showing that COX-2–selective NSAIDs may have a protective effect on human chondrocytes in early osteoarthritis.[38] In dogs, carprofen has been shown to reduce the severity of early structural changes and histologic lesions in experimental models of osteoarthritis.[39,40] Rofecoxib had a protective effect on cartilage in experimental trials in rats, and meloxicam did not cause further cartilage damage in a trial of calcium pyrophosphate crystal–induced osteoarthritis in dogs.[37,41]

Potential effects of NSAIDs on the rate of bone healing are also a concern. Long-term carprofen administration may reduce bone healing after fracture, and meloxicam has also been shown to reduce fracture healing in a mouse model.[42,43]

In general, experimental trial results vary, and outcomes differ based on the type, dose, and duration of the NSAID given to the subject as well as the species of the subject. Controversy remains regarding the impact of long-term NSAID use in osteoarthritis and bone healing, and further *in vivo* studies and clinical trials are necessary.[36]

Neurologic Effects

The most common adverse effect of NSAIDs in the central nervous system (CNS) of people is aseptic meningitis. A number of drugs have been reported to cause this, including meloxicam, diclofenac, naproxen, and ibuprofen.[44-47] There are no published cases of neurologic side effects of NSAID administration in veterinary medicine; however, anecdotal reports suggest that high doses of ibuprofen can cause seizures in dogs.[48]

DRUG INTERACTIONS WITH NSAIDs

Concurrent administration of two NSAIDs or an NSAID with a corticosteroid significantly increases the risk of gastrointestinal and renal injury and can impede healing of ulcers.[10,13,14,26,49] Aspirin in particular increases the risk of GI bleeding when administered with other NSAIDs or corticosteroids.[6,11,49]

NSAIDs are highly protein bound in the plasma and displace other protein-bound drugs, increasing their bioavailability and potentially leading to toxic plasma concentrations. These drugs include other antiinflammatory agents, warfarin, phenytoin, penicillins, and sulfonamide antibiotics. NSAIDs can also increase plasma levels of digoxin and can decrease the efficacy of furosemide.

Use of NSAIDs with other potentially nephrotoxic drugs, such as aminoglycoside antibiotics, is relatively contraindicated, but studies have not been performed to prove a clinical interaction. Diuretic use is not recommended in conjunction with NSAIDs because of the risk of hypovolemia and subsequent renal toxicity.[7] Drugs that induce cytochrome P450 metabolic pathway in the liver (e.g., phenobarbitone) can increase NSAID metabolism, reducing their analgesic efficacy.

TOXIC DOSAGE

The toxic dose of individual NSAIDs can be difficult to determine: it depends on the nature of the ingestion (i.e., acute or chronic), the species and age of the patient, the patient's morbidity, and the administration of any concurrent medications. Furthermore, individual animals vary with regard to the length of time it takes to metabolize some of the NSAIDs, particularly ibuprofen, aspirin, deracoxib, and carprofen.[50-54] Even therapeutic doses of NSAIDs can have adverse effects in any patient with concurrent illness.

Some of the NSAIDs have been studied to determine an acute toxic dose. These doses must be interpreted with care because they were generally extrapolated from only a small number of cases. In one report in dogs, ibuprofen doses of 100 mg/kg caused clinical signs of gastrointestinal disease, whereas renal failure occurred at a dose of 175 mg/kg. In this study, 600 mg/kg of ibuprofen caused acute death.[55] However, ibuprofen at only 8 mg/kg/day has been reported to cause gastrointestinal ulceration after 30 days of therapy.[56] Cats can show adverse effects of ibuprofen administration at approximately half the dose of dogs because of their limited ability to metabolize the drug through glucuronidation.[57]

Aspirin can cause gastrointestinal erosions in dogs at doses of 75 mg/kg/day after 2 days. Acute ingestion of 400 mg/kg can cause toxicity in dogs.[55] In cats, 25 to 100 mg/kg/day can cause gastric ulceration.[58] Doses as low as 5 to 10 mg/kg of naproxen have been reported to cause adverse effects in dogs[59,60] as have doses of greater than 6 mg/kg of deracoxib.[61] Meloxicam can cause gastrointestinal upset in dogs at 0.15 to 0.2 mg/kg/day for 3 days.[36,62] Renal failure has been reported in dogs after 3 days of therapy at 0.6 to 1 mg/kg/day.[62]

CLINICAL SIGNS

The clinical signs associated with gastrointestinal toxicity of NSAIDs are often nonspecific and include inappetence, lethargy, and vomiting. Depending on the location of the mucosal injury, hematemesis, melena, or hematochezia can occur. These signs are seen less commonly in cats with gastrointestinal ulceration than with dogs.[25] Intestinal perforation can cause chemical or septic peritonitis. Signs may include acute pain, hypovolemia, and, in some cases, fever. Animals may be presented in a collapsed state as a result of hypovolemic or septic shock.

Renal injury can result in polyuria or oliguria, dehydration, inappetence, abdominal pain, and vomiting. If NSAIDs cause a clinical coagulopathy, signs of bleeding from mucosal surfaces could be observed, including epistaxis, hematemesis, or melena.

DIAGNOSIS OF NSAID TOXICITY

In most cases NSAID toxicosis is diagnosed by the presence of relevant clinical signs associated with a history of NSAID use. In cases of accidental overdose, patients can be presented before the onset of clinical signs and the diagnosis is based on history alone.

The emergency database may show alterations in acid base and electrolyte concentrations. The most common acid base abnormality seen is metabolic acidosis; however, patients that have vomited a significant volume of gastric fluid can present with a metabolic alkalosis. Vomiting, diarrhea, hypovolemia, and potential renal losses can affect electrolyte concentrations; therefore sodium, potassium, and chloride concentrations can be variable, depending on the location of injury and severity of illness in individual patients.

A hemogram may indicate anemia in patients with gastrointestinal hemorrhage or coagulopathy. Conversely, an increase in packed cell volume and plasma protein concentration is seen in dehydrated animals. There may be leukocytosis if there is gastroenteritis or peritonitis. The platelet count is unlikely to be decreased significantly, even in coagulopathy, because NSAIDs affect the function but not the number of platelets. A buccal mucosal bleeding time can be used to assess platelet function. Coagulation tests, such as prothromin time (PT) and activated partial thromboplastin time (aPTT), can be performed to rule out other causes of coagulopathy; these tests are not affected by NSAID toxicity.

Biochemistry results may show evidence of azotemia that can be prerenal because of dehydration or renal if the patient is in acute renal failure. A patient with gastrointestinal hemorrhage may have an increase in blood urea nitrogen without a concurrent increase in creatinine, indicating digestion of blood. Hepatic toxicity causes an increase in alanine transferase, alkaline phosphatase, and, less frequently, serum bilirubin.

Urinalysis can be used to determine whether renal damage is present and to differentiate between renal and prerenal azotemia. Isosthenuria can be indicative of acute renal insufficiency. NSAIDs cause renal tubular injury, so an early sign of toxicity is the presence of casts in the urine sediment. Proteinuria may be present in cases of glomerular damage secondary to reduced renal perfusion.

In some cases abdominal imaging is indicated to rule out other causes of gastrointestinal injury or to find evidence of peritonitis, such as free fluid or air in the peritoneal cavity. If free fluid is present, abdominocentesis is indicated, and the fluid's glucose, lactate, protein, and cell count and differential should be examined (see Chapter 200).

TREATMENT

Asymptomatic Patients

Asymptomatic patients that are presented after accidental overdose should be treated prophylactically to prevent renal and gastrointestinal injury. Induction of emesis may be beneficial in cases that are presented within 2 to 4 hours of ingestion. Activated charcoal can be administered to adsorb any medication that still is present within the GI tract. Many NSAIDs undergo enterohepatic recycling, so repeated dosing of activated charcoal every 4 to 6 hours is recommended (see Chapters 74 and 76).

Intravenous fluid therapy is vital to maintain perfusion to the gastrointestinal tract and kidneys. In most cases of medication overdose, treatment duration depends on the half-life of the drug that has been ingested; treatment should continue until at least three half-lives have passed (Table 76-1). However, NSAIDs can have a longer half-life in the tissues than in the plasma, so treatment should continue if there is laboratory evidence of abnormality or if clinical signs develop.[63] Urine sediment should be monitored daily, even in asymptomatic animals, to look for evidence of renal casts.

Gastrointestinal protectants are indicated to prevent or treat gastric mucosal injury. Proton pump inhibitors such as omeprazole and pantoprazole are more effective at increasing gastric pH than the histamine-2 receptor antagonists ranitidine and famotidine; however, the proton pump inhibitors have a longer onset of action. Misoprostol is a prostaglandin E2 analog and can be used to counteract the effects of NSAIDs.[64] Oral medications should not be administered while the patient is receiving activated charcoal because the medications will also be adsorbed.

Symptomatic Patients

If patients are showing clinical signs of NSAID toxicity, then decontamination procedures such as emesis or activated charcoal are not beneficial because the medication will already have been absorbed

Table 76-1 Elimination Half-Life of Nonsteroidal Antiinflammatory Drugs in Dogs and Cats

Drug	Dog	Cat
Aspirin	7.5 hr*[51]	37.5 hr* (up to 45 hr)
Carprofen	11-14 hr[54]	21 hr (up to 49 hr)[52]
Deracoxib	3 hr*	8 hr[50]
Firocoxib	6 hr[70]	12 hr[71]
Ibuprofen	5 hr[53]	
Meloxicam	24 hr[72] (up to 36 hr)	15-26 hr[73]
Naproxen	74 hr[74]	

*Half-life is dose dependent and increases with higher or prolonged dosing.

from the gastrointestinal tract. Intravenous fluid therapy is required to treat initial perfusion deficits and dehydration and should be continued to ensure adequate blood flow to the GI tract and kidneys.

Symptomatic treatment of nausea, vomiting, and pain is warranted if these signs are present. Metoclopramide should be avoided because this dopamine antagonist could decrease renal blood flow.[65,66] Gastric protectant drugs and appropriate use of nutrition can be used to accelerate healing and improve function of the gastrointestinal tract. Patients with septic peritonitis or acute renal failure should be treated appropriately (see Chapter 122).

Patients with significant gastrointestinal hemorrhage may require a blood transfusion if the patient is showing clinical signs of anemia. Treatment of platelet abnormalities with platelet products is rarely, if ever, indicated in NSAID toxicity.

PROGNOSIS

The prognosis for patients with NSAID toxicity depends on the organ system affected, how early the toxicity is detected, and the severity of organ injury. The degree of organ injury is generally dose related but can also be affected by age, comorbidity, and concurrent medications. The majority of data in the veterinary literature relates to gastrointestinal injury secondary to NSAID administration. In most cases the prognosis is good for patients with gastrointestinal ulceration or hemorrhage, given appropriate treatment and withdrawal of the NSAID. However, although in some reports patients made a good recovery after surgical repair and appropriate treatment, more than 50% of the published cases of NSAID-induced gastrointestinal perforation died or were euthanized because of the severity of disease or cost of treatment.[23-27]

CLIENT EDUCATION

The relative frequency of NSAID toxicoses in veterinary patients means that client education is vital. If NSAIDs are prescribed for home administration, the dose and duration of treatment must be explained carefully and the potential side effects of the medication described clearly. Clients should be advised not to administer the medications and to seek veterinary advice if their pet is not eating, is vomiting or has diarrhea, or if they see hematochezia or melena. NSAIDs should never be administered concurrently with other NSAIDs or with corticosteroids. When using NSAIDs as long-term therapy, clinicians may find that they can titrate the dose over time to the lowest therapeutic dose. Many NSAIDs have been shown to be effective analgesics and antiinflammatory agents at amounts far lower than the recommended dose, but this may depend on the individual patient.[67-69]

REFERENCES

1. Hampshire VA, Doddy FM, et al: Adverse drug event reports at the United States Food and Drug Administration Center for Veterinary Medicine, J Am Vet Med Assoc 225:533-536, 2004.
2. Khan SA, McLean MK: Toxicology of frequently encountered nonsteroidal anti-inflammatory drugs in dogs and cats, Vet Clin North Am Small Anim Pract 42:289-306, 2012.
3. Stenson W: Prostaglandins and epithelial response to injury, Curr Opin Gastroenterol 23:107-110, 2007.
4. Wooten JG, Blikslager AT, et al: Effect of nonsteroidal anti-inflammatory drugs with varied cyclooxygenase-2 selectivity on cyclooxygenase protein and prostanoid concentrations in pyloric and duodenal mucosa of dogs, Am J Vet Res 70:1243-1249, 2009.
5. Fukata M, Chen A, et al: COX-2 is regulated by toll-like receptor-4 (TLR4) signaling: role in proliferation and apoptosis in the intestine, Gastroenterol 131:862-877, 2006.
6. Lichtenberger L, Romero J, Dial E: Surface phospholipids in gastric injury and protection when a selective cyclooxygenase-2 inhibitor (Coxib) is used in combination with aspirin, Br J Pharmacol 150:913-919, 2007.
7. Surdyk K, Sloan D, Brown S: Evaluation of the renal effects of ibuprofen and carprofen in euvolemic and volume-depleted dogs, Int J Appl Res Vet Med 9:129-136, 2011.
8. Anderson B: Paracetamol (acetaminophen): mechanisms of action, Ped Anesth 18:915-921, 2008.
9. Botting R, Ayoub S: COX 3 and the mechanism of action of paracetamol (acetominophen), Prost Leuk Ess Fatty Acids 72:85-87, 2005.
10. Lascelles B, McFarland J, Swann H: Guidelines for safe and effective use of NSAIDs in dogs, Vet Therap 6:237-251, 2005.
11. Micklewright R, Lane S, et al: Review article: NSAIDs, gastroprotection and cyclo-oxygenase-II-selective inhibitors, Aliment Pharmacol Ther 17:321-332, 2003.
12. Little D, Jones S, Blikslager A: Cyclooxygenase (COS) inhibitors and the intestine, J Vet Intern Med 21:367-377, 2007.
13. Tomlinson J, Blikslager A: Role of nonsteroidal anti-inflammatory drugs in gastrointestinal tract injury and repair, J Am Vet Med Assoc 222:946-951, 2003.
14. Goodman L, Torres B, et al: Effects of firocoxib and tepoxalin on healing in a canine gastric mucosal injury model, J Vet Intern Med 23:56-62, 2009.
15. Fornai M, Antonioli L, et al: Emerging role of cyclooxygenase isoforms in the control of gastrointestinal neuromuscular functions, Pharmacol Therap 125:62-78, 2010.
16. Narita T, Okabe N, et al: Nonsteroidal anti-inflammatory drugs induce hypermotilinemia and disturbance of interdigestive migrating contractions in instrumented dogs, J Vet Pharmacol Ther 29:569-577, 2006.
17. Luna SP, Basilio AC, et al: Evaluation of adverse effects of long-term oral administration of carprofen, etodolac, flunixin meglumine, ketoprofen, and meloxicam in dogs, Am J Vet Res 68:258-264, 2007.
18. Briere CA, Hosgood G, et al: Effects of carprofen on the integrity and barrier function of canine colonic mucosa, Am J Vet Res 69:174-181, 2008.
19. Craven M, Chandler ML, et al: Acute effects of carprofen and meloxicam on canine gastrointestinal permeability and mucosal absorptive capacity, J Vet Intern Med 21:917-923, 2007.
20. Dowers K, Uhrig S, et al: Effect of short term sequential administration of nonsteroidal anti-inflammatory drugs on the stomach and proximal portion of the duodenum in healthy dogs, Am J Vet Res 67:1794-1801, 2006.
21. Punke JP, Speas AL, et al: Effects of firocoxib, meloxicam, and tepoxalin on prostanoid and leukotriene production by duodenal mucosa and other tissues of osteoarthritic dogs, Am J Vet Res 69:1203-1209, 2008.
22. Sennello K, Leib M: Effects of deracoxib or buffered aspirin on the gastric mucosa of healthy dogs, J Vet Intern Med 20:1291-1296, 2006.
23. Case JB, Fick JL, Rooney MB: Proximal duodenal perforation in three dogs following deracoxib administration, J Am Anim Hosp Assoc 46:255-258, 2010.
24. Enberg T, Braun L, Kuzma A: Gastrointestinal perforation in five dogs associated with the administration of meloxicam, J Vet Emerg Crit Care 16:34-43, 2006.
25. Hinton LE, McLoughlin MA, et al: Spontaneous gastroduodenal perforation in 16 dogs and seven cats (1982-1999), J Am Anim Hosp Assoc 38:176-187, 2002.
26. Lascelles B, Blikslager A, et al: Gastrointestinal tract perforation in dogs treated with a selective cyclooxygenase-2 inhibitor: 29 cases (2002-2003), J Am Vet Med Assoc 227:1112-1117, 2005.
27. Reed S: Nonsteroidal anti-inflammatory drug-induced duodenal ulceration and perforation in a mature rottweiler, Can Vet J 43:971-972, 2002.
28. Runk A, Kyles AE, Downs MO: Duodenal perforation in a cat following the administration of nonsteroidal anti-inflammatory medication, J Am Anim Hosp Assoc 35:52-55, 1999.
29. Jones C, Budsberg S: Physiologic characteristics and clinical importance of the cyclooxygenase isoforms in dogs and cats, J Am Vet Med Assoc 217:721-729, 2000.
30. MacPhail C, Lappin M, et al: Hepatocellular toxicosis associated with administration of carprofen in 21 dogs, J Am Vet Med Assoc 212:1895-1901, 1998.
31. Lemke K, Runyon C, Horney B: Effects of preoperative administration of ketoprofen on whole blood platelet aggregation, buccal mucosal bleeding

time, and hematologic indices in dogs undergoing elective ovariohysterectomy, J Am Vet Med Assoc 220:1818-1822, 2002.
32. Kearney PM, Baigent C, et al: Do selective cyclo-oxygenase-2 inhibitors and traditional non-steroidal anti-inflammatory drugs increase the risk of atherothrombosis? Meta-analysis of randomised trials, Br Med J 332:1302-1308, 2006.
33. Brainard B, Meredith C, et al: Changes in platelet function, hemostasis, and prostaglandin expression after treatment with nonsteroidal anti-inflammatory drugs with various cyclooxygenase selectivities in dogs, Am J Vet Res 68:251-257, 2007.
34. Kay-Mugford PA, Grimm KA, et al: Effect of preoperative administration of tepoxalin on hemostasis and hepatic and renal function in dogs, Vet Ther 5:120-127, 2004.
35. Ding CH: Do NSAIDs affect the progression of osteoarthritis? Inflamm 26:139-142, 2002.
36. KuKanich B, Bidgood T, Knesl O: Clinical pharmacology of nonsteroidal anti-inflammatory drugs in dogs, Vet Anaesth Analg 39:69-90, 2012.
37. Rainsford KD, Skerry TM, et al: Effects of the NSAIDs meloxicam and indomethacin on cartilage proteoglycan synthesis and joint responses to calcium pyrophosphate crystals in dogs, Vet Res Comm 23:101-113, 1999.
38. Mastbergen SC, Bijlsma JW, Lafeber FP: Selective COX-2 inhibition is favorable to human early and late-stage osteoarthritic cartilage: a human in vitro study, Osteoarthr Cartil 13:519-526, 2005.
39. Liesegang A, Limacher S, Sobek A: The effect of carprofen on selected markers of bone metabolism in dogs with chronic osteoarthritis, Schweiz Arch Tier 149:353-362, 2007.
40. Pelletier JP, Lajeunesse D, et al: Carprofen simultaneously reduces progression of morphological changes in cartilage and subchondral bone in experimental dog osteoarthritis, J Rheumatol 27:2893-2902, 2000.
41. Chan CC, Boyce S, et al: Rofecoxib [Vioxx, MK-0966; 4-(4′-methylsulfonylphenyl)-3-phenyl-2-(5H)-furanone]: a potent and orally active cyclooxygenase-2 inhibitor. Pharmacological and biochemical profiles, J Pharmacol Exp Ther 290:551-560, 1999.
42. Kürüm B, Pekcan Z, et al: The effects of ketoprofen and meloxicam on bone healing in rat model: a comparative dual energy x-ray absorptiometry study, Kafk Univ Vet Fak Derg 18:671-676, 2012.
43. Ochi H, Hara Y, et al: Effects of long-term administration of carprofen on healing of a tibial osteotomy in dogs, Am J Vet Res 72:634-641, 2011.
44. Aygun D, Kaplan S, et al: Toxicity of non-steroidal anti-inflammatory drugs: a review of melatonin and diclofenac sodium association, Histol Histopathol 27:417-436, 2012.
45. Kepa L, Oczko-Grzesik B, et al: Drug-induced aseptic meningitis in suspected central nervous system infections, J Clin Neurosci 12:562-564, 2005.
46. Moreno-Ancillo A, Gil-Adrados A, Jurado-Palomo J: Ibuprofen-induced aseptic meningoencephalitis confirmed by drug challenge, J Investig Allergol Clin Immunol 21:484-487, 2011.
47. Morgan A, Clark D: CNS adverse effects of nonsteroidal anti-inflammatory drugs: Therapeutic implications, CNS Drugs 9:281-290, 1998.
48. Hopper K: Personal communication, 2012.
49. Narita T, Sato R, et al: The interaction between orally administered non-steroidal anti-inflammatory drugs and prednisolone in healthy dogs, J Vet Med Sci 69:353-363, 2007.
50. Gassel AD, Tobias KM, Cox SK: Disposition of deracoxib in cats after oral administration, J Am Anim Hosp Assoc 42:212-217, 2006.
51. Lipowitz AJ, Boulay JP, Klausner JS: Serum salicylate concentrations and endoscopic evaluation of the gastric mucosa in dogs after oral administration of aspirin-containing products, Am J Vet Res 47:1586-1589, 1986.
52. Parton K, Balmer TV, et al: The pharmacokinetics and effects of intravenously administered carprofen and salicylate on gastrointestinal mucosa and selected biochemical measurements in healthy cats, J Vet Pharmacol Ther 23:73-79, 2000.
53. Scherkl R, Frey HH: Pharmacokinetics of ibuprofen in the dog, J Vet Pharmacol Ther 10:261-265, 1987.
54. Schmitt M, Guentert TW: Biopharmaceutical evaluation of carprofen following single intravenous, oral, and rectal doses in dogs, Biopharm Drug Disp 11:585-594, 1990.
55. Villar D, Buck W: Ibuprofen, aspirin and acetaminophen toxicosis and treatment in dogs and cats, Vet Human Toxicol 40:156-162, 1998.
56. Adams S, Bough R, et al: Absorption, distribution and toxicity of ibuprofen, Toxicol Appl Pharmacol 15:310-330, 1969.
57. Dunayer E: Ibuprofen toxicosis in dogs, cats, and ferrets, Vet Med 99:580-586, 2004.
58. Bugat R, Thompson M, Aures D, et al: Gastric mucosal lesions produced by intravenous infusion of aspirin in cats, Gastroenterol 71:754-759, 1976.
59. Gfeller R, Sandors A: Naproxen-associated duodenal ulcer complicated by perforation and bacteria- and barium sulfate-induced peritonitis in a dog, J Am Vet Med Assoc 198:644-646, 1991.
60. Gilmour MA, Walshaw R: Naproxen-induced toxicosis in a dog, J Am Vet Med Assoc 191:1431-1432, 1987.
61. Roberts ES, Van Lare KA, et al: Safety and tolerability of 3-week and 6-month dosing of Deramaxx (deracoxib) chewable tablets in dogs, J Vet Pharmacol Ther 32:329-337, 2009.
62. Boehringer Ingelheim Vetmedica I: Freedom of information summary new animal drug application Metacam® (meloxicam) 0.5 mg/mL and 1.5 mg/mL oral suspension. 2003. NADA 141-219. Available at: http://wwwfdagov/downloads/animalveterinary/ products/approvedanimal drugproducts/foiadrugsummaries/ucm118026pdf.
63. Pelligand L, King JN, et al: Pharmacokinetic/pharmacodynamic modelling of robenacoxib in a feline tissue cage model of inflammation, J Vet Pharmacol Ther 35:19-32, 2012.
64. Roškar T, Nemec Svete A, et al: Effect of meloxicam and meloxicam with misoprostol on serum prostaglandins and gastrointestinal permeability in healthy beagle dogs, Acta Vet 33, 2011.
65. Munn J, Tooley M, et al: Effect of metoclopramide on renal vascular resistance index and renal function in patients receiving a low-dose infusion of dopamine, Br J Anaesth 71:379-382, 1993.
66. Smit AJ, Meijer S, et al: Effect of metoclopramide on dopamine-induced changes in renal function in healthy controls and in patients with renal disease, Clin Sci 75:421-428, 1988.
67. Gunew M, Menrath V, Marshall R: Long-term safety, efficacy and palatability of oral meloxicam at 0.01-0.03mg/kg for treatment of osteoarthritic pain in cats, J Fel Med Surg 10:235-241, 2008.
68. Hazewinkel HAW, van den Brom WE, et al: Reduced dosage of ketoprofen for the short-term and long-term treatment of joint pain in dogs, Vet Rec 152:11-14, 2003.
69. Wernham BGJ, Trumpatori B, et al: Dose reduction of meloxicam in dogs with osteoarthritis-associated pain and impaired mobility, J Vet Intern Med 25:1298-1305, 2011.
70. McCann ME, Andersen DR, et al: In vitro effects and in vivo efficacy of a novel cyclooxygenase-2 inhibitor in dogs with experimentally induced synovitis, Am J Vet Res 65:503-512, 2004.
71. McCann ME, Rickes EL, et al: *In vitro* effects and in vivo efficacy of a novel cyclooxygenase-2 inhibitor in cats with lipopolysaccharide-induced pyrexia, Am J Vet Res 66:1278-1284, 2005.
72. Poulsen Nautrup B, Horstermann D: Pharmacodynamic and pharmacokinetic aspects of the non-steroidal anti-inflammatory drug meloxicam in dogs, Deutsche Tier Wochen 106:94-100, 1999.
73. Lehr T, Narbe R, et al: Population pharmacokinetic modelling and simulation of single and multiple dose administration of meloxicam in cats, J Vet Pharmacol Ther 33:277-286, 2010.
74. Frey HH, Rieh B: Pharmacokinetics of naproxen in the dog, Am J Vet Res 42:1615-1617, 1981.

CHAPTER 77

SEDATIVE, MUSCLE RELAXANT, AND NARCOTIC OVERDOSE

Annie Malouin Wright, DVM, DACVECC

KEY POINTS

- A sedative overdose causes primarily a dose-dependent central nervous system (CNS) depression.
- Signs of acute toxicity with muscle relaxants are often an amplification of their main therapeutic effects: muscular flaccidity, CNS and respiratory depression, and anticholinergic syndrome.
- Opioid overdose may alter mental status, cause respiratory depression, and produce miosis in dogs and mydriasis in cats.
- Sedatives, muscle relaxants, and opioids undergo hepatic biotransformation with primary excretion of their metabolites in the urine. Thus the metabolism of these drugs may be impaired in patients with hepatic disease or renal impairment, increasing the duration and intensity of their pharmacologic action.
- Treatment of intoxication with sedatives, muscle relaxants, and opioids is based on general supportive measures. Antidotes are available for only the benzodiazepines, α_2 agonists, and opioids.

Dogs and cats may experience toxicity from sedatives, central muscle relaxants, and narcotics, either by iatrogenic overdose by a veterinary health care provider or by consumption of the owner's or pet's prescribed medications. All of the agents discussed in this chapter are dispensed only by prescription, and several are not approved for use in veterinary species. Differential diagnoses to consider include the ingestion of other neurotoxins and drugs, as well as primary central nervous system (CNS) disorders. Blood and urine concentration of many of these drugs can be measured. The clinical picture and treatment of overdose for each of these drug categories are discussed separately.

SEDATIVE OVERDOSE

Sedatives include a variety of agents that have the capacity to depress the function of the CNS and result in sedation. They also may contain hypnotic (sleep aid), muscle relaxant, anxiolytic, and anticonvulsant properties. Some euthanasia solutions are formulated with highly concentrated barbiturate products, and acute intoxication with these agents may occur after ingestion of meat from an animal recently euthanized (relay toxicosis). However, studies of clinical use or toxicity for several of the drugs discussed in this section have been conducted only in humans.[1-4] Therefore it is unknown whether the pharmacokinetics and clinical signs of overdose reported for individual agents apply equally to veterinary species.

Mechanism of Action

The sedative agents have various modes of action, which are summarized in Table 77-1.[1-4]

Pharmacokinetics

Table 77-2 describes the pharmacokinetics of the agents listed in Table 77-1.[1-8] All of these sedatives undergo hepatic biotransformation, with excretion of metabolites primarily in the urine. As a result, their metabolism may be impaired in patients with hepatic disease, and their metabolites may accumulate in patients with renal impairment. Benzodiazepines require significant hepatic microsomal enzyme metabolism, and barbiturates stimulate the hepatic microsomal enzyme system.

Clinical Signs

For most sedative overdoses, the clinical picture is nonspecific. All of these drugs cause progressive CNS depression in proportion to the quantity of the agent consumed. Also, concurrent administration or ingestion of other CNS depressants (opioids, anesthetics) has compounding effects. CNS signs vary from mental depression, ataxia, stupor, and surgical anesthesia to coma. Finally, death occurs with sufficient depression of medullary neurons to disrupt coordination of cardiovascular function and respiration. Phenothiazines block α-adrenergic receptors and, if given concurrently with epinephrine, the β-activity prevails, causing vasodilation and an increased heart rate. Zolpidem may cause a paradoxic excitation reaction before the sedation phase.[9] Clinical signs of overdoses with sedatives and possible interactions with various medications are summarized in Table 77-3.[1,3,7,10,11]

Treatment

Treatment of intoxications with sedatives is based on general supportive measures. Antidotes (reversal agents) are available only for benzodiazepines and α_2 agonists (see Chapters 164 and 165). Decontamination is performed as described in Chapter 74 if oral ingestion of a toxic dosage is suspected. Table 77-4 describes the treatment for each class of drugs.[1,3,12] In patients with severe mental depression, oxygen is administered and a patent airway maintained to prevent aspiration pneumonia, hypercarbia, or hypoxemia. Mechanical ventilation is initiated when indicated. Continuous electrocardiographic and blood pressure monitoring is required for patients manifesting cardiovascular instability. Administration of intravenous crystalloid fluids promotes diuresis and therefore hastens the elimination of the metabolites of each of these drugs. Hypotension is managed initially with intravenous fluids, followed by vasopressors if required. Seizures are controlled with standard anticonvulsants (see Chapter 166). The patient's body temperature requires regular monitoring and appropriate measures must be taken to maintain euthermia. Aggressive supportive and nursing care helps prevent complications in recumbent animals.[9,13-15]

MUSCLE RELAXANT OVERDOSE

Muscle relaxants reduce skeletal muscle tension without abolishing voluntary motor control. Most of their effects occur at various levels of the CNS (cortex, brainstem, spinal cord, or all three areas), but some also act directly within the muscle. This clinical grouping of

Table 77-1 **Mechanism of Action of Sedatives**[1-8,10-14,16-18]

Generic Name	Brand Name	Mechanism of Action
Benzodiazepines		
Alprazolam	Xanax	Benzodiazepine receptors are located on the $GABA_A$- receptor complex, a chloride ion channel in the brain and spinal cord. Their activation promotes binding of GABA to its receptor, thereby enhancing chloride currents through these channels (by increasing the frequency of channel openings). The cell membrane becomes hyperpolarized and resistant to excitatory stimuli, explaining the sedative, anticonvulsant, and muscle relaxant effects of benzodiazepines.
Clorazepate	Tranxene	
Chlordiazepoxide	Librium	
Clonazepam	Klonopin	
Diazepam	Valium	
Estazolam	ProSom	
Flurazepam	Dalmane	
Lorazepam	Ativan	
Midazolam	Versed	
Oxazepam	Serax	
Quazepam	Doral	
Temazepam	Restoril	
Triazolam	Halcion	
Imidazopyridines		
Zolpidem	Ambien	Potentiates GABA-ergic transmission by selectively modulating certain subunits of the $GABA_A$- receptor complex in the central nervous system (primarily in the cerebellum). This results in the inhibition of neuronal excitation, slowing the activity in the brain to allow sleep (hypnosis) with fewer side effects.
Pyrazolopyrimidines		
Zaleplon	Sonata	Potentiates GABA-ergic transmission by selectively modulating certain subunits of the $GABA_A$- receptor complex in the central nervous system (mostly the brain). This results in the inhibition of neuronal excitation, slowing the activity in the brain to allow sleep (hypnosis) with fewer side effects.
Cyclopyrrolones		
Eszopiclone	Lunesta	Potentiates GABA-ergic transmission by selectively modulating certain subunits of the $GABA_A$- receptor complex in the central nervous system (mostly the brain). This results in the inhibition of neuronal excitation, slowing the activity in the brain to allow sleep (hypnosis) with fewer side effects.
Phenothiazines		
Acepromazine	Atravet	Blocks postsynaptic dopamine and α_1-adrenergic receptors
α_2-Agonists		
Medetomidine	Domitor	α_2-Adrenoreceptor agonists
Xylazine	Rompun	
Barbiturates		
Phenobarbital	Luminal	Augment GABA responses by promoting the binding of GABA to its receptor $GABA_A$ and by increasing the length of time that chloride channels are open and open the chloride channels in the absence of GABA at higher doses
Pentobarbital	Nembutal	

GABA, γ-Aminobutyric acid.

therapeutic agents accommodates a heterogeneous assembly of medications (Table 77-5) that differ in their chemical, pharmacologic, pharmacokinetic, and toxicologic properties. As a result, the type and severity of clinical effects after an overdose may be diverse. A number of agents are used to alleviate musculoskeletal pain and spasms caused by a variety of neurologic conditions in human patients, but little is known about their clinical application in veterinary medicine. Neuromuscular blockers are muscle relaxants as well and are discussed in Chapter 143. Benzodiazepines were discussed in the previous section and are discussed further in Chapter 164).

Mechanism of Action

Spasmolytic agents work by either enhancing the level of inhibition or reducing the level of myocyte excitation. Table 77-5 summarizes the skeletal muscle relaxants of clinical and toxicologic importance and their modes of action.[3,16-22]

Pharmacokinetics

A detailed discussion of muscle relaxant pharmacokinetics is beyond the scope of this chapter. The reader is encouraged to consult suggested references for further information.[3,16-23] Limited pharmacokinetic data are available for many of these drugs in veterinary species, and thus elimination in dogs and cats may be unpredictable. In humans, most muscle relaxants have peak absorption within 1 to 6 hours and are distributed throughout the body. Therefore clinical effects are seen rapidly after oral ingestion. All of the muscle relaxants are metabolized in the liver, and their metabolites are eliminated mostly in the urine.[16]

Clinical Signs

In most cases of muscle relaxant overdose, the clinical features are exaggerations of their main therapeutic effects. Muscular flaccidity, CNS and respiratory depression, adverse cardiovascular effects, and an anticholinergic syndrome from the agents with antimuscarinic effects often are seen in patients with acute toxicity. Additive sedation may occur when given with other CNS depressant agents. In the veterinary literature, only a few reports are available to describe the clinical course seen with muscle relaxant overdose. Table 77-6 summarizes the clinical signs of acute toxicity with muscle relaxants in humans and in veterinary species.*

Treatment

Because of the potential for a rapid absorption and onset of clinical signs, decontamination should be attempted without delay. General

*References 3, 16, 18-20, 24-27.

Table 77-2 **Pharmacokinetics of Sedatives**[16,22]

Generic Name	Route	Half-Life (hr)	LD_{50}
Benzodiazepines			
Alprazolam	PO	12 ± 2	—
Clorazepate	PO	2.0 ± 0.9	—
Chlordiazepoxide	PO, IV, IM	10 ± 3.4	—
Clonazepam	PO	23 ± 5	—
Diazepam	PO, IV, IM, PR	2.5-2.3	>20 mg/kg (dog)
Estazolam	PO	10-24	—
Flurazepam	PO	74 ± 24	—
Lorazepam	PO, IV, IM	14 ± 5	—
Midazolam	IV, IM	1.9 ± 0.6	IV: 1600 mg/kg
Oxazepam	PO	8.0 ± 2.4	—
Quazepam	PO	39	—
Temazepam	PO	11 ± 6	—
Triazolam	PO	2.9 ± 1.0	—
Imidazopyridines			
Zolpidem	PO	2.6	—
Pyrazolopyrimidines			
Zaleplon	PO	1.0	—
Cyclopyrrolones			
Eszopiclone	PO	5.8	—
Phenothiazines			
Acepromazine	PO, IV, IM, SC	3	PO: 257 mg/kg IV: 61 mg/kg (mice)
α_2-Agonists			
Medetomidine	IV, IM	0.96 ± 0.25	80 mg/kg (rat)
Xylazine	IV, IM, SC	0.5	—
Barbiturates			
Phenobarbital	PO, IV	48	PO: 150 mg/kg IV: 83 mg/kg (rat)
Pentobarbital	PO, IV, IM, PR	8	PO: 85 mg/kg IV: 50 mg/kg (dog)

IM, Intramuscular; *IV*, intravenous; *LD_{50}*, lethal dose; *PO*, per os; *PR*, per rectum; *SC*, subcutaneous.

Table 77-3 **Clinical Signs of Toxicity of Sedatives and Potential Drug Interactions**[1,3,7,10,11]

Drug Class	Clinical Signs of Toxicity	Drug Interactions
Benzodiazepines	Toxicity of these drugs is low CNS depression, ataxia and, uncommonly, respiratory depression and hypotension may occur Cats may develop hepatic failure after oral administration of diazepam	Cimetidine, fluoxetine, erythromycin, isoniazid, ketoconazole, propranolol, metoprolol, valproic acid: may inhibit the metabolism of benzodiazepines and cause excessive sedation
Imidazopyridines	Agitation, sedation, ataxia, anorexia, hypersalivation, vomiting	
Pyrazolopyrimidines	Agitation, sedation, ataxia, anorexia, hypersalivation, vomiting	
Cyclopyrrolones	Agitation, sedation, ataxia, anorexia, hypersalivation, vomiting	
α_2-Agonists	CNS depression, bradycardia, atrioventricular blocks, decreased myocardial contractility, decreased cardiac output, initially arterial hypertension followed by hypotension, decreased respiratory rate, apnea, cyanosis, vomiting, recurrence of sedation after initial recovery, occasional spontaneous muscle contractions (twitching), hypothermia, hyperglycemia, death from circulatory failure with severe pulmonary congestion, increased hepatic or renal enzymes	Decrease dosage of general anesthetics Concurrent use of epinephrine may induce ventricular arrhythmias
Barbiturates	Progressive CNS depression: stupor to coma, ataxia, respiratory depression, hypotension, decreased cardiac contractility, noncardiogenic pulmonary edema, aspiration pneumonia, renal failure, hypothermia, decreased GI motility, anemia, hypoglycemia Cats particularly sensitive to respiratory depressant effects	Accelerate the clearance of other drugs metabolized via hepatic microsomal enzymes Chloramphenicol may increase clinical effects

CNS, Central nervous system; *GI*, gastrointestinal.

Table 77-4 **Treatment of Sedative Overdoses**[1,3,12,14]

Drug	Management
Benzodiazepines Imidazopyridines Pyrazolopyrimidines Cyclopyrrolones	Flumazenil (Romazicon) is a benzodiazepine antagonist binding with high affinity to specific sites on the $GABA_A$-receptor, where it competitively antagonizes benzodiazepines binding and allosteric effects. It also can reverse effects of imidazopyridines, pyrazolopyrimidines, and cyclopyrrolones. Flumazenil has a higher clearance and shorter elimination half-life (1 hr) than all clinically used benzodiazepine agonists. Recurrent benzodiazepine toxicity or resedation is therefore likely once the effects of flumazenil have worn off, and repeated administration may be necessary. Flumazenil is administered only by rapid IV injection because it is highly irritating, and care should be taken to avoid extravasation. Dosage: 0.05 mg/kg IV Elimination is not enhanced by hemodialysis or hemoperfusion.
α_2-Agonists	Atipamezole (Antisedan) is an α_2-adrenergic antagonist that selectively and competitively inhibits α_2-adrenergic receptors, causing sympathetic outflow to be enhanced. It can reverse effects of medetomidine and xylazine. The onset of arousal is apparent usually within 5 to 10 minutes of intramuscular injection, depending on the depth and duration of sedation. Atipamezole also produces a rapid improvement of bradycardia and respiratory depression. Atropine or glycopyrrolate should not be used to prevent or manage bradycardia, because tachycardia and hypertension may result. Atipamezole should be administered intramuscularly regardless of the route used for the α_2-agonist. The dosage is calculated based upon body surface area: 1 mg/m^2, or give IM an equal volume of atipamezole hydrochloride (Antisedan) and medetomidine (Dormitor) (milliliter per milliliter). Yohimbine or tolazoline also can be used to reverse the effects of xylazine but are less specific antagonists with more side effects than atipamezole.
Barbiturates	Promote diuresis to increase the urinary flow rate. Also, alkalinizing the urine (pH > 7) by intravenous administration of sodium bicarbonate enhances the rate of excretion of unchanged drug in its ionized form. Hemodialysis and hemoperfusion can be used to maximize barbiturate elimination.

GABA, γ-Aminobutyric acid; *IV,* intravenous.

Table 77-5 **Summary of Muscle Relaxants and Their Mechanisms of Action**[3,16-22]

Generic Name	Trade Name	Site of Action	Mechanism of Action
Baclofen	Lioresal	CNS	GABA-agonist
Carisoprodol	Soma	CNS	Indirect GABA-agonist
Cyclobenzaprine	Flexeril	CNS	Tricyclic analog: decreases amplitude of monosynaptic reflex potentials by inhibiting descending serotonergic systems in spinal cord
Chlorzoxazone	Parafon Forte	CNS	Exact mechanism unknown; sedation
Dantrolene	Dantrium	Peripheral	Blocks calcium liberation from sarcoplasmic reticulum of skeletal muscle by binding to ryanodine receptor
Methocarbamol	Robaxin	CNS	Unknown; structurally related to guaifenesin
Metaxalone	Skelaxin	CNS	Not established; thought to be related to its sedative properties
Orphenadrine	Norflex	CNS	Directly causes dopamine release; NMDA receptor antagonist; blocks norepinephrine uptake; peripheral antimuscarinic action
Tizanidine	Zanaflex	CNS	Central α_2-adrenergic agonist

CNS, Central nervous system; *GABA,* γ-aminobutyric acid; *NMDA,* N-methyl-D-aspartic acid.

guidelines for decontamination can be found in Chapter 74. For patients that ingest baclofen or carisoprodol, only one dose of activated charcoal with a cathartic is necessary because these drugs do not undergo enterohepatic circulation. For the remaining muscle relaxants, efficacy of multidose activated charcoal regimens has not been established.[16] Gastric lavage should be performed in cases of large ingestions, and the anesthetic protocol used must not compound the CNS depression. A short-acting induction agent such as propofol, followed by inhalant anesthesia, is recommended. The airway must be protected at all times with a cuffed endotracheal tube.

Because no antidote exists for centrally acting muscle relaxant overdose, aggressive supportive care and intensive monitoring are imperative. The patient's ventilation and oxygenation should be monitored closely. Endotracheal intubation and positive-pressure ventilation should be considered in select patients (see Chapter 30).

Animals manifesting cardiovascular instability require continuous electrocardiographic and blood pressure monitoring. Bradycardia from baclofen toxicity is responsive to atropine in human patients.[24,28] Hypotension should be treated initially with intravenous crystalloid or colloid fluids (see Chapter 60), followed by vasopressors if needed (see Chapters 157 and 158). Hypertension should be treated with vasodilators (e.g., nitroprusside, amlodipine) if necessary (see Chapter 159). Baclofen and carisoprodol are excreted by the kidneys; therefore adequate diuresis is important to prevent acute kidney injury and enhance elimination of the drugs. In addition, hemodialysis or hemoperfusion can be used to reduce the

Table 77-6 Clinical Signs of Acute Muscle Relaxant Toxicity[3,6,16,18-20,24-30]

Drug	Clinical Signs
Baclofen	Vomiting, salivation, sedation, ataxia, vocalization, hypotension or hypertension, bradycardia, tachycardia, cardiac conduction abnormalities, coma, dyspnea, respiratory arrest Deaths in dogs have occurred at doses between 8 and 16 mg/kg[18]
Carisoprodol	Coma, hypotension, seizure, shock, respiratory depression, pulmonary edema, respiratory arrest and eventually cardiac arrest, nystagmus, vomiting, urticaria, pruritus, ataxia, tremors, agitation, myoclonus, tachycardia
Cyclobenzaprine	Anticholinergic toxidrome, lethargy, sinus tachycardia, agitation, hypertension or hypotension
Chlorzoxazone	CNS depression, GI upset, hypotonia, areflexia, hypotension, hepatotoxicity
Dantrolene	Hypotonia, sedation, hepatotoxicity
Methocarbamol	Sedation, lethargy, weakness, ataxia, salivation, emesis
Metaxalone	Sedation, GI upset, hepatotoxicity, nephrotoxicity
Orphenadrine	Anticholinergic toxidrome, mydriasis, tachycardia, coma, seizures, hypothermia, shock, cardiac arrest

CNS, Central nervous system; *GABA*, γ-aminobutyric acid; *GI*, gastrointestinal.

elimination half-life of baclofen and carisoprodol.[16,24] Administration of intravenous lipid emulsion is another emerging therapy for animals with lipid-soluble drug toxicities.[29,30]

Agitation can be treated with benzodiazepines. Seizures require prompt treatment with standard anticonvulsants. However, if carisoprodol has been ingested, barbiturates are not recommended for seizure control because they may compound the CNS depression. Diazepam, despite also being a γ-aminobutyric acid agonist, is the drug of choice for baclofen- and carisoprodol-induced seizures.[18-20,24] Flumazenil and physostigmine have been used to help reverse comatose states in cases of baclofen toxicosis in humans.[24,31] Flumazenil had varied results because it may be a proconvulsant when combined with a potential γ-aminobutyric acid antagonist such as baclofen.[24] Temperature regulation may be deranged in recumbent or comatose patients; therefore close monitoring and heat support (or cooling measures), if necessary, are recommended.

Prognosis

Asymptomatic patients having ingested any of these drugs should be observed for a minimum of 24 hours. The prognosis for toxicity with most of these muscle relaxants in veterinary medicine is unknown. For symptomatic patients with baclofen toxicity, resolution of clinical signs may take several days in severe cases, but if adequate supportive care and monitoring are available, the prognosis is generally good.[18] The vast majority of human patients recover after prompt recognition of the toxic condition and rapid institution of supportive care.[32]

NARCOTIC OVERDOSE

Narcotics (opioids) have been the mainstay of pain management for thousands of years, and they remain so today in human and veterinary medicine. These drugs derived from opium, and they include the natural products morphine and codeine, as well as many synthetic derivatives such as fentanyl, methadone, hydrocodone, hydromorphone, and heroin.[33]

Table 77-7 Functions or Side Effects of Opioid Receptors

Opiate Receptor	Function
Mu	Analgesia Respiratory depression Euphoria Bradycardia Constipation Vomiting Physical dependence Temperature change (hypothermia in dogs, hyperthermia in cats)
Delta	Analgesia
Sigma	Autonomic stimulation Dysphoria Hallucinations
Kappa	Analgesia Sedation
Epsilon	Analgesia

Mechanism of Action

Opioids produce their effects by interacting with specific receptors distributed throughout the central and peripheral nervous systems, the gastrointestinal (GI) tract, the urinary tract, and other smooth muscles.[33] Five receptors have been identified: mu (μ), kappa (κ), delta (δ), sigma (σ), and epsilon (ε), and each is associated with certain clinical effects, as described in Table 77-7.[3] Opioid receptor activation results in inhibition of adenyl cyclase activity, activation of receptor-operated potassium currents, and suppression of voltage-gated calcium currents. These effects cause hyperpolarization of the cell membrane, decreased neurotransmitter release, and reduced pain transmission.[33]

Functionally, opioids can be classified into four groups: morphine-like opioid agonists, opioid antagonists, mixed agonist-antagonists, and partial agonists (see Chapter 163).

Pharmacokinetics

An in-depth discussion of opioid pharmacokinetics is beyond the scope of this chapter (see Chapter 163).[3,33,34] However, several points require emphasis. Morphine, oxymorphone, hydromorphone, butorphanol, and buprenorphine are well absorbed after intravenous, intramuscular, subcutaneous, oral, and rectal administration. However, first-pass metabolism is significant and results in low bioavailability and a less predictable effect after oral ingestion.

Distribution of opioids from the blood to the CNS is variable. Generally, with the highly lipid-soluble drugs (e.g., codeine, fentanyl, and heroin), onset of action occurs more rapidly, and the pharmacologic effects resolve earlier. Drugs that are less lipid soluble, such as morphine, move less rapidly and therefore take longer to be effective and may have a longer duration of action. The clinical effects of most opioids persist for 2 to 8 hours; exceptions are fentanyl, which lasts for 15 minutes.[3,33-35] All opioids are metabolized primarily in the liver via glucuronidation. Cats are deficient in this metabolic pathway, and therefore the half-life of certain drugs may be prolonged. Elimination is primarily renal.[3] Patients with severe hepatic and/or renal insufficiency are theoretically at increased risk of toxicity because of the accumulation of active metabolites. In normal dogs, the lethal dose for morphine is 100 mg/kg.[3]

Opiate administration may obscure the clinical course and physical examination findings in some animals and therefore should be used cautiously in patients with intracranial disease, increased intracranial pressure, acute respiratory dysfunction, and acute conditions of the abdomen. Opioids may lead to hypoventilation and hypercapnia, which cause cerebral vasodilation and increased intracranial pressure. In patients with respiratory dysfunction and decreased carbon dioxide sensitivity, opioid drug administration may exacerbate the hypercapnia, necessitating endotracheal intubation and mechanical ventilation. Neonatal and geriatric patients are more susceptible to the effects of opioids and require lower dosages. In the developing fetus, opiates pass more easily into the CNS because the blood-brain barrier is not fully developed. Therefore a fetus may suffer severe depression, although the mother has no evidence of side effects. Small amounts of opioids also are distributed into the milk of nursing mothers.[33,34]

Opioids can interact with many drugs that may potentiate their effects. Morphine is contraindicated in human patients receiving monoamine oxidase inhibitors (MAOIs) because they may exhibit signs of opiate overdose after receiving therapeutic doses of morphine while taking MAOIs.[3,36] Also, fentanyl, meperidine, tramadol, methadone, and dextromethorphan are weak serotonin reuptake inhibitors and have been involved in serotonin toxicity reactions with MAOIs.[36] Interactions between other opioids and MAOIs have not been shown in dogs[37] (see Chapter 79).

Phenothiazines potentiate opioids, possibly by interfering with their metabolism.[33] Cimetidine may increase opioid effects by increasing the duration of action. Erythromycin also may enhance opioid effects.[38]

Clinical Signs

The clinical signs seen with opioid overdose are caused by an amplification of their action at the receptors discussed earlier. The μ receptor, which mediates many of the life-threatening effects, including respiratory depression, principally is affected. There is a classic triad seen with opioid toxicity: CNS depression, respiratory depression, and miosis in dogs. Cats typically develop mydriasis. Multiple organ systems also can be affected. Patients may be hyporeflexic, hypothermic, hypotensive, and have decreased borborygmi. These toxic effects are mediated primarily through stimulation of the μ, κ, and δ receptors.[3,33,34] The miosis in dogs results from μ-related stimulation of the visceral nuclei of the oculomotor nuclear complex and the parasympathetic nerve that innervates the pupil.[39]

The patient's level of consciousness can vary from excitement to dysphoria and from mild sedation to coma.[40,41] Profound CNS depression, impaired gag response, cough suppression, and centrally mediated nausea and vomiting place the animal at high risk for pulmonary aspiration of gastric contents.[3] Seizures can occur with high doses of agonist opioids. This is well recognized in humans[33]; however, its occurrence in small animals is unknown. Intrathecal administration of morphine can cause myoclonus.[42] Opioids may alter the thermoregulatory response. Hypothermia is seen commonly in dogs, whereas hyperthermia may occur in cats.[43]

The most significant adverse side effect of opioids is respiratory depression. It is caused by a reduction in responsiveness to carbon dioxide in the brainstem respiratory center, as well as the centers that regulate respiratory rhythm. Areas of the medulla oblongata that control ventilation (nucleus tractus solitarius and nucleus ambiguus) have many opioid binding sites, and these respiratory neurons are inhibited by opioid receptor agonists. Attenuation of normal chemoreceptor-mediated ventilatory responses to hypercapnia and hypoxia by opioids also may lead to ventilatory depression. Dogs and cats seem to be less sensitive than humans, in whom respiratory arrest is responsible for most opioid-related deaths.[3,33]

Initially, respiratory depression may be subtle in some patients because small decreases in tidal volume may occur before the respiratory rate declines. With further progression, the rate, tidal volume, and minute volume decrease. Therefore the rate alone can be an unreliable measure of ventilation. Because hypoventilation is defined as an inability of the respiratory system to eliminate metabolically produced carbon dioxide, the finding of hypercarbia on arterial (or venous) blood gas analysis is the most objective determinant of the presence and degree of respiratory depression. Opioids also may induce panting indirectly in dogs by resetting the thermoregulatory center, so the animal attempts to lose heat by increasing the respiratory rate, despite a normal to low body temperature.

The effects of opioids on the cardiovascular system are minimal at therapeutic or toxic doses. Pure opioid agonist interactions with μ receptors may result in bradycardia and cardiac conduction abnormalities. The systemic vascular resistance remains relatively stable after opioid administration, although morphine may decrease peripheral vascular tone.[44] Morphine and meperidine, when given intravenously, may cause histamine release leading to peripheral dilation (arterial and venous) and bradycardia; this drug should be avoided in animals with suspected or confirmed mast cell disease or after envenomation. Cutaneous signs include itching, warmth, and urticaria.[34]

Opioids cause a variety of direct gastrointestinal (GI) effects. They decrease the tone of the lower esophageal sphincter. Intestinal tone is increased while propulsive activity is reduced. Opioids also lower small intestinal secretions (pancreatic, biliary, and electrolytes and fluid) and enhance intestinal fluid absorption. These actions may result in constipation. Morphine has been associated with spasm of the sphincter of Oddi; therefore it is not used in people suffering from obstructive biliary or pancreatic diseases. In addition, opioids can directly stimulate the chemoreceptor triggering zone and thus may cause nausea and vomiting.[33] At high doses, opioids may increase ureteral tone, bladder tone, and external sphincter tone, leading to urinary retention. Morphine, as well as other μ-agonist drugs, is reported to increase antidiuretic hormone release and thus reduce urine production and cause an increase in specific gravity.[34]

Treatment

The mainstays of therapy for opioid overdose include providing a means for adequate ventilation and the administration of naloxone, an opioid antagonist (see Chapter 163). Patients whose respiratory status is compromised sufficiently should be intubated and supported with 100% oxygen and positive-pressure ventilation while naloxone is administered. Mechanical ventilation with positive end-expiratory pressure may be required if there is no response to the naloxone or if adequate oxygenation and ventilation cannot be achieved (see Chapter 30). Intubation and cuff inflation provides optimal airway control, decreases the risk of aspiration if vomiting or regurgitation occurs, allows access for airway suctioning and institution of positive pressure ventilation, and enables the administration of naloxone via the endotracheal route if intravenous access cannot be obtained.

GI decontamination should be considered in patients that have had oral exposure to opioids, particularly those drugs that can have delayed absorption such as loperamide and sustained-release morphine products. Concomitant use of naloxone may facilitate GI decontamination by decreasing GI atony (increasing GI tone). Although they occur rarely, seizures, hypotension, and cardiac arrhythmias should be treated with standard therapies. Body temperature should be monitored and euthermia maintained.

Naloxone is a synthetic derivative of oxymorphone (see Chapter 163). It is the opioid antagonist of choice because it competitively binds opioid receptors κ, δ, and, particularly, μ. It has a greater affinity for receptors than do the agonists. It is highly lipophilic and moves rapidly into the CNS. Naloxone usually has an onset of action of 1 to 2 minutes when given intravenously. The duration of action typically persists from 45 to 90 minutes. The dosage of naloxone for dogs and cats to reverse adverse opioid effects is 0.01 to 0.04 mg/kg. It may be given by the intravenous, intramuscular, intraosseous, subcutaneous, or endotracheal routes. Naloxone administration is generally safe in patients with opioid overdose, but very high dosages can initiate seizure activity. In animals with no initial response, repeat doses should be administered and titrated to each patient's response.[3,45]

Naloxone may have a shorter duration of action than most opioids, and repeated doses or a continuous infusion may be necessary. A continuous infusion is administered by determining the amount of naloxone required to reverse respiratory depression, then administering two thirds of this dose every hour as a continuous infusion. Half of the loading dose should be administered 15 minutes after the initial dose because of a transient decline in the naloxone level 20 to 30 minutes after the initial bolus. The rate of the infusion should be titrated to maintain adequate ventilation.

Naloxone can be mixed in most intravenous fluids in varying concentrations.[44] The infusion is continued for the typical duration of effect of the involved opioid then gradually reduced while the patient's respiratory and mental status are monitored closely. Continuous infusions have been used safely in adults and children.[46,47] Larger-than-customary doses may be required to reverse the effects of codeine, methadone, propoxyphene, pentazocine, butorphanol, buprenorphine, and nalbuphine.[48]

PROGNOSIS

Asymptomatic patients overdosed with any of these drugs should be observed for a minimum of 24 hours. The prognosis for toxicity with most of these drugs is unknown, but as with other intoxications, the outcome depends on the quantity of drug ingested and the severity of clinical signs demonstrated on admission. Early decontamination and good supportive care can prevent serious CNS, respiratory, and cardiovascular depression or complications.

REFERENCES

1. Hobbs WR, Rall TW, Verdoorn TA: Hypnotics and sedatives. In Brunton LL, Lazo JS, Parker KL, et al, editors: Goodman & Gilman's the pharmacological basis of therapeutics, ed 11, New York, 2006, McGraw-Hill.
2. Bosse JM: Benzodiazepine. In Tintinalli JE, Kelen GD, Stapczynski JS, et al, editors: Tintinalli's emergency medicine: a comprehensive study guide, ed 6, New York, 2004, McGraw-Hill.
3. Plumb DC: Plumb's veterinary drug handbook, ed 5, Ames, Iowa, 2005, Blackwell.
4. Gross ME, Booth NH: Tranquilizers, α_2-adrenergic agonists and related agents. In Adams HR, editor: Veterinary pharmacology and therapeutics, ed 7, Ames, Iowa, 1995, Iowa State University Press.
5. Material Safety Data Sheet, Diazepam injection, USP, issued September 1, 1999, www.accessbutler.com/msdimages/A0001053.pdf. Accessed November 16, 2007.
6. Material Safety Data Sheet Safety Information, http://www.statkit.com/images/Midazolam-Roche.pdf, issued May 13, 1991. Accessed November 16, 2007.
7. Murrell JC, Hellebrekers LJ: Medetomidine and dexmedetomidine: a review of cardiovascular effects and antinociceptive properties in the dog, Vet Anaesth Analg 32:117, 2005.
8. Material Data Safety Sheet, issued December 13, 2006, issued December 13, 2006, www.mylabonline.com/mds/cobas/tdm/04876/7190.pdf. Accessed November 16, 2007.
9. Giorgi M, Portela DA, Breghi G, et al: Pharmacokinetics and pharmacodynamics of zolpidem after oral administration of a single dose in dogs, Am J Vet Res 73:1650, 2012.
10. Hughes D, Moreau RE, Overall KL, et al: Acute hepatic necrosis and liver failure associated with benzodiazepine therapy in six cats (1986-1995), J Vet Emerg Crit Care 6:13, 1996.
11. Garnier R, Guerault E, Muzard D, et al: Acute zolpidem poisoning—analysis of 344 cases, J Toxicol Clin Toxicol 32:391, 1994.
12. Tranquilli WJ, Lemke KA, Williams LL, et al: Flumazenil efficacy in reversing diazepam or midazolam overdose in dogs, J Vet Anaesth 19:65, 1992.
13. Richardson JA, Gwaltney-Brant SM, Albretsen JC, et al: Clinical syndrome associated with zolpidem ingestion in dogs: 33 cases (January 1998-July 2000), J Vet Intern Med 16:208, 2002.
14. Lancaster AR, Lee JA, Hovda LR, et al: Sleep aid toxicosis in dogs: 317 cases (2004-2010), J Vet Emerg Crit Care 21:658, 2011.
15. Drover DR: Comparative pharmacokinetics and pharmacodynamics of short-acting hypnosedatives: zaleplon, zolpidem and zopiclone, Clin Pharmacokinet 43:227, 2004.
16. Schauben JL: Muscle relaxants. In Delaney KA, Ling LJ, Erickson T, Ford MD, editors: Clinical toxicology, St Louis, 2001, WB Saunders.
17. Martinez EA, Mealey KA: Muscle relaxants. In Boothe DM, editor: Small animal clinical pharmacology and therapeutics, St Louis, 2001, WB Saunders.
18. Wismer T: Baclofen overdose in dogs, Vet Med 99:406, 2004.
19. Hecht DV, Allenspach K: Presumptive baclofen intoxication in a dog, J Vet Emerg Crit Care 8:49, 1998.
20. Lane GS, Mazzaferro E: SOMA (carisoprodol) toxicity in a dog, J Vet Emerg Crit Care 15:48, 2005.
21. Honda M, Nishida T, Ono H: Tricyclic analogs cyclobenzaprine, amitriptyline and cyproheptadine inhibit the spinal reflex transmission through 5-HT(2) receptors, Eur J Pharmacol 458:91, 2003.
22. Wagstaff AJ, Bryson HM: Tizanidine: a review of its pharmacology, clinical efficacy and tolerability in the management of spasticity associated with cerebral and spinal disorders, Drugs 53:435, 1997.
23. Douglas JF, Ludwig BJ, Schlosser A: The metabolic fate of carisoprodol in the dog, J Pharmacol Exp Ther 138:21, 1962.
24. Shannon MW: Muscle relaxants. In Haddad LM, Shannon MW, Winchester JF, editors: Clinical treatment of poisoning and drug overdose, ed 3, Philadelphia, 1998, WB Saunders.
25. Adams HR, Kerzee T, Morehead CD: Carisoprodol-related death in a child, J Forensic Sci 20:200, 1975.
26. Spiller HA, Winter ML, Mann KV, et al: Five-year multicenter retrospective review of cyclobenzaprine toxicity, J Emerg Med 13:781, 1995.
27. Sangster B, Van Heijst ANP, Zimmerman ANE: Treatment of orphenadrine overdose, N Engl J Med 296:1006, 1977.
28. Cohen MB, Gailey R, McCoy GC: Atropine in the treatment of baclofen overdose, Am J Emerg Med 4:552, 1986.
29. Torre DM, Labato MA, Rossi T, et al: Treatment of a dog with severe baclofen intoxication using hemodialysis and mechanical ventilation, J Vet Emerg Crit Care 18:312, 2008.
30. Scott NE, Francey T, Jandrey K: Baclofen intoxication in a dog successfully treated with hemodialysis and hemoperfusion coupled with intensive supportive care, J Vet Emerg Crit Care 17:191, 2007.
31. Muller-Schwartz G, Penn R: Physostigmine in the treatment of intrathecal baclofen overdose, J Neurosurg 71:273, 1989.
32. Watson WA, Litovitz TL, George C, et al: 2004 Annual report of the American Association of Poison Control Centers Toxic Exposure Surveillance System, Am J Emerg Med 23:589, 2005.
33. Gutstein HB, Akil H: Opioid analgesics. In Brunton LL, Lazo JS, Parker KL, et al, editors: Goodman & Gilman's the pharmacological basis of therapeutics, ed 11, New York, 2006, McGraw-Hill.
34. Boothe DM: Control of pain in small animal: opioid agonists and antagonists and other locally and centrally acting analgesics. In Boothe DM, editor: Small animal clinical pharmacology and therapeutics, ed 1, St Louis, 2001, WB Saunders.
35. Murphy MR, Olson WA, Hug CC Jr: Pharmacokinetics of 3H-fentanyl in the dog anesthetized with enflurane, Anesthesiology 50:13, 1979.
36. Gillman PK: Monoamine oxidase inhibitors, opioid analgesics and serotonin toxicity, Br J Anaesth 95:434, 2005.

37. Dodam JR, Cohn LA, Durham HE, Szladovits B: Cardiopulmonary effects of medetomidine, oxymorphone, or butorphanol in selegiline-treated dogs, Vet Anaesth Analg 31:129, 2004.
38. Maurer PM, Bartkowski RR: Drug interactions of clinical significance with opioid analgesics, Drug Safety 8:30, 1993.
39. Lee HK, Wang SC: Mechanism of morphine-induced miosis in the dog, J Pharmacol Exp Ther 192:415, 1975.
40. Hofmeister EH, Herrington JL, Mazzaferro EM: Opioid dysphoria in three dogs, J Vet Emerg Crit Care 16:44, 2006.
41. Golder FJ, Wilson J, Larenza MP, et al: Suspected acute meperidine toxicity in a dog, Vet Anaesth Analg 37:471, 2010.
42. da Cunha AF, Carter JE, Grafinger M, et al: Intrathecal morphine overdose in a dog, J Am Vet Med Assoc 231:1665, 2007.
43. Branson KR, Gross ME, Booth NH: Opioid agonists and antagonists. In Adams HR, editor: Veterinary pharmacology and therapeutics, ed 7, Ames, Iowa, 1995, Iowa State University Press.
44. Zelis R, Mansour EJ, Capone RJ, Mason DT: The cardiovascular effects of morphine. The peripheral capacitance and resistance vessels in human subjects, J Clin Invest 54:1247, 1974.
45. Freise KJ, Newbound GC, Tudan C, et al: Naloxone reversal of an overdose of a novel, long-acting transdermal fentanyl solution in laboratory Beagles, J Vet Pharmacol Ther 35:45, 2012.
46. Goldfrank L, Weisman RS, Errick JK, Lo M: A dosing nomogram for continuous infusion intravenous naloxone, Ann Emerg Med 15:566, 1986.
47. Lewis JM, Klein-Schwartz W, Benson BE, et al: Continuous naloxone infusion in pediatric narcotic overdose, Am J Dis Child 138:944, 1984.
48. Chamberlain JM, Klein BL: A comprehensive review of naloxone for the emergency physician, Am J Emerg Med 12:650, 1994.

CHAPTER 78

CALCIUM CHANNEL BLOCKER AND β-BLOCKER DRUG OVERDOSE

Annie Malouin Wright, DVM, DACVECC • Lesley G. King, MVB, DACVECC, DACVIM

KEY POINTS

- Close regulation of intracellular calcium is essential for many physiologic processes, including excitation-contraction coupling, impulse formation and conduction, and maintenance of vascular tone.
- Calcium channel blockers and β-blockers inhibit L-type voltage sensitive calcium channels.
- The main physiologic derangements caused by overdose with any of these medications are negative inotropy and chronotropy, leading to decreased cardiac output, hypotension, tissue hypoperfusion, and cardiovascular shock.
- No single pharmacologic agent has been consistently effective in the management of critically ill patients with these toxicities. A combination of antidotes may be necessary until the clinical signs are resolved.
- The prognosis depends on the quantity of drug ingested and the severity of signs at presentation. Early aggressive decontamination and intensive supportive care and monitoring can prevent the onset of serious hemodynamic failure.

Calcium channel blockers and β-blockers are among the most frequently prescribed drugs for the treatment of cardiovascular disease in humans and small animals. These drugs have proven effective for people suffering from hypertension, angina pectoris and cardiac arrhythmias, migraines, tremors, and bipolar disorders.[1] In veterinary medicine, calcium channel β-blockers are used to treat cardiac arrhythmias, hypertrophic cardiomyopathy, hypertension, and oligoanuric acute kidney injury.[2-3]

Calcium plays a role in many physiologic processes, including impulse formation and conduction, excitation-contraction coupling, and maintenance of vascular tone. Close regulation of intracellular calcium is essential to accomplish these cardiovascular functions.[4] Several types of calcium channels include three different voltage-operated calcium channels, designated as neuronal (N-type), transient (T-type), and long-lasting (L-type). The L-type channels are the most sensitive to the commercially available calcium channel blockers. β-Blockers inhibit the effects of the adrenergic system on the heart and indirectly modify these voltage-sensitive channels via a second messenger system. The L-type channels are located in various tissues, but they are found in highest concentration in atria, vascular smooth muscle, and skeletal muscle. In cardiac and skeletal muscle the density of L-type calcium channels is higher in the t-tubules than in the surface sarcolemma. L-type voltage regulated calcium channels are activated as the transmembrane potential of the cell becomes progressively less negative during the upstroke of the action potential (phase 0). These channels have a prolonged opening time and are high conductance. As a result, large amounts of calcium can pass rapidly through them and cause sudden changes in intracellular calcium.[5]

Both types of drugs therefore lead to decreased intracellular calcium, depressing cardiovascular function, and in the most severe situations, cause cardiovascular collapse.[5] Although calcium channel blockers and β-blockers have different mechanisms of action, their physiologic effects are similar.[3] Thus signs and symptoms of toxicity, as well as management strategies, are nearly identical for both drug classes.

Table 78-1 **Expected Cardiovascular Effects of Calcium Channel Blocking Agents in Healthy Animals and After Overdose**[2,3]

Class	Trade Name	Chronotropic (HR)	Dromotropic (AV conduction)	Inotropic (Strength)	Systemic Vascular Resistance	Coronary Resistance	Signs of Toxicity
Phenylalkylamines							
Verapamil	Calan, Verelan, Isoptin Covera-HS	0 or +	++	+	+	+	Sinus bradycardia Bradyarrhythmias (all degrees of heart block, QT interval prolongation, or junctional rhythms) Hypotension Reduced myocardial contractility
Benzothiazepines							
Diltiazem	Cardiazem, Dilacor	0 or ++	++	0 or +	+	+	Same as for verapamil
Dihydropyridines							
Nifedipine	Procardia, Adalat	0	0	0	++	++	Hypotension Sinus tachycardia
Nicardipine	Cardene	0	0	0	++	++	Same as for nifedipine
Amlodipine	Norvasc	0	0	0	++	+	Same as for nifedipine

0 = no change, + = mild to moderate decrease, ++ = moderate to marked decrease. This effect is rate dependent and more pronounced at higher heart rates.

METHOD OF ACTION

Calcium Channel Blockers

Currently available calcium channel blockers block transmembrane flow of calcium ions through voltage-gated L-type channels, thus decreasing intracellular calcium concentration. Calcium channel blockers are classified into three major groups based on their structure. These include the phenylalkylamines (e.g., verapamil), the benzothiazepines (e.g., diltiazem) and the dihydropyridines (e.g., amlodipine). The structural differences between the classes allow them to associate with distinct binding sites on the calcium channel, resulting in varying potency and tissue affinities (Table 78-1). All three types of calcium channel blockers exert the majority of their effects on cardiac myocytes, pacemaker cells, and vascular smooth muscle. However, their structural heterogeneity leads to functional differences, particularly with regard to their vasodilator potency, and inotropic, chronotropic, and dromotropic effects on the heart.[1-3]

Cardiac effects

The calcium ion is essential for impulse conduction through the cardiomyocytes. Pacemaker cells of the sinoatrial (SA) and atrioventricular (AV) nodes rely on the inward calcium current through L-type and T-type channels to initiate depolarization (phase 4). Calcium channel blockers inhibit this inward flow through the L-type channel, leading to slow SA activity, decreased conduction of impulses through the AV node, and, as a result, a drop in the heart rate.[5] The negative chronotropic effect occurs primarily with the phenylalkylamines and benzothiazepines. This effect may be attenuated or even abolished by stimulation of the sympathetic nervous system with some calcium channel blockers.[2]

Calcium also plays an important function during excitation-contraction coupling in cardiac and vascular smooth muscles. Within Purkinje cells and myocytes, opening of the L-type calcium channels in response to membrane depolarization increases calcium conductance (phase 2 of the action potential). This inward flow of calcium triggers the release of additional calcium into the cytoplasm from the sarcoplasmic reticulum. Intracellular calcium binds to troponin, changing its conformation and enabling cross bridging of actin and myosin and subsequent contraction of the muscle to occur. By decreasing the magnitude and rate of increase of intracellular calcium, the calcium channel blockers reduce calcium release from the sarcoplasmic reticulum and thus cause a decrease in the force of contraction.[2,5] This negative inotropic effect is seen most commonly with the phenylalkylamines and to a lesser extent with the benzothiazepines.[2] The majority of the calcium channel blockers have a negative inotropic effect at high doses.[3]

Vascular effects

In vascular smooth muscle cells, opening of calcium channels increases the cytosolic calcium concentration. This calcium interacts with calmodulin, leading to phosphorylation of the myosin light chain and subsequent actin-myosin binding. This results in smooth muscle contraction and vasoconstriction. Calcium channel blockers prevent the rise in intracellular calcium needed for formation of the calcium-calmodulin complex and thus cause dilatation of systemic and coronary arteries and arterioles.[5] Veins have less smooth muscle in their wall, thus, at therapeutic concentrations, calcium channel blockers have minimal effects on the venous system. Each class of calcium channel blockers has different tissue specificities. The phenylalkylamines are less selective and affect vascular and cardiac tissue. The benzothiazepines have intermediate selectivity, and the dihydropyridines exert a greater effect on vascular tissue.[2]

Pancreatic effects

The beta cells of the pancreatic islets, which produce insulin, also contain L-type calcium channels. Calcium influx into pancreatic islet cells via L-type channels is required for insulin release. High doses of calcium channel blockers may induce insulin resistance, which causes serum glucose levels to rise, while intracellular glucose stores fall. In all tissues, including the heart, the cell then may have to switch to inefficient fatty acid metabolism to make energy. This lack of intracellular glucose is another mechanism by which calcium channel blocker overdose may impair cardiovascular function, leading to cellular metabolic shock.[6-8]

β-Blockers

Two types of β-receptors are present in the body. The β_1-receptors are located primarily within the heart, kidney, and adipose tissue.

Stimulation of these receptors within the heart results in increases in heart rate, myocardial contractility, atrioventricular conduction velocity, and automaticity of subsidiary pacemakers. They are present in the sinus and atrioventricular nodes, where, if stimulated, they contribute to an increase in heart rate and conduction velocity. In addition, they are in the myocardium, where stimulation results in increased contractility.[4] The β_2-receptors are located primarily in the smooth muscle of the bronchial and vascular walls (e.g., coronary, hepatic, and skeletal arteries), where they produce relaxation. They also are located in the pancreas and gastrointestinal and reproductive tract smooth muscle (details below). Numerous β-adrenergic blocking agents are marketed for pharmacologic use and they differ in their ability to block β-receptor types.[9] In veterinary medicine, the four most commonly used drugs are propranolol (β_1- and β_2-receptor blocker), atenolol (specific β_1-receptor blocker), esmolol (specific β_1-receptor blocker), and sotalol (β_1- and β_2-receptor blocker).[3]

Cardiac effects

The interaction of catecholamines with a β-receptor in the cardiac nodal cell membrane or in the cardiomyocyte cell membrane stimulates the membrane-bound enzyme, adenyl cyclase, which raises the intracellular concentration of cyclic AMP. Cyclic AMP activates protein kinases that phosphorylate the L-type calcium channel, increasing myocellular calcium entry, which then triggers the release of more calcium from the sarcoplasmic reticulum. This calcium interacts with the myocardial contractile machinery and produces systole. At the same time, protein kinases phosphorylate a protein, phospholamban, which causes the sarcoplasmic reticulum to take up calcium more rapidly, allowing relaxation (diastole).[5] Cardiac β-sympathetic blockade decreases transmembrane calcium flow by decreasing cyclic AMP synthesis, thereby decreasing atrial and ventricular contractility, slowing the heart rate, and slowing the spread of excitation through the AV node and ventricles.[3]

Pulmonary, pancreatic, gastrointestinal, vascular, and renal effects

In the lung, stimulation of β_2-receptors promotes bronchodilation and their blockade leads to bronchoconstriction or bronchospasm in susceptible patients. In the pancreas, β_2-receptors mediate insulin release and their blockade inhibits insulin release and leads to decreased glycogenolysis, lipolysis, and gluconeogenesis. In the smooth muscle of the gastrointestinal tract and vascular system, inhibition of β_2-receptors results in contraction. In the kidney, β_1-receptors mediate renin release; inhibition suppresses catecholamine-stimulated renin release, thus decreasing aldosterone synthesis.[4]

PHARMACOKINETICS

Calcium Channel Blockers

Calcium channel blockers are rapidly and almost completely absorbed from the gastrointestinal tract but have extensive first-pass metabolism. Times to peak serum concentration are rapid; 20 to 45 minutes for immediate-release forms and 4 to 12 hours for sustained-release formulations and amlodipine besylate (which has a slower absorption rate), in dogs and cats.[2] The onset of action varies with the formulation and the way it is ingested. An animal that bites into and swallows a sustained-release product can show signs within 5 minutes, whereas one that swallows the product whole may not show signs for several hours. In addition, sustained-release products may have prolonged toxicity because of slower absorption.[10] Distribution is extensive in all classes, and calcium channel blockers are approximately 80% protein bound. Therefore interaction with other highly protein-bound drugs may result in competition for binding sites. In people, calcium channel blockers are metabolized in the liver by oxidative pathways, predominantly by cytochrome P450 CYP3A. Therefore their clearance is decreased with impaired hepatic function or reduced hepatic blood flow.[1] Similarly, their elimination can be slowed by drugs that inhibit hepatic enzymes (e.g., cimetidine), potentially increasing their cardiovascular effects and producing toxicity.[10,11] In addition, the phenylalkylamines and benzothiazepines can interact with many drugs, because they are strong inhibitors of hepatic microsomal enzymes. Elimination half-lives depend on the formulation (i.e., immediate vs. sustained-release), and in dogs and cats vary from 2 to 30 hours. Excretion is primarily through urine and, to a lesser extent, bile and feces.[2]

β-Blockers

The pharmacokinetics of β-blockers, although well established in people, remain unclear in small animals. The more lipid-soluble compounds (e.g., propranolol) require hepatic biotransformation before excretion and therefore can accumulate in animals with decreased hepatic blood flow or hepatic insufficiency. The lipid-soluble compounds have a large volume of distribution and enter the central nervous system faster and more extensively than the water-soluble β-blockers. In contrast, the water-soluble compounds (e.g., atenolol) are excreted by the kidney and can accumulate in patients with renal insufficiency. Esmolol is water soluble but does not accumulate in animals with renal disease because it is metabolized by erythrocyte esterases.[12]

Channel selectivity and any concurrent diseases should be considered when prescribing these medications. For example, β_1-selective agents are safer than nonselective agents for diabetic patients or cats with asthma. In patients with heart failure, chronic increases in circulating catecholamine concentrations and increased sympathetic nervous system activity cause down-regulation of β-adrenergic receptors. Fewer receptors are present to which a β-blocker may bind. Despite decreased numbers of receptors, many patients with compromised myocardial function rely on stimulation of remaining β-receptors to maintain myocardial contractility. In these circumstances, acute administration of medium to high doses of a β-blocker can result in lethal decreases in contractility and heart rate.[3]

DIAGNOSIS OF OVERDOSE

Clinical signs associated with calcium channel and β-blocker toxicity generally reflect an extension of the therapeutic effects of these drugs.[13,14] In Table 78-1, cardiovascular signs of overdose specific to calcium channel blocker classes are described. Table 78-2 displays the therapeutic dose ranges of the calcium channel and β-blockers most commonly used in dogs and cats.[2,3,12] The main physiologic derangements caused by acute overdose with any of these medications are negative inotropy and chronotropy leading to decreased cardiac output, hypotension, tissue hypoperfusion, and cardiovascular shock. Most calcium channel and β-blocker overdoses are evident within 6 hours of ingestion in humans, but clinical signs may be delayed when sustained-release preparations or sotalol are ingested.[9]

Although calcium channel and β-blocker overdoses often present in a similar fashion, subtle differences in presentation may suggest poisoning with one class over another. After calcium channel blocker toxicity, the drug's usual selectivity for cardiac versus vascular is decreased but not eliminated. Vasodilation, particularly associated with agents (e.g., dihydropyridines) that have more pronounced effects on the vascular smooth muscles, results in hypotension, decreased systemic vascular resistance, and vasodilatory shock. In contrast to calcium channel blockers, distinctions among the various β-blockers classes tend to disappear in overdose situations.[15]

The most common ECG findings in patients with significant calcium channel blocker ingestion are sinus bradycardia,

Table 78-2 **Therapeutic Dose Ranges of Calcium Channel Blockers and β-Blockers Most Commonly Used in Dogs and Cats**[2,3,12]

Drugs	Therapeutic Doses: Dogs	Therapeutic Doses: Cats
Calcium Channel Blocker		
Phenylalkylamines		
Verapamil hydrochloride	0.1-5 mg/kg PO q8-12h 0.15 mg/kg IV over 2 min	*
Benzothiazepines		
Diltiazem hydrochloride	0.5-1.5 mg/kg PO, q8h 0.25 mg/kg IV over 5 min	1.75-2.5 mg/kg PO q8h
Dihydropyridines		
Amlodipine besylate	0.05-0.25 mg/kg PO q24h	0.625 mg/cat PO q24h
Nifedipine	0.5 mg/kg PO q8h	—
Nicardipine	0.5-5 mcg/kg/min IV CRI	—
β-Blockers		
Propranolol	If severe cardiac disease: 0.1-0.5 mg/kg PO q8h If normal myocardial function: 2 mg/kg PO q8h	2.5-10 mg PO q8h
Atenolol	6.25 to 50 mg PO q12h	6.25 mg PO q12h
Esmolol	Loading dose: 0.25-0.5 mg/kg IV Followed by constant rate infusion: 10-200 mcg/kg/min IV	
Metoprolol	0.25-1 mg/kg PO q12-24h	2-15 mg (total dose) PO q8h
Carvedilol	—	—

References 2, 3, 12.
*Verapamil is not recommended for use in cats because of safety concerns.[12,16]

atrioventricular block, and junctional rhythms.[10,16] β-Blocker toxicity also causes bradycardia, but ventricular conduction defects tend to be more common in humans.[17]

Mild hyperkalemia may be observed with toxic levels of β-blockers. This stems from two mechanisms: (1) lower aldosterone levels as a result of β-blocker–induced suppression of the catecholamine-induced renin release and (2) decreased cellular uptake of potassium by the cells. Normally, agonist binding to the β_2-adrenergic receptor stimulates the formation of cyclic AMP, which acts through protein kinase A to phosphorylate and activate the Na^+/K^+-ATPase pump, leading to the influx of potassium into cells. Competitive inhibition of the β_2-receptor by β-blockers decreases Na^+/-K^+-ATPase function and thus reduces potassium uptake by cells resulting in hyperkalemia.[4] Hypocalcemia occasionally is reported in patients with calcium channel blocker toxicity.[9] These electrolyte disturbances may further lower the threshold for serious cardiac rhythm abnormalities. Hyperglycemia is a common finding in patients with calcium channel blocker toxicity because of inhibition of insulin release from pancreatic beta cells.[6]

Noncardiogenic pulmonary edema has been reported in association with high doses of calcium channel and β-blockers.[18] A number of theories have been proposed regarding the pathophysiology of noncardiogenic pulmonary edema. Studies have shown that calcium blockage inhibits alveolar fluid clearance by interfering with transepithelial sodium and potassium transport.[19] Combined with excessive fluid therapy during resuscitation, selective precapillary vasodilation may result in pulmonary transudation.[18] A massive sympathetic discharge may occur secondary to the sudden bradycardia and hypotension.[20-21] Dyspnea caused by bronchospasm is reported rarely after β-blocker overdose, although patients with pre-existing asthma may experience more severe pulmonary effects after β_2-receptor antagonist ingestion or administration.

People who overdose on highly lipid-soluble β-blockers, such as propranolol, frequently present with central nervous system depression and seizures.[9] Seizures after ingestion of verapamil are rare but have been reported in animals[16] and people.[11]

Terminal events after either calcium channel or β-blocker toxicity include a worsening of the shock state, multiple organ failure (e.g., myocardial infarction, mesenteric ischemia, acute kidney injury, coma), and ultimately cardiac arrest.

THERAPY

Asymptomatic Patients

Decontamination

Gastrointestinal decontamination should be performed in all asymptomatic animals that have ingested large amounts of calcium channel blockers or β-blockers. If the ingestion was recent (within the last 2 hours) and the patient is stable, emesis is recommended. In cases of massive ingestion or in patients with altered levels of consciousness, gastric lavage should be performed. Activated charcoal (1 to 3 g/kg PO for dogs and cats) with a cathartic should be given to absorb and hasten the excretion of any remaining toxicant. The patient must be stable before receiving activated charcoal; care should be taken to protect the patient's airway and closely monitor hemodynamic parameters, as indicated.[22] The cathartic is to be used only once with the first charcoal dose. Activated charcoal can be administered every 4 to 6 hours for two to four repeated doses if a sustained-release product was ingested.[10-12,23] Also, a warm water enema (2.5 to 5 mL/kg) could be considered to facilitate evacuation of intestinal contents.

The first 24 hours after presentation are critical. The patient's cardiovascular function should be monitored closely with serial or continuous electrocardiograms, blood pressure measurements, and evaluation of blood glucose and serum electrolyte concentrations.

Table 78-3 Dosages of Pharmacologic Options for Treatment of Patients with Calcium Channel or β-Blocker Toxicity

Drugs	Dosages for Dogs and Cats
Calcium gluconate 10%	Bolus of 0.5 to 1.5 ml/kg (50-150 mg/kg) IV over 10-20 min Possibly followed by a CRI of 10-15 mg/kg/hr
Atropine	0.02-0.05 mg/kg IV
Epinephrine	0.005 to 1 mcg/kg/min IV CRI
Norepinephrine	0.05 to 2 mcg/kg/min IV CRI
Dopamine	5 to 20 mcg/kg/min IV CRI
Dobutamine	2 to 20 mcg/kg/min IV CRI in dogs. 1 to 5 mcg/kg/min IV CRI in cats
Vasopressin	0.5 to 5 mU/kg/min IV CRI for dogs; dosage for cats is unknown
Glucagon	Bolus of 0.15 mg/kg IV followed by a CRI of 0.05-0.10 mg/kg/hr titrated to effect
Regular insulin	Bolus of 1.0 U/kg IV followed by an infusion of 1.0 U/kg/hr for the first hour, followed by 0.5 U/kg/hr until toxicity resolves
Intravenous lipid: lipid solutions 20%	Bolus of 1.5 ml/kg over 2-3 minutes IV followed by a CRI of 0.25 ml/kg/min for 30-60 minutes

Elimination of calcium channel blockers and lipid-soluble β-blockers (e.g., propranolol) via extracorporeal removal procedures (e.g., hemodialysis, hemoperfusion) is ineffective because these compounds are highly protein bound and have large volumes of distribution. It may be possible to remove water-soluble β-blockers (e.g., atenolol and esmolol) using hemodialysis.[9] The use of intravenous lipid emulsion is a more recent therapy for the treatment of lipid-soluble drugs; this is discussed later in this chapter.

Symptomatic Patients

Controlling the clinical signs of the symptomatic animal is the priority. As with any emergent patient, initial evaluation of cardiovascular and respiratory function should determine whether it is necessary to establish an airway and/or provide ventilatory and circulatory support. The patient must be stable before any type of decontamination is performed. After venous access is obtained, hypotensive animals should receive intravenous fluids (i.e., isotonic crystalloids and/or synthetic colloids) for volume expansion (see Chapter 60). Pharmacologic options for treatment of patients with calcium channel or β-blocker toxicity include calcium, atropine, catecholamine vasopressors, vasopressin, glucagon, hyperinsulinemia/euglycemia, and intravenous lipid emulsions (Table 78-3 and Figure 78-1).* All of these drugs have been tested in dog trials of cardiogenic shock induced by overdose with calcium channel or β-blockers.[7,8,25,30,31] No single agent has been consistently effective in the management of critically ill patients with these toxicities; therefore a combination of antidotes may be necessary. The animal should be treated and monitored continuously until the clinical signs are resolved.

Calcium salts

Administration of calcium intravenously is the initial treatment for calcium channel blocker and β-blocker overdose.[24] It is a reasonable first antidote because it is readily available and easily administered through a peripheral or central catheter. Exogenous calcium administration increases the extracellular calcium concentration and the free (unbound) calcium. This increase in calcium availability stimulates the sarcoplasmic reticulum to release more calcium into the cytoplasm, which is then available for diverse cellular functions. Intravenous calcium may improve cardiac conduction, inotropy, and blood pressure.[24,25]

The exact dose of calcium that should be used is unclear. Hariman, et al showed that in dogs increasing the serum calcium by 1 to 2 mEq/L resulted in a reversal of the negative inotropic effects of verapamil, and even greater increases in serum calcium resulted in improvement of depressed atrioventricular conduction and sinus node function.[24] A continuous infusion titrated to a desirable heart rate and blood pressure also has been suggested.[9,26] In general, the treatment protocol for calcium consists of an initial bolus dose of calcium salts followed by a continuous infusion with measurement of serum calcium at least twice daily. Initially, calcium gluconate 10% should be given at a dose of 0.5 to 1.5 ml/kg (50 to 150 mg/kg) IV over 10 to 20 minutes to stabilize cardiovascular parameters. Excessively rapid injection can cause hypotension, cardiac arrhythmias, and cardiac arrest. Continuous infusions of calcium gluconate also have been used at 10 to 15 mg/kg/hr. Calcium chloride is an alternative to calcium gluconate; however, this preparation is more irritating to extravascular tissues than the other parenteral calcium salts.[12] The calcium concentration should be maintained at a normal level; there is no evidence to support supraphysiologic calcium levels. Careful maintenance of patent intravenous access sites is important to prevent injury secondary to extravasation of calcium solution. Although treatment with intravenous calcium salts is successful in many cases, other modes of therapy should be added if the patient is refractory to calcium treatment.

Parasympatholytics and sympathomimetics

Atropine is a vagolytic drug that can be given in an attempt to reverse bradycardia and atrioventricular blockade. However, it has shown an inconsistent benefit in the treatment of calcium channel blocker and β-blocker intoxications.[11,27] The dosage of atropine is 0.02 to 0.04 mg/kg IV.[12]

Adrenergic agents such as dopamine, dobutamine, norepinephrine, epinephrine, and isoproterenol may be needed either alone or in combination with other drugs to counter the hypotension secondary to drug overdose. These agents act by stimulating α- and β-adrenergic receptors. As previously reviewed, β-adrenergic receptor stimulation causes the formation of adenyl cyclase and subsequently cAMP. Direct α-adrenergic receptor agonists promote calcium release from the sarcoplasmic reticulum through receptor-operated calcium channels and bypass L-channel blockade.[5] The choice of agents depends on the hemodynamic picture of the patient and the responses to specific antidotes (see Chapter 157). Based on their pharmacologic profiles, β-adrenergic receptor agonist such as dobutamine would be a logical choice when the toxicity affects primarily cardiac chronotropy and inotropy. Direct α-adrenergic receptor agonists may be a better choice if the toxicity is related primarily to decreased systemic vascular resistance. Furthermore, combining α- and β-adrenergic receptor agonists (such as dobutamine and norepinephrine) or using agents with α- and β-adrenergic effects (such as epinephrine or dopamine) may ameliorate cardiac dysfunction and increase systemic vascular resistance.

However, treatment with adrenergic drugs may yield a poor response in patients with moderate to severe overdose. β-Agonists bind only receptors that are not occupied by a β-blocker. In animals with moderate to severe β-blocker intoxication, β-agonist drugs may not be effective because most adrenergic receptors are blocked.[27]

*References 7, 8, 11, 13, 14, 24, 25, 27-32.

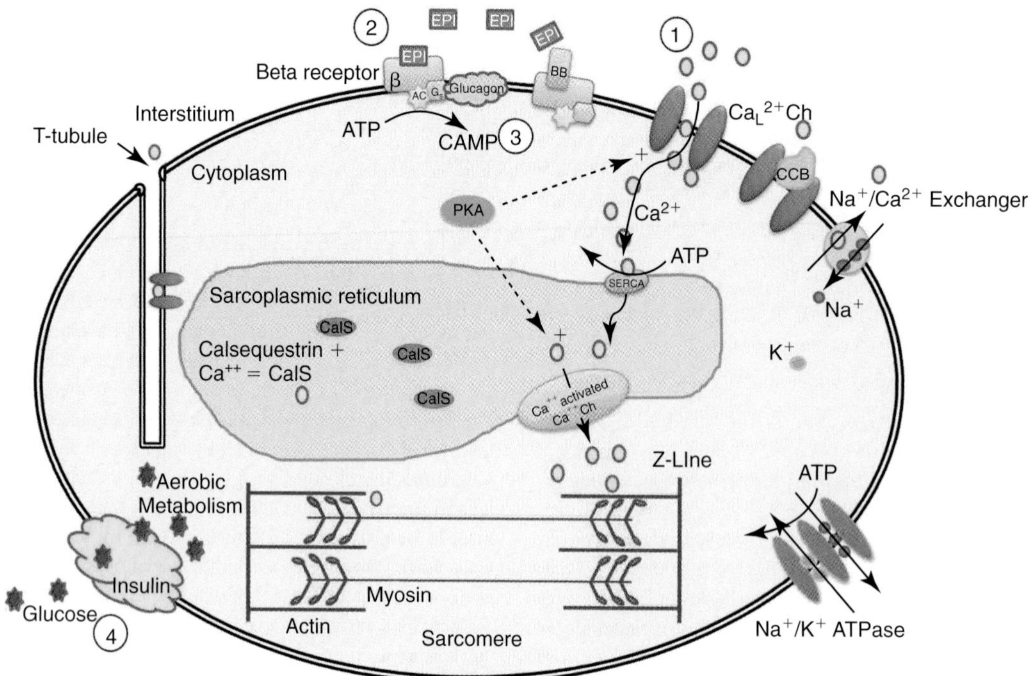

FIGURE 78-1 Schematic of a cardiomyocyte during treatment of β-blocker (BB) and calcium channel blocker (CCB) toxicity with calcium (Ca^{2+}), epinephrine (EPI), glucagon, and insulin. (1) Ca^{2+} enters the cell through voltage gated L-type Ca^{2+} channels. It is then pumped into the sarcoplasmic reticulum via the sarcoplasmic endoplasmic reticulum Ca^{2+}-ATPase (SERCA). In the sarcoplasmic reticulum the Ca^{2+} becomes bound to the high-capacity Ca^{2+} binding protein calsequestrin (CalS). The stored Ca^{2+} is released from the sarcoplasmic reticulum when the Ca^{2+} activated Ca^{2+} channel is opened. The released Ca^{2+} pairs with troponin to cause muscle contraction via actin and myosin fibers. (2) EPI (epinephrine) binds and stimulates β-receptors that are not occupied or blocked by a β-blocker (BB). This in turn activates the attached G_s protein that activates adenylate cyclase (AC). AC catalyzes the conversion of adenosine triphosphate (ATP) to cyclic adenosine monophosphate (cAMP). This then activates protein kinase A (PKA), which stimulates the opening of dormant Ca^{2+} channels thus enhancing the release of Ca^{2+} from the sarcoplasmic reticulum. (3) Glucagon bypasses the β-receptor and acts directly on the G_s protein, stimulating conversion of ATP to cAMP. Thus glucagon can enhance myocardial contractility, heart rate, and atrioventricular conduction. (4) Insulin improves the outcomes of β-blocker and calcium channel blocker toxicity via its positive inotropic effects and its positive effects on myocardial carbohydrate metabolism. During non-stress conditions the cardiac cells prefer to use free fatty acid as their primary energy substrate. During toxicity events the myocardial energy substrate switches to carbohydrates. *(Figure illustrated by David M. Wright, MD.)*

Vasopressin

Vasopressin has been used anecdotally to treat refractory hypotension from calcium channel blocker and β-blocker overdoses. Vasopressin stimulates V1-receptors in smooth muscle and increase vascular tone (see Chapter 158). The extrapolated dose for dogs with vasodilatory shock is 0.5 to 5 mU/kg/min. The dosage for cats is unknown.[28-31]

Glucagon

Glucagon is a polypeptide hormone secreted from the pancreatic islets. Its efficacy in the treatment of calcium channel and β-blocker toxicity is attributed to the fact that glucagon binds to receptor sites that are distinct from L-type calcium channels and adrenergic receptors. It then stimulates adenyl cyclase, which results in the formation of cyclic adenosine monophosphate (cAMP), promoting calcium influx and stimulating the release of calcium from the sarcoplasmic reticulum. Glucagon's effects on adenyl cyclase also cause stimulation of the SA and AV nodes. As a result, glucagon has inotropic, chronotropic, and dromotropic properties.[32]

Several animal model studies evaluated the efficacy of high dose glucagon for treatment of calcium channel blocker and β-blocker overdoses and have shown that it increased heart rate and cardiac output and reversed second- and third-degree AV blocks. However, there was no effect on mean arterial blood pressure and it did not appear to change survival rate. The dose of glucagon suggested by the animal models and used to treat people is an intravenous bolus dose of 0.05 to 0.150 mg/kg given over 1 to 2 minutes. This initial dose will have a transient effect that should occur within approximately 5 minutes. If a benefit is seen, the initial dose should be followed by an intravenous continuous rate infusion of 0.05 to 0.10 mg/kg/hr. The infusion rate can then be tapered downward as the patient improves. If improvement is not seen with the initial bolus dose, consider increasing the initial dose. Glucagon is lyophilized powder for injection that requires reconstitution; consult the manufacturer's recommendations for preparation of the infusion.[13,14,32] Glucagon-treated patients should be monitored for side effects of nausea, vomiting, hypokalemia, and hyperglycemia.

Hyperinsulinemia and euglycemia

Calcium channel blockers inhibit insulin secretion, resulting in hyperglycemia and alterations of myocardial fatty acid oxidation.[8] Similarly, blockade of β_2-adrenergic receptors in β-blocker toxicity impairs lipolysis, glycogenolysis, and insulin release.[33] Insulin is presumed beneficial because of its ability to increase simultaneously lactate oxidation while switching myocardial cell metabolism from fatty acids to carbohydrates during shock, thus restoring calcium fluxes and improving cardiac contractility.[7,34-36] Second, insulin has inotropic properties.[37,38]

In an unstressed state, myocytes oxidize free fatty acids for metabolic energy. However, in a state of shock, such as that associated with overdose of calcium channel and β-blockers, myocytes use glucose for energy. It is known that hypoinsulinemia prevents the uptake of glucose by myocytes, thus decreasing inotropy. Therefore insulin therapy may improve inotropy and increase peripheral vascular resistance by improving the uptake of glucose by cardiomyocyte smooth muscle cells.[35]

Lactic acidosis from toxicity-induced circulatory shock is partially a manifestation of poor tissue perfusion but also is due to mitochondrial dehydrogenase inhibition. In high concentrations, calcium channel blockers inhibit mitochondrial calcium entry at the sarcolemma and mitochondrial membrane, which in turn can decrease pyruvate dehydrogenase activity. Pyruvate cannot enter the Krebs cycle and lactate accumulates, producing a metabolic acidosis. Insulin can increase myocardial pyruvate dehydrogenase activity, enhancing lactate oxidation and reversing the acidosis.[7]

The recommended dosage regimen is a regular insulin bolus of 1.0 U/kg, followed by an infusion of 1.0 U/kg/hr for the first hour, followed by 0.5 U/kg/hr until toxicity resolves.[36] Blood glucose should be monitored at least hourly and supplemented as needed concurrently during the insulin infusion. Depending on the severity of overdose, resistance to insulin-mediated glucose clearance may be significant.[33] Electrolyte abnormalities such as hypokalemia, hypophosphatemia, and hypomagnesaemia also may occur, and their serum levels should be monitored at least every 12 hours (see Chapters 51 and 53). These ions should be supplemented according to standard medical indications.

Intravenous lipid emulsion

Calcium channel and β-blockers are variably fat soluble; propranolol and verapamil are the most soluble. Extra-label use of intravenous lipid emulsion (ILE) has been reported for the management of a lipophilic drug toxicity, when general supportive measures and recognized antidotes are not effective (see Chapter 74).[39-42] ILE is the injectable lipid portion of parenteral nutrition formulations, which typically contains triglycerides and a phospholipid emulsifier. The specific mechanism by which ILE may increase the rate of recovery for diverse drug toxicoses is currently unknown. It may improve directly cardiac performance and/or serve as a separate intravascular compartment or "sink," which would sequester lipid soluble drugs and therefore reduce the amount of free toxic drug in circulation.

Several ILE infusion protocols for the management of lipophilic drug toxicity in dogs and cats are published. All use 20% lipid solutions (e.g., Intralipid, Liposyn), which can be infused via a peripheral or central venous catheter, although sterile technique is imperative. Before administration of ILE, decontamination and efforts to maximize the patient's oxygenation and perfusion should be performed. ILE can be given initially as a slow bolus (1.5 ml/kg over 2 to 3 minutes) followed by a CRI (0.25 ml/kg/min) for 30 to 60 minutes. The patient should be monitored closely until clinical signs of the toxicity have resolved and the serum is no longer lipemic. If no improvement is noted after three consecutive doses (bolus and CRI), ILE therapy should be discontinued. The safety of using bolus ILE therapy has not been established. Possible complications may include pancreatitis, fat emboli, hemolysis, hypersensitivity reactions, interference with concurrent drug administration (e.g., anticonvulsants), and interference with laboratory tests resulting from lipemia.

Mechanical support

Mechanical supportive measures may be necessary in the setting of failure of pharmacologic therapy. Electrical cardiac pacing, intraaortic balloon counterpulsation, and extracorporeal cardiopulmonary bypass are treatments that have been used with variable success rates in human patients with calcium channel blocker overdose.[9,43]

Supportive Care

Supportive care may include airway protection and management, ensuring adequate ventilation and oxygenation, and hemodynamic monitoring. Endotracheal intubation may prevent pulmonary aspiration of stomach contents if the patient vomits or regurgitates while recumbent and after enteral charcoal administration. Control of the airway also facilitates achieving adequate oxygenation and ventilation and may improve cardiac output and survival. A central venous catheter should be inserted to provide a portal for pulmonary artery catheterization (if needed to measure pulmonary capillary wedge pressures and cardiac output), to monitor central venous pressure while adjusting fluid therapy, and to administer calcium salts, which are irritating to peripheral veins. A urinary catheter should be placed to monitor urine production and the nutritional status should be addressed as soon as possible.

CONCLUSION

The flow of calcium across cell membranes is necessary for cardiac automaticity, conduction, and contraction, as well as maintenance of vascular tone and insulin secretion. Calcium channel and β-blockers impede calcium fluxes across cell membranes through different mechanisms; however, they share common cardiovascular pharmacologic effects if overdosed. In general, they depress myocardial contractility, sinus and atrioventricular nodal conduction, and cause vasodilatation. The prognosis for each individual patient depends on the quantity of drug ingested and the severity of signs at presentation. An understanding of the drugs' basic mechanisms of action and the resulting pathophysiology of their misuse is essential for the development of a rational approach to treating toxicity. Early aggressive decontamination and intensive supportive care can prevent the onset of serious hemodynamic failure and organ dysfunction.

REFERENCES

1. Abernethy DR, Schwartz JB: Calcium-antagonist drugs, N Engl J Med 341:1447, 1999.
2. Cooke KL, Snyder PS: Calcium channel blockers in veterinary medicine, J Vet Intern Med 12:123, 1998.
3. Kittleson MD, Kienle RD: Small animal cardiovascular medicine, ed 1, St Louis, 1998, Mosby.
4. Guyton AC, Hall JE: Textbook of medical physiology, ed 11, Philadelphia, 2006, WB Saunders.
5. Berne RM, Levy MN: Cardiovascular physiology, ed 8, St Louis, 2001, Mosby.
6. Kline JA, Raymond RM, Schroeder DJ, Watts JA: The diabetogenic effects of acute verapamil poisoning, Toxicol Appl Pharmacol 145:357, 1997.
7. Kline JA, Raymond RM, Leonova ED, et al: Insulin improves heart function and metabolism during nonischemic cardiogenic shock in awake canines, Cardiovasc Res 34:289, 1997.
8. Shepherd G, Klein-Schwartz W: High-dose insulin therapy for calcium channel blocker overdose, Ann Pharmacother 39:923, 2005.
9. DeWitt CR, Waksman JC: Pharmacology, pathophysiology and management of calcium channel blocker and β-blocker toxicity, Toxicol Rev 23:223, 2004.
10. Holder T: Calcium channel blocker toxicosis, Vet Med 95:912, 2000.
11. Salhanick SD, Shannon MW: Management of calcium channel antagonist overdose, Drug Saf 26:65, 2003.
12. Plumb DC: Plumb's veterinary drug handbook, ed 7, Ames Iowa, 2011, Blackwell.
13. Hayes CL, Knight M: Calcium channel blocker toxicity in dogs and cats, Vet Clin Small Anim 42:263, 2012.
14. Costello M, Syring RS: Calcium channel blocker toxicity, J Vet Emerg Crit Care 18:54, 2008.

15. Newton CRH, Delgado JH, Gomez HF: Calcium and β-receptor antagonist overdose: a review and update of pharmacological principles and management, Semin Respir Crit Care Med 23:19, 2002.
16. MacPhail C, Hackett TB: Verapamil toxicity in a cat, Feline Pract 26:16, 1998.
17. Love JN, Enlow B, Howell JM, et al: Electrocardiographic changes associated with β-blocker toxicity, Ann Emerg Med 40:603, 2002.
18. Humbert VHJ, Munn NJ, Hawkins RF: Noncardiogenic pulmonary edema complicating massive diltiazem overdose, Chest 99:258, 1991.
19. Han DY, Nie HG, Gu X, et al: K+ channel openers restore verapamil-inhibited lung fluid resolution and transepithelial ion transport, Respir Res 11:65, 2010.
20. Gustafsson D: Microvascular mechanism involved in calcium antagonist edema formation, J Cardiovasc Pharmacol 10:S121, 1987.
21. Brass BJ, Winchester-Penny S, Lipper BL: Massive verapamil overdose complicated by noncardiogenic pulmonary edema, Am J Emerg Med 14:459, 1996.
22. Rosendale ME: Decontamination strategies, Vet Clin Small Anim Small Anim Pract 32:311, 2002.
23. Laine K, Kivisto KT, Neuvonen PJ: Effect of delayed administration of activated charcoal on the absorption of conventional and slow-release verapamil, Clin Toxicol 37:263, 1997.
24. Hariman RJ, Mangiardi LM, McAllister RG, et al: Reversal of the cardiovascular effects of verapamil by calcium and sodium: differences between electrophysiologic and hemodynamic responses, Circulation 59:797, 1979.
25. Love JN, Hanfling D, Howell JM: Hemodynamic effects of calcium chloride in a canine model of acute propranolol intoxication, Ann Emerg Med 28:1, 1996.
26. Howarth DM, Dawson AH, Smith AJ, et al: Calcium channel blocking drug overdose: an Australian series, Hum Exp Toxicol 13:161, 1994.
27. Weinstein RS: Recognition and management of poisoning with β-adrenergic blocking agents, Ann Emerg Med 13:1123, 1984.
28. Kanagarajan K, Marraffa JM, Bouchard NC, et al: The use of vasopressin in the setting of recalcitrant hypotension due to calcium channel blocker overdose, Clin Toxicol 45:56-9, 2007.
29. Holger JS, Engebretsen KM, Obetz CL, et al: A comparison of vasopressin and glucagon in beta-blocker induced toxicity, Clin Toxicol 44(1):45-51, 2006.
30. Sztajnkrycer MD, Bond GR, Johnson SB, et al: Use of vasopressin in a canine model of severe verapamil poisoning: a preliminary descriptive study, Acad Emerg Med 11: 1253-61, 2004.
31. Barry JD, Durkovich DW, Richardson W, et al: Vasopressin treatment of verapamil toxicity in the porcine model, J Med Toxicol 1:3-10, 2005.
32. Bailey B: Glucagon in β-blocker and calcium channel blocker overdose: a systematic review, J Toxicol Clin Toxicol 41:595, 2003.
33. Megarbane B, Karyo S, Baud FJ: The role of insulin and glucose (hyperinsulinemia/euglycaemia) therapy in acute calcium and β-blocker poisoning, Toxicol Rev 23:215, 2004.
34. Kerns W, Schroeder D, Williams C, et al: Insulin improves survival in a canine model of acute β-blocker toxicity, Ann Emerg Med 29:748, 1997.
35. Kline JA, Leonova E, Raymond RM: Beneficial myocardial metabolic effects of insulin during verapamil toxicity in the anesthetized canine, Crit Care Med 23:1251, 1995.
36. Engebretsen KM, Kaczmarek KM, Morgan J, et al: High-dose insulin therapy in beta-blocker and calcium channel blocker poisoning. Clin Toxicol 49:277, 2011.
37. Whitehurst VE, Vick JA, Alleva FR, et al: Reversal of propranolol blockade of adrenergic receptors and related toxicity with drugs that increase cyclic AMP, Proc Soc Exp Biol Med 221:382, 1999.
38. Farah AE, Alousi AA: The actions of insulin on cardiac contractility, Life Sci 29:975, 1981.
39. Fernandez AL, Lee JA, Rahilly L, et al: The use of intravenous liquid emulsion as an antidote in veterinary toxicology, J Vet Emerg Crit Care 21:309, 2011.
40. Gwaltney-Brant S, Meadows I: Use of intravenous lipid emulsions for treating certain poisoning cases in small animals, Vet Clin Small Anim 42:251, 2012.
41. Tebbutt S, Harvey M, Nicholson T, et al: Intralipid prolongs survival in a rat model of verapamil toxicity, Acad Emerg Med 13:134, 2006.
42. Jamaty C, Bailey B, Larocque A, et al: Lipid emulsions in the treatment of acute poisoning: a systematic review of human and animal studies, Clin Toxicol 48:1, 2010.
43. Syring RS, Costello MF: Temporary transvenous pacing in a dog with diltiazem intoxication, J Vet Emerg Crit Care 18:75, 2008.

CHAPTER 79
SEROTONIN SYNDROME

Erica L. Reineke, VMD, DACVECC

KEY POINTS

- Serotonin (5-hydroxytryptamine [5-HT]) syndrome is a drug-induced condition resulting from excess serotonergic agonism of the central and peripheral nervous system serotonin receptors.
- Serotonin syndrome can result from overdoses of serotonin reuptake inhibitors, monoamine oxidase inhibitors, tricyclic antidepressant medications, lithium, dietary supplements, or administration of multiple serotonergic medications.
- Clinical signs reported in companion animals resulting from accidental ingestion of serotonergic medications include nervous system signs (seizures, depression, tremors, hyperesthesia, ataxia, paresis, disorientation, coma, hyperreflexia, mydriasis, blindness), gastrointestinal tract symptoms (vomiting, diarrhea, abdominal pain, ptyalism, flatulence, bloat), hyperthermia, and death.
- Treatment of symptomatic animals consists primarily of supportive measures and correction of nervous system and cardiovascular abnormalities but also could include administration of a 5-HT_{2A} receptor antagonist such as cyproheptadine.

Over the past 10 years, with mental depression and other psychiatric disorders becoming more prevalent, numerous drugs have been developed to manipulate neurotransmitters in the brain. With the increasing use of these antidepressant medications in humans and animals, the incidence of intentional and accidental ingestions of these medications also is increasing.

The history of antidepressant medications began in 1951 with the introduction of the drug isoniazid and its isopropyl derivative iproniazid to manage tuberculosis.[1,2] Doctors quickly discovered that patients treated with this drug exhibited signs of elevated mood. This psychotropic effect was found to result from iproniazid's ability to inhibit the enzyme monoamine oxidase, responsible for the breakdown of serotonin, resulting in increased amounts of serotonin in the brain.[1,2] Since that time, evidence has accumulated to support the hypothesis that the diminished formation of neurotransmitters, serotonin in particular, may be responsible for mental depression.[3] This has led to the development of novel drugs designed to increase the levels of serotonin in the brain by inhibiting the breakdown of serotonin (monoamine oxidase inhibitors [MAOIs]), increasing serotonin release (amphetamines), and blocking the reuptake of serotonin (selective serotonin reuptake inhibitors [SSRIs] and tricyclic antidepressants [TCAs]). These medications may be prescribed by veterinarians to treat behavior problems in small animals.

DEFINITION

Serotonin syndrome refers to a drug-induced condition resulting from excess serotonergic agonism of the central and peripheral nervous system serotonin receptors. This life-threatening syndrome is characterized by a clinical triad of mental status changes, autonomic instability, and neuromuscular abnormalities.[4] In humans this syndrome can occur after initial administration of an SSRI or more commonly results from the concurrent administration of two serotonergic medications. One of the most common and lethal interactions is the combination of an SSRI with an MAOI.[4,5] In companion animals, this syndrome has been reported only secondary to accidental ingestion but also could occur secondary to therapeutic dosages of serotonergic medications and drug interactions.[6]

SEROTONIN AND PATHOPHYSIOLOGY OF SEROTONIN SYNDROME

Serotonin exerts its effects in the peripheral and central nervous systems. Most of the serotonin in the body is synthesized and stored in the enterochromaffin cells and myenteric plexus in the gastrointestinal (GI) tract.[7] Serotonin produced by the enterochromaffin cells in the GI mucosa is scavenged and stored by platelets through an active uptake mechanism. Serotonin also is removed from the circulation by the lungs and either stored there or transferred to platelets.[7]

The effects of serotonin in the peripheral nervous system include vasoconstriction, platelet aggregation, uterine contraction, intestinal peristalsis, and bronchoconstriction.[7,8] Serotonin cannot cross the blood-brain barrier, so it must be synthesized in the central nervous system. Most serotonin-producing neurons in the brain are located on the midline raphe nuclei of the lower pons and medulla and project fibers to many areas of the brain and spinal cord.[3] Centrally, serotonin exerts influences on mood, aggression, thermoregulation, sleep, vomiting, and pain perception.[3,8]

Serotonin is formed in the body by hydroxylation and decarboxylation of the essential amino acid tryptophan by tryptophan hydroxylase. Increased intake of tryptophan in the diet can increase brain serotonin levels because the tryptophan hydroxylase normally does not reach saturation levels.[7] Serotonin is synthesized in the cytosol in neurons, stored in vesicles at the nerve terminal, and released into the synaptic cleft, where it binds to the postsynaptic receptor, mediating neurotransmission. After release, much of the serotonin is recaptured by an active reuptake mechanism and subsequently inactivated by monoamine oxidase to form 5-hydroxyindoleacetic acid. This substance is then eliminated in the urine (Figure 79-1).[7]

Seven families of serotonin receptors have been identified (5-HT_1 to 5-HT_7), several of which have multiple members.[4] No single receptor appears to be responsible for serotonin syndrome, although several lines of evidence suggest that the 5-HT_1 and 5-HT_{2A} receptors contribute substantially to the condition.[2,4] Severe serotonin excess can lead to activation of other pathways through the release of noradrenaline, dopamine, and glutamine from the anterior hypothalamus.[9]

Drug classes that have been implicated in serotonin syndrome include serotonin precursors, serotonin agonists, serotonin releasing agents (SRAs), serotonin reuptake inhibitors, MAOIs, lithium, and herbal medications (Box 79-1).[4]

CLINICAL SIGNS

In humans the serotonin syndrome encompasses a wide range of clinical findings ranging from tremor and diarrhea in mild cases to delirium, neuromuscular rigidity, and severe hyperthermia in life-threatening cases. The clinical findings in 2222 serotonergic drug self-poisonings in humans included neuromuscular signs such as hyperreflexia, inducible clonus, myoclonus, ocular clonus, spontaneous clonus, peripheral hypertonicity, and shivering.[10] Autonomic manifestations included tachycardia, mydriasis, diaphoresis, increased bowel sounds, and diarrhea.[10] The mental status abnormalities included agitation and delirium.[10] In severe cases of serotonin syndrome, cardiac arrhythmias, disseminated intravascular coagulation, respiratory compromise, and rhabdomyolysis causing pigment nephropathy may occur.[8]

Clinical signs associated with accidental ingestion of antidepressant medication in companion animals mirror those seen in humans with serotonin syndrome. In a retrospective study of 456 companion animal cases of TCA ingestion that were reported to the Animal Poison Control Center, hyperexcitability and vomiting were the most common initial signs, followed by ataxia, lethargy, and muscle tremors.[11] Bradycardia and other cardiac arrhythmias were seen during the late stages of toxicity secondary to the disruption of the sodium-potassium pump by TCAs.[11] Of the cases reported to the Animal Poison Control Center, death occurred in more than 7% of the animals that displayed adverse signs.[11]

Similar signs in dogs have been reported in several retrospective studies describing serotonin toxicosis and serotonin-reuptake inhibitor toxicosis.[6-8] The first study reported on 21 dogs with serotonin toxicosis secondary to 5-hydroxytryptophan ingestion.[6] Tryptophan can be found in an over-the-counter dietary supplement and is converted rapidly to serotonin after absorption from the GI tract. Clinical signs developed within 10 minutes to 4 hours after ingestion in 19 of the 21 dogs.[6] Again, neurologic and GI signs were seen most commonly. The neurologic signs consisted of mydriasis, transient blindness, depression, disorientation, hyperesthesia, hyperreflexia, tremors, ataxia, paresis, seizures, and coma.[6] The GI signs consisted of vomiting, diarrhea, abdominal pain, ptyalism, flatulence, and bloat.[6] Seven dogs developed hyperthermia (103.7° to 108° F rectally) and death occurred in three dogs.[6] In two more recent retrospective studies of serotonin reuptake inhibitor toxicosis in 189 dogs[7] and 313 dogs[8] similar clinical signs were reported, including lethargy, neurologic signs (mydriasis, restlessness, agitation, hyperactivity, ataxia, somnolence, tremors, disorientation), gastrointestinal tract signs,

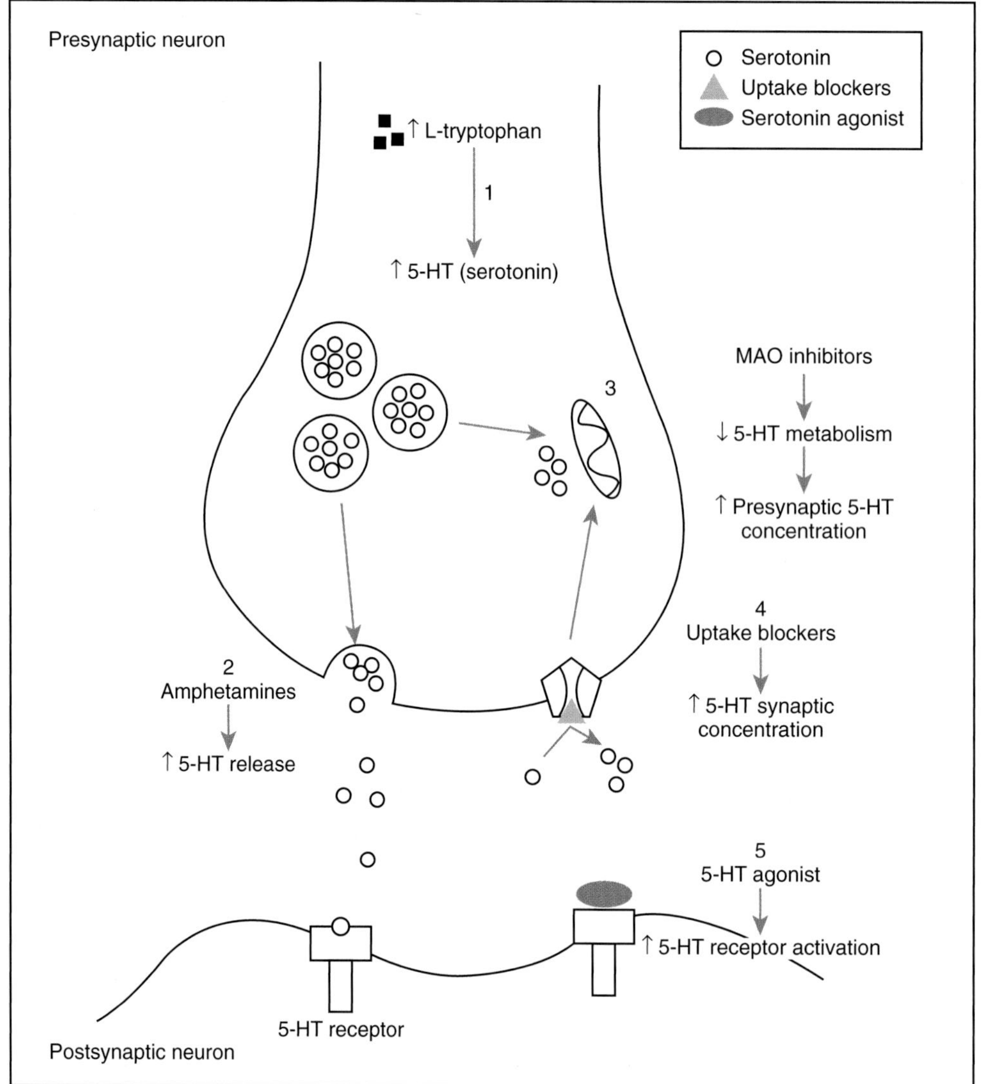

FIGURE 79-1 Mechanisms of serotonin syndrome. (1) Increased L-tryptophan increases serotonin. (2) Amphetamines and other drugs increase the release of stored serotonin. (3) Inhibition of serotonin metabolism by monoamine oxidase inhibitors (MAOIs) increases presynaptic serotonin concentrations. (4) Impairment of serotonin transport into presynaptic neurons by uptake blockers (i.e., SSRI, TCA) increases synaptic serotonin concentration. (5) Direct serotonin agonists can stimulate postsynaptic serotonin receptors. *5-HT,* Serotonin; *MAO,* monoamine oxidase.

cardiovascular signs (tachycardia), respiratory signs, and hyperthermia. The majority of the animals in the study of 313 dogs were reported to have no clinical signs (239 out of 313, or 76.3%) as a result of the SSRI ingestion; however, it is unclear how many of these dogs received decontamination procedures. The animals with follow-up information demonstrated a 100% survival rate.[8]

Although much less common compared with ingestion in dogs, ingestion of serotonergic medications can also occur in cats. In a 2013 retrospective study of 33 cats with SSRI toxicosis, the majority of cats were also asymptomatic for the ingestion, with only 8 cats developing clinical signs (8/33; 24%). The most common clinical signs were sedation and gastrointestinal signs, although central nervous system signs, cardiovascular signs, and hyperthermia were seen in 1 cat. Of the ingested medications, venlafaxine caused clinical signs more often than other medications. All symptomatic cats had resolution of clinical signs and survived to discharge.[11a]

TOXICITY

SSRIs, TCA inhibitors, and MAOIs are absorbed rapidly from the GI tract after oral ingestion. TCAs have a narrow margin of safety with a therapeutic dosage generally falling in the range of 2 to 4 mg/kg and a toxic dose of 15 mg/kg.[13,14] MAOIs are also considered extremely toxic; however, the lethal dose in dogs and cats has yet to be published. In humans, an MAOI dose of only 2 mg/kg is considered extremely toxic.[1] On the other hand, SSRIs are considered relatively safe, with the minimum lethal dose reported to be greater than 100 mg/kg in dogs and 50 mg/kg in cats.[12] However, clinical signs consistent with serotonin toxicosis have been observed in dogs at doses ranging from 0.3 to 50 mg/kg[7,8,15] with lower doses (1 to 3 mg/kg) associated with mild clinical signs such as lethargy and salivation, moderate doses (8 to 10 mg/kg) associated with more severe signs such as tremors and lethargy, and very high doses (>25 mg/kg) associated with seizures.[7] This dose-dependent response may not be seen with all types of SSRIs, and lower doses of certain medications (i.e., paroxetine) may be associated with more severe clinical signs.[8]

DIAGNOSIS AND TREATMENT

The diagnosis of serotonin syndrome typically is based on the history of ingestion of serotonergic drugs and compatible clinical signs. In an animal with no known history of ingestion, urine, blood, and

BOX 79-1 *Serotonergic Medications*

Increase in Serotonin Production

L-tryptophan
1-5-Hydroxytryptophan

Inhibition of Metabolism of Serotonin

MAO inhibitors: tranylcypromine
MAO-A inhibitors: moclobemide
MAO-B inhibitors: selegiline, clorgyline

Serotonin-Releasing Agents

Amphetamines
MDMA (Ecstasy)
Cocaine

Serotonin Reuptake Inhibitors

SSRIs: fluoxetine, citalopram, paroxetine, sertraline, venlafaxine
Tramadol, fentanyl, pethidine, methadone, meperidine
Dextromethorphan
TCAs: amitriptyline, clomipramine, doxepin, imipramine, mirtazipine, trazodone

Stimulation of Serotonin Receptors

LSD
Lithium
Buspirone
Sumatriptan

LSD, Lysergic acid diethylamide; *MAO,* monoamine oxidase; *MDMA,* 3,4-methylenedioxymethamphetamine; *SSRIs,* selective serotonin reuptake inhibitors; *TCAs,* tricyclic antidepressants.

gastric contents can be submitted to a toxicology laboratory for drug screening.

Any animal with a suspected overdose of serotonergic medication should undergo prompt decontamination (see Chapter 74). Emesis or gastric lavage should be performed in a clinically normal animal within 15 minutes of ingestion. This should be followed by administration of activated charcoal to further minimize drug absorption. Repeated doses of activated charcoal every 6 hours are necessary with TCAs or other medications that undergo enterohepatic recirculation.[13] A cathartic, such as sorbitol, could be administered concurrently with the first dose of activated charcoal. However, magnesium-containing cathartics should be avoided in animals that have ingested TCAs because of decreased GI motility, which may lead to toxic blood levels of magnesium.[13] Gastric lavage and administration of activated charcoal should not be performed in animals with severe clinical signs because of the risk of aspiration pneumonia.

In animals with clinical signs of toxicosis, emergency treatment should be aimed at assessing airway patency, breathing, and circulatory and neurologic status (see Chapter 1).[5] Life-threatening problems that can occur from serotonergic medication overdose include seizures, hyperthermia, and autonomic instability (tachycardia, bradycardia, hypertension, and hypotension). The intensity of therapy employed depends on the amount of drug ingested and severity of clinical signs. For example, in animals with mild neurologic and GI tract signs, supportive therapy should include intravenous fluids to correct and maintain hydration in addition to controlling GI tract signs. Diuresis does not enhance excretion because these drugs are highly protein bound.

Animals with neurologic signs, such as agitation, tremors, and seizures, should be treated with intravenous diazepam (Valium) at 0.25 to 1 mg/kg as a bolus or 0.25 to 1 mg/kg/hr as a constant rate infusion (CRI).[16] If seizures cannot be controlled with diazepam, phenobarbital should be administered at 2 to 20 mg/kg IV[17] (see Chapters 164 and 166). Hyperthermic animals should receive active and passive cooling measures. Antipyretic agents are not indicated because hyperthermia is a result of excessive muscular activity.[4] In severe, refractory cases, general anesthesia with or without neuromuscular paralysis and mechanical ventilation should be considered (see Chapters 30 and 143).[4,5]

Animals should be monitored closely for autonomic instability with continuous electrocardiographic and blood pressure monitoring (either direct or indirect). Hypotension should be managed with direct-acting sympathomimetics (such as norepinephrine, phenylephrine, or epinephrine; see Chapter 157). Indirect agents, such as dopamine, have to be metabolized to epinephrine and norepinephrine.[4] In many overdose patients, such as occurs with TCAs, catecholamine depletion occurs and renders dopamine ineffective. On the other hand, tachycardia and hypertension may occur in MAOI overdose because of excessive concentrations of epinephrine and norepinephrine.[4] These animals should be treated with either a short-acting β-blocker such as esmolol (200 to 500 mcg/kg IV followed by a CRI at 25 to 200 mcg/kg/min) or nitroprusside (0.5 to 3 mcg/kg/min) (see Chapters 171 and 159).[4,18,19]

Serotonin receptor antagonists, such as cyproheptadine and chlorpromazine, may have utility in the management of serotonin syndrome. Cyproheptadine, a nonspecific 5-HT_{1A} and 5-HT_2 receptor antagonist, has been shown to prevent the onset of clinical signs in animal models of serotonin syndrome.[20,21] However, evidence for its usefulness in human cases of serotonin syndrome is limited primarily to case reports, and its efficacy has not been established fully.[2,20] Cyproheptadine is available only in oral formulations and is well absorbed. It may be administered at dosages of 1.1 mg/kg in dogs or 2 to 4 mg in cats PO q 4-6h.[6,7,22,23] When oral dosing is not possible or if there has been a recent administration of activated charcoal, cyproheptadine may be crushed and administered rectally.[7,21]

Chlorpromazine is also a 5-HT_2 receptor antagonist and may be used as an antidote in animals with serotonergic medication overdose (0.2 to 0.5 mg/kg IV, IM, or SC q6h).[24] The main side effects of this medication are sedation and hypotension. Therefore close blood pressure monitoring is indicated before and after administration. A study performed to evaluate the effects of serotonin receptor antagonists in a rat model of serotonin syndrome concluded that cyproheptadine (10 mg/kg) was more effective than chlorpromazine (20 to 40 mg/kg).[24] Nevertheless, both drugs prevented death at the higher dosages.[25] Other serotonin receptor antagonists investigated in animal models include ritanserin, pipamperone, risperidone, and ketanserin.[25,26]

Finally, intravenous lipid emulsion (ILE) recently has been described in several case reports for treatment of human patients with serotonin syndrome secondary to TCA and SSRI overdoses.[27,28] Several reports in the veterinary literature have been published on the successful and safe use of ILE for treatment of moxidectin, ivermectin, lidocaine, and permethrin toxicosis in dogs and cats, although its use in animals with serotonergic medication toxicosis has not been reported (see Chapter 174).[29-32] ILE is composed of neutral medium- to long-chain triglycerides derived from a combination of plant oils and has been used historically as a source of essential fatty acids for patients requiring parenteral nutrition.[33] The effectiveness of lipid therapy results in part from the rapid formation of an expanded lipid compartment, or "lipid sink," within the intravascular space that draws tissue-bound drug off cellular receptor sites and into the plasma, where it becomes trapped in the transiently expanded lipid phase.[34-36] At this time, this unproven therapy should be considered only in animals with severe clinical signs that do not respond to standard initial treatment measures until more evidence for its use in treatment of patients with serotonin syndrome is available. If used, a sterile peripheral or central intravenous catheter should be placed and a bolus of 1.5 ml/kg of 20% Liposyn should be administered over 10 minutes followed by 0.25 ml/kg/hr of 20% Liposyn infused over 1 hour.[35] The infusion may be repeated in cases that have recurrent clinical signs and no evidence of ongoing lipemia. No adverse effects have been reported from the use of ILE in animals other than transient lipemia. However, potential adverse effects to lipid infusion reported in people include acute allergic reactions, fat embolism, thrombocytopenia, prolonged clotting times, sepsis, neurologic signs, and thrombophlebitis.[37,38]

PROGNOSIS

The prognosis for animals with serotonin syndrome is variable depending on the quantity ingested, clinical signs, treatment, and concurrent administration of other highly protein-bound medications.[16] Animals with minimal signs generally have a good prognosis, but animals with severe neurologic signs, hyperthermia, and GI signs have a more guarded prognosis.

REFERENCES

1. Brent J: Monoamine oxidase inhibitors and the serotonin syndrome. In Haddad LM, Shannon MW, Winchester JF, editors: Clinical management of poisoning and drug overdose, Philadelphia, 1998, Saunders.
2. Gillman PK: Monoamine oxidase inhibitors, opioid analgesics and serotonin toxicity, Br J Anaesth 95:434, 2005.
3. Guyton AC, Hall JE: Textbook of medical physiology, ed 11, Philadelphia, 2006, Saunders.
4. Boyer EW, Shannon M: The serotonin syndrome, N Engl J Med 352:1112, 2005.
5. Isibister GK, Buckley NA: The pathophysiology of serotonin toxicity in animals and humans, Clin Neuropharmacol 28:205, 2005.
6. Gwaltney-Brant SM, Albretson JC, Khan SA: 5-Hydroxytryptophan toxicosis in dogs: 21 cases (1989-1999), J Am Vet Med Assoc 216:1937, 2000.
7. Mohammed-Zadeh LF, Moses L, Gwaltney-Brant SM: Serotonin: a review, J Vet Pharmacol Therap 31:187-199, 2008.
8. Thomas DE, Lee JA, Hovda LR: Retrospective evaluation of toxicosis from selective serotonin reuptake inhibitor antidepressants: 313 dogs (2005-2010), J Vet Emerg Crit Care 22(6):674-681, 2012.
9. Ganong WF: Review of medical physiology, ed 21, New York, 2003, McGraw Hill Companies.
10. Ener RA, Meglathery SB, Van Decker WA, et al: Serotonin syndrome and other serotonergic disorders, Pain Med 4:63, 2003.
11. Shioda K, Nisijima K, Yoshino T, et al: Extracellular serotonin, dopamine and glutamate levels are elevated in the hypothalamus in a serotonin syndrome animal model induced by tranylcypromine and fluoxetine, Neuropsychopharmacology 28:633, 2004.

11a. Pugh CM, Sweeney JT, Block CP, et al: Selective serotonin reuptake inhibitor (SSRI) toxicosis in cats: 33 cases (2004-2010), J Vet Emerg Crit Care 23(5):565-570, 2013.

12. Dunkley EJC, Isbister GK, Sibbritt D, et al: The Hunter serotonin toxicity criteria: simple and accurate diagnostic decision rules for serotonin toxicity, Q J Med 96:635, 2003.
13. Johnson LR: Tricyclic antidepressant toxicosis, Vet Clin North Am Small Anim Pract 20:393, 1990.
14. Stark P, Fuller RW, Wong DT: The pharmacologic profile of fluoxetine, J Clin Psychiatry 46(3):7-13, 1985.
15. Koe BK, Weissman A, Welch WM, et al: Sertraline, IS, 4S-N-methyl-4-(3,4-dichlorophenyl)-1,2,3,4-tetrahydro-1-naphthylamine, a new uptake inhibitor with selectivity for serotonin, J Pharmacol Exp Ther 226:686, 1983.
16. Plumb DC: Diazepam. In Plumb's Veterinary drug handbook, Stockholm, Wis, 2005, Pharma Vet.
17. Plumb DC: Phenobarbital. In Plumb's veterinary drug handbook, Stockholm, Wis, 2005, Pharma Vet.
18. Plumb DC: Esmolol. In Plumb's veterinary drug handbook, Stockholm, Wis, 2005, Pharma Vet.
19. Plumb DC: Sodium nitroprusside. In Plumb's veterinary drug handbook, Ames, Stockholm, Wis, 2005, Pharma Vet.
20. Graudins A, Stearman A, Chan B: Treatment of serotonin syndrome with cyproheptadine, J Emerg Med 16:615, 1998.
21. Mills KC: Serotonin syndrome: a clinical update, Crit Care Clin 13:763, 1997.
22. Wismer TA: Antidepressant drug overdose in dogs, Vet Med 95:520, 2000.
23. Plumb DC: Cyproheptadine. In Plumb DC: Veterinary drug handbook, Ames, Iowa, 2002, Iowa State University Press.
24. Plumb DC: Chlorpromazine. In Plumb DC: Veterinary drug handbook, Ames, Iowa, 2002, Iowa State University Press.
25. Nisijima K, Yoshino T, Yui K, et al: Potent serotonin (5-HT)2A receptor antagonists completely prevent the development of hyperthermia in an animal model of the 5-HT syndrome, Brain Res 899:23, 2001.
26. Nisijima K, Shioda K, Yoshino T, et al: Memantine, an NMDA antagonist, prevents the development of hyperthermia in an animal model for serotonin syndrome, Pharmacopsychiatry 37:57, 2004.
27. Dagtekin O, Markus H. Muller C, et al: Lipid therapy for serotonin syndrome after intoxication with vanlafaxin, lamotrigine and diazepam, Minerva Anesthesiol 77:93-95, 2011.
28. Castaneres-Zapatero D, Wittebole X, Huberlant V, et al: Lipid emulsion as a rescue therapy in lamotrigine overdose, J Emerg Med 42(1):4851, 2011.
29. Crandell DE, Weinberg GL: Moxidectin toxicosis in a puppy successfully treated with intravenous lipids, J Vet Emerg Crit Care 19:181-186, 2009.
30. O'Brien TQ, Clark-Price SC, Evans EE, et al: Infusion of a lipid emulsion to treat lidocaine intoxication in a cat, J Am Vet Med Assoc 237(12):1455-1458, 2010.
31. Clarke DC, Lee JA, Murphy L, et al: Use of an intravenous lipid emulsion to treat ivermectin toxicosis in a Border Collie, J Am Vet Med Assoc 239(10):1328-1333, 2011.
32. Haworth MD, Smart L: Use of intravenous lipid emulsion therapy in three cases of feline permethrin toxicosis, J Vet Emerg Crit Care 22(6):697-702, 2012.
33. Krieglstein J, Meffert A, Neimeyer DH: Influence of emulsified fat on chlorpromazine availability in rabbit blood, Experientia 30:924-926, 1974.
34. Weinberg G, Ripper R, Feinsetin DL, et al: Lipid emulsion infusion rescues dogs from bupivacaine-induced cardiac toxicity, Reg Anesth Pain Med 28:198-202, 2003.
35. Weinberg G: Lipid rescue resuscitation from local anesthetic toxicity, Toxicol Rev 25:139-45, 2006.
36. Weinberg GL, Di Gregorio G, Ripper R, et al: Resuscitation with lipid versus epinephrine in a rate model of bupivacaine overdose, Anesthesiology 108:907-13, 2008.
37. Driscoll DF: Lipid injectable emulsions: pharmacopeial and safety issues, Pharm Res 23:1959-1969, 2006.
38. Geyer RP: Parenteral nutrition, Physiol Rev 40:150-186, 1960.

PART IX NEUROLOGIC DISORDERS

CHAPTER 80
DETERIORATING MENTAL STATUS

Marguerite F. Knipe, DVM, DACVIM (Neurology)

KEY POINTS

- Consciousness is maintained by the cerebral cortex and the brainstem's reticular activating system.
- Abnormalities in mentation may be seen with metabolic disease, drug administration or toxicity, and structural brain disease.
- Metabolic disease, drugs, or toxins usually cause signs of diffuse or bilateral brain dysfunction.
- Structural disease or injuries typically result in lateralized brainstem or lateralized cerebrothalamic signs.
- Five patient evaluation parameters that aid in lesion localization and prognosis for recovery include (1) level of consciousness, (2) motor activity, (3) respiratory patterns, (4) pupil size and reactivity, and (5) oculocephalic reflex.
- Frequent reassessment of the patient with deteriorating mental status permits detection of changes that may require intervention.

Altered mentation in patients, whether rapidly or slowly progressive, is of particular concern to the clinician in the intensive care unit (ICU). It is seen with primary neurologic disease, neurologic complications of other diseases, many systemic diseases, and some drugs.[1] A decline in mental status is characterized by decreasing responsiveness and interaction with the environment, although agitation and hyperreactivity also can indicate neurologic dysfunction. Rapid neurologic assessment of the declining patient, coupled with knowledge of underlying disease and medication, permits the formulation of a list of possible causes and diagnostic and therapeutic plans, as well as an estimation of prognosis.

STATES OF CONSCIOUSNESS

Normal

The animal has a normal demeanor and interaction with its environment. "Normal" varies among animals, and the clinician relies on the client's knowledge of the pet's behavior, as well as the initial neurologic evaluation. For example, docile behavior in a cat, which most clinicians would consider desirable, may be abnormal if the owner reports the cat is typically fearful and aggressive.

Obtunded

Obtundation is a state of decreased responsiveness or alertness and is graded as mild, moderate, or severe. Lethargy is similar, reflecting decreased level of consciousness with listlessness and drowsiness. Other terms commonly used to describe altered mentation in humans, such as confusion, delirium, and dementia, are difficult to extrapolate to veterinary medicine because these states are characterized by disorientation to time and place, loss of memory, and disorganized speech, which are difficult to impossible to evaluate in the veterinary patient.[2,3]

Stupor or Semicoma

The patient responds only to vigorous or painful stimuli.

Coma

The patient does not respond consciously to any stimuli. Segmental spinal reflexes are present (in the absence of additional lesions) and possibly exaggerated, and cranial nerve reflexes may be present, depending on the location of the lesion causing the coma.[3,4]

NEUROANATOMY

Abnormalities in mentation indicate either dysfunction of the reticular activating system in the brainstem or dysfunction of the cerebrum.

Cerebrum

The cerebrum is the region of the brain responsible for the integration of sensory information from the entire body, planning of motor activity, and appropriate responses to this information, emotion, and memory. Functionally distinct regions are present in the cerebral cortex (e.g., occipital lobe associated with vision; temporal lobe associated with auditory function).[5]

Reticular Activating System

The ascending reticular activating system (RAS), or reticular formation, is a network of anatomically and physiologically distinct nuclei in the brainstem that function to "activate" the cerebral cortex and maintain consciousness.[6] Experimentally, stimulation of the RAS in anesthetized cats produced electroencephalogram patterns consistent with the conscious state.[7]

Numerous nuclei in the reticular activating system have projections to the cerebrum, but those in the midbrain, rostral pons, and thalamus are the most important for maintaining consciousness.[2,8] In anesthetized cats, transection of the brainstem at the level of the pons and midbrain produced coma, but transection at the junction of the medulla and cervical spinal cord did not.[9]

ETIOLOGY OF LESIONS

Lesions causing changes in mentation are structural, metabolic, or toxic in origin. Clinical signs of diffuse cerebral disease with normal

BOX 80-1 *Common Metabolic Diseases That May Cause Altered Mentation*[2,6]

- Hypoxia (anemia, pulmonary disease, methemoglobinemia)
- Ischemia (cardiac disease, post-arrest, hyperviscosity, systemic embolic disease)
- Hypoglycemia
- Hepatic disease (hepatic encephalopathy)
- Renal failure (uremic encephalopathy)
- Endocrine dysfunction (hyperfunction or hypofunction)
    - Pituitary (apoplexy)
    - Thyroid
    - Adrenal (hypoadrenocorticism, pheochromocytoma)
    - Pancreas (diabetes mellitus, especially hyperosmolar)
- Sepsis
- Hyperbilirubinemia (kernicterus)
- Hyperthermia or hypothermia
- Pain
- Central nervous system diseases
    - Continuous seizure activity
    - Postictal state
    - Diffuse meningitis or encephalitis
- Electrolyte or acid-base abnormalities
    - Sodium or water
    - Magnesium
    - Calcium
    - Acidosis (metabolic or respiratory)
    - Alkalosis (metabolic or respiratory)

BOX 80-2 *Common Drugs That May Cause Altered Mentation*[1,2,10]

- Anticonvulsants (barbiturates, bromides)
- Benzodiazepines
- Opiates
- Anesthetic drugs
- Atropine
- Antibiotics (penicillin, cephalosporins, quinolones, aminoglycosides, metronidazole)
- Steroids
- Histamine-2 receptor blockers
- Cardiac glycosides (digitalis)
- Antihypertensives (hydralazine, ACE inhibitors)
- Illicit substances (cannabis, cocaine, amphetamines)

ACE, Angiotensin-converting enzyme.

brainstem function are most common with metabolic disease, toxins, or drugs affecting the cerebrum globally (Boxes 80-1 and 80-2). Seizures indicate cerebral cortical dysfunction caused by either extracranial or intracranial disease (see Chapter 82). Impairment of the brainstem or thalamus, as well as lateralized cerebral dysfunction (e.g., compulsive circling in one direction, unilateral cortical blindness), is more likely the result of structural disease or injury (Box 80-3).

EVALUATION

Basic neurologic evaluation of the patient with altered mentation includes assessment of five physiologic variables: (1) level of consciousness or mentation, (2) motor activity, (3) respiratory patterns, (4) pupil size and reactivity, and (5) oculocephalic movements.[2] Coma scales are based on information obtained from these assessments (see Chapter 81), and knowledge of the pathophysiology

BOX 80-3 *Structural Lesions That May Alter Mentation*

- Neoplasia (primary, secondary)
- Infection (e.g., bacterial, fungal, protozoal, viral)
- Inflammation, noninfectious
    - Granulomatous meningoencephalomyelitis
    - Necrotizing encephalitis
    - Necrotizing meningoencephalitis
- Trauma (hemorrhage, edema)
- Vascular lesions (infarction, hemorrhage)
- Hydrocephalus, especially if resulting from acute obstruction of cerebrospinal fluid
- Shifts of intracranial structures (herniation), secondary to any of the above

affecting these variables aids in lesion localization and determining progression of disease.

Level of Consciousness

As discussed previously, mentation abnormalities result from structural or metabolic disease affecting the cerebrum or reticular activating system or both. Grading of mentation from normal to comatose and any details specific to the individual patient should be described (e.g., readily opens eyes when name is called).

Motor Activity

The patient may be ambulatory or nonambulatory and may have generalized ataxia, hemiparesis, tetraparesis, or hemiplegia. Obvious gait abnormalities with paresis or paralysis are more indicative of a lesion at, or caudal to, the midbrain, and deficits are ipsilateral to the lesion. Patients with mild or moderate lesions rostral to the midbrain often have minimal gait abnormalities or paresis, although contralateral proprioceptive reactions are absent.[4]

Decerebrate and decerebellate postures are associated with lesions in specific brain regions. Decerebrate rigidity is seen with lesions of the rostral pons and midbrain. Opisthotonus with extensor rigidity of all four limbs is present, and mentation is stuporous to comatose. Decerebellate rigidity may occur with acute cerebellar lesions. Opisthotonus with extensor rigidity of the thoracic limbs and either extension or flexion of the pelvic limbs is present, depending on the location of the cerebellar lesion; the patient should be responsive and have voluntary movement, unless additional lesions are present.[3,4]

Respiratory Patterns

Some respiratory patterns are associated with lesions in certain areas of the brain (Box 80-4). Animals with brainstem lesions causing respiratory changes have a guarded to poor prognosis.[4] Abnormal respiratory patterns may include apneustic, Cheyne-Stokes, and ataxic patterns. Other diseases must be considered in patients with abnormal ventilation. Hyperventilation can be seen with diabetic ketoacidosis, uremia, hepatic failure, sepsis, and pneumonia. Hypoventilation may result from administration of sedative drugs (especially opiates), generalized neuromuscular disease, and pulmonary disease.[2]

Pupil Size and Reactivity

Pupil size is the result of balance between sympathetic and parasympathetic innervation to the eye. Parasympathetic innervation is particularly important when evaluating for neurologic deterioration because it is mediated through the midbrain and cranial nerve III (loss of parasympathetic innervation results in mydriasis).[4] Most abnormalities of pupil size and pupillary light reflexes are the result

BOX 80-4 *Respiratory Patterns Associated with Intracranial Lesions*[1,2,6]

Cheyne-Stokes breathing: Periods of hyperpnea alternating with periods of apnea; can be seen with diffuse cerebral or thalamic disease and metabolic encephalopathies
Central neurogenic hyperventilation: Persistent hyperventilation that may result in respiratory alkalosis; associated with midbrain lesions
Apneusis: Breathing pauses for a period at full inspiration; associated with pontine lesions
Irregular or "ataxic" breathing: Irregular frequency and depth of respiration that typically precedes complete apnea; associated with lesions of lower pons and medulla

BOX 80-5 *Pupillary Abnormalities and Lesion Localization*[1,4]

Unilateral mydriatic, unresponsive pupil: Loss of parasympathetic innervation to the eye; indicates destruction or compression of the ipsilateral midbrain or cranial nerve III, often associated with increased intracranial pressure and unilateral cerebral herniation; rule out unilateral topical ophthalmic atropine or tropicamide
Bilateral miosis: Can be seen with metabolic encephalopathies or diffuse midbrain compression with increased intracranial pressure and may precede mydriatic, unresponsive pupils
Bilateral, mydriatic, unresponsive pupils: Fixed and dilated pupils; severe, bilateral compression or destruction of the midbrain or cranial nerve III, typically from bilateral cerebral herniation; grave prognosis

of structural lesions of the brain,[6] but metabolic encephalopathies and some drugs (benzodiazepines, opiates) can cause bilateral miosis, whereas parasympatholytic agents (atropine) may cause mydriasis[1,4] (Box 80-5).

Oculocephalic Reflex

Physiologic nystagmus, or "doll's eye" reflex, consists of conjugate eye movements in response to vestibular input (turning the head from side to side). Loss of the oculocephalic reflex occurs with lesions of the medial longitudinal fasciculus in the pons and midbrain, which coordinates functions of cranial nerves III, IV, and VI innervating the extraocular eye muscles, and usually indicates a poor prognosis.[4] Lesions of the individual nuclei or cranial nerves III, IV, or VI also result in an abnormal oculocephalic reflex, but a persistent, nonpositional strabismus is present in the affected eye.[3] Extreme caution should be taken when manipulating the heads of patients with a history of trauma, until cervical fractures or luxations have been ruled out.

DIAGNOSTIC APPROACH

In all patients with abnormal mentation, the clinician initially should assess systemic and metabolic stability. When patients arrive in the ICU acutely ill, physical examination and historical information such as drug exposure, previous or ongoing illness, and possible trauma are invaluable to determining the cause of mentation abnormalities. Routine blood work evaluates acid-base status, electrolyte values, hematocrit, and liver and kidney function. Additional tests or blood work should be done based on suspicion of underlying disease. Once systemic disease is ruled out and a lesion is localized to the brain, specific neurodiagnostic tests, particularly intracranial imaging with magnetic resonance imaging or computed tomography, and cerebrospinal fluid analysis should be pursued as indicated.

For patients in the ICU with nonneurologic disease that experience a deterioration in mentation, the status of their underlying disease and metabolic state must be reassessed for any recent changes. If no changes have occurred, then neurologic complications of the primary disease should be considered (e.g., vascular event such as ischemia or hemorrhage).

For patients in the ICU with known structural brain disease, the most life-threatening cause for a decline in mentation is increased intracranial pressure and herniation of brain structures. Infarction or hemorrhage secondary to the underlying brain lesion is also possible.

TREATMENT

Because so many systemic and neurologic diseases can cause abnormal mentation, treatment is based on the underlying cause. If toxin exposure or drug reaction is suspected, supportive care and withdrawal of medication is indicated. The patient's metabolic parameters should be maintained within normal ranges, and in patients with brain disease and suspected increased intracranial pressure, aggressive medical therapy should be instituted (see Chapters 84 and 191). Most importantly, vigilant and repeated assessment of the patient with altered mental status by the ICU clinicians and staff permits early detection of changes so that appropriate diagnostic and therapeutic intervention can be implemented.

REFERENCES

1. Haymore J: A Neuron in a haystack: advanced neurologic assessment, AACN Clin Issues 15:568, 2004.
2. Plum F, Posner JB: The diagnosis of stupor and coma, ed 3, Philadelphia, 1980, FA Davis.
3. Lorenz MD, Kornegay JN: Handbook of veterinary neurology, ed 4, St Louis, 2004, Saunders.
4. DeLahunta A: Veterinary neuroanatomy and clinical neurology, ed 2, St Louis, 1983, Saunders.
5. Saper C, Iversen S, Frackowiak R: Integration of sensory and motor function: the association areas of the cerebral cortex and the cognitive capabilities of the brain. In Kandel E, Schwartz JH, Jessel TM, editors: Principles of neural science, ed 4, New York, 2000, McGraw-Hill.
6. Saper C: Brain stem modulation of sensation, movement, and consciousness. In Kandel E, Schwartz JH, Jessel TM, editors: Principles of neural science, ed 4, New York, 2000, McGraw-Hill.
7. Moruzzi G, Magoun HW: Brain stem reticular formation and activation of the EEG, Electroencephalogr Clin Neurophysiol 1:455, 1949.
8. Parvizi J, Damasio A: Neuroanatomical correlates of brainstem coma, Brain 126:1524, 2003.
9. Bremer F: Cerveau "isole" et physiologie du sommeil, C R Soc Biol 118:1235, 1935.
10. Small S, Mayeux R: Delirium and dementia. In Rowland L, editor: Merritt's neurology, ed 11, Philadelphia, 2005, Lippincott Williams & Wilkins.

CHAPTER 81

COMA SCALES

Simon R. Platt, BVM&S, MRCVS, DACVIM (Neurology), DECVN

KEY POINTS

- Coma can result from many causes affecting the intracranial nervous system.
- Severe head trauma is a common cause of coma in veterinary medicine, and victims commonly have a poor prognosis.
- The prognosis for a patient with head trauma depends on the severity of the neurologic injury at the time of hospital admission.
- Neurologic injury can be categorized numerically based on the abnormalities detected on examination.
- The numeric scoring system developed for animals with head injury is the modified Glasgow Coma Scale.
- The scoring system is based on specific abnormalities of mentation, motor function, and neuroophthalmologic examination.

Although coma can be caused by an array of direct and indirect neurologic disorders affecting the intracranial structures in small animals, the development of coma scales has focused on dogs and cats with head trauma.

An ideal coma scale would be reliable (measures what it is supposed to measure), valid (yields the same results with repeated testing), linear (gives all components equal weight), and easy to use. In addition, these scales may predict outcome, although mortality rates in veterinary medicine are confounded by euthanasia. These scales can be used objectively to decide when to initiate aggressive treatment, to monitor the success of therapy and, in some cases, provide a prognosis. Such scoring systems are still in their infancy in veterinary medicine and are meant to be only a guide to management. They can be used to monitor patients with any cause of coma based on this premise. This chapter is focused on coma scales as they specifically relate to head trauma.

Appropriate therapy for patients with head trauma remains controversial in veterinary medicine (see Chapter 137). Treatment must be immediate if the animal is to recover to a level that is functional and acceptable to the owner. Therefore clinicians must be aware of the optimal way to assess these patients; many dogs and cats can recover from severe brain injuries if the clinician is able to identify treatable systemic and neurologic abnormalities in a timely manner.

Intracranial Pressure After Head Trauma

Increases in intracranial pressure (ICP) are often responsible for the clinical decline seen in many animals that sustain head trauma.[1] After traumatic brain injury, the volume of the brain tissue compartment increases, usually a result of edema or hemorrhage. As this tissue compartment increases, the cerebrospinal fluid (CSF) and blood compartments must decrease in a compensatory manner to prevent an increase in ICP. Compensation for increased brain tissue volume initially involves shifting of cerebrospinal fluid out of the skull, decreased production of CSF, and eventually decreased cerebral blood flow.[2] These compensatory mechanisms prevent increases in ICP for an undetermined period. In general, the compensation is more effective when the increases in ICP are slow. Once the capacity for compensation is exhausted, a further small increase in intracranial volume results in dramatic elevations of ICP, with an immediate onset of clinical signs.[2] Unfortunately, the clinical signs of a significantly increased ICP often become evident too late in small animals for any therapy to be effective. A clear understanding of what clinical signs necessitate immediate intervention, those that indicate a grave prognosis, and those that need to be monitored closely helps with the successful treatment of patients after head trauma.

NEUROLOGIC ASSESSMENT

Initial neurologic assessment should include an evaluation of the patient's state of consciousness, breathing pattern, size and responsiveness of pupils, ocular position and movements, and least of all, appendicular motor responses. Motor dysfunction rarely is associated with cerebral disease but may result from brainstem injury. A concurrent spinal cord should be considered during this evaluation. The neurologic evaluation should be repeated at least every 30 to 60 minutes in patients with severe head injuries to assess for deterioration and/or to monitor the effectiveness of therapy. This would require an objective mechanism to "score" the patient's condition so that treatment decisions could be made logically.

MODIFIED GLASGOW COMA SCORING SYSTEM

In humans, traumatic brain injury is graded as mild, moderate, or severe on the basis of the level of consciousness or the Glasgow Coma Scale.[3] Mild traumatic brain injury in humans usually is due to a concussion, and full neurologic recovery routinely occurs. A patient with moderate traumatic brain injury is lethargic or stuporous, and a patient with severe injury is comatose. Patients with severe traumatic brain injury have a high risk of hypotension, hypoxemia, and brain swelling.[3] If these sequelae are not prevented or managed properly, they can exacerbate the existing brain damage and increase the risk of death.[3] The clinical point at which to initiate therapy for a veterinary patient with head trauma, the extent of appropriate therapy, and the length of time that such treatment is necessary are documented poorly. The effectiveness of specific treatment and the prognosis for any given animal always is difficult to assess because of the multifactorial nature of the injury.

A modification of the Glasgow Coma Scale used in humans has been proposed for use in veterinary medicine.[4] This scoring system enables grading of the initial neurologic status and serial monitoring of the patient. Such a system can facilitate the assessment of prognosis, which is crucial information for the veterinarian and owner.[4] An almost linear correlation between this scoring system and the immediate or short-term survival of dogs with head trauma has been evaluated (Figure 81-1).[5] Long-term survival and functional outcome have not been evaluated using these scales in dogs or cats.

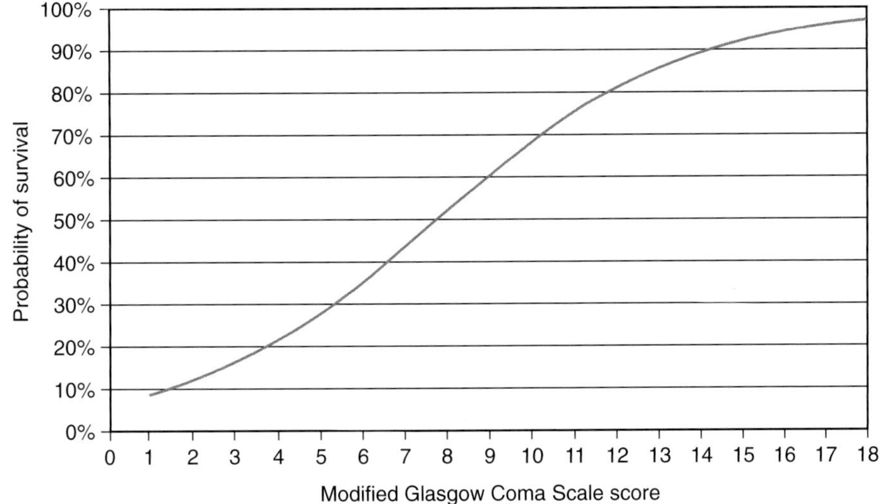

FIGURE 81-1 Probability of survival for patients with head trauma based on their individual modified Glasgow Coma Scale score at admission. *(Reprinted with permission from Platt SR, Radaelli ST, McDonnell JJ: The prognostic value of the modified Glasgow Coma Scale in head trauma in dogs, J Vet Intern Med 15:581, 2001.)*

Each of the three categories of the examination (i.e., level of consciousness, motor activity, brainstem reflexes) is assigned a score from 1 to 6 (Table 81-1). The level of consciousness provides information about the functional capabilities of the cerebral cortex and the ascending reticular activating system in the brainstem.[6]

Levels of Consciousness

The level of consciousness is the most reliable empiric measure of impaired cerebral function after head injury. Impairment of consciousness is stratified in terms of the responses to external stimuli, and serial records of these responses are an important clinical guide to treatment.

The level of consciousness is also a valuable index of injury severity. In the early evaluation, the depth of impairment can be used as a measure of cerebral dysfunction and therefore injury (assuming perfusion parameters are adequate). Levels of consciousness range from normal, depressed, or delirious to stuporous or comatose. Depression is a reduced state of mental function. A delirious animal manifests a reduced state of consciousness with profound disorientation. Stupor is partial or nearly complete unconsciousness, manifested by response only to vigorous or noxious stimulation. Coma is a state of unconsciousness from which the patient cannot be aroused.

Decreasing levels of consciousness indicate abnormal function of the cerebral cortex or interference with transmission of sensory stimuli by the brainstem ascending reticular activating system. Patients that arrive in a state of coma generally have bilateral or global cerebral abnormalities or severe brainstem injury and have a guarded prognosis.[7]

Limb Movements, Posture, and Reflexes

Spontaneous and evoked limb movements are studied as part of the coma scale examination.[5] The clinician must determine whether spinal cord injury or severe orthopedic abnormalities are present before extensive manipulation of the patient. Motor activity may be affected by the animal's level of consciousness; the best motor response the animal is capable of is the most important. Animals that are not comatose but have an altered state of consciousness usually maintain some voluntary motor activity.

Muscle tone is assessed by putting the limbs through a full range of passive movement, keeping in mind the possibility of a long bone

Table 81-1 Small Animal Modified Glasgow Coma Scale[5]

Assessment Parameter	Score
Motor Activity	
Normal gait, normal spinal reflexes	6
Hemiparesis, tetraparesis, or decerebrate activity	5
Recumbent, intermittent extensor rigidity	4
Recumbent, constant extensor rigidity	3
Recumbent, constant extensor rigidity with opisthotonus	2
Recumbent, hypotonia of muscles, depressed or absent spinal reflexes	1
Brainstem Reflexes	
Normal pupillary light reflexes and oculocephalic reflexes	6
Slow pupillary light reflexes and normal to reduced oculocephalic reflexes	5
Bilateral, unresponsive miosis with normal to reduced oculocephalic reflexes	4
Pinpoint pupils with reduced to absent oculocephalic reflexes	3
Unilateral, unresponsive mydriasis with reduced to absent oculocephalic reflexes	2
Bilateral, unresponsive mydriasis with reduced to absent oculocephalic reflexes	1
Level of Consciousness	
Occasional periods of alertness and responsiveness to environment	6
Depression or delirium, capable of responding but response may be inappropriate	5
Semicomatose, responsive to visual stimuli	4
Semicomatose, responsive to auditory stimuli	3
Semicomatose, responsive only to repeated noxious stimuli	2
Comatose, unresponsive to repeated noxious stimuli	1

A score is given to each of three categories of the neurologic examination: motor activity, brainstem reflexes, and level of consciousness. Within each category, a score of 1 to 6 exists, representing the most severe to the mildest of clinical pictures. A total score can then be helpful (1) in estimating the severity of the initial condition, which determines the most appropriate level of therapy, (2) assessing the prognosis for survival within the first 72 hours, and (3) assessing the effect of therapy.

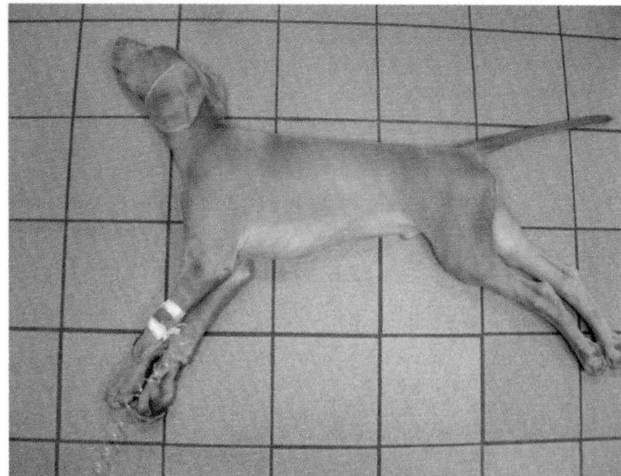

FIGURE 81-2 An 18-month-old male neutered Weimaraner exhibiting decerebrate rigidity after a head injury; note the hyperextension of all four limbs. The dog is unconscious when demonstrating this posture.

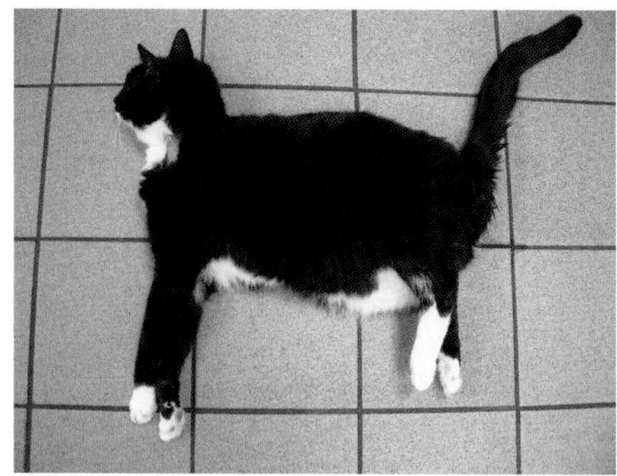

FIGURE 81-3 Decerebellate rigidity in a 6-year-old domestic shorthaired cat. Note the flexion in the pelvic limbs. The animal is conscious.

Table 81-2 **Anatomic Interpretation of Pupillary Abnormalities**

Injury	Ipsilateral Pupil	Associated Findings
Oculomotor nerve	Dilated and fixed to direct light No consensual constriction from contralateral light but normal consensual constriction in contralateral pupil	Ptosis and ventrolateral strabismus
Optic nerve	Fixed to direct light Absent consensual constriction in contralateral pupil Normal consensual constriction from contralateral light	Spontaneous fluctuations in pupil size
Oculomotor and optic nerve	Dilated and fixed to direct light No consensual constriction from contralateral light and no consensual constriction in contralateral pupil	Ptosis and ventrolateral strabismus
Iris or ciliary body	Dilated and fixed to direct light No consensual constriction from contralateral light but normal consensual constriction in contralateral pupil	Often signs of orbital injury No strabismus
Cervical sympathetic pathway	Constricted and fixed or sluggish to direct light and contralateral light but normal consensual constriction in contralateral pupil	Ptosis

fracture. The tendon reflexes are elicited; these reflexes have little value in the diagnosis of acute cerebral injuries, but localized absence of tendon jerks may disclose a peripheral nerve injury. Exaggerated reflexes are often present in all four limbs in most patients with cerebral injury (or cervical spinal cord trauma), but severely (terminally) affected comatose animals frequently lose muscle tone and reflex activity.

Opisthotonus with hyperextension of all four limbs is suggestive of decerebrate rigidity (Figure 81-2), whereas variable flexion and rigid extension of the hind limbs is seen in animals with cerebellar injury (Figure 81-3).[7,8] Decerebrate rigidity, occasionally seen in animals recumbent as a result of craniocerebral trauma, can provide further information about the severity of the brain injury.[4]

Neuroophthalmologic Examination

Pupils

This is the basis of the brainstem reflexes category. Pupil size, shape, and reactivity are recorded routinely during the initial examination and should be checked at frequent intervals thereafter. If the pupillary light reflex is impaired on one side, the contralateral light reflex is tested to see whether the impaired pupil reacts consensually. In the unconscious patient, changes in the pupillary light reflexes often provide diagnostic information regarding the cerebral injury and the animal's prognosis.[6] The pupillary light reflex also may be the only available test of optic nerve function (Table 81-2). It is necessary to use a strong light source and shield the opposite eye when testing for a consensual response.

Pupillary abnormalities may be bilateral or unilateral; they may be present from the time of the injury or may appear later. Mild size discrepancy between the two pupils (<3 mm) has not been associated significantly with patient outcome in humans.[9] Pupils that are dilated widely at the time of initial examination may indicate an irreparable primary midbrain (rostral brainstem) lesion or advanced herniation. However, other causes should be ruled out. These include the following: the early postictal period, inadequate cerebral perfusion,[10] local trauma to the iris or its innervation on both sides before administration of opioid (cats only) or anticholinergic therapy, or the use of a mydriatic agent to view the fundus. Previous ocular disease may be associated with bilateral or unilateral pupillary abnormalities. In humans, bilateral optic nerve injury may result in bilaterally fixed or sluggish pupils, sometimes with autonomic balance fluctuations causing spontaneous fluctuations in diameter (also known as hippus).[10]

Pupils that respond appropriately to light, even if miotic, indicate adequate function of the rostral brainstem, optic chiasm, optic nerves, and retinas. In the absence of concurrent ocular trauma, miosis may indicate a diencephalic lesion, particularly in the hypothalamus, because this area represents the origin of the sympathetic pathway.[4,7,8] Bilateral miosis in human head trauma patients also has been associated infrequently with pontine lesions.[10]

Pupils that are initially miotic and then become mydriatic are indicative of a progressive brainstem lesion, whereas bilateral mydriasis with no response to light is usually indicative of irreversible midbrain damage, herniation of the cerebellum through the foramen magnum, or both.[7] Unilateral mydriasis may indicate unilateral cerebellar herniation or brainstem hemorrhage but also may indicate ocular damage resulting from the trauma.[6,7] However, a unilateral mydriasis and loss of direct light reflex in one eye commonly implies a cranial nerve III paralysis and commonly is accompanied by ptosis and ventrolateral strabismus (see Table 81-2). In humans, this can be a sign associated with extradural bleeding and warrants immediate advanced imaging.[11]

Eye movements

In the unconscious patient, spontaneous ocular movements should be assessed.[5] If there are none, the oculocephalic reflexes (i.e., physiologic nystagmus) are tested by rotating the head in vertical and horizontal planes. This can be done only when a cervical spinal injury has been excluded. Oculocephalic reflexes may be impaired in animals with brainstem lesions as a result of either involvement of cranial nerve nuclei that innervate the extraocular muscles or the interconnecting ascending medial longitudinal fasciculus within the pons and midbrain.[11]

In addition to their localizing value, the eye movements have been considered indices of head injury severity. The ability of the patient to fix its eyes on a target and follow it is a favorable finding, and absence of eye movements is an ominous finding. Absence of eye movements upon irrigation of the external auditory canal with ice-cold water (oculovestibular reflex) is indicative of profound brainstem failure and is an accepted criterion of brain death in humans.[10] However, such a test should not be performed if there is any suspicion of a cranioaural fistula or a skull base fracture. Between the presence and absence of inducible eye movements, there are many ill-defined disturbances with unknown diagnostic and prognostic implications.[10]

COMA SCALES AND LONG-TERM FUNCTIONAL OUTCOME

No long-term functional outcome studies have been performed in dogs or cats after head trauma, so the use of coma scales for long-term prognosis is not documented. An accurate assessment of outcome obviously is needed because patients surviving head trauma may be left with multiple neurologic deficits that markedly affect the quality of life (or at least the owner's perception of the animal's quality of life). Exceptional owner commitment may enable some very disabled patients to return home, but minor neurologic deficits may be viewed by some owners as unacceptable.

A standardized outcome scale used in human medicine is the Glasgow Outcome Scale.[12] This scale is based on the overall social capability of the patient, which takes into account specific mental and neurologic deficits. It was devised for victims of brain damage in general because it was required for studies of head injury and of atraumatic coma. Four categories of survival are recognized and are listed as good recovery, moderate disability (independent but disabled), severe disability (conscious but dependent), and vegetative state.[12] Each category contains variation, but much of this may not be applicable to veterinary patients because it is based on the ability of the patient to communicate and be self-sufficient. However, the modified Glasgow Coma Scale should be correlated with an outcome scale in veterinary medicine, because this would truly assist with defining a prognosis in small animal patients. Until this time, coma scales can be used only as a guide of the immediate success of therapy and, more important, when to initiate this treatment.

THE FUTURE OF COMA SCALES

The use of coma scales or head trauma scoring systems in veterinary medicine is still crude and has a lot of potential for interrater variability. The use of the MGCS in isolation could lead to misinterpretation of the prognosis or potential response to aggressive treatment. Evaluation of concurrent systemic injuries and the results of the minimum database and imaging evaluations also must be taken into consideration. Further modification of the MGCS is likely in the near future in an effort to decrease variability in patient scoring and to improve its accuracy as a measure of short- and long-term prognosis.

A new coma scale recently has been introduced in human medicine named the Full Outline of UnResponsiveness (FOUR) score.[13] The FOUR score is based on the bare minimum of tests necessary for assessing a patient with altered consciousness but also includes much important information not assessed by the human GCS, including the measurement of brainstem reflexes; determination of eye opening, blinking, and tracking; and the presence of abnormal breath rhythms and a respiratory drive.

The FOUR score has four components: eye responses, motor responses, brainstem reflexes, and respiratory pattern. Each component has a maximal value of 4. As expected, some of the evaluations that make up this scoring system are not translated easily into a veterinary scoring system. However, this scoring system has proven to be simpler, more accurate, and more consistently used in human medicine.[13] Most likely a similar improved scoring system will be available in veterinary medicine in the near future.

REFERENCES

1. Freeman C, Platt SR: Head trauma. In Platt SR, Garosi L: Small animal neurological emergencies, London, 2012, Mansun.
2. Bagley RS: Intracranial pressure in dogs and cats, Comp Cont Educ Pract Vet 18:605, 1996.
3. Ghajar J: Traumatic brain injury, Lancet 356:923, 2000.
4. Shores A: Craniocerebral trauma. In Kirk RW, editor: Current veterinary therapy X, St Louis, 1989, Saunders.
5. Platt SR, Radaelli ST, McDonnell JJ: The prognostic value of the modified Glasgow Coma Scale in head trauma in dogs, J Vet Intern Med 15:581, 2001.
6. Dewey CW: Emergency management of the head trauma patient, Vet Clin North Am Small Anim Pract 30:207, 2000.
7. Winter CD, Adamides AA, Lewsi PM, et al: A review of the current management of severe traumatic brain injury, Surgeon 3:329, 2005.
8. Johnson JA, Murtaugh RJ: Craniocerebral trauma. In Bonagura JD, editor: Kirk's current veterinary therapy XIII, St Louis, 2000, Saunders.
9. Chesnut RM, Gautille T, Blunt BA, et al: The localizing value of asymmetry in pupillary size in severe head injury: relation to lesion type and location, Neurosurgery 34:840, 1994.
10. Simpson DA: Clinical examination and grading. In Reilly PL, Bullock R, editors: Head injury: pathophysiology and management, ed 2, London, 2005, Hodder Arnold.
11. Jones NR, Molloy CJ, Kloeden CN, et al: Extradural hematoma: trends in outcome over 35 years, Br J Neurosurg 7:465, 1993.
12. Jennett B: Outcome after severe head injury. In Reilly PL, Bullock R, editors: Head injury: pathophysiology and management, ed 2, London, 2005, Hodder Arnold.
13. Fischer M, Rüegg S, Czaplinski A, et al: Inter-rater reliability of the full outline of unresponsiveness score and the Glasgow Coma Scale in critically ill patients: a prospective observational study, Crit Care 14:R64, 2010.

CHAPTER 82

SEIZURES AND STATUS EPILEPTICUS

Karen M. Vernau, DVM, MAS, DACVIM (Neurology)

KEY POINTS

- Epilepsy refers to recurrent seizures of any type resulting from an intracranial cause and may be subdivided into true epilepsy (inherited, acquired, and idiopathic) and symptomatic epilepsy.
- Seizures are classified as partial or generalized; generalized seizures are the most common.
- Status epilepticus is a life-threatening neurologic emergency, and a common initial complaint at the emergency hospital.
- Status epilepticus may cause serious systemic problems such as hypoxia, hyperthermia, systemic lactic acidosis, shock, and acute renal failure.
- Disorders that induce seizures and status epilepticus are either extracranial or intracranial.
- A complete history, physical examination, neurologic examination, and minimum diagnostic database are recommended for all animals with a seizure disorder.
- Further investigation of intracranial diseases using electroencephalography, magnetic resonance imaging, or computed tomography imaging, cerebrospinal fluid analysis, serology, and biopsy may be indicated.
- Seizure management is based on control of seizures by selection and appropriate administration of an anticonvulsant drug. When an underlying disease is present, it should be treated concurrently. Seizures associated with status epilepticus should be stopped as quickly as possible.

The epidemiology of seizures in cats and dogs is unknown, despite reports of the rate,[1] prevalence,[2] and incidence.[3] Population-based animal studies are difficult to execute, thus most studies are based on data from groups of veterinary hospitals or referral-based veterinary teaching hospitals.[2] The epidemiology of seizures in groups of purebred dogs or colonies of research dogs[1] with epilepsy has been reported. For example, one population-based study reported the lifetime prevalence of epilepsy in the Danish Labrador as 3.1% (95% confidence interval 1.6% to 4.6%).[4] Although these studies are interesting, the information cannot be extrapolated beyond the research colony, hospital, or specific purebred dog geographic setting.

Despite the lack of prevalence or incidence data, it is accepted that seizure disorders are common in dogs and cats and that seizures occur more frequently in dogs than in cats. Estimates of lifetime seizure frequencies are 0.5% to 5.7% in dogs and 0.5% to 1.0% in cats.[5]

Status epilepticus (SE) is a life-threatening neurologic emergency and a common presenting complaint at an emergency hospital. Although the population prevalence of SE is not known, in one report the prevalence of SE and cluster seizures in dogs was 0.44% of all hospital admissions.[6]

Although many different types of seizures occur in dogs and cats, a classification system that is accepted universally by veterinary neurologists has not been established.[7-9] To diagnose and treat effectively dogs and cats with seizure disorders, including SE, it is important to understand the terminology, pathophysiology, and causes of seizures.

Definitions

A *seizure* is the clinical manifestation of a paroxysmal cerebral disorder, caused by a synchronous and excessive electrical neuronal discharge, originating from the cerebral cortex.[5]

Cluster seizures are two or more seizures within a 24-hour period.[6]

Epilepsy is recurrent seizures of any type resulting from an intracranial cause.[5] There are three types of epilepsy:

1. Idiopathic: seizures caused by a genetically determined intracranial disorder
2. Symptomatic: seizures caused by underlying intracranial disorder
3. Cryptogenic: cause of the seizures is suspected to be symptomatic, but an underlying cause is not found[10,11]

Status epilepticus is a neurologic emergency requiring immediate therapy. A universally accepted definition for SE in humans or animals does not exist.[6,10] The authors recommend the definition "continuous seizures, or two or more discrete seizures between which there is incomplete recovery of consciousness, lasting at least 5 minutes."[11]

CLASSIFICATION

Seizures in dogs and cats may be classified as partial or generalized, based on clinical observations rather than EEG characteristics. Partial seizures originate from a focus in one cerebral hemisphere and usually manifest localized clinical signs. Partial seizures usually have an acquired cause and may be subdivided into simple partial seizures or complex partial seizures. In simple partial seizures there is no alteration in consciousness, and the clinical signs during the seizure are limited to isolated muscle groups (e.g., tonus or clonus of a limb). Additional clinical signs (e.g., autonomic signs) may be present during a simple partial seizure. Complex partial seizures are accompanied by an alteration in consciousness. There may be involuntary or compulsive actions such as chewing, licking, and defensive or aggressive behavior. Complex partial seizures have been referred to as psychomotor seizures. Both types of partial seizures may spread throughout the brain, causing generalized seizures.[5]

Generalized seizures are the most commonly recognized seizures in dogs and cats. The most common type is the tonic-clonic seizure. Other types of generalized seizures such as tonic, clonic, or myoclonic seizures are recognized. In tonic-clonic seizures, animals lose consciousness. In the tonic phase, increased muscle tone results in limb and head extension, causing the animal to fall to the side. In the clonic phase, alternating extension and flexion of the limbs, and exaggerated chewing movements, occur. The animal usually urinates, defecates, and salivates.[5]

PATHOPHYSIOLOGY

The normal brain is capable of seizures in response to a variety of intracranial and extracranial stimuli. When the brain's homeostasis is overcome, cerebrocortical excitability is altered and the seizure threshold is decreased. Normal animals with a low seizure threshold may be induced to have a seizure by many factors, including fatigue, fever, estrus, and photic stimulation.

Experimentally, repeated stimulation of the rat cerebral cortex by a subconvulsive electrical stimulus caused generalized seizures over time. This phenomenon is referred to as *kindling*.[12] Following establishment of a focal seizure focus, abnormal electrical activity may be recorded over the contralateral cerebral cortex. This secondary seizure focus is termed a *mirror focus*.[13] Either the primary or secondary focus, or both, may cause seizures. The mirror focus may cause seizures even if the primary seizure focus is removed.[14] Although kindling and mirror foci are observed as experimental phenomena, they may be relevant clinically in the therapy of animals with seizure disorders.

In SE there is failure of the normal brain homeostasis mechanisms that work to stop seizures. Proposed mechanisms for the development of SE include persistent neuronal excitation, inadequate neuronal inhibition, or both.[11] Extrasynaptic factors may be important in spreading and maintaining the seizure. An excess of excitatory neurotransmitters such as glutamate, aspartate, or acetylcholine, or antagonists of γ-aminobutyric acid (GABA) (an inhibitory neurotransmitter) may cause SE.

SE lasting 30 to 45 minutes results in brain injury in experimental animals.[15] However, brain injury likely occurs in clinical patients after a much shorter time. SE may cause neuronal necrosis, particularly in brain regions with high metabolic rates.

In early SE, an increase in cerebral blood flow may be protective for the brain. In late SE, cerebral blood flow decreases simultaneously as blood pressure decreases and cerebral metabolic rate (e.g., glucose and oxygen use) increases. This leads to adenosine triphosphate depletion and lactate accumulation, which contribute to neuronal necrosis. SE may be associated with systemic problems, including hypoxemia, hyperthermia, aspiration pneumonia, systemic lactic acidosis, hyperkalemia, hypoglycemia, shock, cardiac arrhythmias, neurogenic pulmonary edema, and acute renal failure.

ETIOLOGY

Disorders that induce seizures and SE arise either outside the nervous system (extracranial) or within the nervous system (intracranial). Extracranial causes may be divided into those that originate outside the body (e.g., toxins) and those that originate within the body but outside the nervous system (e.g., liver disease). Intracranial causes of seizures are divided into progressive and nonprogressive diseases.[5]

Extracranial causes may result in generalized seizures because they affect the brain globally. Causes of progressive intracranial disease include inflammation (e.g., granulomatous meningoencephalitis), neoplasia, nutritional alterations (e.g., thiamine deficiency), infection, anomalous entities (e.g., hydrocephalus), and trauma. Most animals with progressive intracranial disease are clinically abnormal between seizures and usually have progression of clinical signs. However, seizures may be the only clinical sign for a prolonged time, before others become apparent.

Examples of nonprogressive causes of seizures include inherited epilepsy, and previously active cerebral diseases such as infections, and traumatic lesions, that are no longer active. Dogs with inherited epilepsy usually are 6 months to 5 years of age. Many dogs breeds are known or suspected to have inherited epilepsy.[17] In animals with idiopathic epilepsy, the seizures are caused by a functional problem with the brain and are therefore are generalized and symmetric.

Very few veterinary studies have evaluated the clinical features of SE; therefore it is not possible to make generalizations concerning underlying causes or concerning short-term and long-term outcomes. One study[18] evaluated a cohort of 50 dogs with SE. Of those, 28% had idiopathic epilepsy, 32% had symptomatic epilepsy, and 12% had seizures secondary to a systemic insult or to physiologic stress; 44% had not had SE previously. Many dogs were euthanized, and thus a mortality rate was not reported.[18] In another study[19] of SE in dogs with idiopathic epilepsy, 59% of the dogs had one or more episodes of SE. Survival time was shorter in dogs with both idiopathic epilepsy and SE than in those with idiopathic epilepsy alone.[19] In another study of SE or cluster seizures in dogs, a poor outcome was reported in dogs with granulomatous meningoencephalitis, poor seizure control after 6 hours of hospitalization, or SE manifest by partial seizures. Of the dogs in this study, 59% died or were euthanized.[6]

It is essential to distinguish between extracranial and intracranial (progressive and nonprogressive) diseases that cause seizures. Therapy for extracranial and progressive intracranial diseases requires not only control of seizures but also therapy for the underlying disease.

DIAGNOSTIC PLAN

A seizure disorder is essentially a manifestation of an underlying disease; therapy is most effective when the underlying disease is diagnosed and treated. Therefore an accurate diagnosis should be established in a timely manner. In some animals an underlying cause may not be identified, as with idiopathic epilepsy. A complete history and physical and neurologic examination are necessary for all animals with a seizure disorder (Figure 82-1).

History

A complete general history should be obtained from the owner, as well as a specific seizure history: age at onset, frequency, and description of seizures, behavior between seizures, and temporal associations (e.g., associated with eating or not eating). A videotape of a seizure may be useful, as an adjunct to the owner's description of the event.

Age and Breed

The age at onset is necessary to determine the most likely cause of a seizure disorder. Dogs 5 years and older usually have an acquired seizure disorder, such as a primary brain tumor. The breed is important, because inherited epilepsy is reported in certain breeds such as Beagles, German Shepherds, Poodles, and others.[17] Some breeds may have a higher prevalence of intracranial tumors (Boxers) or inflammatory disease (Maltese dogs).

Physical Examination

A complete physical examination is important in all animals with seizures, to recognize systemic problems or local problems (e.g., skull mass) that may affect the brain.

Neurologic Examination

A complete neurologic examination should be done in *all* animals with seizures. In animals with idiopathic epilepsy, neurologic examination findings between seizures most often are normal. Dogs and cats with extracranial or progressive intracranial disease may have neurologic abnormalities between seizures.

Animals may be abnormal neurologically for days after a seizure. Therefore multiple, serial neurologic examinations may be necessary before neurologic deficits can be attributed to a progressive intracranial disorder.

Minimum Database

A minimum database (complete blood count, serum chemistry panel, 24-hour fasting blood glucose, urinalysis) is recommended on admission for all animals with seizures. In some animals, serum

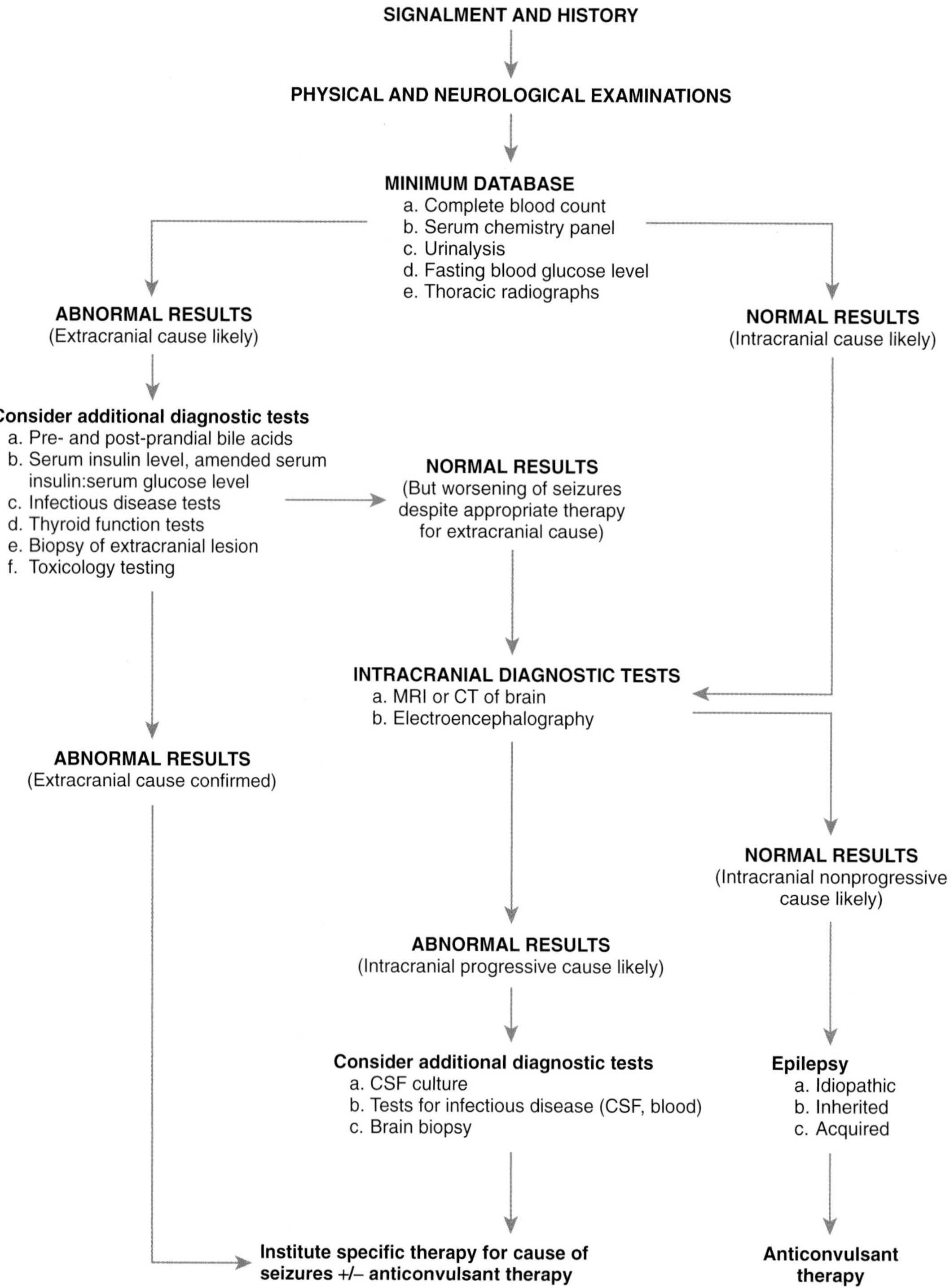

FIGURE 82-1 Diagnostic approach to seizure disorders in dogs and cats. CSF, *Cerebrospinal fluid;* CT, *computed tomography;* MRI, *magnetic resonance imaging.*

triglycerides and preprandial and postprandial bile acid levels should be obtained to evaluate the possibility of a portosystemic shunt and hypertriglyceridemia. If systemic disease or intracranial disease is suspected, thoracic radiography and abdominal ultrasonography should be performed to screen further for secondary neoplastic and systemic infectious disease.

Diagnostic Tests for Intracranial Disease

Further investigation of intracranial diseases, including electroencephalography (EEG), MRI (or CT if MRI is not available), CSF analysis, biopsy (for cytology, histopathology, or both), and serology, may be indicated after a minimum database is completed. EEG is useful in some animals. When a seizure disorder is a possible cause for a paroxysmal event, abnormal findings on EEG may help to distinguish the presence of seizures from other paroxysmal nonseizure events. EEG findings may help the clinician to evaluate the anticonvulsant therapy, particularly in a patient undergoing treatment for SE, because the external manifestations of seizures may be abolished by drugs.[20] In the future, EEG may be useful in the classification of canine and feline seizure disorders. If continuous intracranial EEG monitoring technology is adopted in clinical patients, this technology may change the way that veterinarians and owners monitor and treat dogs with seizure disorders.[22]

MRI is preferred over CT imaging, unless acute head trauma or an acute intracranial hemorrhage is suspected. MRI and CT imaging are noninvasive, yielding the most diagnostic information with respect to location, extent, and type of disease in animals with progressive intracranial problems. The results of advanced imaging may help to define the underlying cause of the seizure disorder.

Ideally, CSF is collected after MRI or CT imaging has been done. Usually CSF is collected from the cisterna magna (see Chapter 207). Because there is risk to the patient undergoing CSF puncture, CSF is not collected in all animals with intracranial disease (see Chapter 84). Usually CSF analysis results are supportive of a diagnosis, rather than providing a definitive diagnosis. However, CSF occasionally provides diagnostic information with some infections (e.g., *Cryptococcus neoformans*) and with some neoplasms (e.g., lymphoma) and is therefore an essential part of an intracranial workup in most animals.

TREATMENT PLAN

Regardless of the underlying cause, seizure control is based on selection and administration of an appropriate anticonvulsant drug. Underlying disease, if present, should be treated concurrently. Adverse effects may limit the usefulness of a particular anticonvulsant drug; therefore knowledge of the mechanisms of action and drug interactions is essential. Selection of an anticonvulsant drug should be based on results of pharmacokinetic studies in the species in which the drug is to be used.

The ultimate goal of anticonvulsant therapy is to eradicate all seizure activity; however, this goal rarely is achieved. A more realistic goal is to reduce the severity, frequency, and duration of seizures to a level that is acceptable to the owner, without intolerable or unacceptable adverse effects on the animal. A general guideline is to consider anticonvulsant drug therapy when the seizure frequency is greater than once every 6 weeks.

Immediate, short-term (acute) anticonvulsant therapy is required to manage SE, cluster seizures, and seizures resulting from some toxicities. Chronic (or maintenance) anticonvulsant therapy is used to manage epilepsy. Seizure control with anticonvulsant drugs is most effective when started early in the course of a seizure disorder, because each seizure may increase the probability of additional seizures secondary to effects such as kindling and mirror focus development.

Status Epilepticus

The goal of therapy for patients with SE is to stop the seizure as soon as possible. In veterinary medicine, EEG monitoring is not routine in the intensive care unit, so effectiveness of SE therapy is evaluated by the cessation of the outward physical manifestations. Therefore, in some animals, although no clinical signs of SE are obvious, the brain still may have ongoing seizure activity that may affect outcome negatively. As with many disorders in veterinary medicine, there are no controlled, double-blinded, placebo-controlled clinical trials for patients with SE that may be used to guide therapy. Therefore recommended treatments are guidelines only (Table 82-1).

Treatment should be divided into the (1) immediate emergency evaluation and treatment (such as airway, breathing, cardiovascular function, body temperature, glucose concentration, and blood pressure) (see Chapter 1) and (2) pharmacologic treatment (see Table 82-1). Animals that are admitted in SE or with cluster seizures may have cerebral edema, and mannitol administration should be considered (see Chapter 84).

Pharmacologic Therapy for Status Epilepticus

Benzodiazepines

Diazepam and midazolam are the first-line drugs for treatment of SE in dogs and cats. Diazepam is lipid soluble and enters the brain

Table 82-1 Anticonvulsant Drugs for Status Epilepticus in Dog and Cats

Drug	Dose	Comments
Diazepam (first-line)	IV bolus: 0.5-1.0 mg/kg may be repeated 2-3 times Constant rate infusion: 0.5-1 mg/kg/hr Per rectum: 0.5-1 mg/kg (2 mg/kg if receiving concurrent phenobarbital) Intranasal: 1 mg/kg	IV injections and infusions should be administered into a central vein.
Midazolam	IV bolus: 0.2 mg/kg; may be repeated 2-3 times. Constant rate infusion: 0.2-0.4 mg/kg/hr IM/IN: 0.2 mg/kg	Per rectum route not recommended IN: gel may achieve higher plasma concentrations than solution.
Phenobarbital (use concurrently with diazepam or midazolam)	2-4 mg/kg IV every 20-30 minutes to a total of 18-20 mg/kg	Administer concurrently with diazepam or midazolam to prevent recurrence of seizures once diazepam brain levels reduce. This dose may be repeated every 20-30 minutes until a cumulative dose of 18-20 mg/kg has been given. Once seizures are controlled a maintenance dose of phenobarbital is used (3-5 mg/kg IV or IM q12h for 24-48 hr). Oral anticonvulsant therapy should be resumed or initiated every 12 hours as soon as the animal is able to swallow.
Levetiracetam	30-60 mg/kg IV	Administer once status epilepticus treated, to prevent cluster seizures or additional episodes of status epilepticus.
Pentobarbital (second-line)	6-15 mg/kg IV slow bolus, followed by a constant rate infusion of 0.5-2 mg/kg/hr	Strict monitoring of physiologic parameters is required.
Propofol (third-line)	2-8 mg/kg slow IV bolus, given as 25% of the total dose every 30 seconds until desired effect achieved	Constant rate infusion should be considered (0.1-0.4 mg/kg/min). Strict monitoring of physiologic parameters is required.

IM, Intramuscular; *IV*, intravenous; *IN*, intranasal.

rapidly when given intravenously, intranasally (IN), or per rectum (PR). It binds to the GABA receptor and enhances neuronal hyperpolarization, reducing neuronal firing. The duration of action is short, so a maintenance anticonvulsant (such as phenobarbital) should be administered concurrently to avoid recurrence of seizures or SE when diazepam levels in the brain decrease. (For animals not currently receiving phenobarbital, a loading dosage is administered.) Owners may be trained to administer PR diazepam to their animals at home. Midazolam is a water-soluble benzodiazepine and may be used to manage SE. Although the IV route is preferred, midazolam may be given IN and IM if IV access cannot be obtained. A gel formulation of midazolam (0.4% hydroxypropyl methylcellulose) given IN to dogs had a higher peak plasma concentrations when compared with the midazolam solution given IN and PR but has not been evaluated yet for efficacy.[23] Because of variable and erratic plasma concentrations with PR administration of midazolam, the PR route of administration is not recommended for the treatment of status epilepticus.[24]

If SE continues or further seizures occur, additional boluses of diazepam or midazolam may be given, or a constant rate infusion (CRI) may be used. If the SE does not stop, or recurs multiple times, then barbiturates (pentobarbital), or injectable levetiracetam may be used.[25] The dosage of phenobarbital should be reviewed at this point in time to ensure that an adequate dose has been administered. With the manufacturer delays and resulting backorders of both intravenous diazepam and midazolam preparations continuing to plague veterinarians, alternative drugs to treat status epilepticus must be evaluated for their safety and efficacy to treat this potentially life-threatening emergency.

Barbiturates

Barbiturates potentiate the action of GABA by interfering with sodium and potassium transmission in the neuronal membrane. Because the half-life of most drugs used to manage SE is short, a maintenance anticonvulsant *must* be part of the treatment regimen. Phenobarbital and levetiracetam are administered most commonly because both drugs can be given intravenously.

Pentobarbital is used as a second-line drug if benzodiazepines fail to treat status epilepticus, but the drug has a limited anticonvulsant effect. Pentobarbital is administered as a bolus, followed by a CRI. Pentobarbital may cause sedation, respiratory depression, hypotension, and death. Animals that are sedated heavily or anesthetized should be intubated so that an open airway is maintained. Other physiologic parameters (e.g., heart rate, blood pressure, oxygenation) should be monitored regularly or continuously. Therefore the dosage should be titrated carefully to stop or reduce the motor activity from the seizure but to avoid anesthesia if possible. During recovery, it may be difficult to determine if the animal is recovering from the pentobarbital or still is having seizures.

Propofol

Propofol is a rapid-acting, lipid-soluble general anesthetic agent. It is a third-line drug for the management of SE in dogs and cats. The anticonvulsant effect of propofol is likely because of its GABA agonist activity.[21] There are case series describing its use in animals and humans with SE.[21,22,26-29] However, propofol use is controversial because seizures are associated with its use in humans[23] and in a dog.[24] In one study, humans with SE who were treated with propofol had a higher mortality rate than those treated with midazolam.[22]

Chronic Seizure Disorders

Successful anticonvulsant therapy depends on the maintenance of plasma concentrations of appropriate anticonvulsant drugs within a therapeutic range defined for the species in which the drug is to be administered. Therefore anticonvulsant drugs that are eliminated slowly should be employed. The elimination half-life of anticonvulsant drugs varies considerably between species. Few anticonvulsant drugs used in humans are suitable for use in dogs and cats, largely because of species differences in pharmacokinetics. Pharmacokinetic data for and clinical experience with many anticonvulsant drugs are lacking in cats. Selection should be based on the known pharmacokinetic properties of a drug in the species in which it is to be administered (see Chapter 166 for further discussion of anticonvulsant drugs).

Phenobarbital and bromide are the first-line of anticonvulsant drugs recommended for chronic seizure disorders in dogs. Phenobarbital is the first-line anticonvulsant in cats.

REFERENCES

1. Bielfelt SW, Redman HC, McClellan RO: Sire- and sex-related differences in rates of epileptiform seizures in a purebred Beagle dog colony, Am J Vet Res 32:2039, 1971.
2. Schwartz-Porsche D: Epidemiological, clinical, and pharmacological studies in spontaneously epileptic dogs and cats, Proceedings of the 4th Forum of the American College of Veterinary Internal Medicine, Washington, DC, May 22-24, 1986.
3. Bunch SE: Anticonvulsant therapy in companion animals. In Kirk RW, editor: Current veterinary therapy IX, St Louis, 1986, Saunders.
4. Berendt M, Gredal H, Pedersen LG et al: A cross-sectional study of epilepsy in Danish Labrador Retrievers: prevalence and selected risk factors, J Vet Intern Med 16:262, 2002.
5. LeCouteur RA, Child G: Clinical management of epilepsy of dogs and cats, Probl Vet Med 1:578, 1989.
6. Bateman SW, Parent JM: Clinical findings, treatment, and outcome of dogs with status epilepticus or cluster seizures: 156 cases (1990-1995), J Am Vet Med Assoc 215:1463, 1999.
7. Podell M: Epilepsy and seizure classification: a lesson from Leonardo, J Vet Intern Med 13:3, 1999.
8. Chandler K: Canine epilepsy: what can we learn from human seizure disorders? Vet J 172:207, 2006.
9. Berendt M, Gram L: Epilepsy and seizure classification in 63 dogs: a reappraisal of veterinary epilepsy terminology, J Vet Intern Med 13:14, 1999.
10. Schwartz M, Munana KR, Nettifee-Osborne J: Assessment of the prevalence and clinical features of cryptogenic epilepsy in dogs: 45 cases (2003-2011), J Am Vet Med Assoc 242:651-657, 2013.
11. Commission on Classification and Terminology of the International League Against Epilepsy, Epilepsia 30(4):389-399, 1989.
12. International League Against Epilepsy: Glossary; http://www.ilae-epilepsy.org/Visitors/Centre/ctf/glossary Accessed November 14, 2007.
13. Lowenstein DH, Bleck T, Macdonald RL: It's time to revise the definition of status epilepticus, Epilepsia 40:120, 1999.
14. Goddard GV, McIntyre DC, Leech CK: A permanent change in brain function resulting from daily electrical stimulation, Exp Neurol 25:295, 1969.
15. Morrell F: Secondary epileptogenic lesions, Epilepsia 1:538, 1960.
16. Reference deleted in pages.
17. Sloviter RS: "Epileptic" brain damage in rats induced by sustained electrical stimulation of the perforant path. I. Acute electrophysiological and light microscopic studies, Brain Res Bull 10:675, 1983.
18. Lorenz MD, Kornegay JN: Seizures, narcolepsy and cataplexy. In Lorenz MD, Kornegay JN, editors: Handbook of veterinary neurology, ed 4, St Louis, 2004, Saunders.
19. Platt SR, Haag M: Canine status epilepticus: a retrospective study of 50 cases, J Small Anim Pract 43:151, 2002.
20. Saito M, Munana KR, Sharp NJ, et al: Risk factors for development of status epilepticus in dogs with idiopathic epilepsy and effects of status epilepticus on outcome and survival time: 32 cases (1990-1996), J Am Vet Med Assoc 219:618, 2001.
21. Markand ON: Pearls, perils, and pitfalls in the use of the electroencephalogram, Semin Neurol 23:7, 2003.

22. Davis KA, Sturges BK, Vite CH, et al: A novel implanted device to wirelessly record and analyze continuous intracranial canine EEG, Epilepsy Res 96:116-122, 2011.
23. Eagelson JS, Platt SR, Elder Strong DL, et al: Bioavailability of a novel midazolam gel after intranasal administration in dogs, Am J Vet Res 73:539-545, 2012.
24. Schwartz M, Muana KR, Nettiffee-Osborne JA: The pharmacokinetics of midazolam after intravenous, intramuscular and rectal administration in healthy dogs, J Vet Pharmacol Therap 36:471-477, 2013. doi: 10.1111/jvp.12032.
25. Hardy BT, Patterson EE, Cloyd JM, et al: Double-masked, placebo-controlled study of intravenous levetiracetam for the treatment of status epilepticus and acute repetitive seizures in dogs, J Vet Intern Med 26:334-340, 2012.
26. Steffen F, Grasmueck S: Propofol for treatment of refractory seizures in dogs and a cat with intracranial disorders, J Small Anim Pract 41:496, 2000.
27. Prasad A, Worrall BB, Bertram EH, et al: Propofol and midazolam in the treatment of refractory status epilepticus, Epilepsia 42:380, 2001.
28. Makela JP, Iivanainen M, Pieninkeroinen IP, et al: Seizures associated with propofol anesthesia, Epilepsia 34:832, 1993.
29. Smedile LE, Duke T, Taylor SM: Excitatory movements in a dog following propofol anesthesia, J Am Anim Hosp Assoc 32:365, 1996.

CHAPTER 83
SPINAL CORD INJURY

Emily Davis, DVM • Charles H. Vite, DVM, PhD, DACVIM (Neurology)

KEY POINTS

- Any animal with suspected spinal cord instability or fractures should be restrained on a flat board or in a small cage until further diagnostic tests can be performed.
- An accurate history and lesion localization lead to a reliable list of differential diagnoses.
- The presence of upper motor neuron (UMN) signs, lower motor neuron (LMN) signs, or a combination of both (i.e., LMN to the thoracic limbs and UMN to the pelvic limbs) should be identified to determine accurately the location of the spinal cord lesion.
- Prognosis for recovery ranges from excellent to grave; time is the only certain determinant of the extent of return of function.

Injury to the spinal cord is common in domestic animals and may result from vascular, infectious, inflammatory, degenerative, neoplastic, and/or traumatic processes. Animals with disease of the spinal cord may be presented with only a focal area of spinal pain, or with anesthesia and paralysis at the level of, and extending caudal to the lesion. Signs of neurologic dysfunction that fall between these two extremes include spinal ataxia, limping or leg-carrying lameness (a "root signature"), ambulatory or nonambulatory paresis, or paralysis. Animals should be evaluated and their deficits graded using one of several available scoring systems (Table 83-1).[1,2]

This chapter focuses on traumatic spinal cord injuries, including intervertebral disk herniation, and mentions only briefly other causes of spinal cord disease. The emergency and critical care veterinarian must be able to recognize neurologic dysfunction, accurately localize the lesion, generate a list of differential diagnoses, institute appropriate acute therapy, and recognize the prognosis of animals with injuries to the spinal cord. Ideally, appropriate diagnostic testing should be performed quickly to obtain a definitive diagnosis and specific therapy instituted.

PATHOPHYSIOLOGY

Two stages of spinal cord injury follow trauma: initial primary tissue damage from direct mechanical disruption followed by secondary damage via biochemical and vascular events.[4,5] When cellular membrane integrity is disrupted, a complex cascade of biochemical reactions is initiated, including the release of excitotoxic amino acids, free fatty acids, oxygen free radicals, and vasoactive agents. N-methyl-D-aspartate (NMDA) receptors are activated and voltage-sensitive calcium and sodium channels open.[6] These membrane changes result in increased intracellular calcium and sodium, decreased intracellular potassium, and increased extracellular potassium. In addition to changes in ionic concentrations, a decrease in blood flow occurs as a result of direct mechanical compression and/or loss of autoregulation, vasospasm, and hemorrhage, leading to spinal cord ischemia.[4,6] Ischemia results in cytotoxic edema, axonal degeneration, demyelination, abnormal impulse transmission, conduction block, and cellular death.[4,6]

LOCALIZATION

When the animal is presented to the veterinarian, a thorough history should be obtained. If a fracture or luxation is suspected, the goal is

Table 83-1 Neurologic Scoring System[3]

Neurologic Grade	Neurologic Description
Grade 1	No deficits
Grade 2	Paresis, walking
Grade 3	Paresis, nonambulatory
Grade 4	Paralysis
Grade 5	Paralysis, no deep pain

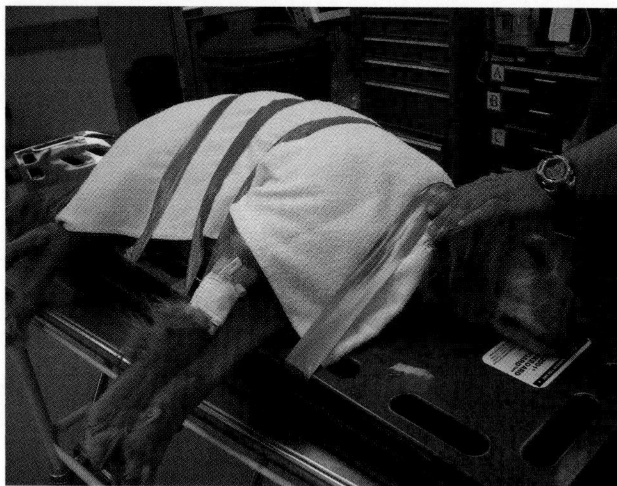

FIGURE 83-1 A dog with suspected spinal injury is secured on a back board to prevent further trauma.

to decrease activity that could damage the spinal cord further. A nonambulatory animal should be placed on a flat board and strapped down; sedation and/or analgesia may be required in anxious or painful patients (Figure 83-1). Strict cage rest to restrict activity may be all that the ambulatory animal tolerates. When external trauma to the spinal cord has occurred secondary to a motor vehicle accident, fall from a height, or severe bite wound(s), it may be necessary to radiograph the entire spinal column immediately after a limited general and neurologic examination.

A complete neurologic examination should be performed unless it is likely to injure the patient further. The goal of the examination is to identify neurologic dysfunction and determine functional integrity. Interpretation of the neurologic examination allows the clinician to localize the site of spinal cord injury based on specific signs of dysfunction. For localization of lesions, the spinal cord often is divided into five regions, with disease of each region resulting in a characteristic group of signs. These regions include cervical cord segments one through cervical five (C1-C5), cervical six through thoracic two (C6-T2), thoracic three through lumbar three (T3-L3), lumbar four through sacral one (L4-S1), and sacral one through sacral three (S1-S3). Only spinal cord segments C1, C2, and the last thoracic and first two lumbar segments are located in the vertebral body with the same vertebral number in the dog.[7] More caudally along the spine, the spinal cord segments lie in the spinal canal cranial to the vertebrae with the same number. [8] The presence of spinal cord segments within vertebral bodies of different numbers is important to consider when evaluating images of the spine, particularly in the lower lumbar spine, where, for example in dogs, spinal cord segments L7, S1, S2, S3, and Cd1 may be present within the fifth lumbar vertebral body.[9]

If a spinal fracture or luxation is not suspected and the patient is capable of walking, then examination should begin with gait analysis. The thoracic and pelvic limbs should be evaluated separately. First, the presence or absence of proprioceptive (spinal) ataxia should be determined. Spinal ataxia is recognized by incoordination and a "wobbly" gait characterized by an increased stride length, dragging or scuffing the toes, walking on the dorsum of the paw, or crossing over of the limbs. At the same time, the animal is evaluated for paresis (incomplete paralysis characterized by the inability to support weight fully while standing or walking, shuffling of the paws, or trembling when bearing weight) or paralysis (loss of the voluntary ability to move a body part) of one or multiple limbs. Posture is assessed by noting the position of the head and limbs when the animal is at rest and when walking. Once this portion of the examination is completed, postural reactions (replacement of a knuckled over paw, hopping, placing, wheelbarrowing, extensor postural thrust, hemistanding or hemiwalking) and segmental reflexes (stretch reflexes [extensor carpi radialis, triceps, biceps, quadriceps, cranial tibial, and gastrocnemius] and withdrawal reflexes) should be evaluated. Assessment for the presence of muscle atrophy, sensation (presence or absence of conscious response to pinch, as well as evidence of spinal or limb pain), and normal mental status and cranial nerve function should be performed. Signs of dysfunction of each of the five the spinal cord regions, beginning caudally and moving cranially, are discussed next.

Spinal Cord Segments S1-S3

The sacral spinal cord segments give rise to the lower motor neurons (LMNs) and sensory fibers that contribute to the sciatic, pelvic, pudendal, and perineal nerves and also connect the caudal spinal cord segments to the spinal cord. General signs of LMN dysfunction are flaccidity, diminished segmental reflexes, and rapidly progressing muscle atrophy (1 to 2 weeks). LMN signs associated with injury to S1-S3 spinal cord segments include paresis/paralysis of the sciatic nerve, anal sphincter, and bladder. If sciatic nerve dysfunction is present, the paws of the pelvic limbs may shuffle when walking, a plantigrade posture may be evident (i.e., tarsocrural joint in close proximity to the ground), the knuckled-over paw may fail to be replaced, and the segmental reflexes (i.e., cranial tibial, gastrocnemius, and withdrawal of the distal limb) may be decreased. The femoral nerve is spared with an injury to this area, and therefore the withdrawal reflex is not completely absent but instead manifests with coxofemoral joint flexion without flexion of the tarsocrural joint. Muscle atrophy of the hamstrings and distal limb muscles may be observed. Denervation of the anal sphincter and bladder results in decreased anal sphincter tone and a flaccid bladder, and the appearance of fecal and/or urinary incontinence. In addition, the ability to wag the tail volitionally can be lost (with damage to the caudal spinal cord segments, flaccid paralysis of the tail results). Sensation may be diminished to the perineum, tail, and lateral and caudal skin of the distal pelvic limbs.

Spinal Cord Segments L4-S1

Spinal cord segments L4-S1 include the lumbar intumescence and give rise to the spinal nerves that contribute to the femoral, obturator, sciatic, pelvic, and pudendal nerves.[2] A lesion of L4-S1 may show dysfunction of the pelvic limbs, tail, and anus with normal thoracic limb function. The pelvic limb gait may be short-strided, and the paws may shuffle as seen with an S1-S3 lesion. Paresis or paralysis may result in a plantigrade stance or inability to stand or support weight because of femoral nerve involvement. Other signs include absent to decreased pelvic limb postural reactions, absent to decreased segmental reflexes (femoral, cranial tibial, gastrocnemius, and withdrawal), decreased pelvic limb tone, and rapidly progressing muscle atrophy of the limbs. Anal sphincter tone may be normal or decreased. Sensation may be decreased in all digits, as well as in the skin at the level of, and caudal to, the lesion.

The upper motor neuron (UMN) system originates in the cerebral cortex and brainstem, is confined to the central nervous system, and terminates on the LMN. The UMN results in movement and muscle tone through its actions on the LMN.[10] Urinary incontinence may be accompanied by a large bladder because of either LMN paralysis or increased urethral sphincter tone (a UMN sign); the more caudal the lesion, the more evidence of LMN involvement.

Spinal Cord Segments T3-L3

A T3-L3 lesion results in so-called UMN signs caudal to the level of the lesion. Diminished UMN influence can result in paresis or

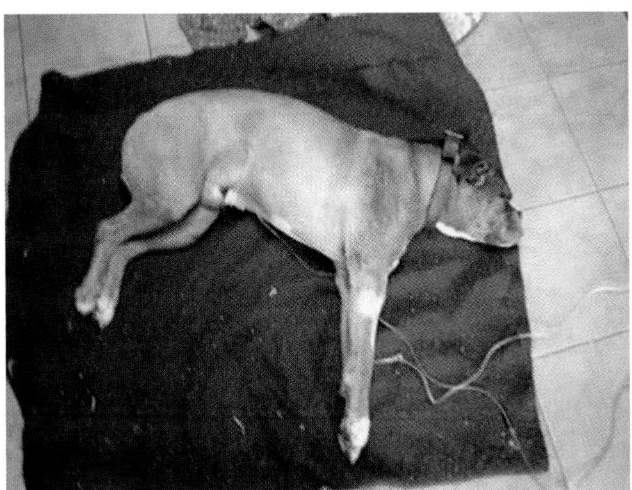

FIGURE 83-2 Note the increased extensor tone present in the thoracic limbs consistent with Schiff-Sherrington phenomenon. Although the etiology of this posture is an acute T3-L3 myelopathy, the presence of this phenomenon is not associated with a worse prognosis.

paralysis, spasticity, exaggerated segmental reflexes, crossed extensor reflex, and diminished to absent postural reactions. These signs are restricted to the pelvic limbs in animals with a T3-L3 lesion. In addition, urinary retention, a moderate-sized firm bladder, and fecal incontinence (despite normal anal tone) may occur.

A T3-L3 lesion also may result in incoordination of the pelvic limbs characterized by crossing over of the limbs, increased stride length, abduction or circumduction, or walking on the dorsal surface of the paw. These signs are recognized as proprioceptive (spinal) ataxia and are due to dysfunction of ascending proprioceptive tracts.

More precise lesion localization can be made by evaluating the cutaneous trunci reflex and assessing the animal for spinal pain. This cutaneous trunci reflex is tested by pinching or pricking the skin lateral to the dorsal midline from the thorax to the level of the L5 vertebral body and observing the movement of the cutaneous trunci muscle. Abnormalities in this reflex are seen as a lack of muscle movement that is caused by the interruption of sensory input from the stimulated dermatome. The sensory nerve from the dermatome being pinched enters the spinal cord approximately two vertebrae cranial to the level of the stimulated skin. Therefore absence of a cutaneous trunci reflex when the skin is pinched at the level of the L3 vertebral body is consistent with a lesion of the spinal nerves or spinal cord at approximately the L1 vertebral body. Further confidence in the correct lesion localization is gained if the animal also appears painful at the site.

A T3-L3 lesion also can result in increased tone to the thoracic limbs (Figure 83-2). This *Schiff-Sherrington phenomenon* results from a lack of ascending inhibitory input to the thoracic limbs originating from the border cells located in the lower thoracic and lumbar spinal cord. Border cells are responsible for tonic inhibition of extensor muscle α-motor neurons in the cervical intumescence.[6] Increased thoracic limb tone caused by the Schiff-Sherrington phenomenon is not accompanied by proprioceptive deficits or deficits in voluntary motor function.

Spinal Cord Segments C6-T2

The cervical intumescence gives rise to spinal nerves that make up the subscapular, suprascapular, musculocutaneous, axillary, radial, median, and ulnar nerves.[2] A lesion in the C6-T2 region causes UMN signs to the pelvic limbs (spastic paresis/paralysis, exaggerated segmental reflexes, and diminished to absent postural reactions) and LMN signs to the thoracic limbs (short-strided gait, flaccidity, diminished segmental reflexes, diminished to absent postural reactions, and rapidly progressing muscle atrophy). The animal also may limp or carry a thoracic limb because of nerve root compression (root signature). This neuropathic lameness often is confused with orthopedic disease. A neurogenic cause of the lameness frequently can be ascertained by identifying proprioceptive deficits, nonuniform muscle atrophy over the limb, or by electrodiagnostic testing. Additional signs may include absence of the cutaneous trunci reflex, Horner's syndrome, and decreased thoracic wall movement when breathing. The cutaneous trunci reflex may be absent (unilateral or bilateral) as a result of damage to the LMNs that contribute to the lateral thoracic nerve. Horner's syndrome (miosis, ptosis, and enophthalmos) results from damage to the sympathetic fibers that leave the spinal cord at this level. Decreased movement of the thoracic wall with respiration occurs because of the inability of the brainstem to control intercostal nerve function. If only the phrenic nerve is functioning properly, diaphragmatic (abdominal) breathing may be seen.

A characteristic gait can occur with lesions of the C6-T2 spinal cord segments. The pelvic limbs may show spinal ataxia and the thoracic limbs a short-strided gait. This mix of signs often is referred to as a *two-engine gait*.

Spinal Cord Segments C1-C5

Last, a lesion of spinal cord segments C1 to C5 may show UMN signs in the pelvic and thoracic limbs. Respiration may be shallow or absent because of the loss of phrenic and intercostal nerve function. Spinal ataxia of all limbs is seen, characterized by a long-strided or "floating" thoracic and pelvic limb gait.

Spinal Shock

In animals examined soon after spinal cord injury, a phenomenon called *spinal shock* may be present, leading to inaccurate neurolocalization. Spinal shock is a profound depression of segmental reflexes caudal to a lesion, despite reflex arcs remaining physically intact. In dogs, these signs often occur transiently, with evidence of areflexia lasting up to 12 to 24 hours after an injury.[11] This exemplifies the importance of performing serial neurologic examinations after a spinal cord injury to ensure accurate neurolocalization.

DIAGNOSIS

Once the neurologic examination is completed and a lesion or lesions are localized, a list of differential diagnoses should be formulated.[12] Differential diagnoses for spinal cord lesions include trauma (spinal fracture, luxation, or subluxation; bruise; compression by intervertebral disk), vascular diseases (hemorrhage, fibrocartilaginous emboli, infarct), neoplasia, malformations (compression from atlantoaxial subluxation or caudal cervical spondylomyelopathy; arachnoid cyst; syrinx) and, less commonly, infectious (toxoplasmosis, Rocky Mountain spotted fever, neosporosis, ehrlichiosis, feline infectious peritonitis, fungal, bacterial), inflammatory (granulomatous meningomyelitis), and degenerative disease (degenerative myelopathy). History, patient age and breed, onset and progression of signs, and presence or absence of pain help to generate a likely list of differential diagnoses (Table 83-2).

At this point, additional diagnostic tests should be performed. In cases of acute onset of clinical signs, plain radiographs of the spinal column, including lateral and ventrodorsal (or dorsoventral) views, or a CT scan should be obtained. Radiographs can show obvious fractures, displacement of vertebrae, narrowing of the intervertebral disk space, articular facets or intervertebral foramen, lytic lesions, or sclerotic lesions. However, as a means to diagnose intervertebral disk herniation, plain radiographs are inaccurate. The most useful

Table 83-2 **Differential Diagnoses for Spinal Cord Lesions Based on Signalment, History, and Physical Examination**

	Young	Old	Acute Onset	Insidious Onset	Progressive	Painful
Trauma	++	+	+	–	–	+
IVDD type 1	+	+	+	–	+	+
IVDD type 2	–	+	–	+	+	±
Vascular disease	+	+	+	–	–	–
Infectious and inflammatory disease	++	+	+	–	+	±
Degenerative disease	–	+	–	+	+	–
Anomalous or malformation	+	–	+	+	–	±
Neoplastic disease	+	++	+	+	+	±

IVDD, Intervertebral disk disease.
++, More likely; +, yes; –, no; ±, sometimes.

radiographic sign, a narrowed intervertebral space, had only moderate sensitivity (range 64% to 69%) and moderate predictive value (range 63% to 71%) for intervertebral disk protrusion.[13] CT is an accurate imaging modality for diagnosing intervertebral disk herniation, especially in the chondrodystrophoid patient that commonly develops intervertebral disk mineralization. Overall sensitivity for detection of disk herniation is similar for myelography (84%) versus CT (82%), although CT was more accurate in chronically affected dogs and dogs weighing more than 5 kg.[14] CT and CT myelography also may be the preferred imaging modalities for the diagnosis of vertebral fractures.[15] Finally, high-field MRI (1.5 T or greater), when available, is a suitable imaging modality for almost all causes of myelopathy. Intramedullary lesions or noncompressive nuclear pulposus extrusions may be missed if imaging modalities other than MRI are employed.[16] If inflammatory or infectious myelitis is a possibility, cerebrospinal fluid collection via lumbar puncture and analysis also is indicated.

TREATMENT

Emergency treatment of spinal cord injury may vary depending on the diagnosis. For all acute spinal cord injuries, intravenous fluid therapy is indicated because of presumed compromise of spinal cord vasculature that inhibits the normal autoregulation of arteriolar blood flow (see Chapters 59 and 60, respectively). As a result, blood flow to the damaged spinal cord is dependent on mean arterial blood pressure, so cardiovascular stability therefore must be optimized.[3,6]

If a fracture or displacement of the vertebral column is detected, the animal should be heavily sedated or anesthetized to place a splint that immobilizes the spine. In the case of a cervical fracture or displacement, the splint should be placed on the neck, extending from the rostral portion of the mandible to the manubrium of the sternum. Bandaging material can be used to hold the splint in place and should start just caudal to the ears and extend beyond the caudal aspect of both scapulae. If surgical management is not pursued and long-term cervical splint treatment is attempted, frequent changing of the bandage material and monitoring are essential. This is because soiling of the bandage during eating and drinking, frequent pyoderma, and pressure necrosis along the ventral mandible are commonly seen complications.

If surgery is required, the animal should be referred to an experienced surgeon. Surgical fixation has been indicated as the treatment of choice in animals with atlantoaxial subluxation to prevent recurrence of signs.[17] Fractures can be complicated. If the fracture incorporates the articular facets, the vertebral body, or both, internal fixation is recommended.[18] Luxations or subluxations that have compromised the ventral buttress (vertebral body, dorsal and ventral longitudinal ligaments, and intervertebral disks) are susceptible to rotation and require surgical repair to inhibit this movement.[18] However, for animals in which the neurologic status is not deteriorating, external support and strict rest are the treatments of choice for displaced or unstable fractures of the cervical spine.[19] This is due to the high incidence of mortality (approximately 40%) associated with surgical intervention for cervical fractures.[19] Smaller dogs may be splinted along the ventral cervical region, whereas larger dogs often need dorsal and ventral, or even circumferential splinting. Fiberglass splinting is an effective medium because it is rigid yet lightweight. Splinting the thoracic or lumbar vertebral column is more challenging because of the anatomic location. When available, surgical stabilization is recommended for displaced or unstable fractures of the thoracic or lumbar vertebrae. Intervertebral disk disease resulting in Grade 3 or greater deficits (see Table 83-1), recurrent episodes, and episodes unresponsive to medical treatment should be treated with surgical decompression.

Sacrococcygeal or intracoccygeal fractures or luxations are a common injury after trauma in cats, most likely because of a tractional injury to the tail. Neurologic deficits resulting from injuries in this location can be especially devastating in cats because of extension of the spinal cord more caudally (to the level of the sacrum) compared with dogs. Prognosis depends on the extent of the injury. Prompt surgical stabilization and tail amputation are recommended to prevent further spinal cord and/or cauda equina injury.[20]

Pain control for animals with spinal cord injury often requires pure opioid agonists (fentanyl, hydromorphone, oxymorphone, or morphine) or a partial opioid agonist (buprenorphine). If these medications are used, the patient should be monitored closely for respiratory depression (see Chapter 144).

Treatment for spinal cord edema and lipid peroxidation is a controversial subject. Methylprednisolone sodium succinate at 30 mg/kg IV has been shown to improve some aspects of neurologic outcome in humans if given within 8 hours of the injury,[21] although similar studies have not been performed in the dog or cat. Subsequent doses of methylprednisolone sodium succinate at 10 mg/kg IV can be given at 2 hours and 6 hours, and then once every 8 hours for up to 48 hours after trauma. Gastrointestinal protectants such as histamine-2 blockers (e.g., famotidine) can be given for 24 to 48 hours postinjury to decrease the likelihood gastric irritation or ulcers induced by injury and steroid administration (see Chapter 161). However, it is unlikely that antacid therapy will prevent gastrointestinal complications.[22]

Novel treatment therapies for improving functional recovery after subacute spinal injury are being explored within the research setting.

Transplantation of mesenchymal stem cells into the spinal parenchyma has proven to be a safe procedure with histologic improvements seen in treated cords. However, to date, no functional improvements have been shown after this type of therapy in the experimental model.[23] This treatment is one of several that has shown potential to improve outcomes in human and veterinary patients after spinal cord injury. Future investigation likely will reveal additional therapeutic options for clinical research.

PROGNOSIS

The prognosis for animals with spinal cord injury is variable and often difficult to predict. Many factors play a role in outcome including age, size, and breed of the animal, etiology, onset of clinical signs, severity of signs, location of disease, and type of therapy. Animals with cervical spinal cord injury caused by trauma, atlantoaxial subluxation, and intervertebral disk herniation have differing prognoses. Dogs with cervical spinal trauma have been reported to have a good prognosis (recovery rate of 82%) if the animal does not suffer from pulmonary complications.[19] Animals with atlantoaxial subluxations resulting in severe neurologic deficits that are treated conservatively (i.e., splint stabilization) are reported to have a good to guarded prognosis for recovery (good outcome in 62.5% of dogs), but approximately 25% relapse at a later date.[17] Those treated with surgical stabilization also are reported to have a good to guarded prognosis for recovery,[17] with success rates ranging from 61% to 91%.[24-26] The treatment of cervical intervertebral disk herniation (IVDH) with ventral slot surgery in animals with tetraparesis or tetraplegia led to a 56% chance of recovery in 1 to 6 weeks in one study; animals with only pelvic limb paresis had a 75% chance of recovery in 3 to 8 weeks.[27] Another study reported better outcomes in patients with high cervical intervertebral disk herniation (C2-C3 and C3-C4); long-term resolution after ventral decompression was seen in 66% of dogs. However, in animals with caudal cervical sites of intervertebral disk herniation (IVDH) (C4-C5, C5-C6, and C6-C7), long-term resolution of signs was seen in only 21% of cases.[28] Dogs that are presented because of cervical spondylomyelopathy (Wobbler's syndrome) are often large- to giant-breed dogs. Even with surgical correction, patients presenting with a nonambulatory tetraparesis may have prolonged recovery until unassisted ambulation is achieved. In one study, dogs that were presented with nonambulatory tetraparesis took an average of 2½ months to regain unassisted ambulation after dorsal laminectomy.[29] The most common postoperative complications include vertebral instability and subluxation. Another important complication is hypoventilation requiring ventilatory support. This was seen in 4.9% of dogs that underwent surgery for cervical spinal cord disorders but carries a good prognosis after short-term mechanical ventilation.[30]

Thoracolumbar spinal cord injuries also have shown varying reports of success. In a study of nine cases of traumatic injuries (car accidents or falls from height) that resulted in the loss of deep pain sensation, none of the dogs regained deep pain sensation with treatment (six treated conservatively and the remaining three treated surgically). However, two dogs did regain the ability to walk (spinal walking).[31] Another report indicated that loss of deep pain sensation because of thoracolumbar luxation or fracture resulted in a less than 10% recovery rate (i.e., motor ability).[2,32] A loss of deep pain for more than 12 to 24 hours after injury and severe luxation or displacement of vertebral bodies also carries a poor to grave prognosis.[33] Overall, the prognosis for recovery after trauma to the thoracolumbar spinal cord that results in the loss of deep pain sensation is grave. In animals with thoracolumbar disk herniation, many studies have revealed varying rates of recovery (25% to 76%) for dogs that did not have deep pain sensation in the pelvic limbs.[25,34-38] In a study examining dogs presented for acute intervertebral disk herniation with lack of deep pain perception (DPP) that were treated surgically via decompressive hemilaminectomy, 58% regained the ability to walk and DPP, 11% regained the ability to walk but not DPP, 17% remained paraplegic without DPP, and 14% were euthanized.[39] In contrast, the recovery rate for dogs that have retained deep pain sensation in the pelvic limbs is good (86% to 96% success).[37,38] In a study of 36 dogs presenting for acute paraplegia with loss of nociception resulting from severe, acute thoracolumbar disk herniation treated with decompressive hemilaminectomy, cranial progression of the cutaneous trunci reflex was examined as a potential prognostic indicator. All dogs with caudal progression of the cutaneous trunci reflex showed improvement by 12 to 20 weeks. Five of six dogs with cranial progression of the cutaneous trunci reflex developed ascending myelomalacia and were euthanized. This underscores the importance of continued serial neurologic evaluation in the postsurgical patient.

ACKNOWLEDGMENT

The authors would like to acknowledge and thank Kersten Johnson, MS, DVM, DACVIM-Neurology, for her original contribution as an author of the first edition of this chapter.

REFERENCES

1. Olby NJ, De Risio L, Muñana KR, et al: Development of a functional scoring system in dog with acute spinal cord injuries, Am J Vet Res 62:1624, 2001.
2. Sharp NJ, Wheeler SJ: Small animal spinal disorders, ed 2, Edinburgh, 2005, Mosby.
3. Davies JV, Sharp JH: A comparison of conservative treatment and fenestration for thoracolumbar intervertebral disc disease in the dog, J Small Anim Pract 24:12, 1983.
4. Olby NJ: Current concepts in the management of acute spinal cord injury, J Vet Intern Med 13:399, 1999.
5. Park EH, White GA, Tieber LM: Mechanisms of injury and emergency care of acute spinal cord injuries in dogs and cats, J Vet Emerg Crit Care 22:1, 2012.
6. Jeffry ND, Blakemore WF: Spinal cord injury in small animals: 1. Mechanisms of spontaneous recovery, Vet Rec 144:407, 1999.
7. Evans HE: Miller's anatomy of the dog, ed 3, Philadelphia, 1993, Saunders.
8. DeLahunta A: Veterinary neuroanatomy and clinical neurology, ed 3, St Louis, 2011, Saunders.
9. Kot W, Partlow GD, Parent J: Anatomical survey of the cat's lumbosacral spinal cord, Prog Vet Neurol 5:162, 1994.
10. Rowland LP: Diseases of the motor unit. In Kandell ER, Schwartz JH, Jessell TM, editors: Principles of neural science, ed 4, New York, 2000, McGraw-Hill.
11. Smith PM, Jeffery ND: Spinal shock: comparative aspects and clinical relevance, J Vet Intern Med 19:788, 2005.
12. Marioni K, Vite CH, Newton AL, et al: Prevalence of diseases of the spinal cord of cats, J Vet Intern Med 18:851, 2004.
13. Lamb CR, Nicholls A, Targett M, et al: Accuracy of survey radiographic diagnosis of intervertebral disc protrusion in dogs, Vet Radiol Ultrasound 43:3, 2005.30.
14. Israel SK, Levine JM, Kerwin SC, et al: The relative sensitivity of computed tomography and myelography for identification and thoracolumbar intervertebral disc herniations in dogs, Vet Radiol Ultrasound 50:3, 2009.
15. Robertson I, Thrall DE: Imaging dogs with suspected disc herniation: pros and cons of myelography, computed tomography, and magnetic resonance, Vet Radiol Ultrasound 52:1, 2011.
16. Henke D, Gorgas D, Flegel T, et al: Magnetic resonance imaging findings in dogs with traumatic intervertebral disk herniations with and without spinal cord compression: 31 cases (2006-2010), J Am Vet Med Assoc 242:2, 2013.

17. Havig ME, Cornell KK, Hawthorne JC, et al: Evaluation of nonsurgical treatment of atlantoaxial subluxation in dogs: 19 cases, J Am Vet Med Assoc 227:257, 2005.
18. Patterson RH, Smith GK: Backsplinting for treatment of thoracic and lumbar fracture/luxation in the dog, Vet Comp Orthop Traumatol 5:179, 1992.
19. Hawthorn JC, Blevins WE, Wallace LJ, et al: Cervical vertebral fractures in 56 dogs: a retrospective study, J Am Anim Hosp Assoc 35:135, 1999.
20. Eminaga S, Palus V, Cherubini G: Acute spinal cord injury in the cat: causes, treatment and prognosis, J Fel Med Surg 13:850, 2011.
21. Bracken MB, Shephard MJ, Holford TR, et al: Administration of methylprednisolone for 24 or 48 hours or tirilazad mesylate for 48 hours in the treatment of acute spinal cord injury. Results of the third national acute spinal cord injury randomized controlled trial, J Am Med Assoc 277:1597, 1997.
22. Neiger R, Gaschen F, Jaggy A: Gastric mucosal lesions in dogs with acute intervertebral disc disease: Characterization and effects of omeprazole or misoprostol, J Vet Intern Med 14:33, 2000.
23. Ryu H, Kang B, Kim Y, et al: Comparison of mesenchymal stem cells derived from fat, bone marrow, Wharton's jelly, and umbilical cord blood for treating spinal cord injuries in dogs, J Vet Med Sci 74:12, 2012.
24. McCarthy RJ, Lewis DD, Hosgood G: Atlantoaxial subluxation in dogs, Compend Contin Educ Vet Pract 17:215, 1995.
25. Denny HR, Gibbs C, Waterman A: Atlantoaxial subluxation in the dog: a review of 30 cases and an evaluation of treatment by lag screw fixation, J Small Anim Pract 29:37, 1988.
26. Thomas WB, Sorjonen DC, Simpson ST: Surgical management of atlantoaxial subluxation in 23 dogs, Vet Surg 20:409, 1991.
27. Denny HR: The surgical treatment of cervical disc protrusions in the dog: a review of 40 cases, J Small Anim Pract 19:251, 1978.
28. Fitch RB, Kerwin SC, Hosgood G: Caudal cervical intervertebral disk disease in the small dog: role of distraction and stabilization in ventral slot decompression, J Am Anim Hosp Assoc 36:68, 2000.
29. Risio LD, Munana K, Murray M, et al: Dorsal laminectomy for caudal cervical spondylomyelopathy: Post-operative recovery and log-tern follow-up in 20 dogs, Vet Surg 31:5, 2002.
30. Beal MW, Paglia DT, Griffin GM, et al: Ventilatory failure, ventilator management, and outcome in dogs with cervical spinal disorders: 14 cases (1991-1999), J Am Vet Med Assoc 218:1598, 2001.
31. Bagley RS: Spinal fracture or luxation, Vet Clin North Am Small Anim Pract 30:133, 2000.
32. Brown NO, Helphrey ML, Prata RG: Thoracolumbar disc disease in the dog: a retrospective analysis of 187 cases, J Am Anim Hosp Assoc 13:665, 1977.
33. Olby NJ, Levine J, Harris T, et al: Long-term functional outcome of dogs with severe injuries of the thoracolumbar spinal cord: 87 cases (1996-2001), J Am Vet Med Assoc 222:762, 2003.
34. Gambardella PC: Dorsal decompressive laminectomy for treatment of thoracolumbar disc disease in dogs: a retrospective study of 98 cases, Vet Surg 9:24, 1980.
35. Anderson SM, Lippincot CL, Gill PJ: Hemilaminectomy in dogs without deep pain perception, Calif Vet 45:24, 1991.
36. Scott HW, Mckee WM: Laminectomy for 34 dogs with thoracolumbar intervertebral disc disease and loss of deep pain perception, J Small Anim Pract 40:417, 1999.
37. Brisson BA, Moffatt SL, Swayne SL, et al: Recurrence of thoracolumbar intervertebral disk extrusion in chondrodystrophic dogs after surgical decompression with or without prophylactic fenestration: 265 cases (1995-1999), J Am Vet Med Assoc 224:1808, 2004.
38. Ferreira AJ, Correira JH, Jaggy A: Thoracolumbar disc disease in 71 paraplegic dogs: influence of rate of onset and duration of clinical signs on treatment results, J Small Anim Pract 43:158, 2002.
39. Olby N, Levine J, Harris T, et al: Long-term functional outcome of dogs with severe injuries of the thoracolumbar spinal cord: 87 cases (1996-2001), J Am Vet Med Assoc 222:6, 2003.

CHAPTER 84

INTRACRANIAL HYPERTENSION

Beverly K. Sturges, DVM, MS, DACVIM (Neurology) •
Richard A. LeCouteur, BVSc, PhD, DACVIM (Neurology), DECVN

KEY POINTS

- Intracranial hypertension (ICH) is the persistent elevation of intracranial pressure (ICP) above the normal range of 5 to 12 mm Hg.
- Causes include trauma, hemorrhage, infarction, ischemia, edema, masses, encephalopathy, and status epilepticus.
- Intracranial hypertension develops when the volume of the intracranial contents exceeds the accommodation of compensatory mechanisms.
- Intracranial hypertension damages the brain through its deleterious effects on cerebral blood flow (CBF) and oxygen delivery, causing hypoxia, ischemia, and brain herniation.
- The primary treatment goals are maintenance of cerebral blood flow and tissue oxygenation without contributing to intracranial hypertension.
- Effective management of intracranial hypertension includes critical maintenance of cerebral perfusion pressure (CPP) and often requires hyperosmolar therapy.

PHYSIOLOGY OF INTRACRANIAL PRESSURE

Intracranial Fluid Dynamics

The collective volume of intracranial contents is the major determinant of intracranial pressure (ICP). The cranial space may be divided into four distinct physiologic compartments, each with separately regulated water content: blood, cerebrospinal fluid (CSF), intracellular fluid (ICF), and extracellular fluid (ECF).

Cerebrospinal Fluid Flow

Most CSF is formed by ultrafiltration of fluid from the blood vessels of the choroid plexus lining the ventricles and drains into the subarachnoid space, from where it is absorbed. When ventricular pressure is elevated, the flow of fluid may be reversed, back into the brain parenchyma.[2] As compensation for intracranial hypertension (ICH), CSF production falls, absorption increases, and a greater volume of CSF is displaced into the spinal subarachnoid space.[1,3]

Brain Water Movement

The blood-brain barrier (BBB) tightly regulates the entry of solutes into the brain but is permeable to water. Changes in effective osmolality across the BBB are accompanied by water movement to equalize osmolality, but at the expense of changes in cell volume. With increases in the osmolality of intravascular fluid or ECF, ICF may shift to the extracellular environment. With persistence of hyperosmolar conditions in the ECF for many hours, brain cells, having lost volume, compensate by generating intracellular osmolytes (idiogenic osmoles) to raise the osmotic draw intracellularly and restore cell volume. Breakdown of these idiogenic osmoles occurs over several days. Rapid decreases in ECF osmolality should be prevented, because the intracellular osmolytes may draw water into the cell, causing cell swelling, membrane disruption, and exacerbation of ICH.[4]

Cerebral Blood Flow

The high metabolic demands of the brain require maintaining cerebral blood flow (CBF) in the normal range at all times. CBF is dependent on cerebral perfusion pressure (CPP), which is calculated as mean arterial pressure (MAP) minus ICP[4-6]:

$$CPP = MAP - ICP$$

The volume of blood in the brain (cerebral blood volume [CBV]) is affected by factors that change CBF, such as altered vascular tone or blood viscosity, and those that impair venous outflow, such as head-down posture, jugular vein compression, or increased intrathoracic pressure.[1,4,5] Cerebrovascular vasodilation increases CBF and thereby CBV, leading to increased ICP; cerebral vasoconstriction decreases CBF, CBV, and therefore ICP but may result in hypoxia and neuronal ischemia.[1,4,5]

INTRACRANIAL PRESSURE

ICP is the pressure inside the cranial vault exerted by the tissues and fluids against the encasing bone. Normal ICP in the dog is 5 to 12 mm Hg. This is similar to that of humans, for whom 20 mm Hg is an arbitrary upper limit, beyond which treatment for ICH may be instituted[1,3] (see Chapter 191). The upper limit of ICP, above which treatment is indicated for ICH, has not been defined in dogs and cats. It seems reasonable to use the human guidelines for ICH until species-specific information is available.

Homeostatic Responses of the Brain

Three primary homeostatic mechanisms maintain ICP within a range at which the brain is functional. These include volume buffering, autoregulation, and the Cushing response.[1,4-6]

Volume buffering

The brain is relatively noncompressible and is encased in bone, causing the volume of the intracranial contents to be fixed. Increase in the volume of one component requires a compensatory decrease in one or more of the others if ICP is to remain unchanged (Monro-Kellie doctrine). Sources of added volume include tumor, hemorrhage, CSF accumulation, vascular congestion, cerebral edema, and decreases in venous outflow. Immediate volume buffering responses, specifically displacement of blood and CSF extracranially, are reflected by the pressure-volume curve that relates the temporal change in ICP to expanding intracranial volume (Figure 84-1).

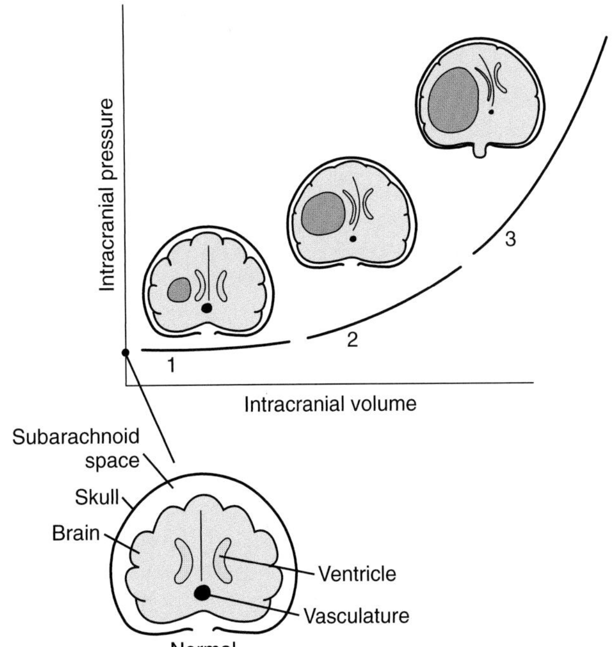

FIGURE 84-1 Pressure-volume curve. An idealized elastance curve that illustrates changes in intracranial pressure (ICP) accompanying the progressive addition of intracranial volume. *First segment:* Compliance is high, compensatory mechanisms are functioning well, primarily a result of expansion of the dura mater in the cranial and cervical spinal space, allowing for added volume with no or little increase in ICP. *Second segment:* As volume is added to the system, displacement of cerebrospinal fluid and blood allow for further volume additions with progressive changes in ICP. *Third segment:* The vertical portion of the elastance curve shows the high-pressure, low-compliance situation that occurs when the volume buffering capacity is exhausted. Further displacement of intracranial fluids is not possible and addition of more volume causes an exponential rise in ICP. Decompensation is occurring and any volume buffering at this point is due to distention, compression, and eventual herniation of neural tissues.

Autoregulatory mechanisms

Pressure autoregulation

Autoregulation of CBF results from a vascular (myogenic) reflex that changes resistance of cerebral arterioles in response to changes in transmural pressure. The purpose is to prevent underperfusion or overperfusion of the brain. Normally this mechanism operates at perfusion pressures between 50 and 150 mm Hg. Outside this range, CBF becomes linear with MAP (Figure 84-2).[1,4,5]

Chemical autoregulation

Chemical regulation of cerebral vascular resistance is influenced by three factors: partial pressure of arterial carbon dioxide ($PaCO_2$), partial pressure of arterial oxygen (PaO_2), and cerebral metabolic rate of oxygen consumption.[1,4,5]

Partial Pressure of Arterial Carbon Dioxide. Cerebral vascular resistance is directly responsive to changes in $PaCO_2$ concentrations, because carbon dioxide combines with water to form hydrogen ions, which, when increased in concentration, stimulate cerebral vasodilation and when decreased, may cause vasoconstriction. Therefore, in the normal brain, hyperventilation decreases $PaCO_2$, causing vasoconstriction, reduced cerebral blood volume, and lowering of ICP.

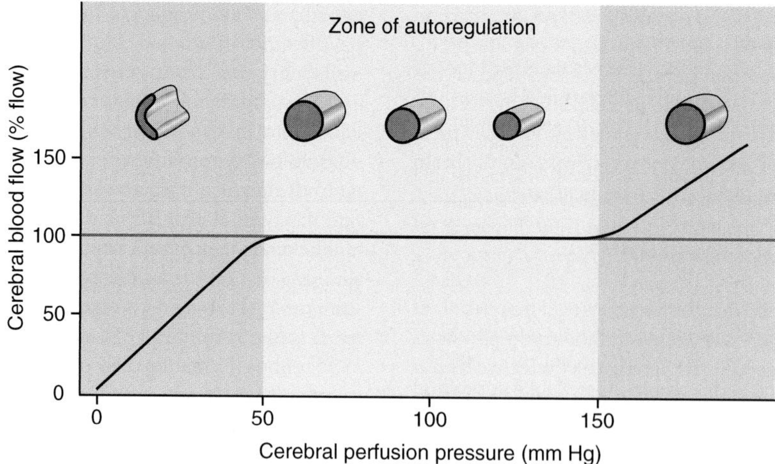

FIGURE 84-2 Classic cerebral pressure autoregulation curve. Cerebral autoregulation maintains a relatively constant rate of cerebral blood flow across a wide of range of cerebral perfusion pressures as shown (50 to 150 mm Hg). With intact autoregulation, cerebrovascular tone appears to respond to transmural pressure, which is approximately the same as cerebral perfusion pressure. Note the marked rise and fall in cerebral blood flow as cerebral perfusion pressure changes above and below, respectively, the normal limits of autoregulation. With impairment of autoregulation in the injured brain, cerebral blood flow passively follows systemic arterial blood pressure.

Partial Pressure of Arterial Oxygen. Decreases in PaO_2 cause vasodilation, resulting in increased CBF, CBV, and ICP.

Cerebral Metabolic Rate of Oxygen Consumption. CBF is coupled to local cerebral metabolism. In regions of high cerebral metabolic activity, pH alterations in the perivascular environment have a direct influence on cerebral vascular tone. Increased hydrogen ion concentration, as seen with lactic acidosis or accumulation of other acids formed during the course of cerebral metabolism, causes an increase in CBF. When cerebral metabolic rate of oxygen consumption is decreased, low levels of hydrogen ion concentration result in decreased CBF locally as a result of arteriolar constriction.

Cushing Response

Autoregulation often is impaired in animals with intracranial disease, in which pressure autoregulation generally is affected first and chemically mediated regulation is increasingly affected as brain injury progresses. When volume buffering and autoregulatory adjustments are exhausted, ICH leads to decreased CBF, cerebral ischemia, and accumulation of carbon dioxide. Decreased CBF and elevated carbon dioxide levels can stimulate the release of catecholamines, which may cause systemic vasoconstriction and increased cardiac output. Baroreceptors sense this hypertensive state and cause a vagally mediated bradycardia. Hypertension and bradycardia secondary to ICH is known as the *Cushing response.* The catecholamine release also may result in cardiac arrhythmias because of myocardial ischemia, the so-called "brain-heart syndrome."

CAUSES OF INTRACRANIAL HYPERTENSION

In general terms, causes of ICH can be classified as vascular or nonvascular. Vascular mechanisms of ICH include cerebral vasodilation caused by increased $PaCO_2$, distention of cerebral vessels resulting from loss of vascular tone, or venous outflow obstruction. Nonvascular mechanisms include increased brain water (interstitial edema or intracellular swelling), masses, or obstruction of CSF outflow.

Pressure gradients associated with ICH may result in movement of neural tissues within and between anatomic compartments (brain herniation) that may perpetuate injury and ischemia by distorting or fracturing brain tissue, and by compression and shearing of cerebral vasculature.[1,7]

CLINICAL ASPECTS OF INTRACRANIAL HYPERTENSION

A complete history and physical examination are essential in the assessment of patients suspected to have ICH. A careful neurologic examination is required for accurate clinical diagnosis, institution of therapy, and determination of a baseline to which results of future examinations may be compared. Aspects of the neurologic examination that are of particular importance include level of consciousness, brainstem reflexes, respiratory pattern, motor responses, abnormal postures, and breathing patterns. Papilledema identified on fundic examination is a reliable sign of ICH.

Level of Consciousness

Four levels of consciousness are recognized:

1. *Alert and responsive:* normal responses to sensory stimuli; expected behavior
2. *Obtunded (depressed):* slow or inappropriate response to sensory stimuli
3. *Stuporous (semicomatose):* generally unresponsive, except to vigorous or painful stimuli
4. *Comatose:* complete unresponsiveness to repeated noxious stimulation

The mechanisms responsible for consciousness are located in the rostral brainstem, the ascending reticular activation system (ARAS; reticular formation), and diffusely throughout the cerebrum.

Progression from a higher to a lower level of consciousness often is caused by elevation of ICP. Although focal loss of autoregulation may not be recognized clinically, unconscious animals are likely to have global impairment of autoregulatory responses.[1,4]

Brainstem Reflexes

Size and reactivity of pupils

The midbrain and efferent parasympathetic fibers of the oculomotor nerve (cranial nerve III [CN III]) are responsible for pupillary constriction. In the absence of ophthalmic injury, abnormalities in pupil size or reactivity indicate brainstem dysfunction. Several patterns of pupillary abnormality are commonly recognized in patients with ICH:

1. *Mydriasis* usually denotes a lesion (ipsilateral or bilateral) of the midbrain or the CN III.
2. *Miosis* may occur ipsilateral to severe brainstem injury or as part of Horner's syndrome (ptosis, enophthalmos, third eyelid protrusion), indicating a lesion affecting the sympathetic pathway to the eye.
3. *Severe bilateral miosis* is a sign of acute, extensive brain disturbance and probably occurs as a result of functional disturbance of higher centers, with release of CN III efferents from cerebral inhibition.
4. *Severe, unresponsive bilateral mydriasis* generally indicates a grave prognosis, and it often accompanies brain herniation.

The return of pupils to normal size and responsiveness to light is a favorable prognostic sign.

Resting eye position, eye movements, and oculovestibular reflexes

1. Resting eye position and presence of spontaneous nystagmus should be noted. Eye abduction may be caused by medial rectus muscle paresis because of CN III damage. Adduction may be caused by lateral rectus muscle paresis resulting from abducens nerve (CN VI) damage, or damage to the rostral medulla oblongata or pons.
2. Oculovestibular movements are elicited by moving the head from side to side or vertically. Conjugate oculovestibular movements require integrity of the brainstem pathways from the cranial cervical spinal cord and medulla oblongata rostrally to the nuclei of CN III, CN IV (trochlear nerve), and CN VI, via the medial longitudinal fasciculus. Thus the oculovestibular maneuver is a convenient method for examination of the functional integrity of large areas of the brainstem and the cranial nerves involved in eye movements.

Corneal reflexes

Although evaluation of corneal reflexes alone rarely is useful, findings may corroborate eye movement abnormalities. Touching the cornea with a wisp of cotton should cause bilateral eyelid closure. The corneal reflex may be absent when the afferent trigeminal nerve (CN V), the efferent facial nerve (CN VII), or their reflex connections within the pons and medulla oblongata are damaged.

Respiration

Breathing is regulated principally by respiratory centers in the caudal brainstem between the midpons and cervicomedullary junction. Respiratory patterns have proven useful but inconsistent in localizing brain injury.

1. *Cheyne-Stokes respiration* consists of phases of hyperpnea regularly alternating with apnea. Its presence implies a lesion deep in the cerebral hemispheres or in the rostral brainstem.[1]
2. *Central neurogenic hyperventilation* consists of sustained, rapid, fairly deep, and regular respirations at a rate of approximately 25 breaths/min, with hypocapnia. This respiratory pattern may indicate a lesion in the caudal midbrain and pons.[1]
3. *Neurogenic pulmonary edema* may occur almost instantaneously after rostral brainstem injury in the absence of direct pulmonary trauma.[1] ICH occasionally may result in neurogenic pulmonary edema.
4. *Gasping or chaotic respirations* reflect caudal brainstem damage and represent the terminal respiratory pattern of severe ICH. The appearance of, or progression to, abnormal respiratory patterns, strongly suggests that the animal is deteriorating and mandates more aggressive medical therapy or surgery.[1]

Motor Responses

Ataxia and paresis may determined by observing the gait and response to testing of postural reactions. If an animal is nonambulatory, voluntary movement of the limbs is determined based on response to noxious stimuli.

Posture

Decerebrate rigidity occurs with midbrain lesions and is characterized by unconsciousness, recumbency, opisthotonos, and rigid extension of all limbs. This posture signifies a grave prognosis and must be distinguished from decerebellate posture, which is caused by a lesion in the cerebellum characterized by extensor rigidity in the thoracic (and sometimes all) limbs in a conscious animal, and Schiff-Sherrington phenomenon, in which extensor rigidity is present in the thoracic limbs but the pelvic limbs show signs of severe myelopathy due to a lesion in the thoracolumbar spinal cord (brain not involved).

DIAGNOSIS OF INTRACRANIAL HYPERTENSION

In the absence of direct ICP monitoring, a clinical diagnosis of ICH usually is based on results of serial neurologic examinations. Ultimately, if ICH is not controlled, significant shifts in brain parenchyma occur, leading to forcible movement of brain tissue, or herniation. CT or MR imaging may be more sensitive than clinical examination in detecting brain herniation in animals. For example, a slow-growing brain tumor may cause significant cerebellar herniation in a patient without clinical signs of ICH.

Brain death usually is indicated clinically by coma, absence of spontaneous respiration, and loss of brainstem reflexes (e.g., fixed, dilated pupils). Additional criteria used in human patients include an isoelectric electroencephalogram and absence of CBF on arteriographic evaluation.[1]

TREATMENT OF INTRACRANIAL HYPERTENSION

Appropriate treatment of ICH is often more important to the short-term survival of the patient than primary treatment of the underlying brain disease. Treatment goals include reduction of intracranial volume and prevention of secondary brain injury by restoration and maintenance of circulating blood volume, blood pressure, oxygenation, and ventilation[4-6,8] (Box 84-1).

BOX 84-1 ***Concepts in Management of Intracranial Hypertension***

Reduction of Intracranial Volume

Reducing brain size and edema
Reducing CSF volume and obstruction to flow
Reducing cerebral blood volume
Reducing the size of pathologic process (tumor, hematoma, inflammation)
Increasing the space for expansion of structures by decompressive craniectomy

Prevention of Secondary Brain Injury

Preventing hypoxia
Preventing hypotension
Maintaining euvolemia, euglycemia
Maintaining electrolyte and acid-base balance
Managing seizures, fever, SIRS, MODS

CSF, Cerebrospinal fluid; *MODS,* multiple organ dysfunction syndrome; *SIRS,* systemic inflammatory response syndrome.

General Supportive Care

The initial step is to recognize and correct life-threatening, nonneural injuries, especially in the case of brain trauma.[8,9] Shock most often is due to tissue damage and blood loss from other organs; intracranial disease alone, including head trauma, rarely results in shock.

Prevent hypoxia

The animal should be placed in an oxygen-rich environment with its head elevated and a clear airway. Oxygen supplementation does not prevent hypercapnia in a hypoventilating animal. Tracheal intubation and mechanical ventilation are indicated in apneic or hypoventilating patients.[8,9]

Prevent hypotension

Prevention and management of hypotension are central to the treatment of ICH; therefore intensive monitoring of arterial blood pressure is essential.[4,8,9]

Guidelines for Specific Therapy of Intracranial Hypertension

After general supportive measures have been completed, medical treatment is instituted to reduce brain edema, decrease ICP, and maintain cerebrovascular perfusion and tissue oxygenation. The patient should be assessed (at least) every 15 to 30 minutes until stabilized. A response to therapy should be seen within 2 hours; if a response does not occur, medical therapy should be reassessed, and surgical therapy considered (Box 84-2).

Maintain adequate cerebral perfusion pressure

Maintenance of adequate CPP is the theoretical basis for managing ICH.[1,10,11] For CPP to remain constant, the MAP must increase when ICP increases. If the ICP cannot be controlled after adequate fluid resuscitation, vasopressors may be considered to increase MAP.[10] However, in the absence of cerebral ischemia, attempts to maintain CPP at more than 70 mm Hg with pressors should not be pursued aggressively.[10,11] CPP in dogs and cats ideally is maintained at 50 to 90 mm Hg. When it is not possible to monitor ICP, mean arterial blood pressure should be maintained at or above 80 mm Hg.

BOX 84-2 Suggested Protocols for Initiating Management of Intracranial Hypertension

Management for ICH

All patients with evidence of ICH or at risk of developing ICH

Prevention of hypercapnia with a target $PaCO_2$ of 30 to 35 mm Hg
Oxygen supplementation as needed to maintain a $PaO_2 >$ 80 mm Hg
Head elevation (30 degrees) and prevention of jugular compression
Removal of causes of increased intrathoracic pressure
Control of systemic factors

- Prevent hypotension
- Prevent hypoxemia
- Prevent electrolyte and acid-base imbalances
- Maintain euvolemia and euglycemia

Clinical Evidence of Marked ICH: Deteriorating Neurologic Status

All of the above therapies
Hyperosmolar agents
Ventricular CSF drainage if feasible

Clinical Evidence of Severe ICH: Comatose Mental State, or Rapid Neurologic Deterioration

All of the above therapies
Hyperventilation therapy
Barbiturate coma
Decompressive craniectomy

CSF, Cerebrospinal fluid; *ICH,* intracranial hypertension; *$PaCO_2$,* partial pressure of arterial carbon dioxide; *PaO_2,* partial pressure of arterial oxygen.

Decrease cerebral venous blood volume

Head elevation promotes drainage of venous blood to reduce ICP. Neck wraps, improper positioning of the head and neck, or positive end-expiratory pressure may impair venous drainage, causing an increase in brain volume.

Control $PaCO_2$

The most important factor controlling CBF and CBV is $PaCO_2$.[5] Controlled ventilation, used judiciously, can lower ICH by vasoconstriction and reduced CBF. The target $PaCO_2$ is 30 to 35 mm Hg. Lower values may lead to neuronal ischemia and exacerbation of ICH.[5,11,12]

Control PaO_2

CBF begins to increase when PaO_2 falls below 60 mm Hg. However, the brain is even more sensitive to arterial oxygen content. For example, in humans, halving the hematocrit doubles the CBF, even if PaO_2 is higher than 60 mm Hg.[5]

Reduce cerebral edema with hyperosmolar fluid therapy

Reduction of brain water content has long been theorized to be an effective means of controlling ICP. To this end, the misguided practice of dehydrating patients by using diuretics or restricting fluids was used initially to manage ICH. In more recent years, hyperosmolar agents, primarily mannitol or hypertonic saline, have been used widely.[8,10,11] The superiority of either mannitol or hypertonic saline for the treatment of ICH is unknown.[13-16] A recent meta-analysis concluded that hypertonic saline was more effective in treating ICH when compared with mannitol.[15] Despite this, numerous studies support the use of mannitol, and the topic remains controversial in the literature. The patient's fluid and electrolyte balance should be determined before starting hyperosmolar therapy.

Mannitol

The short-term beneficial effects of mannitol on ICH, CPP, and CBF are accepted widely.[8,10,11,17] A comparison of the action of equimolar doses of mannitol versus hypertonic saline in normal rats found that mannitol reduced brain water by a greater extent for a period of 5 hours.[16] Although the mechanism of action is controversial, mannitol probably has two effects: (1) an immediate (within minutes) plasma-expanding effect that reduces blood viscosity, thus increasing CBF and the delivery of oxygen to the brain, and (2) a delayed osmotic effect that occurs 15 to 30 minutes after administration when gradients are established between plasma and cells, causing a reduction in brain water content. An osmotic increase of at least 10 mOsm is thought to be required for this effect to be seen. This delayed effect persists for 1 to 3 hours. It is considered best not to exceed a plasma osmolality of 320 mOsm/kg. However, the authors have used hyperosmolar therapy routinely in animals with blood osmolalities higher than this, without adverse effects, in situations of severe ICH. Strict monitoring and maintenance of fluid and electrolyte balance are essential during mannitol therapy. The recommended dosage is 20% mannitol solution 0.5 to 1 gm/kg IV over 20 minutes.

Mannitol should be administered as repeated doses, not as a continuous infusion. Dangers of repeated dosage are related to effects on

BOX 84-3 ***Precautions for Use of Mannitol***

1. Maintain euvolemia. Correct hypovolemia before use, but do not overhydrate. A catheter placed in the urinary bladder to monitor urine output facilitates this aspect of treatment.
2. Use a fluid line filter when administering mannitol or dissolve visible crystals in solution before use.
3. Administer as a slow bolus over 20 minutes.
4. If possible, monitor and maintain serum osmolality at or below 320 mOsm/L, particularly when there is concern for renal failure.
5. Monitor serum electrolytes and acid base balance and maintain in normal range.
6. Monitor urine output. If urine is not produced within 15 minutes of mannitol administration, give furosemide to induce diuresis.
7. Do not use when clear evidence of ongoing intracranial hemorrhage is present, for example, imaging evidence.

blood volume and electrolytes rather than specific toxicity. Mannitol may accumulate in the brain parenchyma, especially in an injured area, possibly leading to a rebound effect of increasing ICP when it is discontinued. Preventing hypovolemia after mannitol administration may reduce this complication[8,17] (Box 84-3).

Hypertonic Saline

Hypertonic saline is a useful therapy for ICH.[8,10,18,19] Animal models have shown it to be as effective as mannitol in reducing cerebral water content.[18] Since the sodium is reabsorbed in the kidneys, there is less likelihood of causing hypotension than with mannitol, making hypertonic saline a safe choice for patients with ICH and systemic hypotension. It also may have beneficial effects on excitatory neurotransmitters, as well as on the immune system.

The recommended dosage is sodium chloride 7.5% solution 4 ml/kg IV over 10 minutes. There is no specific serum sodium concentration that should be targeted with hypertonic saline therapy.[20] Repeated doses can be administered if necessary and have been found to be beneficial in cases of refractory ICH in human patients with traumatic brain injury but it may not be without risk.[21] Prolonged dosing of hypertonic saline in human pediatric patients has been associated with adverse events including acute kidney injury, neutropenia, thrombocytopenia, and acute respiratory distress syndrome.[22]

Furosemide

Furosemide therapy can be given in addition to mannitol or hypertonic saline in an effort to increase the degree of brain water loss. Furosemide is a loop diuretic that may reduce brain water by promoting a diuresis of hypoosmotic urine, in addition to other undetermined ICP-lowering effects. Administration of furosemide simultaneously with mannitol reportedly has been synergistic in reducing ICP.[4] The addition of furosemide therapy to hypertonic saline resulted in a similar degree of brain water loss in normal rats as that of mannitol.[16]

The recommended dose of furosemide is 0.7 to 2 mg/kg IV. Furosemide takes effect within 30 minutes after IV administration. Maintenance of fluid and electrolyte balance is required.

Glucocorticoids

A beneficial role for glucocorticoids in the treatment of head trauma remains unproven, and their routine use is discouraged until such time as appropriate studies support the use of glucocorticoids in the treatment of ICH caused by traumatic brain injury.[11] Primary infectious and noninfectious inflammatory diseases and tumor-associated edema are indications for considering glucocorticoids in the treatment of ICH.[23]

The recommended dose of dexamethasone sodium phosphate is 0.1 to 0.25 mg/kg IV.

Other Drugs

Although the authors do not recommend usage of additional drugs for the treatment of ICH, several drugs have been recommended. Dimethyl sulfoxide (DMSO) and opioid antagonists (e.g., naloxone) have been used to treat brain edema, although there is no evidence to support their use in place of osmotic diuretics. Tirilazad mesylate has shown promise as a neuroprotectant in experimental models of focal cerebral ischemia and subarachnoid hemorrhage. Research is ongoing concerning use of agents such as tromethamine (an alkalinizing agent), superoxide dismutase, allopurinol, thyrotropin-releasing hormone, fluosol, and calcium channel–blocking drugs.[17]

Cerebral metabolic rate of oxygen consumption

CBF and cerebral metabolic rate (CMR) are coupled so that an increase CMR is accompanied by a rise in CBF. Reducing the oxygen requirement of the brain may reduce ICP by reducing cerebral blood volume. Hyperthermia, fever, and hallucinogenic drugs (e.g., ketamine) increase the oxygen requirements of the brain. Measures to reduce CMR include sedation with barbiturates, anesthesia, and hypothermia.[10,11]

Surgical therapy

Craniectomy should be considered in animals with ICH refractory to medical decompression. Other indications for surgery include debulking of mass lesions, drainage of intracranial abscesses, and treatment of open skull fractures, depressed skull fractures, or fractures involving a venous sinus or middle meningeal artery.[1,17] Durotomy appears to be significantly more effective than skull removal in lowering ICP experimentally in dogs and cats.[17]

In humans, aspiration of CSF via intraventricular catheterization is used frequently to treat ICH.[10] It may be possible to aspirate CSF from animals with ventriculomegaly, and ultrasound-guided CSF aspiration may be considered in animals with fontanelles.

Other considerations

Intensive supportive care, as discussed in various sections of this manual, is essential. Factors such as frequent turning, prevention of pressure sores, nutritional support, and attention to bladder and bowel function are of paramount importance in preventing complications associated with recumbency. Most animals with ICH have depressed swallowing and gag reflexes, so oral feeding should be avoided, because aspiration pneumonia may result. Alternative methods of nutritional support, such as a feeding tube or total parenteral nutrition, should be considered early in the course of treatment.

PROGNOSIS

In general, animals with brainstem lesions, especially persistent coma, abnormal respiration, or progressive loss of cranial nerve reflex function, have a poorer prognosis than those with cerebrocortical involvement. Patience and persistence are essential in treatment, because recovery may require a prolonged time for resolution of edema, necrosis, and hemorrhage. Also, compensatory mechanisms of the central nervous system often require many months for maximum development. Even animals with residual deficits may be functional pets.

REFERENCES

1. Lee KR, Hoff JT: Intracranial pressure. In Youmans JR, editor: Neurological surgery, ed 4, Philadelphia, 1996, Saunders.
2. Vandevelde M, Zurbriggen A, Bailey CS, et al: Pathophysiology of the central nervous system. In Dunlop RH, Malbert CH, editors: Veterinary pathophysiology, Philadelphia, 2004, Blackwell.
3. Marmarou AM, Beaumont A: Physiology of the cerebrospinal fluid and intracranial pressure. In Winn HR, editor: Neurological surgery, ed 5, Philadelphia, 2004, Saunders.
4. Bagley RS: Pathophysiology of nervous system disease. In Bagley RS, editor: Fundamentals of veterinary clinical neurology, Oxford, 2005, Blackwell.
5. Khurana VG, Benarroch EE, Katusic ZS, et al: Cerebral blood flow and metabolism. In Winn HR, editor: Neurological surgery, ed 5, Philadelphia, 2004, Saunders.
6. Proulx J, Dhupa N: Severe brain injury. Part I. Pathophysiology, Comp Cont Educ Pract Vet 20:897, 1998.
7. Fishman RA: Brain edema and disorders of intracranial pressure. In Rowland LP, editor: Merritt's neurology, ed 11, Philadelphia, 2005, Lippincott Williams & Wilkins.
8. Proulx J, Dhupa N: Severe brain injury. Part II. Therapy, Comp Cont Educ Pract Vet 20:993, 1998.
9. Sinson G, Reilly PM, Grady MS: Moderate and severe traumatic brain injury: initial resuscitation and patient evaluation. In Winn HR, editor: Neurological surgery, ed 5, Philadelphia, 2004, Saunders.
10. Vincent JL, Berre J: Primer on medical management of severe brain injury, Crit Care Med 33:1392, 2005.
11. Bullock MR, Povlishock JT, editors: Guidelines for the management of severe traumatic brain injury, J Neurotrauma 24:1, 2007.
12. Stocchetti N, Maas AI, Chieregato A, et al: Hyperventilation in head injury: a review, Chest 127:1812, 2005.
13. Wakai A, McCabe A, Roberts I, Schierhout G: Mannitol for acute traumatic brain injury, Cochrane Database Syst Rev 8:CD001049, 2013.
14. Diringer MN: New trends in hyperosmolar therapy? Curr Opin Crit Care 19:77-82, 2013
15. Kamel H, Navi BB, Nakagawa K, et al: Hypertonic saline versus mannitol for the treatment of elevated intracranial pressure: a meta-analysis of randomized clinical trials, Crit Care Med 39:554-559, 2011.
16. Wang LC, Papangelou A, Lin C, et al: Comparison of equivolume, equiosmolar solutions of mannitol and hypertonic saline with or without furosemide on brain water content in normal rats, Anesthesiology 118:903-913, 2013.
17. Bagley RS: Treatment of important and common diseases involving the intracranial nervous system of dogs and cats. In Bagley RS, editor: Fundamentals of veterinary clinical neurology, Oxford, 2005, Blackwell.
18. Ogden AT: Hyperosmolar agents in neurosurgical practice: the evolving role of hypertonic saline, Neurosurgery 58:1003, 2006.
19. Ogden AT, Mayer SA, Connolly ES Jr: Hyperosmolar agents in neurosurgical practice: the evolving role of hypertonic saline, Neurosurgery 57:207, 2005.
20. Wells DL, Swanson JM, Wood GC, et al: The relationship between serum sodium and intracranial pressure when using hypertonic saline to target mild hypernatremia in patients with head trauma, Crit Care 16:R193, 2012.
21. Eskandari R, Filtz MR, Davis GE, et al: Effective treatment of refractory intracranial hypertension after traumatic brain injury with repeated boluses of 14.6% hypertonic saline, J Neurosurg 119:338-346, 2013.
22. Gonda DD, Meltzer HS, Crawford JR, et al: Complications associated with prolonged hypertonic saline therapy in children with elevated intracranial pressure, Pediatr Crit Care Med 14:610-620, 2013.
23. Sarin R, Murthy V: Medical decompressive therapy for primary and metastatic intracranial tumours, Lancet Neurol 2:357, 2003.

CHAPTER 85

DISEASES OF THE MOTOR UNIT

Christiane Massicotte, DVM, PhD, DACVIM (Neurology)

KEY POINTS

- The motor unit consists of the lower motor neuron (LMN), the neuromuscular junction (NMJ), and its skeletal muscle fiber.
- Disease of the motor unit results in poor muscle tone, decreased segmental reflexes, and progressive muscle atrophy.
- Acute neuropathies or myopathies may result from immune-mediated, infectious, metabolic, vascular, toxic, traumatic or idiopathic causes. Neoplasia occasionally presents acutely. Botulism, tick paralysis, acquired myasthenia gravis, or aminoglycoside intoxication may cause diffuse junctionopathies.
- Clinical signs, clinical pathology, electrodiagnostic assessment, muscle and nerve biopsy with molecular analysis when available, and multiple imaging methods can be used to identify the location of the disease within the motor unit.

Lower motor neurons (LMNs) consist of the cell body found in the brainstem or spinal cord, and their motor axons within cranial or spinal nerves, respectively. They terminate on skeletal muscle fibers at the neuromuscular junction (NMJ). The LMN, NMJ, and skeletal muscle fibers together form the motor unit.[1]

The neurologic examination and its interpretation are the first and most important steps in localizing the lesion.[2] This chapter describes how to identify motor unit disorders, diagnostic tests available to localize the lesion anatomically within the motor unit, and available treatments for a number of motor unit diseases.

IDENTIFYING NEUROPATHIES, JUNCTIONOPATHIES, AND MYOPATHIES

Clinical Signs

Recognizing features associated with motor unit diseases and gathering information about its clinical course and lesion distribution are essential in reaching a final diagnosis.[3] Disease of the motor unit results in flaccid paresis or paralysis. A short-strided gait is apparent when appendicular muscles are involved. Postural reactions and segmental reflexes frequently are diminished. Muscle atrophy is common, although involvement of specialized striated muscle groups may result in more specific dysfunction such as incontinence, dysphagia, dysphonia, regurgitation, and abnormal facial expressions. Clinical signs may suggest specific involvement of the nerve, NMJ, or skeletal muscle. For instance, proprioceptive deficits and diminished tactile or pain sensation may be recognized in patients with neuropathies when sensory fibers also are affected, but these deficits seldom are seen with NMJ or muscle diseases. However, diseases of the NMJ and muscles are associated more frequently with muscle pain, swelling, and exercise intolerance, which are uncommon features of neuropathies. In addition to knowing the clinical characteristics associated with motor unit disorders, reaching a final diagnosis requires a comprehensive combination of information obtained from clinicopathologic tests, electrodiagnostic testing, muscle and nerve biopsies, and occasionally more sophisticated methods of imaging, as described in the following section.

Clinicopathologic Testing

A complete blood count and chemistry profile should be performed when metabolic disorders that can affect the motor end unit are suspected (i.e., hypokalemia, diabetes mellitus and hypoglycemia). In addition, increased serum enzyme activities specific to muscles such as creatine kinase, serum glutamic aspartate aminotransferase, and lactate dehydrogenase can indicate damage to muscle fibers resulting from myopathies. These tests results must be interpreted with caution because damage to muscle may occur also from prolonged recumbency and trauma to specific muscle groups. Other, more specific endocrine disorders such as hyper- or hypoadrenocorticism and hypothyroidism can be identified by performing resting cortisol, ACTH stimulation, and thyroid hormone panel, respectively. More specific titers can be submitted when infectious diseases such as toxoplasmosis or neosporosis are suspected, or to confirm masticatory muscle myositis and myasthenia gravis, as discussed later in this chapter.

Cerebrospinal fluid (CSF) analysis may be useful to identify nerve root disease and more centralized nervous system disorders associated with inflammatory processes and demyelination. Radiculopathies caused by degenerative, neoplastic, or inflammatory processes can result in elevations in CSF protein and pleocytosis. These elevations are not expected in most animals with myopathies, junctionopathies and/or neuropathies, where nerve roots are not affected by the disease process.

Electrophysiologic Testing

Electrodiagnostic testing, including electromyography (EMG) and evoked response testing, are useful to better localize the lesion within the motor unit. In most cases, these tests are conducted under general anesthesia. Electromyography can detect abnormal spontaneous electrical discharges of muscle fibers that are independent of neural control. Fibrillation potentials, positive sharp waves, and complex repetitive discharges are some of the most common abnormal spontaneous electrical activities recorded from damaged (myopathy) or denervated muscles (neuropathy) but rarely are found with junctionopathies. These spontaneous discharges do not discriminate myopathies from neuropathies.

Nerve fibers can be stimulated electrically to produce compound muscle action potentials (CMAPs). The amplitude and duration of these evoked potentials can be measured to differentiate neuropathy from myopathies or junctionopathies, or to localize a focal lesion along a nerve or nerve root. Small-amplitude evoked responses are found in neuropathies in which axonal dysfunction is present and also may be seen with some junctionopathies and myopathies. A prolonged duration of the CMAP and a significant decrease in nerve conduction velocity can occur in neuropathies in which myelin dysfunction occurs, or when axonal degeneration is severe. Repetitive nerve stimulation and single muscle fiber stimulation can be used to identify junctionopathies. F waves and cord dorsum potentials are additional advanced evoked responses capable of detecting a lesion within the ventral and dorsal nerve roots, respectively. Electrophysiology is helpful to rapidly quantify the extent of PNS involvement and to localize a focal lesion within the motor unit but remains a nonspecific finding common to many diseases. Electrophysiology remains a powerful tool which helps the clinician generating a list of suitable differential diagnoses and judiciously selects the proper additional test(s) required to make a final diagnosis.

Nerve and Muscle Biopsy

Nerve and muscle biopsies are often necessary to complete studies of the motor unit and achieve a final diagnosis. Nerve biopsy may reveal degeneration or inflammation of the axon or myelin associated with the neuropathy. Although most muscles can be biopsied easily, nerve studies are usually limited to fascicular biopsies of the ulnar or peroneal nerves to prevent further deficits. Common and nonspecific muscle changes associated with neuropathies may include muscle fiber degeneration, inflammation, or infiltration with fat and connective tissue. More specific changes such as type I or type II muscle fiber grouping and group atrophy of adjacent muscle fibers of similar type also can be seen with neuropathies. In contrast, primary myopathies are characterized by muscle necrosis, regeneration, and/or inflammation distributed in a more random pattern.[2] Immunochemistry can complete clinical pathology findings in the case of myasthenia gravis, masticatory muscle myositis, and some genetic disorders.

Imaging

Sophisticated methods of imaging such as magnetic resonance imaging (MRI) and computed tomography (CT) scan may be required to visualize the lesion when neoplasia or inflammation are suspected within the nerve roots, the brachial or lumbar plexus, or with more subtle nonpalpable lesions along the cranial and spinal nerves. A MRI can be useful to determine the size and invasiveness of a peripheral nerve lesion, and the study can be extended easily to evaluate the integrity of the spinal cord or brainstem/medulla.

CAUSES OF ACUTE NEUROPATHY, MYOPATHY, OR JUNCTIONOPATHY

Acute Neuropathies

Neuropathies can affect one or multiple cranial or spinal nerve(s) or nerve root(s). A mononeuropathy may later progress to a more generalized polyneuropathy. Specific cranial nerve(s) initially may be the only affected structure(s) or may be an indication of a more diffuse subclinical polyneuropathy. Neoplastic or inflammatory lesions involving the central nervous system (brainstem, medulla, and thoracic and lumbar intumescences) also may present as unilateral or bilateral dysfunction of multiple cranial or spinal nerves. Rabies encephalitis always must be considered as a cause of acute cranial nerve deficits, especially with trigeminal nerve involvement. Common neuropathies seen in dogs and cats are described in the following section.

Neuropathies Associated with Specific Cranial Nerves

Trigeminal neuritis

Trigeminal neuritis causes bilateral mandibular muscle paralysis and sometimes decreases facial sensation or triggers facial hyperesthesia.

As a result, dogs present with an acute inability to close the mouth, difficulty eating and drinking, and severe ptyalism. Horner's syndrome occasionally may be seen as sympathetic fibers adjacent to the ophthalmic branch of the trigeminal nerve also may become inflamed. Other differential diagnoses for mandibular paralysis are rabies encephalitis, round cell neoplasia, and polyneuritis.[4] Treatment is supportive and the animal is fed by placing small meatball-shaped foods in the mouth with the head elevated. Tape muzzle also may be useful. Recovery usually occurs in 2 to 4 weeks, although longer recovery times also have been described.

Trigeminal nerve sheath tumor

The most common cranial nerve affected by nerve sheath tumor is the trigeminal nerve. Unilateral and rapid temporal, masseter, pterygoid, and digastric muscle atrophy may occur, with unilateral facial hyperesthesia or analgesia as sensory fibers become involved. As the mass grows and compresses the brain, signs of brainstem dysfunction may occur; hemiparesis and vestibular system dysfunction are particularly common. Malignant nerve sheath tumors also can affect spinal nerves and nerve roots (as described in the following section). Diagnosis generally is made by CT or MRI. Surgery and radiation therapy have been attempted and may slow the progression of signs.[5]

Facial nerve paralysis

Facial nerve paralysis most commonly causes a unilateral, but sometimes bilateral, paralysis of the muscles responsible for facial expression. Patients often present unable to move the lip or blink and with a droopy ear and severe ptyalism. Signs may be due to inflammatory, neoplastic, traumatic, or idiopathic causes.[6] The idiopathic form occurs commonly in older dogs, with Cocker Spaniels and Beagles being overrepresented. It is a diagnosis made by exclusion of other conditions associated with facial nerve paralysis. Although no specific treatment is available, spontaneous recovery may occur but often takes weeks to months.

Facial nerve paralysis resulting from otitis media/interna is indistinguishable from the idiopathic form unless accompanied by Horner's syndrome or evidence of ear disease identified by otoscopic examination, brainstem auditory evoked response testing, or advanced imaging. Several months of antimicrobial therapy, based on culture and susceptibility testing, may be adequate treatment for facial nerve paralysis associated with middle ear infections. Surgical bulla osteotomy and drain placement may be required if medical management fails to restore facial nerve function.

Lymphosarcoma or nerve sheath tumors also may cause unilateral facial nerve paralysis. In these cases, the major petrosal nerve also may be affected intracranially, resulting in decreased tear production.[7] Imaging and biopsies are required for final diagnosis. Prognosis for functional facial nerve recovery is poor.

Laryngeal paralysis

Dogs and cats with increased inspiratory sounds, dysphonia, gagging, cyanosis, panting, and collapse may have disorders of the vagus or recurrent laryngeal nerves. Laryngeal paralysis may be unilateral or bilateral and may be due to trauma, degeneration (hypothyroid, polyneuropathy), toxic (lead, organophosphates) or idiopathic causes, and has a genetic basis in Siberian Huskies, Bouvier des Flandres, Dalmatians, Rottweilers, Bull Terriers, German Shepherds, and Pyrenean Mountain Dogs (IVIS).[8,9]

The diagnosis is made under light sedation as abduction of one or both vocal folds is decreased with inspiration. Electromyography may reveal spontaneous electrical activity in the cricoarytenoideus dorsalis muscle, and in many cases, similar changes are observed in distal appendicular muscles, suggesting a more generalized polyneuropathy.[10] Treatment consists of exercise restriction, tranquilization, and cooling the patient. Intubation may be necessary in extreme cases, and arytenoid lateralization surgery also may be indicated for long-term management.

Traumatic Neuropathies

Acute neuropathies resulting from trauma may be classified into three categories based on lesion severity. Neurapraxia, the loss of nerve conduction without structural change, occurs from transient loss of blood supply and usually resolves over weeks to months. Axonotmesis, axonal damage without loss of supporting structures, requires regeneration of the axons toward its specific muscle target before functional recovery. In the case of axonotmesis, axonal regeneration occurs at a rate of approximately 1 mm per day. Neurotmesis is the complete severance of the nerve and is seen with severe trauma. Direct trauma to nerves is frequent in small animals after fractures or lacerations. Injections also can inflict direct trauma to nerves or cause damage secondary to diffusion of irritant/toxic substances around the nerves. Traction injuries, known as brachial or pelvic plexus avulsion, are common in animals that sustain severe trauma. The avulsion may be partial, causing only stretch and swelling of the nerve roots, or can result in complete severance of the nerve(s) from the spinal cord. It results in acute flaccid paralysis of the limb or muscle groups innervated by the damaged nerves or nerve roots.

Lesion severity may be determined by visual inspection, repeated clinical examinations, and electrodiagnostic testing.[1,7,11] Electrodiagnostic testing may be normal up to 4 days after proximal nerve injury and the results therefore must be interpreted with caution during the first week after injury. In general, severe and more proximal nerve damage is associated with a less favorable prognosis for complete functional recovery. Although sharp transections may respond well to surgical intervention, effective therapy for traction injuries has not yet been described.

Acute Polyneuropathies

Metabolic causes

Metabolic disorders generally are associated with insidious onset of polyneuropathies but can sometimes present with acute clinical signs. Dogs with hypoadrenocorticism may manifest signs ranging from rear limb paresis to complete recumbency. Diabetic animals may have a plantigrade stance. In both instances hyporeflexia occurs. Hypothyroid neuropathy also is described with generalized weakness, muscle atrophy, hyporeflexia, facial nerve paresis, vestibular system dysfunction, laryngeal paralysis, and megaesophagus.[12] Control of these metabolic diseases most commonly results in resolution of neurologic dysfunctions. However, hypoglycemia resulting from an insulin-secreting tumor carries a poor long-term prognosis. Insulinomas cause flaccid paresis or paralysis, hyporeflexia, lethargy, bradycardia, muscle tremors, hypothermia, and disorientation, with or without seizures. Medical management with specific diets containing high protein, fat and complex carbohydrates, diazoxide and/or prednisone is often beneficial. Surgical removal of neoplastic tissues is not curative but may increase survival time and improve response to further medical management.[13,14]

Neoplasia

Round cell tumors and malignant peripheral nerve sheath tumors (MPNSTs) are the most common tumors affecting cranial and spinal peripheral nerves and nerve roots. Both tend to affect proximal motor nerves. Clinical signs associated with MPNSTs are usually unilateral because the tumor affects one or adjacent ipsilateral nerves near the spinal cord and favors nerves of the thoracic limbs. In contrast, round cell tumors may cause bilateral paresis or paralysis without location specificity. Both tumors are sometimes palpable and painful and can be diagnosed with MRI or CT and biopsy. MPNSTs may be treated with radical resection of the nerves because incomplete resected tumors have the tendency to regrow towards the spinal cord, ultimately invading and compressing the spinal cord.[15] Radiation therapy also can reduce tumor size in 50% of patients with nonresectable masses.[16] Lymphoma can be treated with radiation and/or chemotherapy with variable success rates.[17]

Toxoplasmosis and neosporosis

These protozoal diseases initially present with flaccid paraparesis that may progress to a chronic state of extreme increase extensor tone, which completely restricts flexion of these joints. Signs of neuropathy and myopathy often occur, and retinitis may accompany these signs. The diagnosis is made by finding protozoa in muscle or nerve biopsies or by finding rising serum antibody titers. Several weeks of antimicrobial therapy, such as trimethoprim-sulfadiazine and clindamycin, used alone or in combination, are required to improve clinical signs associated with these infectious agents. However, once hind limb rigidity has developed, clinical improvement no longer occurs.[18,19]

Acute polyradiculoneuritis

Affected dogs may have a history of exposure to raccoons, recent vaccination, or neither. Flaccid tetraparesis or paralysis and hyporeflexia develop within 1 to 3 days of the onset of signs. Facial muscle paresis and a change in bark may occur. Clinical signs may progress rapidly to respiratory paralysis, requiring mechanical ventilation. Tail and neck motion, swallowing, and fecal and urinary continence often are maintained. The animal may develop hyperesthesia if dorsal nerve roots become inflamed. CSF analysis may show an increase in protein as demyelination of the ventral nerve roots occurs. Early after onset of clinical signs, nerve conduction velocity and F-wave latencies are slower and CMAP amplitudes are decreased.[20] Electromyographic changes follow, with diffuse fibrillation potentials and positive sharp waves occurring 4 to 7 days after the onset of clinical signs. Biopsy of the nerve or nerve root may show inflammatory cell infiltrates, demyelination, and axonal loss.

Treatments with immunosuppressive drugs are controversial because most of them do not affect the progression of this disease. However, treatment with human IV immunoglobulin may shorter its clinical course.[21] In most cases, aggressive supportive care is necessary to prevent and treat decubital ulcers and urinary tract infections. Close observation for respiratory muscle paresis is important, and the patient may require intubation and mechanical ventilation if the respiratory function becomes severely compromised (see Chapter 30). Partial or complete recovery may take 2 to 3 weeks, although signs can recur. Respiratory paralysis is a poor prognostic indicator for recovery.[22]

Aortic thromboembolism

Animals may have a peracute onset of unilateral or bilateral paraparesis/plegia as peripheral nerves and muscles become ischemic. In most severe cases, anesthesia also may accompany the paralysis. Limbs are painful and cool, pulses are weak or absent, and muscles are initially painful and often firm. Abdominal ultrasonography may identify a thrombus in the distal aorta. Analgesics, intravenous fluids, heparin, vasodilators, aspirin, and clopidogrel may be beneficial. Thromboembolism has been associated with cardiomyopathy, hyperadrenocorticism and with protein-losing nephropathy/enteropathy (see Chapter 104).[23,24]

Intoxications

Drugs that may result in neuropathies include vincristine, thallium, and organophosphates. In most cases, clinical signs have an insidious onset and are associated with drug administration or exposure to toxins.

MYOPATHIES

Inflammatory Myopathies

Generalized polymyositis

Dogs and cats of any age may develop generalized polymyositis of striated skeletal muscles, which is characterized by a weak, stiff, and short-strided gait that may worsen with exercise.[25] In addition, involvement of skeletal muscles within the pharynx and esophagus, and extraocular or masticatory muscles occasionally can result in dysphagia, dysphonia, regurgitation, and megaesophagus. In the acute phase, pain and swelling are present upon palpation of appendicular muscles and animals are often febrile and lethargic. Increases in creatine kinase, serum glutamic aspartate aminotransferase, lactate dehydrogenase, and antinuclear antibody titers may occur. Electromyography shows fibrillation potentials, positive sharp waves, and complex repetitive discharges in many muscles.

Most cases of polymyositis are caused by immune-mediated disorders, although infectious etiologies such as toxoplasmosis and neosporosis should be ruled out with serology and/or muscle biopsies. Muscle biopsy shows lymphoplasmacytic inflammation and muscle necrosis with immune-mediated disease. Immunosuppressive doses of glucocorticoids are necessary to control the initial clinical signs. Doses are tapered slowly as long as the patient is not symptomatic. Other immunosuppressive drugs such as azathioprine and cyclosporine also have been used in addition to glucocorticoids with variable success. Antimicrobial therapy may be essential in some cases when pharyngeal and esophageal muscle involvement results in aspiration pneumonia.

Masticatory myositis

Swelling and pain upon palpation of the temporalis, masseter, and pterygoid muscles are features of the acute phase of this disease. As a result, manipulation of the jaw causes the patient great discomfort. If left untreated, the condition may progress to atrophy of the masticatory muscles, reducing mandibular range of motion and causing difficulty prehending food. Masticatory myositis may be confirmed by muscle biopsy or serum titers for antibodies against type IIM muscle fibers. Immunosuppressive doses of glucocorticoids tapered over several months usually result in improvement of clinical signs. However, severe muscle atrophy and a decreased range of motion of the jaw still occur frequently. Other immunosuppressive drugs also may be added if clinical signs are not well controlled with glucocorticoid alone (as previously described with polymyositis).

Noninflammatory generalized myopathies

Acute noninflammatory and more generalized forms of myopathies usually are associated with endocrine or metabolic disturbances. They cause generalized muscle weakness without pain and swelling (in contrast to inflammatory myopathies). These conditions may be present concomitantly with neuropathies and may produce dysphagia, dysphonia, and megaesophagus. A thorough diagnostic plan consists of a comprehensive thyroid hormone panel, resting cortisol level (+/– ACTH stimulation), electrolytes and muscle biopsies, when indicated. Vascular events also can result in acute painful paralysis secondary to muscle and nerve necrosis; this most frequently occurs in the hind limbs. This condition is seen mainly in cats, and prognosis is poor, especially with loss of deep pain perception in the affected limb(s) and/or coexisting cardiomyopathy.

Megaesophagus

Dysfunction of esophageal muscles can result in megaesophagus. Animals with megaesophagus present with regurgitation, ptyalism, and/or aspiration pneumonia. Megaesophagus is often part of more generalized disease processes, such as neuropathies, polymyopathies, and junctionopathies (e.g., myasthenia gravis, botulism); it also may be associated with paraneoplastic syndromes. However, it also may be seen as a sole clinical sign with idiopathic conditions. Idiopathic megaesophagus may be congenital or acquired, and although disease of the vagus nerve is suspected, this has not been confirmed. A diagnosis of idiopathic megaesophagus is made by clinical and radiographic findings, and by ruling out obstruction, toxic exposures, infectious diseases, endocrine disorders, and myasthenia gravis. Small, frequent and elevated feedings may help food reach the stomach by gravity, and patients also may be held in an upright position shortly after to further prevent regurgitation (see Chapter 120). Smooth muscle prokinetic agents such as metoclopramide and cisapride are used frequently but rarely improve esophageal motility in dogs. Aspiration pneumonia is common, often reoccurs, and requires long-term management to prevent regurgitation (as described in the following section for myasthenia gravis).

Junctionopathies

Acquired myasthenia gravis

Acquired myasthenia gravis (MG) is rare in cats but has been reported in many breeds of dogs more than 8 months of age, with German Shepherds, Labrador Retrievers, and Akitas overrepresented. At least three clinical pictures may occur: (1) focal MG, (2) generalized MG, and (3) acute fulminating MG.[26-28]

Animals with the focal form show facial, pharyngeal, or laryngeal dysfunction without appendicular muscle involvement. Megaesophagus may occur as a sole clinical sign or may be associated with aspiration pneumonia secondary to regurgitation. Frequently ptyalism, dysphagia, dysphonia, coughing, and retching are also present.

Generalized MG is characterized by appendicular muscle weakness, with or without signs of facial, pharyngeal, or laryngeal dysfunction. Strength may return after periods of rest, or the animal may show continuous weakness; the rear limbs often are affected more severely. The animal has a stiff, short-strided gait and may develop passive ventroflexion of the head and neck. Postural reactions are usually normal if the animal is supported. Spinal reflexes and sensation are unaffected.

Acute, fulminating MG is the most severe form of the disease.[26,27] Signs include a sudden, rapid progression of severe appendicular muscle weakness; this results in recumbency (that is unabated by rest), frequent regurgitation (associated with megaesophagus), and facial, pharyngeal, and/or laryngeal dysfunction. Varying degrees of apparent dyspnea are frequently present, most likely the result of aspiration pneumonia and loss of respiratory muscle strength.

Definitive diagnosis of acquired MG may be made by identifying increased circulating acetylcholine receptor antibody in blood (>0.6 nm/L in dogs; >0.3 nm/L in cats). Antibodies are detectable in 80% to 90% of dogs with acquired disease. Intercostal muscle biopsy also may be used to identify acetylcholine receptor antibodies at the NMJ. If a more immediate diagnosis is necessary, edrophonium response testing may be performed. Dramatic gait improvement occurs in some cases for the first 2 minutes after edrophonium injection. This positive response rarely is seen with acute fulminating MG. Pretreatment with atropine is recommended to decrease salivation, defecation, urination, bronchial secretions, and bronchoconstriction that may be seen after edrophonium administration. Electrodiagnostic testing also may be performed. A 10% or greater decremental response of the fourth or fifth compound action potential recorded from the interosseous muscle after repetitive stimulation of the tibial or ulnar nerve at 3 Hz may be observed. Single muscle fiber stimulation is the electrodiagnostic test of choice in humans and also may be helpful for the diagnosis of MG in dogs.

Animals affected with generalized MG may be treated with oral pyridostigmine bromide (0.2 to 2 mg/kg q8-12h; IV infusions of 0.01 to 0.03 mg/kg/hr also have been used). Intramuscular neostigmine bromide or methylsulfate (0.04 mg/kg q6-8h) may be given to animals with significant dysphagia and regurgitation, or in cases of fulminating MG. A low dosage is begun and titrated upward over 2 to 3 days until clinical signs resolve or signs of cholinergic toxicity occur. Although appendicular muscle weakness improves with treatments, pharyngeal, laryngeal, and esophageal dysfunction are more resistant to therapy and may become permanent.

Management of animals with severe dysphagia and megaesophagus secondary to focal and/or generalized MG must include feeding the animal from a raised height and keeping the head elevated for 10 minutes afterward to facilitate passage of food into the stomach. Frequently, a gastrostomy tube is necessary to provide nutritional support until dysphagia improves and regurgitation frequency decreases. Frequent auscultation and radiographs of the thorax are recommended to determine whether aspiration pneumonia is present; treatment includes broad-spectrum antimicrobial therapy, IV fluids, and oxygen support (see Chapter 23).

Treatment of acquired MG with prednisone is controversial because it results in further appendicular muscle weakness and compromises respiratory function. In addition, the immunosuppressive effects of corticosteroid therapy may lead to rapid respiratory deterioration in patients with aspiration pneumonia. However, immunomodulation with azathioprine and mycophenolate mofetil has proven useful when aspiration pneumonia is not present.[29-31]

The acquired disease is usually a temporary state and may resolve over many months of supportive care. The most common cause of death or euthanasia is aspiration and pneumonia. Acute, fulminating MG carries a poor prognosis for recovery because a large proportion of dogs are euthanized or die secondary to respiratory failure and aspiration pneumonia, despite anticholinesterase inhibitor therapy.[22,27] Plasmapheresis and intravenous gamma-globulins are useful in treating acute, fulminating disease in humans but are not yet readily available or studied in small animals.[28]

In approximately 15% of dogs with acquired MG, the disease is related to a thymoma. In these cases, resolution of clinical signs occurs after thymectomy. Paraneoplastic syndromes associated with osteogenic sarcoma or biliary carcinoma also can cause myasthenia gravis. Hypothyroidism has been reported concomitantly with MG and polymyositis as part of a more generalized immune-mediated disorder; thyroid hormone levels should be tested in these cases. [32]

Botulism

Dogs present hours to days after ingestion of a toxin produced by *Clostridium botulinum.* The toxin interferes with the release of acetylcholine at the NMJ. A stiff and short-strided gait is noted initially, rapidly progressing to flaccid tetraplegia and diminished-to-absent spinal reflexes. Cranial nerves often are affected, resulting in facial paresis, dysphagia, dysphonia, and megaesophagus. Autonomic signs such as mydriasis, decreased tear production, constipation, and urinary retention occasionally are seen. In more severely affected animals, respiratory paresis or paralysis ultimately may develop.

Patients usually are treated based on history and compatible clinical signs because a definitive diagnosis is difficult to reach. The toxin is identified rarely in food, serum, stomach contents, or feces because it is present only early in the course of the disease. Incremental CAMP amplitudes after repetitive nerve stimulation also may be seen with botulism. Supportive care often results in complete resolution of signs within 2 to 3 weeks. The patient should be monitored for aspiration pneumonia. A gastrostomy tube or parenteral nutrition may be necessary to provide nutritional support. If acute exposure occurs and signs are progressing, type C antitoxin may be administered (see Chapter 174).[33]

Tick paralysis

The clinical signs seen in animals with tick paralysis in the United States are due to a toxin present in tick saliva that interferes with the release of acetylcholine at the NMJ. Clinical signs occur 3 to 5 days after the tick is attached and consist of ataxia or paresis that may progress rapidly to recumbency and complete flaccid tetraplegia within 24 to 72 hours. Clinical features may be similar to those found with botulism. Slow nerve conduction velocities may be found, in addition to decreased CMAP amplitudes. In all patients developing a sudden onset of flaccid tetraparesis, a thorough examination for ticks and application of a topical tick treatment should be performed. Resolution of clinical signs occurs within 24 to 72 hours of tick removal.[34] Tick paralysis in Australia causes a more severe and prolonged course of disease.

Snake bites

Venom from Elapid snakes (Coral snakes of North America) and Mojave rattlesnakes (Southwest United States and Mexico) causes postsynaptic neuromuscular blockade, CNS depression, muscle paralysis, and vasomotor instability with only mild tissue reaction at the bite site.[35] Clinical signs usually occur within 24 hours after the bite. No definitive diagnostic tests are available to confirm the exposure. Supportive care is essential and must be established promptly for better outcome and may involve mechanical ventilation and prevention of aspiration pneumonia. Compressive bandages may be helpful. Monitoring hemostasis is also important in these patients. Antivenom is available for Mojave rattlesnake and Elapid species, and it must be given promptly (see Chapter 174). Prognosis depends on the amount of venom delivered and size of the patient and supportive care.

Aminoglycoside intoxication

Aminoglycosides cause acute of LMN disorders resulting from neuromuscular blockade or by triggering peripheral neuropathies. The condition is usually reversible once aminoglycosides are discontinued. Consequently, aminoglycosides should be used very cautiously in patients suffering from LMN disorders because they potentially can exacerbate weakness associated with these conditions.

REFERENCES

1. DeLahunta A: Veterinary neuroanatomy and clinical neurology, ed 2, St Louis, 1983, Saunders.
2. Rowland LP: Diseases of the motor unit. In Kandell ER, Schwartz JH, Jessell TM, editors: Principles of neural science, ed 4, New York, 2000, McGraw-Hill.
3. Dyck PJ, Dyck JB, Grant IA, et al: Ten steps in characterizing and diagnosing patients with peripheral neuropathy, Neurology 47:10, 1996.
4. Mayhew PD, Bush WW, Glass EN: Trigeminal neuropathy in dogs: a retrospective study of 29 cases (1991-2000), J Am Anim Hosp Assoc 38:262, 2000.
5. Bagley RS, Wheeler SJ, Klopp L, et al: Clinical features of trigeminal nerve sheath tumor in 10 dogs, J Am Anim Hosp Assoc 34:19, 1998.
6. Kern TJ, Erb HN: Facial neuropathy in dogs and cats: 95 cases (1975-1985), J Am Vet Med Assoc 191:1604, 1987.
7. Oliver JE, Hoerlein BF, Mayhew IG: Veterinary neurology, Philadelphia, 1987, Saunders.
8. Mahony OM, Knowles KE, Braund KG, et al: Laryngeal paralysis-polyneuropathy complex in young Rottweilers, J Vet Intern Med 12:330, 1998.
9. Braund KG: Braund's clinical neurology in small animals: localization, diagnosis and treatment, 2005, International Veterinary Information Service. Available at: http://www.ivis.org. Accessed March 21, 2006.
10. Thieman KM, Krahwinkel DJ, Sims MH, et al: Histopathological confirmation of polyneuropathy in 11 dogs with laryngeal paralysis, J Am Anim Hosp Assoc 46:161, 2010.
11. Kapatkin AS, Vite CH: Neurosurgical emergencies, Vet Clin North Am Small Anim Pract 30:627, 2000.
12. Jaggy A, Oliver JE, Ferguson DC, et al: Neurological manifestations of hypothyroidism: a retrospective study of 29 dogs, J Vet Intern Med 8:328, 1994.
13. Goutal CM, Brugmann BL, Ryan KA: insulinoma in dogs: a review, J Am Anim Hosp Assoc 48:151, 2012.
14. Polton GA, White RN, Brearley MJ, et al: Improved survival in a retrospective cohort of 28 dogs with insulinoma, J Small Anim Pract 48(3):151-156, 2007.
15. Brehm DM, Vite CH, Steinberg HS, et al: A retrospective evaluation of 51 cases of peripheral nerve sheath tumors in the dog, J Am Anim Hosp Assoc 31:349, 1995.
16. McChesney SL, Withrow SJ, Gilette EL: Radiotherapy of soft tissue sarcomas in dogs, J Am Vet Med Assoc 194:60, 1989.
17. Noonan M, Kline KL, Meleo K: Lymphoma of the central nervous system: a retrospective study of 18 cats, Compend Contin Educ Pract Vet 3:203, 1997.
18. Knowler C, Skerritt G: Canine neosporosis and toxoplasmosis, Prog Vet Neurol 5:167, 1994.
19. Braund K, Blagburn B, Toivio-Kinnucan M, et al: Toxoplasma polymyositis/polyneuropathy: a new clinical variant in two mature dogs, J Am Anim Hosp Assoc 24:93, 1988.
20. Cuddon PA: Electrophysiologic assessment of acute polyradiculoneuropathy in dogs: comparison with Guillain-Barré syndrome in people, J Vet Intern Med 12:294, 1998.
21. Hirschvogel K, Jurina K, Steinberg TA, et al: Clinical course of acute canine polyradiculoneuritis following treatment with human IV immunoglobulin, J Am Anim Hosp Assoc 48:299, 2012.
22. Rutter CR, Rozanski EA, Sharp CR, et al: Outcome and medical management in dogs with lower motor disease undergoing mechanical ventilation: 14 cases (2003-2009), J Vet Emerg Crit Care 21:531, 2011.
23. Flanders JA: Feline aortic thromboembolism, Compend Contin Educ Vet Pract 8:473, 1986.
24. Van Winkle TJ, Liu SM, Hackner SG: Clinical and pathological features of aortic thromboembolism in 36 dogs, J Vet Emerg Crit Care 3:13, 1993.
25. Evans J, Levesque D, Shelton GD: Canine inflammatory myopathies: a clinicopathologic review of 200 cases, J Vet Intern Med 18:679, 2004.
26. Dewey CW, Bailey CS, Shelton GD, et al: Clinical forms of acquired myasthenia gravis in dogs: 25 cases (1988-1995), J Vet Intern Med 11:50, 1997.
27. King LG, Vite CH: Acute fulminating myasthenia gravis in five dogs, J Am Vet Med Assoc 212:830, 1998.
28. Khorzad R, Whelan M, Sisson A, et al: Myasthenia gravis in dogs with an emphasis on treatment and critical care management, J Vet Emerg Crit Care 21:193, 2011.
29. Dewey CW, Coates JR, Ducoté JM: Azathioprine therapy for acquired myasthenia gravis in five dogs, J Am Anim Hosp Assoc 35:396, 1999.
30. Abelson AL, Shelton D, Whelan MF, et al: Use of mycophenolate mofetil as a rescue agent in the treatment of severe generalized myasthenia gravis in three dogs, J Vet Emerg Crit Care 19:369, 2009.
31. Dewey CW, Cerda-Gonzalez S, Fletcher DJ, et al: Mycophenolate mofetil treatment in dogs with serologically diagnosed acquired myasthenia gravis: 27 cases, J Am Vet Med Assoc 236:664, 2010.
32. Dewey CW, Shelton GD, Bailey CS, et al: Neuromuscular dysfunction in five dogs with acquired myasthenia gravis and presumptive hypothyroidism, Prog Vet Neurol 6:117, 1995.
33. Barsanti JA: Botulism. In Greene CE, editor: Clinical microbiology and infectious diseases of the dog and cat, Philadelphia, 1984, Saunders.
34. Malik R, Farrow BR: Tick paralysis in North America and Australia, Vet Clin North Am Small Anim Pract 21:157, 1991.
35. Peterson ME: Snake bite: coral snakes. In Peterson ME, Talcott PA, editors: Small animal toxicology, St Louis, 2006, Elsevier Saunders.

CHAPTER 86

TETANUS

Simon R. Platt, BVM&S, MRCVS, DACVIM (Neurology), DECVN

KEY POINTS

- Tetanus is the result of a bacterial infection by *Clostridium tetani* after a skin wound, surgery, or parturition.
- The clinical signs are due to the effects of an exotoxin produced by the bacillus that prevents neurotransmitter release.
- Common signs include spasms of the masticatory, pharyngeal, and facial muscles, but the whole body can be involved.
- Definitive diagnosis is difficult in many cases unless serum antibodies can be associated with the bacterial toxin.
- Treatment is initiated immediately upon suspicion of the disease based on clinical signs.
- Tetanus antitoxin can prevent further patient deterioration from unbound toxin at the time of administration, but improvement relies on regrowth of axons and nerve terminals.
- Broad-spectrum anaerobic antimicrobial therapy, wound cleansing, muscle relaxants, and sedatives are the important constituents of medical management.
- A quiet environment and intensive nursing care are essential for success of the treatment regimens.

ETIOLOGY

Tetanus is caused by the neurotoxins released by *Clostridium tetani,* a motile, gram-positive, nonencapsulated, anaerobic, spore-forming bacterium. The toxin is produced during vegetative growth of the organism in a suitable environment.[1] The deoxyribonucleic acid for this toxin is contained in a plasmid and is antigenically homogenous. The organism's resistant spores are ubiquitous, with a natural habitat in moist, fertile soil; however, they can survive indefinitely in dusty indoor environments. The spores are resistant to boiling water and an autoclave temperature of 120° C for up to 20 minutes.[2] However, the vegetative phase of this bacterium is susceptible to chemical and physical inactivation. Organisms can be isolated from the feces of dogs, cats, and humans, but presence of the organism does not indicate infection because not all strains possess the plasmid.[1]

Cats and dogs are considered to be relatively resistant to infection by the bacterium, especially compared with horses and humans. Cats are approximately 10 times more resistant to infection than dogs; dogs are 600 times more resistant to tetanus than horses. The resistance in these species is due in part to the inability of the toxin to penetrate and bind to nervous tissue.[2]

PATHOGENESIS

Tetanus develops when spores are introduced into wounds or via penetrating injuries. Most cases develop after skin wounds, but infection can follow teething, parturition, or ovariohysterectomy.[3-6] Under anaerobic conditions found in necrotic or infected tissue, the tetanus bacillus secretes two exotoxins: tetanospasmin and tetanolysin. Tetanolysin is capable of locally damaging otherwise viable tissue surrounding the infected area and optimizing the conditions for bacterial multiplication.[1]

Tetanospasmin leads to the clinical syndrome of tetanus. This toxin may constitute more than 5% of the weight of the organism.[1] It is a two-chain polypeptide of 150,000 daltons that is initially inactive, made up of a light and a heavy chain. The light chain acts presynaptically to prevent neurotransmitter release from affected neurons. Tetanospasmin binds to the membranes of the local motor nerve terminals. If toxin load is high, some may enter the bloodstream from where it diffuses to bind to nerve terminals throughout the body and may even enter the central nervous system (CNS) through an intact blood-brain barrier. The toxin then is internalized and transported intraaxonally and in a retrograde fashion to the cell body at a speed of 75 to 250 mm per day.[1,2] Transport occurs first in motor and later in sensory and autonomic nerves. Further retrograde intraneural transport occurs with toxin spreading to the brainstem in a bilateral fashion, up the spinal cord. This passage includes retrograde transfer across synaptic clefts by a mechanism that is unclear.

The light chain becomes activated after internalization into inhibitory neurons; at this stage the toxin is no longer accessible for neutralization by antitoxin.[7,8] It prevents neurotransmitter release by cleaving and inactivating synaptobrevin, a membrane or "docking" protein necessary for the export of intracellular vesicles containing the neurotransmitter.[9] In addition to disrupting docking proteins, the toxin may lead to cross-linking of synaptic vesicles to the cytoskeleton, further preventing neurotransmitter release.[10]

The toxin predominantly affects inhibitory interneurons, inhibiting release of glycine and γ-aminobutyric acid (GABA).[1,8] Interneurons inhibiting α-motor neurons are first affected, and the motor neurons lose inhibitory control. The disinhibitory effect on the motor neuron may cause diminution of function at the neuromuscular junction; therefore the clinical effect is dissimilar to that of the related botulinum toxin. Medullary and hypothalamic centers also may be affected. Disinhibited autonomic discharge leads to disturbances in autonomic control, with sympathetic overactivity and excessive plasma catecholamine levels.

Neuronal binding of toxin is thought to be irreversible. Recovery requires the growth of new nerve terminals, which explains the long duration of tetanus.[11]

CLINICAL PRESENTATION

Tetanus most commonly affects young large breed dogs but is rare in cats.[12] Clinical signs can take up to 3 weeks from the onset of infection to be apparent, although most cases exhibit symptoms within 5 to 12 days.[3,12,13] The clinical signs initially can be localized or generalized, with the former more common in dogs and cats. Only a few cats with tetanus have been documented in the literature; most had predominantly localized clinical signs.[14-17] A study of 38 dogs with tetanus revealed that ocular and facial changes were the most common initial signs.[3] Localized signs begin proximal to the site of introduction of the infection and can include single muscle rigidity, entire limb rigidity, and facial muscle spasms. However, cats may be more likely to experience carpal flexion, whereas dogs exhibit extension.[14,15] The clinical signs may progress with more extensive muscle involvement.[18] Generalized signs include a stiff gait affecting all limbs, increased muscle tone, dyspnea, an elevated tail and a "sawhorse stance," although the animal may become uncomfortable standing with such excessive muscle activity. At least 50% of dogs progress within a median of 4 days (range 0 to 14 days) to recumbency with severe muscle spasms.[3,12,13]

Involvement of the head can lead to spasms of the masticatory and pharyngeal muscles, causing trismus (lockjaw) and dysphagia. This can be exacerbated functionally by increased salivation, increased bronchial secretions, and increased respiratory rate resulting from involvement of the parasympathetic and somatic cranial nerve nuclei. Regurgitation and gastroesophageal reflux can result rarely from esophageal hiatal hernia and megaesophagus, which may lead to aspiration pneumonia when combined with the problems described earlier.[19] Excessive contraction of the facial muscles causes erect ears and a wrinkled forehead (Figure 86-1) and gives the animal a characteristic sneering of the lips known as *risus sardonicus,* or the *sardonic grin* (Figure 86-2).[8] In addition, the patient can exhibit protrusion of the third eyelid and enophthalmos resulting from retraction of the globe because of hypertonus of the extraocular muscles.[2] Reflex muscle spasms can occur in animals with generalized tetanus or intracranial involvement; these may be painful and resemble seizure activity, affecting agonist and antagonist muscle groups together.[2] Severe progression of signs can cause recumbency, opisthotonus, seizure-like activity, respiratory paralysis, and central respiratory arrest, potentially causing death if not rapidly recognized and managed.[8] Death ranged between 8% and 50% of dogs in three recent retrospective studies, and many of these dogs demonstrated concurrent autonomic signs.[3,12,13]

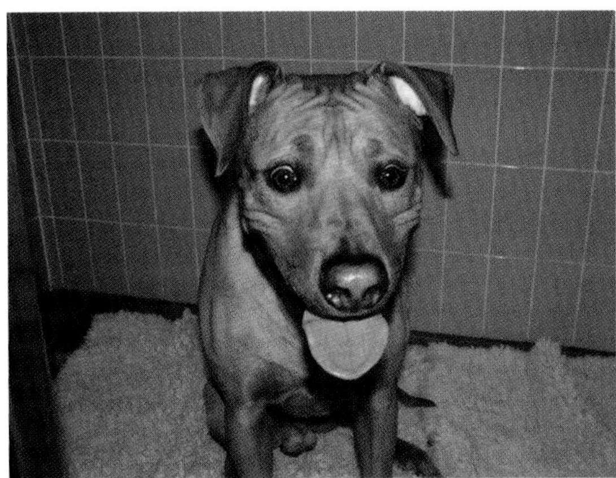

FIGURE 86-1 A 2-year-old female Rhodesian Ridgeback with tetanus demonstrates classic spasms of facial musculature.

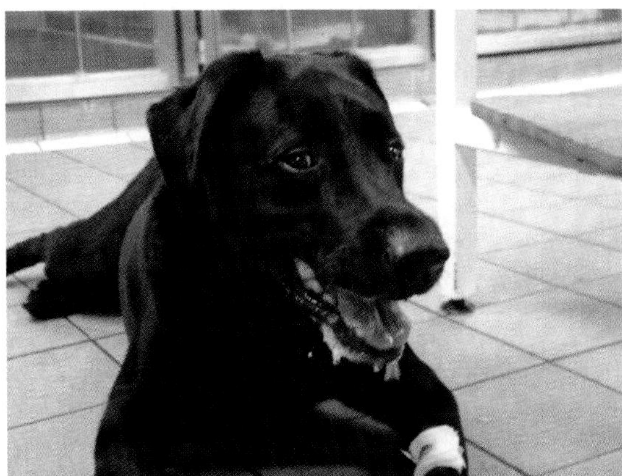

FIGURE 86-2 A 6-year-old female spayed Labrador Retriever with tetanus exhibiting marked accumulation of saliva and a facial grimace often seen with this disease.

It is possible to see an effect on the autonomic system evidenced by episodes of bradycardia and tachycardia, hypertension, marked vasoconstriction, and pyrexia.[12,14,15] A study of 38 dogs with tetanus revealed that 37% demonstrated abnormalities of blood pressure or rectal temperature, or both, consistent with autonomic disturbance.[3] In the mild generalized cases, autonomic involvement may be manifested by dysuria and urinary retention, constipation, and gaseous distention. In humans, "autonomic storms" occur, causing marked cardiovascular instability, severe hypertension alternating with profound hypotension, and even recurrent cardiac arrest.[1] During these "storms," plasma catecholamine levels are raised to tenfold, similar to levels seen in animals with a pheochromocytoma.[1]

A neurologic examination of these patients can reveal normal initiation of a response to postural reaction testing but a stiff and reduced motor response.[2] Myotatic reflexes generally are accentuated and flexor reflexes depressed, but both may be difficult to assess because of the extreme rigidity of the limbs. Although a complete neurologic examination is always ideal, animals can become sensitive to tactile, visual, or auditory stimulation that can exacerbate clinical signs, occasionally causing a mild, generalized form of the disease to progress to a crisis situation.

A tetanus severity classification system has been proposed in dogs[3]: class I dogs have only facial signs of tetanus; class II dogs have generalized rigidity or dysphagia, with or without class I signs; class III dogs have class I or II signs and are recumbent or have seizures; and class IV dogs have class I, II, or III signs as well as abnormal heart rate, respiratory rate, or blood pressure measurements.[3]

DIAGNOSIS

The patient's history and clinical signs are usually sufficient to make a presumptive diagnosis of tetanus. Differential diagnoses considered in patients with tetanus could include immune-mediated polymyositis, strychnine toxicity, spinal trauma, hypocalcemia, or meningoencephalitis. The differential diagnoses for "lockjaw" should include temporomandibular joint (TMJ) ankylosis, which can be secondary to fracture, masticatory muscle myositis, neoplasia, TMJ luxation and dysplasia, osteoarthritis, retrobulbar abscess, and severe ear disease.[20]

If general anesthesia is used for diagnostic tests such as cerebrospinal fluid acquisition, the muscle spasms can be reduced but rarely are abolished. Intubation may be difficult in patients with trismus, and a stylet-assisted intubation should be anticipated in severely affected animals (see Supportive Intensive Care).

A complete blood count may suggest an infectious process from a wound, whereas serum biochemistry (with the exception of muscle enzymes) and cerebrospinal fluid analysis findings are normal.[2] Muscle enzymes may be elevated in patients with tetanus because of the persistent muscle spasticity; high activities of creatine kinase (1599-18405 U/L [reference range 61 to 394 U/L]) have been documented in more than 50% of dogs.[13] Radiographs may be helpful to identify involvement of the esophagus, diaphragm, and secondary changes in the lungs resulting from aspiration pneumonia.

Electrodiagnostic abnormalities in patients with tetanus are nonspecific and consist of prolonged electric discharges after needle insertion on electromyography. There is a subsequent persistence of motor unit discharges occurring as "doublets," which are double discharges of the same motor unit at short intervals and often simultaneous activity of agonist and antagonist muscles. Nerve conduction velocities are normal.[21]

Measurement of serum antibodies to tetanospasmin can be performed by some laboratories and used for a definitive diagnosis.[8] Values have to be compared with those of control animals.

Attempts to isolate *C. tetani* from wounds often fails because of the low concentration of organisms and the requirement for strict anaerobic culture conditions at 37° C for at least 2 weeks.[8] A Gram stain of a smear from an open wound may identify gram-positive rods and dark-staining spheric endospores, but the morphology of the bacterium is nonspecific and similar to that of many other bacteria.[2]

TREATMENT

Treatment strategies involve three principles: toxins present in the body outside of the CNS should be neutralized; organisms present in the body should be destroyed to prevent further toxin release; and the effects of the toxin already in the CNS should be minimized. Intensive care management is also paramount. A detailed discussion on antitoxin can be found in Chapter 174, but a brief review and dosing follows.

Neutralization of Unbound Toxin

Antitoxin neutralizes any toxin that is unbound to the CNS or yet to be formed. Therefore the timing of administration in relation to the onset of the disease is essential to its effectiveness. The antitoxin used can be either antitetanus equine serum or human tetanus immune globulin. The latter may be more likely to produce reactions if given intravenously.[22] Early intervention has been recommended as a matter of routine, but there are no prospective studies objectively evaluating antitoxin use in dogs or cats, and its efficacy in cases with no evidence of a recent wound is unknown. A recent retrospective of 20 dogs with tetanus reported that antitoxin was used in 16 (80%).[12] There were no statistically significant differences in survival, severity of clinical signs, or duration of clinical signs between dogs treated with antitoxin and those that did not receive antitoxin.[12] Another retrospective of 38 dogs documented antitoxin use in 29 cases; there was no association between earlier administration of antitoxin and progression of clinical signs (i.e., worsening tetanus severity classification) or 28-day mortality rate.[3]

The recommended dosage of equine antitoxin for dogs and cats is 100 to 1000 U/kg (maximum 20,000 U/kg) IV, SC, or IM.[2] Intravenous administration is preferred to intramuscular or subcutaneous administration (see Chapter 174). Although intravenous use of antitoxin is associated with a higher incidence of anaphylaxis, the reported rate of hypersensitivity reactions in dogs is relatively low.[2] Epinephrine (0.1 ml/kg IV of the 1 : 10,000 dilution), glucocorticoids, and an antihistamine (e.g., diphenhydramine) should be readily available in case of an adverse reaction (see Chapter 152). Repeated doses of antitoxin are more likely to cause adverse reactions and are not recommended or necessary because therapeutic levels persist for approximately 14 days. The use of intradermal testing or intramuscular injections near the wound site is not well substantiated in the literature and therefore not recommended at this time. See Chapter 174 for further details.

Removal of Source of Infection

Any obvious wounds should be radically debrided after the administration of antitoxin. Flushing the wound with hydrogen peroxide increases oxygen tension, which inhibits anaerobic organisms, although wound healing also may be impaired[2] (see Chapter 139).

Antimicrobials are essential to kill vegetative *C. tetani* organisms and thereby reduce the amount of circulating toxin. Although local administration of antimicrobials at the wound site has been advised, parenteral administration is recommended more routinely.[2] Classically, penicillin G has been the drug of choice, either intravenously as an aqueous potassium or sodium salt or intramuscularly as the procaine salt (20,000 to 100,000 U/kg q6-12h for 10 days in cats and dogs). However, metronidazole (7 to 10 mg/kg PO or IV q8-12h for 10 days) has been shown superior to penicillin G in clinical tetanus because it achieves bactericidal therapeutic concentrations in anaerobic tissues.[2] Other options include clindamycin (10 mg/kg PO, IV, or IM q8-12h) and tetracycline (22 mg/kg PO or IV q8h) or doxycycline (5 to 10 mg/kg PO or IV q12h).[2]

Control of Rigidity and Spasms

See Anesthesia and Pain Management for more details on specific therapies.

Prevention of unnecessary stimulation is mandatory, but the mainstay of treatment is sedation with a benzodiazepine (see Chapter 164). Benzodiazepines augment GABA agonism at the $GABA_A$ receptor. Diazepam (0.5 to 1 mg/kg PO q8h in dogs [maximum 10 mg], 0.25 to 0.5 mg/kg in cats [maximum 5 mg, caution with oral diazepam in cats because of hepatotoxicity], or a continuous intravenous infusion of 0.1 to 1 mg/kg/hr in dogs and cats) or clorazepate (0.5 to 1 mg/kg PO q8h in dogs; 0.2 to 0.5 mg/kg PO q12-24h in cats) can be used in this regard, although both may cause oversedation in some patients. As an alternative, midazolam can be used as a continuous intravenous infusion (0.2 to 0.5 mg/kg/hr).

Additional sedation can be provided with anticonvulsant therapy, particularly phenobarbital (1 to 4 mg/kg PO or IV q12h or IM q6h), which further enhances GABAergic activity. Phenothiazines may be highly effective in controlling the hyperexcitable state; chlorpromazine (0.1 to 0.5 mg/kg IM, IV, or PO q6-12h) is the drug of choice, although acetylpromazine (0.005 to 0.05 mg/kg IV q2h as needed [maximum 3 mg in any dog]) is a useful substitute.

With severe signs such as generalized tonic-clonic seizure activity, generalized body stiffness, and opisthotonus, a propofol (or pentobarbital, if available) infusion may be necessary, but cardiovascular parameters should be monitored closely and careful consideration should be given to whether the patient should be intubated and placed on positive-pressure ventilation. Sedation with propofol has been shown to assist with muscle spasm and rigidity control in humans, without the use of neuromuscular-blocking drugs.[24] Neuromuscular blocking agents may be an option for the most severely affected veterinary patients, but assisted ventilation is imperative. Recently, the use of magnesium sulfate ($MgSO_4$) infusions or supraphysiologic magnesium therapy has been documented as a potential adjunct therapy in the management of spastic paralysis in dogs with tetanus.[25] However, a recent human metaanalysis of tetanus patients treated with magnesium could not detect a difference in mortality.[26] A dose of 70 mg/kg over 30 minutes followed by an initial constant rate infusion of 100 mg/kg/day has been recommended for dogs based on human literature. The goal of this treatment is to increase total serum magnesium to 2 to 4 mmol/L (4.86 to 9.73 mg/dl) based on a target therapeutic range derived from the human literature.[25] Clinical signs of magnesium toxicity range from lethargy and nausea to respiratory depression, bradycardia, and hypotension. Recommended methods to monitor for early signs of toxicity include assessing serum magnesium concentrations every 4 to 6 hours, checking the patella tendon reflex every hour for hyporeflexia, continuous electrocardiogram, pulse oximetry, and noninvasive blood pressures. The beneficial effects of magnesium in tetanus patients are likely multifactorial. It is thought that magnesium's beneficial activity stems primarily from its action as a nonspecific calcium channel blocker. At the neuromuscular junction, magnesium decreases calcium entry into presynaptic terminals resulting in decreased acetylcholine (ACh) release. In addition, it decreases the sensitivity of postsynaptic motor endplates to Ach, with the net result being muscle relaxation. Magnesium has been reported to decrease catecholamine release from adrenal glands and peripheral adrenergic nerve terminals as well as reduce sensitivity of receptors to these neurotransmitters.[25]

The use of botulinum toxin for tetanus-induced rigidity in humans recently has been suggested.[27] Botulinum toxins enter nerve terminals of lower motor neurons.[27] The toxins are zinc metalloproteinases that attack synaptic vesicle proteins, but they do so differentially: botulinum toxin A cleaves synaptosomal-associated protein (SNAP-25), botulinum toxins B, D, F, and G cleave synaptobrevin (which also is attacked by tetanus toxin); botulinum toxin C cleaves SNAP-25 and syntaxin.[27] The effects of botulinum toxins remain fairly confined to the nerve terminals of lower motor neurons, inhibiting release of acetylcholine and activation of voluntary muscles. For this reason they may have a role in reducing the muscular hyperactivity in tetanus patients.

Narcotics and parasympatholytics such as atropine should be used with caution. In severe human forms of tetanus, atropine infusions have helped to control autonomic dysfunction, although close monitoring for adverse advents is advised.[28]

Supportive Intensive Care

Intensive nursing care is essential for successful treatment of patients with tetanus. The dog or cat should be isolated in a dark and quiet environment, with cotton wool balls placed in the external ear canals (Figure 86-3). Minimal handling is optimal, and all treatments therefore should be coordinated to occur together at set times through the day. A recent study of 13 dogs with tetanus documented the complications that occurred in these dogs during treatment; these included aspiration pneumonia, upper respiratory tract obstruction requiring tracheostomy, hiatal hernia, hyperthermia, and coxofemoral luxation.[13]

Weight loss and dehydration are common in patients with tetanus resulting from poor prehending, mastication, and swallowing capabilities, reduced gastrointestinal function in the presence of autonomic dysfunction, increased metabolic rate, and hyperthermia from the muscular activity and prolonged critical illness. Nutrition and fluid therapy therefore should be established as early as possible. Enteral nutrition may be associated with a lower incidence of complications and is less expensive than parenteral nutrition, but the latter may be necessary in select cases. The risk of vomiting and subsequent aspiration pneumonia must be considered when making this decision (see Chapters 129 and 130, respectively).

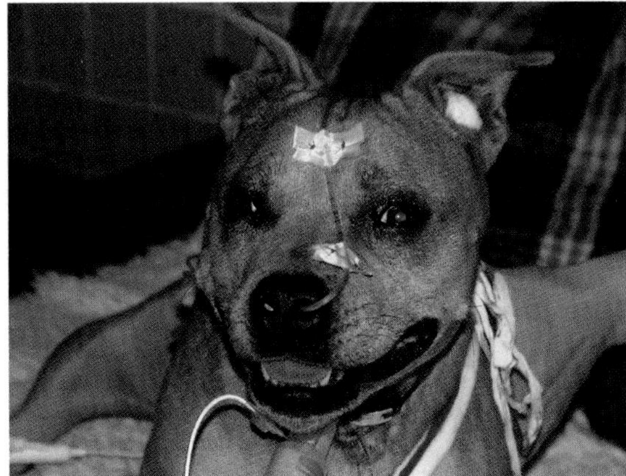

FIGURE 86-3 A dog with tetanus that has a nasoesophageal feeding tube for enteral nutritional support and tracheostomy for airway protection and ventilator support, if needed. Note the cotton in the external ear canals to help prevent noise-induced titanic spasms.

Percutaneous gastrostomy tube placement may prevent the complications associated with nasogastric tube feeding, particularly the stress that may be associated with an indwelling intranasal tube. Gastrostomy- or gastrojejunostomy-assisted tube feeding also can reduce the risk of aspiration pneumonia, a potential complication in dogs with severe forms of tetanus and those that are recumbent for a prolonged period.

If airway obstruction develops because of laryngeal spasm or a buildup of saliva or tracheal secretions, intubation and mechanical ventilation may be necessary. A tracheostomy often is performed in these patients to decrease the need for continuous anesthesia (see Chapter 197). A stylet may be inserted into the airway and the endotracheal tube fed over the stylet for intubation of dogs with severe laryngospasm. A tracheostomy requires meticulous care to prevent introduction of infection but allows intermittent tracheal suction to be performed with little stress to the animal. Oxygen supplementation may be administered via tracheostomy flow-by, intratracheally, or with mechanical ventilation.

Urinary and fecal retention occur in some patients with hypertonic anal and urinary sphincters. An indwelling urinary catheter may be beneficial in these patients, although the urine should be analyzed regularly for evidence of nosocomial infection.

Pressure sores or decubital ulcers should be prevented with appropriate soft or padded bedding and frequent turning and physiotherapy. However, the balance between frequent physiotherapy and isolated rest is difficult to achieve, and pharmacologic sedation may be necessary before physical manipulation is possible in some patients.

PROGNOSIS

Recovery in dogs with tetanus depends on successful support of the animal while new axonal terminals form. Most dogs that recover (58% to 77%) show some improvement within 5 to 12 days, although the presence of autonomic abnormalities is a poor prognostic indicator.[3,12] Median length of hospitalization for dogs has been reported to be 13 days (range 6 to 42 days). One study estimated the mortality rate to be approximately 18% in affected dogs, but it also has been reported as high as 50%.[25] Mortality is likely related to the severity of clinical signs; one study reveals that all dogs with class I or II clinical signs survived and only 58% of class III or IV signs survived.[3] However, actual mortality may be difficult to estimate given the fact that long-term intensive management of these cases is associated with a significant financial burden for the owners; therefore many animals are euthanized humanely.

Dogs with surgical wounds manifest a more severe clinical course than those with external wounds, but wound type has not been associated with mortality. Young dogs are also more likely to develop more severe treatment.[3] Currently there is no documented association between earlier wound treatments, antimicrobial drug therapy, or antitoxin administration and either progression of signs or survival.[3] However, prospective trials are necessary to further investigate the value of these therapeutic options. A full recovery may not be possible in at least 15% of dogs that survive, but continued improvement may be seen for 3 to 5 months.[3,12,13]

A tetanus vaccine has not been developed for dogs because of their relative resistance to the disease. Natural infection does not provide effective, long-lasting immunity. The best way to prevent tetanus is through rapid and appropriate wound management and appropriate antimicrobial selection.

Cats are reported to recover well from localized tetanus with some residual deficits remaining several months later[14-17]; there are no large studies assessing the prognosis in cats with generalized tetanus.

REFERENCES

1. Cook TM, Protheroe RT, Handel JM: Tetanus: a review of the literature, Br J Anaesth 87:477, 2001.
2. Greene CE: Tetanus. In Greene CE, editor: Infectious diseases of the dog and cat, ed 4, St Louis, 2011, Saunders.
3. Burkitt JM, Sturges BK, Jandrey KE, Kass PH: Risk factors associated with outcome in dogs with tetanus: 38 cases (1987-2005), J Am Vet Med Assoc. 230:76, 2007.
4. Arthur JE, Studdert VP: Parturition in a bitch with tetanus, Aust Vet J 61:126, 1984.
5. Bagley RS, Dougherty SA, Randolph JF: Tetanus subsequent to ovariohysterectomy in a dog, Prog Vet Neurol 5:63, 1994.
6. Lee EA, Jones BR: Localized tetanus in two cats after ovariohysterectomy, N Z Vet J 44:105, 1996.
7. Montecucco C, Schiavo G: Mechanism of action of tetanus and botulinum neurotoxins, Mol Microbiol 13:1, 1994.
8. Coleman ES: Clostridial neurotoxins: tetanus and botulism, Comp Cont Educ Small Anim Pract 20:1089, 1998.
9. Schiavo G, Benfenati F, Poulain B, et al: Tetanus and botulinum-B neurotoxins block neurotransmitter release by proteolytic cleavage of synaptobrevin, Nature 359:832, 1992.
10. Facchiano F, Valtorta F, Benfenati F, et al: The transglutaminase hypothesis for the action of tetanus toxin, Trends Biochem Sci 18:327, 1993.
11. Sandford JP: Tetanus: forgotten but not gone, N Engl J Med 332:812, 1995.
12. Bandt C, Rozanski EA, Steinberg T, Shaw SP: Retrospective study of tetanus in 20 dogs: 1988-2004, J Am Anim Hosp Assoc 43:143, 2007.
13. Adamantos S, Boag A: Thirteen cases of tetanus in dogs, Vet Rec 161:298, 2007.
14. Langner KF, Schenk HC, Leithaeuser C, et al: Localised tetanus in a cat, Vet Rec 169:126, 2011.
15. De Risio L, Gelati A: Tetanus in the cat—an unusual presentation, J Feline Med Surg 5:237, 2003 .
16. Baral RM, Catt MJ, Malik R: What is your diagnosis? Localised tetanus in a cat, J Feline Med Surg 4:221, 2002.
17. Polizopoulou ZS, Kazakos G, Georgiadis G, et al: Presumed localized tetanus in two cats, J Feline Med Surg 4:209, 2002.
18. Dieringer TM, Wolf AM: Esophageal hiatal hernia and megaesophagus complicating tetanus in two dogs, J Am Vet Med Assoc 199:87, 1991.
19. Panciera DL, Baldwin CJ, Keene BW: Electrocardiographic abnormalities associated with tetanus in two dogs, J Am Vet Med Assoc 192:225, 1988.
20. Gatineau M, El-Warrak AO, Marretta SM, et al: Locked jaw syndrome in dogs and cats: 37 cases (1998-2005), J Vet Dent 25:16, 2008.
21. De Risio L, Zavattiero S, Venzi C, et al: Focal canine tetanus: diagnostic value of electromyography, J Small Anim Pract 47:278, 2006.
22. Bleck T: Pharmacology of tetanus, Clin Neuropharmacol 9:103, 1986.
23. Reference deleted in pages.
24. Borgeat A, Popovic V, Schwander D: Efficiency of a continuous infusion of propofol in a patient with tetanus, Crit Care Med 19:295, 1991.
25. Simmonds EE, Alwood AJ, Costello MF: Magnesium sulfate as an adjunct therapy in the management of severe generalized tetanus in a dog, J Vet Emerg Crit Care 21:542, 2011.
26. Rodrigo C, Samarakoon L, Fernando SD, Rajapakse S: A meta-analysis of magnesium for tetanus, Anaesthesia 67:1370, 2012.
27. Hassel B: Tetanus: pathophysiology, treatment, and the possibility of using botulinum toxin against tetanus-induced rigidity and spasms, Toxins 5:73, 2013.
28. Dolar D: The use of continuous atropine infusion in the management of severe tetanus, Intensive Care Med 18:26, 1992.

CHAPTER 87
VESTIBULAR DISEASE

Simon R. Platt, BVM&S, MRCVS, DACVIM (Neurology), DECVN

KEY POINTS

- Patients with vestibular disease have dysfunction of the vestibular system and often are presented for treatment on an emergent basis.
- The vestibular system is comprised of a peripheral component within the structures of the inner ear and central components in the brainstem and cerebellum.
- The common clinical signs of vestibular disease include head tilt, ataxia, and nystagmus.
- Peripheral vestibular disease can be accompanied by Horner's syndrome and facial nerve paresis.
- Central vestibular disease typically is accompanied by loss of proprioceptive and motor function, in addition to multiple cranial nerve deficits and mentation changes.
- The differential diagnosis for the cause of vestibular disease depends on the localization of the lesion to the peripheral or central compartments.
- Treatment of vestibular disease is determined by the underlying etiology, but supportive care is extremely important, especially during the initial stages of the disease.

Dogs and cats have the ability to control posture and movements of the body and eyes relative to the external environment. The vestibular system mediates these activities through a network of receptors and neural elements. Disease leading to dysfunction of the vestibular system can lead to dramatic signs of disequilibrium. The investigation, treatment, and prognosis of the cause of the disequilibrium can differ depending on whether the peripheral or central components of the system are affected.

This chapter outlines the relevant anatomy of the vestibular system and how this influences the clinical signs of its dysfunction, in addition to the diseases that are most commonly responsible for the acute onset of clinical signs.

NEUROANATOMY OF THE VESTIBULAR SYSTEM

The vestibular system can be divided into (1) peripheral components located in the inner ear and (2) central nervous system (CNS) components. Three major CNS areas receive projections from the peripheral sensory receptors of the vestibular system: the cerebral cortex, the spinal cord, and the cerebellum. The projection to the cerebral cortex incorporates extensions to the extraocular muscles.

Nerve Pathways to the Extraocular Muscles

Two neurons make up the pathway responsible for the sensory input of the head to the cerebral cortex (Figure 87-1).

Neuron 1

The cell location for the first neuron is within the vestibular ganglion of the eighth cranial or vestibulocochlear nerve, and the axon projects into the ipsilateral vestibular nuclei. These neurons receive input from the vestibular receptors in the membranous labyrinth contained within a bony labyrinth in the petrous temporal bone. The sensory neurons are incorporated into the vestibulocochlear nerve, which leaves the petrous temporal bone via the internal acoustic meatus, along with the facial nerve, and enters the medulla of the brainstem.[1]

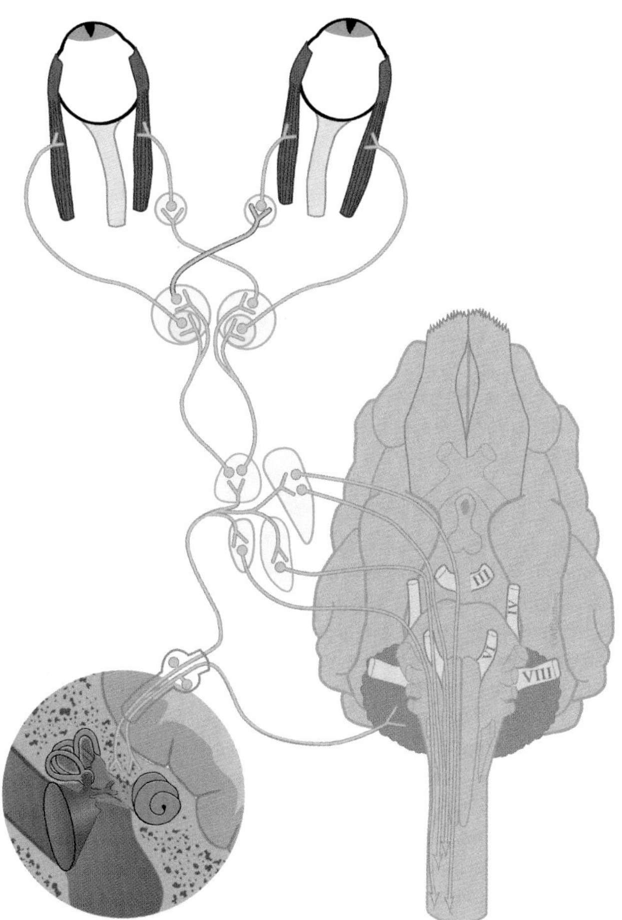

FIGURE 87-1 Diagrammatic overview of the neuroanatomy of the vestibular system. *(From Platt S, Olby N, editors: Manual of canine and feline neurology, ed 4, Gloucester, 2012, British Small Animal Veterinary Association. A. Wright, illustrator.)*

Neuron 2

The cell location for the second neuron is in the vestibular nuclei, which are situated in the medulla oblongata. From these nuclei, axons travel in the medial longitudinal fasciculus within the brainstem. The ascending axons within the fasciculus give off numerous side branches to the motor nuclei of cranial nerves III, IV, and VI, thereby providing coordinated conjugated eyeball movements associated with changes in position of the head. Some axons project from the nuclei into the reticular formation and go on to provide afferents to the vomiting center located there.[1]

Nerve Pathways to the Spinal Cord

The vestibulospinal tract descends from the vestibular nuclei and projects mainly onto α-neurons or extensor motor neurons throughout the length of the cord via interneurons in the ventral grey column.[1] This pathway is strongly facilitatory to the ipsilateral alpha and gamma motor neurons to extensor muscles.

Nerve Pathways to the Cerebellum

The vestibular nuclei project directly to the cortex of the ipsilateral flocculonodular lobe (the flocculus of the hemisphere and the nodulus of the caudal vermis), as well as the fastigial nucleus of the cerebellum.[1] The return pathway from a cerebellar nucleus to the vestibular nuclei is also ipsilateral; this is an extremely large projection, providing the cerebellum with a strong influence over the activity of the vestibular nuclei. These pathways between the cerebellum and the vestibular nuclei travel in the caudal cerebellar peduncle.

CLINICAL SIGNS

Unilateral vestibular disease produces asymmetric signs, often on or toward the side of the disease. The most common clinical signs of vestibular disease are head tilt, nystagmus, and ataxia; these may be single entities or a combination of signs.[2] The primary aim of the neurologic examination is to determine if these vestibular signs are due to a peripheral vestibular system (inner ear) disease or a central vestibular system (brainstem and cerebellum, or both) disease. Localization of the disease determines the most appropriate diagnostic tests, the differential diagnoses, and the prognosis.

The essential determination of whether these signs are due to a peripheral or central disease may be possible by the identification of associated neurologic signs that are present only with central disease.[2] Signs of central vestibular syndrome suggest damage to the brainstem and are not present in patients with inner ear disease unless there has been extension of the inner ear disease into the brainstem, such as can be seen with otitis media, otitis interna, and neoplasia.[3]

Specific Signs of Vestibular Dysfunction

Signs of vestibular dysfunction are outlined in Table 87-1.

Head tilt

Loss of equilibrium is most commonly represented clinically as a head tilt that may be present with either central or peripheral vestibular disease. The head tilt is always toward the side of the lesion with peripheral disease but may be toward either side with central disease. When the head tilt is opposite to the side of the lesion, it is termed *paradoxical*.[2] This can be seen with lesions of the flocculonodular lobe of the cerebellum or the supramedullary part of the caudal cerebellar peduncle, with sparing of the vestibular nuclei in the rostral medulla; the head tilt often is accompanied by ipsilateral cerebellar signs, paresis, and proprioceptive deficits.[3]

Table 87-1 Neurologic Examination Findings in Animals with Peripheral and Central Vestibular Dysfunction

Clinical Signs	Peripheral Vestibular Disease	Central Vestibular Disease
Head tilt	Toward the lesion	Toward the lesion, or away from the lesion with paradoxical disease
Spontaneous nystagmus	Horizontal or rotatory with the fast phase away from the side of the lesion Rarely positional	Horizontal, rotatory, vertical, and/or positional with the fast phase toward or away from the lesion
Paresis and proprioceptive deficits	None	Commonly ipsilateral to the lesion
Mentation	Normal to disoriented	Depressed, stuporous, obtunded, or comatose
Cranial nerve deficits	Ipsilateral CN VII deficit	Ipsilateral CN V, VII, IX, X, and XII
Horner's syndrome	Common ipsilateral to the lesion	Uncommon
Head tremors	None	Can occur with concurrent cerebellar dysfunction
Circling	Infrequent but can be seen toward the side of the lesion	Usually toward the side of the lesion

CN, Cranial nerve.

Bilateral peripheral vestibular disease does not produce asymmetric lesions such as a head tilt. A characteristic side-to-side head movement is seen instead.

Nystagmus

Pathologic or spontaneous nystagmus is an involuntary rhythmic oscillation of both eyes, occurs when the head is still, and is a sign of altered vestibular input to the neurons that innervate the extraocular eye muscles.[2] This is in contrast to physiologic nystagmus, which can be induced in normal animals. Pathologic nystagmus may be horizontal, rotatory, or vertical. Vertical nystagmus implies a central vestibular lesion but it is not a definitive localizing sign. If nystagmus of any direction is induced only when the head is placed in an unusual position, it is known as *positional nystagmus,* which may be more common with, but not specific for, central disease; this term also may refer to nystagmus that changes its predominant direction with altered head positions.[2]

Nystagmus occurs with the fast phase away from the damaged side; the slow phase commonly is directed toward the affected side. In acute and or aggressive nystagmus, the eyelids may be seen to contract at a rate corresponding to that of the nystagmus. Nystagmus may disappear with chronicity of the underlying lesion, particularly with peripheral disease, but its presence usually indicates an active disease process within the vestibular apparatus. Animals with bilateral vestibular disease do not have pathologic or physiologic nystagmus.[4]

Ataxia

Ataxia is a failure of muscular coordination or an irregularity of muscle action. It generally is associated with a cerebellar, vestibular, or proprioceptive pathway abnormality. Animals with vestibular dysfunction assume a wide-based stance and may lean or drift toward the side of a lesion if the dysequilibrium is not too severe.[4]

Signs That May Be Associated with Vestibular Dysfunction

Facial paresis, paralysis, and hemifacial spasm

Cranial nerve VII, the facial nerve, is involved commonly in the same disease processes that cause peripheral vestibular disease.[5] The resulting signs are those of facial paresis, paralysis or, more rarely, spasm.

Horner's syndrome

Horner's syndrome (miosis, ptosis, enophthalmos, and protrusion of the third eyelid) of the ipsilateral eye may be present with either middle or inner ear disease causing peripheral vestibular dysfunction.[6] This association is seen because the vagosympathetic trunk synapses in the cranial cervical ganglion deep to the tympanic bulla. Horner's syndrome rarely is associated with central vestibular disease.[1]

Conscious proprioception deficits

Animals with central vestibular dysfunction often have ipsilateral proprioceptive deficits manifested by abnormal postural reactions such as hopping and proprioceptive placing. These deficits are due to the concurrent disturbance of the ascending proprioceptive pathways located in the brainstem.

Hemiparesis or tetraparesis

Paresis suggests abnormal neurologic function (weakness) without complete paralysis, which implies that some voluntary motion remains. Locomotion is thought to be initiated in the brain stem of animals, so paresis usually is seen with any lesion within the neuraxis caudal to the level of the red nucleus in the midbrain.[3] With unilateral focal central vestibular diseases, paresis of the ipsilateral limbs (hemiparesis) may be seen if the motor pathways in the medulla oblongata also are affected. A large lesion or multifocal lesions may cause an asymmetric tetraparesis. Paresis does not occur with peripheral vestibular disease.

Circling, leaning, and falling

With unilateral vestibular dysfunction, dogs or cats may exhibit an ipsilateral reduction in extensor tone, and contralateral hypertonicity, causing them to lean, fall, and circle toward the side of the lesion.[2] Falling may occur when the animal shakes its head if there is aural irritation.

Altered mental state

Disorders causing central vestibular dysfunction may be accompanied by altered mentation. The reticular activating system of the brainstem facilitates the alert and awake state in animals.[1] Damage to this area may cause the animal to become disoriented, stuporous, or comatose.[3] Although peripheral vestibular disease does not cause stupor or coma, it may cause disorientation, which can make the assessment of the animal's mental status difficult.

Multiple cranial nerve dysfunction

Central vestibular syndrome may be accompanied by other cranial nerve dysfunction as well. Clinical signs can include ipsilateral facial hypalgesia, atrophy of the masticatory muscles, reduced jaw tone, facial paralysis, tongue weakness, and loss of the swallow or gag reflex.

Decerebellate posturing

In severe forms of central vestibular dysfunction, the underlying disease also may cause decerebellate posturing or rigidity; this is characterized by opisthotonus with thoracic limb extension, normal mentation, and flexion of the pelvic limbs.[3] This posture can occur intermittently and be accompanied by vertical nystagmus, the combination being confused by owners as some type of seizure activity. Dorsiflexion of the neck sometimes elicits this posture.

Vomiting

The vomiting center is located within the reticular substance of the medulla, and there are direct connections to it from the vestibular nuclei.[1] Vomiting may be seen in animals affected acutely by vestibular disease.[2]

DIFFERENTIAL DIAGNOSIS OF ACUTE VESTIBULAR DISEASE

Tables 87-2 and 87-3 outline the overall etiologies and infectious causes of acute vestibular disease, respectively.

DIAGNOSTIC APPROACH TO THE ANIMAL WITH ACUTE VESTIBULAR DISEASE

The approach to an animal with vestibular disease can depend on whether a peripheral or central lesion is suspected (Figure 87-2). To determine this, a complete history and a thorough physical and neurologic examination are essential.

The following tests can be performed in sequence, advancing in expense and invasive nature until satisfactory information is acquired. All of the tests may be necessary if central disease is suspected, whereas cerebrospinal fluid (CSF) analysis and advanced imaging may not be necessary if peripheral disease is responsible for the vestibular dysfunction.

Minimum Database

Hematology, a comprehensive serum biochemistry, thyroid function analysis, urinalysis with culture and susceptibility, thoracic radiographs, and abdominal ultrasonography or radiographs should be analyzed in all cases of acute vestibular dysfunction to evaluate the patient for multisystemic or concurrent disease.

Otoscopy and Pharyngeal Examination

General anesthesia is necessary to examine thoroughly the ears and pharynx for abnormalities such as exudates and soft tissue masses. Both ears should be examined with an otoscope. The tympanum should be examined for color, texture, and integrity; it is usually dark gray or brown in cases of otitis. An intact tympanum does not rule out otitis media, and diagnosing otitis media on the sole basis of a ruptured tympanum is also unreliable.[5]

Radiography

Radiography is useful for evaluating the osseous tympanic bulla. Skull radiographs should be performed under general anesthesia to achieve adequate positioning. This may not be possible always, particularly in the trauma patient. Assessment of the tympanic bulla can

Table 87-2 Etiologies of Peripheral and Central Vestibular Diseases[1,2,13]

	Specific Diseases	
Disease Mechanism	**Peripheral Disease**	**Central Disease**
Degenerative	—	Cerebellar cortical abiotrophy Lysosomal storage diseases
Anomalous	Congenital vestibular disease	Hydrocephalus Intracranial intra-arachnoid cysts
Metabolic	Hypothyroidism	Hypothyroidism[17]
Nutritional	—	Thiamine deficiency
Neoplasia	Squamous cell carcinoma Fibrosarcoma Osteosarcoma Ceruminous gland or sebaceous gland adenocarcinoma	Meningioma Oligodendroglioma Medulloblastoma Lymphoma Extension of middle ear neoplasia Metastasis
Inflammatory or infectious	Bacterial otitis interna or labyrinthitis Cryptococcosis Nasopharyngeal polyps (Cuterebra larval migration)	See Table 87-3
Idiopathic	Idiopathic vestibular syndrome	—
Toxic	Aminoglycosides Furosemide Chlorhexidine 10% fipronil solution (aural administration)	Metronidazole Lead
Traumatic	Iatrogenic: external middle ear flushing or bulla osteotomy Bulla fracture or hemorrhage	Head trauma
Vascular	—	Infarction or hemorrhage Feline ischemic encephalopathy Cuterebra larval migration

Table 87-3 Infectious and Inflammatory Central Nervous System Disorders That May Cause Vestibular Dysfunction[1,12,13]

Class of Etiologic Agent	Disease
Viral	Feline infectious peritonitis Feline immunodeficiency virus Feline leukemia virus Rabies Pseudorabies Borna disease virus Distemper virus
Protozoal	Toxoplasmosis, neosporosis Encephalitozoonosis
Bacterial	Aerobes Anaerobes
Rickettsial	*Rickettsia rickettsii* *Ehrlichia* spp.
Fungal	Cryptococcosis Blastomycosis Histoplasmosis Coccidioidomycosis Aspergillosis Phaeohyphomycosis
Parasitic	*Angiostrongylus vasorum* Cuterebra larval myiasis Dirofilaria immitis
Agent unknown	Nonsuppurative meningoencephalomyelitis (presumed viral) Eosinophilic meningoencephalitis Granulomatous meningoencephalitis Necrotizing meningoencephalitis (Pug, Maltese, Terrier, Chihuahua) Necrotizing leukoencephalitis (Yorkshire Terrier)

be made using lateral, dorsoventral, or ventrodorsal, lateral-20 degree ventral-laterodorsal oblique, and rostral-30 degree ventral-caudodorsal open-mouth oblique radiographic images.[7]

Myringotomy

Myringotomy is the deliberate puncture or incision of an intact, although not necessarily healthy, tympanic membrane.[8] Needle puncture and subsequent aspiration through the ventrocaudal part of the tympanic membrane allows for collection of fluid from the tympanic cavity for cytologic examination and microbial culture and susceptibility testing.

Brainstem Auditory Evoked Potentials

Brainstem auditory evoked potentials testing, also known as *brainstem auditory evoked response testing,* can be used to assess the integrity and function of the peripheral and central auditory pathways, which allows for indirect evaluation of the vestibular pathways because of their close association.[9] Brainstem auditory evoked potentials are recordings of sound-evoked electrical changes in portions of the auditory pathway between the cochlea and the auditory cortex. Because of the level of patient cooperation required, sedation or a light plane of general anesthesia often is needed to perform and interpret this test properly.[9]

Cerebrospinal Fluid Analysis

CSF analysis is a useful adjunctive test for determining the cause of central vestibular disease, although results are rarely specific. Although serum and CSF antibody titers have been used previously to diagnose infectious diseases, polymerase chain reaction analysis of CSF can now be performed in specialized laboratories to evaluate for the presence of infectious antigens (rather than antibody titers).[10] The risk of iatrogenic CNS trauma or cerebellar herniation after cisterna magna puncture in animals with space-occupying lesions should not be underestimated. It is preferable to obtain advanced imaging studies of the brain (see the following section) before performing CSF tap, especially if a caudal fossa lesion is suspected.

Advanced Imaging

Computed tomography (CT) and magnetic resonance imaging (MRI) have revolutionized the diagnosis of vestibular diseases. CT evaluation of the peripheral vestibular system is particularly useful if radiographs have not determined an underlying cause, if nasopharyngeal polyps and neoplasia are considerations and they cannot be visualized on physical examination, and if the extent of the lesion needs accurate demarcating and the animal is a potential surgical candidate. CT evaluation for animals with central vestibular diseases may be less helpful because of the artifacts relating to the density of the petrous temporal bones surrounding the medulla (e.g., beam hardening).[11]

MRI of the peripheral and central vestibular systems provides excellent multiplanar soft tissue resolution when compared with CT.[11] The improved soft tissue contrast provided by this modality allows better assessment of neoplastic and inflammatory conditions that result in vestibular dysfunction (Figure 87-3). A typical MRI study consists of T1-weighted, T2-weighted, and proton density–weighted transverse images made before contrast medium administration.[11] Post-contrast sequences have been recommended if a mass is present in the tympanic bulla or the external ear canal.

TREATMENT AND PROGNOSIS

The damaged vestibular system can compensate over time with central reprogramming of eye movements and postural responses, as well as reliance on visual and other sensory input that replaces lost vestibular input.[2,14] If the underlying disease process can be determined, the prognosis for a functional recovery can be good. Residual signs, such as a head tilt, are always possible. Recurrences can occur at times of stress, recurrent disease, or after anesthesia.

Supportive care is essential, especially because these animals are frequently anorexic; feeding tubes and fluid therapy can be vital initially until the patient can self-maintain. Vomiting, salivation, and nausea associated with vestibular disease can be treated with antiemetic medications. Drugs commonly used include the phenothiazine derivative chlorpromazine (0.5 mg/kg IV, IM, SC q-6-8h in dogs, 0.2 to 0.4 mg/kg IM, SC q6-8h in cats), serotonin receptor antagonists dolasetron (0.6 to1 mg/kg IV, SC, or PO q12-24h) and ondansetron (0.1 to 1 mg/kg IV, PO q8-12h), metoclopramide, an antidopaminergic serotonin receptor antagonist and chemoreceptor trigger zone inhibitor (0.1 to 0.5 mg/kg IV, IM, SC, or PO q6-12h or as an IV infusion of 1 to 2 mg/kg q24h), or the antihistamines diphenhydramine (2 to 4 mg/kg PO or IM q8h) and meclizine (12.5 mg PO q24h; see Chapter 162).[2] Recently, maropitant, a novel neurokinin type-1 receptor antagonist, has been described as a good choice to prevent vomiting in dogs and cats (1 mg/kg SC q24h or 2 mg/kg PO q24h),[15,16] and anecdotally has been effective as an adjunctive treatment in animals affected by vestibular disease.

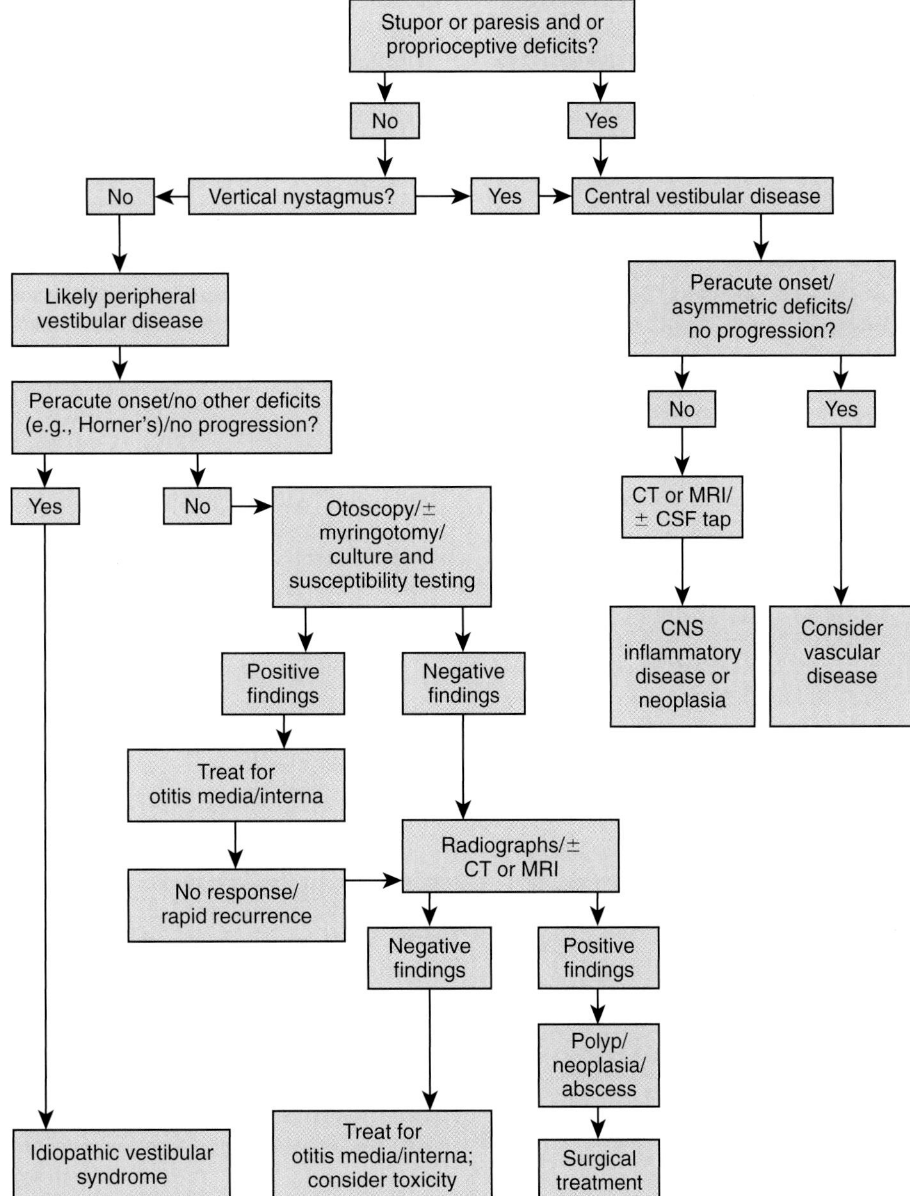

FIGURE 87-2 Algorithm detailing the approach to the patient with acute vestibular disease. *CNS,* Central nervous system; *CSF,* cerebrospinal fluid; *CT,* computed tomography; *MRI,* magnetic resonance imaging.

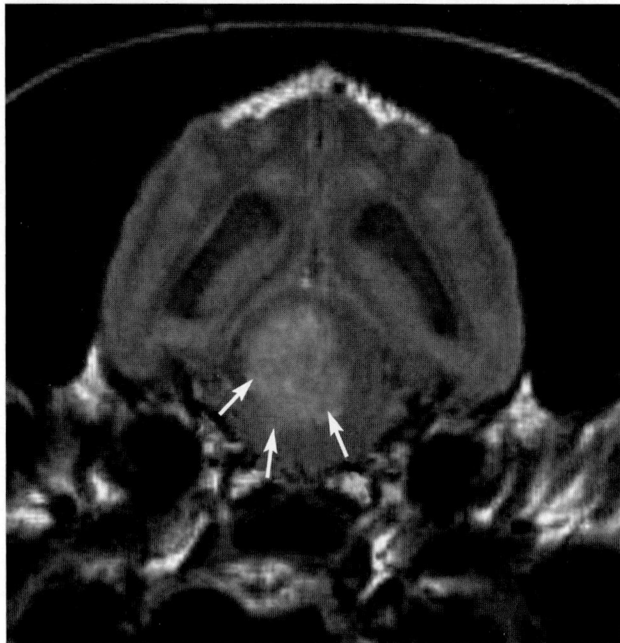

FIGURE 87-3 Transverse T2-weighted fluid-attenuated inversion recovery magnetic resonance study of a 4-year-old mixed breed dog with central vestibular disease and multiple cranial nerve involvement. A large irregular lesion hyperintense to the surrounding brainstem is identified *(arrows)*. Pathologic examination confirmed granulomatous meningoencephalomyelitis.

REFERENCES

1. DeLahunta A: Vestibular system: special proprioception. In DeLahunta A, Glass E: Veterinary neuroanatomy and clinical neurology, ed 3, St Louis, 2009, Saunders.
2. Rossmeisl JH Jr: Vestibular disease in dogs and cats, Vet Clin North Am Small Anim Pract 40:81, 2010.
3. Bagley RS: Recognition and localization of intracranial disease, Vet Clin North Am Small Anim Pract 26:667, 1996.
4. Kent M, Platt SR, Schatzberg SJ: The neurology of balance: function and dysfunction of the vestibular system in dogs and cats, Vet J 185:247, 2010
5. Garosi LS, Lowrie ML, Swinbourne NF: Neurological manifestations of ear disease in dogs and cats, Vet Clin North Am Small Anim Pract 42(6):1143, 2012.
6. Gelatt KN: Comparative neuroophthalmology. In Gelatt KN: Essentials of veterinary ophthalmology, ed 2, Philadelphia, 2008, Blackwell.
7. Bischoff MG, Kneller SK: Diagnostic imaging of the canine and feline ear, Vet Clin North Am Small Anim Pract 34:437, 2000.
8. Harvey RG, Harari J, Delauche AJ: The normal ear. In Harvey RG, Harari J, Delauche AJ: Ear diseases of the dog and cat, Ames, Iowa, 2001, Iowa State University Press.
9. Sims MH: Electrodiagnostic evaluation of hearing and vision. In August JR, editor: Consultations in feline internal medicine, ed 3, Philadelphia, 1997, Saunders.
10. Schatzberg SJ, Haley NJ, Barr SC, et al: Use of a multiplex polymerase chain reaction assay in the antemortem diagnosis of toxoplasmosis and neosporosis in the central nervous system of cats and dogs, Am J Vet Res 64:1507, 2003.
11. Tidwell AS, Jones JC: Advanced imaging concepts: a pictorial glossary of CT and MRI technology, Clin Tech Small Anim Pract 14:65, 1999.
12. Munana K: Inflammatory disorders of the central nervous system. In August JR, editor: Consultations in feline internal medicine, ed 4, Philadelphia, 2001, Saunders.
13. Garosi L: Head tilt and ataxia. In Platt S, Garosi L, editors: Small animal neurological emergencies, London, 2012, Manson.
14. Tighilet B, Trottier S, Mourre C, et al: Changes in the histaminergic system during vestibular compensation in the cat, J Physiol 573:723, 2006.
15. Ramsey DS, Kincaid K, Watkins JA, et al: Safety and efficacy of injectable and oral maropitant, a selective neurokinin 1 receptor antagonist, in a randomized clinical trial for treatment of vomiting in dogs, J Vet Pharmacol Ther 31:538, 2008.
16. Hickman MA, Cox SR, Mahabir S, et al: Safety, pharmacokinetics and use of the novel NK-1 receptor antagonist maropitant (Cerenia) for the prevention of emesis and motion sickness in cats, J Vet Pharmacol Ther 31:220, 2008.
17. Higgins MA, Rossmeisl JH Jr, Panciera DL: Hypothyroid-associated central vestibular disease in 10 dogs: 1999-2005, J Vet Intern Med 20:1363, 2006.

CHAPTER 88

HEPATIC ENCEPHALOPATHY

David Holt, BVSc, DACVS

KEY POINTS

- Hepatic encephalopathy is associated with moderate to severe liver insufficiency and may be secondary to a portosystemic shunt(s), end-stage liver disease, or a congenital urea cycle enzyme deficiency.
- The pathophysiology of hepatic encephalopathy is complex and incompletely understood; however, recent work has reemphasized the importance of elevated levels of ammonia.
- Clinical signs may include depression, dementia, stupor, coma, muscle tremors, motor abnormalities, excessive salivation, and focal or generalized seizures.
- Medical management includes strategies to minimize ammonia absorption from the intestine and control seizure activity, if present.
- Definitive treatment involves correcting treatable underlying causes, such as surgical treatment of a portosystemic shunt.

Hepatic encephalopathy (HE) is a spectrum of neurologic abnormalities associated with moderate to severe liver insufficiency. In dogs and cats, it occurs most commonly because of portosystemic shunting of blood. Fulminant hepatic failure is an important cause of HE in humans but is seen less commonly in veterinary medicine. Congenital urea cycle enzyme deficiencies also may lead to HE.

CAUSES

In dogs and cats, congenital extrahepatic or intrahepatic portal-to-systemic venous communications are the most frequent cause of HE; up to 95% of affected animals demonstrate neurologic clinical signs.[1] These communications are generally a single vessel, but multiple extrahepatic[2] and intrahepatic[3] congenital portosystemic shunts have been reported. Hepatic arteriovenous malformations cause portal hypertension, multiple extrahepatic portosystemic shunts, and ascites and may lead to clinical signs of HE. In young dogs, hepatic microvascular dysplasia[4] and, rarely, congenital urea cycle deficiencies[5] also can cause HE. In older animals, portosystemic shunts develop secondary to portal hypertension that results from chronic liver disease. Hepatic lipidosis often is associated with clinical signs of HE in cats. Other causes of chronic and acute hepatic failure that can result in HE are discussed in Chapter 116.

PATHOPHYSIOLOGY

In 1893 Marcel Nencki and Ivan Pavlov described the physiologic consequences of a surgically created, end-to-side portocaval shunt ("Eck's fistula") and showed that clinical signs worsened after a meat meal in this canine model, linking HE to the concept of "meat intoxication."[7] Ever since this description, HE has been considered a condition caused by gut-derived toxins that are not metabolized by a diseased or failing liver. Research over the last century has elaborated on this concept and demonstrated the complexity of this condition. However, recent work on several aspects of HE including cerebrospinal fluid amino acid alterations,[8,9] glutamate neurotoxicity,[10] the generation of reactive oxygen species,[11] and the mitochondrial permeability transition[12] emphasizes the central role of elevated ammonia concentrations in HE. Other substances considered synergistic to ammonia toxicity include mercaptans, free fatty acids, phenols, and bile salts.[13] Please see Chapter 116, Table 116-2, for a summary of implicated toxins causing HE.

Ammonia is produced in the intestinal tract as the end product of amino acid, purine and amine breakdown by bacteria, the metabolism of glutamine by enterocytes, and the breakdown of urea by bacterial urease.[14] It then is absorbed into the portal blood and rapidly converted to urea or glutamine in the normal liver. In animals with portosystemic shunting of blood or significant liver disease, high levels of ammonia are present in the systemic circulation. The permeability of the blood-brain barrier to ammonia increases in HE and experimental studies suggest that HE coma is associated with brain ammonia concentrations in the low millimolar range.[15] These concentrations of ammonia decrease excitatory neurotransmission, in part by down-regulating the N-methyl-D-aspartate (NMDA, excitatory) receptors,[10] yet at the same time, also block chloride extrusion from the postsynaptic neuron, decreasing inhibitory neurotransmission.[16]

The brain has no urea cycle; consequently, ammonia in the CNS is removed by transamination of glutamate into glutamine in astrocytes.[17] Glutamine concentrations in the cerebrospinal fluid are elevated in dogs with HE[8] and frequently are correlated with the degree of neurologic dysfunction in humans with HE.[10] Glutamine is exchanged across the blood-brain barrier for tryptophan, leading to increased levels of tryptophan and tryptophan metabolites in the central nervous system (Figure 88-1).[8] The tryptophan metabolites serotonin and quinolinate are important agonists in inhibitory and excitatory neurotransmission, respectively, although the exact alterations in both of these systems in HE are complex and incompletely understood. Glutamine also is transported from astrocytes into neurons, where it is converted to glutamate.[18] Overstimulation of the NMDA receptors by glutamate and ammonia can cause seizures and neurotoxicity, in part because of free radical formation.

γ-Aminobutyric acid (GABA) is the most important inhibitory neurotransmitter in the CNS. Alterations in GABA neurotransmission have been proposed as an important component of HE. In spite of several different observations implicating "increased GABAergic tone" in HE, increased amounts of GABA in the CNS, changes in the number of GABA receptors, or affinity of the receptor for its ligands

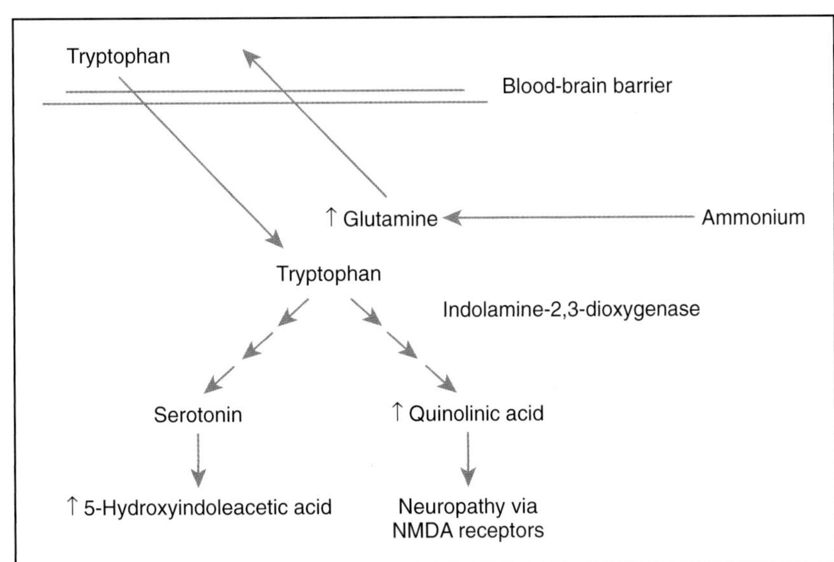

FIGURE 88-1 Diagram of the proposed effect of ammonia on tryptophan metabolism. Ammonia is metabolized to glutamine that shares an antiport transport mechanism across the blood-brain barrier with tryptophan. An increase in tryptophan transport leads to an increased flux through the serotonin and quinolinic acid pathways. *NMDA,* N-Methyl-D-aspartic acid.

have not been found in patients with HE.[19] It is likely that if increased GABA neurotransmission exists in patients with HE, it is due to increased brain concentrations of endogenous GABA ligands, including endogenous benzodiazepines and neurosteroids. Increased levels of endogenous benzodiazepine receptor ligands have been found in the portal blood and systemic circulation of some dogs with portosystemic shunts.[20] Elevated levels of ammonia and manganese (also seen in liver disease) increase the expression of "peripheral-type" benzodiazepine receptors (PTBR), a heterooligomeric protein complex on the outer mitochondrial membrane of astrocytes. Activation of the PTBR increases mitochondrial cholesterol uptake and the synthesis of neurosteroids that then may act on GABA receptors.[21]

Recent investigations have focused on the role of microglial cell activation in rodent models of liver disease. Microglial cell activation and the production of proinflammatory cytokines (TNF-α, IL-1β) within the brain occurs in the early stages of encephalopathy.[22] Treatment with N-acetylcysteine and minocycline has been shown to ameliorate CNS inflammation and brain edema in experimental studies.[22] To the author's knowledge, these therapies have not been assessed in either human or veterinary HE patients.

Evidence demonstrates that amino acid imbalances may play a role in hepatic encephalopathy. Dogs with portocaval shunts have a decreased ratio of branched-chain (valine, leucine, isoleucine) to aromatic (phenylalanine, tyrosine, tryptophan) amino acids.[23] This relative increase in the concentration of aromatic amino acids facilitates their preferential transport across the blood-brain barrier. This leads to an increased synthesis of false neurotransmitters and a reduction in the synthesis of dopamine and norepinephrine. Normal dogs infused with the aromatic amino acids tryptophan and phenylalanine became comatose; addition of the branched chain amino acids to the infusion prevented coma.[24]

CLINICAL SIGNS

The clinical signs associated with HE are often subtle and episodic initially. A new puppy may be mildly lethargic or depressed and "first time" owners may not recognize this as abnormal behavior. Other clinical signs include disorientation, personality change, stupor, pacing, head pressing, "star gazing," amaurotic blindness, coma, and occasionally seizures. In general, signs of central nervous system depression predominate over signs associated with hyperexcitability. In cats, ptyalism is common, and is often the only clinical sign associated with HE. In dogs, polydipsia and polyuria is also a common clinical finding. It is presumed to be secondary to hypercortisolemia, the subsequent partial inhibition of vasopressin's action on the renal tubules,[6] and ineffective medullary concentrating because of low urea levels. Clinical signs of gastrointestinal (vomiting, anorexia) and urinary tract (stranguria, hematuria, secondary to ammonium biurate calculi) disease also can occur with portosystemic shunting of blood. Although these signs are not unique to HE, it is important that they alert the veterinarian to investigate the possibility of moderate to severe liver disease or insufficiency.

Clinical signs can be precipitated or worsened by the ingestion of a high protein meal, gastrointestinal bleeding, systemic infection, and several medications, including narcotics and other anesthetic agents. Other precipitating factors include electrolyte imbalances (hyponatremia, hypokalemia), hypoglycemia, acidosis or alkalosis, and constipation.

DIAGNOSIS

The diagnosis of HE is made when an animal has clinical signs compatible with the condition, and alterations on a biochemical panel and liver function tests confirming moderate to severe liver disease (see Chapter 116 for further details). At the same time, none of the clinical signs described are specific for HE and other potential diagnoses, including other metabolic disorders, toxin or drug ingestion, and intracranial lesions should be excluded. Routine lab work (CBC, biochemical profile, urinalysis) and liver function testing often are indicated. Possible liver function tests include blood ammonia levels (+/− ammonia tolerance, but may precipitate seizures in animals with HE), pre- and postprandial bile acids, and the sulfobromophthalein (BSP) dye retention test. Samples for blood ammonia concentrations are useful only if processed immediately. Canine samples for blood ammonia determination stored frozen for any period of time give erroneous results.[25] Additional diagnostic testing that may prove beneficial includes rectal portal scintigraphy and liver histopathology.

TREATMENT

See Chapter 116, Table 116-3, for a summary of treatments.

Animals that are presented with or develop focal or generalized seizures require immediate cessation of the seizures (see Chapter 166). The use of diazepam is controversial because of the possibility of increased levels of endogenous benzodiazepines. (see above). The dose of diazepam is typically 0.5 mg/kg IV. Alternatively, the seizure activity may be treated with propofol (0.5 to 1 mg kg IV bolus, then 0.05 to 0.1 mg/kg/min constant rate infusion), although careful respiratory monitoring is essential. Mannitol therapy also may prove beneficial if cerebral edema is present (0.5 to 1 gm/kg IV over 10 to 20 minutes). Antiepileptic therapy can be administered in an attempt to prevent further seizure activity. Potassium bromide is given commonly as a loading dose initially (400 to 600 mg/kg/day divided into four doses on day 1), then maintenance therapy is continued at 40 mg/kg/day PO or rectally. Sodium bromide has been suggested as a parenteral bromide formulation in dogs and cats, although few data support it at this time. The drug generally is dosed at 15% of the potassium bromide dose, including the loading dose on day 1. Phenobarbital also may be given parenterally, with a loading dose of 16 mg/kg IV divided into four doses given on day 1, followed by 2 to 4 mg/kg IV q12h thereafter. The bromide drugs and phenobarbital may lead to excessive sedation and close monitoring is therefore essential.

Animals that are comatose or seizuring should have any predisposing factors treated as soon as possible. For example, in the case of benzodiazepine sedation, flumazenil (0.02 mg/kg IV) should be administered. Intubation of comatose animals or those recovering from seizure activity may be necessary to protect the airway from aspiration and ensure adequate ventilation. Intravenous fluids are often necessary, but the animal's serum albumin, glucose, electrolyte, and acid-base status should be evaluated carefully before and during administration. Affected animals are often hypoproteinemic and hypoglycemic; alkalosis increases ammonia diffusion into the central nervous system and hypokalemia stimulates renal ammonia production. Colloid administration (synthetic or natural/plasma), and potassium and glucose supplementation are often necessary. Should a red blood cell transfusion be necessary, fresh whole blood or fresh packed red blood cells are used because blood storage increases the ammonia concentration of the products. A lactulose enema (1 to 3 ml/10 kg BW diluted 1 : 1 to 1 : 3 with warm water) is administered to minimize ammonia production in, and absorption from, the colon. Lactulose (beta galactosidofructose) is a nonabsorbable disaccharide that exerts an osmotic cathartic action. In addition, intestinal bacteria hydrolyze lactulose-producing organic acids that lower colonic pH. Acidification traps ammonia in its NH_4^+ form, preventing absorption by nonionic diffusion and also resulting in the net movement of ammonia from the blood into the bowel lumen.

Fulminant hepatic failure (FHF) is uncommon in animals but often fatal. Death in humans with FHF often is associated with cerebral edema, hemorrhage, and sepsis. Therapy is similar to that described for hepatic coma and seizures. Assisted ventilation is used to prevent hypo- or hyperventilation and minimize changes in intracranial pressure. Twenty-five percent mannitol (0.5 to 1 g/kg IV over 30 minutes) is administered to minimize cerebral edema. Glucose is supplemented as necessary, although hyperglycemia should be avoided. Animals with FHF may be coagulopathic; fresh frozen plasma (10 to 20 ml/kg IV q6-12h) is administered to supplement coagulation factors, if needed. Animals with suspected sepsis should be given empirically with broad-spectrum antimicrobial therapy and bacterial cultures (blood, urine) obtained (see Chapter 91).

The general treatment goals for stable animals with HE or those that have been stabilized after treatment for emergent conditions include reducing ammonia levels, decreasing GABA, and lowering endogenous benzodiazepines. Clinical signs of HE typically can be managed with diet modification, oral administration of lactulose, and antimicrobial therapy. The diet should be moderately protein restricted (14% to 17% protein on a dry matter basis in dogs; 30% to 35% protein in cats) and high in carbohydrates. A high-quality protein source with an increased level of branched-chain amino acids is preferred. The diet should be a low-residue, easily digestible food to minimize the amount of material reaching the colon. It must contain adequate amounts of arginine for cats because is an essential amino acid necessary for the urea cycle. Lactulose (1 to 3 ml/10 kg BW diluted 1 : 1 to 1 : 3 with warm water q6-8h) is administered orally or rectally, and the dose rate and interval are titrated to produce two to four moderately soft stools daily.

Antimicrobial therapy is administered to decrease numbers of urease-producing bacteria in the intestines. Neomycin sulfate (20 mg/kg PO q6-8h) generally is considered nonabsorbable but should be avoided in animals with concurrent renal disease. Metronidazole (7 to 10 mg/kg PO or IV q12h) is a reasonable alternative, but neurotoxicity may occur more commonly in animals with hepatic disease. Rifaximin is an oral antimicrobial recently approved for the treatment of humans with hepatic encephalopathy.[26] It appears to be at least as effective as other oral antimicrobials but has a better safety profile. Information on its use in small animals is limited at this time and cost may be a limiting factor for many owners. The effect of long-term therapy with antimicrobials on the intestinal flora of dogs and cats is not clear. Because the therapeutic effect of lactulose depends in part on its metabolism by colonic bacteria, the benefit of combined lactulose and antimicrobial therapy is open to question in small animals. Although the two treatments often are considered synergistic, oral neomycin inhibits lactulose metabolism in 25% to 30% of human patients.

Enemas also have been used to decrease the colonic bacterial numbers and substrates. The following types of enemas have been recommended:

- Warm water enemas at 10 ml/kg q4-6h until signs improve, lactulose enemas at 1 to 3 ml/10 kg BW diluted 1 : 1 to 1 : 3 with warm water q6-8h
- Neomycin enemas at 15 to 20 ml of 1% solution q8-12h
- Metronidazole enemas at 7.5 mg/kg (systemic dose) mixed with water q12h
- Betadine enemas given by diluting 1 : 10 with warm water and giving 10 ml/kg q8h and flushing out with warm water after 10 to 15 minutes
- Activated charcoal enemas using the liquid suspension q8h
- Vinegar enemas made by diluting the vinegar 1 : 4 with warm water and administering at 10 ml/kg q8h

Other therapies that have been tried in humans but not companion animals include ornithine, aspartate, zinc supplementation, branched chain amino acid solutions, flumazenil, and levodopa administration.[27] Inhibitors of the glutamine synthetase enzyme and serotonin receptor antagonists have been associated with a high rate of side effects and are not recommended for treatment of clinical HE in humans. The use of "probiotics" to repopulate the digestive tract with lactose fermenting, non–urease-containing bacteria has been reported extensively. A large meta-analysis of human trails concluded that, although probiotics appeared to reduce plasma ammonia levels compared with placebo treatment or no intervention, there was no firm evidence that they made a clinically relevant difference to patient outcomes.[28]

In cases of HE secondary to portosystemic shunting of blood, surgical correction of the portosystemic shunt often permanently resolves the clinical signs of HE in dogs. However, a variable percentage of surgically treated cats may have residual or recurrent neurologic signs.[29] Treatment of extrahepatic shunts usually involves either complete suture ligation or placement of either an ameroid ring or cellophane band to occlude gradually the shunting vessel. Intrahepatic shunts are treated either surgically or with interventional radiographic techniques. All of these procedures require general anesthesia; the metabolism of anesthetic agents and their effects on the central nervous system are far from clear in animals with HE. Although controlled clinical trials are lacking, general clinical opinion favors a period of medical treatment to stabilize animals with HE before anesthesia.

Animals with liver insufficiency commonly experience clinical or subclinical gastrointestinal hemorrhage and the digested blood serves as a protein source that may cause or contribute to HE. It therefore is recommended that these animals receive gastrointestinal protectant therapy (see Chapter 161). Drugs such as famotidine (0.5 to 1 mg/kg PO or IV q12-24h), omeprazole (1.0 to 2.0 mg/kg q12-24h) or esomeprazole (0.5 to 1.0 mg/kg/day IV q24h), misoprostol (2 to 5 mcg/kg PO q6-12h), and sucralfate (0.25 to 1 gm PO q6-8h) are used commonly.

REFERENCES

1. Breznock EM, Whiting PG: Portocaval shunts and anomalies. In Slatter DH, editor: Textbook of small animal surgery, Philadelphia, 1985, WB Saunders.
2. Suter PF: Portal vein anomalies in the dog: their angiographic diagnosis, Vet Radiol 16:84, 1975.
3. Hunt GB, Youmans KR, Sommerlad S, et al: Surgical management of multiple congenital intrahepatic shunts in two dogs: case report, Vet Surg 27(3):262, 1998.
4. Christiansen JS, Hottinger HA, Allen L, et al: Hepatic microvascular dysplasia in dogs: a retrospective study of 24 cases (1987-1995), J Am Anim Hosp Assoc 36:385, 2000.
5. Strombek DR, Meyer DJ, Freedland RA: Hyperammonemia due to a urea cycle enzyme deficiency in two dogs, J Am Vet Med Assoc 166:1109, 1975.
6. Rothuizen J, Mol JA: The pituitary-adrenocortical system in canine hepato-encephalopathy, Front Horm Res 17:28, 1987.
7. Shawcross DL, Olde Damink SWM, Butterworth RF, Jalan R: Ammonia and hepatic encephalopathy: the more things change, the more they stay the same, Metabol Brain Dis 20:169, 2005.
8. Holt DE, Washabau RJ, Djali S, et al: Cerebrospinal fluid glutamine, tryptophan, and tryptophan metabolite concentrations are altered in dogs with portosystemic shunts, Am J Vet Res 63:1167, 2002.
9. Butterworth J, Gregory CR, Aronson LR: Selective alterations of cerebrospinal fluid amino acids in dogs with congenital portosystemic shunts, Metabol Brain Dis 12:299, 1997.
10. Albrecht J, Jones EA: Hepatic encephalopathy: molecular mechanisms underlying the clinical syndrome, J Neurol Sci 170:138, 1999.
11. Konsenko E, Venediktova N, Kaminsky Y, et al: Sources of oxygen radicals in brain in acute ammonia intoxication in vivo, Brain Res 981:193, 2003.

12. Bai G, Rama Rao KV, Murthy CR, et al: Ammonia induces the mitochondrial permeability transition in primary cultures of rat astrocytes, J Neurosci Res 66(5):981, 2001.
13. Maddison JE: Hepatic encephalopathy. Current concepts and pathogenesis, J Vet Intern Med 6:341, 1992.
14. Dimski DS: Ammonia metabolism and the urea cycle: functional and clinical implications, J Vet Intern Med 8:73, 1994.
15. Hindfelt B, Plumb F, Duffy TE: Effects of acute ammonia intoxication on cerebral metabolism in rats with portacaval shunts, J Clin Invest 59:386, 1977.
16. Raabe WA: Neurophysiology of ammonia intoxication. In Butterworth RF, Layrargues GP, editors: Hepatic encephalopathy: pathophysiology and treatment, Clifton, NJ, 1989, Humana Press.
17. Butterworth RF: Hepatic encephalopathy. In Arias IM, Boyer JL, Fausto N, et al, editors: The liver: biology and pathobiology, New York, 1994, Raven Press Ltd.
18. Raghavendra Rao VL, Murthy ChRK, Butterworth RF: Glutamatergic synaptic dysfunction in hyperammonemic syndromes, Metabol Brain Dis 7:1, 1992.
19. Ahboucha S, Butterworth RF: Pathophysiology of hepatic encephalopathy: a new look at GABA from the molecular standpoint, Metabol Brain Dis 19:331, 2004.
20. Aronson LR, Gacad RC, Kaminsky-Russ K, et al: Endogenous benzodiazepine activity in the peripheral and portal blood of dogs with congenital portosystemic shunts, Vet Surg 26(3):189, 1997.
21. Butterworth RF: Neurotransmitter dysfunction in hepatic encephalopathy: new approaches and new findings, Metabolic Brain Dis 16:55, 2001.
22. Butterworth RF: Hepatic encephalopathy: a central neuroinflammatory disorder? Hepatology 53:1372, 2011.
23. Strombeck DR, Rogers Q: Plasma amino acid concentrations in dogs with hepatic disease, J Am Vet Med Assoc 173:93, 1978.
24. Rossi-Fanelli F, Freund H, Krause R, et al: Induction of coma in normal dogs by the infusion of aromatic amino acids and its prevention by the addition of branched-chain amino acids, Gastroenterol 83:664, 1982.
25. Hitt ME, Jones BD: Effects of storage temperatures and time on canine plasma ammonia concentrations, Am J Vet Res 47:363, 1986.
26. Eltawil KM, Laryea M, Peltekian K, et al: Rifaximin vs. conventional oral therapy for hepatic encephalopathy: a meta-analysis, World J Gastroenterol 18:767:2012.
27. Riordan SM, Williams R: Current concepts: treatment of hepatic encephalopathy, New Engl J Med 337:473, 1997.
28. McGee RG, Bakens A, Wiley K, et al: Probiotics for patients with hepatic encephalopathy, Cochr Database Syst Rev (11):CD008716, 2011.
29. Havig M, Tobias KM: Outcome of ameroid constrictor occlusion of single congenital extrahepatic portosystemic shunts in cats: 12 cases (1993-2000), J Am Vet Med Assoc 220:337, 2002.

PART X INFECTIOUS DISORDERS

CHAPTER 89
NOSOCOMIAL INFECTIONS AND ZOONOSES

Shelley C. Rankin, BSc (Hons), PhD

KEY POINTS

- Nosocomial (hospital-acquired) infection is defined as any infection that is neither present nor incubating when a patient is admitted to a hospital.
- Risk factors for nosocomial infection in intensive care unit (ICU) patients include severity of underlying illness, prolonged length of stay, mechanical ventilation, indwelling devices, and antibiotic use.
- Multiple antibiotic resistance is common among nosocomial pathogens.
- Methicillin-resistant *Staphylococcus* spp. are emerging in dogs and cats.
- The reservoirs of nosocomial pathogens include people, animals, fomites, air currents, water, food sources, insects, and rodents. The spread of pathogens in hospitals occurs primarily via the hands of personnel.
- Establishment of biosecurity nosocomial infection control programs must become a priority in veterinary hospitals.
- Zoonosis is a disease that can be transmitted from animals to humans. A more technical definition is a disease that normally exists in animals but that can infect humans. Many organisms can cause zoonotic disease.

In human health care settings, nosocomial infection is defined as any infection that is neither present nor incubating when a patient is admitted to a hospital. In 1988 the Centers for Disease Control and Prevention proposed more specific definitions, and it now is accepted generally that infections are considered to be nosocomial if they develop at least 48 hours after hospital admission without proven prior incubation.[1] In addition, if infections occur up to 3 days after discharge or within 30 days of a surgical procedure, they are attributed to the admitting hospital.[1] These definitions are accepted in human health care and, although they may require refinement in veterinary medicine, they stand unchallenged.

Hospitalization of sick animals can lead to an increased risk of infection, and various policies have been proposed to reduce the risk of nosocomial infection in veterinary medicine.[2-4] In addition to patient care concerns, many nosocomial pathogens are well recognized as zoonotic agents, so infection control policies should address the issue of animal-to-human transmission.[2]

NOSOCOMIAL INFECTIONS IN DOGS AND CATS

One of the first published reports of nosocomial infection in a veterinary hospital described *Klebsiella* infection in dogs and one cat in the intensive care unit (ICU) at the New York State College of Veterinary Medicine in 1978.[5] Since that time there have been a few well-characterized studies, but many of these have centered on large animal facilities with various *Salmonella enterica* serotypes as the causative organisms.[6-8] Specific reports of nosocomial infection in dogs and cats remain limited.[5] Since 1978 organisms such as *Serratia marcescens, Salmonella* species, *Clostridium perfringens, Acinetobacter baumannii, Escherichia coli,* and *Clostridium difficile* have been implicated as causes of nosocomial infection in dogs and cats.[6,9-13] The bacteria responsible for nosocomial infection in ICUs originate either from the patient's own endogenous flora or from exogenous sources. Nosocomial infections derived from endogenous flora may occur in patients receiving chemotherapy, glucocorticoid therapy, or antimicrobial therapy. In contrast to endogenous infections, exogenous infections are prevented more easily by standard or specific precautions devised to reduce the overall rate of transmission.[14] Reviews of nosocomial infections in veterinary medicine provide data on the pathogenesis, diagnosis, treatment, and strategies for the prevention of urinary tract infections, surgical site infections, bloodstream infections, pneumonia, and diarrhea.[15,16]

RISK FACTORS

Although ill-defined in veterinary medicine, independent risk factors for nosocomial infection acquisition in the critically ill patient can be extrapolated from human studies. Prolonged length of hospital stay, mechanical ventilation, and indwelling devices (i.e., intravascular or urinary catheters and nasogastric or endotracheal tubes) are well-recognized risk factors.[1] Many intrinsic, patient-related factors also have been identified and include patient demographics (e.g., age, gender), comorbidities, and severity of underlying illness, which is the most widely reported risk factor. Patient-specific risk factors are related to general health and immune status, respiratory status, neurologic status, and fluid status. The most significant risk factors in the ICU are trauma, especially when associated with open fractures and antimicrobial use. Risk factors for dogs becoming carriers of multidrug-resistant (MDR) *E. coli* during hospitalization have been shown to include hospitalization for more than 6 days, treatment with cephalosporins before admission, treatment with cephalosporins for less than 1 day, and treatment with metronidazole while hospitalized.[17] Several less well-acknowledged factors also have been suggested as contributing factors. Among them, understaffing and overcrowding in the ICU have been well documented as causes of cross-transmission of nosocomial infections.[1]

MULTIPLE ANTIBIOTIC–RESISTANT NOSOCOMIAL PATHOGENS

In an excellent review of the problem of antimicrobial drug use and resistance in veterinary medicine, Prescott and colleagues state that,

"Despite a possible wealth of data in filing cabinets in veterinary clinical microbiology laboratories around the world, there have been virtually no systematic investigations of changes in antimicrobial drug resistance in bacteria isolated from companion animals over time, using standard methodologies for assessing resistance."[18] The situation has changed little since that statement was made in 2002.

Although it often is speculated that organisms isolated from nosocomial infection outbreaks in veterinary patients now have an increasingly broad spectrum of antimicrobial resistance, there are no active nosocomial infection surveillance systems in this field. Much of the antibiotic resistance data are derived from "local" surveillance, and a lack of standardization results in data that are incomparable from one setting to another.[19,20] In terms of the impact of multidrug-resistant (MDR) bacteria with regard to nosocomial infection, the data that have been published agree that resistant bacteria can reduce the effectiveness of management.[18]

Data on trends in resistance patterns among nosocomial pathogens from veterinary sources are few, but the wealth of surveillance data from human health care systems often can be used as a predictor of what to expect from nosocomial pathogens in veterinary patients.[21-23] Local surveillance of antibiotic resistance in animal isolates is preferred, but in the absence of such data, extrapolation from human surveillance data is encouraged.

Bacterial resistance to β-lactam antibiotics and the β-lactamase inhibitors is becoming increasingly common and threatens to reduce the clinical spectrum of these drugs. In particular, organisms that produce extended-spectrum β-lactamases (ESBLs) and plasmid-mediated AmpC enzymes are posing unique challenges in clinical situations.[20] Although the prevalence of ESBLs is not known, it is thought to be increasing, and in many parts of the world 10% to 40% of strains of *E. coli* and *K. pneumoniae* produce such enzymes. Novel β-lactamases also are becoming especially important among diverse gram negative pathogens such as *Pseudomonas aeruginosa, S. enterica* serotype Typhimurium, *Proteus mirabilis,* and *A. baumannii.*[24] The source of these novel enzymes is unknown, but their presence on plasmids and ready transferability among pathogens of different genera is of concern. Organisms that produce ESBLs are found commonly in those areas of the hospital environment where antimicrobial use is frequent and the patient's condition is critical, and these resistant organisms cause increased morbidity and mortality.[24]

ZOONOSES

The simplest definition of a zoonosis is a disease that can be transmitted from animals to humans. A more technical definition is a disease that normally exists in animals but that can infect humans. Some authors further subdivide the concept into zooanthroponosis, infections that humans can acquire from animals, and anthropozoonosis, a disease of humans that is transmissible to other animals. A comprehensive literature review has identified 1415 species of infectious organism known to be pathogenic to humans and out of these, 868 (61%) are zoonotic.[25] Overall, 19% are viruses or prions, 31% are bacteria or rickettsia, 13% are fungi, 5% are protozoa, and 32% are helminths. Thirty-five percent of zoonoses can be transmitted by direct contact, 61% by indirect contact, 22% by vectors, and for 6% the transmission route is unknown. Only 33% of zoonotic species are known to be transmissible between humans and only 3% are considered to have their main reservoir in human populations; the main reservoir of the remainder is in animal populations. Zoonoses are more likely to be transmitted by indirect contact or vectors and are less likely to be transmitted by direct contact when compared with all pathogens.

The list of zoonoses found in animals in the ICU is long, but because some organisms are generally more prevalent, they have a greater potential for transfer to humans and result in disease.[25a] The enteric pathogens, such as *Campylobacter, Salmonella, C. difficile,* and *E. coli* commonly are isolated from animals in the ICU, and all of these organisms have been responsible for nosocomial outbreaks in that setting.[7,8,13] *Campylobacter* species can occur in large numbers as commensals in companion animals, and there is a strong correlation between diarrhea and the ability to recover *C. jejuni* from healthy dogs. *Salmonella* spp., on the other hand, are not normal commensals of dogs and cats, and the presence of *Salmonella* in feces likely indicates infection. Enteropathogenic *E. coli* (EPEC) have been isolated from dogs and cats with enteritis, and strains have emerged as important causes of diarrhea in puppies. *E. coli* is also the most common cause of urinary tract infections in dogs and cats in the ICU, and many strains are now resistant to a wide spectrum of antimicrobial agents. Zoonotic transmission of resistant urinary isolates of *E. coli* from companion animals to humans has been suggested.[26] *C. difficile* and *Enterococcus* species are now considered emerging zoonotic agents, and this is also true of some veterinary staphylococci, particularly methicillin-resistant *S. pseudintermedius* (MRSP) and methicillin-resistant *S. schleiferi* (MRSS).[27,28]

Pathogenic *Leptospira* species have the potential to infect humans and also cause nosocomial infections in animals housed with infected or shedding animals (see Chapter 124). Leptospires often colonize proximal convoluted kidney tubules and may be excreted in urine for extended periods by dogs that show no clinical symptoms. The carrier state may be as short as a few days or may extend throughout the life of the animal. The primary routes of infection for dogs are direct contact (oral, conjunctival), venereal and placental transfer, bite wounds, and ingestion of contaminated water or meat.

The cutaneous mycoses of animals are caused primarily by *Microsporum* and *Trichophyton* species and are well-recognized zoonotic agents that cause ringworm in humans and can be acquired from contact with infected animals or fomites. Dermatophyte spores gain entry into the skin through minor trauma such as abrasions.

Uncommon, but perhaps emerging, zoonotic agents that may be found in veterinary patients also include a variety of *Mycobacterium* species, *Malassezia pachydermatis, Candida albicans, Brucella canis,* and MDR strains of *P. aeruginosa* and *Klebsiella pneumoniae.* Undoubtedly, as veterinary nosocomial infection surveillance systems improve, a host of additional pathogenic or MDR organisms will be reclassified as zoonotic.

EMERGING NOSOCOMIAL INFECTIONS IN DOGS AND CATS

Consistent with a generalized increase in β-lactam resistance, several reports in the veterinary literature have described an increase in the prevalence of MRSA strains isolated from dogs and cats.[29,30] In 1998 a Korean veterinary hospital representative reported three small nosocomial clusters of MRSA infection in hospitalized dogs. Isolates were obtained from 12 dogs and were recovered from the anterior nares, catheters, conjunctiva, a postoperative wound, and a skin lesion.[31] A further description of MRSA infection in dogs from the United Kingdom reported that in 8 of 11 dogs the infection likely was contracted during surgical procedures, most commonly during repair of traumatic fractures.[32] Of the 11 dogs, three suffered from chronic pyoderma that was not responsive to routine antimicrobial management. The MRSA infection resolved or improved in nine of those cases after appropriate antimicrobial therapy. Management of individual MRSA cases must begin with review of the antibiotic susceptibility profile of individual isolates, and selective antimicrobial therapy should be based upon those results.

In addition to MRSA, methicillin-resistant *S. pseudintermedius* and *S. schleiferi* may present a more pressing threat to veterinary patients. In a survey done at the Matthew J. Ryan Veterinary Hospital of the University of Pennsylvania, the rates of methicillin resistance in these three pathogens isolated between 2003 and 2004 was 32%, 17%, and 49%, respectively.[33]

C. difficile was implicated as the causative organism in an outbreak of diarrhea in dogs at a small animal veterinary teaching hospital.[13] No cases were identified in the ICU, and this was attributed to stringent infection control measures. *C. difficile*–associated disease (CDAD) occurs as a result of intestinal colonization and toxin production by toxigenic strains. A diagnosis of CDAD is made after detection of an enterotoxin, designated Toxin A, and a cytotoxin, designated Toxin B, in fecal specimens. Some animals are known to carry toxigenic strains of *C. difficile* without toxin production, so demonstration of the organism in feces by anaerobic culture is not confirmatory. Sources of nosocomial *C. difficile* include colonized or infected animals, indirect contact via hospital personnel, or environmental reservoirs of potentially pathogenic spores that are known to be resistant to commonly used disinfectants. Management of CDAD depends on a number of factors, especially if coinfection with additional enteric pathogens is suspected or confirmed. Metronidazole or vancomycin is generally the antimicrobial of choice for uncomplicated CDAD.

Vancomycin-resistant *Enterococcus faecium* (VRE) has not been implicated yet in nosocomial infections of dogs and cats. However, VRE has been identified in a canine urinary tract infection, and monitoring at veterinary teaching hospitals in the United States and Europe has revealed VRE carriage in healthy dogs.[34,35] Dogs treated with antimicrobials for 2 to 9 days in a veterinary ICU were shown to carry a large drug-resistant population of enterococci.[36] Most enterococci, (especially VRE) isolates are highly resistant to many other antimicrobial classes, and the gene responsible for vancomycin resistance is resident on a transposable element; the exchange of this element has been demonstrated between human and canine *E. faecium*. Therefore the use of vancomycin alone may not be a necessary prerequisite for selection of VRE in small animals.[34]

Overall, the number of reports of infection or colonization in animal species of pathogens that traditionally have been thought to have a reservoir only in humans has increased since the earliest reports of MRSA in the 1960s and 1970s. This trend can be considered a significant public health concern given the potential for direct spread of MDR pathogens between humans and animals. A reasonable assumption is that infected dogs and cats can serve as reservoirs for these pathogenic organisms. However, the alternative hypothesis, that humans also can be a reservoir for MDR infectious agents that can be transmitted to dogs and cats, now seems equally feasible.

NOSOCOMIAL INFECTION PREVENTION AND CONTROL

The reservoirs of nosocomial pathogens include people, animals, fomites, air currents, water and food sources, insects, and rodents; it has long been known that the spread of pathogens in hospitals occurs primarily via the hands of personnel.[1] Therefore frequent hand washing is of the utmost importance and the use of gloves when handling patients also may help to decrease the incidence of nosocomial infections. In 1989 Murtaugh and Mason proposed that nosocomial infection control committees be established in veterinary hospitals, especially at the larger teaching and referral centers.[37] Some veterinary institutions were receptive to this proposal, but there are still no national or international standards for veterinary hospital infection control. A survey of veterinary teaching hospitals in the United States indicated that only 42% of these hospitals required personnel to complete a biosecurity training program, but 40% of respondents indicated that they believed that their hospital ranked among the top 10% in regard to rigor of infection control efforts.[38] Much of what is done is borrowed from human health care guidelines, and worldwide surveillance statistics of veterinary nosocomial infection rates are not available.

The guidelines for prevention and control of nosocomial infection are simple and comprise three main strategies. First, methods are needed to prevent cross-contamination and to control potential sources of pathogenic microorganisms that can be transmitted from patient to patient or from hospital personnel to patient. Second, guidelines are needed to direct the appropriate use of prophylactic, empiric, and therapeutic antimicrobial use. Finally, strategies to limit the emergence or spread of MDR pathogens should be developed and targeted against organisms known to be prevalent in individual institutions. Some of these approaches may at first seem to be restrictive, but infection control guidelines are intended only to improve the process of care. Infection control measures when instituted in human health care settings have been unpopular, and compliance is difficult to maintain. It has been suggested that noncompliance is connected with many aspects of human behavior, including the yearning of human beings for liberty, the false perception of an invisible risk, and the underestimation of individual responsibility in the epidemiology of the institution.[1]

CONCLUSION

In conclusion, the importance of nosocomial transmission of infectious organisms, particularly in the ICU, cannot be overemphasized. Although the intrinsic risk factors of individual animal patients for the development of nosocomial infection are difficult to assess, the risk of transmission of pathogenic and MDR organisms can and should be reduced to a minimum whenever possible.

REFERENCES

1. Eggimann P, Pittet D: Infection control in the ICU, Chest 120(6):2059-2093, 2001.
2. Morley PS: Biosecurity of veterinary practices, Vet Clin North Am Food Anim Pract 18(1):133-155, 2002.
3. Weese JS: Barrier precautions, isolation protocols, and personal hygiene in veterinary hospitals, Vet Clin North Am Equine Pract 20(3):543-549, 2004.
4. Portner JA, Johnson JA: Guidelines for reducing pathogens in veterinary hospitals: disinfectant selection, cleaning protocols and hand hygiene, Compend Contin Educ Vet 32:5, E1-E12, 2010.
5. Glickman LT: Veterinary nosocomial (hospital acquired) Klebsiella infections, J Am Vet Med Assoc 179(12):1389-1392, 1989.
6. Sanchez S, McCrackin Stevenson MA, Hudson CR, et al: Characterization of multidrug-resistant Escherichia coli isolates associated with nosocomial infections in dogs, J Clin Microbiol 40(10):3586-3595, 2002.
7. Cherry B, Burns A, Johnson GS, et al: *Salmonella typhimurium* outbreak associated with a veterinary clinic, Emerg Infect Dis 10(12):2249-2251, 2004.
8. Wright JG, Tengelsen LA, Smith KE, et al: Multidrug-resistant *Salmonella typhimurium* in four animal facilities, Emerg Infect Dis 11(8):1235-1241, 2005.
9. Fox JG, Beaucage CM, Folta CA, et al: Nosocomial transmission of *Serratia marcescens* in a veterinary hospital due to contamination by benzalkonium chloride, J Clin Microbiol 14(2):157-160, 1981.
10. Uhaa IJ, Hird DW, Hirsch DC, et al: Case-control study of risk factors associated with nosocomial *Salmonella krefeld* infection in dogs, Am J Vet Res 49:1501-1505, 1988,
11. Kruth SA, Prescott JF, Welch MK, et al: Nosocomial diarrhea associated with enterotoxigenic *Clostridium perfringens* infection in dogs, J Am Vet Med Assoc 195(3):331-334, 1989.
12. Francey T, Gaschen F, Nicolet J, et al: The role of *Acinetobacter baumannii* as a nosocomial pathogen for dogs and cats in an intensive care unit, J Vet Intern Med 14:177-183, 2000.

13. Weese JS, Armstrong J: Outbreak of *Clostridium difficile*-associated disease in a small animal veterinary teaching hospital, J Vet Intern Med 17:813-816, 2003.
14. Grundmann H, Barwolf S, Tami A, et al: How many infections are caused by patient to patient transmission in intensive care units? Crit Care Med 23(5):946-951, 2005.
15. Johnson JA: Nosocomial infections, Vet Clin North Am Small Anim Pract 32(5):1101-1126, 2002.
16. Nakamura RK, Tompkins E: Nosocomial infections, Compend Contin Educ 34: 4, E1-E11, 2012.
17. Gibson JS, Morton JM, Cobbold RN, et al: Risk factors for dogs becoming rectal carriers of multidrug-resistant *Escherichia coli* during hospitalization, Epidemiol Infect 139:1511-1521, 2011.
18. Prescott JF, Brad Hanna WJ, Reid-Smith R, Drost K: Antimicrobial drug use and resistance in dogs, Can Vet J 43:107-110, 2002.
19. Brooks MB, Morley PS, Dargatz DA, et al: Survey of antimicrobial susceptibility testing practices of veterinary diagnostic laboratories in the United States, J Am Vet Med Assoc 222(2):168-174, 2003.
20. Wieler LH, Ewers C, Guenther S, et al: Methicillin-resistant staphylococci (MRS) and extended-spectrum beta-lactamases (ESBL)-producing *Enterobacteriaceae* in companion animals: Nosocomial infections as one reason for the rising prevalence of these potential zoonotic pathogens in clinical samples, Int J Med Microbiol 301:635-641, 2011.
21. Normand EH, Gibson NR, Reid SWJ, et al: Antimicrobial-resistance trends in bacterial isolates from companion-animal community practice in the UK, Prev Vet Med 46:267-278, 2000.
22. Normand EH, Gibson SR, Taylor DJ, et al: Trends of antimicrobial resistance in bacterial isolates from a small animal referral hospital, Vet Record 146:151-155, 2000.
23. Jones RN: Resistance patterns among nosocomial pathogens. Trends over the past few years, Chest 119(2):397S-404S, 2001.
24. Shah AA, Hasan F, Ahmed S, et al: Characteristics, epidemiology and clinical importance of emerging strains of Gram-negative bacilli producing extended-spectrum beta-lactamases, Res Microbiol 155:409-421, 2004.
25. Taylor LH, Latham SM, Woolhouse MEJ: Risk factors for human disease emergence, Phil Trans R Soc Lond B 356:983-989, 2001.
25a. Epp T, Waldner C: Occupational health hazards in veterinary medicine: zoonoses and other biological hazards, Can Vet J 53(2):144-150, 2012.
26. Johnson JR, Stell AL, Delavari P, et al: Phylogenetic and Pathotypic Similarities between Escherichia coli isolates from urinary tract infections in dogs and extraintestinal infections in humans, J Infect Dis 183:897-906, 2001.
27. Morris DO, Boston RC, O'Shea K, et al: The prevalence of carriage of methicillin-resistant staphylococci by veterinary dermatology practice staff and their respective pets, Vet Dermatol 21:400-407, 2010.
28. Damborg P, Top J, Hendrickx APA, et al: Dogs are a reservoir of ampicillin resistant *Enterococcus faecium* lineages associated with human infections, Appl Env Microbiol 75:2360-2365, 2009.
29. Duquette RA, Nuttall TJ: Methicillin-resistant *Staphylococcus aureus* in dogs and cats: an emerging problem? J Small Anim Pract 45:591-597, 2004.
30. Weese JS: Methicillin-resistant *Staphylococcus aureus*: an emerging problem in small animals, J Am Anim Hosp Assoc 41:150-157, 2005.
31. Pak SI, Han HR, Shimizu A: Characterization of methicillin-resistant *Staphylococcus aureus* isolated from dogs in Korea, J Vet Med Sci 61(9):1013-1018, 1999.
32. Tomlin J, Pead MJ, Lloyd DH, et al: Methicillin-resistant *Staphylococcus aureus* infections in 11 dogs, Vet Record 1:60-64, 1999.
33. Morris DO, Rook KA, Shofer FS, et al: Screening of *Staphylococcus aureus*, *Staphylococcus intermedius*, and *Staphylococcus schleiferi* isolates obtained from small companion animals for antimicrobial resistance: a retrospective review of 749 isolates (2003-2004), Vet Dermatol 17:332-337, 2006.
34. Simjee S, White DG, McDermott PF, et al: Characterization of Tn1546 in vancomycin-resistant *Enterococcus faecium* isolated from canine urinary tract infections: evidence of gene exchange between human and animal enterococci, J Clin Microbiol 40(12):4659-4665, 2002.
35. Pressel MA, Fox LE, Apley MD, et al: Vancomycin for multi-drug resistant *Enterococcus faecium* cholangiohepatitis in a cat, J Feline Med Surg 7:317-321, 2005.
36. Ghosh A, Dowd SE, Zurek L: Dogs leaving the ICU carry a very large multi-drug resistant enterococcal population with capacity for biofilm formation and horizontal gene transfer, PLoS ONE 6(7):e22451, 2011.
37. Murtaugh RJ, Mason GD: Antibiotic pressure and nosocomial disease, Vet Clin North Am Small Anim Pract 19(6):1259-1274, 1989.
38. Benedict KM, Morley PS, Van Metre DC: Characteristics of biosecurity and infection control programs at veterinary teaching hospitals, J Am Vet Med Assoc 233:767-773, 2008.

CHAPTER 90
FEBRILE NEUTROPENIA

Melissa A. Claus, DVM, DACVECC

KEY POINTS

- Neutropenia is defined broadly as less than 2900 cells/μl in dogs and less than 2000 cells/μl in cats.
- Three primary mechanisms by which febrile neutropenia can develop include increased tissue use of neutrophils, decreased egress of neutrophils from the bone marrow, and immune-mediated destruction of neutrophils.
- Diagnostic tests to consider performing in a patient with febrile neutropenia include blood cultures, a urine culture, chest radiographs, abdominal ultrasound, cardiac ultrasound, and bone marrow aspiration or core biopsy.
- Animals with febrile neutropenia should receive broad-spectrum antibiotics using an antipseudomonal β-lactam. Neutropenic patients in septic shock should receive an antipseudomonal β-lactam coupled with an aminoglycoside. These regimens should be de-escalated with receipt of the susceptibility profiles of cultured organisms.
- Recombinant human and canine granulocyte-colony stimulating factors (rhG-CSF and rcG-CSF) should not be used in Parvovirus infection–induced neutropenia because of poor efficacy (rh-GCSF) and lack of safety data (rcG-CSF).

- Recombinant canine G-CSF has been demonstrated effective at generating myelopoiesis in dogs with chemotherapy-induced neutropenia and cyclic hematopoiesis.
- Meticulous hand washing before and after handling neutropenic patients and using alcohol-based hand sanitizer and donning gloves before handling any indwelling devices is imperative to decrease incidence of nosocomial infection in these patients.

Febrile neutropenia in dogs and cats has multiple etiologies. Regardless of the underlying cause, insufficient numbers of circulating neutrophils can affect significantly patient morbidity and mortality. Without these vital cells of the innate immune system, patients with febrile neutropenia have little protection against invading pathogens and are even at risk of developing life-threatening infections from their own commensal microflora. This chapter discusses the normal processes and production of neutrophils, the etiologies of febrile neutropenia, and diagnostic tests and recommended treatments for patients with this condition.

NEUTROPHIL PHYSIOLOGY

Neutrophil Function

Neutrophils are the most abundant leukocyte in dogs and cats. They are a crucial part of the innate immune system because they are often the first phagocytes to recognize and destroy invading pathogens, including bacteria and fungi. Recognition of invading pathogens occurs when pattern recognition receptors (PRRs) present on the neutrophil membrane bind pathogen-associated molecular patterns (PAMPs) on the cell wall of pathogens. Binding of PRRs activates the neutrophil. Neutrophils also become activated when PRRs bind damage-associated molecular patterns (DAMPs), released from necrotic and apoptotic tissues. Via this mechanism, the neutrophilic response that occurs with sterile inflammation can mimic that occurring with infection.

Neutrophils kill invading pathogens with two main mechanisms: phagocytosis followed by degranulation or formation of neutrophil extracellular traps (NETs). When an organism expressing PAMPs is phagocytosed, cytoplasmic granules containing lethal proteases and peptides fuse with an intracytoplasmic phagosome in a process known as degranulation. These cytotoxic molecules coupled with the production of reactive oxygen species via an intraphagosomal oxidative burst destroy the organism and trigger apoptosis of the neutrophil. The other mechanism by which neutrophils help eradicate foreign organisms is a newly recognized process called *NET formation*. During this process, nuclear material including DNA and histones combine with cytotoxic molecules from cytoplasmic granules and are expelled from the cell into the extracellular space. This web of deadly material ensnares and kills microorganisms while limiting the spread of cytotoxic molecules to prevent damage to regional tissues. The entire process leads to death of the neutrophil via a process termed NETosis, a programmed cell death that appears to have different characteristics from necrosis and apoptosis.[1-3]

Neutrophil Production

The driving factors behind myelopoiesis and neutrophil homeostasis are not understood completely. The production of neutrophils depends in part on the presence of the cytokine granulocyte-colony stimulating factor (G-CSF). G-CSF is produced primarily by bone marrow stromal cells but also is secreted from a variety of other cells, including macrophages, monocytes, endothelial cells, and fibroblasts.[4,5] It is the most important cytokine responsible for maintaining neutrophil homeostasis. It promotes progenitor differentiation into committed production of neutrophils, increases cell division, decreases the time to maturation, and increases release of neutrophils from the bone marrow.[4,5] One stimulus for G-CSF release by bone marrow stromal cells is an elevated level of cytokine IL-17.[6] This cytokine is produced by specific lymphocytes under the stimulation of cytokine IL-23, a cytokine released by tissue macrophages.[7] This pathway of G-CSF production is the underpinning of the main theory for the homeostatic maintenance of neutrophils. When neutrophils reach the end of their life span in the tissues, they undergo apoptosis and are phagocytized by IL-23–producing tissue macrophages. The act of ingesting apoptotic neutrophils decreases the secretion of IL-23 by the macrophage, thus in turn decreasing the secretion of IL-17 by lymphocytes and downregulating the secretion of G-CSF by the bone marrow stromal cells.[8] Once the neutrophil population is depleted and fewer neutrophils are phagocytized in the tissues, the secretion of IL-23 increases. This, in turn, increases IL-17 by lymphocytes and then increases G-CSF concentrations in the plasma to promote further neutrophil production.

Emergency myelopoiesis is a term used to describe the ramping up of leukocyte production that occurs outside of a more steady-state production of neutrophils. It is driven by cytokine stimulation and PAMP/DAMP binding to PRRs on hematopoietic stem cells. These molecules promote proliferation of progenitor cells and directed differentiation into the granulocyte cell line. Recent research suggests that myelopoiesis more likely exists along a continuum, rather than in a switched on (emergency) or switched off (steady-state) form. This is due to the constant presence of PRR signaling in hematopoietic stem cells and progenitors stimulated by commensal microflora. This idea was exemplified in a study of germ-free mice living in a pathogen-free environment. These mice were healthy but demonstrated a markedly attenuated neutrophil steady state with 10% of normal circulating neutrophil counts along with a low serum G-CSF concentration, demonstrating no stimulation to increase myelopoiesis.[9]

Neutrophils are present in several different locations in the body, including the bone marrow, the blood vessels, marginated in the microcirculation, and in the tissues. Neutrophils are produced by progenitor cells in the bone marrow. It is here that they mature into segmented neutrophils. In dogs and cats, the bone marrow houses a fairly large reserve pool of mature neutrophils. Under the stimulation of growth factors and cytokines including G-CSF, GM-CSF, TNF-α, TNF-β, and complement 5a, neutrophils are released from the bone marrow.[10] Once they enter the circulation, they are found in one of two pools: the circulating pool or the marginated pool. The circulating pool neutrophils travel rapidly through the center of larger vessels along with the red blood cells. These neutrophils are the ones that are sampled and counted in a complete blood count. The marginated pool neutrophils roll slowly along the endothelium of smaller vessels and capillaries and tend to stagnate in postcapillary venules. In dogs, about half of the neutrophils in circulation are in the circulating pool and half are in the marginated pool. In cats, only about a quarter of neutrophils are in the circulating pool, whereas three quarters are in the marginated pool. This distinction affects the definition of neutropenia in dogs versus cats. Neutropenia is defined broadly as less than 2900 cells/μl.[11] However, it may be more appropriate to consider a different definition for neutropenia in cats because the majority of neutrophils in circulation are marginated and thus are not actually within the blood collected when assessing a complete blood count. For this reason, neutropenia in cats may be better defined as less than 2000 cells/μl.[12]

PATHOPHYSIOLOGY OF NEUTROPENIA

Neutropenia places a patient at high risk of developing overwhelming infections and thus can contribute significantly to patient morbidity.

Severe neutropenia usually is accompanied by a fever because of the systemic inflammatory response elicited by opportunistic invading pathogens. Febrile neutropenia can occur because of a multitude of different disease processes. Animals may become neutropenic during hospitalization, or severe febrile neutropenia may be the reason they are admitted to the ICU. Febrile neutropenia develops by three main mechanisms, including increased use of neutrophils, decreased egress from bone marrow, and immune-mediated destruction.

Increased Utilization

Infectious microorganisms in the tissues as well as DAMP-expressing endogenous tissues trigger a host inflammatory cascade. Cytokines and chemokines are generated by tissue macrophages and neutrophils. These molecules promote the margination and then extravasation of circulating neutrophils into the tissues, where they depopulate the invading pathogens or necrotic tissue via the two mechanisms described above, phagocytosis with degranulation or NETosis. The larger the population of infectious organisms or the more extensive the quantity of necrotic tissue, the stronger the inflammatory response and the higher the concentration of secreted cytokines. Acutely, the tissue recruitment of neutrophils depletes the neutrophils in circulation. Low levels of circulating neutrophils decrease the concentration of specific chemokines in the bone marrow that retain neutrophils. This allows the stored mature neutrophils to egress into circulation.[9] Ultimately, this can deplete the reserve pool of mature neutrophils in the bone marrow. If the inflammation is overwhelming and persistent, it can exceed the ability of the bone marrow to generate new neutrophils, thus leading to neutropenia.

The severity of neutropenia may not be due entirely to increased extravasation but also may be due to decreased bone marrow production. A 2009 study in a septic mouse model demonstrated the ability of the bone marrow to replete the population of circulating neutrophils is compromised during sepsis by precluding the hematopoietic stem and progenitor cells from differentiating into committed myeloid progenitor cells.[13] Decreasing the differentiating capacity of the bone marrow maximally affects the neutrophil concentration because this cell line has the shortest half-life of the blood cells, especially during a period of increased extravasation. Other studies have shown similar effects on granulopoiesis in the presence of the inflammatory cytokine IFN-γ, as well as in murine models of sepsis and thermal injury.[14-16]

Decreased Egress from the Bone Marrow

Depletion of granulocyte progenitor cells and ineffective granulopoiesis are two bone marrow-centric causes of circulating neutropenia. Generalized bone marrow hypoplasia reduces quantities of granulocyte progenitor cells along with the other hematopoietic cell lines. Bone marrow hypoplasia can occur because of a variety of processes, including infectious diseases, exposure to some drugs and toxicants, radiation, myelophthisis, and cyclic hematopoiesis (gray collie syndrome). Ineffective granulopoiesis is the term used to describe the presence of adequate granulocyte precursors in the bone marrow coupled with a peripheral neutropenia. This can be due to maturational arrest of the neutrophil cell line or retention and/or destruction of mature neutrophils in the bone marrow. Ineffective granulopoiesis can occur with infectious diseases (feline leukemia virus, feline immunodeficiency virus), myelodysplasia, lithium administration in cats, acute myeloid leukemia, and trapped neutrophil syndrome of Border Collies.[17,18]

Depletion of granulocyte progenitor cells

Infectious diseases

Parvovirus in dogs and cats infects rapidly dividing cell populations, including hematopoietic precursor cells. This leads to apoptosis of the cells, depopulation of the bone marrow, and severe leukopenia results.[19] Neutrophils are affected early and severely because of the short half-life of this cell population. This is especially significant in the presence of increased extravasation and use of neutrophils in the gut, where Parvovirus causes severe compromise to the gut mucosal barrier, allowing invasion from gut flora.[20,21]

Although not consistently present, neutropenia may be seen with different rickettsial infections. It is reported more consistently with *Ehrlichia canis*, a monocyte-infecting bacterium, than with *Anaplasma phagocytophilum* and *Ehrlichia ewingii*, granulocytic ehrlichioses. The mechanism by which neutropenia is induced in acute infections is unknown, although severe generalized bone marrow hypoplasia with secondary pancytopenia is described to occur with chronic infections.[22]

Cats infected with one of the retroviruses, feline leukemia virus or feline immunodeficiency virus, have an increased risk of developing neutropenia, although neither disease routinely leads to neutropenia.[23] Underlying causes for the development of neutropenia are varied and depend on the virus involved. Cats with feline leukemia virus tend to develop myelophthisis and myelodysplastic disorders secondary to round cell neoplasms infiltrating the bone marrow.[23] One mechanism for the development of neutropenia in cats with feline immunodeficiency virus is that infected bone marrow stromal cells secrete myelosuppressing factors that depress granulopoiesis.[24] Neutropenia also may develop in feline immunodeficiency virus–infected cats as a result of myelodysplasia occurring with infection of bone marrow and stromal cells.[25]

Medications, toxicants, and radiation

Several drugs, including antiinfective agents, antiepileptics, colchicine, captopril, methimazole, and phenylbutazone, have been reported to induce neutropenia idiosyncratically.[10,26-28] The mechanisms by which neutropenia develops vary between different drugs and often are understood incompletely. Potential causes may include bone marrow necrosis or fibrosis, suppression of granulopoiesis, immune-mediated destruction of granulocytic precursors or mature granulocytes, or a combination of these effects.[28-30]

Chemotherapeutic drugs are the most common drugs associated with the development of severe neutropenia. In one retrospective observational assessment of the causes of neutropenia in dogs and cats, two thirds of cases of dogs with suspected drug-induced neutropenia and the only case of a cat with suspected drug-induced neutropenia were due to antineoplastic agents.[12] These drugs are effective in the treatment of neoplasia because they primarily decimate colonies of rapidly dividing cells. Thus myelotoxicity is a common side effect of administration of these agents.[10] Likewise, radiation as a treatment for cancer can induce mitotic failure and apoptosis of hematopoietic progenitor cells, leading to bone marrow failure and severe neutropenia.[31]

Estrogens have been demonstrated to be myelotoxic in mice, rats, ferrets, and dogs.[32-35] Dogs are exposed to this steroid hormone by ingestion of an estrogen analog, or from estrogen-secreting tumors (Sertoli cell tumors). Doses at which depressed granulopoiesis is seen are variable in dogs, but significant neutropenia is not seen typically until the dose ingested exceeds the recommended therapeutic dose. Studies in dogs and mice demonstrate no direct effect of estrogen on the hematopoietic progenitor cells. Instead, in both species some evidence suggests that a myelopoiesis inhibitory factor is produced by thymic stromal cells exposed to estrogen.[34,36-38]

Myelophthisis

Myelophthisis is the failure of bone marrow to continue normal hematopoiesis because of its decimation by infiltrating abnormal tissue, typically neoplastic cells or collagen (myelofibrosis), and rarely osteoid (osteosclerosis) or diffuse intramedullary inflammation (e.g., fungal osteomyelitis).[39] Neoplasms associated with myelophthisis are usually round cell neoplasms, including leukemias, lymphomas, multiple myeloma, and histiocytic sarcoma.[12,32] Myelofibrosis has been found in dogs with a variety of diseases, including immune-mediated hemolytic anemia, medullary lymphoma, and extramedullary neoplasia. It has also been documented in dogs receiving chronic treatment with different medications. Of 19 dogs reported to have myelofibrosis in one retrospective study, only two were reported to be neutropenic, despite all dogs displaying a poorly regenerative anemia.[28] The main mechanism by which neutropenia develops with myelophthisis is due to a loss of granulocytic progenitor cells coupled with a loss of the nurturing marrow microenvironment that occurs as a result of destruction of the bone marrow stromal cells.[40,41]

Cyclic hematopoiesis

Canine cyclic hematopoiesis is an autosomal recessive genetic disorder also known as gray collie syndrome because it is found in Collies with a diluted (gray) coat color. The disease is characterized by severe neutropenia developing every 10 to 14 days. Assessment of the bone marrow before a neutropenic episode shows a drastic decline in the myeloid lines, whereas myeloid hyperplasia prefaces the recovery of circulating neutrophil numbers.[42] The disease in gray Collies is associated with a genetic mutation that decreases the neutrophil elastase activity within the neutrophil. How this mutation specifically leads to the clinical presentation of the disease is unclear, but it is postulated that neutrophil elastase must be involved with normal feedback inhibition during granulopoiesis.[41,43]

Ineffective granulopoiesis despite normal to excessive quantities of progenitor cells

Dysgranulopoiesis describes the presence of dysplastic granulocyte progenitor cells that lead to a peripheral circulating neutropenia. This neutropenia occurs in the presence of normal to excessive quantities of progenitor cells in the bone marrow. Dysmyelopoiesis is a more general term used to describe the presence of dysplastic hematopoietic cells, not just granulocyte precursors. Three major classifications of dysmyelopoiesis include myelodysplastic syndrome (MDS), secondary dysmyelopoiesis, and congenital dysmyelopoiesis (which will not be discussed further).[44]

Myelodysplastic syndrome ultimately arises as a result of clonal expansion of a mutated hematopoietic progenitor cell. The cells arising from the mutant cell do not follow the normal maturation pathway and ultimately undergo apoptosis before they are released from the marrow. Thus the bone marrow appears hyperplastic and contains an abnormally high number of blasts, but there are insufficient cells in circulation.[44] Myelodysplastic syndrome can be one cause of neutropenia in cats with feline leukemia virus.[45]

Secondary dysmyelopoiesis is similar to MDS with the exception that the number of blasts present in the marrow is not increased from normal. Secondary dysmyelopoiesis can occur secondary to different diseases, including immune-mediated hemolytic anemia, immune-mediated thrombocytopenia, and lymphoma. Secondary dysmyelopoiesis also can be seen with the administration of some drugs, including antineoplastic drugs, estrogen, phenobarbital, cephalosporins, chloramphenicol, and colchicine, as well as lithium in cats.[17,44,46] Many of these drugs also lead to hypoplastic bone marrow, as described above.

Separate to dysmyelopoiesis, a heritable disease has been described in Border Collies, in which the bone marrow displays hyperplastic granulopoiesis and no evidence of maturation arrest or dysplasia but a severe circulating neutropenia.[47] This disease is known as trapped neutrophil syndrome (TNS). Although the gene mutation that causes TNS has been identified, the underlying mechanism by which this mutation leads to decreased release of segmented neutrophils into circulation remains unknown.[48]

Immune-Mediated Destruction

Applicable to small animal veterinary patients are two main types of immune-mediated destruction of neutrophils: (1) primary or idiopathic immune-mediated neutropenia and (2) immune-mediated neutropenia that occurs secondary to an underlying trigger including infection, drugs, or neoplasia. Idiopathic immune-mediated neutropenia occurs when antibodies are produced against neutrophil surface proteins. These antibodies bind to the surface proteins and either activate complement-mediated death of the neutrophil or opsonize the cell for phagocytosis by macrophages.[49] The veterinary literature includes few reports of patients with confirmed immune-mediated neutropenia: the standard for definitive diagnosis is to demonstrate the presence of antineutrophil antibodies in the serum of the patient. Although successful detection of antineutrophil antibodies has been reported in dogs with immune-mediated neutropenia using flow cytometry, this test is not readily and widely available.[50-52] Instead, diagnosis often is based on exclusion of the other causes of neutropenia discussed above, in conjunction with improvement in neutrophil counts when treated with immune-suppressive agents.[12,53-58]

CLINICAL PRESENTATION AND DIAGNOSTIC TESTS

The clinical signs exhibited by the patient with febrile neutropenia ultimately depend on the underlying cause for neutropenia. Animals with an increased tissue demand and extravasation of neutrophils often demonstrate signs of severe sepsis or septic shock, typically with a marked suppurative exudate at the focus of infection or inflammation. In addition, these patients would likely display a marked degenerative left shift on a complete blood count. If neutropenia is secondary to decreased egress from bone marrow or immune-mediated destruction, patients may have opportunist infections of their skin (e.g., IV catheter site) or in their lungs or urinary tract but show minimal pathologic changes on visual inspection, thoracic radiographs, or urinalysis because of marked suppression of the normal inflammatory response.[59,60] Some animals, despite being profoundly neutropenic, may not have a fever on presentation. For example, many septic cats and very ill septic dogs are hypothermic on presentation to the emergency clinic. In addition, neutropenic patients that have received glucocorticoids or nonsteroidal antiinflammatory drugs may have suppression of their fever because of inhibition of prostaglandin formation.

Determining the underlying cause of neutropenia helps to develop an appropriate treatment plan. In many cases, the underlying cause for neutropenia may be clear: an obvious septic focus or a recent history of chemotherapy administration. In other cases, exhaustive diagnostics may be necessary to determine the underlying cause. Diagnostic tests to consider in a patient with neutropenia include blood cultures, urinalysis and culture, radiographs of the thorax and abdomen, ultrasound of the abdomen, and a bone marrow evaluation.

Blood cultures should be performed in febrile neutropenic patients as early as possible and ideally before administering antimicrobials. The 2012 Surviving Sepsis Guidelines recommend taking at least two 10- to 20-ml blood samples from different sites before starting antimicrobial therapy. Blood cultures allow for conclusive diagnosis of sepsis, and the susceptibility profile allows for appropriate de-escalation of antimicrobial therapy.[61] A urinalysis may have benign sediment in the face of a severe infectious process because of lack of the patient's ability to mount an immune response. A urine culture, like a blood culture, is important to evaluate to determine if antimicrobial therapy is appropriate and can allow de-escalation of these drugs.

Imaging of the thorax and abdomen using radiographs and ultrasound can help determine if there is a septic focus that has led to neutropenia. It also can help assess for other causes of neutropenia or for the presence of multiple organ dysfunction as a result of neutropenia (e.g., acute respiratory distress syndrome). Imaging of the cardiac valves also may be indicated in a neutropenic patient with a new murmur because vegetative endocarditis may be the septic source.

Bone marrow aspiration and/or a core biopsy are required to diagnose many of the causes of neutropenia, including infiltrative neoplasia, myelofibrosis, osteosclerosis, and dysmyelopoiesis. Evidence of maturation arrest in a bone marrow aspirate also may help support a presumptive diagnosis of immune-mediated neutropenia.[10] Bone marrow aspiration is a test that may help a clinician determine if the patient is responding to therapy and may help assess the likelihood of recovery from neutropenia.

TREATMENT AND SUPPORTIVE CARE

Most of the literature assessing treatment for febrile neutropenic patients consists of studies assessing care of oncology patients that are febrile secondary to their chemotherapy or radiation treatments. This group of neutropenic patients is different than patients that develop neutropenia for any of the other reasons mentioned previously, thus not all recommendations apply to all neutropenic patients.

Broad-spectrum antimicrobial therapy should be initiated in all febrile neutropenic patients. Decisions as to which antimicrobial therapy to choose should be based on the individual patient's characteristics, including previous antimicrobial exposure, previous culture results, suspected pathogen based on clinical signs, and regional microbe infection patterns. In people, monotherapy using an antipseudomonal β-lactam (e.g., ceftazidime, piperacillin-tazobactam, ticarcillin-clavulanate) has been shown to be efficacious in stable febrile neutropenic patients. In neutropenic people exhibiting signs of septic shock, the recommendation is to combine a β-lactam with an aminoglycoside (e.g., amikacin).[62] If infection with a fungal organism is suspected, antifungals also are recommended.[61] Once the susceptibility results of blood culture and urine culture are available, the antimicrobial therapy is changed to target specifically the pathogen(s) cultured. This can decrease the risk for the development of secondary infections with microorganisms that are multidrug resistant.[61] It also can help decrease the risk of organ damage that can develop with the use of some antimicrobials.

Any patient that is neutropenic and has clinical signs of sepsis, severe sepsis, or septic shock should be resuscitated aggressively using intravenous crystalloids and vasopressors as needed, and broad-spectrum antimicrobial therapy should be initiated as soon as possible.[61,63] If present and identified, source control of the septic focus should occur. Intensive monitoring for the development of multiple organ dysfunction syndrome and meticulous supportive care has to be provided to these patients. See Chapters 5, 6, and 7 for further information on this topic.

Another medication recommended for the treatment of febrile neutropenia is recombinant G-CSF. G-CSF increases the differentiation of progenitor cells into neutrophils and acts on mature neutrophils to increase chemotaxis, enhance the respiratory burst, and improve IgA-mediated phagocytosis.[64] In specific situations, recombinant human G-CSF (rhG-CSF) is recommended as a prophylactic treatment to people receiving chemotherapy because it has been shown to decrease the incidence of febrile neutropenia and secondary infection in this population.[65-68] Recombinant human G-CSF has been reported effective at stimulating granulopoiesis in dogs and cats.[69,70] However, it was shown to be ineffective in treating dogs with neutropenia secondary to Parvovirus.[71,72] In addition, administration of this human protein to dogs may lead to the development of antibodies against rhG-CSF. These antibodies cross-react with and neutralize canine G-CSF, which causes a chronic neutropenia.[73]

Recombinant canine G-CSF (rcG-CSF) was developed and has been used effectively to increase granulopoiesis in dogs and cats.[74-78] It has been demonstrated effective in dogs to accelerate recovery from neutropenia resulting from Parvovirus, chemotherapeutics, and cyclic hematopoiesis.[64,76,77,79] Some questions remain regarding its safety, however. In one study, dogs with Parvovirus treated with rcG-CSF had a higher mortality rate than dogs with Parvovirus that were not treated with this drug.[64] In addition, no studies have been performed in cats to determine if long-term or repeat rcG-CSF use may induce antibody formation and lead to chronic neutropenia as seen with rhG-CSF use in dogs. Evidence suggests that this outcome does occur in rabbits receiving rcG-CSF.[80] Use of this medication to treat dogs with neutropenia should be at the discretion of the clinician. Given lack of safety data, it is not recommended to use rcG-CSF in dogs with Parvovirus infections, or in alternate species.

Frequently recommended nursing practices include isolating severely neutropenic patients from other hospitalized animals and practicing barrier nursing, in which the carer dons a gown, gloves, and a mask before handling the patient. No literature reviews the efficacy of these practices in veterinary medicine, and the studies available regarding people tend to be small and uncontrolled with multiple interventions occurring simultaneously, making their results difficult to interpret.[81] Arguments against going to these lengths include the cost associated with maintaining a clean isolation ward and providing disposable barrier clothing, in addition to the potential for a decreased level of nursing care given the increased work required to prepare to care for these patients.[82] The current recommendation is to focus on meticulous hand hygiene, ensuring thorough washing of the hands before and after handling a neutropenic patient, in addition to using alcohol-based hand sanitizer and donning gloves before handling any indwelling devices including intravenous catheters, urinary catheters, feeding tubes, or tracheostomy tubes. Because these patients are at risk of developing infections secondary to their own commensal flora, keeping these patients clean and dry is critical. Preventing fecal and urine contamination of skin and indwelling devices is imperative.

REFERENCES

1. Seeley EJ, Matthay MA, Wolters PJ: Inflection points in sepsis biology: from local defense to systemic organ injury, Am J Physiol Lung Cell Mol Physiol 303:L355-363, 2012.
2. Borregaard N: Neutrophils, from marrow to microbes, Immunity 33:657-670, 2010.
3. Hostetter SJ: Neutrophil function in small animals, Vet Clin North Am Small Anim Pract 42:157-171, 2012.
4. Bugl S, Wirths S, Muller MR, et al: Current insights into neutrophil homeostasis, Ann N Y Acad Sci 1266:171-178, 2012.
5. Panopoulos AD, Watowich SS: Granulocyte colony-stimulating factor: molecular mechanisms of action during steady state and "emergency" hematopoiesis, Cytokine 42:277-288, 2008.
6. Schwarzenberger P, Huang W, Ye P, et al: Requirement of endogenous stem cell factor and granulocyte-colony-stimulating factor for IL-17-mediated granulopoiesis, J Immunol 164:4783-4789, 2000.
7. Aggarwal S, Ghilardi N, Xie MH, et al: Interleukin-23 promotes a distinct CD4 T cell activation state characterized by the production of interleukin-17, J Biol Chem 278:1910-1914, 2003.
8. Stark MA, Huo Y, Burcin TL, et al: Phagocytosis of apoptotic neutrophils regulates granulopoiesis via IL-23 and IL-17, Immunity 22:285-294, 2005.
9. Bugl S, Wirths S, Radsak MP, et al: Steady-state neutrophil homeostasis is dependent on TLR4/TRIF signaling, Blood 121:723-733, 2013.
10. Schnelle AN, Barger AM: Neutropenia in dogs and cats: causes and consequences, Vet Clin North Am Small Anim Pract 2012;42:111-122.

11. Schultze AE: Interpretation of canine leukocyte responses. In Weiss DJ, Wardrop KJ, editor: Schalm's veterinary hematology, ed 6, Ames, Iowa, 2010, Blackwell, pp 321-334.
12. Brown MR, Rogers KS: Neutropenia in dogs and cats: a retrospective study of 261 cases, J Am Anim Hosp Assoc 37:131-139, 2001.
13. Rodriguez S, Chora A, Goumnerov B, et al: Dysfunctional expansion of hematopoietic stem cells and block of myeloid differentiation in lethal sepsis, Blood 114:4064-4076, 2009.
14. de Bruin AM, Libregts SF, Valkhof M, et al: IFNgamma induces monopoiesis and inhibits neutrophil development during inflammation, Blood 119:1543-1554, 2012.
15. Santangelo S, Gamelli RL, Shankar R: Myeloid commitment shifts toward monocytopoiesis after thermal injury and sepsis, Ann Surg 233:97-106, 2001.
16. Shoup M, Weisenberger JM, Wang JL, et al: Mechanisms of neutropenia involving myeloid maturation arrest in burn sepsis, Ann Surg 228:112-122, 1998.
17. Dieringer TM, Brown SA, Rogers KS, et al: Effects of lithium carbonate administration to healthy cats, Am J Vet Res 53:721-726, 1992.
18. Tvedten HaRRE: Leukocytic disorders. In Small animal clinical diagnosis by laboratory methods, ed 5, St Louis, 2012, Elsevier Saunders, pp 63-91.
19. Breuer W, Stahr K, Majzoub M, et al: Bone-marrow changes in infectious diseases and lymphohaemopoietic neoplasias in dogs and cats—a retrospective study, J Comp Pathol 119:57-66, 1998.
20. Goddard A, Leisewitz AL, Christopher MM, et al: Prognostic usefulness of blood leukocyte changes in canine parvoviral enteritis, J Vet Intern Med 22:309-316, 2008.
21. Kruse BD, Unterer S, Horlacher K, et al: Prognostic factors in cats with feline panleukopenia, J Vet Intern Med 24:1271-1276, 2010.
22. Little SE: Ehrlichiosis and anaplasmosis in dogs and cats, Vet Clin North Am Small Anim Pract 40:1121-1140, 2010.
23. Gleich S, Hartmann K: Hematology and serum biochemistry of feline immunodeficiency virus-infected and feline leukemia virus-infected cats, J Vet Intern Med 23:552-558, 2009.
24. Tanabe T, Yamamoto JK: Phenotypic and functional characteristics of FIV infection in the bone marrow stroma, Virology 282:113-122, 2001.
25. Fujino Y, Horiuchi H, Mizukoshi F, et al: Prevalence of hematological abnormalities and detection of infected bone marrow cells in asymptomatic cats with feline immunodeficiency virus infection, Vet Microbiol 136:217-225, 2009.
26. Jacobs G, Calvert C, Kaufman A: Neutropenia and thrombocytopenia in three dogs treated with anticonvulsants, J Am Vet Med Assoc 212:681-684, 1998.
27. Brazzell JL, Weiss DJ: A retrospective study of aplastic pancytopenia in the dog: 9 cases (1996-2003), Vet Clin Pathol 35:413-417, 2006.
28. Weiss DJ, Smith SA: A retrospective study of 19 cases of canine myelofibrosis, J Vet Intern Med 16:174-178, 2002.
29. Weiss DJ: Bone marrow necrosis in dogs: 34 cases (1996-2004), J Am Vet Med Assoc 227:263-267, 2005.
30. Garbe E: Non-chemotherapy drug-induced agranulocytosis, Expert Opin Drug Saf 6:323-335, 2007.
31. Kulkarni S, Ghosh SP, Hauer-Jensen M, et al: Hematological targets of radiation damage, Curr Drug Targets 11:1375-1385, 2010.
32. Weiss DJ, Evanson OA, Sykes J: A retrospective study of canine pancytopenia, Vet Clin Pathol 28:83-88, 1999.
33. Hart JE: Endocrine pathology of estrogens: species differences, Pharmacol Ther 47:203-218, 1990.
34. Crandall TL, Joyce RA, Boggs DR: Estrogens and hematopoiesis: characterization and studies on the mechanism of neutropenia, J Lab Clin Med 95:857-867, 1980.
35. Sontas HB, Dokuzeylu B, Turna O, et al: Estrogen-induced myelotoxicity in dogs: a review, Can Vet J 50:1054-1058, 2009.
36. Luster MI, Boorman GA, Korach KS, et al: Mechanisms of estrogen-induced myelotoxicity: evidence of thymic regulation, Int J Immunopharmacol 6:287-297, 1984.
37. Farris GM, Benjamin SA: Inhibition of myelopoiesis by serum from dogs exposed to estrogen, Am J Vet Res 54:1374-1379, 1993.
38. Farris GM, Benjamin SA: Inhibition of myelopoiesis by conditioned medium from cultured canine thymic cells exposed to estrogen, Am J Vet Res 54:1366-1373, 1993.
39. Topper MJ: Hemostasis. In Latimer KS, Mahaffey EA, Prasse KW, editors: Duncan & Prasse's veterinary laboratory medicine clinical pathology, ed 4, Ames, Iowa, 2003, Blackwell Publishing Company, pp 99-135.
40. Makoni SN, Laber DA: Clinical spectrum of myelophthisis in cancer patients, Am J Hematol 76:92-93, 2004.
41. Harvey JW: Evaluation of leukocytic disorders. In Veterinary hematology: a diagnostic guide and color atlas, St Louis, 2012, Elsevier Saunders, pp 122-176.
42. Dale DC, Ward SB, Kimball HR, et al: Studies of neutrophil production and turnover in grey collie dogs with cyclic neutropenia, J Clin Invest 51:2190-2196, 1972.
43. Horwitz MS, Corey SJ, Grimes HL, et al: ELANE mutations in cyclic and severe congenital neutropenia: genetics and pathophysiology, Hematol Oncol Clin North Am 27:19-41, 2013.
44. Weiss DJ: Recognition and classification of dysmyelopoiesis in the dog: a review, J Am Vet Med Assoc Am Coll Vet Int Med 19:147-154, 2005.
45. Weiss DJ: Evaluation of dysmyelopoiesis in cats: 34 cases (1996-2005), J Am Vet Med Assoc 228:893-897, 2006.
46. Weiss DJ, Aird B: Cytologic evaluation of primary and secondary myelodysplastic syndromes in the dog, Vet Clin Pathol 30:67-75, 2001.
47. Allan FJ, Thompson KG, Jones BR, et al: Neutropenia with a probable hereditary basis in Border Collies, New Z Vet J 44:67-72, 1996.
48. Shearman JR, Wilton AN: A canine model of Cohen syndrome: trapped neutrophil syndrome, BMC Genomics 12:258, 2011.
49. Chickering WR, Prasse KW: Immune mediated neutropenia in man and animals: a review, Vet Clin Pathol 10:6-16, 1981.
50. Weiss DJ: An indirect flow cytometric test for detection of anti-neutrophil antibodies in dogs, Am J Vet Res 68:464-467, 2007.
51. Weiss DJ: Evaluation of antineutrophil IgG antibodies in persistently neutropenic dogs, J Vet Int Med 21:440-444, 2007.
52. Weiss DJ, Henson M: Pure white cell aplasia in a dog. Veterinary clinical pathology, Am Soc Vet Clin Pathol 36:373-375, 2007.
53. Brown CD, Parnell NK, Schulman RL, et al: Evaluation of clinicopathologic features, response to treatment, and risk factors associated with idiopathic neutropenia in dogs: 11 cases (1990-2002), J Am Vet Med Assoc 229:87-91, 2006.
54. Snead E, Vargo C, Myers S: Glucocorticoid-dependent hypoadrenocorticism with thrombocytopenia and neutropenia mimicking sepsis in a Labrador retriever dog, Can Vet J 52:1129-1134, 2011.
55. Fidel JL, Pargass IS, Dark MJ, et al: Granulocytopenia associated with thymoma in a domestic shorthaired cat, J Am Anim Hosp Assoc 44:210-217, 2008.
56. McManus PM, Litwin C, Barber L: Immune-mediated neutropenia in 2 dogs, J Vet Intern Med 1999;13:372-374.
57. Vargo CL, Taylor SM, Haines DM: Immune mediated neutropenia and thrombocytopenia in 3 giant schnauzers, Can Vet J 48:1159-1163, 2007.
58. Perkins MC, Canfield P, Churcher RK, et al: Immune-mediated neutropenia suspected in five dogs, Aus Vet J 82:52-57, 2004.
59. Bodey GP: Unusual presentations of infection in neutropenic patients, Int J Antimicrob Agents 16:93-95, 2000.
60. Sipsas NV, Bodey GP, Kontoyiannis DP: Perspectives for the management of febrile neutropenic patients with cancer in the 21st century, Cancer 103:1103-1113, 2005.
61. Dellinger RP, Levy MM, Rhodes A, et al: Surviving Sepsis Campaign: international guidelines for management of severe sepsis and septic shock, 2012, Intens Care Med 39:165-228, 2013.
62. Tam CS, O'Reilly M, Andresen D, et al: Use of empiric antimicrobial therapy in neutropenic fever. Australian Consensus Guidelines 2011 Steering Committee, Intern Med J 41:90-101, 2011.
63. Kumar A, Roberts D, Wood KE, et al: Duration of hypotension before initiation of effective antimicrobial therapy is the critical determinant of survival in human septic shock, Crit Care Med 34:1589-1596, 2006.
64. Duffy A, Dow S, Ogilvie G, et al: Hematologic improvement in dogs with parvovirus infection treated with recombinant canine granulocyte-colony stimulating factor, J Vet Pharmacol Ther 33:352-356, 2010.
65. Aapro MS, Bohlius J, Cameron DA, et al: 2010 update of EORTC guidelines for the use of granulocyte-colony stimulating factor to reduce the incidence of chemotherapy-induced febrile neutropenia in adult patients with lymphoproliferative disorders and solid tumours, Eur J Cancer 47:8-32, 2011.

66. Liang DC: The role of colony-stimulating factors and granulocyte transfusion in treatment options for neutropenia in children with cancer, Paediatr Drugs 5:673-684, 2003.
67. Sung L, Nathan PC, Lange B, et al: Prophylactic granulocyte colony-stimulating factor and granulocyte-macrophage colony-stimulating factor decrease febrile neutropenia after chemotherapy in children with cancer: a meta-analysis of randomized controlled trials, J Clin Oncol 22:3350-3356, 2004.
68. Sung L, Nathan PC, Alibhai SM, et al: Meta-analysis: effect of prophylactic hematopoietic colony-stimulating factors on mortality and outcomes of infection, Ann Intern Med 147:400-411, 2007.
69. Fulton R, Gasper PW, Ogilvie GK, et al: Effect of recombinant human granulocyte colony-stimulating factor on hematopoiesis in normal cats, Exper Hematol 19:759-767, 1991.
70. Lothrop CD Jr, Warren DJ, Souza LM, et al: Correction of canine cyclic hematopoiesis with recombinant human granulocyte colony-stimulating factor, Blood 72:1324-1328, 1988.
71. Rewerts JM, McCaw DL, Cohn LA, et al: Recombinant human granulocyte colony-stimulating factor for treatment of puppies with neutropenia secondary to canine parvovirus infection, J Am Vet Med Assoc 213:991-992, 1998.
72. Mischke R, Barth T, Wohlsein P, et al: Effect of recombinant human granulocyte colony-stimulating factor (rhG-CSF) on leukocyte count and survival rate of dogs with parvoviral enteritis, Res Vet Sci 70:221-225, 2001.
73. Hammond WP, Csiba E, Canin A, et al: Chronic neutropenia. A new canine model induced by human granulocyte colony-stimulating factor, J Clin Invest 87:704-710, 1991.
74. Obradovich JE, Ogilvie GK, Powers BE, et al: Evaluation of recombinant canine granulocyte colony-stimulating factor as an inducer of granulopoiesis. A pilot study, J Vet Intern Med 5:75-79, 1991.
75. Zinkl JG, Cain G, Jain NC, et al: Haematological response of dogs to canine recombinant granulocyte colony stimulating factor (rcG-CSF), Comp Haematol Int 2:151-156, 1992.
76. Ogilvie GK, Obradovich JE, Cooper MF, et al: Use of recombinant canine granulocyte colony-stimulating factor to decrease myelosuppression associated with the administration of mitoxantrone in the dog, J Vet Intern Med 6:44-47, 1992.
77. Mishu L, Callahan G, Allebban Z, et al: Effects of recombinant canine granulocyte colony-stimulating factor on white blood cell production in clinically normal and neutropenic dogs, J Am Vet Med Assoc 200:1957-1964, 1992.
78. Obradovich JE, Ogilvie GK, Stadler-Morris S, et al: Effect of recombinant canine granulocyte colony-stimulating factor on peripheral blood neutrophil counts in normal cats, J Vet Intern Med 7:65-67, 1993.
79. Yamamoto A, Fujino M, Tsuchiya T, et al: Recombinant canine granulocyte colony-stimulating factor accelerates recovery from cyclophosphamide-induced neutropenia in dogs, Vet Immunol Immunopathol 142:271-275, 2011.
80. Reagan WJ, Murphy D, Battaglino M, et al: Antibodies to canine granulocyte colony-stimulating factor induce persistent neutropenia, Vet Pathol 32:374-378, 1995.
81. Larson E, Nirenberg A: Evidence-based nursing practice to prevent infection in hospitalized neutropenic patients with cancer, Oncol Nurs Forum 31:717-725, 2004.
82. Mank A, van der Lelie H: Is there still an indication for nursing patients with prolonged neutropenia in protective isolation? An evidence-based nursing and medical study of 4 years experience for nursing patients with neutropenia without isolation, Eur J Oncol Nurs 7:17-23, 2003.

CHAPTER 91

SEPSIS AND SEPTIC SHOCK

Elise Mittleman Boller, DVM, DACVECC • Cynthia M. Otto, DVM, PhD, DACVECC

KEY POINTS

- Sepsis is a clinical syndrome of systemic inflammation in response to infection. Much of the morbidity and mortality associated with sepsis is a result of the host's inflammatory response.
- Alterations in the regulation of vasomotor tone, increased vascular permeability, dysfunctional microcirculation, and coagulation abnormalities are hallmarks of sepsis.
- Microcirculatory abnormalities are often present in the face of normal macrohemodynamics.
- Treatment should be directed at targeted resuscitation, early administration of antimicrobials if bacterial sepsis is suspected, and controlling the source of infection.
- Untreated sepsis can progress to septic shock, which is characterized by hypotension, vascular leak, and microvascular dysfunction. This macrocirculatory and microcirculatory impairment leads to tissue and global oxygen debt, organ failure, and possibly death.

Sepsis, severe sepsis, and septic shock are common causes of morbidity and mortality: The incidence of severe sepsis in humans in the United States is high, killing one in four patients or approximately 215,000 people each year.[1,2] The incidence of sepsis in veterinary medicine is unknown, but the mortality rates appear to be similar, ranging from 20% to 68%.[3-8] The incidence of sepsis is increasing in human health care, likely because of advanced and invasive treatments, widespread use of antimicrobials, increased incidence of resistant infections, and an increasing number of elderly, debilitated, and immunocompromised patients.[9] Recognition, early and aggressive intervention, and intensive supportive care are key to the treatment of sepsis and septic shock.

DEFINITIONS AND CLINICAL MANIFESTATIONS

In 2001 the International Sepsis Definitions Conference produced consensus guidelines for definitions and terminology for syndromes

BOX 91-1 *Definitions*[10,90]

Bacteremia: The presence of live bacterial organisms in the bloodstream.

Sepsis: The clinical syndrome caused by infection and the host's systemic inflammatory response to it; may be of bacterial (gram positive or gram negative), viral, protozoal, or fungal origin.

Severe sepsis: Sepsis complicated by dysfunction of one or more organs.

Septic shock: Acute circulatory failure and persistent arterial hypotension (despite volume resuscitation) associated with sepsis. In people, hypotension is defined by a systolic arterial pressure less than 90 mm Hg, a mean arterial pressure less than 60, or a reduction in systolic pressure of greater than 40 mm Hg from baseline despite adequate volume resuscitation, in the absence of other causes of hypotension.[10]

Systemic inflammatory response syndrome (SIRS): The clinical signs of systemic inflammation in response to infectious or noninfectious insults (e.g., trauma, pancreatitis, burns, snakebites, neoplasia, and heat stroke).

Multiple organ dysfunction syndrome (MODS): Physiologic derangements of the endothelial, cardiopulmonary, renal, nervous, endocrine, and gastrointestinal (GI) systems associated with the progression of uncontrolled systemic inflammation and disseminated intravascular coagulation (DIC).

Table 91-1[5] Systemic Inflammatory Response Syndrome Criteria for Dogs and Cats

Species	Dogs	Cats
Temperature (Celsius/Fahrenheit)	<37.2/99, >39.2/102.5	<37.8/100.4, >40/104
Heart rate (beats/min)	>140	<140, >225
Respiratory rate (breaths/min)	>30	>40
WBC × 10^3/µl	<6, >19	<5, >19

WBC, White blood cells.

associated with microbial infection and the subsequent host response called systemic inflammatory response syndrome, or SIRS (Box 91-1 and Table 91-1; see Chapter 6).[5,10] SIRS has been previously described in veterinary patients.[5] Studies in both human and veterinary medicine are seeking to identify reliable and specific biomarkers of inflammation that can be used to assess the host inflammatory response to infection. Currently it is more feasible to use deviations in heart rate, respiratory rate, body temperature, and white blood cell count as markers of systemic inflammation. These clinical parameters are most valuable for screening sick patients for eligibility to participate in clinical studies of sepsis. The SIRS criteria lack specificity (many nonseptic patients can fit the criteria) and rarely dictate interventions but can help increase the index of suspicion for sepsis. In human medicine, *sepsis* is defined as a documented or suspected infection with one or more general or inflammatory variables that suggest the presence of SIRS (Table 91-2).[10] *Severe sepsis* is defined as a documented or suspected infection and signs of organ dysfunction such as those listed in Table 91-3.[10] Multiple organ dysfunction syndrome (MODS) involves the physiologic derangements of the endothelial, cardiopulmonary, renal, nervous, endocrine, microcirculatory, and gastrointestinal systems associated with progression of uncontrolled systemic inflammation and disseminated intravascular coagulation (DIC). *Septic shock* is defined as acute circulatory failure and persistent arterial hypotension despite volume resuscitation. Acute circulatory failure (in people) is defined as a systolic blood pressure of less than 90 mm Hg, mean arterial pressure of less than 60 mm Hg, or a reduction in systolic blood pressure greater than 40 mm Hg from baseline despite adequate volume.[10] In veterinary patients there are no studies to define critical blood pressures, but it is reasonable to consider that similar blood pressure values are appropriate.[11]

Table 91-2 Diagnostic Criteria for Sepsis in People (Defined as Known or Suspected Infection and Some of the Following)[10]

	Human Parameters
General Variables	
Fever	Core temperature >38.3° C
Hypothermia	Core temperature <36° C
Heart rate	>90/min or >2 SD above the normal value for age
Tachypnea	
Altered mental status	
Significant edema or positive fluid balance	>20 ml/kg over 24 hrs
Hyperglycemia	Plasma glucose >120 mg/dl in the absence of diabetes
Inflammatory Variables	
Leukocytosis	WBC count >12,000/µl
Leukopenia	WBC count <4000/µl
Normal WBC count with >10% immature forms	Normal WBC count with >10% immature forms
Plasma C-reactive protein	>2 SD above the normal value
Plasma procalcitonin >2 SD above the normal value	>2 SD above the normal value
Tissue Perfusion Variables	
Hyperlactatemia	(>1 mmol/L)
Decreased capillary refill or mottling	
Other Variables	
$ScvO_2$	>70%
Cardiac index	>3.5 L/min

SD, Standard deviation; *WBC*, white blood cells.

Table 91-3 Diagnostic Criteria for Severe Sepsis in People (Defined as Sepsis with Organ Dysfunction)[10]

Organ Dysfunction Variables:	
Arterial hypoxemia	PaO_2/FiO_2 <300
Acute oliguria	Urine output <0.5 ml/kg/hr or 45 mmol/L for at least 2 hours
Creatinine	>2 mg/dl
Coagulation abnormalities	INR >1.5 or aPTT >60 seconds
Thrombocytopenia	Platelet count <100,000/µl
Hyperbilirubinemia	Plasma total bilirubin >2 mg/dl or 35 mmol/L

aPTT, Activated partial thromboplastin time; *INR*, international normalized ratio.

Sepsis is a clinical syndrome characterized by a systemic inflammatory response to a bacterial, viral, protozoal, or fungal infection. Bacteremia, defined by the presence of live organisms in the bloodstream, may be variably present in septic patients. The syndrome of sepsis includes the continuum of severity from uncomplicated (SIRS with an infection) to severe (where organ failure becomes a component) to septic shock (the development of hypotension despite volume resuscitation). The prognosis for survival decreases with progression along this continuum and the associated progressive systemic inflammation, organ dysfunction, and ultimately cardiovascular collapse. Dysregulation of vasomotor tone, increased vascular permeability, dysfunctional microcirculation, and coagulation abnormalities are hallmarks of sepsis. The clinical manifestations and course of disease in patients with sepsis ultimately depend on the location of infection; virulence of the organism; size of inoculums; host nutritional status, comorbidities, age, immune response, and organ function; and genetic host response, including coding for cytokine genes, immune effector molecules, and receptors. After the 2001 International Sepsis Definitions Conference, a concept called *PIRO* was adopted to stage sepsis and to describe clinical manifestations of the infection and host response to it.[10] In this model, PIRO is an acronym for *p*redisposition, *i*nsult or *i*nfection, *r*esponse, and *o*rgan dysfunction. This conceptual and clinical framework attempts to incorporate patient factors with the microbial insult in order to stage the disease process and identify factors that may contribute to morbidity and mortality. The PIRO approach may employ advanced diagnostic techniques not yet available in veterinary medicine, but hopefully it can serve as a guideline until similar methods are available and validated.

PATHOGENESIS OF THE SEPTIC SYSTEMIC INFLAMMATORY RESPONSE

Microbial Factors

Sources for gram-negative sepsis commonly include the gastrointestinal (GI) and genitourinary systems. The gram-negative bacterial cell wall contains a potent molecule, lipopolysaccharide (LPS). This pathogen-associated molecular pattern (PAMP) is recognized as one of the most potent stimuli of the host immune response. Host recognition and reaction involves binding of LPS to lipopolysaccharide binding protein (LBP), followed by the LPS-LBP complex binding to membrane-bound CD14 on macrophages.[12,13] This binding activates the macrophage and initiates signaling transduction via the Toll-like receptors to the nucleus to start transcription of inflammatory cytokines,[14] most notably tumor necrosis factor-α (TNF-α), interleukin (IL) 1, IL-6, IL-8, and interferon γ. In addition to proinflammatory mediators, the response also generates production of counterinflammatory mediators (IL-4, IL-10, IL-13, transforming growth factor β, and glucocorticoids), also referred to as the compensatory antiinflammatory response syndrome, or CARS.[13]

Common sources for gram-positive sepsis include skin, injured soft tissue, and intravenous catheters.[15] Activation of the inflammatory cascade by gram-positive bacteria occurs in response to cell wall components (lipoteichoic acid, peptidoglycan, peptidoglycan stem peptides) or bacterial DNA or via elaboration of soluble bacterial exotoxins. Gram-positive bacterial exotoxins can act as "superantigens" and induce widespread activation of T cells, leading to uncontrolled release of inflammatory cytokines such as interferon γ and TNF-α.[13] In both gram-negative and gram-positive sepsis, interaction with these PAMPS largely drives the host response and clinical manifestations of sepsis.

Host Response to Bacterial Infection

Activation of macrophages initiates the sepsis-induced systemic inflammatory response, and TNF-α production is a key factor in the early phase of sepsis.[2] LPS is the most potent stimulus for the release of TNF-α, which acts as an early central regulator of interactions among cytokines. Macrophage-derived cytokines, such as TNF-α, activate other inflammatory cells (i.e., neutrophils, monocytes), and chemokines serve to attract other cells to the affected area. Neutrophil responses to cytokine signaling can result in extensive host tissue damage secondary to the release of products such as reactive oxygen species, proteases, lysozymes, lactoferrin, cathepsins, and defensins. Neutrophils produce relatively small amounts of TNF-α, IL-1, and platelet-activating factor.

A controlled inflammatory response is beneficial to the host. Such a response is localized and represents a balance between activation of the inflammatory cascade and host CARS. An excessive inflammatory response results from disproportionate activation of the proinflammatory mediators or lack of regulatory counterparts. On the other extreme, "immune paralysis" results from excessive antiinflammatory activity. Additionally there may be regional and temporal differences in proinflammatory versus antiinflammatory activity.[16]

LOSS OF HOMEOSTATIC MECHANISMS IN SEPSIS

Many of the pathophysiologic derangements and subsequent clinical signs in septic patients are related to derangements of normal homeostatic mechanisms responsible for regulating vasomotor tone, inflammation, coagulation, endothelial permeability, and microvascular perfusion.

Loss of vasomotor tone

In patients with severe sepsis and septic shock, loss of the normal homeostatic balance between endogenous vasoconstrictors and vasodilators occurs, resulting in dysregulation of vasomotor tone. Overproduction of nitric oxide (NO) during sepsis is a major contributing factor.[17] NO is a powerful vascular smooth muscle relaxant that contributes to the vasodilatory state of patients with septic shock, leading to clinical signs such as hyperemic mucous membranes, short capillary refill time, and tachycardia in dogs and in people.[5,17-20] Cats do not typically display the hyperemic, hyperdynamic state.[20-22] In response to stimulation with endotoxin, TNF-α, IL-1, or platelet activating factor (PAF), inducible nitric oxide synthase (iNOS) accumulates and generates high levels of nitric oxide (NO), thereby contributing to signs of vasodilatory shock.[17,23] In one prospective, observational study in dogs, the NO breakdown products nitrate/nitrite in plasma were was significantly greater in septic dogs or in dogs with SIRS compared with healthy controls.[24]

Dysregulation of inflammation and coagulation

Bacterial infection and host inflammatory cytokines upregulate tissue factor (TF) levels; TF then combines with factor VIIa to initiate the coagulation cascade.[25] The TF-fVIIa complex and its downstream products (i.e., thrombin) can also trigger the elaboration of inflammatory cytokines and platelet activation.[25] Normally, initiation of the coagulant pathway causes a counterregulatory activation of fibrinolytic and anticoagulant pathways to maintain hemostasis without excessive thrombosis. In septic patients, however, natural anticoagulant and fibrinolytic processes (as well as other complex processes) are inhibited via downregulation of antithrombin, tissue factor pathway inhibitor, and tissue plasminogen activator (tPA) and increased plasminogen activator inhibitor (PAI-1).[25] The protein C/S pathway is also inhibited, leading to a reduction of the normal activated protein C anticoagulant and antiinflammatory effects. Platelets also play a major role in this procoagulant state. Platelets exacerbate expression of procoagulant products such as TF, factor Va, and VIIIa; express the fibrinogen receptor; recruit additional platelets; and serve as part of the support structure of clots.[26] The hemostatic balance in septic patients, therefore, favors the procoagulant and antifibrinolytic state initially. Progression over time to a hypocoagulable state depends on host protein synthesis, effectiveness of natural coagulation inhibitors, virulence of the invading organism, and resolution of the inflammatory source.

Hemostatic dysfunction has been reported in septic dogs.[26,27] One study showed that septic dogs had significantly lower protein C levels and antithrombin (AT) activities and higher prothrombin time, partial thromboplastin time, D-dimer, and fibrin(ogen) degradation products than did controls.[4] In a study of dogs with septic peritonitis, coagulation abnormalities, lower AT activity, lower protein C, higher fibrinogen, and less hypercoagulable thromboelastograms were associated with poor outcomes.[28] Dogs with naturally occurring parvoviral enteritis had decreased AT activity and increased maximum amplitude on the thromboelastogram, consistent with hypercoagulability (see Chapter 104).[29] Commonly available laboratory testing may elucidate these hematologic and hemostatic changes (see Table 91-2).[18,26,30]

Endothelial, microcirculatory, and mitochondrial abnormalities

Alterations in the endothelium, increased vascular permeability, and microcirculatory derangements can be caused by many different and complicated mechanisms, including endothelial dysfunction,[31] alterations and damage to the endothelial glycocalyx layer,[32] rheologic changes to red blood cells,[33] leukocyte activation, microthrombosis, and loss of vascular smooth muscle autoregulation.[34] The overall regulation of vascular permeability is complicated (see Chapter 11). The decreased functional capillary density, increased diffusional distance for oxygen, and heterogenous microvascular blood flow all lead to alterations in tissue oxygen extraction and tissue hypoxia.[35-37] Importantly, serious microcirculatory disturbances can occur despite normal macrohemodynamic variables (e.g., blood pressure); this disconnect between systemic hemodynamics and microcirculatory perfusion, also known as cryptic shock, is characteristic of both septic human and canine patients.[35,36]

One prospective observational study in critically ill dogs evaluated vascular endothelial growth factor (VEGF) levels and edema formation in critically ill dogs. VEGF is a hypoxia-responsive angiogenic factor that is also associated with increasing vascular permeability. Although VEGF levels were not correlated to presence of edema on physical examination, dogs that had markedly elevated VEGF levels were less likely to survive.[37] Increased vascular permeability causes efflux of water, proteins and solutes into the interstitial space, thereby causing an increased distance from the red blood cells within the capillaries to the target cell mitochondria, and consequently impairment of oxygen transport and delivery to the mitochondria.[35] One can think of the endothelium itself as an "organ," subject to dysfunction and failure in sepsis, just as the heart, kidneys and brain (and others) can become dysfunctional. There are likely regional and temporal differences in microcirculatory function and dysfunction. Areas that are very dysfunctional contribute to arteriovenous shunting as a result of functional and mechanical obstruction; the associated tissue suffers from a hypoxic insult. The dysfunctional endothelium has been proposed as the "motor" of MODS. New technology such as sidestream darkfield imaging enables visualization and assessment of microcirculatory derangements during sepsis and in response to therapy.

Even if the microcirculation is functional, mitochondrial changes still occur secondary to sepsis.[35] Mitochondria themselves can become dysfunctional in septic patients (termed *cytopathic hypoxia*), which contributes further to heterogenous hypoxic tissue beds.[33,38] In addition to their critical role in oxidative phosphorylation, mitochondria are also involved in apoptotic pathways and cell death.

EPIDEMIOLOGY

Septic Foci, Diseases, and Pathogens Associated with Sepsis

The available epidemiologic information describing the septic foci and common pathogens in small animals can be found in Table 91-4. Although there are numerous possible septic sources (see Table 91-4 and Chapters 23, 97 to 102, 117, 122, and 126), septic peritonitis is a common cause of sepsis, particularly in dogs. Leakage of contents from the GI tract occurs secondary to GI neoplasia, ingestion of foreign bodies (and subsequent perforation), dehiscence of biopsy sites, enterotomies or resected intestine,

Table 91-4 Septic Foci in Cats and Dogs and Pathogens Involved[4,19,21,22,40-45,89-92]

Site	Disease Examples	Dogs (%)	Cats (%)	Pathogens
Peritoneal cavity	GI perforation	35%-36%[2,4,8]	47%[10]	Coagulase-negative *Staphylococcus* spp, *Enterococcus* spp, B-hemolytic *Streptococcus* spp, *Escherichia coli, Klebsiella* spp, *Enterobacter* spp, *Pasteurella* spp, *Corynebacterium* spp[4,40,42,43]
Pulmonary parenchymal, pleural	Pneumonia	20%[4,41]	24% (pyothorax) + 14% (pneumonia)[21]	B-hemolytic *Streptococcus* spp, *E. coli, Bordetella bronchiseptica, Staphylococcus* spp, *E. coli, Klebsiella* spp, *Pseudomonas* spp, *Enterococcus faecalis, Acinetobacter* spp, *Pasteurella* spp[4,44]
Gastrointestinal	Enteritis, bacterial translocation	4%	5%[21]	*E. coli*[21]
Reproductive	Pyometra Prostatitis	25%[4,6]		Group G *Streptococcus* spp, *Enterococcus* spp, B-hemolytic *Streptococcus* spp, *E. coli, Klebsiella* spp[4]
Urinary tract	Pyelonephritis Bacterial cystitis	4%-10%[4]	8%,[22] 7%[21]	B-hemolytic *Streptococcus* spp, *E. coli, Acinetobacter* spp, *Enterococcus* spp[4,22]
Soft tissue, bone	Trauma, osteomyelitis, bite wounds	29%	16%,[22] 3% (osteomyelitis) + 3% (bite wounds[21]; 3%-50%[6,21,22]	*E. coli, Enterobacter* spp[4]
Cardiovascular	Endocarditis		14%[21]	*Staphylococcus lugdunensis, Bartonella* spp, *S. aureus, E. faecalis, Granulicatella* spp, *Streptococcus* spp, *Brucella* spp[45]

nonsteroidal antiinflammatory drug (NSAID)–associated ulcers, perforation of megacolon, and severe colitis. Other reported causes of septic peritonitis include contamination from the urinary bladder, gallbladder, or uterine rupture; GI disease such as salmonellosis or parvoviral enteritis; and hepatic, pancreatic, splenic, and mesenteric lymph node abscess formation.[6,22,40] Aside from septic peritonitis, other less common causes of sepsis include pyelonephritis, pneumonia, septic arthritis, deep pyoderma, bacterial endocarditis, tick-borne diseases, vasculitis, septic meningitis, pyothorax, trauma, bite wounds, osteomyelitis, septic prostatitis, and immune suppression.[*]

Gram-negative enteric bacteria are the most commonly implicated organisms in sepsis in dogs and cats; however, mixed infections and gram-positive infections are also described.[4,22,40,42-45] Culture of infected tissue should be obtained whenever possible (i.e., safe for the patient) because early and appropriate antimicrobial selection is essential for preventing bacterial replication and reducing the host inflammatory response to infection. Knowledge of common isolates and the hospital antibiogram may help guide empiric antimicrobial selection (see Chapter 175).

RESUSCITATION AND TREATMENT OF SEPSIS, SEVERE SEPSIS, AND SEPTIC SHOCK

Introduction to the Bundle Concept

Major improvements in outcome in septic human patients have been accomplished through use of sepsis treatment "bundles." A *bundle of care* refers to a group of therapies that, when instituted together, result in better outcomes than if each individual component were to be implemented alone.[46] For sepsis, evidence-based guidelines for sepsis management are published in the Surviving Sepsis campaign international guidelines. Hospitals[47] that have implemented the guidelines report decreased mortality rates.[48-50] Bundle recommendations and the current guidelines were born out of earlier landmark studies in early goal-directed resuscitation.[51] Although there is still controversy regarding the best individual bundle components, numerous studies have since shown that implementation of a sepsis bundle reduces mortality.[52] Enthusiasm remains for the bundle approach (even in veterinary medicine), and it stands to reason that the same approach may improve outcomes in veterinary patients.[†]

Bundle Element: Lactate

Lactate production is a result of anaerobic metabolism, most commonly as a result of hypoperfusion. High initial lactate levels are associated with poorer outcomes, particularly if the hyperlactatemia persists and if accompanied by hypotension.[55-62] However, lactate clearance as it relates to traditional (e.g., blood pressure) and more recent (e.g., $ScvO_2$) parameters remain unclear. Lactate kinetics in the individual patient probably depends on the phase of sepsis; lactate together with $ScvO_2$ may provide complementary information about the efficacy of resuscitation (see Chapter 183).[58,63] The Surviving Sepsis campaign guidelines recommend measuring lactate within the first 6 hours of admission and promptly initiating fluid resuscitation for patients with lactate concentrations 4 mmol/L or greater.[38] The available veterinary literature supports this recommendation (see Chapter 56).[36,53,55]

Bundle Element: Samples for Culture (Blood, Tissue, or Fluid Cultures)

In human health care, obtaining blood cultures in patients with sepsis or suspected sepsis is very much the standard of care and blood cultures are positive in 30% to 50% of patients with severe sepsis or septic shock.[1,48] In veterinary medicine, blood cultures may be less routinely performed. In one study, however, 49% of critically ill dogs and cats had positive blood cultures.[64] Another study reported that 43% of dogs with gastric dilation and volvulus developed positive blood cultures. The importance of obtaining samples for culture to aid in selection (and deescalation) of antimicrobials cannot be overemphasized; however, obtaining the samples should not cause a delay in initiating resuscitation nor put the patient at risk.

Bundle Element: Early Source Control and Early Antibiotic Administration (see Chapters 175 to 182)

Of paramount importance in treating the septic patient is the identification and removal of the septic focus ("source control") and early administration of antimicrobials. In human patients with septic shock, elapsed time from shock recognition and qualification for early goal-directed therapy to appropriate antimicrobial therapy is a primary determinant of mortality; there is no reason to think that the same is not true in veterinary patients.[65-67] Early antimicrobial therapy is now conceptually "bundled" with more traditional aspects of sepsis resuscitation such as hemodynamic stabilization.[68] Empiric selection of appropriate antimicrobials can be challenging and should consider the location of the infection (and the ability of the antibiotic to penetrate the site), the suspected bacterial flora, community versus nosocomial source, duration of hospitalization, and previous exposure to antimicrobials (see Chapter 175). Bactericidal rather than bacteriostatic antimicrobials are preferred. In both veterinary and human studies, administration of inappropriate antimicrobials is associated with increased mortality.[6,67] In patients who have been hospitalized for some time, the chances of infection with multidrug-resistant bacteria increase, so careful consideration of hospital antibiograms should be employed when choosing empiric antimicrobials therapy.[69] In some patients, sample collection may be impossible because of cardiopulmonary instability or coagulopathy; however, the inability to gather samples for culture and susceptibility testing should never cause a delay in the administration of antimicrobials to patients with sepsis, severe sepsis, or septic shock. Septic patients require a broad-spectrum bactericidal antimicrobial regimen that is administered via the intravenous route (see Chapters 175 and 182). Following are some examples of four-quadrant therapy (i.e., therapies that are effective against gram-positive and gram-negative aerobes and anaerobes). All dosages are listed for the *intravenous* route, except when indicated otherwise:

- Ampicillin (22 mg/kg q8h) and enrofloxacin (10 to 20 mg/kg q24h; 5 mg/kg q24h in cats)
- Ampicillin (22 mg/kg q8h) and amikacin (15 mg/kg q24h [dog], 10 mg/kg q24h [cat])
- Ampicillin (22 mg/kg q8h) and gentamicin (10 mg/kg q24h [dog], 6 mg/kg q24h [cat])
- Cefazolin (22 mg/kg q8h) and amikacin (15 mg/kg q24h [dog], 10 mg/kg q24h [cat])
- Cefazolin (22 mg/kg q8h) and gentamicin (10 mg/kg q24h [dog], 6 mg/kg q24h [cat])
- Ampicillin (22 mg/kg q8h) and cefoxitin (15 to 30 mg/kg q4-6h)
- Ampicillin (22 mg/kg q8h) and cefotaxime (25 to 50 mg/kg q4-6h)
- Ampicillin (22 mg/kg q8h) and ceftazidime (30 to 50 mg/kg q6-8h)
- Clindamycin (8 to 10 mg/kg q8-12h) and enrofloxacin (5 to 20 mg/kg q24h; 5 mg/kg q24h in cats)
- Clindamycin (8 to 10 mg/kg q8-12h) and amikacin (15 mg/kg q24h [dog], 10 mg/kg q24h [cat])
- Clindamycin (8 to 10 mg/kg q8-12h) and gentamicin (10 mg/kg q24h [dog], 6 mg/kg q24h [cat])

*References 4, 6, 21, 22, 29, 41.
†References 18, 36, 48, 50, 53, 54.

Table 91-5 **Circulatory Support in Severe Sepsis and Septic Shock**[20]

Fluid Therapy	Indications	Dose	Comments
Isotonic crystalloids	Intravascular volume replacement Interstitial fluid deficits Maintenance	*Dog:* Up to 60 to 90 ml/kg* *Cat:* Up to 40 to 60 ml/kg*	May precipitate interstitial edema in patients with capillary leak or a low colloid osmotic pressure
Synthetic colloids (e.g., hydroxyethyl starch)	Volume replacement Colloid osmotic support	*Dog:* 5 to 20 ml/kg* *Cat:* 5 to 10 ml/kg*	Dose-related coagulopathies and acute kidney injury (humans) have been documented An arbitrary recommendation is ≤20 ml/kg q24h
Human albumin solution (HSA)	Colloid osmotic pressure support Volume replacement Albumin supplementation	2 ml/kg/hr of 25% HSA for 1 to 2 hours followed by 0.1 to 0.2 ml/kg/hr × 10 hours Or, calculate albumin deficit: Alb deficit (in grams) = 10 × (desired Alb − patient Alb) × wt (kg) × 0.3 and replace over 4 to 6 hours	Doses extrapolated from human literature Monitor closely for reactions
Fresh frozen plasma	Coagulopathies Factor deficiencies Supplemental volume and colloid osmotic support	10 to 15 ml/kg as needed	Not effective at increasing albumin concentration
Packed red blood cells	Anemia	10 to 15 ml/kg will raise PCV by ~10%	—
Fresh whole blood	Anemia Thrombocytopenia Coagulopathies and factor deficiencies Volume replacement	20 ml/kg will raise PCV by ~10%	—

Alb, Albumin; *HSA,* human albumin serum; *PCV,* packed cell volume.
*Listed intravenous fluid doses are "shock doses." Generally, a fraction of the listed dose is given (e.g., one fourth to one half) and response is assessed; the dose is repeated as necessary or until fluid tolerance is reached. Cats seem to have a poor pulmonary tolerance to volume resuscitation; therefore smaller doses may be tried first.

- Ticarcillin and clavulanic acid (50 mg/kg q6h) and enrofloxacin (10 to 20 mg/kg q24h; 5 mg/kg q24h in cats)
- Imipenem (5 to 10 mg/kg q6-8h)
- Meropenem (24 mg/kg q24h or 12 mg/kg SC q8-12h)
- Chloramphenicol (25 to 50 mg/kg q8h; 12.5 to 20 mg/kg q12h in cats)

Bundle Element: Treat Hypotension with Fluids and Possibly Vasopressors

Assessment of volume status and responsiveness

Because septic shock patients are, by definition, in circulatory collapse despite volume resuscitation, cardiovascular support is of key importance. Fluid therapy is essential to maintain adequate tissue oxygen delivery and to prevent the development of MODS and death (see Chapter 60). Assessment of volume status and the potential for volume responsiveness can be difficult. Traditionally, static measures to indirectly measure preload, such as pulmonary artery occlusion pressure (PAOP) and central venous pressure (CVP), have been used. However, they can be cumbersome (PAOP) and not predictive of volume responsiveness (CVP).[70] Dynamic measures of fluid responsiveness may include echocardiographic evaluation of cardiac function and arterial waveform variation in ventilated patients. More simple yet still dynamic measures may include administering serial small fluid boluses or (in people) passive leg elevation and evaluation of the hemodynamic response.[52,71] Accurate monitoring of body weight and urine output via an indwelling urinary catheter is also helpful in assessing total fluid balance as well as monitoring for oligoanuric renal failure. It should be noted, however, that urinary output is a result of the balance between preglomerular and postglomerular resistance. Thus a marked increase in postglomerular resistance can induce an increase in urinary output in the presence of renal hypoperfusion.

Fluid choice

The first line of resuscitation in septic patients is fluid therapy. Isotonic crystalloids, hypertonic crystalloid solutions, synthetic colloids, and blood component therapy may be used for fluid therapy in the septic patient (Table 91-5). The choice of fluids depends on the overall clinical and clinicopathologic picture (see Chapters 58 and 60). Recent studies in human septic patients have called into question the safety of synthetic colloids, specifically hydroxyethyl starches, which now have a black box warning for this population of human patients.[72,73] Synthetic colloids have been a staple of fluid resuscitation in veterinary medicine; however, human studies have shown that resuscitation with these fluids in people is associated with an increased incidence of acute kidney injury and need for renal replacement therapy and, in the case of the Perner et al study, an increased risk of death at day 90. The results of other studies regarding the safety of synthetic colloids were mixed, and no safety studies to date are available in veterinary patients.[74-76] The current recommendation in human critical care is to avoid synthetic colloids in septic patients, especially when other fluid therapy options such as albumin, plasma, or crystalloids are available, or until more rigorous data on the safety of synthetic colloids are published.[52]

Patients with severe sepsis and septic shock are very often hypoalbuminemic.[77,78] Unfortunately, large volumes of fresh frozen plasma are required for albumin replacement (i.e., 22 ml/kg of plasma to raise the albumin concentration by 0.5 g/dl).[78] Fresh frozen plasma is therefore generally only used to prevent a further decline in albumin in severely hypoalbuminemic patients and for correction of

Table 91-6 **Commonly Used Constant Rate Infusion Vasopressor Therapy**

Vasopressor	Dose rate
Norepinephrine	0.1-2 mcg/kg/min IV
Vasopressin	0.5-5 mU/kg/min IV
Dopamine	5-15 mcg/kg/min IV

coagulopathies and factor deficiencies. Human serum albumin (5% or 25%) is still in the early stages of clinical use in veterinary medicine and research is ongoing. The 25% human serum albumin solution is hyperoncotic (colloid osmotic pressure = 100 mm Hg) and should be used judiciously in patients with limited fluid tolerance (see Chapter 58 for further details). Although it does seem effective in raising albumin concentration, questions regarding its safety exist.[79-81] Coagulopathies, anemia, and thrombocytopenia may prompt the use of blood component therapy (e.g., fresh frozen plasma, packed red blood cells, fresh whole blood, respectively).

Hypotension despite volume resuscitation (septic shock)

Hypotension that persists after restoration of intravascular volume is an indication for vasopressors or inotropic agents to support flow to tissues (see Chapters 8, 157, and 158). The decision to use a vasopressor or cardiotonic drug depends on the clinical presentation and objective information obtained from the septic patient (e.g., assessment of cardiac contractility). Vasopressors such as norepinephrine, vasopressin, dopamine, and phenylephrine are most commonly used in patients with peripheral vasodilation (Table 91-6). Norepinephrine is preferred to dopamine in septic human patients, and vasopressin is also considered a reasonable first-line vasopressor.[52,82,83] Studies in septic veterinary patients are ongoing. Although vasopressors may maintain arterial blood pressure, they can also result in excessive vasoconstriction, particularly to the splanchnic and renal circulation, thereby causing GI and renal ischemia. Particularly in the dog, splanchnic vasoconstriction may exacerbate the septic state by promoting loss of gut barrier function and bacterial translocation of bacteria to the bloodstream.

Positive inotropic agents such as dobutamine are generally used in patients with evidence of impaired myocardial contractility (decreased fractional shortening on M-mode echocardiography, decreased cardiac output per invasive or noninvasive measurements). They might also be combined with more selective vasoconstrictors such as vasopressin or phenylephrine.

Bundle Element: Target Central Venous Pressure and Central Venous Pressure and $ScvO_2$

Venous oxygen saturation is a measure of the saturation of hemoglobin with oxygen in the venous blood; it is reflective of the difference between oxygen delivery (DO_2) and oxygen consumption (VO_2). Venous oximetry is monitored intermittently via blood sampling or co-oximetry, or continuously using fiberoptics (spectrophotometry).[84] Mixed venous oxygen saturation (SvO_2) refers to venous blood in the pulmonary artery. Mixed venous blood is pooled blood from the entire body, including blood from the caudal half of the body (i.e., the abdomen and lower extremities) and the coronary circulation. SvO_2 can be viewed as the result of the overall difference in oxygen delivery (DO_2) and oxygen consumption (VO_2) and therefore is a marker of global oxygen debt. Central venous oxygen saturation ($ScvO_2$) generally refers to the saturation of blood in the cranial vena cava, reflective of oxygen delivery and utilization in the head and upper body. In health, $ScvO_2$ is slightly lower than SvO_2 by about 2% to 3%, in part because of the high metabolic rate of the brain and cranial half of the body and also because of the contribution of vascular circuits that use blood for nonoxidative phosphorylation needs in the caudal half of the body (e.g., the renal blood flow).[84] In shock states the relationship between central and mixed saturation can reverse; $ScvO_2$ can be much higher than SvO_2; this likely is due to redistribution of blood flow from the splanchnic circulation to the coronary and cerebral vascular beds.[85-87] Consensus and the international guidelines state that measuring $ScvO_2$ in lieu of SvO_2 (because it technically easier) can be used successfully during sepsis resuscitation.[48]

In health much more oxygen is delivered than is extracted; however, when delivery decreases to a critical threshold, extraction decreases in concert and the patient experiences oxygen debt and lactic acidosis. Monitoring venous oxygen saturation and using it as a therapeutic target is a recommendation in the Surviving Sepsis guidelines.[48] The few veterinary studies that have evaluated $ScvO_2$ as a therapeutic goal suggest its potential value in resuscitating septic and critically ill veterinary patients.[53,88] In both studies, $ScvO_2$ was associated with prognosis.[53,88] These veterinary studies mirror a large body of work in human medicine that resulted in a recommendation in the Surviving Sepsis campaign to resuscitate to an $ScvO_2$ of 70% or greater or an SvO_2 65% or greater.[48]

CONCLUSION

Sepsis is an important and very common problem in both veterinary and human health care. Hallmark pathophysiologic changes include widespread endothelial disruption, microcirculatory failure, progressive inflammation or immune paralysis, and activation of the coagulation cascade. Throughout the progression from sepsis to septic shock, there is extensive interplay between the coagulation and immune systems. Ultimately, circulatory collapse (both macro- and micro-) leads to hypoperfusion, tissue ischemia, organ failure, and death. Treatment of septic patients critically depends on early recognition, early antimicrobial therapy, and aggressive hemodynamic support. Bundled care appears to be very effective in human septic patients, and studies in veterinary medicine are starting to suggest the same.

REFERENCES

1. Angus DC, Linde-Zwirble WT, Lidicker J, et al: Epidemiology of severe sepsis in the United States: Analysis of incidence, outcome, and associated costs of care, Crit Care Med 29(7):1303, 2001.
2. Li J, Carr B, Goyal M, et al. Sepsis: The inflammatory foundation of pathophysiology and therapy, Hosp Pract (Minneap) 39(3):99, 2011.
3. Parsons KJ, Owen LJ, Lee K, et al: A retrospective study of surgically treated cases of septic peritonitis in the cat (2000-2007), J Small Anim Pract 50(10):518, 2009.
4. de Laforcade AM, Freeman LM, Shaw SP, et al: Hemostatic changes in dogs with naturally occurring sepsis, J Vet Intern Med 17(5):674, 2003.
5. Hauptman JG, Walshaw R, Olivier NB: Evaluation of the sensitivity and specificity of diagnostic criteria for sepsis in dogs, Vet Surg 26(5):393, 1997.
6. King LG: Postoperative complications and prognostic indicators in dogs and cats with septic peritonitis: 23 cases (1989-1992), J Am Vet Med Assoc 204(3):407, 1994.
7. Greenfield CL, Walshaw R: Open peritoneal drainage for treatment of contaminated peritoneal cavity and septic peritonitis in dogs and cats: 24 cases (1980-1986), J Am Vet Med Assoc 191(1):100, 1987.
8. Wan L, Bellomo R, May CN: The effect of normal saline resuscitation on vital organ blood flow in septic sheep, Intensive Care Med 32(8):1238, 2006.
9. Martin GS: Sepsis, severe sepsis and septic shock: changes in incidence, pathogens and outcomes, Expert Rev Anti Infect Ther 10(6):701, 2012.

10. Levy MM, Fink MP, Marshall JC, et al: 2001 SCCM/ESICM/ACCP/ATS/SIS international sepsis definitions conference, Crit Care Med 31(4):1250, 2003.
11. Silverstein DC, Wininger FA, Shofer FS, et al: Relationship between Doppler blood pressure and survival or response to treatment in critically ill cats: 83 cases (2003-2004), J Am Vet Med Assoc 232(6):893, 2008.
12. Dobrovolskaia MA, Vogel SN: Toll receptors, CD14, and macrophage activation and deactivation by LPS, Microbes Infect 4(9):903, 2002.
13. Van Amersfoort ES, Van Berkel TJ, Kuiper J: Receptors, mediators, and mechanisms involved in bacterial sepsis and septic shock, Clin Microbiol Rev 16(3):379, 2003.
14. Jiang Q, Akashi S, Miyake K, et al: Lipopolysaccharide induces physical proximity between CD14 and toll-like receptor 4 (TLR4) prior to nuclear translocation of NF-kappa B, J Immunol 165(7):3541, 2000.
15. Martin GS: Sepsis, severe sepsis and septic shock: changes in incidence, pathogens and outcomes, Expert Rev Anti Infect Ther 10(6):701, 2012.
16. Bone RC, Grodzin CJ, Balk RA: Sepsis: a new hypothesis for pathogenesis of the disease process, Chest 112(1):235, 1997.
17. Fernandes D, Assreuy J: Nitric oxide and vascular reactivity in sepsis, Shock 30(Suppl 1):10, 2008.
18. Aird WC: The hematologic system as a marker of organ dysfunction in sepsis, Mayo Clin Proc 78(7):869, 2003.
19. Reference deleted in pages.
20. Brady CA, Otto CM: Systemic inflammatory response syndrome, sepsis, and multiple organ dysfunction, Vet Clin North Am Small Anim Pract 31(6):1147, v-vi, 2001.
21. Brady CA, Otto CM, Van Winkle TJ, et al: Severe sepsis in cats: 29 cases (1986-1998), J Am Vet Med Assoc 217(4):531, 2000.
22. Costello MF, Drobatz KJ, Aronson LR, et al: Underlying cause, pathophysiologic abnormalities, and response to treatment in cats with septic peritonitis: 51 cases (1990-2001). J Am Vet Med Assoc. 2004;225(6):897-902.
23. De Kock I, Van Daele C, Poelaert J: Sepsis and septic shock: pathophysiological and cardiovascular background as basis for therapy, Acta Clin Belg 65(5):323, 2010.
24. Osterbur K, Whitehead Z, Sharp CR, et al: Plasma nitrate/nitrite concentrations in dogs with naturally developing sepsis and non-infectious forms of the systemic inflammatory response syndrome, Vet Rec 169(21):554, 2011.
25. Levi M, van der Poll T, Schultz M: New insights into pathways that determine the link between infection and thrombosis, Neth J Med 70(3):114, 2012.
26. Brainard BM, Brown AJ: Defects in coagulation encountered in small animal critical care, Vet Clin North Am Small Anim Pract 41(4):783, vii, 2011.
27. de Laforcade A: Diseases associated with thrombosis, Top Companion Anim Med 27(2):59, 2012.
28. Bentley A, Mayhew P, Culp W, et al: Alterations in the hemostatic profiles of dogs with naturally occurring septic peritonitis, J Vet Emerg Crit Care (San Antonio) 2013 (in press).
29. Otto CM, Rieser TM, Brooks MB, Russell MW: Evidence of hypercoagulability in dogs with parvoviral enteritis, J Am Vet Med Assoc 217(10):1500, 2000.
30. Aird WC: Endothelium in health and disease, Pharmacol Rep 60(1):139, 2008.
31. Vallet B, Wiel E: Endothelial cell dysfunction and coagulation, Crit Care Med 29(7 Suppl):S36-S41, 2001.
32. Chappell D, Westphal M, Jacob M: The impact of the glycocalyx on microcirculatory oxygen distribution in critical illness, Curr Opin Anaes 22(2):155-162, 2009.
33. Reggiori G, Occhipinti G, De Gasperi A, et al: Early alterations of red blood cell rheology in critically ill patients, Crit Care Med 37(12):3041-3046, 2009.
34. De Backer D, Creteur J, Preiser JC, et al: Microvascular blood flow is altered in patients with sepsis, Am J Resp Crit Care Med 166(1):98-104, 2002.
35. De Backer D, Donadello K, Cortes DO: Monitoring the microcirculation, J Clin Monit Comput 26(5):361, 2012.
36. Silverstein D: Tornadoes, sepsis, and goal-directed therapy in dogs, J Vet Emerg Crit Care (San Antonio) 22(4):395, 2012.
37. Silverstein DC, Montealegre C, Shofer FS, et al: The association between vascular endothelial growth factor levels and clinically evident peripheral edema in dogs with systemic inflammatory response syndrome, J Vet Emerg Crit Care (San Antonio), 19(5):459, 2009.
38. Fink MP: Cytopathic hypoxia: mitochondrial dysfunction as mechanism contributing to organ dysfunction in sepsis, Crit Care Clin 17(1):219, 2001.
39. Reference deleted in pages.
40. Bonczynski JJ, Ludwig LL, Barton LJ, et al: Comparison of peritoneal fluid and peripheral blood pH, bicarbonate, glucose, and lactate concentration as a diagnostic tool for septic peritonitis in dogs and cats Vet Surg 32(2):161, 2003.
41. Weiss DJ, Welle M, Mortiz A, et al: Evaluation of leukocyte cell surface markers in dogs with septic and nonseptic inflammatory diseases, Am J Vet Res 65(1):59, 2004.
42. Son TT, Thompson L, Serrano S, et al: Surgical intervention in the management of severe acute pancreatitis in cats: 8 cases (2003-2007), J Vet Emerg Crit Care (San Antonio) 20(4):426, 2010.
43. Parsons KJ, Owen LJ, Lee K, et al: A retrospective study of surgically treated cases of septic peritonitis in the cat (2000-2007), J Small Anim Pract 50(10):518, 2009.
44. Radhakrishnan A, Drobatz KJ, Culp WT, et al: Community-acquired infectious pneumonia in puppies: 65 cases (1993-2002), J Am Vet Med Assoc 230(10):1493, 2007.
45. Meurs KM, Heaney AM, Atkins CE, et al: Comparison of polymerase chain reaction with bacterial 16s primers to blood culture to identify bacteremia in dogs with suspected bacterial endocarditis, J Vet Intern Med 25(4):959, 2011.
46. Cinel I, Dellinger RP: Guidelines for severe infections: are they useful? Curr Opin Crit Care 12(5):483, 2006.
47. Dellinger RP, Levy MM, Rhodes A, et al: Surviving Sepsis campaign: international guidelines for management of severe sepsis and septic shock, 2012, Intensive Care Med 39(2):165, 2013.
48. Dellinger RP, Levy MM, Carlet JM, et al: Surviving sepsis campaign: International guidelines for management of severe sepsis and septic shock: 2008, Crit Care Med 36(1):296, 2008.
49. Nguyen HB, Corbett SW, Steele R, et al: Implementation of a bundle of quality indicators for the early management of severe sepsis and septic shock is associated with decreased mortality, Crit Care Med 35(4):1105, 2007.
50. Levy MM, Dellinger RP, Townsend SR, et al: The surviving sepsis campaign: results of an international guideline-based performance improvement program targeting severe sepsis, Crit Care Med 38(2):367, 2010.
51. Rivers E, Nguyen B, Havstad S, et al: Early goal-directed therapy in the treatment of severe sepsis and septic shock, N Engl J Med 345(19):1368, 2001.
52. Puskarich MA: Emergency management of severe sepsis and septic shock, Curr Opin Crit Care 18(4):295, 2012.
53. Conti-Patara A, de Araujo Caldeira J, de Mattos-Junior E, et al: Changes in tissue perfusion parameters in dogs with severe sepsis/septic shock in response to goal-directed hemodynamic optimization at admission to ICU and the relation to outcome, J Vet Emerg Crit Care (San Antonio) 22(4):409, 2012.
54. Butler AL: Goal-directed therapy in small animal critical illness, Vet Clin North Am Small Anim Pract 41(4):817, vii, 2011.
55. Stevenson CK, Kidney BA, Duke T, et al: Serial blood lactate concentrations in systemically ill dogs, Vet Clin Pathol 36(3):234, 2007.
56. Puskarich MA, Trzeciak S, Shapiro NI, et al: Prognostic value and agreement of achieving lactate clearance or central venous oxygen saturation goals during early sepsis resuscitation. Acad Emerg Med 19(3):252, 2012.
57. Mikkelsen ME, Miltiades AN, Gaieski DF, et al: Serum lactate is associated with mortality in severe sepsis independent of organ failure and shock, Crit Care Med 37(5):1670, 2009.
58. Napoli AM, Seigel TA. The role of lactate clearance in the resuscitation bundle, Crit Care 15(5):199, 2011.
59. Nguyen HB, Loomba M, Yang JJ, et al: Early lactate clearance is associated with biomarkers of inflammation, coagulation, apoptosis, organ dysfunction and mortality in severe sepsis and septic shock, J Inflamm (Lond) 7:6, 2010.

60. Nguyen HB, Rivers EP, Knoblich BP, et al: Early lactate clearance is associated with improved outcome in severe sepsis and septic shock, Crit Care Med 32(8):1637, 2004.
61. Puskarich MA, Trzeciak S, Shapiro NI, et al: Association between timing of antibiotic administration and mortality from septic shock in patients treated with a quantitative resuscitation protocol, Crit Care Med 39(9): 2066, 2011.
62. Tian HH, Han SS, Lv CJ, et al: The effect of early goal lactate clearance rate on the outcome of septic shock patients with severe pneumonia, Zhongguo Wei Zhong Bing Ji Jiu Yi Xue 24(1):42, 2012.
63. Rivers EP, Elkin R, Cannon CM: Counterpoint: should lactate clearance be substituted for central venous oxygen saturation as goals of early severe sepsis and septic shock therapy? No, Chest 140(6):1408; discussion 1413, 2011.
64. Dow SW, Curtis CR, Jones RL, et al: Bacterial culture of blood from critically ill dogs and cats: 100 cases (1985-1987), J Am Vet Med Assoc 195(1):113, 1989.
65. Gaieski DF, Mikkelsen ME, Band RA, et al: Impact of time to antibiotics on survival in patients with severe sepsis or septic shock in whom early goal-directed therapy was initiated in the emergency department, Crit Care Med 38(4):1045, 2010.
66. Kumar A, Roberts D, Wood KE, et al: Duration of hypotension before initiation of effective antimicrobial therapy is the critical determinant of survival in human septic shock, Crit Care Med 34(6):1589, 2006.
67. Kumar A, Ellis P, Arabi Y, et al: Initiation of inappropriate antimicrobial therapy results in a fivefold reduction of survival in human septic shock, Chest 136(5):1237, 2009.
68. Mikkelsen ME, Gaieski DF: Antibiotics in sepsis: timing, appropriateness, and (of course) timely recognition of appropriateness, Crit Care Med 39(9):2184, 2011.
69. Black DM, Rankin SC, King LG: Antimicrobial therapy and aerobic bacteriologic culture patterns in canine intensive care unit patients: 74 dogs (January-June 2006), J Vet Emerg Crit Care (San Antonio) 19(5):489, 2009.
70. Marik PE, Baram M, Vahid B: Does central venous pressure predict fluid responsiveness? A systematic review of the literature and the tale of seven mares, Chest 134(1):172, 2008.
71. Cavallaro F, Sandroni C, Marano C, et al: Diagnostic accuracy of passive leg raising for prediction of fluid responsiveness in adults: Systematic review and meta-analysis of clinical studies, Intensive Care Med 36(9):1475, 2010.
72. Perner A, Haase N, Guttormsen AB, et al: Hydroxyethyl starch 130/0.42 versus Ringer's acetate in severe sepsis, N Engl J Med 367(2):124, 2012.
73. Bayer O, Reinhart K, Sakr Y, et al: Renal effects of synthetic colloids and crystalloids in patients with severe sepsis: a prospective sequential comparison, Crit Care Med 39(6):1335, 2011.
74. Sakr Y, Payen D, Reinhart K, et al: Effects of hydroxyethyl starch administration on renal function in critically ill patients, Br J Anaesth 98(2):216, 2007.
75. Schortgen F, Lacherade JC, Bruneel F, et al: Effects of hydroxyethylstarch and gelatin on renal function in severe sepsis: a multicentre randomised study, Lancet 357(9260):911, 2001.
76. Falco S, Bruno B, Maurella C, et al: In vitro evaluation of canine hemostasis following dilution with hydroxyethyl starch (130/0.4) via thromboelastometry, J Vet Emerg Crit Care (San Antonio) 22(6):640, 2012.
77. Declue AE, Delgado C, Chang CH, et al: Clinical and immunologic assessment of sepsis and the systemic inflammatory response syndrome in cats, J Am Vet Med Assoc 238(7):890, 2011.
78. Sganga G, Siegel JH, Brown G, et al: Reprioritization of hepatic plasma protein release in trauma and sepsis, Arch Surg 120(2):187, 1985.
79. Vigano F, Perissinotto L, Bosco VR: Administration of 5% human serum albumin in critically ill small animal patients with hypoalbuminemia: 418 dogs and 170 cats (1994-2008), J Vet Emerg Crit Care (San Antonio) 20(2):237, 2010.
80. Mathews KA: The therapeutic use of 25% human serum albumin in critically ill dogs and cats, Vet Clin North Am Small Anim Pract 38(3):595, xi, 2008.
81. Trow AV, Rozanski EA, Delaforcade AM, et al: Evaluation of use of human albumin in critically ill dogs: 73 cases (2003-2006), J Am Vet Med Assoc 233(4):607, 2008.
82. De Backer D, Aldecoa C, Njimi H, et al: Dopamine versus norepinephrine in the treatment of septic shock: a meta-analysis*, Crit Care Med 40(3):725, 2012.
83. Vasu TS, Cavallazzi R, Hirani A, et al: Norepinephrine or dopamine for septic shock: systematic review of randomized clinical trials, J Intensive Care Med 27(3):172, 2012.
84. Marx G, Reinhart K: Venous Oximetry, Curr Opin Crit Care 12(3):263, 2006.
85. Scheinman M, Brown M, Rapaport E: Critical assessment of use of central venous oxygen saturation as a mirror of mixed venous oxygen in severely ill cardiac patients, Circulation 40:165, 1969.
86. Lee J, Wright F, Barber R: Central venous oxygen saturation in shock: A study in man. Anesthesiology 36:472, 1972.
87. Reinhart K, Kuhn H, Hartog C, et al: Continuous central venous and pulmonary artery oxygen saturation monitoring in the critically ill, Intensive Care Med 30:1572, 2004.
88. Hayes GM, Mathews K, Boston S, et al: Low central venous oxygen saturation is associated with increased mortality in critically ill dogs, J Small Anim Pract 52(8):433, 2011.
89. Case JB, Fick JL, Rooney MB: Proximal duodenal perforation in three dogs following deracoxib administration, J Am Anim Hosp Assoc 46(4):255, 2010.
90. Hickey MC, Magee A: Gastrointestinal tract perforations caused by ingestion of multiple magnets in a dog, J Vet Emerg Crit Care (San Antonio) 21(4):369, 2011.
91. Rossmeissl EM, Palmer KG, Hoelzler MG, et al: Multiple magnet ingestion as a cause of septic peritonitis in a dog, J Am Anim Hosp Assoc 47(1):56, 2011.
92. Humm KR, Adamantos SE, Benigni L, et al: Uterine rupture and septic peritonitis following dystocia and assisted delivery in a great dane bitch, J Am Anim Hosp Assoc 46(5):353, 2010.

CHAPTER 92

MYCOPLASMA, ACTINOMYCES, AND *NOCARDIA*

Christina Maglaras, DVM • Amie Koenig, DVM, DACVIM (Internal Medicine), DACVECC

KEY POINTS

- Mycoplasmas should be considered as a differential diagnosis in cats and dogs with disease of the respiratory or urinary tracts. The organism lacks a cell wall, thus cannot be visualized by cytology, and is resistant to β-lactam antimicrobials.
- *Actinomyces* spp. are normal inhabitants on mucous membranes of animals and rely on disruption of the mucosa to cause disease. Prognosis is good with long-term antimicrobial therapy. The empiric drug of choice for treating *Actinomyces* spp. is penicillin.
- *Nocardia* spp. are found normally in the environment, and opportunistic infection arises after inhalation or direct inoculation. Therapy involves surgical debridement and long-term treatment with antimicrobials; the empiric drug of choice is trimethoprim sulfa. Prognosis is guarded to poor for patients with nocardiosis.

Although *Mycoplasma, Actinomyces*, and *Nocardia* spp. belong to different genera, they share the potential to cause life-threatening infection. They also can pose diagnostic dilemmas because of difficulty in isolating the organisms via culture, their presence in mixed infections, and their lack of cell wall (*Mycoplasma* spp.), which inhibits cytologic identification. This chapter focuses on infections caused by nonhemotropic *Mycoplasmas, Actinomyces*, and *Nocardia* spp. that may be encountered in the critical care setting.

NONHEMOTROPIC MYCOPLASMAS

Etiology and Clinical Syndromes

Mycoplasmas are prokaryotes within the class Mollicutes and are the smallest free-living, self-replicating microorganisms.[1,2] All members of the class lack a protective cell wall; thus they are damaged easily when outside of the host and are difficult to identify with most staining techniques. The small genome of mycoplasmas limits their metabolic capacity and requires the organisms to derive nutrients from the mucosal surfaces on which they colonize. Mycoplasmas can be categorized into nonhemotropic and hemotropic forms. Hemotropic forms include *Mycoplasma haemocanis* and *Mycoplasma haemofelis* (see Chapter 110). Nonhemotropic forms include *Mycoplasma canis, Mycoplasma cynos, Mycoplasma felis, Mycoplasma gateae*, and *Ureaplasma* spp. This section focuses on the nonhemotropic forms, which is referred to generically as "mycoplasmas" for the remainder of the chapter.

Canine and feline mycoplasmas encompass a relatively small portion of the veterinary literature when compared with other types of infections.[3] The role of mycoplasmas in disease is somewhat controversial, although interest regarding their role as either commensal, primary, or opportunistic pathogens in dogs and cats continues. Mycoplasmas have been implicated in infections of the respiratory, ocular, urogenital, and nervous systems, in addition to systemic infections.

Respiratory Infections

Mycoplasmas are found as normal flora in the upper respiratory tract of dogs and cats[3]; they have been isolated from the lungs of healthy dogs but not healthy cats.[1,2,4] Mycoplasmas (including ureaplasmas) were isolated from lungs of ill and healthy dogs at equivalent rates in one study[5]; *M. canis* was isolated more frequently from lungs of dogs with respiratory disease (24% versus 13% of healthy dogs) in another.[6] Ureaplasmas rarely are isolated from healthy or diseased cat lungs.[7] Although it is unclear whether mycoplasmas are primary or opportunistic pathogens, their contribution to upper and lower respiratory disease in veterinary species cannot be overlooked.

In the cat, mycoplasma has been implicated as an important contributor to feline upper respiratory disease[8] and has been identified in up to 80% of nasal and pharyngeal samples from cats with respiratory disease.[9] In shelter cats that were euthanized with signs of upper respiratory disease, feline herpes virus-1 (FHV-1) was identified most commonly; however, *M. felis* was the next most common isolate (in approximately 30% of the cats).[8] *M. felis* is associated with feline conjunctivitis and has been isolated more commonly from cats with conjunctivitis than clinically normal cats.[10,11] In one study of 41 cats with conjunctivitis and upper respiratory disease, 49% had *Mycoplasma* spp. amplified from PCR testing of conjunctival swabs.[11] Of those cats that tested positive for mycoplasma conjunctivitis, 50% had co-infections with *Chlamydophila felis* and 25% had coinfections with FHV-1 and *C. felis.*[11] Although several *Mycoplasma* spp. have been isolated from canine conjunctiva, they have not been associated conclusively with canine conjunctivitis.[12] Common clinical signs of *Mycoplasma* infection of the feline upper respiratory tract include serous to purulent oculonasal discharge, conjunctivitis, blepharospasm, chemosis, and hyperemic conjunctiva.[11]

Mycoplasmas also have been identified in mixed bacterial infections and as the sole pathogen associated with lower airway disease. Mycoplasmas may invade the lower respiratory tract as secondary opportunistic pathogens in patients with impaired mucociliary function secondary to a primary bacterial or viral infection or because of ciliary dyskinesia.[1,13] Inflammatory airway disease, concurrent respiratory infections, aspiration of oropharyngeal contents, and/or immunosuppression also can facilitate mycoplasmal infections of the lower airway.[3,4] *Mycoplasma cynos* has been isolated from dogs with naturally occurring respiratory disease, including puppies with lethal neonatal respiratory infections and dogs in kennel settings.[14,15] In cats, mycoplasmosis has caused rare cases of bronchopneumonia and was reported in two young cats and one older cat with chronic coughing,[16] one cat with bronchopneumonia with associated respiratory failure,[17] as well as a pyothorax case in conjunction with *Arcanobacterium* spp.[18] Commonly reported clinical signs of mycoplasma infections of the lower respiratory tract include coughing (spontaneous and on tracheal palpation), labored breathing, tachypnea, dyspnea, and nasal discharge. Secondary signs, such as weakness, anorexia, and fever, may or may not be seen.[4]

Urogenital Associated Infections

As with the respiratory tract, mycoplasmas are normal inhabitants of the human and canine urinary and urogenital mucosa.[1,19] Currently, urogenital mycoplasmas are considered opportunistic bacteria; however, more research is needed to define their role further.[1,3] Ureaplasmas require urea for a carbon source and thus are associated more commonly with the urogenital tract epithelium than other locations.[20] *M. canis* has been cultured from dogs with urinary tract infections and from the mucosa of the lower urogenital tract in healthy dogs.[21]

There are also important species differences regarding urogenital mycoplasmal infections. *Ureaplasma* spp. can be transmitted from human mothers to their newborns through various routes, and these infections can cause pneumonia in human neonates.[19] Thus far, similarly acquired infections have not been documented in the small animal literature. A litter of Golden Retriever puppies infected with *M. canis* was thought to acquire the infection via oral translocation from the bitch because the pathogen was not isolated from vaginal swabs.[15]

Mycoplasma infections infrequently are associated with the lower urinary tract but may manifest as pollakiuria, stranguria, hematuria, pyuria, and/or vulvar discharge. Only a small number of mycoplasmas may be needed to induce clinical disease[21,22]; therefore, in a dog with compatible clinical signs, identifying mycoplasmas in a urine sample obtained by cystocentesis is likely significant. In comparison, traditional canine bacterial urinary tract infections are considered significant if urine cultures obtained via cystocentesis have more than 1000 colony-forming units per milliliter.[23] In one study of 100 dogs with signs of lower urinary tract disease, 41% had a positive aerobic culture, but only 4% had *Mycoplasma* spp. isolated (one with a mixed infection and three with only *Mycoplasma* spp.).[24] All dogs with *Mycoplasma* spp. infections from this study were azotemic.[24] In another study, mycoplasma was cultured from 60 urine samples obtained from 41 dogs with lower urinary tract infections.[22] Of the cultures, 68% had mycoplasma grown in pure culture and 32% had mycoplasma mixed with other bacteria. *M. canis* was the most common mycoplasma species isolated.[22]

Normal feline urine seems to be relatively impervious to mycoplasmas, and no current evidence suggests that *Mycoplasma* spp. cause lower urinary tract disease in cats.[20,25,26] Because of their lack of a cell wall, mycoplasmas are at high risk for osmotic damage by the normally highly concentrated feline urine.[20] During *in vitro* studies, *M. felis* and *M. gateae* seemingly were unable to tolerate the hyperosmotic conditions presented by synthetic feline urine.[20]

Other Infections

Nonhemotropic mycoplasmas also have been associated with other infections, including polyarthritis, bite wound abscesses, and meningoencephalitis.[1,27-30] *Mycoplasma* spp. also have been isolated from blood cultures in one postoperative dog with suspected hyperadrenocorticism-induced immunosuppression that presented 5 days after a bilateral adrenalectomy with fever, vomiting, diarrhea, and shifting leg lameness with associated joint effusion.[31] The exact cause of the infection was unclear.[31] Identification of such unusual cases associated with mycoplasma suggests that the organism may be more common than recognized.

Diagnosis

Cytology of infected tissue or fluids yields neutrophilic inflammation (and possibly presence of coinfecting bacteria)[13] (Figure 92-1). Mycoplasmas lack a protective cell wall, preventing cytologic identification with Gram stain and other staining methods that target cell wall components.[19] Although the small size and lack of cell wall make visualization of the organism via light microscopy difficult, negative staining with electron microscopy has been proven highly sensitive.[32] Histopathology of *Mycoplasma*-infected tissues are unlikely useful as the sole diagnostic for this organism. In cats with upper respiratory disease, histopathology of nasal and oropharyngeal tissues commonly showed severe rhinitis and ulceration in cases of a coinfection with FHV-1.[8] However, in the cases of solitary *M. felis* infections, the lesions were nonspecific and showed mild to moderate inflammatory changes.[8]

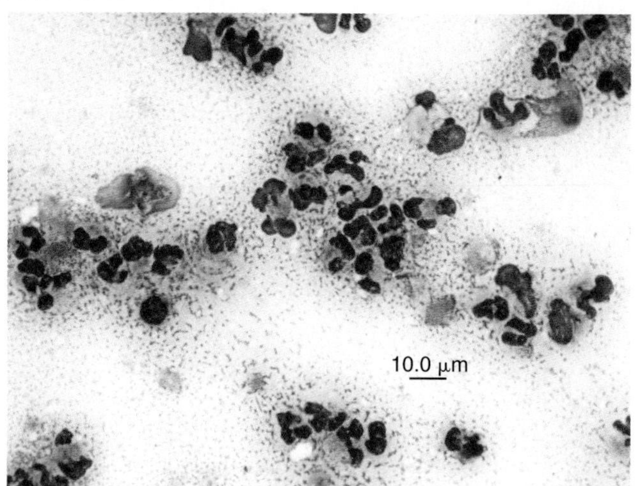

FIGURE 92-1 Suppurative transtracheal wash from a patient with mycoplasmosis. *(Photo courtesy Dr. B. Garner, University of Georgia.)*

Culture with *Mycoplasma*-specific media still is considered the standard diagnostic test, although PCR is fast becoming the preferred method.[11,14,33,34] Appropriate culture and PCR samples should be taken from the affected organ system and may include biopsy samples, conjunctival swabs, exudates, blood, and urine. To prevent contamination of voided samples with normal flora of the distal urogenital tract, urine samples should be obtained via a sterile cystocentesis.

Ideal diagnostic specimens depend on the location of the infection (Table 92-1). Contact with a diagnostic lab before sample collection helps ensure appropriate collection, handling, and transport of samples for successful mycoplasma culture.[1] Mycoplasmas are osmotically fragile microorganisms, and they require specialized culture media such as Hayflick broth, Amies medium, or modified Stuart bacterial-transport medium.[1,19] In the absence of specialized media, samples can be placed in a sterile, red-topped tube.[4] Samples should be refrigerated if the culture will not be plated for 2 to 3 days or frozen if plating the culture will take longer.[1] Mycoplasmas are slow growing and often are cultured for 1 to 2 weeks before finalizing a "negative" culture. At this time, species identification and antimicrobial sensitivities are not available in all laboratories.[4]

Because of the fragile state of most mycoplasmas outside of their hosts, the diagnosis of mycoplasma could be missed as a result of improper sample handling, prolonged transport time, or collection errors[34,35] Polymerase chain reaction (PCR) methods are used for identification and speciation of mycoplasmal DNA. PCR is valued for its rapidity of test results, improved sensitivity compared with culture, and ability to identify nonviable organisms that may not have survived transport or have been killed by antimicrobial agents.[35] However, if only DNA is detected and the organisms are not cultured, then the potential for contamination by commensals must be considered.[35] In one study of cats and dogs with respiratory disease, 15.0% of all samples yielded discordant results between culture and PCR; mailed samples were more likely discordant than samples

Table 92-1 **Diagnostic Options for Mycoplasma**[1,8,11,14,19,32-35]

Diagnostic Test	Utility as a Diagnostic for *Mycoplasma* Species Tool	Additional Information
Cytology or Gram stain	Low utility	Lack of cell wall precludes identification with standard stains Useful to confirm presence of suppurative inflammation and any co-infections
Transmission electron microscopy (TEM)	Useful	Negative staining is sensitive for identification of mycoplasmas Expensive, not widely available
Histopathology	Low utility	Should identify compatible suppurative inflammatory response
Culture	Extremely useful Current gold standard	Typically slow growing; organism may die before culturing, specialized transport and growth media recommended Contact laboratory before sample collection for protocol
Polymerase chain reaction (PCR)	Extremely useful	Improved sensitivity over culture, able to identify nonviable organisms Faster results than culture

hand-carried to the diagnostic lab immediately after acquisition (31.6% versus 9.3%, respectively).[34] Another study demonstrated that PCR and culture were equivalent at detecting *Mycoplasma* spp. in nasal and pharyngeal swabs in cats with signs of acute upper respiratory tract disease.[9] Use of PCR and culture, along with monitoring response to therapy while waiting for test results, may optimize diagnosis. In addition, unresponsive infections that have been treated with antimicrobial drugs targeting cell wall synthesis may be another clinical clue to prompt testing for mycoplasma.

Ancillary diagnostic tests, including complete blood count (CBC), serum chemistry, urinalysis, and imaging studies such as thoracic and abdominal radiographs, are important to rule out underlying disease and to assess the severity and extent of the infection. Common CBC abnormalities in dogs and cats with mycoplasma respiratory disease include neutrophilia, leukocytosis, lymphopenia, and eosinophilia; however, CBC and serum chemistry analyses also may be unremarkable.[4,16] Thoracic radiographs of patients with mycoplasmal respiratory disease commonly reveal patterns consistent with pneumonia, such as lung lobe consolidation and bronchoalveolar patterns; collapsing trachea and bronchi also were noted in one study.[4,16]

Treatment

Antimicrobials commonly used to treat mycoplasmal infections include tetracyclines, macrolides, lincosamides, fluoroquinolones, and chloramphenicol (Table 92-2).[1,36,37] Species of the patient, location of the infection within the body, and presence of any coinfections may influence drug selection. Because the lack of a cell wall renders mycoplasmas resistant to β-lactam antimicrobials, therapy with this drug class should be avoided unless it is used to treat susceptible coinfections. Information regarding prognosis and response to treatment is limited and may vary depending on the type of infection. One study demonstrated that 14.3% of patients with respiratory disease that had mycoplasma as the sole isolate via culture had complete resolution with no recurrence, 42.9% of cases improved but then experienced a recurrence, and the remainder of cases had no response to therapy.[4] Treatment is complicated by the bacteriostatic nature of most of the effective drugs, necessitating weeks to months of therapy, and the lack of antimicrobial sensitivity data for isolates.[1]

ACTINOMYCOSIS AND NOCARDIOSIS

Actinomycosis and nocardiosis share similar clinical presentations, but there are some important differences between these organisms and their disease manifestations (Table 92-3).

Etiology and Clinical Syndromes

Actinomycosis is an infection caused by organisms belonging to the genus *Actinomyces* or *Arcanobacterium.* These anaerobic or microaerophilic, gram-positive organisms are normal inhabitants on the mucous membranes of the oral cavity and gastrointestinal and urogenital tracts in humans and animals.[1,38] These organisms are opportunists, have never been cultured from the environment,[1] and are dependent upon disruption of the mucosa (i.e., direct inoculation) to cause disease. In dogs, infection seems to occur more commonly in large breed, outdoor, or hunting/working dogs, which have increased exposure to plant material such as migrating grass awns.[1,39] Such material likely becomes contaminated with *Actinomyces* spp. when passing through the oropharynx as it is inhaled or ingested,[1,40] then acts as a nidus for infection as it migrates through the body. In cats, exposure seems to stem more commonly from bite wounds.[41]

Actinomycosis in dogs often manifests as cervicofacial, cutaneous/subcutaneous, or thoracic forms.[1] Cats may have a higher incidence of the thoracic form (i.e., pyothorax) but also may be presented with peritonitis or cellulitis after a bite or puncture wound.[1,42] Cervicofacial actinomycosis may result from dental disease, oral foreign bodies, or penetrating wounds to the head or oral cavity. This infection can manifest as an acute to chronic infection of the head and neck, causing swellings, abscesses, or mass effects.[1,39] Cutaneous/subcutaneous infections may present as single or multiple mass lesions with draining tracts and can occur anywhere on the body, including tracking into body cavities.[1,39] Thoracic, abdominal, and retroperitoneal actinomycosis can manifest with intracavitary effusions, external draining tracts connecting to the respective body cavity, spinal pain, or palpable abdominal mass or with more vague presenting complaints of weight loss, fever, and weakness.[1,39,40] Actinomycosis infections can cause periosteal new bone formation and osteomyelitis if the infection is occurring near or on a bony structure,[1] such as when retroperitoneal infections spread to the vertebral bodies. Actinomycosis also has been reported in the central nervous system (CNS).[43]

Nocardiosis is an opportunistic infection caused by the aerobic gram-positive bacteria of the family Nocardiaceae.[1,41,44] Unlike *Actinomyces* spp., *Nocardia* spp. are not part of the normal flora of mammals; they are ubiquitous environmental saprophytes found in soil, grasses, and other organic material.[1,41] Animals can carry this organism on their claws or skin after environmental exposure,[41] and infection may arise from inhalation of the organism or direct inoculation from a penetrating wound.

Nocardiosis is reported less commonly than *Actinomyces* infections.[1] Immunosuppression may predispose to infections in humans

Table 92-2 **Common Antimicrobials for Mycoplasmosis, Actinomycosis, Nocardiosis**[1,36,37]

Drug	Organism Targeted	Species	Dose, Route, Frequency
Amikacin	*Nocardia*	Dog Cat	15 mg/kg IV, SC, IM q24h 10 mg/kg IV, SC, IM q24h
Ampicillin, Ampicillin/sulbactam	*Actinomyces,* Nocardia*	Dog Cat	20-40 mg/kg IV, SC q8h 20-40 mg/kg IV, SC q8h
Azithromycin	*Mycoplasma*	Dog Cat	5-10 mg/kg PO, IV q24h 5-10 mg/kg PO, IV q24h
Cefotaxime	*Nocardia*	Dog Cat	20-80 mg/kg IV, SC, IM q6-8h 20-80 mg/kg IV, SC, IM q6-8h
Chloramphenicol	*Mycoplasma, Actinomyces*	Dog Cat	40-50 mg/kg PO, IV q6-8h 25-50 mg/kg PO, IV q12h
Clindamycin	*Mycoplasma, Actinomyces*	Dog Cat	10 mg/kg PO, IV q12h 10 mg/kg PO, IV q12h
Doxycycline	*Mycoplasma,† Actinomyces*	Dog Cat	5-10 mg/kg PO or IV q12h 5-10 mg/kg PO or IV q12h
Enrofloxacin	*Mycoplasma†*	Dog Cat	10-15 mg/kg PO, IV, IM q24h 5 mg/kg PO q24h
Erythromycin	*Mycoplasma, Actinomyces, Nocardia*	Dog Cat	10-20 mg/kg PO, IV q8h 10-20 mg/kg PO, IV q8h
Imipenem	*Nocardia*	Dog Cat	5-10 mg/kg IV q6-8h 5-10 mg/kg IV q6-8h
Meropenem	*Nocardia*	Dog Cat	24 mg/kg IV q24h or 12 mg/kg SC q8-12h 24 mg/kg IV q24h or 12 mg/kg SC q8-12h
Penicillin G	*Actinomyces**	Dog Cat	100,000 U/kg IV, SC, IM q6-8h or 40 mg/kg PO q8h 100,000 U/kg IV, SC, IM q6-8h or 40 mg/kg PO q8h
Pradofloxacin	*Mycoplasma*	Dog Cat	5 mg/kg PO q24h 5 mg/kg PO q24h
Trimethoprim-sulfa	*Nocardia**	Dog Cat	30 mg/kg PO, IV q12h 30 mg/kg PO, IV q12h

*Indicates drug of choice for that microbe.
†Common/preferred drug for *Mycoplasma.*

Table 92-3 **Comparison of Actinomycosis and Nocardiosis**[1,38-41,44,45,56-59]

	Actinomycosis	Nocardiosis
Predisposition	Outdoor, male dogs; fight wounds in cats	Immunocompromised patients; fight wounds in cats
Biologic requirements	Facultative or obligate anaerobe	Aerobic
Staining and morphology	Gram positive, rod-shaped, non-acid fast	Gram positive, rod-shaped, partially acid fast
Culture	Challenging to culture; often seen with mixed infections	Typically isolated in pure culture
Preferred empiric antimicrobial	Penicillins	Trimethoprim-sulfamethoxazole
Prognosis	Good, when treated appropriately	Guarded to poor

and veterinary species,[41,44] and nocardiosis has been reported in canines with distemper virus–induced immunosuppression.[45] In dogs, infections occur more commonly in the young, whereas in cats, there is a strong predisposition (up to 75%) for males to contract the disease, mostly likely through scratches and bites.[41] Disease occurs in cats of all ages and infected cats may or may not be immunosuppressed as well (i.e., retroviral infections).[41,46]

Nocardiosis causes acute to chronic suppurative inflammation and most commonly presents in cutaneous/subcutaneous, pulmonary, and disseminated (involving two or more body systems) forms.[1,41,44] When *Nocardia* spp. initially enter the host through skin inoculation, the inflammation may resemble a localized pyoderma and often is treated as such.[41] The cutaneous form is by far the most common type of infection in feline patients and eventually may manifest as multiple draining tracts or sinuses within the skin that spread outwards from the central lesion.[40,41] Pulmonary nocardiosis may manifest as either pneumonia or pyothorax; this form is the most common type of infection in humans, particularly in immunocompromised patients,[1,44] and has been reported in more commonly in dogs than in cats.[1] Disseminated nocardiosis and systemic disease forms are rare. They may stem from systemic spread of cutaneous/subcutaneous or pulmonary forms and typically involve abscessation

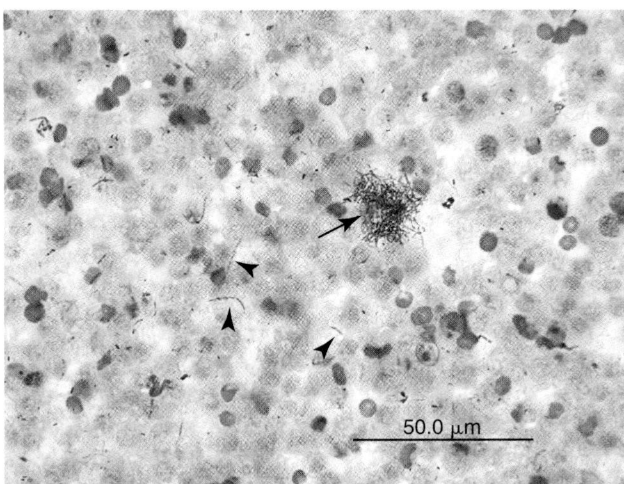

FIGURE 92-2 A focal aggregate of mixed bacteria *(arrow)*, including filamentous beaded rods, is seen against a background of poorly preserved, poorly staining leukocytes admixed with low number of erythrocytes. Individual bacteria *(arrowheads)* also are observed scattered in the background. Wright's stain. 1000× magnification. *(Photo courtesy Dr. B. Flatland, University of Tennessee.)*

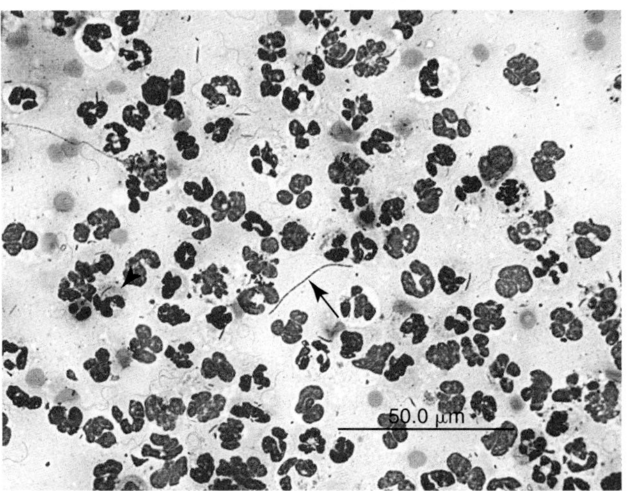

FIGURE 92-3 Mixed bacteria of varying morphology, including beaded filamentous rods *(arrow)*, admixed with numerous neutrophils. Neutrophils exhibit nondegenerate and degenerate morphology; rare neutrophils *(arrowhead)* contain phagocytosed bacteria. Wright's stain. 1000× magnification. *(Photo courtesy Dr. Bente Flatland, University of Tennessee.)*

of two or more noncontiguous sites within the body, such as the eyes, bones, joints, spleen, liver, peritoneum, CNS, and lymph nodes.[1,43]

Clinical Signs

Clinical signs of actinomycosis or nocardiosis depend on the location of infection and also may include anorexia, fever, dyspnea, tachypnea, coughing, and depression.[1,47] Historical findings may reveal lethargy, weight loss, an outdoor lifestyle (actinomycosis), or a history of bite wounds. Physical examination may reveal decreased heart or lung sounds if pleural effusion is present, draining tracts, abscesses, oral cavity lesions, palpable abdominal mass effect, or spinal pain, depending on the area of the body affected.[1,39,40,48]

Diagnosis

Blood work typically is consistent with an inflammatory response; patients with either disease also may show anemia, hypoalbuminemia, and hyperglobulinemia.[1,39] Nocardiosis may manifest with an ionized hypercalcemia secondary to the granulomatous response[49] but has not been documented yet in the literature for actinomycosis. Radiographic findings can include cavitary effusions, alveolar or interstitial lung patterns, lymphadenopathy, mass effects in any area of the body (i.e., mediastinum, abdomen), as well as periosteal bone growth or osteomyelitis if lesions are adjacent or affecting bones.[39,40,48] Ultrasound findings of the thorax or abdomen may show free fluid accumulation in the chest or abdomen or mass effects within the cavity examined.[50]

The characteristic cytologic finding of exudates from *Actinomyces* spp. and *Nocardia* spp. lesions is suppurative to pyogranulomatous inflammation.[1] Both organisms appear as dense mats of gram-positive filamentous rods that may be branched; and actinomycosis infections often are accompanied by a population of mixed bacteria (Figures 92-2 and 92-3). In addition, *Nocardia* spp. are partially acid fast staining, whereas *Actinomyces* spp. are not.[1] Effusions and exudates may contain malodorous, macroscopic sulfur granules, which appear as tan/grey aggregates[1] (Figure 92-4). Histopathology of mass lesions and affected lymph nodes with either actinomycosis or nocardiosis infections show pyogranulomatous inflammation and fibrosis and may contain tissue granules of variable diameter. Special stains, such as Brown-Brenn Gram stain, may be needed to visualize further the filamentous structures.[1,39]

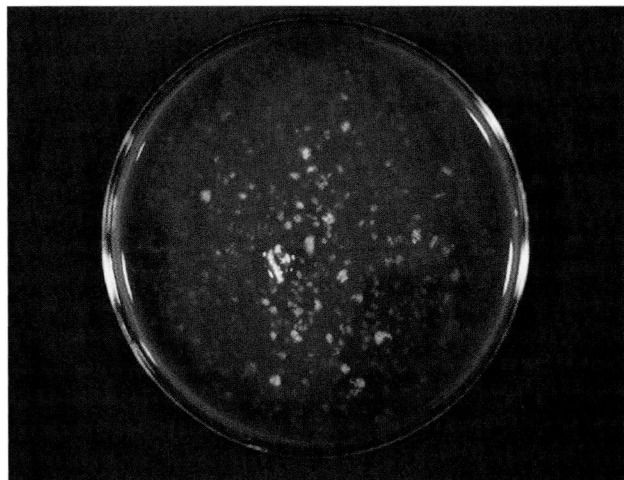

FIGURE 92-4 Sulfur granules present in pleural fluid from a dog with nocardiosis. *(Photo courtesy Noah's Arkive™ at The University of Georgia. Image by Dr. J.A. Ramos-Vara, Purdue University, copyright 1993. University of Georgia Research Foundation, Inc. Noah's Arkive™ is a trademark of the University of Georgia Research Foundation, Inc.)*

Exudates, sulfur granules, needle aspirates of mass-like lesions, airway wash fluid, and cavitary effusions may be submitted for culture, although both organisms are difficult to grow. If either nocardiosis or actinomycosis are suspected, obtaining aerobic and anaerobic cultures optimizes the chance of isolating the organism because some species of actinomycosis are aerotolerant.[1] Pure cultures of *Nocardia* spp. usually are isolated from lesions, although it may take several days to weeks to grow.[1] *Actinomyces* spp. have specific growth requirements (ranging from facultative to obligate anaerobes) and also may require 2 to 4 weeks of incubation.[1] Despite their presence, however, *Actinomyces* spp. may not be isolated, and co-infecting bacteria, such as *Escherichia coli, Pasturella multocida,* or *Streptococcus* spp., may be cultured instead.[1] Because *Actinomyces* is a commensal organism of the oropharynx, isolation does not confirm infection; positive culture results are a more reliable indicator of disease if one or more of the following criteria are present: compatible clinical signs, surrounding pyogranulomatous inflammation, and growth of associated co-infectious organisms.

Species identification can be obtained for both organisms, but it is particularly important to speciate *Nocardia* spp. because susceptibility to antimicrobial agents varies by species.[1,46] Polymerase chain reaction (PCR) methods can be used to speciate *Nocardia*, although DNA-DNA hybridization is considered the standard method.[52] Speciating *Actinomyces* can be difficult, and sequencing of the 16D rRNA gene may be required.[1] PCR has been used to diagnose bacterial endocarditis and also was used to identify an *Actinomyces* species that did not grow on blood culture.[53] Cell wall deficient variants of actinomyces (L-forms) have been identified, albeit infrequently.[51]

Treatment

The mainstay of successful therapy for *Actinomyces* infections is prolonged high-dose antimicrobials; surgery also may be indicated, depending on the nature of the infection.[1] Penicillin is the drug of choice: no *Actinomyces* spp. have shown resistance to penicillins.[1] For patients unable to take penicillins, other antimicrobials have been used successfully (see Table 92-2).[1,36,37] Drugs reportedly ineffective for *Actinomyces* include metronidazole, aztreonam, trimethoprim sulfamethoxazole (TMS), penicillinase-resistant penicillins (e.g., methicillin, nafcillin, oxacillin, cloxacillin), cephalexin, and aminoglycosides, although *Arcanobacterium* spp. are sensitive to aminoglycosides (except streptomycin).[1,54] For all antibiotics, prolonged therapy (6 to 12 months) is necessary, even after resolution of clinical disease, to ensure penetration of the dense mats of bacteria and pyogranulomatous inflammation and reduce the chance of recurrence. In addition to antimicrobials, treatment always should include drainage of any abscessed areas and cavitary effusions; continuous and intermittent suction techniques have proven effective.[55,56] Surgery may be indicated for actinomycosis infections that are nonresponsive to appropriate medical management or for isolated lesions such as lung abscesses or solitary body wall masses; even these patients should be followed up with long-term antibiotic therapy. With appropriate management, patients with actinomycosis usually have a good therapeutic response, with reported cure rates of more than 90% in the dog.[1,39,55] The prognosis for feline cutaneous and pyothorax *Actinomyces* infections generally is considered good with appropriate management; however, large clinical or retrospective studies involving feline cases of actinomycosis have not been published.[1]

Nocardiosis is more difficult to treat and achieve complete resolution of disease. Treatment should include prolonged antibiotic therapy as well as surgical drainage or debulking of lesions to optimize response to treatment.[57,58] Sulfonamides (e.g., trimethoprim sulfamethoxazole, or TMS) are the empiric drugs of choice for nocardiosis because most isolates are sensitive to this drug (see Table 92-2).[1] However, antimicrobial susceptibility is dependent on the infecting species of *Nocardia*, so isolates ideally should be speciated,[1,46,58] especially if antimicrobial therapy is failing or side effects, such as myelosuppression from the TMS, prohibit its long-term use. Although each *Nocardia* species has a relatively predictable antibiogram,[1] organisms may not be equally susceptible to all drugs within the same class. Combination therapy often is used in patients with severe illness or central nervous system infections, and certain combinations work synergistically.[1,59] A combination of TMS and a β-lactam should be effective against most isolates.[52,61] For CNS infections, drugs with good penetration include third-generation cephalosporins, imipenem/meropenem, and linezolid, although use of linezolid use has been discouraged to prevent development of resistance to this relatively new antimicrobial.[1,52,61] Antimicrobial therapy for nocardiosis is prolonged; durations of therapy range from 1 to 3 months for a simple cutaneous infection or at least 1 year for severe systemic infections or immunocompromised patients.[1] Prognosis for patients with nocardiosis is guarded: one study reported a 50% mortality rate from the disease and a 38.5% euthanasia rate resulting from a lack of clinical response.[61] Underlying disease, delayed diagnosis, and inappropriate or inadequate therapy likely contribute to this poor outcome.[61] Prognosis appears to be equally as guarded in cats, especially those with disseminated disease.[41]

REFERENCES

1. Greene CE: Infectious diseases of the dog and cat, ed 4, St Louis, 2012, Elsevier-Saunders.
2. Waites KB, Talkington DF: Mycoplasma pneumonia and its role as a human pathogen, Clin Microbiol Rev 17:697, 2004.
3. Chalker VJ: Canine mycoplasmas, Res Vet Sci 79:1, 2005.
4. Chandler JC, Lappin MR: Mycoplasmal respiratory infections in small animals: 17 cases (1988-1999), J Am Anim Hosp Assoc 38:111, 2002.
5. Randolph JF, Moise NS, Scarlett JM, et al: Prevalence of mycoplasmal and ureaplasmal recovery from tracheobronchial lavages and prevalence of mycoplasmal recovery from pharyngeal swab specimens in dogs with or without pulmonary disease, Am J Vet Res 54:387, 1993.
6. Chalker VJ, Owen WM, Paterson C, et al: Mycoplasmas associated with canine infectious respiratory disease, Microbiology 150:3491, 2004.
7. Randolph JF, Moise NS, Scarlett JM, et al: Prevalence of mycoplasmal and ureaplasmal recovery from tracheobronchial lavages and prevalence of mycoplasmal recovery from tracheobronchial lavages and of mycoplasmal recovery from pharyngeal swab specimens in cats with or without pulmonary disease, Am J Vet Res 54:897, 1993.
8. Burns RE, Wagner DC, Leutenegger CM, et al: Histologic and molecular correlation in shelter cats with acute upper respiratory infection, J Clin Microbiol 49:2454, 2011.
9. Veir JK, Ruch-Gallie R, Spindel ME, et al: Prevalence of selected infectious organisms and comparison of two anatomic sampling sites in shelter cats with upper respiratory tract disease, J Feline Med Surg 10:551, 2008.
10. Low HC, Powell CC, Veir JK, et al: Prevalence of feline herpesvirus 1, *Chlamydophila felis*, and *Mycoplasma* spp DNA in conjunctival cells collected from cats with and without conjunctivitis, Am J Vet Res 68:643, 2007.
11. Hartmann AD, Hawley J, Werckenthin C, et al: Detection of bacterial and viral organisms from the conjunctiva of cats with conjunctivitis and upper respiratory tract disease, J Feline Med Surg 12:775, 2010.
12. Campbell LH, Okuda HK: Cultivation of mycoplasma from conjunctiva and production of corneal immune response in guinea pigs, Am J Vet Res 36:893, 1975.
13. Bernis DA: Bordetella and mycoplasma respiratory infections in dogs and cats, Vet Clin North Am Sm Anim Pract 22:1173, 1992.
14. Hong S, Kim O: Molecular identification of *Mycoplasma cynos* from laboratory beagle dogs with respiratory disease, Lab Anim Res 28:61, 2012.
15. Zeugswetter F, Weissenbock H, Shibly S, et al: Lethal bronchopneumonia caused by *Mycoplasma cynos* in a litter of golden retriever puppies, Vet Rec 161:626, 2007.
16. Foster SF, Barrs VR, Martin P, et al: Pneumonia associated with *Mycoplasma* spp. in three cats, Aus Vet J 76:460, 1998.
17. Trow AV, Rozanski EA, Tidwell AS: Primary mycoplasma pneumonia associated with reversible respiratory failure in a cat, J Feline Med Surg 10:398, 2008.
18. Gulbahar M, Gurturk K: Pyothorax associated with a *Mycoplasma* sp. and *Arcanobacterium pyogenes* in a kitten, Aus Vet J 80:344, 2002.
19. Waites KB, Katz B, Schelonka RL: Mycoplasmas and ureaplasmas as neonatal pathogens, Clin Microbiol Rev 18:757, 2005.
20. Brown MB, Stoll M, Maxwell J, et al: Survival of feline mycoplasmas in urine, J Clin Microbiol 29:1078, 1991.
21. L'Abee-Lund TM, Heiene R, Friis NF, et al: Mycoplasma canis and urogenital disease in dogs in Norway, Vet Rec 153:231, 2003.
22. Jang SS, Ling GV, Yamamoto R, et al: Mycoplasma as a cause of canine urinary tract infection, J Am Vet Med Assoc 185: 45, 1984.
23. Lulich JP, Osborne CA: Bacterial urinary tract infections. In Ettinger SJ, Feldman EC, editors: Textbook of veterinary internal medicine, ed 4, Philadelphia, 1999, WB Saunders.
24. Ulgen M, Cetin C, Senturk S, et al: Urinary tract infections due to *Mycoplasma canis* in dogs, J Vet Med A Physiol Pathol Clin Med 53:379, 2006.

25. Senior DF, Brown MB: The role of mycoplasma species and ureaplasma species in feline lower urinary tract disease, Vet Clin North Am Sm Anim Pract 26:305, 1996.
26. Abou N, Houwers DJ, van Dongen AM: PCR-based detection reveals no causative role for mycoplasma and ureaplasma in feline lower urinary tract disease, Vet Microbiol 116:246, 2006.
27. Walker RD, Walshaw R, Riggs CM, et al: Recovery of two mycoplasma species from abscesses in a cat following bite wounds from a dog, J Vet Diagn Invest 7:154, 1995.
28. Ilha MRS, Rajeev S, Watson C, et al: Meningoencephalitis caused by *Mycoplasma edwardii* in a dog, J Vet Diagn Invest 22:805, 2010.
29. Beauchamp DJ, da Costa RC, Premanandan C, et al: *Mycoplasma felis*–associated meningoencephalitis in a cat, J Feline Med Surg 13:139, 2011.
30. Zeugswetter F, Hittmair KM, de Arespacochaga AG, et al: Erosive polyarthritis associated with *Mycoplasma gateae* in a cat, J Feline Med Surg 9:226, 2007.
31. Stenske KA, Bernis DA, Hill K, et al: Acute polyarthritis and septicemia from *Mycoplasma edwardii* after surgical removal of bilateral adrenal tumors in a dog, J Vet Intern Med 19:768, 2005.
32. Barth OM, Majerowica S: Rapid detection by transmission electron microscopy of mycoplasma contamination in sera and cell cultures, Mem Inst Oswaldo Cruz 83:63, 1988.
33. Johnson LR, Drazenovich NL, Foley JE: A comparison of routine culture with polymerase chain reaction technology for the detection of mycoplasma species in feline nasal samples, J Vet Diagn Invest 16:347, 2004.
34. Cruse AM, Sanchez S, Ratterree W, et al: Comparison of culture and polymerase chain reaction assay for the detection of *Mycoplasma* species in canine and feline respiratory tract samples, Research Abstract Program of the 26th Annual ACVIM Forum, 2008.
35. Reed N, Simpson K, Ayling R, et al: Mycoplasma species in cats with lower airway disease: Improved detection and species identification using a polymerase chain reaction assay, J Feline Med Surg 14:833, 2012.
36. Plumb D: Plumb's veterinary drug handbook, ed 7, St Paul, 2011, PharmaVet Inc.
37. Papich MG: Saunders handbook of veterinary drugs, ed 3, St Louis, 2011, Elsevier-Saunders.
38. Acevedo F, Baudrand R, Letelier LM, et al: Actinomycosis: a great pretender. Case reports of unusual presentations and review of the literature, Int J Infect Dis 12:358, 2008.
39. Kirpensteijn J, Fingland RB: Cutaneous actinomycosis and nocardiosis in dogs: 48 cases (1980–1990), J Am Vet Med Assoc 201:917, 1992.
40. Edwards DF, Nyland TG, Weigel JP: Thoracic, abdominal and vertebral actinomycosis: diagnosis and long-term therapy in three dogs, J Vet Intern Med 2:184, 1988.
41. Malik R, Krockenberger MB, O'Brien CR, et al: Nocardia infections in cats: a retrospective multi-institutional study of 17 cases, Aust Vet J 84:235, 2006.
42. Love DN, Jones RF, Bailey M, et al: Isolation and characterization of bacteria from pyothorax (empyaemia) in cats, Vet Microbiol 7:455, 1982.
43. Radaelli ST, Platt SR: Bacterial meningoencephalomyelitis in dogs: retrospective study of 23 cases (1990-1999), J Vet Intern Med 16:159, 2002.
44. Ambrosioni J, Lew D, Garbino J: Nocardiosis: updated clinical review and experience at a tertiary center, Infection 38:89, 2010.
45. Ribero MG, Salerno T, Mattos-Guaraldi AL, et al: Nocardiosis: an overview and additional report of 28 cases in cattle and dogs, Rev Inst Med Trop Sao Paulo 50:177, 2008.
46. Hirsh DG, Jang SS: Antimicrobial susceptibility of *Nocardia nova* isolated from five cats with nocardiosis, J Am Vet Med Assoc 215:815, 1999.
47. Ackerman N, Grain E, Castleman W: Canine nocardiosis, J Am Vet Anim Hosp Assoc 18:147, 1982.
48. Marino DJ, Jaggy A: Nocardiosis, a literature review with selected case reports in two dogs, J Vet Intern Med 7:4, 1993.
49. Mealey KL, Willard MD, Nagode LA, et al: Hypercalcemia associated with granulomatous disease in a cat, J Am Vet Med Assoc 215:959, 1999.
50. Boothe, HW, Howe LM, Boothe DM, et al: Evaluation of outcomes in dogs treated for pyothorax: 46 cases (1983-2001), J Am Vet Med Assoc 236:657, 2010.
51. Buchanan AM, Scott JL: Actinomyces hordeovulneris, a canine pathogen that produces L-phase variants spontaneously with coincident calcium deposition, Am J Vet Res 45:2552, 1984.
52. Brown-Elliott BA, Ward SC, Crest CJ, et al: In vitro activities of linezolid against multiple nocardia species, Antimicrob Agents Chemother 45:1295, 2001.
53. Meurs KM, Heaney AM, Atkins CE, et al: Comparison of polymerase chain reaction with bacterial 16s primers to blood culture to identify bacteremia in dogs with suspected bacterial endocarditis, J Vet Intern Med 25:959, 2011.
54. Guérin-Faublée V, Flandrois JP, Broye E, et al: Actinomyces pyogenes: Susceptibility of 103 clinical animal isolates to 22 antimicrobial agents, Vet Res 24:251, 1993.
55. Turner WD, Breznock EM: Continuous suction drainage for management of canine pyothorax: a retrospective study, J Am Anim Hosp Assoc 24:5-94, 1988.
56. Frendin J: Pyogranulomatous pleuritis with empyema in hunting dogs, Zentralbl Veterinarmed A 44:167, 1997.
57. Lerner PI: Nocardiosis, Clin Infect Dis 22:891, 1996.
58. McNeil MM, Brown JM: The medically important aerobic actinomycetes: epidemiology and microbiology, Clin Microbiol Rev 7:357, 1994.
59. Gombert ME, Aulicino TM: Synergism of imipenem and amikacin in combinations with other antibiotics against *Nocardia asteroides*, Antimicrob Agents Chemother 24:810, 1983.
60. Gomez-Flores A, Welsh O, Said-Fernández S, et al: In vitro and in vivo activities of antimicrobials against *Nocardia brasiliensis*, Antimicrob Agents Chemother 48:832, 2004.
61. Beaman BL, Sugar AM: Nocardia in naturally acquired and experimental infections in animals, J Hygiene 91:393, 1983.

CHAPTER 93

GRAM-POSITIVE INFECTIONS

Reid P. Groman, DVM, DACVIM (Internal Medicine), DACVECC

KEY POINTS

- Most gram-positive infections are caused by normal resident microflora of the skin, mucous membranes, and gastrointestinal tract.
- Critically ill hospitalized patients are at increased risk for infections with opportunistic gram-positive bacteria.
- *Streptococcus canis* is a well-recognized cause of various suppurative infections in animals, including toxic shock syndrome.
- Enterococci, traditionally viewed as commensal bacteria in the alimentary tract of animals, are known to be capable of causing life-threatening, multidrug-resistant infections in dogs and cats.
- As antibiotic-resistant staphylococci evolve, the ability to treat staphylococcal infections in companion animals with cephalosporins, penicillins, and fluoroquinolones is decreasing.

Since the early 1990s the epidemiology of pathogenic bacteria isolated from critically ill patients has shifted from gram-negative organisms to an increasing number of nosocomial infections caused by gram-positive isolates.[1,2] Increasing numbers of pathogenic, multidrug-resistant (MDR) gram-positive organisms now are being isolated from dogs and cats, paralleling the trend in antibiotic-resistant nosocomial and community-acquired infections in humans.[3-6] Awareness of emerging trends of resistance, particularly in *Enterococcus faecium* and various strains of staphylococci, militates against indiscriminate antimicrobial use and provides a basis for appropriately treating critically ill patients suffering from such infections.[7,8]

GRAM-POSITIVE CELL STRUCTURE AND PATHOGENICITY

Morphologically, gram-positive bacteria are composed of a cell wall, a single cytoplasmic membrane, and cytosol.[9-11] The cell wall is a thick, coarse structure that serves as an exoskeleton. Buried within the cell wall are enzymes called *transpeptidases,* commonly referred to as *penicillin-binding proteins (PBPs)*. PBPs are a group of enzymes responsible for the building and maintenance of the cell wall.[9,10]

In addition to a thick cell well, most gram-positive bacteria have other protective mechanisms. One of these mechanisms is an outer capsule or biofilm that extends beyond the cell wall and interfaces with the external milieu.[9,10] Hydrolase enzymes located within the cytoplasmic membrane, called *β-lactamases,* serve a protective role for the bacteria.[9,10] Once attacked by the hydrolases, the β-lactam antibiotics are no longer capable of binding to PBPs in normally susceptible bacteria.

Peptidoglycan is the basic structural component of the cell wall of gram-positive bacteria, accounting for 50% to 80% of the total cell wall content. Like endotoxin, peptidoglycan is released by bacteria during infection, reaches the systemic circulation, and exhibits proinflammatory activity.[9,10] Lipoteichoic acids found in the gram-positive cell wall have structural and epithelial adherence functions. Lipoteichoic acid induces a proinflammatory cytokine response, the production of nitric oxide, and may lead to cardiovascular compromise.

In addition to structural components, gram-positive organisms produce soluble exotoxins that may play a role in the pathogenesis of sepsis. Much attention is focused on the roles of superantigenic exotoxins that promote the massive release of cytokines, potentially leading to shock and multiorgan failure in human and veterinary patients.[6,9]

STREPTOCOCCAL INFECTIONS

The genus *Streptococcus* consists of gram-positive cocci arranged in chains.[11,12] These are fastidious bacteria that require the addition of blood or serum to culture media. They are nonmotile and non–spore forming. Most are facultative anaerobes and may require enriched media to grow.[9,12] Streptococci are generally commensal organisms found on the skin and mucous membranes and are ecologically important as part of the normal microflora in pets and humans.[11,12] However, several species of streptococci are capable of causing localized or widespread pyogenic infections in companion animals.[11]

Streptococci may be grouped superficially by how they grow on blood agar plates as either hemolytic or nonhemolytic.[9,13] The type of hemolytic reaction displayed on blood agar has been used to classify the bacteria as either α-hemolytic or β-hemolytic. β-Hemolytic species are generally pathogenic, and nonhemolytic or α-hemolytic members of the genera have been viewed traditionally as contaminants or unimportant invaders when isolated.

Streptococci also are classified serologically based on species-specific carbohydrate cell wall antigens, with groups designated A through L.[9,11,12] Group A streptococci *(Streptococcus pyogenes)* cause pharyngitis, glomerulonephritis, and rheumatic fever in humans.[11-13] Although dogs may become colonized transiently with this organism, group A streptococci rarely cause illness in dogs and cats.[11] Therapy generally is not indicated, but these organisms are susceptible to most β-lactam agents, macrolides, and chloramphenicol.

The group B streptococci, which are all strains of *Streptococcus agalactiae,* infrequently cause infections in dogs and cats.[11] Rare infections with *S. agalactiae* have been associated with metritis, fading puppy syndrome, and neonatal sepsis in dogs, and septicemia and peritonitis in parturient cats.[11] Similarly, group C streptococci are rare causes of illness in immunocompetent pets. Species included in this serologic group include *Streptococcus equi* ssp. *zooepidemicus* and *Streptococcus dysgalactiae.* Sporadic cases of endometritis, wound infections, pyelonephritis, lymphadenitis, and neonatal sepsis resulting from infection with β-hemolytic group C streptococci have been reported in dogs and cats. The number of reports of outbreaks of hemorrhagic pneumonia in dogs caused by *S. equi* ssp. *zooepidemicus* is limited but increasing. This acute, highly contagious, and often fatal disease most often is reported in dogs housed in shelters and research kennels. Clinical findings include moist cough, sanguinous nasal discharge, fever, and acute respiratory distress.[6] Postmortem findings reveal fibrinosuppurative, hemorrhagic, and necrotizing pneumonia. Pleural effusion is also common.[6,11] As with most streptococci, isolates frequently were susceptible to ampicillin and amoxicillin. Some isolates were susceptible to doxycycline. Isolates of *S. equi* ssp. *zooepidemicus* were found to be susceptible in vitro to enrofloxacin.[6] However, many streptococci are intrinsically resistant to second-generation fluoroquinolones, and thus single-agent therapy with enrofloxacin is not recommended for any streptococcal infections.[14] The combination of penicillin and an aminoglycoside was found to be effective in one study.[15]

Group G streptococci are common resident microflora and are the cause of most streptococcal infection in dogs and cats.[9,11] The most common isolate is *Streptococcus canis*.[9,11] The main source of infection with this pathogen in dogs is the anal mucosa; young cats more commonly acquire infection from the vagina of the queen or via the umbilicus.[11] Infection spreads rapidly in neonatal kittens and is often fatal during the first week of life in affected cats. *S. canis* may be isolated from adult cats with abscesses, pyelonephritis, sinusitis, arthritis, metritis, or mastitis, and from kittens with lymphadenitis, pneumonia, or neonatal septicemia.

S. canis is generally an opportunistic pathogen of dogs and is isolated from an array of nonspecific infections, including wounds, mammary tissues, urogenital tract, skin, and ear canal.[10,11] *S. canis* is a cause of canine prostatitis, mastitis, abscesses, infective endocarditis, cholangiohepatitis, pericarditis, pyometra, sepsis, discospondylitis, and meningoencephalomyelitis.[11] *S. canis* has also been implicated in cases of fading puppy syndrome, causing polyarthritis and septicemia in affected pups.[11]

Despite 50 years of penicillin use in animals, no mechanism of resistance to the drug in β-hemolytic group G streptococci has been documented; penicillin G and ampicillin are therefore effective for most infections.[2,10,11] Erythromycin, clindamycin, potentiated sulfonamides (TMP-SMZ), and most cephalosporins are also usually efficacious. Susceptibility to veterinary-approved fluoroquinolones is negligible, and their use generally is discouraged for streptococcal infections.[14,16] *Streptococcus* spp. generally are not considered susceptible to aminoglycosides, owing to poor transport across the cytoplasmic membrane.[2] However, combination therapy with a β-lactam agent and an aminoglycoside is an appropriate treatment strategy for critically ill animals with streptococcal bacteremia or endocarditis.[2,14] Combination therapy is also recommended for cases of infective necrotizing fasciitis and myositis (NFM) (see Empiric Antibiotic Strategies), endocarditis, or when polymicrobial infections are suspected. Although long-term (at least 6 weeks) therapy is recommended for treating unstable patients with disseminated infection, in most clinical settings aminoglycosides are rarely prescribed for this duration due to concerns for drug-associated nephrotoxicity.

Over the past decade, streptococcal toxic shock syndrome (STTS), with or without necrotizing fasciitis and myositis (NFM) resulting from infection with *S. canis*, has emerged as a recognized syndrome in dogs (see Chapter 101).[9,11,17] The most common source for infection in animals with STTS appears to be the lung, with occasional reports of affected dogs suffering from acute or peracute suppurative bronchopneumonia. Some case histories have included failed attempts to treat patients with enrofloxacin and nonsteroidal antiinflammatory agents.[11,18] Cases of STTS-associated septicemia are often fatal, whereas most dogs with NFM alone survive with prompt, appropriate medical therapy and aggressive surgical resection (see Chapter 139).[11,18]

The most likely pathogenesis for STTS and NFM starts with minor trauma. The dog then licks its wounds and seeds *S. canis* from the oral mucosa into the wound. The bacteria proliferate, typically resulting in painful, rapidly developing cellulitis, skin discoloration, and often signs of systemic illness.[17] Prompt recognition and aggressive surgical debridement are imperative. Clindamycin has proven to be effective therapy in affected animals.[11,17] Aminopenicillins, erythromycin, and β-lactam antibiotics also may be effective.[11] Culture and susceptibility testing is important because similar toxic shock–like diseases in dogs may be caused by bacteria other than streptococci. Gram staining of tissues or fluids should be helpful in ascertaining the morphology of the infecting agent, particularly in acute infections. A similar syndrome in young cats with suppurative lymphadenopathy and multifocal ulcerative skin lesions caused by group G streptococci has been reported.[11]

ENTEROCOCCAL INFECTIONS

Enterococcus species are facultative anaerobic cocci that demonstrate intrinsic and acquired resistance to multiple antibiotics. Unlike streptococci and staphylococci, most enterococci do not produce reliably a set of proinflammatory toxins, but they are equipped with many genes that mediate adhesion to host tissues.[7] Enterococci (previously group D streptococci), as the name implies, are commensal bacteria that inhabit the alimentary tract of animals and humans.[9,12] Enterococcal infections previously were considered rare, and not especially virulent, in companion animals. Presently, enterococcal infections are a leading cause of nosocomial disease in human health care, and pathogenic and multidrug resistant (MDR) enterococci are recovered increasingly from hospitalized veterinary patients.[1,11]

Postoperative wound and urogenital infections are seen most commonly; however, enterococcal cholangiohepatitis, peritonitis, vegetative endocarditis, mastitis, and blood-borne infections have been reported in companion animals.[11,19] Many enterococci are intrinsically resistant to numerous antibiotics, and the development of MDR enterococci is thought to result from inappropriate antimicrobial usage and poor infection control measures in hospitalized patients.[11,12,19] The majority of clinical isolates belong to the species *Enterococcus faecalis,* although *Enterococcus faecium* remains the species that exhibits a disproportionately greater resistance to multiple antibiotics.[11,19]

E. faecium is increasingly resistant to vancomycin, which was effective for almost all penicillin-resistant enterococci until recently.[9,11,19] Strains that remain susceptible to vancomycin may be resistant to a wide range of drugs that are selected empirically for managing bacterial infection in critically ill patients.[11,19] *E. faecium* often possesses inherent and acquired resistance to many drug classes, including the fluoroquinolones, lincosamides, macrolides, and potentiated sulfonamides (TMP-SMZ).[7,11,19] Unlike most streptococci, enterococci are often inhibited, but not killed, by penicillins and are generally resistant to cephalosporins.[2] Moreover, although enterococci do not often intrinsically produce β-lactamases, production of these enzymes by the bacteria may be induced by exposure to β-lactamase–inhibitor drugs. As such, it is not appropriate to prescribe amoxicillin-clavulanate or ampicillin-sulbactam for an enterococcal isolate that is reported to be susceptible to ampicillin. Until recently, aminopenicillin monotherapy was successful for many enterococcal infections. However, this is no longer predictable. Presently, many isolates are resistant to aminopenicillins and many other antimicrobials that were previously effective in managing gram-positive infections.[2,11,19] One of the few effective modes of therapy takes advantage of antibiotic synergy. Penicillins alone only arrest bacterial growth, and aminoglycosides are without effect against enterococci, except at very high concentrations, but the combination of both drugs effectively kills the organism.[2,14] This high-dosage synergy approach is among the most effective pharmacologic means to clear infection. Unless there is documentation that other potentially safer antibiotic regimens are effective in vivo and in vitro, the co-administration of gentamicin (but not amikacin) with a cell wall–active agent (generally ampicillin) is standard of care for serious enterococcal infections in critically ill patients and in those with osteomyelitis, endocarditis, sepsis or joint infections.[11,14,17]

Unfortunately, some enterococci are resistant to aminoglycosides, even when coadministered with ampicillin, leaving few alternatives for treating these infections.[7,11] In some cases, the only effective drugs are glycopeptides, such as vancomycin, but this drug should be viewed as a therapy of absolute last resort.[2] Vancomycin has a narrow spectrum and is potentially nephrotoxic (see Chapter 181). Clinical experience with vancomycin is limited in veterinary medicine.

STAPHYLOCOCCAL INFECTIONS

The broad distribution of staphylococci as normal flora of domestic animals is perhaps the most important epidemiologic factor in staphylococcal infections.[1,5,20,21] These organisms are often not inherently invasive and colonize intact epithelium of healthy animals without causing disease.[9,21] Subsequently, isolation of these bacteria may signify the presence of transient or long-term colonization of epithelial surfaces.[10,22]

Disease pathogenesis and lesion development are not fully understood but likely involve a breach of the host's mucosal barrier or other means of immunocompromise, in conjunction with numerous bacterial virulence factors such as staphylococcal toxins and enzymes that permit them to withstand phagocytosis by neutrophils.[5,11,21,22] Biofilm formation has been demonstrated for many staphylococci, increasing bacterial resistance to stressful environmental conditions and antimicrobial exposure. Biofilm formation may be particularly important for infections associated with implants and invasive devices such as indwelling catheters.[2,20,23] For many years, production of coagulase by staphylococci has been associated with virulence and tissue tropism. Almost all infections in humans, dogs, and cats were caused by coagulase-positive species, with coagulase-negative staphylococci viewed invariably as contaminants.[5,10,20] More recent studies implicate coagulase-negative staphylococci as a cause of significant morbidity in humans and companion animals.[1,2,20]

Pathogenic staphylococci may affect any organ system and are responsible for community-acquired and nosocomial infections.[5,20,21] Of approximately 35 species of staphylococcal organisms, three are of clinical importance in companion animals: *Staphylococcus pseudintermedius, Staphylococcus aureus,* and *Staphylococcus schleiferi* ssp. *coagulans.*[20,22,24] *Staphylococcus intermedius* previously was considered the most important staphylococcal species in dogs and cats. What was recognized previously as *S. intermedius* now is known to be the closely related *S. pseudintermedius.*[4,5,20,22] *S. pseudintermedius* is a common canine commensal, with colonization rates of 31% to 68% in healthy dogs, and is the leading pyogenic bacterium of dogs.[4,20,22] Although it is recognized as the most common etiologic agent of bacterial skin and ear infections, it also may cause systemic infections, including arthritis, osteomyelitis, cystitis, mastitis, wound infections, and bacteremia.[9,20,22] Sites of infection are similar in cats, although reports of disseminated disease are less numerous.[20]

Until recently, *S. pseudintermedius* isolates were generally susceptible to β-lactamase–resistant β-lactam antibiotics.[20] Infections with strains of *S. pseudintermedius* that are resistant to multiple antibiotics are becoming common, and since 2006 methicillin-resistant *S. pseudintermedius* (MRSP) has emerged as a significant health problem in veterinary medicine.[4,20,21,24,25] As with other staphylococci, the methicillin resistance of *S. pseudintermedius* is mediated by the *mecA* gene that encodes production of a modified penicillin binding protein (PBP).[4,21] Normally, β-lactam antibiotics bind to *S. pseudintermedius* to prevent cell wall development by the bacterium. The modified PBP of *S. pseudintermedius* has a low affinity for β-lactams, and therefore cell wall synthesis is not inhibited by these antimicrobials.

The treatment of infections with MRSP is a new challenge in veterinary medicine.[4,20,21,25] Determination of methicillin resistance for all staphylococci is based on in vitro resistance to oxacillin. Oxacillin is used as a surrogate for methicillin because it is sensitive and more stable. If staphylococci are resistant to oxacillin, they are inherently resistant to all other β-lactams, including cephalosporins and amoxicillin-clavulanate, regardless of the results of in vitro susceptibility testing.[4,24] MRSP isolates are often resistant to many other antimicrobials, including all of those licensed for use in companion animals.[3,20,24,25] Most *S. pseudintermedius* infections are not caused by MRSP, and infections with MRSP are clinically indistinguishable from infections caused by methicillin-susceptible *S. pseudintermedius* (MSSP).[20] Further, there is currently no indication that MRSP is more virulent than MSSP, and most reported MRSP infections have been treated successfully, albeit with fewer options for antimicrobial therapy.[3,21,25] Based on in vitro testing, the most useful systemic antibiotics include rifampicin, amikacin, chloramphenicol, and/or minocycline (see Empiric Selection).[4,20,25]

Similar antibiotic resistance patterns have emerged for pyoderma and systemic infections caused by *S. schleiferi.* Although this bacterium appears to be a less frequent cause of disseminated infections, results of clinical studies reveal that tissue tropism and antimicrobial susceptibility data are not predictable for this relatively novel species.[20]

S. aureus is well established as a significant community-acquired and nosocomial pathogen in humans, and infection with methicillin-resistant *S. aureus* (MRSA) is a relatively recent development in veterinary medicine.[1,20,21,26] The emergence of MRSA in dogs and cats appears to be a direct reflection of MRSA in the human population.[20,21] Unlike *S. pseudintermedius, S. aureus* is not a true commensal organism in dogs and cats.[20,27] Although dogs and cats are not natural reservoirs of *S. aureus,* they can become colonized, in all likelihood from humans.[20,21] Once colonized, pets may clear the organism, go on to develop infection, or remain asymptomatic carriers for an indeterminate period. *S. aureus* produces a similar range of infections as those caused by *S. pseudintermedius.*[20,21,27]

Infected animals should be isolated, and barrier contact precautions should be used when handling patients, food bowls, bandages, and all associated materials. Hand washing between patients is imperative. Such guidelines must be enforced (1) to minimize the risk of patient-to-patient spread of resistant clones and (2) to limit the likelihood of animal-to-human transmission. There is increasing evidence that interspecies transmission of MRSA occurs and that it may emerge as an important zoonotic and veterinary disease.[20,21,27]

In human hospitals, transmission of MRSA occurs mainly via the transiently colonized hands of health care workers.[2,20,26] Colonized veterinary personnel are thought to be the most likely vectors of MRSA in veterinary hospitals.[27,28] All personnel in contact with patients should be advised of appropriate precautions once MRSA infection is confirmed. Like other staphylococci, MRSA can survive for long periods on inanimate objects such as bedding and cages, and it is relatively resistant to heat. Thus it may be difficult to eliminate once introduced to the hospital environment. MRSA infections most often remain treatable, albeit by a small number of antibiotics.[20] Because MRSA may be transmitted between animals and humans, owners of infected or colonized animals should be informed of this potential. However, veterinarians are discouraged from making any recommendations regarding the diagnosis or treatment of MRSA, or any disease, in humans.

Treatment of deep or disseminated staphylococcal infections requires prompt systemic therapy. Drug choices should be based on in vitro susceptibility testing in combination with other factors (e.g., drug penetration, site of infection). Historically, uncomplicated methicillin-susceptible staphylococcal infections were predictably susceptible to β-lactam-β-lactamase inhibitor combination drugs (e.g., amoxicillin-clavulanic acid) and first-generation cephalosporins (e.g., cephalexin, cefazolin).[20] These agents remain appropriate for treating uncomplicated and/or first-time staphylococcal infections in otherwise stable pets. This level of confidence does not extend to hospitalized patients with risk factors for MDR, such as those with a history of recent antibiotic use, indwelling devices, exposure to nosocomial pathogens, and protracted hospital stays. Clindamycin, potentiated sulfonamides (TMP-SMZ), doxycycline, and aminoglycosides are frequently, although not uniformly, effective for treating staphylococcal infections.[5,20,25] The role of fluoroquinolones in critically ill pets with staphylococcal infections is controversial, particularly with methicillin-resistant strains, as emergence of resistance and treatment failures are reported.[4,14,20] Inducible resistance to clindamycin is documented and generally is not identified with culture and susceptibility testing. However, *S. aureus* reported as susceptible to clindamycin but resistant to erythromycin should be inferred to be resistant to clindamycin.[4,20] Inducible clindamycin resistance is rare in *S. pseudintermedius*, but erythromycin-resistant strains similarly should not be managed with clindamycin.[20]

Commercial veterinary laboratories should test all β-lactam–resistant staphylococci for susceptibility to chloramphenicol, aminoglycosides, tetracyclines, TMP-SMZ, erythromycin, and clindamycin.[20,24,25] Duration of therapy depends on the site of infection and comorbid conditions that may impair host defenses or delay healing. When tolerated, therapy generally extends 2 weeks beyond the resolution of clinical signs of infection.

Vancomycin, linezolid, tigecycline, and daptomycin remain the only effective antimicrobials for resistant strains of staphylococcus in human health care settings; these drugs should be used only in exceptional circumstances in veterinary medicine.[20,25] It is argued that their use should be restricted in dogs and cats because avoidance of antibiotic use is a valid strategy to curtail antibiotic resistance.

Table 93-1 **Antibiotics Used to Treat Gram-Positive Infections**

Drug	Dosage
Amikacin	15 mg/kg IV q24h (dogs) 10 mg/kg IV q24h (cats)
Ampicillin	22 mg/kg IV q6-8h
Ampicillin-sulbactam	22 mg/kg IV q8h
Azithromycin	5 to 10 mg/kg IV q24h
Cefazolin	22 mg/kg IV q6-8h
Cefotetan	30 mg/kg IV q8h
Cefoxitin	30 mg/kg IV q6-8h
Chloramphenicol	25 to 50 mg/kg IV q8h (dogs) 15 to 20 mg/kg IV q12h (cats)
Clindamycin	10 mg/kg IV q12h
Enrofloxacin	15 to 20 mg/kg IV q24h (dogs) 5 mg/kg IV q24h (cats)
Gentamicin	10 mg/kg IV q24h (dogs) 6 mg/kg IV q24h (cats)
Imipenem-cilastatin	5 to 10 mg/kg IV q6-8h
Meropenem	8 to 12 mg/kg IV q8-12h
Ticarcillin-clavulanate	50 mg/kg IV q6-8h
Trimethoprim-sulfamethoxazole or trimethoprim-sulfadiazine	15 to 30 mg/kg PO/IV q12h
Vancomycin	15 mg/kg IV q8h (dogs) 10 to 15 mg/kg IV q8-12h (cats)

IV, Intravenous.

EMPIRIC ANTIBIOTIC STRATEGIES

In critically ill patients, prompt administration of broad-spectrum injectable antimicrobials is warranted when a polymicrobial infection is suspected or when the causative agent causing an infection is not known (Table 93-1). Wright-Giemsa and Gram-stained cytologic preparations of aspirates or impression smears should be examined to evaluate the morphologic and staining characteristics of bacterial pathogens.

Clinicians should be familiar with the gram-positive pathogens associated with severe infections in their hospital and choose therapy based on the prevalence and susceptibility patterns of these bacteria, as well as the site(s) of infection. Once culture and susceptibility data are available, therapy is streamlined to ensure eradication of the pathogen without promoting resistance secondary to inappropriate antimicrobial treatment.[14]

Although bacterial resistance to previously effective antibiotics is an ever-increasing concern in patients with gram-positive infections, first-choice recommendations for first time and non–life-threatening infections include a first-generation cephalosporin (e.g., cefazolin) or a β-lactam- β-lactamase inhibitor combination (e.g., amoxicillin-clavulanic acid, ampicillin-sulbactam). The first-generation cephalosporins have a similar spectrum of activity to ampicillin, with the notable difference that β-lactamase–producing staphylococci often remain susceptible to the cephalosporins.[14,20] However, methicillin-resistant, coagulase-positive staphylococci are resistant to all cephalosporins.[4,22,25] Sulbactam, like clavulanic acid, is an inhibitor of β-lactamases (the latter is more potent). β-Lactamase inhibitors have weak antibacterial activity by themselves, but they show extraordinary synergism when co-administered with ampicillin, amoxicillin, or ticarcillin owing to the irreversible binding of the β-lactamase enzymes of many resistant bacteria.[14] The aminopenicillins and first-generation cephalosporins have relatively short half-lives, and in the absence of renal impairment, they may be administered every 6 hours to take advantage of the well-described pharmacodynamic properties of most β-lactam agents. This recommendation is particularly relevant for patients with altered volumes of distribution (i.e., patients receiving intravenous fluids, parenteral nutrition, or blood products, and those with vascular leak or third-spacing syndromes).[14]

Alterations in drug clearance can occur rapidly. The clinician must consider these and other pharmacokinetic principles when determining dosages of all antibiotics to achieve the desired pharmacodynamic effects. Similarly, individualization of regimens based on prior antibiotic use may reduce the risk of therapeutic failure.

An important exception to the above therapeutic recommendations exists when a new infection is documented in a patient currently receiving antibiotics. Similarly, critically ill patients with a history of recent antibiotic use or presumed polymicrobial infection should be managed with broader-spectrum antibiotics, such as a carbapenem, alone or in conjunction with an aminoglycoside or fluoroquinolone, while culture and susceptibility results are pending. For treatment of infections caused by some enterococci or methicillin-resistant staphylococci, evaluation of susceptibility data is imperative to avoid treatment failures.[2,11,20,29]

Fluoroquinolones and aminoglycosides remain effective treatment for some staphylococci. Neither drug class is predictably active against streptococci. However, they are often active against gram-negative pathogens that may be contributing to patient morbidity.

These agents generally are administered once daily at the upper end of the dosage range. In cats, enrofloxacin should not be prescribed at a dose exceeding 5 mg/kg/day because its administration has been associated with temporary or permanent blindness in domestic felids.[14]

Among the aminoglycosides, gentamicin is reported to be more effective than amikacin for treatment of staphylococcal infections in humans.[25] The clinical relevance of this distinction among veterinary isolates is not clear. Both amikacin and gentamicin are associated with potential renal dysfunction, but both are frequently prescribed without incident for short-term therapy (<10 days) in well-hydrated patients without preexisting renal disease. Gentamicin, when administered with ampicillin, is effective for many serious enterococcal infections. This combination results in synergistic bactericidal activity against susceptible strains. Treatment options for enterococcal isolates with high-level gentamicin resistance are limited, since amikacin is not effective against enterococci. Clindamycin demonstrates in vitro activity against some staphylococci and streptococci, and may be particularly useful for managing patients with cellulitis or bone infections caused by susceptible strains.[1,20] All pathogenic enterococci are inferred to be intrinsically resistant to clindamycin.

Carbapenems, such as imipenem and meropenem, are highly active against most *Streptococcus* and *Staphylococcus* spp. However, they are uniformly ineffective for the treatment of methicillin-resistant pathogens and vancomycin-resistant enterococci. They are prescribed based on culture and susceptibility data or administered empirically to patients with risk factors for infection with MDR organisms. However, they should not be used liberally because excessive use of carbapenems is associated with β-lactamase production against other β-lactam antibiotics, especially cephalosporins.[2,30]

Chloramphenicol and potentiated sulfonamides generally are not used empirically in the critically ill patient, but some MDR staphylococci are susceptible to these agents. Both have been available for many years, and practitioners are encouraged to familiarize (or refamiliarize) themselves with the spectrum of activity of these medications and with the uncommon but potentially serious adverse events that may occur with their use. All enterococci are inherently resistant to potentiated sulfonamides. Vancomycin seldom is required to treat isolates of any of the gram-positive cocci in small animal veterinary medicine.

Pharmaceutical companies are devoting fewer resources to the development of new antimicrobials, and few novel drugs are in the pipeline. Therefore there are no known indications for veterinarians to prescribe any of the antibiotics for virulent MDR enterococci or staphylococci recently approved for human medicine. Daptomycin, quinupristin-dalfopristin, linezolid, ceftaroline, telithromycin, and tigecycline are the last lines of defense for patients with life-threatening infections[2,26] (see Chapter 181). A small number of human *E. faecium* and *S. aureus* isolates already possess documented resistance to some of these drugs, and clinicians thus are urged to use antibiotics rationally and wisely.

REFERENCES

1. Menichetti F: Current and emerging serious Gram-positive infections, Clin Microbiol Infect 11(suppl 3):22-28, 2005.
2. Woodford N: Biological counterstrike: antibiotic resistance mechanisms of Gram-positive cocci, Clin Microbiol Infect 11(suppl 3):2-21, 2005.
3. Weese JS, Sweetman K, Edson H, Rousseau J: Evaluation of minocycline susceptibility of methicillin-resistant *Staphylococcus pseudintermedius*, Vet Microbiol 162:968-971, 2013.
4. Frank LA, Loeffler A: Methicillin-resistant *Staphylococcus pseudintermedius*: clinical challenge and treatment options, Vet Dermatol 23:283-291, 2012.
5. Bond R, Loeffler A: What's happened to *Staphylococcus intermedius*? Taxonomic revision and emergence of multi-drug resistance, J Small Anim Pract 53:147-154, 2012.
6. Priestnall S, Erles K: *Streptococcus zooepidemicus*: an emerging canine pathogen, Vet J 188:142-148, 2011.
7. Arias CA, Murray BE: The rise of the Enterococcus: beyond vancomycin resistance, Nat Rev Microbiol 10:266-278, 2012.
8. Cain CL: Antimicrobial resistance in staphylococci in small animals, Vet Clin North Am Small Anim Pract 43:19-40, 2013.
9. Hirsch DC, MacLachlan NJ: Veterinary microbiology, Ames, Iowa, 2004, Blackwell.
10. Quinn PJ, et al: Veterinary microbiology and microbial disease, Chichester, West Sussex, UK, 2011, Wiley-Blackwell.
11. Greene CE, Prescott JF: In Infectious diseases of the dog and cat, St Louis, 2012, Elsevier, pp 326-333.
12. Hardie JM, Whiley RA: Classification and overview of the genera Streptococcus and Enterococcus, J Appl Microbiol 83:1S-11S, 1997.
13. Winn WC, Janda WM, Woods GL: Koneman's color atlas and textbook of diagnostic microbiology, Philadelphia, 2006, Lippincott Williams and Wilkins.
14. Boothe DM, Greene CE: In Infectious diseases of the dog and cat, St Louis, 2012, Elsevier Saunders, pp 291-302.
15. Kim MK, Jee H, Shin SW, et al: Outbreak and control of haemorrhagic pneumonia due to *Streptococcus equi* subspecies zooepidemicus in dogs, Vet Rec 13;161(15):528-530, 2007.
16. Ingrey KT, Ren J, Prescott JF: A fluoroquinolone induces a novel mitogen-encoding bacteriophage in *Streptococcus canis*, Infect Immun 71:3028-3033, 2003.
17. Naidoo SL, Campbell DL, Miller LM, et al: Necrotizing fasciitis: a review, J Am Anim Hosp Assoc 41(2):104-109 2005.
18. Prescott JF, Miller CW, Mathews KA, et al: Update on canine streptococcal toxic shock syndrome and necrotizing fasciitis, Can Vet J 38:241-242, 1997.
19. Tendolkar PM, Baghdayan AS, Shankar N, et al: Pathogenic enterococci: new developments in the 21st century, Cell Molecular Life Sci 60:2622-2636, 2003.
20. Weese JS: In Infectious diseases of the dog and cat, St Louis, 2012, Elsevier Saunders, pp 341-346.
21. Weese JS, van Duijkeren E: Methicillin-resistant *Staphylococcus aureus* and *Staphylococcus pseudintermedius* in veterinary medicine, Vet Microbiol 140:418-429, 2010.
22. Bannoehr J, Guardabassi L: *Staphylococcus pseudintermedius* in the dog: taxonomy, diagnostics, ecology, epidemiology and pathogenicity, Vet Dermatol 23:253-66, e51-2, 2012.
23. Greene CE, Weese JS, Calpin JP: In Infectious diseases of the dog and cat, St Louis, 2012, Elsevier Saunders, pp 1085-1095.
24. van Duijkeren E, et al: Review on methicillin-resistant *Staphylococcus pseudintermedius*, J Antimicrob Chemother 66:2705-2714, 2011.
25. Papich MG: Selection of antibiotics for meticillin-resistant *Staphylococcus pseudintermedius*: time to revisit some old drugs? Vet Dermatol 23:352-360, 2012.
26. Gould IM, David MZ, Esposito S, et al: New insights into methicillin-resistant *Staphylococcus aureus* (MRSA) pathogenesis, treatment and resistance, Int J Antimicrob Agents 39(2):96-104, 2012.
27. Baptiste KE, et al: Methicillin-resistant staphylococci in companion animals, Emerg Infect Dis 11, 1942, 2005.
28. Leonard FC, et al: Methicillin-resistant *Staphylococcus aureus* isolated from a veterinary surgeon and five dogs in one practice, Vet Rec 158:155-159, 2006.
29. Seol B: Comparative in vitro activities of enrofloxacin, ciprofloxacin and marbofloxacin against *Staphylococcus intermedius* isolated from dogs, Vet Arh 75:189, 2005.
30. Weston JS: Treatment of gram-positive infections: past, present, and future, Crit Care Nurs Clin North Am 14:17-29, 2002.

CHAPTER 94

GRAM-NEGATIVE INFECTIONS

Reid P. Groman, DVM, DACVIM (Internal Medicine), DACVECC

KEY POINTS

- Lipopolysaccharides are the major constituents of the outer membrane of most gram-negative bacteria.
- Endotoxin is a lipopolysaccharide and potent stimulator of the inflammatory response; it is believed to initiate the pathology of gram-negative sepsis.
- Immunosuppression, hospitalization, invasive procedures, and prior antimicrobial administration are suspected risk factors for colonization and infection with multidrug-resistant gram-negative bacteria.
- Increasing rates of antibiotic resistance among gram-negative pathogens threaten the effectiveness of empiric antibiotic therapy in veterinary medicine.
- Antimicrobial selection should be guided by culture and susceptibility results, especially for patients that do not respond to empiric therapy.
- Initial antimicrobial therapy for first-time gram-negative infections includes a β-lactam/β-lactamase inhibitor, alone or in combination with a fluoroquinolone.
- Therapy for life-threatening infections caused by resistant or nosocomial gram-negative pathogens should include a third-generation cephalosporin, extended-spectrum β-lactam/β-lactamase inhibitor, and/or an aminoglycoside
- Fourth-generation cephalosporins, aztreonam, and polymyxin are prescribed for select highly resistant gram-negative infections in human hospitals. Relevance to treatment in dogs and cats is not established and caution should be exercised.

Infections resulting from gram-negative organisms are a significant cause of morbidity and mortality in critically ill patients.[1-3] Important aerobic or facultatively anaerobic gram-negative infections are often due to an opportunistic invasion by commensal intestinal flora, including *Escherichia coli, Proteus* spp., *Pseudomonas aeruginosa,* and *Klebsiella* spp.[2,4] Less commonly, opportunistic infections are caused by environmental saprophytes that enter the body through wounds or the respiratory tract .[5]

GRAM-NEGATIVE CELL STRUCTURE AND PATHOGENICITY

In addition to having a cytoplasmic membrane and peptidoglycan layer similar to that found in gram-positive organisms, gram-negative bacteria possess unique factors that contribute to their ability to cause disease.[1,2,5] Among the bacterial products commonly implicated in the pathogenesis of gram-negative infections is endotoxin, a unique lipopolysaccharide (LPS) that accounts for 75% of the outer surface of the gram-negative cell membrane.[5,6] The role of LPS in triggering the cellular and physiologic host response is well established.[5-8]

Structurally, endotoxin consists of an outer polysaccharide chain that is bound to lipid A.[2] Although it is buried deep in the bacterial cell wall, lipid A is known to be the toxic moiety of endotoxin.[5,8] Lipid A induces a wide range of proinflammatory responses (i.e., release of cytokines and activation of the compliment cascade) and endothelial dysfunction.[5-9] During minor or local infections with small numbers of bacteria, small amounts of LPS are released, leading to controlled cytokine production. The cytokines released promote body defenses by stimulating inflammation, fever, and appropriate protective immunologic responses.[5,8] However, during severe systemic infections with large numbers of bacteria, increased amounts of LPS are released, resulting in excessive, and sometimes maladaptive, cytokine production by monocytes and macrophages (see Chapter 6).[2] Harmful effects of endotoxin include vasodilation, enhanced vascular permeability, tissue destruction, and activation of coagulation pathways.[5,7,9]

Gram-negative organisms also possess cellular structures that often are recognized as virulence factors.[2,5,6,9,10] Flagella are protein filaments that extend from the cell membrane and allow for locomotion. They undulate in a coordinated manner to move the bacteria toward or away from a chemical gradient, a process called *chemotaxis.* Pili (also called *fimbriae)* are straight filaments arising from the bacterial cell wall and most often serve as adherence factors, in which case they are referred to *adhesins.*[10] For many bacteria, adhesins are vital to their ability to cause disease. Capsules are protective walls, generally composed of simple sugar residues that surround the cell membranes.[5,10] Encapsulation enhances virulence by preventing bacterial phagocytosis by host neutrophils and macrophages.[10]

Failure to contain or eradicate gram-negative pathogens may result in further damage due to the inexorable progression of inflammation and infection.[8-10] Thus, of the many therapeutic interventions, early initiation of appropriate antimicrobial therapy is critical to ensure a favorable outcome.[1,11]

IDENTIFICATION OF GRAM-NEGATIVE BACTERIA OF MEDICAL IMPORTANCE

The classification of gram-negative bacteria is based on several criteria, including their appearance on selective media, use of carbohydrates (e.g., lactose), production of certain end products (e.g., acids and alcohols), and the presence or absence of specialized enzymes (e.g., oxidase).[5,10] Although the clinical relevance of these categories is a point for contention among clinicians, taxonomic schemes permit the microbiology laboratory to distinguish rapidly among commonly encountered bacteria.[5,10] For example, facultatively anaerobic oxidase-negative, gram-negative rods that grow on MacConkey agar are presumed to be members of the Enterobacteriaceae.[5,6,10] As more information accumulates, reclassification of bacteria among genera and species and the creation of new designations must be accepted as part of scientific progress.[3,11]

ENTEROBACTERIACEAE

Members of the family Enterobacteriaceae are the most frequently encountered gram-negative isolates recovered from clinical specimens.[1,3,5] These commensal organisms are found in soil and water, on plants and, as the family name implies, within the intestinal tract of animals and humans.[2,5]

Before the advent of antimicrobials, chemotherapy, and immunosuppressive measures, the infectious diseases caused by the Enterobacteriaceae were relatively well defined and typically characterized by diarrhea and other gastrointestinal syndromes.[2,10] However, members of the Enterobacteriaceae now are incriminated in virtually any type of infectious disease and may be recovered from any tissue or fluid specimen submitted to the laboratory.[4-6,10] By definition, commensal organisms colonize an individual without causing disease. However, in a vulnerable host, these "pathogenic commensals" have the capacity to produce disease.[2,3,11] Generally, enhanced bacterial virulence factors or damage to the mucosal barrier or immune system of the host is required for infection to occur.[2,5,6,9,10] Critically ill and immunocompromised patients are susceptible to hospital-acquired infections after colonization with environmental strains or invasive procedures such as catheterization, endoscopy, and surgery.[9-11]

E. coli is the most commonly encountered bacteria in clinical microbiology laboratories and is thought to be the most important of the facultative aerobic gram-negative species that comprise the normal flora of the alimentary tract in most dogs and cats.* Most strains of *E. coli* are of low virulence, but they may cause opportunistic infections in extraintestinal sites.[1,2,6,10]

Pathogenic *E coli* have been classified based on their virulence properties into pathovars (e.g., enterotoxigenic, enteroinvasive, and uropathogenic strains). Such molecular typing may be performed to differentiate among different isolates.[2] However, this is not offered routinely by commercial veterinary laboratories and seldom warranted for *E. coli* isolates causing extraintestinal infection. *E. coli* organisms were previously susceptible to select drugs. However, multidrug-resistant (MDR) *E. coli* have emerged as a cause of opportunistic infections in companion animals.[2,4,12] The proportion of *E. coli* resistant to aminopenicillins, fluoroquinolones, and cephalosporins is increasing in human and veterinary medicine.[4,11,13,16] Indiscriminate use of antimicrobials, inadequate hygiene, and extended hospital stays are among the proposed reasons for resistance to these commonly used agents (see Chapter 175).[11-14]

Infections with serovars of *Salmonella enterica* are uncommon in dogs and cats. *S. enterica* can survive for relatively long periods in the environment, and transmission through food, water, or fomites contaminated by fecal material likely plays a role in disease pathogenesis.[15] The diagnosis of salmonellosis is traditionally made based on isolation of the organism in fecal samples, in conjunction with clinical signs and assessment for risk factors, such as hospitalization, age, and antibiotic exposure. Importantly, the prevalence of *Salmonella* spp. in canine fecal samples varies and does not correlate with clinical disease. Young dogs are more susceptible to infection and clinical illness.[15] Factors that increase susceptibility to salmonellosis include poor nutrition, anesthesia, overcrowding, concurrent disease, and prior or current antibacterial therapy. The severity of signs varies from none to subacute diarrhea and septic shock. Fever, lethargy, and anorexia may be followed by abdominal pain, vomiting, hemorrhagic diarrhea, and dehydration. Central nervous system (CNS) signs, polyarthritis, and pneumonia may be seen.[15] Only a small proportion of infected animals (less than 10%) die during the acute stages of salmonellosis. Recovered animals generally shed organisms for up to 6 weeks.[15] Salmonellosis is a zoonotic disease. Although most cases in humans are associated with food-borne outbreaks, dogs and cats are recognized as vectors for infection. Aggressive supportive care is the cornerstone of therapy. The use of plasma, probiotics, and polyclonal antiserum is controversial. Antimicrobial therapy is generally not advocated for uncomplicated *Salmonella* enteritis, as fecal shedding may be prolonged with injudicious antibiotic use. Antimicrobial therapy only is recommended for animals with severe extraintestinal signs. Aminopenicillins, chloramphenicol, and potentiated sulfonamides are generally effective, while aminoglycosides and carbapenems are reserved for immunosuppressed animals or those with overwhelming sepsis.[15]

Among the 16 species included in the genus *Enterobacter, Enterobacter aerogenes* and *Enterobacter cloacae* are the species most commonly encountered in clinical infections. *Enterobacter* species cause severe infections that can originate in virtually any body compartment. MDR *E. cloacae* have been recovered from the urinary tract, respiratory tract, and surgical wounds of veterinary patients.[2] *E. cloacae* strains are inherently resistant to amoxicillin, amoxicillin-clavulanate, narrow-spectrum cephalosporins, and cefoxitin. In addition, *E. cloacae* may acquire resistance to broad-spectrum β-lactams, especially when they are subjected to antibiotic pressure.[1] Carbapenems and fourth-generation cephalosporins (e.g., cefepime) are the most reliable antimicrobials for severe *Enterobacter* infections. Aminoglycosides, fluoroquinolones, and the potentiated sulfonamides are frequently, although less predictably, effective.[1] Third-generation cephalosporins frequently show in vitro activity against these organisms, but *Enterobacter* spp are known to develop resistance to these drugs during therapy. Thus third-generation cephalosporins are not considered drugs of choice. Because of the inherent resistance of *Enterobacter* strains to many antibiotics, and their propensity for resistance to develop during treatment, prompt submission of samples for culture and susceptibility testing is especially important for therapeutic success.

Klebsiella spp. are ubiquitous and may be regarded as normal flora in the alimentary canal, biliary tract, and pharynx in dogs and cats.[22] Of the pathogenic *Klebsiella, K. pneumoniae* is the most prevalent and clinically important; this is thought to be related to its large antiphagocytic capsule. Patients with *K. pneumoniae* infection frequently have predisposing conditions, including immunosuppression, indwelling devices, chronic respiratory disease, or extended hospital stays.[2,7] Although *K. pneumoniae* can cause severe pneumonia, it is more commonly the cause of hospital-acquired wound or urinary tract infections.[16] Antimicrobials with high intrinsic activity against *K. pneumoniae* include third-generation cephalosporins, carbapenems, and aminoglycosides. Fluoroquinolone susceptibility is less predictable. Extensive use of broad-spectrum antimicrobials in hospitalized patients has led to the development of resistant strains that produce extended-spectrum β-lactamases (ESBLs).[11,13] The bowel is the most common site of colonization, with secondary infection of the urinary tract, respiratory tract, peritoneal cavity, biliary tract, wounds, and bloodstream.[2,16]

Proteus includes five species. The most common clinical isolates are *Proteus vulgaris* and *Proteus mirabilis.* Both may be recovered from infected sites in immunocompromised hosts, and are associated with respiratory tract, wound, and genitourinary infections.[13] *Proteus* play an important role in urinary tract infections, utilizing fimbriae to mediate attachment to uroepithelium. *Proteus* organisms have the ability to produce urease and alkalinize urine by hydrolyzing urea to ammonia. This occasionally leads to precipitation of organic and inorganic compounds, promoting struvite stone formation. Most infections are caused by *P. mirabilis. P. vulgaris* is isolated less frequently, causing sporadic infections in hospitalized patients. The recovery of an indole-negative *Proteus* spp. can be identified presumptively as *P. mirabilis.* This is clinically important because different *Proteus* species differ in their susceptibility to different antibiotics. *P. mirabilis* isolates are typically more susceptible to antimicrobials

*References 2, 5, 6, 9, 10, 13.

than *P. vulgaris. P. mirabilis* is inherently resistant to tetracyclines, but unlike *P. vulgaris,* most strains are susceptible to aminopenicillins and first-generation cephalosporins. Susceptibility of *P. vulgaris* to fluoroquinolones is variable. Most veterinary isolates remain susceptible to sulfonamides and aminoglycosides. Rare strains of *P. vulgaris* possess inducible β-lactamases (not found in *P. mirabilis*) . Infections caused by these organisms may be treated with carbapenems and most third-generation cephalosporins.

Serratia species are widespread in the environment but are not common resident flora. *S. marcescens* is the primary pathogenic species responsible for surgical wound, urinary, and lower respiratory tract infections. Hospitalization is a well-described risk factor for infection. Mechanical ventilation and placement of intravenous and urinary catheters are known risk factors for *Serratia* infection in human ICUs, and *Serratia* bacilli have been linked to nosocomial infections in dogs and cats.[2,16] *S. marcescens* is naturally resistant to ampicillin, macrolides, and first-generation cephalosporins. The most reliable antimicrobials for *S. marcescens* infection are carbapenems and amikacin. There is increasing resistance to other aminoglycosides, including gentamicin and tobramycin. Fluoroquinolones are highly active against most strains. Definitive therapy should be based on results of susceptibility testing because MDR strains are common.

NONFERMENTING GRAM-NEGATIVE BACTERIA

The nonfermenting gram-negative bacteria are a group of aerobic, non–spore-forming bacilli that either do not use carbohydrates as a source of energy or degrade them through metabolic pathways other than fermentation.[2,5] Unlike the Enterobacteriaceae, the nonfermenting gram-negative bacilli do not fit conveniently into a single family of well-characterized genera, and the correct taxonomic placement of many of these organisms remains unresolved.[5,6]

Most often, gram-negative nonfermenters are niche pathogens that cause opportunistic infections in critically ill or immunocompromised patients.[2,11,16] Unlike the Enterobacteriaceae, gram-negative nonfermenters are intrinsically resistant to common antibiotics such as ampicillin, most cephalosporins, and macrolides.[2,11] These bacteria, most notably *Pseudomonas aeruginosa,* are also capable of rapidly acquiring resistance to other classes of drugs, and MDR is common.[3,11,16,17] Recent exposure to broad-spectrum antibiotics and invasive diagnostic procedures represent important risk factors for acquisition of these pathogens.[3,11,16]

P. aeruginosa is an obligate aerobic organism that is ubiquitous in the environment, particularly in decaying soil and vegetation.[2,18] It can be cultured from normal tissues of healthy animals, including the alimentary tract, urethra, nasal cavity, mouth, tonsils, upper airways, and conjunctivae. Purulent exudates with a grapelike odor are characteristic of this bacteria. *P. aeruginosa* is the prototypic opportunistic pathogen in that it seldom causes disease in immunocompetent animals but can cause serious infection in almost any tissue when immune function is impaired.[12,16,18,22,23] *P. aeruginosa* expresses a variety of virulence factors that confer resistance to a broad array of antimicrobial agents.[11] *P. aeruginosa* also possesses a repertoire of exotoxins and enzymatic products designed to evade host defenses.[2,3,17,18] In animals, it has been incriminated as the causative agent of many infections, including otitis, urethrocystitis, endocarditis, surgical wound infections, conjunctivitis, pneumonia, intravenous catheter site colonization, endocardial valve infections, prostatitis, and osteomyelitis.[2,18] Most strains are resistant to chloramphenicol and retain susceptibility to aminoglycosides, particularly amikacin. The fluoroquinolones once were considered effective for *P. aeruginosa* infections, but strains are increasingly resistant to this drug class.[11,17] Indeed, exposure to fluoroquinolones causes *P. aeruginosa* to develop resistance more rapidly than occurs with other bacteria.[1,2,11] Many strains also retain susceptibility to enhanced spectrum β-lactam/β-lactamase inhibitors (e.g., piperacillin-tazobactam and ticarcillin-clavulanate) Of the third-generation cephalosporins, only ceftazidime is active against *P. aerugenosa.*[19] Amikacin, prescribed in combination with an antipseudomonal β-lactam, is effective for most infections.[1,10,19,22] The traditional approach of combining a β-lactam with an aminoglycoside to treat *P. aeruginosa* infections is fundamentally based on in vitro synergistic activity and the potential to prevent emergence of resistance. Although in vitro studies support the use of a β-lactam/fluoroquinolone combination for the treatment of *P. aeruginosa,* development of MDR phenotypes during fluoroquinolone therapy has been documented. The carbapenems (imipenem and meropenem) are reserved for serious infections resistant to other antibiotics.[17] The monobactams (e.g., aztreonam) and fourth-generation cephalosporins (e.g., cefepime) are effective, albeit last-line antipseudomonal agents.[19] The sporadic use of polymyxin E (colistin) in humans is relegated to therapy of *P. aeruginosa* infections that are resistant to all other antibiotics.

Acinetobacter spp. (principally *A. baumannii*) have emerged during the past few decades as one of the most difficult nosocomial microorganisms to control and treat.[1,11] *Acinetobacter* spp. colonize multiple sites and can persist on environmental surfaces for extended periods.[2,3,17,20] *A. baumannii* is a water organism and preferentially colonizes moist environments. *A baumannii* colonization is particularly common in intubated patients or in patients that have multiple intravenous lines, surgical drains, urinary catheters, and monitoring devices. Although colonization with *Acinetobacter* always precedes infection, colonization does not always result in infection. The recovery of the organism from a nonsterile body site (e.g., endotracheal secretions) does not indicate or imply an infectious pathogenic role. When infection occurs, it usually involves organ systems that have a high fluid content. *A. baumannii* is an important cause of nosocomial pneumonia, and it increasingly is associated with infections of the urinary tract and peritoneal cavity .[2,3,11,20] Infections occur predominantly in select patients with risk factors such as mechanical ventilation, extended intensive care unit (ICU) stays, and prior antimicrobial use.[2,3,11,17,20] *A. baumannii* is intrinsically resistant to several classes of antimicrobials, and it is able to develop and transfer resistance quickly.[2,11,16] Cephalosporins and penicillins have little or no activity against *Acinetobacter.* Most isolates of *A. baumannii* are effectively treated with carbapenems (particularly meropenem), amikacin, minocycline, and colistin. Although carbapenems and aminoglycosides are considered to be the most effective agents, *A. baumannii* strains that possess aminoglycoside-modifying enzymes and carbapenemases are reported increasingly in human ICUs, rendering these "last-line" antibiotics ineffective in such cases.[3,11] Every attempt should be made to isolate patients colonized with *Acinetobacter* in order to prevent transmission among hospitalized patients.

Other nonfermentative gram-negative organisms implicated in hospital-acquired infections in human and veterinary medicine include *Burkholderia cepacia, Aeromonas* spp., *Chryseobacterium* spp., and *Stenotrophomonas maltophilia.*[10,16] These opportunistic organisms are generally of low virulence but colonize and multiply in aqueous hospital environments such as intravenous fluids, irrigation solutions, respiratory tubing, and urine. They are generally contaminants and not considered primary pathogens. Antibiotic treatment of colonized patients is not always necessary and may be harmful unless or until infection is proven. Although infections are of low prevalence, these organisms survive in the environment for extended periods and are increasingly found to cause bacteremia, pneumonia, urethrocystitis, and surgical wound infections in humans and companion animals.[10,16] The increased incidence of infection is likely a consequence of impaired host defenses, and the selective pressure caused by overuse of broad-spectrum β-lactams and fluoroquinolones.* Prospective epidemiologic studies of infections by these pathogens are lacking in veterinary medicine.

RESISTANCE AMONG GRAM-NEGATIVE PATHOGENS

The frequency of antibiotic resistance is increasing dramatically, particularly among gram-negative bacteria, and antibiotics that were once formidable weapons are now commonly ineffective.[1-3,11,13,17] Resistance among gram-negative pathogens may be due to alterations of the target binding site on the bacteria, decreased penetration of the antimicrobial drug into the bacteria, and enzymatic degradation of the target antibiotic by enzymes such as β-lactamases, the single most common cause of gram-negative bacterial resistance to β-lactam drugs (see Chapter 175).[3,11,14,16]

Acquired resistance to antibiotics occurs by either a mutation in the bacterial chromosomal DNA or acquisition of new genetic material. Mutations are uncommon events but may result in the development of resistance during therapy in organisms that are initially susceptible. Of greatest concern is the development of resistance by acquisition of new genetic material. Genes mediating antibiotic resistance are found on transposons and plasmids. These mobile genetic elements may be transferred from organism to organism and even from one bacterial species to another.[1,11,12] This mechanism of resistance is best exemplified by the β-lactamase family of enzymes, which act by hydrolyzing the β-lactam ring of penicillins, cephalosporins, and carbapenems. There are hundreds of β-lactamase enzymes that may be distinguished by their substrate profiles and activities.[12]

Plasmid-mediated β-lactamases such as those exhibited by *E. coli, K. pneumoniae,* and *B. fragilis* generally can be overcome with β-lactamase inhibitors such as clavulanic acid, sulbactam, or tazobactam. *P. aeruginosa, Serratia* spp., and *Enterobacter* spp. have chromosomal β-lactamase genes and can increase β-lactamase production if induced by penicillins or cephalosporins.

Third-generation cephalosporins were developed to circumvent β-lactam hydrolysis, but *Enterobacteriaceae* that produce extended-spectrum β-lactamases (ESBL) have emerged. ESBLs are a heterogenous group of enzymes encoded by plasmid-borne genes. There is no consensus on the precise definition of ESBLs. A commonly used working definition is that ESBLs are β-lactamases capable of conferring bacterial resistance to the penicillins; first-, second-, and third-generation cephalosporins; and aztreonam by hydrolysis of these antibiotics, and which are inhibited by β-lactamase inhibitors such as clavulanic acid.[1,3,12,13] The most common ESBL-producing organisms in human and veterinary medicine are strains of *E. coli, P. mirabilis,* and *K. pneumoniae.* [1,11]

Screening for ESBL-producing organisms is not challenging for microbiology laboratories, and veterinary diagnostic laboratories are encouraged to follow Clinical Laboratory Standards Institute (CLSI) guidelines.[23a]

Disk-diffusion and broth microdilution methods can be used to screen *Enterobacteriaceae* for ESBL production. Resistance to aztreonam, cefpodoxime, or ceftazidime should raise suspicion for ESBL production and is an indication that phenotypic confirmatory testing should be performed. According to CLSI guidelines, isolates with a positive confirmatory test should be reported as resistant to aztreonam, penicillins, and all cephalosporins regardless of results reported on standard antibiograms. Significantly, ESBL producing organisms exhibit co-resistance to many other classes, including aminoglycosides, chloramphenicol, sulfonamides, tetracyclines, and fluoroquinolones, often resulting in limited therapeutic options.[2,4] Although increased carbapenem use is associated with the development of resistant strains of bacteria, carbapenems are the treatment of choice for serious infections due to ESBL-producing organisms.[3,11,12,17] Accordingly, empiric prescription of carbapenems for non–life-threatening infection is discouraged. Combinations of β-lactams and β-lactamase inhibitors may represent an alternative for treating infections resulting from susceptible ESBL-producing *Enterobacteriaceae* in dogs and cats. There may be poor correlation with susceptibility results when routine published break points are applied to ESBL-producing bacteria; thus veterinarians should ensure that their microbiology laboratory of choice is performing to the standards put forward by the CLSI subcommittee on veterinary susceptibility testing (VAST) to limit therapeutic failures in their patients.

Implanted materials have significant potential for incurring biofilm infection with gram-negative pathogens.[14] Biofilms are antibiotic-resistant colonizations of bacteria that attach to surfaces and form a slimelike barrier that acts as a formidable defense mechanism, protecting the bacteria from eradication.[14,16] The biofilm matrix offers bacterial protection and thereby increases resistance to humoral immunologic responses and the phagocytic activity of host neutrophils and tissue macrophages.[14,16] Significantly, biofilms provide a suitable environment for the spread of resistance to several antibiotics that encode for multidrug resistance.[14,16] In addition to rational prescription of antimicrobial agents in the ICU, emphasis should be placed on adequate infection control procedures to prevent transmission among hospitalized patients. ICUs must implement a thorough disinfection protocol and have in place a means of identifying and handling patients with MDR or nosocomial infections.[2,12,14,16]

THERAPY FOR GRAM-NEGATIVE INFECTIONS

Veterinarians are faced with the dilemma of selecting an antibiotic on two occasions during life-threatening bacterial infections. Initially the clinician must prescribe empiric antimicrobial coverage when the causative pathogen and its susceptibilities are unknown. Broad-spectrum antimicrobial therapy is advocated at this time for most critically ill patients with documented or suspected bacterial infections.[9,12,14] The second decision point occurs when the causative pathogen is identified; the transition should be made to treat the patient with the most narrow-spectrum agent once the pathogen's susceptibility profile is determined. These basic tenets of pharmacotherapy are expected to reduce selective pressure for resistance to the more extended-spectrum antibiotics (see Chapter 175).[12,14] The choice of antibiotics for most serious gram-negative infections is ideally based on culture and susceptibility testing. Although therapy is not withheld until results are reported, careful sampling of representative samples (e.g., urine, blood, respiratory secretions, macerated tissue) should be performed before antimicrobial therapy is begun. Among the disadvantages of culture and susceptibility testing is the time that elapses between sample collection and pathogen identification. The utility of Gram staining in the selection of an antimicrobial should not be overlooked. Direct Gram staining of relevant fluid or tissue specimens often allows rapid confirmation of bacterial infection and aids in the initial selection of antibiotics. When slides are stained appropriately and examined promptly, gram-positive bacteria will retain crystal violet dye and stain blue, whereas gram-negative bacteria stain pink or red. Although Wright-Giemsa stain is most often used to evaluate peripheral blood smears, it can also aid in the diagnosis of bacterial infection. Giemsa-stained slides often reveal microorganisms and help classify bacteria based on morphologic characteristics. The observation of intracellular rods from an otherwise normally sterile site is supportive of infection with a gram-negative pathogen.

*References 10, 11, 14, 16, 17, 21.

Not all gram-negative infections require culture and susceptibility testing to be effectively treated. Many first-time or uncomplicated gram-negative infections in antibiotic-naïve patients are treated empirically, and are often successfully treated with amoxicillin, ampicillin, amoxicillin-clavulanic acid, or a fluoroquinolone, depending on regional resistance patterns and location of the infection. Infections in "hard to penetrate" tissues (e.g., eye, prostate, CNS), should be treated with a lipid-soluble drug such as a fluoroquinolone or trimethoprim-sulfamethoxazole (TMP-SMZ). Skin infections are commonly caused by β-lactamase producing strains of *Staphylococcus*. Thus amoxicillin-clavulanate, but not amoxicillin, would be a suitable choice in an otherwise healthy patient.

Life-threatening infections invariably require immediate and aggressive intravenous administration of antibiotics to achieve high concentrations of the drug at the site of infection. Subcutaneous or intramuscular administration of antibiotics is generally discouraged for managing infections in most critically ill patients. Parenteral antimicrobials used to treat aerobic or facultatively anaerobic gram-negative infections in dogs and cats include the cephalosporins, aminoglycosides, fluoroquinolones, and β-lactam/β-lactamase inhibitor combinations (e.g., ampicillin-sulbactam, piperacillin-tazobactam, ticarcillin-clavaulanic acid) (Table 94-1). The monobactams (aztreonam) and polymyxin (colistin) are viewed as drugs of last resort for treating MDR gram-negative pathogens. While both are life-saving drugs in human ICUs, dosing recommendations and indications for their use have not been established in veterinary medicine.

The first-generation cephalosporins (e.g., cefazolin) have a spectrum of activity that includes wild-type strains of some enteric bacteria (see Chapter 176). However, resistance among gram-negative bacteria develops easily, primarily by synthesis of β-lactamase enzymes capable of hydrolyzing the parent drug.[1,11,12] Until recently, first-generation cephalosporins were often effective for treating first-time, community-acquired skin, soft tissue, and lower urinary tract infections caused by *P. mirabilis* and *E. coli* in otherwise stable animals. However, resistance of most gram-negative enteric pathogens toward cefazolin and other members of its class has increased significantly and susceptibility is no longer predictable. Moreover, cefazolin is not active against *P. aeruginosa* or other opportunistic gram-negative organisms. Second-generation cephalosporins are characterized by enhanced activity toward *Enterobacter* spp., *Klebsiella* spp., *E. coli*, and *Proteus* spp., but they are similarly ineffective against *P. aeruginosa*. The cephamycins, cefoxitin and cefotetan, the most frequently prescribed members of this group in veterinary medicine, are very effective for most anaerobic organisms, including *Bacteroides* spp. Cefoxitin is often used to treat mixed aerobic/anaerobic infections, including abscesses and perioperative and postoperative management of intraabdominal sepsis associated with bacterial translocation or intestinal perforation. The intravenous third-generation cephalosporins (ceftriaxone, ceftazidime, and cefotaxime) are very active against most gram-negative bacteria. Cefotaxime is effective for anaerobic infections, whereas others (ceftazidime, ceftriaxone) are not. Among cephalosporins, only ceftazidime and cefepime (a fourth-generation cephalosporin) have activity against *P. aeruginosa*. There is little information on cefepime use in veterinary patients.

Table 94-1 Intravenous Antibiotics for Gram-Negative Infections in Dogs and Cats

Drug	Recommended Dosage
Amikacin	15 mg/kg IV q24h (dogs) 10 mg/kg IV q24h (cats)
Ampicillin-sulbactam	22 mg/kg IV q8h
Azithromycin	5 to 10 mg/kg IV q24h
Cefazolin	22 mg/kg IV q6-8h
Cefotaxime	25 to 50 mg/kg IV q6-8h
Cefotetan	30 mg/kg IV q8h
Cefoxitin	30 mg/kg IV q6-8h
Ceftazidime	30 mg/kg IV q6h
Enrofloxacin	15 to 20 mg/kg IV q24h (dogs) 5 mg/kg IV q24h (cats)
Gentamicin	10 mg/kg IV q24h (dogs) 6 mg/kg IV q24h (cats)
Imipenem-cilastatin	5 to10 mg/kg IV q6-8h
Meropenem	8 to 12 mg/kg IV q8-12h
Piperacillin-tazobactam	40 mg/kg IV q6h
Ticarcillin-clavulanate	50 mg/kg IV q6h
Trimethoprim-sulfamethoxazole or trimethoprim-sulfadiazine	15 to 30 mg/kg IV q12h

Despite their potential nephrotoxicity, the aminoglycosides remain the cornerstone of therapy for complicated or serious gram-negative infections. Gentamicin and amikacin are predictably effective against most gram-negative aerobic pathogens, including many MDR and nosocomial strains (see Chapter 177). Amikacin is more effective than gentamicin for many gram-negative pathogens and is used preferentially over other aminoglycosides to treat life-threatening infections with nosocomial gram-negative bacteria, including *P. aeruginosa* and many Enterobacteriaceae.[2] The prevalence of resistance remains relatively low compared with that of fluoroquinolones and cephalosporins, and emergence of resistance during treatment is uncommon. However, low-level resistance has been identified in MDR *P. aeruginosa*, *Burkholderia* spp., *Acinetobacter*, and *E. coli*.

Aminopenicillins (e.g., ampicillin and amoxicillin) are active against some gram-negative pathogens, including *Salmonella*, *Proteus*, and *E coli*. The aminopenicillins are β-lactamase susceptible and monotherapy with ampicillin or amoxicillin is inadequate for treating serious gram-negative infections. Combination with a β-lactamase inhibitor (e.g., clavulanic acid or sulbactam) broadens the spectrum to include organisms that have acquired resistance through β-lactamase production, including strains of *E. coli*, *Klebsiella*, *Proteus*, and *Bacteroides* spp. However, many pathogenic *E. coli* are no longer susceptible to amoxicillin-clavulanate. *Pseudomonas* spp. and other gram-negative organisms remain resistant. The affinity of clavulanic acid toward β-lactamases is much greater than that of sulbactum. Thus an organism resistant to amoxicillin-clavulanate is always inferred to be resistant to ampicillin-sulbactam. Ampicillin-sulbactam is available in the United States and most countries. Injectable formulations of amoxicillin-clavulanic acid are available and widely used in many countries outside the United States. The extended-spectrum penicillins, piperacillin and ticarcillin, generally have greater activity than aminopenicillins against gram-negative bacteria due to their enhanced penetration through the cell wall of susceptible pathogens. Their major advantage is their excellent activity toward *P. aeruginosa*. Like other penicillins, they contain a β-lactam ring that can be cleaved by β-lactamase enzymes. Piperacillin and ticarcillin are manufactured and sold as fixed combinations with a β-lactamase inhibitor (tazobactam and clavulanic acid, respectively) that protects the parent drugs from degradation and expands their utility. Imipenem and meropenem, members of the carbapenem class of β-lactam antibiotics, are among the most broadly active agents available against gram-positive and gram-negative bacteria.[12] As a result they are often used as "last line" agents in patients infected with highly resistant bacteria. They are prescribed for mixed bacterial infections and for organisms that are not susceptible to other antibiotics, including most nonfermenting gram-negative organisms and the Enterobacteriaceae. Meropenem is slightly more effective than imipenem against the *P. aeruginosa.* Both agents are active against almost all anaerobic bacteria, including *B. fragilis.* Imipenem administration may be associated with CNS toxicity (e.g., seizure activity). In contrast, meropenem has a greater margin of safety. In addition, meropenem is more water-soluble and thus can be administered more flexibly, as short infusions or bolus injections. Ertapenem and doripenem are newer members of this drug class approved for use in humans. Classified as a monobactam, aztreonam is a β-lactam drug with a spectrum of activity restricted to gram-negative aerobic bacteria. It has few known side effects and has been used extensively in human medicine for more than 20 years. It is often active against MDR gram-negative pathogens including nonfermenting gram-negative bacteria as well as many Enterobacteriaceae. It may be a therapeutic consideration in rare circumstances when fluoroquinolones or aminoglycosides are ineffective or relatively contraindicated. Dosages are not established in veterinary medicine, and reports of its use for managing clinical infections in dogs and cats have not been published.

The fluoroquinolones are considered "broad-spectrum" drugs when referring to their gram-negative spectrum. Organisms particularly susceptible include *Klebsiella* spp., *E. cloacae, P. mirabilis,* and *S. marcescens.* While *E. coli* and *P. aeruginosa* are included in their spectrum, fluoroquinolone-resistant strains are occasionally retrieved from critically ill animals and from pets with a history of recent antibiotic therapy. Enrofloxacin is the only approved parenteral fluoroquinolone for use in companion animals. Although it is administered intravenously to dogs and cats, enrofloxacin is licensed for intramuscular injection in dogs only (see Chapter 178). Intravenous ciprofloxacin is marketed for use in human medicine, but clinical use of this formulation has not been reported in animals. Enrofloxacin is metabolized partially to ciprofloxacin, which may account for 30% to 40% of the peak fluoroquinolone concentration.[22] Fluoroquinolones display largely concentration-dependent kill characteristics, and inappropriately low dosing of fluoroquinolones is associated with the emergence of resistant bacterial strains, particularly *P. aeruginosa.*[17,23]

Polymyxin E (colistin) is a polypeptide antibiotic (see Chapter 181). In addition to its ability to neutralize endotoxin, it is active against many gram-negative pathogens, including *P. aeruginosa, E. coli, Acinetobacter* spp., and *Stenotrophomonas maltophilia.*[23,24] Because of its nephrotoxicity, its use was abandoned as less toxic antimicrobials became available, but the emergence of MDR pathogens has prompted reevaluation of its utility in human ICUs.[7,23,24] Relevance to treatment of clinical infections in dogs or cats is not established.

Empiric recommendations for managing infections with gram-negative bacteria vary based on geography and prior exposure to antimicrobials.[2] In general, most Enterobacteriaceae are not susceptible to chloramphenicol, tetracyclines, first-generation cephalosporins, aminopenicillins, or TMP-SMZ.[2,12] Thus appropriate initial therapy for animals with first-time and non–life-threatening infections caused by gram-negative enteric organisms may include amoxicillin-clavulanate, ampicillin-sulbactam, or a fluoroquinolone. Pathogen retrieval should be initiated preferably before the first dose of antibiotic is given, but should not delay therapy in critically ill patients. Empiric antibiotic therapy must be comprehensive and cover all likely pathogens. Definitive therapy should be based on results of susceptibility testing. Pending such results, patients with life-threatening infections presumptively ascribed to *Proteus, E. coli,* or *Klebsiella* may be treated with a third-generation cephalosporin, fluoroquinolone, extended-spectrum β-lactam/β-lactamase inhibitor or amikacin.[2] *P. aeruginosa* is notorious for its intrinsic resistance to multiple antibiotics. Initial recommendations for life-threatening infections with *Pseudomonas* and other nonfermentative gram-negative bacteria include ticarcillin-clavulanic acid, as a single agent or in combination with amikacin or a fluoroquinolone. Optimal treatment with aminoglycosides and fluoroquinolones requires achieving high plasma and tissue concentrations for a successful clinical outcome. Although the fluoroquinolones are generally safer than aminoglycosides, the latter are predictably more effective for the treatment of gram-negative pathogens and less likely to contribute to antibiotic resistance.* Nosocomial, recurrent, or recalcitrant infections with *P. aeruginosa, Acinetobacter* spp., or other opportunistic pathogen suggest acquired resistance and should be aggressively treated with a combination of two antipseudomonal agents. Carbapenems and ceftazidime are stable against hydrolysis by various β-lactamases and generally kept in reserve. However, therapy with either drug should not be delayed when cultures from initial specimens grow strains that are resistant to other antibiotics or when patients are deteriorating in the face of therapy with other broad-spectrum agents. Individualization of regimens based on prior antibiotic use may reduce the risk of inadequate therapy.

The escalating number of infections caused by MDR and ESBL producing strains of *E. coli, Klebsiella,* and other Enterobacteriaceae in veterinary and human hospitals is accompanied by rising rates of antibiotic resistance. Treatment options to meet this challenge are increasingly limited. Selection of an antibiotic lacking activity against the causative organism can have dire consequences for patients and underscores the need for early, appropriate antibiotic therapy. Empiric combination therapy with two drugs directed at gram-negative pathogens is a logical approach when selecting therapy for critically ill animals, particularly when there are risk factors for acquiring MDR organisms (e.g., prior antibiotic therapy, extended hospitalization, wounds, invasive devices or procedures such as mechanical ventilation, urinary catheters, or surgery). Combination therapy is also indicated for mixed infections or those of unknown etiology to ensure coverage of gram-positive and anaerobic pathogens. Ultimately, the clinical utility of combination therapy rests on reducing the likelihood of inappropriate treatment or microbiologic failure. There is, however, considerable debate over the role of monotherapy versus combination therapy when treating gram-negative infections, particularly those caused by *P. aeruginosa, A. baumannii,* and MDR Enterobacteriaceae.[1,11,12,21] Combination therapy has several theoretic advantages, including *in vitro* bacterial killing superior to the simple additive activity of each antibiotic alone, a phenomenon termed *synergism,* as well as reducing the emergence of subpopulations of microorganisms resistant to the antibiotics.[1,12,21] Interest in monotherapy has increased, particularly since the introduction of broad-spectrum β-lactam antibiotics effective against *P. aeruginosa.*. Although both fluoroquinolones and aminoglycosides demonstrate in vitro synergy with β-lactams, some of the proposed advantages of combining an aminoglycoside or fluoroquinolone with a broad-spectrum β-lactam agent for treating gram-negative infections are not substantiated in the clinical setting.[1,21] The importance of initial combination therapy is well established, although de-escalation to a single agent once susceptibility data are available is often recommended. Despite in vitro and animal models demonstrating a beneficial effect of continued combination therapy, convincing clinical data that demonstrate a need for combination therapy once susceptibilities are known are lacking. Similarly, superiority of combination therapy has not been prospectively examined in critically ill veterinary patients.[2,12,22]

---

*References 10, 11, 14, 16, 17, 21.

Newer classes of antimicrobial agents with activity against many MDR gram-negative pathogens include the glycylcyclines (e.g., tigecycline) and the monobactams (e.g., aztreonam) (see Chapter 181). To curtail the development of drug resistance among small animal patients, veterinarians are cautioned against prescribing these agents. If existing antibiotics are used appropriately for gram-negative bacteria, veterinarians may be able to avoid the expense of newer and highly valuable antimicrobials developed for use in humans. Consultation with a pharmacologist or veterinary microbiologist is recommended before concluding that a dog or cat requires therapy with these agents.

REFERENCES

1. Boyd N, Nailor MD: Combination antibiotic therapy for empiric and definitive treatment of gram-negative infections: insights from the society of infectious diseases pharmacists, Pharmacotherapy 31:1073-1084, 2011.
2. Koenig A: In Infectious diseases of the dog and cat, St Louis, 2012, Elsevier Saunders, pp 349-357.
3. Giamarellou H, Poulakou G: Multidrug-resistant Gram-negative infections: what are the treatment options? Drugs 69:1879-1901, 2009.
4. Boothe D, Smaha T, Carpenter DM, et al: Antimicrobial resistance and pharmacodynamics of canine and feline pathogenic *E. coli* in the United States, J Am Anim Hosp Assoc 48:379-389, 2012.
5. Quinn PJ, et al: Veterinary microbiology and microbial disease, Chichester, West Sussex, UK, 2012, Wiley-Blackwell.
6. Hirsch DC, MacLachlan NJ: Veterinary microbiology, Ames, Iowa, 2004, Blackwell.
7. Şentürk S: Evaluation of the anti-endotoxic effects of polymyxin-E (colistin) in dogs with naturally occurred endotoxic shock, J Vet Pharmacol Ther 28:57-63, 2005.
8. Llewelyn M, Cohen J: New insights into the pathogenesis and therapy of sepsis and septic shock, Curr Clin Top Infect Dis 21:148-171, 2001.
9. Silverstein D, Otto CM: In Infectious diseases of the dog and cat, St Louis, 2012, Elsevier Saunders, pp 369-368.
10. Winn WC, Janda WM, Woods GL: Koneman's color atlas and textbook of diagnostic microbiology, Philadelphia, 2006, Lippincott Williams and Wilkins.
11. Slama TG: Gram-negative antibiotic resistance: there is a price to pay, Crit Care 12:S4, 2008.
12. Boothe DM, Greene CE: In Infectious diseases of the dog and cat, St Louis, 2012, Elsevier Saunders, pp 291-302.
13. Savard P, Perl TM: A call for action: managing the emergence of multidrug-resistant Enterobacteriaceae in the acute care settings, Curr Opin Infect Dis 25:371-377, 2012.
14. Ogeer-Gyles JS, Mathews KA, Boerlin P: Nosocomial infections and antimicrobial resistance in critical care medicine, J Vet Emerg Crit Care 16:1-18, 2006.
15. Greene CE: In Infectious diseases of the dog and cat, pp 383-388, St Louis, 2012, Elsevier Saunders, pp 383-388.
16. Greene CE, Weese JS, Calpin JP: In Infectious diseases of the dog and cat, St Louis, 2012, Elsevier Saunders, pp 1085-1095.
17. McGowan Jr JE: Resistance in nonfermenting gram-negative bacteria: multidrug resistance to the maximum, Am J Infect Control 34:S29-S37, 2006.
18. Šeol B, Naglić T, Madić J, Bedeković M: In vitro antimicrobial susceptibility of 183 Pseudomonas aeruginosa strains isolated from dogs to selected antipseudomonal agents, J Vet Med B 49:188-192, 2002.
19. Burgess DS, Nathisuwan S: Cefepime, piperacillin/tazobactam, gentamicin, ciprofloxacin, and levofloxacin alone and in combination against *Pseudomonas aeruginosa*, Diagn Microbiol Infect Dis 44:35-41, 2002.
20. Francey T, Gaschen F, Nicolet J, Burnens AP: The role of *Acinetobacter baumannii* as a nosocomial pathogen for dogs and cats in an intensive care unit, J Vet Intern Med 14:177-183, 2000.
21. Kollef MH: Gram-negative bacterial resistance: evolving patterns and treatment paradigms, Clin Infect Dis 40(suppl 2):S85-88, 2005.
22. Boothe DM, Boeckh AI, Simpson RB, Dubose K: Comparison of pharmacodynamic and pharmacokinetic indices of efficacy for 5 fluoroquinolones toward pathogens of dogs and cats, J Vet Intern Med 20:1297-1306, 2006.
23. Roberts JA, Lipman J: Pharmacokinetic issues for antibiotics in the critically ill patient, Crit Care Med 2009.

23a. Performance Standards for Antimicrobial Disk and Dilution Susceptibility Tests for Bacteria Isolated From Animals; Approved Standard-Fourth Edition and Supplement. CLSI document Vet01A4 and Vet01S2, Wayne, PA, 2012, Clinical and Laboratory Standards Institute.

24. Nation RL, Li J: Colistin in the 21st century, Curr Opin Infect Dis 22:535, 2009.

CHAPTER 95

FUNGAL INFECTIONS

Marie E. Kerl, DVM, MPH, DACVIM, DACVECC

KEY POINTS

- Fungal infections typically are slowly progressive diseases; however, respiratory, ocular, and gastrointestinal involvement can cause an emergency situation.
- Diagnosis is made most commonly with direct visualization of fungal organisms.
- Treatment includes antifungal drug therapy and supportive measures for specific organ involvement.

Systemic fungal infections cause significant morbidity and mortality in dogs and cats in most regions of the United States. These pathogens gain entry through a single portal and disseminate to affect multiple body systems. Although affected individuals frequently present with chronic illness, fungal infections can precipitate emergency presentations for acute respiratory distress, severe gastrointestinal (GI) disease, central nervous system (CNS) disease, or acute blindness. This chapter focuses on clinical signs, diagnosis, and prognosis of the most common systemic mycoses of dogs and cats, including blastomycosis, histoplasmosis, coccidiomycosis, and cryptococcosis, and addresses treatment of fungal infections.

BLASTOMYCOSIS

Blastomycosis is caused by infection with fungal spores of *Blastomyces dermatitidis,* most commonly via inhalation and respiratory colonization. Environmental conditions favoring fungal growth include moist, acidic soil with decaying vegetation or animal feces. Geographic regions with the greatest prevalence of blastomycosis include the Mississippi, Missouri, and Ohio River valleys and the Great Lakes areas of the United States and Canada.[1]

Infection typically occurs when an animal inhales conidiophores from the environment, but inoculation by penetration can cause localized disease. Dogs are affected more commonly than cats.[1,2] After inhalation, infective conidia are phagocytized by macrophages and transformed to the thick-walled yeast phase (8 to 12 μm) that bud to form daughter cells with broad-based attachments (Figure 95-1, *A*). Yeast may produce a localized infection or may disseminate to distant sites.[1]

Clinical Signs

Affected dogs are typically young adult, large breed, and of either gender.[3] Clinical signs develop weeks to months after exposure to the organism and include anorexia, depression, lethargy, weight loss, cachexia, and fever. Physical examination findings include respiratory signs (tachypnea, dyspnea, cyanosis, respiratory distress, pulmonary thromboembolism), lymphadenopathy, ocular changes (uveitis, retinal detachment, secondary glaucoma), dermal nodules, bone lesions, and CNS abnormalities.[1,3-5] Pyogranulomatous inflammation occurs as a result of stimulation of cell-mediated immunity.

Blastomycosis is an uncommon fungal disease in cats.[2] Clinical signs are similar to those in dogs and include respiratory signs (dyspnea, increased bronchovesicular signs), weight loss, ocular manifestation, draining skin lesions, CNS disease, and dermal abscesses.[2,6]

Diagnosis

Complete blood count (CBC) may reveal mild nonregenerative anemia, mature neutrophilia, or neutrophilia with left shift. Possible abnormalities on serum biochemical profile include hypoalbuminemia, hyperglobulinemia, and hypercalcemia.[1,3] Thoracic radiographs reveal a diffuse or nodular interstitial pattern, alveolar infiltrates, hilar lymphadenopathy, or a combination of these in 70% of cases.[5] Bone involvement most commonly affects the appendicular skeleton. Radiographic lesions (osteolysis with periosteal proliferation and soft tissue swelling) are similar to those seen in primary osteosarcoma.[1,3]

The most straightforward method of diagnosis is to identify the characteristic thick-walled, budding organisms retrieved from affected sites. The site of involvement dictates the method of sampling. Aspirating affected lymph nodes, dermal lesions, and/or eyes (vitreous) yields organisms reliably. Lung aspirate, tracheal wash, and bronchoalveolar lavage (BAL) are frequently nondiagnostic because of the interstitial location of the organisms.[1,3] Culture is unnecessary if cytologic or histopathologic examination demonstrates characteristic organisms. Caution should be exercised when handling infected tissues because the yeast form is infective to humans.[1]

Serologic testing should be considered when multiple attempts to identify the organism have failed. Agar gel immunodiffusion (AGID) is the serologic test that historically has been reported to identify antibodies to *Blastomyces* organisms, with sensitivity reported to be 41% to 90%, and specificity of 90% to 100%.[7,8] AGID is often negative early in the course of disease and may remain positive even with clinical resolution of disease. AGID in cats is unrewarding.

Antigen testing for *Blastomyces dermatitidis* has replaced AGID antibody detection as the serologic test of choice (MiraVista Diagnostics, Indianapolis, IN).[9] This test in an enzyme immunoassay that can be performed on serum or urine from affected dogs, has greater sensitivity (serum sensitivity 87%, urine sensitivity 93%) than antibody testing, and has a low rate of false-positive results in uninfected dogs.[9] There is cross-reactivity of the antigen test between *Histoplasma* and *Blastomyces* spp. Serial monitoring of the urine antigen test may be helpful to monitor response to treatment.[9]

Prognosis

The prognosis of a patient with blastomycosis is generally good unless there is CNS or severe pulmonary involvement.[1] Approximately 70% to 75% of dogs receiving antifungal therapy survive.

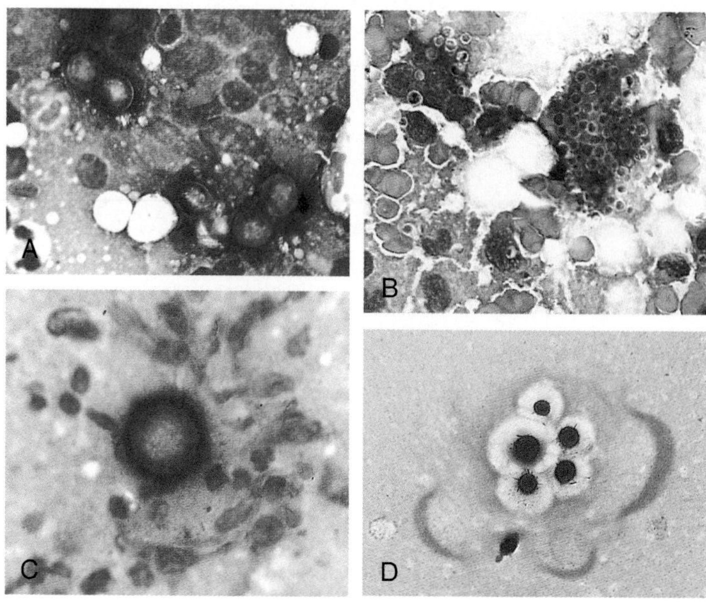

FIGURE 95-1 Microscopic appearance of common systemic fungal organisms. **A,** *Blastomyces* spp. **B,** *Histoplasma* spp. **C,** *Coccidioides* spp. **D,** *Cryptococcus* spp.

Dogs with severe respiratory infections or multiple body system involvement are more likely to die within the first week of therapy. Brain involvement is associated significantly with treatment failure. Most animals that die during or soon after treatment do so because of the subsequent inflammatory response associated with sudden death of many fungal organisms.

HISTOPLASMOSIS

Histoplasmosis is caused by infection with the soil-borne, dimorphic fungus *Histoplasma capsulatum.* This organism survives wide temperature variations. Moist soil containing bird or bat waste favors growth. Regions of the United States with greatest prevalence are the Ohio, Missouri, and Mississippi river valleys.[10-12]

Soil contaminated with *H. capsulatum* contains free-living microconidia (2 to 5 μm) or macroconidia (5 to 18 μm) that cause mammalian infection. Route of entry is typically respiratory. Oral exposure may occur because some animals have only GI signs; however, experimental studies have failed to produce gastrointestinal histoplasmosis after oral administration of the organism.[12] Dissemination occurs to any organ. Lungs, GI tract, lymph nodes, spleen, liver, bone marrow, eyes, and adrenal glands are affected most commonly. The incubation period is 12 to 16 days in dogs, but clinical signs may be absent or insidious.[12] Exposure to highly contaminated environments may cause point-source outbreaks in dogs and humans. Cats and dogs are equally likely to develop histoplasmosis.[12] Histoplasmosis has been reported in dogs and cats from nonendemic regions.[13,14]

Clinical Signs

Most affected dogs are large breed, young adults. Males are slightly predisposed, and hunting breeds are overrepresented.[11,12] Disseminated histoplasmosis with GI involvement accounts for most clinical presentations.[12] GI signs include small and large intestinal diarrhea, weight loss, hypoalbuminemia, intestinal bleeding (melena or hematochezia), and tenesmus. Hepatosplenomegaly occurs in up to 50% of dogs. Coughing, tachypnea, dyspnea, or pleural effusion occurs with pulmonary involvement. Less specific findings include fever, anorexia, and depression. In contrast to blastomycosis, histoplasmosis is associated less frequently with bone, ocular, or dermal lesions.[12]

Cats with histoplasmosis have slightly different clinical signs than dogs. In a recent retrospective case series, median age of affected cats was 9 years, and females were overrepresented.[15] This is in contrast to prior case series reporting that younger cats were affected more commonly and no breed or gender predilection.[12,16] Clinical signs include weakness, lymphadenopathy, weight loss, and anorexia, and anemia. Specific GI signs are identified less commonly than in dogs. Pulmonary involvement results in dyspnea, tachypnea, and abnormal lung sounds. Lymphadenopathy and hepatosplenomegaly occur with dissemination. Bone marrow involvement can cause various blood cell deficiencies. Dermal, ocular, urinary, and oral lesions also occur.[15,17]

Diagnosis

No pathognomonic findings on routine laboratory evaluation are consistent with histoplasmosis. Nonregenerative anemia is the most common CBC abnormality, occurring as a result of chronic inflammation, GI blood loss, and bone marrow infection.[12] Thrombocytopenia commonly occurs. Serum biochemical profile abnormalities include hypoalbuminemia, elevated hepatic enzymes and total bilirubin, and hypercalcemia.[12] Thoracic radiographs reveal diffuse or nodular interstitial infiltrates, or hilar lymphadenopathy.[12,15]

Definitive diagnosis is established by identification of *H. capsulatum* via cytology or histopathology. Organisms typically are found clustered within mononuclear phagocytes. *H. capsulatum* organisms are 2 to 4 μm in diameter, with a thin, clear halo surrounding basophilic cytoplasm (Figure 95-1, *B*). Diagnostic samples may be obtained from rectal mucosal scraping, lymph node aspirate, dermal nodule cytology, fluid analysis, bone marrow, liver or splenic aspirate, or BAL.[12]

Serologic tests to diagnose histoplasmosis are unreliable; false-negative results occur in active disease and false-positive results occur in animals without active disease. Serum antibody testing (AGID, complement fixation) is available for identification of histoplasmosis in companion animals; however, results are unreliable, with frequent false-positive and false-negative results.[18] Antigen detection testing is available for humans (MiraVista Diagnostics, Indianapolis, IN).[12] This assay detects cell wall galactomannan antigen in blood, urine, or other body fluid and has demonstrated diagnostic accuracy in human beings. A recent report in cats evaluated performance of urine antigen assay for *H. capsulatum* compared with cytologic or histologic diagnosis and found that antigen testing correctly identified 17 of 18 cats with histoplasmosis.[19] The blastomycosis antigen test is cross-reactive with histoplasmosis.[9]

Prognosis

In the author's experience, prognosis is guarded to good, depending on the nature of systemic involvement of organ systems and response to antifungal therapy. In case series of cats treated with itraconazole or fluconazole, survival to discharge or clinical resolution of disease was 55% to 66%. Treatment with itraconazole or fluconazole appears to result in similar outcomes.[14]

COCCIDIOIDOMYCOSIS

Coccidioidomycosis is a systemic fungal infection caused by *Coccidioides immitis,* a soil saprophyte that grows in semiarid conditions (Figure 95-1, *C*). Growth of *C. immitis* is limited to the southwestern United States, Mexico, and Central and South America.[20] In the environment, *C. immitis* grows as a mycelium with thick-walled, barrel-shaped arthroconidia, 2 to 4 μm wide and 3 to 10 μm long. After exposure by inhalation, the arthroconidia form a spherule 20 to 200 μm in diameter. The disease has been reported in most mammals, but dogs are infected more frequently than cats.[20]

Exposure and infection occur via the respiratory route. Inhaled arthrospores migrate through the pleural tissue to the subpleural space.[20] The incubation period ranges from 1 to 3 weeks in dogs. An intense inflammatory response develops, causing clinical respiratory signs. If dissemination occurs, involvement of other organ systems includes bones, eyes, heart, pericardium, testicles, brain, spinal cord, and visceral organs.[20]

Clinical Signs

Young adult, large breed outdoor dogs are predisposed to these infections. Clinical signs primarily occur in the respiratory system and may be unapparent after exposure. In animals with ineffective immunity, signs become severe. Chronic cough is the most common initial complaint. Fever, weight loss, and anorexia are also common.[20] Bone involvement occurs in 65% of dogs, sometimes causing draining skin nodules over bone lesions. Myocardial or pericardial infection causes cardiac arrhythmias, heart-base masses, or restrictive pericarditis.[20,21] CNS signs include seizures, behavior change, or coma. Ocular involvement is less common with coccidiomycosis than with other systemic fungal infections.[4]

Cats are resistant to coccidioidomycosis compared with dogs.[22] No obvious age, breed, or gender predilection exists. Skin lesions from dermal inoculation with fungus are the most common manifestation. Lesions may form masses or be associated with abscess formation and drainage.[22] Fever, inappetence, and weight loss commonly occur in affected cats. Respiratory signs occur in only 25% of affected cats.[22] Ocular involvement has been reported in cats. Clinical signs include conjunctival masses and fluid-filled periorbital swellings, chorioretinitis, uveitis, and retinal detachment.[23]

Diagnosis

Changes on CBC include normocytic, normochromic, nonregenerative anemia, neutrophilia with left shift, and monocytosis. Serum biochemical profile commonly reveals hypoalbuminemia and hyperglobulinemia, hepatic transaminases elevation, and azotemia. Hypercalcemia can occur.

Thoracic radiographs reveal a diffuse interstitial or peribronchial pattern, frequently with hilar lymphadenopathy. Alveolar infiltrate can occur. Pleural involvement includes pleural thickening, effusion, and fibrosis. Hypertrophic osteopathy has been reported with pulmonary involvement.[20]

Demonstration of organisms provides a conclusive diagnosis for coccidioidomycosis. Locating organisms is often difficult because of relatively low organism numbers and difficulty obtaining samples from inaccessible locations.[20] Fungal culture is not clinically useful, because definitive identification requires inoculation into animals to induce spherule formation.

Serologic diagnosis of coccidioidomycosis often is used when organisms are not found. A variety of serologic tests may be used to detect immunoglobulin M and immunoglobulin G antibodies. Serologic testing should be interpreted in light of signs consistent with active infection to confirm diagnosis. Obtaining negative serologic results in affected animals is possible. Repeat testing in 2 to 4 weeks to demonstrate increasing titer is warranted in questionable cases.[20] Although galactomannan antigen testing has demonstrated usefulness in diagnosing other systemic fungal infections and coccidioidomycosis in human cases, urine or serum antigen testing for coccidioidomycosis has shown poor sensitivity and specificity in dogs with clinical suspicion and positive antibody test results.[24] This difference between coccidioidomycosis and other fungal antigen testing in dogs may be due to the comparatively low numbers of *Coccidioides* organisms present in canine infections compared with people.[24]

Prognosis

Coccidioidomycosis remains a challenge to diagnose and treat, and it is difficult to cure compared with other systemic mycoses. Localized respiratory infections may resolve spontaneously and generally carry a good prognosis. Disseminated infections result in death if not treated. An overall recovery rate of 60% has been noted with ketoconazole therapy; however, multiple bone or CNS involvement carries a worse prognosis.[20]

CRYPTOCOCCOSIS

Cryptococcosis is caused by a variety of species of *Cryptococcus; Cryptococcus neoformans* and *Cryptococcus gatti* are the most clinically significant because they thrive at mammalian body temperature.[25,26] *Cryptococcus* is a saprophytic, round, yeast-like fungus 3.5 to 7 μm in diameter, with a capsule of 1 to 30 μm that does not take up cytologic stains.[25] *Cryptococcus* spp. reproduce by budding from the parent cell. Buds can break off at different stages of growth, resulting in size variation of organisms (Figure 95-1, *D*). Environmental sources are near avian habitats or in litter of eucalyptus trees. Cryptococcosis does not occur in a defined geographic region.[25]

Cryptococcosis occurs with greater frequency in cats than in dogs.[25] The most likely route for infection is the respiratory tract. *Cryptococcus* spp. are unencapsulated in the environment and may be as small as 1 μm, enhancing respiratory colonization. After tissue deposition, organisms colonize either the upper or lower respiratory tract and regenerate their capsules. The capsule prevents normal host immune response and organism elimination. CNS involvement is common in cats and dogs and may occur as a result of extension from nasal cavity disease.[25-29]

Clinical Signs

Cryptococcosis is the most common systemic fungal infection of cats. There is no obvious gender predilection, and age range of infection is broad.[25] Upper respiratory infection is evident in 50% to 60% of cases.[26] Clinical signs include nasal or facial deformity, mass protruding from nares, nasal discharge, skin lesions, sneezing, respiratory noise, or change of voice. Ocular and CNS signs occur in approximately 15% of cases. Ocular signs consist of blindness resulting from retinal detachment and granulomatous chorioretinitis.[30] Neurologic signs include depression, temperament changes, ataxia, vestibular signs, and blindness.[25,31]

Affected dogs are generally less than 4 years of age. Great Danes, Doberman Pinschers, Labrador Retrievers, and American Cocker Spaniels are overrepresented.[25] Clinical signs most often are localized to the CNS, with seizure, ataxia, central vestibular disease, papilledema, cervical pain, tetraparesis, or multifocal cranial nerve involvement.[28] Dogs also may have ocular lesions to include granulomatous chorioretinitis, retinal hemorrhage, and optic neuritis.[4]

Diagnosis

Results of CBC and serum biochemical profile are usually unremarkable. Thoracic radiographs occasionally reveal nodular interstitial infiltrates, hilar lymphadenopathy, or pleural effusion. Skull radiographs or computed tomography can demonstrate nasal bone destruction and soft tissue swelling.[25] With CNS involvement, cerebrospinal fluid commonly exhibits increased protein and mixed mononuclear and neutrophilic pleocytosis.[28]

The most reliable method to diagnose cryptococcosis is direct organism visualization on cytologic or histopathologic evaluation (see Figure 95-1, *D*). Cytologic examination may be performed on nasal discharge, skin exudates, cerebrospinal fluid, tissue aspirate, or samples obtained by ocular paracentesis. Dogs may have subclinical renal infection; therefore microscopic evaluation of urine sediment is warranted. Wright stain may cause some distortion of *Cryptococcus* spp. and Gram stain may facilitate visualization.

Serologic testing is available and useful to aid diagnosis. Recommended testing consists of latex agglutination testing to identify capsular antigen. Antigen testing is considered positive at a titer of 1:16 or greater. Response to treatment is correlated with declining titer results. Testing cerebrospinal fluid for cryptococcal antigen can confirm diagnosis with CNS involvement when the organism cannot be visualized.[27] Histopathology of affected tissue is indicated if cytology results are negative; however, impression smears always should be made of biopsy samples because of the comparative ease of cytologic diagnosis. Histopathologically, the large capsule differentiates *Cryptococcus* spp. from *Blastomyces* spp., and budding and lack of endospores differentiate it from *Coccidioides immitis.* Fungal isolation is not clinically useful because of prolonged growing time.

Prognosis

Cats have a good prognosis when disease occurs outside of the CNS.[27] Progressive decrease of antigen titer by tenfold over 2 months has been associated with favorable prognosis in cats. Dogs with any form of disease, and cats with CNS disease, have a guarded prognosis.[27] In cats, concurrent feline leukemia virus and feline immunodeficiency virus infections decrease response to treatment.

TREATMENT

In general, treatment for fungal infections can be separated into definitive antifungal therapy for long-term control or cure of the disease and supportive care to minimize the acute signs associated with specific organ involvement. There are a limited number of antifungal drugs and treatment regimens, which are discussed in detail in Chapter 180.

Respiratory Supportive Therapy

Respiratory decompensation is the most common reason for emergency presentation of fungal disease. Although any fungal organism can cause respiratory infection, blastomycosis is the most common pulmonary fungal pathogen, followed by coccidioidomycosis and histoplasmosis. Supportive therapy for hypoxemic patients includes supplemental oxygen. Respiratory rate, effort, and oxygenation status (arterial blood gas, pulse oximetry) should be monitored as frequently as needed to address patient changes. Respiratory arrest can occur with severe infection, necessitating cardiopulmonary resuscitation and mechanical ventilation. Pulmonary thromboembolism has been reported with fungal infections and would cause acute deterioration in respiratory function. Antibiotics can be prescribed if secondary bacterial infection is suspected.[1,32] Handling should be kept to a minimum to reduce stress-induced respiratory effort. Short-term antiinflammatory glucocorticoids have been advocated for initiating antifungal chemotherapy in patients with respiratory compromise to minimize the effects of rapid fungal death and subsequent inflammatory response.[33,34]

Gastrointestinal Supportive Therapy

Histoplasmosis is the fungal pathogen that most commonly affects the GI tract, causing signs consistent with small or large bowel diarrhea. Ancillary therapy includes dietary modification and antibiotic therapy to control concurrent small intestinal bacterial overgrowth. Antidiarrheal therapy may be helpful in conjunction with antifungal therapy for symptomatic relief.[12] Loss of body condition is often dramatic as a result of prolonged anorexia, malabsorption, and malnutrition, and affected animals often are debilitated at the time of diagnosis. Partial or total parenteral nutrition support can be prescribed until normal GI function resumes. With severe intestinal disease, GI absorption of oral antifungal medications may not occur normally, causing treatment failure.

Ocular Supportive Therapy

Fungal ocular infection causes moderate to marked bilateral uveitis, with secondary glaucoma in some instances. Retinal detachment is common with fungal disease, and permanent vision loss can result. Ocular changes are associated with pain and discomfort. Ancillary therapy for uveitis or glaucoma can be prescribed, to include topical glucocorticoids and carbonic anhydrase inhibitors as needed.[4] Enucleation may be recommended in blind, painful eyes, and histopathology can be performed on the tissue for definitive diagnosis if not yet established.

Other Supportive Therapy

Orthopedic pain from bone lesions can be treated with nonsteroidal antiinflammatory medications pending resolution of infection. Dermal wounds should be shaved and kept clean and dry. Personnel who handle animals with draining wounds should exercise caution to avoid accidental infection.[35]

REFERENCES

1. Legendre AM: Blastomycosis. In Greene CE: Infectious disease of the dog and cat, ed 4, St Louis, 2012, Elsevier.
2. Miller PE, Miller LM, Schoster JV: Feline blastomycosis: a report of three cases and literature review (1961-1988), J Am Anim Hosp Assoc 26:417, 1990.
3. Arceneaux KA, Taboada J, Hosgood G: Blastomycosis in dogs: 115 cases (1980-1995), J Am Vet Med Assoc 213:658, 1998.
4. Krohne SG: Canine systemic fungal infections, Vet Clin North Am Small Anim Pract 30:1063, 2000.
5. Crews LJ, Feeney DA, Jessen CR, et al: Utility of diagnostic tests for and medical treatment of pulmonary blastomycosis in dogs: 125 cases (1989-2006), J Am Vet Med Assoc 232:222, 2008.
6. Gilor C, Graves TK, Barger AM, et al: Clinical aspects of natural infection with Blastomyces dermatitidis in cats: 8 cases (1991-2005), J Am Vet Med Assoc 229:96, 2006.
7. Legendre AM, Becker PU: Evaluation of the agar-gel immunodiffusion test in the diagnosis of canine blastomycosis, Am J Vet Res 41:2109, 1980.
8. Phillips WE Jr, Kaufman L: Cultural and histopathologic confirmation of canine blastomycosis diagnosed by an agar-gel immunodiffusion test, Am J Vet Res 41:1263, 1980.
9. Spector D, Legendre AM, Wheat J, et al: Antigen and antibody testing for the diagnosis of blastomycosis in dogs, J Vet Intern Med 22:839, 2008.
10. Clinkenbeard KD, Cowell RL, Tyler RD: Disseminated histoplasmosis in cats 12 cases 1981-1986, J Am Vet Med Assoc 190:1445, 1987.
11. Clinkenbeard KD, Cowell RL, Tyler RD: Disseminated histoplasmosis in dogs: 12 cases (1981-1986), J Am Vet Med Assoc 193:1443, 1988.
12. Brömel C, Greene CE: Histoplasmosis. In Greene CE: Infectious diseases of the dog and cat, ed 4, St Louis, 2012, Elsevier.
13. Pratt CL, Sellon RK, Spencer ES, et al: Systemic mycosis in three dogs from nonendemic regions, J Am Anim Hosp Assoc 48:411, 2012.
14. Reinhart JM, KuKanich KS, Jackson T, et al: Feline histoplasmosis: fluconazole therapy and identification of potential sources of Histoplasma species exposure, J Feline Med Surg 14:841, 2012.
15. Aulakh HK, Aulakh KS, Troy GC: Feline histoplasmosis: a retrospective study of 22 cases (1986-2009), J Am Anim Hosp Assoc 48:182, 2012.
16. Clinkenbeard KD, Wolf AM, Cowell RL, et al: Feline disseminated histoplasmosis, Comp Cont Ed Pract Vet 11:1223, 1989.
17. Taylor AR, Barr JW, Hokamp JA, et al: Cytologic diagnosis of disseminated histoplasmosis in the wall of the urinary bladder of a cat, J Am Anim Hosp Assoc 48:203, 2012.
18. Hodges RD, Legendre AM, Adams LG, et al: Itraconazole for the treatment of histoplasmosis in cats, J Vet Intern Med 8:409, 1994.
19. Cook AK, Cunningham LY, Cowell AK, et al: Clinical evaluation of urine Histoplasma capsulatum antigen measurement in cats with suspected disseminated histoplasmosis, J Feline Med Surg 14:512, 2012.
20. Greene RT: Coccidiomycosis and paracoccidiodmycosis. In Greene CE, editor: Infectious diseases of the dog and cat, ed 4, St Louis, 2012, Elsevier.
21. Ajithdoss D, Trainor K, Snyder K, et al: Coccidioidomycosis presenting as a heart base mass in two dogs, J Comp Pathol 145:132, 2011.
22. Greene RT, Troy GC: Coccidioidomycosis in 48 cats: a retrospective study (1984-1993), J Vet Intern Med 9:86, 1995.
23. Tofflemire K, Betbeze C: Three cases of feline ocular coccidioidomycosis: presentation, clinical features, diagnosis, and treatment, Vet Ophthalmol 13:166, 2010.
24. Kirsch EJ, Greene RT, Prahl A, et al: Evaluation of coccidioides antigen detection in dogs with coccidioidomycosis, Clin Vaccine Immunol 19:343, 2012.
25. Sykes JE, Malik R: Cryptococcosis. In Greene CE: Infectious diseases of the dog and cat, ed 4, St Louis, 2012, Elsevier.
26. Gerds-Grogan S, Dayrell-Hart B: Feline cryptococcosis: a retrospective evaluation, J Am Anim Hosp Assoc 33:118, 1997.
27. Berthelin CF, Bailey CS, Kass PH, et al: Cryptococcosis of the nervous system in dogs, 1. Epidemiologic, clinical, nad neruopathological features, Prog Vet Neurol 5:88, 1994.
28. Berthelin CF, Legendre AM, Bailey CS, et al: Cryptococcosis of the nervous system in dogs, 2. Diagnosis, treatment, monitoring, and prognosis, Prog Vet Neurol 5:136, 1994.

29. Tiches D, Vite CH, Dayrell-Hart B, et al: A case of canine central nervous system cryptococcosis: management with fluconazole, J Am Anim Hosp Assoc 34:145, 1998.
30. Gionfriddo JR: Feline systemic fungal infections, Vet Clin North Am Small Anim Pract 30:1029, 2000.
31. Beatty JA, Barrs VR, Swinney GR, et al: Peripheral vestibular disease associated with cryptococcosis in three cats, J Feline Med Surg 2:29, 2000.
32. Greene CE: Antifungal chemotherapy. In Greene CE: Infectious diseases of the dog and cat, ed 4, St Louis, 2012, Elsevier.
33. Legendre AM, Toal RL: Diagnosis and treatment of fungal diseases of the respiratory system. In Bonagura JD: Kirk's current veterinary XIII small animal practice, Philadelphia, 2000, WB Saunders.
34. Schulman RL, McKiernan BC, Schaeffer DJ: Use of corticosteroids for treating dogs with airway obstruction secondary to hilar lymphadenopathy caused by chronic histoplasmosis: 16 cases (1979-1997), J Am Vet Med Assoc 214:1345, 1999.
35. Cote E, Barr SC, Allen C: Possible transmission of Blastomycosis dermatitidis via culture specimen, J Am Vet Med Assoc 210:479, 1997.

CHAPTER 96

VIRAL INFECTIONS

Jane E. Sykes, BVSc(Hons), PhD, DACVIM

KEY POINTS

- A number of viral infections may be associated with acute and severe illness, leading to presentation of affected dogs and cats to emergency and critical care veterinarians.
- Treatment of viral infections is generally supportive and includes intravenous fluid therapy, early nutrition, antiemetic therapy, supplemental oxygen therapy, and antibiotics for secondary bacterial infections. Hospitalization in isolation may be required.
- The feline leukemia virus and feline immunodeficiency virus status of all cats should be known.
- The use of antiviral medications is limited, and few controlled studies evaluate their effectiveness in dogs and cats. Famciclovir can be effective for treatment of severe infections by feline herpesvirus 1.
- The range of diagnostic tests for viral infections in dogs and cats has increased with the availability of nucleic acid–based assays, such as the polymerase chain reaction (PCR). Quality control for PCR assays can be problematic. The use of laboratories that perform real-time (fluorogenic) PCR and that include a quality assurance program can lessen the chance of false-positive results.

A large number of viruses can cause acute and severe illness in dogs and cats (Table 96-1). The most common or important viral infections that may come to the attention of emergency and critical care veterinarians are canine parvovirus (CPV), canine distemper virus (CDV), canine influenza virus (CIV), feline panleukopenia virus, feline herpesvirus 1 (FHV-1), feline calicivirus (FCV), feline infectious peritonitis virus (FIPV), feline immunodeficiency virus (FIV), feline leukemia virus (FeLV), and rabies virus infection. The FIV and FeLV status of all cats should be determined on arrival by questioning the owner or testing using in-house enzyme-linked immunosorbent assays for FeLV antigen and FIV antibody. Because cats may be infected subclinically by these viruses and because some cats subsequently undergo regressive FeLV infections, positive test results alone are not reason for euthanasia. CPV infection is covered in the following chapter. Other viral diseases that may present to emergency and critical care veterinarians include enteric viral infections such as rotavirus and coronavirus infections, feline paramyxovirus infection, pseudorabies virus infection, vector-borne viral infections such as West Nile virus infection, infectious canine viral hepatitis, and canine herpesvirus infection.

An extensive discussion of the etiology, clinical signs, diagnosis, treatment, and prevention of every one of these infections is beyond the scope of this chapter. Instead, the purpose of this chapter is to provide the reader with an update on selected common and important viral infections in dogs and cats that may be evaluated by emergency and critical care veterinarians. Treatment of viral infections is largely supportive and usually includes intravenous fluid therapy, early enteral or parenteral nutrition, antiemetics, analgesia, and oxygen therapy when pulmonary disease is present. Blood products may be needed for cats with retroviral infections. Antibiotics may be needed for secondary bacterial infections. Attempts to culture secondary bacterial invaders and determine sensitivity to antimicrobial agents should be considered before commencing antimicrobial therapy. Use of antiviral medications is still limited in dogs and cats, but famciclovir can be effective for treatment of severe infections with feline herpesvirus 1.

CANINE DISTEMPER VIRUS INFECTION

CDV infection is a contagious disease of dogs that may involve the gastrointestinal (GI), respiratory, or neurologic systems. Distemper still occurs sporadically, even in vaccinated dog populations. Disease most commonly occurs in dogs 3 to 6 months of age, when maternal antibody level is declining, but can occur in older dogs that have been vaccinated infrequently or improperly, especially after stress, immunosuppression, or contact with other affected dogs.[1]

CDV is an enveloped ribonucleic acid (RNA) virus that belongs to the family Paramyxoviridae. The virus survives for about 3 hours at room temperature and is highly susceptible to routine hospital disinfectants such as quaternary ammonium compounds. Several strains of CDV exist and vary in pathogenicity. Some, such as the Snyder Hill strain, are more likely to produce neurologic disease than others. A study has documented the existence of CDV strains that differ from vaccine strains and from those previously documented in the United States.[2]

Table 96-1 **Viral Infections to Be Included on the List of Differential Diagnosis in Dogs and Cats with Respiratory, Gastrointestinal, or Neurologic Symptoms**

	Affected Body System		
Species	**Respiratory**	**Gastrointestinal**	**Neurologic**
Dog	Canine distemper Influenza viruses Canine parainfluenza Canine adenovirus Canine herpesvirus Canine respiratory coronavirus Possibly other viruses such as canine pneumovirus	Canine distemper Canine parvovirus Canine enteric coronavirus Rotaviruses, astroviruses, adenoviruses, caliciviruses, and several other novel viruses such as norovirus	Canine distemper Rabies Arthropod-borne infections (togaviruses, bunyaviruses, and flaviviruses)*
Cat	Feline calicivirus Feline herpesvirus Feline infectious peritonitis Influenza viruses Retroviruses†	Feline panleukopenia Feline coronavirus Rotavirus Retroviruses[1]	Feline panleukopenia Feline infectious peritonitis Rabies FIV Retroviruses† Paramyxoviruses

FIV, Feline immunodeficiency virus.
*These also have the potential to cause disease in cats, but disease has been reported more often in dogs. Most animals are infected subclinically.
†Feline retrovirus infections also may be associated with these signs through induction of neoplastic disease or secondary infections resulting from immunosuppression.

CDV is shed in respiratory secretions for up to 90 days after infection. Initial replication of CDV is in lymphoid tissue, and viral destruction of lymphocytes results in lymphopenia and pyrexia. Approximately 1 week after infection the virus spreads to epithelial tissues (lungs, GI tract, kidney, bladder) and the central nervous system (CNS), and virus shedding begins. Poor cell-mediated immunity (CMI) is associated with spread of the virus to a variety of tissues, severe respiratory and GI signs with or without CNS involvement, and death. Dogs with an intermediate or delayed CMI response may develop persistent infection of the uvea, CNS, and footpad and nasal epithelium, leading to neurologic, cutaneous (hard pad), and ocular signs such as chorioretinitis. Infection with CDV is highly immunosuppressive, and secondary infections with opportunistic pathogens such as *Nocardia* and *Salmonella* spp. may occur.

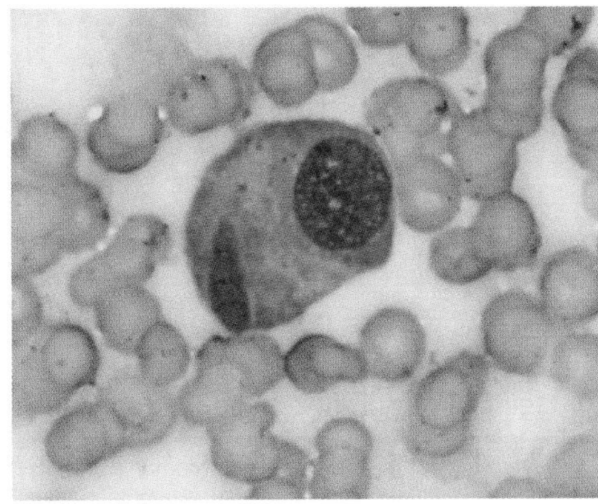

FIGURE 96-1 Distemper virus inclusion within the cytoplasm of a conjunctival epithelial cell. Diff-Quik stain.

Distemper should be high on the list of differential diagnoses for any dog with respiratory and/or CNS signs. Mild signs are common and resemble those of kennel cough. Severe, generalized distemper may begin with a serous to mucopurulent conjunctivitis and rhinitis and progress to include signs of lower respiratory disease, lethargy, anorexia, vomiting and diarrhea, severe dehydration, and death. Neurologic signs then occur in some dogs, either with systemic illness or after a several-week delay. Neurologic signs are frequently progressive despite treatment and are a poor prognostic sign. Myoclonus, an involuntary twitching of various muscle groups, can be most pronounced when affected dogs are at rest and is virtually pathognomonic for CDV infection. Ocular signs may consist of sudden blindness resulting from optic neuritis, chorioretinitis, or retinal detachment. Cutaneous signs may be useful for prognostication. Footpad and nasal hyperkeratosis often are accompanied by neurologic complications, whereas the presence of vesicular and pustular dermatitis implies a good CMI response and rarely is associated with neurologic complications.

Physical examination of dogs suspected to have distemper should include a fundic examination, careful inspection of the skin, including the nose and footpads, and careful thoracic auscultation. Any dog suspected to have distemper should be placed in isolation if possible. This may be complicated by a requirement for oxygen therapy.

The most commonly used diagnostic test for distemper is cytologic examination of conjunctival scrapings. Acutely, these may show cytoplasmic inclusions in epithelial cells when stained with Wright or Diff-Quik stain (Figure 96-1). The sensitivity of cytology is increased after application of immunofluorescent antibody to smears by regional diagnostic laboratories. Smears should be air dried and, if possible, fixed in acetone for 5 minutes before transport. Intracytoplasmic inclusions also may be seen in erythrocytes, lymphocytes, other white blood cells, and cells within the cerebrospinal fluid (CSF). Thoracic radiography may reveal an interstitial pattern or an alveolar pattern with secondary bacterial bronchopneumonia. Analysis of CSF may show increased protein and cell count, and measurement of anti-CDV antibody in the CSF also can be useful for diagnosis in dogs with neurologic signs. Other antemortem diagnostic tests for distemper include immunohistochemistry for CDV antigen on biopsies of nasal mucosa, footpad epithelium, and haired skin of the dorsal neck, and reverse transcriptase–polymerase chain reaction (RT-PCR) testing for viral nucleic acid. Specimens suitable for RT-PCR testing include buffy coat cells, whole blood, serum, CSF, and urine.[3] With any PCR assay, quality control can be problematic, and the use of laboratories that perform real-time (fluorogenic) PCR and that have a quality assurance program is recommended. Virus isolation is difficult and is not used widely for diagnosis.

Attenuated live vaccines can prevent canine distemper and should provide at least partial protection even in the face of variant strains. The interested reader is referred to a comprehensive review of vaccination for CDV for further information on the topic.[1]

CANINE INFLUENZA VIRUS INFECTION

Canine influenza first appeared in racing Greyhounds in Florida between 1999 and 2003.[4] At the time of writing, evidence of CIV infection has been detected in dogs in animal shelters, adoption groups, pet stores, boarding kennels, and veterinary clinics in at least 38 U.S. states. The most significant outbreaks of disease resulting from CIV have occurred in Florida, New England, Colorado, Wyoming, and Texas. Sequence analysis has indicated that the virus isolated from dogs shares more than 96% homology with equine influenza A. All the genes from the canine isolates are of equine influenza virus origin, providing evidence that the virus crossed the species barrier. Concern has been raised by scientists that this virus also may have the potential to cross the dog-human species barrier, as occurs with avian influenza viruses. Influenza viruses are enveloped viruses that are susceptible to routine hospital disinfection practices.

Clinical signs occur 2 to 5 days after exposure to the virus. As with distemper, canine influenza virus causes a syndrome that may mimic kennel cough, although fever may be more likely to occur with influenza virus than with parainfluenza virus, adenovirus, or *Bordetella bronchiseptica* infections. Nearly 80% of exposed dogs develop clinical signs, which consist of a cough that persists for 2 to 3 weeks despite therapy, serous to mucopurulent nasal discharge, and a low-grade fever. Some dogs develop more severe pneumonia with a high fever (104° to 106° F), tachypnea, and respiratory distress. The overall mortality has been less than 5%. Shedding of virus occurs for 7 to 10 days after the onset of clinical signs.

Dogs with these signs should be placed in isolation. Findings on thoracic radiography are the same as those described above for distemper. Antemortem diagnosis of CIV infection relies on serology using hemagglutination inhibition, RT-PCR, or virus isolation. To distinguish past exposure from recent infection, serology should be performed on samples collected at the time of presentation and 2 to 3 weeks later. Because most dogs have not yet been exposed positive results in a single specimen collected 7 days after onset of clinical signs may be suggestive of current infection.

Nucleic acid testing using RT-PCR is offered by a few laboratories and can be performed on pharyngeal swab specimens. Pharyngeal swabs should be kept refrigerated and transported as soon as possible on ice to the laboratory performing nucleic acid testing. Detection of virus appears to be difficult beyond 3 to 4 days after the onset of clinical signs; the same is true for virus isolation.[5] Virus isolation and RT-PCR also can be successful when performed on lung tissue from dogs that have died within 2 to 3 days of the onset of clinical signs. Swabs for virus isolation must be placed in virus transport medium.

Treatment of serious influenza virus infection in human patients has involved use of the neuraminidase inhibitor oseltamivir phosphate, which inhibits spread of the virus from cell to cell.[6] Anecdotal reports exist regarding treatment of dogs with this drug, but no published studies are available, and nothing is known regarding the optimal dosage in dogs to inhibit viral replication. Until the results of such studies become available, use of this drug to treat dogs that have been diagnosed definitively with CIV infection is not recommended.

OTHER EMERGING RESPIRATORY VIRAL INFECTIONS OF DOGS

Other emerging respiratory viral pathogens of dogs include canine respiratory coronavirus (CRCoV), other influenza virus types, and canine pneumovirus. CRCoV was reported first in 2003 in a group of dogs with respiratory disease in a rehoming facility in England that had been vaccinated against canine adenovirus-2, CDV, and canine parainfluenza virus.[7] It is distinct from canine enteric coronavirus. Alone, CRCoV causes subclinical infections or mild respiratory disease, but like human respiratory coronaviruses, it may cause reversible damage to, or loss of, the respiratory epithelial cell cilia. As a result, infected dogs become predisposed to secondary infections. Serologic evidence of exposure to CRCoV appears to be widespread in dogs from North America, Great Britain and continental Europe, Japan, Korea and New Zealand, and the virus has been detected widely using PCR-based methods in dogs with respiratory disease from many of these countries. Canine pneumovirus is a parainfluenza virus that belongs to the genus *Pneumovirus*. It was isolated first from dogs with acute respiratory disease in shelters in the United States in 2010.[8] The extent to which this virus causes disease in dogs remains to be investigated.

FELINE PANLEUKOPENIA

Feline panleukopenia is caused by a small, single-stranded deoxyribonucleic acid (DNA) virus closely related to CPV. Cats with feline panleukopenia also may be infected with CPV strains 2a, 2b, and 2c.[9] Although most cats shed virus for just a few days after infection, it may be shed for as long as 6 weeks, and viral persistence in the environment plays an important role in disease transmission. The virus can survive for a year at room temperature on fomites and survives disinfection with routine hospital disinfectants; inactivation generally requires a 1:30 dilution of household bleach, potassium peroxymonosulfate, or concentrated accelerated hydrogen peroxide solutions.

Feline panleukopenia should be suspected in poorly vaccinated kittens with acute illness including fever, lethargy, anorexia, vomiting and, less commonly, diarrhea. Oral ulceration and icterus may be noted in complicated infections. Death may result from severe dehydration, secondary bacterial infections, and disseminated intravascular coagulation. Cats between 3 and 5 months of age may be most susceptible to severe disease, which is exacerbated by concurrent gastrointestinal infections.

Cats suspected to have feline panleukopenia should be placed in isolation. Supportive treatment is similar to that recommended for CPV. Diagnosis is based on clinical signs along with the finding of leukopenia on a complete blood count. Leukopenia is not always present and may occur with other diseases such as salmonellosis. Severe panleukopenia may be associated with concurrent infection with FeLV.[10] In-house fecal enzyme-linked immunosorbent assays for CPV are suitable for diagnosis of feline panleukopenia, although false-negative results may occur, so a negative test result does not rule out feline panleukopenia. Sensitivity in one study ranged from 50% to 80% depending on the kit used, and specificity ranged from 94% to 100%. False-positive fecal antigen assay results after vaccination with attenuated live viral vaccines appear to be uncommon but vary with the test used.[11] PCR assays are also available for detection of viral DNA in fecal and tissue specimens from affected cats. Cats with panleukopenia that survive the first 5 days of treatment usually recover, although recovery is often more prolonged than it is for dogs with parvoviral enteritis. In 244 cats with feline panleukopenia from Europe, the survival rate was 51%.[12] Nonsurvivors had lower leukocyte and platelet counts than survivors, and cats with white cell counts below 1000/μl were almost twice as likely to die than those with white cell counts above 2500/μl. Only total leukopenia, and not lymphopenia, was correlated with mortality. Hypoalbuminemia and hypokalemia also were associated with an increased risk of mortality.

FELINE RESPIRATORY VIRAL DISEASE

The most common causes of feline respiratory viral disease are FHV-1 and FCV. FHV-1 is an enveloped DNA virus. It survives a maximum of 1 day at room temperature and is susceptible to destruction by common disinfectants. FCV is a nonenveloped RNA virus, which survives up to 10 days at room temperature. Inactivation requires hypochlorite solutions, concentrated accelerated hydrogen peroxide solutions, or potassium peroxymonosulfate; quaternary ammonium compounds are not effective.[13]

FHV-1 and FCV infections may be acquired by contact with acutely infected cats, contact with organisms in the environment, or by contact with carrier cats. The chance of infection is increased when large numbers of cats are housed together. Both viruses replicate mainly in the tonsils and respiratory tissues. In addition to the nasal, conjunctival, and oral shedding common to both viruses, FCV also is shed in the feces and occasionally in the urine.

Almost all cats infected with FHV-1 develop latent infections, whereby the virus persists in tissues such as the trigeminal ganglia for the life of the animal. Reactivation of virus shedding occurs in roughly 50% of infected cats, with or without concurrent clinical signs. This may occur spontaneously or after stressful events. Shedding occurs 4 to 11 days after the stress and lasts 1 to 2 weeks. In contrast, shedding of FCV by persistently infected cats is continuous and not affected by stress. In some cats, shedding is lifelong; in others, it ceases after several weeks.

Acute disease caused by FCV and FHV-1 occurs after an incubation period of 2 to 10 days. The most severe signs tend to occur in very young and elderly debilitated cats. Concurrent immunosuppressive illness or infection with other respiratory pathogens and opportunistic bacteria can influence dramatically the severity of disease. Clinical signs common to both infections include conjunctivitis, serous or mucopurulent nasal discharge and sneezing and, less commonly, coughing and dyspnea. Lethargy, anorexia, hypersalivation, and pyrexia also may be present in acute infections. FHV-1, but not FCV, may be associated with corneal ulceration and keratitis. Ulcerative glossitis is more common and severe with FCV infection but may be associated with FHV-1 infection. A small proportion of FCV carriers develop chronic lymphoplasmacytic or chronic ulceroproliferative stomatitis, which is often refractory to therapy. Transient lameness and pyrexia have been reported in association with acute FCV infection and after FCV vaccination.

Highly virulent strains of FCV have been isolated from outbreaks of severe systemic febrile illness.[14,15] This condition is characterized by a high mortality, fever, anorexia, ulcerative facial dermatitis, and diffuse cutaneous edema (Figure 96-2). Coagulopathies also can develop, along with hypoproteinemia and mild hyperbilirubinemia. The suspected or confirmed outbreaks of infection reported shared several significant features: (1) in every outbreak in which a suspected index case was identified, a hospitalized shelter cat appeared to be the source of infection, (2) otherwise healthy, adult, vaccinated cats have been affected prominently, whereas kittens tended to show less severe signs, (3) spread occurred very readily, including via fomites to cats belonging to hospital employees and clients, (4) spread of disease was limited to the affected clinic(s) or shelter, with no spread within the community reported, and (5) the outbreak resolved within approximately 2 months.[14,15]

Attempts to make a diagnosis in cases of feline respiratory viral illness are encouraged especially in catteries because knowledge of the causative organism can assist with treatment strategies. Because of the communicability and high mortality associated with virulent FCV infection, microbiologic testing is essential for cats suspected to have the systemic febrile syndrome, and suspect cats should immediately be handled as if they were infected with the organism. Infection with FCV and FHV-1 can be diagnosed using virus isolation or PCR assays from nasal, conjunctival, or oropharyngeal swabs, although oropharyngeal swabs are most likely to yield a diagnosis. For virus isolation, swabs should be transported on ice in a viral transport medium containing antibiotics to prevent bacterial overgrowth; commercial swabs are available for this purpose. PCR assays may be more reliable for diagnosis of FHV-1 than of FCV infection. However, because apparently healthy cats commonly have positive results using sensitive PCR assays for FHV-1, it may not be possible to prove an association with a particular disease.[16] Results should be interpreted carefully in light of the clinical signs present.

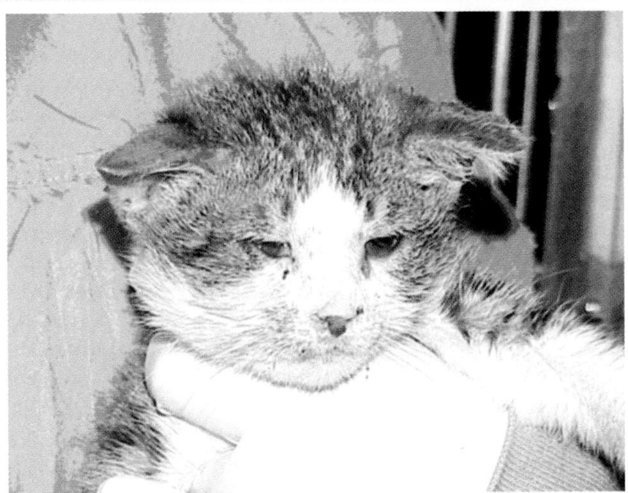

FIGURE 96-2 A kitten suffering from virulent systemic calicivirus disease (FCV-Kaos strain) showing characteristic signs of facial edema and crusting and alopecia of the face and pinnae. *(From August J: Consultations in feline internal medicine, vol 5, St Louis, 2006, Elsevier.)*

Cats with severe upper respiratory tract signs and suspected or confirmed FHV-1 infection may benefit from treatment with systemic or topical antiherpesviral drugs. The most effective and safe systemic antiherpesviral drug is famciclovir. Famciclovir is a prodrug that is converted to penciclovir. The latter is a guanosine analog that inhibits the viral DNA polymerase. Famciclovir is extremely well tolerated and has been used safely in kittens as young as 12 days of age.[17] The dosage of famciclovir is 40 to 90 mg/kg PO q8h. Cats with herpetic keratitis can be treated with topical ophthalmic antivirals such as trifluridine, idoxuridine, vidarabine, or a 0.5% solution of cidofovir. Although more expensive, cidofovir has the advantage of requiring only twice daily administration, whereas idoxuridine, trifluridine, and vidarabine must be administered 5 to 6 times a day. Trifluridine is irritating and may not be well tolerated by cats.

The outbreaks of systemic febrile caliciviral disease have demonstrated the importance of control measures to limit the spread of feline respiratory viruses because of the high mortality, poor efficacy of vaccines, and lack of specific treatments. Quick recognition and implementation of effective control measures, including disinfection, quarantine, and testing procedures, are critical to reduce the impact of this disease. These have been described in detail elsewhere.[18] An adjuvanted, inactivated vaccine for virulent systemic disease that contains a single hypervirulent strain was introduced in the United States in 2007. However, the degree to which this vaccine cross-protects against other hypervirulent strains is unknown, and in every outbreak, the strain involved has differed, and the outbreak has ceased when infection control measures were implemented. Because of this and the increased risk of sarcoma formation with adjuvanted vaccines, the usefulness of the vaccine has been questioned.

FELINE INFECTIOUS PERITONITIS

FIPV infection is caused by feline coronavirus, an enveloped RNA virus. Feline coronaviruses mutate readily, and researchers hypothesize that a relatively nonpathogenic feline coronavirus that replicates within the gastrointestinal tract (FCoV) mutates within the host to form virulent FIPV. Mutation occurs soon after infection with FCoV, or years later. Spread of FIP from cat to cat does not occur, so affected cats do not have to be isolated.

The prevalence of antibodies to feline coronavirus in single-cat households is approximately 25%, whereas in some multicat households, all cats may have positive titers. In contrast, FIP affects 1 in 5000 cats in single-cat households and approximately 5% of cats in catteries. The incidence of FIP is related to levels of virus in the environment, immunosuppression resulting from overcrowding and other stressors, and genetic factors. Purebred cats are more susceptible, and affected cats are usually 3 months to 3 years of age. Occasionally geriatric cats are affected, perhaps because of waning immune function.

Feline coronavirus is highly infectious and is spread via the fecal-to-oral route. FCoV replicates in enterocytes and destroys the villus tips, sometimes resulting in mild gastrointestinal signs. Mutation to virulent FIPV is associated with the ability to replicate within macrophages and possibly loss of the ability to replicate in enterocytes. Cats with a poor CMI response develop pyogranulomatous vasculitis because of deposition of antigen-antibody complexes within the venular epithelium. Pleural and peritoneal effusions develop (effusive FIP). Cats with a partial CMI response are able to slow replication of the virus, with subsequent granuloma formation in a variety of tissues (noneffusive FIP). This may deteriorate to effusive FIP if the CMI response wanes.

Cats with FIP often are evaluated for fever, weight loss, anorexia, and lethargy. Other signs and physical examination abnormalities may include respiratory distress resulting from pleural effusion or pneumonia, abdominal distention because of ascites, abdominal masses, icterus, splenomegaly, irregular renomegaly, anterior uveitis, retinal detachments, multifocal neurologic signs, and GI signs relating to organ failure or obstructive intestinal masses.

FIP remains an antemortem diagnostic challenge. The presence of hyperglobulinemia on the complete blood count may increase suspicion for FIP, but it is not present in all cats and may occur with other diseases. The presence of high-protein (5 to 12 g/dl), low-cellularity (predominantly neutrophils) effusion fluid is also supportive of the diagnosis. However, tests such as the serum or effusion albumin-to-globulin ratio, effusion γ-globulin concentration, and the Rivalta test can be associated with false-positive and false-negative results, especially in populations in which the prevalence of FIP is low.[19] Serologic tests that detect anti-FCoV antibody are not FIP tests. Positive test results mean only exposure to a coronavirus, and many healthy cats have positive titers but never develop FIP. In one study, titers of 1 : 1600 or greater in cats that were suspected to have FIP had a 94% chance of truly having FIP, but cats that had any coronavirus antibody titer had a 44% chance of truly having FIP.[19] However, considerable interlaboratory variation in assay results occurs, so this may not be true for serology performed at all laboratories. The same study also showed that immunocytochemistry for feline coronavirus on macrophages in effusion fluid had a specificity of 100% for diagnosis of FIP, although the sensitivity was only 57%. The mutation that occurs when FCoV becomes virulent FIPV is not predictable, and there is no way to distinguish the viruses based on nucleotide sequence. Because FCoV may be found within tissues and body fluids, false-positive results may occur when testing tissues or fluids using RT-PCR. The standard for diagnosis of FIP is detection of pyogranulomatous vasculitis on histopathologic examination of biopsy specimens, with intralesional virus antigen as detected using immunostaining techniques.

Treatment of FIP remains a challenge, and controlled studies of antiviral drug use are few. Although treatment with feline recombinant interferon-ω (1 million U/kg SC q72h until remission, then weekly thereafter) and prednisolone (1 mg/kg PO q12h then tapered to q72h) showed promise in a preliminary study,[20] in which 4 of 11 cats with effusive disease survived as long as 2 years, a subsequent placebo-controlled clinical trial showed no benefit of the treatment. Currently the only medication that appears to slow the progression of the disease in cats is prednisolone. Although most cats typically live only a few months after diagnosis, occasionally survival times of up to 2 years have been documented when the disease has been detected early.

REFERENCES

1. Greene CE, Vandevelde M: Canine distemper. In Greene CE, editor: Infectious diseases of the dog and cat, ed 4, St Louis, 2012, Elsevier.
2. Pardo ID, Johnson GC, Kleiboeker SB: Phylogenetic characterization of canine distemper viruses detected in naturally infected dogs in North America, J Clin Microbiol 43:5009, 2005.
3. Saito TB, Alfieri AA, Wosiacki SR, et al: Detection of canine distemper virus by reverse transcriptase-polymerase chain reaction in the urine of dogs with clinical signs of distemper encephalitis, Res Vet Sci 80:116, 1996.
4. Crawford PC, Dubovi EJ, Castleman WL, et al: Transmission of equine influenza virus to dogs, Science 310:482, 2005.
5. Cornell University College of Veterinary Medicine Animal Health Diagnostic Center web site: Emerging issues: canine influenza virus; http://www.diaglab.vet.cornell.edu/issues/civ.asp. Accessed January 22, 2007.
6. Oxford J: Oseltamivir in the management of influenza, Expert Opin Pharmacother 6:2493, 2005.
7. Erles K, Toomey C, Brooks HW, et al: Detection of a group 2 coronavirus in dogs with canine infectious respiratory disease, Virology 310:216-223, 2003.
8. Renshaw RW, Zylich NC, Laverack MA, et al: Pneumovirus in dogs with acute respiratory disease, Emerg Infect Dis 16:993-995, 2010.
9. Ikeda Y, Nakamura K, Miyazawa T, et al: Feline host range of canine parvovirus: recent emergence of new antigenic types in cats, Emerg Infect Dis 8:341, 2002.
10. Lutz H, Castelli I, Ehrensperger F, et al: Panleukopenia-like syndrome of FeLV caused by coinfection with FeLV and feline panleukopenia virus, Vet Immunol Immunopathol 46:21, 1995.
11. Patterson EV, Reese MJ, Tucker SJ, et al: Effect of vaccination on parvovirus antigen testing in kittens, J Am Vet Med Assoc 230:359-363, 2007.
12. Kruse BD, Unterer S, Horlacher K, et al: Prognostic factors in cats with feline panleukopenia, J Vet Intern Med 24:1271-1276, 2010.
13. Doultree JC, Druce JD, Birch CJ, et al: Inactivation of feline calicivirus, a Norwalk virus surrogate, J Hosp Infect 41:51, 1999.
14. Hurley KF, Sykes JE: Update on feline calicivirus: new trends, Vet Clin North Am Small Anim Pract 33:759, 2003.
15. Hurley KF, Pesavento PA, Pedersen NC, et al: An outbreak of virulent systemic feline calicivirus disease, J Am Vet Med Assoc 224:241, 2004.
16. Maggs DJ, Clarke HE: Relative sensitivity of polymerase chain reaction assays used for detection of feline herpesvirus type 1 DNA in clinical samples and commercial vaccines, Am J Vet Res 66:1550, 2005.
17. Sykes JE, Papich MJ: Antiviral and immunomodulatory drugs. In Sykes JE, editor: Canine and feline infectious diseases, St Louis, 2014, Elsevier.
18. Sykes JE: Feline respiratory viral infections. In Sykes JE, editor: Canine and feline infectious diseases, St Louis, 2014, Elsevier.
19. Hartmann K, Binder C, Hirschberger J, et al: Comparison of different tests to diagnose feline infectious peritonitis, J Vet Intern Med 17:781, 2003.
20. Ishida T, Shibanai A, Tanaka S, et al: Use of recombinant feline interferon and glucocorticoid in the treatment of feline infectious peritonitis, J Feline Med Surg 6:107, 2004.

CHAPTER 97
CANINE PARVOVIRUS INFECTION

Ronald Li, BSc, DVM, MVetMed, MRCVS • Karen R. Humm, MA, VetMB, CertVA, FHEA, MRCVS, DACVECC

KEY POINTS

- Canine parvovirus is a common pathogen in young dogs, generally causing disease between the ages of 6 and 20 weeks.
- Canine parvovirus is a highly pathogenic virus that can cause severe vomiting and diarrhea and may be fatal.
- Vaccination against canine parvovirus is practiced widely, but maternal antibodies can prevent a normal response to vaccination.
- A fecal enzyme-linked immunosorbent assay allows for a rapid in-house diagnosis, but a negative result does not rule out naturally occurring infection.
- Treatment is mainly supportive with fluid therapy, nutritional support, antiemetics, and antibiotics.
- Reported survival rates for dogs treated for CPV infection vary widely (64% to 92%), but prompt and aggressive treatment maximizes the chances of success; the first few days are crucial.
- Parvoviridae are very stable, surviving a pH range of 3 to 9 and temperatures of 60° C for 60 minutes. They also can survive for 5 to 7 months in the environment; therefore isolation of affected patients and thorough decontamination is vital to decrease the risk of transmission.

EVOLUTION OF CANINE PARVOVIRUS 2

Canine parvovirus (CPV-1) was discovered in 1967 and was found to cause mild diarrhea.[1] A completely new species of the genus Parvoviridae, later named CPV-2, was recognized in 1978; it caused a much more severe disease, resembling panleukopenia in cats. A sudden death syndrome resulting from myocarditis and congestive heart failure was also seen.[2] CPV-2 is genetically distinct from CPV-1 but is related closely to feline and mink parvoviruses, differing by only a few deoxyribonucleic acid (DNA) bases.[3] It therefore is presumed to have evolved from another parvovirus by mutation. It infects feline cells in culture but does not infect cats. It is suspected to have evolved in Europe; DNA analysis suggests that this occurred approximately 10 years before discovery.[3] It spread around the world rapidly because of the immunologically naive population of domesticated and wild members of the family Canidae. Subtypes of CPV-2 were recognized in 1979 and 1984 and named CPV-2a and CPV-2b, respectively. CPV-2b is thought to be more pathogenic in some dogs; a study in 1991 showed that it had replaced CPV-2a as the cause of parvovirosis in many regions of the United States.[4] CPV is undergoing continual genetic evolution, and large phenotypic variations can result from single nucleotide substitutions.[5] More recent mutations in the viral capsid protein sequence have been identified, leading to the development of a new variant named CPV-2c. Conventional type 2 vaccines appear to provide adequate protection in dogs that were challenged experimentally with CPV-2c.[6,7]

SIGNALMENT

CPV is seen most commonly in dogs less than 6 months of age, generally between the ages of 6 and 20 weeks. Susceptibility occurs because of failure of passive transfer or early waning of maternal antibodies, because of lack of vaccination, or because of passive maternal immunity preventing an efficacious response to vaccination. This latter mechanism means that CPV can infect and cause clinical signs in vaccinated animals.[8] In dogs less than 6 months of age CPV shows no gender predilection, but in those more than 6 months old, male intact dogs were overrepresented in one study.[8] Doberman Pinschers, Rottweilers, American Pit Bull Terriers, and German Shepherd Dogs are thought to be more susceptible than other breeds.[9] Rottweilers and Doberman Pinschers may have an increased susceptibility because of increased monocyte TNF-α production compared with other breeds. This possibly could affect host immunity and response to infection, although no clinical link to CPV infection has been shown.[10] Breed, gender, age, and body weight were not shown to be associated with duration of hospitalization and outcome in one study.[11]

PATHOGENESIS

CPV is a small, nonenveloped, single-stranded DNA virus that replicates in the nucleus of dividing cells in late the S phase or early G2 phase of the cell cycle. This leads to the preferential infection of rapidly dividing cells, hence the effects of the virus on the bone marrow and the gastrointestinal tract. CPV is spread by ingestion of virus-containing material from the environment.[1] The virus replicates initially in oropharyngeal lymphoid tissue and then enters the bloodstream. Intestinal crypt epithelium usually is infected by day 4 after infection. Antibodies start to appear approximately 5 days after infection and increase to maximal levels by days 7 to 10.[12] Clinical signs appear 4 to 10 days after infection.

When CPV first appeared, myocarditis was common because passively acquired maternal antibodies were not present. However, these antibodies are now nearly universal and they cover the period of rapid myocardial cell division (completed within the first 2 weeks of life), so myocarditis is now an extremely rare manifestation of CPV infection.

CLINICAL SIGNS

The most common clinical presentation of CPV infection involves acute onset vomiting, malaise, abdominal pain, anorexia, and pyrexia, followed 12 to 48 hours later by diarrhea. Antibody titer measurement in unvaccinated dogs suggests that many dogs experience an asymptomatic parvoviral infection or have only mild signs. Diarrhea may not be seen in mild cases, especially in adult dogs.[12] This later appearance or absence of diarrhea should be remembered when considering the differential diagnosis for a vomiting dog. Vomiting can be profuse and can lead to a secondary esophagitis.

The viral destruction of the intestinal crypts leads to intestinal bleeding, and hematochezia is common. The intestinal pathology coupled with the neutropenia makes infected puppies vulnerable to translocation of bacteria and endotoxin. Systemic inflammatory response syndrome (SIRS), sepsis, septic shock, and multiple organ dysfunction syndrome (MODS) may occur in severe cases. Hypoperfusion is usually present to varying degrees and can result in clinical evidence of shock, including tachycardia, poor pulse quality, prolonged capillary refill time, cold extremities, and depression. Mucous membranes are usually pale but may be injected in a dog with concurrent SIRS. Dogs with severe CPV enteritis that fulfilled three of the four SIRS criteria were shown to have a mortality rate of up to 55% according to one study.[11] When myocarditis does occur, puppies usually die suddenly from pulmonary edema because of congestive heart failure. Retching and dyspnea may precede death. If death does not occur, the focal myocardial necrosis that results can progress to fibrosis or dilated cardiomyopathy.

DIAGNOSIS

In-house enzyme-linked immunosorbent assay (ELISA) test kits are available that detect fecal antigen via an immunochromatographic assay, allowing for a rapid and inexpensive diagnosis. The sensitivities of ELISA for detection of CPV-2b and CPV-2c do not differ significantly.[13] Other external laboratory tests are available, including electron microscopy (although CPV-1 is morphologically identical), virus isolation, hemagglutination, and polymerase chain reaction (PCR). PCR is the most sensitive of these and is the test of choice for a dog with suspicious clinical signs that has a negative in-house ELISA result. A new real-time PCR (RT-PCR) test was developed with improved sensitivity and specificity, allowing for rapid detection and quantitation of CPV-2.[14] When RT-PCR was used as a gold standard, ELISA had a sensitivity between 56.16% to 81.8% and a specificity of 100%.[13,15] This high number of false-negative results may be due to test failure when samples are taken very early in the disease when fecal antigen levels are low or when large numbers of antibodies are present, binding the antigen. For that reason, ELISA testing should be repeated 36 to 48 hours later if clinical signs are suggestive of parvovirosis despite a negative result.[15] In the past, serology (immunoglobulins G and M) was used to diagnose parvovirosis, but this now has been surpassed by the aforementioned methods because it is not possible to differentiate between previous subclinical infection, active infection, or the result of vaccination.

The diagnosis of CPV in recently vaccinated dogs that have suggestive clinical signs can be challenging. Because the vaccine-modified live virus also replicates in the mucosal epithelium, the presence of low levels of antigen theoretically can be detected by various diagnostic tests resulting in false-positive results. A recent study showed that the administration of various types of modified live CPV-2 vaccines did not produce levels of CPV-2 antigen in the feces detectable by the SNAP ELISA Parvo antigen test on day 0 to 7 postvaccination.[16] Given the high specificity of ELISA and its improbability of producing false-positive results secondary to vaccination, a positive result likely indicates true infection. The RT-PCR assays using type-specific minor groove binder probe technology have been established to discriminate between vaccine strains available in the European market and type 2a/2b field strains.[17]

CLINICOPATHOLOGIC FINDINGS

A lymphopenia is seen initially as a result of direct lymphocytolysis. Other mechanisms that can lead to profound lymphopenia include endogenous release of cortisol, resulting in trapping and redistribution of lymphocytes, direct injury and destruction of the lymphoproliferative organs, and loss of lymphocyte-rich lymph as seen in protein-losing enteropathy.[18] The lymphopenia then usually is followed by a neutropenia because of peripheral consumption and destruction of white blood cell precursors in the bone marrow. Because the duration of monocyte production is shorter than the time required for neutrophil production within the bone marrow, the monitoring of monocyte count may aid in the evaluation of myelopoiesis within the bone marrow.[19] Leukopenia may serve as a significant negative prognostic indicator. The lack of a lymphopenia (at least 1.0×10^3/ul) in infected dogs on admission and at 24 and 48 hours postadmission was found to have a positive predictive value of 100% for survival in one study.[20] Nonsurvivors in the same study failed to develop a degenerate left shift and continued to have significant leukopenia, lymphopenia, eosinopenia, and monocytopenia at 24 and 48 hours after admission. However, severe neutropenia is not a useful prognostic indictor.[20]

Biochemical changes may include hypoproteinemia, hyperbilirubinemia, elevated liver enzymes, hypokalemia, hypoglycemia, and a prerenal azotemia.[21] Serum triglyceride, and high- and low-density lipoprotein cholesterol also have been shown to be elevated. Dogs with lower levels of total cholesterol and high-density lipoprotein cholesterol may have a better outcome. This may be explained by the binding of lipoproteins to lipopolysaccharide (LPS), which prevents the interaction of LPS and LPS-responsive cells and in turn diminishes the release of inflammatory cytokines such as TNF-α.[22] Thrombocytopenia, prolonged activated clotting time, prothrombin time, activated partial thromboplastin time, and increased D-dimer levels can be seen in severe cases, suggesting disseminated intravascular coagulation (DIC). Hypercoagulability also has been noted in dogs suffering from CPV enteritis without DIC, possibly because of hyperfibrinogenemia and a reduction in antithrombin activity.[23]

Changes in serum cortisol and thyroxine concentrations in critically ill puppies with CPV enteritis were described in one study. Nonsurvivors in the study were shown to have persistently lower thyroxine concentrations and higher cortisol concentrations during hospitalization, indicating that the pituitary-thyroid axis is suppressed by cortisol and other factors such as interleukin-6.[24] Further studies are required to evaluate the use of thyroxine concentrations as a predictor of outcome in dogs with CPV.

Acute phase proteins such as C-reactive protein (CRP), haptoglobin, and ceruloplasmin are found to be elevated in dogs with CPV enteritis. In one study, a serum CRP concentration greater than 92.4 mg/l was shown to predict mortality with a sensitivity and specificity of 91% and 61%, respectively.[25] The procalcitonin gene (CALCA) in dogs with CPV was documented to be expressed in nonthyroidal tissues, such as spleen, lung, and liver. This ubiquitous expression of CALCA is likely secondary to systemic inflammation and sepsis.[26] Plasma citrulline, a marker for global enterocyte mass, is decreased significantly in dogs with CPV enteritis but fails to offer any prognostic value.[27]

DIAGNOSTIC IMAGING

Diagnostic imaging can be useful to rule out other causes of vomiting and diarrhea, such as intestinal obstruction; however, radiography often reveals a dilated small bowel ileus that is sometimes difficult to differentiate from intestinal obstruction. Thoracic radiographs may be required if aspiration pneumonia is suspected. Abdominal ultrasonographic findings that are indicative of CPV enteritis may include altered wall layering of the duodenum and jejunum with hyperechoic mucosal speckling and undulation of the luminal-mucosal interface, thinning of the duodenal and jejunal mucosa without significant decrease of the overall wall thickness, and generalized hypomotility to immotility with a fluid-filled lumen. However, these findings are not pathognomonic for CPV enteritis and may occur in other diseases such as peritonitis and pancreatitis.[27a] Intussusception is an important differential diagnosis for parvovirus and a potential sequela that is readily detectable using ultrasonography.

TREATMENT

Symptomatic supportive treatment with fluids, antibiotics, and antiemetics forms the mainstay of therapy for CPV.

Fluid Therapy

The majority of animals with symptomatic parvovirus infection are dehydrated. Recognition of dehydration can be difficult, however; skin tenting is insensitive in puppies because they have mobile skin (see Chapter 155), and puppies grow quickly so that even if a recent weight were obtained, the full extent of fluid loss may be underestimated. Except for the mildest of cases, intravenous fluid therapy is necessary.

Intravenous fluid therapy always should address hypoperfusion first and then dehydration. An isotonic, balanced electrolyte solution should be chosen, such as Normosol-R, Plasmalyte 148, 0.9% sodium chloride, or lactated Ringer's solution (see Chapters 59 and 60). Aggressive fluid rates may be necessary initially and the response to therapy closely assessed. In patients with septic shock, hypoalbuminemia, or vasculitis, response to isotonic crystalloid fluid therapy can be inadequate and colloid therapy may be necessary (see Chapter 58). The larger molecules present in hydroxyethylated starches may be preferable because vasculitis could result in extravasation of albumin. The use of plasma for volume expansion and treatment of hypoalbuminemia is controversial. In most cases, plasma is reserved for cases with symptomatic coagulopathy, such as prolonged enteral bleeding or DIC. Whole blood may be necessary if the puppy is severely anemic. Plasma lactate measurement can aid in guiding fluid resuscitation, although very young puppies normally have higher lactate values (see Chapter 155). Once hypoperfusion is controlled, dehydration is corrected over 6 to 24 hours, and fluid rates should be titrated each day to account for ongoing losses. Frequent monitoring is necessary to assess the fluid therapy plan.

If the animal is anorexic or if hypokalemia is present, potassium chloride should be added to the fluids but only after hypoperfusion has been corrected (see Chapter 51). Gastrointestinal losses also can result in hyponatremia and hypochloremia. Blood glucose levels are often low as a result of immature hepatic function, sepsis, inadequate glycogen stores, and decreased caloric intake. Dextrose supplementation may be required, potentially exacerbating any concurrent hypokalemia.

Maintaining catheter sterility can be difficult in puppies with CPV when they are vomiting and producing copious volumes of diarrhea. Careful bandaging and regular checking of catheter sites are required. Although a more durable jugular catheter may appear desirable, the hypercoagulability seen in CPV-infected puppies can lead to jugular thrombosis. In mildly affected animals, treatment at home with subcutaneous fluid administration can be attempted; however, this is suboptimal in the majority of animals because it will not restore circulating volume in a timely and effective manner.

Antibiotics

Dogs with evidence of sepsis or that are pyrexic or severely neutropenic require antibiotic therapy. Afebrile, neutropenic dogs should be treated with a broad-spectrum antibiotic, but if evidence of sepsis is present, antibiotics such as potentiated amoxicillin or combinations such as ampicillin and amikacin or enrofloxacin with activities against gram-positive, gram-negative, and anaerobic organisms are recommended (see Chapter 175). With the use of amikacin, care must be taken to ensure renal perfusion is optimized and urine sediment should be monitored daily for proteinuria, glucosuria, or casts. The adverse effects of enrofloxacin on the cartilage of growing animals have been shown histologically, so it usually is avoided in puppies. Ideally, antibiotic choice is guided by blood culture, but this rarely is performed. Subsequent infection by multidrug-resistant bacteria may occur in some cases. Parenteral administration is preferred because vomiting and delayed gastric emptying may result in poor reliability of absorption of oral preparations. Intravenous administration is ideal because dehydration and hypovolemia can lead to decreased uptake of subcutaneous drugs.

Antiemetics

Vomiting leads to dehydration, electrolyte and acid-base disturbances, and esophagitis. Nausea causes increased morbidity and anorexia. Maropitant, metoclopramide, and ondansetron or dolasetron can be effective (see Chapter 162). Although the latter two are expensive, they are useful when vomiting is unresponsive to other drugs. A retrospective study found that the use of antiemetics in dogs with CPV was associated significantly with longer hospitalization; however, whether this was due to merely differing drug regimens in more severely affected animals was not clear.[28]

Nutrition

Once vomiting has been controlled, dogs should be encouraged to eat small, frequent meals of a low-fat, easily digestible diet (see Chapter 129). It is not necessary to withhold food from animals with diarrhea. A nasoesophageal tube can be placed if the patient is anorexic. One study suggested that even if an animal is still vomiting, nasoesophageal feeding is well tolerated and results in earlier clinical improvement.[29] Great care must be taken to monitor these patients for aspiration of ingesta, especially because they often are located in an isolation ward and lack frequent patient observation. Nasogastric tubes can be used to allow gastric decompression, which may decrease nausea and lessen the risk of aspiration pneumonia in animals with refractory vomiting. In smaller puppies the bore of the nasogastric tube may be so narrow that decompression is not possible. Electrolytes and acid-base status must be monitored closely to allow early detection and management of hypochloremia, hypokalemia, or metabolic alkalosis. Enteral nutrition is preferred because it helps maintain intestinal mucosal integrity and decreases bacterial translocation. Total or partial parenteral nutrition can be administered when needed, but meticulous catheter asepsis and monitoring should be performed because these animals are commonly immunosuppressed and coagulopathic.

Antiviral Drugs

Feline interferon (type omega) is licensed for treatment of parvovirus in dogs in Europe, Japan, Australia, and New Zealand but can be imported only by special permits in the United States of America and Canada. In one study of 94 clinical cases, administration of feline interferon at 2.5 mU/kg q24h for 3 consecutive days was found to decrease mortality rates by 4.4-fold, although the mortality rate was as high as 50% in the placebo group.[30] Similar results were demonstrated in another study, which showed that the administration of 1.0 mU/kg q24h for 3 consecutive days was just as effective as the 2.5 mU/kg dose.[31]

Although oseltamivir, a neuraminidase inhibitor for treating human influenza virus, does not have direct antiviral effects on CPV, benefits such as decrease of bacterial translocation and alleviating endotoxemia, SIRS, and sepsis have been reported anecdotally. One clinical trial evaluating the use of oseltamivir in dogs with CPV enteritis showed that the treatment group had a greater average in-hospital weight gain compared with the placebo group. The trial failed to demonstrate the proposed benefits of its use such as improvement of clinical outcome and shortening of hospital stay.[32]

Gastric Protectants

Histamine-2 receptor antagonists such as ranitidine, cimetidine, and famotidine can be used in animals with esophagitis or gastritis; however, the efficacy of ranitidine in significantly altering gastric pH has been questioned.[35] Sucralfate also can be administered if vomiting is controlled adequately. If upper GI tract ulceration is suspected (e.g., if melena or hematemesis is seen), omeprazole (or injectable esomeprazole) may be more effective than other agents at promoting healing (see Chapter 161).[33]

Controversial Treatments

Antiendotoxin has been suggested for the treatment of parvovirosis. It is used diluted 1:1 with crystalloid fluids, administered over 30 to 60 minutes, and should be given before antibiotics that can cause endotoxin release from bacterial cell walls. Because the endotoxin is of equine origin, it can cause anaphylaxis and should not be used for repeated dosing more than 7 days apart. Conflicting results have been published, with one study suggesting increased mortality rates associated with antiendotoxin, but another found that survival rates increased with its use.[34,35] Granulocyte colony-stimulating factor may increase the white blood cell count in severely leukopenic patients, but it is expensive and has not been shown to improve CPV survival rates.[36]

Passive immunotherapy using CPV-immune plasma has been reported previously. A clinical trial evaluating the use of a single dose of pooled, anti-CPV plasma with a mean anti-CPV titers of 1:7000 in CPV infected dogs did not show any significant differences of leukocyte counts, duration of hospitalization, cost of overall treatment, and magnitude of viremia among the treatment and placebo groups.[37] The timing and frequency of administration and the use of the same dose regardless of each of the patient's body weight may be some of the factors resulting in a lack of treatment effect in that study. Serum from recovered dogs also has been used (1.1 to 2.2 ml/kg IV) to provide antibodies, but this information is anecdotal and no controlled clinical trials have been reported.

VACCINATION

Most adult dogs are immune to CPV, either via juvenile infection, subclinical adult infection, or immunization.[12] Susceptible animals are therefore mainly puppies. Pups with seronegative nursing dams or pups that do not get any colostrum are obviously susceptible to infection. If the dam has low antibody titers, pups may acquire protection for only 4 to 6 weeks after birth. Dams with high antibody titers may pass on protection from parvovirus that lasts for 12 to 20 weeks.[38]

Despite vaccination, dogs can still suffer from parvovirus infection: 12% of dogs with CPV brought to a referral hospital were vaccinated, although this compared with 64% of dogs with nonenteric illness during the same period.[8] Live vaccines generally are used, but killed virus vaccines are available and advised for use in unvaccinated pregnant bitches.

Earlier vaccines were sometimes ineffective because preexisting maternal antibodies neutralized vaccinal antigens. This led to protocols of vaccination every 2 to 3 weeks beginning at 6 to 8 weeks of age until 18 to 20 weeks of age. Vaccines were then developed in the mid-1990s that had higher antigen levels and also were more effective immunostimulants, obviating the need for such frequent administration.[39,40] A recent study suggests that the window of susceptibility may be shortened by seroconversion when puppies with high maternal antibody levels are vaccinated with a high titer vaccine at 4 weeks of age.[41] Some newer vaccines may provide protective titers for up to 3 years.[42]

The antibody response to vaccination and the requirement for boosters can be assessed by hemagglutination inhibition. The commonly used so-called *protective titer* of at least 1:80 is incompletely protective in some cases, although signs are less severe in affected animals.[43] Vaccine efficacy also may be determined by the precise duration and amount of viral shedding by RT-PCR.[17]

PREVENTION OF TRANSMISSION

CPV-infected dogs should be isolated and barrier nursed to avoid the risk of transmission to other patients in the hospital. They shed virus into the surrounding environment, so thorough cleaning is required with agents that kill parvovirus, such as bleach (dilute 1 part bleach to 32 parts water) or alkyl dimethyl benzyl ammonium chloride. Soft furnishings can be difficult to clean effectively, so if the environment cannot be sterilized effectively, such as in a home, breeding should be discontinued and no unvaccinated, naive animals should be introduced for 1 year. An animal that has recovered should be kept away from other dogs initially, because they have been shown to shed virus for up to 39 days postinfection. Careful disposal of feces is required.

ACKNOWLEDGEMENT

The authors would like to acknowledge the work of Dez Hughes, BVSc Dip ACVECC, co-author of this chapter in the first edition of SACCM.

REFERENCES

1. Binn LN, Lazar EC, Kajima A: Recovery and characterization of a minute virus of canines, Infect Immun 1:503, 1970.
2. Shackelton LA, Parrish CR, Truyen U, et al: High rate of viral evolution associated with the emergence of carnivore parvovirus, Proc Natl Acad Sci U S A 102:379, 2005.
3. Tratschin JD, McMaster GK, Kronauer G, et al: Canine parvovirus: relationship to wild-type and vaccine strains of feline panleukopenia virus and mink enteritis virus, J Gen Virol 61:33, 1982.
4. Parrish CR, Aquadro CF, Strassheim ML, et al: Rapid antigenic-type replacement and DNA sequence evolution of canine parvovirus, J Virol 65:6544, 1991.
5. Martella V, Cavalli A, Decaro N, et al: Immunogenicity of an intranasally administered modified live canine parvovirus type 2b vaccine in pups with maternally derived antibodies, Clin Diagn Lab Immunol 12:1243, 2005.
6. Markovich J, Stucker K, Carr A, et al: Effects of canine parovirus strain variations on diagnostic test results and clinical management of enteritis in dogs, J Am Vet Med Assoc 241:66, 2012.
7. Siedek EM, Schmidt H, Sture GH, et al: Vaccination with canine parvovirus type 2 (CPV-2) protects against challenge with virulent CPV-2b and CPV-2c, Berl Munch Tierarztl Wochenschr 124:58, 2011.
8. Houston DM, Ribble CS, Head LL: Risk factors associated with parvovirus enteritis in dogs: 283 cases (1982-1991), J Am Vet Med Assoc 208:542, 1996.
9. Glickman LT, Domanski LM, Patronek GJ, et al: Breed-related risk factors for canine parvovirus enteritis, J Am Vet Med Assoc 187:589, 1985.
10. Nemzek JA, Agrodnia D, Hauptman JG: Breed-specific pro-inflammatory cytokine production as a predisposing factor for susceptibility to sepsis in the dog, J Vet Emerg Crit Care 17:368, 2007.
11. Kalli I, Leontides L, Mylonakis M, et al: Factors affecting the occurrence, duration of hospitalization and final outcome in canine parvovirus infection, Res Vet Sci 89:174, 2010.
12. Bohm M, Thompson H, Weir A, et al: Serum antibody titres to canine parvovirus, adenovirus and distemper virus in dogs in the UK which had not been vaccinated for at least 3 years, Vet Rec 154:457, 2004.

13. Markovich J, Stucker K, Carr A, et al: Effects of canine parvovirus strain variations on diagnostic test results and clinical management of enteritis in dogs, J Am Vet Med Assoc 241:66, 2012.
14. Decaro N, Elia G, Martella V, et al: A real-time PCR assay for rapid detection and quantitation of canine parvovirus type 2 in the feces of dogs, Vet Microbiol 105:19, 2005.
15. Desario C, Decaro N, Campolo M, et al: Canine parvovirus infection: which diagnostic test for virus? J Virol Methods 126:179, 2005.
16. Schultz R, Larson L, Lorentzen L: Effects of modified live canine parvovirus vaccine on the SNAP ELISA antigen assay (Abstract International Veterinary Emergency and Critical Care Symposium 2008).
17. Decaro N, Buonavoglia C: Canine parvovirus—A review of epidemiological and diagnostic aspects, with emphasis on type 2c, Vet Micobiol 155:1, 2012.
18. Woods CB, Pollack RVH, Carmichael LE: Canine parvovirus enteritis, J Am Anim Hosp Assoc 16:171, 1980.
19. Decardo N, Altamura M, Pratelli A, et al: Evaluation of the innate immune response in pups during canine parvovirus type 1 infection, New Microbiol 25:291, 2002.
20. Goddard A, Leisewitz AL, Chistopher MM, et al: Prognostic usefulness of blood leukocyte changes in canine paroviral enteritis, J Vet Intern Med 22:309, 2008.
21. McCaw, DL, Harrington DP, Jones BD: A retrospective study of canine parvovirus gastroenteritis, J Vet Intern Med 10:157, 1996.
22. Yilmaz Z, Senturk S: Characterisation of lipid profiles in dogs with parvoviral enterits, J Small Anim Pract 48:643, 2007.
23. Otto CM, Rieser TM, Brooks MB et al: Evidence of hypercoagulability in dogs with parvoviral enteritis, J Am Vet Med Assoc 217:1500, 2000.
24. Schoeman JP, Goddard A, Herrtage ME: Serum cortisol and thyroxine concentrations as predictors of death in critically ill puppies with parvoviral diarrhea, J Am Vet Med Assoc 231:1534, 2007.
25. Kocaturk M, Martinez S, Eralp O, et al: Prognostic value of serum acute-phase proteins in dogs with parvoviral enteritis, J Small Anim Pract 51:478, 2010.
26. Guinti M, Peli A, Battilani M, et al: Evaluation of CALC-I gene (CALCA) expression in tissues of dogs with signs of the systemic inflammatory response syndrome, J Vet Emerg Crit Care 20:523, 2010.
27. Dossin O, Rupassar SI, Weng HY, et al: Effects of parvoviral enteritis on plasma citrulline concentration in dogs, J Vet Intern Med 25:215, 2011.
27a. Stander N, Wagner WM, Goddard A, et al: Ultrasonographic appearance of canine parvoviral enteritis in puppies, Vet Radiol Ultrasound 51:69, 2010.
28. Mantione NL, Otto CM: Characterization of the use of antiemetic agents in dogs with parvoviral enteritis treated at a veterinary teaching hospital: 77 cases (1997-2000), J Am Vet Med Assoc 227:1787, 2005.
29. Mohr AJ, Leisewitz AL, Jacobson LS, et al: Effect of early enteral nutrition on intestinal permeability, intestinal protein loss, and outcome in dogs with severe parvoviral enteritis, J Vet Intern Med 17:791, 2003.
30. de Mari K, Maynard L, Eun HM, et al: Treatment of canine parvoviral enteritis with interferon-ω in a placebo-controlled field trial, Vet Rec 152:105, 2003.
31. Uchino T, Matsumoto H, Sakamoto T, et al: Treatment of canine parvovirus infection with recombinant feline interferon-ω, J Vet Clin Sci 1:130, 2008.
32. Savigny MR, Macintire DK: Use of oseltamivir in the treatment of canine parvoviral enteritis, J Vet Emerg Crit Care 20:132, 2010.
33. Bersenas AM, Mathews KA, Allen DG, et al: Effects of ranitidine, famotidine, pantoprazole, and omeprazole on intragastric pH in dogs, Am J Vet Res 66:425, 2005.
34. Mann FA, Boon GD, Wagner-Mann CC, et al: Ionized and total magnesium concentrations in blood from dogs with naturally acquired parvoviral enteritis, J Am Vet Med Assoc 212:1398, 1998.
35. Dimmitt R: Clinical experience with cross-protective antiendotoxin antiserum in dogs with parvoviral enteritis, Canine Pract 16:23, 1991.
36. Rewerts JM, McCaw DL, Cohn LA, et al: Recombinant human granulocyte colony-stimulating factor for treatment of puppies with neutropenia secondary to canine parvovirus infection, J Am Vet Med Assoc 213:991, 1998.
37. Bragg RF, Duffy AL, DeCecco FA: Clinical evaluation of a single dose of immune plasma for treatment of canine parvovirus infection, J Am Vet Med Assoc 240:700, 2012.
38. Bohm M, Thompson H, Weir A, et al: Serum antibody titres to canine parvovirus, adnovirus and distemper virus in dogs in the UK which had not been vaccinated for at least 3 years, Vet Rec 154:457, 2004.
39. Larson LJ, Schultz RD: Comparison of selected canine vaccines for their ability to induce protective immunity against parvovirus infection, Am J Vet Res 58:360, 1997.
40. Mockett APA, Stahl MS: Comparing how puppies with passive immunity respond to three canine parvovirus vaccines, Vet Med 90:430, 1995.
41. De Crammer KG, Stylianides E, van Vuuren M: Efficacy of vaccination at 4 and 6 weeks in the control of canine parvovirus, Vet Microbiol 149:126, 2011.
42. Gore TC, Lakshmanan N, Duncan KL, et al: Three-year duration of immunity in dogs following vaccination against canine adenovirus type 1, canine parvovirus, and canine distemper virus, Vet Ther 6:5, 2005.
43. Elia G, Cavalli A, Cirone F, et al: Antibody levels and protection to canine parvovirus type 2, J Vet Med B Infect Dis Vet Public Health 52:320, 2005.

CHAPTER 98

INFECTIVE ENDOCARDITIS

Kristin A. MacDonald, DVM, PhD, DACVIM (Cardiology)

KEY POINTS

- Infective endocarditis (IE) is an uncommon clinical disease associated with high mortality.
- Diagnosis is challenging because the signs are nonspecific and a variety of organ systems can be affected.
- Using criteria extrapolated from human medicine may improve diagnostic capabilities.
- The vegetative lesions associated with infective endocarditis make eradication of the infectious organism difficult.
- Antimicrobial therapy should consist of long-term bactericidal administration.
- The prognosis for patients with infective endocarditis is poor.
- Antimicrobial prophylaxis should be considered in high-risk patients (i.e., patients with subaortic stenosis) that are undergoing surgical or dental procedures.

Infective endocarditis (IE) is an uncommon, often fatal disease in dogs that typically involves the mitral and/or the aortic valves. Medium to large breed, male dogs are affected most commonly. Severe pathophysiologic sequelae to IE may include congestive heart failure; immune-mediated diseases, including polyarthritis or glomerulonephritis; thromboembolism (sterile or septic); or severe cardiac arrhythmias. Echocardiographic evidence of a vegetative valvular lesion and valvular insufficiency is the mainstay in diagnosis of IE, and additional criteria help support a clinical diagnosis. Although blood cultures are important to submit to identify a bacterial cause and assess microbial susceptibility, unfortunately they are often negative because of concurrent antibiotic use or infection with a fastidious organism. Treatment includes long-term broad-spectrum antibiotics for 6 to 8 weeks; the first week of therapy ideally is given intravenously.

PATHOPHYSIOLOGY

Microbial Adherence and Endothelial Invasion

The inciting event in formation of IE is bacterial adherence to the disrupted endothelial surface of a cardiac valve (Figure 98-1). Mechanical lesions (i.e., subaortic stenosis, cardiac catheterization procedure) or inflammatory disease can promote bacterial seeding within the endothelium. Extracellular matrix proteins, thromboplastin, and tissue factor are exposed by the damaged endothelium, which trigger coagulation. A coagulum containing fibrinogen, fibrin, and platelet proteins forms and avidly binds bacteria. Fibrinogen binding mediates the primary attachment of bacteria to the disrupted endothelium, and subsequent fibronectin binding triggers endothelial cell internalization and local proinflammatory and procoagulant responses. Inflammation induces endothelial cell expression of integrins that bind bacteria and fibronectin to the extracellular matrix. Some bacteria (i.e., *Staphylococcus aureus*) carry fibronectin-binding proteins and also can trigger active internalization by host cells. Organisms that commonly cause IE are those that have the greatest ability to adhere to damaged valves because of expression of special receptors called *microbial surface components* recognizing adhesive matrix molecules (MSCRAMMS); these include *Staphylococcus* and *Streptococcus* spp.[1] These bacteria can trigger tissue factor production and induce platelet aggregation. Platelets release bactericidal proteins, but many of the bacteria that cause IE are resistant to these proteins. Bacteria such as *S. aureus* and *Bartonella* spp. may become internalized within the endothelial cells and escape detection by the immune system. Bacteria also can excrete enzymes that lead to destruction of valve tissue and proliferation of the vegetative lesion. A therapeutic sanctuary of bacteria clustered within the fibrinous vegetative lesion with little access to phagocytes limits host-mediated defenses and provides a formidable obstacle for antibiotic penetration.

Congestive Heart Failure

Congestive heart failure (CHF) is the most common sequela of IE and is the most common cause of death. Acute heart failure is a common feature of this rapidly progressive, virulent disease. Damage to either mitral or aortic valve leads to valvular insufficiency, which is typically severe, and causes volume overload to the left heart and increases left ventricular end diastolic volume and pressure. In experimental models, cardiogenic pulmonary edema develops once the left ventricular end diastolic pressure rises above 20 to 25 mm Hg.[2] Edema formation in chronic cardiac disease occurs first in the pulmonary interstitium and radiographically appears as interstitial infiltrates in the perihilar region of the lungs, with concurrent cardiomegaly, left atrial dilation, and pulmonary venous distention. However, most cases of IE result in acute and severe valvular insufficiency and a rapid increase in left ventricular filling pressure, which results in fulminant pulmonary edema with alveolar flooding, often before the development of left atrial dilation. Typically, pulmonary veins are distended despite the lack of marked radiographic cardiomegaly. Measurement of pulmonary capillary wedge pressure may be useful to document left heart failure in these acute cases.

Immune-Mediated Disease

Patients with IE tend to develop high antibody titers against causative microorganisms, and there is continuous formation of circulating immune complexes consisting of IgM, IgG, and C3 (complement).[3] Factors such as rheumatoid factor may impair the ability of complement to solubilize immune complexes and may lead to formation of large immune complexes. Extracardiac disease manifestations are caused by immune complex deposition and further complement activation and tissue destruction in the glomerular basement membrane, joint capsule, or dermis. Shortly after antibiotic therapy, circulating immune complexes are reduced greatly in people with IE. Immune-mediated disease, including polyarthritis and glomerulonephritis, is seen commonly in dogs with IE (75% and 36%, respectively).[4] Joint fluid analysis and culture should be performed in any dog with lameness to evaluate for immune-mediated polyarthritis or septic arthritis.

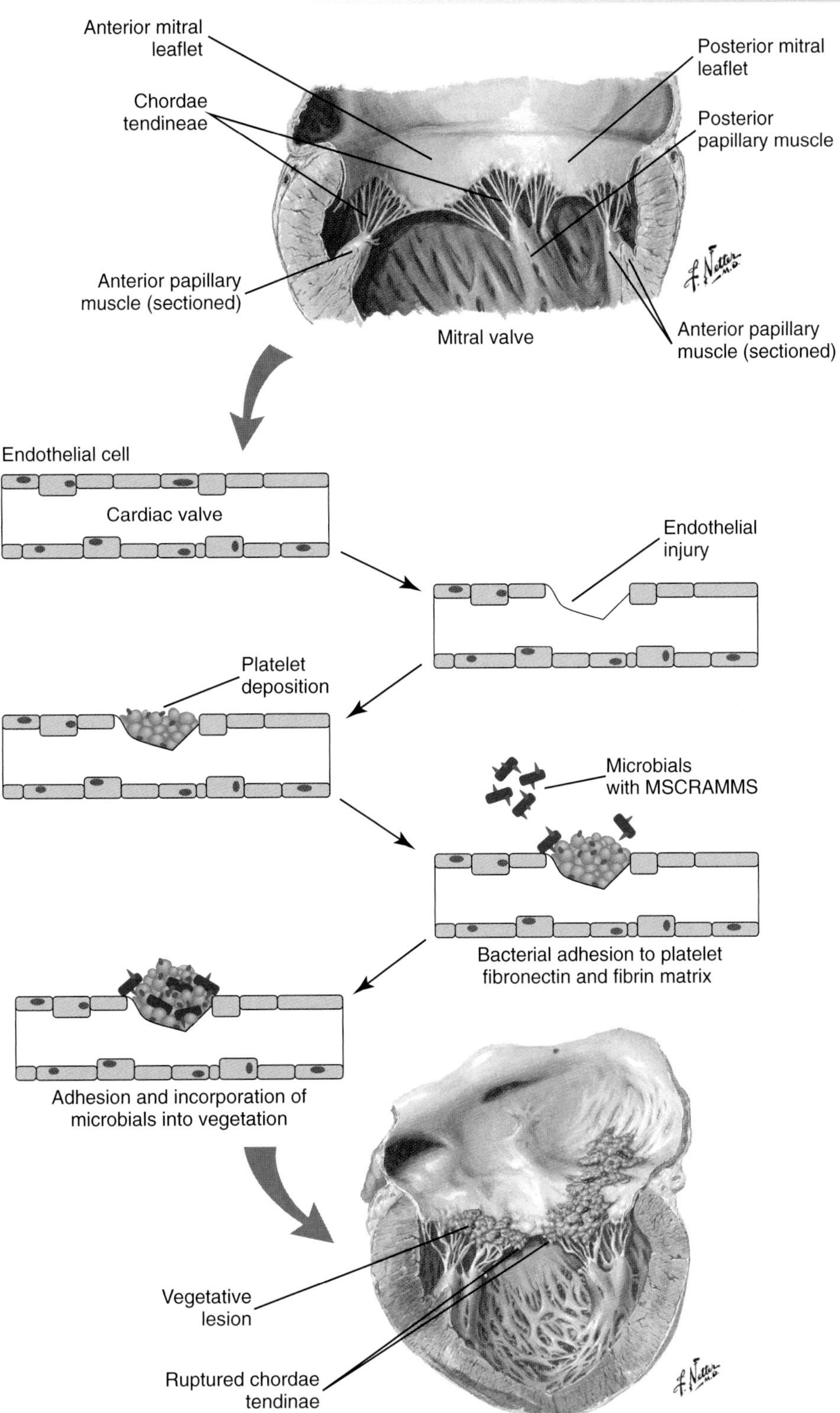

FIGURE 98-1 Pathophysiologic mechanisms of infective endocarditis. A normal mitral valve (including leaflets and chordae tendineae) is represented *(top)* and a magnified view shows intact normal endothelium *(bottom)*. The initiating step in development of infective endocarditis is an injury to the endothelium, which exposes extracellular matrix proteins. A coagulum of platelets (yellow), fibrinogen, fibronectin, and fibrin (orange) develops. The fibronectin receptor on platelets and extracellular matrix proteins avidly bind bacteria that contain microbial surface components recognizing adhesive matrix molecules (MSCRAMMs). The microorganism becomes embedded and incorporated into a vegetative lesion, and multiplies. The vegetative lesion may extend to chordae tendineae, opposing leaflet, or atrial endothelium and may cause rupture of chordae tendineae. The result is severe mitral regurgitation and congestive heart failure. *(From MacDonald K: Infective endocarditis in dogs: diagnosis and therapy, Vet Clin North Am Small Anim Pract 40(4):665-684, 2010.)*

A urine protein : creatinine ratio should be evaluated in any dog with proteinuria to support the diagnosis of glomerulonephritis.

Thromboembolism

Thromboembolism (septic and aseptic) is a common sequelae to IE in dogs, was documented on pathology in 70% to 80% of dogs, and was suspected clinically antemortem in 44% of dogs with IE.[4,5] Like people, dogs are more likely to suffer from thromboembolic disease with mitral valve IE.[5] The highest risk factors for thromboembolic disease in people with IE include mitral valve involvement, large mobile vegetative lesions more than 1 to 1.5 cm, or increasing lesion size during antibiotic therapy.[6,7] Infarction of the kidneys and spleen are most common in dogs, followed by myocardium, brain, and limbs. Vascular encephalopathy occurs in approximately one third of people with IE and is uncommon in dogs. Central nervous system thromboembolism most commonly occurs in the middle cerebral artery in people and dogs and results in brain ischemia and possibly ischemic necrosis if persistent.

INCIDENCE, SIGNALMENT, AND PRESENTING COMPLAINT

IE is an uncommon disease in dogs, with an estimated incidence of 0.05% to 6.6% in dogs referred to a veterinary teaching hospital and rarely is seen in cats.[4,5,8] Most dogs are medium to large breed dogs weighing more than 15 kg and are typically middle-age to old (more than 5 years in more than 75% of cases in one study), with a male sex predisposition.[5] Overrepresented breeds include Labrador Retriever, German Shepherd, Boxer, and Golden Retriever. The most common presenting complaint is lameness, followed by nonspecific signs, including lethargy, anorexia, respiratory abnormalities, weakness, and collapse. Neurologic abnormalities (i.e., seizures, ataxia, deficits of conscious proprioception, obtundation, cranial nerve deficits, and vestibular signs), vomiting, and epistaxis are less common presenting complaints.

PREDISPOSING FACTORS

Presence of bacteremia and endothelial disruption are necessary for development of IE. Subaortic stenosis is the only structural heart disease that significantly predisposes dogs to development of IE, and no other cardiac disease has been identified statistically as a predisposing cause.[9,10] Myxomatous valve degeneration is the most common heart disease in dogs, but it occurs most frequently in small breed, aged dogs that rarely develop IE, making it unlikely to be a predisposing factor for IE. Common sources of bacteremia in dogs include diskospondylitis, prostatitis, pneumonia, urinary tract infection, pyoderma, periodontal disease, and long-term indwelling central venous catheters. The role of immunosuppression as a predisposing factor for IE is controversial: in one study, only 1 of 18 dogs (5%) recently had been administered immunosuppressive therapy, yet another earlier study reported 17 of 45 dogs (38%) had received corticosteroids at some time during the course of disease.[4,8] Dental prophylaxis has long been suspected anecdotally as a predisposing factor, which has been rejected by a study showing no association of IE and dental procedures, oral surgical procedures, or oral infection in the preceding 3 months.[10]

ETIOLOGIC AGENTS

In order of frequency, the most common causes of IE in dogs include *Staphylococcus* spp. (aureus, intermedius, coagulase positive, and coagulase negative), *Streptococcus* spp. (*S. canis*, *S. bovis*, and β-hemolytic streptococci), and *Escherichia coli* (Box 98-1). Less common bacterial isolates include *Enterococcus* spp., *Pseudomonas* spp., *Erysipelothrix rhusiopathiae, Enterobacter* spp., *Pasteurella* spp., *Corynebacterium* spp., and *Proteus* spp. Rare causes of IE include *Bordetella avium*-like organism, *Erysipelothrix tonsillarum, Actinomyces turicensis, Blastomyces dermatitidis*, and *Mycobacterium* spp.[4,11,12]

Bartonella spp. have emerged as an important cause of culture-negative IE in people and in dogs and was the cause of IE in 28% of dogs living in Northern California, including 45% of dogs with negative blood cultures.[4,13] This may be an unusually high prevalence of IE caused by *Bartonella* spp. compared with other parts of the country but highlights the importance of testing for bartonellosis in dogs with IE. *Bartonella vinsonii* ssp. *berkhoffii* is the most important species of *Bartonella* causing IE in dogs.[4,14] Other, less common *Bartonella* species that cause IE in dogs include *B. clarridgeiae, B. washoensis, B. quintana, B. rochalimae, B. clarridgeiae*-like, and *B. koehlerae.*[15,16] In dogs, *Bartonella* spp. affect primarily the aortic valve and less commonly affect the mitral valve. The clinical characteristics of dogs with IE resulting from *Bartonella* spp. are not different than dogs with IE resulting from traditional bacteria. In the author's experience, dogs with IE resulting from traditional bacteria do not have coinfections with *Bartonella* spp.[4,17] Several epidemiologic studies have suggested that ticks and fleas may be vectors for *Bartonella* spp. Concurrent seroreactivity to *Anaplasma phagocytophilum, Ehrlichia canis*, or *Rickettsia rickettsii* is common in dogs with IE resulting from *Bartonella* spp., and titers should be submitted for

BOX 98-1 *Suggested Criteria for Diagnosis of Infective Endocarditis in Dogs*

Major Criteria

1. Positive echocardiogram
   Vegetative, oscillating lesion
   Erosive lesion
   Abscess
2. New valvular insufficiency
3. >Mild AI in absence of subaortic stenosis
4. Positive blood culture
   ≥2 positive blood cultures
   ≥3 with common skin contaminant

Minor Criteria

1. Fever
2. Medium to large dog (>15 kg)
3. Subaortic stenosis
4. Thromboembolic disease
5. Immune-mediated disease
   Polyarthritis
   Glomerulonephritis
6. Positive blood culture not meeting major criteria
7. *Bartonella* serology ≥ 1 : 1024

Diagnosis

Definite

Pathology of the valve
Two major criteria
One major and two minor criteria

Possible

One major and one minor criterion
Three minor criteria

Unlikely

Other diagnosis made
Resolved in <4 days of treatment
No evidence at necropsy

AI, Aortic insufficiency.

tick-borne diseases in any dog that is seroreactive to *Bartonella* spp. antigens.[4,13]

CLINICAL ABNORMALITIES

A murmur is ausculted in a majority of dogs with IE (89% to 96%).[4,9] Presence of a new or changing (i.e., increased intensity) murmur is the prototypical auscultation abnormality, but in one study only 41% of dogs with IE had a new murmur.[8] Clinical findings of a diastolic murmur and bounding femoral pulses should trigger a high level of suspicion of aortic valve IE, although diastolic murmurs can be challenging to identify because they are typically a low intensity. Fever is often, but not always, present (50% to 74%) but may be masked by concurrent antibiotic therapy in 80% of dogs in one study.[4] Dogs infected with *Bartonella* spp. are less likely to have a fever compared with other causative agents.[11] Arrhythmias are common (40% 70%) with dogs with IE and include, in order of frequency: ventricular arrhythmias, supraventricular tachycardia, third-degree atrioventricular block (because of periannular abscess from aortic IE), and atrial fibrillation. Dogs with IE of the aortic valve appear to be prone particularly to develop arrhythmias, including 62% of dogs having ventricular arrhythmias reported in one study.[9] CHF is present in almost half of patients and is diagnosed by identification of perihilar to caudodorsal pulmonary infiltrates, often in the absence of left atrial dilation in 75% of cases in one study because of the acute nature of the disease.[4] The occurrence of CHF does not differ between IE of the mitral or aortic valves.[4]

CLINICOPATHOLOGIC ABNORMALITIES

The most common clinicopathologic abnormality is leukocytosis, which occurred in 89% of dogs in a case series.[5] Typically there is a mature neutrophilia and monocytosis. Mild to severe thrombocytopenia and/or anemia (typically mild and nonregenerative) are seen commonly in half of dogs.[5] There is often evidence of a procoagulable state in dogs with IE, including an elevated D-dimer or fibrin degradation products in 87% of dogs, in which they were measured, as well as hyperfibrinogenemia in 83% of dogs, in which it was measured in one study.[5] Serum chemistry often shows hypoalbuminemia (95% of dogs), elevated hepatic enzyme activity, and acidosis. Renal complications are seen in at least half of dogs with IE and include prerenal or renal azotemia, glomerulonephritis, pyelonephritis, and renal thrombosis. Moderate to severe renal failure was present in approximately one third of dogs in a case series.[4] The most common abnormalities on urinalysis include cystitis (60% of dogs), proteinuria (50% to 60% of dogs), and hematuria (18% to 62%). Urine protein:creatinine ratio (UPC) is a necessary test in dogs with proteinuria to establish if there is excess protein loss from the kidneys, which may lead to a hypercoagulable state by loss of antithrombin III. Anticoagulant or antiplatelet therapy may be indicated in patients with evidence of a hypercoagulable state. An increased UPC ratio was present in 77% of dogs, in which it was measured and was moderate or severely elevated in 58% of these dogs.[5]

DIAGNOSIS

Echocardiography

The cornerstone of diagnosing IE in dogs is identification of a vegetative valvular lesion on echocardiography (ECHO) or at necropsy. The pathognomonic echocardiographic lesion is a hyperechoic, oscillating, irregular-shaped (i.e., shaggy) mass adherent to, yet distinct from, the endothelial cardiac surface (Figure 98-2). The term *oscillating* means that the lesion is mobile with high-frequency movement independent from the underlying valve structure; this finding highly supports the echocardiographic diagnosis of a vegetative lesion. The mitral and aortic valves are almost exclusively affected in small animals. Erosive and minimally proliferative lesions are less common and may be challenging to visualize on ECHO. Valvular insufficiency of the affected valve (i.e., mitral insufficiency and/or aortic insufficiency) is always present and is identified using color flow Doppler (Figure 98-2, *F*). Presence of moderate or severe aortic insufficiency on color flow Doppler should raise the suspicion of aortic IE, and careful interrogation of the aortic cusps is necessary. Severity of aortic insufficiency may be estimated by the length of the insufficiency jet on color flow Doppler and the slope of the aortic insufficiency on continuous wave Doppler of the left apical five-chamber view (i.e., steep slope, severe aortic insufficiency), and in chronic cases the severity of the left ventricular eccentric hypertrophy (Figure 98-2, *D*). Left atrial enlargement or eccentric hypertrophy of the left ventricle may not be present if the IE is acute. Myocardial failure often occurs secondary to chronic severe aortic insufficiency in dogs with aortic IE, if they survive long enough (Figure 98-2, *C*). A myocardial abscess may appear as a heterogenous, thickened, hyperechoic region or mass in the myocardium or annulus. A fistula or septal defect may be seen between two chambers if the abscess has ruptured.

Blood Culture

Blood and urine cultures are important to obtain but are frequently negative (60% to 70%) because of concurrent antibiotic use in a majority (80%) of dogs.[4] Three or four blood samples (5 to 10 ml each) should be collected aseptically from different venous sites at least 30 minutes to 1 hour apart and submitted for aerobic and anaerobic culture. If antibiotics have been given, the blood collection should be done at the estimated trough of the drug level. Lysis centrifugation tubes (Isolator, Isostat microbial system, Wampole Laboratories, Cranbury, NJ) may increase diagnostic yield. It is important to collect adequate volumes of blood (if clinically appropriate based on patient size) because the concentration of bacteria in blood is very low (less than 5 to 10 bacteria/ml).[18] *Bartonella* spp. are fastidious organisms that rarely grow on culture medium, so routine culture is not recommended. The combination of blood cultures and aseptically collected blood for polymerase chain reaction (PCR) with bacterial 16s primers identified bacteria in 61% of dogs with suspected IE compared with either test alone (33% and 39%, respectively), making this combination an attractive option to increase diagnostic yield in suspected IE cases.[19]

Modified Duke Criteria for Diagnosis of Infective Endocarditis

The modified Duke criteria have been developed to identify humans at high risk for IE and have been modified further use in dogs evaluated for possible IE (see Box 98-1). Cases of possible IE with high clinical suspicion should undergo transesophageal ECHO if available to better evaluate the valve morphology, or transthoracic ECHO should be repeated in a few days. Based on the veterinary literature, high seroreactivity to *Bartonella* spp. (greater than 1:1024) may be an additional minor criterion for diagnosis of IE caused by *Bartonella* spp. in dogs. Because *Bartonella* spp. commonly live within endothelial cells or erythrocytes, PCR on serum may have limited yield and frequent false negatives. For example, direct PCR on serum was positive in only 8 of 61 dogs (13%) with bartonellosis, but when performed after prolonged incubation (for up to 1 month) in special enrichment media, 40 of 61 dogs were PCR positive.[20]

TREATMENT

Along with aggressive (broad-spectrum, bacteriostatic) intravenous antibiotics, in human medicine up to half of patients require surgery

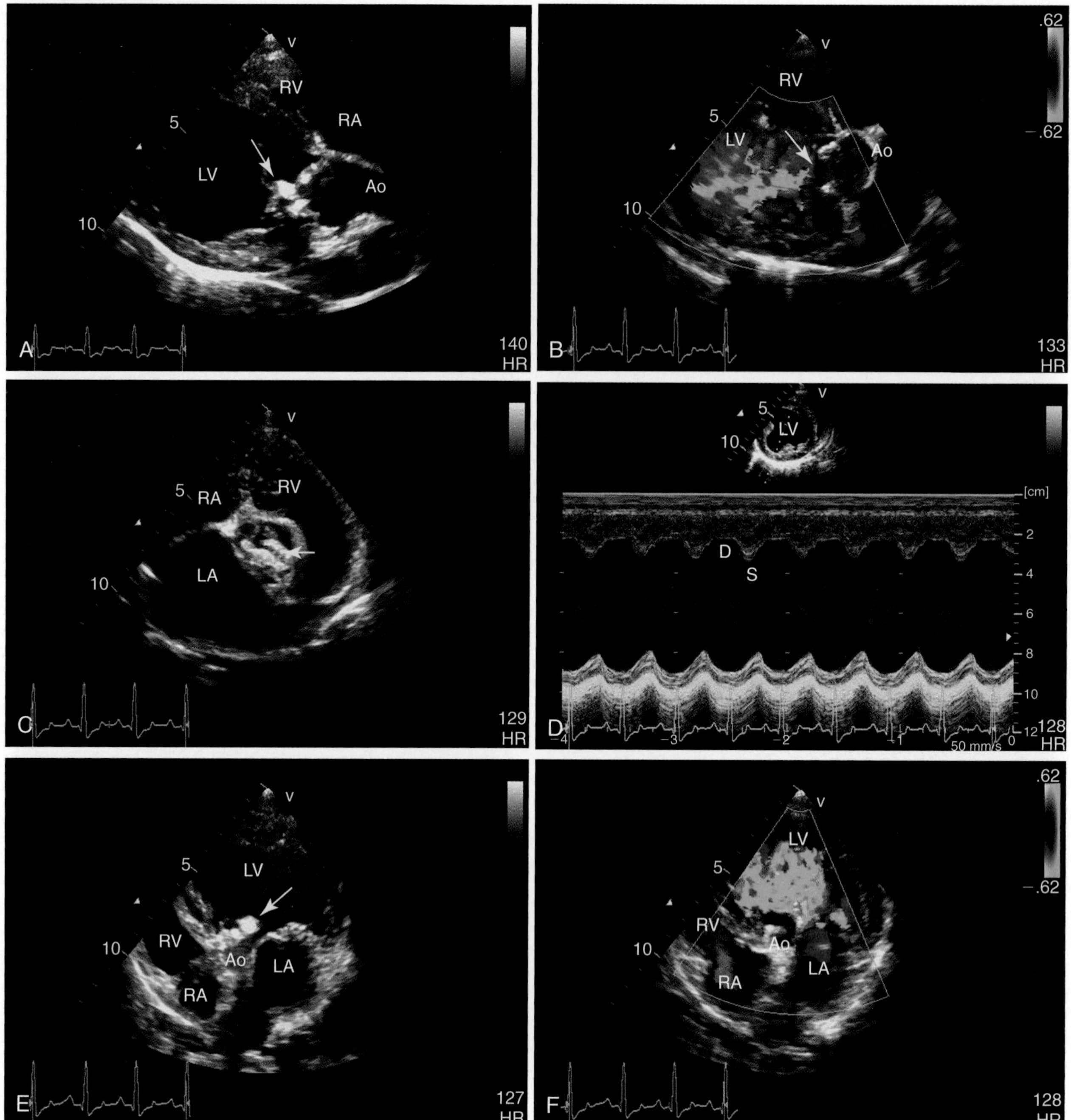

FIGURE 98-2 Echocardiogram of a dog with infective endocarditis of the aortic valve. There is a large vegetative lesion on the aortic valve seen in multiple views including the right parasternal left ventricular outflow tract view **(A),** the short axis view of the aortic valve at the heart base **(C)**, and the left apical five chamber view **(E)**. The aortic valve is severely thickened with a hyperechoic, shaggy, oscillating mass lesion *(arrow)* that extends backwards into the left ventricular outflow tract. Color flow Doppler interrogation of the aortic valve from the right parasternal long axis left ventricular outflow tract view **(B)** and the left apical five chamber view **(F)** shows severe aortic insufficiency (AI, green), which is turbulent blood flow leaking back from the aorta into the left ventricle during diastole. Severe AI causes a severe volume overload and eccentric hypertrophy of the left ventricle (increased end diastolic diameter) and secondary myocardial failure (increased end systolic diameter) on M-mode echocardiography **(D)**. The left atrial to aortic dimension is only mildly increased despite presence of severe AI and left heart failure due to the acute nature of the IE **(C)**. Continuous wave Doppler measurement of the aortic blood flow velocity identifies the AI as a high velocity turbulent flow backwards into the left ventricle during diastole (above the line), and normal systolic aortic blood flow velocity (below the line) **(G)**. The severe AI causes a rapid increase in the left ventricular diastolic pressure and a rapid decrease in the aortic to left ventricular pressure difference, creating a steep slope of the AI jet on CW Doppler. *AI,* Aortic insufficiency; *Ao,* aorta; *LA,* left atrium; *LV,* left ventricle; *RA,* right atrium; *RV,* right ventricle.

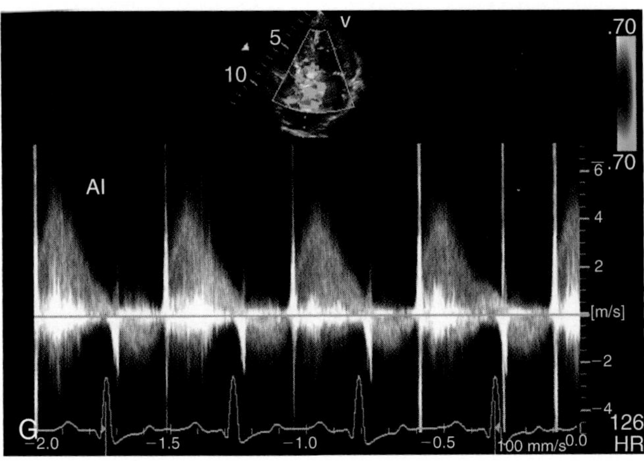

FIGURE 98-2, cont'd

for valve replacement.[1] Valve replacement is performed rarely in dogs with IE, which limits treatment to chronic antibiotics and likely contributes to the high mortality rate seen in dogs with IE.[21] Long-term bactericidal antibiotics are the mainstay therapy of IE. Empiric broad-spectrum antibiotic therapy is started while blood and urine cultures are pending and may be continued in cases with no identifiable pathogen. High serum concentration of antibiotics that have good tissue and intracellular penetrating properties is needed to penetrate within the vegetative lesion to kill the bacteria. Antibiotic doses used are on the high end of the range to achieve high blood levels. The optimal antibiotic treatment depends on culture of the microorganism and minimum inhibitory concentration (MIC) of the antibiotics, which is often impossible because of culture-negative cases from previous antibiotic use. Common etiologic agents, their typical sensitivity profile, and therapeutic regimens are included in Table 98-1. Therapeutic recommendations were derived from the UC Davis VMTH microbiological service database of antimicrobial sensitivity of microorganisms and were based on *at least* 90% of the cultured isolates sensitive to the particular antibiotic. However, general antibiotic sensitivities and resistance profiles may vary depending on the hospital, and choice of the optimal antibiotic may be more challenging in secondary or tertiary referral hospitals. There is significant resistance of many bacteria isolated from IE cases at UC Davis to enrofloxacin and ampicillin, making those questionable choices for empiric, acute first line of defense when an MIC is unavailable. Although aminoglycosides possess potent bactericidal properties and are an attractive choice for treatment of IE, they may be limited to dogs without acute heart failure because furosemide potentiates their nephrotoxicity.

Typically 1 to 2 weeks of intravenous antibiotic therapy is necessary for acute aggressive treatment of IE. This may be challenging to owners because it involves chronic hospitalization and expensive treatment and monitoring for this period of time. Placement of an indwelling chronic vascular access port is an option in these patients that ideally should be treated with intravenous antibiotics for several weeks. After the first 1 to 2 weeks of intravenous antibiotics, chronic long-term oral antibiotics are needed for at least 6 to 8 weeks or longer. Subcutaneous administration of antibiotics on an outpatient basis rather than oral antibiotics has been suggested by some clinicians, but this has no clear advantage over chronic oral treatment using antibiotics with high bioavailability and blood levels. One exception is in the chronic treatment of resistant infections using a carbapenem such as imipenem administered subcutaneously after an initial 1- to 2-week course administered intravenously, although subcutaneous administration may cause discomfort with this drug.[22]

Often it is challenging to decide when chronic antibiotic therapy may be discontinued because the affected valve often has residual thickening even with a sterile lesion. Serial monitoring of echocardiograms, as well as other parameters such as CBC, recheck of urine or blood cultures (if previously positive), and body temperature are needed to follow the response to antibiotics. Lack of improvement in an oscillating vegetative lesion after the first week of antibiotic therapy in an animal without a previous bacterial isolate and MIC may indicate a more aggressive, resistant bacterium that may require switching antibiotics or starting additional antibiotics. During chronic therapy, the presence of an oscillating mass, recurrent fever, leukocytosis, or positive follow-up urine or blood cultures necessitates continued chronic therapy, possibly with a different antibiotic combination.

The superior antibiotic for treatment of *Bartonella* spp. infections in dogs has not been defined, but an assortment of antibiotics have been used, including doxycycline, azithromycin, fluoroquinolones, amoxicillin/clavulanate, and aminoglycosides.[23] However, an *in vitro* study found that only gentamicin, and not ciprofloxacin, streptomycin, erythromycin, ampicillin, or doxycycline, exerted bactericidal activity against *Bartonella* spp.[24] Azithromycin appears to have the least minimum bactericidal activity compared with the other medications listed above and is susceptible to rapid development of resistance.[25] Therefore azithromycin should not be a first-line sole antibiotic treatment for bartonellosis. Treatment with at least 2 weeks of aminoglycosides has been shown to improve survival in people with *Bartonella* IE.[26] In dogs with severe life-threatening IE resulting from *Bartonella* spp., aggressive treatment with aminoglycosides may be necessary, with careful monitoring of renal values and cautiously administered intravenous fluids. Measurement of pulmonary capillary wedge pressure with an indwelling Swan Ganz catheter may be helpful in these cases to monitor serially left heart filling pressure and manage heart failure.

Anticoagulant therapy currently is not recommended because there has been a trend of increased bleeding episodes and no benefit in vegetation resolution or reduced embolic events in humans with IE treated with aspirin.[3] Although the use of antithrombotic therapy in IE in humans is somewhat controversial, a recent summary of European guidelines for IE in people stated, "There is no indication for the initiation of antithrombotic drugs (thrombolytic drugs, anticoagulant, or antiplatelet therapy) during the active phase of IE" because of increased risk of intracranial hemorrhage.[27] An early diagnosis, prompt antibiotic treatment, and a careful selection of patients who benefit from early surgical intervention remain essential in the prevention of embolic complications in people with IE.[28] Surgery is often the therapy of choice in human patients at high risk for thromboembolism, including patients with vegetative lesions larger than 10 mm or patients with recurrent thromboembolism despite antimicrobial therapy. Because there is no data regarding effects of anticoagulants on thromboembolic complications of IE in dogs, the author tends to extrapolate human results and does not recommend anticoagulants in dogs with IE, much like anticoagulants are not recommended for dogs with heartworm disease to lessen thromboembolic complications.

Standard heart failure therapy including furosemide, an ACE inhibitor, and pimobendan is appropriate in dogs with IE of the mitral or aortic valves (see Chapter 40 for more information regarding heart failure therapy). Afterload reduction with amlodipine (0.2 to 0.5 mg/kg PO q12-24h) may be needed in dogs with heart failure because of severe aortic insufficiency, or in dogs with severe mitral regurgitation and refractory heart failure. Systolic arterial blood pressure should be maintained less than 140 mm Hg (but more than 95 mm Hg), and 10 to 15 mm Hg lower than baseline blood pressure.

Table 98-1[29] **Common Etiologic Agents, Typical Antimicrobial Sensitivity Profiles, and Treatment Recommendations for Dogs With Infective Endocarditis**

Etiological Agent and Bacteremia Source	Typical Sensitivity Profile	Recommended Antibiotic
Staphylococcus intermedius Pyoderma	Usually sensitive	Acute: timentin IV q6h or enrofloxacin IV q12h × 1-2 wk Chronic: amoxicillin with clavulanic acid or enrofloxacin ≥ 6-8 wk
Staphylococcus aureus	Often resistant If methicillin resistance, avoid β-lactam antibiotics	Individually dependent, evaluate MIC Acute: amikacin or vancomycin and oxacillin, nafcillin or cefazolin IV × 1-2 wk Chronic: if not methicillin resistant, high-dose first-generation cephalosporin PO ≥ 6-8 wk
Streptococcus canis Urogenital, skin, respiratory tract	Usually sensitive	Acute: ampicillin IV q6-8h or ceftriaxone IV q12h × 1-2 wk If resistant, amikacin and high-dose penicillin Chronic: amoxicillin with or without clavulanic acid PO ≥ 6-8 wk
Escherichia coli GI tract, peritonitis, urinary tract	Often resistant (β-lactamase production)	Individually dependent, evaluate MIC Acute: amikacin and/or carbapenem IV q8h × 1-2 wk Chronic: carbapenem SC ≥ 6-8
Pseudomonas spp. Chronic wounds, burns	Resistant, need extended MIC	Acute: amikacin, timentin, or carbapenem × 1-2 wk Chronic: carbapenem SC or amoxicillin with clavulanic acid ≥ 6-8 wk
Bartonella spp.	MIC not predictive of MBC	Acute: amikacin 20 mg/kg IV ×1-2 wk Chronic: doxycycline AND enrofloxacin > 6-8 wk; may add azithromycin 5 mg/kg PO q24h × 7 days then EOD if lack of response
Culture negative	Unknown	Acute: amikacin and timentin IV × 1-2 wk Chronic: amoxicillin with clavulanic acid PO ≥ 6-8 wk and enrofloxacin PO ≥ 6-8 wk

Specific drug doses should be based on the high end of the recommended range with consideration of patient factors such as renal disease. Typical MIC profiles derived from UC Davis VMTH microbial service database of antimicrobial sensitivity of cultured microorganisms. Recommended antibiotics for particular bacteria were chosen based on ≥ 90% of the cultured isolates sensitive to the particular antibiotic. *d,* Day; *EOD,* every other day; *MBC,* minimum bactericidal concentration; *MIC,* minimum inhibitory concentration; *wk,* week.

Nitroprusside may be necessary in patients with acute fulminant heart failure resulting from severe mitral or aortic IE.

PROGNOSIS

Dogs with aortic IE have a grave prognosis, and median survival in one study was only 3 days compared with a median survival of 476 days for dogs with mitral valve IE.[4] Likewise, dogs with *Bartonella* IE have short survival times because the aortic valve is affected almost exclusively. Another case series of dogs with aortic IE reported similar outcomes, including 33% mortality in the first week and 92% mortality within 5 months of diagnosis.[9] Other risk factors for early cardiovascular death include glucocorticoid administration before treatment, presence of thrombocytopenia, high serum creatinine concentration, renal complications, and thromboembolic disease.[5,8] Death occurring soon after diagnosis most often is due to CHF or sudden cardiac death from a lethal arrhythmia. Other causes of death within the first week of treatment in dogs with IE include renal failure, pulmonary hemorrhage, and severe neurologic disease.

REFERENCES

1. Que YA, Moreillon P: Infective endocarditis, Nat Rev Cardiol 8:322-336, 2011.
2. Guyton AC, Lindsay AW: Effect of elevated left atrial pressure and decreased plasma protein concentration on the development of pulmonary edema, Circ Res 7:649-657, 1959.
3. Baddour LM, Wilson WR, Bayer AS, et al: Infective endocarditis: diagnosis, antimicrobial therapy, and management of complications: a statement for healthcare professionals from the Committee on Rheumatic Fever, Endocarditis, and Kawasaki Disease, Council on Cardiovascular Disease in the Young, and the Councils on Clinical Cardiology, Stroke, and Cardiovascular Surgery and Anesthesia, American Heart Association: endorsed by the Infectious Diseases Society of America, Circulation 111:e394-e434, 2005.
4. MacDonald KA, Chomel BB, Kittleson M, et al: A prospective study of canine infective endocarditis in northern California (1999-2001): emergence of *Bartonella* as a prevalent etiologic agent, J Vet Intern Med 18:56-64, 2004.
5. Sykes JE, Kittleson MD, Chomel BB, et al: Clinicopathologic findings and outcome in dogs with infective endocarditis: 71 cases (1992-2005), J Am Vet Med Assoc 228:1735-1747, 2006.
6. Mugge A, Daniel WG, Frank G, Lichtlen PR: Echocardiography in infective endocarditis: reassessment of prognostic implications of vegetation size determined by the transthoracic and the transesophageal approach, J Am Coll Cardiol 14:631-638, 1989.
7. Macarie C, Iliuta L, Savulescu C, et al: Echocardiographic predictors of embolic events in infective endocarditis, Kardiol Pol 60:535-540, 2004.
8. Calvert CA: Valvular bacterial endocarditis in the dog, J Am Vet Med Assoc 180:1080-1084, 1982.
9. Sisson D, Thomas WP: Endocarditis of the aortic valve in the dog, J Am Vet Med Assoc 184:570-577, 1984.
10. Peddle GD, Drobatz KJ, Harvey CE, et al: Association of periodontal disease, oral procedures, and other clinical findings with bacterial endocarditis in dogs, J Am Vet Med Assoc 234:100-107, 2009.
11. Sykes JE, Kittleson MD, Pesavento PA, et al: Evaluation of the relationship between causative organisms and clinical characteristics of infective endocarditis in dogs: 71 cases (1992-2005), J Am Vet Med Assoc 228:1723-1734, 2006.
12. Schmiedt C, Kellum H, Legendre AM, et al: Cardiovascular involvement in 8 dogs with blastomyces dermatitidis infection, J Vet Intern Med 20:1351-1354, 2006.

13. Breitschwerdt EB, Hegarty BC, Hancock SI: Sequential evaluation of dogs naturally infected with *Ehrlichia canis, Ehrlichia chaffeensis, Ehrlichia equi, Ehrlichia ewingii*, or *Bartonella vinsonii*, J Clin Microbiol 36:2645-2651, 1998.
14. Breitschwerdt EB, Atkins CE, Brown TT, et al: Bartonella vinsonii subsp. berkhoffii and related members of the alpha subdivision of the Proteobacteria in dogs with cardiac arrhythmias, endocarditis, or myocarditis, J Clin Microbiol 37:3618-3626, 1999.
15. Chomel BB, Kasten RW, Williams C, et al: Bartonella endocarditis: a pathology shared by animal reservoirsand patients, Ann N Y Acad Sci 1166:120-126, 2009.
16. Ohad DG, Morick D, Avidor B, et al: Molecular detection of *Bartonella henselae* and *Bartonella koehlerae* from aortic valves of Boxer dogs with infective endocarditis, Vet Microbiol 141:182-185, 2010.
17. Pesavento PA, Chomel BB, Kasten RW, et al: Pathology of bartonella endocarditis in six dogs, Vet Pathol 42:370-373, 2005.
18. Peddle G, Sleeper MM: Canine bacterial endocarditis: a review, J Am Anim Hosp Assoc 43:258-263, 2007.
19. Meurs KM, Heaney AM, Atkins CE, et al: Comparison of polymerase chain reaction with bacterial 16s primers to blood culture to identify bacteremia in dogs with suspected bacterial endocarditis, J Vet Intern Med 25:959-962, 2011.
20. Perez C, Maggi RG, Diniz PP, et al: Molecular and serological diagnosis of *Bartonella* infection in 61 dogs from the United States, J Vet Intern Med 25:805-810, 2011.
21. Arai S, Wright BD, Miyake Y, et al: Heterotopic implantation of a porcine bioprosthetic heart valve in a dog with aortic valve endocarditis, J Am Vet Med Assoc 231:727-730, 2007.
22. Barker CW, Zhang W, Sanchez S, et al: Pharmacokinetics of imipenem in dogs, Am J Vet Res 64:694-699, 2003.
23. Breitschwerdt EB, Blann KR, Stebbins ME, et al: Clinicopathological abnormalities and treatment response in 24 dogs seroreactive to *Bartonella vinsonii (berkhoffii)* antigens, J Am Anim Hosp Assoc 40:92-101, 2004.
24. Rolain JM, Maurin M, Raoult D: Bactericidal effect of antibiotics on *Bartonella* and *Brucella* spp.: clinical implications, J Antimicrob Chemother 46:811-814, 2000.
25. Biswas S, Maggi RG, Papich MG, et al: Molecular mechanisms of *Bartonella henselae* resistance to azithromycin, pradofloxacin and enrofloxacin, J Antimicrob Chemother 65:581-582, 2010.
26. Raoult D, Fournier PE, Vandenesch F, et al: Outcome and treatment of Bartonella endocarditis, Arch Intern Med 163:226-230, 2003.
27. Tornos P, Gonzalez-Alujas T, Thuny F, et al: Infective endocarditis: the European viewpoint, Curr Probl Cardiol 36:175-222, 2011.
28. Vanassche T, Peetermans WE, Herregods MC, et al: Anti-thrombotic therapy in infective endocarditis, Expert Rev Cardiovasc Ther 9:1203-1219, 2011.
29. From MacDonald KA: Infective endocarditis. In Bonagura J, editor: Current Veterinary Therapy XIV, St. Louis, 2005, Saunders.

CHAPTER 99
UROSEPSIS

Lillian R. Aronson, VMD, DACVS

KEY POINTS

- Urosepsis is an uncommonly diagnosed condition in the small animal patient.
- *E. coli* is the most frequently diagnosed uropathogen in patients with urosepsis.
- In most animals with urosepsis, bacteria from the rectum, genital, and perineal areas serve as the principle source of infection.
- Patients with a urinary tract infection and risk factors, including the presence of an anatomic abnormality, a urinary tract obstruction, nephrolithiasis, prior urinary tract disease, renal failure, neurologic disease, diabetes mellitus, hyperadrenocorticism, and immunosuppression, are more prone to the development of urosepsis.
- Causes of urosepsis that have been identified in the veterinary patient include pyelonephritis, bladder rupture, prostatic infection, testicular and vaginal abscessation, pyometra, and catheter-associated urinary tract infections.
- Treatment should be instituted as soon as possible and often includes a combination of intravenous fluid and broad-spectrum antimicrobial therapy, correction of the underlying condition, as well as attempting to correct any predisposing or complicating factors.

Urosepsis, an uncommonly reported condition in veterinary medicine, refers to sepsis associated with a complicated urinary tract infection (UTI). In humans, the source of the infection can be the kidney, bladder, prostate, or genital tract.[1] More specifically, urosepsis in humans has been associated with acute bacterial pyelonephritis, emphysematous pyelonephritis, pyonephrosis, renal abscessation, fungal infections, bladder perforation, and prostatic and testicular infections.[2-5] In addition in human patients, urinary catheter-associated infections also have resulted in sepsis.[6-8] Although many of these conditions often are diagnosed in the veterinary patient, little information currently exists in the veterinary literature regarding the incidence of urosepsis as a complication of these conditions. In one retrospective study looking at sepsis in small animal surgical patients, the urogenital tract was identified as the source of infection in approximately 50% of the cases.[9] Of 61 dogs included in the study, sources of urosepsis included a pyometra (14), prostatic abscessation or suppuration (12), testicular abscessation (3), renal abscessation (3; see Figure 99-1) and vaginal abscessation (1). Of four cats included in the study, one cat had a pyometra and a second cat had a ruptured uterus. This chapter discusses pathogenesis and reviews the current veterinary literature to determine what conditions in veterinary medicine have been associated with urosepsis. Accurate recognition

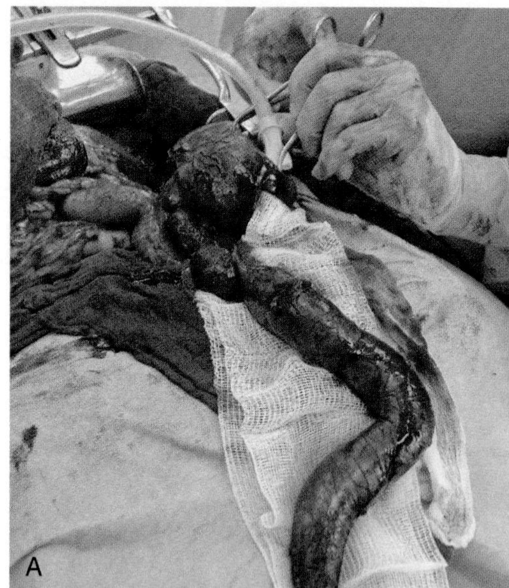

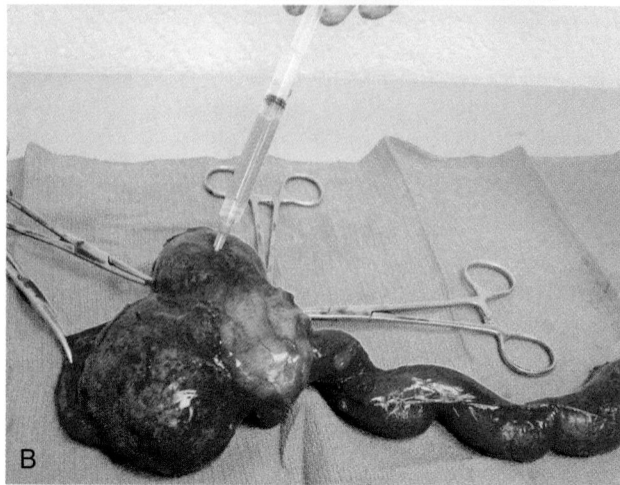

FIGURE 99-1 A, Renal and ureteral abscessation in a dog that presented with urosepsis. **B,** The kidney was not salvageable and a nephrectomy was performed. Purulent fluid was aspirated from the kidney.

of these complicated UTIs and appropriate treatment are necessary to prevent morbidity and mortality.

PATHOGENESIS

Urosepsis is a clinical condition that occurs secondary to a systemic bacterial infection originating from the urogenital tract and the associated inflammatory response. In most cases of urosepsis, bacteria isolated from the rectum, genital, and perineal area are the principle source of infection.[10] These bacteria then can migrate from the genital tract to the lower and then upper urinary tract.[10] Similar to human patients, *E. coli* is the most common uropathogen affecting dogs and cats and accounts for up to 50% of the urine isolates.[10-16] Gram-positive cocci, including staphylococci, streptococci, and enterococci account for up to one third of bacteria isolated and, although uncommonly diagnosed, *Pseudomonas, Klebsiella, Pasteurella, Corynebacterium,* and *Mycoplasma* spp. account for the remaining isolates.[12,17-19] In humans, gram-negative sepsis frequently is caused by infections originating from the urinary tract.[6,13]

E. coli is the most common pathogen affecting the urinary tract of human and veterinary patients and consequently the most commonly isolated pathogen in patients with urosepsis; therefore its virulence has been investigated extensively. Most *E. coli* UTIs are caused by pathogenic *E. coli* from the phylogenetic group B2, and to a lesser extent, group D.[20] Although several hundred serotypes of *E. coli* are known, fewer than 20 account for most bacterial UTIs.[21] In dogs and humans, the majority of strains associated with urovirulence belong to a small number of serogroups (O, K, and H; see Chapter 94).[13] Certain properties that may enhance the bacterial virulence include the presence of a particular pilus that mediates attachment to the uroepithelium; the presence of hemolysin and aerobactin; resistance to the bactericidal action of serum; and the rapid replication time in urine.[10-13] In mouse models of human disease, uropathogenic *E. coli* have been shown to possess multiple adaptations, allowing them to survive and persist in the urinary tract.[22-26] In patients with structural or functional abnormalities of the urinary tract or those with altered defenses, infections can be caused by gram-negative aerobic bacilli other than *E. coli*, gram-positive cocci including staphylococci and enterococci, and by bacterial strains that normally lack uropathogenic properties.[5,14] In patients that have a septic peritonitis associated with a urinary tract disorder, the visceral and parietal peritoneum provide a large surface area for absorption of bacteria and endotoxins, resulting in septic shock (see Chapter 91).[27]

The development of a UTI and subsequent urosepsis in human and veterinary patients often represents a balance between the quantity and pathogenicity of the infectious agents and host defenses. The following local host defense mechanisms typically prevent ascending UTIs: normal micturition, extensive renal blood supply, normal urinary tract anatomy (i.e., urethral length and high pressure zones within the urethra), urethral and ureteral peristalsis, mucosal defense barriers, antimicrobial properties of the urine, and systemic immunocompetence.[10,12] Systemic defenses are most important for the prevention of hematogenous spread from the urinary tract.[10] Patients with a UTI and risk factors including the presence of an anatomic abnormality, a urinary tract obstruction, nephrolithiasis, prior urinary tract disease, renal failure, neurologic disease, diabetes mellitus, hyperadrenocorticism, and/or immunosuppression should be considered to have a complicated UTI and are more prone to the development of urosepsis.[2,5,10,28-30] In addition, a UTI diagnosed in pregnant or intact dogs and cats also should be considered complicated.

Clinical and laboratory findings in patients with urosepsis are often similar to patients whose sepsis originated from another source; these may include lethargy, fever, hypothermia, hyperemic mucous membranes, tachycardia, tachypnea, bounding pulses, a positive blood culture, and a leukogram that reveals a leukocytosis or leukopenia with or without a left shift (see Chapter 91).[31] However, patients with urosepsis may display early laboratory changes that identify abnormalities specifically related to the urinary tract, including azotemia, an active urine sediment, and a positive urine bacterial culture. A positive urine culture is extremely important in these patients to confirm the results of the blood culture by isolation of the same organism(s) with identical antimicrobial profiles.[6] In cases of severe sepsis, multiple organ dysfunction can be present along with pale mucous membranes, weak pulses, and a prolonged capillary refill time (see Chapter 7). In addition, in cats, diffuse abdominal pain, bradycardia, anemia, and icterus may be identified.[31]

Aggressive treatment is necessary and typically includes a combination of intravenous fluids and broad-spectrum antimicrobial therapy. However, specific treatment protocols vary depending on the source of the infection and the complications resulting from sepsis. Once the culture and susceptibility testing results are available, antimicrobial coverage should be modified to treat the isolated organism(s). Veterinary professionals have continued concerns regarding the increasing resistance of canine urinary tract isolates to common antimicrobials, including fluoroquinolones, clavulanic acid–potentiated β-lactams, and third-generation cephalosporins.[32-35]

Similar to humans, canine *E. coli* isolates resistant to fluoroquinolones have a lower prevalence for many of the virulence genes and are more likely to be from phylogenetic groups A and B1 and less likely from phylogenetic group B2.[36] Prudent use of antimicrobials is critical to reduce the incidence of antimicrobial resistance. In addition, the clinician should address the underlying condition and attempt to correct any complicating factors.[14] Although different causes of urosepsis in the veterinary patient somewhat overlap, some clinical findings, laboratory results, and treatments are unique to each condition. The rest of this chapter discusses the different causes of urosepsis that have been identified in small animals.

CAUSES OF UROSEPSIS

Pyelonephritis

The kidneys and ureters are affected most commonly by ascending bacteria rather than via hematogenous infections. Renal trauma or the presence of a urinary tract obstruction may increase the incidence of hematogenous spread of infection to the urinary tract because of interference with the renal microcirculation.[37,38] In human patients, hematogenous pyelonephritis occurs most commonly in patients debilitated from either chronic illness or those receiving immunosuppressive therapy.[13] Urosepsis resulting from pyelonephritis has been reported uncommonly in the veterinary literature. In a retrospective study evaluating 61 dogs with severe sepsis, a renal abscess in conjunction with pyelonephritis was the source of the infection in only three dogs.[9] In a second retrospective study evaluating 29 cats with sepsis, pyelonephritis was the cause in only two cats.[31] The author has identified seven cats with obstructive calcium oxalate urolithiasis that also were diagnosed with a pyelonephritis based upon a positive bacteriologic culture result from urine collected by pyelocentesis. None of the cats identified were clinically septicemic, but this can be difficult to diagnose definitively in feline patients. Human patients with infected stones or renal pelvic urine were found to be at a greater risk for the development of urosepsis than those with a lower UTI.[39]

Dogs and cats with pyelonephritis and urosepsis may be febrile, anorexic, lethargic, and dehydrated and have a history of recent weight loss. If the disease is acute, one or both kidneys may be enlarged and painful, and the animal may have signs of polyuria, polydipsia, and vomiting. Azotemia secondary to acute kidney injury may be present, and blood work often reveals a neutrophilic leukocytosis with a left shift and a metabolic acidosis. In acute and chronic cases, abdominal ultrasound and/or intravenous pyelography may reveal mild to moderate pelvic dilation and ureteral dilation. The renal cortex as well as the surrounding retroperitoneal space may appear hyperechoic. Renal enlargement often is identified in cases of acute pyelonephritis; poor corticomedullary definition, distortion of the renal collecting system, irregular renal shape, and reduced kidney size may be seen with chronic cases. The urinalysis may reveal impaired urine concentrating ability, bacteriuria, pyuria, proteinuria, hematuria, and/or granular casts.[10,40]

As previously mentioned, treatment includes the removal of predisposing factors, intravenous fluid therapy, and broad-spectrum antimicrobial administration until a specific organism is identified. Antimicrobial therapy targeted against the isolated organism should continue for 4 to 8 weeks. A urinalysis and bacterial culture should be performed after 1 week of treatment and before discontinuation of antimicrobial therapy to determine whether the infection has resolved. In addition, a urine culture should be performed 2 to 3 days after therapy has been discontinued. In cases of unilateral advanced pyelonephritis, pyonephrosis, or the presence of a renal abscess, a total nephrectomy in addition to antimicrobial therapy is often the preferred treatment.[41] Cases of pyonephrosis have been treated successfully at the author's institution with the temporary placement of a ureteral stent to allow for continued drainage of the kidney. This is done in conjunction with antimicrobial therapy based on culture and susceptibility.

Bladder Rupture

Although rare, urosepsis may result from a bladder and/or a proximal urethral rupture in a patient with a lower UTI.[42] Urosepsis is not identified typically in patients with an intact lower urinary tract.[10] Rupture of the urinary tract in dogs and cats most commonly occurs after blunt trauma resulting from being hit by a car. Other causes include penetrating injuries, aggressive catheterization, rupture secondary to prolonged urethral obstruction, or excessive force during bladder expression. Physical examination may reveal dehydration, lack of a bladder on palpation, fluid accumulation within the peritoneal cavity, and ventral abdominal bruising. Clinical signs are often vague initially but can worsen as the uremia and inflammation/sepsis progress. Signs may include vomiting, anorexia, depression, abdominal pain, and systemic inflammation (see Chapter 6). Abdominocentesis and abdominal fluid to peripheral blood creatinine and/or potassium ratios are often diagnostic of uroperitoneum,[43,44] and the presence of bacteria on cytology confirms a septic peritonitis (for further details, see Chapter 122).[45] Urosepsis after bladder rupture is reported uncommonly in the veterinary literature. In a retrospective study evaluating 23 dogs and cats with septic peritonitis, only one cat had septic peritonitis associated with intestinal herniation and bladder rupture.[46] In a second study evaluating 26 cases of uroperitoneum in cats, five patients had aerobic bacterial cultures performed from the peritoneum or bladder, and of those, three were positive. Organisms isolated included *Enterococcus* spp., *Staphylococcus* spp., and alpha-streptococcus.[43]

If septic peritonitis is confirmed, early repair and/or urinary diversion is recommended to halt continued accumulation of septic urine in the abdominal cavity. The bladder defect is debrided of any devitalized tissue and then closed using a single-layer appositional suture pattern. If the viability of the bladder wall is a concern, a closed indwelling urinary catheter system can be used to maintain bladder decompression postoperatively. Treatment options for patients with urethral trauma include primary urethral repair, placement of a urethral catheter to stent the urethra, placement of a cystostomy tube for urinary diversion until the urethra heals, or the combination of a cystostomy tube and a urethral catheter.

Prostatic Infection

In addition to normal host defense mechanisms previously mentioned, prostatic fluid contains a zinc-associated antibacterial factor, which serves as an important natural defense mechanism. Despite these defense mechanisms, bacterial colonization of the prostate can occur through ascension of urethral flora or by the hematogenous route.[47] Suppurative prostatitis and prostatic abscessation are some of the most common causes of urosepsis in canine surgical patients, with 12 out of 61 cases diagnosed in one study.[9] Dogs with suppurative prostatitis usually have a history of an acute onset of illness. Patients often are presented with signs of anorexia, vomiting, tenesmus, lethargy, fever, dehydration, injected mucous membranes, weight loss, pain upon rectal examination, caudal abdominal discomfort and/or pain in the pelvic and lumbar region, a stiff or stilted gait, and an unwillingness to breed.[48-50] In addition, hematuria, pyuria, stranguria, hemorrhagic preputial discharge, urinary incontinence, or the inability to urinate also may be identified. If the infection is not treated, microabscesses can form and eventually coalesce into a large abscess. A complete blood count often reveals a mature neutrophilia and evidence of a left shift. Septicemia and endotoxemia quickly develop, particularly if the abscess has ruptured into the abdominal cavity.[51] After rupture of a prostatic abscess, the peritoneal surface provides a large surface area for absorption of bacteria and bacterial by-products, thus leading to the development of septic shock. Hindlimb edema also has been identified in these patients and can result from altered vascular permeability that commonly occurs with sepsis as well as the presence of an abscess interfering with normal lymphatic and venous drainage from the peripheral lymph nodes.

A definitive diagnosis is confirmed after identification of a septic exudate from an ejaculated sample, prostatic wash, traumatic catheterization, urethral discharge, or fine-needle aspirate (although this can be dangerous). Inflammatory changes identified in prostatic fluid are associated with histologic inflammation in more than 80% of the cases.[52] Because of the potential of inducing septicemia during prostatic palpation or rupturing an abscess on fine-needle aspiration, it can be difficult and even clinically dangerous to collect prostatic fluid using some of the above-mentioned techniques from dogs with acute prostatitis.[49] In dogs, similar to humans with acute bacterial prostatitis, bacteremia may result from manipulation of the inflamed gland.[13,49] Because the infectious agent often can be identified on a Gram stain of the urine and bacterial culture collected via cystocentesis, vigorous prostatic palpation generally is avoided.[13] Abdominal radiographs often reveal prostatomegaly; the area near the bladder neck may have poor detail resulting from localized peritonitis. Abdominal ultrasound may reveal varying echogenicity with symmetric or asymmetric enlargement of the gland. Cyst like structures as well as hypoechoic areas also may be present and could represent abscess formation. Rectal examination may reveal fluctuant areas when the abscess is near the dorsal periphery of the gland. Dogs with prostatitis may have a normal ultrasound examination, underscoring the need to make a definitive diagnosis using the previously mentioned techniques.

Suppurative prostatitis and prostatic abscessation are serious life-threatening disorders. In patients with acute suppurative prostatitis, treatment involves fluid therapy to correct dehydration and treat cardiovascular shock and antimicrobial therapy based on culture and susceptibility of urine or prostatic fluid. Because of the risks of obtaining prostatic fluid in this patient population, a urine sample for a urinalysis as well as culture and susceptibility testing should be obtained first to determine if a diagnosis can be made. Antimicrobials should be administered for a minimum of 4 to 6 weeks, then the urine or prostatic fluid should be cultured after discontinuation of antimicrobial therapy and again in 2 to 4 weeks to determine if the infection is eliminated completely.[47-49] If the infection is not eliminated, resistant bacterial infections of the prostate and urinary tract can develop. Castration also is recommended once the infection is controlled and appears to be beneficial in the resolution of chronic bacterial prostatitis in an experimental model.[49,52,53]

In addition to the above-mentioned treatments, surgical drainage or excision is often the treatment of choice in a patient with a prostatic abscess. Antimicrobial therapy in conjunction with castration alone has been ineffective at resolving abscesses.[50] Before surgery, ultrasonography is used to determine the location(s) of the abscess(es). Surgical techniques that have been described to treat prostatic abscessation include prostatic omentalization, placement of Penrose drains, marsupialization of the abscess, ultrasound-guided percutaneous drainage, and subtotal or excisional prostatectomy.[42,54,55] In one study, of the three dogs that were presented with prostatic abscessation, two already had signs of sepsis.[54] In a second study, 15 out of 92 dogs died in the postoperative period because of sepsis. *E. coli* was the most common bacteria isolated.[51] Sepsis and shock were common postoperative complications developing in 33% of the dogs surviving surgery. Absorption of bacteria and toxins from an infected prostate gland and inflamed peritoneal surface contributed to the development of septic shock.[51] Approximately half of the dogs that died had rupture of the abscess and secondary septic peritonitis and shock before surgery.

Pyometra

Pyometra is a serious condition affecting older dogs in the luteal stage of the estrus cycle. It has been associated with neutrophilia and impaired immune function, including a decrease in lymphocyte activity.[56] Urosepsis can occur in dogs and cats diagnosed with pyometra with or without uterine rupture. In the largest retrospective study to date evaluating sepsis in the small animal surgical patient, pyometra was the most common source of urosepsis, with 14 out of 61 dogs reported. Of four cats included in the study, urosepsis occurred secondary to a pyometra in one cat and a ruptured uterus in a second cat.[9] In a review of 80 cases of pyometra, 3 out of 73 dogs developed complications from generalized septicemia and thromboembolic disease in the immediate postoperative period, and one dog died from endotoxic shock resulting from a ruptured uterus.[57] In a second retrospective study evaluating 183 cats diagnosed with pyometra, uterine rupture was present in seven cats. Four of seven cats died of septic peritonitis after uterine rupture.[58] Many aerobic and some anaerobic bacteria have been identified in dogs and cats with pyometra, including *Staphylococcus*, *Streptococcus*, *Pasteurella*, *Klebsiella*, *Proteus*, *Pseudomonas*, *Aerobacter*, *Haemophilus*, and *Moraxella* spp. and *Serratia marcescens*. However, *E. coli* is the most common bacteria isolated. Strains of *E. coli* in cases of canine pyometra display a strong similarity to isolates obtained from UTIs, likely because of the similar pathogenesis (i.e., ascending from the host's intestinal or vaginal flora).[59] UTIs are common complications of pyometra. Although culture results are rarely negative in the dog, aerobic culture results are negative in 15% to 31% of affected cats.[58,60] Dogs diagnosed with a pyometra often are presented systemically sick with signs of anorexia, lethargy, depression, polydipsia, vomiting, diarrhea, and, if the cervix is patent, vaginal discharge. When abdominal pain is present, septic peritonitis is likely.[58] *E. coli* pyometra has been associated commonly with renal dysfunction in dogs, albeit typically transient.[61-65] A recent study evaluating urinary biomarkers in these patients has identified the glomerulus and proximal tubules of the nephron as the main sites of injury.[66] Body temperature may be normal, elevated, or subnormal. Clinical signs in cats are similar but often more subtle.

Clinicopathologic abnormalities in both species can occur to varying degrees and may include anemia, leukocytosis, or leukopenia with a left shift, azotemia, hypoalbuminemia, hypoglycemia or hyperglycemia, hyperglobulinemia, increased alkaline phosphatase, and metabolic acidosis.[58,67-69] Before surgery, medical therapy should be instituted and include intravenous fluid and antimicrobial therapy to correct deficits and concurrent metabolic derangements (see Chapters 60 and 91). Surgery is not postponed in the very sick animals for more than a few hours because of worsening septicemia. Treatment for pyometra is ovariohysterectomy. If the uterus ruptures at surgery, the abdomen is lavaged and the patient treated for septic peritonitis (see Chapter 122).

Catheter-Associated Urinary Tract Infection

In human patients, bacteriuria occurs in up to 20% of hospitalized patients with indwelling urinary catheters and, of these patients, 1% to 2% develop gram-negative bacteremia.[13] The catheterized urinary tract has been demonstrated repeatedly to be the most common source of gram-negative sepsis in human patients[13] and, although rare, the mortality rate in these patients can reach 30%.[13] In human patients, bacteremia can occur immediately as a result of mucosal trauma associated with catheter placement and removal or secondary to mucosal ulceration.[13] Many infecting strains, including *E. coli* and

Proteus, Pseudomonas, Klebsiella, and *Serratia* spp., show marked antimicrobial resistance compared with organisms identified in uncomplicated UTIs.

Although nosocomial UTIs after the use of an indwelling urinary catheter in dogs and cats is reported to be a common complication by some authors, the subsequent development of urosepsis is uncommon. Bacterial UTIs developed in 20% of healthy adult female dogs after intermittent catheterization; in 33% of male dogs during repeated catheterization and in 65% of healthy male cats within 3 to 5 days of open indwelling catheterization.[10,70]

A few studies in the veterinary literature have looked at the incidence of UTIs in dogs and cats when a closed catheter system was used. In one study, 11 out of 21 (52%) animals and in a second study, 9 out of 28 animals (32%) developed catheter-associated infections.[71,72] Both of these studies suggested that the risk of infection increased with duration of catheterization and that antimicrobial therapy was associated with increasingly resistant gram-negative organisms. Although the incidence of catheter-associated infections was high in both studies, urosepsis was not identified. In the most recent study looking at the incidence of catheter-associated UTIs in 39 dogs in a small animal intensive care unit, only 4 of 39 dogs (10.3%) developed a UTI.[72] The lower incidence reported in this study was attributed to a shorter duration of catheterization, stricter definition of infection, different indications for catheterization, urine sample collection technique, and the protocol for catheter placement and maintenance. Urosepsis was not a reported complication.

In veterinary and in human hospitals, pathogens can be introduced from the hands of hospital staff, via instrumentation or contaminated disinfectants. The most common location for bacteria to enter the system can occur at the catheter-collecting tube junction or at the drainage bag portal. Intestinal flora also can migrate along the catheter into the bladder from the perineal area of the patient.[13] In a study evaluating multidrug-resistant (MDR) *E. coli* isolates from urine collected from dogs with an indwelling urinary catheter, the electrophoresis pattern of the MDR isolate from one dog was similar to the rectal isolate from the same dog.[73] To prevent or minimize the incidence of catheter-associated infections, clinicians should avoid indiscriminate use of catheters. In addition, catheters should be used cautiously in patients with preexisting urinary tract disease, cats or female dogs with voluminous diarrhea, or those whose immune system is compromised. Appropriate antimicrobial therapy should be instituted rapidly should an infection occur.

Many veterinary hospitals use used intravenous fluid bags as part of their urine collection system, resulting in an open system. In a recent study, 95 properly stored (at least 7 days), used intravenous bags were cultured to see if they were a potential source of contamination for the patient. No aerobic bacterial contamination or growth was identified in the system.[74] Recently, the use of an open versus closed collection system for a short duration of catheterization (at least 7 days) was evaluated with regard to the development of nosocomial bacteriuria. The study included 51 dogs and found an overall incidence of bacteriuria of 9.8%; the type of collection system (open vs. closed) was not associated with the development of bacteriuria. The authors concluded that the low incidence of bacteriuria likely was associated with a strict standard protocol of catheter placement and maintenance as well as the short duration of indwelling catheterization.[75] Another study found that the risk of infection increased by 27% for each 1-day increase in catheterization.[76] Because a longer duration of catheterization has been associated with antimicrobial resistant bacteria and the duration of catheterization is unpredictable, prophylactic use of antimicrobials is not recommended.[72] In addition, diagnostic and therapeutic procedures that may result in the introduction of bacteria into the urinary system also should be minimized.[10,13]

CONCLUSION

Urosepsis is an uncommonly diagnosed but serious problem that can affect dogs and cats. Conditions in veterinary medicine that have been associated with urosepsis include bacterial pyelonephritis and renal abscessation, bladder rupture in patients with a UTI, prostatic suppuration and abscessation, testicular and vaginal abscessation, pyometra, and catheter-associated UTIs. Risk factors that may cause patients to be more prone to the development of urosepsis or complicate treatment include the presence of an anatomic abnormality, a urinary tract obstruction, nephrolithiasis, prior urinary tract disease, acute kidney injury, neurologic disease, diabetes, Cushing's disease, and immunosuppression. Accurate recognition and aggressive therapy addressing the underlying condition, complicating risk factors, and the associated inflammatory response are necessary to prevent significant morbidity and mortality.

REFERENCES

1. Kunin CM: Definition of acute pyelonephritis vs the urosepsis syndrome, Arch Intern Med 163:2393-2394, 2003.
2. O'Donnell MA: Urological sepsis. In Zinner SR, editor: Sepsis and multi-organ failure, Baltimore, 1997, Williams & Wilkins, pp 441-449.
3. Stamm WE: Urinary tract infections and pyelonephritis. In Harrison's principles of internal medicine, ed 15, New York, 2001, McGraw-Hill, pp 1620-1626.
4. Opal SM: Urinary tract infections. In Irwin RS, Cerra FB, Rippe JM: Intensive care medicine, Philadelphia, 1999, Lippincott-Raven, pp 1117-1126.
5. Melekos MD, Naber KG: Complicated urinary tract infections, Int J Antimicrob Agents 15:247-256, 2000.
6. Paradisi F, Corti G, Mangani V: Urosepsis in the critical care unit, Crit Care Clin 14:166-181, 1998.
7. Rosser CJ, Bare RL, Meredith JW: Urinary tract infections in the critically ill patient with a urinary catheter, Am J Surg 177:287-290, 1999.
8. Reed RL: Contemporary issues with bacterial infection in the intensive care unit, Surg Clin North Am 80:1-12, 2000.
9. Hardie EM, Rawlings CA, Calvert CA: Severe sepsis in selected small animal surgical patients, J Small Anim Pract 44:13-16, 2003.
10. Bartges JW: Urinary tract infections. In Ettinger SC, Feldman EC: Textbook of veterinary internal medicine, ed 6, St Louis, 2005, Elsevier, pp 1800-1808.
11. Senior DF: Management of difficult urinary tract infections. In Bonagura JD: Kirk's current veterinary therapy XIII: small animal practice, Philadelphia, 1999, WB Saunders, pp 883-888.
12. Bartges JW, Barsanti JE: Bacterial urinary tract infections in cats. In Bonagura JD: Kirk's current veterinary therapy XIII: small animal practice, Philadelphia, 1999, WB Saunders, pp 880-886.
13. Stamm WE, Turck M: Urinary tract infections and pyelonephritis. In Harrison JR, Wilson JD, Isselbacher KJ, et al, editors: Harrison's Principles of internal medicine, ed 12, New York, 1991, McGraw-Hill, pp 538-544.
14. Wagenlehner FME, Naber KG: Hospital-acquired urinary tract infections, J Hosp Infect 46:171-181, 2000.
15. Feldman EC: Urinary tract infections. In Nelson RW, Couto CG, editors: Small animal internal medicine, ed 4, St Louis, 2009, Mosby, pp 624-630.
16. Olszyna DP, Prins JM, Dekkers PEP: Sequential measurements of chemokines in urosepsis and experimental endotoxemia, J Clin Immunol 19:399-405, 1999.
17. Lees GE: Epidemiology of naturally occurring feline bacterial urinary tract infections, Vet Clin North Am Small Anim Pract 14:471-479, 1984.
18. Ling GV, Norris CR, Franti CE, et al: Interrelations of organism prevalence, specimen collection method, and host age, sex, and breed among 8,354 canine urinary tract infections (1969-1995), J Vet Intern Med 15:341-347, 2001.
19. Wooley RE, Blue JL: Quantitative and bacteriological studies of urine specimens from canine and feline urinary tract infections, J Clin Microbiol 4:326-329, 1976.

20. Thompson MF, Litster AL, Platell JL, et al: Canine bacterial urinary tract infections: new developments in old pathogens, Vet J 190:22-27, 2011.
21. Oluoch AO, Kim CH, Weisiger RM, et al: Nonenteric *Escherichia coli* isolates from dogs: 674 cases (1990-1998), J Am Vet Med Assoc 218:381-384, 2001.
22. Kau AL, Hunstad DA, Hultgren SJ: Interaction of uropathogenic Escherichia coli with host uroepithelium, Curr Opin Microbiol 8:54-59, 2005.
23. Garofalo CK, Hooton TM, Martin SM, et al: Escherichia coli from the urine of female patients with urinary tract infections is competent for intracellular bacterial community formation, Infect Immun 75:52-60, 2007.
24. Mulvey MA, Schilling JD, Hultgren SJ: Establishment of a persistent *Escherichia coli* reservoir during the acute phase of a bladder infection, Infect Immun 69:4572-4579, 2001.
25. Justice SS, Hung C, Theriot JA, et al: Differentiation and development pathways of uropathogenic *Escherichia coli* in urinary tract pathogenesis, Proc Natl Acad Sci USA 101:1333-1338, 2004.
26. Bower JM, Eto DS, Mulvey MA: Covert operations of uropathogenic *Escherichia coli* within the urinary tract, Traffic 6:18-31, 2005.
27. Matthiessen DT, Marretta SM: Complications associated with the surgical treatment of prostatic abscessation, Probl Vet Med 1:63-73, 1989.
28. Stewart C: Urinary tract infections. In Howell JM: Emergency medicine, Philadelphia, 1998, WB Saunders, pp 859-868.
29. Karunajeewa H, Mcgechie D, Stuccio G, et al: Asymptomatic bacteriuria as a predictor of subsequent hospitalization with urinary tract infection in diabetic adults: The Fremantle Diabetic Study, Diabetologia 48:1288-1291, 2005.
30. Farley MM: Group B Streptococcal disease in nonpregnant adults, Emerg Infect 33:556-561, 2001.
31. Brady CA, Otto CM, Van Winkle TJ, et al: Severe sepsis in cats: 29 cases (1986-1998), J Am Vet Med Assoc 217:531-535, 2000.
32. Gibson JS, Morton JM, Cobbold RN, et al: Multidrug resistant *E. coli* and Enterobacter extraintestinal infection in 37 dogs, J Vet Intern Med 22:844-850, 2008.
33. Cooke CL, Singer RS, Jang SS, et al: Enrofloxacin resistance in *Escherichia coli* isolated from dogs with urinary tract infections, J Am Vet Med Assoc 220:190-192, 2002.
34. Cohn LA, Gary AT, Fales WH, et al: Trends in fluoroquinolone resistance of bacteria isolated from canine urinary tracts, J Vet Diag Invest 15:338-343, 2003.
35. Prescott JF, Hanna WJB, Reid-Smith R, et al: Antimicrobial drug use and resistance in dogs, Can Vet J 43:107-116, 2002.
36. Johnson JR, Kuskowski MA, Owens K, et al: Virulence genotypes and phylogenetic background of fluoroquinolone-resistance and susceptible *Escherichia coli* urine isolates from dogs with urinary tract infections, Vet Microbiol 136:108-114, 2009.
37. Bartges JW, Finco DR, Polzin DJ, et al: Pathophysiology of urethral obstruction, Vet Clin North Am Small Anim Pract 26:255-264, 1996.
38. Finco DR, Barsanti JA: Bacterial pyelonephritis, Vet Clin North Am 9:645, 1979.
39. Mariappan P, Smith G, Bariol SV, et al: Stone and pelvic urine culture and sensitivity are better than bladder urine as predictors of urosepsis following percutaneous nephrolithotomy: a prospective clinical study, J Urol 173:1610-1614, 2005.
40. Dibartola SP, Rutgers HC: Diseases of the kidney. In Sherding RG: The cat: diseases and clinical management, St Louis, 1994, Saunders, pp 1353-1395.
41. Rawlings CA, Bjorling DE, Christie BA: Kidneys. In Slatter D, editor: Textbook of small animal surgery, ed 3, Philadelphia, 2003, Saunders, pp 1606-1619.
42. McGrotty Y, Doust R: Management of peritonitis in dogs and cats, Companion Anim Pract Jul/Aug, pp 360-367, 2004.
43. Aumann M, Worth LT, Drobatz KJ: Uroperitoneum in cats: 26 cases (1986-1995), J Am Anim Hosp Assoc 34:315-324, 1998.
44. Schmiedt C, Tobias KM, Otto CM: Evaluation of abdominal fluid: peripheral blood creatinine and potassium ratios for diagnosis of uroperitoneum in dogs, J Vet Emerg Crit Care 11:275-280, 2001.
45. Kirby BM: Peritoneum and peritoneal cavity. In Slatter D: Textbook of small animal surgery, ed 3, Philadelphia, 2003, Saunders, pp 414-445.
46. King LG: Postoperative complications and prognostic indicators in dogs and cats with septic peritonitis: 23 cases (1989-1992), J Am Vet Med Assoc 204:407-413, 1994.
47. Johnson C: Reproductive system disorders. In Nelson RW, Couto CG, editors: Small animal internal medicine, St Louis, 2003, Mosby, pp 930-932.
48. Basinger RR, Robineete CL, Spaulding KA: Prostate. In Slatter D, editor: Textbook of small animal surgery, ed 3, Philadelphia, 2003, Saunders, pp 1542-1557.
49. Krawiec DR: Canine prostate disease, J Am Vet Med Assoc 204:1561-1563, 1994.
50. Kutzler MA, Yeager A: Prostatic diseases. In Ettinger SG, Feldman EC, editor: Textbook of veterinary internal medicine, St Louis, 2005, Elsevier, pp 1809-1819.
51. Mullen HS, Matthiesses DT, Scavelli TD: Results of surgery and postoperative complications in 92 dogs treated for prostatic abscessation by a multiple Penrose drain technique, J Am Anim Hosp Assoc 26:370-379, 1990.
52. Barsanti JA, Finco DR: Canine prostatic disease, Vet Clin North Am 16:587-599, 1986.
53. Cowan LA, Barsanti JA, Crowell W, et al: Effects of castration on chronic bacterial prostatitis in dogs, J Am Vet Med Assoc 199:346-350, 1991.
54. Apparicio M, Vicenti WRR, Pires EA, et al: Omentalisation as a treatment for prostatic cysts and abscesses, Aust Vet Pract 34:157-159, 2004.
55. Boland LE, Hardie RJ, Gregory SP, et al: Ultrasound-guided percutaneous drainage as the primary treatment for prostatic abscesses and cysts in dogs, J Am Anim Hosp Assoc 39:151-159, 2003.
56. Faldyna M, Laznicka A, Toman M: Immunosuppression in bitches with pyometra, J Small Anim Pract 42:5-10, 2001.
57. Wheaton LG, Johnson AL, Parker AJ, et al: Results and complications of surgical treatment of pyometra: a review of 80 cases, J Am Anim Hosp Assoc 25:563-568, 1989.
58. Kenney KJ, Matthiessen DT, Brown NO, et al: Pyometra in cats: 183 cases (1979-1984), J Am Vet Med Assoc 191:1130-1131, 1987.
59. Hagman R, Kuhn I: *E. coli* strains isolated from the uterus and urinary bladder of bitches suffering from pyometra: comparison by restriction enzyme digestion and pulsed filed gel electrophoresis, Vet Microbiol 84:143-153, 2002.
60. Dow C: The cystic hyperplasia-pyometra complex in the cat, Vet Rec 74:141, 1962.
61. Asheim A: Pathogenesis of renal damage and polydipsia in dogs with pyometra, J Am Vet Med Assoc 147:736-745, 1965.
62. Heiene R, Kristiansen V, Teige J, et al: Renal histomorphology in dogs with pyometra and control dogs, and long term clinical outcome with respect to signs of kidney disease, Acta Vet Scand 49:13-22, 2007.
63. Heiene R, Moe L, Molmen G: Calculation of urinary enzyme excretion, with renal structure and function in dogs with pyometra, Res Vet Sci 70:129-137, 2001.
64. Obel AL, Nicander L, Asheim A: Light and electron microscopic studies of the renal lesions in dogs with pyometra, Acta Vet Scand 5:93-125, 1964.
65. Stone EA, Littman MP, Robertson JL, et al: Renal dysfunction in dogs with pyometra, J Am Vet Med Assoc 193:457-464, 1988.
66. Maddens B, Daminet S, Smets P, et al: Escherichia coli pyometra induces transient glomerular and tubular dysfunction in dogs, J Vet Intern Med 24:1263-1270, 2010.
67. Marretta SM, Matthiessen DT, Nichols R: Pyometra and its complications, Probl Vet Med 1:50-61, 1989.
68. Hardy RM, Osborne CA: Canine pyometra: a polysystemic disorder. J Am Anim Hosp Assoc 10:245-268, 1974.
69. Stone EA, Littman MP, Robertson JL, et al: Renal dysfunction in dogs with pyometra, J Am Vet Med Assoc 193:457-464, 1988.
70. Smarick SD, Haskins SC, Aldrich J, et al: Incidence of catheter-associated urinary tract infection among dogs in a small animal intensive care unit, J Am Vet Med Assoc 224: 1936-1940, 2004.
71. Lippert AC, Fulton RB, Parr AM: Nosocomial infection surveillance in a small animal intensive care unit. J Am Anim Hosp Assoc 24:627-636, 1988.
72. Barsanti JA, Blue J, Edmunds J: Urinary tract infection due to indwelling bladder catheters in dogs and cats, J Am Vet Med Assoc 187:384-387, 1985.

73. Ogeer-Gyles J, Mathews K, Weeses S, et al: Evaluation of catheter-associated urinary tract infections and multi-drug resistant *Escherichia coli* isolates from the urine of dogs with indwelling urinary catheters, J Am Vet Med Assoc 229:1584-1590, 2006.
74. Barrett M, Campbell VL: Aerobic bacterial culture of used intravenous fluid bags intended for use as urine collection reservoirs, J Am Anim Hosp Assoc 44:1-6, 2008.
75. Sullivan LA, Campbell VL, Onuma SC: Evaluation of open versus closed urine collection systems and development of nosocomial bacteriuria in dogs, J Am Vet Med Assoc 237:187-190, 2010.
76. Bubenik LJ, Hosgood GL, Waldron DR, et al: Frequency of urinary tract infection in catheterized dogs and comparison of bacterial culture and susceptibility testing results for catheterized and non-catheterized dogs with urinary tract infections, J Am Vet Med Assoc 231:893-899, 2007.

CHAPTER 100
MASTITIS

Margret L. Casal, DrMedVet, PhD, DECAR

KEY POINTS

- After parturition, the mammaries should be evaluated twice daily for signs of mastitis until the puppies or kittens are weaned.
- Clinical signs of acute mastitis are painful, erythematous, edematous, and swollen mammaries that may turn dark red to purple, abscess, and become gangrenous.
- Causes are trauma to the nipples by nursing puppies or kittens, poor environmental conditions, and concurrent disease.
- The most common bacteria found are *E. coli*, *Streptococcus* spp., and *Staphylococcus* spp.; in the absence of culture and susceptibility, antibiotics should be chosen to treat these infectious agents.
- Despite immediate treatment, abscesses and gangrene often develop, which spontaneously rupture or should be drained and usually heal on secondary intention.

Mastitis (mammary inflammation or mammitis) is defined as inflammation of the mammary gland tissue that generally occurs during lactation during either the postpartum period or pseudopregnancy.[1-4] Infections are common but need not be present.[5] Mastitis may be localized within a single gland, or diffuse inflammation may be present in one or more mammary glands.[2-4] Acute inflammation is characterized by local clinical signs, which may be accompanied by systemic signs. The frequency of subclinical or chronic mastitis is not known, and clinical signs are generally not present in this form. The diagnosis is made by physical examination, culture and susceptibility of the affected tissue and/or milk from the affected gland, blood work, and potentially ultrasound. Treatment includes appropriate antibiotics, debridement of the affected tissue, or removal of the affected gland if necessary.[2-4]

ANATOMY: BRIEF OVERVIEW

In dogs and cats, one pair of mammary glands refers to a left gland and its corresponding right gland. Neither blood nor lymphatic vessels communicate between the two. Most dogs have five pair of mammary glands, although four pair are more common in smaller breed dogs, but six pair also have been described in mid-size to larger dogs. In dogs, the glands are named according to their location: two pairs of thoracic glands, two pairs of abdominal glands, and one pair of inguinal glands. In cats, each pair of glands is numbered 1 to 4 from cranial to caudal (older texts refer to the feline glands as axial, thoracic, abdominal, and inguinal). The parenchyma is prominent only during the second half of pregnancy, lactation, and pseudopregnancy (in the dog), and regresses by 50 days after weaning. Milk is produced in the parenchyma and collected in sinuses from which the milk exits via the teat through 4 to 8 ducts in cats and 7 to 16 in dogs. Arterial blood is supplied to the cranial glands from the cranial superficial epigastric artery that branches off of the internal thoracic artery. The caudal glands receive their blood supply from the caudal superficial epigastric artery that branches off of the external pudendal artery. In the dog, the two cranial (thoracic) mammary glands on each side drain into the respective axillary lymph nodes and also may drain into the cranial sternal lymph node along with the middle (cranial abdominal) gland. The two pairs of caudal (caudal abdominal and inguinal) glands drain into their respective superficial inguinal lymph nodes, and the middle gland on each side can drain into either the axillary or superficial inguinal lymph node.[6]

ETIOLOGY

The primary cause of mastitis is an ascending infection after trauma to the nipples by nursing puppies or kittens. Hematogenous infections may occur in bitches with concurrent disease such as endometritis, but this is less common. Predisposing factors include skin disease, contamination of the mammaries with lochia, poor environmental conditions, overcrowding, and galactostasis shortly before birth, after weaning, or after the loss of a litter.[1-4,7] Various pathogens that have been isolated from infected mammaries include *Klebsiella* spp., *Proteus* spp., *Pasteurella* spp., *Pseudomonas* spp., and others.[8,9] However, *Staphylococcus* spp., *Streptococcus* spp., and in particular *E. coli* are the most common offenders.[5,8-11] If culture and susceptibility are not available for diagnosis, as a rule of thumb staphylococcal infections lead to abscesses and gangrene, streptococcal infections are generally diffuse and spread into other glands, and *E. coli* lead to abscessation and septic mastitis.

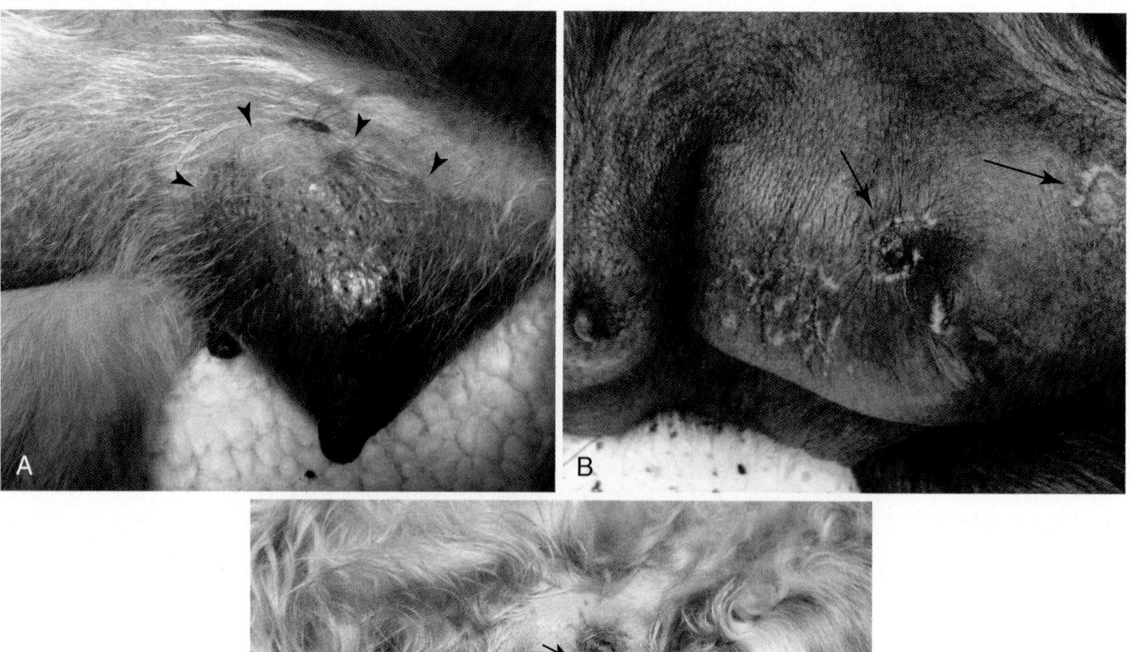

FIGURE 100-1 **A,** Acute mastitis with areas of distinct demarcation *(arrowheads).* **B,** Formation of abscesses with development of necrotic tissue resulting in tearing of the skin *(arrows).* **C,** Acute mastitis with ruptured abscesses and gangrene *(arrows). (**A,** Courtesy Dr. Lauren Jones, Country Companion Animal Hospital, Morgantown, Penn. **B,** Courtesy Dr. Kit Kampschmidt, Brittmoore Animal Hospital, Inc., Houston, Tex. **C,** Courtesy Dr. B. J. Parsons, Kanuga Animal Clinic, Hendersonville, NC.)*

CLINICAL FINDINGS

Acute Mastitis

Acute mastitis is characterized by extremely painful, hot, swollen, erythematous, and edematous mammary tissue. The skin over the affected area generally is discolored and has a dark red to purple appearance with distinct areas of demarcation (Figure 100-1, *A*). The caudalmost mammaries are most likely to be affected during the acute phase. Systemic signs such as lethargy, fever, vomiting, dehydration, and inappetence are common and, if left untreated, bitches may become septic.[1-4,6,11,12] Bitches or queens with mastitis may neglect their puppies or kittens, which may fade and die. Secretions from the affected gland can look almost normal but are more commonly purulent, brownish, bloody, or malodorous. As the disease progresses, abscesses may form (Figure 100-1, *B*), and the gland may rupture, exposing the necrotic tissue underneath the skin (Figure 100-1, *C*). The gangrenous gland(s) must be treated immediately to avoid severe sepsis in the bitch or queen.

Chronic or Subclinical Mastitis

Chronic or subclinical mastitis is a poorly defined condition. Bitches and queens with subclinical mastitis do not present with systemic signs other than perhaps fading offspring. The affected glands and the expressed milk generally appear macroscopically normal, but the parenchyma of the affected gland may palpate thickened and hardened. Bitches and queens may have offspring that fail to gain weight, that lose weight, or that die.[5,8]

Neonatal death is not necessarily linked to the type of bacteria found in the mother's infected mammary, regardless of acute or subclinical mastitis.[5,8] Studies have shown that bacteria are present in 10% to 50% of milk from normal bitches or older queens.[8,13] In one study, cultures were obtained from 25 puppies that died of sepsis within the first week of life and from their seven dams that were affected with acute mastitis.[5] Only one of these deceased puppies had the same bacteria as its mother with mastitis.

DIAGNOSIS

The case history and the typical clinical signs provide the basis for a diagnosis. Milk samples should be obtained for cytology and microbial culture and susceptibility before antibiotic therapy is initiated. To avoid contamination by the surrounding skin, vaginal discharge, and other environmental contaminants, the affected gland should be cleaned gently with a dilute chlorhexidine solution before expressing milk for diagnostics. Gloves should be worn and the first drop of expressed milk discarded before collecting the milk for analysis. In one study, cytology of milk from the affected gland during the early stages of acute mastitis revealed macrophages and large numbers of neutrophils with engulfed bacteria. Three days after onset of disease, the neutrophils became degenerate, and by day 6 lymphocytes began to invade the affected gland and were present in the corresponding milk. As the disease progressed, lymphocytes increased in number and by 2 weeks after onset, they made up the majority of cells on cytologic evaluation of the milk.[11] Cell counts can be highly variable between the individual glands in a single bitch and between bitches with and without disease.[11,13] High cell counts have been observed in normal bitches at weaning or at the end of pseudopregnancy when the mammaries begin to involute.[11,13] Typically, some neutrophils are present, and a large number of macrophages with vacuolated cytoplasm predominate. A diagnosis of mastitis should not be made by cytology alone. Complete blood cell counts may reveal neutrophilia with a left shift in acute mastitis. One dog with gangrenous mastitis resulting from *S. aureus* presented with leukocytosis and thrombocytopenia.[14] Alternatively, neutropenia may be present in advanced stages of the disease.

Ultrasound is a useful adjunct in determining the extent of the mastitis. Normal inactive and active glands are characterized by layers that are different from each other. In active glands, the parenchyma is mildly coarse grained and echogenic, whereas distinctive layering was absent in inflamed tissues, which also demonstrated a loss in echogenicity.[15] Using a Doppler to assess vascularity of the inflamed tissue may allow for prognosis: dogs with decreased vessel density in the inflamed tissue appeared to have a poorer outcome as opposed to those with increased vascularity.[15] This can be explained by having increased vascularity during the beginning stages of inflammation, and as the disease progresses necrosis sets in, thereby decreasing vascularity.

DIFFERENTIAL DIAGNOSES

Any dog or cat that is presented with a swollen, painful, and inflamed mammary gland after having given birth most likely has mastitis. However, mammary cancers may mimic the clinical signs, and thus every attempt should be made to confirm the diagnosis. Other differentials include trauma (overzealous neonatal nursers), galactostasis, severe pyoderma, or fibroadenomatous mammary hyperplasia, a benign condition of young cats. Other clinical signs and unusual pathogens such as blastomycosis in three dogs[16] and toxoplasmosis in a cat[17] also have been reported as causes of mastitis.

TREATMENT

Therapy depends on the severity of disease. In dogs or cats with acute mastitis and sepsis, hospitalization and treatment for sepsis/shock are required. The puppies or kittens must be removed from their mothers and fostered to another or hand-raised. Antibiotics are required and initially have to be administered intravenously. In dogs or cats with septic mastitis, a combination of antibiotics such as ampicillin/enrofloxacin (see below) provides excellent coverage. For any mastitis being treated, a course of 3 to 4 weeks of antibiotics is recommended.

Antibiotics that are weak bases get trapped in the slightly acidic milk.[2,3,9,12,18] However, the blood milk barrier breaks down in the face of severe inflammation. Thus the pH of the milk approaches that of the plasma. In the absence of microbial culture results, antibiotics should be chosen according to the cytology results. If predominantly cocci are noted in the milk sample, cephalosporins or amoxicillin–clavulonic acid are preferred antibiotics. On the other hand, if rods are primarily present, enrofloxacin and marbofloxacin are generally better.

In dogs or cats with subclinical mastitis, the blood milk barrier is generally intact. Treatment is based on culture and susceptibility results and long-term therapy is required. The choice of drugs has to be based on pH, lipid solubility, and the amount of drug bound to proteins. The more drug that is protein bound, the less is transferred into the milk. Finally, treatment also depends on the presence or absence of nursing offspring.

If the bitch or queen with acute mastitis is not septic, antibiotic therapy can be initiated without removing the puppies or kittens. The choice of antibiotics has to take into consideration that they will be present in the milk and therefore will be passed to the offspring. All of the penicillins, cephalosporins, and macrolides are safe to use in bitches and queens that are still nursing offspring. Most other drugs have side effects in the neonates and should be avoided. These include chloramphenicol, tetracyclines, and aminoglycosides. Fluoroquinolones are debatable because most of the damage to cartilage occurs in puppies when they are ambulatory. Thus, if a fluoroquinolone is required, any ambulatory puppies should be removed. If the puppies are younger than 2 weeks of age, they need not be removed if their dam is being treated with a fluoroquinolone. Side effects seen in puppies receiving fluoroquinolones do not appear to occur in kittens.[19,20] The most common side effect in any of the offspring of a mother with mastitis receiving antibiotics is diarrhea.[12]

In addition to antibiotic therapy, the affected gland should be treated with hot compresses several times daily to encourage drainage. The offspring may be allowed to nurse if the mother is not septic or in shock; often the bitch or queen does not allow them to nurse from the affected gland.[12] However, once the dam is being treated, there does not appear to be a detriment to the offspring that are nursing from an affected mammary gland.[5]

Demarcation in a mammary gland with mastitis indicates imminent abscessation and/or gangrene and drainage will likely be necessary.[2,12] The affected gland should be cleaned carefully and prepared as if for sterile surgery. A scalpel blade can be used to lance the abscess, which is then left to drain. Necrotic tissue should be debrided and the cavity irrigated with sterile saline until the fluid runs clear. Anesthesia is generally not required because the tissue is already dead and necrotic. The wound should be cleaned at least two to three times daily and is left to heal by secondary intention. In severe cases, the affected gland should be removed surgically in its entirety.

Non-steroidal antiinflammatory drugs such as meloxicam or carprofen for 3 to 4 days have been recommended. However, these drugs will be present in the milk and may result in side effects in the offspring. In the author's experience, opiates, including tramadol, are a safer choice. Dopamine agonists decrease prolactin resulting in decreased milk production and thus prevent galactostasis in the other mammary glands. If offspring are present, dopamine agonists may be given for 2 to 3 days, and for 8 or more days if the offspring have been weaned. Cabergoline is the drug of choice and is given at 5 mcg/kg once daily.[9]

REFERENCES

1. Feldman EC, Nelson RW: Periparturient diseases. In Feldman EC, Nelson RW, editors: Canine and feline endocrinology and reproduction, Philadelphia, 1996, Saunders.
2. Kitchell BE, Loar AS: Diseases of the mammary glands. In Morgan RV, editor: Handbook of small animal practice, Philadelphia, 1997, Saunders.
3. Olson PN: Periparturient diseases of the bitch. In Proceedings, Annual Meeting of the Society for Theriogenology, Orlando, 1988.
4. Wheeler SL, Magne ML, Kaufman PW, et al: Postpartum disorders in the bitch, Comp Cont Educ Pract 6:493-500, 1984.
5. Schäfer-Somi S, Spergser J, Breitenfellner J, et al: Bacteriological status of canine milk and septicaemia in neonatal puppies—a retrospective study, J Vet Med B 50:343-6, 2003.
6. Johnston SD, Root Kustritz MV, Olson PNS: In Canine and feline theriogenology, Philadelphia, 2001, Saunders.
7. Walser K, Henschelchen O: [Contribution to the etiology of acute mastitis in the bitch], Berliner und Münchener tierarztliche Wochenschrift 96:195-197, 1983.
8. Sager M, Remmers C: [Perinatal mortality in dogs. Clinical, bacteriological and pathological studies], Tierarztliche Praxis 18:415-419, 1990.

9. Wiebe VJ, Howard JP: Pharmacologic advances in canine and feline reproduction, Top Companion Anim Med 24:71-99, 2009.
10. Kuhn G, Pohl S, Hingst V: [Elevation of the bacteriological content of milk of clinically unaffected lactating bitches of a canine research stock]. Berliner und Münchener tierarztliche Wochenschrift 104:130-133, 1991.
11. Ververidis HN, Mavrogianni VS, Fragkou IA, et al: Experimental staphylococcal mastitis in bitches: clinical, bacteriological, cytological, haematological and pathological features, Vet Microbiol 124:95-106, 2007.
12. Biddle D, Macintire DK: Obstetrical emergencies, Clin Tech Small Anim Pract 15:88-93, 2000.
13. Olson PN, Olson AL: Cytologic evaluation of canine milk, Vet Med Small Anim Clin 79:641-646, 1984.
14. Hasegawa T, Fujii M, Fukada T, et al: Platelet abnormalities in a dog suffering from gangrenous mastitis by *Staphylococcus aureus* infection, J Vet Med Sci 55:169-71, 1993.
15. Trasch K, Wehrend A, Bostedt H: Ultrasonographic description of canine mastitis, Vet Radiol Ultrasound 48:580-584, 2007.
16. Ditmyer H, Craig L: Mycotic mastitis in three dogs due to *Blastomyces dermatitidis*, J Am Anim Hosp Assoc 47:356-358, 2011.
17. Park CH, Ikadai H, Yoshida E, et al: Cutaneous toxoplasmosis in a female Japanese cat, Vet Pathol 44:683-687, 2007.
18. Greene CE, Schultz RD: Immunoprophylaxis. In Greene CE, editors: Infectious diseases of the dog and cat, Philadelphia, 2006, WB Saunders.
19. Altreuther P: Safety and tolerance of enrofloxacin in dogs and cats. In 1st International Symposium on Baytril, Bonn, Germany, 1992.
20. Brown SA: Fluoroquinolones in animal health, J Vet Pharmacol Ther 19:1-14, 1996.

CHAPTER 101
NECROTIZING SOFT TISSUE INFECTIONS

Elke Rudloff, DVM, DACVECC • Kevin P. Winkler, DVM, DACVS

KEY POINTS

- Necrotizing soft tissue infections (NSTI) and toxic shock syndrome can be rapidly fatal if not identified and treated aggressively.
- Signs of circulatory shock must be treated rapidly using fluid resuscitation and analgesia.
- Because of the lack of obvious skin changes in many cases of necrotizing soft tissue infections, a high index of suspicion is necessary for diagnosis.
- Broad-spectrum intravenous antimicrobial therapy should be instituted early.
- Surgery is the cornerstone of treatment in necrotizing soft tissue infections, and radical debridement including amputation may be necessary to eliminate the infection.
- Antibiotic therapy should be broad spectrum until directed by culture and susceptibility results.

Necrotizing soft tissue infection (NSTI) is the term used to describe a subset of soft tissue infections involving skin, subcutaneous tissue, muscle, and fascia that cause vascular occlusion, ischemia, and necrosis. NSTIs are associated with virulent bacterial and fungal organisms and encompass syndromes including Fournier's gangrene, Ludwig's angina, flesh-eating disease, hemolytic streptococcal gangrene, necrotizing fasciitis (NF), and myonecrosis.[1,2] In contrast to uncomplicated soft tissue infections, NSTIs are progressive and rapidly spread along tissue planes. Uncontrolled NSTIs are lethal. The term severe soft tissue infection (SSTI) also has been used to describe lesions with or without necrosis.[3]

Toxic shock syndrome (TSS) is an acute, severe, systemic inflammatory response initiated by a microbial infection at a normally sterile site, usually exotoxin-releasing *Staphylococcus* or *Streptococcus* spp. Unlike other invasive infections, TSS manifests as an acute, early occurrence of circulatory shock and multiorgan dysfunction that can include renal and/or hepatic dysfunction, coagulopathy, acute respiratory distress syndrome, and/or an erythematous rash.[4] In people, TSS commonly is associated with NF and pleuropulmonary infection.[5] NSTI and STTI have been described in dogs and cats and are associated with virulent *Streptococcus* spp. and other bacterial organisms.[3,6-18]

Human mortality rates for NSTI are reported to be between 12% and 41.6%.[19,20] An increased awareness and knowledge of the importance of early debridement has resulted in a trend toward an improved outcome. The mortality rate for TSS in people is reported to be more than 35%.[21] A report of 47 dogs with NSTI found a 53% mortality rate, but the majority of deaths were due to euthanasia, so this result is difficult to interpret.[3] Risk factors identified in human medicine include age more than 50 years, atherosclerosis or peripheral vascular disease, obesity, trauma, hypoalbuminemia, diabetes mellitus, and glucocorticoid usage.[1,22,23]

NSTI can be stratified into four categories based on type of infection (Box 101-1). Type I NSTI is polymicrobial, Type II NSTI is monomicrobial, Type III NSTI is associated with gram-negative, often marine-related organisms, and Type IV NSTI is associated with fungal infection.[23,24] Most of the veterinary cases reported could be categorized as Type II NF[3] associated with a history of minor trauma and inoculation with virulent bacteria. Infection can spread rapidly, and seemingly limited infections can cause limb-threatening and life-threatening systemic sequelae. Fibrous attachments between the subcutaneous and fascial tissue can form a boundary to limit spread of organisms; however, such boundaries do not exist in the extremities or truncal regions, making these areas more susceptible to widespread infection and NF.[26,27]

Despite their severity and rapid progression, relatively little actually is known about the pathophysiology of TSS and NSTI. Enhanced toxicity of virulent streptococci through the release of exotoxin superantigens, cell envelope proteinases, hyaluronidase, complement inhibitor, M protein, protein F, and streptolysins amplifies cytokine release and induction of a systemic inflammatory response and septic shock. Clostridial toxins can cause hemolysis, platelet aggregation, leukocyte destruction, and histamine release, in addition to damage vascular endothelium, collagen, and hyaluron. Angiothrombotic microbial invasion with liquefactive necrosis of the superficial fascia and soft tissue is a key pathologic process of NSTI. Occlusion of nutrient vessels can lead to extensive undermining of apparently normal-appearing skin, followed by gangrene of the subcutaneous fat, dermis, and epidermis, evolving into ischemic necrosis.[1] Preliminary diagnosis is based initially on clinical suspicion, because definitive diagnosis requires tissue sampling and time for test results to return.

DIAGNOSIS

The clinical signs of NSTI and TSS can be nonspecific. Skin changes, fever, respiratory signs, increased urination frequency, or signs of malaise may be described by the pet owner. Surgery or a recent traumatic event may be included in the history.

TSS and NSTI are associated with circulatory shock. NSTI may be associated with signs of bruising, edema, cellulitis, or crepitus from subcutaneous emphysema (Figure 101-1). Cutaneous bullae are considered an important indicator of impending dermal necrosis in humans; however, this has not been a frequent finding in veterinary patients.[8] Although a skin wound or discoloration is obvious, the epidermis can appear unscathed with deep tissue necrosis. When skin lesions are seen, they should be outlined with a marker so that progression of the discoloration can be followed. Rapid progression (extension within a few hours) and disproportionate localized pain are hallmark signs of NSTI; however, NSTI associated with postoperative, gut flora-associated infection may progress more slowly (hours to days).[24] Protective gloves should be worn during examination of the lesions and patient handling to prevent inadvertent contamination of a cut on the examiner's hand or another patient with potentially virulent pathogens.

BOX 101-1 *Categories of Necrotizing Soft Tissue Infections*[24,25]

Type I Infections: Polymicrobial

- Mixed anaerobes and aerobes
- Usually isolate four or more organisms

Type II Infections: Monomicrobial

- β-hemolytic *Streptococcus* commonly

Type III Infections: Gram-Negative Monomicrobials

- Such as *Clostridia* infections
- Includes marine organisms

Type IV Infections: Fungal

- Such as *Candida* infections

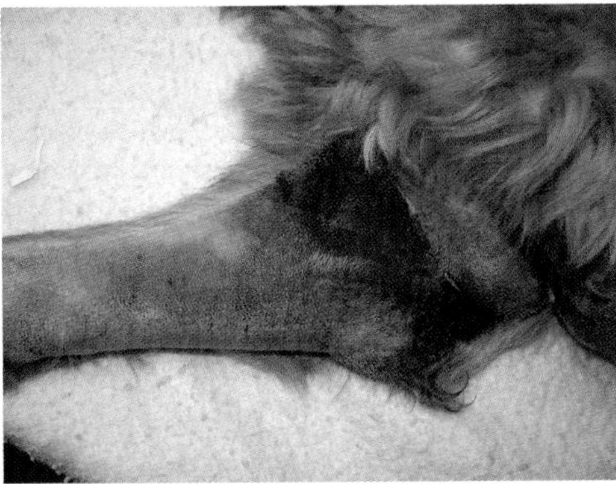

FIGURE 101-1 Necrotizing soft tissue infection of the medial aspect of the elbow of a dog.

Laboratory Findings

Laboratory findings cannot be used to diagnose NSTI or TSS, but they may reflect changes associated with infection and a systemic inflammatory response syndrome. These may include hemoconcentration, anemia, hypoalbuminemia, neutrophilia or neutropenia, left shift (often severe), hyperlactatemia, coagulation alterations consistent with DIC, hypoglycemia, elevated creatinine phosphokinase levels, and organ dysfunction (elevated serum alanine transaminase, alkaline phosphatase, bilirubin, creatinine levels). Hypocalcemia can occur when extensive fat necrosis has developed with NF.[22]

TSS is associated with bacterial toxins invading the circulatory system through the skin barrier or via organ infections, such as pneumonia or urinary tract infections. Urinalysis may show evidence of infection confirmed with culture analysis. When thoracic radiographs suggest pneumonia, transtracheal wash samples may indicate infection. Blood cultures may yield positive growth. Fine-needle aspirate from an affected tissue site or organ may reveal a discharge, and cytology and Gram stain may identify chains of gram-positive cocci.

A diagnostic scoring system called the laboratory risk indicator for necrotizing fasciitis (LRINEC) score, based on measurement of C-reactive protein, white blood cell count, hemoglobin, sodium, creatinine, and glucose has been used in human patients, although it has been reported to fail to detect some cases and its role is currently under debate.[28,29]

Imaging

Imaging studies are suggestive but not specific for NSTI. On plain film radiographs, subcutaneous air is rare but characteristic of necrotizing lesions with gas-producing organisms (Figure 101-2). Computed tomography features suggestive of NSTI include asymmetric fascial thickening, hypodermal fat inflammation, and gas in the soft tissue planes.[30,31] Magnetic resonance imaging (MRI) may prove helpful in determining the extent of deep tissue infections not readily identified from the skin surface because of its soft tissue and multiplanar imaging capabilities. Thickened fascia with high signal intensity in T2 images is seen commonly on MRI.[31] Absence of deep fascial involvement can exclude NF. However, MRI cannot differentiate necrotizing infections from nonnecrotizing problems, and the time involved in obtaining test results may delay surgery.[32] Diagnostic imaging should never delay time to surgical intervention.

Definitive Diagnosis

Definitive diagnosis of TSS requires positive streptococcal or staphylococcal culture findings and evidence of septic shock. Definitive diagnosis of NSTI is based on the histopathologic findings, including fascial necrosis and myonecrosis. Pathologic descriptions also include deep angiothrombotic microbial invasion and liquefactive necrosis.[33,34] Frozen section biopsy can provide a rapid diagnosis at the time of surgical exposure.[35] Because of the rapid progression of disease and the time in obtaining results, rapid treatment and immediate surgical evaluation is necessary when there is a clinical suspicion of a NSTI.

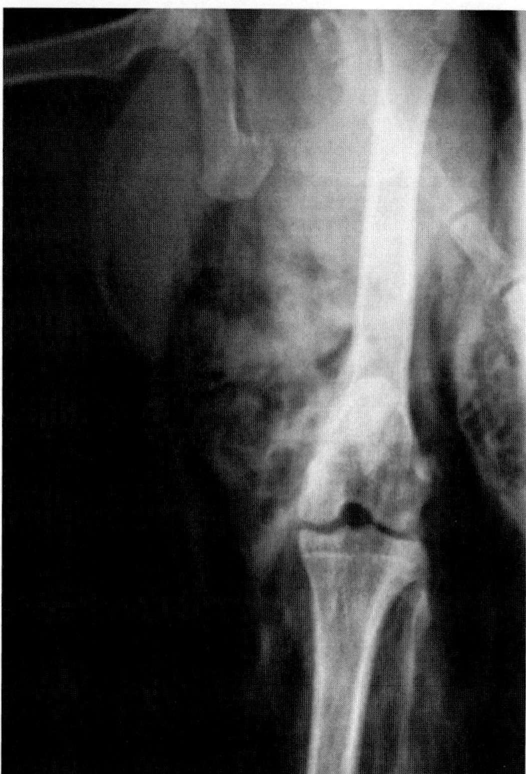

FIGURE 101-2 Radiographs of necrotizing fasciitis may demonstrate soft tissue swelling and occasionally subcutaneous emphysema. The extent of the necrosis may not be reflected by the size of the skin lesion.

TREATMENT

Successful management of TSS and NSTI is based on treatment of the entire patient, not just the infected site, although cardiovascular stabilization may be difficult without surgical intervention. Patients in circulatory shock are resuscitated rapidly using large-volume resuscitation techniques with a combination of balanced isotonic crystalloid fluids and synthetic colloids (e.g., hydroxyethyl starch).[36] Recent reports have identified an increased risk of acute kidney injury in people with severe sepsis who have received hydroxyethyl starch; however, this problem has yet to be recognized in small animals.[37] Fluids are titrated to perfusion end points, namely, normal heart rate, arterial blood pressure, mucous membrane color, and capillary refill time (see Chapter 60). Heart rate may not return to normal until analgesics are administered. Because there may be a high degree of pain associated with NSTI, strong analgesic intervention is necessary (see Chapter 144). Injectable opioid agonists (e.g., hydromorphone, oxymorphone) in combination with regional or local anesthesia may be adequate. Opioids can be continued as a constant rate infusion in combination with low-dose ketamine and lidocaine to provide continuous analgesia. Nonsteroidal antiinflammatory analgesic medications are not recommended until signs of circulatory shock have been alleviated and debridement has been successful. Circulatory shock unresponsive to fluid infusion may require vasopressor therapy (see Chapter 8).

If hypoglycemia occurs, glucose is administered as a bolus followed by a constant rate infusion (see Chapter 66). Calcium is administered when plasma ionized calcium levels are decreased significantly (see Chapter 52).

Antimicrobial Therapy

Rapid administration of appropriate antimicrobial therapy is an essential part of treatment. Samples for cytology and Gram stain are collected and immediately evaluated. Samples for aerobic, anaerobic, and fungal culture and susceptibility testing of the affected area are submitted before injectable broad-spectrum antibiotic coverage is instituted. A second set of culture and susceptibility samples always should be acquired during the debridement procedure. Penicillin G, aminopenicillins (ampicillin, amoxicillin), and cephalosporins target gram-positive and many gram-negative organisms and should be part of the initial antimicrobial therapy plan. However, high tissue concentrations of Group A streptococcal organisms can put them in a stationary phase, causing penicillins to become ineffective.[38] Clindamycin remains effective during the stationary phase and turns off exotoxin synthesis, inhibits streptococcal M-protein synthesis (which facilitate mononuclear phagocytosis), and suppresses lipopolysaccharide-induced monocyte synthesis of tumor necrosis factor.[39] It also provides coverage for anaerobic organisms. Aminoglycosides and third-generation cephalosporins may increase gram-negative organism coverage. Gentamicin has a synergistic effect with penicillin against streptococci. For broad-spectrum coverage in the compromised patient, the authors would recommend clindamycin in combination with an aminoglycoside or third-generation cephalosporin. Fluoroquinolone administration, specifically enrofloxacin, is not recommended, because it may have limited activity against streptococcal infection and may cause bacteriophage-induced lysis of *S. canis*, enhancing its pathogenicity.[39] In the severely immunocompromised patient, antifungal therapy also may be considered pending fungal culture results.

Surgical Debridement

Necrosis and underlying loss of blood supply limit tissue penetration of systemic antibiotics. Necrotic tissue serves as a culture medium, creating an anaerobic environment that impairs polymorphonuclear cell activity. Therefore the most important part of treatment of NSTI is surgical debridement. Inadequate debridement promotes continuing spread of infection and may result in an inoperable condition or death. Surgical intervention should occur within 4 to 6 hours of presentation, once the cardiovascular system is stabilized as best as possible. Higher amputation and mortality rates have been documented in humans when surgery was delayed more than 12 hours.[40,41]

Surgical preparation should include a generous area surrounding the affected tissue because significant undermining of the tissue planes may not be evident until surgical exposure. Because of the lack of purulent discharge, typical drainage techniques are ineffective. With no large pockets of purulent material for drainage, appropriate debridement frequently requires removal of large amounts of tissue, including skin and open wound management. Successful debridement may require multiple procedures, not just a single surgery.

Removal of nonviable tissue may involve resection of muscle and tendons. Muscle viability can be tested by its response to stimulation from an electrocautery device. When contraction is absent, the muscle may not be viable and should be debrided. If the wound is on the limb, debridement can result in loss of limb function. Therefore amputation may be the best option for limiting morbidity and mortality in addition to minimizing postoperative cost of treatment. This is a difficult emotional decision for the owner. Often the pet has deteriorated in such a rapid fashion that the owner may not understand the necessity for an amputation. Because a delay can result in loss of the pet, appropriate client communication to emphasize the severity and rapid progression of an NSTI is essential.

Postoperative Care

Postoperative monitoring should follow Kirby's Rule of 20.[42] Crystalloid and colloid fluids are continued to maintain intravascular volume and replace ongoing fluid losses. The cardiovascular system is monitored closely for decompensation, and frequent evaluation of glucose, albumin, and electrolyte levels uncover any abnormalities that require intervention. Bandage removal for evaluation of the wound edges is done frequently (initially every 30 to 60 minutes) to determine if necrosis is continuing to spread despite surgery, indicating the need for repeat debridement. Antimicrobial therapy is adjusted once culture and susceptibility results are available. Special attention is paid to providing adequate nutrition and analgesia.

Nutritional support is an important consideration, because these patients have increased protein loss in the exudates and increased demands of healing (see Chapter 127). There also may be a decrease in voluntary food intake associated with pain or fever. Partial parenteral nutrition and/or enteral feeding via nasogastric or esophagostomy tube facilitates protein metabolism and limits protein catabolism during recovery. Caloric requirements should be calculated and then nutritional supplementation started immediately postoperatively, with full caloric supplementation reached within 48 hours.

High-dose intravenous immunoglobulin G therapy has shown some benefit in clinical improvement and reduction in mortality in treated versus control human patients.[43] It also may reduce the need for radical debridement in cases of NSTI by augmenting immune clearance of streptococcal organisms, neutralizing superantigens, as well as providing an immunomodulating effect.[44-45] Positive benefits have been recognized with group A streptococcal NF but not gram-negative infection. Its use in veterinary medicine for TSS or NSTI has not been established.

Hyperbaric Oxygen

Hyperbaric oxygen therapy is the delivery of oxygen at higher than atmospheric pressure to compromised tissue. Hyperbaric oxygen therapy may enhance host antimicrobial activity and the action of various antibiotic agents by facilitating their transport across the bacterial cell wall.[46] Unfortunately, most reports are either anecdotal or have yielded conflicting results.[8,47-49] There are no prospective, controlled veterinary studies demonstrating efficacy of hyperbaric oxygen in NSTI, but it has been described in a single canine case of limb NF.[8]

CONCLUSION

NSTI and TSS can be treated successfully if medical and surgical therapy is provided rapidly. A delay in therapy worsens the prognosis. Circulatory shock and laboratory abnormalities must be corrected immediately and aggressive analgesia provided. Broad-spectrum intravenous antimicrobial therapy should be administered as soon as possible. Prompt surgery with radical debridement and appropriate antimicrobial therapy is required for successful treatment of NSTI. The extent of the lesion may not be appreciated fully until surgery is performed. Amputation or multiple surgical procedures may be necessary to remove diseased tissue. Major reconstructive procedures may be required once diseased tissue has been removed successfully.

REFERENCES

1. Wong CH, Chang HC, Pasupathy S, et al: Necrotizing fasciitis: clinical presentation, microbiology, and determinants of mortality, J Bone Joint Surg Am 85:1454, 2003.
2. Phan HH, Cocanour CS: Necrotizing soft tissue infections in the intensive care unit, Crit Care Med 38:S460, 2010.
3. Buriko Y, Van Winkle TJ, Drobatz KJ, et al: Severe soft tissue infections in dogs: 47 cases (1996-2006), J Vet Emerg Crit Care 18:608, 2008.
4. Defining the group A streptococcal toxic shock syndrome. Rationale and consensus definition. The Working Group on Severe Streptococcal Infections, J Am Med Assoc 269:390, 1993.
5. Plainvert C, Doloy A, Loubinoux J, et al: CNR-Strep network. Invasive group A streptococcal infections in adults, France (2006-2010), Clin Microbiol Infect 18:702, 2012.
6. Prescott JF, Miller CW, Mathews KA, et al: Update on canine streptococcal toxic shock syndrome and necrotizing fasciitis, Can Vet J 38:241, 1997.
7. Miller CW, Prescott, JF, Mathews KA, et al: Streptococcal toxic shock syndrome in dogs, J Am Vet Med Assoc 209:1421, 1996.
8. Jenkins CM, Winkler K, Rudloff E, et al: Necrotizing fasciitis in a dog, J Vet Emerg Crit Care 11:299, 2001.
9. DeWinter LM, Low DE, Prescott JF: Virulence of *Streptococcus canis* from canine streptococcal toxic shock syndrome and necrotizing fasciitis, Vet Microbiol 70:95, 1999.
10. Declercq, J: Suspected toxic shock-like syndrome in a dog with closed-cervix pyometra, Vet Dermatol 18:41, 2007.
11. Sura R, Hinckley LS, Risatti GR, et al: Fatal necrotising fasciitis and myositis in a cat associated with *Streptococcus canis*, Vet Record 162:450, 2008.
12. Crosse PA, Soares K, Wheeler JI, et al: *Chromobacterium violaceum* infection in two dogs, J Am Anim Hosp Assoc 42:154, 2006.
13. Slovak J, Parker VJ, Deitz KL: Toxic shock syndrome in two dogs, J Am Anim Hosp Assoc 48:434–438, 2012.
14. Taillefer M, Dunn M: Group G streptococcal toxic shock-like syndrome in three cats, J Am Anim Hosp Assoc 40:418, 2004.
15. Worth AJ, Marshal N, Thompson KG: Necrotising fasciitis associated with *Escherichia coli* in a dog, N Z Vet J 53:257, 2005.
16. Kulendra E, Corr S: Necrotising fasciitis with sub-periosteal *Streptococcus canis* infection in two puppies, Vet Comp Orthop Traumatol 21:474, 2008.
17. Weese JS, Poma Rr, James F, et al: *Staphylococcus pseudintermedius* necrotizing fasciitis in a dog, Can Vet J 50:655, 2009.
18. Csiszer AB, Towle HA, Daly CM: Successful treatment of necrotizing fasciitis in the hind limb of a Great Dane, J Am Anim Hosp Assoc 46:433, 2012.
19. Mills MK, Faraklas I, Davis C, et al: Outcomes from treatment of necrotizing soft tissue infections: results from the National Surgical Quality Improvement Program database, Am J Surg 200:790, 2010.
20. George SMC, Harrison DA, Welch CA, et al: Dermatological conditions in intensive care: a secondary analysis of the Intensive Care National Audit & Research Centre (ICNArc) Case Mix Programme Database, Crit Care 12:S1, 2008.
21. Group A streptococcal disease. Centers for Disease Control and Prevention. Update April 3 2008. http://www.cdc.gov/ncidod/dbmd/diseaseinfo/groupastreptococcal_t.htm.
22. McHenry CR, Piotrowski JJ, Petrinic D, et al: Determinants of mortality for necrotizing soft tissue infections, Ann Surg 221:558, 1995.
23. Sarani B, Strong M, Pascual J, et al: Necrotizing fasciitis: Current concepts and review of the literature, J Am Coll Surg 208:279, 2009.
24. Morgan MS: Diagnosis and management of necrotising fasciitis: a multiparametric approach, J Hosp Infect 5:249, 2010.
25. Ustin JS, Sevransky JE: Necrotizing soft tissue infection, Crit Care Med 39:2156, 2011.
26. Hill MK, Sanders CV: Necrotizing and gangrenous soft tissue infections. In Nesbitt LT Jr, Saunders CV, editors: The skin and infection: a color atlas and text, Baltimore, 1995, Williams & Wilkins.
27. Bosshardt TL, Henderson VJ, Organ CH Jr: Necrotizing soft tissue infections, Arch Surg 131:846, 1996.
28. Wall DB, Klein SR, Black S, et al: A simple model to help distinguish necrotizing fasciitis from nonnecrotizing soft tissue infection, J Am Coll Surg 191:227, 2000.
29. Wilson MP, Schneir AB: A case of necrotizing fasciitis with a LRINEC score of zero: clinical suspicion should trump scoring systems, J Emerg Med 44(5):928, 2013.
30. Wysoki MG, Santora TA, Shah RM, et al: Necrotizing fasciitis: CT characteristics, Radiology 203:859, 1997.
31. Malghem J, Lecouvet FE, Omoumi P, et al: Necrotizing fasciitis: contribution and limitations of diagnostic imaging, Joint Bone Spine 80(2):146, 2013.
32. Loh NN, Ch'en IY, Cheung LP, et al: Deep fascial hyperintensity in soft-tissue abnormalities as revealed by T2-weighted MR imaging, AJR Am J Roentgenol 168:1301, 1997.
33. Wong CH, Wang YS: The diagnosis of necrotizing fasciitis, Curr Opin Infect Dis 18:101, 2005.

34. Umbert IJ, Winkelmann RK, Oliver GF, et al: Necrotizing fasciitis: a clinical, microbiological, and histopathological study of 14 patients, J Am Acad Dermatol 20:774, 1989.
35. Stamenkovic I, Lew PD: Early recognition of potentially fatal necrotizing fasciitis. The use of frozen-section biopsy, N Engl J Med 310:1689, 1984.
36. Kirby R, Rudloff E: Crystalloid and colloid fluid therapy. In Ettinger SJ, Feldman EC, editors: Textbook of veterinary internal medicine, ed 6, St Louis, 2005, Saunders.
37. Perner A, Haase N, Guttormsen AB, et al: Hydroxyethyl starch 130/0.42 versus Ringer's acetate in severe sepsis, N Engl J Med 367:124-134, 2012.
38. Theis JC, Rietweld J, Danesh-Clough T: Severe necrotising soft tissue infections in orthopaedics surgery, J Orthop Surg 10:108, 2012.
39. Ingrey KT, Ren J, Prescott JF: A fluoroquinolone induces a novel mitogen-encoding bacteriophage in *Streptococcus canis*, Infect Immun 71:3028, 2003.
40. Sudarsky LA, Laschinger JC, Coppa GF, Spencer FC: Improved results from standardized approach in treating patients with necrotizing fasciitis, Ann Surg 206:661, 1987.
41. Kaiser RE, Cerra FB: Progressive necrotizing surgical infections: a unified approach, J Trauma 21:349, 1981.
42. Purvis D, Kirby R: Systemic inflammatory response syndrome: septic shock, Vet Clin North Am Small Anim Pract 24:1225, 1994.
43. Darenberg J, Ihendyane N, Sjolin J, et al: Intravenous immunoglobulin G therapy in streptococcal toxic shock syndrome: a European randomized, double-blind, placebo-controlled trial, Clin Infect Dis 37:333, 2003.
44. BarryW: Intravenous immunoglobulin therapy for toxic shock syndrome, J Am Med Assoc 267:3315, 1992.
45. Norrby-Teglund A, Haul R, Low DE, et al: Evidence for the presence of streptococcal-superantigen neutralising antibodies in normal polyspecific immunoglobulin, Infect Immun 64:5395, 1996.
46. Hosgood G, Kerwin SC, Lewis DD, et al: Clinical review of the mechanism and applications of hyperbaric oxygen therapy in small animal surgery, Vet Comp Orthop Traumatol 5:31, 1992.
47. Kerwin SC, Hosgood G, Strain GM, et al: The effect of hyperbaric oxygen treatment on a compromised axial pattern flap in the cat, Vet Surg 22:31, 1993.
48. Cooper NA, Unsworth IP, Turner DM, et al: Hyperbaric oxygen used in the treatment of gas gangrene in a dog, J Small Anim Pract 17:759, 1976.
49. George ME, Rueth NM, Skarda DE, et al: Hyperbaric oxygen does not improve outcome in patients with necrotizing soft tissue infection, Surg Infect (Larchmt) 10:21, 2009.

CHAPTER 102
CATHETER-RELATED BLOODSTREAM INFECTION

Sean Smarick, VMD, DACVECC • Melissa Edwards, DVM, DACVECC

KEY POINTS

- Intravenous catheters may become contaminated and can lead to local and distal infectious complications. Septicemia caused by a colonized catheter is referred to as a *catheter-related bloodstream infection (CRBSI).*
- The diagnosis of a catheter-related bloodstream infection includes culturing the catheter and blood, but any fever of unknown origin, bacteremia, or infection at the insertion site should prompt the clinician to consider this type of infection.
- Treatment of known catheter-related bloodstream infection includes removing the catheter and administering systemic antibiotics.
- Frequency of catheter-related bloodstream infection may be reduced by aseptically placing and maintaining catheters and educating caretakers involved in catheter placement and maintenance.

DEFINITION

Intravenous catheters often are used in critically ill patients, but they can become contaminated with microorganisms. Skin contaminants may be introduced during placement or may migrate along the external surface of the catheter. In addition, contamination of the catheter hub or infusate may lead to colonizing of the internal surface. Some bacteria and fungi produce biofilm, a matrix of microorganisms and their produced glycocalyces along with host salts and proteins that provide protection from the host's defenses. Catheter contamination may lead to local signs of phlebitis; when catheter colonization leads to septicemia, the resultant infection is referred to as a *catheter-related bloodstream infection (CRBSI).*[1,2] The majority of CRBSIs are bacterial; however, fungal causes play an important role in people but are not well documented in veterinary medicine.[3]

INCIDENCE

CRBSI has been reported in dogs and cats. In small animal intensive care units, CRBSIs have been implicated as a cause of morbidity and mortality.[4-8] In veterinary medicine the incidence of catheter contamination has been reported as 10.4% to 24% in peripheral catheters[3,4,8-10] and from 0 to 26% in jugular catheters, which is consistent with human reports.[7,8,10,11] CRBSI is well studied in humans, and the incidence is approximately 1.5% with central venous catheters.[12] In a few studies in dogs and cats looking at catheter contamination rates, 4 in 304 cases were identifiable as CRBSI in a combination of peripherally and centrally placed venous catheters.[4,7,8,11] This suggests a combined rate of 1.3% (1.3 bloodstream infections per 100 catheters). This rate likely underestimates the current and future incidence of CRBSI because peripheral venous catheters have a lower rate of CRBSI, and the use of central venous and arterial catheters is increasing in veterinary medicine. Indwelling catheters that are tunneled through the subcutaneous tissues have been described for long-term use (weeks to months) in veterinary patients. Some of these catheters have access ports also placed subcutaneously. The combined reported rate of CRBSI for these types of catheters of 6 in 244 is consistent with rates reported in people for similar catheter types, despite a decreased duration of catheterization in the veterinary patients. The veterinary population was overrepresented by patients undergoing radiation therapy or chemotherapy for neoplasia, and that group included all of the patients that developed CRBSI.[12-17]

DIAGNOSIS

CRBSI should be considered in febrile patients that have an intravascular catheter in place when no other source of infection is obvious. Phlebitis and especially purulent discharge at the catheter site may indicate that catheter colonization has resulted in a localized infection that may lead to a CRBSI; however, the lack of localized reaction does not rule out a CRBSI; close to 50% of humans show no local signs. Because clinical signs are not reliable, cultures are required for the diagnosis of a CRBSI.[1,10,18] A CRBSI differs from a catheter-associated bloodstream infection. In a CRBSI, the catheter is the primary source of the bloodstream infection as determined by cultures of the catheter and blood, whereas in a catheter-associated bloodstream infection, a catheter is present in the face of a bloodstream infection but is unable to be cultured, and no other source of infection can be identified. The lack of another identifiable or suspected source of infection and critical interpretation of cultures are needed to diagnose a CRBSI.[19]

Considering the relatively low incidence of CRBSI, routine screening of qualitative (i.e., positive versus negative) catheter tip or segment cultures is not recommended because of the number of false-positive results.[18-20] Numerous culturing methods of diagnosing a CRBSI have been reported, and the source (intraluminal versus extraluminal) of the infection, number of lumens of the catheter, availability of culturing methods, ability to aspirate the catheter, and need to keep the present catheter in place may dictate which method is to be used in individual patients. Because infections identified soon after catheter placement tend to originate on the external surface, and infections of long-term catheters tend to originate on the internal lumen, culturing blood from the lumen may be a source of false-negative cultures in short-term catheterization.[18] Multilumen catheters pose a challenge in that one or multiple lumens may be colonized, leading to false-negative results if only one lumen is cultured. In humans, sampling only one lumen of a triple-lumen catheter correctly identified less than two thirds of the CRBSIs.[21,22] Catheters do not necessarily have to be removed to diagnose a CRBSI. Considering the low number of true CRBSIs in febrile patients, catheters in such patients may remain unless they are no longer needed, they have a purulent discharge, or the patient is decompensating.[1,18,23]

Ideally, quantitative cultures of blood obtained percutaneously and through the catheter are submitted. A positive result is one in which the catheter-obtained culture(s) has three to five times more bacterial concentration than the culture obtained percutaneously. Alternatively, qualitative cultures in which positive blood culture results from the catheter precede results from the percutaneous culture by more than 2 hours can be used if the quantitative methods are unavailable. If neither method is available or if the catheter is removed, a semiquantitative culture obtained by rolling a 5-cm section of the catheter four times over a blood agar plate and finding more than 15 colony-forming units (CFU) is also a method with good sensitivity and specificity in humans. Qualitative or quantitative (more than 100 CFU/ml) blood cultures drawn from the catheter and quantitative cultures (more than 1000 CFU/ml) of broth that was flushed through or sonicated with the catheter also have been described for diagnosing CRBSI. Staining lysed cells from catheter-obtained blood samples with acridine orange to look for organisms and performing cultures of endoluminal brushing of the catheter are additional methods of diagnosis.[1,18,20]

For obtaining blood cultures, the catheter and percutaneous site should undergo aseptic preparation, equal volumes for each sample site should be collected, and the samples should be obtained within 10 minutes of each other. Ideally, cultures are obtained before instituting empiric antibiotic therapy.[1,18,20]

TREATMENT

Treatment of known CRBSI consists of removal of the catheter and appropriate antimicrobial therapy; however, in febrile patients with a catheter in place without local signs of infection, "watchful waiting" is an effective strategy. In humans, leaving the catheter in place awaiting culture results led to a 60% reduction in the number of catheters removed with no significant change in outcome. The risks of catheter replacement versus having a potential nidus of infection must be weighed in each patient; deteriorating patients should be treated more aggressively. When a suspected infected catheter is left in place, an antibiotic lock consisting of concentrated amounts of antibiotics, ethanol, or other substances occupying the lumen dead space has been shown in humans to effectively eliminate many bacterial infections and spares the patient the catheter removal. The concentrated amount of antibiotic allows biofilm penetration unattainable with systemic administration. If replacement of a catheter suspected to be infected is necessary, it should not be replaced with an over-the-wire technique; a separate insertion site should be used. Systemic antibiotics guided by culture and susceptibility should be continued for 10 to 14 days after catheter removal. As with many infections, the best treatment of CRBSI is prevention.[1,20,23]

PREVENTION

Recommendations for the prevention of CRBSI have been published in the veterinary literature and include caregiver hand washing, placement of catheters by trained personnel, aseptic catheter placement, use of the most bioinert catheter material (i.e., polyurethane versus Teflon), and monitoring for CRBSI. Scheduled catheter replacement is no longer recommended. These recommendations were based on limited veterinary observational studies and guidelines for human patients.[2,7,8]

In the absence of well-controlled and well-powered veterinary studies, it is reasonable to adopt human recommendations to prevent CRBSI formulated on evidence-based guidelines. In 2011 the Centers for Disease Control and Prevention (CDC) published (and made available online) the "Guidelines for the Prevention of Intravascular Catheter-Related Infections."[19] A checklist adapted to veterinary patients to decrease the incidence of CRBSI is presented in Box 102-1. Educating caregivers about the indications, proper catheter selection and placement, maintenance, and nosocomial surveillance of vascular catheters is considered paramount in preventing CRBSI. As with all nosocomial infections, hand washing is crucial for prevention; wearing gloves augments the preventive effect of but does not replace hand washing. Other recommendations from the CDC include not to administer prophylactic antibiotics and not to replace catheters routinely for infection control. However, catheters that were placed under less-than-ideal emergency conditions should be replaced within 48 hours, and peripheral catheters may be replaced every 72 to 96 hours to prevent phlebitis.[19]

BOX 102-1 ***Checklist for Placement and Maintenance of Intravascular Catheters to Prevent Catheter-Related Bloodstream Infections***

- Wash hands with soap and water or alcohol-based hand rub.
- Wear clean gloves.
- Provide aseptic insertion and care of catheter.
- Use a 2% chlorhexidine skin preparation.
- For peripheral intravenous catheters, use three to seven cycles of scrub, then wipe with alcohol, and do not touch the insertion site after preparation.
- Use sterile gloves for arterial and central venous catheters and maximum barrier protection (sterile gown and drape, mask) when placing central venous catheters. Change gloves for the new catheter when rewiring.
- Minimize cut down approaches for catheter placement.
- Dress the catheter with a sterile gauze (or Band-Aid) and bandage or sterile, transparent, semipermeable dressing.
- Avoid ointments at the catheter site.
- Monitor regularly: visualize when dressing changed, palpate through dressing, look for discomfort, phlebitis, or fever without another source.

Catheter Dressings

Inspect dressing daily.

- Change gauze dressings every 48 hours or if moist or soiled and transparent dressings every 7 days, sooner if loose or concerns arise.
- Wipe injection ports with alcohol before using; stopcocks should be capped.
- Change administration sets (aseptically) every 4 to 7 days.
- Change arterial line administration sets and transducers (aseptically) every 96 hours.
- Change administration sets (aseptically) every 6 to 12 hours if propofol infused.
- Change administration sets (aseptically) every 24 hours if lipid-containing TPN solutions or blood products are infused.
- Evaluate the need for the catheter; remove it when it is no longer needed.

TPN, Total parenteral nutrition.

The CDC also recognizes infusates and intravenous admixtures as a source for CRBSI. Blood products and lipid-containing parenteral nutrition solutions should not be infused for longer than 4 hours and 24 hours, respectively.[24] The administration sets through which blood products and lipid-containing emulsions are given should also be changed within 24 hours.[19] In addition, the sterility of administered drugs and intravenous admixtures should be maintained by using single-dose vials, swabbing multidose vials with alcohol before aspiration, and discarding any suspected compromised solution.[19,25]

In the war against device-associated nosocomial infections, catheters impregnated with antiseptics and antibiotics have been introduced. In humans, studies support a reduction in the incidence of CRBSI with the use of these catheters; however, the debate over their use continues. Current recommendations are for using these catheters only in areas in which comprehensive strategies (e.g., education, hand washing) have been unsuccessful in decreasing CRBSI rates and not for routine use because of reported allergic reactions, potential for the development of resistant organisms, and the additional expense.[1,19]

The current trend is toward the use of needleless intravascular catheter systems in the prevention of needlestick injuries. These systems come in several forms, such as stopcocks, split septum connectors, and mechanical valve systems, and can contribute to catheter contamination and CRBSI. Stopcocks should be capped at all times when not in use and their use avoided if possible. Some evidence suggests that mechanical valve needleless connector systems also may increase risk over split septum connector designs in some cases.[19,26,27]

REFERENCES

1. Slaughter SE: Intravascular catheter-related infections. Strategies for combating this common foe, Postgrad Med 116:59, 2004.
2. Tan RH, Dart AJ, Dowling BA: Catheters: a review of the selection, utilisation and complications of catheters for peripheral venous access, Aust Vet J 81:136, 2003.
3. Seguela J, Pages JP: Bacterial and fungal colonisation of peripheral intravenous catheters in dogs and cats, J Small Anim Pract 52:531, 2011.
4. Burrows CF: Inadequate skin preparation as a cause of intravenous catheter-related infection in the dog, J Am Vet Med Assoc 180:747, 1982.
5. Francey T, Gaschen F, Nicolet J, et al: The role of Acinetobacter baumannii as a nosocomial pathogen for dogs and cats in an intensive care unit, J Vet Intern Med 14:177, 2000.
6. Glickman LT: Veterinary nosocomial (hospital-acquired) Klebsiella infections, J Am Vet Med Assoc 179:1389, 1981.
7. Lippert AC, Fulton RB, Parr AM: Nosocomial infection surveillance in a small animal intensive care unit, J Am Anim Hosp Assoc 24:627, 1988.
8. Mathews KA, Brooks MJ, Valliant AE: A prospective study of intravenous catheter contamination, J Vet Emerg Crit Care 6:33, 1996.
9. Lobetti RG, Joubert KE, Picard J, et al: Bacterial colonization of intravenous catheters in young dogs suspected to have parvoviral enteritis, J Am Vet Med Assoc 220:1321, 2002.
10. Marsh-Ng ML, Burney DP, Garcia J: Surveillance of infections associated with intravenous catheters in dogs and cats in an intensive care unit, J Am Anim Hosp Assoc 43:13, 2007.
11. Martin GJ, Rand JS: Evaluation of a polyurethane jugular catheter in cats placed using a modified Seldinger technique, Aust Vet J 77:250, 1999.
12. Dudeck MA, Horan TC, Peterson KD, et al: National Healthcare Safety Network (NHSN) Report, data summary for 2010, device-associated module, Am J Infect Control 39:798, 2011.
13. Abrams-Ogg AC, Kruth SA, Carter RF, et al: The use of an implantable central venous (Hickman) catheter for long-term venous access in dogs undergoing bone marrow transplantation, Can J Vet Res 56:382, 1992.
14. Evans KL, Smeak DD, Couto CG, et al: Comparison of two indwelling central venous access catheters in dogs undergoing fractionated radiotherapy, Vet Surg 23:135, 1994.
15. Blaiset MA, Couto CG, Evans KL, et al: Complications of indwelling, silastic central venous access catheters in dogs and cats, J Am Anim Hosp Assoc 31:379, 1995.
16. Culp WT, Mayhew PD, Reese MS, et al: Complications associated with use of subcutaneous vascular access ports in cats and dogs undergoing fractionated radiotherapy: 172 cases (1996-2007), J Am Vet Med Assoc 236:1322, 2010.
17. Valentini F, Fassone F, Pozzebon A, et al: Use of totally implantable vascular access port with mini-invasive Seldinger technique in 12 dogs undergoing chemotherapy, Res Vet Sci 94:152, 2013.
18. Safdar N, Fine JP, Maki DG: Meta-analysis: methods for diagnosing intravascular device-related bloodstream infection, Ann Intern Med 142:451, 2005.
19. O'Grady NP, Alexander M, Burns LA, et al: Guidelines for the prevention of intravascular catheter-related infections, Clin Infect Dis 52:e162, 2011.
20. Mermel LA, Allon M, Bouza E, et al: Clinical practice guidelines for the diagnosis and management of intravascular catheter-related infection: 2009 Update by the Infectious Diseases Society of America, Clin Infect Dis 49:1, 2009.
21. Dobbins BM, Catton JA, Kite P, et al: Each lumen is a potential source of central venous catheter-related bloodstream infection, Crit Care Med 31:1688, 2003.
22. Guembe M, Rodriguez-Creixems M, Sanchez-Carrillo C, et al: How many lumens should be cultured in the conservative diagnosis of catheter-related bloodstream infections? Clin Infect Dis 50:1575, 2010.

23. Sherertz RJ: Update on vascular catheter infections, Curr Opin Infect Dis 17:303, 2004.
24. O'Grady NP, Alexander M, Dellinger EP, et al: Guidelines for the prevention of intravascular catheter-related infections, Infect Control Hosp Epidemiol 23:759, 2002.
25. Macias AE, Huertas M, de Leon SP, et al: Contamination of intravenous fluids: a continuing cause of hospital bacteremia, Am J Infect Control 38:217, 2010.
26. Rupp ME, Sholtz LA, Jourdan DR, et al: Outbreak of bloodstream infection temporally associated with the use of an intravascular needleless valve, Clin Infect Dis 44:1408, 2007.
27. Jarvis WR, Murphy C, Hall KK, et al: Health care-associated bloodstream infections associated with negative- or positive-pressure or displacement mechanical valve needleless connectors, Clin Infect Dis 49:1821, 2009.

CHAPTER 103
MULTIDRUG-RESISTANT INFECTIONS

Steven Epstein, DVM, DACVECC

KEY POINTS

- Multidrug-resistant pathogens are increasingly common in veterinary medicine, and early culture and susceptibility testing is crucial to their diagnosis.
- Regional knowledge of likely pathogens and their susceptibility patterns is helpful in guiding empiric therapy.
- Consultation with an infectious disease specialist can be helpful in optimizing success for multidrug- resistant infections.

Multidrug-resistant (MDR) pathogens are an increasing concern in veterinary medicine in the hospitalized and outpatient populations. In human hospitalized patients, the intensive care unit (ICU) has the highest rate of antimicrobial resistance.[1,2] These pathogens also are identified frequently in the veterinary ICU.[3-5] Within veterinary teaching hospitals, MDR pathogens are also commonly found on multiple other surfaces.[6-8] The possibility of MDR pathogens in the ICU is a major factor in the empiric selection of antimicrobials for these patients, creating numerous challenges. ICU clinicians are more commonly faced with treating infections caused by organisms with limited (MDR or extensively drug resistant [XDR]) or no viable treatment options (pandrug-resistant [PDR]).

DEFINITIONS

Antimicrobial resistance is a measure of an antimicrobial agent's decreased ability to kill or inhibit the growth of a microorganism. This is determined practically by testing a bacterial isolate in an *in vitro* system against various antimicrobials. From this testing a minimum inhibitory concentration (MIC) can be determined. A MIC is the lowest concentration of an antimicrobial that inhibits growth of a microorganism. An organism is said to be susceptible to that antimicrobial if the MIC is below the breakpoint for that antimicrobial. The Clinical and Laboratory Standards Institute has established many breakpoints based on large numbers of isolates that determine resistance or susceptibility. A breakpoint is the highest MIC achievable (usually a serum concentration of antimicrobial given at routine doses) that still inhibits growth of that microorganism. These are based on achievable serum concentrations, not necessarily the concentration of the antimicrobial of the infected tissue, which are typically slightly less than the serum.

Bacteria may exhibit three different types of resistance. Intrinsic resistance is an inherent feature of a microorganism that results in lack of activity of an antimicrobial drug or class of drugs. One example of this is *Pseudomonas aeruginosa,* which shows resistance to the majority of β-lactam antimicrobials, except for the few specifically designed as anti-*Pseudomonas* drugs. Another example is that all gram-negative organisms are resistant to vancomycin, which cannot penetrate their cell membrane. Circumstantial resistance is when an *in vitro* test predicts susceptibility, but *in vivo* the antimicrobial lacks clinical efficacy. This may be due to lack of the drug to penetrate the site of infection (CNS, prostate, bone) or inability to work because of local pH (inactivation in acidic urine). Acquired resistance is a change in the phenotypic characteristics of a microorganism, compared with the wild type, which confers decreased effectiveness of an antimicrobial against that microorganism.

Acquired resistance can occur via many different mechanisms, and a full review of this topic is beyond the scope of this chapter. One of the most important mechanisms is exposure to prior antimicrobials; this is a known risk factor in veterinary medicine.[9] This acquired resistance is what leads to the development of many MDR microorganisms. The European Centre for Disease Prevention and Control and the U.S. Centers for Disease Control and Prevention published standardized terminology for grading antimicrobial resistance.[10] MDR organisms are defined as those not susceptible to at least one agent in three or more classes of antimicrobials to which they are usually susceptible. XDR organisms are susceptible to only one or two classes of antimicrobials. PDR organisms are not susceptible to all known or licensed antimicrobials currently available.

RISK FACTORS FOR MULTIDRUG-RESISTANT PATHOGENS

The identification of patients at risk for having a MDR infection is paramount for the selection and treatment of empiric antimicrobials in critical care. In human medicine some of the major risk factors associated with either MDR gram-negative or gram-positive infections are previous antimicrobial use, admission to an ICU, infection control lapses, prolonged length of hospital stay, recent surgery or invasive procedures, mechanical ventilation, or colonization or exposure to a patient with colonization of a MDR pathogen.[11-13]

Minimal information is available on this topic in veterinary medicine, but the risk factors are likely the same as in human medicine. In dogs, predisposing diseases, prior antimicrobial use, duration of hospitalization, duration of ICU hospitalization, surgical procedure, and mechanical ventilation have been associated with increased MDR pathogen identification.[4,14-16] Evaluating a patient for these risk factors helps the clinician to decide whether an escalation or de-escalation approach to antimicrobial therapy is appropriate for the patient.

ESCALATION VERSUS DE-ESCALATION THERAPY

Escalation therapy involves selecting an antimicrobial with a narrow spectrum of activity that likely covers the pathogen causing the suspected infection. When culture and susceptibility results are available, the antimicrobial agent may be continued if susceptibility is predicted or switched if resistance is documented. De-escalation therapy consists of the empiric administration of broad-spectrum antimicrobials aimed to cover all pathogens most frequently related to the infection, including MDR and XDR pathogens. The coverage selected usually is limited to bacterial infections, unless life-threatening fungal infections are suspected. When culture and susceptibility results are available, the spectrum of activity of the antimicrobials is then narrowed if possible.

The rationale for using de-escalation therapy is to lower mortality by early achievement of appropriate empiric antimicrobial coverage in addition to prevention of the development of MDR pathogens. Human patients in which a de-escalation approach is recommended include patients with pneumonia at risk for MDR pathogens[17] and patients with severe sepsis or septic shock.[18] This recommendation is based on results of a study that found that, for every 1 hour that appropriate antimicrobial therapy is not given after the first 6 hours a patient is diagnosed with septic shock, mortality increased by 7.6%. This means that 24 hours of ineffective antimicrobials would reduce the chance of survival to approximately 20%.[19] De-escalation therapy has been demonstrated to be feasible in human ICUs with de-escalation rates of 32% to 51%.[20-22] In addition, de-escalation has not been shown to increase the level of MDR carriage.[21,22]

The majority of patients in veterinary medicine should have an escalation approach to antimicrobial therapy taken. In veterinary critical care, a de-escalation approach usually is reserved for patients who have severe sepsis/septic shock or for patients that have acquired an infection in hospital while on antimicrobials. Practically speaking, for a critically ill patient the clinician must consider, "Does this patient appear sick enough, that if I choose the wrong antimicrobial, it might die of its infection/sepsis in the next 24 hours?" When the answer is yes, then a de-escalation approach should be instituted. If a de-escalation approach is used, then obtaining a culture from the infected tissue should be considered mandatory, if it can be accomplished without compromising patient safety. This allows for Gram stain and cytology, which help guide empiric therapy.

SPECIFIC MULTIDRUG-RESISTANT PATHOGENS

Methicillin-Resistant Staphylococcus

Staphylococcal infections in small animals are most likely to be *Staphylococcus pseudintermedius* (SP), whereas *Staphylococcus aureus* (SA) is rare. Various coagulase-negative *Staphylococcus* species are clinically important. The primary mechanism of resistance is the acquisition of the mecA gene, which confers methicillin resistance. This encodes an altered penicillin-binding protein, making it resistant to all members of the β-lactam family regardless of susceptibility testing. Laboratory testing may be to oxacillin instead of methicillin; however, they are equivalent in determining resistance to all members of the β-lactams group.

If a methicillin-resistant *Staphylococcus* (MRS) is suspected, culture and susceptibility testing is imperative because more than 90% of canine isolates of MRSP were resistant to representatives of at least four additional antimicrobial drug classes.[23] Along with resistance to the β-lactam group of antimicrobials, MRS is frequently resistant to clindamycin, fluoroquinolones, macrolides, and trimethoprim-sulfonamides. Given the high rates of co-resistance in MRS, if a de-escalation approach is to be taken, the antimicrobial typically used empirically would be vancomycin (see Chapter 181). Vancomycin is the drug of choice for MRSA in human medicine, although the frequency of vancomycin-intermediate and vancomycin-resistant *S. aureus* is increasing. In the author's ICU, if empiric vancomycin therapy is used, culture and susceptibility testing as well as therapeutic drug monitor typically are initiated to help prevent resistance from developing. Serum levels of vancomycin when steady state has been reached, typically just before the fourth dose, are recommended and dosing altered to maintain trough concentrations higher than 10 mg/L to avoid development of resistance.[24]

An alternative to vancomycin for MRS in veterinary medicine are the aminoglycosides (amikacin and gentamicin, primarily). Aminoglycosides have efficacy against many MRS. Potential disadvantages to aminoglycoside therapy are that with extended use or concurrent hypotension, the risk of acute kidney injury increases; they must be administered parentally; and they have decreased activity in purulent material or cellular debris. Despite these disadvantages, they are an acceptable alternative to vancomycin for empiric therapy for suspected MRS.

Other antimicrobials that may have efficacy against MRS are bacteriostatic and may be useful with an escalation approach (e.g., healthy patient with superficial infection). These antimicrobials include the tetracyclines (doxycycline and minocycline), chloramphenicol, and rifampin. Prior knowledge of the common resistance patterns of MRS in the practice location helps clinicians decide which of these is most likely to be efficacious (e.g., at the author's institution, the majority of MRS are resistant to doxycycline).

If a MRS is identified that is also a vancomycin-resistant *Staphylococcus* sp., human medicine offers multiple alternatives for antimicrobials, but few have been used in veterinary medicine. These antimicrobials include daptomycin, linezolid, quinupristin/dalfopristin, tigecycline, and a fifth-generation cephalosporin ceftaroline fosamil. Consultation with an infectious disease specialist is recommended before starting therapy with any of these medications.

Enterococcus

Enterococci are gram-positive cocci found normally in the gastrointestinal tract. The two species most commonly identified are *Enterococcus faecalis* and *Enterococcus faecium*. They are an important source of nosocomial infection and have been isolated frequently from surfaces in one veterinary study.[6] *E. faecalis* is isolated more commonly; however, *E. faecium* is more often MDR.

Enterococci have a high level of intrinsic resistance to many antimicrobials, including all cephalosporins, clindamycin, and aminoglycosides at serum concentrations achievable without toxicity. Fluoroquinolones also exhibit poor activity against *Enterococcus* spp. Third-generation cephalosporin use and fluoroquinolone use have been associated with the development of vancomycin-resistant *Enterococcus* spp. in humans.[25,26] Acquired resistance in enterococci is related primarily to acquisition of aminoglycoside-modifying enzymes (AME) or alterations in penicillin-binding protein (PBP5), which confer resistance to high levels of aminoglycosides (HLAR) and all penicillins and carbapenems, respectively.

Because enterococci are not highly pathogenic organisms, isolation from a culture does not always necessitate treatment of the organism. In cases in which colonization, not infection, is suspected (e.g., superficial wound or asymptomatic bacteriuria), the patient may be monitored and not treated. When MDR *Enterococcus* spp. co-exist with other pathogens, clinical resolution of disease is possible without treating the *Enterococcus* spp. and directing therapy at the other microorganisms. This has been shown in humans with intraabdominal sepsis treated with surgery but no enterococcal antimicrobial, although no veterinary studies evaluate this.[27]

Treatment of MDR *Enterococcus* spp. typically involves one of two options: (1) the combination of ampicillin and gentamicin or (2) vancomycin.[28] The combination of ampicillin and gentamicin rely on the synergistic activity of these two drugs. This combination of agents allows for bacterial killing with differing mechanisms with ampicillin disturbing the cell wall, which then facilitates the entry of gentamicin into the cytoplasmic space affecting protein synthesis. This synergistic combination can be achieved even if routine susceptibility testing predicts resistance to both drugs. Specialized testing for high-level resistance is needed to determine if this combination would be effective *in vivo*. If MICs are 64 mg/L or less for ampicillin and at least 500 mg/L for gentamicin, this combination can be used. Amikacin or tobramycin should not be used for the treatment of *Enterococcus* spp. because no synergy with ampicillin exists.

If this combination is not possible, then treatment of MDR *Enterococcus* spp. with vancomycin is recommended. As with MRS, if a vancomycin-resistant *Enterococcus* sp. is encountered, treatment may involve linezolid, daptomycin, quinupristin/dalfopristin, or ceftaroline (for *E. faecalis* not *E. faecium*).

Pseudomonas aeruginosa

P. aeruginosa is a nonfermenting gram-negative pathogen found widely in the health care environment, and outbreaks of clonal infections have been seen in ICUs.[29] *P. aeruginosa* is a pathogen that has a very high level of intrinsic resistance. It is resistant to the majority of β-lactam antimicrobial with the exception of ticarcillin, piperacillin, ceftazidime, and the carbapenems. Other classes of antimicrobials with known efficacy are aminoglycosides and the fluoroquinolones.

Acquired resistance to *P. aeruginosa* occurs frequently. The three main mechanisms behind acquired resistance include a decrease in intracellular drug entry from efflux pumps or altered membrane structure, enzymes that modify or destroy antimicrobials, or modification of the target of the antimicrobials (DNA gyrase mutation). These mechanisms frequently lead to resistance against aminoglycosides, fluoroquinolones, and the β-lactams. Production of carbapenemases is uncommon unless previous use in that patient exists.

Treatment of MDR *P. aeruginosa* often involves the use of amikacin or a carbapenem. In a large-scale human study the highest susceptibility rates for *P. aeruginosa* were to amikacin (90%), whereas only 83% to meropenem.[30] As such amikacin or a carbapenem can be used empirically when *P. aeruginosa* is suspected. The ideal carbapenem for use is not clear; meropenem[31] and imipenem[32] have been associated with the development of resistance to carbapenems. The role for combination therapy for MDR or XDR *P. aeruginosa* is not clear because some studies show synergistic effects, whereas others show antagonistic effects; therefore combination therapy is not recommended routinely.

For XDR *P. aeruginosa*, the use of colistin, an old antimicrobial previously known as polymyxin E, is more frequently being administered in human medicine. It is used primarily as a rescue treatment with inconsistent results; however, 92% of MDR *P. aeruginosa* were susceptible to colistin.[33] The ideal dosing is not known and nephrotoxicity is a possibility, potentially limiting its use in veterinary medicine.

β-Lactamase–Producing Gram-Negative Bacteria

Acquisition of a β-lactamase is one the most frequent mechanisms of acquired resistance in gram-negative organisms. β-Lactamase is an enzyme that hydrolyzes and disrupts the β-lactam ring in the β-lactam group of antimicrobials (see Chapter 176). This confers resistance to penicillins, aminopenicillins, carboxypenicillins and narrow-spectrum cephalosporins. β-Lactams combined with a β-lactamase inhibitor (sulbactam, clavulanic acid) retain efficacy against these pathogens. Many third-generation cephalosporins and the carbapenems are also stable in the presence of this enzyme.

Multiple other forms of this resistance mechanism have developed in recent decades. Extended-spectrum β-lactamases (ESBLs) occur in more than 300 different varieties and now are being seen in veterinary patients. In addition to hydrolyzing the above antimicrobials, the ESBLs hydrolyze third-generation cephalosporins. However, carbapenems are stable in the presence of this enzyme. ESBLs primarily have been identified from *E. coli*, *Klebsiella pneumoniae*, and *Enterobacter* spp. Their isolation has been shown to be as much as twice as frequent in an ICU versus a non-ICU population.[2] There are no data from a randomized controlled trial for the treatment of ESBL-producing bacteria; however, carbapenems are considered the preferred treatment. Alternatively, fluoroquinolones or aminoglycosides can be used if shown to be susceptible from culture results.

Enterobacteriaceae also have evolved carbapenemases as a form of acquired resistance. These bacteria are considered XDR and are resistant to the *entire* class of β-lactam antimicrobials. There are no reports of carbapenemase producing bacteria in dogs and cats. Treatment options are often limited because co-resistance to fluoroquinolones (90% to 100% of isolates), aminoglycosides (45% to 90% of isolates), and trimethoprim-sulfamethoxazole are frequent.[34,35] Polymyxins such as colistin with or without rifampin are often the only option to treat these infections. Consultation with an infectious disease specialist is recommended if one of these pathogens is encountered.

REFERENCES

1. Archibald L, Phillips L, Monnet D, et al: Antimicrobial resistance in isolates from in-patients nd outpatients in the United States: increasing importance of the intensive care unit, Clin Infect Dis 24:211, 1997.
2. Badal RE, Bouchillon SK, Lob SH, et al: Etiology, extended-spectrum β-lactamase rates and antimicrobial susceptibility of gram-negative bacilli causing intra-abdominal infections in patients in general pediatric and pediatric intensive care units-global data from the study for monitoring antimicrobial resistance trends from 2008 to 2010, Pediatr Infect Dis J 32:636, 2013.
3. Black DM, Rankin SC, King LG: Antimicrobial therapy and aerobic bacteriologic culture patterns in canine intensive care unit patients: 74 dogs (January-June 2006), J Vet Emerg Crit Care 19:489, 2009.
4. Ogeer-Gyles J, Mathews K, Sears W, et al: Development of antimicrobial drug resistance in rectal Escherichia coli isolates from dogs hospitalized in an intensive care unit, J Am Vet Med Assoc 229:694, 2006.
5. Ghosh A, Dowd SE, Zurek L: Dogs leaving the ICU carry a very large multi-drug resistant enterococcal population with the capacity for biofilm formation and horizontal gene transfer, PLoS ONE 6:e22451, 2011.
6. Hamilton E, Kaneene JB, May KJ, et al: Prevalence and antimicrobial resistance of *Enterococcus* spp and *Staphylococcus* spp isolated from

surfaces in a veterinary teaching hospital, J Am Vet Med Assoc 240:1463, 2012.

7. Kukanich KS, Ghosh A, Skarbek JV, et al: Surveillance of bacterial contamination in small animal veterinary hospitals with special focus on antimicrobial resistance and virulence traits of enterococci, J Am Vet Med Assoc 240:437, 2012.
8. Julian T, Singh A, Rousseau J, et al: Methicillin-resistant staphylococcal contamination of cellular phones of personnel in a veterinary teaching hospital, BMC Res Notes 5:193, 2012.
9. Baker SA, Ban-Balen J, Lu B, et al: Antimicrobial drug use in dogs prior to admission to a veterinary teaching hospital, J Am Vet Med Assoc 241:210, 2012.
10. Magiorakos AP, Srinivasan A, Carey RB, et al: Multi-drug resistant, extensively drug-resistant and pandrug-resistant bacteria: an international expert proposal for interim standard definitions for acquired resistance, Clin Microbiol Infect 18:268, 2012.
11. Maragakis LL: Recognition and prevention of multidrug-resistant gram-negative bacteria in the intensive care unit, Crit Care Med 38:s345, 2010.
12. Lin MY, Hayden MK: Methicillin-resistant *Staphylococcus aureus* and vancomycin-resistant *Enterococcus*: recognition and prevention in intensive care units, Crit Care Med 38:s335, 2010.
13. Ogeer-Gyles JS, Mathews KA, Boerlin P: Nosocomial infections and antimicrobial resistance in critical care medicine, J Vet Emerg Crit Care 16:1, 2006.
14. Epstein SE, Mellema MS, Hopper K: Airway microbial culture and susceptibility patterns in dogs and cats with respiratory disease of varying severity, J Vet Emerg Crit Care 20:587, 2010.
15. Gibson JS, Morton JM, Cobbold RN, et al: Multi-drug resistant *E. coli* and Enterobacter extraintestinal infection in 37 dogs, J Vet Int Med 22:844, 2008.
16. Gibson JS, Morton HM, Cobbold RN, et al: Risk factors for multidrug-resistant *Escherichia coli* rectal colonization of dogs on admission to a veterinary hospital, Epidemiol Infect 139:197, 2011.
17. American Thoracic Society: Guidelines for the management of adults with hospital-acquired, ventilator-associated, and healthcare-associated pneumonia, Am J Resp Crit Care Med 171:388, 2005.
18. Dellinger RP, Levy MM, Rhodes A, et al: Surviving sepsis campaign: international guidelines for management of severe sepsis and septic shock, Intens Care Med 39:165, 2013.
19. Kumar A, Roberts D, Wood KE, et al: Duration of hypotension before initiation of effective antimicrobial therapy is the critical determinant of survival in human septic shock, Crit Care Med 34:1589, 2006.
20. Joung MK, Lee J, Moon S, et al: Impact of de-escalation therapy on clinical outcomes for intensive care unit-acquired pneumonia, Crit Care 15:R79, 2011.
21. Gonzalez L, Cravoisy A, Barraud D, et al: Factors influencing the implementation of antibiotic de-escalation and impact of this strategy in critically ill patients, Crit Care 17:R140, 2013.
22. Morel J, Casoetto J, Jospe R, et al: De-escalation as part of a global strategy of empiric antibiotherapy management. A retrospective study in a medico-surgical intensive care unit, Crit Care 14:R225, 2010.
23. Bemis DA, Jones RD, Frank LA, et al: Evaluation of susceptibility rest breakpoints used to predict mecA-mediated resistance in *Staphylococcus pseudintermedius* isolated from dogs, J Vet Diagn Invest 21:53, 2009.
24. Rybak MJ, Lomaestro BM, Rotscahfer JC, et al: Vancomycin therapeutic guidelines: a summary of consensus recommendations from the infectious diseases society of America, the American society of health-system pharmacists, and the society of infectious diseases pharmacists, Clin Infect Dis 49:325, 2009.
25. Hayakawa K, Marchaim D, Palla M, et al: Epidemiology of vancomycin-resistant Enterococcus faecalis: a case-case-control study, Antimicrob Agents Chemother 57:49, 2013.
26. Fridkin SK, Edwards JR, Courval JM, et al: The effect of vancomycin and third-generation cephalosporin's on prevalence of vancomycin-resistant enterococci in 126 U.S. adult intensive care units, Ann Intern Med 135:175, 2001.
27. Chatterjee I, Iredell JR, Woods M, et al: The implications of enterococci for the intensive care unit, Crit Care Resusc 9:69, 2007.
28. Arias CA, Contreras GA, Murray BE: Management of multidrug-resistant enterococcal infections, Clin Microbial Infect 16:555, 2010.
29. Koutsogiannou M, Drougka E, Liakopoulos A, et al: Spread of multidrug-resistant *Pseudomonas aeruginosa* clones in a university hospital, J Clin Microbiol 51:665, 2013.
30. Zhanel GG, Adam JH, Baxter MR, et al: Antimicrobial susceptibility of 22746 pathogens from Canadian hospitals: results of the CANWARD 2007-2011 study, J Antimicrob Chemother 68(suppl):i7, 2013.
31. Ong DS, Jongerden IP, Buiting AG, et al: Antibiotic exposure and resistance development in Pseudomonas aeruginosa and Enterobacter species in intensive care units, Crit Care Med 39:2458, 2011.
32. Carmeli Y, Troillet N, Eliopoulos GM, et al: Emergence of antibiotic-resistant *Pseudomonas aeruginosa*: comparison of risks associated with different antipseudomonal agents, Antimicrob Agents Chemother 43:1279, 1999.
33. Walkty A, DeCorby M, Nichol K, et al: In vitro activity of colistin (polymyxin E) against 3,480 isolates of gram-negative bacilli obtained from patients in Canadian hospitals of the CANWARD study, 2007-2008, Antimicrob Agents Chemother 53:4924, 2009.
34. Bratu S, Tolany P, Karumudi U, et al: Carbapenemase-producing *Klebsiella pneumoniae* in Brooklyn, NY: molecular epidemiology and in vitro activity of polymyxin B and other agents, J Antimicrob Chemother 53:5046, 2005.
35. Endimiani A, Huger AM, Perez F, et al: Characterization of blaKPC-containing *Klebsiella pneumoniae:* isolates detected in different institutions in the eastern USA, J Antimicrob Chemother 63:427, 2009.

CHAPTER 104
HYPERCOAGULABLE STATES

Alan G. Ralph, DVM, DACVECC • Benjamin M. Brainard, VMD, DACVECC, DACVAA

KEY POINTS

- Thrombophilia is a propensity for pathologic thrombus formation.
- Thrombophilia may be inherited (congenital causes) or acquired.
- Many acquired thrombophilias exist in veterinary medicine.
- Causes may include increases in procoagulant elements, altered blood flow, endothelial barrier disruption, or decreases in endogenous anticoagulants or fibrinolysis.

Hypercoagulability, or thrombophilia, describes a propensity for inappropriate thrombus formation. In vivo, coagulation is kept in check by a delicate balance of endogenous factors that either promote or decrease blood clot formation. Many of the factors that reduce clot formation are activated by the products of procoagulant factors.[1] Hypercoagulability indicates that the balance has been tipped in favor of coagulation, which may arise because of a variety of perturbations in the coagulation system (increased procoagulant elements, decreased anticoagulant elements, or diminished fibrinolysis), ultimately culminating in an increased risk of thrombosis or thromboembolism (TE). Thrombotic disease can increase morbidity, duration of hospital stay, cost of hospitalization, and potentially mortality.

Thrombophilia is a result of inherited or acquired causes. Inherited conditions reported in people include the factor V Leiden mutation or protein C deficiency, among others. No inherited forms of thrombophilia have been described in veterinary medicine.

Three major areas of predisposition to thrombotic disease are described as "Virchow's triad" and include endothelial dysfunction, hypercoagulability of blood, and blood stasis or altered blood flow. In most clinical scenarios, these contributors overlap. For instance, endothelial dysfunction leads to numerous alterations (e.g., loss of thrombomodulin function [TM], release of von Willebrand [vWF] multimers) that ultimately affect the coagulability of blood. Nonetheless, this model provides a meaningful template for understanding prothrombotic conditions.

Activation of coagulation is a central theme throughout many inflammatory disease states, such as sepsis. Likewise, widespread coagulation perpetuates the inflammatory response by direct activation of inflammatory mediators (e.g., thrombin, which can induce directly inflammatory cytokine production, and microthrombosis, which leads to tissue hypoxia and possible reperfusion injury).[2] Inflammation and coagulation are intertwined inextricably, and both processes proceed in a bidirectional fashion.

MECHANISMS OF THROMBOPHILIA

Endothelial Disturbances

In health, the endothelium exhibits an anticoagulant phenotype, maintaining normal blood flow and organ perfusion. Upon activation or injury, the endothelium transitions to a prothrombotic phenotype. The endothelial barrier is comprised of vascular endothelial cells (EC) and a thin, carbohydrate-rich luminal glycocalyx that localizes many key anticoagulant elements.

The glycocalyx comprises a large network of negatively charged glycosaminoglycans (GAGs), proteoglycans, and glycoproteins. Heparan sulfate accounts for 50% to 90% of the proteoglycans and facilitates the binding of antithrombin (AT),[3,4] which increases the efficiency of AT-mediated inhibition of thrombin.[5] Other important anticoagulants bind the glycocalyx, including heparin cofactor II and TM. Tissue factor pathway inhibitor (TFPI) localizes to the glycocalyx, although the exact binding mechanism is debatable, occurring either via heparan sulfate[6,7] or via a glycosylphosphatidylinositol-lipid anchor.[8] The glycocalyx also serves as a mechanoreceptor, sensing altered blood flow and releasing nitric oxide during conditions of increased shear stress to maintain appropriate organ perfusion. Nitric oxide (NO) has important effects on the inflammatory response, leukocyte adhesion to the endothelium, and inhibition of platelet aggregation.[10-12]

With inflammation, synthesis of the GAGs is decreased: these comprise the glycocalyx, decreasing the function of key anticoagulants that rely on the glycocalyx (e.g., TM and protein C, TFPI).[9] The glycocalyx also buffers EC by preventing the binding of inflammatory cytokines to cell surface receptors.[13,14-16]

EC can be activated by tumor necrosis factor-α (TNF-α), bradykinin, thrombin, histamine, and vascular endothelial growth factor (VEGF).[17-20] Once activated or injured, EC release ultralarge multimers of vWF (UL-vWF) from the Weibel-Palade bodies (which also contain P-selectin, IL-8, tissue plasminogen activator [tPA], and factor VIII [fVIII]).[21] UL-vWF can bind platelet GP Ibα receptors, initiate platelet tethering and activation, and are more active for platelet adhesion and activation than smaller vWF multimers.[22] In health, UL-vWF quickly are cleaved into smaller multimers by a disintegrin-like and metalloproteinase with thrombospondin type 1 repeats (ADAMTS13).[23] These smaller vWF molecules circulate freely in association with fVIII and have considerably less platelet aggregatory activity than the UL-vWF molecules. The UL-vWFs usually remain tethered at sites of endothelial activation or injury, bound to the cell surface or to exposed collagen. A decrease or absence of ADAMTS13 may result in high concentrations of UL-vWF, which then can cause systemic platelet aggregation, thrombosis, and a subsequent consumptive thrombocytopenia (thrombotic thrombocytopenic purpura [TTP], reported in people). Acquired TTP has been reported in human patients who have developed antibodies against ADAMTS13 and in patients exposed to certain drugs such as clopidogrel or cyclosporine. Patients with certain malignancies and systemic lupus erythematosus are also at risk. Lower ADAMTS13 levels resulting from inflammatory disease may contribute to pathologies seen with other coagulopathies (e.g., disseminated intravascular coagulation [DIC]).[24,25]

Increased Procoagulant Elements

Endothelial disruption exposes procoagulant substances such as tissue factor (TF) to the circulating blood. Our current understanding suggests that virtually all coagulation in vivo is initiated through the interaction of TF with activated factor VII (fVIIa).[26,27] TF may be expressed on monocytes/macrophages that have been activated by inflammation[28] and also has been identified on the surface of various neoplastic cells.[29] Like many procoagulant elements, TF perpetuates inflammation through the activation of nuclear factor κB, leading to the production of TNF-α.[30]

Platelets also may serve as a source of procoagulant membrane. Upon activation, platelets undergo shape change and shuffle negatively charged phospholipids (phosphatidylserine and phosphatidylethanolamine) to the surface. These provide the catalytic surface essential for the tenase and prothrombinase complexes for the propagation phase of clot formation.[1] With activation, platelets activate and greatly increase the number of copies of the active fibrinogen receptor (glycoprotein IIbIIIa [GP IIbIIIa], also known as integrin $\alpha_{IIb}\beta_3$) on their surface. The contents of alpha and dense granules also are secreted, releasing procoagulant elements such as calcium, factor Va, serotonin, fibrinogen, P-selectin, and ADP. Feline alpha granules also release vWF.[31]

Microparticles (MPs) are circulating small vesicles (membrane blebs) released from activated or apoptotic cells. MPs may be derived from platelets, ECs, leukocytes, erythrocytes, and neoplastic cells.[32,33] Like platelets, MPs also can provide an asymmetric phospholipid membrane for thrombin generation. MPs can express TF on their surface, and those expressing phosphatidylserine and TF are characterized as procoagulant MPs.[34] TF-bearing MPs originating from granulocytes and platelets have been identified in people with sepsis.[35] Moreover, TF-bearing MPs have been shown to induce coagulation in vitro through the VIIa-TF pathway.[36] Some evidence suggests the presence of increased circulating TF activity in dogs with IMHA, which may be a result of TF-bearing MPs.[37] Other procoagulant MPs may display vWF-binding sites and UL-vWF multimers, which can tether and activate circulating platelets.[38,39]

Decreased Endogenous Anticoagulants

Endogenous (natural) anticoagulants are essential to restricting coagulation to the site of vascular insult. The nearly simultaneous activation of anticoagulant factors, even while clot propagation is still occurring, helps to prevent a procoagulant state or the systemic dissemination of coagulation. The three primary anticoagulant proteins are AT, protein C, and TFPI. Many other anticoagulant factors exist, with an anticoagulant described for nearly every procoagulant element. The endothelium is where all three major systems are most active, underscoring the importance of an intact endothelial barrier. AT, TFPI, and the protein C system are directly or indirectly antiinflammatory.

Antithrombin acts primarily to inhibit thrombin and factor Xa and has lesser inhibitory effects on factors IXa and the fVIIa-TF complex. AT is most effective when bound to heparin-like GAGs of the glycocalyx (e.g., heparan sulfate), or when exposed to exogenous heparins, increasing the inhibition of thrombin greater than 1000-fold from non-bound AT.[40] In the absence of heparins, AT's inhibition of thrombin can be enhanced (nearly eightfold) by the binding of AT to TM in the presence of thrombin.[41]

Antithrombin typically is decreased in systemic inflammation or critical illness by one of three mechanisms: consumption (because of thrombin generation), decreased production (negative acute phase protein), or degradation by neutrophil elastase.[42-44] Urinary loss of AT also may occur in animals with glomerulonephritis.[45]

The protein C system is an important inhibitor of factors Va and VIIIa. Protein C is activated (to activated protein C, APC) when trace amounts of thrombin bind TM located on the endothelium, predominantly in the microcirculation.[46] This reaction is accelerated in the presence of the endothelial protein C receptor (EPCR). In the presence of the cofactor protein S, APC's inhibition of Va and VIIIa is accelerated nearly twentyfold.[47,48] By binding thrombin, TM helps generate APC and prevents thrombin from acting on fibrinogen and platelets. This reaction also generates thrombin activatable fibrinolysis inhibitor (TAFI), which inhibits fibrinolysis.

The protein C system is less functional during systemic inflammation resulting from decreased hepatic synthesis of protein C and S. The activation of protein C also is hindered by the effects of inflammatory cytokines on the endothelium and TM. TNF-α can downregulate the expression of TM,[49] whereas elastase from endotoxin-activated neutrophils can cleave TM from the endothelium.[50,51] Circulating or soluble TM is less effective than when it is complexed with the EPCR on the endothelium. Soluble TM is increased in people with sepsis and independently predicts the presence of DIC, multiorgan dysfunction syndrome (MODS), and mortality.[52]

TFPI is released primarily from ECs and acts to inhibit fVIIa-TF complexes and factor Xa (fXa); in essence, all components of the TF- or extrinsic pathway.[53] Other sources of TFPI include platelets,[54] mononuclear cells,[55] vascular smooth muscle and cardiac myocytes,[56] fibroblasts,[56] and megakaryocytes.[57] Protein S serves as a cofactor for the inhibition of fXa by TFPI, and a decrease in TFPI activation contributes to the thrombophilia associated with protein S deficiency in people.[58,59]

Perturbations in Fibrinolysis

Fibrinolysis is the final protective step to prevent vascular occlusion. Thrombi that remain in the macro- or microvasculature can impair organ perfusion and oxygen delivery and may be an important contributor to secondary injury that leads to MODS. Circulating plasminogen is incorporated into forming clots and is converted to plasmin by fibrinolytic activators, including tissue-type (tPA) and urinary-type plasminogen activator (urokinase). Plasmin breaks down the fibrin meshwork of the formed clot and allows for recannulation of blood vessels. tPA and urokinase are derived largely from the endothelium and released upon activation or injury. The effects of plasminogen are decreased by endogenous plasminogen activator inhibitor (PAI-1). In the presence of TNF-α and IL-1β, there is a delayed but more sustained increase in PAI-1 than tPA, decreasing fibrinolysis and resulting in the persistence of thrombi.[61]

DIAGNOSTICS

The identification of a hypercoagulable state before the development of a consumptive coagulopathy or thrombotic complications can be challenging. Often in clinical veterinary medicine, a hypercoagulable state is not identified until a thrombotic event occurs or the patient develops DIC, limiting the opportunity to intervene with specific therapies. In fact, detecting the presence of a thrombus or thromboembolus is one of the only means for a clinician to learn definitively that pathologic coagulation is occurring.

Traditional coagulation tests, such as platelet count, activated partial thromboplastin time (aPTT), and prothrombin time (PT), are most accurate for the demonstration of hypocoagulability and do not reliably identify a predisposition towards hypercoagulability. Prolongations of aPTT/PT and decreased platelet count may appear in patients with hypercoagulability, although this usually is due to consumption of platelets and coagulation factors after unregulated thrombin generation. In practice, a drop in circulating platelet count accompanied by a prolongation of at least 20% in baseline aPTT in an at-risk patient should raise concern of consumptive coagulopathy and prompt further investigation.[62]

Documentation of a hypercoagulable state relies on identifying a rise in procoagulant elements (e.g., MPs, fV, or VIII activities, or fibrinogen), a decrease in endogenous anticoagulants (e.g., AT, protein S and C, or TFPI), or a decrease in fibrinolysis (decreased tPA; increased α2-antiplasmin, PAI-1, TAFI). Testing that assesses more than one aspect (e.g., viscoelastic coagulation [thromboelastography] or calibrated automated thrombography [CAT]) also may be useful. In addition, markers of ongoing thrombin generation (e.g., thrombin-AT complex [TAT], prothrombin activation fragment [F1+2], or fibrinopeptides A and B) or lysis of fibrin clots (fibrin [-ogen] degradation product [FDP] or D-dimer) may be used (Box 104-1).

Procoagulant factor (fV and fVIII) activities and many anticoagulant and fibrinolytic components can be evaluated at specialty reference laboratories, such as the Comparative Coagulation Laboratory at Cornell University. Many sensitive assays are available for documenting activation of specific coagulation components in people (e.g., activation of the contact pathway by factor XIIa or factor XII-C1 inhibitor complex); however, these have not been validated for veterinary species.[63] Other markers of thrombin generation, such as fibrinopeptide A and F1+2, have been evaluated in dogs, although poor cross-reactivity to the reagents in the human-based assay was noted.[64]

Tests to assess coagulation globally are becoming more widely available in veterinary medicine and are unique in the information they provide. Commonly available tests include viscoelastic coagulation devices (thromboelastography [TEG] or rotational thromboelastometry [ROTEM]) or CAT. Viscoelastic testing evaluates the time to initial fibrin cross-linking, rate of clot formation, and the viscoelastic characteristics of the clot formed,[65] whereas CAT focuses on the thrombin generation potential (endogenous thrombin potential, ETP) in a sample. These tests may help to suggest a hypercoagulable state. Hypercoagulable samples clot more quickly, with a faster rate of clot formation, and greater clot strength (viscoelastic tests); or exhibit a greater ETP for CAT.

Platelet contributions to a hypercoagulable state may be inferred by assessing markers of platelet activation (e.g., P-selectin expression, platelet-neutrophil aggregates) (Box 104-2) or documentation of hyperfunctional platelets in response to standard stimuli (see Chapter 107). Although whole blood viscoelastic testing does integrate platelet function, detection of specific proteins on platelets or other circulating cells requires advanced techniques such as flow cytometry. Flow cytometric techniques also can be used to document the presence of procoagulant MPs, although standardization of techniques is necessary because of the small size of the MPs (less than 1.5 microns). The Advia 120 hemostasis analyzer (Bayer Healthcare, Shawnee Mission, KS) reports a parameter called *mean platelet component (MPC)*, which is related to the granularity of the circulating platelets. After activation, the granularity of platelets decreases, and thus a decreased MPC may represent circulating activated platelets, although further study is necessary to apply this technology to veterinary medicine.

BOX 104-1 ***Laboratory Markers of a Hypercoagulable State***

Ongoing Thrombin Generation

Thrombin-antithrombin complex (TAT)[141]
Prothrombin fragment (F1+2)[226]
Fibrinopeptides A + B[227,228]
D-dimer (lysis of cross-linked fibrin by plasmin)

Supportive of Hypercoagulable State

Hyperfibrinogenemia
Elevated factor V or VIII activities
Activation of specific factors (e.g., factor IX activation peptide)[229]
Elevated tissue factor (TF) expression (e.g., fX-dependent chromogenic assay)[230]
Elevated von Willebrand multimers (particularly ultralarge multimers)
Deficiency of disintegrin and metalloproteinase with thrombospondin type-1 repeats, member 13 (ADAMTS-13)
Elevated fibrin(ogen) degradation products (fibrin or fibrinogen lysis by plasmin)
Whole blood coagulation assessed viscoelastic coagulation tests (e.g., TEG)
Enhanced thrombin generation (calibrated automated thrombography)[231]
Presence of lupus anticoagulants or anticardiolipin antibodies
Presence of procoagulant microparticles (e.g., Bearing TF or phosphatidylserine)
Decreased endogenous anticoagulants
Antithrombin
Protein C, S, or Z
Decreased activation of protein C
Activated protein C[232]
Protein C peptide[233]
Protein C-inhibitor complex[234]
Activated protein C-α2-macroglobulin complex[235]
Activated protein C-α1-antitrypsin complex[235]
Tissue factor pathway inhibitor
Suppressed fibrinolysis
Hypoplasminogenemia[236]
Decreased tissue-type plasminogen activator[236]
Increased thrombin activatable fibrinolysis inhibitor (carboxypeptidase-B2)[237]
Increased plasminogen activator inhibitor-1[238]
Increased α-2 antiplasmin[239]
Decreased Bβ1-42 or Bβ15-42 fragment (cleaved from amino terminus of Bβ chain of fibrin I or fibrin II, respectively, by plasmin)[240,241]
Prolonged euglobulin lysis time (estimate of overall fibrinolysis using the euglobulin fraction of plasma)
Fibrinolysis assessed by viscoelastic coagulation testing

COMMON CONDITIONS IN VETERINARY MEDICINE

Systemic Inflammation

Our current understanding of the coagulopathy associated with systemic inflammation describes a complex process involving increased expression of TF, activation of ECs and disruption of the glycocalyx, impairment of anticoagulant systems, and abatement of fibrinolysis.[66-68]

BOX 104-2 *Markers of Platelet Activation*

Platelet Membrane Expression

Conformational changes in the GPIIb/IIIa Complex (also termed $\alpha_{IIb}\beta_3$)

Monoclonal antibody (mAb) PAC1 (binds only to the exposed fibrinogen-binding
site of GPIIb/IIIa after activation [conformational change])[242]
mAb targeting ligand-induced binding sites (LIBS) of GPIIb/IIIa (e.g. LIBSa, LIBS6)[243-245]
mAb against receptor-induced binding sites (RIBS): changes induced by receptor-ligand (fibrinogen) binding (e.g., 2G5, F26, canine activated platelet 1 [CAP1])[244-246]

Granule membrane protein exposure

P-selectin from alpha granules[247]
GMP-33 (α granule membrane protein)[248]
Lectin-like oxidized LDL receptor-1 (LOX-1)[249]
Lysosomal-associated membrane proteins (e.g., LAMP-1)[250]
CD63 (lysosomal glycoprotein)[251]

Platelet-leukocyte aggregates

Binding of platelets (via P-selectin) to leukocytes via the P-selectin glycoprotein
Ligand-1 counter-receptor on leukocytes[252]

Surface binding of secreted proteins

CD40L (transmembrane protein of the tumor necrosis family)[253]
Multimerin (large alpha granule glycoprotein involved in factor V/Va binding)[254]
Thrombospondin (alpha granule protein involved in platelet aggregation)[255]

Procoagulant platelet surface

Factor Va binding[256]
Factor VIIIa binding[257]
Factor Xa binding[258]

Platelet-Derived Microparticles

Flow cytometry evaluated[259]
Procoagulant assays[260]

Soluble Markers

Soluble P-selectin[261]
Platelet factor 4[262]
β-Thromboglobulin[262]
Soluble GP V[263]
Plasma and urine thromboxane A_2 metabolites[264]
Soluble CD40L[265,266]

Many of the processes by which inflammation affects coagulation are interrelated: glycocalyx shedding and EC activation leads to compromised production of local regulators (e.g., NO) and increased expression of procoagulant molecules (e.g., UL-vWF or TF) and adhesion molecules (e.g., P-selectin),[69,70] with derangement of anticoagulant defenses. TM may be damaged by multiple mechanisms (leading to decreased activation of protein C), and AT is less effective because of decreased concentrations and impaired interactions with an endothelium that has been denuded of GAGs.[9] TFPI similarly may have impaired EC localization. In addition, an exuberant release of PAI-1 resulting from inflammatory cytokine release can slow fibrinolysis and further impede coagulation defenses.[61]

Patients with sepsis develop an initial hypercoagulable phase, followed by a much longer hypocoagulable phase resulting from consumption. The majority of patients described in the veterinary literature display a hypocoagulable phenotype with evidence of prior clot formation. In dogs with septic peritonitis, the presence of coagulopathy (defined by prolongations of PT or aPTT, or a platelet count of 100,000/μl or less) is associated independently with increased odds of death.[71] Although less is known about coagulopathy in cats, inflammatory conditions (pancreatitis and sepsis) are recognized as two of the top three identified causes of DIC in cats.[72] Dogs with sepsis have significantly prolonged aPTT and/or PT, along with higher FDP and D-dimer concentrations than control dogs. Septic dogs also have lower protein C and AT activities, further supporting a consumptive coagulopathy.[73] Septic dogs with continually decreasing levels of protein C and AT proteins had a worse outcome.[74] TAFI is increased in dogs with bacterial sepsis and other inflammatory conditions (e.g., neoplasia), resulting in downregulation of fibrinolysis.[75]

Studies in dogs with induced endotoxemia have demonstrated a decrease in fibrinogen concentration and platelet count, as well as a prolongation in PT, aPTT, and a rise in D-dimer concentration, consistent with a consumptive coagulopathy. TEG testing in this cohort showed progressively hypocoagulable tracings after endotoxemia. A dramatic decrease in protein C and S also were noted in these dogs, consistent with a tendency towards hypercoagulability, although this was more likely a response to the widespread activation of coagulation.[76] Other studies of canine platelet activity during endotoxemia (using the PFA-100 [see Chapter 107]) showed increased activity within 30 minutes of lipopolysaccharide (LPS) administration, which then decreased to activity values less than baseline.[77] The initial shortening of the PFA closure time may indicate platelet hyperactivity in response to the LPS and may provide a plausible origin for the consumptive coagulopathy seen at later time points.

Protein-Losing Nephropathy

Dogs with glomerular disease and significant proteinuria with or without nephrotic syndrome (NS) are at a heightened risk of thrombotic complications and are represented in nearly every study describing pathologic thrombus formation or TE.[78-82] One case series reported the rate of thrombosis or TE to be 22.2%,[83] and nearly half of the protein-losing nephropathy (PLN) patients in a recent study were diagnosed with thrombi ante- or postmortem.[45]

In people, the thrombophilia associated with PLN appears to be multifactorial. Platelets are hyperaggregable and exhibit increased markers of activation (e.g., P-selectin).[84,85] Soluble factors show increases in fVIII activity and fibrinogen concentration, whereas vWF levels and fV are elevated variably.[86-88] The loss of endogenous anticoagulant potential centers on low AT activity, which occurs in people and dogs.[87,89] Despite this consistent finding, AT activity fails to uniformly predict thrombotic risk across studies in people.[90,91] Protein C levels are variable in patients with PLN,[92,93] and several studies have documented elevated levels of TFPI, suggesting that this anticoagulant is not likely a significant component of the thrombophilia.[94] In people, levels of TAFI can be increased,[95] along with PAI-1, suggesting a decreased fibrinolytic state.[96] People have a propensity toward development of renal vein thrombosis, and increased markers of endothelial activation have been documented.[95,97] These suggest some involvement of a local mechanism (e.g., endothelial activation or abnormal renal blood flow) contributing to the overall thrombophilia.

Coagulation abnormalities have been investigated thoroughly in a group of seven dogs with marked proteinuria compared with dogs with nonproteinuric renal failure and dogs presenting for other systemic illness. TEG tracings were more hypercoagulable in PLN and renal failure compared with systemically ill and healthy dogs, and fibrinogen activity was elevated in PLN dogs. AT activity was lower in PLN than systemically ill dogs, and higher α2-antiplasmin and protein C activities were identified.[45] Hyperfibrinogenemia and low AT activity were described in a previous study of three dogs, which also identified elevated fVIII activity.[98] All of these factors could contribute to increased procoagulant potential.

Immune-Mediated Hemolytic Anemia

Thrombi have been identified in up to 46% to 80% of nonsurvivors[99,100] and DIC in 45% of dogs suffering from immune-mediated hemolytic anemia (IMHA).[101] The majority of deaths in dogs with IMHA occur within the first 2 weeks, primarily because of anemia and/or thrombotic complications.[99,100] A postmortem evaluation of dogs suffering from IMHA found lesions consistent with coagulopathy (macro- and microthrombi, widespread fibrin deposition, and hemorrhage) in 73.5% of dogs.[102] Coagulation abnormalities consistent with a hypercoagulable state (low AT activity, elevated FDPs and D-dimer, and markedly elevated fibrinogen concentration) are commonly reported in this population.[101] TEG studies also have documented hypercoagulability, primarily on the basis of an increased clot strength (maximal amplitude or MA).[103-105] The cause of an increased MA is difficult to tease apart in this population; fibrinogen, platelet count and function, and hematocrit are key contributors to the MA. Nonetheless, the hypercoagulable changes reflected in these dogs are often striking (see Chapter 110).

Circulating TF is also a likely contributor to the procoagulant state of IMHA, with upregulation of TF gene expression in whole blood, although the source of the TF has not been determined.[37] Increased TF could come from numerous sources (e.g., platelet, MPs, mononuclear cells); or from stimulation of EC TF expression by cell-free heme.[106] Free heme can also decrease the bioavailability of NO and upregulate EC adhesion molecules (e.g., E-selectin).[107-110] Hemolyzed erythrocytes augment thrombin generation in vitro, an effect attributed to erythrocyte-derived MPs or procoagulant erythrocyte membrane.[111]

Platelet activation in canine IMHA has been evaluated in two studies, reaching disparate conclusions. In one study, increased platelet P-selectin expression was identified,[112] whereas another found no significant changes in P-selectin expression, fibrinogen binding (representing GP IIb/IIIa expression), or platelet-leukocyte aggregates when dogs with IMHA were compared with healthy controls.[113] An increase in MPs was also reported, although no further characterizations (e.g., cellular origin) were made.[113] A survival benefit was observed in dogs with IMHA who were receiving aspirin as part of their therapy in one retrospective study.[114]

Antiphospholipid syndrome (APS) refers to the thrombophilia associated with a broad family of autoantibodies that are detected by lupus anticoagulant tests (LA), or by ELISA for anticardiolipin antibodies (aCL) or antibodies directed against other phospholipids or phospholipid-binding proteins.[115,116] Currently available studies suggest that APS does not likely play a significant role in dogs with IMHA.[117,101] There have been healthy Bernese Mountain Dogs detected with aCLs and LAs in Europe,[118] and LAs were found in a dog suffering from hemolysis and thrombosis.[119]

Hypercortisolemia

Hyperadrenocorticism (HAC) in people is associated with a significantly increased risk of thrombotic complications, with rates comparable to those following major orthopedic surgery (rates of venous TE up to 5%).[120] Changes identified in people with HAC include elevated activities of fVIII and vWF,[121,122] heightened levels of PAI-1,[123] and elevated activities of factors IX, XI, and XII.[120,124-127] In contrast to veterinary patients, many people with HAC suffer from comorbidities (e.g., obesity, diabetes mellitus, and hypertriglyceridemia) that are also prothrombotic conditions.

Dogs with HAC are represented in most case series describing thrombotic conditions (e.g., aortic thrombosis, pulmonary TE [PTE], splenic or portal vein thrombosis).[78-81,128] Despite these observations, a consistent cause or definable procoagulant state has not been identified. In an early study of 56 dogs with HAC, increased activities of factors II, V, VII, IX, X, and XII, in addition to decreased AT and elevated TAT complexes were noted. There were no differences in plasminogen or PAI-1 compared with healthy control dogs.[129] An earlier study found increased activities of factors V, XI, AT, and elevated plasminogen in 12 dogs.[130] A more recent study evaluated platelet count, mean platelet volume, AT, PT, aPTT, fibrinogen, and TEG. No differences were noted between age-matched controls and 28 dogs with naturally occurring HAC.[131] TEG and thrombin generation have been used to assay for a procoagulant state in six healthy beagles given 1 or 4 mg/kg/day oral prednisone for 2-week periods. TEG revealed changes consistent with a procoagulant state in both prednisone groups, whereas the CAT measure of thrombin generation was increased only in the 1 mg/kg/day treatment group.[132]

Cardiomyopathies

Arterial thromboembolism (ATE) in cats is associated most commonly with cardiac disease; many cats are asymptomatic before experiencing an ATE.[133,134] Thrombosis secondary to cardiac disease is reported infrequently in dogs but has been associated with dilated cardiomyopathies and atrial fibrillation (AF).[135]

Left atrial (LA) and LA appendage enlargement is associated with numerous structural changes, culminating in a procoagulant phenotype, such as increased TF and vWF on areas of denuded or damaged endothelium.[136] Growth hormones (e.g., VEGF), which are increased in people with AF, may promote the upregulation of TF.[137] Through atrial enlargement, shear stress is decreased (stasis), reducing the release of NO.[138] There is a direct link between inflammation and AF development in humans and experimental dogs.[139,140]

A systemic hypercoagulable state occurs in 50% of cardiomyopathic cats with spontaneous echocardiographic contrast (or "smoke") with or without a LA thrombus, and in 56% of cats with ATE and LA enlargement.[141] vWF:Ag concentrations were elevated in only the cats with ATE, and the presence of hypercoagulability was not related to LA size or the presence of congestive heart failure.[141] These results are echoed by an earlier study that revealed changes consistent with a hypercoagulable state in 45% of cats with hypertrophic cardiomyopathy (HCM).[142]

Platelets from cats with cardiomyopathy required significantly lower doses of ADP to result in irreversible aggregation compared with control cats.[143] In a small group of cats with predominantly thyrotoxic cardiomyopathy, platelets were less responsive to ADP and more responsive to collagen for aggregation.[144] Many of these cats were receiving medications to treat hyperthyroidism or heart disease, and it is unclear if these may have interfered with aggregation responses. A more recent study evaluated platelet function in cats with HCM compared with healthy control cats and did not show significant differences in platelet activity.[145] Many of the cats in this study had less severe disease, and cats with ATE were excluded.

Neoplasia

Coagulopathic complications are common in many dogs and cats with neoplasia.[146-155] DIC has been described in 9.6% of dogs with malignancies; the highest rates occur in dogs with hemangiosarcoma, mammary carcinoma, and adenocarcinoma of the lung.[156] The criteria of DIC were fulfilled in 50% of dogs with hemangiosarcoma,[157] and malignancies were among the top three most common reasons for DIC in cats.[72]

Coagulation components are both contributors to thrombosis and important in cancer behavior: in particular, tumor growth, angiogenesis, and metastasis. TF has been identified on malignant cells and in tumor vasculature,[158,159] and tumor cells have the ability to shed TF-bearing MPs.[159] TF supports thrombophilia and also plays a key role in regulation of integrin function responsible for tumor angiogenesis. In mice, TF blockade results in decreased angiogenesis and tumor growth, through modulation of VEGF.[160,161] Moreover, TF expression on histopathology samples is an independent predictor of poor overall or relapse-free survival for many tumor types in people.[162-165] TF expression has been evaluated in canine cell lines of mammary tumors, pancreatic carcinoma, pulmonary adenocarcinoma, prostatic carcinoma, and sarcomas (osteosarcoma and fibrosarcoma). TF was highly expressed in all but osteosarcoma; tumors of epithelial origin (mammary carcinoma and pulmonary adenocarcinoma) expressed the highest levels. These tumors also shed TF-bearing microparticles into tissue culture supernatants.[29]

A recent investigation in dogs with various neoplasms showed a hypercoagulable TEG tracing in 70.4%, with 4.2% having a hypocoagulable tracing. All three dogs with hypocoagulable tracings were suffering from disseminated neoplasia, a finding also noted in another TEG study of 49 dogs with cancer.[166] Patients with distant metastasis commonly have a higher fibrinogen and D-dimer compared with locally invasive or noninvasive disease.[167] In canine patients with carcinomas, thrombocytosis and hyperfibrinogenemia were found more commonly (compared with healthy controls). TEG-derived thrombus generation (TEG_{TG}), revealed a faster TEG_{TG} in dogs with carcinoma (46% of these dogs being hypercoagulable on other testing). PAI-1 activity was decreased in this population.[168]

The most common hemostatic abnormalities in dogs with untreated mammary carcinoma included hyperfibrinogenemia, elevated fV, and decreased fVIII activities; these hemostatic abnormalities are more common with increasing tumor stage.[169] Platelet and fibrinogen survival in dogs with metastatic disease are decreased, further supporting ongoing consumption.[170] In a broad evaluation of AT activities in dogs, a low AT was frequently present in dogs with neoplasia and was associated with a greater risk of mortality.[171]

Platelet aggregometry was assessed in dogs with untreated multicentric lymphoma; affected dogs had a greater maximum aggregation than controls.[172] Another study of dogs with various malignancies showed that platelets from affected dogs had shorter delays in aggregation response, higher maximum aggregation, greater ATP secretion, and a tendency to aggregate in response to lower concentrations of weak agonists (e.g., ADP).[173]

Isolated Brain Injury

A state of intravascular coagulation resembling DIC has been recognized in people suffering traumatic brain injury (TBI), with significant impacts on outcome in adults and children.[174-176] For TBI patients who are coagulopathic on presentation, there is an approximately doubled rate (85% vs. 31%) of hemorrhagic progression of neuronal lesion(s) or development of new ischemic lesions.[177] Coagulopathy upon hospital presentation is associated with higher rates of craniotomy, single and multiple organ failures, less intubation-free days, and longer ICU and hospital stays, compared with noncoagulopathic TBI patients. The overall mortality for TBI patients with coagulopathy was 50.4%, compared with 17.3% in patients without coagulopathy.[178] The coagulopathy can develop up to 4.5 days post-trauma (mean of 68 ± 7.4 hours), with a faster onset with worsening injury severity.[179]

The brain is rich in TF, suggesting TF is likely the initiator of coagulation in TBI patients.[180] TBI patients have elevated monocyte TF expression for the first 24 hours, which then quickly returns to normal.[181] Enhanced thrombin generation has been documented as blood passes the vasculature of the brain. In a study of people with severe isolated TBI, patients had prolonged aPTT and PT; elevated D-dimer, TAT, and F1+2; and low AT, platelets, and fibrinogen upon presentation. Complement C5b-9 and IL-6 also were elevated, with IL-6 levels at least 100-fold greater than controls. A transcranial gradient (arterial vs. jugular venous blood) of TAT, F1+2, and IL-6 was present, representing brain vasculature-initiated thrombin generation.[182] Similar results were found in another study comparing internal jugular, peripheral venous, and arterial samples of coagulation markers.[183]

Procoagulant MPs after TBI are increased significantly in CSF and blood. These MPs were primarily of EC and platelet origin, adding evidence to the likely contribution of cerebrovascular endothelial activation or injury.[184] Although local procoagulant factors initiate coagulation, inflammatory cytokines and procoagulant MPs provide a means for dissemination of the condition, leading to a systemic response.

Studies have suggested a state of platelet hypofunction in brain injured patients.[182,185] This is opposed to non–brain-injured trauma patients who generally have increased platelet reactivity.[186] A subset of TBI patients in this study also showed an increase in flow-cytometric markers of platelet activation (e.g., P-selectin expression, activated conformation of GPIIb/IIIa), despite exhibiting decreased aggregation responses. The cause of the platelet dysfunction in TBI patients has not been identified; however, this pattern would be most consistent with platelets that are partially activated in vivo (e.g., acted on by thrombin).

Eight experimental cats with TBI-induced coagulopathy secondary to bullet-inflicted brain injury showed a decreased platelet count and decreased platelet clumping, possibly suggesting a decreased reactivity of the cats' platelets. A decreasing fibrinogen was also present throughout the experiment.[187]

MANAGEMENT OF HYPERCOAGULABLE CONDITIONS

Treatment of the Underlying Condition

The management of hypercoagulable states should be focused on eliminating the underlying condition or trigger. This can include appropriate antimicrobials, source control (including surgery if necessary), and aggressive supportive care. Maintenance of oxygen delivery to tissues is paramount to avoid ischemia and tissue acidosis, which may worsen inflammation.

Recombinant Anticoagulant Therapy

Endogenous anticoagulant replacement therapy has long been investigated as a means to address complex coagulopathies while simultaneously decreasing inflammation. These therapies, although logical given the decrease in endogenous anticoagulants in many disease states (e.g., decreased protein C or AT), have failed thus far to improve survival in large clinical trials.

AT supplementation has been effective at reversing apparent heparin resistance in cardiopulmonary patients with low AT activities.[188] In a study of people with severe sepsis, AT supplementation did not improve survival, but subgroup analysis of patients who were not administered concomitant heparin showed an improvement in survival at 90 days for those receiving AT.[189] A study of AT without heparin for severe sepsis found an improved survival in human patients with DIC but no difference (compared to placebo) for patients that did not display DIC.[190]

Recombinant APC (rAPC) has been shown to have numerous benefits in sepsis and inflammatory conditions. It has been documented to prevent TNF-α-mediated hypotension in rats with septic shock,[191] improve microvascular perfusion in people with sepsis,[192] and result in dramatic improvements in survival in baboons with *Escherichia coli* septicemia.[193] Recent large trials have failed to confirm a survival benefit in people with sepsis, and the patented product (Xigris) was removed from the market in October of 2011.[194]

Recombinant TFPI (rTFPI) has been proven an effective antithrombotic agent in experimental models of sepsis and DIC,[195-197] coronary artery disease, and thrombosis in animal models, and it was shown to reduce the mortality rate in sepsis-induced DIC.[197] More extensive human trials have failed to prove a survival benefit to date.[198-200]

Recombinant soluble TM recently has garnered considerable attention and has shown promise for attenuating DIC,[201-203] with a survival benefit seen in septic patients requiring mechanical ventilation.[204]

Antithrombotic Therapy

Exogenous antithrombotic therapy can consist of drugs that inhibit platelet function (e.g., aspirin or clopidogrel) or drugs that facilitate the inhibition of thrombin (e.g., unfractionated [UFH] or low molecular weight heparins [LMWH]). Exogenous antithrombotics should be used when a patient has an identified risk for thrombotic complications, and the risks of thrombosis outweigh possible adverse effects of the therapy. Much of the decision on therapy depends on the underlying condition, perceived length of therapy, and underlying hemostatic status of the patient. Although oral platelet inhibitors are typically easier for long-term administration by owners, heparin may be more advantageous for in-hospital use because many conditions (e.g., sepsis) may be accompanied by thrombocytopenia. Although commonly prescribed for people with thrombophilia, warfarin therapy can prove challenging for the clinician not experienced in its behavior in small animals. It has the added disadvantage of being dosed orally, a hindrance in some critically ill patients (see Chapters 167 and Chapter 168).

Inflammatory conditions

Although dogs and cats with inflammatory conditions have a known risk for thrombotic complications, no veterinary studies are currently available to help identify specific populations in which thromboprophylaxis may prove most advantageous. Coagulation testing should be evaluated frequently in these patients, with particular attention paid to those exhibiting more than one significant predisposition (e.g., a patient with cancer that develops a source of sepsis or hypoxemia). A drop in circulating platelet count or at least 20% prolongation in aPTT should raise concerns for the early stages of a consumptive coagulopathy.

In a study of thromboplastin-induced DIC in dogs, high doses of LMWH (0.9 ± 0.07 anti-FXa U/ml) were required to decrease further consumptive coagulopathy when administered 2 hours after initiation.[205] This highlights the difficulty in slowing the consumption of coagulation components once DIC is initiated. Unfortunately, high-dose heparin therapy after initiation of a consumptive coagulopathy may worsen the clinical picture, and the identification of the hypercoagulable phase when heparin therapy may be most useful remains difficult.

Protein-losing nephropathy

Despite the long-standing association of thrombosis with PLN, no studies have assessed antithrombotic interventions. Any patient with PLN or NS, and likely those with significant proteinuria, may benefit from some form of thromboprophylaxis (unless contraindicated). Given the broad nature of this thrombophilia and lack of utility for AT as a sole indicator, this should not be the only measure of a patient's risk for thrombotic complications. Historically, these patients have been treated with platelet inhibitors such as aspirin[206]; however, more aggressive therapy may be warranted. In cases of markedly decreased AT activity, heparins may have less efficacy and other anticoagulants (e.g., warfarin) may be needed for more substantial anticoagulation. Larger studies are needed to better define the risk of thrombotic complications in the face of antithrombotics.

Immune-mediated hemolytic anemia

Various thromboprophylactics have been reported for use in IMHA, including aspirin,[114,207] clopidogrel,[207] and heparin.[208] In one retrospective study, aspirin was associated with a survival benefit in IMHA dogs. Heparin was also evaluated in this study, but a lower dose was used compared with current recommendations.[114]

UFH was given at 300 IU/kg SC q6h to 18 dogs with IMHA. Half (three of six) of necropsied nonsurvivors had thrombi identified. One of these dogs was 2 months postdiagnosis and no longer receiving any antithrombotics. Only 8 out of 18 dogs attained target anti-Xa at this dosing protocol.[208] Adjusted-dose heparin therapy (targeting an anti-Xa activity of 0.35 to 0.7 U/ml) may improve survival from IMHA by limiting thrombotic complications.[209]

Clopidogrel recently was evaluated alone and with aspirin in dogs with primary IMHA.[206] There was one dog in each group receiving aspirin or clopidogrel (monotherapy) with thrombotic complications. None of the patients on the combination therapy developed apparent thrombotic disease.

Hypercortisolemia

Given the conflicting evidence regarding hypercortisolemia-associated thrombophilia, testing for markers to support a prothrombotic state seems prudent before anticoagulation. Clinicians should be vigilant when other procoagulant insults (e.g., surgery or systemic infection) occur in patients with hypercortisolemia because it is more likely that multiple contributors are involved with thrombosis in these patients.

Cardiomyopathies

Long-term thromboprophylaxis in cats with cardiomyopathies traditionally has been with an oral platelet inhibitor. There was no difference in survival times for cats with ATE treated with high-dose (at least 40 mg per cat q24-72h) or low-dose aspirin (5 mg per cat q72h) therapy, although there were fewer side effects in the low-dose group, and cats in both groups suffered a second ATE.[134] The most effective dose of aspirin for inhibition of platelet aggregation in cats remains unclear,[210] but clopidogrel does result in decreased platelet aggregation and platelet serotonin release in cats.[211,212] Clopidogrel is also effective in dogs when administered at 1 mg/kg PO q24h.[213]

LMWH (dalteparin or enoxaparin) have been administered to cats with cardiomyopathy, but the effective doses, dosing interval, and anti-Xa ranges for these drugs have yet to be determined definitively.[214-216]

Thrombolysis may be considered for any recent onset ATE with signs of ischemia. Studies of cats undergoing thrombolysis suggest a similar survival compared with conservative management, with a heightened risk of complications.[134,217-219] More recently, tPA administration resulted in pulse restoration for 53% of affected limbs within 24 hours.[217]

Neoplasia

The risk of thrombotic complications in veterinary patients with neoplasia is similar to that for people. Despite the known risk, prediction of thrombotic complications in animals with particular tumor types remains challenging. Tumors of epithelial cell origin and hemic neoplasms (e.g., lymphoma, leukemia, histiocytic sarcoma, hemangiosarcoma) are among the most commonly implicated; however, any cancer may promote thrombus formation resulting from alterations in vascular flow, endothelial damage, inflammation, or a combination of all three.

Various antithrombotics (e.g., warfarin[220] and aspirin[221]) have been implicated in decreasing the rate of metastasis with cancer, presumably by preventing metastasis on thrombi, activated platelets, or possibly MPs. The role of antithrombotics in veterinary species requires further study to determine whether a benefit or detriment in tumor behavior may exist.

Coagulation testing is advised in patients with known predilections (e.g., hemic neoplasms or carcinoma), especially in those with greater tumor burdens (e.g., disseminated or metastatic disease). Antithrombotics should be considered when testing suggests a risk for (or ongoing) thrombin generation (e.g., elevated D-dimer or TAT) in concert with a clinical suspicion.

Isolated brain injury

Hypertonic saline (HTS)/dextran administration decreases leukocyte cell-surface adhesion molecules, degranulation markers on neutrophils and monocytes, vascular and intercellular adhesion molecules, TNF-α, TF, and D-dimer in severely brain injured patients given HTS/dextran before hospital presentation.[222] Many of these benefits are attributed to the immunomodulatory effects of HTS and from earlier restoration of normal cerebral perfusion pressure.

Recombinant factor VIIa (rVIIa) has been shown to attenuate the hemorrhagic phenotype of the TBI-induced coagulopathy in people. Patients receiving rFVIIa used less plasma, required fewer days of mechanical ventilation, and had a decreased cost of hospitalization.[223] rFVIIa use also may allow shorter times to neurosurgical intervention[224] and lower mortality rates when patients need transfer to another hospital for definitive care.[225]

The TBI-induced coagulopathy described in humans has not been described in clinical veterinary cases. Given the nature of this disorder, clinicians should be diligent in assessing the hemostatic status of TBI patients, particularly those with more severe injury. Most people exhibit significant coagulopathy at the time of hospital presentation, suggesting that the management in veterinary patients would be aimed largely at directed therapy for consumptive coagulopathy.

CONCLUSION

Hypercoagulability or thrombophilia describes a tendency for pathologic thrombus formation. Acquired thrombophilias exist in veterinary medicine and can be caused by commonly recognized conditions (e.g., proteinuria). Any perturbation in the delicate balance of coagulation may beget a thrombophilia. Early recognition of risk relies on an index of clinical suspicion and laboratory testing, although a thrombophilia is noted in many patients after exhibiting thrombotic complications or a consumptive coagulopathy. Despite the prevalence of these conditions, large prospective studies to guide intervention are lacking.

REFERENCES

1. Smith SA: The cell-based model of coagulation, J Vet Emerg Crit Care 19(1):3-10, 2009.
2. Coughlin SR: Thrombin signaling and protease-activated receptors, Nature 407(6801):258-264, 2000.
3. Reitsma S, Slaaf DW, Vink H, et al: The endothelial glycocalyx: composition, functions, and visualization, Pflügers Archiv 454(3):345-359, 2007.
4. Ihrcke NS, Wrenshall LE, Lindman BJ, et al: Role of heparan sulfate in immune system-blood vessel interactions, Immunol Today 14(10):500-505, 1993.
5. Shimada K, Kobayashi M, Kimura S, et al: Anti-coagulant heparin-like glycosaminoglycans on endothelial cell surface, Jpn Circ J 55(10):1016-1021, 1991.
6. Kato H: Regulation of functions of vascular wall cells by tissue factor pathway inhibitor: basic and clinical aspects, Arterioscler Thromb Vasc Biol 22(4):539-548, 2002.
7. Ho G, Broze GJ Jr, Schwartz AL: Role of heparan sulfate proteoglycans in the uptake and degradation of tissue factor pathway inhibitor-coagulation factor Xa complexes, J Biol Chem 272(27):16838-16844, 1997.
8. Lupu C, Goodwin CA, Westmuckett AD, et al: Tissue factor pathway inhibitor in endothelial cells colocalizes with glycolipid microdomains/caveolae. Regulatory mechanism(s) of the anticoagulant properties of the endothelium, Arterioscler Thromb Vasc Biol 17(11):2964-2974, 1997.
9. Kobayashi M, Shimada K, Ozawa T: Human recombinant interleukin-1 beta- and tumor necrosis factor alpha-mediated suppression of heparin-like compounds on cultured porcine aortic endothelial cells, J Cell Physiol 144(3):383-390, 1990.
10. Ignarro LJ, Buga GM, Wood KS, et al: Endothelium-derived relaxing factor produced and released from artery and vein is nitric oxide, Proc Natl Acad Sci USA 84(24):9265-9269, 1987.
11. Bath PM, Hassall DG, Gladwin AM, et al: Nitric oxide and prostacyclin: divergence of inhibitory effects on monocyte chemotaxis and adhesion to endothelium in vitro, Arterioscler Thromb 11(2):254-260, 1991.
12. Loscalzo J, Welch GN: Nitric oxide and its role in the cardiovascular system, Prog Cardiovasc Dis 38(2):87-104, 1995.
13. Bode L, Eklund EA, Murch S, et al: Heparan sulfate depletion amplifies TNF-alpha-induced protein leakage in an in vitro model of protein-losing enteropathy, Am J Physiol Gastrointes Liver Physiol 288(5):G1015-1023, 2005.
14. Henry CB, Duling BR: TNF-α increases entry of macromolecules into luminal endothelial cell glycocalyx, Am J Physiol Heart Circ Physiol 279(6):H2815-2823, 2000.
15. Rehm M, Bruegger D, Christ F, et al: Shedding of the endothelial glycocalyx in patients undergoing major vascular surgery with global and regional ischemia, Circulation 116(17):1896-1906, 2007.
16. Kozar RA, Peng Z, Zhang R, et al: Plasma restoration of endothelial glycocalyx in a rodent model of hemorrhagic shock, Anesth Analg 112(6):1289-1295, 2011.
17. Rotundo RF, Curtis TM, Shah MD, et al: TNF-alpha disruption of lung endothelial integrity: reduced integrin mediated adhesion to fibronectin, Am J Physiol Lung Cell Mol Physiol 282(2):L316-329, 2002.
18. Aschner JL, Lum H, Fletcher PW, et al: Bradykinin- and thrombin-induced increases in endothelial permeability occur independently of phospholipase C but require protein kinase C activation, J Cell Physiol 173(3):387-396, 1997.
19. Andriopoulou P, Navarro P, Zanetti A, et al: Histamine induces tyrosine phosphorylation of endothelial cell-to-cell adherens junctions, Arterioscler Thromb Vasc Biol 19(10):2286-2297, 1999.
20. Hippenstiel S, Krull M, Ikemann A, et al: VEGF induces hyperpermeability by a direct action on endothelial cells, Am J Physiol 274 (5 Pt 1):L678-684, 1998.
21. Ribes JA, Francis CW, Wagner DD: Fibrin induces release of von Willebrand factor from endothelial cells, J Clin Invest 79(1):117-123, 1987.
22. Haberichter SL, Montgomery RR: Structure and function of von Willebrand factor. In Colman RW, Marder VJ, Clowes AW, et al, editors: Hemostasis and thrombosis: basic principles and clinical practice, ed 5, Philadelphia, 2006, Lippincott, Williams & Wilkins, pp 707-718.
23. Bernardo A, Ball C, Nolasco L, et al: Effects of inflammatory cytokines on the release and cleavage of the endothelial cell-derived ultralarge von Willebrand factor multimers under flow, Blood 104(1):100-106, 2004.
24. Martin K, Borgel D, Lerolle N, et al: Decreased ADAMTS-13 (a disintegrin-like and metalloprotease with thrombospondin type 1 repeats) is associated with a poor prognosis in sepsis-induced organ failure, Crit Care Med 35(10):2375-2382, 2007.
25. Claus RA, Bockmeyer CL, Budde U, et al: Variations in the ratio between von Willebrand factor and its cleaving protease during systemic inflammation and association with severity and prognosis of organ failure, Thromb Haemost 101(2):239-247, 2009.
26. Creasey AA, Chang AC, Feigen L, et al: Tissue factor pathway inhibitor reduces mortality from Escherichia coli septic shock, J Clin Invest 91(6):2850-2860, 1993.
27. Warr TA, Rao LV, Rapaport SI: Disseminated intravascular coagulation in rabbits induced by administration of endotoxin or tissue factor: effect of anti-tissue factor antibodies and measurement of plasma extrinsic pathway inhibitor activity, Blood 75(7):1481-1489, 1990.

28. Aird WC: The role of the endothelium in severe sepsis and multiple organ dysfunction syndrome, Blood 101(10):3765-3777, 2003.
29. Stokol T, Daddona JL, Mubayed LS, et al: Evaluation of tissue factor expression in canine tumor cells, Am J Res 72(8):1097-1106, 2011.
30. Morrissey JH: Tissue factor: a key molecule in hemostatic and nonhemostatic systems, Int J Hematol 79(2):103-108, 2004.
31. Brooks MB, Catalfamo JL: Von Willebrand disease. In Weiss DJ, Wardop KJ, editors: In Shalm's veterinary hematology, ed 6, Ames, Iowa, 2010, Blackwell Publishing Ltd, pp 612-618.
32. Berckmans RJ, Nieuwland R, Boing AN, et al: Cell-derived microparticles circulate in healthy humans and support low grade thrombin generation, Thromb Haemost 85(4):639-646, 2001.
33. Mallat Z, Benamer H, Hugel B, et al: Elevated levels of shed membrane microparticles with procoagulant potential in the peripheral circulating blood of patients with acute coronary syndromes, Circulation 101(8):841-843, 2000.
34. Key NS: Analysis of tissue factor positive microparticles, Thromb Res suppl 1:S42-S45, 2010.
35. Nieuwland R, Berckmans RJ, McGregor S, et al: Cellular origin and procoagulant properties of microparticles in meningococcal sepsis, Blood 95(3):930-935, 2000.
36. Combes V, Simon AC, Grau GE, et al: In vitro generation of endothelial microparticles and possible prothrombotic activity in patients with lupus anticoagulant, J Clin Invest 104(1):93-102, 1999.
37. Piek CJ, Brinkhof B, Teske E, et al: High intravascular tissue factor expression in dogs with idiopathic immune-mediated haemolytic anaemia, Vet Immunol Immunopathol 144(3-4):346-354, 2011.
38. Jy W, Jimenez JJ, Mauro LM, et al: Endothelial microparticles induce formation of platelet aggregates via a von Willebrand factor/ristocetin dependent pathway, rendering them resistant to dissociation, J Thromb Haemost 3(6):1301-1308, 2005.
39. Horstman LL, Jy W, Jimenez JJ, Ahn YS: Endothelial microparticles as markers of endothelial dysfunction, Front Biosci 9:1118-1135, 2004.
40. Olson ST, Bjork I: Predominant contribution of surface approximation to the mechanism of heparin acceleration of the antithrombin-thrombin reaction. Elucidation from salt concentration effects, J Biol Chem 266(10):6353-6364, 1991.
41. Preissner KT, Delvos U, Muller-Berghaus G: Binding of thrombin to thrombomodulin accelerates inhibition of the enzyme by antithrombin III. Evidence for a heparin-independent mechanism, Biochemistry 26(9):2521-2528, 1987.
42. Levi M, Marder VJ: Coagulation abnormalities in sepsis. In Colman RW, Marder VJ, Clowes AW, et al, editors: Hemostasis and thrombosis: basic principles and clinical practice, ed 5, Philadelphia, 2006, Lippincott, Williams & Wilkins, pp 1601-1611.
43. Vary TC, Kimball SR: Regulation of hepatic protein synthesis in chronic inflammation and sepsis, Am J Physiol 262(2 Pt 1): C445-C452, 1992.
44. Seitz R, Wolf M, Egbring R, et al: The disturbance of hemostasis in septic shock: role of neutrophil elastase and thrombin, effects of antithrombin III and plasma substitution, Eur J Haematol 43(1):22-28, 1989.
45. Donahue SM, Brooks M, Otto CM: Examination of hemostatic parameters to detect hypercoagulability in dogs with severe protein-losing nephropathy, J Vet Emerg Crit Care 21(4):346-355, 2011.
46. van de Wouwer M, Collen D, Conway EM: Thrombomodulin-protein C-EPCR system: integrated to regulate coagulation and inflammation, Arterioscler Thromb Vasc Biol 24(8):1374-1383, 2004.
47. O'Brien LM, Mastri M, Fay PJ: Regulation of factor VIIIa by human activated protein C and protein S: inactivation of cofactor in the intrinsic factor Xase, Blood 95(5):1714-1720, 2000.
48. Rosing J, Hoekema L, Nicolaes GA, et al: Effects of protein S and factor Xa on peptide bond cleavages during inactivation of factor Va and factor VaR506Q by activated protein C, J Biol Chem 270(46):27852-27858, 1995.
49. Conway EM, Rosenberg RD: Tumor necrosis factor suppresses transcription of the thrombomodulin gene in endothelial cells, Mol Cell Biol 8(12):5588-5592, 1988.
50. Liaw PC, Esmon CT, Kahnamoui K, et al: Patients with severe sepsis vary markedly in their ability to generate activated protein C, Blood 104(13):3958-3964, 2004.
51. Takano S, Kimura S, Ohdama S, et al: Plasma thrombomodulin in health and diseases, Blood 76(10):2024-2029, 1990.
52. Lin SM, Wang YM, Lin HC, et al: Serum thrombomodulin level relates to the clinical course of disseminated intravascular coagulation, multiorgan dysfunction syndrome, and mortality in patients with sepsis, Crit Care Med 36(3):683-689, 2008.
53. Rao LV, Rapaport SI: Studies of a mechanism inhibiting the initiation of the extrinsic pathway of coagulation, Blood 69(2):645-651, 1987.
54. Maroney SA, Haberichter SL, Friese P, et al: Active tissue factor pathway inhibitor is expressed on the surface of coated platelets, Blood 109(5):1931-1937, 2007.
55. van der Logt CP, Dirven RJ, Reitsma PH, et al: Expression of tissue factor and tissue factor pathway inhibitor in monocytes in response to bacterial lipopolysaccharide and phorbolester, Blood Coagul Fibrinolysis 5(2): 211-220, 1994.
56. Bajaj MS, Steer S, Kuppuswamy MN, et al: Synthesis and expression of tissue factor pathway inhibitor by serum-stimulated fibroblasts, vascular smooth muscle cells and cardiac myocytes, Thromb Haemost 82(6):1663-1672, 1999.
57. Werling RW, Zacharski LR, Kisiel W, et al: Distribution of tissue factor pathway inhibitor in normal and malignant human tissues, Thromb Haemost 69(4):366-369, 1993.
58. Hackeng TM, Sere KM, Tans G, et al: Protein S stimulates inhibition of the tissue factor pathway by tissue factor pathway inhibitor, Proc Natl Acad Sci USA 103(9):3106-3111, 2006.
59. Castoldi E, Simioni P, Tormene D, et al: Hereditary and acquired protein S deficiencies are associated with low TFPI levels in plasma, J Thromb Haemost 8(2):294-300, 2010.
60. Reference deleted in text.
61. van der Poll T, Levi M, Buller HR, et al: Fibrinolytic response to tumor necrosis factor in healthy subjects, J Exp Med 174(3):729-732, 1991.
62. Brainard BM, Brown AJ: Defects in coagulation encountered in small animal critical care, Vet Clin North Am Small Anim Pract 41(4):783-803, 2011.
63. Bauer CA: Laboratory markers of coagulation and fibrinolysis. In Colman RW, Marder VJ, Clowes AW, et al, editors: Hemostasis and thrombosis: basic principles and clinical practice, ed 5, Philadelphia, 2006, Lippincott Williams & Wilkins, pp 835-850.
64. Ravanat C, Freund M, Dol F, et al: Cross-reactivity of human molecular markers for detection of prothrombotic states in various animal species, Blood Coagul Fibrinolysis 6(5):446-455, 1995.
65. Donahue SM, Otto CM: Thromboelastography: a tool for measuring hypercoagulability, hypocoagulability, and fibrinolysis, J Vet Emerg Crit Care 15(1):9-16, 2005.
66. Taylor FB, Chang A, Ruf W, et al: Lethal Escherichia coli septic shock is prevented by blocking tissue factor with monoclonal antibody, Circ Shock 33(3):127-134, 1991.
67. Levi M, ten Cate H, Bauer KA, et al: Inhibition of endotoxin-induced activation of coagulation and fibrinolysis by pentoxifylline or by monoclonal anti-tissue factor antibody in chimpanzees, J Clin Invest 93(1):114-120, 1994.
68. Osterud B, Flaegstad T: Increased tissue thromboplastin activity in monocytes of patients with meningococcal infection: related to an unfavorable prognosis, Thromb Haemost 49(1):5-7, 1983.
69. Szotowski B, Antoniak S, Poller W, et al: Procoagulant soluble tissue factor is released from endothelial cells in response to inflammatory cytokines, Circ Res 96(12):1233-1239, 2005.
70. Sugama Y, Tiruppathi C, Janakidevi K, et al: Thrombin-induced expression of endothelial P-selectin and intercellular-adhesion molecule-1: a mechanism for stabilizing neutrophil adhesion, J Cell Biol 119(4): 935-944, 1992.
71. Kenney EM, Rozanski EA, Rush JE, et al: Association between outcome and organ system dysfunction in dogs with sepsis: 114 cases (2003-2007), J Am Vet Med Assoc 236(1):83-87, 2010.
72. Estrin MA, Wehausen CE, Jessen CR, et al: Disseminated intravascular coagulation in cats, J Vet Intern Med 20(6):1334-1339, 2006.

73. de Laforcade AM, Freeman LM, Shaw SP, et al: Hemostatic changes in dogs with naturally occurring sepsis, J Vet Intern Med 17(5):674-679, 2003.
74. de Laforcade AM, Rozanski EA, Freeman LM, et al: Serial evaluation of protein C and antithrombin in dogs with sepsis, J Vet Intern Med 22(1):26-30, 2008.
75. Jesser LR, Wiinberg B, Kjelgaard-Hansen M, et al: Thrombin-activatable fibrinolysis inhibitor activity in healthy and diseased dogs, Vet Clin Pathol 39(3):296-301, 2010.
76. Eralp O, Yilmaz Z, Failing K, et al: Effect of experimental endotoxemia on thrombelastography parameters, secondary and tertiary hemostasis in dogs, J Vet Intern Med 25(3):524-531, 2011.
77. Yilmaz Z, Ilcoi YO, Ulus IH: Investigation of diagnostic importance of platelet closure times measured by Platelet Function Analyzer—PFA 100 in dogs with endotoxemia, Berl Munch Tierztl Wochenschr 118(7-8):341-348, 2005.
78. Winter RL, Sedacca CD, Adams A, et al: Aortic thrombosis in dogs: presentation, therapy, and outcome in 26 cases, J Vet Cardiol 14(2):333-342, 2012.
79. Laurenson MP, Hopper K, Herrera MA, et al: Concurrent diseases and conditions in dogs with splenic vein thrombosis, J Vet Intern Med 24(6):1298-1304, 2010.
80. Respess M, O'Toole TE, Taeymans O, et al: Portal vein thrombosis in 33 dogs: 1998-2011, J Vet Intern Med 26(2):230-237, 2012.
81. Lake-Bakaar GA, Johnson EG, Griffiths LG: Aortic thrombosis in dogs: 31 cases (2000-2010), J Am Vet Med Assoc 241(7):910-915, 2012.
82. Johnson LR, Lappin MR, Baker DC: Pulmonary thromboembolism in 29 dogs: 1985-1995, J Vet Intern Med 1913(4):338-345, 1999.
83. Cook AK, Cowgill LD: Clinical and pathological features of protein-losing glomerular disease in the dog: a review of 137 cases (1985-1992), J Am Anim Hosp Assoc 32(4):313-322, 1996.
84. Remuzzi G, Mecca G, Marchesi D, et al: Platelet hyperaggregability and the nephrotic syndrome, Thromb Res 16(3-4):345-354, 1979.
85. Sirolli V, Ballone E, Garofalo D, et al: Platelet activation markers in patients with nephrotic syndrome. A comparative study of different platelet function tests, Nephron 91(3):424-430, 2002.
86. Thomson C, Forbes CD, Prentice CR, et al: Changes in blood coagulation and fibrinolysis in the nephrotic syndrome, Q J Med 43(171):399-407, 1974.
87. Vaziri ND, Branson HE, Ness R: Changes in coagulation factors IX, VIII, VII, X, and V in nephrotic syndrome, Am J Med Sci 280(3):167-171, 1980.
88. Kanfer A: Coagulation factors in nephrotic syndrome, Am J Nephrol 10(suppl 1):63-68, 1990.
89. Kauffman RH, Veltkamp JJ, Van Tilburg NH, et al: Acquired antithrombin III deficiency and thrombosis in the nephrotic syndrome, Am J Med 65(4):607-613, 1978.
90. Robert A, Olmer M, Sampol J, et al: Clinical correlation between hypercoagulability and thrombo-embolic phenomena, Kidney Int 31(3):830-835, 1987.
91. Mehls O, Andrassy K, Koderisch J, et al: Hemostasis and thromboembolism in children with nephrotic syndrome: differences from adults, J Pediatr 110(6):862-867, 1987.
92. Cosio FG, Harker C, Batard MA, et al: Plasma concentration of the natural anticoagulants protein C and protein S in patients with proteinuria, J Lab Clin Med 106(2):218-222, 1985.
93. Mannucci PM, Valsecchi C, Bottasso B, et al: High plasma levels of protein C activity and antigen in the nephrotic syndrome, Thromb Haemost 55(1):31-33, 1986.
94. Ariens RA, Moia M, Rivolta E, et al: High levels of tissue factor pathway inhibitor in patients with nephrotic proteinuria, Thromb Haemost 82(3):1020-1023, 1999.
95. Malyszko J, Malyszko JS, Mysliwiec M: Markers of endothelial cell injury and thrombin activatable fibrinolysis inhibitor in nephrotic syndrome, Blood Coagul Fibrinolysis 13(7):615-621, 2002.
96. Yoshida Y, Shiiki H, Iwano M, et al: Enhanced expression of plasminogen activator inhibitor 1 in patients with nephrotic syndrome, Nephron 88(1):24-29, 2001.
97. Zhang Q, Zeng C, Fu Y, et al: Biomarkers of endothelial dysfunction in patients with primary focal segmental glomerulosclerosis, Nephrology 17(4):338-345, 2012.
98. Green RA, Kabel AL: Hypercoagulable state in three dogs with nephrotic syndrome: role of acquired antithrombin III deficiency, J Am Vet Med Assoc 181(9):914-917, 1982.
99. Thompson MF, Scott-Moncrieff JC, Brooks MB: Effect of a single plasma transfusion on thromboembolism in 13 dogs with primary immune-mediated hemolytic anemia, J Am Anim Hosp Assoc 40(6):446-454, 2004.
100. Carr AP, Panciera DL, Kidd L: Prognostic factors for mortality and thromboembolism in canine immune-mediated hemolytic anemia: a retrospective study of 72 dogs, J Vet Intern Med 16(5):504-509, 2002.
101. Scott-Moncrieff MA, McCullough SM, Brooks MB: Hemostatic abnormalities in dogs with primary immune-mediated hemolytic anemia, J Am Anim Hosp Assoc 37(3):220-227, 2001.
102. McManus PM, Craig LE: Correlation between leukocytosis and necropsy findings in dogs with immune-mediated hemolytic anemia: 34 cases (1994-1999), J Am Vet Med Assoc 218(8):1308-1313, 2001.
103. Sinnott VB, Otto CM: Use of thromboelastography in dogs with immune-mediated hemolytic anemia: 39 cases (2000-2008), J Vet Emerg Crit Care 19(5):484-488, 2009.
104. Goggs R, Wiinberg B, Kjelgaard-Hansen M, et al: Serial assessment of the coagulation status of dogs with immune-mediated haemolytic anaemia using thromboelastography, Vet J 191(3):347-353, 2012.
105. Fenty RK, de Laforcade AM, Shaw SP, et al: Identification of hypercoagulability in dogs with primary immune-mediated hemolytic anemia by means of thromboelastography, J Am Vet Med Assoc 238(4):463-467, 2011.
106. Setty BN, Betal SG, Zhang J, et al: Heme induces endothelial tissue factor expression: potential role in hemostatic activation in patients with hemolytic anemia, J Thromb Haemost 6(12):2202-2209, 2008.
107. Reiter CD, Wang X, Tanus-Santos JE, et al: Cell-free hemoglobin limits nitric oxide bioavailability in sickle-cell disease, Nat Med 8(12):1383-1389, 2002.
108. Minneci PC, Deans KJ, Zhi H, et al: Hemolysis-associated endothelial dysfunction mediated by accelerated NO inactivation by decompartmentalized oxyhemoglobin, J Clin Invest 115(12):3409-3417, 2005.
109. Kato GJ, McGowan V, Machado RF, et al: Lactate dehydrogenase as a biomarker of hemolysis-associated nitric oxide resistance, priapism, leg ulceration, pulmonary hypertension and death in patients with sickle cell disease, Blood 107(6):2279-2285, 2006.
110. Wagener FA, Feldman E, deWitte T, et al: Heme induces the expression of adhesion molecules ICAM-1, VCAM-1, and E-selectin in vascular endothelial cells, Proc Soc Exp Biol Med 216(3):456-463, 1997.
111. Horne MK III, Cullinane AM, Merryman PK, et al: The effect of red blood cells on thrombin generation, Br J Haematol 133(4):403-408, 2006.
112. Weiss DJ, Brazzell JL: Detection of activated platelets in dogs with primary immune-mediated hemolytic anemia, J Vet Intern Med 20(3):682-686, 2006.
113. Ridyard AE, Shaw DJ, Milne EM: Evaluation of platelet activation in canine immune-mediated haemolytic anaemia, J Small Anim Pract 51(6):296-304, 2010.
114. Weinkle TK, Cener SA, Randolph JF, et al: Evaluation of prognostic factors, survival rates, and treatment protocols for immune-mediated hemolytic anemia in dogs: 151 cases (1993-2002), J Am Vet Med Assoc 226(11):1869-1880, 2005.
115. Rand JH, Senzel L: Antiphospholipid antibodies and the antiphospholipid syndrome. In Hemostasis and thrombosis: basic principles and clinical practice, ed 5, Philadelphia, 2006, Lippincott, Williams & Wilkins, pp 1621-1636.
116. Levin JS, Branch DW, Rauch J: The antiphospholipid syndrome, New Engl J Med 346(10):752-763, 2002.
117. Miller AG, Dow S, Long L, et al: Antiphospholipid antibodies in dogs with immune mediated hemolytic anemia, spontaneous thrombosis, and hyperadrenocorticism, J Vet Intern Med 26(3):614-623, 2012.
118. Nielson LN, Wiinberg B, Kjelgaard-Hansen M, et al: The presence of antiphospholipid antibodies in healthy Bernese Mountain Dogs, J Vet Intern Med 25(6):1258-1263, 2011.

119. Stone MS, Johnstone IB, Brooks M, et al: Lupus-type "anticoagulant" in a dog with hemolysis and thrombosis, J Vet Intern Med 8(1):57-61, 1994.
120. Van Zaane B, Nur E, Squizzato A, et al: Hypercoagulable state in Cushing's syndrome: a systematic review, J Clin Endocrinol Metab 94(8):2743-2750, 2009.
121. Dal Bo Zanon R, Fornasiero L, Boscaro M, et al: Increased factor VIII associated activities in Cushing's syndrome: a probable hypercoagulable state, Thromb Haemost 47(2):116-117, 1982.
122. Casonato A, Pontara E, Boscaro M, et al: Abnormalities of von Willebrand factor are also part of the prothrombotic state of Cushing's syndrome, Blood Coagul Fibrinol 10(3):145-151, 1999.
123. Erem C, Nuhoglu I, Yilmaz M, et al: Blood coagulation and fibrinolysis in patients with Cushing's syndrome: increased plasminogen activator inhibitor-1 and unchanged thrombin-activatable fibrinolysis inhibitor levels, J Endocrinol Invest 32(2):169-174, 2009.
124. Brotman DJ, Girod JP, Posch A, et al: Effects of short-term glucocorticoids on hemostatic factors in healthy volunteers, Thromb Res 118(2):247-252, 2006.
125. Fatti LM, Bottasso B, Invitti C, et al: Markers of activation of coagulation and fibrinolysis in patients with Cushing's syndrome, J Endocrinol Invest 23(3):145-150, 2000.
126. Franchini M, Lippi G, Manzato F, et al: Hemostatic abnormalities in endocrine and metabolic disorders, Eur J Endocrinol 162(3):439-451, 2010.
127. Sjoberg HE, Blomback M, Granberg PO: Thromboembolic complications, heparin treatment and increase in coagulation factors in Cushing's syndrome, Acta Med Scand 199(1-2):95-98, 1976.
128. Boswood A, Lamb CR, White RN: Aortic and iliac thrombosis in six dogs, J Small Anim Pract 41(3):109-114, 2000.
129. Jacoby RC, Owings JT, Ortega T, et al: Biochemical basis for the hypercoagulable state seen in Cushing syndrome, Arch Surg 136(9):1003-1006, 2001.
130. Feldman BF, Rasedee A, Feldman EC: Haemostatic abnormalities in canine Cushing's syndrome, Res Vet Sci 41(2):228-230, 1986.
131. Klose TC, Creevy KE, Brainard BM: Evaluation of coagulation status in dogs with naturally occurring canine hyperadrenocorticism, J Vet Emerg Crit Care 21(6):625-632, 2011.
132. Rose LJ, Dunn ME, Allegret V, et al: Effects of prednisone administration on coagulation variables in healthy Beagle dogs, Vet Clin Pathol 40(4):426-434, 2011.
133. Schoeman JP: Feline distal aortic thromboembolism: a review of 44 cases (1990-1998), J Feline Med Surg 1(4):221-231, 1999.
134. Smith SA, Tobias AH, Jacob KA, et al: Arterial thromboembolism in cats: acute crisis in 127 cases (1992-2001) and long-term management with low-dose aspirin in 24 cases, J Vet Intern Med 17(1):73-83, 2003.
135. Usechak PJ, Bright JM, Day TK: Thrombotic complications associated with atrial fibrillation in three dogs, J Vet Cardiol 14(3):453-458, 2012.
136. Nakamura Y, Nakamura K, Fukushima-Kusano K, et al: Tissue factor expression in atrial endothelia associated with nonvalvular atrial fibrillation: possible involvement in intracardiac thrombogenesis, Thromb Res 111(3):137-142, 2003.
137. Armesilla AL, Lorenzo E, Gomez del Arco P, et al: Vascular endothelial growth factor activates nuclear factor of activated T cells in human endothelial cells: a role for tissue factor gene expression, Mol Cell Biol 19(3):2032-2043, 1999.
138. Davis ME, Cai H, Drummond GR, et al: Shear stress regulates endothelial nitric oxide synthase expression through c-Src by divergent signaling pathways, Circ Res 89(11):1073-1080, 2001.
139. Conway DS, Buggins P, Hughes E, et al: Prognostic significance of raised plasma levels of interleukin-6 and C-reactive protein in atrial fibrillation, Am Heart J 148(3):462-466, 2004.
140. Zhang Z, Zhang C, Wang H, et al: N-3 polyunsaturated fatty acids prevents atrial fibrillation by inhibiting inflammation in a canine sterile pericarditis model, Int J Cardiol 153(1):14-20, 2011.
141. Stokol T, Brooks M, Rush JE, et al: Hypercoagulability in cats with cardiomyopathy, J Vet Intern Med 22(3):546-552, 2008.
142. Bedard C, Lanevschi-Pietersma A, Dunn M: Evaluation of coagulation markers in the plasma of healthy cats and cats with asymptomatic hypertrophic cardiomyopathy, Vet Clin Pathol 36(2):167-172, 2007.
143. Helenski CA, Ross JN: Platelet aggregation in feline cardiomyopathy, J Vet Intern Med 1(1):24-28, 1987.
144. Welles EG, Boudreaux MK, Crager CS, et al: Platelet function and antithrombin, plasminogen, and fibrinolytic activities in cats with heart disease, Am J Vet Res 55(5):619-627, 1994.
145. Jandrey KE, Norris JW, MacDonald KA, et al: Platelet function in clinically healthy cats and cats with hypertrophic cardiomyopathy: analysis using the platelet function analyzer-100, J Vet Clin Pathol 37(4):385-388, 2008.
146. Wray JD, Bestbier M, Miller J, et al: Aortic and iliac thrombosis associated with angiosarcoma of skeletal muscle in a dog, J Small Anim Pract 47(5):272-277, 2006.
147. Ledieu D, Palazzi X, Marchal T, et al: Acute megakaryoblastic leukemia with erythrophagocytosis and thrombosis in a dog, Vet Clin Pathol 34(1):52-56, 2005.
148. Saridomichelakis MN, Koutinas CK, Souftas V, et al: Extensive caudal vena cava thrombosis secondary to unilateral renal tubular cell carcinoma in a dog, J Small Anim Pract 45(2):108-112, 2004.
149. Santamarina G, Espino L, Vila M, et al: Aortic thromboembolism and retroperitoneal hemorrhage associated with a pheochromocytoma in a dog, J Vet Intern Med 17(6):917-922, 2003.
150. LaRue MJ, Murtaugh RJ: Pulmonary thromboembolism in dogs: 47 cases (1986-1987), J Am Vet Med Assoc 197(10):1368-1372, 1990.
151. Schermerhorn T, Pembleton-Corbett JR, Kornreich B: Pulmonary thromboembolism in cats, J Vet Intern Med 18(4):533-535, 2004.
152. Currao RL, Buote NJ, Flory AB, et al: Mesenteric vascular thrombosis associated with disseminated abdominal visceral hemangiosarcoma in a cat, J Am Anim Hosp Assoc 47(6):168-172, 2011.
153. Rogers CL, O'Toole TE, Keating JH, et al: Portal vein thrombosis in cats: 6 cases (2001-2006), J Vet Intern Med 22(2):282-287, 2008.
154. Norris CR, Griffey SM, Samii VF: Pulmonary thromboembolism in cats: 29 cases (1987-1997), J Am Vet Med Assoc 215(11):1650-1654, 1999.
155. Sottiaux J, Franck M: Cranial vena caval thrombosis secondary to invasive mediastinal lymphosarcoma in a cat, J Small Anim Pract 39(7):352-355, 1998.
156. Maruyama H, Miura T, Sakai M, et al: The incidence of disseminated intravascular coagulation in dogs with malignant tumor, J Vet Med Sci 66(5):573-575, 2004.
157. Hammer AS, Couto CG, Swardson C, et al: Hemostatic abnormalities in dogs with hemangiosarcoma, J Vet Intern Med 5(1):11-14, 1991.
158. Contrino J, Hair G, Kreutzer DL, et al: In situ detection of tissue factor in vascular endothelial cells: correlation with the malignant phenotype of human breast disease, Nat Med 2(2):209-225, 1996.
159. Rak J: Microparticles in cancer, Semin Thromb Hemost 36(8):888-906, 2010.
160. Zhang Y, Deng Y, Luther T, et al: Tissue factor controls the balance of angiogenic and antiangiogenic properties of tumor cells in mice, J Clin Invest 94(3):1320-1327, 1994.
161. Hembrough TA, Swartz GM, Papathanassiu A, et al: Tissue factor/factor VIIa inhibitors block angiogenesis and tumor growth through a nonhemostatic mechanism, Cancer Res 63(11):2997-3000, 2003.
162. Regina S, Valentin JB, Lachot S, et al: Increased tissue factor expression is associated with reduced survival in non-small cell lung cancer and with mutations of TP53 and PTEN, Clin Chem 55(10):1834-1842, 2009.
163. Ryden L, Grabau D, Schaffner F, et al: Evidence for tissue factor phosphorylation and its correlation with protease-activated receptor expression and the prognosis of primary breast cancer, Int J Cancer 126(10):2330-2340, 2010.
164. Yamashita H, Kitayama J, Ishikawa M, et al: Tissue factor expression is a clinical indicator of lymphatic metastasis and poor prognosis in gastric cancer with intestinal phenotype, J Surg Oncol 95(4):423-431, 2007.
165. Poon RT, Lau CP, Ho JW, et al: Tissue factor expression correlates with tumor angiogenesis and invasiveness in human hepatocellular carcinoma, Clin Cancer Res 9(14):5339-5345, 2003.
166. Kristensen AT, Wiinberg B, Jessen LR, et al: Evaluation of human recombinant tissue factor-activated thrombelastography in 49 dogs with neoplasia, J Vet Intern Med 22(1):140-147, 2008.
167. Andreasen EB, Tranholm M, Wiinberg B, et al: Haemostatic alterations in a group of canine cancer patients are associated with cancer type and disease progression, Acta Veterinaria Scandinavica 54:3, 2012.

168. Saavedra PV, Garcia AL, Lopez SZ, et al:Hemostatic abnormalities in dogs with carcinoma: a thromboelastographic characterization of hypercoagulability, Vet J 190(2):e78-83, 2011.
169. Stockhaus C, Kohn B, Rudolph R, et al: Correlation of haemostatic abnormalities with tumour stage and characteristics in dogs with mammary carcinoma, J Small Anim Pract 40(7):326-331, 1999.
170. O'Donnell MR, Slichter SJ, Weiden PL, et al: Platelet and fibrinogen kinetics in canine tumors, Cancer Res 41(4):1379-1383, 1981.
171. Kuzi S, Segev G, Haruvi E, et al: Plasma antithrombin activity as a diagnostic and prognostic indicator in dogs: a retrospective study of 149 dogs, J Vet Intern Med 24(3):587-596, 2010.
172. Thomas JS, Rogers KS: Platelet aggregation and adenosine triphosphate secretion in dogs with untreated multicentric lymphoma, J Vet Intern Med 13(4):319-322, 1999.
173. McNiel EA, Ogilvie GK, Fettman MJ, et al: Platelet function in dogs with malignancies, J Vet Intern Med 11(3):178-182, 1997.
174. Laroche M, Kutcher ME, Huang MC, et al: Coagulopathy after traumatic brain injury, Neurosurgery 70(6):1334-1345, 2012.
175. Stein SC, Chen XH, Sinson GP, et al: Intravascular coagulation: a major second insult in nonfatal traumatic brain injury, J Neurosurg 97(6): 1373-1377, 2002.
176. Chiaretti A, Piastra M, Pulitano S, et al: Prognostic factors and outcome of children with severe head injury: an 8-year experience, Child's Nerv Syst 18(3-4):129-136, 2002.
177. Stein SC, Young GS, Talucci RC, et al: Delayed brain injury after head trauma: significance of coagulopathy, Neurosurgery 30(2):160-165, 1992.
178. Wafaisade A, Lefering R, Tjardes T, et al: Acute coagulopathy in isolated blunt traumatic brain injury, Neurocrit Care 12(2):211-219, 2010.
179. Lustenberger T, Talving P, Kobayashi L, et al: Time course of coagulopathy in isolated severe traumatic brain injury, Injury 41(9):924-928, 2010.
180. Eddleston M, de la Torre JC, Oldstone MB, et al: Astrocytes are the primary source of tissue factor in the murine central nervous system: a role for astrocytes in cerebral hemostasis, J Clin Invest 92(1):349-358, 1993.
181. Utter GH, Owings JT, Jacoby RC, et al: Injury induces increased monocyte expression of tissue factor: factors associated with head injury attenuate the injury-related monocyte expression of tissue factor, J Trauma 52(6):1071-1077, 2002.
182. Nekludov M, Bellander BM, Blomback M, et al: Platelet dysfunction in patients with severe traumatic brain injury, J Neurotrauma 24(11): 1699-1706, 2007.
183. Murshid WR, Gader AG: The coagulopathy in acute head injury: comparison of cerebral versus peripheral measurements of haemostatic activation markers, Br J Neurosurg 16(4):362-369, 2002.
184. Morel N, Morel O, Petit L, et al: Generation of procoagulant microparticles in cerebrospinal fluid and peripheral blood after traumatic brain injury, J Trauma 64(3):698-704, 2008.
185. Davis KP, Musunuru H, Walsh M, et al: Platelet dysfunction is an early marker for traumatic brain injury-induced coagulopathy, Neurocrit Care 18(2):201-208, 2013.
186. Jacoby RC, Owings JT, Holmes J, et al: Platelet activation and function after trauma, J Trauma 51(4):639-647, 2001.
187. Awasthi D, Rock WA, Carey ME, et al: Coagulation changes after an experimental missile wound to the brain in the cat, Surg Neurol 36(6):441-446, 1991.
188. Avidan MS, Levy JH, Scholz J, et al: A phase III, double-blinded, placebo-controlled, multicenter study on the efficacy of recombinant human antithrombin in heparin-resistant patients scheduled to undergo cardiac surgery necessitating cardiopulmonary bypass, Anesthesiology 102(2):276-284, 2005.
189. Warren BL, Eid A, Singer P, et al: Caring for the critically ill patient. High-dose antithrombin III in severe sepsis: a randomized controlled trial, J Am Med Assoc 286(15):1869-1878, 2001.
190. Kienast J, Juers M, Wiedermann CJ, et al: Treatment effects of high-dose antithrombin without concomitant heparin in patients with severe sepsis with or without disseminated intravascular coagulation, J Thromb Haemost 4(1):90-97, 2006.
191. Isobe H, Okajima K, Uchiba M, et al: Activated protein C prevents endotoxin-induced hypotension in rats by inhibiting excessive production of nitric oxide, Circulation 104(10):1171-1175, 2001.
192. De Backer D, Verdant C, Chierego M, et al: Effects of drotrecogin alfa activated on microcirculatory alterations in patients with severe sepsis, Crit Care Med 34(7):1918-1924, 2006.
193. Taylor FBJ, Chang A, Esmon CT, et al: Protein C prevents the coagulopathic and lethal effects of Escherichia coli infusion in the baboon, J Clin Invest 79(3):918-925, 1987.
194. Ranieri VM, Thompson BT, Barie PS, et al: Drotrecogin alfa (activated) in adults with septic shock, N Eng J Med 366(22):2055-2064, 2012.
195. Holst J, Lindblad B, Bergqvist D, et al: Antithrombotic effect of recombinant truncated tissue factor pathway inhibitor (TFPI1-161) in experimental venous thrombosis- a comparison with low molecular weight heparin, Thromb Haemost 71(2):214-219, 1994.
196. Abendschein DR, Meng Y, Torr-Brown S, et al: Maintenance of coronary patency after fibrinolysis with tissue factor pathway inhibitor, Circulation 92(4):944-949, 1995.
197. Camerota AJ, Creasey AA, Patla V, et al: Delayed treatment with recombinant human tissue factor pathway inhibitor improves survival in rabbits with gram-negative peritonitis, J Infect Dis 177(3):668-676, 1998.
198. Abraham E, Reinkart K, Opal S, et al: Efficacy and safety of tifacogin (recombinant tissue factor pathway inhibitor) in severe sepsis: a randomized controlled trial, J Am Med Assoc 290(2):238-247, 2003.
199. Abraham E, Reinkart K, Svoboda P, et al: Assessment of the safety of recombinant tissue factor pathway inhibitor in patients with severe sepsis: a multicenter, randomized, placebo-controlled, single-blind, dose escalating study, Crit Care Med 29(11):2081-2089, 2001.
200. Wunderink RG, Laterre PF, Francois B, et al: Recombinant tissue factor pathway inhibitor in severe community-acquired pneumonia: a randomized trial, Am J Respir Crit Care Med 183(11):1561-1568, 2011.
201. Yagasaki H, Kato M, Shimozawa K, et al: Treatment responses for disseminated intravascular coagulation in 25 children treated with recombinant thrombomodulin: a single institutional experience, Thromb Res 130(6):e289-293, 2012.
202. Ikezoe T, Takeuchi A, Isaka M, et al: Recombinant human soluble thrombomodulin safely and effectively rescues acute promyelocytic leukemia patients from disseminated intravascular coagulation, Leuk Res 36(11):1398-1402, 2012.
203. Saito H, Maruyama I, Shimazaki S, et al: Efficacy and safety of recombinant human soluble thrombomodulin (ART-123) in disseminated intravascular coagulation: results of a phase III, randomized, double-blinded clinical trial, J Thromb Haemost 5(1):31-41, 2007.
204. Ogawa Y, Yamakawa K, Ogura H, et al: Recombinant human soluble thrombomodulin improves mortality and respiratory dysfunction in patients with severe sepsis, J Trauma Acute Care Surg 72(5):1150-1157, 2012.
205. Mischke R, Fehr M, Nolte I: Efficacy of low molecular weight heparin in a canine model of thromboplastin-induced acute disseminated intravascular coagulation, Res Vet Sci 79(1):69-76, 2005.
206. Grauer GF, Greco DS, Getzy DM, et al: Effects of enalapril versus placebo as a treatment for canine idiopathic glomerulonephritis, J Vet Intern Med 14(5):526-533, 2000.
207. Mellett AM, Nakamura RK, Bianco D: A prospective study of clopidogrel therapy in dogs with primary immune-mediated hemolytic anemia, J Vet Intern Med 25(1):71-75, 2011.
208. Breuhl EL, Moore G, Brooks MB, et al: A prospective study of unfractionated heparin therapy in dogs with primary immune-mediated hemolytic anemia, J Am Anim Hosp Assoc 45(3):125-133, 2009.
209. Helmond SE, Polzin DJ, Armstrong PJ, et al: Treatment of immune-mediated hemolytic anemia with individually adjusted heparin dosing in dogs, J Vet Intern Med 24(3):597-605, 2010.
210. Cathcart CJ, Brainard BM, Reynolds LR, et al: Lack of inhibitory effect of acetylsalicylic acid and meloxicam on whole blood platelet aggregation in cats, J Vet Emerg Crit Care 22(1):99-106, 2012.
211. Hogan DF, Andrews DA, Green HW, et al: Antiplatelet effects and pharmacodynamics of clopidogrel in cats, J Am Vet Med Assoc 225(9):1406-1411, 2004.

212. Hamel-Jolette A, Dunn M, Bedard C: Plateletworks: a screening assay for clopidogrel therapy monitoring in healthy cats, Can J Vet Res 73(1):73-76, 2009.
213. Brainard BM, Kleine SA, Papich MG, et al: Pharmacodynamic and pharmacokinetic evaluation of clopidogrel and the carboxylic acid metabolite SR 26334 in healthy dogs, Am J Vet Res 71(7):822-830, 2010.
214. Smith CE, Rozanski EA, Freeman LM, et al: Use of low molecular weight heparin in cats: 57 cases (1999-2003), J Am Vet Med Assoc 225(8):1237-1241, 2004.
215. Vargo CL, Taylor SM, Carr A, et al: The effect of a low molecular weight heparin on coagulation parameters in healthy cats, Can J Vet Res 73(2):132-136, 2009.
216. Alwood AJ, Downend AB, Brooks MB, et al: Anticoagulant effects of low-molecular-weight heparins in healthy cats, J Vet Int Med 21(3):378-387, 2007.
217. Welch KM, Rozanski EA, Freeman LM, et al: Prospective evaluation of tissue plasminogen activator in 11 cats with arterial thromboembolism, J Feline Med Surg 12(2):122-128, 2010.
218. Moore KE, Morris N, Dhupa N, et al: Retrospective study of streptokinase administration in 46 cats with arterial thromboembolism, J Vet Emerg Crit Care 10(4):245-257, 2000.
219. Laste NJ, Harpster NK: A retrospective study of 100 cases of feline distal aortic thromboembolism 1977-1993, J Am Anim Hosp Assoc 31(6):492-500, 1995.
220. Maat B, Hilgard P: Anticoagulants and experimental metastases-evaluation of antimetastatic effects in different model systems, J Cancer Res Clin Oncol 101(3):275-283, 1981.
221. Gastpar H: Platelet-cancer cell interaction in metastasis formation: a possible therapeutic approach to metastasis prophylaxis, J Med 8(2):103-114, 1977.
222. Rhind SG, Crnko NT, Baker AJ, et al: Prehospital resuscitation with hypertonic saline-dextran modulates inflammatory, coagulation and endothelial activation marker profiles in severe traumatic brain injured patients, J Neuroinflammation 7:5, 2010.
223. Stein DM, Dutton RP, Kramer ME, et al: Reversal of coagulopathy in critically ill patients with traumatic brain injury: recombinant factor VIIa is more cost-effective than plasma, J Trauma 66(1):63-72, 2009.
224. Stein DM, Dutton RP, Kramer ME, et al: Recombinant factor VIIa: decreasing time to intervention in coagulopathic patients with severe traumatic brain injury, J Trauma 64(3):620-627, 2008.
225. Brown CV, Sowery L, Curry E, et al: Recombinant factor VIIa to correct coagulopathy in patients with traumatic brain injury presenting to outlying facilities before transfer to the regional trauma center, Am Surg 78(1):57-60, 2012.
226. Teitel JM, Bauer KA, Lau HK, et al: Studies of the prothrombin activation pathway utilizing radioimmunoassays for the F_2/F_{1+2} fragment and thrombin-antithrombin complex, Blood 59(5):1086-1097, 1982.
227. Nossel HL, Yudelman I, Canfield RE, et al: Measurement of fibrinopeptide A in human blood, J Clin Invest 54(1):43-53, 1974.
228. Bilezikian SB, Nossel LH, Butler BP Jr, et al: Radioimmunoassay of human fibrinopeptide B and kinetics of cleavage by different enzymes, J Clin Invest 56(2):438-445, 1975.
229. Bauer KA, Kass BL, ten Cate H, et al: Factor IX is activated in vivo by the tissue factor mechanism, Blood 764(4):731-736, 1990.
230. Stokol T, Daddona JL, Choi B: Evaluation of tissue factor procoagulant activity on the surface of feline leukocytes in response to treatment with lipopolysaccharide and heat-inactivated fetal bovine serum, Am J Vet Res 71(6):623-629, 2010.
231. Cate H: Thrombin generation in clinical conditions, Thromb Res 129(3):367-370, 2012.
232. Gruber A, Griffin JH: Direct detection of activated protein C in blood from human subjects, Blood 79(9):2340-2348, 1992.
233. Bauer KA, Kass BL, Beeler DL, et al: Detection of protein C activation in humans, J Clin Invest 74(6):2033-2041, 1984.
234. Espana F, Griffin JH: Determination of functional and antigenic protein C inhibitor and its complexes with activated protein C in plasma by ELISAs, Thromb Res 55(6):671-682, 1989.
235. Scully MF, Toh CH, Hoogendoorn H, et al: Activation of protein C and its distribution between its inhibitors, protein-C inhibitor, alpha 1-antitrypsin and alpha 2-macroglobulin, in patients with disseminated intravascular coagulation, Thromb Haemost 69(5):448-453, 1993.
236. Brandt JT: Plasminogen and tissue-type plasminogen activator deficiency as risk factors for thromboembolic disease, Arch Pathol Lab Med 126(11):1376-1381, 2002.
237. Heylen E, Miljic P, Willemse J, et al: Procarboxypeptidase U (TAFI) contributes to the risk of thrombosis in patients with hereditary thrombophilia, Thromb Res 124(4):427-432, 2009.
238. Lau HK, Teitel JM, Cheung T, et al: Hypofibrinolysis in patients with hypercoagulability: the roles of urokinase and of plasminogen activator inhibitor, Am J Hematol 44(4):260-265, 1993.
239. Levi M, Roem D, Kamp AM, et al: Assessment of the relative contribution of different protease inhibitors to the inhibition of plasmin in vivo, Thromb Haemost 69(2):141-146, 1993.
240. Weitz JI, Koehn JA, Canfield RW, et al: Development of a radioimmunoassay for the fibrinogen-derived peptide Bβ1-42, Blood 67(4):1014-1022, 1986.
241. Kudryk B, Rohoza A, Ahadi M, et al: Specificity of a monoclonal antibody for the NH2-terminal region of fibrin, Mol Immunol 21(1):89-94, 1984.
242. Shattil SJ, Hoxie JA, Cunningham M, et al: Changes in the platelet membrane glycoprotein IIb/IIIa complex during platelet activation, J Biol Chem 260(20):11107-11114, 1985.
243. Frelinger AL, Lam SC, Plow EF, et al: Selective inhibition of integrin function by antibodies specific for ligand-occupied receptor conformers, J Biol Chem 265(11):6346-6352, 1990.
244. Michelson AD: Laboratory markers of platelet activation. In Colman RW, Marder VJ, Clowes AW, et al, editors: Hemostasis and thrombosis: basic principles and clinical practice, ed 5, Philadelphia, 2006, Lippincott Williams & Wilkins, pp 825-834.
245. Gralnick HR, Williams SB, McKeown L, et al: Endogenous platelet fibrinogen: its modulation after surface expression is related to size-selective access to and conformational changes in the bound fibrinogen, Br J Haematol 80(3):347-357, 1992.
246. Boudreaux MK, Panangala VS, Bourne C: A platelet activation-specific monoclonal antibody that recognizes a receptor-induced binding site on canine fibrinogen, Vet Pathol 33(4):419-427, 1996.
247. Sharp KS, Center S, Randolph JF, et al: Influence of treatment with ultralow-dose aspirin on platelet aggregation as measured by whole blood impedance aggregometry and platelet P-selectin expression in clinically normal dogs, Am J Vet Res 71(11):1294-1304, 2010.
248. Metzelaar MJ, Heijnen HF, Sixma JJ, et al: Identification of a 33-kD protein associated with the alpha-granule membrane (GMP-33) that is expressed on the surface of activated platelets, Blood 79(2):372-379, 1992.
249. Chen M, Kakutani M, Naruko T, et al: Activation-dependent surface expression of LOX-1 in human platelets, Biochem Biophys Res Commun 282(1):153-158, 2001.
250. Febbraio M, Silverstein RL: Identification and characterization of LAMP-1 as an activation-dependent platelet surface glycoprotein, J Biol Chem 265(30):18531-18537, 1990.
251. Nieuwenhuis HK, van Oosterhout JJ, Rozemuller E, et al: Studies with a monoclonal antibody against activated platelets: evidence that a secreted 53,000-molecular weight lysome-like granule protein is exposed on the surface of activated platelets in the circulation, Blood 70(3):838-845, 1987.
252. McEver RP: P-selectin/PSGL-1 and other interactions between platelets, leukocytes, and endothelium. In Michelson AD, editor: Platelets, New York, 2002, Academic Press/Elsevier Science.
253. Andre P, Nannizzi-Alaimo L, Prasad SK, et al: Platelet-derived CD40L, the switch hitting player of cardiovascular disease, Circulation 106(8):896-899, 2002.
254. Hayward CP, Bainton DF, Smith JW, et al: Multimerin is found in the alpha-granules of resting platelets and is synthesized by a megakaryocytic cell line, J Clin Invest 91(6):2630-2639, 1993.
255. Aiken ML, Ginsberg MH, Plow EF: Mechanisms for expression of thrombospondin on the platelet cell surface, Semin Thromb Hemost 13(3):307-316, 1987.

256. Sims PJ, Faioni EM, Wiedmer T, et al: Complement proteins C5b-9 cause release of membrane vesicles from the platelet surface that are enriched in the membrane receptor for coagulation factor Va and express prothrombinase activity, J Biol Chem 263(34):18205-18212, 1988.
257. Gilbert GE, Sims PJ, Wiedmer T, et al: Platelet-derived microparticles express high affinity receptors for factor VIII, J Biol Chem 266(26):17261-17268, 1991.
258. Holme PA,Brosstad F, Solum NO: Platelet-derived microvesicles and activated platelets express factor Xa activity, Blood Coagul Fibrinolysis 6(4):302-310, 1995.
259. Michelson AD, Rajasekhar D, Bednarek FJ, et al: Platelet and platelet-derived microparticle surface factor V/Va binding in whole blood: differences between neonates and adults, Thromb Haemost 84(4):689-694, 2000.
260. McMichael M, Smith SA, Herring JM, et al: Quantification of procoagulant phospholipid in erythrocyte concentrates stored with and without leukoreduction [abstract], J Vet Emerg Crit Care 21(suppl 1): S8, 2011.
261. Chong BH, Murray B, Berndt MC, et al: Plasma P-selectin is increased in thrombotic consumptive platelet disorders, Blood 83(6):1535-1541, 1994.
262. Levine SP: Secreted platelet proteins as markers for pathological disorders. In Phillips DR, Shuman MA, editors: Biochemistry of platelets, Orlando, 1986, Academic Press, pp 378-415.
263. Blann AD, Lanza F, Galajda P, et al: Increased platelet glycoprotein V levels in patients with coronary and peripheral atherosclerosis—the influence of aspirin and cigarette smoking, Thromb Haemost 86(3):777-783, 2001.
264. Oates JA, FitzGerald GA, Branch RA, et al: Clinical implications of prostaglandin and thromboxane A2 formation, N Engl J Med 319(11):689-698, 1988.
265. Henn V, Steinbach S, Buchner K, et al: The inflammatory action of CD40 ligand (CD154) expressed on activated human platelets is temporally limited by coexpressed CD40, Blood 98(4):1047-1054, 2001.
266. Prasad KS, Andre P, Yan Y, et al: The platelet CD40L/GPIIb/IIIa axis in atherothrombotic disease, Curr Opin Hematol 10(5):356-361, 2003.

CHAPTER 105

BLEEDING DISORDERS

Susan G. Hackner, BVSc, MRCVS, DACVIM, DACVECC •
Alexandre Rousseau, DVM, DACVIM (Internal Medicine), DACVECC

KEY POINTS

- Patients with subclinical hemostatic defects may not demonstrate evidence of bleeding until an invasive procedure or contributory event occurs. The clinician should be suspicious of bleeding disorders in certain patient populations to identify the patient at risk.
- Bleeding disorders occur as a result of disorders of primary hemostasis, disorders of secondary hemostasis, hyperfibrinolysis, or combinations of these.
- Diagnosis begins with determining if the bleeding is due to local factors or to a systemic bleeding disorder and, in case of the latter, characterization of the hemostatic defect(s).
- Characterization of the disorder is achieved via careful history taking, a thorough physical examination, and routine coagulation testing.
- Massive trauma or surgery can cause an acute coagulopathy. This is exacerbated by shock, hypothermia, acidemia, and aggressive fluid therapy, which can result in profound coagulopathy and exacerbation of bleeding.
- Management relies on early recognition and reversal of life-threatening events and contributing factors, the provision of plasma or platelet products and, when possible, therapy targeted at the inciting cause. The use of prohemostatic agents is indicated in certain conditions.

Bleeding disorders are conditions that result in inappropriate hemostasis, causing or predisposing to bleeding. Some coagulopathies result in spontaneous bleeding, but many are subclinical and hemorrhage occurs only after an invasive procedure. This is particularly true in cats, in whom subclinical hemostatic defects are relatively common with underlying disease, such as hepatopathy, viral disease, or neoplasia.[1]

Bleeding disorders always should be considered life threatening. Even the stable patient can decompensate rapidly from massive hemorrhage, or hemorrhage into a vital organ. Therefore, rapid diagnosis is paramount. Recognizing patients at risk, identifying the hemostatic disorder, and initiating rational therapy are necessary steps for successful outcomes.

HEMOSTASIS AND FIBRINOLYSIS

Hemostasis and fibrinolysis maintain the integrity of a closed, high-pressure circulatory system after vascular damage.[2] Vascular injury provokes a complex response in the endothelium and the blood that culminates in the formation of a thrombus to seal the breach. Hemostasis can be divided into two distinct but overlapping phases: primary hemostasis, involving the interaction between platelets and endothelium resulting in the formation of a platelet plug, and secondary hemostasis, a system of proteolytic reactions involving coagulation factors and resulting in the generation of fibrin polymers, which stabilize the platelet plug to form a mature thrombus. These phases occur concomitantly and, under normal physiologic conditions, intrinsic regulatory mechanisms contain thrombus formation temporally and spatially. Fibrinolysis is the dissolution of the fibrin clot to restore vascular patency. The delicate balance between proteolytic and inhibitory reactions in hemostasis and fibrinolysis can be disrupted, by inherent or acquired defects, to result in abnormal bleeding.

Primary hemostasis immediately follows vascular damage. Platelets adhere to subendothelial collagen via the platelet glycoprotein VI

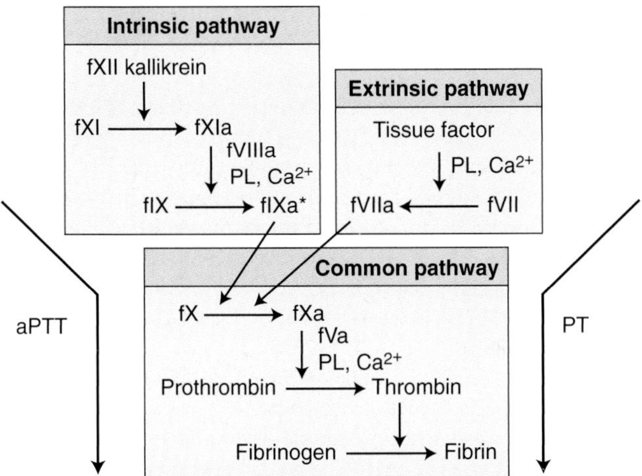

FIGURE 105-1 The cascade model of coagulation. The intrinsic pathway was considered to be initiated through contact activation of factor XII, and the extrinsic system by exposure to extravascular tissue factor (TF). Either pathway results in the activation of factor X in the common pathway, leading to thrombin production. The aPTT tests the intrinsic and common pathways; the PT tests the extrinsic and common pathways. *aPTT,* Activated partial thromboplastin time; *PL,* platelet phospholipid; *PT,* prothrombin time. *(From Hackner SG, White CR: Bleeding and hemostasis. In Tobias KM, Johnston SA, editors: Veterinary surgery small animal, St Louis, 2012, Elsevier, p 95.)*

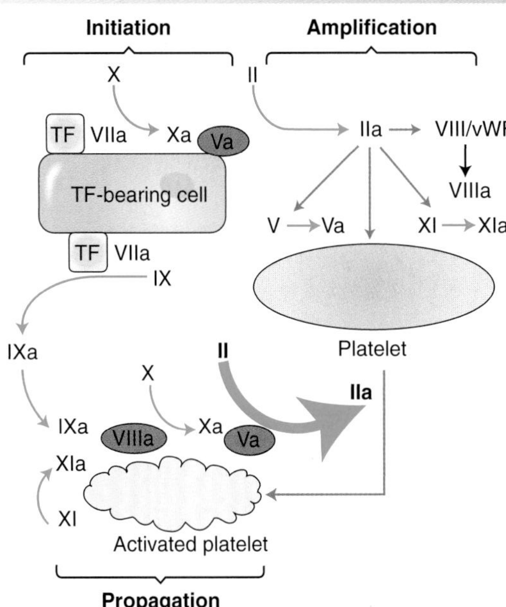

FIGURE 105-2 A cell-based model of coagulation. Coagulation is initiated through tissue factor (TF) on the surface of TF-bearing cells, leading to the generation of small amounts of thrombin (IIa) from prothrombin (II) (initiation phase). Thrombin amplifies the initial signal by activating platelets and cofactors (fVa, fVIIIa) on the platelet surfaces (amplification phase). Large-scale thrombin generation occurs on the surface of the activated platelet (propagation phase). *(From Hackner SG, White CR: Bleeding and hemostasis. In Tobias KM, Johnston SA, editors: Veterinary surgery small animal, St Louis, 2012, Elsevier, p 96.)*

receptor, or to collagen-bound von Willebrand factor (vWF) via the glycoprotein Ib receptor.[2] Adherence triggers a cascade of cytosolic signaling that stimulates platelet arachidonic acid metabolism and the release of granular contents (activation). Thrombin, generated by secondary hemostasis, is also a powerful platelet agonist. Activated platelets release secondary agonists, notably thromboxane A_2 (TxA_2), adenosine diphosphate (ADP), and serotonin, which recruit and activate additional platelets, thus amplifying and sustaining the initial response.[2,3] The final common pathway for all agonists is the activation of the platelet integrin $\alpha_{IIb}\beta_3$ receptor (formerly known as glycoprotein IIbIIIa receptor).[2,3] Agonist binding induces a conformational change in the receptor, exposing binding domains for fibrinogen. Binding results in interplatelet cohesion and aggregation. Aggregated platelets constitute the primary hemostatic plug and provide a stimulus and framework for secondary hemostasis.

Secondary hemostasis culminates in the formation of fibrin. The traditional model of coagulation consisted of a cascade of enzymatic reactions, in which enzymes cleaved substrates to generate the next enzyme in the cascade (Figure 105-1).[4] This model was divided into two pathways: the "extrinsic" pathway, initiated by tissue factor (TF), and the "intrinsic" pathway, initiated through contact activation of fXII. These two pathways converge into a final common pathway of thrombin generation and fibrin formation. Although this model is valid for interpretation of traditional in vitro coagulation testing, it does not adequately explain coagulation in vivo.[2,5] For example, although deficiencies of fXII cause marked coagulation test prolongation, they do not result in a bleeding tendency. In contrast, isolated deficiencies of the intrinsic pathway, such as hemophilia, result in profound bleeding in spite of an intact extrinsic pathway.

A cell-based model of coagulation more accurately reflects coagulation in vivo.[2,5,6] This model includes two fundamental paradigm shifts: that TF is the primary physiologic initiator of coagulation (contact activation playing no role in vivo); and that coagulation is localized to, and controlled by, cellular surfaces.[2,5] Coagulation occurs in three overlapping phases: initiation (on TF-bearing cells), amplification, and propagation (on platelets) (Figure 105-2).[5,6] The initiation phase is the TF-initiated ("extrinsic") pathway that generates small amounts of thrombin. TF is a membrane protein, expressed on endothelial cells, fibroblasts, and other extravascular cells under physiologic conditions. Coagulation is initiated when vascular damage or inflammation enables contact between plasma and TF-bearing cells. Plasma fVII binds to TF and is activated, generating small amounts of thrombin, which, in turn, activate platelets that are adhered at the site of vascular damage. During the activation phase, platelets are activated and have activated cofactors V and VIII bound to their surfaces. In this manner, thrombin amplifies the initial signal, acting on the platelet to "set the stage" for procoagulant complex assembly. During the propagation phase, complexes are assembled on the surface of the activated platelet, and large-scale thrombin generation occurs (similar to the previously-named "intrinsic" pathway). This provides the burst of thrombin necessary to produce large quantities of fibrin. Fibrin monomers are then complexed to form fibrin polymers and a stable thrombus.

Fibrinolysis is the enzymatic dissolution of fibrin. Plasminogen activators, most notably tissue-type plasminogen activator (tPA) proteolytically convert plasminogen to plasmin, which, in turn, degrades fibrin into soluble degradation products (fibrin split products, FSPs).

HEMOSTATIC TESTING

Hemostatic testing is essential for the identification and characterization of hemostatic defects. However, in vitro tests do not accurately reflect in vivo hemostasis. Moreover, hemostatic testing makes high demands on sampling procedure; improper technique leads to artifactual results.[7] Tests should always be performed and interpreted carefully, along with the clinical findings, and with their limitations in mind. Normal values are presented in Table 105-1.

Platelet Enumeration and Estimation

Platelet counts detect quantitative platelet disorders (thrombocytopenia). Enumeration is performed via automated cell counter or

Table 105-1 **Normal Values for Common Coagulation Tests**

Diagnostic Test	Dog	Cat
Platelet count (× 10^3/µl)	200-500	200-600
Buccal mucosal bleeding time (min)	1.7-4.2	1.4-2.4
Prothrombin time (sec)	6-11	6-12
Activated partial thromboplastin time (sec)	10-25	10-25
Fibrin split products (mcg/ml)	<10	<10
D-dimer (ng/dl)	<250	<250
Fibrinogen (mg/dl)	150-400	150-400

manually (by hemocytometer). Pseudothrombocytopenia is a common artifact that occurs when platelets in blood are not adequately counted. This usually results from platelet aggregation during sample collection and is especially common in cats (reported in 71% of feline blood samples).[8] Even in the absence of platelet clumping, pseudothrombocytopenia is frequent with automated platelet counts in cats because of the considerable overlap between erythrocyte and platelet volumes in this species, and in dogs and cats when large platelets are present.[9] For these reasons, low platelet counts should always be confirmed by blood smear examination.

Examination of a blood smear allows for rapid estimation of platelet numbers as well as assessment of other blood cell lines. The feathered edge of the smear should be examined for platelet clumps that indicate pseudothrombocytopenia and the need for repeat sampling. (The use of an EDTA-rinsed syringe for venipuncture may help to reduce clumping.) In the absence of platelet clumping, the platelet count can be estimated by multiplying the average number of platelets per high-power field (within the monolayer of the blood film) by 15,000/µl.[10]

Buccal Mucosal Bleeding Time

The bleeding time is the duration of hemorrhage resulting from the infliction of a small standardized injury involving only microscopic vessels and reflects in vivo primary hemostasis.[11] The buccal mucosal bleeding time (BMBT) is the only reliable and reproducible method in small animals.[11,12] Sedation is generally not required, except in cats and nervous dogs. The patient is restrained in lateral recumbency and a strip of gauze is tied around the maxilla to fold up the upper lip, sufficiently tight to cause moderate mucosal engorgement. A spring-loaded device (SurgiCutt, ITC, Edson, NJ; Simplate II, Organon Teknika, Austria) is used to make two 1-mm–deep incisions in the mucosa of the upper lip. The incisions should be made at a site devoid of visible vessels and inclined so that the blood flows toward the mouth. Shed blood is blotted carefully with filter paper, taking extreme care not to disturb the incisions. The BMBT is the time from incision to cessation of bleeding.

The BMBT test is indicated in patients with a suspected primary hemostatic defect when the platelet count is adequate. It is prolonged in dogs with von Willebrand disease (vWD) and nonsteroidal antiinflammatory drug (NSAID)–induced thrombopathia. The BMBT also is used for the preoperative screening of patients considered at risk for vWD or other thrombopathias. However, the test has significant limitations. It is influenced by hematocrit and blood viscosity and has appreciable inter- and intraoperator variability (up to 2 minutes).[13] Moreover, it is a poor predictor of surgical bleeding.[14]

The Prothrombin Time and Activated Partial Thromboplastin Time

The prothrombin time (PT) and the activated partial thromboplastin time (aPTT) assess secondary hemostasis via reagents that activate the extrinsic or the intrinsic pathway, respectively (see Figure 105-1).[15] The PT evaluates the extrinsic and common pathways, specifically factors VII, X, V, II and fibrinogen. Because of the short half-life of factor VII, the PT is sensitive to vitamin K deficiency or antagonism. The APTT evaluates the intrinsic and common pathways; only factors VII and XIII are not evaluated. It is more sensitive to heparin than is the PT.

A point-of-care (POC) coagulometer (e.g., CoagDx, Idexx, ME) is invaluable for patient-side coagulation testing. However, it is not equivalent to conventional laboratory testing. In canine patients, sensitivities of the aPTT and PT were 100% and 86%, respectively; specificities were 83% and 96%, respectively.[16] In the authors' experience, clinically significant defects are reliably identified; marked prolongations are generally accurate, whereas mild prolongations should be interpreted with caution. Results that do not correlate with clinical findings should be verified via conventional testing.

Although the PT and aPTT are invaluable in the diagnosis of disorders of secondary hemostasis, they are in vitro plasma-based tests, represented by the cascade model of coagulation, and do not accurately represent in vivo hemostasis. As such, they are not predictive of bleeding.

Fibrin Split Products

Fibrin/fibrinogen split products (FSPs, also known as fibrin/fibrinogen degradation products or FDPs) are generated when fibrinogen, soluble fibrin, or cross-linked fibrin is lysed by plasmin. Commercial latex agglutination kits enable rapid, semiquantitative FSP determination.[17] Elevated concentrations indicate increased fibrinolysis and/or fibrinogenolysis. Because clearance is by hepatic metabolism and the mononuclear phagocytic system, disorders of these systems also result in elevated FSP concentrations. FSPs can inhibit coagulation and induce platelet dysfunction, contributing to a bleeding tendency. Elevated FSP concentrations are commonly detected with disseminated intravascular coagulation (DIC) but are not specific for the condition; elevated concentrations are also described in dogs with thromboembolism (TE), neoplasia, immune-mediated hemolytic anemia (IMHA), hepatic dysfunction, neoplasia, sepsis and the systemic inflammatory response syndrome (SIRS), heat stroke, trauma, heart failure, and gastric-dilatation volvulus.[18]

D-dimers

D-dimer is a neo-epitope produced when soluble fibrin is cross-linked by fXIIIa. The D-dimer epitope is exposed by plasmin-induced cleavage of cross-linked fibrin. In contrast to other FSPs, which indicate only the activation of plasmin, D-dimers indicate the activation of thrombin and plasmin and are specific for active coagulation and fibrinolysis.[19,20] The half-life of D-dimers is short (approximately 5 hours); therefore elevated concentrations indicate recent or ongoing fibrinolysis.[20]

Several D-dimer assays have been validated in dogs, including the semiquantitative Accuclot D-dimer latex agglutination assay (Sigma Chemical), the immunometric POC NycoCard assay (Axis shield PoC), the Tina-Quant (a) immunoturbidometric D-dimer assay (Boehringer), and the canine-specific immunochromatographic AGEN canine D-dimer test (Sigma Chemical).[19,21-26] The latex agglutination test is validated for feline use.[19] Assay must be considered when interpreting results because methodologies are not comparable. Moreover, few human assays crossreact with canine or feline

D-dimer, so it is important to ensure that the test has been validated in the species.

D-dimers are a sensitive indicator of thrombotic conditions, such as disseminated intravascular coagulation (DIC) and thromboembolism (TE), and are more sensitive than are FSPs.[26] They have good negative predictive value, but the absence of elevated D-dimers does not preclude a diagnosis of DIC.[24] Conversely, elevated D-dimer concentrations are not specific; elevated concentrations are demonstrated in dogs with DIC, TE, neoplasia, hepatic disease, renal failure, cardiac failure, internal hemorrhage, and after surgical procedures.[19,24-26] D-dimers should be considered an ancillary diagnostic test; the diagnosis of DIC relies on the appropriate constellation of clinical findings and abnormal results of hemostatic testing. The diagnostic utility of D-dimers in cats remains uncertain. Specificity and sensitivity were low (56% and 67%, respectively) when cats with DIC were compared with cats with other conditions.[27]

Fibrinogen Concentration

Fibrinogen concentration is usually determined via the Clauss method, a functional assay based on the time for fibrin clot formation after the addition of excess thrombin.[28,29] Decreased concentrations (hypofibrinogenemia) can be inherited or acquired. Acquired disorders are described with hemodilution, massive transfusion, hepatic dysfunction, DIC, and sepsis and after thrombolytic therapy. Hypofibrinogenemia generally does not result in prolongation of standard coagulation tests (PT, aPTT) until fibrinogen is markedly decreased (less than 50 to 100 mg/dl).

Thrombin Time

The thrombin time (TT) tests functional fibrinogen, via measure of the time taken for a standardized thrombin solution to convert fibrinogen to fibrin.[30] The TT is prolonged with hypofibrinogenemia, dysfibrinogenemia, or in the presence of factors that inhibit fibrin polymerization (e.g., heparin, FSPs).

Thromboelastography and Thromboelastometry

Thromboelastography (TEG) and thromboelastometry (TEM) enable point-of-care global assessment of hemostasis in whole blood. The viscoelastic properties of the blood clot are evaluated, from initiation of coagulation, through amplification and propagation, to fibrinolysis.[31] Information is generated regarding the strength and stability of the clot and the dynamics of its formation and breakdown. Compared with routine hemostatic tests, these methodologies provide global assessment of hemostasis as determined by the interplay of plasma and cellular components, more closely reflecting in vivo hemostasis.[31]

The thromboelastograph (Haemoscope Corporation, Niles, IL) consists of a plastic cup and a pin suspended by a torsion wire.[32,33] A sample of citrated blood is placed in the cup with calcium chloride (at 37° C), and the cup is elevated so that the pin hangs in the sample. The cup is then oscillated around the vertical axis. When fibrin strands form between the pin and the cup, the torque generated is transmitted to a transducer, which converts the signal data for computer display of the TEG tracing (Figure 105-3). Testing is routinely performed 30 minutes after sampling. Reliable and reproducible results also can be obtained at 120 minutes, but results are statistically different from 30 minutes.[33]

TEG generates several parameters.[32,34] The reaction time (R) represents the enzymatic portion of coagulation (secondary hemostasis). The clotting time (K) represents clot kinetics, largely determined by clotting factors, fibrinogen, and platelets. The angle (α) depends largely on fibrinogen, as well as platelets and factors. The maximum amplitude (MA) represents the ultimate strength of the fibrin clot, dependent primarily on platelet aggregation (platelet number and function) and, to a lesser extent, fibrinogen. MA is used to derive the clot shear elastic modulus G, where

$$G = 5000 \times MA/(100 - MA)$$

and is a measure of the overall coagulant status. Fibrinolysis is measured by the extent of clot lysis at 30 and 60 minutes after MA (LY30 and LY60, respectively).

TEG has been demonstrated to reliably identify hypocoagulability and hypercoagulability in canine patients, using either native citrated samples or samples activated with recombinant human TF.[32,33,35-43] In a prospective study, TEG correctly identified bleeding, with a positive predictive value (PPV) of 89% and a negative predictive value (NPV) of 98%, based on G alone.[42] In contrast, the routine coagulogram had a PPV of 50% to 81% and a NPV of 92% to 93%. In human patients,

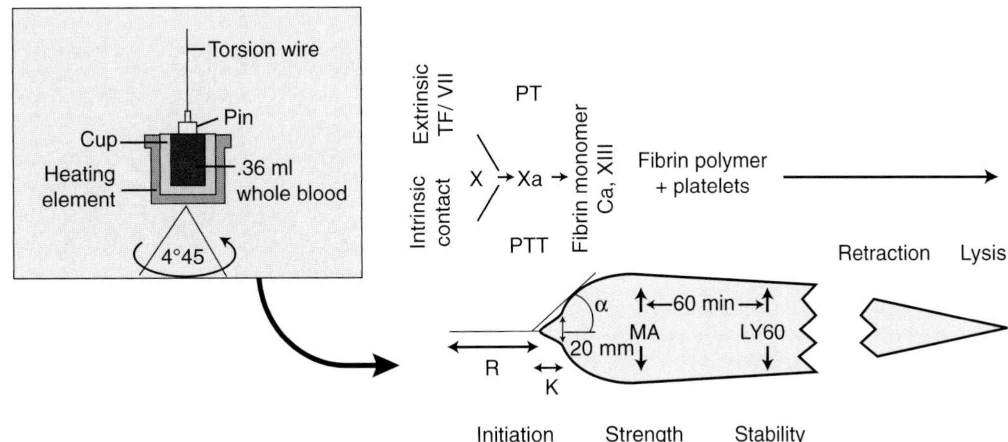

FIGURE 105-3 The thromboelastogram. The thromboelastography tracing (thromboelastogram) provides a visual representation of hemostasis. Reaction time *(R)* represents the time of latency from test initiation until beginning of fibrin formation, measured as an increase in amplitude of 2 mm. The clotting time *(K)* is the time to clot formation, measured from the end of R until an amplitude of 20 mm is reached. The angle *(α)* represents the rapidity of fibrin accumulation and cross-linking. Maximum amplitude *(MA)* represents clot strength. LY60 reflects fibrinolysis, determined by the percentage decrease in amplitude 60 minutes after MA. *(From Hackner SG, White CR: Bleeding and hemostasis. In Tobias KM, Johnston SA, editors: Veterinary surgery small animal, St Louis, 2012, Elsevier, p 100.)*

BOX 105-1 ***Disorders of Primary Hemostasis***

Thrombocytopenia

Decreased production

- Drug-induced disorders
- Immune-mediated megakaryocytic hypoplasia
- Viral (FeLV, FIV)
- Chronic rickettsial disease (ehrlichiosis)
- Estrogen-secreting neoplasm
- Myelodysplasia
- Megakaryocytic leukemia
- Cyclic thrombocytopenia *(Anaplasma platys)*
- Radiation
- Idiopathic bone marrow aplasia
- Postvaccination

Increased Destruction

- Immune-mediated thrombocytopenia (ITP)
  - Primary
    - Idiopathic
    - Evan's syndrome (ITP and IMHA)
    - Systemic lupus erythematosus (SLE)
  - Secondary
    - Drugs
    - Live virus vaccination
    - Tick-borne disease
    - Neoplasia
    - Bacterial infection
- Nonimmune disorders
  - Drug-induced
  - Ehrlichiosis
  - Rocky Mountain spotted fever
  - Dirofilariasis

Consumption and/or Sequestration

- Disseminated intravascular coagulation
- Microangiopathies
- Splenic torsion, hypersplenism
- Sepsis
- Hepatic disease
- Severe acute hemorrhage
- Severe hypothermia
- Hemolytic uremic syndrome

Nonpathologic

- Inherited macrothrombocytopenia (Cavalier King Charles Spaniel)

Thrombopathia

Acquired

- Drugs
  - NSAIDs (aspirin, non-aspirin)
  - Antibiotics (carbenicillin, cephalothin, moxalactam, sulfonamides)
  - Cardiac, respiratory drugs (calcium channel blockers, methylxanthines, β-blockers)
  - Miscellaneous (barbiturates, heparin, hydroxyethyl starch)
- Uremia
- Anemia
- Hepatic disease
- Hypothermia
- Colloid hemodilution
- Myeloproliferative disorders and paraproteinemias
- Ehrlichiosis
- Snake venom
- DIC

Inherited

- Von Willebrand disease (many dog breeds, rare in cats)
- Signal transduction disorders (Basset Hound, Eskimo Spitz)
- Glanzmann's thrombasthenia (Otterhound, Great Pyrenees)
- Chediak-Higashi syndrome (grey Persian cats)
- Selective ADP deficiency (American Cocker Spaniel)
- Cyclic hematopoiesis (grey Collie)
- Procoagulant expression disorders, Scott syndrome (German Shepherd dog)
- Macrothrombocytopenia (Cavalier King Charles Spaniel)

Vascular Disorders

Acquired

- Vasculitis
- Hyperadrenocorticism
- Atherosclerosis

Inherited

- Ehlers-Danlos syndrome

FeLV, Feline leukemia virus; *IMHA,* immune-mediated hemolytic anemia; *ITP,* immune-mediated thrombocytopenia; *NSAID,* nonsteroidal antiinflammatory drug.

TEG has shown clinical utility in predicting bleeding and guiding transfusion therapy.[44-47] These applications have yet to be evaluated further in small animals. The usefulness of TEG in veterinary practice is limited by the few institutions that have the technology, and the need to run tests within a short, finite period after sampling.

Similar to TEG, ROTEM (PentaPharm, Munich, Germany) provides information on initial fibrin formation (clotting time, CT), kinetics of fibrin formation (clotting formation time, CFT; angle, α), maximum fibrin clot strength (maximum clot firmness, MCF), and clot lysis at 30 and 60 minutes (CL30 and CL60).[48]

Limitations of TEG and ROTEM are the inability to detect vWD and insensitivity to antiplatelet drugs. The methodologies are also affected by blood viscosity; polycythemia results in hypocoagulable tracings and anemia produces hypercoagulable tracings.[49,50]

ETIOLOGY

Bleeding disorders are classified as disorders of primary or secondary hemostasis, or both, based on the pathophysiology of the hemostatic defect. Disorders of primary hemostasis result from decreased circulating platelet numbers (thrombocytopenia), from platelet dysfunction (thrombopathia) or, rarely, from a vascular anomaly (vasculopathy) (Box 105-1). Disorders of secondary hemostasis result from low concentration or activity of coagulation factors (Box 105-2). Inherited disorders are almost invariably a single defect in the hemostatic mechanism. Acquired disorders, which are more common, frequently affect more than one aspect of hemostasis. Disorders of fibrinolysis (hyperfibrinolysis) can also cause, or contribute to, clinical bleeding. Hyperfibrinolysis is demonstrated in DIC and in massive trauma and is suspected to be the primary mechanism of delayed postoperative bleeding in Greyhound dogs.

HYPOCOAGULABILITY IN THE CRITICALLY ILL OR INJURED PATIENT

Coagulation anomalies, ranging from isolated thrombocytopenia or prolonged coagulation times to complex derangements, are relatively common in critically ill patients. Thrombocytopenia is a frequent finding in human ICU patients; some degree of thrombocytopenia occurs in 35% to 44% of patients, and 12% to 15% have severe

BOX 105-2 ***Disorders of Secondary Hemostasis***

Acquired

- Vitamin K deficiency
- Hepatic failure
- Disseminated intravascular coagulation
- Pharmacologic anticoagulants
- Hemodilution (dilutional coagulopathy)
- Severe hypothermia
- Acidemia
- Shock
- Massive trauma (Acute Coagulopathy of Shock-Trauma)

Inherited Factor Deficiencies

- I: Hypofibrinogenemia and dysfibrinogenemia (Bernese, Borzoi, Lhasa Apso, Vizsla, Saint Bernard, other dog breeds)
- II: Hypoprothrombinemia (Boxer, Otter Hound, English Cocker Spaniel)
- VII: Hypoproconvertinemia (Beagle, Malamute, Boxer, Bulldog, Miniature Schnauzer, mixed breed dogs)
- VIII: Hemophilia A (German Shepherd, other dog breeds, mixed breed dogs, cats)
- IX: Hemophilia B (numerous dog breeds, cats)
- X: Stuart-Prower trait (American Cocker Spaniel, Jack Russell Terrier, mixed breed dogs)
- XI: Plasma thromboplastin antecedent deficiency (English Springer Spaniel, Kerry Blue Terrier, Great Pyrenees)
- Vitamin K-dependent factor deficiency (Devon Rex cats)
- Prekallikrein deficiency (several dog breeds)

Nonpathologic

- XII: Hageman factor deficiency (Miniature Poodle, Standard Poodle, German Shorthair Pointer, Shar Pei, cats)

thrombocytopenia (less than 50,000/μl).[51,52] New-onset thrombocytopenia is an independent predictor of ICU mortality, and the severity of thrombocytopenia and the extent of decrease in platelet count are inversely related to survival.[51-55] The prognostic implications of thrombocytopenia in critical small animals patients have yet to be determined.

Many critical patients have underlying conditions that can result in hypocoagulability, either directly (such as hepatic disease) or by inducing DIC (such as sepsis, SIRS, or neoplasia). An acute trauma-induced coagulopathy associated with massive trauma or surgery is also described (see Specific Conditions). Moreover, a host of secondary factors in the critical ill or injured patient can cause or contribute to a bleeding tendency. These factors include hemodilution, hypothermia, and acidemia.

Dilutional Coagulopathy

Dilutional coagulopathy refers to the syndrome resulting from blood loss, consumption of coagulation factors and platelets, and intravascular volume replacement. During hypovolemic shock, reduced intravascular hydrostatic pressure results in shifts of coagulation factor-deficient interstitial fluids into the plasma. This is compounded by aggressive resuscitation with IV fluids and/or massive red blood cell transfusion and further exacerbated by synthetic colloids, particularly hydroxyethyl starches (e.g., hetastarch).[56-58] (The term *massive transfusion* is defined as the transfusion of blood components that is greater than the patient's blood volume within a 24-hour period, or the transfusion of half the blood volume within 3 hours.)[59] Studies in humans have found that 40% to 60% hemodilution is required to produce a coagulopathy and that coagulopathy increases with increasing volumes of intravenous fluid administration.[56] The incidence of coagulopathy is more than 40% in human patients receiving 2 L of crystalloid fluids, more than 50% in patients receiving 3 L of fluids, and more than 70% in patients receiving 4 L of fluids.[60]

The mechanisms of dilutional coagulopathy are multiple. Fibrinogen is the first factor to become critically reduced.[61] Fibrinogen is required in substantially higher concentrations than other factors, but the limited increase in synthesis cannot compensate for increased breakdown.[62] The resultant hypofibrinogenemia decreases thrombin formation and fibrin polymerization, decreasing the speed, strength, and stability of clot formation.[61] This effect is seen with even moderate blood loss and hemodilution. The magnitude of effect is determined by the severity of the hypofibrinogenemia and the type of resuscitative fluid used. At fibrinogen levels below 50 mg/dl no clot is formed; clot formation occurs almost linearly up to 300 mg/dl.[63] Hetastarch demonstrates the most pronounced hemodilution effects because it also affects vWF and fVIII.[61,64,65]

Thrombocytopenia and the dilution of coagulation factors affect coagulation at a later point in resuscitation than does hypofibrinogenemia. After replacement of one blood volume of platelet-deficient fluid, only 35% to 40% of platelets remain in the circulation.[66] In the patient with a normal platelet count before resuscitation, this dilution may not be clinically significant. In 15 massively transfused dogs, moderate thrombocytopenia was recorded in all dogs in which platelet counts were measured, but none developed counts below 50,000/μl.[67] Prolongation of PT and aPTT occurs in human patients after replacement of two blood volumes.[68] Prolongations were demonstrated in 70% of dogs after massive transfusion, but a correlation to transfused volumes was not made.[67]

Fibrinolysis is affected by hemodilution. Progressive dilution of α_2-antiplasmin and fXIII reduces fibrin cross-linking and prolongs the half-life of plasmin.[69] Plasminogen activator inhibitor is also decreased, resulting in prolonged tPA activity.[70] The net result is enhanced fibrinolysis.

Hypothermia

Hypothermia, as results from hypoperfusion, evaporation from exposed body cavities during surgery, or the infusion of cold resuscitation fluids, leads to a reversible hypocoagulability. Platelets are extremely temperature sensitive. Evidence suggests that the bleeding tendency observed in humans at mildly reduced temperatures (33° to 37° C) results primarily from decreased vWF-mediated platelet adhesion.[71] At temperatures below 33° C, reduced platelet function and enzyme activity occur, with TF-fVIIa complex activity decreasing linearly.[71,72] Because conventional coagulation tests are performed at 37° C hypothermia-induced coagulopathy may be difficult to detect.[73]

Acidemia

Acidemia, as occurs with hypoperfusion or massive transfusion of CPDA-stored red cells, results in increased fibrinogen degradation and impaired coagulation protein activity.[74,75] fXa-Va complex activity is decreased by 50% at pH 7.2, and 70% at pH 7.0.[72] At a pH of 7.0, factor VIIa activity is also decreased by more than 90%.[72] The coagulopathy is not reversed with correction via buffer administration.[76]

DIAGNOSIS

A rapid and systematic diagnostic approach is paramount. The clinician should strive to answer three initial questions: (1) Does the patient have a bleeding disorder or is bleeding the result of local factors? (2) If the patient does have a bleeding disorder, what is the nature of the hemostatic defect: primary hemostasis, secondary hemostasis, fibrinolysis, or a combination of these? (3) Is the defect inherited or acquired? These questions usually can be answered easily based on information gleaned from the history, physical examination, and routine hemostatic testing.

History

The patient may present for bleeding that is evident to the owner, but this is not always the case.

Hemorrhage into the eyes, joints, lungs, or brain generally presents for signs related to these systems. Acute severe hemorrhage into the gastrointestinal tract or a body cavity can result in hypovolemia, whereas slower hemorrhage may result only in signs related to anemia.

The signalment of the patient can be informative. Severe inherited disorders are generally apparent within the first 6 months of life. Milder forms, such as vWD, may not be diagnosed until surgery, trauma, or concurrent disease intervenes. A history of repeated bleeding episodes suggests an inherited disorder.

The owner should be purposefully questioned regarding any evidence of bleeding in more than one site, suggesting a bleeding disorder. The clinician should try to determine whether bleeding episodes occurred spontaneously or were precipitated by injury or surgery. Some inherited disorders (e.g., hemophilia) and many acquired disorders (e.g., thrombocytopenia, vitamin K deficiency) produce spontaneous bleeding, whereas other conditions (e.g., vWD, factor VII deficiency, fibrinolytic disorders) more commonly require some form of trauma to make the impairment apparent. The patient's response to prior trauma or surgery may allow the clinician to date the onset of the disorder; a patient that has tolerated surgery is unlikely to have a severe inherited bleeding disorder.

The history should include specific enquiries about current and previous illnesses and medications (prescription and over-the-counter), as well as the environment and patient behavior that may reveal the potential of exposure to infectious agents, toxins, or trauma. Where possible, information should be sought concerning family members and their current medications.

Physical Examination

Evaluation of the distribution and extent of hemorrhage requires careful examination of all body systems including the skin, mucous membranes, eyes, and joints, as well as the urine and feces. The presence of hemorrhage in more than one site is suggestive of a bleeding disorder, but single-site hemorrhage does not exclude this possibility. With spontaneous hemorrhage, the nature of the bleeding may help to characterize the hemostatic defect. Defects of primary hemostasis are characterized by ecchymosis and/or spontaneous bleeding from mucosal surfaces (e.g., epistaxis, gingival bleeding, hyphema, hematuria, melena). Petechiae are typical of thrombocytopenia rather than thrombopathia.[77] Defects of secondary hemostasis are usually characterized by single or multiple hematomas and bleeding into subcutaneous tissue, body cavities, muscles, or joints. Some acquired disorders, such as DIC, defy this classification because multiple hemostatic defects are present. vWD usually has the characteristics of a primary hemostatic defect but, in its most severe form, may mimic a secondary hemostatic disorder.

Physical examination also should be aimed at seeking evidence of an underlying disease that can be associated with a bleeding disorder (e.g., hepatopathy, neoplasia, immune-mediated disease). The presence of shock or hypothermia should raise suspicion that these may be contributing to a bleeding diathesis.

Hemostatic Testing

Laboratory tests are essential to confirm and characterize the hemostatic defect. An initial diagnostic panel should include, at minimum, platelet enumeration/estimation, PT, and aPTT. D-dimer (or FSP) and fibrinogen concentrations are also recommended. This testing is generally sufficient to confirm a hemostatic defect and to characterize the defect as a disorder of primary hemostasis, secondary hemostasis, or both. With characterization of the hemostatic defects, a concise list of differential diagnoses can be constructed (see Boxes 105-1 and 105-2) and further diagnostic workup efficiently pursued (see Specific Conditions).

PRINCIPLES OF MANAGEMENT

The basic principles of management are as follows:

1. Recognize and treat shock and any other life-threatening conditions.
2. Control local bleeding, if possible.
3. Restore normal hemostasis via blood product transfusion, medications, reversal of hypothermia, and/or control of other precipitating or contributing factors.
4. Monitor for stability of coagulation parameters; correct as needed.
5. Monitor for new or ongoing sources of blood loss.
6. Monitor for complications associated with new or ongoing blood loss (e.g., intrapulmonary hemorrhage).

The early recognition and arrest of shock is a management priority. Because shock and fluid resuscitation can exacerbate coagulopathy, all attempts should be made to limit the duration of shock and to aggressively correct the coagulopathy while reducing hypoperfusion, hemodilution, and hypothermia. Recent management paradigms in human patients include permissive hypotension and the early use of plasma products (see Trauma-Induced Coagulopathy). Local causes of bleeding should be addressed as soon as possible. In the case of postsurgical bleeding, urgent reexploration is indicated if operative events or postoperative imaging suggests that a technical cause is plausible. Reexploration is essential if appropriate coagulation testing fails to reveal a coagulopathy, or if bleeding continues after reversal of hemostatic defects.

Restoration of normal hemostasis is an important goal of management. Directed therapy via medications and/or blood products depends on the cause (see Specific Conditions). Where a specific cause has not yet been established, characterization of the hemostatic defect guides transfusion. Aggressive rewarming measures should be employed to correct and limit hypothermia, including warm air blankets and the use of warmed IV fluids and blood products. The acid-base and electrolyte status should be closely monitored and abnormalities addressed. Where above measures fail to correct bleeding, the use of prohemostatic agents may be considered.

The hemostatic derangements that occur in critically ill or injured patients can change rapidly relating to either disease progression or intervention. The dynamic nature of these patients underscores the importance of vigilant monitoring and periodic reassessment.

Plasma and Platelet transfusion

Blood components and transfusion principles are addressed in Chapters 61 and 62.

Fresh frozen plasma (FFP) is most commonly used in veterinary practice. It contains hemostatic factors equivalent to the plasma from which it was obtained and is indicated for the treatment and prevention of bleeding associated with acquired and inherited disorders of secondary hemostasis. An exception is heparin-induced bleeding, because the hemorrhagic diathesis is caused by factor inhibition, not deficiency; moreover, antithrombin in FFP may enhance heparin effects. Cryoprecipitate (CP) is prepared from FFP and contains fVII, vWF, fibrinogen, and fibronectin in 10% of the original plasma volume.[78] CP is indicated for the management of patients with vWD, factor VII deficiency, hypofibrinogenemia, and dysfibrinogenemia. Strong evidence in human patients indicates a beneficial role of CP in the management of dilutional coagulopathy and trauma-induced coagulopathy (see Trauma-Induced Coagulopathy).

Platelet transfusion poses many challenges in veterinary practice. Short shelf-lives and an inability to administer sufficient platelet numbers to meet the patient's needs are major difficulties encountered. Because the use of platelet-rich plasma (PRP) and platelet concentrate (PC) is limited primarily to institutions where they are produced, fresh whole blood (FWB) remains the primary means of platelet transfusion in veterinary practice. Preserved platelet products have been developed to provide extended storage and immediate availability for transfusion. Cryopreserved platelets (in DMSO) are commercially available for dogs.[79] In spite of demonstrated in vitro platelet function and reduced in vivo recovery and half-life, evidence indicates that cryopreserved platelets retain the ability to become activated and survive in the circulation for sufficient time (approximately 2 days) to be of clinical benefit.[79-81]

Platelet transfusion in veterinary medicine is usually therapeutic, indicated for the management of uncontrolled or life-threatening bleeding resulting from severe thrombocytopenia or thrombopathia. Even with immune-mediated thrombocytopenia (ITP), in which transfused platelets are rapidly destroyed, a negligible increase in platelet count may provide adequate, life-saving hemostasis.[82] Prophylactic platelet transfusions should be considered in dogs with severe thrombocytopenia or thrombopathia before surgery. Human recommendations are a platelet trigger of 5,000 to 10,000 cells/µl if the patient is not bleeding and not undergoing an invasive procedure and 50,000 cells/µl if the patient is to undergo surgery.[83,84] The efficacy of platelet transfusion should be assessed by measurement of platelet count 1 hour after transfusion. As with all blood products, the administration of platelet products or FWB may be associated with adverse events; general guidelines for transfusion compatibility and monitoring apply.

Prohemostatic Agents

Desmopressin

Desmopressin (de-amino D-arginine vasopressin, DDAVP) is a synthetic vasopressin analog that induces, via V2 receptors, the release of subendothelial vWF stores (see Chapter 158).[85] DDAVP is used for the management of thrombopathia of various causes in humans.[86] In dogs, DDAVP is used as adjunctive treatment of bleeding associated with canine type 1 vWD, as well as for presurgical prophylaxis (administered 30 minutes before surgery). The successful use of IV DDAVP has been described in dogs to reverse aspirin-induced BMBT prolongation.[87] Injectable or intranasal DDAVP is administered at 1 to 4 mcg/kg SC or IV.[88,89] Onset of action is delayed approximately 30 minutes, and duration of effect is usually 2 hours. The effects of repeated doses are diminished because vWF stores are depleted. The efficacy of DDAVP is variable and its effects short-lived; the patient should be closely monitored and blood products made available.

Antifibrinolytics

Aprotinin, are clinically used antifibrinolytics. Aprotinin directly inhibits plasmin and contributes to platelet function.[85] Epsilon-aminocaproic acid (EACA) and tranexamic acid (TEA) are lysine analogs; they block the binding and activation of plasminogen and also exert antiinflammatory effects through interleukin inhibition.[85] TEA is approximately 10 times more potent than EACA. These agents, particularly aprotinin, have been used widely in human medicine, with demonstrated efficacy in decreasing blood loss and reducing transfusion requirements.[90,91] However, concerns regarding the safety of aprotinin have resulted in the suspension of its clinical use.[92,93] TEA and EACA appear to have comparable efficacy with minimal risk of adverse events.[90,91]

EACA neutralizes experimentally induced hyperfibrinolysis in dogs and has a wide therapeutic index.[94-96] However, the precise clinical application in small animals remains to be determined. EACA has been shown to reduce postoperative bleeding in Greyhound dogs when administered preemptively at 15 to 40 mg/kg q8h (see Delayed Postoperative Bleeding of Greyhound dogs).[98,99] Its use in other bleeding conditions has not been described.

SPECIFIC CONDITIONS

Thrombocytopenia

Thrombocytopenia is the most common primary hemostatic defect, resulting from decreased platelet production, increased destruction, or increased platelet consumption/sequestration (see Box 105-1). Thrombocytopenia is confirmed by a low platelet count, verified by blood smear examination. The bleeding threshold is not predictable from the count alone and depends on factors such as platelet function, secondary hemostasis, and the presence of precipitating trauma. Spontaneous bleeding generally does not occur until platelet counts fall below 30,000 to 50,000/µl, unless a concomitant bleeding disorder exists. In the patient with spontaneous bleeding, a platelet count of more than 50,000/µl should prompt investigation for another contributing hemostatic defect. Platelet counts as low as 5000/µl can occur without bleeding.[97] Patients with ITP tend to bleed less than patients with equivalent counts from other causes because of the presence of young, hyperfunctional platelets.[100,101] Thrombocytopenia associated with splenic torsion, although it can be profound, is not associated with bleeding.[102] Nonpathologic thrombocytopenia is reported in Cavalier King Charles Spaniels and Greyhound dogs and should not be overinterpreted.[103]

The diagnosis and management of thrombocytopenia is detailed in Chapter 106.

Thrombopathia

Vascular disorders are an uncommon cause of bleeding. In the patient with a primary hemostatic disorder and adequate platelet numbers, a platelet function defect is likely. A prolonged BMBT in a patient with adequate platelet count confirms thrombopathia. The drug history should be carefully appraised because numerous drugs can cause or contribute to thrombopathia.[70,104] Diseases known to affect platelet function should be excluded (see Box 105-1). If no obvious cause of acquired thrombopathia can be found, a hereditary disorder is suspected. The diagnosis and management of thrombopathia is detailed in Chapter 107.

Inherited Coagulopathies

Inherited deficiencies of all coagulation factors are reported, usually involving a single factor. A rare combined deficiency of vitamin K–dependent coagulation factors (II, VII, IX, X) has been described in Devon Rex cats.[105] Most inherited coagulopathies cause bleeding within the first year of life. Mildly affected animals, and those with factor VII deficiency, may not bleed until later in life, particularly if they do not undergo surgery or trauma.[106]

Inherited coagulopathies should be suspected in younger animals, breeds associated with factor deficiencies, and animals with a history of recurrent bleeding, and if acquired causes are ruled out or deemed unlikely. A deficiency of factor VII prolongs only the PT, whereas factor VIII and IX deficiencies (hemophilia A and B) cause prolongation of the PTT. Both parameters are prolonged with deficiencies of factors I, II, or X, and with inherited vitamin-K dependent factor deficiency. Diagnostic confirmation requires specific factor assays.

The management of patients with inherited coagulopathies adheres to general principles of bleeding control. If bleeding is severe or unrelenting, factors can be provided via transfusion of plasma products. Cryoprecipitate is ideal for deficiencies of factors VIII and fibrinogen, whereas cryosupernatant is indicated for deficiencies of factors II, VII, IX, X, and XI.[106,107] Where these products are not available, fresh frozen plasma is an acceptable option.

Factor XII deficiency is an asymptomatic condition of dogs and cats. It is the most common factor deficiency in cats, with a reported prevalence of 2.1%.[108] Because fXII is involved in contact factor activation but is not essential for in vivo hemostasis, deficiency results in significant prolongation of the aPTT but no hemorrhagic tendency. fXII deficiency is usually diagnosed incidentally and must be distinguished from pathologic causes of aPTT prolongation.

Vitamin K Deficiency

Vitamin K is required for the activation of factors II, VII, IX, and X; deficiency results in disordered secondary hemostasis. After activation of coagulation proteins, vitamin K is recycled via the enzyme, vitamin K epoxide reductase. An absolute or relative vitamin K deficiency occurs in several conditions.[109] Dietary insufficiency is rare but has been reported in neonates or with prolonged TPN administration. Broad-spectrum oral antimicrobial drugs can inhibit vitamin K synthesis. Decreased absorption can result from severe gastrointestinal disease, hepatopathy, pancreatic insufficiency, or biliary obstruction. Vitamin K antagonism occurs with warfarin therapy or anticoagulant rodenticide toxicity. These compounds inhibit vitamin K epoxide reductase, leading to a relative vitamin K deficiency.

Spontaneous bleeding is universal with anticoagulant rodenticide toxicity, whereas subclinical hemostatic defects are common with disease- or drug-related deficiency. PT prolongation occurs first, reflecting the short half-life of fVII (4 to 6 hours). Prolongation of the aPTT follows when other factors are depleted (approximately 2 days).[110] FSP, D-dimer, and fibrinogen concentrations are generally normal. The platelet count is usually normal but may be mildly to moderately decreased as a result of hemorrhage-related consumption. Diagnosis is based on the coagulogram anomalies, a history of toxin ingestion, drugs or disease that may be associated with deficiency, exclusion of other causes of a secondary hemostatic defect, and, in some cases, response to vitamin K supplementation. Testing for rodenticides or for proteins induced by vitamin K antagonism (PIVKA) may confirm an uncertain diagnosis.[109] Treatment of vitamin K deficiencies are covered in detail in Chapter 111.

Hepatic Failure

The liver plays a pivotal role in hemostasis by synthesizing clotting factors, coagulation inhibitors (antithrombin, protein C), and fibrinolytic proteins, as well as by clearing activated factors, enzyme-inhibitor complexes, and FSPs. Hepatic disease can result in complex and variably severe disorders of hemostasis; the spectrum of defects includes impaired factor synthesis, vitamin K deficiency, hyperfibrinolysis, thrombocytopenia, thrombopathia, and DIC (see Chapter 116).

Because of the large reserve capacity of the liver, decreased factor synthesis occurs only with significantly decreased functional hepatic mass (more than 70%), fVII showing earliest reduction.[109,111] Vitamin K deficiency, because of malabsorption of fat-soluble vitamins or biliary obstruction, can contribute.[111] Approximately 30% of human patients with cirrhosis have low-grade hyperfibrinolysis but an exaggerated response to surgery, leading to a burst of fibrinolytic activity and bleeding.[112] Thrombocytopenia can occur, primarily because of impaired hepatic synthesis of thrombopoietin.[109,111] Qualitative platelet defects have been attributed to decreased thromboxane synthesis as well as circulating inhibitors (FSPs).[111,113]

Up to 93% of dogs and 82% of cats with hepatic disease have some degree of hemostatic dysfunction.[114,115] Spontaneous hemorrhage occurs in less than 2%, but bleeding is common in response to a hemostatic challenge, such as surgery, liver biopsy, or gastrointestinal ulceration.[109,114,116,117] The myriad hemostatic anomalies vary with the severity of disease and the individual and cannot be predicted. In dogs with hepatic disease, 50% and 75% had an abnormal PT and aPTT, respectively.[117] In cats, PT prolongations were more common (73%).[115] Thrombocytopenia is reported uncommonly. In canine reports, the prevalence of thrombocytopenia is 0 to 10%, and platelet counts were significantly lower in dogs with chronic hepatitis and cirrhosis than those with other hepatopathies.[114,118,119] In 22 cats with hepatic disease, thrombocytopenia was reported in only one case.[115] Elevated FSP and D-dimer concentrations occur but are not invariably present and are usually not severe.[114,117] Severe hypofibrinogenemia is uncommon. DIC rarely occurs secondary to hepatic disease.[119] Because of the similar hemostatic defects and pattern of laboratory anomalies, distinguishing these conditions can be challenging. Fibrinogen levels tend to be lower, and D-dimer concentrations higher, in DIC compared with hepatic disease.[111]

Correction of hemostatic defects is indicated in patients who are actively bleeding or are to undergo an invasive procedure. Therapy should be tailored to the individual, based on serial hemostatic testing. Prolongation of coagulation times is an indication for FFP transfusion, directed at achieving hemostatically effective factor levels.[111] Although this is successful in most cases, the duration of effect is transient and repeated transfusion every 8 to 12 hours may be required. Because coagulation tests do not distinguish between vitamin K deficiency and coagulation factor deficiency, a vitamin K trial is valid, particularly in the patient with cholestatic disease.[109,111] Although this is rarely the primary cause of hepatic coagulopathy, a brief course (2 to 3 days) will exclude it as a contributing factor. Hyperfibrinolysis should be considered in the patient with unrelenting hemorrhage after correction of other measurable parameters. In human patients, antifibrinolytic agents are considered in selected patients unresponsive to other modalities and after the exclusion of DIC.[112] rFVIIa has been employed successfully with cirrhosis-associated bleeding.[120,121]

Trauma-Induced Coagulopathy

The syndrome of trauma-induced coagulopathy occurs in humans after massive trauma and hypovolemia and accounts for more than 50% of trauma-related deaths within the first 48 hours of admission.[122,122a,122b] Until recently, it was believed that traumatic coagulopathy, which invariably accompanies major hemorrhage, was a late consequence of hemodilution, acidemia, hypothermia, and loss of coagulation proteins through bleeding and consumption. The recent identification of an endogenous coagulopathy, occurring early in the clinical course, has led to the development of new resuscitation paradigms in human trauma and surgical patients.

Approximately 25% of severely injured patients are presented with a clinically significant coagulopathy that develops minutes after the initial traumatic insult.[123-125] This coagulopathy, termed the *acute coagulopathy of trauma and shock* (ACoTS), is associated with a fourfold increase in mortality.[60] Resuscitation-associated coagulopathy (RAC) develops later in the posttraumatic period secondary to hypothermia, worsening acidosis, and hemodilution resulting from the administration of intravenous fluids and/or blood transfusion.[122]

ACoTS is caused by tissue trauma, shock, sympathoadrenal activation, and inflammation.[126,127] Shock with tissue hypoperfusion appears to be the major driver of ACoTS, with the extent of hypoperfusion directly correlated with the degree of coagulopathy.[126,128] Higher injury severity increases the incidence and severity of coagulopathy in hypoperfused patients. Fibrinolysis is activated early after injury. Hypoperfusion is believed to result in increased expression of thrombomodulin on the surface of endothelial cells. The resultant increases in activated protein C (APC) inactivate fVIIa and fVa and promote fibrinolysis through the inhibition of plasminogen activator inhibitor-1 (PAI-1).[122,129] In addition, endothelial activation and injury lead to the release of tPA, endogenous heparinization from glycocalyx shedding, and increased vascular permeability. Recent studies show that fibrinogen concentrations are decreased in injured patients on admission, even preceding significant fluid resuscitation, and are associated with poor outcomes.[130-132]

RAC occurs in the period after injury, as a result of persistent hypothermia, acidemia, and hemodilution. These effects result in multiple hemostatic derangements that include hypofibrinogenemia, platelet dysfunction, thrombocytopenia, and decreased enzymatic activity (see Hypocoagulability in the Critically Ill or Injured Patient).

Diagnosis of trauma-induced coagulopathy is challenging. Traditional plasma-based coagulation tests, such as the PT and aPTT, do not accurately reflect the in vivo coagulopathy. The PT appears to be more sensitive than the aPTT in identifying enzymatic disorders in these patients, but these tests do not detect hyperfibrinolysis or platelet dysfunction and are not prolonged until fibrinogen falls to exceedingly low levels. However, viscoelastic testing (TEG and ROTEM) have proved superior in predicting coagulopathy and in guiding plasma and platelet transfusions.[122,133]

Recent understanding of the pathogenesis of trauma-induced coagulopathy has prompted revision of traditional resuscitation protocols in human trauma victims. Newer protocols, termed "damage control resuscitation," focus on the prevention of coagulopathy through permissive hypotension, limiting fluids, and delivering higher ratios of plasma and platelets.[122,134] The goal of permissive hypotension is to minimize dilutional coagulopathy secondary to fluid administration by maintaining a lower systemic blood pressure. In humans with penetrating injuries, maintaining a target mean arterial pressure (MAP) of 50 mm Hg, compared with 65 mm Hg, was associated with a decreased incidence of coagulopathy, decreased blood product use, and improved survival.[135] Intravascular volume support is achieved preferentially via red cell and FFP transfusion, with plasma administered as early as possible. Several studies have shown the clinical benefit of aggressive hemostatic resuscitation using the empiric transfusion ratio of FFP:RBC over 1:1.[133,136,137]

The administration of fibrinogen, via transfusion of CP or fibrinogen concentrate, has been shown to reverse the coagulopathy, to decrease transfusion requirements, and to improve survival of humans after massive trauma or surgery.[132,134,138-141] One unit of CP per 7 to 10 kg body weight is estimated to increase plasma fibrinogen by 50 mg/dl in the absence of bleeding.[65,69] No clear guidelines exist regarding a critical threshold for fibrinogen. Traditional transfusion algorithms do not treat fibrinogen levels unless they are less than 100 to 150 mg/dl, but studies have shown concentrations less than 200 mg/dl to be highly predictive for hemorrhage.[142] Current recommendations are that treatment decisions be based on TEG-determined clot strength, rather than fibrinogen concentrations.[61]

Trauma-induced coagulopathy is rarely reported in the veterinary literature.[142a] The recent prospective, multicenter observational study found that 15% of 40 dogs had acute traumatic coagulopathy within 12 hours of severe blunt or penetrating trauma; aPTT was the best indicator of nonsurvival. However, until more data are available, human medical experience may provide valuable diagnostic and treatment guidance. Namely, the veterinary clinician should be vigilant regarding coagulopathy after trauma or surgery with massive hemorrhage, anticipate a coagulopathy even in the absence PT and aPTT prolongation, and consider damage control resuscitation with the early transfusion of FFP and, possibly, CP. CP was reported to control bleeding in three dogs with hypocoagulable DIC and postoperative hemorrhage when administered at 50 to 70 ml/10 kg.[143]

Disseminated Intravascular Coagulation

DIC is characterized by the systemic activation of coagulation, leading to widespread microvascular thrombosis, which compromises organ perfusion and can contribute to organ failure.[144,145] The ongoing activation of coagulation may exhaust platelet and coagulation factors, resulting in a hypocoagulable state and bleeding. DIC invariably occurs as a complication of an underlying disorder; sepsis and the systemic inflammatory response syndrome (SIRS) are the most common causes in humans and dogs.[144-146] Clinical signs vary considerably and range from asymptomatic (nonovert DIC) to signs of organ failure associated with microvascular thrombosis to fulminant bleeding (overt DIC).[145,147] Bleeding occurs in a minority of patients with DIC; organ dysfunction is more common. Hemostatic evaluation via TEG showed that the majority of dogs with DIC were hypercoagulable; only 22% were hypocoagulable.[43] In a feline study, only 15% of cats with DIC had evidence of bleeding.[148] Bleeding tendencies reflect disorders of primary and/or secondary hemostasis and may manifest as prolonged bleeding from venipuncture sites, ecchymoses, epistaxis, hematoma formation, and/or gastrointestinal, urinary, or intracavitary hemorrhage.

The diagnosis of DIC can be challenging. DIC represents a dynamic continuum, and findings depend on where that patient lies on the continuum at that point in time. Moreover, hemostatic tests are not specific for DIC. Neither a gold standard nor consensus for the diagnosis of DIC exists in animals. Hemostatic tests are best evaluated together, and in light of clinical findings. Diagnosis is generally based on the presence of an underlying condition that could trigger DIC, together with three or more of the following anomalies: thrombocytopenia, prolongation of the PT, aPTT or TT, elevated D-dimers, hypofibrinogenemia, reduced antithrombin activity, and/or evidence of red blood cell fragmentation (schistocytes) on blood smear examination.[1,19,148,149] The International Society on Thrombosis and Hemostasis (ISTH) recommends a diagnostic scoring algorithm for human patients.[145,150] If the patient has underlying disease known to be associated with DIC, then routine hemostatic tests are assigned a score of 0 to 3 based on the extent of abnormality, and cumulative scores of 5 or greater are considered compatible with overt DIC. A prospective evaluation of this scoring system in ICU patients revealed high sensitivity and specificity and a strong correlation between an increasing DIC score and mortality. A similar scoring system has been developed and evaluated in dogs with DIC-associated conditions.[151] This model, which establishes a score based on PT, aPTT, fibrinogen, and D-dimers, was shown to have a good sensitivity and specificity, with positive and negative predictive values of approximately 80%. The diagnosis of DIC by routine laboratory testing is restricted to identification of the overt coagulopathic stage of the disease. TEG enables identification of the more common hypercoagulable phase. Differentiation between hypercoagulable and hypocoagulable patients has been demonstrated; higher mortality rates occur in hypocoagulable dogs.[43]

The diagnostics, pathophysiology, etiology, and management of DIC are detailed in Chapter 104.

Delayed Postoperative Bleeding in Greyhound Dogs

The prevalence of postoperative bleeding in Greyhound dogs far exceeds that of other breeds. Bleeding rates of 26% have been reported in Greyhounds after routine gonadectomy, compared with 0 to 2% in other dog breeds.[152-154] Bleeding is delayed 36 to 72 hours after surgery. In some dogs, bleeding progresses to a generalized bleeding disorder associated with clinical signs of illness, profuse widespread bleeding, mild thrombocytopenia, hemolysis, and increased hepatic and muscle enzyme activities. Hemorrhagic complications result in increased transfusion needs, hospital stays, and costs.

No significant differences have been identified between bleeders and nonbleeders with respect to platelet count, platelet function, PT, aPTT, fibrinogen concentration, D-dimer, factor XIII, and plasminogen. Antiplasmin and antithrombin activities have been shown to be significantly lower in dogs that bled compared with those that did not.[153] These findings, together with the delayed onset of the bleeding suggest anomaly of the fibrinolytic system or endothelial dysfunction, rather than a primary or secondary hemostatic disorder. In human patients, hyperfibrinolysis is suggested by decreased fibrinogen concentrations and elevated fibrin split products.[155] These have not been shown to occur in this population of Greyhound dogs, although some degree of enhanced fibrinolysis is suggested on TEG.[153]

Postoperative bleeding in Greyhound dogs is reduced by the prophylactic use of EACA. Dogs that did not receive preemptive EACA after limb amputation were 5.7 times more likely to bleed than dogs that did receive EACA.[98] Of 100 elective gonadectomies in retired racing Greyhound dogs, bleeding occurred in 30% of the placebo group compared with only 10% of the EACA group.[99] In both studies, EACA was administered at 500- to 1000-mg total dose (15 to 40 ml/kg) every 8 hours for 5 days, beginning immediately or soon after surgery. An increased likelihood of bleeding associated with body weight suggests that higher dose rates may be more effective.[99]

REFERENCES

1. Peterson JL, Couto CG, Wellman ML: Hemostatic disorders in cats: a retrospective study and review of the literature, J Vet Intern Med 9:298, 1995.
2. Furie B, Furie BC: Mechanisms of thrombus formation, N Engl J Med 359:938, 2008.
3. Davi G, Patrono C: Platelet activation and atherothrombosis, N Engl J Med 357:2482, 2007.
4. MacFarlane RG: An enzyme cascade in the blood clotting mechanism, and its function as a biologic amplifier, Nature 202:498, 1964.
5. Hoffman M, Monroe DM: A cell-based model of hemostasis, Thromb Haemost 85:958, 2001.
6. Roberts HR, Hoffman M, Monroe DM: A cell-based model of thrombin generation, Semin Thromb Hemost 32:32, 2006.
7. Herring J, McMichael M: Diagnostic approach to small animal bleeding disorders, Top Companion Anim Med 27:73, 2012.
8. Norman EJ, Barron RC, Nash AS, et al: Prevalence of low automated platelet counts in cats: comparison with prevalence of thrombocytopenia based on blood smear estimation, Vet Clin Pathol 30:137, 2001.
9. Knoll JS: Clinical automated haematology systems. In Feldman BF, Zinkl JG, Jain NJ, editors: Schalm's veterinary hematology, ed 5, Philadelphia, 2000, Lippincott Williams & Wilkins.
10. Séverine T, Cripps PJ, Mackin AJ: Estimation of platelet counts on feline blood smears, Vet Clin Pathol 28:42, 1999.
11. Brooks M, Catalfamo J: Buccal mucosal bleeding time is prolonged in canine models of primary hemostatic disorders, Thromb Haemost 70:777, 1993.
12. Jergens AE, Turrentine MA, Kraus KH, et al: Buccal mucosal bleeding times of healthy dogs and of dogs in various pathologic states, including thrombocytopenia, uremia, and von Willebrand's disease, Am J Vet Res 48:1337, 1987.
13. Sato I, Anderson GA, Parry BW: An interobserver and intraobserver study of buccal mucosal bleeding time in greyhounds, Res Vet Sci 68:41, 2000.
14. Lind SE: The bleeding time does not predict surgical bleeding, Blood 77:2547, 1991.
15. Angelos MG, Hamilton GC: Coagulation studies: prothrombin time, partial thromboplastin time, bleeding time, Emerg Med Clin North Am 4:95, 1986.
16. Tseng LW, Hughes D, Giger U: Evaluation of a point-of-care coagulation analyzer for measurement of prothrombin time, activated partial thromboplastin time, and activated clotting time in dogs, Am J Vet Res 62:1455, 2001.
17. Stokol T, Brooks M, Erb H, et al: Evaluation of kits for the detection of fibrin(ogen) degradation products in dogs, J Vet Intern Med 13:478, 1999.
18. Boisvert AM, Swenson CL, Haines CJ: Serum and plasma latex agglutination tests for detection of fibrin(ogen) degradation products in clinically ill dogs, Vet Clin Pathol 30:133, 2001.
19. Stokol T, Brooks MB, Erb HN, et al: D-dimer concentrations in healthy dogs and dogs with disseminated intravascular coagulation, Am J Vet Res 61:393, 2000.
20. Stokol T: Plasma D-dimer for the diagnosis of thromboembolic disorders in dogs, Vet Clin North Am Sm Anim Pract 33:1419, 2003.
21. Boutet P, Heath F, Archer J, et al: Comparison of quantitative immunoturbidometric and semiquantitative latex-agglutination assays for D-dimer measurement in canine plasma, Vet Clin Pathol 38:78, 2009.
22. Caldin M, Furlanello T, Lubas G: Validation of an immunoturbidometric D-dimer assay in canine citrated plasma, Vet Clin Pathol 29:51, 2000.
23. Dewhurst E, Cue S, Crawford E, et al: A retrospective study of canine D-dimer concentrations measured using an immunometric "point-of-care" test, J Small Anim Pract 49:344, 2008.
24. Griffin A, Callan MB, Shofer ES, et al: Evaluation of a canine D-dimer point-of-care test kit for use in samples obtained from dogs with disseminated intravascular coagulation, thromboembolic disease, and hemorrhage, Am J Vet Res 64:1562, 2003.
25. Lanevschi-Pietersma C, Bedard L, Kohlbrenner L: D-dimer, thrombin-antithrombin complex and fibrinogen degradation product levels measured in dogs with different systemic diseases, Vet Clin Pathol 32:225, 2003.
26. Nelson OL, Andreasen C: The utility of plasma D-dimer to identify thromboembolic disease in dogs, J Vet Intern Med 17:830, 2003.
27. Tholen I, Weingart C, Kohn B: Concentration of D-dimers in healthy cats and sick cats with and without disseminated intravascular coagulation, J Feline Med Surg 11:842, 2009.
28. Doolittle RF: Fibrinogen and fibrin, Sci Am 245:126, 1981.
29. Mosesson MW: The roles of fibrinogen and fibrin in hemostasis and thrombosis, Semin Hematol 29:177, 1992.
30. Palmer RL: Laboratory diagnosis of bleeding disorders: basic screening tests, Postgrad Med 76:137, 1984.
31. Mallet SV, Cox DJA: Thromboelastography, Br J Anaesth 69:307, 1992.
32. Donahue SM, Otto CM: Thromboelastography: a tool for measuring hypercoagulability, hypocoagulability, and fibrinolysis, J Vet Emerg Crit Care 15:9, 2005.
33. Wiinberg B, Jensen AL, Rojkjaer, et al: Validation of human recombinant tissue factor-activated thromboelastography on citrated whole blood from clinically healthy dogs, Vet Clin Pathol 34:389, 2005.
34. Traverso CI, Caprini JA, Arceles JI: Application of thromboelastography in other medical and surgical states, Semin Thromb Haemost 21:50, 1995.
35. Brainard BM, Meredith CP, Callan MB, et al: Changes in platelet function, hemostasis, and prostaglandin expression after treatment with nonsteroidal anti-inflammatory drugs with various cyclooxygenase selectivities in dogs, Am J Vet Res 68:251, 2007.
36. Couto CG, Lara A, Iazbik MC, et al: Evaluation of platelet aggregation using a point-of-care instrument in retired racing Greyhounds, J Vet Intern Med 20:365, 2006.
37. Kristensen AT, Wiinberg B, Jenssen LR, et al: Evaluation of human recombinant tissue factor-activated thromboelastography in 49 dogs with neoplasia, J Vet Intern Med 22:140, 2008.
38. Mischke R: Alterations of the global haemostatic function test "resonance thrombography" in spontaneously traumatized dogs, Pathophysiol Haemost Thromb 33:214, 2003.
39. Otto CM, Rieser TM, Brooks MB, et al: Evidence of hypercoagulability in dogs with parvoviral enteritis, J Am Vet Med Assoc 217:1500, 2000.
40. Vilar P, Couto CG, Westendorf N, et al: Thromboelastographic tracings in retired racing greyhounds and in non-greyhound dogs, J Vet Intern Med 22:374, 2008.

41. Wagg CR, Boysen SR, Bedard C: Thromboelastography in dogs admitted to an intensive care unit, Vet Clin Pathol 38:453, 2009.
42. Wiinberg B, Jensen AL, Rozanski E, et al: Tissue factor activated thromboelastography correlates to clinical signs of bleeding in dogs, Vet J 179:121, 2007.
43. Wiinberg B, Jensen AL, Johansson PI, et al: Thromboelastographic evaluation of hemostatic function in dogs with disseminated intravascular coagulation, J Vet Intern Med 22:357, 2008.
44. Ganter MT, Hofer CK: Coagulation monitoring: current techniques and clinical use of viscoelastic point-of-care coagulation devices, Anesth Analg 106:1366, 2008.
45. Johansson PI: Treatment of massively bleeding patients: introducing real-time monitoring, transfusion packages and thromboelastography (TEG), ISBT Science Series 2:159, 2007.
46. Bolliger D, Seeberger MD, Tanaka KA: Principles and practice of thromboelastography in clinical coagulation management and transfusion practice, Transfus Med Rev, 26:1, 2012.
47. Shore-Lesserson L, Manspeiser HE, DePerio M, et al: Thromboelastography-guided transfusion algorithm reduces transfusions in complex cardiac surgery, Anesth Analg 88:312, 1999.
48. McMichael MA, Smith SA: Viscoelastic coagulation testing: technology, applications, and limitations, Vet Clin Pathol 40:140, 2011.
49. Brooks AC, Guillaumin J, Cooper ES, et al: Effects of hematocrit and red blood cell-independent viscosity on canine thromboelastographic tracings, Transfusion epub, 2013.
50. Smith SA, McMichael M, Gilor S: Results of thromboelastometry on canine whole blood correlate with hematocrit, platelet concentration, and plasma coagulation factors, Am J Vet Res 73:789, 2009.
51. Levi M, Opal SM: Coagulation abnormalities in critically ill patients, Crit Care 10:222, 2006.
52. Strauss R, Wehler M, Mehler K, et al: Thrombocytopenia in patients in the medical intensive care unit: bleeding prevalence, transfusion requirements, and outcome, Crit Care Med 30:1765, 2002.
53. Ngyuyen TC, Carcillo JA: Bench-to-bedside review: thrombocytopenia-associated multiple organ failure—a newly appreciated syndrome in the critically ill, Crit Care 10:235, 2006.
54. Acka S, Haji MP, de Medonca A, et al: The time course of platelet counts in critically ill patients, Crit Care Med 30:753, 2002.
55. Vanderschueren S, De Weerdt A, Malbrain M, et al: Thrombocytopenia and prognosis in intensive care, Crit Care Med 28:1871, 2000.
56. Coats TJ, Brazil E, Heron M, et al: Impairment of coagulation by commonly used resus citation fluids in human volunteers, Emerg Med J 23:846, 2006.
57. Ho AM, Karmakar MK, Dion PW: Are we giving enough coagulation factors during major trauma resuscitation? Am J Surg 190:479, 2005.
58. Kheirabadi BS, Crissey JM, Deguzman R, et al: Effects of synthetic versus natural colloid resuscitation on inducing dilutional coagulopathy and increasing hemorrhage in rabbits, J Trauma 64:1218, 2008.
59. Holcomb JB, Wade CE, Michalek JE, et al: Increased plasma and platelet to red blood cell ratios improves outcome in 466 civilian trauma patients, Ann Surg 248:447, 2008.
60. Maegele M, Lefering R, Yucel N, et al: Early coagulopathy in multiple injury: an analysis from the German Trauma Registry of 8724 patients, Injury 38:298, 2007.
61. Mittermayr M, Streif W, Haas T, et al: Hemostatic changes after crystalloid or colloid administration during major orthopedic surgery: the role of fibrinogen administration, Anesth Analg 105:905, 2007.
62. Martini WZ, Chinkes DL, Pusateri AE, et al: Acute changes in fibrinogen metabolism and coagulation after hemorrhage in pigs, Am J Physiol Endocrinol Metab 289:E930, 2005.
63. Nielsen VG, Cohen BM, Cohen E: Effects of coagulation factor deficiency on plasma coagulation kinetics determined via thromboelastography: critical roles of fibrinogen and factors II, VII, X and XII, Acta Anaesthesiol Scand 49:222, 2005.
64. Brummel-Zieldins K, Whelihan MF, Zieldins EG, et al: The resuscitative fluid you choose may potentiate bleeding, J Trauma 61:1350, 2006.
65. Fenger-Eriksen C, Tonnesen E, Ingerslev J, et al: Mechanisms of hydroxyethyl starch induced dilutional coagulopathy, J Thromb Haemost 7:1099, 2009.
66. Marietta M, Facchini L, Pedrazzi P, et al: Pathophysiology of bleeding in surgery, Transplant Proc 38:812, 2006.
67. Jutkowitz LA, Rozanski EA, Moreau J, et al: Massive transfusion in dogs: 15 cases (1997-2002), J Am Vet Med Assoc 220:1664, 2002.
68. Miller RD, Robbins TO, Barton SL: Coagulation defects associated with massive transfusions, Ann Surg 174:794, 1971.
69. Bollinger D, Szlam F, Levy JH, et al: Haemodilution-induced profibrinolytic state is mitigated by fresh frozen plasma: implications for early haemostatic intervention in massive haemorrhage, Br J Anaesth 104:318, 2010.
70. Boudreaux MK: Acquired platelet dysfunction. In Feldman BF, Zinkl JG, Jain NC, editors: Schalm's veterinary hematology, ed 5, Philadelphia, 2000, Lippincott Williams & Wilkins.
71. Wolberg AS, Meng ZH, Monroe DM, et al: A systematic evaluation of the effect of temperature on coagulation enzyme activity and platelet function, J Trauma 56:1221, 2004.
72. Meng ZH, Wolberg AS, Monroe DM III, et al: The effect of temperature and pH on the activity of factor VIIa: implications for the efficacy of high-dose factor VIIa in hypothermic and acidotic patients J Trauma 55:886, 2003.
73. Zimmerman LH: Causes and consequences of critical bleeding and mechanisms of blood coagulation, Pharmacotherapy 27:45S, 2007.
74. Cosgriff N, Moore EE, Sauaia A, et al: Predicting life-threatening coagulopathy in the massively transfused trauma patient: hypothermia and acidosis revisited, J Trauma 58:1002, 1997.
75. Rutherford EJ, Morris JA, Reed GW, et al: Base deficit stratifies mortality and determines therapy, J Trauma 33:417, 1992.
76. Martini WZ, Dubick MA, Wade CE, et al: Does bicarbonate correct coagulation function impaired by acidosis in swine, J Trauma 61:99, 2006.
77. Nachman RL, Rafii S: Platelets, petechiae, and preservation of the vascular wall, N Engl J Med 359:1261, 2008.
78. Brooks M: Transfusion of plasma and plasma derivatives. In Feldman BF, Zinkl JG, Jain NC, editors: Schalm's veterinary hematology, ed 5, Philadelphia, 2000, Lippincott Williams and Wilkins.
79. Callan MB, Appleman EH, Sachais BS: Canine platelet transfusions, J Vet Emerg Crit Care 19:401, 2009.
80. Appleman EH, Sachaias BS, Patel R, et al: Cryopreservation of canine platelets, J Vet Intern Med 23:138, 2009.
81. Currie LM, Livesey SA, Harper JR, et al: Cryopreservation of single donor platelets with a reduced dimethyl sulfoxide concentration by the addition of second messenger effectors: enhanced retention of in vitro functional activity, Transfusion 38:160, 1998.
82. Carr JM, Kuskall MS, Kaye JA, et al: Efficacy of platelet transfusions in immune thrombocytopenia, Am J Pathol 80:1051, 1986.
83. Rebulla P, Finazzi G, Marangoni F, et al: The threshold for prophylactic platelet transfusions in adults with acute myeloid leukemia, N Engl J Med 337:1870, 1997.
84. Slichter SJ: Background, rationale, and design of a clinical trial to assess the effects of platelet dose on bleeding risk in thrombocytopenic patients, J Clin Apheresis 21:78, 2006.
85. Mannucci PM: Hemostatic drugs, N Engl J Med 339:245, 1998.
86. Despotis GJ, Levine V, Saleem R, et al: Use of point-of-care test in identification of patients who can benefit from desmopressin during cardiac surgery: a randomized controlled trial, Lancet 354:106, 1999.
87. Di Mauro FM, Holowaychuk MK: Intravenous administration of desmopressin acetate to reverse acetylsalicylic acid-induced coagulopathy in three dogs, J Vet Emerg Crit Care, 23:455, 2013.
88. Carr AP, Nibblett BM, Panciera DL: Von Willebrand's disease and other hereditary coagulopathies. In Bonagura JD, Twedt DC, editors: Kirk's current veterinary therapy, ed 14, St Louis, 2009, Saunders Elsevier.
89. Kraus KH, Turrentine MA, Jergens AE, et al: Effect of desmopressin acetate on bleeding times and plasma von Willebrand factor in Doberman pinchers with vWD, Vet Surg 18:103, 1989.
90. Henry D, Carless P, Fergusson D, et al: The safety of aprotinin and lysine-derived antifibrinolytic drugs in cardiac surgery: a meta-analysis, CMAJ 180:183, 2009.
91. Schouten ES, van de Pol AC, Schouten AN, et al: The effect of aprotinin, tranexamic acid, and aminocaproic acid on blood loss and use of blood

products in major pediatric surgery: a meta-analysis, Pediatr Crit Care Med 10:182, 2009.
92. Murkin JM: Lessons learned in antifibrinolytic therapy: the BART trial, Semin Cardiothorac Vasc Anesth 13:127, 2009.
93. Takagi H, Manabe H, Kawai N, et al: Aprotinin increases mortality as compared with tranexamic acid in cardiac surgery: a meta-analysis of randomized head-to-head trials, Interact Cardiovascul Thor Surg 9:98, 2009.
94. Belko JS, Warren R, Regan EE, et al: Induced fibrinolytic activity and hypofibrinogenemia—effect of epsilon-amino-caproic acid, Arch Surg 86:396, 1963.
95. Pokorny F: Toxicological experiments with cyclohexamine oxine, e caprolactein and e aminocaproic acid; mutual biological comparison, Sb Lek 54:28, 1952.
96. Sherry S, Fletcher A, Alkjaerisg N, et al: E-amino-caproic aci— "a potent antifibrinolytic agent," Trans Assoc Am Physicians 72:62, 1959.
97. Lewis DC, Myers KM: Canine idiopathic thrombocytopenic purpura, J Vet Intern Med 10:207, 1996.
98. Marín LM, Iazbik MC, Zaldivar-Lopez S, et al: Retrospective evaluation of the effectiveness of epsilon aminocaproic acid for the prevention of postamputation bleeding in retired racing Greyhounds with appendicular bone tumors: 46 cases (2003-2008), J Vet Emerg Crit Care 22:332, 2012.
99. Marín LM, Iazbik MC, Zaldivar-Lopez S, et al: Epsilon aminocaproic acid for the prevention of delayed postoperative bleeding in retired racing greyhounds undergoing gonadectomy, Vet Surg 41:594, 2012.
100. Abrams-Ogg ACG: Triggers for prophylactic use of platelet transfusions and optimal platelet dosing in thrombocytopenic dogs and cats, Vet Clin N Am Small Anim 33:1401, 2003.
101. Neel JA, Birkenheuer AJ, Grindem CB: Thrombocytopenia. In Bonagura JD, Twedt DC, editors: Kirk's current veterinary therapy, ed 14, St Louis, 2009, Saunders Elsevier.
102. Russell KE, Grindem CB: Secondary thrombocytopenia. In Feldman BF, Zinkl JG, Jain NC, editors: Schalm's veterinary hematology, ed 5, Philadelphia, 2000, Lippincott Williams and Wilkins.
103. Smedile LE, Houston DM, Taylor SM, et al: Idiopathic asymptomatic thrombocytopenia in Cavalier King Charles spaniels: 11 cases (1983-1993), J Am Anim Hosp Assoc 33:411, 1997.
104. Brooks MB, Catalfamo JL: Platelet dysfunction. In Bonagura JD, Twedt DC, editors: Kirk's current veterinary therapy, ed 14, St Louis, 2009, Saunders Elsevier.
105. Maddison JE, Watson AD, Eade IG, et al: Vitamin K-dependent multifactor coagulopathy in Devon Rex cats, J Am Vet Med Assoc 197:1495, 1990.
106. Dodds WJ: Other hereditary coagulopathies. In Feldman BF, Zinkl JG, Jain NJ, editors: Schalm's veterinary hematology, ed 5, Philadelphia, 2000, Lippincott Williams and Wilkins.
107. Mansell P: Hemophilia A and B. In Feldman BF, Zinkl JG, Jain NJ, editors: Schalm's veterinary hematology, ed 5, Philadelphia, 2000, Lippincott Williams and Wilkins.
108. Brooks M, Spagnoletti-DeWilde LS: Feline Factor XII deficiency, Comp Cont Ed 28:148, 2006.
109. Prater MR: Acquired coagulopathy II: liver disease. In Feldman BF, Zinkl JG, Jain NC, editors: Schalm's veterinary hematology, ed 5, Philadelphia, 2000, Lippincott Williams and Wilkins.
110. Mount M: Diagnosis and therapy of anticoagulant rodenticide intoxications, Vet Clin North Am Small Anim Pract 18:115, 1988.
111. Kujovich JL: Hemostatic defects in end stage liver disease, Crit Care Clin 21:563, 2005.
112. Hu KQ, Yu AS, Tiyyagura L, et al: Hyperfibrinolytic activity in hospitalized cirrhotic patients in a referral liver unit, Am J Gastroenterol 96:1581, 2001.
113. Willis SE, Jackson ML, Meric SM, et al: Whole blood platelet aggregation in dogs with liver disease, Am J Vet Res 50:1893, 1989.
114. Badylak SF, Dodds WJ, Van Vleet JF, et al: Plasma coagulation factor abnormalities in dogs with naturally occurring hepatic disease, Am J Vet Res 44:2336, 1983.
115. Lisciandro SC, Hohenhaus A, Brooks M: Coagulation abnormalities in 22 cats with naturally occurring liver disease, J Vet Intern Med 12:71, 1998.
116. Badylak SF: Coagulation disorders and liver disease, Vet Clin North Am Small Anim Pract 18:87, 1988.
117. Webster CL: History, clinical signs, and physical findings in hepatobiliary disease. In Ettinger SJ, Feldman EC, editors: Textbook of veterinary internal medicine, ed 6, St Louis, 2005, Elsevier Saunders.
118. Kummeling A, Teske E, Rothuizen J, et al: Coagulation profiles in dogs with congeital portosystemic shunts before and after surgical attenuation, J Vet Intern Med 20:1319, 2006.
119. Prins M, Schellens CJ, van Leeuwen MW, et al: Coagulation disorders in dogs with hepatic disease, Vet J 185:163, 2010.
120. Ejlersen E, Melsen T, Ingerslev J, et al: Recombinant activated factor VII (rFVIIa) acutely normalizes prothrombin time in patients with cirrhosis during bleeding from esophageal varices, Scand J Gastroenterol 36:1081, 2001.
121. Franchini M, Zaffanello M, Veneri D: Recombinant factor VIIa: an update on its clinical use, Thromb Haemost 93:1027, 2005.
122. Noel P, Cashen S, Patel B: Trauma-induced coagulopathy: from biology to therapy, Semin Hematol 50:259, 2013.
122a. Palmer L, Martin L: Traumatic coagulopathy. Part 1: Pathophysiology and diagnosis, J Vet Emerg Crit Care 24(1):63-74, 2014.
122b. Palmer L, Martin L: Traumatic coagulopathy. Part 2: Resuscitative strategies, J Vet Emerg Crit Care 24(1):75-92, 2014.
123. Brohi K, Singh J, Heron M, et al: Acute traumatic coagulopathy, J Trauma 54:1127, 2003.
124. Brohi K, Cohen MJ, Ganter MT, et al: Acute coagulopathy of trauma: hypoperfusion induces systemic anticoagulation and hyperfibrinolysis, J Trauma 64:1211, 2008.
125. Hess JR, Brohi K, Dutton RP, et al: The coagulopathy of trauma: a review of mechanisms, J Trauma 65:748, 2008.
126. Brohi K, Cohen MJ, Ganter MT, et al: Acute traumatic coagulopathy: initiated by hypoperfusion, modulated through the protein C pathway? Ann Surg 245:812, 2007.
127. Johansson PL, Stensballe J, Rasmussen LS, et al: A high admission syndecan-1 level, a marker of endothelial glycocalyx degradation, is associated with inflammation, protein C depletion, fibrinolysis, and increased mortality in trauma patients, Ann Surg 254:194, 2011.
128. Frith D, Brohi K: The acute coagulopathy of trauma shock: clinical relevance, Surgeon 8:159, 2010.
129. Anastasiou G, Gialeraki A, Merkouri E, et al: Thrombomodulin as a regulator of the anticoagulant pathway: implication in the development of thrombosis, Blood Coagul Fibrinolysis 23:1, 2012.
130. Frith D, Brohi K: The pathophysiology of trauma-induced coagulopathy, Curr Opin Crit Care 18:631, 2012.
131. Levy JH, Szlam F, Tanaka KA, et al: Fibrinogen and hemostasis: a primary hemostatic target for the management of acquired bleeding, Anesth Analg 114:261, 2012.
132. Rourke C, Curry N, Khan S, et al: Fibrinogen levels during trauma hemorrhage, response to replacement therapy, and association with patient outcomes, J Thromb Haemost 10:1342, 2012.
133. Holcomb JB, Minei KM, Scerbo ML, et al: Admission rapid thromboelastography can replace conventional coagulation tests in the emergency department, Ann Surg 256:476, 2012.
134. Bollinger D, Gorlinger K, Tanaka KA: Pathophysiology and treatment of coagulopathy in massive hemorrhage and hemodilution, Anesthesiology 113:1205, 2010.
135. Morrison CA, Carrick MM, Norman MA, et al: Hypotensive resuscitation strategy reduces transfusion requirements and severe postoperative coagulopathy in trauma patients with hemorrhagic shock: preliminary results of a randomized controlled trial, J Trauma 70:652, 2011.
136. Golzalez EA, Moore FA, Holcomb JB, et al: Fresh frozen plasma should be given earlier to patients requiring massive transfusion, J Trauma 62:112, 2007.
137. Shaz BH, Dente CJ, Nicholas J, et al: Increased number of coagulation products in relation to red blood cell products transfused improves mortality in trauma patients, Transfusion 50:493, 2009.
138. Stinger HK, Spinella PC, Perkins JG, et al: The ratio of fibrinogen to red cells transfused affects survival in casualties receiving massive transfusions at an army combat support hospital, J Trauma 64:S79, 2008.
139. Fenger-Eriksen C, Lindberg-Larsen M, Christensen AQ, et al: fibrinogen concentrate substitution therapy in patients with massive

hemorrhage and low plasma fibrinogen concentrations, Br J Anaesth 101:769, 2008.
140. Fenger-Eriksen C, Ingerslev J, Sorensen B: Fibrinogen concentrate—a potential universal hemostatic agent, Expert Opin Biol Ther 9:1325, 2009.
141. Fenger-Eriksen C, Jensen TM, Kristensen BS, et al: Fibrinogen substitution improves whole blood clot firmness after dilution with hydroxyethyl starch in bleeding patients undergoing radical cystectomy: a randomized, placebo-controlled trial, J Thromb Haemost 7:795, 2009.
142. Charbit B, Mandelbrot L, Samain E, et al: PPH study group: the decrease of fibrinogen is an early predictor of the severity of postpartum hemorrhage, J Thromb Haemost 5:266, 2007.
142a. Holowaychuk MK, Hanel RM, Wood RD, et al: Prospective multicenter evaluation of coagulation abnormalities in dogs following severe acute trauma, J Vet Emerg Crit Care 24(1):93-104, 2014.
143. Vilar P, Ball R, Westendorf N, et al: Hemostatic effects of cryoprecipitate in dogs with disseminated intravascular coagulation (abstract), J Vet Intern Med 23:692, 2009
144. Levi M: Disseminated intravascular coagulation, Crit Care Med 35:2191, 2007.
145. Taylor FB, Toh CH, Hoots WK, et al: Towards definition, clinical and laboratory criteria, and a scoring system for disseminated intravascular coagulation, Thromb Haemost 86:1327, 2001.
146. de Laforcade AA, Freeman LA, Shaw SP, et al: Hemostatic changes in dogs with naturally occurring sepsis, J Vet Intern Med 17:674, 2003.
147. Bick RL, Arun B, Frenkel EP: Disseminated intravascular coagulation: clinical and pathophysiologic mechanisms and manifestations, Haemostasis 29:111, 1999
148. Estrin MA, Wehausen CE, Jessen CR, et al: Disseminated intravascular coagulation in cats, J Vet Intern Med 20:1334, 2006.
149. Bateman SW, Mathews KA, Abrams-Ogg AC, et al: Diagnosis of disseminated intravascular coagulation in dogs admitted to an intensive care unit, J Am Vet Med Assoc 215:798, 1999.
150. Levi M, Toh CH, Thachil J, et al: Guidelines for the diagnosis and management of disseminated intravascular coagulation. British committee for standards in haematology, Br J Haematol 145:24, 2009.
151. Wiinberg B, Jensen AL, Johansson PI, et al: Development of a model based scoring system for diagnosis of canine disseminated intravascular coagulation with independent assessment of sensitivity and specificity, Vet J 185:292, 2010.
152. Burrow R, Batchelor D, Cripps P: Complications observed during and after ovariohysterectomy of 142 bitches at a veterinary teaching hospital, Vet Rec 157:829, 2005.
153. Lara-García A, Couto CG, Iazbik MC, et al: Postoperative bleeding in retired racing greyhounds, J Vet Intern Med 22:525, 2008.
154. Pollari F, Bonnett B, Bamsey S, et al: Postoperative complications of elective surgeries in dogs and cats determined by examining electronic and paper medical records, J Am Vet Med Assoc 208:1882, 1996.
155. Hunt BJ, Segal H: Hyperfibrinolysis, J Clin Pathol 49:958, 1996.

CHAPTER 106
THROMBOCYTOPENIA

Andrea Wang, DVM, MA, DACVIM • Benjamin M. Brainard, VMD, DACVAA, DACVECC

KEY POINTS

- Thrombocytopenia can occur by four general mechanisms: (1) decreased production of platelets, (2) consumption of circulating platelets, (3) sequestration of platelets, and (4) increased destruction of circulating platelets or megakaryocytes.
- Clinical bleeding may be seen at platelet counts less than 25,000 to 50,000/μl.
- Goals of treatment are to address underlying causes and ameliorate clinical signs related to thrombocytopenia.
- Transfusions containing platelets can be considered in animals with a platelet count less than 10,000/μl, thrombocytopenic animals that require surgery, and those with life-threatening clinical signs of thrombocytopenia.

Thrombocytopenia has been reported in 5.2% and 1.2% of the total dog and cat population, respectively, that are presented to a veterinary referral hospital. It is a far more common occurrence in critically ill patients.[1,2] Normal platelet count in small animals ranges between 200 and 800 × 10^9/L, with some variation between diagnostic laboratories.[3]

In human intensive care patients, thrombocytopenia has been associated with sepsis, neoplasia, and the acute respiratory distress syndrome (ARDS).[4] In addition, human patients may develop antibodies to unfractionated heparin bound to platelets that may result in severe thrombocytopenias (heparin-induced thrombocytopenia [HIT]) during hospitalization. HIT has not been reported in small animal veterinary medicine. Two other common causes for thrombocytopenia recognized in human ICUs are thrombocytic thrombocytopenic purpura and hemolytic uremic syndrome (the thrombotic microangiopathies), which have not been reported widely in veterinary medicine.[5,6]

In human medicine, thrombocytopenia has been associated with decreased survival in a mixed medical and surgical ICU population.[7] Similar findings were seen in a cohort of human patients with septic shock, in whom 55% of patients developed thrombocytopenia, and low platelet count was associated with higher SOFA (Sequential Organ Failure Assessment) score, vasopressor requirements, and mortality.[8] The presence of thrombocytopenia in veterinary medicine has been associated with decreased survival in patients with immune-mediated hemolytic anemia,[9] neoplasia,[10-12] and feline panleukopenia.[13]

CAUSES

In a population of thrombocytopenic dogs admitted to a teaching hospital, the underlying diseases identified included immune-mediated thrombocytopenia (5%); neoplasia-associated thrombocytopenia(13%); inflammatory or infectious causes (23%); and other causes or combined causes of thrombocytopenia (59%).[1] This general distribution was similar to other studies that have evaluated dogs with thrombocytopenia, with some variability in the number of cases with infectious disease.[14,15] A study of dogs with neoplasia of various cytologic origins documented a 10% incidence of thrombocytopenia; lymphoid neoplasia made up 29% of the cases, and carcinomas made up 28%.[16] Dogs with lymphoma, hemangiosarcoma, and melanoma were at an increased risk for development of thrombocytopenia, but this also may have been a result of cytotoxic therapy.[16] In 41 cats with thrombocytopenia presenting to a veterinary referral hospital, causes included infectious disease (29%), neoplasia (20%), cardiac disease (7%), and only one cat with primary immune-mediated disease; eight of the cats (20%) did not have a definitive diagnosis.[2] Thrombocytopenia characteristic of a consumptive coagulopathy secondary to inflammatory disease or neoplasia (i.e., vasculitis, disseminated intravascular coagulopathy [DIC]) has been reported in dogs and cats.[5,17]

Infectious causes of thrombocytopenia include tickborne infections such as Rocky Mountain spotted fever,[3] anaplasmosis,[18,19] babesiosis,[20,21] and ehrlichiosis.[22] Other commonly incriminated infectious causes include leishmaniasis,[23] leptospirosis,[24] heartworm disease,[3] feline immunodeficiency virus (FIV),[25,26] feline leukemia virus (FeLV),[2,26] feline infectious peritonitis (FIP), and sepsis. Systemic inflammatory diseases, including neoplasia and subsequent DIC, and systemic thrombosis can cause thrombocytopenia.[5,27] Immune-mediated mechanisms, in general, cause the most severe form of thrombocytopenia.[14,28] One study has identified platelet-bound antibodies in thrombocytopenic dogs with a multitude of underlying conditions, including infectious and neoplastic causes, pancreatitis, hepatitis, and SIRS. This suggests many conditions can cause immune-mediated destruction of circulating platelets.[29]

Clinically significant bleeding as a result of low platelet numbers can be observed when platelet count drops below 25 to 50 × 10^9/L.[30] Clinical signs of thrombocytopenia include petechiae and ecchymoses, frequently seen on oral mucous membranes, ear pinnae, or in the inguinal area. Mucosal bleeding is also common, causing epistaxis, hyphema, hematemesis, melena, hematochezia, and hematuria. Central nervous system signs resulting from cerebral and spinal cord bleeds may be seen, and prolonged bleeding or excessive bruising may follow venipuncture or trauma.

Thrombocytopenia in the Critically Ill

In critically ill human patients, thrombocytopenia has been associated with decreased survival; moreover, a decrease in platelet count, even if the platelet count remains within normal range, serves as an independent predictor of mortality.[7,31] Causes of thrombocytopenia in critically ill patients are multifaceted. Exclusion of the aforementioned mechanisms is imperative to initiate appropriate specific treatment (i.e., therapy for infectious diseases such as ehrlichiosis and dirofilariasis, or for inflammatory, DIC, or drug-induced causes). Many conditions that may cause a patient to need intensive care (e.g., those resulting in hypoxemia or hypotension) are associated with decreased oxygen delivery to tissues and inflammation, either as a trigger or consequence of physiologic instability. Prolonged clinical or subclinical inflammation may trigger coagulation responses, in particular DIC, so that even in the absence of an overt inflammatory condition, patients with critical illness can develop a consumptive coagulopathy and thrombocytopenias. Maintenance of vascular integrity in cases of inflammation and endothelial injury also may consume platelets and cause mild to moderate thrombocytopenias.[32]

DIAGNOSTIC TECHNIQUES FOR THROMBOCYTOPENIA

To confirm a diagnosis of thrombocytopenia, technical or laboratory error should be ruled out. A manual platelet count performed on a blood smear is an easy and cost-effective method to estimate platelet count. It is particularly useful in situations in which the clinician requires a quick platelet estimate before invasive procedures if an automated complete blood count is not immediately available, and to verify the accuracy of an automated platelet count. In particular, cats and dogs with inflammatory diseases tend to have platelets that form clumps (especially with traumatic venipuncture) and that may be miscounted by automated analyzers, resulting in a falsely lowered platelet count (Figure 106-1).[33] In addition, the large size of feline platelets may result in miscounting by automated impedance analyzers because of the overlap in size with feline red blood cells.[33]

On review of peripheral blood smears, a high-powered field (hpf, 100×) should contain 8 to 15 platelets, which corresponds to 120,000 to 225,000/µl (each platelet representing about 15,000/µl).[34] Evaluation of a blood smear also allows the clinician to evaluate platelet size, red blood cell number and morphology, and white blood cell number and distribution. The presence of large platelets (macrothrombocytes) may be supportive of increased production and generally reflect a regenerative response by the bone marrow when indexed to platelet count,[28,35] although some breeds have been described to have a nonclinical macrothrombocytopenia.[28,36]

Advanced testing, such as assays for reticulated platelets to assess thrombopoiesis, has been described in the literature but is currently available only using flow cytometry or certain automated analyzers.[37] Advanced hematology analyzers such as the Advia 120 (Bayer Healthcare, Shawnee Mission, KS generate additional platelet indices based on the size and complexity of the platelet. The mean platelet component (MPC) has been investigated in dogs[38] and cats[39] and is thought to reflect platelet activation.[40] In patients with macrothrombocytopenia and in other diseases, the measurement of plateletcrit (reflecting the packed cell volume of the platelet component) has been advocated as a more accurate marker of platelet capacity.[36]

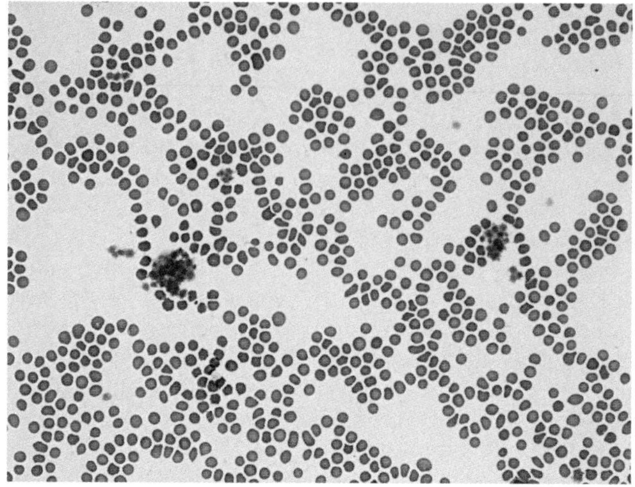

FIGURE 106-1 Cat blood smear with platelet clumps, Diff-Quik stain 50×.

Mild, nonregenerative anemia can accompany infectious, inflammatory, or neoplastic diseases. A full diagnostic work-up for a thrombocytopenic dog or cat also should include complete blood count, a biochemistry panel, clotting profiles, thoracic and abdominal imaging, in addition to infectious disease testing.

MECHANISMS OF THROMBOCYTOPENIA

Thrombocytopenia is a result of one or more of these four generalized categories of causes: (1) decreased production, (2) consumption, (3) sequestration, and (4) increased destruction.

Decreased Production

Suppression or destruction of megakaryocytes may be caused by immune-mediated disease, drugs or toxins, infectious agents, irradiation, hypoadrenocorticism, neoplasia, and myelophthisis. Drug induced thrombocytopenia can be categorized as (1) decreased production via bone marrow suppression and/or (2) increased platelet destruction by immune-mediated processes. Non–immune-mediated thrombocytopenia develops more gradually as megakaryocytes are suppressed and replacement of senescent platelets falters. Immune-mediated thrombocytopenia likely develops more quickly.[41]

Drugs can induce immune-mediated destruction of platelets by several proposed mechanisms. The first is hapten-dependent antibody formation, caused by the drug binding covalently to platelet membrane proteins, causing antibody production and drug-specific immune reaction. Examples of drugs that use this mechanism include penicillins and cephalosporins. Other drugs can induce production of antibodies that bind to platelet membrane proteins (most commonly glycoprotein [GP] IIbIIIa/integrin αIIbβ3) in the presence of the drug, or optimize interactions between antibodies and platelet antigen. Examples of drugs that use this mechanism include quinine, vancomycin, sulfonamides, rifampin, and fluoroquinolones. Still other drugs induce production of auto-antibodies that react with platelets even in the absence of the drug, such as sulfonamides.[42] Non–immune-mediated mechanisms include bone marrow suppression or toxicity; examples include phenobarbital, chloramphenicol, penicillins, cephalosporins, cancer chemotherapeutics, methimazole, azathioprine, and albendazole.[30,43]

A bone marrow aspirate should be performed for dogs and cats with thrombocytopenia that does not respond to treatment, pancytopenias, and in those animals with signs suspicious for neoplasia.[44] Bone marrow cytology and histopathology allow for assessment of megakaryocyte population and distribution as well as myeloid and erythroid precursors, submission for FeLV testing, and detection of fibrosis or neoplastic cell populations.

Consumption

Platelet counts decrease with excessive consumption, such as during significant hemorrhage and DIC. Blood loss leading to platelet consumption and loss can be due to coagulopathies, such as vitamin K antagonist rodenticide toxicity and massive trauma. DIC is a syndrome characterized by systemic microthrombosis caused by systemic infection or inflammation, tissue necrosis and trauma, capillary stasis, vascular damage, or release of pro-coagulant factors. In addition to moderate thrombocytopenia, laboratory findings consistent with DIC include prolongation of the prothrombin and activated partial thromboplastin times, elevated fibrinogen and fibrinogen degradation products, and elevated D-dimers (see Chapter 104).[45,46]

Sequestration

Splenomegaly and splenic congestion, neoplasia, and severe hypothermia can cause sequestration of platelets in the spleen. Splenic sequestration usually causes a mild thrombocytopenia.

Increased Destruction

Immune-mediated thrombocytopenia (ITP) is an autoimmune disorder in dogs that can be primary (idiopathic) or secondary to neoplastic, infectious, toxic, or inflammatory causes. Vaccines have been cited as a cause in children and implicated as an inciting cause in dogs; however, the relation is tenuous in veterinary medicine.[47] Type II hypersensitivity results in destruction of platelets and/or megakaryocytes after antiplatelet and/or antimegakaryocyte antibody attachment,[42,48] and immunoglobulin opsonization and subsequent phagocytosis by the reticuloendothelial system. Idiopathic ITP is a diagnosis of exclusion and is reported in 5% of all thrombocytopenic dogs and 2% of thrombocytopenic cats.[49] Reported mortality rates for idiopathic ITP range from 25% to 30%.[50] Primary ITP appears to be rare in cats.[2,48]

THERAPEUTIC APPROACHES TO THROMBOCYTOPENIA

In humans, there is no consensus for initiating medical treatment for thrombocytopenia. In children, ITP is often a self-limiting disease; therefore medical treatment often is not recommended, even if the platelet count is severely low (below 10×10^9/L). In adults, because of a higher prevalence of comorbidities and increased mortality, treatment often is recommended for patients with platelet counts less than 30×10^9/L.[51]

DIC is a secondary disease entity, caused by inflammatory, severe infectious, or neoplastic diseases; therefore treatment for thrombocytopenia associated with DIC is centered on correcting the underlying cause while providing supportive care, which may include appropriate fluids and blood products, oxygen therapy, and anticoagulant therapy.[45,46]

The mainstay of treatment for ITP is immunosuppression; glucocorticoids are the cornerstone of treatment. Glucocorticoids have a broad range of actions, down-regulating Fc receptors on macrophages, preventing release of the proinflammatory cytokines IL-1 and IL-6, reducing antigen presenting and processing, reducing antibody adhesion onto epitopes, and directly inhibiting T-cell function.[52] Immunosuppressive doses of prednisone range from 2 to 4 mg/kg, divided into two doses per day. Secondary immunosuppressive agents that may be used include human intravenous immunoglobulin (IVIG), cyclosporine, azathioprine, mycophenolate mofetil, and leflunomide.[53] Vincristine is an antitubular agent, which increases platelet counts by causing release of platelets from megakaryocytes (the microtubule system of the megakaryocyte controls the release of new platelets into circulation) and impairing phagocytosis of opsonised platelets by impairing microtubule assembly in macrophages. At a dose of 0.02 mg/kg IV once given with standard doses of glucocorticoids, vincristine decreased hospitalization duration without changing prognosis in dogs with ITP.[54]

Human IVIG is the mainstay of immunosuppressive treatment for children with ITP in the United States.[51,55] A prospective study in dogs with primary ITP found that those dogs given glucocorticoids and human IVIG at a dose of 0.5 g/kg IV once, showed a more rapid increase in platelet count and had a shorter duration of hospitalization compared with dogs given only glucocorticoids.[56,57] For human patients, splenectomy is a second-line treatment if response to immunosuppression is not effective. However, in small animals splenectomy generally is considered as a last resort because of the possibility of exacerbation of hemoparasitic infections such as babesiosis and hemotropic mycoplasmosis. Splenectomy has resulted in the resolution of clinical signs in some veterinary patients with immune-mediated hematologic disease.[58,59] Rituximab (an anti-CD-20 monoclonal antibody targeting B cells that produce antiplatelet antibodies) and the thrombopoietic agents, romiplostim (AMG 531) and eltrombopag, are recently developed treatments for chronic human ITP.[60,61] These therapies can be splenectomy-sparing, but investigation into their use in veterinary medicine is needed.

PLATELET TRANSFUSIONS

Platelet transfusions are indicated when life-threatening bleeding occurs as a result of severe thrombocytopenia.[62] In dogs with ITP, which is the most common cause of severe thrombocytopenia, platelet transfusions are given uncommonly because of the belief that transfused platelets are marked rapidly for destruction, and the resultant increase in platelet count is negligible.[63] In the case of life-threatening hemorrhage, however, a platelet transfusion may help to slow or stop bleeding.

In people, platelet transfusions are recommended for any patients with a platelet count below 10×10^9/L (10,000/μl) and patients with a platelet count less than 50×10^9/L (50,000/μl) requiring invasive procedures.[60] Platelet concentrate obtained by plateletpheresis is the recommended form of platelet transfusion in human medicine resulting from the viability of the platelets, and the low-volume and high concentration of platelets that can be obtained with this technique.[63]

Platelet transfusion products in veterinary medicine include fresh whole blood (FWB), platelet-rich plasma (PRP), fresh platelet concentrate (PC), cryopreserved platelets, and lyophilized platelets.[63] Canine PRP is harvested from fresh whole blood after centrifugation at $1000 \times g$ for 4 minutes (i.e., a relatively slow spin compared with that necessary for separation of fresh frozen plasma). The supernatant PRP can be used for platelet transfusion, or it then can be expressed into a satellite bag and centrifuged further at $2000 \times g$ for 10 minutes to produce a platelet concentrate. PC is obtained either by sequential centrifugations of PRP or by plateletpheresis. This product contains a high concentration of platelets ($1475 \pm 430 \times 10^9$/L) in a relatively small volume and thus differs from PRP, which generally contains a lower number of platelets in a larger volume.[64] In one study, a mean of 3.3×10^{11} platelets in 246 ± 15 ml were collected successfully from 20-kg dogs,[64] and other PC products can have a minimum platelet count of 550×10^3 in a volume of 50 to 60 ml (personal communication, UC Davis Veterinary Blood Bank).

One unit of whole blood-derived PRP or PC (~8×10^{10} platelets)/10 kg dog results in a maximum platelet increase by 40×10^9/L. Fresh whole blood is indicated for thrombocytopenic patients that are concurrently anemic. A dose of 10 ml/kg of FWB results in a maximum platelet increase of 10×10^9/L.[63,65] The efficacy of platelet transfusion can be monitored by checking platelet counts 1 and 24 hours posttransfusion, as well as by monitoring the severity of clinical bleeding or other markers of hemorrhage.[32,62,63]

In veterinary patients, the cost and logistics involved in providing fresh platelet concentrate make it impractical in most clinical settings. Fresh platelet products have a short shelf life; fresh whole blood can be stored at room temperature (22°C) for up to 8 hours, whereas PRP and PC can be stored at room temperature for up to 5 days under continuous gentle agitation. Cryopreserved platelets in DMSO solution are commercially available. Although posttransfusion recovery and half-life are less than PC, they may be stored at -20°C for up to 6 months. Laboratory studies have demonstrated effectiveness in lethally irradiated thrombocytopenic dogs in reducing clinical bleeding, but the cryopreserved product has significantly lower activity than fresh platelets.[66] Clinical studies of the cryopreserved platelet product are still lacking.[66] It is estimated that approximately 2.5 units of cryopreserved PCs must be given to achieve the same level of platelet increment as that achieved by 1 unit of fresh PC. This is due to loss of platelet function and number after cryopreservation.

Freeze-dried or lyophilized platelets are fixed by a cross-linking agent so that they can withstand the processes of dehydration and rehydration. A lyophilized canine platelet product, which can be stored at 4°C for up to 12 months, has been studied for canine patients. One study found it to be safe and easy to use.[62] Because of the shorter lifespan of lyophilized platelets (minutes), their indication is for arresting active hemorrhage rather than for preventing future hemorrhage or raising platelet count.

Platelet refractoriness, defined as a failure to achieve an expected increase in platelet count in response to a platelet transfusion, can be caused by immune or nonimmune reasons, including splenic sequestration, continued bleeding, fever, and infection. Alloimmunization can occur after repeated platelet transfusions as a result of development of lymphotoxic antibodies in the recipient. Although the necessity for repeat platelet transfusions is uncommon in veterinary patients, leukoreduction of platelet products can remove the donor's antigen presenting cells (APC) and decrease the incidence of alloimmunization.[63] Serious adverse events associated with platelet transfusions occur in 2% of human platelet transfusions.[63] These are potential adverse reactions that may occur in veterinary patients and are manifested as an increase in body temperature more than 2°C, chills, dyspnea, cyanosis, bronchospasm, and extensive urticaria.[65] Two major causes of platelet transfusion reactions are leukocyte and platelet proinflammatory mediators and bacterial sepsis (see Chapter 61).[62,63]

REFERENCES

1. Grindem CB, Breitschwerdt EB, Corbett WT, et al: Epidemiologic survey of thrombocytopenia in dogs: a report on 987 cases, Vet Clin Pathol 20:38, 1991.
2. Jordan HL, Grindem CB, Breitschwerdt EB: Thrombocytopenia in cats: a retrospective study of 41 cases, J Vet Intern Med 7:261, 1993.
3. Prater R, Tvedten H: Hemostatic Abnormalities In Willard MD, Tvedten H, editors: Small animal clinical diagnosis by laboratory methods, St Louis, 2004, Saunders, p 92.
4. Parker RI: Etiology and significance of thrombocytopenia in critically ill patients, Crit Care Clin 28:399, 2012.
5. Russell KE, Grindem CB: Secondary thrombocytopenia In Feldman BF, Zinkl JG, Jain NC, editors: Schalm's veterinary hematology, ed 5, Philadelphia, 2000, Lippincott Williams & Wilkins, p 487.
6. Thomas JS: Non-immune-mediated thrombocytopenia In Weiss DJ, Wardrop KJ, editor: Schalm's veterinary hematology, Ames, Iowa, 2010, Wiley-Blackwell, p 596.
7. Crowther MA, Cook DJ, Meade MO, et al: Thrombocytopenia in medical-surgical critically ill patients: prevalence, incidence, and risk factors, J Crit Care 20:348, 2005.
8. Sharma B, Sharma M, Majumder M, et al: Thrombocytopenia in septic shock patients—a prospective observational study of incidence, risk factors and correlation with clinical outcome, Anaesth Intens Care 35:874, 2007.
9. Goggs R, Boag AK, Chan DL: Concurrent immune-mediated haemolytic anaemia and severe thrombocytopenia in 21 dogs, Vet Rec 163:323, 2008.
10. Moore AS, Cotter SM, Rand WM, et al: Evaluation of a discontinuous treatment protocol (VELCAP-S) for canine lymphoma, J Vet Intern Med 15:348, 2001.
11. Zemann BI, Moore AS, Rand WM, et al: A combination chemotherapy protocol (VELCAP-L) for dogs with lymphoma, J Vet Intern Med 12:465, 1998.
12. Schwartz P, Kovak JR, Koprowski A, et al: Evaluation of prognostic factors in the surgical treatment of adrenal gland tumors in dogs: 41 cases (1999-2005), J Am Vet Med Assoc 232:77, 2008.
13. Kruse BD, Unterer S, Horlacher K, et al: Prognostic factors in cats with feline panleukopenia, J Vet Intern Med 24:1271, 2010.

14. Botsch V, Kuchenhoff H, Hartmann K, et al: Retrospective study of 871 dogs with thrombocytopenia, Vet Rec 164:647, 2009.
15. Shelah-Goraly M, Aroch I, Kass PH, et al: A prospective study of the association of anemia and thrombocytopenia with ocular lesions in dogs, Vet J 182:187, 2009.
16. Grindem CB, Breitschwerdt EB, Corbett WT, et al: Thrombocytopenia associated with neoplasia in dogs, J Vet Intern Med 8:400, 1994.
17. Estrin MA, Wehausen CE, Jessen CR, et al: Disseminated intravascular coagulation in cats, J Vet Intern Med 20:1334, 2006.
18. Heikkila HM, Bondarenko A, Mihalkov A, et al: Anaplasma phagocytophilum infection in a domestic cat in Finland: case report, Acta Vet Scand 52:62, 2010.
19. Ravnik U, Tozon N, Strasek K, et al: Clinical and haematological features in *Anaplasma phagocytophilum* seropositive dogs, Clin Microbiol Infect 15(suppl 2):39, 2009.
20. Rafaj RB, Matijatko V, Kis I, et al: Alterations in some blood coagulation parameters in naturally occurring cases of canine babesiosis, Acta Vet Hung 57:295, 2009.
21. Schetters TP, Kleuskens JA, Van De Crommert J, et al: Systemic inflammatory responses in dogs experimentally infected with Babesia canis; a haematological study, Vet Parasitol 162:7, 2009.
22. Gaunt S, Beall M, Stillman B, et al: Experimental infection and co-infection of dogs with Anaplasma platys and Ehrlichia canis: hematologic, serologic and molecular findings, Parasit Vectors 3:33, 2010.
23. Cortese L, Sica M, Piantedosi D, et al: Secondary immune-mediated thrombocytopenia in dogs naturally infected by Leishmania infantum, Vet Rec 164:778, 2009.
24. Sykes JE, Hartmann K, Lunn KF, et al: 2010 ACVIM small animal consensus statement on leptospirosis: diagnosis, epidemiology, treatment, and prevention, J Vet Intern Med 25:1, 2011.
25. Fujino Y, Horiuchi H, Mizukoshi F, et al: Prevalence of hematological abnormalities and detection of infected bone marrow cells in asymptomatic cats with feline immunodeficiency virus infection, Vet Microbiol 136:217, 2009.
26. Gleich S, Hartmann K: Hematology and serum biochemistry of feline immunodeficiency virus-infected and feline leukemia virus-infected cats, J Vet Intern Med 23:552, 2009.
27. Palmer KG, King LG, Van Winkle TJ: Clinical manifestations and associated disease syndromes in dogs with cranial vena cava thrombosis: 17 cases (1989-1996), J Am Vet Med Assoc 213:220, 1998.
28. Bommer NX, Shaw DJ, Milne EM, et al: Platelet distribution width and mean platelet volume in the interpretation of thrombocytopenia in dogs, J Small Anim Pract 49:518, 2008.
29. Dircks BH, Schuberth HJ, Mischke R: Underlying diseases and clinicopathologic variables of thrombocytopenic dogs with and without platelet-bound antibodies detected by use of a flow cytometric assay: 83 cases (2004-2006), J Am Vet Med Assoc 235:960, 2009.
30. Zimmerman KL: Drug-induced thrombocytopenias In Feldman BF, Zinkl JG, Jain NC, editors: Schalm's veterinary hematology, ed 5, Philadelphia, 2000, Lippincott Williams & Wilkins, p 472.
31. Moreau D, Timsit JF, Vesin A, et al: Platelet count decline: an early prognostic marker in critically ill patients with prolonged ICU stays, Chest 131:1735, 2007.
32. Hux BD, Martin LG: Platelet transfusions: treatment options for hemorrhage secondary to thrombocytopenia, J Vet Emerg Crit Care 22:73, 2012.
33. Granat F, Geffre A, Braun JP, et al: Comparison of platelet clumping and complete blood count results with Sysmex XT-2000iV in feline blood sampled on EDTA or EDTA plus CTAD (citrate, theophylline, adenosine and dipyridamole), J Feline Med Surg 13:953, 2011.
34. Weiss D, Tvedten H: The complete blood count and bone marrow examination: general comments and selected techniques. In Willard MD, Tvedten H, editors: Small animal clinical diagnosis by laboratory methods, St Louis, 2004, Saunders, p 14.
35. Sullivan PS, Manning KL, McDonald TP: Association of mean platelet volume and bone marrow megakaryocytopoiesis in thrombocytopenic dogs: 60 cases (1984-1993), J Am Vet Med Assoc 206:332, 1995.
36. Tvedten H, Lilliehook I, Hillstrom A, et al: Plateletcrit is superior to platelet count for assessing platelet status in Cavalier King Charles Spaniels, Vet Clin Pathol 37:266, 2008.
37. Pankraz A, Bauer N, Moritz A: Comparison of flow cytometry with the Sysmex XT2000iV automated analyzer for the detection of reticulated platelets in dogs, Vet Clin Pathol 38:30, 2009.
38. Flatland B, Fry MM, LeBlanc CJ, et al: Leukocyte and platelet changes following low-dose lipopolysaccharide administration in five dogs, Res Vet Sci 90:89, 2011.
39. Zelmanovic D, Hetherington EJ: Automated analysis of feline platelets in whole blood, including platelet count, mean platelet volume, and activation state, Vet Clin Pathol 27:2, 1998.
40. Ahnadi CE, Sabrinah Chapman E, Lepine M, et al: Assessment of platelet activation in several different anticoagulants by the Advia 120 Hematology System, fluorescence flow cytometry, and electron microscopy, Thromb Haemost 90:940, 2003.
41. Lachowicz JL, Post GS, Moroff SD, et al: Acquired amegakaryocytic thrombocytopenia–four cases and a literature review, J Small Anim Pract 45:507, 2004.
42. Lavergne SN, Trepanier LA: Anti-platelet antibodies in a natural animal model of sulphonamide-associated thrombocytopaenia, Platelets 18:595, 2007.
43. Loo AS, Gerzenshtein L, Ison MG: Antimicrobial drug-induced thrombocytopenia: a review of the literature, Semin Thromb Hemost, 2012.
44. Miller MD, Lunn KF: Diagnostic use of cytologic examination of bone marrow from dogs with thrombocytopenia: 58 cases (1994-2004), J Am Vet Med Assoc 231:1540, 2007.
45. Lobetti RG, Joubert K: Retrospective study of snake envenomation in 155 dogs from the Onderstepoort area of South Africa, J S Afr Vet Assoc 75:169, 2004.
46. Willey JR, Schaer M: Eastern Diamondback Rattlesnake (Crotalus adamanteus) envenomation of dogs: 31 cases (1982-2002), J Am Anim Hosp Assoc 41:22, 2005.
47. Huang AA, Moore GE, Scott-Moncrieff JC: Idiopathic immune-mediated thrombocytopenia and recent vaccination in dogs, J Vet Intern Med 26:142, 2012.
48. Wondratschek C, Weingart C, Kohn B: Primary immune-mediated thrombocytopenia in cats, J Am Anim Hosp Assoc 46:12, 2010.
49. Neel J, Birkenheuer AJ, Brindem CB: Thrombocytopenia. In Bonagura JD, Twedt, David C, editor: Kirk's current veterinary therapy, ed XIV, St Louis, 2006, Saunders Elsevier, p 281.
50. O'Marra SK, Shaw SP, deLaforcade AM: Investigating hypercoagulability during treatment for immune-mediated thrombocytopenia: a pilot study, J Vet Emerg Crit Care 22:126, 2012.
51. Pels SG: Current therapies in primary immune thrombocytopenia, Semin Thromb Hemost 37:621, 2011.
52. Sousa CA: Glucocorticoids in veterinary dermatology. In Bonagura JD, Twedt DC, editors: Kirk's current veterinary therapy XIV, ed XIV, St Louis, 2009, Saunders Elsevier, p 400.
53. Whitley NT, Day MJ: Immunomodulatory drugs and their application to the management of canine immune-mediated disease, J Small Anim Pract 52:70, 2011.
54. Rozanski EA, Callan MB, Hughes D, et al: Comparison of platelet count recovery with use of vincristine and prednisone or prednisone alone for treatment for severe immune-mediated thrombocytopenia in dogs, J Am Vet Med Assoc 220:477, 2002.
55. Bianco D, Armstrong PJ, Washabau RJ: Treatment of severe immune-mediated thrombocytopenia with human IV immunoglobulin in 5 dogs, J Vet Intern Med 21:694, 2007.
56. Spurlock NK, Prittie JE: A review of current indications, adverse effects, and administration recommendations for intravenous immunoglobulin, J Vet Emerg Crit Care 21:471, 2011.
57. Bianco D, Armstrong PJ, Washabau RJ: A prospective, randomized, double-blinded, placebo-controlled study of human intravenous immunoglobulin for the acute management of presumptive primary immune-mediated thrombocytopenia in dogs, J Vet Intern Med 23:1071, 2009.
58. Horgan JE, Roberts BK, Schermerhorn T: Splenectomy as an adjunctive treatment for dogs with immune-mediated hemolytic anemia: ten cases (2003-2006), J Vet Emerg Crit Care 19:254, 2009.
59. Vargo CL, Taylor SM, Haines DM: Immune mediated neutropenia and thrombocytopenia in 3 giant schnauzers, Can Vet J 48:1159, 2007.

60. Stasi R: Immune thrombocytopenia: pathophysiologic and clinical update, Semin Thromb Hemost 38:454, 2012.
61. Arnold DM: Positioning new treatments in the management of immune thrombocytopenia, Pediatr Blood Cancer 2012.
62. Davidow EB, Brainard B, Martin LG, et al: Use of fresh platelet concentrate or lyophilized platelets in thrombocytopenic dogs with clinical signs of hemorrhage: a preliminary trial in 37 dogs, J Vet Emerg Crit Care 22:116, 2012.
63. Callan MB, Appleman EH, Sachais BS: Canine platelet transfusions, J Vet Emerg Crit Care 19:401, 2009.
64. Callan MB, Appleman EH, Shofer FS, et al: Clinical and clinicopathologic effects of plateletpheresis on healthy donor dogs, Transfusion 48:2214, 2008.
65. Brooks MB, Catalfamo JL: Platelet dysfunction. In Bonagura JD,Twedt DC, editors: Kirk's current veterinary therapy, ed XIV, St Louis, 2009, Saunders Elsevier.
66. Guillaumin J, Jandrey KE, Norris JW, et al: Analysis of a commercial dimethyl-sulfoxide-stabilized frozen canine platelet concentrate by turbidimetric aggregometry, J Vet Emerg Crit Care 20:571, 2010.

CHAPTER 107
PLATELET DISORDERS

Karl E. Jandrey DVM, MAS, DACVECC

KEY POINTS

- Thrombocytopathies most commonly are inherited but also may be acquired.
- Intrinsic thrombocytopathies are more common than extrinsic thrombocytopathies in small animals.
- von Willebrand's disease is the most common thrombocytopathy and is seen in many breeds, whereas most of the other intrinsic platelet disorders are breed specific.
- Clinical signs of bleeding can vary in severity and location, depending on the type of platelet dysfunction and extent of injury.
- Treatment for von Willebrand's disease requires transfusion with a plasma product rich in concentration of von Willebrand factor.
- Platelet concentrates are used to treat dogs with clinical bleeding resulting from an inherited intrinsic platelet defect.

Platelet disorders in dogs and cats are identified more frequently as point-of-care and laboratory testing has become more commonplace in veterinary practice. This chapter highlights the more common thrombocytopathies encountered in small animal critical care, inclusive of their pathophysiology and treatments. These platelet function defects generally cause a loss in function so that abnormal bleeding occurs. Some hyperactivity of platelet function, and thus thrombosis, also may occur in select disease states. Those topics are reviewed elsewhere in this text (see Chapter 104). The therapy of thrombocytopathies also is summarized in Table 107-1.

INHERITED DISORDERS

Extrinsic Disorders

Extrinsic platelet disorders are characterized by the lack of a functional protein needed for platelet adhesion and aggregation. The platelets are normal in structure and function. The most common thrombocytopathy is *von Willebrand's disease (vWD)* in dogs[1-3] and humans.[4,5] vWD is an inherited extrinsic platelet disorder. vWD in dogs is caused by a deficiency or dysfunction of von Willebrand factor (vWF), a plasma protein of variably sized multimers that mediates platelet hemostatic function, as well as circulates with and stabilizes Factor VIII (FVIII). Platelets contain only a small amount of vWF in dogs, whereas the richest source is in the endothelial cells.

vWD in dogs is classified into three separate types.[6] Type I is a quantitative reduction in vWF. All multimers are present; however, the concentration is less than adequate for appropriate hemostasis. Type II vWD patients have measurable reductions in vWF, but the subset of large multimers is scant. This causes a qualitative reduction in vWF because the large multimers are essential for effective hemostatic function. Type III vWD patients have an absolute lack of vWF altogether. Inheritance is autosomal dominant or recessive in type I but autosomal recessive in types II and III. No sex predilection has been found.

Animals with vWD typically show mucosal bleeding (epistaxis, melena, hematuria, gingival hemorrhage) or excessive cavity bleeding

Table 107-1 Treatment Choices for Small Animal Patients with Bleeding Resulting from Thrombocytopathies

Treatment	Condition
Plasma containing vWF (fresh frozen plasma, cryoprecipitate, fresh whole blood) 10-20 ml/kg fresh frozen plasma or 1 unit cryoprecipitate/10 kg IV	Inherited or acquired vWD
Platelet concentrate (fresh or cryopreserved) 1 unit/10 kg (treat to effect)	Inherited intrinsic platelet disorders
DDAVP 1-3 μg/kg SC	Type I vWD, acquired drug-induced platelet dysfunction
Remove drugs associated with thrombocytopathies	All conditions

DDAVP, Desmopressin acetate; *vWD*, von Willebrand's disease; *vWF*, von Willebrand factor.

after surgery (hemoabdomen, scrotal hematoma) or trauma.[7,8] Petechiae and ecchymoses are uncommon. The clinical signs are worse with type III dogs and can be variable with type I. In general, the lower the vWF concentration, the higher the risk of bleeding. However, type II dogs can have severe bleeding because the lack of the high molecular weight vWF multimers is essential to support platelet adhesion.

Diagnosis of vWD usually begins with suspicious bleeding after vascular injury. The typical physical examination finding in a known breed affected with vWD leads the clinician to measure a manual and automated platelet count. Thrombocytopenia must be ruled out before continuation through the ensuing coagulation work-up. The buccal mucosal bleeding time (BMBT) is the best in vivo assessment of primary hemostasis. However, it is not specific for vWD. Normal BMBT results are less than 3 minutes.[9] Variables in people that may alter the reference range (which is typically 6 to 11 minutes) include skin thickness, skin temperature, age, gender, hematocrit, and vascular pattern.[10] A prolonged result is consistent with intrinsic thrombocytopathia or von Willebrand's disease.[11] This test of primary hemostasis is highly operator dependent; variable results have been reported in animals and in humans. Therefore the measurement of the vWF:antigen concentration is essential to prove the diagnosis of vWD.

Treatment for a patient with a confirmed diagnosis of vWD is completed with plasma products rich in vWF. Cryoprecipitate (1 unit/10 kg body weight IV within 8 hours of thaw) is the best choice for transfusion therapy. Manufacturers have variably sized units, but in general 1 unit equates to cryoprecipitate from 200 ml fresh frozen plasma.[6] Fresh frozen plasma is also an effective therapy for vWD. Fresh whole blood can be used if the vWD patient is also profoundly anemic in an effort to provide red blood cells and vWF. However, the use of red blood cell–free products prevents sensitization to red blood cell antigens and reduces the risk of volume overload. For therapy outside of transfusions, avoidance of injury or use of drugs that can impair platelet function is a must. Desmopressin acetate (deamino 8-d-arginine vasopressin, DDAVP) is used to stimulate endothelial V2 receptors to release intracellular stores of vWF. Type 1 vWD patients have some response to DDAVP. Types II and III have little to no response to DDAVP.

Intrinsic Disorders

Intrinsic platelet disorders are those inherent to platelets. *Chediak-Higashi syndrome (CHS)* is an autosomal recessive disease that manifests as prolonged bleeding times in the presence of normal platelet concentrations. It is reported in humans and cats but not dogs and is classified as an intrinsic platelet storage pool deficiency. Patients with CHS have altered lysosomal granule formation and abnormal degranulation in neutrophils and platelets. Platelet dense granules and/or their constituents are lacking in this disease. Because of this, aggregation response to collagen is absent.[12] Treatment with platelet concentrates has been shown to correct abnormal oral mucosal bleeding times.[13]

Glanzmann's thrombasthenia is an inherited, intrinsic platelet functional defect found in humans and dogs. It has been characterized in Otterhounds and Great Pyrenees dogs.[14] The primary defect leads to a deficiency in the number of the $\alpha_{IIb}\beta_3$ integrin. Mucosal bleeding (epistaxis, gingival and gastrointestinal hemorrhages) and prolonged bleeding times are present because of the lack of fibrinogen binding to this essential integrin. This mutation has been mapped, and the disease has been corrected successfully with experimental bone marrow transplantation and gene therapy.[15-17] Successful therapy with perioperative platelet-rich plasma administration has been published in a dog with Glanzmann's thromboasthenia.[18]

Diagnostic evaluation requires extensive platelet functional testing, often limited to research laboratories. However, the clot retraction assay can be used as a screening tool in any practice for patients with normal red blood cell and platelet concentrations because clot retraction is impaired by thrombocytopathia, abnormalities in fibrinogen, and some coagulation defects.[19] Clot retraction is determined by the placement of 5 ml of whole blood into a sterile glass tube (without any anticoagulant). A wooden applicator is inserted into the tube and blood. The tube then is sealed with plastic paraffin film before incubation at 37° C. The assessment of clot formation and clot retraction is noted over 8 to 24 hours. Within 2 to 4 hours a normal clot retracts markedly. Results are recorded as complete clot retraction (retraction occurred and serum was found surrounding the clot) or failed clot retraction (no serum was found surrounding the clot).

Another platelet membrane receptor disorder recently was found in the Greater Swiss Mountain Dog.[20] This inherited intrinsic platelet functional defect is the first documented mutation of the *$P2Y_{12}$ receptor* in domestic animals. The sentinel patient in this study bled excessively after an ovariohysterectomy; neither this dog nor her relations were known to have prior bleeding problems. The lack of a functional $P2Y_{12}$ receptor prevents activation via ADP-induced outside-in signaling for fibrinogen binding on the platelet surface at the $\alpha_{IIb}\beta_3$ integrin. This is important because of the growing use of clopidogrel as an antithrombotic agent. Clopidogrel blocks ADP from binding at the $P2Y_{12}$ receptor, reducing platelet activation.

Another mutation that reduces platelet function and creates abnormal bleeding tendencies (epistaxis, gingival bleeding, petechiation) is found within the *calcium-diacylglycerol guanine nucleotide exchange factor 1 gene (CalDAG-GEF1)*. This mutation alters a protein involved in signal transduction that is crucial to inside-out and outside-in integrin signaling events. This intrinsic inherited thrombocytopathy has been reported in Landseers, Basset Hounds, and Spitz dogs.[21]

Canine Scott syndrome (CSS) is a more recently diagnosed and understood, rare intrinsic platelet disorder[22,23] that mimics the human disease. This has been found in related and unrelated German Shepherd Dogs (GSD).[24] In a pedigree study, the mutation was found to be autosomal recessive. The defect lies in the inability for phosphatidylserine to be externalized for the creation of a procoagulant surface. These dogs also have a decreased microparticle release compared with nonaffected GSD. The clinical findings from CSS dogs include epistaxis, postoperative hemorrhage, and spontaneous soft tissue hemorrhage. Diagnosis requires flow cytometry because typical coagulation testing and point-of-care analysis with the Platelet Function Analyzer-100 or thromboelastography did not show a difference between platelet function of affected and nonaffected dogs. Spontaneous hemorrhage in these dogs cannot be prevented by treatment; however, perioperative dimethylsulfoxide cryopreserved platelet-rich plasma transfusions plus a postoperative antifibrinolytic agent has been used with success.

Idiopathic asymptomatic macrothrombocytopenia in Cavalier King Charles Spaniels (CKCS) is another inherited autosomal recessive platelet defect.[25] A mutation in β1-tubulin likely leads to altered proplatelet formation in megakaryocytes.[26] It also has been reported in related Norfolk Terriers.[27] CKCS have not been found to have any clinical bleeding[28,29] or any abnormalities on platelet aggregation testing.[29]

ACQUIRED DISORDERS

Drugs

Platelet dysfunction in people has been found secondary to aspirin, ticlopidine, clopidogrel, as well as some antibiotics and nonsteroidal antiinflammatory drugs.[30] These findings may be similar in dogs and cats; however, not all antiinflammatory drugs have a similar effect on laboratory measurements of hemostasis. DDAVP has been used IV to reverse acquired acetylsalicylic acid-induced coagulopathy in three dogs.[31]

von Willebrand's Disease

vWD is encountered less commonly as an acquired disorder[5,6] and is caused by defects in vWF concentration, structure, or function that is not directly inherited. They are the result of other medical conditions in humans (and likely in animals), such as autoimmune clearance or inhibition of vWF (i.e., myeloproliferative diseases, some cancers, immune-mediated diseases), increased shear-induced proteolysis of vWF (i.e., cardiovascular lesions or pulmonary hypertension), or increased binding of vWF to platelets and other cell surfaces. In veterinary patients, as well as in people, hypothyroidism and treatment with hydroxyethyl starch and dextran solutions also have been implicated in acquired vWD. Other drugs reported to lead to the syndrome of acquired von Willebrand's disease in humans include ciprofloxacin, griseofulvin, and valproic acid.

Uremia

Uremic patients are well recognized to have prolonged mucosal bleeding times and delayed formation of the primary hemostatic plug. These abnormalities are due to defects in platelet adhesion, secretion, and aggregation.[32,33] Defects in vWF function (probably receptor binding) are thought to play a major role. Uremic patients have been found to have normal to increased vWF levels, but platelet function can be improved in the uremic patient by transfusion of cryoprecipitate or administration of DDAVP.[34] In addition uremic patients produce increased levels of nitric oxide and prostacyclin that can alter vascular tone and platelet function. Acquired platelet storage pool deficiencies have been demonstrated as well as a reduced ability to produce thromboxane A_2. Some of the uremic toxins are believed to act as direct platelet inhibitors by competing for receptor binding. Anemia, a common finding in uremic patients, also is believed to play an important role in altering platelet interactions with the vessel walls and reduced nitric oxygen scavenging ability. References 32 and 33 contain further discussion of the pathophysiology of bleeding in uremic patients. Many of these platelet function defects can be reversed by dialysis, suggesting that much of the acquired thrombocytopathy of uremia is due to circulating uremic toxins.

TREATMENT SUMMARY

Avoidance of traumatic situations for patients with any platelet dysfunction is not completely feasible. When a patient with a known platelet disorder is presented to the emergency room or critical care unit, the treatment is based on the underlying cause of the defect in primary hemostasis. The most common primary platelet defect is vWD. Therefore treatment with fresh frozen plasma or cryoprecipitate would be efficacious.[35] Current dosing recommendations are 10 to 20 ml/kg fresh frozen plasma or 1 unit cryoprecipitate/10 kg IV over no more than 4 hours. Desmopressin (DDAVP, 1 µg/kg SC) may be advantageous if the patient had type I vWD.[36,37]

To investigate the underlying cause for a patient with a bleeding problem, quick action must be taken to rule out disorders of secondary hemostasis while ensuring the patient is not thrombocytopenic. When a primary hemostatic disease is suspected because of a primary thrombopathy other than vWD, treatment should involve fresh platelet concentrates[38,39] or dimethyl sulfoxide cryopreserved platelets.[39,40]

REFERENCES

1. Mattoso CRS, Takahira RK, Beier SL, et al: Prevalence of von Willebrand disease in dogs from Sao Paolo State, Brazil, J Vet Diagn Invest 22(1):5-60, 2010.
2. Gavazza A, Prescuittini S, Keuper H, et al: Estimated prevalence of canine type 2 von Willebrand disease in Deutsch-Dratthaar (German Wirehaired Pointer) in Europe, Res Vet Sci 93(3):1462-6, 2012.
3. van Dongen AM, van Leeuwen M, Slappendel RJ: Canine von WIllebrand's disease type 2 in German wirehair pointers in the Netherlands, Vet Rec 148(3):80-82, 2001.
4. James PD, Lillicrap DP: The diagnosis and management of von Willebrand disease in Canada, Sem Thromb Haemost 37(5):522-527, 2011.
5. Nichols WL, Hultin MB, James AH, et al: von Willebrand disease (VWD): evidence-based diagnosis and management guidelines, the National Heart, Lung, and Blood Institute (NHLBI) Expert Panel report (USA), Haemophlia 14(2):171-232, 2008.
6. Brooks MB, Catalfamo JL: Von Willebrand disease. In Weiss DJ, Wardrop KJ, editor: Schalm's veterinary hematology, ed 6, Ames, Iowa, 2010, Wiley-Blackwell, pp 612-618.
7. Brooks MB, Dodds WJ, Raymond SL: Epidemiologic features of von Willebrand's disease in Doberman pinschers, Scottish terriers, and Shetland sheepdogs: 280 cases (1984-1988), J Am Vet Med Assoc 200(8):1123-1127, 1992.
8. Burgess HJ, Woods JP, Abrams-Ogg ACG, et al: Use of a questionnaire to predict von Willebrand disease status and characterize hemorrhagic signs in a population of dogs and evaluation of a diagnostic profile to predict risk of bleeding, Can J Vet Res 73(4):241-251, 2009.
9. Jergens AE, Turrentine MA, Kraus KH, et al: Buccal mucosal bleeding times ofhealthy dogs and dogs in various pathologic states, including thrombocytopenia, uremia, and von Willebrand's disease, Am J Vet Res 48(9):1337-1342, 1987.
10. Harrison P, Mumford A: Screening tests of platelet function: update on their appropriate uses for diagnostic testing, Semin Thromb Hemost 35(2):150-157, 2009.
11. Marks SL: The buccal mucosal bleeding time, J Am Anim Hosp Assoc 36(4):289-290, 2000.
12. Colgan SP, Thrall MA, Gasper PW: Platelet aggregation and ATP secretion in whole blood of normal cats and cats homozygous and heterozygous for Chediak-Higashi syndrome, Blood Cells 15(3):585-595, 1989.
13. Cowles BE, Meyers KM, Wardrop KJ, et al: Prolonged bleeding time of Chediak-Higashi cats corrected by platelet transfusion, Thromb Haemost 67(6):708-712, 1992.
14. Boudreaux MK, Lipscomb DL: Clinical, biochemical, and molecular aspects of Glanzmann's thrombasthenia in humans and dogs, Vet Pathol 38(3):249-260, 2001.
15. Lipscomb DL, Bourne C, Boudreaux MK: Two genetic defects in α_{IIb} are associated with type I Glanzmann's thrombasthenia in a Great Pyrenees dog: a 14-base insertion in exon 13 and a splicing defect of intron 13, Vet Pathol 37(6):581-588, 2000.
16. Niemeyer GP, Boudreaux MK, Goodman-Martin SA, et al: Correction of a large animal model of type I Glanzmann's thrombasthenia by nonmyeloablative bone marrow transplantation, Exp Hematol 31(12):1357-1362, 2003.
17. Fang J, Jensen ES, Boudreaux MK, et al: Platelet gene therapy improves hemostatic function for integrin $\alpha_{IIb}\beta_3$-deficient dogs, Proc Natl Acad Sci 108(23): 9583-9588, 2011.
18. Brdecka DJ, Adin CA, Boudreaux MK, et al: Successful ovariectomy in a dog with Glanzmann thrombasthenia, J Am Vet Med Assoc 224(11):1796-1798, 2004.
19. Cole EH: Hemostasis and coagulation of blood. In Cole EH, ed: Veterinary clinical pathology, Philadelphia, 1980, WB Saunders, p 150.
20. Boudreaux MK, Martin M: $P2Y_{12}$ receptor gene mutation associated with postoperative hemorrhage in a Greater Swiss Mountain dog, Vet Clin Pathol 40(2):202-206, 2011.
21. Boudreaux MK, Catalfamo JL, Klok M: Calcium-diacylglycerol guanin nucleotide exchange factor 1 gene mutations associated with loss of function in canine platelets, Transl Res 150(2):81-92, 2007.
22. Brooks MB, Randolph J, Warner K, et al: Evaluation of platelet function screening tests to detect platelet procoagulant deficiency in dogs with Scott Syndrome, Vet Clin Pathol 38(3):306-315, 2009.

23. Brooks M, Etter K, Catalfamo J, et al: A genome-wide linkage scan in German shepherd dogs localizes canine platelet procoagulant deficiency (Scott Syndrome) to canine chromosome 27, Gene 450(1-2):70-75, 2010.
24. Jandrey KE, Norris JW, Tucker M, et al: Clinical characterization of canine platelet procoagulant deficiency (Scott Syndrome), J Vet Int Med 26(2):1402-1407, 2012.
25. Pedersen HD, Haggstrom J, Olsen LH, et al: Idiopathic asymptomatic thrombocytopenia in Cavalier King Charles Spaniels is an autosomal recessive trait, J Vet Int Med 16(2):169-173, 2002.
26. Davis B, Toivio-Kinnucan M, Schuller S, et al: Mutation of β1-tubulin correlates with macrothrombocytopenia in Cavalier King Charles Spaniels, J Vet Int Med 22(3):540-545, 2008.
27. Gelain ME, Tutino GF, Pogliani, et al: macrothrombocytopenia in a group of related Norfolk terriers, Vet Rec 167:493-494, 2010.
28. Cowan SM, Bartges JW, Gompf RE, et al: Giant platelet disorder in the Cavalier King Charles Spaniel, Exp Hematol 32(4):344-350, 2004.
29. Olsen LH, Kristensen AT, Haggstrom J, et al: Increased platelet aggregation response in Cavalier King Charles Spaniels with mitral valve prolapse, J Vet Int Med 15(3):209-216, 2001.
30. Scharf RE, Rahman MM, Seidel H: The impact and management of acquired platelet dysfunction, Haemostaseologie 31(1):28-40, 2011.
31. DiMauro FM, Holowaychuk MK: Intravenous administration of desmopressin acetate to reverese acetylsalicylic acid-induced coagulopathy in three dogs, J Vet Emerg Crit Care 23(4):455-8, 2013.
32. Kow D, Malhotra D: Platelet dysfunction and end-stage renal disease, Semin Dialysis 19:317-322, 2006.
33. Sohal AS, Gangji AS, Crowther MA, et al: Uremic bleeding: pathophysiology and clinical risk factors, Thrombosis Res 118:417-422, 2006.
34. Hedges SJ, Dehoney SB, Hooper JS, et al. Evidence-based treatment recommendations for uremic bleeding. Nat Clin Pract Nephrol 3:138-153, 2007.
35. Stokol T, Parry BW: Efficacy of fresh-frozen plasma and cryoprecipitate in dogs with von Willebrand's disease or hemophilia A, J Vet Int Med 12(2):84-92, 1998.
36. Callan MB, Giger U: Effect of desmopressin acetate administration on primary hemostasis in Doberman Pinschers with type 1 von Willebrand disease as assessed by a point-of-care instrument, Am J Vet Res 63(12):1700-1706, 2002.
37. Callan MB, Giger U, Catalfamo JL: Effect of desmopressin on von Willebrand factor multimers in Doberman Pinschers with type 1 von Willebrand disease, Am J Vet Res 66(5):861-867, 2005.
38. Davidow EB, Brainard B, Martin LG, et al: Use of fresh platelet concentrate or lyophylyzed platelets in thrombocytopenic dogs with clinical signs of hemorrhage: a preliminary trial in 37 dogs, J Vet Emerg Crit Care 22(1):116-125, 2012.
39. Callan MB, Appleman EH, Sachais BS: Canine platelet transfusion, J Vet Emerg Crit Care 19(5):401-415, 2009.
40. Guillaumin J, Jandrey KE, Norri JW, et al: Assessment of a dimethyl sulfoxide-stabilized frozen canine platelet concentrate, Am J Vet Res 69(12):1580-1586, 2008.

CHAPTER 108

ANEMIA

Urs Giger, PD, DrMedVet, MS, FVH, DACVIM, DECVIM-CA, DECVCP

KEY POINTS

- Anemia is one of the most common problems in critically ill patients and, although not always an acute abnormality, it often requires immediate consideration and supportive care.
- Although a patient's clinical signs may be suggestive of anemia, routine and specific laboratory tests generally are needed to further define the severity, type, and cause.
- Although (peracute) acute external blood loss anemias are generally easy to identify, internal hemorrhage, hemolysis, and bone marrow failure are other important mechanisms that may not be readily evident.
- The specific underlying cause(s) of any anemia should be determined to formulate an accurate prognosis and therapeutic plan; however, supportive care often begins immediately.
- Whenever possible, appropriate blood samples (EDTA, serum, and citrate tubes filled with adequate blood volumes) should be collected before any therapeutic intervention. This helps to determine a definitive diagnosis for the anemia.
- A low packed cell volume and total protein level classically are seen after external blood loss. Animals with hemolysis typically have a normal to high serum total protein level and hyperbilirubinemia and hyperbilirubinuria, with or without hemoglobinemia or hemoglobinuria.
- A microscopic evaluation of a blood smear can provide clues readily regarding the cause of the anemia and always should be part of an emergency minimum database.
- Although there is no specific trigger, transfusions are given based on the assessment of clinical signs, rapidity of onset, severity, progression, and underlying cause(s) of the anemia.
- Severely anemic animals with serious clinical signs likely benefit from blood type–compatible packed red blood cells (RBCs) or whole blood transfusions.

Anemia is defined as a reduction in the oxygen-carrying capacity of blood resulting from decreases in hemoglobin (Hb) concentration and red blood cell (RBC) mass. It is certainly one of the most common laboratory test abnormalities in small animals, particularly in an intensive care unit (ICU) setting. However, anemia is not a final diagnosis and thus further clinical investigation is indicated to define the underlying cause. The three primary mechanisms leading to anemia are blood loss, hemolysis, and reduced erythropoiesis (Figure 108-1).[1-3]

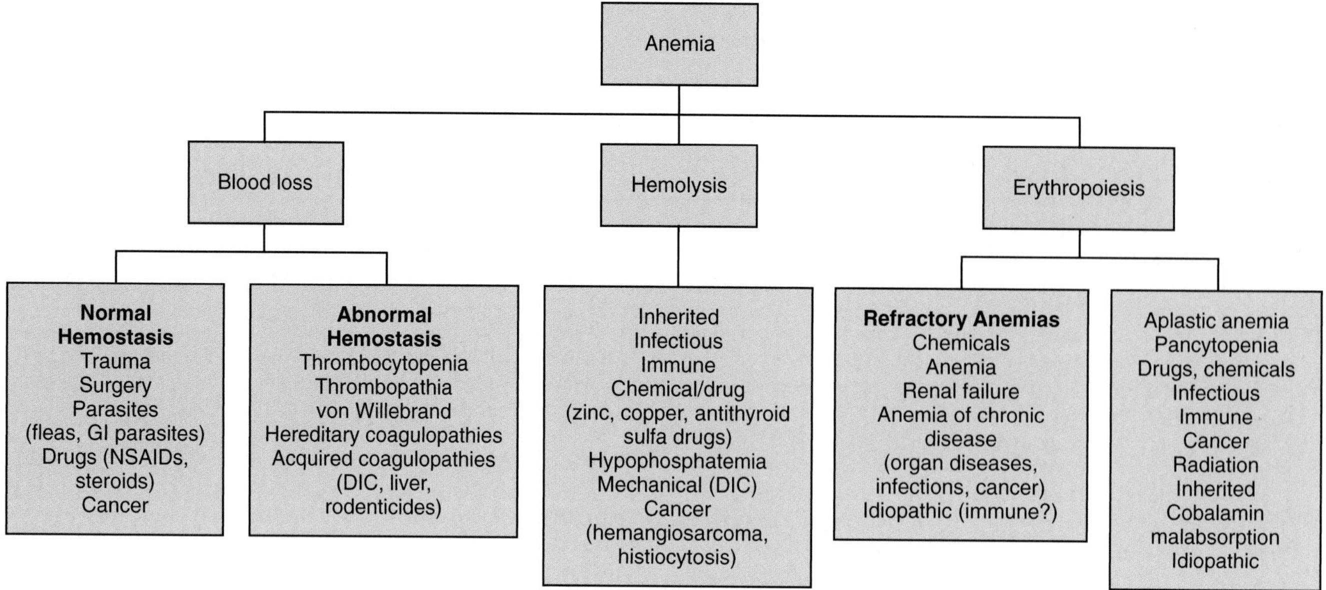

FIGURE 108-1 Classification of anemias (also see other chapters in Part XI for more details). *DIC,* Disseminated intravascular coagulation; *GI,* gastrointestinal; *NSAIDs,* nonsteroidal antiinflammatory drugs.

Although anemia may result from primary hematologic disorders, it more often is associated with other organ disorders. This chapter discusses the clinical approach to and general therapeutic principles of an anemic animal for the critical care clinician. Specific hematologic disorders or abnormalities are addressed in more depth in other chapters (see Hematologic Disorders).

SIGNALMENT AND HISTORY

The breed of the patient may be of particular importance now that many hereditary blood diseases (e.g., pyruvate kinase deficiency in many cat and dog breeds, phosphofructokinase deficiency in several canine breeds) and genetic predispositions in certain breeds have been recognized (e.g., immune-mediated hemolytic anemia [IMHA] in Cocker Spaniels). Although many hereditary erythrocyte defects,[2,3] coagulopathies (e.g., hemophilia A and B, factor VII or XI deficiency), von Willebrand disease, and thrombopathias lead to anemia in juvenile animals, some may be recognized only in the older animal after acute, and possibly recurrent, episodes of bleeding, hemolysis, and secondary anemia have been documented.[2,4,5] Furthermore, most hereditary disorders are observed in equal proportions in both genders, although hemophilia A and B, two serious coagulopathies, affect only male animals (X-chromosomal recessive trait).

A carefully taken history and review of previous laboratory test results often can provide clues to the duration and cause of the anemia. For instance, depending on the geographic location and travel history, exposure to a certain infectious agent such as *Babesia, Ehrlichia, Anaplasma, Mycoplasma, Leishmania,* and *Leptospira* spp. in dogs and various viral (feline leukemia virus, feline immunodeficiency virus, and feline infectious peritonitis), bacterial (*Mycoplasma haemofelis,* other *Mycoplasma* spp.), and parasitic *(Cytauxzoon felis)* infections in cats (as well as other emerging infectious diseases) may require diagnostic testing by serology, antigen assay, or DNA/RNA polymerase chain reaction testing. There are heavy metals (zinc and copper [but not lead]) and other chemicals (anticoagulant rodenticides), drugs (e.g., antithyroid drugs [cat], estrogens [dog], heparin, warfarin, aspirin), and even food components (onions, garlic) that represent known triggers of anemia (see Intoxications). A history of anemia, hemorrhage, icterus, or requirement for transfusion therapy may indicate a recurrent or chronic problem. Finally, some concurrent chronic illnesses and organ disorders, such as renal and hepatic failure, diabetes mellitus, or adverse effects of medical therapy (e.g., chemotherapeutics and many other drugs, hypophosphatemia induced by insulin administration or refeeding syndrome) may lead to severe anemia.

CLINICAL SIGNS

The clinical signs of anemia vary greatly depending on the rapidity of onset, type, and underlying cause. Determining whether the cause of anemia is hemorrhage, hemolysis, or a hematopoietic production disorder is critical. Any form of anemia may be associated with pallor, and this may be the only sign in some animals. However, characteristic signs such as hemorrhage with blood loss-induced anemia (Table 108-1) or icterus or pigmenturia with hemolytic anemia may help the clinician determine the cause.

In animals with peracute blood loss, the clinical signs are related mostly to hemorrhage and hypovolemia (e.g., normal PCV initially with hypovolemic shock), and animals with acute and chronic anemias display more typical signs (e.g., lethargy, pallor, tachycardia). Although anemia by itself does not cause tachypnea, there are common coexisting abnormalities that may lead to an increased respiratory rate via stimulation of the carotid body chemoreceptors (e.g., acidemia or hypoxemia). External blood loss is often readily evident, except for animals with gastrointestinal (GI) hemorrhage originating from the nasopharynx to the rectum. In contrast, internal hemorrhage may be hard to localize, especially in animals with retroperitoneal or deep muscle hemorrhage. A single site of hemorrhage may occur secondary to a local process such as trauma or surgery (e.g., a single lacerated vessel, hematoma) but also may be caused by an underlying bleeding tendency. Surface hemorrhage, such as petechiations and ecchymoses, suggests a thrombocytopenia or vasculopathy, whereas multiple or recurrent hematomas and intracavitary hemorrhage indicate a coagulopathy. Von Willebrand disease and hereditary coagulopathies occur commonly in dogs but rarely in cats (the common factor XII deficiency in cats does not cause clinical bleeding).

Table 108-1 Hematologic and Physical Examination Changes with Anemia from External Blood Loss

Parameter	Peracute	Acute	Chronic
Onset	Minutes to hours	Hours to days	Weeks to months
Hct/PCV	N	↓	↓↓↓
MCV	N	N to T ↑	↓↓
MCHC	N	N to T ↑	↓↓
Reticulocytes, polychromasia	N	N to ↑↑	↑↑
Capillary refill time	↑↑	↑↑ to N	N
Skin turgor	N	↓ to N	N
Serum iron*	N	N	↓↓
WBCs	↑	↑	N or ↓
Platelets	N to ↓	↓ to ↑	↑↑

Hct, Hematocrit; *MCHC,* mean corpuscular hemoglobin concentration; *MCV,* mean cell volume; *N,* normal; *PCV,* packed cell volume; *WBC,* white blood cell; ↓, decreased; ↑, increased/prolonged.
*With internal blood loss, some changes related to iron values are not observed.

Icterus may be observed the day after substantial hemolysis if the serum bilirubin concentration exceeds 2 mg/dl. However, pigmenturia resulting from hyperbilirubinuria, and less commonly hemoglobinuria, are noted earlier in the disease process, even with mild hemolysis. Animals with IMHA may have a combination of cholangiohepatic and hemolytic processes that often result in severe icterus. Finally, cyanosis is not a clinical sign of anemia except in the presence of methemoglobinemia (more than 20%) associated with oxidative injury to the RBCs, such as acetaminophen or onion toxicity. There must be approximately 5 g/dl of unoxygenated Hb in the capillaries for cyanosis to be appreciated clinically; therefore severely anemic animals with severe hypoxemia may not appear cyanotic despite severe concurrent hypoxemia when having concurrent cardiopulmonary disease. The tissue hypoxia caused by anemia also activates a series of compensatory mechanisms that result in the typical signs of anemia and include the following[1]:

- Immediate shunting of blood away from tissues with low oxygen demand (e.g., skin) and toward the vital organs (i.e., brain, kidney, and heart) is accomplished by selective peripheral vasoconstriction and splenic contraction (in dogs). This contributes to pale mucous membranes and delayed capillary refill time in patients with acute or peracute blood loss-induced anemia. In contrast, patients with chronic anemia appear vasodilated from adaptation to local tissue hypoxia and compensatory volume expansion.
- Cardiac output is augmented, initially via an increase in heart rate and contractility and eventually leading to cardiomegaly. This increases the supply of well-oxygenated blood to hypoxic tissue. A mild systolic flow murmur may be heard as a result of changes in blood rheology.
- Oxygen delivery is enhanced by a reduction in Hb-oxygen affinity (i.e., a right shift in the Hb-oxygen dissociation curve) caused by increased metabolic acidity (Bohr effect), and also an increased concentration of 2,3-diphosphoglyceride in RBCs (dogs only).
- Animals with any kind of anemia, but particularly those with acute anemias, show decreased activity levels, exercise intolerance, lethargy, and possibly even collapse; stress should be minimized, and they should be handled gently because they may decompensate rapidly.
- Finally, the erythropoietin-mediated accelerated erythropoiesis takes its maximal effect after about 5 to 7 days (see Laboratory Tests).

Although the signs of acute anemia generally are caused by blood loss or hemolysis and can be dramatic, signs associated with chronic anemia are more subtle. This is because these animals have had time to compensate and adapt to the lower oxygen-carrying capacity, at least until they are stressed (e.g., admission to a veterinary hospital; see Table 108-1). Furthermore, the signs of anemia may be characterized by specific signs of the underlying disease. Dogs with IMHA to may have an acute history of GI signs, recent vaccination, or fever.

LABORATORY TESTS

Clinical signs may be strongly suggestive of anemia, but laboratory tests generally are needed to further define the severity, type, and cause of the disorder.[3,6,7] The minimal laboratory database obtained in an emergency or critical care setting certainly provides a lot of information, but additional tests often are needed. Therefore, whenever possible, collecting more samples than are immediately necessary is advisable before instituting therapy. However, it is important not to delay critical life support, induce major stress to the patient, or cause significant additional blood loss in the severely hypovolemic, anemic animal.

In any case of suspected anemia, it is advisable to draw blood into a serum, citrate, and ethylenediaminetetraacetic acid (EDTA) tube (tilt 5 to 10 times immediately upon collection) and to provide adequate hemostasis at the site of venipuncture (*at least* 5 minutes) in case a hemorrhagic tendency is present. Samples from a catheter line are prone to dilution with heparin-saline flush, which particularly affects coagulation study results. Therefore adequate presample volumes (at least 6 ml for most catheters) and proper technique are paramount when obtaining blood samples from indwelling catheters.

Microhematocrit tubes that generally can be used even in the tiniest patients provide invaluable information, such as PCV, buffy coat, total protein concentration, and plasma color. Furthermore, before centrifugation of the microhematocrit tube, a drop of blood can be placed on a slide or whole blood may be used for chemistry analyses. In cases of acute anemia, various hematologic parameters do not change for hours to days, until fluid shifts from extravascular compartments have occurred or fluid therapy has corrected the hypovolemia. However, a low PCV and total protein level typically are seen with external blood loss; animals with hemolysis have a normal or high total protein level and hyperbilirubinuria, with or without hemoglobinemia or hemoglobinuria.

Microscopic examination of a blood smear can provide readily important clues regarding the type and cause of the anemia and should therefore be part of any emergency minimum database (see Chapter 196).[6] Many clinicians rely solely on an instrument complete blood cell count (CBC) determination, when in fact much of the necessary (and even additional) information can be gleaned from a quick blood smear review. Abnormal instrument CBC results always should be confirmed by a blood film review.

Although any form of anemia is nonregenerative initially, polychromasia typically is seen soon after blood loss or hemolysis. The degree of polychromasia can be confirmed by obtaining a reticulocyte count. Several point-of-care instruments offer reticulocyte counts in dogs and cats. An absolute reticulocyte count of less than 40,000/μl clearly indicates a nonregenerative anemia, although a true regenerative response is reflected by more than 100,000/μl. Moreover, the reticulocyte response varies depending on the duration and degree of anemia. Mild anemias may be associated with only slight increases in reticulocyte counts, whereas patients with hemolytic anemias of at least 5 days' duration may have reticulocyte counts up to a million/µl. The aggregate reticulocytes in cats are considered equal to the typical canine reticulocytes. However, nucleated RBCs are not a good parameter for assessing regeneration in small animals, because they are seen in diseases without anemia or regenerative bone marrow response, such as with lead poisoning, sepsis, heatstroke, neoplasia (hemangiosarcoma), and hyperadrenocorticism.

Depending on the presence or absence of a concurrent leukopenia and thrombocytopenia, the truly nonregenerative anemias (not just because of the lack of time to respond) can be separated into refractory versus aplastic anemias (pancytopenias) or extramedullary versus intramedullary disorders.[2] These additional cytopenias require confirmation by careful review of the blood film at the feathered edge because clumping can result in pseudothrombocytopenia and pseudoleukopenia. Typically 8 to 15 platelets are seen per microscopic high-power oil field (1 platelet reflecting 15,000/µl), and serious bleeding concerns arise when there are *three* platelets or less per high-power field (less than 40,000/µl). One neutrophil should be identified microscopically on every third field, and although high white blood cell counts are expected with infection, they also can be seen with inflammation, immune-mediated disorders, and neoplasia (e.g., leukemoid response; paraneoplastic syndrome).

A variety of RBC changes may be helpful in guiding the diagnosis. Severe hypochromasia is nearly diagnostic for chronic blood loss anemia that often is associated with leukopenia and thrombocytosis (unless thrombocytopenia is the cause of hemorrhage), and mild hypochromasia can be seen with any regenerative anemia because of the incomplete hemoglobinization of juvenile RBCs. The presence of schistocytes (disseminated intravascular coagulation [DIC], hemangiosarcoma), many Heinz bodies (toxic or oxidative Hb and RBC damage), RBC organisms *(Babesia, Cytauxzoon, Mycoplasma),* and marked spherocytosis (more than 20/microscopic high power field with IMHA) are characteristic for certain hemolytic disorders (see Chapter 196).

Autoagglutination of RBCs is found commonly either directly in an EDTA tube or on a stained blood film from any sick dog but is not necessarily diagnostic for IMHA. It could be caused by rouleaux formation (stacked up RBCs, rather than clumps) that often breaks up with the addition of equal amounts of saline on the slide. However, other nonspecific RBC agglutination may disperse only after carefully "washing" the blood sample (using 5 to 10 parts of [buffered] physiologic saline added to one part EDTA and blood), a process that typically is done before the direct antiglobulin (Coombs') and crossmatch testing in the laboratory. The diluted blood sample is mixed gently and centrifuged. The supernatant is discarded, and the RBC pellet is resuspended in saline, mixed, and centrifuged two more times to then examine the blood for agglutination. If the agglutination persists, it is considered "true" or "persistent" autoagglutination, which is strongly suggestive of IMHA and precludes further Coombs' and crossmatch testing, and possibly blood typing if the test is agglutination-based. Furthermore, the presence of persistent agglutination or spherocytosis, or both, is seen with primary (idiopathic) and secondary IMHA (see Chapter 110).[1]

An instrument-derived CBC with reticulocyte count and a microscopic blood film evaluation are desirable for any critically ill animal to expand on and confirm the initial findings. Furthermore, a number of additional tests may prove helpful to determine the cause of the anemia. Although performing a cystocentesis may not be advisable in an animal with a bleeding tendency, a free catch urine sample may reveal pigmenturia resulting from hematuria (intact RBCs rarely cause major blood loss), hemoglobinuria (free Hb [intravascular hemolysis]), or hyperbilirubinuria (hemolysis/hepatopathy). A chemistry screen likely will identify an underlying hepatic or renal disorder and reveal the degree of hyperbilirubinemia or hypoalbuminemia. If hypophosphatemia is present, it should be recognized as the cause of, or contributing factor to, the anemia. Animals receiving insulin or suffering from refeeding syndrome are at particular risk of developing hypophosphatemia.

Fecal examinations are done primarily to identify parasites such as blood-sucking hookworms and whipworms, but they also reveal hematochezia and melena, which can be a source of major blood loss. Occult fecal blood tests rarely are needed to confirm GI blood loss, but some animals have only intermittent blood loss. Moreover, a radiograph of the abdomen may discover a coin (U.S. pennies contain zinc if minted as of 1982) or other foreign metal in the stomach causing copper-induced or zinc-induced hemolysis. However, lead is generally not a cause of anemia, but rather increased numbers of nucleated RBCs, GI cramping/apparent pain, and neurologic signs. Toxicologic blood analysis can diagnose definitively a heavy metal, rodenticide, or other suspected toxin as the cause of anemia, when indicated.

In addition to the evaluation of platelet count and size, further hemostatic studies often are indicated in anemic animals, particularly those with signs of multisystemic disease or excessive hemorrhage (see Chapter 105).[4,5] Overall hemostasis can be evaluated by a cuticle bleeding time, but this is a relatively crude and slightly painful procedure, and thus specific blood tests for primary and secondary hemostasis are preferred. An assessment of coagulation cascades is performed easily with the inexpensive activated coagulation time (ACT) tube test or activated partial thromboplastin time (aPTT) test and prothrombin time (PT). Point-of-care instruments enable the assessment of aPTT and PT on fresh whole citrated blood. The ACT or aPTT screening tests are prolonged by any single hereditary (e.g., hemophilia A and B) or combined coagulation factor deficiencies (liver disease, rodenticide toxicity, heparin), except isolated hereditary factor VII deficiency, which causes a prolongation of the PT only. Hereditary factor VII deficiency has been identified in many Beagles, Alaskan Klee Kais, and Scottish Deerhounds and causes a mild bleeding tendency.

Animals bleeding as a result of anticoagulant rodenticide intoxication have a severely (more than two times) prolonged PT as well as aPTT and also may be moderately thrombocytopenic secondary to toxicity (see Chapter 111). The historically used PIVKA test (proteins induced by vitamin K antagonism or absence) is a modified PT test but is neither more sensitive nor specific for rodenticide intoxication and thus does not offer any additional value to diagnose rodenticide-induced coagulopathies. Mild prolongations in coagulation times of 25% above a normal control or just slightly out of the normal range can be clinically important if caused by diseases such as hemophilia and other hereditary coagulopathies, vitamin K malabsorption, or even DIC (reference laboratories often have very large reference ranges for coagulation times). Using a veterinary laboratory or in-clinic instrument validated for use in companion animals with established normal coagulation times (human coagulation times are longer) is crucial.

Because von Willebrand disease is so common in dogs screening of an EDTA blood sample for von Willebrand factor deficiency with an enzyme-linked immunosorbent assay (ELISA) certainly may be indicated (see Chapter 105). Because these results are generally not immediately available a buccal mucosal bleeding time may be performed. However, the buccal mucosal bleeding time is prolonged in animals with von Willebrand disease and other thrombopathias, including those associated with renal failure and animals that recently have received nonsteroidal agents such as aspirin. This test should be performed only if the platelet count is higher than 100,000/µl because lower platelet counts cause longer bleeding times. Finally, in addition to schistocytosis and thrombocytopenia, an increased D-dimer or fibrin split product concentration and low or falling plasma fibrinogen concentration are suggestive of intravascular thrombosis, such as DIC. These findings are prognostically important because they may be associated with many underlying disorders including neoplasia, sepsis, systemic inflammation, and immune-mediated disease. Thromboelastography has become a valuable tool to indicate hyper- and hypocoagulable states but does not eliminate the need of the other conventional hemostatic tests.

Other diagnostic tests for underlying causes of anemia include a search for infectious agents and neoplasia. In some cases of nonregenerative anemia, a bone marrow aspirate for cytology may be warranted.

THERAPEUTIC PRINCIPLES

Depending on the cause, severity, and progression of the anemia, the indicated therapies vary greatly, and the recommendations for specific disease conditions are found in the correlating chapters. A few therapeutic principles related to the critically ill patient requiring emergent treatment are stated here. Whenever possible, the triggering agent is removed and the identified underlying disease is treated. Until the underlying disease is treated and the bone marrow has responded, supportive care is provided as needed.[1,4,5] Animals that are cardiovascularly unstable or have evidence of tachypnea will likely benefit from oxygen therapy.

Animals with (peracute) acute blood loss generally benefit from aggressive fluid therapy to ensure vital organ perfusion before the administration of blood products to improve oxygen-carrying capacity (see Chapter 60). This should be accomplished immediately, and an associated drop in PCV is anticipated and of lesser concern until normovolemia is reached. Local hemostasis should be provided immediately if indicated (e.g., compression, hemostat clamping, thrombin, and other hemostatic agents). Surgical correction of hemorrhage likely should be delayed until a hemostatic defect has been excluded and the bleeding tendency and anemia have been controlled adequately to permit safe surgery.

Animals that have been poisoned with an anticoagulant rodenticide, but whose bleeding is not life threatening, respond rapidly to parenteral or oral (as long as there is no vomiting) vitamin K1 administration (2 to 5 mg/kg q12h), depending on the specific toxin, amount ingested, and response to treatment (see Chapter 111). In dogs with von Willebrand disease, desmopressin at a dosage of 1 to 4 mcg/kg SC q3-4h has helped to control minor hemorrhage. This drug is likely less helpful in treating other bleeding disorders (see Chapter 158). Another underused agent is ε-aminocaproic acid, which inhibits fibrinolysis, is inexpensive, and may stop bleeding from vasculopathies such as seen in Greyhounds.

No specific transfusion trigger is established; therefore the need to provide RBCs or hemostatic blood components is a clinical judgment. Generally, transfusions are administered when the patients PCV drops rapidly, reaches values of 20% or less, and the animal is showing signs of tissue hypoxia related to anemia. In animals with peracute blood loss, it is often difficult to transfuse RBCs fast enough because of the high viscosity of the blood. Blood product replacement is not required to restore completely normal hematologic values but rather to return them to levels that ensure adequate oxygen carrying capacity and hemostasis. A rise in PCV to 20% to 25% and the most deficient coagulation factors to 20% of normal is often sufficient to achieve adequate oxygen content and hemostasis, respectively. The utility of "resuscitation bundles" that use lactate clearance and central venous oxygen saturation for goal-directed therapy, rather than a specific transfusion trigger, has shown benefits in human and animals, but further research is necessary (see Chapter 183). The product selection for anemic or bleeding animals, the volume to transfuse, frequency of administration, and required blood compatibility testing procedures are described in detail in Chapter 61.

Hemolytic anemia is not necessarily IMHA; many other differential diagnoses include the following:

- Chemical-induced or oxidative-induced hemolysis by drugs, copper, zinc, onions, and hypophosphatemia
- Hereditary erythrocyte defects such as:
  Phosphofructokinase deficiency (severe intermittent anemia: English Springer and Cocker Spaniels, Whippet, Wachtelhund, and mixed breeds)
  Pyruvate kinase deficiency (persistent anemia: many canine breeds; and intermittent anemia: Abyssinian, Somali, Bengal, Singapura, and domestic shorthair cats)
- Infectious hemolytic anemias (see Signalment and History in this chapter)
- Hemolysis caused by neoplasia, such as malignant histiocytosis and hemangiosarcoma

Because some of the diagnostic modalities may not be immediately available and IMHA also may occur secondary to other disorders or triggers, hemolytic patients often are treated initially with prednisolone (2 to 4 mg/kg PO q12h; or an equivalent parenteral dose of dexamethasone) and antibiotics (e.g., doxycycline) until the triggering agents are removed and a definitive diagnosis is reached. In the initial treatment of IMHA, there is no need to use other immunosuppressive agents because none of them has proven beneficial and some may cause major side effects and increase cost. Nevertheless, when IMHA is confirmed and no response is seen with glucocorticosteroid medications or their side effects are intolerable, consideration may be given to the use of cyclosporine, human intravenous immunoglobulin, or mycophenolate. In a critical review of published data, none of the immunosuppressive agents other than glucocorticosteroids have been safe and effective in dogs with IMHA[8] (see Chapter 110).

In any case of intoxication, the causative agent should be removed immediately. Zinc-containing coins or other objects lodged in the stomach may be removed endoscopically or surgically. There are few antidotes, such as acetylcysteine and methylene blue, for acetaminophen and other methemoglobin-inducing intoxications.

Intoxicated animals need aggressive supportive care. Antimicrobial therapy should be selected carefully to target the likely organisms and prevent antibiotic resistance or perpetuate immune-mediated drug reactions (e.g., sulfonamides, cephalosporin classes). Some parasites, such as *Babesia canis, Babesia gibsoni,* and *Cytauxzoon felis,* require treatment with specific antiparasitic agents, and the animals still may remain carriers indefinitely. Flea-infested young animals that are severely anemic are handled cautiously with a flea comb and supportive care (possibly a transfusion) before using topical insecticides. Fleas and flea dirt also may transmit other infectious diseases. Similarly, anemic oncology patients may require a slow and more conservative diagnostic and therapeutic approach to prevent causing massive tumor lysis or cytopenias.

Last, animals with chronic, but decompensated, poorly or nonregenerative anemias require supportive care for longer periods because the bone marrow probably will not respond quickly, even with specific treatment. They are generally normovolemic and their heart works at maximal capacity; hence any fluid and blood administration has to occur slowly so as not to cause volume overload. Human erythropoietin can be beneficial in animals with anemia because of chronic renal failure and some other disorders. This drug may have effects beyond causing a rise in PCV; it often results in rapidly improved well-being. However, this is a human product that may cause neutralizing antibodies with ensuing pure red blood cell aplasia (less so with darbepoetin alpha).

SUMMARY

A careful approach to the anemic animal with appropriate clinical and laboratory examinations allows the clinician to identify the cause and in return provide rewarding targeted and supportive therapy in a critical care setting.

REFERENCES

1. Giger U: Regenerative anemias caused by blood loss and hemolysis. In Ettinger SJ, Feldman EC, editors: Textbook of veterinary internal medicine, ed 6, St Louis, 2005, Saunders, pp 1886-1907.
2. Feldman BF: Nonregenerative anemia. In Ettinger SJ, Feldman EC, editors: Textbook of veterinary internal medicine, ed 6, St Louis, 2005, Saunders.
3. Feldman BF, Zinkl JG, Jain NC, editors: Schalm's veterinary hematology, ed 5, Philadelphia, 2000, Lippincott Williams & Wilkins.
4. Brooks M: Coagulopathies and thrombosis. In Ettinger SJ, Feldman EC, editors: Textbook of veterinary internal medicine, ed 6, St Louis, 2005, Saunders.
5. Brooks MB, Catalfamo JL: Platelet disorders and von Willebrand disease. In Ettinger SJ, Feldman EC, editors: Textbook of veterinary internal medicine, ed 6, St Louis, 2005, Saunders.
6. Rebar AH, MacWilliams PS, Feldman BF, et al: A guide to hematology in dogs and cats, Jackson, WY, 2001, Teton NewMedia.
7. Villiers E, Blackwood L: BSAVA manual of canine and feline clinical pathology, Gloucester, England, 2005, British Small Animal Association.
8. Swann JW, Skelly BJ: Systematic review of evidence relating to the treatment of immune-mediated hemolytic anemia in dogs, J Vet Intern Med 27(1):1-9, 2013.

CHAPTER 109

METHEMOGLOBINEMIA

Louisa J. Rahilly, DVM, DACVECC • Deborah C. Mandell, VMD, DACVECC

KEY POINTS

- Methemoglobin (metHb) is hemoglobin in which the ferrous (Fe^{2+}) molecule is oxidized to the ferric (Fe^{3+}) form. Methemoglobin is incapable of carrying oxygen, and high levels (more than 20%) can cause cellular hypoxia and shock.
- Clinical methemoglobinemia occurs when erythrocyte defense systems are overwhelmed and cannot reduce methemoglobin to hemoglobin fast enough to keep up with the oxidative damage. Methemoglobin reductase deficiency is a rare condition in small animals that leads to inefficient reduction of methemoglobin in the body but may or may not lead to clinical signs of methemoglobinemia.
- Substances that can cause clinical methemoglobinemia in small animals include acetaminophen, topical benzocaine formulations, phenazopyridine (a urinary tract analgesic), nitrites, nitrates, hydroxycarbamide, and skunk musk.
- Many substances that cause methemoglobinemia also can cause the body to form clinically significant numbers of Heinz bodies (HzBs), aggregations of denatured hemoglobin that can lead to immune-mediated red blood cell destruction and anemia.
- Treatment for methemoglobinemia involves augmentation of endogenous glutathione levels with N-acetylcysteine (NAC), methylene blue administration (in severe cases), antioxidant therapy, increased clearance or decreased metabolism of any toxins present, blood transfusions (if required), and supportive care.

Hemoglobin, the molecule that confers oxygen-carrying capacity to erythrocytes, is composed of four polypeptide chains (globins); each is attached to a heme molecule.[1,2] Heme is made up of a tetrapyrrole with a central iron molecule.[1,2] The iron molecule must be maintained in the ferrous (Fe^{2+}) state for the hemoglobin to bind oxygen.[1-3] Methemoglobin (MetHb) is an inactive form of hemoglobin created when the iron molecule of hemoglobin is oxidized to the ferric (Fe^{3+}) state because of oxidative damage within the red blood cell.[1-6] It gives the red blood cell a darker brown color and results in dusky cyanotic or chocolate-colored mucous membranes.[1-3,5] MetHb increases the affinity for oxygen in the remaining ferrous moieties of the hemoglobin molecule, decreasing release of oxygen to the tissues and shifting the oxyhemoglobin dissociation curve to the left.[5,7,8] Approximately 0.5% to 3% of hemoglobin is oxidized to metHb each day in normal animals.[2-4] However, numerous mechanisms prevent oxidative injury in erythrocytes, and metHb is reduced to functional hemoglobin rapidly, so metHb accounts for less than 3% of total hemoglobin in normal dogs and cats.[9,10] Exogenous substances that overwhelm the antioxidant defenses, or a congenital or acquired abnormality within the adaptive response, can result in elevated levels of metHb.[2,3,5]

PATHOPHYSIOLOGY

Oxidation in the Erythrocyte

Reactive species derived from oxygen can cause oxidative damage within the body by transferring or extracting an unpaired electron to or from another molecule.[1] Protective mechanisms that prevent or reverse oxidative damage include proteins that act as free radical scavengers and reducing agents that can remove the unpaired electron from an oxidized molecule.[1]

Erythrocytes are especially vulnerable to oxidative damage because they carry oxygen, are exposed to various chemicals in plasma, and have no nucleus or mitochondria.[1,4] The lack of cellular organelles renders the membrane the deformability necessary to

BOX 109-1 ***Chemical Reactions Resulting in Free Radical Formation, Their Removal, and Methemoglobin Reduction***

Free Radical Formation

Superoxide anion: $O_2 + e^- \rightarrow O_2^-$
Ferric production: $Fe^{2+} + H_2O_2 \rightarrow Fe^{3+} + OH^- + OH^{\cdot}$

Mechanisms of Free Radical Removal

Superoxide dismutase reaction: $2O_2^- + 2H^+ \rightarrow H_2O_2 + O_2$

Catalase reaction: $O_2^{-\cdot} + H_2O_2 \xrightarrow{CAT} O_2 + OH^- + OH^{\cdot}$

Glutathione Peroxide and Glutathione Reductase Reactions

$H_2O_2 + 2GSH \xrightarrow{GP} 2H_2O + GSSG$

$GSSG + H^+ + NADPH \xrightarrow{GR} 2GSH + NADP^+$

Methemoglobin Reduction

$MetHb\text{-}Fe^{3+} \xrightarrow{MR} HbFe^{2+} + O_2$

NADH ↷ NAD^+

Modified from Engelking LR: Textbook of veterinary physiological chemistry, Jackson Hole, Wyo, 2004, Teton NewMedia.

CAT, Catalase; *GP*, glutathione peroxidase; *GR*, glutathione reductase; *GSH*, glutathione; *GSSG*, oxidized glutathione; *HbFe*$^{2+}$, ferrous hemoglobin; *MR*, methemoglobin reductase; *NAD*, nicotinamide adenine dinucleotide; *NADH*, nicotinamide adenine dinucleotide; *NADPH*, nicotinamide adenine dinucleotide phosphate; *SOD*, superoxide dismutase.

navigate capillary beds but results in a cell that is incapable of producing proteins or performing efficient energy production.[1] Therefore they have a finite number of cell proteins and rely on anaerobic respiration to generate energy and reducing agents.[1] Oxidants continuously generated *in vivo* include hydrogen peroxide (H_2O_2), superoxide free radicals (O_2^-), and hydroxyl radicals (OH^-) (Box 109-1).[1,3,4] Hemoglobin can undergo auto-oxidation as an electron is pulled off the hemoglobin onto an oxygen molecule, resulting in the generation of metHb and O_2^-.[1,3,6] Free radicals also may extract electrons by oxidizing deoxyhemoglobin.[3] In contrast, oxidant toxins can donate an electron to oxyhemoglobin, creating metHb and hydrogen peroxide (see Box 109-1).[3]

Despite their limited capacity to produce energy and proteins, erythrocytes have many mechanisms to protect themselves from oxidative damage. These include superoxide dismutase, catalase, glutathione peroxidase, glutathione, and metHb reductase (also known as cytochrome b_5 reductase or nicotinamide adenine dinucleotide diaphorase) (see Box 109-1).[1-4] Glutathione (GSH) is a tripeptide produced in erythrocytes and composed of glutamic acid, cysteine, and glycine and contains an easily oxidizable sulfhydryl (SH) group.[3] It is a powerful antioxidant that operates as a free radical scavenger. Reducing agents such as nicotinamide adenine dinucleotide phosphate (NADPH) and nicotinamide adenine dinucleotide (NADH) are instrumental in reducing oxidized glutathione and metHb back to functional molecules (see Box 109-1).[1,3,4]

Heinz Bodies

Heinz bodies (HzBs) are aggregates of denatured, precipitated hemoglobin within erythrocytes that form as hemoglobin with oxidative damage is metabolized.[1-4] Oxidation of the SH groups of hemoglobin, either through auto-oxidation, free radical extraction of an electron, or oxidant toxin donation of an electron, causes conformational changes in the globin chains that result in precipitation of the denatured globin.[3,4] Aggregates of denatured globin and metabolized metHb clump into HzBs and continue to coalesce until visible, pale structures can be seen within the red blood cell cytoplasm (see Figure 109-2, *B*).[4] Formation of metHb is thought to be necessary for the development of HzBs.[3,4] Feline hemoglobin is more susceptible to oxidative damage because it has eight SH groups on the globin part of the molecule rather than four, as the canine counterpart does.[3,4,8,11]

HzBs have an affinity for membrane proteins.[4] Binding of a HzB to these proteins causes disruption of anion transport, decreased membrane deformability, and aggregations of membrane protein complexes that may act as autoantibodies.[4,8] Numerous HzBs can disrupt the membrane sufficiently to result in "ghost" cells, empty red blood cells with just a cell membrane and HzB remaining, which are associated with oxidation-induced intravascular hemolysis.[8] However, more commonly erythrocytes that have undergone oxidative damage are removed by the mononuclear phagocyte system, particularly within the spleen.[4,8] Rigid cells or cells with large HzBs protruding from the surface become lodged in the narrow openings between splenic endothelial cells and undergo phagocytosis by the splenic macrophages.[3] In most animals, the spleen can perform pitting functions and remove the HzBs from the erythrocyte.[3] However, feline spleens have an ultrastructural variation and impaired ability to catch and remove oxidized red blood cells.[3,8,12] As a result of the combination of more SH groups available for oxidation on feline hemoglobin and the unique spleen in this species, healthy cats often have notable HzBs in circulation (with reports up to 96%).[12] The reasons are still unknown why some cats undergo hemolysis with HzB percentages lower than 96%, but other cats have no clinical signs with most of their erythrocytes affected.[8,12] However, various agents and disease processes induce oxidative damage in different ways and to varying extents, and the nature of the damage, the amount of affected hemoglobin within a cell, and individual variations seem to determine whether a given cat develops clinically significant hemolysis.[8]

SPECIFIC CAUSES OF ERYTHROCYTE OXIDATION

Methemoglobinemia has been documented in small animals in association with acetaminophen ingestion, topical benzocaine products,[13] phenazopyridine (a urinary tract analgesic) ingestion, nitrites, nitrates, skunk musk,[14] hydroxycarbamide,[15-17] aniline (a chemical intermediate used in dyes),[18] and metHb reductase deficiency.[3,19] Agents that have resulted in metHb in humans (and may be used in veterinary medicine) include dapsone, metoclopramide, sulfonamides, nitroglycerin, and nitroprusside.[5,6] Regardless of the toxic agent, metHb often is formed within minutes to hours of exposure. Substances that cause metHb production are likely to cause HzB production, and potentially hemolytic anemia, in the days after the exposure. Numerous substances that cause an increase in HzBs are thought to cause some degree of methemoglobinemia, but associated clinical signs typically are attributable to a hemolytic anemia secondary to the HzBs rather than the metHb. These substances include *Allium* plants (onions and garlic), propylene glycol, zinc, methylene blue, crude oils, naphthalene (ingredient in moth balls),[20] repeated use of propofol in cats,[12] phenothiazine, phenylhydrazine, methionine (a urinary acidifier) in cats, menadione (vitamin K_3) in dogs, and copper (particularly in animals with copper storage diseases).[3,4] Depending on the individual patient's metabolism, the dose, and the period over which the drug or chemical was ingested, these substances cause varying degrees of HzB formation, and anemia does not occur usually until HzB formation is moderate to severe.

Some disease states are known to increase oxidative stress in the body and are associated with oxidative damage to erythrocytes. Low levels of metHb have been documented in humans with sepsis resulting from increased levels of nitric oxide.[21] Certain disease states in cats have been associated with increased levels of HzB and mild to moderate anemia; these include diabetes mellitus, particularly those with ketoacidosis, hyperthyroidism, and lymphoma.[4,22,23] The clinical significance of these red blood cell changes depends on the extent of erythrocytes affected as well as comorbid conditions (i.e., cardiovascular dysfunction, hypoxemia and anemia) that negatively affect oxygen delivery.[7]

Acetaminophen

Acetaminophen (Tylenol) is an analgesic and antipyretic drug used widely in human medicine.[7,11] It is present in many pain and cold medications.[7] Although considered safe in humans, this drug can be toxic to small animals, causing acute hepatotoxicity and/or life-threatening methemoglobinemia.[7,11] Most phenacetin, a component of over-the-counter drug formulations, is metabolized rapidly to acetaminophen and also could result in toxicity in small animals.[7] A dose of as little as 10 mg/kg of acetaminophen is toxic for cats, and 150 to 200 mg/kg is toxic for dogs.[7] Unfortunately, the vast majority of acetaminophen toxicities in small animals are due to intentional administration by the owner in an attempt to treat pain or malaise in their pets.[7,11]

Acetaminophen is metabolized in the liver via one of several pathways: (1) it is conjugated to a sulfate compound by a phenol sulfotransferase, (2) it is conjugated to a glucuronide compound by a uridine diphosphate-glucuronosyl transferase, or (3) it can be transformed and oxidized by the cytochrome P-450 system that converts it to the reactive intermediate N-acetyl-P-benzoquinone-imine (NAPQI).[7] The glucuronide and sulfate conjugations are nontoxic and are excreted in the bile and urine in most species other than the cat.[7,11] GSH reacts with NAPQI to form a nonreactive molecule, mercapturic acid, which is excreted in the urine.[11] An additional metabolite of acetaminophen, *para*-Aminophenol (PAP), is produced by deacylation of acetaminophen by hepatic microsomal carboxyesterases.[24] PAP is removed by biotransformation through N-acetylation with N-acetyltransferase (NAT), conjugation with GSH, or sulfation.[24] Low doses of acetaminophen are metabolized readily to nontoxic products, but higher doses can overwhelm the sulfate and glucuronide conjugate systems of the liver and deplete GSH stores.[7] Ultimately, the metabolites NAPQI and PAP build up and unmetabolized acetaminophen accumulates.[7,24] Thus the half-life of acetaminophen becomes longer with higher dosages.[7]

Cats are limited in their ability to conjugate glucuronide because they lack a specific form of the enzyme glucuronyl transferase needed to conjugate acetaminophen.[7,11] Unfortunately, cats also have a somewhat limited sulfate binding capacity.[7,11] Therefore cats are estimated to have one tenth the capacity to eliminate acetaminophen compared with dogs.[7] In addition, humans have multiple NAT enzymes, whereas cats have only one and dogs have none. This leads to decreased biotransformation and elimination of PAP in both species compared with humans.[24]

NAPQI oxidizes hepatic proteins, resulting in hepatocellular damage.[7] Historically NAPQI was believed to cause intracellular damage in erythrocytes as well, but recent research demonstrates that PAP may play a more significant role in erythrocyte oxidative damage.[24] PAP co-oxidizes with oxyhemoglobin forming metHb and an oxidized PAP intermediate.[24] This intermediate is reduced by GSH and the metHb is reduced primarily by metHb reductase.[24] Lower levels of metHb reductase in dogs and cats relative to other species further increase potential erythrocyte oxidative toxicity associated with acetaminophen in these patients.[24,25] Methemoglobinemia becomes overt when metHb reductase and necessary reducing equivalents (i.e., NADH and GSH) become depleted in erythrocytes. NAPQI and PAP theoretically can cause intracellular oxidative damage, converting hemoglobin to metHb, but PAP may be more the culprit because the enzymes necessary to form NAPQI are not present in erythrocytes and circulating NAPQI is either inactive or protein-bound.[24]

After the acute episode of metHb production, HzBs begin to form and aggregate into larger structures, eventually causing enough changes in the erythrocyte to trigger hemolysis.[7] Although cats tend to develop metHb and HzB anemia and dogs undergo a significant hepatic insult with acetaminophen toxicity, there is much individual variation, and many animals have evidence of both.[7] The prognosis for acetaminophen toxicity is guarded; evidence in veterinary and human literature demonstrates that time from ingestion to treatment is the most important factor in determining morbidity and survival.[7,11] If the animal is not showing any clinical signs, no contraindications exist, and ingestion was recent (less than 60 minutes), emesis should be induced (see Chapter 74).

Topical Benzocaine

Benzocaine sprays for laryngeal spasm in cats and over-the-counter creams for pruritus in dogs and cats have been associated with methemoglobinemia.[2,3,13] An experimental study evaluating a 2-second spray of aerosolized 14% benzocaine (approximately 56 mg) demonstrated an increase in metHb levels in cats and dogs; cats were affected more severely than dogs.[13] However, dogs did develop a more significant reaction if they received the benzocaine intravenously.[13] Metabolites of benzocaine are likely responsible for oxidative damage to hemoglobin.[13] The effects of HzBs associated with benzocaine toxicity are generally mild and rarely associated with hemolysis.[2]

Skunk Musk

There is one case report of methemoglobinemia and HzB hemolytic anemia in a dog after exposure to skunk musk.[14] The toxic substances in skunk musk are thought to be thiols, which can react with oxyhemoglobin to form metHb, a thiyl radical, and hydrogen peroxide.[14] The dog in this report was treated successfully with intravenous fluids and antibiotics. Three days later she required a whole blood transfusion for treatment of the HzB anemia. The authors mention that N-acetylcysteine could have been considered because of the severe methemoglobinemia initially present.

Nitrites and Nitrates

Unlike most substances that cause methemoglobinemia, nitrites and nitrates are not documented to cause HzB production.[3] Exposure to these substances could occur in small animals that receive vasodilatory drugs that release nitric oxide, including nitroglycerin and sodium nitroprusside.[26] Nitric oxide is decomposed in vivo by interacting with oxyhemoglobin to form metHb and nitrate.[26,27] The metHb is reduced by metHb reductase in red blood cells, but some evidence indicates that nitric oxide decreases metHb reductase activity.[27] Nitric oxide also interacts with oxygen to form nitrogen dioxide (NO_2), which dissolves in solution and yields nitrite and nitrate.[26,27] Nitrite also can convert oxyhemoglobin to metHb.[26] Although significant methemoglobinemia has not been reported in the veterinary literature associated with nitroglycerin or nitroprusside, it is a potential complication of these agents and may contribute to the morbidity of patients requiring therapy with these drugs. Toxicity should be considered in animals receiving these drugs and developing an unexplained hyperlactatemia.

Hydroxycarbamide

One case report of methemoglobinemia was caused by hydroxycarbamide (hydroxyurea) ingestion in a dog,[15] and reports of methemoglobinemia, cyanosis, and signs consistent with methemoglobinemia in canine cases of hydroxycarbamide toxicity have been reported to animal poison centers.[16,17] Hydroxycarbamide inhibits ribonucleoside diphosphate reductase. It is used to treat polycythemia vera and other neoplastic conditions in small animals and humans. Acute toxicity in humans can lead to methemoglobinemia, myelosuppression, pneumonitis, and hepatotoxicity.[15]

Methemoglobin Reductase Deficiency

MetHb reductase deficiency is a rare congenital abnormality.[19] Affected animals cannot efficiently reduce metHb (see Box 109-1) and therefore have elevated blood levels of metHb (18% to 41%), exhibit mild to moderate cyanosis of the mucous membranes (present in 100% of cases), and may suffer from exercise intolerance (present in less than 50% of cases).[19] A definitive diagnosis is obtained by measuring erythrocyte metHb reductase enzyme activity at a research laboratory.[2,19] The defect has been documented in one domestic shorthaired cat and several breeds of dogs, including the Chihuahua, Borzoi, English Setter, Terrier mix, Cockapoo, Poodle, Corgi, Pomeranian, and toy American Eskimo dogs.[2]

In humans this disorder is an inherited, autosomal recessive defect, but familial studies in dogs have not been done. This condition is typically fairly benign, rarely requires treatment, and affected dogs have a normal life span.[2,19] Indications for treatment include clinical signs of metHb such as lethargy, tachycardia, and/or tachypnea, and as preparation for animals that require general anesthesia.[4]

DIAGNOSIS

Clinical Signs

The clinical presentation of patients with methemoglobinemia is consistent with decreased oxygen-carrying capacity, cellular hypoxia, and shock.[3] These signs begin with a metHb level of 20% and include tachycardia, tachypnea, dyspnea, lethargy, anorexia, vomiting, weakness, ataxia, stupor, hypothermia, ptyalism, and convulsions in cats, and coma and death if metHb levels reach 80%.[5,7,11,19] Chocolate-brown mucous membranes and cyanosis are common findings, with cyanosis appearing at metHb levels of 12% to 14% or more (Figure 109-1).[19] Small animals can develop head, neck, and limb edema associated with acetaminophen toxicity,[7,11,28,29] but this is more common in cats. Facial edema also has been reported with repeated administration of propofol in cats.[12]

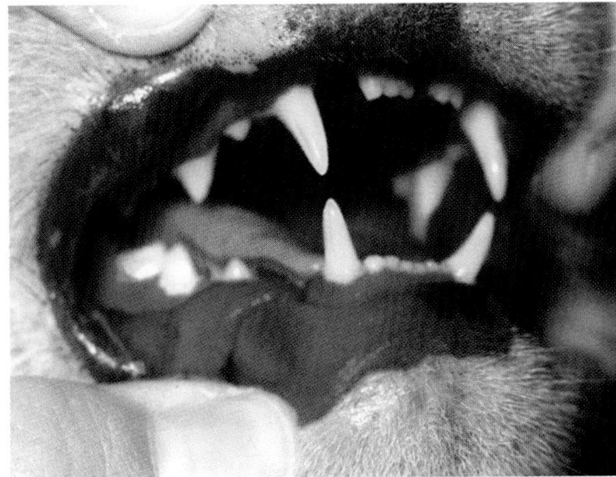

FIGURE 109-1 Chocolate brown mucous membranes of a cat with acetaminophen toxicity.

Determining Methemoglobin Presence and Levels

Methemoglobinemia is apparent on blood sampling because the blood has a chocolate-brown discoloration. A simple qualification test can be performed by placing a drop of venous blood from the patient onto a white piece of paper next to a drop of control blood. After exposure to oxygen in the air, the control blood has a distinctly red appearance, but blood with more than 10% metHb remains dark with a brown discoloration.[2,5,19] Similarly, one can observe blood in a tube containing ethylenediaminetetraacetic acid (EDTA).[19] If the blood contains deoxyhemoglobin as a result of cardiac or respiratory disease, it turns red when exposed to room air for 15 minutes. However, if the blood contains elevated levels of metHb, it remains dark.

Definitive diagnosis and quantification of metHb levels require direct measurement via a co-oximeter or assay.[5,10] A co-oximeter is a machine used to measure hemoglobin content, oxygen saturation, percentage of carboxyhemoglobin, and percentage of metHb (see Chapter 186). An assay for metHb can be performed at some veterinary and human laboratories and involves spectrophotometrically quantifying the change in absorbance at 630 nm before and after the addition of cyanide to the sample.[30,31] The cyanide converts metHb to cyanmethemoglobin, which has a different absorbance than metHb.[30]

Comparing pulse oximeter oxygen saturation to arterial blood gas saturation (saturation gap) also can be helpful in diagnosing methemoglobinemia.[5] The pulse oximeter determines the ratio of oxyhemoglobin to deoxyhemoglobin. The presence of metHb distorts this ratio. If metHb levels exceed 30% the pulse oximeter reading plateaus at about 85% regardless of the true oxygen content.[5] Methemoglobinemia should be suspected if the saturation gap is greater than 5%.[5] Carboxyhemoglobinemia also can cause this gap.[32,33] Broadband diffuse optical spectroscopy as a method of quantifying metHb in vivo using the different absorbance spectra of various hemoglobins has been evaluated experimentally in rabbits but is not yet used commonly in the clinical setting in human or veterinary medicine.[34]

Examining a peripheral blood smear for HzBs, eccentrocytes, and "ghost" cells also can be helpful when looking for evidence of oxidative damage (Figure 109-2, *A*). Feline HzBs may appear as pale inclusions within red blood cells or as projections from the surface of the cell (see Figure 109-2, *B*).[2,30] However, canine HzBs are often small and scattered throughout the cell. These may require stains such as new methylene blue, with which they appear as dark, refractile inclusions, or a reticulocyte stain with which they appear as light blue inclusions.[2] "Ghost" cells contain HzBs seen as red inclusions within an erythrocyte membrane or "ghost."[2] Eccentrocytes are cells with hemoglobin concentrated at one side of the cell and are formed by the adhesion of the erythrocyte membrane from opposing sides of the cell.[2,4]

TREATMENT

Treatment of animals with methemoglobinemia initially involves recognition, careful history acquisition, and elimination of the source of oxidative damage, if possible. Although oxygen therapy increases the amount of dissolved oxygen in the blood and is often the first line of therapy until a full assessment and treatment plan are established, the hemoglobin capable of carrying oxygen usually is maximally saturated, and supplemental oxygen is not sufficient as a sole therapy.[2,7] Therapy for methemoglobinemia often involves diuresis or medications to increase the rate of elimination or decrease the production of toxic metabolites.[7] Induction of vomiting followed by the administration of activated charcoal should be considered if the

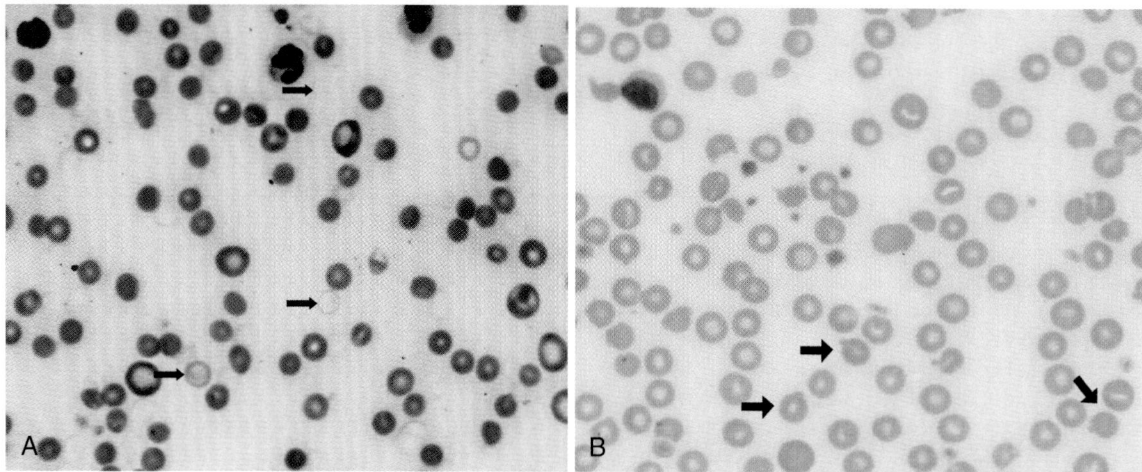

FIGURE 109-2 A, Ghost cells in a dog after suffering an oxidative insult. **B,** Heinz bodies on red blood cells in a dog that ingested onions.

animal has a history of recently ingesting a toxic substance and is not yet clinically ill (see Chapter 74).[7,11] Supportive care is also important to correct volume status, hydration, and electrolyte or acid-base disturbances.[7]

N-Acetylcysteine

N-Acetylcysteine (NAC) is considered the preferred treatment for the treatment of acetaminophen toxicity.[35] NAC augments the endogenous glutathione stores as it is hydrolyzed to cysteine (one of the components of GSH).[7,11,35] GSH therapy is of minimal value to these patients, because it is not capable of penetrating cells and must be synthesized within the cell. NAC also interacts directly with NAPQI to form a nontoxic conjugate and increases the fraction of acetaminophen excreted as the sulfate conjugate.[7,35] The half-life of acetaminophen is halved in cats treated with NAC.[35] NAC is most effective if administered within 12 hours of ingestion of acetaminophen but still is recommended up to 36 to 80 hours after ingestion.[7,35]

The recommended regimen is an initial dose of 140 mg/kg IV (280 mg/kg in severe toxicosis) followed by 70 mg/kg q6h for seven additional treatments.[7,11] NAC typically causes nausea and vomiting when given orally, hypotension and bronchospasm if given rapidly intravenously, and phlebitis if it leaks perivascularly.[35] Because of these adverse effects the recommended route of administration is a slow intravenous infusion of a 5% solution (10% or 20% NAC solution diluted with 5% dextrose or physiologic saline) over 30 to 60 minutes through a 0.2-μm filter (only if the product is not formulated for intravenous use).[11,35]

Methylene Blue

Methylene blue increases the rate of reduction of metHb through use of another reducing system within the erythrocyte, NADPH dehydrogenase.[3] Methylene blue is administered as a 1% solution intravenously over several minutes at a dosage of 1 mg/kg once.[2] Improvement in clinical parameters should be noted within 30 minutes of administration.[2] However, methylene blue causes oxidative damage in red blood cells, particularly in cats, and can potentiate a HzB anemia caused by the original oxidative insult.[2,3] A delayed reaction may occur (days after drug administration); therefore the hematocrit and blood smear should be monitored closely for 3 to 4 days after administration.[2] One study comparing the effectiveness of methylene blue with that of NAC for the treatment of acetaminophen toxicity in cats demonstrated minimal effect on the half-life of metHb with methylene blue therapy and possible attenuation of the beneficial effects of NAC on the half-life of acetaminophen in male cats when both drugs were given.[36]

Adjunctive Treatments

Multiple other treatment modalities have been used to treat methemoglobinemia, HzB anemia, and acetaminophen toxicity. These include ascorbic acid (vitamin C),[2,7,11] cimetidine,[7,11] S-adenosylmethionine (SAMe),[37] bioflavonoids,[3,38] and blood transfusions.[7,6,15] Ascorbic acid is used at a dosage of 30 mg/kg IV q6h as an antioxidant and can augment metHb conversion to hemoglobin through nonenzymatic reduction.[7,11] Cimetidine, a histamine-2 receptor antagonist, is theoretically useful in cases of acetaminophen toxicity because it inhibits the P-450 oxidation system in the liver, limiting the production of NAPQI.[7,11] Studies evaluating the efficacy of cimetidine-induced alterations of acetaminophen metabolism in humans, however, have not been able to demonstrate consistent benefits.[11] The suggested dosage is 5 mg/kg IV q8h as adjunctive therapy in patients with acetaminophen toxicity.[7,11] SAMe is an essential metabolite that is vital to hepatocytes and has been reported to be hepatoprotective, have antioxidant properties, and decrease the osmotic fragility of erythrocytes.[38,39] An experimental, prospective study evaluating the effects of SAMe for the treatment of acetaminophen intoxication in cats revealed no apparent effect on metHb formation but some efficacy in decreasing the number of HzBs formed and the degree of anemia.[37] Bioflavonoids are antioxidants that work by increasing the activity of the NADPH reductase system, an alternative physiologic metHb system that uses flavins as substrates for reduction.[3] A prospective, experimental trial evaluating cats that were subjected to acetaminophen toxicity demonstrated a significantly decreased number of HzBs formed in the cats that received bioflavonoids.[37] However, as with the therapeutic effects of SAMe, the amount of metHb produced was not significantly different.[37] Blood transfusion may be necessary in patients with severe hemolytic anemia secondary to HzB production (see Chapters 61 and 62).[7]

REFERENCES

1. Engelking LR: Textbook of veterinary physiological chemistry, ed 2, Oxford, 2011, Elsevier.
2. Harvey JW: Methemoglobinemia and Heinz body hemolytic anemia. In Bonagura J, editor: Kirk's current veterinary therapy XII, Philadelphia, 1995, WB Saunders.

3. Harvey JW: The erythrocyte: physiology, metabolism and biochemical disorders. In Kaneko JJ, Harvey JW, Bruss ML, editors: Clinical biochemistry of domestic animals, ed 6, London, 2008, Elsevier.
4. Thrall MA: Regenerative anemia. In Thrall MA, Weiser G, Allison RW, et al, editors: Veterinary hematology and clinical chemistry, ed 2, Oxford, 2012, Wiley-Blackwell.
5. Skold A, Cosco DL, Klein R: Methemoglobinemia: pathogenesis, diagnosis and management, So Med J 104:757, 2011.
6. Mansouri A, Lurie AA: Concise review: methemoglobinemia, Am J Hematol 42:7, 1993.
7. Taylor NS, Dhupa N: Acetaminophen toxicity in cats and dogs, Compend Contin Educ Vet Pract 22:160, 2000.
8. Christopher MM, White JG, Eaton JW: Erythrocyte pathology and mechanisms of Heinz body–mediated hemolysis in cats, Vet Pathol 27:299, 1990.
9. Herfmann K, Haskins S: Determination of P_{50} for feline hemoglobin, J Vet Emerg Crit Care 15:26, 2005.
10. Zaldivar-Lopez S, Chisnell HK, Couto CG, et al: Blood gas analysis and cooximetry in retired racing Greyhounds, J Vet Emerg Crit Care 21:24, 2011.
11. Aronson LR, Drobatz K: Acetaminophen toxicity in 17 cats, J Vet Emerg Crit Care 6:65, 1996.
12. Andress JL, Day TK, Day DG: The effects of consecutive day propofol anesthesia on feline red blood cells, Vet Surg 24:277, 1995.
13. Davis JA, Greenfield RA, Brewer TG: Benzocaine-induced methemoglobinemia attributed to topical application of the anesthetic in several laboratory species, Am J Vet Res 54:1322, 1993.
14. Zaks KL, Tan EO, Thrall MA: Heinz body anemia in a dog that had been sprayed with skunk musk, J Am Vet Med Assoc 226:1516, 2005.
15. Wray JD: Methaemoglobinaemia caused by hydroxycarbamide (hydroxyurea) ingestion in a dog, J Small Anim Pract 49:211-215, 2008.
16. Bates N: Letter: hydroxycarbamide (hydroxyurea) toxicity in dogs, J Small Anim Pract 49:216, 2008.
17. Khan SA: Toxicology brief: hydroyurea toxicosis in dogs and cats. dvm360.com, Industry Matter: Comprehensive information for professionals. Accessed Aug. 11, 2011.
18. Pauluhn J: Concentration-dependence of aniline-induced methemoglobinemia in dogs: a derivation of an acute reference concentration, Toxicology 214:140-150, 2005.
19. Fine DM, Eyster GE, Anderson LK, et al: Cyanosis and congenital methemoglobinemia in a puppy, J Am Anim Hosp Assoc 35:33-35, 1999.
20. Todisco V, Lamour J, Finberg L: Hemolysis from exposure to naphthalene mothballs, New Engl J Med 325:1660, 1991.
21. Ohashi K, Yukioka H, Hayashi M, et al: Elevated methemoglobin in patients with sepsis, Acta Anaesthesiol Scand 42:713-716, 1998.
22. Christopher MM: Relation of endogenous Heinz bodies to disease and anemia in cats: 120 cases (1978-1987), J Am Vet Med Assoc 194(8):1089-1095, 1989.
23. Christopher MM, Broussard JD, Peterson ME: Heinz body formation associated with ketoacidosis in diabetic cats, J Vet Intern Med 9:24, 1995.
24. McConkey SE, Grant DM, Cribb AE: The role of para-aminophenol in acetaminophen induced methemoglobinemia in dogs and cats, J Vet Pharmacol Therap 32:585-595, 2009.
25. Rockwood GA, Armstrong KR, Baskin SI: Species comparison of methemoglobin reductase,. Exp Biol Med 228:79-83, 2003.
26. Zhang P, Ohara A, Mashimo T, et al: Cardiovascular effects of an ultrashort-acting nitric oxide–releasing compound, zwitterionicdiamine/NO adduct, in dogs, Circulation 94:2235, 1996.
27. Kosaka H, Uozumi M, Tyuma I: The interaction between nitrogen oxides and hemoglobin and endothelium-derived relaxing factor, Free Radic Biol Med 7:653, 1989.
28. Schlesinger DP: Methemoglobinemia and anemia in a dog with acetaminophen toxicity, Can Vet J 36:515-517, 1995.
29. Mariani CL, Fulton RB: Atypical reaction to acetaminophen intoxication in a dog, J Vet Emerg Crit Care 11(2):123-126, 2001.
30. Christopher MM, Harvey JW: Specialized hematology tests, Semin Vet Med Surg (Small Anim) 7:301, 1992.
31. Evelyn KA, Malloy HT: Microdetermination of oxyhemoglobin, methemoglobin, and sulfhemglobin in a single sample of blood, J Biol Chem 126:655-662, 1938.
32. Haymond S, Cariappa R, Eby CS, et al: Laboratory assessment of oxygenation in methemoglobinemia, Clin Chem 51(2):434-444, 2005.
33. El-Husseini A, Azarov N: Is the threshold for treatment of methemoglobinemia the same for all? A case report and literature review, Am J Emerg Med 28:748e5-e10, 2010.
34. Lee J, El-Abaddi J, Duke A, et al: Noninvasive in vivo monitoring of methemoglobin formation and reduction with broadband diffuse optical spectroscopy, J Appl Physiol 100: 615-622, 2006.
35. Bahri LE, Lariviere N: Pharm profile: N-acetylcysteine, Compend Contin Educ Vet Pract 25:276, 2003.
36. Rumbeiha WK, Yu-Shange L, Oehme W, et al: Comparison of N-acetylcysteine and methylene blue, alone or in combination, for treatment of acetaminophen toxicosis in cats, Am J Vet Res 56:1529, 1995.
37. Webb CB, Twedt DC, Fettman MJ, et al: S-adenosylmethionine (SAMe) in a feline acetaminophen model of oxidative injury, J Feline Med Surg 5:69, 2003.
38. Allison RW, Lassen ED, Burkhard MJ, et al: Effect of bioflavonoid dietary supplementation on acetaminophen-induced oxidative injury to feline erythrocytes, J Am Vet Med Assoc 217:1157, 2000.
39. Center SA, Randolph JF, Warner J, et al: The effects of S-adenosylmethionine on clinical pathology and redox potential in the red blood cell, liver, and bile of clinically normal cats, J Vet Intern Med 19:303, 2005.

CHAPTER 110

ACUTE HEMOLYTIC DISORDERS

Leah A. Cohn, DVM, PhD, DACVIM

KEY POINTS

- Not all hemolytic anemia (HA) is immunologically mediated; treatment depends on proper identification of the cause of hemolysis.
- Hemolysis can be caused by red blood cell (RBC) fragmentation, toxin-induced RBC damage, inherited RBC defects, infection, immune-mediated RBC destruction, or a variety of other causes.
- Distinguishing intravascular from extravascular hemolysis can be useful diagnostically and prognostically.
- Proper therapy for HA includes supportive care (e.g., transfusion) and treatment aimed at the underlying cause of hemolysis.
- Immune-mediated hemolytic anemia (IMHA) may be a primary or secondary disease process. Recognition of inciting causes for secondary IMHA (e.g., infection, drugs, neoplasia) is important.

Hemolysis is the destruction of red blood cells (RBCs). All RBCs are destroyed eventually, but pathologic hemolysis occurs when the rate of destruction is increased and the life span of RBCs thus is shortened. Hemolytic anemia (HA) results when regeneration of RBCs from precursor cells is inadequate to replenish the destroyed cells. HA is caused by several immunologically and nonimmunologically mediated mechanisms (Box 110-1). The veterinarian must distinguish among these causes of hemolysis to provide appropriate therapy.

Anemia can be classified as either regenerative or nonregenerative. Blood loss and HA are the two main causes of regenerative anemia. Realistically, regeneration of RBCs requires time, and hemolysis is often an acute process. Therefore hemolysis that has been present for less than 3 to 5 days (dog and cat, respectively) is unlikely to be regenerative. Although hemolysis may be chronic and low grade, a drop in packed cell volume (PCV) of more than 1% per day suggests either blood loss or hemolysis. Once blood loss is ruled out (typically by the absence of detectable bleeding, a normal coagulation profile, and the presence of a normal total protein level), hemolysis becomes more likely the cause of a rapidly progressive anemia.

Evaluation of the Patient with Hemolysis

The clinical presentation of the dog or cat with HA is nonspecific and may relate to hemolysis and an underlying disease process. Although anemia resulting from defective or deficient RBC production is insidious in onset, HA frequently results in an acute illness. As a result of the anemia and decrease in oxygen content and delivery to the tissues, owners may notice exercise intolerance, anorexia, general malaise, syncope or collapse, and/or pallor. Upon physical examination, pale mucous membranes are a characteristic finding and icterus often is noted. Other findings may include tachycardia, tachypnea, bounding pulses, and a soft, systolic basilar heart murmur.

Many causes of hemolysis occur predominantly extravascularly, but RBC destruction also may occur inside the vascular space. Either way, breakdown of RBCs leads to release of bilirubin; bilirubinemia and bilirubinuria occur with either intravascular or extravascular pathologic hemolysis.[1] Hemoglobinemia and hemoglobinuria are found only with intravascular hemolysis. Several disease states cause intravascular and extravascular hemolysis. When intravascular hemolysis predominates, the disease process often carries a poorer prognosis for recovery than diseases associated with predominantly extravascular hemolysis.[1]

Hemolysis is associated with numerous changes in RBC appearance, and these changes are often helpful in identifying the cause.[1] There is no substitute for a thorough evaluation of a well-stained blood smear using oil immersion and high magnification; blood cell counts alone are inadequate for the evaluation of an animal with

BOX 110-1 *Causes of Hemolysis*

Fragmentation Hemolysis

Disseminated intravascular coagulation
Caudal caval syndrome
Splenic torsion
Heart valve disease
Hemangiosarcoma
Vasculitis

Toxicant-Induced Hemolysis

Foodstuffs and additives

Onion
Garlic
Propylene glycol

Drugs

Acetaminophen
DL-methionine
Vitamin K
Methylene blue
Benzocaine
Dimethylsulfoxide
Various antimicrobials

Chemicals

Zinc
Copper
Naphthalene
Skunk musk

Immune-Mediated Hemolysis

Idiopathic primary
Secondary (neoplasia, infection, drugs)
Neonatal isoerythrolysis
Transfusion

Heritable Hemolysis

Phosphofructokinase deficiency
Pyruvate kinase deficiency
Osmotic fragility syndromes
Nonspherocytic HA of Beagles

Infection-Related Hemolysis

Red blood cell infection
- *Mycoplasma haemofelis*
- *Mycoplasma haemocanis*
- Candidatus *M. haemominutum*
- Candidatus *M. haematoparvum*
- Candidatus *M. turensis*
- *Babesia canis*
- *Babesia gibsoni*
- *Babesia conradae*
- Other *Babesia* spp.
- Cytauxzoon felis

Systemic infection
- Feline leukemia virus
- Feline immunodeficiency virus
- Leptospirosis
- Bartonellosis
- *Ehrlichia canis*

Miscellaneous Causes of Hemolysis

Hypophosphatemia
Hemolytic-uremic syndrome
Iatrogenic changes in osmolarity
Envenomation
Histiocytic neoplasia
Intravenous administration of hypotonic fluids

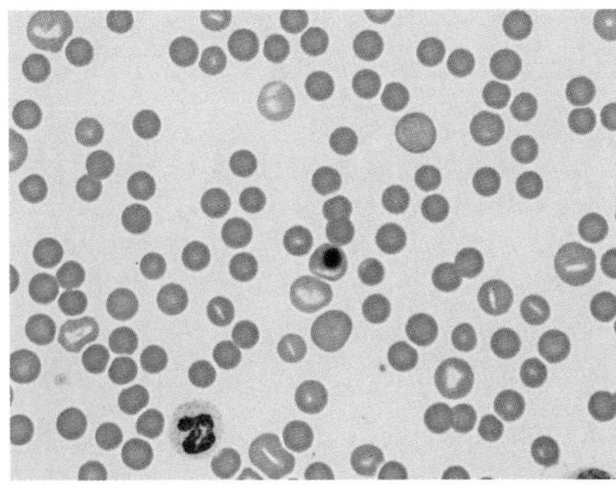

FIGURE 110-1 Marked spherocytosis is seen on the blood smear of a dog with immune-mediated hemolytic anemia. Notice the loss of red blood cell central pallor on this Wright-Giemsa–stained smear; original magnification, ×1000. *(Courtesy Angela Royal, University of Missouri, Columbia, MO.)*

suspected hemolysis. Shape changes may point to a specific cause. For example, schistocytes suggest fragmentation, spherocytes suggest immune-mediated destruction (Figure 110-1), and Heinz bodies suggest oxidative damage (see Figure 196-6). In addition, erythrocytic parasites may be observed microscopically.

A serum biochemical profile can provide useful information regarding causation of anemia and to gauge comorbid or complicating disease(s). For example, increased BUN with normal creatinine and low serum proteins should prompt investigation of GI bleeding as a cause of anemia rather than hemolysis, whereas severe hypophosphatemia may explain the cause of a hemolytic crisis.[2] Regardless of the cause of hemolysis, certain therapeutic principles apply. Heme pigments released by hemolysis can cause nephrotoxicity in humans. Although acute kidney injury resulting from hemolysis is not reported in small animals, adequate renal perfusion should be maintained to minimize this risk. Supportive care for animals with severe or rapid-onset anemia includes provision of transfused RBCs. The need for transfusion should be based on not merely an RBC count, hemoglobin measurement, or PCV but on clinical assessment (e.g., mental state, activity level, heart and respiratory rates, pulse quality). A packed RBC transfusion provides oxygen-carrying capacity with less volume than whole blood and often is preferred in animals with hemolysis (see Chapters 61 and 62). Transfusion in cats must follow blood typing of donor and recipient; blood typing of recipient dogs is not required for first-time transfusions, and DEA 1.1-negative blood is preferred. Although transfusion of cross-matched blood is ideal, first transfusions in dogs and transfusion of blood-type compatible cats are usually successful without cross-matching.[3] Transfused RBCs may be susceptible to the same cause of hemolysis as native RBCs. Although currently not commercially available, purified hemoglobin solutions do not require cross-matching or blood typing.

FRAGMENTATION HEMOLYSIS

Fragmentation of RBCs results from numerous processes but is most commonly the result of shearing of the RBC membrane in the small vessels (microangiopathic hemolysis) or from altered rheologic forces. Because shearing typically occurs inside the vascular space, hemoglobinemia and hemoglobinuria commonly result. The observation of schistocytosis on a peripheral blood smear provides supportive evidence of fragmentation; keratocytes and acanthocytes also are identified frequently.[1] When fragmentation is suspected, diagnostic testing is aimed at identification of the underlying pathology. In a dog with a prominent heart murmur, this may include an echocardiographic examination to rule out caudal caval syndrome, whereas the presence of marked splenomegaly would prompt ultrasonographic examination to rule out splenic torsion or neoplasia. Assays of coagulation usually are indicated because disseminated intravascular coagulation (DIC) is a common cause of fragmentation hemolysis, and several of the conditions that lead to fragmentation hemolysis can precipitate DIC.[1] Fragmentation hemolysis is a mechanical process, and management must be aimed at correction of the underlying disease. Supportive care includes provision of adequate oxygen-carrying capacity (e.g., RBC transfusion) and prevention of complications of hemolysis (e.g., nephrotoxicosis, DIC).

TOXICANT-INDUCED HEMOLYSIS

Much toxicant-induced hemolysis is related to oxidative injury. Oxidation of hemoglobin iron results in formation of methemoglobin, which, although unable to bind oxygen, does not shorten RBC life span (see Chapter 109). However, oxidative membrane damage can lead to intravascular hemolysis (resulting from membrane rupture) or extravascular destruction (resulting from premature phagocytosis). Oxidation of hemoglobin causes Heinz body formation, which, in turn, leads to removal of RBCs. Unlike dogs, cats may have some Heinz bodies without anemia. Eccentrocytes and pyknocytes are additional morphologic changes indicative of oxidative injury.

A variety of substances can result in toxicant-induced hemolysis (see Box 110-1). Cats are more susceptible to chemical oxidant injury than dogs for several reasons, including differences in drug metabolism and hemoglobin structure. Therapy for toxicant-induced HA involves removal of the toxicant (when possible) combined with supportive care. Clinicians should be especially alert for the presence of metallic foreign bodies within the gastrointestinal (GI) tract (e.g., pennies minted after 1982), especially in puppies and young dogs with HA, because removal of the object(s) with or without chelation therapy is curative.[4] For some oxidant toxins, other therapies are possible. For instance, N-acetylcysteine (140 mg/kg PO, then 70 mg/kg q6h for seven treatments) is recommended for treatment of acetaminophen toxicity.[5] A therapeutic role for additional antioxidants (e.g., S-adenosyl-L-methionine) in other toxicant-induced hemolytic diseases is defined less clearly.[6]

HERITABLE HEMOLYSIS

Although heritable HA is relatively uncommon, heritable defects may be common in a given breed (Table 110-1) or family. Not all hereditary erythrocyte defects lead to HA.[1,7] When present, hemolysis is more likely to be detected in young adults than in puppies or kittens. Clinical severity of hemolysis can range from mild and well compensated to a life-threatening crisis. Inherited erythrocyte defects should be considered in animals with a Coombs'-negative HA when causes of fragmentation, toxins, and infection are not identified, or in breeds known to have a high incidence of heritable hemolysis. Often changes in RBC shape are absent except for anisocytosis, signifying a regenerative anemia.[1,7]

Erythrocyte defects leading to hemolysis are associated with membrane abnormalities or enzyme deficiencies. The most common of these include syndromes of increased osmotic fragility, pyruvate kinase deficiency, and phosphofructokinase deficiency.[7-9] Specific testing for these causes of hereditary hemolysis can be divided into physical and functional tests of the RBC or molecular genetic tests. Physical and functional tests are available from only a few laboratories (e.g., Josephine Deubler Genetic Disease Testing Laboratory for Companion Animals at the School of Veterinary Medicine, University of Pennsylvania). Genetic tests identify breed-specific mutations. These tests are most valuable in identification of heterozygous

Table 110-1 Heritable Conditions Predisposing to Hemolysis

Defect	Reported Breed Associations	Typical Clinical Picture
Osmotic fragility	Abyssinian and Somali cats, English Springer Spaniel	Intermittent moderate to severe anemia with splenomegaly (cats)
Phosphofructokinase deficiency	English Springer Spaniel, Cocker Spaniel, canine mixed breed	Exercise or excitement (panting)-induced hemolytic crises and exertional myopathy characterized by hemoglobinuria
Pyruvate kinase deficiency	Basenji, Beagle, miniature Poodle, Toy Eskimo, Dachshund, Chihuahua, Pug, West Highland White Terrier, Labrador Retriever, Somali cats, Abyssinian cats	Initial extremely regenerative mild anemia becomes nonregenerative as a result of osteosclerosis and myelofibrosis Hemosiderosis-associated hepatic failure also occurs

carriers (most erythrocyte defects in dogs and cats are autosomal recessive traits). Treatment usually entails supportive care and includes cross-matched transfusion as needed. Other therapies, such as splenectomy for cats with increased osmotic fragility, may be beneficial.[9]

INFECTION-RELATED HEMOLYSIS

Infection may lead to hemolysis, either as a result of direct cell damage, through initiation of an immunologically mediated response to infection, or both. Systemic infections also can lead to microangiopathic hemolysis. The importance of recognizing infection-induced hemolysis cannot be overstated because appropriate therapy offers the potential for a cure and may avoid unnecessary and potentially harmful treatment strategies (e.g., immunosuppression).

Infection of Red Blood Cells

Few important RBC infections cause hemolysis of dogs or cats in the United States. These include hemotropic *Mycoplasma* spp. (formerly known as *Haemobartonella)* and protozoan parasites *Cytauxzoon felis* and *Babesia* spp.

Mycoplasma haemofelis (the causative agent of feline infectious anemia) should be a differential diagnosis for any cat with HA.[10] Presumably transmitted by fleas, the resulting hemolysis is variable in severity, cyclic in nature, and often Coombs' positive. The smaller Candidatus *Mycoplasma haemominutum* and *Mycoplasma turicensis* seem to be less virulent than their larger cousins.[10,11] Although routine microscopy often allows for identification of RBC parasites, parasite burden waxes and wanes, and hemotropic *Mycoplasma* may "fall off" RBCs *in vitro*. For these reasons, polymerase chain reaction testing is preferred to rule out infection. Doxycycline (5 mg/kg PO q12h for 21 days) is the preferred treatment, but the immune-mediated component of severe hemolysis may respond to a short course of prednisolone (2 to 4 mg/kg PO q24h). Hemotropic canine *Mycoplasma haemocanis* and Candidatus *Mycoplasma haematoparvum* rarely cause significant hemolysis unless in cases of prior splenectomy or immune suppression.[12]

Although multiple species of *Babesia* can infect dogs, the species of *Babesia* most likely to cause HA in dogs and cats in the United States are *B. canis* subspecies *vogeli* and *B. gibsoni.*[13,14] Breed associations include Greyhounds and Pit Bull Terriers, respectively, so hemolysis in these breeds should result in a high index of suspicion.[13,15] Although both organisms are transmitted by ticks, perinatal infection, fighting, and transfusion are additional means of infection in the United States. Hemolysis, thrombocytopenia, and hyperglobulinemia are common findings but are not universally present; many infected dogs appear healthy. As with *M. haemofelis,* microscopy is specific but not sensitive for diagnosis; polymerase chain reaction testing and serology are also available. The therapy of choice for *B. canis* is imidocarb dipropionate (6.6 mg/kg IM once, repeat in 2 weeks), but *B. gibsoni* is treated with a combination of atovaquone and azithromycin (13.5 mg/kg PO q8h and 10 mg/kg PO q24h, respectively, both for 10 days).

Cytauxzoon felis causes a tick-transmitted infection endemic to the southeastern, midwestern, and mid-Atlantic regions of the United States.[16] Cats typically become sick in the spring or summer seasons with an acute febrile illness that often is accompanied by icterus and pancytopenia. Although HA is a part of the illness, death results from multiple organ failure as a result of vascular occlusion by schizont-laden monocytes. When monocytes rupture, they release merozoites that then are taken up by RBCs, where they are identified as *piroplasms.* Sometimes death precedes the findings of hemolysis or RBC piroplasms. In addition, recovered carrier cats may harbor microscopically identifiable piroplasms without anemia. Treatment with a 10-day course of atovaquone (15 mg/kg PO q8h) and azithromycin (10 mg/kg PO q24h) offers the best response, but prognosis is guarded even with appropriate therapy.[17]

Systemic Infections

Systemic infections may lead to hemolysis through a variety of mechanisms. Feline leukemia virus infection often leads to anemia because of ineffective RBC production, but HA also may occur in feline leukemia-infected cats. In some cases, hemolysis may be due to hemotropic mycoplasmosis, but in others hemolysis remains idiopathic and likely immune mediated.[18,19] Likewise, feline immunodeficiency virus can lead to hemolysis.[20] Although *Ehrlichia canis* frequently causes a nonregenerative anemia, it is an infrequent cause of severe hemolysis.[21] Bartonellosis may result in HA in dogs.[22] Any infection leading to DIC or severe vasculitis may precipitate fragmentation hemolysis. Although extremely rare, certain *E. coli* infections may cause hemolytic-uremic syndrome, a condition characterized by hemolysis, acute kidney injury, and thrombocytopenia.[23]

IMMUNE-MEDIATED HEMOLYSIS

Most dogs and many cats with hemolysis will eventually be determined to have immune-mediated hemolytic anemia (IMHA), wherein destruction of RBCs is mediated by antibody-triggered or complement-triggered events.[1] In some cases, an infection, drug, or cancer is determined to have initiated the aberrant immune attack on the RBCs (i.e., secondary IMHA). Identification of such triggers profoundly affects treatment and prognosis. Signalment, history, and physical examination guide the direction and intensity of a search for triggers of IMHA. Hemolysis in cats, in very young or old dogs, in animals with concurrent disease or drug histories, or in animals with physical examination findings not directly related to hemolysis and anemia should prompt added vigilance for explanations other than idiopathic primary IMHA.

Findings Suggestive of Immune-Mediated Hemolytic Anemia

IMHA occurs more commonly in dogs than cats.[18] Certain dog breeds (e.g., Cocker Spaniel) are overrepresented, as are female dogs, but any breed and either gender may be affected.[24,25] Most dogs with idiopathic IMHA are young or middle-aged adults. Unless the immune attack includes RBC precursors, IMHA becomes a regenerative anemia within a few days. Leukocytosis and thrombocytopenia are common findings in dogs with IMHA, as are hyperbilirubinemia and hyperbilirubinuria. Although several tests confirm the immune-mediated nature of hemolysis, secondary as well as primary IMHAs are detected by these methods. The most common form of IMHA results from an immunoglobulin-mediated type II hypersensitivity reaction causing extravascular hemolysis. Phagocytic damage to the RBC membrane results in formation of highly characteristic spherocytes, as seen in Figure 110-1 (difficult to detect in cats because of a normal lack of central RBC pallor). Less commonly, immunoglobulin mediates RBC autoagglutination in patients with IMHA.[26] Agglutination can be seen grossly and microscopically but must be differentiated from rouleaux formation. Often simply adding an equal volume of saline to whole blood disperses rouleaux; if it does not, the RBCs should be washed with saline and reexamined. True autoagglutination persists despite washing; this finding confirms an immunologic component (Figure 110-2). The Coombs' test is helpful when spherocytosis is minimal and autoagglutination absent to confirm the immune-mediated nature of hemolysis, as may be the case in animals with intravascular hemolysis.[27] Species-specific antisera containing antibody to IgG, IgM, and complement are combined for reaction with the patient's washed RBCs; if the antibody or complement is attached to the RBC, agglutination results. Because false-positive and false-negative results are possible, more sophisticated tests have been developed, including flow cytometric assays for the presence of RBC-bound antibody.[28]

Treatment of Immune-Mediated Hemolytic Anemia

Unfortunately, few randomized, prospective evaluations of any effective therapy exist for treatment of patients with IMHA. Despite aggressive treatments many patients die.[24,29,30] Therapies can be divided into those aimed at suppression of the aberrant immunologic response, those providing supportive care, and those aimed at prevention of complications.

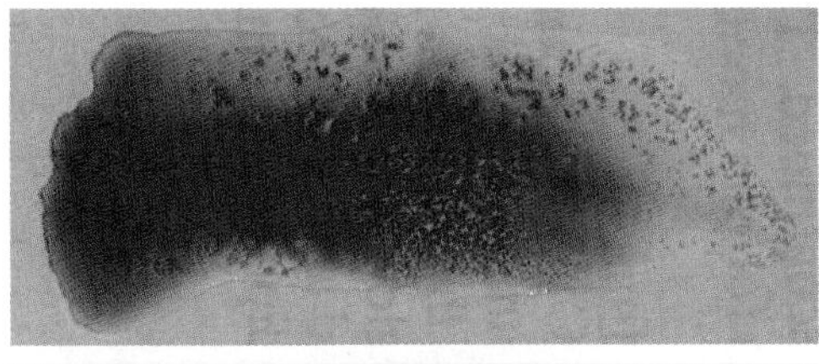

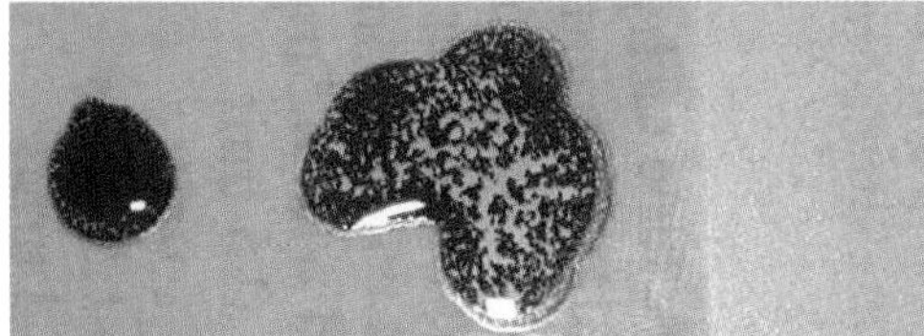

FIGURE 110-2 Macroscopic autoagglutination. The bottom slide represents a drop of blood collected in ethylenediaminetetraacetic acid; notice the icteric plasma and the clumping of red blood cells. The top slide is the same sample after the addition of an equal volume of saline. Note the persistence of red blood cell clumping.

Immune suppression

Glucocorticoids (GC) are the mainstay of treatment for IMHA. High-dose glucocorticoids exert multiple actions to slow immunologically mediated destruction of RBCs, but positive response requires several days (approximately 5 days). Initially, prednisone or prednisolone (cats) is given at a dosage of 1 to 2 mg/kg PO q12h. Medium to large dogs generally should be treated with the lower end of the dose range (e.g., 1 mg/kg PO q12h or 50 mg/m^2), whereas cats may require higher dosages. Equivalent dosages of parenteral glucocorticoids (e.g., 0.2 to 0.6 mg/kg q24h IV of dexamethasone) may be substituted (e.g., when gastrointestinal disease is present). Glucocorticoids are continued at high doses until the RBC count has normalized. Then the dosage is tapered slowly (with frequent reevaluations of RBC numbers) as long as hemolysis does not recur. Although tapering has no definitive rule, twice daily doses usually are consolidated into a single daily dose, and the total dosage is decreased by increments of 20% to 25% every few weeks until reaching 0.5 mg/kg q24h. At that point, the dose is unaltered but frequency is changed to every other day to spare the hypothalamic-pituitary-adrenal axis. Tapering can continue until the lowest effective dosage is attained or GC treatment is discontinued altogether. Depending on initial disease severity and response to therapy, the entire course of treatment may last from 4 to 9 months or more.

Because glucocorticoids require several days to slow hemolysis and may not halt hemolysis adequately and because they often are associated with pronounced adverse effects, other forms of immune suppression have been used (Table 110-2); for most, no evidence supports or refutes efficacy. However, cyclophosphamide has fallen out of favor as a result of potentially worsened outcome.[31-33] Cyclosporine is an alternative immune suppressant believed to have a rapid onset of action, but no positive impact on survival has been demonstrated yet.[30] Intravenous immunoglobulin also acts rapidly and has been used when other treatments have failed; it does not seem to improve long-term survival.[34] The most popular adjunctive immunosuppressive drugs may be azathioprine and the less myelotoxic/hepatotoxic but similarly acting agent mycophenolate mofetil; unfortunately, proof of efficacy is still lacking for either drug.[25,30,35,36]

Supportive care

Supportive care for animals with hemolysis often includes the provision of adequate oxygen-carrying capacity via transfusion of RBCs. The rapidity of onset of anemia may have more to do with clinical signs than the absolute degree of anemia. Tachycardia, tachypnea, weakness, bounding pulses, and hyperlactatemia are relative indicators that oxygen-carrying support is required. In the past, practitioners were often reluctant to transfuse patients with IMHA for fear that transfused cells may blunt the drive to a regenerative response, or that RBC breakdown products may damage the renal tubules. The former concern seems to have little merit, and the latter is also unlikely and further outweighed by the need to prevent tissue hypoxia. Unless plasma is required for other reasons, packed RBCs are preferred to whole blood transfusions.

Prevention of complications

Dogs treated for IMHA typically die because they are euthanized or from complications (such as pulmonary thromboembolism or DIC) rather than from anemia.[24] Prevention of pulmonary thromboembolism using a standardized dose of heparin alone has shown little success, but individually adjusted dosing may have better results (see Chapter 168).[37,38] Oral anticoagulants, either ultralow-dose aspirin (0.5 mg/kg PO q24h) or clopidogrel (loading dose 10 mg/kg PO once, followed by 2 to 3 mg/kg q24h), have similar effects but do not always prevent thromboembolism.[38] Although hypercoagulability in

Table 110-2 Immunosuppressive Drug Regimens Used to Manage IMHA in Dogs and Cats

Drug	Starting Dosage	Important and Common Adverse Effects	Comments
Prednisone	2 to 4 mg/kg PO q12h; medium to large dogs typically treated with 1 mg/kg q12h; cats may require up to 8 mg/kg per 24 hr	PU and PD, polyphagia, panting, altered behavior, loss of muscle mass, hypercoagulability, thinning coat	Initial dosage is tapered slowly as allowed by clinical condition
Azathioprine	2.2 mg/kg PO q24h	GI upset, myelotoxicity, hepatopathy	Initial dosage is halved in 7 to 10 days, slowly tapered
Cyclosporine	Oil-based: 10 to 25 mg/kg PO divided q12h Emulsified: 5 to 10 mg/kg PO divided q12h	GI upset, gingival hyperplasia, rarely nephrotoxicity	Trough levels must be monitored to adjust dosage
Cyclophosphamide	50 mg/m^2 q72h, PO q8-12h or 200 mg/m^2 IV once/week	GI upset, myelotoxicity, sterile hemorrhagic cystitis	Not recommended
Chlorambucil	0.1 to 0.2 mg/kg q24h	GI upset, myelotoxicity	Not recommended
Leflunomide	4 mg/kg q24h	GI upset, anemia, lymphopenia	Trough levels monitored to adjust dosage
Danazol	5 mg/kg q8-12h	Virilization, hepatotoxicity	Not recommended
Mycophenolate mofetil	20 to 40 mg/kg PO divided q8-12h	GI upset	Little veterinary experience
IVIG	0.5 to 1.5 g/kg infused IV over 6 to 12 hr	Hypersensitivity reaction	Single-use treatment in crisis

GI, Gastrointestinal; *IMHA,* immune-mediated hemolytic anemia; *IV,* intravenous; *IVIG,* intravenous immunoglobulin; *PD,* polydipsia; *PO,* per os; *PU,* polyuria.

dogs with IMHA is the norm, the condition is associated with DIC. Prognosis for survival is worse in dogs demonstrating hypocoagulability at presentation.[39] Because high-dose GC use can result in GI ulceration, consideration should be given to the use of GI protectants in dogs with IMHA receiving GC (see Chapter 161).

Other Causes of Immune-Mediated Hemolytic Anemia

Transfusion reactions and neonatal isoerythrolysis result from immunologically mediated but nonaberrant attack against RBCs. Animals have unique blood types, and transfusion of unmatched blood can result in a normal hemolytic response by the host against the transfused cells. In dogs, preformed antibodies to RBC antigens are uncommon, as are hemolytic complications of non–blood typed, non–cross-matched initial transfusions. However, subsequent transfusions may result in hemolysis.[3] Because cats have preformed antibodies to RBC antigens other than their own, even first transfusion of non–blood-typed, non–cross-matched blood may result in severe hemolysis (especially type B cats receiving type A blood).[3,40] These same preformed antibodies mediate feline neonatal isoerythrolysis. Type A or type AB kittens born to type B queens can develop HA after absorption of alloantibodies via colostrum.[41] Although most cats in the United States are type A, British Shorthair, Devon Rex, Abyssinian, and Somali cats have a high prevalence of type B blood.[40] In addition, evidence suggests that the prevalence of type B cats varies by country and region (i.e., type B cats are seen more frequently in the western United States compared with the eastern United States).

REFERENCES

1. Stockham SL, Scott MA: Erythrocytes. In Stockham SL, Scott MA, editors: Fundamentals of veterinary clinical pathology, Ames, Iowa, 2008, Blackwell Publishing, pp 107-222.
2. Adams LG, Hardy RM, Weiss DJ, et al: Hypophosphatemia and hemolytic anemia associated with diabetes mellitus and hepatic lipidosis in cats, J Vet Intern Med 7:266-271, 1993.
3. Tocci LJ: Transfusion medicine in small animal practice, Vet Clin North Am Small Anim Pract 40:485-494, 2010.
4. Hammond GM, Loewen ME, Blakley BR: Diagnosis and treatment of zinc poisoning in a dog, Vet Hum Toxicol 46:272-275, 2004.
5. Taylor NS, Dhupa N: Acetaminophen toxicity in cats and dogs, Comp Cont Ed Pract Vet 22:160, 2000.
6. Hill AS, O'Neill S, Rogers QR, et al: Antioxidant prevention of Heinz body formation and oxidative injury in cats, Am J Vet Res 62:370-374, 2001.
7. Giger U: Hereditary erythrocyte disorders. In Bonagura J, editor: Kirk's current veterinary therapy XIII, Philadelphia, 2000, WB Saunders.
8. Owen JL, Harvey JW: Hemolytic anemia in dogs and cats due to erythrocyte enzyme deficiencies, Vet Clin North Am Small Anim Pract 42:73-84, 2012.
9. Kohn B, Goldschmidt MH, Hohenhaus AE, et al: Anemia, splenomegaly, and increased osmotic fragility of erythrocytes in Abyssinian and Somali cats, J Am Vet Med Assoc 217:1483-1491, 2000.
10. Tasker S: Haemotropic mycoplasmas: what's their real significance in cats? J Feline Med Surg 12:369-381, 2010.
11. Novacco M, Boretti FS, Wolf-Jackel GA, et al: Chronic "*Candidatus Mycoplasma turicensis*" infection, Vet Res 42:59, 2011.
12. Warman SM, Helps CR, Barker EN, et al: Haemoplasma infection is not a common cause of canine immune-mediated haemolytic anaemia in the UK, J Small Anim Pract 51:534-539, 2010.
13. Irwin PJ: Canine babesiosis, Vet Clin North Am Small Anim Pract 40:1141-1156, 2010.
14. Solano-Gallego L, Baneth G: Babesiosis in dogs and cats–expanding parasitological and clinical spectra, Vet Parasitol 181:48-60, 2011.
15. Birkenheuer AJ, Correa MT, Levy MG, et al: Geographic distribution of babesiosis among dogs in the United States and association with dog bites: 150 cases (2000-2003), J Am Vet Med Assoc 227:942-947, 2005.
16. Cohn LA, Birkenheuer AJ: Cytauxzoonosis. In Greene DE, editor: Infectious disease of the dog and cat, St Louis, 2012, Elsevier Saunders, pp 764-770.
17. Cohn LA, Birkenheuer AJ, Brunker JD, et al: Efficacy of atovaquone and azithromycin or imidocarb dipropionate in cats with acute cytauxzoonosis, J Vet Intern Med 25:55-60, 2011.
18. Kohn B, Weingart C, Eckmann V, et al: Primary immune-mediated hemolytic anemia in 19 cats: diagnosis, therapy, and outcome (1998-2004), J Vet Intern Med 20:159-166, 2006.

19. Hartmann K: Feline leukemia viurs infection. In Greene CE, editor: Infectious disease of the dog and cat, St Louis, 2012, Elsevier Saunders, pp 108-136.
20. Sellon RK, Harmann K: Feline immunodeficiency virus infection. In Greene CE, editor: Infectious diseases of the dog and cat, St Louis, 2012, Elsevier Saunders, pp 136-148.
21. Cohn LA: Ehrlichiosis and related infections, Vet Clin North Am Small Anim Pract 33:863-884, 2003.
22. Breitschwerdt EB, Blann KR, Stebbins ME, et al: Clinicopathological abnormalities and treatment response in 24 dogs seroreactive to *Bartonella vinsonii* (*berkhoffii*) antigens, J Am Anim Hosp Assoc 40:92-101, 2004.
23. Caprioli J, Remuzzi G, Noris M: Thrombotic microangiopathies: from animal models to human disease and cure, Contrib Nephrol 169:337-350, 2011.
24. Carr AP, Panciera DL, Kidd L: Prognostic factors for mortality and thromboembolism in canine immune-mediated hemolytic anemia: a retrospective study of 72 dogs, J Vet Intern Med 16:504-509, 2002.
25. Weinkle TK, Center SA, Randolph JF, et al: Evaluation of prognostic factors, survival rates, and treatment protocols for immune-mediated hemolytic anemia in dogs: 151 cases (1993-2002), J Am Vet Med Assoc 226:1869-1880, 2005.
26. Harkin KR, Hicks JA, Wilkerson MJ: Erythrocyte-bound immunoglobulin isotypes in dogs with immune-mediated hemolytic anemia: 54 cases (2001-2010), J Am Vet Med Assoc 241:227-232, 2012.
27. Wardrop KJ: The Coombs' test in veterinary medicine: past, present, future, Vet Clin Pathol 34:325-334, 2005.
28. Kucinskiene G, Schuberth HJ, Leibold W, et al: Flow cytometric evaluation of bound IgG on erythrocytes of anaemic dogs, Vet J 169:303-307, 2005.
29. Piek CJ, Junius G, Dekker A, et al: Idiopathic immune-mediated hemolytic anemia: treatment outcome and prognostic factors in 149 dogs, J Vet Intern Med 22:366-373, 2008.
30. Swann JW, Skelly BJ: Evaluation of immunosuppressive regimens for immune-mediated haemolytic anaemia: a retrospective study of 42 dogs, J Small Anim Pract 52:353-358, 2011.
31. Mason N, Duval D, Shofer FS, et al: Cyclophosphamide exerts no beneficial effect over prednisone alone in the initial treatment of acute immune-mediated hemolytic anemia in dogs: a randomized controlled clinical trial, J Vet Intern Med 17:206-212, 2003.
32. Burgess K, Moore A, Rand W, et al: Treatment of immune-mediated hemolytic anemia in dogs with cyclophosphamide, J Vet Intern Med 14:456-462, 2000.
33. Grundy SA, Barton C: Influence of drug treatment on survival of dogs with immune-mediated hemolytic anemia: 88 cases (1989-1999), J Am Vet Med Assoc 218:543-546, 2001.
34. Whelan MF, O'Toole TE, Chan DL, et al: Use of human immunoglobulin in addition to glucocorticoids for the initial treatment of dogs with immune-mediated hemolytic anemia, J Vet Emerg Crit Care 19:158-164, 2009.
35. Piek CJ, van Spil WE, Junius G, et al: Lack of evidence of a beneficial effect of azathioprine in dogs treated with prednisolone for idiopathic immune-mediated hemolytic anemia: a retrospective cohort study, BMC Vet Res 7:15, 2011.
36. Whitley NT, Day MJ: Immunomodulatory drugs and their application to the managmenet of canine immune-mediated disease, J Small Anim Pract 52:70, 2011.
37. Helmond SE, Polzin DJ, Armstrong PJ, et al: Treatment of immune-mediated hemolytic anemia with individually adjusted heparin dosing in dogs, J Vet Intern Med 24:597-605, 2010.
38. Mellett AM, Nakamura RK, Bianco D: A prospective study of clopidogrel therapy in dogs with primary immune-mediated hemolytic anemia, J Vet Intern Med 25:71-75, 2011.
39. Goggs R, Wiinberg B, Kjelgaard-Hansen M, et al: Serial assessment of the coagulation status of dogs with immune-mediated haemolytic anaemia using thromboelastography, Vet J 191:347-353, 2012.
40. Knottenbelt CM: The feline AB blood group system and its importance in transfusion medicine, J Feline Med Surg 4:69-76, 2002.
41. Silvestre-Ferreira AC, Pastor J: Feline neonatal isoerythrolysis and the importance of feline blood types, Vet Med Int 2010:753726, 2010.

CHAPTER 111
RODENTICIDES

Andrew J. Brown, MA, VetMB, MRCVS, DACVECC • Lori S. Waddell, DVM, DACVECC

KEY POINTS

- Rodenticide intoxication is common in the dog and is seen occasionally in the cat.
- The clinician must identify which rodenticide has been consumed.
- Unless contraindicated, decontamination techniques should be performed immediately after acute ingestion to reduce absorption and prevent development of clinical signs.
- Anticoagulant rodenticide exposure most commonly causes body cavity or pulmonary parenchymal bleeding.
- Treatment of patients with rodenticide-induced coagulopathy consists of providing active clotting factors with fresh frozen plasma or fresh whole blood, vitamin K_1 to enable production of endogenous active coagulation factors, and supportive care.
- Coagulopathy resulting from anticoagulant rodenticide exposure has an excellent prognosis if treated appropriately and promptly.
- Bromethalin intoxication leads to cerebral edema and severe neurologic signs and is associated with a poor prognosis once clinical signs are evident.
- Cholecalciferol intoxication results in hypercalcemia. This can lead to soft tissue mineralization, acute kidney injury, and cardiac arrhythmias.
- Zinc phosphide and strychnine intoxications are less common, although secondary intoxication from the ingestion of poisoned rodents is possible.

Rodenticide ingestion is a common intoxication in dogs. Anticoagulant rodenticide intoxications traditionally have been the most frequent type presented to the emergency veterinarian, but legislation introduced in the United States in 2011 banned the use of second-generation anticoagulants (including brodifacoum, bromadiolone, and difenacoum) in consumer products; they are available only for commercial use. Subsequently, the number of cases of intoxication with either bromethalin or cholecalciferol may increase. Rodenticides now are formulated typically in bars and must include bait stations, which are plastic housing units that should reduce accidental ingestion by pets and children. Loose bait such as pellets should no longer be produced for sale in the United States according to Environmental Protection Agency risk mitigation rules. However, at least one company is under scrutiny for continued production of products that have been banned by the EPA; veterinarians may continue to see toxicity from loose bait consumption and the second-generation anticoagulants for the next few years.

As with any toxicity, the correct rodenticide must be identified rapidly; treatment for the wrong intoxication could lead to the death of the animal. Owners should be encouraged to bring in rodenticide packaging for determination of the active ingredient. Animal Poison Control Center can give excellent advice to help identify the rodenticide and recommend specific treatment for these patients. In many cases the ingestion has been witnessed and the dog or cat is taken immediately to the emergency clinic before the onset of clinical signs. Other animals are presented with clinical signs of intoxication; this typically occurs when the owner was unaware that the pet ingested a rodenticide. Presenting complaints and clinical signs vary with the type of rodenticide ingested. Careful questioning of the owner during the history is critical. Asking, "Is there any rat poison on your property?" rather than "Is there any chance that your pet has gotten into rat poison?" often results in a more useful response.

The goal of treatment depends on how soon after ingestion the animal is presented. Decontamination of the animal to prevent rodenticide absorption is key after acute ingestion, whereas treatment and supportive care are needed for patients that have clinical evidence of intoxication.

The mechanism of action, pathologic consequences, and published lethal dose[1] of common rodenticides are shown in Table 111-1.

ANTICOAGULANT RODENTICIDES

Pathophysiology and Clinical Signs

Animals that consume a sufficient amount of an anticoagulant rodenticide develop clinical signs secondary to a coagulopathy. Activation of coagulation factors II, VII, IX, and X (the vitamin K–dependent factors) requires reduced vitamin K (hydroquinone) for posttranslational γ-carboxylation. Activation of these factors leads to oxidation of reduced vitamin K to inactive epoxide. The enzyme vitamin K reductase catalyzes the conversion of inactive epoxide back to active hydroquinone. Anticoagulant rodenticides antagonize the action of vitamin K epoxide reductase, so levels of hydroquinone decrease. Activation of the vitamin K–dependent coagulation factors cannot occur (Figure 111-1), and levels of active factors II, VII, IX, and X decrease. Depleted levels of these factors result in a coagulopathy and associated clinical signs. Usually a lag period of 3 to 5 days occurs between exposure and appearance of clinical signs as the vitamin K–dependent factors become depleted. Coagulopathies typically are characterized by lung and body cavity bleeding, but bleeding at other sites (e.g., joints and trachea) has been reported. Fatal hemorrhage in the central nervous system (CNS) may occur.

There used to be many commercial, warfarin-based anticoagulant rodenticide products available for rodent control. However, the

Table 111-1 Mechanism of Action, Pathologic Consequences, and Lethal Dose of Rodenticides

Rodenticide	Class	Mechanism of Action	Pathologic Consequences	Lethal Dose (mg/kg)	
				Dog	Cat
Brodifacoum	Second-generation hydroxycoumarin	Inhibition of vitamin K epoxide reductase	Clinical bleeding because of coagulopathy	0.2 to 4	25
Bromadiolone	Second-generation hydroxycoumarin	Inhibition of vitamin K epoxide reductase	Clinical bleeding because of coagulopathy	11 to 15	>25
Chlorophacinone	Indandione	Inhibition of vitamin K epoxide reductase	Clinical bleeding because of coagulopathy	NK	NK
Diphacinone	Indandione	Inhibition of vitamin K epoxide reductase	Clinical bleeding because of coagulopathy	0.9 to 8	15
Warfarin	First-generation hydroxycoumarin	Inhibition of vitamin K epoxide reductase	Clinical bleeding because of coagulopathy	20 to 300	5 to 30
Cholecalciferol	Cholecalciferol	Increased gastrointestinal absorption and decreased renal calcium loss	Hypercalcemia leading to acute kidney injury	1.5 to 8	NK
Bromethalin	Bromethalin	Uncoupling of oxidative phosphorylation	Neurologic signs from intramyelinic edema	2.5 to 5	0.5 to 1.5
Zinc phosphide	Zinc phosphide	Disruption of mitochondrial respiration and free radical production	Gastrointestinal signs, lethargy, neurologic abnormalities, respiratory distress, and cardiovascular compromise	NK	NK
Strychnine	Strychnine	Prevents uptake of glycine at inhibitory synapses of Renshaw cells in the CNS (disinhibition)	Muscle contractions, convulsions, extensor rigidity, and death	0.5 to 1.0	2

NK, Not known.

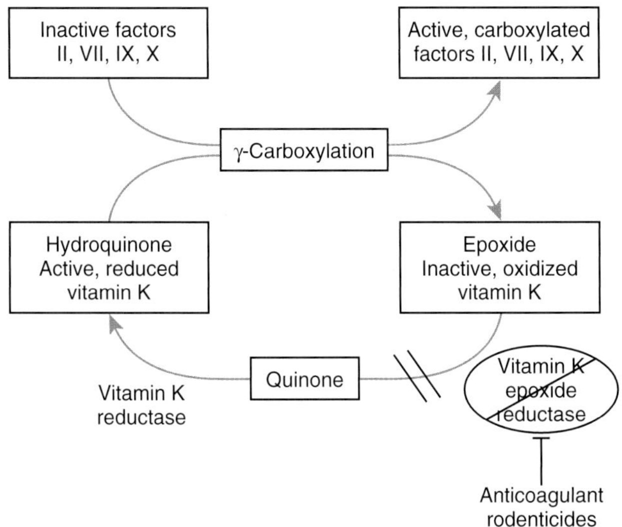

FIGURE 111-1 Mechanism of action of anticoagulant rodenticides.

warfarin-based rodenticides now are used rarely; they have been replaced by the second-generation anticoagulants. The second-generation anticoagulants retain the same basic nucleus, but the chemical structures were selected for increased potency (single lethal feeding potential), longer duration of activity, and efficacy against resistant rodents. Second-generation anticoagulants include the coumarin-based generics: brodifacoum, difenacoum, and bromadiolone and the indandiones: diphacinone (also called diphenadione) and chlorophacinone. The use of these longer-acting anticoagulants affects the treatment of patients; treatment with vitamin K_1 must be administered for only 2 weeks after ingestion for the first-generation anticoagulants but must be administered for 4 weeks after ingestion of the second-generation anticoagulants. The most common anticoagulants ingested by dogs in two retrospective studies from the United States are brodifacoum, bromadiolone, and diphacinone, all of which are second-generation anticoagulants.[2,3] However, these data were gathered before enforcement of the recent changes in EPA legislation and may be subject to change.

Case Management

Acute ingestion

Animals commonly are presented to the emergency clinician after a recent witnessed ingestion of anticoagulant rodenticide. If a patient is presented within 4 hours of ingestion and there is no contraindication to emesis (seizures, depression, problems with airway), then vomiting should be induced immediately with apomorphine (0.03 mg/kg IV or 0.04 mg/kg IM) or hydrogen peroxide (1 to 2 ml/kg of 3% solution PO) for dogs. Hydrogen peroxide should only be used if apomorphine is not available. Cats preferably are given xylazine (0.44 mg/kg IM or SC, followed by reversal with yohimbine at a dose of 0.25 to 0.5 mg/kg IM or SC) for induction of emesis. Activated charcoal (1 to 4 g/kg PO) also should be administered to adsorb remaining rodenticide in the gastrointestinal (GI) tract. This is most effective when given within an hour of ingestion. Dogs that ingest rodenticide typically are not fastidious eaters and likely will eat a charcoal and canned dog food slurry mix. Sodium sulfate (250 mg/kg in dogs and cats) or a 70% sorbitol solution (1 to 2 ml/kg) may be administered as a cathartic (see Chapter 74).

A prothrombin time (PT) should be obtained for all patients 48 hours after ingestion if they have not received any doses of vitamin K. The PT is a measure of the extrinsic pathway, including factor VII. Factor VII has the shortest half-life of all the vitamin K–dependent coagulation factors (6.2 hours), and as a result, the PT will be prolonged before the activated partial thromboplastin time (aPTT) and before the development of clinical signs. Factor VII levels will be depleted after 48 hours, resulting in a prolongation of the PT; however, this is not enough time for depletion of the other factors that would result in clinical bleeding. If the PT is prolonged 48 hours after ingestion, oral vitamin K_1 (also known as phytonadione) should be administered at a dosage of 2.5 mg/kg PO q12h. Almost all anticoagulant rodenticide toxicities are currently second-generation[2,3] products, and therefore treatment should be continued for 4 weeks. However, this may change in the United States as new regulations are enforced. Forty-eight hours after the last dose of vitamin K_1, the PT should be rechecked to ensure that an adequate course of therapy has been given. If the PT still is prolonged, vitamin K_1 therapy should be continued for an additional 1 to 2 weeks, then the PT checked again 48 hours after the last dose. An alternative treatment option is to empirically give vitamin K_1 for 4 weeks at the above dose, then check the PT 48 hours after the last dose. Because of the cost of vitamin K_1, checking the PT 48 hours after ingestion generally is preferred. A retrospective study evaluated the incidence of PT prolongation in 151 dogs receiving gastrointestinal decontamination within 6 hours of anticoagulant rodenticide ingestion. Only 8.3% of dogs required vitamin K_1 therapy, and none of them had adverse events develop during the time period between ingestion and starting vitamin K_1 therapy.[3]

Coagulopathies

If the patient has evidence of clinical bleeding, presenting complaints may include lethargy, anorexia, dyspnea, hemoptysis, and/or lameness.[2,4] Physical examination typically shows abnormalities consistent with the location of the bleed. Auscultation may reveal dull lung sounds if there is pleural effusion, or dull heart sounds because of pericardial effusion. Episcleral hemorrhage or subcutaneous hematomas also may be seen. Palpation of the abdomen, kidneys, or joints may be painful. Differential diagnoses for animals with a severe coagulopathy include anticoagulant rodenticide intoxication, disseminated intravascular coagulation (secondary to the systemic inflammatory response), neoplasia, severe thrombocytopenia, hemophilia, and liver failure (see Chapter 105).

A minimum database may be consistent with acute hemorrhage (low total solids with low or normal packed cell volume). Blood gas analysis may reveal a metabolic acidosis (typically a lactic acidosis secondary to hypovolemia and decreased perfusion), hypoxia, and an elevated alveolar-arteriolar gradient if there is pleural or pulmonary parenchymal hemorrhage. A blood smear should be evaluated for erythrocyte morphology and adequacy of platelets. Patients with anticoagulant rodenticide intoxication are often severely thrombocytopenic; this is thought to be a result of profound consumption secondary to the massive hemorrhage that can occur. Every patient with evidence of severe bleeding should be evaluated for objective measures of coagulation.

Anticoagulant rodenticides induce a prolongation of the PT before the aPTT. The aPTT becomes prolonged as factors II, IX, and X are depleted and from consumption of other factors once bleeding has occurred. The activated clotting time also reflects the intrinsic pathway and therefore will not be prolonged until factor depletion is severe. If a patient has a greater elevation in the PT relative to the increase in aPTT, then anticoagulant rodenticide intoxication is likely.[2] Similarly, anticoagulant rodenticide intoxication is unlikely in a patient with a severe prolongation of the aPTT and a mild prolongation of the PT. If the PT and the aPTT are both prolonged severely, then a diagnosis of anticoagulant rodenticide intoxication is more difficult to confirm.

The PIVKA (proteins induced by vitamin K antagonism) was thought previously to be a more specific test for diagnosing anticoagulant rodenticide intoxication. However, it can be elevated with other disease processes, particularly severe liver disease and/or malabsorption and maldigestion syndromes. One study found that performing a PT and a PIVKA simultaneously added no additional diagnostic information.[5] Definitive diagnosis is possible with anticoagulation rodenticide screens using spectrophotometry (available at veterinary laboratories), which can demonstrate quantitatively the presence of the toxin in whole blood. The concentration of rodenticide detected does not correspond with the severity of the change in PT or aPTT.[2] Although it takes 3 to 5 days to obtain results of this screen, the clinician can obtain a definitive diagnosis of anticoagulant rodenticide intoxication and learn the type of rodenticide ingested. This is especially useful when the owner insists the animal has not been exposed to rodenticide. Unless the patient is receiving coumadin therapeutically, there is no possibility of a false-positive test result.

Radiography may reveal loss of body cavity detail, and effusion may be seen on thoracic and abdominal ultrasonography. If no pleural hemorrhage is present, a patchy to diffuse pulmonary alveolar to interstitial pattern consistent with alveolar hemorrhage may be noted.

Treatment of the symptomatic patient is based on correcting the coagulopathy, providing exogenous vitamin K_1 for regeneration of coagulation factors, and supportive care. Clotting factors in the form of fresh frozen plasma (typically 10 to 20 ml/kg) or fresh whole blood (20 to 40 ml/kg) should be administered to the patient until clotting times have normalized. Animals with less severe clinical signs and a normal PTT may benefit from frozen plasma that no longer contains labile clotting factors but retains functional vitamin K–dependent clotting factors. Red blood cells may be needed if a significant anemia develops; they can be given as packed red blood cells if fresh frozen plasma was used to provide clotting factors. Patients in respiratory distress require oxygen therapy, and if hemorrhagic pleural effusion is present, thoracocentesis may be necessary. This ideally should be performed after correction of the coagulopathy but depends ultimately on the clinical status of the animal. Pericardiocentesis also may become necessary in animals with hemorrhagic pericardial effusion, but only in extremely critical cases and after providing active clotting factors. Animals with life-threatening hemorrhage may benefit from auto-transfusion to maintain the hematocrit above dangerous levels and fresh frozen plasma therapy to provide active clotting factors and to stop the bleeding (see Chapters 61 and 62).

Exogenous vitamin K_1 should be administered at an initial dose of 5 mg/kg SC using a small-gauge needle. There is a high frequency of anaphylaxis after intravenous administration of vitamin K_1, so this route is not recommended. There is better bioavailability of vitamin K_1 when ingested, so therapy should be switched from subcutaneous to the oral route as soon as possible. Oral vitamin K_1 should be administered at 2.5 mg/kg PO with food q12h for 4 weeks, with a recheck PT performed 48 hours after cessation of therapy (as described earlier in the section Acute Ingestion). Supportive care, including correcting the anemia and supplying oxygen therapy, is necessary while the blood is resorbed and clinical signs resolve.

Outcome

Patients with a witnessed anticoagulant rodenticide ingestion that are treated rapidly by induction of emesis, activated charcoal, and a PT performed 48 hours after ingestion (+/-vitamin K_1 therapy as needed) have an excellent prognosis. Those patients with a severe coagulopathy and clinical evidence of bleeding also carry an excellent prognosis when treated aggressively, appropriately, and promptly.[2,6] Of all the causes of a severe coagulopathy, anticoagulant rodenticide intoxication has the best prognosis. In a recently published retrospective study, 98.6% (74 of 75) of dogs that had a positive anticoagulant rodenticide screen survived,[2] emphasizing the importance of a timely and accurate diagnosis and treatment.

CHOLECALCIFEROL

Pathophysiology and Clinical Signs

Intoxication from cholecalciferol rodenticide results in hypercalcemia and associated clinical signs. After ingestion of the bait, cholecalciferol (vitamin D_3) is absorbed rapidly and transported to the liver by specific binding proteins. It first is converted within the hepatocytes to 25-hydroxycholecalciferol and then to 1,25-dihydroxycholecalciferol within the kidney, which increases GI absorption of calcium, reduces renal excretion of calcium, and increases resorption of calcium from the bone. The primary pathologic effects of the hypercalcemia are acute kidney injury and cardiac arrhythmias (see Chapter 52).

Clinical signs can develop between 4 and 36 hours after ingestion. Initial signs are related to the hypercalcemia and include polyuria and polydipsia (through inhibition of ADH), lethargy, anorexia, and vomiting. Acute kidney injury develops secondary to the hypercalcemia and soft tissue mineralization. Dehydration quickly ensues because of decreased fluid intake caused by nausea from the uremia and increased GI and renal losses. Cardiac arrhythmias often are present because of mineralization of the heart or changes in the ratio of intracellular-to-extracellular ion concentrations and an increase in the depolarization threshold.

Case Management

Acute ingestion

Many patients are presented for treatment after recent witnessed ingestion of the rodenticide. As with acute anticoagulant ingestion, GI decontamination strategies should be performed unless there is a contraindication to doing so (see Chapter 74). A serum calcium level should be checked 48 hours after acute ingestion.

Hypercalcemia

In patients with hypercalcemia, cholecalciferol intoxication always should be considered and owners questioned accordingly. Other differential diagnoses for increased ionized calcium levels include hypercalcemia of malignancy, hypoadrenocorticism, chronic kidney disease, primary hyperparathyroidism, osteolytic bone disease, and ingestion of vitamin D ointments (psoriasis creams) or supplements. Physical examination may reveal depression, weakness, dehydration, and cardiac arrhythmias. Blood work reveals severe hypercalcemia (total and ionized) and hyperphosphatemia. As the toxicosis progresses, hyperproteinemia, azotemia, hyperkalemia, and metabolic acidosis also may develop. Histopathology commonly reveals diffuse soft tissue mineralization.

Therapy for hypercalcemic patients is directed toward reducing blood calcium levels and preventing acute kidney injury. Intravenous isotonic saline (0.9% NaCl) should be administered to correct dehydration and provide moderate volume expansion. The high sodium concentration of 0.9% NaCl (154 mEq/L) induces a calciuresis. Renal calcium loss also is enhanced by furosemide, glucocorticoids, salmon calcitonin, and bisphosphonate therapy (e.g., pamidronate).[7] However, furosemide should be administered only after fluid deficits are corrected and glucocorticoids given only after other diagnoses of hypercalcemia have been excluded. In addition to inducing a calciuresis, salmon calcitonin inhibits osteoclast activity and thus reduces the resorption of calcium from bones. However, there is a risk of anaphylaxis with salmon calcitonin therapy and therefore bisphosphonate therapy typically is preferred over calcitonin. Pamidronate disodium is a commonly used bisphosphonate that also inhibits osteoclastic bone resorption and reduces calcium concentrations within 48 hours of administration (see Chapters 52 and 124).

Outcome

Dogs with cholecalciferol intoxication and mild to no azotemia have a fair to good prognosis with aggressive medical therapy; in four published case reports, four out of six dogs survived.[7-10] Three cats with hypercalcemia associated with cholecalciferol toxicity were reported to have survived in one published case series.[11] Once hypercalcemia and acute kidney injury have developed, prognosis is poor. Rapid and aggressive therapy to reduce the calcium concentration and prevent soft tissue mineralization leads to a better chance of survival.

BROMETHALIN

Pathophysiology and Clinical Signs

The toxic effects of bromethalin are due to the uncoupling of oxidative phosphorylation with a resultant decrease in adenosine triphosphate (ATP) production. This decrease in cellular energy leads to an inability of the ATP-dependent membrane transport pumps to function. The nonfunctioning Na^+/K^+-ATPase transport pump causes a buildup of intracellular sodium, which allows water to move into the cells. Although many organs can be affected, clinical signs are associated predominantly with cerebral edema and the resultant elevated intracranial pressure.

Clinical signs and their onset vary with the dose ingested. Ingestion of doses larger than the LD_{50} (the dose of the drug that causes death in 50% of experimental animals; dogs 4.7 mg/kg and cats 1.8 mg/kg) results in severe muscle tremors, hyperthermia, extreme hyperexcitability, and focal or generalized seizures within 24 hours. Clinical signs with lower doses may manifest between 1 and 3 days; signs include hind limb ataxia, paresis or paralysis, and CNS depression.

Case Management

Acute ingestion

Animals that are presented after acute ingestion require immediate and aggressive decontamination. This includes emesis induction or general anesthesia, intubation, and gastric lavage if the patient is unable to protect its airway and is at risk of aspiration. Repeated doses of activated charcoal should be administered (3 to 5 g/kg q6-8h) for 48 hours because of enterohepatic circulation of the toxin. Sodium sulfate or magnesium sulfate (250 mg/kg in dogs and cats) or a 70% sorbitol solution (1 to 2 ml/kg) may be administered as a cathartic (see Chapter 74).

Neurologic complications

Treatment of animals with neurologic signs is based on seizure control and supportive care (see Chapters 84 and 166). Attempts to maintain cerebral perfusion pressure and oxygen delivery should be made. These strategies include the administration of mannitol to reduce cerebral edema, elevation of the head at a 15- to 30-degree incline, prevention of jugular compression, and maintenance of normocapnia. Strategies to ensure normoglycemia and prevent hyperthermia also should be considered. Treatment of bromethalin-induced neurologic signs with glucocorticoids has been cited commonly.[12] However, no evidence supports this recommendation. Considering the known side effects of steroids, including hyperglycemia, and only a theoretic benefit, glucocorticoid use in animals with bromethalin intoxication is not recommended.

Unfortunately, a definitive diagnosis can be made only postmortem. Histopathologic examination of the cerebrum, cerebellum, brainstem, and spinal cord may support a diagnosis of bromethalin intoxication. Diffuse white matter vacuolation (spongy degeneration) with microgliosis is described consistently.[13] Gas chromatography with electron capture can be used to detect bromethalin in samples of kidney, liver, fat, or brain.

Outcome

Animals with severe signs have a poor prognosis. To the authors' knowledge, no reports exist of dogs ingesting more than 5 mg/kg bromethalin, developing neurologic signs, and surviving. However, there is a report of a dog that survived after ingesting a lower dose of bromethalin (less than 2.5 mg/kg), which led to tremors, ataxia, and muscle weakness.[14] GI decontamination with induction of emesis and repeated doses of activated charcoal after acute ingestion to prevent signs is therefore essential to patient survival.[12]

MISCELLANEOUS RODENTICIDES

Zinc phosphide is a restricted use pesticide, although formulations using lower concentrations are available to the public for control of moles and gophers. Commercial use is increasing and secondary intoxication of dogs (i.e., from consumption of poisoned rodents) is possible.[15] After ingestion and contact with gastric acid, zinc phosphide is hydrolyzed to phosphine gas and free radicals. Enhanced susceptibility to zinc phosphide occurs when it is ingested with food because of gastric acid secretion. The kinetics for hydrolysis are favored at a lower pH, and the rate of phosphine gas generated is enhanced markedly in these conditions. Phosphine causes toxicity by disrupting mitochondrial respiration as well as producing free radicals such as reactive oxygen species. The onset of clinical signs is variable but is usually evident 15 minutes to 4 hours after ingestion of a toxic dose. Gastrointestinal signs are most common, but clinical signs also may include lethargy, neurologic abnormalities (e.g., seizures, paralysis, incoordination and coma), respiratory distress, and cardiovascular compromise.[16] Once clinical signs are observed, the prognosis is guarded. The unpleasant odor of phosphine (smells like acetylene, garlic, or rotting fish) may be detectable on the breath, vomitus, or carcass, although the absence of this odor should not be used to exclude zinc phosphide exposure.

Caution is recommended strongly because veterinary hospital staff treating animals can be poisoned from phosphine gas.[17] The AVMA has drawn up guidelines for veterinarians and pet owners.[18] No specific antidote exists, and treatment is based on decontamination and supportive care. These include moving the animal outside, inducing vomiting, and standing upwind of and above animal level to reduce exposure to phosphine gas. The animal then should be removed from the vicinity and the area flushed with copious amounts of water (while remaining upwind). If the animal vomits in an enclosed area, the area should be vacated and the fire department contacted. If practical, windows and doors should be opened, and if personnel are exposed to the phosphine gas, they should seek medical attention immediately if they are experiencing symptoms.

Thirty years ago, strychnine was used commonly as a rodenticide, and accidental or malicious intoxication occurred frequently. It is now a restricted use pesticide and canine or feline exposure is rare, although secondary intoxication is more likely to occur than with zinc phosphide. Strychnine prevents the uptake of glycine at inhibitory synapses of Renshaw cells in the CNS. This inhibition of an inhibitory pathway is termed *disinhibition* and results in a net excitatory effect from an excessive afferent input and efferent response. Onset of stimulant activity, including apprehension and muscle contractions, occurs within minutes to hours of ingestion. Signs progress to convulsions, extensor rigidity, and death. Confirmation of strychnine exposure can be made from stomach contents or postmortem tissue samples.[19] Decontamination strategies are recommended unless clinical signs are apparent. Therapy to prevent seizures and provide muscle relaxation and supportive care should be instituted. Animals often die from respiratory muscle paralysis and hypoventilation; mechanical ventilation of the paralyzed patient therefore may prove lifesaving.

REFERENCES

1. Murphy MJ: Rodenticides, Vet Clin Am Small Anim Pract 32:469, 2002.
2. Waddell LS, Poppenga RH, Drobatz KJ: Anticoagulant rodenticide screening in dogs and cats: 123 cases (1996-2003), J Am Vet Med Assoc 15:516, 2013.
3. Pachtinger GE, Otto CM, Syring RS: Incidence of prolonged prothrombin time in dogs following gastrointestinal decontamination for acute anticoagulant rodenticide ingestion, J Vet Emerg Crit Care 18:285, 2008.
4. Sheafor SE, Couto CG: Anticoagulant rodenticide toxicity in 21 dogs, J Am Anim Hosp Assoc 35:38, 1999.
5. Rozanski EA, Drobatz KJ, Hughes D, et al: Thrombotest (PIVKA) test results in 25 dogs with acquired and hereditary coagulopathies, J Vet Emerg Crit Care 9:73, 1999.
6. Kohn B, Weingart C, Giger U: Haemorrhage in seven cats with suspected anticoagulant rodenticide intoxication, J Feline Med Surg 5:295, 2003.
7. Dougherty SA, Center SA, Dzanis DA: Salmon calcitonin as adjunct treatment for vitamin D toxicosis in a dog, J Am Vet Med Assoc 196:1269, 1990.
8. Garlock SM, Matz ME, Shell LG: Vitamin D3 rodenticide toxicity in a dog, J Am Anim Hosp Assoc 27:356, 1991.
9. Fooshee SK, Forrester SD: Hypercalcemia secondary to cholecalciferol rodenticide toxicosis in two dogs, J Am Vet Med Assoc 196:1265, 1990.
10. Livezay L, Dorman DC: Hypercalcemia induced by vitamin D_3 toxicosis in two dogs, Canine Pract 16:26, 1991.
11. Moore FM, Kudisch M, Richter K, et al: Hypercalcemia associated with rodenticide poisoning in three cats, J Am Vet Med Assoc 193:1099, 1988.
12. Dorman DC, Parker AJ, Buck WB: Bromethalin toxicosis in the dog. Part II: selected treatments for the toxic syndrome, J Am Anim Hosp Assoc 26:595, 1990.
13. Dorman DC, Simon J, Harlin KA, et al: Diagnosis of bromethalin toxicosis in the dog, J Vet Diagn Invest 2:123, 1990.
14. Dorman DC, Parker AJ, Buck WB: Bromethalin toxicosis in the dog. Part I: clinical effects, J Am Anim Hosp Assoc 26:589, 1990.
15. Casteel SW, Bailey EM: A review of zinc phosphide poisoning, Vet Hum Toxicol 28:151, 1986.
16. Gray SL, Lee JA, Hovda LR, et al: Potential zinc phosphide rodenticide toxicosis in dogs: 362 cases (2004-2009), J Am Vet Med Assoc 239:646, 2011.
17. Centers for Disease Control and Prevention: Occupational phosphine gas poisoning at veterinary hospitals from dogs that ingested zinc phosphide—Michigan, Iowa, and Washington, 2006-2011, MMWR Morb Mortal Wkly Rep 61: 286, 2012
18. AVMA Phosphine Gas Precautions: https://www.avma.org/KB/Resources/Reference/Pages/Phosphine-product-precautions.aspx
19. Blakley BR: Epidemiologic and diagnostic considerations of strychnine poisoning in the dog, J Am Vet Med Assoc 184:46, 1984.

PART XII INTRAABDOMINAL DISORDERS

CHAPTER 112

ACUTE ABDOMINAL PAIN

Kenneth J. Drobatz, DVM, MSCE, DACVIM, DACVECC

KEY POINTS

- The principles of emergency and critical care should be applied initially to any patient with a painful abdomen (stabilize respiratory and cardiovascular systems).
- Any portion of the abdomen or lumbar and sacral spine could be a source of apparent abdominal pain.
- The general causes of abdominal pain include distention of a hollow viscus or organ capsule, ischemia, traction, and inflammation secondary to a variety of causes.
- If the underlying cause of abdominal pain can be identified quickly and treated, the occurrence of more serious complications such as septic peritonitis or systemic inflammatory response syndrome and multiorgan dysfunction syndrome can be minimized.

Animals with an acute condition of the abdomen are characterized primarily as having abdominal pain. Vomiting and/or diarrhea often accompany this abdominal pain. As with any patient suffering from an emergent condition, the basic principles of stabilization of the four most important body systems (respiratory, cardiovascular, neurologic, and renal systems) should be applied when initially assessing and stabilizing these patients (see Chapter 1).

After initial stabilization, a thorough diagnostic evaluation should be performed to determine the underlying cause as soon as possible so that definitive care can be provided. The general causes of abdominal pain include distention of a hollow viscus or organ capsule, ischemia, traction, and inflammation secondary to a variety of causes. If left untreated, any of these causes could result in necrosis of tissue and loss of function; therefore the underlying cause must be identified quickly. Prompt identification and treatment of the underlying abnormality minimize the occurrence of more serious complications, such as septic peritonitis or systemic inflammatory response syndrome and multiorgan dysfunction syndrome.

DIAGNOSTIC EVALUATION

The diagnostic evaluation of animals with abdominal pain begins with signalment, medical history, and physical examination, followed by a complete blood count, biochemical profile, urinalysis, radiographs, abdominal ultrasound, radiographic contrast studies, abdominocentesis, peritoneal lavage, response to treatment, and/or exploratory laparotomy. The list of specific causes of abdominal pain is extensive because any portion of the abdomen could be a source of pain. Intervertebral disk disease also may simulate a painful abdomen, but direct palpation of the area of spinal pain usually elicits a more diagnostic response.

Signalment and History

Signalment can be a clue to the cause of abdominal pain or vomiting. For example, young animals commonly swallow foreign bodies or contract infectious diseases. An older, intact male dog may have a painful prostate. Abdominal pain in an intact female dog with a pyometra should raise concern of a possible uterine rupture and septic peritonitis. Young adult German Shepherd Dogs with pancreatic exocrine insufficiency are predisposed to mesenteric volvulus. String foreign bodies are common in cats. Acute pancreatitis commonly occurs in middle-aged, obese female dogs.

An accurate history may be the most important diagnostic clue in the assessment of animals with acute abdominal pain. Questions should include the potential for exposure to toxins or dietary indiscretion. In addition, is ingestion of a foreign body a possibility? Are any other animals affected? Has the animal had any major medical problems in the past? Is the patient currently receiving any medications, including over-the-counter drugs such as aspirin or other nonsteroidal antiinflammatory medications? Is there a possibility of trauma? Could the patient have been exposed to any other animals? Is the patient current on all vaccinations? The clinician should determine when the animal's condition was last normal, what the first abnormal sign was, and how clinical signs have progressed since the problem began.

The progression of the clinical signs also can help determine the urgency of diagnosing the underlying cause. Chronic abdominal pain that has remained relatively static in its progression is not usually an emergency, although the problem could become an emergency at any time. An animal that has a chronic problem and deteriorates rapidly, or an animal with an acute problem that is or is not deteriorating rapidly, warrants a more aggressive and expedient approach to define the underlying cause of the painful abdomen.

Physical Examination

A full physical examination should be performed, with initial attention given to the cardiovascular, respiratory, central nervous, and renal systems, as for any critically ill patient. More specifically for the animal with acute abdominal pain, a careful and detailed abdominal palpation occasionally may locate the specific area of pain (e.g., a loop of intestine, the prostate, or the kidneys), and this may help in the diagnostic approach. Many times, a specific area cannot be identified and diagnosing the underlying cause requires assimilation of information from a variety of diagnostic tests; these include clinical pathology, abdominal imaging, abdominocentesis, diagnostic peritoneal lavage (see Chapter 200), response to treatment, and/or exploratory laparotomy.

Emergency Clinical Pathology

An extended database that includes a packed cell volume (PCV), total solids (TS), glucose, dipstick blood urea nitrogen (BUN), blood smear, venous blood gas, and electrolyte levels (including sodium, potassium, chloride, and ionized calcium) helps to provide rapidly a relatively well-rounded metabolic assessment of the patient and sometimes can point toward the underlying cause.

The PCV and TS always should be assessed together. Parallel increases in both (hemoconcentration) suggest dehydration. A normal or increased PCV with a normal to low TS indicates protein loss from the vasculature. In animals with an acute condition of the abdomen, this clinicopathologic picture often is associated with protein loss from peritonitis. Hemorrhagic gastroenteritis (HGE) is associated with a high PCV (60% to 90%) and normal or low TS in dogs presenting with an acute onset of vomiting and bloody diarrhea.

Hemorrhage most commonly results in a parallel decrease in the PCV and TS, although in animals with acute hemorrhage these changes may not be recognized initially until intravenous fluid therapy has been provided. Acute hemorrhage in dogs can lead to a normal or increased PCV and normal or decreased TS. Splenic contraction in dogs makes TS a more sensitive indicator of acute blood loss than PCV. The most common causes of hemorrhage in dogs with acute conditions of the abdomen are splenic rupture (usually secondary to neoplasia) and severe hemorrhage from gastrointestinal (GI) ulceration. The most common causes of hemoabdomen in cats are nonneoplastic conditions (54%) and abdominal neoplasia (46%). Blood glucose measurement is obtained easily and rapidly by dipstick methods and a glucometer. Increased blood glucose in a dog with an acute condition of the abdomen may be caused by diabetes or transient diabetes associated with severe pancreatitis. Blood glucose is rarely more than 200 mg/dl in dogs with extreme hypovolemia secondary to severe abdominal or GI hemorrhage, presumably a result of the effects of catecholamines on glycogenolysis and gluconeogenesis. Physical examination findings of extremely poor tissue perfusion are evident, and the animal may die imminently if the hypovolemia is not corrected rapidly. Increased blood glucose levels in cats may be associated with stress or diabetes; therefore hyperglycemia in cats is not as useful diagnostically as it is in dogs.

Decreased blood glucose often is associated with sepsis and warrants an aggressive approach to find the underlying cause of the acute abdominal pain, particularly if septic peritonitis may be present. Rarely, extremely low blood glucose levels may occur as a result of sepsis, but more typically it falls in the 40 to 60 mg/dl range. Hypoadrenocorticism also may be a cause of low blood glucose levels (see Chapter 66).

Dipstick BUN provides an estimate of azotemia in an animal with an acute condition of the abdomen. Increased BUN may be due to prerenal, renal, or postrenal causes. Increased BUN also may be noted in animals with acute abdominal pain caused by pyelonephritis or ureteral or urethral obstruction. Disproportionately high BUN compared with creatinine levels should prompt the clinician to rule out GI hemorrhage.

Reliable assessment of a blood smear depends on a good-quality sample. All cell lines should be evaluated systematically, including the red blood cells, white blood cells, and platelets. The average number of platelets per monolayer field under oil immersion should be estimated (see Chapter 196). The smear first should be screened at low power to search for platelet clumps that may result in a falsely low platelet estimate before evaluating the counting area under oil immersion. In normal dogs and cats, there are 8 to 15 platelets per oil immersion field (100×); each platelet in a monolayer field is equivalent to approximately 15,000 platelets/μl. If there are more than two to three platelets per field, it is unlikely that the bleeding is strictly the result of thrombocytopenia. Most patients with spontaneous bleeding resulting from thrombocytopenia have less than two platelets per oil immersion field. A decreased number of platelets is one of the most consistent findings in animals with disseminated intravascular coagulation (DIC). Animals with acute conditions of the abdomen may have DIC secondary to systemic inflammation or massive peritoneal inflammation.

Red blood cell morphology should be examined. Anisocytosis, macrocytosis, and polychromasia indicate regeneration. Schistocytes or fragments of red blood cells suggest DIC. Heinz bodies often are seen in systemically ill cats. The smear should be scanned at lower power to get an estimate of the number of white blood cells and then at higher power to assess the character of the white blood cells. Leukocytosis with a mature neutrophilia suggests an inflammatory or infectious process, although excessive numbers of any cell line may indicate neoplasia. Band cells indicate a more severe inflammatory or infectious process. The absence of a leukocytosis or a left shift does not rule out an inflammatory or infectious process. Leukopenia can be due to decreased production or sequestration of white blood cells, a viral infection such as parvovirus, or immunosuppressive drugs.

A venous blood gas provides an evaluation of the metabolic acid-base status. Animals that have severe vomiting because of GI foreign bodies may have a hypochloremic metabolic alkalosis as well as hypokalemia and hyponatremia.[1] Often, a metabolic acidosis is also present because of severe diarrhea or lactic acidosis from hypoperfusion.[1]

Abdominal Radiographs

A full description of all radiographic and ultrasonographic findings in an animal with acute abdominal pain is beyond the scope of this chapter, but specific points regarding plain abdominal radiographs are provided. Abdominal radiographs should be obtained in any animal with abdominal pain. A systematic and detailed review of all abdominal and extraabdominal structures should be performed. All organs in the abdominal cavity should be evaluated for density, shape, size, and location. Abnormalities in any organ may help localize the cause of the abdominal pain. Extraabdominal structures should be examined for completeness of evaluation and further diagnostic clues. The retroperitoneal space should be assessed as well. Loss of detail of the kidneys, a "streaky" appearance, or distention of the retroperitoneal space suggests fluid accumulation, a space-occupying mass, or sublumbar lymphadenopathy. The structures that make up the abdominal compartment "walls" should be assessed carefully for integrity to rule out herniation or rupture.

Evidence of free gas in the peritoneum without prior abdominocentesis or recent abdominal surgery suggests intestinal perforation or the presence of gas-forming organisms within the abdominal cavity. Free gas is detected most commonly between the stomach or liver and the diaphragm on the lateral radiograph. A horizontal beam radiograph with the animal in left lateral recumbency and focused at the least dependent area can increase the sensitivity for identifying free gas in the peritoneal space. A large volume of free gas in the peritoneum often is associated with pneumocystography of a ruptured urinary bladder, a ruptured vagina, recent abdominal surgery, ruptured gastric dilatation-volvulus, pneumoperitoneography, or extension of a pneumomediastinum. Pneumomediastinum is associated most often with pneumoretroperitoneum, although on rare occasions, pneumoperitoneum can occur. A small volume of free gas in the peritoneal space is associated most often with rupture of the GI tract or infection with a gas-forming organism. Gas in the gallbladder wall, liver, or spleen is associated most often with a *Clostridia* spp. infection.

Segmental gaseous or fluid distention of the small bowel suggests an intestinal obstruction. The normal diameter of the small intestine in the dog is approximately two to three times the width of a rib, or less than the width of an intercostal space. In addition, all of the small bowel loops should have a similar diameter, and it is abnormal for one segment to be 50% larger than other portions. Feline small intestines should not exceed twice the height of the central portion of L4 vertebral body, or 12 mm.[2]

Generalized small bowel distention suggests generalized small bowel ileus or a distal GI obstruction. Localized small bowel distention is not always a definitive finding for intestinal obstruction but should prompt further investigation if an obvious foreign body is not evident. One option is to repeat plain radiographs 3 hours later. If the bowel remains distended in the same area, this suggests a bowel obstruction. A more definitive diagnosis for intestinal obstruction can be obtained by performing an upper GI positive contrast study with barium. Severe intraperitoneal inflammation and granuloma formation can occur if barium leakage occurs as a result of a bowel rupture. This problem can be minimized if abdominal surgery with peritoneal lavage is done immediately, as indicated after the diagnosis of small bowel rupture. Therefore upper GI contrast study with barium is not contraindicated if the clinician is attempting to diagnose GI perforation. Abdominal ultrasound by an experienced, trained ultrasonographer is becoming the standard for ruling out GI obstruction and has been found to be more sensitive and specific than abdominal radiography.[3]

Loss of abdominal detail on plain abdominal radiographs may be due to lack of fat in the abdomen (puppies or very thin animals), free abdominal fluid, pancreatitis, large mass(es), or carcinomatosis.

Abdominal Fluid Analysis

Obtaining free abdominal fluid for analysis is important if it is present in an animal with a painful abdomen. Abdominal fluid analysis can help rule out septic peritonitis and also may provide a diagnosis or help direct further diagnostic investigation. Fluid may be obtained by abdominocentesis (blindly or by ultrasound guidance). If fluid cannot be obtained but still is suspected to be present, a diagnostic peritoneal lavage is indicated (see Chapter 200).

Free abdominal fluid should be analyzed for creatinine and/or potassium and compared with peripheral blood concentrations if urinary tract leakage is suspected (see Chapter 122). Creatinine and potassium are higher in the abdominal fluid if a uroperitoneum is present.[4,5] Measurement of fluid glucose and lactate concentrations may be helpful in diagnosing a bacterial peritonitis. These measurements can be compared with simultaneously collected peripheral blood glucose and lactate concentrations. A glucose gradient greater than 20 mg/dl of peripheral blood to abdominal fluid was 100% sensitive and 100% specific in diagnosing septic peritonitis in dogs (86% sensitive and 100% specific in cats) in one study. In addition, a blood-to-abdominal fluid lactate gradient of 2 mmol/L or more was also 100% sensitive and 100% specific in diagnosing septic peritonitis in dogs.[6] If bile peritonitis is suspected, abdominal bilirubin concentration often is higher than simultaneously collected blood bilirubin concentration.[7]

A pure transudate is grossly clear and is characterized by a total protein less than 2.5 g/dl and low cell count (fewer than 500 cells/μl). Of the few cells present, most are either nondegenerate neutrophils or reactive mesothelial cells. The most common causes of a pure transudate in the abdomen include hypoalbuminemia and portal venous obstruction.

A modified transudate is usually serous to serosanguineous, with a total protein level between 2.5 and 5 g/dl and a moderate total cell count (300 to 5500 cells/μl). Depending on the cause, there may be variable numbers of red blood cells, nondegenerate neutrophils, mesothelial cells, macrophages, and lymphocytes. This type of effusion often is due to passive congestion of the liver and viscera and impaired drainage of the lymphatic vessels. The most common causes include right-sided heart failure, dirofilariasis, neoplasia, and liver disease.

An exudate is often cloudy and has a total protein concentration greater than 3 g/dl and a cell count greater than 5000 to 7000 cells/μl. The predominant cell type is usually the neutrophil, although numerous other cells may be present as well. This is the most common type of free abdominal fluid associated with acute abdominal pain. Exudates can be septic or nonseptic, but making this classification can be challenging at times. Septic exudates are characterized by the presence of intracellular and extracellular bacteria. In most animals with septic peritonitis, cytologic evidence of bacteria can be found, particularly if the clinician has patience and explores numerous microscopic fields and examines the cytology of the sediment of the abdominal fluid. Rarely, septic peritonitis can be present despite the absence of cytologic evidence of bacteria in the fluid.

Table 112-1 summarizes some objective diagnostics in the patient with an acute abdomen.

SURGICAL VERSUS MEDICAL MANAGEMENT

One of the most challenging decisions regarding animals with acute abdominal pain is deciding whether immediate surgery is indicated. Clear indications for immediate surgery include abdominal wall perforation, septic peritonitis, persistent abdominal hemorrhage, intestinal obstruction, intestinal foreign body causing pain or bowel obstruction, uroperitoneum, free abdominal gas (not associated with previous surgery, pneumomediastinum, or invasive procedures), abdominal abscess, ischemic bowel, gastric dilation volvulus, mesenteric volvulus, and bile peritonitis. Without these clear indications, the clinician must use all information that can be obtained quickly to determine if exploratory surgery is warranted, including signalment, history, physical examination, clinicopathology, imaging modalities, response to medical therapy, informed discussion with the owner, and clinical intuition. Using all this information, the clinician can make the correct decision whether to perform exploratory surgery.

Table 112-1 **Summary of Some Objective Diagnostics Used in the Approach to the Acute Abdomen***

Test	Diagnostic Criteria	Sensitivity	Specificity
Blood glucose minus peritoneal glucose for diagnosis of septic peritonitis	>20 mg/dl	Dogs: 100% Cats: 86%	Dogs: 100% Cats: 100%
Peritoneal fluid lactate minus blood lactate for diagnosis of septic peritonitis	>2.0 mmol/L	Dogs: 100% Cats: not reported	Dogs: 100% Cats: not reported
Dogs abdominal ultrasound: small intestinal lumen dilation	Jejunal luminal diameter of >1.5 cm with normal wall layering	Not reported but should aggressively investigate for intestinal obstruction	Not reported but luminal diameter not dilated then intestinal obstruction not likely
Fluid to blood potassium ratio for diagnosis of uroabdomen	Dogs: ratio of 1.4:1 Cats: ratio 1.9:1	Dogs: 100% Cats: unknown	Not reported but considered diagnostic for uroabdomen
Fluid to blood creatinine ratio for diagnosis of uroabdomen	Dogs: ratio 2:1 Cats: ratio 2:1	Dogs: 86% Cats: unknown	Dogs: 100% Cats: unknown
Fluid to blood bilirubin ratio for diagnosis of bile peritonitis (also may see bile pigment/crystals in abdominal fluid)	>2:1	Dogs: 100% Cats: unknown	Not reported
Dogs: ratio of maximal small intestinal diameter to the narrowest width of L5 on lateral radiograph	Ratio > 1.6	Not reported but suggestive of small intestinal obstruction.	Not reported but suggestive of small intestinal obstruction
Cats: ratio of maximal small intestinal diameter to the height of cranial endplate of L2	Ratio > 2.0	Not reported but suggestive of small intestinal obstruction.	Not reported but suggestive of small intestinal obstruction
Specific cPLI (serum) for diagnosis of pancreatitis	<200 mcg/L: pancreatitis unlikely 200-400 mcg/L: gray zone >400 mcg/L: pancreatitis likely	82% with severe pancreatitis, 63.6% with less severe pancreatitis	96.8%
Specific fPLI (serum) for diagnosis of pancreatitis	<3.5 mcg/L: pancreatitis unlikely 3.5-5.3 mcg/L: gray zone >5.3 mcg/L: pancreatitis likely	67% in all cats with pancreatitis and 100% in cats with moderate to severe pancreatitis	100%
SNAP cPLI (serum) for diagnosis of pancreatitis	Spot intensity test	92%-94%	71%-78%
SNAP fPLI (serum) for diagnosis of pancreatitis	Spot intensity test	79%	80%

*Confidence intervals for the diagnostic characteristics (sensitivity and specificity) have not been reported. Therefore the numbers are point estimates and should be considered to have some degree of variation.

REFERENCES

1. Boag AK, Coe RJ, Martinez TA, et al: Acid-base and electrolyte abnormalities in dogs with gastrointestinal foreign bodies, J Vet Intern Med 19:816, 2005.
2. Owens JM, Biery DN: Radiographic interpretation for the small animal clinician, ed 2, Media, Penn, 1999, Williams & Wilkins.
3. Sharma A, Thompson S, Scrivani PV, et al: Comparison of radiography and ultrasonography for diagnosing small-intestinal mechanical obstruction in vomiting dogs, Vet Radiol Ultras 52(3):248-255, 2011.
4. Schmiedt C, Tobias KM, Otto CM: Evaluation of abdominal fluid: peripheral blood creatinine and potassium ratios for diagnosis of uroperitoneum in dogs, J Vet Emerg Crit Care 11:4, 275, 2001.
5. Aumann M, Worth LT, Drobatz KJ: Uroperitoneum in cats: 26 cases (1986-1995), J Am Anim Hosp Assoc 34:315, 1998.
6. Bonczynski JJ, Ludwig LL, Barton BJ, et al: Comparison of peritoneal fluid and peripheral blood pH, bicarbonate, glucose, and lactate concentration as a diagnostic tool for septic peritonitis in dogs and cats, Vet Surg 32:161, 2003.
7. Ludwig LL, McLoughlin MA, Graves TK, et al: Surgical treatment of bile peritonitis in 24 dogs and 2 cats: a retrospective study (1987-1994), Vet Surg 26:90, 1997.

CHAPTER 113
ACUTE PANCREATITIS

Alison R. Gaynor, DVM, DACVIM, DACVECC

KEY POINTS

- Acute pancreatitis is a dynamic inflammatory disease, with episodes ranging in severity from mild and self-limiting to severe fulminant disease with extensive necrosis, systemic inflammation, and multiorgan failure.
- Clinical signs, physical examination findings, and results of diagnostic evaluation are variable and often nonspecific in dogs and cats with acute pancreatitis.
- Suggested risk factors associated with increased morbidity and mortality include older age, obesity, gastrointestinal disease, and concurrent endocrinopathies in dogs, and ionized hypocalcemia in cats. Hepatic lipidosis and other concurrent diseases also are associated with more severe disease in cats.
- Evaluation of serum amylase and lipase concentrations is not useful for diagnosis of acute pancreatitis in dogs and cats.
- Early, aggressive intravascular volume resuscitation and intensive monitoring are crucial for patients with severe acute pancreatitis.
- Early enteral nutrition and aggressive pain control are important aspects of therapy, whereas prophylactic antibiotic therapy and surgical intervention are infrequently indicated.
- Development of clinical and histopathologic consensus definitions, prognostic scoring systems, and other objective means of determining and stratifying severity of acute pancreatitis in veterinary patients is greatly needed.

Pancreatitis, broadly classified as acute, recurrent, or chronic, is a fairly common disease in dogs and has become more widely recognized in cats.[1,2] Acute and recurrent acute pancreatitis (AP) are characterized by episodes of pancreatic inflammation with a sudden onset and variable course. Episodes may range in severity from mild and self-limiting to severe fulminant disease with extensive necrosis, systemic inflammation and/or sepsis, multiorgan failure, and death. In addition to these systemic complications, moderately severe acute pancreatitis (MSAP) and severe acute pancreatitis (SAP) may include local complications (acute peripancreatic fluid collection, acute necrotic collection, pancreatic pseudocyst, or walled-off necrosis), which may be sterile or infected.[3] In veterinary medicine there is no universally accepted classification scheme for pancreatitis, with most current schemes based on variable terminology and histopathologic descriptions. However, these usually are not available at the time of diagnosis and do not necessarily correlate well with clinical severity and disease progression.[1,4-7] Therefore a clinically based classification system, simplified and adapted from consensus definitions in human medicine,[8] recently revised,[3] and used by other authors,[1,4,9-11] may be more appropriate to our patient population and is used in this chapter.

PATHOPHYSIOLOGY

A number of factors have been implicated as potential etiologic factors of pancreatitis. In humans, most cases of AP are caused by biliary calculi or alcohol exposure. Most cases in dogs and cats, however, are considered to be idiopathic, because a direct causal relationship is infrequently demonstrated.* Regardless of the underlying etiology, AP involves intrapancreatic activation of digestive enzymes with resultant pancreatic autodigestion. Studies of animal models suggest that initial events occur within the acinar cell by abnormal fusion of normally segregated lysosomes with zymogen granules (catalytically inactive forms of pancreatic enzymes), resulting in premature activation of trypsinogen to trypsin, and may involve changes in signal transduction, intracellular pH, and increases in intracellular ionized calcium (iCa) concentrations.[14] Trypsin in turn activates other proenzymes, setting in motion a cascade of local and systemic effects that are responsible for the clinical manifestations of AP.†

Local ischemia, phospholipase A_2, and reactive oxygen species (ROS) (produced in part from activation of xanthine oxidase by chymotrypsin) disrupt cell membranes, leading to pancreatic hemorrhage and necrosis, increased capillary permeability, and initiation of the arachidonic acid cascade. Elastase can cause increased vascular permeability secondary to degradation of elastin in vessel walls. Phospholipase A_2 degrades surfactant, promoting development of pulmonary edema, acute lung injury (ALI), and acute respiratory distress syndrome (ARDS) (see Chapter 24). Trypsin may activate the complement cascade, leading to an influx of inflammatory cells and production of multiple cytokines and more ROS. Trypsin also can activate the kallikrein-kinin system, resulting in vasodilation, hypotension, and possibly acute renal failure, and the coagulation and fibrinolytic pathways, resulting in microvascular thromboses and disseminated intravascular coagulation (DIC). Local inflammation and increases in pancreatic and peripancreatic microvascular permeability may cause massive fluid losses, further compromising perfusion and stimulating additional recruitment of inflammatory cells and mediators, leading to a vicious cycle culminating in the systemic inflammatory response syndrome (SIRS) and multiple organ dysfunction syndrome (MODS) (see Chapters 6 and 7).

CLINICAL PRESENTATION

Clinical signs and presentation associated with AP are variable and often nonspecific, particularly in cats, and may be difficult to distinguish from those of other acute abdominal disorders. Dogs with AP are usually presented because of anorexia, vomiting, weakness, depression, and sometimes diarrhea.[1,4,17,18] They may be febrile, dehydrated, and icteric, and often exhibit signs of abdominal discomfort, sometimes with abdominal distention and absent bowel sounds from associated peritonitis and intestinal ileus. Dogs that are middle-aged and older, those that are overweight, those that have a history of prior or recurrent gastrointestinal (GI) disturbances, and those

*For more in-depth reviews of etiologies see references 1, 2, and 4 (veterinary patients) and 12 and 13 (humans).

†See references 1, 2, and 13 through 16 for more in-depth reviews of pathophysiology.

with concurrent endocrinopathies (diabetes mellitus [DM], hypothyroidism, or hyperadrenocorticism) have been suggested to be at increased risk for development of fatal SAP.[9,18,19] Yorkshire Terriers, Miniature Schnauzers, and other terrier breeds also may be at increased risk.[18,19] Common clinical findings in cats with AP include lethargy, anorexia, dehydration, and hypothermia; vomiting and abdominal pain appear to be reported less frequently.[20-22] Icterus and pallor often are noted as well.[5,22] Concurrent conditions such as hepatic lipidosis, inflammatory bowel disease (IBD), interstitial nephritis or other kidney disease, DM, and cholangitis-cholangiohepatitis occur frequently, and signs of these conditions may predominate.[5,6,20-23] In either species, patients with MSAP or SAP may present with signs of systemic complications including dyspnea, bleeding disorders, cardiac arrhythmias, oliguria, shock, and collapse.

DIAGNOSIS

Diagnosis of AP requires careful integration of historical, physical examination, laboratory, and diagnostic imaging findings combined with a high degree of suspicion. Because many of these findings may be nonspecific and disease severity varies widely, diagnosis can be challenging. It is important to note that the absence of specific findings in any one diagnostic test does not rule out the possibility of AP.

Laboratory Assessment

Initial hemogram and serum chemistry profile abnormalities are variable and nonspecific, and may reflect concurrent extrapancreatic disease. Neutrophilic leukocytosis with a left shift is reported most commonly,[1,17,20] although neutropenia also has been reported in dogs[17] and may be more common in cats.[2] Thrombocytopenia also appears to be common.[17] The hematocrit and red blood cell counts may be normal, but anemia also may be seen, especially in cats.[5,20,21] An elevated hematocrit reflecting hemoconcentration and dehydration may be present; in human patients with AP this is associated with more severe disease. Elevations in hepatic enzyme activities and total bilirubin are often noted,[5,6,17,20,21] which may reflect ischemic and/or toxic hepatocellular injury or concurrent hepatobiliary disease. Patients are frequently azotemic, usually from prerenal causes, although acute renal failure also may be present.[17,19,20] Hyperglycemia is common[17,20] and is thought to be secondary to stress-related increases in endogenous cortisol and catecholamine levels, to hyperglucagonemia, or to overt DM. However, hypoglycemia may be seen if concurrent hepatic dysfunction, severe SIRS, or sepsis is present. Hypercalcemia has been reported in some dogs with SAP.[17] Mild to moderate hypocalcemia and hypomagnesemia are not uncommon, possibly as a result of pancreatic and peripancreatic fat saponification, although multiple mechanisms have been proposed.[22] Ionized hypocalcemia appears to be common in cats with AP and is associated with a poorer outcome.[22] Other common findings include hypokalemia, hypercholesterolemia, hypertriglyceridemia, and hypoalbuminemia, which may be secondary to GI losses, sequestration, and shifting of protein production to acute phase proteins. Hyperlipemia may be grossly apparent and may interfere with determination of other serum chemistry values.[17,19]

Increased activities of serum lipase and amylase historically have been used as markers of pancreatitis, but are of limited diagnostic value because elevations also may occur from extrapancreatic sources such as azotemia and glucocorticoid administration.[1,17] Furthermore, lipase and amylase activities are often within normal limits in animals with confirmed pancreatitis, particularly cats.[1,17,20,24,25]

Elevations in trypsin-like immunoreactivity (TLI) may suggest a diagnosis of pancreatitis, but also occurs with azotemia, and with GI disease in cats[6]; TLI may be normal in some patients with AP.[6,26,27] Although it is neither sensitive nor specific, evaluation of TLI may have some clinical utility in cats in combination with diagnostic imaging,[26] but is not considered useful in dogs.[1]

Elevations in pancreatic elastase-1 (cPE-1) also have been demonstrated in dogs with AP. A recent study suggested that evaluation of serum cPE-1 may be useful for diagnosis of SAP in dogs, but not for mild AP[28]; however, further evaluation is needed.

Species-specific pancreatic lipase immunoreactivity (fPLI, cPLI) assays have been validated for use in cats and dogs, respectively; data suggest that PLI is sensitive and specific for AP in experimental and spontaneous cases of AP in both species, and does not appear to be affected by renal disease or glucocorticoid administration.[1,27,29] PLI is currently the most useful serum marker available for the diagnosis of AP in cats and dogs.[29,30]

Diagnostic Imaging

Abdominal radiographs are neither sensitive nor specific for AP but may provide supportive evidence, and are especially valuable in helping to rule out other causes of acute abdominal disease such as intestinal obstruction or perforation. In dogs radiographic signs may include increased density and loss of detail in the right cranial abdomen, displacement of the descending duodenum to the right with widening of the angle between the proximal duodenum and the pylorus, and caudal displacement of the transverse colon. Gastric distention and static gas patterns suggestive of ileus may be noted in the descending duodenum and transverse colon.[1,17] Abdominal radiographs in cats typically are nonspecific, with decreased peritoneal detail most commonly reported; hepatomegaly, a mass effect in the cranial abdomen, and small intestinal dilation also have been reported.[5,20,21,31]

Abdominal ultrasonography (US) is particularly helpful as a diagnostic tool, for monitoring progression of the disease, and for evaluating the extent of associated complications and concurrent disorders. The pancreas may appear enlarged and hypoechoic, suggesting edema or necrosis, with hyperechoic peripancreatic tissue. More subtle changes such as pancreatic duct dilation, thromboses, and organ infarcts also may be detected.[17,22,27,31,32] US is also valuable for identifying and guiding sampling of masses, localized inflammation, and focal or regional fluid accumulations.* US-guided fine-needle aspiration (FNA) of pancreatic necrosis is used routinely in humans with AP to identify infected pancreatic necrosis[3,12,34,35] and has been described in dogs[32] and cats.[25]

Contrast-enhanced computed tomography (CECT) is considered the gold standard in human patients with AP for identifying pancreatic/peripancreatic necrosis and other local complications, and is used frequently as a guide for FNA.[3,12,34-36] Preliminary studies in veterinary patients suggested that CT was not particularly sensitive for diagnosis of AP in cats,[26,27] although a more recent study showed promising results.[37] CECT has been used to identify pancreatic necrosis in two dogs with AP.[32]

Cytology and Histopathology

FNA of the pancreas is minimally invasive, relatively safe, and can be used as a diagnostic aid, although this may be unnecessary in many clinical cases, and as mentioned below, focal lesions can be missed.[1,7] However, as discussed elsewhere in this chapter, cytology may be more valuable for evaluating local complications, infected necrosis, and for monitoring disease progression than for diagnosis of AP per se.

Although histopathology is the gold standard for diagnosis of AP in veterinary patients, this is infrequently obtained antemortem, may be too invasive for critically ill patients, and may be unnecessary for

*References 6, 17, 21, 22, 32, 33.

most clinical cases.[1,30] Determining the significance of histopathologic findings may be challenging because these may not correlate with clinical severity.[1,4-7] Inflammatory lesions are often focal or multifocal and easily can be missed, necessitating multiple biopsies, and it appears that histopathologic evidence of pancreatic inflammation is common in both species, even in patients with no corresponding clinical signs.[1,7,29] Histopathology has been described elsewhere.[1,2,7,20]

Additional Diagnostic Evaluation

Additional diagnostic evaluation not specific for AP but to help determine patient status and provide baseline information for subsequent monitoring may include urinalysis, urine culture and susceptibility, thoracic radiographs, evaluation of venous and arterial blood gases, lactate and iCa concentrations, and a complete coagulation profile. Coagulation abnormalities reflecting DIC and thromboses appear to be common in dogs and cats with SAP.* If focal or regional fluid accumulations (including pleural effusions) are detected, these should be sampled, with fluid analysis, cytology, and cultures evaluated as indicated. Serial cytologic and imaging evaluation may be helpful in monitoring disease progression. A recent preliminary investigation suggested that elevated cPLI concentration and lipase activity in peritoneal fluid may support a diagnosis of AP in dogs.[38]

DETERMINING SEVERITY

Because of the variability in presentation, early determination of disease severity and identification of those patients at risk for more severe disease would help guide earlier, more aggressive goal-oriented monitoring and therapy. In human medicine, various clinical and radiologic scoring systems and biochemical markers have been evaluated as objective methods for early determination of severity. In addition to selecting patients for earlier admission to an intensive care unit, these allow objective stratification of patients for prognostic purposes, for evaluating disease progression, and for clinical research including evaluation and comparison of various treatment protocols.

Clinical scoring systems include generalized predictors of severity such as the Acute Physiology and Chronic Health Evaluation (APACHE) II score, and pancreatitis-specific scoring systems including Ranson's Criteria, the Glasgow (Imrie) score, and Balthazar's CT index, as well as newer, more simplified systems such as the Bedside Index for Severity in AP (BISAP) and Harmless AP Score (HAPS).† The updated clinical classification system mentioned previously[3] incorporates the modified Marshall (MODS) scoring system,[41] and also defines local and systemic complications.

Of the many biochemical markers evaluated, pancreas-specific ones such as trypsinogen activation peptides (TAP) and carboxypeptidase, and more global markers of systemic inflammation such as C-reactive protein (CRP), interleukin-6, interleukin-8, and neutrophil elastase seem most promising. CRP is currently the best established and most widely available biochemical marker for predicting severity.‡

In veterinary medicine, in addition to the potential risk factors previously described, a simplified scoring system based on organ involvement[43] and a clinical severity index[10] have been proposed for dogs with AP; a survival prediction index has been developed for critically ill dogs (see Chapter 13). Increases in CRP[10,44] and urinary TAP-to-creatinine ratios[9] have been demonstrated in dogs with spontaneous AP, although further evaluation is needed to determine their clinical utility.

*References 9, 17, 20-22, 25, 32.

†See references 11, 12, 35, 36, 39, and 40 for more in-depth reviews of clinical scoring systems.

‡See references 11, 12, 39, and 42 for more in-depth reviews of biochemical markers.

TREATMENT

Therapy for patients with AP involves elimination of any identifiable underlying cause, if possible, symptomatic and supportive therapy, and anticipation of and early aggressive intervention against systemic complications. Although severity scoring systems and prognostic indicators are valuable, these do not replace the need for intensive monitoring and therapy on an individual basis. Patients that initially appear stable can decompensate rapidly; therefore close monitoring and frequent reassessment are critical. Throughout this section the reader is referred to related chapters in this book for more specific details on various therapies and monitoring.

Resuscitation, Fluid Therapy, and Monitoring

Patients with severe disease may be hemodynamically unstable and in need of rapid resuscitation with shock-rate replacement fluids. A recent preliminary study in human AP patients suggested that resuscitation with lactated Ringer's solution reduced systemic inflammation at 24 hours when compared with normal saline; however, there were no significant differences between treatment groups for other outcomes.[45] Resuscitation fluid types and rates of administration have not been evaluated in veterinary patients with AP.

Maintenance fluid requirements also may be substantial, to combat massive ongoing fluid losses from the vascular space due to vomiting and third spacing into the peritoneal cavity, GI tract, and the interstitium. Balanced electrolyte solutions are appropriate for maintenance needs, but should be modified based on frequent evaluation of electrolyte and acid-base status. Potassium supplementation is usually necessary. Calcium should not be supplemented unless clinical signs of tetany are observed, because of the potential for exacerbation of free radical production and cellular injury. Concurrent use of a synthetic colloid is often necessary for patients with severe disease. This will reduce the volume of crystalloids needed, and may help maintain intravascular volume and improve microcirculatory perfusion and oxygen delivery.

Frequent monitoring of vital signs, arterial blood pressure, central venous pressure, and urine output may help guide rates and types of intravenous fluids while avoiding overhydration. Other parameters that require frequent monitoring include hematocrit and total plasma solids; venous blood gas and electrolytes; blood glucose, albumin, and lactate; oxygenation and ventilation; an electrocardiogram; coagulation status; renal function; and mentation.

Patients that are hypotensive despite adequate volume replacement will need pressor therapy; dopamine may be used, although in some instances other agents may be necessary. In experimental feline models of AP, low-dose dopamine (5 mcg/kg/min) has been shown to reduce the degree of pancreatic inflammation by decreasing microvascular permeability,[46] although there have been no controlled studies in cats or dogs with spontaneous disease.

Supplemental oxygen is indicated for patients with evidence of hypovolemic shock and/or respiratory abnormalities. Patients that present with or develop tachypnea or dyspnea should be evaluated for ALI and ARDS, as well as aspiration pneumonia, pleural effusion, pulmonary thromboembolism, overhydration, and preexisting cardiopulmonary disease, and appropriate therapy instituted. Systemic causes of tachypnea such as metabolic acidosis, pain, and hyperthermia should also be considered. Patients with significant anemia may require packed red blood cell transfusions; this may be more of a problem in cats and small dogs, in part as a result of repeated blood sampling.

Use of fresh frozen plasma (FFP) often is advocated for patients with SAP to provide a source of α_2-macroglobulins, important protease inhibitors that help to clear activated circulating proteases. However, studies in human patients with SAP have not shown any improvement in morbidity or outcome with use of plasma.[47] A recent retrospective study in dogs with AP also suggested no benefit,[48] but there have been no prospective controlled studies in veterinary patients. FFP administration may be indicated for treatment of coagulopathies, including DIC.

Pain Management

Aggressive analgesic therapy is indicated for all patients with AP, including those that may not exhibit overt signs of pain. Adequate analgesic therapy is critical for maintaining patient comfort and will help decrease levels of stress hormones, will improve ventilation, and may improve GI motility if ileus is due in part to pain. Systemic opioids are the mainstay of therapy, and may be supplemented with low-dose ketamine or lidocaine, or both, in patients with more severe pain. Low-dose lidocaine has promotility effects and may be particularly beneficial for patients with severe ileus. Epidural and intraperitoneal analgesia also may be effective in select patients. Nonsteroidal antiinflammatory agents are not recommended unless patients are hemodynamically stable, not azotemic, and are well perfused.

Nutrition

The traditional recommendation to withhold food and water for patients with AP is no longer recommended; the current standard of care is to initiate enteral nutrition early, ideally within 24 hours of hospitalization.[1,34,49,50] Although there is no agreement about the timing of feeding for patients with mild AP, patients with MSAP and SAP are in a hypercatabolic state and for these patients early enteral nutrition is definitely indicated.*

Potential benefits of early enteral nutrition in patients with MSAP and SAP include improved gut mucosal structure and function and decreased bacterial translocation, thus attenuating stimuli for propagation of SIRS.[34,36,49-51] Compared with parenteral nutrition, early enteral feeding is associated with fewer complications including fewer infections, decreased risk of MODS, decreased mortality rates, less expense, and shorter duration of hospitalization.[12,34,49,52] Use of a jejunostomy tube to deliver nutrients to the jejunum is thought to minimally stimulate exocrine pancreatic secretion; however, it is not clear how exocrine pancreatic function is altered during AP, or whether stimulation of these secretions is actually detrimental. Because jejunostomy tube placement can be technically difficult and usually requires general anesthesia and special equipment, many veterinary clinicians have used other routes of enteral feeding including nasogastric and esophagostomy tubes, particularly in cats with AP because of the risk for hepatic lipidosis.[1,2] Preliminary studies suggest that early nasogastric tube feeding in cats[23] and human patients[53] and esophagostomy tube feeding in dogs[50] with SAP is well tolerated and feasible. Although additional studies are needed, thus far no differences in outcome compared with nasojejunal feeding have been noted in human patients.[49] Patients with severe ileus or intractable vomiting may tolerate low-volume enteral nutrition (trickle feeding or microenteral nutrition); however, supplemental total or partial parenteral nutrition should be considered when nutritional requirements cannot be met with enteral nutrition alone. Elemental or partial-elemental diets usually are recommended; although the ideal composition is unknown, supplementation with glutamine currently is recommended.[4,34] Cats, particularly those with concurrent GI tract disease, may require parenteral cobalamin supplementation.[1] Close monitoring for complications associated with refeeding is critical, and overfeeding should be avoided.

Considering the benefits of early enteral nutrition in patients with more severe disease as well as the fact that patient status at presentation can change rapidly, early enteral nutrition (within 24 hours) is also recommended for patients with mild AP.[1,49] This can be accomplished by oral feeding (if the patient is able and willing to eat), or by tube feeding, with vomiting controlled as needed.

*References 1, 12, 34, 35, 49, 50.

Additional and Supportive Therapy

Other therapies that do not necessarily influence the outcome of AP but do provide patient comfort include the use of GI protectants, thermal support, and physical therapy. Antiemetics and promotility agents are useful for patients that are vomiting and for those with GI ileus. It has been suggested that dopaminergic antagonists such as metoclopramide may be less effective or should be avoided.[1,2,4] Intermittent nasogastric decompression also may be helpful for patients with severe ileus; this will improve patient comfort, decrease nausea, and may decrease the risk of aspiration.

Treatment of concurrent diseases and of any inciting factors that may be identified is also important. Patients with overt DM, diabetic ketoacidosis (DKA), and those with persistent hyperglycemia should receive regular insulin, because strict glycemic control is important in the treatment of any critically ill patient. Cats with concurrent IBD may require glucocorticoid therapy.

Antibiotic Therapy

Routine use of prophylactic antibiotic therapy is controversial and is not recommended in most cases of AP because of the risk of inducing resistant bacterial strains and fungal infections.[1,12,34-36] For patients with documented infections, broad-spectrum antibiotics with activity against gram-negative species can be started while awaiting results of culture and susceptibility testing. In human patients with SAP, there is an increased risk for pancreatic/peripancreatic infection with greater than 30% necrosis, and infected pancreatic necrosis is a major risk factor for MODS and death; the incidence of infection appears to peak later during the course of the disease and is rare in the first week.[3,12,34,36] Despite numerous studies, however, it has not been shown convincingly that prophylactic antibiotic therapy improves outcome and, although conflicting, most of the recent consensus statements and meta-analyses recommend against routine antibiotic prophylaxis.[12,34-36,54] In the veterinary literature antibiotic therapy is frequently recommended despite a lack of supporting evidence, but in fact the incidence of infection is thought to be low.* The actual incidence is unknown.

Empiric antibiotic therapy may be reasonable for those patients that do not respond to other therapy and for those that initially respond but later deteriorate. However, every attempt to document infection in these patients should be made, including serial US or CECT-guided FNA of areas of pancreatic and peripancreatic necrosis. Development of infection in extrapancreatic sites such as the urinary tract or respiratory tract also may occur.

Surgery

Indications for surgery in patients with SAP are not always clear, and in the veterinary literature usually include those patients with infected pancreatic necrosis, those with extrahepatic biliary obstruction (EHBO), and those who continue to deteriorate despite aggressive medical therapy.[1,4,11,25,55] However, these patients are also very poor anesthetic risks, so the decision for surgical intervention should be made on an individual basis. In human medicine the trend in

*References 1, 4, 10, 11, 33, 55.

recent years has been away from early aggressive surgical intervention to more conservative treatment strategies, and it is generally agreed that surgery is not indicated for most cases involving sterile pancreatic necrosis.[12,34,35,56] Debridement and/or drainage is indicated for patients with infected necrosis, although whenever possible delayed and/or staged therapy is recommended to allow time for better demarcation of necrotic from viable tissue. This may also allow for use of less invasive interventions, including percutaneous, endoscopic, and laparoscopic techniques. Successful US-guided percutaneous drainage of pancreatic pseudocysts[33] and US-guided percutaneous cholecystocentesis[57] have been described in veterinary patients with AP.

OUTCOME

Patients that survive an episode of pancreatitis may be normal, or may continue to have episodic flare-ups. Those that improve but again become ill several weeks to months after the initial presentation should be evaluated closely for development of local complications such as pancreatic pseudocyst or walled-off necrosis, as well as for EHBO. Some patients may develop DM, chronic pancreatitis, and/or exocrine pancreatic insufficiency. Development of pancreatic exocrine and/or endocrine dysfunction is not uncommon in human patients.[12]

CONCLUSION

Specific therapies using direct inhibitors of pancreatic secretion (atropine, somatostatin, glucagon, calcitonin) or using protease and other pancreatic enzyme inhibitors generally have proved unsuccessful; despite decades of research, therapy for AP remains primarily supportive. With the increasing recognition of the importance of inflammatory mediators in the progression to systemic organ dysfunction, much ongoing research is focused on the use of free radical scavengers, cytokine antagonists, and other forms of immunomodulation.

Continued advances in biochemical and diagnostic imaging modalities will help improve our ability to more rapidly and definitively diagnose AP in our patients, and may provide improved and objective means for determining and monitoring severity of disease. Decreases in morbidity and mortality in human patients with AP in the recent past have been attributed in part to development of consensus definitions, scoring systems, and other predictors of severity, as previously discussed. In order to have meaningful evaluation of different therapies and to better understand the pathophysiologic mechanisms involved in canine and feline patients with AP, development of consensus definitions for clinical and histopathologic classification of AP and validation of severity scoring systems should be encouraged.

REFERENCES

1. Xenoulis PG, Steiner JM: Pancreas-diagnostic evaluation; necrosis and inflammation: canine. In Washabau RJ, Day MJ, editors: Canine and feline gastroenterology, St Louis, 2013, Elsevier.
2. Washabau RJ: Pancreas-necrosis and inflammation: feline. In Washabau RJ, Day MJ, editors: Canine and feline gastroenterology, St Louis, 2013, Elsevier.
3. Banks PA, Bollen TL, Dervenis C, et al: Classification of acute pancreatitis—2012: revision of the Atlanta classification and definitions by international consensus, Gut 62:102-111, 2013. Originally published online October 25, 2012: doi:10.1136/gutjnl-2012-302779.
4. Mansfield C: Acute pancreatitis in dogs: advances in understanding, diagnostics, and treatment, Topics Companion Anim Med 27:123-132, 2012.
5. Ferreri J, Hardam E, Kimmel SE, et al: Clinical differentiation of acute necrotizing from chronic nonsuppurative pancreatitis in cats: 63 cases (1996-2001), J Am Vet Med Assoc 223:469-474, 2003.
6. Swift NC, Marks SL, MacLachan NJ, et al: Evaluation of serum feline trypsin-like immunoreactivity for the diagnosis of pancreatitis in cats, J Am Vet Med Assoc 217:37-42, 2000.
7. Newman S, Steiner J, Woosley K, et al: Localization of pancreatic inflammation and necrosis in dogs, J Vet Intern Med 18:488-493, 2004.
8. Bradley EL: A clinically based classification system for acute pancreatitis. Summary of the International Symposium on Acute Pancreatitis, Atlanta, GA, September 11 through 13, 1992, Arch Surg 128:586-590, 1993.
9. Mansfield CS, Jones BR, Spillman T: Assessing the severity of canine pancreatitis, Res Vet Sci 74:137-144, 2003.
10. Mansfield CS, James FE, Robertson ID: Development of a clinical severity index for dogs with acute pancreatitis, J Am Vet Med Assoc 233:936-944, 2008.
11. Holm JL, Chan DL, Rozanski EA: Acute pancreatitis in dogs, J Vet Emerg Crit Care 13:201-213, 2003.
12. Lipsett PA: Acute pancreatitis. In Vincent JL, Abraham E, Moore FA, et al, editors: Textbook of critical care, ed 6, Philadelphia, 2011, Elsevier.
13. Elfar M, Gaber LW, Sabek O, et al: The inflammatory cascade in acute pancreatitis: relevance to clinical disease, Surg Clin N Am 87:1325-1340, 2007.
14. Halangk W, Lerch MM: Early events in acute pancreatitis, Gastroenterol Clin N Am 33:717-731, 2004.
15. Mansfield C: Pathophysiology of acute pancreatitis: potential application from experimental models and human medicine to dogs, J Vet Intern Med 26:875-887, 2012.
16. Isenmann R, Henne-Bruns D, Adler G: Shock and acute pancreatitis, Best Pract Res Clin Gastroenterol 17:345-355, 2003.
17. Hess RS, Saunders HM, Van Winkle TJ, et al: Clinical, clinicopathologic, radiographic, and ultrasonographic abnormalities in dogs with fatal acute pancreatitis: 70 cases (1986-1995), J Am Vet Med Assoc 213:665-670, 1998.
18. Hess RS, Kass PH, Shofer FS, et al: Evaluation of risk factors for fatal acute pancreatitis in dogs, J Am Vet Med Assoc 214:46-51, 1999.
19. Cook AK, Breitschwerdt EB, Levine JF, et al: Risk factors associated with acute pancreatitis in dogs: 101 cases (1985-1990), J Am Vet Med Assoc 203:673-679, 1993.
20. Hill RC, Van Winkle TJ: Acute necrotizing pancreatitis and acute suppurative pancreatitis in the cat. A retrospective study of 40 cases (1976-1989), J Vet Intern Med 7:25-33, 1993.
21. Akol KG, Washabau RJ, Saunders HM, et al: Acute pancreatitis in cats with hepatic lipidosis, J Vet Intern Med 7:205-209, 1993.
22. Kimmel SE, Washabau RJ, Drobatz KJ, et al: Incidence and prognostic value of low plasma ionized calcium concentration in cats with acute pancreatitis: 46 cases (1996-1998), J Am Vet Med Assoc 219:1105-1109, 2001.
23. Klaus JA, Rudloff E, Kirby R: Nasogastic tube feeding in cats with suspected acute pancreatitis: 55 cases (2001-2006), J Vet Emerg Crit Care 19:337-346, 2009.
24. Parent C, Washabau RJ, Williams DA, et al: Serum trypsin-like immunoreactivity, amylase and lipase in the diagnosis of feline acute pancreatitis (abstract), J Vet Intern Med 9:194, 1995.
25. Son TT, Thompson L, Serrano S, et al: Surgical intervention in the management of severe acute pancreatitis in cats: 8 cases (2003-2007), J Vet Emerg Crit Care 20:426-435, 2010.
26. Gerhardt A, Steiner JM, Williams DA, et al: Comparison of the sensitivity of different diagnostic tests for pancreatitis in cats, J Vet Intern Med 15:329-333, 2001.
27. Forman MA, Marks SL, De Cock HEV, et al: Evaluation of serum feline pancreatic lipase immunoreactivity and helical computed tomography versus conventional testing for the diagnosis of feline pancreatitis, J Vet Intern Med 18:807-815, 2004.
28. Mansfield C, Watson PD, Jones BR: Specificity and sensitivity of serum canine pancreatic elastase-1 concentration in the diagnosis of pancreatitis, J Vet Diag Invest 23:691-697, 2011.
29. Xenoulis PG, Steiner JM: Canine and feline pancreatic lipase immunoreactivity, Vet Clin Pathol 41:312-324, 2012.
30. McCord K, Morley PS, Armstrong J, et al: A multi-institutional study evaluating the diagnostic utility of the Spec cPL™ and SNAP

cPL™ in clinical acute pancreatitis in 84 dogs, J Vet Intern Med 26:888-896, 2012.

31. Saunders HM, Van Winkle TJ, Drobatz K, et al: Ultrasonographic findings in cats with clinical, gross pathologic, and histologic evidence of acute pancreatic necrosis: 20 cases (1994-2001), J Am Vet Med Assoc 221:1724-1730, 2002.
32. Jaeger JQ, Mattoon JS, Bateman SW, et al: Combined use of ultrasonography and contrast enhanced computed tomography to evaluate acute necrotizing pancreatitis in two dogs, Vet Radiol Ultrasound 44:72-79, 2003.
33. Van Enkevort BA, O'Brien RT, Young KM: Pancreatic pseudocysts in 4 dogs and 2 cats: ultrasonographic and clinicopathologic findings, J Vet Intern Med 13:309-313, 1999.
34. Nathens AB, Curtis JRC, Beale RJ, et al: Management of the critically ill patient with severe acute pancreatitis, Crit Care Med 32:2524-2536, 2004.
35. Hasibeder WR, Torgersen C, Rieger M, et al: Critical care of the patient with acute pancreatitis, Anaesth Intensive Care 37:190-206, 2009.
36. Banks PA, Freeman ML, Practice Parameters Committee of the American College of Gastroenterology: Practice guidelines in acute pancreatitis, Am J Gastroenterol 101:2379-2400, 2006.
37. Head LL, Daniel GB, Becker TJ, et al: Use of computed tomography and radiolabeled leukocytes in a cat with pancreatitis, Vet Radiol Ultrasound 46:263-266, 2005.
38. Chartier M, Hill S, Sunico S, et al: Evaluation of canine pancreas-specific lipase (Spec cPL) concentration and, amylase and lipase activities in peritoneal fluid as complementary diagnostic tools for acute pancreatitis in dogs (abstract), J Vet Intern Med 27:696, 2013.
39. Mofidi R, Patil PV, Suttie SA, et al: Risk assessment in acute pancreatitis, Br J Surg 96:137-150, 2009.
40. Mounzer R, Langmead CJ, Wu BU, et al: Comparison of existing clinical scoring systems to predict persistent organ failure in patients with acute pancreatitis, Gastroenterology 142:1476-1482, 2012.
41. Marshall JC, Cook DJ, Christou NV, et al: Multiple organ dysfunction score: a reliable descriptor of a complex clinical outcome, Crit Care Med 23:1638-1652, 1995.
42. Papachristou GI, Clermont G, Sharma A, et al: Risk and markers of severe acute pancreatitis, Gastroenterol Clin N Am 36:277-296, 2007.
43. Ruaux CG, Atwell RB: A severity score for spontaneous canine acute pancreatitis, Aust Vet J 76: 804-808, 1998.
44. Holm JL, Rozanski EA, Freeman LM, et al: C-reactive protein concentrations in canine acute pancreatitis, J Vet Emerg Crit Care 14:183-286, 2004.
45. Wu BU, Hwang JQ, Gardner TL, et al: Lactated ringer's solution reduces systemic inflammation compared with saline in patients with acute pancreatitis, Clin Gastroenterol Hepatol 9:710-717, 2011.
46. Karanjia ND, Lutrin FJ, Chang YB, et al: Low dose dopamine protects against hemorrhagic pancreatitis in cats, J Surg Res 48:440-443, 1990.
47. Lees T, Holliday M, Watkins M, et al: A multicentre controlled clinical trial of high-volume fresh frozen plasma therapy in prognostically severe acute pancreatitis, Ann R Coll Surg Engl 73:207-214, 1991.
48. Weatherton LK, Streeter EM: Evaluation of fresh frozen plasma administration in dogs with pancreatitis: 77 cases (1995-2005), J Vet Emerg Crit Care 19:617-622, 2009.
49. Olah A, Romics L: Evidence-based use of enteral nutrition in acute pancreatitis, Langenbecks Arch Surg 395:309-316, 2010.
50. Mansfield CS, James FE, Steiner JM, et al: A pilot study to assess tolerability of early enteral nutrition via esophagostomy tube feeding in dogs with severe acute pancreatitis, J Vet Intern Med 25:419-425, 2011.
51. Qin HL, Su ZD, Hu LG: Effect of early intrajejunal nutrition on pancreatic pathological features and gut barrier function in dogs with acute pancreatitis, Clin Nutr 21:469-473, 2002.
52. Al-Omran M, AlBalawi ZH, Tashkandi MF, et al: Enteral versus parenteral nutrition for acute pancreatitis (Review), Cochrane Database Syst Rev 1:CD002837, 2010.
53. Eatock FC, Chong P, Menezes N, et al: A randomized study of early nasogastric versus nasojejunal feeding in severe acute pancreatitis, Am J Gastroenterol 100:432-439, 2005.
54. Wittau M, Mayer B, Scheele J, et al: Systematic review and meta-analysis of antibiotic prophylaxis in severe acute pancreatitis, Scand J Gastroenterol 46:261-270, 2011.
55. Thompson LJ, Seshadri R, Raffe MR: Characteristics and outcomes in surgical management of severe acute pancreatitis: 37 dogs (2001-2007), J Vet Emerg Crit Care 19:165-173, 2009.
56. Freeman ML, Werner J, van Santvoort HC, et al: Interventions for necrotizing pancreatitis: summary of a multidisciplinary consensus conference, Pancreas 41:1176-1194, 2012.
57. Herman BA, Brawer RS, Murtaugh RJ, et al: Therapeutic percutaneous ultrasound-guided cholecystocentesis in three dogs with extrahepatic biliary obstruction and pancreatitis, J Am Vet Med Assoc 227:1782-1786, 2005.

CHAPTER 114

ACUTE CHOLECYSTITIS

Mark P. Rondeau, DVM, DACVIM (Internal Medicine)

KEY POINTS

- Although clinical findings in dogs and cats with cholecystitis are often nonspecific, clinical pathologic and abdominal ultrasound findings are often essential for localizing the gallbladder as the source of disease.
- Gallbladder mucocele is the most common disease of the gallbladder in dogs. However, the presence of cholecystitis is variable and depends on the degree of injury or vascular compromise to the gallbladder wall.
- Ultrasonographic appearance of echogenic fluid within the gallbladder fossa or generalized throughout the abdomen, echogenic reaction in the pericholecystic region, and radiographic evidence of decreased peritoneal detail are each sensitive indicators of gallbladder rupture and warrant surgical intervention regardless of the underlying cause of gallbladder disease.

Cholecystitis implies inflammation of the gallbladder; however, the term has been used to describe gallbladder-related symptoms in humans without confirmation of inflammation.[1] In dogs and cats, two main histologic types of cholecystitis have been described: neutrophilic cholecystitis and lymphoplasmacytic, follicular cholecystitis.[2] Most clinical descriptions in the veterinary literature involve neutrophilic cholecystitis. Cholecystitis may be caused by infectious agents, duct obstruction, blunt trauma, or systemic disease.[3]

Some common and significant gallbladder disease is not always associated with inflammation. In dogs, gallbladder mucocele is a major cause of clinical disease, and the presence of inflammation is variable depending on the degree of injury or vascular compromise to the gallbladder wall.[2] Gallbladder infarction in dogs is thought to be a vascular disease that is not associated with inflammation of the gallbladder.[4] Because these diseases may mimic cholecystitis clinically they are discussed in this chapter.

CLINICAL FINDINGS

In general, patient signalment, history, and physical examination findings are nonspecific in dogs and cats with cholecystitis. Affected patients can be of any age, breed, or sex. Shetland Sheepdogs are predisposed to gallbladder disorders in general, and gallbladder mucocele in particular.[5] Cocker spaniels also are overrepresented in surveys of dogs with gallbladder mucocele.[6-8] Common historical findings include anorexia, lethargy, vomiting, and diarrhea. Some physical examination findings are similarly nonspecific (i.e., fever). However, many patients have abdominal pain, which helps to localize the disease to the abdominal cavity. Some patients are visibly icteric, which suggests that the hepatobiliary system may be the source of the problem. However, in most cases clinical pathologic data raise the suspicion of a hepatobiliary disorder and imaging (particularly abdominal ultrasound) is most useful for identifying the gallbladder as the source of the problem.

Clinical pathologic findings consistent with hepatobiliary disease are common in dogs and cats with gallbladder disease. Serum biochemical analysis commonly reveals increased activity of hepatocellular and biliary epithelial enzymes, including alanine aminotransferase (ALT), aspartate aminotransferase (AST), alkaline phosphatase (ALP), and γ-glutamyltransferase (GGT). In cases with significant cholestasis or biliary obstruction, elevation in serum total bilirubin and cholesterol may be present. Hematologic analysis often reveals an inflammatory leukogram characterized by leukocytosis and neutrophilia. Once a suspicion of hepatobiliary disease is raised by the clinical findings, abdominal ultrasound is recommended to characterize the disease further. Specific imaging findings are discussed in the following sections.

COMMON CAUSES OF CHOLECYSTITIS IN DOGS AND CATS

Infectious Agents

Bacteria

Bacterial infection is the most commonly reported infectious cause of cholecystitis in dogs and cats. Bacterial cholecystitis may be a component of neutrophilic cholangitis in cats (see Chapter 115). Bacterial species isolated from dogs and cats with cholecystitis are typically of enteric origin, most commonly *Escherichia coli*, *Enterococcus* spp., *Bacteroides* spp. and *Clostridium* spp.[9-11] The underlying cause of bacterial infection in the bile often is unknown. Although the biliary tracts of dogs and cats are normally sterile, transient presence of low numbers of bacteria has been reported.[12] Bacterial colonization of bile may occur via reflux of duodenal bacteria or by hematogenous spread through the portal vasculature. The presence of bacteria within the bile, combined with increased biliary pressure as a result of an obstructive process, leads to infection of the bile and cholecystitis.[12]

The limited clinical descriptions of cholecystitis in the veterinary literature focus mainly on the canine disease.[10,11] Clinical findings are nonspecific as described above but often include vomiting, lethargy, and anorexia. Abdominal ultrasound findings in dogs with cholecystitis may include hyper- or hypoechoic thickening of the gallbladder wall, distention of the gallbladder, and/or cystic duct and echogenic bile.[10,11] The presence of gas within the lumen or wall of the gallbladder implies emphysematous cholecystitis, which is associated with infection by gas producing bacteria such as *Escherichia coli* and *Clostridium* spp.[3] Necrotizing cholecystitis has been described to occur in three types: type I involves areas of necrosis without gallbladder rupture; type II involves acute inflammation with rupture; type III involves chronic inflammation with adhesions and/or fistulae to adjacent organs.[10] The majority of dogs reported with necrotizing cholecystitis have had bacterial infection,[10] although it can occur in the absence of infection secondary to gallbladder mucocele (see below). Recognition of existing or impending gallbladder rupture is critical because prompt surgical intervention is required. The ultrasonographic presence of echogenic fluid within the gallbladder fossa or generalized throughout the abdomen, echogenic reaction in the pericholecystic region, and radiographic evidence of decreased peritoneal detail are sensitive indicators of gallbladder rupture.[13] In cases with peritoneal effusion, an effusion bilirubin concentration greater than twice the serum bilirubin confirms bile peritonitis (see Chapter 122).[14] If gallbladder rupture is considered unlikely, cholecystitis may be treated medically.[11] Ideally, this would involve antimicrobial selection based on culture and susceptibility testing results from bile obtained via ultrasound-guided cholecystocentesis. Empiric antimicrobial therapy should be directed at aerobic and anaerobic enteric flora. Although little information exists regarding the outcome of medically managed patients with cholecystitis, the prognosis for surgical intervention is guarded. High perioperative mortality is reported, with overall long-term survival ranging from 61% to 82% for dogs with bacterial cholecystitis undergoing surgery.[10,13]

Parasites

Trematode parasites may inhabit the gallbladder and bile ducts of cats and rarely dogs, leading to cholecystitis and/or cholangitis.[15,16] The most commonly identified organisms are the feline parasites *Platynosomum concinnum* and *Amphimerus pseudofelineus*. Both organisms have a similar life cycle, with their eggs ingested by a land snail, then entering a second intermediate host (fish or arthropod). Cats acquire infection by ingesting the second intermediate host. Adult worms develop in the gallbladder or bile ducts, causing varying degrees of illness ranging from nonspecific signs (anorexia, lethargy) to complete bile duct obstruction. Praziquantel appears to be the most effective treatment. Patients with severe infestations have a grave prognosis, with long-term survival rarely reported.

Obstruction

Any obstruction to bile flow from the gallbladder leads to cholecystitis. Complete extrahepatic bile duct obstruction (EHBDO) results in dilation of the gallbladder and cystic duct within 24 hours, and dilation of intrahepatic bile ducts within 5 to 7 days.[3] With more chronic obstruction, hepatic changes can occur, including hepatocyte necrosis, cholangitis, and periportal fibrosis.[3] Potential causes of EHBDO are listed in Box 114-1.

Cholelithiasis uncommonly is associated with cholecystitis in dogs and cats. Most choleliths are incidental findings. However, choleliths can cause cholecystitis by mechanical trauma or duct obstruction. Choleliths also may develop secondary to cholecystitis; increased

BOX 114-1 *Causes of Extrahepatic Bile Duct Obstruction in Dogs and Cats*

Hepatobiliary Disorders	Duodenal Disorders
Cholangitis/cholecystitis/ choledochitis	Neoplasia
Gallbladder mucocele	Intraluminal foreign body
Cholelithiasis	**Miscellaneous Disorders**
Neoplasia	Regional mass or lymphadenopathy
Cysts	Local peritonitis
Biliary trematode infestation	Iatrogenic (surgical ligation)
Inspissated bile	Trauma (stricture/fibrosis)
Pancreatic Disorders	
Pancreatitis, acute or chronic	
Neoplasia	

gallbladder mucin production and decreased gallbladder motility associated with inflammation may promote cholelith formation.[17,18] Choleliths in dogs and cats are composed most commonly of calcium carbonate and bilirubin pigments (bilirubin or calcium bilirubinate), as opposed to the cholesterol stones that predominate in humans.[3] Clinical signs may be absent in many cases. However, in cases with concurrent cholecystitis or bile duct obstruction, the clinical signs associated with those conditions are present. Abdominal ultrasound is the preferred imaging modality for identification of choleliths because radiopaque choleliths are reported in only 48% of dogs and 83% of cats with symptomatic cholelithiasis.[17,18] Radiopaque stones may be less prevalent in asymptomatic patients. Although identification of choleliths during abdominal ultrasound may represent an incidental finding, the concurrent presence of bile duct distention and/or clinical signs and clinicopathologic evidence of cholecystitis warrants suspicion of gallbladder disease. In such cases, abdominal exploratory surgery is indicated and cholecystectomy may be the treatment of choice. Samples of liver, gallbladder, and bile should be obtained for biopsy and aerobic and anaerobic culture and susceptibility testing. Prognosis likely depends on the presence or absence of concurrent disease, bacterial infection, and/or gallbladder rupture. Reported long-term survival rates after surgery are 78% for cats and 41% for dogs.[17,18]

Gallbladder Mucocele

Gallbladder mucocele is a condition exclusive to dogs that has been recognized at an increasing rate as the use of diagnostic abdominal ultrasound has become more common. The condition involves the accumulation of thick, mucin-laden bile within the gallbladder and bile ducts leading to varying degrees of obstruction to bile flow. Progressive distention of the gallbladder can lead to ischemic necrosis of the wall and resultant gallbladder rupture. Development of gallbladder mucocele is thought to result from a combination of increased mucin production and decreased gallbladder motility,[3] although the cause of these changes is unknown. A genetic susceptibility to gallbladder mucocele must be considered because Shetland Sheepdogs, Cocker Spaniels, and Miniature Schnauzers appear to be at increased risk.[5-8] An insertion mutation on the ABCB4 gene, which encodes for a protein that translocates phosphatidylcholine from the hepatocyte to the biliary canalicular lumen, has been associated with gallbladder mucocele formation in Shetland Sheepdogs and other breeds.[19] The condition also has been associated with dsylipidemias and glucocorticoid excess. Dogs with hyperadrenocorticism have a significantly increased risk of developing gallbladder mucocele.[20] Histopathologic examination of the gallbladder in affected dogs routinely reveals cystic mucinous hyperplasia (in addition to secondary changes such as necrotizing cholecystitis),[6-8] which may be an incidental finding in older dogs and has been induced by administration of progestational compounds in the study that first described gallbladder mucoceles in dogs.[21]

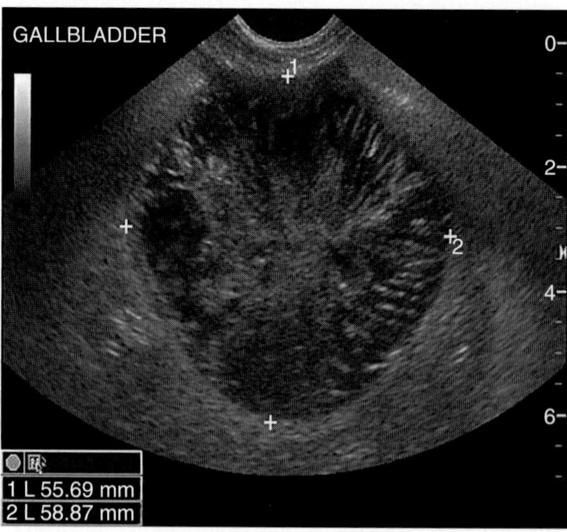

FIGURE 114-1 Ultrasonographic appearance of gallbladder mucocele in a dog.

Because the development of a gallbladder mucocele likely occurs gradually and the time of progression to necrotizing cholecystitis and/or gallbladder rupture is unknown, affected dogs may be identified incidentally. Increased activity of liver enzymes, hypercholesterolemia, and/or hyperbilirubinemia may be identified on routine screening serum biochemical analysis. Alternatively, the mucocele may be identified during abdominal ultrasound examination to evaluate another problem. Affected dogs are typically middle age to older, with a median age of 9 to 11 years, but dogs as young as 3 years of age have been reported.[6-8] When clinical signs do occur as a result of gallbladder mucocele, they are often nonspecific, as described above for other forms of gallbladder disease. Vomiting, lethargy, and decreased appetite are seen most commonly. When present, these clinical signs are usually present for 1 week or less.[6-8] Gallbladder mucocele usually is suspected on the basis of its hallmark ultrasonographic appearance (Figure 114-1). Echogenic, nonmobile material fills the distended gallbladder in either a stellate (resembling the cut surface of a kiwi fruit) or finely striated pattern, often with a hypoechoic rim along the wall.[6] In contrast to nonpathologic bile sludge, the echogenic contents of the gallbladder mucocele do not move as the patient's position is changed. As discussed previously, concurrent identification of echogenic fluid within the gallbladder fossa or generalized throughout the abdomen, or an echogenic reaction in the pericholecystic region suggests possible gallbladder rupture. Bacterial infection of the gallbladder or bile appears to be uncommon in dogs with gallbladder mucocele; it was reported in fewer than 10% of cases in most studies,[7,8,13] with the exception of positive aerobic bile cultures in six of nine cases in one study.[6]

The optimal treatment plan for gallbladder mucocele in dogs is unknown. Most would agree that surgical intervention clearly is indicated in cases with ultrasonographic suspicion of gallbladder rupture.[3,8] Surgical intervention also may be appropriate in dogs with clinicopathologic evidence of biliary obstruction (hyperbilirubinemia, hypercholesterolemia) and/or clinical signs consistent with cholecystitis and no other apparent cause aside from the mucocele. Some clinicians recommend surgical intervention as a preventive measure in any dog having an ultrasonographically identified gallbladder mucocele, even if the dog is asymptomatic.[3] When surgical intervention is pursued, cholecystectomy is the preferred treatment.

Cholecystotomy to remove gallbladder contents is contraindicated because the underlying cause of mucocele formation is not being addressed (resulting in recurrence of mucocele), and there may be areas of gallbladder necrosis, even in the absence of gross rupture (resulting in postoperative leakage). Biliary diversion techniques have been associated with a worse prognosis and also should be avoided.[22] At the time of cholecystectomy, the common bile duct must be catheterized and thoroughly flushed to ensure patency. The excised gallbladder should be submitted for histopathologic examination as well as aerobic and anaerobic bacterial culture. Concurrent liver biopsy is recommended to evaluate for underlying disease.

Medical management and strict patient surveillance may be considered in lieu of surgery for asymptomatic dogs. Nonsurgical resolution of gallbladder mucocele within 3 months has been reported in two dogs.[23] Both of these dogs had hypothyroidism and were treated with ursodeoxycholic acid (UDCA) and levothyroxine after the mucocele was identified. One of the two also was treated with S-adenosylmethionine (SAMe), amoxicillin, and omega fatty acid supplementation. Although these two cases do not provide enough information to make recommendations regarding medical management, the use of UDCA has several potential benefits: it causes choleresis, has immunomodulatory properties, may decrease mucin secretion, and may improve gallbladder motility.[3] UDCA is dosed at 10 to 15 mg/kg orally once to twice daily. SAMe also has hepatoprotective effects as a glutathione precursor and antioxidant and may have choleretic effects (shown at higher doses in cats).[3] SAMe is given on an empty stomach for optimal absorption at a dose of 20 to 40 mg/kg daily. Antimicrobial therapy aimed at enteric flora also may be considered to treat potential bacterial cholangitis associated with the mucocele, although bacterial infection is uncommon, as discussed above. Ultimately, it should be stressed that gallbladder mucocele is a surgical disease, and attempting medical resolution assumes a risk of necrotizing cholecystitis and gallbladder rupture. Medical management should be undertaken only with intensive follow-up patient monitoring and client communication.

The prognosis for dogs with gallbladder mucocele is guarded. The progression with medical management is unknown. Surgery carries a high perioperative mortality of 20% to 40%.[6-8,23] However, dogs surviving the immediate postoperative period appear to have good long-term survival. Although the presence of gallbladder rupture may not be associated with a worse prognosis,[7,8,13] septic bile peritonitis does carry a worse prognosis than sterile bile peritonitis.[14]

Gallbladder Infarction

Gallbladder infarction is another condition of dogs that does not result in gallbladder inflammation but can present with clinical signs that mimic cholecystitis. This disease has been described in a small group of 12 dogs.[4] Affected dogs ranged in age from 4 to 14 years. Clinical signs of fewer than 2 weeks' duration include vomiting, anorexia, and diarrhea. Clinicopathologic findings also mimic cholecystitis with increased activity of liver enzymes, hyperbilirubinemia, and leukocytosis in more than 50% of cases. The diagnosis is confirmed by histopathology, and no hallmark diagnostic findings allow for a presurgical diagnosis. All 12 of the described dogs were treated by cholecystectomy. Gallbladder rupture was present at the time of surgery in 50% of the cases. Bacterial infection was documented in 25% of the cases, with isolation of enteric organisms (*Escherichia coli*, *Clostridium* spp.). Postoperative survival rate was 67%.

Histologic findings in affected gallbladders include transmural coagulative necrosis with minimal to absent inflammation. Thrombi were identified in an artery supplying the gallbladder in 2 of 12 cases. An additional case had atherosclerotic changes in arterioles adjacent to the gallbladder. Another two dogs had evidence of distant thrombosis of the spleen. Therefore the authors suggest that the gallbladder necrosis in affected dogs is a result of infarction that may be a sign of a more generalized hypercoagulable state. Three of the 12 dogs described were receiving treatment for hypothyroidism and another for hyperadrenocorticism. The role of these concurrent diseases in the pathogenesis of gallbladder infarction is unknown. Gallbladder infarction represents an uncommon condition in dogs that can mimic cholecystitis and can result in gallbladder rupture.

REFERENCES

1. Aguirre A: Diseases of the gallbladder and extrahepatic biliary system. In Ettinger SJ, Feldman EC, editors: Textbook of veterinary internal medicine, St Louis, 2010, Saunders Elsevier.
2. Cullen JM: Hepatobiliary histopathology. In Washabau RJ, Day MJ, editors: Canine and feline gastroenterology, St Louis, 2013, Elsevier Saunders.
3. Center SA: Diseases of the gallbladder and biliary tree, Vet Clin North Am Small Anim Pract 39:543-598, 2009.
4. Holt DE, Mehler SE, Mayhew PD, et al: Canine gallbladder infarction: 12 cases (1990-2003), Vet Pathol 41:416-418, 2004.
5. Aguirre AL, Center SA, Randolph JF, et al: Gallbladder disease in Shetland Sheepdogs: 38 cases (1995-2005), J Am Vet Med Assoc 231:79-88, 2007.
6. Besso JG, Wrigley RH, Gliatto JM, et al: Ultrasonographic appearance and clinical findings in 14 dogs with gallbladder mucocele, Vet Radiol Ultrasound 41:261-271, 2000.
7. Worley DR, Hottinger HA, Lawrence HJ: Surgical management of gallbladder mucoceles in dogs: 22 cases (1999-2003), J Am Vet Med Assoc 225:1418-1422, 2004.
8. Pike FS, Berg J, King NW, et al: Gallbladder mucocele in dogs: 30 cases (2000-2002), J Am Vet Med Assoc 224:1615-1622, 2004.
9. Wagner KA, Hartmann FA, Trepanier LA: Bacterial culture results from liver, gallbladder or bile in 248 cats and dogs evaluated for hepatobiliary disease: 1998-2003, J Vet Intern Med 21:417-424, 2007.
10. Church EM, Matthiesen DT: Surgical treatment of 23 dogs with necrotizing cholecystitis, J Am Anim Hosp Assoc 24:305-310, 1988.
11. Rivers BJ, Walter PA, Johnston GR, et al: Acalculous cholecystitis in four canine cases: ultrasonographic findings and use of ultrasonographic-guided, percutaneous cholecystocentesis in diagnosis, J Am Anim Hosp Assoc 33:207-214, 1997.
12. Neel JA, Tarigo J, Grindem CB: Gallbladder aspirate from a dog, Vet Clin Pathol 35:467-470, 2006.
13. Crews LJ, Feeney DA, Jessen CR, et al: Clinical, ultrasonographic and laboratory findings associated with gallbladder disease and rupture in dogs: 45 cases (1997-2007), J Am Vet Med Assoc 234:359-366, 2009.
14. Ludwig LL, McLoughlin MA, Graves TK, et al: Surgical treatment of bile peritonitis in 24 dogs and 2 cats: a retrospective study (1987-1994), Vet Surg 26:90-98, 1997.
15. Bowman DD, Hendrix CM, Lindsay DS, et al: Feline clinical parasitology, Ames, Iowa, 2002, Iowa State University Press.
16. Foley RH: Platynosomum concinnum infection in cats, Compend Contin Educ Pract Vet 16:1271-1274, 1994.
17. Kirpensteijn J, Fingland RB, Ulrich T, et al: Cholelithiasis in dogs: 29 cases (1980-1990), J Am Vet Med Assoc 202:1137-1142, 1993.
18. Eich CS, Ludwig LL: The surgical treatment of cholelithiasis in cats: a study of 9 cases, J Am Anim Hosp Assoc 38:290-296, 2002.
19. Mealey KL, Minch JD, White SN, et al: An insertion mutation in ABCB4 is associated with gallbladder mucocele formation in dogs, Comp Hepatol 9:6, 2010.
20. Mesich MLL, Mayhew PD, Paek M, et al: Gallbladder mucoceles and their association with endocrinopathies in dogs: a retrospective case-control study, J Small Anim Pract 50:630-635, 2009.
21. Kovatch RM, Hildebrandt PK, Marcus LC: Cystic mucinous hypertrophy of the mucosa of the gallbladder in the dog, Pathol 2:574-584, 1965.
22. Amsellem PM, Seim HB, MacPhail CM, et al: Long-term survival and risk factors associated with biliary surgery in dogs: 34 cases (1994-2004), J Am Vet Med Assoc 229:1451-1457, 2006.
23. Walter R, Dunn ME, d'Anjou M, et al: Nonsurgical resolution of gallbladder mucocele in two dogs, J Am Vet Med Assoc 232:1688-1693, 2008.

CHAPTER 115

HEPATITIS AND CHOLANGIOHEPATITIS

Mark P. Rondeau, DVM, DACVIM (Internal Medicine)

KEY POINTS

- Hepatitis is defined as any inflammatory cell infiltrate within the hepatic parenchyma; the term *cholangiohepatitis* describes the extension of that inflammation to include the intrahepatic bile ducts.
- Although many causes of hepatitis and cholangiohepatitis have been described in dogs and cats, the cause in many cases remains unknown.
- A suspicion of hepatitis or cholangiohepatitis may be based on supportive historical, physical examination, and clinicopathologic findings that are similar for most causes of hepatic disease. A diagnosis of hepatitis or cholangiohepatitis is made ultimately via histopathologic evaluation of hepatic tissue.
- The mechanisms of hepatocellular injury in animals with hepatitis and cholangiohepatitis are poorly understood. Elucidation of these mechanisms may provide the basis for future therapeutic options.
- Successful treatment of the patient with hepatitis or cholangiohepatitis involves addressing the underlying disease or inciting cause and providing aggressive symptomatic therapy and supportive care.

Hepatitis is defined as any inflammatory cell infiltrate within the hepatic parenchyma, and the term *cholangiohepatitis* describes extension of that inflammation to include the intrahepatic bile ducts.[1] A diagnosis of these conditions is based on histopathologic examination of hepatic biopsy specimens. The histopathologic appearance gives clues regarding the duration of the inflammation. Acute hepatitis is characterized by a combination of inflammation, hepatocellular apoptosis, necrosis, and possibly regeneration, but a lack of fibrosis. The relationship between the development of hepatitis and necrosis is complex, and it can be difficult to determine which abnormality was the initial lesion.[1] Chronic hepatitis, on the other hand, is identified by the presence of fibrosis, proliferation of ductular structures, and regenerative nodules in addition to an inflammatory infiltrate, apoptosis, and/or necrosis.[2] The type of inflammatory cellular infiltrate may give the clinician some clues regarding the cause. Occasionally, causative agents are identified within biopsy specimens. However, the cause remains unknown for many cases of hepatitis and cholangiohepatitis in dogs and cats. This chapter discusses the clinical presentation of animals with hepatitis and cholangiohepatitis and outlines the most commonly recognized clinical syndromes with respect to diagnosis and treatment of the specific disease. Effective treatment of patients with hepatitis or cholangiohepatitis includes specific therapy of any identified inciting cause and aggressive symptomatic and supportive therapy. A discussion of symptomatic treatment and supportive therapy for the sequelae of hepatitis and cholangiohepatitis can be found in Chapter 116.

HISTORICAL FINDINGS

In general, the historical findings associated with hepatitis are nonspecific, as with most types of liver disease. Exposure to certain etiologic agents or toxins may be ascertained from the client history and thus raise the suspicion for hepatic involvement. Because of the large reserve capacity of the liver, a short duration of clinical signs does not necessarily indicate acute disease. Animals with cholangiohepatitis (CH) may not show outward clinical signs until a significant portion of hepatic function is affected. Presenting owner complaints for animals with hepatitis may include vomiting, diarrhea, anorexia, lethargy, polyuria, polydipsia, abdominal distention, dysuria, neurologic abnormalities associated with hepatic encephalopathy or vascular accidents, and icterus.

PHYSICAL EXAMINATION FINDINGS

Similar to historical findings, the physical examination findings in animals with hepatitis are often nonspecific. Icterus, when present in the absence of hemolytic anemia, suggests disease of the hepatic parenchyma or extrahepatic biliary system. Animals with acute hepatitis are more likely to have fever and abdominal pain, and those with CH are more likely to have ascites. Hepatomegaly may be present in some patients, especially those with acute hepatitis. Many animals with hepatitis do not have any of these physical abnormalities present on the initial examination, and serum biochemical changes in those cases are likely to direct the clinician toward the liver as the site of disease.

MECHANISMS OF HEPATOCELLULAR INJURY

The pathogenesis by which hepatitis and cholangiohepatitis lead to hepatocellular necrosis and apoptosis is not understood completely. Experimental studies have suggested many mechanisms of hepatocellular injury, but their specific evaluation in dogs and cats with hepatitis is lacking. Mechanisms of hepatocellular injury that are not specific to hepatitis include tissue hypoxia, lipid peroxidation, intracellular cofactor depletion, intracellular toxin production, cholestatic injury, endotoxic insults, and hepatocyte plasma membrane injury.[3]

Hepatocytes are especially susceptible to anoxia because the liver receives a mixture of venous and arterial blood. Hypoxic damage quickly leads to plasma membrane and cytosolic organelle injury secondary to adenosine triphosphate (ATP) depletion. Free radicals may cause oxidative cellular injury that can result in lipid peroxidation and subsequent plasma membrane damage.

Cellular toxins may bind to nucleic acids and inhibit protein synthesis. Cholestasis causes retention of bile acids that directly damage cellular organelles. Endotoxins work via various mechanisms, most of which involve stimulation of inflammatory cells to produce inflammatory mediators (cytokines such as prostaglandins and leukotrienes) that perpetuate inflammation within the liver parenchyma. Experimental work in mouse models suggests an important role for tumor necrosis factor-α (TNF-α) in the initiation and perpetuation of hepatitis. TNF-α, produced secondary to the interaction of the costimulatory molecules CD154 on T cells and

CD40 on hepatocytes and Kupffer cells, stimulates hepatocyte apoptosis through the Fas-Fas ligand pathway.[4] A better understanding of the complex mechanisms of hepatocellular injury in animals with hepatitis may encourage the development of novel therapeutic modalities for affected patients.

CAUSES OF HEPATITIS AND CHOLANGIOHEPATITIS IN DOGS AND CATS

Box 115-1 lists the reported causes of hepatitis and cholangiohepatitis in dogs and cats. A complete discussion of all disease entities is beyond the scope of this chapter. A discussion of the most common clinical syndromes follows.

Idiopathic Causes

Feline cholangitis complex

The feline cholangitis complex is one of the most common hepatobiliary disorders in cats.[5] This syndrome has been reported in dogs[6] but is primarily a feline disease. Several classification schemes have been proposed to define the various elements of this syndrome. The World Small Animal Veterinary Association (WSAVA) Liver Standardization Group has proposed a classification system that divides feline cholangitis into two main categories: neutrophilic cholangitis and lymphocytic cholangitis.[7]

BOX 115-1 *Causes of Hepatitis and Cholangiohepatitis in Dogs and Cats*

Idiopathic	**Parasitic**
Canine chronic hepatitis	Visceral larval migrans
Feline cholangitis complex	Dirofilariasis (caudal vena caval syndrome)
Nonspecific reactive hepatitis	Liver fluke migration
Lobular dissecting hepatitis	Schistosomiasis
Viral	*Echinococcus* cysts
Infectious canine hepatitis (adenovirus type I)	**Fungal**
Acidophil cell hepatitis	Histoplasmosis
Herpesvirus (neonates)	Blastomycosis
Feline infectious peritonitis	Coccidioidomycosis
Bacterial	Aspergillosis (disseminated)
Feline cholangitis complex	Phycomycosis
Leptospirosis	**Algal**
Bartonellosis	Protothecosis
Tyzzer's disease *(Clostridium piliforme)*	**Hepatotoxins**
Salmonellosis	Acetaminophen
Listeriosis	Aflatoxin
Tularemia	Amiodarone
Brucellosis	Aspirin
Yersiniosis	Azathioprine
Helicobacter spp.	Azole antifungals
Mycobacteria	Carprofen
Septicemia	Cycads (e.g., Sago palm)
Rickettsial	Diazepam (oral)
Ehrlichiosis	Halothane
Rocky Mountain spotted fever	Lomustine
Protozoal	Methimazole
Toxoplasmosis	Phenobarbital
Neosporosis	Phenytoin
Leishmaniasis	Primidone
Cytauxzoonosis	Tetracyclines
Hepatozoonosis	Trimethoprim/sulfadiazine or sulfamethoxazole
Coccidiosis	Xylitol
	Zonisamide

Neutrophilic Cholangitis

Histologically, neutrophilic cholangitis (NC) is characterized by infiltration of neutrophils within the wall or lumen of intrahepatic bile ducts. This disease can be seen in acute and chronic stages. In acute neutrophilic cholangitis (ANC), edema and neutrophilic inflammation may extend into the portal areas. In chronic neutrophilic cholangitis (CNC), a mixed inflammatory infiltrate may be noted in portal areas, along with varying degrees of fibrosis and bile duct hyperplasia.[7] This syndrome was referred to previously as *acute cholangiohepatitis* or *suppurative cholangitis-cholangiohepatitis.*[8,9] NC can occur in cats of any age, breed, or sex. Clinical signs are nonspecific and include anorexia, lethargy, vomiting, and weight loss. The duration of these clinical signs ranges from a few days to a few months and may be shorter in cats with ANC than in those with CNC,[8] but this is not a consistent finding.[10,11] Physical examination findings commonly include dehydration and icterus. Fever is present in 19% to 37.5% of cases.[10,12] Some reports suggest that fever is associated more commonly with ANC than CNC,[12] whereas others recognize no difference.[10,11] Hepatomegaly is seen in fewer than half of the cases and abdominal pain is noted occasionally.[8,10,11] Biochemical analysis commonly reveals increased activity of alanine aminotransferase (ALT), aspartate aminotransferase (AST), alkaline phosphatase (ALP), and γ-glutamyltransferase (GGT) ranging in severity from mild to severe. However, increased liver enzyme activity may be absent in some cases.[13] Cholangitis in cats has been associated with inflammatory bowel disease (IBD) and pancreatitis,[12] and many investigators believe that NC is the result of an ascending bacterial infection from the gastrointestinal (GI) tract. However, rates of bacterial isolation using traditional methods have varied greatly, from less than 20% to more than 60% in affected cats.[8,10] When isolated, common bacterial species include *Escherichia coli, Enterococcus* spp., *Clostridium* spp., and *Staphylococcus* spp. Samples for aerobic and anaerobic bacterial cultures should be obtained in any cat suspected of having cholangitis; gallbladder bile is preferred to liver tissue as the culture source.[14] Treatment with a broad-spectrum antimicrobial therapy, focusing on enteric flora, is recommended pending results of culture and susceptibility testing. Prognosis for cats with NC is typically good with aggressive treatment, although sequelae may include bile duct obstruction, acute necrotizing pancreatitis, sepsis, and multiple organ dysfunction.

Lymphocytic Cholangitis

Lymphocytic cholangitis (LC) is a chronic form of disease that is characterized histologically by a mixed inflammatory infiltrate (typically small lymphocytes, or lymphocytes and plasma cells) within portal areas and is associated with varying degrees of fibrosis and bile duct hyperplasia.[7] Inflammation within the walls or lumens of intrahepatic bile ducts may be present but is not a specific hallmark of the disease. LC likely includes a wide spectrum of clinical diseases with varying severity and clinical significance.[14] LC likely includes syndromes that have been referred to previously as *chronic cholangiohepatitis, nonsuppurative cholangitis-cholangiohepatitis,* and *lymphocytic portal hepatitis.*[5,8,9,12] The clinical picture of cats with LC varies widely and has significant overlap with other forms of hepatobiliary disease in cats, including NC.[10,11] Nonspecific clinical signs, including anorexia, lethargy, vomiting, and weight loss, may be chronic and intermittent.[8] Physical examination findings may include icterus, hepatomegaly, or ascites, but none are consistent findings. Signs of hepatic encephalopathy (dullness, ptyalism, seizures) may develop in severely affected cats. Definitive diagnosis is made by liver biopsy. As discussed for NC, ancillary diagnostics provide information to support hepatobiliary disease but are not specific for LC. Activity of serum liver enzymes is increased in many but not all cases and varies in severity. Abdominal radiographic and ultrasonographic findings are nonspecific but may aid in the recognition of concurrent disease. The cause of LC is unknown, although a chronic response to an ascending bacterial infection from GI flora and an association with IBD and pancreatitis (as seen with NC) has been suggested.[8,9] Immunohistochemical analysis of hepatic biopsy specimens from cats with LC has shown a predominance of CD3+ T cells infiltrating the bile duct epithelium and periportal areas, a smaller proportion of B cells forming discrete aggregates in the portal regions, and expression of major histocompatibility complex class II on the biliary epithelium.[15,16] These findings, combined with anecdotal response to glucocorticoid therapy and the fact that active infection has been documented rarely in cats with LC, have led to the suspicion that LC is an immune-mediated disease. Treatment typically involves immunosuppressive glucocorticoid therapy in animals with no evidence of infection. Treatment with ursodeoxycholic acid (10 to 15 mg/kg PO q24h) has anecdotal and theoretic benefits, although no clinical studies examining its efficacy in cats have been published. Prognosis is typically good with appropriate management, although concurrent disease is common and may affect prognosis.

Canine chronic hepatitis

Although many causes of chronic hepatic inflammation in dogs have been identified, the term *canine chronic hepatitis* (CCH) describes an idiopathic, progressive necroinflammatory disease of unknown cause that is common in the canine population.[1] Evidence supports an immune-mediated process as the perpetuating factor,[1,17,18] although it is unclear whether the disease is a primary or secondary immune response. Because of the chronic nature of the disease and the large reserve capacity of the liver, many affected animals are not identified until the onset of fulminant hepatic failure. However, increasing numbers of cases are now being identified at an earlier asymptomatic stage as a result of increased hepatic enzyme activity that is noted on routine serum biochemical screening.

Animals of any age and sex are affected, although middle-age female dogs may be overrepresented. CCH is seen with increased frequency in certain breeds (Box 115-2), suggesting a familial predisposition. No specific diagnostic findings separate CCH from other causes of hepatitis. Ultimately, the diagnosis is based on histopathologic examination of liver tissue revealing inflammation (usually lymphocytic and plasmacytic, occasionally neutrophilic), necrosis and/or apoptosis, evidence of regeneration, fibrosis and/or hyperplasia of ductular structures and the absence of an identifiable underlying cause.[1] The optimal treatment protocol for animals with CCH has not been well studied, but immunosuppressive therapy is the mainstay of treatment. Corticosteroids are the only class of drug shown potentially to provide benefit[19] and their use is indicated in patients with signs of hepatic failure. Other immunomodulatory drugs that may be used include ursodeoxycholic acid, metronidazole, azathioprine, and cyclosporine. Colchicine may delay progression of hepatic fibrosis. Copper chelation may be beneficial when copper retention is a significant contributing factor. The overall prognosis is difficult to ascertain because asymptomatic animals may have a slowly progressive course and excellent prognosis. However, once hepatic failure and/or cirrhosis develops, the prognosis is poor.

BOX 115-2 *Breeds Predisposed to Chronic Hepatitis*

American Cocker Spaniel
Bedlington Terrier*
Dalmatian*
Doberman Pinscher*
English Cocker Spaniel
English Springer Spaniel
Labrador Retriever*
Skye Terrier*
Standard Poodle
West Highland White Terrier*

*Proven or suspected copper-associated hepatopathy.

Role of Copper

The role of copper in the pathogenesis of CCH is unclear. Elevated hepatic copper levels have been identified in many dogs with CCH, but because biliary excretion is the major mechanism of maintaining copper homeostasis, any cause of cholestasis would be expected to increase hepatic copper levels.[18] However, it has been shown in the Bedlington Terrier that elevated copper levels (caused by an inherited defect in excretion) lead to chronic hepatitis and cirrhosis.[1] However, it may be difficult to determine which came first, the copper accumulation or the hepatitis. A propensity for increased hepatic copper levels in association with CCH has been described for many breeds in addition to the Bedlington Terrier, and these are listed in Box 115-2.

A suspected primary hepatic copper storage disorder also has been reported in one cat.[20] Whether the copper accumulation is a primary or secondary event, the excessive copper is damaging to hepatocytes. Copper chelation treatment has improved or resolved the hepatic pathologic findings in a group of Doberman Pinschers with elevated hepatic copper levels and subclinical CCH.[21] Hepatic tissue should be harbored for copper quantification in any dog undergoing liver biopsy. If elevated levels are identified, a reduction of dietary copper and chelation with d-penicillamine (10 to 15 mg/kg q12h, given 1 to 2 hours before feeding) or trientine (10 to 15 mg/kg q12h, given 1 to 2 hours before feeding) are likely to be beneficial.

Nonspecific reactive hepatitis

Nonspecific reactive hepatitis is a histologic diagnosis that describes the liver's response to a variety of extrahepatic disease processes. The lesion is characterized by widespread inflammatory infiltrates (usually lymphocytes and plasma cells) in the portal areas and parenchyma in the absence of hepatocellular necrosis.[2] Identification of this lesion should alert the clinician that a liver-specific problem is unlikely and that further investigation into the underlying disease process is necessary.

Viral Causes

Viral hepatitis is uncommon in dogs and cats. Most viral infections carry a poor prognosis. Specific therapy is not available or has not been evaluated. Symptomatic therapy and supportive care are therefore the primary therapeutic options.

Infectious canine hepatitis

Infectious canine hepatitis is caused by canine adenovirus type I. This disease has become rare because of extensive vaccination protocols using the cross-reacting adenovirus type II vaccine. As such, the disease is seen only in young, unvaccinated dogs. The degree of antibody response determines the severity of disease, with a poor response resulting in an acutely fatal syndrome. Animals that mount an appropriate response may recover or develop CH. Corneal edema and anterior uveitis may develop in animals that recover from acute illness. The diagnosis is made by histopathologic identification of large basophilic to amphophilic intranuclear inclusion bodies within hepatocytes and Kupffer cells that are identified during the first week of infection.[15] Histopathology also reveals multifocal coagulative necrosis and a neutrophilic inflammatory infiltrate that may not be present in animals with severe acute infection.

Feline infectious peritonitis

Feline infectious peritonitis (FIP) is caused by the feline enteric coronavirus. FIP can affect any organ in the body. Cats with hepatic involvement often have increased activities of ALT and AST and develop hyperbilirubinemia as the disease progresses. Histologic lesions include multifocal necrosis (often around blood vessels) with associated infiltration with neutrophils and macrophages. Pyogranulomatous lesions may be noted on the liver capsule.[17] Immunohistochemistry can be performed on liver biopsy specimens to confirm the presence of virus.[22] When hepatic involvement occurs, the disease is uniformly fatal. Because there is no definitive treatment, supportive care is the mainstay of therapy.

Bacterial Causes

Leptospirosis

Leptospirosis is caused by any one of several serovars of spiral bacteria belonging to the species *Leptospira interrogans* sensu lato. The commonly isolated serovars in small animals include *Leptospira icterohaemorrhagiae, Leptospira canicola, Leptospira pomona, Leptospira hardjo, Leptospira grippotyphosa,* and *Leptospira bratislava.* Infection in dogs most commonly results in acute renal failure, although hepatic involvement may occur in 20% to 35% of cases.[3,23] Other clinical manifestations of infection include pulmonary hemorrhage, uveitis, and acute fever.[24] Infection in young animals and infection with serovars *L. icterohaemorrhagiae* and *L. pomona* are more likely to result in hepatic involvement.[25] Affected dogs may show acute hepatitis or develop chronic hepatitis with subclinical acute infection. Although cats are generally resistant to leptospirosis, experimental infection with *L. pomona* has caused hepatic lesions in this species.[3] Patients with hepatic involvement show increased activity of hepatic enzymes (ALT, AST, ALP), although ALP often is affected most severely. Hyperbilirubinemia and signs of hepatic failure may occur. Diagnosis of leptospirosis usually is based on clinical suspicion because of renal and hepatic involvement combined with serologic evidence of infection. However, antibody titers may be negative during the first week of infection, and antibody production may persist for only 2 to 6 weeks.[3] Suspected patients with negative antibody titers and a short duration of illness should be treated as though they have leptospirosis, and antibody titers should be repeated in 2 weeks. Histopathologic changes in the liver of affected animals may include coagulative necrosis and infiltration of lymphocytes and plasma cells with lesser numbers of neutrophils and macrophages. Organisms may be identified in biopsy specimens with silver staining, but this is an insensitive diagnostic test. Polymerase chain reaction (PCR) techniques to detect organisms in blood and urine samples are available. These techniques have not been well studied in dogs with clinical disease, but they are likely to make this diagnosis less challenging in the future. Historically, treatment recommendations have included penicillin to eliminate the leptospiremic stage, followed by doxycycline to eliminate the carrier state. However, treatment with doxycycline alone is effective for the leptospiremic stage and carrier state (5 mg/kg PO/IV q12h).[24] Penicillins may be used in animals that do not tolerate doxycycline. Alternative antibiotic choices include azithromycin, ceftriaxone, and cefotaxime.[24] Prognosis is typically good, but patients often require intensive supportive care, including hemodialysis in animals with oliguric or anuric renal failure. Pulmonary involvement worsens prognosis.

Bartonellosis

Bartonella species are arthropod-transmitted bacteria that have been associated with multiple clinical syndromes in veterinary medicine.[26] *Bartonella henselae* and *Bartonella clarridgeiae* have been identified as causes of hepatic disease in dogs.[27] Clinical findings are similar to those of dogs with other causes of hepatitis. Histologic examination of hepatic tissue from dogs with *B. henselae* infection has revealed peliosis hepatis[28] and granulomatous hepatitis,[27] both of which have been described in infected humans. Diagnosis was made via identification of *Bartonella* DNA using PCR techniques on hepatic biopsy specimens. This is the preferred method of diagnosis because serologic assays impart information only regarding exposure, and granulomatous hepatitis may be caused by other agents. The cause of granulomatous hepatitis in dogs frequently is unknown, although reported causes include fungal infection, mycobacterial infection, dirofilariasis, lymphoma, histiocytosis, and intestinal lymphangiectasia.[29] Azithromycin is the antibiotic of choice for treatment of bartonellosis, although its use in dogs with hepatic disease caused by *Bartonella* spp. has not been evaluated thoroughly. Other antibiotics that may be effective include doxycycline (high dose, 10 to 15 mg/kg q12h), enrofloxacin, and rifampin (in combination with doxycycline or enrofloxacin).[26]

Septicemia

An important cause of hepatitis in critically ill dogs and cats is bacterial seeding of the liver secondary to bacteremia or via translocation from the GI tract. Commonly isolated aerobic bacteria include *Staphylococcus* spp., *Streptococcus* spp., and enteric gram-negative organisms. Commonly identified anaerobes include *Bacteroides* spp., *Clostridium* spp., and *Fusobacterium* spp.[3] The diagnosis of bacteremia can be difficult in veterinary patients (see Chapter 91). Septicemia-induced hepatitis should be suspected in critically ill animals that develop clinicopathologic evidence of hepatic disease while hospitalized, especially those in which bacterial infection or severe GI disease have been documented. Treatment with broad-spectrum antimicrobials (pending sensitivity testing), along with aggressive supportive care, are vital to a successful outcome.

Drugs and Toxins

The liver is particularly susceptible to toxic injury because it receives blood from the portal circulation. Histologic changes in the liver secondary to toxic injury vary and may include no changes, hepatocellular swelling, steatosis, necrosis, cholestasis, inflammation, and/or fibrosis.[2] Several substances reported to cause hepatotoxicity are noted in Box 115-1, but this is by no means an exhaustive list. Because of the varying and nonspecific nature of histologic changes, diagnosis of hepatotoxicity often is made on the basis of clinical suspicion (biochemical alterations, such as marked increases in liver enzyme activity) with or without a history of known exposure. Treatment involves removal of the offending agent and aggressive supportive care. S-Adenosylmethionine (SAMe) (20 mg/kg PO q24h) has been effective in treating acetaminophen toxicity.[30,31] Although its effectiveness against other forms of hepatotoxicity has not been evaluated, it is a logical choice for supportive care in animals suffering any hepatotoxic insult, mainly because of its ability to increase hepatic glutathione levels, which may increase antioxidant and repair abilities.

REFERENCES

1. Johnson SE: Parenchymal disorders. In Washabau RJ, Day MJ, editors: Canine and feline gastroenterology, St Louis, 2013, Elsevier Saunders.
2. van den Ingh TSGAM, Van Winkle T, Cullen JM, et al: Morphological classification of the parenchymal disorders of the canine and feline liver. In Rothuizen J, Bunch SE, Charles JA, et al, editors: WSAVA standards for clinical and histological diagnosis of canine and feline liver disease, Edinburgh, 2006, Saunders Elsevier.
3. Center SA: Acute hepatic injury: hepatic necrosis and fulminant hepatic failure. In Guilford WG, et al, editors: Strombeck's small animal gastroenterology, ed 3, Philadelphia, 1996, WB Saunders Company.
4. Zhou F, Ajuebor MN, Beck PL, et al: CD154-CD40 interactions drive hepatocyte apoptosis in murine fulminant hepatitis, Hepatology 42:372-380, 2005.
5. Gagne JM, Weiss DJ, Armstrong PJ: Histopathologic evaluation of feline inflammatory liver disease, Vet Pathol 33:521-526, 1996.
6. Forrester SD, Rogers KS, Relford RL: Cholangiohepatitis in a dog, J Am Vet Med Assoc 200:1704-1706, 1992.
7. van den Ingh TSGAM, Cullen JM, Twedt DC, et al: Morphological classification of biliary disorders of the canine and feline liver. In Rothuizen J, Bunch SE, Charles JA, et al, editors: WSAVA standards for clinical and histological diagnosis of canine and feline liver disease, Edinburgh, 2006, Saunders Elsevier.
8. Center SA: The cholangitis/cholangiohepatitis complex in the cat. In Proceedings, 12th Am Coll Vet Intern Med, 766-771, 1994.
9. Weiss DJ, Gagne JM, Armstrong PJ: Relationship between inflammatory hepatic disease and inflammatory bowel disease, pancreatitis, and nephritis in cats, J Am Vet Med Assoc 209:1114-1116, 1996.
10. Rondeau MP: WSAVA classification and role of bacteria in feline inflammatory hepatobiliary disease. In Proceedings, Forum Am Coll Vet Intern Med, 590-591, 2009.
11. Morgan M, Rondeau M, Rankin S, et al: A survey of feline inflammatory hepatobiliary disease using the WSAVA classification, J Vet Intern Med 22:860A, 2008.
12. Gagne JM, Armstrong PJ, Weiss DJ, et al: Clinical features of inflammatory liver disease in cats: 41 cases (1983-1993), J Am Vet Med Assoc 214:513-516, 1999.
13. Callahan Clark JE, Haddad J, Brown DC, et al: Feline cholangitis: a necropsy study of 44 cats (1986-2008), J Feline Med Surg 13:570-576, 2011.
14. Rondeau MP: Intrahepatic biliary disorders. In Washabau RJ, Day MJ, editors: Canine and feline gastroenterology, St Louis, 2013, Elsevier Saunders.
15. Day MJ: Immunohistochemical characterization of the lesions of feline progressive lymphocytic cholangitis/cholangiohepatitis, J Comp Pathol 119:135-147, 1998.
16. Warren A, Center S, McDonough S, et al: Histopathologic features, immunophenotyping, clonality, and eubacterial fluorescence in situ hybridization in cats with lymphocytic cholangitis/cholangiohepatitis, Vet Pathol 48:627-641, 2011.
17. Center SA: Chronic hepatitis, cirrhosis, breed-specific hepatopathies, copper storage hepatopathy, suppurative hepatitis, granulomatous hepatitis, and idiopathic hepatic fibrosis. In Guilford WG, et al, editors: Strombeck's small animal gastroenterology, ed 3, Philadelphia, 1996, WB Saunders Company.
18. Boisclair J, Doré M, Beauchamp G, et al: Characterization of the inflammatory infiltrate in canine chronic hepatitis, Vet Pathol 38:628-635, 2001.
19. Strombeck DR, Miller LM, Harrold D: Effects of corticosteroid treatment on survival time in dogs with chronic hepatitis: 151 cases (1977-1985), J Am Vet Med Assoc 193:1109-1113, 1988.
20. Meertens NM, Bokhove CA, van den Ingh TSGAM: Copper-associated chronic hepatitis and cirrhosis in a European Shorthair cat, Vet Pathol 42:97-100, 2005.
21. Mandigers PJ, van den Ingh TSGAM, Bode P, et al: Improvement in liver pathology after 4 months of D-penicillamine in 5 Doberman Pinschers with subclinical hepatitis, J Vet Int Med 19:40-43, 2005.
22. Giori L, Giordano A, Giudice C, et al: Performances of different diagnostic tests for feline infectious peritonitis in challenging clinical cases, J Small Anim Pract 52:152-157, 2011.
23. Adin CA, Cowgill LD: Treatment and outcome of dogs with leptospirosis: 36 cases (1990-1998), J Am Vet Med Assoc 216:371-375, 2000.
24. Sykes JE, Hartmann K, Lunn KF, et al: 2010 ACVIM small animal consensus statement on leptospirosis: diagnosis, epidemiology, treatment and prevention, J Vet Intern Med 25:1-13, 2011
25. Greene CE, Sykes LE, Moore GE, et al: Leptospirosis. In Greene CE, editor: Infectious diseases of the dog and cat, ed 4, St Louis, 2012, Elsevier Saunders.
26. Breitschwerdt EB, Chomel BB: Canine bartonellosis. In Greene CE, editor: Infectious diseases of the dog and cat, ed 4, St Louis, 2012, Elsevier Saunders.
27. Gillespie TN, Washabau RJ, Goldschmidt MH, et al: Detection of *Bartonella henselae* and *Bartonella clarridgeiae* DNA in hepatic specimens from two dogs with hepatic disease, J Am Vet Med Assoc 222:47-51, 2003.
28. Kitchell BE, Fan TM, Kordick D, et al: Peliosis hepatic in a dog infected with *Bartonella henselae*, J Am Vet Med Assoc 216:519-523, 2000.
29. Chapman BL, Hendrick MJ, Washabau RJ: Granulomatous hepatitis in dogs: nine cases (1987-1990), J Am Vet Med Assoc 203:680-684, 1993.
30. Wallace KP, Center SA, Hickford FH, et al: S-adenosylmethionine (SAMe) for the treatment of acetaminophen toxicity in a dog, J Am Anim Hosp Assoc 38:246-254, 2002.
31. Song Z, McClain CJ, Chen T: S-Adenosylmethionine protects against acetaminophen-induced hepatotoxicity in mice, Pharmacology 71:199-208, 2004.

CHAPTER 116
HEPATIC FAILURE

Allyson Berent, DVM, DACVIM (Internal Medicine)

KEY POINTS

- Hepatic failure typically holds a poor prognosis; a prompt diagnosis, search for an underlying cause, and rapid and appropriate treatment are critical for survival.
- Hepatic encephalopathy and coagulopathy are typically the main clinical consequences of hepatic failure and should be treated accordingly.
- Therapy should be aimed at minimizing signs of encephalopathy and treating the underlying pathology, thereby allowing the liver to regenerate.
- Researchers currently are exploring adipose-derived mesenchymal stem cell therapy and liver replacement therapy. This has potential promise for veterinary medicine.

Liver failure occurs as a result of severe hepatocyte injury or dysfunction, regardless of the cause,[1-3] manifesting as an acute or chronic process. The loss of hepatic function leads to a spectrum of metabolic derangements, which results in devastating clinical consequences and most commonly the clinical onset of hepatic encephalopathy and coagulopathy. Other complications associated with this state include gastrointestinal ulceration, bacterial sepsis, cardiopulmonary dysfunction, and ascites. Before the development of hepatic transplantation, liver failure had a mortality rate greater than 90% in people.[1,2] Early detection, treatment, and aggressive supportive care is critical to embracing the regenerative capacity of the liver because it is capable of regenerating 75% of its functional capacity in only a few weeks. Common causes of liver disease that can result in failure in dogs and cats are listed in Table 116-1.[4-6]

PATHOPHYSIOLOGY

The histologic changes seen in the liver of patients with acute or chronic liver failure are variable and depend on the underlying cause. Acute liver diseases are likely to display hepatocellular necrosis as the prominent lesion. Fat accumulation or hepatocellular drop-out also may be noted. A chronically diseased liver also may demonstrate hepatocellular necrosis, but fibrosis, inflammation, and hyperplasia of ductular structures are often present as well.

Patients with hepatic failure display common physiologic clinical features, regardless of the cause. These include hypotension, lactic acidosis resulting from the poor oxygen uptake by muscles and peripheral tissues combined with decreased hepatic lactate metabolism, electrolyte alterations, hepatic encephalopathy, and coagulopathy. Over time, dysfunction of multiple organ systems can occur. In people, acute kidney injury is a common sequela to liver failure (hepatorenal syndrome),[7] although this is described rarely in veterinary patients.[5]

Hepatic Encephalopathy

Hepatic encephalopathy (HE), the hallmark feature of hepatic failure, is a neuropsychiatric syndrome involving many neurologic abnormalities. The pathogenesis of HE is understood incompletely in veterinary and human medicine and typically occurs when more than 70% of hepatic function is lost.[2,4,8-11] This results in the central nervous system (CNS) entering an encephalopathic state. More than 20 different compounds have been found in excess in the circulation when liver function is impaired, including ammonia, aromatic amino acids, endogenous benzodiazepines, γ-aminobutyric acid (GABA), glutamine, short-chain fatty acids, tryptophan, and others (Table 116-2).[4,8,9,11,12] These substances may impede neuronal and astrocyte function, causing cell swelling, inhibition of membrane pumps or ion channels, an elevation in intracellular calcium concentrations, depression of electrical activity, and interference with oxidative metabolism.[8-10]

Ammonia often is considered the most important neurotoxic substance. Increased concentrations trigger a sequence of metabolic events that have been implicated in HE in rats, humans, and dogs.[8,9,11,13,14] Ammonia is produced by the gastrointestinal flora and then converted in the normal liver to urea and glutamine via the urea cycle. Ammonia is excitotoxic and associated with an increased release of glutamate, the major excitatory neurotransmitter of the brain. Overactivation of the glutamate receptors, mainly N-methyl-D-aspartate (NMDA) receptors, has been implicated as one of the causes of HE-induced seizures. With chronicity, inhibitory factors such as GABA and endogenous benzodiazepines surpass the excitatory stimulus, causing signs more suggestive of coma or CNS depression.[8,9,13] Long-standing metabolic dysfunction, as seen in patients with chronic liver failure, also results in alterations in neuronal responsiveness and energy requirements.[9,14]

Acute liver failure may result in a form of HE that leads to cerebral edema, increased intracranial pressure, and possible herniation of the brain.[8,9] Edema is described in up to 80% of humans with hepatic failure, and 33% can develop fatal herniation.[3,8,9] Clinical signs associated with HE are variable, with most being suggestive of neuroinhibition. Excitatory activity such as seizures, aggression, and hyperexcitability also occur. A combination of complex metabolic derangements that occur in patients with hepatic insufficiency (e.g., hypoglycemia, dehydration, hypokalemia, azotemia, alkalemia) and systemic toxins (see Table 116-2) are responsible for a variety of signs that can be exacerbated by exogenous substances such as nonsteroidal antiinflammatory drugs (NSAIDs), high-protein meals, gastrointestinal ulcerations, constipation, stored blood transfusions (because of ammonia levels), and drugs (sedatives, analgesics, benzodiazepines, antihistamines). Recently inflammation and elevated manganese levels also have been proven to be associated with HE in people and dogs.[15,16] These factors, in addition to an altered permeability of the blood brain barrier, impair cerebral function in various ways.[4,8,9,15,16]

Treatments that decrease ammonia concentrations, which are measured easily in animals, seem to reduce the signs of HE. In humans, the degree of encephalopathy is not well correlated with the blood ammonia levels,[17] suggesting that other suspected neurotoxins are also important in pathophysiology of HE. Ammonia

Table 116-1 **Causes of Hepatic Failure**[4-6]

	Dog	Cat
Infectious agents	Canine adenovirus-1 Acidophil cell hepatitis virus Canine herpes virus Clostridiosis Bartonellosis Leptospirosis Liver abscess Tularemia Hepatozoonos*is* *Rickettsia rickettsii* Histoplasmosis Coccidiomycosis/blastomycosis Leishmaniasis Toxoplasmosis *Dirofilaria immitis* *Ehrlichia canis*	Feline infectious peritonitis Clostridiosis Liver abscesses Histoplasmosis Cryptococcosis Toxoplasmosis
Drugs	Acetaminophen Aspirin Phenobarbital Phenytoin Carprofen Tetracycline Macrolides Trimethoprim-sulfa Griseofulvin Thiacetarsemide Ketoconazole/itraconazole Halothane	Acetaminophen Aspirin Diazepam Halothane Griseofulvin Ketoconazole/itraconazole Methimazole Methotrexate Phenobarbital Phenytoin
Chemical agents/toxins	Industrial solvents Plants: sago palm Envenomation Heavy metals (Cu, Fe, P) Mushrooms *(Amanita phalloides)* Aflatoxins Blue-green algae Cycad seeds Carbon tetrachloride Dimethylnitrosamine Zinc phosphide Xylitol (dogs only)	Same as for dogs
Miscellaneous	Chronic hepatitis/cirrhosis-idiopathic, copper storage disease, leptospirosis induced,idiosyncratic drug reaction, lobular dissecting hepatitis Granulomatous hepatitis Hepatic amyloidosis (Chinese Shar-Pei) Hepatic neoplasia (primary or metastatic disease) Portosystemic shunting Portal venous hypoplasia/microvascular dysplasia (Yorkshire and Cairn Terrier)	Feline hepatic lipidosis Inflammatory bowel disease Pancreatitis Cholangitis/cholangiohepatitis Septicemia/endotoxemia Hemolytic anemia Neoplasia: lymphoma, mastocytosis Metastasis Amyloidosis (Abyssinian, Oriental, and Siamese cats)
Traumatic/thermal/hypoxic	Diaphragmatic hernia Shock Liver torsion Heat stroke Massive ischemia	

concentrations do not correlate always with signs of HE in veterinary patients either, and on rare occasions, dogs with normal ammonia concentrations have obvious HE signs. In addition, many dogs with high ammonia levels appear neurologically normal.

Coagulation Disorders

Coagulation abnormalities that develop in patients with liver failure are multifactorial, depending on the interactions of the coagulation, anticoagulation, and fibrinolytic systems. Spontaneous hemorrhage is uncommon. Hemorrhagic complications usually are induced with associated factors such as gastrointestinal ulceration, invasive procedures (aspiration, biopsy, surgery), or other concurrent medical problems. Suggested causes of coagulopathy in liver failure patients include decreased factor synthesis, increased factor utilization, decreased factor turnover, increased fibrinolysis and tissue thromboplastin release, synthesis of abnormal coagulants (dysfibrinogenemia), decreased platelet function and numbers, vitamin K deficiency (particularly in patients with bile duct obstruction), and increased production of anticoagulants.[4,18]

Table 116-2 **Toxins Implicated in Hepatic Encephalopathy**[4,6,8-12,15,16]

Toxins	Mechanisms Suggested in the Literature
Ammonia	Increased brain tryptophan and glutamine; decreased ATP availability; increased excitability; increased glycolysis; brain edema; decreased microsomal Na^+/K^+-ATPase in brain
Aromatic amino acids	Decreased DOPA (dihydroxyphenylalanine) neurotransmitter synthesis; altered neuroreceptors; increased production of false neurotransmitters
Bile acids	Membranocytolytic effects alter cell/membrane permeability; blood-brain barrier more permeable to other HE toxins; impaired cellular metabolism because of cytotoxicity
Decreased alpha-ketoglutaramate	Diversion from Krebs cycle for ammonia detoxification; decreased ATP availability
Endogenous benzodiazepines	Neural inhibition: hyperpolarize neuronal membrane
False Neurotransmitters	
Tyrosine → Octapamine	Impairs norepinephrine action
Phenylalanine → Phenylethylamine	Impairs norepinephrine action
Methionine → Mercaptans	Synergistic with ammonia and SCFA
	Decreases ammonia detoxification in brain urea cycle; GIT derived (fetor hepaticus-breath odor in HE); decreased microsomal Na^+/K^+-ATPase
GABA	Neural inhibition: hyperpolarize neuronal membrane; increase blood-brain barrier permeability to GABA
Glutamine	Alters blood-brain barrier amino acid transport
Manganese	Elevated manganese levels seen with hepatic failure and HE and results in neurotoxicity. Its toxicity is associated with disruption of the glutamine (Gln)/glutamate (Glu)-γ-aminobutyric acid (GABA) cycle (GGC) between astrocytes and neurons, thus leading to changes in Glu-ergic and/or GABAergic transmission and Gln metabolism
Phenol (from phenylalanine and tyrosine)	Synergistic with other toxins; decreases cellular enzymes; neurotoxic and hepatotoxic
Short chain fatty acids (SCFA)	Decreased microsomal Na^+/K^+-ATPase in brain; uncouple oxidative phosphorylation, impairs oxygen use, displaces tryptophan from albumin, increasing free tryptophan
Tryptophan	Directly neurotoxic; increases serotonin: neuroinhibition

ATP, Adenosine triphosphate *DOPA,* dihydroxyphenylalanine, *GABA,* γ-aminobutyric acid.

Other

In addition to altered mentation and coagulation disorders, hepatic failure has been associated with an increased susceptibility to infection, systemic hypotension, pulmonary abnormalities, acid-base disturbances, renal dysfunction, and portal hypertension. Bacterial infection occurs in 80% of human patients, and this may be due to various mechanisms.[1,3,4,18] Inhibition of the metabolic activity of granulocytic cells, cell adhesion, and chemotaxis, as well as decreased hepatic synthesis of plasma complement, has been described.[1,3,4,18] Kupffer cells also have shown reduced phagocytic ability, allowing pathogens to translocate from the portal circulation into the systemic circulation. Hypotension is seen in most people with hepatic failure and may be due to systemic vasodilation. This is likely a centrally mediated phenomenon and may be linked to systemic infection, inflammation, cytokine release, cerebral edema, or circulating toxins. Approximately 33% of humans with hepatic failure develop pulmonary edema. Altered permeability of pulmonary capillaries leading to vascular leak, as well as decreased albumin/colloid osmotic pressure and vasodilation, has been implicated in the development of edema. This may be associated with endotoxemia as well.[1,3]

Tissue oxygen extraction decreases in patients with hepatic failure, resulting in tissue hypoxia and the development of lactic acidosis. Hypoxemia (which can occur with pulmonary edema) further exacerbates cerebral dysfunction in patients with HE, accelerating cerebral hypotension and additional cerebral edema. Ventilatory support may be needed if respiratory distress or arrest occurs. This may be of central origin or secondary to muscle weakness.[1,18] The development of acute kidney injury has been well described in humans and rarely suggested in dogs.[5] Hypovolemia and hypotension, secondary to vasodilation, can diminish renal blood flow and glomerular filtration rate.[1-3] Some hepatotoxins (nonsteroidal drugs) and infectious agents (leptospirosis, feline infectious peritonitis) also cause acute and chronic kidney injury.

Portal hypertension, typically secondary to cirrhosis, is a common sequela of chronic liver failure. It has been seen in some acute patients and typically holds a poor prognosis. Massive sinusoidal collapse can block intrahepatic flow, causing portal pressure elevations. In addition, portal vein thrombosis can be seen.[19] This may lead to severe congestion of the splanchnic vasculature, exacerbating gastrointestinal bleeding and diarrhea.[3-5]

CLINICAL SIGNS

Most of the clinical signs seen in dogs and cats with hepatic failure are nonspecific and include anorexia, vomiting, diarrhea, weight loss, and dehydration. Icteric mucous membranes, sclera, hard palate, and skin, are seen commonly in patients with liver failure associated with intrahepatic cholestasis. If icterus is documented, prehepatic (hemolysis), hepatic (intrinsic hepatic injury/failure), and/or posthepatic (functional or mechanical bile duct obstruction) causes should be discerned. Dogs and cats with liver failure secondary to congenital portosystemic shunting should not be icteric. Polyuria and polydipsia are common findings, which may be due to failure of the liver to produce urea, resulting in defective renal medullary concentrating ability, and a decreased release and/or responsiveness of the renal collecting ducts to antidiuretic hormone (ADH). Primary polydipsia, resulting from the central effects of hepatotoxins, also has been hypothesized. Other theories include increased renal blood flow and increased adrenocorticotropic hormone (ACTH) secretion with associated hypercortisolism.[20,21]

Clinical signs associated with HE include behavioral changes, ataxia, blindness, circling, head pressing, panting, pacing, seizures, coma, and ptyalism (especially cats). The clinical manifestations of HE range from minimal behavior and motor activity changes, to overt deterioration of mental function, decreased consciousness, coma, and/or seizure activity. Bleeding diathesis, melena (resulting from gastroduodenal ulceration), and ascites (resulting from portal hypertension and/or hypoalbuminemia) are also common findings.

DIAGNOSIS

Fulminant hepatic failure is diagnosed when a patient shows signs of HE, changes in the liver function parameters on blood chemistry, possible evidence of coagulopathy, and associated historical and physical examination findings. Hematologic abnormalities may include the presence of target cells, acanthocytes, and anisocytosis. A nonregenerative anemia may be noted in association with chronic disease, chronic GI bleeding, or portosystemic/microvascular shunting. A regenerative anemia may be noted in association with blood loss from gastroduodenal ulceration. A leukocytosis or leukopenia may be seen with infectious causes or bacterial translocation, depending on the agent and severity of infection. A consumptive thrombocytopenia may occur in animals that develop disseminated intravascular coagulation and an immune-mediated thrombocytopenia can be associated with infectious or immune causes of liver failure.

Serum biochemical analysis reveals elevated activities of hepatic enzymes in most cases. Alanine aminotransferase (ALT) and aspartate aminotransferase (AST) are found in the cytosol of hepatocytes and leak from the cell after disruption of the cell membrane. ALT is the more liver specific of these enzymes and has a short half-life (24 to 60 hours).[4,6,22,23] AST is present in many tissues (liver, muscle, red blood cells) and has a shorter half-life than ALT. Alkaline phosphatase (ALP) has many clinically significant isoenzymes (bone, liver, and steroid induced [in the dog only]). The hepatic isoenzyme is located on the membranes of hepatocyte canalicular cells and biliary epithelial cells. Its activity increases in association with cholestatic disease. ALP has a short half-life in cats, making any elevation suggestive of active liver disease. γ-Glutamyltransferase (GGT) also is found in many tissues, although most of the biochemically measured enzyme is located on membranes of hepatocyte canalicular cells and biliary epithelial cells. GGT is useful in the diagnosis of cholestatic disease and is more specific and less sensitive than ALP (particularly in feline patients). The presence of normal or only mildly elevated liver enzyme activity does not eliminate hepatic failure as a possible diagnosis because animals with end-stage hepatic failure or portal-systemic vascular anomalies may have normal, or near normal, enzyme activities.

Serum biochemical analysis also may reveal hyperbilirubinemia in animals with hepatic failure. Bilirubin is one of the breakdown metabolites of hemoglobin, myoglobin, and cytochromes. With significant cholestasis, bile duct obstruction, or canalicular membrane disruption, bilirubin escapes into the systemic circulation, resulting in hyperbilirubinemia and the typical icteric appearance to the skin, mucous membranes, and organs (visible when values are at least 2.3 to 3.3 mg/dl).[6,22,23]

The liver functional parameters that are noted classically when hepatic failure is present include hypoalbuminemia with normal to increased globulins, hypocholesterolemia, hypoglycemia, and decreased blood urea nitrogen (BUN). Albumin is produced only in the liver, representing approximately 25% of all proteins synthesized by the liver. Altered albumin synthesis is not detected until more than 66% to 80% of liver function is lost.[23] Because of its long half-life (8 days in dogs and cats) hypoalbuminemia is a hallmark of chronic liver dysfunction (although concomitant disease processes also may contribute to its loss, including protein-losing nephropathy (PLN), protein-losing enteropathy (PLE), and third-spacing protein loss). Cholesterol is synthesized in many tissues, although up to 50% of its synthesis occurs in the liver. In patients with hepatic failure, hypocholesterolemia is observed commonly. With extrahepatic bile duct obstruction or pancreatitis, cholesterol elimination is altered and hypercholesterolemia can develop. Because the liver helps to maintain glucose homeostasis via gluconeogenesis and glycogenolysis, hypoglycemia may develop when less than 30% of normal hepatic function is present.[4,6]

Urine sediment examination may show ammonium biurate or urate crystals, particularly in animals with portal-systemic vascular anomalies. Dogs have the ability to produce and conjugate bilirubin in their renal tubules, accounting for a small amount of bilirubinuria in a healthy state (males more than females). Cats, on the other hand, do not have this ability and have a higher threshold (9 times higher) than dogs to reabsorb bilirubin rather than eliminate it in the urine.[4,22] Therefore bilirubinuria in the cat is always inappropriate and indicative of abnormal bilirubin metabolism.

Additional testing may be performed to assess hepatic function. Coagulopathies are seen classically in animals with hepatic failure. Prolongation of the activated partial thromboplastin time (aPTT), prothrombin time (PT), activated clotting time (ACT), and buccal mucosal bleeding time (BMBT) may be observed. Increased fasting and postprandial serum bile acids are indicative of hepatic dysfunction and classically seen in animals with hepatic failure. They also may play a role in inciting inflammatory liver disease.[4,6] Plasma fasting ammonia, 6-hour postprandial ammonia, or ammonia tolerance testing are sensitive tests of liver function. The ammonia tolerance test is contraindicated in animals with encephalopathy and may precipitate seizure activity.[4-6,22]

Electrolyte abnormalities also may be seen in patients with hepatic failure. Hypokalemia may develop because of inadequate intake, vomiting, or the use of potassium-wasting diuretics for treatment of ascites. Centrally induced hyperventilation and respiratory alkalosis may encourage renal potassium excretion, worsening the hypokalemia, and a decrease in potassium levels may exacerbate HE. In addition, hypocapnia results in a shift of intracellular carbon dioxide into the extracellular space, raising intracellular pH and accelerating the use of phosphate to phosphorylate glucose. This may result in hypophosphatemia, which ultimately can cause hemolysis of red blood cells.

Diagnostic imaging is often useful to determine the underlying cause of hepatic failure. Abdominal radiographs are useful for determining liver size and contour, identifying mass lesions and evaluating abdominal detail, which may be decreased in the presence of ascites. Abdominal ultrasonography is valuable for the evaluation of hepatic parenchymal architecture, the biliary tract, and vascular structures. It also can help to guide diagnostic sampling procedures, when indicated. Computed tomography with angiography is a great tool to diagnose portosystemic shunting but requires general anesthesia, which carries considerable risk in patients with clinical HE.

Ultimately cytologic or histologic evaluation is necessary to determine the underlying cause of hepatic failure if a congenital PSS is not found. Fine-needle aspiration cytology is useful for diagnosing infiltrative neoplasia such as lymphoma but gives little information about the hepatic parenchymal changes needed for a definitive diagnosis of the inflammatory/infectious, necrotic, fibrosing, and microvascular diseases. Aspiration has been proven insensitive in making a definitive diagnosis.[24] Histopathologic evaluation of liver tissue is more useful and should be obtained whenever possible. Liver biopsies can be performed with ultrasound guidance, laparoscopy, or surgery. In humans, a transjugular approach, under fluoroscopic guidance, is used commonly, particularly in coagulopathic patients, to avoid penetrating the hepatic capsule and cause third space bleeding.[1] This currently is not recommended in veterinary patients. A blood type and coagulation profile should be obtained before liver biopsy in all animals. A small amount of liver tissue should be stored so that further testing can be performed, if indicated, after histopathology is complete, such as aerobic and anaerobic culture, copper analysis (dogs), or PCR testing for certain infectious agents.

THERAPY

Successful management of patients with hepatic failure requires treatment of the underlying liver disease, therapy aimed at the complications of hepatic failure (HE and coagulopathy), and routine supportive care. Fortunately, hepatocytes have an immense ability to regenerate if given appropriate support and time. Treatment of the primary disease process, if possible, is critical. However, a discussion of the treatment recommendations for each specific liver disease is beyond the scope of this chapter. Supportive care is required to maintain the normal physiologic functions of the patient while the liver recovers from the insult (Table 116-3).

Animals that are presented with, or develop, focal or generalized seizure activity require immediate anticonvulsant therapy (see Table 116-3 and Chapters 82, 88, and 166). Propofol (0.5 to 1 mg/kg IV bolus, then 0.05 to 0.1 mg/kg/min constant rate infusion) generally is recommended for rapid control of seizures resulting from hepatoencephalopathy. More recently the use of levetiracetam has been shown to prevent postanesthetic seizures in dogs with portosystemic shunts, so prophylactic loading and maintenance therapy now is performed commonly.[25] Endotracheal intubation should be performed in patients that are hypoventilating because hypercapnia further increases intracranial pressure. Animals that lose their gag reflex also should be intubated to protect the airway from aspiration. Mannitol therapy also may prove beneficial if cerebral edema is present (0.5 to 1 g/kg IV over 20 to 30 minutes), especially because cerebral edema is associated with herniation in people (see Chapter 84).[1-3]

The use of diazepam for the treatment of HE-associated seizures in animals is controversial. GABA and its receptors are implicated in the pathogenesis of HE, and the use of a benzodiazepine antagonist, such as flumazenil, has been proven beneficial in humans with HE-induced comas.[8,9] Flumazenil therapy for HE has not been evaluated yet in veterinary patients, however.

Symptomatic therapy for patients with HE may include withholding food, cleansing enemas with warm water and/or lactulose, oral lactulose therapy, and antimicrobial therapy.[4-6,10] Antimicrobials such as metronidazole, neomycin, or ampicillin decrease GI bacterial numbers, thus reducing ammonia production. Metronidazole and ampicillin also help decrease the risk of bacterial translocation and systemic bacterial infections. However, neurotoxicity from

Table 116-3 Therapies for Hepatic Failure

Symptom	Therapy
Bacterial translocation	Cleansing enemas with warm water or 30% lactulose solution at 5-10 ml/kg (see Chapter 88 for further details) Antibiotics: Metronidazole: 7.5 mg/kg IV or PO q12h Ampicillin: 22 mg/kg IV q8h Neomycin: 22 mg/kg PO q12h (avoid if any evidence of intestinal bleeding, ulcerations, or renal failure)
Gastrointestinal ulceration	Antacid[20]: Famotidine: 0.5-1.0 mg/kg/day IV or PO q12-24h Omeprazole: 0.5-1.0 mg/kg/day q12h PO Esomeprazole: 0.5-1 mg/kg IV q24h Misoprostol: 2-5 mcg/kg PO q6-12h Protectant: Sucralfate: 0.25-1 g PO q6-12h Correct coagulopathy
Coagulopathy	Fresh frozen plasma (10-15 ml/kg over 2-3 hours) Vitamin K1: 1.0-2.0 mg/kg SC q12h for three doses, then once daily
Control seizures	Avoid benzodiazepines: consider propofol 0.5-1 mg/kg IV bolus + IV CRI at 0.05-0.4 mg/kg/min OR IV phenobarbital (16 mg/kg IV, divided into 4 doses over 12-24 hours), or potassium bromide/sodium bromide loading (see Chapter 166) OR IV levetiracetam: 30-60 mg/kg once, then 20 mg/kg q8h
Decrease cerebral edema	Mannitol (0.5-1.0 g/kg IV over 20-30 min)
Hepatoprotective therapy	SAMe (Denosyl): 17-22 mg/kg PO q24h Ursodeoxycholic acid (Actigall): 10-15 mg/kg/day Vitamin E: 15 IU/kg/day Milk thistle: 8-20 mg/kg divided q8h L-Carnitine: 250-500 mg/cat q24h Vitamin B complex: 1 ml/L of IV fluids
Antifibrotic therapy	D-Penicillamine: 10-15 mg/kg PO q12h Colchicine: 0.03 mg/kg/day Prednis(ol)one: 1 mg/kg/day
Nutritional support	Moderate protein restriction: 18% to 22% dogs and 30% to 35% cats; dairy or vegetable proteins; vitamin B supplementation; multivitamin supplementation

metronidazole therapy may occur more commonly in animals with hepatic disease.

Symptomatic therapy is necessary for bleeding patients. Those with gastric ulceration should be treated with acid receptor blockade (H_2 blocker, proton pump inhibitor, prostaglandin analog) and sucralfate (see Chapter 161). Recent evidence suggests that ranitidine may not be as effective as famotidine in reducing gastric acid in dogs.[26] Coagulopathic patients with signs of active bleeding should be treated with fresh frozen plasma or fresh whole blood and subcutaneous vitamin K_1 (especially if the coagulopathy is thought to be due to cholestasis and fat malabsorption).[4-6] Patients that are significantly anemic benefit from packed red blood cell or whole blood transfusions. If HE is evident, fresh whole blood is preferred because stored blood has increased levels of ammonia (see Chapter 61).

Ascites and hepatic fibrosis may be seen in patients with chronic, severe liver disease. If ascites is due to low oncotic pressure, then synthetic colloidal therapy should be considered (see Chapters 58 and 59). If the ascites is due to portal hypertension, the use of diuretics and a low-sodium diet should be considered. Spironolactone is the initial diuretic of choice for its aldosterone antagonism and subsequent potassium-sparing effects. Furosemide may be necessary as well but should be used with caution because it may potentiate hypokalemia. A number of drugs theoretically decrease connective tissue formation and may be helpful in patients with hepatic fibrosis (i.e., prednisone, D-penicillamine, and colchicines; see Table 116-3).[4-6,23]

Fluid therapy and nutritional support are the cornerstones of supportive therapy. Fluid therapy is indicated to maintain hydration and provide cardiovascular (and occasionally oncotic) support. Lactated Ringer's solution often is avoided because of the need for hepatic conversion of lactate to bicarbonate. Supplementation with potassium and glucose often are required. Nutritional management is important in patients with acute and chronic liver failure, particularly cats with hepatic lipidosis. The diet should be readily digestible, contain a protein source of high biologic value (enough to meet the animal's need, but not worsen HE), supply enough essential fatty acids, maintain palatability, and meet the minimum requirements for vitamins and minerals. Low-protein diets should be avoided unless HE is noted. Milk and vegetable proteins are lower in aromatic amino acids and higher in branched chain amino acids (valine, leucine, isoleucine) than animal proteins and are considered less likely to potentiate HE.[4,6,23] In the patient with hepatic failure, total parenteral or partial parenteral nutrition should be considered if enteral intake cannot be tolerated (see Chapter 130). If the animal is not vomiting or regurgitating and temperature and systemic blood pressure are stable but the patient will not eat voluntarily, a feeding tube should be considered to allow for localized enterocyte nutrition (see Chapter 129).

Supportive nutraceutical therapy has been recommended for a variety of liver diseases. Drugs in this class include S-adenosylmethionine (SAMe), vitamin E, and milk thistle.[26] SAMe has hepatoprotective, antioxidant, and antiinflammatory properties. It also serves as a precursor to the production of glutathione, which plays a critical role in detoxification of the hepatocyte. Vitamin E is another antioxidant and should be considered to prevent and minimize lipid peroxidation within the hepatocytes. Silymarin is the active extract in milk thistle. An abundance of in vivo animal and in vitro experimental data show the antioxidant and free radical scavenging properties of silymarin.[27] Specifically, it inhibits lipid peroxidation of hepatocyte and microsomal membranes. Silymarin increases hepatic glutathione content and appears to retard hepatic collagen formation.[26]

Ursodeoxycholic acid, another hepatoprotective medication, is recommended for most types of inflammatory, oxidative, and cholestatic liver disease. It has antiinflammatory, immunomodulatory, and antifibrotic properties, as well as promoting choleresis and decreasing the toxic effects of hydrophobic bile acids on hepatocytes. This medication is contraindicated in patients with biliary duct outflow obstruction until after the obstruction is relieved.

Zinc is an essential trace mineral involved in many metabolic and enzymatic functions of the body and is an important intermediary involved in enhanced ureagenesis, glutathione metabolism, copper chelation, and immune function. Zinc appears to have antifibrotic activities as well. Zinc deficiency occurs in many humans with liver disease, and this decrease seems to correlate with hepatic encephalopathy, demonstrating its importance in ureagenesis. Please refer to Chapter 88 and other sources for further explanation.[26-29]

PROGNOSIS

The prognosis for animals with hepatic failure is generally poor. Few published guidelines are established to predict outcome. Some factors suggested to be poor prognostic indicators include PT of greater than 100 seconds, very young or very old animals, viral or idiosyncratic drug reaction as the underlying cause, and a markedly increased bilirubin.[4] When a known hepatotoxin is involved, the use of an appropriate antidote can improve survival markedly, although most do not have an antidote. Better survival rates likely are attained in a hospital where aggressive and intensive supportive therapy is available. The prognosis for hepatic failure associated with congenital portosystemic shunting is considered good if the patient is medically managed appropriately and the shunt ultimately can be occluded.

FUTURE THERAPIES

People with severe HE are placed immediately on a liver transplant list, which may be an option for veterinary patients in the future. Substitution of hepatocytes with various forms of artificial liver support has been promoted over the past 10 years in human medicine. A multicenter randomized trial using a bio-artificial liver showed no benefit over traditional therapy while awaiting transplantation in overall outcome, although more advanced equipment is showing great promise. More recently research has shown the benefit of this modality, especially in acute-on-chronic liver failure.* This may be something for the future in veterinary medicine.

Over the past 5 years great advances have been made in the area of stem cell therapy for the treatment of liver failure in various animal models. Mesenchymal stem cells (MSC) have been used in veterinary medicine for osteoarthritis and kidney disease,[31-33] with the goal of autogenous multipotent stem cells acting in a paracrine manner to improve the regenerative environment of an organ undergoing inflammation, fibrosis, and necrosis. More recently the use of MSC for chronic and acute inflammatory liver disease in dogs is being investigated. Studies in mice have shown that undifferentiated MSC have the ability to improve hepatic function in mice with acute liver injury.[34] In a rabbit model[35] of acute-on-chronic liver failure, those who received adipose-derived MSC had improved biochemical parameters, histomorphologic scoring, and survival rates when compared with those that did not. This holds great promise for the future of veterinary medicine.

Overall, hepatic failure is a severe life-threatening disease that holds a poor prognosis. With aggressive intensive care, avid supportive therapy, and early diagnosis, the regenerative capacity will improve, as will the outcome.

*References 1-3, 8, 9, 28, 30.

REFERENCES

1. Gill RQ, Sterling RK: Acute liver failure, J Clin Gastroenterol 33:191-198, 2001.
2. Atillasoy E, Berk PD: Fulminant hepatic failure: pathophysiology, treatment and survival, Ann Rev Med 46:181-191, 1995.
3. D'Agata ID, Balistreri WFF: Pediatric aspects of acute liver failure. In Lee WM, Williams R, editors: Acute liver failure, Cambridge, 1997, Cambridge University Press.
4. Center SA: Acute hepatic injury: hepatic necrosis and fulminant hepatic failure. In Guilford WG, et al, editors: Strombeck's small animal gastroenterology, ed 3, Philadelphia, 1996, WB Saunders.
5. Walton RS: Severe liver disease. In Wingfield WE, Raffe MR, editors: The Veterinary ICU book, Jackson Wyo, 2002, Teton NewMedia.
6. Webster CR: History, clinical signs, and physical findings in hepatobiliary disease. In Ettinger SJ, Feldman EC, editors: Textbook of veterinary internal medicine, ed 6, St Louis, 2005, Elsevier Saunders.
7. Sandhu BS, Sanyal AJ: Hepatorenal syndrome, Curr Treat Options Gastroenterol 8:443-450, 2005.
8. Jalan R, Shawcross D, Davies N: The molecular pathogenesis of hepatic encephalopathy, Intern J Biochem Cell Biol 35:1175-1181, 2003.
9. Jalan R: Pathophysiological basis of therapy of raised intracranial pressure in acute liver failure, Neurochem Intern 47:78-83, 2005.
10. Shawcross D, Jalan R: Dispelling myths in the treatment of hepatic encephalopathy, Lancet 365:431-433, 2005.
11. Holt DE, Washabau RJ, et al: Cerebrospinal fluid glutamine, tryptophan, and trypophan metabolite concentrations in dogs with portosystemic shunts, Am J Vet Res 63:1167-1171, 2002.
12. Albrecht J, Jones EA: Hepatic encephalopathy: molecular mechanisms underlying the clinical syndrome, J Neurol Sci 170:138-146, 1999.
13. Berent AC, Rondeau M: Hepatic failure. In Silverstein DC, Hopper K, editor: Small animal critical care medicine, St Louis, 2009, Saunders Elsevier.
14. Center SA: Hepatic vascular diseases. In Guilford WG, editor: Strombeck's small animal gastroenterology, ed 3, Philadelphia, 1996, WB Saunders, 1996, p 802.
15. Gow AG, Marques AI, Yool DA, et al: Dogs with congenital porto-systemic shunting (cPSS) and hepatic encephalopathy have higher serum concentrations of C-reactive protein than asymptomatic dogs with cPSS, Metab Brain Dis 27(2):227-229, 2012.
16. Gow AG, Marques AI, Yool DA, et al: Whole blood manganese concentrations in dogs with congenital portosystemic shunts, J Vet Intern Med 24(1):90-96, 2010.
17. Fischer J: On the occurrence of false neurochemical transmitters. In Williams R, Murray-Lyons I, editors: Artificial liver support, Tunbridge Wells, UK, 1975, Pitman Medical.
18. Fingerote RJ, Bain VG: Fulminant hepatic failure, Am J Gastroenterol 88(7):1000-1010, 1993.
19. Respess M, O'Toole TE, Taeymans O, et al: Portal vein thrombosis in 33 dogs: 1998-2011, J Vet Intern Med 26(2):230-237, 2012.
20. Center SA: Serum bile acids in companion animal medicine, Vet Clin North Am Small Anim Pract 23:625, 1993.
21. Berent A, Weisse C: Hepatic vascular Anomalies. In Ettinger SJ, Feldman ED, editor: Textbook of veterinary internal medicine: diseases of the dog and cats, ed 7, St Louis, 2010, Elsevier Saunders.
22. Willard MD, Twedt DC: Gastrointestinal, pancreatic, hepatic disorders. In Willard MD, Tvedten H, Turnwald G, editors: Small animal clinical diagnosis by laboratory methods, ed 3, Philadelphia, 1999, WB Saunders.
23. Taboada J: Hepatic pathophysiology. In Proceedings: International Veterinary Emergency and Critical Care Symposium, 2003.
24. Wang KY, Panciera DL, Al-Rukibat RK, et al: Accuracy of ultrasound-guided fine needle aspiration of the liver and cytologic findings in dogs and cats: 97 cases (1990-2000), J Am Vet Med Assoc 224(1):75-78, 2004.
25. Fryer KJ, Levine JM, Peycke LE, et al: Incidence of postoperative seizures with and without levetiracetam pretreatment in dogs undergoing portosystemic shunt attenuation, J Vet Intern Med 25(6):1379-1384, 2011.
26. Flatland B: Botanicals, vitamins, and minerals and the liver: therapeutic applications and potential toxicities, Comp Cont Ed 25(7):514-524, 2003.
27. Flora K, Hahn M, Rosen H, et al: Milk thistle (Silybum marianum) for the therapy of liver disease, Am J Gastroenterol 93(2):139, 1998.
28. Williams R, Gimson AE: Intensive liver care and management of acute hepatic failure, Digest Dis Sci 36(6):820-826, 1991.
29. Bersenas, AM, Mathews, KA, Allen DG, et al: Effects of ranitidine, famotidine, pantoprazole, and omeprazole on intragastric pH in dogs, Am J Vet Res 66:425-431, 2005.
30. Bañares R, Catalina MV, Vaquero J: Liver support Systems: will they ever reach prime time? Curr Gastroenterol Rep 15(3):312, 2013.
31. Black LL, Gaynor J, Adams C, et al: Effect of intraarticular injection of autologous adipose-derived mesenchymal stem and regenerative cells on clinical signs of chronic osteoarthritis of the elbow joint in dogs, Vet Ther 9(3):192-200, 2008.
32. Quimby J, Webb TL, Gibbons DS, et al: Evaluation of intrarenal MSC injection for treatment of chronic kidney disease in cats: a pilot study, J Fel Med Surg 13:418-426, 2011.
33. Berent A, Weisse C, Langston C, et al: Selective renal intra-arterial and nonselective IV Delivery of autologous mesenchymal-derived stem cells for kidney disease in dogs and cats: pilot study. Abstract, ACVS 2012, Washington, DC.
34. Kim SJ, Park KC, Lee JU, et al: Therapeutic potential of adipose tissue-derived stem cells for liver failure according to the transplantation routes, J Korean Surg Soc 81(3):176-186, 2011.
35. Zhu W, Shi XL, Xiao JQ, et al: Effects of xenogeneic adipose-derived stem cell transplantation on acute-on-chronic liver failure, Hepatobiliary Pancreat Dis Int 12(1):60-67, 2013.

CHAPTER 117
GASTROENTERITIS

Tara K. Trotman, VMD, DACVIM (Internal Medicine)

KEY POINTS

- Clinical signs of acute gastroenteritis typically involve vomiting, diarrhea, and partial or complete anorexia.
- Physical examination findings are often nonspecific but may include abdominal discomfort, dehydration, and hypovolemia.
- Gastroenteritis has a variety of causes, and determination of an underlying cause is often not possible. Fecal samples should be evaluated for parasitic and bacterial infections in most animals. Systemic diseases are often diagnosed based on the results of a complete blood cell count, biochemical profile, and urinalysis.
- Supportive care is the mainstay of therapy if an underlying cause is not found. Prognosis for most dogs and cats with gastroenteritis is excellent.

Gastroenteritis is a broad term used to indicate inflammation of the stomach and the intestinal tract. It is a common cause for acute-onset vomiting, anorexia, and diarrhea in dogs and cats but should be differentiated from other problems that may cause similar clinical signs, such as pancreatitis, azotemia, hepatitis, and intestinal obstruction (see additional chapters in Intraabdominal Disorders section).[1] Inflammation of the alimentary tract may occur in dogs and cats and can be due to a wide variety of underlying causes, including dietary indiscretion, infectious organisms, toxins, immune dysregulation, and metabolic disorders (see Chapters 120 and 121). A thorough history and physical examination may aid in uncovering an underlying cause, but often a specific cause is not identified. In most cases, supportive therapy, including appropriate fluid support, dietary modification, antiemetics, and gastric protectant agents, are sufficient for resolution of clinical signs. However, acute decompensation can occur in severe cases. This is usually secondary to volume depletion, fluid losses, electrolyte imbalances and acid-base disturbances that occur because the intestinal tract cannot perform its normal hemostatic functions.

ANATOMY AND PHYSIOLOGY

The stomach is the compartment between the esophagus and small intestine that functions as a storage reservoir for food and a vessel for mixing and grinding food into smaller components that then enter the small intestine.[2] The stomach is made up of muscular layers, glandular portions, and a mucosal barrier. The muscular layers grind food into smaller particles and move it forward into the small intestine through the pyloric sphincter. Of equal importance are the glandular portions of the stomach, which include parietal cells (for secretion of hydrochloric acid), chief cells (for secretion of pepsinogen), and mucus-producing cells (which also secrete bicarbonate). Normally, the gastric mucosal barrier keeps hydrochloric acid and digestive enzymes within the lumen and prevents loss of plasma constituents into the stomach.[2] Once the food particles are ground into small enough components, they pass through the pyloric sphincter into the beginning of the small intestine, known as the *duodenum.*

The small intestine of cats and dogs functions in digestion and absorption of food and its nutrients and is divided arbitrarily into the duodenum, jejunum, and ileum.[3] The mucosa of the small intestine is involved in secretory and absorptive functions and contains a single layer of epithelial cells called *enterocytes.* The mucosa along the length of the small intestine is formed into villi, which are fingerlike projections into the intestinal lumen that enlarge the surface of the small intestine. Microvilli then form the "brush border" to further increase the surface area available for digestion and absorption of nutrients. Enzymes within the brush border aid in digestion of larger food molecules into smaller, more readily absorbable particles. Absorption may occur via specific transport mechanisms or by pinocytosis. The epithelial cells also are involved with absorption and secretion of electrolytes and water.[3] Enterocytes are connected to each other by tight junctions, limiting absorption between cells, as well as preventing backflow of nutrients from the interstitium into the intestinal lumen. The enterocytes start at the crypt (base of the villus) and migrate toward the intestinal lumen where they are shed, with a lifespan of approximately 2 to 5 days. A healthy, intact mucosal lining is important for the integrity of the intestine. Any type of inflammation that disrupts this layer can lead to significant intestinal disease.[4] The gastrointestinal (GI) tract absorbs approximately 99% of the fluid presented to it; therefore any damage can cause significant alterations in acid-base and fluid balances.[5,5a]

HISTORY AND CLINICAL SIGNS

A thorough history is critical to identifying an underlying cause for gastroenteritis. Questions may be related to the patient's current diet, recent change in diet, and exposure to unusual food, foreign materials, garbage, or toxins. It is also important to find out about the patient's environment, including exposure to other animals, and if other exposed animals have similar signs or a history of similar signs. Vaccination status, deworming history, and medication use are also important.

Clinical signs of gastroenteritis are often similar regardless of the underlying cause. Vomiting, diarrhea, and anorexia are most common, and certain combinations of these signs may make one cause more or less likely than another. Severe inflammation or ulceration, depending on the cause, can lead to hematemesis or melena.

Physical examination is often unrewarding towards finding an underlying cause. Patients may have varying degrees of dehydration, as well as abdominal pain. In severe cases, such as those animals with hemorrhagic gastroenteritis (HGE) or parvoviral enteritis, patients may have signs of hypovolemia and shock because of the severe fluid losses and acid-base disturbances.

CAUSES

Infectious Gastroenteritis

A variety of infectious agents can affect the GI tract. Viruses, bacteria, parasites, protozoa, and fungi have been shown to cause

BOX 117-1 ***Infectious Causes of Gastroenteritis in Dogs and Cats***

Bacterial

Campylobacter spp.
Clostridium spp.
Escherichia coli
Salmonella spp.
Helicobacter spp.

Viral

Parvovirus
Rotavirus
Enteric coronavirus
Feline infectious peritonitis
Canine distemper virus
Feline leukemia virus
Feline immunodeficiency virus

Fungal, Algal, and Oomycoses

Histoplasmosis
Protothecosis
Pythiosis

Parasitic

Ascarids *(Toxocara canis, Toxocara cati, Toxascaris leonina)*
Hookworms (*Ancylostoma* spp., *Uncinaria stenocephala*)
Strongyloides stercoralis
Whipworms (*Trichuris vulpis*)
Coccidiosis (*Isospora canis* or *felis*, *Toxoplasma gondii*, *Cryptosporidium parvum*)
Giardia
Tritrichomonas
Balantidium coli

Rickettsial

Neorickettsia helminthoeca (salmon poisoning)

gastroenteritis of varying severity. The descriptions in the text are limited to the most common. Please see Box 117-1 for a more complete list of potential infectious causes of gastroenteritis.

Viral enteritis

Canine parvovirus-2 (CPV-2) is one of the most common infectious diseases in dogs and may be characterized by severe enteritis, vomiting, hemorrhagic diarrhea, and shock.[4] The pathophysiology and treatment of CPV-2 are discussed in Chapter 97. Other viral diseases that can lead to severe GI inflammation include coronavirus and rotavirus infection, although clinical manifestations of these viral diseases are typically milder than those of CPV-2, possibly because they affect the tips of the villi, whereas CPV-2 affects the crypts.[6] Feline panleukopenia, also caused by a parvovirus, can cause similar signs of severe gastroenteritis in cats.

Bacterial enteritis

The bacterial organisms most commonly associated with acute gastroenteritis in dogs and cats include *Clostridium perfringens* and *Clostridium difficile*, *Campylobacter jejuni* and *Campylobacter upsaliensis*, *Salmonella* spp., *Helicobacter* spp., and enterotoxigenic *E. coli.*[7-10] Controversy continues regarding whether some of these organisms truly cause clinical disease because some of them can be found in nondiarrheic patients as well as animals with diarrhea. With emerging and improved diagnostic techniques such as ELISA and PCR testing, newer recommendations for definitive diagnosis rely on a multimodal evaluation for some of these organisms.[11] Evidence does support the role of *Clostridium* spp. in gastroenteritis.[8-9,12] However, because many dogs have *C. perfringens* and its CPE toxin in their GI tracts without developing clinical signs, evaluation of the roles of these organisms, as well as those of *Campylobacter* and *Helicobacter* spp. in GI disease of companion animals, is ongoing.[13]

Although the majority of Salmonella infections in dogs are self-limiting and resolved by the host's local immune response, bacterial translocation and septicemia can occur, leading to systemic inflammatory response and multi-organ dysfunction in some patients (see Chapters 6 and 7). Those most at risk are the young or immunocompromised, those that have concurrent infections, or those that have received prior antibiotic or glucocorticoid therapy. As is the case with many bacterial organisms, Salmonella can be found in a population of healthy, nonclinical patients, so its documentation in the GI tract should be correlated with clinical signs.[13]

In addition to the aforementioned more commonly diagnosed bacterial infections, evidence is beginning to suggest that histiocytic ulcerative colitis in Boxer dogs may be due to invasive *E. coli* organisms within the colonic mucosa of affected dogs.[14,15] Fluoroquinolones have become the standard treatment for these patients, with the use of fluorescent in situ hybridization (FISH) to confirm the presence of these organisms.[14,15] Culture and susceptibility testing of colonic tissue can be used to isolate and guide therapy because antimicrobial resistance has become of increasing concern.[14,15]

Parasitic gastroenteritis

Although most dogs and cats with GI parasites have mild clinical signs, ascarids (*Toxocara* spp., *Toxascaris leonina, Ollulanus tricuspis,* and *Physaloptera* spp.), hookworms *(Ancylostoma* spp., *Uncinaria stenocephala),* and whipworms *(Trichuris* spp.) can cause significant GI tract inflammation, vomiting, and diarrhea. GI blood loss is also common with severe hookworm infestations. Protozoans that cause canine and feline gastroenteritis include *Giardia* spp., coccidia, and *Cryptosporidia* spp. *Tritrichomonas foetus* infection is another protozoal cause of diarrhea in cats (primarily large bowel) with waxing and waning signs. Although patients may appear unthrifty, it is rarely the cause of critical illness.[6]

Fungal gastroenteritis

Fungal disease can affect the GI tract of dogs and cats, although the likelihood greatly depends on the animal's geographic location or recent travel destinations. Histoplasmosis is the fungal pathogen that most commonly affects the GI tract, causing a severe protein-losing enteropathy (PLE). *Pythium* spp., an oomycete, also can cause similar disease.

Hemorrhagic Gastroenteritis

Hemorrhagic gastroenteritis (HGE) is a disease of unknown cause. It typically affects young to middle-age, small breed dogs, and its clinical course usually includes a peracute onset of clinical signs that can progress rapidly to death without appropriate therapy.[7,16] Affected animals are often previously healthy dogs with no pertinent historical information. The syndrome is characterized by acute onset of bloody diarrhea, often explosive, along with an elevated packed cell volume (PCV) (at least 60%).[7,16] Although the cause remains unknown, it has been suggested that abnormal immune responses to bacteria, bacterial endotoxin, or dietary ingredients may play a role.[17] *C. perfringens* has been isolated from cultures of GI contents in dogs with HGE; however, its exact role in the syndrome has not been determined. Fatal acute HGE was reported in a dog with large numbers of enterotoxin-positive A *C. perfringens* isolated from the intestinal tract.[12]

Clinical signs of vomiting and depression, progressing to explosive, bloody diarrhea and anorexia are classic, and the diarrhea often is described as having the appearance of raspberry jam.[7] Thorough investigation to rule out other causes of hemorrhagic diarrhea such as parvovirus, bacterial infections, or GI parasites should be undertaken before arriving at a diagnosis of HGE. Along with hemoconcentration, the total protein concentration typically increases little or not at all (it may actually decrease). The elevated PCV occurs because of hemoconcentration and/or splenic contraction, whereas GI loss of serum proteins or redistribution of body water into the vascular space explains the lack of rise in total protein levels.[7]

Aggressive therapy is warranted in these animals because rapid decompensation may occur. Adequate replacement of fluid volume is essential; more specific fluid management strategies can be found in Chapters 59 and 60. General goals are to replace quickly the fluid deficits from the acute diarrhea and vomiting then adjust fluid rates to maintain proper hydration. The GI tract is a "shock organ" in the dog, and lack of proper perfusion to the GI tract can lead to worsening GI inflammation, bacterial translocation, sepsis, and disseminated intravascular coagulation (see Chapter 91).[18,19] Because serum proteins are lost through the intestinal tract, close attention should be paid to the patient's colloid osmotic pressure and colloidal support given when necessary. Fluid therapy is the mainstay of treatment for patients with HGE. Antiemetic and gastric protectant drugs should be used as indicated. Although antimicrobials may be warranted in patients with suspected bacterial translocation, caution is advised because inappropriate use of these drugs may promote antimicrobial resistance or other unwanted side effects. In some dogs with HGE but no signs of sepsis, antimicrobial therapy may not be indicated.[20] With rapid and appropriate therapy, the prognosis for full recovery from HGE is excellent.

Dietary Indiscretion

Gastroenteritis caused by ingestion of toxins (i.e., organophosphates), foreign materials, or garbage is common in dogs, and less so in cats. Some toxins lead directly to inflammation of the GI tract, although ingestion of other foreign materials may lead to direct GI trauma or an osmotic diarrhea secondary to nondigestible substances within the intestinal tract. Ingestion of excessive fatty products also may cause pancreatitis in these animals. Many drugs are associated with vomiting and diarrhea (antimicrobials, antineoplastics, anthelminthics), and garbage ingestion can lead to exposure of the intestinal tract to preformed bacterial toxins. Most commonly, dietary indiscretion leads to acute onset of vomiting, diarrhea, and anorexia. The patient's history is useful because the owner may be aware of exposure to a specific toxicant or garbage. The diagnosis is usually presumptive, and treatment involves supportive care such as fluid therapy to maintain hydration, antiemetic drugs, and gastric protectants as needed. The prognosis is excellent, and most animals recover within 24 to 72 hours.

Protein-Losing Enteropathy

Protein-losing enteropathy (PLE) is a broad diagnosis that includes any cause of GI disease that results in excessive loss of plasma proteins. The diseases most commonly associated with PLE are severe lymphocytic-plasmacytic, eosinophilic, or granulomatous inflammatory bowel diseases, lymphangiectasia, diffuse GI fungal disease, and diffuse neoplasia such as lymphosarcoma. Some of the aforementioned GI diseases can cause PLE if the inflammation and damage to the intestinal mucosa are severe enough.

The mechanism of protein loss may be related to inflammation or loss of the GI barrier.[21] Protein loss likely arises because of disruption to the normal enterocyte function, as well as deranged permeability through the tight junctions.[21] Clinical signs of PLE usually are associated with chronic wasting because of lack of nutrient integration into the body. However, the proteins lost into the intestinal tract can include large proteins such as albumin and antithrombin, both of which have important roles in homeostasis. Albumin, with a molecular weight of 69,000 daltons, contributes significantly to oncotic pressure. Loss of albumin through the GI tract can lead to a reduced colloid osmotic pressure and subsequent loss of fluid from the intravascular space. Although this is typically a gradual process, it can cause significant changes in the compartmentalization of fluids in some patients. If third spacing has occurred, it may be necessary to use colloidal fluids such as hydroxyethyl starch or human albumin, in addition to crystalloids, to prevent further intravascular fluid losses (see Chapter 58).[22]Albumin also has additional beneficial effects, such as its antioxidant and antiinflammatory properties.[23]

Antithrombin plays a critical role in the coagulation and fibrinolytic cascade by inactivating thrombin and other clotting factors. Even a small reduction in antithrombin levels can cause a large propensity toward thrombosis and thromboembolism. This becomes important in patients with PLE that lose large amounts of protein and are predisposed to developing thromboemboli in various parts of the body, including the pulmonary vessels, portal vein, or coronary or cerebral vessels. Therapy for PLE often involves glucocorticoids, which also increase the risk of thromboembolic disease. Therefore anticoagulant or antiplatelet therapy, or both, may be warranted in these cases.

Therapy for PLE is aimed at treating the underlying cause. Animals with diffuse neoplasia such as lymphosarcoma should be treated with chemotherapy, and those with severe inflammatory bowel disease may benefit from antiinflammatory drugs and a hypoallergenic diet. Lymphangiectasia may be primary or secondary, and administration of a diet low in fat may be more important than feeding a hypoallergenic diet, depending on the degree of inflammation.

Extraintestinal Diseases

Hypoadrenocorticism, liver or kidney disease, acute pancreatitis, and peritonitis are common extraintestinal causes of gastroenteritis in small animals.

DIAGNOSIS

The extent of diagnostic testing in a dog that is presented with signs of acute gastroenteritis depends on factors such as historical information, prior occurrence of similar clinical signs, and stability of the patient. Fecal samples should be evaluated for parasitic diseases and bacterial infections in most animals with clinical signs of acute gastroenteritis. A culture and Gram stain evaluation also should be performed. Feces should be tested at least three times before a negative result is confirmed. Testing for clostridial enterotoxins may include use of a *C. perfringens* enterotoxin enzyme-linked immunosorbent assay (ELISA), or an ELISA that detects *C. difficile* toxins A and B. Recent developments with real PCR testing have provided another diagnostic method for detection of many organisms that are seen commonly in small animals. A *Giardia* antigen test also exists. If parvovirus is suspected, a fecal antigen test (ELISA) should be performed.

Systemic evaluation should include a complete blood count, chemistry screen, and urinalysis. Typically results of these tests are normal and do not aid in determining an underlying cause for the gastroenteritis. However, in certain circumstances such as HGE (in which the PCV is elevated with a normal to decreased total protein concentration), PLE (which may cause a decrease in total protein, globulin, albumin, and cholesterol levels), these tests can aid in making a diagnosis. Electrolytes should be checked regularly to confirm adequate fluid management.

Abdominal radiographs may be unrewarding or may show signs of fluid-filled bowel loops. Radiographs are indicated if a GI obstruction (i.e., foreign body, neoplasia) is suspected. Abdominal ultrasonography is an excellent tool to evaluate all abdominal organs, including the thickness and layering of the stomach and small intestine. These findings may be insensitive and nonspecific, however, and always should be used in conjunction with other diagnostic tests.

If PLE is suspected and biopsies of the stomach and intestine are required, there are two main ways of achieving this. Endoscopy is a noninvasive method for visualizing the esophageal, gastric, and duodenal mucosa, as well as for obtaining small (1.8- to 2.4-mm) biopsy samples. Disadvantages of this method are that the samples are small and biopsies cannot be obtained distal to the duodenum. Ileal samples can be obtained if colonoscopy is performed, but this requires patient preparation (i.e., administration of cleansing enemas), which can cause decompensation in unstable animals resulting from fluid and electrolyte shifts. Another method for obtaining samples is via exploratory laparotomy. This is an excellent method for acquiring full-thickness biopsy samples of multiple areas of the GI tract (and other organs if they are found to be abnormal). The disadvantages are that it is much more invasive, and poor wound healing may be a concern in patients with reduced albumin levels. This has been reported in human surgical patients as well as canine surgical patients.[24-26] In addition, diseased gastric and intestinal walls may heal poorly. Laparoscopy is another technique that can be used to obtain excellent visualization of the abdominal cavity along with full-thickness biopsies of the GI tract (and other organs as needed). Laparoscopy is less invasive than exploratory laparotomy and may be associated with less morbidity because of smaller incisions; however, healing of gastric and intestinal biopsy sites would remain a concern in patients with low albumin levels or diseased walls.

The most common clinical signs of gastroenteritis are vomiting, diarrhea, and anorexia. These are common to a variety of diseases; therefore gastroenteritis is often a diagnosis of exclusion. Differential diagnosis may include systemic diseases such as kidney disease, liver disease, hypoadrenocorticism, complicated diabetes mellitus (diabetic ketoacidosis), vestibular disease or other neurologic abnormalities, pancreatitis, pyometra, prostatitis, and peritonitis. Additional primary GI diseases to consider include intussusception, foreign body or mass obstruction, infiltrative disease (neoplasia, infectious), or ischemia. It is important to rule out these other disorders, as indicated, before making a diagnosis of gastroenteritis.

TREATMENT

Most cases of gastroenteritis respond well to supportive care. Aggressiveness of treatment depends on the severity of clinical signs and the underlying cause. Because the most common clinical signs of gastroenteritis, regardless of underlying cause, are vomiting, diarrhea, and anorexia, dehydration is a common occurrence, and initial therapy should be aimed at addressing the patient's hydration status and perfusion parameters (see Chapters 57, 59, and 60).

Other treatments can be divided into specific or symptomatic therapies. Specific drugs can be used to treat some of the underlying causes of disease. For the most part, drugs used to eradicate many of the infectious causes for gastroenteritis are available. GI parasites may be treated with fenbendazole or other antihelminthic drugs. *Campylobacter* spp. have responded well to such drugs as erythromycin, enrofloxacin, and cefoxitin,[27] and *Clostridium* spp. may respond to metronidazole or ampicillin.[28] The choice of drug depends on many factors, including patient age and ability to take oral medications. Few antiviral drugs are effective in veterinary medicine; therefore diseases such as parvoviral enteritis are treated supportively. As stated before, the aims of therapy for animals with PLE are to treat the underlying cause, commonly with diet change and antiinflammatory agents.

Many of the drugs used to treat gastroenteritis are nonspecific. In addition to fluids, most animals respond well to resting the GI tract by withholding food for 24 to 48 hours. When food is offered, a wet, easily digestible diet is recommended. Addition of GI protectants (see Chapter 161) or antiemetics (see Chapter 162), or both, may hasten recovery of the enterocyte damage, give the GI tract time to heal, and decrease nausea. In animals with severe GI damage, in which bacterial translocation is a concern (especially in puppies with parvoviral enteritis), antimicrobials may be indicated and should aim at treating the common organisms expected in the intestinal tract. This usually consists of drugs with good gram-negative and anaerobic coverage. More recently, use of probiotics has been evaluated in veterinary medicine for treatment of acute and chronic GI disease. Two recent prospective studies have shown that the use of probiotics in acute gastroenteritis may hasten recovery and reduce the severity of diarrhea in affected patients. Although specific mechanisms for their benefit still are poorly understood, probiotics may compete with pathogenic organisms for nutrition, they may produce antimicrobial substances, and they may stimulate the immune system.[29,30]

CONCLUSION

Prognosis for animals with mild to moderate gastroenteritis is typically excellent. However, early diagnosis and timely therapy are important to prevent multiple organ involvement and maximize outcome.

REFERENCES

1. Guilford WG, Strombeck DS: Acute gastritis. In Guilford WG, Center SA, Strombeck DR, et al, editors: Strombeck's small animal gastroenterology, ed 3, Philadelphia, 1996, Saunders.
2. Guilford WG, Strombeck DS: Gastric structure and function. In Guilford WG, Center SA, Strombeck DR, et al, editors: Strombeck's small animal gastroenterology, ed 3, Philadelphia, 1996, Saunders.
3. Strombeck DS: Small and large intestine: normal structure and function. In Guilford WG, Center SA, Strombeck DR et al, editors: Strombeck's small animal gastroenterology, ed 3, Philadelphia, 1996, Saunders.
4. Macintire DK, Smith-Carr S: Canine parvovirus. Part II. Clinical signs, diagnosis, and treatment, Comp Cont Educ Pract Vet 19:291, 1997.
5. Simpson KW, Birnbaum N: Fluid and electrolyte disturbances in gastrointestinal and pancreatic disease. In DiBartola SP, editor: Fluid, electrolyte, and acid-base disorders in small animal practice, ed 3, St Louis, 2006, Saunders.

5a. Center SA: Fluid, electrolyte, and acid-base disturbances in liver diseases. In DiBartola SP, editor: Fluid, electrolyte, and acid-base disorders in small animal practice, ed 3, St Louis, 2006, Saunders.

6. Greene CE, Decaro N: Canine viral enteritis. In Greene CE, editor: Infectious diseases of the dog and cat, St Louis, 2012, Elsevier Saunders.
7. Triolo A, Lappin MR: Acute medical diseases of the small intestine. In Tams TR, editor: Handbook of small animal gastroenterology, St Louis, 2003, Saunders.
8. Marks SL, Kather EJ, Kass PH, et al: Genotypic and phenotypic characterization of *Clostridium perfringens* and *Clostridium difficile* in diarrheic and healthy dogs, J Vet Intern Med 16:533, 2002.
9. Weese JS, Staempfli HR, Prescott JF, et al: The roles of *Clostridium difficile* and enterotoxigenic *Clostridium perfringens* in diarrhea in dogs, J Vet Intern Med 15:374, 2001.
10. Bender JB, Shulman SA, Averbeck GA, et al: Epidemiologic features of *Campylobacter* infection among cats in the upper Midwestern United States, J Am Vet Med Assoc 226:544, 2005.
11. Marks SL, Rankin SC, Byrne BA, et al: Enteropathogenic bacteria in dogs and cats: diagnosis, epidemiology, treatment, and control, J Vet Intern Med 25:1195-1209, 2011.

12. Schlegel BJ, Van Dreumel T, Slavic D, et al: *Clostridium perfringens* type A fatal acute gastroenteritis in a dog, Can Vet J 53(5):555-557, 2012.
13. Lappin MR: Infection (small intestine). In Washabau RJ, Day MJ: Canine and feline gastroenterology, St Louis, 2013, Elsevier Saunders.
14. Simpson KW, Dogan B, Rishniw M, et al: Adherent and invasive *Escherichia coli* is associated with granulomatous colitis in boxer dogs, Infect Immun 74(8):4778-4792, 2006.
15. Mansfield CS, James FE, Craven M, et al: Remission of histiocytic ulcerative colitis in boxer dogs correlates with eradication of invasive intramucosal *Escherichia coli*, J Vet Intern Med 23:964-969, 2009.
16. Guilford WG, Strombeck DS: Acute hemorrhagic enteropathy (hemorrhagic gastroenteritis: HGE). In Guilford WG, Center SA, Strombeck DR, et al, editors: Strombeck's small animal gastroenterology, ed 3, Philadelphia, 1996, Saunders.
17. Spielman BL, Garvey MS: Hemorrhagic gastroenteritis in 15 dogs, J Am Anim Hosp Assoc 29:341, 1993.
18. Guilford WG, Strombeck DS: Classification, pathophysiology, and symptomatic treatment of diarrheal disease. In Guilford WG, Center SA, Strombeck DR, et al, editors: Strombeck's small animal gastroenterology, ed 3, Philadelphia, 1996, Saunders.
19. Hackett T: Acute hemorrhagic diarrhea. In Wingfield WE, Raffe MR, editors: The veterinary ICU book, Jackson Hole, Wyo, 2002, Teton NewMedia.
20. Unterer S, Strohmeyer K, Kruse BD, et al: Treatment of aseptic dogs with hemorrhagic gastroenteritis with amoxicillin/clavulanic acid: a prospective blinded study, J Vet Intern Med 25(5):973-9, 2011.
21. Williams DA: Malabsorption, small intestinal bacterial overgrowth, and protein losing enteropathy. In Guilford WG, Center SA, Strombeck DR et al, editors: Strombeck's small animal gastroenterology, ed 3, Philadelphia, 1996, Saunders.
22. Vigano F, Perissinotto L, Bosco VRF: Administration of 5% human serum albumin in critically ill small animal patients with hypoalbuminemia: 418 dogs and 170 cats (1994-2008), J Vet Emerg Crit Care April 20(2):237-243, 2010.
23. Powers KA, Kapus A, Khadaroo RG, et al: Twenty-five percent albumin prevents lung injury following shock/resuscitation, Crit Care Med 31:2355, 2003.
24. Gibbs J, Cull W, Henderson W, et al: Preoperative serum albumin level as a predictor of operative mortality and morbidity, Arch Surg 134:36, 1999.
25. Ralphs SC, Jessen CR, Lipowitz AJ: Risk factors for leakage following intestinal anastomosis in dogs and cats: 115 cases (1991-2000), J Am Vet Med Assoc 223:73, 2003.
26. Grimes JA, Schmiedt CW, Cornell KK, et al: Identification of risk factors for septic peritonitis and failure to survive following gastrointestinal surgery in dogs, J Am Vet Med Assoc 238(4):486-494, 2011.
27. Fox JG: *Campylobacter* infections. In Greene CE, editor: Infectious diseases of the dog and cat, ed 4, St Louis, 2012, Elsevier Saunders.
28. Marks SL: *Clostridium perfringens*- and *Clostridium difficile*-associated diarrhea. In Greene CE, editor: Infectious diseases of the dog and cat, ed 4, St Louis, 2012, Elsevier Saunders.
29. Herstad HK, Nesheim BB, L'Abée-Lund T, et al: Effects of a probiotic intervention in acute canine gastroenteritis—a controlled clinical trial, J Small Anim Pract 51(1):34-38, 2010.
30. Bybee SN, Scorza AV, Lappin MR: Effect of the probiotic Enterococcus faecium SF68 on presence of diarrhea in cats and dogs housed in an animal shelter, J Vet Intern Med 25(4):856-860, 2011.

CHAPTER 118
MOTILITY DISORDERS

Patricia M. Dowling, DVM, MSc, DACVIM, DACVP

KEY POINTS

- Treatment of canine congenital and acquired megaesophagus is symptomatic, with protectants and histamine-2 blockers or serotonergic drugs for esophageal reflux and esophagitis.
- Gastric emptying disorders can be treated with metoclopramide, serotonergic drugs, ghrelin mimetics, motilin receptor agonists, and acetylcholinesterase inhibitors.
- Intestinal transit disorders can be treated with serotonergic drugs, ghrelin mimetics, motilin receptor agonists, and acetylcholinesterase inhibitors.
- Megacolon in cats can be treated with serotonergic drugs.

Gastrointestinal (GI) motility disorders are common yet challenging to diagnose and treat in humans and animals. Therapy is directed at correcting predisposing factors and using prokinetic drugs to promote normal GI motility.

MEGAESOPHAGUS

Etiology and Clinical Signs

Congenital megaesophagus is seen in a number of breeds of dogs, including Wire-haired Fox Terriers, Miniature Schnauzers, German Shepherd Dogs, Great Danes, Irish Setters, Labrador Retrievers, Newfoundlands, and Chinese Shar Peis. It is rare in cats, but Siamese cats may be predisposed. Congenital megaesophagus in dogs is due to organ specific sensory dysfunction, in which the distention sensitive vagal afferent system innervating the esophagus is defective, whereas other contiguous and physiologically similar distention sensitive vagal afferent systems are unaffected.[1] Acquired megaesophagus can develop in association with a number of primary diseases in dogs and cats, but most adult-onset cases are idiopathic.[2] Myasthenia gravis accounts for the majority of cases with a known cause. Other causes of acquired megaesophagus include hypoadrenocorticism, lead and thallium poisoning, lupus, esophageal neoplasia, and severe esophagitis. Inflammatory myopathies associated with megaesophagus in dogs include immune-mediated polymyositis infectious and preneoplastic myositis and dermatomyositis. Dogs with peripheral neuropathies, laryngeal paralysis, myasthenia gravis, esophagitis, and chronic or recurrent gastric dilatation with or without volvulus are at an increased risk of developing megaesophagus. German Shepherd Dogs, Golden Retrievers, and Irish Setters and Abyssinians and Somali cats are predisposed to acquired megaesophagus.[2,3] Esophageal dysmotility without overt megaesophagus occurs in young terriers and is thought to be a syndrome of delayed esophageal maturation.[4] Affected dogs can be symptomatic or asymptomatic, and normal esophageal motility develops with time in some dogs. Although often blamed as a cause, a clear link between hypothyroidism and megaesophagus cannot be demonstrated.

Regurgitation is the predominant clinical sign associated with megaesophagus and a careful history can help distinguish between passive regurgitation and active vomition. The frequency of episodes and relation to time of feeding vary considerably. Puppies with congenital megaesophagus typically begin regurgitating when started on solid foods. Emaciation from malnutrition and aspiration pneumonia are the most common complications of megaesophagus.

Diagnosis and Treatment

Plain survey radiographs are often diagnostic, but contrast radiography may be useful to confirm the diagnosis and evaluate motility. Endoscopy also confirms the diagnosis and can identify esophagitis, which often occurs in dogs with megaesophagus. Routine hematology, serum biochemistries, and urinalysis should be performed to investigate primary disorders that can result in secondary megaesophagus. Additional diagnostic tests for acquired megaesophagus include serology for nicotinic ACH receptor antibody and antinuclear antibody, adrenocorticotropic hormone stimulation, serum creatine phosphokinase activity, electromyography and nerve conduction velocity, and nerve and muscle biopsies.

Treatment of congenital megaesophagus is symptomatic; traditional prokinetic drugs such as metoclopramide or cisapride have not proven beneficial. Because of the high incidence of esophagitis, affected animals should be treated with sucralfate (1 g q8h for large dogs, 0.5 g q8h for smaller dogs and 0.25 g q8-12h for cats), a histamine-2 blocker (cimetidine, 5 to 10 mg/kg q8-12h PO; ranitidine, 1 to 2 mg/kg q12h PO; famotidine, 0.5 to 1 mg/kg q12h PO), or a proton pump inhibitor (omeprazole, 1 to 2 mg/kg q24h PO). Animals with secondary megaesophagus should be treated appropriately for the primary disease. Myasthenia gravis in dogs is treated with pyridostigmine (1 to 3 mg/kg q12h PO), prednisone (1 to 2 mg/kg q12h PO), or azathioprine (2 mg/kg q24h PO initially). Mycophenolate mofetil, a new immunosuppressant drug, does not improve clinical outcome when added to pyridostigmine therapy in dogs with acquired myasthenia gravis.[5] Affected animals should be fed small amounts of high-calorie diet at frequent intervals from an elevated position to allow gravity to assist passage into the stomach. The "Bailey Chair" is an example of a positioning device that may be helpful for affected dogs; images and directions on how to build the chair are available on the Internet. If dogs are unable to maintain adequate nutritional intake with positioning, a temporary or permanent gastrostomy tube can be placed. Without a definitive diagnosis, most cases of megaesophagus typically do not do well long term, and affected patients should be given a poor prognosis because of recurrent complications.

GASTRIC EMPTYING DISORDERS

Etiology and Clinical Signs

Gastric emptying disorders from mechanical obstruction or defective propulsion frequently occur in dogs and cats.[6] Defective propulsion is caused by abnormalities in myenteric neuronal or gastric smooth muscle function or antropyloroduodenal coordination. In cats, hair balls can be caused by and be the cause of gastric obstruction or disturbed motility.[7] Primary problems known to cause defective propulsion include infectious or inflammatory diseases, ulcers, and postsurgical gastroparesis. Delayed gastric emptying also occurs secondarily to electrolyte imbalances, metabolic derangements, drugs (cholinergic antagonists, adrenergic and opioid agonists), and peritonitis. In critically ill animals, delayed gastric emptying limits enteral nutrition, and the effects of severe disease further deplete caloric reserves, impairing wound healing, decreasing immune function, and increasing morbidity and mortality.[8]

Diagnosis and Treatment

The most common presenting complaint is chronic, intermittent vomiting that occurs more than 8 hours after eating. Gastric distention may be discernible after eating and is relieved by vomiting. In addition, some patients are presented with weight loss. Although diagnosis and management of mechanical obstruction is straightforward, disorders of propulsion are more challenging. Imaging studies are used to confirm delayed gastric emptying, the most common gastric motility disorder. Survey films, barium contrast studies, and fluoroscopy may be used to document abnormal gastric emptying. Barium impregnated polyspheres (BIPS) can be administered to evaluate the passage of different size beads. Endoscopy is used to rule out gastritis or obstructive disease. If no underlying cause is determined, a functional disorder of gastric emptying is diagnosed presumptively. Treatment consists of dietary management and gastric prokinetic agents.[6] Animals should be fed frequent small meals that are low in fat and protein and high in carbohydrate (e.g., cottage cheese, rice, pasta).

SMALL INTESTINAL TRANSIT DISORDERS

Etiology and Clinical Signs

Causes of small intestinal transit disorders include enteritis, postsurgical ileus, nematode impaction, intestinal sclerosis, and radiation enteritis.[9] Pseudo-obstructions are functional obstructions caused by hypomotility and ileus; most are idiopathic. Intestinal stasis can result in bacterial overgrowth, and the absorption of endotoxin and bacteria can lead to endotoxemia and septicemia. Clinical signs depend on the location and cause of the disorder but typically include vomiting, diarrhea, and weight loss. Abdominal pain and distention may be noted.

Diagnosis and Treatment

With pseudo-obstruction, survey radiographs show dilated bowel loops without evidence of a physical obstruction. Contrast studies or BIPS demonstrate delayed transit through the small intestine. The hemogram is typically normal, but changes in the serum biochemical profile may be seen with protracted vomiting and/or diarrhea. Mechanical obstructions always should be ruled out before treatment with prokinetic drugs. Additional therapy is based on the primary cause of the transit disorder and may include corticosteroids and/or antimicrobials.

MEGACOLON

Etiology and Clinical Signs

Idiopathic megacolon with constipation or obstipation is a common clinical condition in middle-age cats.[10,11] Less common causes of constipation in cats are pelvic canal stenosis, dysautonomia, nerve injury, and Manx sacral spinal cord deformities. The underlying cause of megacolon in cats appears to be a generalized dysfunction of colonic smooth muscle.[12]

Cats with megacolon typically are presented for reduced, absent, or painful defecation. The owner usually notices the cat making numerous unproductive attempts to eliminate in the litter box. When passed, feces are often dry and hard, and hematochezia may be present. Prolonged constipation may also cause anorexia, vomiting, and weight loss.

Diagnosis and Treatment

Colonic impaction is usually obvious on physical examination. Depending on the severity and duration of the condition, other clinical signs can include weight loss, abdominal pain, dehydration, and mesenteric lymphadenopathy. Results of complete blood counts and serum chemistries are typically normal, but metabolic causes of constipation, such as dehydration, hypokalemia, or hypocalcemia, occasionally can be detected. Abdominal radiography can document the extent of fecal impaction and identify exacerbating factors including foreign material (e.g., bones), intraabdominal masses, pelvic fractures, and spinal column abnormalities. Digital rectal examination should be performed carefully but may be helpful in identifying pelvic fractures, rectal diverticula, or neoplasia.

Therapy of constipation depends on the severity and the underlying cause. Mild to moderate cases typically are managed with dietary modification, laxatives, and colonic prokinetic agents. Subtotal colectomy with preservation of the ileocolic junction should be considered in cats that are refractory to medical therapy.[13] Cats have a generally favorable prognosis for recovery after colectomy, although mild to moderate diarrhea may persist for weeks to months postoperatively in some cases.

PROKINETIC DRUGS FOR GASTROINTESTINAL MOTILITY DISORDERS

Serotonergic Drugs

The enteric nervous system (ENS) of the GI tract can function independently of the central nervous system (CNS) to control bowel function.[14] Because no nerve fibers actually penetrate the intestinal epithelium, the ENS uses enteroendocrine cells such as the enterochromaffin cells as sensory transducers. More than 95% of the body's serotonin (also known as 5-hydroxytryptamine, 5-HT) is located in the GI tract, and more than 90% of that store is in the enterochromaffin cells that are scattered in the enteric epithelium from the stomach to the colon. The remaining serotonin is located in the ENS, where 5-HT acts a as a neurotransmitter. From the enterochromaffin cells, serotonin is secreted into the lamina propria in high concentrations, with overflow into the portal circulation and intestinal lumen. The effect of serotonin on intestinal activity is coordinated by 5-HT receptor subtypes. The 5-HT_{1P} receptor initiates peristaltic and secretory reflexes, and so far no drugs have been developed to target this specific receptor. The 5-HT_3 receptor activates extrinsic sensory nerves and is responsible for the sensation of nausea and induction of vomiting from visceral hypersensitivity. Therefore specific 5-HT_3 antagonists such as ondansetron and granisetron are used to treat the nausea and vomiting seen with chemotherapy. Stimulation of the 5-HT_4 receptor increases the presynaptic release of acetylcholine (ACH) and calcitonin gene-related peptide, thereby enhancing neurotransmission. This enhancement promotes propulsive peristaltic and secretory reflexes. Specific 5-HT_4 agonists such as cisapride enhance neurotransmission and depend on natural stimuli to evoke peristaltic and secretory reflexes. This makes these drugs safe because they do not induce perpetual or excessive motility. It is also the reason for the limitations of these drugs because they will not be effective if enteric nerves have degenerated or become nonfunctional.

Cisapride

Cisapride was introduced in 1993 and was the most efficacious prokinetic drug in the treatment of human GI motility disorders. It also became popular for treating motility disorders in dogs and cats. Cisapride is related chemically to metoclopramide, but unlike metoclopramide, it does not cross the blood-brain barrier or have antidopaminergic effects. Therefore it does not have antiemetic action and it does not cause the extrapyrimidal effects seen with metoclopramide. Cisapride is more potent and has broader prokinetic activity than metoclopramide, increasing the motility of the colon, as well as that of the esophagus, stomach, and small intestine. Cisapride is useful in managing gastric stasis, idiopathic constipation, gastroesophageal reflux, and postoperative ileus in dogs and cats. Cisapride is useful in managing cats with megacolon; in many cases, it alleviates or delays the need for subtotal colectomy.[15]

Initially, the only adverse side effects reported in humans were increased defecation, headache, abdominal pain, cramping, and flatulence, and cisapride appeared to be well tolerated by dogs and cats. As cisapride became widely used in the management of gastroesophageal reflux in humans, cases of heart rhythm disorders and deaths were reported. These cardiac problems in humans were associated highly with concurrent drug therapy or specific underlying conditions. Cisapride is metabolized by the liver by the cytochrome P450 enzyme system. Cardiac abnormalities in humans were associated with concomitant administration of other drugs that inhibit cisapride's metabolism, thereby increasing cisapride blood concentrations. Drugs known to inhibit the metabolism of cisapride include clarithromycin, erythromycin, troleandomycin, nefazodone, fluconazole, itraconazole, indinavir, and ritonavir. Because of the human cardiovascular adverse effects, the manufacturer of cisapride withdrew the product from sale in North America. Currently, cisapride can be obtained only from compounding pharmacies in the United States and Canada and is formulated from active pharmaceutical ingredient. Because of the lack of standardized products, efficacy may vary, but a suggested dose is 2.5 to 5 mg/cat q8-12h PO. Oral absorption increases with food, so cisapride should be administered 15 minutes before feeding.

Because of the adverse effects of cisapride, alternative 5-HT_4 receptor agonists have been developed. The most promising is mosapride, which has shown prokinetic and anti-ulcerogenic properties in dogs.[16-18] However, mosapride is currently not available in North America.

METOCLOPRAMIDE

Metoclopramide (Reglan, Schwarz Pharma) is a central dopaminergic antagonist and peripheral 5-HT_3 receptor antagonist and 5-HT_4 receptor agonist with GI and CNS effects. Metoclopramide stimulates and coordinates esophageal, gastric, pyloric, and duodenal motor activity. It increases lower esophageal sphincter tone and stimulates gastric contractions, while relaxing the pylorus and duodenum. Metoclopramide is administered to control nausea and vomiting associated with chemotherapy and as an antiemetic for dogs with parvoviral enteritis. Metoclopramide is effective in treating postoperative ileus in dogs, which is characterized by decreased GI myoelectric activity and motility.[19] Metoclopramide has little or no effect on colonic motility, so it is not useful in cats with megacolon.

Metoclopramide readily crosses the blood-brain barrier, where dopamine antagonism at the chemoreceptor trigger zone produces an antiemetic effect. However, dopamine antagonism in the striatum causes adverse effects known collectively as extrapyramidal signs, which include involuntary muscle spasms, motor restlessness, and inappropriate aggression. Many practitioners can relate stories of frenzied dogs and cats with resulting human injuries after metoclopramide administration. If recognized in time, the extrapyramidal signs can be reversed by restoring an appropriate dopamine to ACH balance with the anticholinergic action of diphenhydramine hydrochloride (Benadryl, Johnson & Johnson, Inc.) administered at a dose of 1.0 mg/kg IV.

Metoclopramide is available in 5- and 10-mg tablets, as 1 mg/ml oral solution, and as a 5 mg/ml injectable formulation. In dogs and cats, it is dosed at 0.2 to 0.5 mg/kg q8h, PO or SC, at least 30 minutes before a meal and at bedtime. It also can be given by continuous IV infusion at 0.01 to 0.02 mg/kg/hr.

Ghrelin Mimetics and Motilin Receptor Agonists

Ghrelin and motilin participate in initiating the migrating motor complex in the stomach and stimulate gastrointestinal motility, accelerate gastric emptying, and induce "gastric hunger." Ghrelin mimetics and motilin agonists currently are being developed to reverse gastrointestinal hypomotility disorders.

Rikkunshito is a kampo herbal medicine that is used widely in Japan for the treatment of the upper gastrointestinal disorders by potentiating ghrelin. In dogs, intragastric administration of rikkunshito stimulated gastrointestinal contractions in the interdigestive state through cholinergic neurons and 5-HT type 3 receptors and increased plasma ghrelin levels.[20]

Macrolide antibiotics, including erythromycin and clarithromycin, are motilin receptor agonists. At microbially ineffective doses, they stimulate migrating motility complexes and antegrade peristalsis in the proximal GI tract. They also appear to stimulate cholinergic and noncholinergic neuronal pathways that increase motility. Erythromycin increases gastroesophageal sphincter pressure in dogs and cats, so it should be useful in treating gastroesophageal reflux and reflux esophagitis.[21] Erythromycin increases gastric emptying rate in normal dogs; however, large food chunks may enter the small intestine and be digested inadequately.[6] Erythromycin accelerates colonic transit in the dog and stimulates canine but not feline colonic smooth muscle in vitro.[21]

Human pharmacokinetic studies indicate that erythromycin suspension is the ideal dosage form for administration of erythromycin as a prokinetic agent. The suggested prokinetic dose is 0.5 to 1.0 mg/kg q8h. Nonantibiotic derivatives of erythromycin are being developed as prokinetic agents. Mitemcinal is a motilin agonist derived from erythromycin that accelerated gastric emptying in dogs with normal and delayed gastric emptying better than cisapride.[22] In a dose-dependent manner, mitemcinal also stimulated antroduodenal motility in the interdigestive and digestive states. Oral administration of mitemcinal (0.3 to 3 mg/kg) stimulated colonic motility and accelerated bowel movement after feeding without inducing diarrhea in dogs.[23] Mitemcinal is currently in development as a treatment for diabetic gastroparesis in humans.

Acetylcholinesterase Inhibitors

Ranitidine (Zantac, Boehringer Ingelheim) and nizatidine (Axid, Braintree Laboratories) are histamine H_2 receptor antagonists that are prokinetics in addition to inhibiting gastric acid secretion.[24,25] Their prokinetic activity is due to acetylcholinesterase inhibition, with the greatest activity seen in the proximal GI tract. Cimetidine and famotidine are not acetylcholinesterase inhibitors and do not have prokinetic effects. Ranitidine and nizatidine stimulate GI motility by increasing the amount of acetylcholinesterase available to bind smooth muscle muscarinic cholinergic receptors. However, oral ranitidine had no detectable effect on gastrointestinal transit times in normal dogs using a wireless motility capsule system,[26] and it does not reduce the incidence of gastroesophageal reflux when given before anesthesia in dogs.[27]

Ranitidine is available as 75-mg (available over the counter in the United States and Canada), 150-mg and 300-mg tablets, a 15 mg/ml syrup, and a 25 mg/ml injectable solution. An oral dose of 1 to 2 mg/kg every 12 hours inhibits gastric acid secretion as well as stimulating gastric emptying. Nizatidine is available as 75-mg (available over the counter in the United States only), 150-mg, and 300-mg capsules. Like ranitidine, at gastric antisecretory doses of 2.5 to 5 mg/kg, nizatidine also has prokinetic effects. Ranitidine causes less interference with cytochrome P450 metabolism of other drugs than cimetidine and nizatidine does not affect hepatic microsomal enzyme activity, so both drugs have a wide margin of safety.

Acotiamide is a novel selective acetylcholinesterase inhibitor that has gastroprokinetic action in the dog via cholinergic pathways.[28] It currently is undergoing clinical trials for the treatment of functional dyspepsia in people.

REFERENCES

1. Holland CT, Satchell PM, Farrow BR: Selective vagal afferent dysfunction in dogs with congenital idiopathic megaoesophagus, Auton Neurosci 99:18-23, 2002.
2. Gaynor AR, Shofer FS, Washabau RJ: Risk factors for acquired megaesophagus in dogs, J Am Vet Med Assoc 211:1406-1412, 1997.
3. Shelton GD, Ho M, Kass PH: Risk factors for acquired myasthenia gravis in cats: 105 cases (1986-1998), J Am Vet Med Assoc 216:55-57, 2000.
4. Bexfield NH, Watson PJ, Herrtage ME: Esophageal dysmotility in young dogs, J Vet Intern Med 20:1314-1318, 2006.
5. Dewey CW, Cerda-Gonzalez S, Fletcher DJ, et al: Mycophenolate mofetil treatment in dogs with serologically diagnosed acquired myasthenia gravis: 27 cases (1999-2008), J Am Vet Med Assoc 236:664-668, 2010.
6. Hall JA, Washabau RJ: Diagnosis and treatment of gastric motility disorders, Vet Clin North Am Small Anim Pract 29:377-395, 1999.
7. Cannon M: Hair balls in cats: a normal nuisance or a sign that something is wrong? J Feline Med Surg 15:21-29, 2013.
8. Woosley KP: The problem of gastric atony, Clin Tech Small Anim Pract 19:43-48, 2004.
9. MacPhail C: Gastrointestinal obstruction, Clin Tech Small Anim Pract 17:178-183, 2002.
10. Bertoy RW: Megacolon in the cat, Vet Clin North Am Small Anim Pract 32:901-915, 2002.
11. Washabau RJ, Holt D: Pathogenesis, diagnosis, and therapy of feline idiopathic megacolon, Vet Clin North Am Small Anim Pract 29:589-603, 1999.
12. Washabau RJ, Stalis IH: Alterations in colonic smooth muscle function in cats with idiopathic megacolon, Am J Vet Res 57:580-587, 1996.
13. White RN: Surgical management of constipation, J Feline Med Surg 4:129-138, 2002.
14. Gershon MD: Review article: serotonin receptors and transporters—roles in normal and abnormal gastrointestinal motility, Aliment Pharmacol Ther 20(suppl)7:3-14, 2004.
15. Hasler AH, Washabau RJ: Cisapride stimulates contraction of idiopathic megacolonic smooth muscle in cats, J Vet Intern Med 11:313-318, 1997.
16. Matsunaga Y, Tanaka T, Yoshinaga K, et al: Acotiamide hydrochloride (Z-338), a new selective acetylcholinesterase inhibitor, enhances gastric motility without prolonging QT interval in dogs: comparison with cisapride, itopride, and mosapride, J Pharmacol Exp Ther 336:791-800, 2011.
17. Tsukamoto A, Ohno K, Maeda S, et al: Prokinetic effect of the 5-HT4R agonist mosapride on canine gastric motility, J Vet Med Sci 73:1635-1637, 2011.
18. Tsukamoto A, Ohno K, Tsukagoshi T, et al: Ultrasonographic evaluation of vincristine-induced gastric hypomotility and the prokinetic effect of mosapride in dogs, J Vet Intern Med 25:1461-1464, 2011.
19. Graves GM, Becht JL, Rawlings CA: Metoclopramide reversal of decreased gastrointestinal myoelectric and contractile activity in a model of canine postoperative ileus, Vet Surg 18:27-33, 1989.
20. Yanai M, Mochiki E, Ogawa A, et al: Intragastric administration of rikkunshito stimulates upper gastrointestinal motility and gastric emptying in conscious dogs, J Gastroenterol, 2012.
21. Washabau RJ: Gastrointestinal motility disorders and gastrointestinal prokinetic therapy, Vet Clin North Am Small Anim Pract 33:1007-1028, vi, 2003.
22. Onoma M, Yogo K, Ozaki K, et al: Oral mitemcinal (GM-611), an erythromycin-derived prokinetic, accelerates normal and experimentally

delayed gastric emptying in conscious dogs, Clin Exp Pharmacol Physiol 35:35-42, 2008.
23. Ozaki K, Sudo H, Muramatsu H, et al: Mitemcinal (GM-611), an orally active motilin receptor agonist, accelerates colonic motility and bowel movement in conscious dogs, Inflammopharmacology 15:36-42, 2007.
24. Bertaccini G, Coruzzi G, Poli E: Histamine H2 receptor antagonists may modify dog intestinal motility independently of their primary action on the H2 receptors, Pharmacol Res Commun 17:241-254, 1985.
25. Ueki S, Matsunaga Y, Yoneta T, et al: Gastroprokinetic activity of nizatidine during the digestive state in the dog and rat, Arzneimittelforschung 49:618-625, 1999.
26. Lidbury JA, Suchodolski JS, Ivanek R, et al: Assessment of the variation associated with repeated measurement of gastrointestinal transit times and assessment of the effect of oral ranitidine on gastrointestinal transit times using a wireless motility capsule system in dogs, Vet Med Int 2012:938417, 2012.
27. Favarato ES, Souza MV, Costa PR, et al: Evaluation of metoclopramide and ranitidine on the prevention of gastroesophageal reflux episodes in anesthetized dogs, Res Vet Sci 93:466-467, 2012.
28. Nagahama K, Matsunaga Y, Kawachi M, et al: Acotiamide, a new orally active acetylcholinesterase inhibitor, stimulates gastrointestinal motor activity in conscious dogs, Neurogastroenterol Motil 24:566-574, e256, 2012.

CHAPTER 119
GASTROINTESTINAL HEMORRHAGE

Søren R. Boysen, DVM, DACVECC

KEY POINTS

- Gastrointestinal hemorrhage is an important cause of blood loss anemia.
- In dogs and cats gastrointestinal ulceration is the most commonly reported cause of gastrointestinal hemorrhage.
- Nonsteroidal antiinflammatory drugs and hepatic disease are frequent causes of gastrointestinal ulceration in dogs.
- Neoplasia is a common cause of gastrointestinal ulceration in cats.
- Severe thrombocytopenia should not be overlooked as a cause of gastrointestinal hemorrhage in dogs.
- Hematemesis and melena suggest gastrointestinal hemorrhage but are not always noted.
- With acute severe gastrointestinal hemorrhage, the primary objective is to assess rapidly the patient's cardiovascular status and institute resuscitative efforts if shock is present.
- It is reasonable to administer gastrointestinal protectants before confirming the cause of gastrointestinal hemorrhage.
- Most cases of gastrointestinal hemorrhage respond well to medical treatment, although surgery may be indicated in others.

Gastrointestinal (GI) hemorrhage is an important cause of blood loss anemia and a potentially life-threatening condition in dogs.[1] It is reported less frequently in cats. It may be acute or chronic, occult (no visible blood) or overt (grossly visible blood), and can vary from mild, self-limiting states to severe life-threatening conditions. Significant GI hemorrhage often can be detected during history and physical examination. However, on occasion even acute severe GI hemorrhage may be overlooked if signs localizing blood loss to the GI tract are not present or if concurrent disease obscures the diagnosis.[2,3] In addition, because even mild cases may progress to life-threatening events, it is important to identify rapidly patients with GI hemorrhage and institute therapies to prevent their deterioration.

ETIOLOGY

GI hemorrhage in dogs and cats can be the result of a primary insult to the GI tract or may be secondary to a systemic disease process. It may originate in the esophagus, stomach, small intestine, or large intestine. As such, a number of pathologic processes have been associated with GI hemorrhage. In general, these can be divided into three broad categories: diseases causing ulcers, diseases causing coagulopathies, and diseases associated with vascular anomalies. Some diseases are difficult to classify into one of the above categories, and animals may have single or multiple predisposing causes.[1,4] Diseases associated with GI ulceration and/or GI hemorrhage in dogs and cats are listed in Box 119-1.

The most common cause of GI hemorrhage in dogs and cats is GI ulceration.[3-6] The severity of GI hemorrhage associated with ulcers varies with the degree and extent of mucosal erosion. With erosion into an underlying artery, the magnitude of bleeding is related to the size of the arterial defect and the diameter of the artery.[7] Nonsteroidal antiinflammatory drugs (NSAIDs) and hepatic disease are the most commonly reported risk factors for ulcers in dogs (Figure 119-1).[4] Neoplasia is a common risk factor for ulcers in cats; systemic mastocytosis, gastrinoma, intestinal lymphosarcoma, and adenocarcinoma are the most commonly reported tumors.[3] Inflammatory bowel disease also may be an important nonneoplastic cause of GI ulceration in cats and dogs.[3,8] Stress ulcers are a frequent cause of GI hemorrhage in critically ill human patients and have been reported in dogs and cats after hypovolemia and surgery.[3,9] The true incidence and significance of stress ulcers in critically ill cats and dogs has not been determined but should be considered in patients that develop GI hemorrhage while in the hospital.

Coagulation disorders associated with GI hemorrhage include rodenticide toxicity, disseminated intravascular coagulation, coagulation factor deficiencies (factor XII and prekallikrein deficiency), and thrombocytopenia.[1,5] Thrombocytopenia is the most common coagulation disorder resulting in GI hemorrhage in dogs and should

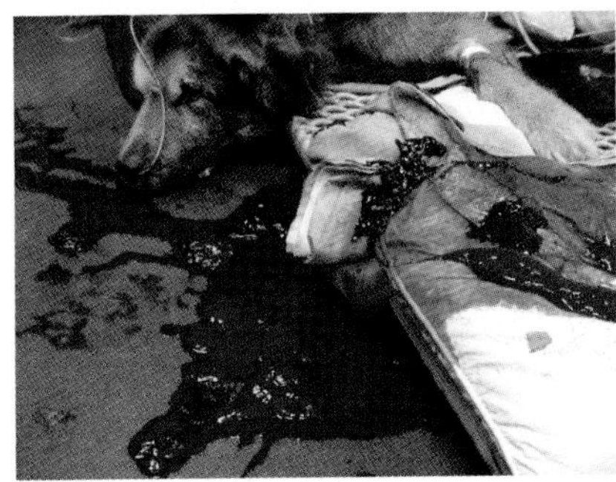

FIGURE 119-1 Severe hematemesis in a dog subsequent to ingestion of naproxen, a nonselective nonsteroidal anti-inflammatory drug used in humans. Although this case involved accidental ingestion, gastrointestinal hemorrhage has been reported in animals after administration of nonsteroidal antiinflammatory drugs at recommended therapeutic dosages.

BOX 119-1 *Diseases Associated with Gastrointestinal Ulceration and Hemorrhage in Dogs and Cats*

Drug Administration

NSAIDs
Glucocorticoids

Systemic and Metabolic Diseases

Hepatic disease
Uremia
Pancreatitis
Hypoadrenocorticism

Ischemic Events

GDV
Mesenteric volvulus
Mesenteric thrombosis
Intussusception

Neurologic Disease

Head trauma
IVDD
Mucosal trauma
Foreign bodies

Fungal Infections

Pythium
Histoplasma

Bacterial Infections

Salmonella
Clostridium spp.
Campylobacter
Helicobacter (controversial)

Parasitic Infections

Hookworms
Whipworms
Coccidia
Roundworms

Viral Infections

Parvovirus
Coronavirus

Algal Infections

Protothecosis

Systemic neoplasia

Mastocytosis
Gastrinoma

Gastrointestinal Neoplasia

Lymphoma
Adenocarcinoma
Leiomyoma
Leiomyosarcoma
Hemangioma

Stress of Critical Illness

Major surgery
Hypovolemia
Sepsis

Miscellaneous

IBD
Polyps
Idiopathic eosinophilic masses
HGE

GDV, Gastric dilatation-volvulus; *GI,* gastrointestinal; *HGE,* hemorrhagic gastroenteritis; *IBD,* inflammatory bowel disease; *IVDD,* intervertebral disk disease; *NSAIDs,* nonsteroidal antiinflammatory drugs.

not be overlooked.[1] Coagulation disorders resulting in GI hemorrhage appear to be less common in cats.

Vascular anomalies, because of the high incidence of varices, are a common cause of GI hemorrhage in humans. In contrast, only a few cases of vascular anomaly have been reported in the veterinary literature, and it appears to be an infrequent cause of GI hemorrhage in dogs and cats.[10] It should be considered when more common causes of GI hemorrhage have been ruled out.

HISTORY AND PHYSICAL EXAMINATION

With extensive hemorrhage, vomiting, diarrhea, or ulcer perforation, patients with GI hemorrhage may be presented in a state of shock resulting from blood loss, hypovolemia, endotoxemia, or sepsis. Examination findings consistent with shock include tachycardia, diminished or thready arterial pulses (particularly peripheral), cool extremities, prolonged capillary refill time, and pale mucous membranes. Immediate resuscitative therapies to reverse the state of shock take precedence (see Chapters 5 and 60), and localization of the site of hemorrhage and tailored therapies may have to be delayed until the cardiovascular system is stable.

Once resuscitative efforts have commenced, a complete history and physical examination should be performed. Hematemesis (vomitus with the appearance of coffee grounds or frank blood), hematochezia (passage of bright red or frank blood with or without stool), or melena (black, tarry stool) suggests the GI tract as a source of hemorrhage. However, these signs are not always evident clinically and may not appear until significant GI hemorrhage has occurred.[3,4,11] With duodenal hemorrhage, if reflux of duodenal contents into the stomach is insufficient, blood may not be visible in the vomitus.[12] However, when it is present, hematemesis suggests ongoing blood loss.[13] Diseases of the nasal cavity and oropharynx occasionally can cause hematemesis and melena from swallowing blood of epistaxis or hemoptysis (coughing of blood). In addition, activated charcoal, metronidazole, bismuth (Pepto-Bismol), and diets high in iron (liver, unsweetened baking chocolate) can result in dark stools and should not be confused with melena.[14]

A history of aspirin or other NSAID administration is not uncommon.[4,11,15] Case reports exist of GI ulceration, hemorrhage, and GI perforation occurring in veterinary patients that have received selective cyclooxygenase inhibitors at recommended therapeutic dosages.[11] Decrease or loss of appetite with or without other signs of GI disease should prompt consideration of GI side effects in any patients receiving NSAIDs. The medication should be discontinued and the patient should be examined. In cases of thrombocytopenia or coagulation disorders, there may be a history of bleeding from other sites of the body, including the nasal cavities or urinary tract. Thorough examination of the mucosal surfaces may reveal petechiae in severely thrombocytopenic patients. A search for subcutaneous nodules or masses may detect underlying mast cell tumors.

Because GI hemorrhage may be insidious in onset, especially when chronic, the abdomen should be examined carefully. Abdominal palpation may localize areas of pain (tenderness, voluntary or involuntary guarding) or induce nausea, identify masses or foreign objects, or detect abdominal distention or a fluid wave. Splenomegaly or hepatomegaly may be identified in patients with mastocytosis, other neoplasia, or hepatic diseases. A careful rectal examination should be performed to detect frank blood or melena and to look for masses or foreign bodies.

Localizing the site of GI hemorrhage is important because the cause, diagnostic tests, and therapies for upper and lower GI hemorrhage may vary.[5,14] Although hemorrhage from any site in the GI tract can be serious, upper GI hemorrhage tends to be more severe.[13,14] Hematemesis or melena suggests upper GI hemorrhage.[14] However, it is the amount of time the blood remains in the GI tract and not necessarily the site of bleeding that determines its color.[14,15] Delayed GI transit time and retention of blood in the colon could result in melena associated with a lower GI tract lesion.[14,16] Hematochezia is usually reflective of large intestinal, rectal, or anal hemorrhage;

however, severe acute intestinal hemorrhage can act as a cathartic, significantly decreasing GI transit time.[13-15] This may result in the passage of frank blood in the stool after significant blood loss into the upper GI tract.[13,15]

DIAGNOSTIC TESTS

GI hemorrhage is confirmed when a source of bleeding is localized to the GI tract. Patients with signs of shock should have emergency minimum blood tests performed (hematocrit, total protein, blood urea nitrogen [BUN], glucose and, if available, pH, lactate, and electrolytes) while resuscitative efforts and a search for the underlying cause are undertaken. In cases suspected to have hemoabdomen or septic peritonitis, abdominocentesis, emergency abdominal sonography, and possibly diagnostic peritoneal lavage are warranted and may be performed during initial resuscitation of the patient. Once resuscitative efforts have commenced or the patient's condition has stabilized, other diagnostic modalities should be considered.

Tests to Help Detect Presence of Gastrointestinal Hemorrhage

Certain hematologic and biochemical abnormalities are suggestive of GI hemorrhage. Anemia of undetermined origin should prompt consideration of GI hemorrhage. The finding of microcytic, hypochromic anemia (iron deficiency anemia) is reported with chronic GI hemorrhage.[4] However, because iron deficiency anemia takes time to develop, normocytic normochromic anemia is more common in cases of recent GI hemorrhage.[1,4] A high BUN-to-creatinine ratio (greater than 20) has been reported with GI hemorrhage.[16] This phenomenon has been explained by volume depletion and intestinal absorption of proteins, including digested blood, into the circulatory system.[16] However, diseases resulting in increased protein metabolism (fever, burns, infections, starvation, and administration of glucocorticoids) also may result in an increased BUN-to-creatinine ratio.[1,16] Large bowel hemorrhage reportedly has little effect on BUN levels, and many dogs with GI hemorrhage do not have an elevation in the BUN concentration.[1,16,17]

In equivocal cases of GI hemorrhage a fecal occult blood test (most of which rely on the peroxidase activity of hemoglobin) may be performed. Although helpful for detecting occult GI hemorrhage, diets containing red meat or having high peroxidase activity, such as fish, fruits, or vegetables, can cause false-positive results.[18] Animals should be fed a meat-free diet for at least 72 hours before a fecal occult blood test.[19] The presence of peroxidase-producing bacteria within the GI tract also may cause false-positive results.[18] Despite false-positive results a negative fecal occult blood test result does rule out significant GI hemorrhage.[2] When significant gastric hemorrhage is suspected, passage of a nasogastric tube and aspiration of the stomach contents may confirm and help localize the site of GI hemorrhage. However, this procedure may cause discomfort, and false-negative results have been reported.[12,17]

Tests to Help Identify Underlying Causes

A coagulation profile, complete blood count, routine biochemistry profile, electrolytes, adrenocorticotropic hormone stimulation testing, imaging, and endoscopy often are indicated to try to identify the underlying cause of GI hemorrhage.

The coagulation profile may identify coagulopathies such as rodenticide intoxication or clotting factor deficiencies. It also may detect prolonged bleeding times that are not the direct cause of GI hemorrhage. The platelet count is important, because immune-mediated thrombocytopenia is a common cause of moderate to severe GI hemorrhage in dogs.[1] An elevated hematocrit in a patient with acute hemorrhagic diarrhea and a relatively normal plasma protein concentration is suggestive of hemorrhagic gastroenteritis.[19]

Biochemical markers reflective of hepatic and renal disease may be evident (alkaline phosphatase, alanine aminotransferase, aspartate aminotransferase, and bilirubin in cases of hepatic disease; and urea, creatinine, and phosphorus in cases of renal disease). Because hypoadrenocorticism has been reported as a cause of severe GI hemorrhage in the dog, electrolyte levels should be evaluated and an adrenocorticotropic hormone (ACTH) stimulation test performed if another cause for GI hemorrhage cannot be found.[20] Fecal smears, cultures, and parvovirus testing may be indicated if infectious disease is suspected. Measurement of gastrin levels is recommended in cases of recurrent GI ulceration and in cases that fail to respond to medical therapy.[4]

Radiographs may detect foreign bodies, masses, or free air in the peritoneal cavity. Pneumoperitoneum is suggestive of GI perforation in a patient that has not undergone recent abdominal surgery. Although contrast radiographs may identify gastrointestinal mucosal defects, they generally have been replaced by ultrasonography and endoscopy.[4,17] Ultrasonography may identify foreign bodies and masses and may help to identify concurrent GI perforation when present.[21,22] The use of ultrasonography to identify ulcers in dogs has been described. It allows evaluation of the intestinal wall structure and thickness and can detect the presence of a defect or crater.[22] When used serially, it may help determine changes in response to therapy and has suggested the need for surgery in some instances.[22] Ultrasonography also has been reported in the assessment of cats with GI ulceration.[3]

Endoscopy is considered the most sensitive test to evaluate upper GI tract hemorrhage and ulcers, although patients must be resuscitated optimally before the procedure.[7,17] It often provides a diagnosis, helps assess prognosis, and may have therapeutic benefits (i.e., foreign body retrieval). In addition to allowing direct visualization of the mucosa, it permits biopsies for histology and culture, which may be required to identify lesions and infectious diseases (i.e., neoplasia, inflammatory bowel disease, protothecosis). The disadvantages of endoscopy include the need for anesthesia, its limitation to the proximal GI tract and colon, the potential to exacerbate GI hemorrhage, and the possibility of causing iatrogenic ulcer perforation.[15]

If the above diagnostic procedures fail to identify the cause of significant ongoing GI hemorrhage, abdominal exploratory surgery, scintigraphy using technetium-labeled red blood cells, and arteriography should be considered.[2,17,19] Scintigraphy has been demonstrated to aid in localization of GI hemorrhage in dogs, and arteriography may help identity GI vascular anomalies.[2,10,19]

TREATMENT

The treatment priority in patients with GI hemorrhage is to stabilize the cardiovascular system, control ongoing hemorrhage, treat existing ulcers, prevent bacterial translocation, and to identify and address the underlying cause. Because of the large number of disease conditions that can result in GI hemorrhage, therapy directed toward correcting the underlying cause is variable (i.e., surgery for foreign bodies or tumors, steroids for hypoadrenocorticism, immunosuppressives for immune-mediated thrombocytopenia, discontinuation of NSAIDs). In considering the underlying cause, it is important to consider related or unrelated coagulation abnormalities (i.e., liver disease causing ulceration and a clotting factor deficiency) and to address concurrent diseases that may exacerbate GI hemorrhage (i.e., uremia in a patient on NSAIDs).

Medical Management

The initial priority is to identify rapidly and reverse any signs of shock (see Chapters 5 and 60). Depending on the duration and extent of blood loss, administration of packed red blood cells, whole blood, or hemoglobin-based oxygen-carrying solution may be indicated. In the patient with severe acute GI hemorrhage, this often is implemented as part of the initial resuscitation protocol. Guidelines regarding when to transfuse patients with GI hemorrhage that are anemic but cardiovascularly stable are not well established in veterinary medicine and are controversial in human medicine.[23] The hematocrit at which a patient requires a transfusion varies depending on the degree and rate of blood loss, hemodynamic status, initial and subsequent hematocrits, presence of concurrent illness, and severity of clinical signs.[24] If the patient displays clinical signs attributable to a decrease in oxygen delivery (i.e., tachycardia, hyperlactatemia, tachypnea) or if serial measurements reveal a decreasing hematocrit after initiating therapy, a blood transfusion is indicated.[24] The need for general anesthesia and surgery also may influence the decision of when to transfuse.

If GI hemorrhage is the result of a primary coagulopathy or is exacerbated by a secondary coagulopathy (i.e., disseminated intravascular coagulation, hepatic failure, shock, or dilution with aggressive fluid therapy), fresh frozen plasma should be considered. In patients with persistent GI hemorrhage as a result of thrombocytopenia, vincristine may increase the release of platelets from the bone marrow, although the function of these platelets has been questioned.[25]

The use of iced saline gastric lavage to decrease GI hemorrhage is no longer recommended[5,6]; it has not been proven to slow hemorrhage, is known to cause discomfort and rapidly can lower core body temperature, which prolongs bleeding in experimental canine studies.[6,15]

Animals with hematemesis and melena should be treated for GI ulcers until proven otherwise. Medications known to cause ulcers should be discontinued (i.e., NSAIDs). Given the association between GI hemorrhage and steroids in dogs, unless they are considered essential to therapy (i.e., hypoadrenocorticism, immune-mediated diseases), they also should be discontinued.

It is reasonable to administer GI protectants before confirming the cause of GI hemorrhage, given that ulcers are the most common cause of GI hemorrhage in dogs and cats, and GI protectants have a wide safety margin. In addition, intraluminal gastric acid neutralization may slow GI hemorrhage by promoting mucosal homeostasis.[7,26] Commonly used GI protectants include acid suppressants such as histamine-2 receptor antagonists (cimetidine, ranitidine, famotidine) and proton pump inhibitors (omeprazole, pantoprazole), mucosal binding agents such as sucralfate, and synthetic prostaglandins such as misoprostol. There are no veterinary studies to conclude which gastroprotectants or combination of gastroprotectants is most efficacious in the management of GI ulcers. However, a study demonstrated that famotidine (0.5 mg/kg IV q12h), omeprazole (1 mg/kg PO q24h), and pantoprazole (1 mg/kg IV q24h) significantly suppressed gastric acid secretion in dogs, but ranitidine (2 mg/kg IV q24h) failed to show significant gastric acid suppression at the dosage evaluated.[26] In cases of NSAID toxicity, misoprostol may provide additional benefit (see Chapters 76 and 161).

In deciding which medications to use, clinicians should give consideration to the route of drug administration because absorption of medications administered orally in critically ill patients has been questioned, particularly if GI hypoperfusion is present. Many dogs with GI hemorrhage are also vomiting, which may further limit the utility of oral medications. In patients that have persistent vomiting, antiemetics can be used. Metoclopramide, given as a constant intravenous infusion (1 to 2 mg/kg q24h), often is tried initially. Cases refractory to metoclopramide may benefit from additional antiemetics such as ondansetron. Because many causes of GI hemorrhage are associated with discomfort and pain, analgesics such as an opioid should be considered.

Although controversial, in cases with significant GI hemorrhage and suspected GI mucosal barrier compromise, broad-spectrum antibiotics (i.e., a penicillin and an aminoglycoside or fluoroquinolone, or a combination of a cephalosporin, metronidazole, and an aminoglycoside or fluoroquinolone) are warranted because of the risk of bacterial translocation. Broad-spectrum antibiotics also are recommended in patients that are septic. Ideally, samples for culture and susceptibility (i.e., urine and blood) should be collected before starting antibiotic therapy. In cases in which GI mucosal barrier compromise is not believed to be a factor (i.e., idiopathic immune mediated thrombocytopenia) and there is no evidence of sepsis, supportive therapy and addressing the underlying cause supersedes the administration of broad-spectrum antibiotics. A recent study evaluating the efficacy of amoxicillin/clavulanic acid in dogs with aseptic idiopathic acute hemorrhagic gastroenteritis found no difference in morbidity or mortality in patients treated with antibiotics compared with those given a placebo.[27]

Endoscopy, Interventional Radiology, and Surgery

Most cases of GI hemorrhage can be managed medically. In cases of severe GI ulceration and hemorrhage refractory to medical treatment, endoscopic hemostasis may be beneficial. Upper GI endoscopy is recommended for the diagnosis and treatment of upper GI bleeding in people: the source of bleeding can be identified in up to 95% of cases and endoscopic therapy is reported to be effective in 80% to 90% of patients.[28] Ulcer hemostasis has been described by injecting epinephrine or 98% alcohol through an endoscope sclerotomy needle into the base of an ulcer.[7,29] The combination of epinephrine injection and use of either endoclips, endoscopic cautery (thermal, electric, or laser), or fibrin/thrombin injections currently is recommended in people to control GI hemorrhage unresponsive to medical management.[7,12,30] In people, endoscopic therapy also is indicated for active arterial bleeding as well as visualization of a nonbleeding vessel or an adherent blood clot because both findings are associated with high risk of rebleeding (50% and 25% to 30%, respectively).[30] Surgery can be avoided in most cases but is indicated for preexisting surgical disease (foreign body, tumor, septic abdomen) in patients at risk of exsanguination or perforation (based on endoscopy or serial sonographic evaluation), or if the patient fails to respond to medical therapy. An equally efficacious alternative to surgery with lower morbidity in human studies is percutaneous angiography and embolization, which may be applicable to veterinary patients.[30,31]

PROGNOSIS

Many cases of GI hemorrhage are self-limiting and the prognosis varies with the underlying cause. In cases of moderate to severe GI hemorrhage requiring a blood transfusion, the prognosis is reportedly fair to poor, with a mortality rate of 29% to 45%.[1]

REFERENCES

1. Waldrop JE, Rozanski EA, Freeman LM, et al: Packed red blood cell transfusions in dogs with gastrointestinal hemorrhage: 55 cases (1999-2001), J Am Anim Hosp Assoc 39:523, 2003.
2. Washabau RJ: Acute gastrointestinal hemorrhage. Part I. Approach to patients, Comp Cont Educ Pract Vet 1:1317, 1996.

3. Liptak JM, Hunt GB, Barrs VRD, et al: Gastroduodenal ulceration in cats: eight cases and a review of the literature, J Feline Med Surg 4:27, 2002.
4. Stanton ME, Ronald BM: Gastroduodenal ulceration in dogs: retrospective study of 43 cases and literature review, J Vet Intern Med 3:238, 1989.
5. Washabau RJ: Acute gastrointestinal hemorrhage. Part II. Causes and therapy, Comp Cont Educ Pract Vet 1:1327, 1996.
6. Kirk RW, Bonagura JD, editors: Kirk's current veterinary therapy XI, St Louis, 1992, Saunders.
7. Palmer K: Management of haematemesis and melaena, Postgrad Med J 80:399, 2004.
8. Lyles SE, Panciera GK, Saunders GK, et al: Idiopathic eosinophilic masses of the gastrointestinal tract in dogs, J Vet Intern Med 23:818-823, 2009.
9. Hinton LE, McLoughlin MA, Johnson SE, et al: Spontaneous gastroduodenal perforation 16 dogs and 7 cats (1982-1999), J Am Anim Hosp Assoc 38:176, 2002.
10. Gelens HCJ, Moreau RE, Stalis IH, et al: Arteriovenous fistula of the jejunum associated with gastrointestinal hemorrhage in a dog, J Am Vet Med Assoc 202:1867, 1993.
11. Enberg TB, Braun LD, Kuzma AB: Gastrointestinal perforation in five dogs associated with the administration of meloxicam, J Vet Emerg Crit Care 16:34, 2006.
12. Kupfer Y, Cappell MS, Tessler S: Acute gastrointestinal bleeding in the intensive care unit, Gastroenterol Clin North Am 29:275, 2000.
13. Zuckerman GR: Acute gastrointestinal bleeding: clinical essentials for the initial evaluation and risk assessment by the primary care clinician, J Am Osteopath Assoc 100:S4, 2000.
14. Case VL: Melena and hematochezia. In Ettinger SJ, Feldman EC, editors: Textbook of veterinary internal medicine, ed 7, St Louis, 2010, Saunders.
15. Shaw N, Burrows CF, King RR: Massive gastric hemorrhage induced by buffered aspirin in a Greyhound, J Am Anim Hosp Assoc 33:215, 1997.
16. Prause LC, Grauer GF: Association of gastrointestinal hemorrhage with increased blood urea nitrogen and BUN/creatinine ratio in dogs: a literature review and retrospective study, Vet Clin Pathol 27:107, 1998.
17. Steiner J, editor: Small animal gastroenterology, Hannover, 2008, Schluetersche (distributed by Manson publishing).
18. Tuffli SP, Gaschen F, Neiger R: Effect of dietary factors on the detection of fecal occult blood in cats, J Vet Diagn Invest 13:177, 2001.
19. Hall EJ, German AJ: Diseases of the small intestine. In Ettinger SJ, Feldman EC, editors: Textbook of veterinary internal medicine, ed 7, St Louis, 2010, Saunders.
20. Medinger TL, Williams DA, Bruyette DS: Severe gastrointestinal tract hemorrhage in three dogs with hypoadrenocorticism, J Am Vet Med Assoc 202:1869, 1993.
21. Boysen SR, Tidwell AS, Penninck DG: Ultrasonographic findings in dogs and cats with gastrointestinal perforation, Vet Radiol Ultrasound 44:556, 2003.
22. Penninck DG, Matz M, Tidwell AS: Ultrasonographic detection of gastric ulceration, Vet Radiol Ultrasound 38:308, 1997.
23. Villanueva C, Colomo A, Bosch A, et al: Transfusion strategies for acute upper gastrointestinal bleeding, N Eng J Med 368(1):11-21, 2013.
24. Maltz GS, Siegel JE, Carson JL: Hematologic management of gastrointestinal bleedings, Gastroenterol Clin North Am 29:169, 2000.
25. Rozanski EA, Callan MB, Hughes DH, et al: Comparison of platelet count recovery with use of vincristine and prednisone or prednisone alone for treatment of severe immune-mediated thrombocytopenia in dogs, J Am Vet Med Assoc 220:477, 2002.
26. Bersenas AM, Mathews KA, Allen DG, et al: Effects of ranitidine, famotidine, pantoprazole, and omeprazole on intragastric pH in dogs, Am J Vet Res 66:425, 2005.
27. Unterer S, Strohmeyer BD, Kruse C, et al: Treatment of aseptic dogs with hemorrhagic gastroenteritis with amoxicillin/clavulanic acid: a prospective blinded study, J Vet Intern Med 25:973-979, 2011.
28. Millward S: ACR appropriateness criteria on treatment of acute nonvariceal gastrointestinal tract bleeding, J Am Coll Radiol 5:550-554, 2008.
29. Matz ME: Endoscopy. In Wingfield WE, Raffe MR, editors: The veterinary ICU book, Jackson Hole, Wyo, 2002, Teton NewMedia.
30. Dineson L, Benson M: Managing acute upper gastrointestinal bleeding in the acute assessment unit, Clin Med 12(6):589-593, 2012.
31. Ripoll C, Banares R, Baceiro I, et al: Comparison of transcatheter arterial embolization and surgery for treatment of bleeding peptic ulcer after endoscopic treatment failure, J Vasc Radiol 15:447-550, 2004.

CHAPTER 120

REGURGITATION AND VOMITING

Peter S. Chapman, BVetMed, DECVIM-CA, DACVIM (Internal Medicine), MRCVS

KEY POINTS

- Differentiation between vomiting and regurgitation is important before proceeding with further diagnostic testing or therapy.
- Idiopathic megaesophagus is the most common cause of persistent regurgitation in the adult dog. Myasthenia gravis is the most common cause of secondary megaesophagus, accounting for 20% to 30% of all cases. Aspiration pneumonia is the most important cause of morbidity in the regurgitating patient.
- The multitude of differential diagnoses for vomiting can be subdivided into primary gastrointestinal and other causes.
- Abdominal imaging is critical in the evaluation of the patient with persistent vomiting. Radiographs have reasonable sensitivity for the identification of obstruction, but ultrasonography may be preferred, if available, given its higher sensitivity.

DIFFERENTIATION OF VOMITING AND REGURGITATION

Before formulating a diagnostic and therapeutic plan, clinicians must define the patient's clinical problem. Most importantly, vomiting and regurgitation must be distinguished. Pet owners may not differentiate between the two problems, but the diagnostic investigation and treatment options differ significantly. It also may be necessary to differentiate respiratory signs from gastrointestinal (GI) signs because some pet owners mistake the harsh coughing and retching of from diseases such as canine infectious tracheobronchitis for attempts at vomiting. In most cases the problem can be defined accurately after taking a thorough history. Historic findings likely to assist in the differentiation between vomiting and regurgitation are presented in

Table 120-1 **Comparison of the Key Features of Vomiting and Regurgitation**

Vomiting	Regurgitation
Premonitory signs (nausea) often seen (hypersalivation, depression, discomfort)	No premonitory signs
Active abdominal contractions	Passive ejection of food
May occur at any time	Typically occurs shortly after ingestion of food
Digested food	Undigested food, may conform to the cylindric shape of the esophagus
Bile may be present	No bile

Table 120-1. Premonitory signs, active abdominal contractions, and the presence of bile in the vomitus are the characteristics that are most useful for distinguishing vomiting because they are seen uncommonly in regurgitating patients. However, regurgitating animals may stretch and arch their necks, mimicking abdominal contractions, and the response to pain from an inflamed or ulcerated esophagus may resemble the classic signs of nausea. Ptyalism is commonly seen secondary to nausea in vomiting patients or as a result of pooling and/or inability to swallow saliva effectively in animals with regurgitation.

True bile must be distinguished from the froth and saliva that animals with esophageal disease may regurgitate. Frequency of the episodes also can help define the problem; animals with esophageal disease may regurgitate saliva frequently (e.g., hourly) yet remain bright and systemically healthy. A vomiting animal is unlikely to sustain this frequency of vomiting without developing further systemic signs of illness, such as dehydration and lethargy.

BOX 120-1 *Important Differential Diagnoses for Regurgitation*

Pharyngeal Disease

Cricopharyngeal achalasia
Focal or generalized neuromuscular disease
Foreign body
Neoplasia

Esophageal Disease

Hypomotility: megaesophagus

Congenital
Idiopathic (primary)
Secondary
- Myasthenia gravis (20% to 30% of cases)
- Generalized neuromuscular disease
- Hypoadrenocorticism
- Lead toxicity
- Hypothyroidism
- Dysautonomia

Inflammation: esophagitis

Drug: chemical-induced
Gastroesophageal reflux
- General anesthesia
- Hiatal hernia
- Idiopathic

Lupus myositis
Spirocerca lupi infection

Mechanical obstruction

Esophageal stricture
Foreign body
Neoplasia
Vascular ring anomalies
Extraluminal compression (e.g., mediastinal mass)
Hiatal hernia
Gastroesophageal intussusception

REGURGITATION

Definition

Regurgitation is the passive ejection of food, water, or saliva associated with esophageal or, less commonly, pharyngeal disease.

Clinical Consequences of Regurgitation

The most significant clinical complication of regurgitation is aspiration pneumonia, which has been proven to be a significant negative prognostic indicator in patients with megaesophagus.[1] Regardless of the underlying disease, any patient with persistent regurgitation is at risk of aspiration pneumonia, and measures to reduce its occurrence such as appropriate feeding strategies, amended anesthetic protocols, and elevation of the head in recumbent patients should be instigated. Aspiration pneumonia is the most likely indication for hospitalization and intensive treatment of regurgitating patients. In the absence of aspiration pneumonia or other disease, most patients are able to maintain good hydration, although persistent regurgitation of undigested food may lead to marked weight loss.

Differential Diagnoses

Regurgitation is associated with esophageal or pharyngeal disease. It is more common in dogs than in cats. In most cases the problem is localized to the esophagus or pharynx, but it is sometimes a manifestation of systemic disease. Common differential diagnoses are provided in Box 120-1. Idiopathic megaesophagus is the most common cause of regurgitation in the adult dog, and most middle-age to older patients with uncomplicated regurgitation have this disease.[2] However, a significant subset of dogs with megaesophagus have focal myasthenia gravis in the absence of other neurologic signs.[3]

Many other concurrent diseases, such as hypothyroidism, have been reported to cause megaesophagus, but epidemiologic evidence supporting an association is lacking.[3] It is reasonable to exclude these diseases from the differential diagnosis if other clinical and clinicopathologic changes are lacking and the problem list is limited to regurgitation.

Diagnostic Approach

History

Important historic information includes access to drugs or caustic substances and recent drug therapy or anesthesia that may have precipitated esophagitis. Most cases of drug-induced esophagitis are a result of doxycycline administration, but many drugs have the potential to cause this side effect. Animals with esophagitis also may show signs of apparent esophageal discomfort, such as pain on swallowing (odynophagia), repeated swallowing attempts, lip smacking, and arching of the neck. These signs are seen less often in patients with megaesophagus, most of which regurgitate without premonitory signs and show no odynophagia.

Most animals that do not have odynophagia maintain a good appetite and often attempt to eat the regurgitated ingesta. Other systemic signs such as lethargy, anorexia, vomiting, and diarrhea are not seen in patients with uncomplicated esophageal disease and suggest a concurrent disease process or an underlying cause for the esophageal disease. Coughing or a sudden deterioration in the patient's clinical status should alert the clinician to the possibility of aspiration pneumonia.

Physical examination

The physical examination should include a thorough oral examination and palpation of the neck. Abnormalities in the neck may include masses, palpable esophageal dilation, or pain. In some cases, palpation of the esophagus may elicit regurgitation or discomfort. Any crackles ausculted over the lung fields should be noted, but these should be differentiated from sounds of fluid in the esophagus.

Clinical pathology

Routine hematology and biochemistry may show evidence of an underlying cause of megaesophagus. Results are unremarkable in most patients with uncomplicated idiopathic megaesophagus.

Diagnostic imaging

Thoracic radiography is the most important and useful imaging modality for evaluating patients with regurgitation. Plain radiographs are diagnostic in most cases of megaesophagus resulting from a foreign body obstruction. Plain radiographs also may show evidence of secondary aspiration pneumonia, mediastinal masses, or congenital abnormalities (e.g., vascular ring anomaly). Two lateral radiographs and an orthogonal view should be obtained to evaluate all lung fields. If plain radiographs do not show any abnormalities, contrast studies or endoscopy may be indicated. Abdominal ultrasonography rarely provides useful information in animals with regurgitation.

Further diagnostic testing

Serum should be submitted for acetylcholine receptor antibody assay on all patients with megaesophagus. Additional tests to consider based on clinical suspicion include an adrenocorticotropic hormone stimulation test, serology for antinuclear antibody, serum creatine phosphokinase activity, lead levels in the blood, electromyography and nerve conduction velocity, and muscle and nerve biopsy. Evidence for an association with hypothyroidism is lacking, but thyroid function (thyroid stimulating hormone assay, thyroid stimulating hormone stimulation, free and total thyroid hormone levels) testing may be warranted in individual patients with other suspicious signs.[3] Most patients with megaesophagus secondary to hypoadrenocorticism have electrolyte changes and other systemic signs.

General Treatment Guidelines

Most animals with regurgitation are stable and well hydrated and do not require emergent therapy before a definitive diagnosis is made. In the absence of concurrent disease, these patients can be treated on an outpatient basis and do not require hospitalization. Empiric treatment with a histamine-2 receptor antagonist or proton pump inhibitor is indicated to reduce the risk of secondary esophagitis (see Chapter 161). The addition of sucralfate may be warranted in patients with suspected active esophageal ulceration. The canine esophagus is comprised almost exclusively of striated muscle, so smooth muscle prokinetic agents such as metoclopramide and cisapride have no beneficial effect. Moreover, these agents could decrease the transit of ingesta to the stomach by increasing lower esophageal sphincter tone. Anecdotal reports show that the parasympathomimetic agent, bethanechol, is a useful prokinetic agent in dogs with megaesophagus, but data are lacking. The caudal third of the feline esophagus comprises smooth muscle. However, although prokinetics such as cisapride theoretically may be more useful in this species, primary esophageal dysmotility is uncommon in the cat.

Animals with secondary aspiration pneumonia require more intensive therapy and monitoring. These patients should be treated with broad-spectrum antimicrobials (see Chapter 23) and may require supplemental oxygen (see Chapter 14). Prolonged or repeated courses of antimicrobial agents may be required and, when possible, airway samples should be collected for cytology and culture before initiating antimicrobial therapy. If regurgitating animals require hospitalization, the priority should be to prevent aspiration pneumonia by feeding a high-calorie diet in small, frequent meals from an elevated or upright position, and dietary consistency should be tailored to the animal. Although intuitively a firm diet would appear to reduce the risk of aspiration, many patients have less frequent regurgitation when fed a more liquid ration. Animals that cannot maintain adequate nutritional balance with oral intake should be fed using a temporary or permanent gastrostomy tube (see Chapter 129). Esophagostomy and nasoesophageal tube placement is contraindicated.

Prognosis

Animals with congenital idiopathic megaesophagus have a fair prognosis. With adequate attention to caloric needs and prevention of aspiration pneumonia, many animals develop improved esophageal motility over several months. Pet owners must be committed to a prolonged period of physical therapy and nutritional support. The morbidity and mortality associated with acquired idiopathic megaesophagus continues to be unacceptably high. Patients with megaesophagus or other causes of regurgitation where a specific underlying disease can be identified and treated may have a better prognosis.

VOMITING

Definition

Vomiting is the forceful ejection of upper GI tract contents and may occur as a result of gastric, intestinal, or systemic disease.

Physiology of Vomiting

The vomiting reflex is mediated by the vomiting center in the medulla.[4] Vagal and sympathetic afferent pathways from the GI tract transmit impulses to the vomiting center when stimulated by inflammation or overdistention. The vomiting center also receives stimulation from within the brain: the vestibular system, cerebrum, and chemoreceptor trigger zone provide input to the vomiting center. The latter is a specialized region (area postrema) that is located on the floor of the fourth ventricle and lacks an intact blood-brain barrier. The chemoreceptor trigger zone is sensitive to several common drugs and toxins. The pathways involved in vomiting and the receptors involved are shown schematically in Figure 120-1.

Sufficient stimulation of the vomiting center results in the initiation of vomiting. A period of intestinal antiperistalsis is followed by a highly coordinated sequence of events, beginning with a deep inspiration and ending with a strong simultaneous contraction of the diaphragm and abdominal wall musculature and relaxation of the lower esophageal sphincter.

Clinical Consequences of Vomiting

The principal deleterious consequence of vomiting is dehydration as a result of fluid loss in the vomitus and a reduced fluid intake. The loss of GI contents compounded by dehydration may lead to electrolyte and acid-base disturbances. A hypochloremic metabolic alkalosis, primarily resulting from the loss of gastric contents rich in hydrogen and chloride ions, with or without a contraction alkalosis, is the most common finding in dogs with GI foreign bodies, regardless of their location.[5] Patients with more chronic vomiting may be more prone to developing metabolic acidosis as a result of dehydration, and mixed acid-base disorders may be seen. Hypokalemia is the

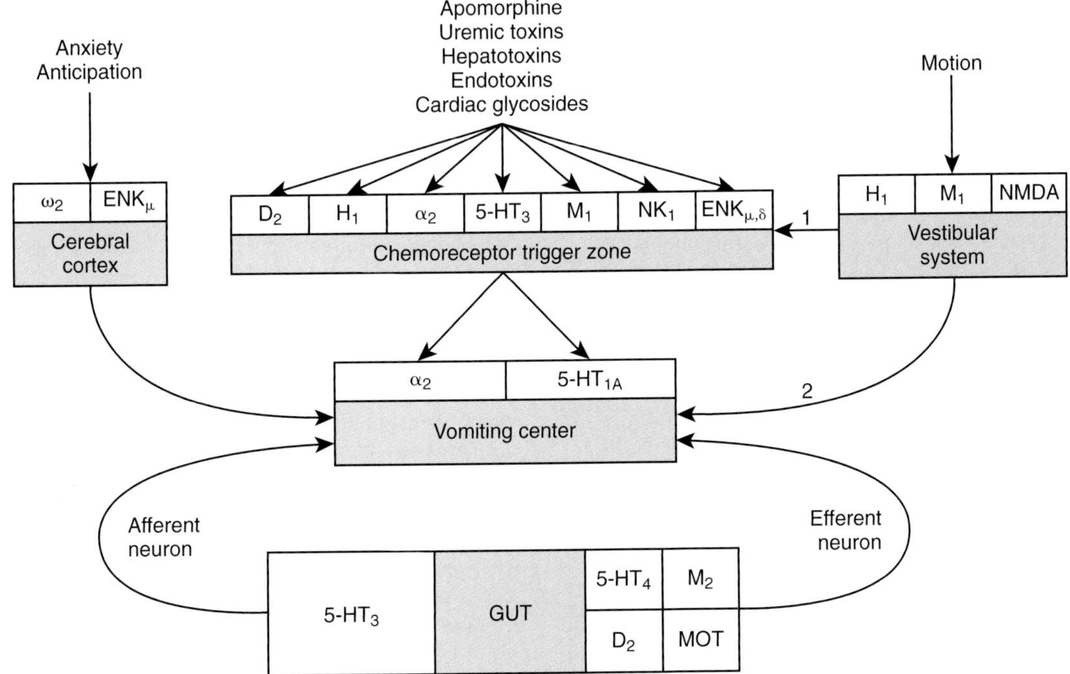

FIGURE 120-1 Schematic representation of the receptors and pathways involved in vomiting. *1,* Pathway more important in dogs; *2,* pathway more important in cats. Receptors: *D,* dopaminergic; *H,* histaminergic; *M,* acetylcholine (muscarinic); *NK,* neurokinin; *5-HT,* serotonin; *α,* α-adrenergic; *ω,* benzodiazepine; *ENK,* enkephalinergic opioid; *MOT,* motilin; *NMDA,* N-methyl-D-aspartate (glutamate receptor).

most common electrolyte disturbance in vomiting patients. Aspiration pneumonia is a less common complication of vomiting than it is of regurgitation because reflex closure of the glottis occurs during emesis. It is a greater risk in animals with impaired laryngeal function, typically a result of primary laryngeal disease or a decreased level of consciousness.

Differential Diagnoses

Many differential diagnoses for vomiting exist; therefore subdividing the causes is useful to assist in the diagnostic investigation and treatment plan. One commonly used subdivision is between those diseases in which the primary pathology is in the GI tract and those in which the primary pathology is outside the GI tract. Other systemic signs such as polydipsia or weight loss are often present in patients with extra-GI causes, but vomiting (and/or diarrhea) is likely to be the major presenting complaint in patients with primary GI disease. Thus an animal that is vomiting but lacks other signs is more likely to have primary GI disease, and an animal that vomits only occasionally but has marked systemic signs is more likely to have an extra-GI problem. It also can be useful to distinguish between those diseases that are more likely to cause acute vomiting and those that are more likely to cause chronic vomiting. The most common and important differential diagnoses for vomiting are shown in Box 120-2.

BOX 120-2 ***Important Differential Diagnoses for Vomiting***

Gastrointestinal

Obstruction

Foreign body*
Intussusception*
Neoplasia
Torsion or volvulus

Dietary

Allergy†
Intolerance†
Indiscretion*

Infectious

Viral (parvovirus)*
Parasitic†
Bacterial (salmonellosis)*

Other

Neoplasia†
Inflammatory bowel disease†
Gastrointestinal ulceration
Drug-induced (e.g., chemotherapy, NSAIDs, antibiotics)
Uremic gastritis
Liver disease

Extragastrointestinal

Uremia
Pancreatitis*
Diabetic ketoacidosis*
Liver disease
Peritonitis*
Pyometra*
Prostatitis
Drug or toxin induced*
Hypoadrenocorticism†
Hyperthyroidism
Vestibular disease
Heartworm disease (cats)

*More commonly acute.
†More commonly chronic.
NSAID, Nonsteroidal antiinflammatory drug.

Diagnostic Approach

History

A description of the character of the vomiting should be obtained and, as described above, should be distinguished from regurgitation. The approximate frequency and duration of vomiting should be determined because the chronicity and severity of signs help the clinician formulate a diagnostic and therapeutic plan. Fresh blood or digested blood ("coffee grounds") is suggestive of gastric ulceration, but bleeding also may be present in animals with acute infectious conditions (see Chapter 119). Other important information from the patient's history includes vaccination status, travel history, medication history, dietary indiscretion or recent diet changes, drug or toxin exposure, and any possibility of foreign body ingestion. As noted above, systemic signs should raise the possibility of an extra-GI cause for the vomiting.

Physical examination

Vital signs and a thorough physical examination are important in the vomiting patient. The most important part of the physical examination is a thorough palpation of the abdomen. Attention should be paid to any abdominal pain or discomfort and the presence of any palpable effusion, organ distention, masses, or foreign bodies. The mouth should be examined for evidence of systemic disease (uremic or ketotic odor, ulcers) or a linear foreign body. In cats, the thyroid gland should be palpated to check for a goiter. A rectal examination should be performed for additional information (hematochezia, worms, prostatomegaly with or without pain), and an examination of the central nervous system may be indicated in difficult cases. Assessment of hydration and hemodynamic status helps the clinician formulate an appropriate treatment plan.

Clinical pathology

A full hematology and biochemistry panel should be performed in any persistently vomiting patient. In most animals with an extra-GI cause, the biochemistry panel results have notable abnormalities. Normal biochemical and hematologic parameters are more strongly suggestive of primary GI disease. The hematology and biochemistry panels also allow evaluation of abnormalities in electrolytes and acid-base status, which may be complications of protracted vomiting. A sample for urinalysis should be obtained at the earliest opportunity to aid in differentiating prerenal from renal azotemia. A fecal sample should be submitted for zinc sulfate flotation in all cases, and also for selective bacterial culture or analyses in patients with acute vomiting. Further testing should be performed based on clinical suspicions.

Diagnostic imaging

Abdominal imaging is vital in the investigation of persistent vomiting. The choice of abdominal radiographs or ultrasound depends on the nature of the complaint. In the acutely vomiting patient, the priority is to establish whether medical or surgical management is indicated (i.e., rule out a GI obstruction). Abdominal radiographs have reasonable specificity in identifying the presence of obstruction and the wide availability of abdominal radiography makes them an acceptable first line test.[6] However, in the hands of an experienced operator, abdominal ultrasonography has been shown to have greater accuracy for identifying small intestinal obstruction than radiographs and is indicated in patients with equivocal radiographs or persistent vomiting.[6] Abdominal ultrasound also may assist in the identification of neoplastic obstructions and allows evaluation of the other abdominal organs to help exclude extra-GI cause of the vomiting. If ultrasonography is not available, administration of barium and sequential abdominal radiographs may be helpful.

Patients with chronic vomiting are less likely to suffer from intestinal obstruction than those that are vomiting acutely, and abdominal radiography therefore has a lower diagnostic yield. Abdominal ultrasonography generally is preferred in these patients. It allows an evaluation of the intestinal wall thickness and layering along with a thorough evaluation of the extraintestinal structures. It therefore proves useful in helping to decide whether medical management, endoscopy, or surgery would be the most appropriate management strategy.

Thoracic radiographs should also be obtained in vomiting patients. Their role is multifold. They may show evidence of esophageal disease if the history has led to an incorrect identification of the primary problem; they aid in the detection of neoplastic involvement in the thorax and allow for assessment of the heart and pulmonary vasculature; and they may show evidence of pulmonary disease such as aspiration pneumonia.

General Treatment Guidelines

The important factors to consider when treating a vomiting patient are (1) treatment of the underlying cause, (2) treatment and prevention of electrolyte and acid-base disturbances, and (3) symptomatic control of further vomiting, when appropriate. Fluid therapy and supportive care for the vomiting patient are discussed in Chapters 57, 59, 161, and 162. The general recommendation for stable animals with recent onset of vomiting is to withhold food for 24 to 48 hours.[7] The rationale behind this recommendation is to avoid stimulating further vomiting and let the GI tract rest, to prevent the development of food aversions in nauseated patients, and to reduce the risk of aspiration pneumonia.

Food always should be withheld from patients with suspected GI obstruction or any patient whose signs worsen after feeding. However, some vomiting patients may have a significantly quicker recovery when early enteral nutrition is instigated, and dogmatic enforcement of starvation may be unnecessary for some canine and feline patients.[8] Animals with persistent vomiting may not be good candidates for feeding tubes, and parenteral nutrition may be necessary (see Chapter 130).

CONCLUSION

A wide variety of underlying diseases may cause regurgitation or vomiting. Successful management of these patients requires an accurate definition of the clinical problem and determination of whether the disease is primarily gastrointestinal or systemic in origin. An appropriate treatment plan then may be initiated.

REFERENCES

1. McBrearty AR, Ramsey IK, Courcier EA, et al: Clinical factors associated with death before discharge and overall survival time in dogs with generalized megaesophagus, J Am Vet Med Assoc 238:1622, 2011.
2. Washabau RJ: Gastrointestinal motility disorders and gastrointestinal prokinetic therapy, Vet Clin North Am Small Anim Pract 33:1007, 2003.
3. Gaynor AR, Shofer FS, Washabau RJ: Risk factors for acquired megaesophagus in dogs, J Am Vet Med Assoc 211:1406, 1997.
4. Guyton AC, Hall JE: Vomiting. In Guyton AC, Hall JE, editors: The textbook of medical physiology, ed 12, Philadelphia, 2010, Saunders/Elsevier.
5. Boag AK, Coe RJ, Martinez TA, et al: Acid-base and electrolyte abnormalities in dogs with gastrointestinal foreign bodies, J Vet Intern Med 19:816, 2005.
6. Sharma A, Thompson MS, Scrivani PV, et al: Comparison of radiography and ultrasonography for diagnosing small-intestinal mechanical obstruction in vomiting dogs, Vet Radiol Ultrasound 52:248, 2011.
7. Webb C, Twedt DC: Canine gastritis, Vet Clin North Am Small Anim Pract 33:969, 2003.
8. Mohr AJ, Leisewitz AL, Jacobson LS, et al: Effect of early enteral nutrition on intestinal permeability, intestinal protein loss, and outcome in dogs with severe parvoviral enteritis, J Vet Intern Med 17:791, 2003.

CHAPTER 121
DIARRHEA

Daniel Z. Hume, DVM, DACVIM (Internal Medicine), DACVECC

KEY POINTS

- Diarrhea is a common clinical finding in critically ill animals.
- Diarrhea can lead to abnormalities in nutrient, acid-base, and electrolyte balance.
- Diarrhea may result from iatrogenic causes, primary gastrointestinal diseases, or other disease processes.

Diarrhea is a common clinical sign observed in critically ill canine and feline patients. Diarrhea is defined as an increase in fecal mass caused by an increase in fecal water or solid content. This usually is associated with an increase in frequency, fluidity, or volume of feces. In a 20-kg dog, approximately 2.5 L of fluid enters the duodenum each day, and about 98% of the fluid entering the intestine is absorbed.[1] Diarrhea in the critical care setting often is overlooked and overshadowed by the primary disease process. However, diarrhea can lead to severe aberrations in nutrient, acid-base, fluid, and electrolyte balance. Without proper attention it can lead to deterioration of the patient's condition. Diarrhea may be associated with patient discomfort, local dermatitis, catheter or catheter site infections, and potentially bacterial translocation if the integrity of the intestinal mucosa is altered. Consideration of the most likely cause is important because it allows the clinician to decide which diagnostic modalities are indicated for proper workup of the diarrhea. Three broad etiologic categories may be used when considering the potential cause of diarrhea in a given patient: iatrogenic causes, primary gastrointestinal (GI) causes, and other diseases secondarily causing diarrhea.

PATHOPHYSIOLOGIC MECHANISMS OF DIARRHEA

The several categorization schemes for diarrhea have great overlap among the classifications. One of the most commonly used classification schemes arranges the pathophysiologic mechanisms underlying diarrhea as follows: osmotic diarrhea, secretory diarrhea, diarrhea resulting from altered permeability, and diarrhea resulting from deranged motility.

Osmotic diarrhea is caused by the presence of excess luminal osmoles, drawing fluid into the intestinal lumen. Most causes of a diarrhea have an osmotic component.

Secretory diarrhea is caused by a net increase in intestinal fluid secretion. This results from either an absolute increase in intestinal secretion or a relative increase caused by a decrease in intestinal absorption.

Normal intestinal physiology and systemic health depend on the semipermeable nature of the intestinal mucosa. Nutrients, electrolytes, and fluid are absorbed and secreted, and the mucosa and immune system of the intestine inhibit translocation of bacteria and bacterial toxins. However, microscopic and macroscopic damage to either the epithelial cells or epithelial cell junctions can lead to altered intestinal permeability. Vital substances are lost into the intestinal lumen, and the altered permeability leaves the intestine vulnerable to translocation of potentially fatal bacteria and their products.

Alterations in intestinal motility are probably the least understood of the causes of diarrhea. Motility alterations leading to diarrhea include either increased peristaltic contractions or decreased segmental contractions.[1] Even within this classification scheme, significant overlap occurs among the groups.

In animals with primary GI causes of diarrhea, historical questions may provide evidence that allows anatomic localization of the disease to either the small or large bowel. This differentiation allows a more accurate formation of differential diagnoses and subsequent diagnostic testing. Historical and clinical differences usually noted between small and large bowel diarrhea are illustrated in Table 121-1.

IATROGENIC CAUSES OF DIARRHEA

Iatrogenic causes of diarrhea are likely more common than is realized and should be ruled out to facilitate clinical improvement. Diarrhea is a common side effect of several classes of drugs used in critically ill patients (Box 121-1). Antimicrobial agents may cause diarrhea as a direct result of drug formulation or properties, or as a result of alterations in intestinal microbacterial flora. Most of the chemotherapeutic agents have direct toxic effects against the rapidly dividing cells of the intestinal crypts, leading to villous blunting and altered absorption. Other classes of drugs, such as antiarrhythmic agents, lactulose, and proton pump inhibitors, also may be associated with diarrhea.

Acute or abrupt changes in the diet are not uncommon in hospitalized or critically ill patients. Anorexic animals often are coaxed to eat with canned diets and other potentially novel foods. Enteral tube feeding also is employed commonly in critically ill patients. The osmotic and caloric properties of these diets may exceed the digestive and absorptive capacities of the intestine and lead to osmotic

Table 121-1 **Differentiation of Diarrhea Based on Anatomic Location**

Characteristic	Small Bowel	Large Bowel
Mucus	Uncommon	Common
Hematochezia	Uncommon	May be present
Stool volume	Increased to normal	Normal to decreased
Melena	May be present	Absent
Frequency	May be increased to normal	Increased
Urgency	Uncommon	Common
Tenesmus	Uncommon	Common

BOX 121-1 *Medications Commonly Associated with Diarrhea*[20,21]

Antimicrobial Agents	Endocrine Medications
Gastrointestinal medications	Mitotane
Histamine-2 antagonists	Trilostane
Misoprostol	Methimazole
Proton pump inhibitors	Acarbose
Oral antacids	**NSAIDs**
Chemotherapeutic Agents	***Miscellaneous agents***
Cardiac medications	Amitriptyline
Quinidine	Parasiticides
Procainamide	Bethanechol
Digoxin	Clomipramine
Antihypertensive Agents	Colchicine
β-adrenergic antagonists	Acetazolamide
ACE inhibitors	
Immunomodulatory Agents	
Azathioprine	
Cyclophosphamide	
Cyclosporine	

ACE, Angiotensin-converting enzyme; *NSAIDs,* nonsteroidal antiinflammatory drugs.

diarrhea. Furthermore, prolonged quiescence of the intestine from either anorexia or parenteral nutrition can lead to villous atrophy and decreased absorptive function when enteral feeding is initiated (see Chapter 129).

PRIMARY GASTROINTESTINAL CAUSES OF DIARRHEA

Adverse reactions to foods can result from immunologic reactions (food allergy) or nonimmunologic reactions (food intolerance) to a dietary substance.[2] Although true food allergies are rare, food intolerance is probably one of the more common causes of acute diarrhea in the small animal patient. Intolerance can result from dietary indiscretion or gluttony, but often the exact cause is unknown. The resultant diarrhea is short term and self-limiting.

Infectious disease is a common cause of diarrhea in canine and feline patients. Gastrointestinal parasitism (e.g., *Ancylostoma* spp., *Toxocara* spp., *Toxascaris* spp., *Trichuris* spp.) is another common cause of diarrhea but rarely is associated with debilitation except in young or small patients. The exact role of various infectious bacterial organisms as the cause of diarrhea is controversial. Gastrointestinal disease and diarrhea may be associated with a variety of bacteria, including *Salmonella* spp., *Campylobacter* spp., enteropathogenic *Escherichia coli, Clostridium difficile,* and *Clostridium perfringens.*[3-8] Although diarrhea has been associated with clostridial organisms in the dog and cat,[3-8] the direct role remains unclear given that *C. difficile* toxin and *C. perfringens* enterotoxin can be found in the feces of animals with normal stool quality and no clinical GI signs.[6-8]

Systemic viral infections such as canine parvovirus and feline panleukopenia commonly are associated with diarrhea. Feline panleukopenia and canine parvovirus are caused by similar, but not identical, nonenveloped DNA parvoviruses.[9,10] Transmission occurs via oronasal exposure and the organism subsequently spreads to the bone marrow, lymphoid organs, and intestinal crypts, leading to a peripheral leukopenia and intestinal villus blunting and collapse.[9,10]

Fungal (*Histoplasma, Pythium,* and *Cryptococcus* spp.), algal (*Prototheca* spp.), protozoal (*Tritrichomonas foetus, Giardia, Cryptosporidium, Isospora* spp.), and rickettsial (*Neorickettsia* spp.) induced gastroenteritis may be seen depending on the geographic location and husbandry of the patient. Intussusceptions may occur secondary to infectious or idiopathic causes and may lead to severe diarrhea.

The role of small intestinal bacterial overgrowth (SIBO) or antibiotic-responsive diarrhea (ARD) is a controversial subject in small animal gastroenterology. Debate exists regarding whether the disease occurs as a primary condition, how it should be defined, and how it is diagnosed best. Some authors have divided the disease into either secondary SIBO (in cases in which an accompanying or primary intestinal disease can be identified) or idiopathic ARD in cases, in which no underlying disease can be found.[11] Examples of secondary SIBO can be seen with exocrine pancreatic insufficiency and inflammatory bowel disease (IBD). The exact cause of ARD has yet to be identified, but local intestinal immunodeficiency may play a role in the pathogenesis.[12]

Neoplastic disease also may lead to diarrhea in small animal patients; GI adenocarcinoma, alimentary lymphosarcoma, mast cell tumor, and GI stromal tumors are examples. These tumors may cause significant intestinal leakage and loss of protein and blood.

IBD is one of the more common causes of chronic diarrhea in cats and dogs. Loss of local immune tolerance to normal dietary and bacterial components leads to up-regulation of immune and inflammatory responses and establishment of an inflammatory focus within the intestine. Infiltration with inflammatory cells leads to thickening of the intestinal absorptive surface and decreased absorptive capacity. Different types of IBD are found in the dog and cat, and classification is based on the primary type of inflammatory cell infiltrate. Lymphocytic-plasmacytic is the most common form of IBD, but eosinophilic and granulomatous forms also are reported. Prolonged or extensive bowel disease can lead to severe metabolic derangements, including panhypoproteinemia and hypocholesterolemia. The diagnosis of IBD is based on histopathologic evidence of moderate to severe GI inflammation coupled with the exclusion of an underlying cause of the inflammation.

Lymphangiectasia can occur as a primary disease (Yorkshire Terrier, Norwegian Lundehund, and Maltese Terrier) or secondary to other infiltrative processes such as IBD. Alterations of intestinal lymphatic permeability lead to leakage of protein-rich and fat-rich chyle into the intestinal lumen and loss of these dietary components into the feces. Resultant clinical signs include chronic diarrhea and severe weight loss.

EXTRAGASTROINTESTINAL DISEASES CAUSING DIARRHEA

Extragastrointestinal causes of diarrhea include hepatobiliary disease, pancreatic disease, endocrine disease, or other miscellaneous abnormalities. Diarrhea may occur in dogs and cats with hepatobiliary disease for several reasons. Concurrent inflammatory GI disease may be seen in the dog and is common in the cat.[13-15] End-stage cirrhosis may be associated with elevated portal hydrostatic pressures, and functional hepatic failure may lead to hypoalbuminemia and GI wall edema. Both of these conditions often lead to altered absorptive properties of the GI tract. Diseases affecting the biliary tree also may hinder delivery of bile salts to the intestine, leading to fat maldigestion.

Diarrhea is seen commonly as a sequela of pancreatic disease. Exocrine pancreatic insufficiency may result from pancreatic acinar atrophy (primarily dogs) or chronic pancreatitis (primarily cats). Lack of exocrine pancreatic function leads to maldigestion and malabsorption of dietary substrates and culminates in diarrhea and weight loss. Acute and chronic pancreatitis also may lead to diarrhea. Pancreatic inflammation may cause local inflammation of the duodenum and colon, interfere with pancreatic acinar secretion, and result in decreased bile salt delivery to the small intestine via obstruction of biliary flow.

Congestive heart failure, particularly right-sided failure, can lead to intestinal and hepatic venous congestion and ascites. Congestion of the splanchnic vasculature may cause alteration in the absorptive capacities of the intestine.

Several endocrine disorders may be associated with diarrhea. Diarrhea is noted in some cats with hyperthyroidism. The diarrhea in these cases may be a result of increased food intake as well as intestinal hypermotility. Waxing and waning GI signs are seen frequently in dogs and less commonly in cats with hypoadrenocorticism. Cortisol is vital for maintenance of normal GI function, motility, and integrity, as well as vascular tone and subsequent perfusion. The lack of mineralocorticoids may be associated with alterations in electrolyte balance, leading to altered GI motility and absorption. Diarrhea is an uncommonly reported clinical sign associated with hypothyroidism.

Various other diseases may be associated with diarrhea. Idiopathic noncirrhotic portal hypertension may interfere with absorption within the intestinal tract. The role of hypoalbuminemia as a direct cause of diarrhea is debated. The decreased oncotic draw resulting from hypoalbuminemia leads to alterations in Starling forces and decreased absorption of fluid across the intestinal lumen. Hemorrhagic diarrhea is seen commonly in critically ill patients suffering from, or after resuscitation from, various causes of cardiovascular shock (e.g., heat-induced illness). GI complications are common in animals with acute and chronic renal disease, but diarrhea is not reported commonly. Systemic infections (including sepsis) may affect secondarily the GI tract and cause diarrhea. Experimental canine studies have shown that bacterial endotoxin impairs colonic water and sodium absorption and increases small and large intestinal motility, at least partially explaining the diarrhea noted in septic patients.[16,17]

DIAGNOSTIC EVALUATION

The diagnostic evaluation of patients with diarrhea is guided best by the historical, clinicopathologic, and physical examination findings. The physical condition of the patient and the duration and clinical course of the diarrhea help determine how aggressive the clinician should be in attempting to find a cause.

Results of a complete blood count, serum chemistry profile, and urinalysis are indicated in all critically ill patients and often help to differentiate between GI and non-GI causes of diarrhea. Based on these findings, additional tests may be needed to screen for hyperthyroidism, hypoadrenocorticism, or occult liver disease. Fecal flotation (including zinc sulfate for *Giardia* spp.) and direct cytologic examination of the feces is recommended in most cases. Although cytologic examination of the feces may help indirectly to point toward a particular pathogen, isolation or amplification of toxin or enterotoxin may provide a more specific diagnosis in the case of clostridial infection. Bacterial culture (*Salmonella* spp., *Campylobacter* spp., enteropathogenic *E. coli*), enterotoxin screening (*Clostridium* spp.), and enzyme-linked immunosorbent assay (ELISA) (parvovirus) of the feces may be indicated when an infectious cause is suspected. Specific tests for other infectious agents also may prove helpful depending on the geographic location and husbandry of the patient. Exfoliative rectal cytology may be useful in diagnosing fungal, algal, inflammatory, and neoplastic diseases. Trypsin-like immunoreactivity testing is indicated in any patient with suspected exocrine pancreatic insufficiency. Folate and cobalamin testing may be helpful in animals with suspected SIBO. Although abdominal radiographs are of limited value in animals affected primarily with diarrhea, abdominal ultrasound often is indicated and useful for assessing integrity, architecture, and thickness of the GI system and other abdominal organs. Last, GI endoscopy or exploratory laparotomy often is needed for direct visualization of the intestinal tract and procurement of diagnostic samples.

TREATMENT

Iatrogenic causes of diarrhea should be considered in all patients, especially those in which diarrhea was not part of the presenting complaint. If the diarrhea is severe, current medications may have to be discontinued or modified. Although diarrhea is associated commonly with enteral feeding, the diet formulation may require alteration if the diarrhea is severe or adversely affecting the patient's quality of life.

Treatment of diarrhea associated with primary GI diseases or diseases secondarily causing diarrhea is achieved best after careful diagnostic evaluation of the underlying cause. Once a definitive diagnosis has been achieved, direct treatment can be initiated. Rarely, medications directed toward symptomatic treatment of the diarrhea are used (see Chapter 161). Intestinal transit time is effectively a result of the balance between propulsive peristalsis and segmental contractions.[1] Contrary to historical belief, diarrhea rarely results from increased peristalsis but more commonly is the result of decreased segmental contractions.[1] Anticholinergic agents generally are contraindicated because they decrease propulsive peristalsis and segmental contractions and predispose the patient to ileus. Conversely, opioid-containing medications such as loperamide, diphenoxylate, and opium tincture can decrease propulsive contractions and increase segmental contractions; water and fluid absorption also is augmented.[1] These medications may be indicated in some cases of diarrhea in which infectious causes have been excluded. Kaolin, pectin, and bismuth subsalicylate are used occasionally for symptomatic treatment.[1] However, this rarely is indicated because treatment of the primary disease process provides the best means for eliminating diarrhea. Indications for symptomatic therapy include diarrhea that adversely affects the patient's quality of life, causes severe fecal scalding of the skin, or predisposes to secondary infection (e.g., urinary or intravenous catheter infections in recumbent animals).

In animals with IBD, treatment often is tailored to the individual patient based on the severity of the clinical signs and histopathologic lesions. Dogs and cats with intermittent clinical signs, good body condition, and mild histologic lesions may respond to dietary therapy alone. This may be due to a loss of immunologic tolerance to normal dietary proteins and subsequent GI inflammation in patients with IBD. Dietary therapy for pets with IBD usually relies on either a novel protein diet or a diet with a hydrolyzed protein source. Animals with some degree of lymphangiectasia may benefit from a low-fat diet.

However, most animals with moderate to severe disease need some degree of immunomodulation to obtain clinical remission. Glucocorticoids (prednisone, prednisolone, and dexamethasone) are the mainstay of immunomodulatory therapy. The locally active steroid, budesonide, undergoes significant first-pass metabolism, thereby limiting systemic absorption and potentially lessening the side effects compared with glucocorticoids. Azathioprine, chlorambucil, or other immunomodulating agents may be necessary for dogs with refractory disease or those unable to tolerate glucocorticoid therapy. Aminosalicylates (sulfasalazine, mesalamine) can be prescribed for dogs with primarily large bowel disease. Metronidazole often is used for its antimicrobial and antiinflammatory effects.

Antimicrobial therapy may be useful in many other diarrheal diseases of dogs and cats (Table 121-2). Primary (idiopathic) or

Table 121-2 Formulary of Commonly Used Drugs for the Treatment of Diarrhea in Small Animals

Drug	Canine	Feline
Prednisone	1 to 2 mg/kg PO q12h	1 to 4 mg/kg PO q12h
Budesonide	<5 kg: 1 mg PO q24h 5 to 15 kg: 2 mg PO q24h >15 kg: 3 mg PO q24h	1 mg PO q24h
Azathioprine	2 mg/kg PO q24h	Not routinely used
Chlorambucil	Not routinely used	2 mg/m^2 PO q48h
Sulfasalazine	10 to 15 mg/kg PO q8-12h	10 to 20 mg/kg PO q24h
Metronidazole	10 to 15 mg/kg PO q12h	10 to 15 mg/kg PO q12h
Oxytetracycline	22 mg/kg PO q8h	10 to 15 mg/kg PO q8h
Tylosin	10 to 20 mg/kg PO q8-12h	10 to 20 mg/kg PO q8-12h
Erythromycin	10 to 20 mg/kg PO q8h	10 to 20 mg/kg PO q8h
Enrofloxacin	10 to 20 mg/kg PO q24h	5 mg/kg PO q24h

PO, Per os.

secondary ARD often respond well to antimicrobial agents. Those most often prescribed include metronidazole, oxytetracycline, and tylosin.[4] The drug of choice for treatment of *Campylobacter* spp. is the macrolide erythromycin. However, its use is associated with GI side effects (typically vomiting and/or diarrhea). Other antimicrobial drugs that may be considered include azithromycin, enrofloxacin, tetracyclines, chloramphenicol, cefoxitin, and tylosin. Animals with diarrhea of suspected clostridial origin may be treated with metronidazole, ampicillin, macrolides, or tetracyclines.[4] In stable, immunocompetent animals, the routine empiric use of antimicrobials may not be beneficial. A recent study showed no significant difference in outcome parameters in a group of aseptic dogs with hemorrhagic gastroenteritis treated with a broad-spectrum antimicrobial.[18]

Probiotic supplementation is becoming increasingly more popular in human and veterinary medicine. Specific indications for probiotic use include antibiotic-associated diarrhea and diarrhea resulting from alterations of the normal GI flora. Numerous mechanisms have been proposed, but they likely exert their effects through modulation of the immune system and direct competition for, or antagonism of, pathogenic bacteria. In at least one veterinary report, probiotic therapy has been shown to shorten the duration of clinical signs in dogs with acute gastroenteritis.[19]

REFERENCES

1. Guilford WG, Strombeck DR: Classification, pathophysiology, and symptomatic treatment of diarrheal diseases. In Strombeck's small animal gastroenterology, Philadelphia, 1996, WB Saunders.
2. Guilford WG: Adverse reactions to food. In Strombeck's small animal gastroenterology, Philadelphia, 1996, WB Saunders.
3. Cave NJ, Marks SL, Kass PH, et al: Evaluation of a routine diagnostic fecal panel for dogs with diarrhea, J Am Vet Med Assoc 221:52, 2002.
4. Fox JG, Greene CE, Marks SL: Enteric bacterial infections. In Greene CL, editor: Infectious diseases of the dog and cat, ed 4, St Louis, 2012, Elsevier Saunders.
5. Weese JS, Wesse HE, Bourdeau TL, et al: Suspected *Clostridium difficile*-associated diarrhea in two cats, J Am Vet Med Assoc 218:1436, 2001.
6. Marks SL, Kather EJ, Kass PH, et al: Genotypic and phenotypic characterization of *Clostridium perfringens* and *Clostridium difficile* in diarrheic and healthy dogs, J Vet Intern Med 16:533, 2002.
7. Weese JS, Staempfli HR, Prescott JF, et al: The roles of *Clostridium difficile* and enterotoxigenic *Clostridium perfringens* in diarrhea in dogs, J Vet Intern Med 15:374, 2001.
8. Marks SL, Rankin SC, Byrne BA, et al: Enteropathogenic bacteria in dogs and cats: Diagnosis, epidemiology, treatment, and control: ACVIM Consensus Statement, J Vet Intern Med 25:1195, 2011.
9. Green CL: Canine viral enteritis. In Greene CL, editor: Infectious diseases of the dog and cat, ed 4, St Louis, 2012, Elsevier Saunders.
10. Greene CE: Feline panleukopenia. In Greene CL, editor: Infectious diseases of the dog and cat, ed 4, St Louis, 2012, Elsevier Saunders.
11. Hall EJ: Small intestine. In Washabau RJ, Day MJ, editors: Canine and feline gastroenterology, St Louis, 2013, Elsevier Saunders.
12. German AJ, Hall EJ, Day MJ: Chronic intestinal inflammation and intestinal disease in dogs, J Vet Intern Med 17:8, 2003.
13. Weiss DJ, Gagne JM, Armstrong PJ: Relationship between inflammatory hepatic disease and inflammatory bowel disease, pancreatitis, and nephritis in cats, J Am Vet Med Assoc 209:1114, 1996.
14. Baez JL, Hendrick MJ, Walker LM, et al: Radiographic, ultrasonographic, and endoscopic findings in cats with inflammatory bowel disease of the stomach and small intestine: 33 cases (1990-1997), J Am Vet Med Assoc 215:349, 1999.
15. Ferreri JA, Hardam E, Kimmel SE, et al: Clinical differentiation of acute necrotizing from chronic nonsuppurative pancreatitis in cats: 63 cases (1996-2001), J Am Vet Med Assoc. 223:469, 2003.
16. Spates ST, Cullen JJ, Ephgrave KS, et al: Effect of endotoxin on canine colonic motility and transit, J Gastrointest Surg 2:391, 1998.
17. Cullen JJ, Spates ST, Ephgrave KS, et al: Endotoxin temporarily impairs canine colonic absorption of water and sodium, J Surg Res 74:34, 1998.
18. Unterer S, Strohmeyer K, Kruse, et al: Treatment of aseptic dogs with hemorrhagic gastroenteritis with amoxicillin/clavulanic acid: a prospective blinded study, J Vet Intern Med 25, 973, 2011.
19. Herstad, HK, Nesheim BB, et al: Effects of a probiotic intervention in acute canine gastroenteritis- a controlled clinical trial, J Small Anim Pract 51:34, 2012.
20. Ringel AF, Jameson GJ, Foster ES: Diarrhea in the intensive care patient, Crit Care Clin 11:465, 1995.
21. Plumb DC: Plumb's veterinary handbook, ed 7, Ames, Iowa, 2011, Wiley-Blackwell.

CHAPTER 122
PERITONITIS

Susan W. Volk, VMD, PhD, DACVS

KEY POINTS

- Peritonitis is inflammation of the peritoneal cavity and is most commonly the result of gastrointestinal rupture, perforation, or dehiscence in small animals.
- Clinical signs in patients with peritonitis may be mild to severe and are often nonspecific.
- Abdominocentesis is the preferred diagnostic method for confirming peritonitis.
- When abdominal fluid cytology reveals degenerative neutrophils and intracellular bacteria, confirming a diagnosis of septic peritonitis, emergency surgical exploration of the abdomen is indicated.
- Open peritoneal drainage or closed suction drainage should be considered for management of septic peritonitis in which the source of contamination cannot be controlled completely, or if significant contamination or inflammation remains after surgical debridement and lavage.
- Prognosis is guarded for patients with peritonitis. Reported survival rates are highly variable and depend on the cause, presence of infection, and development of systemic inflammatory response syndrome and/or organ dysfunction.

Peritonitis is defined as inflammation of the peritoneal cavity and may be classified according to the underlying cause (primary or secondary), extent (localized or generalized), or the presence of infectious agents (septic or nonseptic). Primary peritonitis refers to a spontaneous inflammatory condition in the absence of underlying intraabdominal pathology or known history of penetrating peritoneal injury. Secondary peritonitis occurs more commonly in the dog and cat and is the consequence of a preexisting aseptic or septic pathologic intraabdominal condition. Because of the multitude of conditions that may lead to peritonitis the types of clinical signs and their severity vary.

Hematogenous dissemination of infectious agents has been postulated as the mechanism of development of primary peritonitis and likely is facilitated by impaired host immune defenses. The most common form of primary peritonitis is the effusive form of feline infectious peritonitis, caused by feline coronavirus, which should be included on any differential diagnosis list for cats with peritoneal effusion. Other infectious agents reported to cause primary peritonitis in dogs and cats include *Salmonella typhimurium, Chlamydia psittaci, Clostridium limosum, Mesocestoides* spp., *Bacteroides* spp., *Actinomyces* spp., *Blastomyces* spp., and *Candida* spp. Given the common occurrence of isolated *Bacteroides* and *Fusobacterium* spp. from cats with primary septic peritonitis, these bacteria may be translocating from the oral cavity through either unrecognized direct penetration (bites) or a hematogenous route.[1]

Inflammation of the abdominal cavity in the absence of infectious pathogens (aseptic peritonitis) most commonly occurs in response to exposure of the peritoneum to sterile fluids (i.e., gastric, biliary, or urine), pancreatic enzymes, or foreign material. Aseptic bile and urine cause minimal peritoneal inflammation, whereas gastric fluid and pancreatic enzyme leakage lead to a more intense peritoneal reaction. Microscopic and macroscopic foreign material, including surgical glove powder, surgical materials (suture, cotton swabs, surgical sponges), hair, and impaled objects (sticks, plant material, metal) may elicit a granulomatous response. To minimize iatrogenic causes of aseptic peritonitis, surgeons should rinse surgical gloves preoperatively with sterile saline or use powder-free gloves, perform a surgical sponge count before opening and closing a celiotomy, and use surgical sponges with radiopaque markers.

More commonly, secondary peritonitis is identified as a septic process, most commonly secondary to contamination from the gastrointestinal (GI) tract. Leakage of GI contents may occur through stomach and intestinal walls that have been compromised by ulceration, foreign body obstruction, neoplasia, trauma, ischemic damage, or dehiscence of a previous surgical incision. Spontaneous gastroduodenal perforation may be associated with nonsteroidal antiinflammatory drug administration but also may be seen with corticosteroid administration, neoplastic and nonneoplastic GI infiltrative disease, gastrinoma, and hepatic disease.[2,3] Neoplasia was found to be the underlying pathology in 25% of cats with septic peritonitis secondary to GI leakage in one study, with adenocarcinoma and lymphosarcoma the most common types.[4] Septic peritonitis secondary to surgical site dehiscence occurs in 6% to 16% of postoperative patients requiring intestinal enterotomy or resection and anastomosis.[5-8] GI linear foreign bodies in dogs have been reported as the inciting cause of peritonitis in 41% of cases, higher than that previously reported for cats.[9] One canine study found that two or more of the following conditions increased the risk for leakage after intestinal anastomosis: preoperative peritonitis, intestinal foreign body, and a serum albumin concentration of 2.5 g/dl or less.[8] In addition, a recent study suggests that intraoperative hypotension is also a risk factor for the development of septic peritonitis after gastrointestinal surgery.[5] Interestingly, this retrospective of 225 surgeries found the presence of a foreign body to be a protective factor. Other causes of septic peritonitis can be found in Box 122-1.

CLINICAL SIGNS

Historical information may provide clues regarding the underlying cause of peritonitis. Previous and current maladies and surgical procedures (including neutering), current medications (particularly those that may predispose to GI ulceration), and duration of current clinical signs should be investigated. Owners should be questioned specifically regarding the potential for trauma exposure and foreign body ingestion. A history of recent abdominal surgery should raise suspicion for septic peritonitis, particularly if gastrointestinal surgery was performed.

Clinical signs of dogs and cats with peritonitis vary in type and intensity and may reflect the underlying disease process. Peritoneal effusion is a consistent finding but may be difficult to appreciate on physical examination if only a small volume of fluid is present; it also

BOX 122-1 *Differential Diagnoses of Septic Peritonitis in Dogs and Cats*

Primary

Feline coronavirus (feline infectious peritonitis)
Salmonella typhimurium
Chlamydia psittaci
Clostridium limosum
Mesocestoides spp.
Blastomyces spp.
Candidiasis spp.

Secondary

Penetrating abdominal wounds
Surgical peritoneal contamination
Peritoneal dialysis
Gastrointestinal conditions
Gastric rupture secondary to GDV, neoplasia, perforating ulcer
Intestinal leakage
Perforating foreign body, ulcer, or neoplasia
Bacterial translocation secondary to obstruction (foreign body, neoplasia, intussusception, or bowel incarceration)
Dehiscence of intestinal surgical wound
Ischemic intestinal injury
Hepatobiliary condition
Liver abscess
Liver lobe torsion with abscess formation
Ruptured biliary tract with bacterobilia
Pancreatitis or pancreatic abscess
Hemolymphatic conditions
Splenic abscess
Splenic torsion with anaerobic bacterial colonization
Mesenteric lymph node abscess formation
Urogenital conditions
Renal abscess
Septic uroabdomen
Pyometra (ruptured or with mural bacterial translocation)
Uterine torsion
Prostatic abscess formation

GDV, Gastric dilatation-volvulus.

may be difficult to detect sonographically in animals that are dehydrated. Abdominal pain may be appreciated on palpation, with a small number of dogs exhibiting the "prayer position" in an attempt to relieve their abdominal discomfort. Abdominal pain is a less consistent finding in feline peritonitis patients (38% to 62%).[4,10] Most animals with septic peritonitis are systemically ill and exhibit nonspecific clinical signs such as anorexia, vomiting, mental depression, and lethargy. These patients may arrive in progressive states of hypovolemic and cardiovascular shock, with either injected or pale mucous membranes, prolonged capillary refill time, tachycardia with weak pulses, and with either hyperthermia or hypothermia reflecting poor peripheral perfusion. A significant number of cats (16%) with septic peritonitis exhibited bradycardia (see Chapters 6 and 91).[4] In fact, the combination of bradycardia and hypothermia in cats with primary septic peritonitis has been established as a negative prognostic indicator.[1] Animals with uroperitoneum may continue to urinate with concurrent leakage into the peritoneal cavity.

DIAGNOSTIC TESTS

Although the preoperative diagnosis of peritonitis is confirmed by identification of a septic or aseptic inflammatory process in peritoneal fluid obtained by abdominocentesis, patients with suspected or confirmed peritonitis should have routine hematologic, biochemical, and coagulation analyses performed. A marked neutrophilia with a left shift is the predominant hematologic finding, although a normal or low neutrophil count may be present. Animals recovering without incident from GI surgery also may have a transient inflammatory leukogram; however, the overall peripheral white blood cell counts typically fall within normal limits.[11] An increasingly left-shifted neutrophilia (or neutropenia) paired with clinical signs of peritonitis may raise the clinician's index of suspicion for postoperative intestinal dehiscence (which typically occurs 3 to 5 days after surgery).

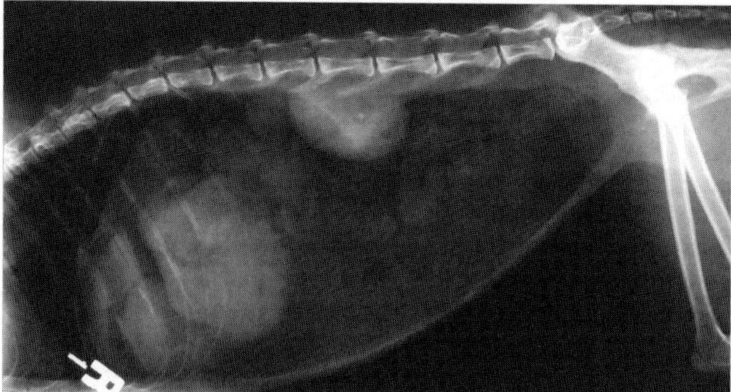

FIGURE 122-1 Lateral abdominal radiograph showing free peritoneal gas and possibly ingesta free within the abdomen. Pneumoperitoneum, without a history of recent surgery or open-needle abdominocentesis, indicates the need for abdominal exploratory surgery. This cat was diagnosed with a ruptured gastric mass at surgery.

Furthermore, acid-base and electrolyte abnormalities may be noted. Hyperkalemia (and azotemia) may indicate uroperitoneum, particularly if trauma or urinary tract dysfunction has been noted historically. Hypoproteinemia may be a result of the loss of protein within the peritoneal cavity. Patients with a concurrent septic process may be hypoglycemic. Hepatic enzymes, creatinine, and blood urea nitrogen may be elevated, indicating primary dysfunction of these organs or perhaps reflecting a state of decreased perfusion or dehydration. The serum of patients with bile peritonitis is often icteric if the total bilirubin is elevated. Recently, the prevalence of ionized hypocalcemia in cats and dogs with septic peritonitis has been recognized and a failure to normalize calcium levels during hospitalization associated with negative prognosis.[12,13]

Plain radiographs may reveal a focal or generalized loss of detail that also is known as the *ground glass appearance.* A pneumoperitoneum (Figure 122-1) suggests perforation of a hollow viscous organ, penetrating trauma (including recent abdominal surgery) or, less commonly, the presence of gas-producing anaerobic bacteria. Intestinal tract obstruction or bowel plication should be ruled out. Prostatomegaly in male dogs and evidence of uterine distention in female dogs should be noted. Thoracic radiographs should be performed to rule out concurrent illness (infectious, neoplastic, or traumatic). The presence of bicavitary effusion increased the mortality rate of patients 3.3-fold compared with that of patients with peritoneal effusions alone.[14] Ultrasonography may be useful for defining the underlying cause of peritonitis, in addition to its use in localizing and aiding retrieval of peritoneal effusion. In the case of a confirmed uroabdomen, preoperative contrast radiography (excretory urography or cystourethrography) is recommended to localize the site of urine leakage and aid in surgical planning. All patients should be stabilized hemodynamically and medically before diagnostic imaging is performed.

Patients with suspected peritonitis should be evaluated for peritoneal effusion. Little or no fluid may be detected initially if patients arrive early in the disease process or before fluid resuscitation if they are dehydrated (see Table 112-1). Large volumes of effusion may be obtained via blind abdominocentesis or, alternatively, via ultrasonographic guidance (see Chapter 200). Single paracentesis attempts are successful in only 20% of patients with low volumes of peritoneal effusion (3 ml/kg) and in only 80% with larger volumes (10 ml/kg). Ultrasonographic guidance facilitates the retrieval of smaller volumes of peritoneal fluid. If single-site sampling is negative for fluid, four-quadrant sampling should be performed.

A diagnostic peritoneal lavage (DPL, see Chapter 200) should be performed when peritonitis is suspected despite the absence of detectable effusion or when a minimal volume of effusion makes it difficult to obtain a sample. DPL ideally is performed using a peritoneal dialysis catheter but also can be performed using an over-the-needle, large-bore (14- to 16-gauge) catheter. The technique is performed by placing a catheter sterilely into the abdomen, infusing 22 ml/kg of a warmed, sterile isotonic saline solution, then retrieving a sample for analysis and culture and susceptibility testing. The lavage solution dilutes the sample and therefore alters the fluid analysis. A repeated DPL may increase accuracy of the technique when results of the first procedure are equivocal.

Whether obtained by paracentesis or DPL, cytologic, biochemical, and microbiologic analyses are useful in diagnosing peritonitis and further classifying type (septic or aseptic) and potential underlying cause (see Table 112-1 for overview). Leukocyte morphology has been suggested to be more reliable than cell counts in diagnosing peritonitis.[15] In an experimental study, DPL samples obtained before and after abdominal surgery suggest a nucleated cell count less than 1000 cells/µl (predominantly segmented neutrophils and macrophages) in dogs without intraabdominal pathology, whereas nucleated cell counts increased significantly in postoperative samples.[11] In a second experimental study, DPL cell counts between 500 and 10,500 cells/µl consisting predominantly of nondegenerate neutrophils are seen within the first 3 days after uncomplicated intestinal anastomosis.[15] Peritoneal leukocyte counts in animals with experimentally induced peritonitis exceed 5000 cells/µl (consistent with an exudate), with primarily degenerative neutrophils. Early in the disease process, lower cell numbers or an absence of degenerate neutrophils may occur in the face of septic peritonitis. The presence of intracellular bacteria, plant material/GI ingesta with associated inflammation, and/or free biliary crystals supports the diagnosis of peritonitis. Furthermore, increasing inflammation (numbers of neutrophils or morphologic features of toxicity in these cells) observed in serial samples and correlated with clinical findings may prove more useful than single leukocyte counts in abdominal fluid samples when deciding whether reoperation is indicated. Dogs receiving antimicrobial therapy may have no observable bacteria in peritoneal fluid samples, despite having peritoneal contamination.

In addition to the presence of bacteria and a high nucleated cell count with the presence of degenerate neutrophils, the glucose concentration of abdominal effusion is a useful predictor of bacterial peritonitis in dogs. A concentration difference of more than 20 mg/dl between paired samples for blood and peritoneal fluid glucose is a reliable predictor of a bacterial peritonitis; intravenous administration of dextrose or the presence of a hemoperitoneum may decrease the accuracy of this test. In addition, an abdominal fluid lactate concentration that is 2.0 mmol/L or greater than the blood lactate is predictive of septic peritonitis in dogs but has not been as useful in cats.[16,17] These parameters have been shown to be unreliable indicators of septic peritonitis in the evaluation of postoperative cases in which closed suction drains have been placed.[18] Samples for aerobic and anaerobic cultures should be obtained at the time of initial sampling so that additional samples are not required after confirming the presence of a septic process and initiating antimicrobial therapy.

The diagnosis of uroperitoneum in dogs can be made if the peritoneal fluid creatinine or potassium concentration exceeds that of the serum creatinine (more than 2:1) or potassium concentration (more than 1.4:1).[19] Similarly, biliary rupture leads to a bilirubin concentration that is higher in the peritoneal fluid than in the serum. In addition, bile pigment or crystals may be visible on cytologic examination of the peritoneal effusion in animals with bile peritonitis (Figure 122-2). These changes may not be seen in patients with bile peritonitis secondary to a ruptured gallbladder mucocele because the gelatinous bile often fails to disperse throughout the abdomen.

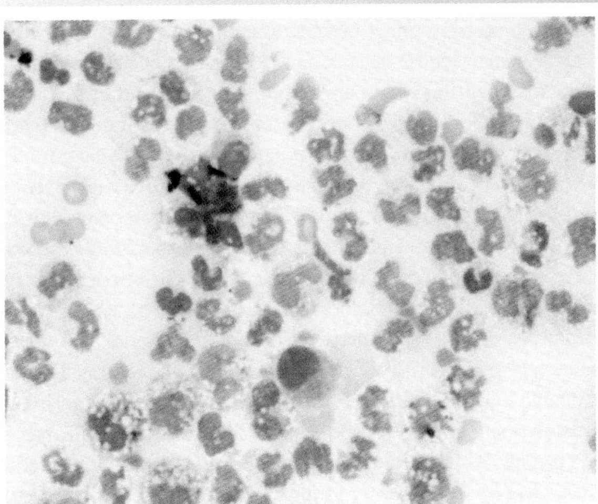

FIGURE 122-2 Microscopic examination of Wright-stained peritoneal fluid reveals markedly degenerative neutrophils, activated macrophages, and extracellular gold-brown pigment. One neutrophil in this high-powered field contains large bacterial rods (lower right hand side). This cytologic evaluation, together with elevated total bilirubin concentration in the peritoneal fluid relative to the serum concentration, confirms a diagnosis of a septic bile peritonitis.

TREATMENT

Medical Stabilization

The goals for animals with septic peritonitis are to identify and address the source of contamination to resolve the infection and treat the systemic consequences as quickly as possible (i.e., fluid and electrolyte abnormalities and hypoperfusion). Before surgical intervention, a decision must be made whether additional hemodynamic stabilization is indicated before proceeding, or whether this additional time and continued contamination of the abdominal cavity will result in further clinical decline that outweighs the benefits of additional medical treatment.

The goals of medical therapy are to restore normal fluid and electrolyte balance and minimize ongoing contamination. Fluid resuscitation is initiated after obtaining pretherapy blood samples for a minimum database (packed cell volume, total solids, BUN, dextrose), hematology, serum chemistry, and coagulation evaluation. Urine should be collected, if possible, for analysis with or without culture and susceptibility testing. Shock doses of crystalloids (up to 90 ml/kg in the dog, 50 ml/kg in the cat) or a combination of isotonic crystalloids (up to 20 to 40 ml/kg) and synthetic colloids (hydroxyethyl starch up to 20 ml/kg in the dog or up to 10 ml/kg in the cat; or 7% to 7.5% hypertonic saline in synthetic colloid solution (1 part 23.4% hypertonic saline to 2 parts synthetic colloid), 3 to 5 ml/kg IV over 5 to 15 minutes) should be administered to effect (see Chapter 60). Because significant amounts of protein are lost into the peritoneal cavity, plasma and/or albumin administration also may be warranted. Judicious fluid therapy is recommended to avoid volume overload. Electrolytes and glucose should be supplemented if indicated (see Electrolyte and Acid-Base Disturbances, Chapters 50 through 56, and Chapter 66). After appropriate volume resuscitation, vasopressor therapy may be necessary to alleviate hypotension further. A urinary catheter may aid in diversion of infected urine in the case of a ruptured bladder or proximal urethra and allow time for the necessary correction of any metabolic derangements (typically hyperkalemia and acidosis) before surgery. Analgesia is an important component of preoperative management for peritonitis patients. Opioids often are used as a first-line choice for pain management; however, they must be used with caution because of their negative effects on GI motility, as well as their dose-dependent respiratory depression (see Chapters 144 and 163).

Broad-spectrum antimicrobial therapy should be initiated immediately after confirming the diagnosis of septic peritonitis (see Chapters 93 and 94). *Escherichia coli, Clostridium* spp., and *Enterococcus* spp. are common isolates. A second-generation cephalosporin such as cefoxitin (30 mg/kg IV q6-8h) may be used as a single agent or combination antimicrobial therapy such as ampicillin or cefazolin (22 mg/kg IV q8h) administered concurrently with either enrofloxacin (10 to 20 mg/kg IV q24h [dog], 5 mg/kg IV q24h [cat]) or an aminoglycoside (amikacin 15 mg/kg IV, IM, SC q24h [dog], 10 mg/kg IV, IM, SC q24h [cat] or gentamicin 10 mg/kg IV, IM, SC q24h [dog], 6 mg/kg IV, IM, SC q24h [cat]). If extended anaerobic coverage is necessary, metronidazole (10 mg/kg IV q12h) may be considered. Aminoglycosides usually are avoided until renal insufficiency or acute kidney injury has been ruled out and the patient is well hydrated. Antimicrobial therapy should be tailored to the results of culture and susceptibility testing.

Surgical Treatment

The goals of surgical treatment for patients with septic peritonitis include resolving the cause of the infection, diminishing the infectious and foreign material load, and promoting patient recovery with aggressive supportive care and nutritional supplementation, if indicated. A ventral midline celiotomy from xiphoid to pubis allows a thorough exploratory laparotomy to determine the underlying cause. Monofilament suture material is advocated in animals with a septic process, and surgical gut is avoided because of its shortened half-life in this environment. Placement of nonabsorbable suture material or mesh within the abdominal cavity is not recommended in cases of septic peritonitis because these materials may serve as a nidus for infection. If possible, the surgeon should isolate the offending organ from the rest of the abdomen with laparotomy sponges to prevent further contamination during correction of the problem.

Surgical treatment is tailored to the individual case and the underlying cause of the septic peritonitis. If a GI leakage is identified, adjunctive procedures such as serosal patching or omental wrapping of the repaired site are recommended to reduce the incidence of postoperative intestinal leakage or dehiscence. Although heavily contaminated or necrotic omentum may necessitate partial omentectomy, preservation of as much omentum as possible is advised to promote venous and lymphatic drainage from the peritoneal cavity. In addition, potential benefits of surgical applications of the omentum (e.g., intracapsular prostatic omentalization for prostatic abscess formation[20] pancreatic abscess omentalization,[21] omentalization of enterotomy or intestinal resection and anastomosis sites, and around gastrostomy or enterostomy tube sites) relate to its immunogenic, angiogenic, and adhesive properties. Because enteral nutrition directly nourishes enterocytes and decreases bacterial translocation across the intestinal wall, feeding tube placement (gastrostomy or jejunostomy) should be considered during initial surgical exploration.

After addressing the underlying cause to prevent further contamination of the peritoneum, clinicians must reduce the infectious and foreign material load by a combination of debridement and lavage. Localized peritonitis should be treated with lavage of the affected area initially to minimize dissemination of the infection. A thorough lavage of the entire abdominal cavity with sterile isotonic fluid (warmed to body temperature) is warranted to remove bacteria, as well as GI contents, urine, or bile. The addition of antiseptics and antibiotics to lavage fluid is not beneficial and actually may be detrimental by inducing a superimposed chemical peritonitis. Lavage of the abdominal cavity is continued until the retrieved fluid is clear. All lavage fluid should be retrieved because fluid accumulation in the abdominal cavity impairs bacterial opsonization and clearance.[22]

If debridement and lavage can resolve gross foreign material or GI spillage and the source of contamination can be controlled, the abdomen should be closed primarily because of the potential complications associated with continued abdominal drainage (described below). All patients with open abdominal drainage are susceptible to superinfection with nosocomial bacteria and may experience massive fluid and protein losses.

Open peritoneal drainage is accomplished with a simple continuous pattern of nonabsorbable suture material in the rectus abdominis muscle, placed loosely enough to allow drainage through a gap of 1 to 6 cm in the body wall (Figure 122-3). A preassembled, sterile bandage that comprises a nonadherent contact layer, laparotomy sponges or gauze pads, roll cotton or surgical towels, roll gauze, and an outer water-impermeable layer is placed to absorb fluid and protect the abdominal contents from the environment. Initially, this bandage is replaced twice during the first 24 hours and daily thereafter, although the amount of drainage produced by an individual patient may dictate more frequent changes. A sterile-gloved finger may have to be inserted through the incision to break down adhesions and to allow thorough drainage of the peritoneal cavity. Alternatively, patients with severely contaminated tissues may require daily general anesthesia for repeated abdominal exploration and lavage before reapplying the bandage. The quantity of fluid can be estimated by the difference in weight of the bandage before application and after removal. Abdominal closure typically is performed 3 to 5 days after the initial surgery. The placement of a urinary catheter and collection system helps to limit urine soaking of the bandage and underlying exposed tissues.

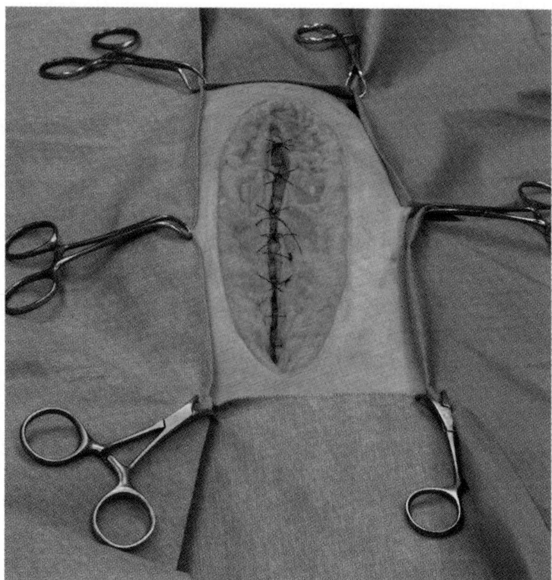

FIGURE 122-3 Open abdominal drainage incision. The incision should be closed with a single layer of nonabsorbable suture material to provide an opening that allows drainage but does not allow abdominal viscera or omentum to herniate through the open incision. A preassembled sterile bandage is placed over this incision and is changed daily, or more frequently as required to prevent strike-through.

The use of vacuum-assisted peritoneal drainage (VAPD) recently has been described as a means to provide continued postoperative abdominal drainage (see Chapter 139). Although the caudal one third to two thirds of the abdominal incision is closed primarily, the remainder of the incision is reapposed loosely (as described earlier in the chapter) and subatmospheric pressure applied to the cranial portion of the incision. This approach has been used successfully in human patients and its success demonstrated by significant reductions in open abdominal drainage duration times, number of dressing changes, re-exploration rate, and successful abdominal closure rates.[23,24] Superiority of this approach has yet to be established in small animal surgical patients. Survival rates for canine and feline septic peritonitis patients treated with VAPD has been reported as 37.5% (3/8)[25] and 50% (3/6),[26] which is similar to that seen with other abdominal drainage techniques. However, at this time, insufficient case numbers have been examined to draw conclusions as to whether the success of VAPD seen in human patients can be achieved in veterinary medicine. Dressings are available commercially that provide a barrier between the abdominal wall and viscera to protect the abdominal organs.

Alternatively, the abdomen may be closed primarily and drainage accomplished with closed suction (e.g., Jackson-Pratt) drains.[27] Closed suction drainage has been advocated for treatment of patients with generalized peritonitis because it has several advantages over open abdominal drainage, including a decreased risk of nosocomial infection, less intensive nursing care and bandaging requirements, decreased risk for evisceration, and the need for only one surgical procedure.[27] Disadvantages are that the drains may induce some fluid production and may become occluded, although active drainage was maintained for up to 8 days with this technique in 30 dogs and 10 cats in one study.[27] In addition, closed suction drains allow daily quantitative and qualitative assessment of retrieved fluid for evaluating the progression of the peritonitis. Typically, one drain placed between the liver and diaphragm is sufficient for small dogs and cats, whereas two drains are more appropriate for larger dogs (the fenestrated portion of second drain is placed in the caudal abdomen along the ventral body wall). The drain tubes exit the body wall through a paramedian stab incision and are sutured to the abdominal skin with a pursestring and Chinese finger-trap sutures (Figure 122-4). After routine closure of the abdomen, the suction reservoir bulb is attached to the tubing with vacuum (negative pressure) applied. A protective abdominal bandage is placed with sterile contact material around the tube-skin interface and is changed daily to allow assessment of this site. Fluid collected within the bulbs is emptied using aseptic technique, and the volume is recorded every 4 to 6 hours, or more frequently if needed. Drains are removed by applying gentle traction when the volume of fluid production has decreased significantly and cytologic analysis suggests resolution of the peritonitis (i.e., decreasing cell numbers and nondegenerative neutrophils, absence of bacteria). A sterile bandage is reapplied to cover the drain exit site for 24 hours.

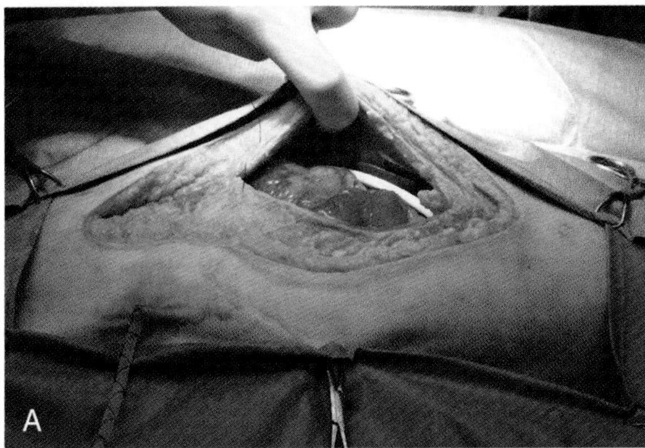

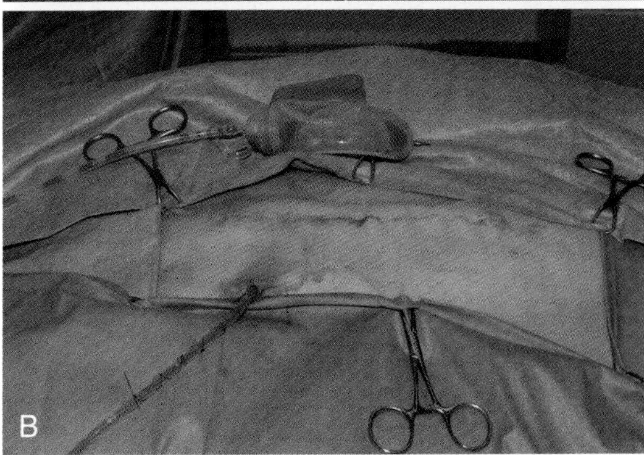

FIGURE 122-4 A, Closed suction drainage may be accomplished by placing a single Jackson-Pratt drain cranial to the liver (a second drain also may be placed in the caudal abdomen along the ventral body wall in large dogs), exiting paramedian to the abdominal incision. **B,** The tubing is secured to the body wall with a purse-string and Chinese finger trap sutures. Once the abdomen is routinely closed, the suction reservoir is attached and a vacuum is created by compressing the bulb. An abdominal bandage is placed to allow attachment of the drainage tubing and reservoir to prevent entanglement and premature removal by the patient.

Postoperative Care

Postoperative care for patients with peritonitis is typically intense because these patients are critically ill and subject to a variety of complications (see Chapter 131).[28] Aggressive intravenous fluid therapy is a necessity, particularly in patients with continued fluid losses from the inflamed peritoneal cavity. Electrolytes and acid-base status should be assessed routinely during the postoperative period and corrected as needed. Because anemia and hypoproteinemia are common complications in these patients, blood component therapy and synthetic colloidal support are often necessary, with a goal of maintaining a packed cell volume greater than 20% to 25%, serum protein over 3.5 g/dl, and colloid osmotic pressure higher than 16 mm Hg.

Proper nutrition provides a much-needed source of protein and energy in these patients. Failing to meet nutritional demands, either with parenteral or enteral nutrition, may contribute to impaired wound healing and immune defenses. In fact, early nutritional support is associated with shorter hospitalization in dogs.[29] Enteral feeding is preferred over parenteral feeding but may be stymied by the anorectic patient unless GI feeding tubes were placed at the time of surgery. If this was not done, a nasoesophageal tube can be placed easily in patients unable to tolerate repeated anesthesia. Alternatively, an esophagostomy tube may prove beneficial in patients that can tolerate general anesthesia. Animals with refractory vomiting typically require parenteral nutrition (see Chapters 129 and 130).

Postoperative hypotension may be treated with vasopressor therapy but only after addressing any underlying hypovolemia (see Chapters 8, 157, and 158). Proper analgesia is required to ensure patient comfort and to diminish the negative cardiovascular effects associated with overactive sympathetic stimulation (see Chapter 144). Other complications, including cardiac arrhythmias, disseminated intravascular coagulation, and systemic inflammatory response syndrome can be found in other chapters (see Chapters 6 and 91).

PROGNOSIS

The prognosis for animals with peritonitis depends on the underlying cause and whether infection is present. Studies in which patients have benefited from advances in critical care management cite overall survival rates of 44% to 71%.* Cats were reported to have a lower survival rate than dogs in two studies[3,30]; however, two studies focusing on feline septic peritonitis found an approximate 70% survival in animals in which treatment was pursued.[1,4] Poor prognostic indicators for animals with septic peritonitis have included refractory hypotension, cardiovascular collapse, disseminated intravascular coagulation, and respiratory disease.[27,34] The combination of hypothermia and bradycardia on presentation in feline patients appears to be a negative prognostic indicator.[1] Mortality rates in patients with septic peritonitis secondary to GI leakage have been reported to vary between 30% and 85%.[2,3,7,8] Bacterial contamination was associated significantly with mortality in animals with bile peritonitis.[36] Although survival in dogs with aseptic bile peritonitis was between 87% and 100%, those with septic bile peritonitis had survival rates of only 27% to 45%.[32,36] Overall survival rate in cats with uroperitoneum was 62%.[31] Survival rates appear to be similar in patients with septic peritonitis treated with primary closure, open peritoneal drainage, closed suction drainage, or vacuum-assisted drainage.[25-27,33,35]

REFERENCES

1. Ruthrauff CM, Smith J, Glerum L: Primary bacterial septic peritonitis in cats: 13 cases, J Am Anim Hosp Assoc 45:268-276, 2009.
2. Lascelles BDX, Blikslager AT, Fox SM, et al: Gastrointestinal tract perforation in dogs treated with a selective cyclooxygenase-2 inhibitor: 29 cases (2002-2003), J Am Vet Med Assoc 227:1112-1117, 2005.
3. Hinton LE, McLoughlin MA, Johnson SE, et al: Spontaneous gastroduodenal perforation in 16 dogs and seven cats (1982-1999), J Am Anim Hosp Assoc 38:176-187, 2002.
4. Costello MF, Drobatz KJ, Aronson LR, et al: Underlying cause, pathophysiologic abnormalities, and response to treatment in cats with septic peritonitis, J Am Vet Med Assoc 225:897-902, 2004.
5. Grimes JA, Schmeidt CW, Cornell KK, et al: Identification of risk factors for septic peritonitis and failure to survive following gastrointestinal surgery in dogs, J Am Vet Med Assoc 238:486-494, 2011.
6. Allen DA, Smeak DD, Schertel ER: Prevalence of small intestinal dehiscence and associated clinical factors: a retrospective study in 121 dogs, J Am Anim Hosp Assoc 28:70-75, 1992.
7. Wylie KB, Hosgood G: Mortality and morbidity of small and large intestinal surgery in dogs and cats: 115 cases (1991-2000), J Am Anim Hosp Assoc 30: 469-474, 1994.
8. Ralphs SC, Jessen CR, Lipowitz AJ: Risk factors for leakage following intestinal anastomosis in dogs and cats: 115 cases (1991-2000), J Am Vet Med Assoc 223:73-77, 2003.
9. Evans KL, Smeak DD, Biller DS: Gastrointestinal linear foreign bodies in 32 dogs: a retrospective evaluation and feline comparison, J Am Anim Hosp Assoc 30:445-450, 1994.
10. Parsons KJ, Owen LJ, Lee K, et al: A retrospective study of surgically treated cases of septic peritonitis in the cat (2000-2007), J Small Anim Pract 50:518-524, 2009.
11. Bjorling DE, Latimer KS, Rawlings CA, et al: Diagnostic peritoneal lavage before and after abdominal surgery in dogs, Am J Vet Res 44:816-820, 1983.
12. Kellett-Gregory LM, Boller EM, Brown DC, et al: Ionized calcium concentrations in cats with septic peritonitis: 55 cases (1990-2008), J Vet Emerg Crit Care 20(4):398-405, 2010.
13. Luschini MA, Fletcher DJ, Schoeffler GL: Incidence of ionized hypocalcemia in septic dogs and its association with morbidity and mortality: 58 cases (2006-2007), J Vet Emerg Crit Care 20(3):303-312, 2010.
14. Steyn PF, Wittum TE: Radiographic, epidemiologic, and clinical aspects of simultaneous pleural and peritoneal effusions in dogs and cats: 48 cases (1982-1991), J Am Vet Med Assoc 202:307-312, 1993.
15. Botte RJ, Rosin E: Cytology of peritoneal effusion following intestinal anastomosis and experimental peritonitis, Vet Surg 12(1):20-23, 1983.
16. Bonczynski JJ, Ludwig LL, Barton LJ, et al: Comparison of peritoneal fluid and peripheral blood pH, bicarbonate, glucose, and lactate concentration as a diagnostic tool for septic peritonitis in dogs and cats, Vet Surg 32:161-166, 2003.
17. Levin GM, Bonczynski JJ, Ludwig LL, et al: Lactate as a diagnostic test for septic peritoneal effusion in dogs and cats, J Am Vet Med Assoc 40:364-371, 2004.
18. Szabo SD, Jermyn K, Neel J, et al: Evaluation of postceliotomy peritoneal drain fluid volume, cytology, and blood-to-peritoneal fluid lactate and glucose differences in normal dogs, Vet Surg 40:444-449, 2011.
19. Schmiedt CW, Tobias KM, Otto CM: Evaluation of abdominal fluid: peripheral blood creatinine and potassium ratios for diagnosis of uroperitoneum in dogs, J Vet Emerg Crit Care 11(4):275-280, 2001.
20. White RAS, Williams JM: Intracapsular prostatic omentalization: a new technique for management of prostatic abscesses in dogs, Vet Surg 24:390-395, 1995.
21. Johnson MD, Mann FA: Treatment of pancreatic abscesses via omentalization with abdominal closure versus open peritoneal drainage in dogs: 15 cases (1994-2004), J Am Vet Med Assoc 228:397-402, 2006.
22. Platell C, Papadimitriou JM, Hall JC: The influence of lavage on peritonitis, J Am Coll Surg 191(6):672-680, 2000.
23. Pliakos I, Papavramidis TS, Michalopoulos N, et al: The value of vacuum-assisted closure in septic patients treated with laparotomy, Am Surgeon 78:957-961, 2012.
24. Perez D, Wildi S, Demartines N, et al: Prospective evaluation of vacuum-assisted closure in abdominal compartment syndrome and severe abdominal sepsis, J Am Coll Surg 205:586-592, 2007.
25. Cioffi KM, Schmiedt CW, Cornell KK, et al: Retrospective evaluation of vacuum-assisted peritoneal drainage for the treatment of septic peritonitis in dogs and cats: 8 cases (2003-2010), J Vet Emerg Crit Care 22(5):601-609, 2012.
26. Buote NJ, Havig ME: The use of vacuum-assisted closure in the management of septic peritonitis in six dogs, J Am Anim Hosp Assoc 48:164-171, 2012.
27. Mueller MG, Ludwig LL, Barton LJ: Use of closed-suction drains to treat generalized peritonitis in dogs and cats: 40 cases (1997-1999), J Am Vet Med Assoc 219:789-794, 2001.
28. Hardie EM: Life threatening bacterial infection, Comp Cont Educ Pract 17:763, 1995.
29. Liu DT, Brown DC, Silverstein DC: Early nutritional support is associated with decreased length of hospitalization in dogs with septic peritonitis: a retrospective study of 45 cases (2000-2009), J Vet Emerg Crit Care 224(453):459, 2012.
30. Culp WTN, Zeldis TE, Reese MS, et al: Primary bacterial peritonitis in dogs and cats: 24 cases (1990-2006), J Am Vet Med Assoc 234:906-913, 2009.
31. Aumann M, Worth LT, Drobatz KJ: Uroperitoneum in cats: 26 cases (1986-1995), J Am Anim Hosp Assoc 34:315-324, 1998.
32. Ludwig LL, McLoughlin MA, Graves TK, et al: Surgical treatment of bile peritonitis in 24 dogs and 2 cats: a retrospective study (1987-1994), Vet Surg 26:90-98, 1997.
33. Lanz OI, Ellison GW, Bellah JR, et al: Surgical treatment of septic peritonitis without abdominal drainage in 28 dogs, J Am Anim Hosp Assoc 37:87-92, 2001.
34. King LG: Post-operative complications and prognostic indicators in dogs and cats with septic peritonitis: 23 cases (1989-1992), J Am Vet Med Assoc 204:407-414, 1994.
35. Staatz AJ, Monnet E, Seim HB. Open peritoneal drainage versus primary closure for the treatment of septic peritonitis in dogs and cats, Vet Surg 31:174-180, 2002.
36. Mehler SJ, Mayhew PD, Drobatz KJ, et al: Variables associated with outcome in dogs undergoing extrahepatic biliary surgery: 60 cases (1988-2002), Vet Surg 33(6):644-649, 2004.

*References 1, 3-5, 8, 10, 27, 30-35.

CHAPTER 123

GASTRIC DILATATION-VOLVULUS

Claire R. Sharp, BSc, BVMS(Hons), MS, DACVECC

KEY POINTS

- Gastric dilatation-volvulus is a life-threatening condition that requires aggressive emergency medical stabilization, surgical intervention, and intensive postoperative care to optimize management.
- The pathogenesis of gastric dilatation-volvulus is complex and has genetic and environmental influences.
- Distention and displacement of the stomach cause cardiorespiratory dysfunction and gastrointestinal compromise.
- Potential life-threatening postoperative complications include cardiac arrhythmias, persistent hypotension, disseminated intravascular coagulation, peritonitis, and multiple organ dysfunction syndrome.
- Client education is key and promotes early intervention and decreased incidence of this condition through breeding and home management practices.
- Despite often challenging case management, the overall survival rate for dogs treated appropriately for gastric dilatation-volvulus approaches 85%.

Gastric dilatation–volvulus syndrome, commonly referred to as bloat, includes acute gastric dilatation (GD), acute gastric dilatation with gastric volvulus (GDV), and chronic gastric volvulus (cGV)[1], of which GDV is documented most thoroughly in the literature. GDV is a common condition associated with high morbidity and the potential for mortality in large and giant breed dogs presented for emergency care. The pathogenesis of GDV is complex and incompletely understood, although certain predispositions have now been well characterized. An index of suspicion for the condition is vital to direct appropriate and timely diagnostics and facilitate early medical and surgical intervention to restore hemodynamic stability and decompress and derotate the stomach. Given the potential for numerous perioperative complications, close monitoring and critical care treatment is indicated. An understanding of the pathogenesis, pathophysiology, and clinical features of this syndrome is important to ensure preparedness to manage this life-threatening condition optimally.

PATHOGENESIS

The pathogenesis of GDV is complex and multifactorial, with apparent genetic and environmental influences. GDV is predominantly a syndrome of large and giant breed dogs, although small dogs, cats, and other small mammals can develop GDV. Predisposed breeds include the Great Dane, Weimaraner, Saint Bernard, Gordon Setter, Irish Setter, and Standard Poodle.[2] GDV is also common in military working dogs such as German Shepherds.[3,4] Most dogs with GDV are adults, and older dogs are at greatest risk.

Several large studies have investigated risk factors for the development of GDV in affected breeds. Although different studies have slightly different findings, generally considered risk factors for developing GDV include first-degree relatives that have had GDV; higher thoracic depth-to-width ratio; lean body condition; advancing age; eating quickly (in large but not giant breed dogs); stressful events (e.g., boarding, traveling, or a vet visit); fearful, nervous, or aggressive temperament; and several diet-related factors, including having a raised food bowl, being fed only dry food, and/or a single large meal each day.[5-8]

Genetic predisposition to GDV may occur through inheritance of some of the aforementioned risk factors, such as conformation, personality, and/or temperament. In addition, failure of normal eructation and pyloric outflow mechanisms may be a prerequisite for gastric dilatation.[9] Laxity or agenesis of the perigastric ligaments, a well-characterized cause of GDV in children, also has been proposed a potential contributor to GDV in dogs. However, in a case control study, dogs with GDV had longer hepatogastric ligaments than control dogs because measurements were performed after GDV, the investigators were unable to determine if this was present pre-GDV (and hence potentially causative) or a consequence of GDV.[10] Stretching or transection of perigastric ligaments, as may occur with splenic masses or torsion and splenectomy, respectively, was suggested in earlier studies to increase risk for GDV,[11,12] although more recent studies have failed to confirm this association.[13,14] Similarly postprandial exercise, once thought to contribute to GDV risk, was not corroborated as a risk factor in subsequent studies,[6] and in fact has even been suggested to be beneficial in an Internet survey–based study.[15] A recent study suggested that gastric foreign body is a significant risk factor for GDV in at-risk breeds.[16]

Based on the available data current recommendations are that, as with other polygenic disorders, the breadth of the pedigree increases selective pressure against the condition. Breeders are encouraged to select dogs for breeding with lower thoracic depth-width ratios and whose littermates have not had GDV.[17]

PATHOPHYSIOLOGY

Although whether dilatation or volvulus occurs first in GDV syndrome has been debated, it is plausible that either may occur primarily because isolated cases of both conditions are documented. Regardless of the sequence of events, once gastric distention and malpositioning occur, cardiovascular compromise ensues, leading to decreased tissue oxygen delivery (DO_2) and the clinical manifestations of shock. Significant gastric distention results in the compression of the low-pressure intraabdominal veins (i.e., the caudal vena cava, portal vein, and splenic veins), leading to decreased caudal vena cava flow rate, decreased venous return, and subsequently decreased cardiac output and mean arterial pressure. Decreased DO_2 has multisystemic effects, including cardiovascular, respiratory, central nervous system, gastrointestinal (GI), and renal compromise. Decreased venous return and increased venous pressure also results in splanchnic pooling and portal hypertension that can contribute to interstitial edema and loss of intravascular volume. Shock is the life-threatening abnormality in dogs with GDV, and an understanding of the cause of this state allows rational treatment.

Respiratory compromise is common in dogs with GDV and is likely multifactorial. Gastric distention and increased intraabdominal pressure decrease total thoracic volume, prevent normal caudal diaphragmatic excursion, and may result in partial lung lobe collapse resulting in decreased tidal volumes and ventilation-perfusion (V/Q) mismatching. To compensate, respiratory rate and effort increase, although these compensatory efforts may become inadequate and both hypercapnia and hypoxemia may result.

Aspiration pneumonia is also likely to contribute to respiratory compromise in a proportion of dogs with GDV. Postoperative aspiration pneumonia has long been recognized as a complication of GDV, contributing to mortality.[1,18] A more recent study documented that 14% of dogs with GDV, in which preoperative thoracic radiographs were taken, had evidence of aspiration pneumonia.[19] Aspiration of pharyngeal contents preoperatively resulting in subclinical pneumonia preoperatively but contributing to morbidity and mortality postoperatively should be a consideration in the management of these dogs and may warrant preemptive screening thoracic radiographs and antimicrobial coverage.

Gastric necrosis is a feared complication of GDV because it is associated with increased morbidity and mortality.[20] In dogs with GDV, gastric blood flow likely is decreased because of a combination of factors including compression, thrombosis, or avulsion of the splenic and/or short gastric arteries, elevated intragastric pressure (gastric wall tension that exceeds driving pressure in the gastric wall arterioles and capillaries), and reduced cardiac output. Thus the degree of dilatation and degree and duration of volvulus likely contribute to the risk of gastric necrosis. Clinically, gastric necrosis in dogs with GDV follows a predictable pattern, with the gastric fundus most commonly affected, and progression to the body of the stomach. Necrosis of the cardia also occurs and is likely the result of direct vascular occlusion. Decreased gastric blood flow and gastric venous obstruction initially manifest as gastric mucosal, submucosal, and serosal edema and hemorrhage. Susceptibility of the mucosa to damage by hypoperfusion may be exacerbated by the acidic environment of the gastric lumen as well as its high metabolic demands. Left untreated, severe compromise to the gastric wall results in necrosis and ultimately perforation, with resultant peritonitis.

Intestinal blood flow also is compromised in dogs with GDV, resulting from direct compression of the portal vein and decreased cardiac output. Experimental models of GDV have documented intestinal villous injury and mucosal barrier compromise, leading to translocation and increased circulating concentrations of bacterial lipopolysaccharide, which in turn can contribute to systemic inflammation in these dogs. In combination with perioperative variables, such as anesthetic and analgesic drugs, this may contribute to postoperative GI ileus.

Given the close anatomic association between the stomach and spleen, splenic compromise is not uncommon in dogs with GDV and also is associated with a worse outcome. Splenic vascular avulsion, intravascular thrombosis, splenic torsion, and infarction have been reported in dogs with GDV, and thus intraoperative assessment of splenic viability and consideration of splenectomy is imperative. Rupture of the short gastric arteries commonly results in hemoabdomen and is another important surgical consideration.

Cardiac arrhythmias, mainly ventricular in origin, occur in approximately 40% of dogs with GDV.[1,18] Several factors have been implicated in the cause of cardiac arrhythmias. Coronary blood flow in experimentally induced GDV is decreased by 50%.[21] Histologic lesions compatible with myocardial ischemia are seen in experimental and spontaneous GDV and may establish ectopic foci of electrical activity. Circulating cardiostimulatory substances, such as epinephrine, and cardioinhibitory substances, such as proinflammatory cytokines (e.g., tumor necrosis factor-α and interleukin-1β), also have been implicated in the generation of arrhythmias. Consistent with the suspicion of myocardial injury, cardiac troponins have been proven elevated in dogs with GDV and are associated with the severity of ECG abnormalities and outcome.[22]

Abnormalities of acid-base status commonly are seen in dogs with GDV. Mixed acid-base disorders occur frequently, and primary abnormalities may include a high anion gap (lactate) metabolic acidosis (resulting from low DO_2), a hypochloremic metabolic alkalosis (resulting from sequestration of gastric HCl acid), and respiratory acidosis (resulting from hypoventilation and hypercapnia). Because of the potential for concurrent and opposing primary disorders pH may be normal.[23]

Electrolyte abnormalities also occur variably in dogs with GDV. Several pathophysiologic events may promote the development of hypokalemia, including the administration of a large volume of low-potassium fluids, sequestration of potassium within the stomach or loss through vomiting or lavage, hyperchloremic metabolic alkalosis with transcellular shifting, activation of the renin-angiotensin-aldosterone system, and catecholamine-induced intracellular shifting of potassium.

Disseminated intravascular coagulation (DIC) is another of the organ dysfunctions seen frequently in dogs with GDV.[11] Likely contributing factors include pooling of blood in the caudal vena cava, portal vein, or splanchnic circulation, tissue hypoxia, acidosis, systemic inflammation, endotoxemia, and potentially sepsis.

HISTORY AND CLINICAL SIGNS

Typically, the onset of clinical signs in dogs with GDV is acute, with affected dogs appearing restless, uncomfortable, and anxious. Most affected dogs salivate and may retch unproductively or attempt to vomit. As the condition progresses, they may be found collapsed. The owners may note a distended abdomen, although this can be difficult to appreciate in deep-chested, well-muscled, or obese dogs.

PHYSICAL EXAMINATION

Physical examination parameters are manifestations of the circulatory and respiratory compromise that results from acute GDV. Dogs often present in early decompensated shock, with depressed mentation, pale mucous membranes, prolonged capillary refill time, tachycardia, and weak pulses. Irregular cardiac rhythms and pulse deficits may be present. Increased respiratory rate and/or effort may be associated with discomfort and the aforementioned respiratory compromise. The abdomen can vary from unremarkable on palpation, through distended and firm, to tympanic. Splenic congestion may lead to the finding of splenomegaly and the spleen may be displaced caudally. If presentation has been delayed, dogs can be collapsed and comatose.

DIAGNOSIS

GDV generally is diagnosed based on a single right lateral abdominal radiograph.[24] Abdominal radiography is used to differentiate simple GD from GDV and to rule out other conditions. The pylorus in a dog with GDV moves cranial and dorsal to, and is separated by a soft tissue opacity from, the gastric fundus (called a *reverse C, double bubble,* or *Popeye sign*) in the right lateral projection (Figure 123-1). In comparison, the pylorus lies ventral to the fundus in a dog without volvulus.

If the presence or nature of gastric malpositioning is unclear based on the right lateral projection, a dorsoventral or ventrodorsal view may be taken to help delineate gastric position. In dogs with GDV the pylorus is to the left of midline on the dorsoventral view.

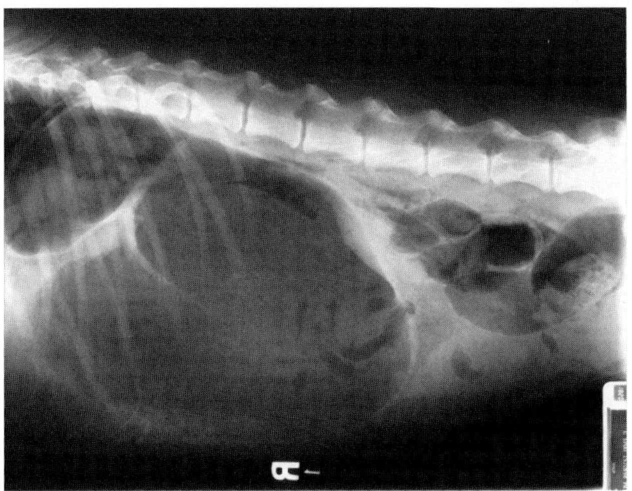

FIGURE 123-1 The right lateral recumbent view is the radiographic view of choice for diagnosis of gastric dilatation-volvulus. In this view, the pylorus moves to a cranial position in a dog with gastric dilatation-volvulus and is separated by a soft tissue opacity from the body of the stomach. In addition, in this example, enlargement of the spleen is evident and the serosal surfaces of the stomach, small intestine, and diaphragm are well defined, indicating a pneumoperitoneum.

In comparison, the pylorus lies to the right of midline in a dog without volvulus. Ventrodorsal positioning may lead to further cardiovascular compromise and may predispose to aspiration pneumonia should the dog regurgitate or vomit. Although gastric pneumatosis (intramural gas) and pneumoperitoneum suggest gastric necrosis and possibly perforation, gastric air may be introduced when a trocar is used in the emergency stabilization of the dog before radiographs are taken.[25]

Thoracic radiographs also may be indicated in dogs with GDV. Indications include to detect aspiration pneumonia, especially in those with hypoxemia, in older animals that may have coexisting disease, as a check for metastatic disease, or dogs suspected of having concurrent cardiac disease.[19]

A minimum database should include at least a packed cell volume (PCV), total protein (TP), and lactate measurement. The PCV and TP may be increased because of hemoconcentration. Hyperlactatemia is often present and failure of severe hyperlactatemia to improve with stabilization is a predictor of nonsurvival in dogs with GDV.[19,26-28]

A complete blood count and biochemical profile may be performed, especially in older animals, or to establish a baseline. Hematologic abnormalities may include hemoconcentration and a stress leukogram. Platelet consumption and/or loss may lead to thrombocytopenia.

Although dogs with GDV rarely have bleeding complications, baseline evaluation of coagulation status may be performed. The presence of three or more abnormal hemostatic parameters (prolonged prothrombin or activated partial thromboplastin time, hypofibrinogenemia, thrombocytopenia, elevated fibrin degradation products concentration, and antithrombin depletion), consistent with DIC, has been shown to correlate with gastric necrosis in one study.[11] DIC is also a negative prognostic indicator for survival.[29]

Biochemical abnormalities may include elevated hepatic transaminases (associated with hepatocellular damage) and/or azotemia (generally prerenal).

TREATMENT GOALS

The most important initial goal of treatment is to improve the cardiovascular status of the dog. After initial stabilization, treatment goals for dogs with GDV include gastric decompression, followed by surgery to reposition and pexy the stomach. Fluid resuscitation usually is performed through two large-bore (14- to 18-gauge) cephalic venous catheters. Resuscitation from shock involves administration of large volumes of isotonic crystalloids (with or without synthetic isotonic colloids) to effect (see Chapter 60), with the understanding that the maldistributive and/or obstructive component of shock cannot be resolved completely until the GDV is resolved. After appropriate volume resuscitation, vasopressor therapy may be necessary to manage hypotension. Continuous electrocardiographic (ECG) monitoring should be performed and arrhythmias (typically ventricular) treated if they interfere with cardiac output (see Chapter 48). It is unclear whether antimicrobial therapy is warranted in dogs with GDV; however, indications include evidence of aspiration pneumonia on preoperative radiographs, concern regarding GI bacterial translocation, and perioperative concerns, especially with regard to surgery of prolonged duration.

Gastric decompression should be attempted only after cardiovascular resuscitation has begun. Decompression further improves cardiorespiratory function; however, additional cardiovascular insult can occur associated with reperfusion injury. Gastric decompression ideally is accomplished with orogastric intubation after administration of opioid analgesia, rapid sequence anesthesia induction, and intubation. The smooth-surfaced orogastric tube should be marked to a length of the distance from the nares to the caudal edge of the last rib and the lubricated tube not passed beyond this point. In the event that the orogastric tube cannot be passed easily, trocar insertion should be performed using a large-gauge, short needle or over-the-needle catheter in a region of the left or right cranial, dorsolateral abdomen. This should be performed in an area that exhibits the greatest tympany and that has been clipped and aseptically prepared. Successful trocar placement is confirmed by a hissing sound as gas is released from the distended stomach. Splenic laceration and gastric perforation can occur as potential complications of attempted trocarization.

Immediate surgical intervention then is indicated for animals with GDV. Dogs with GD alone typically do not require immediate surgical intervention, although gastropexy is recommended to help prevent the development of GDV in the future. Conservative treatment in these dogs is tailored to the individual dog and may consist of intravenous fluid therapy and orogastric intubation as needed. In addition, simethicone (2 to 4 mg/kg PO q6h) and metoclopramide (0.2 to 0.4 mg/kg SC q8h) may be considered to decrease the amount of gas and promote gastric emptying, respectively. Even in the absence of radiographic evidence of gastric volvulus, surgical exploration should be recommended for GD patients that are unresponsive to medical treatment (repeated bloating, persistent hypotension, and/or tachycardia).

SURGICAL TREATMENT

The goals for surgery are to decompress and reposition the stomach, assess viability of the stomach and spleen, remove irreversibly compromised tissue, and create a permanent adhesion between the stomach and body wall to help prevent recurrence of gastric volvulus.

A large ventral midline incision is made, taking care not to damage abdominal viscera pushed up to the linea by gastric distention. Typically, the pylorus has moved from its normal position next to the right body wall toward the left body wall, in a clockwise direction. The rotation may be 90 to 360 degrees but most commonly is 180 to 270 degrees. With this type of rotation, the greater omentum is found draped over the cranial abdominal organs.

The stomach is decompressed by orogastric intubation (by the anesthetist with guidance by the surgeon) or via gastrocentesis and is rotated back into its normal position. The pylorus can be located by tracing the duodenum (identifiable by the attached pancreas) forward from the duodenocolic ligament. By gently bringing the pylorus back to the right of midline using one hand and using the other hand to push the body of the stomach dorsally, the stomach is derotated. An orogastric tube may be used to decompress the stomach completely and empty ingesta. Gastrotomy is not recommended for the removal of suspected food particles but is warranted if potentially obstructive material is present within the gastric lumen.

Next, the stomach and the spleen should be assessed for viability and gastric resection or splenectomy performed as needed. The spleen should be removed only if it has thrombosed or been damaged by the gastric volvulus. Partial gastrectomy is required when gastric necrosis has occurred, usually along the greater curvature. Gastric viability is assessed by examination of serosal color, palpation of gastric wall thickness, and evidence of arterial bleeding if incised. Gray or black coloration and palpable thinning of the stomach are signs of necrosis. Serosal coloration within areas of viable tissue may improve dramatically within minutes of decompression and repositioning. Gastric resection may be accomplished by preplacing stay sutures to minimize or prevent additional abdominal contamination, followed by resection of the devitalized area until bleeding tissue is reached and then closure.

Whether sutures or stapling (TA-90 or GIA-50) is used for closure, a second inverting suture line is recommended.[30] Invagination of necrotic tissue also has been used to treat gastric necrosis. Because this technique does not require opening of the gastric lumen, it is technically less demanding and is theoretically less likely to result in peritoneal contamination through gross spillage during partial gastrectomy or because of suture dehiscence; however, invaginated tissue may be prone to ulcer formation.[31,32] Although risks are associated with gastric resection and invagination, the devastating sequelae of perforation and peritonitis resulting from necrotic tissue that is not excised make it advisable to remove or invaginate any gastric tissue of questionable viability. Gastric necrosis has been associated with the development of several life-threatening complications, including peritonitis, DIC, sepsis, and arrhythmias.[29] Although two large retrospective studies examining postoperative outcome in dogs surgically treated for GDV (295 and 166 cases) did not agree whether gastric resection was a risk factor for death, these studies suggest that with aggressive preoperative and postoperative management, 70% to 74% of dogs with gastric resections may survive to discharge.[1,28,29]

Many procedures have been described to pexy the pyloric antral region of the stomach to the right body wall. These include the tube, incisional, muscular flap, circumcostal, and belt loop gastropexies, as well as various modifications of the above. The aim is to create a permanent adhesion between the antral region of the stomach and the right body wall. An incisional gastropexy is accomplished easily and quickly by making an incision about 5 cm long in the transversus abdominis muscle just caudal to the last rib, and a corresponding incision is made in the gastric seromuscular layer (taking care not to enter the gastric lumen). The orientation of the incisions reflects an attempt to preserve a relatively normal gastric position when the two edges of each incision are sutured together using either polypropylene or polydioxanone. The pexy site should not be incorporated into the abdominal closure because the stomach could be damaged if cranial abdominal surgery is required at a future date.

Although strength of the adhesions formed using the various techniques when tested in vitro varies somewhat, recurrence rates are similar for all of the above techniques when performed properly (percutaneous endoscopic gastrostomy tubes are not recommended because of inconsistent adhesion formation).[33] The tube gastropexy may be associated with a higher morbidity because of premature tube removal and peristomal cellulitis; however, it may be useful for continued gastric decompression of air and gastric secretions and for administration of medications and nutritional support to anorexic patients postoperatively.

The surgical technique used is probably less important than the surgeon's familiarity with one of the established techniques and the surgeon's ability to perform it proficiently and efficiently.

POSTOPERATIVE CARE

The aim of postoperative management is to maintain DO_2. Because of substantial fluid loss into the peritoneal cavity and GI tract, reasonably high fluid rates often are required for the first 48 to 72 hours. Mucous membrane color, capillary refill time, PCV, TP, urine output, ECG, blood pressure, and acid-base balance should be monitored closely postoperatively. Dogs recovering well from surgery can be offered food as soon as they are adequately awake from anesthesia. If nausea is present it can be treated with an antiemetic (see Chapter 162). These dogs can be weaned gradually off their intravenous fluids over 1 to 2 days. Because of the high incidence of gastric mucosal compromise, nonsteroidal antiinflammatory drugs are to be avoided, and histamine-2 receptor antagonists (e.g., famotidine) and gastric-coating agents (sucralfate) should be considered.

Cardiac arrhythmias often begin 12 to 24 hours after surgery. Continuous ECG monitoring is ideal. If arrhythmias occur, the aforementioned contributing factors should be sought and treated if present. Antiarrhythmic therapy should be considered if cardiac output is impaired or if serious electrical changes are evident (such as R on T phenomenon, multiform ventricular premature contractions, or when sustained ventricular tachycardia occurs with a heart rate of more than 180 beats/min) because this rate probably impairs ventricular filling and therefore cardiac output (see Chapters 47 and 48). Reports have been conflicting regarding whether the presence of arrhythmias negatively affects the prognosis.[1,18,29]

Perioperative risk factors significantly associated with death before suture removal include hypotension at any time during hospitalization, combined splenectomy and partial gastrectomy, peritonitis, sepsis, and DIC.[29] Dogs with GDV often fulfill criteria of the systemic inflammatory response syndrome and multiple organ dysfunction syndrome may occur in critically ill patients postoperatively (see Chapters 6 and 7).

OWNER RECOMMENDATIONS

Based on available information, veterinarians should discuss preventive strategies with owners of large and giant breed dogs. These include not feeding dogs from a raised food bowl and trying to ensure that large breed dogs eat more slowly (although this may be contraindicated in giant breed dogs). This may involve supervising feedings and separating dogs in households with multiple pets to decrease competition at feeding time. On the basis of the findings of Glickman and colleagues,[5] one of the strongest recommendations to prevent GDV is to remove from the breeding pools dogs that have a first-degree relative that has had a GDV. Prophylactic gastropexy, either laparoscopically or via a conventional approach, has been shown to reduce the lifetime probability of death resulting from GDV in at-risk breeds and therefore should be offered to owners of these dogs.[29,34,35]

REFERENCES

1. Brockman DJ, Washabau RJ, Drobatz KJ: Canine gastric dilatation/volvulus syndrome in a veterinary critical care unit: 295 cases (1986-1992), J Am Vet Med Assoc 207(4):460-464, 1995.

2. Glickman LT, Glickman NW, Perez CM, et al: Analysis of risk factors for gastric dilatation and dilatation-volvulus in dogs, J Am Vet Med Assoc 204(9):1465-1471, 1994.
3. Moore GE, Burkman KD, Carter MN, et al: Causes of death or reasons for euthanasia in military working dogs: 927 cases (1993-1996), J Am Vet Med Assoc 219(2):209-214, 2001.
4. Jennings PB, Jr., Butzin CA: Epidemiology of gastric dilatation-volvulus in the military working dog program, Mil Med 157(7):369-371, 1992.
5. Glickman LT, Glickman NW, Schellenberg DB, et al: Incidence of and breed-related risk factors for gastric dilatation-volvulus in dogs, J Am Vet Med Assoc 216(1):40-45, 2000.
6. Glickman LT, Glickman NW, Schellenberg DB, et al: Non-dietary risk factors for gastric dilatation-volvulus in large and giant breed dogs, J Am Vet Med Assoc 217(10):1492-1499, 2000.
7. Schellenberg DB, Yi Q, Glickman NW, et al: Influence of thoracic conformation and genetics on the risk of gastric dilatation-volvulus in Irish Setters, J Am Anim Hosp Assoc 34(1):64-73, 1998.
8. Raghavan M, Glickman NW, Glickman LT: The effect of ingredients in dry dog foods on the risk of gastric dilatation-volvulus in dogs, J Am Anim Hosp Assoc 42(1):28-36, 2006.
9. Brockman DJ, Holt DE, Washabau RJ: Pathogenesis of acute gastric dilatation-volvulus syndrome: is there a unifying hypothesis? Comp Cont Ed Pract Vet 22:1108, 2000.
10. Hall JA, Willer RL, Seim HB, et al: Gross and histologic evaluation of hepatogastric ligaments in clinically normal dogs and dogs with gastric dilatation-volvulus, Am J Vet Res 56(12):1611-1614, 1995.
11. Millis DL, Nemzek J, Riggs C, et al: Gastric dilatation-volvulus after splenic torsion in two dogs, J Am Vet Med Assoc 207(3):314-315, 1995.
12. Marconato L: Gastric dilatation-volvulus as complication after surgical removal of a splenic haemangiosarcoma in a dog, J Vet Med A Physiol Pathol Clin Med 53(7):371-374, 2006.
13. Goldhammer MA, Haining H, Milne EM, et al: Assessment of the incidence of GDV following splenectomy in dogs, J Small Anim Pract 51(1):23-28, 2010.
14. Grange AM, Clough W, Casale SA: Evaluation of splenectomy as a risk factor for gastric dilatation-volvulus, J Am Vet Med Assoc 241(4):461-466, 2012.
15. Pipan M, Brown DC, Battaglia CL, et al: An Internet-based survey of risk factors for surgical gastric dilatation-volvulus in dogs, J Am Vet Med Assoc 240(12):1456-1462, 2012.
16. de Battisti A, Toscano MJ, Formaggini L: Gastric foreign body as a risk factor for gastric dilatation and volvulus in dogs, J Am Vet Med Assoc 241(9):1190-1193, 2012.
17. Bell JS: Risk Factors for Canine Bloat. Paper presented at: Tufts' Canine and Feline Breeding and Genetics Conference, 2003, Tufts Cummings School of Veterinary Medicine.
18. Brourman JD, Schertel ER, Allen DA, et al: Factors associated with perioperative mortality in dogs with surgically managed gastric dilatation-volvulus: 137 cases (1988-1993), J Am Vet Med Assoc 208(11):1855-1858, 1996.
19. Green JL, Cimino Brown D, Agnello KA: Preoperative thoracic radiographic findings in dogs presenting for gastric dilatation-volvulus (2000-2010): 101 cases, J Vet Emerg Crit Care 22(5):595-600, 2012.
20. Mackenzie G, Barnhart M, Kennedy S, et al: A retrospective study of factors influencing survival following surgery for gastric dilatation-volvulus syndrome in 306 dogs, J Am Anim Hosp Assoc 46(2):97-102, 2010.
21. Horne WA, Gilmore DR, Dietze AE, et al: Effects of gastric distention-volvulus on coronary blood flow and myocardial oxygen consumption in the dog, Am J Vet Res46(1):98-104, 1985.
22. Schober KE, Cornand C, Kirbach B, et al: Serum cardiac troponin I and cardiac troponin T concentrations in dogs with gastric dilatation-volvulus., J Am Vet Med Assoc 221(3):381-388, 2002.
23. Wingfield WE, Twedt DC, Moore RW, et al: Acid-base and electrolyte values in dogs with acute gastric dilatation-volvulus, J Am Vet Med Assoc 180(9):1070-1072, 1982.
24. Hathcock JT: Radiographic view of choice for the diagnosis of gastric volvulus: the right lateral recumbent view, J Am Anim Hosp Assoc 20, 1984.
25. Fischetti AJ, Saunders HM, Drobatz KJ: Pneumatosis in canine gastric dilatation-volvulus syndrome, Vet Radiol Ultrasound 45(3):205-209, 2004.
26. Beer KA, Syring RS, Drobatz KJ: Evaluation of plasma lactate concentration and base excess at the time of hospital admission as predictors of gastric necrosis and outcome and correlation between those variables in dogs with gastric dilatation-volvulus: 78 cases (2004-2009), J Am Vet Med Assoc 242(1):54-58, 2013.
27. Zacher LA, Berg J, Shaw SP, et al: Association between outcome and changes in plasma lactate concentration during presurgical treatment in dogs with gastric dilatation-volvulus: 64 cases (2002-2008), J Am Vet Med Assoc 236(8):892-897, 2010.
28. de Papp E, Drobatz KJ, Hughes D: Plasma lactate concentration as a predictor of gastric necrosis and survival among dogs with gastric dilatation-volvulus: 102 cases (1995-1998), J Am Vet Med Assoc 215(1):49-52, 1999.
29. Beck JJ, Staatz AJ, Pelsue DH, et al: Risk factors associated with short-term outcome and development of perioperative complications in dogs undergoing surgery because of gastric dilatation-volvulus: 166 cases (1992-2003), J Am Vet Med Assoc 229(12):1934-1939, 2006.
30. Hedlund C, Fossum TW: Surgery of the digestive tract. In Fossum TW, editor: Small animal surgery, St Louis, 2007, Mosby.
31. MacCoy DM, Kneller SK, Sundberg JP, et al: Partial invagination of the canine stomach for treatment of infarction of the gastric wall, Vet Surg 15(3):237-245, 1986.
32. Parton AT, Volk SW, Weisse C: Gastric ulceration subsequent to partial invagination of the stomach in a dog with gastric dilatation-volvulus, J Am Vet Med Assoc 228(12):1895-1900, 2006.
33. Waschak MJ, Payne JT, Pope ER, et al: Evaluation of a percutaneous gastrostomy as a technique for permanent gastropexy, Vet Surg 26(3):235-241, 1997.
34. Rawlings CA, Mahaffey MB, Bement S, et al: Prospective evaluation of laparoscopic-assisted gastropexy in dogs susceptible to gastric dilatation, J Am Vet Med Assoc 221(11):1576-1581, 2002.
35. Ward MP, Patronek GJ, Glickman LT: Benefits of prophylactic gastropexy for dogs at risk of gastric dilatation-volvulus, Prev Vet Med 60(4):319-329, 2003.

CHAPTER 124
ACUTE KIDNEY INJURY

Catherine E. Langston, DVM, DACVIM • Adam E. Eatroff, DVM, DACVIM

KEY POINTS

- Acute kidney injury (AKI) resulting from hemodynamic compromise can be reversed rapidly, whereas animals with intrinsic parenchymal injury may take weeks to months to recover.
- Aggressive intravenous fluid therapy, beyond that which is necessary to restore and maintain normal renal perfusion, is more likely to result in complications associated with fluid overload than to improve renal function.
- Renal replacement therapy is the most is the most efficient means of managing uremic, acid-base, electrolyte, and fluid-related sequelae of fulminant acute kidney injury.
- Polyuric acute kidney injury can be associated with extreme fluid losses from high-volume urine output.
- Mortality rates for AKI are high (approximately 50%). Anuric and oliguric AKI carry a worse prognosis than polyuric acute kidney injury.
- Small increases in serum or plasma creatinine concentrations may be associated with a worse clinical outcome in hospitalized dogs.

Acute renal failure is a term often used to characterize an abrupt decline in renal function that leads to retention of uremic toxins and dysregulation of fluid, electrolyte, and acid-base balance. However, recent recognition of the wide spectrum of disease (ranging from clinically undetectable, subcellular damage to fulminant, excretory failure) and the association of small decreases in glomerular filtration rate (GFR) with worse clinical outcomes has led to a shift in terminology. The term *acute kidney injury (AKI)* currently is recognized as the preferred nomenclature for this clinical syndrome because it reflects the entire continuum of clinically relevant disease. Recently, in human medicine, staging schemes that characterize AKI according to minor, relative changes in GFR and serum or plasma creatinine concentrations, as well as quantification of urine output, have been developed and validated. The two most widely accepted schemes include the Risk Injury Failure End Stage Kidney Disease (RIFLE) scheme[1] and the Acute Kidney Injury Network (AKIN),[2] the latter of which was developed by modification of the former, with the intent to improve the sensitivity of detection of AKI. Both schemes appear to perform equally well when sensitivity for detection of AKI and predictive ability of adverse outcomes are considered. A recent study evaluating AKI in hospitalized cats and dogs, using a modified version of the AKIN scheme (Table 124-1), has confirmed a similar relationship between small increases in plasma creatinine concentrations and poor clinical outcomes.[3] Most notably, the authors showed that relative increases in plasma creatinine of at least 150% or 0.3 mg/dl from baseline concentrations are associated with increased in-hospital mortality.[3] These findings suggest that biomarkers of renal function (e.g., serum or plasma creatinine concentration) should be monitored closely in hospitalized patients. However, currently, most cases of AKI recognized in small animal practice are community-acquired and are characterized by severely increased serum or plasma creatinine concentrations, representing severe renal dysfunction.

ETIOLOGY

AKI classically has been categorized into hemodynamic (prerenal), renal parenchymal (intrinsic), and postrenal causes. Hemodynamic causes include decreases in renal perfusion or excessive vasoconstriction and are characterized as rapidly reversible if the inciting cause is eliminated. However, prolonged ischemia can contribute to renal parenchymal injury. Additional intrinsic causes of AKI include infectious diseases, toxins, or systemic diseases with renal manifestations. Removal of the inciting cause of parenchymal injury is often the only means of directly addressing this type of insult. Box 124-1[4] lists substances with a nephrotoxic potential. Postrenal AKI is due to obstruction or diversion of urine flow, including urethral obstruction, bilateral ureteral obstruction, or unilateral obstruction with a nonfunctional contralateral kidney, or rupture of any portion of the urinary tract. Restoration of urine flow may rapidly reduce the concentrations of circulating uremic toxins. However, prolonged obstruction of urine flow may lead to renal parenchymal injury.[5] Obstructive calcium oxalate nephroliths and ureteroliths are encountered in cats with increasing frequency. This condition commonly has many features of AKI, although frequently includes a significant component of chronic kidney disease. The classic causes of AKI frequently produce insults that encompass more than one of the hemodynamic, intrinsic, or postrenal processes. A specific cause is not identified in every case of AKI.

PATHOPHYSIOLOGY

The pathophysiologic process of AKI is often multifactorial, with overlapping ischemic, inflammatory, toxic, and septic components. Classically, the clinical course of AKI proceeds through four phases. These phases are defined by experimental models of ischemic acute kidney injury and may not be representative of the multifactorial nature of the disease. The initiation phase is characterized by the first

Table 124-1 Veterinary Acute Kidney Injury Staging Scheme for Dogs[3]

VAKI Stage	Criteria
Stage 0	Creatinine increase <150% from baseline
Stage 1	Creatinine increase of 150% to 199% from baseline OR Creatinine increase of 0.3 mg/dl from baseline
Stage 2	Creatinine increase of 200% to 299% from baseline
Stage 3	Creatinine increase of ≥300% from baseline OR An absolute creatinine value of >4.0 mg/dl

VAKI, Veterinary acute kidney injury.

stages of renal injury. Intervention at this phase may prevent progression to more severe injury, but injury at this stage occurs on a subcellular level and may not be biochemically evident. During the extension phase, cellular injury progresses to cell death. At this stage, biochemical derangements and clinical manifestations of disease manifest. During the maintenance phase, cell death and regeneration occur simultaneously, and the potential for and length of recovery from this phase may be determined by the balance between these processes. Removal of the initiating cause at this stage does not alter the existing damage but may allow for the balance to shift in favor of parenchymal regeneration. The recovery phase is characterized by improvement in GFR and tubular function; this final phase may last weeks to months.

BOX 124-1 ***Substances with Nephrotoxic Potential[4]***

Therapeutic Agents

Antimicrobial Agents

Aminoglycosides
Aztreonam
Carbapenems
Cephalosporins
Penicillins
Polymyxins
Quinolones
Rifampin
Sulfonamides
Tetracyclines
Vancomycin

Antifungal Agents

Amphotericin B

Cancer Chemotherapy

Cisplatin and carboplatin
Doxorubicin
Methotrexate

Antiviral Agents

Acyclovir
Foscarnet

Antiprotozoal Agents

Dapsone
Pentamidine
Sulfadiazine
Thiacetarsamide
Trimethoprim-sulfamethoxazole

Miscellaneous Therapeutic Agents

Acetaminophen
Allopurinol
Angiotensin-enzyme converting inhibitors
Antidepressants
Apomorphine
Cimetidine
Deferoxamine
Dextran-40
Diuretics
ε-Aminocaproic acid
EDTA
Lipid-lowering drugs
Lithium
Methoxyflurane
Nonsteroidal antiinflammatory drugs
Penicillamine
Phosphorus-containing urinary acidifiers
Streptokinase
Tricyclic antidepressants
Vitamin D analogs

Immunosuppressive Drugs

Azathioprine
Calcineurin inhibitors (e.g., cyclosporine, tacrolimus)
Interleukin-2

Nontherapeutic Agents

Endogenous Compounds

Hemoglobin
Myoglobin

Heavy Metals

Antimony
Arsenic
Bismuth salts
Cadmium
Chromium
Copper
Gold
Lead
Mercury
Nickel
Silver
Thallium
Uranium

Organic Compounds

Carbon tetrachloride and other chlorinated hydrocarbons
Chloroform
Ethylene glycol
Herbicides
Pesticides
Solvents

Miscellaneous Nontherapeutic Agents

Bee venom
Diphosphonate
Calcium antagonists
Gallium nitrate
Grapes or raisins
Illicit drugs
Lilies
Mushrooms
Radiocontrast agents
Snake venom
Sodium fluoride
Superphosphate fertilizer
Vitamin D-containing rodenticides

CLINICAL PRESENTATION

History

Listlessness, vomiting, diarrhea, and anorexia are common historical findings but are nonspecific and may be the result of a variety of extrarenal diseases. Oliguria, anuria, or polyuria may be reported. When a patient is polyuric, compensatory polydipsia may be present, or it may be overshadowed by anorexia. Less common historical findings include seizures, syncope, ataxia, and dyspnea.

Physical Examination

Dehydration is a common finding at the time of initial presentation. However, inaccurate assessment of hydration status by physical examination parameters is common, and many euhydrated and overhydrated patients are categorized erroneously as dehydrated. Other findings specific (but not exclusive) to uremia include halitosis, oral ulceration, tongue tip necrosis, scleral injection, bradycardia, cutaneous bruising, and peripheral edema. A hallmark of AKI is enlarged, painful kidneys. Melena or diarrhea may be present from uremic gastritis or enteritis. Signs of the primary ailment causing AKI (e.g., disseminated intravascular coagulation, vasculitis) may predominate.

DIAGNOSIS

Laboratory Tests

Care must be taken to examine urine shortly after collection to avoid artifactual changes in composition. The urine specific gravity is frequently isosthenuric (1.007 to 1.015) in cases of intrinsic failure. A urine dipstick may reveal any combination of glucosuria (without hyperglycemia), proteinuria, bilirubinuria, and hemoglobinuria, depending on the underlying etiology. The urine pH is usually acidic, unless there is a concurrent bacterial urinary tract infection. Careful microscopic assessment of urine sediment may disclose dysmorphic red blood cells (suggestive of glomerular disease), pyuria, or casts (most frequently granular, but red and white blood cell casts are observed uncommonly). Calcium oxalate crystals in large numbers are supportive of ethylene glycol intoxication, although a few oxalate crystals may be present in the urine of healthy patients. An in-house variation of a Romanowsky stain is frequently useful for detailed assessment of red and white blood cell morphology, as well as for the identification of bacteria. A bacterial urine culture is important to confirm the presence of a urinary tract infection and guide antimicrobial therapy.

The hematocrit may be increased from hemoconcentration or decreased from gastrointestinal blood loss or hemolysis. The platelet count may be normal or low, although uremia and various infectious diseases (e.g., leptospirosis) induce a thrombocytopathy, prolonging the buccal mucosal bleeding time despite a normal coagulation profile. An infectious cause or complications should be suspected when severe leukocytosis is present.

The severity of azotemia depends on the cause and duration of AKI. The ratio of blood urea nitrogen to creatinine can be high from GI bleeding or dehydration, or it can be low in early stages of AKI. Ionized calcium concentrations are normal or low (provided that hypercalcemia is not a cause of AKI). Ethylene glycol intoxication causes a profound ionized hypocalcemia, because of severe hyperphosphatemia and chelation of calcium by oxalate. The anion gap is usually high secondary to retained organic and inorganic acids that the injured kidney is unable to excrete but can be normal early in the course of disease, or if hypoalbuminemia is present. A high anion gap without (or before) the presence of azotemia is supportive of intoxication in cases of suspected ethylene glycol exposure. The anion gap is calculated by the formula

$$\text{Anion gap} = (Na^+ + K^+) - (HCO_3^- + Cl^-)$$

where Na^+ = sodium, K^+ = potassium, HCO_3^- = bicarbonate, and Cl^- = chloride. The normal anion gap is approximately 12 to 26 mEq/L; the average anion gap is 5 mEq/L higher in cats versus dogs.

Imaging

Survey abdominal radiographs may show a normal renal silhouette or renomegaly. Nephroliths or ureteroliths may be readily apparent, although obstructing ureteroliths may be smaller than the limit of detection. Abdominal ultrasonography usually shows normal or enlarged kidneys with normal parenchymal architecture. Perirenal fluid is seen commonly with a variety of causes.[6] Obstruction is characterized by renal pelvic dilation and lymphosarcoma by a diffusely thickened cortex and perirenal hypoechoic halo. Historically, pyelonephritis has been associated with renal pelvic dilation. However, this ultrasonographic sign is associated with various other lesions and is not pathognomonic for renal infection.[7] With ethylene glycol intoxication, oxalate crystal deposition in the kidneys increases the echogenicity, making the renal cortices and, to a lesser extent, the medulla hyperechoic. An intravenous pyelogram can aid in the identification of pelvic, ureteral, and cystic disease processes, especially obstructive renal lesions that are not readily apparent with survey radiography or ultrasound. In addition it can provide information regarding renal function in the contralateral kidney (i.e., if uptake of radiocontrast is not detectable in the renal parenchyma or collecting system, the likelihood of a substantial GFR in that kidney is low). If the GFR in an obstructed kidney is below a certain threshold, an intravenous pyelogram results in inadequate study quality because of poor uptake of contrast. Antegrade pyelography may be a better choice for ureteroliths because this technique does not rely on an adequate GFR. Computed tomography or magnetic resonance imaging can add information about renal architecture and better characterize obstruction but typically requires general anesthesia.

Other Diagnostic Modalities

Measurement of GFR (e.g., iohexol clearance, endogenous creatinine clearance, scintigraphy) can be expensive and some techniques are subject to limited availability. These studies have limited applicability in the initial treatment of AKI because the degree of impairment in GFR is almost always detectable by surrogate markers, such as serum or plasma creatinine concentration. Ethylene glycol intoxication is an emergency situation requiring immediate, specific therapy, which makes accurate and timely diagnosis crucial. Commercially available in-house test kits are available.

Leptospira serology detects an antibody production in response to organism or vaccine exposure. Care must be taken with interpretation of this test because there are multiple limitations. There is considerable cross-reactivity among different *Leptospira* serovars, but most available assays are limited in the number of serovars tested. Titers also may be negative within the first 7 to 10 days of illness; a fourfold rise after 2 to 4 weeks is used to confirm exposure when initial titers are negative. A single titer of 1:800 or greater, with appropriate clinical signs and in the absence of recent vaccination is also suggestive of *Leptospira* spp. exposure. However, there is a high degree of discordance in interpretation of leptospirosis among different commercial laboratories, potentially affecting interpretation of borderline results.[8] A strong clinical suspicion for leptospirosis must be present with titers in excess of 1:800 for serovar Autumnalis because titers often increase parallel to vaccinal serovars and with other diseases. Polymerase chain reaction assays for blood and urine have been developed for rapid, early diagnosis in dogs, but data on their clinical usefulness are lacking. Serologic tests for other infectious diseases known to cause AKI, such as Rocky Mountain spotted fever *(Rickettsia rickettsii), Ehrlichia canis,* Lyme disease *(Borrelia burgdorferi), Babesia* spp., or *Leishmania* spp., may be useful in certain areas or in cases of other consistent clinical or pathologic signs, although a positive titer does not prove causality of AKI.

Cytology of tissue acquired by fine-needle aspirates can confirm the presence of lymphosarcoma but frequently provides false-negative results. The risk of bleeding secondary to this procedure is low but possible. Histopathology can be assessed via percutaneous, ultrasonographically guided needle biopsy, laparoscopy, or surgical wedge biopsy. Histopathology may confirm a suspected cause (e.g., ethylene glycol intoxication, renal lymphosarcoma) or it may disclose nonspecific findings. When AKI cannot be distinguished clinically from end-stage chronic kidney disease, histopathology (particularly Masson's trichrome stain) can aid in assessment of the severity of fibrosis and provide insight into the potential for renal recovery. The risk of significant hemorrhage secondary to renal biopsy is high when uremia is severe.

TREATMENT

Treatment of AKI is directed primarily at the underlying disease process (when identified) and supportive measures to minimize the clinical sequelae of uremia.

Fluid Therapy

To ensure normal perfusion of the kidneys, extracellular fluid deficits should be corrected with a balanced polyionic solution. Ultimately, the type of fluid administered must be guided by monitoring of serum or plasma concentration of electrolytes because the degree of solute and free water balance varies widely in patients with AKI. Colloidal support also may be considered to reduce the total amount of fluid administered, if oliguria or anuria is suspected, although no benefit over crystalloid therapy has been documented in human or veterinary medicine.[9,10] Avoidance of fluid overload (typically defined as fluid accumulation more than 10% of baseline body weight) is essential because ample evidence documents the association between fluid overload and worse clinical outcomes.[11,12]

The formula used to calculate the volume of fluid to administer for replacement of deficits (percentage of dehydration × body weight [kg] = fluid deficit in liters) can result in administration of inadequate or excess volumes of fluid. Therefore, although this formula can be an initial guide, goal-directed therapy to restore surrogate markers of perfusion (e.g., blood pressure, venous lactate concentration, venous oxygen saturation) should be employed with endpoints set to be reached within 24 hours, if not sooner (see Chapter 59). If oliguria or anuria persists despite achievement of normal surrogate markers of perfusion, additional fluid administration is more likely to result in fluid overload than urine production.

Maintenance fluid administration (volume and composition) should be guided by the volume and composition of urine produced, as well as ongoing, sensible losses (vomitus, diarrhea, and yield from gastric suction) and insensible loss (respiration, formed stool). Urine volume can be determined by a variety of methods, including (1) indwelling urinary catheter and closed collection system, (2) collection of naturally voided urine, (3) metabolic cage, (4) weighing cage bedding and litter pans (1 ml of urine = 1 g), and (5) using body weight before and immediately after urination. Urine production can be categorized as anuria (none to negligible amount), oliguria (less than 0.5 ml/kg/hr), or polyuria (more than 2 ml/kg/hr). Ancillary monitoring techniques of urine output include measurement of urine sodium concentration with point of care analyzers. Insensible losses can be estimated between 12 and 29 ml/kg/day and depend on a variety of factors, such as species, patient activity, and body temperature.

Once the patient's fluid deficit has been corrected and maintenance fluid therapy is initiated, care must be taken to maintain a neutral fluid balance, as well as normal surrogate markers of perfusion. Attempts at fluid diuresis to improve GFR are often futile and frequently result in fluid overload, a condition that has been associated with a higher mortality rate in human and veterinary patients. Careful attention must be given to serial changes in the patient's body weight because peracute fluctuations in weight are most likely the result of changes in fluid balance rather than changes in lean muscle or fat content. Consideration of the fluid load incurred by administration of parenteral medications, parenteral and enteral nutrition, and catheter flushes (to maintain patency and for techniques such as central venous pressure monitoring) is essential to maintain a neutral fluid balance.

An anuric, euhydrated patient should receive intravenous fluid therapy to replace insensible loss only. Frequently, this requirement is met in excess by administration of medications, nutrition, and catheter flushes. If the patient is diagnosed with fluid overload, all fluid therapy should be withheld. Fluid overload with concurrent oliguria or anuria is a clear indication for renal replacement therapy.

Monitoring fluid status is an ongoing process that must be repeated frequently. Efforts should be made to adhere to objective monitoring parameters (e.g., body weight, venous lactate concentration) of fluid status because subjective parameters, (e.g., skin turgor, saliva production) are inaccurate and often affected by variables other than hydration status. Body weight should be measured at least twice daily. Central venous pressure measurement traditionally has been recommended as a surrogate marker of cardiac preload, and thus fluid status. However, a thorough understanding of the limitations of this technique is necessary for appropriate interpretation because the correlation between central venous pressure and clinical manifestations of fluid overload is not perfect.

Diuretics

Many of the benefits of the most commonly used diuretics in veterinary AKI, furosemide and mannitol, have been only theorized or demonstrated in experimental models of AKI. In fact, little or no clinical evidence in human or veterinary medicine, respectively, demonstrates that diuretics improve outcome in established AKI. A recent meta-analysis of randomized controlled clinical trials of loop diuretic use in human AKI showed a statistically insignificant trend towards an association with increased mortality.[13]

Some nephrologists have postulated that the ability to respond to diuretics is a marker of less severe renal injury associated with a better prognosis. However, an increase in urine output after diuretic administration does not necessarily preclude the need for renal replacement therapy if severe uremia or acid-base and electrolyte abnormalities persist. In veterinary medicine, because renal replacement therapy is not readily available, diuretic administration plays a primary role in volume management. Conversion from an oliguric or anuric state to normal urine production or polyuria may enhance the clinician's ability to prevent or manage fluid overload and thus allow administration of necessary parenteral medications and nutrition that would otherwise contribute to fluid overload, (see Chapter 160).

Acid-Base and Electrolyte Balance

Metabolic acidosis is a frequent complication in AKI of varying severities. When tubular function is compromised, the ability to reabsorb bicarbonate and excrete hydrogen ions is diminished. Lactic acidosis secondary to compromised tissue perfusion (i.e., either volume deficit or excess) also may contribute. Treatment is directed at restoring perfusion and provision of supplemental alkali, usually in the form of parenteral sodium bicarbonate. Hydrogen ions combine with the bicarbonate to form carbonic acid, which quickly dissociates to water and carbon dioxide, the latter of which is removed via gas exchange in the lungs. If the patient is hypoventilating, carbon dioxide accumulates. Bicarbonate administration in this situation can increase the partial pressure of carbon dioxide and can lead to paradoxical CNS acidosis. This phenomenon is due to the ability of carbon dioxide to diffuse across the blood-brain barrier, whereas the charged bicarbonate molecule diffuses across this barrier less readily. An additional consideration when administering parenteral sodium bicarbonate is that most formulations have high osmolality (e.g., 8.4% solution = 1 mEq/ml = 2000 mOsm/L). Therefore this solution must be diluted before administration, and the total volume administered must be factored into the fluid therapy plan. Sodium bicarbonate therapy usually is reserved for patients with a pH less than 7.2 or bicarbonate level less than 12 mEq/L. The bicarbonate dosage can be calculated from the formula

$$0.3 \times \text{body weight (kg)} \times \text{base deficit} = \text{bicarbonate (mEq/L)}$$

where the base deficit = 24 mEq/L - patient bicarbonate concentration. One fourth to one third of the dose should be given intravenously as a slow bolus, and an additional one fourth over the next 4 to 6 hours. Subsequent doses should be based on serial venous blood gas analyses. Provision of bicarbonate with renal replacement therapy is as effective in restoring extracellular acid-base status as sodium bicarbonate infusion and has the added advantage of avoiding the fluid load necessary with the latter treatment. Although no evidence in the form of randomized controlled trials supports supplementation of alkali in human AKI,[14] it is recommended in veterinary AKI when renal replacement therapy is not available.

Hyperkalemia can be an immediately life-threatening complication of AKI and is secondary to a decline in excretory function. The increase in extracellular potassium concentration makes excitable cells refractory to repolarization, thus resulting in decreased conduction of cardiac and neuromuscular tissue. Typical electrocardiographic changes include bradycardia, tall T waves, shortened QT intervals, wide QRS complexes, and small, wide, or absent P waves. Severe hyperkalemia can lead to sine waves, ventricular fibrillation, or standstill. A variety of pharmacologic treatments are available for emergent hyperkalemia (see Chapter 51), but these therapies act to translocate potassium to the intracellular space or increase the resting membrane potential to allow repolarization of excitable cells, rather than enhance excretion of potassium. Therefore the efficacy of these treatments is modest and transient. Only provision of renal replacement therapy or restoration of native renal excretory function can reduce significantly the potassium burden in fulminant AKI.

Although ionized hypocalcemia occurs frequently in AKI, clinical signs (e.g., tetany) associated with this problem are rare. When manifestations of hypocalcemia do occur, the minimum dose of supplemental calcium that controls clinical signs should be used to prevent precipitation with phosphorus. Calcium gluconate 10% can be used at a dosage of 0.5 to 1.5 ml/kg IV over 20 to 30 minutes. As with the treatment of hyperkalemia, the electrocardiogram should be monitored closely during infusion.

Management of Gastrointestinal Signs

Antiemetic therapy is recommended in all patients with severe AKI, regardless of whether they are vomiting (see Chapter 162). Metoclopramide is used frequently for this purpose, but reduced clearance associated with compromised renal function and resultant adverse effects (primarily neurologic) must be considered. Metoclopramide was found to be inferior to the 5-HT_3 antagonist, ondansetron, in prevention of vomiting and nausea in uremic human patients.[15] In addition, in a study of vomiting dogs with presumably normal renal function, metoclopramide was less efficacious than maropitant in preventing emesis.[16] The use of antisecretory drugs (e.g., histamine-2-receptor antagonists, proton pump inhibitors; see Chapter 161) historically has been recommended for patients with AKI. Although uremic gastritis and stress-related mucosal disease is a concern in human AKI patients, gastric acid output and intragastric pH are not compatible with a hypersecretory state.[17] Nonetheless, because of the high incidence of hemorrhage from the gastrointestinal tract in human AKI patients (presumably related to a combination of uremic injury and stress-related mucosal disease) and its association with mortality,[18] antisecretory drugs should be considered in high-risk patients. A recent meta-analysis showed superiority of proton pump inhibitors versus histamine-2 receptor antagonists in the prevention of stress related mucosal bleeding.[19] These results, in combination with the potential for accumulation of histamine-2 receptor antagonists in patients with diminished renal function favor the use of proton pump inhibitors.

Nutritional Support

Nutritional support for AKI has been shown to improve nitrogen balance and thus survival in oliguric or anuric humans.[20] Similar results for nitrogen balance (but not survival) have been shown for patients with preserved urine production.[21] Enteral feeding is the preferred method of nutrient delivery but often is limited by vomiting and ileus. For those patients that are not vomiting, esophageal, gastric, and jejunal feeding devices can be used. If vomiting cannot be controlled, partial or total parenteral nutrition should be considered. In patients who are anuric or oliguric, the volume and osmolality of nutritional product, whether administered enterally or parenterally, must be taken into consideration and may constitute a relative contraindication unless there is a method of excess fluid and solute removal (e.g., renal replacement therapy). Phosphate binders (e.g., aluminum hydroxide) administered concurrently with enteral feedings may decrease phosphate absorption. However, the benefits of phosphate control in regard to outcome in AKI have not been determined.

Renal replacement therapy

Renal replacement therapy (see Chapter 205) is the most efficient means of managing uremic, acid-base, electrolyte, and fluid-related sequelae of AKI. In fulminant cases, available pharmacologic therapies are, at best, incompletely effective at reversing the aforementioned complications, and their effects are transient. However, the cost and limited availability of renal replacement therapy make it impractical for most owners and veterinarians.

Fluid administration during recovery phase polyuria

During renal recovery, the patient may convert from oliguria or anuria to a polyuric state. This phenomenon may occur with any cause of AKI, but most commonly occurs in cases of leptospirosis or obstructive disease. Careful monitoring of urine volume, body weight, and surrogate markers of perfusion is necessary to guide fluid administration and avoid fluid depletion. Intravenous fluids often are administered at sustained delivery rates higher on a per-weight basis than any other situation in veterinary medicine. Once the patient's azotemia and body weight are stable on a fixed delivery rate of intravenous fluids, the rate can be decreased by 10% per day. If the urine output diminishes by a corresponding degree and the patient's weight and surrogate markers of perfusion remain stable, tapering of the intravenous fluid rate should continue. Recovery phase polyuria can last for weeks, until tubular function returns to a level sufficient to control solute and water losses.

Specific Treatments

In many cases of AKI, the exact cause is not determined, and therapy is aimed at controlling the sequelae of uremia, as well as acid-base, electrolyte, and fluid-related disorders. However, some causes of AKI have specific treatments. Penicillin G or ampicillin (22 mg/kg q8h) is the antibiotic of choice for leptospiremia, although doxycycline is also effective in the leptospiremic phase. The carrier state can be eliminated using doxycycline (5 mg/kg q12h for 2 weeks). Intervention by surgical or endoscopy-guided stent placement is indicated for obstruction of the upper (and less frequently, lower) urinary tract, although ureteral obstructions can resolve spontaneously. Few antidotes are available for nephrotoxic injuries. Antidotes for ethylene glycol (4-methylpyrazole [4-MP, Antizol-Vet] or alcohol) must be administered shortly after ingestion to be effective.

PROGNOSIS

The overall mortality rate for AKI in dogs is approximately 60%.[22] In the dogs that survive, approximately 60% have chronic kidney disease, and only 40% recover normal renal function.[22] In cats, mortality is approximately 40% to 50%, with approximately 50% of survivors left with chronic kidney disease.[23] Certain subsets of patients have better prognoses. Approximately 82% to 86% of dogs with leptospirosis survived in one series.[24] Patients with polyuria have a better outcome than those with oliguria or anuria.[23,25]

REFERENCES

1. Bellomo R, Ronco C, Kellum JA, et al: Acute renal failure—definition, outcome measures, animal models, fluid therapy and information technology needs: the Second International Consensus Conference of the Acute Dialysis Quality Initiative (ADQI) Group, Crit Care 8:R204-212, 2004.
2. Mehta RL, Kellum JA, Shah SV, et al: Acute Kidney Injury Network: report of an initiative to improve outcomes in acute kidney injury, Crit Care 11:R31, 2007.
3. Thoen ME, Kerl ME: Characterization of acute kidney injury in hospitalized dogs and evaluation of a veterinary acute kidney injury staging system, J Vet Emerg Crit Care (San Antonio) 2011;21:648-657.
4. Langston CE: Acute uremia. In Ettinger SJ, Feldman EC, editors: Textbook of veterinary internal medicine, St Louis, 2010, Saunders.
5. Wen JG, Frokiaer J, Jorgensen TM, et al: Obstructive nephropathy: an update of the experimental research, Urol Res 27:29-39, 1999.
6. Holloway A, O'Brien R: Perirenal effusion in dogs and cats with acute renal failure, Vet Radiol Ultrasound 48:574-579, 2007.
7. D'Anjou MA, Bedard A, Dunn ME: Clinical significance of renal pelvic dilatation on ultrasound in dogs and cats, Vet Radiol Ultrasound 52:88-94, 2011.
8. Miller MD, Annis KM, Lappin MR, et al: Variability in results of the microscopic agglutination test in dogs with clinical leptospirosis and dogs vaccinated against leptospirosis, J Vet Intern Med 25:426-432, 2011.
9. Myburgh J, Cooper DJ, Finfer S, et al: Saline or albumin for fluid resuscitation in patients with traumatic brain injury, N Engl J Med 357:874-884, 2007.
10. Myburgh JA, Finfer S, Bellomo R, et al: Hydroxyethyl starch or saline for fluid resuscitation in intensive care, N Engl J Med 367(20):1901-1911, 2012.
11. Bouchard J, Soroko SB, Chertow GM, et al: Fluid accumulation, survival and recovery of kidney function in critically ill patients with acute kidney injury, Kidney Int 76:422-427, 2009.
12. Sutherland SM, Zappitelli M, Alexander SR, et al: Fluid overload and mortality in children receiving continuous renal replacement therapy: the prospective pediatric continuous renal replacement therapy registry, Am J Kidney Dis 55:316-325, 2010.
13. Bagshaw SM, Delaney A, Haase M, et al: Loop diuretics in the management of acute renal failure: a systematic review and meta-analysis, Crit Care Resusc 9:60-68, 2007.
14. Hewitt J, Uniacke M, Hansi NK, et al: Sodium bicarbonate supplements for treating acute kidney injury, Coch Database Syst Rev 6:CD009204, 2012.
15. Ljutic D, Perkovic D, Rumboldt Z, et al: Comparison of ondansetron with metoclopramide in the symptomatic relief of uremia-induced nausea and vomiting, Kidney Blood Press Res 25:61-64, 2002.
16. de la Puente-Redondo VA, Siedek EM, Benchaoui HA, et al: The antiemetic efficacy of maropitant (Cerenia) in the treatment of ongoing emesis caused by a wide range of underlying clinical aetiologies in canine patients in Europe, J Small Anim Pract 48:93-98, 2007.
17. Wesdorp RI, Falcao HA, Banks PB, et al: Gastrin and gastric acid secretion in renal failure, Am J Surg 141:334-338, 1981.
18. Fiaccadori E, Maggiore U, Clima B, et al: Incidence, risk factors, and prognosis of gastrointestinal hemorrhage complicating acute renal failure, Kidney Int 59:1510-1519, 2001.
19. Barkun AN, Bardou M, Pham CQ, et al: Proton pump inhibitors vs. histamine 2 receptor antagonists for stress-related mucosal bleeding prophylaxis in critically ill patients: a meta-analysis, Am J Gastroenterol 107:507-520, 2012.
20. Scheinkestel CD, Kar L, Marshall K, et al: Prospective randomized trial to assess caloric and protein needs of critically Ill, anuric, ventilated patients requiring continuous renal replacement therapy, Nutrition 19:909-916, 2003.
21. Singer P: High-dose amino acid infusion preserves diuresis and improves nitrogen balance in non-oliguric acute renal failure, Wien Klin Wochenschr 119:218-222, 2007.
22. Vaden SL, Levine J, Breitschwerdt EB: A retrospective case-control of acute renal failure in 99 dogs, J Vet Intern Med 11:58-64, 1997.
23. Worwag S, Langston CE: Acute intrinsic renal failure in cats: 32 cases (1997-2004), J Am Vet Med Assoc 232:728-732, 2008.
24. Adin CA, Cowgill LD: Treatment and outcome of dogs with leptospirosis: 36 cases (1990-1998), J Am Vet Med Assoc 216:371-375, 2000.
25. Behrend EN, Grauer GF, Mani I, et al: Hospital-acquired acute renal failure in dogs: 29 cases (1983-1992), J Am Vet Med Assoc 208:537-541, 1996.

CHAPTER 125

CHRONIC KIDNEY DISEASE

Catherine E. Langston, DVM, DACVIM • Adam E. Eatroff, DVM, DACVIM

KEY POINTS

- Chronic kidney disease (CKD) has a high prevalence in geriatric cats and dogs but also occurs in juvenile animals.
- Although inciting and perpetuating causes of chronic kidney disease should be investigated, the underlying cause rarely is identified.
- Intravenous and subcutaneous fluid therapy should be directed toward the restoration and maintenance, respectively, of normal hydration status. Many cats require large volumes of parenteral fluid to achieve these goals.
- Early initiation of enteral nutritional support and treatment with erythropoiesis stimulating agents should be considered in cases of decompensated, end-stage chronic kidney disease.
- Clients should be counseled on the progressive and irreversible course of chronic kidney disease.

In recent years the veterinary community has supplanted the term *chronic renal failure*, which was used previously to describe the multitude of chronic nephropathies that affect cats and dogs, with a new designation, chronic kidney disease. The word *failure*, which may imply end-stage disease, was eschewed for the more inclusive description, disease, with the intent of emphasizing the broad spectrum of clinically relevant disease that may be present in various types of chronic nephropathies. This paradigm shift was reflected by the four-stage classification system proposed by the International Renal Interest Society (IRIS), which includes two stages of disease severity defined by plasma or serum creatinine concentrations within the normal range of many reference laboratories.[1] This classification scheme is depicted in Table 125-1. Despite the growing appreciation for the long-term metabolic and clinical sequelae that may arise from less severe, possibly even biochemically undetectable, ongoing injury, the objective of this chapter is to address the clinical aspects of decompensated or end-stage chronic kidney disease (CKD).

ETIOLOGY

In cats and dogs, the underlying cause of CKD rarely is determined. Histopathologic renal lesions consist primarily of inflammatory infiltrates in the tubulointerstitium, in the glomeruli, or in both nephron subunits simultaneously. Concurrent fibrosis is almost always present to varying degrees. Additional findings include tubular atrophy and glomerular sclerosis or senescence. The typical location and specific characteristics of the histopathologic lesions vary with species. In cats, lymphoplasmacytic tubulointerstitial nephritis and fibrosis is the most common morphologic diagnosis, noted in 70.4% of cases in one study.[2] In dogs, glomerular lesions appear more commonly, with estimates as high as 52% in one study.[3] Another study identified interstitial nephritis as the most common lesion (58.3%).[2] It is hypothesized that, in many cases, these lesions are not due to any specific underlying cause but are more likely the final point in a pathway common to a variety of renal insults. However, for many congenital forms of CKD (of genetic and other origins), the inciting and ongoing insult is known. These diseases include renal dysplasia, polycystic kidney disease, and amyloidosis (Box 125-1).[4] Additional discernible, inciting, and perpetuating causes of CKD include pyelonephritis, nephrolithiasis or ureterolithiasis, infarctions, lymphoma, glomerulonephritis, and incomplete resolution of acute renal failure.

PATHOPHYSIOLOGY

CKD progression is speculated to be the result of an ongoing insult or secondary to compensatory changes of surviving nephrons that may be maladaptive in the long-term. Ongoing injury may manifest in the glomerulus, tubulointerstitium, or in both nephron subunits. However, because each nephron operates as a unit, if the glomerulus is damaged irreversibly, the associated tubule degenerates, and vice versa. As functional renal mass is lost, the remaining nephrons hypertrophy. Although initially adaptive, glomerular hyperfiltration damages the surviving nephrons. After a certain amount of damage

Table 125-1 International Renal Interest Society Staging Scheme for Chronic Kidney Disease[1]

	Dogs	Cats
Plasma Creatinine (mg/dl)		
Stage I	<1.4	<1.6
Stage II	1.4-2.0	1.6-2.8
Stage III	2.1-5.0	2.8-5.0
Stage IV	>5.0	>5.0
Substage Based on Urine Protein-to-Creatinine Ratio		
Nonproteinuric (NP)	<0.2	<0.2
Borderline proteinuric (BP)	0.2-0.5	0.2-0.4
Proteinuric (P)	>0.5	>0.4
Substage Based on Arterial Blood Pressure (same parameters for cats and dogs)		
	Systolic blood pressure (mm Hg)	**Diastolic blood pressure (mm Hg)**
Minimal risk (AP0)	<150	<95
Low risk (AP1)	150-159	95-99
Moderate risk (AP2)	160-179	100-119
High risk (AP3)	≥180	≥120
No evidence of end organ damage/ complications		No complications (NC)
Evidence of end organ damage/ complications		Complications (C)
Blood pressure not measured		Risk not determined (RND)

has been sustained, kidney injury may be and often is irreversible and progressive regardless of whether the initiating cause is resolved. Once a threshold of dysfunction has been reached, complications associated with decreased functional mass become clinically evident.

CLINICAL PRESENTATION

CKD affects cats and dogs of any age but is more common in the geriatric population. The highest prevalence (31%) was reported in cats older than 15 years of age.[5] The canine population has a bimodal distribution of prevalence because of a high frequency of CKD in the juvenile population as a result of congenital disease, as well as a high frequency of CKD in the geriatric population. Several reports exist of breed or familial associations with specific structural and functional lesions. A summary of these associations is presented in Box 125-1.[4]

Mild clinical signs (especially polyuria, polydipsia, and weight loss) may be present but go unrecognized for months to years before decompensation or the development of end-stage CKD. When patients finally are presented with decompensated or end-stage CKD, the clinical presentation is frequently remarkable. Commonly reported clinical signs (in addition to those described above) include anorexia, vomiting, lethargy or somnolence, halitosis, dysphagia or oral discomfort, and weakness. Common physical examination findings include muscle atrophy and depleted fat stores, dehydration, small and irregular kidney shape, heart murmur, oral ulceration, halitosis, hypothermia, and pale mucous membranes. Severely affected animals may suffer from altered consciousness, seizures, or bleeding problems, and they may be presented moribund or comatose.

BOX 125-1 *Congenital/Familial Nephropathies in Cats and Dogs*[4]

Dogs

Renal dysplasia

Lhasa Apso
Shih Tzu
Standard Poodle
Soft-Coated Wheaten Terrier
Chow Chow
Alaskan Malamute
Miniature Schnauzer
Dutch Kooiker (Dutch Decoy) Dog

Primary glomerulopathies

Samoyed kindred
Navasota kindred
English Cocker Spaniel
English Springer Spaniel
Bull Terrier
Dalmatian
Doberman Pinscher
Bullmastiff
Newfoundland
Rottweiler
Pembroke Welsh Corgi
Beagle
Soft-Coated Wheaten Terrier

Polycystic kidney disease

Bull Terrier
Cairn Terrier
West Highland White Terrier

Amyloidosis

Shar Pei
English Foxhound
Beagle

Immune-mediated glomerulonephritis

Bernese Mountain Dog (autosomal recessive, suspected)
Brittany Spaniel (autosomal recessive)

Miscellaneous

Boxer—reflux nephropathy with segmental hypoplasia
Basenji—Fanconi syndrome
German Shepherd—multifocal cystadenocarcinoma
Pembroke Welsh Corgi—telangiectasia

Cats

Polycystic kidney disease

Persian

Amyloidosis

Abyssinian
Siamese and Oriental

DIAGNOSIS

The combination of historical and physical examination findings frequently leads to a clinical suspicion of decompensated or end-stage CKD. Clinicopathologic and imaging testing can confirm the diagnosis, occasionally indicate the underlying cause, and detect potentially treatable complications of uremia.

Laboratory Tests

Common laboratory abnormalities include azotemia, hyperphosphatemia, hypokalemia, metabolic acidosis, hypercalcemia (total calcium), and an increased creatinine kinase concentration. Less commonly, hyperkalemia and ionized hypocalcemia are noted. Serum or plasma concentrations of total calcium should not be used to predict the concentration of the biologically active fraction, ionized calcium, because the results of these two tests are frequently discordant.[6] Venous blood gas analyses may aid in determining the requirement for alkali therapy.

The combination of decreased red blood cell life span and inadequate production of erythropoietin, a hematopoietic hormone, lead to nonregenerative anemia. Chronic inflammation or iron deficiency from chronic gastrointestinal blood loss also may contribute to anemia. Some animals have become acutely anemic secondary to acute blood loss from gastrointestinal mucosal injury. The platelet count is usually normal, although platelet function may be impaired in the uremic state. A buccal mucosal bleeding time may be prolonged, but coagulation panel (prothrombin time and partial thromboplastin time) results are expected to be normal.

Historically, poorly concentrated urine (urine specific gravity less than 1.035 in cats, less than 1.030 in dogs) with concurrent azotemia has been the hallmark of CKD. However, a subset of cats and, less frequently, dogs may be presented with azotemia and concentrated urine (urine specific gravity of at least 1.030). This phenomenon has been referred to as "glomerulotubular imbalance," although the pathophysiologic process leading to this phenomenon has not been determined. Active urine sediment (white blood cells, red blood cells, bacteria) may indicate urinary tract infection as a cause or, more commonly, a consequence of CKD. Routine urinalysis and bacterial urine culture is recommended even in the absence of lower urinary tract signs because many cats with CKD have clinically silent urinary tract infections.[7] Although a positive bacterial urine culture result may support the presence of pyelonephritis, there is no evidence that pyelonephritis is a common cause or modifier of CKD. It is the authors' experience, however, that many cats with CKD and obstructive nephrolithiasis or ureterolithiasis have negative urine cultures when specimens are obtained from the bladder, but positive urine cultures are obtained from the upper urinary tract (at the time of surgery or necropsy). Whether bacterial colonization of the upper urinary tract actually contributes to deterioration of renal function has not been investigated.

The urine protein-to-creatinine ratio should be evaluated in all cats and dogs with CKD because it has shown prognostic utility[8-10] and may help the clinician to determine the microanatomic, morphologic lesion (glomerular versus exclusively tubulointerstitial). Typically, dogs with a urine protein-to-creatinine ratio of at least 2 are likely to have glomerular disease.[11] No data implicate a urine protein-to-creatinine ratio threshold to indicate glomerular disease in cats, but it is accepted that values higher than 1 are likely to be associated with glomerular disease. In the acutely ill patient, urine protein-to-creatinine ratios must be measured on multiple occasions to confirm the presence of persistent, pathologic proteinuria because a single measurement may be affected by factors that may resolve as the acute illness stabilized. Microalbuminuria is defined as a quantity of albuminuria that is abnormal but below the detection limit of standard urine dipstick assays. The role of microalbuminuria in the treatment, monitoring, or prognostication of CKD has not been determined because identification of this degree of proteinuria has not been shown to be prognostically superior to urine protein-to-creatinine ratios.

Imaging

Abdominal ultrasonography frequently reveals diminished renal architecture resulting from progressive fibrosis. Other changes that may be identified readily include renal pelvic mineralization, nephroliths or ureteroliths, polycystic kidney disease, and perinephric pseudocysts. Abdominal radiographs may show abnormal kidney size or shape. Approximately 33% of cats with CKD have small kidneys, 40% have normal-size kidneys, and 27% have large kidneys.[5] Nephroliths or ureteroliths may be readily apparent, although the presence of uroliths in the upper urinary tract is not always associated with azotemia.[12] Frequently, obstructive ureteroliths and other obstructive lesions may be undetectable by radiography and ultrasonography. In these cases, a diagnosis of obstructive kidney disease is supported ultrasonographically by the presence of hydronephrosis[13] or a progressive dilation in the width of the renal pelvis. Historically, pyelonephritis has been associated with renal pelvic dilation of varying severity. However, this ultrasonographic sign is noted frequently in polyuric cats and dogs. Furthermore, this sign is associated with various other kidney diseases and is not pathognomonic for renal infection.[13]

Other Diagnostic Modalities

Hypertension occurs in approximately 20% of cats[14] and 31% of dogs[15] with CKD, although many patients with decompensated or end-stage CKD are hypotensive because of dehydration and hypovolemia. Microscopic assessment of renal tissue (either aspirates and cytology or needle/wedge biopsy and histopathology) is indicated when renomegaly is present to rule out lymphoma or feline infectious peritonitis. In addition, renal biopsy can be useful for the differentiation of acute and chronic kidney diseases, when historical and clinical data does not allow for determination of chronicity. The diagnostic yield of these procedures must be weighed against the potential risks because uremic inhibition of platelet function increases the risk of hemorrhage secondary to renal tissue sampling. Measurement of glomerular filtration rate rarely is used when azotemia is present because it can be assumed that this test shows severely diminished excretory function. Parathyroid hormone concentration may be elevated if renal secondary hyperparathyroidism is present.

TREATMENT

The goal of therapy for decompensated or end-stage CKD is to address specifically the insult that resulted in deterioration of the patient's status (if it can be identified) and/or remedy the accumulated sequelae of the deterioration in renal function. Because of the nearly invariably terminal nature of this disease, the clinician should strive to improve the patient's quality of life, while minimizing hospitalization time.

Fluid Therapy

A markedly dehydrated patient with decompensated or end-stage CKD likely needs hospitalization for intensive intravenous fluid therapy. Cats with CKD of any stage are frequently polyuric, whereas the volume of urine (relative to body mass) produced by dogs is more variable. Consequently, cats with decompensated or end-stage CKD commonly are presented with severe dehydration and hypovolemia. The large volume of fluid administration required by cats in a uremic crisis mandates the intravenous route. A balanced polyionic fluid is generally appropriate, provided that serum or plasma electrolyte concentrations are within or close to the normal range. The fluid deficit is calculated (% dehydration × body weight [kg] = volume of deficit in liters) and usually replaced over 6 to 24 hours, although some situations may necessitate more rapid replacement (e.g., hemodynamic instability or collapse, uncertain urine production capability) or slower replacement (e.g., cardiac disease). In addition to replacing the fluid deficit, ongoing losses (e.g., vomiting, diarrhea) should be replaced, and a maintenance rate of fluid administration should be added to the total fluid rate.

Frequently, cats hospitalized for decompensated or end-stage CKD require intravenous fluids at administration rates far exceeding fluid requirements of an anorectic cat with extrarenal disease. The purpose of continued, large volume fluid administration for cats with decompensated chronic kidney disease is not to induce a diuresis because these patients are experiencing diuresis independent of fluid administration, as a consequence of impaired renal concentrating ability. Rather, these patients commonly are enduring massive urinary fluid losses and, more variably, solute losses for which they are unable to compensate with enteral intake. For this reason, fluid therapy should be directed towards normalization of hydration status and improvement in acid-base and electrolyte abnormalities, rather than towards inducing diuresis for the purpose of improving azotemia. Achievement of the former goal almost always results in achievement of the latter. However, if intravenous fluid is administered at volumes in excess of what is required to maintain normal fluid status, the patient will be at greatest risk for volume overload (most frequently manifested as congestive heart failure).

Once the patient's hydration status is normalized, the plasma or serum creatinine concentration usually decreases by at least 1 mg/dl per day. When the creatinine concentration reaches a baseline value (i.e., it is no longer decreasing despite normal hydration status), intravenous fluid rates should be tapered over the course of 2 to 3 days in preparation for patient discharge. Slowly decreasing the intravenous fluid rate allows the clinician to assess the patient's ability to maintain normal hydration with enteral intake of water and food and aids in the determination of whether the patient requires administration of subcutaneous fluid therapy to maintain hydration.

Acid-Base and Electrolyte Balance

Because hypokalemia is a common manifestation of CKD, most cats and many dogs benefit from potassium supplementation in the intravenous fluids. The amount of potassium supplemented can be based on calculations of potassium deficit determined from serum potassium levels or, more simply, standard concentrations can be added to intravenous fluids based on serum potassium concentration. Guidelines for potassium supplementation of intravenous fluids can be found in Chapter 51. Frequently, the original amount of potassium supplemented to intravenous fluid formulations must be altered as dictated by regular monitoring of plasma or serum potassium concentrations and assessment of trends towards hypokalemia or hyperkalemia. It has been suggested that a potassium supplementation rate of 0.5 mEq/kg/hr should not be exceeded, to avoid adverse cardiac effects. In the authors' experience, however, supplementation rates in excess of 0.5 mEq/kg/hr are occasionally necessary for repletion of potassium stores (plasma or serum potassium less than 2 mEq/L). If this rate is exceeded, plasma or serum potassium concentrations and electrocardiogram changes should be monitored closely, and the rate of potassium supplementation should be reduced when the plasma or serum potassium concentration increases (usually to more than 2.5 to 3 mEq/L). When potassium is supplemented intravenously at high rates, consideration should be given to using a separate infusion line so that intravenous fluid rates can be altered independently of potassium supplementation rates. Because of the high osmolality of potassium chloride (typically supplied in concentrations of 2 mEq/mL, 4000 mOsm/L), infusion through central venous catheters may be necessary to prolong catheter life and avoid thrombophlebitis. If hypokalemia is refractory to aggressive supplementation, additional electrolyte abnormalities (e.g., hypomagnesemia, hypocalcemia) and/or endocrinopathies (e.g., hyperaldosteronemia) should be investigated. Frequently, patients that initially are presented with severe hypokalemia require enteral potassium supplementation (e.g., potassium gluconate or potassium citrate) after hospital discharge.

Patients with decompensated or end-stage CKD are frequently acidemic at the time of initial presentation. Although the degree of acidemia frequently improves after correction of volume deficits and perfusion abnormalities, it rarely normalizes in cases of end-stage CKD. If the blood pH remains below 7.2 after restoration of normal hydration status, intravenous sodium bicarbonate supplementation should be considered (see Chapter 124). For patients requiring intravenous sodium bicarbonate therapy, enteral alkali therapy (e.g., sodium bicarbonate or potassium citrate) should be considered for long-term management.

Management of Gastrointestinal Signs

Acute management of the gastrointestinal manifestations of decompensated or end-stage CKD does not differ from that of acute kidney injury (see Chapter 124). However, although there is evidence for hypergastrinemia in cats with CKD,[16] it is uncertain whether these patients have a lower gastric luminal pH, predisposing them to ulceration. The authors are unaware of any evidence in the veterinary literature that shows a clinical benefit for the use of antisecretory drugs (e.g., histamine-2 receptor antagonists, proton pump inhibitors) in the chronic management of these patients. In the author's experience, the administration of these medications provides no benefit over the use of antiemetic drugs alone for chronic management of end-stage CKD but does add to the daily pill burden administered, which may negatively affect the animal-human bond.

Nutritional Support

In cases of decompensated or end-stage CKD, assisted feeding is indicated frequently. During stabilization of a uremic crisis, a previously anorectic patient may begin to show an interest in food, but consumption frequently falls short of nutritional requirements. Placement of a feeding tube can ensure that nutritional requirements are met and can facilitate administration of fluids and medications by the owner. Nasogastric or nasoesophageal tubes can be placed easily without the need for general anesthesia or sedation and can provide appropriate short-term support (1 to 2 weeks). Esophagostomy tubes and percutaneous endoscopic gastrostomy (PEG) tubes are also relatively easy to place and have several advantages over nasal feeding tubes (see Chapter 129). Use of these types of feeding tubes in cats has been met with owner satisfaction.[17] However, placement of esophagostomy and PEG tubes requires general anesthesia, so prior restoration of hydration, acid-base, and electrolyte abnormalities is recommended, if possible.

Cats and, less frequently, dogs may respond to appetite-stimulating drugs, including cyproheptadine (1 to 2 mg/cat, 0.3 to 1.1 mg/kg in dogs PO q12h, 30 minutes before meals) and mirtazapine. Although a recent pharmacokinetic study has demonstrated a safe and effective dose and dosing interval for mirtazapine for cats with chronic kidney disease (1.88 mg/cat PO q48h),[18] the same information is not currently available for dogs with CKD. Although an immediate increase in voluntary food consumption often is witnessed in cats after administration of mirtazapine, the appetite-stimulating effects of this medication are often inadequate to result in a sustained increase in nutritional intake that would preclude the requirement of assisted feeding. Nonetheless, appetite-stimulating drugs can be beneficial by temporarily increasing voluntary food ingestion, thus providing partial nutritional support and improving a patient's candidacy for sedation or anesthesia, should feeding tube placement be elected.

The optimal composition of the diet fed to cats and dogs with decompensated or end-stage is not known. Although diets with restricted quantities of protein and phosphorus content have been shown to both prolong survival and decrease signs of uremia in patients with stable CKD,[19,20] it is unclear whether these diets are appropriate for patients suffering from end-stage disease. Several points of controversy exist. Firstly, the patient may develop a food aversion to this type of diet if it is fed before stabilization, making long-term voluntary intake less likely. Second, many patients with end-stage CKD are in a catabolic state and are severely cachectic. Provision of the most calorically dense diets available may offer the highest probability of weight gain and improvement of muscle mass. Secondly, renal diets are less calorically dense than some prescription recovery diets (e.g., Iams Veterinary Formula Maximum-Calories) and must be blended with large amounts of water to facilitate passage through feeding tubes with smaller luminal diameter, resulting in reduction of caloric density and an increase in the total volume of food necessary to meet caloric requirements. Many patients cannot tolerate the total volume of blended food necessary to achieve a neutral or positive energy balance and therefore catabolism continues despite nutritional support. Third, the low sodium content of renal diets can predispose patients to severe hyponatremia and neurologic sequelae, if large volumes of water are administered after being blended with the diet or separately for maintenance of hydration. Careful attention must be given to plasma or serum electrolyte concentrations, especially in small patients, or in those patients for which parenteral fluid therapy (a source of large amounts of sodium) is being tapered or discontinued. Provision of supplemental sodium may be necessary in these cases. The benefits of a renal diet have not been demonstrated in cats with stage IV CKD and have been demonstrated only in a small number of dogs with stage IV CKD; thus it is uncertain whether these patients, with an expected survival time of months, benefit more from a renal diet or a more calorically dense diet. Although traditionally, transition to a renal diet is recommended for all animals with CKD, the potential disadvantages of these diets in cats with decompensated or end-stage CKD must be weighed against the potential advantages.

Management of Anemia

If the patient is severely anemic (hematocrit less than 20%) and clinical signs associated with anemia (weakness, tachycardia, tachypnea) are present, transfusion (whole blood, packed red blood cells, or hemoglobin based oxygen carrier) may be necessary for immediate stabilization. Given the high probability that the patient's ability to synthesize and secrete endogenous erythropoietin is impaired, consideration should be given to administration of an erythropoiesis stimulating agent (ESA) early in the course of hospitalization. Epoetin alpha (Epogen or Procrit) traditionally has been used in veterinary medicine for this problem and is effective in stimulating erythropoiesis in cats and dogs. However, its use has been associated with the formation of antibodies directed against the exogenous ESA and endogenous erythropoietin in up to 25% of cats and dogs thus treated.[21] Once antibodies develop, the patient is typically transfusion dependent and can require blood transfusions as frequently as once weekly.

A newer recombinant erythropoietin product, darbepoetin α (Aranesp), has become the preferred treatment for cats and dogs with anemia of renal disease. Darbepoetin α is hyperglycosylated, which prolongs the circulating half-life of the molecule and may reduce immunogenicity. Anecdotal reports suggest a lower rate of anti-erythropoietin antibody development in cats and dogs compared with recombinant human erythropoietin. Because of the perceived safety of darbepoetin alpha compared with erythropoietin, early initiation of this treatment should be considered even if the patient does not require a blood transfusion.

The optimal starting dose of darbepoetin alpha has not been determined. However, a retrospective case series describing the use of darbepoetin alpha in cats with CKD concluded that a starting dose of 1 U/kg SC once weekly resulted in an erythropoietic response in 13 of 14 patients.[22] The authors currently use the following dosing schedules for cats and dogs: 6.25 U/cat SC or IV once weekly until the hematocrit is greater than 25%, then the same dose administered every 2 to 3 weeks as determined by serial hematocrit measurements; 1 U/kg up to 25 U per dog SC or IV once weekly until the hematocrit is more than 35%, then the same dose administered every 2 to 3 weeks as determined by serial hematocrit measurements. The hematocrit should initially be measured before each injection until the interval between administrations has stabilized between 2 and 3 weeks. Hypertension is a frequently recognized complication of epoetin α and darbepoetin α, so blood pressure should be monitored regularly during treatment.

Adequate iron stores are necessary for an optimal response, and iron administration usually is required during the initial treatment period. Iron sources include iron dextran (50 mg/cat; 10 to 20 mg/kg in dogs, deep IM injection monthly), ferrous sulfate (50 to 100 mg/cat, 100 to 300 mg/dog PO q24h). Cats and dogs with CKD that are administered ESAs generally show a response (increased hematocrit, reticulocytosis) after 2 weeks of treatment, unless extraneous factors causing resistance are present (e.g., gastrointestinal hemorrhage, infection, or chronic inflammation).

Long-Term Management

Once the patient has been stabilized and can be managed on an outpatient basis, long-term care generally is undertaken by the primary veterinarian or a veterinary internist. A detailed discussion of long-term management of CKD is beyond the scope of this chapter. However, the following considerations should be made.

Dietary Therapy

With the caveats discussed above, a diet with restricted quantities of protein and phosphorus should be introduced gradually.

Fluid Therapy

Pets with chronic dehydration may benefit from SC fluid therapy. Owners can be taught to administer fluids at home. Dosage is empiric, based on subjective assessment of patient's well-being and hydration status. Lactated Ringer's solution and 0.9% saline are used most frequently. A typical starting dosage for a cat is 100 to 125 ml q24-72h. Animals that do not require ongoing SC fluid therapy may benefit from intermittent treatment during times of stress (exacerbation of uremia, other illness, boarding, traveling).

Additional Considerations

If a diet restricted in phosphorus content is not sufficient to control hyperphosphatemia, a phosphate binding drug should be administered with food. As discussed above, the human or veterinary literature contains no evidence that long-term administration of antisecretory drugs (e.g., histamine-2 receptor antagonists and proton pump inhibitors) has any clinical benefit. However, administration of an antiemetic drug is recommended empirically and can be used at the discretion of the owner, for symptomatic control of the gastrointestinal manifestations of uremia.

Hypertension can be managed with amlodipine in cats and dogs. This medication can be used with or without an angiotensin converting enzyme (ACE) inhibitor (e.g., enalapril, benazepril). An ACE inhibitor is recommended if proteinuria is present. See Chapter 159 for further discussion of antihypertensive therapy.

A low dosage of calcitriol decreases mortality in dogs with CKD, possibly by normalizing parathyroid hormone concentrations.[23] A similar benefit has yet to be demonstrated in cats but is likely to exist. Administration of calcitriol to a patient with hyperphosphatemia or ionized hypercalcemia is contraindicated because of the risk of soft tissue mineralization. Plasma or serum phosphorus and ionized calcium concentrations should be monitored closely if this drug is used.

Advanced Therapeutic Modalities

Renal transplantation may be appropriate for some cats, depending on availability. The best candidates for renal transplantation are those cats with stage II to III CKD, without concurrent illness or infection. Renal transplantation should be considered before end-stage CKD, rather than as an emergency or salvage procedure. However, decompensated or end-stage CKD is not an absolute contraindication for transplantation. The availability and success of canine renal transplantations is limited and, thus it is not recommended in dogs. Chronic hemodialysis is available in a limited number of veterinary hospitals. Because of the need for frequent treatments (minimum of two to three times a week for the remainder of the patient's life) and cost associated with these treatments, chronic hemodialysis is not commonly used for dogs or cats with CKD, but excellent results may be obtained in select cases. Complications associated with peritoneal dialysis (especially catheter occlusion and peritonitis) have limited its use to acute settings.

PROGNOSIS

CKD is a progressive disease, but the rate of progression is highly variable. Multiple studies have been conducted to determine predictors of decompensation or mortality for cats with CKD. These studies have demonstrated that the following variables are associated with these end-points: plasma creatinine concentration, urine protein-to-creatinine ratio, urine albumin-to-creatinine ratio, leukocytosis, and hyperphosphatemia.[9,10,24] A Kaplan-Meier survival curve for cats with CKD, stratified by IRIS stage is displayed in Figure 125-1. In the canine studies that investigated predictors of decompensation or mortality, the urine protein-to-creatinine concentration, hypoalbuminemia, and hypertension were positively associated with the decompensation or mortality, whereas body condition score was associated negatively with mortality.[8,15,25] Although not independently associated with mortality, creatinine is the primary means of determining the severity of and prognosis for canine CKD in clinical practice. Kaplan-Meier survival curves for dogs with CKD, stratified

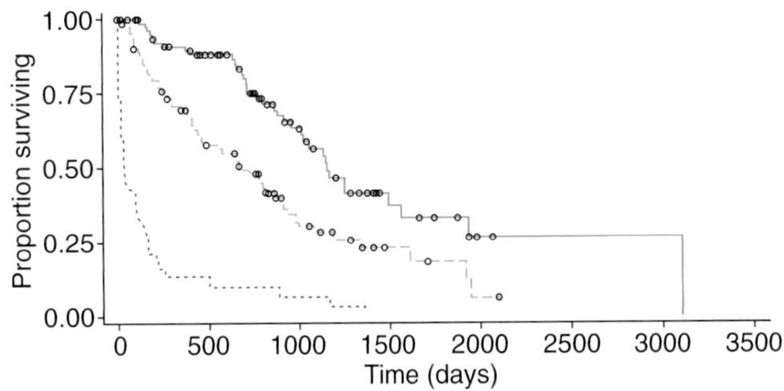

FIGURE 125-1 Kaplan-Meier survival curve of cats with CKD, stratified by IRIS stage (stage IIb = green line, stage III = blue line, stage IV red line; circles indicate patients censored for nonrenal deaths).[24]

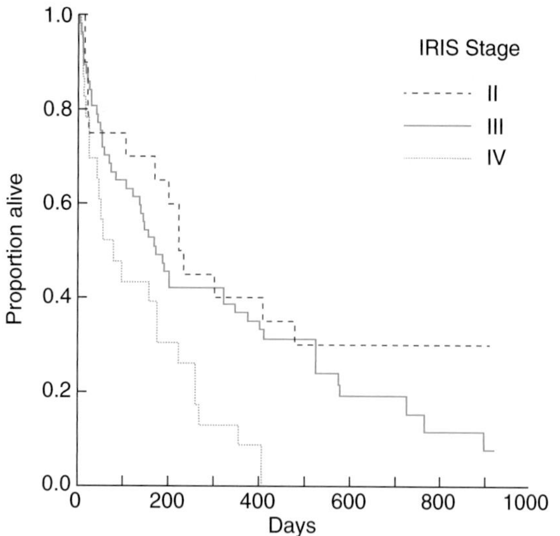

FIGURE 125-2 Kaplan-Meier survival curve of dogs with CKD, stratified by IRIS stage (a) and body condition score (b).[25]

by IRIS stage and body condition score are displayed in Figure 125-2. Most animals eventually die of CKD or related complications, although some maintain stable renal function and die of unrelated causes (such as neoplasia).

REFERENCES

1. Elliot J, Watson ADJ: Chronic kidney disease: staging and management. In Bonagura JD,Twedt DC, editors: Kirk's current veterinary therapy, St Louis, 2009, Saunders, pp 883-892.
2. Minkus G, Reusch C, Horauf A, et al: Evaluation of renal biopsies in cats and dogs - histopathology in comparison with clinical data, J Small Anim Prac 35:465-472, 1994.
3. Macdougall DF, Cook T, Steward AP, et al: Canine chronic renal disease: prevalence and types of glomerulonephritis in the dog, Kidney Int 29:1144-1151, 1986.
4. Lees GE: Congenital kidney diseases. In Bartges J, Polzin D, editors: Nephrology and urology of small animals, West Sussex, 2011, Wiley-Blackwell.
5. Lulich JP, Osborne CA, O'Brien TD, et al: Feline renal failure: questions, answers, questions, Compend Contin Educ Pract Vet 14:127-153, 1992.
6. Schenck PA, Chew DJ: Prediction of serum ionized calcium concentration by serum total calcium measurement in cats, Can J Vet Res 74:209-213, 2010.
7. Mayer-Roenne B, Goldstein RE, Erb HN: Urinary tract infections in cats with hyperthyroidism, diabetes mellitus and chronic kidney disease, J Feline Med Surg 9:124-132, 2007.
8. Jacob F, Polzin DJ, Osborne CA, et al: Evaluation of the association between initial proteinuria and morbidity rate or death in dogs with naturally occurring chronic renal failure, J Am Vet Med Assoc 226:393-400, 2005.
9. Syme HM, Markwell PJ, Pfeiffer D, et al: Survival of cats with naturally occurring chronic renal failure is related to severity of proteinuria, J Vet Intern Med 20:528-535, 2006.
10. King JN, Tasker S, Gunn-Moore DA, et al: Prognostic factors in cats with chronic kidney disease, J Vet Intern Med 21:906-916, 2007.
11. Center SA, Wilkinson E, Smith CA, et al: 24-Hour urine protein/creatinine ratio in dogs with protein-losing nephropathies, J Am Vet Med Assoc 187:820-824, 1985.
12. Kyles AE, Hardie EM, Wooden BG, et al: Clinical, clinicopathologic, radiographic, and ultrasonographic abnormalities in cats with ureteral calculi: 163 cases (1984-2002), J Am Vet Med Assoc 226:932-936, 2005.
13. D'Anjou MA, Bedard A, Dunn ME: Clinical significance of renal pelvic dilatation on ultrasound in dogs and cats., Vet Radiol Ultrasound 52:88-94, 2011.
14. Syme HM, Barber PJ, Markwell PJ, et al: Prevalence of systolic hypertension in cats with chronic renal failure at initial evaluation, J Am Vet Med Assoc 220:1799-1804, 2002.
15. Jacob F, Polzin DJ, Osborne CA, et al: Association between initial systolic blood pressure and risk of developing a uremic crisis or of dying in dogs with chronic renal failure, J Am Vet Med Assoc 222:322-329, 2003.
16. Goldstein RE, Marks SL, Kass PH, et al: Gastrin concentrations in plasma of cats with chronic renal failure, J Am Vet Med Assoc 213:826-828, 1998.
17. Ireland LM, Hohenhaus AE, Broussard JD, et al: A comparison of owner management and complications in 67 cats with esophagostomy and percutaneous endoscopic gastrostomy feeding tubes, J Am Anim Hosp Assoc 39:241-246, 2003.
18. Quimby JM, Gustafson DL, Lunn KF: The pharmacokinetics of mirtazapine in cats with chronic kidney disease and in age-matched control cats, J Vet Intern Med 25:985-989, 2011.
19. Jacob F, Polzin DJ, Osborne CA, et al: Clinical evaluation of dietary modification for treatment of spontaneous chronic renal failure in dogs, J Am Vet Med Assoc 220:1163-1170, 2002.
20. Ross SJ, Osborne CA, Kirk CA, et al: Clinical evaluation of dietary modification for treatment of spontaneous chronic kidney disease in cats, J Am Vet Med Assoc 229:949-957, 2006.
21. Cowgill LD, James KM, Levy JK, et al: Use of recombinant human erythropoietin for management of anemia in dogs and cats with renal failure, J Am Vet Med Assoc 212:521-528, 1998.
22. Chalhoub E, Frinak S, Zasuwa G, et al: De novo once-monthly darbepoetin alpha treatment for the anemia of chronic kidney disease using a computerized algorithmic approach, Clin Nephrol 76:1-8, 2011.
23. Polzin D, Ross SJ, Osborne CA, et al: Clinical benefit of calcitriol in canine chronic kidney disease, J Vet Intern Med 19:433, 2005.
24. Boyd LM, Langston C, Thompson K, et al: Survival in cats with naturally occurring chronic kidney disease (2000-2002), J Vet Intern Med 22:1111-1117, 2008.
25. Parker VJ, Freeman LM: Association between body condition and survival in dogs with acquired chronic kidney disease, J Vet Intern Med 25:1306-1311, 2011.

CHAPTER 126

PYOMETRA

M. Bronwyn Crane, DVM, MS, DACT

KEY POINTS

- Pyometra affects primarily older, intact bitches and queens.
- The pathogenesis of pyometra is hormone dependent and often preceded by cystic endometrial hyperplasia (CEH).
- Bitches have signs of endotoxemia and may or may not have vaginal discharge.
- Diagnosis is based on a combination of clinical signs, laboratory findings, abdominal radiographs, and ultrasonography.
- The recommended treatment for bitches not intended for breeding is ovariohysterectomy.
- Depending on the severity of the condition, valuable bitches intended for breeding may be treated medically. These cases have a strong likelihood of reoccurrence.

Cystic endometrial hyperplasia (CEH)-pyometra describes a spectrum of uterine pathology that is the most common uterine disease in middle-aged and older intact bitches and queens. Many authors prefer to consider these two diseases separately because of their different clinical and histopathologic presentation. CEH is mostly a subclinical disease with no clinical signs other than infertility; histologically there is no inflammation. Pseudoplacentational endometrial hyperplasia (PEH) is another recently described condition of the uterus, in which the hyperplastic endometrium remodels into histology similar to normal placentation sites.[1]

Pyometra often is preceded by CEH but can develop independently of CEH. It is an endocrine disease occurring during diestrus, when corpora lutea are present and serum progesterone concentrations are high. Severity of the disease varies greatly and depends on its stage of progression; a bitch with pyometra may present stable with mild clinical signs, or near death because of sepsis. Pyometra can be classified further as open-cervix or closed-cervix pyometra, with the latter condition resulting in more severe clinical signs. Once diagnosed, pyometra may be treated by ovariohysterectomy (OHE) or medically with prostaglandin $F_{2\alpha}$ ($PGF_{2\alpha}$), progesterone receptor antagonists and antibiotics.

INCIDENCE

Pyometra is a disease of intact, older females, and the number of cases observed in a population depends on the number of intact females. In a study of intact bitches under 10 years of age in Sweden the average lifetime risk for pyometra was 23% to 24%,[2] whereas in colony-raised Beagle bitches, the incidence of CEH was 15.2%.[3] Risk factors for pyometra include increasing age, nulliparity,[4] breed, and exogenous estrogen or progesterone administration. When medroxyprogesterone acetate was used for population control, the prevalence of pyometra increased in treated bitches to 45%, over a prevalence of only 5% in untreated bitches.[5]

PATHOGENESIS

CEH is a subclinical disease characterized by the proliferation and hypersecretion of endometrial glands, resulting in the formation of fluid-filled cysts and accumulation of glandular fluid within the uterine lumen. Alone, CEH is not associated with any signs other than infertility. CEH is generally considered the initiating stage that progresses to pyometra after uterine bacterial colonization. Pyometra is a life-threatening illness involving the accumulation of intraluminal purulent exudate within the uterus and inflammatory cell infiltration into the layers of the endometrium and myometrium. Although CEH generally precedes pyometra, the latter can occur without CEH.

Pyometra typically occurs during diestrus when progesterone stimulates endometrial growth and glandular secretory activity after the uterus has been primed by estrogen. Progesterone also reduces myometrial contractility and maintains cervical closure. A comparison of the distribution of progesterone and estrogen receptors within the cervix between normal bitches and bitches with pyometra found that receptors were not influenced by the stage of the estrous cycle in bitches with pyometra, as they were in normal bitches.[6] These findings suggest that cervical dilation may be controlled by different mechanisms in bitches with uterine pathology. In addition, progesterone diminishes immune function by decreasing neutrophil chemotaxis and phagocytosis and increases endometrial bacterial adherence. Despite this, peripheral serum progesterone concentrations in bitches with pyometra are not higher than those of normal diestrual bitches.[7,8] Estrogens also have a role in the pathogenesis of CEH through the up-regulation of endometrial progesterone and estrogen receptors. Administration of estrogens followed by progesterone, or progesterone alone, induces CEH.[9]

Bacteria gain access to the uterus via ascension during cervical dilation that occurs with estrus. Bacteria found in healthy uteri and the uteri of bitches with pyometra are representative of the normal microflora of the vagina and cervix.[10] Many bitches with pyometra also have a concurrent urinary tract infection (22% to 72%).[11] The most common bacterium isolated in cases of pyometra is *Escherichia coli*.[8] Infusion of E. *coli* isolates obtained from bitches with pyometra into the uteri of healthy bitches resulted in the development of pyometra.[12,13] Other less common bacteria isolated from cases of pyometra include *Streptococcus* spp., *Enterobacter* spp., *Proteus* spp., *Klebsiella* spp., and *Pseudomonas* spp. The mechanical irritation caused by bacteria within the endometrium is a sufficient stimulus for CEH. Any stimulus, from an embryo to a piece of silk thread,[14] induces local proliferation of endometrial glands and hyperplastic changes within the endometrium.[9,15] The inflammatory cells present in the uteri of bitches with pyometra express high levels of transforming growth factor-α (TGFα), TGFα plays an important role in cell proliferation and differientation.[16] The high levels of TGFα produced by inflammatory cells may be involved in the aberrant growth of endometrial glands, contributing to the development of CEH.

DIAGNOSIS

Presumptive diagnosis of pyometra is made based on the history, clinical signs, abdominal palpation of an enlarged uterus, diagnostic imaging, hematology, and biochemistry results. Differentiating CEH with mucometra from pyometra is often an important aspect of the diagnosis because treatment recommendations may be different for valuable breeding bitches.

Signalment

The median age of dogs with pyometra in various studies is 8 to 9 years.[3,17] CEH is diagnosed infrequently in dogs less than 4 years old and occurs more often in maiden bitches. In a retrospective study of pyometra in cats, the mean age was 32 months.[18] Although a breed predisposition has not been established for pyometra, studies examining the breed risk found an increased incidence in rough-coated Collies, Rottweilers, Cavalier King Charles Spaniels, and Golden Retrievers.[2,17]

History and Physical Examination

Most bitches and queens with pyometra have a history of recent estrus. The average interval from the onset of proestrus to diagnosis of CEH-pyometra is 35 days (range 20 to 70 days). In cats, most cases of pyometra occurred within 8 weeks of estrus and most of those queens were known to have been bred.[18] Although pyometra is considered a disorder of diestrus, it also can occur during anestrus when progesterone is at baseline concentrations. Cases that occur during anestrus may be due to the persistence of abnormal events that occurred during diestrus, a nonovarian source of progesterone, or incomplete luteolysis resulting in prolonged low levels of progesterone. Frequently bitches with pyometra have a history of treatment with exogenous progestins for contraception[5] or exogenous estrogens for pregnancy termination.[17] Many cases concurrently have estrogen-secreting cystic follicles, ovarian neoplasia, or a history of prolonged estrus.

The clinical signs of pyometra include vaginal discharge (80%), fever (47%), polydipsia, polyuria, and vomition.[19] Other signs include lethargy, anorexia, dehydration, tachycardia, tachypnea, and pale or hyperemic mucous membranes. Abdominal palpation may elicit pain or reveal a large tubular structure. Uterine exudate in the form of vaginal discharge may be purulent, mucoid, or hemorrhagic. Pyometras are classified further as open-cervix or closed-cervix, based on the presence of vaginal discharge. Cytology of the cranial vagina is a useful first step in the diagnosis and often reveals degenerate neutrophils and bacteria. Before obtaining the cytology specimen, the clinician should swab the cranial vagina using a guarded swab for culture and antibiotic susceptibility testing. A vaginal speculum examination also is warranted to rule out a vaginal abnormality or foreign body as the source of vulvar discharge. Advanced cases of pyometra may arrive in decompensatory septic shock with hypotension. Signs that are more likely to be present in cases of pyometra than in CEH include polyuria and polydipsia, lethargy, and vomiting or inappetence.[20] The more severe signs associated with pyometra are due to the effects of bacterial toxins.

Clinical signs observed in queens with pyometra include vaginal discharge, anorexia, lethargy, weight loss, unkempt appearance, and polyuria and polydipsia.[18] A palpably enlarged uterus is a more common physical examination finding in cats than dogs, perhaps a result of the pliability of a cat's abdomen.

Diagnostic Imaging

Ultrasonography is the most useful diagnostic imaging modality for pyometra. It can be used to examine for uteromegaly and is particularly useful because it can evaluate endometrial integrity, uterine wall thickness, uterine distention, and cystic endometrial glands. Ultrasonography can be used to differentiate pregnancy (more than 28 days) and neoplasia from pyometra. Ultrasonography of a uterus with pyometra reveals convoluted tubular horns containing an anechoic or hypoechoic fluid; the fluid also may have a slow, swirling pattern. In cases of CEH without pyometra, endometrial glands are increased in size and number, appearing as 1- to 2-mm anechoic areas within the endometrium.[19]

Abdominal radiographs may reveal uteromegaly. Uterine enlargement can be recognized by the presence of a fluid-filled convoluted or tubular structure between the bladder and the colon. Other potential conditions to rule out include pregnancy less than 42 days (more than 42 days after the luteinizing hormone surge, fetal skeletons should be visible), mucometra, hydrometra, CEH, and uterine neoplasia. If the cervix is open and the uterus is draining, uteromegaly may not be present. If abdominal radiographs reveal a generalized loss of detail, it is possible that uterine rupture has occurred already.

Laboratory Findings

Neutrophilia is a common hematologic finding, ranging from 15,000 to 60,000 cells/ml. Patients with pyometra often have an increased percentage of band neutrophils. They often have an anemia of chronic disease (70% of cases)[11] that is characterized as nonregenerative, normochromic, and normocytic and may be due to red blood cell diapedesis into the uterus or toxic suppression of erythropoiesis. Hyperproteinemia and hyperglobulinemia occur secondary to dehydration and antigenic stimulation. Hypoalbuminemia is another common finding[20] and may be due to sepsis.[11]

Approximately 12% to 37% of bitches with pyometra have elevated creatinine and blood urea nitrogen levels.[11] Azotemia may be due to dehydration (prerenal) or reversible renal tubular damage. *E. coli* lipopolysaccharide (LPS) endotoxin causes insensitivity to antidiuretic hormone at the distal convoluted tubules and collecting ducts, which impairs concentrating ability and results in isosthenuria or hyposthenuria. This is usually reversible, but a poor prognosis is indicated if the blood urea nitrogen level is greater than 60 mg/dl. Cytotoxic necrotizing factor–positive *E. coli* also causes reversible hepatocellular damage or hypoxia because of dehydration resulting in increased aspartate aminotransferase, alkaline phosphatase, and alanine amino transferase.

When fluid in the uterus is detected, pyometra may be differentiated from CEH with mucometra by measuring percentage of band neutrophils, alkaline phosphatase, C-reactive protein (an inflammatory marker used in human medicine), or circulating prostaglandin-F metabolites (PGFM). The percentage of band neutrophils is the most sensitive single parameter for differentiating pyometra (more than 19.9% band neutrophils is 94.2% sensitive and 70% specific).[20] Mean alkaline phosphatase in bitches with pyometra (362 IU/L) was significantly higher than in bitches with CEH (133 IU/L) and control dogs (81 UI/L).[20] Concentrations of PGFM of 3054 pmol/L or greater indicate a 95% probability of pyometra.[21] Combining PGFM results with percentage of band neutrophils increases the sensitivity of differentiating pyometra from mucometra to 100%.[21] Bitches with more than 19.9% band neutrophils and more than 260.2 mg/L C-reactive protein had a 95% probability of having pyometra versus CEH.[20] However, neither PGFM nor canine C-reactive protein determination is readily available at most clinics.

Many bitches with pyometra also have a concurrent urinary tract infection, although performing a cystocentesis is not recommended because of the risk of perforating the uterus and inducing peritonitis.

TREATMENT

The decision to treat a bitch or queen surgically or medically depends on the severity of clinical and laboratory findings and intended purpose of the animal. The ideal treatment for any case of pyometra is OHE. If the patient is a valuable breeding bitch and only mildly affected, then medical treatment is an option. If medical treatment does not result in significant improvement within 48 hours or the condition of the patient deteriorates, then OHE should be performed as soon as possible.

Stabilizing the Patient

The patient should be stabilized appropriately and rapidly before surgical or medical management. Fluid therapy should be initiated to correct shock, hypoglycemia, electrolyte, and acid-base abnormalities if present (see Chapters 60, 66, and 91).

The patient should be started on broad-spectrum antibiotics that are effective against gram-negative pathogens until culture and susceptibility results are available. Because approximately 60% to 70% of cases are infected with *E. coli*,[8,22] antibiotic therapy should target this organism initially. Preferred antibiotics for pyometra include amoxicillin, amoxicillin/clavulanate, enrofloxacin, gentamicin, streptomycin, sulfamethoxazole, tetracycline, and trimethoprim. Caution is important with the use of aminoglycoside antibiotics in animals with known renal dysfunction because of the risk of further renal damage. A study examining antimicrobial resistance among *E. coli* strains isolated from naturally occurring pyometra cases found minimal resistance (10% or less) to the commonly used antibiotics listed above.[22] Antibiotic therapy should be continued for at least 10 days in surgical cases[11] or 30 days in medically treated cases.[23]

Endotoxemia is present in pyometra because of the toxic effects of LPS released from bacteria. LPS may reach toxic or lethal levels of 0.7 to 1 ng/ml in bitches with pyometra.[24] Antibiotics can increase the concentration of LPS up to 2000-fold and potentially worsen the signs of endotoxemia. To augment treatment of endotoxemia, treatment of dogs with polyvalent equine antiendotoxin hyperimmune plasma (anti-LPS) has been reported. The reported dose is 0.5 mg/kg SC when surgery can be delayed 24 hours, or diluted in 100 to 300 ml lactated Ringer's solution and infused intravenously when surgery must be performed immediately.[24] No side effects were observed in the one study using this treatment, but it is likely that antibodies will be formed against the foreign proteins found in equine plasma, especially if repetitive treatments are required. The efficacy of this therapy remains unknown.

Progesterone receptor antagonists such as aglepristone (RU 534; Alizin, Virbac Animal Health) can be used to convert a closed-cervix pyometra into an open-cervix pyometra. Aglepristone competes for uterine receptors at a fixating rate three-fold that of progesterone[25] and has virtually no reported side effects. When aglepristone was administered on days 1 and 2 after diagnosis, the mean time to cervical opening was 25.1 hours after the first injection (range 4 to 48 hours).[26] Cervical opening was associated with evacuation of large volumes of purulent exudate and an immediate improvement in general condition, with an increase in appetite.[26] Unfortunately, aglepristone is not commercially available in the United States or Canada but is marketed for veterinary use in Europe and other countries. It also can be used for medical management of pyometra and is discussed later.

Surgical Management

OHE is the preferred treatment for bitches and queens with pyometra. Surgery should be performed as soon as they are stable and surgical risk is minimized. Depending on the condition of the patient, surgical outcome may be improved if surgery is delayed for 24 hours while the patient receives fluid therapy, antibiotics and, if available, anti-LPS plasma and aglepristone.[27]

If uterine rupture is evident at the time of surgery or peritonitis is present, the abdomen should be lavaged with copious amounts of warm saline, and management as an open abdomen may be indicated[27] (see Chapter 122). Cystocentesis should be performed for urine culture before the abdomen is closed, because a high percentage of animals with pyometra also have a urinary tract infection. After surgery, patients have a 92% survival rate; the most common complication is peritonitis.[11]

Medical Management

For less severe cases of pyometra in animals intended for breeding, patients can be treated medically with combinations $PGF_{2\alpha}$ or $PGF_{2\alpha}$ analogs, progesterone receptor antagonists, and dopamine agonists. Additional supportive therapy, such as systemic antibiotics, intravenous fluid therapy, and anti-LPS plasma (if available), should be administered in all cases of pyometra. The goal of medical management is to improve the general condition of the animal, remove the source of progesterone by inducing luteolysis, stimulate uterine contractions to aid evacuation, and eliminate the infection. Various protocols for the medical management of pyometra are outlined in Table 126-1; recovery rate in these studies is strongly influenced by case selection.

$PGF_{2\alpha}$ causes myometrial contractility, which expels the luminal contents. It also causes luteolysis, which decreases progesterone concentrations. Side effects of $PGF_{2\alpha}$ are associated with the dosage and include panting, salivation, anxiety, vomiting, diarrhea, urination, abdominal contractions, and ataxia within 15 minutes of administration. Additional side effects of $PGF_{2\alpha}$ treatment in queens that were not observed in dogs included vocalization, grooming, kneading, mydriasis, and lordosis.[18] Side effects may last for up to 120 minutes. Tolerance, in the form of fewer side effects, develops after repeated treatments. $PGF_{2\alpha}$ analogs, such as cloprostenol, are longer acting and more potent than natural $PGF_{2\alpha}$. They have the advantage of less-frequent administration because of their prolonged period of effectiveness. Less severe side effects are observed with cloprostenol, and dosages of 1 mcg/kg have been associated with mild nausea, diarrhea, and vomiting in 31% to 55% of patients.[28,29]

Medically managed patients with pyometra should be hospitalized because of the frequent side effects, potential toxicity, and frequency of treatments. Fewer side effects can be achieved by using protocols with lower and more frequent prostaglandin doses,[29] intravaginal administration of prostaglandin,[30] combining prostaglandin with other agents such as antiprogestins[26] or dopamine agonists,[28] administering prostaglandin 1 to 2 hours from feeding, and walking the patient immediately afterward for 20 to 40 minutes. A low-dose prostaglandin protocol, such as outlined in Table 126-1, is highly effective and is associated with minimal side effects. It is ideal to begin $PGF_{2\alpha}$ treatment with a low dose (0.02 mg/kg dinoprost SC q2-4h), monitor side effects and progress to a higher dose if it is well tolerated. Protocols using high dosages of $PGF_{2\alpha}$ with infrequent treatment schedules are associated with the most severe side effects. The therapeutic index for $PGF_{2\alpha}$ in dogs is narrow, with a lethal dose of 5.13 mg/kg for dinoprost (natural $PGF_{2\alpha}$). Although various prostaglandin protocols are published with finite treatment periods, it is best to monitor uterine diameter ultrasonographically and continue treatment until uterine diameter returns to normal and until a purulent vulvar discharge is no longer present (up to 2 to 3 weeks).[31]

Progesterone receptor antagonists or antiprogestins, such as aglepristone, result in better recovery rates when they are used in conjunction with prostaglandins (see Table 126-1). Interestingly, a

Table 126-1 Protocols for the Medical Management of Pyometra in Bitches, Used in Addition to Antibiotic and Fluid Therapy

Protocol	Drug and Dosage	Frequency	Recovery Rate	Reference
Low $PGF_{2\alpha}$	Dinoprost 0.02 to 0.1 mg/kg SC	q2-4h until uterine evacuation or luteolysis	75% (9 of 12)	31, 29
Medium $PGF_{2\alpha}$	Dinoprost 0.1 to 0.25 mg/kg SC	q24h	Not reported	11, 23
High $PGF_{2\alpha}$	Dinoprost 0.25 to 0.5 mg/kg SC	q24h for 3 days	100% (10 of 10)	33
$PGF_{2\alpha}$ in queens	0.1 mg/kg SC	q12-24h for 3 to 5 days	95.2% (20 of 21)	18
Intravaginal $PGF_{2\alpha}$	Dinoprost 0.15 mg/kg intravaginally at 0.3 ml/kg	q12h for 3 to 12 days	81.8% (9 of 11)	30
$PGF_{2\alpha}$ analog	Cloprostenol 1 to 5 mcg/kg SC	q12-24h	Not reported	31, 23
$PGF_{2\alpha}$ analog + dopamine agonist	Cloprostenol 1 mcg/kg SC Cabergoline 5 mcg/kg PO	Both q24h for 7 days, cloprostenol q24h for up to 14 days	83% (24 of 29)	28
Antiprogestin	Aglepristone 10 mg/kg SC	Once on days 1, 2, 8, 14, and 28*	45% (9 of 20) by day 28 60% (12 of 20) by day 90	26
Antiprogestin + $PGF_{2\alpha}$ analog	Aglepristone 10 mg/kg SC Cloprostenol 1 mcg/kg SC	Aglepristone once on days 1, 3, 8, and 15* Cloprostenol once on days 3 and 8	100% (8 of 8)	25
	Aglepristone 10 mg/kg SC Cloprostenol 1 mcg/kg SC	Aglepristone once on days 1, 3, 8, and 15* Cloprostenol once on days 3, 5, 8, 10, 12, and 15*	100% (7 of 7)	25
	Aglepristone 10 mg/kg SC Cloprostenol 1 mcg/kg SC	Aglepristone once on days 1, 2, 8, 14, and 28* Cloprostenol once on days 3, 4, 5, 6, and 7	72% (23 of 32) by day 28 84% (27 of 32) by day 90	3

*Treatment was continued beyond day 8 only if necessary.
PGF, Prostaglandin F; *PO,* per os; *SC,* subcutaneous.

positive effect of aglepristone alone also has been found in bitches with basal progesterone concentrations[25] and may be due to an increased sensitivity of receptors. Aglepristone also can be used to prevent reoccurrence of pyometra in treated bitches that are not inseminated at a subsequent estrus.[32] Aglepristone is unique in that it offers a safe method of converting a closed pyometra into an open pyometra for medical management.[26] Because of the delay (4 to 48 hours) before the cervix opens, medical treatment of a closed pyometra should not be attempted in bitches with compromised liver or kidney function. Prostaglandin therapy may be successful in patients with closed pyometras but is generally not recommended because of the risk of uterine rupture or expulsion of uterine contents from the oviducts into the peritoneal cavity.[32]

Dopamine agonists, such as cabergoline, cause luteolysis by reducing prolactin concentrations. Prolactin is a major source of luteotropic support in the bitch. Dopamine agonists should be used in combination with prostaglandin (see Table 126-1), because together they result in more complete luteolysis. Meanwhile, prostaglandin exerts a uterotonic effect. The combined use of these drugs allows a lower dose of prostaglandin and reduces the side effects.

Once recovered, the bitch should be reevaluated between 10 and 20 days after her last treatment and the need for additional treatment determined at that time.[32] The recurrence rate of pyometra within 1 to 2 years in medically managed cases is between 20% and 77%.[28,33] A slightly lower recurrence rate (3 of 21) was observed in queens treated with PGF_{2a}.[18] To prevent reoccurrence during the next cycle, the bitch should undergo ovulation timing and be bred to a male with known fertility during her most fertile period. Prophylactic antibiotics may be given during proestrus and estrus. If the owners choose not to breed the bitch, antibiotics and aglepristone[31] can be given to prevent recurrence. Approximately 40% to 90% of bitches whelp a normal litter after medical management.[23,33] Young bitches or those developing pyometra as a result of exogenous estrogen or progesterone therapy are more likely to maintain a pregnancy after treatment.

UTERINE STUMP PYOMETRA

Uterine stump pyometra has a pathogenesis similar to that of pyometra, with the exception that the patient previously was believed to have had the uterus and ovaries completely removed. In patients with a uterine stump pyometra, remnants of ovarian tissue with a variable amount of uterine tissue have been left behind after OHE.[23] The clinical signs are similar to those of pyometra and include vulvar discharge, depression, and anorexia. Diagnosis is made by retrograde vaginography and ultrasonography that reveal single or multiple fluid-filled areas adjacent to the bladder. Other methods of diagnosis include abdominal palpation, laboratory evaluation, radiography, and exploratory laparotomy. Management involves surgical resection of all remaining uterine and ovarian tissue.

REFERENCES

1. Schlafer DH, Gifford AT: Cystic endometrial hyperplasia, pseudo-placentational endometrial hyperplasia, and other cystic conditions of the canine and feline uterus, Theriogenology 70:349, 2008.
2. Egenvall A, Hagman R, Bonnett BN, et al: Breed risk of pyometra in insured dogs in Sweden, J Vet Intern Med 15:530, 2001.
3. Fukuda S: Incidence of pyometra in colony-raised Beagle dogs, Exp Anim 50:325, 2001.

4. Hagman R, Lagerstedt A-S, Hedhammar A, et al: A breed-matched case-control study of potential risk-factors for canine pyometra, Theriogenology 75:1251, 2011.
5. Von Berky A, Townsend WL: The relationship between the prevalence of uterine lesions and the use of medroxyprogesterone acetate for canine population control, Aust Vet J 70:249, 1994.
6. Kunkitti P, Srisuwatanasagul S, Chatdarong K: Distribution of estrogen receptor alpha and progesterone receptor, and leukocyte infiltration in the cervix of cyclic bitches and those with pyometra, Theriogenology 75:979, 2011.
7. Ververidis HN, Boscos CM, Stefanakis A, et al: Serum estradiol-17β, progesterone and respective uterine cytosol receptor concentrations in bitches with spontaneous pyometra, Theriogenology 62:614, 2004.
8. Noakes DE, Dhaliwal GK, England GCW: Cystic endometrial hyperplasia-pyometra in dogs: a review of the causes and pathogenesis, J Reprod Fertil Suppl 57:395, 2001.
9. Chen YMM, Wright PJ, Lee CS: A model for the study of cystic endometrial hyperplasia in bitches, J Reprod Fertil Suppl 57:407, 2001.
10. Hagman R, Kuhn I: *Escherichia coli* strains isolated from the uterus and urinary bladder of bitches suffering from pyometra: comparison by restriction enzyme digestion and pulsed-field gel electrophoresis, Vet Microbiol 84:143, 2002.
11. Jutkowitz LA: Reproductive emergencies, Vet Clin North Am Small Anim Pract 35:397, 2005.
12. Tsumagari S, Ishinazaka T, Kamata H, et al: Induction of canine pyometra by inoculation of *Escherichia coli* into the uterus and its relationship to reproductive features, Anim Reprod Sci 87:301, 2005.
13. Arora N, Sandford J, Browning GF, et al: A model for cystic endometrial hyperplasia/pyometra complex in the bitch, Theriogenology 66:1530, 2006.
14. De Bosschere H, Ducatelle R, Tshamala M: Is mechanically induced cystic endometrial hyperplasia (CEH) a suitable model for study of spontaneously occurring CEH in the uterus of the bitch? Reprod Domest Anim 37:152, 2002.
15. Dhaliwal GK, England GCW, Noakes DE: The effects of endometrial scarification on uterine steroid receptors, bacterial flora and histological structure in the bitch, Anim Reprod Sci 69:238, 2002.
16. Kida K, Maezono Y, Nawate N, et al: Epidermal growth factor, transforming growth factor-α, and epidermal growth factor receptor expression and localization in the canine endometrium during the estrous cycle and in bitches with pyometra, Theriogenology 73:36, 2010.
17. Niskanen M, Thrusfield MV: Associations between age, parity, hormonal therapy and breed, and pyometra in Finnish dogs, Vet Rec 143:493, 1998.
18. Davidson AP, Feldman EC, Nelson RW: Treatment of pyometra in cats, using prostaglandin F_2-a: 21 cases (1982-1990), J Am Vet Med Assoc 200:825, 1992.
19. Bigliardi E, Parmigiani E, Cavirani S, et al: Ultrasonography and cystic hyperplasia-pyometra complex in the bitch, Reprod Domest Anim 39:136, 2004.
20. Fransson BA, Karlstam E, Bergstrom A, et al: C-reactive protein in the differentiation of pyometra from cystic endometrial hyperplasia/mucometra in dogs, J Am Anim Hosp Assoc 40:391, 2004.
21. Hagman R, Kindahl H, Fransson B, et al: Differentiation between pyometra and cystic endometrial hyperplasia/mucometra in bitches by prostaglandin F_2-a metabolite analysis, Theriogenology 66:198, 2006.
22. Hagman R, Greko C: Antimicrobial resistance in Escherichia coli isolated from bitches with pyometra and from urine samples from other dogs, Vet Rec 157:193, 2005.
23. Johnston SD, Root Kustritz MV, Olson PNS: Disorders of the canine uterus and uterine tubes (oviducts). In Johnston SD, Root Kustritz MV, Olson PNS, editors: Canine and feline theriogenology, Philadelphia, 2001, Saunders.
24. Wessels BC, Wells MT: Antiendotoxin immunotherapy for canine pyometra endotoxemia, J Am Anim Hosp Assoc 25:455, 1989.
25. Gobello C, Castex G, Klima L, et al: A study of two protocols combining aglepristone and cloprostenol to treat open cervix pyometra in the bitch, Theriogenology 60:901, 2003.
26. Fieni F: Clinical evaluation of the use of aglepristone, with or without cloprostenol, to treat cystic endometrial hyperplasia-pyometra complex in bitches, Theriogenology 66:1550, 2006.
27. Swalec Tobias KM, Wheaton LG: Surgical management of pyometra in dogs and cats, Semin Vet Med Surg (Small Anim) 10:30, 1995.
28. Corrada Y, Arias D, Rodriguez R, et al: Combination of dopamine agonist and prostaglandin agonist treatment of cystic endometrial hyperplasia-pyometra complex in the bitch, Theriogenology 66:1557, 2006.
29. Arnold S, Hubler M, Casal M, et al: Use of a low-dose prostaglandin for the treatment of canine pyometra, J Small Anim Pract 29:303, 1988.
30. Gabor G, Siver L, Szenci O: Intravaginal prostaglandin F_2a for the treatment of metritis and pyometra in the bitch, Acta Vet Hung 47:103, 1999.
31. Romagoli S: Canine pyometra: pathogenesis, therapy and clinical cases, Proc 27th World Small Anim Vet Assoc Congress, 2002.
32. Threlfall WR: Diagnosis and medical management of pyometra, Semin Vet Med Surg (Small Anim) 10:21, 1995.
33. Meyers-Wallen V, Goldschmidt M, Flickinger G: Prostaglandin $F_{2\alpha}$ treatment of canine pyometra, J Am Vet Med Assoc 189:1557, 1986.

PART XIV NUTRITION

CHAPTER 127
NUTRITIONAL ASSESSMENT

Cecilia Villaverde, BVSc, PhD, DACVN, DECVCN • Jennifer A. Larsen, DVM, PhD, DACVN

KEY POINTS

- Nutritional assessment is an important aspect of the management of hospitalized veterinary patients because malnutrition is a common yet often overlooked feature.
- Using nutritional assessment tools can help standardize protocols in the clinic.
- Nutritional support may help reduce complications and improve outcomes, and proactive implementation is the goal.
- In critical care settings, patients often have new or ongoing disease processes and altered physiology that complicate recovery and limit nutritional support options.

Hospitalized veterinary patients are often malnourished or are consuming inadequate diets, and preventing or reversing this problem should be a goal of all clinicians. One study showed that provision of adequate calories was only achieved 27% of the time in 276 hospitalized dogs over a total of 821 days.[1] Malnutrition in people is associated with increased complication rates, increased mortality, and longer hospital stays.[2,3] Similarly, poor outcomes in veterinary patients receiving inadequate nutritional support can be expected. To appropriately address this problem and minimize adverse effects of malnutrition in hospitalized dogs and cats, clinicians and staff should proactively ensure adequate documentation and monitoring so that adequate interventions are pursued as needed.

IMPACTS OF NUTRITIONAL SUPPORT DURING CRITICAL ILLNESS

Compared with that in human medicine, there is a dearth of data describing the impact of nutritional support on hospitalized veterinary patients. However, one study showed that hospitalized dogs and cats that received less than one third of their target energy requirements were more likely to have a poor outcome.[4]

In addition, illness and other physiologic stressors are associated with a hypermetabolic state characterized by increases in circulating cytokines, catecholamines, and other stress mediators.[5] These ultimately result in an inflammatory response with undesirable effects including increased protein catabolism and impaired healing ability.[6,7] This preferential catabolism of lean body mass over glycogen and fat stores in animals that are critically ill has a profoundly negative effect on healing, immune function, and recovery from disease and trauma. As such, intervention and provision of appropriate and adequate nutritional support are necessary to promote positive outcomes in veterinary patients. However, proactive assessment of individual patients is necessary to more accurately identify those with the most immediate needs as well as those at risk for greater complications.

SCREENING SYSTEMS USED FOR NUTRITIONAL ASSESSMENTS

Assessing the nutritional status of human patients is now routinely done in hospital settings and is important to identify patients suffering from or at risk of malnutrition. Several studies have shown that early nutritional intervention is necessary to achieve positive outcomes,[8] and efforts should be made to identify these patients before malnutrition is overt.

To do this in a completely objective way is currently not feasible, which is why a variety of screening assessment tools have been developed.[9-11] These include the Subjective Global Assessment (SGA) and the Malnutrition Universal Screening Tool (MUST) among others, and they use information from the medical and diet history, physical examination, anthropomorphic measures, and laboratory data to assign a subjective score to a patient. This assessment usually addresses four main aspects: recent weight loss, recent food intake, current body mass index, and disease severity. The goal is to identify patients that require monitoring or moderate to intensive nutritional intervention. Some of these screening systems are specific for disease conditions (e.g., geriatric, postsurgical, or hemodialysis patients) to make them as accurate as possible, despite their intrinsic subjectivity.

Nutritional assessment in veterinary patients historically has not been standard practice; however, published information and guidelines have recently become available[12,13] that aim to identify the nutritional status of the patient using data from the signalment, medical history, diet history, physical examination, and laboratory data. These guidelines were first published by the American Animal Hospital Association (AAHA)[12] and were subsequently adopted by the World Small Animal Veterinary Association (WSAVA).[13] The guidelines propose that the nutritional assessment should be the fifth vital sign of the examination of small animals (after temperature, pulse, respiration, and pain assessment). The goal is to recognize patients at risk of nutritional problems; these patients are then identified as candidates for an extended nutritional evaluation. The evaluation focuses on three aspects:

- Animal factors
- Diet factors
- Environmental factors (including feeding method)

For critically ill patients, the most important information to be collected comes from the physical examination (including body weight and body composition) and the medical history (in particular the diet history). In all cases, patients with higher nutrient needs (such as growing, reproducing, or geriatric animals) are more at risk than adult patients at maintenance.

BODY WEIGHT

Body weight is unquestionably valuable in evaluating the nutritional status of a patient. Specifically, serial and historical body weights are very important. During hospitalization, serial daily body weight will help determine if the energy intake is adequate or not. The goal for hospitalized patients is always to maintain body weight, regardless of whether the patient is an ideal body weight or overweight. Similarly, a historical record of body weights for a particular patient will be very helpful to determine if the current body weight is normal or not. Patients that have lost more than 10% of their previous body weight involuntarily should be considered malnourished because of negative energy balance. However, body weight alone, despite being very useful, will not provide information about the body composition of the dog or cat and can be affected by hydration status, fluid accumulation, organomegaly, or mass growth, so it is important to also assess and consider body composition.

BODY COMPOSITION

Measures of body composition such as dual-energy x-ray absorptiometry (DEXA) or deuterium oxide dilution (D_2O) are available at some academic institutions but are unlikely to be used at most primary and secondary referral clinics. Therefore objectively assessing the proportions of adipose and lean body mass is not possible in most cases, and subjective assessments are commonly employed.

Adipose Tissue

Although an increasing proportion of veterinary patients suffer from obesity, this condition is not necessarily correlated with adequate food intake during hospitalization. In fact, they may be more likely to suffer malnutrition from a deficiency of intake of energy and other nutrients, because of both clinician perception and the challenge of accurately assessing body weight and muscle mass changes. For example, clinical staff may not perceive any urgency in nutritional assessment and intervention for overweight or obese patients, with the assumption that such animals have a "reserve" of energy or even a need for acute weight loss. Further, because of the abundant subcutaneous adipose accumulation in many of these cases, assessment of lean body mass is very difficult.

Body condition score systems

There are several body condition score (BCS) systems in veterinary medicine that are used primarily to assess body fat in dogs and cats.[14] The most commonly used are the 5-point scale and the 9-point scale. The 9-point BCS system has been validated, showing very good correlation with objective measures (DEXA) of body fat mass in both cats[15] and dogs.[16] There are BCS charts for both dogs and cats in the Nutrition Toolkit produced by the World Small Animal Veterinary Association (WSAVA).[17]

The BCS systems use visual and palpable data from the patient to evaluate the fat depots and assign a corresponding numerical score. Important places to examine visually and to palpate are over the ribs, above the spine, at the waistline, and at the abdominal tuck. On the 9-point scale, a score 4 or 5 out of 9 for dogs and 5 out of 9 for cats is considered ideal, equivalent to 3 on a 5-point scale. Scores below ideal are underweight to emaciated and scores above ideal are overweight to obese (Figure 127-1). For the 9-point scale, each point differing from 5 represents a 10% to 15% excess or deficit of body fat. Patients with lower BCS are at more immediate risk in the ICU setting than those with higher scores (Figure 127-2), partly because of the likely chronic nature of the malnutrition; however, both are abnormal and require more detailed nutritional assessment and intervention.

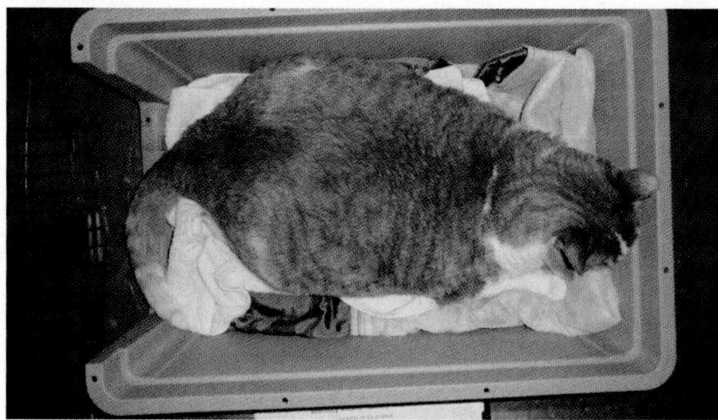

FIGURE 127-1 Overweight cat with a body condition score of 8 out of 9.

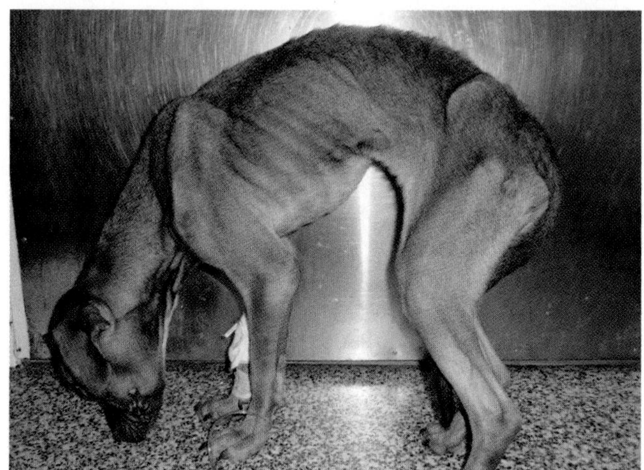

FIGURE 127-2 Malnourished dog with a body condition score of 1 out of 9.

Lean Body Mass

The loss of lean body mass associated with various disease processes (cachexia) and with aging (sarcopenia) has been linked to increased morbidity and mortality in people, and these syndromes are an area of interest and active research in both humans and animals.[18,19] Although negative nitrogen balance is likely common in hospitalized veterinary patients, more data are needed to identify causative or contributory factors and to establish relationships with specific outcomes for dogs and cats. In addition, enabling clinicians to predict risk for individual patients or populations as well as guide specific interventions would have significant value.

Besides measuring lean body mass with DEXA and D_2O methodology, the protein balance of a patient can be estimated by measuring urea nitrogen loss in the urine, because urea is the major protein breakdown product[20]; increased losses indicate a negative nitrogen balance. However, this method may not be practical in the ICU setting.

Muscle condition scoring

Of primary importance is the need to develop a system with guidelines to enable accurate assessment of clinical patients. Preliminary data have been presented for a muscle condition scoring system; however, these remain to be validated.[21,22] The AAHA and WSAVA

Table 127-1 Proposed Muscle Condition Scoring System Based on Palpation of Muscles Over the Spine, Scapulae, Skull, or Wings of the Ilia[21]

Cachexia Score	Description
3	Good muscle tone with no evidence of muscle wasting
2	Mild muscle wasting
1	Moderate muscle wasting
0	Marked muscle wasting as evidenced by atrophy of all muscle groups

BOX 127-1 *Resting Energy Requirement*

Formula for calculation of resting energy requirement:

$$70 \times [\text{body weight (kg)}]^{0.75}$$

guidelines propose a 4-point system, from normal muscle mass to mild, moderate, and severe atrophy, determined subjectively by visual and tactile examination of muscles over the temporal bone, scapulae, ribs, and pelvic bones. A proposed scoring system is shown in Table 127-1, and a muscle condition score chart with visual examples is included in the WSAVA Nutrition Toolkit.[17] Despite not yet being fully developed, it is important to include these data in the assessment of each critical care patient because moderate and severe muscle atrophy are clear indications for nutritional intervention.

DIET HISTORY

Current intake

It is important to account for all components of diet, including food given as meals as well as snacks, treats, or supplements. Specifically inquiring about how medications are administered often reveals additional food items that owners don't always consider part of the pet's diet, some of which contribute significant proportions of energy. A thorough diet history includes the exact brand and formula of food, the exact amounts of treats or any human foods provided, and the frequency of meals and treats.

Quantifying the energy intake of the hospitalized patient should be done daily, and thus should have a dedicated space in the daily hospitalization chart, in order to actively monitor and intervene if necessary. The goal is for patients to eat enough calories to maintain body weight during hospitalization, independent of the BCS. Weight gain would be desired in patients with low BCS and muscle atrophy, but it might not be possible in the critical care setting while any underlying diseases are still not under control.

There is a lack of knowledge on the effect that disease has on energy requirements.[23] At this time the consensus is that ICU patients should eat at least their resting energy requirement (RER) determined as kcal per day (Box 127-1).The RER is lower than maintenance energy requirements because of less physical activity during hospitalization. Adjustments should be made as needed; however, starting no higher than RER can help avoid problems related with overfeeding (including gastrointestinal distress, hyperglycemia, and hyperlipidemia). Tools to assist in the nutritional management of hospitalized veterinary patients, such as a feeding guide, feeding instructions, and a monitoring chart, are available in the WSAVA Nutrition Toolkit.[17]

Historical intake

In many human nutritional assessment systems, historical food intake is a very important piece of information because of its high predictive value for poor food intake during hospitalization. The exact duration of anorexia or hyporexia should be noted while taking the history. In cases where the appetite is reduced but not absent it is important to quantify it. This may be challenging in cases of patients fed ad libitum or when the diet is highly variable on a regular basis or to address inappetence. Often the fact that the patient is eating "something" delays nutritional intervention in patients that require it; however, a more targeted and quantitative guideline is indicated. A patient eating less than 75% of its RER should be considered hyporexic. In general the recommendation is to institute nutritional support in patients that are anorexic for more than 3 to 5 days and hyporexic for more than 1 week.

LABORATORY DATA

Few data from the clinicopathologic database can support generalized or specific causes of malnutrition; however, hypoalbuminemia together with inadequate lean body mass can indicate poor long-term protein status.[24] Certain types of anemia may support suspicions of poor B vitamins or trace minerals status. Differentiating abnormalities caused by poor intake (e.g., hypokalemia in cats with chronic kidney disease and poor appetite) from those resulting from malabsorption (e.g., hypocobalaminemia with inflammatory enteropathy) or abnormal losses (e.g., hypoalbuminemia with lymphangiectasia) can be challenging in some cases. However, these abnormalities are common with a variety of other disease processes.

More commonly these data are used to guide nutritional interventions or to assess individual patient tolerance of specific nutrients. For example, hyperglycemia is commonly noted in critically ill cats[25] and may preclude the use of dextrose-containing parenteral nutrition solutions or necessitate administration of insulin. Likewise, hyperkalemia sometimes develops in dogs with kidney disease and will significantly influence dietary options,[26] as will fasting hyperlipidemia in both dogs and cats. Correlating concurrent dietary intake with clinicopathologic data is necessary for developing a customized and rational nutritional management plan for individual patients.

CONCLUSION

Nutritional evaluation is very important in critically ill patients, which are at high risk of malnutrition secondary to their inappetence and their hypermetabolic state, which may result in a worse outcome. This assessment will help decide if careful monitoring or nutritional intervention is needed. As a general rule, patients that have been anorectic for more than 3 days or hyporectic for more than a week, have lost 10% of their body weight involuntarily, or have a low BCS or moderate to severe muscle atrophy are candidates for nutritional intervention. Readers are directed to Chapters 129 and 130 for further discussion of the nutritional support of critically ill patients.

REFERENCES

1. Remillard RL, Darden DE, Michel KE, et al: An investigation of the relationship between caloric intake and outcome in hospitalized dogs, Vet Ther 2:301, 2001.
2. Stratton RJ, Elia M: Deprivation linked to malnutrition risk and mortality in hospital, Br J Nutr 96:870, 2006.
3. Koretz RL, Avenell A, Lipman TO, et al: Does enteral nutrition affect clinical outcome? A systematic review of the randomized trials, Am J Gastroenterol 102:412, 2007.

4. Brunetto MA, Gomes MOS, Andre MR, et al: Effects of nutritional support on hospital outcome in dogs and cats, J Vet Emer Crit Care 20:224, 2010.
5. Coss-Bu JA, Klish WJ, Walding D, et al: Energy metabolism, nitrogen balance, and substrate utilization in critically ill children, Am J Clin Nutr 74:664, 2001.
6. Michel KE, King LG, Ostro E: Measurement of urinary urea nitrogen content as an estimate of the amount of total urinary nitrogen loss in dogs in intensive care units, J Am Vet Med Assoc 210:356, 1997.
7. Hasselgren PO, Fischer JE: Muscle cachexia: current concepts of intracellular mechanisms and molecular regulation, Ann Surg 233:9, 2001.
8. Kreymann KG: Early nutritional support in critical care: a European perspective, Curr Opin Clin Nutr Metab Care 11:156, 2008.
9. Skipper A, Ferguson M, Thompson K, et al: Nutrition screening tools: an analysis of the evidence, J Parent Enteral Nutr 36:292, 2012.
10. Kondrup J, Rasmussen HH, Hamberg O, et al: Nutritional risk screening (NRS 2002): a new method based on an analysis of controlled clinical trials, Clin Nutr 22:321, 2003.
11. Rasmussen HH, Holst M, Kondrup J: Measuring nutritional risk in hospitals, Clin Epidemiol 21:209, 2010.
12. Baldwin K, Bartges J, Buffington T, et al: AAHA nutritional assessment guidelines for dogs and cats, J Am Anim Hosp Assoc 46:285, 2010.
13. Freeman L, Becvarova I, Cave N, et al: WSAVA Nutritional Assessment Guidelines, J Small Anim Pract 52:385, 2011.
14. Burkholder WJ: Use of body condition scores in clinical assessment of the provision of optimal nutrition, J Am Vet Med Assoc 217:650, 2000.
15. Laflamme D: Development and validation of a body condition score system for cats: a clinical tool, Feline Pract 25:13, 1997.
16. Laflamme D: Development and validation of a body condition score system for dogs, Canine Pract 22:10, 1997.
17. http://www.wsava.org/nutrition-toolkit (accessed 2/14/14), Nutrition Toolkit, World Small Animal Veterinary Association Global Nutrition Committee.
18. Freeman LM: Cachexia and sarcopenia: emerging syndromes of importance in dogs and cats, J Vet Intern Med 26:3, 2012.
19. Hutchinson D, Sutherland-Smith J, Watson AL, et al: Assessment of methods of evaluating sarcopenia in old dogs, Am J Vet Res 73:1794, 2012.
20. Michel KE, King LG, Ostro E: Measurement of urinary urea nitrogen content as an estimate of the amount of total urinary nitrogen loss in dogs in intensive care units, J Am Vet Med Assoc 210:356, 1997.
21. Michel KE, Anderson W, Cupp C, et al: Validation of a subjective muscle mass scoring system for cats, J Anim Physiol Anim Nutr 93:806, 2009.
22. Michel KE, Anderson W, Cupp C, et al: Correlation of a feline muscle mass score with body composition determined by dual-energy X-ray absorptiometry, Br J Nutr 106:S57, 2011.
23. Burkholder WJ: Metabolic rates and nutrient requirements of sick dogs and cats, J Am Vet Med Assoc 206:614, 1995.
24. Michel KE: Prognostic value of clinical nutritional assessment in canine patients, Vet Emer Crit Care 3:96, 1993.
25. Chan DL, Freeman LM, Rozanski EA, et al: Alternations in carbohydrate metabolism in critically ill cats, J Vet Emerg Crit Care 16:s7, 2006.
26. Segev G, Fascetti AJ, Weeth LP, et al: Correction of hyperkalemia in dogs with chronic kidney disease consuming commercial renal therapeutic diets by a potassium-reduced home-prepared diet, J Vet Intern Med 24:546, 2010.

CHAPTER 128
NUTRITIONAL MODULATION OF CRITICAL ILLNESS

Daniel L. Chan, DVM, DACVECC, DACVN, FHEA, MRCVS

KEY POINTS

- Nutrients such as certain vitamins, amino acids, and polyunsaturated fatty acids have been shown to modulate inflammation and the immune response.
- Nutritional modulation of diseases, dubbed *therapeutic nutrition,* may be a useful strategy for companion animals; however, until trials can elucidate which specific nutrients and what dosages confer beneficial effects to particular patient populations, a certain degree of caution is advised.
- There may be significant species differences in the efficacy of therapeutic nutrition that may reduce the usefulness of some of these approaches in veterinary patients.
- Therefore further research in veterinary patients is warranted to evaluate possible novel strategies for modulating various diseases in critically ill small animals.

In critically ill animals, the role of nutritional support in the overall management of patients is well established. However, nutrition is most often simply regarded as a supportive measure. Recently, further understanding of the underlying mechanisms of various disease processes and the recognition that certain nutrients possess pharmacologic properties have led to investigations into how nutritional therapies themselves could modify the behavior of various conditions and improve patient outcomes; this has been dubbed *therapeutic nutrition.*[1] Nutrients such as certain vitamins, amino acids, and polyunsaturated fatty acids and even dextrose content can modulate inflammation and the immune response.[2,3] A major focus of nutrition in critically ill human patients now involves the development of strategies that target or modulate metabolic pathways, inflammation, and the immune system.[3] Exploiting pharmacologic effects of certain nutrients to modulate disease processes and patient outcomes has been the subject of various clinical trials in people; however, a similar focus on clinical veterinary patients has of yet not taken place. The use of nutritional strategies in ameliorating animal diseases has been shown to be beneficial in the areas of chronic kidney disease[4,5] (e.g., protein and phosphorous restriction) and cardiac disease[6,7] (e.g., taurine, omega-3 fatty acids). In people there is mounting evidence that certain nutrients such as glutamine, omega-3 fatty acids, and antioxidants can positively affect both morbidity and mortality in critically ill populations. It is hoped that a greater understanding of how these nutrients impart such beneficial effects may lead to developments of novel strategies for modulating various diseases in small animals. To this end, a review how nutritional strategies could be used to modulate disease, especially in critically ill animals, is the focus of this chapter and is discussed in greater detail.

OMEGA-3 FATTY ACIDS

Because inflammation plays a crucial role in many diseases, modulation of the inflammatory response has become an important target of therapy. Inflammation yields several lipid mediators that are involved in a complex regulatory array of the inflammatory process. Lipid mediators are synthesized by three main pathways—namely the cyclooxygenase, 5-lipoxygenase, and cytochrome P450 pathways—and they each use polyunsaturated fatty acids (PUFA) such as arachidonic acid (AA), eicosapentaenoic acid (EPA) and γ-linolenic acid (GLA) as substrates.[8] Potent proinflammatory eicosanoids, leukotrienes, and thromboxanes of the 2 and 4 series are produced from AA metabolism. Classically, modulation of inflammation was thought to result from greater substitution of omega-6 fatty acids (i.e., AA) with the omega-3 fatty acids (i.e., EPA and DHA) in cell membranes, such that when these PUFAs were cleaved by phospholipases and oxidized by several enzymes it led to less inflammatory eicosanoids of the 3 and 5 series.[8]

However, it is now clear that the biologic antiinflammatory activities of omega-3 fatty acids are far beyond the simple regulation of eicosanoid production. Namely, these PUFAs can affect immune cell responses through the regulation of gene expression, subsequent downstream events by acting as ligands for nuclear receptors, and through control of some key transcription factors.[9] EPA can also inhibit the activity of the proinflammatory transcription nuclear factor kappa B (NF-κB) at several levels, which regulates the expression of many proinflammatory mediators (e.g., cytokines, chemokines) and other effectors of the innate immune response system.[9] In addition, recent research has revealed that free EPA and DHA also inhibit the activation of Toll-like receptor 4 by endotoxin and thereby further inhibit the inflammatory response.[10] Finally, recent discoveries have identified that EPA and DHA are also substrates of two novel classes of mediators called resolvins and protectins, which are involved in the inhibition and resolution of the inflammatory process, which now appears to be a well-orchestrated, complex, active process involving these mediators.[9,11] Therefore, in the context of disease modulation, omega-3 fatty acids help reduce the production of inflammatory mediators and are incorporated in the synthesis of antiinflammatory and "pro-resolution" factors, which serve to attenuate the inflammatory response and the innate immune response.

In regard to the clinical use of omega-3 fatty acids in critically ill populations, the evidence is exclusively from human medicine. Enteral supplementation of EPA/DHA with concurrent antioxidants has been well established in ventilated patients with acute lung injury,[12] and more recently it has been shown to improve outcome in patients with early sepsis.[13] However, the data are not entirely conclusive, especially when omega-3 fatty acids are administered intravenously via parenteral nutrition. In a recent meta-analysis of studies evaluating supplemental omega-3 fatty acids in parenteral nutrition, no statistically significant benefits were identified in regard to mortality, infection, or intensive care unit (ICU) stay and only weak evidence that such supplementation shortens overall hospitalization.[14] However, the analysis should be considered preliminary because there are fewer than 10 trials included in the analysis and 6 of these trials contained fewer than 50 patients; therefore the conclusions regarding the utility of parenteral omega-3 fatty acids should be reserved until more data are available.[14] It is worth noting that the analysis did possibly uncover that timing of supplementation (i.e., early versus late in the disease process) may have a large effect on results. Many of the trials included in the analysis recruited patients in septic shock, and therefore the ability to demonstrate treatment benefit would be extremely difficult.[14] The recent results of the INTERSEPT study[13] using enteral EPA/DHA support this hypothesis because researchers recruited patients with early sepsis without organ dysfunction and were able to demonstrate various improvements in outcome. Currently, no data are available on the use of omega-3 fatty acids in critically ill veterinary populations. Given the number of potential benefits in modulation inflammation and patient outcome, further research in this area is warranted.

ANTIOXIDANTS

Similar to inflammation, oxidative stress is also recognized to be a prominent and common feature of many disease processes, including neoplasia, cardiac disease, trauma, burns, severe pancreatitis, sepsis, and critical illness. During various pathophysiologic states, particularly those typified by an inflammatory response, cells of the immune system such as neutrophils, macrophages, and eosinophils substantially contribute to the production of reactive oxygen species (ROS) and reactive nitrogen species (RNS). With the depletion of normal antioxidant defenses, the host is more vulnerable to free radical species and prone to cellular and subcellular damage (e.g., DNA, mitochondrial damage).[15] The degree of antioxidant depletion appears to reflect severity of illness in human patient populations.[16] Oxidative stress is believed to be not only a promoter of inflammation but also a key factor leading to multiple organ failure.[15]

Replenishment of antioxidant defenses attempts to lessen the intensity of the injury caused by ROS and RNS. Antioxidants can be classified in three different systems: (1) Antioxidant proteins such as albumin, haptoglobin, and ceruloplasmin; (2) enzymatic antioxidants such as superoxide dismutase, glutathione peroxidase, and catalase; and (3) nonenzymatic or small molecule antioxidants such as ascorbate (vitamin C), alpha-tocopherol (vitamin E), glutathione, selenium, lycopene, and beta-carotene. N-acetylcysteine is a powerful progenitor of glutathione and has been associated with some positive results in several patient populations. Treatment with N-acetylcysteine not only scavenges ROS but also enables continual production of glutathione and even blocks transcription of inflammatory cytokines.[15]

In regard to clinical evidence in critically ill people, a number of meta-analyses have indicated that the administration of antioxidant micronutrients (both as in monotherapy or combination therapy or antioxidant cocktails) is associated with a mortality risk reduction and reduced mechanical ventilator dependence but only a trend for reduced infectious complications.[15,17,18] It is interesting to note that the effect on mortality reduction was most apparent in populations with expected highest mortality rates, but a difference could not be detected when the mortality rate between the critically ill population and control population was less than 10%.[15] However, not all of the data regarding the use of antioxidants in the critically ill are positive. In a recent Cochrane review[19] of the use of N-acetylcysteine for sepsis and systemic inflammatory response syndrome (SIRS) in adult human patients, the authors concluded that their analysis casts "doubt on the safety and utility of intravenous N-acetylcysteine as an adjuvant therapy in SIRS and sepsis.[19] At best, N-acetylcysteine is ineffective in reducing mortality and complications in this patient population."[19] The analysis also highlighted concern that administration of N-acetylcysteine after 24 hours of onset of symptoms could lead to cardiovascular depression.[19] Typically, Cochrane reviews are very conservative in their analytical methods and seldom support novel interventions in critically ill populations. It is clear that further research is required to identify the most appropriate approach in modulating oxidative stress in the critically ill patients.

Despite the clear importance of oxidative stress in various diseases in veterinary species, investigations evaluating the effect of antioxidants on disease processes are limited. Positive results have been demonstrated in experimental models of oxidative stress including in conditions such as congestive heart failure,[20] acute pancreatitis,[21] gastric dilatation-volvulus,[22] renal transplantation,[23] gentamicin-induced nephrotoxicity,[24] and acetaminophen toxicity.[25,26] Supplementation of vitamin E alone did not prevent oxidative injury (i.e., development of Heinz body anemia), in cats fed onion powder or propylene glycol, but the same group of investigators later showed that supplementation of vitamin E with cysteine in cats decreased the production of methemoglobinemia after acetaminophen challenge.[26]

In naturally occurring disease such as chronic valvular disease[7] and renal insufficiency[27] there have also been some positive results that support the need for further evaluation. Unfortunately, the use of antioxidants in the setting of critically ill veterinary patients has not been published.

IMMUNE-MODULATING NUTRIENTS

Amino acids fulfill a vast array of functions in the body. They primarily serve as building blocks for protein synthesis and participate in various chemical reactions. Certain amino acids have immune-modulating properties, and they help maintain the functional integrity of immune cells and aid in wound healing and tissue repair. They may also serve as an energy source for certain cells, perhaps the most pertinent example being glutamine, which is the preferred fuel source for enterocytes and cells of the immune system. During disease states, the body undergoes marked alterations in substrate metabolism that could lead to a deficiency in these amino acids. In response to stress there may be a dramatic increase in demand by the host of particular amino acids such as arginine and glutamine. In health these amino acids are adequately synthesized by the host. However, during periods after severe trauma, infection, or inflammation, the demand for these amino acids cannot be met by the host and they become "conditionally essential" and must be obtained from the diet. Given the importance of these amino acids, the sudden depletion in these important substrates led to the hypothesis that dietary supplementation of these amino acids during disease would improve outcome. In addition, in times of injury and tissue repair and rapid cellular proliferation, nucleotide availability may become depleted and rate-limiting for the synthesis of nucleotide-derived compounds.[3]

Arginine

Arginine is a conditionally essential amino acid that is required for polyamine synthesis (for cell growth and proliferation) and proline synthesis (for wound healing) and is a precursor for nitric oxide (signaling molecule for immune cells). After extensive injury or surgery, immature cells of myeloid origin produce arginase-1, an enzyme that breaks down arginine. The ensuing arginine deficiency is associated with suppression of T-lymphocyte function.[28] When steps are taken to replenish arginine along with omega-3 fatty acids, T cell number and function improve. There are also data that demonstrate a significant treatment benefit following supplementation after major surgery. Clinical benefits included fewer infectious complication rates and decreased overall length of stay when compared with standard nutritional support.[3]

The one population in whom arginine therapy is likely to be contraindicated is patients with severe sepsis.[3] Likely causes of this detrimental effect relate to promotion of excessive nitric oxide synthesis, worsening of cardiovascular tone, and decreasing organ perfusion.[3]

Glutamine

Glutamine, another conditionally essential amino acid, is the most abundant free amino acid in circulation; however, stores are rapidly depleted during critical illness in people. A deficiency in glutamine has been documented to impair several important defense mechanisms of the host. Supplementation of glutamine during critical illness is believed to confer beneficial effects on patient outcomes. The evidence has been so strong that nutritional guidelines for critically ill people have included recommendations for supplemental glutamine to any patient receiving parenteral nutrition.[29-31] The proposed mechanisms by which glutamine improves outcomes involve the following[1]:

1. Tissue protection (e.g., heat shock protein expression, maintenance of gut barrier integrity and function, and decreased apoptosis)
2. Antiinflammatory and immune modulation (e.g., decreased cytokine production, inhibition of NF-κB)
3. Preservation of metabolic function (e.g., improved insulin sensitivity, adenosine triphosphate [ATP] synthesis)
4. Antioxidant effects (i.e., enhance glutathione generation)
5. Attenuation of inducible nitric oxide synthase activity

The evidence supporting the use of glutamine in critically ill human patients had been overwhelmingly positive until the publication of the largest randomized, placebo-controlled, double-blinded clinical trial evaluating high-dose glutamine and antioxidants in severely ill patients.[32] In this seminal study, more than 1200 critically ill patients with at least two failing organ systems and requiring mechanical ventilation were randomly allocated to glutamine versus placebo treatment and antioxidants versus placebo treatment. Unexpectedly the result was a trend for increased mortality associated with glutamine use.[32] There was no effect of glutamine on rates of organ failure or infectious complications, and antioxidants had no discernible effects.[32] The exact reasons for the observed trend in increased mortality was not identified, but it is worth noting that the dose of glutamine used in this study was much higher than any previous study to date and also that this study population included patients in shock being treated with nutritional support before achieving hemodynamic stability. Most recommendations for nutrition support (both enteral and parenteral) in the critically ill patient stipulate that cardiovascular stability must be achieved before commencing nutritional support.[30] These confounding factors may explain the differences in outcome observed compared with previous studies.

Despite ample evidence guiding treatment recommendations in people, there are no equivalent recommendations in the veterinary literature pertaining to glutamine use. This likely is due to the lack of supporting data and limited availability of parenteral glutamine. To date, only a few published veterinary trials have evaluated the use of glutamine (enteral or parenteral) in dogs and cats. In a trial of cats treated with methotrexate, enteral glutamine offered no intestinal protection in terms of reducing intestinal permeability or improving severity of clinical signs.[33] Another trial evaluating the effects of enteral glutamine on plasma glutamine concentrations and prostaglandin E_2 concentrations in radiation-induced mucositis showed no measurable benefit.[34] Possible reasons for the apparent failures in both these trials could be attributed to inadequate doses used or because of the form used, enteral, was not effective in these conditions. In contrast, a recent experimental canine model of postoperative ileus by Ohno et al[35] evaluated the effects of glutamine on restoration of interdigestive migrating contraction in the intestines, and they were able to demonstrate a statistically significant reduction in the time to restore contractions in the glutamine-treated group. Authors hypothesized that the benefit was derived from glutamine's ability to maintain glutathione concentration and thereby counteract the deleterious effects from surgical injury, inflammation, and oxidative stress. The authors concluded that administration of glutamine after gastrectomy could shorten the duration of ileus (a major postoperative problem in critically ill people) and may protect against surgical stress in general.[35] Given these positive results, further studies should evaluate the possible beneficial effects of glutamine supplementation in treating ileus and other gastrointestinal motility disorders in dogs with naturally occurring disease.

Most recently Kang et al[36] demonstrated that the immune suppression induced by high-dose methylprednisolone sodium succinate therapy can be ameliorated by parenteral administration of L-alanyl-L-glutamine.[36] The study was designed to address a common concerns associated with high-dose glucocorticoid therapy, namely, immune suppression. The model employed did demonstrate that such high doses of glucocorticoid can suppress oxidative burst activity and phagocytic capacity of neutrophils. Although the study used an experimental model, it does suggest that parenteral glutamine does have immunomodulatory effects in dogs and that in the future more clinically applicable uses should be explored. Unfortunately, parenteral glutamine is not routinely available in North America and the majority of studies evaluating parenteral glutamine are performed in Europe and Asia.

Nucleotides

Nucleotides, low-molecular-weight intracellular compounds (i.e., pyrimidine and purine), are the basic building blocks for the synthesis of DNA, RNA, ATP, and key coenzymes involved in essential metabolic reactions. Similarly to amino acids, nucleotides can be synthesized de novo or can be salvaged and recycled from other molecules. The reason nucleotides are included in this discussion of therapeutic nutrition is that during disease states and injury, the rapid cell proliferation required for tissue healing leads to nucleotide depletion.[3] Dietary supplementation can compensate for such depletions and support cell proliferation and differentiation. Because the cell types most affected by shortfalls in nucleotides are cells of the immune systems and of the gastrointestinal tract, nucleotide supplementation is often included in "immune-enhancing diets." The evidence for the beneficial effects of dietary nucleotides are mostly from preclinical trials and rodent models; therefore further research is still warranted.[37] From the pathophysiologic point of view, supplementation of dietary nucleotides may be particularly important in animals with prolonged anorexia because supplementation in rodent models enhances intestinal repair, restores brush-border enzyme activity, and improves gut barrier function.[37] Additional benefits of dietary nucleotides include positive effects on gut flora, gastrointestinal microcirculation, immune function, and inflammation.[37] Given the plethora of potential beneficial effects without clear detrimental effects, it is not surprising that nucleotides have been included in some immune-enhancing diet cocktails despite the lack of definitive results. Although results of trials using these immune-enhancing cocktails are encouraging and mostly positive, it is unknown if these effects are synergistic or whether they result from the summation of the individual components. To date, no veterinary studies have evaluated the potential utility of supplementing nucleotides to critically ill patients.

PROBIOTICS

Probiotics are live microorganisms that, when ingested in sufficient amounts, have a positive effect on the health of the host. Some of the benefits purportedly related to probiotics include reduced production of toxic bacterial metabolites, increased production of certain vitamins, enhanced resistance to bacterial colonization, and reinforced host natural defenses. Probiotics are also believed to shorten duration of infections or decrease host susceptibility to pathogens.[38] The proposed mechanisms underlying the positive effects include restoration of gastrointestinal barrier function; modification of the gut flora by inducing host cell antimicrobial peptides (i.e., defensins, cathelicidins), releasing probiotic antimicrobial factors (e.g., bacteriocins, microsins) competing for epithelial adherence; and immunomodulation.[38] Probiotics are therefore believed to have a role in balancing gut microflora and increasing host resistance to pathogenic bacteria. It is worth bearing in mind that the effects of probiotics are not only dose dependent but also both strain and species specific.[39] In people, probiotics used include various species of *Lactobacillus*, *Bifidobacterium*, and *Streptococcus*.[38] Microorganisms approved for use in animal feeds include strains belonging to the *Bacillus*, *Enterococcus*, and *Lactobacillus* bacterial groups.

The mechanism by which probiotics enhance gut barrier function may involve how certain bacteria (e.g., *Lactobacillus*) stimulate mucin production and thereby inhibit pathogenic bacteria from invading and attaching to the gut epithelium.[38] Concerns about the use of probiotics include the risk that certain microorganisms, such as enterococci, may harbor transmissible antimicrobial resistance determinants (i.e., plasmids), thus contributing to the problem of antimicrobial resistance. The use of probiotics in the critically ill is controversial, and guidelines recommend additional safety trials before further use in critically ill patients.[39]

In human critical care, probiotics have been used to combat antimicrobial-associated diarrhea, *Clostridium difficile* infections, and ventilator-associated pneumonia.[38] The probiotic yeast *Saccharomyces boulardii* apparently produces a protease that degrades *C. difficile* toxins and may also stimulate immunoglobulin A (IgA) secretions against *C. difficile* toxins.[39] The only meta-analysis evaluating probiotics to prevent ventilator-associated pneumonia demonstrated a significant reduction in incidence of ventilator-associated pneumonia and length of ICU stay.[40] Thus far, trials evaluating probiotics in critically ill patients have only demonstrated a trend toward reduced ICU mortality.[39]

Probiotics have the theoretical risk of transferring antibiotic resistance genes, translocating from the intestine to other areas or developing adverse reactions via interactions with host's microflora. Although bacteremia has not been documented with probiotic use in critically ill people, there are single case reports detailing infections with probiotic strains in immune-suppressed patients.[41]

In veterinary medicine there are no trials evaluating the use of probiotics in a critically ill patient population. However, there have been trials in dogs with gastrointestinal signs. A prospective placebo-controlled probiotic trial using a canine-specific probiotic cocktail containing three different *Lactobacillus spp* strains in addition to novel protein diet was able to demonstrate a dramatic improvement in clinical signs after dietary change but no additional benefit attributed to the addition of a probiotic.[42] Other studies have documented some positive effects such as improvements in immunologic markers or desirable changes in microbiota; however, these trials have mostly been performed on healthy dogs. It is uncertain whether these benefits would improve clinical signs in dogs with critical illness.

CONCLUSION

Despite the many pitfalls discussed, nutritional modulation of diseases appears to be potentially useful strategy for companion animals. However, until trials can elucidate which specific nutrients and what dosages confer beneficial effects to particular patient populations, a certain degree of caution is advised. Of particular concern is the distinct possibility that significant species differences may reduce the usefulness of some of these approaches in veterinary patients. Before general recommendations for the use of immunomodulating nutrients in veterinary patients can be made, many questions must be answered. Central issues of safety, purity, and efficacy must be addressed. However, as our understanding of the interactions between nutrients and disease processes grows, we may yet identify specific nutrients that could modulate serious diseases. Based on the progress being made in the area of clinical nutrition, it is quite evident that there should be a greater appreciation for the role nutrients play in ameliorating diseases and how treatment strategies for certain conditions in companion animals may one day heavily depend on nutritional therapies.

REFERENCES

1. Wischmeyer PE, Heyland DK: The future of critical care nutrition therapy, Crit Care Clin 26:433, 2010.
2. Cahill NE, Dhaliwal R, Day AG, et al: Nutrition therapy in the critical care setting: what is "best achievable" practice? An international multicenter observational study, Crit Care Med 38:395, 2010.
3. Hegazi RA, Wischmeyer PE: Clinical review: optimizing enteral nutrition for critically ill patients—a simple data-driven formula, Crit Care 15:234, 2011.
4. Bauer JE, Markwell PJ, Rauly JM, et al: Effects of dietary fat and polyunsaturated fatty acids in dogs with naturally developing chronic renal failure, J Am Vet Med Assoc 215:1588, 1999.
5. Brown SA, Brown CA, Crowel WA, et al: Beneficial effects of chronic administration of dietary omega-3 polyunsaturated fatty acids in dogs with renal insufficiency, J Lab Clin Med 131:447,1998.
6. Freeman LM, Rush JE, Khayias JJ, et al: Nutritional alterations and effect of fish oil supplementation in dogs with heart failure, J Vet Inter Med 12:440, 1998.
7. Smith CE, Freeman LM, Rush JE, et al: Omega-3 fatty acids in Boxer dogs with arrhythmogenic right ventricular cardiomyopathy, J Vet Inter Med 21:265, 2007.
8. Mayer K, Schaefer MB, Seeger W: Fish oil in the critically ill: from experimental to clinical data, Curr Opin Clin Nutr Metab Care 9:140, 2006.
9. Singer P, Shapiro H, Theilla M, et al: Anti-inflammatory properties of omega-3 fatty acids in critical illness: novel mechanisms and an integrative perspective, Intensive Care Med 34:1580, 2008.
10. Lee JY, Hwang DH: The modulation of inflammatory gene expression by lipids: mediation through Toll-like receptors, Mol Cell 21:176, 2006.
11. Willoughby DA, Moore AR, Colville-Nash PR, et al: Resolution of inflammation, Int J Immunopharmacol 22:1131, 2000.
12. Pontes-Arruda A, Demichele S, Seth A, et al: The use of an inflammation-modulating diet in patients with acute lung injury or acute respiratory distress syndrome: a meta-analysis of outcome data, JPEN J Parenter Enteral Nutr 32:596, 2008.
13. Pontes-Arruda A, Martins LF, de Lima SM, et al: Enteral nutrition with eicosapentaenoic acid, gamma-linolenic acid and antioxidants in the early treatment of sepsis: results from a multicenter, prospective, randomized, double-blinded, controlled study: the INTERSEPT Study, Crit Care 15:R144, 2011.
14. Palmer AJ, Ho CKM, Ajinola O, et al: The role of omega-3 fatty acid supplemented parenteral nutrition in critical illness in adults: a systemic review and meta-analysis, Crit Care Med 41:307, 2013.
15. Manzanares W, Dhaliwal R, Jiang X, et al: Antioxidant micronutrients in the critically ill: a systemic review and meta-analysis, Crit Care 16:R66, 2012.
16. Alonso de Vega JM, Serrano E, Carbonell LF: Oxidative stress in critically ill patients with systemic inflammatory response syndrome, Crit Care Med 30:1782, 2002.
17. Heyland DK, Dhaliwal R, Suchner U, et al: Antioxidants nutrients: a systematic review of trace elements and vitamins in the critically ill patient, Intensive Care Med 31:327, 2005.
18. Visse J, Labadarios D, Blaauw R: Micronutrient supplementation for critically ill adults: a systemic review and meta-analysis, Nutrition 27:745, 2011.
19. Szakmany T, Hauser B, Radermacher P: N-acetylcysteine for sepsis and systemic inflammatory response in adults, Cochrane Database Syst Rev 9:CD006616, 2012.
20. Amado LC, Saliaris AP, Raju SV, et al: Xanthine oxidase inhibition ameliorates cardiovascular dysfunction in dogs with pacing induced heart failure, J Mol Cell Cardiol 39:531, 2005.
21. Marks JM, Dunkin BJ, Shillingstad BL, et al: Preteratment with allopurinol diminishes pancreatography-induced pancreatitis in a canine model, Gastr Endos 48:180, 1998.
22. Badylak SF, Lanz GC, Jeffries M: Prevention of reperfusion injury in surgical induced gastric dilatation volvulus in dogs, Am J Vet Res 51:294, 1990.
23. Lee JI, Son HY, Kim MC: Attenuation of ischemia-reperfusion injury by ascorbic acid in the canine renal transplantation, J Vet Sci 7:375, 2006.
24. Varzi HN, Esmailzadeh S, Morovvati H, et al: Effect of silymarin and vitamin E on gentamycin-induced nephrotoxicity in dogs, J Vet Pharmacol Ther 30:477, 2007.
25. Webb CB, Twedt DC, Fettman MJ, et al: S-adenosylmethionine (SAMe) in a feline acetaminophen model of oxidative injury, J Fel Med Surg 5:69, 2003.
26. Hill AS, Rogers QR, O'Neill SL, et al: Effects of dietary antioxidant supplementation before and after oral acetaminophen challenge in cats, Am J Vet Res 66:196, 2005.
27. Plevraki K, Koutinas AF, Kaldrymidou H, et al: Effects of allopurinol treatment on the progression of chronic nephritis in Canine leishmaniosis (Leishmania infantum), J Vet Intern Med 20:228,2006.
28. Popovic PJ, Zeh HJ, Ochoa JB: Arginine and immunity, J Nutr 136:1681S, 2007.
29. Wernerman J: Glutamine supplementation, Ann Intensive Care 1:25, 2011.
30. McClave SA, Martindale RG, Vanek VW, et al: Guidelines for the provision and assessment of nutritional support therapy in adult critically ill patient: Society of Critical Care Medicine (SCCM) and the American Society for Parenteral and Enteral Nutrition (ASPEN), J Parenter Enteral Nutr 33:277, 2009.
31. Kreymann KG, Berger MM, Deutz NE, et al: ESPEN guidelines on enteral nutrition: intensive care, Clin Nutr 25:210, 2006.
32. Heyland D, Muscedere J, Wischmeyer PE, et al: A Randomized trial of glutamine and antioxidants in critically ill patients, N Eng J Med 368:1489, 2013.
33. Marks SL, Cook AK, Reader R, et al: Effects of glutamine supplementation of an amino acid-based purified diet on intestinal mucosal integrity in cats with methotrexate-induced enteritis, Am J Vet Res 60:755, 1999.
34. Lana SE, Hansen RA, Kloer L, et al: The effects of oral glutamine supplementation on plasma glutamine concentrations and PGE2 concentrations in dogs experiencing radiation-induced mucositis, J Appl Res Vet Med 1:259, 2003.
35. Ohno T, Mochiki E, Ando H, et al: Glutamine decreases the duration of postoperative ileus after abdominal surgery: an experimental study of conscious dogs, Dig Dis Sci 54:1208, 2009.
36. Kang JH, Kim SS, Yang MP: Effect of parenteral L-alanyl-L-glutamine administration on phagocytic responses of polymorphonuclear neutrophilic leukocytes in dogs undergoing high-dose methylprednisolone sodium succinate treatment, Am J Vet Res 73:1410, 2011.
37. Hess JR, Greenberg NA: The role of nucleotides in the immune and gastrointestinal systems: potential clinical applications, Nutr Clin Pract 27:281, 2012.
38. Morrow LE, Gogineni V, Malesker MA: Probiotics in the intensive care unit, Nutr Clin Pract 27:235, 2012.
39. Petrof EO, Dhaliwal R, Manazanares W, et al: Probiotics in the critically ill: a systematic review of the randomized trial evidence, Crit Care Med 40:3290, 2012.
40. Siempos I, Ntaidou TK, Falagas ME: Impact of the administration of probiotics on the incidence of ventilator-associated pneumonia: a metaanalysis of randomized, controlled trials, Crit Care Med 38:954, 2010.
41. Boyle RJ, Robbins-Browne RM, Tang MLK: Probiotic use in clinical practice: what are the risks? Am J Clin Nutr 83:1256, 2006.
42. Sauter SN, Benyacoub J, Allenspach K, et al: Effects of probiotic bacteria in dogs with food responsive diarrhoea treated with an elimination diet, J Anim Phys Anim Nutr 90:269, 2006.

CHAPTER 129

ENTERAL NUTRITION

Laura Eirmann, DVM, DACVN • Kathryn E. Michel, DVM, MS, DACVN

KEY POINTS

- The goal of enteral nutrition is to provide the patient with adequate caloric and nutrient intake to prevent the adverse consequences of malnutrition.
- Every critically ill patient must have an assessment performed to determine an appropriate nutrition plan. Patient reevaluation and nutrition plan reassessment need to occur throughout the hospitalization.
- As a general guideline, enteral feeding as far proximal as possible in the gastrointestinal (GI) tract is the preferred route of delivering nutritional support.
- Feasibility of enteral nutrition is based on patient factors such as GI function and ability to protect the airway, as well as nonpatient factors such as cost, predicted length of hospitalization, technical expertise, and level of patient monitoring.
- The daily caloric goal for most critically ill patients will be the resting energy requirement (RER). Evaluating whether a patient achieves this level of intake requires detailed feeding orders and documentation of patient intake.
- Potential complications of enteral nutrition include patient factors such as inadequate intake, GI side effects, metabolic derangements, and infectious complications, as well as nonpatient factors such as mechanical complications related to the feeding device.

The goal of enteral nutrition is to provide the patient with adequate caloric and nutrient intake via the gastrointestinal (GI) tract in order to prevent the adverse consequences of malnutrition (see later). Hospitalized patients often have decreased caloric intake for many reasons, including patient factors such as nausea, pain, and anxiety and nonpatient factors such as poorly written feeding orders. At the same time, critically ill patients have metabolic alterations mediated by catecholamines, corticosteroids, and inflammatory mediators such as interleukin 1 and tumor necrosis factor-α, which alter metabolism, resulting in a catabolic state.[1] Decreased voluntary intake coupled with a catabolic state places critically ill patients at high risk for malnutrition, necessitating nutritional support. Malnutrition in the critically ill patient leads to depletion of endogenous proteins, which may have serious adverse effects on tissue synthesis, immunocompetence, maintenance of GI tract integrity, and intermediary drug metabolism.[2] Malnutrition in humans is associated with increased complication rates, duration of hospitalization, and cost.[3] Extensive studies have not been conducted in veterinary medicine, but in one prospective study, puppies with parvoviral enteritis receiving early enteral nutrition showed earlier clinical improvement and significant weight gain compared with puppies who remained NPO until vomiting ceased for 12 hours.[4] Two retrospective studies also provide evidence for nutritional support in veterinary medicine. One study demonstrated a positive association between energy intake and hospital discharge.[5] The second retrospective made a positive association between dogs with septic peritonitis receiving early enteral or parenteral support and a shorter length of hospitalization.[6]

DETERMINING THE ROUTE OF NUTRITIONAL SUPPORT

Enteral Versus Parenteral

Nutritional support can be delivered via the GI tract (enteral route), intravenously (parenteral route), or using a combination of the two. Hypotensive or hypothermic patients likely have poor gut motility and perfusion and so should first be stabilized before initiating enteral feeding. The route of nutrient delivery is determined by patient factors such as GI function and ability to protect the airway, and nonpatient factors such as cost, predicted length of hospitalization, technical expertise, and level of patient monitoring. Enteral feeding is preferable to parenteral feeding because it is more physiologic, less costly, and safer.[7] The physiologic benefits of enteral feeding include prevention of intestinal villous atrophy, maintenance of intestinal mucosal integrity (which decreases the risk of bacterial translocation), and preservation of GI immunologic function. Contraindications for enteral feeding are uncontrolled vomiting, GI obstruction, ileus, malabsorption or maldigestion, or inability to protect the airway. However, if the patient is unable to protect the airway, the clinician may select a route of nutrient delivery distal to the pharynx or esophagus if the concern is aspiration during swallowing or distal to the pylorus if the concern is aspiration during vomiting or regurgitation. Figure 129-1 outlines the decision process for selecting an appropriate enteral feeding route.

Oral Intake Versus Enteral Feeding Device

When enteral feeding is appropriate, the clinician selects the mode of nutrient delivery, sets a caloric goal, and chooses an appropriate diet. Enteral feeding as far proximal in the GI tract as the patient can tolerate is preferred. Voluntary oral intake has distinct advantages. It requires no special equipment or techniques and allows the owner to participate in patient care. If the oral route is selected, the clinician must write specific feeding orders. The technical staff offers the amount written on the feeding orders and records the amount consumed. The clinician then determines if the nutrition goal was met. If intake does not meet the goal, the clinician reassesses the patient, diet, and environment. The clinician may change the diet (e.g., more palatable diet, warming the food) or change the environment (e.g., quieter ward, owner feeding the pet). Syringe feeding a liquid or blenderized pet food may be attempted for 1 to 2 days but often becomes too stressful and time consuming. If the patient shows any signs of nausea, oral feeding should be discontinued immediately, because this can lead to a learned food aversion. Medication to ameliorate nausea and an alternative feeding method should be considered. Appetite stimulants such as cyproheptadine or mirtazapine may be considered after careful patient assessment. The effectiveness of the treatment must be closely monitored by recording daily caloric intake and any possible side effects. Pharmacologic stimulation of appetite does not replace the need for daily nutritional assessment nor negate consideration of enteral feeding devices. If adequate intake is not achieved or side

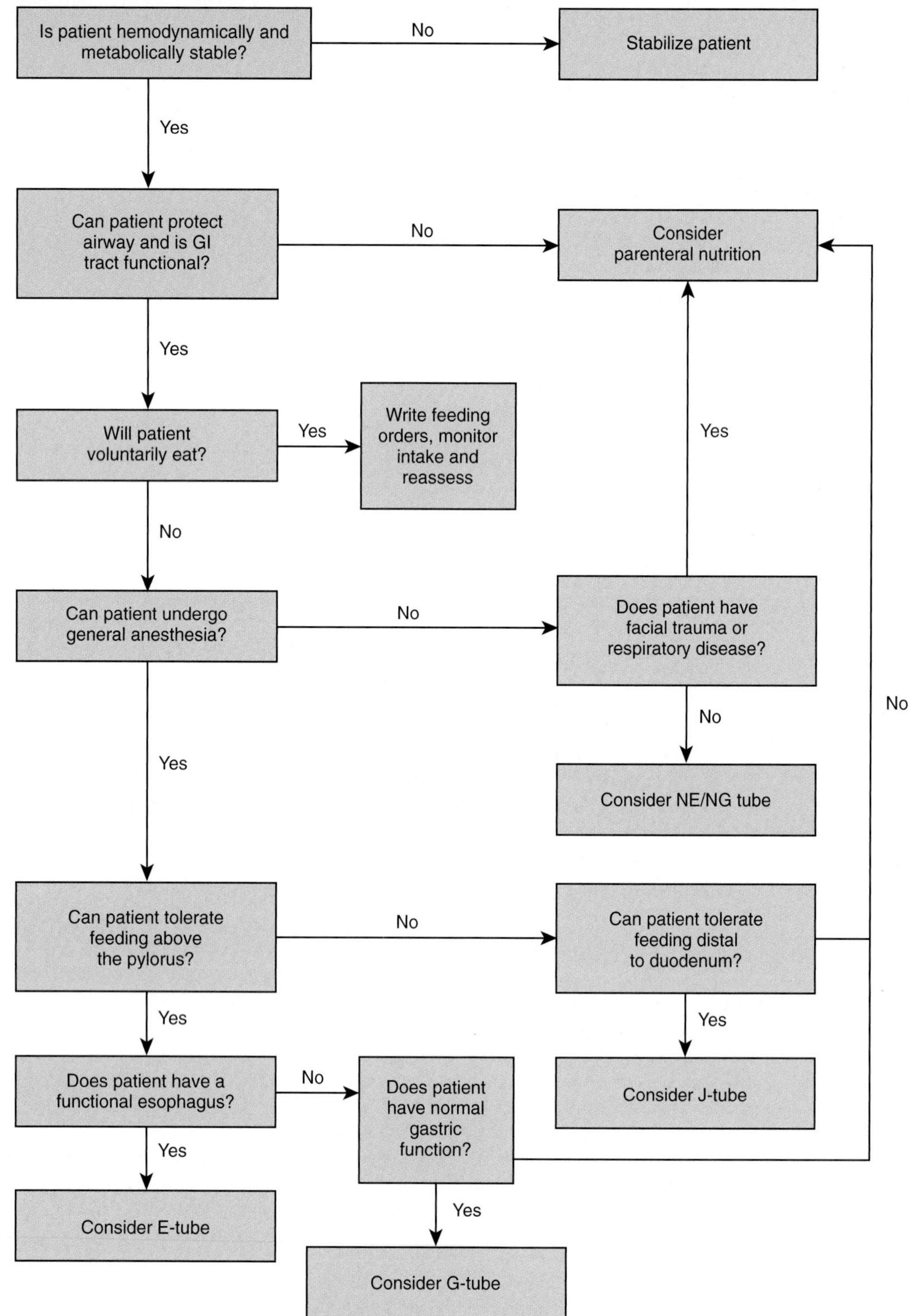

FIGURE 129-1 Decision tree for selecting enteral feeding route. *CRI,* Constant rate infusion; *GI,* gastrointestinal; *NE,* nasoesophageal; *NG,* nasogastric; *E,* esophagostomy; *G,* gastrostomy; *J,* jejunostomy..

effects occur, the plan must be revised to meet the patient's nutritional needs.

An enteral feeding tube removes the variable of voluntary intake. The technical staff delivers a prescribed amount of a specific diet via the feeding tube according to orders written by the veterinarian. These tubes are well tolerated by veterinary patients and, when anticipated, can be placed while the patient is sedated or anesthetized for a diagnostic or therapeutic procedure. A retrospective owner survey concluded that owners were comfortable managing their cats at home with esophagostomy and percutaneous endoscopic gastrostomy tubes.[8] Enteral feeding device placement usually requires sedation or anesthesia and technical skill. Technicians and owners must be taught how to use feeding devices and monitor for complications. Table 129-1 outlines advantages and disadvantages of the various forms of enteral access used in veterinary patients.

Table 129-1 **Advantages and Disadvantages of Enteral Feeding Devices**

Enteral Feeding Device	Advantages	Disadvantages
NE or NG tube	Ease of placement No general anesthesia NG tube allows for gastric decompression	Limited to liquid diets Short term (<14 days) Can be irritating; requires E-collar Can dislodge if patient sneezes or vomits Contradicted in facial trauma or respiratory disease NG tube may create incompetence of lower esophageal sphincter
Esophagostomy tube	Blenderized pet foods or liquid diets can be used Well tolerated by patient Ease of placement Can feed as soon as patient awakens from anesthesia Can be removed at any time Good long-term option	Requires general anesthesia Risk of cellulitis or infection at site Can dislodge if patient vomits Can cause esophageal irritation or reflux if malpositioned
Gastrostomy tubes	Blenderized pet foods or liquid diets can be used Well tolerated by patient Good long-term option	Requires general anesthesia Risk of cellulitis or infection at site Risk of peritonitis Must wait 24 hours after placement before feeding Must wait 10 to 14 days before removing
Jejunostomy tube	Able to feed distal to pylorus and pancreatic duct	Requires general anesthesia Limited to liquid diets Technically more difficult to place Risk of cellulitis or infection at site Risk of peritonitis Risk of tube migration with secondary GI obstruction Must wait 24 hours after placement before feeding Requires CRI feeding Requires very close monitoring Short-term option

CRI, Constant rate infusion; *GI,* gastrointestinal; *NE,* nasoesophageal; *NG,* nasogastric.

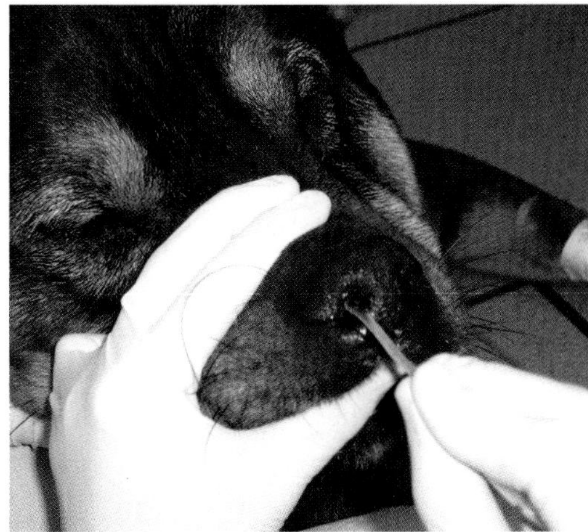

FIGURE 129-2 Placement of a nasoesophageal tube in a dog. Note that the nose is being pushed upward to facilitate passage of the tube into the ventral meatus.

ENTERAL FEEDING TUBES

Nasoesophageal or Nasogastric Tubes

A 3.5 to 8 Fr silicone or polyurethane feeding tube may be placed through the nares into the distal esophagus (nasoesophageal [NE]) or into the stomach (nasogastric [NG]) (Figure 129-2). NE tubes have historically been recommended because the risk of gastric reflux increases if the tube passes through the lower esophageal sphincter, compromising sphincter competence. However, one small retrospective study failed to demonstrate a difference in recorded complication rates between a group of dogs fed via NE versus NG tubes.[9] NG tubes allow for gastric decompression and measurement of gastric residual volume. Radiographic confirmation of correct placement for all tube types is recommended.

An advantage of NE and NG tubes is that they can be placed easily using a local anesthetic or light sedation.[10] This is a good option for patients that are poor candidates for general anesthesia. Facial trauma or coagulopathy may preclude placement of this type of tube, and it should not be used in patients with respiratory disease because it may exacerbate respiratory compromise by occluding a nares. Any patient that receives enteral nutrition must have a functional GI tract and the ability to guard the airway if vomiting or regurgitation occurs.

Because only small-bore tubes are used, diet selection is limited to liquids. NE and NG tubes are best for short-term (7 to 14 days) feeding because they can be irritating. An Elizabethan collar (E-collar) and close monitoring are required because the pet may attempt to dislodge the tube. In addition, sneezing or vomiting may dislodge the tube, requiring reassessment for correct placement. Complications associated with NE or NG tubes include epistaxis, rhinitis, sinusitis, dacryocystitis, inadvertent placement or dislodgement of the tube into the airway, esophageal irritation, reflux, or clogging of the tube. One prospective[11] and two retrospective[12,13] studies evaluating nasoenteric feeding tubes compared bolus versus constant rate infusion and reported differing results with respect to time required to achieve targeted caloric intake. However, all three studies concluded that the nasoenteral feeding was well tolerated.

Esophagostomy Tube

A larger feeding tube (usually a 12 to 14 Fr tube for cats and up to a 22 Fr for larger dogs) can be placed in the proximal esophagus at the mid-cervical level, with the tip positioned in the distal esophagus (Figure 129-3). The esophagostomy tube (E-tube) has several

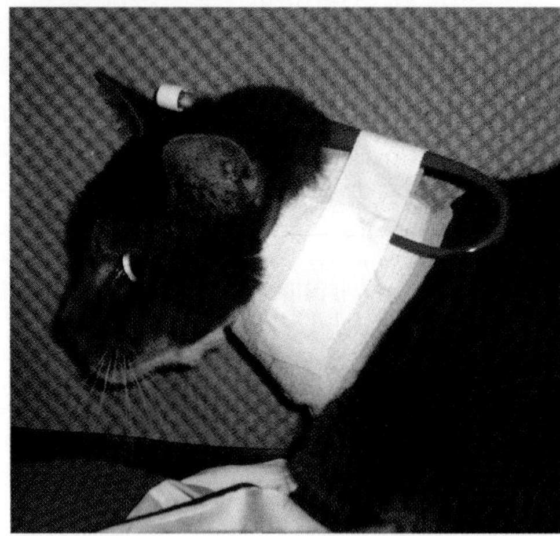

FIGURE 129-3 A cat with an esophagostomy tube in place.

advantages. Veterinary patients appear to tolerate them quite well. They can be used for fairly long periods (weeks to months) in both the hospital and outpatient settings. The larger tube allows for a wider selection of diets, including blenderized canned pet foods. The tube can be used in patients with facial or oral disease that precludes NE tube placement. As with the NE tube, the patient must have normal GI function, including normal esophageal function and the ability to protect the airway.

Placement of this tube requires general anesthesia and technical skill, although the procedure is relatively simple and well described.[14-18] E-tubes can be used for feeding as soon as the patient recovers from anesthesia and can be removed by the clinician when the patient has resumed adequate voluntary intake. Risks associated with E-tubes include placement in the airway or mediastinum, pneumomediastinum, pneumothorax, and damage to cervical vascular structures or nerves. As with the NE tube, a lateral radiograph should be taken to verify placement. Complications after placement include cellulitis or infection at the tube site, patient dislodgement, esophageal irritation and reflux, displacement during vomiting or regurgitation, and clogging of the tube.

Gastrostomy Tube

Larger (usually 16 to 22 Fr mushroom-tipped) feeding tubes can be placed directly in the stomach via surgical placement,[2,19] endoscopic guidance,[2,20] or blind technique using a gastrostomy tube placement device.[2,21] All techniques require longer time under anesthesia and more technical skill than is needed for E-tube placement. The percutaneous endoscopic gastrostomy and blind technique avoid doing a laparotomy, but if the patient is undergoing abdominal surgery, surgical placement is preferable because the surgeon can visualize placement and "-pexy" the stomach to the abdominal wall. Endoscopic placement is preferred over a blind technique because it allows visualization of the gastric placement site and decreases the risk of iatrogenic injury to abdominal viscera during placement.[18]

The gastrostomy tube (G-tube) provides nutrients distal to the esophagus, providing enteral feeding to patients with esophageal disease. The G-tube is well tolerated, permits bolus meal feedings, and is appropriate for long-term at-home feeding.[8,22] As with the E-tube, the option of blenderized pet foods allows a wider diet selection. The patient must tolerate feeding above the pylorus without vomiting. The tube cannot be used for the first 24 hours after placement to allow return of gastric motility and formation of a fibrin seal at the stoma. The tube should not be removed until the stomach has adhered to the body wall to prevent stomach content leakage and secondary peritonitis. The tube is typically left in place for at least 10 to 14 days or longer in more severely compromised or malnourished patients. Major complications associated with G-tubes include abdominal visceral injury during percutaneous placement or peritonitis if stomach contents leak into the abdominal cavity secondary to tube displacement or dehiscence. As with any surgically placed feeding device, cellulitis or infection at the stoma site is possible. Pressure necrosis can occur if the external flange places too much pressure on the stoma site. Improperly placed G-tubes may cause a pyloric outflow obstruction. A G-tube requires closer monitoring and is more costly than techniques previously described.

Jejunal Tubes

A small-bore feeding tube (usually 5 to 8 Fr) can be placed directly in the proximal jejunum (J-tube). Nasojejunal, gastrojejunal, and jejunostomy tubes permit enteral feeding distal to the pylorus for patients unable to tolerate gastric feedings. Indications include gastroparesis, uncontrolled vomiting, proximal GI obstruction (i.e., secondary to neoplasia), massive proximal GI resection, and inability to protect the airway. Jejunal feeding is often recommended for the treatment of acute canine pancreatitis to decrease stimulation of pancreatic secretion, although early enteral feeding proximal to the pylorus may be well tolerated in these patients.[23] A J-tube can be placed surgically during laparotomy or laparascopy,[24-27] and transpyloric placement techniques via nasojejunal or gastrojejunal feeding tubes using surgical, endoscopic, or fluoroscopic techniques have been described.[27-33] Surgical placement allows visualization of tube position and a pexy of the bowel to the abdominal wall. Transpyloric techniques are less invasive, with nasojejunal tubes eliminating the risk of bowel content leakage into the peritoneum. However, transpyloric placement requires advanced technical skill and either endoscopic or fluoroscopic guidance. J-tubes can be used for a moderately short period (days to weeks). Surgically placed J-tubes placed using the purse string, inverted serosal, or simple jejunopexy techniques or endoscopically placed gastrojejunal tubes cannot be removed for a minimum of 5 to 7 days, until a fibrin seal has formed at the body wall, to avoid the risk of peritonitis.

The small diameter of J-tubes limits diet selection to liquids. To minimize the risk of abdominal cramping and vomiting, constant infusion is preferred over bolus feeding. This requires more diligent patient monitoring and does not allow for at-home feeding under most circumstances.

Complications associated with J-tubes include peristomal cellulitis or infection, peritonitis secondary to leakage, retrograde migration of the J-tube, intestinal obstruction secondary to tube migration, and clogging of the tube.

DETERMINING THE AMOUNT TO BE FED

Hospitalized patients should initially be fed to meet the RER, defined as the amount of energy (calories) needed to maintain homeostasis in the fed state in a thermoneutral environment.[2] "Illness factors" are no longer widely used in critical care nutrition.[34] Calorimetry is not used in the clinical veterinary setting, so estimates of RER can be calculated by allometric formulas such as $70(BW_{kg})^{0.75}$. Calculations for obese patients should be based on optimal body weight to prevent overfeeding. Calculations for growing puppies and kittens start with an initial caloric goal of RER to ensure tolerance. However, as with any patient, the pediatric patient must have frequent assessments. Caloric intake may need to be increased, especially if hospitalization is prolonged, provided the patient is tolerating the prescribed feeding amount. All patients must be reassessed to see if the initial caloric estimate is appropriate. The goal during hospitalization is to maintain body weight (excluding fluctuations as a result of hydration status) and lean body mass. Overfeeding is associated with GI and metabolic complications. Certain disease conditions such as sepsis, head trauma, increased muscle activity (e.g., tremors, seizures) or burns may require increased caloric intake if the previously stated goals are not met by RER. In patients with prolonged anorexia, gastrointestinal compromise, or metabolic derangements, the caloric goal should be achieved over several days. Typical feeding protocols might provide 25% to 50% RER on day 1, with the goal of reaching full RER over the next 1 to 3 days.

SELECTING THE DIET

Patient Variables

Highly digestible nutrients from high-quality sources should be selected for critical care patients. A patient with a poor appetite may benefit from a more calorie-dense diet because a smaller volume of food will meet the caloric goal. A more calorie-dense slurry may also be indicated for patients who are volume intolerant such as those at risk of congestive heart failure. The clinician must determine if any macronutrients or micronutrients should be altered because of the patient's disease condition. For example, enteral protein intake should be 4 to 6 g of protein per 100 kcal (15% to 25% of total energy) for dogs and 6 g or more of protein per 100 kcal (25% to 35% of total energy) for cats.[34] Certain disease conditions, such as hepatic encephalopathy, may require the clinician to select diets closer to the minimum protein requirement to help prevent worsening of the clinical signs of encephalopathy. However, when a lower protein diet is fed, adequate calorie and protein intake is essential in order to minimize the risk of protein malnutrition. Conversely, disease conditions associated with a high degree of protein loss may require a diet replete with protein. Other examples of nutrient modulation include sodium in patients with congestive heart failure and fat in patients with hyperlipidemia, canine pancreatitis, and GI diseases leading to fat malassimilation. Certain patients with known dietary hypersensitivities may need to avoid products containing certain ingredients. In addition to veterinary enteral products, there is a vast array of enteral products formulated for humans. However, these formulas typically are not balanced for veterinary patients and often require modification such as additional protein, arginine, taurine, and B vitamins for cats.

Nonpatient Variables

Nonpatient variables contribute to diet selection. Small-diameter NE, NG, or J-tubes require liquid diets. Financial constraints and cost of diets may factor into the selection process. Choices are limited by availability (i.e., the hospital inventory) and the clinician's knowledge of various products.

MONITORING THERAPY

Nutritional assessment should occur at least daily. The clinician reviews past feeding orders to determine if the appropriate diet plan was instituted and if the patient achieved the set goals. If the patient did not meet the dietary goal, the clinician must determine whether the cause was related to patient issues (e.g., nausea, unpalatable diet) or nonpatient issues (e.g., improperly written orders, orders not followed, feeding withheld for procedures). The clinician then updates the plan. Patients unable to meet desired nutritional goals enterally may benefit from supplemental parenteral nutrition (see Chapter 130).[35] Monitoring of body weight (at least every 12 to 24 hours), hydration status, and laboratory values such as blood glucose, total solids, triglycerides, serum lipemia, blood urea nitrogen, and electrolytes must be done to assess the response to, or complications from, dietary intervention. The frequency and specifics of monitoring depend on the patient's disease condition, the mode of dietary intervention, and financial constraints. Patients that are critically ill and those receiving aggressive dietary intervention require the closest monitoring.

PREVENTING AND MANAGING COMPLICATIONS

Patient-Related Complications

Many feeding complications can be prevented by proper patient evaluation, selection of the appropriate route and amount of nutrient delivery, an understanding of the risks associated with the specific feeding plan, and close patient monitoring. Most enteral feeding complications are minor, but aspiration, premature dislodgement of a gastrostomy or enterostomy tube, and certain metabolic abnormalities can be life threatening.[36] GI intolerance may manifest as vomiting, diarrhea, or ileus. This complication can compromise the ability to continue enteral feeding. The clinician should assess the feeding plan to confirm that daily intake does not exceed the patient's energy requirements (approximately RER in most cases) and that the day's feeding is divided into multiple small meals. Food should be warmed to body temperature for tube feeding. The patient's disease condition or medications may contribute to nausea, vomiting, ileus, or diarrhea. Altering medications or providing antiemetics or prokinetic agents may allow for continued enteral feeding.

Metabolic complications can arise if a patient is unable to assimilate certain nutrients. For example, a patient with glucose intolerance may need a dietary formulation low in simple carbohydrates to modulate hyperglycemic episodes. Anticipating specific intolerances during nutritional assessment and setting conservative caloric goals will minimize the risk.[36] Refeeding syndrome is a life-threatening metabolic complication that may occur in patients after prolonged anorexia or in certain catabolic states, such as hepatic lipidosis. In this syndrome, upon reintroduction of feeding, there is a rapid shift of key intracellular electrolytes from the vascular to the intracellular space causing life-threatening hypokalemia, hypophosphatemia, or hypomagnesemia. This electrolyte abnormality can occur within days of resuming enteral (or parenteral) feeding.[37] At-risk patients should be fed conservative amounts initially with close monitoring and correction of any electrolyte abnormalities via parenteral or enteral replacement.

Aspiration is a potentially life-threatening complication that can be minimized by careful patient selection and close monitoring. Infections may occur at the peristomal site, along fascial planes, or within the peritoneum. Infectious complications can be minimized with proper tube placement, careful monitoring of tube sites, and basic hygiene during the preparation and delivery of food.

Non–Patient-Related Complications

Mechanical complications include obstructed tubes or tube migration. Clogging can be prevented by proper management such as flushing with warm water before and after every use. One should avoid using the feeding tube to administer medications. If the tube becomes obstructed, flushing with warm water under alternating pressure and suction may dislodge the debris.[38] Assessment of various solutions to dissolve in vitro feeding tube clogs caused by a veterinary critical care diet revealed that the injection of a solution of ¼ tsp pancreatic enzyme and 325 mg sodium bicarbonate in 5 ml warm water was most effective.[38] Proper technique in placing and suturing tubes will minimize the risk of tube migration and dislodgement. E-collars, bandages, and patient monitoring help prevent the patient from removing a tube. The tube should be marked with indelible ink where it exits the body so that migration can be detected. Radiographs should be performed to confirm placement of NE, NG, and E-tubes, especially if tube migration is suspected. If leakage of enteral contents into the peritoneum is suspected, a water-soluble contrast study can also be performed. Dislodged or migrated tubes should never be used for feeding without verifying placement.

REFERENCES

1. Thatcher CD: Nutritional needs of critically ill patients, Compend Contin Educ Vet Pract 18:1303, 1996.
2. Saker KE, Remillard RL: Critical care nutrition and enteral-assisted feeding. In Hand MS, Thatcher CD, Remillard RL, et al, editors: Small animal clinical nutrition, ed 5, Topeka, KS, 2010, Mark Morris Institute.
3. Giner M, Laviano A, Meguid MM, Gleason JR: In 1995 a correlation between malnutrition and poor outcome in critically ill patients still exists, Nutrition 12:23, 1996.
4. Mohr AJ, Leisewitz AL, Jacobson LS, et al: Effect of early enteral nutrition on intestinal permeability, intestinal protein loss, and outcome in dogs with severe parvoenteritis, J Vet Intern Med 17:791, 2003.
5. Brunetto MA, Gomes MOS, Andre MR, et al: Effects of nutritional support on hospital outcome in dogs and cats, J Vet Emerg Crit Care 20:224, 2010.
6. Liu DT, Brown DC, Silverstein DC: Early nutritional support is associated with decreased length of hospitalization in dogs with septic peritonitis: a retrospective study in 45 cases (2000-2009), J Vet Emerg Crit Care 22:453, 2012.
7. Prittie J, Barton L: Route of nutrient delivery, Clin Tech Small Anim Pract 1:6, 2004.
8. Ireland LM, Hohenhaus AE, Broussard JD, Weissman BL: A comparison of owner treatment and complications in 67 cats with esophagostomy and percutaneous endoscopic gastrostomy feeding tubes, J Am Anim Hosp Assoc 39:241, 2003.
9. Freeman L: Personal communication, 2012.
10. Abood SK, Buffington CA: Improved nasogastric intubation technique for administration of nutritional support in dogs, J Am Vet Med Assoc 199:577, 1991.
11. Holahan M, Abood S, Hauptman J, et al: Intermittent and continuous enteral nutrition in critically ill dogs: a prospective randomized trial, J Vet Emerg Crit Care 24:520, 2010.
12. Klaus JA, Rudloff E, Kirby R: Nasogastric tube feeding in cats with suspected acute pancreatitis: 55 cases (2001-2006), J Vet Emerg Crit Care 19:337, 2009.
13. Campbell JA, Jutkowitz LA, Santoro KA, et al: Continuous versus intermittent delivery of nutrition via nasoenteric feeding tubes in hospitalized canine and feline patients: 91 patients (2002-2007), J Vet Emerg Crit Care 20:232, 2010.
14. von Werthern CJ, Wess G: A new technique for insertion of esophagostomy tubes in cats, J Am Anim Hosp Assoc 37:140, 2001.
15. Devitt CM, Seim HB: Clinical evaluation of tube esophagostomy in small animals, J Am Anim Hosp Assoc 33:55, 1997.
16. Rawlings CA: Percutaneous placement of a midcervical esophagostomy tube: new technique and representative cases, J Am Anim Hosp Assoc 29:526, 1993.
17. Rawlings CA, Bartges JW: Esophagostomy tube placement: alternative technique. In Borjab MJ, editor: Current techniques in small animal surgery, Baltimore, 1998, Williams & Wilkins.
18. Han E: Esophageal and gastric feeding tubes in ICU patients, Clin Tech Small Anim Pract 1:22, 2004.
19. Seim HB, Willard MD: Postoperative care of the surgical patient. In Fossum TW, editor: Small animal surgery, ed 2, St Louis, 2002, Mosby.
20. Mauterer JV: Endoscopic and nonendoscopic percutaneous gastrostomy tube placement. In Bonagura JD, editor: Kirk's current veterinary therapy XIII, St Louis, 2000, Saunders.
21. Fulton RB, Dennis JS: Blind percutaneous placement of a gastrostomy tube for nutritional support in dogs and cats, J Am Vet Med Assoc 201:697, 1992.
22. Elliot DA, Riel DL, Rodgers QR: Complications and outcomes associated with the use of gastrostomy tubes for nutritional treatment of dogs with renal failure, J Am Vet Med Assoc 217:1337, 2000.
23. Mansfield CS, James FE, Steiner JM, et al: A pilot study to assess tolerability of early enteral nutrition via esophagostomy tube feeding in dogs with severe acute pancreatitis, J Vet Intern Med 25:419, 2011.
24. Crowe DT, Devey JJ: Clinical experience with jejunostomy feeding tubes in 47 small animal patients, J Vet Emerg Crit Care 7:7, 1997.
25. Daye RM, Huber ML, Henderson RA: Interlocking box jejunostomy: a new technique for enteral feeding, J Am Anim Hosp Assoc 35:129, 1999.
26. Hewitt SA, Brisson BA, Sinclair MD, et al: Evaluation of laparoscopic-assisted placement of jejunostomy feeding tubes in dogs, J Am Vet Med Assoc 225:65, 2004.
27. Heuter K: Placement of jejunal feeding tubes for postgastric feeding, Clin Tech Small Anim Pract 1:32, 2004.
28. Cavanaugh RP, Kovak JR, Fischetti AJ, et al: Evaluation of surgically placed gastrojejunostomy feeding tubes in critically ill dogs, J Am Vet Med Assoc 232:380, 2008.
29. Jergens AE, Morrison JA, Miles KG, et al: Percutaneous endoscopic gastrojejunostomy tube placement in healthy dogs and cats, J Vet Intern Med 21:18, 2007.
30. Jennings M, Center SA, Barr SC, et al: Successful treatment of feline pancreatitis using an endoscopically placed gastrojejunostomy tube, J Am Anim Hosp Assoc 37:145, 2001.
31. Papa K, Psader R, Sterczer A, et al: Endoscopically guided nasojejunal tube placement in dogs for short-term postduodenal feeding, J Vet Emerg Crit Care 19:554, 2009.
32. Wohl JS: Nasojejunal feeding tube placement using fluoroscopic guidance: technique and clinical experience in dogs, J Vet Emerg Crit Care 16:S27, 2006.
33. Beal MW, Brown AJ: Clinical experience utilizing a novel fluoroscopic technique for wire-guided nasojejunal tube placement in the dog: 26 cases (2006-2010), J Vet Emerg Crit Care 21:151, 2011.
34. Chan DL: Nutritional requirements of the critically ill patient, Clin Tech Small Anim Pract 1:1, 2004.
35. Chan DL, Freeman LM, Labato MA, et al: Retrospective evaluation of partial parenteral nutrition in dogs and cats, J Vet Intern Med 16:440, 2002.
36. Michel KE: Preventing and managing complications of enteral nutritional support, Clin Tech Small Anim Pract 1:49, 2004.
37. Justin RB, Hohenhaus AE: Hypophosphatemia associated with enteral alimentation in cats, J Vet Intern Med 9:228, 1995.
38. Parker VJ, Freeman LM: Comparison of various solutions to dissolve critical care diet clots, J Vet Emerg Crit Care 23(3):344, 2013.

CHAPTER 130
PARENTERAL NUTRITION

Kathryn E. Michel, DVM, MS, DACVN • Laura Eirmann, DVM, DACVN

KEY POINTS

- Parenteral nutrition (PN) is provided by the intravenous route and is used when nutritional support is indicated for a patient but enteral delivery is not feasible or intake is insufficient.
- The three basic requirements that must be met for parenteral nutritional support are (1) the ability to obtain and maintain appropriate vascular access aseptically; (2) the ability to provide 24-hour nursing care and monitoring, including basic point-of-care serum chemistry evaluation; and (3) the means and the expertise to formulate the PN prescription and compound the nutrient admixture.
- Special considerations for the nutritional assessment of a candidate for PN include assessing vascular access, fluid tolerance, and preexisting conditions that may affect the patient's nutrient tolerance or predispose it to metabolic complications.
- Particular attention should be paid to the venous catheter site for signs of phlebitis or infection. Daily monitoring of hydration status, fluid tolerance, blood glucose concentration, serum electrolyte values, and evidence of lipemia are indicated.

Parenteral nutrition (PN) is provided by the intravenous route. The intraosseous route can also be used for very small patients such as neonatal dogs and cats. Parenteral delivery is used when nutritional support is indicated for a patient but the enteral route is not feasible. Most commonly this happens because per os feeding is contraindicated, as with a patient experiencing nausea and vomiting or a patient unable to guard its airway and thereby at risk for aspirating stomach contents. PN is also indicated in patients that need nutritional support but are experiencing gastrointestinal malassimilation and are unable to absorb adequate nutrients by the enteral route.

Although enteral nutrition has many advantages over the parenteral route (see Chapter 129), PN can be life sustaining until enteral nutrition can be effectively and safely initiated. In fact, combining PN with enteral feeding has been shown to improve outcome in companion animal patients.[1,2] Regardless, PN has been used successfully in many species, including humans, dogs, cats, horses, cattle, birds, and various exotic species.[1-7]

TECHNICAL REQUIREMENTS

Parenteral nutritional support may not be feasible in every veterinary practice, but the associated technology and equipment is becoming increasingly accessible and affordable for many small animal hospitals. Three basic requirements must be met in order to provide parenteral nutritional support to a patient. First, it must be possible to obtain and maintain appropriate vascular access aseptically. Second, 24-hour nursing care must be available, along with the ability to do at least basic point-of-care serum chemistry evaluation. And third, there must be the means and the expertise to formulate the PN prescription and compound the nutrient admixture in-house or at a nearby facility.

Vascular Access

To minimize the risk of line sepsis or drug-nutrient interactions, PN must be delivered through a dedicated venous catheter, although a single dedicated port of a multilumen catheter will suffice. A dedicated line is one that is not used for any other purpose, including blood sampling, hemodynamic monitoring, or delivery of other intravenous (IV) fluids or medications. Because some of the nutrient solutions used to formulate the PN admixture are hyperosmolar, central venous access is preferred. The hyperosmolar PN admixture will be diluted by the rapid blood flow in central vessels, thus greatly reducing the risk of phlebitis. However, both centrally and peripherally inserted central venous catheters can be used. It is possible to dilute solutions sufficiently to enable delivery through a peripheral venous catheter, but the resulting increased volume that must be delivered may preclude meeting nutritional goals in patients with limited fluid tolerance.

Catheters should be composed of nonthrombogenic materials such as polyurethane or silicone, and peripheral catheters should be as long as practically possible. The line placement should be treated as a surgical procedure, with surgical preparation of the catheter site, draping, and sterile gloves. The catheter site should be covered with a sterile dressing that is inspected and changed daily.

Monitoring and Nursing Care

The best setting for delivering PN is an intensive care or fluid ward that has 24-hour staffing and the capability of doing basic in-house serum chemistry analysis. Most patients requiring PN are critically ill and will need intensive care and monitoring. Even a relatively stable patient receiving PN needs to be in a facility that can provide expert nursing care to properly maintain the central venous catheter and monitor the patient. Although PN can be delivered cyclically, it is best delivered as a constant rate infusion. It is necessary to monitor various serum chemistry values, sometimes multiple times within 24 hours, depending on the patient's underlying condition (e.g., electrolytes, glucose, blood urea nitrogen [BUN], albumin). This is greatly facilitated by having in-house laboratory equipment.

Formulating and Compounding Nutrient Admixtures

Veterinary patients usually are rarely supported with PN for longer than 1, or at most 2, weeks. Therefore it is rare that a patient would receive a nutrient admixture that was formulated to provide complete nutrition. Generally PN solutions provide energy, protein, and water-soluble vitamins, with the optional addition of electrolytes and some of the trace elements. In addition to knowing how to formulate the PN prescription, it is necessary to have ready access to the special nutrient solutions and knowledge of how to compound these solutions for the nutrient admixture (Figure 130-1). Nutrient solutions must be combined in the proper order to prevent components from precipitating out of solution or suspension, and the entire process must be done under sterile conditions to prevent microbial contamination. Therefore, unless PN is used frequently in a practice, it is far

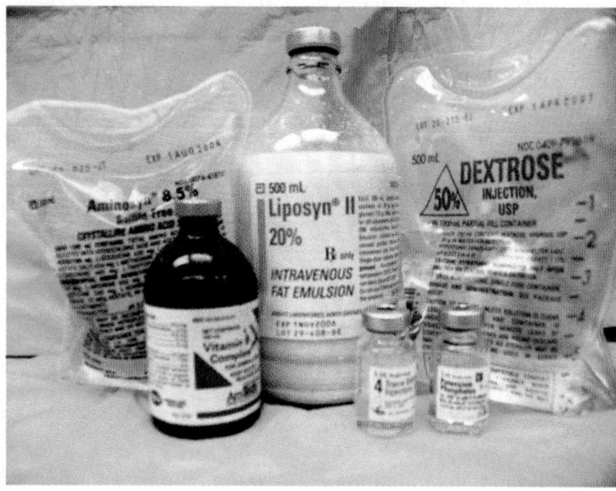

FIGURE 130-1 Parenteral nutrient admixtures typically provide energy from dextrose solutions and lipid emulsions, protein from amino acid solutions and water-soluble vitamins with the optional addition of electrolytes and some trace elements

Table 130-1 **Conditions that Can Predispose Patients Receiving PN to Metabolic Complications.**

Complication	Predisposing Conditions
Hyperglycemia	Diabetes mellitus, hyperadrenocorticism
Lipemia	Pancreatitis, idiopathic hyperlipidemia, diabetes mellitus, hyperadrenocorticism
Azotemia	Renal failure
Hyperammonemia	Hepatic failure, portosystemic shunt
Refeeding syndrome (hypokalemia, hypophosphatemia and/or hypomagnesemia)	Prolonged starvation or catabolic disease, diabetes mellitus

more practical to find a human hospital or home transfusion service that will compound the solutions on request.

There are commercially available ready-to-use products containing dextrose and amino acids that can be infused via a peripheral IV catheter. The drawback of such products is that they have a low energy density, and although they can provide sufficient protein to most patients, the patients' caloric needs will not necessarily be met because of fluid volume considerations. These types of products are most useful as a short-term intervention until a more tailored compounded solution can be obtained, or in combination with enteral nutritional support.

NUTRITIONAL ASSESSMENT

The task of evaluating a patient for nutritional support has been covered in detail in Chapter 127. Additional considerations for candidates requiring PN include assessing vascular access, fluid tolerance, and preexisting conditions that may affect the patient's nutrient tolerance or predisposition for metabolic complications.

Ideally PN should be delivered via a dedicated central line; however, central venous access may be unobtainable or contraindicated. For example, central catheter placement via a jugular vein is contraindicated in patients with head trauma or other conditions predisposing to increased intracranial pressure, those at risk of thromboembolic disease (e.g., protein-losing nephropathy or enteropathy, disseminated intravascular coagulation [DIC], hyperadrenocorticism, or those receiving high-dose glucocorticoids), or patients with severe coagulopathies. Fortunately, central vascular access can still be obtained in most patients by using a peripherally inserted central venous catheter (PICC).

Patients should be evaluated for their ability to tolerate the additional fluids that they will receive from the PN admixture. This will not be a problem for most patients, especially because a majority of the fluid administered contains metabolizable energy and water; however, animals experiencing heart failure or oliguria will be at risk of volume overload. Patients with reduced fluid tolerance should have central venous access to allow the most concentrated nutrient solutions to be used for formulation of the PN admixture (and CVP monitoring if possible). It may be possible to reduce the volume of the other IV fluids that the patient is receiving to accommodate that of the PN. Even so, occasionally there will be patients for whom it will not be possible to meet nutritional goals with parenteral nutritional support because of fluid intolerance.

Metabolic complications of PN are common,[1-5] but most can be minimized, if not avoided, by evaluating each patient for predisposing conditions such as an impaired ability to metabolize a specific nutrient or eliminate its metabolites. Table 130-1 lists some of the more common metabolic complications seen with PN and the conditions that may predispose to them. By anticipating complications, the PN admixture can be formulated in such a way as to reduce the likelihood or magnitude of PN-related problems.

PRESCRIPTION FORMULATION

Calculation of Energy Requirements

Evidence suggests that while critically ill patients are in a catabolic state their energy needs are not necessarily increased above normal.[8,9] Furthermore, excessive calories and nutrients in the form of PN can have adverse consequences, including many of the metabolic complications described in Table 130-1 as well as fatty infiltration of the liver and hypercapnia.[3,10] For these reasons, caloric goals for parenterally fed patients should be conservative and, in most cases, based on an estimate of a patient's resting energy expenditure: $70(BW_{kg})^{0.75}$. The caloric goal can then be adjusted based on the patient's response (see Chapter 129).

Calculation of Protein Requirements

There has been limited investigation regarding the protein requirements of companion animals receiving PN.[10,11] Most recommendations call for 4 to 6 g of protein per 100 kcal for dogs and 6 or more g of protein per 100 kcal for cats. Some have advocated meeting the patient's energy requirements with nonprotein calories from dextrose and lipids in addition to providing the required protein. This approach has the potential of supplying excessive calories, particularly in patients deemed to have high protein requirements. A more conservative approach is to subtract the required protein calories from the patient's total energy requirement and provide the balance as nonprotein calories. Using the recommendations given earlier, this roughly translates into 15% to 25% of calories for dogs and 25% to 35% of calories for cats delivered as protein. Patients that are protein depleted or have high ongoing losses will require PN admixtures containing protein amounts in the upper ranges. For patients with conditions that impair protein tolerance (e.g., renal insufficiency or failure, see Table 130-1), it may be necessary to restrict the amount of protein in the PN admixture below the lower end of these ranges.

Amino acid solutions are available in concentrations ranging from 3% to 15%. Because of increasing osmolarity, solutions more concentrated than 6% should not be used for peripherally infused PN. The electrolyte content of these products varies. Because the less concentrated products are used for peripherally infused PN, they often have higher concentrations of electrolytes to preclude the need for further supplementation. The more concentrated solutions can be obtained with or without additional electrolytes. Greater flexibility can be obtained by using the amino acid solutions without supplements for PN formulation and providing electrolytes in the patient's IV fluids.

Calculation of Lipid and Carbohydrate Requirements

Once the percentage of protein calories has been established, it is necessary to decide how to apportion the remaining calories between carbohydrate and fat. Although it is possible to provide all nonprotein calories as carbohydrate using dextrose solutions, lipid emulsions have the advantage of being isoosmolar and a more concentrated form of calories. Also, patients are at greater risk of becoming hyperglycemic when fed PN admixtures containing large amounts of dextrose. This is especially a concern in cats or those with diabetes mellitus.[3,5] Conversely, concerns have been raised about the potential for lipid emulsions to have proinflammatory and immunosuppressive effects because they contain high concentrations of omega-6 fatty acids.[12] Lipid emulsions composed of structured lipids containing medium chain triglycerides or omega-3 fatty acids have the potential to provide a lipid source less likely to cause these adverse effects. These alternative lipid emulsions are not available in the United States at present. Therefore, unless there is a preexisting condition that would suggest fat intolerance, conventional lipid emulsions are still considered an acceptable and beneficial component of PN and can be used to provide 50% to 70% of the nonprotein calories, with the balance delivered as dextrose. Total lipid intake should be taken into account when animals are receiving either a constant rate infusion or multiple doses of drugs that contain lipid emulsions (e.g., propofol).

Lipid emulsions are available in 10% (1.1 kcal/ml), 20% (2.0 kcal/ml), and 30% (3.0 kcal/ml) concentrations. They are composed of emulsified soybean or safflower oils with a particle size equivalent to a chylomicron. Dextrose is available in concentrations ranging from 5% to 70%. For centrally infused PN, 50% dextrose (1.7 kcal/ml, 2500 mOsm/L) is typically used. For peripherally infused PN lower concentrations must be used (e.g., 10%, 0.34 kcal/ml, 500 mOsm/L; or 20%, 0.68 kcal/ml, 1000 mOsm/L) to keep final osmolarity less than 700 mOsm/L.

Calculation of Micronutrient Requirements

Although parenteral forms of all essential micronutrients are available, typically only injectable B complex and certain electrolytes (phosphorus and magnesium) are included in PN admixtures that are used for companion animals. Some clinicians also add trace element preparations containing zinc because there is evidence that this nutrient can be depleted rapidly in critically ill patients.[13] Table 130-2 contains dosage guidelines for these nutrients and Box 130-1 contains a sample prescription formulation.

Table 130-2 Guidelines for Micronutrient Dosages in PN Admixtures

Micronutrient	Dosage
Vitamin B complex*	0.2 to 0.5 ml/100 kcal
Potassium phosphate	8 to 10 mmol/1000 kcal
Magnesium sulfate	0.8 to 1.0 mEq/100 kcal
Zinc	1 mcg/kcal

*Injectable vitamin B complex does not contain folate because of compatibility issues; thus patients receiving PN for more than a few days may become deficient and should be supplemented with this nutrient via a route other than the PN admixture.

DELIVERY AND MONITORING

A patient starting PN should receive 50% of goal nutrients the first day as a constant rate infusion over 24 hours and, if that is well tolerated, can receive 100% of its goal the following day. The PN admixture should be delivered via a dedicated catheter or port of a multilumen catheter using a 1.2-μm filter (to prevent lipid embolization) and a fluid pump. The PN admixture should be disconnected only when changing the bottle or bag, and the administration set should also be changed at that time. Gloves should be worn in performing catheter care and changing bottles and administration sets. Ideally patients should be weaned off PN over the course of several hours once they are receiving at least 50% of their goal calories through voluntary intake or enteral feeding. If it becomes necessary to abruptly discontinue PN, 5% dextrose should be added to the patient's IV fluids to prevent hypoglycemia.

Monitoring of patients receiving nutritional support has been reviewed in Chapter 129. For patients receiving parenteral nutritional support, particular attention should be paid to the catheter site and associated vessel for signs of infection or phlebitis, respectively. Hydration status and fluid tolerance should be assessed regularly. Although the exact amount of fluid that remains in the vascular space after PN administration is not easily calculated, it is presumably less than 100% because most of the solution is metabolizable energy and free water. Blood glucose, serum sodium, and potassium concentrations should be monitored at least once daily. Insulin administration may be indicated if persistent hyperglycemia occurs (0.1 U/kg regular insulin intravenously, intramuscularly [IM], or subcutaneously [SC] as needed; continuous IV infusion may be necessary in severely affected animals). Whenever a packed cell volume determination is performed, the serum or plasma in the hematocrit tube should be examined for evidence of lipemia. Serum phosphorus and magnesium concentrations should be checked after the first day of PN infusion. If serum levels of these electrolytes have decreased significantly, further monitoring is warranted so that patients can receive appropriate supplementation if necessary. Complete blood cell counts and serum chemistry analysis should be performed as indicated but at least once weekly while patients are receiving PN. Measurement of ammonia levels may be indicated in animals with hepatic insufficiency or clinical signs of hepatic encephalopathy.

PREVENTING AND MANAGING COMPLICATIONS

Catheter and Parenteral Nutrition Admixture Complications

Catheter complications include loss of vascular access because of catheter malposition, thrombosis, thrombophlebitis, or catheter-associated infection. The incidence of complications can be reduced greatly with appropriate catheter selection and adherence to strict guidelines for catheter care.

Complications involving the PN admixture include microbial contamination, precipitation of admixture components, and drug-nutrient interactions. These problems can be avoided by proper compounding of the admixture under sterile conditions and infusion of the admixture through a dedicated line. The particles making up a lipid emulsion can come out of suspension in an improperly compounded admixture. Lipid-containing admixtures should be inspected periodically during infusion for signs of separation or layering. An in-line filter will prevent fat embolism in patients receiving lipid-containing PN.

BOX 130-1 ***Centrally Administered PN Example: High-Protein Formulation for a Cat***

Weight: 4.5 kg RER = 216 kcal/day
Day 1 Goal: 50% RER = (0.5)(216) = 108 kcal
Day 2 Goal: 100% RER = 216 kcal

Protein Calories

35% from amino acids

Nonprotein Calories

70% from lipid
30% from dextrose

Solutions

8.5% amino acids (without electrolytes)
50% dextrose
20% lipid emulsion
Zinc (1 mg/ml)
Potassium phosphate (3 mmol/ml)
Injectable vitamin B complex

Day 1 Calculations

1. Amino acids
   (0.35)(108 kcal) = 38 kcal from protein
   There are 4 kcal/g in protein.
   Therefore 9.5 g of protein is needed (38 kcal ÷ 4 kcal/g = 9.5 g).
   8.5% amino acid solution = 0.085 g protein/ml
   Therefore 112 ml of 8.5% amino acid solution is needed (X ml = 9.5 g ÷ 0.085 g/ml).
2. Nonprotein calories
   (0.65) (108 kcal) = 70 kcal
   (a) 50% dextrose to provide 30% nonprotein calories = 21 kcal
   50% dextrose solution = 1.7 kcal/ml
   Therefore 12 ml 50% dextrose solution is needed (X ml = 21 kcal ÷ 1.7 kcal/ml).
   (b) 20% lipid emulsion to provide 70% nonprotein calories = 49 kcal
   20% lipid emulsion = 2 kcal/ml
   Therefore 25 ml 20% lipid emulsion is needed (X ml = 49 kcal ÷ 2.0 kcal/ml).
3. Zinc
   Zinc prescribed at 1 mcg/kcal delivered.
   Zinc solution contains 1.0 mg/ml.
   Therefore 0.1 ml of trace element solution is needed (X ml = 108 kcal ÷ [1.0 mg/ml × 1000]).
4. Potassium phosphate
   Potassium phosphate prescribed at 8 mmol/1000 kcal delivered.
   Therefore 0.9 mmol potassium phosphate is needed.
   (X mmol = [8 mmol × 108 kcal] ÷ 1000 kcal)
   Potassium phosphate solution = 3 mmol/ml
   Therefore 0.3 ml potassium phosphate is needed.
   (X ml = 0.9 mmol ÷ 3 mmol/ml)
5. Vitamin B complex
   Vitamin B complex prescribed at 0.2 ml/100 kcal delivered.
   Therefore 0.2 ml vitamin B complex is needed (X ml = [0.2 ml × 108 kcal] ÷ 100 kcal).
6. Infusion rate
   149 ml/24 hr = 6.2 ml/hr

Day 2 Calculations

Same as for Day 1—just substitute 216 kcal for 108 kcal.

Metabolic Complications

Most metabolic complications can be anticipated based on the patient's nutritional assessment and can be avoided or minimized by formulating the PN admixture accordingly. Most metabolic disturbances are less likely to occur if estimates of caloric needs are conservative.[3,10] "Refeeding syndrome" (see Chapter 129) has been described in patients receiving PN.[3-5] Those at increased risk of the electrolyte abnormalities seen with this condition are patients that have experienced a period of prolonged starvation or catabolism or patients with uncontrolled diabetes mellitus. In correcting electrolyte abnormalities, supplementation in the IV fluids as opposed to the PN admixture allows greater flexibility. Once the amount of electrolyte supplementation for maintenance is established, it can be included in the PN formulation.

REFERENCES

1. Queau Y, Larsen JA, Kass PH, et al: Factors associated with adverse outcomes during parenteral nutrition administration in dogs and cats, J Vet Intern Med 25:446, 2011.
2. Chan DL, Freeman LM, Labato MA, et al: Retrospective evaluation of partial parenteral nutrition in dogs and cats, J Vet Intern Med 16:440, 2002.
3. Crabb SE, Freeman LM, Chan DL, et al: Retrospective evaluation of total parenteral nutrition in cats: 40 cases (1991-2003), J Vet Emerg Crit Care 16:S21, 2006.
4. Reuter JD, Marks SL, Rogers QR, et al: Use of total parenteral nutrition in dogs: 209 cases (1988-1995), J Vet Emerg Crit Care 8:210, 1996.
5. Pyle SC, Marks SL, Kass PH: Evaluation of complications and prognostic factors associated with administration of total parenteral nutrition in cats: 75 cases (1994-2001), J Am Vet Med Assoc 225:242, 2004.
6. Durham AE, Phillips TJ, Walmsley JP, et al: Study of the clinical effects of postoperative parenteral nutrition in 15 horses, Vet Rec 153:493, 2003.
7. Degernes L, Davidson G, Flammer K, et al: Administration of total parenteral nutrition in pigeons, Am J Vet Res 55:660, 1994.
8. O'Toole E, Miller CW, Wilson BA, et al: Comparison of the standard predictive equation for calculation of resting energy expenditure with indirect calorimetry in hospitalized and healthy dogs, J Am Vet Med Assoc 225:58, 2004.
9. Walton RS, Wingfield WE, Ogilvie GK, et al: Energy expenditure in 104 postoperative and traumatically injured dogs with indirect calorimetry, J Vet Emerg Crit Care 6:71, 1998.
10. Lippert AC, Faulkner JE, Evans AT, et al: Total parenteral nutrition in clinically normal cats, J Am Vet Med Assoc 194:669, 1989.
11. Michel KE, King LG, Ostro E: Measurement of urinary urea nitrogen as an estimate of total urinary nitrogen loss in dogs, J Am Vet Med Assoc 210:356, 1997.
12. Kang JH, Yang MP: Effect of a short-tem infusion with soybean oil-based lipid emulsion on phagocytic responses of canine peripheral blood polymorphonuclear neutrophilic leukocytes, J Vet Intern Med 22:1166, 2008.
13. Iriyama K, Mori T, Takenaka T, et al: Effect of serum zinc level on amount of collagen hydroxyproline in the healing gut during total parenteral nutrition: an experimental study, JPEN J Parenter Enteral Nutr 6:416, 1982.

CHAPTER 131

PERIOPERATIVE EVALUATION OF THE CRITICALLY ILL PATIENT

Elisa M. Mazzaferro, MS, DVM, PhD, DACVECC

KEY POINTS

- A systematic approach to any critically ill patient is necessary to improve anesthetic and surgical outcome.
- An animal's airway, breathing, and circulatory status should be examined and stabilized first, before other vital organ systems are evaluated.
- Evaluation of the coagulation status and possible requirement for blood product administration is essential in the preoperative evaluation of the critically ill patient.

Careful assessment of the critically ill small animal patient can make the difference between surgical success or failure and, in particular, the difference between the animal's life and death. In the perioperative patient there is particular focus on stabilization for the anesthetic period, support during anesthetic recovery and intensive monitoring until the patient is no longer considered critical.

PREOPERATIVE PATIENT EVALUATION

The primary objective of evaluation of the preoperative patient is to recognize and treat any conditions that will increase the risk of anesthetic and surgical complications.[1] In addition, preoperative evaluation may provide some indication of the likely outcome for the patient (see Chapter 13).

Evaluation of the animal's signalment, history, physical examination, diagnostic tests, and presumed anesthetic risk are essential. Triage and physical examination are of particular importance when evaluating the critically ill patient (see Chapters 1 and 2). The respiratory, cardiovascular and hematologic systems are of primary importance when considering anesthetic and surgical risks. The clinician should use a step-by-step approach to each patient to ensure that all necessary information regarding these systems is obtained before anesthesia induction.

Part of the assessment of the preoperative patient is the choice of an appropriate anesthetic protocol (see Chapter 143).

Respiratory Resuscitation

Any sign of respiratory distress and hypoxemia should be corrected with supplemental oxygen therapy. If arterial blood gas analysis is not feasible and/or considered too stressful for the critically ill patient, noninvasive evaluation of respiratory status with pulse oximetry and visualization of the animal's respiratory effort can be used to determine response to oxygen therapy. Once the animal is able to tolerate the procedure, thoracic radiographs should be performed to determine whether pulmonary parenchymal (hemorrhage, pneumonia, edema), pleural space (pneumothorax, diaphragmatic hernia), or thoracic cage (rib fractures) abnormalities are present. Thoracic radiographs are always recommended before a major surgical procedure to rule out abnormalities that may affect the patient's ability to tolerate anesthesia, as well as to look for evidence of neoplasia that may alter the prognosis and hence the owner's expectations for the animal (see the Respiratory Disorders section of this text).

Cardiovascular Resuscitation

Hypovolemic shock is the most common cause of cardiovascular compromise in the critically ill patient and needs to be resolved before anesthesia induction. Clinical signs of hypovolemic shock include prolonged capillary refill time, tachycardia or bradycardia, hypotension, pale mucous membranes, and decreased urine output. A more thorough explanation regarding clinical signs and treatment of various forms of shock are listed elsewhere in this text. If pulse deficits, bradycardia, tachycardia, or an irregular heart rhythm is noted on physical examination, an electrocardiogram is indicated and specific therapy administered as appropriate (see Chapters 46, 47, and 48).

Pain

Pain has numerous systemic consequences, slows recovery, and can prevent adequate assessment of the patient. Adequate analgesia is an essential aspect of stabilization of the critically ill patient. A variety of pain scoring systems have been used to document the severity of pain in animals.[2] In some cases pain assessment is easy, when the animal exhibits obvious signs of distress such as yelping, splinting or guarding of the injured site, or lameness. Some individuals, however, appear more stoic and, rather than display abnormal behaviors, demonstrate a lack of normal behaviors as their only sign of discomfort (see Chapter 141). Analgesic drugs should never be withheld, even in the most critically ill patient. Opioid drugs are cardiovascularly sparing and are generally safe to use in even the most critically ill animals. Administration of a preanesthetic drug not only acts as an analgesic but also decreases the total dosage of drugs required for anesthesia induction and maintenance (see Chapters 142 and 143).

ASA Scoring

The American Society of Anesthesiologists (ASA) uses a classification scheme to score a patient's physical status before induction of anesthesia.[2,3] Patients with a grade 1 score are normal and healthy with no obvious clinical signs of disease, and patients with grade V are extremely critical, moribund or comatose, and are not expected to live with or without surgical intervention.[3] In all cases it is important to attempt cardiovascular and respiratory stabilization before induction of general anesthesia and surgery.

GLOBAL ASSESSMENT

After adequate stabilization of the respiratory and cardiovascular systems and effective analgesia, a more detailed evaluation of the patient can be performed. The patient's neurologic status should be evaluated. Seizure activity requires immediate anticonvulsant therapy and, when present, is of higher priority than the ABCs (airway, breathing, circulation). Seizures can be associated with a metabolic disorder such as hypoglycemia, or they can be associated with an increase in intracranial pressure, cerebral edema, or a primary brain disorder. If a spinal injury is suspected, the patient should be immobilized immediately. The neck and pelvis are immobilized with tape, with the patient secured on a flat hard surface, to prevent further spinal cord destabilization, which can cause further injury. Neurologic abnormalities in the preoperative patient may influence the anesthetic and surgical management, in addition to the prognosis, and should be discussed with the owner. For example, if increased intracranial pressure is of concern, inhalant anesthetics should be avoided and mechanical ventilation is indicated to tightly control the partial pressure of carbon dioxide (PCO_2).

Obvious orthopedic fractures or luxations should be stabilized after provision of adequate analgesia and sedation. Penetrating injuries or open fractures should be treated as soon as possible, although this must wait until the cardiovascular and respiratory systems have been stabilized. In the meantime, administration of a first-generation cephalosporin should provide sufficient antimicrobial coverage to prevent infection until definitive surgical repair can be performed.

Global assessment of organ function can be obtained by evaluating serum biochemical analyses and a complete blood cell count, if available. Abdominal ultrasound will further aid in identifying organ abnormalities, may be readily available on an emergency basis, and may help determine the nature of surgery required, the risks, and the associated prognosis.

LABORATORY TESTING

Part of the assessment of the critically ill patient is evaluation of key laboratory parameters. This is particularly important in the preoperative patient before anesthesia induction. Recommended minimal laboratory evaluation before surgery includes a packed cell volume, total protein, blood glucose, lactate, electrolyte, and acid-base evaluation. A full serum biochemistry panel and a complete blood cell count are ideal but may not be feasible in an emergency situation. In the absence of this information, evaluation of a blood smear for an estimated platelet and neutrophil counts may be beneficial.

Serum electrolyte and acid-base abnormalities should be corrected before anesthesia induction. Hyperkalemia, hypocalcemia, and hypoglycemia are of particular concern and require immediate intervention (see Chapters 51, 52, and 66). Serum lactate can be used as an indicator of global organ perfusion. An elevation in serum lactate concentration is often observed in cases of organ ischemia, hypovolemic shock, and septic shock. Reports have demonstrated a positive correlation between hyperlactatemia and mortality,[4-6] and serial measurements of serum lactate after administration of intravenous fluids can be used to determine how an animal is responding to treatment. Correction of hyperlactatemia is ideal. Worsening hyperlactatemia after volume correction is a poor prognostic indicator in the critically ill patient (see Chapter 56).

Coagulation

Coagulation status should be determined before surgery. Activated partial thromboplastin time, prothrombin time, and buccal mucosal bleeding time measurement may be indicated depending on the history, signalment, and current disease processes. An activated clotting time can be measured if activated partial thromboplastin and prothrombin times are not readily obtainable. A baseline platelet count should also be performed. If severe thrombocytopenia is present (platelet counts less than 20,000 to 30,000 cells/ml) preoperatively, administration of platelet-containing blood products may be indicated. If hypocoagulability is present, replenishment of clotting factors with fresh frozen plasma and vitamin K should be considered (see Chapters 61, 62, and 63).

Blood Type and Crossmatch

Even during the most routine surgeries, blood loss is possible. Critically ill patients maybe at greater risk of blood loss, and they are likely to be less tolerant of hemorrhage. Ideally, animals should be given only appropriately crossmatched red blood cell products, but this may not be feasible in the emergency setting. When crossmatching cannot be performed, assessment of blood type compatibility between the recipient and donor is recommended. In life-threatening hemorrhagic shock it may be necessary to administer unmatched, untyped blood products. Oxygen delivery is optimal with a packed cell volume (PCV) of approximately 30%. If an animal has clinically apparent anemia, with signs of lethargy, inappetence, tachycardia, or tachypnea, administration of whole blood or packed red blood cells should be considered before induction of anesthesia and surgery. Induction of anesthesia can be expected to cause a drop in the PCV of 4% to 5% and preoperative evaluation of anemia needs to take this change into consideration. In the emergency patient, hemoglobin-based oxygen carriers can also be administered until type-specific blood products are available. In general, the "Rule of Ones" states that administration of 1 ml of whole blood per 1 lb (~2 ml blood/kg) will raise the recipient's PCV by 1%.[7] If the calculated dosage is insufficient to cause the predicted rise in the animal's PCV, blood loss may be ongoing (see Chapter 61).

KIRBY'S RULE OF TWENTY

Evaluation of the critical patient before and after surgery must be approached in a careful, step-by-step manner. Although a number of methods have been suggested to predict prognosis in the critical small animal patient, one approach is to make use of a checklist so that no organ system is inadvertently overlooked. Kirby's "Rule of Twenty" is an excellent tool with which to approach any critical patient, in both the preoperative and postoperative periods.[8]

THE POSTOPERATIVE PERIOD

Getting a critical patient through surgery is just one of many hurdles that the clinician and animal will face before discharge from the hospital. In the immediate postsurgical period, careful patient assessment, monitoring, and nursing care can make the difference between life and death. Anesthesia is essentially administration of substances that, when controlled, cause analgesia, amnesia, and sleep. The same substances, even at minute doses, can also cause cardiovascular and respiratory compromise that ultimately can lead to impaired tissue oxygen delivery. Postoperative care focuses on anesthetic recovery and monitoring and support of all major organ functions.

Airway and Breathing

Similar to the preoperative period, careful monitoring of the patient's airway, breathing, oxygenation, and ventilation should continue throughout and after anesthetic recovery. During prolonged anesthesia and recumbency, dependent lung lobes can be atelectic and can cause intrapulmonary shunting of blood. If possible, a Wright's respirometer can be used to assess the animal's tidal volume (normal 10 to 15 ml/kg) during anesthesia. The patient's airway should remain intubated with a cuffed endotracheal tube until the patient can actively swallow and is actively fighting the endotracheal tube. Vomiting or regurgitation of gastric contents is common in the immediate postoperative period. If this occurs, the airway should be suctioned and the esophagus flushed with sterile saline in an effort to prevent aspiration pneumonia and esophagitis.

Ventilation and Oxygenation[9]

Anesthetic gases and pain can predispose a patient to hypoventilation. While still intubated, end-tidal carbon dioxide ($ETCO_2$) monitoring, or capnography, can be performed to noninvasively assess the animal's ventilatory status. An animal's respiratory rate and character should be carefully monitored. If rapid shallow respirations are present, differential diagnoses include pain, pulmonary parenchymal disease, or pleural space disease. Oxygenation can be assessed by noninvasive pulse oximetry or arterial blood gas analysis. If hypoxemia with a PaO_2 less than 70 mm Hg or an SpO_2 less than 92% is present, administration of oxygen supplementation is recommended until the patient is able to oxygenate on room air.

Oxygen Delivery

Oxygen delivery is largely dependent on arterial oxygenation, hematocrit, and the ability of the heart and circulatory system to deliver vital oxygen to end-organs, including peripheral tissues. Factors that influence cardiac output include anything that affects heart rate, stroke volume, preload, afterload, or contractility. Therefore bradyarrhythmias or tachyarrhythmias, inadequate circulating intravascular fluid volume, inadequate hemoglobin or oxygen-carrying capacity, inadequate hemoglobin saturation of oxygen, peripheral vasoconstriction that increases vascular afterload, hypothermia and inadequate offloading of oxygen at the level of the tissues, and depressed myocardial contractility all affect delivery of oxygen to tissues. Until anesthetic drugs have worn off or have been metabolized, inappropriate vasodilation, hypoventilation, and decreased myocardial contractility may be present. Careful monitoring of cardiac rhythm, blood pressure, oxygen saturation, and core body temperature should be performed until all have normalized.

Arrhythmias, Decreased Myocardial Contractility, and Hypotension

Cardiac arrhythmias should be treated with supplemental oxygen and administration of appropriate antiarrhythmic drugs to effect. Tachyarrhythmias can be associated with inadequate circulating intravascular volume, inadequate myocardial oxygenation, or increased circulating catecholamines from pain. If hemoglobin concentration is decreased during states of anemia, administration of type-specific packed red blood cells or hemoglobin-based oxygen carriers should be considered to increase oxygen-carrying capacity. A suggested target PCV in the cardiovascularly stable patient is 20% to 25%, whereas cardiovascularly unstable patients may benefit from a higher PCV in the order of 30%. Hypotension should be treated with a combination of intravenous crystalloid and colloid fluids, positive inotropic drugs, and vasopressors as indicated.

Analgesia

In the immediate postoperative period, pain control is of paramount importance. Multimodal analgesia with opioids, nonsteroidal antiinflammatory drugs (if not contraindicated), and intrapleural or local administration of anesthetic agents can be performed to minimize patient discomfort and maximize analgesia without causing adverse side effects. Physical examination parameters such as heart rate and blood pressure can be increased with pain or can be increased because of anxiety, dysphoria, or an animal's need to urinate or defecate in an area away from its immediate environment.

Hypothermia

Hypothermia is a leading postoperative complication that can interfere with tissue offloading of oxygen from hemoglobin, cardiac performance, elimination of anesthetic wastes, coagulation, and wound healing.[10-11] Hypothermia can be potentially avoided or minimized intra- and postoperatively by use of circulating warm water blankets, circulating warmed forced-air blankets, intravenous fluid warmers, and lavage of body cavities with warmed sterile fluids.[12] Electric blankets and electric heating pads should never be used because of the risk of causing severe thermal burns.[13] In the immediate postoperative period, anesthetic drugs may prevent the body's normal physiologic mechanisms that create shivering. Once the animal's core body temperature has been increased to 99.5° F (37.5° C), active and passive rewarming efforts should stop to avoid accidental hyperthermia.[14]

LABORATORY PARAMETERS

Coagulation

Preoperative and intraoperative administration of large volumes of intravenous crystalloid or colloid fluids,[15] blood products,[16] and hypothermia can all lead to coagulation abnormalities. Anticoagulants used in blood products can bind with calcium and lead to poor muscular responsiveness. In animals with refractory perianesthetic hypothermia and hypotension that have received blood products, ionized calcium concentration should be measured because hypocalcemia can interfere with arteriolar constriction and vascular tone. When present, hypocalcemia can be corrected with intravenous administration of calcium gluconate (50 to 150 mg/kg intravenously [IV] slowly over 20 minutes) and careful infusion of calcium-containing crystalloid fluids, such as lactated Ringer's solution. True coagulopathies that have been documented by prolonged prothrombin time (PT), activated partial thromboplastin time (aPTT), or thrombocytopenia can be partially reversed with administration of activated clotting factors in fresh frozen plasma. Serial measurements of the animal's hematocrit can be performed to document and then treat ongoing blood loss and anemia. In animals whose serial coagulation profiles document worsening thrombocytopenia, elevations in fibrin degradation products or D-dimers and prolonged aPTT or PT disseminated intravascular coagulation should be suspected.

Acid-Base and Electrolyte Status

Acid-base, electrolyte, and glucose abnormalities are common in the immediate postoperative period. The animal's acid-base and electrolyte status should be evaluated at least once every 12 to 24 hours. Metabolic acidosis can be associated with decrease organ perfusion and can usually be corrected once intravascular circulating volume and hypothermia have been corrected. Severe metabolic acidosis with a pH less than 7.1 may require intervention with supplemental bicarbonate therapy. Bicarbonate therapy is further discussed in Chapter 54.

PATIENT CLEANLINESS, WOUND AND CATHETER CARE, AND BANDAGING

Patient cleanliness is of paramount importance in the postoperative period. Contamination of surgical sites with wound exudates, feces, urine, or vomitus or from the external environment can promote delayed wound healing and infection. Wounds and surgical sites should be covered to prevent nosocomial contamination from the outside. Moisture or strike-through of blood or wound exudates can promote wicking of bacteria from the environment into the wound.[17,18] Further, a large percentage of nosocomial infections are acquired from direct contact with the hands of hospital personnel. For this reason, gloves should be worn at all times when handling catheters and wounds, to prevent iatrogenic infection. Bandages should be checked frequently for evidence of soilage or strike-through and changed immediately when present. Surgical, wound, and catheter sites should be checked at least once to twice daily for evidence of erythema, tenderness, pain, thrombosis, or discharge. Immobile animals should have a urinary catheter in place to prevent urination into bedding and urine scald. Bedding should be well padded, soft, clean, and dry to prevent urine scalding, pressure necrosis, and the formation of decubital ulcers.

PATIENT IMMOBILIZATION AND PHYSICAL THERAPY

Immobile animals are at particular risk for atelectasis, pneumonia, and decubital ulcer formation. Nonambulatory or immobile animals should be turned from side to side and placed in sternal recumbency at least every 4 to 6 hours to prevent atelectasis and reduce the likelihood of pressure sores. Padding around pressure points (elbows, shoulders, hips, and stifles) should be thick and adequate to prevent pressure necrosis. Deep tissue massage and passive range-of-motion exercises should be performed three to four times daily to prevent disuse atrophy and edema.

NUTRITION

Nutritional support is one of the most important aspects of promoting healing. Inadequate enteral nutrition can promote delayed wound healing and bacterial translocation from the gastrointestinal tract and thus increase patient morbidity, length of hospital stay, and potentially mortality. At the time of surgery, esophagostomy, gastrostomy, or jejunostomy tubes should be placed if an animal has been inappetent or is at risk for inappetence in the postoperative period.[19-23] If enteral nutrition is impossible and the patient experiences a prolonged period of inappetence, parenteral nutrition can be provided.[23] Supplemental feeding can be discontinued once the animal is able and willing to voluntarily consume its daily caloric requirements.

SUMMARY

In conclusion, careful monitoring and assessment of the critical patient is challenging in the immediate postoperative period. Although the immediate time of anesthetic recovery is very critical, other criteria, including nutrition, cleanliness, and physical therapy, are necessary to maximize the animal's well-being and promote wound healing. Analgesia and sedation should be maximized without causing dysphoria and agitation. Wound and bandage care is optimal in preventing postoperative infection. Kirby's Rule of 20 checklist can provide even the most astute clinician with a source of potential complication in the critically ill patient.

REFERENCES

1. Syring RE, Drobatz KJ: Preoperative evaluation and management of the emergency surgical small animal patient, Vet Clin North Am Small Anim Pract 30(3):473, 2000.
2. Thurmon JC, Tranquilly WJ, Benson GJ, et al: Considerations for general anesthesia. In: Lumb WV, Jones EW, editors: Veterinary anesthesia, Baltimore, 1991, Williams and Wilkins, p 22.
3. Hardie EM, Jayawickrama J, Duff LC, et al: Prognostic indicators of survival in high-risk canine surgery patients, J Vet Emerg Crit Care 5:42, 1995.
4. de Papp E, Drobatz KJ, Hughes D: Plasma lactate concentration as a predictor of gastric necrosis and survival among dogs with gastric dilatation-volvulus: 102 cases (1995-1998), J Am Vet Med Assoc 215:49, 1999.
5. Green TI, Tonozzi CC, Kirby R, et al: Evaluation of initial plasma lactate values as a predictor of gastric necrosis and initial and subsequent plasma lactate values as a predictor of survival in dogs with gastric dilatation-volvulus: 84 dogs (2003-2007), J Vet Emerg Crit Care 21(1):36, 2011.
6. Santoro-Beer KA, Syring RS, Dronatz KJ: Evaluation of plasma lactate concentration and base excess at the time of hospital admission as predictors of gastric necrosis and outcome and correlation between those variables in dogs with gastric dilatation-volvulus: 78 cases (2004-2009), JAVMA 242(1):54, 2013.
7. Wagner AE, Dunlap CI: Anesthetic and medical management of acute hemorrhage during surgery, J Am Vet Med Assoc 203(1):40, 1993.
8. Purvis D, Kirby R: Systemic inflammatory response syndrome: septic shock, Vet Clin North Am Small Anim Pract 24(6):1225, 1994.
9. Hackett TB: Pulse oximetry and end-tidal carbon dioxide monitoring, Vet Clin Small Anim 32:1021, 2002.
10. Oncken AK, Kirby R, Rudloff E: Hypothermia in critically ill dogs and cats, Compendium Contin Educ Pract Vet 23(6):506, 2001.
11. Beal MW, Brown DC, Shofer FS: The effects of perioperative hypothermia and the duration of anesthesia on postoperative wound infection rates in clean wounds: a retrospective study, Vet Surg 29:123, 2000.
12. Armstrong SR, Roberts BK, Aronsohn M: Perioperative hypothermia, J Vet Emerg Crit Care 15(1):32, 2005.
13. Kirby R, Rudloff E: The critical need for colloids: selecting the right colloid, Comp Cont Educ Pract Vet 19(6):705, 1997.
14. Swaim S, Lee A, Hughes K: Heating pads and thermal burns in small animals, J Am Anim Hosp Assoc 25(2):156, 1989.
15. Jutkowitz LA, Rozanski EA, Moreau JA, et al: Massive transfusion in dogs: 15 cases (1997-2001), J Am Vet Med Assoc 220(11):1664, 2002.
16. Burrows CF: Inadequate skin preparation as a cause of intravenous catheter-related infection in the dog, J Am Vet Med Assoc 180:747, 1982.
17. Mathews KA, Brooks MJ, Valliant AE: A prospective study of intravenous catheter contamination, J Vet Emerg Crit Care 6:33, 1996.
18. Seim HB, Willard MD. Postoperative care of the surgical patient. In Fossum TW, editor: Small animal surgery, ed 2, St Louis, 2002, Mosby, pp 69-91.
19. Brady CA, King LG: Postoperative management of the emergency surgery small animal patient, Vet Clin North Am Small Anim 30:681, 2000.
20. Mazzaferro EM: Esophagostomy tubes: don't underutilize them! J Vet Emerg Crit Care 11(2):153, 2001.
21. Han E: Esophageal and gastric feeding tubes in ICU patients, Clin Tech Small Anim Pract 19(1):22, 2004.
22. Heuter K: Placement of jejunal feeding tubes for post-gastric feeding, Clin Tech Small Anim Pract 19(1):32, 2004.
23. Otto CM, Kaufman GM, Crowe DT: Intraosseous infusion of fluids and therapeutics, Comp Cont Educ Pract Vet 11:421, 1989.

CHAPTER 132

PORTOSYSTEMIC SHUNT MANAGEMENT

Margo Mehl, DVM, DACVS

KEY POINTS

- Clinical signs of animals with portosystemic shunts (PSS) include neurologic, gastrointestinal, and urinary abnormalities and can manifest as other signs, such as prolonged recovery from anesthesia.
- Intrahepatic PSS are more common in large breed dogs and extrahepatic PSS usually occur in small dogs and cats.
- The goal of preoperative PSS stabilization and medical management is to control signs of hepatic encephalopathy (HE) and prevent progression of neurologic signs.
- The treatment of choice is surgical attenuation of the shunting vessel.
- Perioperative morbidity and mortality is higher with intrahepatic PSS attenuation compared with surgical correction of extrahepatic PSS.
- The major postoperative complications of PSS attenuation include hemorrhage, hypoglycemia, seizures, and portal hypertension.
- Several predictors of clinical outcome have been identified for surgical treatment of extrahepatic and intrahepatic PSS in dogs.

Portosystemic shunts (PSS) are vascular anomalies that connect the portal circulation with systemic circulation, diverting portal blood away from the liver. These vascular anomalies are most commonly categorized as extrahepatic or intrahepatic. Extrahepatic PSS can be further categorized as congenital or acquired and often described based on the supplying and draining vessel, such as portocaval or portoazygous. Intrahepatic PSS are usually classified based on the branch of the portal vein supplying the shunt and divides intrahepatic PSS into left-, central-, and right-divisional.

Single extrahepatic PSS are the most commonly reported type of PSS in dogs and cats, are congenital, and primarily are seen in small breed dogs.[1-3] Clinical signs are related to hepatic dysfunction, including gastrointestinal signs, central nervous system disturbances, and urolithiasis. Some patients will require intensive therapy to stabilize them before surgical correction of the PSS. Postoperative complications can occur in an unpredictable and precipitous manner and can range in severity from ascites to life-threatening hemodynamic and neurologic abnormalities, making these patients challenging to manage after surgery.

PREOPERATIVE STABILIZATION

Animals with PSS commonly will present with neurologic abnormalities, gastrointestinal signs, urinary signs, and other signs such as prolonged recovery from a previous anesthesia.[3] Preoperative stabilization depends on the animal's status at presentation and often includes fluid therapy and anticonvulsants to stop the progression of neurologic signs. If a patient presents for mild signs of hepatic encephalopathy (HE) and is stable, treatment may include initiating medical management (i.e., low-protein diet, anticonvulsants, antibiotics, and cathartics). When a patient presents with moderate to severe signs of HE, more aggressive therapy is required. A major contributing factor to the worsening of HE in these patients can be hemorrhage into the gastrointestinal tract, which acts as a large protein source for more ammonia production. Therefore the treatment plan includes immediate removal of this protein source with lactulose enemas and reducing ongoing ammonia production and absorption with antibiotic therapy and lactulose. See Chapter 88 for further discussion of the management of HE.

Gastrointestinal signs in PSS patients often include vomiting and diarrhea, which can lead to fluid and electrolyte imbalances. These fluid and electrolyte imbalances should be corrected before surgical correction of the PSS. Pica is a common clinical sign reported in PSS patients, and therefore these patients may present for vomiting secondary to a gastrointestinal foreign body.

Occasionally animals can present with a urinary emergency secondary to PSS, such as a urethral obstruction. Initial treatment may include correcting fluid and electrolyte abnormalities followed by unblocking the urinary system.

MEDICAL MANAGEMENT

As long as portal blood flow is being shunted away from the liver, hepatic function will continue to decline. Both surgical and medical treatment of PSS can lead to long-term survival, although dogs treated with surgery live longer than those treated medically.[4] Surgery is the treatment of choice and offers the opportunity to redirect portal blood back to liver.[1] Medical management should be initiated before surgical correction of the PSS in animals with signs of HE, and anticonvulsant therapy may be beneficial in PSS patients preoperatively.

The goal of medical therapy is to decrease production and absorption of ammonia and includes dietary modification, antibiotic therapy, and cathartics. Typically, a diet high in carbohydrates and low in protein decreases the building blocks for ammonia production. Dairy and vegetable protein sources are less likely to cause clinical signs of HE compared with meat-source proteins. Antibiotics that concentrate in the gastrointestinal tract, such as amoxicillin, neomycin, and metronidazole, reduce the number of bacteria responsible for producing ammonia. Cathartics, such as lactulose, increase transit time in the gastrointestinal tract and trap ammonium ions in the lumen, reducing ammonia absorption. Acid-base, electrolyte abnormalities, and hypoglycemia should be identified and corrected before surgery.

Hypoalbuminemia is a consistent finding in PSS patients. Because this hypoalbuminemia is due to chronic disease, generally it is not associated with clinical signs in the stable patient and as such it does not warrant specific therapy. Hypoalbuminemia will, however, be a concern in the patient that requires significant fluid resuscitation, a common requirement of the perioperative PSS patient. Large volumes of crystalloid fluid administration will cause hemodilution and worsen the hypoalbuminemia, making maintenance of intravascular volume challenging. Hemodynamically compromised hypoproteinemic patients generally require support of serum colloid osmotic pressure (COP). Although synthetic colloids such as hetastarch are very effective at increasing COP, they do interfere with coagulation. Because PSS patients are known to have coagulation deficits, cautious use of synthetic colloids is advised.[5,6] The hydroxyethyl starch product VetStarch interferes less with coagulation than the higher molecular weight hetastarch and may be preferable in these patients. Plasma transfusions will support intravascular volume, help maintain COP and provide coagulation factors. For this reason plasma can be an invaluable therapy in the perioperative stabilization of the PSS patient.

The benefit of preoperative anticonvulsant therapy was evaluated by Tisdall et al, who reported that the use of prophylactic anticonvulsants did not significantly reduce the risk of postoperative neurologic signs but may have reduced their severity.[7] An additional study by Fryer et al demonstrated that the use of levetiracetam was protective against the development of postoperative seizures.[8] In this study the suggested dosing for levetiracetam in dogs was 20 mg/kg PO q8h with therapy being initiated at least 24 hours before surgery. In general most surgeons elect to have patients on an anticonvulsant therapy before or at the time of PSS attenuation. There are variable protocols for routine use of prophylactic anticonvulsant therapy in dogs with PSS. Reported anticonvulsant drugs used include potassium bromide, phenobarbital, and levetiracetam. The author typically uses potassium bromide as a preoperative anticonvulsant at a loading dose (100 mg/kg PO q6h for 24 hours) or maintenance dose (40 mg/kg PO q12h for 15 days) (Table 132-1).

SURGICAL OPTIONS

The treatment of choice is complete attenuation of the shunting vessel.[1] The traditional surgical technique involves placement of a ligature around the anomalous vessel, which is gradually tightened while measuring portal pressure and observing the splanchnic viscera. If the ligature is placed too tight, there is significant risk of inducing portal hypertension, which can be a severe and fatal complication. Criteria for judging the safe degree of PSS attenuation include an increase in portal pressure with temporary complete PSS attenuation of no greater than 10 cm of H_2O.[9-12]

Gradual, rather than acute, PSS occlusion has been advocated as a safer surgical technique.[13,14] It is proposed that gradual occlusion allows the development of the hepatic architecture in response to the increased vascular supply, while avoiding fatal portal hypertension. The ameroid ring constrictor (ARC) and the cellophane band are both designed to produce gradual vascular occlusion. Intravascular occlusion of both extrahepatic and intrahepatic PSS has been performed successfully. These techniques require specialized equipment and specific case selection that allows for more acute closure of the PSS or necessitates multiple procedures.[15]

Surgical access, localization, and attenuation of an intrahepatic PSS can be challenging. A number of techniques, both intravascular and extravascular, have been reported for accessing an intrahepatic PSS, some of which require a caudal sternotomy. Intrahepatic PSS are often large vessels shunting sizeable volumes of portal blood away from the liver, and there is a significant risk of portal hypertension with excessive attenuation. Therefore, patients with an intrahepatic PSS may only tolerate partial PSS ligation.

POSTOPERATIVE MONITORING

General critical care principles apply to the postoperative management of PSS patients, and close observation is extremely important because their status can deteriorate rapidly. The most optimal outcome occurs when clinicians identify life-threatening complications early and treat aggressively. Several parameters should be monitored in these patients after surgery, including arterial blood pressure, heart rate, and respiratory rate. These patients are often young small breed dogs that can be hypothermic after surgery and benefit from continuous temperature monitoring and active rewarming. Box 132-1 provides a comprehensive list of parameters for postoperative monitoring.

Hypovolemia is a common postoperative issue as a result of venous congestion of the splanchnic viscera, gastrointestinal losses, and hypoproteinemia, which may be more severe after intraoperative hemodilution. Signs of hemodynamic compromise such as evidence of poor perfusion or systemic hypotension should be considered as secondary to hypovolemia unless proven otherwise. Central venous pressure monitoring may be advantageous to guide fluid therapy. When choosing a fluid for volume resuscitation it is important to consider that these patients will have both a low COP and coagulation defects. As a result plasma transfusions are often the fluid of

Table 132-1 Possible Preoperative Anticonvulsant Therapy in Dogs and Cats With PSS[8,29,30]

Drug	Canine and Feline Dosage	Therapeutic Blood Levels
Phenobarbital	1 to 3 mg/kg PO q12h	15 to 45 mcg/ml
Levetiracetam	20 mg/kg PO q8h	Unknown
Potassium bromide	Loading dosage*: 100 mg/kg PO q6h × 4 doses (total dosage of 400 mg/kg in 24 hours) Maintenance dosage: 60 to 100 (canine) mg/kg once a day	2 to 3 mg/ml when used as a sole agent 1 to 2 mg/ml when used in conjunction with phenobarbital

*A loading dose is recommended if therapeutic levels are required quickly. This is one of several protocols for potassium bromide loading. A maintenance dose given longer than 15 days in dogs will provide adequate blood levels as an alternative to giving the loading dose.[30] Phenobarbital and potassium bromide can be associated with neurologic and respiratory depression and patients should be monitored accordingly. Loading doses of potassium bromide can cause gastrointestinal disturbances. *PO*, Per os, *PSS*, portosystemic shunts.

BOX 132-1 *Recommended Clinicopathologic Parameters to Monitor in the Postoperative PSS Patient*

Clinical Parameters	Laboratory Parameters
Heart rate	Packed cell volume
Respiratory rate	Total protein
Temperature	Glucose
Direct arterial pressure*	Lactate
Central venous pressure	Electrolytes
Electrocardiogram	Acid-base status
Urine output	
Abdominal circumference	
Intraabdominal pressure	
Mentation and neurologic status	

*When direct arterial pressure is unavailable, indirect arterial pressure should be measured.
PSS, Portosystemic shunt.

choice in combination with isotonic crystalloids. Synthetic colloids should be used judiciously. Clinicopathologic parameters to evaluate at regular intervals after surgery include packed cell volume, total protein, lactate, glucose, and electrolytes (see Box 132-1). Monitoring intraabdominal pressure using a urinary catheter can provide useful information, which may assist in determining development of life-threatening portal hypertension (see Chapter 188). Severity and progression of abdominal distention can also be monitored with serial measurements of abdominal circumference using a measuring tape or string. Some of these patients may require a continuous electrocardiogram to detect any cardiac arrhythmias that may need treatment.

POSTOPERATIVE COMPLICATIONS

The three major postoperative complications seen in PSS patients are portal hypertension, coagulopathy, and neurologic abnormalities.

Portal Hypertension

Portal hypertension describes any process that increases the vascular pressure in the portal circulation and is categorized anatomically as prehepatic, hepatic, or posthepatic in origin.[16] Surgical attenuation of a PSS will increase the blood flow in the portal vein and can create a prehepatic cause for portal hypertension. This increase in portal venous pressure can lead to venous congestion of the abdominal organs normally drained by the portal system. Vascular fluid loss in the form of ascites, organ edema, and intestinal fluid losses (including hemorrhage) can follow and may be associated with significant hemodynamic compromise. The major clinical signs of an animal with portal hypertension are abdominal pain, abdominal distention, melena, diarrhea, and hypovolemia. The degree of portal hypertension can vary from minor to severe. Although most patients can be stabilized with fluid therapy, including blood products, and opioid-based pain management, animals with signs of severe portal hypertension that are not responsive to aggressive medical therapy may require emergency surgery to remove the occlusion device from the shunting vessel. The interested reader is referred to reference 16 for further information on portal hypertension.

Coagulopathy

The portal vein supplies the liver with 50% of its oxygen requirements and other essential hepatotrophic factors.[3] In PSS patients, portal venous blood is bypassing the liver, resulting in reduced hepatic mass and decreased production and activation of coagulation factors.[6] Canine patients with PSS have been reported to have prolonged activated partial thromboplastin times compared with healthy dogs.[5,6] These coagulation abnormalities are likely to be exacerbated during surgery by dilution from fluid therapy and possible coagulation changes associated with hydroxyethyl starch products. As a result plasma therapy may be indicated as part of the fluid therapy plan for the surgical and postoperative period and is likely to be necessary if overt hemorrhage develops. Clinical signs of a PSS patient with a coagulopathy can range from minor oozing from catheter and surgical sites to life-threatening hemorrhage into body cavities. See Chapter 61 for further discussion of transfusion therapy.

Neurologic Complications

Postoperative seizures can occur in the immediate postoperative period and have been reported to occur up to 72 hours after surgery.[17] In dogs undergoing surgery for PSS attenuation, the risk for the development of postoperative neurologic complications has been reported to range from 5% to 12%.[7,8,18] In some dogs neurologic signs, such as vocalization, disorientation, and ataxia, are observed before seizures. Dogs with mild clinical signs of partial seizures, such as disorientation, vocalization, salivation, or focal twitching, may resolve after administration of anticonvulsant therapy, whereas postoperative grand mal seizures are associated with a high mortality rate.[19,20] Cats appear to have a higher rate of postoperative seizure after PSS attenuation.[21-23] In a study by Lipscomb et al, 37% of cats developed neurologic complications after surgical attenuation of the shunting vessel.[23] The institution of treatment and the ideal treatment choice for postoperative neurologic complications in cats are debatable. In the study by Lipscomb et al, of cats that developed postoperative seizure after PSS attenuation, 56% had resolution of the neurologic signs.

The cause of neurologic signs after attenuation of a PSS has not been fully defined and is likely to be multifactorial. Increased blood ammonia levels are generally considered part of the pathophysiology of HE and can occur subsequent to gastrointestinal hemorrhage. Because gastrointestinal hemorrhage may occur as a consequence of portal hypertension, this may be a cause of changes in neurologic state after surgery. Other proposed mechanisms include the production of neurotransmitter substances by the gastrointestinal tract such as γ-aminobutyric acid (GABA), aromatic amino acids, and endogenous benzodiazepine receptor ligands that are normally removed from the portal blood by the liver. In PSS patients this fails to occur and the brain is exposed to higher levels of these substances. One study in dogs with PSS demonstrated elevated levels endogenous benzodiazepine receptor ligands in the peripheral and portal blood compared with control animals.[24] This could contribute to central nervous system depression in these animals, and it has been suggested that attenuation of the PSS could lead to an abrupt decrease in the level of these compounds as a possible contribution to postoperative neurologic complications. There is growing evidence for the role of systemic inflammation and oxidative stress in the pathophysiology of HE in people. This may also be relevant to veterinary patients because a study in dogs with PSS found increased levels of C-reactive protein compared with normal dogs and a significant difference between PSS dogs with HE compared with those without.[25]

Currently there are several recommendations for the treatment of seizure activity after surgical attenuation of PSS in dogs, including a single agent or a combination of the following intravenous agents: diazepam, phenobarbital, pentobarbital, or propofol (Table 132-2). Anticonvulsant therapy protocols in PSS patients have not been scientifically evaluated and as such there is no proven benefit of any one agent or agents over another. Gommerenk et al reported the successful use of propofol and phenobarbital in the treatment of status epilepticus in three dogs after PSS attenuation.[26] These patients should be monitored closely because many of these therapies used as a sole agent or in combination can necessitate mechanical ventilation. Treatment recommendations include avoiding hypoglycemia and other electrolyte abnormalities and treating seizure activity early. Postoperatively, dogs and cats with neurologic signs of partial or focal seizures should be treated aggressively with anticonvulsant therapy to prevent the progression of clinical signs to grand mal seizures, which carry a very grave prognosis.

PROGNOSIS

A number of studies have reported the mortality rate after surgical repair of both extrahepatic and intrahepatic PSS. The perioperative mortality rate for extrahepatic PSS repaired using a method for slow attenuation, cellophane banding or ameroid ring constrictor placement, has been reported between 5.5% and 7.1%.[18,27] Among several factors that predict surgical mortality in dogs with single extrahepatic PSS treated by ameroid ring constrictor placement were the occurrence of postoperative complications and preoperative white blood cell count.[18] Similarly, the mortality rate and predictive factors for

Table 132-2 **Recommended Treatment for Neurologic Dysfunction in Patients with PSS[29]**

Agent	Mode of Administration	Canine and Feline Dosage
Diazepam	Bolus	0.2 to 2 mg/kg IV to effect
	CRI	0.2 to 1.0 mg/kg/hr IV to effect
Midazolam	Bolus	0.1 to 0.5 mg/kg IV to effect
	CRI	0.1 to 0.5 mg/kg/hr IV to effect
Propofol	Bolus	1 to 4 mg/kg IV to effect
	CRI	0.1 to 0.4 mg/kg/min IV to effect
Phenobarbital	Bolus	2 to 5 mg/kg IV; can repeat at 20-min intervals up to a total dosage of 20 mg/kg
	Maintenance	2 to 4 mg/kg IV q12h
Pentobarbital	Bolus	3 to 15 mg/kg IV SLOWLY to effect
	CRI	0.5 to 5 mg/kg/hr to effect

NOTE: All these drugs are associated with moderate to profound neurologic and respiratory depression. Intensive monitoring is essential; patients may require intubation and mechanical ventilation.
CRI, Constant rate infusion; *IV,* intravenous; *PSS,* portosystemic shunts.

surgical mortality have been reported after surgical treatment of intrahepatic PSS. Papazoglou et al reported a surgical mortality rate of 12.5% in 32 dogs with intrahepatic PSS repair, and this study reported several predictors for short-term outcome for dogs with intrahepatic PSS, including body weight, total protein, albumin, and blood urea nitrogen.[28] A number of studies have reported higher surgical mortality rates in the treatment of intrahepatic PSS compared with extrahepatic PSS. Although the surgical repair of PSS carries a significant risk of postoperative mortality, it is more likely to allow for a normal lifespan.

REFERENCES

1. Johnson CA, Armstrong PJ, Hauptman JG: Congenital portosystemic shunts in dogs: 46 cases (1979-1986), J Am Vet Med Assoc 191:1478, 1987.
2. Bostwick DR, Twedt DC: Intrahepatic and extrahepatic portal venous anomalies in dogs: 52 cases (1982-1992), J Am Vet Med Assoc 206:1181, 1995.
3. Tobias TM: Portosystemic shunts and other hepatic vascular anomalies. In Slatter DH, editor: Textbook of small animal surgery, ed 3, St Louis, 2003, Saunders.
4. Greenhalgh SN, Dunning MD, McKinley TJ, et al: Comparison of survival after surgical or medical treatment in dogs with a congenital portosystemic shunt, J Am Vet Med Assoc 236:1215, 2010.
5. Kummeling A, Teske E, Rothuizen J, et al: Coagulation profiles in dogs with congenital portosystemic shunts before and after surgical attenuation, J Vet Intern Med 20:1319, 2006.
6. Niles JD, Williams JM, Cripps PJ: Hemostatic profiles in 39 dogs with congenital portosystemic shunts, Vet Surg 30:97, 2001.
7. Tisdall PLC, Hunt GB, Youmans KR, et al: Neurological dysfunction in dogs following attenuation of congenital extrahepatic portosystemic shunts, J Small Anim Pract 41:539, 2000.
8. Fryer KJ, Levine JM, Peycke LE, et al: Incidence of postoperative seizures with and without levetiracetam pretreatment in dogs undergoing portosystemic shunt attenuation, J Vet Intern Med. 25:1379, 2011.
9. Watson PJ, Herrtage ME: Medical management of congenital portosystemic shunts in 27 dogs: a retrospective study, J Small Anim Pract 39:62, 1998.
10. Swalec KM, Smeak DD: Partial versus complete attenuation of single portosystemic shunts, Vet Surg 19:406, 1990.
11. Mathews K, Gofton N: Congenital extrahepatic portosystemic shunt occlusion in the dog: gross observations during surgical correction, J Am Anim Hosp Assoc 24:387, 1988.
12. Lawrence D, Bellah JR, Diaz R: Results of surgical management of portosystemic shunts in dogs: 20 cases (1985-1990), J Am Vet Med Assoc 201:1750, 1992.
13. Vogt JC, Krahwinkel DJ, Bright RM et al: Gradual occlusion of extrahepatic portosystemic shunts in dogs and cats using the ameroid constrictor, Vet Surg 25:495, 1996.
14. Swalec Tobias KM, Seguin B, Johnston G: Surgical approaches to single extrahepatic portosystemic shunts, Compend Contin Educ Vet Pract 20:593, 1998.
15. Hogan DF, Benitez ME, Parnell NK, et al: Intravascular occlusion for the correction of extrahepatic portosystemic shunts in dogs, J Vet Intern Med 24:1048, 2010.
16. Buob S, Johnston AN, Webster CRL: Portal hypertension: Pathophysiology, diagnosis and treatment, J Vet Intern Med 25:169, 2011.
17. Matushek KJ, Bjorling D, Mathews K: Generalized motor seizures after portosystemic shunt ligation in dogs: five cases (1981-1988), J Am Vet Med Assoc 196:2014, 1990.
18. Mehl ML, Kyles AE, Hardie EM, et al: Evaluation of ameroid ring constrictors for treatment for single extrahepatic portosystemic shunts in dogs: 168 cases (1995-2001), J Am Vet Med Assoc 226:2020, 2005.
19. Hardie EM, Kornegay JN, Cullen JM: Status epilepticus after ligation of portosystemic shunts, Vet Surg 19:412, 1990.
20. Ahboucha S, Butterworth RF: Role of endogenous benzodiazepine ligands and their GABA-A–associated receptors in hepatic encephalopathy, Metab Brain Dis 20:425, 2005.
21. Havig M, Tobias KM: Outcome of ameroid constrictor occlusion of single congenital portosystemic shunts in cats: 12 cases (1993-2000), J Am Vet Med Assoc 220:337, 2002.
22. Kyles AE, Hardie EM, Mehl M, et al: Evaluation of ameroid ring constrictors for the management of single extrahepatic portosystemic shunts in cats: 23 cases (1996-2001), J Am Vet Med Assoc 220:1341, 2002.
23. Lipscomb VJ, Jones HJ, Brockman DJ: Complications and long-term outcomes of the ligation of congenital portosystemic shunts in 49 cats, Vet Rec 160:465, 2007.
24. Aronson LR, Reynaldo GC, Kaminsky-Russ K, et al: Endogenous benzodiazepine activity in the peripheral and portal blood of dogs with congenital portosystemic shunts, Vet Surg 26:189, 1997.
25. Gow AG, Marques AI, Yool DA, et al: Dogs with congenital portosystemic shunting (cPSS) and HE have higher serum concentrations of C-reactive protein with asymptomatic dogs with Cpss, Metab Brain Dis 27:227, 2012.
26. Gommeren K, Claeys S, de Rooster H, et al: Outcome from status epilepticus after portosystemic shunt attenuation in 3 dogs treated with propofol and Phenobarbital, J Vet Emer Crit Care 20:346, 2010.
27. Hunt GB, Kummeling A, Tisdall PLC, et al: Outcomes of cellophane banding for congenital portosystemic shunts in 106 dogs and 5 cats, Vet Surg 33:25, 2004.
28. Papazoglou LG, Monnet E, Seim II HB: Survival and prognostic indicators for dogs with intrahepatic portosystemic shunts: 32 cases (1990-2000), Vet Surg 31:561, 2002.
29. Plumb DC: Plumb's veterinary drug handbook, ed 7, Stockholm, WI, 2011, PharmaVet.
30. March PA, Podell M, Sam RA: Pharmacokinetics and toxicity of bromide following high-dose oral potassium bromide administration in healthy Beagles, J Vet Pharmacol Ther 25:425, 2002.

CHAPTER 133
PERITONEAL DRAINAGE TECHNIQUES

Matthew W. Beal, DVM, DACVECC

KEY POINTS

- A variety of medical and surgical disease processes necessitate the evacuation of fluid from the peritoneal cavity.
- When combined with source control, peritoneal drainage is a critical component in the management of chemical and septic peritonitis.
- Peritoneal drainage techniques may be used to facilitate preoperative stabilization of the patient with life-threatening hyperkalemia and azotemia secondary to urinary tract disruption.
- The peritoneal cavity may be drained initially using needle paracentesis or catheter paracentesis. When sustained drainage is indicated, closed suction drains or open peritoneal drainage techniques are employed.

Sampling and evacuation of fluid from the peritoneal cavity are both diagnostic and therapeutic cornerstones for the treatment of the dog or cat with an acute condition of the abdomen and a host of other medically and surgically managed disease processes. A number of medical and surgical procedures maybe used to facilitate peritoneal drainage, and each has specific indications, contraindications, advantages, and disadvantages. A thorough knowledge of peritoneal drainage strategies allows for appropriate medical and surgical decision making and will maximize the likelihood of a positive clinical outcome.

INDICATIONS FOR PERITONEAL DRAINAGE

Septic Peritonitis

Septic peritonitis is by far the most common indication for sustained peritoneal drainage. It is generally accepted that the removal of fluid that may contain infectious agents, inflammatory mediators, and foreign material (e.g., bile, ingesta) is beneficial to resolution of the infection within the peritoneal space. Furthermore, fluid within an infected cavity may significantly impair humoral and cell-mediated immune mechanisms.[1] Despite a lack of prospective, randomized controlled studies in dogs and cats to definitively document decreased morbidity and improved outcome when peritoneal drainage is established, open peritoneal drainage (OPD) or closed suction peritoneal drainage (CSD) are the standard of care for generalized septic peritonitis. Vacuum-assisted drainage (VAD) is an established human technique that is currently under investigation for use in the small animal patient.[2,3]

Recommendations for abdominal drainage techniques in dogs and cats with septic peritonitis are shown in Box 133-1. In clinical practice the author prefers to use CSD, even when criteria are met for primary closure. CSD allows not only for drainage of abdominal fluid that may accumulate but also for sampling of the abdominal fluid for cytologic analysis and confirmation that the inflammatory reaction and infectious process are indeed subsiding. Detailed descriptions of OPD, CSD, and VAD techniques may be found later in this chapter.

Chemical Peritonitis

Uroperitoneum and bile peritonitis account for two common sources of chemical peritonitis. Although most commonly sterile, both conditions may be associated with sepsis. Cytological examination and biochemical analysis (glucose and lactate) of abdominal fluids may aid in differentiating between sterile and septic processes.

Bile peritonitis is associated with an intense inflammatory response. Bile salts are toxic to mesothelial cells in the peritoneal cavity, and the presence of bile alters host defense mechanisms and may reduce phagocytic abilities of inflammatory cells in the peritoneal space.[4,5] Just as in septic peritonitis, source control is of paramount importance in the management of bile peritonitis. OPD is probably unnecessary in sterile bile peritonitis and may predispose to nosocomial colonization of the peritoneal cavity. The author has found CSD to be valuable for maintaining peritoneal cavity decompression and facilitating ongoing removal of small bile particulate matter in dogs with sterile bile peritonitis.

Peritoneal drainage plays important roles in both the preoperative and postoperative management of the dog or cat with uroperitoneum. In the preoperative setting, in addition to standard therapeutic measures to manage hypovolemia and hyperkalemia (see Chapters 51, 60, and 205) a fenestrated catheter in the peritoneal space will facilitate the evacuation of urine from the peritoneal cavity and the diversion of urine that continues to leak from the disrupted urinary tract until the patient is stable and surgical intervention can be performed. In the postoperative setting, because the likelihood of large particulate debris in the peritoneal space concurrent with uroperitoneum is unlikely, CSD (rather than OPD) will facilitate the

BOX 133-1 ***Guidelines for the Choice of Abdominal Drainage in Dogs and Cats with Septic Peritonitis***

Open Peritoneal Drainage

Source control accomplished
Severe generalized peritonitis
Severe contamination that cannot be resolved completely with debridement and lavage

Closed Suction Drainage

Source control accomplished
Moderate to severe generalized peritonitis
Severe contamination that can or cannot be resolved completely with debridement and lavage
Localized peritonitis

Primary Closure

Source control accomplished
Local or focal peritonitis of nongastrointestinal origin
Minimal contamination that is resolved completely with debridement and lavage

BOX 133-2 ***Possible Indications for Peritoneal Drainage***

- Septic peritonitis
- Bile peritonitis
- Uroperitoneum
- Pancreatitis-associated peritonitis
- Peritoneal dialysis
- Increased intraabdominal pressure
- Abdominal effusion compromising ventilation
- Abdominal effusion compromising patient comfort

evacuation of inflammatory exudates from the peritoneal cavity and should be necessary for only 1 to 3 days postoperatively in dogs and cats with moderate to severe generalized chemical peritonitis.

Other Indications for Peritoneal Drainage

Peritoneal dialysis requires reliable cannulae for infusion and drainage of fluid from the peritoneal space. Two CSD catheters or a long-term peritoneal dialysis catheter may be placed laparoscopically or through a small laparotomy incision. Partial omentectomy may be required to help prevent CSD obstruction. Renal biopsy may be performed during the procedure. The increasing availability of continuous renal replacement therapy (CRRT) and intermittent hemodialysis (HD) has decreased the necessity for peritoneal dialysis in veterinary patients. For additional information, please see Chapter 205.

Increased intraabdominal pressure has been documented in conditions including, but not limited to, portal hypertension, repair of chronic diaphragmatic hernia, abdominal counterpressure bandages, hemoperitoneum, and gastric dilation-volvulus.[6] Elevated intraabdominal pressure has generalized deleterious effects on the cardiovascular system, primarily mediated through decreased venous return and subsequent decreases in cardiac output. Local cardiovascular effects include decreased end-organ perfusion, both dependent and independent of the aforementioned effect on cardiac output. Increased intraabdominal pressure is also transmitted to the thoracic cavity via the diaphragm and may result in hypoxemia and hypoventilation (see Chapter 188 for more information). Peritoneal drainage may be indicated for animals with abdominal hypertension.[6] Box 133-2 lists conditions for which peritoneal drainage might be employed. Routine drainage of peritoneal fluid accumulations caused by right-sided heart failure, portal hypertension, or other noninflammatory or noninfectious processes is not indicated in the absence of significantly increased intraabdominal pressure, respiratory embarrassment, or interference with quality of life.

TECHNIQUES FOR PERITONEAL DRAINAGE

Needle or Catheter Paracentesis

Abdominal drainage via a hypodermic needle or over-the-needle catheter is a minimally invasive technique. However, it is very inefficient and does not allow for sustained abdominal drainage. Additionally, clogging of the needle or catheter with omentum or other visceral structures may preclude effective evacuation. This technique is more useful for sampling of abdominal fluid for diagnostic purposes or one-time decompression in a patient exhibiting signs of respiratory compromise or discomfort secondary to abdominal fluid accumulation.

Necessary supplies include a 14- to 20-gauge hypodermic needle or over-the-needle catheter of a length appropriate for the anticipated thickness of the body wall. If an over-the-needle catheter is used, a small 1- to 3-mm side hole may be created using a no. 11 scalpel blade approximately one fourth of the way from the tip of the catheter to the hub. The side hole increases the surface area for the retrieval of fluid and makes occlusion of the catheter with omentum less of a problem. Additional equipment will include a 60-ml syringe, three-way stopcock, and intravenous extension tubing to attach to the needle or catheter. The author prefers to use a closed collection system to minimize the likelihood of contamination of the peritoneal cavity and to minimize the introduction of air into the peritoneal space.

The patient is positioned in left lateral recumbency to allow the spleen to fall away from the proposed site of needle insertion. The abdomen should be liberally clipped of hair and aseptically prepared as if for a surgical procedure and draped using a fenestrated sterile drape. The proposed insertion site is located 2 to 3 cm caudal to the umbilicus, either on or slightly to the left of midline. Infusion of local anesthetic or sedation may improve patient comfort if drainage is likely to take an extended time. The needle should be inserted perpendicular to the surface of the body and advanced through the skin. The stopcock may then be opened and the syringe aspirated. The needle is then advanced in 1- to 2-mm increments and the syringe aspirated intermittently until fluid is retrieved. In circumstances in which only a small volume of peritoneal fluid is present and single-quadrant paracentesis is unsuccessful, four-quadrant paracentesis may be performed. Ultrasonography may be used to guide the sampling needle to very small volume fluid accumulations. Samples should always be saved for cytologic analysis, culture (if indicated), and chemical analysis, if indicated. For additional information, please see Chapter 200.

Paracentesis with a Fenestrated Catheter per the Mini-Laparotomy Method

In contrast to paracentesis with a needle or over-the-needle catheter, use of a catheter with multiple fenestrations will facilitate both rapid and sustained decompression of larger volume abdominal effusions. This technique might be used during stabilization of a dog with bladder rupture and uroperitoneum in preparation for surgical intervention.

A number of commercially available catheters may be used.* Many of these are designed to be placed via a completely closed method using a trochar within the catheter; however, it is the author's experience and recommendation that placing these catheters using a small laparotomy incision will optimize the likelihood of successful placement, while minimizing risk of injury to intraabdominal organs that may occur during closed placement.

The patient should be given sedatives and analgesics appropriate for the cardiovascular and respiratory status. First, the bladder should be emptied via catheterization or gentle expression. The patient should be prepared as described previously (Needle or Catheter Paracentesis). Local anesthesia techniques focusing on the skin, subcutaneous tissues, and the body wall are critical to performing this procedure with a minimum of discomfort to the patient.

Strict asepsis must be practiced. The patient should be placed in dorsal recumbency, and a 1-cm skin incision should be made on the ventral midline approximately 2 cm caudal to the umbilicus. Blunt dissection to the linea alba should be performed using a hemostat. The linea should be grasped at one or both ends of the incision using hemostats or forceps allowing for the creation of tension. A number 11 scalpel blade is then used to create a 2- to 3-mm incision in the linea. The catheter should be placed through a separate skin incision 2 cm lateral to the insertion site. This creates a small subcutaneous

*10.2 to 12 Fr 30-cm Thoracic Two-Part Drainage Catheter Set, SurgiVet/Smiths Medical, Dublin, OH; Pigtail Drainage Catheter Set, Infinitimedical LLC, Menlo Park, CA.

tunnel, making the collection system less susceptible to contamination. When using this technique in the postoperative setting, the catheter should never be inserted through the laparotomy incision and instead should be placed 3 to 4 cm off midline. If the catheter is of a type in which the trochar protrudes from the tip of the catheter, it should be withdrawn to just inside the catheter. The trochar and catheter may then be inserted into the peritoneal cavity in a dorsocaudal direction (toward the pelvic inlet). After the trochar and catheter are 2 to 3 cm inside the peritoneal cavity, the catheter may be advanced over the trochar. Dead space in the subcutaneous tissues should be eliminated and the skin incision closed routinely. A purse-string and finger-trap suture should be used to secure the catheter to the skin at the insertion site. A sterile dressing should be applied and changed at regular intervals.

Paracentesis with a Fenestrated Catheter Using the Seldinger Technique

Abdominal paracentesis may also be performed using a fenestrated catheter placed via the Seldinger technique.* The patient should be sedated and prepared as described previously, positioned in dorsal recumbency, and the urinary bladder evacuated. Landmarks are similar to those described earlier. Local anesthetic usage will facilitate this procedure. Briefly, a small incision is made in the skin and subcutaneous tissues using a number 11 scalpel blade. A puncture needle is used to penetrate the body wall and a guidewire is introduced into the peritoneal space. Serial dilation of the tract is performed over the wire and then the fenestrated catheter is placed over the wire with or without use of a peel-away introducer. Once in place, the catheter may be secured and dressed as described earlier.

Surgical Placement of Closed Suction Drains

CSD has allowed surgeons to find a middle ground between the sometimes risky method of primary closure of the abdominal cavity and the labor-intensive method of providing OPD in the patient with acute, effusive, surgically treated abdominal disease (e.g., septic peritonitis).[7]

Numerous types of closed suction drains exist, ranging from flat drains with multiple fenestrations (Jackson-Pratt†) to those that are fluted (Blake‡) (Figure 133-1), designs that are resistant to obstruction by omentum, tissue, and cellular debris. Most closed suction drains are made out of silicone. Closed suction drains are placed as the last step before abdominal closure. In a cat or small dog, a single 10-Fr drain maybe placed in a craniocaudal direction. In larger dogs, dual 10- or 15-Fr drains may be placed parallel to one another in a craniocaudal direction, or with one drain located cranially and the other located more caudal. The drains may exit the skin 2 to 3 cm lateral to midline.

Most drains come swaged onto a steel trochar that is used to pass the drain tubing from the intraabdominal space to the drain exit site. The drains should never exit from the laparotomy incision. Ideally the trochar/drain is passed through the abdominal wall and into the subcutaneous tissues and then tunneled approximately 2 cm before exiting the skin. They should be secured with a purse-string and finger-trap suture at the exit point. Once the abdomen is closed, the drains should be connected to the negative pressure reservoirs that have an integrated antireflux valves.§ The drain exit sites should be covered with sterile dressings and an abdominal bandage. The negative pressure reservoir may then be attached to the abdominal bandage. The sterile dressing and abdominal bandage should be replaced daily and the ostomy site and surgical incision evaluated for evidence of infection.

Drain reservoirs should be evacuated at regular intervals, not just when they are full, because drainage systems vary in their rate of loss of suction during filling.[8] Drain effluent should be evaluated every 24 to 48 hours to ensure that the underlying disease process is resolving. The author prefers to collect these samples for cytologic analysis from the drain tubing rather than the reservoir. Routine precautions to prevent contamination of the drain tubing or reservoir should be performed. The drains may be removed when the drainage declines to acceptable levels (5 to 10 ml/kg q24h), patient condition is improving, and cytologic characteristics of the drain fluid show a resolving inflammatory response and no evidence of infection. The presence of indwelling drains may place the patient at risk for hospital-acquired infection, but this hazard may be minimized by strict attention to aseptic technique while handling the drains and while changing the dressings. Overall advantages of CSD over OPD include reduced labor, elimination of the risk of visceral herniation, easy quantification of drain output, and elimination of the need for another surgical intervention for abdominal closure in the resolving peritonitis case.[3]

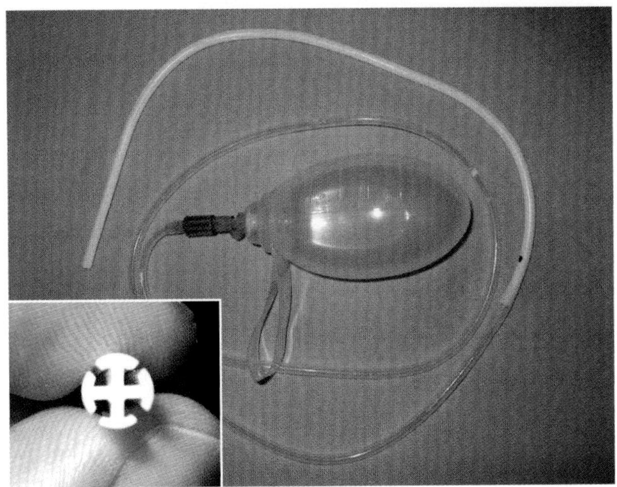

FIGURE 133-1 Blake drain (Blake Drain Kit, Ethicon Inc., Somerville, NJ). Note cross-sectional view illustrating channels for fluid retrieval. After placement, the negative pressure reservoir is attached (J-Vac, Ethicon Inc., Somerville, NJ).

Open Peritoneal Drainage Technique

OPD was the original alternative to primary closure in patients with septic peritonitis.[9,10] Once source control has been established and the abdominal cavity lavaged thoroughly, the OPD technique may be performed. In male dogs the parapreputial aspect of the ventral midline incision is closed routinely. A urinary catheter should be placed in all dogs to prevent urine from soiling the abdominal dressing and to help quantify urine output. The technique for providing OPD involves placement of a monofilament suture (most often 2-0 or 0 polypropylene) in the external rectus sheath as is routine for closure of a ventral midline abdominal incision. However, the sutures are not pulled tight, leaving a gap for drainage of approximately 2 to 4 cm. Sutures prevent evisceration during bandage changes (Figure 133-2). A sterile, nonadherent dressing* is then placed over the abdominal incision. This is followed by a large layer of highly absorbent sterile dressing† and a sterile hand towel. The entire bandage is

*Tenckhoff Acute Peritoneal Dialysis Catheters, Cook Medical, Bloomington, IN; Pigtail Drainage Catheter Set, Infinitimedical LLC, Menlo Park, CA.
†Jackson-Pratt Wound Drainage Systems, Cardinal Health, Dublin OH.
‡Blake Drain Kit, Ethicon Inc., Somerville, NJ.
§J-Vac, Ethicon Inc., Somerville, NJ.

*Adaptic, Johnson & Johnson Medical, Gargrave, Skipton, UK.
†SteriRoll, Franklin-Williams, Lexington, KY.

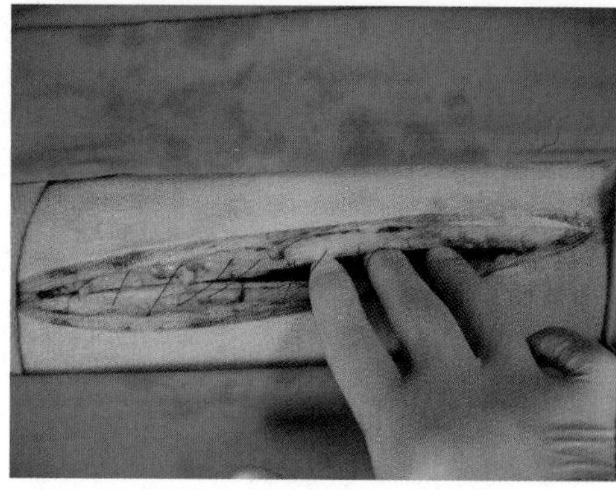

FIGURE 133-2 Suture placement technique for open peritoneal drainage.

secured using cast padding,* stretchable roll gauze,† and additional bandaging materials as needed. The external bandage material should extend far cranial and caudal to the abdominal incision to ensure that it will remain covered in the event of bandage migration.

The abdominal dressing should be changed a minimum of 1 to 2 times daily and always when strike-through is evident. Weighing the abdominal dressing before placement and after removal may help quantify fluid losses and thus help direct fluid therapy. During bandage change, sterile-gloved fingers may be inserted into the abdominal cavity between sutures to ensure that fibrin and abdominal organs are not precluding effective abdominal drainage. Abdominal fluid should be evaluated daily or every 48 hours.

Once abdominal drainage has decreased and cytologic characteristics of the drainage fluid show evidence of resolving inflammatory response and no evidence of infection, the abdomen may be closed. The author advocates reexploration and lavage of the abdomen at the time of closure. Cultures may be collected from the abdominal cavity. The subcutaneous and skin layers are debrided as needed, lavaged, and closed routinely. OPD may place the patient at risk for hospital-acquired infection, but this hazard may be prevented by strict attention to aseptic technique while performing dressing changes. Advantages of OPD include effective drainage and the ability to reexplore the abdomen at the time of closure. Finally, OPD helps create an aerobic environment in the peritoneal space.[11]

Vacuum-Assisted Drainage

VAD involves the application of controlled, evenly distributed subatmospheric pressure to the peritoneal space via a reticulated polyurethane foam. VAD has been thoroughly evaluated in humans with septic peritonitis and the technique is generally applied for 48 to 72 hours before changing the system. In veterinary medicine, two techniques have been described.[2,3] using a noncommercial VAD system. Briefly, the abdomen is partially closed, similar to the method described for OPD. Then a reticulated polyurethane foam is positioned over the open portion of the abdomen between the subcutaneous tissues and skin. Next, a 14- to 18-Fr red rubber catheter is inserted into the foam and an impermeable, adherent dressing is applied. The catheter was then secured to a vacuum pump with 75 to 125 mm Hg negative pressure. In these studies, bandage changes were planned every 48 hours but often were required every 24 hours.[3] In humans a visceral protective layer is placed between the foam and the viscera to prevent adhesion to the foam and pressure-induced trauma to the viscera. VAD will require further investigation in dogs before it can be considered a safe, effective method with similar outcomes to CSD and OPD methods for the management of septic peritonitis in dogs and cats.

*Specialist Cast Padding, BSN Medical, Rutherford College, NC.
†Curity Stretch Bandages, Covidien, Mansfield, MA.

COMPLICATIONS OF PERITONEAL DRAINAGE

Volume and Albumin Loss

All surgical procedures have inherent disadvantages and complications. A knowledge and expectation of certain complications inherent to peritoneal drainage techniques will allow the clinician to anticipate and modulate these.

Injury to internal structures during nonsurgical placement of drainage devices could result in acute hemorrhage, leakage of urine, or septic peritonitis. With attention to appropriate technique, these complications are rare.

Anytime the peritoneum is evacuated of fluid, the patient will suffer a volume loss as well as potential loss of albumin and other proteins. Appreciation that abdominal fluid is in flux with the extracellular fluid volume and that significant volumes of fluid can be lost as a result of ongoing drainage will allow the clinician to replace fluid volumes and provide oncotic support as necessary.

One advantage of the CSD technique is easy quantification of volume loss. Comparing the weight of the dry OPD bandage with its weight after removal can give an estimate of fluid losses through the OPD site. Close attention should be paid to total volume losses as well as patient albumin concentration, colloid osmotic pressure, and evidence of peripheral edema when choosing a fluid therapy regimen. Early nutritional support should be strongly considered in patients with acute abdominal illness.

CONCLUSION

A variety of peritoneal drainage techniques are available to allow clinicians to provide one-time, intermittent, or sustained drainage for patients requiring evacuation of fluid from the peritoneal cavity. Attention to indications, contraindications, and aseptic technique will allow these techniques to be employed with minimal complications.

REFERENCES

1. Alexander JW, Korelitz J, Alexander NS: Prevention of wound infections, a case for closed suction drainage to remove wound fluids deficient in opsonic proteins, Am J Surg 132:59, 1976.
2. Buote NJ, Havig ME: The use of vacuum-assisted closure in the management of septic peritonitis in six dogs, J Am Anim Hosp Assoc 48:164, 2012.
3. Cioffi KM, Schmiedt CW, Cornell KK, et al: Retrospective evaluation of vacuum-assisted peritoneal drainage for the treatment of septic peritonitis in dogs and cats: 8 cases (2003-2010), J Vet Emerg Crit Care 22:601, 2012.
4. Walker EM, Ellis H: Relationship of the constituents of bile to biliary peritonitis in the rat, Gut 19:827, 1978.
5. Andersson R, Schalen C, Tranberg KG: The effect of intraperitoneal bile on growth, peritoneal absorption and blood clearance of Escherichia coli in E. coli peritonitis, Arch Surg 126:773, 1991.
6. Conzemius MG, Sammarco JL, Holt DE, et al: Clinical determination of preoperative and postoperative intra-abdominal pressures in dogs, Vet Surg 24:195, 1995.
7. Mueller MG, Ludwig LL, Barton LJ: Use of closed-suction drains to treat generalized peritonitis in dogs and cats: 40 cases (1997-1999), J Am Vet Med Assoc 219:789, 2001.
8. Halfacree ZJ, Wilson AM, Baines SJ: Evaluation of in vitro performance of suction drains, Am J Vet Res 70:283, 2009.
9. Woolfson JM, Dulisch ML: Open abdominal drainage in the treatment of generalized peritonitis in 25 dogs and cats, Vet Surg 15:27, 1986.
10. Greenfield CL, Walshaw R: Open peritoneal drainage for treatment of contaminated peritoneal cavity and septic peritonitis in dogs and cats: 24 cases (1980-1986), J Am Vet Med Assoc 191:100, 1987.
11. Culp WTN, Holt DE: Septic peritonitis, Comp Cont Ed Vet Oct E1, 2010.

CHAPTER 134
POSTTHORACOTOMY MANAGEMENT

Julien Guillaumin, DrVet, DACVECC • Christopher A. Adin, DVM, DACVS

KEY POINTS

- Postoperative management of the patient after thoracotomy requires intensive monitoring of pulmonary and cardiovascular function.
- Optimization of oxygen delivery is the primary goal during the postoperative period.
- Hypoxemia, hypotension, and arrhythmias are very common after thoracotomy.
- Aggressive pain control to improve comfort and ventilation is essential.

Thoracotomy is routinely performed in numerous veterinary patients; both as an elective and emergency intervention. As technical capabilities in anesthesia and surgery have advanced, demands for intensive care after thoracotomy have also expanded and postoperative care is now one of the major areas of focus for the intensivist. Complications after thoracic surgery are common and often life threatening; as such, intensive care monitoring is essential to maintain acceptable outcomes.

Specific conditions treated with thoracic surgery include chest wall diseases (e.g., penetrating bite wounds, impalement); cardiac conditions (e.g., pericardectomy, surgical correction of patent ductus arteriosus [PDA], open-chest cardiopulmonary resuscitation [CPR]); pathologic lung conditions (e.g., lung mass resection, pulmonary abscess); pleural space abnormalities (e.g., pyothorax, pneumothorax, neoplastic effusion); and esophageal, mediastinal, and diaphragmatic diseases. Because of the complex nature of these conditions, animals that are undergoing thoracotomy are often affected by comorbidities that complicate postoperative management. This chapter reviews the common complications in companion animals undergoing thoracic surgery, focusing on early recognition and prevention.

IMMEDIATE POSTTHORACOTOMY ASSESSMENT

The assessment of the patient recovering from surgery after thoracotomy involves three major areas: postoperative pain, lung function (i.e., ventilation and oxygenation), and volume status. A minimum database begins with a thorough physical examination: rectal temperature, perfusion parameters, chest auscultation, and assessment of pain (see Chapter 1). Diagnostic tests should include packed cell volume/total protein (PCV/TP), blood pressure, and pulse oximetry on all patients after thoracotomy. Additionally, an arterial blood gas measurement with special attention to PaO_2, $PaCO_2$, and lactate may be indicated (see Chapter 186). Other monitoring tools include electrocardiogram (ECG) with arrhythmia monitoring, urine production, serial monitoring of physical examination and blood work, and qualitative and quantitative assessment of thoracic drainage. Table 134-1 presents some examples of common postthoracotomy complications, their potential causes, and steps to diagnose and treat those complications.

ANALGESIA

The intensity of pain after thoracotomy is reported to be high in humans, and there are no reasons to believe it should be different in small animals.[1] Noxious input from the skin incision, cut or retracted muscle, fractured or excised ribs, and damaged parietal pleura are transmitted along the intercostal nerves.[1] Noxious stimuli from the lung may be carried by the vagus nerve, and those from the mediastinum, diaphragm, and pericardial pleura may be relayed by the phrenic nerve.[1] Pain impairs ventilation and may result in hypoxemia. Pain also affects catecholamine levels and coagulation and activates the stress response, which is implicated in excessive thrombosis and systemic inflammatory response syndrome (SIRS).[1]

There is conflicting evidence regarding the surgical technique used and subsequent pain, although most clinicians believe that a median sternotomy is associated with a higher need for postoperative analgesia than a lateral thoracotomy.[2,3] Altering the method of wire cerclage closure or limiting the extent of the sternotomy in order to preserve the manubrium, the xiphoid, or both can improve mechanical stability of the sternum after surgery and seems to play a role in immediate pain management.[4] Similarly, muscle-sparing approaches, alternative closure techniques for lateral thoracotomy, and the use of minimally invasive surgery are reported as methods to decrease postoperative pain.[5,6]

Several pain control strategies are available for postthoracotomy patients. It is commonly believed that a multimodal approach is beneficial, with the expectation that the effect of each will be at least additive, if not synergistic, and side effects of each will be minimized.[1]

It is important to realize that even though local analgesia provides additional pain control, it only stops pain from tissues supplied by the blocked nerves. It is therefore imperative that additional intravenous analgesia is provided (see Chapter 144). Most surgeons, anesthesiologists and intensivists recommend the use of fentanyl for its analgesic potency and ability to quickly titrate to effect, although other μ agonists (e.g., oxymorphone, hydromorphone, morphine) can be used. Buprenorphine has also been recommended, although its lower analgesic potential and longer effect impair the ability to titrate analgesic effects and are regarded as undesirable.

The classic recommended dose of fentanyl is 1 to 5 mcg/kg/hr, although fentanyl research is scarce in veterinary medicine. However, in dogs an average plasma fentanyl concentration of 1.18 ng/ml was found to be as analgesic as approximately 0.05 mg/kg intramuscular oxymorphone.[7] This analgesic plasma concentration of 1.01 to 1.25 ng/ml has been obtained in conscious dogs receiving a single fentanyl injection (10 mcg/kg intravenously [IV]) followed by a constant rate infusion (CRI) of 10 mcg/kg/hr. Although there were wide interindividual variations, it is possible that the recommended dose

Table 134-1 Type of Complications, Potential Causes, Monitoring, and Therapeutic Options for Patients Recovering from Thoracotomy Surgery

Complication Type	Potential Causes	Monitoring Option	Therapeutic Options
Hypoxemia	V/Q mismatch Hypoventilation Severe pleural space disease Pain PTE	Respiratory rate and effort Chest auscultation SpO_2 Arterial blood gas	Oxygen supplementation Positive pressure ventilation Mobilization of patient (if deemed safe) (See Hypoventilation)
Hypoventilation	Pain Sensitivity to pain medication Pleural space disease	Respiratory rate Chest auscultation Venous/arterial blood gas Capnometry	Addition of pain medication Reversal of pain medication Mobilization of patient (if deemed safe) Evacuation of pleural space cavity using chest tube or thoracocentesis
Immediate postoperative dysphoria/hyperreactivity	Drug-associated dysphoria Pain Hypersensitivity to tight bandage (cat especially)	Not applicable	Fast- and short-acting sedation (e.g., acepromazine, dexmedetomidine) Reassessment of pain regimen Reassessment of bandage strategy
Anemia/hemorrhage	Primarily caused by surgery Hemostatic disorders Hypothermia	Platelet count Clotting times Buccal mucosal bleeding time Other platelet function assays (e.g., PFA 100)	Transfusion of FFP and PRBCs as needed Use of hemostatic agents (e.g., aminocaproic acid, tranexamic acid) Administration of DDAVP for thrombocytopathia Surgical exploration
Postoperative pain caused by surgical incision and chest drain	Various	None	Paravertebral block Interpleural block Possible addition of NSAIDs, intravenous ketamine CRI, intravenous dexmedetomidine CRI
Potential postoperative chest infection or postoperative pyothorax	Surgical Caused by primary disease Caused by chest tube	Complete blood cell count Blood culture Pleural fluid culture	Administration of intravenous antimicrobials Removal of chest tube
Wound complications	Dead space present because of surgical intervention Surgical technique Surgical asepsis	Complete blood cell count Wound culture PCV-TP Albumin Oncotic pressure	Use of antimicrobials if indicated Bandage (including pressure bandage) Vacuum-assisted closure device

CRI, Constant rate infusion; *FFP,* fresh frozen plasma; *NSAIDs,* nonsteroidal antiinflammatory drugs; PRBC, packed red blood cells; *PTE,* pulmonary thromboembolism; *V/Q,* ventilation-perfusion.

of fentanyl CRI may be insufficient for a number of dogs.[8] See Chapter 144 for more details on doses for analgesic medications.

In recent years, it has been a clinical choice to use a multimodal approach of intravenous analgesia for severe pain, including in postthoracotomy patients, with a continuous intravenous infusion of a "cocktail" of morphine, lidocaine, and ketamine, also known as the MLK protocol. It should be noted that a MLK protocol (morphine 3.3 mcg/kg/min, lidocaine 50 mcg/kg/min, and ketamine 10 mcg/kg/min) showed no difference in lowering the isoflurane minimum alveolar concentration (MAC) compared with morphine alone (45% versus 48%, respectively).[9] Along with the increased use of fentanyl, combinations of intravenous fentanyl, lidocaine, and ketamine CRI (sometimes called FLK) have become popular among veterinarians, although there is no evidence to suggest that FLK is more beneficial that fentanyl alone. Lidocaine as a continuous infusion should be avoided in cats, or the dosage reduced to decrease potential toxicity and cardiovascular depression.

Using ketamine as a continuous infusion in addition to an opioid also adds some antagonism to N-methyl-D-aspartate and may be beneficial for lowering postoperative pain, especially when combined with local or epidural analgesia.[1] The use of low doses of an α_2 agonist (medetomidine or dexmedetomidine) may be considered as an alternative method for supplemental analgesia, despite their side effects (e.g., increase peripheral resistance as a result of vasoconstriction, bradycardia, and decreased cardiac output).

Intercostal nerve blocks can be used for relieving pain after thoracotomy. A minimum of 2 adjacent intercostal spaces on both side of the incision should be blocked because of overlap of nerve supply. The site for needle placement is the caudal border of the rib near the intervertebral foramen. Depending on the size of the dog, 0.25 to 1 ml of 0.5% bupivacaine can be instilled per site and may control postthoracotomy pain for 3 to 6 hours after a successful block.[10] Although not commonly used in veterinary medicine, a paravertebral catheter (which can be placed during surgery) allows for continuous analgesia and is as effective as epidural analgesia in humans.[11]

Interpleural analgesia with bupivacaine can be administered, especially if a thoracostomy tube has been placed. Because the pain from the thoracotomy arises from intercostal nerves on the dorsal aspect of the dog, the use of analgesia instilled into the interpleural space has been questioned, and conflicting reports regarding interpleural analgesia exist in human medicine.[11,12] Three possible mechanisms of analgesia are proposed, although full mechanisms are not well understood: retrograde diffusion of anesthetic causing intercostal nerve block, unilateral block of the thoracic sympathetic chain and splanchnic nerves, and diffusion of anesthetic into the ipsilateral brachial plexus.

There is evidence in dogs to suggest that interpleural infusion has some benefits compared with systemic administration of opioids. Interpleural analgesia with bupivacaine (1.5 mg/kg q4h) has been shown to provide better analgesia than buprenorphine (10 mcg/kg

IV q6h) in dogs. Interestingly, it also improved PaO_2 and oxygen saturation, probably through improved ventilation and decreased atelectasis.[13] Bolus interpleural bupivacaine is effective in relieving postthoracotomy pain for 3 to 12 hours.[14] Interpleural administration of bupivacaine may be contraindicated if the pericardium has been disrupted.

The protocol used at the author's institution is briefly described here (for dogs):

1. The dose is 1.5 mg/kg (0.3 ml/kg using bupivacaine 0.5%).
2. Dilute bupivacaine with 3 parts 0.9% NaCl.
3. One part sodium bicarbonate 8.4% can be added to 9 parts of the diluted solution to decrease pain at the time of administration
4. The solution should be administered slowly and should remain in the pleural space for at least 30 minutes; the patient should be kept with the incision side down
5. This treatment can be repeated q4-6h with a maximum dose of bupivacaine of 9 mg/kg/day.

Animals with effusive pleural space disease are not good candidates for interpleural analgesia because of dilution of the drug that renders it ineffective.

Epidural analgesia with an epidural catheter is considered the standard for postthoracotomy analgesia in humans.[1] However, its use is limited in veterinary medicine because of perceived or real technical difficulty in small dogs, potential damage to the spinal cord and meninges, risk of infection, and other catheter-related problems. However, with practice, epidural catheter placement is feasible, especially in large dogs, and complications can be minimized with proper protocols for placement and care.[10] Opioids (usually preservative-free morphine) or local anesthetics such as lidocaine or bupivacaine are commonly used for epidural analgesia, although other drugs and analgesics have been used.[10,15,16] Epidural analgesia can also be achieved by bolus injection without placing a catheter, although the analgesic effects will be limited in duration (usually less than 24 hours with a morphine-bupivacaine combination).[16] Hemostatic disorders are an absolute contraindication for epidural catheter placement. Complications of epidural catheter are reported to be around 20% in small animals, with catheter dislodgement and catheter site contamination being the most common complications.[17]

In summary, the best analgesic strategy aims at multiple anatomic and pharmacologic sites of actions, such as using combinations of (1) neuronal blockade by local anesthetics; (2) infusion of opioids intravenously; (3) nonsteroidal antiinflammatory drugs (NSAIDs) if toxicity is not of concern; and (4) other analgesic agents if refractory (e.g., ketamine, lidocaine, or dexmedetomidine), taking into account potential benefits and known side effects.[1,15]

Postthoracotomy Pain Syndrome in Humans

In humans, long-term pain associated with thoracotomy has been recognized for several decades and is called *postthoracotomy pain syndrome (PTPS)*. In humans, published data suggest that PTPS can affect more than 50% of thoracotomy patients. It is a chronic condition, and a large proportion of patients may experience pain for years after surgery. Most patients experience pain along the general area of the thoracotomy scar, but pain can also occur elsewhere in the body. Allodynia, the sensation of pain in response to a normally nonpainful stimulus, is a common feature of PTPS. The exact pathogenesis of PTPS is unclear, but cumulative evidence suggests a combination of neuropathic and nonneuropathic pain. Pain intensity 24 hours after surgery, analgesic consumption during the first postoperative day and week, female gender, chest wall resection, and pleurectomy have been proven risk factors for PTPS. Since reports of a predictive relationship between an immediate postoperative intense pain and PTPS, it has been suggested that adopting an aggressive and effective postoperative analgesic regimen might reduce the incidence of PTPS, although few studies are available to date.

Treatment is symptomatic and, as with most forms of neuropathic pain, is also difficult and often unsatisfactory. First-line management includes physical therapy, NSAIDs, electrical nerve stimulation, tricyclic antidepressants, antiepileptics, sodium channel blockers, and opioids.[18] The authors are not aware of a description of PTPS in veterinary medicine, and the ability to consistently recognize this condition may be confounded by a number of factors that are unique to veterinary patients and by a lack of awareness among veterinary clinicians.

VENTILATION

Ventilatory drive can be depressed by anesthetic drugs, pleural space diseases, tight thoracic bandages, or somatic pain (see Chapter 16).[2] Hypoventilation can be perpetuated and aggravated by pleural space and chest wall disorders such as pneumothorax or pleural effusion resulting from the surgical procedure, thoracostomy tube placement, or the primary disease process (e.g., chylothorax, pyothorax).

Respiratory rate should be monitored and changes investigated and treated. Thoracic auscultation may be used to detect decreased lung sounds, especially unilateral, which may indicate pleural space disease. Hypoventilation can be detected using capnometry in the intubated patient. Recently, monitoring of end-tidal CO_2 was described using nasal catheters in spontaneously breathing critically ill dogs, although caution should be exercised in animals with respiratory disease or those receiving oxygen supplementation.[19] Alternatively, direct measurement of venous PCO_2 is of equal value to arterial blood samples for detecting hypoventilation in animals with normal perfusion.

Strategies for treating hypoventilation in the postoperative patient are dependent on the cause and could include evacuation of pleural contents, use of alternative bandaging techniques to decrease thoracic compression, addition of pain medications to allow lung expansion, or reversal of analgesic agents in the case of excessive ventilatory drive suppression.

HYPOXEMIA

The effect of thoracotomy on lung function has been well studied. After thoracotomy, even with analgesia, dogs had significant decreases in arterial pH, PaO_2, and SaO_2 and significant increases in $PaCO_2$ and alveolar-arterial oxygen differences in the postoperative period. After surgery, a decrease in lung compliance (up to 50%), an increase in work of breathing (up to 200%), and an increase in pulmonary resistance (up to almost 400%) may be observed.[20]

The cause of those changes is multifactorial. Penetration into the pleural space results in loss of negative interpleural pressure, which causes atelectasis and V/Q mismatch (see Chapter 15). This V/Q mismatch can be further aggravated by surgical manipulation of the lungs during the surgical procedure. Even after surgical closure and reestablishment of negative pleural pressure, atelectasis may be present because of recumbency or insufficient analgesia causing pain during inspiration.

Other causes for postoperative hypoxemia include hypoventilation, lung edema (e.g., reexpansion pulmonary edema), acute lung injury (ALI), and acute respiratory distress syndrome (ARDS) or a primary disease process (e.g., pneumonia, neoplasia) (see Respiratory Disorders section for further details).

Although oxygenation and ventilation issues are usually well controlled during general anesthesia with the help of 100% inspired oxygen, assisted intraoperative ventilation, and intraoperative analgesia, the transition to the intensive care unit (ICU) can result in a severe decrease oxygenation and hypoventilation. Changes in respiratory rate and effort may be the first indications of pulmonary insufficiency. An acute change may be an indication of chest wall (e.g., pain), pleural space (e.g., hemothorax or pneumothorax), or parenchymal (e.g., atelectasis, hemorrhage, edema) disease. Many of these issues can be addressed with additional analgesia, emptying of the pleural cavity using the chest tube, or providing supplemental oxygen. Thoracic auscultation findings (e.g., decreased lung sounds, pulmonary crackles, or increased lung sounds) can help direct the clinician toward suspicion for parenchymal versus pleural space disease. Respiratory rate and effort and thoracic auscultation should be performed regularly on each postthoracotomy patient.

Pulse oximetry is a noninvasive and readily available method to assess oxygen saturation. It can be used to assess oxygenation ability in the respiratory distress patient and, when normal, can quickly raise suspicion for nonrespiratory causes of distress (e.g., pain, anxiety, anemia, hypovolemia). When hypoxemia is suggested by pulse oximetry, arterial blood gases should be used to confirm hypoxemia when possible (see Chapter 186). In patients with confirmed hypoxemia, additional diagnostics include thoracic focused assessment with sonogram for trauma (TFAST scan), diagnostic thoracocentesis, or chest tube aspiration and chest radiographs.

Treatment for hypoxemia involves identifying and treating the underlying cause if possible. For example, proper nursing care, analgesia, and early mobilization decrease atelectasis and improve oxygenation. Oxygen supplementation is always indicated for patients with respiratory distress while waiting for test results. Oxygen supplementation can be provided by using an oxygen cage, mask, or hood or nasal catheter. If noninvasive management is insufficient, anesthesia, intubation, and positive pressure ventilation are indicated (see Chapter 30).

HYPOVOLEMIA

Direct blood loss during thoracic surgery is an obvious cause of hypovolemia; however, relative hypovolemia can also occur during thoracotomy because of decreased venous return associated with the collapse of large intrathoracic veins after entering the chest cavity and loss of negative interpleural pressure. Evaporative losses during surgery can also contribute to hypovolemia.

Assessment of organ perfusion is performed at the time of patient admission to the ICU and should be followed by careful and targeted serial physical examinations until full recovery. Shock is a physical examination diagnosis and should be investigated using an examination that is targeted to six perfusions parameters: tachycardia (can be bradycardia in cats), poor pulse quality, pale mucous membranes, prolonged capillary refill time (CRT), cold extremities, and a decreased mental state (see Chapter 5). In animals showing evidence of shock, treatment with fluid immediately should be initiated. Fluid choice depends on additional parameters and clinician's preference and includes crystalloid, synthetic colloids, and blood products (see Chapters 58, 60, and 61).

COMPLICATIONS AND MORTALITY AFTER THORACOTOMY

There is a paucity of literature regarding outcome and complications of thoracotomy in dogs and cats, especially in the immediate postoperative period, because some authors exclude from statistical analysis patients who died within 2 to 7 days.[21,22] Overall mortality rates for patients recovering from thoracotomy are reported between 11% and 44% but seem to be highly dependent on the indication for thoracotomy, with higher mortality rate for thoracic neoplasia and lower for surgical correction of PDA.[22-25]

Postoperative complications are common after thoracic surgery in dogs. Retrospective studies indicate that between 36% and 47% of animals experience complications in the postoperative period.[21,22,25] Complications (especially related to wound healing) may be more common for pyothorax (45%) and after median sternotomy (71%).[21]

Complications of thoracotomy can be divided into several categories based on etiology. Complications from the surgical approach are most common (between 22% and 71% of patients) and include seroma, ventral edema, wound inflammation, wound discharge, incision dehiscence, and ipsilateral thoracic limb lameness.[2,6,21,22] Complications related to the thoracostomy tube are also common (22% in one study) and include pneumothorax, pain, inflammation, and infection.[21] Complications associated with the surgery itself (hemothorax, hypoventilation, reexpansion pulmonary edema, hypothermia, shock, SIRS, and multiorgan dysfunction syndrome) are less common but often life threatening, and early recognition is crucial.[3,22] Finally, some patients develop complications that are related to their primary disease, such as aspiration pneumonia, pulmonary contusions, coagulopathy, arrhythmia, infection, or neoplasia.

Hypothermia

Hypothermia results from a loss of heat from the large surface area within the thoracic cavity that is exposed to room air and therefore is dependent on length of surgery. Hypothermia is associated with disturbances in cardiovascular function, respiratory function, and coagulation (see Chapter 148). Because of the known risks of hypothermia, proactive patient warming is crucial in animals undergoing thoracotomy and should be performed continuously throughout the anesthetic and immediate postoperative recovery period, as indicated by temperature monitoring. In many hospitals, anesthesiologists use circulating water blankets underneath the patient to prevent convective heat loss, with additional circulating warm air blankets placed over the animal recovering in ICU.

Thoracostomy Tube Care

Thoracostomy tube placement before closure is almost always indicated after thoracic surgery.[2,3] Maintenance of a postoperative thoracostomy tube allows drainage of air or fluid from the interpleural space and maintains negative interpleural pressure. In certain elective cardiac procedures (e.g., PDA ligation), accumulation of air or fluid after surgery is rare and surgeons may elect to remove the thoracostomy tube or catheter before recovery from anesthesia.

Multiple protocols exist for management of thoracostomy tubes, and frequency of aspiration must be tailored to the needs of the individual patient (see Chapter 199). Chest tube evacuation is typically performed every 1 to 4 hours, depending on breathing pattern of the patient and recent fluid/air production. The tube can be removed when two or more consecutive evacuations are "negative." Historically it was believed that the presence of a thoracostomy tube resulted in the production of 1 to 2 ml/kg body weight (BW)/day of pleural fluid, although recent evidence is lacking on that subject. Air and liquid should be recorded and monitored. Analysis of the pleural fluid is common, although controversial, and interpretations should be made in light of the overall patient status and accompanying diagnostic tests.[26]

The incidence of infection associated with closed placement of chest drains in human medicine is 9% to 12%. In a 2010 abstract, 61 dogs and 8 cats were included in a prospective cohort study after thoracostomy tube placement.[26] The mean volume of pleural fluid produced at the time of tube removal was 0.57 ml/kg/hr. Microbial culture yielded a positive result in 19% of the cases, and the duration the tube was in place was significantly and positively associated with an increased risk of a positive bacterial culture. Of the 13 patients with positive microbial culture results, three developed clinical signs of septic pleuritis, of which two died.[26]

If the surgeon expects chronic filling of the chest cavity by air or chylous or neoplastic infusion, a pleural access port and drainage catheter can be placed at the time of surgery.[27] Aspiration of the thorax is performed using a specially adapted Huber needle to puncture a subcutaneous access port. Similar to a standard thoracostomy tube, this device can also be used to instill local analgesics, antimicrobials, or chemotherapy agents after surgery. Because of the nature of this long-term implant, strict aseptic technique is required when accessing the subcutaneous port.

CONCLUSION

Thoracotomy patients can be challenging and the perioperative mortality can be significant. Knowledge of possible complications and integration of all aspects of anesthesia (e.g., perioperative pain control), surgery (e.g., wound and thoracostomy tube management), and critical care (e.g., blood gas analysis, fluid resuscitation, oxygenation and ventilation) are important to ensure the best possible outcome for these patients.

REFERENCES

1. Ochroch EA, Gottschalk A: Impact of acute pain and its management for thoracic surgical patients, Thorac Surg Clinics 15(1):105, 2005.
2. Radlinsky MG: Thoracic cavity. In Tobias KM, Johnston SA, editors: Veterinary surgery: small animal, vol 2, St Louis, 2011, Saunders, pp 1787-1812; 105.
3. Hunt GB: Thoracic wall. In Tobias KM, Johnston SA, editors: Veterinary surgery: small animal, vol 2, St Louis, 2011, Saunders, pp 1769-1786; 104.
4. Davis KM, Roe SC, Mathews KG, et al: Median sternotomy closure in dogs: a mechanical comparison of technique stability, Vet Surg 35(3):271, 2006.
5. Rooney MB, Mehl M, Monnet E: Intercostal thoracotomy closure: transcostal sutures as a less painful alternative to circumcostal suture placement, Vet Surg 33(3):209, 2004.
6. Walsh PJ, Remedios AM, Ferguson JF, et al: Thoracoscopic versus open partial pericardectomy in dogs: Comparison of postoperative pain and morbidity, Vet Surg 28(6):472, 1999.
7. Kyles AE, Hardie EM, Hansen BD, et al: Comparison of transdermal fentanyl and intramuscular oxymorphone on post-operative behaviour after ovariohysterectomy in dogs, Res Vet Sci 65(3):245, 1998.
8. Sano T, Nishimura R, Kanazawa H, et al: Pharmacokinetics of fentanyl after single intravenous injection and constant rate infusion in dogs, Vet Anaesth Analg 33(4):266, 2006.
9. Muir WW 3rd, Wiese AJ, March PA: Effects of morphine, lidocaine, ketamine, and morphine-lidocaine-ketamine drug combination on minimum alveolar concentration in dogs anesthetized with isoflurane, Am J Vet Res 64(9):1155, 2003.
10. Skarda RT, Tranquili WJ: Local and regional anesthetic and analgesic techniques: dogs. In Tranquilli WJ, Thurmon JC, Grimm KA, editors: Lumb & Jones' veterinary anesthesia and analgesia, ed 4, vol 1, Ames, IA, 2007, Wiley-Blackwell, pp 561-594; 20.
11. Silomon M, Claus T, Huwer H, et al: Interpleural analgesia does not influence postthoracotomy pain, Anesth Analg 91(1):44, 2000.
12. McIlvaine WB: Pro: intrapleural anesthesia is useful for thoracic analgesia, J Cardiothorac Vasc Anesth 10(3):425, 1996.
13. Conzemius MG, Brockman DJ, King LG, et al: Analgesia in dogs after intercostal thoracotomy: a clinical trial comparing intravenous buprenorphine and interpleural bupivacaine, Vet Surg 23(4):291, 1994.
14. Thompson SE, Johnson JM: Analgesia in dogs after intercostal thoracotomy. A comparison of morphine, selective intercostal nerve block, and interpleural regional analgesia with bupivacaine, Vet Surg 20(1):73, 1991.
15. Pavlidou K, Papazoglou L, Savvas I, et al: Analgesia for small animal thoracic surgery, Compend Contin Educ Vet 31(9):432, 2009.
16. Hendrix PK, Raffe MR, Robinson EP, et al: Epidural administration of bupivacaine, morphine, or their combination for postoperative analgesia in dogs, J Am Vet Med Assoc 209(3):598, 1996.
17. Swalander DB, Crowe DT Jr, Hittenmiller DH, et al: Complications associated with the use of indwelling epidural catheters in dogs: 81 cases (1996-1999), J Am Vet Med Assoc 216(3):368, 2000.
18. Karmakar MK, Ho AM: Postthoracotomy pain syndrome, Thorac Surg Clin 14(3):345, 2004.
19. Kelmer E, Scanson LC, Reed A, et al: Agreement between values for arterial and end-tidal partial pressures of carbon dioxide in spontaneously breathing, critically ill dogs, J Am Vet Med Assoc 235(11):1314, 2009.
20. Stobie D, Caywood DD, Rozanski EA, et al: Evaluation of pulmonary function and analgesia in dogs after intercostal thoracotomy and use of morphine administered intramuscularly or intrapleurally and bupivacaine administered intrapleurally, Am J Vet Res 56(8):1098, 1995.
21. Moores AL, Halfacree ZJ, Baines SJ, et al: Indications, outcomes and complications following lateral thoracotomy in dogs and cats, J Small Anim Pract 48(12):695, 2007.
22. Tattersall JA, Welsh E: Factors influencing the short-term outcome following thoracic surgery in 98 dogs, J Small Anim Pract 47(12):715, 2006.
23. Bellenger CR, Hunt GB, Goldsmid SE, et al: Outcomes of thoracic surgery in dogs and cats, Aust Vet J 74(1):25, 1996.
24. Burton CA, White RN: Review of the technique and complications of median sternotomy in the dog and cat, J Small Anim Pract 37(11):516, 1996.
25. Ringwald R: Complications of median sternotomy in the dog and cat, J Am Anim Hosp Assoc 25:430, 1989.
26. Cariou M, Lipscomb V, Baines SJ: Bacteria-related complications associated with thoracostomy tube use in dogs and cats: analysis of incidence and risk factors: Preliminary results. Oral presentation at the British Small Animal Veterinary Association Congress, Birmingham, April 2010.
27. Cahalane AK, Flanders JA: Use of pleural access ports for treatment of recurrent pneumothorax in two dogs, J Am Vet Med Assoc 241(4):467, 2012.

CHAPTER 135
KIDNEY TRANSPLANTATION

Lillian R. Aronson, VMD, DACVS

KEY POINTS

- Kidney transplantation is a viable option for cats suffering from acute kidney injury or chronic renal failure.
- Careful case selection of a potential recipient is critical to prevent both short- and long-term complications.
- Fractious cats or those with a history of recurrent urinary tract infections or significant cardiac disease are not typically good candidates for the procedure.
- Lifelong immunosuppression is necessary and consists of a combination of the calcineurin inhibitor, cyclosporine, and the glucocorticoid, prednisolone.
- Risk factors associated with survival after discharge include increasing age, intraoperative hypotension, and length of anesthesia.
- Successful treatment of complications secondary to chronic immunosuppressive therapy (i.e., infectious complications, diabetes mellitus, and neoplasia) still remains a significant challenge for the clinician.

Kidney transplantation, which was first introduced to the veterinary community in 1987 by Drs. Clare Gregory and Ira Gorley from the University of California at Davis School of Veterinary Medicine, continues to remain an accepted treatment option for cats with acute kidney injury or chronic renal failure. Since its introduction, it is estimated that between 400 and 500 cases of feline renal transplantation have been performed at various centers around the country. Recent evaluation of both published and unpublished information suggests that survival to discharge and long-term survival is improving; this is likely related to more stringent case selection, improved surgical experience, and the clinician's ability to better recognize early and treat successfully perioperative and long-term complications. Although some question whether there is justification for the technique as a treatment for cats suffering from kidney failure, in a recent report comparing survival time of cats that had undergone a renal transplant to a control population of medically treated cats, renal transplantation appeared to prolong survival times and improve the quality of life of these patients compared with those receiving medical management.[1] Despite lessons learned over the years with regards to short- and long-term management of these cases, they still remain a challenge for the veterinary clinician. This chapter discusses the most up-to-date information with regard to appropriate case selection, pre- and postoperative care, anesthetic and surgical management, and treatment of the most common long-term complications. The procedure has been performed predominantly in felines and thus that is the focus of this chapter. However, canine kidney transplantation is performed at selected facilities around the United States and further information is presented at the end of this chapter.

INDICATIONS

The most common histopathologic diagnosis identified from native kidney biopsy samples of cats necessitating a renal transplant is chronic interstitial nephritis. Other underlying conditions for which transplantation has been performed include oxalate nephrosis, polycystic kidney disease, renal fibrosis, pyelonephritis, membranous glomerulonephropathy, ethylene glycol and lily toxicity, amyloidosis, and renal dysplasia. It is unclear if patients with pyelonephritis or amyloidosis are appropriate candidates for the procedure because of the potential long-term effect on the allograft. Patients with acute kidney injury secondary to a ureteral obstruction or toxicosis often require hemodialysis for stabilization. Additionally, hemodialysis may be necessary for the removal of ethylene glycol and its toxic metabolites before transplantation.

CASE SELECTION

Thorough screening of a potential feline renal transplant recipient is critical to decrease morbidity and mortality that can occur after the procedure. Although the best time to intervene with surgery is still subjective, clinicians with experience managing these patients suggest that surgical intervention should be performed in cats with early decompensated chronic kidney disease or irreversible acute kidney injury.[2,3] Clinical signs that indicate decompensation include worsening of the azotemia and anemia as well as continued weight loss in the face of medical therapy. It is important to be aware that some candidates that are clinically stable can rapidly deteriorate and die without prior evidence that decompensation was present. At one center, indications for transplantation additionally include a serum creatinine (Cr) more than 4 mg/dl or significant aberrations in calcium and phosphorus levels.[4] Some clinicians have been successful in preventing the physical deterioration of individual patients for up to 2 years by the placement of either a percutaneous endoscopic gastrostomy (PEG) or esophagostomy feeding tube.[3]

Both physical and biochemical parameters need to be evaluated carefully to determine a cat's candidacy. The animal should be free of other disease conditions, including significant heart disease, recurrent urinary tract infections, uncontrolled hyperthyroidism, and underlying neoplasia. Cats with a fractious temperament are also often declined as candidates. Although the presence of inflammatory bowel disease (IBD) has been a concern for some clinicians, patients with IBD have been successfully transplanted at the author's facility. There are insufficient data to determine if cats with diabetes should be declined as potential candidates. More recently, additional risk factors have been associated with morbidity and mortality in this patient population. In one study, the degree of azotemia before transplantation was found to be a risk factor. Cats with a Cr greater than 10 and an increased blood urea nitrogen (BUN) were more likely to suffer mortality before discharge.[1] In a second study, the level of azotemia was not related to long-term survival but did significantly increase the risk of neurologic complications in the perioperative period.[5] It is possible that the use of preoperative hemodialysis in these patients may be warranted. Additionally, in two separate studies recipient age was identified as a factor associated with survival after discharge. In the first study cats older than 10 years had a higher

BOX 135-1 *Preoperative Screening for a Potential Feline Renal Transplant Recipient*

Complete blood cell count
Serum chemistry profile
Blood type and major and minor crossmatch to donor
Thyroid hormone level (T_4)
Urinalysis, urine culture, urine protein/creatinine ratio
Abdominal radiography
Abdominal ultrasonography
Thoracic radiography
Electrocardiography, echocardiography, arterial blood pressure
Feline leukemia virus and feline immunodeficiency virus testing
Toxoplasmosis titer (IgG and IgM)

mortality in the first 6 months after transplantation, and in the second study median survival times decreased with increasing age, with median survival times of 1423, 613, and 150 days, respectively, for cats younger than 5 years, between 5 and 10 years, and older than 10 years.[1,5] To date, the oldest cat that has been transplanted at our facility was 18 years of age. Finally, both preoperative blood pressure (BP) and weight have also been shown to influence overall survival.[1] Preoperative examination involves various laboratory tests including a complete blood cell count, biochemical evaluation, blood type and thyroid evaluation, evaluation of the urinary tract (urinalysis, urine culture, urine protein/creatinine ratio, abdominal radiographs, abdominal ultrasound), evaluation for cardiovascular disease (thoracic radiography, electrocardiography, echocardiography, blood pressure), and screening for infectious disease (feline leukemia virus/feline immunodeficiency virus [FeLV/FIV], *Toxoplasma* IgG and IgM titers)[4,6] (Box 135-1). There is currently no age restriction for a potential transplant recipient. The feline recipient must also have compatible blood (via crossmatch) to a prospective kidney donor and to two or three blood donor cats.

Evaluation of the Urinary Tract

Evaluation of the urinary tract is essential, particularly to rule out any underlying infection or neoplastic disease. If ultrasound findings are suggestive of feline infectious peritonitis or neoplasia, a fine needle aspirate or biopsy is recommended. If a patient has recently been treated for a urinary tract infection or if a patient has had recurrent urinary tract infections but at the time of presentation has a negative urine culture, then a cyclosporine (CsA; Neoral, Novartis, East Hanover, NJ) challenge is recommended before transplantation to determine if the cat will "break" with an infection after immunosuppression. To perform this challenge, CsA is administered for approximately a 2-week period at the recommended dose for transplantation immunosuppression. The urine is evaluated for the presence of an infection after therapeutic CsA blood levels have been obtained and at the end of the 2-week period. It is important to note that a negative urine culture result after a challenge will not guarantee that a patient will remain infection-free after surgery and chronic immunosuppressive therapy. Another option is to place all potential candidates on CsA for 2 weeks before surgery to attempt to identify an occult infection.[3]

Finally, if unilateral or bilateral hydronephrosis is identified in any patient during the screening process, a pyelocentesis and culture is recommended before transplantation. Immunosuppression in a patient harboring an infection can not only potentiate the rejection process but also lead to increased morbidity and mortality.

Cardiovascular Disease

Limited information currently exists regarding the effect of pre- and postoperative hypertension on outcomes. In one feline study, preoperative blood pressure did influence overall survival.[1] In a second report, preoperative hypertension did not predict postoperative episodes of hypertension and the administration of antihypertensive medication preoperatively did not significantly decrease the postoperative incidence of hypertension.[5] At the time of presentation for transplantation, a systolic murmur may be ausculted on physical examination. These murmurs may be a physiologic murmurs associated with the anemia of chronic renal failure and not represent significant heart disease.[2] However, in a study from the University of California at Davis evaluating cardiac abnormalities in 84 potential transplant recipients, 78% of patients had abnormalities including both papillary muscle and septal muscle hypertrophy. The authors suggested that these changes may be related to hypertension, chronic uremia, age, or early changes of hypertrophic cardiomyopathy.[7] An analysis of preoperative echocardiographic changes in that study found no significant predictors of 1-month survival. Another study found that duration of intraoperative hypotension and increased left ventricular wall thickness were risk factors for perioperative mortality.[1] Cats with diffuse hypertrophic cardiomyopathy are declined as candidates for renal transplantation at our facility. A decision is made on a case to case basis in those cats with less severe cardiac disease.

Infectious Disease

If a cat is FeLV positive or has an active FIV infection, they are declined as candidates for transplantation. Additionally, all potential donor and recipients currently undergo serologic testing (IgG and IgM) for toxoplasmosis. *Toxoplasma gondii* can cause significant morbidity and mortality in immunocompromised human and veterinary patients. As a matter of policy at our facility, seropositive recipients are placed on lifelong prophylactic clindamycin (25 mg PO q12h), which is started when immunosuppression is initiated. Trimethoprim-sulfamethoxazole (15 mg/kg PO q12h) has also been used in cats that do not tolerate clindamycin. Although we no longer use seropositive donors for seronegative recipients, we have successfully used a seropositive donor for a seropositive recipient.

DONOR SELECTION

Kidney donors are typically between 1 and 3 years of age and in excellent health. Standard evaluation includes a complete blood cell count and blood type, serum chemistry profile, urinalysis and culture, FeLV and FIV testing and a toxoplasmosis titer (IgG and IgM). The feline kidney donor must also have a compatible blood crossmatch to the recipient and be of a similar size. Although a method for a lymphocytotoxic crossmatch test for feline renal transplantation has been described to investigate antilymphocyte antibodies in cats, it has not been used clinically.[8] Rarely, incompatible crossmatch tests between AB compatible donor and recipient pairs have been identified. The absence of a novel red cell antigen identified as Mik has resulted in naturally occurring anti-Mik alloantibodies after an AB-matched blood transfusion (see Chapter 61).[9] Additionally, we currently perform computed tomography (CT) angiography on all of the donors to evaluate the renal vasculature as well as the renal parenchyma for any abnormalities that may preclude successful transplantation.[10] The donor cat is adopted by the owner of the recipient and a suitable home is found for any donor that fails the screening process. Currently, there is only 1 published study evaluating the long-term effects of performing a unilateral nephrectomy in feline kidney donors. In that study, 16 donors were followed between 24 and 67 months postoperatively.[11] Fifteen of the 16 cats were clinically normal and serum Cr concentrations for these cats remained within the reference range. One cat was diagnosed with chronic renal insufficiency 52 months after donation. Although a unilateral nephrectomy does not appear to affect normal life expectancy in cats, long-term monitoring is recommended.

PREOPERATIVE MANAGEMENT

Upon admission to the transplant facility, the recipient is placed on intravenous fluid therapy of a balanced or maintenance electrolyte solution at 1.5 to 2 times the daily maintenance requirements (see Chapter 59). This rate may vary in cases of severe dehydration or in cats with underlying cardiac disease. In one study, cats that died before discharge were more likely to have received Hetastarch as part of their therapeutic protocol.[1] At some centers, hemodialysis is performed before transplantation for cats that are anuric or those with severe azotemia (BUN > 100 mg/dl, Cr > 8 mg/dl).[6] Additionally, if the cat is hypertensive, the calcium channel blocker amlodipine (Norvasc, 0.625 mg/cat PO q24h) may be indicated before surgery. Anemia is typically corrected at the time of surgery with crossmatch-compatible whole blood or packed red cell transfusions. The first unit that is administered is one that has been previously collected from the kidney donor. If the patient has evidence of decreased oxygen delivery from the anemia, blood products can be given at the time of admission to the transplant facility. If the patient will be traveling a long distance to the transplant clinic, it is worthwhile to have a blood sample sent before arrival to identify a compatible donor as well as potential blood donors. If a delay in the transplant procedure is expected, erythropoietin (100 IU/kg SC 2 to 3 times per week until the packed cell volume [PCV] is approximately 30%, then decrease to 1 to 2 times per week) or darbepoetin (6.25 mcg/kg q1wk for 2 to 4 weeks until PCV is approximately 25%, then every other week) can be administered and may greatly reduce the need for blood products at the time of surgery. Phosphate binders and gastrointestinal protectants are given if deemed necessary. If the cat is anorectic, a nasogastric, esophagostomy or PEG tube may be placed to administer nutritional support before (or at the time of) surgery.

Immunosuppression for the Feline Renal Transplant Recipient

The immunosuppressive protocol currently used at our facility consists of a combination of the calcineurin inhibitor CsA and the glucocorticoid prednisolone. Cyclosporine prevents the activation of a number of transcription factors that regulate cytokine genes with a role in allograft rejection, including interleukin 2 (IL-2), IL-4, interferon γ (IFN-γ), tumor necrosis factor-α (TNF-α), and granulocyte-macrophage colony-stimulating factor (GM-CSF).[12-14] Corticosteroids also inhibit these cytokines, but the exact mechanism of action is not fully understood. The effects of current therapy on feline cytokine production in vitro have recently been evaluated. In the first report, using real-time polymerase chain reaction (PCR), CsA inhibited the expression of mRNA for IL-2, IL-4, IFN- γ, and TNF-α in a dose-dependent manner.[15] In the second report, CsA resulted in a significant decrease in the production of IFN-γ, IL-2, and GM-CSF.[16] Dexamethasone alone only suppressed the production of GM-CSF; however, when dexamethasone was combined with CsA, a significant decrease in the production of IFN-γ, IL-2, and GM-CSF occurred.[16]

Because of the small dose of cyclosporine that cats often require for immunosuppression, the liquid microemulsified formulation, Neoral (100 mg/ml), is recommended so the dose can be titrated for each individual cat. Neoral can be diluted in water or other oral solutions but must be administered immediately after dilution.[2] Cyclosporine administration is begun 72 to 96 hours before transplantation at a dose of 1 to 5 mg/kg PO q12h (depending on the cat's appetite). In the author's experience, cats that are anorexic or are eating a minimal amount have a much lower drug requirement to obtain appropriate drug levels before surgery. Additional drugs that inhibit P-450 hepatic enzymes may alter drug concentrations and should be used with caution in these patients. A 12-hour whole-blood trough concentration is obtained the day before surgery so that the dose can be adjusted before surgery if necessary. The drug level is measured using the technique of high-pressure liquid chromatography (HPLC). The goal is to obtain a trough concentration of 300 to 500 ng/ml before surgery.[6] This level is maintained for approximately 1 to 3 months after surgery and is then tapered to approximately 250 ng/ml for maintenance therapy. Prednisolone is administered beginning the morning of surgery. Prednisolone is preferred over prednisone for immunosuppression. In an abstract evaluating the bioavailability and activity of these two drugs in cats, serum prednisolone levels were significantly greater for oral prednisolone than oral prednisone.[17] At our facility, prednisolone is started at a dose range of 0.5 to 1 mg/kg q12h orally for the first 3 months and then tapered to q24h. It is important to note that protocols for both CsA and prednisolone vary between transplantation facilities.

A second protocol used by some clinicians for feline immunosuppression combines the antifungal medication ketoconazole (10 mg/kg PO q24h) with the CsA and prednisolone.[18,19] Ketoconazole can affect CsA metabolism by inhibiting both hepatic and intestinal cytochrome P450 oxidase activity, resulting in increased blood CsA concentrations.[19] Once ketoconazole is added to the immunosuppressive protocol, CsA and prednisolone are administered once a day and CsA doses are adjusted into the therapeutic range by measuring q24h whole-blood trough levels. This protocol may reduce the cost of CsA and be more appealing for owners whose work schedule does not permit twice a day dosing of medication. If signs of hepatotoxicity are identified, ketoconazole administration should be discontinued. In two separate studies, the effect of multiple oral dosing of itraconazole and single oral dosing of clarithromycin on the pharmacokinetics of cyclosporine were evaluated in normal cats. Itraconazole, an antifungal with less toxicity than ketoconazole, and the macrolide antibiotic clarithromycin were each found to decrease the required cyclosporine dosage that would be necessary for renal transplantation.[20,21] Clarithromycin, known to have immunosuppressive properties, has been used successfully in conjunction with cyclosporine and prednisolone for one feline renal transplant recipient.[21]

ANESTHETIC MANAGEMENT

At the time of anesthetic induction, both the donor cat and the recipient are given cephalexin (22 mg/kg IV q2h). Additionally, an epidural is given to both cats (bupivacaine [0.1 mg/kg] and morphine [0.15 mg/kg]) for analgesia. In addition to a peripheral catheter, a double (or triple) lumen indwelling jugular catheter is placed in the recipient, preferably using the right jugular vein. The left side of the neck is preserved in animals that need an esophagostomy tube. Using this catheter, blood products can be given as needed; blood sampled regularly for evaluation of blood gases, electrolytes, packed cell volume and total protein; and central venous pressure monitored, if needed. Because the procedure can last up to 6 hours, hypothermia is of serious concern. A Bair Hugger and heating pads are used throughout the procedure and esophageal temperatures are monitored continuously. Systemic arterial blood pressure is monitored regularly throughout the procedure in both cats using a Doppler technique. Intraoperative hypertension is treated with the subcutaneous (SC) administration of hydralazine (2.5 mg SC for a 4-kg cat) and intraoperative hypotension corrected by decreasing the concentration of inhalant anesthetic or by the administration of fluid boluses, blood products, or dopamine (starting at 5 mcg/kg/min). In a recent report evaluating the influence of anesthetic variables on long-term survival of 94 cats undergoing renal transplantation, intraoperative hypotension and the duration of anesthesia for the recipient negatively affected long-term survival.[22]

SURGERY

Currently at our facility each transplant procedure involves a team of three surgeons. The donor cat is brought into the surgical suite approximately 30 to 45 minutes before the recipient. During this time, the donor kidney will be prepared for the nephrectomy. At the time of the abdominal incision, the donor is given a dose of mannitol (0.25 g/kg intravenously [IV] over 15 minutes) to help prevent renal arterial spasms, improve renal blood flow, and protect against injury that can occur during the warm ischemia period. Some surgeons also recommend the administration of the α-adrenergic agonist acepromazine (0.01 mg/kg IV).[18] The renal artery and vein are cleared of as much fat and adventitia as possible, and the ureter is dissected free to the point where it joins the bladder. The left kidney is preferred because it has a longer vein. If two renal veins are present, the smaller vein can be sacrificed. Before sacrificing a vein, however, the surgeon needs to identify the ureteral vein and determine that it is not draining into the vein that is being sacrificed. It is essential, however, to harvest a donor kidney with a single renal artery at the point where the artery joins the aorta. A minimal length of 0.5 cm of single renal artery is necessary for the arterial anastomosis.[2] The nephrectomy will be performed when the recipient is prepared to receive the kidney. Fifteen minutes before nephrectomy, an additional dose of mannitol (1 g/kg IV) is given to the donor cat.

The majority of the recipient surgery is performed using an operating microscope. The renal artery is anastomosed end-to-side to the abdominal aorta (proximal to the caudal mesenteric artery), and the renal vein is anastomosed end-to-side to the caudal vena cava. Partial occlusion clamps are used to obstruct blood flow in both the aorta and the caudal vena cava. Holes are created in both the aorta and vena cava to match the size of the renal artery and vein. Both aorta and vena cava are flushed with a heparinized saline solution. The allograft is flushed with a phosphate-buffered sucrose organ preservation solution. The renal artery is anastomosed to the aorta using 8-0 nylon in a simple continuous pattern and the renal vein is anastomosed to the vena cava using 7-0 silk in a simple continuous pattern. Once the anastomosis is complete, the venous clamp is removed first and then the arterial clamp. A small amount of hemorrhage usually occurs and is controlled with pressure. Any significant leaks may need to be repaired with the placement of additional single interrupted sutures.

An alternative technique that requires only one surgical team is the use of hypothermic storage to preserve the donor kidney until the recipient surgery is performed. After donor kidney preparation and nephrectomy, the graft is flushed with a phosphate-buffered sucrose organ preservation solution and then placed in a stainless steel bowl containing the same solution.[18] The bowl is floated in an ice slush, the kidney agitated until cold to the touch, and then the bowl covered with a sterile drape until the recipient surgery is performed.[18,23] This technique reduces personnel and resources needed for the transplantation procedure. Additionally, the cold preservation has been found to minimize ischemic injury that can occur to the kidney.

Once the vascular anastomosis is complete, a ureteroneocystotomy is performed using an intravesicular mucosal apposition technique. A ventral midline cystotomy is performed and then the end of the ureter brought directly into the bladder lumen through a hole created at the bladder apex. The bladder is everted, the distal end of

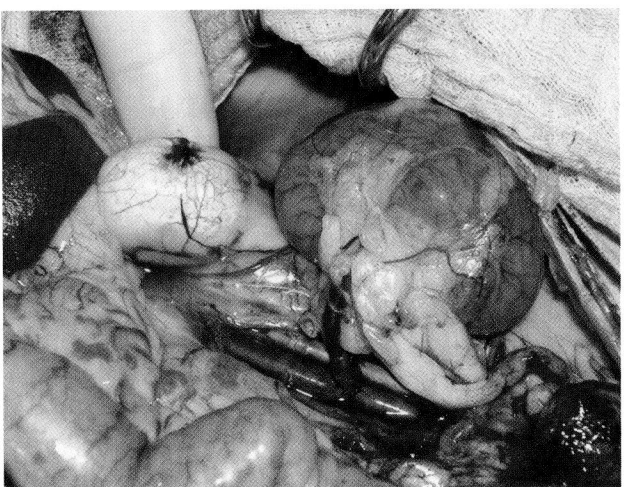

FIGURE 135-1 Image showing the venous anastomosis between the allograft renal vein and the recipient's vena cava. Both the allograft and native kidney are shown. A biopsy of the native kidney was taken at the time of transplantation. The recipient's native kidneys are usually left in place to act as a reserve in case graft function is delayed.

the ureter is excised, periureteral fat is removed, and the end of the ureter is spatulated. The ureteral mucosa is sutured to the bladder mucosa using either 8-0 nylon or 8-0 vicryl in a simple interrupted pattern. After completion of the anastomosis, the bladder is inverted and closed routinely.

Two extravesicular techniques for ureteral implantation have also been described. In the first technique, a 1-cm incision is made on the ventral surface of the bladder through the seromuscular layer, allowing the mucosa to bulge through the incision.[2,24] A smaller incision (3 to 4 mm) is made through the mucosal layer. The distal end of the ureter is prepared as previously described, and the ureteral mucosa is sutured to bladder mucosa using 8-0 nylon. Once complete, the seromuscular layer is apposed in a simple interrupted pattern over the ureter with 4-0 absorbable suture. In the second technique, the entire ureter and ureteral papilla is harvested from the donor and sutured using an extravesicular technique.[25]

Before closure, a biopsy of one of the native kidneys is performed and the allograft pexied to the abdominal wall using six interrupted sutures of 4-0 polypropylene. The recipient's native kidneys are usually left in place to act as a reserve in case graft function is delayed (Figure 135-1). Patients with polycystic kidney disease (or a kidney abscess/infection) are an exception because at least one of the native kidneys often needs to be removed at the time of the transplantation procedure in order to create space in the abdomen for the allograft.

POSTOPERATIVE MANAGEMENT AND PERIOPERATIVE COMPLICATIONS

After surgery the recipient is maintained on intravenous fluid therapy, which should be adjusted as needed based on the cat's renal function, urine output, hydration status, and oral intake of water. Blood transfusions are given only if necessary. Minimal stress and handling and prevention of hypothermia are critical during the early postoperative period. While a catheter is in place, the cat is maintained on intravenous antibiotic therapy (cefazolin 22 mg/kg IV q8h). Once all catheters are removed, the cat is then maintained on oral antibiotic therapy (amoxicillin plus clavulanic acid 62.5 mg PO q12h) for another 2 to 3 weeks or until the feeding tube is removed and CsA levels regulated. If the cat is *Toxoplasma* positive, clindamycin (25 mg

PO/IV q12h) is administered in conjunction with the immunosuppression and continued for the lifetime of the cat. Postoperative pain has been controlled successfully at our facility using buprenorphine (0.005 to 0.02 mg/kg IV q4-8h), hydromorphone (0.05 to 0.2 mg/kg IV, IM, or SC q4-6h), methadone (0.15 to 0.3 mg/kg IV q4-6h), or a constant rate infusion (CRI) of butorphanol (0.1 to 0.5 mg/kg/hr). Initially, blood work is performed twice daily to evaluate acid-base status, packed cell volume, total protein, electrolytes, and blood glucose; these are tapered gradually depending on the stability of the cat. A renal panel is checked every 24 to 48 hours and a blood CsA level is checked every 3 to 4 days and the dose adjusted accordingly. Voided urine is weighed and recorded when possible (urinary catheters should be avoided). Abdominal palpation is not performed during the postoperative period. With improvement in the azotemia and appropriate pain control, most cats will start eating within 24 to 48 hours after the surgical procedure. In some cases in which continued anorexia is thought to be associated with altered gastric motility after surgery, metoclopramide administration (0.2 mg/kg SC q6-8h or 1 to 2 mg/kg/24 hours as an IV CRI) has been successful in improving a cat's appetite. If the cat remains anorexic, a feeding tube may be necessary, if not already placed.

Because of the association identified between postoperative hypertension and postoperative central nervous system (CNS) disorders (i.e., seizure activity), indirect blood pressure is measured every 1 to 2 hours during the first 48 to 72 hours after surgery to monitor for the development of hypertension.[26] If the systolic blood pressure is equal to or greater than 180 mm Hg and the animal appears comfortable, hydralazine (2.5 mg SC for a 4-kg cat) is administered. The hydralazine dose can be repeated if the systolic pressure has not decreased within 15 to 30 minutes. If the cat is refractory to hydralazine, acepromazine (0.005 to 0.01 mg/kg IV) has also been effective. It is important to note that the incidence of hypertension and CNS disorders is not seen with equal frequency between transplant centers and thus the cause of CNS disorders in cats after renal transplantation still remains a challenge for some clinicians.[18] In one recent study, an increase of 1 mg/dl in serum Cr or 10 mg/dl in BUN increased the likelihood of postoperative CNS disease by 1.6- and 1.8-fold, respectively.[5] In addition to monitoring patients for postoperative hypertension, complications can also arise if postoperative hypotension occurs. Systolic blood pressure is commonly maintained at 100 mm Hg or greater. Sustained hypotension can lead to poor graft perfusion and must be treated aggressively to prevent acute tubular necrosis and delayed graft function.

If surgery is technically successful, azotemia typically resolves within the first 24 to 72 hours after surgery. If improvement does not occur during this time or if improvement in renal function is initially identified but then worsens, an ultrasonographic examination of the allograft is recommended. The allograft should be evaluated for adequate blood flow as well as any signs of a ureteral obstruction, including hydronephrosis or hydroureter. If repeat ultrasonographic evaluations reveal worsening of the hydronephrosis, a ureteral obstruction should be suspected. Another laparotomy is performed so that the allograft can be evaluated. In some cases, the ureter may need to be reimplanted into the urinary bladder. If graft perfusion is adequate and no signs of obstruction are present, then delayed graft function should be considered.

Cats are discharged from the hospital when graft function appears adequate and the cat is clinically stable. Cats with delayed graft function can also be discharged if the patient is otherwise clinically stable. In these cases, improvement in function often occurs within the first few weeks after surgery. Medical management of the renal failure can be continued in this subset of patients until graft function returns to normal. If the transplanted kidney fails to function, the kidney should be biopsied before retransplantation.

LONG-TERM MANAGEMENT AND COMPLICATIONS

Patients should be evaluated by their veterinarian once a week for the first 6 to 8 weeks, then monthly rechecks depending on the cat's condition. During each examination, the cat should be weighed and blood work performed, including a renal panel (e.g., BUN, creatinine, phosphorus total carbon dioxide [TCO_2], and magnesium), packed cell volume, total protein, cyclosporine level, and a urinalysis (only if a free-catch urine sample is available). Because of intra- and interpatient variability in the absorption of oral cyclosporine and its metabolism, it is essential that blood levels are checked regularly to maintain therapeutic concentrations and minimize toxic side effects. It is recommended that a complete blood cell count and serum chemistry panel are run at least every 3 to 4 months and, if the cat had been diagnosed with underlying cardiac disease, an echocardiogram performed every 6 to 12 months. If there are any concerns about allograft function, an abdominal ultrasound should be performed as an initial investigative step to identify any evidence of a urinary obstruction or vascular thrombosis. If a feeding tube has been placed, it should be removed once oral intake of food and water is deemed appropriate (or at least 7 to 10 days after placement).

Renal complications after transplantation that have been reported include allograft rejection, calcium oxalate (CaOx) nephrosis, ureteral complications, hemolytic uremic syndrome, allograft rupture, retroperitoneal fibrosis, delayed graft function, and vascular pedicle complications. Acute rejection can occur at any time but is most common within the first few months after surgery.[1,27] Cats that are experiencing a rejection episode may or may not have overt clinical signs including polyuria/polydipsia, lethargy, depression, and anorexia. For this reason, weekly blood sampling is essential during the early postoperative period. Histopathologic as well as sonographic and scintigraphic examination of allograft rejection in cats has recently been described.[28,29] Sonographic examination often reveals a significant increase in cross-sectional area to the allograft of at least 10% (mean 34%), a subjective increase in echogenicity, and a decrease in corticomedullary demarcation.[29] Although normal allograft enlargement is expected during the first week postoperatively, a gradual decline should then occur. In a study evaluating renal autografts in normal cats, cross-sectional area of the grafts increased by 63% at 1 week and remained at 60% above baseline by day 13.[30] In a second study, an increase in cross-sectional area occurred between 1 and 3 days postoperatively, then declined over the next 3 weeks but did not return to baseline.[31] Neither resistive index (RI) nor glomerular filtration rate were sensitive indicators in normal grafts or those undergoing allograft rejection.[29-31] In an ultrasonographic study of 69 clinical renal allografts, graft volume was a better indicator than RI of graft disease, including ureteral obstruction and those experiencing rejection episodes.

If possible, before starting the rejection protocol a urine sediment should be evaluated to rule out an underlying infection. Suspected acute rejection episodes are treated with intravenous administration of cyclosporine (CsA; 6.6 mg/kg q24h given over 4-6h) and prednisolone sodium succinate (Solu Delta Cortef, 10 mg/kg IV q12h). Each milliliter of the intravenous cyclosporine is diluted with 20 to 100 ml of either 0.9% NaCl or 5% dextrose.[32] The infusion of CsA can be repeated. However, another potential cause for the azotemia should be considered if the creatinine concentration does not improve within 24 to 48 hours. Chronic rejection is characterized by gradual loss of organ function over months to years, often without evidence of a rejection episode. Histopathology of these grafts reveals severe narrowing of numerous arteries and thickening of the glomerular capillary basement membrane. The cause of chronic rejection is unknown at this time. Hemolytic uremic syndrome is a rare but fatal side effect of CsA therapy. Patients develop hemolytic anemia and thrombocytopenia with rapid deterioration of renal function secondary to glomerular and renal arteriolar platelet and fibrin thrombi.[33] In the author's experience, the mortality rate has been 100%.

Renal transplantation is a treatment option for cats whose underlying cause of renal failure is associated with calcium oxalate urolithiasis. In a study evaluating these patients, no difference in long-term outcome was found between a group of cats with stones and a control group of cats whose underlying cause of renal failure was not related to urolithiasis.[34] Additionally, in specifically evaluating 19 stone formers, 5 cats formed calculi within the allograft between 4 and 22 months postoperatively. Although formation of calculi in the allograft of 5 cats did not significantly reduce survival, the power of the study was low and there was a trend toward worse survival in cats that formed calculi in the allograft. Four of the 5 cats had calculi attached to the 8-0 nylon suture used to perform the ureteroneocystostomy and two cats that formed calculi were diagnosed with a urinary tract infection. Based on these findings, absorbable suture material is now used to perform the ureteroneocystostomy in cats known to form stones. Additionally, thorough screening for infection is recommended.

Another potential cause of recurrence of azotemia within the first few months after surgery is the development of retroperitoneal fibrosis.[35] Abdominal ultrasound in these patients reveals hydronephrosis (often without the presence of hydroureter because of the compression of the ureter from scar tissue). Occasionally, a capsule can be identified surrounding the allograft, resulting in a partial or complete ureteral obstruction. Surgery has been successful in relieving the obstruction and restoring normal renal function; however, reformation of scar tissue resulting in a second obstruction has been identified in some patients (Figure 135-2). The exact cause is unclear at this time.

Finally, complications can occur secondary to chronic immunosuppressive therapy. These have included the development of infections including opportunistic infections, diabetes mellitus (DM), and neoplasia.

In a large retrospective study evaluating the prevalence of infection in 169 cats that had undergone transplantation, 47 infections developed in 43 of 169 cats. The most common infections encountered were bacterial (25/47), followed by viral (13/47), fungal (6/47), and protozoal (3/47) infections.[36] Infections not only cause direct morbidity and mortality from the infection itself but may also activate the rejection process. Half of the infectious complications occurred within the first 2.5 months after surgery, when immunosuppression was kept at its highest level. The development of DM in this patient population significantly increased the risk of developing an infection.[36] In these patients, a reduction in CsA dosage as well as a tapering of the steroid dose should be performed while carefully monitoring renal function.

The prevalence of malignant neoplasia in cats after renal transplantation has been reported. In one study, the prevalence in cats was 9.5% with a median survival time of 14 months.[37] This compares to a median survival time of 22 months for a group of 66 feline renal transplant recipients from the same facility that did not develop neoplasia. In a second report, malignant neoplasia after transplantation occurred in 24% of the cases (median survival time was 1020 days [34 months] compared with 1146 days [38 months] for the control population).[38] In this study, the development of neoplasia did not significantly affect overall survival. Additionally, CsA-based therapy in conjunction with transplantation was significantly associated with the development of neoplasia and these cats had a 6.1 times higher odds of developing a malignancy compared with a control group.[38] Similar to this report, recent work from our facility found a 22.5% incidence of malignant neoplasia in a group of 111 cats.[39] In

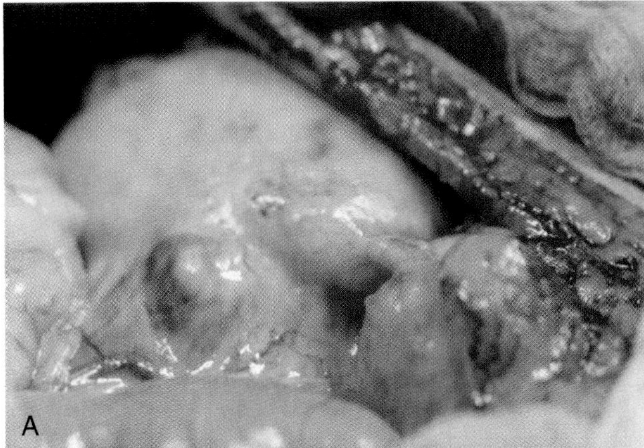

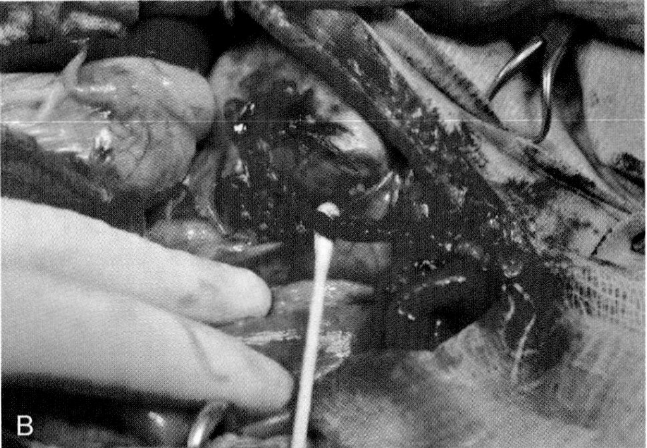

FIGURE 135-2 A, Retroperitoneal fibrosis. Note the white scar tissue surrounding the renal allograft and bladder and the shortened length of the ureter because it is encased in fibrotic tissue. **B,** Surgical resection of the fibrotic tissue surrounding the allograft ureter allows the ureter to become unobstructed.

all three studies, lymphoma was the predominant type of neoplasia identified. Additionally, histopathologic review of either necropsy (5 cats) or biopsy (2 cats) samples from 7 cats with lymphoma revealed that all samples were classified as mid- to high-grade, diffuse large B-cell lymphoma, similar to what is identified in human renal transplant recipients.[40]

In a multicenter study investigating the incidence and risk factors for the development of DM in a group of 187 feline renal transplant recipients, 13.9% of cats developed DM after transplantation and these patients were 5.45 times as likely to develop DM compared with cats with chronic renal failure.[41] Glycemic control in these cats has been done successfully with dietary management, tapering immunosuppressive therapy, glipizide or insulin treatment, and in some cases, a combination of techniques. The mortality rate in this group of cats was 2.38 times the mortality rate of feline renal transplant recipients that did not develop DM.

CANINE TRANSPLANTATION

Canine renal transplantation is an uncommonly performed procedure. At our facility, canine transplantation has been performed successfully between mixed lymphocyte response (MLR) matched donor and recipient pairs to treat animals with membranous glomerulonephropathy and renal dysplasia. Because the donor dog is a relative, the donor typically already has a home. Similar physical and biochemical parameters need to be evaluated carefully in order to determine if a dog is a suitable candidate for transplantation. The ideal immunosuppressive regimen for canine transplant recipients still remains a challenge, particularly in unrelated donor and recipient pairs. A number of immunosuppressive protocols are being used in both unrelated and related donor and recipient pairs with varying results.[42,43] Currently at our facility, a combination of cyclosporine and prednisolone is being used. The recommended dosage of cyclosporine is 2.5 to 5 mg/kg PO q12h to attain a 12-hour whole-blood trough concentration of 300 to 500 ng/ml. This level is maintained for approximately 1 to 3 months after surgery and is then tapered to approximately 250 ng/ml for maintenance therapy. The cyclosporine is given in combination with prednisolone at a dose of 0.5 to 1 mg/kg q12h orally for the first 3 months and then tapered to q24h. Similar to cats, ketoconazole can be added to the cyclosporine protocol to decrease the cost of therapy, particularly in medium and large breed dogs. Potential adverse effects in dogs include hepatotoxicity and cataract formation.

The canine anesthetic protocol is similar to the feline protocol with a few exceptions. Because of the high incidence of intussusceptions after renal transplantation in the dog, morphine is used as a premedication, during the procedure (0.5 mg/kg IV as a bolus when the abdomen is entered), and for pain management postoperatively. Additionally, because of complications associated with thromboembolic disease, enoxaparin (0.5 to 1 mg/kg subcutaneously q24h) is started the day before surgery and continued for 7 days after surgery.

The surgical techniques described for renal transplantation in the dog are similar to those described previously for the cat with a few minor differences. In addition to anastomosing the renal vasculature to the caudal aorta and vena cava, the iliac vessels of the recipient can also be used for the anastomosis. Recently, a novel technique for vascular anastomosis has been described in the dog. In this technique, both the renal artery and vein are anastomosed using an end to side technique to the recipient's ipsilateral external iliac artery and vein.[44] Magnification may not be necessary and often depends on the size of the patient.[1] Suture material used for the vascular anastomosis is generally larger than that used in cats and includes 4-0 to 6-0 silk for the venous anastomosis and 5-0 to 8-0 nylon or polypropylene for the arterial anastomosis. Because of the high incidence of intussusceptions after the procedure, enteroplication is performed before closure.

Limited information currently exists regarding complications in clinical canine patients. Infection (bacterial, fungal, protozoal) involving the urinary tract, nasal cavity, CNS, and skin, allograft rejection, and thromboembolic disease have been reported.[45-47] The majority of canine transplantation studies involve experimental animals and evaluate different immunosuppressive protocols. Complications reported in healthy animals are similar to those reported in clinical patients. Additionally, intussusception, hepatotoxicity, ocular toxicity, cardiac failure, neurotoxicity, and gingival hyperplasia have been reported.[48-52]

CONCLUSION

Renal transplantation offers a unique method of treatment for renal failure in cats (and dogs). Compared with medical management, transplantation does appear to prolong the life expectancy in cats with end-stage renal disease. Based on both published and unpublished information, 70% to 93% of cats have been discharged from the hospital after transplantation and median survival times have ranged from 360 to 616 days. Continued clinical experience with short- and long-term management, as well as the ability to identify specific risk factors both pre- and postoperatively, will hopefully continue to improve long-term outcome in these patients. Clients need to understand the risks involved with the procedure and that it is a commitment for the life of the animal. Although renal transplantation is the treatment of choice for cats suffering from renal failure, the lack of an effective immunosuppressive protocol in unrelated dogs has limited its application in clinical practice.

REFERENCES

1. Schmeidt CW, Holzman G, Schwarz T, et al: Survival, complications and analysis of risk factors after renal transplantation in cats, Vet Surg 37:683, 2008.
2. Gregory CR, Bernsteen L: Organ transplantation in clinical veterinary practice. In Slatter DH, editor: Textbook of small animal surgery, Philadelphia, 2000, WB Saunders, pp 122-136.
3. Mathews KG: Renal transplantation in the management of chronic renal failure. In August JR, editor: Consultations in feline internal medicine, ed 4, Philadelphia, 2001, WB Saunders, pp 319-327.
4. Katayama M, McAnulty: Renal transplantation in cats: patient selection and preoperative management, Compend Contin Educ Pract Vet 24:868, 2002.
5. Adin CA, Gregory CR, Kyles AE, et al: Diagnostic predictors and survival after renal transplantation in cats, Vet Surg 30:515, 2001.
6. Bernsteen L, Gregory CR, Kyles AE, et al: Renal transplantation in cats, Clin Tech Small Anim Pract 15:40, 2000.
7. Adin DB, Thomas WP, Adin CA, et al: Echoardiographic evaluation of cats with chronic renal failure (abstract), ACVIM Proc, May 25, 2000, p 714.
8. Kuwahara Y, Kobayashi R, Iwata J, et al: Method of lymphocytotoxic crossmatch test for feline renal transplantation, J Vet Med Sci 61:481, 1999.
9. Weinstein NM, Blais MC, Harris K, et al: A newly recognized blood group in domestic shorthair cats: the Mik red cell antigen, J Vet Intern Med 21:287, 2007.
10. Bouma JL, Aronson LR, Keith DM, et al: Use of computed tomography renal angiography for screening feline renal transplant donors, Vet Radiol Ultrasound 44:636, 2003.
11. Lirtzman RA, Gregory CR: Long-term renal and hematological effects of uninephrectomy in healthy feline kidney donors, J Am Vet Med Assoc 207:1044, 1995.
12. Halloran PF, Leung Lui S: Approved immunosuppressants. In Primer on transplantation, Thorofare, NJ, 1998, American Society of Transplant Physicians, pp 93-102.
13. Kahan BD, Yoshimura N, Pellis, NR, et al: Pharmacodynamics of cyclosporine, Transplantation Proc 238-251, 1986.
14. Kim W, Cho ML, Kim SI, et al: Divergent effects of cyclosporine on Th1/Th2 Type cytokines in patients with severe, refractory rheumatoid arthritis, J Rheumatol 27:324-331, 2000.
15. Kuga K, Nishifuji K, Iwasaki T: Cyclosporine A inhibits transcription of cytokine genes and decreases the frequencies of IL-2 producing cells in feline mononuclear cells, J Vet Med Sci 70:1011, 2008.
16. Aronson LR, Stumhofer J, Drobatz KJ, et al: Affect of cyclosporine, dexamethasone and CTLA4-Ig on production of cytokines in normal cats and those undergoing renal transplantation, Am J Vet Res 72:541, 2011.
17. Graham-Mize CA, Rosser EJ: Bioavailability and activity of prednisone and prednisolone in the feline patient, Dermatol Abstracts 15:9, 2004.
18. Katayama M, McAnulty JF: Renal transplantation in cats: techniques, complications, and immunosuppression, Compend Contin Educ Pract 24:874, 2002.
19. McAnulty JF, Lensmeyer GL: The effects of ketoconazole on the pharmacokinetics of cyclosporine A in cats, Vet Surg 28:448, 1999.
20. Katayama M, Katayama R, Kamishina H: Effects of multiple oral dosing of itraconazole on the pharmacokinetics of cyclosporine in cats, J Fel Med Surg 12:512, 2010.
21. Katayama M, Nishijima N, Okamura Y, et al: Interaction of clarithromycin with cyclosporine in cats: pharmacokinetic study and case report, J Fel Med Surg 14:257, 2012.
22. Snell W, Aronson LR, Larenza P: Influence of anesthetic variables on long-term survival in 94 cats undergoing renal transplantation surgery. Not yet submitted.
23. McAnulty JF: Hypothermic storage of feline kidneys for transplantation: successful ex vivo storage up to 7 hours, Vet Surg 27:312, 1998.
24. Mehl ML, Kyles AE, Pollard R, et al: Comparison of 3 techniques for ureteroneocystostomy in cats, Vet Surg 34:114, 2005.

25. Hardie RJ, Schmiedt C, Phillips L, et al: Ureteral papilla implantation as a technique for neoureterocystotomy in cats, Vet Surg 34:393, 2005.
26. Kyles AE, Gregory CR, Wooldridge JD, et al: Management of hypertension controls postoperative neurological disorders after renal transplantation in cats, Vet Surg 28:436, 1999.
27. Mathews KG, Gregory CR: Renal transplants in cats: 66 cases (1987-1996), J Am Vet Med Assoc 211:1432, 1997.
28. Kyles AE, Gregory CR, Griffey SM, et al: Evaluation of the clinical and histological features of renal allograft rejection in cats, Vet Surg 31:49, 2002.
29. Halling KB, Graham JP, Newell SP, et al: Sonographic and scintigraphic evaluation of acute renal allograft rejection in cats, Vet Radiol Ultrasound 44:707, 2003.
30. Pollard R, Nyland TG, Bernsteen L, et al: Ultrasonagraphic evaluation of renal autografts in normal cats, Vet Radiol Ultrasound 40:380, 1999.
31. Halling KB, Graham JP, Newell SP, et al: Sonographic and scintigraphic evaluation of acute renal allograft rejection in cats, Vet Radiol Ultrasound 44:707, 2003
32. Gregory CR. In Bojrab MJ, editor: Renal Transplantation. Current techniques in small animal surgery, ed 4, Baltimore, 1998, Williams and Wilkins.
33. Aronson LR, Gregory CR: Possible hemolytic uremic syndrome in three cats after renal transplantation and cyclosporine therapy, Vet Surg 28:135, 1999.
34. Aronson LR, Kyles AE, Preston A, et al: Renal transplantation in cats diagnosed with calcium oxalate urolithiasis: 19 cases (1997-2004), J Am Vet Med Assoc 228:743, 2006.
35. Aronson LR: Retroperitoneal fibrosis in four cats following renal transplantation, J Am Vet Med Assoc 221:984, 2002.
36. Kadar E, Sykes JE, Kass PH, et al: Evaluation of the prevalence of infections in cats after renal transplantation:169 cases (1987-2003), J Am Vet Med Assoc 227:948, 2005.
37. Wooldridge J, Gregory CR, Mathews KG, et al: The prevalence of malignant neoplasia in feline renal transplant recipients, Vet Surg 31:94, 2002.
38. Schmeidt CW, Grimes JA, Holzman G: Incidence and risk factors for development of malignant neoplasia after feline renal transplantation and cyclosporine-based immunosuppression, Vet Compar Oncol 7:45, 2009.
39. Wormser C, Aronson LR, Donnahue A, et al: Malignant neoplasia following renal transplantation in cats: 28 cases (1998-2010) (in progress).
40. Durham A, Mariano AD, Holmes E, et al: Characterization of post transplantation lymphoma in feline renal transplant recipients J of Comparative Pathology. In Press. (in progress).
41. Case JB, Kyles AE, Nelson RW, et al: Incidence of and risk factors for diabetes mellitus in cats that have undergone renal transplantation: 187 cases (1986-2005), J Am Vet Med Assoc 230:880, 2007.
42. Gregory CR, Kyles AE, Bernsteen L, et al: Results of clinical renal transplantation in 15 dogs using triple drug immunosuppressive therapy, Vet Surg 35:105, 2006.
43. Lirtzman RA, Gregory CR, Levitski RE, et al: Combined immunosuppression with Leflunomide and Cyclosporine prevents MLR-mismatched renal allograft rejection in a mongrel canine model, Transplantation Proc 28:945, 1996.
44. Phillips H, Aronson LR: Novel vascular technique for renal transplantation in dogs, J Am Vet Med Assoc 240:298, 2012.
45. Gregory CR, Gourley IM, Taylor NJ, et al: Preliminary results of clinical renal allograft transplantation in the dog and cat, J Vet Intern Med 1:53, 1987.
46. Mathews KA, Holmberg DL, Miller CW: Kidney transplantation in dogs with naturally occurring end stage renal disease, J Am Anim Hosp Assoc 36:294, 2000.
47. Bernsteen L, Gregory CR, Kyles AE, et al: Microemulsified cyclosporine-based immunosuppression for the prevention of acute renal allograft rejection in unrelated dogs: preliminary experimental study, Vet Surg 32:219, 2003.
48. Broaddus KD, Tillson DM, Lenz SD, et al: Renal allograft histopathology in dog leukocyte antigen mismatched dogs after renal transplantation, Vet Surg 35:125, 2006.
49. Kyles AE, Gregory CR, Griffey SM, et al: An evaluation of combined immunosuppression with MNA 715 and microemulsified cyclosporine on renal allograft rejection in mismatched mongrel dogs, Vet Surg 31:358, 2002.
50. Kyles AE, Gregory CR, Griffey SM, et al: Modified noble placation for the prevention of intestinal intussusception after renal transplantation in dogs, J Invest Surg 16:161, 2003.
51. Milovancev M, Schmeidt CW, Bentley E, et al: Use of capecitabine to prevent acute renal allograft rejection in dog erythrocyte antigen-mismatched mongrel dogs, Vet Surg 36:10, 2007.
52. Schmeidt C, Penzo C, Schwab M, et al: Use of Capecitabine after renal allograft transplantation in dog erythrocyte antigen matched dogs, Vet Surg 35:113, 2006.

CHAPTER 136
MINIMALLY INVASIVE PROCEDURES

Dana L. Clarke, VMD, DACVECC • William T.N. Culp, VMD, DACVS

KEY POINTS

- Following the trend in human medicine, minimally invasive procedure options in veterinary medicine have grown in popularity and availability.
- Minimally invasive and interventional treatment procedures often require specialized equipment and advanced training to be performed safely and with proficiency.
- Careful patient selection and appropriate discussions about the procedural risks and benefits compared with traditional options are essential to successful outcomes and client satisfaction.
- While there are limited laparoscopic and thoracoscopic indications in emergency and critical care medicine, some interventional procedures, such as tracheal and urethral stenting and vascular access techniques, may be needed emergently.

The use of minimally invasive procedures in the critical care setting has historically been limited; however, increased accessibility to more advanced technology and an explosion in the available endoscopic and interventional radiology treatment options have made these procedures more readily obtainable. Currently, minimally invasive procedures play a major role in the treatment of critically ill veterinary patients, and that role is likely to continue expanding.

INSTRUMENTATION

The use of more advanced imaging modalities and novel categories of instrumentation has allowed clinicians to decrease the morbidity that has traditionally been encountered with certain diagnostics and treatments. Endoscopic procedures use a camera that transmits an image onto a monitor. The endoscope is designed to be relatively small to decrease the invasiveness of the procedure, while image transmission to a monitor still allows the clinician to perform procedures with excellent visualization. Endoscopes are created in both flexible and rigid forms and can be equipped with working channels to allow for fluid or contrast infusion and precise instrument placement.

Nearly all instruments that are currently available for use in open surgery have been modified for use in laparoscopic and thoracoscopic procedures. Ports are used for the passage of instrumentation after being introduced into the appropriate body cavity. Scissors, hemostats, retractors, vessel-sealing devices, and many other instruments have been designed for passage through a small port. Stapling devices and bags for the removal of samples help to prevent seeding of cells or infection to adjacent tissue and are used on a regular basis. Suction and cautery devices have also been specifically designed for use during minimally invasive procedures.

Interventional radiology (IR) involves the use of imaging modalities and minimally invasive equipment for the purpose of performing diagnostic and therapeutic procedures. Clinicians performing IR procedures need to develop a strong understanding of different imaging modalities, particularly fluoroscopy, ultrasound, and computed tomography, as well as when each modality is indicated for a given patient. The instrumentation used during IR procedures is often unique to a particular procedure and has a specific role. Some examples of common IR instruments include guide wires, selective and guiding catheters, vascular introducers and guiding sheaths, stents, balloons and embolic agents.

APPROACHES/ACCESS

Many minimally invasive procedures use a natural orifice as an access point for the region of the body that requires evaluation or treatment. Esophagoscopy, gastroscopy, duodenoscopy, tracheoscopy, and retroflex rhinoscopy can all be performed through the mouth, as can tracheal and esophageal stenting. The nares are an entry point for procedures such as nasopharyngeal balloon dilation and stenting, as well as antegrade rhinoscopy. Access to the urethra and bladder is obtained via the penis in male dogs and the vulva in female dogs.

For procedures such as laparoscopy and thoracoscopy, small incisions must be made into the particular body cavity that is being evaluated. Additional incisions for the placement of extra ports are often also necessary to perform particular techniques. For procedures such as renal biopsy and laparoscopic-guided cholecystocentesis, only the camera port is necessary because the instrumentation needed for sample acquisition can be passed percutaneously. However, other procedures (e.g., liver biopsy, ovariohysterectomy to treat pyometra, laparoscopic foreign body retrieval) require additional incisions for the placement of more ports.

Vascular access is necessary for emergent management of hemorrhage or vascular obstructions. Arterial or venous access can be achieved percutaneously or through a surgical approach to the vessel. Patients suffering from severe hemorrhage that is refractory to traditional treatment options can be treated with embolization after a vascular introducer and sheath are placed. For many small animals with intravascular foreign bodies, access to the appropriate vessel must be obtained with a large introducer sheath to allow for extraction of the foreign body. Foreign bodies occurring in the peripheral or central venous system often lodge in the great veins, heart, or pulmonary arteries, and access through the jugular vein is usually recommended.[1]

Scope-Guided Procedures

Laparoscopic/thoracoscopic procedures

Currently the indications for laparoscopy and thoracoscopy in a critical care setting are limited. Laparoscopy and thoracoscopy can be used as a means of initial evaluation in cases where a large exploration may not be necessary. These procedures can be useful in assessing patients with pleural and abdominal effusions to determine an underlying cause[2]; however, suctioning of the cavity is likely indicated to allow for more thorough investigation. If a biopsy of a thoracic or abdominal organ is needed to guide case management, laparoscopy and thoracoscopy offer a fast and minimally invasive means of obtaining these biopsy samples.[2,3] However, in all cases where laparoscopic or thoracoscopic procedures are performed, clinicians performing these techniques must be comfortable with conversion to a laparotomy or thoracotomy in the event of procedural complications such as hemorrhage, significant organ damage, inadequate visualization, or extensive pathology.

A few specific emergent conditions can be treated with these techniques. The removal of both thoracic and abdominal foreign bodies with thoracoscopic- or laparoscopic-guidance, respectively, has been described.[4,5] In the study evaluating laparoscopic foreign body retrieval, 20 dogs underwent a laparoscopic gastrotomy with subsequent closure performed using manual suturing or linear staples.[5] The outcome of the procedure in all dogs was deemed satisfactory.[5]

A recent report documented the use of laparoscopy for the treatment of canine pyometra in 10 dogs.[6] In these dogs a wound retraction device was placed in the caudal incision to allow for exteriorization of the uterus and uterine horns via a laparoscopic-assisted technique. The wound retraction device also protected the body wall and helped to diminish the chance of tearing the diseased reproductive tract. Overall, the outcome with this procedure was excellent; however, a major complication occurred in one case when a uterine horn was torn during manipulation. In this case, conversion to an open procedure was performed.[6,7]

Pericardial effusion may result in cardiac tamponade, hypotension, and eventual death. A thoracoscopic pericardial window and subtotal pericardectomy have become established techniques in veterinary medicine for management of pericardial effusion.[7] These procedures enable the pericardial fluid to drain into the pleural space to prevent the development of cardiac tamponade and resultant cardiovascular dysfunction.

Tracheoscopy/bronchoscopy

Tracheoscopy and bronchoscopy are helpful adjunctive diagnostics when evaluating animals with tracheal, bronchial, and lower airway disease. Depending on the size of the patient, endoscopic airway evaluation while maintaining intubation may not be possible and extubation during tracheoscopy/bronchoscopy may be required. In these patients, oxygen insufflation through a red rubber catheter in the trachea or via the working channel of the scope can help maintain oxygenation during evaluation. Alternatively, high-frequency jet ventilation can also be useful in patients that require extubation. In patients large enough to maintain intubation during these procedures, the use of a bronchoscope adaptor allows for passage of the scope into a closed system while maintaining oxygen within the circuit.

If a foreign body is aspirated, subsequent airway inflammation or obstruction may result.[8,9] In a recent study evaluating the bronchoscopic removal of foreign bodies in the airway, the most common culprit was plant material.[9] In that cohort of dogs and cats, bronchoscopy was successfully used to retrieve the foreign body in 76% of animals (Figure 136-1).[9]

Esophagoscopy/gastroscopy/duodenoscopy

Gastrointestinal endoscopic procedures are regularly performed in many practices and are often used in the diagnosis and treatment of intestinal disease. Gastrointestinal endoscopy can be used as a tool to obtain biopsies of the esophagus, stomach, and duodenum, as well as to assess these organs for the presence of disease such as ulcerations, neoplasia, and foreign bodies. Certain procedures such as percutaneous endoscopic gastrostomy (PEG) tube placement and endoscopic-assisted gastropexy can also be performed.[10,11]

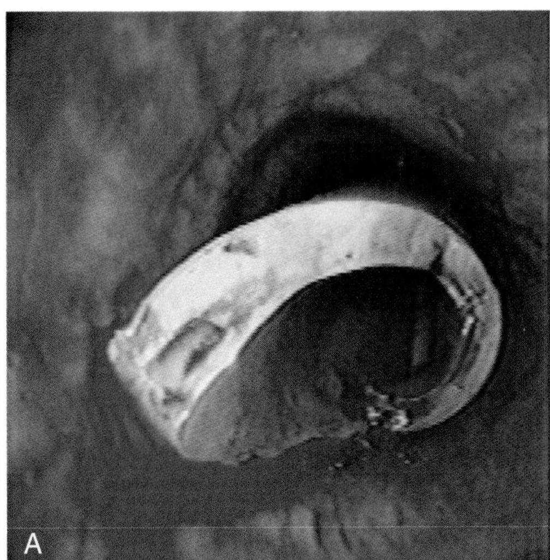

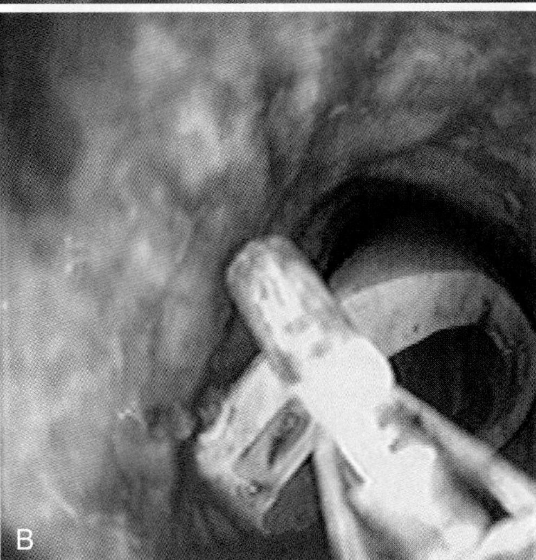

FIGURE 136-1 A, Chewed end of an endotracheal tube lodged in the distal trachea of a young German Shepherd after general anesthesia for wound debridement. **B,** Endoscopic alligator forceps placed in the working channel of the bronchoscope facilitated removal.

The ingestion of foreign bodies that lead to intestinal obstruction is common in canine and feline patients; the removal of these foreign bodies is often considered an emergent procedure. Several studies have evaluated the effectiveness of the use of endoscopy to facilitate removal of these foreign bodies.[12,13] Endoscopy has successfully removed esophageal or gastric foreign bodies in up to 90% of dogs.[12] However, a separate study evaluating only dental chew esophageal foreign bodies noted a success rate of approximately 25%.[14] In those cases where endoscopic removal is not possible, foreign bodies can often be pushed into the stomach to allow for removal via gastrotomy; most consider a laparotomy and gastrotomy to be technically easier and to result in less morbidity than a thoracotomy and esophagotomy.

Cystourethroscopy

Cystourethroscopy, much like gastrointestinal endoscopy, has tremendous diagnostic and treatment potential. The performance of cystourethroscopy on an emergent basis is occasionally necessary to assess patients with urethral obstruction from both malignant and benign (e.g., urethritis and calculi) disease and to assist with management of the obstruction.[15-17] Cystourethroscopy may be used for visualization during laser lithotripsy with the goal of breaking a stone into small enough fragments for extraction.[15] Cystourethroscopy can also be used to assist with catheter placement in patients that are difficult to catheterize in a typical retrograde fashion and to remove urethral or bladder foreign bodies.[18]

Interventional Radiology Procedures

Urethral stenting

Bladder, urethral, and prostatic neoplasia can result in obstruction of the urethra and prevent the voiding of urine. As a result of this obstruction, postrenal azotemia, electrolyte imbalances, and hyperkalemia-induced life-threatening arrhythmias may result. Long-term strategies for managing the urethral obstruction in these patients include cystostomy tube placement or urethral stenting. Chemotherapy, including nonsteroidal antiinflammatory drugs, and radiation therapy may be considered as primary tumor treatment; however, these procedures are generally not effective in an acute setting and are pursued only after the urethral obstructions have been relieved and the patient is hemodynamically stable.

In cases of malignant urethral obstruction, urine drainage can be accomplished on an immediate basis via cystocentesis or urethral catheterization. When retrograde catheterization cannot be performed, percutaneous antegrade urethral access can be performed using cystocentesis and fluoroscopic-guided guide wire passage through the bladder in an antegrade direction out of the urethra. A catheter can then be placed retrograde over the guide wire and positioned in the bladder for drainage until definitive therapy can be performed.

Placing a stent within the urethra to restore luminal patency can allow for voiding of urine and immediately improve a patient's clinical status and comfort. This procedure is easily and quickly performed by someone experienced in stent placement. Although this treatment will not alter the course of the primary disease process (e.g., transitional cell carcinoma), it will alter the immediate clinical course and likely improve the quality of life for the patient.

Three retrospective studies have evaluated the outcomes associated with stent placement for malignant urethral obstruction in dogs.[19-21] The median survival times after stent placement have ranged from 20 to 78 days[19-21]; however, the administration of adjuvant therapy such as chemotherapy significantly prolonged survival in one study.[19] In the current studies most owners have demonstrated satisfaction with their decision to pursue stent placement.[18,21]

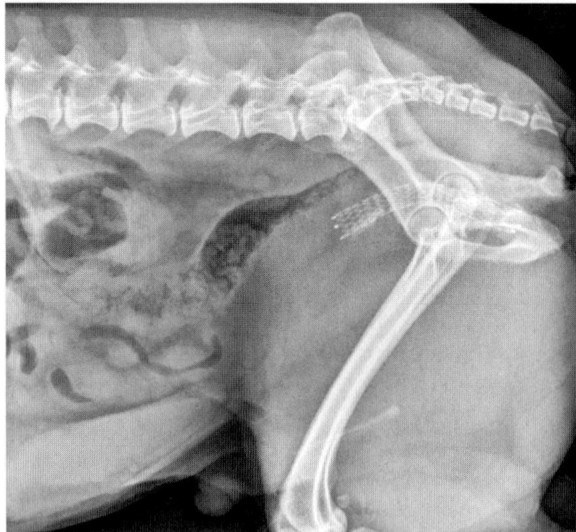

FIGURE 136-2 Self-expanding nitinol stent in the urethra of a male dog with urethral obstruction secondary to transitional cell carcinoma.

Although complications such as incontinence, stent migration, and in-growth of disease through the stent are possible after urethral stenting, clinical improvement in urinary stream and comfort is noted in the majority of cases. At this time no predictive factors have been identified for the development of incontinence, and owners must be prepared to accept an approximately 25% risk of severe urinary incontinence as a complication of this permanent procedure.[19-21] Because the procedure can be performed in a minimally invasive fashion through a natural orifice (except male cats; see the next paragraph), many clients elect to pursue urethral stenting to improve the quality of life of their pet (Figure 136-2).

Benign urethral obstructions occur less commonly in dogs than malignant obstructions; however, cats may develop benign urethral strictures secondary to a previous traumatic catheterization or prior stone passage.[22] Feline urethral stenting has been documented in several case reports, and successful outcomes have been achieved.[20,23-25] In male cats it is necessary to perform urethral stenting from an antegrade approach (because of the size of the urethral orifice) unless a previous perineal urethrostomy has been performed.

Ureteral stenting

Ureteral obstructions are a complex problem affecting both dogs and cats. One study suggested that most cases of proximal ureteral obstruction are treated by ureterotomy, whereas most cases of distal ureteral obstruction are treated by partial ureterectomy or ureteroneocystostomy.[26] However, cases of ureteral obstruction are often not straightforward, because some stones may not be noted on radiographs or ultrasound, and some dogs and cats may have multiple stones, an accumulation of crystals, dried solidified blood clots, or strictures resulting in ureteral obstruction. Many animals with ureteral obstruction are azotemic and critically ill at the time of initial evaluation, and decompression of the kidney is often recommended to prevent destruction of the parenchyma.[27]

Ureteral stenting has been advocated as a means of allowing urine to pass from the kidney into the bladder in cases of obstruction.[28] Ureteral stenting involves the placement of a stent within the ureter that is anchored both within the renal pelvis and the bladder by the pigtail design of the stent. Ureteral stents are placed either surgically or with the assistance of cystoscopy. These stents may be removed at a future date, but the clinical status of the patient may alter this course. Over time, these stents cause passive dilation of the ureter around the stent, allowing urine and potentially calculi to pass.[29] Complications associated with ureteral stenting include injury to the ureter during stent placement, urine leakage, infection, stent migration, encrustation and reobstruction, hematuria, and stranguria.[29-31]

Currently, ureteral stenting for benign and malignant disease in dogs and cats is performed regularly.[28,32] In most feline cases, ureteral stents are placed surgically and access to the ureter may be antegrade (through the kidney) or retrograde (from the ureteral orifice). In female dogs, many stents can be placed with cystoscopic-guidance and surgery is therefore not necessary. A technique for placement of ureteral stents for malignant ureteral obstruction via percutaneous access has been described.[32] The procedure was found to be safe and effective, and all patients experienced improvement in the severity of hydroureter and hydronephrosis.[32]

In azotemic patients, significant postobstructive diuresis can follow relief of the ureteral obstruction. These patients require intensive management of fluid and electrolyte balance during diuresis. Frequent monitoring of body weight, hydration, central venous pressure, and urine output is essential.

Tracheal stenting

Dogs with tracheal collapse may be presented with minor signs, such as occasional coughing, or may display severe respiratory distress to the point of requiring endotracheal intubation. When possible, medical management with oral therapies (e.g., anxiolytics and antitussives) is attempted first for the treatment of animals with tracheal collapse; however, this approach is not always successful in controlling clinical signs. Several procedures have been advocated when medical management fails; general categories include surgery and stent placement within the trachea.

Tracheal stenting can be performed quickly by an experienced individual and in many cases allows for immediate relief of clinical signs. However, long-term medical management is often necessary after stent placement and owners should be well prepared for this when electing to pursue tracheal stenting. Stent placement can be performed with either endoscopic or fluoroscopic guidance (Figure 136-3).[33-35]

Several studies have focused on the use of intraluminal tracheal stents and the outcomes associated with this procedure in dogs.[34-37] Although many clients are pleased with the animal's improvement after tracheal stenting, several complications can occur, including stent fracture, excessive granulation tissue formation, tracheitis, pneumonia, and incorrect deployment.[34-36] Currently, only one case series of intraluminal tracheal stenting to treat feline tracheal stenosis (benign and malignant) has been documented in the veterinary literature. In all three cats, there were no complications associated with the stenting procedure, and all cats had resolution of respiratory difficulty upon recovery from the procedure. The cat with tracheal neoplasia developed respiratory distress secondary to pulmonary parenchymal disease 6 weeks after stenting and the two cats with benign disease were symptom free at 32 weeks and 44 months.[33]

Cavity effusions and percutaneous drainage

Body cavity effusions can occur for many reasons, and the underlying cause should be treated whenever possible. In certain scenarios (e.g., idiopathic chylothorax), cavitary effusions may continue despite appropriate therapy and other options must be considered. Additionally, the percutaneous drainage of effusions may be beneficial in particular cases before pursuing definitive therapy (e.g., uroperitoneum). The goal of the drainage in those cases is not to provide long-term treatment but to stabilize the animal before undergoing a long anesthetic event.

Locking-loop catheters are a good option for short-term drainage and often require only sedation for placement. The placement of a locking-loop catheter can be performed percutaneously (with

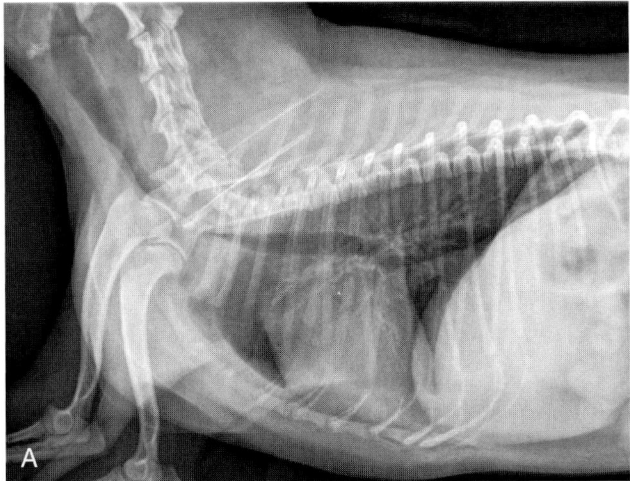

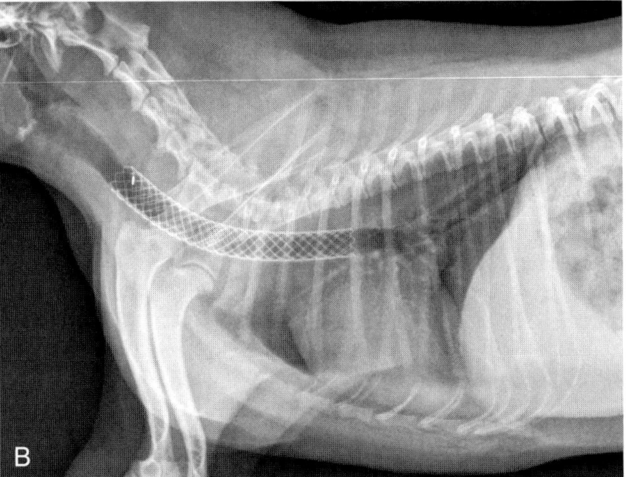

FIGURE 136-3 A, Thoracic radiographs from a 3-year-old spayed female Yorkshire Terrier presenting for respiratory distress showing severe tracheal collapse of the caudal cervical through cranial intrathoracic trachea. **B,** Postoperative radiographs from the same dog after placement of an intraluminal tracheal stent.

fluoroscopic guidance), and the clinician can elect to use guide wire guidance or place the catheter over the associated stylet and needle that are provided with the drainage catheter. The catheter should be placed in a dependent region of the chest or abdomen, and all fenestrations must be located intracavitary.

Drainage catheters can also be attached to a port for long-term drainage; general anesthesia is required for this procedure because of the increased incision necessary for port placement. The catheter component can still be placed percutaneously. When the catheter is exited from the body cavity, it is attached to a port that is sutured in an accessible and proximal subcutaneous space to allow for periodic aspiration. This option is recommended for effusions that may be suspected to persist such as chylothorax or neoplastic effusions.

In one recent study a modified Seldinger technique was used to place small-bore chest drains in the thorax.[38] Anesthesia was not necessary for drain placement in any of the cases, and the drains were placed easily and effectively by people with varying levels of experience.[38]

Percutanous drainage of organs can also be performed; cystostomy, nephrostomy, and cholecystostomy drainage catheters allow for temporary drainage of these particular organs. The chance of accidental removal is decreased when using locking-loop catheters. A combination of ultrasound and fluoroscopic guidance can be used during placement.

Intravascular foreign body removal

One complication of intravascular catheterization includes breakage or dislodgement of a component or components of the catheter that results in an intravascular foreign body. Complication rates as high as 71%, and even death, have been reported in human cases.[39,40]

Although intravascular foreign bodies are still an uncommon entity, the use of more minimally invasive interventional techniques in veterinary medicine will likely lead to increased encounters. A recent report documented the percutaneous removal of intravascular foreign bodies in five dogs, a goat, and a horse.[1] All devices were successfully removed with the use of a snare that was manipulated under fluoroscopic guidance.[1]

Epistaxis

Several causes of epistaxis have been described, including severe rhinitis, neoplasia, trauma, periapical abscessation, coagulopathy, hypertension, and vasculitis; however, idiopathic epistaxis is reported in a large number of cases.[41,42] Historically, treatments such as packing the nasal passage with sponges, injection of vasoconstrictive medications into the nasal passages, and ligation of a carotid artery or arteries have been attempted with mixed success.

An alternative to these options involves the delivery of an embolic agent to the blood vessels that are contributing to bleeding and epistaxis. This is performed by catheterizing the arterial system and visualizing the nasal vasculature with intravenous contrast and fluoroscopy. Digital subtraction angiography and roadmapping are especially useful for procedures involving small vasculature. When the supplying vessels have been localized, an embolic agent is delivered via the catheter to cause cessation of blood flow. This treatment allows for a more specific treatment directed at the blood supply causing the epistaxis and decreases the likelihood of collateral blood vessels causing continued epistaxis. Reports of this treatment in animals are rare, but this treatment has been reported to be successful in three dogs with intractable epistaxis.[43]

Vascular obstructions

Vascular obstructions secondary to thrombosis are reported relatively commonly in veterinary medicine; however, the true incidence is probably underestimated because they can be difficult to diagnose. Management of patients with confirmed thromboembolic disease can be challenging. Vascular obstruction can also occur secondary to neoplastic vascular compression or invasion. Surgical therapy for vascular obstructions can be technically challenging and dangerous, which is why interventional management options to remove or palliate the obstruction are gaining popularity.[44-46]

Venous thrombi are primarily composed of fibrin and red blood cells and are generally considered secondary to stasis of blood flow or hypercoagulability.[44] Obstruction of the cranial vena cava (caval syndrome) can result from thrombi, heartworm disease, cranial mediastinal masses, and pacemaker leads. Obstruction of the caudal vena cava (Budd-Chiari syndrome) can be secondary to thrombi, stenosis (congenital or acquired), fibrous obstruction, falciform entrapment, and intrathoracic caudal vena cava kinking.[46-53] A case report of local tissue plasminogen activator (tPA) administration in a dog with caval syndrome and chylothorax secondary to pacemaker leads was ineffective for resolution of the obstruction, and balloon dilation of the vessel was required.[54] Systemic tPA given to a Maltese with catheter-associated thrombosis of the cranial vena cava and secondary chylothorax decreased the size of the thrombus and resolved the chylothorax but resulted in hemorrhage from the jugular catheter and esophagostomy tube sites.[55] The use of a self-expanding nitinol stent in the caudal vena cava of a kitten with refractory ascites and caudal vena cava stricture that did not respond to dilation has been described.[56] Endovascular stenting of a hepatic vein with or without caval stenting for treatment of Budd-Chiari syndrome in three dogs with suspected or confirmed neoplastic obstructions of the caudal vena cava and hepatic veins has been described. The minimally invasive therapy resulted in long-term (7 to 20 months) resolution of clinical signs in patients for whom there were limited options for palliation.[57]

Arterial thrombi are composed primarily of platelets. Because arterial thromboembolic events are often emergencies that result in pain, ischemia, and tissue damage, antiplatelet drugs are of limited value for treatment of acute arterial thromboembolic events in veterinary patients.[44,46]

Systemic urokinase, streptokinase, and tPA have been used with varying effectiveness in cats with aortic thromboembolism (ATE), in dogs with ATE, and in a femoral arterial obstruction in a dog.[58-70] Local administration of tPA in a cat with ATE and a Greyhound with ATE secondary to protein-losing nephropathy has been described, with both cases having return of motor function in their limbs and survival to discharge.[71,72] Rheolytic therapy with AngioJet technology (requiring general anesthesia) has been described in six cats with ATE. The AngioJet uses high-velocity jets of saline directed at the catheter tip to create a vacuum that pulls pieces of thrombus into the collection system. Five of the six cats had successful clot dissolution, but only three of the six survived to discharge, which is similar to other management strategies.[73]

REFERENCES

1. Culp WT, Weisse C, Berent AC, et al: Percutaneous endovascular retrieval of an intravascular foreign body in five dogs, a goat, and a horse, J Am Vet Med Assoc 232:1850, 2008.
2. Kovak JR, Ludwig LL, Bergman PJ, et al: Use of thoracoscopy to determine the etiology of pleural effusion in dogs and cats: 18 cases (1998-2001), J Am Vet Med Assoc 221:990, 2002.
3. Monnet E, Twedt DC: Laparoscopy, Vet Clin North Am Small Anim Pract 33:1147, 2003.
4. Grand JG, Bureau SC: Video-assisted thoracoscopic surgery for pneumothorax induced by migration of a K-wire to the chest, J Am Anim Hosp Assoc 47:268, 2011.
5. Lew M, Jalynski M, Brzeski W: Laparoscopic removal of gastric foreign bodies in dogs—comparison of manual suturing and stapling viscerosynthesis, Pol J Vet Sci 8:147, 2005.
6. Adamovich-Rippe KN, Mayhew PD, Runge JJR, et al: Evaluation of laparoscopic-assisted ovariohysterectomy for treatment of canine pyometra, Vet Surg 42(5):572, 2013
7. Monnet E: Interventional thoracoscopy in small animals, Vet Clin North Am Small Anim Pract 39:965, 2009.
8. Lotti U, Niebauer GW: Tracheobronchial foreign bodies of plant origin in 153 hunting dogs, Compendium 14:900, 1992.
9. Tenwolde AC, Johnson LR, Hunt GB, et al: The role of bronchoscopy in foreign body removal in dogs and cats: 37 cases (2000-2008), J Vet Intern Med 24:1063, 2010.
10. Dujowich M, Reimer SB: Evaluation of an endoscopically assisted gastropexy technique in dogs, Am J Vet Res 69:537, 2008.
11. Salinardi BJ, Harkin KR, Bulmer BJ, et al: Comparison of complications of percutaneous endoscopic versus surgically placed gastrostomy tubes in 42 dogs and 52 cats, J Am Anim Hosp Assoc 42:51, 2006.
12. Gianella P, Pfammatter NS, Burgener IA: Oesophageal and gastric endoscopic foreign body removal: complications and follow-up of 102 dogs, J Small Anim Pract 50:649, 2009.
13. Thompson HC, Cortes Y, Gannon K, et al: Esophageal foreign bodies in dogs: 34 cases (2004-2009), J Vet Emerg Crit Care (San Antonio) 22:253, 2012.
14. Leib MS, Sartor LL: Esophageal foreign body obstruction caused by a dental chew treat in 31 dogs (2000-2006), J Am Vet Med Assoc 232:1021, 2008.
15. Lulich JP, Osborne CA, Albasan H, et al: Efficacy and safety of laser lithotripsy in fragmentation of urocystoliths and urethroliths for removal in dogs, J Am Vet Med Assoc 234:1279, 2009.
16. Messer JS, Chew DJ, McLoughlin MA: Cystoscopy: techniques and clinical applications, Clin Tech Small Anim Pract 20:52, 2005.
17. Hostutler RA, Chew DJ, Eaton KA, et al: Cystoscopic appearance of proliferative urethritis in 2 dogs before and after treatment, J Vet Intern Med 18:113, 2004.
18. Cherbinsky O, Westropp J, Tinga S, et al: Ultrasonographic features of grass awns in the urinary bladder, Vet Radiol Ultrasound 51:462, 2010.
19. Blackburn AL, Berent AC, Weisse CW, et al: Evaluation of outcome following urethral stent placement for the treatment of obstructive carcinoma of the urethra in dogs: 42 cases (2004-2008), J Am Vet Med Assoc 242:59, 2013.
20. McMillan SK, Knapp DW, Ramos-Vara JA, et al: Outcome of urethral stent placement for management of urethral obstruction secondary to transitional cell carcinoma in dogs: 19 cases (2007-2010), J Am Vet Med Assoc 241:1627, 2012.
21. Weisse C, Berent A, Todd K, et al: Evaluation of palliative stenting for management of malignant urethral obstructions in dogs, J Am Vet Med Assoc 229:226, 2006.
22. Anderson RB, Aronson LR, Drobatz KJ, et al: Prognostic factors for successful outcome following urethral rupture in dogs and cats, J Am Anim Hosp Assoc 42:136, 2006.
23. Christensen NI, Culvenor J, Langova V: Fluoroscopic stent placement for the relief of malignant urethral obstruction in a cat, Aust Vet J 88:478, 2010.
24. Hadar EN, Morgan MJ, Morgan OD: Use of a self-expanding metallic stent for the treatment of a urethral stricture in a young cat, J Feline Med Surg 13:597, 2011.
25. Newman RG, Mehler SJ, Kitchell BE, et al: Use of a balloon-expandable metallic stent to relieve malignant urethral obstruction in a cat, J Am Vet Med Assoc 234:236, 2009.
26. Kyles AE, Hardie EM, Wooden BG, et al: Management and outcome of cats with ureteral calculi: 153 cases (1984-2002), J Am Vet Med Assoc 226:937, 2005.
27. Roberts SF, Aronson LR, Brown DC: Postoperative mortality in cats after ureterolithotomy, Vet Surg 40:438, 2011.
28. Nicoli S, Morello E, Martano M, et al: Double-J ureteral stenting in nine cats with ureteral obstruction, Vet J 194:60, 2012.
29. Lennon GM, Thornhill JA, Grainger R, et al: Double pigtail ureteric stent versus percutaneous nephrostomy: effects on stone transit and ureteric motility, Eur Urol 31:24, 1997.
30. Auge BK, Preminger GM: Ureteral stents and their use in endourology, Curr Opin Urol 12:217, 2002.
31. Liatsikos E, Kallidonis P, Stolzenburg JU, et al: Ureteral stents: past, present and future, Expert Rev Med Devices 6:313, 2009.
32. Berent AC, Weisse C, Beal MW, et al: Use of indwelling, double-pigtail stents for treatment of malignant ureteral obstruction in dogs: 12 cases (2006-2009), J Am Vet Med Assoc 238:1017, 2011.
33. Culp WT, Weisse C, Cole SG, et al: Intraluminal tracheal stenting for treatment of tracheal narrowing in three cats, Vet Surg 36:107, 2007.
34. Durant AM, Sura P, Rohrbach B, et al: Use of nitinol stents for end-stage tracheal collapse in dogs, Vet Surg 41:807, 2012.
35. Sura PA, Krahwinkel DJ: Self-expanding nitinol stents for the treatment of tracheal collapse in dogs: 12 cases (2001-2004), J Am Vet Med Assoc 232:228, 2008.
36. Moritz A, Schneider M, Bauer N: Management of advanced tracheal collapse in dogs using intraluminal self-expanding biliary wallstents, J Vet Intern Med 18:31, 2004.
37. Sun F, Uson J, Ezquerra J, et al: Endotracheal stenting therapy in dogs with tracheal collapse, Vet J 175:186, 2008.
38. Valtolina C, Adamantos S: Evaluation of small-bore wire-guided chest drains for management of pleural space disease, J Small Anim Pract 50:290, 2009.
39. Fisher RG, Ferreyro R: Evaluation of current techniques for nonsurgical removal of intravascular iatrogenic foreign bodies, AJR Am J Roentgenol 130:541, 1978.
40. Richardson JD, Grover FL, Trinkle JK: Intravenous catheter emboli. Experience with twenty cases and collective review, Am J Surg 128:722, 1974.

41. Bissett SA, Drobatz KJ, McKnight A, et al: Prevalence, clinical features, and causes of epistaxis in dogs: 176 cases (1996-2001), J Am Vet Med Assoc 231:1843, 2007.
42. Strasser JL, Hawkins EC: Clinical features of epistaxis in dogs: a retrospective study of 35 cases (1999-2002), J Am Anim Hosp Assoc 41:179, 2005.
43. Weisse C, Nicholson ME, Rollings C, et al: Use of percutaneous arterial embolization for treatment of intractable epistaxis in three dogs, J Am Vet Med Assoc 224:1307-1311, 1281, 2004.
44. Dunn ME: Thrombectomy and thrombolysis: the interventional radiology approach, J Vet Emerg Crit Care 21(2):144, 2011.
45. Weisse CW: Introduction to interventional radiology for the criticalist, J Vet Emerg Crit Care 21(2):79, 2011.
46. Scansen BA: Interventional cardiology for the criticalist, J Vet Emerg Crit Care 21(2):123, 2011.
47. Lisciandro GR, Harvey HJ, Beck KA: Automobile-induced obstruction of the intrathoracic caudal vena cava in a dog, J Small Anim Pract 36(8):368, 1995.
48. Langs LL: Budd-Chiari-like syndrome in a dog due to liver lobe entrapment with falciform ligament, J Am Anim Hosp Assoc 45(5):253, 2009.
49. Macintire DK: Budd-Chiari syndrome in a kitten, caused by membranous obstruction of the caudal vena cava, J Am Anim Hosp Assoc 31(6):484, 1995.
50. Schoeman JP, Stidworthy MF: Budd-Chiari-like syndrome associated with an adrenal phaeochromocytoma in a dog, J Small Anim Pract 42(4):191, 2001.
51. Whelan MF, O'Toole TE, Carlson KR, et al: Budd–Chiari-like syndrome in a dog with a chondrosarcoma of the thoracic wall, J Vet Emerg Crit Care 17(2)175, 2007.
52. Pelosi A, Prinsen JK, Eyster GE, et al: Caudal vena cava kinking in dogs with ascites, Vet Rad Ultrasound 53(3):233, 2012.
53. Van De Wiele CM, Hogan DF, Green HW, et al: Cranial vena caval syndrome secondary to transvenous pacemaker implantation in two dogs, J Vet Cardiol 10(2):155, 2008.
54. Cunningham SM, Ames MK, Rush JE, et al: Successful treatment of pacemaker-induced stricture and thrombosis of the cranial vena cava in two dogs by use of anticoagulants and balloon venoplasty, J Am Vet Med Assoc 235(12):1467, 2009.
55. Bliss SP, Bliss SK, Harvey HJ: Use of recombinant tissue-plasminogen activator in a dog with chylothorax secondary to catheter-associated thrombosis of the cranial vena cava, J Am Anim Hosp Assoc 38(5):431, 2002.
56. Haskal ZJ, Dumbleton SA, Holt D: Percutaneous treatment of caval obstruction and Budd-Chiari syndrome in a cat, J Vasc Interv Radiol 10(4):487, 1999.
57. Schlicksup MD, Weisse CW, Berent AC, et al: Use of endovascular stents in three dogs with Budd-Chiari syndrome, J Am Vet Med Assoc 235(5):544, 2009.
58. Luis Fuentes V: Arterial thromboembolism risks, realities and a rational first-line approach, J Feline Med Surg 14(7):459, 2012.
59. Pion P: Feline aortic thromboemboli and the potential utility of thrombolytic therapy with tissue plasminogen activator, Vet Clin North Am Small Anim Pract 18(1):79, 1988.
60. Pion P: Feline aortic thromboemboli t-PA thrombolysis followed by aspirin therapy and rethrombosis, Vet Clin North Am Small Anim Pract 18(1):262, 1988.
61. Boswood A, Lamb CR, White RN: Aortic and iliac thrombosis in six dogs, J Small Anim Pract 41(3):109, 2000.
62. Lake-Bakaar GA, Johnson EG, Griffiths LG: Aortic thrombosis in dogs: 31 cases (2000-2010), J Am Vet Med Assoc 241(7):910, 2012.
63. Guillaumin J, Hmelo S, Farrell K, et al: Canine aortic thromboembolism (2005-2011): a retrospective study of 50 cases. Abstract from IVECCS 2012, J Vet Emerg Crit Care 22(s2):s6, 2012.
64. Morris B, O'Toole T, Rush J: Aortic thromboembolism in dogs: retrospective evaluation of 51 cases. Abstract from IVECCS 2012, J Vet Emerg Crit Care 22(s2):s8, 2012.
65. Killingsworth CR, Eyster GE, Adams T, et al: Streptokinase treatment of cats with experimentally induced aortic thrombosis, Am J Vet Res 47(6):1351, 1986.
66. Moore KE, Morris N, Dhupa N, et al: Retrospective study of streptokinase administration in 46 cats with arterial thromboembolism, J Vet Emerg Crit Care 10(4):245, 2000.
67. Ramsey CC, Burney DP, Macintire DK, et al: Use of streptokinase in four dogs with thrombosis, J Am Vet Med Assoc 209(4)780, 1996.
68. Tater KC, Drellich S, Beck K: Management of femoral artery thrombosis in an immature dog, J Vet Emerg Crit Care 15(1):52, 2005.
69. Clare AC, Kraje BJ: Use of recombinant tissue-plasminogen activator for aortic thrombolysis in a hypoproteinemic dog, J Am Vet Med Assoc 212(4):539, 1988.
70. Welch KM, Rozanski EA, Freeman LM, et al: Prospective evaluation of tissue plasminogen activator in 11 cats with arterial thromboembolism, J Feline Med Surg 12(2):122, 2010.
71. Koyama H, Matsumoto H, Fukushima RU, et al: Local intra-arterial administration of urokinase in the treatment of a feline distal aortic thromboembolism, J Vet Med Sci 72(9):1209, 2010.
72. Dunn ME, Weisse CW, Berent AC: Minimally invasive management of distal aortic thrombosis in a dog. Abstract, Key Largo, FL, 2009, Veterinary Endoscopy Society.
73. Reimer SB, Kittleson MD, Kyles AE: Use of rheolytic thrombectomy in the treatment of feline distal aortic thromboembolism, J Vet Intern Med 20(2):290, 2006.

PART XVI TRAUMA

CHAPTER 137
TRAUMATIC BRAIN INJURY

Daniel J. Fletcher, PhD, DVM, DACVECC • Rebecca S. Syring, DVM, DACVECC

KEY POINTS

- Identification and management of extracranial disorders, such as systemic hypotension, hypoxemia, and hypoventilation, should be the first priority when treating patients with acute traumatic brain injury (TBI).
- Mannitol is effective in treating intracranial hypertension, but it can compromise cerebral perfusion if its osmotic diuretic effects are not ameliorated rapidly with intravascular volume replacement.
- Hypertonic saline (7% to 8%) is effective in treating intracranial hypertension and is less likely to lead to hypovolemia and decreased cerebral perfusion.
- Corticosteroids are not recommended for the treatment of TBI.
- Prognosis varies, but even patients with severe neurologic deficits can recover with aggressive supportive care.

INCIDENCE AND PREVALENCE OF HEAD INJURY

Traumatic brain injury (TBI) is common in dogs and cats, with motor vehicle accidents, animal interactions, and unknown etiologies being the most common causes seen in a multicenter study of 1099 dogs and 191 cats.[1] In that study 26% of dogs and 42% of cats had evidence of head injury on physical examination. Other common causes of head injury in dogs and cats include falls from heights, blunt trauma, gunshot wounds, and other malicious human activity.[2] The overall prevalence and incidence of head injury in veterinary medicine have not been well studied, but a retrospective study from a large, urban veterinary hospital reported an average of 145 cases of confirmed TBI per year from 1997 to 1999.[3]

GENERAL APPROACH TO THE PATIENT WITH A HEAD INJURY

When treating a patient with an acute head injury, both extracranial and intracranial priorities must be considered. Identification of life-threatening extracranial injuries such as hemorrhage, penetrating thoracic or abdominal wounds, airway obstruction, and compromised oxygenation, ventilation, or volume status is of paramount importance. Once life-threatening extracranial factors have been addressed, intracranial priorities should include maintenance of adequate cerebral perfusion pressure (CPP), ensuring adequate oxygen delivery to the brain, and treatment of acute intracranial hypertension, as well as continued monitoring of neurologic status.

PATHOPHYSIOLOGY

The underlying injuries that result from head trauma can be separated into two categories: primary injury and secondary injury. Primary injury occurs as an immediate result of the traumatic event. Secondary injury occurs during the hours to days after trauma and is caused by a complex series of biochemical events, including release of inflammatory mediators and excitatory neurotransmitters, and changes in cellular membrane permeability.

Primary Injury

The least severe primary brain injury is concussion, characterized by a brief loss of consciousness. Concussion is not associated with an underlying histopathologic lesion.[4] Brain contusion consists of parenchymal hemorrhage and edema and clinical signs can range from mild to severe. Contusions can occur in the brain directly under the site of impact ("coup" lesions), in the opposite hemisphere ("contrecoup" lesions), or both, as a result of displacement of the brain within the skull. Although mild contusions can be difficult to differentiate from a concussion, unconsciousness for more than several minutes is most consistent with contusion.[2]

Laceration is the most severe type of primary brain injury and is characterized by physical disruption of the brain parenchyma. Axial hematomas within the brain parenchyma and extraaxial hematomas in the subarachnoid, subdural, and epidural spaces can occur, causing compression of the brain and leading to severe localizing signs or diffuse neurologic dysfunction.[5] The older literature suggests that extraaxial hemorrhage is rare in dogs and cats after head injury; however, there is mounting evidence that this type of hemorrhage occurs in up to 10% of animals with mild head injury and more than 80% of dogs and cats with severe head injury.[5,6]

Secondary Injury

TBI triggers a series of biochemical events that ultimately result in neuronal cell death. Box 137-1 provides a list of the most common types of secondary injury. These secondary injuries are caused by a combination of intracranial and systemic insults that occur in both independent and dependent ways.

Systemic insults that contribute to secondary brain injury include hypotension, hypoxemia, systemic inflammation, hyperglycemia, hypoglycemia, hypercapnia, hypocapnia, hyperthermia, electrolyte imbalances, and acid-base disturbances. Intracranial insults include increased intracranial pressure (ICP), compromise of the blood-brain barrier, mass lesions, cerebral edema, infection, vasospasm, and seizures. All these factors ultimately lead to neuronal cell death.[7]

BOX 137-1 *Most Common Factors Leading to Secondary Brain Injury*

- Excitotoxicity
- Ischemia
- Inflammation
- ATP depletion
- Production of reactive oxygen species
- Accumulation of intracellular sodium and calcium
- Nitric oxide accumulation
- Cerebral lactic acidosis

ATP, Adenosine triphosphate.

Table 137-1 Interpretation of Pupil Size and Pupillary Light Response in Head Trauma

Pupil Size	Response to Light	Level of Lesion	Prognosis
Midposition	Normal	—	Good
Bilateral miosis	Poor to none	Cannot localize	Variable
Unilateral mydriasis	Poor to none	Cranial nerve III	Guarded to poor
Unilateral mydriasis and ventrolateral strabismus	Poor to none	Midbrain	Guarded to poor
Midposition	None	Pons, medulla	Poor to grave
Bilateral mydriasis	Poor to none	—	Poor to grave

Immediately after brain injury there is massive release of excitatory neurotransmitters that causes influx of sodium and calcium into neurons, resulting in depolarization and further release of excitatory neurotransmitters. Increased influx of calcium overwhelms mechanisms for removal, causing severe intracellular damage and ultimately neuronal cell death.[8] Excessive metabolic activity also results in depletion of adenosine triphosphate (ATP) stores in the brain.

Several factors favor the production of reactive oxygen species after TBI, including hypoperfusion and local tissue acidosis. Hemorrhage provides a source of iron, which favors the production of hydroxyl radicals. Catecholamines may also contribute to the production of free radicals by direct and indirect mechanisms. These reactive oxygen species then oxidize lipids, proteins, and deoxyribonucleic acid (DNA), resulting in further destruction of neurons. Because the brain provides a lipid-rich environment, it is particularly susceptible to oxidative injury.

Nitric oxide has been associated with perpetuation of secondary brain injury after trauma, most likely because of its vasodilatory effects and its participation in free radical reactions, but the exact mechanism is not well understood.[8]

TBI is associated with production of inflammatory mediators.[9] These mediators perpetuate secondary brain injury via a number of mechanisms, including inducing nitric oxide production, triggering influx of inflammatory cells, activating the arachidonic acid and coagulation cascades, and disrupting the blood-brain barrier. Because studies have shown both neuroprotective and neurotoxic effects of inflammation, research is focusing on the development of targeted antiinflammatory agents that preferentially affect the more acute, destructive inflammatory processes.[9]

Primary and secondary intracranial injuries, in combination with systemic effects of the trauma, ultimately result in worsening of cerebral injury as a result of a compromised CPP, the force driving blood into the calvarium and providing the brain with essential oxygen and nutrients. CPP is defined as the difference between mean arterial blood pressure (MAP) and ICP.

Blood flow to the brain per unit time, or cerebral blood flow (CBF), is a function of CPP and cerebrovascular resistance. The normal brain is capable of maintaining a constant CBF over a wide range of MAP (50 to 150 mm Hg) via autoregulatory mechanisms. However, the traumatized brain often loses much of this autoregulatory capacity, making it susceptible to ischemic injury with even small decreases in MAP.

The following equation summarizes the "Monro-Kellie Doctrine," developed in the early nineteenth century to describe intracranial dynamics:

$$V_{\text{intracranial}} = V_{\text{brain}} + V_{\text{CSF}} + V_{\text{blood}} + V_{\text{mass lesion}}$$

where V = volume. Sudden increases in any of these volumes as a result of primary and secondary brain injuries can lead to dramatic increases in ICP.

Initially, increases in ICP will trigger the Cushing's reflex, or central nervous system (CNS) ischemic response, a characteristic rise in MAP and reflex decrease in heart rate (see Chapter 84). The CNS ischemic response in a patient with head trauma is a sign of a potentially life-threatening increase in ICP and should be treated promptly.

NEUROLOGIC ASSESSMENT

Initial neurologic examination should focus on the level of consciousness, posture, and pupil size and response to light (Table 137-1). A more detailed neurologic examination can be performed once stabilizing therapy has been instituted. Based on findings from this examination, a numeric score can be assigned to grade the severity of injury using the modified Glasgow Coma Scale, a system developed for animals with head injuries[10] (see Chapter 81). The initial neurologic examination should be interpreted in light of the cardiovascular and respiratory system because shock can have a significant effect on neurologic status, reducing the patient's level of consciousness and pupillary responses.

DIAGNOSTIC TESTS AND MONITORING

Because of the likelihood of multisystemic injury associated with head trauma, initial diagnostic tests and patient monitoring should focus upon a global assessment of patient stability. Emergency blood screening should consist of a packed cell volume and total solids determination to assess for hemorrhage, blood glucose to assess the severity of injury,[3] and a blood gas (venous or arterial) to assess ventilation, perfusion, and acid-base status. When available, electrolyte, lactate, renal values, and markers of hepatic damage should also be evaluated before therapy is instituted. Serial monitoring of these values is essential because dramatic changes can occur with therapy. Jugular venipuncture should be avoided because occlusion of the jugular vein can result in marked increases in ICP as a result of decreased venous outflow from the brain.

Diligent monitoring of the cardiovascular and respiratory systems is imperative to minimize the risk of secondary brain injury. With each episode of hypoxemia or hypotension, the prognosis for neurologic recovery dramatically decreases in human patients with TBI.[11] Basic monitoring of the cardiovascular system focuses on maintenance of adequate tissue perfusion (pink mucous membranes, capillary refill time of 1 to 2 seconds, good peripheral pulse quality, and a normal heart rate). In addition, systemic blood pressure should be monitored routinely. MAP should be maintained at or above 80 mm Hg in order to maintain CPP. Blood pressure as measured with the Doppler technique should be maintained above 100 mm Hg. Heart rate should be assessed when hypertension (MAP > 120 mm Hg or systolic > 140 mm Hg) is present. If evidence of the central nervous system ischemic response is present, therapy directed toward lowering ICP should be instituted. Alternatively, hypertension associated with tachycardia suggests pain or anxiety, which should be treated as indicated.

Monitoring of the respiratory system focuses on maintenance of oxygenation and ventilation. Oxygenation can be assessed via pulse oximetry, with a goal of maintaining saturation above 94%. When arterial sampling is possible, oxygen tension should be maintained above 80 mm Hg. If oxygenation cannot be monitored, oxygen supplementation should be provided. Failure to maintain oxygenation above these levels may warrant intubation and positive pressure ventilation (see Chapter 30).

Ventilation can be assessed by blood gas analysis or end-tidal capnometry (see Chapter 186). Although arterial blood gas sampling is the gold standard for assessing carbon dioxide tension, a venous blood gas can be substituted if tissue perfusion is normal. Venous carbon dioxide concentrations will exceed arterial by 2 to 5 mm Hg; however, this difference is exacerbated with poor tissue perfusion. End-tidal capnometry tends to underestimate arterial carbon dioxide tension by 5 mm Hg, and changes in cardiac output can significantly alter the value obtained.

Radiographs of the skull in patients that have sustained head trauma are an insensitive diagnostic tool and rarely provide valuable information. Computed tomography (CT) is the preferred imaging method. CT scans are superior to magnetic resonance imaging (MRI) for assessing bone and areas of acute hemorrhage or edema. As the time from injury increases, or when subtle neurologic deficits are present, MRI becomes a more useful tool.[12] Advanced imaging provides information about mass lesions (epidural, subdural, or intraparenchymal hemorrhage) or depressed skull fractures that may require surgical intervention. Such studies should be considered in patients with moderate to severe neurologic abnormalities on presentation, lateralizing signs, failure to improve significantly within the first few days, or those with an acute deterioration in neurologic status.

TREATMENT

When formulating a treatment plan for a patient with TBI, both intracranial and extracranial concerns must be addressed. Extracranial priorities include ventilation, oxygenation, and maintenance of normal blood pressure, and intracranial priorities include treatment of intracranial hypertension and control of cerebral metabolic rate.

Extracranial Therapy

The first priority in treating a patient with head trauma is extracranial stabilization. As with any severely injured patient, the basics of airway, breathing, and circulation should be evaluated and addressed if necessary. Patency of the airway should be assessed as soon as possible and treated with endotracheal intubation or emergency tracheostomy, if indicated. The pharynx and larynx should be inspected visually and suctioned as needed to maintain airway patency. Hypoxia is also common, and supplemental oxygen is indicated in the initial treatment of all patients with significant head injury. Increases in the blood CO_2 concentration can lead to cerebral vasodilation and increased intracranial blood volume, worsening ICP (see Secondary Injury section). Conversely, hypocapnia caused by hyperventilation can lead to cerebral vasoconstriction, decreasing cerebral blood flow and leading to cerebral ischemia. Therefore CO_2 should be maintained at the low end of the normal range in patients with head trauma (e.g., venous CO_2 40 to 45 mm Hg, arterial CO_2 35 to 40 mm Hg).[13] In some patients this will require mechanical ventilation (see Chapter 30).

Patients with head trauma commonly present in hypovolemic shock, and volume resuscitation goals should be aggressive (MAP of 80 to 100 mm Hg; see Chapter 60). For patients without electrolyte disturbances, normal saline (0.9%) is the best initial choice for fluid resuscitation because it contains the smallest amount of free water (sodium concentration 154 mEq/L) of the isotonic fluids and is therefore least likely to contribute to cerebral edema. Synthetic colloid resuscitation may also prove beneficial. For hydrated patients with evidence of hypovolemia and increased ICP, a combination colloid and hyperosmotic (hypertonic saline) solution is recommended (see Intracranial Therapy later in this chapter and Table 137-2). Patients that do not respond to volume resuscitation require vasopressor support (see Chapter 157).

Intracranial Therapy

Hyperosmotic agents

Mannitol has been shown to decrease ICP, increase CPP and CBF, and have a beneficial effect on neurologic outcome in patients with head injury.[14] Mannitol may also possess free radical scavenging properties. Its positive effects can be seen clinically within minutes of administration, most likely a result of its rheologic its effects (decreased blood viscosity) causing an increase in CBF and cerebral oxygen delivery. Within 15 to 30 minutes, its osmotic effects predominate, drawing water out of the brain parenchyma (primarily normal tissue) and into the intravascular space. These effects can last from 1.5 to 6 hours. In humans, mannitol may induce acute renal failure if serum osmolarity exceeds 320 mOsm/L, suggesting that serial measurement of serum osmolality may be useful in patients receiving repeated doses.[15] Mannitol may cause increased permeability of the blood-brain barrier, allowing it to leak into the brain parenchyma where it can exacerbate edema. Because this effect is most pronounced when mannitol remains in the circulation for long periods, the drug should be administered as repeated boluses rather than as a constant rate infusion.[14] Mannitol boluses of 0.5 to 1.5 g/kg have been recommended for the treatment of increased ICP in dogs and cats.[16] Treatment must be followed with isotonic crystalloid or colloid solutions, or both, to maintain intravascular volume.

Hypertonic saline is an alternative hyperosmotic solution that may have advantages over mannitol in some patients with head injury. Because sodium does not freely cross the blood-brain barrier, hypertonic saline has similar rheologic and osmotic effects to mannitol. In addition, it improves hemodynamic status and has beneficial vasoregulatory and immunomodulatory effects.[17] Because sodium is redistributed within the body and reabsorbed in the kidneys, hypotension is a less likely sequela than with mannitol, making it a better choice for patients with increased ICP and systemic hypotension. Hypertonic saline can be administered with a colloid in such cases to allow for a more prolonged volume expansion effect (see Table 137-2).

Corticosteroids

Corticosteroids are potent antiinflammatory agents and have historically been used extensively in human and veterinary medicine to treat patients that have sustained head trauma. A clinical trial evaluating more than 10,000 human adults with head injury showed that corticosteroid treatment was associated with worse outcomes at 2 weeks and 6 months after injury.[18,19] The Brain Trauma Foundation

Table 137-2 **Drugs, Fluids, and Dosages for the Treatment of Patients with Head Trauma**

Indication	Drug or Fluid	Dosage	Notes
Any patient with evidence of head trauma and hypotension	Isotonic crystalloid solution (0.9% saline preferred)	Administer boluses of one fourth to one third of the shock dose (shock dose 90 ml/kg for dogs, 50 ml/kg for cats)	May repeat as needed Consider colloid boluses if no response after 2 to 3 crystalloid boluses
Increased ICP in normotensive or hypertensive patients	Mannitol 25%	0.5 to 1.0 g/kg IV over 15 minutes May repeat	Use filter during administration; can lead to severe dehydration; follow with isotonic crystalloids or synthetic colloids to prevent dehydration and hypovolemia Closely monitor intake and output
Increased ICP in hypovolemic or hypotensive patients	HTS (7%)* plus hydroxyethyl starch	3 to 5 ml/kg IV over 15 minutes May repeat	Do not use in hyponatremic patients Monitor serum sodium levels
Increased ICP in normotensive, hypertensive, or hypotensive patients	HTS (7% to 7.8%)†	3 to 5 ml/kg IV over 15 minutes May repeat	Do not use in hyponatremic patients Monitor serum sodium levels
Seizures	Diazepam	0.5 mg/kg IV May repeat Consider CRI 0.2-1.0 mg/kg/hr if refractory	Monitor ventilation, may lead to profound sedation and hypoventilation Protect from light
	Levetiracetam	20 mg/kg IV	May repeat as needed; very low toxicity potential Minimal sedation or ventilatory side effects

HTS, Hypertonic saline; *ICR*, intracranial pressure; *IV*, intravenous.
*If using 23.4% HTS, dilute 1 part HTS with 2 parts sterile water.
†If using 23.4% HTS, dilute 1 part HTS with 2 parts hydroxyethyl starch. If using 7% to 7.5% HTS, administer separate doses of HTS and colloid (3 to 5 ml/kg HTS, 2 to 3 ml/kg artificial colloid).

recommends against corticosteroid administration in patients with TBI.[13]

Furosemide

Furosemide has been used in patients with head trauma either as a sole agent to reduce cerebral edema or in combination with mannitol to decrease the initial increase in intravascular volume and hydrostatic pressure associated with the drug. However, the use of this drug as a sole agent in patients with head trauma has been called into question because of the potential for intravascular volume depletion and systemic hypotension, leading to decreased CPP.[20] The Brain Trauma Foundation guidelines do not recommend the administration of furosemide in combination with mannitol.[14] Therefore it should be reserved for those patients in whom it is indicated for reasons other than cerebral edema, such as those with pulmonary edema or oligoanuric renal failure.

Decreasing cerebral blood volume

Techniques to decrease cerebral blood volume (CBV) have been proposed as methods for lowering increased ICP. Elevation of the head by 15 to 30 degrees reduces CBV by increasing venous drainage, decreasing ICP, and increasing CPP without deleterious changes in cerebral oxygenation.[21] A slant board should be used instead of pillows or towels to prevent occlusion of the jugular veins by bending of the neck. Higher elevations of the head may cause a detrimental decrease in CPP.

Prevention of hypoventilation, as described earlier, can reduce cerebral vasodilation and decrease CBV; the goal should be normocapnia (arterial carbon dioxide of 35 to 40 mm Hg). In animals with acute intracranial hypertension, short-term hyperventilation to an arterial carbon dioxide of 25 to 35 mm Hg may be used to reduce CBV and ICP, but long-term hyperventilation is not recommended based on evidence that the decrease in CBF leads to cerebral ischemia and worsens outcome.[14]

Seizure treatment/prophylaxis

Post-TBI seizures are common in people, occurring within 3 years in 4.4% of patients with mild TBI, 7.6% of patients with moderate TBI, and 13.6% of patients with severe TBI in one recent study.[22] Recent veterinary studies have documented a similar phenomenon, with seizure rates of 6.8% in dogs and 0% in cats (although the 95% confidence interval was 0% to 5.6%).[23,24] Unfortunately, prophylactic anticonvulsant therapy has not been shown to reduce development of delayed seizures after TBI in people.[25] However, aggressive treatment of seizures while animals are hospitalized is recommended. Suggested anticonvulsant drugs and doses are listed in Table 137-2 (further details can be found in Chapter 166).

Decreasing cerebral metabolic rate

Increased cerebral metabolic rate because of excitotoxicity and inflammation after head injury can lead to cerebral ischemia and cellular swelling, thus increasing ICP. Interventions that decrease cerebral metabolic rate may lessen secondary brain injury. Although rarely used in veterinary medicine, induction of a barbiturate coma and therapeutic hypothermia have been used in experimental studies and clinical trials in humans and can be effective in decreasing ICP and improving outcome in patients with refractory intracranial hypertension.[26] There is a single case report in the veterinary literature of successful use of therapeutic hypothermia to treat refractory seizures in a dog after TBI.[27] The Brain Trauma Foundation states that there is insufficient evidence to publish treatment standards on the use of barbiturates, but this therapy may be considered in patients with elevated ICP that is refractory to medical and surgical therapy.[14] A recent systematic review concluded that mild to moderate therapeutic hypothermia for 48 hours after injury is beneficial in human patients with severe TBI[28]; further study evaluating the efficacy and practicality of these measures in veterinary medicine is needed.

PROGNOSIS

The prognosis is difficult to predict after TBI. Although the initial neurologic status may be helpful in predicting outcome, reassessment after stabilizing therapy is recommended because the level of consciousness may improve once tissue perfusion has been corrected. Pupillary dilation, loss of pupillary light responses, and deterioration in the level of consciousness during therapy are poor prognostic indicators (see Table 137-1). It is likely that younger animals, particularly kittens, can make remarkable recoveries despite severe dysfunction immediately after trauma, although definitive research is lacking. Owners should be aware that animals that survive severe TBI may have persistent neurologic deficits for an indefinite period. These animals can also develop delayed seizure disorders.

The Small Animal Coma Scale was developed to quantitatively assess functional impact of brain injury (see Chapter 81). This scale assesses three major categories: motor activity, level of consciousness, and brainstem reflexes. Although this scale has not been validated prospectively in animals, it has been shown retrospectively to correlate with 48-hour outcome in dogs with head trauma.[6] This may be most useful when evaluated serially in patients to determine if there has been improvement or deterioration after treatment.

In human medicine, hyperglycemia at admission and persistence of hyperglycemia have been associated with worsened mortality and outcome.[29] In a meta-analysis of the utility of admission laboratory parameters as prognostic indicators for people with TBI, increasing glucose concentrations and decreasing hemoglobin concentrations were the strongest with poor neurologic outcome.[30] Hyperglycemia has been associated with more severe injury in head-injured veterinary patients[3] but has not been validated as an independent predictor of outcome.

REFERENCES

1. Kolata RJ: Trauma in dogs and cats: an overview, Vet Clin North Am Small Anim Pract 10(3):515, 1980.
2. Shores A: Craniocerebral trauma. In Kirk RW, ed: Current Veterinary Therapy X, Philadelphia, 1989, WB Saunders, pp 847-854.
3. Syring RS, Otto CM, Drobatz KJ: Hyperglycemia in dogs and cats with head trauma: 122 cases (1997-1999), J Am Vet Med Assoc 218(7):1124, 2001.
4. Dewey C, Budsberg S, Oliver J: Principles of head trauma management in dogs and cats. Part II, Compend Contin Educ Pract Vet 15(2):177, 1993.
5. Dewey C, Downs M, Aron D, et al: Acute traumatic intracranial haemorrhage in dogs and cats, Vet Comp Ortho Trauma 6:153, 1993.
6. Platt SR, Radaelli ST, McDonnell JJ: Computed tomography after mild head trauma in dogs, Vet Rec 151(8):243, 2002.
7. Chesnut RM: The management of severe traumatic brain injury, Emerg Med Clin North Am 15(3):581, 1997.
8. Zink BJ: Traumatic brain injury, Emerg Med Clin North Am 14(1):115, 1996.
9. Dietrich WD, Chatzipanteli K, Vitarbo E, et al: The role of inflammatory processes in the pathophysiology and treatment of brain and spinal cord trauma, Acta Neurochir Suppl 89:69, 2004.
10. Platt SR, Radaelli ST, McDonnell JJ: The prognostic value of the modified Glasgow Coma Scale in head trauma in dogs, J Vet Intern Med 15:581, 2001
11. Chesnut RM, Marshall LF, Klauber MR, et al: The role of secondary brain injury in determining outcome from severe head injury, J Trauma 34(2):216, 1993.
12. Lee B, Newberg A: Neuroimaging in traumatic brain imaging, NeuroRx 2(2):372, 2005.
13. Winter CD, Adamides AA, Lewis PM, et al: A review of the current management of severe traumatic brain injury, Surgeon 3(5):329, 2005.
14. Brain Trauma Foundation: Management and prognosis of severe traumatic brain injury, New York, 2000, Brain Trauma Foundation.
15. Dorman HR, Sondheimer JH, Cadnapaphornchai P: Mannitol-induced acute renal failure, Medicine (Baltimore) 69(3):153, 1990.
16. Plumb D: Plumb's veterinary drug handbook, ed 7, Oxford, UK, 2011, Wiley-Blackwell.
17. Ware ML, Nemani VM, Meeker M, et al: Effects of 23.4% sodium chloride solution in reducing intracranial pressure in patients with traumatic brain injury: a preliminary study, Neurosurgery 57(4):727; discussion 727-736, 2005.
18. Edwards P, Arango M, Balica L, et al: Final results of MRC CRASH, a randomised placebo-controlled trial of intravenous corticosteroid in adults with head injury-outcomes at 6 months, Lancet 365(9475):1957, 2005.
19. Roberts I, Yates D, Sandercock P, et al: Effect of intravenous corticosteroids on death within 14 days in 10008 adults with clinically significant head injury (MRC CRASH trial): randomised placebo-controlled trial, Lancet 364(9442):1321, 2005.
20. Chesnut RM, Gautille T, Blunt BA, et al: Neurogenic hypotension in patients with severe head injuries, J Trauma 44(6):958; discussion 963-964, 1998.
21. Ng I, Lim J, Wong HB: Effects of head posture on cerebral hemodynamics: its influences on intracranial pressure, cerebral perfusion pressure, and cerebral oxygenation, Neurosurgery 54(3):593; discussion 598, 2004.
22. Ferguson PL, Smith GM, Wannamaker BB, et al: A population-based study of risk of epilepsy after hospitalization for traumatic brain injury, Epilepsia 51(5):891, 2010.
23. Friedenberg SG, Butler AL, Wei L, et al: Seizures following head trauma in dogs: 259 cases (1999-2009), J Am Vet Med Assoc 241(11):1479, 2012.
24. Grohmann KS, Schmidt MJ, Moritz A, et al: Prevalence of seizures in cats after head trauma, J Am Vet Med Assoc 241(11):1467, 2012.
25. Temkin NR: Preventing and treating posttraumatic seizures: the human experience, Epilepsia 50 Suppl:210, 2009.
26. Vincent J-L, Berré J: Primer on medical management of severe brain injury, Crit Care Med 33(6):1392, 2005.
27. Hayes GM: Severe seizures associated with traumatic brain injury managed by controlled hypothermia, pharmacologic coma, and mechanical ventilation in a dog, J Vet Emerg Crit Care (San Antonio) 19(6):629, 2009.
28. Fox JL, Vu EN, Doyle-Waters M, et al: Prophylactic hypothermia for traumatic brain injury: a quantitative systematic review, CJEM 12(4):355, 2010.
29. Lam AM, Winn HR, Cullen BF, et al: Hyperglycemia and neurological outcome in patients with head injury, J Neurosurg 75(4):545, 1991.
30. Van Beek JGM, Mushkudiani NA, Steyerberg EW, et al: Prognostic value of admission laboratory parameters in traumatic brain injury: results from the IMPACT study, J Neurotrauma 24(2):315, 2007.

CHAPTER 138

THORACIC AND ABDOMINAL TRAUMA

William T.N. Culp, VMD, DACVS • Deborah C. Silverstein, DVM, DACVECC

KEY POINTS

- The extent of thoracic and abdominal trauma is often not known at first evaluation, and extensive diagnostics are typically necessary to fully assess the status of a particular patient.
- Many different disease states can occur secondary to thoracic and abdominal trauma and the performance of diagnostic testing, particularly fluid analysis, is essential.
- While some animals experiencing thoracic and abdominal trauma can be managed conservatively, surgery is often necessary to correct associated problems.

Thoracic and abdominal trauma is common, and the clinical manifestations of these injuries can range widely. Clinicians faced with these cases should be prepared for the potential diagnostic and treatment options that may need to be considered, as well as the variable prognoses that may be altered according to what is found during surgery, if pursued. General categories of trauma affecting the thorax and abdomen include blunt and penetrating trauma. The internal injuries associated with both categories can be similar; however, it is important to make the distinction because further exploration of skin, muscle, and subcutaneous space over these cavities may be necessary. Additionally, more potentially life-threatening injuries (e.g., brain trauma) may be occurring simultaneously, and these need to be addressed immediately.

TRAUMA CATEGORIES

Blunt Trauma

Motor vehicle accidents, high-rise falls, and intentional physical injuries are often encountered in an emergency setting, and the effect these events may have on the abdomen and thorax of a patient is immense. When blunt trauma to the thorax or abdomen does occur, the severity of the injury often is not recognized immediately while other life-threatening injuries are being assessed and treated.

Recently injuries that can occur secondary to blunt trauma were evaluated.[1-3] In a study of 235 canine cases of blunt trauma, 91.1% of all blunt trauma cases were secondary to motor vehicular accidents.[1] Common chest injuries included pulmonary contusions (58%), pneumothorax (47%), hemothorax (18%), and rib fractures (14%), and common abdominal injuries included hemoperitoneum (23%), abdominal hernias (5%), and urinary tract ruptures (3%).[1]

A retrospective study of 600 dogs that were struck with a motor vehicle has also been performed. The most common thoracic injuries were pulmonary contusions, pneumothorax, and hemothorax, and nearly 12% of dogs experienced thoracic trauma.[4] That study also noted that when skeletal injuries were found in cases of thoracic trauma, 63% of these were cranial to T13.[4] Abdominal trauma was noted in 5% of dogs (as diagnosed by surgery or necropsy).[4] The liver was the abdominal organ most often damaged (31% of the abdominal organ injuries), with injuries ranging from fissures of the capsule or parenchyma to fragmentation of a hepatic lobe. Other commonly injured organs included the urinary bladder, diaphragm, and kidney. Of the 33 dogs that died from their injuries, 8 (24%) had abdominal injury alone and 13 (39%) had both abdominal and thoracic injury.

High-rise falls in dogs and cats result in abdominal injuries in 15% and 7% of cases, respectively.[5,6] Dogs falling from a height of greater than three stories are more likely to experience abdominal injury than those falling less than or equal to three stories. Also, dogs that fall accidentally more often experience abdominal and hind limb injury than dogs that jump from a height. In both dogs and cats, thoracic trauma was diagnosed more commonly than abdominal trauma, perhaps because of the readily apparent respiratory compromise.

In a study evaluating high-rise falls in 119 cats, approximately 34% were noted to have thoracic trauma.[7] Pneumothorax and pulmonary contusions were regularly diagnosed, being documented in 60% and 40% of cats with thoracic trauma, respectively.[7] Additionally, hemothorax was diagnosed in 10% of cats. Although injury to the chest and bones was common, nearly 97% of cats survived the fall. Falls from the seventh story or higher were more likely to result in thoracic trauma.[7] Abdominal injuries were uncommon in this cohort of cats, and the authors hypothesized that this was secondary to the forelimbs absorbing the impact of the landing.[7] However, a separate study described pancreatic rupture in four cats,[8] and treating clinicians should be aware of abdominal trauma that cannot be externally visualized.

Unfortunately, human abuse of companion animals is another cause of blunt trauma. In a study investigating intentional injury[9] to animals, internal injury to the abdomen was documented less often than superficial injuries or fractures. However, 13 of 217 (6%) dogs in this study experienced rupture of an organ, including spleen, liver, bladder, and kidney. Cats tended to experience abdominal muscle rupture. Kicking of the animal was the cause of the abdominal injury in most cases.

Penetrating Trauma

Penetrating trauma most commonly occurs secondary to bite wounds in companion animals; however, reports of missile injuries, impalement/stab injuries, and evisceration exist. Bite wounds can result in both blunt and penetrating trauma. Exploration of superficial wounds is often necessary to fully recognize the organ damage that has occurred.[10] The thorax is the body region most likely to experience trauma from a bite wound in dogs; it is second only to the back region in cats.[11]

Wounds that do not appear to penetrate the thorax or abdomen still often require surgical exploration because bacteria from the biting animal's mouth or environment will likely contaminate the wound and result in abscess formation. Additionally, it may not always be obvious if a wound has entered a body cavity.[11] In one large retrospective study evaluating bite wounds in dogs and cats, mortality only occurred in those cases with intrathoracic or intra-abdominal injury.[11]

Gunshot wounds have been reviewed in several animal studies.[12-14] Of 84 animals reported in one retrospective study,[13] 32 thoracic and 14 abdominal injuries were encountered. Animals with thoracic injury were managed conservatively in the majority of cases.[13] Animals with abdominal injury also tended to have more cardiovascular compromise on arrival than those that did not have abdominal injury. In a separate study of dogs exposed to high-caliber, high-velocity weapons, only 38% survived the gunshot injury.[12] The thorax was the most common site of injury in that study with 50% of dogs afflicted with a thoracic wound.[12]

Other types of penetrating abdominal wounds include stab wounds, impalement injuries (from sticks or other devices), or after a high-rise fall.[9,15] Some of these injuries are self-induced, and others are the result of mismanagement. Either way, early intervention is likely required to maximize a good outcome.

DIAGNOSTICS

Clinical Laboratory Tests

Blood work is essential in all cases of thoracic and abdominal trauma to assess organ status as well as the ability to undergo anesthesia, should it be necessary. The red blood cell, white blood cell, and platelet counts are assessed by the complete blood count. Bleeding often occurs secondary to trauma, and this can be reflected in the red blood cell count; animals may be anemic on presentation depending on the severity of trauma and the amount of time since the traumatic event. Leukocytosis (specifically neutrophilia) can be increased secondary to stress, inflammation, or infection, all of which may occur with trauma. Thrombocytopenia secondary to consumption of platelets with bleeding may also be encountered.

A biochemistry panel should be evaluated, with particular attention paid to the liver and renal values as well as the electrolyte and acid-base balance. Alanine aminotransaminase (ALT) and aspartate transaminase (AST) can be increased when liver trauma has occurred. In cases of biliary trauma and subsequent bile leakage, increases in alkaline phosphatase (ALP), γ-glutamyl transferase (GGT), and bilirubin are often present. Abnormalities of electrolytes may be seen secondary to clinical signs such as vomiting or anorexia or because of specific conditions such as uroabdomen. Similarly, azotemia is often noted in animals with a uroabdomen or those suffering from dehydration or acute kidney injury. Measurement of urine specific gravity before fluid therapy may help the clinician assess renal function.

Imaging

Chest radiographs are essential for several reasons. When an abdominal trauma has occurred, the chest radiographs may reveal a diaphragmatic rupture or body wall herniation; herniation of organs such as stomach and intestine may be life threatening. Additionally, pneumothorax, pleural effusion, and pulmonary contusions can be detected with chest radiographs. Some injuries to the skin and subcutaneous tissue can be severe enough that a flail chest may not be noted. Chest radiographs often help the clinician to assess for the presence of rib fractures.

Abdominal radiographs are useful in the diagnosis of intra-abdominal pathologic conditions, but identifying a specific diagnosis may not always be possible. The presence of intra-abdominal gas suggests that abdominal wall penetration or organ perforation has occurred and requires immediate attention. The general loss of serosal detail in the abdomen is suggestive of the presence of fluid in the peritoneal space, retroperitoneal space, or both. Animals with traumatic pancreatitis or very young or thin animals may also have poor serosal detail on radiographs.

Fluid in the peritoneal space may originate from a bleeding organ or ruptured vessel, urine from the distal ureter, bladder or proximal urethral rupture, bile from a rupture in the biliary system, or a septic exudate in cases of septic peritonitis. Fluid in the retroperitoneal space is most commonly urine from damage to the kidney or proximal ureter or blood. Subcutaneous emphysema can be seen when gas accumulates in the subcutaneous spaces, with or without intra-abdominal injury (i.e., tracheal or esophageal perforation may also lead to subcutaneous emphysema).

Diaphragmatic and body wall ruptures are commonly diagnosed with radiographs.[16-18] Both thoracic and abdominal radiographs should be taken in suspected cases of diaphragmatic rupture. Characteristic changes seen on radiographs in animals with a diaphragmatic rupture include loss of continuity of the diaphragm, loss of intrathoracic detail (specifically cardiac silhouette), and the presence of gas-filled bowel loops or a mass effect in the thorax. These changes are not always present, and further imaging may be necessary to confirm the diagnosis.

Ultrasonography is useful in specific cases of abdominal trauma. As with radiographs, ultrasonography can diagnose the presence of air or gas in the abdomen (see Chapter 189). One study found that abdominal ultrasound correctly diagnosed a diaphragmatic hernia in 93% of cases.[18] A suspected body wall rupture can be definitively diagnosed with an ultrasound examination, and the organs displaced through the rupture may be assessed. An ultrasonographic modality that is now regularly used in veterinary medicine is the focused assessment with sonography for trauma (FAST) technique.[19,20] The early description of the FAST technique was for the evaluation of the abdomen and involved quickly assessing four specific areas (just caudal to the xiphoid process, just cranial to the pelvis, and over the right and left flanks caudal to the ribs at the most gravity-dependent location of the abdomen) with two views (transverse and longitudinal).[19] This technique was found to be useful at detecting intra-abdominal fluid, even when used by veterinarians with minimal ultrasonographic experience.[19]

A more recent study evaluated the use of a FAST technique for evaluation of thoracic trauma cases (see Chapter 189).[21] In this study, the thoracic FAST (TFAST) procedure is described with the patient placed in right lateral or sternal recumbency.[21] There are three main views obtained: bilateral chest tube site views, pericardial site views, and a diaphragmatico-hepatic view.[21] This study demonstrated that the TFAST has tremendous potential to diagnose pneumothorax as well as pleural and pericardial effusion and to do so in a short period (median time for TFAST was 3 minutes).[21]

Other imaging modalities employed in animals with abdominal trauma include fluoroscopy and computed tomography (CT) scans. Both are useful in the diagnosis of urinary tract injuries and body wall or diaphragmatic ruptures, and CT scans are commonly used for surgical planning in human patients that have experienced abdominal trauma.[22,23]

Fluid Analysis

When an abdominal effusion is suspected on physical examination, radiographs, or ultrasound, it is important to obtain a sample of the fluid for evaluation. For a detailed description of abdominocentesis, see Chapter 200. Several analyses should be performed on the fluid sample, including hematocrit, total solids, bilirubin, creatinine, potassium, and glucose (see Chapter 122 for further details). Other potential tests may include PaO_2, carbon dioxide, lactate, amylase, and lipase. In addition, a slide of the sample should be obtained for cytologic examination.

The presence of red blood cells in an abdominal effusion does not necessarily confirm a hemoperitoneum. With a true hemoperitoneum, red blood cells are usually observed within macrophages, signifying erythrophagocytosis (although this may not be present in the acute stages).[24] Hemosiderin from the broken down red blood cells usually fills the cytoplasm of the involved phagocyte.[24] Alternatively, if the packed cell volume (PCV) of the fluid is increasing or nears the PCV found in the peripheral blood, ongoing hemorrhage should be suspected. Another guideline is that the fluid PCV should be at least 10% to 25% of the peripheral blood PCV to be considered a hemorrhagic effusion.[24]

Using an abdominal FAST technique (described earlier), one study evaluated an abdominal fluid scoring system, or AFS.[3] When using the AFS, clinicians were able to determine a semiquantitative measure of free abdominal fluid.[3] Additionally, the AFS was associated with severity of injury; dogs with AFS scores of 3 or 4 were more likely to have a significantly lower PCV and total plasma protein as well as increased serum concentrations of ALT.[3]

The comparison of the concentration of creatinine and potassium in an abdominal effusion has been shown to be a useful indicator of uroperitoneum in both dogs and cats (see Chapters 112 and 122). In cats, mean serum/abdominal fluid creatinine ratio and mean serum/abdominal potassium ratio have been found to be 1:2 and 1:1.9, respectively, in cases of uroperitoneum.[25] Therefore a cat with a creatinine or potassium concentration in the abdominal effusion that is 2 times or more the peripheral blood likely has a uroperitoneum. In dogs, the sensitivity and specificity were both 100% when using a ratio of greater than 1.4:1 in comparing abdominal fluid potassium concentration with peripheral blood potassium concentration for the diagnosis of uroperitoneum. Similarly, using abdominal fluid creatinine concentration (compared with peripheral blood creatinine concentration) was beneficial, in that a ratio of more than 2:1 was 86% sensitive and 100% specific in the diagnosis of uroperitoneum.[26]

A bilirubin concentration in an abdominal effusion greater than twice that of the peripheral blood is diagnostic for bile leakage (see Chapters 112 and 122). This abdominal effusion generally has a yellow-green to brown tint, and bile crystals are occasionally evident upon cytologic examination.[24] Biliary effusions can be septic, especially in animals with cholecystitis, and cytologic evaluation may reveal the presence of bacteria.[24]

Chylothorax/chylous ascites occur uncommonly secondary to trauma, but suspicion is raised when an opaque effusion is noted. Chylous effusions generally have a triglyceride concentration greater than 100 mg/dl and are considered modified transudates.[24] Most of the cells obtained in a chylous effusion are mononuclear (lymphocytes); however, the white cell population can change over time because of the associated inflammatory response.[24]

The importance of abdominal fluid analysis in the diagnosis of septic peritonitis has been well documented. Cytologic examination is especially important in the diagnosis of septic peritonitis, and the presence of intracellular bacteria confirms the diagnosis as long as gastrointestinal aspiration has not occurred.[24] The glucose and lactate concentrations of the peritoneal fluid should also be compared with the respective concentrations in the blood.[27,28] A detailed description of the importance of these analyses is found in Chapters 112 and 122.

STABILIZATION

Monitoring

When thoracic trauma is suspected, an electrocardiogram (ECG) should be performed to assess the patient for signs of traumatic myocarditis. Arrhythmias that require treatment are occasionally encountered. Blood pressure monitoring is also very important in all trauma cases. Animals with hemothorax/hemoperitoneum/hemoretroperitoneum may develop hypotension secondary to hypovolemia, although patients with pyothorax or septic peritonitis are also often hypotensive. A combination of fluid therapy, blood product administration, and vasopressors may be necessary in severely affected cases.

Antimicrobial Therapy

Antimicrobial therapy may be indicated in trauma cases depending on the organ that is traumatized and the extent of injury to the skin, subcutaneous tissue, and muscles. If a penetrating injury has occurred, antimicrobials should be initiated; all wounds should be cultured and broad-spectrum antimicrobials administered pending the results of the susceptibility. For cases of bowel perforation and pyothorax, antimicrobial therapy should be started immediately with broad-spectrum drugs that also have anaerobic coverage (see Antimicrobial Therapy section, Chapters 175 to 182).[29]

Fluid Therapy/Blood Product Administration

In the initial treatment of these patients, it is essential to treat hemorrhagic shock and improve perfusion by administering isotonic crystalloids (up to 50 ml/kg in cats and 90 ml/kg in dogs) or synthetic colloids (5 to 20 ml/kg; see Chapter 60). A recent study evaluated the effectiveness of intravenous fluid resuscitation in an emergency setting.[30] In that cohort of dogs, bolus fluid therapy resulted in increased systolic arterial blood pressure in all dogs and patients that demonstrated a normalized blood pressure within the first hour of fluid therapy were more likely to be discharged alive compared with those that remained hypotensive.[30]

"Hypotensive resuscitation"[31,32] to a mean arterial pressure of 60 mm Hg or systolic blood pressure of 90 mm Hg may prevent excessive bleeding or disruption of clot formation and function. Some animals may also require the use of blood transfusions (see Chapter 61) during the resuscitation period (i.e., whole blood, packed red blood cells, and plasma). Animals that are unresponsive to crystalloid and synthetic colloid fluid resuscitation and have evidence of severe hemorrhage should be given fresh whole blood or packed red blood cells and fresh frozen plasma in an attempt to stabilize the clinical signs of shock, maintain the hematocrit above 25%, and sustain the clotting times within the normal range. Packed red blood cells and fresh frozen plasma are administered at a dose of 10 to 15 ml/kg and fresh whole blood at a dose of 20 to 25 ml/kg (a blood type and crossmatch should be performed if possible).

External Wound Care

Although the injuries that are present in the thorax and abdomen often require emergency consideration, any entry wounds or wounds away from those cavities (e.g., limbs, neck, head), should also be evaluated closely. Sterile lubricating jelly or sterile bandaging material can be placed in the wound in an attempt to keep the wound clean before clipping and anesthetic preparation. As soon as the patient is stable, fur should be removed from the wound area and the skin surrounding the wound. Any obvious foreign material should be removed and the wounds flushed with sterile saline (see Chapter 139).

It is essential that bite wounds be explored for the presence of more severe disease deeper to the externally located punctures. When a dog or cat sustains bite wounds, there is commonly tearing of the underlying tissue and elevation of the skin away from the body wall.[14] Drains are usually required to address these wounds because fluid accumulation in these regions is common; when fluid is left to accumulate, abscess formation is more likely to occur.

SPECIFIC CONDITIONS

Diaphragmatic Rupture

Trauma is the most common cause of diaphragmatic ruptures in small animals.[33,34] Therefore a diaphragmatic rupture should be suspected in any dog or cat with respiratory distress after a traumatic event. Furthermore, other obvious clinical lesions may not be present in 48% of cases of traumatic diaphragmatic ruptures.[34]

These animals may have signs of shock upon presentation, and early stabilization and oxygen therapy should be initiated (see Chapter 1). After stabilization, surgery is indicated to repair the rupture. If any gastrointestinal organs are displaced into the thoracic cavity or respiratory stability is unachievable, surgery is indicated on an emergency basis (see Chapter 28). The outcome associated with surgical intervention is good, with an approximate 90% perioperative survival rate in dogs and cats treated on an acute or chronic basis.[33]

Body Wall Rupture/Abdominal Evisceration

Rupture of the body wall with subsequent organ exteriorization can occur secondary to trauma. Organ exteriorization from the thoracic cavity is uncommon as the ribs play a protective role for the intrathoracic organs; additionally, intrathoracic organs are anchored, preventing easy dislodgement. Abdominal evisceration can occur when penetrating trauma results in an opening of the abdominal cavity and subsequent herniation of abdominal contents. Cases of abdominal evisceration should be treated as emergencies and surgery pursued as quickly as possible. The injury causing the development of an abdominal rupture will likely also result in additional trauma to the intra-abdominal organs and treatment of myriad injuries may be indicated. A full abdominal exploration should be performed to evaluate all intra-abdominal organs for injury or compromise.

In a study of 12 animals (8 dogs and 4 cats) with major abdominal evisceration, 4 were secondary to trauma (2 motor vehicular accidents, 1 bite wound, 1 penetration by glass shard).[35] Although all the study animals had exposure of the intestines with gross contamination, there was 100% survival to discharge from the hospital after a thorough surgical exploration was performed.[35] The median duration of hospitalization among all dogs was 4 days; however, dogs developing abdominal evisceration secondary to trauma had a significantly longer hospital stay as compared with dogs developing evisceration after postsurgical dehiscence.[35]

Eighty-six percent to 88% of cases of abdominal body wall rupture in dogs occur secondary to bite wounds or vehicular trauma.[16,36] These patients should also be carefully evaluated for bony trauma because fractures may be the source of the rupture. The timing of the stabilization of fractures will depend on the extent of the injury to the thorax and abdomen, and a staged procedure may be required.

Body wall ruptures are generally surgical emergencies, especially if caused by bite wounds. Organs can be entrapped in the defect, resulting in strangulation and rapid demise of the patient. Intestines have been reported to be displaced through the rupture in as many as 54% of cases[36] and often require a resection and anastomosis because of devitalized tissue. Other organs commonly displaced include the omentum, liver, and urinary bladder.[16,36] In one study 73% of dogs and 80% of cats survived to discharge from the hospital after surgical repair of a body wall rupture.[16]

Chylothorax/Chylous Ascites

Chylothorax is characterized by the accumulation of a chylous effusion (consisting of triglycerides and mononuclear cells) in the thorax. Although the cause of chylothorax in the majority of animals is unknown, and therefore labeled as idiopathic, trauma has been documented to cause chylothorax.[37,38] Clinical signs of chylothorax are generally nonspecific (e.g., lethargy, weight loss, anorexia) or related to the respiratory system (e.g., coughing, exercise intolerance, respiratory distress).

Several treatment options have been developed for the treatment of chylothorax in companion animals, and mixed results have been achieved.[39-43] Most recommendations for treatment include a combination of the following potential surgical options: thoracic duct ligation, pericardectomy, omentalization of the thoracic cavity, and cisterna chyli ablation. Less invasive options (via thoracoscopy and interventional radiology) are developing and early results are promising.[39,44,45] Chylous ascites has been documented in both dogs and cats, but a traumatic etiology has not been noted.

Pyothorax

Pyothorax, an inflammatory exudate in the pleural cavity, is generally septic. As with most disease affecting the pleural cavity, the clinical signs often associated with pyothorax include respiratory distress and tachypnea[46-48]; pyrexia is diagnosed in approximately half of animals with a pyothorax.[46,47] In a recent study, 4 of 10 animals with pyothorax were suspected to be secondary to trauma.[47] It is difficult to determine the inciting cause in many cases of pyothorax, so the true incidence of traumatically induced pyothorax is unknown.

Both medical and surgical treatment of pyothorax may be indicated.[29,47,48] Medical management often consists of bilateral thoracostomy tube placement, intravenous antimicrobials, and, potentially, intrapleural lavage. In order to determine the origin of a pyothorax and plan the best surgical approach, advanced imaging with CT is recommended.

Septic Peritonitis

Gunshot wounds, bite wounds, and vehicular trauma to the abdomen can result in septic peritonitis either from direct contamination with bacteria or leakage from an intra-abdominal organ. In a retrospective canine study evaluating gunshot and bite wounds to the abdomen, peritonitis was noted in 40% of the dogs with gunshot wounds and 14% of the dogs with bite wounds.[49] Another study in cats found that 8 of 51 cases of septic peritonitis occurred secondary to trauma (gunshot wounds, bite wounds, and motor vehicle trauma).[50]

Animals presenting with septic peritonitis often present in shock and have a palpable abdominal effusion. Initial treatment should target the cardiovascular and respiratory systems. Fluid resuscitation and broad-spectrum antimicrobial therapy are essential (see Chapters 60 and 122).

When the patient has been stabilized, surgical exploration should be performed and the inciting cause must be found and eliminated. Postoperative management with either open abdominal drainage or primary closure with closed-suction drains should be performed.[51] If drains are placed, the amount of effusion produced should be monitored and recorded every 2 to 6 hours. Cytology of the fluid should be checked regularly to monitor for evidence of recurrence of a septic effusion or a secondary infection.

Bile Peritonitis

Leakage of bile from the gallbladder or biliary ducts can occur secondary to blunt or penetrating abdominal trauma.[52] It is reportedly more common for blunt trauma to result in ductal rupture than gallbladder rupture, usually just distal to the last hepatic duct.[52]

Bile leakage should be addressed surgically as soon as possible. Bile in the peritoneal cavity can cause severe peritonitis because bile acids are toxic to most living tissues. In addition, many biliary effusions are septic and may prove life threatening (see Chapter 122). Appropriate antimicrobial therapy and supportive care are vital.

Hemothorax/Hemoperitoneum/ Hemoretroperitoneum

The diagnosis of a hemorrhagic effusion may prove challenging on physical examination. However, many of these cases will be presented in shock with obvious signs of blood loss and cardiovascular compromise (i.e., mental depression, pale mucous membranes, prolonged capillary refill time, poor pulse quality, and tachycardia; see Chapter 5).

After initial stabilization, the decision to manage these cases conservatively (medically) or surgically must be made. External counterpressure can be attempted for control of abdominal hemorrhage via the placement of an abdominal bandage; the use of external counterpressure in stabilizing blood pressure and improving survival has been advocated.[53] Other conservative management options include internal counterpressure and autotransfusion.[54] The decision to perform surgery is case dependent, but if a patient is not responding to fluid resuscitation efforts, has a rising intra-abdominal PCV, or is continuing to effuse based on ultrasonographic evaluation or physical examination, surgery should be performed.

In a retrospective study[55] evaluating cases of traumatic hemoperitoneum, the spleen, liver, and kidney were bleeding in 58%, 50%, and 23% of cases, respectively (determined during surgery or necropsy). Of the 28 cases evaluated in that study, 9 underwent exploratory laparotomy; 4 cases survived to discharge, 2 died, and 3 were euthanized. Discounting the euthanized cases, the mortality rate for the animals managed surgically was 33% and the mortality rate for the cases managed medically was 25%.[55]

Uroperitoneum/Uroretroperitoneum

After rupture of the urinary tract, urine can accumulate both in the peritoneal space and in the retroperitoneal space, depending on the location of rupture; if trauma to the distal urethra is severe enough, urine can also be noted in the perineal region. Trauma has been found to be the most likely cause of uroperitoneum in cats (85%), with 59% of cases occurring secondary to blunt trauma.[25] In both dogs and cats the bladder is the urinary tract organ most likely to be ruptured after blunt trauma.[25]

Dogs and cats with urine leakage often are presented azotemic, and these cases should be stabilized as much as possible before undergoing anesthesia or pursuing surgery. Additionally, severe electrolyte abnormalities (in particular, hyperkalemia) can cause arrhythmias, further compromising a patient that is already a high anesthetic risk. Characteristic ECG abnormalities noted in cases of hyperkalemia may include tall, tented T waves, absence of P waves, and bradycardia. If not addressed immediately, this can become life threatening. Medical management may include the administration of drugs such as calcium gluconate, insulin/glucose, bicarbonate, or β agonist therapy (see Chapters 51 and 122).

Definitive surgical treatment for cases of uroperitoneum secondary to renal or ureteral injury is generally necessary for a successful outcome and may result in an ureteronephrectomy. Bladder ruptures often require surgical correction, although small leaks may heal with the placement of a urinary catheter and collection system for continuous decompression (see Chapter 208). Surgical correction is typically accomplished by placing sutures over the rupture site. Bladder resection may be necessary if the bladder tissue appears severely damaged. Urethral trauma is managed conservatively in some cases by placing a urethral catheter or a cystostomy tube. If conservative management is unsuccessful, surgical closure of the urethral defect is necessary. Postoperative supportive care and intensive monitoring is important in these animals to ensure a positive outcome. Fluid therapy and urine output must be closely monitored and cessation of azotemia is expected if the injury has been properly addressed.

PROGNOSIS

The prognosis for animals that sustain blunt trauma can be good if they receive proper and timely medical attention.[1] Several factors have been identified that may negatively affect survival, however, and include corresponding head trauma, cranium fractures, recumbency at admission, hematochezia, suspicion of acute respiratory distress syndrome, disseminated intravascular coagulation, multiorgan dysfunction syndrome, development of pneumonia, positive pressure ventilation, vasopressor use, and cardiopulmonary arrest.[1] Further, hypocalcemia has been investigated as a prognostic indicator after trauma.[56] Dogs in the study that demonstrated ionized hypocalcemia were significantly more likely to require therapy with oxygen, colloids, blood products, and vasopressors and spent significantly longer in the hospital and intensive care unit than dogs without hypocalcemia. Dogs with ionized hypocalcemia also had a higher mortality rate.[56]

The animal trauma triage (ATT) scoring system has been created to aid in the assessment of veterinary trauma patients.[57] The score is based on an assessment of six categories, including perfusion, cardiac, respiratory, eye/muscle/integument, skeletal, and neurologic status; a score of 0 to 3 is given to each category with 0 indicating slight or no injury and 3 indicating severe injury (highest possible score would be 18).[57] In this study, the mean ATT was significantly lower for survivors than nonsurvivors.[57] This finding was corroborated in a more recent study evaluating animals involved in motor vehicle accidents.[2]

Overall, although several factors affect prognosis and the potential conditions that can occur after blunt and penetrating trauma are vast, many dogs and cats can survive if properly treated. Clinical signs may be vague and the true extent of the disease unknown at the time of first evaluation, and clinicians should be cognizant of the potential diagnostic and treatment options available. Aggressive resuscitation may be required, and surgical exploration of the thorax or abdomen is often an important part of treatment.

REFERENCES

1. Simpson SA, Syring R, Otto CM: Severe blunt trauma in dogs: 235 cases (1997-2003), J Vet Emerg Crit Care (San Antonio) 19:588, 2009.
2. Streeter EM, Rozanski EA, Laforcade-Buress A, et al: Evaluation of vehicular trauma in dogs: 239 cases (January-December 2001), J Am Vet Med Assoc 235:405, 2009.
3. Lisciandro GR, Lagutchik MS, Mann KA, et al: Evaluation of an abdominal fluid scoring system determined using abdominal focused assessment with sonography for trauma in 101 dogs with motor vehicle trauma, J Vet Emerg Crit Care (San Antonio) 19:426, 2009.
4. Kolata RJ, Johnston DE: Motor vehicle accidents in urban dogs: a study of 600 cases, J Am Vet Med Assoc 167:938, 1975.
5. Gordon LE, Thacher C, Kapatkin A: High-rise syndrome in dogs: 81 cases (1985-1991), J Am Vet Med Assoc 202:118, 1993.
6. Whitney WO, Mehlhaff CJ: High-rise syndrome in cats, J Am Vet Med Assoc 191:1399, 1987.
7. Vnuk D, Pirkic B, Maticic D, et al: Feline high-rise syndrome: 119 cases (1998-2001), J Feline Med Surg 2004;6:305, 2004.
8. Liehmann LM, Dorner J, Hittmair KM, et al: Pancreatic rupture in four cats with high-rise syndrome, J Feline Med Surg 14:131, 2012.
9. Munro HM, Thrusfield MV: 'Battered pets': non-accidental physical injuries found in dogs and cats, J Small Anim Pract 42:279, 2001.
10. Holt DE, Griffin G: Bite wounds in dogs and cats, Vet Clin North Am Small Anim Pract 2000;30:669-679, viii, 2000.
11. Shamir MH, Leisner S, Klement E, et al: Dog bite wounds in dogs and cats: a retrospective study of 196 cases, J Vet Med A Physiol Pathol Clin Med 49:107, 2002.
12. Baker JL, Havas KA, Miller LA, et al: Gunshot wounds in military working dogs in Operation Enduring Freedom and Operation Iraqi Freedom: 29 cases (2003-2009), J Vet Emerg Crit Care (San Antonio) 23:47, 2013.
13. Fullington RJ, Otto CM: Characteristics and management of gunshot wounds in dogs and cats: 84 cases (1986-1995), J Am Vet Med Assoc 210:658, 1997.

14. Risselada M, de Rooster H, Taeymans O, et al: Penetrating injuries in dogs and cats. A study of 16 cases, Vet Comp Orthop Traumatol 21:434, 2008.
15. Pratschke KM, Kirby BM: High rise syndrome with impalement in three cats, J Small Anim Pract 43:261, 2002.
16. Shaw SR, Rozanski EA, Rush JE: Traumatic body wall herniation in 36 dogs and cats, J Am Anim Hosp Assoc 39:35, 2003.
17. Worth AJ, Machon RG: Traumatic diaphragmatic herniation: pathophysiology and management, Compend Contin Educ Vet 27:178, 2005.
18. Spattini G, Rossi F, Vignoli M, et al: Use of ultrasound to diagnose diaphragmatic rupture in dogs and cats, Vet Radiol Ultrasound 44:226, 2003.
19. Boysen SR, Rozanski EA, Tidwell AS, et al: Evaluation of a focused assessment with sonography for trauma protocol to detect free abdominal fluid in dogs involved in motor vehicle accidents, J Am Vet Med Assoc 225:1198, 2004.
20. Lisciandro GR: Abdominal and thoracic focused assessment with sonography for trauma, triage, and monitoring in small animals, J Vet Emerg Crit Care (San Antonio) 21:104, 2011.
21. Lisciandro GR, Lagutchik MS, Kelly KA, et al: Evaluation of a Thoracic Focused Assessment with Sonography for Trauma (TFAST) protocol to detect pneumothorax and concurrent thoracic injury in 145 traumatized dogs, J Vet Emerg Crit Care 18:258, 2008.
22. Akoglu H, Akoglu EU, Evman S, et al: Utility of cervical spinal and abdominal computed tomography in diagnosing occult pneumothorax in patients with blunt trauma: computed tomographic imaging protocol matters, J Trauma Acute Care Surg 73:874, 2012.
23. Chatoorgoon K, Brown RL, Garcia VF, et al: Role of computed tomography and clinical findings in pediatric blunt intestinal injury: a multicenter study, Pediatr Emerg Care 28:1338, 2012.
24. Alleman AR: Abdominal, thoracic, and pericardial effusions, Vet Clin North Am Small Anim Pract 33:89, 2003.
25. Aumann M, Worth LT, Drobatz KJ: Uroperitoneum in cats: 26 cases (1986-1995), J Am Anim Hosp Assoc 34:315, 1998.
26. Schmiedt CW, Tobias KM, Otto CM: Evaluation of abdominal fluid: peripheral blood creatinine and potassium ratios for diagnosis of uroperitoneum in dogs, J Vet Emerg Crit Care 11:275, 2001.
27. Bonczynski JJ, Ludwig LL, Barton LJ, et al: Comparison of peritoneal fluid and peripheral blood pH, bicarbonate, glucose, and lactate concentration as a diagnostic tool for septic peritonitis in dogs and cats, Vet Surg 32:161, 2003.
28. Levin GM, Bonczynski JJ, Ludwig LL, et al: Lactate as a diagnostic test for septic peritoneal effusions in dogs and cats, J Am Anim Hosp Assoc 40:364, 2004.
29. Scott JA, Macintire DK: Canine pyothorax: clinical presentation, diagnosis, and treatment, Compend Contin Educ Vet 25:2003, 2003.
30. Silverstein DC, Kleiner J, Drobatz KJ: Effectiveness of intravenous fluid resuscitation in the emergency room for treatment of hypotension in dogs: 35 cases (2000-2010), J Vet Emerg Crit Care (San Antonio) 22:666, 2012.
31. Bickell WH, Wall MJ, Jr., Pepe PE, et al: Immediate versus delayed fluid resuscitation for hypotensive patients with penetrating torso injuries, N Engl J Med 331:1105, 1994.
32. Dutton RP: Haemostatic resuscitation, Br J Anaesth 109(Suppl 1):i39, 2012.
33. Gibson TW, Brisson BA, Sears W: Perioperative survival rates after surgery for diaphragmatic hernia in dogs and cats: 92 cases (1990-2002), J Am Vet Med Assoc 227:105, 2005.
34. Wilson GP, 3rd, Hayes HM Jr: Diaphragmatic hernia in the dog and cat: a 25-year overview, Semin Vet Med Surg (Small Anim) 1:318, 1986.
35. Gower SB, Weisse CW, Brown DC: Major abdominal evisceration injuries in dogs and cats: 12 cases (1998-2008), J Am Vet Med Assoc 234:1566, 2009.
36. Waldron DR, Hedlund CS, Pechman R: Abdominal hernias in dogs and cats: a review of 24 cases, J Am Anim Hosp Assoc 22:817, 1986.
37. Birchard SJ, Smeak DD, McLoughlin MA: Treatment of idiopathic chylothorax in dogs and cats, J Am Vet Med Assoc 212:652, 1998.
38. Fossum TW, Birchard SJ, Jacobs RM: Chylothorax in 34 dogs, J Am Vet Med Assoc 188:1315, 1986.
39. Allman DA, Radlinsky MG, Ralph AG, et al: Thoracoscopic thoracic duct ligation and thoracoscopic pericardectomy for treatment of chylothorax in dogs, Vet Surg 39:21, 2010.
40. Carobbi B, White RA, Romanelli G: Treatment of idiopathic chylothorax in 14 dogs by ligation of the thoracic duct and partial pericardiectomy, Vet Rec 163:743, 2008.
41. Fossum TW, Mertens MM, Miller MW, et al: Thoracic duct ligation and pericardectomy for treatment of idiopathic chylothorax, J Vet Intern Med 18:307, 2004.
42. McAnulty JF: Prospective comparison of cisterna chyli ablation to pericardectomy for treatment of spontaneously occurring idiopathic chylothorax in the dog, Vet Surg 40:926, 2011.
43. Stewart K, Padgett S: Chylothorax treated via thoracic duct ligation and omentalization, J Am Anim Hosp Assoc 46:312, 2010.
44. Mayhew PD, Culp WT, Mayhew KN, et al: Minimally invasive treatment of idiopathic chylothorax in dogs by thoracoscopic thoracic duct ligation and subphrenic pericardiectomy: 6 cases (2007-2010), J Am Vet Med Assoc 241:904, 2012.
45. Radlinsky MG, Mason DE, Biller DS, et al: Thoracoscopic visualization and ligation of the thoracic duct in dogs, Vet Surg 31:138, 2002.
46. Barrs VR, Allan GS, Martin P, et al: Feline pyothorax: a retrospective study of 27 cases in Australia, J Feline Med Surg 7:211, 2005.
47. Boothe HW, Howe LM, Boothe DM, et al: Evaluation of outcomes in dogs treated for pyothorax: 46 cases (1983-2001), J Am Vet Med Assoc 236:657, 2010.
48. Rooney MB, Monnet E: Medical and surgical treatment of pyothorax in dogs: 26 cases (1991-2001), J Am Vet Med Assoc 2002;221:86-92.
49. Bjorling DE, Crowe DT, Kolata RJ, et al: Penetrating abdominal wounds in dogs and cats, J Am Anim Hosp Assoc 1982:742, 1982.
50. Costello MF, Drobatz KJ, Aronson LR, et al: Underlying cause, pathophysiologic abnormalities, and response to treatment in cats with septic peritonitis: 51 cases (1990-2001), J Am Vet Med Assoc 225:897, 2004.
51. Mueller MG, Ludwig LL, Barton LJ: Use of closed-suction drains to treat generalized peritonitis in dogs and cats: 40 cases (1997-1999), J Am Vet Med Assoc 219:789, 2001.
52. Neer TM: A review of disorders of the gallbladder and extrahepatic biliary tract in the dog and cat, J Vet Intern Med 6:186, 1992.
53. McAnulty JF, Smith GK: Circumferential external counterpressure by abdominal wrapping and its effect on simulated intra-abdominal hemorrhage, Vet Surg 15:270, 1986.
54. Vinayak A, Krahwinkel DJ Jr: Managing blunt trauma-induced hemoperitoneum in dogs and cats, Compend Contin Educ Vet 26:276, 2004.
55. Mongil CM, Drobatz KJ, Hendricks JC: Traumatic hemoperitoneum in 28 cases: a retrospective review, J Am Anim Hosp Assoc 31:217, 1995.
56. Holowaychuk MK, Monteith G: Ionized hypocalcemia as a prognostic indicator in dogs following trauma, J Vet Emerg Crit Care (San Antonio) 21:521, 2011.
57. Rockar RA, Drobatz KJ, Shofer FS: Development of a scoring system for the veterinary trauma patient, J Vet Emerg Crit Care 4:77, 1994.

CHAPTER 139
WOUND MANAGEMENT

Caroline K. Garzotto, VMD, DACVS, CCRT

KEY POINTS

- The patient should always be stabilized and assessed for internal trauma before treating external wounds.
- In the first aid care of wounds, it is important to keep the wound moist, clean, and covered until definitive treatment can be performed.
- Open wounds containing penetrating foreign bodies or projecting bone should not be manipulated until the patient has been stabilized.
- Once the patient is stable, all wounds should be cleaned and debrided, even if the animal will eventually be transferred to a surgical specialist. Surgical exploration is indicated for all penetrating wounds.
- Most wounds can be managed successfully with appropriate technique, close follow-up, cooperative owners, and minimal materials.
- Although wet-to-wet or wet-to-dry bandaging has been a mainstay of wound management, consideration of moist wound management techniques including newer dressings and negative pressure wound therapy should be considered.
- The diagnosis and prognosis for full return to function should be discussed with the owner as soon as possible. In addition, the patient's predicted treatment regimen (e.g., daily bandage changes) and total cost estimate should also be discussed.

Most traumatic wounds seen in the small animal veterinary patient include bite wounds, abrasions or shearing injuries resulting from motor vehicle trauma, degloving, lacerations, and punctures. Wounds can also result from decubitus ulcers in the recumbent animal secondary to poor nursing care, or wounds can appear in postoperative surgical incisions that dehisce or become infected.

WOUND HEALING PRINCIPLES

Wound Classification

Wounds are classified based on degree of contamination as follows[1-3]:

- *Clean:* Atraumatic, surgically created under aseptic conditions (e.g., incisions)
- *Clean contaminated:* Minor break in aseptic surgical technique (e.g., controlled entry into the gastrointestinal [GI], urogenital, or respiratory tracts) in which the contamination is minimal and easily removed
- *Contaminated:* Recent wound related to trauma with bacterial contamination from street, soil, or oral cavity (e.g., shearing or bite wound); can also be a surgical wound with major breaks in asepsis (e.g., spillage from the GI or urogenital tracts)
- *Dirty or infected:* Older wound with exudate or obvious infection (e.g., abscess in a bite wound, puncture wound, or traumatic wound with retained devitalized tissue); contains more than 10^5 organisms per gram of tissue

If a wound is associated with a broken bone, this is called an *open fracture,* and these can be classified as follows[4]:

- *Grade I:* Small break in the skin caused by the bone penetrating through
- *Grade II:* Soft tissue trauma contiguous with the fracture, often caused by external trauma (e.g., bite wound, low-velocity gunshot injuries)
- *Grade III:* Extensive soft tissue injury, commonly in addition to a high degree of comminution of the bone (e.g., distal extremity shearing wounds, high-velocity gunshot injuries)

Although definitive repair of an open fracture should be done as soon as possible for patient comfort, initial care of the soft tissues should not be delayed if a surgeon is not immediately available or if the patient is not stable enough to undergo general anesthesia for several hours. Any exposed bone should be covered with sterile lubricating jelly and a sterile bandage but should not be pushed back below the skin surface because this can cause deeper contamination of the wound or further injury to the tissues. Similar guidelines exist for wounds with penetrating foreign bodies such as arrows, large wooden splinters, or knives. The foreign body may be tamponading a large vessel, and removal could lead to severe hemorrhage. These objects should be removed only under controlled surgical conditions.

Other wound classifications describe the length of time that the wound has been open because this relates to how quickly bacteria can multiply in a wound. Although this is important to know, it is not as vital as assessing the patient and wound directly. It is more important to understand the local and systemic defenses of the patient and the types and virulence of bacteria that may be present in the wound so that appropriate treatment can be initiated.[1]

Phases of Healing

A basic understanding of the phases of wound healing gives the clinician an idea of how long it will take for a wound to improve in appearance and for making wound management decisions. Wound healing can be described in four phases: (1) inflammation, (2) debridement, (3) repair/proliferation, and (4) maturation.[1] The phases overlap and the transitions are not visible to the naked eye.

The inflammatory phase occurs during the first 5 days after injury. Immediately after trauma there is hemorrhage caused by disruption of blood vessels, and then vasoconstriction and platelet aggregation limit the bleeding. Vasodilation follows within 5 to 10 minutes, allowing fibrinogen and clotting elements to leak from the plasma into the wound to form a clot and eventually a scab. The clot serves as scaffolding for invading cells such as neutrophils, monocytes, fibroblasts, and endothelial cells. Also contained in the plasma are inflammatory mediators (cytokines) such as histamine, prostaglandins, leukotrienes, complement, and growth factors.

The debridement phase occurs almost simultaneously with the inflammatory phase. It is marked by the entry of white blood cells into the wound. Neutrophils are the first to appear in the wound approximately 6 hours after injury. They remove extracellular debris via enzyme release and phagocytosis. Monocytes appear approximately 12 hours after trauma, and they become macrophages within 24 to 48 hours. The monocytes stimulate fibroblastic activity, collagen synthesis, and angiogenesis. Macrophages remove necrotic tissue, bacteria, and foreign material.

The repair phase, also called the *proliferative phase*,[5,6] begins 3 to 5 days after injury and lasts about 2 to 4 weeks. This is the most dramatic healing phase and is characterized by angiogenesis, granulation tissue formation, and epithelialization. Fibroblasts proliferate and start synthesizing collagen, and then capillary beds grow in to form granulation tissue. Granulation tissue provides a surface for epithelialization and is a source of myofibroblasts that play a role in wound contraction. New epithelium is visible 4 to 5 days after injury and occurs faster in a moist environment.[1] Wound contraction is first noticeable by 5 to 9 days after injury and continues into the maturation phase.[6]

Finally, the maturation phase occurs once adequate collagen deposition is present and is marked by wound contraction and remodeling of the collagen fiber bundles. It starts at about 17 to 20 days after injury and may continue for several years. Healed wounds are never as strong as the normal tissue; a scar is only about 80% as strong as the original tissue.[6]

INITIAL PATIENT ASSESSMENT

Before handling the patient, the clinician and patient should be protected by the use of examination gloves. Initial stabilization of the patient should address the cardiac and respiratory system to ensure adequate oxygen delivery to the tissues (see Chapter 1). Intravenous catheter placement, fluid therapy, and supplemental oxygen may be required for severely traumatized patients or patients in shock (see Chapters 14 and 60). A complete blood cell count, biochemical analysis, urinalysis, and venous or arterial blood gas analysis should be performed upon admission.

Direct pressure should be applied to any bleeding wounds. If bleeding cannot be controlled by direct pressure, emergent surgical intervention is required. Bleeding from appendages can be controlled with tourniquets by using a pneumatic blood pressure cuff inflated to 200 mm Hg for up to 1 hour.[7] It is important to remember that bite wounds commonly result from the penetration of both the upper and lower teeth. If bite marks are seen only on one side of the limb or trunk, then the other side should be shaved to search for the corresponding wounds. Wounds should be kept clean and moist and protected from the hospital environment. A sterile, water-soluble lubricant and saline-soaked sponges can be applied to the wounds initially and then covered with a sterile towel and soft padded bandage if the patient must be moved. It is important that the damaged tissue remain moist because desiccation impairs wound healing.

If the animal has wounds associated with trauma, ultrasound is often indicated to assess for other more immediate, life-threatening injuries (see Chapter 189). Radiographs of the spine, chest, abdomen, and pelvic region, in addition to appendages if there is suspicion of a fracture, may also prove beneficial. Blunt trauma, such as motor vehicle trauma or falling from heights, warrants chest and abdominal radiographs or ultrasound to assess for pulmonary contusions, pneumothorax or hemothorax, diaphragmatic hernia, and peritoneal effusion secondary to blood or urinary tract trauma. A thorough neurologic assessment is also important to rule out spinal or neurologic injury. Assessment of perfusion and sensation to the digits is important when severe trauma to peripheral blood supply and nerves might preclude a successful outcome.

DEBRIDEMENT AND LAVAGE

Once the patient has been thoroughly examined and stabilized and all diagnostic tests performed, and if sedation or anesthesia can be administered safely, initial assessment and debridement of the wound should be done. The primary goal in the management of all wounds is to create a healthy wound bed with a good blood supply that is free of necrotic tissue and infection in order to promote healing.[5] Most wounds will require daily debridement and bandage changes, and the clinician should not be discouraged if the wound cannot be closed initially. The following summarizes the steps for daily wound evaluation:

1. Assess need for or response to antimicrobial therapy.
2. Debride, removing necrotic tissue, and then lavage the wound.
3. Determine if the wound can be closed.
4. Protect the wound with a bandage, Elizabethan collar, or both.

Initial debridement will require general anesthesia, local anesthesia, or neuroleptanalgesia. For future wound evaluations, the patient may require only sedation or analgesia and restraint if surgical debridement is minimal. Local anesthetics are ideal in unstable patients that cannot tolerate general anesthesia but have significant injuries to the limbs. In these cases wounds of the pelvic limbs can be debrided using epidural analgesia (see Chapter 144) and thoracic limb wounds can be debrided using a brachial plexus block.[8]

Sterile lubricating jelly should be applied to the exposed wound to protect it from further contamination and a wide area of fur clipped from the skin around the wound. Gross dirt from the skin around the wound should be cleaned by applying surgical scrub solution (chlorhexidine or povidone-iodine) to unbroken skin, but *not* to the surface of the wound because these solutions are damaging to exposed tissues.

Debridement should be done using aseptic technique: sterile gloves, sterile gown, and cap and mask, and the wound should be draped with sterile towels or water-impermeable drapes. At the time of initial assessment and subsequent bandage changes, necrotic tissue should be excised. All bite wounds should be explored, even if they look minor, because teeth exert a macerating or crushing force that can damage tissues deep below the skin surface (Figure 139-1). The hole around the bite wound should be trimmed and then tented up to evaluate the subcutaneous tissues. A probe, such as a mosquito or Kelly forceps, can be used to assess for dead space or pockets under the skin that could form hematomas, seromas, and abscesses.

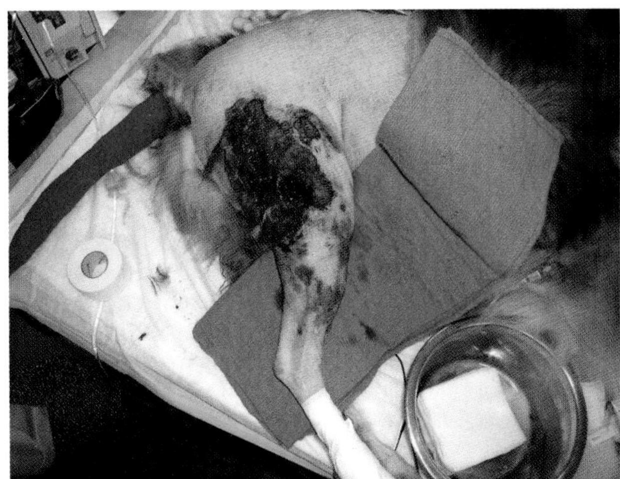

FIGURE 139-1 This 12-year-old Sheltie was bitten on the right hind limb by a Pit Bull and suffered extensive destruction of the skin and muscle on the lateral surface of the limb. *(Courtesy O. Morgan.)*

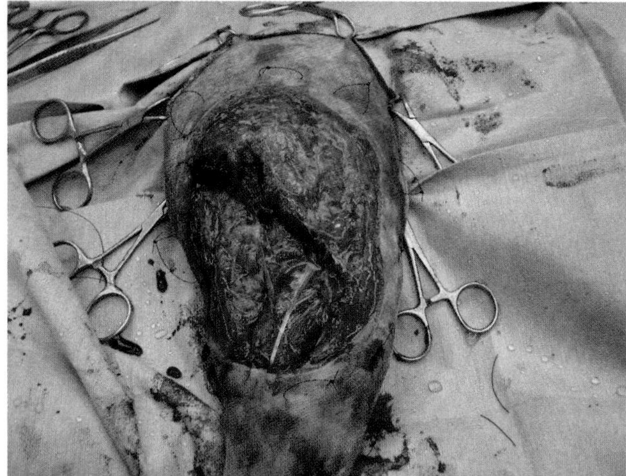

FIGURE 139-2 The wound from Figure 139-1 after initial surgical debridement. Only the necrotic tissues were removed initially. Note the loops of sutures surrounding the wound used for a tie-over dressing.

Obviously necrotic tissue (black, green, or gray) is removed first. In areas that have ample skin for closure, initial trimming of skin can be done more aggressively. In areas such as the distal limbs, trimming of skin should be done conservatively and questionable tissues given time to "declare" themselves (Figure 139-2). Bone, tendons, nerves, and vessels are preserved as much as possible unless segments of these vital structures are completely separated from the tissue and obviously nonviable.

The wound can be lavaged with a variety of solutions. Wounds that are heavily contaminated with road dirt or soil can be cleaned of debris using lukewarm tap water with a spray nozzle.[1] Maggots should be removed from severely necrotic wounds manually or with aggressive flushing. Chlorhexidine and povidone-iodine can be used in dilute form (chlorhexidine 0.05% solution: 1 part chlorhexidine 2% to 40 parts sterile water; povidone-iodine 1% solution: 1 part povidone-iodine 10% to 9 parts sterile saline) as initial lavage in contaminated and infected wounds because of their wide spectrum of antimicrobial activity. Povidone-iodine is more irritating to tissues, toxic to cells needed for wound healing, and inactivated by organic debris,[1] so it may not be the preferred lavage solution. Lactated Ringer's solution or 0.9% saline are the most commonly used lavage solutions. An in vitro study demonstrated that normal saline and tap water cause mild and severe cytotoxic effects on fibroblasts, respectively, whereas lactated Ringer's solution did not cause significant fibroblast injury.[9]

Lavage is performed by flushing with a bulb syringe or a 60-ml syringe with an 18-gauge needle. In order to facilitate refilling, the syringe and needle setup are connected to a three-way stopcock and an intravenous fluid bag.

Sugar and Honey

Sugar and honey have been used to treat wounds for hundreds of years. They are advantageous because they are readily available, are inexpensive, can be used both for debridement and to treat infections, and adhere to moist wound management principles.

Sugar has a bactericidal effect through its osmotic action, and it draws macrophages to the wound, which accelerates sloughing of devitalized tissue.[10] It is especially advantageous because it is effective and economical for large wounds. Indications include degloving and shearing injuries, infected wounds (*Streptococcus, Escherichia coli,* and *Pseudomonas* spp), burns, and other wounds that require further debridement. The wound is first debrided and lavaged. The area is then patted dry with a sterile towel before applying a coating (up to 1 cm thick) of granulated sugar. Sterile towels or lap sponges are used as the dressing in the primary layer, and then a thick, absorbent secondary layer is applied. Bandages are changed at least daily, or more frequently if strikethrough occurs. Sugar application is stopped when healthy granulation tissue appears. One disadvantage of sugar is that it may cause greater effusion in wounds, thus requiring more frequent bandage changes.[11]

BOX 139-1 *Materials for Dressing Changes*

- Sterile lubricating jelly, sterile gauze, umbilical tape, sterile impermeable drape material, cast padding, 18-gauge needles, 35- to 60-ml syringe, Vetrap or Elastikon
- Triple antibiotic ointment, silver sulfadiazine
- Isotonic crystalloids such as lactated Ringer's solution or 0.9% saline
- 4-0 to 0 monofilament, absorbable and nonabsorbable suture material
- A variety of splints for forelimb and hind limb stabilization

Honey, in the form of Manuka honey or medicinal honey (Medihoney, Derma Sciences, Princeton, NJ), has many favorable properties in the management of wounds, including burn wounds. Healing properties of honey are varied; honey decreases edema, accelerates sloughing of necrotic tissue, and provides a rich cellular energy source, promoting a healthy granulation bed. In addition, honey has antibacterial properties because of its high osmolarity, acidity, and hydrogen peroxide content. The hydrogen peroxide is present in levels that are harmless to healthy tissue. Honey can be used during the debridement phase and also over infected granulation tissue.[12] It has been shown to be more effective in some cases than more expensive commercial products, including silver sulfadiazine and conventional dressings (i.e., impregnated gauze, polyurethane films).[13,14]

Honey is applied to the wound after hydrotherapy and debridement of necrotic tissue. Gauze sponges soaked in honey are placed directly on the wound as the primary layer, then covered with an absorbent second layer to prevent it from leaking through the bandage. As with sugar, dressings may need to be changed one to three times a day, and the wound should be lavaged and reassessed before each application of honey.

DRESSING AND BANDAGING

Good bandaging practice is essential to maintaining and protecting the wound. Ideally a bandage should cover all open wounds. A bandage consists of three layers: (1) primary, (2) secondary, and (3) tertiary. The necessary supplies are listed in Box 139-1.

The primary layer is the dressing applied directly to the wound. This layer determines the purpose of the bandage by whether it is an adherent or nonadherent dressing. The secondary layer is composed of padded material that aids in absorption of exudates. The tertiary layer is the outermost protective layer that holds the others in place.[15]

An *adherent dressing* is used when the wound is in the debridement phase, providing mechanical debridement. The most common of these is the *wet-to-dry dressing,* in which sterile gauze sponges soaked with sterile lactated Ringer's solution or 0.9% saline are wrung out and applied directly to the surface of the wound, then covered with dry, sterile gauze sponges. The dry sponges soak up moisture from the wet ones, and this wicking action causes necrotic tissue and debris to adhere to the sponges when they are removed. It is often necessary to wet the dressing slightly with sterile lactated Ringer's solution or 0.9% saline to allow easier removal and to make it less uncomfortable for the patient.

During the debridement phase, it is necessary to change the wet-to-dry dressing and bandage at least once daily. Sometimes it will be necessary to change it up to three times a day initially, depending on how dirty the wound is or if moisture quickly "strikes through" to the outer layer of the bandage.

Although adherent dressings are still in common use in veterinary medicine during the debridement phase, they have received criticism because they nonselectively remove both necrotic and healthy tissue alike. Moist wound management principles are becoming increasingly popular in veterinary medicine because of improved wound understanding and technologic advances in wound products. The idea of moist wound healing was first promoted during the early 1960s after research conducted by Winter first demonstrated the benefit of a moist environment in optimizing wound healing by increasing epithelialization compared with leaving wounds open to air.[16] By providing a moist wound environment, the process of autolytic debridement can be more effective, which means that the body's own phagocytic processes will take care of wound debridement.[3,17]

Alginates, foams, hydrogels, hydrocolloids, and transparent films are examples of some newer types of *nonadherent* dressings that can be selected based on their specific benefits to promote moist wound management through all phases of wound healing (Table 139-1). These products are more expensive than traditional gauze, but an overall cost savings can be realized because frequency of bandage changes decreases from several times a day to once every 1 to 3 days and improved wound healing leads to faster healing times.[17] The more commonly used nonadherent dressings such as Telfa pads (Kendall, Mansfield, MA) and Adaptic (Johnson & Johnson, New Brunswick, NJ) are most appropriately used once a healthy, pink granulation bed has covered the surface of the wound and it is no longer infected.

Once the primary layer is applied, the next layer can be either a soft padded bandage or a tie-over bandage. Soft padded bandages are used to protect soft tissue wounds on the limbs, and a splint can be incorporated between the second and third layers to stabilize distal fractures or ligamentous injuries. The secondary layer is most commonly rolled cotton that is held in place with rolled gauze. The splint is placed over the cotton and under the gauze. The tertiary layer is often Vetrap (3M, St. Paul, NJ) or Elastikon (Johnson & Johnson, New Brunswick, NJ) and is placed over the secondary layer but without compression of the bandage or wound.

The *tie-over bandage* is used for wounds on areas of the body that are not amenable to soft padded bandages, such as the flank, perineum, or hip areas.[5] Materials include 2-0 to 0 nylon, umbilical tape, gauze, and water-impermeable drape material. Loose suture loops are applied circumferentially around the wound (see Figure 139-2). The secondary layer consists of several layers of dry gauze squares or laparotomy sponges that are applied for padding and moisture absorption. The tertiary layer is a water-impermeable drape cut to fit the wound, and then all three layers are held in place by the umbilical tape that is looped through the sutures in a shoelace fashion.

The bandage should be protected from the patient by judicious use of an Elizabethan collar. If the bandage is on a limb, the foot should be covered with a strong plastic bag taped to the bandage

Table 139-1 **Dressings**[3,17]

Type	Uses	Contraindications	Examples
Gauze	Inexpensive, readily available Wet-to-wet; wet-to-dry nonselective debridement	Not appropriate when healthy granulation tissue is present or when trying to get wound to epithelialize.	Surgical sponges
Impregnated gauze	Added zinc, iodine, or petrolatum nonadherent and help prevent desiccation Absorbs bacteria and exudate	Although it increases wound contraction, it can delay epithelialization.	Adaptic (J&J)
Polyester film with cotton	Used primarily during epithelialization phase on surgical wounds, wounds with good granulation tissue and with minimal exudate	May promote excessive granulation tissue.	Telfa pads (Kendall)
Calcium alginates	Absorbs heavy exudate Pad, ribbon or fiber forms gel when absorbing exudate Hemostatic, favors epithelialization and granulation	Do not use over exposed tendon, bone, or necrotic tissue.	Curasorb (Kendall)
Hydrogels	Absorbs minimal exudate Autolytic debridement Rehydrates to soften dry wounds	Discontinue after healthy granulation tissue is present because it can promote exuberant granulation.	Curafil (Kendall) BioDres (DVM Pharmaceuticals) Carravet (Carrington Labs)
Hydrocolloids	Autolytic debridement Increases epithelialization and comfort Promotes granulation	Not for use in exudative or infected wounds. Can promote exuberant granulation.	DuoDERM (Convatec)
Foams	Absorbent and comfortable Used in deep wounds with minimal exudate Promotes epithelialization and contraction	Reduces granulation. May cause maceration.	Hydrasorb (Kendall) Copa Plus (Kendall)
Polyurethane films	Occlusive but permeable to air and water vapor, but impermeable to fluid and microorganisms Autolytic debridement Covering for sutured wounds	Because of occlusive, adherent property, may cause bacterial proliferation and tissue maceration. Should be changed every 1-3 days.	Tegaderm (3M)

when the patient is taken outside to keep it from getting wet or dirty. The bandage should be changed immediately when it gets wet, dirty, or slips, or when there is strikethrough from the wound.

Exposed Bone

Exposed bone is prone to slow healing and must be covered with a granulation bed before skin graft or flap application. Injuries with exposed bone are seen most often with carpal or tarsal shearing injuries caused by motor vehicle trauma. In most cases exposed bone is eventually covered by advancing granulation tissue from surrounding healthy soft tissues when proper moist wound management techniques are applied.

Bone perforation can enhance wound healing by encouraging growth of granulation tissue over the exposed bone.[1,5,18] Once the wound has entered the repair phase, a Jacob's chuck and 0.045- to 0.062-inch K-wires may be used to perforate the surface of exposed bone through to the medullary cavity. Blood should not be wiped away. A nonadherent dressing with antibiotic ointment should be applied as the primary layer of the bandage. Bandage changes are done at 3- to 5-day intervals. Once a complete layer of granulation tissue is present (approximately 7 to 10 days), a free skin graft is applied or ongoing wound management continued until second-intention healing is complete.

Negative pressure wound therapy has also been shown to improve coverage of exposed bone in the case of distal extremity shearing wounds in dogs.[19]

WOUND CLOSURE

The decision as to when and how to close a wound depends on the cleanliness and extent of the wound.

Clean, fresh wounds, small, contaminated wounds or even infected wounds that can be excised completely should be closed primarily. Monofilament absorbable suture should be used in subcutaneous tissue and muscle, and nonabsorbable suture should be used on the skin. Avoid tight sutures and tension on the suture line.

Closure should be delayed for contaminated wounds or large wounds with questionable viability. Closure can be performed when a healthy granulation bed is present, which occurs during the repair phase of healing. Healthy granulation tissue should be pink, smooth, or slightly bumpy, should cover the entire wound, and should bleed on the cut surface or when an adhered dressing is removed. If in doubt, the wound should be treated as an open infected wound until the granulation bed is more definitively healthy.

Delayed primary closure of a wound is performed 2 to 5 days after the injury. Secondary closure of a wound is defined as closure of a wound 5 or more days after the inciting injury and is usually selected for wounds that were initially classified as dirty (Figure 139-3). If the wound is at least 5 days old, granulation tissue and epithelialized skin edges may need to be excised to allow closure.[2] If the wound is too large to be closed, the clinician should consider a skin graft or flap, or closure by second-intention healing. Second-intention healing occurs over a healthy granulation bed by the processes of wound contraction and epithelialization, which continue until the two epithelialized edges of the wound meet. Second-intention healing, even of very large wounds, can often be successful and does not require anything more than diligent bandaging and wound care.

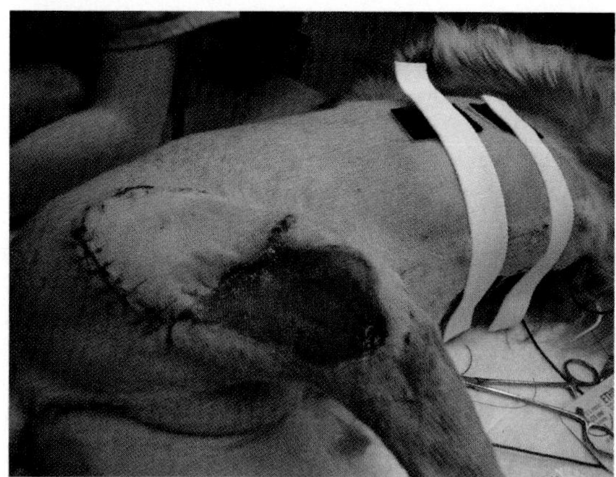

FIGURE 139-3 The wound from Figure 139-2 2 weeks after a caudal superficial epigastric flap was performed. Note the healthy granulation bed in the distal half of the wound. Skin stretchers were applied to allow harvest of the opposite caudal superficial epigastric flap to cover the distal half of the wound. However, by the time the flap surgery was scheduled, the remainder of the wound contracted enough to allow primary closure by trimming the epithelialized skin edges and undermining the skin circumferentially.

Drains

Drain placement is indicated during wound closure in areas with excessive dead space, areas with potential for fluid accumulation, or infected or contaminated areas (e.g., abscess, bite wound). The drain should exit from the dependent portion of the wound via a separate stab incision, not through the suture line. Ideally the drain should be covered with a bandage to prevent removal by the patient, to further compress dead space, and to keep the area clean. Drains are removed when drainage is clear or minimal (2 to 7 days).

There are two types of drains, passive and active. A Penrose drain is the best means of passive gravitational drainage. This type of drain can be secured at the proximal extent of the wound pocket with a simple interrupted suture through the skin that catches the flimsy rubber tubing while it is held in position with a hemostat. A separate opening to secure a Penrose drain proximally should never be made because this allows bacteria to migrate into the wound. The Penrose drain should exit the wound pocket at its most dependent location and be secured with a simple interrupted or cruciate suture to the skin edge of the opening where it exits the wound pocket (Figure 139-4).

There are many types of active or closed-suction drains, which consist of a vacuum-generating reservoir connected to fenestrated tubing. These can be used only in areas that can be closed completely because a vacuum must be created within the wound. There are numerous commercially available closed-suction drains such as the J-VAC (Johnson & Johnson, Arlington, TX) and the Sil-Med vacuum drain (Sil-Med Corp., Taunton, MA), which has a grenade-type reservoir. There are also several ways to make closed suction devices.[1,15] A butterfly catheter and red-top blood collection tube can be used for small spaces. For larger areas of dead space, a drain can be made of intravenous tubing with additional fenestrations cut out of the segment to be placed in the wound using a number 15 scalpel blade. The tubing is then connected to a 60-ml syringe, and the plunger is held open with a needle or pin.

An alternative to a closed suction drain that is especially appropriate for very large or very hard to immobilize areas is negative pressure wound therapy (see the next section).

Negative Pressure Wound Therapy

Topical negative pressure (TNP) and *negative pressure wound therapy (NPWT)* are the generic terms used to describe the application of a vacuum to a wound to promote and hasten healing by second intention and to prepare wounds for closure with skin flaps or grafts. *Vacuum-assisted closure (VAC)* refers to a commercially available device (V.A.C., Kinect Concepts Inc., San Antonio, TX) that was used in some of the earliest published studies[20,21] and is also used in the majority of published controlled clinical trials.[22] Commercial units

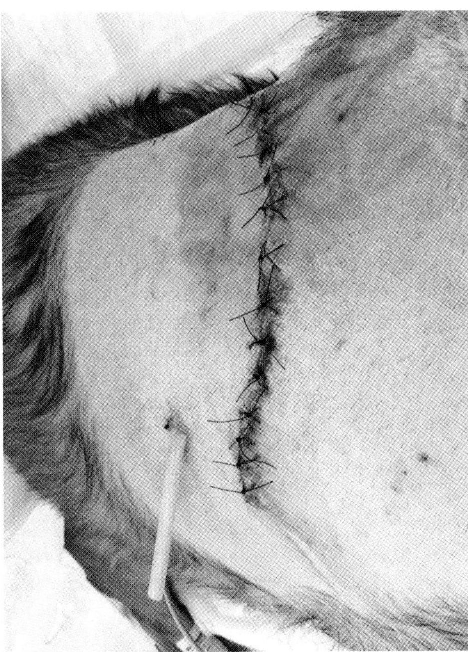

FIGURE 139-4 This dog had a skin laceration over its right scapula after a run through the woods. This fresh wound was cleaned and closed primarily. A Penrose drain is seen exiting a wound pocket distal and caudal to the incision. It is secured in place with a tacking suture to the skin edge where it exits distally. Proximally the Penrose is secured also with a tacking suture; however, the drain does *not* exit the skin.

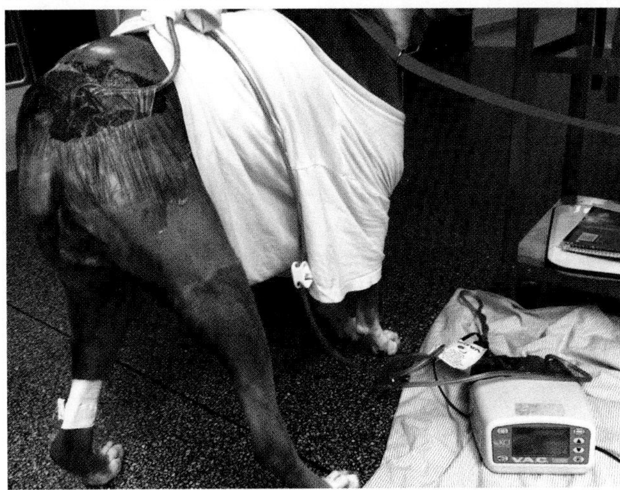

FIGURE 139-5 This 7-year-old female spayed Boxer developed a large abscess over her right and left dorsal pelvic regions while on chemotherapy (prednisone and vinblastine) 1 month after complete excision of a high-grade mast cell tumor from this area. The wounds were opened, cultured, lavaged, and debrided and a VAC (as seen in photo) was applied to decrease dead space, improve removal of exudate, and attain healthy granulation tissue. Interestingly, 24 hours after VAC application, swelling and hematoma formation were noted around the dressing. Tests for possible coagulopathy were negative, and biopsies showed no evidence of remaining mast cell disease. Although the VAC did help initially to clean up the wound, it is important to monitor for such complications. *(Courtesy T. Hamilton.)*

as well as homemade versions of these devices are used in veterinary medicine. The basic materials needed include open-pore polyurethane foam or open-weave gauze sponges for the contact layer, suction tubing, adhesive occlusive film, and a suction device with a canister to hold the evacuated fluid. The contact layer is fitted to the contours of the wound and then sealed with the adhesive occlusive film that overlaps the wound edges by at least 5 cm[21] and that must form a leakproof seal to maintain the vacuum. A drainage tube is connected to the foam dressing through an opening in the adhesive film. The drainage tube is then connected to a vacuum source most commonly set at −125 mm Hg[23] (Figure 139-5).

Clinical use of NPWT has outpaced appropriate randomized clinical trials to demonstrate efficacy and superiority to traditional methods.[24] Evidence-based reviews of the human literature looking at mechanisms of action of NPWT agree on the following mechanisms of action[22,25]: increased vascularization, improved granulation tissue formation, and a reduction in the wound volume/size. Clinical advantages of NPWT include more optimal fixation of skin grafts, better management of highly exudative wounds, and decreased costs because of the need for less frequent bandage changes.[22,25,26] Many studies have attempted to prove that NPWT can decrease bacteria and edema in wounds; however, these studies are contradictory.[22]

A prospective, controlled veterinary study[27] found that NPWT in dogs promoted earlier and less exuberant granulation tissue; however, prolonged use led to decreased wound contraction (at >7 days), higher bacterial load (at day 7), and decreased percent epithelialization (at >11 days) compared with a standard absorbent foam wound dressing (Copa Foam Dressing, Kendall Tyco Healthcare, Mansfield, MA).

Contraindications for NPWT as reported by the FDA include the following[28]:

- Necrotic tissue with eschar present
- Untreated osteomyelitis
- Nonenteric and unexplored fistulas
- Malignancy in the wound
- Exposed vasculature
- Exposed nerves
- Exposed anastomotic site
- Exposed organs

Patients with active bleeding, bleeding disorders, or those that are receiving anticoagulant therapy should not be treated with NPWT. Deaths have been reported with the use of NPWT as a result of bleeding and worsening of wound infections.[28] NWPT should only be applied after appropriate debridement to minimize the potential for fatal infections.[24]

Reports in the veterinary wound literature have described VAC use in distal limb injuries,[19] to decrease the size of large wounds and bolster bandaging of skin grafts,[29,30] in cases of surgical dehiscence/infection over orthopedic implants, in degloving wounds, in chronic nonhealing wounds, and for postoperative edema and seroma prevention.[30] Other uses include in cases of peritonitis, for open management of bite wounds over the thorax, and in compartment syndrome.[30]

Although there are many applications of NPWT for wounds, it is not proven to be a more effective treatment option in all cases. Important considerations include lack of progress with conventional wound management methods, the need for suction/drainage in particularly difficult to bandage locations (axillary, flank, and inguinal wounds or large mass removals), wounds that don't require daily assessment, patients in which daily sedation/anesthesia may be contraindicated, and patients that will cooperate for the treatment. Further research investigating optimal pressure settings, intermittent versus continuous modes of operation, and optimal materials for the wound contact layer will undoubtedly prove beneficial.[22]

ADDITIONAL WOUND MANAGEMENT MODALITIES

There are many additional strategies to advance wound healing that have been around for decades. Examples of treatments gaining increasing attention in veterinary medicine include hyperbaric oxygen therapy, low level laser-light therapy, and shockwave therapy. These treatment modalities are often attempted for management of difficult, chronic nonhealing wounds.

Hyperbaric oxygen therapy involves placing patients in a chamber that replaces room air with 100% oxygen under pressure. This creates a gradient that increases the partial pressure of oxygen dissolved in the plasma (PaO_2) and that subsequently diffuses across capillary membranes, into the interstitial space and ultimately into peripheral tissues.[31] Hyperbaric oxygen therapy has not been well studied in dogs and cats but may promote angiogenesis (which is fostered by the increased oxygen gradient), increased proliferation of fibroblasts, and increased leukocyte oxidative killing of bacteria. In addition, decreased edema after hyperbaric therapy allows better diffusion of oxygen and nutrients to the affected tissues while relieving pressure on surrounding vessels and structures.[17,31] Currently there is limited access to hyperbaric oxygen chambers for dogs and cats, but they may become more commonplace in the future.[31] Animals that are most likely to benefit include those with crush injuries, compromised skin grafts, severe burns, and infections with anaerobic organisms.

Low level laser-light therapy (LLLT), or "cold" laser, is better described by the name photobiomodulation. This technology uses low levels of red and near-infrared light to penetrate tissue and increase ATP production in the mitochondria of chromophores, as well as promote healing via the activation of fibroblasts.[32] Initial rodent studies in the 1960s showed that laser light stimulated hair growth and wound healing. LLLT is used routinely in human medicine,[32] and more recently in veterinary medicine,[33] to reduce inflammation and promote healing of wounds and deeper tissues. Although there appears to be clinical evidence supporting the use of LLLT, good randomized controlled trials are lacking and results are often not repeatable because of differences in laser technology (e.g., LED vs. class 3B vs. class IV lasers) and the need to specify variable parameters, including wavelength, power density, pulse structure, and timing of the applied light. Dosing guidelines for treatments are currently set by the World Association of Laser Therapy (WALT, www.waltza.co.za), which is considered the authoritative body overseeing laser research.

Shockwave therapy is a treatment modality that generates acoustic waves that travel through tissue to induce perturbations at the cellular level, which reportedly upregulates immunomodulatory mechanisms.[34] Although there is limited evidence in both experimental and clinical studies that shockwave therapy may promote wound healing, there is still no consensus regarding expected results and specific protocols for various types of wounds that might benefit from this treatment modality.

Before using one of these devices, the veterinarian must undergo specialized training in order to understand proper use of the equipment, indications, contraindications, and safety concerns. Although there is ongoing research and limited use of these technologies in private and specialty veterinary hospitals, fortunately a majority of wounds will heal uneventfully by following basic wound care principles and techniques.

ANTIMICROBIAL THERAPY

The most common bacterial wound pathogens include gram-positive *Staphylococcus* spp and *Streptococcus* spp and gram-negative organisms such as *Escherichia coli, Enterococcus, Proteus* spp, and *Pseudomonas* spp.[3,4,35,36] When humans (or animals) are bitten by dogs and cats, *Pasteurella multocida* is a common oral pathogen.[35] The most common anaerobic isolates in bite wounds include *Bacillus* spp, *Clostridium* spp, and *Corynebacterium* spp.[36] Often *Pseudomonas* will be an acquired infection on the surface of the granulation bed, noticeable by the wound's slimy feel and obvious pungent odor. Rarely does this organism cause systemic infection and thus it does not necessitate systemic antimicrobial therapy.

Antimicrobial drug therapy is not an excuse for inappropriate wound care. Debridement, lavage, and bandaging are the most important parts of wound management, promoting healing of the tissues and creating an environment that negatively affects the ability of bacteria to proliferate. Systemic antimicrobials are indicated for contaminated and infected wounds to help eliminate bacteria and promote healing.[37] Some clean, recent wounds, such as sharp lacerations, do not require microbial evaluation,[1] and superficial wounds that are easily debrided and closed may require only perioperative antimicrobial use (Table 139-2).

Table 139-2 Antimicrobial Use Recommendations in Wound Management[1,37]

Antimicrobial Use	Situation
Indicated	Obvious local or systemic signs of infection
	Wounds older than 6 hours
	Deep tissue injury involving muscle, fascia, bone, tendon
	Wounds likely to become infected such as bite wounds, penetrating wounds, and wounds involving body orifices
	Wounds requiring staged debridement, wet-to-dry bandaging
	Prophylactic use to prevent contamination of surrounding normal tissues
	To keep bacterial numbers low when planning a flap or graft
	Chronic nonhealing wounds
	Immunocompromised patient or one that has other condition that might jeopardize healing (e.g., diabetes or Cushing's disease)
May not be indicated	Clean wounds
	Superficial wounds less than 6 hours old
	A contaminated wound that can be converted easily to a clean wound with primary closure
	Wounds with a mature, healthy granulation bed

If a wound appears infected on presentation, a Gram stain can be performed to determine the predominant bacterial population and guide the initial antimicrobial selection. Culture and susceptibility testing of the wound should be done *after* initial debridement and lavage.

Superficial wounds in systemically stable animals are best treated with a bactericidal antimicrobial that is effective against gram-positive bacteria, such as cefazolin or cephalexin, pending culture and susceptibility results (see Chapter 175). Infected, deeper wounds may require a broader-spectrum antimicrobial such as amoxicillin with a β-lactamase inhibitor such as clavulanic acid. In one study the most commonly cultured bacteria from bite wounds (*Staphylococcus, E. coli, Enterococcus* spp) were 100% sensitive to amoxicillin and clavulanic acid.[36] Published recommendations for treatment of dog-bite wounds[36] suggests that initial antimicrobial coverage for severe bite wounds include intravenous ampicillin and either a fluoroquinolone or aminoglycoside. If the wound becomes infected, reculturing the wound is recommended because cultures taken during the first surgical debridement are of little value in predicting the organism involved. These antimicrobial recommendations can also apply to most other types of severe wounds or trauma, resulting in extensive deep tissue disruption, including necrotizing soft tissue infections.[38]

When systemic antimicrobials are administered, they should be started as soon as possible after the injury, given for a minimum of 5 to 7 days, and changed if necessary based on culture and susceptibility results and clinical resolution.[1] Wounds can be sampled for repeat culture after 3 to 4 days to determine the effectiveness of antimicrobial therapy. If wound healing is not progressing after the first 2 to 3 days or the animal's condition is worsening, a change in antimicrobial therapy may be indicated. Once mature granulation tissue has become established, antimicrobial usage is usually unnecessary because this tissue is resistant to infection.[1]

Topical antimicrobial drugs are often used to decrease bacterial populations on the wound, but they should always be used in conjunction with debridement and lavage.[1] The following medications are best used by spreading a thin layer onto a sterile nonadherent pad that serves as the primary layer of the bandage. Triple antibiotic ointment is more effective for preventing infection than treating it, and it has poor activity against *Pseudomonas.* Silver sulfadiazine cream has a favorable broad-spectrum coverage and is the agent of choice for burn wounds. Nanocrystalline silver dressings (e.g., Acticoat, Smith & Nephew, Andover, MA) have been developed to achieve sustained release of silver into the wound to decrease frequency of dressing changes from daily to every 3 days.[17] Nitrofurazone is a broad-spectrum antimicrobial agent with hydrophilic properties; it dilutes thick exudates for better absorption into bandages. Topical gentamicin sulfate preparations are effective treatment of wounds infected with *Pseudomonas* and are often used on open wounds before skin grafting is done.[1]

PATIENT CARE

Patients with extensive wounds that require daily debridement and bandage care often require intensive care initially (see Chapter 131). They also require pain management (see Chapter 144) and nutritional therapy (see Chapters 129 and 130) while recovering from trauma. Table 139-3 lists some of the commonly used analgesics and antimicrobials with their dosages.

COMPLICATIONS

The major concern for the clinician managing a patient with severe wounds is poor wound healing. Anemia, severe trauma, or hypovolemia can delay wound healing because of poor oxygen delivery to

Table 139-3 Drugs Commonly Used During Wound Management

Key Drug	Drug Class	Dosage Range	Frequency	Route	Indications
Amoxicillin or ampicillin	Extended-spectrum penicillin antimicrobial	22 mg/kg	q6-8h	PO (amoxicillin) or IV or IM (ampicillin)	Infection, dirty wounds
Amoxicillin-clavulanic acid	Extended-spectrum penicillin antimicrobial with β-lactamase inhibitor	22 mg/kg	q8-12h	PO	Superficial wounds
Amoxicillin-sulbactam	Extended-spectrum penicillin antimicrobial with β-lactamase inhibitor	22 mg/kg	q8-12h	IV, IM	Superficial wounds
Cefazolin	First-generation cephalosporin antimicrobial	22 mg/kg	q6-8h; for perioperative use give 20 min before surgery and then q2h until surgery is complete	IV, SC	Infection, dirty wounds
Cefovecin	Third-generation extended-spectrum cephalosporin	8 mg/kg	Once but can repeat after 14 days	SC	Efficacy comparable to cefadroxil for abscesses and infected wounds[40]
Enrofloxacin	Fluoroquinolone antimicrobial	5-20 mg/kg (do not exceed 5 mg/kg q24h in cats)	q24h (or divided q12h)	IM (IV use is off-label)	Infection, dirty wounds
Metronidazole	Antimicrobial	7-10 mg/kg	q8-12h	PO, IV	Anaerobic infection, dirty wounds
Methadone	Opioid	0.1-0.5 mg/kg	q2-6h	IV, IM, SC	Pain management
Hydromorphone	Opioid	0.05-0.1 mg/kg	q4-6h	IV, IM, SC	Pain management
Acepromazine	Phenothiazine anxiolytic	0.005-0.02 mg/kg	As needed	IV, IM, SC	Used with opioids for restraint during bandage changes
Fentanyl patch (Duragesic)	Opioid	<10 kg: 25 mcg 10-20 kg: 50 mcg 20-30 kg: 75 mcg >30 kg: 100 mcg	12 hrs to peak effect, lasts 72 hrs	Dermal	Pain management
Fentanyl	Opioid	1-3 mcg/kg bolus, then 2-5 mcg/kg/hr CRI	Short-acting analgesia	IV	Pain management

Continued

Table 139-3 **Drugs Commonly Used During Wound Management—cont'd**

Key Drug	Drug Class	Dosage Range	Frequency	Route	Indications
Epidural morphine (Duramorph)	Opioid	0.1 mg/kg diluted in 0.1 ml/kg 0.9% saline, not to exceed 6 ml	Produces pain relief in 30-60 min and lasts 10-24 hrs	Epidural	Pain management; local analgesia if combined with bupivacaine (use 0.1 ml/kg of 0.5% bupivacaine instead of saline)
Bupivicaine 0.5%	Local anesthetic	1.5 mg/kg maximum dose	Duration of effect 4-6 hrs	Local block	Pain management, early assessment, aid in restraint during debridement
Vitamin A	Vitamin	10,000 IU/dog	Once a day	PO	Antagonizes the effect of corticosteroids on wound healing

CRI, Constant rate infusion; *IM,* Intramuscular; *IV,* intravenous; *PO,* per os; *SC,* subcutaneous.

the wound. Poor perfusion and nutritional status can also have detrimental effects on healing. Serum total protein levels less than 2 g/dl impede wound repair by decreasing fibrous tissue deposition.[6] Infection and foreign bodies cause intense inflammatory reactions that interfere with healing. Patients with cancer that are receiving chemotherapy or those who have had radiation therapy to the area of the wound will also be prone to delayed wound healing. Patients with diabetes, uremia, liver disease, or hyperadrenocorticism are susceptible to infection or delayed healing as well. Corticosteroids decrease the inflammatory phase of healing and the rate of protein synthesis; however, vitamin A (10,000 IU/dog PO q24h) can antagonize these detrimental effects of corticosteroids.[6]

Most wounded patients are dogs; however, cats often present the more challenging cases. Axillary wounds in cats can be particularly difficult to manage. An experimental study found that cats have significant differences in wound healing compared with dogs.[39] Sutured wounds in cats are only half as strong as those in dogs by day 7, and cats demonstrate significantly less granulation tissue production than dogs in wounds that were evaluated for second-intention healing.

Lack of bleeding or negative sensation in a limb indicates a poor prognosis and may necessitate amputation. These changes may not be predictable at the time of initial evaluation.

As with any surgery other complications can include infection, dehiscence, and scarring. Contracture of limb wounds that are allowed to close by second intention can result in decreased mobility and may require referral to a specialized surgeon for skin reconstruction.

PROGNOSIS

Owners should be advised as early as possible of the prognosis, extent of care involved, and cost. Prognosis depends on the extent of injury and the location. Some wounds may be irreparable, leading to the loss of a limb. Cost depends on the extent of the injury and increases with multiple injuries and if fracture repair or abdominal or thoracic exploration is required. Length of hospitalization depends on the extent of debilitation, whether intravenous fluids or a feeding tube is required, and whether daily bandage changes and wound debridement are needed. Costs of $5000 or more are common if injuries require daily bandage changes and wound debridement, and expenses can reach $10,000 or more if fracture repair or additional surgery is required. In some cases, patients can be treated on an outpatient basis with bandage changes every other day. Complicated wound healing can take several months and require multiple surgical procedures.

REFERENCES

1. Swaim SF, Henderson RA: Small animal wound management, ed 2, Baltimore, 1997, Williams & Wilkins.
2. Waldron DR, Zimmerman-Pope N: Superficial skin wounds. In Slatter DH, editor: Textbook of small animal surgery, ed 3, St Louis, 2003, Saunders.
3. Fossum TW, Hedlund CS, Hulse DA, et al: Surgery of the integumentary system. In Fossum TW, editor: Small animal surgery, ed 3, St Louis, 2007, Mosby.
4. Anson LW: Emergency management of fractures. In Slatter D, editor: Textbook of small animal surgery, ed 2, St Louis, 1993, Saunders.
5. Pavletic MM: Basic principles of wound healing. In Atlas of small animal wound management and reconstructive surgery, ed 3, Ames, IA, 2010, Wiley-Blackwell.
6. Hosgood G: Wound repair and specific tissue response to injury. In Slatter DH, editor: Textbook of small animal surgery, ed 3, St Louis, 2003, Saunders.
7. Crowe DT: Emergency care of wounds, DVM Best Practices Feb:11, 2002.
8. Muir WM, Hubbell JAE, Skarda RT, et al: Handbook of veterinary anesthesia, ed 3, St Louis, 2000, Mosby.
9. Buffa EA, Lubbe AM, Verstraete FJM et al: The effects of wound lavage solutions on canine fibroblasts: an in vitro study, Vet Surg 26:460, 1997.
10. Mathews KA, Binnington AG: Wound management using sugar, Compend Contin Educ Pract Vet 24:41, 2002.
11. Tobias KM, Ayers J: Wound management in action: case presentations, Proc Pro/NAVC Clinicians Brief, November 2012.
12. Mathews KA, Binnington AG: Wound management using honey, Compend Contin Educ Pract Vet 24:53, 2002.
13. Subrahmanyam M: A prospective randomised clinical and histological study of superficial burn wound healing with honey and silver sulfadiazine, Burns 24:157, 1998.
14. Jull AB, Rodgers A, Walker N: Honey as a topical treatment for wounds (review). In The Cochrane Collaboration, Hoboken, NJ, 2009, John Wiley & Sons.
15. Davidson DB: Managing bite wounds in dogs and cats. Part II, Compend Contin Educ Pract Vet 20:974, 1998.
16. Winter GD: Formation of the scab and the rate of epithelisation of superficial wounds in the skin of the young domestic pig, 1962, Nature 4:366, 1995.
17. Murphy PS, Evans GRD: Advances in wound healing: a review of current wound healing products, Plast Surg Int 190436, 2012.
18. Clark GN: Bone perforation to enhance wound healing over exposed bone in dogs with shearing injuries, J Am Anim Hosp Assoc 37:215, 2001.
19. Ben-Amotz R, Lanz OI, et al: The use of vacuum-assisted closure therapy for the treatment of distal extremity wounds in 15 dogs, Vet Surg 36:684, 2007.
20. Morykwas MJ, Argenta LC, Shelton-Brown EI, et al: Vacuum-assisted closure: a new method for wound control and treatment: animal studies and basic foundation, Ann Plast Surg 38:553, 1997.

21. Argenta LC, Morykwas MJ: Vacuum-assisted closure: a new method for wound control and treatment: clinical experience, Ann Plast Surg 38:563, 1997.
22. Mouës CM, Heule F, Hovius SER: A review of topical negative pressure therapy in wound healing: sufficient evidence? Am J Surg 201:544, 2011.
23. Morykwas MJ, Faler BJ, Pearce DJ, et al: Effects of varying levels of subatmospheric pressure on the rate of granulation tissue formation in experimental wounds in swine, Ann Plast Surg 47:547, 2001.
24. Orgill DP, Bayer LR: Update on negative-pressure wound therapy, Plast Reconstr Surg 127(Suppl 1):105S, 2011.
25. Hunter JE, Teot L, Horch R, et al: Evidence-based medicine: vacuum-assisted closure in wound care management, Int Wound J 4:256, 2007.
26. Schneider AM, Morykwas MH, Argenta LC: A new and reliable method of securing skin graft to the difficult recipient bed, Plast Reconstr Surg 102:1195, 1998.
27. Demaria M, Stanley BJ, Hauptman JG, et al: Effects of negative pressure wound therapy on healing of open wounds in dogs, Vet Surg 40:658, 2011.
28. Division of Small Manufacturers, International and Consumer Assistance (DSMICA), U.S. Food and Drug Administration: Update on serious complications associated with negative pressure wound therapy systems, Silver Spring, MD, February 24, 2011, U.S. Dept. of Health and Human Services. Available at: http://www.fda.gov/MedicalDevices/Safety/AlertsandNotices/ucm244211.htm.
29. Guille AE, Tseng LW, Orsher RJ: Use of vacuum-assisted closure for the management of a large skin wound in a cat, J Am Vet Med Assoc 230:1669, 2007.
30. Kirby K, Wheeler JL, Farese JP, et al: Vacuum-assisted wound closure: clinical applications, Compend Contin Educ Vet 32:E1, 2010.
31. Braswell C, Crowe DT: Hyperbaric oxygen therapy, Compend Contin Educ Vet, 34:E1, 2012.
32. Chung H, Dai T, Sharma SK, et al: The nuts and bolts of low-level laser (light) therapy, Ann Biomed Eng 40:516, 2012. doi: 10.1007/s10439-011-0454-7
33. Lucroy MD, Edwards BJ, Madewell BR: Low-intensity laser light-induced closure of a chronic wound in a dog, Vet Surg 28:292, 1999.
34. Qureshi AA, Ross KM, Ogawa R, Orgill DP: Shock wave therapy in wound healing, Plast Reconstruct Surg 128(6):721, 2011.
35. Davidson DB: Managing bite wounds in dogs and cats. Part I, Compend Contin Educ Pract Vet 20:811, 1998.
36. Griffin GM, Holt DE: Dog-bite wounds: bacteriology and treatment outcome in 37 cases, J Am Anim Hosp Assoc 37:453, 2001.
37. Walshaw R: Current concepts in antimicrobial therapy in the wounded patient, Proceedings of the ACVS Veterinary Symposium, San Diego, October 27-30, 2005.
38. Buriko Y, Van Winkle TJ, et al: Severe soft tissue infections in dogs: 47 cases (1996-2006). J Vet Emerg Crit Care 18(6): 608, 2008.
39. Bohling MW, Henderson RA, Swaim SF, et al: Cutaneous wound healing in the cat: a macroscopic description and comparison with cutaneous wound healing in the dog, Vet Surg 33:579, 2004.
40. Six R, Cherni J, et al: Efficacy and safety cefovecin in treating bacterial folliculitis, abscesses or infected wounds in dogs. J Am Vet Med Assoc 233: 433, 2008.

CHAPTER 140
THERMAL BURN INJURY

Caroline K. Garzotto, VMD, DACVS, CCRT

KEY POINTS

- Electric heating pads, motor vehicles with hot mufflers, and fire exposures are the most common sources of burn injuries seen in the small animal veterinary patient.
- If the injury is from a fire exposure, the patient should be assessed for evidence of pulmonary dysfunction caused by smoke inhalation.
- If more than 20% of the total body surface area is involved, cardiovascular shock, major metabolic derangements, and sepsis may occur. These patients will need intensive medical and surgical treatment.
- Burn wounds may take several days to "declare" themselves because heat dissipates slowly from burned skin.
- The eschar should be removed early to help establish a healthy granulation bed and prevent infection.
- Silver sulfadiazine is the mainstay of topical treatment for most burn wounds.
- Cost of treatment and prognosis, especially in animals with severe metabolic derangements that necessitate intensive care, should be thoroughly discussed with owners.

Thermal burn wounds are relatively uncommon in veterinary medicine. The most common sources of burns in small animals include electric heating pads, fire exposure, scalding water, stovetops, radiators, heat lamps, automobile mufflers, improperly grounded electrocautery units, and radiation therapy.[1] Most burn wounds can be managed the same as traumatic wounds (see Chapter 139). Like traumatic wounds, burn wounds can be labor intensive and expensive for the owner. In addition, numerous metabolic derangements can adversely affect the patient, prolong hospitalization, and complicate recovery.

DEFINITIONS

Burn wounds are assessed using two major parameters: the degree of the injury and the percentage of body surface area involved. First, a review of skin anatomy is helpful.[1] The most superficial layer of skin is the epidermis and the deeper layer of skin is the dermis. The dermis is composed of a superficial plexus and a middle plexus, where hair and glandular structures arise. Below the dermis lies the hypodermis, which contains the deep or subdermal plexus and the panniculus muscle. The subdermal plexus brings the blood supply to overlying skin through the superficial and middle plexus. Capillary loops in the

Table 140-1 Burn Wound Assessment and Healing

Degree	Depth	Appearance	Healing
First	Superficial—epidermis only	Erythematous Painful to touch	Healing is rapid; reepithelializes in 1 week with topical wound management No systemic affects
Second	Epidermis and superficial part of dermis	Epidermis will be charred and sloughs; plasma leakage occurs Hair follicles spared Painful to touch	Healing by epithelialization from the wound margin with minimal scar in 10 to 21 days May have systemic effects
Second	Epidermis and deeper part of dermis	Skin appears black or yellow-white Hair follicles destroyed Decreased pain sensation	Healing by contraction and epithelialization but scarring is significant without surgical intervention Significant systemic effects expected
Third	Full thickness—entire epidermis and dermis	Skin is black, leathery; eschar insensitive to touch	Healing often requires extensive surgical intervention, possible skin grafts and flaps May have life-threatening systemic effects
Fourth	Full thickness—with extension to muscle, tendon, and bone	Same as above	Skin grafts and flaps usually required to prevent scarring that could restrict joint movements.

superficial plexus supply the epidermis; however, they are poorly developed in the dog and cat compared with humans, thus leading to less severe erythema and blisters than human burn victims.[1,2]

Although these are now considered older terms, many physicians still like to refer to burn wounds as *first-degree, second-degree, third-degree,* and *fourth-degree injuries* (Table 140-1).[1-3] First-degree burn wounds are superficial and are confined to the outermost layer of the epidermis. The skin will be reddened, dry, and painful to touch.

Second-degree burn wounds are partial-thickness injuries that involve the epidermis and a variable amount of the dermis. If only the superficial part of the dermis is affected, there will be thrombosis of blood vessels and leakage of plasma. The hair follicles are spared. In deeper partial-thickness burns, hair follicles are usually destroyed, the skin appears yellow-white or brown, and there is decreased sensation except to deep pressure.[1]

Third-degree burn wounds are full-thickness injuries that have destroyed the epidermis and entire dermis. The skin is leathery and charred and lacks sensation. Fourth-degree burn wounds have the same characteristics as third-degree burn wounds but also affect deeper tissues such as muscle, tendon, and bone.[1-3]

When burned, skin retains heat, so an accurate assessment of the degree of the wound may not be apparent initially.[1] It can take up to 3 days for the burn to "declare" itself, and during that time thermal injury and circulatory compromise from thrombosed vessels can continue.

Patients with burns involving more than 20% of their total body surface area (TBSA) can have serious metabolic derangements. Patients with more than 50% of their TBSA involved have a poor prognosis, and euthanasia should be discussed with the owners as a humane alternative. TBSA can be estimated in animals using percentages allotted to body area using the rule of nines as described in Table 140-2.[1,4,5]

When skin is severely burned, it forms an eschar within 7 to 10 days. Eschar is a deep cutaneous slough of tissue composed of full-thickness degenerated skin.[6] It appears as a black, firm, thick movable crust that separates from the surrounding skin. Purulent exudates often lie beneath the eschar, particularly if it covers deep or extensive injuries, and sepsis can result if not treated promptly (Figure 140-1).

Table 140-2 Estimating Total Body Surface Area Burned

Area	Percentage (%)	Total %
Head and neck	9	9
Each forelimb	9	18
Each rear limb	18	36
Dorsal trunk	18	18
Ventral trunk	18	18
TOTAL		99

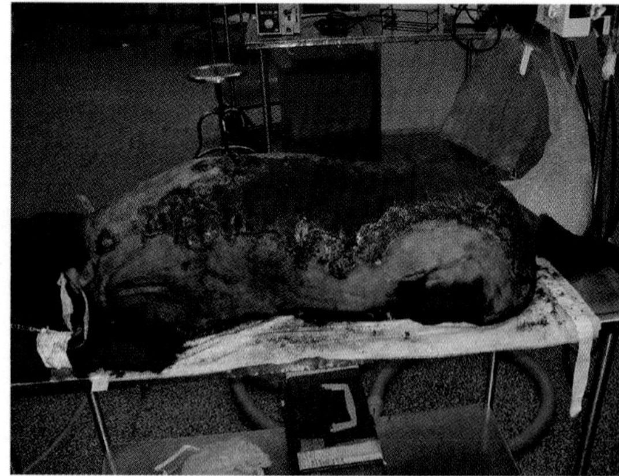

FIGURE 140-1 This dog was burned by a hot paint can that exploded in a fire. Note the large eschar on the dorsum of the patient. This large area of full-thickness necrotic skin impedes granulation tissue formation and allows purulent exudates to accumulate beneath it. The dog was anesthetized to remove the eschar. *(Courtesy M. Nicholson.)*

PATIENT ASSESSMENT AND MEDICAL MANAGEMENT

The patient should be assessed immediately for airway, breathing, and circulatory compromise, as with all trauma patients (see Chapter 1). After a full physical examination, including inspection of the patient from head to foot pads, an assessment of the degree and TBSA of the burn wounds should be performed to help determine prognosis and the extent of treatment necessary. Blood should be collected initially for evaluation of packed cell volume, total solids, electrolyte values, and blood gas parameters at the very minimum.

Metabolic Derangements

If more than 20% of a patient's TBSA is burned or if the wounds are classified as second or third degree, hypovolemic shock often occurs. As a result of capillary thrombosis and plasma leakage, massive amounts of fluid are retained in the wound, often leading to burn wound edema.[5] This results in the loss of fluid and electrolytes, with the most dramatic losses occurring within the first 12 hours. Systemic abnormalities should be anticipated, including anemia, hypoproteinemia, hypernatremia or hyponatremia, hyperkalemia or hypokalemia, acidosis (metabolic and respiratory), oliguria, and prerenal azotemia. The course of the systemic abnormalities changes with time.[4]

Hemoconcentration will be noted initially because of the dramatic loss of plasma; however, red blood cell hemolysis also occurs from both direct damage and destruction through the damaged microcirculation. The patient should be monitored for disseminated intravascular coagulation (DIC), upper airway edema, and oliguria. Between days 2 and 6, the patient should be assessed for anemia, DIC, immune dysfunction, systemic inflammatory response syndrome, and early burn wound infection. From day 7 and on, the clinician should watch for hyperthermia, hypoxemia, pneumonia, sepsis, and wound demarcation.

Fluid losses can result in hypovolemic shock (see Chapter 60). After initial shock resuscitation with isotonic crystalloids (up to 90 ml/kg intravenously [IV] in dogs and 50 ml/kg in cats) and synthetic colloids or blood products, if needed, total fluid delivery rate during the first 24 hours should be 1 to 4 ml/kg body weight × % TBSA burned.[4] After 12 to 24 hours, when vascular permeability is stabilized, a constant rate infusion (CRI) of synthetic colloids (e.g., hydroxyethyl starch) may be beneficial at a rate of 20 to 40 ml/kg/day (see Chapter 58). Fresh frozen plasma is given at 0.5 ml/kg body weight × % TBSA burned in humans, although this has not been investigated in dogs and cats. By 48 hours after injury, plasma volume is mostly restored, and thus patients are at high risk for generalized edema and fluid overload from the high initial demands for fluid replacement.[5] Ideally, fluid therapy should be tailored to the individual patient based on hemodynamic and perfusion indices (see Chapter 183).

Nutrition

Because of their fragile metabolic state, the importance of adequate nutrition cannot be overemphasized in patients with healing burn wounds. Nutritional requirements should be based on the patient's needs; an initial estimate is made by calculating the resting energy requirement. The diet should be high calorie and high protein, and the quantity of food can be increased as tolerated by the patient.

It is best if the patient can eat voluntarily, but if the animal is not consuming adequate nutrition, an esophagostomy tube should be placed or total parenteral nutrition commenced (see Chapters 129 and 130). Gastrointestinal (GI) protectants (famotidine at 0.5 to 1 mg/kg per os [PO], subcutaneously [SC], intramuscularly [IM], or IV q12-24h) are recommended to manage GI ulceration secondary to GI hypoperfusion (see Chapter 161).

Patient Comfort

Although severely damaged skin is often numb, deeper viable tissues and surrounding areas are often hypersensitive and thermal damage may be ongoing; thus one should assume that burn patients experience extreme pain (see Chapters 144 and 163). Good systemic analgesics include methadone (0.1 to 0.5 mg/kg IV q2-6h), hydromorphone (0.05 to 0.1 mg/kg IV q4-6h) or fentanyl as a CRI (2 to 5 mcg/kg/hr IV +/− 1 to 3 mcg/kg bolus). A fentanyl patch may not be appropriate in animals with more than 20% TBSA burned or who are still being treated for hypovolemic shock because of altered absorption. Good nursing care is important, and animals should be turned every 4 hours if recumbent to prevent decubitus ulcers. Passive range-of-motion limb exercises can help prevent edema and maintain mobility.[4]

Antimicrobial Therapy

Sepsis is one of the greatest threats to burn patients with extensive TBSA involvement, because bacteria can colonize and proliferate in wounds that have lost the protective skin barrier (see Chapter 182). The best way to prevent local and systemic infection is to protect the wound from contamination in the hospital environment, and to remove all necrotic tissue and purulent exudates from the wound surface as aggressively as possible through serial debridement. Systemic antimicrobials are not indicated unless the patient is immunocompromised, has pneumonia or pulmonary injury, or sepsis is suspected (see Chapter 175). Topical antibiotics are the antimicrobial treatment of choice (see Burn Wound Management in the following section). Because most invasive burn wound infections are caused by *Pseudomonas* or other gram-negative organisms, antimicrobials against these bacteria are administered empirically until culture and susceptibility testing results are available (see Chapters 93 and 94).[5]

BURN WOUND MANAGEMENT

Although early wound closure is the primary goal to decrease further electrolyte, protein, and fluid losses, this is not usually performed for at least 3 to 7 days while the wound is "declaring" itself. Daily wound care, however, is critical. Once systemically stable, the patient is sedated with neuroleptanalgesia or placed under general anesthesia and the fur is liberally clipped to assess the damage. If fur pulls easily out of the skin, the wound is likely a deep partial-thickness or full-thickness burn[1] (see Table 140-1).

If the patient presents within 2 hours of the burn injury (which is usually not the case), cold water lavage for 30 minutes will often help to release heat from the skin and limit the depth of injury.[1] The temperature of the water should not be below 3° C, and if large body surface areas require treatment, it is important to prevent iatrogenic hypothermia. The affected area can be submerged in a cold water bath if it is on a limb, and cool towels or cool water from a spray nozzle can be applied to other areas.

Treatment of the wound then depends on its depth. In patients with superficial burns or superficial partial-thickness burns, it may be appropriate to use daily lavage and topical agents alone until the extent and depth of the wound is determined.[1] Deep partial-thickness and full-thickness burns require debridement, which can be done in three ways: conservatively, enzymatically, or surgically.[1] Conservative debridement is often used for the first 3 to 7 days as the wound declares itself and the patient stabilizes; then more aggressive surgical debridement can be performed. In human burn patients, prompt removal of burn eschar is positively correlated with improved survival and reduced morbidity because of control of sepsis and reduced scarring.[7,8]

Daily treatment of burn wounds with conservative debridement involves hydrotherapy, removal of necrotic tissue, topical therapy, and bandaging. This may need to be done more than once a day initially for wounds that are necrotic or exudative. Hydrotherapy consists of gentle lavage of the wound with room temperature sterile saline or lactated Ringer's solution. This helps to loosen and separate any nonviable or necrotic tissue from the surface of the burn. The lavage solutions should be delivered using a 35-ml syringe and a 19-gauge needle to create a pressure of 8 psi. Higher pressures may induce tissue trauma and cause deeper seeding of bacteria into the burn. A wet-to-wet dressing under a bandage can also be placed on

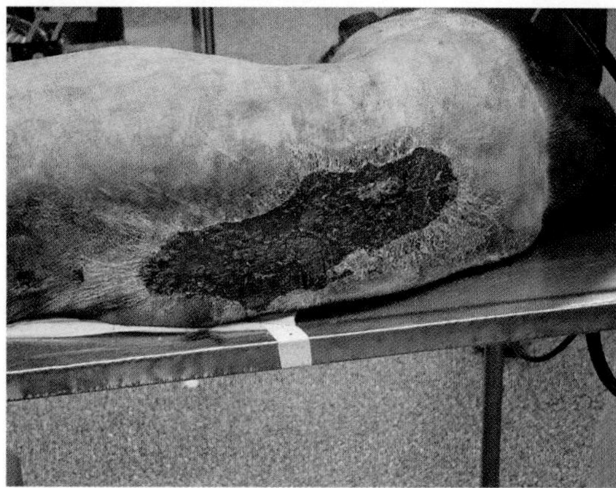

FIGURE 140-2 This is the dog from Figure 140-1, 4 weeks after escharectomy. Note the healthy granulation tissue and how the wound has become smaller via contraction and epithelialization. *(Courtesy M. Nicholson.)*

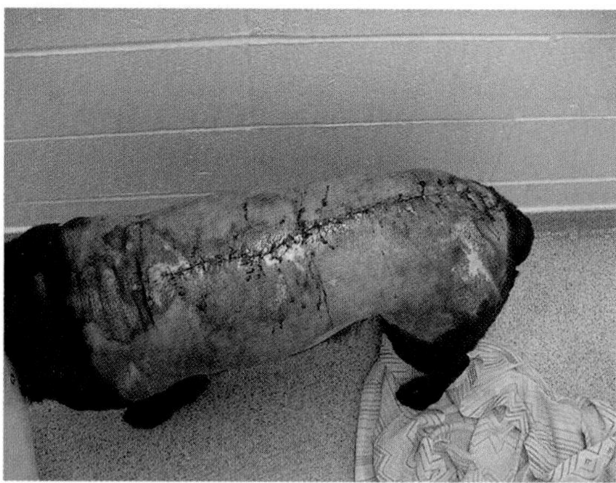

FIGURE 140-3 Postoperative view of the burn wound of the dog from Figures 158-1 and 158-2; it was closed primarily by elevating the skin edges and taking advantage of the loose, elastic skin over the body of the dog. *(Courtesy M. Nicholson.)*

burns for several hours at a time to slowly loosen the necrotic tissue and facilitate debridement.[1,6]

Conservative debridement is characterized by the daily serial piecemeal removal of necrotic tissue (black and hard, burned skin) using aseptic technique, with either sterile gauze or sterile scissors and thumb forceps. Because necrotic tissue is without sensation, this may not require daily general anesthesia; however, manipulation of deeper viable tissues and surrounding hyperemic areas likely will be painful during lavage. This form of debridement is acceptable initially, when there is no clear definition of nonviable tissue, or when it is prudent to be conservative in areas overlying tendons, ligaments, and bone.[1]

Enzymatic debridement is the use of topical agents to soften, loosen, and digest necrotic tissue, facilitating removal with gentle lavage. The advantages are that it does not require general anesthesia and also spares healthy tissue. Because some of the commercially available agents are expensive, it is most cost effective to use them on small limb wounds. The most commonly used enzymatic topical agent contains trypsin, balsam Peru, and castor oil (Granulex, UDL Laboratories, Inc., Canonsburg, PA). This product should be applied only in the early stages of wound therapy, then discontinued once a healthy bed of granulation tissue has been established.[6]

Aggressive surgical excision of an entire burn wound requires general anesthesia and is indicated in deep partial-thickness and full-thickness burn wounds that may otherwise take days or weeks with conservative debridement. This is done most easily on large areas of the trunk or small areas of the limbs, which can then be closed primarily (Figures 140-2 and 140-3). If the area cannot be closed primarily, it will take about 5 to 7 days for a healthy granulation bed to form, at which time flap or skin graft surgery can be performed.[1]

Topical Agents

After hydrotherapy and debridement, topical agents, dressings, and bandages are applied. Aloe vera and silver sulfadiazine are the most commonly used and readily available topical compounds for burn wounds.

Aloe vera cream has antithromboxane effects that prevent vasoconstriction and thromboembolic seeding of the dermal vasculature.[2,6] Ideally, using it within the first 24 hours can help prevent progression of superficial partial-thickness burns. Aloe vera is applied liberally to the surface of the wound with a sterile gloved finger while the patient is sedated, because these wounds are painful when touched. The wound should then be covered with a nonadherent hydrophilic dressing and bandage.

After the first 24 hours, silver sulfadiazine should be applied.[2] It has a wide spectrum of bactericidal activity against gram-positive and gram-negative bacteria and *Candida*. The cream is placed directly on the wound under the contact layer of a bandage using sterile gloves. For very large areas that are not amenable to bandaging, silver sulfadiazine should be slathered over the wound and the patient confined within a low-fomite environment (empty clean cage with no blankets or stuffed toys).[1,6] If needed, the cream can be rinsed off gently before reapplication, up to 2 to 3 times a day. Silver sulfadiazine can be used during both the early debridement stage under wet-to-wet dressings and through the repair stages of healing using nonadherent bandages. Alternatively, nanocrystalline silver dressings that allow for slow sustained release of silver are a slightly more expensive option that can be left on the wound for up to 3 to 7 days.[2,9]

Medicinal honey and sugar can also be used in the treatment of burn wounds; they are beneficial during debridement and help to control secondary infections (see Chapter 139).

Closure Options and Healing

Superficial and partial-thickness burn wounds have a favorable outcome with no surgical intervention. These wounds reepithelialize quickly and can heal within 1 to 3 weeks with open wound management. If only the superficial layer of the dermis is involved in partial-thickness burns, healing is often rapid. The overlying burned epidermis will slough, and healthy epithelium will be apparent below. Deeper burns involving the hair follicles, especially if they are large, will heal more slowly (up to 3 weeks). Deep dermal partial-thickness and full-thickness burns heal by contraction and epithelialization once a healthy granulation bed has been created by diligent debridement. Eventually, these wounds can be closed primarily. Full-thickness burns covering large areas of the body, or those on the limbs, may require skin grafts or skin flaps for complete closure.

Improvement in the healing of extensive burn wounds has been investigated using newer treatment strategies including negative pressure wound therapy and hyperbaric oxygen therapy (see Chapter 139).

Complications

Scarring and wound contracture are the biggest complications in patients with burn wounds left to heal by second intention. This is particularly a concern for patients with burn wounds in the axillary or inguinal areas, or around joints, which can lead to decreased mobility and range of motion of the limbs. Wounds in these areas should be managed by someone experienced in reconstructive surgery because they will likely require skin grafts or flaps.

REFERENCES

1. Pavletic MM: Management of specific wounds: Burns. In Atlas of small animal wound management and reconstructive surgery, ed 3, Ames, IA, 2010, Wiley-Blackwell.
2. Fossum TW, Hedlund CS, Hulse DA, et al: Burns and other thermal injuries. In Fossum TW, editor: Small animal surgery, ed 3, St Louis, 2007, Mosby.
3. Bohling MW: Burns. In Tobias KM, Johnston SA, editors: Veterinary surgery small animal, St Louis, 2012, Elsevier Saunders.
4. Dhupa N, Pavletic MM: Burns. In Morgan R, editor: Handbook of small animal practice, ed 4, 2003, Saunders.
5. Pope ER: Burns: thermal, electrical, and chemical burns and cold injuries. In Slatter DH, editor: Textbook of small animal surgery, ed 3, St Louis, 2003, Saunders.
6. Swaim SF, Henderson RA: Small animal wound management, ed 2, Baltimore, 1997, Williams & Wilkins.
7. Scaffle JR: Critical care management of the severely burned patient. In Parrillo JE, Dellinger RP, editors: Critical care medicine—principles of diagnosis and management in the adult, ed 3, Philadelphia, 2008, Mosby Elsevier.
8. Gallager JJ: Burn wound management. In Cameron JL, Cameron AM, editors: Current surgical therapy, ed 3, Philadelphia, 2011, Elsevier Saunders.
9. Murphy PS, Evans GRD: Advances in wound healing: a review of current wound healing products, Plastic Surg Int 190436, 2012.

PART XVII ANESTHESIA AND PAIN MANAGEMENT

CHAPTER 141

PAIN AND SEDATION ASSESSMENT

Sandra Perkowski, VMD, PhD, DACVA

KEY POINTS

- Pain is considered the fifth vital sign in human medicine (along with temperature, pulse, respiration, and blood pressure), which emphasizes the importance of an effective approach to pain management in the critical care patient.
- Pain assessment in the veterinary patient is inherently difficult, especially within the confines of a hospital setting where anxiety and stress can confound the accurate assessment of changes in patient status.
- Physiologic changes, although an integral part of the overall patient assessment, are not always reliable indicators of pain.
- Observational measures of behavior are an essential part of pain assessment, although they are subject to misinterpretation, especially in the anxious or dysphoric patient.
- No single pain scoring system has been universally adopted in veterinary medicine as the gold standard, although descriptions of many systems have been published and some systems have been validated.
- Before any assessment tool is applied, it is important to recognize the limits of the technique.
- The effectiveness of any treatment should be reevaluated regularly and pain management therapy adjusted as needed.
- A return to normal behavior and/or improvement in quality of life are the ultimate goals of any pain management strategy.

The multimodal use of analgesics has become an integral part of small animal practice over the last several years as the awareness of the complexity of pain pathways and the potential for long-term detrimental effects in veterinary patients has increased. Traditionally, it has been believed that some pain persisting into the postoperative period may be helpful to encourage immobility and, in turn, healing and recovery. Similarly, acute pain occurring at the area of injury in the trauma patient can serve to help protect the body part or system, minimizing further injury. However, acute pain also causes significant negative endocrine and metabolic effects that are known to delay recovery. These include immobility, decreased pulmonary function and atelectasis, decreased immune function, higher incidence of pneumonia, catecholamine release leading to increased metabolic rate and oxygen consumption, increased blood pressure and heart rate, cardiac arrhythmias, peripheral vasoconstriction, stress hormone release, inappetence, and insomnia. Most importantly, pain leads to patient suffering. The use of analgesics is especially important in critically ill patients in which any negative physiologic effects may have a profound impact on outcome. Although analgesia may be postponed for a severely injured patient due to the need for immediate lifesaving interventions, adequate pain control is ultimately essential to offset further detrimental effects.

Increased comfort with the use of constant rate infusions and a better understanding of the pharmacokinetic and pharmacodynamics differences between the many veterinary species and humans has led to new and synergistic combinations of multiple analgesic drugs (multimodal analgesia), which allows for decreased doses and reduced adverse effects in the critically ill patient.

DEFINITION OF PAIN

Aristotle first envisioned pain as originating from specific types of stimulation, including heat, cold, toxins, and crush, leading to acute awareness of the need to escape. Pain has more recently been defined by the International Association for the Study of Pain as "an unpleasant sensory and emotional experience associated with actual or potential tissue damage or described in terms of such damage."[1] By definition, pain is a subjective event and cannot truly be measured in an accurate fashion by an outside objective observer.

The perception of pain and response to a noxious stimulus are determined not only by the degree of injury but also by the individual's unique experience. Pain assessment becomes inherently more difficult in veterinary patients due to the obvious limitations in verbal communication, with attempts to anthropomorphize the animal's behavior potentially increasing the degree of error in our assessment. As a result, a number of assessment techniques have been described in the veterinary literature over the past several years, some of which are currently undergoing validation using strict criteria.

Nociception involves the series of electrochemical events that start at the site of tissue injury and result in the perception of pain. First, *transduction* of the noxious stimulus into an electrical stimulus (action potential) occurs in a discrete set of receptors (nociceptors) that detect tissue-injuring stimuli. Second, *transmission* of the nervous impulse occurs along the primary afferent fibers (A-delta and C-polymodal fibers) from the periphery through the spinal cord and ascending relay neurons in the thalamus to the somatosensory cortex. As the signal travels through the dorsal horn of the spinal cord, *modulation* (amplification or inhibition) of the message helps determine the strength of the signal reaching higher centers in the brain. In addition, projections to the reticular formation and hypothalamus increase alertness and autonomic functions (e.g., heart rate and respiratory rate) and increase catecholamine and glucocorticoid release. Finally, integration of the aforementioned processes with the unique psychology of the individual results in the final experience of pain *perception*.

Knowledge of these processes has stimulated considerable research into endogenous circuits, neurotransmitters, and interactions that either facilitate or inhibit the perception of pain. These processes are no longer viewed as a static system. Long-term anatomic, genetic expression, and circuit changes occur within the peripheral and central nervous system following acute and chronic stimulation. This has led to an emphasis on preemptive analgesia. Patients under anesthesia during surgery may be unconscious and unable to feel pain, but that does not necessarily attenuate the processing of nociceptive input and altered perception upon awakening.

The pharmacology of analgesics is different in patients with chronic pain and those with acute pain. For example, opioids appear to be more effective for patients with acute rather than chronic, neuropathic pain. In addition, opioid use rapidly (within hours) leads to the development of opioid tolerance and opioid-induced hyperalgesia, both of which may be attenuated by the addition of an *N*-methyl-d-aspartate receptor antagonist (e.g., ketamine or methadone) or gabapentin.

PAIN VERSUS STRESS

In general, physiologic and behavioral responses to pain have been used to develop a number of pain assessment tools or rating scales to determine the level of pain and/or sedation in the veterinary patient. These scales may change depending on the circumstances under which the scale is being used (e.g., acute pain after trauma or surgery vs. chronic pain of orthopedic or neuropathic origin), the underlying disease process (e.g., cancer vs. orthopedic disease), as well as the location (somatic vs. visceral, deep vs. superficial) and severity of the inciting stimulus. Consideration must also be given to differences in behavior with age, species, breed, and environment. It is important to recognize that these pain scoring systems have little value in optimizing analgesic therapy unless the person applying them has a basic understanding of pain physiology and pathways. Understanding mechanisms of pain transmission and antinociceptive mechanisms allows a logical choice to be made in prescribing analgesics for patients. Analgesia may be directed at minimizing inflammatory changes at the site of injury, inhibiting transduction or transmission of the nerve impulse (both at peripheral and spinal endings), or increasing the activity of descending inhibitory pathways acting at the central nervous system. For example, opioids have traditionally been viewed as centrally acting drugs and are most frequently given systemically. However, opioids may also be given epidurally or intrathecally, stimulating opioid receptors found at the level of the spinal cord to produce analgesia. In addition, there is evidence for the activation of peripheral opioid receptors (e.g., within the joint capsule) following tissue damage or chronic inflammation.

Another confounding factor in assessing pain in veterinary patients is that it is frequently accompanied by *stress and anxiety.* The stress response may occur in the absence of injury and in response to any number of environmental factors, including restraint, new surroundings, the presence of other animals, or other perceived threats to the animal. Stress, anxiety, and sleeplessness can all amplify the animal's perception of pain. Because anxiety increases the stress response to a painful stimulus, the responses themselves begin to impact the individual negatively. These responses include behavioral changes associated with "fight or flight"; neuroendocrine responses such as cortisol release, hyperglycemia, and catecholamine release; physiologic changes associated with sympathetic nervous system stimulation (e.g., tachycardia, hypertension, vasoconstriction); immunosuppression; and hypercoagulability. In terms of pain assessment, many of the physiologic changes seen during the stress response are similar to those seen in the pain response. The patient may not eat or sleep well. In conjunction with the neurohormonal responses, this sets up an overall catabolic state in the patient. Although it is incumbent upon the medical provider to treat the animal on the assumption that it may be in pain, frequently it is not possible to quiet the animal using analgesics alone, and administration of a sedative agent such as a benzodiazepine tranquilizer (midazolam 0.1 mg/kg), a phenothiazine tranquilizer (acepromazine 0.005 to 0.01 mg/kg) or a low-dose α_2 agonist (e.g., dexmedetomidine 0.5 to 1 mcg/kg) is necessary to reduce the anxiety and allow the animal to rest and recuperate. Midazolam or dexmedetomidine may be given as a constant rate infusion, if needed. In addition, those who interact with the animal should remember to use a soothing tone and gentle demeanor.

PAIN ASSESSMENT

Behavior

As stated previously, the perception of pain is clearly a subjective experience and can be quite difficult to quantify, especially in veterinary patients. However, there are some basic strategies that may help to assess accurately pain in these patients. First of all, it is important to observe the patient. This should be done with the patient both on its own and while interacting with people. Is the patient displaying one or more signs indicative of pain? These include both physiologic signs associated with sympathetic nervous system stimulation and behavioral signs (Box 141-1).

It is apparent that physiologic responses related to catecholamine release and sympathetic nervous system stimulation may be very difficult to differentiate from changes seen in response to anxiety. Therefore physiologic changes are not always reliable indicators of pain. In one study comparing subjective and objective measures for determining the severity of pain after cruciate repair in dogs,[2] changes in physiologic parameters did not correspond well with pain threshold testing and correlated only poorly with subjective measures of pain (visual analog or numerical rating scale; see later in

BOX 141-1 *Signs Associated with Acute Pain in Dogs and Cats*

Physiologic Signs

Increased heart rate with or without arrhythmias
Increased respiratory rate (often with decreased tidal volume)
Increased blood pressure
Increased temperature
Salivation
Dilated pupils

Behavioral Signs

Vocalization: growling, whining, whimpering, groaning (dogs); purring, growling (cats)
Restlessness or agitation
Resentment of handling of painful area
Depression or inactivity
Insomnia or reluctance to lie down
Inappetence
Increased aggression or timidity
Abnormal posturing (hunched, prayer position)
Alterations in gait, disuse or guarding
Licking or chewing at painful area
Trembling, increased muscle tension
Altered facial expression (fixed stare, squinting)
Failure to groom (cats)
Increased or decreased urination, failure to use litter box (cats)

chapter). Similar findings have been reported by others in both children[3] and dogs.[4] In addition, pain produces other neuroendocrine responses similar to those produced in stress situations, including stress hormone (cortisol) release and hyperglycemia. Furthermore, immunocompetency is decreased and a stress leukogram may be present.

Observational measures of behavior are also an essential part of pain assessment, although they are subject to limitation, especially in the anxious or dysphoric patient. Most people tend to focus on vocalization and agitation as signs of pain. Unfortunately, these two behaviors are frequently the least specific, especially after administration of opioid analgesics or in the postoperative period when many animals are disoriented or excited due to the anesthetic drugs that were used. Many animals show few outward signs of pain in the presence of other animals or humans. The species, breed, and age of the animal may also affect the signs exhibited. For example, cats are especially difficult to assess for pain. The need for analgesia is frequently overlooked in feline patients, since they tend not to vocalize. One study examining analgesic use in dogs and cats after major surgery in a veterinary teaching hospital[5] found that only 1 in 15 cats received any postoperative analgesia and that only one dose of medication was administered. Although much has changed over the ensuing years, this example demonstrates how easy it may be to confuse pain with mental depression in many feline patients. Most cats will merely sit quietly in the back of the cage and not move when they are in pain. They frequently stop grooming. They may be inappetent, insomnolent, or mildly pyrexic. A dramatic improvement in attitude and appetite is often seen after administration of analgesics.

Tools

A number of different pain scoring systems are currently in use in both human and veterinary medicine. The large number of these systems is testament to the fact that no one system has yet been universally adopted as the gold standard. It also should be recognized that pain scales used in the acute setting may not be appropriate for use in the chronic setting, in which owner involvement and quality-of-life assessment become increasingly more important.[6]

However, use of a pain assessment form may be helpful in raising awareness of an individual patient's pain and/or distress and increasing the use of appropriate analgesic and/or sedative therapy in the hospital setting. In the acute setting, quantification of pain behaviors is often done using variations of a simple descriptive scale, a visual analog scale (VAS), or a numerical rating scale (NRS), which may or may not incorporate changes in physiologic parameters.

The simple descriptive scale typically rates pain as "none," "mild," "moderate," or "severe." Each rating is then assigned a number (e.g., from 1 to 4), which becomes the patient's score. Although relatively simple to use, such a scale lacks sensitivity due to the relatively small number of categories. In contrast, a human study found that a 10- to 20- point scale was required to provide sufficient sensitivity to assess pain intensity in a group of patients with chronic pain.[7]

Visual analog (Figure 141-1) and numerical rating scales have been used to evaluate pain in human infants, in laboratory animals, and in several veterinary clinical studies. These scales can give reproducible results, even when used by multiple observers.[2,8] In pediatric medicine, a strong correlation exists between ratings provided by patients and ratings of their caregivers when either scale is used.[9]

The VAS is typically a straight line, 100 mm in length. One end of the line (0 mm) represents no pain and the other end (100 mm) represents the worst pain possible. The observer (or patient) is asked to mark where along the scale the patient's perceived pain would fall and a measurement is then taken and a number recorded, which allows the observer to track changes over time. Advantages of the VAS are that it avoids the use of descriptive terms and the need to assign a number to the pain. In the hands of an experienced observer, it can be a sensitive tool with reproducible results and has been considered the gold standard pain measurement tool in humans.[10] Similarly, owners can be easily taught to track changes in their animal at home. Disadvantages of the technique include observer variability in the interpretation of the term "worst pain possible." For example, does this mean the worst pain possible for this particular injury or disease, or for any injury or disease? Another disadvantage is that the VAS may be unduly influenced by signs that are easily detectable. For example, one study found that VAS scores were significantly and consistently correlated with increases in vocalization and respiratory rate in dogs after cruciate repair, both of which are easy to recognize at a quick glance.[2,11] Although both of these signs may increase in response to pain, they may also increase in response to anxiety or drug-induced dysphoria. These other factors must then be identified and taken into account when using a VAS. Similarly, the clinical significance of a given amount of change in the VAS may change depending on the patient and the disease process. Therefore the VAS is often used in conjunction with other pain assessment tools.

The NRS consists of multiple categories with which to evaluate the patient's behavior. Within each category, different levels of that behavior are given and assigned a whole number. In addition to these specific behaviors, changes in physiologic parameters may also be included. For example, an increase in heart rate or respiratory rate from 0% to 10% of baseline in the postsurgical patient may be assigned a value of 0, a change of 10% to 20% a value of 1, a change of 20% to 30% a value of 2, and so forth, and these scores added to the total. However, it should be noted that multiple studies have shown that changes in heart rate, respiratory rate, and blood pressure correlate poorly or not at all with pain threshold or subjective measures of pain in dogs in the postoperative setting.[2,12] A simple NRS is shown in Table 141-1.

One disadvantage of the NRS is that it provides an ordinal measurement and assumes that a change from 1 to 2 is equivalent in

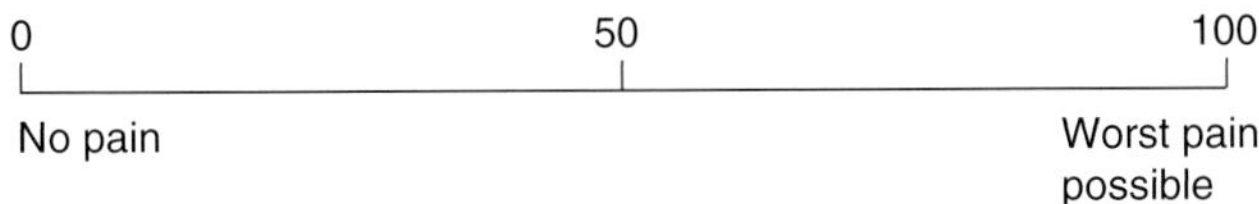

FIGURE 141-1 Example of a visual analog scale (VAS) used to assess severity of pain by making a mark along a 100-mm line to indicate the patient's estimated level of pain.

Table 141-1 Example of a Numerical Rating Scale Used to Assess Severity of Pain in Dogs

Observed Behavior	Score	Criteria
Vocalization	0	No vocalizing
	1	Vocalizing, responds to calm voice and stroking
	2	Vocalizing, does not respond to calm voice and stroking
Movement	0	None
	1	Frequent position changes
	2	Thrashing
Agitation	0	Asleep or calm
	1	Mild agitation
	2	Moderate agitation
	3	Severe agitation

SHORT FORM OF THE GLASGOW COMPOSITE PAIN SCALE

Dog's name ____________________________

Hospital Number__________ **Date** / / **Time**

Surgery Yes/No (delete as appropriate)

Procedure or Condition ____

____

In the sections below please circle the appropriate score in each list and sum these to give the total score.

A. Look at dog in kennel

Is the dog?

(i)		(ii)	
Quiet	0	Ignoring any wound or painful area	0
Crying or whimpering	1	Looking at wound or painful area	1
Groaning	2	Licking wound or painful area	2
Screaming	3	Rubbing wound or painful area	3
		Chewing wound or painful area	4

In the case of spinal, pelvic, or multiple limb fractures. or where assistance is required to aid locomotion do not carry out section **B** and proceed to **C**
Please tick if this is the case ☐ then proceed to C.

B. Put lead on dog and lead out of the kennel.

When the dog rises/walks is it?

(iii)	
Normal	0
Lame	1
Slow or reluctant	2
Stiff	3
It refuses to move	4

C. If it has a wound or painful area including abdomen, apply gentle pressure 2 inches around the site.

Does it?

(iv)	
Do nothing	0
Look around	1
Flinch	2
Growl or guard area	3
Snap	4
Cry	5

D. Overall

Is the dog? *(v)*		*Is the dog?* *(vi)*	
Happy and content or happy and bouncy	0	Comfortable	0
Quiet	1	Unsettled	1
Indifferent or nonresponsive to surroundings	2	Restless	2
Nervous or anxious or fearful	3	Hunched or tense	3
Depressed or nonresponsive to stimulation	4	Rigid	4

Total Score (i+ii+iii+iv+v+vi) = ______

FIGURE 141-2 Short form of a validated pain questionnaire developed for assessment of acute pain in dogs. Descriptors are ranked numerically according to the associated severity of pain. The assessment should be performed following closely the procedure described in the questionnaire. The pain score is the sum of the rank scores; the maximum possible score is 24 or 20, depending on whether or not mobility is possible to assess. The recommended analgesic intervention level is 6 out of 24 or 5 out of 20.

degree to a change from 2 to 3. Similarly, the categories themselves are not weighted and instead are assigned equal importance in determining the overall score. Another problem with the simple descriptors used in some NRS systems is their lack of specificity. In an unpublished survey involving the clinically active veterinarians and nurses at the University of Pennsylvania (S.Z. Perkowski, unpublished data, 1992), vocalization was the most commonly cited indicator of pain in dogs. However, vocalization also occurs nonspecifically with a high incidence in the postsurgical patient and can contribute to a falsely high pain score.

Clearly, behavioral changes indicative of pain may be difficult to recognize reliably in the acute clinical setting given the time frame. One study comparing use of an NRS and a quantitative behavioral scoring system over a 24-hour period found that dogs receiving adequate opioid analgesia after ovariohysterectomy had a more rapid return to normal greeting behaviors than dogs that received placebo.[13] However, the NRS used was unable to differentiate between the two groups of dogs. A pain scoring system was developed by the University of Melbourne (University of Melbourne Pain Scale) to assess postoperative pain in dogs by comparing preoperative and postoperative behavior, and an improved degree of interobserver agreement was found using this method.[14] This suggests that increased familiarity with the animal can help in overall pain assessment and management. In dogs with osteoarthritis, the owner assessment of the degree of pain correlates better with force plate evaluation than the assessment by veterinarians. Similarly, in cats with osteoarthritis, a subjective assessment by owners performed using a simple yes/no questionnaire to determine changes in activity associated with pain relief correlated well with changes in activity objectively measured using activity counts generated by an accelerometer.[15]

The Glasgow Composite Measures Pain Scale is among the most completely validated multidimensional pain scale system for use in dogs with acute postoperative pain.[16,17] This tool takes the form of a questionnaire, and the behaviors included in the scale fall into several basic categories: posture, comfort, vocalization, attention to wound, demeanor, mobility, and response to touch. Assessment includes both observation from a distance and interaction with the patient. A short form of this scale has been developed that takes only a few minutes to complete (Figure 141-2).

SUMMARY

Veterinary patients frequently require analgesics for a period of time after acute trauma or surgery. Before any assessment tool is applied, it is important to recognize the limits of the technique. Learning to anticipate when a patient will be in pain is extremely helpful, since pain is much easier to manage if the patient is treated *before* it experiences pain and becomes upset than if it is treated afterward. Frequently, knowing what the patient's underlying disorder is, whether or not a procedure has recently been performed on the animal, and, if so, what type of procedure can guide the appropriate use of analgesics. Usually, analgesics are given before any invasive procedure to take advantage of preemptive analgesia and minimize "wind-up." It should be remembered that very young and very old patients, as well as critically ill patients, tend to be less tolerant of pain and the neurohormonal and autonomic changes associated with pain. Close attention should be paid as to whether the initial treatment provides adequate analgesia and how long the analgesic effect lasts. Reevaluate the effectiveness of treatment regularly! Response to therapy can help enormously in guiding overall pain management. Do not wait for obvious signs of pain before repeating the treatment, unless the adverse effects are excessive. Individualize the treatment approach. Before administering any drug, carefully observe the animal and consider the underlying disease process. If any expected adverse effects are undesirable or potentially life threatening, the analgesic technique should be modified. It is important to remember that a return to normal behavior is the ultimate goal of pain management.

REFERENCES

1. Bonica JJ: The need of a taxonomy, Pain 6(3):247-248, 1979.
2. Conzemius MG, Hill CM, Sammarco JL, et al: Correlation between subjective and objective measures used to determine severity of postoperative pain in dogs, J Am Vet Med Assoc 210:1619-1622, 1997.
3. Anand KJ, Hickey PR: Pain and its effects in the human neonate and fetus, N Engl J Med 317:1321-1329, 1987.
4. Holton L, Scott EM, Nolan AM, et al: Relationship between physiological factors and clinical pain in dogs scored using a numerical rating scale, J Small Anim Pract 39:469-474, 1998.
5. Hansen B, Hardie E: Prescription and use of analgesics in dogs and cats in a veterinary teaching hospital: 258 cases (1983-1989), J Am Vet Med Assoc 202:1485-1494, 1997.
6. Yazbek KVB, Fantoni DT: Validity of a health-related quality-of-life scale for dogs with signs of pain secondary to cancer, J Am Vet Med Assoc 226:1354-1358, 2005.
7. Jensen MP, Turner JA, Romano JM: What is the maximum number of levels needed in pain intensity measurement? Pain 58:387-392, 1994.
8. Welsh EM, Gettinby G, Nolan AM: Comparison of visual analogue scale and a numerical rating scale for assessment of lameness, using sheep as a model, Am J Vet Res 54:976-983, 1993.
9. Manne SL, Jacobsen PB, Redd WH: Assessment of acute pediatric pain: do child self report, parent ratings and nurse ratings measure the same phenomenon? Pain 48:45-52, 1992.
10. De Williams AC, Davies HT, Chadury Y: Simple pain ratings scales hide complex idiosyncratic meanings, Pain 85:457-463, 2000.
11. Sammarco JL, Conzemius MG, Perkowski SZ, et al: Postoperative analgesia for stifle surgery: a comparison of intra-articular bupivacaine, morphine, or saline, Vet Surg 25:59-69, 1996.
12. Holton L, Scott EM, Nolan AM, et al: Comparison of three methods used for assessment of pain in dogs, J Am Vet Med Assoc 212:61-66, 1998.
13. Hardie EM, Hansen BD, Carroll GS: Behavior after ovariohysterectomy in the dog: what's normal? Appl Anim Behav Sci 51:111-128, 1997.
14. Firth AM, Haldane SL: Development of a scale to evaluate postoperative pain in dogs, J Am Vet Med Assoc 214:651-659, 1999.
15. Lascelles BDX, Hansen BD, Roe S, et al: Evaluation of client-specific outcome measures and activity monitoring to measure pain relief in cats with osteoarthritis, J Vet Intern Med 21:410-416, 2007.
16. Holton L, Reid J, Scott EM, et al: Development of a behaviour-based scale to measure acute pain in dogs, Vet Rec 148:525-531, 2001.
17. Morton CM, Reid J, Scott EM, et al: Application of a scaling model to establish and validate an interval level pain scale for assessment of acute pain in dogs, Am J Vet Res 66:2154-2166, 2005.

CHAPTER 142

SEDATION OF THE CRITICALLY ILL PATIENT

Sandra Perkowski, VMD, PhD, DACVA

KEY POINTS

- Evaluation and preparation of the critically ill patient are essential before any drug is administered. The choice of sedative agent depends on the patient's current physical status, preexisting conditions, reason for presentation, current treatment, and procedure to be performed.
- Most sedative techniques in the critically ill patient, especially those with cardiovascular compromise, involve using a sedative or tranquilizer in combination with an opioid analgesic.
- Critically ill patients are often depressed and require lower doses of drug to achieve the desired sedative effect; drugs should be titrated to effect carefully to minimize further compromise.
- Respiratory depressants, such as opioids, should be used judiciously in patients with severe hypoxemia or upper airway obstruction.
- Due to its short duration of action, propofol is ideal for short procedures requiring heavy sedation. However, it may cause significant cardiovascular depression in patients with volume depletion or cardiovascular compromise.

Sedation of critically ill veterinary patients is often required to permit minor surgical procedures and diagnostic measures. Advantages over general anesthesia include flexibility and ease of drug administration as well as avoidance of the need for intubation and inhalant anesthetics (although oxygen supplementation is generally recommended). Significant cardiovascular and respiratory depression may result, however, leading to life-threatening compromise of the patient's status. To minimize the influence of preexisting conditions and the extent of crises that may occur, a thorough evaluation and adequate preparation of the patient are essential before any drug is administered.

PATIENT EVALUATION AND MANAGEMENT

On arrival of the patient to the intensive care unit, immediate attention should be paid to the ABCs (airway, breathing, and circulation; see Chapter 1). These should be deemed adequate before proceeding. Evaluation of neurologic status, including assessment for mental status and evidence of head trauma, should be included. A complete history should be obtained if possible, including presenting complaint, known medical conditions, any current medications, and previous anesthetic history.

Oxygen supplementation and ventilatory support are provided as necessary. Indications for securing an airway early include poor ventilation or oxygenation, deteriorating mental status, lack of a gag reflex, and signs of developing airway obstruction. Stabilization of fluid balance and cardiovascular function is also essential before drug administration, although assessing the adequacy of intravascular volume can be difficult (see Chapter 60). The impact of inadequate intravascular volume will be accentuated by the peripheral vasodilation caused by many sedative agents, including acepromazine and propofol, and the generalized decrease in sympathetic tone that occurs with sedation. Adequate intravascular access is essential.

Cardiac arrhythmias, especially premature ventricular contractions, are commonly seen in critically ill patients, including those with gastric dilatation or volvulus, hemoabdomen, and thoracic trauma. In addition, they can occur secondary to electrolyte abnormalities, hypoxemia, or hypercarbia. Before sedation, the type and significance of any arrhythmias present should be determined and the underlying cause treated, if possible. Indications for antiarrhythmic therapy before drug administration include frequent, multifocal premature ventricular contractions and paroxysmal ventricular tachycardia that adversely affects blood pressure or perfusion parameters (see Chapter 171).

When time and the animal's condition permit, any electrolyte abnormalities should be corrected before drug administration. Severe hyperkalemia (potassium $[K^+] > 6.0$ mEq/L) is frequently seen in patients with renal compromise, urinary obstruction or rupture, massive tissue trauma, or severe dehydration with acidosis. Drug administration can exacerbate the cardiac effects of hyperkalemia, including arrhythmias and cardiac arrest, and therefore management should be instituted before proceeding. Hypocalcemia may be seen transiently after citrated blood product administration, although this generally resolves once administration is finished.

CHOICE OF AGENT

The choice of sedative agent depends on the patient's current physical status, reason for presentation, pertinent history, and procedure to be performed. Special attention should be paid to both cardiovascular and respiratory effects of these agents, but specific contraindications to drug use should also be considered. Intravenous administration allows titration of the drugs and is generally preferred. Intramuscular administration may be helpful, especially in the fractious patient or one with severe respiratory distress that does not have an intravenous catheter and becomes easily stressed with restraint.

OPIOIDS

Most sedative techniques in the critically ill patient involve the use of a sedative or tranquilizer in combination with an opioid analgesic. This "neuroleptanalgesic" combination generally produces a greater degree of sedation and analgesia with less cardiovascular depression than that achieved by comparable doses of either drug alone.

Most of the clinically used pure opioid agonists (morphine, oxymorphone, hydromorphone, methadone, fentanyl, remifentanil) bind primarily to the μ-receptor in the central nervous system, although they interact with the others (κ, δ), especially at higher doses.[1] In healthy animals, opioids cause behavioral changes ranging from sedation to excitement; however, in critically ill patients, opioids usually cause sedation (see Chapter 163). Cardiovascular function, including left ventricular function, cardiac output, and systemic blood pressure, is well maintained. Although morphine may be a useful sedative, histamine release with subsequent vasodilation and hypotension may occur, especially if higher doses are given intravenously (IV).[2] In contrast, no increase in plasma histamine level is seen after hydromorphone or oxymorphone administration. The incidence of nausea and vomiting, a risk factor for the development of aspiration pneumonia, is less after oxymorphone (33%) than after hydromorphone (44% to 66%) or morphine (50% to 75%).[3,4] Nausea and vomiting are rarely seen after administration of methadone, fentanyl, or remifentanil. A recent report found a significant decrease in the incidence of nausea and vomiting in dogs given the neurokinin-1 receptor antagonist maropitant, 1 mg/kg subcutaneously [SC]) 1 hour before hydromorphone is administered intramuscularly (IM).[4] Oxymorphone, hydromorphone, methadone, fentanyl, and remifentanil are all useful intravenous agents, especially in combination with benzodiazepine tranquilizers (midazolam, diazepam), since they provide the most cardiovascular stability (see Chapter 164).[5,6] Vagally mediated bradycardia or second-degree atrioventricular block is often seen after opioid administration and can be treated with anticholinergics (atropine, glycopyrrolate) as indicated. Fentanyl and remifentanil are short-acting agents and may be given as a constant rate infusion (CRI). They are often used in combination with a propofol CRI for total intravenous anesthesia (also known as TIVA).[7] A low-dose ketamine CRI may be added to provide additional analgesia.

Although opioids are relatively sparing of the cardiovascular system, they may act as respiratory depressants, causing a decreased ventilatory response to increased CO_2 concentrations. Respiratory depression may be exacerbated by concomitant administration of other sedatives. Therefore opioids should be used judiciously and at decreased doses if respiratory depression and hypoventilation are contraindicated, as in patients with airway obstruction or increased intracranial pressure. Remifentanil is especially potent as a respiratory depressant, although it has a short elimination half-life of about 7 minutes, so spontaneous ventilation usually resumes soon after the infusion is turned off.[7] It is important not to mistake panting for effective ventilation; therefore the clinician must look carefully at the depth of each breath as well as the rate.

Methadone is being used with increasing frequency in the critical care setting because it is associated with a lower incidence of nausea and vomiting relative to the other available drugs. In addition to its effects at the opioid receptor, methadone has *N*-methyl-d-aspartate (NMDA) receptor antagonistic properties (similar to ketamine), which can help prevent the development of opioid tolerance and opioid-induced hyperalgesia.[8]

Butorphanol, a κ agonist and μ antagonist, and buprenorphine, a partial μ agonist, may cause less respiratory depression and are preferred in some cases. Other clinically significant adverse effects such as vomiting and decreased gastrointestinal motility may also be less pronounced with these drugs, although they also tend to provide less analgesia. If undesirable side effects should occur, the opioid drug can be reversed using naloxone (0.01 to 0.02 mg/kg IV, IM, SC). The effects of buprenorphine may be difficult to reverse, and up to 10 times the naloxone dose may be required. Opioid reversal with naloxone will also remove the analgesia. Alternatively, small doses of butorphanol (0.05 mg/kg IV, IM, SC) may be titrated to reverse some of the sedative effect of a pure μ agonist while retaining part of the analgesia by enhancing the κ effects.

Before an opioid (or any other drug) is administered, the animal should be observed carefully and the underlying disease process considered (Tables 142-1 and 142-2).

SEDATIVES AND TRANQUILIZERS

Benzodiazepines (see Chapter 164 for further details)

Benzodiazepines (diazepam, midazolam) are mild tranquilizers and cause minimal cardiopulmonary depression.[8] They are not generally used alone for sedation since the result may be unpredictable and the animal may become more difficult to handle. Benzodiazepines are most commonly given in combination with other drugs to increase their effect. Diazepam and midazolam have similar effects and are given at similar dosages (0.1 to 0.5 mg/kg IV or IM), although midazolam is preferred for intramuscular use since it is water soluble and readily absorbed. In critically ill patients, small intravenous doses of either drug can cause profound sedation. In

Table 142-1 **Suggested Doses of Opioids in Small Animals**

Drug	Dose	Route	Duration of Effect (hr)	Comments
Opioid Agonists*				
Methadone	0.1-0.5 mg/kg	IV	1-2	
	0.5-1.0 mg/kg	IM, SC		
Morphine	0.1 mg/kg (dogs)	IV	2-4	May cause excitement or hypotension in dogs IV
	0.2-1.0 mg/kg (dogs)	IM, SC	2-6	Vomiting may occur
	CRI: 0.1 mg/kg/hr			
Oxymorphone	0.02-0.1 mg/kg	IV	1-2	Good CV stability
	0.05-0.2 mg/kg	IM, SC	2-4	
Hydromorphone	0.05-0.2 mg/kg	IM, IV	1-4	Good CV stability
Fentanyl	2-10 mcg/kg	IV		
	CRI: 0.03-0.2 mcg/kg/min			Bradycardia
Remifentanil	CRI: 0.03-0.2 mcg/kg/min			Respiratory depression
Opioid Agonists-Antagonists or Partial Agonists				
Butorphanol	0.1-0.5 mg/kg	IV, IM, SC	1-4	κ Agonist μ Antagonist (partial agonist?)
Buprenorphine	0.005-0.02 mg/kg	IV, IM, SC	4-12	μ Partial agonist Effects may be difficult to reverse

CRI, Constant rate infusion; *CV*, cardiovascular; *IM*, intramuscularly; *IV*, intravenously; *SC*, subcutaneously.
*Doses in cats are generally half those used in dogs for any of the opioids listed. Cats may be more prone to excitement after opioid administration.

Table 142-2 Doses of Drugs Commonly Used in Sedation in Small Animals

Drug*	Dose† (mg/kg)	Route
Anticholinergics		
Atropine	0.02	IM, SC
	0.01	IV
Glycopyrrolate	0.01	IM
	0.005	IV
Sedatives and Tranquilizers		
Acepromazine	0.005-0.02	IM, IV
Diazepam	0.1-0.3	IV
Midazolam	0.1-0.3	IM, IV
Flumazenil (reversal agent)	0.01-0.02	IV
Dexmedetomidine	0.0005-0.002	IM, IV
Atipamezole (reversal agent)	Given in equivalent volume	IM
Opioid Agonists/Partial Agonists‡		
Buprenorphine	0.005-0.02	IM, IV
Butorphanol	0.1-0.5	IV
	0.5	IM
Fentanyl	0.002-0.01	IV
Hydromorphone	0.05-0.2	IM, IV
Methadone	0.1-0.5	IV
	0.5-1.0	IM
Morphine	0.2-1.0	IM
Oxymorphone	0.05-0.2 (0.02-0.1)	IM(IV)
Naloxone (reversal agent)	0.02-0.04	IM, IV
Other Agents		
Ketamine	2.0-4.0	IM (cats only)
	2.0-4.0	IV
Propofol	1.0-4.0	IV (titrate slowly to effect)

IM, Intramuscularly; *IV*, intravenously; *SC*, subcutaneously.
*Many of these drugs can be given as a constant rate infusion by taking the IV dose listed and administering it over the dosing interval time. Start with the lowest dose and titrate to effect as needed.
†All IM doses may be given SC.
‡Doses in cats are generally half those used in dogs for any of the opioids listed. Cats may be more prone to excitement after opioid administration.

addition, diazepam is metabolized to active metabolites that can have a prolonged duration of action in some animals.[9] These effects are readily reversed using the benzodiazepine antagonist flumazenil (0.01 to 0.02 mg/kg IV).

Phenothiazine Tranquilizers

Phenothiazine tranquilizers (acepromazine) are commonly used in healthy veterinary patients to provide calming.[10] They are generally avoided or used at very low doses in patients with questionable cardiovascular stability since they act as α antagonists, causing peripheral vasodilation and possible hypotension in hypovolemic patients. Acepromazine may be useful in cases of airway obstruction in which calming of the patient may decrease respiratory effort and actually improve ventilation. Respiratory depression is minimal, and intramuscular injection is usually effective if given sufficient time to work (20 to 30 minutes after injection). Lower doses should be used (0.005 to 0.01 mg/kg IV or 0.02 to 0.05 mg/kg IM), especially if a physical examination has been difficult to perform due to the animal's respiratory status.

α_2 Agonists *(see Chapter 165 for further details)*

The α_2 agonists (xylazine, medetomidine, dexmedetomidine) produce sedation, muscle relaxation, and analgesia.[10] However, they may cause profound changes in cardiac output and blood pressure, even at very low doses. Cardiac output decreases after drug administration due to decreased heart rate, direct myocardial depression, and increased afterload (decreased stroke volume). In addition, coronary vasoconstriction can lead to myocardial hypoxia and dysfunction. Several surveys have suggested that use of xylazine is associated with a higher incidence of morbidity and mortality than use of other anesthetic agents, and newer α_2 agonists are preferred.[11]

Medetomidine and dexmedetomidine are more specific for the α_2 (vs. α_1) receptor than xylazine but also have a longer duration of action. Medetomidine is the racemic mixture of dextro and levo isomers, whereas dexmedetomidine contains only the active dextro isomer. Doses for dexmedetomidine are generally half that for medetomidine. Notable adverse effects following their administration include bradycardia (heart rate < 40 beats/min) and peripheral vasoconstriction. Administration of an anticholinergic drug either in combination with the α_2-agonist sedative or as a treatment for bradycardia is not recommended because it provides only a minimal increase in cardiac output and leads to an increased myocardial workload and increased incidence of cardiac arrhythmias. Reversal of the drug's effects with atipamezole is the preferred treatment. Other adverse effects of α_2-agonist administration include respiratory depression, vomiting, inhibition of insulin release, and diuresis.

The recommended dose range for medetomidine (in the drug insert) is 10 to 40 mcg/kg IV or IM and is associated with moderate to profound sedation and analgesia. However, hemodynamic changes are qualitatively similar irrespective of dose when the drug is administered at between 1 and 20 mcg/kg IV, although less of an effect is seen at 1 to 2 mcg/kg (*note:* the effect is near maximal at 5 mcg/kg). Administration of medetomidine (1 mcg/kg IV) in dogs decreased cardiac output to less than 40% of resting values and it remained almost 50% below normal for 1 hour.[12] Medetomidine and dexmedetomidine may be useful when given as a low-dose CRI as an adjunct sedative in the dysphoric or anxious patient. When given as a low-dose CRI (0.5 to 5 mcg/kg/hr) in combination with fentanyl, medetomidine infusion reduced cardiac index, heart rate, and oxygen delivery compared with fentanyl alone in healthy dogs.[13] Doses as low as 1 mcg/kg dexmedetomidine in anesthetized dogs increased coronary vascular resistance, decreased coronary blood flow in all myocardial layers, and increased oxygen extraction. Low-dose infusions also have been shown to decrease blood flow to the splanchnic organs (including the pancreas) and to decrease oxygen delivery to the renal vasculature, which may be of concern in critically ill patients. Therefore in the critically ill patient these drugs should be used only after careful consideration.

OTHER ANESTHETIC AGENTS

Ketamine

Ketamine is a dissociative anesthetic with a variable effect on the cardiovascular system, depending on the patient's status. The increases in heart rate, cardiac output, and blood pressure seen with ketamine depend on a centrally mediated sympathetic response and endogenous catecholamine release.[14] Due to the potential for increased myocardial contractility and oxygen consumption, ketamine should be used only after careful consideration in patients with underlying cardiac disease (e.g., hypertrophic cardiomyopathy). Catecholamine release may also predispose to arrhythmias. Ketamine has a direct myocardium-depressant effect, and in debilitated patients with a poor catecholamine response, destabilization of the cardiovascular system and hypotension may occur.

Although ketamine causes dose-dependent respiratory depression, this is usually transient and ketamine may be useful in patients in which maintenance of spontaneous ventilation is desirable. Ketamine also has bronchodilator activity and may be considered for use in patients with asthma or other causes of bronchoconstriction. Ketamine is an NMDA receptor antagonist and is a useful adjunct to other analgesic therapy. Ketamine has been shown to prevent the development of opioid tolerance and opioid-induced hyperalgesia and is often given as a low-dose CRI (0.1 to 0.5 mg/kg/hr) in combination with an opioid such as fentanyl. Ketamine increases both intracranial and intraocular pressure and is therefore contraindicated in patients with head or ocular trauma.

Ketamine has a rapid onset of action after intramuscular injection and is often used for intramuscular sedation in cats. Ketamine is rarely used IM in dogs, and should not be used alone since it may cause seizure-like activity. More commonly, ketamine is administered IV and is generally given in combination with a benzodiazepine (or other tranquilizer) to minimize the possibility of ketamine-induced seizures and muscle rigidity. Ketamine is metabolized by the liver in most species other than the cat, in which it is eliminated unchanged by the kidneys. Doses should be adjusted accordingly in patients with liver or renal disease. For a recalcitrant feline patient in which sedation is required but a decrease in ketamine dose is desired, a combination of ketamine (2 to 4 mg/kg), oxymorphone (0.05 mg/kg) or methadone (0.2 to 0.5 mg/kg), and midazolam or diazepam (0.1 to 0.3 mg/kg) provides excellent restraint.

Telazol is a combination of tiletamine (a dissociative anesthetic) and zolazepam (a benzodiazepine) and has effects similar to those seen with a ketamine-diazepam combination, although recoveries may be prolonged or otherwise unsatisfactory.

Propofol

Propofol is an ultrashort-acting intravenous anesthetic with a 5- to 10-minute duration of anesthesia after induction, with the patient being remarkably alert on recovery. Due to its short duration of action, it is ideal for short procedures and sedations. Propofol is a peripheral vasodilator and myocardial depressant and may cause significant cardiovascular depression in patients with volume depletion or cardiovascular compromise.[15,16] Propofol should not be used (or used only used after careful consideration) in these cases. Cardiovascular depression is especially pronounced if propofol is given as a large, rapidly delivered bolus, and smaller, slowly administered boluses (1 mg/kg IV) or induction via low-dose infusion (1 mg/kg/min as a loading dose followed by 0.1 to 0.2 mg/kg/min) is preferred. Propofol can also cause significant respiratory depression—again more pronounced with large, rapidly administered boluses. Animals should receive supplemental oxygen via a face mask before and during propofol administration.

Propofol may be given in combination with other cardiovascular system–sparing drugs such as fentanyl, midazolam, or ketamine, which decreases the amount of propofol required for induction. Midazolam or diazepam (0.1 to 0.3 mg/kg IV) also helps to control the myoclonic twitching occasionally seen after propofol administration. Propofol can be given as a CRI (0.1 to 0.2 mg/kg/min) for long-term sedation. Cats occasionally have a prolonged recovery, and Heinz body formation has been reported after repeated or prolonged propofol sedation in cats.[17,18] Propofol is provided in a soybean oil–lecithin emulsion and should be handled using strict aseptic technique. The manufacturer states that propofol should not be refrigerated and that once the container is opened, the contents should be used within 6 to 12 hours due to the potential for significant bacterial contamination. More recently, a formulation of propofol was released for use in dogs that can be used for 28 days after the bottle is opened and also does not require refrigeration.

SEDATION OF ANIMALS WITH SPECIFIC CONDITIONS

Cardiovascular Instability

Systemic blood pressure depends on cardiac output and systemic vascular resistance and must be kept above the minimum level required to maintain cerebral, coronary, and renal perfusion. Mean arterial blood pressures of less than 65 to 70 mm Hg are generally considered inadequate for maintaining blood flow to the tissues. In patients that are in hemodynamically unstable condition due to hypovolemia, neural and neurohormonal mechanisms can increase systemic vascular resistance and minimize apparent changes in blood pressure, while decreasing blood flow and oxygen delivery to the tissues. In addition, although some animals may have primary cardiac disease at presentation, many have cardiac dysfunction secondary to sepsis or have cardiac signs (e.g., arrhythmias) secondary to trauma or significant metabolic disease. The choice of agent depends on the underlying disease, volume status, presence or absence of heart failure and degree of heart failure, and presence or absence of arrhythmias. Ideally, the patient should undergo fluid resuscitation before drug administration. Stress during patient handling should be avoided if possible to minimize catecholamine release, tachycardia, and increased myocardial work. If sedation is necessary, opioids are generally the drug of choice because cardiovascular function is well maintained. Anticholinergics are not used unless indicated. A combination of an opioid agonist (e.g., oxymorphone 0.05 to 0.1 mg/kg, hydromorphone 0.05 to 0.1 mg/kg, or methadone 0.1 to 0.5 mg/kg) or agonist-antagonist (e.g., butorphanol 0.1 mg/kg or buprenorphine 0.005 to 0.01 mg/kg) and a benzodiazepine tranquilizer (diazepam or midazolam 0.1 to 0.3 mg/kg) or low-dose acepromazine (0.0025 to 0.01 mg/kg) may be used to sedate patients for chest radiography or echocardiography. This combination provides sedation with minimal cardiovascular depression. Some patients may pant if a pure opioid agonist is used, so butorphanol may be preferred. The combination may be repeated IV if necessary or the dosage doubled and given IM. Reversal may be accomplished by using an opioid antagonist such as naloxone (0.01 to 0.02 mg/kg IV) and/or a benzodiazepine antagonist such as flumazenil (0.01 to 0.02 mg/kg IV). Acepromazine should be avoided in hypovolemic or hypotensive patients. However, acepromazine *in very low doses* may be beneficial in some circumstances because it calms the patient, decreases afterload, and decreases the incidence of arrhythmias. It should be used only after careful consideration, however, since the α blockade may lead to peripheral vasodilation, hypotension, and decreased preload. The α_2 agonists are generally avoided. Ketamine should be used only after careful consideration because it can cause catecholamine release, which increases heart rate and contractility and myocardial oxygen demand.

Respiratory Disease

Respiratory diseases requiring emergency anesthesia include upper airway diseases that result in the inability to ventilate and primary lung diseases that lead to hypoxemia (see Part II of this book). In addition, some animals with intrathoracic disease (e.g., diaphragmatic hernia) have difficulty both ventilating and oxygenating. Animals will be handled slightly differently depending on whether the primary problem is an inability to ventilate or to oxygenate. Manipulations in both groups should occur with a minimum of stress or excitement. Many patients need supplemental oxygen.

All anesthetic agents depress respiration to some degree, and this should be taken into account before administration. Respiratory depressants, such as opioids, should be used judiciously in a patient with severe hypoxemia or upper airway obstruction. The animal should always be closely monitored after administration of any drug. Premedication with acepromazine is very useful in patients with upper airway obstruction. Low doses (0.005 to 0.01 mg/kg IM) should be used if a complete physical examination cannot be performed without stressing the patient, although it should be given sufficient time to act (15 to 20 minutes). Ketamine or propofol also may be used. Patient positioning may be important (e.g., in a patient with diaphragmatic hernia). The least affected side should be kept up (or at least an attempt should be made to maintain sternal recumbency) to aid ventilation.

Sedating an animal that cannot ventilate due to airway obstruction is among the most potentially catastrophic of all procedures. The clinician should never assume that intubation is possible. The clinician should have available an assortment of endotracheal tubes (which occasionally requires some ingenuity), as well as stylets, a laryngoscope (ideally), and a tracheostomy set (see Chapter 17). Potent respiratory depressants should be avoided when intubation may be difficult or impossible. Induction with low-dose boluses of propofol (to minimize respiratory effects) and midazolam (0.1 to 0.3 mg/kg) may be useful. Alternatively, ketamine (2 to 4 mg/kg) and diazepam may be used. In animals with hypoxemia but no airway obstruction, opioids may be used (see Table 142-2).

CONCLUSION

Anesthesia is both an art and a science. The exact choice of drugs and the sequence in which they are given is determined by both knowledge and experience. The specific agent, dose, and route of administration depends in large part on the patient's overall demeanor and cardiopulmonary profile, including underlying disease process, volume status, presence or absence of cardiac or airway disease, and presence or absence of arrhythmias. In addition, the procedure to be performed must be taken into consideration. Any drug should be titrated carefully to help avoid further compromise in the critically ill patient.

REFERENCES

1. Reisine T, Pasternak G: Opioid analgesics and antagonists. In Hardman JG, Limbird LE, editors: Goodman and Gilman's The pharmacological basis of therapeutics, ed 9, New York, 1996, McGraw-Hill, pp 521-555.
2. Robinson EP, Faggella AM, Henry DP, et al: Comparison of histamine release induced by morphine and oxymorphone administration in dogs, Am J Vet Res 49:1699-1701, 1988.
3. Valverde A, Cantwell S, Hernandez J, et al: Effects of acepromazine ion the incidence of vomiting associated with opioid administration in dogs, Vet Anaesth Analg 31:40-45, 2004.
4. Hay Kruse BL: Efficacy of maropitant in preventing vomiting in dogs premedicated with hydromorphone, Vet Anaesth Analg 40:28-34, 2013.
5. Copland VS, Haskins SC, Patz JD: Oxymorphone: cardiovascular, pulmonary, and behavioral effects in dogs, Am J Vet Res 48:1626-1630, 1987.
6. Eisele JH, Reitan JZ, Torten M, et al: Myocardial sparing effect of fentanyl during halothane anaesthesia in dogs, Br J Anaesth 47:937-940, 1975.
7. Gimenes AM, Aguiar AJA, Perri SHV, et al: Effect of intravenous propofol and remifentanil on heart rate, blood pressure and nociceptive response in acepromazine premedicated dogs, Vet Anaesth Analg 38:54-62, 2011.
8. Jones DJ, Stehling LC, Zauder HL: Cardiovascular responses to diazepam and midazolam maleate in the dog, Anesthesiology 51:430-434, 1979.
9. Driessen JJ, Vree TB, Van de Pol F, et al: Pharmacokinetics of diazepam and four 3-hydroxy-benzodiazepines in the cat, Eur J Drug Metab Pharmacokinet 12:219-224, 1987.
10. Lemke KA: Anticholinergics and sedatives. In Tranquilli WJ, Thurmon JC, Grimm KA, editors: Lumb and Jones' veterinary anesthesia, ed 4, Ames, Ia, 2007, Blackwell, pp 209-245.
11. Dyson DH, Maxie MG: Morbidity and mortality associated with anesthetic management in small animal veterinary practice in Ontario, J Am Anim Hosp Assoc 34:325-335, 1998.
12. Pypendop BH, Vergenstegen JP: Hemodynamic effects of medetomidine in the dog: a dose titration study, Vet Surg 27:612-622, 1998.
13. Grimm KA, Tranquilli WJ, Gross DR, et al: Cardiopulmonary effects of fentanyl in conscious dogs and dogs sedated with a continuous rate infusion of medetomidine, Am J Vet Res 66:1222-1226, 2005.
14. Lin HC: Dissociative anesthetics. In Tranquilli WJ, Thurmon JC, Grimm KA, editors: Lumb and Jones' veterinary anesthesia, ed 4, Ames, Ia, 2007, Blackwell, pp 304-356.
15. Ilkiw JE, Pascoe PJ, Haskins SC, et al: Cardiovascular and respiratory effects of propofol administration in hypovolemic dogs, Am J Vet Res 53:2323-2327, 1992.
16. Quandt JE, Robinson EP, Rivers WJ, et al: Cardiorespiratory and anesthetic effects of propofol and thiopental in dogs, Am J Vet Res 59:1137-1143, 1998.
17. Branson KR: Injectable and alternative anesthetic techniques. In Tranquilli WJ, Thurmon JC, Grimm KA, editors: Lumb and Jones' veterinary anesthesia, ed 4, Ames, Ia, 2007, Blackwell, pp 277-303.
18. Andress JL, Day TK, Day D: The effects of consecutive day propofol anesthesia on feline red blood cells, Vet Surg 24(3):277-282, 1995.

CHAPTER 143

ANESTHESIA IN THE CRITICALLY ILL PATIENT

Jane Quandt, BS, DVM, MS, DACVAA, DACVECC

KEY POINTS

- Appropriately stabilizing the condition of the critically ill animal before anesthesia is imperative to minimize anesthesia-related complications.
- Problems should be anticipated and an appropriate and efficient treatment and therapeutic plan developed before induction of anesthesia.
- The use of a balanced anesthesia technique should be considered to minimize potential deleterious effects of single-drug therapy.
- The use of positive pressure ventilation is mandatory with the administration of neuromuscular blocking agents.
- Neuromuscular blocking agents do not have anesthetic or analgesic properties.

In the critically ill patient a thorough preoperative assessment is necessary to define what type of trauma or compromise the patient is undergoing. The critically ill patient has altered physiology and decreased reserves, which will affect the pharmacokinetic and pharmacodynamic behavior of anesthetic drugs. These patients benefit from minimization of stress and optimization of oxygen delivery.

Stabilizing the condition of the critically ill patient before anesthetic drug exposure is essential because induction of anesthesia in a patient in unstable condition increases the risk of anesthesia-related complications.

STABILIZATION

A thorough diagnostic assessment, including serial physical examinations, diagnostic imaging, blood chemistry testing, complete blood count, determination of coagulation profile, and measurement of acid-base status, blood glucose level, and lactate level should be performed as indicated before anesthesia. A dehydrated or hypovolemic state along with fluid, acid-base, and electrolyte deficits should be corrected before anesthesia induction.

Maintaining venous access is imperative in managing and anesthetizing the critical care patient because it is not uncommon for the critically ill animal to experience hypotension during the anesthesia period. Intravenous administration of drugs is usually preferred because drugs administered by the intramuscular or subcutaneous routes may have delayed absorption, particularly when the patient is dehydrated, hypovolemic, poorly perfused, or hypothermic. Critically ill patients often benefit from placement of more than one intravenous catheter; either a peripheral or central line can be used. The intravenous catheter provides a port not only for drug administration but also for antibiotic delivery, vasopressor and inotropic support, and fluid therapy. Because of different fluid rate requirements and possible incompatibility of various agents, such as vasopressors, sodium bicarbonate, and blood transfusion products, a minimum of two intravenous catheters should be placed before anesthesia induction in patients in unstable condition. Blood products should be administered via a dedicated catheter, and no other fluids or drugs should be administered in the same line during the transfusion due to concerns of possible contamination and potential for bacterial growth. This is also true for those patients that are receiving total parenteral nutrition (TPN). The catheter for TPN should be a dedicated line; it should never be disconnected, and no other fluid should be run through the same line due to the risk of sepsis. TPN solution is considered a hyperosmotic crystalloid and should be accounted for as part of the crystalloid fluid volume. It is also important to provide warm intravenous fluids before and during anesthesia to help maintain organ perfusion and body temperature. If fluids need to be given at a rapid, shock bolus rate, use of the shortest, largest-bore catheter (e.g., peripheral cephalic catheter) will allow for the most rapid fluid administration. Placement of an arterial catheter once the animal is under general anesthesia is recommended. An arterial catheter allows for direct arterial blood pressure measurement and can be used to collect samples for arterial blood gas analysis.

A packed cell volume (PCV) greater than 25% is necessary for adequate oxygen-carrying capacity and oxygen delivery. During anesthesia the PCV can decrease by 3% to 5%; therefore even a small volume of blood loss may be significant in the anesthetized animal and may warrant a blood transfusion.[1] Similarly, patients with hypoproteinemia (total protein ≤ 3.5 g/dl and/or albumin level ≤ 2 g/dl) may benefit from the use of colloids to help maintain normal colloid osmotic pressure (COP; normal = 18 to 24 mm Hg) and to prevent edema formation or vascular leak.[2,3] Measurement of COP before anesthesia is helpful in determining the need for colloid support and deciding when to terminate colloid therapy. If patients are hypoproteinemic, colloid options include Hetastarch, VetStarch, 25% human serum albumin, or even Oxyglobin. High-molecular-weight hydroxyethyl starch synthetic colloids such as hetastarch impair coagulation in a dose dependent manner, and this may limit their use in hypocoagulable, hypoproteinemic surgical patients. VetStarch is a low-molecular-weight tetrastarch that has far fewer coagulation effects than the hetastarches. As a result it may have a role in the support of COP in the surgical patient, although it would seem prudent to minimize its use in high-risk patients with hypocoagulability (see Chapter 58).

In small, hypocoagulable, or hypoalbuminemic patients, the use of fresh frozen plasma (FFP) at 6 to 20 ml/kg is warranted. Unfortunately, size, dosing, and cost become a limiting factor in the use of FFP to treat hypoalbuminemia in larger patients because it takes a dose on the order of 45 ml/kg of FFP to increase the albumin level by 1 g/dl.[4] The use of 25% human serum albumin has recently been implemented in veterinary medicine, but adverse effects such as polyarthritis, future transfusion reaction, glomerulonephritis, and other immune-mediated effects warrant cautious use.[3] (For more information see Chapter 58.)

Finally, patients should be carefully evaluated for underlying metabolic disease before anesthesia because this may affect the anesthetic protocol. In patients with renal insufficiency, a higher fluid rate may be required to maintain renal perfusion, and urine output should be monitored carefully during anesthesia.[5] In addition, drugs excreted by the kidney (e.g., ketamine in cats) may have delayed excretion and should be used cautiously. In patients with liver disease, anesthetic protocols and monitoring may be affected due to decreased glucose and albumin production, altered drug metabolism via cytochrome P-450 enzymes, and decreased production of coagulation factors.[5] Patients with heart murmurs may have decreased ability to compensate under anesthesia, and fluid overload should be avoided. Blood pressure should also be carefully monitored because anesthesia-induced hypotension may result in decompensation. Finally, one should always determine whether the patient is currently receiving any drug therapy, such as nonsteroidal antiinflammatory drugs, diuretics, anticonvulsants, or cardiac medications.

PREMEDICATION

Premedication may not be necessary unless the animal is in severe pain or is extremely fractious. If it is decided that the critically ill patient would benefit from premedication, μ-agonist opioids such as morphine, hydromorphone, or oxymorphone in combination with a tranquilizer such as midazolam or low-dose acepromazine (0.005 to 0.01 mg/kg) can be given intramuscularly to provide analgesia and sedation. If given to the critically ill, acepromazine should be used at lower doses than in a normal animal due to the profound hypotension that can result. A μ agonist is preferred because the κ agonist butorphanol and the partial μ agonist buprenorphine may not be sufficient for severe pain. Although a μ-agonist narcotic can be combined with an α_2 agonist and/or a dissociative drug and administered intramuscularly in an animal that is in severe pain or is extremely fractious, this is rarely indicated in a critically ill patient, which is usually obtunded and easily handled. Anticholinergics are not routinely used unless there is a need to treat bradycardia. Protocols should be implemented to minimize the amount of time the animal is under anesthesia; therefore steps such as preclipping the surgical site with the animal awake should be performed if possible. Preoxygenation of the animal before induction will allow for additional time that may be needed to intubate the animal; this is especially helpful for animals that are in respiratory distress or have a difficult airway. Finally, electrocardiographic and blood pressure monitoring should be in place before induction to detect evidence of arrhythmias, hypotension, or cardiovascular collapse that may occur during induction in the critically ill animal. In the severely compromised animal, arrest drugs such as atropine and epinephrine should be close at hand during the induction and anesthetic period.

INDUCTION

In the compromised, critically ill patient, the anesthetic drug doses often can be reduced to half of those for a normal, healthy patient (Table 143-1). Induction drugs should be slowly titrated intravenously (IV) to effect, and the minimal amount of drug necessary to

Table 143-1 Anesthetic Agents and Their Dosages

Drugs	Dose	Comments
Anticholinergic agents	Atropine 0.04 mg/kg IM, 0.02 mg/kg IV Glycopyrrolate 0.01 mg/kg IM, IV	May make secretions more viscous Increase anatomic dead space Increase heart rate Can increase myocardial work and oxygen consumption Glycopyrrolate does not cross blood-brain barrier or the placenta
Opioids		
μ Agonists	Morphine 0.2 to 2 mg/kg IM, SC; CRI: 0.1 to 0.3 loading dose, then 0.1 mg/kg/hr Oxymorphone 0.05-0.2 mg/kg IM, IV, SC Meperidine 2-5 mg/kg IM, SC Hydromorphone 0.05-0.2 mg/kg IV, IM, SC; CRI: 0.025-0.05 mg/kg IV loading dose, then 0.01-0.04 mg/kg/hr Fentanyl 0.005-0.05 mg/kg IM, IV, SC; CRI for dogs: loading dose 5-10 mcg/kg, then 0.7-1 mcg/kg/min; CRI for cats: loading dose 5 mcg/kg, then 0.3-0.4 mcg/kg/min Remifentanil 3 mcg/kg IV; CRI: 0.1-0.3 mcg/kg/min	Complete reversal with naloxone Analgesic Cause respiratory depression Cause bradycardia Minimal effect on CV performance Give anticholinergic drug before starting CRI Monitor for hyperthermia in cats
Partial μ agonist	Buprenorphine 0.005-0.02 mg/kg IM, IV	Slow onset, effects difficult to reverse Good for moderate pain
κ agonist/ μ antagonist	Butorphanol 0.1-0.8 mg/kg IM, IV, SC; CRI: 0.1-0.2 mg/kg IV loading dose, then 0.1-0.2 mg/kg/hr	Partial reversal of μ-agonist drugs Minimal CV effects Not good for severe pain
Opioid antagonist	Naloxone 0.002-0.02 mg/kg IM, IV	Complete reversal of μ agonist effects
Dissociative agents	Ketamine 4-11 mg/kg IV, IM; CRI: 0.5 mg/kg IV loading dose, then 0.1-0.5 mg/kg/hr Tiletamine and zolazepam (Telazol) 2-4 mg/kg IM, IV	Cause salivation Increase heart rate Increase ICP and intraocular pressure Analgesic Renal elimination in cat
Benzodiazepines	Diazepam 0.2-0.5 mg/kg IM, IV; CRI: 0.1-0.5 mg/kg/hr Midazolam 0.07-0.4 mg/kg IM, IV; CRI: 0.1-0.5 mg/kg/hr	Can decrease required dose of other drugs Mild sedative and muscle relaxant Anticonvulsant Not analgesic Diazepam formulation contains propylene glycol

Table 143-1 **Anesthetic Agents and Their Dosages—cont'd**

Drugs	Dose	Comments
Phenothiazine	Acepromazine 0.01-0.1 mg/kg IM, IV; no more than 3 mg total dose	Vasodilatory Long duration of action Not analgesic
Barbiturates	Thiopental 4-20 mg/kg IV Methohexital 4-10 mg/kg IV	Cause cardiovascular depression Cause respiratory depression Provide rapid induction Decrease ICP and intraocular pressure Effects may be potentiated by concurrent acidosis or hypoproteinemia
Propofol	2-8 mg/kg IV; CRI: 0.05-0.4 mg/kg/min	Rapidly acting with short duration of action Causes respiratory depression Causes peripheral vasodilation Myocardial depressant Not analgesic Use with caution in patients with volume depletion or cardiovascular compromise; can cause significant depression Can cause Heinz body anemia in cats
Etomidate	0.5-4 mg/kg IV	Maintains cardiovascular stability Not used alone Suppresses adrenocortical function for 2-6 hr following single bolus dose Contains propylene glycol
α_2 Agonist	Dexmedetomidine 3-40 mcg/kg IM, IV; CRI: 1 mcg/kg IV loading dose, then 0.5-2 mcg/kg/hr	Causes cardiovascular depression Can cause vomiting Provides good sedation and analgesia Can be combined with butorphanol or ketamine
Antagonist	Atipamezole 0.04-0.5 mg/kg IM, IV	
Neuroleptanalgesic	Combination of opioid and tranquilizer	Analgesic Causes noise sensitivity Maintains cardiovascular stability
Alfaxalone	2-5 mg/kg IV	Sedation may be needed to improve recovery
Lidocaine	CRI: 1-2 mg/kg IV loading dose, then 1-3 mg/kg/hr	Not recommended in cats
Inhalants	Isoflurane Nitrous oxide Sevoflurane	Produce dose-dependent cardiovascular depression and peripheral vasodilation Anesthesia depth can be adjusted rapidly Potential for hypoxemia Isoflurane and sevoflurane show rapid uptake and recovery Nitrous oxide should be used with caution with closed gas spaces
Neuromuscular blocking agents	Atracurium 0.1 mg/kg IV; or CRI: 3-8 mcg/kg/min IV Cisatracurium 0.1 mg/kg IV; incremental doses of 0.02-0.04 mg/kg IV	
Reversal agents	Neostigmine 0.04-0.06 mg/kg IV Edrophonium 0.5 mg/kg IV	

CRI, Constant rate infusion; *CV*, cardiovascular; *ICP*, intracranial pressure; *IM*, intramuscularly; *IV*, intravenously; SC, subcutaneously.

intubate the patient should be used. In addition, use of a balanced anesthetic technique helps to minimize the adverse effects from any single agent. One can consider the use of local anesthetic blocks and epidural anesthetics if appropriate to decrease the amount of general anesthetic that is required. Intubation should always be performed to control the airway to provide the ability to ventilate the patient and to protect the airway from aspiration. The emergent patient should be considered to have a full stomach and therefore to be at risk of aspiration. A laryngoscope, endotracheal tubes in a variety of sizes, and a breathing circuit that matches the patient's size should all be readily available. All supplies and machinery should be checked thoroughly before induction and intubation. One should be ready to implement positive pressure ventilation if the patient hypoventilates, becomes apneic, or is to undergo a thoracic procedure.

Ideally there should be a slow transition to general anesthesia that would allow time for the cardiovascular and nervous systems to respond and accommodate appropriately.[6] However, the critically ill patient may not be able to respond appropriately, and therapeutic intervention must be available to prevent the demise of the patient. For example, a patient in respiratory distress will require a rapid-sequence intubation to gain control of the airway and provide ventilation with 100% oxygen.

Thiopental and Propofol

A rapid-sequence induction can be accomplished with agents that have a short onset time, such as thiopental or propofol. These agents have an onset time of approximately 30 seconds and need to be given IV. Their duration of action is also short, with thiopental lasing 10 to 15 minutes and propofol lasting 5 to 10 minutes; propofol may be the preferred agent due to its shorter duration of action. Both of these drugs can be used in combination with diazepam or midazolam to improve relaxation and to decrease the overall dose needed. Both agents are capable of creating cardiac arrhythmias, hypotension, and apnea; hence intermittent positive pressure ventilation may be necessary.[7] Neither agent provides analgesia, so additional analgesics must be given (using inhalant or injectable agents) before the surgical procedure. Thiopental and propofol do decrease intracranial and intraocular pressure and would be indicated for induction in a patient with head trauma.[8] The new formulation of propofol, PropoFlo 28, is not labeled for use in cats. The new formulation contains the preservative benzyl alcohol, which can be toxic to cats when given in large doses. Cats have a low capacity for glucuronic acid conjugation and therefore have limited ability to metabolize benzoic acid. However, PropoFlo 28 has been used safely in healthy cats, with no indications of toxicity and with normal recoveries.[9] Propofol as an agent is less well tolerated in cats than in dogs, with slower metabolism and excretion, and repeated doses or infusions are associated with prolonged recoveries. It has also been shown that propofol can increase the presence of Heinz bodies.[9] It may be prudent to avoid the use of PropoFlo 28 in cats that are debilitated or have liver impairment.

Alfaxalone

A new induction agent, alfaxalone, may be useful for anesthesia induction in the critically ill animal. Alfaxalone is a synthetic neuroactive steroid. It is rapidly metabolized and eliminated from the body. Alfaxalone, like thiopental and propofol, is associated with dose-dependent changes such as hypoventilation and apnea but has a wide margin of safety. It can also be used as a constant rate infusion (CRI) and provides good muscle relaxation and rapid recovery. There may be some excitement on recovery, with paddling and muscle twitching or even violent movements; sedation improves recovery. Alfaxalone has a short duration of action, 14 to 50 minutes.[10] In dogs that were considered a poor anesthetic risk, alfaxalone administered at 1 to 2 mg/kg IV over 60 seconds was shown to be an acceptable induction agent with smooth recovery.[11] Alfaxalone can be safely combined with a fentanyl CRI. Use of alfaxalone in cats results in a smooth induction, but there may be paddling and trembling in recovery, and the quality of recovery worsens as the dose of alfaxalone increases. Cats recovering from alfaxalone induction may be more disoriented and nervous than those recovering from propofol induction.[12]

Etomidate

The use of etomidate for anesthesia induction in critically ill patients is appealing due to its minimal cardiovascular effects, which would be helpful in the patient with cardiovascular instability. Etomidate should not be used as the sole induction agent because it may lead to retching and myoclonus. These adverse effects are minimized by giving a benzodiazepine or opioid IV before etomidate is administered. Repeated use of etomidate in cats may lead to hemolysis due to the propylene glycol vehicle.[13] The use of etomidate in critically ill human patients is controversial due to its ability to cause adrenal dysfunction, which may lead to an increase in morbidity and mortality. The duration of the adrenal dysfunction can range from 24 to 48 hours in the critically ill patient.[14] The use of hydrocortisone to treat the etomidate-induced adrenal insufficiency had no effect on outcome.[15] The recommendation in human medicine is to use etomidate cautiously in patients with septic shock.

Ketamine

Ketamine may be used IV as part of an induction protocol; it is commonly administered with a benzodiazepine. Ketamine has the potential to induce seizures when given as a sole agent.[8] Ketamine increases heart rate, blood pressure, and cardiac output via a centrally mediated sympathetic response and endogenous catecholamine release. Because of the potential for increased cardiac contractility, it should be used cautiously in animals with hypertrophic cardiomyopathy. Ketamine can have direct myocardial-depressant effects, and in debilitated patients with a decreased endogenous catecholamine response there may be hypotension and cardiovascular instability. As an *N*-methyl-d-aspartate receptor agonist, ketamine provides analgesia peripherally and somatically.[16]

Opioids

In critically ill patients in stable condition, a more gradual induction technique can be implemented. This may be accomplished with the use of neuroleptanalgesics such as hydromorphone, oxymorphone, or fentanyl and diazepam or midazolam with the addition of either propofol or ketamine to facilitate induction. In dogs and cats with severe liver compromise, remifentanil may be considered for analgesia during general anesthesia. Remifentanil is a synthetic opioid that has a direct action on the μ receptors and an ultrashort duration of action. The elimination of remifentanil is independent of hepatic or renal function, which makes it an attractive agent for use in animals with hepatic or renal compromise. It is metabolized by nonspecific esterases in blood and tissues. Recovery from remifentanil effects is very rapid even following long-term intravenous infusions.[17] It has been used in dogs at an initial dose of 3 mcg/kg IV and then a CRI of 0.1 to 0.3 mcg/kg/min, with the drug diluted in normal saline.[17,18] Due to the drug's short duration of action an additional analgesic must be administered upon termination of the remifentanil effects if the painful condition persists. The clinical effects of remifentanil are rapidly dissipated upon discontinuation of the infusion, with dogs recovering in 5 to 20 minutes regardless of the duration of the infusion. Remifentanil administered by CRI, like other opioid CRIs, is a potent respiratory depressant, and therefore mechanical ventilation may be required; however, this respiratory depression does not persist following recovery. Remifentanil has been used in cats. A dose higher than 1 mcg/kg/min was associated with dysphoric behavior and frenetic locomotor activity.[19]

The use of multiple agents (e.g., hydromorphone, diazepam, ketamine, and lidocaine) is an example of balanced anesthesia. This protocol produces a slower onset but provides analgesia and is more sparing of the cardiovascular system.[20] Ketamine may be used to enhance analgesia and increases heart rate and blood pressure.[21] When these drugs are used for induction, the dose also serves as the loading dose before their administration as a CRI. Morphine (3.3 mcg/kg/min), lidocaine (50 mcg/kg/min), and ketamine (10 mcg/kg/min) can be administered as a CRI analgesic combination in dogs.[20] In addition lidocaine may retard the effects of compromised viscera, reperfusion injury, or ventricular arrhythmias due its free radical scavenging abilities, analgesic effects, and antiarrhythmic properties.[22] Use of a lidocaine CRI is not recommended to use a lidocaine CRI in cats due to its depressive effects on the cardiovascular system.[23]

Propofol is not recommended for use as a single agent for major surgical procedures because it does not prevent hemodynamic responses to noxious stimulation. It can be used in combination with other agents such as lidocaine and ketamine in dogs for total intravenous anesthesia. Propofol has negative chronotropic and inotropic effects and also causes venodilation, which can lead to a decrease in blood pressure.[24]

In animals with splenic disease such as a tumor or splenic fracture, the use of an appropriate induction agent is indicated because some agents are known to increase splenic size, which could lead to tumor rupture or increased hemorrhage. The administration of acepromazine, thiopental, and propofol can result in splenomegaly. It may be best to avoid these agents in animals with splenic disease or if laparoscopy is planned. Hydromorphone and dexmedetomidine were found not to result in increased splenic size. There was also a reduction in hematocrit in those dogs receiving acepromazine, thiopental, and propofol, which may be of concern in the anemic patient.[25]

MAINTENANCE

Inhalants

Once the animal is intubated, anesthesia can be maintained via an inhalant agent such as isoflurane or sevoflurane. These two agents are the most commonly used, but both agents cause cardiovascular and respiratory depression. Both agents have a rapid onset and recovery time, and allow for rapid changes in anesthetic concentration.[26]

Constant Rate Infusion

Maintenance anesthesia can also be achieved with a CRI if an animal cannot tolerate the hypotensive effects of inhalant anesthesia. Ketamine-propofol and ketamine-propofol-dexmedetomidine infusions have been used in cats during ovariectomy. Cats were given one of the two combinations IV for induction and then maintained on a ketamine-propofol infusion for the surgery. No adverse effects were seen with either group, but sedation was more profound in the group receiving dexmedetomidine.[27]

As stated previously, morphine, lidocaine, and ketamine can be used as a CRI to provide analgesia and to decrease the amount of inhalant required in dogs. Additional μ agonists that can be used as a CRI include fentanyl, oxymorphone, and hydromorphone.[8] An α_2 agonist can also be used as a CRI to enhance analgesia and minimize the amount of inhalant needed.[28] Such CRIs that have been used during surgery can be carried over into recovery to provide titratable analgesia, and the dose can usually be lower once surgical stimulation is over.

Neuromuscular Blocking Agents

Neuromuscular blocking agents (NMBs) can be used to facilitate positive pressure ventilation as part of a balanced anesthetic technique or as part of an anesthetic technique for animals undergoing intensive care unit mechanical ventilation. Neuromuscular blockade helps to prevent respiratory dysynchrony, stop spontaneous respiratory efforts and muscle movement, improve gas exchange, and facilitate inverse-ratio ventilation. NMBs may also be useful in managing increased intracranial pressure and the muscle spasms of tetanus, drug overdose, or seizures.[29] Their use in surgery is to enhance skeletal muscle relaxation, to facilitate control of respiratory efforts during intrathoracic surgery, to immobilize the eye for ocular surgery, and to facilitate intubation of a difficult airway.[30]

These agents do not have anesthetic or analgesic properties, and therefore it is imperative that they be given only when the animal is adequately insensible to pain and awareness.[31] Positive pressure ventilation is mandatory with their use. The duration of action of NMBs can be altered by hypothermia, acid-base abnormalities, and electrolytes disturbances, conditions commonly seen in critically ill patients. NMBs can be given by intermittent intravenous bolus or CRI. Intermittent bolus administration may offer some advantages, including control of tachyphylaxis, monitoring for accumulation, provision of analgesia and amnesia, and limiting of complications related to prolonged or excessive blockade.[29] There must be constant supervision when an animal is receiving an NMB because the patient would be incapable of spontaneous respiration should a malfunction of the mechanical breathing circuit occur, and this would lead to death of the animal.

The preferred relaxing agent is a nondepolarizing NMB. There are two types of nondepolarizing NMB: aminosteroidal and benzylisoquinolinium compounds. There are several different NMB drugs in each of these classes. The details of each class are beyond the scope of this chapter. For a full review of NMB drugs the interested reader is directed to Hall et al[31] and Lukasik.[32]

Benzylisoquinolinium agents

The benzylisoquinolinium compounds are more commonly used and include atracurium, cisatracurium, doxacurium, and mivacurium. Atracurium is intermediate acting and has minimal cardiovascular effects.[29] Atracurium is unusual in that its degradation process is independent of enzymatic function; it is inactivated in the plasma by ester hydrolysis and Hofmann elimination, with spontaneous degradation occurring at body temperature and pH.[29,31,33] Atracurium is indicated for use in neonates and patients with significant hepatic or renal impairment.[31]

Atracurium blockade occurs within 3 to 5 minutes of administration and has a duration of 20 to 30 minutes.[31] Atracurium can be redosed at 0.1 mg/kg IV or given as a CRI of 3 to 8.0 mcg/kg/min IV.[8] Recovery of normal neuromuscular activity usually occurs within 1 to 2 hours after discontinuance of a CRI and is independent of organ function. Long-term CRIs have been associated with the development of tolerance, requiring dose increases or switching to another NMB.[29] Atracurium can be used as part of an anesthetic induction protocol. It may be considered when it is desirable to avoid increases in intraocular, intracranial, or intraabdominal pressure caused by patient coughing or a Valsalva maneuver. It may also be used to provide faster control of ventilation in an animal in unstable condition.[31] There are two induction techniques. In one method atracurium is given in divided doses of one tenth to one sixth of the calculated dose initially, and then 3 to 6 minutes later the rest of the calculated dose is given along with the induction agent. This method accelerates relaxation after induction. The second technique is to give a single bolus of atracurium and 3 minutes later, at the onset of muscle weakness, to give the induction agent.[31]

Potential adverse effects that may occur with the use of atracurium include laudanosine formation and histamine release. Laudanosine is a breakdown product of Hofmann elimination that has been associated with central nervous system excitement. This may be a concern in patients that have received extremely high doses of atracurium or that have hepatic failure because laudanosine undergoes liver metabolism.[29] At clinically useful doses, 0.1 to 0.30 mg/kg IV, the potential for histamine release does not appear to be a problem.[34] Long-term use of atracurium and other NMBs has been associated with persistent neuromuscular weakness.[29] A study in dogs in which neuromuscular blockade was produced by atracurium and either sevoflurane or propofol CRI was used for anesthesia demonstrated that the duration of neuromuscular blockade was approximately 15 minutes longer when sevoflurane was used than when propofol was used.[34]

Cisatracurium is an isomer of atracurium. It is similar in duration of action, elimination profile, and production of laudanosine.[29] It produces few if any cardiovascular effects and has a lesser tendency to produce histamine release, and is more potent than atracurium.[29,33] As with atracurium, prolonged weakness may occur following long-duration use of cisatracurium.[29] The dose is 0.1 mg/kg IV, with incremental doses of 0.02 to 0.04 mg/kg IV in the dog to maintain the blockade. The initial dose has a duration of effect of 27.2 ± 9.3 minutes, the incremental doses appear to be noncumulative, and no adverse effects have been noted. The kidney and liver excrete the metabolites of laudanosine, but the hepatic excretion is less important in the dog. Laudanosine can cause hypotension and seizures, but this may be more likely in dogs with kidney or liver disease.[33]

Monitoring of neuromuscular blocking agents

Monitoring of NMB effects using a peripheral nerve stimulator is recommended. Monitoring the depth of the blockade allows the lowest dose of NMB to be used and therefore minimizes adverse effects. It will also help to confirm that adequate neuromuscular function has returned before discontinuation of ventilator support and anesthesia. Monitoring is done by observing skeletal muscle movement and respiratory efforts and measuring the twitch response to transcutaneous delivery of electric current to induce peripheral nerve stimulation.[29] The peripheral nerves most commonly used include the facial, ulnar, tibial, and superficial peroneal nerves.[30]

When NMB effects begin to diminish the animal may show decreased chest wall compliance and increased resistance to ventilation and greater peak inspiratory pressure will be generated at the same tidal volume.[31] Nystagmus, papillary dilation, and palpebral reflex may be noted. To evaluate the recovery from NMB one should asses the tidal volume using a Wright respirometer as well as the character of ventilation, the ability to swallow, the adequacy of pulse oximetry readings, and end-tidal carbon dioxide. If there is residual weakness, this can be serious and potentially life-threatening. If doubt exists about the strength of recovery, a reversal agent can be given.

Reversal Agents for neuromuscular blocking agents

Reversal of the effects of nondepolarizing neuromuscular blocking agents is possible, although not always necessary. Reversal may be considered in the critically ill patient to improve respiratory muscle function. An anticholinesterase inhibitor, edrophonium or neostigmine, is used for reversal. Reversal should not be attempted when no twitches are seen with the train-of-four monitor. Twitch height must be a minimum of 10% of the baseline height for reversal to be successful.[31] The accumulation of acetylcholine also produces muscarinic effects such as bradycardia, salivation, increased bronchial secretion, smooth muscle contraction, defecation, urination, and hypotension.[30,31] These adverse effects can be minimized by concurrent administration of an anticholinergic agent such as atropine or glycopyrrolate.

Neostigmine has peak effects at 7 to 10 minutes after administration and a duration of action of 60 to 70 minutes and is dosed at 0.04 to 0.06 mg/kg IV combined with glycopyrrolate 0.01 mg/kg IV to combat bradycardia.[8,31] Edrophonium reaches peak effect within 1 to 2 minutes and has a duration of action of approximately 66 minutes; it is dosed at 0.5 mg/kg IV and combined with atropine 0.01 to 0.02 mg/kg IV.[34] It is combined with atropine due to their similar times of onset and duration. The atropine should be given 5 minutes before the edrophonium.[8] For further information on reversal of NMB agents, the interested reader is directed to Hall et al[31] and Lukasik.[32]

MONITORING

Maintenance anesthesia requires careful and constant monitoring to avoid excessive depth of anesthesia and to preserve cardiovascular function. The electrocardiogram should be monitored closely for changes in heart rate and rhythm, and for the presence of malignant arrhythmias, which may be more prevalent in patients with trauma, splenic disease, septic peritonitis, hypoxia, or gastric dilatation-volvulus. Additional monitoring during the maintenance phase of anesthesia includes maintaining the mean arterial blood pressure above 60 mm Hg to maintain renal perfusion. Physical examination parameters indicative of perfusion, such as capillary refill time, mucous membrane color, and pulse quality, should also be monitored continuously. Depth of anesthesia should be frequently assessed by monitoring eye position, pupil size, jaw tone, response to stimulus, heart rate, blood pressure, and respiratory rate throughout the duration of anesthesia. Other monitoring techniques should be implemented, both during and after anesthesia, to enhance the quality of care and increase survival. The use of pulse oximetry adds information on hemoglobin saturation and oxygenation.[35] It is important to remember that patients maintained on pure oxygen (fraction of inspired oxygen of 100%) may have a "normal" pulse oximetry reading despite having abnormal oxygenating ability. The pulse oximeter (assuming it is accurate) will read less than 100% only when the arterial partial pressure of oxygen falls below approximately 140 mm Hg. As a result patients, breathing 100% oxygen can have significant decreases in oxygenating ability that the pulse oximeter cannot recognize. Because of this, arterial blood gas monitoring may be necessary as the gold standard in critically ill patients under anesthesia. Arterial blood gas values will provide information on oxygenation, ventilation, hemoglobin saturation, acid-base balance, and electrolyte levels.

Capnography allows monitoring of the adequacy of ventilatory function and provides an indication of adequate cardiac output. Capnography is also used to monitor for the occurrence of esophageal intubation, breathing circuit disconnection, and cardiac arrest, circumstances where in which it will not register any carbon dioxide.[35] (For further information see Chapter 190.)

Urine output should be monitored carefully, and goals to achieve normal urine output of 1 to 2 ml/kg/hr should be achieved.[5] The use of an indwelling urinary catheter can be considered to measure urinary output adequately in patient's with renal impairment or inadequate blood volume (in which one would clinically see decreased urine output). Fluid balance can be assessed by comparing the volume of fluid administered during anesthesia with the measured losses during the same time period. Preexisting fluid deficits must be considered when making this evaluation. The measurement of central venous pressure may help in the evaluation of fluid therapy but assesses only the right side of the heart.[5] (Chapter 183 discusses hemodynamic monitoring in more detail.) Packed cell volume, total protein, and COP should be monitored frequently because rapid changes can occur in the surgical patient. In the absence of colloid osmometry the total protein measurements can be evaluated, although these do not reflect the presence of synthetic colloids accurately. Blood glucose levels should be closely monitored in pediatric animals and those with sepsis, diabetes, or severe liver disease. Finally, body temperature should be continuously monitored because anesthetic drugs disrupt normal thermoregulatory mechanisms and hypothermia leads to prolongation of recovery.[36]

INTRAOPERATIVE HYPOTENSION

Because critically ill patient are often hypotensive during anesthesia, a mean arterial blood pressure of less than 60 mm Hg or a systolic pressure of less than 90 mm Hg requires prompt treatment to maintain appropriate organ perfusion.[37] The initial step should be to decrease the administration of inhalant anesthetic agents due to their depressant and vasodilatory properties. Next, administration of a fluid bolus should be initiated. Either a crystalloid (without potassium supplementation) delivered at a rate of 10 to 20 ml/kg IV over 15 to 20 minutes or a colloid bolus of 5 to 10 ml/kg IV administered over 10 to 20 minutes should be given. If no effect is observed, administration of multiple small boluses can be attempted, with consideration of the total volume of fluids that have been given. If the hypotension persists during fluid therapy there may be a need for inotropic and/or vasopressor support in the form of dopamine or dobutamine. Because of their short half-life these agents are given as a CRI at 2 to 10 mcg/kg/min IV.[37] Dopamine and dobutamine can be used concurrently. Patients receiving inotropes and vasopressors should be monitored carefully for tachycardia, which may necessitate a decrease in the rate of the infusion or the addition of another inotrope. Other agents that may be used are ephedrine (0.05 to 0.5 mg/kg IV as a single bolus), norepinephrine (0.1 to 1 mcg/kg/min IV as a CRI), and vasopressin (1 to 5 mU/kg/min IV as a CRI).[37,38] If the initial inotrope is not successful in correcting the hypotension, a second agent is added while continuing administration of the first agent. For example, norepinephrine is most often used in combination with dopamine or dobutamine, and vasopressin can be used in combination with these agents as well. (See Chapters 8, 157, and 158 for more information on the treatment of hypotension.)

If the animal continues to remain hypotensive even after appropriate fluid therapy and inotropic and vasopressor support, it may be necessary to consider discontinuing the inhalant anesthetic agent to eliminate the hypotensive effects of the inhalant and continuing the anesthesia maintenance using an injectable drug. This may involve administration of a CRI of a μ agonist such as fentanyl or morphine in combination with ketamine and lidocaine. Some patients may need only fentanyl as an intermittent intravenous bolus or as a CRI. Recent research suggests that a lidocaine CRI should not be used in the anesthetized cat due to its depressant effects on the cardiovascular system.[23]

RECOVERY

In critically ill patients, continuous cardiovascular support, monitoring, supportive care, and analgesia are imperative during the recovery period. The recovering patient may still require inotropic and/or vasopressor support, which should be continued in the intensive care unit upon recovery. The patient should be kept dry and warm, and should recover in a quiet, stress-free place where the patient can be continuously and carefully monitored. A shivering animal has greatly increased demands for glucose and oxygen, and oxygen supplementation and heat support should be given until the animal is no longer shivering.[7] Acid-base, electrolyte, PCV, total protein, and blood glucose levels should also be monitored in the recovering and shivering animal. The use of forced warm air heating blankets can help in the treatment of hypothermia. Finally, the use of analgesics is imperative in these critically ill patients in pain. Although these patients may not exhibit classic pain response symptoms due to their debilitated state, they should be carefully but appropriately treated with analgesics. Pain can lead to catabolism and complications such as delayed wound healing, sepsis, and nosocomial disease.[39] (See Chapter 144.)

SUMMARY

The condition of critically ill patients should be stabilized aggressively before anesthesia. Appropriate monitoring should be performed at all times to ensure that these delicate patients survive their emergent surgery. Postoperative care includes continued vasopressor and inotropic support, appropriate fluid therapy, analgesic support, oxygen therapy, blood pressure monitoring, and nursing care to improve survival in this critically ill patient population.

REFERENCES

1. Trim CM: Anesthetic considerations and complications. In Paddleford RR, editor: Manual of small animal anesthesia, ed 1, New York, 1999, Churchill Livingstone.
2. Chan DL, Rozanski EA, Freeman LM, et al: Colloid osmotic pressure in health and disease, Compend Contin Educ Pract Vet 23:896, 2001.
3. Mathews KA, Barry M: The use of 25% human serum albumin: outcome and efficacy in raising serum albumin and systemic blood pressure in critically ill dogs and cats, J Vet Emerg Crit Care (San Antonio) 15:110-118, 2005.
4. Mazzaferro EM, Rudloff E, Kirby R: the role of albumin replacement in the critically ill veterinary patient, J Vet Emerg Crit Care (San Antonio) 12:113-124, 2002.
5. Raffe MR: Pre-operative and post-operative management of the emergency surgical patient. In Murtaugh RJ, Kaplan PM, editors: Veterinary emergency and critical care medicine, St Louis, 1992, Mosby–Year Book.
6. Jacobson JD: Sedating and anesthetizing patients that have organ system dysfunction, Vet Med 518-524, 2005.
7. Hall LW, Clarke KW, Trim CM: General pharmacology of the injectable agents used in anaesthesia. In Hall LW, Clarke KW, Trim CM, editors: Veterinary anaesthesia, ed 10, London, 2001, Saunders. A good basic anesthesia textbook
8. Macintire DK, Drobatz KJ, Haskins SC, et al: Anesthetic protocols for short procedures. In Macintire DK, Drobatz KJ, Haskins SC, et al, editors: Manual of small animal emergency and critical care, Philadelphia, 2005, Lippincott Williams & Wilkins, pp 38-54.
9. Taylor PM, Chengelis CP, Miller WR, et al: Evaluation of propofol containing 2% benzyl alcohol preservative in cats, J Feline Med Surg 14(8):516-526, 2012.
10. Jimenez CP, Mathis A, Mora SS, et al: Evaluation of the quality of the recovery after administration of propofol or alfaxalone for induction of anaesthesia in dogs anaesthetized for magnetic resonance imaging, Vet Anaesth Analg 39:151-159, 2012.
11. Psastha E, Alibhai HIK, Jimenez-Lozano A, et al: Clinical efficacy and cardiorespiratory effects of alfaxalone, or diazepam/fentanyl for induction of anaesthesia in dogs that are a poor anaesthetic risk, Vet Anaesth Analg 38:24-36, 2011.
12. Mathis A, Pinelas R, Brodbelt DC, et al: Comparison of quality of recovery from anaesthesia in cats induced with propofol or alfaxalone, Vet Anaesth Analg 39:282-290, 2012.
13. Carroll G, Martin DD: Trauma and critical patients. In Tranquilli WJ, Thurmon JC, Grimm KA, editors: Lumb and Jones' veterinary anesthesia and analgesia, ed 4, Ames, Ia, 2007, Blackwell, pp 969-984.
14. de la Granville B, Arroyo D, Walder B: Etomidate in critically ill patients. Con: do you really want to weaken the frail? Eur J Anaesthesiol 29:511-514, 2012.
15. Cutherbertson BH, Sprung CL, Annane D, et al: The effects of etomidate on adrenal responsiveness and mortality in patients with septic shock, Intensive Care Med 35:1868-1876, 2009.
16. Perkowski S: Sedation of the critically ill patient. In Silverstein DC, Hopper K, editors: Small animal critical care medicine, ed 1, St Louis, 2009, Saunders pp 700-704.
17. Anagnostou TL, Kazakos GM, Savvas I, et al: Remifentanil/isoflurane anesthesia in five dogs with liver disease undergoing liver biopsy, J Am Anim Hosp Assoc 47:e103-e109, 2011.
18. Allweiler S, Brodbelt DC, Borer K, et al: The isoflurane-sparing and clinical effects of a constant rate infusion of remifentanil in dogs, Vet Anaesth Analg 34:388-393, 2007.
19. Brosnan RJ, Pypendop BH, Siao KT, et al: Effects of remifentanil on measures of anesthetic immobility and analgesia in cats, Am J Vet Res 70:1065-1071, 2009.
20. Muir WW, Wiese AJ, March PA: Effects of morphine, lidocaine, ketamine, and morphine-lidocaine-ketamine drug combination on minimum alveolar concentration in dogs anesthetized with isoflurane, Am J Vet Res 64(9):1155-1160, 2003.
21. Wagnor AE, Walton JA, Hellyer PW, et al: Use of low doses of ketamine administered by constant rate infusion as an adjunct for postoperative analgesia in dogs, J Am Vet Med Assoc 221(1):72-75, 2002.
22. Cassutto BH, Gfeller RW: Use of intravenous lidocaine to prevent reperfusion injury and subsequent multiple organ dysfunction syndrome, J Vet Emerg Crit Care (San Antonio) 13:137-148, 2003.
23. Pypendop BH, Ilkiw JE: Assessment of the hemodynamic effects of lidocaine administered IV in isoflurane anesthetized cats, Am J Vet Res 66:661-668, 2005.
24. Mannarino R, Luna SPL, Monteiro ER, et al: Minimum infusion rate and hemodynamic effects of propofol, propofol-lidocaine and propofol-lidocaine-ketamine in dogs, Vet Anaesth Analg 39:160-173, 2012.

25. Baldo CF, Garcia-Pereira FL, Nelson NC, et al: Effects of anesthetic drugs on canine splenic volume determined via computed tomography, Am J Vet Res 73:1715-1719, 2012.
26. Hall LW, Clarke KW, Trim CM: General pharmacology of the inhalation anesthetics. In Hall LW, Clarke KW, Trim CM, editors: Veterinary anaesthesia, ed 10, London, 2001, Saunders.
27. Ravasio G, Gallo M, Beccaglia M, et al: Evaluation of a ketamine-propofol drug combination with or without dexmedetomidine for intravenous anesthesia in cats undergoing ovariectomy, J Am Vet Med Assoc 241:1307-1313, 2012.
28. Quandt JE, Lee JA: Analgesia and constant rate infusions. In Silverstein DC, Hopper K, editors: Small animal critical care medicine, ed 1, St Louis, 2009, Saunders. pp 710-716.
29. Murray MJ, Cowen J, DeBlock H, et al: Clinical practice guidelines for sustained neuromuscular blockade in the adult critically ill patient, Crit Care Med 30:142-156, 2002.
30. Hall LW, Clarke KW, Trim CM: Relaxation of the skeletal muscle. In Hall LW, Clarke KW, Trim CM, editors: Veterinary anaesthesia, ed 10, London, 2001, Saunders.
31. Lukasik VM: Neuromuscular blocking drugs and the critical care patient, J Vet Emerg Crit Care 5:99-113, 1995.
32. Martinez EA, Keegan RD: Muscle relaxants and neuromuscular blockade. In Tranquilli WJ, Thurman JC, Grimm KA, editors: Lumb and Jones' veterinary anesthesia and analgesia, ed 4, Ames, Ia, 2007, Blackwell, pp 419-437.
33. Adams WA, Robinson KJ, Senior JM, et al: The use of the nondepolarizing neuromuscular blocking drug cis-atracurium in dogs, Vet Anaesth Analg 28:156-160, 2001.
34. Kastrup MR, Marsico FF, Ascoli FO, et al: Neuromuscular blocking properties of atracurium during sevoflurane or propofol anaesthesia in dogs, Vet Anaesth Analg 32:222-227, 2005.
35. Wright B, Hellyer PW: Respiratory monitoring during anesthesia: pulse oximetry and capnography, Compend Contin Educ Pract Vet 18:1083-1097, 1996.
36. Hall LW, Clarke KW, Trim CM: Patient monitoring and clinical measurement. In Hall LW, Clarke KW, Trim CM, editors: Veterinary anaesthesia, ed 10, London, 2001, Saunders.
37. Hall LW, Clarke KW, Trim CM: Anaesthesia of the dog. In Hall LW, Clarke KW, Trim CM, editors: Veterinary anaesthesia, ed 10, London, 2001, Saunders.
38. Pablo LS. The use of vasopressin in critical care patients. In: Proceedings North American Veterinary Conference. Gainesville FL: 2006, p. 280-282.
39. Muir WW: Physiology and pathophysiology of pain. In Gaynor JS, Muir WW, editors: Handbook of veterinary pain management, ed 1, St Louis, 2002, Mosby.

CHAPTER 144

ANALGESIA AND CONSTANT RATE INFUSIONS

Jane Quandt, BS, DVM, MS, DACVAA, DACVECC • Justine A. Lee, DVM, DACVECC, DABT

KEY POINTS

- There are several general drug classes, administration routes, and techniques by which analgesia can be achieved.
- The clinician should be able to develop an appropriate analgesic therapeutic plan that addresses the type and severity of pain.
- Patients should be frequently evaluated for response to treatment and treated appropriately with additional analgesics if necessary.
- Multimodal or combination analgesic drug therapy may be beneficial in the critically ill patient.

ANALGESIA

The critically ill patient benefits from analgesia because it promotes an animal's overall well-being and has a positive effect on the speed and quality of recovery.[1] The goal of pain control is to achieve a state in which the pain is bearable but some of the protective aspects of pain, such as inhibiting use of a fractured leg, still remain.[1] There are several general drug classes, administration routes, and techniques by which analgesia can be achieved. General drug classes that are commonly used include the following: opioids, nonsteroidal antiinflammatory drugs (NSAIDs), α_2-adrenergic agonists (see Chapter 165 for more information on α_2 agonists and antagonists), local anesthetics, *N*-methyl-d-aspartate (NMDA) antagonists, benzodiazepines, and phenothiazines. Analgesics can be administered by various methods including the intravenous, subcutaneous, intramuscular, epidural, transmucosal, transdermal, oral, intraarticular, intrapleural, and intraperitoneal routes as well as by local infiltration. The type of treatment may depend on the severity of pain and the nature of the animal. Specific dosages of analgesic drugs are provided in Table 144-1.

In intensive care unit (ICU) patients, analgesics should be administered as soon as possible after patient assessment and appropriate patient resuscitation to provide a significant benefit.[2] It is vital, however, that the underlying disease process be addressed while pain relief is provided because analgesic therapy may mask the underlying disorders or the hemodynamic status of a patient. Ideally analgesics should be administered before pain develops (e.g., preemptive analgesia) because less drug therapy may be necessary to control pain. This is especially important before surgery or other invasive procedures; however, this is not always feasible in trauma or emergent cases.[2,3]

Pain development and sensation may involve a multiplicity of pathways; therefore it is important to develop an analgesic therapeutic plan that assesses the type and severity of the pain and the response to treatment. Because pain pathways are complex, it is often unlikely that one agent alone will completely alleviate pain, regardless of how high the dose is.[4] The use of more than one class of drug can improve analgesia because the drugs affect multiple receptor types and such

Table 144-1 Analgesics and Their Dosages

Generic Name	Dosage
Acetylpromazine, acepromazine	0.01-0.05 mg/kg IM, IV q3-6h; do not exceed a total of 3 mg in large dogs
Atipamezole (reverses α_2-adrenergic agonist drugs)	0.05-0.2 mg/kg IM, IV, SC
Bupivacaine	Nerve block: 1-2 mg/kg SC q6h
Buprenorphine	0.005-0.02 mg/kg IM, IV q6-8h *Cats:* 0.01-0.02 mg/kg q6-8h PO
Butorphanol	0.1-0.4 mg/kg IM, IV q1-4h Partial reversal of μ-opioid agonist: 0.05-0.1 mg/kg IV Loading dose for CRI: 0.1 mg/kg IV Maintenance for CRI: 0.03-0.4 mg/kg/hr IV
Carprofen	2-4 mg/kg SC (single dose)
Cyproheptadine	*Dogs:* 0.3-2 mg/kg PO q12h *Cats:* 2 mg/cat PO q12h
Deracoxib	*Dogs:* 1-2 mg/kg PO q24h Postoperative pain: 3-4 mg/kg PO q24h; do not give for >7 days
Dexmedetomidine	1-5 mcg/kg IV q4h Loading dose: 1 mcg/kg IV Maintenance: 0.5-3 mcg/kg/hr IV CRI
Etodolac	*Dogs:* 5-15 mg/kg PO q24h
Fentanyl	*Dogs:* Loading dose: 2 mcg/kg IV Maintenance: 2-5 mcg/kg/hr CRI *Cats:* Loading dose: 1 mcg/kg IV Maintenance: 1-4 mcg/kg/hr CRI
Fentanyl patch	Cats, dogs < 5 kg: 25-mcg patch Dogs 5-10 kg: 25-mcg patch Dogs 10-20 kg: 50-mcg patch Dogs 20-30 kg: 75-mcg patch Dogs > 30 kg: 100-mcg patch
Gabapentin	1.25-4 mg/kg PO q24h
Hydromorphone HCl	*Dogs:* 0.05-0.2 mg/kg IM or SC; 0.05-0.1 mg/kg IV q2-4h *Cats:* 0.05-0.1 mg/kg IM or SC q3-4h; 0.03-0.05 mg/kg IV q3-4h
Indomethacin	No safe dose established
Ketamine	Analgesia without sedation: 0.1-1 mg/kg IV Loading dose: 0.5 mg/kg IV Maintenance during surgery: 10 mcg/kg/min IV CRI Maintenance after surgery: 2 mcg/kg/min CRI for 24 hr
Lidocaine	Nerve block: 1-2 mg/kg SC Loading dose: 1-2 mg/kg IV Maintenance: 2-3 mg/kg/hr IV CRI
2% Lidocaine	Nerve block: 1-2 mg/kg SC
Lidocaine patch	No animal dose established, but patch contains 700 mg of lidocaine. Significant systemic absorption has not been found to occur. Patch should be cut to fit size of area.
Meloxicam	0.1-0.2 mg/kg IV or SC (single dose)
Morphine	*Dogs:* 0.25-1 mg/kg IM q4-6h
Morphine sulfate	*Dogs:* 0.5-2 mg/kg IM, SC q4h *Cats:* 0.05-0.4 mg/kg IM, SC q3-6h Loading dose: 0.15-0.5 mg/kg IV administered slowly to avoid histamine release Maintenance: 0.1-1 mg/kg/hr CRI
Naloxone (opioid reversal)	0.002-0.1 mg/kg IM, IV, or SC
Oxymorphone	*Dogs:* 0.03-0.1 mg/kg IM or IV q2-4h *Cats:* 0.01-0.05 mg/kg IM or IV q2-4h
Remifentanil	3 mcg/kg IV, then CRI of 0.1-0.3 mcg/kg/min
Tepoxalin	*Dogs:* 10 mg/kg PO q24h
Morphine-lidocaine-ketamine infusion	Morphine: 3.3 mcg/kg/min Lidocaine: 50 mcg/kg/min Ketamine: 10 mcg/kg/min Preparation: Mix 10 mg of morphine sulfate, 150 mg of 2% lidocaine, and 30 mg of ketamine into a 500-ml bag of lactated Ringer's solution Administration rate: 10 ml/kg/hr

CRI, Constant rate infusion; *IM,* intramuscularly; *IV,* intravenously; *PO,* per os; *SC,* subcutaneously.

combination therapy may also overcome the problem of varying onset times and durations of action of different drug classes. Examples of effective combinations of analgesic therapy are the administration of opioids with NSAIDs, local anesthetics (e.g., lidocaine patches) with opioids, and an epidural analgesic with systemic opioid therapy. Regardless of what type of analgesic or combination of analgesics is used, patients should be reassessed frequently to ensure that the analgesic regimen is adequate and appropriate. Finally, administration of analgesics may be diagnostic when pain behavior is difficult to recognize in stoic patients.[4]

OPIOIDS

Opioids act centrally to limit the input of nociceptive information to the central nervous system (CNS), which reduces central hypersensitivity.[5] Receptors in the brain and dorsal horn of the spinal cord receive impulses from peripheral nerves, which are modulated before being transmitted to higher centers.[6] Opioids are commonly used in critically ill patients because they have a rapid onset of action and are safe, reversible, and potent analgesics. As with all analgesic therapy in critically ill patients, opioids should be slowly titrated intravenously (IV) to effect, due to altered drug pharmacokinetics.[7] Opioid analgesics vary in effectiveness, depending on which receptor is stimulated and which class of opioid is being administered.

The four classes of opioids are pure agonists, partial agonists, agonists-antagonists, and antagonists. Pure receptor agonist stimulation results in a pronounced analgesic effect, whereas partial agonists bind at the same receptor but produce a less pronounced effect.[6] Agonists-antagonists have mixed effects, with an agonist effect at one type of receptor and an antagonist effect at a different type of receptor. This results in an analgesic effect at one receptor and no effect (or a less pronounced effect) at the other receptor. Opioid antagonists (e.g., naloxone) bind to the same receptor as agonists but cause no effect and can competitively displace the agonist from the receptor and therefore reverse the agonist effect.[6] The partial agonist buprenorphine and mixed agonist-antagonist butorphanol reach maximal effect at the upper end of the dose range. If the pain is severe or the analgesia is inadequate, additional doses of partial or mixed agonists-antagonists are unlikely to be effective. Using a pure μ agonist (e.g., morphine, hydromorphone, fentanyl, oxymorphone, remifentanil) would be more effective because there is no upper limit to the analgesia provided by a pure μ agonist.[5]

Potent adverse effects such as respiratory depression and bradycardia may be seen at the higher end of the dose range with a pure μ agonist; therefore the higher doses should be used cautiously in critically ill patients.[5,6] Additional adverse effects of some μ agonists (e.g., morphine and meperidine) include histamine release, which is of particular concern when these agents are given rapidly IV because this can lead to severe hypotension due to vasodilation.[6] Opioids can lead to gastroparesis and ileus, which may result in vomiting, regurgitation, and aspiration of gastrointestinal (GI) contents, particularly in depressed, sedated, weak, or critically ill patients. Gastric distention caused by opioids may also be a concern in patients with abdominal disease (e.g., pancreatitis) because stimulation of pancreatic secretions may occur. Patients at risk of pancreatitis or gastroparesis may require intermittent or constant gastric decompression (via nasogastric, esophagostomy, or gastrostomy tube) if they are treated with opioids for longer than 12 to 24 hours or may require motility drug therapy (e.g., metoclopramide) for treatment of ileus.[8]

Opioids can be safely administered to cats to provide analgesia.[5] Morphine, hydromorphone, or oxymorphone can be administered for analgesia; however, adverse effects such as hyperexcitability or agitation may occur. It has been shown that the onset of mydriasis following administration of opioids correlates with adequate analgesia in cats; continual dosing after mydriasis is achieved may result in adverse effects such as dysphoria and agitation.[8] Another option for cats is the mixed partial μ agonist buprenorphine, which has been shown to be an effective analgesic.[6]

The newest μ agonist, remifentanil, may offer some advantages over the more commonly used μ opioids. In dogs and cats with severe liver compromise, remifentanil may be considered for analgesia during general anesthesia and as a constant rate infusion (CRI) to provide analgesia in the ICU. Remifentanil is a synthetic opioid with direct action on the μ receptors. It has an ultrashort duration of action, which allows a rapid recovery even after long-term IV infusion. The elimination of remifentanil is independent of hepatic or renal function because the drug is metabolized by nonspecific esterases in blood and tissues, which makes it an attractive agent for use in patients with hepatic or renal compromise.[9] Remifentanil has been used in dogs at an initial dose of 3 mcg/kg IV followed by a CRI of 0.1 to 0.3 mcg/kg/min. The clinical effects of remifentanil are rapidly dissipated upon discontinuation of the CRI, with dogs recovering within 5 to 20 minutes regardless of the duration of the infusion.[9,10] Due to the drug's short duration of action, additional analgesic therapy is necessary upon termination of the CRI if clinical signs of pain persist. Like other opioids, remifentanil is a potent respiratory depressant when used as a CRI, and the patient should be monitored for hypoventilation. If depression is severe, the use of naloxone or mechanical ventilation may be required. The respiratory depression associated with remifentanil typically does not persist following recovery.[10] In cats, the use of remifentanil at dosages higher than 1 mcg/kg/min has been associated with dysphoric behavior and frenetic locomotor activity.[11]

Fentanyl, another pure μ agonist, is commonly used in veterinary medicine, both in injectable form and in transdermal patches (Duragesic). The newest formulation of fentanyl is Recuvyra, which has been developed for transdermal application in dogs only. (This product is not to be used in cats.) The canine dose is a single application of 2.6 mg/kg delivered via a specialized syringe to the dorsal scapular area 2 to 4 hours before surgery, with analgesia lasting a minimum of 4 days.[12] If accidental overdose occurs, naloxone (40 or 160 mcg/kg intramuscularly [IM] q1h as needed) can be used to reverse any signs of excessive sedation, bradycardia, or hypothermia. The shorter duration of action of naloxone relative to that of transdermal fentanyl may necessitate repeated injections of naloxone.[13]

One advantage of opioid administration in critically ill patients is that their effects can be reversed if necessary with a pure antagonist such as naloxone. Naloxone can reverse the CNS depression, respiratory depression, and bradycardia associated with the opioid; however, reversal of the sedative effect and analgesia effect can cause acute pain, excitement, emergence delirium, aggression, and hyperalgesia.[14] Low-dose naloxone (0.004 mg/kg titrated slowly IV) has been recommended to reverse CNS depression without affecting analgesia.[8] The duration of effect for naloxone is relatively short (20 to 30 minutes) because of its rapid metabolism in dogs and cats, which may predispose patients to renarcotization when the drug is used to reverse long-acting opioids.[14,15] Agonists-antagonists such as butorphanol (0.05 to 0.1 mg/kg IV) may also be used to reverse sedation and respiratory depression from μ agonists.[8,14] The benefit of using butorphanol as a reversal agent is that complete reversal of analgesia does not occur due to the κ-agonist effects of butorphanol. Butorphanol administered as a reversal agent may produce additive analgesia with the μ agonist.[14] In contrast, buprenorphine is not as easily reversed as butorphanol because it is difficult to displace from the receptor.[6]

NONSTEROIDAL ANTIINFLAMMATORY DRUGS

Inflammation plays a significant role in the pain process, and therefore the use of NSAIDs to reduce or eliminate peripheral inflammation may be helpful. NSAIDs decrease the pain input to the CNS, which may aggravate central hypersensitivity.[2] There are several commercially available veterinary NSAIDs, including carprofen (Rimadyl), deracoxib (Deramaxx), meloxicam (Metacam), etodolac (Etogesic), tepoxalin (Zubrin), and robenacoxib (Onsior). The analgesic and antiinflammatory effects associated with NSAIDs are related to inhibition of cyclooxygenase (COX) enzyme isoforms. COX-1 is primarily responsible for basal prostaglandin production for normal homeostatic processes within the body, including gastric mucus production, platelet function, and, indirectly, hemostasis, whereas COX-2 is found at sites of inflammation (although COX-2 is responsible for some basal production of constitutive prostaglandins as well). Ideally, selective inhibition of prostaglandins produced primarily by COX-2 would provide analgesic and antiinflammatory effects without the unwanted adverse effects of COX-1 inhibition.[16] At present, there is no pure COX-2 inhibitor; rather, certain NSAIDs have varying degrees of COX-1 inhibition. For this reason, NSAIDs should be used cautiously in patients with hypotension, hypovolemia, preexisting renal disease (due to the increased potential for renal vascular vasoconstriction, which would lead to worsening of renal insufficiency), and GI disease or gastric ulceration.[5,7,17]

Ideally, enteral NSAIDs should be given with food when possible to decrease the incidence of gastric ulceration. In addition, NSAIDs should be used cautiously in the perioperative period because decreased platelet function may increase the incidence of operative hemorrhage. Injectable NSAIDs (e.g., carprofen, meloxicam) have an advantage over oral NSAIDs because injectable drug therapy can be administered to patients that cannot tolerate oral administration due to preoperative fasting for anesthesia, nausea, vomiting, or decreased mentation.[5] Finally, although NSAIDs have a slow onset of action (requiring up to 45 to 60 minutes to take effect), they provide analgesia for an extended period of time.[18] Carprofen has a 12-hour dosing frequency, whereas other NSAIDs (e.g., deracoxib, meloxicam, etodolac) are labeled for once-daily dosing.[16] The new feline-specific NSAID Onsior contains robenacoxib and is a COX-2 inhibitor with a high safety index in cats.[19] It has analgesic, antiinflammatory, and antipyretic effects in cats and selectively distributes to inflamed tissues, while sparing COX-1 at the clinically recommended dose.[20] It can be given subcutaneously (SC) between the shoulder blades (2 mg/kg) or orally (PO) (6 mg per cat q24h for cats weighing 2.5 to 6 kg and 12 mg per cat q24h for cats weighing 6.1 to 12 kg for 3 days).[20,21] Robenacoxib has a terminal half-life of 1.9 hours in cats, with efficacy persisting for 22 hours.[20]

As mentioned previously, NSAIDs can be used in combination with opioids for a combined therapeutic effect. However, the concurrent use of NSAIDs and corticosteroids is not recommended due to the potentiated adverse GI effects of COX-1 inhibition.[5]

α_2-ADRENERGIC AGONISTS

The α_2-adrenergic agonists bind to receptors in the CNS, which leads to sedation, peripheral vasoconstriction, bradycardia, respiratory depression, diuresis, muscle relaxation, and analgesia.[8,22] Dexmedetomidine is the most common α_2-adrenergic agonist administered to small animals. Dexmedetomidine is the dextrorotatory enantiomer of medetomidine, which is the active form. The clinical effects of both drugs are similar, and any comments made about medetomidine in the remainder of this discussion can be applied equally to dexmedetomidine. It is approved for use in dogs and cats,[22] and both dexmedetomidine and medetomidine can be given IM or IV. These drugs are biotransformed by the liver, with inactive metabolites excreted in the urine. Both of these α_2-adrenergic agonists have a rapid onset of action.[23] The sedative effects of medetomidine have a longer duration of action than do the analgesic effects, which last approximately 30 to 90 minutes.[24] Low-dose medetomidine (1 to 10 mcg/kg IV) can be safely used in patients in stable condition or administered in conjunction with opioids to produce analgesic synergism and increase the duration of analgesia up to 4 hours.[8,24] At higher doses, medetomidine can be used for sedation of distressed animals and for minor procedures (e.g., restraint and analgesia for radiographic positioning).[8] In patients in stable cardiovascular condition, medetomidine can be used as a CRI for analgesia (initial loading dose of 1 mcg/kg IV then a CRI of 1 to 3 mcg/kg/hr).[25] One should note that the dose range for dexmedetomidine is half that for medetomidine. As with opioids, the effects of α_2-adrenergic agonists can be reversed. Atipamezole is a specific α_2-adrenergic antagonist that reverses analgesia, sedation, and respiratory depression. Intramuscular or subcutaneous administration is preferred for reversal because intravenous administration can lead to abrupt hypotension and/or aggression.[14] See Chapter 165 for more information on α_2 agonists and antagonists.

TRANSDERMAL ANALGESICS

Administration of topical analgesics in conjunction with other analgesic therapy is well tolerated by patients and has minimal systemic effects.[26] Fentanyl patches can be used to provide long-term analgesia but may vary in time to onset of effects and steady-state concentrations.[7,18,27] Because of this variability, systemic analgesia must be provided until the patch becomes effective (typically up to 24 hours in dogs).[8] Fentanyl uptake is affected by dermal blood flow, hair, and obesity and may be greatly altered in hypovolemic or hypothermic patients. In cats the drug may reach therapeutic levels in 6 to 12 hours, and steady states can be maintained for approximately 5 days.[18,27] It should be noted that therapeutic levels may not be reached with the patch in all animals. If the patient still appears to be in pain 12 to 24 hours after patch application, additional analgesic treatment may be necessary.[8] Fentanyl patches are currently available in 25-, 75-, and 100-mcg formulations. Fentanyl patches should not be cut or otherwise altered because this may affect the amount of absorption or drug loss. The pet owner should be specifically instructed regarding the proper disposal of used fentanyl patches because there is potential for human abuse.

Lidoderm, a 5% lidocaine patch, was recently introduced to the human and veterinary markets. Lidoderm was approved in 1999 by the U.S. Food and Drug Administration for treatment of postherpetic neuralgia in humans.[26] Lidoderm is a nonwoven, polyester, felt-backed patch covered with a polyethylene terephthalate film release liner that should be removed before the patch is applied to the skin. Each 10- × 14-cm adhesive patch contains 700 mg of lidocaine (50 mg per gram of adhesive) in an aqueous base. Lidocaine penetration into intact skin is sufficient to produce an analgesic effect but does not result in complete sensory block. The Lidoderm patch can be safely worn for as long as 24 hours and provides analgesia without numbness or loss of sensitivity to touch or temperature. Therapeutic levels are achieved via absorption within 30 minutes. Unlike the fentanyl patch, the lidocaine patch can be cut to fit patient size without affecting drug delivery. Lidocaine patches can be used back to back for continuous analgesia because toxic blood levels do not develop; however, the skin needs to be monitored for development of localized dermatitis because the most common adverse effects in humans are transient dermal reactions such as localized rash and pruritus.[28]

For application of analgesic patches in veterinary patients, the hair must be clipped and cleaned. The lidocaine patch can be stapled in place with surgical staples to ensure appropriate contact with skin.[29] The use of staples to aid in adherence of fentanyl patches has not been evaluated. Anecdotally, the Lidoderm patch has been used in dogs and cats to provide analgesia for severe skin abrasions, bruising, and surgical incisions; no apparent toxic effects have been noted thus far. In addition, multimodal analgesia can be initiated with both the lidocaine patch and fentanyl patch applied simultaneously. The lidocaine patch will provide local analgesia, whereas the fentanyl patch will provide systemic analgesia.

N-METHYL-D-ASPARTATE RECEPTOR ANTAGONISTS

NMDA receptor antagonists work by blocking multiple binding sites at this receptor, which results in analgesic, amnestic, and psychomimetic effects as well as neuroprotection.[30] Ketamine, a noncompetitive NMDA receptor antagonist, can reverse central hypersensitivity by preventing the exaggerated response, wind-up activity, and central sensitization of wide-dynamic-range neurons in the dorsal horn of the spinal cord.[5] Ketamine can be administered PO, SC, IM, or IV. Ketamine prevents the response to nociceptive stimuli carried by afferent pain neurons (e.g., C fibers).[31,32] Ketamine causes minimal cardiovascular depression, does not depress laryngeal protective reflexes, and produces less ventilatory depression than opioids; however, adverse effects include tremors and sedation along with increased cardiac output due to increased sympathetic tone.[32] Subanesthetic or low doses in dogs and cats (0.1 to 1 mg/kg IV, followed by a CRI of 2 mcg/kg/min) may produce analgesic effects without causing anesthesia or profound sedation.[5,32] Oral ketamine can also be used (8 to 12 mg/kg PO q6h in dogs) to provide pain relief following burn injuries.[7]

ACEPROMAZINE

The phenothiazine acepromazine (0.01 to 0.05 mg/kg IV, not to exceed a total dose of 3 mg) does *not* provide analgesia alone and should not be administered as a single agent if analgesia is desired. Rather, it should be used in combination with opioids as an anxiolytic and sedative. However, in the critically ill patient it should be used with caution due to the potential for vasodilation and resultant profound hypotension and hypothermia. Even with IV administration, up to 15 minutes may be required before the sedative effect of acepromazine is clinically observed; therefore repeated doses should be avoided until the full effect is evident.[8] Acepromazine can be safely administered to ICU patients if given at low doses (0.005 to 0.01 mg/kg) in patients in hemodynamically stable condition with adequate respiratory function.[33]

INFILTRATIVE AND LOCAL ANESTHETICS

Local anesthetics (e.g., lidocaine, bupivacaine) provide analgesia by blocking both specific nerve pathways and action potential transmission in nerve fibers (including nociceptive fibers).[5] Local anesthetics can be used for local injection (e.g., small bite wounds), intercostal nerve blocks, and intrathoracic or intraperitoneal administration. In addition, 0.5% bupivacaine (2 mg/kg q6h) can be administered to provide analgesia for painful diseases and conditions (e.g., fractures, pancreatitis) or for procedures (e.g., thoracotomy, placement of a thoracostomy tube).[5,18] Intercostal nerve blockade can be used to provide analgesia for rib fractures. Bupivacaine (1 to 1.5 mg/kg q6h, not to exceed 4 mg/kg on day 1) can be injected into the area of the intervertebral foramen on the caudal border of the rib to block the intercostal nerves.[5] Bupivacaine can also be administered into the pleural space via a thoracostomy tube to provide analgesia following thoracic surgery or tube placement because the presence of the tube itself may be painful. In cases of pancreatitis or abdominal pain, bupivacaine (2 mg/kg diluted in saline q6h intraperitoneally) can be administered via an aseptically placed, temporary butterfly catheter to provide analgesia. However, it may be ineffective when ascites is present due to dilution of the topical analgesic.

When local anesthetics are used, use of an aseptic technique is imperative. The patient should be appropriately positioned so that the medication disperses over the desired site to enhance analgesia.[5] In addition, sodium bicarbonate (1 mEq/ml) may be added to lidocaine (at a ratio of 1 to 2 parts bicarbonate to 8 to 9 parts lidocaine) to decrease the burning sensation caused by the administration of lidocaine alone, which is due to the acidity of the local anesthetic.[8] When bupivacaine is used, a 1:30 ratio of sodium bicarbonate to bupivacaine is sufficient.

Potential adverse effects of bupivacaine include arrhythmias and reduced cardiac output; therefore the drug should not be administered to animals with preexisting life-threatening arrhythmias. Also, because bupivacaine is selectively cardiotoxic, only half the canine dose should be administered to cats.[8] Certain contraindications to bupivacaine administration exist and warrant the use of alternative analgesics. In patients undergoing pericardectomy, intrapleural bupivacaine should be used judiciously due to the potential risk of cardiotoxicity.[5] Although intrapleural bupivacaine has been used safely in healthy dogs with and without an open pericardium, its use in patients with underlying cardiovascular instability or other disease has not been assessed.[34] Intrapleural bupivacaine may also interfere with ventilation by inducing diaphragmatic paralysis. Animals with good respiratory reserve capacity rarely develop clinically significant compromise, but administration of intrapleural anesthetics should be avoided in animals with marginal respiratory function.[8] Finally, toxicity may occur with higher doses of lidocaine (>10 to 20 mg/kg) and bupivacaine (>4 mg/kg). Clinical signs of toxicosis may include seizures, cardiac arrhythmias, tachycardia, and cardiovascular collapse. The maximum safe dose for most species is 4 mg/kg of lidocaine and 1 to 2 mg/kg of bupivacaine.[5] Administration of epinephrine, which normally enhances the duration of effect of local anesthetics, should be avoided in critically ill patients because it may lead to cardiac stimulation or ischemia from vasoconstriction.[5]

EPIDURAL ANALGESICS

Epidural analgesia is an alternative way of delivering analgesia to the caudal half of the body. Depending on the dose or volume of drug used, analgesia of the forelimbs can also be achieved: an injected volume of 1 ml/5 kg blocks to the first lumbar vertebra, and use of a larger volume results in a cranial spread of the analgesia. Lower concentrations of local anesthetics can provide analgesia without secondary motor deficits. Complete anesthesia can be achieved with higher doses of local anesthetics, which result in motor paralysis of the rear limbs. Epidural opioids can provide analgesia without affecting motor function; nociceptive input is reduced but not completely abolished. Higher doses may also lead to vasodilation and subsequent hypotension.[5] In critically ill patients, lower doses of local anesthetics should be used epidurally to avoid inducing hypotension. In general, critically ill patients often benefit from epidural analgesia because it decreases anesthetic requirements and provides analgesia without cardiorespiratory effects or excessive sedation.

The technique for epidural analgesia has been described elsewhere,[5] and readers are referred to those sources for further information on technique. Contraindications for the use of epidural analgesia or epidural catheter placement include trauma over the pelvic region (with loss of appropriate landmarks), sepsis, coagulopathy, CNS disease, skin infection over the site of injection, hypovolemic shock, and severe obesity.[5,18,35,36] Epidural catheters can also be used to help maintain long-term analgesia, although stringent aseptic protocol must be followed; in addition, these catheters may be technically difficult to place. An epidural catheter can be placed using the same landmarks as those for administration of a single injection. The advantage of epidural catheterization is the ability to provide continuous analgesia without the need for repeated epidural needle punctures. In addition, the catheter can be advanced cranially to improve analgesia to the front limbs or thoracic structures. Catheters must be placed aseptically under anesthesia or heavy sedation and maintained with sterility and care. Proper location of the epidural catheter can be confirmed via lateral radiography or fluoroscopy after catheter placement. If the epidural catheter is not radiopaque, a low dose of myographic contrast agent can be injected into the catheter to allow evaluation and ensure appropriate placement. Catheters have been safely left in place from 1 to 332 hours.[36] With epidural catheters, the total volume injected should be limited to 6 ml in a large dog.[36] See Table 144-2 for epidural dosing.

Adverse effects of epidural anesthesia include vomiting, urinary retention, pruritus, and delayed hair growth at the clipped epidural site.[35] Additional complications associated with epidural catheters include catheter dislodgement, discharge from the site, fecal contamination, line or filter breakage, and localized dermatitis.[37] When complications occur, removal of the epidural catheter is recommended. Adverse effects of epidural anesthesia should be treated symptomatically. Urinary retention can be treated or prevented by manually expressing the bladder or placing an indwelling urinary catheter.

Another complication is inadvertent injection of drug into the subarachnoid space. In dogs, the dural sac ends before the lumbosacral space, so inadvertent injection into the subarachnoid space is less likely. In cats, however, the dural sac ends past the lumbosacral space; therefore care must be taken to avoid subarachnoid injection when administering epidural drugs. If the subarachnoid space is penetrated, the nonpreservative formulation of the drug may still be given; however, a significantly reduced dose (50% to 75% of the original dose) should be administered.[36] The lower dose is sufficient for an analgesic response because the roots of the spinal cord are more accessible within the subarachnoid space, where they are not protected by the dura.[38]

CONSTANT RATE INFUSIONS

The administration of analgesics as a CRI has the advantage of maintaining effective plasma concentrations for continued pain relief. Anesthesia can also be maintained with a CRI if the animal cannot tolerate the hypotensive effects of inhalant anesthesia. The CRIs that have been administered during surgery can be carried over into recovery to provide titratable analgesia; the dose can usually be lower once surgical stimulation is over. All CRIs should be delivered by syringe pump for accurate dosing.[32] To avoid histamine release, which may occur with rapid IV morphine administration, a morphine CRI (0.1 to 1 mg/kg/hr) should be started after administration of an initial loading dose (0.15 to 0.5 mg/kg IV, diluted and delivered slowly over 5 to 10 minutes).[7,39] A CRI of morphine (0.12 mg/kg/hr) reportedly induces effects similar to those of intramuscular morphine (1 mg/kg q4h) in dogs undergoing laparotomy.[40] Regardless of how morphine is administered, its use may result in bradycardia, hypothermia, and panting. Other opioids (e.g., fentanyl, oxymorphone, hydromorphone) can also be administered as a CRI if undesirable adverse effects of morphine occur.[3] In critically ill animals that are poor anesthetic candidates, fentanyl, in conjunction with propofol, can provided adequate, safe, cardiovascular system–sparing anesthesia and therefore reduce or minimize the amount of inhalant anesthesia necessary. Adverse effects such as bradycardia may require treatment with an anticholinergic.[41]

Butorphanol has been administered at a loading dose of 0.1 mg/kg followed by 0.03 to 0.4 mg/kg/hr IV CRI.[7] Lidocaine can also be administered for pain control at an initial loading dose of 1 to 2 mg/kg followed by 0.025 mg/kg/min IV CRI.[39] Lidocaine doses as high as 2 to 3 mg/kg/hr IV have been reported.[17] The α_2 agonists can also

Table 144-2 Epidural Dosing[33]

Epidural Drug	Dog Dose and Duration of Action	Cat Dose and Duration of Action	Benefits	Cautions
Morphine (preservative free for epidural use)	0.1-0.4 mg/kg, with maximum volume of 6 ml[33] Onset of action: 20-60 min Duration of action: 6-24 hr[5,36]	0.16 mg/kg Duration of action: 20 hr[33]	Lipid soluble Long acting Longer duration of action than systemic dosing[5] Can reverse with naloxone	Use preservative-free formulation when administering
Buprenorphine	0.003-0.006 mg/kg	0.003-0.006 mg/kg	Preservative free Not a schedule II drug High lipid solubility	Difficult to reverse
Bupivacaine	0.5-2 mg/kg; higher end of dose range may result in transient paralysis[33] Onset of action and duration similar to those of morphine	0.5-1 mg/kg Duration of action: 20 hr[33]	Less likely to result in urinary retention than morphine[5,7,35,36]	
Epidural catheter dosing	When an epidural catheter is used the following drugs and doses are recommended: Morphine 0.1 mg/kg Bupivacaine 0.05-0.12 mg/kg Buprenorphine 0.003-0.006 mg/kg[35] When the agent is injected through the epidural catheter, the injection should be given slowly because rapid injection may precipitate vomiting. A CRI of morphine (0.3 mg/kg q24h) or bupivacaine (0.2-0.3 mg/kg q24h) can be given slowly into the epidural space using a syringe pump. Bupivacaine may be administered via CRI through an epidural catheter, but this may result in muscle weakness. If the weakness is excessive, the infusion should be promptly discontinued and the dose of bupivacaine reduced.[35]			

be administered as a CRI to enhance analgesia and minimize the level of inhalant needed.[42] The reader is directed to Table 144-1 for more information on drug dosing.

Low doses of ketamine can be used perioperatively to prevent wind-up, do not have undesirable side effects such as dysphoria or hallucination, and can be used for intraoperative and postoperative analgesia in dogs. A loading dose of ketamine (0.5 mg/kg IV) should be immediately followed by a CRI of 10 mcg/kg/min. This should then be reduced to 2 mcg/kg/min during the recovery phase and postoperative phase.[32]

Combinations of multiple types of analgesics can also be used as a CRI to provide analgesia and to decrease the amount of inhalant required in dogs. Some examples include morphine-lidocaine-ketamine and fentanyl-lidocaine-ketamine, which are described further in the following sections.

MORPHINE-LIDOCAINE-KETAMINE

Morphine (3.3 mcg/kg/min), lidocaine (50 mcg/kg/min), and ketamine (10 mcg/kg/min) can be administered as a CRI analgesic combination in dogs.[31] These agents can be given separately or mixed together in a single bag. Use of a combination of agents may result in enhanced analgesia through synergism and multiple receptor activation. Ketamine has been found to attenuate and reverse morphine tolerance in rodents and humans, thereby yielding an opioid-sparing effect and providing superior analgesia compared with either drug alone.[31] Recent work in the cat has shown that CRIs of lidocaine should be used cautiously (if at all) in this species due to cardiopulmonary depression; this would be an especially important consideration in the critically ill animal.[43]

Lidocaine has been used as a CRI along with fentanyl to provide analgesia in dogs undergoing ovariectomy. The intravenous dose of lidocaine was 2 mg/kg over 5 minutes followed by a CRI of 50 mcg/kg/min, with fentanyl dosed at 4 mcg/kg over 5 minutes followed by a CRI of 8 mcg/kg/hour. The lidocaine did not enhance the analgesia but did not adversely affect recovery.[44] Lidocaine may be more useful in those dogs that are suspected to have ischemia-reperfusion injury. Lidocaine may help diminish the level of reperfusion injury by inhibiting Na^+/Ca^{2+} exchange and Ca^{2+} accumulation during ischemia, scavenging hydroxyl radicals, decreasing the release of superoxide from granulocytes, and decreasing polymorphonuclear leukocyte activation, migration into ischemic tissues, and subsequent endothelial dysfunction.[45]

CONCLUSION

Administering analgesics in critically ill animals should be considered as an integral part of a treatment regimen. Critically ill patients may present a challenge when clinicians assess the presence of pain and evaluate the response to analgesic therapy. Because of the potential physiologic effects of some analgesics, the class of analgesic and route of administration should be chosen carefully for ICU patients. Using multimodal therapy that emphasizes lower doses of different classes of drugs may be a safer and more effective way of achieving analgesia in critically ill patients.

REFERENCES

1. Hellebrekers LJ: Pathophysiology of pain in animals and its consequences for analgesic therapy. In Hellebrekers LJ, editor: Animal pain in a practice-oriented approach to an effective pain control in animals, Utrecht, The Netherlands, 2000, Van Der Wees, pp 71-83.
2. Muir WW: Choosing and administering the right analgesic therapy. In Gaynor JS, Muir WW, editors: Handbook of veterinary pain management, St Louis, 2002, Mosby, pp 329-345.
3. Muir WW, Birchard SJ: Questions and answers on analgesia, anesthesia, and sedation. In Proceedings of the North American Veterinary Conference, Orlando, Fla, June 11-15, 1997, pp 1-24.
4. Lamont LA, Tranquilli WJ, Grimm KA: Physiology of pain, Vet Clin North Am Small Anim Pract 30(4):703-728, 2000.
5. Dobromylskyj P, Flecknell PA, Lascelles BD, et al: Management of postoperative and other acute pain. In Flecknell P, Waterman-Pearson A, editors: Pain management in animals, Philadelphia, 2000, Saunders, pp 81-145.
6. Wagnor A: Opioids. In Gaynor JS, Muir WW, editors: Handbook of veterinary pain management, St Louis, 2002, Mosby, 164-183.
7. Pascoe PJ: Problems of pain management. In Flecknell P, Waterman-Pearson A, editors: Pain management in animals, Philadelphia, 2000, Saunders, pp 161-177.
8. Hansen B: Acute pain management, Vet Clin North Am Small Anim Pract 30(4):899-916, 2000.
9. Anagnostou TL, Kazakos GM, Savvas I, et al: Remifentanil/isoflurane anesthesia in five dogs with liver disease undergoing liver biopsy, J Am Anim Hosp Assoc 47:e103-e109, 2011.
10. Allweiler S, Brodbelt DC, Borer K, et al: The isoflurane-sparing and clinical effects of a constant rate infusion of remifentanil in dogs, Vet Anaesth Analg 34:388-393, 2007.
11. Brosnan RJ, Pypendop BH, Siao KT, et al: Effects of remifentanil on measures of anesthetic immobility and analgesia in cats, Am J Vet Res 70:1065-1071, 2009.
12. Freise KJ, Newbound GC, Tudan C, et al: Pharmacokinetics and the effect of application site on a novel, long-acting transdermal fentanyl solution in healthy laboratory Beagles, J Vet Pharmacol Ther 35(Suppl 2):27-33, 2012.
13. Freise KJ, Newbound GC, Tudan C, et al: Naloxone reversal of an overdose of a novel, long-acting transdermal fentanyl solution in laboratory Beagles, J Vet Pharmacol Ther 35(Suppl 2):45-51, 2012.
14. Muir WW: Drug antagonism and antagonists. In Gaynor JS, Muir WW, editors: Handbook of veterinary pain management, St Louis, 2009, Mosby, pp 391-401.
15. Plumb DC: Naloxone. In Plumb DC, editor: Veterinary drug handbook, ed 4, Ames, Ia, 2002, Iowa State University Press, pp 575-576.
16. Budsberg S: Nonsteroidal anti-inflammatory drugs. In Gaynor JS, Muir WW, editors: Handbook of veterinary pain management, St Louis, 2009, Mosby, pp 183-209.
17. Hellebrekers LJ: Practical analgesic treatment in canine patients. In Hellebrekers LJ, editor: Animal pain: a practice-oriented approach to an effective pain control in animals, Utrecht, The Netherlands, 2000, Van Der Wees, pp 117-129.
18. Mathews KA: Management of pain in cats. In Hellebrekers LJ, editor: Animal pain: a practice-oriented approach to an effective pain control in animals, Utrecht, The Netherlands, 2000, Van Der Wees, pp 131-144.
19. Sano T, King JN, Seewald W, et al: Comparison of oral robenacoxib and ketoprofen for the treatment of acute pain and inflammation associated with musculoskeletal disorders in cats: a randomized clinical trial, Vet J 193(2):397-403, 2012.
20. Kamata M, King JN, Seewald W, et al: Comparison of injectable robenacoxib versus meloxicam for peri-operative use in cats: results of a randomized clinical trial, Vet J 193(1):114-118, 2012.
21. Onsior (robenacoxib) (package insert). Basel, Switzerland, 2012, Novartis Animal Health.
22. Plumb DC: Dexmedetomidine HCL. In Plumb DC, editor: Veterinary drug handbook, ed 7, Ames, Ia, 2011, Iowa State University Press, pp 298-300.
23. Muir WW, McDonell WN, Kerr CL, et al: Anesthetic physiology and pharmacology. In Grimm KA, Tranquilli WJ, Lamont LA, editors: Essentials of small animal anesthesia and analgesia, ed 2, Ames, Ia, 2011, Wiley-Blackwell, pp 15-81.
24. Lamont L: α_2 Agonists. In Gaynor JS, Muir WW, editors: Handbook of veterinary pain management, St Louis, 2009, Mosby, pp 210-230.
25. Campbell VL: Injectable anesthetic techniques. In Proceedings of the 11th International Veterinary Emergency and Critical Care Symposium, 2005, pp 21-24.
26. Gammaitoni AR, Alvarez NA, Galer BS: Safety and tolerability of the lidocaine patch 5%, a targeted peripheral analgesic: a review of the literature, J Clin Pharmacol 43:111-117, 2003.

27. Lee DD, Papich MG, Hardie EM: Comparison of pharmacokinetics of fentanyl after intravenous and transdermal administration in cats, Am J Vet Res 61(6):672-677, 2000.
28. Pasero C: Lidocaine patch 5%: how to use a topical method of controlling localized pain, Am J Nurs 103(9):75-78, 2003.
29. Bidwell LA, Wilson DV, Caron JP: Systemic lidocaine absorption after placement of Lidoderm patches on horses: preliminary findings. In Proceedings of the Veterinary Midwest Anesthesia and Analgesia Conference, 2004, pp 15.
30. Lamont LA, Tranquilli WJ, Mathews KA: Adjunctive analgesic therapy, Vet Clin North Am Small Anim Pract 30(4):805-813, 2000.
31. Muir WW, Wiese AJ, March PA: Effects of morphine, lidocaine, ketamine, and morphine-lidocaine-ketamine drug combination on minimum alveolar concentration in dogs anesthetized with isoflurane, Am J Vet Res 64(9):1155-1160, 2003.
32. Wagnor AE, Walton JA, Hellyer PW, et al: Use of low doses of ketamine administered by constant rate infusion as an adjunct for postoperative analgesia in dogs, J Am Vet Med Assoc 221(1):72-75, 2002.
33. Flecknell P, Waterman-Pearson A, editors: Pain management in animals, Philadelphia, 2000, Saunders.
34. Bernard F, Kudnbig ST, Monnet E: Hemodynamic effects of interpleural lidocaine and bupivacaine combination in anesthetized dogs with and without an open pericardium, Vet Surg 35:252-258, 2006.
35. Troncy E, Junot S, Keroack S, et al: Results of preemptive epidural administration of morphine with or without bupivacaine in dogs and cats undergoing surgery: 265 cases (1997-1999), J Am Vet Med Assoc 221(5):666-672, 2002.
36. Hansen BD: Epidural catheter analgesia in dogs and cats: technique and review of 182 cases (1991-1999), J Vet Emerg Crit Care (San Antonio) 11(2):95-103, 2001.
37. Swalander DB, Crowe DT, Hittenmiller DH, et al: Complications associated with the use of indwelling epidural catheters in dogs: 81 cases (1996-1999), J Am Vet Med Assoc 216(3):368-370, 2000.
38. Muir WW, Skarda RT: Pain management in the horse. In Gaynor JS, Muir WW, editors: Handbook of veterinary pain management, St Louis, 2002, Mosby, pp 420-444.
39. Smith LJ, Bentley E, Shih A, et al: Systemic lidocaine infusion as an analgesic for intraocular surgery in dogs: a pilot study, Vet Anaesth Analg 31(1):53-63, 2004.
40. Lucas AN, Firth AM, Anderson GA, et al: Comparison of the effects of morphine administered by constant-rate intravenous infusion or intermittent intramuscular injection in dogs, J Am Vet Med Assoc 218(6):884-891, 2001.
41. Mendes GM, Selmi AL: Use of a combination of propofol and fentanyl, alfentanil, or sufentanil for total intravenous anesthesia in cats, J Am Vet Med Assoc 223(11):1608-1613, 2003.
42. Quandt JE, Lee JA: Analgesia and constant rate infusions. In Silverstein DC, Hopper K, editors: Small animal critical care medicine, ed 1, St Louis, 2009, Saunders, pp 710-716.
43. Pypendop BH, Ilkiw JE: Assessment of the hemodynamic effects of lidocaine administered IV in isoflurane anesthetized cats, Am J Vet Res 66:661-668, 2005.
44. Columbano N, Secci F, Careddu GM, et al: Effects of lidocaine constant rate infusion on sevoflurane requirement, autonomic responses, and postoperative analgesia in dogs undergoing ovariectomy under opioid-based balanced anesthesia, Vet J 193:448-455, 2012.
45. Cassutto BH, Gfeller RW: Use of intravenous lidocaine to prevent reperfusion injury and subsequent multiple organ dysfunction syndrome, J Vet Emerg Crit Care (San Antonio) 13:137-148, 2003.

CHAPTER 145

REHABILITATION THERAPY IN THE CRITICAL CARE PATIENT

Ann M. Caulfield, VMD, CCRP, CVA

KEY POINTS

- Rehabilitation therapy should be included in the treatment plan for most critically ill veterinary patients.
- Rehabilitation therapy must be prescribed and performed by (or under the direct supervision of) a trained and experienced rehabilitation therapist.
- Patients must be frequently assessed and treatment plans modified based on the current medical status of the patient.
- A team approach involving the critical care patient's primary care veterinarian, nursing staff, and rehabilitation therapist is of absolute necessity in ensuring safe and effective rehabilitation therapy for each patient.

Rehabilitation therapy is a new and rapidly expanding discipline in modern veterinary medicine. Rehabilitation recommendations for a variety of orthopedic and neurologic conditions are now considered standard of care. The veterinary critical care patient is less commonly considered a candidate for rehabilitation therapy. It is well documented that the human critical care patient may experience any number of debilitating multisystem comorbidities associated with serious illness, pharmacologic adverse effects, and especially immobility.[1] These include, but are not limited to, neuromuscular disorders, atelectasis, ileus, malnutrition, protein wasting, and depression.[2] In the human intensive care unit (ICU), physical therapists specializing in critical care are integral members of a multidisciplinary team working together to optimize outcomes in patient recovery.[2,3] Veterinary critical care patients are surviving catastrophic injuries and disease thanks to dramatic advances in critical care medicine.

BOX 145-1 *Goals for Range-of-Motion Exercises*

Maintain or improve pain-free range of motion
Maintain or improve flexibility, extensibility, and strength of periarticular soft tissues
Maintain or improve synovial fluid diffusion across the articulating surface
Prevent joint contracture
Improve blood and lymphatic flow
Promote proprioceptive responses and facilitate neuromuscular reeducation

The critically ill small animal patient is equally at risk of many of the same comorbidities seen in the human counterpart. Incorporating an individualized rehabilitation therapy program into the critical care patient's overall treatment plan will enhance the animal's recovery by minimizing systemic complications associated with immobility, reducing adverse effects of some pharmacologic interventions, improving pain management, and mitigating stress and anxiety associated with ill health and hospitalization.

The aim of this chapter is to introduce the concept of rehabilitation therapy for the veterinary critical care patient and discuss the benefits of some basic, easily implemented therapies. The intent is not to provide a "how to" on the details of carrying out a specific treatment but rather to educate the reader on the important role that a comprehensive rehabilitation therapy program has in improving the quality of patient care in the modern veterinary critical care unit. Critically ill patients are in a dynamic physiologic state, and each patient is unique in its pathologic conditions, temperament, and tolerance of therapeutic interventions. To optimize treatment outcomes and ensure the safety of the patient, the importance of a trained and experienced rehabilitation therapist working in close communication with the animal's primary clinician cannot be overemphasized.

MUSCULOSKELETAL SYSTEM

Range-of-Motion Exercise

Critical care patients often have or quickly develop range-of-motion (ROM) limitations due to preexisting conditions such as osteoarthritis or orthopedic, neurologic, or soft tissue trauma or disease, or as a consequence of sustained disuse or immobilization.[4,5] All joints have a given range through which they normally move. Movement may be passive, active assisted, or active. Normal ROM for any joint is influenced by a number of factors, including flexibility of the periarticular soft tissue structures (joint capsule, muscles, tendons, ligaments, and skin) as well as the structure and health of the joint itself. Limitations in normal joint ROM result from conditions affecting any of these structures. The goals for ROM exercises are provided in Box 145-1.[5]

Passive Range-of-Motion Exercise

Passive range-of-motion (PROM) exercises are passive movements of a joint through its available range. PROM movement incorporates an external force to move the joint and therefore does not involve active muscle contraction.[5] Performed regularly, PROM exercises may help prevent joint contracture as well as soft tissue shortening. PROM exercises can also maintain movement across fascial planes and augment lymphatic flow. PROM sessions should be incorporated early in the course of treatment for any animal that is unable or not permitted to actively move its joints on its own. Since PROM exercises do not involve active muscle contraction, they do not prevent muscle atrophy or increase muscle strength. Guidelines for safe, effective administration of PROM exercises and stretching are listed in Box 145-2.

BOX 145-2 *Guidelines for Performing Passive Range-of-Motion Exercises and Stretching Safely and Effectively*

Exercises should be performed in a calm, quiet environment with the animal resting in lateral recumbency.
Patient comfort is of the highest priority. Movements should be slow and gentle and limited to the patient's comfortable range. Overaggressive passive range-of-motion exercises result in pain, cause reflex inhibition, and may promote the formation of fibrous tissue around the joint.
Care should be taken to avoid disturbing any peripheral intravenous or arterial lines, indwelling urinary catheters, or electrocardiograph leads or other monitoring equipment.
Movement should be limited to a single joint by stabilizing with one hand placed proximal to the joint and producing movement with the opposite hand placed just distal to the joint. To minimize forces being applied, the hands should be placed close to the joint being moved.

Generally, PROM exercises are performed three to five times per day for all peripheral joints, including the digits. Each movement is repeated 10 to 15 times.

Active Assisted and Active Range-of-Motion Exercise

Active assisted and active ROM exercises encourage movement of a joint through active muscle contraction. In active assisted ROM, the therapist initiates or guides joint movement as the animal participates with active muscle contraction. Active ROM movement achieves joint motion solely through the animal's muscle contraction.[5] Active assisted or active ROM exercises are ideal for animals that are beginning to transition from PROM or those that are weak but capable of independent joint movement. Like PROM exercises, active assisted and active ROM exercises help counter the effects of immobilization and disuse on joints and periarticular structures. However, because they involve active muscle contraction, they can increase muscle strength and even bone strength at the sites of muscle attachment. Active and active assisted ROM exercises improve proprioception and balance. By coordinating movement of the various muscle groups they also facilitate reeducation of normal movement patterns. There are a variety of active assisted and active ROM exercises that can be used in the appropriate critical care patient.

Therapeutic Exercise and the Importance of Early Mobilization

In human ICU patients early-intervention mobilization and exercise improve function by increasing oxygenation, strength, and endurance.[4,6] Early mobilization has been shown to reduce length of stay in the hospital and in the ICU in particular.[7,8] Immobility in the human model has been associated with a number of physiologic changes, including rapid loss of muscle mass and transformation of skeletal muscle fibers resulting in reduced aerobic capacity. Loss of muscle strength was greatest during the first 7 days of immobilization, with as much as a 40% reduction in strength.[1] Also contributing to loss of muscle mass and strength in the human critical care patient are the direct effects of hypercapnia, hypoxia, malnutrition, and hemodynamic instability.[9] The most profound loss of muscle strength was seen in the elderly and, not surprisingly, the chronically ill (e.g. patients with congestive heart failure).[4]

Although there is a paucity of studies investigating the effects of early-intervention mobilization in veterinary critical care patients, it is reasonable to assume that its benefits extend to nonhuman patients. For the stable patient, early mobilization through assisted standing and/or facilitated walking should be a priority in the rehabilitation treatment plan.

Assisted Standing

Standing requires sophisticated neuromuscular coordination. Standing, even if assisted with a sling or therapy ball, promotes muscular strength in both the supporting peripheral limb muscles and the core muscles. In addition, it improves circulation and respiratory function, stimulates proprioceptive input, and promotes neuromuscular reeducation.[5] To be upright and standing often improves a recumbent animal's sense of well-being and can reduce frustration and associated anxiety. Sessions should be short, with careful attention paid to the patient's fatigue level as well as any vital parameters of special concern to that individual such as respiratory rate and effort. When the animal is in a normal standing position, an attempt can be made to introduce weight shifts by gently and slowly rocking the animal front to back and side to side. Standing weight shifts are an excellent way to stimulate balance and proprioception as well as promote limb and core muscle strength.

Walking (Assisted and Unassisted)

Walking is one of the most important therapeutic exercises prescribed for a rehabilitation therapy patient, including those in the critical care unit.[7] Common sense dictates that this be an activity reserved for stable patients with no medical conditions precluding such movement. Walking provides a controlled, low-impact form of active exercise that enhances muscle strength, benefits articular cartilage, and promotes connective tissue health while at the same time improving cardiac, lymphatic, and respiratory system functions. A basic walking program facilitates normal balance and proprioceptive function and enhances a patient's emotional well-being. There are a variety of mobility aids designed to assist a patient in walking. They range from simple booties that can improve traction on a slippery surface to slings and therapy carts that an ambulatory but weak patient can use as a "walker." Regardless of the level of assistance an individual patient may need, it is critical that the walks be kept to short sessions several times a day. Careful monitoring of the patient's status immediately before, during, and after the walk is important to ensure that the patient is not showing signs of weakness, fatigue, or respiratory compromise. Walk lengths can gradually be increased on a regular basis as the patient shows signs of improvement.

Individual exercises should be prescribed by a trained rehabilitation therapist working in collaboration with the critical care team. As always, careful assessment of the patient's current medical status and degree of debilitation should be made before any therapy session.

Neuromuscular Electrical Stimulation and Transcutaneous Electrical Stimulation

In human critical care medicine, complications from severe illness and immobilization frequently lead to debilitating and persistent neuromuscular abnormalities.[7] These observations have led physical therapists to develop early intervention treatment programs for the human critical care patient. Once a patient is deemed physiologically stable, appropriate rehabilitation therapy is initiated. One modality used in patients at risk of developing muscle weakness is neuromuscular electrical stimulation. Neuromuscular electrical stimulation is easily adapted to the veterinary critical care patient at risk of muscle wasting. Additionally, other electrical current therapy, like transcutaneous electrical stimulation, can be used as an adjunct to pain management in the critical care animal patient.

Neuromuscular electrical stimulation

Neuromuscular electrical stimulation (NMES) uses low-voltage electrical current transmitted through electrodes placed on the skin to stimulate passive muscle contraction.[7] In some ways, NMES simulates repetitive contractions of mild exercise since NMES-stimulated muscles have increased blood flow, maximal force output, and force endurance.[9,10] There is a difference, however, in the order of motor unit recruitment between a physiologically initiated and an electrically induced muscle contraction. Electrical stimulation recruits the larger, fast twitch muscle fibers before the smaller, slow twitch fibers. This is the opposite of the order in which physiologically initiated recruitment occurs.[5,11] Clinically, this is important because fast twitch fibers fatigue more quickly than slow twitch fibers; therefore longer rest periods are required between contractions to prevent muscle fatigue in the patient.[11] Another important clinical consideration when using NMES for preventing disuse atrophy and strengthening muscles is that electrically stimulated muscle contractions likely recruit different motor units within a muscle than those recruited during a normal physiologic contraction. To optimize muscle strengthening, it is best to combine NMES with physiologic contractions if the patient is capable of some low-level assisted or active assisted exercise.[11]

Transcutaneous electrical stimulation

Transcutaneous electrical stimulation (TENS) uses electrical current to modulate pain, most likely by interfering with transmission of noxious stimuli along A-delta and unmyelinated C nerve fibers. TENS activates nonnociceptor A-beta fibers. When more A-beta fibers are activated than C fibers and A-delta fibers, pain sensation is diminished. TENS may also produce analgesia by stimulating the production and release of endogenous opioids.[11]

Massage

Massage is a highly effective, underutilized treatment in the veterinary critical care patient. Medical massage is recognized in the human medical community for its success in treating muscle, nerve, and fascia disorders as well as disruptions in the normal neurophysiology of the enteric nervous system with consequential disturbances in gastrointestinal motility.[12] Specific training in medical massage therapy is now part of the curricula of many physical therapy training programs and medical schools. The benefits of gentle and caring touch delivered by a trained therapist can be wide ranging, from direct effects of increasing blood and lymphatic flow, improving gastrointestinal motility, and reducing muscle spasm to the more indirect effects of stress and anxiety reduction. Massage can easily be incorporated into the treatment plan of nearly every critical care patient in stable condition.

Massage is the manual application of pressure to the body though a variety of specific maneuvers such as effleurage (stroking), tapotement (tapping or percussion), vibration, friction, and pétrissage (kneading).[13] Fundamentally, therapeutic massage works through direct mechanical effects on muscle fibers, connective tissue, and vessel walls and through neuromodulation of peripheral sensory nerve receptors that relay information to the spinal cord for further processing and projection to higher centers.[14] Peripheral stimulation of autonomic nerve fibers within the fascia may modulate the high sympathetic tone that occurs in many animal patients experiencing pain, illness, and/or emotional distress.[13,15] Sustained increased sympathetic tone results in a physiologically maladaptive "vicious cycle," which is counterproductive to healing and contributes to increased morbidity, central hypersensitization, and chronic pain states.[13] Therapeutic massage techniques can decrease heart rate and blood pressure, which supports the idea that, in these patients, stimulation of peripheral sensory receptors with vagal nerve affiliation can dial down abnormally high sympathetic tone and dial up the parasympathetic system (which is more conducive to healing). As a result, heart rate, blood pressure, and cortisol levels decrease, vessels vasodilate and muscles relax, gastrointestinal motility becomes more normalized, and, at least for a while, the animal may disassociate from its current distressed state and gain a healing advantage.

In both human and animal ICU patients it is common to see alterations in gastrointestinal motility caused by immobility, adverse effects of some medications, stress, and pain.[12] It is interesting to note that in many human ICU patients ileus, nausea, and constipation are frequently mitigated through the use of specific abdominal massage techniques that promote improved gastrointestinal motility by stimulating dermal and subdermal vagal afferent nerves as well as gastrointestinal mechanoreceptors.[12,15]

One of the great advantages of properly performed therapeutic massage is the relative safety and low incidence of adverse effects associated with its use, even in a critically ill patient. However, there are contraindications that should be considered. Massage is contraindicated in areas of active infection or acute inflammation, near a tumor, in cases of deep vein thrombosis or coagulopathies, in patients with unstable fractures, and of course in animals intolerant of this type of hands-on therapy.

RESPIRATORY SYSTEM

Respiratory system disease and dysfunction are leading contributors to increased morbidity and mortality in both human and veterinary critical care patients. Immobility and prolonged recumbency, mechanical ventilation, pain from chest wall or abdominal surgery or trauma, and sedation and altered states of consciousness secondary to head trauma or seizures can all interfere with the normal respiratory pattern and potentially reduce chest wall and lung expansion.[16] Often animals in pain adopt a characteristic rapid and shallow breathing pattern that reduces tidal volume and lung compliance. The end result can be hypoventilation, atelectasis, accumulation of respiratory secretions, and pneumonia. Hypoxemia secondary to hypoventilation, ventilation-perfusion mismatch, or even intrapulmonary shunting necessitates treatment, thus prolonging hospital stays and further compromising an already debilitated patient.[16]

Respiratory therapists manage these patients daily in the human ICU. Adaptations of the techniques of these professionals can be incorporated into the veterinary treatment model so that the critically ill animal patient is at reduced risk of developing serious respiratory complications while in the critical care unit. It must be remembered that patients with compromised respiratory systems are in a precarious position and can easily decompensate. The following sections provide an overview of some basic techniques that can improve pulmonary function by helping to eliminate secretions, expand lung volume and open atelectatic lung fields, improve oxygenation, and reduce the work of breathing.[17] It is critical that the trained therapist work closely with the patient's primary clinician and be fully knowledgeable about any and all disease processes and health concerns, medications, and treatments for that patient. Constant objective and subjective assessment and reassessment before, during, and after a therapy session is important.

Positioning

Proper positioning can positively influence lung function and is an effective treatment for animals with lung disease or a treatment strategy to prevent pulmonary complications in immobile patients. Simply alternating from opposite sides and sternal recumbency every 2 to 4 hours can increase chest wall expansion and lung volume, prevent atelectasis, improve oxygenation and perfusion, prevent respiratory secretions from settling in dependent lung lobes, and improve patient comfort.[18] Regularly changing a recumbent patient's body position holds benefits beyond the respiratory system that include reduced muscle and joint stiffness, improved skin perfusion, and reduction in the formation of pressure sores, as well as prevention of dependent limb edema.[17]

Postural Drainage

Retention of respiratory secretions interferes with proper oxygenation and ventilation. Postural drainage is a technique employed commonly by respiratory therapists treating human patients with pulmonary disease.[18] It uses the force of gravity to aid in removing tracheal and bronchial secretions from a diseased lung segment by placing the patient into specific body positions. The patient is positioned so that the segmental bronchi are vertical to the diseased lung lobe.[17] This positioning allows drainage of the secretions into the larger airways so that they are more easily expelled when a cough is elicited. Imaging studies are necessary to determine which lung segments are affected and therefore which positions should be used. It may be beneficial to nebulize the patient just before a treatment.[5] Generally, the most affected lung segments are treated first and in the earlier part of the day. Treatment times range from 5 to 10 minutes in each position and treatments are performed several times a day. Following a treatment, the patient is encouraged to cough to aid in removal of the mobilized secretions.[18] In animal patients, gentle digital pressure at the larynx or proximal trachea often elicits a cough. In some patients, it may take 30 to 60 minutes following a treatment for the secretions to be mobilized.

There are certain patients in which postural drainage is contraindicated or should be approached with increased caution. Administration of supplemental oxygen before a treatment may be beneficial. In some patients, the standard postural drainage positions can actually worsen the animal's condition. In these cases, postural drainage may not be an option or the standard drainage positions may need to be modified. Box 145-3 lists the conditions that may preclude the use of postural drainage as a treatment option.

Postural drainage should be reserved for those patients that are immobile and have no contraindications to this treatment. Movement and exercise are superior to postural drainage in mobilizing respiratory secretions. Regular standing and walking should be used first in all patients that are capable of active mobility.

Percussion (Coupage) and Vibration

Percussion and vibration are two chest rehabilitation techniques that can be quite effective in loosening bronchial secretions and then moving them from smaller to larger airways where they are more easily expelled via coughing.[17,18] In percussion, the therapist uses cupped hands to gently tap over the diseased lung lobe in an even and steady rhythm. The cupping should produce a hollow tapping rather than a slapping sound and should be done between 100 and

BOX 145-3 ***Conditions That May Preclude the Use of Postural Drainage***

Active pulmonary edema
Congestive heart failure
Severe obesity
Increased intracranial pressure or head trauma
Hemodynamic instability
Recent cervical, cranial thoracic, or ocular surgery
Vertebral body instability
Patient intolerance of the procedure

BOX 145-4 *Contraindications to the Use of Percussion and Vibration*

Rib fractures, flail chest, or other thoracic trauma
Coagulopathy
Pneumothorax, pulmonary contusions, or other chest trauma
Cervical or cranial thoracic subcutaneous emphysema
Pulmonary embolism
Frequent regurgitation
Patient intolerance of the procedure

400 times per minute for 2 to 4 minutes. Percussion is done throughout the entire respiratory cycle.

Vibration is performed following each percussion cycle and only during the exhalation phase of respiration. The therapist uses full hand contact on the animal's chest to oscillate or shake the chest wall throughout the entire expiration. The hands should lie flat and remain placed over the area of diseased lung field. Vibration should be done during four to six consecutive exhalations following each set of percussions. Percussion and vibration are contraindicated in the conditions listed in Box 145-4.

SUMMARY

Veterinary rehabilitation therapy offers highly effective, noninvasive treatment options for the unique subset of veterinary patients that are critically ill. Early intervention with comprehensive, individualized programs should be considered standard of care for every critical care patient.

REFERENCES

1. Genc A: Early mobilization of the critically ill patients: toward standardization, Crit Care Med 40(4):1346-1347, 2012.
2. Bemis-Dougherty AR, Smith JM: What follows survival of critical illness? Physical therapists' management of patients with post-intensive care syndrome, Phys Ther 93:179-185, 2013.
3. Denely L, Bernay S: Physiotherapy in the intensive care unit, Phys Ther Rev 11(1):49-56, 2006.
4. Cirio S, Piaggi GS, DeMattia E, et al: Muscle retraining in ICU patients, Minerva Anestesiol 68(5):341-345, 2003.
5. Millis DL, Levine D, Taylor R: Canine rehabilitation and physical therapy, St Louis, 2004, Saunders.
6. Llano-Diez M, Renaud G, Anderson M, et al: Mechanisms underlying intensive care unit muscle wasting and effects of passive mechanical loading, Crit Care 16(5):R209, 2012.
7. Kress J: Clinical trials of early mobilization of critically ill patients, Crit Care Med 37(10):S442-S447, 2009.
8. Morris P, Goad A, Thompson C, et al: Early intensive care unit mobility therapy in the treatment of acute respiratory failure, Crit Care Med 36(8):2238-2243, 2008.
9. Needham DM: Mobilizing patients in the intensive care unit: improving neuromuscular weakness and physical function, JAMA 300:1685-1690, 2008.
10. Needham D, Trvong A, Fan E: Technology to enhance physical rehabilitation of critically ill patients, Crit Care Med 3(10):S436-S441, 2009.
11. Cameron M: Physical agents in rehabilitation: from research to practice, ed 2, St Louis, 2003, Saunders.
12. Robinson N: Acupuncture, massage can get the gut going, Vet Pract News, pp 36-38, February 2011.
13. Robinson N: Small animal manual therapy. In Proceedings Pennsylvania Veterinary Medical Association, 2012, pp 570-575.
14. Beck M: Theory and practice of therapeutic massage, ed 3, New York, 1999, Milady.
15. Tappan F: Healing massage techniques: holistic, classic, and emerging methods, ed 2, Norwalk, Conn, 1988, Appleton & Lange.
16. Powell L: Respiratory support for acute intensive care, NAVC Clin Brief, pp 13-16, April 2007.
17. Dunning D, Halling K, Ehrhart N: Rehabilitation of medical and acute care patients, Vet Clin North Am Small Anim Pract 35(6):1411-1426, 2005.
18. Davis LC: Personal communication, April 2012.

CHAPTER 146
COMPLEMENTARY AND ALTERNATIVE MEDICINE

Narda G. Robinson, DO, DVM, MS, FAAMA

KEY POINTS

- Several complementary and alternative medical approaches such as acupuncture, massage, laser therapy, and music therapy provide clinically meaningful benefits for hospitalized patients; for this reason, these modalities warrant consideration for early inclusion into treatment plans for critical care patients.
- Herbal remedies, like medications, can help or harm. Unlike medications, however, their pharmacologic and safety profiles are lacking for veterinary patients. In addition, inadequate regulatory enforcement allows product sales without demonstration of product purity and full disclosure of the types and quantities of contents. These factors present hurdles when prescribing plant-based drugs in veterinary medicine.
- Aromatherapy (essential oil therapy) has shown value to promote relaxation in dogs but risks subjecting staff and other patients to potentially soporific, epileptogenic, or allergy-provoking substances. In small quantities and in limited sections of the clinic, however, aromatherapy could benefit some patients.
- High-velocity chiropractic adjustments and other forceful manipulative therapy maneuvers may injure debilitated patients

and should generally be avoided in critically ill animals unless clearly justified.
- Homeopathy and flower essences have no proven value beyond the placebo effect.

The intensive care unit (ICU) can seem frightening, lonely, and stressful to patients. In addition to the illness that caused their admission, ICU inhabitants face mounting stress induced by pain, tension, lack of sleep, loneliness, anxiety, and the inability to communicate their needs adequately.[1] According to one of the leading researchers in the ethics of human critical care, "Alleviating the stresses and symptoms of critically ill patients will enhance the quality of their ICU stay, which itself achieves an important beneficial and ethical outcome, an outcome that should be a priority of every intensivist."[2]

Sleep deprivation and immobilization impair recovery. They sensitize the central nervous system, causing "wind-up," which amplifies pain and stress. As a result, cardiac demand, vasoconstriction, blood viscosity, platelet aggregation, and cellular catabolism increase. In fact, "in many patients with severe posttraumatic or postsurgical pain, the ensuing neuroendocrine responses are sufficient to initiate or maintain a state of shock."[3] Pharmaceutical analgesics and sedatives may contribute to constipation and disorientation, however. Certain complementary and alternative medical interventions can offer safe and effective nonpharmacologic alternatives.[4]

ICU personnel often welcome complementary and alternative medical interventions that support the animals' quality of life and potentially improve survival. In human medicine, a 2005 survey published in the *American Journal of Critical Care* indicated that over 90% of critical care nurses reported eagerness or openness regarding the use of complementary and alternative medical interventions in the ICU setting.[5]

ACUPUNCTURE

Acupuncture works by stimulating nerve endings near acupuncture points and improving blood flow and tissue cytokine balance locally, while also impelling afferent signals toward the central nervous system; that is, the spinal cord and brain. Once there, they serve to neuromodulate brain function toward a restorative, "wound-down" functional state that affects both somatic and visceral structures. Autonomic neuromodulations help to restore the balance between the sympathetic and parasympathetic divisions, augmenting blood flow and reducing inflammatory states in internal organs and the myofascia. Acupuncture improves neurotransmitter and hormone profiles in the central nervous system, activating endogenous analgesic pathways and decreasing anxiety.[6]

Box 146-1 lists the types of conditions that acupuncture may be of benefit to in patients in the ICU.[7,8] Mechanisms that improve internal organ function include reflex neuromodulation[8,9] of autonomic function. That is, peripheral nerves supplying acupuncture points link to spinal cord loci that connect somatic and autonomic neurons as well as somatoautonomic convergence centers in the brainstem, such as the nucleus tractus solitarius and the rostroventrolateral medulla.

BOX 146-1 *Conditions for Which Acupuncture May Be Beneficial in Intensive Care Unit Patients*

Cardiac Conditions

- Adjunct to cardiopulmonary resuscitation measures
- Arrhythmias
- Peripheral edema
- Acupuncture-assisted anesthesia for high-risk patients

Respiratory Conditions

- Nasal blockage
- Sinusitis
- Bronchospasm
- Hiccoughs
- Chest wall pain inhibiting diaphragmatic excursion

Acute and Chronic Pain

- Neuropathic pain (central or peripheral)
- Arthritis pain
- Back pain
- Postsurgical pain
- Phantom limb pain
- Abdominal pain
- Pain associated with cancer and its treatment
- Ocular discomfort
- Facial and dental pain

Orthopedic Problems

- Muscle tension and restriction
- Contractures
- Tendonitis, bursitis
- Posttraumatic discomfort
- Ligamentous injury
- Sprain
- Fracture
- Contusions

Neurologic Issues

- Anxiety
- Peripheral or cranial neuropathy, neuritis, or nerve trauma
- Cerebrovascular accident
- Seizures
- Cognitive disorder
- Spinal cord injury
- Disk disease
- Autonomic dysregulation

Gastrointestinal Disorders

- Nausea
- Vomiting
- Inappetence
- Esophageal spasm
- Ileus (posttraumatic and postsurgical)
- Gastric hyperacidity
- Intestinal motility disorders, including diarrhea, constipation, obstipation, megacolon

Urinary Dysfunction

- Renal impairment
- Urinary retention or incontinence

Patients with spinal cord injury (SCI) should receive acupuncture early after admission and during their stay. Evidence demonstrates the benefit of acupuncture for dogs with SCI in both acute and chronic settings.[10] Such treatment not only promotes spinal cord health but improves concomitant sequelae of SCI such as voiding dysfunction and pain. Researchers at São Paulo State University's School of Veterinary Medicine and Animal Science compared the effectiveness of decompressive surgery, low-frequency electroacupuncture (at 2 and 15 Hz), and a combination of the two for treatment of thoracolumbar intervertebral disk disease (IVDD) in dogs with severe neurologic deficit of longer than 48 hours' duration.[11] Using a retrospective control group, they found electroacupuncture alone or in combination with surgery to be more effective than surgery alone for improving neurologic outcomes. Although this was not an ideal study methodologically, it builds on other work that found similar results.

A 2009 review pointed to the accelerated improvements made possible in sensory, motor, and functional outcomes with acupuncture. One study showed a "much larger effect of electroacupuncture on ultimate neurologic recovery from acute SCI than any pharmacologic intervention to date."[12] Another study reported that electroacupuncture cut the time for recovery of proprioception in half and stimulated an even quicker return of motor control when combined with corticosteroid treatment.[13]

Electroacupuncture combined with conventional approaches for treatment of IVDD shortened the time needed to recover deep pain perception and ambulation compared with standard of care alone in dogs with thoracolumbar IVDD according to a report published in the *Journal of the American Veterinary Medical Association* in 2007.[14] Acupuncture stimulates neuronal regeneration, possibly through stem cell mobilization and differentiation[15-17]; it also reduces apoptotic cell death after SCI.[18] Although some practitioners claim that steroids negate the benefits of acupuncture, a 2003 study in Korea demonstrated the opposite; that is, the combination produced synergistic effects in pain relief, inflammation control, and edema resolution.[13]

Relative contraindications to acupuncture include severe immune compromise or coagulopathy, widespread skin infections, and pregnancy.

MASSAGE THERAPY

Massage, or gentle, rhythmic stroking, can reduce stress, alleviate discomfort stemming from tension and immobility, and help normalize physiologic function.[19-23] The comfort massage provides can promote sleep, a vital restorative process.[24] Pulmonary function may improve after vibratory massage.[25] Patients with burn injuries and scarring may also benefit from massage.[26,27]

For patients nearing death, massage is gaining recognition as a reliable way to reduce pain, medication requirements, and isolation.[28] End-of-life patients who receive massage on a regular basis become more peaceful and comfortable.[29,30] Massage alleviates constipation and encourages the elimination of metabolic end products from tissues.[31,32] It also benefits circulation, relaxes muscle tension, settles the nervous system, and relieves psychologic strain.[31] Along with aromatherapy, massage reduced both anxiety and depression for up to 2 weeks after treatment in a study published in the *Journal of Clinical Oncology*.[33]

Dying can be lonely, frightening, and painful. Humans regard pain as one of the most fearful aspects of dying[34]; what they want is to spend time with family and friends, have pain well controlled, breath comfortably, maintain dignity and self-respect, have peace with dying, be touched, avoid strain on loved ones, and side-step the need for artificial life support.[35] With this in mind, massage can and should become routine in veterinary critical care as well as animal hospice. One human group noted, "Incorporating a 5-minute massage of hands or feet into a schedule of nursing care should be within the capabilities of all palliative care nurses."[36] Regular hands-on treatment yields important opportunities to detect precipitous declines in quality of life, typically more common in patients with cancer.[37] The growing veterinary hospice movement commonly extrapolates principles and practices from the human side to animals.[38,39] As noted by Downing in a compelling series of articles on veterinary hospice care,[28,38] "Our obligation as veterinary health care providers is to advocate on behalf of beings that cannot advocate for themselves."[40] Although medications and subcutaneous fluids may extend lives, sick and dying patients' emotional, physical, and psychologic needs for touch and movement frequently remain unassessed and unmet, as often happens in human medicine.[31] Families feel helpless when watching a loved one linger between life and death. A slow, gentle back rub or neck massage may coax a dying patient to relax[41] and shift the autonomic nervous system from fight/flight to rest/restore. Many clients express eagerness to learn simple and safe massage techniques; acquiring a skill to provide a treatment that their animal accepts allows them to regain a sense of purpose and connection. Massage practitioners in a veterinary clinic may also identify environmental and other sources of stress for the patient, such as noise (radio, television, pumps, alarms, loud voices, barking dogs), hygiene and skin-related concerns, patient bedding or mobility issues, and previously unrecognized areas of tenderness or dysfunction.[42] When death seems imminent, or in anticipation of a scheduled euthanasia, clients may ask their dog's or cat's massage therapist to accompany them during the process to treat the animal and ease the transition from life to death. This final act of loving kindness leaves a cherished memory in the hearts and minds of those left in this world, who are reassured that their treasured companion's first step on the journey to the beyond was made that much more peaceful through massage.

How does massage work? Moderate-pressure massage affects the nervous system through pressure-sensitive mechanoreceptors in the skin, subcutaneous tissue, and myofascia. Signals from treated tissue travel to the spinal cord and brain where neuromodulation occurs that in many ways is similar to that from acupuncture and laser therapy.[43] Moderate-pressure massage slows the heart rate, lowers blood pressure, and reduces cortisol levels through its modulatory effects on the autonomic nervous system, specifically the vagal nerve network.[44] Investigations eventually identified the vagal nerve network as the final common pathway. This tenth cranial nerve and the associated brainstem nuclei affect nearly every bodily function, serving as a neural expressway mediating the tightly orchestrated, restorative parasympathetic nervous system. Some of the most compelling research on massage and the vagus nerve involves term and preterm infants. For example, massage allows preterm infants to better autoregulate their body temperature.[45] Properly massaged infants show less physiologic stress and reactivity,[46] higher vagal tone, and significantly less fussing, crying, and stress behavior such as hiccups.

Contraindications to massage depend on the patient's medical status and receptivity to touch. Patients with cardiovascular instability or severe, uncontrolled hypertension may become overstimulated.[19,47] Massage should be avoided near sites of fractures, contusions, thrombi, inflammation, pain, and/or infection.

LASER THERAPY

The ability of laser therapy to reduce pain, swelling, tissue necrosis, and inflammation is making this therapy a popular adjunctive treatment in the critical care setting (e.g., in cases of snake envenomation).[48] Laser therapy supports soft tissue and muscle healing after acute injury (e.g., trauma, surgery) through its effects on circulation, inflammation, growth factors, and cytokines.[49] Photobiomodulation through laser therapy causes tissue changes that accelerate wound healing through both local and systemic mechanisms.[50]

Laser therapy has been used in a variety of patients, including patients with pain and inflammatory diseases, neurologic injury (e.g., traumatic brain disorders, SCI, peripheral nerve damage),[51] and organ dysfunction.[52,53]

Because laser therapy speeds cell division, promotes new vessel formation, and limits apoptosis, the safety of laser therapy in patients with cancer remains unknown.[54] However, moderate to strong evidence has been gathered in favor of its use for the prevention and treatment of cancer therapy–induced mucositis.[55,56]

MUSIC THERAPY

Therapeutic music has been applied in the human medical setting since the 1800s after the invention of the phonograph, and sound was used to encourage sleep and stimulate endogenous analgesia.[57] Currently, music therapy is experiencing a resurgence in human medicine and entering the realm of veterinary medicine; evidence is accruing about its neurophysiologic benefits and suitable applications.[58] For instance, playing soothing music in the postanesthesia care unit improves comfort and reduces pain.[59] Music reduces anxiety in patients receiving mechanical ventilation and in older adults undergoing cardiovascular surgery.[60,61] Listening to classical music reduces potentially detrimental physiologic and psychologic responses to percutaneous coronary interventions, and results in lower pain scores.[62] Relaxing music reduces pain after dressing changes for vascular wounds.[63] Both classical and self-selected relaxing music reduce negative emotional states and levels of sympathetic nervous system arousal (e.g., pulse and respiratory rates) after stress compared with heavy metal music or complete silence.[64] The main adverse effects of music therapy arise from either incorrect selection of music or tempo for the listener's specific problem, or stimulation of musicogenic seizures (reported only in humans).[65]

How does music therapy work? Music causes changes in brain activity and in neurohumoral, cardiovascular, and immune responses, although the genre and tempo influence the direction of those changes.[66-69] Music listening during the early period after stroke improves cognitive recovery and buoys the mood.[70] Functional brain imaging studies demonstrate that listening to music induces brain-wide alterations in processing functions related to attention and semantic, music-syntactic, memory, and motor functions.[70] Thus researchers are finding that, instead of allowing brain-injured patients to languish in silence for most of the day without any interaction or activity, one could instead fill the neural plasticity window in the postinjury phase with auditory provocation that reduces depression and improves brain function.[71] Even during brain development and maturation, exposure to music modifies protein expression in key brain areas associated with verbal learning, mood, and memory.[72]

HERBS

Critical care clinicians should ask clients to provide a complete list of supplements, herbs, and homeopathic compounds their animal receives, along with a full list of ingredients. Veterinarians treating critically ill patients often find themselves in the difficult position of either accommodating or denying clients' requests to give herbs and supplements, with little substantive information on which to base the decision. In some cases, the decision to decline administering herbs seems obvious, as in the case of proprietary Chinese herbal mixtures for which a manufacturer refuses to disclose the amount of toxic ingredients such as strychnine (a known neurotoxin) or aconite (a known cardiotoxin).[73] In addition, the interactions of strychnine and aconite with conventional pharmaceuticals, combined with the lack of evidence regarding safety or effectiveness, may raise concern as to why veterinarians continue to sell and prescribe these mystery mixtures capable of causing harm.[74] Properly educating clients about the risks posed by these products is therefore paramount.

The precise ingredients in the popular Chinese herbal formulation known as *Yunnan Paiyao* (or Yunnan Baiyao) have also been withheld until recently on the grounds that it is an "ancient Chinese secret" and "protected Chinese herbal medicine."[75] In fact, in 2013 the producer and distributors of Yunnan Paiyao were sued for failing to disclose all of the product's ingredients.[76] Problems resulting from the aconite (Kusnezoff monkshood root) found in the formula include kidney damage, allergic reactions, and death. The preparation, administered either orally or topically, has gained widespread acceptance as a treatment or preventative agent for bleeding disorders.[77] Research is beginning to emerge that is elucidating its hemostatic effects,[78-80] contents,[81] and applications in other conditions, including inflammatory bowel disease,[82] rheumatoid arthritis,[83] and aphthous stomatitis.[84] However, although some aspects of Yunnan Paiyao look promising, problems with Chinese herbs persist, including their secret ingredients and suspect manufacturing practices.

Herbs pose additional hazards due to the unknowns stemming from unique species-specific metabolism, altered pharmacodynamics and pharmacokinetics in the critically ill patient, and unanticipated drug-herb interactions.[85] Botanical substances that affect neurotransmitters, such as serotonin in the case of St. John's wort and γ-aminobutyric acid in the case of valerian root, can cause excessive sedation when combined with barbiturates, opiates, or other psychoactive medications. Common herbs such as ginkgo, ginseng, garlic, and dong quai may promote bleeding by inhibiting platelet function. Trauma victims or postoperative patients that have been receiving these herbs before entering the clinic may exhibit unexpectedly heavy bleeding. Unanticipated potentiation of anticoagulants is another potential outcome.[86] Various Western and Asian plant products affect blood sugar levels; these include *Gymnema*, psyllium, fenugreek, bilberry, garlic, ginseng, dandelion, burdock, prickly pear cactus, and bitter melon.[87] Clinicians also need to take into account any prior coadministration of herbs with insulin to optimize glucose control during hospitalization.

Untoward reactions to phytomedicinals commonly involve the liver. As an illustration of how conflicting information can confuse herbal prescribing, one of the Chinese herbs most commonly used for liver disease, *Radix bupleurum*, or bupleurum, has now been shown actually to *cause* hepatitis. Traditional Chinese veterinary medicine herbal texts and handbooks have called for the use of bupleurum as a hepatoprotectant, antipyretic, and antiinflammatory agent.[88] Despite the concerns, many veterinary herbalists continue to recommend it for patients with acute and chronic hepatitis and even hepatic lymphoma.[89]

Bupleurum's role in actually inducing hepatitis rather than remedying it is drawing closer attention, whether the botanical is included in a popular formula such as Xiao Chai Hu Tang (also known as *Minor Bupleurum*) or tested as the sole saponin in rodent models.[90] Xiao Chai Hu Tang is "the most common traditional drug in Asian countries for patients with chronic hepatitis and liver cirrhosis."[90] The revelation that humans have been injured and/or killed by the plant drug comes as a rude awakening. Not only is there obscure language surrounding traditional Chinese veterinary medicine practice, but many of the products veterinary practitioners sell to clients contain undisclosed and unverified amounts of each ingredient. This complicates investigations as to the potential cause of liver injury in a dog or cat receiving these medications. Labels also lack warnings. Because of this, clients may fail to report their use to an emergency physician examining a jaundiced cat or dog. As a group of Hong Kong toxicologists put it so well, "Herbal products should be used cautiously and enhanced pharmacovigilance is necessary."[91]

Part of the reason why the harmful effects of bupleurum are now coming to light may be the growing study of Kampo medicine, a traditional Japanese herbal system that takes a more scientific approach than does traditional Chinese medicine. Both systems may use similar plant combinations, but Kampo's emphasis on evidence from clinical and laboratory studies brings to light adverse effects of Asian herbs.[92,93] For example, "it has been well demonstrated that several potential side effects such as allergic reactions, cramps, diarrhoea, fever, gastrointestinal disturbances, headaches, haematuria, nausea, photosensitization and vomiting may be experienced when administering Kampo medicine or herbal medicines. In addition, it has been reported that Kampo medicine or herbal medicine may have antagonistic or synergistic interactions with western drugs or with some foods."[93]

Many herbs cause adverse effects or drug-herb interactions; underreporting of injury to animals from botanical mixtures makes it impossible to realistically assess the dangers of these products.[94]

AROMATHERAPY

Aromatherapy may play a supportive role in the ICU, although subjecting all animals and staff to volatile substances may be problematic. For example, some inhaled oils such as lavender and passion flower induce relaxation in the short term,[95,96] but overexposure (>1 hour) may increase blood pressure and heart rate.[97] Oils with high levels of camphor can reportedly promote seizures and for this reason should be avoided near epileptic patients.[98] Asthmatic cats may develop bronchoconstriction in response to aromatherapy.

HOMEOPATHY AND FLOWER ESSENCES

As Overall and Dunham noted concerning homeopathy, "When an approach declares itself outside the accepted methodologies of science, it should not and cannot be taken seriously by scientists. Hypothesis testing and falsification are at the very core of the scientific approach. If homeopathy and other complementary and alternative medical approaches wish to be considered by scientists, they must be shown to be valid using methods that science uses to evaluate all treatment modalities. If these fields are not willing to comply with these rules they cannot be considered scientific and cannot be used in any set of scientific and medical best practices."[99] Both homeopathy and flower essence therapy use highly diluted "remedies" made from plants, animals, and minerals, or, in the case of flower essences, only flower petals and other plant parts. Neither approach has withstood rigorous scientific testing or been shown to confer therapeutic value beyond the placebo effect. Indeed, as has been noted with parents trying to treat temper tantrums in their 2- to 5-year-old children, the results some claim to witness following administration of these "vibrational medicine compounds" may amount to nothing more than "placebo by proxy."[100,101]

CONCLUSION

Physical medicine approaches including acupuncture, massage, and laser therapy deserve consideration for most critical care patients, barring specific contraindications. Their ability to support healing, induce relaxation, and relieve pain raises the question of why some practitioners advise waiting before integrating these quality of life–enhancing maneuvers, especially when experience indicates that patients recover faster with the inclusion of these modalities. Although botanical medicine may one day accrue enough evidence in animals to play a more prominent role in critical care medicine, at this point the attention herbs receive in the ICU needs to focus more on their possible adverse effects and herb-drug interactions. Neither homeopathy nor flower essence therapy belongs in the ICU because researchers have not shown them superior to placebo. Nevertheless, now that clinicians have a range of scientifically verified integrative approaches from which to choose, opting to include them earlier in the critical care setting (rather than as a last-ditch effort before euthanasia) can provide patients the opportunity to recover with more functionality and comfort.

REFERENCES

1. Rotondi AJ, Chelluri L, Sirio C, et al: Patients' recollections of stressful experiences while receiving prolonged mechanical ventilation in an intensive care unit, Crit Care Med 30:746, 2002.
2. Silverman HJ: Symptom management in the intensive care unit: toward a more holistic approach, Crit Care Med 30:936, 2002.
3. Lamont LA, Tranquilli WJ, Grimm KA: Physiology of pain, Vet Clin North Am Small Anim Pract 30:703, 2003.
4. Chlan L: Integrating nonpharmacological, adjunctive interventions into critical care practice: a means to humanize care? Am J Crit Care 11:14, 2002.
5. Tracy MF, Lindquist R, Savik K, et al: Use of complementary and alternative therapies: a national survey of critical care nurses, Am J Crit Care 14:404, 2005.
6. Wang S-M, Kain ZN, White P: Acupuncture analgesia: I. The scientific basis, Pain Med 106(2):602-610, 2008.
7. American Academy of Medical Acupuncture: Conditions for which medical acupuncture may be indicated in a hospital setting. Available at http://www.medicalacupuncture.org/ForPatients/GeneralInformation/HealthConditions.aspx. Accessed July 23, 2007.
8. Robinson N: Evidence-based medicine: neuromodulation and kidney disease, Vet Pract News, September 2011. Available at http://www.veterinarypracticenews.com/vet-dept/small-animal-dept/neuromodulation-and-kidney-disease.aspx. Accessed June 18, 2013.
9. Takahashi T: Mechanism of acupuncture on neuromodulation in the gut—a review, Neuromodulation 14(1):8-12, 2011.
10. Dorsher PT, McIntosh PM: Acupuncture's effects in treating the sequelae of acute and chronic spinal cord injuries: a review of the allopathic and Traditional Chinese Medicine literature, Evid Based Complement Alternat Med 2011:428108, 2011.
11. Joaquim JGF, Luna SPL, Brondani JT, et al: Comparison of decompressive surgery, electroacupuncture, and decompressive surgery followed by electroacupuncture for the treatment of dogs with intervertebral disk disease with long-standing severe neurologic deficits, J Am Vet Med Assoc 236:1225-1229, 2010.
12. Wong AM, Leong CP, Su TY, et al: Clinical trial of acupuncture for patients with spinal cord injuries, Am J Phys Med Rehabil 82:21-27, 2003. Cited by Dorsher PT, McIntosh PM: Acupuncture's effects in treating the sequelae of acute and chronic spinal cord injuries: a review of the allopathic and Traditional Chinese Medicine literature, Evid Based Complement Alternat Med 2011:428108, 2011.
13. Yang JW, Jeong SM, Seo KM, et al: Effects of corticosteroid and electroacupuncture on experimental spinal cord injury in dogs, J Vet Sci 4:97-101, 2003.
14. Hayashi AM, Matera JM, Fonseca Pinto AC: Evaluation of electroacupuncture treatment for thoracolumbar intervertebral disk disease in dogs, J Am Vet Med Assoc 231:913-918, 2007.
15. Moldenhauer S, Burgauner M, Hellweg R, et al: Mobilization of $CD133^+CD34^-$ cells in healthy individuals following whole-body acupuncture for spinal cord injuries, J Neurosci Res 88(8):1645-1650, 2010.
16. Yan Q, Ruan JW, Ding Y, et al: Electro-acupuncture promotes differentiation of mesenchymal stem cells, regeneration of nerve fibers and partial recovery after spinal cord injury, Exp Toxicol Pathol 63(1-2):151-156, 2011.

17. Sun Z, Li X, Su Z, et al: Electroacupuncture-enhanced differentiation of bone marrow stromal cells in to neuronal cells, J Sports Rehabil 18(3):398-406, 2009.
18. Choi DC, Lee JY, Moon YJ, et al: Acupuncture-mediated inhibition of inflammation facilitates significant functional recovery after spinal cord injury, Neurobiol Dis 39:272-282, 2010.
19. Richards KC, Gibson R, Overton-McCoy AL: Effects of massage in acute and critical care, AACN Clin Issues 11:77, 2000.
20. Hill CF: Is massage beneficial to critically ill patients in intensive care units? A critical review, Intensive Crit Care Nurs 9:116, 1993.
21. Keegan L: Therapies to reduce stress and anxiety, Crit Care Nurs Clin North Am 15:321, 2003.
22. Hansen G: The role of massage in the care of the critically ill, N Z Nurs 8:14, 2002.
23. Hayes J, Cox C: Immediate effects of a 5-minute foot massage on patients in critical care, Intensive Crit Care Nurs 15:77, 1999.
24. Richards KC: Effect of a back massage and relaxation intervention on sleep in critically ill patients, Am J Crit Care 7:288, 1998.
25. Doering TJ, Fieguth HG, Steuernagel B, et al: External stimuli in the form of vibratory massage after heart or lung transplantation, Am J Phys Med Rehabil 78:108, 1999.
26. Field T, Peck M, Krugman S, et al: Burn injuries benefit from massage therapy, J Burn Care Rehabil 19:241, 1998.
27. Roques C: Massage applied to scars, Wound Repair Regen 10:126, 2002.
28. Downing R: The role of physical medicine and rehabilitation for patients in palliative and hospice care, Vet Clin North Am Small Anim Pract 41:591-608, 2011.
29. Polubinski JP, West L: Implementation of a massage therapy program in the home hospice setting, J Pain Symptom Manage 30(1):104-106, 2005.
30. Hodgson NA, Lafferty D: Reflexology versus Swedish massage to reduce physiologic stress and pain and improve mood in nursing home residents with cancer: a pilot trial, Evid Based Complement Alternat Med 2012:456897, 2012.
31. Gray RA: The use of massage therapy in palliative care, Complement Ther Nurs Midwifery 6:77-82, 2000.
32. Preece J: Introducing abdominal massage in palliative care for the relief of constipation, Complement Ther Nurs Midwifery 8:101-105, 2002.
33. Wilkinson SM, Love SB, Westcombe AM, et al: Effectiveness of aromatherapy massage in the management of anxiety and depression in patients with cancer: a multicenter randomized controlled trial, J Clin Oncol 25(5):532-539, 2007.
34. Gorman G, Forest J, Stapleton SJ, et al: Massage for cancer pain: a study with university and hospice collaboration, J Hosp Palliat Nurs 10(4):191-197, 2008.
35. Downey L, Engelberg RA, Curtis JR, et al: Shared priorities for the end-of-life period, J Pain Symptom Manage 37(2):175-188, 2009.
36. Buckley J: Massage and aromatherapy massage: nursing art and science, Int J Palliat Nurs 8(6):276-280, 2002.
37. Downey L, Engelberg RA: Quality-of-life trajectories at the end of life: assessments over time by patients with and without cancer, J Am Geriatr Soc 58:472-479, 2010.
38. Downing R, Adams VH, McClenaghan AP: Comfort, hygiene, and safety in veterinary palliative care and hospice, Vet Clin North Am Small Anim Pract 41:619-634, 2011.
39. Villalobos A: Qualify of life scale. Available at http://www.veterinarypracticenews.com/images/pdfs/Quality_of_Life.pdf. Accessed October 4, 2012.
40. Downing R: Pain management for veterinary palliative care and hospice patients, Vet Clin North Am Small Anim Pract 41:531-550, 2011.
41. Meek SS: Effects of slow stroke back massage on relaxation in hospice clients, Image J Nurs Sch 25(1):17-21, 1993.
42. Smith MC, Yamashita TE, Bryant LL, et al: Providing massage therapy for people with advanced cancer: what to expect, J Altern Complement Med 15(4):367-371, 2009.
43. Robinson NG: The benefits of medical massage, Vet Pract News, August 2010. Accessed at http://www.veterinarypracticenews.com/vet-practice-news-columns/complementary-medicine/the-benefits-of-medical-massage.aspx on 01-30-14.
44. Diego MA, Field T: Moderate pressure massage elicits a parasympathetic nervous system response, Int J Neurosci 119:630-638, 2009.
45. Diego MA, Field T, Hernandez-Reif M: Temperature increases in preterm infants during massage therapy, Infant Behav Dev 31(1):149-152, 2008.
46. Feldman R, Singer M, Zagoory O: Touch attenuates infants' physiological reactivity to stress, Dev Sci 13(2):271-278, 2010.
47. Tyler DO, Winslow EH, Clark AP, et al: Effects of a 1-minute back rub on mixed venous oxygen saturation and heart rate in critically ill patients, Heart Lung 19:562, 1990.
48. Nadur-Andrade N, Barbosa AM, Carlos FP, et al: Effects of photobiostimulation on edema and hemorrhage induced by *Bothrops moojeni* venom, Lasers Med Sci 27(1):65-70, 2012.
49. Fernandes KP, Alves AN, Nunes FD, et al: Effect of photobiomodulation on expression of IL-1β in skeletal muscle following injury, Lasers Med Sci 28(3):1043-1046, 2013.
50. Vilela DDC, Chamusca FV, Andrade JCS, et al: Influence of the HPA axis on the inflammatory response in cutaneous wounds with the use of 670-nm laser photobiomodulation, J Photochem Photobiol B 116:114-120, 2012.
51. Hashmi JT, Huang Y-Y, Osmani BZ, et al: Role of low-level laser therapy in neurorehabilitation. PM R 2(12 Suppl 2):S292-S305, 2010.
52. Hentschke VS, Jaenisch RB, Schmeing LA, et al: Low-level laser therapy improves the inflammatory profile of rats with heart failure, Lasers Med Sci 28(3):1007-1016, 2013.
53. Yang Z, Wu Y, Zhang H, et al: Low-level laser irradiation alters cardiac cytokine expression following acute myocardial infarction: a potential mechanism for laser therapy, Photomed Laser Surg 29(6):391-398, 2011.
54. e Lima MT, e Lima JG, de Andrade MF, et al: Low-level laser therapy in secondary lymphedema after breast cancer: systematic review, Lasers Med Sci Epub November 29, 2012.
55. Bensadoun RJ, Nair RG: Low-level laser therapy in the prevention and treatment of cancer therapy-induced mucositis: 2012 state of the art based on literature review and meta-analysis, Curr Opin Oncol 24(4):363-370, 2012.
56. Bjordal JM, Bensadoun R-J, Tuner J, et al: A systematic review with meta-analysis of the effect of low-level laser therapy (LLLT) in cancer therapy-induced oral mucositis, Support Care Cancer 19:1069-1077, 2011.
57. Barrera ME, Rykov MH, Doyle SL: The effects of interactive music therapy on hospitalized children with cancer: a pilot study, Psychooncology 11:379-388, 2002.
58. Kogan LR, Schoenfeld-Tacher R, Simon AA: Behavioral effects of auditory stimulation on kenneled dogs, J Vet Behav 7:268-275, 2012.
59. Shertzer KE, Keck JF: Music and the PACU environment, J Perianesth Nurs 16(2):90-102, 2001.
60. Lee OKA, Chung YFL, Chan MF, et al: Music and its effect on the physiological responses and anxiety levels of patients receiving mechanical ventilation: a pilot study, J Clin Nurs 14(5):609-620, 2005.
61. Twiss E, Seaver J, McCaffrey R: The effect of music listening on older adults undergoing cardiovascular surgery, Nurs Crit Care 11(5):224-231, 2006.
62. Chan MF: Effects of music on patients undergoing a C-clamp procedure after percutaneous coronary interventions: a randomized controlled trial, Heart Lung 36:431-439, 2007.
63. Kane FM, Brodie EE, Coull A, et al: The analgesic effect of odour and music upon dressing change, Br J Nurs 13:S4-S12, 2004.
64. Labbe E, Schmidt N, Babin J, et al: Coping with stress: the effectiveness of different types of music, Appl Psychophysiol Biofeedback 32:163-168, 2007.
65. Avanzini G: Musicogenic seizures, Ann N Y Acad Sci 999:95-102, 2003.
66. Leardi S, Pietroletti R, Angeloni G, et al: Randomized clinical trial examining the effect of music therapy in stress response to day surgery, Br J Surg 94:943-947, 2007.
67. Nakamura T, Tanida M, Niijima A, et al: Auditory stimulation affects renal sympathetic nerve activity and blood pressure in rats, Neurosci Lett 416:107-112, 2007.
68. Conrad C, Niess H, Jauch K-W, et al: Overture for growth hormone: requiem for interleukin-6, Crit Care Med 35(12):2709-2713, 2007.

69. Angelucci F, Ricci E, Padua L, et al: Music exposure differentially alters the levels of brain-derived neurotrophic factor and nerve growth factor in the mouse hypothalamus, Neurosci Lett 429:152-155, 2007.
70. Sarkamo T, Terveniemi M, Laitinen S, et al: Music listening enhances cognitive recovery and mood after middle cerebral artery stroke, Brain 131:866-876, 2008.
71. Thaut MH: Neural basis of rhythmic timing networks in the human brain, Ann N Y Acad Sci 999:364-373, 2003.
72. Xu F, Cai R, Xu J, et al: Early music exposure modifies GluR2 protein expression in rat auditory cortex and anterior cingulated cortex, Neurosci Lett 420:179-183, 2007.
73. Robinson NG: TCVM's silk road may lead to detour, Vet Pract News, April 2010. Available at http://www.veterinarypracticenews.com/vet-practice-news-columns/complementary-medicine/tcvm-silk-road-may-lead-to-detour.aspx. Accessed December 1, 2012.
74. Xie H: TCVM treatment of intervertebral disk disease, TCVM News (14):1, 2011. Available at http://www.tcvm.com/doc/TCVMNews2011MayR.pdf. Accessed June 18, 2013.
75. Chang L: TCM med secrets exposed in US. Global Times, December 20, 2010. Available at http://www.globaltimes.cn/china/society/2010-12/602827.html. Accessed June 18, 2013.
76. Yunnan Baiyao sued for not listing "secret" ingredients, WantChinaTimes.com website, January 30, 2013. Available at http://www.wantchinatimes.com/news-print-cnt.aspx?id=20130130000117&cid=1103. Accessed June 18, 2013.
77. Robinson NG: Chinese herb known for hemostatic abilities, Veterinary Practice News website. Available at http://www.veterinarypracticenews.com/vet-practice-news-columns/complementary-medicine/chinese-herb-known-for-hemostatic-abilities.aspx. Accessed June 18, 2013.
78. Lenaghan SC, Xia L, Zhang M: Identification of nanofibers in the Chinese herbal medicine: Yunnan Baiyao, J Biomed Nanotechnol 5(5):472-476, 2009.
79. Ladas EJ, Karlik JB, Rooney D, et al: Topical Yunnan Baiyao administration as an adjunctive therapy for bleeding complications in adolescents with advanced cancer, Support Care Cancer 20(12):3379-3383, 2012.
80. Tang ZL, Wang X, Yi B, et al: Effects of the preoperative administration of Yunnan Baiyao capsules on intraoperative blood loss in bimaxillary orthognathic surgery: a prospective, randomized, double-blind, placebo-controlled study, Int J Oral Maxillofac Surg 38(3):261-266, 2009.
81. Shmalberg J, Hill RC, Scott KC: Nutrient and metal analyses of Chinese herbal products marketed for veterinary use, J Anim Physiol Anim Nutr (Berl) 97:305-314, 2013.
82. Li R, Alex P, Ye M, et al: An old herbal medicine with a potentially new therapeutic application in inflammatory bowel disease, Int J Clin Exp Med 4(4):309-319, 2011.
83. He H, Ren X, Wang X, et al: Therapeutic effect of Yunnan Baiyao on rheumatoid arthritis was partially due to regulating arachidonic acid metabolism in osteoblasts, J Pharm Biomed Anal 59:130-137, 2012.
84. Liu X, Guan X, Chen R, et al: Repurposing of Yunnan Baiyao as an alternative therapy for minor recurrent aphthous stomatitis, Evid Based Complement Alternat Med 2012:284620, 2012.
85. Lu Y: Herb use in critical care. What to watch for, Crit Care Nurs Clin North Am 15:313, 2003.
86. Rogers EA, Gough JE, Brewer KL: Are emergency department patients at risk for herb-drug interactions? Acad Emerg Med 8:932, 2001.
87. Cicero AFG, Derosa G, Gaddi A: What do herbalists suggest to diabetic patients in order to improve glycemic control? Evaluation of scientific evidence and potential risks, Acta Diabetol 41:91, 2004.
88. Xie H, Preast V, editors: Xie's Chinese veterinary herbology, Ames, Ia, 2010, Wiley-Blackwell.
89. Marsden S: Chinese herbal treatment of cancer in small animals. Small animal and exotics. In Proceedings of the North American Veterinary Conference, Orlando, Florida, January 16-20, 2010. Gainesville, Fla, 2010, The North American Veterinary Conference, pp 45-52 (AN: 20103181461).
90. Hsu L-M, Huang Y-S, Tsay S-H, et al: Acute hepatitis induced by Chinese hepatoprotective herb, Xiao-Chai-Hu-Tang, J Chin Med Assoc 69(2):86-88, 2006.
91. Cheung WI, Tse ML, Ngan T, et al: Liver injury associated with the use of Fructus Psoraleae (Bol-gol-zhee or Bu-gu-zhi) and its related proprietary medicine, Clin Toxicol (Phila) 47:683-685, 2009.
92. Yu F, Takahashi T, Moriya J, et al: Traditional Chinese Medicine and Kampo: a review from the distant past for the future, J Int Med Res 34:231-239, 2006.
93. Ikegami F, Sumino M, Fujii Y, et al: Pharmacology and toxicology of *Bupleurum* root-containing Kampo medicines in clinical use, Hum Exp Toxicol 25:481-494, 2006.
94. Gompf RE: Nutritional and herbal therapies in the treatment of heart disease in cats and dogs, J Am Anim Hosp Assoc 41:355, 2005.
95. Barocelli E, Calcina F, Chiavarini M, et al: Antinociceptive and gastroprotective effects of inhaled and orally administered *Lavandula hybrida Reverchon "Grosso"* essential oil, Life Sci 76:213, 2004.
96. Wheatley D: Medicinal plants for insomnia: a review of their pharmacology, efficacy and tolerability, J Psychopharmacol 19:414, 2005.
97. Chuang KJ, Chen HW, Liu IJ, et al: The effect of essential oil on heart rate and blood pressure among solus por aqua workers, Eur J Prev Cardiol Epub November 29, 2012.
98. Betts T: Use of aromatherapy (with or without hypnosis) in the treatment of intractable epilepsy: a 2-year follow-up study, Seizure 12:534, 2003.
99. Overall KL, Dunham AE: Homeopathy and the curse of the scientific method, Vet J 180:141-148, 2009.
100. Whalley B, Hyland ME: Placebo by proxy: the effect of parents' belief on therapy for children's temper tantrums, J Behav Med 36(4):341-346, 2013.
101. American Veterinary Medical Association: 2013 HOD resolutions and proposed bylaw amendments. Available at https://www.avma.org/About/Governance/Pages/2013-HOD-Resolutions-and-Proposed-Bylaw-Amendments.aspx?utm_source=avma-at-work&utm_medium=web. Accessed December 1, 2012.

PART XVIII ENVIRONMENTAL EMERGENCIES

CHAPTER 147

SMOKE INHALATION

Shailen Jasani, MA, VetMB, MRCVS, DACVECC

KEY POINTS

- The relative lack of clinical veterinary information on smoke inhalation likely reflects a very high incidence of preadmission mortality. Hypoxia from carbon monoxide poisoning is presumed to be the most common cause of immediate death.
- Direct thermal injury to the upper respiratory tract can cause laryngeal obstruction. Lower respiratory tract injury from irritant gases and superheated particulate matter can result in atelectasis, pulmonary edema, decreased lung compliance, and acute respiratory distress syndrome.
- Bacterial bronchopneumonia typically occurs later in the course of the condition and is usually secondary to therapeutic interventions or sepsis.
- Acute neurologic dysfunction may be seen initially or as a delayed syndrome.
- Significant dermal burn injury exacerbates morbidity and mortality.
- Aggressive oxygen supplementation is the immediate priority to hasten carbon monoxide elimination. Supportive measures for respiratory and neurologic complications follow.
- If carbon monoxide poisoning resolves, the prognosis is good in the absence of significant dermal burn injury, bronchopneumonia, or acute neurologic signs.

A significant number of dogs and cats are likely to be involved in residential fires each year, yet little information is available regarding actual clinical cases. This dearth of information is most likely due to a very high incidence of preadmission mortality. A recent case series describing 21 dogs trapped in a kennel fire has increased the available information to some extent.[1]

PATHOPHYSIOLOGY

Carbon Monoxide

Carbon monoxide is a nonirritant gas that competitively and reversibly binds to hemoglobin at the same sites as oxygen but with an affinity that is 230 to 270 times greater and results in marked anemic hypoxia.[2,3] It is produced by incomplete combustion of carbon-containing materials and is therefore most significant in enclosed fires because there is increasingly less oxygen available.[4] The resultant carboxyhemoglobin (COHb) also shifts the oxygen-hemoglobin dissociation curve to the left, which results in less offloading at the tissue level.[2] There are three possible outcomes in pure, uncomplicated carbon monoxide poisoning: (1) complete recovery with possible transient hearing loss but no permanent effects, (2) recovery with permanent central nervous system abnormalities, and (3) death.[2,5-9] Carbon monoxide poisoning is the main cause of immediate death from smoke inhalation in humans, and death is due to cerebral and myocardial hypoxia.[6,7]

Hydrogen Cyanide

Hydrogen cyanide (HCN) is most prevalent in fires involving wools, silks, and synthetic nitrogen-containing polymers (e.g., urethanes, nylon). It is a nonirritant gas that interferes with the utilization of oxygen by cellular cytochrome oxidase and thereby causes histotoxic hypoxia.[3,6] The incidence and significance of cyanide toxicity in veterinary smoke inhalation victims remain undefined.[4,10]

Thermal Injury

Direct thermal injury caused by hot, dry air is highly unusual distal to the larynx because heat is dissipated effectively by the thermal regulatory system of the nasal and oropharyngeal areas.[6,11] Thermal injury can manifest as mucosal edema, erosions, and ulceration. Of greatest concern is the potential for laryngeal edema, which may result in fatal upper respiratory tract obstruction. Although these changes may not be apparent initially, they can be progressive. In one study, a tracheostomy was required because of laryngeal obstruction in 2 of 27 dogs with smoke exposure and was performed 24 and 72 hours after admission.[8] Steam has a much greater heat capacity than dry air and is therefore likely to produce more extensive injury throughout the respiratory tract.[6] Inhalation of superheated particulate matter (mainly soot) can result in thermal injury to the trachea and lower respiratory tract.

Irritant Gases and Superheated Particulate Matter

A variety of irritant noxious gases can be inhaled during a fire, depending on the nature of the materials undergoing combustion. These include short-chain aldehydes, gases that are converted into acids in the respiratory tract (e.g., oxides of sulfur and nitrogen), highly water-soluble gases (e.g., ammonia, hydrogen chloride), and benzene (from plastics).[6,11] Particulate matter acts as a vehicle by which these gases can be carried deep into the respiratory tract. The pathophysiologic consequences depend on the types of gases and particulate matter inhaled, the duration of exposure, and underlying host characteristics.[6,12]

Reduced lung compliance

Lung compliance may be markedly reduced as a result of alveolar atelectasis due to impaired pulmonary surfactant activity, as well as pulmonary edema caused by increased permeability (see Chapter 21).[3,6,13,14] Pulmonary edema can occur within minutes of smoke inhalation, although it typically develops over a period of up to 24 hours.[6] Ventilation-perfusion alterations also occur, and acute lung injury and acute respiratory distress syndrome are potential sequelae (see Chapter 24). A recent case report described the successful management of a dog that developed acute respiratory distress syndrome following smoke inhalation.[14a]

Airway damage and obstruction

The mucociliary escalator is significantly impaired following smoke inhalation. Progressive mucosal edema may be accompanied by mucosal sloughing over several hours, and the damaged epithelium gives rise to pseudomembranous casts.[6,14] Marked tracheobronchitis, necrotizing bronchiolitis, alveolar hyaline membrane formation, and intraalveolar hemorrhage all may follow.[6,14] Smoke inhalation induces a reflex bronchoconstriction, and airway obstruction is exacerbated by the copious secretions and edema fluid.[6]

Bacterial pneumonia

Smoke inhalation may increase the likelihood of bacterial pneumonia by impairment of alveolar macrophage function. In addition, the stagnant luminal contents create a milieu conducive to bacterial colonization. Nevertheless, bacterial pneumonia is thought typically to occur as a secondary phenomenon following therapeutic interventions such as endotracheal intubation and tracheostomy, or due to sepsis associated with dermal burn injuries.[12,15] Infection usually is not seen for at least 12 to 24 hours and is associated with a higher incidence of respiratory failure.[6,12,15] *Pseudomonas aeruginosa, Staphylococcus* spp, and *Streptococcus* spp are most commonly involved in humans, but it is unknown if the same is true in dogs and cats.

Dermal Burn Injury

The morbidity and mortality associated with smoke inhalation are much greater when significant concurrent dermal burn injury is present.[8,10,11] This is due to both the pulmonary pathophysiology associated with dermal burns (pulmonary edema, bacterial pneumonia, acute lung injury, and acute respiratory distress syndrome) and to burn management requirements, including more aggressive fluid therapy and repeated general anesthesia (see Chapter 140).[10,11]

HISTORY

If owner contact is possible, a full medical history should be obtained at the appropriate time. The current illness is usually related to being involved in an enclosed-space fire, and the duration of exposure and types of materials involved in the fire should be ascertained. The patient's neurologic status at the scene predominantly reflects the degree of carbon monoxide poisoning. Paroxysmal or intractable coughing may suggest the inhalation of more irritating gases.

PHYSICAL EXAMINATION

Physical examination findings depend on a number of factors, including the type, severity, and duration of smoke inhalation; the presence of dermal burn injuries; the use or nonuse of oxygen supplementation by human paramedics; the delay in arrival at the hospital; and the patient's preexisting health status.

Neurologic abnormalities on admission may include reduced mental status, from depression through coma, as well as anxiety, agitation, ataxia, and convulsions. In one case series dogs with altered mental status at the time of presentation had a significantly increased COHb concentration at presentation compared with normal dogs.[1] New neurologic signs have been reported after 2 to 6 days in dogs that had neurologic dysfunction initially.[16,17] Lethargy may be a common finding in cats.[18]

Respiratory signs may be absent initially and can take 24 hours or more to develop; however, two studies found that animals without respiratory abnormalities at admission typically did not go on to develop any significant problems.[8,14,18] Clinical signs include tachypnea, panting (dogs), open-mouth breathing, dyspnea, inspiratory stridor, harsh lung sounds, expiratory wheezes, and crackles.[1,6,8] In one report dogs with increased respiratory effort and abnormal auscultation findings had significantly greater carboxyhemoglobinemia than normal dogs.[1]

Cardiovascular findings may or may not be normal and depend on both the myocardial effects of carbon monoxide and HCN toxicity and the coexistence of significant dermal burn injury. Cardiovascular status tends to normalize quickly in uncomplicated cases, but complicated cases are more likely to show a range of cardiovascular abnormalities that persist for a longer period.[6,12,18] The cherry red appearance of mucous membranes (and skin) attributed to carboxyhemoglobinemia is rarely witnessed in clinical cases. This probably reflects a high level of preadmission mortality in patients that would fall into this category.[7] Individuals that live long enough to be treated are more likely to have either normal or hyperemic mucous membranes. Hyperemia may be due to carboxyhemoglobinemia, cyanide toxicosis, systemic vasodilation, and local vasodilation due to mucosal irritation, and this may mask both concurrent perfusion abnormalities and cyanosis.[8]

Rectal temperature may be normal, decreased, or increased.[1,8] The animal's coat is likely to smell of smoke. Ptyalism may be present and there may be evidence of soot in the oral cavity (or on microscopic examination of saliva). Mucosal edema and burns inside the oral cavity as well as on the face and lips may suggest smoke inhalation injury to the respiratory tract, but such findings are associated with a high incidence of false positives in humans.[14] In two retrospective veterinary studies of smoke exposure, only 1 of the 27 dogs and none of the 22 cats had a major dermal burn injury; minor injuries such as singed hair and skin lacerations were more common in dogs.[8,18] Evidence of ocular irritation and injury may be present.

CLINICAL EVALUATION

Arterial Blood Gas Analysis

Initially, when carbon monoxide (and HCN) poisoning is likely to be the predominant cause of morbidity, arterial partial pressure of oxygen (PaO_2) may remain within normal limits.[2,3,6] Oxygen saturation based on pulse oximetry may also appear normal because these devices do not differentiate between COHb and oxyhemoglobin.[4] Co-oximetry allows direct measurement of oxyhemoglobin and COHb (see Chapter 186).[10] A reduction in the arterial-venous oxygen gradient may be suggestive of significant HCN toxicity.[10,19] Repeated arterial blood gas measurements are invaluable in detection and monitoring of the potentially progressive respiratory complications of smoke inhalation and may reveal impaired oxygenation and/or ventilation.

Acid-Base Status

Acidemia is likely and may be of respiratory, metabolic, or mixed origin.[6,11,12] Hyperlactatemia may be present as a result of tissue hypoxia, and excessively high plasma lactate levels at admission are a sensitive indicator of HCN intoxication (independent of hypoxemia) in humans.[19]

Thoracic Radiography

Thoracic radiographic abnormalities may be absent initially when injury is confined to the airways but usually appear within the first 24 hours and can be expected in 70% to 80% of affected dogs and cats.* Radiographic changes do not always correlate with either the severity of respiratory tract injury or patient morbidity; serial studies may be needed.[6,8,18] An asymmetric radiographic pattern consistent with pulmonary edema is typical with alveolar, interstitial, and peribronchial changes.[6,8,18,20] Diffuse coalescing consolidation, collapse of the right middle lung lobe, and pleural effusion (especially in cats) have all been reported.[6,8,18] If bacterial pneumonia develops, a more pronounced alveolar pattern with air bronchograms can be expected.[6] Computed tomography is likely to offer a more sensitive means of detecting lung injury earlier, but currently there is only limited published information on this topic for human patients and experimental animals.

Laryngoscopy, Bronchoscopy, and Transtracheal Aspiration

Laryngoscopy is useful in sedated or unconscious animals to detect potentially progressive laryngeal obstruction. Fiberoptic bronchoscopy is used widely in humans to examine the lower airway. The presence of carbonaceous particulate matter in the airway confirms the diagnosis, and direct visualization of the anatomic level and extent of airway injury is possible along with sample collection.[4] Serial examinations may need to be performed as respiratory changes progress.[10] General anesthesia is required in veterinary patients in the absence of a tracheostomy, so a risk-benefit assessment must be made in considering this procedure. Transtracheal aspiration may be used in veterinary patients. Samples may reveal carbonaceous particulate matter as well as cytologic changes consistent with thermal injury affecting the ciliated epithelial cells in particular.[21] This technique is also useful for the diagnosis of bacterial bronchopneumonia and for the procurement of samples for culture and susceptibility testing.

DIAGNOSIS

Smoke inhalation is suspected in a patient with a history of involvement in an enclosed-space fire along with facial burns, especially if carbonaceous particulate matter is present in the oral cavity or on microscopic examination of saliva. The results of physical examination and clinical evaluation support the diagnosis. In animals with significant dermal burn injury, and in the absence of a COHb measurement, the use of a transtracheal wash or bronchoscopy may be necessary to diagnose smoke inhalation as the cause of respiratory abnormalities.

TREATMENT

Smoke inhalation victims can be divided broadly into the following groups: (1) those that have no clinical signs and are assessed to be at low risk of progression, (2) those that have only mild signs but are assessed to be at high risk of progression, and (3) those that require intensive treatment from the outset.[4] Treatment must be tailored to this initial assessment and adapted thereafter based on regular patient evaluation.

Oxygen Supplementation

Oxygen supplementation is the immediate priority for presumed carbon monoxide toxicity and may cause significant clinical improvement within minutes.[8,15,17] The half-life of carbon monoxide is approximately 250 minutes in patients with normal respiratory exchange breathing room air but is reduced to 26 to 148 minutes at a fraction of inspired oxygen (FiO_2) of 100%.[6,22] In one case series the change in COHb 24 hours following presentation was significantly greater in dogs that received oxygen therapy (78% reduction; range, 59% to 84%) than in dogs that did not (48% reduction; range, 32% to 68%).[1] The use of hyperbaric oxygen therapy to potentially reduce the half-life of carbon monoxide still further has been reported in humans; other beneficial effects are also postulated. However, a recent Cochrane review evaluated seven randomized controlled trials that used hyperbaric oxygen therapy in carbon monoxide poisoning and concluded that there was insufficient evidence to support its use in human patients for this purpose.[23] Providing an FiO_2 of 100% via endotracheal tube is an effective, readily available alternative that allows access to the patient. Treatment periods ranging from 30 minutes to 6 hours have been described.[6,24,25] Oxygen supplementation clearly has a crucial therapeutic role in treating the respiratory complications that may develop subsequently.

Cyanide Toxicity

Usual treatment of cyanide toxicity involves administration of intravenous sodium nitrite followed by intravenous sodium thiosulfate. However, sodium nitrite may not be appropriate in smoke inhalation victims because it results in the formation of methemoglobin and further compromises oxygen-carrying capacity.[6] Sodium thiosulfate should therefore be used alone.

Airway Management

A tracheostomy may be required to treat laryngeal obstruction; strict aseptic technique must be maintained during the procedure, with regular suctioning and humidification thereafter, because secondary infection may be life-threatening. The empiric use of bronchodilators is indicated, especially in patients with wheezes on auscultation. Options include terbutaline (0.01 mg/kg intravenously [IV] or intramuscularly in both dogs and cats), aminophylline (dogs: 10 mg/kg slowly IV, diluted; cats: 4 mg/kg slowly IV, diluted), and inhaled albuterol. Supplemental oxygen must be humidified, and regular saline nebulization followed by coupage should also be performed. Human clinical studies have suggested that coupage is contraindicated in the presence of bacterial pneumonia (see Chapter 22). Gentle activity is to be encouraged if possible, and mucolytics such as bromhexine and acetylcysteine may also be helpful. Antitussives are best avoided because they reduce airway clearance.

Sedation

Animals that are agitated at initial contact may be exhibiting neurologic symptoms associated with carbon monoxide (and HCN) toxicity. Use of appropriate chemical restraint to allow more aggressive oxygen supplementation is empirically justified in such cases. Thereafter, sedation may be required to minimize anxiety associated with dyspnea. Low-dosage opioids may be adequate, and additional sedation (e.g., acepromazine) may be necessary, especially in patients with upper respiratory tract compromise (see Chapter 142).

Mechanical Ventilation

Assisted ventilation may be required due to either inadequate spontaneous ventilation or respiratory failure (see Chapter 30).[10] A lung-protective strategy is warranted. Continuous positive airway pressure, provided to spontaneously breathing patients, may be an alternative in the absence of hypoventilation, but this usually necessitates orotracheal intubation or tracheostomy.[26,27]

Intravenous Fluid Therapy

Fluid requirements are significantly increased in patients with dermal burns (see Chapter 140), but this is not necessarily the case in isolated smoke inhalation injury. Moreover, overresuscitation may increase pulmonary microvascular pressures and edema formation under the high-permeability conditions in early lung injury. Both overzealous

*References 4, 6, 8, 10, 18, 20.

fluid administration and excessive fluid restriction may potentially be harmful in patients with isolated smoke inhalation injury.[10,14,28,29]

Additional Therapies

Prophylactic antibiotics are not recommended due to the risk of selecting for resistant organisms. In animals with suspected bacterial pneumonia, antibiotic selection should be based on culture and susceptibility testing of samples collected by transtracheal wash or bronchoscopy. Gram stain examination of these samples can guide drug selection while results are awaited. Otherwise, broad-spectrum coverage for both gram-negative and gram-positive infections should be instituted and then amended if necessary once test results are obtained. Blood cultures are recommended in animals that are thought to have developed bacterial pneumonia due to sepsis.[4]

The use of glucocorticoids following smoke inhalation has been widely investigated. Experimental studies report variable effects associated with this treatment, but the vast majority of clinical reports point to an increased incidence of bacterial pneumonia with no clear clinical benefit.[4,8,11,14,30] The use of glucocorticoids is therefore not recommended in these patients.[4,10,14]

The permeability edema following smoke inhalation was said to be less responsive to standard diuretic therapy than high-pressure edema. However, there is more recent evidence in support of multimodal beneficial effects of judicious furosemide administration in such cases in the absence of hypovolemia or dehydration (see Chapter 21).

A variety of inhaled drugs are under investigation in human patients and/or experimental animals. Nebulized heparin and N-acetylcysteine have been used in some human patients; topical antiinflammatory drugs, nitric oxide inhibitors, and antioxidants are other agents being explored.[31]

PROGNOSIS

Mortality rates in people following admission for smoke inhalation have been reported to be less than 10% without and 25% to 65% with dermal burn injury.[10] Of the 27 dogs with smoke exposure in one retrospective canine study, 4 died and a further 4 were euthanized. In uncomplicated cases, dogs recovering from the initial carbon monoxide poisoning had a favorable prognosis, with improvements in respiratory signs over 24 hours. However, dogs that were clinically worse the following day were more likely to die, to be euthanized, or to require prolonged hospitalization.[8] In one retrospective case series of 21 dogs trapped in a kennel fire, 5 dogs had worsening of respiratory or neurologic signs following admission, but only 1 of the dogs failed to survive to discharge (euthanized after developing pneumonia).[1] In another study, smoke-exposed dogs admitted with acute neurologic signs had an overall mortality rate of 46%.[16] Despite initial improvement, acute, delayed neurologic signs developed in 46% of the dogs within 2 to 6 days. Mortality rate for this group was 60%.[16] In a retrospective feline study, none of the 22 cats with smoke exposure died, but 2 were euthanized due to severe respiratory or neurologic signs.[18] Animals with concurrent dermal burn injury should be given a more guarded prognosis from the outset. Although smoke inhalation can result in permanent changes to lung structure, any long-term effects on lung function are unlikely to be clinically significant.[4,6,8,10]

REFERENCES

1. Ashbaugh EA, Mazzaferro EM, McKierman BC, et al: The association of physical examination abnormalities and carboxyhemoglobin concentrations in 21 dogs trapped in a kennel fire, J Vet Emerg Crit Care (San Antonio) 22:361, 2012.
2. Winter PM, Miller JN: Carbon monoxide poisoning, JAMA 236:1502, 1976.
3. West JB: Respiratory physiology: the essentials, ed 9, Baltimore, 2012, Lippincott Williams & Wilkins.
4. Ruddy RM: Smoke inhalation injury, Pediatr Clin North Am 41:317, 1994.
5. Berent AC, Todd J, Sergeeff J, et al: Carbon monoxide toxicity: a case series, J Vet Emerg Crit Care (San Antonio) 15:128, 2005.
6. Fitzgerald KT, Flood AA: Smoke inhalation, Clin Tech Small Anim Pract 21:205, 2006.
7. Thom SR: Smoke inhalation, Emerg Med Clin North Am 7:371, 1989.
8. Drobatz KJ, Walker LM, Hendricks JC: Smoke exposure in dogs: 27 cases (1988-1997), J Am Vet Med Assoc 215:1306, 1999.
9. Rozanski E: Acute lung injury: near-drowning and smoke inhalation. In Proceedings of 10th International Veterinary Emergency and Critical Care Symposium, San Diego, Calif, September 2004.
10. Clark WR: Smoke inhalation: diagnosis and treatment, World J Surg 16:24, 1992.
11. Trunkey DD: Inhalation injury, Surg Clin North Am 58:1133, 1978.
12. Stephenson SF, Esrig BC, Polk HC Jr, et al: The pathophysiology of smoke inhalation injury, Ann Surg 182:652, 1975.
13. Nieman GF, Clark WR Jr, Wax SD, et al: The effect of smoke inhalation on pulmonary surfactant, Ann Surg 191:171, 1980.
14. Herndon DN, Langner F, Thompson P, et al: Pulmonary injury in burned patients, Surg Clin North Am 67:31, 1987.
14a. Guillaumin J, Hopper K: Successful outcome in a dog with neurological and respiratory signs following smoke inhalation, J Vet Emerg Crit Care 33(3):328-334, 2013.
15. Zikria BA, Weston GC, Chodoff M, et al: Smoke and carbon monoxide poisoning in fire victims, J Trauma 12:641, 1972.
16. Jackson CB, Drobatz KJ: Neurologic dysfunction associated with smoke exposure in dogs, J Vet Emerg Crit Care (San Antonio) 12:193, 2002.
17. Mariani CL: Full recovery following delayed neurologic signs after smoke inhalation in a dog, J Vet Emerg Crit Care (San Antonio) 13:235, 2003.
18. Drobatz KJ, Walker LM, Hendricks JC: Smoke exposure in cats: 22 cases (1986-1997), J Am Vet Med Assoc 215:1312, 1999.
19. Band FJ, Bairiot P, Toffis V, et al: Elevated blood cyanide concentrations in victims of smoke inhalation, N Engl J Med 325:1761, 1991.
20. Teixidor HS, Rubin E, Novick G, et al: Smoke inhalation: radiologic manifestations, Radiology 149:383, 1983.
21. Tams TR: Aspiration pneumonia and complications of inhalation of smoke and toxic gases, Vet Clin North Am Small Anim Pract 15:971, 1985.
22. Weaver LK, Howe S, Hopkins R, et al: Carboxyhemoglobin half-life in carbon monoxide-poisoned patients treated with 100% oxygen at atmospheric pressure, Chest 117:801, 2000.
23. Buckley NA, Juurlink DN, Isbister G, et al: Hyperbaric oxygen for carbon monoxide poisoning, Cochrane Database Syst Rev (4):CD002041, 2011.
24. Piantadosi CA: Hyperbaric oxygen for acute carbon monoxide poisoning, N Engl J Med 347:1053, 2002.
25. Hart GB, Strauss MB, Lennon PA, et al: Treatment of smoke inhalation by hyperbaric oxygen, J Emerg Med 3:211, 1985.
26. American Association for Respiratory Care: Application of continuous positive airway pressure to neonates via nasal prongs, nasopharyngeal tube, or nasal mask: 2004 revision and update, Respir Care 49:1100, 2004.
27. Orton CE, Wheeler SL: Continuous positive airway pressure therapy for aspiration pneumonia in a dog, J Am Vet Med Assoc 188:1437, 1986.
28. Clark WR, Nieman GF, Goyette D, et al: Effects of crystalloids on lung fluid balance after smoke inhalation, Ann Surg 208:56, 1988.
29. Hughes D: Fluid therapy with lung disease: is wetter better or drier desired? In Proceedings of the 9th International Veterinary Emergency and Critical Care Symposium, 2003.
30. Nieman GF, Clark WR, Hakim T: Methylprednisolone does not protect the lung from inhalation injury, Burns 17:384, 1991.
31. Toon MH, Maybauer MO, Greenwood JE, et al: Management of acute smoke inhalation injury, Crit Care Resusc 12:53, 2010.

CHAPTER 148
HYPOTHERMIA

Jeffrey M. Todd, DVM, DACVECC

KEY POINTS

- Hypothermia causes severe cardiovascular, respiratory, electrolyte, nervous system, acid-base, and coagulation abnormalities.
- Early and aggressive treatment can decrease morbidity and mortality in the critically ill patient.
- Rewarming shock is a common complication resulting from peripheral vasodilation when the periphery is warmed before the core.

Hypothermia is the end result of an animal's inability to maintain thermoregulatory homeostasis. It occurs when the individual or combined effects of excessive heat loss, decreased heat production, or a disruption of the normal thermoregulatory functions permit the core (vital organ) body temperature (CBT) to drop below species-specific physiologic parameters. The sequelae of hypothermia can disrupt the normal physiologic processes of all organ systems. Although this disruption negatively affects the majority of functions, it can be positively applied in a small subset of clinical conditions and disease states.

Hypothermia is a relatively common complication in both acutely ill or injured patients and chronically ill critical care patients. Deleterious effects may be observed on the cardiovascular, respiratory, and nervous systems as well as on acid-base balance, coagulation, and electrolyte levels. Although the normal behavioral thermoregulatory defense mechanisms, such as huddling or heat seeking, may be enough in healthy patients, critically ill patients must depend on their autonomic defenses and caretakers.[1]

The goal of therapy is to provide early and aggressive treatment to prevent further decreases in core temperature, stabilize the vital cardiopulmonary functions, and provide a means of achieving normothermia at a safe rewarming rate.

CLASSIFICATION

Hypothermia is defined as either a primary or secondary condition in which the CBT is less than 37° C (see conversion table in the inside cover for conversion of Celsius values to Fahrenheit). Primary hypothermia, or "accidental" hypothermia, is a subnormal temperature caused by excessive exposure to low environmental temperatures. Secondary hypothermia is a result of disease, trauma, surgery, or drug-induced alteration in heat production and thermoregulation.[2] Although the underlying causes may differ, the clinical consequences associated with hypothermia are similar.

Hypothermia traditionally has been classified as "mild," "moderate," or "severe" based purely on the CBT (Table 148-1). Although this classification is simple, it does not capture the functional changes that characterize the differing levels of symptoms not directly related to a specific CBT. Therefore some have proposed classifying the severity of hypothermia based on the clinical consequences at each stage, not strictly on the CBT (see Table 148-1).

Briefly, in mild hypothermia the thermoregulatory mechanisms, such as shivering and heat-seeking behavior, are still intact, but ataxia may be observed. Moderate hypothermia brings about the progressive loss of the thermoregulatory system, with decreasing levels of consciousness and initial cardiovascular instability. Further progression into severe hypothermia is marked by complete loss of the thermoregulatory system, an inability to shiver, comatose states and susceptibility to ventricular fibrillation.[2,3]

REVIEW OF THERMOREGULATION

A normal CBT is maintained by an intricate balance of metabolic heat production and heat loss. The main thermostat of the body is the hypothalamus, with temperature changes sensed by the preoptic and anterior hypothalamic nuclei. Secondary temperature sensors are located within the skin and deep body tissues; namely, the spinal cord, abdominal viscera, and great veins.[4] Temperature is sensed by the transient receptor potential family of ion channels, which are activated at distinct temperature thresholds.[1] This peripheral input from the skin travels to the spinal cord or trigeminal dorsal horn for passage to the midbrain and thalamus. This thermal information is then output to the sensory cortex, producing the sensation of hot and cold. The behavioral and autonomic responses are linked to the reticular inputs in the brainstem.[5] This system is so precise that, in humans, changes in CBT of fractions of a degree Celsius result in autonomic thermoregulatory responses. Amazingly, this can lead to a change from sweating to shivering within a span of 0.6° C.[6]

The core is defined by well-perfused tissues in which the temperature remains relatively uniform, such as within the abdominal and thoracic cavities, or the cerebrum.[7]

The peripheral temperatures can vary significantly based on activity, distance from areas of thermal production, environmental temperature, and vascular responses. This can lead to dramatic

Table 148-1 Classification of Hypothermia Based on Temperature and Clinical Signs

Core Temperature[9]	Severity of Hypothermia	Clinical Signs[3,9]
32°-37° C	Mild	Shivering, ataxia, vasoconstriction
28°-32° C	Moderate	Decreased level of consciousness, hypotension, ± shivering
<28° C	Severe	Loss of shivering, dysrhythmias, profound central nervous system deficits
Normal Temperatures[50]		
Canine	37.5°-39.2° C (99.5°-102.5° F)	
Feline	37.8°-39.5° C (100°-103.1° F)	

core/peripheral temperature gradients, which makes accurate CBT measurements important.

Heat production is secondary to the chemical metabolism of energy substrates within cells. The majority of heat production occurs by the most metabolically active systems: the brain, truncal organs, and active muscles.[4,7,8] The rate of heat production therefore depends on the metabolic rate of the body. In a normal body, this rate is determined by activity, environmental temperature, age, food ingestion, and circulating levels of thyroid hormones, epinephrine, and norepinephrine.[4] As heat is produced, it distributes rapidly to core tissues but more slowly to the peripheral tissues via convective heat transfer through blood and conductive heat transfer through adjacent tissues.[7]

As hypothermia develops, the normal thermoregulatory response is to produce and retain heat, and thereby maintain the CBT. This is accomplished by both behavioral responses such as huddling and curling, and reflex physiologic changes such as piloerection, peripheral vasoconstriction, and shivering.[9] The initial autonomic response causes specialized anastomoses, linking arterioles with veins, to open as the CBT nears 37° C, which prevents heat loss to the distal extremities. Dogs have recently been found to have an additional mechanism of CBT protection in their footpads, in which the veins are intimately associated with the arteries, so that the blood is heated before it is returned to the core.[10] This is followed by shivering, which is typically noted at a degree lower than the vasoconstrictive response. This is important because it can be metabolically inefficient and much of the heat can be lost to the environment.[5] Shivering is characterized by involuntary oscillatory skeletal muscular activity and can increase the metabolic rate by a factor of four to ten.[1,7] The energy substrate for shivering is usually carbohydrate oxidation, but in glycogen-depleted patients, lipid and protein reserves need to be used.[11] Therefore this method of heat production may be diminished in the cachectic, the very old, and the very young.

Heat loss is required to maintain normothermia but when in excess it leads to hypothermia. There are four primary mechanisms of heat loss in the veterinary patient:

- *Convection* is the transfer of heat from the body surfaces to air surrounding the body. This heat transfer is maximized when the air is circulated, as evidenced by the "wind chill factor" (perceived decrease in temperature with wind exposure).
- *Conduction* is the transfer of heat from body surfaces to objects that come into contact with the body, such as the ground, examination tables, and kennels. Immersion hypothermia can cause a profound heat loss via this mechanism.
- *Radiation heat transfer* is the loss of heat to surrounding structures that do not come into direct contact with the body, such as walls. Electromagnetic waves (photons) are emitted from any object that has a temperature above absolute zero, and this energy transfers heat.[5] This heat transfer occurs regardless of the temperature of the intermediary substance, such as air. Athletes commonly wear reflective blankets after extremely strenuous activities to limit this form of heat loss.
- *Evaporative heat transfer* is the loss of heat from moisture on the body surfaces or through the respiratory tract to the environment. Although dogs and cats have minimal perspiration, this loss can be significant if the patient is wet, either incidentally or in preparation for surgery.[2,7,12]

Many factors contribute to the degree of heat loss and require special consideration. For example, neonates have a large surface area, which allows for accelerated heat loss. Cachectic patients have decreased fat and muscle stores, which permits faster heat transfer and loss. Finally, severely debilitated patients may be less able to respond to hypothermia due to the inability either to seek and retain heat or to mount an appropriate physiologic response.

PHYSIOLOGIC EFFECTS OF HYPOTHERMIA

Cardiovascular and Hemodynamic Effects

The primary detrimental cardiovascular changes found in hypothermia include bradycardia, hypotension, cardiac dysrhythmias, decreased cardiac output, and ultimately asystole. The initial response to hypothermia includes a mild sinus tachycardia and an increase in arterial blood pressure secondary to catecholamine release via the autonomic nervous system.[8,13] The vasoconstriction of the peripheral arteries leads to an increase in the central venous pressure.[14] This, in addition to a left shift in the oxygen-hemoglobin dissociation curve, may lead to peripheral tissue hypoxia or dysoxia, causing an increase in systemic vascular resistance.[8] As the hypothermia progresses, vascular responsiveness to norepinephrine at the α_1-receptor begins to decrease, which leads to a loss of vasoconstriction and subsequent arterial vasodilation contributing to hypotension.[2]

Sinus bradycardia follows the initial tachycardia secondary to a decrease in the rate of diastolic repolarization in the cells of the sinus node.[14] This makes the bradycardia nonresponsive to atropine administration. Although the bradycardia causes a decrease in cardiac output, the accompanying hypothermic decrease in metabolic rate may allow for a balance between oxygen delivery and oxygen consumption.[15] Cardiac contractility has been shown to be dependent on heart rate in hypothermic human patients. If the patient's heart rate is allowed to remain low, the systolic function can actually increase, whereas the diastolic function decreases. Yet, when the heart rate is artificially elevated, this protective benefit was lost.[14] This protection was found only in mild and moderate hypothermia; severe hypothermia leads to a decrease in myocardial contractility.[15]

Other electrocardiographic changes include prolongation of the action potential duration and a decrease in the rate of myocardial conduction. This leads to prolongation of the PR interval, widening of the QRS complex, and, in humans, pathognomonic Osborn waves. These waves, sometimes called *J waves,* are an acute ST-segment elevation at temperatures of 32° to 33° C and have rarely been documented in small animals.[9] As severe hypothermia develops there is an increased risk of dysrhythmias. The initial dysrhythmia is atrial fibrillation, which can progress to ventricular tachycardia and fibrillation.[16] As CBT approaches 23.5° C, 50% of dogs demonstrate ventricular fibrillation.[9] A canine ventricular wedge preparation demonstrated that cooling to 26° C profoundly increased the transmural dispersion of repolarization. This dispersion of repolarization is known to be a prerequisite for reentrant excitation and arrhythmogenesis and may be directly linked to the mechanism of ventricular fibrillation in severe hypothermia.[17]

Respiratory Effects

The respiratory effects of hypothermia include decreases in respiratory rate and depth (with CBT < 28° C), pulmonary tissue injury, and oxygen dissociation disturbances.[2] Initial mild hypothermia results in tachypnea followed by a reduction in minute ventilation, bronchospasm, and bronchorrhea.[18] As the hypothermia progresses, decreased cellular metabolism and lowered carbon dioxide production reduce the stimulus for respiration, which leads to lower tidal volumes and respiratory rates.[8] Loss of airway protective reflexes and a reduction in ciliary clearance may predispose the patient to aspiration pneumonia. At temperatures below 34° C, the sensitivity to partial pressure of carbon dioxide decreases, and carbon dioxide production decreases by 50% with an 8° C fall in body temperature.[9] A degree of ventilation-perfusion mismatch may also occur as physiologic and anatomic dead space is increased secondary to bronchodilation. Finally, as the hypothermia becomes severe, apnea or in rare cases noncardiogenic pulmonary edema may develop.[18,19]

Neuromuscular Effects

Human patients display progressive central neurologic effects with hypothermia, such as confusion, apathy, impaired judgment, and depression of consciousness culminating in coma at temperatures below 30° C. These signs are secondary to a progressive decrease in cerebral blood flow of 6% to 10% for each 1° C decrease in CBT.[9,15,18] Although the early signs are difficult to assess in the veterinary patient, ataxia, hyporeflexia, and decreased level of consciousness may be observed in latter stages.

Mild hypothermia activates shivering, and ataxia may be noted. As the CBT continues to decline into moderate hypothermia, there may be a loss of shivering, which in humans can occur at a wide range of temperatures (24° to 35° C). Synovial fluid becomes more viscous and stiffness in muscles and joints appear, as well as hyporeflexia and pupillary sluggishness. Severe hypothermia brings about muscle rigidity, pupillary dilation, and areflexia at temperatures below 28° C. Below 25° C, there is loss of cerebrovascular autoregulation with a marked reduction in metabolic rate. This reduction in metabolic demand allows a degree of tolerance to cerebral ischemia, and an electroencephalogram will be flat at 20° C.[18]

Acid-Base Effects

The primary effect on acid-base status is an acidosis, frequently a mixed respiratory and metabolic acidosis. A respiratory alkalosis may initially be present secondary to tachypnea, but as the hypothermia progresses, the respiratory drive decreases and a respiratory acidosis occurs. The solubility of carbon dioxide is increased in cooled blood, which leads to further increases in blood carbon dioxide content. The metabolic acidosis that occurs is secondary to a decrease in hepatic metabolism, a decrease in acid excretion from the kidneys, an increase in lactate generation secondary to shivering and decreased tissue perfusion, and a decreased buffering capacity of cold blood.[19]

Coagulation Effects

Hypothermia has dramatic effects on normal coagulation mechanisms. The changes are associated with an apparent thrombocytopenia, platelet and coagulation factor activity dysfunction, and disruption of fibrinolytic equilibrium.

Primary hemostasis abnormalities include sequestration of platelets by the liver and spleen, which accounts for the quantitative platelet decrease. This is accompanied by decreased platelet aggregation secondary to decreased production of thromboxane B_2, decreased platelet granule secretion, attenuation of P selectin expression, and diminished expression of the von Willebrand factor receptor. Ying et al demonstrated this defect by noting prolonged closure times on platelet function assays.[20,21]

Secondary hemostasis abnormalities develop due to the depressed enzymatic activity of the activated clotting factors in hypothermia. This may include prolongation of prothrombin time and activated partial thromboplastin time. Of significance is the disparity between the clinically observed coagulopathy and the "normal" result obtained on a coagulation assay. This is due to the fact that kinetic coagulation tests are performed on warmed blood. Therefore the standard clotting tests performed in the laboratory at 37° C will not reflect the effects of hypothermia on the patient's clotting cascade.[9,19,20] Thromboelastography (TEG) studies on hypothermic blood have resulted in mixed outcomes. In a recent study, blood from healthy dogs was cooled ex vivo to a range of hypothermic temperatures. The subsequent in vitro assay revealed a significant association between hypothermia and coagulation parameters related to clot kinetics and the speed of fibrin buildup and cross-linking.[22] These data suggest that the clots may form more slowly but that the ultimate clot strength was unaffected. Ao et al evaluated TEG changes in the blood of dogs kept hypothermic for 72 hours and found that a platelet dysfunction led to poor aggregation and ultimately to prolonged coagulation times.[23] A study of human hypothermic blood revealed no change in initial clot formation but a decrease in ultimate clot strength.[24] Therefore, although coagulation abnormalities exist, the underlying pathophysiology is still unclear, and coagulation testing should be performed with this in mind.

Alternatively, the coagulation abnormality may include a physiologic hypercoagulability and disseminated intravascular coagulation. This may be caused by circulatory collapse, thromboplastin release from cold tissues, or release of catecholamines and steroids. An increase in blood viscosity due to hemoconcentration and red blood cell stiffening and decreased deformability may also play a part because hematocrit increases by about 2% for every 1° C decline in temperature.[18,19]

Renal and Metabolic Effects

Renal, hepatic, and immunologic complications may be encountered in the hypothermic patient.

The initial renal effect observed in mild to moderate hypothermia is diuresis, regardless of hydration status. This is often referred to as *cold diuresis* and can cause significant hypovolemia and subsequent hypotension. The diuresis occurs as a result of an initially sensed increase in blood volume caused by peripheral vasoconstriction and begins before a drop in CBT.[8,18] As the CBT drops, there is a decreased response to vasopressin (antidiuretic hormone) at the level of the distal tubule. This causes an inability to resorb water and a loss of electrolytes. In moderate hypothermia, the glomerular filtration rate decreases secondary to decreases in cardiac output and renal blood flow. This reduction in tubular function causes a reduction in renal clearance of glucose as well as the capacity for H^+ ion secretion, which contributes to hyperglycemia and acidosis. In humans, acute renal failure is seen in over 40% of patient admitted into an intensive care unit because of accidental hypothermia.[25]

Hyperglycemia may be identified in hypothermia due to renal changes and a combination of decreased insulin sensitivity and reduced insulin secretion from the pancreatic islet cells. This may be important because the dosage of insulin required to correct a profound hyperglycemia will be increased. It is important to note that, although sustained hyperglycemia is associated with adverse outcomes in critically ill humans, what the ideal glucose is and how aggressive glucose management should be are still quite controversial.[14,15]

Electrolyte levels are frequently decreased due to the renal tubular dysfunction, which permits excess electrolyte loss, as well as a hypothermia-induced intracellular shift. Hypophosphatemia, hypomagnesemia, and hypokalemia may have negative consequences on the cardiac, nervous, and respiratory systems.[14,15]

The hepatic consequence of hypothermia is related to the decreased hepatic enzyme activity and reduced perfusion of the liver.[2,14] This leads to decreased metabolism of substances and prolonged drug clearances. Common medications that have been shown to have either increased potency or decreased clearance in hypothermia are fentanyl, pentobarbital, morphine, midazolam, phenobarbital, propofol, and volatile anesthetics.[14,26] In a prospective human study, postanesthetic recovery time was lengthened by 40 minutes for each 2° C decrease in CBT.[27]

Hypothermia also causes direct impairment of primary immune functions, including impairment of chemotaxis and phagocytosis of granulocytes, leukocyte depletion, decreased mobility of macrophages, and impaired oxidative killing by neutrophils.[18,28] This could predispose the patient to infection, although in a retrospective study in veterinary patients a correlation was not found between mild hypothermia and wound infection, at least for clean surgical wounds.[29]

Table 148-2 **Rewarming Techniques***

	Passive External	Active External	Active Core
Recommended for	Mild hypothermia	Moderate/severe hypothermia	Moderate/severe hypothermia
Basis	Augmentation of patient's own intrinsic heat production mechanisms	Application of exogenous heat to the skin	Application of exogenous heat directly to the core organs
Applications	Insulated blankets Reflective blankets	Warm air convection Warm water blanket Radiant heat Warm water bottles	Heated infusions Warmed humidified air Peritoneal lavage with heated fluid Thoracic lavage with heated fluid
Complications	Slow rewarming	Relative hypovolemia due to vasodilation Afterdrop Rewarming acidosis	Potentially invasive Hemorrhage

*See text for details.

CORE BODY TEMPERATURE MEASUREMENT

An accurate CBT measurement is needed to determine the overall status of the thermoregulatory system as well as to monitor therapy. The pulmonary artery and thoracic esophageal temperatures are excellent references for CBT, but these measurements are technically difficult or impractical to obtain unless the patient is anesthetized. Rectal temperatures are useful in steady-state conditions but are slow to change and can read slightly high (by 0.4° C).[5] A comparison of auricular, rectal, and pulmonary artery thermometry in dogs found a strong correlation among the temperatures obtained by three methods, but measurements were evaluated only in mild hypothermia (36.6° C).[30] Therefore the rectal temperature can be used as a guide but with the knowledge that it may not be the true CBT.

REWARMING

The technique used for rewarming depends on the degree of hypothermia and the stability of the patient's condition (Table 148-2). A thorough understanding of the basis of the available techniques allows the clinician to choose applications that are most appropriate for the individual patient, not simply the CBT. Lack of evidence-based treatment guidelines requires therapy to be instituted based on the patient's pathophysiology as well as the resources available.[19]

Passive external rewarming is simply augmentation of the patient's own heat generation by minimizing loss of the generated heat to the environment. This is accomplished through insulation with cloth or reflective blankets to minimize the heat lost through conduction, convection, radiation, and evaporation. This technique works well for mildly hypothermic patients, particularly those that are shivering, because the patients will be generating additional heat and can slowly rewarm themselves. If patients are moderately or severely hypothermic, their bodies will be unable to shiver or produce significant endogenous heat, and this technique is applied only to assist in diminishing further CBT drops.

Active rewarming, either through application of exogenous heat directly to the skin (active external warming) or to the vital organs (active core rewarming), is typically required in moderate or severe hypothermia. In these hypothermic stages, the body is no longer able to generate enough heat to rewarm effectively. This may due to the lack of a shivering response or to the underlying environment and pathologic condition that was the cause of the hypothermia.[12,19]

Active external rewarming (AER) is the application of exogenous heat to the skin through a variety of methods. Although AER can help rewarm a moderately hypothermic patient, there are a number of complications that must be considered. Surface rewarming causes peripheral vasodilation, and this can lead to a relative hypovolemia and hypotension termed *rewarming shock.* Along with this is the potential for core temperature *afterdrop,* in which the colder peripheral blood is returned back to vital organs and thereby decreases the CBT further.[2,9,12,19] Finally, the returning colder blood and associated lactic acid are carried back to the core causing a *rewarming acidosis.* These complications are most likely to occur when the extremities are warmed before the core; therefore application of external heat should be focused on the truncal regions of the body, not the extremities. Another consideration in the use of AER is that heat applied to the skin diminishes shivering, an effective source of heat generation. However, a benefit of AER over vigorous shivering is decreased metabolic stress and less afterdrop.[31] Therefore clinical judgment is required to determine whether application of AER will provide more heat than the heat generation lost through cessation of shivering.

- Forced-air surface rewarming (e.g., 3M Bair Hugger) provides forced heated air, circulated through a blanket with apertures, to permit convective transfer of heat to the patient. This system minimizes the risk of thermal injury to hypothermic skin, which may be vasoconstricted and unable to conduct heat away, and may decrease the afterdrop effect.[9,31]
- Resistive heating (e.g., Hot Dog warming blanket) transfers heat to the patient through low-voltage electricity embedded in a fabric. It has been shown to increase CBT in mildly to moderately hypothermic trauma victims.[32] Blankets that circulate warm water can also be used with little risk of thermal injury to the patient.
- Radiant heat, hot water bottles and electric heating pads are other techniques for providing AER, but the risk of thermal injury is higher than with the other techniques listed.

Active core rewarming (ACR) is the application of exogenous heat to core vital organs. In veterinary medicine, this may be accomplished effectively through warmed humidified air, heated infusions, and heated peritoneal or thoracic lavage. In human medicine, additional methods include cardiopulmonary bypass, hemodialysis, and extracorporeal warming. The rates of rewarming achieved using several techniques are shown in Table 148-3.[33] Previously described techniques for gastric, urinary bladder, and colonic lavage for rewarming are relatively ineffective due to the limited surface area involved. ACR is best suited for patients with moderate to severe hypothermia, particularly those patients in cardiovascular arrest.[9,12,19]

- Intravenous infusions of heated crystalloids (warmed to 40° to 42° C) can provide exogenous heat to patients when large volumes of fluids are required. In a swine model of fluid resuscitation in hemorrhagic shock, resuscitation with ambient-temperature fluid worsened hypothermia.[34] Clinically, it is challenging to provide warmed intravenous fluids to the veterinary patient because flow rates are relatively low and the warmed fluids will cool to ambient temperature before reaching the patient. This was demonstrated in a recent study in which a common in-line veterinary fluid warmer was used to heat fluids delivered at low rates.[35] At higher rates of fluid administration and in severely hypothermic patients, however, the results may improve.

- Airway rewarming can be accomplished through delivery of warmed (40° to 45° C) humidified air via a face mask or endotracheal tube. The effectiveness depends on the humidification level, the delivery method, and the temperature of the inhaled air. The benefits of airway rewarming are that it is noninvasive, allows alveolar warming of the blood returning to the heart and conduction to contiguous structures in the mediastinum, prevents further respiratory heat loss, helps ensures adequate oxygenation, and reduces the amount and viscosity of secretions in cold-induced bronchorrhea.[12,19] Although the amount of heat supplied is low (rewarming rate of 1° to 2° C/hr), it is typically applied with other AER or ACR techniques to maximum effect. Most in-hospital humidifiers do not exceed 41° C and would require modification to reach the known maximum safe inhalation temperature of 45° C.[36]
- Peritoneal lavage can be performed with heated (40° to 45° C) isotonic dialysate (normal saline, lactated Ringer's solution, or 1.5% dextrose dialysate solute) infused via a peritoneal catheter at 10 to 20 ml/kg.[37] A dwell time of 20 to 30 minutes is allowed and then the fluid is aspirated and the procedure repeated. This method allows transfer of heat to a large surface area, including great vessels and abdominal viscera. An additional benefit is direct hepatic rewarming, which reactivates detoxification and conversion enzymes.[19] In a hypothermia model of dogs with cardiac arrest, the investigators found that peritoneal dialysis, with appropriate cardiopulmonary resuscitation (CPR), was as effective as partial cardiac bypass.[37] The main disadvantages of peritoneal dialysis are that it is invasive, can complicate ongoing coagulopathies, and can cause electrolyte shifts requiring careful monitoring.
- Thoracic lavage is described in the human literature as an effective method of core rewarming in cardiac arrest.[38] Heated (40° to 41° C) normal saline is infused through large-bore thoracostomy tubes into the hemithorax and then extracted after a 2-minute dwell time. This allows for closed-chest CPR and defibrillation as indicated.
- Extracorporeal blood rewarming can be achieved through cardiopulmonary bypass, continuous arteriovenous warming, venovenous warming, and hemodialysis.[12,19,39] To date, the author knows of no application of these techniques in veterinary medicine for rewarming in hypothermia.

Table 148-3 Rewarming Rates (Degrees Celsius per Hour)[33]

	Passive External Rewarming	Active External Rewarming	Inhalation of Warm Air	Peritoneal Lavage
First hour	1.4	1.5	1.0-2.5	1.5
Second hour	1.4	2.4	2.0	2.5

THERAPY

The aggressiveness of therapy for hypothermia depends on the patient's current clinical consequences. An initial approach is aimed at stabilizing the patient's condition and starting a slow rewarming process as dictated by the severity of signs. Recommended monitoring parameters are listed in Table 148-4.

- *Prevention of further decreases in CBT* is indicated in all cases of hypothermia. This is best accomplished through passive rewarming techniques. Ideally, if the patient is wet, the patient should be dried, contact with cold surfaces should be prevented, and administration of large volumes of ambient-temperature intravenous fluids should be avoided.
- *A safe and steady rewarming rate* should be established, typically 0.5° C/hr to 2.0° C/hr, through use of the appropriate active external and active core rewarming methods.[12,19]
- *Stability of the cardiopulmonary system* should be achieved and maintained through appropriate fluid therapy. Most fluid shifts will be reversed by rewarming, and therefore in mild hypothermia only modest rates of fluid administration will be required. As the severity of hypothermia progresses, the complications of volume shifts and increased blood viscosity, increased vascular permeability, and low-flow states will dictate aggressive fluid resuscitation. It

Table 148-4 Monitoring Recommendations and Potential Errors*

Diagnostic Test	Common Result	Comment
Blood pressure	Hypotension	Peripheral vasoconstriction may make result unreliable; consider direct arterial or Doppler monitoring.[19]
Electrocardiogram	Bradycardia, atrial/ventricular dysrhythmias	
Glucose level	Hyperglycemia, hypoglycemia	Insulin administration may be ineffective until CBT is higher than 30°-32° C.[19]
Electrolyte levels	Hypokalemia	Vigilant monitoring needed for resultant hyperkalemia during rewarming due to extracellular shifts.
Complete blood count	Hemoconcentration	Hematocrit increases by 2% for every 1° C drop in CBT.[18]
Blood gas analysis	Mixed acidosis	
Coagulation panel	Normal or hypocoagulable	Laboratory error is possible due to warming of blood.
Chemistry panel	Elevated levels of liver enzymes and lactate	
Oxygen saturation (by pulse oximetry)	Hypoxemia	Vasoconstriction limits usefulness.[12]

CBT, Core body temperature.
*See text for details.

is important to note that, in severe hypothermia, it may be impossible to achieve complete stability without significant rewarming. Therefore the aggressiveness of rewarming will need to be altered appropriately.

- *Appropriate physiologic support* should be provided as dictated by clinicopathologic findings. Glucose may need to be administered in mild to moderate hypothermia because there can be increased catecholamine and cortisol production.[2] In moderate to severe hypothermia, on the other hand, a profound hyperglycemia may develop secondary to decreased insulin sensitivity and secretion, and insulin therapy may be required. Electrolyte alterations may require supplementation, particularly of potassium. Acid-base alterations typically correct with rewarming, but cardiopulmonary support may require attention in patients with severe acidosis.[13,14]
- *Anticipation and prevention of known hypothermic complications* should be part of the therapeutic plan. Coagulopathies require minimizing the use of invasive procedures. The patient should be monitored carefully for hypovolemia secondary to cold diuresis and natriuresis. The increased incidence of infection may require empirical antibiotic therapy. And dysrhythmias associated with rewarming or overly aggressive handling may require antiarrhythmics.

Cardiopulmonary Resuscitation

There are some unique challenges in hypothermic cardiopulmonary arrest that require consideration. Importantly, in severe hypothermia, the patient may appear pulseless, have a nonauscultable heartbeat, and even have an apparent asystolic rhythm on electrocardiogram. These changes are due to severe bradycardia, peripheral vasoconstriction, and hypotension, which can lead to the erroneous assessment of cardiopulmonary arrest.[9,19] Lack of organized cardiac function can be confirmed with assessment of cardiac wall motion by echocardiogram if possible. Because return of spontaneous circulation may not occur until severe hypothermia has been addressed, the duration of CPR may depend on the length of time it takes to warm the patient. An extreme example is a human patient experiencing accidental hypothermia who was successfully resuscitated after 6.5 hours of closed chest compressions.[40]

THERAPEUTIC HYPOTHERMIA

Induction or prolongation of hypothermia as a therapeutic technique has been shown to be of benefit in a number of disease states.[13] A large body of evidence supports the use of mild therapeutic hypothermia (target temperature, 32° to 34° C) to prevent or limit damage following return of spontaneous circulation after cardiac arrest in humans.[41,42] Of importance for veterinarians, the initial data came from studies in dogs.[43-46] The neuroprotection afforded by hypothermia is thought to be due to the prevention of apoptosis after cellular injury, retardation of destructive enzymatic reactions, suppression of free radical reactions, and reduction in cerebral oxygen demand.[41]

In one experimental study, mild or moderate hypothermia during prolonged CPR in dogs improved outcome and preserved extracerebral organ viability.[47] A case report describes the successful use of therapeutic hypothermia in a dog with intractable seizures following a traumatic brain injury. In this latter case, the patient was cooled to 33° to 35° C for the neuroprotective effects while undergoing mechanical ventilation.[48]

The Reassessment Campaign on Veterinary Resuscitation (RECOVER) initiative examined the evidence for the use of mild therapeutic hypothermia and concluded that the data suggest a beneficial effect on neurologically intact survival when the hypothermia is instituted as soon as possible after restoration of spontaneous circulation and maintained for longer than 12 hours; however, the practical aspects of its clinical application with regard to onset, level, and duration still need to be determined.[49]

REFERENCES

1. Sessler DI: Thermoregulatory defense mechanisms, Crit Care Med 37:S203, 2009.
2. Oncken AK, Kirby R, Rudloff E: Hypothermia in critically ill dogs and cats, Compend Contin Educ Small Anim Pract 23:506, 2001.
3. Giesbrecht GG: Emergency treatment of hypothermia, Emerg Med 13:9, 2001.
4. Guyton AC, Hall JE, editors: The textbook of medical physiology, ed 10, Philadelphia, 2000, Saunders.
5. Crawshaw LI, Nagashima K, Yoda T, et al: Thermoregulation. In Auerbach PS, editor: Wilderness medicine, ed 6, Philadelphia, 2012, Elsevier.
6. Pitoni S, Sinclair HL, Andrews PJ: Aspects of thermoregulation physiology, Curr Opin Crit Care 17:115, 2011.
7. Sessler DI: Perioperative heat balance, Anesthesiology 92:578, 2000.
8. Armstrong SR, Roberts BK, Aronson M: Perioperative hypothermia, J Vet Emerg Crit Care (San Antonio) 15:32, 2005.
9. Wingfield WE: Accidental hypothermia. In Wingfield WE, Raffe MR, editors: Veterinary ICU book, Jackson Hole, Wyo, 2002, Teton NewMedia.
10. Ninomiya H, Akiyama E, Simazaki K, et al: Functional anatomy of the footpad vasculature of dogs: scanning electron microscopy of vascular corrosion casts, Vet Dermatol 22:475, 2011.
11. Haman F, Peronnet F, Kenny GP, et al: Effects of carbohydrate availability on shivering: I. Oxidation of plasma glucose, muscle glucose, muscle glycogen, and proteins, J Appl Physiol 96:32, 2004.
12. Prendergast HM, Erickson TB: Procedures pertaining to hypothermia and hyperthermia. In Roberts JR, Hedges JR, editors: Clinical procedures in emergency medicine, Philadelphia, 2010, Saunders.
13. Polderman KH: Application of therapeutic hypothermia in the intensive care unit, Intensive Care Med 30:757, 2004.
14. Polderman KH, Herold I: Therapeutic hypothermia and controlled normothermia in the intensive care unit: practical considerations, side effects, and cooling methods, Crit Care Med 37:1101, 2009.
15. Polderman KH: Mechanisms of action, physiological effects, and complications of hypothermia, Crit Care Med 37:S186, 2009.
16. Campbell SA, Day TK: Spontaneous resolution of hypothermia-induced atrial fibrillation in a dog, J Vet Emerg Crit Care (San Antonio) 14:293, 2004.
17. Piktel JS, Rosenbaum DS, Wilson LD: Mild hypothermia decreases arrhythmia susceptibility in a canine model of global myocardial ischemia, Crit Care Med 40:2954, 2012.
18. Mallet ML: Pathophysiology of accidental hypothermia, QJM 95:775, 2002.
19. Danzl DF: Accidental hypothermia. In Auerbach PS, editor: Wilderness medicine, ed 6, Philadelphia, 2012, Elsevier.
20. Lynn M, Jeroukhimov I, Klein Y: Updates in the management of severe coagulopathy in trauma patients, Intensive Care Med 28:S241, 2002.
21. Ying CL, Tsang SF, Ng KF: The potential use of desmopressin to correct hypothermia-induced impairment of primary hemostasis—an in vitro study using PFA-100, Resuscitation 76:129, 2008.
22. Taggart R, Austin B, Hans E, et al: In vitro evaluation of the effect of hypothermia on coagulation in dogs via thromboelastography, J Vet Emerg Crit Care (San Antonio) 22:219, 2012.
23. Ao H, Moon JK, Tashiro M, et al: Delayed platelet dysfunction in prolonged induced canine hypothermia, Resuscitation 51:83, 2001.
24. Ramaker A, Meyer P, van der Meer J, et al: Effects of acidosis, alkalosis, hyperthermia, and hypothermia on hemostasis: results of point of care testing with the thromboelastography analyzer, Blood Coagul Fibrinolysis 20:463, 2009.
25. Megarbane B, Axler O, Chary I, et al: Hypothermia with indoor occurrence is associated with a worse outcome, Intensive Care Med 26:1843, 2000.

26. Tortorici MA, Kochanek PM, Poloyac SM: Effects of hypothermia on drug disposition, metabolism, and response: a focus of hypothermia-mediated alterations on the cytochrome P450 enzyme system, Crit Care Med 35:2196, 2007.
27. Lenhardt R, Marker E, Goll V, et al: Mild intraoperative hypothermia prolongs postanesthetic recovery, Anesthesiology 87:1318, 1997.
28. Kurz A, Sessler DI, Lenhardt R: Perioperative normothermia to reduce the incidence of surgical wound infection and shorten hospitalization, N Engl J Med 334:1209, 1996.
29. Beal MW, Brown DC, Shofer FS: The effects of perioperative hypothermia and the duration of anesthesia on postoperative wound infection rate in clean wounds: a retrospective study, Vet Surg 29:123, 2000.
30. Southward ES, Mann FA, Dodam J, et al: A comparison of auricular, rectal and pulmonary artery thermometry in dogs with anesthesia induced hypothermia, J Vet Emerg Crit Care (San Antonio) 16:172, 2006.
31. Giesbrecht GG, Shroeder M, Bristow GK: Treatment of mild immersion hypothermia by forced-air warming, Aviat Space Environ Med 65:803, 1994.
32. Kober A, Scheck T, Fulesdi B, et al: Effectiveness of resistive heating compared with passive warming in treating hypothermia associated with minor trauma, Mayo Clin Proc 76:369, 2001.
33. Danzl DF, Pozos RS, Auerback PS, et al: Multicenter hypothermia survey, Ann Emerg Med 16:1042, 1987.
34. Silbergleit R, Satz W, Lee DC, et al: Hypothermia from realistic fluid resuscitation in a model of hemorrhagic shock, Ann Emerg Med 31:339, 1998.
35. Chiang V, Hopper K, Mellema MS: In vitro evaluation of the efficacy of a veterinary dry heat fluid warmer, J Vet Emerg Crit Care (San Antonio) 21:639, 2011.
36. Wallace W: Does it make sense to heat gases higher than body temperature for the treatment of cold water near-drowning or hypothermia? A point of view paper, Alaska Med 39:75, 1997.
37. Moss JF, Karklin M, Southwick HW, et al: A model for the treatment of accidental severe hypothermia, J Trauma 26:68, 1986.
38. Kjaergaard B, Bach P: Warming of patients with accidental hypothermia using warm water pleural lavage, Resuscitation 68:203, 2005.
39. Farstad M, Andersen KS, Koller ME, et al: Rewarming from accidental hypothermia by extracorporeal circulation, Eur J Cardiothorac Surg 20:58, 2001.
40. Lexow K: Severe accidental hypothermia: survival after 6 hours 30 minutes of cardiopulmonary resuscitation, Arctic Med Res 50:112, 1991.
41. The Hypothermia After Cardiac Arrest Study Group: Mild therapeutic hypothermia to improve the neurologic outcome after cardiac arrest, N Engl J Med 346:549, 2002.
42. Bernard SA, Gray TW, Buist MD, et al: Treatment of comatose survivors of out-of-hospital cardiac arrest with induced hypothermia, N Engl J Med 346:557, 2002.
43. Leonov Y, Sterz F, Safar P, et al: Moderate hypothermia after cardiac arrest of 17 minutes in dogs: effect on cerebral and cardiac outcome, Stroke 21:1600, 1990.
44. Leonov Y, Sterz F, Safar P, et al: Mild cerebral hypothermia during and after cardiac arrest improves neurologic outcome in dogs, J Cereb Blood Flow Metab 10:57, 1990.
45. Sterz F, Safar P, Tisherman S, et al: Mild hypothermic cardiopulmonary resuscitation improves outcome after prolonged cardiac arrest in dogs, Crit Care Med 19:379, 1991.
46. Weinrauch V, Safar P, Tisherman S, et al: Beneficial effect of mild hypothermia and detrimental effect of deep hypothermia after cardiac arrest in dogs, Stroke 23:1454, 1992.
47. Nozari A, Safar P, Stezoski SW, et al: Mild hypothermia during prolonged cardiopulmonary cerebral resuscitation increases conscious survival in dogs, Crit Care Med 32:2110, 2004.
48. Hayes GM: Severe seizures associated with traumatic brain injury managed by controlled hypothermia, pharmacologic coma, and mechanical ventilation in a dog, J Vet Emerg Crit Care (San Antonio) 19:629, 2009.
49. Smarick SD, Haskins SC, Boller M, et al: RECOVER evidence and knowledge gap analysis on veterinary CPR. Part 6: Post-cardiac arrest care, J Vet Emerg Crit Care (San Antonio) 22:S85, 2012.
50. Plumb DC: Plumb's veterinary drug handbook, ed 5, Ames, Ia, 2005, Blackwell.

CHAPTER 149
HEAT STROKE

Kenneth J. Drobatz, DVM, MSCE, DACVIM (Internal Medicine), DACVECC

KEY POINTS

- Heat stroke is the most serious of the heat-induced illnesses.
- Heat stroke can be classified as exertional (overheating while exercising) or nonexertional (classic heat stroke).
- Heat stroke is generally associated with multiorgan derangements, but central nervous system dysfunction (ranging from mild to moderate altered mentation to seizures or coma) is the hallmark of the condition.
- Every body system can be involved, but the major ones affected are the cardiovascular, central nervous, gastrointestinal, renal, and coagulation systems.
- Treatment involves cooling the patient and providing aggressive supportive care.
- In human medicine and experimental dog models, no one cooling method has proved superior to others.
- A worse prognosis in dogs has been associated with hypoglycemia, decreased cholesterol level, increased bilirubin concentration, decreased albumin level, ventricular arrhythmias, increased creatinine values, longer delay from incident to treatment, obesity, seizures, prolonged prothrombin time and activated partial thromboplastin time, disseminated intravascular coagulation, and increased number of nucleated red blood cells.

Three syndromes of heat illness that represent a continuum from the least to the most severe are described in humans. Heat cramp is characterized by muscle spasms resulting from sodium and chloride depletion. When signs such as fatigue, weakness, muscle tremors, vomiting, and diarrhea occur, heat prostration or heat exhaustion is the most likely diagnosis. The hallmark of heat stroke is severe central nervous system (CNS) disturbance, and it is often associated with multiple organ dysfunction. A more recent definition of heat stroke describes it as a form of "hyperthermia associated with a systemic inflammatory response leading to a syndrome of multiorgan dysfunction in which encephalopathy predominates."[1] This latter definition is more physiologically based and gives a more informative description of what is seen clinically in dogs with heat stroke. Generally, clients seek veterinary attention when their pets are demonstrating signs consistent with heat prostration, heat exhaustion, or heat stroke. This chapter focuses primarily on dogs with heat-induced illness because cats rarely experience heat stroke.

PHYSIOLOGY, PATHOGENESIS, AND PATHOPHYSIOLOGY

A hot environment or exercise in a hot environment does not equate to overheating and heat-induced illness. It is the increase in core body temperature that results in heat-induced illness (see Chapter 10). Therefore the body has developed a relatively effective thermoregulation system to protect itself from overheating.

Thermal homeostasis is maintained by a balance between heat load (environmental heat and heat generated through metabolism and exercise) and heat-dissipating mechanisms controlled by temperature-sensitive centers in the hypothalamus. Body temperature increases when heat load exceeds heat dissipation. Heat dissipation may occur via four mechanisms: convection, conduction, radiation, and evaporation. As the body temperature increases, 70% of heat loss in dogs and cats occurs by radiation and convection through the skin. Heat loss is facilitated by increased cutaneous circulation as a result of increased cardiac output and sympathetically mediated peripheral vasodilation.[2] Shunting of blood to the periphery involves a trade-off with blood supply to the viscera (intestines and kidneys). Significant heat loss also occurs as a result of evaporation from the respiratory tract through panting, and this becomes the predominant mechanism of heat loss when ambient temperature is equal to or greater than body temperature.

A warm, humid environment and exercise are the two most common heat loads experienced by dogs that may cause extreme hyperthermia, even in animals with functional heat-dissipating mechanisms. Respiratory evaporative heat loss may be diminished by humid climatic conditions, confinement in a closed space with poor ventilation, and upper respiratory tract abnormalities such as brachycephalic conformation, laryngeal paralysis or airway masses, or collapsing trachea. Additionally, the work of breathing in these latter conditions can contribute substantially to the heat load in these animals. Diminished radiational and convective heat loss from the skin may occur as a result of hypovolemia from any cause, poor cardiac output, obesity, extremely thick hair coat, or lack of acclimatization to heat. Situations that combine high heat load and diminished heat dissipation may result in a rapid and extreme body temperature increase.

Most dogs with heat illness are brought to the veterinarian when the warm, humid weather begins, so the seasonal pattern differs depending on climatic conditions and year-to-year variations in temperature and humidity. In some instances, despite progressively warmer days later in the summer, heat-induced illness becomes less frequent.[3] This may be related to the time available for acclimatization to the change in environmental temperature. In humans, acclimatization to heat can take 2 weeks or longer and is associated with enhanced cardiac performance, salt conservation by the kidney and sweat glands through activation of the renin-angiotensin-aldosterone axis, an increased capacity to sweat, plasma volume expansion, increased glomerular filtration rate, and increased ability to resist exertional rhabdomyolysis.[4]

Increased body heat induces three protective mechanisms: thermoregulation (mentioned previously), an acute-phase response, and increased expression of intracellular heat shock proteins.[1] The acute-phase response involves a variety of proinflammatory and antiinflammatory cytokines. Proinflammatory mediators induce leukocytosis, promote synthesis of acute-phase proteins, stimulate the hypothalamic-pituitary-adrenal axis, and activate endothelial cells and white blood cells. These mediators are protective for the body when balance is maintained between the proinflammatory and antiinflammatory sides.

The heat shock proteins protect the cell and the body against further heat insults; they protect against denaturation of intracellular proteins and help to regulate the baroreceptor response during heat stress, thus preventing hypotension and conferring cardiovascular protection.[5] Heat stroke results from a failure of thermoregulation followed by an exaggerated acute-phase response and alteration of heat shock proteins.[1] Additionally, absorption of endotoxin from the gastrointestinal (GI) tract may fuel the inflammatory response because intestinal mucosal permeability is increased during heat stress.[6] It has been noted that many of the mediators involved in heat stroke are the same mediators associated with sepsis and the systemic inflammatory response syndrome (see Chapters 6 and 91).[1]

The suggested pathophysiologic sequence in heat stroke involves initial production and release of interleukin-1 and interleukin-6 from the muscles into the circulation and increased systemic levels of endotoxin from the GI tract.[1] These factors mediate excessive activation of leukocytes and endothelial cells, which results in release of numerous proinflammatory and antiinflammatory cytokines as well as activation of coagulation and inhibition of fibrinolysis. Direct endothelial cell injury due to the heat, combined with an initial hypercoagulable state, results in microthrombosis and progressive tissue injury. These proinflammatory and procoagulation processes and direct heat injury can lead to multiple organ dysfunction syndrome. Because of the multisystemic problems in patients with heat stroke, these animals should be assessed and monitored for multiple organ failure, with particular attention to the respiratory, cardiovascular, renal, GI, and central nervous systems, as well as the coagulation system.

PHYSICAL EXAMINATION

The physical findings of dogs suffering from heat-induced illness vary with the intensity and duration of the increased body temperature and the individual pathophysiologic responses that are initiated.

Temperature, Pulse, and Respiratory Rate

The rectal temperature may be decreased, normal, or increased depending on tissue perfusion and whether cooling measures have already been implemented. The pulse rate is usually increased as a result of a compensatory sinus tachycardia. The respiratory rate is very rapid, usually in an attempt to improve heat dissipation rather than as a result of primary respiratory disease.

Cardiovascular System

Most dogs arrive for treatment in a hyperdynamic state. The mucous membranes are usually hyperemic and the capillary refill time is very short. The pulses are often weak because of hypovolemia secondary to evaporative fluid loss, vomiting, diarrhea, and vasodilation (causing a relative hypovolemia). Sinus tachycardia is common. Rarely, a dog will have intermittent ventricular arrhythmias, which have been associated with a worse outcome in clinical cases of heat-induced illness.[3] Electrocardiographic evaluation and monitoring should be performed for all patients with severe heat-associated illness.

Respiratory System

Careful evaluation of the respiratory system is warranted because evaporation through the respiratory tract is a major mechanism for heat dissipation. Loud or noisy breathing that is heard without the stethoscope suggests an upper airway abnormality such as laryngeal paralysis or edema, obstruction (e.g., brachycephalic syndrome), or tracheal collapse. Careful auscultation for loud airway or adventitious lung sounds (e.g., pulmonary crackles) should be performed. Many dogs with heat-induced illness have been vomiting; therefore aspiration pneumonia must be considered. Dogs suffering from disseminated intravascular coagulation (DIC; see Coagulation System section and Chapter 104) may have pulmonary parenchymal hemorrhage resulting in crackles or loud airway sounds. However, in a retrospective study of clinical heat stroke cases, respiratory abnormalities were not common.[3] More recently, a necropsy-based study of dogs that died due to heat stroke revealed that the majority had hyperemia, edema, and hemorrhage in the lungs.[7]

Central Nervous System

Mentation may range from alert to comatose, with depression being the most common abnormality. The severely affected dog will be comatose or stuporous at presentation. Pupil size may range from dilated to pinpoint, but pupils are usually responsive to light. Some dogs may be cortically blind when they are brought in, but that may resolve after several hours. Similarly, head bobbing or tremors occur transiently and resolve over hours. Ambulatory dogs may be ataxic. The causes of these neurologic abnormalities may include poor cerebral perfusion, direct thermal damage, cerebral edema, CNS hemorrhage, or metabolic abnormalities such as hypoglycemia or hepatoencephalopathy, although the latter has not been documented in clinical cases of dogs with heat stroke.

Renal System

Physical evaluation of the renal system is very limited. Palpation of bladder size and the change in size as fluid therapy ensues may be helpful in assessing urine production. Acute kidney injury is a potential complication of heat stroke, and monitoring urine production and gross abnormalities (e.g., pigmenturia) is a valuable tool (see Chapter 124).

Gastrointestinal System

Many of the severely affected dogs have protracted vomiting and diarrhea. The diarrhea may range from watery to hemorrhagic with mucosal sloughing. This may occur secondary to DIC or poor visceral perfusion and reperfusion as volume resuscitation is provided. Gastric ulceration may occur as well, resulting in vomiting with or without blood.

Coagulation System

DIC is a relatively common finding in dogs with heat-induced illness. The presence of petechiae and ecchymoses or blood in the urine, vomit, or stool suggests that DIC may be present (see Chapter 104).

LABORATORY EVALUATION

An initial data set including a blood smear, packed cell volume, total solids, dipstick blood urea nitrogen (BUN) level, whole blood glucose concentration, and blood sodium and potassium levels should be obtained, if possible. The packed cell volume and total solids are often elevated because of hemoconcentration. The dipstick BUN value may be increased, likely because of poor renal perfusion, although GI hemorrhage or acute kidney injury must also be considered. The blood glucose concentration may be very low in severely affected patients secondary to increased utilization from hyperthermia and/or early sepsis. Sodium and potassium concentrations are generally normal in these patients on arrival but warrant evaluation, especially if vomiting and diarrhea have occurred or an acidosis or kidney injury is suspected. In addition, excessive panting may quickly lead to hypernatremia due to a loss of free water. An increased number of nucleated red blood cells (NRBCs) may be noted on a blood smear and is associated with a worse outcome.

Urinalysis should be performed, preferably before fluid therapy is initiated, to assess renal function or damage; however, collection by cystocentesis should be avoided because of potential coagulation abnormalities. Urine specific gravity should be interpreted in light of the patient's hydration and perfusion status. Urine assessment by dipstick often yields positive results for protein and hemoglobin. Glucosuria may be detected despite normal or even low blood glucose levels, which may suggest proximal tubular damage or recent hyperglycemia with glucosuria. Urine sediment examination may reveal red blood cells, which indicates renal damage or coagulation abnormalities. The presence of casts in the urine indicates renal damage and warrants close monitoring of urine output and renal function.

Further laboratory evaluation should include a complete blood count, serum chemistry screen, measurement of serum creatinine kinase activity, and coagulation evaluation. The most common complete blood count abnormality reported is an increased number of NRBCs[3]; as noted earlier, this is associated with a worse prognosis. In one canine heat stroke study, a value of 18 or more NRBCs per 100 leukocytes at presentation had a sensitivity and specificity of 91% and 88%, respectively, for predicting death.[8] The NRBC level typically decreases rapidly over the first 24 hours.

Serum alanine aminotransferase and creatinine kinase levels are often elevated and usually peak within 24 to 48 hours. Serum bilirubin level may be increased and serum cholesterol level decreased in more severely affected dogs. Serum creatinine and BUN concentrations may be increased as well. These increases may be a result of dehydration and poor renal perfusion but warrant serial evaluations because renal damage may be present; serial increases in renal clinicopathologic parameters are associated with a worse prognosis.[3]

Activation of the coagulation cascade is initiated by direct thermal injury to the tissues and endothelium and may result in consumption of platelets and coagulation factors. If prothrombin time, partial thromboplastin time, and platelet count measurements cannot be performed, then activated clotting time should be determined, and a blood smear may reveal red blood cell fragments and allow platelet count to be estimated. In general, there should be at least 8 to 15 platelets per 100× oil immersion field on a well-executed blood smear. In patients with DIC, the platelet count is often decreased secondary to increased consumption and/or loss.

TREATMENT AND MONITORING

Cooling Procedures

Cooling measures involve taking advantage of the physics of heat-dissipating mechanisms: evaporation, conduction, convection, and radiation. Evaporative methods include wetting the dog's whole body with tepid water and blowing fans over the body. In humans, ice water is used in this method, but recommendations are to massage the muscles to maintain circulation because extreme cooling of the periphery may result in vasoconstriction and paradoxical inhibition of body cooling. Whole body alcohol bathing should be avoided because not only is this noxious to the animal, but it may present a significant fire hazard should defibrillation be required in dogs that experience cardiac arrest.

Intuitively, wetting the footpads with alcohol seems like an ineffective cooling measure given the small surface area involved, although this technique has not been rigorously evaluated for efficacy. External conduction cooling techniques include application of ice packs over major vessels (e.g., jugular veins), tap water immersion, ice water immersion, and use of cooling blankets. Water immersion methods can be cumbersome, and ice water baths may be uncomfortable and produce peripheral vasoconstriction and thus diminish heat dissipation overall. Internal conduction techniques include iced gastric lavage, iced peritoneal lavage, and cold water enemas, although the latter may interfere with temperature monitoring. These techniques are invasive and can result in serious complications (aspiration pneumonia, septic peritonitis). Pharmacologic techniques such as administration of dantrolene sodium have been evaluated experimentally and have not been effective.[9]

Cooling measures are the only therapies for heat stroke that have been thoroughly evaluated. Many of the techniques already mentioned have been evaluated rigorously, both clinically in humans and experimentally in dogs. No single technique has been proven superior to any other, and in dog experimental studies, rates of temperature decline ranged from 0.15° to 0.23°C (0.27° to 0.41°F) per minute.[10,11] Not surprisingly, many owners recognize that their dogs are overheated and hose them down with water. This is very effective and often results in a normal body temperature by the time of presentation to the veterinarian.[3]

Whole body wetting with water combined with muscle massage and blowing fans is commonly performed. Additionally, administration of room temperature intravenous fluids may be helpful. Rarely, whole body shaving is needed to facilitate cooling in dogs with very thick hair coats. Cooling measures should be discontinued when the rectal temperature reaches 39.4°C (103°F) to prevent rebound hypothermia. Despite this, it is not unusual for dogs to develop body temperatures between 35° and 37.8°C (95° and 100°F) within the first few hours of hospitalization.[3] If hypothermia occurs, warm water bottles or blankets may be necessary to maintain normothermia.

Cardiovascular System

Severely affected dogs often are in hypovolemic shock at presentation. If cardiovascular disease is unlikely, balanced electrolyte fluids of up to 90 ml/kg should be administered intravenously to dogs (up to 50 ml/kg in cats); perfusion status should be assessed continuously and the rate and volume of fluids titrated to effect (see Chapter 60). Excessive volume administration should be avoided. Central venous pressure monitoring can help guide fluid therapy if massive volumes are required, although this usually necessitates jugular venous catheterization, which may be contraindicated in dogs with severe coagulation derangements. If large doses of intravenous fluids do not improve tissue perfusion and blood pressure, administration of synthetic colloids should be considered, with or without positive inotropic or vasopressor agents (e.g., dobutamine, dopamine, or epinephrine; see Chapter 157). Dogs that cannot maintain an adequate blood pressure without pressure support (for prolonged periods) have a poor prognosis. Blood pressure and physical parameters of tissue perfusion should be monitored continuously in severely affected dogs (see Chapter 183).

Respiratory System

Oxygen should be administered at presentation and should be continued until it has been determined that the dog can maintain adequate arterial oxygenation (see Chapters 14 and 186). Serial physical assessments of the respiratory system including thoracic auscultation, observation of respiratory rate and effort, and evaluation of mucous membrane color is warranted in dogs with heat illness. More objective assessments such as arterial blood gas analysis and pulse oximetry may be required, especially in dogs with physical evidence of respiratory compromise.

Central Nervous System

At presentation, a full neurologic examination, including assessment of level of mentation and cranial nerve function, should be performed to establish baseline parameters. More severely affected dogs may be stuporous or comatose at presentation. Serum electrolyte levels, packed cell volume, total solids, and blood glucose measurements should be performed and abnormalities corrected as warranted. Hypoglycemia is not unusual in the severely compromised dog with heat illness. An intravenous bolus of 0.25 to 0.5 g/kg of body weight of a diluted dextrose solution should be administered if hypoglycemia is documented, and dextrose should be added to the intravenous fluids to make a 2.5% to 5% concentration if hypoglycemia is persistent.

Poor tissue perfusion should be corrected and mentation reevaluated after perfusion is improved. If mentation continues to be abnormal after these abnormalities are corrected, then cerebral edema may be present (see Chapter 84). Administration of mannitol (0.5 to 1 g/kg of body weight intravenously over 20 to 30 minutes) should be considered. The head should be elevated 15 to 30 degrees above the horizontal plane of the body while avoiding compression of the jugular veins. Progression of neurologic abnormalities despite therapy carries a poor prognosis.

Renal System

A urinary catheter should be inserted at presentation for monitoring urine output in more severely affected dogs. Complete urinalysis should be performed initially and serially as treatment progresses to detect early signs of renal damage such as the presence of urinary casts. Urine output should be maintained at 2 ml/kg of body weight per hour or more, depending on the amount of fluid being administered. Mean arterial pressure ideally should be at least 80 mm Hg. If urine output remains insufficient despite adequate fluid replacement and blood pressure, then measures to manage oliguria or anuria should be instituted (see Chapter 124). If urine output remains inadequate and renal parameters increase, hemodialysis or peritoneal dialysis may be necessary (see Chapter 205). Serum sodium and potassium concentrations, total solids, BUN, acid-base status, and creatinine should be monitored every 4 to 24 hours as indicated.

Coagulation System

Evaluation of the coagulation system, including measurement of prothrombin time, partial thromboplastin time, platelet count, and levels of D-dimers and fibrin split products, should be performed at presentation and as indicated during therapy. Prolonged coagulation times, decreased platelet count, and increased levels of fibrin split products or D-dimers suggest DIC (see Chapter 104). Thromboelastography may also prove useful, if available.

Gastrointestinal System

Direct thermal damage and poor visceral perfusion and/or reperfusion may result in GI mucosal sloughing and ulceration. This leads to vomiting and diarrhea that may or may not be bloody. Sucralfate (if vomiting is not present) and histamine-2 blockers can help manage gastric ulceration (see Chapters 161 and 162). Breakdown of the mucosal barrier may result in bacteremia or endotoxemia.

Broad-spectrum antimicrobial therapy should be considered in severely affected animals with bloody diarrhea. There are anecdotal reports of the development of small intestinal intussusceptions in some dogs with heat stroke.

PROGNOSIS

The degree of compromise depends on the prior physical health of the dog and the degree and duration of the heat insult. Dogs with multiple organ dysfunction or severe CNS disturbances have a more guarded prognosis.[3] However, many dogs with severe CNS disturbances, DIC, and other organ dysfunction live without any residual problems. Severe heat-induced illness is challenging to treat, but with aggressive medical therapy dogs may recover and do well. Because cats rarely develop heat stroke, there is little information regarding the prognosis and outcome in this species.

REFERENCES

1. Bouchama A, Knochel JP: Heat stroke, N Engl J Med 346:1978, 2002.
2. Flourroy WS, Wohl JS, Macintire DK: Heatstroke in dogs: pathophysiology and predisposing factors, Comp Contin Educ Pract Vet 25:410, 2003.
3. Drobatz KJ, Macintire DK: Heat-induced illness in dogs: 42 cases (1976-1993), J Am Vet Med Assoc 209:1894, 1996.
4. Knochel JP: Catastrophic medical events with exhaustive exercise: "white collar rhabdomyolysis," Kidney Int 38:709, 1990.
5. Moseley PL: Heat shock proteins in heat adaptation of the whole organism, J Appl Physiol 83:1413, 1997.
6. Shapiro Y, Alkan M, Epstein Y, et al: Increase in rat intestinal permeability to endotoxin during hyperthermia, Eur J Appl Physiol Occup Physiol 55:410, 1986.
7. Bruchim Y, Loeb E, Saragusty J, et al: Pathological findings in dogs with fatal heatstroke, J Comp Pathol 140(2/3):97-104, 2009.
8. Aroch I, Segev G, Loeb E, et al: Peripheral nucleated red blood cells as a prognostic indicator in heatstroke in dogs, J Vet Intern Med 23(3):544-551, 2009.
9. Amsterdam JT, Syverud SA, Barker WJ, et al: Dantrolene sodium for the treatment of heatstroke victims: lack of efficacy in a canine model, Am J Med 4:399, 1986.
10. White JD, Kamath R, Nucci R, et al: Evaporative versus iced peritoneal lavage treatment of heatstroke: comparative efficacy in a canine model, Am J Emerg Med 11:1, 1993.
11. Hadad E, Rav-Acha M, Heled Y, et al: Heat stroke: a review of cooling methods, Sports Med 34:501, 2004.

CHAPTER 150

ELECTRICAL AND LIGHTNING INJURIES

F.A. (Tony) Mann, DVM, MS, DACVS, DACVECC

KEY POINTS

- Electrical injury results from the direct effects of the electrical current and from the transformation of electrical energy into heat.
- The severity of electrical injury depends on the resistance of the affected body part, the nature of the current, and the intensity of the current.
- The most common electrical injury in small animals occurs when young dogs and cats chew on household electrical cords.
- Clinical manifestations of electrical injury include surface burns, cardiac arrhythmias, respiratory distress, and neurologic abnormalities, and treatment is tailored to the clinical effects that are evident.
- Dogs and cats are less likely to be struck by lightning than are large animal species, but when struck, dogs might be more susceptible to the effects of lightning than are human beings.

Electrocution may occur by contact with high-voltage or low-voltage electrical sources or by a lightning strike. It is generally accepted that chewing through household electrical cords is the most common cause of electrocution in dogs and cats. From 1968 to 2003, a database compiling patient encounter data from several institutions* recorded that 280 dogs and 92 cats sustained electrical injuries. Of these, 54 dogs and 26 cats had chewed electrical cords, and 4 dogs and no cats had been struck by lightning. It is likely that many of the unspecified electrocutions were low-voltage injuries from chewing household electrical cords.

MECHANISMS OF ELECTRICAL INJURY

The mechanisms of electrical injury are related to the direct effects of the electrical current and the transformation of electrical energy to heat. The electrical current may disrupt electrophysiologic activity, leading to muscle spasms, cardiac arrhythmias, loss of consciousness, and respiratory arrest.[1-3] Direct cellular injury may occur through the process of electroporation. Electroporation is the development of momentary holes in cellular membranes induced by electrical shock. The holes allow passage of macromolecules across membranes, which causes osmotic damage to cells.[4]

*The Veterinary Medical Database (VMDB), Purdue University, West Lafayette, Indiana (http://www.vmdb.org). The VMDB does not make any implicit or implied opinion on the subject of this chapter.

As electrical current is transformed into heat, intracellular and extracellular fluids may become superheated, which results in coagulation of tissue proteins, thrombosis of small vessels, and degenerative changes in small arterial walls.[1,2,4] Ultimately, the result is necrosis of the superheated tissues and those tissues that become ischemic from the vascular consequences. Direct thermal injury may also occur from arcing of a current that leaves the electrical source, crosses an air gap, and strikes tissue.[1]

The severity of electrical injury varies depending on the electrical resistance of the part of the body that is struck, the nature of the current (alternating versus direct), and the intensity of the current (amperage).[1,4] Less energy will be transferred to areas of the body that have high resistance to electrical flow. Dry skin has high resistance; therefore less energy will be transferred in dry skin than in wet skin. Wet skin and moist mucous membranes have low electrical resistance; therefore one can expect high flow of electricity in these tissues and a propensity for maximal tissue damage.

Alternating currents tend to cause more severe injury than direct currents at the same amperage. Higher exposure may occur with alternating current electricity than with direct current because the former elicits muscular contractions that prevent the victim from releasing the power source. For this reason, the exposure time is typically longer with alternating current than with direct current. Direct current electricity does not usually cause muscular tetany.

Given the same resistance, high-voltage electricity can be expected to cause more damage than low-voltage electricity. One might expect more injury from 240-volt outlets used for large household appliances than from standard 120-volt wall outlets. However, current (amperage) is a function of voltage divided by resistance; therefore the magnitude of the current depends on the affected tissue as discussed previously.[1,4]

PREDISPOSITION TO ELECTRICAL INJURY

Young dogs and cats are the most common victims of electrical injury because they are more likely to chew on electrical cords than are older animals. The average age of dogs with electrical injury has been reported to be 3.5 months (range, 5 weeks to 1.5 years; n = 29); the range of ages of seven cats with electrical injury was reported to be 2 months to 2 years.[1] A database compiled by several institutions* revealed that, for 1968 to 2003, the most common age range for electrical injuries was 2 to 12 months; 186 (66%) of 280 dogs and 44 (48%) of 92 cats that had electrical injuries and 38 (70%) of 54 dogs and 12 (46%) of 26 cats that sustained electrical injury from chewing electrical cords were 2 to 12 months old. A seasonal predisposition is generally accepted, but there is some difference of opinion as to what time of year most injuries are seen. Holiday seasons characterized by use of decorative lights (Halloween, Christmas) certainly pose electrical risks,[4] but one study reported that 79% of canine cases occurred during the 6 months from March through August.[1]

CLINICAL FINDINGS

Surface burns may be noted at the point of contact with the electrical source. The thermal injury may be superficial, characterized by mild hyperemia, or may manifest as a severe full-thickness burn. Burns from chewing electrical cords have been noted on the lips, gums, tongue (Figure 150-1), and palate.[1-6] Some oral cavity electrical shocks produce enough trauma to cause dental fractures and oronasal fistulas.[6]

*The Veterinary Medical Database (http://www.vmdb.org).

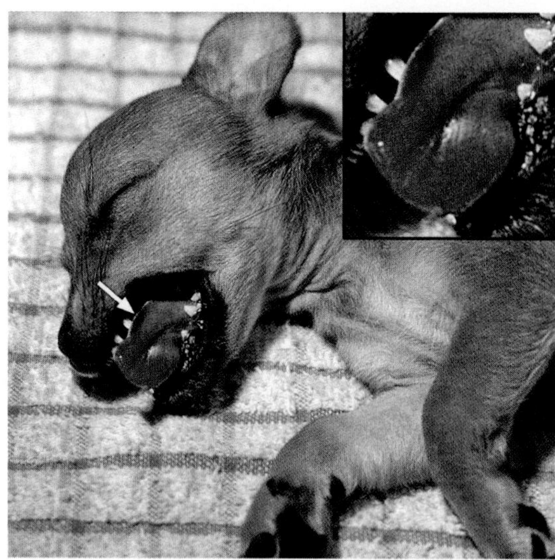

FIGURE 150-1 Puppy brought in dead on arrival after chewing an electrical cord. Note the burn evident on the left lateral tongue margin *(arrow)*.

Cardiac arrhythmias may be present, the severity of which depends on the intensity of the electrical current. Sudden death from electrical shock is likely due to ventricular fibrillation caused by low-voltage current, as with most household exposures.[4,5,7] High-voltage exposure may cause asystole.[4] Animals that survive the initial shock may experience ventricular arrhythmias. Ventricular or sinus tachycardia may be noted on presentation.

Respiratory distress is a common clinical feature noted in the form of tachypnea, cyanosis, orthopnea, coughing, or apnea. Respiratory arrest from tetanic contractions of respiratory muscles occurs during contact with the electrical source, but breathing typically resumes when the victim is separated from the source of electricity.[8]

Causes of respiratory distress include facial or nasopharyngeal edema, diaphragmatic tetany, and neurogenic pulmonary edema. Neurogenic pulmonary edema is a form of noncardiogenic pulmonary edema in which central nervous system (CNS) insult results in massive sympathetic outflow that causes pronounced vasoconstriction and systemic hypertension.[9,10] As a consequence, there is marked elevation of left ventricular afterload and decreased left ventricular stroke volume, which causes blood to accumulate in the pulmonary circulation; this results in increased pulmonary capillary pressure and subsequent edema.[9] The typical radiographic pattern is alveolar infiltration of the caudodorsal quadrant (Figure 150-2).

Respiratory distress is less severe with pulmonary edema induced by electrical cord shock than with other causes of noncardiogenic pulmonary edema. Likewise, there is less radiographic involvement than with other causes of noncardiogenic pulmonary edema,[9] and there is often radiographic evidence of resolving pulmonary infiltrates within 18 to 24 hours (Figures 150-2 and 150-3).[1]

Neurologic injury as a result of direct CNS stimulation may be noted immediately upon electrical contact. Stiffening of the animal has been noted by people who have witnessed a dog or cat biting an electrical cord.[3] The victim usually loses consciousness.[3] There may be focal muscle tremors or seizures, sometimes accompanied by defecation or vomiting.[3,4] Extensor rigidity and death may occur rather rapidly. Tetanic limb contraction has been noted after survival of high-voltage electrical shock.[11] The neurologic manifestations are thought to be due to electrically induced neural activity rather than electroporation and resultant tissue hypoxia, although hypoxia from excess energy consumption could play a role.[12]

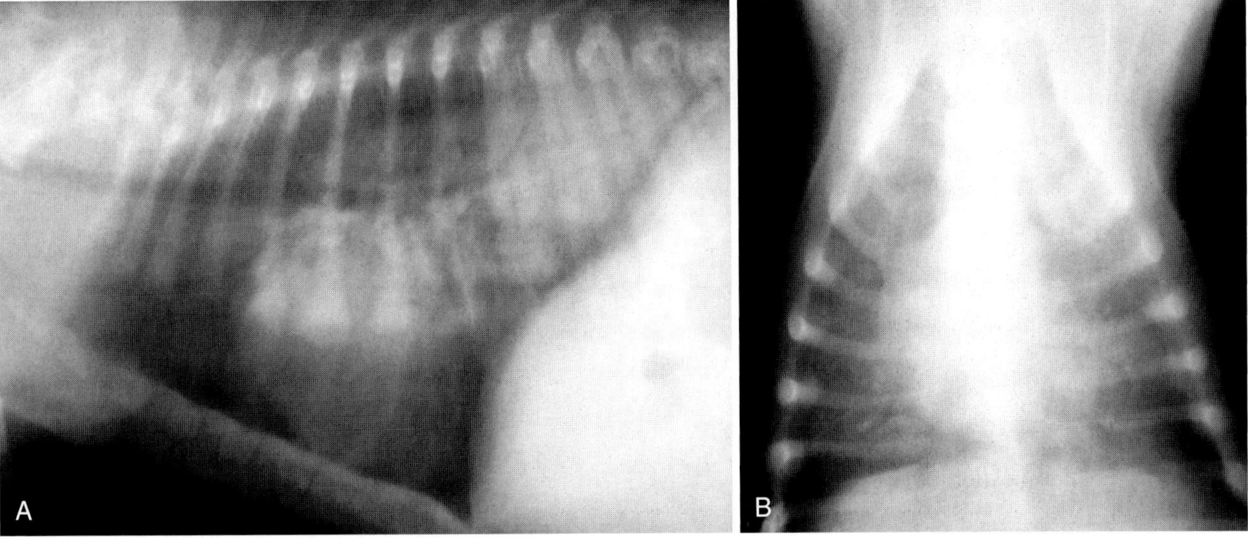

FIGURE 150-2 Lateral **(A)** and ventrodorsal **(B)** thoracic radiographs of a puppy that experienced severe electrical injury by chewing on an electrical cord. Note the prominent infiltration of the caudodorsal lung fields. *(Courtesy Dr. Everett Aronson.)*

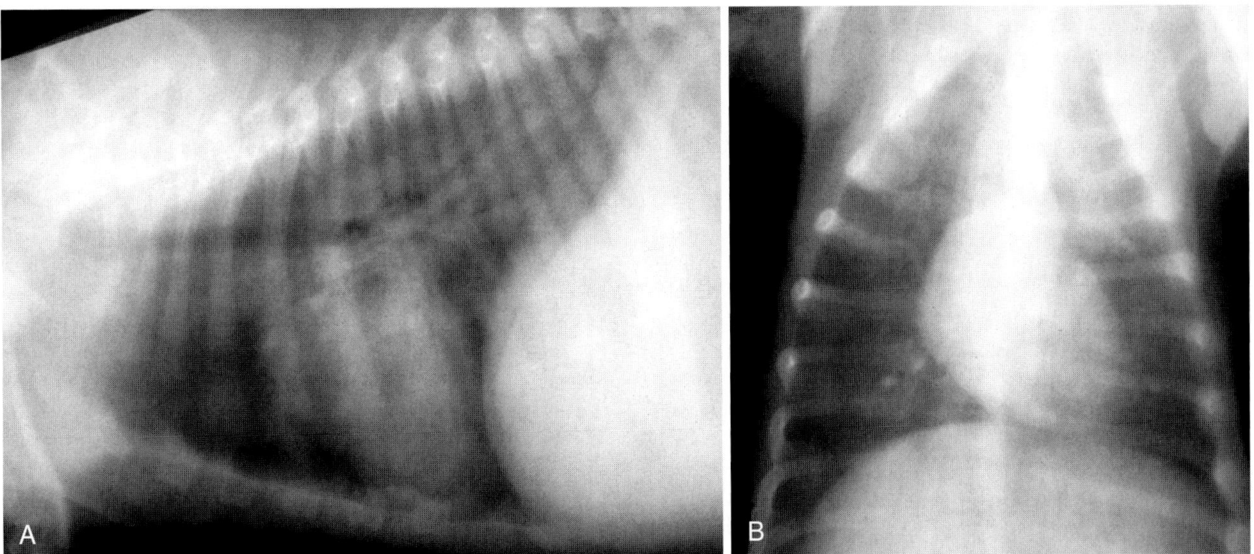

FIGURE 150-3 Lateral **(A)** and ventrodorsal **(B)** thoracic radiographs of the puppy in Figure 150-2 taken approximately 24 hours after the radiographs in Figure 150-2. Note the significant progress in resolution of the pulmonary infiltration. *(Courtesy Dr. Everett Aronson.)*

Gastrointestinal (GI) abnormalities may result from electrical interference with motility. Abdominal radiographs or ultrasonography may show GI gas patterns characteristic of ileus.[4]

Ocular manifestations of electrical injury (cataracts) are usually later findings noted several months after the episode. Cataracts are commonly seen in humans following near-fatal electrical injury and lightning strike and have been reported in a dog that was electrocuted by chewing an electrical cord.[13]

SECONDARY EFFECTS OF ELECTRICAL INJURY

Although complete blood count and serum chemistry results are usually within normal limits, tissue hypoxia from electrically induced ischemia and pulmonary edema may lead to necrosis of the affected tissues and subsequent hematologic changes and additional organ damage. Tissue necrosis may lead to hyperkalemia, myoglobinemia and myoglobinuria, and hemoglobinemia and hemoglobinuria.[4] Hyperkalemia may also result from excessive muscular activity during electrical shock; this muscular activity also contributes to acidemia and hyperlactatemia.[14] Hypoproteinemia may ensue in patients with severe burns.[4]

TREATMENT OF ELECTRICAL INJURY

Initial treatment at the scene of the exposure includes precautions to prevent inadvertent injury to rescuers. The source of electricity should be turned off before the victim is touched. Preferably, the electricity should be turned off at the electrical panel, but alternatively, the offending electrical cord may be unplugged carefully from the outlet. Once the victim is removed from the electrical source, immediate medical attention should be sought regardless of the victim's apparent condition. Victims in cardiopulmonary arrest require cardiopulmonary resuscitation. Better results might be expected in a hospital environment, but lifesaving techniques on the scene may be required if there is any hope of success.

Treatment of animals that survive the initial electrical insult is tailored to the clinical effects. Animals in shock are treated with intravenous fluids to expand intravascular volume because the mechanism of shock is likely a relative hypovolemia. However, because there may be a cardiogenic component to the shock from arrhythmia and subsequently decreased stroke volume, and because neurogenic pulmonary edema may develop quickly, the volume of fluids administered should be strictly controlled. Fluids that typically are given in low volumes (e.g., hypertonic saline, synthetic colloids) are recommended.

Respiratory distress requires prompt attention. Airway obstruction from edematous oropharyngeal tissues may require temporary tracheostomy tube placement. Partial obstructions may be managed conservatively with sedation and, if not contraindicated, antiinflammatory drugs and diuretics. Supplemental oxygen is recommended, but if the respiratory distress is due entirely to obstruction, relief of the obstruction should return oxygenation to normal.

Oxygen supplementation should continue until it is ascertained that neurogenic pulmonary edema has not developed or has resolved. Treatment of pulmonary edema is facilitated by administration of furosemide, particularly if the animal received shock doses of fluids; however, caution should be exercised to prevent creating a state of hypovolemia from excessive diuresis. Bronchodilators may also be useful (see Chapter 21). Positive pressure ventilation may be required if the patient is hypoxic and does not respond to supplemental oxygen (see Chapter 30).

Burned tissues are treated conservatively using standard wound treatment principles. Reconstructive surgery, if indicated, is performed after recovery from the electrical shock when it is determined that the tissues are healthy enough that one can expect good surgical results. Ventricular arrhythmias are managed by administering antiarrhythmic agents and by reversing the underlying pathophysiologic derangements (see Chapters 48 and 171). Seizures are controlled with anticonvulsant therapy (see Chapters 82 and 166). GI abnormalities are best managed with early nutritional support, via an appropriate feeding tube if necessary (see Chapter 129).

Pain management is necessary because burn wounds are painful and because there is likely muscle soreness from excessive activity during the electrical stimulation. Initially, opioids are preferred, but nonsteroidal antiinflammatory drugs may be used when GI integrity and renal function are presumed to be normal.

PROGNOSIS

The prognosis for victims that survive the initial shock episode is generally good, as long as the clinical effects are reversible. Respiratory abnormalities are the clinical effects most likely to alter prognosis. Most cases of electrically induced noncardiogenic pulmonary edema resolve quickly, but one study reported a fatality rate of 38.5%.[1] Some animals will require follow-up surgery to treat residual effects of burns. Recovering victims should be monitored for potential long-term effects. Owners should be instructed to observe for cataract development, which could occur several months after recovery.

LIGHTNING INJURY

Lightning injury is more likely to occur in large animal species[15-17] than in dogs and cats because of their greater outdoor exposure. However, companion animals, especially dogs, share outdoor activities with human beings and therefore may occasionally be exposed. A carefully studied lightning strike at a scene where 2 adults and 26 girls were camping also affected 7 dogs.[18] Fatal injuries occurred in four of the girls and four of the dogs.

Of the surviving dogs, the smallest one, a Maltese-Poodle mix, escaped injury. One of the remaining surviving dogs sustained burns and the other suffered damage to an eye that subsequently became opaque. Because the deceased dogs were farther from the struck tent pole than surviving people, it was speculated that dogs might be more susceptible to the effects of lightning injury than are human beings.[18] It is possible that small dogs, as in the camping site incident, are less susceptible to lightning injury than larger dogs.[18] Among cattle, adults are more likely to be struck by lightning than are calves.[16] Electrical injury from lightning strike has been reported to cause visual impairment in cattle as a result of cerebrocortical necrosis[19] and renal failure in people due to myoglobinuria from muscle damage[20]; these consequences have not been reported in dogs and cats, but are nonetheless possible.

The pathophysiology of lightning injury is similar to that of other electrical injuries, except for the mechanism by which the electricity reaches the victim and the potential for injury from mechanical energy. There are five possible mechanisms by which lightning can deliver electrical energy to a victim: (1) direct lightning strike, (2) direct strike of an object that the victim is touching, (3) side flash from a struck object, (4) step voltages produced by current flowing through the soil beneath, and (5) an upward streamer that does not connect or complete a full lightning strike.[21-24] With the latter mechanism, injury is caused by the upward streamer of charge that is induced from an object on the ground as a lightning leader of flash approaches the ground from a thundercloud.[18,21-24]

In addition to electrical and thermal injury, mechanical energy can be imparted to the lightning victim. A blast effect from rapid air movement caused when superheated air is then cooled may result in physical injury. People are often thrown to the ground and report muscle pain. Lumbosacral fracture with resultant spinal cord injury was the only lesion identified in three pigs in an outdoor pen that was struck by lightning.[17] Spinal fracture due to lightning strike has also been noted in pond fish,[25] and the blast effect of lightning strike has been reported to cause vestibular injury in horses and human beings.[26] Although such injuries have not been reported in dogs and cats, the occurrence of mechanical energy effects similar to those reported in other species should not be surprising.

REFERENCES

1. Kolata RJ, Burrows CF: The clinical features of injury by chewing electrical cords in dogs and cats, J Am Anim Hosp Assoc 17:219-222, 1981.
2. Marks SL: Electrocution, Proc North Am Vet Conf 18:176-177, 2004.
3. Morgan RV: Environmental injuries. In Hoskins J, editor: Veterinary pediatrics: dogs and cats from birth to six months of age, Philadelphia, 1990, Saunders, pp 505-516.
4. Presley RH, Macintire DK: Electrocution and electrical cord injury, Stand Care Emerg Crit Care Med 7(9):7-11, 2005.
5. Decosne-Junot C, Junot S: Electrocuted cats and dogs: diagnosis and treatment, A Hora Veterinária 24:65-68, 2004.
6. Legendre LFJ: Management and long term effects of electrocution in a cat's mouth, J Vet Dent 10:6-8, 1993.
7. Geddes LA, Bourland JD, Ford G: The mechanism underlying sudden death from electric shock, Med Instrum 20(6):303-315, 1986.
8. Bradford A, O'Regan RG: The effects of low-voltage electric shock on respiration in the anaesthetized cat, J Exp Physiol 70:115-127, 1985.
9. Drobatz KJ, Saunders M, Pugh CR, et al: Noncardiogenic pulmonary edema in dogs and cats: 26 cases (1987-1993), J Am Vet Med Assoc 206(11):1732-1736, 1995.

10. Haldane S, Marks SL, Raffe M: Noncardiogenic pulmonary edema, Stand Care Emerg Crit Care Med 5(7):1-5, 2003.
11. Ridgway RL: High-voltage electric shock in a cat, Vet Med Small Anim Clin 70(3):317, 1975.
12. McCreery DB, Agnew WF, Bullara LA, et al: Partial pressure of oxygen in brain and peripheral nerve during damaging electrical stimulation, J Biomed Eng 12:309-315, 1990.
13. Brightman AH, Brogdon JD, Helper LC, et al: Electric cataracts in the canine: a case report, J Am Anim Hosp Assoc 20:895-898, 1984.
14. Bradford A, O'Regan RG: Acidaemia and hyperkalemia following low-voltage electric shock in the anaesthetized cat, Q J Exp Physiol 70:101-113, 1985.
15. Williams MA: Lightning strike in horses, Compend Contin Educ Pract Vet 22(9):860-867, 2000.
16. Tartera P, Schelcher F: Lightning strike in cattle, Point Vétérinaire 32:48-51, 2001.
17. Van Alstine WG, Widmer WR: Lightning injury in an outdoor swine herd, J Vet Diagn Invest 15:289-291, 2003.
18. Carte AE, Anderson RB, Cooper MA: A large group of children struck by lightning, Ann Emerg Med 39:665-670, 2002.
19. Boevé MH, Huijben R, Grinwis G, et al: Visual impairment after suspected lightning strike in a herd of Holstein-Friesian cattle, Vet Rec 154(13):402-404, 2004.
20. Oafur UV: Lightning injuries and acute renal failure: a review, Ren Fail 27(2):129-134, 2005.
21. Anderson RB: Does a fifth mechanism exist for explain lightning injuries? IEEE Eng Med Biol Mag 20:105-113, 2001.
22. Cooper MA: A fifth mechanism of lightning injury, Acad Emerg Med 9(2):172-174, 2002.
23. Cooper MA, Holle RL, Andrews C: Distribution of lightning injury mechanisms. In Proceedings of the 20th International Lightning Detection Conference and 2nd International Lightning Meteorology Conference, Tucson, Ariz, April 24, 2008, pp 1-4.
24. Gomes C: Lightning safety of animals, Int J Biometeorol 56(6):1011-1023, 2012.
25. Barlow AM: "Broken backs" in koi carp *(Cyprinus carpio)* following lightning strike, Vet Rec 133(20):503, 1993.
26. Bedenice D, Hoffman AM, Parrott B, et al: Vestibular signs associated with suspected lightning strike in two horses, Vet Rec 149(17):519-522, 2001.

CHAPTER 151
DROWNING AND SUBMERSION INJURY

Lisa Leigh Powell, DVM, DACVECC

KEY POINTS

- The term *near drowning* is no longer used; the term *drowning* is used to describe any event resulting in primary respiratory impairment from submersion or immersion in a liquid medium, whether it is fatal or not.
- Drowning is a leading cause of morbidity and mortality in humans.
- Reports of drowning in veterinary patients are sparse.
- The primary pathophysiologic abnormality seen in drowning victims is hypoxic tissue damage due to the inability to maintain adequate pulmonary gas exchange.
- Treatment is aimed at providing neuroprotective therapy, cardiovascular support, and an oxygen-rich environment.
- Prognosis in humans depends on submersion time, cardiopulmonary resuscitation time, and severity of acidemia.

DEFINITIONS

Drowning accounts for more than 500,000 human deaths annually worldwide. The number is thought to be grossly underestimated, primarily due to underreporting in less developed countries. Catastrophic natural disasters such as tsunamis, hurricanes, and floods add to the number of injuries and deaths attributable to drowning events. In the United States, in 2002, drowning accounted for 775 deaths in children aged 1 to 14 years and represented the second leading cause of death in this age group.[1] Because of the high incidence of drowning and near-drowning injury, a consensus conference was held to establish guidelines for uniform reporting of data from drowning incidents and to stratify definitions for drowning and its associated pathologic complications.[2] In addition, a systematic review of 43 articles addressing the definition of drowning found 33 different definitions describing drowning incidents: 20 for drowning and 13 for near drowning.[3]

The Consensus Conference on Drowning published its recommended guidelines for uniform reporting of data from drowning in 2003.[2] The following definitions were presented by the consensus conference for use in research and data reporting associated with drowning and near drowning:

- Drowning is a process resulting in primary respiratory impairment from submersion or immersion in a liquid medium. Liquid is present at the victim's airway, preventing respiration of air. The victim may survive or die, but regardless of outcome, the victim has been involved in a drowning incident. This is in contrast to the definition proposed by the American Heart Association in 2000, in which the term *drowning* was reserved for cases in which the victim died from water submersion within 24 hours of the event.[4]
- *Dry drowning* describes cases in which liquid is not aspirated into the lungs, whereas *wet drowning* refers to aspiration of liquid. Victims of dry drowning often experience morbidity from laryngospasm, which results in the same hypoxemic and hypercarbic state seen in those who have aspirated liquid.
- It was concluded in the consensus statement that *near drowning* be abandoned as a term used to describe victims of submersion injury

who ultimately survive because the term *drowning* is inclusive of both survivors and nonsurvivors. The term *submersion victim* was proposed as an alternative to *near-drowning victim* by the American Heart Association and still is in use.

INCIDENCE AND EPIDEMIOLOGY

Humans

The incidence of drowning and submersion injury remains high in humans. Drowning is the third most common cause of accidental death in humans younger than 44 years of age, with 40% of all drowning deaths reported in children younger than 5 years of age.[5] Another 15% to 20% of drowning victims are between the ages of 5 and 20 years, and male victims dominate in all age groups.[5] Most drownings occur in fresh water, with children younger than 1 year of age most often drowning in bathtubs, buckets, or toilets.[6] Drowning occurs most often in residential swimming pools in children aged 1 to 4 years.[7,8] In contrast, adolescents most often drown in rivers, lakes, and canals, and drug or alcohol use is a contributing factor in about 50% of these cases.[9,10] Male individuals are thought to have a higher incidence of drowning, especially during adolescence, because of the tendency toward risky activities and overestimation of their swimming abilities.[11]

Factors associated with a higher risk of drowning in humans include the use of alcohol or recreational drugs, lack of supervision in children, and medical conditions such as epilepsy and long QT syndrome.[12,13]

Veterinary Patients

There are only three published reports of veterinary patients describing submersion injury. The first is a case report of a gelding that recovered from a drowning incident in which he became entangled in a safety line attached to his harness while swimming in a chlorinated swimming pool. The reported adverse effects of the incident included metabolic acidosis, hypoxemia, and pulmonary infiltrates in the dorsocaudal lung fields. Successful therapy included antibiotic administration and bronchoalveolar lavage with surfactant.[14]

The second publication referring to drowning in veterinary patients describes animal abuse cases in a population of dogs and cats in the United Kingdom. In this sample of 243 dogs and 182 cats, drowning accounted for three of the feline abuse cases.[15]

The third veterinary publication is a retrospective study describing fresh water submersion injury in 25 dogs and 3 cats. In this case series, ten patients died, including all three cats, and the total mortality rate was 36%. Respiratory failure was the most common cause of death.[16]

The pathophysiology and clinical course in veterinary patients involved in drowning incidents correlates with the human progression of injury and directs diagnostics, therapy, and outcome in canine and feline drowning victims.

PATHOPHYSIOLOGY OF INJURY

Pulmonary System

Drowning occurs without aspiration of water in about 10% of victims, whereas 90% aspirate fluid into the lungs.[17] All submersion victims experience hypoxemia, either from laryngospasm in which no aspiration occurs or from aspiration of fluid resulting in loss of surfactant that causes atelectasis and intrapulmonary shunt. Most submersion victims (about 85%) that survive are thought to have aspirated less than 22 ml/kg of water.[17]

Hypoxemia in submersion victims results from intrapulmonary shunting of blood. Bronchospasm, atelectasis due to surfactant washout, aspirated water or matter in the alveolar space, infectious or chemical pneumonitis, and acute respiratory distress syndrome (ARDS) all contribute to this shunting in submersion victims.[18]

Submersion victims may experience both ventilation-perfusion mismatch and intrapulmonary shunt from alveolar collapse. In submersion victims that aspirate water into the alveolar space, surfactant washout causes atelectasis. Ventilation-perfusion inequality may be present in submersion victims that aspirate water or particulate matter. Readers are directed to Chapter 15 for further description of the mechanisms of lung disease.

Fluids and Electrolytes

In previous years, medical researchers tried to ascertain the differences in pathologic features when drowning victims aspirated fresh water versus saltwater. It was thought that the hypertonicity of aspirated saltwater would result in an osmotic gradient into the lungs, drawing plasma water into the pulmonary interstitium and alveolar spaces. This shift of plasma water would then result in hypernatremia and a decreased circulating blood volume. In contrast, aspiration of fresh water was hypothesized to shift fluid out of the lung and into circulation, which would result in hypervolemia, hyponatremia, and dilution of other electrolytes.

Studies did not support these hypotheses. One experimental study showed that the amount of aspirated water needed to cause these fluid shifts was far greater than the amount normally aspirated by drowning victims.[19] In another study involving a series of 91 submersion victims, no serious fluid or electrolyte abnormalities were noted.[20] The most prominent pathologic feature in victims of both fresh water and saltwater submersion injury is the washout of surfactant from the alveoli, causing atelectasis, intrapulmonary shunt, and global hypoxia, which may then result in tissue injury, neurologic damage, cardiovascular collapse, and death.

Neurologic and Cardiovascular Systems

In humans, about 10% of drowning victims experience severe neurologic effects.[21] Neurologic abnormalities result from hypoxia-induced brain injury, and the severity of injury is primarily dependent on the duration of hypoxia.

Cardiac arrhythmias and dysfunction may occur in submersion victims as a result of myocardial hypoxia and ischemia, acidemia, electrolyte abnormalities, and hypothermia. Blood pressure is affected by a variety of factors, including catecholamine release, hypercarbia, and hypovolemia from traumatic blood loss during the submersion event. Hypothermia may contribute to hypovolemia caused by inhibition of antidiuretic hormone and induction of diuresis; this results from shunting of blood to core organs, which gives a perception of hypervolemia via arterial stretch receptors.[18]

Effect of Water Temperature

Water temperature has an important effect on the survival of submersion victims. Submersion in ice-cold water (<5° C [41° F]) increases the chances of survival, in part because of the diving reflex that is present in most mammals. Within seconds after a victim's face contacts cold water and before unconsciousness ensues, a reflex mediated by the trigeminal nerve sends impulses to the central nervous system that cause bradycardia, hypertension, and preferential shunting of blood to the cerebral and coronary circulations.[5,22] This reflex acts to protect the brain and heart from hypoxia-induced injury. Hypothermia also causes a decrease in metabolic need, which protects the brain from injury. The effects of this response are evidenced by good neurologic recovery in victims submerged in icy water, despite the initial presence of coma or other negative neurologic prognostic indicators. Hypothermia in patients injured by submersion in warm water, however, is a negative prognostic sign indicating poor peripheral perfusion and longer submersion times.[5]

DIAGNOSTIC TESTS AND MONITORING

On presentation at a hospital, airway, breathing, and circulation should be assessed immediately in the submersion victim. Body temperature should be evaluated and appropriate treatment initiated. In patients with significant neurologic impairment, therapeutic hypothermia may be beneficial in protecting the brain from further injury.[23] A minimum data set, including results of a complete blood count and chemistry panel, should be collected. Arterial blood gas analysis should be performed because many submersion victims experience hypoxemia, respiratory acidosis from hypoventilation, and metabolic acidosis from hypoperfusion and tissue hypoxia.

Monitoring of the drowning victim includes continuous electrocardiography; determination of respiratory rate and effort; lung auscultation; and assessment of body temperature, mentation and pupil responsiveness, arterial blood pressure, serum electrolyte levels, and arterial blood gas concentrations. Continuous pulse oximetry can be used to monitor hemoglobin saturation. Thoracic radiography should be performed when the patient is able to tolerate the procedure.

TREATMENT

Most human submersion victims are pulled from the water and cardiopulmonary resuscitation is attempted at the scene. Cardiopulmonary resuscitation in canine or feline patients at the scene of the accident is much more difficult to perform without proper training. The owner should wrap the pet in a blanket, perform mouth-to-nose breathing if no respirations are noted, and bring the animal to an emergency clinic as quickly as possible.

Therapy for the drowning victim is aimed at improving tissue oxygenation, resolving abnormal serum acid-base status, maintaining tissue perfusion, and stabilizing the cardiovascular and neurologic systems. Hypoxemia and respiratory and metabolic acidosis should be treated as early and aggressively as possible to prevent further organ damage. Oxygen should be administered and, if indicated, the patient should be intubated and mechanically ventilated.[24] Guideline criteria used in human medicine to indicate the need for intubation and mechanical ventilation include an arterial partial pressure of oxygen (PaO_2) of less than 60 mm Hg or an oxygen saturation of less than 90% despite oxygen therapy, worsening hypercapnia, and severe respiratory distress suggestive of impending respiratory failure.[5] See Chapter 30 for further information. Although the initial pulmonary injury of a drowning victim can resemble ARDS, it tends to resolve far more quickly than ARDS, and later pulmonary complications are uncommon in human patients.[25]

Although uncommon, pulmonary complications such as pneumonia or ARDS can occur. In humans, ARDS is defined by the clinical presentation of four features: (1) acute respiratory distress, (2) bilateral pulmonary infiltrates, (3) a PaO_2/fraction of inspired oxygen ratio of less than 200, and (4) a pulmonary artery wedge pressure of less than 18 mm Hg or no evidence of left atrial hypertension (see Chapter 24).[26] These patients often require positive end-expiratory pressure (PEEP) to decrease pulmonary shunt, improve blood oxygenation, and increase lung compliance in atelectatic areas. PEEP is provided through intubation and mechanical ventilation.

Artificial surfactant has been used with some success, and experimental therapies with liquid ventilation, inhaled nitric oxide, and intratracheal ventilation may be employed.[27-30] Finally, submersion victims are prone to develop pneumonia, especially if the submersion medium was grossly contaminated or aspiration of dirt or sand occurred. Antibiotic therapy ideally should be instituted following the culture of bronchoalveolar fluid obtained via bronchoscopy or endotracheal wash. However, in patients in unstable condition, prophylactic use of a broad-spectrum antibiotic may be indicated.

Fluid therapy is necessary in drowning victims to restore circulating volume, correct acid-base abnormalities, and improve tissue perfusion. However, excessive crystalloid administration may worsen noncardiogenic pulmonary edema and cerebral edema. Synthetic colloid therapy used in conjunction with crystalloid therapy can help maintain intravascular volume and decrease the risk of extravasation of excess fluid into interstitial tissue spaces. Fluid therapy should be monitored with serial measurements of body weight, central venous pressure, urine output, and arterial blood pressure.

Neurologic resuscitation is aimed at preventing or decreasing cerebral edema and maintaining normal intracranial pressures. Elevations in arterial partial pressure of carbon dioxide cause cerebral vasodilation, which contributes to an increase in intracranial pressure and creates the potential for cerebral edema. It is recommended that normocapnia be maintained because hyperventilation to create hypocapnia may result in cerebral vasoconstriction and impair cerebral perfusion. Hypertonic therapy such as mannitol may be used in fluid-resuscitated patients if cerebral edema is suspected and neurologic status is deteriorating. Glucocorticoid therapy is not recommended because it has not been shown to improve neurologic outcome, and the resultant hyperglycemia may worsen cerebral cell damage through secondary neuronal injury.[31]

Significant quantities of liquid can be swallowed during a drowning event, and gastric filling volume should be evaluated in all drowning victims. Passage of an orogastric or nasogastric tube to empty the stomach may be indicated.

In the retrospective study of 25 dogs and 3 cats with submersion injury, treatment included supplemental oxygen, antimicrobials, furosemide, glucocorticoids, aminophylline, and, when indicated, assisted ventilation.[16]

OUTCOME

In one study, three factors were associated with 100% mortality in human submersion victims younger than 20 years of age: (1) submersion duration longer than 25 minutes, (2) resuscitation duration longer than 25 minutes, and (3) pulseless cardiac arrest on presentation at the emergency department.[32] Additional factors associated with a poor prognosis included ventricular tachycardia or ventricular fibrillation (93% mortality), fixed pupils (89% mortality), severe acidosis (89% mortality), and respiratory arrest in the emergency department (89% mortality).[32] Patients experiencing acute pulmonary edema had mortality rates ranging from 5% to 19%. Level of consciousness and responsiveness also correlated with survival. Deaths occurred only among victims who remained comatose after presentation to the emergency department. No deaths occurred in patients who arrived alert or depressed but responsive.[33]

As mentioned earlier, mortality was reported as 36% in the study of 25 dogs and 3 cats with submersion injury, with all 3 cats included in the nonsurvivors.[16] Correlation with prognosis in human submersion victims may be made, although in many instances submersion duration may not be known and prehospital therapy, including cardiopulmonary resuscitation, is usually not performed.

Drowning victims with minimal neurologic, respiratory, and cardiovascular abnormalities should have better outcomes; however, intensive treatment of more seriously affected submersion victims can result in a full recovery. The ability to supply adequate inspired oxygen levels, to provide mechanical ventilation if needed, to perform serial evaluations of arterial blood gas concentrations, and to house the patient in a 24-hour intensive care setting may improve the prognosis in severely affected patients.

REFERENCES

1. Centers for Disease Control and Prevention, National Center for Injury Prevention and Control: Web-based Injury Statistics Query and Reporting System (WISQARS). Available at http://www.cdc.gov/ncipc/wisqars. Accessed August 7, 2007.
2. Idris AH, Berg RA, Bierens J, et al: Recommended guidelines for uniform reporting of data from drowning. The "Utstein Style," Circulation 108:2565, 2003.
3. Papa L, Hoelle R, Idris A: Systematic review of definitions for drowning incidents, Resuscitation 65:255, 2005.
4. Part 8: Advanced challenges in resuscitation. Section 3: Special challenges in ECC. 3B: Submersion or near-drowning. European Resuscitation Council, Resuscitation 46:273, 2000.
5. DeNicola LK, Falk JL, Swanson ME, et al: Submersion injuries in children and adults, Crit Care Clin 13:477, 1997.
6. Brenner RA, Trumble AC, Smith GS, et al: Where children drown, United States 1995, Pediatrics 108:85, 2001.
7. Present P: Child drowning study. A report on the epidemiology of drowning in residential pools to children under age five, Washington, DC, 1987, Consumer Product Safety Commission.
8. Wintemute GJ, Kraus JF, Teret SP, et al: Drowning in childhood and adolescence: a population-based study, Am J Public Health 77:830, 1987.
9. Orlowski JP: Drowning, near-drowning, and ice-water submersions, Pediatr Clin North Am 34:75, 1987.
10. Howland J, Hingson R: Alcohol as a risk factor for drownings: a review of the literature (1950-1985), Accid Anal Prev 20:19, 1988.
11. Howland J, Hingson R, Mangione TW, et al: Why are most drowning victims men? Sex differences in aquatic skills and behaviors, Am J Public Health 86:93, 1996.
12. Besag FMC: Tonic seizures are a particular risk factor for drowning in people with epilepsy, BMJ 322:975, 2001.
13. Yoshinaga M, Kamimura J, Fukushige T, et al: Face immersion in cold water induces prolongation of the QT interval and T wave changes in children with nonfamilial long QT syndrome, Am J Cardiol 83:1494, 1999.
14. Humber KA: Near drowning of a gelding, J Am Vet Med Assoc 192:377, 1988.
15. Munro HMC, Thrusfield MV: "Battered pets": nonaccidental physical injuries found in dogs and cats, J Small Anim Pract 42:279, 2001.
16. Heffner GG, Rozanski EA, Beal MW, et al: Evaluation of freshwater submersion in small animals: 28 cases (1996-2006), J Am Vet Med Assoc 232:244-248, 2008.
17. Modell JH: Drowning, N Engl J Med 328:253, 1993.
18. Burford AE, Ryan LM, Stone BJ, et al: Drowning and near-drowning in children and adolescents. A succinct review for emergency physicians and nurses, Pediatr Emerg Care 21:610, 2005.
19. Modell JH: Serum electrolyte changes in near-drowning victims, JAMA 253:557, 1995.
20. Modell JH, Graves SA, Ketover A: Clinical course of 91 consecutive near-drowning victims, Chest 70:231, 1976.
21. Quan L: Near-drowning, Pediatr Rev 20:255, 1999.
22. Levin DL, Morris FC, Toro LO, et al: Drowning and near-drowning, Pediatr Clin North Am 40:321, 1993.
23. Williamson JP, Illing R, Gertler P, et al: Near-drowning treated with therapeutic hypothermia, Med J Aust 181:500, 2004.
24. Szpilman D, Bierens JJ, Handley AL, et al: Drowning, N Engl J Med 366:2102, 2012.
25. Gregorakos L, Markou N, Psalida V, et al: Near-drowning: clinical course of lung injury in adults, Lung 187:93, 2009.
26. Esteban A, Fernandez-Segoviano P, Frutos-Vivar F, et al: Comparison of clinical criteria for the acute respiratory distress syndrome with autopsy findings, Ann Intern Med 141:440, 2004.
27. Norberg WJ, Agnew RF, Brunsvold R, et al: Successful resuscitation of a cold water submersion victim with the use of cardiopulmonary bypass, Crit Care Med 20:1355, 1992.
28. Moller JC, Schailble TF, Reiss I, et al: Treatment of severe nonneonatal ARDS in children with surfactant and nitric oxide in a "pre-ECMO" situation, Int J Artif Organs 18:598, 1995.
29. Arensman RM, Satter MB, Bastawrous AL, et al: Modern treatment modalities for neonatal and pediatric respiratory failure, Am J Surg 172:41, 1996.
30. Burkhead SR, Lally KP, Bristow F, et al: Intratracheal pulmonary ventilation provides effective ventilation in a near-drowning model, J Pediatr Surg 31:337, 1996.
31. Gabrielli A, Layon AJ: Drowning and near-drowning, J Fla Med Assoc 84:452, 1997.
32. Quan L, Kinder D: Pediatric submersions: prehospital predictors of outcome, Pediatrics 90:909, 1992.
33. Quan L, Wentz KR, Gore EJ, et al: Outcome and predictors of outcome in pediatric submersion victims receiving prehospital care in King County, Washington, Pediatrics 86:586, 1990.

PART XIX MISCELLANEOUS DISORDERS

CHAPTER 152

ANAPHYLAXIS

Patricia M. Dowling, DVM, MS, DACVIM, DACVCP

KEY POINTS

- Anaphylaxis is a severe, potentially fatal hypersensitivity reaction that may be triggered by a wide variety of antigens, including venoms, helminths, foods, vaccines, and drugs.
- The classic pathway of anaphylaxis involves immunoglobulin E receptors, mast cells, basophils, histamine, prostaglandins, leukotrienes, serotonin, and platelet-activating factor. The alternative pathway involves immunoglobulin G, Fcγ, macrophages, and platelet-activating factor.
- In dogs, anaphylaxis predominantly affects the gastrointestinal tract, whereas in cats, gastrointestinal and respiratory tract signs frequently occur simultaneously. Dermal and ocular manifestations may occur in both species.
- Although epinephrine is recommended as the treatment of choice for anaphylaxis, its efficacy in reversing the cardiovascular derangements once full-blown shock has developed has been demonstrated only with continuous intravenous administration.
- Antihistamines (histamine-1, histamine-2, and histamine-3 blockers) and glucocorticoids are adjunct treatments, but their effects are delayed, so they are not helpful in patients with cardiovascular collapse or life-threatening bronchoconstriction.
- Administration of albuterol (salbutamol) via metered dose inhaler provides rapid relief of bronchoconstriction.

Anaphylaxis is a severe, potentially fatal hypersensitivity reaction that may involve multiple organ systems, including the skin and eyes, respiratory tract, cardiovascular system, nervous system, and gastrointestinal tract (Box 152-1). Anaphylaxis in dogs and cats can be caused by a variety of antigens but is most commonly triggered by vaccines, drugs, insect and reptile venoms, antimicrobials, nonsteroidal antiinflammatory drugs, glucocorticoids, opiates, foods, and physical factors such as cold and exercise.[1-6] Traditionally, hypersensitivity reactions were classified into four types: type I, or immediate (immunoglobulin E [IgE] dependent); type II, or cytotoxic (IgG, IgM dependent); type III, or immune complex mediated (IgG, IgM complex dependent); and type IV, or delayed (T lymphocyte dependent). Anaphylaxis was attributed to type I reactions, and anaphylactoid reactions were attributed to non–IgE-mediated reactions. However, it is now known that cytotoxic reactions (e.g., blood transfusion reactions) and immune complex–mediated reactions (e.g., reactions to complexes of IgG administered intravenously or intramuscularly) can cause anaphylaxis. An alternate classification system has been proposed based on seven immunopathologic mechanisms with both protective and destructive functions: (1) immune-mediated inactivation/activation reactions involving biologically active molecules; (2) antibody-mediated cytotoxic or cytolytic reactions; (3) immune complex reactions; (4) allergic reactions; (5) T lymphocyte–mediated cytotoxicity; (6) delayed hypersensitivity reactions; and (7) granulomatous reactions.[7] Several of these immunopathologic mechanisms can be operative simultaneously in a given patient. Whether initiated by immune or by nonimmune mechanisms, anaphylaxis results in the activation of mast cells and circulating basophils followed by the release of preformed mediators.

PATHOPHYSIOLOGY

In murine models, two immunologic pathways of anaphylaxis have been identified. The *classic* pathway involves IgE receptors, mast cells, basophils, histamine, prostaglandins, leukotrienes, serotonin, and platelet-activating factor (PAF). An *alternative* pathway involves IgG, Fcγ, macrophages, and PAF.[8] In the classic pathway, when previous exposure to an antigen results in sensitization, IgE is produced and bound to the cell surface of mast cells and basophils by high-affinity receptors for the Fc portion of the immunoglobulin (FcεRIs). With repeated exposure, the antigen causes cross-linkage of two IgE molecules, and the cell is activated to release the anaphylaxis mediators: histamine, heparin, tryptase, kallikreins, proteases, proteoglycans, eosinophilic chemotactic factor of anaphylaxis, and neutrophil chemotactic factor of anaphylaxis. In the IgG-FcγRIII-macrophage pathway, PAF, rather than histamine, is primarily responsible for the development of shock.

Although clinical features associated with the two pathways of anaphylaxis closely resemble each other, there are some important differences. Tachycardia is most likely dependent on IgE and histamine because it is more prominent when anaphylaxis is induced in mast cell–sufficient than in mast cell–deficient mice. Hypothermia induced through the alternative pathway requires 100-fold more antigen than induction of hypothermia through the classic pathway. Anaphylaxis mediated through the alternative pathway also appears to require much more antibody than anaphylaxis mediated through the classic pathway. IgE-mediated anaphylaxis can occur when IgE concentrations are undetectable in serum (although IgE is present on mast cells). In contrast, high concentrations of serum IgG antibody are required for an antigen to induce anaphylaxis through the alternative pathway. These differences are consistent with the much higher affinity of FcεRI for IgE than of FcγRIII for IgG and with the direct binding of antigen to mast cell–associated IgE, whereas antigen-IgG complexes presumably form in blood and lymph before binding to FcγRIII.

Although less antigen is required to trigger the classic pathway in the presence of antigen-specific IgE and the absence of antigen-specific IgG than is required to trigger the alternative pathway when

BOX 152-1 *Clinical Signs of Anaphylaxis*

Dermal

Erythema, pruritus, urticaria, angioedema, maculopapular rash

Gastrointestinal

Nausea, vomiting, diarrhea

Cardiovascular

Tachycardia, hypotension, arrhythmias, myocardial ischemia, cardiac arrest

Respiratory

Nasal congestion, sneezing, stridor, oropharyngeal or laryngeal edema, cough, dyspnea, bronchospasm, tachypnea, abdominal breathing, cyanosis, respiratory arrest

Neurologic

Weakness, syncope, seizures

Ocular

Pruritus, conjunctival injection, lacrimation

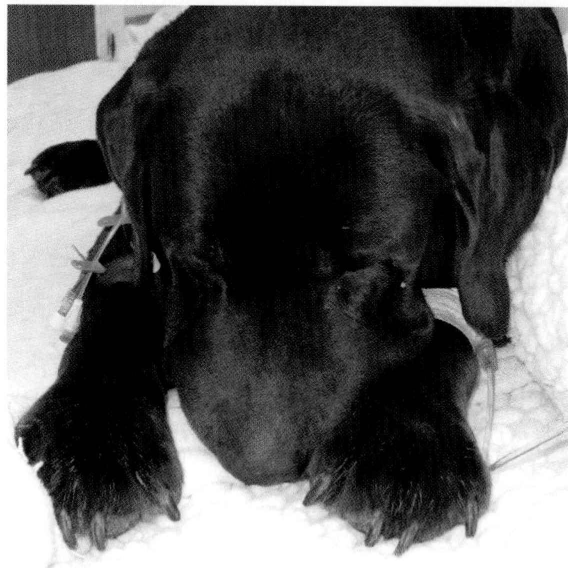

FIGURE 152-1 Urticaria, pruritus, and angioedema in a Chesapeake Bay Retriever that developed anaphylaxis after administration of cephalexin.

antigen-specific IgG is present, responses are dramatically altered in the common situation in which antigen-specific IgE and IgG are both present and there is more IgG than IgE. In this situation, antigen is likely to bind to IgG in blood or lymph before it can bind to mast cell–associated IgE. Consequently, when antigen levels are insufficient to induce IgG-mediated anaphylaxis, high levels of IgG antibodies can prevent the development of anaphylaxis. For a similar reason, larger amounts of antigen trigger anaphylaxis predominantly through the alternative pathway when antigen-specific IgG antibody levels are high. The two anaphylaxis pathways are triggered simultaneously only when the amount of challenge antigen exceeds the capacity of IgG antibody to block antigen binding to mast cell–associated IgE.[8]

Histamine and the leukotrienes are potent vasoactive mediators involved in anaphylaxis, and their release from eosinophils and basophils increases vascular permeability and vasodilation.[9] Histamine acts through histamine-1 (H_1), H_2, and H_3 receptors to promote shock during allergen challenge. H_1 receptors mediate coronary artery vasoconstriction and cardiac depression, whereas H_2 receptors mediate gastric acid production and, when stimulated, produce coronary and systemic vasodilation and increases in heart rate and ventricular contractility. The H_1 receptor activation results in rhinitis, pruritus, and bronchoconstriction. Stimulation of H_1 receptors causes endothelial cells to convert L-arginine into nitric oxide, a potent vasodilator that decreases venous return. The resulting hypotension and hypoxemia/hypercapnia worsens the cardiovascular collapse.[10] H_3 receptors have recently been identified on presynaptic terminals of sympathetic effector nerves that innervate the heart and systemic vasculature. These receptors inhibit endogenous norepinephrine release from sympathetic nerves, so activation accentuates the degree of shock observed during antigen challenge because compensatory neural adrenergic stimulation is blocked.

The response to vasoactive mediators is also regulated through cardiovascular α-adrenergic receptors, which normally increase myocardial contractility and vascular tone to compensate for the decreased intravascular volume, vasodilatation, and myocardial depression that are induced by PAF and histamine.

Interleukin-4 (IL-4) and IL-13 are produced by T cells and basophils and activate phosphatidylinositol 3-kinase in several cell types through the type 1 and type 2 IL-4 receptors. They also act through IL-4 receptors to activate the transcription factor STAT6, which increases responsiveness to several mast cell– and macrophage-generated mediators, including histamine, PAF, serotonin, and leukotriene C_4.[8]

Cross-linking of the FcεRI receptors also activates phospholipase A_2, which sets off production of prostaglandins, thromboxanes, PAF, and leukotrienes. Prostaglandin D_2 is 10 times more potent as a bronchoconstrictor than histamine, and leukotriene D_4 is 1000 times more potent. Cytotoxic events involving IgM or IgG, immune aggregates, activation of complement, kallikrein-kinin, or coagulation systems may also be involved in anaphylaxis.

The systemic anaphylactic response is rapid; release of mediators from activated immune cells occurs within seconds to minutes, the arachidonic cascade is activated within minutes, and cytokine synthesis begins within hours.[11]

DIFFERENTIAL DIAGNOSIS

Anaphylaxis is a clinical diagnosis based on pattern recognition and probability. Systemic diseases that may present with clinical signs similar to anaphylaxis include severe asthma, syncope, pheochromocytoma, and mastocytosis. Inhalation of a foreign body can be potentially misinterpreted as anaphylaxis.

CLINICAL MANIFESTATIONS

Anaphylaxis is a dynamic continuum, beginning with exposure to a trigger followed by rapid onset, evolution, and resolution of symptoms within minutes to hours. There appears to be a correlation between the time of onset of clinical symptoms and the severity of the reaction: the more rapid the onset, the more severe the symptoms.[12] The clinical signs of anaphylaxis vary with the species and route of exposure. In dogs, dermal and gastrointestinal signs predominate, with hepatic vein congestion and portal hypertension leading to vomiting and diarrhea.[1] The reaction may progress to respiratory distress from upper airway obstruction to hypovolemic shock and eventually to death. Dermal reactions in dogs include erythema, urticaria, pruritus, and angioedema (Figure 152-1). Urticarial lesions tend to be generalized, whereas angioedema tends to be localized to the head, extremities, and/or genitalia. Respiratory and gastrointestinal tract signs predominate in cats, with respiratory distress being the typical first sign of anaphylaxis in cats.[3] Dyspnea results from laryngeal and pharyngeal edema, bronchoconstriction, and excessive mucus production. Cats may also develop severe pruritus, vomiting, and diarrhea.

The most severe clinical reactions of respiratory distress and cardiovascular collapse are generally seen when the antigen is administered parenterally. The combination of mediator-induced arrhythmia, coronary artery vasoconstriction, and decreased systemic vascular resistance causes a profound hypotension. A relative hypovolemia occurs as up to 50% of the circulating volume is lost into the tissues by the sudden increase in vascular permeability. Oral ingestion of antigens more frequently causes gastrointestinal distress and dermal reactions. Inhalation typically causes bronchoconstriction and rhinitis. Topical application of an antigen can cause conjunctivitis, urticaria, and pruritus alone or along with systemic signs of anaphylaxis. Urticaria (hives) involves the superficial dermis, whereas angioedema occurs in the deep dermis and subcutaneous tissues.

TREATMENT

Epinephrine

Epinephrine is considered the treatment of choice for anaphylaxis,[13] but mostly on the basis of anecdotal experience (Table 152-1).[14] Spontaneous recovery can occur in individuals because of compensatory mechanisms from endogenous epinephrine release and angiotensin II secretion. The rationale for the administration of epinephrine is that stimulation of β-adrenergic receptors enhances the production of adenyl cyclase and subsequent conversion of adenosine triphosphate to cyclic adenosine monophosphate. The cyclic adenosine monophosphate system inhibits the antigen-induced release of histamine and other anaphylactic mediators. Efficacy was supposed from results of in vitro studies in which epinephrine inhibited mediator release from mast cells when administered before an allergen challenge. But in human patients with anaphylaxis and hypotension, standard therapy with intravenous (IV) epinephrine and fluids did not reverse the hemodynamic abnormalities.[15] Patients experienced a gradual recovery from hypotension that was not attributable to any specific therapeutic intervention. In a canine ragweed anaphylactic shock model, epinephrine was effective in attenuating the circulatory collapse only when given by continuous IV infusion.[11] When epinephrine was administered as a bolus by the IV, intramuscular (IM), or subcutaneous (SC) route, there was no sustained effect on hemodynamic recovery. In this model, endogenous plasma epinephrine concentrations increased from 500 pg/ml at baseline to 4000 pg/ml after antigen challenge. Even with this massive endogenous response, epinephrine concentrations were insufficient to reverse the cardiovascular collapse seen with antigen challenge. As assessed by the area under the plasma concentration–versus–time curve, plasma epinephrine concentrations were significantly higher with epinephrine treatment by any route, but only with bolus administration was there a transient improvement in mean arterial pressure, stroke volume, and pulmonary wedge pressure. The improvement in mean arterial pressure was attributed to the increase in cardiac output from epinephrine's β-adrenergic effects on the heart and not to its α_1 vasoconstrictive effects on the systemic vasculature. Results of the canine ragweed model suggest that in the treatment of anaphylaxis, once the mediators have been released, epinephrine acts primarily as a vasopressor in augmenting hemodynamic recovery and has no special pharmacologic properties that improve immunologic recovery.[3]

From this canine model, it appears that a constant rate infusion of epinephrine is the most effective treatment of cardiovascular collapse when the animal is already in full anaphylactic shock. Epinephrine is supplied as human or veterinary formulations containing either 0.1 mg/ml (1:10,000) or 1.0 mg/ml (1:1000). Although there is no precisely established dosage or regimen for IV epinephrine in anaphylaxis, 2.5 to 5 mcg/kg IV bolus doses are suggested. Continuous low-dose epinephrine infusions might represent the safest and

Table 152-1 Suggested Therapy for Anaphylaxis

Drug	Dose and Route	Comments
Epinephrine	0.05 mcg/kg/min IV via CRI 2.5-5.0 mcg/kg IV 10 mcg/kg IM	
Atropine	0.02-0.04 mg/kg IV	
Glucagon	1-2 mg (human dose) *or* 5-15 mcg/min IV	For patients who are taking β-blockers or are unresponsive to epinephrine.
Albuterol via inhalation	90 mcg per actuation	Repeat as needed for bronchodilation.
Ipratropium via inhalation	18 mcg per actuation	For patients taking β-blockers, repeat as needed for bronchodilation.
Diphenhydramine	0.5-1.0 mg/kg IV, IM, or PO	
Ranitidine	0.5-2.5 mg/kg IV or PO	
Methylprednisolone sodium succinate	30 mg/kg IV	
Dexamethasone	0.1-0.5 mg/kg IV	
Crystalloid fluids	*Dogs:* 90 ml/kg/hr IV *Cats:* 60 ml/kg/hr IV	Tailor to the individual patient.
Dextran or hetastarch	*Dogs:* 10 ml/kg IV *Cats:* 6 ml/kg IV	
Dopamine	5-10 mcg/kg/min IV via CRI	Titrate rate to achieve adequate blood pressure.
Vasopressin	0.03-0.11 U/kg	Administer as small bolus doses over a short time period.

CRI, Constant rate infusion; *IM*, intramuscularly; *IV*, intravenously; *PO*, per os.

most effective form of IV delivery because the dose can be titrated to the desired effect and the potential for accidental administration of large boluses of epinephrine can be avoided. Common, transient adverse effects of epinephrine include pallor, tremor, anxiety, and palpitations. These correlate with epinephrine's pharmacologic activity and are expected. Rapid administration of inappropriately high concentrations of epinephrine can cause myocardial ischemia, which worsens cardiac dysfunction.[13] Although ineffective for treatment of cardiovascular collapse, single IV or IM boluses may be beneficial for bronchoconstriction and laryngeal edema. When given by the IM route, epinephrine may be helpful in reversing mild hypotension. Administration by the SC route should be avoided.

Other Vasopressors

A significant issue is how to proceed if epinephrine and fluid resuscitation do not reverse the effects of anaphylaxis. The available evidence, although largely anecdotal, provides compelling support for the empirical addition of a potent vasoconstrictor bolus to resuscitate patients with severe anaphylaxis. Human patients taking β-blockers have an increased incidence and severity of anaphylaxis and can develop a paradoxic reaction to epinephrine. In these patients, IM or IV administration of glucagon is suggested. Glucagon has inotropic, chronotropic, and vasoactive effects that are independent of β-receptors and causes endogenous catecholamine release.[16] Airway protection must be ensured because glucagon frequently causes emesis. Vasopressin is useful when treating hemorrhagic and septic shock in humans and animals, and appears useful for the treatment of anaphylaxis by vasoconstriction through the V_1 receptors that mediate vasoconstriction via Gq protein activation of phospholipase C.[17,18] Dopamine may be administered as a constant rate infusion in patients with refractory hypotension. Atropine may be administered if bradycardia persists despite the appropriate administration of epinephrine.

Antihistamines

As was seen with epinephrine, even pretreatment with H_1 blockers (chlorpheniramine maleate) or H_2 blockers (ranitidine), a nonsteroidal antiinflammatory drug (indomethacin), or a lipoxygenase inhibitor did not prevent cardiovascular collapse in the canine anaphylactic shock mode. But pretreatment of dogs with the experimental H_3 receptor antagonist thioperamide maleate increased heart rate and improved greater left ventricular systolic function.[19,20] So although they are not useful during the acute phases of anaphylaxis, H_1 and H_2 antihistamines are frequently administered after epinephrine to reduce pruritus and gastric acid secretion.

Glucocorticoids

Rapid-acting glucocorticoids are often administered in acute anaphylaxis, but beneficial effects are not seen for at least 4 to 6 hours. Glucocorticoids block the arachidonic acid cascade and may reduce the severity of the late-phase reaction. Despite their widespread use for treatment of asthma and allergic reactions, glucocorticoids themselves may cause allergic reactions and even anaphylaxis.[21] Because of a strong possibility of cross-reactivity between hydrocortisone, methylprednisolone, and prednisone, any formulation (succinate, acetate, or sodium phosphate) containing these glucocorticoids should be avoided in patients with previous allergic reactions to systemic steroids. Dexamethasone has been suggested as an alternative in such patients.

Potential Therapies

IL-4 receptor antagonists currently being developed for the treatment of asthma are also possible anaphylaxis therapeutics.[8] These agents could work in multiple ways, such as suppressing IgE production, inhibiting helper T cell differentiation, decreasing mast cell differentiation, and blocking the enhancing effects of interleukin on responsiveness to mediators released by mast cells and macrophages.

Fluid Therapy

Aggressive fluid resuscitation should be carried out in patients with hypotension. Isotonic crystalloids (e.g., normal saline) should be administered at shock bolus rates. Severely affected patients may require colloids and vasopressors such as dopamine. Fluid therapy should be guided by heart rate, blood pressure, mucous membrane color, capillary refill time, and respiratory rate and effort.

Ancillary Patient Management

In the early stages of respiratory distress, inhaled bronchodilators have the fastest onset of action. Albuterol (salbutamol) is a β_2-adrenergic agonist bronchodilator and ipratropium bromide is a topical anticholinergic; both are available in metered dose inhalers and can be used with spacers to facilitate administration to dogs and cats. Early elective intubation is recommended in patients with stridor, lingual edema, or laryngeal or oropharyngeal swelling. If delayed, endotracheal intubation may be impossible, and a tracheotomy must be performed. Oxygen should be administered as needed by nasal catheter or oxygen cage.

Patients that respond to therapy require careful observation, but there is no consensus on the observation time needed. Symptoms can reoccur in some patients (biphasic response). In humans, this typically occurs in 1 to 8 hours but has been reported to occur as long as 72 hours after the initial reaction. Avoidance of triggers for anaphylaxis is important, so careful medical history taking is important to identify potential risk factors. Penicillin reactions are the most common antimicrobial-associated reactions documented in veterinary patients. Although this causes concern regarding the use of cephalosporins in dogs and cats with previous reactions to penicillins, the incidence of cross-reactivity is actually low, and a recent review concluded that it is safe to administer cephalosporins to penicillin-allergic people.[22]

PREVENTION

When an animal experiences repeat episodes of clinical signs consistent with anaphylaxis, the role of prevention and first aid therapy may be considered. If the inciting cause is known, then clearly prevention is ideal. First aid in veterinary medicine is limited, and owners should be educated to recognize the early signs of anaphylaxis and to seek veterinary care immediately. Owner administration of epinephrine via an EpiPen (commercially available autoinjectable formulation of epinephrine made for people) has been recommended by some. Before such a recommendation is made, it is important to consider the role of epinephrine and the risks associated with owner administration. Epinephrine is used in human medicine to treat acute bronchospasm and upper airway edema. It would also be beneficial in acute cardiovascular collapse secondary to vasodilation, but this event is rare. Acute airway compromise appears to be uncommon in small animal patients with anaphylaxis. More commonly, hypovolemia and gastrointestinal signs are present, and these require IV fluid administration. Owner-administered epinephrine is not likely to benefit the majority of patients and may delay the immediate transport of the animal to a veterinary facility, and there may be some risk of the owner's being bitten while attempting to administer the drug. Finally, there is the issue of dosing. The adult-size EpiPen contains 0.3 mg of epinephrine and should be used only in animals weighing 30 kg or more. The EpiPen Jr contains 0.15 mg of epinephrine and would be appropriate for dogs of 15 to 30 kg. There is no appropriately dosed EpiPen for animals weighing less than 15 kg.

REFERENCES

1. Miyaji K, Suzuki A, Shimakura H, et al: Large-scale survey of adverse reactions to canine non-rabies combined vaccines in Japan, Vet Immunol Immunopathol 145:447-452, 2012.
2. Moore GE, DeSantis-Kerr AC, Guptill LF, et al: Adverse events after vaccine administration in cats: 2,560 cases (2002-2005), J Am Vet Med Assoc 231:94-100, 2007.
3. Hume-Smith KM, Groth AD, Rishniw M, et al: Anaphylactic events observed within 4 h of ocular application of an antibiotic-containing ophthalmic preparation: 61 cats (1993-2010), J Feline Med Surg 13:744-751, 2011.
4. Armitage-Chan E: Anaphylaxis and anaesthesia, Vet Anaesth Analg 37:306-310, 2010.
5. Walker T, Tidwell AS, Rozanski EA, et al: Imaging diagnosis: acute lung injury following massive bee envenomation in a dog, Vet Radiol Ultrasound 46:300-303, 2005.
6. Mandigers P, German AJ: Dietary hypersensitivity in cats and dogs, Tijdschr Diergeneeskd 135:706-710, 2010.
7. Sell S: Immunopathology. In Rich RR, Fleisher TA, Schwartz BD, et al, editors: Clinical immunology: principles and practice, St Louis, 1996, Mosby, pp 449-477.
8. Finkelman FD: Anaphylaxis: lessons from mouse models, J Allergy Clin Immunol 120:506-515, 2007; quiz 516-507.
9. Kemp SF, Lockey RF: Anaphylaxis: a review of causes and mechanisms, J Allergy Clin Immunol 110:341-348, 2002.
10. Bautista E, Simons FE, Simons KJ, et al: Epinephrine fails to hasten hemodynamic recovery in fully developed canine anaphylactic shock, Int Arch Allergy Immunol 128:151-164, 2002.
11. Mink SN, Simons FE, Simons KJ, et al: Constant infusion of epinephrine, but not bolus treatment, improves haemodynamic recovery in anaphylactic shock in dogs, Clin Exp Allergy 34:1776-1783, 2004.
12. 2005 American Heart Association guidelines for cardiopulmonary resuscitation and emergency cardiovascular care, Circulation 112:IV1-203, 2005.
13. Simons FE, Ardusso LR, Bilo MB, et al: World allergy organization guidelines for the assessment and management of anaphylaxis, World Allergy Organ J 4:13-37, 2011.
14. Sheikh A, Shehata YA, Brown SG, et al: Adrenaline for the treatment of anaphylaxis: Cochrane systematic review, Allergy 64:204-212, 2009.
15. Smith PL, Kagey-Sobotka A, Bleecker ER, et al: Physiologic manifestations of human anaphylaxis, J Clin Invest 66:1072-1080, 1980.
16. Ellis AK, Day JH: Diagnosis and management of anaphylaxis, CMAJ 169:307-311, 2003.
17. Kill C, Wranze E, Wulf H: Successful treatment of severe anaphylactic shock with vasopressin. Two case reports, Int Arch Allergy Immunol 134:260-261, 2004.
18. Hussain AM, Yousuf B, Khan MA, et al: Vasopressin for the management of catecholamine-resistant anaphylactic shock, Singapore Med J 49:e225-e228, 2008.
19. Chrusch C, Sharma S, Unruh H, et al: Histamine H3 receptor blockade improves cardiac function in canine anaphylaxis, Am J Respir Crit Care Med 160:1142-1149, 1999.
20. Mink S, Becker A, Sharma S, et al: Role of autacoids in cardiovascular collapse in anaphylactic shock in anaesthetized dogs, Cardiovasc Res 43:173-182, 1999.
21. Sheth A, Reddymasu S, Jackson R: Worsening of asthma with systemic corticosteroids. A case report and review of literature, J Gen Intern Med 21:C11-C13, 2006.
22. Anne S, Reisman RE: Risk of administering cephalosporin antibiotics to patients with histories of penicillin allergy, Ann Allergy Asthma Immunol 74:167-170, 1995.

CHAPTER 153

AIR EMBOLISM

Bonnie Wright, DVM, DACVAA

KEY POINTS

- Air embolism occurs when a pocket of gas enters or is formed within the vascular compartment and subsequently causes an obstruction to blood flow.
- Intravenous catheter placement and use, laparoscopy, some surgeries, biopsies, and hyperbaric therapies can all be associated with this complication.
- Prevention of air embolism is ideal because detection is difficult and tends to occur late, after the embolism is dangerously large.
- Transesophageal echocardiography is the most sensitive tool for detection of air embolism, but capnography, blood gas analysis, and evaluation for newly arising heart murmurs may also be useful.
- Oxygen administration is recommended after air embolism. Manual reduction involves aspirating the air from the embolus or reducing the size of the air bubble to restore limited perfusion around the bubble. Hyperbaric oxygen therapy, when available, can be beneficial in reducing the size of the air pocket and increasing the amount of dissolved oxygen in the blood.

Because most veterinary patients do not scuba dive, air embolism is almost entirely an iatrogenic phenomenon in veterinary medicine. Simple procedures such as intravenous injection have the potential to cause this calamity, as do more complicated techniques gaining popularity in veterinary medicine such as laparoscopy. The size of bubble, rate of intravenous gas entry, and physiologic status of the patient combine to determine the severity of the pathophysiology.

As small amounts of air enter into the venous circulation the air will lodge either in the right atrium or pulmonary artery in a gravity-dependent location (air weighs less than blood so it "floats" in a direction opposite to gravity). Smaller air emboli wedge into pulmonary vessels, creating ventilation-perfusion mismatching and pulmonary hypertension. Paradoxically, even in the absence of a visible anatomic shunt from the right to left side of the heart (such as in a patent with foramen ovale or septal defect) air emboli may gain entry to the systemic circulation, where they wreak havoc by blocking blood flow and creating hypoxia in critical organs. The cerebral vasculature and coronary artery are vulnerable locations, and emboli in these locations have the most severe consequences. With a continuous influx of air, small emboli coalesce into larger air pockets leading to massive air embolism. Massive air embolism in the heart creates an absolute obstruction to blood flow. The compressible envelope of air contracts and expands with the working of the heart, and no blood gains entry into the air-filled right ventricle, which leads to cardiac failure and arrest. Because the heart is full of air, resuscitation using standard cardiopulmonary resuscitation techniques is not usually successful in the case of air embolism.

When an embolus is discrete enough to allow circulation to persist, gas is absorbed into the tissues, which eventually reduces the volume of the embolus until it is completely dissolved or small enough to move to a more distal tissue bed. For this reason, the type of gas present in the bubble can have a tremendous impact on the amount of ischemia, as does the tissue bed in which the bubble becomes lodged. Administration of extremely insoluble gases (such as nitrous oxide) exacerbates gas emboli because the insoluble gas escapes from the blood supply and diffuses into the air pockets, causing expansion.[1]

Redundant blood flow salvages the lungs from significant damage from many smaller air emboli, and the lungs serve as the primary sponge for venous air emboli. A constant influx of air can overload this "filter" for emboli, however, allowing bubbles to emerge into the arterial system. In dogs, this occurs in 50% of animals when 0.35 ml/kg/min of air (consisting of primarily nitrogen, an insoluble gas) is infused.[2] Furthermore, lodging of air emboli in the lungs is not necessarily benign and may cause focal injury, edema, and the subsequent release of vasoactive mediators. Eventually this can culminate in alveolar collapse, atelectasis, and impaired gas exchange.[3] The vascular changes are prevalent with nitrogen emboli and can include platelet activation, complement response, leukocyte adhesion, and endothelial cell damage, which appear to be mediated by mitochondrial dysfunction.[4]

GAS EMBOLIZATION DUE TO INTRAVENOUS ACCESS MISHAPS

In ordinary-sized patients, it is somewhat difficult to mistakenly introduce enough room air (nitrogen) to create a clinically apparent embolism. Pigs have tolerated 2 ml/kg of air without irreversible hemodynamic collapse.[1] However, pigs have a reduced ability to remove air during infusions compared with dogs. An air delivery rate of only 0.1 ml/kg/min was associated with bubbles breaking through to the arterial system in pigs, whereas dogs tolerated up to 0.35 ml/kg/min[1,5] Extrapolating from the pig single-dose data, a 1-kg dog could probably tolerate up to about 2 ml of air as a single dose before cardiovascular collapse occurred.

Factors that increase the risk of air embolism include use of a venous access site at a level that is gravitationally higher than the heart. This can occur in standing dogs and cats during jugular catheterization or puncture, or when ear catheters are used. This has also been reported in lateral recumbency, although the rate of air entry is reduced due to the smaller gradient above the heart. Nonetheless, great care should be taken when placing jugular catheters in very small patients in which even a small amount of air could rapidly prove fatal.

In larger dogs and cats, embolization generally occurs when elevated catheters are left open to room air or become disconnected from a sealed system. Air moves into the relatively negative intravascular space, causing air entrainment with subsequent coalescence into a complete venous or cardiac obstruction. Because this usually occurs in patients in room air, the bulk of the embolus is composed of nitrogen gas. Nitrogen is relatively poorly soluble in tissues, so it takes several minutes for a nitrogen embolus to dissipate.[6]

Small air bubbles are often administered during intravenous injections and fluid therapy, but these are well tolerated in normal individuals. However, larger volumes of air may be mistakenly administered via intravenous tubing or extension sets that were not appropriately primed before use. Standard intravenous tubing holds more than 10 ml, and a standard extension set holds 4 ml, which is enough air as a bolus to cause arrest in a 5-kg or 2-kg animal, respectively.

Air emboli have also been known to occur when intravenous fluid bags are placed under pressure. Most fluid bags contain a small amount of air, which can be delivered when the entire contents of the bag are pressurized for rapid administration to a patient. Increased caution is warranted in individuals with a right-to-left cardiac shunt because the lungs may not filter out air bubbles; consequently these individuals may experience focal cerebral infarcts when even the smallest air bubbles are administered or allowed to form.

GAS EMBOLIZATION DURING LAPAROSCOPIC PROCEDURES

Laparoscopy has gained enormous popularity as a less invasive method to diagnose or manage many conditions. However, visualization requires the introduction of a sizeable volume of gas into the body cavity of interest. When this gas exists at a pressure midway between venous collapse and the intravenous pressure, it is then free to move into the vascular bed servicing the inflated region. To minimize the impact of gas bubble formation during laparoscopy, carbon dioxide is generally chosen as the inflation gas. For comparison with the reported volumes of nitrogen required to cause fatalities in dogs, when carbon dioxide is used as the carrier gas, a dose of 300 ml was the mean dose to cause death for a 35-kg dog.[7] Carbon dioxide can still form emboli, but because it is absorbed rapidly into tissues, it seldom causes clinical problems (0.001% to 0.59% incidence in humans).[8] Carbon dioxide has an additional advantage over nitrogen: it does not produce bronchoconstriction or changes in pulmonary compliance to the same degree as nitrogen.

With the advent of transesophageal echocardiography for diagnosis of air emboli, it has become evident that a far greater number of patients experience nonlethal emboli than had been realized. In one study, 100% of patients undergoing laparoscopic hysterectomy had emboli form in the right atrium, right ventricle, and right ventricular outflow tract, and 37% of these were grade III (occupying one half of these structures).[9]

Insufflated gas can gain entry into the vascular system by mistaken placement of the needle into an artery, vein, or solid organ. It can also happen simply because of the positive intraabdominal pressure. In theory, for an embolus to enter the venous system during laparoscopy there would have to be a defect in a vein or other vascular bed. If the intraabdominal inflation pressure matched the intravenous pressure, air could gain access to the circulation. If the inflation pressure were high enough to collapse the vein, air entrainment would cease, and if the inflation pressure were lower than venous pressure there would be hemorrhage from the vein without air entrainment. In general, inflation pressures higher than 15 mm Hg are not recommended during laparoscopy.[8] Under normal conditions veins collapse at 20 to 30 mm Hg; this is significantly higher than the recommended intracompartmental pressure. Therefore, when recommended inflation pressures are used, transected vessels should hemorrhage rather than entrain gas.

Another factor that allows early detection of air embolism (and reduced incidence of massive embolism leading to arrest) is slowing the rate of abdominal insufflation to less than 1 L/min.[10] Although this slower speed of insufflation allows more time for pulmonary clearance of air bubbles, it is still very close to the insufflation rate capable of causing arrest in 60% of dogs studied (1.2 ml/kg/min).[11]

Even when these precautions are followed, embolization during laparoscopy occasionally occurs. Massive embolism is fatal in 28% of human patients, and the rate is likely much higher in veterinary patients. Although the use of carbon dioxide limits some of the negative effects of embolism compared with room air, there remains a risk that enough will accumulate to cause an airlock and death. Rapid and complete ligation or cauterization of any injured vein will also limit the access points for gas emboli. Emboli are certainly a risk of laparoscopy, and monitoring for them is important during all laparoscopic procedures.

GAS EMBOLIZATION DURING SURGERY

As during catheterization, gas embolization during surgery is most likely when the surgical site is higher, gravitationally speaking, than the heart. This situation can occur with most forms of neurosurgery (craniotomy and spinal surgeries) and many orthopedic surgeries (fracture repairs). Air entry is permitted via open veins or sometimes through bony routes (sinuses and long bones). Nitrogen is the predominant gas in room air, so slow absorption of entrained air can be anticipated. Nitrogen is far more dangerous than carbon dioxide, and much smaller volumes can cause greater damage and are much slower for the body to clear.

Prevention begins with surgical positioning, with excessive elevation of the surgical site avoided when possible. When this is not possible, keeping the surgical site filled with isotonic fluids will prevent gas from entering the bloodstream. In human neurosurgery, patients are often placed in a sitting position. Elevation of central venous pressures using positive end-expiratory pressure and volume loading reduce the incidence of air embolism in human and animal models.[8,12] Craniotomy positioning in dogs and cats likewise results in surgical site elevation over the level of the heart.

Cardiopulmonary bypass is notorious for the introduction of air into the circulation. This air entry is extremely difficult to reduce because it arises from both the equipment functioning as the circulatory circuit and the surgery itself.[13] In people, a large number of postbypass complications are attributed, in part, to emboli or microemboli. Although unreported, the incidence may be even higher in veterinary patients because their smaller size magnifies the effect of the smallest air bubbles. Furthermore, many of these emboli are arterial, for which heightened consequences include cerebral and coronary artery obstruction.

GAS EMBOLIZATION FROM LUNG BIOPSY

A rarely reported consequence of lung biopsy in humans is air embolism.[14] This is thought to occur due to entry of the biopsy needle into a vascular bed, with entrainment of extrathoracic air or the creation of bronchovenous fistulas. Although not yet reported in veterinary species, it remains an important consideration for biopsy patients because it could easily be missed in the case of a slow leak with delayed onset cardiac arrest.

GAS EMBOLIZATION DURING HYPERBARIC THERAPY

As mentioned before, pet dogs and cats seldom scuba dive or are subjected to dramatic increases in barometric pressure. One exception may be during intentional hyperbaric treatment for conditions such as anaerobic infections and inflammatory disorders. In a hyperbaric setting, gases dissolve more readily into tissues. When the pressure returns to normal these gases rapidly leave the tissues and form bubbles. When hyperbaric therapy is used, careful attention to recommended protocols is key. Even when protocols are followed, some individuals may experience embolism from gases emerging from a dissolved state into the bloodstream or organs. Appropriate evaluation, detection, and decompression therapy by qualified individuals is important to reduce the impact of this sequela. Unfortunately, there is an unpredictable individual variation as to when this occurs.

DETECTION OF AIR EMBOLI

Air emboli should be considered in any situation in which air can be introduced by equipment or error, or when a surgical procedure produces an incised vascular bed with a hydrostatic pressure gradient favoring venous entry. During high-risk procedures, and when TEE is available, constant monitoring is ideal. Other signs of air embolism include neurologic deficits, changes in end-tidal carbon dioxide readings, the development of a distinct murmur, hypotension, and the development of increasing dead space ventilation as indicated by serial blood gas measurements.

Neurologic signs of air embolism are difficult to detect in animals with the exception of seizures, unconsciousness, or poor, prolonged recovery. An astute observer might detect restlessness, agitation, or change in demeanor in a conscious patient. Advanced imaging can show pockets of air in the cerebral vasculature if it is performed before the air pockets have dissolved. Neurologic sequelae will outlast the presence of air due to hypoxic damage to brain tissue.

Carbon dioxide measurement (using capnography) has been reported to detect gas embolism before cardiac arrest. A rapid drop in carbon dioxide when ventilation is held constant may be an early warning sign of air accumulation. However, there are occasional reports of a rise in carbon dioxide rather than a fall when the gas embolus is comprised of carbon dioxide. The advantages of using capnography are that it is continuous and noninvasive.

Distinctive Doppler sounds over the heart or large vessels occur after 0.5 to 2 ml/kg air has entered the venous system, and the sound is described as a *mill-wheel murmur.* Mill-wheel murmurs are described as harsh, churning, splashing, and metallic. They have been reported near the time of cardiac arrest but are inconsistent.[9]

Tachypnea results from air embolism due to vagally and nonvagally mediated mechanisms, and an anesthetized patient that is not paralyzed may become tachypneic or begin to breathe over the ventilator even before the onset of hypoxemia.[6] Unfortunately, air embolism in animals is often detected by the subsequent cardiovascular collapse. Clearly this is a late sign.

With close intraoperative monitoring a classic progression of signs may be observed. In every breath an individual takes, a quantity of the tidal volume never participates in gas exchange. This is known as *dead-space ventilation.* Many things alter the quantity of dead-space ventilation; the normal quantity is generally thought to be around 30% of the tidal volume.[15] When a region of blood flow through the lungs is abolished, a new region of dead space is created, and there will be an acute fall in the end-tidal carbon dioxide ($ETCO_2$) levels and an increase in measured arterial carbon dioxide pressure ($PaCO_2$).[16]

$$\% \text{ Dead space} \approx [(PaCO_2 - ETCO_2)/PaCO_2] \times 100$$

Simultaneously, blood flow will be routed through regions of the lung that are less ventilated, which increases physiologic shunt and decreases oxygenation. If airway pressures are being measured, there will be an acute elevation, and lung compliance will decrease rapidly with an embolism of air.[16] This is recognized as the delivery of lower tidal volumes at inspiratory pressures that previously accomplished normal ventilation. This does not occur if the embolism is comprised of carbon dioxide. Computed tomography and magnetic resonance imaging may be helpful in detecting emboli but are neither guaranteed nor time efficient in a crisis.[17] Therefore clinical assessment is generally preferred.

TEE is an extremely helpful tool for diagnosing intracardiac air embolism before cardiac arrest. Very small amounts of air can be detected by TEE, which has revealed a far greater entrainment of air during laparoscopy than previously recognized.[9] Once the amount of air or carbon dioxide becomes concerning (at grade III, when half of the right ventricle, right atrium, and right ventricular outflow tract are filled with air) definitive action to prevent further entrainment commences. TEE, however, is time consuming, requires constant vigilance by the operator, and is not commonly available in practice. Use of very specific views of the heart improves detection of air emboli, and this requires significant training and practice to master.

MANAGEMENT OF AIR EMBOLISM

Immediate attention toward interrupting further air entrainment is the most important goal of management. This can be a combination of removing insufflated gas from the abdomen, addressing any nonligated vasculature, and increasing central venous pressure (to facilitate bleeding rather than entrainment of air). Once further intravascular gas flow is prevented, a venous air embolism may resolve, and the pulmonary filter may be sufficient to prevent further arterial spillover of air. Administration of 100% oxygen is recommended, and if nitrous oxide is being used it should be discontinued immediately.[1] Positioning the patient so that the heart apex is elevated (head down, dorsal recumbency for most dogs and cats) may allow the remaining blood flow to bypass the air bubble and exit through the outflow tract, maintaining some perfusion if the air block is not complete. However, the use of body position as a treatment for air embolism is controversial. When manual reduction of an air embolism is possible, it can rapidly restore circulation. The goal is to place a catheter in the embolus and aspirate air or foam, a process that is conveniently diagnostic as well as therapeutic.

Oxygen administration can manage hypoxemia and also provide a diffusion gradient if the embolized gas is anything other than oxygen.[1,17] Work in pigs does not support the use of hyperventilation, but ventilatory support is still recommended because of the increased work of breathing associated with pulmonary air embolism.[3] Immediately after embolization, blood pressure may become transiently high, which may facilitate movement of air bubbles into venous locations. Progressive hypotension is lethal, causing increased bubble entrapment and reductions in coronary and cerebral blood flow and thus compromising the organs most susceptible to anoxia.[17] The goal is to establish and maintain normotension.

Some controversy exists as to the utility of hyperbaric oxygen therapy (HBOT) for reversing gas emboli. Animal studies have given mixed results.[3] HBOT can compress the bubble size (more relevant with air than with carbon dioxide due to solubility). Reduction in bubble size may restore circulation, and in the case of nitrogen, limits some of the blood-gas interface inflammatory effects. A reduction in intracranial pressure and increased dissolved oxygen in the plasma are additional positive effects of HBOT. Overall, if HBOT is available, early intervention is necessary for a beneficial effect, but where it is rapidly available it can be used to very good effect.

The use of drugs in gas embolism is controversial. Hemodilution with colloid fluids improves neurologic recovery, with a target packed cell volume of 30%.[18] Crystalloid fluids in excess of one quarter shock dose are not recommended because of their propensity to exacerbate cerebral edema. If seizures occur, barbiturates are recommended in lieu of benzodiazepines because of better inhibition of catecholamines and reduction in oxygen consumption and intracranial pressure.[3] Heparin has a theoretic advantage in preventing platelet clumping after endothelial damage, but mixed results have been reported in the literature.[3] Glucocorticoids are not recommended because they appear to increase vessel occlusion and infarct size. Intravenous lidocaine has been shown to improve cerebral function and decrease infarct size in several studies.[3]

On the cutting edge, fluorocarbons are solutions with high gas-dissolving capability. When administered intravenously these compounds could improve oxygenation and simultaneously help shrink gas emboli.[2] Finally, work is being done to evaluate compounds that alter surface tension because aspheric emboli tend to have higher internal bubble pressure, which speeds their reabsorption time.[9]

Essentially, preventing gas emboli is key. Failing this, early diagnosis using paired $ETCO_2$ and $PaCO_2$ measurements or TEE improves survival. Management targets reduction of bubble size by a variety of mechanisms followed by brain-protective maneuvers.

REFERENCES

1. Kytta J, Tanskanen P, Randell T: Comparison of the effects of controlled ventilation with 100% oxygen, 50% oxygen in nitrogen, and 50% oxygen in nitrous oxide on responses to venous air embolism in pigs, Br J Anaesth 77:658-661, 1996.
2. Butler B, Robinson R, Sutton K, et al: Cardiovascular pressures with venous gas embolism and decompression, Aviat Space Environ Med 66:408-414, 1995.
3. Val Hulst R, Klein J, Lachmann B: Gas embolism: pathophysiology and treatment, Clin Physiol Funct Imaging 23(5):237-246, 2003.
4. Sobolewski P, Kandel J, Eckmann DM: Air bubble contact with endothelial cells causes a calcium-independent loss in mitochondrial membrane potential, PLoS One 7(10):e47254, 2012.
5. Vik A, Brubakk A, Hennessy T, et al: Venous air embolism in swine: transport of gas bubbles through the pulmonary circulation, J Appl Physiol 69:237-244, 1990.
6. Chen J, Kou Y: Vagal and mediator mechanisms underlying the tachypnea caused by pulmonary air embolism in dogs, J Appl Physiol 88:1247-1253, 2000.
7. Dion YM, Lévesque C, Doillon CJ: Experimental carbon dioxide pulmonary embolization after vena cava laceration under pneumoperitoneum, Surg Endosc 9:1065-1069, 1995.
8. Bazin J, Gillart T, Rasson P, et al: Haemodynamic conditions enhancing gas embolism after venous injury during laparoscopy in pigs, Br J Anaesth 78:570-575, 1997.
9. Park EY, Kwon JY, Kim KJ: Carbon dioxide embolism during laparoscopic surgery, Yonsei Med J 53(3):459-466, 2012.
10. Joris J: Anesthesia for laparoscopic surgery. In Miller R, editor: Anesthesia, ed 5, Philadelphia, 2000, Churchill Livingstone.
11. Mayer KL, Ho HS, Mathiesen KA, et al: Cardiopulmonary responses to experimental venous carbon dioxide embolism, Surg Endosc 12:1025-1030, 1998.
12. Pfitzner J, McLean A: Venous air embolism and active lung inflation at high and low CVP: a study in "upright" anesthetized sheep, Anesth Analg 66:1127-1134, 1987.
13. Branger A, Eckmann D: Theoretical and experimental intravascular gas embolism and absorption dynamics, J Appl Physiol 87(4):1287-1295, 1999.
14. Wu YF, Huang TW, Kao CC, et al: Air embolism complicating computed tomography-guided core needle biopsy of the lung, Interact Cardiovasc Thorac Surg 14:771-772, 2012.
15. Kytta J, Randell T, Tanskanene P, et al: Monitoring lung compliance and end-tidal oxygen content for the detection of venous air embolism, Br J Anaesth 75:447-451, 1995.
16. Annane D, Troche G, Delisle F, et al: Kinetics of elimination and acute consequences of cerebral air embolism, J Neuroimag 5:183-189, 1995.
17. Muth C, Shank E: Gas embolism, N Engl J Med 342:476-482, 2000.
18. Reasoner D, Fyu K, Hindman B, et al: Marked hemodilution increases neurologic injury after focal cerebral ischemia in cats, Anesth Analg 81:61-67, 1996.

CHAPTER 154

OCULAR DISEASE IN THE INTENSIVE CARE UNIT

Steven R. Hollingsworth, DVM, DACVO • Bradford J. Holmberg, DVM, MS, PhD, DACVO

KEY POINTS

- Ocular disease is a common manifestation of systemic illness seen in critically ill patients.
- Corneal disease is a possible complication in anesthetized patients, and appropriate preventative therapy should always be provided.
- Identification of ocular disease is accomplished by conducting a thorough ophthalmic examination including indirect ophthalmoscopy, Schirmer tear testing, fluorescein staining, tonometry, and possibly cytologic studies, culture, or biopsy.

Ophthalmic disease can be associated with or secondary to conditions that require a patient to be in a critical care facility. This chapter describes common ocular signs and discusses the appropriate interpretation of these signs and treatment of the ocular disease.

BLEPHAROSPASM

Blepharospasm is a nonspecific sign of ocular pain and may be associated with enophthalmos, elevation of the third eyelid, and spastic entropion. Both surface and intraocular disease can result in blepharospasm. The origin of ocular pain is determined by conducting a thorough ophthalmic examination, including diagnostic tests such as fluorescein staining, Schirmer tear testing, and tonometry. A topical anesthetic (e.g., 0.5% proparacaine) may facilitate examination by eliminating pain related to surface disease.

RED EYE

Veterinary clinicians commonly encounter patients with a "red eye." The redness represents new or congested blood vessels within the episclera, conjunctiva, or cornea. Episcleral vessels are stout, easily identifiable vessels that course perpendicular to the limbus and usually stop before reaching the limbus. Congestion of these vessels is associated most commonly with intraocular disease, specifically uveitis and glaucoma. However, with moderate to severe corneal disease these vessels may become engorged.

Conjunctival blood vessels are extremely fine; without the aid of magnification individual vessels are difficult to identify. When vessels are engorged, a pink-red flush is observable. Mild conjunctival hyperemia may be apparent with intraocular disease, but moderate signs are consistent with surface disease (e.g., conjunctivitis or keratoconjunctivitis). Differential diagnostic considerations for conjunctivitis include infections (canine distemper, feline herpesvirus infection, feline *Chlamydophila* infection, leishmaniasis, onchocerciasis), allergies, postradiotherapy conditions, keratoconjunctivitis sicca (KCS), and exposure. Diagnosis is based on history and the results of Schirmer tear testing, fluorescein staining, cytologic studies, and biopsy.

Conjunctival hyperemia can be easily confused with a conjunctival or subconjunctival infiltrate. This infiltrate may be fluid (chemosis) or cells. Mild chemosis is common with conjunctivitis. Severe chemosis may obstruct visualization of the cornea and intraocular structures. The most common cause of primary chemosis is topical toxicity (from neomycin, atropine, caustic agents). Removing the toxin and treating supportively allows resolution of signs. Rarely, intravenous fluid overload at a rate of two to three times maintenance for a period of 2 days or longer can result in marked chemosis. Tapering the fluid rate allows the chemosis to resolve.

The presence of subconjunctival infiltrates may cause the conjunctiva to appear thickened. The infiltrates may be focal or diffuse. Carefully examining the color of the conjunctiva may help in differentiating an infiltrate from common hyperemia.

A diffuse yellow appearance of the conjunctiva in the absence of thickening is consistent with icterus. This may be the first clinical sign of icterus and should prompt the clinician to pursue further diagnostic tests to assess hepatobiliary status.

Neoplastic cells within the subconjunctiva frequently result in thickening and a yellow to orange hue. Lymphoma is the most common neoplasia presenting in the subconjunctiva, and the subconjunctiva may represent the primary tumor site. Other disorders producing masses in the subconjunctiva include systemic histiocytosis (orange), hemangiosarcoma (red), melanoma (brown), and granulomatous scleritis (pink). A definitive diagnosis can usually be obtained by biopsy. Light sedation and topical anesthesia are typically all that is needed to obtain a diagnostic sample.

Subconjunctival hemorrhage in a critically ill patient, observed as petechiae or ecchymoses, warrants investigation for an underlying coagulopathy. Hemorrhage may be isolated to the subconjunctiva or seen in the anterior chamber (hyphema). Causes of hemorrhage not associated with a coagulopathy include trauma, strangulation (from choke collars), chronic emesis, and rarely constipation.

A blue-green discoloration of the sclera and/or conjunctiva may be noted. This has been observed in dogs receiving mitoxantrone chemotherapy. Signs are temporary and usually resolve within hours to days after cessation of treatment.

TEAR FILM ABNORMALITIES

The tear film is comprised of three layers: an outer lipid layer, a middle aqueous layer, and an inner mucin layer. A deficiency in any of these components may result in decreased tear production or increased tear clearance (evaporation) and may be diagnosed with a Schirmer tear test.

Clinical signs of a tear film abnormality depend on the severity, chronicity, and underlying cause of the tear deficiency. The most consistent and obvious finding is a thick mucoid discharge, commonly accumulated on and around the eyelids. Additional clinical signs include conjunctival hyperemia, a lackluster appearance to the corneal surface, and in chronic cases corneal vascularization and melanosis. Chronic tear film deficiencies lead to thickening of the corneal epithelium, and therefore ulceration is not common. However, the critically ill patient may develop acute KCS resulting in rapid, severe, and potentially globe-threatening corneal ulceration.

There are numerous causes of decreased tear production (KCS) and increased tear clearance. Undoubtedly the most common cause of KCS is immune-mediated destruction of the lacrimal gland and gland of the third eyelid. This will likely be a preexisting disease in critically ill patients, although tear production in canine intensive care unit patients is decreased compared with that in healthy dogs. Treatment with topical cyclosporine or tacrolimus and artificial tear ointments or gels should be initiated to support surface ocular health.

Other causes of decreased tear production include radiation therapy, drug toxicity (sulfonamides, atropine, etodolac), chronic blepharoconjunctivitis, general anesthesia, orbital trauma, neurogenic factors, and congenital lacrimal gland hypoplasia (Yorkshire Terrier, Chinese Crested); rarely, it is secondary to an endocrine disorder (hypothyroidism, diabetes mellitus, hyperadrenocorticism).

In one study megavoltage radiation near the orbit resulted in KCS in 24% of dogs within 1 to 6 months of therapy secondary to direct destruction of glandular tissue.[1] Medical therapy is solely supportive, including the application of artificial tear ointments (petroleum, lanolin, mineral oil base) and gels as frequently as possible.

Sulfa-containing drugs are well known to decrease aqueous tear production, with 65% of patients having decreased tear production, 15% with clinical signs of KCS.[2] Sulfonamides should be used with caution in small breeds, brachycephalic breeds, and those breeds predisposed to KCS. Stopping therapy at the onset of KCS may allow lacrimal function to return in some patients. An idiosyncratic reaction resulting in irreversible, absolute xerophthalmia has been demonstrated in a small percentage (0.0003%) of dogs receiving etodolac. Patients should have a normal Schirmer tear test result before treatment and should be monitored closely during therapy. Any decrease in tear test results warrants cessation of oral therapy and initiation of topical therapy.

General anesthesia, especially with atropine as a premedication, dramatically decreases aqueous tear production, and the decrease may persist for 24 hours.[3] Many patients receive a topical lubricant before anesthesia but rarely afterward. A topical lubricating ointment should be applied at least every 4 hours for 24 hours following anesthesia to decrease ocular surface drying, which may lead to corneal ulceration.

Neurogenic KCS results from disruption of the parasympathetic fibers coursing with the facial and trigeminal nerves to the lacrimal gland. Clinical signs are similar to those of immune-mediated KCS, except that in these cases dysfunction is usually unilateral. If the lesion is near the pterygopalatine ganglion, the caudal nasal nerve will also be affected, and a dry, crusty nose ipsilateral to the dry eye will be noted. Treatment is aimed at stimulating the denervated gland to secrete aqueous tears. Two percent pilocarpine (1 drop/4.4 kg [10 lb] orally [PO] q12h increased slowly to effect) may be effective, although there is a fine line between a therapeutic and a toxic dose. Signs of toxicity include vomiting, diarrhea, and ptyalism. Treatment with topical lubricants and cyclosporine or tacrolimus is also warranted.

Increased tear clearance secondary to evaporation accounts for most cases of dry eye in the intensive care patient. Increased evaporation may be secondary to a tear lipid deficiency, lagophthalmos, or decreased reflex tearing. Meibomianitis, blepharitis, and conjunctivitis damage the meibomian glands or conjunctival goblet cells, which results in instability of the tear film. Treatment with mucinomimetic preparations such as 1% to 2% methylcellulose or sodium hyaluronate helps restore tear film stability.

Lagophthalmos is the inability to completely close the eyelids and may be a conformational disorder (brachycephalic breeds, cicatricial ectropion, eyelid agenesis) or neurologic disorder (facial or trigeminal nerve dysfunction, obtundation). The lack of a consistently complete palpebral reflex is diagnostic. With lagophthalmos, the tear film is exposed and rapidly evaporates, especially in the interpalpebral fissure. Obtunded animals frequently have decreased or absent palpebral reflexes and decreased reflex tearing, which further complicates the tear deficiency. Regardless of the cause, hourly application of an artificial tear ointment or gel is necessary. If the condition is left untreated, progressive corneal ulceration will ensue. Chronic cases (e.g., artificially ventilated patients) may require a lateral temporary tarsorrhaphy.[4]

ABSENT PALPEBRAL REFLEX

Absence of the palpebral reflex is due to either loss of trigeminal nerve function (the afferent arm) or facial nerve paralysis (the efferent arm). Of these, facial nerve paralysis is far more common. In addition to loss of the palpebral reflex, signs associated with facial nerve paralysis in cats and dogs include lowered carriage of the ear, drooping of the eyelids with resultant widening of the palpebral fissure, and increase in scleral visibility on the affected side, as well as "pulling" of the nose toward the normal side (Figure 154-1).

Because the lacrimal nerve runs with the facial nerve over a portion of its course, Schirmer tear test values should be monitored in patients with facial nerve paralysis. Compromise of both facial and lacrimal nerve function can lead to severe corneal disease due to the fact that there is a reduction in both tear production and distribution. This condition is referred to as *neuroparalytic keratitis.*[5] Causes of facial nerve paralysis include trauma, neoplasia, and surgery to the head or neck region. Depending on the cause, the signs of facial nerve paralysis may resolve spontaneously. Because the retractor bulbi muscle is innervated by the abducens nerve, many patients learn to "blink" with their third eyelid by retracting their globes. Facial nerve paralysis can often be managed by frequent application of lubricating ointments (every 4 to 6 hours). However, in severe cases, especially with neuroparalytic keratitis, a partial lateral tarsorrhaphy may be beneficial.

The trigeminal nerve provides sensory innervation to the ocular surface and eyelids. An abnormal palpebral reflex caused by trigeminal dysfunction can be differentiated from that due to facial nerve paralysis by the fact that the patient will blink when menaced.[5] Disruption of this innervation may result in severe keratitis. The most

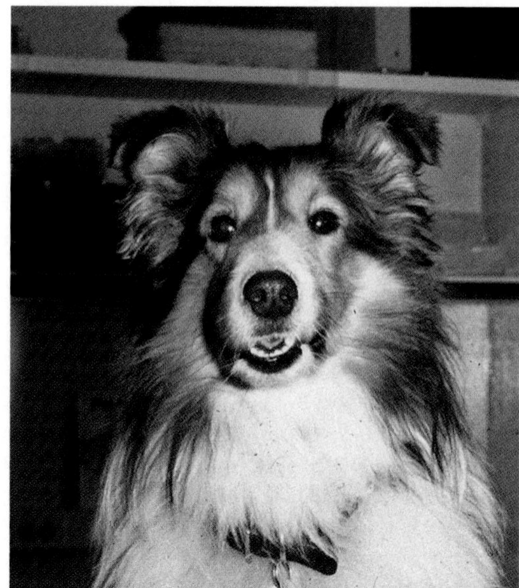

FIGURE 154-1 Right sided facial nerve paralysis in a dog. Note the lowered carriage of the right ear, widening of the right palpebral fissure, and pulling of the nose to the normal, left side.

common cause of trigeminal nerve loss is orbital trauma.[6] Unlike those with facial nerve paralysis, these patients do not "blink" with their third eyelids because they do not have any sensation of ocular surface dryness. Treatment for ocular problems related to trigeminal nerve compromise is supportive care of the cornea with topical lubricants.

CORNEAL CHANGES

Corneal clarity is sacrificed when there is disruption of the normal organization of stromal collagen lamellae, in-growth of blood vessels, or deposition of pigment or cells. Epithelial cell loss usually results in focal corneal edema, although expansive defects can result in diffuse edema. Corneal endothelial cell dysfunction causes diffuse edema and is secondary to intraocular disease, specifically uveitis or glaucoma. A thorough ophthalmic examination including fluorescein staining and tonometry can aid in differentiating the underlying cause.

The normal cornea is avascular and receives nutrition from the tear film and aqueous humor. Therefore the presence of blood vessels indicates an ongoing pathologic process. Superficial corneal blood vessels appear as fine tree branches and are consistent with superficial disease (superficial corneal ulceration, KCS, exposure keratitis, pannus). Deep corneal blood vessels have the appearance of hedges, with individual vessels difficult to identify. These vessels are present with deep corneal (stromal) or intraocular (uveitis, glaucoma) disease. With disease, vessel in-growth is delayed for approximately 2 to 4 days, and then vessels advance approximately 1 mm per day. Therefore length of the vessels can aid in determining the chronicity of disease.

Corneal ulceration is likely the most commonly encountered primary ophthalmic disease in the intensive care patient. Clinical signs include blepharospasm, conjunctival hyperemia, episcleral congestion, mucoid to mucopurulent discharge, focal to diffuse corneal edema, an observable corneal defect, and potentially vascularization, abscess formation, or malacia. Diagnosis is facilitated by application of fluorescein stain. Stromal loss, cellular infiltrate, moderate vascularization, and progression despite medical therapy indicate a complicated corneal ulcer (Figure 154-2).

The leading cause of complicated ulcers is the use of topical steroids in a patient with a corneal defect. Complicated ulcers require strict monitoring and aggressive medical and potentially surgical therapy. Therefore referral to or consultation with an ophthalmologist is recommended.

When one is dealing with a complicated ulcer, determination of the depth of the defect is the first step. This can be accomplished using the slit beam on a direct ophthalmoscope and looking at the change in curvature of the light beam. Other hints include the location of corneal blood vessels (see previous discussion) and fluorescein staining characteristics. If stain is observed only along the walls, but not the floor, a descemetocele is present and immediate referral to an ophthalmologist is recommended.

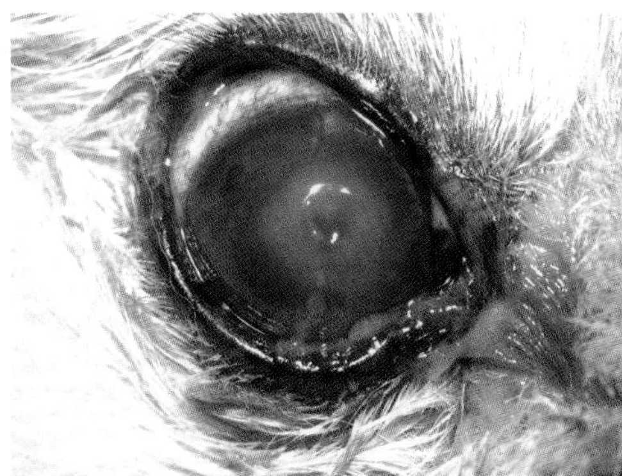

FIGURE 154-2 Infected corneal ulcer in a dog. Note the mucopurulent discharge, conjunctival hyperemia, corneal edema, stomal loss, and cellular infiltrate. This patient also has hypopyon with a few red blood cells intermixed in the ventral aspect of the anterior chamber.

After determination of the depth, samples should be obtained for aerobic bacterial culture and cytologic analysis.[7] Initial therapy should include a broad-spectrum topical antibiotic (dependent on culture and cytology results) at least every 4 hours, topical atropine every 12 hours, and use of an Elizabethan collar. If cellular infiltrate or malacia is present, a more powerful topical antibiotic such as a fourth-generation fluoroquinolone (moxifloxacin or gatifloxacin) should be administered every 2 hours along with topical serum every 2 hours. Serum can be harvested from the patient or a healthy donor of the same species. Serum must be kept refrigerated and a new batch should be harvested once weekly to prevent contamination.

Fortunately, most corneal ulcers are not complicated. A topical triple-antibiotic preparation applied two to four times daily, a single dose of atropine, and use of an Elizabethan collar are usually sufficient. Epithelialization of uncomplicated ulcers occurs within 3 to 5 days. If healing has not occurred within this time, either the ulcer has become complicated or the underlying cause (ectopic cilia, distichiasis, conjunctival or third eyelid foreign body) has not been identified.

Corneal infiltrates other than white blood cells associated with infected ulcers are rare. Notable exceptions include neoplastic cells, mineral, and lipid. Circumferential, severe perilimbal vascularization with a yellow-orange corneal infiltrate along the leading edge of the vessels may represent lymphoma. Cholesterol crystals and lipid may be deposited in an arclike fashion (arcus lipoides) in the anterior corneal stroma. Often this represents a systemic dyslipidemia, and further diagnostic tests to investigate the cause are warranted. Other concurrent signs may include lipemic aqueous or lipemia retinalis. Differential diagnostic considerations include hypothyroidism, diabetes mellitus, hyperadrenocorticism, pancreatitis, and a primary hyperlipidemia.

ANTERIOR CHAMBER ABNORMALITIES

Changes in the appearance of the anterior chamber most often are due to alterations in the composition of the aqueous. The aqueous is essentially modified blood with protein and cells removed in the ciliary body. Under conditions of anterior uveitis, these elements gain entry into the aqueous humor, producing the signs of aqueous flare (protein), keratic precipitates (fibrin and white blood cell aggregates on the posterior cornea), hyphema (red blood cells), and hypopyon (white blood cells) (Figure 154-3).

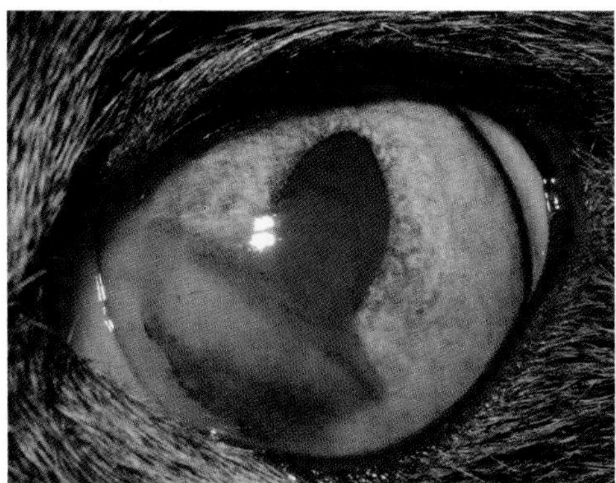

FIGURE 154-3 Fibrin clot in the anterior chamber in a cat with lymphoma.

Although all of these conditions are nonspecific indicators of anterior uveitis, keratic precipitates, hyphema, and hypopyon are seen frequently with certain causes of anterior uveitis. Keratic precipitates are often a sign of feline infectious peritonitis (FIP), lymphoma, or systemic fungal infections. Hyphema frequently is associated with systemic hypertension, coagulopathies, and corneal perforations. Hypopyon is often seen with causes of anterior uveitis that lead to an outpouring of white blood cells, such as systemic fungal or bacterial infections and lymphoma.

Treatment for anterior uveitis should be aimed at both the underlying systemic ailment and the ophthalmic disease. Prednisolone acetate (1% suspension) or dexamethasone (0.1%, either suspension or ointment) administered every 2 to 12 hours depending on severity represent excellent choices for topical therapy. Hydrocortisone is relatively impotent and poorly absorbed when applied topically and is not a suitable antiinflammatory agent for treatment of anterior uveitis.

Topical nonsteroidal ophthalmic medications are also available; namely, flurbiprofen (0.03% solution) and diclofenac (0.1% solution). These are good alternatives to topical steroid preparations if corneal ulceration is present or systemic conditions prevent the use of steroids. Systemically administered steroidal and nonsteroidal drugs reach the anterior uvea and can be helpful adjuncts, especially in severe cases. Topical atropine (1% solution or ointment) may be indicated in the treatment of anterior uveitis to relieve the pain associated with iris sphincter and ciliary body muscle spasms and to prevent posterior synechia. However, it must be used with caution and intraocular pressure must be closely monitored during its use because it can exacerbate glaucoma, especially in dogs.

PUPIL ABNORMALITIES

Pupil abnormalities may or may not be associated with other ophthalmic disease. They are divided into four clinical presentations: anisocoria, miosis, mydriasis, and dyscoria.

Anisocoria

Anisocoria is defined as unequal size of the pupils. Although anisocoria is usually easy to detect, it can be challenging to ascertain which pupil is abnormal. Careful observation of pupil size in ambient light and dim illumination and pupil reaction under stimulation with a bright light source usually allow for this determination. Once it has been determined which is the affected pupil, the next step is to investigate the causes of miosis or mydriasis.

Miosis

Pupil size in mammals is the product of the balance between the parasympathetic tone of the iris sphincter muscle and the sympathetic tone of the iris dilator muscle. Therefore miosis is the result of stimulation of the iris sphincter, loss of sympathetic tone of the iris dilator, or both. Although miosis may be produced with topical medications, such as pilocarpine and latanoprost, there are two clinical conditions that cause miosis: anterior uveitis and Horner's syndrome. Fortunately, these two causes are easily distinguished from one another on the basis of associated ophthalmic signs.

In addition to miosis, signs often associated with anterior uveitis include blepharospasm, epiphora, episcleral injection, 360-degree corneal vascularization, corneal edema, aqueous flare, keratic precipitates, hypopyon, and hyphema. Anterior uveitis is the most common ophthalmic manifestation of systemic disease and is often present in critically ill patients. Common diseases that can cause anterior uveitis in cats and dogs are systemic infectious disease (fungal, bacterial, viral, rickettsial, and algal), primary or secondary neoplasia, blunt or penetrating trauma, and immune-mediated conditions. Treatment for anterior uveitis is covered earlier in the chapter in the section Anterior Chamber Abnormalities.

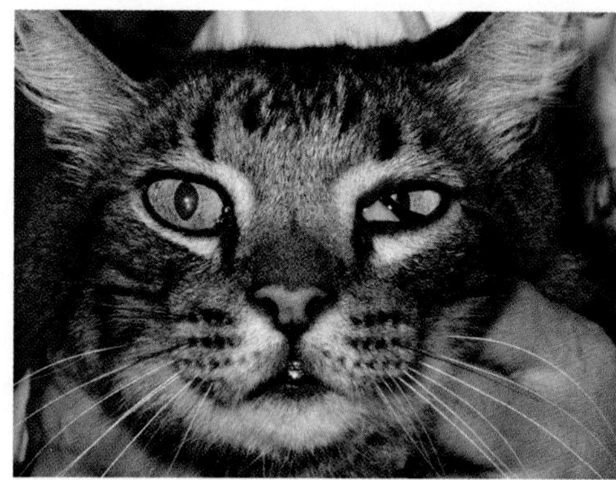

FIGURE 154-4 Left eye of a cat with Horner's syndrome. Note the narrowed palpebral fissure due to drooping of the upper eyelid (ptosis), miosis, and third eyelid protrusion.

The signs associated with Horner's syndrome are secondary to compromise of the sympathetic innervation to the eye and consist of a triad of signs in cats and dogs: ptosis, miosis, and third eyelid protrusion secondary to enophthalmos (Figure 154-4). Although ptosis and third eyelid protrusion can mimic blepharospasm, the eyes of patients with Horner's syndrome are comfortable and noninflamed. Horner's syndrome is frequently idiopathic, but it can occur secondary to otitis interna or media, trauma or surgery to the side of the face or neck, or intracranial or thoracic neoplasia.[8,9] Pharmacologic testing can localize the lesion in Horner's syndrome and is described in detail elsewhere.[10,11] Treatment of Horner's syndrome is accomplished by identifying and addressing the underlying cause, if possible. No specific ophthalmic therapy is indicated.

Mydriasis

Mydriasis is due to stimulation of the iris dilator muscle or compromise of the parasympathetic tone of the iris sphincter muscle, or both. As with miosis, mydriasis can be pharmacologically induced with agents such as atropine. However, unlike miosis, mydriasis is associated with many conditions. Highly stressed patients, particularly cats, can have dilated pupils and poor to absent pupillary light responses (PLRs). Likewise, aged patients with iris atrophy may have mydriasis in one or both eyes. Optic nerve or end-stage retinal disease can also lead to mydriasis. For causes of these conditions, see the Blindness section later.

Mydriasis is a consistent sign of glaucoma, and intraocular pressure should be measured in all patients with dilated pupils. The most common cause of glaucoma in critically ill patients is anterior uveitis. Glaucoma is painful and blinding, and steps should be taken immediately to lower intraocular pressure. If the patient's systemic condition allows it, mannitol (20% to 25% solution) administered slowly intravenously (over the course of about 30 minutes) at a dose of 1 to 2 g/kg can produce a dramatic drop in intraocular pressure. Other effective glaucoma medications include methazolamide (5 mg/kg PO q12-24h), dorzolamide solution (q8-12h topically), and latanoprost solution (q12-24h topically).

Mydriasis is also a consistent finding in dysautonomia (Key-Gaskell syndrome), which is most frequently seen in cats,[12] although a similar syndrome has been reported in dogs.[13] In addition to mydriasis, signs associated with this condition include anorexia, depression, weight loss, dehydration, bradycardia, constipation, protrusion of both third eyelids, and decreased tear production. Pharmacologic testing to verify the diagnosis is described elsewhere.[14] Treatment for the ocular component of dysautonomia consists of topical lubrication.

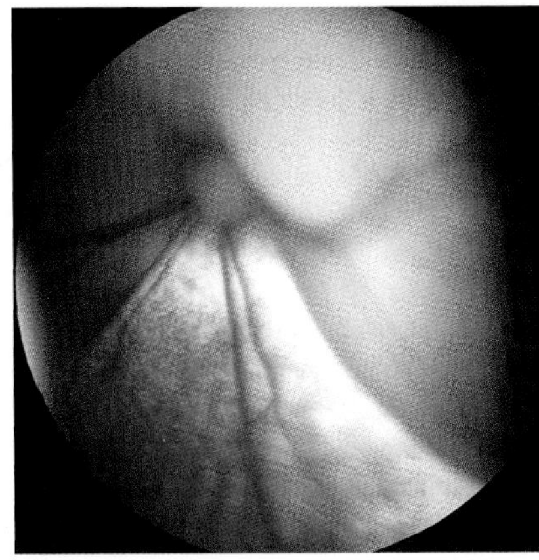

FIGURE 154-5 Exudative retinal separation in a cat.

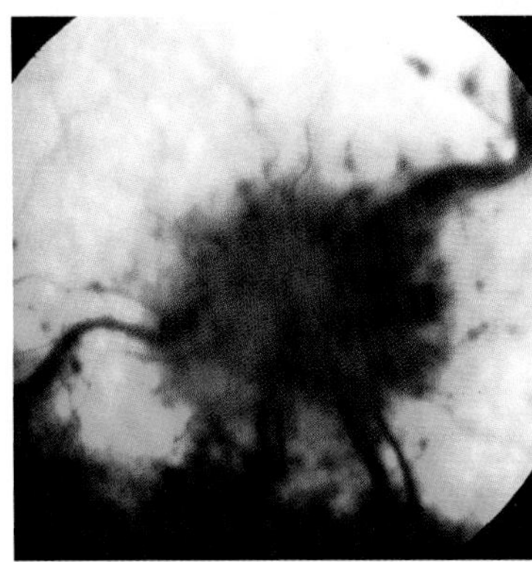

FIGURE 154-6 Optic neuritis resulting from cryptococcosis in a cat. Note the fuzzy, indistinct borders of the optic disc and the peripapillary hemorrhages.

The unique parasympathetic innervation of the feline pupil can produce a variation in mydriasis, the D-shaped or reverse D-shaped pupil in which only one half of the pupil dilates. This defect is due to lesions involving the medial or lateral short ciliary nerve and is commonly associated with feline leukemia virus infection.

Dyscoria

Dyscoria is defined as an irregularly shaped pupil. It is most commonly secondary to posterior synechiae, a result of anterior uveitis.

BLINDNESS

Visual capability commonly is assessed by eliciting a menace response, observing the patient tracking a cotton ball dropped repeatedly within its visual range, or performing a maze test. Unfortunately, verification of visual status is often problematic for the critical care practitioner because many seeing patients appear to fail these routine tests due to either alterations in mentation or inability to ambulate.

Blindness can occur as a result of disease in one of five anatomic locations: (1) cornea, (2) lens, (3) retina, (4) optic nerve or tracts, and (5) brain. Blindness due to corneal changes is readily apparent, and causes of alterations in corneal transparency are covered elsewhere in this chapter. Causes of cataracts associated with serious systemic disease include diabetes mellitus and anterior uveitis. However, neither of these would likely lead to cataract formation over the period that a patient would be hospitalized in a critical care setting.

A number of systemic conditions can lead to retinal disease and vision compromise. PLRs are often present, even in advanced retinal disease. Therefore normal PLRs do not rule out retinal disease as a cause of vision impairment. Retinal conditions associated with vision compromise secondary to systemic disease are manifested most frequently as retinal separation, retinal hemorrhage, or retinal inflammatory cellular infiltrates. Retinal separations frequently are classified by the nature of the subretinal fluid: serous, hemorrhagic, or exudative (Figure 154-5). The type of fluid under the separation can provide clues as to the underlying cause.

Systemic conditions that may manifest with a serous retinal separation include systemic hypertension (early) and autoimmune disease, such as uveodermatologic syndrome in dogs. Typical causes of hemorrhagic retinal separation and intraretinal hemorrhage include systemic hypertension, rickettsial disease (Rocky Mountain spotted fever, ehrlichiosis), toxic coagulopathies due to rodenticides, vasculitis (FIP), immune-mediated hemolytic anemia, and hyperviscosity syndrome. Exudative retinal separation and intraretinal inflammatory cellular infiltrates are commonly an expression of systemic fungal disease, neoplasia (especially lymphoma), toxoplasmosis, viral diseases (canine distemper, feline leukemia virus infection, feline immunodeficiency virus infection, FIP), and protothecosis. Ivermectin toxicity may cause acute blindness in dogs.[15] In addition to blindness, these dogs may be brought to an emergency facility because of neurologic signs such as depression, hypersalivation, ataxia, and tremors.[16,17] A careful history taking often reveals either exposure to horses being wormed with ivermectin or current treatment with ivermectin for *Demodex* infection. Examination of the fundus is either unremarkable or demonstrates focal "cotton wool" areas of retinal edema near the optic disc. Affected dogs usually have a return to vision over the course of a week. Recently, intravenous administration of lipid emulsion has been shown to rapidly reverse the effects of ivermectin toxicity.[18,19]

In cats, acute blindness has been associated with systemic enrofloxacin therapy at dosages as low as 4 mg/kg PO q12h.[20] This is manifested by diffuse tapetal hyperreflectivity and retinal vascular attenuation without signs of retinal separation or retinal cellular infiltration.

The extent of vision impairment with all of these conditions depends on the extent of retinal involvement. For virtually all of these conditions, there is no specific treatment of the ocular component beyond addressing the underlying systemic cause.

Optic nerve disease can lead to blindness and may be associated with a number of systemic illnesses. Unlike retinal causes of vision impairment, blindness due to optic nerve disease usually is accompanied by loss of PLRs and mydriasis. Optic nerve disease may or may not be manifested by changes in the appearance of the optic disc. When present, ophthalmoscopic signs of optic nerve disease include optic disc swelling, fuzzy and indistinct disc borders, and hemorrhages on the disc or in the peripapillary area (Figure 154-6).

Systemic diseases with the potential for optic nerve involvement include granulomatous meningoencephalitis, canine distemper, lymphoma, systemic fungal infection (especially cryptococcosis), meningioma, and hyperviscosity syndrome. Treatment is aimed at the underlying systemic cause.

Blindness secondary to involvement of the visual center in the occipital cortex is rare in cats and dogs. Affected animals usually have marked neurologic deficits.

REFERENCES

1. Roberts SM, Lavach JD, Severin GA, et al: Ophthalmic complications following megavoltage irradiation of the nasal and paranasal cavities in dogs, J Am Vet Med Assoc 190:43, 1987.
2. Berger SL, Scagliotti RH, Lund EM: A quantitative study of the effects of Tribrissen on canine tear production, J Am Anim Hosp Assoc 31:236, 1995.

3. Herring IP, Pickett JP, Champagne ES, et al: Evaluation of aqueous tear production in dogs following general anesthesia, J Am Anim Hosp Assoc 36:427, 2000.
4. Bojrab MJ, Birchard ST, Tomlinson JL, editors: Current techniques in small animal surgery, ed 3, Philadelphia, 1990, Lea & Febiger.
5. Ofri R: Neuroophthalmology. In Maggs DJ, Miller PE, Ofri R, editors: Slatter's fundamentals of veterinary ophthalmology, ed 5, St Louis, 2013, Elsevier.
6. Whitley RD, Gilger BC: Diseases of the canine cornea and sclera. In Gelatt KN, editor: Veterinary ophthalmology, ed 3, Philadelphia, 1999, Lippincott Williams & Wilkins.
7. Morreale RJ: Corneal diagnostic procedures, Clin Tech Small Anim Pract 18:148, 2003.
8. Morgan RV, Zanotti SW: Horner's syndrome in dogs and cats: 49 cases (1980-1986), J Am Vet Med Assoc 194:1096, 1989.
9. Kern TJ, Aromando MC, Erb HN: Horner's syndrome in dogs and cats: 100 cases (1975-1985), J Am Vet Med Assoc 195:369, 1989.
10. Scagliotti RH: Comparative neuroophthalmology. In Gelatt KN, editor: Veterinary ophthalmology, ed 3, Philadelphia, 1999, Lippincott Williams & Wilkins.
11. Slatter D: Neuroophthalmology. In Slatter D, editor: Fundamentals of veterinary ophthalmology, ed 3, Philadelphia, 2001, Saunders.
12. Canton DD, Sharp NJ, Aguirre GD: Dysautonomia in a cat, J Am Vet Med Assoc 192:1293, 1988.
13. Wise LA, Lappin MR: A syndrome resembling feline dysautonomia (Key-Gaskell syndrome) in a dog, J Am Vet Med Assoc 198:2103, 1991.
14. Guilford WG, O'Brien DP, Allert A, et al: Diagnosis of dysautonomia in a cat by autonomic nervous system function testing, J Am Vet Med Assoc 193:823, 1988.
15. Kenny PJ, Vernau KM, Puschner B, et al: Retinopathy associated with ivermectin toxicosis in two dogs, J Am Vet Med Assoc 233:279, 2008.
16. Houston DM, Parent J, Matushek KJ: Ivermectin toxicosis in a dog, J Am Vet Med Assoc 191:78, 1987.
17. Hopkins KD, Marcella KL, Strecker AE: Ivermectin toxicosis in a dog, J Am Vet Med Assoc 197:93, 1990.
18. Clarke DL, Lee JA, Murphy LA, et al: Use of intravenous lipid emulsion to treat ivermectin toxicosis in a Border Collie, J Am Vet Med Assoc 239:1328, 2011.
19. Epstein SE, Hollingsworth SR: Ivermectin-induced blindness treated with intravenous lipid therapy in a dog, J Vet Emerg Crit Care (San Antonio) 23:58, 2013.
20. Gelatt KN, van der Woerdt A, Ketring KL, et al: Enrofloxacin-associated retinal degeneration in cats, Vet Ophthalmol 4:99, 2001.

CHAPTER 155
CRITICALLY ILL NEONATAL AND PEDIATRIC PATIENTS

Maureen McMichael, DVM, DACVECC

KEY POINTS

- There are significant differences in the biochemical, hematologic, radiographic, pharmacologic, and monitoring parameters in neonatal and pediatric animals.
- Dramatic elevations in alkaline phosphatase and γ-glutamyltransferase levels and very low values for serum levels of blood urea nitrogen, albumin, and cholesterol occur in the neonate and can mimic hepatic failure.
- The most common causes of dehydration in the neonate and pediatric patient are gastrointestinal losses and insufficient intake.

There are several crucial differences in the diagnosis, monitoring, and treatment of critically ill neonates and pediatric patients compared with critically ill adult patients, and it is essential for veterinarians with a neonatal and pediatric patient base to become familiar with normal biochemical, hematologic, radiographic, and physical examination values for this age group. In veterinary medicine, the term *neonate* encompasses animals from birth to 2 weeks of age, and the term *pediatric* refers to animals between 2 weeks and 6 months of age. This chapter reviews the hematologic, biochemical, nutritional, imaging, fluid treatment, monitoring, and pharmacologic aspects of the normal and critically ill neonate and pediatric cat and dog. Also included is a brief review of sepsis in the neonate.

PHYSICAL EXAMINATION FINDINGS

Healthy neonates are lively and plump (Box 155-1). Illness is often recognized by incessant crying, lethargy, limpness, and poor muscle tone. Mucous membranes are often hyperemic during the first 4 to 7 days of life and may be pale, cyanotic, or gray in sick neonatal animals. The rectal temperature at birth is normally 35.2° to 37° C (95.4° to 98.6° F) and gradually increases to adult levels over the first 4 weeks of life.

By pediatric stethoscope (ideally), many puppies and kittens will be found to have an innocent murmur until 12 weeks of age. However, other causes of a murmur include a congenital cardiac

BOX 155-1 ***Clinical Values for Normal Puppies and Kittens***

- *Heart rate:* 200 beats/min (puppy) and 250 beats/min (kitten)
- *Respiratory rate:* 15 breaths/min (birth) and 30 breaths/min (by 1 to 3 hours after birth)
- *Temperature:* 35.2° to 37° C (95.4° to 98.6° F) at birth, normalizing to adult values at 4 weeks
- *Mean arterial pressure:* 49 mm Hg at 1 month of age, 94 mm Hg at 9 months (puppies)
- *Central venous pressure:* 8 cm H_2O at 1 month of age, 2 cm H_2O at 9 months (puppies)

defect, stress, fever, sepsis, anemia, and hypoproteinemia. The heart rate in the normal neonatal puppy and kitten is 200 and 250 beats/min, respectively. The heart rate decreases as the animal develops increased parasympathetic tone at 4 weeks of age. The respiratory rate following birth is normally 15 breaths/min but increases to 30 breaths/min within 1 to 3 hours. Because of the small tidal volume and increased interstitial fluid in the normal neonate, assessment of lung sounds is difficult. An increase or decrease in heart rate or respiratory rate should be assessed and rates should be monitored during treatment.

LABORATORY VALUES

The hematocrit (Hct) decreases from 47.5% at birth to 29.9% by day 28 in puppies (Box 155-2).[1] By the end of the first month, the Hct starts to increase again. Kittens also have an Hct nadir at 4 to 6 weeks of 27%.[2] Knowledge of this normal decrease in Hct is essential for assessment of any neonate, and during this period a rise in the Hct is usually indicative of dehydration.

Slight changes are seen in the biochemical profile of newborn puppies and kittens. In dogs there is a mild increase in bilirubin level (0.5 mg/dl; normal adult range, 0 to 0.4 mg/dl) and dramatic increases in serum levels of alkaline phosphatase (3845 IU/L; normal adult range, 4 to 107 IU/L) and γ-glutamyltransferase (1111 IU/L; normal adult range, 0 to 7 IU/L).[3] In kittens, the alkaline phosphatase level (123 IU/L; normal adult range, 9 to 42 IU/L) is threefold higher than that seen in adults.

Lower values of blood urea nitrogen (BUN), creatinine, albumin, cholesterol, and total protein are seen in neonates compared with adults (although the BUN concentration may be slightly elevated during the first week of life). Calcium and phosphorus levels are higher in neonates. Urine is isosthenuric in neonates because the capacity to concentrate or dilute urine is limited in this age group.[4] This becomes important when prescribing fluid therapy because overhydration is just as much a concern as is underhydration.

BOX 155-2 *Normal Laboratory Values for Puppies and Kittens*

Complete Blood Count—Pediatric Canine

Hematocrit: 47% at birth, 29% at 28 days
Leukocyte count: $12.0 \times 10^3/mm^3$, day 7
Band count: $0.5 \times 10^3/mm^3$, day 7
Lymphocyte count: $5 \times 10^3/mm^3$, day 7
Eosinophil count: $0.8 \times 10^3/mm^3$, day 7

Complete Blood Count—Pediatric Feline

Hematocrit: 35% at birth, 27% at 28 days
Leukocyte count: $9.6 \times 10^3/mm^3$ at birth, $23.68 \times 10^3/mm^3$ at 8 weeks
Lymphocyte count: $10.17 \times 10^3/mm^3$ at 8 weeks, $8.7 \times 10^3/mm^3$ at 16 weeks
Eosinophil count: $2.28 \times 10^3/mm^3$ at 8 weeks, $1 \times 10^3/mm^3$ at 16 weeks

Biochemistry Profile—Pediatric Canine*

Bilirubin: 0.5 mg/dl (range, 0.2 to 1; normal adult range, 0 to 0.4)
Alkaline phosphatase: 3845 IU/L (range, 618 to 8760 IU/L; normal adult range, 4 to 107 IU/L)
γ-Glutamyltransferase: 1111 IU/L (range, 163 to 3558 IU/L; normal adult range, 0 to 7 IU/L)
Total protein: 4.1 g/dl (range, 3.4 to 5.2 g/dl; normal adult range, 5.4 to 7.4 g/dl)
Albumin: 1.8 g/dl at 2 to 4 weeks (range, 1.7 to 2 g/dl; normal adult range, 2.1 to 2.3 g/dl)
Glucose: 88 mg/dl (range, 52 to 127 g/dl; normal adult range, 65 to 100 g/dl)

Biochemistry Profile—Pediatric Feline*

Bilirubin: 0.3 mg/dl (range, 0.1 to 1 mg/dl; normal adult range, 0 to 0.2 mg/dl)
Alkaline phosphatase: 123 IU/L (range, 68 to 269 IU/L; normal adult range, 9 to 42 IU/L)
γ-Glutamyltransferase: 1 IU/L (range, 0 to 3 IU/L; normal adult range, 0 to 4 IU/L)
Total protein: 4.4 g/dl (range, 4 to 5.2 g/dl; normal adult range, 5.8 to 8 g/dl)
Albumin: 2.1 g/dl (range, 2 to 2.4 g/dl; normal adult range, 2.3 to 3 g/dl)
Glucose: 117 mg/dl (range, 76 to 129 mg/dl; normal adult range, 63 to 144 mg/dl)

*At birth except where specified.

IMAGING

Normal anatomic differences in the young may be significant and are reviewed briefly. The thymus is located in the cranial thorax on the left side and can mimic a mediastinal mass or lung consolidation on thoracic radiographs. The heart takes up more space in the thorax than it does in adults and can appear enlarged. The lung parenchyma has increased water content and appears more opaque in neonates.[5] There is an absence of costochondral mineralization so that the liver appears to protrude further caudal from under the rib cage than expected, which makes a misdiagnosis of hepatomegaly more likely. There is loss of abdominal detail due to lack of fat and a small amount of abdominal effusion.[5] Radiographic resolution may be improved by reducing the kilovoltage peak value to half of the adult setting and using detailed film or screens.

INTRAVENOUS AND INTRAOSSEOUS CATHETERIZATION

When venous access is required, use of the intravenous route is preferred and should be attempted first. Neonates often require very small-gauge catheters (e.g., 24 or 27 gauge), which can develop burrs easily when advanced through the skin. To avoid this, a small skin puncture can be made with a 20-gauge needle (while the skin is kept elevated), then the catheter can be fed through the skin hole.

If attempts at intravenous catheter placement fail, an intraosseous catheter should be placed (see Chapter 194). An intraosseous catheter can be inserted in the proximal femur or humerus using an 18- to 22-gauge spinal needle or an 18- to 25-gauge hypodermic needle. An intraosseous catheter can be used for fluid and blood administration.[6] The area must be prepared in a sterile manner and the needle inserted into the bone parallel to the long axis. Gentle aspiration will ensure patency, and the needle is secured with a sterile bandage. Intravenous access must be established as soon as possible, ideally within 2 hours, and the intraosseous catheter should be removed to minimize the risk of osteomyelitis or other complications. The incidence of intraosseous catheter complications correlates with duration of use.[7]

FLUID REQUIREMENTS

Neonates have higher fluid requirements than adults because they have a higher percentage of total body water, a higher ratio of surface area to body weight, a higher metabolic rate, more permeable skin, a decreased renal concentrating ability, and less body fat. Both dehydration and overhydration are concerns because neonatal kidneys cannot concentrate or dilute urine as well as adult kidneys can.[4]

A warm isotonic crystalloid bolus (30 to 40 ml/kg in puppies and 20 to 30 ml/kg in kittens) should be administered to moderately dehydrated neonates, followed by a constant rate infusion (CRI) of 80 to 100 ml/kg/day. A liter of fluid warmed to 104° F will cool down to room temperature (70° F) within approximately 10 minutes. A fluid warmer that is placed in line is also a good option. Lactated Ringer's solution may be the ideal fluid because lactate is the preferred metabolic fuel in the neonate with hypoglycemia.[8,9]

Hypoglycemia in neonates commonly occurs as a result of inefficient hepatic gluconeogenesis, inadequate hepatic glycogen stores, and glucosuria. Urinary glucose reabsorption does not normalize until approximately 3 weeks of age in puppies.[10,11] In addition, neonates have greater glucose requirements than do adults. The neonatal brain requires glucose for energy, and brain damage can occur with prolonged hypoglycemia.[11] Fetal and neonatal myocardia use carbohydrate (glucose) for energy rather than the long-chain fatty acids used by the adult myocardium.[12] In summary, neonates have an increased demand for, an increased loss of, and a decreased ability to synthesize glucose compared with adults.

In adults, the counterregulatory hormones (i.e., cortisol, growth hormone, glucagon, and epinephrine) are released in response to low blood glucose levels and facilitate euglycemia by increasing gluconeogenesis and antagonizing insulin. Clinical signs of hypoglycemia can be challenging to recognize in neonates because of inefficient counterregulatory hormone release during hypoglycemia.[11]

Vomiting, diarrhea, infection, and decreased oral intake all contribute to hypoglycemia in neonates. A bolus of 1 to 3 ml/kg of 12.5% dextrose (i.e., 50% dextrose diluted 1:3 with sterile water) followed by a CRI of isotonic fluids supplemented with 2.5% to 10% dextrose is required to treat hypoglycemia. Any continuous supplementation higher than 5% dextrose must be given through a central line. To prevent a rebound hypoglycemia, any bolus should be followed by a dextrose CRI. In addition, some neonates may have refractory hypoglycemia and may respond only to hourly boluses of dextrose in addition to a CRI of crystalloids with supplemental dextrose. Carnitine supplementation may allow maximal utilization of glucose and may be considered as an additional therapeutic option. The recommended dosage is 200 to 300 mg/kg orally q24h for both puppies and kittens.

The most common causes of hypovolemia in neonates are gastrointestinal (GI) disturbances (e.g., vomiting, anorexia, diarrhea) and inadequate oral intake. The most common cause of diarrhea in neonatal puppies and kittens is iatrogenic (owner) overfeeding with formula. In adults with hypovolemia, compensation occurs through an increase in heart rate, concentration of the urine, and a decrease in urine output. In neonates, compensatory mechanisms may not be adequate. Contractile elements make up a smaller portion of the fetal myocardium (30%) than the adult myocardium (60%), which makes it difficult for the fetus to increase cardiac contractility in response to hypovolemia. Neonates also have immature sympathetic nerve fibers in the myocardium and cannot maximally increase heart rate in response to hypovolemia. Complete maturation of the autonomic nervous system does not occur until after 8 weeks in puppies.[13,14] Because neonates have higher fluid requirements and increased losses (less renal concentrating ability, higher respiratory rate, higher metabolic rate), dehydration can progress rapidly to hypovolemia and shock if not treated adequately.

The difficulties associated with assessing hypovolemia in neonates require constant vigilance and continuous monitoring. One must assume that all neonates with severe diarrhea, inadequate intake, or severe vomiting are dehydrated and potentially hypovolemic, and treatment should be initiated immediately. Fluid therapy, monitoring of electrolyte and glucose status, and nutritional support are the mainstays of treatment. The patient should be weighed every 6 to 12 hours. Dehydration is likely when the urine specific gravity reaches 1.020, and this parameter should be monitored as an indicator of rehydration.[15] In severely dehydrated or hypovolemic animals a bolus of 40 to 45 ml/kg (puppies) or 25 to 30 ml/kg (kittens) of warm isotonic fluids is given initially, followed by a CRI of maintenance fluids (80 to 100 ml/kg/day) and replacement of losses. Losses can be estimated (e.g., 2 tablespoons of diarrhea is equal to 30 ml of fluid). If the neonate is hypoglycemic or not able to eat, dextrose is added to the intravenous fluids at the lowest concentration that will maintain normoglycemia (treatment should start with 1.25% dextrose).

TEMPERATURE CONTROL

Neonates are basically poikilothermic for the first 2 weeks of life and are prone to hypothermia because of a higher ratio of surface area to volume, immature metabolism, and immature shivering reflex (this reflex develops at 6 days) and vasoconstrictive ability, and because their temperature is normally lower than that of mature animals. Hypothermic patients should be rewarmed slowly. Animals that are separated from the mother should be placed in a neonatal incubator at a temperature of 85° to 90° F and humidity of 55% to 65%. Heat lamps or heating pads and hot water bottles may also be used, but the neonate should be able to crawl away from the heat source. Heating pads should be covered with a towel to prevent burns.

NUTRITION

Nutrition is crucial to neonatal health, and inadequate caloric intake must be addressed promptly to prevent malnutrition. A surrogate dam is ideal if the biologic dam is unavailable, but this is often difficult to arrange. Weighing the neonate on a pediatric gram scale before and after each feeding can help the clinician to monitor intake.

Bottle and tube feeding are other therapeutic options. Animals that are separated from the mother should be stabilized and rewarmed slowly before feeding because hypothermia prevents digestion and induces ileus. A human infant bottle is preferred for puppies because they often cannot latch onto the smaller kitten-size nipple supplied with most replacement formulas. Tube feeding is done using a 5 Fr red rubber catheter for neonates under 300 g and an 8 to 10 Fr catheter for larger neonates and should be performed only by experienced personnel.[16] It is easy to improperly place the feeding tube in the trachea in neonates because the gag reflex does not develop until 10 days of age.

Up to 10% of body weight may be lost within the first 24 hours following birth; additional weight loss or failure to gain weight is abnormal. Puppies should double their weight within 10 days of birth and gain 5% to 10% of their body weight per day. Nursing kittens should also double their weight within the first 10 days of life, and normal kittens gain 10 to 15 g per day. Formula-fed neonates grow at significantly slower rates, even with identical caloric intake. Although critically ill neonates and pediatric patients may not gain weight normally, weight loss should be prevented.

Recently, the human microbiome project has begun to elucidate the critical nature of our symbiotic relationship with microflora.[17] Intestinal commensal bacteria directly influence the development of the immune functions and differentiation of the epithelium of the GI tract.[18] Microflora produce enzymes that aid in mucus secretion, synthesis of certain vitamins, and absorption of calcium, magnesium, and iron. Protection against invading pathogens occurs via several mechanisms, including release of antibacterials (bacteriocins, lactic acid), competition for adhesion sites and nutrients, and the physical barrier itself.[18] Critical illness combined with long-term medical therapy can disrupt the GI microbiome because of decreases in GI perfusion, antimicrobial drug administration, use of histamine-2 antagonists and proton pump inhibitors, administration of drugs that cause GI stasis, and lack of enteral nutrition. Supplementation with prebiotics (foods that sustain the growth of intestinal microorganisms) and probiotics (microorganism strains that may help recolonize the GI tract) has been shown to be safe and cost effective, in addition to having few known adverse effects. Unfortunately, very little research in this area has been done in veterinary medicine, particularly pediatrics, but this option should be considered in any animal that likely has a compromised GI flora.

MONITORING

Monitoring disease progression and efficacy of treatment can be challenging in neonates because the values of many parameters are significantly different from those in adults. Mean arterial pressure is lower (49 mm Hg at 1 month of age in puppies) and does not normalize (94 mm Hg) until 9 months of age.[19] Central venous pressure is higher (8 cm H_2O) at 1 month of age in puppies but decreases to 2 cm H_2O by 9 months of age[19] (see Box 155-1).

Neonates cannot autoregulate their renal blood pressure with variations in systemic arterial pressure as adults do, so that the glomerular filtration rate decreases as the systemic blood pressure decreases.[19] This makes restoration of intravenous fluid volume critical in neonates.

Appropriate renal concentration and dilution of urine does not occur until approximately 10 weeks of age.[20,21] Simultaneously, BUN and creatinine concentrations are lower in neonates than in adults, which makes monitoring for azotemia very challenging.

The best way to monitor for underhydration or overhydration is to have an accurate pediatric gram scale and weigh the patient three or four times per day. Baseline thoracic radiographs are also helpful because normal neonate lungs have more interstitial fluid than adult lungs, and it can be difficult to diagnose fluid overload without a baseline. Other ways to monitor fluid therapy include checking Hct and total solids. It should be kept in mind that the Hct decreases progressively in normal neonates from day 1 to day 28, and total solids are lower than in adults (see the Laboratory Values section earlier).

Neonatal skin has a lower fat and higher water content than does that of adults, and therefore skin turgor cannot be used to assess dehydration. Mucous membranes remain moist in severely dehydrated neonates and cannot be used for assessment. Lactate level, thought to be a good indicator of perfusion, especially when serial measurements are used, has been shown to be higher in normal puppies than in adult dogs (1.07 to 6.59 mmol/L at 4 days of age and 0.80 to 4.60 mmol/L from 10 to 28 days of age).[22]

Hypothermia 25.6° to 34.4° C (78° to 94° F) is common in neonates and is associated with a depressed respiratory rate, bradycardia, GI paralysis, and coma. Rectal temperature should be monitored using a normal digital thermometer. Temperatures above the normothermic range indicate fever or excessive external warming.

A new therapeutic device that has great potential in veterinary pediatrics is currently being evaluated. Pulse oximetry–based determination of hemoglobin (Hb) level allows measurement of Hb noninvasively.[23] The oximeter uses light absorption to determine levels of total Hb, oxyhemoglobin, and in some cases carboxyhemoglobin and methemoglobin as well. There are still significant issues with the currently approved devices and no published studies in human pediatrics or neonatology using the technology.[23] The current studies reveal problems with accuracy and precision, particularly in patients that are hypotensive or hypoperfused. The benefits of noninvasive Hb measurement are substantial, particularly in the littlest patients.

PHARMACOLOGY

Drug metabolism in neonates differs significantly from that in adults because of differences in levels of body fat, total protein, and albumin (a protein to which many drugs bind). Renal clearance of drugs is decreased in neonates and renal excretion of many drugs (e.g., diazepam, digoxin) is diminished, which increases the half-life of the drug in circulation.[4] Hepatic clearance is more complicated. Drugs requiring activation via hepatic metabolism will have lower plasma concentrations, and drugs requiring metabolism for excretion will have higher plasma concentrations.[24,25]

The oral route of fluid and drug administration should be avoided during the first 72 hours of life because absorption is significantly higher due to increased GI permeability. Intestinal flora is very sensitive to disruption by oral antimicrobial agents. Administration via the intravenous (or intraosseous) route seems to be the most predictable and is preferred over intramuscular or subcutaneous administration in this age group.[4]

One of the safest classes of antimicrobials in neonates is the β-lactam group (i.e., penicillins and cephalosporins), but the dosing interval should be increased to every 12 hours rather than every 8 hours.[4] Metronidazole is the preferred drug for treatment of giardiasis and anaerobic infections. The dose and/or frequency should be decreased in neonates.

Dosages of cardiovascular drugs (e.g., epinephrine, dopamine, dobutamine) can be quite difficult to determine in neonates because of individual variations in maturity of the autonomic nervous system. Assessment of response to treatment and continuous monitoring of hemodynamic variables are essential when these drugs are used. Elevations in heart rate after administration of dopamine, dobutamine, or isoproterenol cannot be predicted until 9 to 10 weeks of age, and response to atropine and lidocaine is decreased in the neonate.[26-28] The blood-brain barrier is more permeable in neonates, allowing drugs to enter that do not normally cross over to the central nervous system.[22]

The normal neonatal respiratory rate is about two to three times higher than the normal adult rate as a result of higher airway resistance and higher oxygen demands. Drugs that depress respiration should be avoided in neonates. Neonates are very dependent on a high heart rate to increase cardiac output, so drugs that depress heart rate should be avoided. Opioids are a good choice for analgesia because of the reversibility of their effects, but the animal must be monitored closely because of the propensity of these drugs to depress heart and respiratory rate.

Caution is advised when using heparinized saline flushes at the same volume (3 ml) used in adults. It is easy to overheparinize young animals; therefore a smaller volume of heparinized saline or plain isotonic saline should be used.

SEPSIS

Wounds such as those from tail docking or umbilical cord ligation as well as respiratory, urinary, and GI tract infections are most commonly implicated in neonatal sepsis. Common bacterial isolates include *Staphylococcus, Streptococcus, Escherichia coli, Klebsiella, Enterobacter, Clostridium,* and *Salmonella.* Additional possible causes of sepsis include brucellosis, viral infections (distemper, panleukopenia, herpesvirus infection, feline infectious peritonitis, and feline leukemia virus infection), and toxoplasmosis. Clinical signs, as with hypovolemia, are often subtle or absent, which makes the diagnosis difficult in this age group. Some clinical signs that may be associated with sepsis are crying and reluctance to nurse, decreased urine output, and cold extremities.

Studies of sepsis in children and several animal models have documented improved survival with rapid, aggressive fluid resuscitation.[29] Large volumes of fluid are often needed in septic patients because of their increased capillary permeability (increased losses) and vasodilation. Resuscitation should be started immediately with a bolus of 30 to 45 ml/kg (puppies) or 25 to 30 ml/kg (kittens) of warm isotonic fluids, followed by a reassessment of the parameters of perfusion (see later in this section).

If perfusion has normalized, a CRI consisting of maintenance fluids plus compensation for estimated dehydration and ongoing losses is begun. If perfusion has not normalized, repeated boluses may be required. Monitoring includes serial checks of perfusion indicators including mucous membrane color, pulse quality, extremity temperature, lactate levels, and mentation. Administration of a CRI of fresh or fresh frozen plasma or subcutaneous administration of serum from a well-vaccinated adult may help to augment immunity.[30] One study in kittens showed that both intraperitoneal and subcutaneous administration of adult cat serum in three 5-ml increments (at birth and at 12 and 24 hours) resulted in immunoglobulin G concentrations equivalent to those seen in kittens that suckled normally.[31] Frequent checks of electrolyte levels, blood glucose concentration, body temperature, and nutrition are done as indicated earlier.

Septic neonates that have undergone adequate fluid resuscitation but that remain in a hypoperfused state (e.g., cold extremities, high lactate levels, low urine output, low blood pressure) may benefit from vasopressor or inotropic support, or both (e.g., dopamine, dobutamine, phenylephrine, norepinephrine). Because of variations in the maturity of the autonomic nervous system, all pressor and inotropic drug therapy needs to be tailored to the individual animal. Acceptable endpoints of therapy to normalize perfusion include increases in extremity temperature, decreases in lactate levels, increased urine production, and improvement in attitude.

Ideally a sample from the area of possible infection is submitted for culture and susceptibility testing before antibiotic treatment is begun. Broad-spectrum antibiotics may be required if the source of infection cannot be identified. Penicillins or first-generation cephalosporins are good choices in the neonate.

If oxygen therapy is needed, the inspired oxygen fraction should be kept at or below 0.4 to avoid oxygen toxicity, which can cause retrolental fibroplasia and lead to permanent blindness.[32]

Sepsis can be very difficult to detect in neonates. A high index of suspicion should be maintained for all neonates with risk factors, and treatment should be instituted rapidly and aggressively. The incidence of pediatric sepsis in humans is highest in premature newborns. Respiratory infections (37%) and primary bacteremia (25%) are the most common infections.[33]

CONCLUSION

The unique anatomic and physiologic characteristics of critically ill neonatal and pediatric patients make diagnosis, monitoring, and treatment of these patients challenging. Parameters used in adults cannot be relied on in very young patients, and an awareness of their unique characteristics is essential. In addition, many laboratory and pharmacologic data differ dramatically in neonates compared with adults of the same species. Familiarity with these variations is essential in the monitoring and treatment of neonatal or pediatric patients that may be experiencing hypovolemia, shock, or sepsis.

REFERENCES

1. Earl FL, Melveger BE, Wilson RL: The hemogram and bone marrow profile of normal neonatal and weanling Beagle dogs, Lab Anim Sci 23:690, 1973.
2. Meyers-Wallen V: Hematologic values in healthy neonatal, weanling and juvenile kittens, Am J Vet Res 45:1322, 1984.
3. Center S, Hornbuckle W, Hoskins JD: The liver and pancreas. In Hoskins JD, editor: Veterinary pediatrics: dogs and cats from birth to six months, ed 3, Philadelphia, 2001, Saunders.
4. Boothe DM, Tannert K: Special considerations for drug and fluid therapy in the pediatric patient, Compend Contin Educ Pract Vet 14:313, 1992.
5. Partington B: The physical examination and diagnostic imaging techniques. In Hoskins JD, editor: Veterinary pediatrics: dogs and cats from birth to six months, ed 3, Philadelphia, 2001, Saunders.
6. Otto C, Kaufman G, Crowe D: Intraosseous infusion of fluids and therapeutics, Compend Contin Educ Vet Pract 11:421, 1989.
7. Fiser DH: Intraosseous infusion, N Engl J Med 322:1579, 1990.
8. Levitsky LL, Fisher DE, Paton JB, et al: Fasting plasma levels of glucose, acetoacetate, D-beta-hydroxybutyrate, glycerol, and lactate in the baboon infant: correlation with cerebral uptake of substrates and oxygen, Pediatr Res 11:298, 1977.
9. Hellmann J, Vannucci RC, Nardis EE: Blood-brain barrier permeability to lactic acid in the newborn dog: lactate as a cerebral metabolic fuel, Pediatr Res 16:40, 1982.
10. Bovie KC: Genetic and metabolic diseases of the kidney. In Bovie KC, editor: Canine nephrology, Philadelphia, 1984, Harel.
11. Atkins C: Disorders of glucose homeostasis in neonatal and juvenile dogs: hypoglycemia: Part 1, Compend Contin Educ Vet Pract 6:197, 1984.
12. Textile D, Hoffman JIE: Coronary circulation and myocardial oxygen consumption. In Glickman PD, Heyman MA, editors: Pediatrics and perinatology: the scientific basis, London, 1996, Arnold.
13. Textile D, Hoffman JIE: Ventricular function. In Glickman PD, Heyman MA, editors: Pediatrics and perinatology: the scientific basis, London, 1996, Arnold.
14. Mace SE, Levy MN: Neural control of heart rate: a comparison between puppies and adult animals, Pediatr Res 17:491, 1983.
15. McIntire D: Pediatric intensive care, Vet Clin North Am Small Anim Pract 29:837, 1999.
16. Hoskins JD: Pediatric health care and management, Vet Clin North Am Small Anim Pract 29:837, 1999.
17. NIH Human Microbiome Project. Available at http://Hmpdacc.org. Accessed August 2013.
18. Papoff P, Ceccarelli G, d'Ettorre G, et al: Gut microbial translocation in critically ill children and effects of supplementation with pre- and pro biotics, Int J Microbiol 2012:151393, 2012.
19. Magrini F: Haemodynamic determinants of the arterial blood pressure rise during growth in conscious puppies, Cardiovasc Res 12:422, 1978.
20. Holster M, Keeler BJ: Intracortical distribution of number and volume of glomeruli during postnatal maturation in the dog, J Clin Invest 50:796, 1971.
21. Fetuin M, Allen T: Development aspects of fluid and electrolyte metabolism and renal function in neonates, Compend Contin Educ Vet Pract 13:392, 1991.
22. McMichael MA, Lees GE, Hennessey J, et al: Serial plasma lactate concentrations in 68 puppies aged 4 to 80 days, J Vet Emerg Crit Care (San Antonio) 15:17, 2005.
23. Holtby H, Skowno JJ, Kor DJ, et al: New technologies in pediatric anesthesia, Pediatr Anesth 22:952-961, 2012.
24. Short CR: Drug disposition in neonatal animals, J Am Vet Med Assoc 184:1161, 1984.
25. Peters E, Farber T, Heider A: The development of drug metabolizing enzymes in the young dog, Fed Proc Am Soc Biol 30:560, 1971.
26. Driscoll DJ, Gillette PC, Lewis RM, et al: Comparative hemodynamic effects of isoproterenol, dopamine, and dobutamine in the newborn dog, Pediatr Res 13:1006, 1979.

27. Mary-Rabine L, Rosen MR: Lidocaine effects on action potentials of Purkinje fibers from neonatal and adult dogs, J Pharmacol Exp Ther 205:204, 1978.
28. Woods WT, Urthaler F, James TN: Progressive postnatal changes in sinus node response to atropine and propranolol, Am J Physiol 234:H412, 1978.
29. Thomas NJ, Carcillo JA: Hypovolemic shock in pediatric patients, New Horiz 6:120, 1998.
30. Poffenbarger EM, Olson PN, Chandler ML, et al: Use of adult dog serum as a substitute for colostrum in the neonatal dog, Am J Vet Res 52:1221, 1991.
31. Levy JK, Crawford PC, Collante WR, et al: Use of adult cat serum to correct failure of passive transfer in kittens, J Am Vet Med Assoc 219:1401, 2001.
32. Jenkinson S: Oxygen toxicity, Crit Care Med 3:137, 1988.
33. Watson RS, Carcillo JA, Linde-Zwirble WT, et al: The epidemiology of severe sepsis in children in the United States, Am J Respir Crit Care Med 167:695, 2003.

CHAPTER 156

CRITICALLY ILL GERIATRIC PATIENTS

Maureen McMichael, DVM, DACVECC

KEY POINTS

- The number of geriatric pet cats and dogs is growing rapidly in many parts of the world, especially the United States and Europe.
- Maintenance energy requirements decrease in older dogs but appear to increase in older cats (>12 years), which affects nutritional requirements in this age group.
- Comorbid conditions are common in this age group and clinicians should maintain an index of suspicion for the ones encountered most frequently.
- Older animals do not appear to possess sufficient physiologic reserves, and acute illness can significantly tax their organ systems.

The number of geriatric pets has increased considerably during the last 10 years. In 1995, 24% of pet cats in the United States were older than 6 years of age. Today the proportion is estimated to be approximately 47%.[1] In Europe the number of geriatric cats increased by over 100% between 1983 and 1995, and the number of geriatric dogs increased by approximately 50% during that time.[2] Unfortunately, this growing subset of the pet population has received little scientific scrutiny, and research pertaining to geriatric critical care is extremely sparse.

In human medicine, gerontology is a distinct specialty, and geriatric competencies have been introduced into emergency and critical care residency programs.[3,4] Older patients tend to have complex clinical presentations that are frequently influenced by comorbid conditions. The goal of the geriatric competencies is to make clinicians more comfortable with the challenges of treating patients in this age group.

Several studies have shown that older age alone does not predict mortality in elderly people. The main determinants of mortality are prior health status and severity of the current disease process(es).[5-7] Although similar studies have not been done in veterinary medicine, it seems prudent to offer aggressive treatment to the older dog and cat once comorbid diseases, quality of life of the pet, and the owner's desires are taken into consideration.

The term *geriatric* is difficult to define in veterinary medicine because it differs between dogs and cats and among breeds (e.g., a Great Dane has a much shorter life span than a Chihuahua). American Animal Hospital Association guidelines suggest that a pet is geriatric when it has entered the last 25% of its expected life span. In the majority of studies small animals older than 7 years are considered geriatric.

A recent prospective screening of 45 geriatric dogs (median age, 11.5 years) elucidated many of the comorbid conditions affecting this age group.[8] Forty-nine percent of owners reported vision and/or hearing loss and 42% reported lameness/stiffness and/or slowing down in their pets.[8] On physical examination 24% of the dogs had decreased range of motion in their joints, 18% had suspected neoplastic masses, and only 34% had a normal urine dipstick. Overall, unrecognized problems were identified in 80% of the dogs in this study, with a mean of 7.8 problems identified per dog. These comorbid conditions may require additional diagnostics, changes in fluid and drug administration, nutritional intervention, and analgesia.

This chapter reviews the physiologic changes that occur as a result of aging as they relate to critical care medicine.

LABORATORY VALUES

In people at rest, the laboratory values for red blood cells, white blood cells, platelets, and hemoglobin do not change with age. However, there is a decrease in the ability of the bone marrow to increase neutrophil production in response to infection and to increase red blood cell production in response to anemia in geriatric humans.[9] Neutrophil function has also been shown to decrease with age in humans.[9]

There are no established reference ranges for geriatric small animal patients, perhaps because the term *geriatric* is difficult to define, and therefore the laboratory values are hard to quantify. Harper and others looked at age-related variations in laboratory values in Beagles and Labrador Retrievers. The dogs were grouped into categories, and the geriatric category included all animals older than 10 years of age. There were no differences between the laboratory values for dogs older than 10 years of age and those for the rest of the adult dogs.[10] Strasser and colleagues[11] investigated age-dependent changes in laboratory values before and after exercise in Beagles. There were no significant differences in the laboratory values for 5-year-old and 10-year-old Beagles at rest. After exercise, however, significant differences were seen in many of the parameters. The older dogs had lower hematocrits, red blood cell counts, and hemoglobin concentrations. They also had a significantly lower venous oxygen saturation and lower plasma glucose levels.[11] In addition, older dogs have a slower hematopoietic response to acute anemia (phlebotomy) than younger dogs.[9]

Although there are limited data for older animals, the research suggests that at-rest laboratory values may not be very different for adult and geriatric animals. However, when stressed by exercise, or perhaps by disease, older animals may show significant differences in laboratory values, and a disease process may place a large burden on their tenuous reserves.

The coagulation system appears to shift toward hypercoagulability as humans age, and the incidence of pulmonary thromboembolism is increased fivefold in humans older than 85 years.[9] Although changes in the coagulation system with age have not been investigated in small animal patients, prophylactic treatment for hypercoagulability may be warranted in this age group, especially in animals with predisposing disease processes.

The human thoracic cage becomes more rigid and the lungs lose elasticity with age. Respiratory muscle strength is decreased by 25%, and the alveolar-arterial gradient increases significantly.[12] Loss of diaphragmatic and intercostal muscle mass are thought to be responsible for the decline in respiratory muscle strength. These aging-related changes may result in a decreased arterial partial pressure of oxygen in older veterinary patients during illness or exertion. One study found no changes in arterial blood gas values in healthy older dogs, but it is not known whether changes occur during illness.[13] Diseases such as pneumonia, pulmonary thromboembolism, and pulmonary edema place great pressure on the limited pulmonary reserves in older patients and may be more difficult to treat for these reasons.

Renal blood flow, glomerular filtration rate, urine concentrating and diluting ability, and creatinine clearance have been shown to decrease with age in people.[12] Inability to conserve sodium or concentrate urine and decreased renal blood flow have been reported in geriatric small animals.[14] This combination leads to the inability of the aged to respond to hypovolemia or hypervolemia and often places severe restrictions on fluid and electrolyte therapy.

Ongoing studies at the University of California, Davis have demonstrated a difference in some aspects of canine endothelial function with age.[15] Older dogs (≥8 years of age) had a greater release of nitric oxide (NO) in response to anesthesia induction with propofol than did younger dogs, even at doses that do not result in clinically apparent hypotension. This was not accounted for by a change in propofol elimination because plasma propofol levels (determined by high-performance liquid chromatography) did not differ between the two age groups. A significant increase in levels of the NO metabolite (i.e., nitrite) was observed in the older age group, which suggests a functional change in endothelial response with age. A similar observation has been made in aged rats.[16] Clinicians should be aware that the reported hypotension with propofol use in older dogs may result, in part, from increased NO release and not just from reduced clearance.

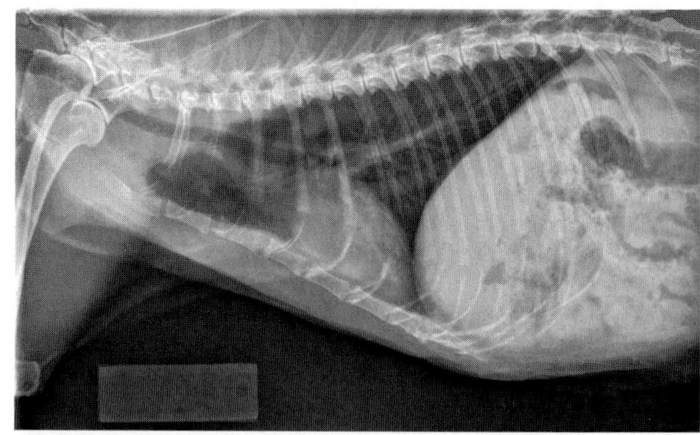

FIGURE 156-1 Thoracic radiograph of a healthy geriatric cat. Note the horizontal heart and prominent aorta. *(Courtesy Dr. Robert O'Brien, DVM, DACVR.)*

IMAGING

Thoracic radiographs of geriatric dogs and cats can show increased lung opacity due to calcification of the bronchial circulation and pulmonary interstitial changes. Mineralized costochondral junctions as well as degenerative changes in the sternebral junctions can also be observed. Heterotopic bone can be seen in the lungs in some older dogs, particularly Collie breeds. Collectively, these changes may be mistaken for pulmonary disease. The heart may appear to lie on the sternum in old cats because it takes on a more horizontal orientation. This can easily be mistaken for cardiomegaly because of increased sternal contact. The aorta may seem more prominent and undulating in older cats due to a "kink" in its appearance (Figure 156-1). The liver may extend beyond the costal arch and appear enlarged in older animals because of stretching of the ligaments that attach it to the diaphragm.

Spondylosis of the vertebrae is common in older dogs, and degenerative joint disease changes may be seen in both dogs and cats as they age.

FLUID THERAPY

Significant changes in multiple organ systems in geriatric animals should be taken into account when the type, dosage, and administration rate of fluids are selected. Additionally, changes in muscle mass and fat stores should be noted since marked changes can affect daily maintenance fluid requirements.

Geriatric animals have increasing amounts of myocardial fibrosis, valvular malfunction, and myocardial fiber atrophy.[14] The decrease in ventricular compliance limits the volume that they can tolerate while paradoxically increasing their dependence on volume. Geriatric animals are highly dependent on end-diastolic volume to increase cardiac output and therefore do not tolerate volume depletion very well during times of stress (e.g., illness, anesthesia).

Renal changes, such as decreased ability to concentrate or dilute urine, decreased renal blood flow, and limited ability to handle sodium, all limit the geriatric animal's capacity to handle volume depletion, volume overload, or electrolyte disturbances. Similarly, the unnecessary use of replacement fluids may lead to hypernatremia in the geriatric patient with moderate or severe renal insufficiency.

Balanced isotonic crystalloids (e.g., lactated Ringer's solution, 0.9% sodium chloride) are ideal for the dehydrated geriatric patient. Both natural colloids (fresh frozen plasma) and artificial colloids (hydroxyethyl starches) are additional options for the treatment of hypovolemia but should be administered at a slower rate in geriatric animals because of their propensity for volume overload.

Supplements such as potassium chloride, vitamin B complex, and dextrose may prove beneficial.

A thorough search for underlying or chronic disease processes (chronic valvular disease, renal failure) is essential when planning fluid therapy. It is imperative that fluid therapy be monitored both diligently and frequently. Monitoring for optimal perfusion includes frequent checks of pulse quality, extremity temperature, venous lactate levels, central venous oxygen saturation, urine output, body weight, and mentation. Monitoring for fluid overload includes frequent checks of respiratory rate, body weight, urine output, central venous pressure, and arterial blood gas concentrations or pulse oximetry readings; frequent thoracic auscultation; and thoracic radiography.

NUTRITION

Maintenance energy requirements decrease with age in dogs but appear to increase after the age of 12 years in cats.[17-19] In addition, there may be a decrease in the ability to digest fat and protein as cats age.[20] These changes can lead to either weight gain (e.g., if an older dog is fed food with the same caloric content as it ages) or weight loss (e.g., if an older cat is fed food with the same caloric content as it ages). The reduced ability to digest fats can lead to deficiencies in fat-soluble vitamins (e.g., vitamin E) as well as water-soluble vitamins (e.g., B vitamins) and electrolytes.[20] There is a high prevalence of malnutrition in elderly humans, and several supplements have been shown to slow cognitive decline, including cobalamin, blueberries, sage, and curcumin.[21] In older dogs with a limited ability to digest fats due to a diminished ability to secrete pancreatic lipase or bile acids, medium-chain triglycerides may be beneficial as a concentrated and highly absorbable energy source.

Adequate protein intake is essential for optimal immune function and is critical in geriatric animals. Protein requirements actually increase in older dogs, and the old dogma recommending protein restriction for kidney protection has been discounted.[22-25]

Antioxidants are essential to combat oxidative stress, which has been shown to increase with age in many species.[26] The free radical/oxidative stress theory of aging suggests that levels of reactive oxygen species increase with age, and amelioration of this increase can retard the aging process.[26] Oxidative stress represents an imbalance between oxidative damage (i.e., free radical damage) and endogenous antioxidant protection. Antioxidants can be administered exogenously and are thought to contribute to decreased levels of oxidative stress and perhaps to increased quality of aging. Some supplements that can be added easily to the treatment regimen include vitamin B complex administered in the intravenous fluids (4 ml/L when given at a maintenance rate), S-adenosyl-L-methionine given orally (20 mg/kg q24h), and N-acetylcysteine given intravenously (50 to 70 mg/kg diluted 1:4 with 0.9% sodium chloride and filtered, administered over 1 hour q6-8h) or orally (50 mg/kg q8-12h). Oral N-acetylcysteine can be found in health food stores in the amino acid section. If the animal develops inappetence or soft stool, the dosage should be decreased.

A relatively new area of study is the effect of gastrointestinal microflora on cognitive decline in the elderly. Probiotics as well as prebiotics appear to be safe, are easily administered, and are potentially helpful, especially in animals receiving antimicrobial therapy.

Anorexia is common in the older critically ill patient and should be treated aggressively after a thorough search for underlying causes. Intravenous midazolam given to anorectic cats caused eating to begin within 2 minutes, and propofol had a similar effect on anorectic dogs.[27,28] Cat food should be delivered in wide, shallow food bowls to prevent the whiskers from touching the sides. Also, smell is an important appetite stimulant in both dogs and cats, and clogged nasal passages (e.g., from bilateral nasal catheters for the delivery of oxygen) may cause decreased appetite. Warming the food and placing a small amount on the tongue may help stimulate the animal to eat.

PHARMACOLOGY

The mantra used most often in geriatric pharmacology is "start low, go slow." Unfortunately, this conflicts with the nature of emergency treatment in many situations, and it is imperative that clinicians take into account the effect of aging on drug dosages. Aging imposes several changes in the absorption, distribution, metabolism, and elimination of many drugs.

Oral absorption may be decreased because gastrointestinal function slows as the animal ages. The loss of lean body mass can alter intramuscular drug absorption.

Distribution of drugs may be altered for several reasons. If fluid retention is present (such as with congestive heart failure, cirrhosis, or renal failure), drugs that are distributed to the extracellular space (e.g., penicillins, nonsteroidal antiinflammatory drugs, aminoglycosides) may have changes in their distribution. Levels of albumin, the protein to which many drugs bind, decrease with age.[29] With less albumin in circulation, more free drug is available, which could lead to an inadvertent increase in active drug. In addition, drug metabolism may change as the geriatric patient experiences a decline in hepatic mass and function. This may result in an increased plasma half-life of drugs that require hepatic excretion, metabolism, or conjugation.[14] Decreased function of phase I metabolic reactions in the liver appear to occur with age and cause decreases in oxidation, reduction, dealkylation, and hydroxylation reactions. Phase II reactions do not appear to be altered.[30]

Drug elimination may be affected by a progressive decline in renal function with age. In geriatric humans there is a steady decline in renal function, with approximately 40% of the nephrons becoming sclerotic and renal blood flow and glomerular filtration rate decreasing by almost 50% by the age of 85.[9] Because of the loss of lean body mass, creatinine levels may remain normal (decreased production and decreased clearance). Approximately 15% to 20% of dogs and cats are thought to suffer from some degree of renal insufficiency as they enter the geriatric years.[31]

There is a progressive decline in ventricular compliance and the number of cardiac myocytes in geriatric humans. Autonomic tissue is replaced by fat and connective tissue and shows decreased responsiveness to autonomic drugs.[9] It is likely that some decline in cardiac function occurs with age in animals, and careful monitoring for specific endpoints is essential when cardiac drugs are prescribed.

Options for appropriate drug dosing in geriatric animals include measurement of renal function, therapeutic drug monitoring with frequent dosage adjustments, and dose or interval reduction based on creatinine concentrations. Examples of drugs that are renally cleared are amoxicillin, allopurinol, and many antifungals. Clinicians should always check renal clearance of specific drugs before dosing. The most practical and cost efficient of the aforementioned options is dose or interval reduction. Dose and interval adjustments based on creatinine concentration use one of the following formulas:

$$\text{Adjusted dosage} = \text{normal dosage} \times (\text{normal serum creatinine} \div \text{patient's serum creatinine})$$

or

$$\text{Adjusted interval} = \text{normal interval } (1 \div [\text{normal serum creatinine} \div \text{patient's serum creatinine}])$$

It is essential to take into account any comorbid diseases (e.g., congestive heart failure, chronic renal failure, hepatic fibrosis) in considering dosage adjustments for geriatric small animals. For example, if an older dog with chronic renal insufficiency requires therapy with angiotensin-converting enzyme inhibitors, the clinician must be aware of the significant likelihood of decreased renal clearance in this animal as a result of both its chronic renal disease and older age.

A good review of general guidelines for dosage adjustments in geriatric small animals can be found in the article by Dowling.[29]

CONCLUSION

Geriatric animals experience a decline of physiologic reserves that may not be apparent at rest. During times of ill health, however, the geriatric animal often cannot mobilize reserves to meet the demands of the disease process, which results in multiple organ failure.

Because of changes in cardiovascular, renal, hepatic, nutritional, and immune function, the older animal will respond differently to both the stress of illness and its treatment than will the young adult. It is essential that the critical care team be familiar with these changes in the older animal and be prepared for vigilant monitoring during diagnostic testing and treatment of the illness.

The severity of illness has the biggest influence on outcome in critically ill geriatric people, and this is likely to be similar in animals. Aggressive and appropriate treatment, careful monitoring, and, of course, tender loving care are essential to a successful outcome in the critically ill geriatric patient.

REFERENCES

1. Stratton-Phelps M: AAFP and AFM panel report of feline senior health care, Comp Cont Educ Pract Vet 21:531, 1999.
2. Kraft W: Geriatrics in canine and feline internal medicine, Eur J Med Res 3:31, 1998.
3. Biese KJ, Roberts E, LaMantia M, et al: Effect of geriatric curriculum on emergency medicine resident attitudes, knowledge, and decision-making, Acad Emerg Med 18:S92-S96, 2011.
4. Hogan TM, Losman ED, Carpenter CR, et al: Development of geriatric competencies for emergency medicine residents using an expert consensus process, Acad Emerg Med 17(3):316-324, 2010.
5. Campion EW, Mulley AG, Goldstein RL, et al: Medical intensive care for the elderly. A study of current use, costs, and outcomes, JAMA 246:2052, 1981.
6. Fedullo AJ, Swinburne AJ: Relationship of patient age to cost and survival in a medical ICU, Crit Care Med 11:155, 1983.
7. Goldstein RL, Campion EW, Thibault GE, et al: Functional outcomes following medical intensive care, Crit Care Med 14:783, 1986.
8. Davies M: Geriatric screening in first opinion practice—results from 45 dogs, J Small Anim Pract 53:507-513, 2012.
9. Rosenthal RA, Kavic SM: Assessment and management of the geriatric patient, Crit Care Med 32:S92, 2004.
10. Harper EJ, Hackett RM, Wilkinson J, et al: Age-related variations in hematologic and plasma biochemical test results in Beagles and Labrador Retrievers, J Am Vet Med Assoc 223:1436, 2003.
11. Strasser A, Simunek M, Seiser M, et al: Age-dependent changes in cardiovascular and metabolic responses to exercise in Beagle dogs, Zentralbl Veterinarmed A 44:449, 1997.
12. Nagappan R, Parkin G: Geriatric critical care, Crit Care Clin 19:253, 2003.
13. King LG, Anderson JG, Rhodes WH, et al: Arterial blood gas tensions in healthy aged dogs, Am J Vet Res 53(10):1744-1748, 1992.
14. Carpenter RE, Pettifer GR, Tranquilli WJ: Anesthesia for geriatric patients, Vet Clin North Am Small Anim Pract 35:571, 2005.
15. Mellema, 2013, unpublished data.
16. Gragasin FS, Davidge ST: The effects of propofol on vascular function in mesenteric arteries of the aging rat, Am J Physiol Heart Circ Physiol 297(1):H466-H474, 2009.
17. Harper EJ: Changing perspectives on aging and energy requirements: aging and energy intakes in humans, dogs and cats, J Nutr 128:2623S, 1998.
18. Kienzle E, Rainbird A: Maintenance energy requirement of dogs: what is the correct value for the calculation of metabolic body weight in dogs? J Nutr 121:S39, 1991.
19. Laflamme DP, Ballam JM: Effect of age on maintenance energy requirements of adult cats, Compend Contin Educ Vet Pract 24:82, 2002.
20. Laflamme DP: Nutrition for aging cats and dogs and the importance of body condition, Vet Clin North Am Small Anim Pract 35:713, 2005.
21. Vauzour D: Dietary polyphenols as modulators of brain functions; biological actions and molecular mechanisms underpinning their beneficial effects, Oxid Med Cell Longev 2012:914273, 2012.
22. Finco DR, Brown SA, Crowell WA, et al: Effects of aging and dietary protein intake on uninephrectomized geriatric dogs, Am J Vet Res 55:1282, 1994.
23. Wannemacher RW Jr, McCoy JR: Determination of optimal dietary protein requirements of young and old dogs, J Nutr 88:66, 1966.
24. Finco DR, Brown SA, Crowell WA: Effects of dietary protein intake on renal functions, Vet Forum 16:34, 1999.
25. Bovee KC: Mythology of protein restriction for dogs with reduced renal function, Compend Contin Educ Vet Pract 21:15, 1999.
26. Bokov A, Chaudhuri A, Richardson A: The role of oxidative damage and stress in aging, Mech Ageing Dev 125:811, 2004.
27. Rangel-Captillo A, Avendano-Carillo H, Reyes-Delgado F: Immediate appetite stimulation of anorexic cats with midazolam, Compend Contin Educ Vet Pract 26:61, 2004.
28. Avendano-Carillo H, Rangel-Captillo A, Reyes-Delgado F: Immediate appetite stimulation of anorexic dogs with propofol, Compend Contin Educ Vet Pract 26:64, 2004.
29. Dowling PM: Geriatric pharmacology, Vet Clin North Am Small Anim Pract 35:557, 2005.
30. Ambrose PJ: Altered drug action with aging, Health Notes 1:12, 2003.
31. Burkholder WJ: Dietary considerations for dogs and cats with renal disease, J Am Vet Med Assoc 216:1730, 2000.

CHAPTER 157
CATECHOLAMINES

†Steve C. Haskins, DVM, MS, DACVAA, DACVECC

KEY POINTS

- Catecholamines are used to support arterial blood pressure, cardiac output, and tissue perfusion in a variety of critical illnesses. Both blood pressure and blood flow parameters must be considered when choosing and monitoring catecholamine therapy.
- Dopamine and dobutamine are the two most commonly used catecholamines for general cardiovascular support. Dopamine is recommended if blood pressure augmentation is necessary; dobutamine, if blood pressure is adequate but forward flow needs to be augmented.
- Norepinephrine, phenylephrine, or vasopressin is used to increase blood pressure and cardiac output if dopamine or dobutamine alone do not work.
- Catecholamines can be mixed and matched in any combination deemed appropriate by the attending clinician.
- Vasoconstrictors may increase or decrease cardiac output and tissue perfusion depending on how they affect venous tone and venous return.
- Adequate plasma cortisol levels are important in the hormonal regulation of cardiovascular function. Cortisol-deficient patients suffer vasoparalysis, impaired myocardial contractility, and impaired responsiveness to endogenous and exogenous catecholamines. Corticosteroid supplementation may improve cardiovascular function while allowing catecholamine therapy to be discontinued.

Catecholamines are used to augment arterial blood pressure, myocardial contractility, and cardiac output in a variety of critical illnesses. The mainstay of treatment of cardiovascular dysfunction is always effective treatment of the underlying disease process (e.g., fluid loading for hypovolemia). But when the underlying problem cannot be identified or cannot be effectively treated, symptomatic catecholamine therapy may be necessary.

HYPOTENSION

In general, treatment of hypotension can be considered when the mean pressure decreases below about 80 mm Hg or the systolic pressure decreases below about 100 mm Hg. Treatment is strongly advised when mean blood pressure decreases below about 60 mm Hg or when systolic pressure decreases below about 80 mm Hg. Since the underlying physiologic cause of the hypotension in diseases like sepsis or end-stage visceral organ failure, or during general anesthesia, often is not clear, the following generic approach to hypotension is suggested.

1. If there is a coexistent sinus bradycardia or first-, second-, or third-degree heart block, administer an anticholinergic (atropine [0.01 to 0.02 mg/kg] or glycopyrrolate [0.005 to 0.01 mg/kg]). It is acceptable to start with a low dose in an attempt to avoid sinus tachycardia, but the low dose of either drug has a tendency to induce a centrally mediated increase in vagal tone and a worsening of the bradyarrhythmia. If this happens, administer more anticholinergic. Move on to catecholamine therapy if the high dose of either drug either does not increase the heart rate or increases the heart rate but does not improve the blood pressure or the tissue perfusion parameter of concern.
2. If a vagotonic agent (α_2 agonist, opioid) has been administered, its action can be partially or completely reversed as long as it does not adversely affect the anesthetic or analgesic regime. If anesthetic depth can be safely decreased, lower the dose of anesthetics being used or switch to drugs with less inherent hypotensive characteristics.
3. If there are serious ventricular arrhythmias, consider an antiarrhythmic.
4. If the case can be made for hypovolemia (physical signs or history of recent fluid loss), implement blood volume restoration therapy. If the case for hypovolemia cannot be made, still administer a volume of fluids rapidly in case there is "silent" hypovolemia, maldistribution, or vasodilation (10 to 20 ml/kg of an isotonic crystalloid or 5 to 10 ml/kg of a colloid).
5. If the preload parameters are deemed adequate, the poor forward flow could be attributed to poor contractility, and a cardiotonic agent should be administered. Usually start with dopamine (5 to 20 mcg/kg/min).
6. If a higher dose of dopamine either does not remedy the hypotension or causes sinus tachycardia or ventricular arrhythmias, administer a vasoconstrictor such as norepinephrine (0.1 to 2.0 mcg/kg/min), phenylephrine (0.5 to 5 mcg/kg/min), or vasopressin (0.5 to 5 mU/kg/min). These agents are usually very effective and one can often "dial" a blood pressure. Higher dosages of vasoconstrictors (norepinephrine and phenylephrine) can cause ventricular arrhythmias and decrease venous return due to venoconstriction. Higher dosages can cause excess arteriolar vasoconstriction and impaired tissue perfusion.

POOR CONTRACTILITY

Poor contractility is suspected when the preload parameters (history of recent fluid loading, ease of jugular vein distention, central venous pressure, postcaval diameter, end-diastolic ventricular volume) suggest normal or high preload and the forward flow parameters

†Deceased.

Table 157-1 **Receptor Activity, Cardiopressor Effects, and Dosages of Commonly Administered Catecholamines**

	Receptor Activity			Effect on*					
	β_1	β_2	α_1 & α_2	Contractility	Heart Rate	Cardiac Output	Vasomotor Tone	Blood Pressure	Dosage
Isoproterenol	+++	+++	0	↑↑↑	↑↑↑	↑↑↑	↓↓↓	↓↓↓	0.02-0.5 mcg/kg/min
Dopexamine	0	++	0	0	↑	↑↑	↓↓	↓↓	1-10 mcg/kg/min
Dobutamine	++	+	+	↑↑	↑	↑↑	↓	Variable	5-20 mcg/kg/min
Dopamine	++	+	++	↑↑	↑↑	Variable	↑↑	↑↑	5-20 mcg/kg/min
Ephedrine	+	+	+	↑	↑	↑	Variable	↑	0.25-1 mg/kg
Epinephrine	+++	+++	+++	↑↑↑	↑↑↑	↑↑	↑↑↑	↑↑↑	0.05-1 mcg/kg/min
Norepinephrine	+	0	+++	↑	Variable	Variable	↑↑↑	↑↑↑	0.1-2 mcg/kg/min
Phenylephrine	0	0	+++	0	↓	↓	↑↑↑	↑↑↑	0.5-5 mcg/kg/min
Vasopressin	0	0	0	0	↓	↓	↑↑	↑↑	0.5-5mU/kg/min
Angiotensin	0	0	0	0	0	↓	↑↑	↑↑	0.01-0.1 mcg/kg/min

*Effects are estimated for the higher dose ranges.
Activity ranges from no activity (0) to maximal activity (+++).
Possible cardiopressor effects include a decrease (↓), mild increase (↑), moderate increase (↑↑), or marked increase (↑↑↑).

(blood pressure, pulse quality, indicators of vasomotor tone [capillary refill time], and indicators of tissue perfusion [appendage temperature, metabolic acidosis, lactate level, central venous oxygen pressure]) suggest poor cardiac out in an animal without organic heart disease (e.g., hypertrophic cardiomyopathy, mitral insufficiency, aortic stenosis, pericardial tamponade, fibrosis). If poor contractility is suspected, administration of a β_1 agonist is indicated. If the animal is also hypotensive, dopamine (5 to 20 mcg/kg/min) is recommended; if blood pressure is acceptable, dobutamine (5 to 20 mcg/kg/min) is recommended.

CATECHOLAMINE CHOICES

Table 157-1 lists the approximate receptor distributions, important cardiovascular effects, and dosages of the available catecholamines (vasopressin is not a catecholamine but is included here because its indications overlap those of the catecholamines; structurally, ephedrine is not a catecholamine either). β_1-Receptor agonists primarily augment heart rate and contractility and ectopic pacemaker activity. β_2-Receptor agonist activity primarily causes vasodilation. Postsynaptic α_1-receptor and presynaptic α_2-receptor agonism cause vasoconstriction and can also cause ectopic pacemaker activity. Arteriolar vasoconstriction increases blood pressure but, if excessive, can increase afterload and impede tissue perfusion. Venular vasoconstriction increases venous return by decreasing venous capacitance but, if excessive, can decrease venous return by increasing resistance to venous return. When a drug exhibits both β_2-receptor vasodilation properties and α_1-receptor vasoconstriction activity (dobutamine, dopamine, epinephrine), the net effect on vasomotor tone and blood pressure will be proportional to the relative power of each effect.

Dopamine

Dopamine is the endogenous precursor to norepinephrine and is an important neurotransmitter in the central nervous system. It has direct β- and α-agonist activity and also releases norepinephrine from the sympathetic nerve endings. It is also a dopamine receptor agonist that induces arterial vasodilation in many vascular beds. Several different dopamine receptors have been identified: D_1 postsynaptic receptors are responsible for the vasodilation, whereas D_2 presynaptic receptors inhibit norepinephrine release from sympathetic nerve endings (which promotes less vasoconstriction). Exogenously administered dopamine does not cross the blood-brain barrier. The effects of dopamine may be dose related, with dopaminergic vasodilatory effects predominating at low dosages (1 to 3 mcg/kg/min), β effects predominating at medium dosages (5 to 10 mcg/kg/min), and α effects predominating at high dosages (>15 mcg/kg/min), although this scaling of effects is difficult to demonstrate clinically. Dopamine has been reported to increase renal blood flow at dosages of less than 5 mcg/kg/min (and to decrease it to baseline at 10 mcg/kg/min) and may increase urine output,[1-3] but dopamine therapy does not appear to provide any low-dose renal-protective efficacy in people.[4,5]

When administered to critically ill people,[6] septic dogs[7] (in the author's experience), anesthetized dogs,[8-10] and anesthetized cats,[11] dopamine generally causes a modest vasoconstriction and increase in blood pressure with little change or modest increases in cardiac output. In one study of anesthetized cats,[12] dopamine was associated with vasodilation and increases in heart rate, cardiac output, and blood pressure.

Dobutamine

Dobutamine is a synthetic analog of dopamine with strong β_1-agonist activity as well as some effects on β_2- and α_1-receptors, but without dopaminergic effects. When dobutamine is given to critically ill humans,[6,13] septic dogs[7] (in the author's experience), anesthetized dogs,[8-10,14] anesthetized cats,[12,15] and anesthetized foals,[16,17] it generally causes modest vasodilation and a marked increase in cardiac output with little change in blood pressure.

Although dopamine is primarily used to raise arterial blood pressure in hypotensive patients, dobutamine is primarily used to increase forward flow when baseline blood pressure is acceptable.

Ephedrine

Ephedrine is a sympathomimetic amine (but not, strictly speaking, a catecholamine) that primarily acts by increasing the release of norepinephrine from the sympathetic nerve endings. It may also have some direct β-agonist effects. Ephedrine is a general cardiovascular stimulant and bronchodilator. Ephedrine can be used as a first-line therapy in cardiovascular support instead of dopamine, but, given its mode of action, it will not be as effective or as reliable. The administration of ephedrine to anesthetized dogs caused a modest decrease in heart rate and an increase in cardiac output, vascular resistance, and arterial blood pressure.[18] The effects of a single dose may last 5 to 15 minutes; it may also be administered as a constant-rate infusion (0.02 to 0.2 mg/kg/min). Prolonged use can deplete norepinephrine stores, which results in tachyphylaxis. Ephedrine crosses the blood-brain barrier and has a mild analeptic effect. In veterinary medicine it is also given orally for urinary incontinence (to increase urethral sphincter tone). In humans it is used topically as a nasal decongestant.

Norepinephrine

Norepinephrine is primarily an α-receptor agonist and is associated with arteriolar and venous constriction. It also exhibits minimal β_1-receptor agonist activity (in contrast to phenylephrine and vasopressin, norepinephrine may increase heart rate and contractility). Norepinephrine generally causes vasoconstriction and increases blood pressure, with variable effects on heart rate; cardiac output may increase,[16,19-24] decrease,[17,24] or remain unchanged.[25,26] These different cardiac output consequences are attributed to differences in baseline effective circulating volume and myocardial contractility, and the relative effect of venoconstriction on venous capacitance (decreased capacitance would tend to increase venous return) and venous resistance to blood flow (increased flow resistance would tend to decrease venous return). Animals with an effective circulating volume but with vasodilation would be expected to experience an increase in cardiac output due to venoconstriction of capacitance vessels. Hypovolemic animals are already vasoconstricted, and further venoconstriction of resistance vessels associated with the administration of a vasoconstrictor would be expected to lead to a further decrease in venous return and cardiac output. Norepinephrine has, in addition, some β_1-receptor activity, which would tend to increase contractility and cardiac output, particularly in patients with poor baseline myocardial contractility.

Norepinephrine is commonly used to raise blood pressure after dopamine therapy alone has proven ineffective. Norepinephrine is usually added to the dopamine infusion but could simply replace the dopamine if the inotropic augmentation provided by dopamine is deemed unnecessary.

Phenylephrine

Phenylephrine is an α-receptor agonist without β-agonist activity. Its administration causes vasoconstriction and an increase in arterial blood pressure, and a decrease in heart rate. Cardiac output may decrease[13,27,28] or increase.[11,12,29] The earlier discussion regarding the different consequences of venoconstriction for norepinephrine apply also to phenylephrine.

Phenylephrine is used to raise blood pressure after dopamine has proven ineffective. Phenylephrine is usually added to the dopamine but can simply replace the dopamine if the inotropic augmentation provided by dopamine is deemed unnecessary. The decision between norepinephrine and phenylephrine is, for the most part, made with a coin toss. Norepinephrine may provide marginally better heart rate and inotropic support.

Vasopressin

Vasopressin is a noncatecholamine vasoconstrictor acting via the vasopressin V_1 receptor that increases intracellular calcium and vasomotor tone (see Chapter 158). It is a pure vasoconstrictor with no direct effect on the heart. Its administration is usually associated with an increase in systemic vascular resistance, a baroreceptor reflex decrease in heart rate, no change in contractility, and no change or a decrease in cardiac output.[13,16,29,30-36] Arterial blood pressure is usually increased. Terlipressin is a long-acting synthetic analog of vasopressin and is associated with increased systemic vascular resistance and arterial pressure, and a decreased heart rate and cardiac output in people[21,37] and in normal and endotoxemic sheep.[38]

The choice between norepinephrine, phenylephrine, and vasopressin is, for the most part, arbitrary. Norepinephrine may provide marginally better heart rate and inotropic support. Vasopressin may be effective in patients hyporesponsive to catecholamines since it operates via different receptors than do the catecholamines.[33,39-41]

Angiotensin

Angiotensin II is a hormone derived from angiotensin I by angiotensin-converting enzyme primarily in the lung but also in many other tissues. Angiotensin II causes vasoconstriction and aldosterone release. Aldosterone increases sodium reabsorption in the collecting tubules of the kidney. The administration of angiotensin II generally results in an increase in systemic vascular resistance, little change in heart rate, no change in contractility, and little change or a decrease in cardiac output.[30,32,42] Angiotensin may be a less potent venoconstrictor than vasopressin, which tends to preserve venous return and cardiac output better than vasopressin.[30,32] Although angiotensin has not been promoted as a therapy for cardiovascular instability, limited evidence suggests that it could be at least as effective as vasopressin.

Epinephrine

Epinephrine is a potent β_1-, β_2-, α_1-, and α_2-receptor agonist. It is a potent inotrope and chronotrope, arteriolar and venular vasoconstrictor, and bronchodilator. It potently increases arterial blood pressure and can cause ventricular ectopic pacemaker activity. Epinephrine administration increases heart rate, systemic vascular resistance, cardiac output, and arterial blood pressure in anesthetized cats[12] and people with sepsis[1] or heart failure.[43]

Epinephrine is used primarily in supraphysiologic doses (5 to 20 mcg/kg) in emergency situations such as anaphylaxis and cardiac arrest in which the sum of its effects are highly important. Epinephrine can be used to support cardiovascular dysfunction in critically ill patients, but its therapeutic margin may not be as liberal as that of the other catecholamines (higher incidence of sinus tachycardia, ventricular arrhythmias, and increased lactate level),[43] and it is a potent vasoconstrictor. Epinephrine is not a first-choice drug in the support of cardiovascular dysfunction in critically ill patients but can be used for rescue therapy when dopamine and other vasoconstrictors have failed to work.

Isoproterenol

Isoproterenol is a potent β-receptor agonist with no α-receptor activity. As such, it is a potent vasodilator and hypotensive agent. In anesthetized dogs, isoproterenol increases heart rate and cardiac output, and decreases blood pressure.[8] If isoproterenol is administered very carefully while blood pressure is monitored and maintained, it can provide potent augmentation of forward blood flow and tissue perfusion.

Dopexamine

Dopexamine is a synthetic analog of dopamine that is a potent β_2 and D_1 receptor agonist without substantial β_1 or α_1 activity. Dopexamine is primarily an arteriolar vasodilator without substantial venous effects and without substantial chronotropic or inotropic impact. Its administration is usually associated with a decrease in systemic vascular resistance and blood pressure, and an increase in cardiac output.[13,44,45] In contrast to other catecholamines, dopexamine is not arrhythmogenic. Dopexamine is not commonly used in veterinary medicine. It is used in humans for short-term support in congestive heart failure, in which the major benefit is attributed to afterload reduction. Although dopexamine is a catecholamine, it might more appropriately be listed under the heading "vasodilator." In this context, its therapeutic siblings are drugs like angiotensin-converting enzyme inhibitors, calcium channel blockers, acepromazine, hydralazine, and nitroprusside. For this reason it has little role as a cardiovascular tonic.

CHOOSING THE RIGHT CATECHOLAMINE

There is much heterogeneity in responses to an individual catecholamine (e.g., norepinephrine may increase or decrease cardiac output). Since catecholamines have different receptor activities and different vasculature beds have varying distributions of receptors, different dosages are expected to have different effects (e.g., low, physiologic doses of epinephrine cause systemic vasodilation, whereas high, pharmacologic doses cause systemic vasoconstriction). In addition to individual and species variations, the underlying disease (or experimental model) and the pretreatment baseline values have much to do with both the direction and the magnitude of the response to therapy. The coadministration of other drugs can also impact responses.

For general cardiovascular support in critically ill patients, the first-choice drug is either dopamine or dobutamine. Ephedrine could also be considered a first-choice drug. These drugs generally increase heart rate and contractility, and may thereby improve cardiac output. They have modest effects on vasomotor tone; dopamine tends to moderately increase systemic vascular resistance (and blood pressure), whereas dobutamine tends to moderately decrease systemic vascular resistance (and increase forward flow).[6,9] Consequently, when hypotension is the problem, dopamine is the drug of choice; dopamine is the "pressure" drug of the two. When blood pressure is acceptable, dobutamine is the drug of choice to augment forward flow; dobutamine is the "flow" drug of the two. Generally, and insofar as is possible, the idea is to identify the specific problem or problems that need to be addressed in the therapy plan (bradycardia, poor contractility, low cardiac output, hypotension, weak pulse quality, poor tissue perfusion) and then to start treatment with either dopamine or dobutamine in increasing dosages until the problem is resolved (or until it is decided that the chosen drug will not solve the problem). When, for instance, higher dosages of dopamine fail to increase blood pressure to acceptable levels, stronger vasoconstrictors such as norepinephrine, phenylephrine, or vasopressin can be added to the therapeutic cocktail.

Isoproterenol and dopexamine are considered too vasodilatory for routine use in critically ill patients with a precariously balanced blood pressure system. If they are used for forward flow augmentation, continuous, accurate, direct blood pressure monitoring is recommended. Norepinephrine, phenylephrine, and vasopressin are considered too vasoconstrictive for primary use, but one should not hesitate to employ them if dopamine or dobutamine fails to correct the identified problems. Epinephrine is used primarily in conditions of serious cardiovascular collapse such as anaphylaxis or cardiac arrest but can be used for cardiovascular support as a last resort when other therapies have failed.

COMBINATION THERAPIES

Combinations of two or more of the sympathomimetics described earlier are often used at the clinician's discretion. When two drugs are used in equipotent dosages, one would expect a net effect approximately midway between that of the two drugs. For instance, one part dopamine plus one part dobutamine would be expected to increase contractility by about the same amount as either two parts dopamine or two parts dobutamine, but with less vasoconstriction than two parts of dopamine and less vasodilation than two parts of dobutamine. Adding dobutamine to dopamine (rather than simply doubling the dose of dopamine) would be expected to further increase contractility and relieve some of the vasoconstriction.[10] The addition of norepinephrine or phenylephrine or vasopressin to dobutamine or dopamine generally increases systemic vascular resistance and blood pressure.[43] One part dopamine and one part norepinephrine would be expected to provide better blood pressure support and fewer arrhythmogenic side effects than two parts of dopamine and better inotropic support than two parts of norepinephrine.

Sympathomimetic drugs can be administered in any combination. The clinician just must be clear about what the treatment is intended to improve (inotropy, cardiac output, blood pressure, tissue perfusion) and select drugs and dosages than seem most likely to achieve those goals.

VASOMOTOR TONE

Of the two determinants of arterial blood pressure—cardiac output and vascular resistance—the latter is the much more powerful contributor. The effect of a drug or disease on blood pressure usually parallels its effect on vasomotor tone. Arteriolar vasomotor tone is also a primary determinant of visceral perfusion. In veterinary medicine, it is common to measure blood pressure and to initiate therapy when it is low. Parameters of tissue perfusion are less precise but no less important than blood pressure and receive less attention during therapy. Focusing therapy on arterial blood pressure without reference to the adequacy of tissue perfusion can be problematic. Vasoconstriction is a good thing to the extent that it supports arterial blood pressure but a bad thing to the extent that it impairs tissue perfusion. Vasodilation, if it could be accomplished without hypotension, would, in fact, be an ideal cardiovascular goal. Dobutamine's claim to fame is specifically that it usually causes a modest, but not excessive, vasodilation coupled with good augmentation of contractility; forward flow is increased, whereas blood pressure does not change much. Although blood pressure is important and continued vigilance of it is imperative, a focused consideration of flow parameters such as cardiac output, pulse quality, and indicators of tissue perfusion is also necessary when choosing and evaluating a cardiotonic/vasoactive therapy plan.

Because vasoconstriction tends to decrease tissue perfusion, vasoconstrictors have a bad reputation embodied in the maxim that "to administer a vasoconstrictor is to impair tissue perfusion and harm the patient." Such an all-or-nothing concept is incorrect. Norepinephrine is commonly used in human intensive care to improve blood pressure and can be administered without adversely affecting visceral tissue perfusion.[22,23,43,46,47] One meta-analysis[47] found that dopamine was associated with an increased relative risk of death compared with norepinephrine. Although vasoconstrictors may not be a first-choice therapy for cardiovascular support because of this concern regarding vasoconstriction, they can, in fact, be very effective in the management of unstable cardiovascular systems (by increasing cardiac output, blood pressure, and visceral tissue perfusion).

Venular vasomotor tone is an important determinant of venous return. Venous return is an important determinant of cardiac output. Veins have two important functions: (1) to store blood volume, and (2) to serve as conduits for venous return. Venoconstrictor drugs have two significant effects: (1) they decrease venous capacitance (which increases venous return and cardiac output), and (2) they increase resistance to venous blood flow (which decreases venous return and cardiac output).[13] Venodilators have the opposite effects. The net effect on venous return and cardiac output depends on the relative strengths of these two opposing influences.[23] Potent vasoconstrictors like norepinephrine and phenylephrine have been variously reported to either increase or decrease cardiac output, and the reason for this disparity is the relative effect on these two opposing processes. The net effect of vasoconstrictors is determined largely by the pretreatment status of the cardiovascular system and drug dosages. From a baseline of venodilation, one might expect an increase in venous return, whereas from a baseline of venoconstriction, one might expect a decrease in venous return. Venodilation might be expected in diseases like anaphylaxis and sepsis and during general anesthesia. Although administration of fluids would "refill" the expanded blood volume capacity and restore venous return in these patients, such therapy would carry the risk of the disadvantageous effects of the particular fluid used (e.g., systemic or pulmonary edema with crystalloid therapy). For this reason, when infusion of a small dose of fluids to first restore cardiovascular homeostasis has failed, vasoconstrictor therapy is commonly initiated. Venoconstriction might be expected to be the normal response to hypovolemia (in which case fluids should be administered) and to excessive administration of a vasoconstrictor (in which case the vasoconstrictor therapy should be reduced). Although vasoconstrictor administration might improve arterial blood pressure in hypovolemic patients as a lifesaving maneuver in the short term, it will most likely diminish venous return, cardiac output, and tissue perfusion in the long term.

CATECHOLAMINES AND CORTISOL

Cortisol has an important regulatory function in the action of the sympathetic nervous system and catecholamine on cardiovascular function; the cardiovascular system does not function well in the absence of cortisol. Acute glucocorticoid deficiency results in cardiovascular collapse and death in as little as a few hours to a few days in the dog[48,49] and cat.[50,51] Cardiovascular changes in such cases are uniformly profound hypotension[48-53] with poor cardiac output and impaired myocardial contractility.[48,50,51,53] Vasodilation and vasoparesis are most common,[48,49,51] although vasoconstriction has been reported in some studies.[50,52] Impaired vasomotor responsiveness to catecholamine and sympathetic nerve stimulation is consistently reported[48,49,53] in acute glucocorticoid deficiency. Humans with heparin-induced thrombocytopenia sometimes experience bilateral adrenal hemorrhage secondary to adrenal venous thrombosis, which leads to acute adrenal insufficiency and hemodynamic collapse characterized by hypotension unresponsive to fluids and catecholamines, and death.[54]

A condition labeled *relative adrenal insufficiency* or critical illness–related adrenal insufficiency has been identified in critically ill people[55,55a] and dogs,[56,57] as well as in patients following resuscitation from cardiac arrest.[58-61] This condition entails a suboptimal cortisol response to stress and to adrenocorticotropic hormone (ACTH) administration and has been reported to have an adverse effect on survival. In addition, inflammatory conditions induce the expression of proinflammatory cytokines that inhibit the expression of genes for receptors for α_1 agonists,[62] angiotensin II,[63] and vasopressin[64] and thereby decrease vasomotor responsiveness to endogenous and exogenous vasoconstrictors. Proinflammatory cytokine expression during sepsis is mediated by the nuclear transcription factor NF-κB.[65] Glucocorticosteroids decrease proinflammatory cytokine production via inhibition of NF-κB activity and tend to reverse vascular hyporeactivity in sepsis.[66-72]

Early studies reported that steroid supplementation in these cortisol-deficient patients improved survival,[67,68,73,74] although a recent study did not confirm this result.[75] One of the findings in the literature on administration of steroids for septic shock, including studies using both high-dose[76] and low-dose[66-68,73] treatment, has been the ability to withdraw catecholamine therapy following the implementation of steroid therapy ("shock reversal"). Dogs with relative adrenal insufficiency were found to be more likely to require catecholamine therapy in one study.[57] This author is aware of a few septic dogs that have experienced dramatic improvement in cardiovascular parameters and general well-being at the same time that sympathomimetic support was reduced or stopped following low-dose hydrocortisone therapy. Although corticosteroid supplementation cannot be universally efficacious, the evidence is suggestive that some critically ill patients requiring exogenous sympathomimetic support of cardiovascular function would benefit from low-dose hydrocortisone therapy (1 mg/kg followed by either 1 mg/kg q6h or an infusion of 0.15 mg/kg/hr, which is then tapered as the patient's condition allows), as evidenced by improved cardiovascular function with reduced or no exogenous catecholamine therapy.

OTHER EFFECTS OF CATECHOLAMINES

Catecholamines have many other effects of which users should be aware. For instance, blood glucose and lactate levels may increase, particularly with epinephrine infusion.[46] The α agonism tends to increase blood glucose levels by decreasing insulin secretion and glycogenolysis. The β agonism contributes to the rise in blood glucose level by increasing glucagon and ACTH secretion (cortisol decreases tissue uptake of glucose) and lipolysis.

The β_2 agonism increases cellular potassium uptake, which reduces plasma potassium concentration.[46,77] This may be important in animals that have severe total-body potassium depletion at presentation. Catecholamines are limited in their effectiveness in the treatment of hyperkalemia by their cardiovascular effects.

Catecholamines increase metabolic oxygen consumption.[78] The increase in oxygen delivery usually is greater than the increase in oxygen consumption, and so this is of limited clinical importance unless therapy fails to increase cardiac output and oxygen delivery.

Exogenous catecholamine therapy may increase shear-induced platelet reactivity.[79,80] This may be important in animals with underlying hypercoagulopathies. There is evidence that this effect may be caused by α_2-receptor agonism and the opening of a sodium-chloride cotransporter in the platelet membrane. Studies suggest that this effect could be diminished by blocking chloride transport with loop[80] or thiazide[81] diuretics.

REFERENCES

1. Day NPJ, Phu NH, Mai NTH, et al: Effects of dopamine and epinephrine infusions on renal hemodynamics in severe malaria and severe sepsis, Crit Care Med 28:1353-1362, 2000.
2. Ichai C, Soubielle J, Carles M, et al: Comparison of the renal effects of low to high doses of dopamine and dobutamine in critically ill patients: a single-blind randomized study, Crit Care Med 28:921-928, 2000.
3. Ichai C, Passeron C, Caries M, et al: Prolonged low-dose dopamine infusion induces a transient improvement in renal function in hemodynamically stable, critically ill patients: a single-blind, prospective, controlled study, Crit Care Med 28:1329-1335, 2000.
4. Holmes CL, Walley KR: Bad medicine: low-dose dopamine in the ICU, Chest 123:1266-1275, 2003.
5. Beale RJ, Hollenberg SM, Vincent JL, et al: Vasopressor and inotropic support in septic shock: an evidence-based review, Crit Care Med 32:S455-S465, 2004.
6. Shoemaker WC, Appel RL, Kram HB, et al: Comparison of hemodynamic and oxygen transport effects of dopamine and dobutamine in critically ill surgical patients, Chest 96:120-126, 1989.
7. Vincent JL, Van der Linden P, Domb M, et al: Dopamine compared with dobutamine in experimental septic shock: relevance to fluid administration, Anesth Analg 66:565-571, 1987.
8. Driscoll DJ, Gillette PC, Fukushige J, et al: Comparison of the cardiovascular action of isoproterenol, dopamine, and dobutamine in the neonatal and mature dog, Pediatr Cardiol 1:307-314, 1980.

9. Abdul-Rasool IH, Chamberlain JH, Swan PC, et al: Cardiorespiratory and metabolic effects of dopamine and dobutamine infusions in dogs, Crit Care Med 15:1044-1050, 1987.
10. Rosati M, Dyson DH, Sinclair MD, et al: Response of hypotensive dogs to dopamine hydrochloride and dobutamine hydrochloride during deep isoflurane anesthesia, Am J Vet Res 68:483-494, 2007.
11. Wiese AJ, Barter LS, Ilkiw JE, et al: Cardiovascular and respiratory effects of incremental doses of dopamine and phenylephrine in the management of isoflurane-induced hypotension in cats with hypertrophic cardiomyopathy, Am J Vet Res 73:906-916, 2012.
12. Pascoe PJ, Ilkiw JE, Pypendop BH: Effects of increasing infusion rates of dopamine, dobutamine, epinephrine, and phenylephrine in healthy anesthetized cats, Am J Vet Res 67:1491-1499, 2006.
13. Funk DJ, Jacobsohn E, Kumar A: The role of venous return in critical illness and shock. Part 1: Physiology, Crit Care Med 41:255-262, 2013.
14. Orchard CH, Chakrabarti MK, Sykes MK: Cardiorespiratory responses to an IV infusion of dobutamine in the intact anaesthetized dog, Br J Anaesth 54:673-679, 1982.
15. Hori Y, Euchi M, Indou A, et al: Changes in the myocardial performance index during dobutamine administration in anesthetized cats, Am J Vet Res 68:385-388, 2007.
16. Valverde A, Giguere S, Sanchez C, et al: Effects of dobutamine, norepinephrine, and vasopressin on cardiovascular function in anesthetized neonatal foals with induced hypotension, Am J Vet Res 67:1730-1737, 2006.
17. Craig CA, Haskins SC, Hildebrand SV: The cardiopulmonary effects of dobutamine and norepinephrine in isoflurane-anesthetized foals, Vet Anesth Analg 14:177-187, 2007.
18. Wagner AE, Dunlop CI, Chapman PL: Effects of ephedrine on cardiovascular function and oxygen delivery in isoflurane-anesthetized dogs, Am J Vet Res 54:1917-1922, 1993.
19. Van Der Linden R, Gilbart E, Engelman E, et al: Adrenergic support during anesthesia in experimental endotoxin shock: norepinephrine versus dobutamine, Acta Anaesthesiol Scand 35:134-140, 1991.
20. Nouira S, Elatrous S, Dimassi S, et al: Effects of norepinephrine on static and dynamic preload indicators in experimental hemorrhagic shock, Crit Care Med 33:2339-2343, 2005.
21. Albanese J, Leone M, Delmas A, et al: Terlipressin or norepinephrine in hyperdynamic septic shock: a prospective, randomized study, Crit Care Med 33:1897-1902, 2005.
22. Jhanji S, Stirling S, Patel N, et al: The effect of increasing doses of norepinephrine on tissue oxygenation and microvascular flow in patients with septic shock, Crit Care Med 37:1961-1966, 2009.
23. Persichini R, Silva S, Teboul JL, et al: Effects of norepinephrine on mean systemic pressure and venous return in human septic shock, Crit Care Med 40:3146-3153, 2012.
24. Maas JJ, Pinsky MR, de Wilde RB, et al: Cardiac output responses to norepinephrine in postoperative cardiac surgery patients: interpretation with venous return and cardiac function curves, Crit Care Med 41:143-150, 2013.
25. Schreuder WO, Schneider AJ, Groeneveld ABJ, et al: Effect of dopamine vs norepinephrine on hemodynamics in septic shock, Chest 95:1282-1288, 1989.
26. Martin C, Eon B, Saux P, et al: Renal effects of norepinephrine used to treat septic shock patients, Crit Care Med 18:282-285, 1990.
27. Crystal GJ, Kim SJ, Salem R, et al: Myocardial oxygen supply/demand relations during phenylephrine infusions in dogs, Anesth Analg 73:283-288, 1991.
28. Nygren A, Thorén A, Ricksten SE: Vasopressors and intestinal mucosal perfusion after cardiac surgery: norepinephrine vs phenylephrine, Crit Care Med 34(3):722-729, 2006.
29. Malay MB, Ashton JL, Dahl K, et al: Heterogeneity of the vasoconstrictor effect of vasopressin in septic shock, Crit Care Med 32:1327-1331, 2004.
30. Heyndrickx GR, Boettcher DH, Vatner SF: Effects of angiotensin, vasopressin, and methoxamine on cardiac function and blood flow distribution in conscious dogs, Am J Physiol 231:1579-1587, 1976.
31. Montani JP, Liard JF, Schoun J, et al: Hemodynamic effects of exogenous and endogenous vasopressin at low plasma concentrations in conscious dogs, Circ Res 47:346-355, 1980.
32. Lee RW, Standaert S, Lancaster LD, et al: Cardiac and peripheral circulatory responses to angiotensin and vasopressin in dogs, J Clin Invest 82:413-419, 1988.
33. Tsuneyoshi I, Yamada H, Kakihana Y, et al: Hemodynamic and metabolic effects of low-dose vasopressin infusions in vasodilatory septic shock, Crit Care Med 29:487-493, 2001.
34. Westphal M, Stubbe H, Sielenkamper AW, et al: Effects of titrated arginine vasopressin on hemodynamic variables and oxygen transport in healthy and endotoxemic sheep, Crit Care Med 31:1502-1508, 2003.
35. Luckner G, Dunser MW, Jochberger S, et al: Arginine vasopressin in 316 patients with advanced vasodilatory shock, Crit Care Med 33:2659-2666, 2005.
36. Luckner G, Mayr VD, Jochberger S, et al: Comparison of two dose regimens of arginine vasopressin in advanced vasodilatory shock, Crit Care Med 35:2280-2285, 2007.
37. Therapondos G, Stanley AJ, Hayes PC: Systemic, portal and renal effects of terlipressin in patients with cirrhotic ascites: pilot study, J Gastroenterol Hepatol 19:73-77, 2004.
38. Scharte M, Meyer J, Van Aken H, et al: Hemodynamic effects of terlipressin (a synthetic analog of vasopressin) in healthy and endotoxemic sheep, Crit Care Med 29:1756-1760, 2001.
39. Silverstein DC, Waddell LS, Drobatz KJ, et al: Vasopressin therapy in dogs with dopamine-resistant hypotension and vasodilatory shock, J Vet Emerg Crit Care 17:399-408, 2007.
40. Lange M, Van Aken H, Westphal M, et al: Role of vasopressinergic V1 receptor agonists in the treatment of perioperative catecholamine-refractory arterial hypotension, Best Pract Res Clin Anaesthesiol 22(2):369-381, 2008.
41. Scroggin RD, Quandt J: The use of vasopressin for treating vasodilatory shock and cardiopulmonary arrest, J Vet Emerg Crit Care 19:145-157, 2009.
42. Lee RW, Lancaster LD, Buckley D, et al: Peripheral circulatory control of preload-afterload mismatch with angiotensin in dogs, Am J Physiol 253:H126-H132, 1987.
43. Levy B, Perez P, Perny J, et al: Comparison of norepinephrine-dobutamine to epinephrine for hemodynamics, lactate metabolism, and organ function variables in cardiogenic shock. A prospective, randomized pilot study, Crit Care Med 39:450-455, 2011.
44. Vincent JL, Reuse C, Kahn RJ: Administration of dopexamine, a new adrenergic agent, in cardiorespiratory failure, Chest 96:1233-1236, 1989.
45. Meier-Hellman A, Bredle DL, Specht M, et al: Dopexamine increases splanchnic blood flow but decreases gastric mucosal pH in severe septic patients treated with dobutamine, Crit Care Med 27:2166-2171, 1999.
46. Bellomo R, Wan L, May C: Vasoactive drugs and acute kidney injury, Crit Care Med 36:S179-S186, 2008.
47. DeBacker D, Aldecoa C, Njimi H, et al: Dopamine versus norepinephrine in the treatment of septic shock: a meta-analysis, Crit Care Med 40:725-730, 2012.
48. Remington JW: Circulatory factors in adrenal crisis in the dog, Am J Physiol 165:306-318, 1951.
49. Brown FK, Remington JW: Arteriolar responsiveness in adrenal crisis in the dog, Am J Physiol 182:279-284, 1955.
50. Weiner DE, Verrier RL, Miller DT, et al: Effect of adrenalectomy on hemodynamics and regional blood flow in the cat, Am J Physiol 213:473-476, 1967.
51. Lefer AM, Verrier RL, Carson WW: Cardiac performance in experimental adrenal insufficiency in cats, Circ Res 22:817-827, 1968.
52. Reidenberg MM, Ohler EA, Sevy RW, et al: Hemodynamic changes in adrenalectomized dogs, Endocrinology 72:918-923, 1963.
53. Lefer AM, Sutfin DC: Cardiovascular effects of catecholamines in experimental adrenal insufficiency, Am J Physiol 206:1151-1155, 1964.
54. Rosenberger LH, Smith PW, Sawyer RG, et al: Bilateral adrenal hemorrhage: the unrecognized cause of hemodynamic collapse associated with heparin-induced thrombocytopenia, Crit Care Med 39:833-838, 2011.
55. Rothwell PM, Udwadia ZF, Lawler PG: Cortisol response to corticotropin and survival in septic shock, Lancet 337:582-583, 1991.
55a. Marik PE: Critical illness-related corticosteroid insufficiency, Chest 135(1):181-193, 2009.
56. Burkitt JM, Haskins SC, Nelson RW, et al: Relative adrenal insufficiency in dogs with sepsis, J Vet Intern Med 21:226-231, 2007.

57. Martin LG, Groman RP, Fletcher DJ, et al: Pituitary-adrenal function in dogs with acute critical illness, J Am Vet Med Assoc 233:87-95, 2008.
58. Miller JB, Donnino MW, Rogan M, et al: Relative adrenal insufficiency in post-cardiac arrest shock is under-recognized, Resuscitation 76:221-225, 2008.
59. Pene F, Hyvernat H, Mallet V, et al: Prognostic value of relative adrenal insufficiency after out-of-hospital cardiac arrest, Intensive Care Med 31:627-633, 2005.
60. Tsai MS, Huang CH, Chang WT, et al: The effect of hydrocortisone on the outcome of out-of-hospital cardiac arrest patients: a pilot study, Am J Emerg Med 25:318-325, 2007.
61. Mentzelopoulos SC, Zakynthinos SG, Tzoufi M, et al: Vasopressin, epinephrine, and corticosteroids for in-hospital cardiac arrest, Arch Intern Med 169:15-24, 2009.
62. Bucher M, Kees F, Taeger K, et al: Cytokines down regulate alpha1-adrenergic receptor expression during endotoxemia, Crit Care Med 31:566-571, 2003.
63. Bucher M, Hobbhahn J, Kurtz A: Nitric oxide-dependent down-regulation of angiotensin II type 2 receptors during experimental sepsis, Crit Care Med 29:1750-1755, 2001.
64. Schmidt C, Höcherl K, Kurt B, et al: Role of nuclear factor-kappaB-dependent induction of cytokines in the regulation of vasopressin V1A-receptors during cecal ligation and puncture-induced circulatory failure, Crit Care Med 36:2363-2372, 2008.
65. Liu SF, Malik AB: NF-kappa B activation as a pathological mechanism of septic shock and inflammation, Am J Physiol 290:L622-L645, 2006.
66. Oppert M, Reinicke A, Graf KJ, et al: Plasma cortisol levels before and during "low-dose" hydrocortisone therapy and their relationship to hemodynamic improvement in patients with septic shock, Intensive Care Med 26:1747-1755, 2000.
67. Briegel J, Kellermann W, Forst H, et al: Low-dose hydrocortisone infusion attenuates the systemic inflammatory response syndrome. The Phospholipase A2 Study Group, Clin Investig 72:782-787, 1994.
68. Briegel J, Forst H, Haller M, et al: Stress doses of hydrocortisone reverse hyperdynamic septic shock: a prospective, randomized, double-blind, single-center study, Crit Care Med 27:723-732, 1999.
69. Briegel J, Jochum M, Gippner-Steppert C, et al: Immunomodulation in septic shock: hydrocortisone differentially regulates cytokine responses, J Am Soc Nephrol 12:870-874, 2001.
70. Annane D, Bellissant E, Sebille V, et al: Impaired pressor sensitivity to noradrenaline in septic shock patients with and without impaired adrenal function reserve, Br J Clin Pharmacol 46:589-597, 1998.
71. Bellissant E, Annane D: Effect of hydrocortisone on phenylephrine—mean arterial pressure dose-response relationship in septic shock, Clin Pharmacol Ther 68:293-303, 2000.
72. Laviolle B, Donal E, Maguet PL, et al: Low doses of fludrocortisones and hydrocortisone, alone or in combination, on vascular responsiveness to phenylephrine in healthy volunteers, Br J Pharmacol 75:423-430, 2012.
73. Bollaert PE, Charpentier C, Levy B, et al: Reversal of late septic shock with supraphysiologic doses of hydrocortisone, Crit Care Med 26:645-650, 1998.
74. Annane D, Sébille V, Charpentier C, et al: Effect of treatment with low doses of hydrocortisone and fludrocortisone on mortality in patients with septic shock, JAMA 288:862-871, 2002.
75. Sprung CL, Annane D, Keh D, et al: Hydrocortisone therapy for patients with septic shock, N Engl J Med 358:111-124, 2008.
76. Sprung CL, Caralis PV, Marcial EH, et al: The effects of high-dose corticosteroids in patients with septic shock, N Engl J Med 311:1137-1143, 1984.
77. Follett DV, Loeb RG, Haskins SC, et al: Effects of epinephrine and ritodrine in dogs with acute hyperkalemia, Anesth Analg 40:400-406, 1990.
78. Scheeren TWL, Arndt JO: Different response of oxygen consumption and cardiac output to various endogenous and synthetic catecholamines in awake dogs, Crit Care Med 28:3861-3868, 2000.
79. Ikarugi H, Taka T, Nakajima S, et al: Norepinephrine, but not epinephrine, enhances platelet reactivity and coagulation after exercise in humans, J Appl Physiol 86:133-138, 1999.
80. Spalding A, Vaitkevicius H, Dill S, et al: Mechanism of epinephrine-induced platelet aggregation, Hypertension 31:603-607, 1998.
81. Vaitkevicius H, Turner I, Spalding A, et al: Chloride increases adrenergic receptor-mediated platelet and vascular responses, Am J Hypertens 15:492-498, 2002.

CHAPTER 158
VASOPRESSIN

Deborah C. Silverstein, DVM, DACVECC

KEY POINTS

- Vasopressin, also known as *antidiuretic hormone,* is a peptide hormone synthesized in the hypothalamus and stored or released from the posterior pituitary gland.
- There are four vasopressin receptors in the body: V_1R, V_2R, V_3R, and the oxytocin receptor.
- In health, vasopressin aids in the regulation of free water balance (via V_2R) in the renal medullary and cortical collecting ducts.
- During states of circulatory shock, vasopressin levels are markedly increased, and vasopressin functions as a potent nonadrenergic vasoconstrictor (via V_1R). Vasopressin also stimulates the release of adrenocorticotropic hormone (via V_3R).
- Vasopressin is used therapeutically for the management of pituitary-dependent diabetes insipidus, von Willebrand disease, vasodilatory hypotension, hemorrhagic shock, and cardiopulmonary resuscitation.
- Long-acting vasopressin analogs and V_1R-specific drugs are currently under investigation.
- The recent clinical and experimental use of vasopressin antagonists for the treatment of various disease states shows early promising results.

PHYSIOLOGY OF VASOPRESSIN

Arginine vasopressin (AVP, also known as *antidiuretic hormone, 8-arginine-vasopressin,* and *β-hypophamine*) is a natural, nine-amino-acid glycopeptide with a disulfide bond that is synthesized in the magnocellular neurons in the hypothalamus before transport down the pituitary stalk for storage in the pars nervosa of the posterior pituitary gland.[1] The entire process of AVP synthesis, transport, and storage in the pituitary takes 1 to 2 hours.

AVP is metabolized rapidly by hepatic and renal vasopressinases, and the half-life of AVP is 10 to 35 minutes. Vasopressin has shown teleologic persistence and is found in more than 120 species spanning four invertebrate phyla and the seven major vertebrate families.[2] In most mammals (dogs, cats, humans), the natural hormone is *arginine* vasopressin, but the porcine species has a lysine in place of arginine, which renders the compound less potent than AVP.

The most potent stimuli for AVP release are increased plasma osmolality, decreased blood pressure, and a decrease in circulating blood volume.[3-5] Additional abnormalities that cause AVP release include pain, nausea, hypoxia, hypercarbia, pharyngeal stimuli, glycopenia, drugs or chemicals (e.g., acetylcholine, high-dose opioids, dopamine, angiotensin II, prostaglandins, glutamine, histamine), certain malignant tumors, and mechanical ventilation.[6-8]

Release of AVP is inhibited by drugs such as glucocorticoids, low-dose opioids, atrial natriuretic factor, and γ-aminobutyric acid. Hyperosmolality is sensed by both peripheral and central osmoreceptors. Central osmoreceptors are located in the third ventricle and detect changes in systemic osmolality. Peripheral osmoreceptors in the mesenteric and portal veins enable early detection of the osmolality of ingested food and liquids. Afferent impulses ascend via the vagus nerve to the paraventricular and supraoptic nuclei in the brain to stimulate AVP release. In addition, plasma hypertonicity depolarizes the magnocellular neurons of the hypothalamus to cause more AVP release.

Decreases in blood volume or pressure also stimulate exponential increases in AVP. Hypovolemia and hypotension shift the osmolality-vasopressin response curve so that higher AVP levels are required to maintain a normal osmolality in hypotensive states.[9] Afferent impulses from the left atrium, aortic arch, and carotid sinus stretch receptors tonically inhibit AVP secretion. Atrial stretch receptors respond to increases in blood volume, and the receptors in the aortic arch and carotid sinuses respond to increases in arterial blood pressure. A decrease in arterial baroreceptor activity causes "disinhibition" of AVP release during hypotensive states and results in increased AVP secretion.

VASOPRESSIN RECEPTORS

Vasopressin receptors are G protein–coupled receptors. The cellular effects of vasopressin are mediated by interactions of the hormone with several types of receptors (Table 158-1).[10] V_1 receptors (V_1Rs), previously known as *V_{1a} receptors,* are found primarily on vascular smooth muscle cells and cause vasoconstriction in most vascular beds that is mediated by G_q protein–coupled activation of the phospholipase C and phosphoinositide pathways. Increased levels of inositol phosphate and diacylglycerol activate voltage-gated calcium channels. This results in increased intracellular calcium levels and subsequent vasoconstriction.

Vasopressin also causes inactivation of the potassium–adenosine triphosphate (ATP) channels in vascular smooth muscle cells. Opening of these channels (as occurs with acidosis or hypoxia) allows an efflux of potassium from the endothelial cells, subsequent hyperpolarization, and prevention of calcium entry into the cells. (An increase in cytosolic calcium is essential for vasoconstriction.) In contrast, inactivation of the potassium–ATP channel by AVP leads to depolarization, opening of the voltage-gated calcium channels, and an increase in cytosolic calcium with subsequent vasoconstriction.

Table 158-1 Vasopressin Receptors, Tissues Affected, and Principal Effects

Receptor	Tissues	Principal Effects
V_1 (V_{1a})	Vascular smooth muscle	Vasoconstriction at high dosages Vasodilation in cerebral, renal, pulmonary, and mesenteric vessels at low dosages
V_2	Renal collecting duct Endothelial cells Platelets Vascular endothelium	Increased water permeability Increased von Willebrand factor release Stimulation of aggregation Vasodilation
V_3 (V_{1b})	Pituitary	Adrenocorticotropic hormone release
Oxytocin	Uterus, mammary gland, Gastrointestinal tract Endothelium	Contraction Vasodilation

Interestingly, vasodilation may occur in some vascular beds, most likely mediated by nitric oxide. V_1Rs are found in the vascular endothelium of the kidney, skin, skeletal muscle, pancreas, thyroid gland, myometrium, bladder, hepatocytes, adipocytes, and spleen. Platelets also express the V_1R, which facilitates thrombosis due to an increase in intracellular calcium upon stimulation. V_1Rs in the kidneys lead to reduced blood flow to the inner medulla, limit the antidiuretic effects of AVP, and selectively cause contraction of the efferent arterioles to increase glomerular filtration rate. There is considerable variation among species with respect to the location and function of the V_1R.

V_2 receptors (V_2Rs) are found primarily on the basolateral membrane of the distal tubule and in the principal cells of the cortical and medullary renal collecting duct. Coupling of the V_2R with the G_s signaling pathway increases intracellular cyclic adenosine monophosphate (cAMP). The increased cAMP triggers fusion of the aquaporin-2–bearing vesicles with the apical plasma membrane of the collecting duct principal cells to increase free water absorption. AVP regulates water homeostasis in two ways: (1) by regulating the fast shuttling of aquaporin-2 to the cell surface, and (2) by stimulating the synthesis of messenger ribonucleic acid–encoding aquaporin-2. Most animals with nephrogenic diabetes insipidus have V_2R gene mutations.

V_2R activation also stimulates the release of platelets from the bone marrow and enhances the release of von Willebrand factor and factor VIII from endothelial cells. It causes a mild increase in the activity of factor VIII–related antigen and ristocetin cofactor. There are also V_2Rs in the vascular endothelium; the potent V_2R agonist 1-deamino-8-D-arginine vasopressin (DDAVP) therefore causes vasodilation in addition to the release of von Willebrand factor and factor VIII.

The V_3 pituitary receptors (V_3Rs, previously known as *V_{1b}Rs*) are located in the anterior pituitary gland and activate G_q protein to release intracellular calcium after activation of phospholipase C and the phosphoinositol cascade. V_3R activation stimulates release of adrenocorticotropic hormone.[11] These receptors are also responsible for the actions of AVP on the central nervous system, where they act as a neurotransmitter or a modulator of memory, blood pressure, body temperature, sleep cycles, and release of pituitary hormones.

The oxytocin receptor is a nonselective vasopressin receptor with equal affinity for both AVP and oxytocin. Activation of the oxytocin receptor leads to smooth muscle contraction, primarily in the myometrium and mammary myoepithelial cells. AVP also acts on oxytocin receptors in the umbilical vein, aorta, and pulmonary artery, where it causes a nitric oxide–mediated vasodilation. Stimulation of cardiac oxytocin receptors leads to the release of atrial natriuretic peptide.

Vasopressin also stimulates the P_2 class of purinoreceptors (ATP receptors), which leads to vasodilation mediated by nitric oxide and prostacyclin. P_2 receptors are also positive inotropic agents without direct effects on heart rate.

PHYSIOLOGIC EFFECTS OF VASOPRESSIN

Vasopressin causes direct systemic vasoconstriction via the V_1Rs. In vitro, AVP is a more potent vasoconstrictor than angiotensin II, norepinephrine, or phenylephrine on a molar basis. It is vital for osmoregulation and maintenance of normovolemia, mediated by the V_2Rs. In addition, AVP maintains hemostasis and assists with temperature modulation, memory, sleep, and secretion of adrenocorticotropic hormone. During normal physiologic states, AVP's primary role is the regulation of free water balance. Vasopressin levels in fasting humans are less than 4 pg/ml. Small increases in plasma osmolality lead to an increase in AVP to 10 pg/ml. A maximum increase in urine osmolality is seen with AVP levels greater than 20 pg/ml.

Vasopressin does not control vascular smooth muscle constriction in normal animals, but it is vital in states of hypotension.[11-13] Plasma AVP levels of 50 pg/ml must be attained before a significant increase in arterial pressure is achieved in humans. The pressor (vasoconstrictive) effects of AVP are nonadrenergic and are thought to be mediated by its direct and indirect effects on arterial smooth muscle. Stimulation of the V_1R leads to vasoconstriction of the skin, skeletal muscles, fat, bladder, myometrium, liver, spleen, pancreas, and thyroid gland. Low levels of AVP lead to vasodilation in the cerebral, pulmonary, mesenteric, and renal vessels. Even with potent stimuli for release, only 10% to 20% of the AVP stored in the pituitary can be readily released, and further release occurs at a much slower rate that results in a biphasic response to vasodilatory shock.[11]

PHARMACOLOGY

Exogenous AVP (8-arginine vasopressin) is sold as a sterile aqueous solution of synthetic AVP for intravenous, intramuscular, or subcutaneous administration. It is destroyed within the gastrointestinal tract and should only be given parenterally. It is not protein bound and has a volume of distribution of 140 ml/kg and a half-life of approximately 24 minutes. The drug is cleared by renal excretion (65%) and metabolism by tissue peptidases (35%). Terlipressin (triglycyl-lysine vasopressin) is a synthetic prodrug that is converted to lysine vasopressin in the circulation and has a greater V_1R selectivity and prolonged duration of action, with an effective half-life of approximately 6 hours. To the author's knowledge, this form of vasopressin has not been used clinically in veterinary medicine, but human and experimental research has advised caution due to potentially detrimental effects.[14-17] Selepressin, a novel selective V_1R, agonist has been studied in humans with septic shock and experimental sheep with sepsis, as well as in healthy research dogs.[18-20] Healthy experimental dogs given selepressin were found to have a reduced risk of coronary ischemia compared with those given AVP.[20]

Desmopressin acetate is a synthetic vasopressin analog that is available in both an intranasal and an injectable form. (An oral tablet form is also manufactured, but the bioavailability following oral ingestion is very low.) It binds primarily to V_2Rs and therefore has more potent antidiuretic and procoagulant activity and less vasopressor action than AVP on a per-weight basis. Both formulations of the drug should be stored in the refrigerator (although the nasal formulation is stable at room temperature for 3 weeks).

Desmopressin acetate causes a dosage-dependent increase in plasma levels of factor VIII and plasminogen factor. It also causes smaller increases in factor VIII–related antigen and ristocetin cofactor activities, but the effect is sustained for only 3 to 4 hours. The onset of antidiuretic action in dogs usually occurs within 2 hour of administration, peaks in 2 to 8 hours, and may persist for up to 24 hours. The metabolism of desmopressin is not well understood. The terminal half-life in humans after intravenous administration ranges from 0.4 to 4 hours.

Tolvaptan, a V_2R *antagonist*, may have therapeutic potential in animals with congestive heart failure. It has been found to elicit a potent aquaretic response and reduce cardiac preload without causing the undesirable effects on systemic or renal hemodynamics, the renin-angiotensin-aldosterone system, or the sympathetic nervous system. Further research is underway.[21-23]

CLINICAL USES

Indications and dosages for the use of vasopressin or DDAVP are summarized in Table 158-2.

Cardiopulmonary Resuscitation

The use of AVP to manage cardiac arrest has been studied extensively in laboratory animals, and a meta-analysis found that AVP was at least equivalent to epinephrine in its ability to aid in the return of spontaneous circulation or survival in humans.[24] A randomized, prospective clinical study in 60 dogs did not reveal an advantage in survival or 6-minute return of spontaneous circulation when AVP (0.5 to 1 U/kg) was compared with low-dose epinephrine (0.01 to 0.02 mg/kg). Further studies would be helpful, especially since the dose of AVP used in most of the dogs was below the recommended dose of 0.8 U/kg and the underlying disease states were extremely variable.[25] Another observational study in canines reported a possible association between the use of AVP therapy and successful resuscitation.[26] Additionally, experimental cardiopulmonary resuscitation studies in pigs showed that AVP improved cerebral oxygen delivery,

Table 158-2 Indications for and Dosages of Vasopressin or DDAVP Therapy

Indication	Dosage
Cardiopulmonary resuscitation	0.4-0.8 U/kg IV ± 1-4 mU/kg/min AVP IV CRI (dogs)*
Vasodilatory shock	0.5-5 mU/kg/min AVP IV CRI (dogs)*
Central diabetes insipidus	0.1 mg/ml intranasal solution DDAVP: 1-4 drops into conjunctival sac q12-24h or 0.01-0.05 ml SC q12-24h Alternatively, aqueous AVP may be used at 3-5 IU/dog or 0.5 IU/kg (cats) SC q4h or as needed
von Willebrand disease	1-4 mcg/kg DDAVP SC q3-4h (dogs)
Gastrointestinal disease, hemorrhagic shock	Unknown

AVP, Arginine vasopressin; *CRI,* constant rate infusion; *DDAVP,* 1-deamino-8-D-arginine vasopressin; *IV,* intravenously; *SC,* subcutaneously.
*Extrapolated from human dosage; dosage in cats is unknown.

resuscitation success, neurologic outcome, and blood flow to major organs, compared with epinephrine. Vasopressin has been listed in the American Heart Association Guidelines for Cardiopulmonary Resuscitation and Emergency Cardiovascular Care for the treatment of unstable ventricular tachycardia and ventricular fibrillation since 2000. The RECOVER veterinary guidelines also list AVP therapy (0.8 U/kg) as an acceptable alternative to epinephrine therapy during cardiopulmonary resuscitation in both dogs and cats.[27] In a large human study comparing AVP with epinephrine, there was a significant increase in survival following asystolic arrest in patients given AVP.[28] A recent pediatric study also revealed an increase in 24-hour survival (80% vs. 30%) in children experiencing cardiopulmonary arrest refractory to 1 dose of epinephrine.[29]

Vasopressin levels are elevated following cardiopulmonary arrest, and levels are significantly higher in humans who are resuscitated than in patients who do not survive.[30] Vasopressin has a shorter duration of effect and produces a greater vasoconstrictive effect during hypoxic and acidemic episodes of cardiopulmonary arrest than does epinephrine. Results of its use in newborn piglets with experimentally induced severe hypoxia and reoxygenation are also very promising.[31] In normal experimental animals, the half-life of AVP is 10 to 20 minutes.[32] Extrapolated doses in dogs are 0.4 to 0.8 U/kg given intravenously, with a constant rate infusion of 1 to 4 mU/kg/min, if needed. Endobronchial administration has been studied in pigs. A systematic review and meta-analysis has been published.[24]

Vasodilatory Shock

Vasopressin deficiency can play an important role in animals with vasoplegia secondary to sepsis, prolonged hemorrhagic shock, or cardiac arrest. Experimentally, exogenous AVP infusions to yield plasma AVP concentrations of 20 to 30 pg/ml can restore blood pressure with minimal adverse effects on organ perfusion. Low-flow states secondary to hypovolemia or septic shock are associated with a biphasic response in serum AVP levels. There is an early increase in the release of AVP from the neurohypophysis in response to hypoxia, hypotension, or acidosis that leads to high levels of serum AVP. This plays a role in the stabilization of arterial pressure and organ perfusion in the initial stages of shock. Agents that block the V_1R lower arterial pressure in both acute hemorrhagic shock and septic shock.

Previous studies in dogs have found concentrations of AVP in the range of 300 to 1000 pg/ml during the early phase of hemorrhagic shock and 500 to 1200 pg/ml following experimentally induced endotoxemia (further details are given later in this chapter). During the later phase of shock, however, the AVP levels are decreased, presumably as a result of degradation of released AVP and depletion of the neurohypophyseal stores, which take time to replenish through resynthesis. The AVP concentration in the experimental dogs decreased to 29 pg/ml during the late phase of hemorrhagic shock.

Humans with advanced vasodilatory shock have both a deficiency of AVP secretion and an enhanced sensitivity to AVP-induced blood pressure changes. Additionally, AVP levels are markedly increased in animal models of acute sepsis, but this increase is followed by a rapid decline over the ensuing few hours. Additional hypotheses to explain the low levels of AVP include a decrease in baroreceptor stimulation of AVP release in hypotensive patients secondary to impaired autonomic reflexes, as seen in sepsis, or tonic inhibition by atrial stretch receptors secondary to volume loading or mechanical ventilation. In addition, AVP release may be inhibited by nitric oxide or high circulating levels of norepinephrine.

Several human studies and reports have demonstrated promising results in the treatment of people with refractory hypotension using an AVP intravenous infusion. Many human patients were subsequently weaned off catecholamine support by the addition of AVP therapy. In addition, there is an increase in urine output, presumably secondary to an increase in renal perfusion pressure due to renal efferent arteriolar constriction, as well as nitric oxide–induced vasodilation; oxytocin receptor stimulation, which increases natriuresis; and an increase in atrial natriuretic peptide. AVP therapy may also reduce the rate of progression of acute kidney injury to renal failure and decrease mortality in people with septic shock.[33] Humans who received AVP therapy before their doses of norepinephrine exceeded 0.5 mg/kg/min had an improved outcome.[34] A recent meta-analysis of publications between 1996 and 2011 showed a reduction in norepinephrine requirement in patients receiving AVP as well as reduced mortality rates in people with septic shock. There was no difference between the AVP treatment group and the control group in adverse events.[35] Interestingly, people who received both physiologic levels of corticosteroids and AVP therapy had decreased mortality compared with those who were treated with norepinephrine and corticosteroids, or with either drug without corticosteroid therapy.[36] Animal trials thus far support the potential benefits of AVP in animals in hypotensive states. However, high-dose therapy is associated with excessive coronary and splanchnic vasoconstriction, as well as a hypercoagulable state. The excessive vasoconstriction can lead to a reduction in cardiac output or even fatal cardiac events, especially in patients with decreased myocardial function.

Guzman et al[37] compared the effects of intravenous norepinephrine with those of intravenous AVP on systemic splanchnic and renal circulation in anesthetized dogs with experimentally induced endotoxic shock. Except for a more pronounced bradycardia in the AVP group, the systemic and splanchnic blood flow changes were comparable. However, the AVP infusion restored renal blood flow and oxygen delivery, but the norepinephrine therapy did not. These types of studies are not representative of patients that have catecholamine-resistant hypotension, but the end-organ results are expected to be similar.

Another canine study by Morales et al[38] examined the effect of AVP administration in dogs with experimental hemorrhagic shock and subsequent requirement for a norepinephrine infusion (3 mcg/kg/min) to maintain a mean arterial pressure of 40 mm Hg. An AVP infusion resulted in an increase in mean arterial pressures from 39 ± 6 mm Hg to 128 ± 9 mm Hg. The serum AVP levels were markedly elevated during the acute hemorrhage but decreased from 319 ± 66 to 29 ± 9 pg/ml before administration of AVP.

Clinically, AVP has been used in dogs with refractory vasodilatory shock.[39] A dosage of 0.5 mU/kg/min was administered intravenously and titrated higher as needed to achieve a mean arterial pressure above 70 mm Hg and a heart rate below 140 beats/min. There was a significant increase in mean arterial pressure with minimal adverse effects. The mean dosage used was 2.1 mU/kg/min. There is no information regarding survival because all of the dogs in this clinical study were euthanized or died.

Hemorrhagic Shock

There have been several experimental animal studies and preliminary human clinical studies evaluating the use of AVP therapy for the treatment of hemorrhagic shock. Its ability to sustain arterial blood pressure and decrease blood loss during hemorrhage deserves further study. Because AVP redirects blood from the skin, skeletal muscle, and periphery, it minimizes blood loss from bleeding extremities. The suggestion that AVP therapy may replace fluid therapy has received much attention; administration of AVP decreased fluid requirements and mortality in one human trauma study,[40] and further studies will be telling.

Central Diabetes Insipidus

Animals with central diabetes insipidus and subsequent deficiency of endogenous AVP can benefit from treatment with either aqueous vasopressin or DDAVP. Caution should be exercised to prevent water intoxication, and serial electrolyte levels should be analyzed during treatment. DDAVP is often preferred because it has more antidiuretic activity and less potential vasopressor properties on a per-weight basis. One to four drops of the 0.1 mg/ml intranasal solution is typically given into the conjunctival sac q24h or q12h. Alternatively, subcutaneous doses of 0.01 to 0.05 ml can be used in dogs q12-24h. Aqueous vasopressin has been administered in subcutaneous doses of 3 to 5 U per dog or 0.5 U/kg in cats q4h or as needed (see Chapter 67).

von Willebrand Disease

DDAVP may be useful in patients with von Willebrand disease, except in those animals with type IIB or platelet-type (pseudo) forms, because platelet aggregation and thrombocytopenia may occur. In addition, treatment with DDAVP is often confounded by its short duration of activity (2 to 4 hours), development of resistance, and expense. It is not effective for dogs with severe type II and III von Willebrand disease. Dosage is 1 to 4 mcg/kg of DDAVP subcutaneously q3-4h. Onset of activity is typically within 30 minutes, and the effects last approximately 2 hours. DDAVP can improve platelet function in a range of disease states in addition to von Willebrand disease (see Chapter 170).

Gastrointestinal and Pulmonary Disease

Several uses of AVP in humans have not yet been studied in dogs. These include the acute treatment of esophageal varices and gastrointestinal hemorrhage, stimulation of peristalsis in patients with postoperative ileus, and dispelling of intestinal gas before abdominal imaging.

AVP has also been shown to improve cardiopulmonary function in ovine acute lung injury secondary to burns and smoke inhalation.[41] This looks like a promising area for further research.

ADVERSE EFFECTS

AVP can cause contraction of the bladder and gallbladder smooth muscle and can increase peristalsis (especially of the colon). The drug may decrease gastric secretions and increase gastrointestinal sphincter pressure. Potential adverse effects of AVP administration include local irritation at the injection site, skin necrosis if extravasated, and skin reactions. Humans treated with AVP for vasodilatory shock have developed an increase in liver enzyme and bilirubin levels, decrease in platelet count, hyponatremia, anaphylaxis, bronchospasm, abdominal pain, hematuria, and urticaria, although the incidence of adverse effects appears to be quite low. Theoretically, because AVP causes a release of von Willebrand factor, it enhances platelet aggregation and may increase the risk of thrombosis. Water intoxication has been reported with high-dose therapy for the treatment of diabetes insipidus. Vasopressin or DDAVP may cause irritation when administered in the conjunctival sac.

VASOPRESSIN ANTAGONISTS

Investigation into vasopressin antagonist therapy is currently underway for a variety of diseases. V_1R antagonists may prove useful for the management of subarachnoid hemorrhage, whereas V_2R antagonists may be preferable to the use of loop diuretics in people and dogs with congestive heart failure.[22,42] A full review of these emerging treatments is beyond the scope of this chapter, but vasopressin antagonists appear to hold great promise for the treatment of a variety of disease states in which elevated endogenous AVP levels are detrimental to the patient.

CONCLUSION

Vasopressin is a drug with many actions, several receptors, and multiple therapeutic uses. It is important to understand the mechanisms of action of the various receptors and the mechanisms of action of the various formulations to treat animals safely and appropriately. The use of this drug in veterinary medicine is expanding as research in people and experimental models continues.

REFERENCES

1. Robinson A, Verbalis J: Posterior pituitary gland. In Larsen P, Kronenberg H, Melmed S, et al, editors: Williams textbook of endocrinology, Philadelphia, 2002, Saunders.
2. Hoyle CH: Neuropeptide families and their receptors: evolutionary perspectives, Brain Res 848:1, 1999.
3. Bourque CW, Oliet SH: Osmoreceptors in the central nervous system, Annu Rev Physiol 59:601, 1997.
4. Quail AW, Woods RL, Korner PI: Cardiac and arterial baroreceptor influences in release of vasopressin and renin during hemorrhage, Am J Physiol 252:H1120, 1987.
5. Norsk P, Ellegaard P, Videbaek R, et al: Arterial pulse pressure and vasopressin release in humans during lower body negative pressure, Am J Physiol 264:R1024, 1993.
6. Holmes CL, Landry DW, Granton JT: Science review: vasopressin and the cardiovascular system. Part 2: Clinical physiology, Crit Care 8:15, 2004.
7. Leng G, Dyball RE, Luckman SM: Mechanisms of vasopressin secretion, Horm Res 37:33, 1992.
8. Day TA, Sibbald JR: Noxious somatic stimuli excite neurosecretory vasopressin cells via A1 cell group, Am J Physiol 258:R1516, 1990.
9. Kam PC, Williams S, Yoong FF: Vasopressin and terlipressin: pharmacology and its clinical relevance, Anaesthesia 59:993, 2004.
10. Holmes CL, Landry DW, Granton JT: Science review: vasopressin and the cardiovascular system. Part 1: Receptor physiology, Crit Care 7:427, 2003.
11. Holmes CL, Patel BM, Russell JA, et al: Physiology of vasopressin relevant to management of septic shock, Chest 120:989, 2001.
12. Graybiel A, Glendy R: Circulatory effects following the intravenous administration of pitressin in normal persons and in patients with hypertension and angina pectoris, Am Heart J 21:481, 1941.
13. Schwartz J, Keil LC, Maselli J, et al: Role of vasopressin in blood pressure regulation during adrenal insufficiency, Endocrinology 112:234, 1983.
14. Singer M: Arginine vasopressin vs. terlipressin in the treatment of shock states, Best Pract Res Clin Anaesthesiol 22(2):359-368, 2008.
15. Lange M, Ertmer C, Westphal M: Vasopressin vs. terlipressin in the treatment of cardiovascular failure in sepsis, Intensive Care Med 34(5):821-832, 2008.
16. Rodriguez-Nunez A, Lopez-Herce J, Gil-Anton J, et al: Rescue treatment with terlipressin in children with refractory septic shock: a clinical study, Crit Care 10(1):R20, 2006.
17. Ishikawa K, Wan L, Calzavacca P, et al: The effects of terlipressin on regional hemodynamics and kidney function in experimental hyperdynamic sepsis, PLoS One 7(2):e29693, 2012.
18. Russell J, Vincent JL, Kjølbye AL, et al: Selepressin, a novel selective vasopressin V1a agonist, reduces norepinephrine requirements and shortens duration of organ dysfunction in septic shock patients, Crit Care Med 40(12):62, 2012.
19. Rehberg S, Ertmer C, Vincent JL, et al: Role of selective V1a receptor agonism in ovine septic shock, Crit Care Med 39(1):119-125, 2011.
20. Boucheix OB, Milano SP, Henriksson M, et al: Selepressin, a new V1A receptor agonist: hemodynamic comparison to vasopressin in dogs, Shock 39(6):533-538, 2013.
21. Laszlo FA, Laszlo F Jr, De Wied D: Pharmacology and clinical perspectives of vasopressin antagonists, Pharmacol Rev 43:73, 1991.

22. Onogawa T, Sakamoto Y, Nakamura S, et al: Effects of tolvaptan on systemic and renal hemodynamic function in dogs with congestive heart failure, Cardiovasc Drugs Ther 25(Suppl 1):S67-S76, 2011.
23. Gheorghiade M, Gattis WA, O'Connor CM, et al: Effects of tolvaptan, a vasopressin antagonist, in patients hospitalized with worsening heart failure: a randomized controlled trial, JAMA 291(16):1963-1971, 2004.
24. Aung K, Htay T: Vasopressin for cardiac arrest: a systematic review and meta-analysis, Arch Intern Med 165:17, 2005.
25. Buckley GJ, Rozanski EA, Rush JE: Randomized, blinded comparison of epinephrine and vasopressin for treatment of naturally occurring cardiopulmonary arrest in dogs, J Vet Intern Med 25(6):1334-1340, 2011.
26. Scroggin RD Jr, Quandt J: The use of vasopressin for treating vasodilatory shock and cardiopulmonary arrest, J Vet Emerg Crit Care (San Antonio) 19(2):145-157, 2009.
27. Rozanski EA, Rush JE, Buckley GJ, et al: RECOVER evidence and knowledge gap analysis on veterinary CPR. Part 4: Advanced life support, J Vet Emerg Crit Care (San Antonio) 22(Suppl 1):S44-S64, 2012.
28. Wenzel V, Krismer AC, Arntz HR, et al: A comparison of vasopressin and epinephrine for out-of-hospital cardiopulmonary resuscitation, N Engl J Med 350:105, 2004.
29. Carroll TG, Dimas VV, Raymond TT: Vasopressin rescue for in-pediatric intensive care unit cardiopulmonary arrest refractory to initial epinephrine dosing: a prospective feasibility pilot trial, Pediatr Crit Care Med 13(3):265-272, 2012.
30. Lindner KH, Strohmenger HU, Ensinger H, et al: Stress hormone response during and after cardiopulmonary resuscitation, Anesthesiology 77:662, 1992.
31. Cheung DC, Gill RS, Liu JQ, et al: Vasopressin improves systemic hemodynamics without compromising mesenteric perfusion in the resuscitation of asphyxiated newborn piglets: a dose-response study, Intensive Care Med 38(3):491-498, 2012.
32. Errington ML, Rocha e Silva M Jr: The secretion and clearance of vasopressin during the development of irreversible haemorrhagic shock, J Physiol 217:43P, 1971.
33. Gordon AC, Russell JA, Walley KR, et al: The effects of vasopressin on acute kidney injury in septic shock, Intensive Care Med 36(1):83-91, 2010.
34. Luckner G, Dunser MW, Jochberger S, et al: Arginine vasopressin in 316 patients with advanced vasodilatory shock, Crit Care Med 33:2659, 2005.
35. Serpa NA, Nassar AJ, Cardoso SO, et al: Vasopressin and terlipressin in adult vasodilatory shock: a systematic review and meta-analysis of nine randomized controlled trials, Crit Care 16(4):R154, 2012.
36. Russell JA, Walley KR, Gordon AC, et al: Interaction of vasopressin infusion, corticosteroid treatment, and mortality of septic shock, Crit Care Med 37(3):811-818, 2009.
37. Guzman JA, Rosado AE, Kruse JA: Vasopressin vs. norepinephrine in endotoxic shock: systemic, renal, and splanchnic hemodynamic and oxygen transport effects, J Appl Physiol 95:803, 2003.
38. Morales D, Madigan J, Cullinane S, et al: Reversal by vasopressin of intractable hypotension in the late phase of hemorrhagic shock, Circulation 100:226, 1999.
39. Silverstein DC, Waddell LS, Drobatz KJ, et al: Vasopressin therapy in dogs with dopamine-resistant hypotension and vasodilatory shock, J Vet Emerg Crit Care 17(4):399-408, 2007.
40. Cohn SM, McCarthy J, Stewart RM, et al: Impact of low-dose vasopressin on trauma outcome: prospective randomized study, World J Surg 35(2):430-439, 2011.
41. Westphal M, Rehberg S, Maybauer MO, et al: Cardiopulmonary effects of low-dose arginine vasopressin in ovine acute lung injury, Crit Care Med 39(2):357-363, 2011.
42. Hockel K, Scholler K, Trabold R, et al: Vasopressin V(1a) receptors mediate posthemorrhagic systemic hypertension thereby determining rebleeding rate and outcome after experimental subarachnoid hemorrhage, Stroke 43(1):227-232, 2012.

CHAPTER 159

ANTIHYPERTENSIVES

Mary Anna Labato, DVM, DACVIM (Internal Medicine)

KEY POINTS

- Clinically, hypertension is divided into two categories: primary and secondary.
- Secondary hypertension accounts for almost all identified cases of elevated blood pressure in veterinary medicine.
- Normal blood pressure values are not identical for dogs and cats. Normal values for dogs are breed specific to some degree.
- Blood pressure values in the dog higher than 150/95 mm Hg (systolic/diastolic) and/or 115 mm Hg (mean) on three separate occasions are consistent with hypertension. For cats, arterial pressures higher than 135/100 mm Hg (mean, 115 mm Hg) on three separate occasions are consistent with hypertension.
- A blood pressure higher than 150/95 mm Hg (mean, 115 mm Hg) on a single occasion in a patient with evidence of organ damage is compatible with hypertension and should be addressed. If the blood pressure exceeds 180/120 mm Hg (mean, 140 mm Hg) , emergent therapy to lower blood pressure should be instituted.
- There are a number of classes of substances used for antihypertensive therapy, and often multiple modalities are necessary.
- Angiotensin-converting enzyme inhibitors and calcium channel blockers are the most commonly used antihypertensive agents in veterinary medicine.

The definition of normal blood pressure in dogs and cats has been quite elusive. It has been the subject of significant research, debate, and confusion.[1] Normal values for dogs have been shown to be somewhat breed specific, whereas for cats blood pressure values are not related to breed.[2]

The pressure defining hypertension has been lowered in recent years. At this time, blood pressure values higher than 150/95 mm Hg (mean, 115 mm Hg) on three separate visits in a patient that demonstrates no clinical signs are considered compatible with hypertension; in addition, a single reading higher than 150/95 mm Hg (mean, >115 mm Hg) in a patient with evidence of clinical disease in those organs susceptible to end-organ damage (e.g., brain, eyes, kidneys) is also deemed to be hypertension requiring treatment. A blood pressure measurement higher than 180/120 mm Hg (mean arterial pressure, >140 mm Hg) is a medical emergency and must be treated as soon as possible.[1,3-5]

ETIOLOGY OF HYPERTENSION

Patients are classified as having primary (essential) or secondary hypertension. In the Seventh Report of the Joint National Committee on Prevention, Detection, Evaluation, and Treatment of High Blood Pressure in humans, a third category termed *prehypertension* was established.[6]

Prehypertension is defined as a systolic blood pressure ranging from 120 to 139 mm Hg and/or a diastolic pressure of 80 to 89 mm Hg. This new designation is intended to identify those individuals in whom early intervention such as changing to a healthy lifestyle and diet could reduce blood pressure or decrease the rate of progression of blood pressure to hypertensive levels.[6]

Primary hypertension is the result of an imbalance in the relationship between cardiac output and systemic vascular resistance. The exact cause has not been determined. Little is known about the prevalence of primary hypertension in animals. There have been reports of both dogs and cats considered to have primary hypertension because secondary causes could not be identified.[7-10]

Secondary hypertension is elevated blood pressure that occurs because of systemic disease or medication. Secondary hypertension accounts for almost all identified cases of elevated blood pressure in veterinary patients. The following disorders have been reported to be associated with a significant risk of developing hypertension: kidney disease, diabetes mellitus, hyperadrenocorticism, hyperthyroidism, and hepatic disease. Additionally, more uncommon causes include pheochromocytoma, hyperaldosteronism, polycythemia, and chronic anemia. The use of drugs such as erythropoietin and glucocorticoids has also been associated with elevations in blood pressure.[8-16]

PROPOSED MECHANISM OF BLOOD PRESSURE ELEVATION

A number of diseases and a variety of causes have been associated with elevations in blood pressure. In patients with hyperadrenocorticism, glucocorticoids induce hepatic production of angiotensinogen, which results in an exaggerated response of the renin-angiotensin system.[11] The hypertension that develops in animals with hyperthyroidism is secondary to the increased cardiac output caused by the effect of thyroid hormone on cardiac muscle.[15-20]

The two predominant mechanisms of renal regulation of blood pressure are pressure natriuresis and the renin-angiotensin-aldosterone system.[5] It has been hypothesized that increased blood volume secondary to either a maladaptive increase in renin secretion or inability of the kidneys to process fluids and electrolytes properly may lead to increased venous return of blood to the heart.[14] Increased levels of endogenous vasoconstrictors such as endothelin, thromboxane, and adrenergic stimuli combined with decreased levels of endogenous vasodilators such as prostacyclin and nitric oxide may also be contributing factors.

The mechanism by which hepatic disease results in hypertension is undetermined. In patients with diabetes mellitus, there are possibly four different mechanisms. In humans with type 1 diabetes, hypertension is thought to develop due to the effects of diabetes on renal function (i.e., diabetic nephropathy characterized by nephritic syndrome and glomerulosclerosis). For type 2 diabetes three different mechanisms have been proposed.[17] One suggested mechanism is that hyperinsulinemia secondary to insulin resistance causes sodium and water retention and increased sympathetic activity. This leads to increased peripheral resistance via changes in blood volume and vasoconstriction, respectively. The second proposed mechanism is that there is hypertrophy of vascular smooth muscle secondary to the mitogenic effects of insulin. The last mechanism that has been proposed is that elevations in insulin levels lead to increased levels of intracellular calcium. The increased calcium results in hyperresponsive vascular smooth muscle contraction and increased peripheral vascular resistance.

Chromocytomas release epinephrine and norepinephrine, which results in vasoconstriction and increased cardiac output (see Chapter 71).[18] The administration of erythropoietin has been associated with the development of hypertension. Anemia leads to chronically dilated capillary beds. With resolution of the anemia, overcompensation of capillary constriction occurs, which results in an increase in peripheral vascular resistance.[19]

ANTIHYPERTENSIVE DRUGS

Angiotensin-Converting Enzyme Inhibitors

Mechanism of action

Angiotensin-converting enzyme (ACE) inhibitors are often used as the initial treatment of choice to control hypertension. ACE inhibitors competitively inhibit the conversion of angiotensin I to angiotensin II. Angiotensin II is one of the most powerful endogenous vasoconstrictors; its inhibition results in systemic vasodilation (Table 159-1).

The primary effects of ACE inhibitors result in a decrease in angiotensin I and II as well as an increase in bradykinin. Drugs in this class induce arterial and venous vasodilation. Since angiotensin II directly stimulates the kidneys to retain sodium, its inhibition results in a reduced plasma volume. In addition, ACE inhibitors prevent aldosterone release, which leads to a decrease in sodium and water retention and decreased blood volume. There is a reduction in both preload and afterload. The other beneficial effect of ACE inhibitors is that they reduce intraglomerular pressure and inhibit growth factors that lead to glomerular hypertrophy and sclerosis.[1,21-26]

Indications

ACE inhibitors are used to reduce blood pressure in all forms of hypertension. They are also used frequently in the treatment of mitral insufficiency and congestive heart failure due to dilated cardiomyopathy. ACE inhibitors also appear to reduce proteinuria by maintaining the heparan sulfate layer of the glomerular basement membrane. For example, benazepril administration has been associated with (1) lowering of glomerular capillary hypertension, (2) decreased release of extracellular matrix and collagen from mesangial and tubular cells, and (3) reduction in the degree of glomerular and interstitial fibrosis.[27,28]

Although there are a number of different ACE inhibitors, the ones used most commonly in veterinary medicine are enalapril, benazepril, ramipril, and lisinopril (Table 159-2). The effects of ACE inhibitors are less predictable in cats. As many as 50% of hypertensive cats do not respond to enalapril, although benazepril has demonstrated a statistically significant antihypertensive effect in cats with kidney disease.[1]

Adverse effects

ACE inhibitors are relatively safe drugs. Adverse effects include weakness and lethargy attributable to a drop in blood pressure. Reversible

Table 159-1 Summary of Antihypertensive Drugs

Drug	Effect	Indications
Angiotensin-converting enzyme inhibitors Benazepril, enalapril, lisinopril, enalaprilat	Arterial and venous vasodilation Decreased preload Decreased afterload	Hypertension Heart failure Proteinuria
Calcium channel blockers Amlodipine, nicardipine	Arterial vasodilation	Hypertension Hypertensive crisis
β-adrenergic antagonists Propranolol, atenolol	Decreased cardiac output Decreased sympathetic outflow Decreased blood pressure Cardiodepression Nonselective (β_1 and β_2) Cardioselective (β_1)	Hypertension Hypertrophic cardiomyopathy Arrhythmias Pheochromocytoma
α-Adrenergic antagonist Prazosin	Balanced vasodilation	Hypertension Pheochromocytoma
Arteriolar vasodilator Hydralazine	Nonspecific arterial vasodilation Reduced peripheral vascular resistance Reduced blood pressure	Hypertension Hypertensive crisis
Arteriolar vasodilator Sodium nitroprusside	Nitric oxide donor Vasodilation	Hypertensive crisis
Angiotensin II receptor blockers Losartan, irbesartan, telmisartan	Arterial and venous vasodilation	Hypertension
Aldosterone blockers Spironolactone, eplerenone	Vasodilation	Hypertension Proteinuria
Dopamine-1 agonist Fenoldopam	Vasodilation Decreased blood pressure Natriuresis Increase in renal blood flow	Hypertension Hypertensive crisis Acute kidney injury

Table 159-2 Commonly Used Antihypertensive Agents and Their Dosages

Drug	Class	Canine Dosage	Feline Dosage
Amlodipine	Calcium channel blocker	0.05-0.2 mg/kg q24h PO or rectally	0.625-1.25 mg q24h PO or rectally
Atenolol	β-Adrenergic blocker	0.25-1 mg/kg q12-24h PO	6.25-12.5 mg q12-24h PO
Benazepril	ACE inhibitor	0.25-0.5 mg/kg q12-24h PO	0.25-0.5 mg/kg q12-24h PO
Enalapril	ACE inhibitor	0.5-1.0 mg/kg q12-24h PO	0.25-0.5 mg/kg q12-24h PO
Enalaprilat	ACE inhibitor	0.1-1.0 mg q6h IV	Unknown
Propranolol	β-Adrenergic blocker	0.04-0.1 mg/kg q8-12h IV or 0.5-1 mg/kg q8-12h PO	0.02-0.06 mg/kg q8-12h IV or 0.2-1.0 mg/kg q8-12h PO
Prazosin	α-Adrenergic blocker	0.5-4 mg q8-12h PO	0.25-0.5 mg/cat q12-24h PO
Spironolactone	Aldosterone inhibitor	1-2 mg/kg q12h PO	1 mg/kg q12h PO
Hydralazine	Arterial vasodilator	0.25-4 mg/kg q12h	0.25-2 mg/kg q12h
Sodium nitroprusside	Nonspecific vasodilator	1-3 mcg/kg/min IV CRI	1-2 mcg/kg/min IV CRI
Losartan	Angiotensin II receptor blocker	0.5 mg/kg q24h	Unknown
Lisinopril	ACE inhibitor	0.25-0.75 mg/kg q24h PO	0.25-0.5 mg/kg q24h PO
Fenoldopam	Dopamine-1 agonist	0.1-0.8 mcg/kg/min IV CRI	0.1-0.8 mcg/kg/min IV CRI
Nicardipine	Calcium channel blocker	0.5-5 mcg/kg/min IV CRI	Unknown
Ramipril	ACE inhibitor	0.125-0.25 mg/kg q24h PO	Unknown
Irbesartan	Angiotensin II receptor blocker	5 mg/kg q24h PO	Unknown
Telmisartan	Angiotensin II receptor blocker	1.0-3.0 mg/kg q24h PO	Unknown

ACE, Angiotensin-converting enzyme; *CRI,* constant rate infusion; *IV,* intravenously; *PO,* per os.

increases in blood urea nitrogen and creatinine levels may result from a reduction in kidney function (which causes reversible elevation of creatinine and blood urea nitrogen levels and decrease in glomerular filtration rate). These effects are especially likely if ACE inhibitors are used in conjunction with diuretics. Hyperkalemia frequently occurs secondary to aldosterone inhibition. A rare adverse effect is the production of a dry cough induced by bradykinin.

Angiotensin II Receptor Blockers

Mechanism of action

Angiotensin II receptor blockers (ARBs) have been shown to be well tolerated, safe, and effective for blood pressure control in humans. Several studies have demonstrated that this class of drugs confers renal benefits in people with diabetic nephropathy. It is controversial whether ARBs are better at protecting the kidney than ACE inhibitors in patients with type 2 diabetes mellitus.[23] Signaling through both angiotensin type 1 receptors (AT_1Rs) and dopamine D_1 receptors (D_1Rs) modulates renal sodium excretion and arterial blood pressure. Thus the antihypertensive effect may be due to both inhibition of AT_1R signaling and enhancement of D_1R signaling.[29]

ARBs displace angiotensin II from its specific AT_1R, antagonizing all of its known effects (i.e., vasoconstriction, sympathetic activation, aldosterone release, renal sodium resorption) and resulting in a dose-dependent fall in peripheral resistance and little change in heart rate or cardiac output.[30]

Indications

In humans, ARBs (losartan, irbesartan, telmisartan) are used to treat hypertension and cardiovascular disease. Their efficacy for the treatment of hypertension in dogs and cats is not known. Losartan, telmisartan, and irbesartan have been used in dogs, but more investigation into their role in the veterinary armamentarium is necessary. Losartan was ineffective as an antihypertensive agent in cats with experimentally induced kidney hypertension.[5,31]

Adverse effects

This class of drugs appears to be safe with few adverse effects. In virtually every human trial, ARBs given to hypertensive patients have been better tolerated than other classes of antihypertensive medications.[30]

Adrenergic Receptor Antagonists

Mechanism of action

Drugs that may be useful in the treatment of hypertension are those that block activation of α- adrenergic or β-adrenergic receptors. Propranolol, a β_1- and β_2-adrenergic receptor antagonist; atenolol, a β_1-selective antagonist; and prazosin, an α_1-adrenergic receptor antagonist have been used to treat hypertension in dogs and cats.

The mechanism of action of β-adrenergic blocking agents includes blockade of renin release, reduction of heart rate and contractility, decrease in peripheral vascular resistance, and reduction in central adrenergic drive.[1,30]

α-Adrenergic blockers exert their antihypertensive effects by selectively antagonizing α-adrenergic receptors on systemic vessels. Prazosin acts as a competitive antagonist of postsynaptic α_1-receptors. It blocks activation of the postsynaptic α_1-receptors by circulating or neurally released catecholamines, an activation that normally induces vasoconstriction. Peripheral resistance falls with minimal changes in cardiac output.[1,30]

Indications

β-Adrenergic blockers are useful in dogs and cats when primary antihypertensive treatment fails to produce the desired decrease in blood pressure. They are also used to manage hypertrophic cardiomyopathy and supraventricular and ventricular tachycardias.

α-Adrenergic antagonists have been used as primary or adjunctive therapy for hypertension in dogs. However, these agents have found greater use in micturition disorders as smooth muscle relaxants of the urethra and for the treatment of hypertension associated with pheochromocytomas.

Adverse effects

Nonselective β-adrenergic blockers, such as propranolol, should not be used in asthmatic cats because they may induce bronchospasm. Additional adverse effects include hyperkalemia, bradycardia, insulin resistance, and depression. Some of these adverse effects occur because the antagonists are not selective for β-receptors or α-receptors.

Prazosin, and other α-adrenergic antagonists, selectively block vascular α_1-receptors and may cause severe hypotension that is unresponsive to α_1-agonist therapy. Consequently, caution should be exercised when anesthetizing patients that are receiving prazosin therapy.

Aldosterone Blockers

Mechanism of action and indications

The aldosterone antagonist spironolactone blocks the effects of aldosterone on the renal distal convoluted tubule and collecting duct and thereby decreases sodium reabsorption and potassium excretion. Its antihypertensive effects arise not only from its action as a weak diuretic but from its effect on the renin-angiotensin-aldosterone system. It is useful in treating hyperaldosteronism, iatrogenic steroid edema, and refractory edema, and may be used in conjunction with other diuretics.

Aldosterone is a mineralocorticoid that regulates sodium and potassium balance in its target tissues (kidney, colon, salivary gland). Mineralocorticoid receptors have been discovered in fibroblasts in cardiac, endothelial, vascular smooth muscle, and brain cells. Aldosterone is considered proinflammatory and profibrotic and causes endothelial dysfunction secondary to vasoconstriction and vascular remodeling. It plays a role in mediating hypertension and kidney injury.[28]

Eplerenone is a novel agent that antagonizes the aldosterone receptor. Its use has been associated with severe hyperkalemia, so potassium levels must be monitored closely. Its major advantage over the nonselective aldosterone receptor antagonist spironolactone is the lack of binding to progesterone and androgen receptors. It has been approved for the treatment of hypertension in people. Aldosterone blockers also have been experimentally shown to reduce proteinuria and attenuate kidney injury by decreasing renal fibrosis and decreasing inflammation.[32,33]

Adverse effects

Hyperkalemia may occur with either spironolactone or eplerenone but is uncommon in the absence of kidney insufficiency or concomitant use of a β-blocker, ACE inhibitor, ARB, or potassium supplements.

Calcium Channel Blockers

Mechanism of action

Calcium channel blockers (CCBs) act by blocking the influx of calcium into vascular smooth muscle cells that is necessary to cause smooth muscle contraction and thereby decreasing systemic vascular resistance.[21] These drugs inhibit the slow transmembrane calcium influx into the cell via voltage-gated L-type calcium channels.[34]

The selectivity of the vascular and cardiac effects of the different CCBs varies. Those drugs that cause vasodilation at arterioles and coronary arteries lead to a reduction of peripheral resistance and a decrease in blood pressure. Those that have negative chronotropic, negative dromotropic, and negative inotropic actions have antiarrhythmic and cardiodepressant effects.[22]

The dihydropyridines (amlodipine, manidipine, nicardipine, nifedipine, nimodipine, nitrendipine) are the family of CCBs that primarily act on blood vessels.[22] They relax the vascular smooth muscles (in arteries, arterioles, and coronary arteries) and exert minimal direct effect on the heart. Dihydropyridines may produce arterial vasodilation and reflex tachycardia.

Indications

The indications for the use of CCBs are hypertension and hypertensive crises. Amlodipine is considered the drug of choice to treat hypertension in cats with chronic kidney disease. Amlodipine is long acting, which allows once-daily dosing, and has a gradual effect that prevents rapid reductions in blood pressure. In animals that cannot tolerate oral medications, rectal amlodipine administration has been used, although the pharmacokinetic data are lacking. A recent study in dogs with acute kidney injury suggested that amlodipine was beneficial in reducing systemic hypertension in this species.[35]

Adverse effects

Adverse effects noted with CCBs are tachycardia, nausea, constipation, and weakness. There is concern about using a CCB as a primary antihypertensive agent. CCBs were thought to have renoprotective effects equivalent to those of the ACE inhibitors. However, studies have shown that the afferent arteriolar vasodilation is greater than the efferent arteriolar vasodilation on the opposite side of the glomerulus, and this decrease in perfusion pressure may actually decrease glomerular filtration and, at higher dosages, lead to kidney damage.[1,21,34]

Arteriolar Vasodilators

Hydralazine

Mechanism of action and indications

Hydralazine is an arteriolar dilator acting directly on the smooth muscle of arterioles by mechanisms that are incompletely understood but result in reduced peripheral vascular resistance and reduced blood pressure. Although not a first-choice antihypertensive drug for patients with chronic kidney disease, hydralazine has been used to treat hypertension in dogs and cats, especially in cases of a hypertensive crisis. Sodium retention and reflex tachycardia may occur. Hydralazine has been known to act as an antioxidant, inhibiting vascular production of reactive oxygen species.[30] Hydralazine may induce arteriolar vasodilation by preventing oxidation of nitric oxide and thereby lowering blood pressure.[30]

Adverse effects

In humans three kinds of adverse effects are seen. The first kind is due to a reflex sympathetic activation. The second type involves a lupus-like reaction. The third kind includes nonspecific problems such as anorexia, nausea, vomiting, diarrhea, muscle cramps, and tremor. In veterinary medicine, adverse effects have primarily included a reflex tachycardia, weakness, and gastrointestinal upset.

Sodium Nitroprusside

Mechanism of action and indications

Sodium nitroprusside is a nonspecific vasodilator and a potent antihypertensive agent that brings about immediate relaxation of resistance and capacitance vessels. This is the result of nitric oxide release, which stimulates the production of cyclic guanine monophosphate (cGMP) in the vascular smooth muscle. cGMP activates a kinase that subsequently leads to the inhibition of calcium influx into the smooth muscle cell and decreased calcium-calmodulin stimulation of myosin light-chain kinase. This in turn decreases the phosphorylation of myosin light chains, which decreases smooth muscle contraction and causes vasodilation. Sodium nitroprusside induces minimal change in renal blood flow and only a slight increase in heart rate. It is indicated for treatment of a hypertensive crisis, rapid reduction of preload and afterload in acute heart failure, and controlled blood pressure reduction during surgery. Because of its high potency, it should be used only if blood pressure can be closely monitored.[1,22,30,36,37]

Adverse effects

Shock and severe hypotension may occur. Cyanide intoxication may be seen in patients who have reduced hepatic function or receive nitroprusside for prolonged periods of time or in high dosages. Upon infusion, sodium nitroprusside oxidizes sulfhydryl groups present in erythrocytes and cell membranes or reacts with hemoglobin to produce methemoglobin. This reaction results in the production of nitric oxide (as well as five cyanide groups), which leads to direct vasodilation through the action on vascular smooth muscle. Free cyanide is converted to thiocyanate by either thiocyanate oxidase within erythrocytes or a transsulfuration reaction with thiosulfate by the rhodanese enzyme in the liver.[38]

Thiocyanate is freely filtered at the glomerulus, which results in definitive elimination. Both cyanide and thiocyanate are toxic and are of concern in patients with renal insufficiency (decreased thiocyanate clearance), patients with liver insufficiency (decreased thiosulfate stores and decreased metabolism), and patients receiving diuretics (decreased thiosulfate and decreased metabolism). In addition, neonatal and geriatric patients may have reduced rhodanese enzyme levels and cyanide metabolism. Due to the greater sensitivity of feline patients to erythrocyte oxidative damage, the total dose and rate of infusion must be lower than in canine patients. Clinical signs of cyanide toxicity include the development of nitroprusside resistance, depression and stupor, seizures, and metabolic acidosis (increased lactate level and increased venous oxygen tension) due to the inhibition of mitochondrial cytochrome c oxidase. Similar clinical signs result from thiocyanate toxicity.[38] Treatment of cyanide toxicity typically includes discontinuation of the drug and hydroxocobalamin therapy. This form of vitamin B_{12} binds to the cyanide in the vascular space and cells to form cyanocobalamin. Exogenous thiosulfate and nitrite administration may be necessary in severe cases, but potential adverse effects limit their use.

When sodium nitroprusside is used, it is imperative to monitor carefully, administer cautiously, or try other options in patients with kidney or liver dysfunction and to give the drug for only short periods of time.

Fenoldopam

Mechanism of action

Fenoldopam is a peripheral dopamine-1 agonist and is a parenteral antihypertensive agent. It maintains or increases renal perfusion while lowering blood pressure. It maintains most of its efficacy for 48 hours as a constant rate infusion without rebound hypertension on discontinuation.[36,37] There is a paucity of data on the use of fenoldopam in clinical veterinary patients, most likely due to the cost of this drug.

Indications

The indications for fenoldopam are severe hypertension and hypertensive crisis. The drug may also be useful in the management and prevention of certain forms of acute kidney injury with oligoanuria.[37]

Adverse effects

Adverse effects include reflex tachycardia and increased intraocular pressure. In humans, headache and flushing is also reported.[37]

HYPERTENSIVE URGENCY

A hypertensive urgency exists when there is a marked elevation in blood pressure but the animal does not demonstrate clinical signs directly attributed to the elevation. The patient is in danger of developing end-organ damage or a vascular accident such as hemorrhage or intravascular coagulation. In these animals it is imperative that blood pressure be lowered, but this should be done in a gradual and controlled fashion.

Treatment of Hypertensive Urgency

Most identified cases of hypertension in veterinary medicine are secondary to other disease processes. The first course of action is to determine the predisposing cause and to institute appropriate therapy. In addition to treatment of the underlying disease, an antihypertensive drug therapy protocol needs to be incorporated for most patients. An important principle in treating hypertension is to allow 1 to 2 weeks before evaluating the efficacy of a particular drug or dosage adjustment.[1] The therapeutic goal is not to normalize blood pressure but rather to lower systolic blood pressure to 170 mm Hg or less, mean arterial pressure to 140 mm Hg or less, and/or diastolic pressure to 100 mm Hg or less.

HYPERTENSIVE EMERGENCY

A hypertensive emergency occurs when the animal has a marked elevation in blood pressure as well as clinical signs directly attributable to hypertension. These patients should be treated quickly and require monitoring in a critical care facility.[11,21] According to the current recommendations for people as outlined in the Seventh Report of the Joint National Committee on Prevention, Detection, Evaluation, and Treatment of High Blood Pressure, the initial goal of therapy in hypertensive emergencies is to reduce mean arterial blood pressure by no more than 25% (within minutes to 1 hour); then, if the patient's condition is stable, to reduce blood pressure to 160/100 to 160/110 mm Hg within the next 2 to 6 hours. Excessive falls in pressure that may precipitate renal, cerebral, or coronary ischemia should be avoided.[6]

Treatment of Hypertensive Emergency

Hypertensive emergencies should be treated at facilities that provide 24-hour critical care. Continuous blood pressure monitoring is imperative, preferably using direct arterial pressure monitoring, although indirect methods are also acceptable (see Chapter 183). Potentially dangerous medications such as nitroprusside and hydralazine may be used. Sodium nitroprusside is a potent arterial and venous dilator that may begin to act in seconds and has a half-life of 2 to 3 minutes. It needs to be administered as a constant rate infusion. Hydralazine is a rapid arteriolar dilator with unpredictable effects and has been associated with profound episodes of hypotension.[1] Nicardipine, a dihydropyridine calcium channel–blocking agent, is another fast-acting, injectable antihypertensive agent with minimal cardiac effects.

Enalaprilat is a parenteral ACE inhibitor similar in action to enalapril; however, it is fast acting. It is used in hypertensive emergencies. The dosage in human medicine is 0.625 to 1.25 mg intravenously over 5 minutes q6h. The dosage has been extrapolated for use in veterinary medicine, and the author uses 0.1 to 1.0 mg q6h intravenously.[37]

REFERENCES

1. Acierno MJ, Labato MA: Hypertension in dogs and cats, Compend Contin Educ Pract Vet 26(5):336, 2004.
2. Egner B: Blood pressure measurement. In Egner B, Carr A, Brown S, editors: Essential facts of blood pressure in dogs and cats, ed 3, Babenhauser, Germany, 2003, BE VetVerlag.
3. Kraft W, Egner B: Causes and effects of hypertension. In Egner B, Carr A, Brown S, editors: Essential facts of blood pressure in dogs and cats, ed 3, Babenhauser, Germany, 2003, BE VetVerlag.
4. Brown S, Atkins C, Bagley R, et al: Guidelines for the identification, evaluation and management of systemic hypertension in dogs and cats, J Vet Intern Med 21(3):542-558, 2007.
5. Syme H: Hypertension in small animal kidney disease, Vet Clin North Am Small Anim Pract 41:63-89, 2011.
6. Chobanian AV, Barkus GL, Black HR, et al: Seventh report of the joint National Committee on Prevention, Detection, Evaluation, and Treatment of High Blood Pressure, Hypertension 42:1206, 2003.
7. Bovee KC, Littman MP, Crabtree GJ, et al: Essential hypertension in a dog, J Am Vet Med Assoc 195(1):81, 1989.
8. Snyder PS, Henik RA: Feline systemic hypertension, Proc Twelfth Annual Vet Med Forum, San Francisco, p 126, 1994.
9. Morgan RV: Systemic hypertension in four cats: ocular and medical findings, J Am Anim Hosp Assoc 22:615, 1986.
10. Jepson R: Feline systemic hypertension: classification and pathogenesis, J Feline Med Surg 13:25-34, 2011.
11. Brown SA, Henik RA: Diagnosis and treatment of systemic hypertension, Vet Clin North Am Small Anim Pract 28(6):1481, 1998.
12. Stiles J, Polzen DJ, Bistmer SL: The prevalence of retinopathy in cats with systemic hypertension and chronic renal failure or hyperthyroidism, J Am Hosp Assoc 30(6):564, 1994.
13. Syme HM, Barber PJ, Markwell PJ, et al: Prevalence of systolic hypertension in cats with chronic renal failure at initial evaluation, J Am Vet Med Assoc 220(12):1799, 2002.
14. Bartges JW, Willis AM, Polzen DJ: Hypertension and renal disease, Vet Clin North Am Small Animal Pract 26(6):1331, 1996.
15. Panciera DC: Cardiovascular complications of thyroid disease. In Bonagura JD, editor: Kirk's current veterinary therapy XIII, ed 13, Philadelphia, 2000, Saunders, p 716.
16. Littman MP: Spontaneous systemic hypertension in 24 cats, J Vet Intern Med 8(2):79, 1994.
17. Struble AL, Feldman EC, Nelson RW, et al: Systemic hypertension and proteinuria in dogs with diabetes mellitus, J Am Vet Med Assoc 213(6):822, 1998.
18. Mellian C, Peterson ME: The incidentally discovered adrenal mass. In Bonagura JD, editor: Kirk's current veterinary therapy XIII, ed 13, Philadelphia, 2000, Saunders p 368.
19. Cowgill LD, James KM, Levy JK, et al: Use of recombinant human erythropoietin for management of anemia in dogs and cats with renal failure, J Am Vet Med Assoc 212(4):521, 1998.
20. Maggio F, DeFrancesco TC, Atkins CE, et al: Ocular lesions associated with systemic hypertension in cats: 69 cases (1985-1998), J Am Vet Med Assoc 217(5):695-702, 2000.
21. Brown SA, Henik RA: Therapy for systemic hypertension in dogs and cats. In Bonagura JD, editor: Kirk's current veterinary therapy XIII, ed 13, Philadelphia, 2000, Saunders, p 838.
22. Ungemach FR: Hypertension. In Egner B, Carr A, Brown S, editors: Essential facts of blood pressure in dogs and cats, ed 3, Babenhauser, Germany, 2003, BE VetVerlag.
23. Messerli FH, Grossman E: Therapeutic controversies in hypertension, Semin Nephrol 25:227, 2005.
24. Steele JL, Henik RA, Stepien RL: Effects of angiotensin-converting enzyme inhibitor on plasma aldosterone concentration, plasma rennin activity, and blood pressure in spontaneously hypertensive cats with chronic renal disease, Vet Ther 3(2):157, 2002.
25. Brown SA, Brown CA, Jacobs G, et al: Effects of the angiotensin converting enzyme inhibitor benazepril in cats with induced renal insufficiency, Am J Vet Res 62(3):375, 2001.
26. Chetboul V, Lefebvre HP, Pinhas C, et al: Spontaneous feline hypertension: clinical and echocardiographic abnormalities, and survival rate, J Vet Intern Med 17:89, 2003.
27. Tenhundefeld J, Wefstaedt P, Nolte IJ: A randomized controlled clinical trial of the use of benazepril and heparin for the treatment of chronic kidney disease in dogs, J Am Vet Med Assoc 234 (8):1031-1037, 2009.

28. Buoncompagni S, Bowles MH: Treatment of systemic hypertension associated with kidney disease, Compend Contin Educ Vet 35(5):E1-E6, 2013.
29. Dong L, Scott L, Crambert S, et al: Binding of losartan to angiotensin AT I receptors increases dopamine D1 receptor activation, J Am Soc Nephrol 23(3):42-48, 2012.
30. Kaplan NM: Treatment of hypertension: drug therapy. In Kaplan's clinical hypertension, ed 9, Philadelphia, 2006, Lippincott Williams & Wilkins, p 217.
31. Reynolds V, Mathur S, Sheldon S, et al: Losartan fails to block angiotensin pressor response in cats. ACVIM Forum, J Vet Intern Med 16(3):341, 2002.
32. Epstein M: Aldosterone as a mediator of progressive renal disease: pathology and clinical implications, Am J Kidney Dis 36:677, 2001.
33. Hostetter TH, Ibrahim HN: Aldosterone in chronic kidney and cardiac disease, J Am Soc Nephrol 14:2395, 2003.
34. Mathur SM, Syme H, Brown CA, et al: Effects of the calcium channel antagonist amlodipine in cats with surgically induced hypertensive renal insufficiency, Am J Vet Res 63(6):833, 2002.
35. Geigy CA, Schweighauser A, Doherr M, et al: Occurrence of systemic hypertension in dogs with acute kidney injury and treatment with amlodipine besylate, J Small Anim Pract 52(7):340-346, 2011.
36. Kaplan NM: Hypertensive crises. In Kaplan's clinical hypertension, ed 9, Philadelphia, 2006, Lippincott Williams & Wilkins, p 311.
37. Fenves AZ, Ram CVS: Drug treatment of hypertensive urgencies and emergencies, Semin Nephrol 25:272, 2005.
38. Proulx J: Intensive management of heart failure. In Proceedings of the 75th Western Veterinary Conference, 2003, Las Vegas, Nevada.

CHAPTER 160
DIURETICS

Thierry Francey, DrMedVet, DACVIM

KEY POINTS

- A thorough clinical and laboratory evaluation is necessary to define clear therapeutic goals for diuretic therapy and to choose the most appropriate drug.
- The main goals for diuretic therapy are the enhanced excretion of retained water, solutes, and toxins; the promotion of urine flow; and a decrease in the urinary concentration of solutes and toxins.
- The most common indications for diuretic use in the critical care patient are oligoanuric acute renal failure, decompensated chronic kidney disease, congestive heart failure, ascites from liver failure, and other fluid and electrolyte disorders.
- The use of diuretics in acute renal failure might improve urine production and the ability to provide therapy, but it does not change the likelihood of renal recovery directly.
- The use of diuretics to treat edema is justified only in cases of fluid retention caused by increased hydrostatic pressure. When vascular permeability is increased, further depletion of the vascular volume with diuretics is rarely indicated and is often detrimental.

Disturbances in the regulation and balance of fluid and electrolytes are very common, and they contribute significantly to the morbidity and mortality of animals treated in the critical care setting. Fluid and solute excesses are often corrected by administering diuretics, a heterogeneous group of drugs acting on various segments of the nephron, where they block the reabsorption of water and solutes and promote their urinary excretion. The correct assessment of electrolyte and mineral disorders is hampered by their compartmentalization, and correction of their serum concentrations is sometimes better achieved by translocation into the proper compartment.

The appropriate use of diuretics in the critical care patient requires a careful clinical and laboratory assessment and a good understanding of the underlying disease and pathophysiology to define clear therapeutic goals for the various fluid compartments, electrolytes, and minerals, and to choose the most appropriate diuretic, its route of administration, and dosage. Because of the complex disease processes in most critically ill animals, the limitations of their clinical assessment, and the limited data from clinical studies in small animals, this therapy remains often empiric and based on pathophysiologic justifications and clinical experience rather than on objective experimental data. Exaggerated diuresis may activate further the renin-angiotensin-aldosterone axis by reducing the intravascular volume and ventricular filling and may subsequently decrease perfusion of peripheral tissues. Careful therapeutic monitoring should therefore aim to assess treatment success more objectively and to anticipate or recognize side effects.

PHYSIOLOGY OF DIURESIS AND ANTIDIURESIS

One of the main characteristics of kidney function is the kidney's ability to regulate the excretion of water and most individual solutes independently of each other.[1] In the normal animal the rate of urine excretion (diuresis) depends mostly on renal handling of water and thus on the concentration of antidiuretic hormone (ADH, or vasopressin). ADH production is increased in response to elevated plasma osmolality or hypovolemia/hypotension and, to a lesser extent, in response to nausea and increased angiotensin II concentration. ADH production is suppressed and diuresis is increased by atrial natriuretic hormone and ethanol.[1]

To perform its antidiuretic function, ADH requires a functional tubular system, a medullary concentration gradient of sodium and urea, and a functional ADH receptor system to use this gradient. Failure of these mechanisms results in an inappropriately increased diuresis. Two additional diuretic mechanisms are involved in pathologic conditions: (1) pressure natriuresis, a negative feedback involved

Table 160-1 **Site of Action and Effect of the Most Commonly Used Diuretics**

Class	Prototype Drug	Site of Action	Global Effect on Water	Electrolytes	Minerals	Acid-Base Balance
Osmotic diuretics	Mannitol	All segments (mostly LH)	↓ TBW ↓ ICF ↑ ECF	↓ Na, K, Cl	↓ Ca, P, Mg	—
Carbonic anhydrase inhibitors	Acetazolamide	PT (+ late DT)	↓ TBW	↓ Na, K, Cl	↓ P	Metabolic acidosis
Loop diuretics	Furosemide	TAL	↓ TBW	↓ Na, K, Cl	↓ Ca, P, Mg	Metabolic alkalosis
Thiazide diuretics	Hydrochlorothiazide	Early DT	↓ TBW	↓ Na, K, Cl	↓ P, Mg ↓ Ca	—
Aldosterone antagonists	Spironolactone	Late DT, CD	↓ TBW	↓ Na, Cl ↑ K	↓ Ca	Metabolic acidosis
Distal diuretics	Amiloride, triamterene	Late DT, CD	↓ TBW	↓ Na, Cl ↑ K	± ↑ Ca	—

↓/↑ Decreased/increased balance; *Ca,* calcium; *CD,* collecting duct; *Cl,* chloride; *DT,* distal tubule; *ECF,* extracellular fluid volume; *ICF,* intracellular fluid volume; *K,* potassium; *LH,* loop of Henle; *Mg,* magnesium; *Na,* sodium; *P,* phosphorus; *PT,* proximal tubule; *TAL,* thick ascending limb of the loop of Henle; *TBW,* total body water.

in hypervolemic hypertensive states leading to increased natriuresis and restoration of normovolemia and normotension; and (2) osmotic diuresis, a passive diuretic mechanism resulting from abnormal urinary concentrations of osmotically active solutes such as glucose or sodium.[1]

Therefore increased diuresis can be achieved therapeutically through exogenous loading with water or salt, administration of poorly reabsorbed solutes, and pharmacologic inhibition of the tubular reabsorption mechanisms for sodium or water. Depending on the mechanisms involved, the diuretic effect will be associated with extracellular fluid (ECF) volume expansion (hypervolemic diuresis) or depletion (hypovolemic diuresis).

PHARMACOLOGY

Diuresis can be induced osmotically or, more commonly, by pharmacologic blockade of sodium reabsorption at various sites along the nephron. The basic rule is that, although proximal diuretics can modulate a greater bulk of sodium, their efficacy may be overcome by distal compensatory increases in sodium reabsorption in the loop of Henle. The efficacy of distal diuretics on the other side is limited by the small amount of sodium actually reaching the distal tubule. Diuretics acting at the loop of Henle are thus most effective because of the large amount of filtrate delivered to this site and the lack of an efficient reabsorptive region beyond their locus of action.[2]

Diuretics are grouped according to their mechanism of action and include, in order of their renal tubular target, osmotic diuretics, carbonic anhydrase (CA) inhibitors, loop diuretics, thiazide diuretics, aldosterone antagonists, and other potassium-sparing distal diuretics (Table 160-1). Mannitol and furosemide are used most frequently in the critical care setting; consequently, the other diuretics are mentioned here only briefly. Usual dosage recommendations are summarized in Table 160-2. In using diuretics it is important to note that fluid therapy should be adjusted closely to the desired goals of the global therapy. For example, if the therapeutic goal is a depletion of the ECF with furosemide in an animal with congestive heart failure (CHF), it does not make sense to administer intravenous fluids concomitantly. Partial free water replacement with 5% dextrose in water may be an exception in this scenario.

All diuretics except spironolactone reach their tubular sites of action through the urinary space. Mannitol is freely filtered in the glomeruli, and the other highly protein-bound diuretics are secreted actively through the organic acid and organic base pathways into the proximal tubule.[2] This explains the decreased efficacy of most diuretics in animals with renal disease. However, the impaired tubular secretion and delivery to the site of action can be compensated partially by a progressive titration to higher plasma concentrations. In animals with proteinuria and nephrotic syndrome, the serum diuretic concentration remains low as a result of hypoproteinemia and results in decreased tubular secretion of the diuretic, which is then partially neutralized by binding to urinary proteins. Dose and frequency adjustments can partially compensate for this and provide sufficient concentrations of the active drugs at the site of action.[2,3] Serial measurements of urinary electrolytes can provide a more objective

Table 160-2 **Dosages of the Most Commonly Used Diuretics**

Drug	Indication/Action	Dosage
Mannitol	Renal failure	0.25-1 g/kg IV q4-6h CRI 1-2 mg/kg/min when diuresis instituted
	Glaucoma	1-3 g/kg IV once
	Cerebral edema	1-1.5 g/kg IV once
Acetazolamide	Glaucoma	50 mg IV once, then 2-10 mg/kg q8-12h PO 7 mg/kg PO q8h in the cat
Furosemide	Diuretic	0.5-4 (max 8) mg/kg IV, IM, SC, PO q8-12h CRI 2-15 mcg/kg/min
Hydrochlorothiazide	Diuretic	0.5-5 mg/kg PO q12-24h
Spironolactone	K-sparing diuretic	1-4 mg/kg PO q12-24h
Amiloride	K-sparing diuretic	0.1-0.3 mg/kg PO q24h
Triamterene	K-sparing diuretic	1-2 mg/kg PO q12h

CRI, Constant rate infusion; *IM,* intramuscularly; *IV,* intravenously; *K,* potassium; *PO,* per os; *SC,* subcutaneously.

assessment of diuretic efficacy to help guide therapeutic decision making, such as adjusting dosage and combining diuretics from different classes.

Tolerance and inefficacy of diuretic therapy can occur after a single dose as a result of depletion of the ECF. In the long term, hypertrophy of the distal nephron reflects increased compensatory solute reabsorption at the distal sites to compensate for proximal tubular blockade. This hypertrophy parallels a progressive loss of drug efficacy and the requirement for higher doses or a sequential blockade of multiple sodium reabsorption sites.[2-4]

Osmotic Diuretics

Mannitol is an osmotically active, nonreabsorbed sugar alcohol that is administered intravenously for its osmotic or diuretic properties, or both. The resulting hyperosmolality of the ECF creates a water shift from the intracellular fluid (ICF) compartment and an initial expansion of the ECF. The contraction of the ICF is used therapeutically in animals with cerebral edema associated with increased ICF and increased intracranial pressure (as in trauma, fluid shifts secondary to a rapid correction of hyperglycemia, hypernatremia, or azotemia).[5-7] Mannitol is freely filtered by the glomerulus (molecular weight, 182 Da) and does not undergo tubular reabsorption, which results in increased tubular flow rate and osmotic diuresis. The increased urine flow reduces the tubular reabsorption of urea, increasing its urinary clearance and thus decreasing its serum concentration.[1,4] This property can be used to intensify fluid diuresis and to accelerate recovery of clinical and metabolic stability in animals with decompensated chronic renal disease, even in nonoliguric states.

Additional potential benefits of mannitol for acute renal injury include decreased renal vascular resistance, decreased hypoxic cellular swelling, decreased renal vascular congestion, decreased tendency of erythrocytes to aggregate, protection of mitochondrial function, decreased free radical damage, and even renoprotection when administered before a toxic or ischemic insult.[1,4,8] There are, however, no data to support a clinical benefit in animals with established renal failure, and its use is based purely on extrapolations and pathophysiologic justifications. Very high doses of mannitol have been described as causing acute tubular injury in humans, and thus it should be used cautiously in oliguric animals to avoid accumulation, volume overload, hyperosmolality, and further renal damage.[1,9]

Carbonic Anhydrase Inhibitors

Acetazolamide inhibits mostly the type II (cytoplasmic) and type IV (membrane) CAs from the proximal tubular epithelium, which leads to a net decrease in the proximal reabsorption of sodium bicarbonate. The resulting metabolic acidosis and natriuresis are self-limiting because progressively less bicarbonate is filtered and the proximal tubular epithelium becomes less responsive to CA inhibition. Furthermore, the proximal site of action of CA inhibitors leads to a compensatory increase in the distal sodium absorption.

CAs are also located in other organs and their inhibition is variable: blockade of ocular and brain CA decreases the production of aqueous humor and cerebrospinal fluid, respectively; blockade of red blood cell CA hampers carbon dioxide removal from the tissues; the gastric CA is affected only minimally by inhibitors. CA inhibitors rarely are used as diuretics except in some combination protocols, and their main clinical application is for the treatment of elevated intraocular pressure in glaucoma.[1,2,4]

Loop Diuretics

The prototypical loop diuretic furosemide binds to and inhibits the Na-K-2Cl cotransporter on the apical membrane of epithelial cells of the thick ascending limb of the loop of Henle. The decreased sodium and chloride reabsorption results in marked natriuresis and diuresis, and rapidly dissipates the medullary osmotic gradient.[10] Increased distal delivery of sodium leads to a sodium-potassium exchange and promotes kaliuresis. The blockade of the secondary active Na-K-2Cl cotransporter decreases the energy expenditure and the oxygen consumption of the tubular epithelial cells and can be beneficial in ischemic conditions. Furosemide further improves the renal parenchymal oxygen supply by decreasing renal vascular resistance and increasing renal blood flow. Blockade of the chloride flux in the macula densa inhibits the important regulatory tubuloglomerular feedback, and the kidney may not be able to adjust its glomerular filtration in response to tubular loss of solutes.[1-4]

The potential concerns about and benefits of furosemide in renal disease are based mostly on pathophysiologic justifications and not on results of controlled clinical studies. The combination of mannitol with furosemide seems to be synergistic in inducing diuresis in dogs with acute renal failure. The use of furosemide for ECF contraction in small animals with CHF is better described. The decreasing responsiveness to loop diuretics in heart failure is mostly a result of the compensatory increase in reabsorption of sodium in the distal tubule, and it commonly requires that the loop diuretic be combined with a more distal diuretic for sequential nephron blockade. The relatively long dosing interval for furosemide compared with its elimination half-life (1 to 1.5 hours in dogs) can result in intermittent rebound sodium retention and diminish its efficacy. Frequent administration or constant rate infusion is required when maximal efficacy is desired.[3,11]

Thiazide Diuretics

Thiazide diuretics exert their action by inhibiting the NaCl cotransporter on the apical membrane of the distal tubule. They have only a few indications in small animal medicine, in which they are used mostly for their anticalciuretic properties in the long-term prevention of calcium-containing uroliths or with other diuretics in combination protocols.[2,12] Thiazides paradoxically reduce urine production in severely polyuric animals with diabetes insipidus by inducing a mild hypovolemia and increasing proximal tubular sodium conservation.[1,13]

Aldosterone Antagonists

Spironolactone and eplerenone competitively antagonize aldosterone by binding to its receptor on the late distal tubule and the collecting duct to increase sodium, calcium, and water excretion and decrease potassium loss. Spironolactone is most efficacious in hyperaldosteronism, and this defines its main clinical applications in liver and heart failure, usually in combination with a more efficient loop diuretic.[1,2,4] Spironolactone also seems to have a positive effect on myocardial remodeling and reduction of cardiac fibrosis.[14] It is commonly combined with other diuretics to reduce their potassium-wasting effects. Recent studies have reported that spironolactone is safe and well tolerated as an adjunctive therapy in dogs with CHF, but there have been contradictory findings with regard to the impact on outcome.[15-17]

Other Potassium-Sparing Distal Diuretics

Amiloride and triamterene inhibit the electrogenic sodium reabsorption in the late distal tubule and the collecting duct, suppressing the driving force for potassium secretion. Their distal site of action gives them only weak diuretic and natriuretic properties, and they are used mostly to enhance the efficacy and counterbalance the potassium-wasting effect of proximal diuretics.[2,4]

Aquaretics

The main mode of action of most diuretics in clinical use is increasing renal sodium excretion, and therefore they can be classified as natriuretics. Aquaretics are a newer class of diuretics that antagonize the vasopressin V_2 receptor in the kidney and promote solute-free water clearance. These vasopressin receptor antagonists, called *vaptans*, include compounds of varying V_1-V_2 receptor selectivity such as conivaptan, tolvaptan, mozavaptan, satavaptan, and lixivaptan. Their main uses are in the treatment of free water retention in hypervolemic hyponatremia (e.g., heart or liver failure) or normovolemic hyponatremia (e.g., syndrome of inappropriate ADH secretion).[18] However, use of these drugs in a clinical setting has not been reported in small animals so far.

INDICATIONS FOR DIURETIC THERAPY

Diuretics are used commonly in the critical care setting, mostly for treatment of urinary and cardiac diseases. A partial list of further indications is provided in Table 160-3.

Urinary Diseases

The use of diuretics to convert the oligoanuria of acute renal failure to a nonoliguric state is controversial. Although successful initiation of diuresis can facilitate or even simply allow the conventional treatment of previously anuric animals, it has no prognostic value and it does not imply further improvements in renal function. Urine production, although necessary, does not equate with renal recovery.

High dosages of furosemide are often combined with mannitol after initial rehydration of the oligoanuric animal. The addition of a so-called renal dosage of dopamine (0.5 to 3 mcg/kg/min) is no longer recommended because of a lack of demonstrable survival benefit and the potential for adverse effects such as vasoconstriction and hypertension.[19,20] When dialytic therapy is available, these diuretic maneuvers are neither indicated nor necessary because the electrolyte and fluid disturbances can be corrected directly by dialysis.

The oliguria of chronic renal disease is rarely an indication for diuresis in animals because most patients in this terminal stage can no longer be managed conventionally. Fluid overload is a feature of end-stage disease and would be treated with dialytic fluid removal and restriction of water intake. The efficacy of diuretics is markedly decreased at this stage because of their poor delivery to the tubular site of action (see previous discussion). However, mannitol is used in animals with decompensated chronic renal disease to intensify the diuretic support (fluid therapy) and temporarily improve the azotemia by decreasing the tubular reabsorption of urea and increasing its urinary clearance. This strategy can accelerate the clinical and metabolic recovery of these animals.

Treatment of the edematous state of nephrotic syndrome is oriented toward decreasing the proteinuria and improving the hypoalbuminemia to correct the disturbances of this overhydrated but hypovolemic condition. In some animals, however, proteinuria is associated to an inappropriate renal tubular sodium retention contributing to nephrotic edema by an overfill mechanism. The use of a natriuretic drug such as furosemide may therefore be indicated when the clinical response is delayed or insufficient to reduce edema and effusions and to improve the quality of life. These drugs need to be titrated to the minimal clinically effective dosage to overcome the decreased efficacy in this disease (see previous discussion) and to avoid further depletion of the vascular volume and renal decompensation.[2-4]

Diuretic therapy is sometimes indicated in lower urinary tract diseases of dogs and cats to decrease the concentration of inflammatory mediators (idiopathic feline lower urinary tract disease in cats) or calculogenic minerals (urolithiasis). This is typically a long-term therapy achieved mostly by hypervolemic diuresis using increased water or salt intake, along with dietary modifications. Thiazide diuretics selectively decrease calciuresis and can be indicated in animals with recurrent calcium oxalate urolithiasis.[12]

Congestive Heart Failure

CHF usually is treated with loop diuretics, if possible, in combination with dietary sodium restriction, despite the potential for activation of the renin-angiotensin-aldosterone system.[21] The progressive tolerance to loop diuretics can be balanced by combining them with distal diuretics, mostly thiazides, although spironolactone is used increasingly for its beneficial effect on myocardial remodeling.[2,14] Serum

Table 160-3 Indications and Goals for Diuretic Therapy

Indication	Main Goal(s)	Diuretic Strategy
Oligoanuria (acute renal failure)	Restore diuresis ↓ Tubular obstruction ↑ Kaliuresis	Furosemide, mannitol (after rehydration)
Uremic crisis (chronic kidney disease)	↓ Blood urea nitrogen	Mannitol (after rehydration) + fluid therapy
Nephrotic syndrome	↓ Interstitial fluid volume	Furosemide
Urinary diseases (urolithiasis, cystitis)	↑ Urine flow	Water, ± salt, thiazides
Congestive heart failure	↓ Preload and extracellular fluid volume ↓ Pulmonary edema or pleural effusion	Furosemide, ± combination with spironolactone
Hypertension	↓ Preload and intravascular volume	Thiazides, furosemide
Liver failure	↓ Interstitial fluid volume	Spironolactone, ± furosemide
Hypercalcemia	↑ Calciuresis	Furosemide + NaCl 0.9%
Hyperkalemia	↑ Kaliuresis	NaCl 0.9%, furosemide
Iatrogenic fluid overload	↓ Total body water	Furosemide
Intracranial pressure	↓ Intracellular fluid volume	Mannitol
Glaucoma	↓ Intraocular pressure	Acetazolamide (mannitol)
Diabetes insipidus	↓ Polyuria	Thiazides

↓/↑ Decrease/increase; *NaCl,* Sodium chloride.

potassium concentration should be monitored carefully when potassium-wasting diuretics are used in patients with cardiac disease because hypokalemia enhances the risk of digoxin toxicity.[2]

Liver Failure

Animals with end-stage liver failure commonly develop ascites and edema as a result of hypoalbuminemia, activation of the renin-angiotensin-aldosterone system, and portal hypertension.[2] Symptomatic relief of the resulting abdominal distention can be obtained by abdominocentesis, but rapid refill of the abdominal cavity can result in hypovolemia and shock. The aldosterone antagonist spironolactone is the first-choice diuretic for this disease process, and it is often combined with loop diuretics for a sustained and progressive reduction of ascites. Because this diuretic effect occurs at the expense of an already depleted intravascular volume, the diuretics should be titrated to the minimally effective dosage necessary to obtain acceptable symptomatic relief of discomfort, as in animals with protein-losing nephropathy and enteropathy.[2]

Electrolyte and Mineral Disorders

Fluid therapy and loop diuretics can help temporarily correct hyperkalemia in an animal with a functional urinary system until the underlying cause can be identified and corrected.[2] Similarly, severe hypercalcemia can be reduced and renal function preserved with high dosages of furosemide and matching rates of physiologic saline infusion until a diagnosis is obtained and a treatment of the cause is instituted. The efficacy of this treatment in severe hypercalcemia is often insufficient, and additional calcium-reducing therapies are required.[2,4]

Systemic Hypertension

Treatment of systemic hypertension in small animals is based mostly on the use of vasodilators, which can activate the renin-angiotensin-aldosterone system over the long term and lead to salt and water retention. Because spontaneous and iatrogenic expansion of the ECF are frequent in hypertensive animals with renal disease, refractory cases commonly require combinations of vasodilators, negative chronotropic drugs, and loop or thiazide diuretics.[2]

REFERENCES

1. Rose BD, Post TW: Clinical physiology of acid-base and electrolyte disorders, ed 5, New York, 2001, McGraw-Hill.
2. Boothe DM: Drugs affecting urine formation. In Boothe DM, editor: Small animal clinical pharmacology and therapeutics, ed 2, St Louis, 2012, Saunders.
3. Brater DC: Diuretic therapy, N Engl J Med 339:387, 1998.
4. Ellison DH, Hoorn EJ, Wilcox CS: Diuretics. In Taal MW, Chertow GM, Marsden PA, et al, editors: Brenner and Rector's the kidney, ed 9, Philadelphia, 2012, Saunders.
5. Qureshi AI, Wilson DA, Traystman RJ: Treatment of elevated intracranial pressure in experimental intracerebral hemorrhage: comparison between mannitol and hypertonic saline, Neurosurgery 44:1055, 1999.
6. Silver P, Nimkoff L, Siddiqi Z, et al: The effect of mannitol on intracranial pressure in relation to serum osmolality in a cat model of cerebral edema, Intensive Care Med 22:434, 1996.
7. Hartwell RC, Sutton LN: Mannitol, intracranial pressure, and vasogenic edema, Neurosurgery 36:1236, 1993.
8. Finn WF: Recovery from acute renal failure. In Molitoris BA, Finn WF, editors: Acute renal failure: a companion to Brenner and Rector's The kidney, Philadelphia, 2001, Saunders.
9. Visweswaran P, Massin EK, DuBose TD Jr: Mannitol-induced acute renal failure, J Am Soc Nephrol 8:1028, 1997.
10. McClellan JM, Goldstein RE, Erb HN, et al: Effects of administration of fluids and diuretics on glomerular filtration rate, renal blood flow, and urine output in healthy awake cats, Am J Vet Res 67:715, 2006.
11. Adin DB, Taylor AW, Hill RC, et al: Intermittent bolus injection versus continuous infusion of furosemide in normal adult greyhound dogs, J Vet Intern Med 17:632, 2003.
12. Lulich JP, Osborne CA, Lekcharoensuk C, et al: Effects of hydrochlorothiazide and diet in dogs with calcium oxalate urolithiasis, J Am Vet Med Assoc 218:1583, 2001.
13. Takemura N: Successful long-term treatment of congenital nephrogenic diabetes insipidus in a dog, J Small Anim Pract 39:592, 1998.
14. Suzuki G, Morita H, Mishima T, et al: Effects of long-term monotherapy with eplerenone, a novel aldosterone blocker, on progression of left ventricular dysfunction and remodeling in dogs with heart failure, Circulation 106:2967, 2002.
15. Lefebvre HP, Ollivier E, Atkins CE, et al: Safety of spironolactone in dogs with chronic heart failure because of degenerative valvular disease: a population-based, longitudinal study, J Vet Intern Med 27(5):1083-1091, 2013. Epub July 19, 2013.
16. Bernay F, Bland JM, Häggström J, et al: Efficacy of spironolactone on survival in dogs with naturally occurring mitral regurgitation caused by myxomatous mitral valve disease, J Vet Intern Med 24:331-341, 2010.
17. Schuller S, Van Israël N, et al: Lack of efficacy of low-dose spironolactone as adjunct treatment to conventional congestive heart failure treatment in dogs, J Vet Pharmacol Ther 34:322-331, 2011.
18. Mahajan S, Sivaramakrishnan R: New weapons for management of hyponatremia: vaptans, Med Update 22:611-614, 2012.
19. Cowgill LD, Francey T: Acute uremia. In Ettinger SJ, Feldmann EC, editors: Textbook of veterinary internal medicine, St Louis, 2005, Saunders.
20. Sigrist NE: Use of dopamine in acute renal failure, J Vet Emerg Crit Care 17:117-126, 2007.
21. Lovern CS, Swecker WS, Lee JC, et al: Additive effects of a sodium chloride restricted diet and furosemide administration in healthy dogs, Am J Vet Res 62:1793, 2001.

CHAPTER 161
GASTROINTESTINAL PROTECTANTS

Michael D. Willard, DVM, MS, DACVIM (Internal Medicine)

KEY POINTS

- Histamine-2 receptor antagonists (H_2RAs) are competitive inhibitors of gastric acid secretion; they lower gastric acid secretion but do not abolish it. They also diminish pepsin secretion.
- Ranitidine and nizatidine are H_2RAs that purportedly have gastric prokinetic activity.
- Cimetidine inhibits hepatic P-450 cytochrome enzyme activity. It can be used therapeutically (e.g., to minimize acetaminophen toxicity) or can cause drug interactions by delaying hepatic metabolism of drugs given concomitantly.
- Proton pump inhibitors are noncompetitive inhibitors of gastric acid secretion. They inhibit gastric acid secretion to a greater extent than H_2RAs. It can take 2 to 5 days for them to achieve maximal effectiveness when given orally, but these drugs still have reasonable effectiveness immediately after therapy is begun.
- Sucralfate is an unabsorbed drug that binds to ulcerated or eroded mucosa. It can adsorb other drugs, delaying or inhibiting their absorption.
- Misoprostol is a prostaglandin analog designed to prevent ulceration and erosion due to nonsteroidal antiinflammatory drug (NSAID) use. It is not as effective or reliable in preventing NSAID-induced ulceration in dogs as it is in humans.
- Orally administered antacids used to neutralize gastric acid have a short duration of action and should not be used to manage or prevent ulcers and erosions in veterinary medicine.

Gastrointestinal ulceration and erosion (GUE) is an important problem in dogs but is less common in cats. Stress (i.e., an event causing substantial hypoperfusion or anoxia of the gastric mucosa) and drug therapy (especially with nonsteroidal antiinflammatory drugs [NSAIDs] and dexamethasone) are especially common causes of GUE in dogs. Prednisolone at commonly administered dosages is rarely ulcerogenic unless there is concurrent gastric hypoxia or hypoperfusion, severe spinal disease, or concurrent use of NSAIDs. Stress ulceration may be due to hypotensive shock, systemic inflammatory response syndrome, severe life-threatening illness, or extreme exertion. Marked hyperacidity (e.g., gastrinoma, mast cell tumor) may cause GUE but more commonly causes duodenal lesions. Hepatic failure, tumors, and, to a lesser extent, foreign bodies may also cause GUE.

Gastrointestinal (GI) protectants are primarily indicated to heal existing gastric ulcers and erosions. Removing the cause of the ulceration or erosion markedly enhances efficacy, as does maintaining GI perfusion. Protectants are often poorly effective at preventing ulceration when the cause (e.g., NSAID use, poor gastric mucosal perfusion) persists. However, when there is a known cause of GUE that cannot be readily alleviated, these drugs are often given in the hope that they will at least retard, if not prevent, ulceration. See Table 161-1 for a list of commonly used GI protectants and dosages.

Proton pump inhibitors (PPIs) and histamine-2 receptor antagonists (H_2RAs) prevent GI ulceration caused by certain forms of stress (probably a combination of poor gastric mucosal blood flow, hypoxia, and possibly other factors) in dogs.[1] There are no drugs that have shown efficacy in preventing GUE caused by the use of steroids (especially dexamethasone).[2-4] Although PPIs are somewhat prophylactic against NSAID-induced GUE, they are not completely effective.[5-9] There is no evidence that combination therapy (e.g., an H_2RA plus sucralfate) is any more effective than administration of just one drug.

Drugs that decrease gastric acid secretion are not antiemetics (i.e., they have no effect on the medullary vomiting center or the chemoreceptor trigger zone); however, they can have an antidyspeptic effect that lessens nausea. They may be used to stimulate appetite or to enhance the efficacy of true antiemetics. When they are used to manage existing ulcers or erosions, evidence of improvement (e.g., less nausea, less bleeding) is expected within 2 to 5 days of beginning therapy, assuming that the initiating cause has been treated or eliminated. If there is no evidence of improvement within that time, endoscopic evaluation and/or surgical removal may be considered.

HISTAMINE-2 RECEPTOR ANTAGONISTS

The most commonly used H_2RAs in dogs and cats are cimetidine, ranitidine, and famotidine. The H_2RAs block the histamine receptor on the gastric parietal cell.[10-12] They are competitive inhibitors of gastric acid secretion, which means that they do not decrease gastric acid secretion as well as the noncompetitive PPIs. Their maximal effect in decreasing gastric acid secretion occurs almost immediately upon initiation of therapy. Nizatidine and ranitidine reportedly have some gastric prokinetic activity, probably via antiacetylcholinesterase activity. However, one study failed to find ranitidine effective in preventing gastroesophageal reflux in anesthetized dogs.[13]

Cimetidine and ranitidine are the least potent H_2RAs and famotidine the most potent, with nizatidine being intermediate. Famotidine has the longest duration of action. With oral administration, cimetidine absorption is delayed by food, but absorption of ranitidine, nizatidine, and famotidine is not. Famotidine, ranitidine, and cimetidine undergo substantial first-pass hepatic metabolism but nizatidine does not. Nizatidine is the most bioavailable and famotidine the least when administered orally. Cimetidine and ranitidine are metabolized extensively by the liver, but famotidine and nizatidine are excreted almost completely unchanged in the urine. It has been suggested that the dosage of cimetidine and famotidine be reduced in patients with renal failure; however, it is not known how important such a dosage reduction is.

Cimetidine markedly inhibits hepatic P-450 enzymes and has been used therapeutically to lessen the severity of acetaminophen intoxication. However, cimetidine also decreases metabolism of theophylline, lidocaine, metronidazole, and many other drugs, which results in higher blood levels that can cause toxicity in some cases. Ranitidine has less effect on these enzymes, and famotidine and nizatidine have almost no such effect. Cimetidine also decreases hepatic blood flow by about 20%.

Table 161-1 **Selected Gastrointestinal Protectants Used in Dogs and Cats**

Drug	Mechanism of Action	Dosage	Special Considerations
Cimetidine	H_2-receptor antagonist	5-10 mg/kg IV, IM, SC, PO q6-8h	Potent inhibitor of hepatic P-450 enzymes Can affect metabolism of toxins or other drugs Decreases hepatic blood flow Food delays absorption
Ranitidine	H_2-receptor antagonist	*Dogs:* 0.5-2 mg/kg IV or 1-4 mg/kg PO q8-12h *Cats:* 2.5 mg/kg IV or 3.5 mg/kg PO q8-12h daily	Has prokinetic activity Has minimal effect on hepatic enzyme function
Famotidine	H_2-receptor antagonist	0.5-1 mg/kg IV, IM, SC, PO q12-24h	Longest acting and most potent H_2-receptor antagonist
Nizatidine	H_2-receptor antagonist	*Dogs:* 2.5-5 mg/kg PO q24h	Exclusively eliminated by the kidneys
Omeprazole	Proton pump inhibitor	1.0-2.0 mg/kg PO q12-24h	Inhibits hepatic P-450 enzymes May cause elevations in liver enzymes Sometimes causes diarrhea
Esomeprazole	Proton pump inhibitor	0.5-1 mg/kg IV q24h*	
Lansoprazole	Proton pump inhibitor	1 mg/kg IV q24h*	Anecdotal
Pantoprazole	Proton pump inhibitor	1 mg/kg IV q24h*	Anecdotal
Misoprostol	Prostaglandin analog	2-5 mcg/kg PO q6-12h	Can cause abortion Often causes transient diarrhea
Sucralfate	Local-acting barrier	*Dogs:* 0.25-1 g PO q6-12h *Cats:* 0.25 g PO q6-12h	Adsorbs many other drugs, slowing their absorption

H_2, Histamine-2; *IM,* intramuscularly; *IV,* intravenously; *PO,* per os; *SC,* subcutaneously.
*Extrapolated dosage.

A new H_2RA, lafutidine, seems unique in that it has additional mechanisms of action (i.e., nitric oxide–mediated and histamine-independent mechanisms).[14] It has a mucosa-protective action that is mediated by capsaicin-sensitive sensory nerves. In one study it was more effective than lansoprazole in inhibiting gastric acid secretion.[15] It also appears to have mild intestinal protective activity.[16]

Adverse effects are uncommon with H_2RAs, with cimetidine tending to be associated with more than ranitidine or famotidine. However, a recent abstract reported a high incidence of apathy, nausea, and vomiting when ranitidine was administered intravenously to healthy dogs.[17] Central nervous system aberrations and cytopenias are reported in humans and are anecdotally reported in dogs. There are anecdotal reports of famotidine's causing hemolytic anemia in uremic cats, but this effect could not be reproduced experimentally. Famotidine administration can be associated with thrombocytopenia in people, which has prompted some to recommend that it not be used in coagulopathic patients.[18] Famotidine administration causes only transient increases in serum gastrin concentrations, which is important to recognize when testing for gastrinomas.[19]

PROTON PUMP INHIBITORS

Omeprazole is the PPI that has been most commonly used in veterinary medicine; there is more limited experience with lansoprazole, pantoprazole, esomeprazole, and dexlansoprazole. In people, lansoprazole has greater bioavailability than omeprazole (80% to 85% vs. 30% to 40%, respectively). Lansoprazole, esomeprazole, and pantoprazole can be given intravenously, an advantage in vomiting patients. Dexlansoprazole is administered orally and is formulated in a dual delayed-release system that produces the longest duration of effect of any PPI; it can be given with food.[20]

The PPI drugs irreversibly inhibit hydrogen-potassium adenosine triphosphatase on the luminal side of the parietal cell, thus stopping secretion of hydrogen ions into the gastric lumen.[10,11] Omeprazole (which is actually a prodrug) is susceptible to destruction by gastric acid, so it is administered as enteric-coated granules that are absorbed in the duodenum. Absorption is diminished by food; therefore this drug should be given on an empty stomach. Once absorbed, omeprazole undergoes first-pass hepatic metabolism, and the rest is selectively sequestered in the acidic environment of the parietal cells, where it is transformed to the active drug. Therefore it is best to administer omeprazole about 1 hour before feeding so as to maximize the acidity of the parietal cell and thereby increase the amount of omeprazole sequestered there.

Because of this complex pharmacologic pathway, it usually takes 2 to 5 days before maximal acid suppression from omeprazole occurs. However, the PPIs are more effective than the H_2RAs[21,22]; in fact, the immediate effects of omeprazole were superior to those of high-dose famotidine when sled dogs were treated.[23] Furthermore, suppression of gastric acid secretion continues for a few days after cessation of PPI therapy because of the irreversible inhibition of the proton pump enzyme.

Historically, H_2RAs were typically administered to patients with uncomplicated GUE first and a PPI used only if the initial therapy failed; however, PPIs are increasingly becoming first-line therapy due to their superior efficacy in lessening gastric acid secretion. Animals with severe esophagitis or duodenal ulceration due to paraneoplastic hyperacidity (e.g., mast cell tumors or gastrinomas) generally should be treated with PPIs as first-line therapy. PPIs are relatively effective in lessening gastric acid reflux during anesthesia, but reflux still occurs in some dogs.[24] In people, PPIs are superior to misoprostol for preventing duodenal but not gastric lesions due to NSAIDs.[25]

Adverse effects associated with PPIs are rare. Toxicologic studies have shown that pantoprazole is relatively safe in dogs.[26] Diarrhea is reported in humans and dogs taking various PPIs.[27] Omeprazole and esomeprazole inhibit hepatic P-450 enzymes. Omeprazole has thus decreased antiplatelet activity by clopidogrel and decreased clearance of diazepam in people (pantoprazole and lansoprazole appear to have fewer such interactions). Hypomagnesemia has been suggested as an adverse effect in people, and elevated liver enzyme levels have been noted. A wide range of hypersensitivity reactions to PPIs (e.g., anaphylaxis, urticaria, angioedema, cutaneous vasculitis, cytopenias, interstitial nephritis) have been reported in people, but they tend to be rare.[28] A markedly increased gastric pH can affect absorption of some drugs such as ketoconazole and digoxin. Currently there is interest in the antineoplastic[29] and antiprotozoal activities[30] of PPIs (pantoprazole and rabeprazole have strong activity against *Giardia* and *Trichomonas in vitro*), but few data are currently available on the clinical relevance of these findings.

SUCRALFATE

Sucralfate is the octasulfate of sucrose combined with aluminum hydroxide.[31] It is a locally acting drug that is administered orally as a tablet or a suspension. It becomes viscous and binds tightly to epithelial cells in the acidic environment of the stomach, especially to the base of erosions and ulcers, where it may remain for 6 hours. It serves as a physical barrier while adhered to the ulcer or erosion and thus protects the ulcer from pepsin and bile acids; it also stimulates local production of prostaglandins and binding to epidermal growth factor (which favors mucosal repair). Sucralfate has almost no adverse effects besides sometimes causing constipation, which can be useful in patients with diarrhea. Sucralfate can adsorb other drugs (e.g., enrofloxacin), which slows their systemic absorption. It should be given before antacid therapy to maximize efficacy and theoretically should not be given with enteral feedings because it may bind the fat-soluble vitamins. Sucralfate can only be given orally, which limits its usefulness in vomiting patients.

PROSTAGLANDIN ANALOGS

Misoprostol is a prostaglandin E_1 analog with both antacid and mucosal protective properties (it stimulates secretion of mucus and bicarbonate and increases gastric mucosal blood flow).[32] The antisecretory effect on gastric acid is probably more important. Misoprostol acts directly on parietal cells to inhibit both nocturnal acid secretion and secretions in response to food, pentagastrin, and histamine. The drug is absorbed rapidly (in the absence of food) and undergoes first-pass metabolism in the liver to the active form. Misoprostol has a short half-life and must be given two to three times daily.

This drug was developed to prevent ulceration caused by NSAIDs. Its greater cost, need for frequent administration, and higher rate of adverse effects usually mean that it is administered only when other therapies for GUE have failed or when patients have difficulty tolerating NSAIDs that they must receive to maintain a good quality of life. It is not as clearly effective in protecting dogs receiving NSAIDs as has been reported in people. Adverse effects include diarrhea and uterine contraction (which can result in abortion in pregnant females). Diarrhea often subsides after 2 to 5 days.

ANTACIDS

Numerous drugs are administered orally to neutralize gastric acid. These drugs are generally not appropriate for treating or preventing GUE because they usually have a relatively short half-life compared with H_2RAs and PPIs. Furthermore, each set of antacid drugs tends to have its own idiosyncrasies. For example, aluminum and magnesium compounds delay or prevent absorption of other drugs.

FUTURE DRUG THERAPY

Troxipide is a new gastric cytoprotective drug.[33] It does not appear to affect gastric acid secretion but was more effective than ranitidine in a preclinical study in people with spontaneous gastritis. Data for dogs are lacking. Another new gastroprotectant that has been studied in people is irsogladine.[34] It seems to protect the gastric mucosa through endogenous nitric oxide and increased cyclic adenosine monophosphate. Irsogladine appears to prevent reduced mucosal blood flow, suppress formation of reactive oxygen radicals, and enhance gap junctional intracellular communication. The drug is currently available only in Japan.

POTENTIAL COMPLICATIONS OF INCREASED GASTRIC pH

Gastric acid is a major defense mechanism that prevents many infectious agents from gaining access to the intestinal tract since few bacteria can withstand the low pH of the stomach. Hence, there is concern that a prolonged increase in gastric pH may result in complications. In critically ill humans,[35,36] it has been hypothesized that patients receiving long-term acid-suppression therapy are at increased risk of bacterial pneumonia following an aspiration event. However, studies have failed to find any consistent risk. Similarly, human patients in such settings have not been found to have an increased risk of gastric carcinoid formation or rebound hyperacidity. There is an increased risk of *Clostridium difficile* infection in some populations, but since dogs and cats are rarely adversely affected by this bacterium, the risk to them appears minimal.

REFERENCES

1. Davis MS, Willard MD, Nelson SL, et al: Efficacy of omeprazole for the prevention of exercise-induced gastritis in racing Alaskan sled dogs, J Vet Intern Med 17:163, 2003.
2. Neiger R, Gaschen F, Jaggy A: Gastric mucosal lesions in dogs with acute intervertebral disc disease: characterization and effects of omeprazole or misoprostol, J Vet Intern Med 14:33, 2000.
3. Rohrer CR, Hill RC, Fischer A, et al: Efficacy of misoprostol in prevention of gastric hemorrhage in dogs treated with methylprednisolone sodium succinate, Am J Vet Res 60:982, 1999.
4. Hanson SM, Bostwick DR, Twedt DC, et al: Clinical evaluation of cimetidine, sucralfate and misoprostol for prevention of gastrointestinal tract bleeding in dogs undergoing spinal surgery, Am J Vet Res 58:1320, 1997.
5. Jenkins CC, DeNovo RC, Patton CS, et al: Comparison of effects of cimetidine and omeprazole on mechanically created gastric ulceration and on aspirin-induced gastritis in dogs, Am J Vet Res 52:658, 1991.
6. Johnston SA, Leib MS, Marini M, et al: Endoscopic evaluation of the stomach and duodenum after administration of piroxicam to dogs, Proc Am Coll Vet Intern Med 15:664, 1997 (abstract).
7. Bowersox TS, Lipowitz AJ, Hardy RM, et al: The use of a synthetic prostaglandin E1 analog as a gastric protectant against aspirin-induced hemorrhage in the dog, J Am Anim Hosp Assoc 32:401, 1996.
8. Ward DM, Leib MS, Johnston SA, et al: The effect of dosing interval on the efficacy of misoprostol in the prevention of aspirin-induced gastric injury, J Vet Intern Med 17:282, 2003.
9. Murtaugh RJ, Matz ME, Labato MA, et al: Use of synthetic prostaglandin E1 (misoprostol) for prevention of aspirin-induced gastroduodenal ulceration in arthritic dogs, J Am Vet Med Assoc 202:251, 1993.
10. Boothe DM: Gastrointestinal pharmacology. In Boothe DM, editor: Small animal clinical pharmacology and therapeutics, ed 2, St Louis, 2012, Saunders, pp 672-739.
11. Wallace JL, Sharkey KA: Pharmacotherapy of gastric acidity, peptic ulcers, and gastroesophageal reflux disease. In Brunton LL, Chabner BA, Knollmann BC, editors: Goodman's and Gilman's The pharmacological basis of therapeutics, ed 12, New York, 2012, McGraw-Hill, pp 1308-1322.
12. McQuaid KR: Drugs used in the treatment of gastrointestinal diseases. In Katzung BG, editor: Basic and clinical pharmacology, ed 9, New York, 2004, Lange Medical Books/McGraw-Hill, pp 1034-1063.
13. Favarato ES, Souza MV, Costa PRS, et al: Evaluation of metoclopramide and ranitidine on the prevention of gastroesophageal reflux episodes in anesthetized dogs, Res Vet Sci 93:466, 2012.

14. Nakano M, Kitano S, Nanri M, et al: Lafutidine, a unique histamine H2-receptor antagonist, inhibits distention-induced gastric acid secretion through an H2 receptor-independent mechanism, Eur J Pharmacol 658:236, 2011.
15. Yamagishi H, Koike T, Ohara S, et al: Stronger inhibition of gastric acid secretion by lafutidine, a novel H2 receptor antagonist, than by the proton pump inhibitor lansoprazole, World J Gastroenterol 14:2406, 2008.
16. Amagase K, Ochi A, Sugihara T, et al: Protective effect of lafutidine, a histamine H2 receptor antagonist, against loxoprofen-induced small intestinal lesions in rats, J Gastroenterol Hepatol 25(Suppl 1):S111, 2010.
17. Cavalcanti GAO, Feliciano MAR, Silveira T, et al: Adverse effects of ranitidine applied in the therapeutic dosage in healthy dogs, Cienc Rural 40:326, 2012.
18. Compoginis JM, Gaspard D, Obaid A: Famotidine use and thrombocytopenia in the trauma patient, Am Surg 77:1580, 2011.
19. Mordecai A, Sellon RK, Mealey KL: Normal dogs treated with famotidine for 14 days have only transient increased in serum gastrin concentrations, J Vet Intern Med 25:1248, 2011.
20. Hershcovici T, Jha LK, Fass R: Dexlansoprazole MR—a review, Ann Med 43:366, 2011.
21. Bersenas A, Mathews K, Allen D, et al: Effects of ranitidine, famotidine, pantoprazole, and omeprazole on intragastric pH in dogs, Am J Vet Res 66:425, 2005.
22. Tolbert K, Bissett S, King A, et al: Efficacy of oral famotidine and 2 omeprazole formulations for the control of intragastric pH in dogs, J Vet Intern Med 25:47, 2011.
23. Williamson KK, Willard MD, Payton ME, et al: Efficacy of omeprazole versus high-dose famotidine for prevention of exercise-induced gastritis in racing Alaskan sled dogs, J Vet Intern Med 24:285, 2010.
24. Panti A, Bennett RC, Corletto F, et al: The effect of omeprazole on oesophageal pH in dogs during anaesthesia, J Small Anim Pract 50:540, 2009.
25. Lazzaroni M, Porro GB: Management of NSAID-induced gastrointestinal toxicity: focus on proton pump inhibitors, Drugs 69:51, 2009.
26. Mansell P, Robinson K, Minck D, et al: Toxicology and toxicokinetics of oral pantoprazole in neonatal and juvenile dogs, Birth Defects Res B Dev Reprod Toxicol 92:345, 2011.
27. Shimura S, Hamamoto N, Yoshino N, et al: Diarrhea caused by proton pump inhibitor administration: comparisons among lansoprazole, rabeprazole, and omeprazole, Curr Ther Res 73:112, 2012.
28. Chang Y: Hypersensitivity reactions to proton pump inhibitors, Curr Opin Allergy Clin Immunol 12:348, 2012.
29. De Milito A, Marino ML, Fais S: A rationale for the use of proton pump inhibitors as antineoplastic agents, Curr Pharm Des 18:1395, 2012.
30. Perez-Villanueva J, Romo-Mancillas A, Hernandez-Campos A, et al: Antiprotozoal activity of proton pump inhibitors, Bioorg Med Chem Lett 21:7351, 2011.
31. Dallwig B: Sucralfate, J Exotic Pet Med 19:101, 2010.
32. Laine L, Takeuchi K, Tarnawski A: Gastric mucosal defense and cytoprotection; bench to bedside, Gastroenterol 135:41, 2008.
33. Dewan B, Balasubramanian A: Troxipide in the management of gastritis: a randomized comparative trial in general practice, Gastroenterol Res Pract 2010:758397, 2010.
34. Akagi M, Amagase K, Murakami, et al: Irsogladine: overview of the mechanism of mucosal protective and healing-promoting actions in the gastrointestinal tract, Curr Pharm Des 19:106, 2013.
35. Abraham NS: Proton pump inhibitors: potential adverse effects, Curr Opin Gastroenterol 28:615, 2012.
36. Moayyedi P, Leontiadis GI: The risks of PPI therapy, Nat Rev Gastroenterol Hepatol 9:132, 2012.

CHAPTER 162
ANTIEMETICS AND PROKINETICS

Michael D. Willard, DVM, MS, DACVIM (Internal Medicine)

KEY POINTS

- The medullary vomiting center (MVC) probably is not a focal, discrete area in the brain; rather, it is spread throughout the medulla.
- Centrally acting antiemetics are more effective than peripherally acting antiemetics. Centrally acting antiemetics that work on the MVC typically are more effective than those that act only at the chemoreceptor trigger zone.
- Maropitant (a neurokinin-1 antagonist) is highly effective in dogs and cats with minimal adverse effects other than pain upon subcutaneous injection.
- The serotonin (5-HT_3) receptor antagonists ondansetron and dolasetron are usually effective in dogs and cats and have few adverse effects.
- Metoclopramide is a dopamine receptor antagonist that works at the chemoreceptor trigger zone and is also a gastric prokinetic. Metoclopramide can sometimes cause abnormal behavior and even vomiting (possibly due to excessive gastric prokinetic activity). It tends to be less effective in cats than in dogs.
- Promazine derivatives (e.g., chlorpromazine, prochlorperazine) are effective centrally acting antiemetics that can cause sedation and hypotension due to α-adrenergic blocking activity.

ANTIEMETICS

Antiemetics are indicated primarily when vomiting makes it difficult to maintain energy, fluid, or electrolyte homeostasis or when quality of life is adversely impacted by nausea (Table 162-1). Not every vomiting patient should receive an antiemetic; sometimes it is more appropriate to allow a patient to vomit once or twice a day to assess the effectiveness of treatment for the underlying disease. Typical indications for antiemetics include pancreatitis, gastritis, enteritis, peritonitis, hepatic disease, renal insufficiency, and motion sickness; they are also used in patients at risk of aspiration pneumonia. With

Table 162-1 **Centrally Acting Antiemetics Commonly Used in Dogs and Cats**

Drug	Dosage	Special Considerations
Maropitant	1 mg/kg SC q24h or 2 mg/kg PO q24h 8 mg/kg PO q24h for up to 2 days for motion sickness in dogs; 1 mg/kg SC, IV, PO q24h in cats	Approved antiemetic for dogs and cats
Ondansetron	0.1-1 mg/kg IV, PO q8-12h	—
Granisetron	0.1-0.5 mg/kg IV q8-24h	—
Dolasetron	0.6-1 mg/kg IV, SC, PO q12-24h	—
Metoclopramide	0.1-0.5 mg/kg IV, IM, PO q8-12h or CRI of 1-2 mg/kg/24 h for nausea	Gastric prokinetic Can cause extrapyramidal effects if overdosed Note: for treatment of gastroesophageal reflux/ileus, 0.3 mg/kg/hr IV after a 0.4 mg/kg loading dose IV
Chlorpromazine	0.5 mg/kg IV, IM, SC q6-8h in dogs 0.2-0.4 mg/kg IM, SC q6-8h in cats	Can cause hypotension and sedation
Prochlorperazine	0.1-0.5 mg/kg IV, IM, SC q8-12h	Can cause hypotension and sedation

CRI, Constant rate infusion; *IM,* intramuscularly; *IV,* intravenously; *PO,* per os; *SC,* subcutaneously.

the exception of the neurokinin-1 (NK-1) receptor antagonists, antiemetic drugs are usually ineffective in patients with gastrointestinal (GI) obstruction. Parenteral administration is typically preferred in actively vomiting patients because oral administration will be ineffective if the drug is vomited before absorption.

Neurokinin-1 Receptor Antagonists

Maropitant is an NK-1 receptor antagonist that blocks the action of substance P in the central nervous system as well as at peripheral NK-1 receptors in the GI tract.[1] It is approved for use in dogs and cats and is considered a safe and effective drug. Dogs are typically treated with 1 mg/kg subcutaneously (SC) or 2 mg/kg orally (PO) q24h for up to 5 consecutive days. Anecdotally, maropitant has been administered intravenously in patients with poor peripheral perfusion and as a way to avoid the pain associated with subcutaneous administration. This appears to be a safe, effective route, but pharmacokinetic studies are lacking. Maropitant often causes pain when injected and is reported to cause bone marrow hypoplasia when administered to puppies younger than 11 weeks old. The drug undergoes extensive first-pass metabolism in the liver; hence, it has a much higher bioavailability when given subcutaneously (90%) than when given orally (23% to 37%, which is not affected by feeding). It can have nonlinear kinetics as the dose is changed.[2] It is effective in preventing vomiting due to motion sickness,[3] vomiting caused by various spontaneous illnesses,[4] and nausea associated with chemotherapy (doxorubicin and cisplatinum)[5] in dogs, as well as motion sickness[6] and xylazine-induced emesis in cats when used at 1 mg/kg SC, PO, or intravenously [IV].

NK-1 antagonists are thought to have many other effects beyond antiemesis (e.g., antiinflammatory, neuroprotectant, hepatoprotectant), although their clinical usefulness for these purposes is as yet unproven.[7] Reduction of diarrhea in patients receiving chemotherapy has been reported, and there is some suggestion that NK-1 antagonists may have antitumor activity. They appear to reduce visceral pain in cats and dogs and reduce the minimum alveolar concentration of sevoflurane during anesthesia if given intravenously.[8,9]

5-HT$_3$ Receptor Antagonists[10]

Ondansetron, granisetron,[11] and dolasetron,[12] were developed to alleviate chemotherapy-associated nausea in people. These drugs are competitive blockers of the serotonin (5-HT$_3$) receptors, which are found both peripherally (where they are responsible for intestinal vagal afferent input) and centrally (in the chemoreceptor trigger zone [CRTZ] and medullary vomiting center [MVC]). Ondansetron has been used off label in veterinary medicine for over a decade and has been anecdotally reported to stop vomiting effectively in patients not responding to metoclopramide or promazine treatment (e.g., puppies with parvoviral enteritis).

Ondansetron is metabolized by the liver and is usually administered at a dosage of 0.1 to 1.0 mg/kg IV q8-12h. It has the unusual characteristic in people of inhibiting emesis at low and high dosages while enhancing emesis at intermediate dosages (the same has been shown for metoclopramide in humans). Dolasetron is metabolized into the active fraction (hydrodolasetron) by the ubiquitous carbonyl reductase. It is eliminated from the body by hepatic P-450 enzymes. It usually is administered to dogs and cats at a dosage of 0.6 to 1 mg/kg SC, IV, or PO q12-24h.

The antiemetic effects of these drugs linger after the drug disappears from the blood; therefore they need to be administered only q8-24h. They are ultimately eliminated in the urine and bile. There is a wide margin of safety in humans, and adverse effects seem to be rare in dogs and cats. Adverse effects in humans may include constipation, diarrhea, and somnolence. Prolongation of the QT interval is reported with dolasetron, but the importance of this in veterinary medicine is doubtful. These drugs have minimal interactions with other drugs. Ondansetron is reported to decrease the efficacy of tramadol.

It has been suggested that because there are many 5-HT$_3$ receptors in the GI tract, administering dolasetron orally might produce both a peripheral and a central antiemetic effect. Dolasetron is reported to have excellent bioavailability when given orally. Combining dolasetron with metoclopramide is often effective for chemotherapy-induced nausea that is resistant to other antiemetics.[11] Ondansetron is effective in preventing emesis caused by dexmedetomidine when the latter is used as a preanesthetic in cats, but it must be given at the same time as the dexmedetomidine.[13]

Metoclopramide

Metoclopramide is a popular antiemetic. Its antidopaminergic activity and ability to block 5-HT$_3$ receptors make it a potent blocker of the CRTZ. However, cats are thought to have a paucity of dopamine receptors, which may explain why the drug seems less effective in that species. Typically given at 0.1 to 0.5 mg/kg IV, SC, or PO, metoclopramide also has gastric prokinetic activity that facilitates gastric emptying and decreases gastroesophageal reflux, although markedly higher dosages may be required in order to achieve these actions. This combination of mechanisms should be very effective; however, clinical practice has shown that metoclopramide is often inadequate in patients with a strong stimulus to vomit (e.g., severe pancreatitis or renal failure). Its effectiveness can be enhanced if it is administered as a constant rate infusion. Intravenous dose recommendations vary and lower dosages are typically adequate for antiemetic actions (1 to 2 mg/kg q24h), but higher doses are necessary to promote gastrokinesis and prevent gastroesophageal reflux (loading dose of 0.4 mg/kg IV, followed by 0.3 mg/kg/hr IV). The drug is sensitive to light, so the intravenous solution should be covered to prevent loss of efficacy. In people undergoing chemotherapy, metoclopramide's effectiveness may be enhanced by concurrent administration of low-dose dexamethasone, but this practice has not been critically evaluated in dogs or cats.

Metoclopramide is excreted by the kidneys, and care must be taken when using it in patients with substantially decreased glomerular filtration. If high blood levels occur due to renal dysfunction or overdosage, extrapyramidal signs (e.g., behavioral changes, apparent hallucinations) may occur. Such patients may display clinical signs similar to those seen with amphetamine intoxication (e.g., hyperactivity, frenzied behavior).

Promazine Derivatives

Promazine derivatives are broad-spectrum, inexpensive, centrally acting antiemetics[14-16] that are effective against most causes of nausea except inner ear problems. They have antidopaminergic and antihistaminic effects that block the CRTZ and, at higher dosages, the MVC. These drugs also have anticholinergic, antispasmodic, and α-adrenergic blocking effects. The promazine derivatives used most commonly as antiemetics in small animal veterinary medicine are chlorpromazine, prochlorperazine,[17] and acepromazine. Chlorpromazine typically is used at 0.1 to 0.5 mg/kg IV, SC, or intramuscularly (IM) q6-8h, and prochlorperazine is used at 0.1 to 0.5 mg/kg IV, IM, or SC q8-12h in dogs. The antiemetic effect of these drugs is typically evident at dosages lower than those causing sedation; however, varying degrees of vasodilation may occur, producing hypotension. Therefore caution is necessary in dehydrated or hypotensive patients; concurrent intravenous fluid therapy may be necessary.

Promazine drugs have been reported to increase central venous pressure and change the heart rate (bradycardia or tachycardia), and they possess antiarrhythmic qualities in the dog. These drugs were once believed to lower the seizure threshold, but this is now doubted.[18] The promazines are metabolized by the liver and can cause central nervous system signs in patients with substantial hepatic insufficiency, especially those with congenital portosystemic shunts. It has been suggested that prochlorperazine and perhaps other promazine derivatives not be used concurrently with metoclopramide because these drugs may potentiate extrapyramidal effects. The clinical importance of this is uncertain.

Anticholinergic Agents

Aminopentamide (0.01 to 0.03 mg/kg IM, SC, or PO q8-12h) is an anticholinergic agent that has been used as an antiemetic in dogs. There are cholinergic receptors in the brain involved in the vomiting center and in the upper GI tract via the vagus nerve. The latter are muscarinic receptors. It is uncertain which receptors aminopentamide affects, but the drug appears to have relatively few of the typical adverse effects that other anticholinergic agents have on the GI tract (e.g., paralysis, distention). Clinically, aminopentamide appears to be less effective than metoclopramide and is certainly inferior to the 5-HT_3 and NK-1 antagonists. Other anticholinergic medications (e.g., atropine, propantheline, glycopyrrolate) tend to be less effective or have more adverse effects (e.g., greater inhibition of GI motility). Aminopentamide should be used with caution in animals with glaucoma, cardiomyopathy, tachyarrhythmias, hypertension, myasthenia gravis, or gastroesophageal reflux.

Other Drugs

Trimethobenzamide has antidopaminergic properties but appears to be a relatively weak antiemetic in dogs. Steroids, especially dexamethasone and methylprednisolone, have been used to prevent nausea in humans undergoing chemotherapy or general anesthesia.[19] There are limited data on the efficacy of steroids in cats,[11,20] but their common use and apparent effectiveness in vomiting cats diagnosed with inflammatory bowel disease at least raises the question of whether they have primary antiemetic actions. In humans, steroids are primarily used as an antiemetic in combination with other drugs such as metoclopramide.

Megestrol acetate[21] and gabapentin[22] have been used as adjuncts in people receiving highly emetogenic chemotherapy protocols in whom vomiting is not adequately controlled with other combination antiemetic therapy. Their use for this purpose has not been reported in veterinary medicine but might be considered in severe cases that are resistant to more traditional therapy. Propofol has a variety of nonanesthetic effects, including antiemesis. Its use for induction and/or maintenance of anesthesia has been associated with less vomiting in human patients.[23] Based on the apparent response of some patients with "limbic epilepsy" and sialomegaly to phenobarbital, there is some thought that phenobarbital might have antiemetic activity.[24] No studies clearly confirm or deny this possibility in dogs or cats. Finally, it may be worth noting that acupuncture has been reported to lessen postoperative nausea in people.[25]

Peripherally Acting Antiemetics

Drugs that soothe inflamed mucosal lesions (e.g., bismuth subsalicylate or barium sulfate) or relieve dyspepsia (e.g., antacid drugs) can be used to alleviate vomiting (see Chapter 161). However, they are typically much less effective than the other drugs that have been discussed.

PROKINETIC DRUGS

Prokinetic drugs promote the orad to aborad movement of intraluminal contents. In veterinary medicine, they are primarily used to promote gastric emptying and colonic emptying.

5-HT_4 Serotonergic Agonists

5-HT_4 serotonergic agonists[26] are the most effective class of prokinetic drugs in veterinary medicine. Cisapride is no longer available for use in people but is available to veterinarians from compounding pharmacies. It has been the primary drug of this class used in veterinary medicine for treating gastroesophageal reflux, poor gastric emptying, and chronic constipation. The drug is well absorbed after oral administration and is primarily eliminated by first-pass metabolism in the liver (hence, elimination may be delayed in animals with severe hepatic insufficiency). Cisapride has approximately 30% bioavailability after oral administration in cats.

Cisapride (0.5 to 1.0 mg/kg PO q8-24h in dogs; 2.5 to 5 mg/cat q8-12h PO in cats) enhances gastric emptying while simultaneously increasing gastroesophageal sphincter pressure.[27,28] It is more effective than metoclopramide in treating patients with gastroesophageal reflux and delayed gastric emptying. Although frequently used to try to enhance esophageal motility in patients with megaesophagus, it is ineffective on striated muscle. The fact that cisapride increases gastroesophageal sphincter tone may make regurgitation worse in such patients (unless gastroesophageal reflux is a major contributing factor to the patient's regurgitation). Cisapride has been effective in treating idiopathic constipation in cats with mild to moderate disease; however, severe disease responds poorly. Finally, cisapride increases small intestinal motility; however, this effect has not found a major application in small animal medicine, probably because many critically ill postoperative patients cannot tolerate oral medications. Cisapride has been responsible for several human deaths due to its effect on cardiac conduction; however, death has not been reported in dogs or cats. Other adverse effects seem rare.

Mosapride (0.25 to 1 mg/kg PO q12h) has recently become available in Japan.[29] It is somewhat similar to cisapride except that it has minimal effects on colonic motility. It can be administered intravenously, which would be advantageous in many critically ill patients. Tegaserod (0.05 to 0.1 mg/kg PO q12h) and prucalopride (0.01 to 0.2 mg/kg PO q12h) are similar drugs currently available in Europe. Tegaserod primarily enhances colonic motility, whereas prucalopride can increase both gastric and colonic motility. There is currently minimal clinical experience with these drugs in veterinary medicine.

Cholinomimetic Drugs

Bethanechol, ranitidine, and nizatidine are the primary examples of the cholinomimetic class of prokinetic drugs. Ranitidine and nizatidine inhibit acetylcholinesterase, whereas bethanechol is a true cholinomimetic drug that binds to muscarinic receptors. Bethanechol (5 to 15 mg/dog PO q8-12h) affects motility throughout the GI tract, whereas ranitidine (1 to 2 mg/kg PO or IV q12h) and nizatidine (2.5 to 5 mg/kg PO or IV q12h) seem more effective for promoting gastric emptying than colonic motility.

Motilin Receptor Agonists

Erythromycin (0.5 to 1 mg/kg PO or IV q8h) stimulates motilin receptors and has been used to promote GI motility in a variety of clinical situations in dogs. It increases lower esophageal sphincter pressure as well as small and large bowel peristalsis.[30] There is some concern that tolerance will develop with sustained use of the drug, rendering it less effective.

Metoclopramide

Metoclopramide is probably the most commonly used prokinetic in veterinary medicine. It was discussed in detail earlier in the section on antiemetics. Metoclopramide's method of action is somewhat debated and appears to involve more than just dopamine receptors; it may increase the sensitivity of the smooth muscle in the small intestine to the effects of acetylcholine. Its primary use in veterinary medicine is as a moderately effective gastric prokinetic. Cisapride is a more effective prokinetic, but metoclopramide can be administered by constant IV infusion, which is advantageous in some patients. Rather high doses are required to cause prokinesis and reduce gastroesophageal reflux: 0.4 mg/kg IV as a loading dose and then 0.3 mg/kg/hr is recommended for this purpose (note this is higher than typically recommended to prevent nausea: 1 to 2 mg/kg/24 h). Intermittent dosing is also possible (0.2 to 0.5 mg/kg PO, SC, or IM q6-8h).

Misoprostol

Misoprostol, a prostaglandin E analog, is discussed in Chapter 161. It appears to enhance colonic motility and has been used in patients with nonresponsive constipation.

REFERENCES

1. Sedlacek HS, Ramsey DS, Boucher JF, et al: Comparative efficacy of maropitant and selected drugs in preventing emesis induced by centrally or peripherally acting emetogens in dogs, J Vet Pharmacol Ther 31:533, 2008.
2. Benchaoui HA, Cox SR, Schneider RP, et al: The pharmacokinetics of maropitant, a novel neurokinin type-1 receptor antagonist, in dogs, J Vet Pharmacol Ther 30:336, 2007.
3. Conder GA, Sedlacek HS, Boucher JF, et al: Efficacy and safety of maropitant, a selective neurokinin1 receptor antagonist, in two randomized clinical trials for prevention of vomiting due to motion sickness in dogs, J Vet Pharmacol Ther 31:528, 2008.
4. Ramsey DS, Kincaid K, Watkins JA, et al: Safety and efficacy of injectable or oral maropitant, a selective neurokinin1 receptor antagonist, in a randomized clinical trial for treatment of vomiting in dogs, J Vet Pharmacol Ther 31:538, 2008.
5. Rau SE, Barber LG, Burgess KE: Efficacy of maropitant in the prevention of delayed vomiting associated with administration of doxorubicin in dogs, J Vet Intern Med 24:1452, 2010.
6. Hickman MA, Cox SR, Mahabir S, et al: Safety, pharmacokinetics and use of the novel NK-1 receptor antagonist maropitant (Cerenia™) for the prevention of emesis and motion sickness in cats, J Vet Pharmacol Ther 31:220, 2008.
7. Munoz M, Covenas R: NK-1 receptor antagonists: a new paradigm in pharmacological therapy, Curr Med Chem 18:1820, 2011.
8. Boscan P, Monnet E, Mama K, et al: Effect of maropitant, a neurokinin 1 receptor antagonist, on anesthetic requirements during noxious visceral stimulation of the ovary in dogs, Am J Vet Res 72:1576, 2011.
9. Alvillar BM, Boscan P, Mama KR, et al: Effect of epidural and intravenous use of the neurokinin-1 (NK-1) receptor antagonist maropitant on the sevoflurane minimum alveolar concentration, Vet Anaesth Analg 39:201, 2012.
10. Machu TK: Therapeutics of 5-HT3 receptor antagonists: current uses and future directions, Pharmacol Ther 130:338, 2011.
11. Rudd JA, Tse JYH, Wai MK: Cisplatin-induced emesis in the cat: effect of granisetron and dexamethasone, Eur J Pharmacol 391:145, 2000.
12. Ogilvie GK: Dolasetron: a new option for nausea and vomiting, J Am Anim Hosp Assoc 36:481, 2000.
13. Santos PCP, Ludders JW, Erb HN, et al: A randomized, blinded, controlled trial of the antiemetic effect of ondansetron on dexmedetomidine-induced emesis in cats, Vet Anaesth Analg 38:320, 2011.
14. Boothe DM: Gastrointestinal pharmacology. In Boothe DM, editor: Small animal clinical pharmacology and therapeutics, ed 2, St Louis, 2012, Saunders, pp 672-739.
15. Sharky KA, Wallace JL: Treatment of disorders of bowel motility and water flux; antiemetics; agents used in pancreatic and biliary tract disease. In Brunton LL, Chabner BA, Knollmann BC, editors: Goodman's and Gilman's The pharmacological basis of therapeutics, ed 12, New York, 2012, McGraw-Hill, pp 1323-1349.
16. McQuaid KR: Drugs used in the treatment of gastrointestinal diseases. In Katzung BG, editor: Basic and clinical pharmacology, ed 9, New York, 2004, Lange Medical Books/McGraw-Hill, pp 1034-1063.
17. Bezek DM: Use of prochlorperazine in treatment of emesis in dogs, Can Pract 23:8, 1998.
18. Tobiad K, Marion-Henry K, Wagner R: A retrospective study on the use of acepromazine maleate in dogs with seizures, J Am Anim Hosp Assoc 42:283, 2006.
19. Grunberg SM: Antiemetic activity of corticosteroids in patients receiving cancer chemotherapy: dosing, efficacy, and tolerability analysis, Ann Oncol 18:233, 2007.
20. Ho CM, Ho ST, Wang JJ, et al: Dexamethasone has a central antiemetic mechanism in decerebrated cats, Anesth Analg 99:734, 2004.
21. Zang J, Hou M, Gou HF, et al: Antiemetic activity of megestrol acetate in patients receiving chemotherapy, Support Care Cancer 19:667, 2011.
22. Cruz FM, Cubero DIG, Taranto P, et al: Gabapentin for the prevention of chemotherapy-induced nausea and vomiting: a pilot study, Support Care Cancer 20:601, 2012.
23. Vasileiou I, Xanthos T, Koudouna E, et al: Propofol: a review of its non-anaesthetic effects, Eur J Pharmacol 605:1, 2009.
24. Boydell P, Pike R, Crossley D, et al: Sialadenosis in dogs, J Am Vet Med Assoc 216:872, 2000.

25. Pettersson PH, Wengstrom Y: Acupuncture prior to surgery to minimize postoperative nausea and vomiting: a systematic review, J Clin Nurs 21:1799, 2012.
26. DeMaeyer JH, Lefebvre RA, Schuurkes JAJ: 5-HT4 receptor agonists: similar but not the same, Neurogastroenterol Motil 20:99, 2008.
27. Washabau RJ, Holt DE: Pathophysiology of gastrointestinal disease. In Slatter D, editor: Textbook of veterinary surgery, ed 3, Philadelphia, 2003, Saunders, pp 530-552.
28. Azcuto AC, Marks SL, Osborn J, et al: The influence of esomeprazole and cisapride on gastroesophageal reflux during anesthesia in dogs, J Vet Intern Med 26:518, 2012.
29. Tsukamoto A, Ohno K, Madea S, et al: Prokinetic effect of the 5-HT4R agonist Mosapride on canine gastric motility, J Vet Med Sci 73:1635, 2011.
30. Melgarejo LT, Simon DA, Washabau RJ: Erythromycin stimulates canine but not feline longitudinal colonic muscle contraction, J Vet Intern Med 15:333, 2001.

CHAPTER 163

NARCOTIC AGONISTS AND ANTAGONISTS

Ralph C. Harvey, DVM, MS, DACVAA

KEY POINTS

- Opioids are an important class of drugs for critically ill veterinary patients because of their effectiveness and relative cardiovascular safety.
- Opioids are most commonly used for analgesia but may also be prescribed for antitussive or sedative therapy.
- The most commonly used opioids include morphine, methadone, fentanyl, hydromorphone or oxymorphone, buprenorphine, and butorphanol.
- It is important that the veterinarian understand the clinical effectiveness, potencies, and potential adverse effects of the various opioids before using them.
- Opioid antagonists include naloxone, nalmefene, and naltrexone. Butorphanol and nalbuphine commonly are used for partial reversal of pure μ-agonist drugs.

Opioids play a variety of roles in veterinary critical care. The foremost of these is as the foundation of analgesic therapy, but they are also used for their sedative and antitussive effects. Less frequent applications include supporting right-sided heart function and controlling compulsive behaviors. In the past, opioids were also used to decrease gastrointestinal (GI) motility.

As analgesics, the opioids are the first line of defense in managing pain due to injury and disease. The remarkable cardiovascular system–sparing effects and inherent safety of opioid therapy in critically ill patients are prominent advantages of this class of drugs. Opioids anchor contemporary balanced or multimodal strategies for pain management (see Chapter 144). Although this chapter deals specifically with the opioids, other publications extend the topic of analgesia in critical care to encompass complementary classes of analgesic drugs and other approaches to pain management.[1,2]

TERMINOLOGY AND HISTORY

Opium

At least 20 distinct alkaloids are derived from the juice of the poppy. Among these, the phenanthrenes are represented by morphine and the benzylisoquinoline derivatives by papaverine.

Opiate

The term *opiate* specifically refers to drugs derived from opium. The first of these was morphine, isolated and recognized in 1803 as the active ingredient in laudanum by Friedrich Wilhelm Adam Ferdinand Serturner, an assistant apothecary. This contribution has been recognized as the beginning of the modern era of pharmacology.

Opioid

The term *opioid* is a more precise, yet broadly inclusive, term for synthetic as well as opium-derived compounds that bind specifically to several opioid receptors and thereby have some morphine-like effects.

Narcotic

The word *narcotic* was derived from a Greek word for sleep or stupor. Because this group of compounds does not readily and reliably produce sleep in all veterinary patients, the term is a less than appropriate descriptor in veterinary medicine. Law enforcement organizations may refer to many substances with a potential for diversion and abuse as *narcotics*. This term includes both opioid and nonopioid controlled substances and often leads to confusion. Controlled substances, including the opioids, must be kept secure under lock and key. Accurate and appropriate inventory control is required, with the level of control for each drug related to the relative potential for abuse.

STRUCTURE-ACTIVITY RELATIONSHIP

The phenanthrene opioid compounds have a three-ring nucleus and a piperidine ring structure with a tertiary amine nitrogen. The levorotatory forms are much more active agonists than the dextrorotary forms.

MECHANISM OF ACTION

Opioids bind to stereospecific opioid receptors located most notably in the central nervous system (CNS) but also in many other sites throughout the body. The receptor affinity correlates well with analgesic potency for the opioids classified as pure agonists only. Receptor binding of endogenous or exogenous ligands activates G proteins as second messengers, modulates adenylate cyclase activity, and thereby alters transmembrane transport of effectors. Opioids also interfere presynaptically with the release of neurotransmitters. These changes result in interruption of the pain message to the brain and a decreased sensation of pain within the brain. Opioids do not alter the responsiveness of afferent nerve endings to noxious stimuli, nor do they impair conduction of nerve impulses along peripheral nerves.

OPIOID RECEPTORS

There are a variety of opioid receptors and subtypes of receptors within many tissues throughout the body. Differential binding and activation at specific receptors (μ-receptor, κ-receptor, δ-receptor, and the more recently recognized opiate-like receptor 1, also known as *OLR-1* or nociceptin receptor), principally in the CNS and the gut, serve to mediate the spectrum of opioid effects. Alternative terminology for the opioid receptors (OP-1 to OP-4) recognizes the order of discovery of the opioid receptor proteins. Another nomenclature, MOP, DOP, KOP, and NOP, has also been suggested, but the traditional μ-, κ-, and δ-receptor designation remains predominant.

PHYSIOLOGIC EFFECTS OF OPIOIDS

The occupation of CNS receptor sites by opioids produces analgesia, sedation, muscle relaxation, and behavior modification. The CNS-depressant action of the opioids results from their effects on the cerebral cortex. In contrast to the more typical sedation and narcosis produced in human patients, disorientation and excitement may also occur in veterinary patients receiving opioid therapy. The excitatory behavioral activity results from the effects of the drug on the hypothalamus. The ability of the opioids to cause depression or excitement is highly drug and species dependent. Excitatory responses may be linked to an indirect activation of dopaminergic receptors. The major tranquilizers, the benzodiazepines and phenothiazines, can block this activation.

Combinations of some opioids and tricyclic antidepressants can produce hypotension. Meperidine, and occasionally other opioids, when administered to patients receiving monoamine oxidase inhibitors (e.g., selegiline hydrochloride, L-deprenyl [Anipryl]) can result in rare but severe and immediate reactions that include excitation, rigidity, hypertension, and severe respiratory depression.

Opioids can be potent respiratory depressants, reducing both respiratory rate and tidal volume. Although this is rarely a clinically significant problem in healthy patients, special attention is warranted in critically ill patients. Animals with increased susceptibility to respiratory effects include those with underlying airway obstruction (e.g., brachycephalic animals) and those with pulmonary disease. The opioids directly depress the pontine and medullary respiratory centers. They also produce a delayed response (altered threshold) and decreased response (altered sensitivity) to arterial carbon dioxide, which leads to retention of carbon dioxide. Tachypnea is sometimes observed after opioid administration and may be due to excitation and/or alteration of the thermoregulation center. Panting in dogs is most notable with oxymorphone and hydromorphone administration.

Bronchoconstriction may also occur. A rare and incompletely understood complication of opioid therapy is a phenomenon known as *wooden chest.* In this syndrome, the patient's chest wall muscles become spastic, which makes ventilation difficult. Treatment involves reversal of the effects of the opioid drug and, if necessary, muscle relaxant therapy.

At therapeutic dosages, the opioids have minimal effects on the cardiovascular system. There is little or no change in blood pressure and myocardial contractility. The opioids can produce a vagally mediated bradycardia that is responsive to atropine or other anticholinergic agents. The decrease in heart rate may also be a manifestation of effective pain relief. The opioids affect the ability of the vascular system to compensate for positional and blood volume changes, although orthostatic hypotension is presumably more problematic in bipedal than quadrupedal patients. Among the opioids, morphine, methadone, and meperidine can cause histamine release, leading to marked hypotension. To minimize histamine-related complications following intravenous administration of morphine, the drug should be diluted with saline and the injection given slowly over 10 to 20 minutes.[1,3] Morphine, methadone, and meperidine are contraindicated in patients with mast cell tumors or other histamine-based diseases. Other opioids are much less likely to cause significant histamine release.

A variety of other physiologic effects may be of interest in the critical care setting. The opioids produce an initial stimulation of the GI tract (vomiting, defecation, or both) followed by a decrease in motility. Most opioids cause release of antidiuretic hormone. Urine retention due to bladder atony is an infrequent, but clinically significant, problem in some animals receiving opioid therapy. Bladder emptying should be verified in all patients.

Some animals receiving opioids may unexpectedly overrespond to noises or sensory stimuli. When this occurs, it can contribute to dysphoria and increase stress in the critically ill patient. The importance of a quiet and calming environment is recognized, but this is challenging to achieve in many critical care settings. Placing cotton balls or foam earplugs in the ears may help to alleviate the noise sensitivity.

Decreased body temperature may be observed in patients receiving opioids because the thermoregulatory center in the hypothalamus is reset to a lower setting. Panting in dogs is one manifestation of altered body temperature regulation. Alternatively, significant increases in body temperature occasionally occur after opioid administration. This appears to be most common in cats and somewhat drug and dosage dependent. Cats receiving higher than usual clinical dosages of morphine, meperidine, and hydromorphone frequently developed increased body temperature (40° to 41.7° C [104° to 107° F]) in one study. Buprenorphine did not result in hyperthermia in feline clinical or research models.[4]

METABOLISM AND EXCRETION

Metabolic elimination of most opioids is accomplished by hepatic conjugation and metabolite excretion in the urine (the exception is remifentanil, which is rapidly metabolized by nonspecific plasma esterases). The principal metabolites can be highly active, as in the case of morphine in humans. The meperidine metabolite normeperidine is a convulsant. Extended therapy with meperidine can lead to neurotoxicity and seizures. Opioid overdoses can effectively change the kinetics of elimination from first order to zero order by saturating the processes responsible for elimination and thereby greatly prolonging the duration of action. This is perhaps most notable with large overdoses of butorphanol, which lead to a prolonged period of sedation but, as a result of the presumed ceiling effect seen with this agonist-antagonist opioid, cause little increase in the magnitude of sedation or analgesia. Independent of any conditions altering elimination, the duration of action of the clinically useful opioids ranges widely, from less than 30 minutes (e.g., remifentanil and fentanyl) to as long as 8 hours (e.g., buprenorphine).

Table 163-1 **Relative Potencies of Opioids**

Opioid	Relative Potency
Morphine	1
Methadone	1
Meperidine (Demerol)	⅕
Codeine	⅒
Butorphanol (Torbugesic)	3-5
Nalbuphine (Nubain)	0.5-0.9
Hydromorphone (Dilaudid)	10
Oxymorphone (Numorphan)	10
Buprenorphine (Buprenex)	50-100
Fentanyl (Sublimaze)	100-150
Remifentanil (Ultiva)	200-300
Pentazocine (Talwin)	⅓
Etorphine (M-99)	1000-80,000

POTENCY AND EFFECTIVENESS OF OPIOIDS

The relative potencies of opioids are compared with the potency of morphine on an "equal-analgesic" basis (Table 163-1). For the pure-agonist opioids, maximum biologic effect (e.g., analgesia or respiratory depression) is relatively dosage dependent. The relative potency and the relative lack of analgesic efficacy of butorphanol, typically classified as a mixed agonist-antagonist opioid, provide an excellent example of the difference between effectiveness and potency. Clinical effectiveness helps identify medications useful for a specific purpose, and potency helps define dosage within the limits of effectiveness. Recommended dosages of several opioids for analgesia in critical care patients are listed in Table 163-2. Dosage ranges are broad for the opioid analgesics, and titration to achieve the desired effect is needed to care for this group of critically ill patients.

EPIDURAL OPIOIDS

Spinal or epidural (neuroaxial) opioid analgesia has been well described and proven effective in veterinary medicine. Epidural morphine analgesia is widely used and is increasingly popular as a method for providing long-lasting profound analgesia. The resultant reduced dosage requirement for systemic opioids decreases dose-dependent undesirable systemic effects, which makes neuroaxial analgesia techniques especially useful in critically ill animals. These techniques are rather simple, are easily implemented using basic clinical skills, and can be cost effective for providing substantial analgesia.

A relatively small dose of morphine (0.1 mg/kg) is typically administered by epidural injection after induction of general anesthesia or heavy sedation. Effective pain relief begins within approximately 30 minutes and persists for 12 to 24 hours. Addition of a local anesthetic, typically bupivacaine (0.5 mg/kg), to the epidural injection further provides a blunting of deleterious postoperative or injury-associated increases in stress hormone levels and the metabolic response to surgery. An epidural catheter can also be placed to facilitate repeated dosing or provide a constant rate infusion (CRI) into the epidural space (see Chapter 144). Contraindications to epidural injection or catheter placement include local infection, coagulopathy, neurologic dysfunction, marked obesity (which increases difficulty), and hypovolemia with hypotension (one should avoid the local anesthetics or compensate with intravenous fluids for volume expansion).

CHARACTERISTICS OF CLINICALLY USEFUL OPIOIDS

Morphine

Morphine, a pure-agonist opioid, is not only the standard of comparison for other opioids but remains one of the most useful analgesic medications. Morphine confers sedation in addition to analgesia, and both effects are dosage dependent, reliable, and effective in many clinical settings. Vomiting, diarrhea, and bradycardia may occur, but these are seen less commonly when morphine is given to treat existing pain than when it is given in the absence of pain. Vomiting may also be less common when diluted morphine is injected slowly intravenously rather than intramuscularly or subcutaneously. There is rapid absorption and almost complete bioavailability of morphine administered by either subcutaneous (if well-hydrated) or intramuscular injection.[5] Dosage recommendations do not differ with the route of injection.

When possible, opioids should be administered by the intravenous rather than the intramuscular or subcutaneous route to reduce trauma and stress in critically ill patients. Hypotension and bronchoconstriction occur in some patients as a result of histamine release, especially in dogs and following intravenous administration. Morphine is contraindicated in patients with mast cell tumors or other histamine-release abnormalities (see earlier section on the physiologic effects of opioids).

A CRI of morphine (with or without other analgesics) is very useful in the treatment of critical care patients experiencing pain. The relatively long plasma half-life of morphine can lead to an increasing plasma concentration when the drug is given as a CRI. This potential problem is minimized by adjusting the infusion as needed to balance analgesia and sedation. The CRI becomes an adjustable rate infusion, with drug dosage titrated to achieve the desired effect. The use of a neuroleptanalgesic (an opioid combined with an anxiolytic drug) or the mixture of morphine, lidocaine, and ketamine delivered as a CRI is effective in many patients.[1,6] One of many recipes for the latter cocktail is given in the next paragraph. See Chapters 142 and 144 for more useful information on sedation and analgesia and CRIs suitable for delivery using controlled syringe or bag-based delivery pumps.

Morphine-lidocaine-ketamine CRI:

1. Remove 73 ml from a 1-L bag of saline or balanced electrolyte fluids.
2. Add 68 ml of 2% lidocaine, 4 ml of morphine (15 mg/ml), and 0.6 ml ketamine (100 mg/ml).
3. Begin CRI at 1 to 2 ml/kg/hr.
4. Adjust as needed for comfort and sedation.

Oral administration of morphine may be effective in some dogs, but the drug is poorly and erratically absorbed from the GI tract.[7] Individual variability in bioavailability following oral dosing suggests that use of the oral route is not to be recommended or at least requires assessment of pharmacodynamics and biologic effectiveness in the individual animal.

Methadone

Methadone acts similarly to morphine in small animals in terms of the degree of analgesia provided and the duration of effect. It is a μ-receptor agonist that also noncompetitively inhibits *N*-methyl-d-aspartate receptors. It is more lipid soluble than morphine but causes less sedation and vomiting.

Hydromorphone and Oxymorphone

Hydromorphone is also a pure-agonist opioid. Vomiting and diarrhea are associated with it less frequently than with morphine, but panting is frequently seen in dogs. Hydromorphone does not

Table 163-2 Opioid Analgesics and Recommended Dosages

Drug	Dosage*	Duration of Effect	Effects/Uses	Adverse Effects	Comments
Morphine	*Dogs:* 0.5-1 mg/kg IV, IM, SC; 0.05-0.5 mg/kg/hr IV CRI, reduce 50% after 24 hr *Cats:* 0.05-0.2 mg/kg IV, IM, SC; 0.025-0.1 mg/kg/hr IV CRI; reduce if agitation develops	4-6 hr	Sedation accompanying analgesia	Vomiting, diarrhea, and bradycardia may occur Hypotension and bronchoconstriction possible (histamine release with rapid IV administration)	Dilute with saline for slow IV injection
Hydromorphone (or oxymorphone)	*Dogs:* 0.05-0.1 mg/kg IV, IM, SC; 0.01-0.05 mg/kg/hr IV CRI *Cats:* 0.05-0.1 mg/kg IV, IM, SC; 0.01-0.025 mg/kg/hr IV CRI; reduce if hyperthermia or agitation develops	4 hr	Useful for managing substantial pain	Panting, vomiting, diarrhea, bradycardia, dysphoria Dosage-dependent sedation or excitement, hyperthermia in cats	
Fentanyl	*Dogs and cats:* 2-10 mcg/kg/hr as CRI after IV loading dose of 2-10 mcg/kg; reduce if hyperthermia or agitation develops (cats more susceptible)	Rapid onset and short duration	Excellent for procedural uses and as a CRI for sustained and titratable analgesia	Dysphoria	May be combined with lidocaine CRI (see text)
Methadone	*Dogs:* 0.1-1.0 mg/kg IV *Cats:* 0.05-0.5 mg/kg IV (up to two times this dose if given IM or SC)	4-6 hr	Sedation accompanying analgesia	Vomiting, diarrhea, bradycardia	Causes less sedation and vomiting than morphine
Butorphanol (Torbutrol, Torbugesic, Stadol)	*Dogs:* 0.1-0.5 mg/kg IV, IM, SC; 0.1-1 mg/kg/hr IV CRI *Cats:* 0.1-0.5 mg/kg IV, IM, SC; 0.1-0.5 mg/kg/hr IV CRI	*Dogs:* 1-2 hr (analgesic effect) for IV, IM, SC *Cats:* 2-4 hr (analgesic effect) for IV, IM, SC	Ceiling effect, limited analgesia, useful for mild sedation and cough suppression, minimal systemic effects	Partial opioid reversal	
Nalbuphine (Nubain)	*Dogs and cats:* 0.2-4 mg/kg IV, IM, SC	30-60 min	Minimal analgesia and minimal sedation, used in combination with sedatives or tranquilizers	Partial reversal of μ-agonist opioids	
Buprenorphine (Buprenex, Temgesic)	*Dogs:* 0.01-0.05 mg/kg IV, IM, SC; 0.02-0.12 mg/kg oral transmucosal *Cats:* 0.005-0.05 mg/kg IV, IM, SC, oral transmucosal	Slow onset and long duration of effect (6-8 hr)		Some ceiling effect on respiratory depression, vomiting not commonly seen	Oral transmucosal absorption is excellent in cats and adequate in dogs for an alternative route to injection

CRI, Constant rate infusion; *IM,* intramuscularly; *IV,* intravenously; *SC,* subcutaneously.
*Rates for IV CRI are from Hansen BD: Analgesia and sedation in the critically ill, J Vet Emerg Crit Care 15:285, 2005, and are recommended analgesic drug dosages used for administration as fluid additives in critical care. Other dosages are taken from the suggested references and the author's experience.

stimulate histamine release. There may be less excitement or dysphoria than with morphine, but the literature and anecdotal reports are mixed on this subject. Hyperthermic reactions are occasionally seen in cats receiving hydromorphone. This is a very useful opioid for managing substantial pain and is quite similar to the formerly popular opioid oxymorphone.

Fentanyl and Remifentanil

Fentanyl has been a useful opioid in veterinary medicine for many years. Fentanyl is combined with droperidol in the preparation Innovar-Vet, a once-popular neuroleptanalgesic. Fentanyl formulated in a controlled-release transdermal patch for human pain treatment has been used (extralabel) in many veterinary species. The pharmacokinetics and pharmacodynamics of transdermal fentanyl have been described for many species, including dogs and cats. This formulation is useful for sustained analgesia in animals with significant trauma (e.g., multiple fractures after vehicular trauma), as part of the treatment of postoperative pain, in critically ill animals with painful systemic disease (e.g., pancreatitis), and in some cancer patients. Fentanyl patches can be useful in cats as well as in dogs. Breakthrough pain may require a supplemental analgesic strategy, often with a complementing class of nonopioid analgesic. Recently, a delayed-release transdermal solution of fentanyl (Recuvyra) that penetrates intact canine skin and serves as a reservoir within the skin has been formulated for use in dogs to provide sustained analgesic action.

The fentanyl patches are available with various rates of drug delivery: 25, 50, 75, and 100 mcg/hr. Effectiveness has been reported for 50-mcg patches in small and medium-sized dogs. The 25-mcg patches have been used extensively in cats and dogs weighing less than 5 kg. The behavioral effects of dysphoria and dementia are unacceptable in some animals and may require tranquilization or removal of the patch. The practice of uncovering only one half of the barrier layer before application has been used to reduce the dosage and minimize this problem, particularly in smaller dogs and cats.

Patches are applied to clipped skin. Uptake is somewhat variable among patients, and clinical efficacy may be related in part to differences in uptake of fentanyl. Onset of analgesia does not occur until 12 to 24 hours after application of the patch. Hence, other options, such as injected opioids or other medications, should be used initially to provide analgesia. It is important to prevent the patient from damaging or ingesting these patches or the contents. Of note, application of a heat source over the area of the patch can greatly increase uptake of the drug, with significant overdose possible. Duration of effectiveness is roughly 4 days.

Fentanyl is a highly abused opioid, and there have been reports of clients removing fentanyl patches from their animals for drug abuse or diversion purposes. Some clinicians use the patches only for hospitalized, closely observed patients. Others find the fentanyl patches a very useful part of managing cancer pain in outpatients, including the terminally ill. The patch can help provide a steady level of opioid for a prolonged period in a way that is cost effective and reasonably convenient for clients. It is essential to emphasize to owners the potential dangers and the importance of protecting other pets and children from ingestion or other possible exposures. Expended (used) patches still contain fentanyl and should be folded onto themselves and flushed down the toilet (in the United States) or returned to a veterinarian for disposal.

Injectable fentanyl has such a short duration of action that a bolus dose, by itself, is of limited benefit for treatment of prolonged (e.g., postoperative) pain, it but may be excellent as a component of procedural pain management (e.g., for bone marrow aspiration or sedation or analgesia for other diagnostic procedures such as radiography). The rapid onset and relatively short duration of action of injected fentanyl make it an excellent choice for administration as a CRI for sustained and titrated analgesia in critical care. For dog and cats, a 2- to 10-mcg/kg/hr intravenous CRI is initiated after an intravenous loading dose of 2 to 10 mcg/kg. As a CRI, fentanyl (50 mg/ml) may be combined with an equal volume of 2% lidocaine as follows: 0.1 to 0.3 ml/kg/hr of a 1 : 1 mixture (by volume) of fentanyl and lidocaine administered as needed for comfort and sedation. After long-term infusion, the recovery from fentanyl is more prolonged. In marked contrast, the fast elimination of remifentanil allows for very reliable and rapid recovery after even a long-term infusion. The very short context-sensitive half-life of remifentanil is preserved during infusions given for analgesia or as a component of sedative or anesthetic combinations. Combined infusions of remifentanil and propofol can provide deep sedation or anesthesia in critically ill patients while preserving the option of rapid recovery.

Butorphanol

Butorphanol was first available in veterinary medicine as an antitussive medication. It can be a useful sedative and cough suppressant, but weak analgesic in the critical care patient and is often combined with nonopioid analgesics and sedatives. There is a recognized ceiling effect that limits the analgesic effectiveness of this mixed-acting agonist-antagonist opioid, and butorphanol has been overused inappropriately to the exclusion of the more effective μ-agonist medications. In many cases a pure-agonist opioid, such as morphine, hydromorphone, or fentanyl, should be selected for more effective analgesia. The analgesic actions of butorphanol are limited not only by its mild contribution to pain relief but also by its short duration of effect, particularly in dogs.

Because the ceiling effect with butorphanol also limits respiratory depression, it has less potential than agonist opioids to cause reflexive increases in intracranial pressure (ICP). This decreased potential for respiratory depression adds a safety component in the use of butorphanol as an opioid sedative for patients with cranial trauma or those that for other reasons are at risk of increased ICP or increased intraocular pressure. Vomiting is rarely a feature of the drug, which avoids another risk factor for increases in ICP or intraocular pressure.

When used for partial reversal of the effects of μ-agonist opioids, butorphanol can provide a gentle reversal of excessive μ-agonist–mediated depression (or dysphoria in cats), yet maintain some effects of weak analgesia and sedation.[8] For this reason, as an alternative to naloxone, it can serve as a very useful partial antagonist in critical care patients.

Nalbuphine

Much like butorphanol, nalbuphine is a weak analgesic that is usually classified as a mixed agonist-antagonist opioid. The sedation provided by nalbuphine is minimal, but it contributes to the sedation afforded by simultaneously administered tranquilizers or sedatives. Nalbuphine is used in combination with acepromazine, benzodiazepines, or α_2 agonists. Like butorphanol, nalbuphine can be used for partial reversal of μ-agonist opioids. Nalbuphine is not currently a scheduled drug in the United States.[9]

Buprenorphine

Buprenorphine typically has been classified as a partial-agonist opioid, with limited agonist activity at μ-receptors. Research suggests that the ceiling effect with this drug may apply more to respiratory depression than to its analgesic actions. Because of this, it provides a relatively moderate analgesic effect. The duration of analgesic action is greater than that of any other clinically available opioids (with the exception of controlled-release formulations and drugs administered by neuroaxial routes). Buprenorphine, like butorphanol, does not stimulate vomiting and similarly may be a good choice for patients at risk of increased ICP or intraocular pressure. Concurrent administration of monoamine oxidase inhibitors with buprenorphine should be avoided. In cats, and to a somewhat lesser degree in dogs, buprenorphine has excellent bioavailability from the oral mucosa. Transmucosal (oral or sublingual but not orogastric) administration of the injectable product is well tolerated and provides a convenient noninjectable option for relatively long-lasting substantial analgesia in cats. It still has useful bioavailability in dogs when give in the cheek pouch or sublingually but not when administered via the orogastric route.[10]

Tramadol

Tramadol provides a mild analgesic effect similar to that of weak opioids and nonsteroidal antiinflammatory drugs (NSAIDs). There is slight μ-opioid binding activity, but the analgesic action is attributed more to interference with both serotonin storage and norepinephrine reuptake. Analgesic action exceeds μ-receptor binding characteristics. The principal metabolite has greater μ binding than does the parent compound. Tramadol may be effective when a weak opioid such as codeine would be chosen and is most useful as an adjunctive analgesic in combination with NSAID analgesics. It is available only as an oral medication in the United States, which might limit its use in critically ill patients.

Codeine

Codeine is a pure μ agonist that has one tenth the potency (analgesic properties) of morphine. It is available only as an oral formulation (which limits its use in the intensive care unit) and is readily absorbed from the GI tract. Codeine is a potent oral analgesic for dogs that require long-term analgesic administration (e.g., as a component of cancer pain management).

OPIOID ANTAGONISTS: NALOXONE, NALMEFENE, NALTREXONE

Three significant opioid antagonists are naloxone (very short acting) and nalmefene and naltrexone (both long acting). These compounds bind with great affinity to the μ, κ, and δ opioid receptors, competitively displacing agonists with lesser affinity and thereby reversing the actions of the agonist agents. The antagonists convey no analgesic activity. Naloxone has been used primarily for reversal of opioid agonist effects but also has been used experimentally in the treatment of shock in dogs.[11] With the infusion of high doses of naloxone in a model of hypovolemic shock, splanchnic capacitance was reduced, which led to an improvement in venous return, mean arterial pressure, and cardiac output.

In displacing morphine and other opioids from receptor sites, the antagonist can reverse all opioid effects. Sedation, respiratory depression, and analgesia can be reversed abruptly, which precipitates acute reactions of severe pain, excitement, and profound stress. If naloxone is used for reversal of adverse or excessive opioid agonist effects in a critical care setting, the diluted drug should be given slowly and titrated by intravenous infusion to the desired effect. Patients should be observed for relapse into sedation or a return of adverse effects (renarcotization). It is difficult to titrate opioid reversal to arouse a patient from excessive sedation and still preserve analgesia.

Partial reversal using butorphanol or nalbuphine is an alternative approach that is suitable for many patients. Buprenorphine binds with great affinity to the receptors and its effects can be difficult to reverse. Fortunately, few critical care patients require complete opioid reversal. Supportive care and treatment of opioid-induced sedation or excessive undesirable effects with partial reversal agents are generally recommended.

Naltrexone and nalmefene (the latter has a longer duration of effect) similarly compete for opioid receptors, displacing agonists, both exogenous and endogenous. For this reason, these drugs have been used to treat compulsive behavior disorders. The lack of any significant naltrexone metabolite in dogs (in contrast to humans) might limit the effectiveness of this strategy.[12]

CONCLUSION

Opioids as a class are among the safest of analgesic medications, with profound usefulness in the critical care setting. Pain relief is the most significant application of the opioids, but they also offer sedation and cough suppression and are essential components of critical care anesthesia. The variety of opioids and the variety of administration routes and strategies available allow for many creative applications to the benefit of critically ill veterinary patients.

REFERENCES

1. Hansen BD: Analgesia and sedation in the critically ill, J Vet Emerg Crit Care 15:285, 2005.
2. Hellyer PW: Pain management. In Wingfield WE, Raffe MR, editors: The veterinary ICU book, Jackson Hole, Wyo, 2002, Teton New Media.
3. Dobromylskyj P, Flecknell PA, Lascelles BD, et al: Pain assessment. In Flecknell P, Waterman-Pearson A, editors: Pain management in animals, London, 2000, Saunders.
4. Niedfeldt RL, Robertson SA: Postanesthetic hyperthermia in cats: a retrospective comparison between hydromorphone and buprenorphine, Vet Anaesth Analg 33:381, 2006.
5. Dohoo S, Tasker RA, Donald A: Pharmacokinetics of parenteral and oral sustained-release morphine sulphate in dogs, J Vet Pharmacol Ther 17:426, 1994.
6. Muir WW, Wiese AJ, March PA: Effects of morphine, lidocaine, ketamine and morphine-lidocaine-ketamine drug combinations on minimum alveolar concentration in dogs anesthetized with isoflurane, Am J Vet Res 64:1155, 2003.
7. Kukanich B, Lascalles BDX, Papich MG: Pharmacokinetics of morphine and plasma concentrations of morphine-6-glucuronide following morphine administration to dogs, J Vet Pharmacol Ther 28:371, 2005.
8. McCrackin MA, Harvey RC, Sackman JE, et al: Butorphanol tartrate for partial reversal of oxymorphone-induced postoperative respiratory depression in the dog, Vet Surg 23:67, 1994.
9. Veterinary Anesthesia and Analgesia Support Group website. Available at http://www.vasg.org. Accessed March 12, 2007.
10. Robertson SA, Taylor PM, Sear J: Systemic uptake of buprenorphine by cats after oral mucosal administration, Vet Record 152:675, 2003.
11. Bell L, Maratea E, Rutlen DL: Influence of naloxone on the total capacitance vasculature of the dog, J Clin Invest 75:1894, 1985.
12. Luescher A: Compulsive behavior in companion animals, IVIS veterinary drug database, Document No. B2410.0403, Ithaca, NY, 2004, International Veterinary Information Service. Available at http://www.ivis.org. Accessed August 7, 2007.

CHAPTER 164
BENZODIAZEPINES

Ralph C. Harvey, DVM, MS, DACVAA

KEY POINTS

- Benzodiazepines are associated with less adverse respiratory and cardiovascular effects than most alternative tranquilizers or sedatives.
- Benzodiazepines are a first line of defense for rapid seizure control.
- Small doses of benzodiazepines are often successful for short-term appetite stimulation in critically ill cats.
- Accidental ingestion of benzodiazepines is treated with supportive care, emetics, and/or activated charcoal. Flumazenil may be administered in severe cases that are associated with marked central nervous system depression.

Benzodiazepines have a wide range of applications in critically ill patients. As a group these drugs offer effects that include sedation, anxiolysis, and anticonvulsant activity, with minor cardiovascular and respiratory effects. They can be used as part of an anesthetic induction protocol for balanced anesthesia, given along with analgesic drugs to enhance patient comfort and sedation, or administered for treatment of status epilepticus. The most commonly used benzodiazepines in veterinary medicine are diazepam and midazolam. Benzodiazepines are considered scheduled substances in the United States (C-IV), and for this reason appropriate storage and documentation is required.[1]

ACTION

Benzodiazepines are believed to act primarily via the inhibitory neurotransmitter γ-aminobutyric acid (GABA); benzodiazepines bind to stereospecific receptors that facilitate the inhibitory actions of GABA.[1,2] The mechanism of action may also involve antagonism of serotonin and diminished release or turnover of acetylcholine in the central nervous system (CNS).[1] Benzodiazepines act at the limbic, thalamic, and hypothalamic level of the CNS with anxiolytic, sedative, hypnotic, skeletal muscle relaxant, and anticonvulsant properties. In humans, benzodiazepines are also recognized to have anterograde amnestic effects, providing amnesia for events that occur subsequent to the administration of the drug.[2] Benzodiazepines are generally considered to provide no analgesia.

Benzodiazepines are metabolized in the liver to active metabolites that, after conjugation, are excreted in the urine.[2]

DIAZEPAM VERSUS MIDAZOLAM

Diazepam and midazolam have similar pharmacologic actions in dogs and cats. The major difference between these drugs is that diazepam is not water soluble; it is formulated in a 40% propylene glycol and 10% alcohol vehicle.[1] Propylene glycol is an irritant to blood vessels and causes phlebitis and thrombosis after repeated or continuous administration through a peripheral vein. For this reason, diazepam should be given only as a constant rate infusion (CRI) or in multiple repeated intermittent doses via a central vein. Prolonged administration of diazepam can also cause propylene glycol toxicity, which may have life-threatening effects including metabolic acidosis, hyperosmolality, neurologic abnormalities, and organ dysfunction.[3] Propylene glycol toxicity is of particular concern in cats; therefore diazepam infusions are not recommended in this species.[4] Diazepam also adsorbs to plastic, so doses should not be stored in plastic syringes for any length of time, and infusion lines may require precoating with the drug before administration. Both diazepam and midazolam should be protected from light. Infusion lines for either diazepam or midazolam should also be tinted or covered to block light exposure.

In contrast to diazepam, midazolam is water soluble and is well absorbed after intramuscular injection. However, midazolam is poorly bioavailable when given per rectum to dogs, so this route of administration is not recommended.[1,5] Diazepam rectal gel is available for human use and may offer a viable alternative for at-home treatment of seizures. Intranasal administration for at-home treatment of seizures is another practical and readily accepted option.[6,7] Midazolam can be given as a CRI through a peripheral vein.

BENZODIAZEPINE EFFECTS

The sedative effects of benzodiazepines are highly variable in dogs and cats. Animals may demonstrate aberrant behavior after benzodiazepine administration, including excitation, irritability, and depression. Patients that are already somewhat obtunded are likely to be effectively sedated, particularly if the benzodiazepine is combined with an opioid. Healthier dogs and cats may demonstrate dysphoria; this is more likely when the drugs are used as sole agents.

BENZODIAZEPINES AND CATS

A rare complication of oral diazepam administration in cats is fulminant hepatic failure. This has been reported as an idiosyncratic reaction resulting in acute hepatic necrosis.[8] This reaction has not been reported in association with other routes of administration.

INDICATIONS

Sedation

As a sole drug, benzodiazepines are rarely sufficient to sedate neurologically normal dogs and cats. Benzodiazepines commonly are combined with opioids to provide sedation for intensive care procedures or to relieve distress and anxiety in critically ill patients when analgesic therapy alone is insufficient.[4] Benzodiazepines are also commonly incorporated into anesthetic protocols for induction and maintenance of anesthesia. These drugs can be given to reduce the required dosage of other anesthetic agents such as propofol or barbiturates in an effort to minimize their adverse effects (see Chapters 142 through 144).

The shorter-acting drug midazolam is often given intravenously (IV) and is generally preferred to diazepam. It can be titrated easily to a desired level to prevent drug accumulation that might delay recovery. Water-soluble midazolam, with its short elimination half-life and duration of action, may be more suitable for continuous infusion in critically ill patients than diazepam. The more slowly eliminated benzodiazepine lorazepam is also water soluble and has been recommended as a more suitable alternative for long term use in human patients, but there is little experience with this drug in veterinary patients.[4,9]

The most important adverse effects of long-term benzodiazepine infusions are dysphoric or excitatory signs and, occasionally, delayed awakening. The antagonist flumazenil and the inverse agonist sarmazenil have each been used to reverse CNS depression or dysphoria due to benzodiazepine agonists in human patients. Significantly delayed recovery or marked dysphoria attributable to benzodiazepines may be responsive to reversal with these agents, but neither can be recommended for routine use in animals in stable condition. Marked excitement and dysphoria can be precipitated by either drug. Significant adverse effects, such as seizures and acute benzodiazepine withdrawal, have been reported.

In most animals in stable condition, the delayed recovery or adverse effects of the benzodiazepines are less problematic than the potential for more severe adverse outcomes with either flumazenil or sarmazenil use. Even in cases of severe benzodiazepine overdose, as from oral ingestion of multiple tablets, the toxic effects generally can be managed with supportive care and administration of emetics and/or activated charcoal (see Chapter 74). Benzodiazepine antagonist therapy with flumazenil is rarely indicated in patients in stable condition, although its use in critically ill patients with cardiovascular or pulmonary instability is more commonly justified.[10] When flumazenil therapy is deemed necessary, a dosage of 0.01 to 0.02 mg/kg IV has been recommended for reversal of benzodiazepine effects in dogs and cats. Alternative routes are effective, with some limitations.[11] Animals requiring frequent redosing may benefit from a temporary IV flumazenil infusion of 0.005 to 0.02 mg/kg/hr.

Anticonvulsant Therapy

Benzodiazepines are the drugs of choice for initial control of status epilepticus in both dogs and cats.[12,13] Midazolam can be given intramuscularly if intravenous access is not available. Intramuscular administration of diazepam is not recommended, and the rectal or intranasal route is preferred in the absence of intravenous access.[1,14,15] Diazepam rectal gel (Diastat) is available, however, for rectal administration in animals having seizures at home or in the hospital before intravenous access is obtained. Its use has not been extensively studied in small animals, but it is expected to act similarly to diazepam given by other routes. For patients with recurrent seizure activity that responds to benzodiazepine administration, an intravenous CRI of diazepam or midazolam may be effective. See Table 164-1 for some suggested anticonvulsant dosages. Chapters 82 and 166 provide a detailed discussion of anticonvulsant therapy and the approach to the patient with seizures.

Appetite Stimulation

Low doses of benzodiazepines can stimulate appetite in many species, especially in cats. The hyperphagic effect is separate from sedation or anxiolysis, involves binding to benzodiazepine receptors, and appears to increase the attraction to tastes. Increases in both the amount of food consumed and the rate of consumption are noted. In experimental models, the hyperphagic response is seen in satiated (fully fed) animals. As an appetite stimulant, diazepam is administered to cats at a dosage of 0.005 to 0.4 mg/kg IV q24h or 1 mg orally q24h (risk of hepatic toxicity in cats should be considered). Food should be readily available because the animal may begin eating within a few seconds of administration.[1]

Table 164-1 Suggested Parenteral Dosages for Benzodiazepines in Dogs and Cats

Use	Diazepam	Midazolam
Sedation	IV: 0.2-0.6 mg/kg CRI: 0.1-1 mg/kg/hr (central vein)	IV, IM: 0.1-0.4 mg/kg CRI: 0.1-0.5 mg/kg/hr
Anticonvulsant therapy	IV, intranasally: 0.5-1 mg/kg; can repeat 2 or 3 times PR: 2 mg/kg CRI: 0.5-1 mg/kg/hr (central vein)	IV, IM: 0.2-0.5 mg/kg; can repeat 2 or 3 times CRI: 0.2-0.5 mg/kg/hr

CRI, Constant rate infusion; *IM,* intramuscularly; *IV,* intravenously; *PR,* per rectum.

HEPATIC ENCEPHALOPATHY

Hepatic encephalopathy (HE) commonly accompanies the syndrome of portosystemic shunting or significant hepatic insufficiency due to other causes (see Chapters 88 and 116). Human patients with HE have occasionally shown arousal following administration of the benzodiazepine antagonist flumazenil. This observation suggests that the syndrome may involve increased endogenous benzodiazepine agonist activity. In contrast, a lack of arousal in other species, including dogs and cats in both clinical and research models of HE, has been interpreted as evidence that endogenous benzodiazepines are not increased in this syndrome.

Administration of the benzodiazepine inverse agonist sarmazenil, but not the antagonist flumazenil, in animal research models of both acute and chronic HE has resulted in improvement of encephalopathic signs. This is consistent with an increased GABAergic constitutive activity in HE, rather than an increase in endogenous benzodiazepine agonist ligands.[16] Although sarmazenil has been useful in elucidating the pathophysiology of HE, it should not be considered part of the therapeutic modality for this disorder. Sarmazenil has also been used for reversal of GABA-mediated toxicity due to moxidectin in a foal. However, this application remains somewhat controversial at this time, as is the use of benzodiazepines for the treatment of HE-induced seizures.

REFERENCES

1. Plumb DC: Diazepam. In Plumb's veterinary drug handbook, ed 5, Ames, Ia, 2005, Blackwell.
2. Charney DS, Mihic SJ, Harris RA: Hypnotics and sedatives. In Hardman JG, Limbird LE, editors: Goodman's and Gilman's The pharmacological basis of therapeutics, ed 10, New York, 2001, McGraw-Hill.
3. Wilson KC, Reardon C, Theodore AC, et al: Propylene glycol toxicity: a severe iatrogenic illness in intensive care unit patients receiving IV benzodiazepines: a case series and prospective, observational pilot study, Chest 128:1674, 2005.
4. Hansen BD: Analgesia and sedation in the critically ill, J Vet Emerg Crit Care (San Antonio) 15:285, 2005.
5. Schwartz M, Muñana KR, Nettifee-Osborne JA, et al: The pharmacokinetics of midazolam after intravenous, intramuscular, and rectal administration in healthy dogs, J Vet Pharmacol Ther 36(5):471-477, 2013.
6. Musulin SE, Mariani CL, Papich MG: Diazepam pharmacokinetics after nasal drop and atomized nasal administration in dogs, J Vet Pharmacol Ther 34(1):17-24, 2011.
7. Eagleson JS, Platt SR, Elder Strong DL, et al: Bioavailability of a novel midazolam gel after intranasal administration in dogs, Am J Vet Res 73(4):539-545, 2012.

8. Center SA, Elston TH, Rowland PH, et al: Fulminant hepatic failure associated with oral administration of diazepam in 11 cats, J Am Vet Med Assoc 209:618, 1996.
9. Notterman DA: Sedation with intravenous midazolam in the pediatric intensive care unit, Clin Pediatr 36:449, 1997.
10. Wismer TA: Accidental ingestion of alprazolam in 415 dogs, Vet Hum Toxicol 44:22, 2002.
11. Unkel JH, Brickhouse TH, Sweatman TWS, et al: A comparison of three routes of flumazenil administration to reverse benzodiazepine-induced desaturation in an animal model, Pediatr Dent 28(4):357-362, 2006.
12. Parent J, Poma R: Single seizure, cluster seizures, and status epilepticus. In Wingfield WE, Raffe MR, editors: The veterinary ICU book, Jackson Hole, Wyo, 2002, Teton NewMedia.
13. Papich MG, Alcorn J: Absorption of diazepam after its rectal administration in dogs, Am J Vet Res 56:1629, 1995.
14. Platt SR, Randell SC, Scott KC, et al: Comparison of plasma benzodiazepine concentrations following intranasal and intravenous administration of diazepam to dogs, Am J Vet Res 61:651, 2000.
15. Meyer HP, Legemate DA, van den Brom W, et al: Improvement of chronic hepatic encephalopathy in dogs by the benzodiazepine-receptor partial inverse agonist sarmazenil, but not by the antagonist flumazenil, Metab Brain Dis 13:241, 1998.
16. Muller JM, Feige K, Kastner SB, et al: The use of sarmazenil in the treatment of a moxidectin intoxication in a foal, J Vet Intern Med 19:348, 2005.

CHAPTER 165

α_2 AGONISTS AND ANTAGONISTS

Bruno H. Pypendop, DrMedVet, DrVetSci, DACVAA

KEY POINTS

- α_2 Agonists can be used to produce sedation and analgesia.
- α_2 Agonists reduce the required analgesic dose of drugs like opioids when used in combination with these drugs.
- α_2 Agonists produce minimal respiratory effects.
- α_2 Agonists have pronounced cardiovascular effects, including bradycardia and vasoconstriction.
- α_2 Agonists should be used with caution in patients with compromised organ blood flow.
- Dexmedetomidine is the α_2 agonist of choice for sedation and analgesia in intensive care; it should be administered as a continuous intravenous infusion when used for purposes other than short-term sedation.
- α_2 Antagonists can be used to reverse the effects of α_2 agonists; atipamezole is suitable for antagonizing the action of dexmedetomidine.

Agonists of α_2-adrenergic receptors (α_2 agonists) produce a variety of effects, some of them potentially beneficial in critically ill patients. They are most often used for sedation and analgesia to facilitate handling and performance of minor procedures. They also inhibit the sympathetic nervous system and therefore decrease autonomic responses. However, their cardiovascular effects may be detrimental, and they have many additional effects of concern in critically ill patients such as the inhibition of insulin and antidiuretic hormone secretion.

α_2 ADRENOCEPTORS

The α_2-adrenergic receptors (α_2-adrenoceptors) are $G_{i/o}$ protein–coupled receptors with seven transmembrane domains of the amine-binding subfamily.[1] There are three receptor subtypes; however, this is currently of little clinical relevance since there is no subtype-selective agonist in clinical use. The interaction of an α_2 agonist with its receptor typically results in the inhibition of adenylyl cyclase, the activation of receptor-operated K^+ channels, the acceleration of Na^+/H^+ exchange, and the inhibition of voltage-gated Ca^{++} channels.[2]

α_2-Adrenoceptors are present on the presynaptic membrane of noradrenergic neurons; their activation inhibits the release of norepinephrine (negative feedback).[3] Postsynaptic α_2-adrenoceptors exist in various tissues, where they exert a distinct physiologic function; these tissues include the vascular smooth muscle, liver, pancreas, platelets, kidney, adipose tissue, and eye. The medullary dorsal motor complex in the brain has a high density of α_2-adrenoceptors.

EFFECTS OF α_2 AGONISTS

Central Nervous System

Stimulation of presynaptic α_2-adrenoceptors in the central nervous system decreases the release of norepinephrine. α_2 Agonists produce sedation by inhibition of noradrenergic neurons in the locus ceruleus (upper brainstem).[4-6] Sedation produced by α_2 agonists is characterized by an increase in stage I and II sleep and a decrease in rapid eye movement sleep, and results from the activation of endogenous sleep pathways; it therefore mimics normal sleep better than sedation produced by other agents.[7,8]

α_2 Agonists produce analgesia via stimulation of receptors in the dorsal horn of the spinal cord[9-16] and in the brainstem, where modulation of nociceptive signals is initiated.[17,18] α_2-Agonist–induced antinociception likely results from inhibition of nociceptive neurons. However, a recent study suggests that direct activation of γ-aminobutyric acid–ergic inhibitory interneurons can be produced by norepinephrine.[19] α_2 Agonists, even when administered at very low doses, have been demonstrated to potentiate opioid-induced analgesia.[15,20-29] The addition of ketamine may further potentiate the effect.[30]

In addition, α_2 agonists decrease the development of tolerance to opioids.[31] α_2-Adrenoceptor agonists administered systemically have been shown to produce synergistic analgesic effects with nonsteroidal antiinflammatory drugs and acetaminophen in models of visceral pain.[32-34]

Administration of α_2 agonists decreases the requirements for anesthetic drugs by up to approximately 80% in dogs and cats and 100% in rats.[35-37] This effect is thought to be mediated by the decrease in norepinephrine release, mainly from the locus ceruleus.[38] However, because minimal alveolar concentration is reduced by a maximum of 40% when noradrenergic transmission is totally abolished, additional mechanisms may be responsible for this anesthetic-sparing effect.[39]

α_2-Adrenoceptor agonists have neuroprotective effects, even though high doses may worsen ischemic brain injury.[40-47] These effects may be due to an α_2-adrenoceptor–mediated decrease in norepinephrine or glutamate, or to the activation of imidazoline receptors.[48,49] Other possible neuroprotective mechanisms include the inhibition of acute expression of immediate early genes involved in cerebral damage and the inhibition of massive norepinephrine release following brain injury.[50,51] α_2 Agonists may prevent vasospasm after subarachnoid hemorrhage.[52] α_2 Agonists also appear to have anticonvulsant effects.[53-59]

α_2-Adrenoceptor agonists induce hypothermia.[60-63] This effect is due to the inhibition, at the hypothalamic level, of central noradrenergic mechanisms responsible for the control of body temperature.[64] α_2 Agonists may also prevent the thermoregulatory response to infection.[65]

Cardiovascular System

The typical cardiovascular response to the administration of an α_2 agonist is biphasic. Initially, blood pressure and systemic vascular resistance increase, whereas heart rate and cardiac output decrease.[66-69] The increase in blood pressure may not be seen after intramuscular administration.[69] These effects are followed by a decrease in arterial pressure; heart rate and cardiac output remain lower than normal. Systemic vascular resistance either declines progressively toward normal or remains elevated, depending on the drug and probably the dose and the species. The bradycardia may be accompanied by other arrhythmias. The cardiovascular effects of α_2 agonists are usually considered to be dose dependent.[70] This typical response is initiated by a vasoconstrictive effect caused by stimulation of α_2-adrenoceptors located on the vascular smooth muscle of both arteries and veins.[71,72] This vasoconstrictive effect results in an increase in arterial blood pressure, which, in turn, causes bradycardia via a baroreceptor response.[73] In addition, bradycardia may also be related to the central sympatholytic action of α_2 agonists that leaves vagal tone unopposed, to an increase in parasympathetic efferent neuronal activity, or to a presynaptically mediated reduction of norepinephrine release in cardiac sympathetic nerves.[73,74] Cardiac output decreases in parallel to heart rate, and stroke volume is usually minimally affected. α_2-Adrenoceptor agonists do not seem to induce direct negative inotrope effects.[75]

Because the decrease in cardiac output appears to be related mainly to the bradycardia, combining these drugs with an anticholinergic agent has been advocated. However, such combinations result in large increases in arterial pressure, with mean blood pressure around 200 mm Hg in dogs in one study.[76] In cats, the addition of glycopyrrolate to xylazine appeared detrimental to cardiovascular performance.[77] Similar results have been reported for the combination of romifidine and glycopyrrolate in dogs.[78]

α_2 Agonists induce blood flow redistribution.[79-81] Blood flow to more vital organs (e.g., heart, brain, kidney) might be partially or totally preserved at the expense of poor blood flow to less vital organs (e.g., skin, muscle, intestine).[79,80,82] It has been reported that, despite its marked cardiovascular effects, dexmedetomidine maintains the balance between myocardial oxygen demand and supply.[83] Cerebral blood flow decreases in response to α_2 agonist administration, and during hypoxia, adequate cerebral oxygenation may not be maintained.[84-86]

α_2 Agonists have historically been reported to be arrhythmogenic or to potentiate the arrhythmogenic effects of other drugs administered concomitantly. These arrhythmias are caused by a number of factors. The reduction in heart rate may reveal foci that are normally inhibited by the impulses coming from the sinoatrial node. Older α_2 agonists such as xylazine activate α_1-adrenoceptors, and stimulation of these receptors is known to sensitize the heart to catecholamine-induced arrhythmias. More recently developed drugs that are more specific for the α_2-adrenoceptors do not appear to induce arrhythmias and may actually increase the threshold for epinephrine-induced arrhythmias. This effect could be mediated by imidazoline receptors, since imidazoline but not nonimidazoline α_2 antagonists reversed this effect.[87,88] α_2-Adrenoceptor stimulation is protective against ventricular tachycardia or fibrillation after ischemia-reperfusion.[89] Similarly, perioperative use of these drugs may decrease the incidence of arrhythmias after cardiac surgery.[90]

Calcium channel blockers may inhibit the peripheral vascular effects of α_2 agonists (i.e., vasoconstriction) while preserving their central effects (i.e., sedation, analgesia), therefore preserving the beneficial effects with fewer hemodynamic changes.[91] More recently, elegant studies have shown that similar results may be obtained by the coadministration of α_2 agonists and the peripheral α_2 antagonist MK-467.[92-94] These studies in dogs also showed that the bradycardic effect of the α_2 agonist was almost entirely abolished, which suggests that, at least in dogs, the bradycardia produced by α_2 agonists is peripherally rather than centrally mediated.

As with most effects, α_2-agonist–induced cardiovascular effects appear to be dose dependent. However, near-maximum effects are likely reached at dosages close to the lower end of the clinically recommended range, which implies that using low dosages in that range minimally reduces these cardiovascular effects.[67,68,95]

Other Effects

In dogs and cats, the effects of α_2 agonists on the respiratory system are considered minimal. Usually, respiratory rate decreases but minute ventilation is maintained. Therefore arterial carbon dioxide and oxygen pressures remain within the normal physiologic range.[96,97] However, α_2 agonists can potentiate the depression induced by other agents such as opioids.[98]

α_2 Agonists inhibit sympathetic outflow and modulate the stress response to anesthesia and surgery.[99] They also decrease the plasma level of circulating catecholamines.[100-102] Stimulation of α_2-adrenoceptors on the beta cells of the islets of Langerhans causes direct inhibition of insulin release, resulting in hyperglycemia.[102-109] The effect appears dose dependent, and 10 to 20 mcg/kg of medetomidine was reported to decrease plasma insulin level without causing significant hyperglycemia in dogs.[110] α_2 Agonists increase the release of growth hormone, which could contribute to the observed hyperglycemia.[111-113] α_2 Agonists inhibit the release of antidiuretic hormone and its effect on renal tubules.[114-117] α_2 Agonists promote diuresis and natriuresis.[109,118] They are thought to inhibit the release of renin and to increase the secretion of atrial natriuretic factor.[119,120]

α_2 Agonists induce a decrease in salivation; gastroesophageal sphincter pressure; esophageal, gastric, and small intestinal motility; and gastric secretion.[121-130] Vomiting after α_2-agonist administration has been reported in 8% to 20% of dogs and up to 90% of cats.[131-137] This effect appears to be related to the stimulation of α_2-adrenoceptors in the chemoreceptor trigger zone.[138]

IMIDAZOLINE RECEPTORS

In addition to binding α_2-adrenoceptors, the α_2 agonists currently in clinical use, with the exception of xylazine, also activate imidazoline receptors. Two types of imidazoline receptors have been identified and are labeled I_1 and I_2. I_1 receptors are involved in blood pressure regulation and may act synergically with α_2-adrenoceptors.[139] Imidazoline receptor agonists seem also to increase sodium excretion and urine flow rate.[140] They may have neuroprotective effects.[141] Stimulation of I_1 receptors may inhibit catecholamine-induced arrhythmias. I_2 receptors have been reported to exert control on central noradrenergic and hypothalamic-pituitary-adrenal axis activity to a greater extent than α_2-adrenoceptors.[142] I_2 receptors also appear to be involved in the regulation of small intestinal motility.[143] They may modulate the effects of opioids.[144,145] Imidazoline receptors could also play a role in the α_2-agonist–induced inhibition of insulin secretion and subsequent hyperglycemia.[146]

DRUGS

The α_2-agonists xylazine, medetomidine, and dexmedetomidine have been approved for use in dogs and cats. Other drugs such as romifidine have been studied in small animal species but have not received regulatory approval.

Xylazine has moderate selectivity for α_2-adrenoceptors and activates α_1-adrenoceptors at clinical doses. This may be responsible for additional adverse effects; its use would therefore not be recommended in critically ill patients.

Medetomidine is highly selective for α_2-adrenoceptors. It is a racemic mixture of dexmedetomidine and levomedetomidine. Within the clinical dosage range, levomedetomidine appears devoid of effects and does not appear to significantly influence the disposition of dexmedetomidine.[147,148] Dexmedetomidine is the active isomer. It is commercially available in many countries; in the United States, only the purified dexmedetomidine isomer is currently available for animal use.

CLINICAL USE

α_2 Agonists are widely used for sedation and analgesia to facilitate handling or performance of minor procedures and for premedication before general anesthesia. As mentioned earlier, in critically ill patients, the agent of choice is (dex)medetomidine.

Dexmedetomidine is used for sedation and analgesia in human critical care patients. Its advantages over other sedative or hypnotic agents include the ability to arouse treated patients quickly when necessary, the lack of respiratory depression, maintenance of hemodynamic stability and sympatholysis, and decreased opioid consumption.[149] It is also used to control delirium.

Although there is no specific literature on the use of dexmedetomidine in small animal intensive care, it is likely that some of the benefits would be similar to those seen in humans. However, the cardiovascular effects, in particular the vasoconstriction, may be more pronounced and/or last longer in dogs and cats than in humans. This may be of concern in many critically ill patients, especially if organ blood flow is already compromised. Because the sedation and the analgesia induced by dexmedetomidine following single administration are of short duration, intravenous infusion is the preferred mode of administration when this drug is used for purposes other than short-term sedation. One study evaluated the use of dexmedetomidine for the management of postoperative pain in dogs[150]; in that study, a loading dose of 25 mcg/m^2 followed by a constant rate infusion of 25 mcg/m^2/hr provided adequate analgesia in some (but not all) patients; the sedation was similar to that produced by a constant rate infusion of morphine. These dosages are based on body surface area, the dosing method often recommended for medetomidine and dexmedetomidine because of the early observations that at similar dosages based on body weight, the level of sedation was lower in smaller dogs than in larger dogs; the dosages used in the study correspond to a 0.9-mcg/kg loading dose and 0.9-mcg/kg/hr infusion in a 20-kg dog. The dose of dexmedetomidine should be titrated to the lowest dose producing the desired effect. See Chapter 144 for further dosage recommendations.

α_2 ANTAGONISTS

The effects of α_2 agonists can be reversed by administration of an α_2 antagonist. Atipamezole is highly selective for α_2-adrenoceptors and is suitable for antagonizing the effects of medetomidine and dexmedetomidine. The recommended dose is 5 and 10 times the administered dose of medetomidine and dexmedetomidine, respectively. After intramuscular administration of atipamezole, the sedative, analgesic, and cardiovascular effects induced by an α_2 agonist are reversed within 5 to 10 minutes. Intravenous administration should be used with caution because it may result in transient but sometimes severe dysphoria. The use of MK-467, an α_2 antagonist that does not cross the blood-brain barrier, has been proposed to prevent the peripheral (i.e., vasoconstrictive) effects of medetomidine and dexmedetomidine in dogs without affecting the central effects (i.e., sedation or analgesia). However, this drug is not commercially available at this time.

CONCLUSION

α_2 Agonists can be used to provide sedation and analgesia in dogs and cats. They do not produce significant respiratory depression but have pronounced cardiovascular effects, including vasoconstriction and bradycardia, and cause hyperglycemia. They should be used with caution in patients in which organ blood flow is compromised.

REFERENCES

1. MacDonald E, Kobilka BK, Scheinin M: Gene targeting—homing in on alpha 2-adrenoceptor-subtype function, Trends Pharmacol Sci 18:211-219, 1997.
2. Limbird LE: Receptors linked to inhibition of adenylate cyclase: additional signaling mechanisms, Faseb J 2:2686-2695, 1988.
3. Langer SZ: Presynaptic regulation of the release of catecholamines, Pharmacol Rev 32:337-362, 1980.
4. Scheinin M, Schwinn DA: The locus coeruleus. Site of hypnotic actions of alpha 2-adrenoceptor agonists? Anesthesiology 76:873-875, 1992.
5. French N: Alpha 2-adrenoceptors and I2 sites in the mammalian central nervous system, Pharmacol Ther 68:175-208, 1995.
6. Nakai T, Hayashi M, Ichihara K, et al: Noradrenaline release in rat locus coeruleus is regulated by both opioid and alpha$_2$-adrenoceptors, Pharmacol Res 45:407-412, 2002.
7. Hossmann V, Maling TJ, Hamilton CA, et al: Sedative and cardiovascular effects of clonidine and nitrazepam, Clin Pharmacol Ther 28:167-176, 1980.
8. Nelson LE, Lu J, Guo T, et al: The alpha2-adrenoceptor agonist dexmedetomidine converges on an endogenous sleep-promoting pathway to exert its sedative effects, Anesthesiology 98:428-436, 2003.
9. North RA, Yoshimura M: The actions of noradrenaline on neurones of the rat substantia gelatinosa in vitro, J Physiol 349:43-55, 1984.
10. Fleetwood-Walker SM, Mitchell R, Hope PJ, et al: An alpha 2 receptor mediates the selective inhibition by noradrenaline of nociceptive responses of identified dorsal horn neurones, Brain Res 334:243-254, 1985.
11. Wikberg JE, Hajos M: Spinal cord alpha 2-adrenoceptors may be located postsynaptically with respect to primary sensory neurons: destruction of primary C-afferents with neonatal capsaicin does not affect the number of [3H]clonidine binding sites in mice, Neurosci Lett 76:63-68, 1987.

12. Sullivan AF, Dashwood MR, Dickenson AH: Alpha 2-adrenoceptor modulation of nociception in rat spinal cord: location, effects and interactions with morphine, Eur J Pharmacol 138:169-177, 1987.
13. Danzebrink RM, Gebhart GF: Antinociceptive effects of intrathecal adrenoceptor agonists in a rat model of visceral nociception, J Pharmacol Exp Ther 253:698-705, 1990.
14. Wang XM, Zhang ZJ, Bains R, et al: Effect of antisense knock-down of $alpha_{2a}$- and $alpha_{2c}$-adrenoceptors on the antinociceptive action of clonidine on trigeminal nociception in the rat, Pain 98:27-35, 2002.
15. Fairbanks CA, Stone LS, Kitto KF, et al: $Alpha_{2c}$-Adrenergic receptors mediate spinal analgesia and adrenergic-opioid synergy, J Pharmacol Exp Ther 300:282-290, 2002.
16. Malmberg AB, Hedley LR, Jasper JR, et al: Contribution of $alpha_2$ receptor subtypes to nerve injury-induced pain and its regulation by dexmedetomidine, Br J Pharmacol 132:1827-1836, 2001.
17. Pertovaara A, Kauppila T, Jyvasjarvi E, et al: Involvement of supraspinal and spinal segmental alpha-2-adrenergic mechanisms in the medetomidine-induced antinociception, Neuroscience 44:705-714, 1991.
18. Pertovaara A: Antinociception induced by alpha-2-adrenoceptor agonists, with special emphasis on medetomidine studies, Prog Neurobiol 40:691-709, 1993.
19. Gassner M, Ruscheweyh R, Sandkuhler J: Direct excitation of spinal GABAergic interneurons by noradrenaline, Pain 145:204-210, 2009.
20. Meert TF, De Kock M: Potentiation of the analgesic properties of fentanyl-like opioids with alpha 2-adrenoceptor agonists in rats, Anesthesiology 81:677-688, 1994.
21. van der Laan JW, Hillen FC: The potentiation of morphine-withdrawal jumping by clonidine is antagonized by m-chlorophenylpiperazine and not by haloperidol, Arch Int Pharmacodyn Ther 283:45-55, 1986.
22. Ossipov MH, Malseed RT, Eisenman LM, et al: Effect of alpha 2 adrenergic agents upon central etorphine antinociception in the cat, Brain Res 309:135-142, 1984.
23. Goodchild CS, Guo Z, Davies A, et al: Antinociceptive actions of intrathecal xylazine: interactions with spinal cord opioid pathways, Br J Anaesth 76:544-551, 1996.
24. Harada Y, Nishioka K, Kitahata LM, et al: Visceral antinociceptive effects of spinal clonidine combined with morphine, [D-Pen^2, D-Pen^5] enkephalin, or U50,488H. Anesthesiology 83:344-352, 1995.
25. Monasky MS, Zinsmeister AR, Stevens CW, et al: Interaction of intrathecal morphine and ST-91 on antinociception in the rat: dose-response analysis, antagonism and clearance, J Pharmacol Exp Ther 254:383-392, 1990.
26. Ossipov MH, Harris S, Lloyd P, et al: Antinociceptive interaction between opioids and medetomidine: systemic additivity and spinal synergy, Anesthesiology 73:1227-1235, 1990.
27. Ossipov MH, Suarez LJ, Spaulding TC: Antinociceptive interactions between alpha 2-adrenergic and opiate agonists at the spinal level in rodents, Anesth Analg 68:194-200, 1989.
28. Roerig SC, Lei S, Kitto K, et al: Spinal interactions between opioid and noradrenergic agonists in mice: multiplicativity involves delta and alpha-2 receptors, J Pharmacol Exp Ther 262:365-374, 1992.
29. Wilcox GL, Carlsson KH, Jochim A, et al: Mutual potentiation of antinociceptive effects of morphine and clonidine on motor and sensory responses in rat spinal cord, Brain Res 405:84-93, 1987.
30. Horvath G, Joo G, Dobos I, et al: The synergistic antinociceptive interactions of endomorphin-1 with dexmedetomidine and/or S^+-ketamine in rats, Anesth Analg 93:1018-1024, 2001.
31. Gursoy S, Ozdemir E, Bagcivan I, et al: Effects of alpha 2-adrenoceptor agonists dexmedetomidine and guanfacine on morphine analgesia and tolerance in rats, Upsala J Med Sci 116:238-246, 2011.
32. Miranda HF, Pinardi G: Isobolographic analysis of the antinociceptive interactions of clonidine with nonsteroidal anti-inflammatory drugs, Pharmacol Res 50:273-278, 2004.
33. Soukupova M, Dolezal T, Krsiak M: Synergistic interaction between rilmenidine and ibuprofen in the writhing test in mice, Neuro Endocrinol Lett 30:215-220, 2009.
34. Soukupova M, Dolezal T, Krsiak M: The synergistic interaction between rilmenidine and paracetamol in the writhing test in mice, Naunyn Schmiedebergs Arch Pharmacol 379:575-580, 2009.
35. Segal IS, Vickery RG, Walton JK, et al: Dexmedetomidine diminishes halothane anesthetic requirements in rats through a postsynaptic alpha 2 adrenergic receptor, Anesthesiology 69:818-823, 1988.
36. Vickery RG, Sheridan BC, Segal IS, et al: Anesthetic and hemodynamic effects of the stereoisomers of medetomidine, an alpha 2-adrenergic agonist, in halothane-anesthetized dogs, Anesth Analg 67:611-615, 1988.
37. Escobar A, Pypendop BH, Siao KT, et al: Effect of dexmedetomidine on the minimum alveolar concentration of isoflurane in cats, J Vet Pharmacol Ther 35:163-168, 2012.
38. Correa-Sales C, Rabin BC, Maze M: A hypnotic response to dexmedetomidine, an alpha 2 agonist, is mediated in the locus coeruleus in rats (see comments), Anesthesiology 76:948-952, 1992.
39. Roizen MF, White PF, Eger EI 2nd, et al: Effects of ablation of serotonin or norepinephrine brain-stem areas on halothane and cyclopropane MACs in rats, Anesthesiology 49:252-255, 1978.
40. Maier C, Steinberg GK, Sun GH, et al: Neuroprotection by the alpha 2-adrenoreceptor agonist dexmedetomidine in a focal model of cerebral ischemia, Anesthesiology 79:306-312, 1993.
41. Jolkkonen J, Puurunen K, Koistinaho J, et al: Neuroprotection by the alpha2-adrenoceptor agonist, dexmedetomidine, in rat focal cerebral ischemia, Eur J Pharmacol 372:31-36, 1999.
42. Riihioja P, Jaatinen P, Haapalinna A, et al: Effects of dexmedetomidine on rat locus coeruleus and ethanol withdrawal symptoms during intermittent ethanol exposure, Alcohol Clin Exp Res 23:432-438, 1999.
43. Wheeler L, WoldeMussie E, Lai R: Role of alpha-2 agonists in neuroprotection, Surv Ophthalmol 48(Suppl 1):S47-51, 2003.
44. Engelhard K, Werner C, Eberspacher E, et al: The effect of the alpha 2-agonist dexmedetomidine and the N-methyl-D-aspartate antagonist S^+-ketamine on the expression of apoptosis-regulating proteins after incomplete cerebral ischemia and reperfusion in rats, Anesth Analg 96:524-531, 2003.
45. Laudenbach V, Mantz J, Lagercrantz H, et al: Effects of $alpha_2$-adrenoceptor agonists on perinatal excitotoxic brain injury: comparison of clonidine and dexmedetomidine, Anesthesiology 96:134-141, 2002.
46. Kuhmonen J, Haapalinna A, Sivenius J: Effects of dexmedetomidine after transient and permanent occlusion of the middle cerebral artery in the rat, J Neural Transm 108:261-271, 2001.
47. Kimura T, Sato M, Nishikawa T, et al: Neuroprotective effect of mivazerol, an alpha 2-agonist, after transient forebrain ischemia in rats, Acta Anaesthesiol Scand 49:1117-1123, 2005.
48. Huang R, Chen Y, Yu AC, et al: Dexmedetomidine-induced stimulation of glutamine oxidation in astrocytes: a possible mechanism for its neuroprotective activity, J Cereb Blood Flow Metab 20:895-898, 2000.
49. Engelhard K, Werner C, Kaspar S, et al: Effect of the alpha2-agonist dexmedetomidine on cerebral neurotransmitter concentrations during cerebral ischemia in rats, Anesthesiology 96:450-457, 2002.
50. Wittner M, Sivenius J, Koistinaho J: Alpha2-adrenoreceptor agonist, dexmedetomidine, alters acute gene expression after global ischemia in gerbils, Neurosci Lett 232:75-78, 1997.
51. Kuhmonen J, Pokorny J, Miettinen R, et al: Neuroprotective effects of dexmedetomidine in the gerbil hippocampus after transient global ischemia, Anesthesiology 87:371-377, 1997.
52. Bunc G, Kovacic S, Strnad S: Attenuation of cerebral vasospasm in rabbits using clonidine hydrochloride, a central adrenergic agonist, Auton Neurosci 105:71-76, 2003.
53. Joy RM, Stark LG, Albertson TE: Dose-dependent proconvulsant and anticonvulsant actions of the alpha 2 adrenergic agonist, xylazine, on kindled seizures in the rat, Pharmacol Biochem Behav 19:345-350, 1983.
54. Wlaz P, Rolinski Z: Xylazine impairs the anticonvulsant activity of conventional antiepileptic drugs in mice, Zentralbl Veterinarmed A 43:495-500, 1996.
55. Spinosa HdS, Gorniak SL, Palermo-Neto J, et al: Pro and anticonvulsant effects of xylazine on convulsion models in rodents, Vet Hum Toxicol 36:12-14, 1994.
56. Miyazaki Y, Adachi T, Kurata J, et al: Dexmedetomidine reduces seizure threshold during enflurane anaesthesia in cats, Br J Anaesth 82:935-937, 1999.
57. Homayoun H, Khavandgar S, Dehpour AR: The role of alpha2-adrenoceptors in the modulatory effects of morphine on seizure susceptibility in mice, Epilepsia 43:797-804, 2002.
58. Tanaka K, Oda Y, Funao T, et al: Dexmedetomidine decreases the convulsive potency of bupivacaine and levobupivacaine in rats: involvement

of alpha2-adrenoceptor for controlling convulsions, Anesth Analg 100:687-696, 2005.
59. Chachua T, Bilanishvili I, Khizanishvili N, et al: Noradrenergic modulation of seizure activity, Georgian Med News 34-39, 2010.
60. Virtanen R, MacDonald E: Comparison of the effects of detomidine and xylazine on some alpha 2-adrenoceptor-mediated responses in the central and peripheral nervous systems, Eur J Pharmacol 115:277-284, 1985.
61. Livingston A, Low J, Morris B: Effects of clonidine and xylazine on body temperature in the rat, Br J Pharmacol 81:189-193, 1984.
62. Talke P, Tayefeh F, Sessler DI, et al: Dexmedetomidine does not alter the sweating threshold, but comparably and linearly decreases the vasoconstriction and shivering thresholds, Anesthesiology 87:835-841, 1997.
63. Quail MT, Shannon M: Severe hypothermia caused by clonidine, Am J Emerg Med 21:86, 2003.
64. Virtanen R: Pharmacological profiles of medetomidine and its antagonist, atipamezole, Acta Vet Scand Suppl 85:29-37, 1989.
65. Tolchard S, Burns PA, Nutt DJ, et al: Hypothermic responses to infection are inhibited by alpha2-adrenoceptor agonists with possible clinical implications, Br J Anaesth 103:554-560, 2009.
66. Yamashita K, Tsubakishita S, Futaok S, et al: Cardiovascular effects of medetomidine, detomidine and xylazine in horses, J Vet Med Sci 62:1025-1032, 2000.
67. Pypendop BH, Verstegen JP: Cardiovascular effects of romifidine in dogs, Am J Vet Res 62:490-495, 2001.
68. Pypendop BH, Verstegen JP: Hemodynamic effects of medetomidine in the dog: a dose titration study, Vet Surg 27:612-622, 1998.
69. Lamont LA, Bulmer BJ, Grimm KA, et al: Cardiopulmonary evaluation of the use of medetomidine hydrochloride in cats, Am J Vet Res 62:1745-1749, 2001.
70. Ebert TJ, Hall JE, Barney JA, et al: The effects of increasing plasma concentrations of dexmedetomidine in humans, Anesthesiology 93:382-394, 2000.
71. Ruffolo RR Jr: Distribution and function of peripheral alpha-adrenoceptors in the cardiovascular system, Pharmacol Biochem Behav 22:827-833, 1985.
72. Talke PO, Lobo EP, Brown R, et al: Clonidine-induced vasoconstriction in awake volunteers, Anesth Analg 93:271-276, 2001.
73. Xu H, Aibiki M, Seki K, et al: Effects of dexmedetomidine, an alpha2-adrenoceptor agonist, on renal sympathetic nerve activity, blood pressure, heart rate and central venous pressure in urethane-anesthetized rabbits, J Auton Nerv Syst 71:48-54, 1998.
74. Penttila J, Helminen A, Anttila M, et al: Cardiovascular and parasympathetic effects of dexmedetomidine in healthy subjects, Can J Physiol Pharmacol 82:359-362, 2004.
75. Flacke WE, Flacke JW, Blow KD, et al: Effect of dexmedetomidine, an alpha 2-adrenergic agonist, in the isolated heart, J Cardiothorac Vasc Anesth 6:418-423, 1992.
76. Alibhai HI, Clarke KW, Lee YH, et al: Cardiopulmonary effects of combinations of medetomidine hydrochloride and atropine sulphate in dogs, Vet Rec 138:11-13, 1996.
77. Dunkle N, Moise NS, Scarlett-Kranz J, et al: Cardiac performance in cats after administration of xylazine or xylazine and glycopyrrolate: echocardiographic evaluations, Am J Vet Res 47:2212-2216, 1986.
78. Sinclair MD, O'Grady MR, Kerr CL, et al: The echocardiographic effects of romifidine in dogs with and without prior or concurrent administration of glycopyrrolate, Vet Anaesth Analg 30:211-219, 2003.
79. Talke PO, Traber DL, Richardson CA, et al: The effect of $alpha_2$ agonist-induced sedation and its reversal with an $alpha_2$ antagonist on organ blood flow in sheep, Anesth Analg 90:1060-1066, 2000.
80. Lawrence CJ, Prinzen FW, de Lange S: The effect of dexmedetomidine on nutrient organ blood flow, Anesth Analg 83:1160-1165, 1996.
81. Bobalova J, Mutafova-Yambolieva VN: Presynaptic alpha2-adrenoceptor-mediated modulation of adenosine 5′ triphosphate and noradrenaline corelease: differences in canine mesenteric artery and vein, J Auton Pharmacol 21:47-55, 2001.
82. Pypendop B, Verstegen J: Effects of a medetomidine-midazolam-butorphanol combination on renal cortical, intestinal and muscle microvascular blood flow in isoflurane anaesthetized dogs: a laser Doppler study, Vet Anaesth Analg 27:36-44, 2000.
83. Lawrence CJ, Prinzen FW, de Lange S: Hemodynamic and coronary vascular effects of dexmedetomidine in the anesthetized goat, Acta Anaesthesiol Scand 41:830-836, 1997.
84. McPherson RW, Koehler RC, Kirsch JR, et al: Intraventricular dexmedetomidine decreases cerebral blood flow during normoxia and hypoxia in dogs, Anesth Analg 84:139-147, 1997.
85. Lei H, Grinberg O, Nwaigwe CI, et al: The effects of ketamine-xylazine anesthesia on cerebral blood flow and oxygenation observed using nuclear magnetic resonance perfusion imaging and electron paramagnetic resonance oximetry, Brain Res 913:174-179, 2001.
86. Prielipp RC, Wall MH, Tobin JR, et al: Dexmedetomidine-induced sedation in volunteers decreases regional and global cerebral blood flow, Anesth Analg 95:1052-1059, 2002.
87. Kamibayashi T, Hayashi Y, Mammoto T, et al: Role of the vagus nerve in the antidysrhythmic effect of dexmedetomidine on halothane/epinephrine dysrhythmias in dogs, Anesthesiology 83:992-999, 1995.
88. Kamibayashi T, Mammoto T, Hayashi Y, et al: Further characterization of the receptor mechanism involved in the antidysrhythmic effect of dexmedetomidine on halothane/epinephrine dysrhythmias in dogs, Anesthesiology 83:1082-1089, 1995.
89. Cai JJ, Morgan DA, Haynes WG, et al: Alpha 2-Adrenergic stimulation is protective against ischemia-reperfusion-induced ventricular arrhythmias in vivo, Am J Physiol Heart Circ Physiol 283:H2606-2611, 2002.
90. Chrysostomou C, Sanchez-de-Toledo J, Wearden P, et al: Perioperative use of dexmedetomidine is associated with decreased incidence of ventricular and supraventricular tachyarrhythmias after congenital cardiac operations, Ann Thorac Surg 92:964-972; discussion 972, 2011.
91. Roekaerts PM, Lawrence CJ, Prinzen FW, et al: Alleviation of the peripheral hemodynamic effects of dexmedetomidine by the calcium channel blocker isradipine, Acta Anaesthesiol Scand 41:364-370, 1997.
92. Honkavaara JM, Restitutti F, Raekallio MR, et al: The effects of increasing doses of MK-467, a peripheral $alpha_2$-adrenergic receptor antagonist, on the cardiopulmonary effects of intravenous dexmedetomidine in conscious dogs, J Vet Pharmacol Ther 34:332-337, 2011.
93. Honkavaara JM, Raekallio MR, Kuusela EK, et al: The effects of L-659,066, a peripheral alpha2-adrenoceptor antagonist, on dexmedetomidine-induced sedation and bradycardia in dogs, Vet Anaesth Analg 35:409-413, 2008.
94. Restitutti F, Honkavaara JM, Raekallio MR, et al: Effects of different doses of L-659′066 on the bispectral index and clinical sedation in dogs treated with dexmedetomidine, Vet Anaesth Analg 38:415-422, 2011.
95. Pypendop BH, Barter LS, Stanley SD, et al: Hemodynamic effects of dexmedetomidine in isoflurane-anesthetized cats, Vet Anaesth Analg 38:555-567, 2011.
96. Haskins SC, Patz JD, Farver TB: Xylazine and xylazine-ketamine in dogs, Am J Vet Res 47:636-641, 1986.
97. Pypendop B, Verstegen J: Cardiorespiratory effects of a combination of medetomidine, midazolam, and butorphanol in dogs, Am J Vet Res 60:1148-1154, 1999.
98. Ho AM, Chen S, Karmakar MK: Central apnoea after balanced general anaesthesia that included dexmedetomidine, Br J Anaesth 95:773-775, 2005.
99. Zalunardo MP, Zollinger A, Spahn DR, et al: Preoperative clonidine attenuates stress response during emergence from anesthesia, J Clin Anesth 12:343-349, 2000.
100. Hokfelt B, Hedeland H, Hansson BG: The effect of clonidine and penbutolol, respectively on catecholamines in blood and urine, plasma renin activity and urinary aldosterone in hypertensive patients, Arch Int Pharmacodyn Ther 213:307-321, 1975.
101. Flacke JW, Flacke WE, Bloor BC, et al: Hemodynamic effects of dexmedetomidine, an alpha 2-adrenergic agonist, in autonomically denervated dogs, J Cardiovasc Pharmacol 16:616-623, 1990.
102. Ranheim B, Horsberg TE, Soli NE, et al: The effects of medetomidine and its reversal with atipamezole on plasma glucose, cortisol and noradrenaline in cattle and sheep, J Vet Pharmacol Ther 23:379-387, 2000.
103. Thurmon JC, Neff-Davis C, Davis LE, et al: Xylazine hydrochloride-induced hyperglycemia and hypoinsulinemia in thoroughbred horses, J Vet Pharmacol Ther 5:241-245, 1982.

104. Tranquilli WJ, Thurmon JC, Neff-Davis CA, et al: Hyperglycemia and hypoinsulinemia during xylazine-ketamine anesthesia in thoroughbred horses, Am J Vet Res 45:11-14, 1984.
105. Hsu WH, Hummel SK: Xylazine-induced hyperglycemia in cattle: a possible involvement of alpha 2-adrenergic receptors regulating insulin release, Endocrinology 109:825-829, 1981.
106. Eichner RD, Prior RL, Kvasnicka WG: Xylazine-induced hyperglycemia in beef cattle, Am J Vet Res 40:127-129, 1979.
107. Symonds HW, Mallinson CB: The effect of xylazine and xylazine followed by insulin on blood glucose and insulin in the dairy cow, Vet Rec 102:27-29, 1978.
108. Cullen LK: Medetomidine sedation in dogs and cats: a review of its pharmacology, antagonism and dose, Br Vet J 152:519-535, 1996.
109. Watson ZE, Steffey EP, VanHoogmoed LM, et al: Effect of general anesthesia and minor surgical trauma on urine and serum measurements in horses, Am J Vet Res 63:1061-1065, 2002.
110. Burton SA, Lemke KA, Ihle SL, et al: Effects of medetomidine on serum insulin and plasma glucose concentrations in clinically normal dogs, Am J Vet Res 58:1440-1442, 1997.
111. Kasuya E, Hodate K, Matsumoto M, et al: Effects of atipamezole, an alpha 2-adrenergic antagonist, and somatostatin on xylazine-induced growth hormone release in calves, Endocr J 43:551-556, 1996.
112. Kasuya E, Hodate K, Matsumoto M, et al: The effects of xylazine on plasma concentrations of growth hormone, insulin-like growth factor-I, glucose and insulin in calves, Endocr J 43:145-149, 1996.
113. Morris AH, Harrington MH, Churchill DL, et al: Growth hormone stimulation testing with oral clonidine: 90 minutes is the preferred duration for the assessment of growth hormone reserve, J Pediatr Endocrinol Metab 14:1657-1660, 2001.
114. Smyth DD, Umemura S, Pettinger WA: Alpha 2-adrenoceptor antagonism of vasopressin-induced changes in sodium excretion, Am J Physiol 248:F767-F772, 1985.
115. Stanton B, Puglisi E, Gellai M: Localization of alpha 2-adrenoceptor-mediated increase in renal Na^+, K^+, and water excretion, Am J Physiol 252:F1016-F1021, 1987.
116. Kimura T, Share L, Wang BC, et al: The role of central adrenoreceptors in the control of vasopressin release and blood pressure, Endocrinology 108:1829-1836, 1981.
117. Peskind ER, Raskind MA, Leake RD, et al: Clonidine decreases plasma and cerebrospinal fluid arginine vasopressin but not oxytocin in humans, Neuroendocrinology 46:395-400, 1987.
118. Saleh N, Aoki M, Shimada T, et al: Renal effects of medetomidine in isoflurane-anesthetized dogs with special reference to its diuretic action, J Vet Med Sci 67:461-465, 2005.
119. Pettinger WA: Renal alpha 2-adrenergic receptors and hypertension, Hypertension 9:3-6, 1987.
120. Chen M, Lee J, Huang BS, et al: Clonidine and morphine increase atrial natriuretic peptide secretion in anesthetized rats, Proc Soc Exp Biol Med 191:299-303, 1989.
121. DiJoseph JF, Taylor JA, Mir GN: Alpha-2 receptors in the gastrointestinal system: a new therapeutic approach, Life Sci 35:1031-1042, 1984.
122. Watkins J, FitzGerald G, Zamboulis C, et al: Absence of opiate and histamine H2 receptor-mediated effects of clonidine, Clin Pharmacol Ther 28:605-610, 1980.
123. Wikberg J: Localization of adrenergic receptors in guinea pig ileum and rabbit jejunum to cholinergic neurons and to smooth muscle cells, Acta Physiol Scand 99:190-207, 1977.
124. Savola M, Savola JM, Puurunen J: Alpha 2-adrenoceptor-mediated inhibition of gastric acid secretion by medetomidine is efficiently antagonized by atipamezole in rats, Arch Int Pharmacodyn Ther 301:267-276, 1989.
125. Maugeri S, Ferre JP, Intorre L, et al: Effects of medetomidine on intestinal and colonic motility in the dog, J Vet Pharmacol Ther 17:148-154, 1994.
126. Nakamura K, Hara S, Tomizawa N: The effects of medetomidine and xylazine on gastrointestinal motility and gastrin release in the dog, J Vet Pharmacol Ther 20:290-295, 1997.
127. Asai T, Mapleson WW, Power I: Differential effects of clonidine and dexmedetomidine on gastric emptying and gastrointestinal transit in the rat, Br J Anaesth 78:301-307, 1997.
128. Wooldridge AA, Eades SC, Hosgood GL, et al: Effects of treatment with oxytocin, xylazine butorphanol, guaifenesin, acepromazine, and detomidine on esophageal manometric pressure in conscious horses, Am J Vet Res 63:1738-1744, 2002.
129. Herbert MK, Roth-Goldbrunner S, Holzer P, et al: Clonidine and dexmedetomidine potently inhibit peristalsis in the Guinea pig ileum in vitro, Anesthesiology 97:1491-1499, 2002.
130. Zullian C, Menozzi A, Pozzoli C, et al: Effects of alpha2-adrenergic drugs on small intestinal motility in the horse: an in vitro study, Vet J 187:342-346, 2011.
131. England GC, Clarke KW: The use of medetomidine/fentanyl combinations in dogs, Acta Vet Scand Suppl 85:179-186, 1989.
132. Nilsfors L, Garmer L, Adolfsson A: Sedative and analgesic effects of medetomidine in dogs—an open clinical study, Acta Vet Scand Suppl 85:155-159, 1989.
133. Vaha-Vahe T: Clinical evaluation of medetomidine, a novel sedative and analgesic drug for dogs and cats, Acta Vet Scand 30:267-273, 1989.
134. Vainio O: Introduction to the clinical pharmacology of medetomidine, Acta Vet Scand Suppl 85:85-88, 1989.
135. Pettifer GR, Dyson DH: Comparison of medetomidine and fentanyl-droperidol in dogs: sedation, analgesia, arterial blood gases and lactate levels, Can J Vet Res 57:99-105, 1993.
136. Amend JF, Klavano PA: Xylazine: a new sedative-analgesic with predictable emetic properties in the cat, Vet Med Small Anim Clin 68:741-744, 1973.
137. Hikasa Y, Takase K, Ogasawara S: Evidence for the involvement of alpha 2-adrenoceptors in the emetic action of xylazine in cats, Am J Vet Res 50:1348-1351, 1989.
138. Colby ED, McCarthy LE, Borison HL: Emetic action of xylazine on the chemoreceptor trigger zone for vomiting in cats, J Vet Pharmacol Ther 4:93-96, 1981.
139. Bousquet P, Greney H, Bruban V, et al: I_1 imidazoline receptors involved in cardiovascular regulation: where are we and where are we going? Ann N Y Acad Sci 1009:228-233, 2003.
140. Li P, Penner SB, Smyth DD: Attenuated renal response to moxonidine and rilmenidine in one kidney-one clip hypertensive rats, Br J Pharmacol 112:200-206, 1994.
141. Regunathan S, Evinger MJ, Meeley MP, et al: Effects of clonidine and other imidazole-receptor binding agents on second messenger systems and calcium influx in bovine adrenal chromaffin cells, Biochem Pharmacol 42:2011-2018, 1991.
142. Finn DP, Lalies MD, Harbuz MS, et al: Imidazoline$_2$ (I_2) binding site- and alpha$_2$-adrenoceptor-mediated modulation of central noradrenergic and HPA axis function in control rats and chronically stressed rats with adjuvant-induced arthritis, Neuropharmacology 42:958-965, 2002.
143. Kaliszan W, Petrusewicz J, Kaliszan R: Imidazoline receptors in relaxation of acetylcholine-constricted isolated rat jejunum, Pharmacol Rep 58:700-710, 2006.
144. Gentili F, Cardinaletti C, Carrieri A, et al: Involvement of I_2-imidazoline binding sites in positive and negative morphine analgesia modulatory effects, Eur J Pharmacol 553(1-3):73-81, 2006.
145. Li JX, Zhang Y, Winter JC: Morphine-induced antinociception in the rat: supra-additive interactions with imidazoline I_2 receptor ligands, Eur J Pharmacol 669:59-65, 2011.
146. Chan SL: Role of alpha 2-adrenoceptors and imidazoline-binding sites in the control of insulin secretion, Clin Sci (Colch) 85:671-677, 1993.
147. Kuusela E, Vainio O, Kaistinen A, et al: Sedative, analgesic, and cardiovascular effects of levomedetomidine alone and in combination with dexmedetomidine in dogs, Am J Vet Res 62:616-621, 2001.
148. Kuusela E, Raekallio M, Anttila M, et al: Clinical effects and pharmacokinetics of medetomidine and its enantiomers in dogs, J Vet Pharmacol Ther 23:15-20, 2000.
149. Afonso J, Reis F: Dexmedetomidine: current role in anesthesia and intensive care, Rev Bras Anestesiol 62:118-133, 2012.
150. Valtolina C, Robben JH, Uilenreef J, et al: Clinical evaluation of the efficacy and safety of a constant rate infusion of dexmedetomidine for postoperative pain management in dogs, Vet Anaesth Analg 36:369-383, 2009.

CHAPTER 166

ANTICONVULSANTS

Adam Moeser, DVM, DACVIM (Neurology) • Sheldon A. Steinberg, VMD, DMSc, DACVIM (Neurology), DECVN

KEY POINTS

- Treatment of seizures in veterinary medicine depends on the underlying cause. Potential causes include reactive seizures, symptomatic epilepsy, and primary (idiopathic) epilepsy.
- The main drugs used to treat seizures in an emergency setting (e.g., cluster seizures, status epilepticus) include benzodiazepines (diazepam, midazolam) and levetiracetam.
- The primary anticonvulsants used in dogs include phenobarbital, potassium bromide, zonisamide, and levetiracetam.
- Less commonly used anticonvulsants in dogs include felbamate, gabapentin, and pregabalin.
- The primary anticonvulsants used in cats include phenobarbital, levetiracetam, and zonisamide.
- A good understanding of potential side effects, drug-related toxicity, and the pharmacokinetics of a particular anticonvulsant should be obtained before using an anticonvulsant.

The treatment of epilepsy in veterinary medicine is based mainly on anecdotal evidence rather than evidence-based medicine. Although phenobarbital and bromide anticonvulsants have been used for many decades, there are still very few well-designed published studies evaluating their effectiveness. Similarly, the number of prospective, randomized, double-blind studies evaluating the use of newer anticonvulsants (e.g., levetiracetam, zonisamide, gabapentin, pregabalin) is also small. Not only is there a paucity of well-designed studies, but most studies involve small numbers of patients that are monitored for short periods of time. Therefore, when reading the information in this chapter, one should keep in mind that most of the referenced sources do not provide definitive evidence for the effectiveness of the different compounds for treating seizures in dogs and cats. Nevertheless, the need for additional therapies for patients with refractory epilepsy is real, and therefore the use of the anticonvulsants discussed here cannot be discouraged based solely on the lack of well-designed studies.

SEIZURES

Seizures and epilepsy are a common presenting complaint of small animal patients seen at veterinary clinics. In fact, 0.6% to 2.3% of all cases reporting to veterinary referral centers have been estimated to involve epilepsy.[1] *Seizure* is defined as a transient and involuntary change in behavior or neurologic status due to the abnormal activity of populations of central nervous system (CNS) neurons.[2] Seizures can be further classified as either generalized or partial seizures. Generalized seizures involve both cerebral hemispheres and typically manifest as either convulsive (motor) or nonconvulsive (behavioral, absence) seizures. Partial seizures are believed to result from a focal electrical event in one hemisphere and are further subdivided into simple partial and complex partial seizures. Simple partial seizure episodes do not result in impairment of consciousness, whereas complex partial seizures do. Partial seizures can develop into generalized seizures. *Epilepsy* refers to the recurrence of seizures over time.[3]

Epilepsy in dogs and cats can be classified by its cause. Symptomatic epilepsy is the result of a known intracranial disease process such as neoplasia, meningoencephalitis, congenital hydrocephalus, or head trauma. When symptomatic epilepsy is suspected but evidence cannot be found, the term *cryptogenic epilepsy* is used. Finally, *idiopathic epilepsy* is the term applied to the seizure state when no cause is discovered and the patient appears otherwise normal. An inherited cause or predisposition has been proposed for such cases. When seizures are due to an extracranial insult such as a toxin or metabolic disturbance, the term *reactive seizures* is used. In addition to the lack of structural CNS disease and lack of an extracranial disease process associated with idiopathic epilepsy, this diagnosis is also typically associated with a particular signalment. Seizures that result from idiopathic epilepsy in dogs usually first occur between the ages of 1 and 5 years, but onset of the disorder has been reported in younger and older dogs.[4] In dogs, idiopathic epilepsy occurs at a higher incidence than reactive and symptomatic seizures whereas in cats reactive and symptomatic seizures are more common than idiopathic epilepsy.[4] Finally, there is no reason to believe that all occurrences of idiopathic epilepsy have the same underlying cause.

Regardless of the cause of the seizures recurrent seizures (epilepsy) should be treated with anticonvulsants. Typically, treatment is strongly recommended if the frequency of seizures is increasing, if symptomatic epilepsy is suspected, or if cluster seizures (more than one seizure in 24 hours) or status epilepticus (any one seizure lasting >5 minutes, or a cluster event without return to normal between seizures) is noted. If an identifiable cause of the seizures (symptomatic epilepsy) is found, treatment of the underlying cause should also be pursued simultaneously with the administration of anticonvulsant therapy. There is some evidence that dogs with idiopathic epilepsy have a better response to treatment if it is started earlier in the course of disease.[5]

The anticonvulsants most commonly used in veterinary medicine include phenobarbital, bromide (potassium bromide, sodium bromide), zonisamide, and levetiracetam. Felbamate is another option but is not used as commonly (see later). Benzodiazepines (diazepam, midazolam, clorazepate, lorazepam) are potent anticonvulsants, but due both to their short half-life and the development of tolerance their use is generally limited to emergency treatment of episodes of cluster seizures or status epilepticus (Table 166-1). Phenytoin, which has a very short half-life in dogs and a very long half-life in cats, is not currently used with any regularity in veterinary medicine.

PHENOBARBITAL

Phenobarbital is a barbiturate that facilitates γ-aminobutyric acid (GABA)-ergic activity by prolonging the opening of the chloride channel associated with the $GABA_A$ receptor.[4,6] In addition to having GABAergic activity, phenobarbital is believed to inhibit glutamate

Table 166-1 Anticonvulsant Drugs and Recommended Dosages for Dogs

Drug	Route	Dosage
Phenobarbital*	PO, IV, IM	3-5 mg/kg q12h
Potassium bromide*	PO, PR	20-40 mg/kg/day
Zonisamide	PO	5-10 mg/kg q12h
Levetiracetam	PO, IV	20 mg/kg q8h (higher dosages tolerated well)
Diazepam†	PO, IV, PR, IN	0.5-1 mg/kg (1-2 mg/kg for rectal administration)
Midazolam†	IV, IM, IN	0.25 mg/kg
Gabapentin	PO	10 mg/kg q8h
Pregabalin	PO	2-4 mg/kg q8h
Felbamate	PO	15 mg/kg q8-12h (dose may be increased every 2 wk by 15 mg/kg/dose until effective or adverse effects noted; toxic dose is 300 mg/kg/day)

IM, Intramuscularly; *IN,* intranasally; *IV,* intravenously; *PO,* per os; *PR,* per rectum.
*May be given via a loading dose to achieve steady-state levels more rapidly.
†Most commonly used for emergency treatment of status epilepticus or cluster seizures due to rapid development of tolerance.

receptors and voltage-gate calcium channels.[6] The mechanism of action is not fully understood. Phenobarbital has a high bioavailability after oral administration (86% to 96%), and about 45% of the drug is protein bound in the plasma.[6] Phenobarbital is metabolized mainly in the liver, with about 25% being excreted unchanged via the kidneys.[6] Therapeutic levels in the CNS are reached after 15 to 20 minutes with intravenous administration.[6] Phenobarbital is considered a primary treatment option for epilepsy in dogs and cats. In dogs, phenobarbital has been reported to lead to a clinical response (≥50% reduction in seizure frequency) in 60% to 80% of dogs with idiopathic epilesy.[7-9] There are very limited data concerning the effectiveness of phenobarbital in cats, but successful treatment has been documented.[10]

The suggested dose of phenobarbital in dogs is 3 to 5 mg/kg by mouth (PO) or intravenously (IV) q12h, and in cats a starting dose of 2.5 mg/kg PO/IV q12h is suggested. If a patient has cluster seizures or status epilepticus at presentation, a 16- to 20-mg/kg IV loading dose can be administered. This dose is usually divided into four to six equal doses and administered over 24 hours. The animal should be closely monitored for extreme sedation (e.g., loss of gag reflex), hypoventilation, and/or hypotension during administration of a loading dose, and the next dose should be delayed if any of these adverse effects are noted. This loading dose is intended to achieve a serum phenobarbital concentration of 20 to 40 mcg/ml. The therapeutic serum concentration referenced in the literature ranges from 15 to 40 mcg/ml.[7,9,11] However, dosing should be based on clinical efficacy and signs of toxicity rather than serum levels alone. The risk of hepatotoxicity appears to increase above a serum level of 40 mcg/ml.[12] The half-life of phenobarbital in dogs varies among dogs and over time in the same dog, which may be due to autoinduction of hepatic enzymes responsible for its metabolism. In dogs, the half-life of phenobarbital has been reported to range from 37 to 89 hours.[8] Consumption of a low-fat and/or low-protein diet may lower the half-life and therefore the serum concentration of phenobarbital.[13] In cats, the half-life of phenobarbital has been reported to range from 34 to 43 hours.[14] Serum drug steady-state levels are reached in 97% of patients after five half-lives.[4] Therefore it is recommended that serum levels of phenobarbital be checked 2 to 3 weeks after a dosage change. Also, due to autoinduction of hepatic enzymes and potential lowering of serum phenobarbital levels with time, serum level should be measured every 6 to 12 months to evaluate the maintenance dosage.

Adverse effects commonly reported in dogs and cats receiving phenobarbital include sedation, ataxia/proprioceptive deficits, polydipsia/polyuria, and polyphagia. The sedation and ataxia/proprioceptive deficits tend to be transient and resolve within 2 to 3 weeks of starting an appropriate dosage of phenobarbital. Less commonly observed adverse effects include excitation, bone marrow suppression, hepatotoxicity, and superficial necrolytic dermatitis. Elevations in alkaline phosphatase level are common in dogs and by themselves do not signify hepatotoxicity. Elevations in alanine transaminase level are less frequent and therefore may be a more specific indicator of hepatotoxicity than elevations in alkaline phosphatase level. Thyroid hormone levels may be decreased in dogs receiving phenobarbital, and therefore therapy for hypothyroidism should not be based on blood levels alone. Elevations in canine pancreatic lipase immunoreactivity have been noted in dogs receiving phenobarbital, but many of these dogs were concurrently receiving potassium bromide.[15]

BROMIDE

Bromide (potassium bromide [KBr] or sodium bromide [NaBr]) is a halide anticonvulsant used in veterinary medicine for the treatment of epilepsy. KBr was first used in the treatment of epilepsy in humans in 1857 but since then has been replaced by newer anticonvulsants with fewer adverse effects.[16] However, KBr is still used as a primary or add-on anticonvulsant in dogs. The suspected mechanism of action of bromide anticonvulsants is hyperpolarization of the neuron via the movement of the bromide ions intracellularly through chloride channels. Bromide is administered as a compounded KBr or NaBr product. Bromide is not metabolized and is excreted unchanged in the urine. KBr has been used with success in veterinary medicine, decreasing seizure frequency in 72% to 74% of epileptic dogs.[16,17] Bromide is not recommended for use in cats due to the risk of development potentially fatal pneumonitis.

The recommended maintenance dosage of KBr is 20 to 40 mg/kg/day; the dosage is reduced by about 15% when the NaBr formulation is used. Patients that have cluster seizures or status epilepticus at presentation can be given a loading dose of KBr of 400 to 600 mg/kg PO or per rectum, divided into equal doses and administered over 1 to 5 days. Rectal administration may cause transient gastrointestinal disturbances. The recommended serum level of bromide is 0.8 to 3.0 mg/ml when bromide is used alone and 0.8 to 2.4 mg/ml when it is used in combination with phenobarbital.[16] However, dosing should be based on clinical efficacy and signs of toxicity rather than serum levels alone. The half-life of KBr in dogs is approximately 25 days, whereas in cats it is approximately 12 days, and can be affected by renal disease or decreased glomerular filtration rate.[6,16] Also, since bromide is reabsorbed in the renal tubules through chloride channels, a change the amount of chloride in the diet can affect the clearance of bromide from the body. Therefore it is generally recommended that patients receiving bromide as an anticonvulsant maintain a relatively constant diet (in terms of chloride intake).

Adverse effects related to bromide therapy include neurologic deficits (sedation, agitation or excitability, caudal paresis, ataxia, decreased pelvic limb flexor withdrawals), polyphagia, polyuria, polydipsia, and vomiting, and bromide use may be associated with the development of pancreatitis. The term *bromism* is used to denote toxic serum concentrations of bromide. Clinical signs of bromism include altered mentation, ataxia, and upper or lower motor neuron paresis. There is no clear serum concentration cutoff value at which bromism occurs, but one study found a mean serum bromide concentration of 3.7 mg/dl in dogs with bromism compared with 1.7 mg/dl in control dogs.[18] However, some dogs without clinical signs of bromism had higher levels than 3.7 mg/dl, and likewise some affected dogs had lower values. Treatment of bromism involves dosage reduction or administration of intravenous 0.9% NaCl. Another potential consequence of KBr administration is pancreatitis. A significant increase in median serum pancreatic lipase immunoreactivity was noted in dogs treated with KBr alone or KBr and phenobarbital together compared with healthy dogs.[15] However, many dogs receiving KBr therapy are polyphagic, which may lead to ingestion of high-fat food and subsequent pancreatitis. Also, KBr can cause gastric irritation resulting in clinical signs similar to those seen with pancreatitis. KBr use in cats has been associated with the development of potentially fatal pneumonitis in 35% to 42% of cats receiving bromide and is therefore not recommended in this species.[19]

ZONISAMIDE

Zonisamide is one of the newer anticonvulsant options available for treatment of epilepsy in dogs and cats. Zonisamide is used both as a primary anticonvulsant and as an add-on therapy for epilepsy. Zonisamide is a sulfonamide drug with multiple reported mechanisms of action, including inhibition of voltage-gated sodium channels, inhibition of T-type calcium channels, modulation of dopaminergic activity, enhancement of GABA activity in the CNS, and inhibition of carbonic anhydrase activity. Zonisamide has a bioavailability of about 70%, with 40% of the drug protein bound in the plasma.[20] Zonisamide is mostly excreted in the urine as metabolites (70%), although approximately 10% is excreted in the urine as the parent compound. Based on studies in humans, hepatic metabolism is important. Zonisamide has not been studied extensively in veterinary medicine, but limited reports suggest that zonisamide is an effective primary or add-on anticonvulsant. One report showed that 60% of patients responded (>50% reduction in seizure frequency) when zonisamide was used as a primary anticonvulsant, and 58% to 82% of dogs responded when zonisamide was used as an add-on anticonvulsant.[21-23] The efficacy of zonisamide in cats has not been well studied, but it appears to be a safe alternative for treatment of epilepsy in cats.

The recommended dosage of zonisamide is 5 to 10 mg/kg PO q12h in dogs and 10 mg/kg PO q24h in cats. Despite these recommendations, higher dosages have been used safely in both species. The recommended therapeutic serum concentrations are adapted from the human literature, and 10 to 40 mcg/ml is usually cited.[22] The half-life of zonisamide in dogs is reported to be about 17 hours.[20] Levels should be measured no sooner than 4 days after initiating or changing the dose of zonisamide in dogs. The coadministration of phenobarbital has been shown to shorten the half-life of zonisamide as well as the maximum serum concentration of zonisamide in healthy dogs; this effect remained for 10 weeks after discontinuation of phenobarbital therapy.[24] It is not completely clear how one should alter the zonisamide dose when both phenobarbital and zonisamide are administered simultaneously. The half-life in cats is reported to be about 32 hours, and therefore once-daily dosing is indicated.[25]

Adverse effects in both species are usually mild, but include ataxia, sedation, and gastrointestinal abnormalities (vomiting, anorexia). Adverse effects in dogs can also include those associated with other sulfonamide drugs like keratoconjunctivitis sicca (KCS) and decreases in the total thyroxine concentration. There are several case reports of an idiosyncratic hepatopathy associated with zonisamide use in dogs.[26,27]

LEVETIRACETAM

Levetiracetam is a novel anticonvulsant that is currently being used as an add-on and primary anticonvulsant in dogs and cats. Levetiracetam's suspected mechanism of action involves binding to the synaptic vesicle protein SV2A. This binding to SV2A is believed to result in decreased release of neurotransmitter into the synapse. The reported bioavailability of orally administered levetiracetam is 100%.[28,29] There is little protein binding (<10%).[6] There is minimal hepatic metabolism of levetiracetam, and about 90% of the drug is excreted in the urine.[6,29] Several open-label studies provide support for levetiracetam's use as an add-on anticonvulsant, but a more recent randomized double-blind study did not show a significant difference between the treatment group and the placebo group in the percentage of responders.[29,30] Levetiracetam also appears to be effective as an add-on anticonvulsant in cats with seizure disorders refractory to phenobarbital, with one study showing a 70% response rate.[31]

The suggested initial maintenance dosage of levetiracetam is 20 mg/kg PO q8h for both cats and dogs. Levetiracetam can be given safely as a bolus at 60 mg/kg IV for the treatment of status epilepticus or cluster seizures.[32] The therapeutic serum level of levetiracetam in dogs and cats has not been established, but the 5 to 45 mcg/ml therapeutic range mentioned in the human literature is often cited in veterinary literature. The half-life of levetiracetam in dogs is 3 to 4 hours, and a similar half-life has been reported in cats.[32,33] The half-life is decreased to 2 hours in dogs that are concurrently receiving phenobarbital.[32] A new extended-release version is available and is being administered by some veterinarians every 12 hours instead of every 8 hours. However, pharmacokinetic information related to the extended-release version is lacking in veterinary patients. Levetiracetam is well tolerated, and doses much higher than 20 mg/kg are often used without significant adverse effects.

Adverse effects related to levetiracetam administration in small animals are uncommon and usually mild. Studies have looked at high-dose levetiracetam therapy and the associated adverse effects, and have noted salivation and vomiting at dosages of 1200 mg/kg/day and ataxia and stiff gait at dosages of 300 mg/kg/day.[30] Sedation is also commonly reported as a possible adverse effect. Changes in blood chemistry values and complete blood count have not been reported to the author's knowledge.

BENZODIAZEPINES

Benzodiazepines are commonly used in veterinary medicine for the treatment of status epilepticus and cluster seizures (see Chapter 164 for additional uses). Diazepam and midazolam are the most commonly used benzodiazepines for the treatment of seizure activity. Although not used frequently in veterinary medicine, lorazepam is commonly used to treat seizures in people. The mechanism of action is believed to be facilitation of GABA-mediated inhibition and therefore increased intracellular chloride flux. Benzodiazepines have good bioavailability and achieve rapid CNS penetration (2 to 3 minutes for diazepam administered intravenously).[6] There is extensive plasma protein binding. Tolerance to diazepam has been observed after 1 week of treatment, and similar findings have been noted during treated with other benzodiazepines.[34,35] Due to the development of tolerance, benzodiazepines are typically used for intravenous treatment of status epilepticus or cluster seizures or for at-home treatment of cluster seizures using oral, rectal, or intranasal preparations.

Diazepam can be administered orally, intravenously, rectally, or intranasally. Midazolam can be administered intravenously,

BOX 166-1 ***Benzodiazepines Commonly Used as Anticonvulsants and Recommended Dosages for Dogs and Cats***[6]

Dogs	Cats
Diazepam • IV: 0.5-1 mg/kg • PR: 1-2 mg/kg • IN: 0.5 mg/kg Midazolam • IV: 0.25 mg/kg • IM: 0.25 mg/kg • IN: 0.25 mg/kg Clorazepate • PO: 0.5-1 mg/kg	Diazepam* • IV: 0.5-1 mg/kg Midazolam • IV: 0.25 mg/kg • IM: 0.25 mg/kg

IM, Intramuscularly; *IN,* intranasally; *IV,* intravenously; *PO,* per os; *PR,* per rectum.
*Severe hepatic adverse effects noted in some cats after oral administration of diazepam.

intramuscularly, or intranasally. Clorazepate is administered orally. The doses are listed in Box 166-1.

Diazepam and midazolam can also be given as a constant rate infusion for the treatment of status epilepticus or cluster seizures. The infusion rate for diazepam is 0.5 to 2.0 mg/kg/hr in dogs and 0.5 to 1.0 mg/kg/hr in cats. Tolerance is noted not only after long-term benzodiazepine therapy but also after administration of several boluses. Therefore, if a response is not noted after administration of three boluses of diazepam or midazolam, another therapy (e.g., levetiracetam) should be instituted for the immediate treatment of seizure activity. The half-life of diazepam (including metabolites) is 3 to 6 hours and that of midazolam is 1 hour.

Adverse effects include sedation, ataxia, weakness, hyperactivity, and an idiosyncratic hepatopathy in cats treated with oral diazepam. Due to the risk of severe hepatic adverse effects associated with long-term oral diazepam therapy in cats, diazepam must be used cautiously as a long-term anticonvulsant in cats.[36]

GABAPENTIN AND PREGABALIN

Gabapentin and pregabalin are two add-on anticonvulsants currently available for the treatment of refractory epilepsy in dogs. Gabapentin and pregabalin are similar structurally, and the proposed mechanism of action is also similar for both. The mechanism of action of these drugs is believed to involve binding to the $\alpha_2\delta$ subunit of neuronal voltage-gated calcium channels, which leads to inhibition of release of excitatory neurotransmitters into the synapse. The bioavailability of gabapentin appears to decrease as the dose increases but is reported to be 80% for a 50 mg/kg/day dose.[37] The bioavailability of pregabalin is believed to be the same or greater based on information in humans.[37] About 34% of gabapentin is metabolized by the liver, and similar hepatic metabolism of pregabalin is suspected based on structural similarities to gabapentin.[37,38] Gabapentin has been shown to be effective as an add-on anticonvulsant in dogs, with a 55% response rate.[39] Pregabalin has also been shown to be an effective add-on anticonvulsant in dogs, with a response rate of 64%.[38]

The suggested oral dosage in dogs for the treatment of seizures is 10 mg/kg q8h for gabapentin and 2 to 4 mg/kg q8h for pregabalin. No studies have been performed establishing a therapeutic serum concentration for either drug in dogs. In dogs the half-life of gabapentin is 3 to 4 hours, and the half-life of pregabalin is 7 hours.[37,38] Drug interactions in dogs receiving gabapentin or pregabalin have not been adequately studied, but in humans receiving gabapentin the half-life of felbamate is increased significantly.[39] The bioavailability of gabapentin is reduced in humans concurrently taking antacids.[39] Both drugs are well tolerated in dogs. There is information available pertaining to the use of gabapentin for analgesia in cats, but the author is unaware of studies examining the use of gabapentin or pregabalin for the treatment of seizure activity in cats.

Adverse effects are similar for both gabapentin and pregabalin. Both drugs may cause sedation and/or ataxia. However, these adverse effects are typically mild and may respond to dosage adjustments (including decreasing the dose of other concurrently administered anticonvulsants such as phenobarbital or KBr). Since both gabapentin and pregabalin undergo significant hepatic metabolism, unlike in humans, abnormalities in blood chemistry values may be noted.[38]

FELBAMATE

Felbamate is an older anticonvulsant that has fallen out of favor in veterinary medicine. The mechanism of action is believed to include inhibition of *N*-methyl-d-aspartate receptor–mediated excitation, along with potentiation of GABAergic activity.[40] The bioavailability appears to be near 100%, with about 22% to 25% of the drug protein bound in plasma.[41] Liver metabolism does occur, with about 30% of the drug excreted unchanged in the urine. Felbamate has been used with reported success in dogs for the treatment of epilepsy.[40]

The recommended oral dosage of felbamate is 15 mg/kg q8h, with a maximum dose of 300 mg/kg/day (toxic dose). A therapeutic serum concentration has not been established for small animals, but in people a range of 60 to 80 mg/L has been reported.[40] The half-life in dogs is 4 to 6 hours.[40] There are no known drug interactions, but care should be used in treating patients receiving other drugs undergoing hepatic metabolism such as phenobarbital. The author is unaware of any information pertaining to the use of felbamate in cats.

Adverse effects are usually not noted at dosages below 300 mg/kg/day and include ataxia, limb rigidity, tremors, salivation, emesis, weight loss, elevation of serum liver enzymes, hepatopathy, and blood dyscrasias.

REFERENCES

1. Podell M, Fenner W: Bromide therapy in refractory idiopathic epilepsy, J Vet Intern Med 7:318, 1993.
2. March P: Seizures: classification, etiologies, and pathophysiology, Clin Tech Small Anim Pract 13:119, 1998.
3. Podell M: Epilepsy and seizure classification: a lesson from Leonardo, J Vet Intern Med 13:3, 1999.
4. Thomas W: Idiopathic epilepsy in dogs and cats, Vet Clin North Am Small Anim Pract 40:161, 2010.
5. Heynold Y, Faissler D, Steffen F, et al: Clinical, epidemiological, and treatment results of idiopathic epilepsy in 54 Labrador retrievers: a long-term study, J Small Anim Pract 38:7, 1997.
6. Vernau K, LeCouteur R: Anticonvulsant drugs. In Maddison J, Page S, Church D, editors: Small animal clinical pharmacology, ed 2, Philadelphia, 2008, Saunders.
7. Schwartz-Porsche D, Loscher W, Frey H: Therapeutic efficacy of phenobarbital and primidone in canine epilepsy: a comparison, J Vet Pharmacol Ther 8:113, 1985.
8. Levitski R, Trepanier L: Effect of timing of blood collection on serum phenobarbital concentrations in dogs with epilepsy, J Am Vet Med Assoc 217:200, 2000.
9. Farnbach G: Serum concentrations and efficacy of phenytoin, phenobarbital, and primidone in canine epilepsy, J Am Vet Med Assoc 184:1117, 1984.
10. Quesnel A, Parent J McDonell W: Clinical management and outcome of cats with seizure disorders: 30 cases (1991-1993), J Am Vet Med Assoc 210:72, 1997.

11. Cunningham JG, Haidukewych D, Jensen HA: Therapeutic serum concentrations of primidone and its metabolites, phenobarbital and phenylethylmalonamide in epileptic dogs, J Am Vet Med Assoc 182:1091, 1983.
12. Dayrell-Hart B, Steinberg S, VanWinkle T, et al: Hepatotoxicity of phenobarbital in dogs: 18 cases (1985-1989), J Am Vet Med Assoc 199:1060, 1991.
13. Maguire P, Fettman M, Smith M, et al: Effects of diet on pharmacokinetics of phenobarbital in healthy dogs, J Am Vet Med Assoc 217:847, 2000.
14. Cochrane S, Parent J, Black W, et al: Pharmacokinetics of phenobarbital in the cat following multiple oral administration, Can J Vet Res 54:309, 1990.
15. Steiner J, Xenoulis P, Anderson J, et al: Serum pancreatic lipase immunoreactivity concentrations in dogs treated with potassium bromide and/or phenobarbital, Vet Ther 9:37, 2008.
16. Trepanier LA, Van Schoick A, Schwark WS, et al: Therapeutic serum drug concentrations in epileptic dogs treated with potassium bromide alone or in combination with other anticonvulsants: 122 cases (1992-1996), J Am Vet Med Assoc 213:1449, 1998.
17. Boothe DM, Dewey C, Carpenter DM: Comparison of phenobarbital with bromide as a first-choice antiepileptic drug for treatment of epilepsy in dogs, J Am Vet Med Assoc 240:1073, 2012.
18. Rossmeisl J, Inzana, K: Clinical signs, risk factor, and outcomes associated with bromide toxicosis (bromism) in dogs with idiopathic epilepsy, J Am Vet Med Assoc 234:1425, 2009.
19. Booth DM, George KL, Couch P: Disposition and clinical use of bromide in cats, J Am Vet Med Assoc 221:1131, 2002.
20. Boothe DM, Perkins J: Disposition and safety of zonisamide after intravenous and oral single dose and oral multiple dosing in normal hound dogs, J Vet Pharmacol Ther 31:544, 2008.
21. Chung JY, Hwang CY, Chae JS, et al: Zonisamide monotherapy for idiopathic epilepsy in dogs, N Z Vet J 60(6):357-359, 2012.
22. Dewey CW, Guiliano R, Booth DM, et al: Zonisamide therapy for refractory idiopathic epilepsy in dogs, J Am Anim Hosp Assoc 40:285, 2004.
23. Von Klopmann T, Rambeck B, Tipold A: Prospective study of zonisamide therapy for refractory idiopathic epilepsy in dogs, J Small Anim Pract 48:134, 2007.
24. Orito K, Saito M, Fukunaga K: Pharmacokinetics of zonisamide and drug interaction with phenobarbital in dogs, J Vet Pharmacol Ther 31:259, 2008.
25. Hasegawa D, Kobayashi M, Kuwabara T, et al: Pharmacokinetics and toxicity of zonisamide in cats, J Feline Med Surg 10:418, 2008.
26. Miller ML, Center SA, Randolph JF: Apparent acute idiosyncratic hepatic necrosis associated with zonisamide administration in a dog, J Vet Intern Med 25:1156, 2011.
27. Schwartz M, Munana KR, Olby NJ: Possible drug-induced hepatopathy in a dog receiving zonisamide monotherapy for treatment of cryptogenic epilepsy, J Vet Med Sci 73:1505, 2011.
28. Moore SA, Mununa KR, Papich MG, et al: Levetiracetam pharmacokinetics in healthy dogs following oral administration of single and multiple doses, Am J Vet Res 71:337, 2010.
29. Munana KR, Thomas WB, Inzana KD, et al: Evaluation of levetiracetam as adjunctive treatment for refractory canine epilepsy: a randomized, placebo-controlled, crossover trial, J Vet Intern Med 26:341, 2012.
30. Volk HA, Matiasek LA, Feliu-Pascual A, et al: The efficacy and tolerability of levetiracetam in pharmacoresistant epileptic dogs, Vet J 176:310, 2008.
31. Bailey KS, Dewey CW, Boothe DM, et al: Levetiracetam as an adjunct to phenobarbital treatment in cats with suspected idiopathic epilepsy, J Am Vet Med Assoc 232:867, 2008.
32. Hardy BT, Patterson EE, Cloyd JM, et al: Double-masked, placebo-controlled study of intravenous levetiracetam for the treatment of status epilepticus and acute repetitive seizures in dogs, J Vet Intern Med 26:334, 2012.
33. Carnes MB, Axlund TW, Boothe DM: Pharmacokinetics of levetiracetam after oral and intravenous administration of a single dose to clinically normal cats, Am J Vet Res 72:1247, 2011.
34. Frey HH, Phillipin HP, Scheuler W: Development of tolerance to the anticonvulsant effect of diazepam in dogs, Eur J Pharmacol 104:27, 1984.
35. Scherkl R, Kurudi D, Frey HH: Clorazepate in dogs: tolerance to the anticonvulsant effect and signs of physical dependence, Epilepsy Res 3:144, 1989.
36. Center SA, Elston TH, Rowland PH, et al: Fulminant hepatic failure associated with oral administration of diazepam in 11 cats, J Am Vet Med Assoc 209:618, 1996.
37. Govendir M, Perkins M, Malik R: Improving seizure control in dogs with refractory epilepsy using gabapentin as an adjunctive agent, Aus Vet J 83:602, 2005.
38. Dewey C, Cerda-Gonzalez S, Levine J, et al: Pregabalin as an adjunct to phenobarbital, potassium bromide, or a combination of phenobarbital and potassium bromide for treatment of dogs with suspected idiopathic epilepsy, J Am Vet Med Assoc 235:1442, 2009.
39. Platt S, Adams V, Garosi L, et al: Treatment with gabapentin of 11 dogs with refractory idiopathic epilepsy, Vet Rec 159:881, 2006.
40. Ruehlmann D, Podell M, March P: Treatment of partial seizures and seizure-like activity with felbamate in six dogs, J Small Anim Pract 42:403, 2001.
41. Adusumalli V, Yang J, Wong K, et al: Felbamate pharmacokinetics in the rat, rabbit, and dog, Drug Metab Dispos 19:1116, 1991.

CHAPTER 167
ANTIPLATELET DRUGS

Benjamin M. Brainard, VMD, DACVAA, DACVECC

KEY POINTS

- Certain disease states may be associated with increased platelet reactivity, and the use of specific platelet antagonist drugs may help to decrease overall platelet activity and aggregation.
- Platelet antagonist drugs are designed to interfere with the release or function of platelet-activating substances or with the integration of platelets into a clot.
- Clopidogrel is an adenosine diphosphate receptor antagonist that effectively decreases platelet aggregation in veterinary species.
- Nonsteroidal antiinflammatory drugs can decrease platelet aggregation by interfering with the production of the potent platelet agonist thromboxane A_2.
- Newer platelet antagonist drugs may also have a role in veterinary medicine, pending further study in clinical patients.

The primary indication for drugs that inhibit platelet function is a real or perceived hypercoagulable state or a state of increased platelet reactivity. In human medicine, platelets are thought to play a major role in arterial thromboembolic disease (e.g., formation and rupture of atherosclerotic plaques), whereas venous thrombosis is generally treated with drugs that inhibit the coagulation cascade.[1] In veterinary medicine, the distinction between arterial and venous thrombotic risk has not been fully described for many diseases, and antiplatelet therapy is frequently used in patients with hypercoagulable tendencies, primarily because of ease of administration, safety, and simplicity of therapeutic monitoring.

PLATELET PHYSIOLOGY

In vivo, platelet activation is initiated by interaction of the platelet with a number of different factors, including von Willebrand factor (vWF), subendothelial collagen, and other activated platelets. Endothelial injury results in exposure of subendothelial collagen and release of vWF from the endothelial Weibel-Palade bodies. The released vWF can bind to the endothelial cell membrane and to exposed collagen, which helps to localize large vWF multimers near sites of vessel injury.[2] The shear stress caused by fast-flowing arterial blood exposes platelet binding sites on vWF that increase the affinity for the platelet glycoprotein Ib (GPIb) receptor.[3] The activation in rapidly flowing blood is one reason that platelets are associated more with arterial thrombosis. After vWF tethering of the platelet, platelet activation is promoted by close association of the platelet with subendothelial collagen, which can activate platelets via specific receptor interactions (e.g., $\alpha_2\beta_1$ and GPVI). Circulating vWF multimers may also associate with exposed collagen after vessel injury, which also promotes platelet recruitment to the area of injury.[4] In the presence of inflammation, changes to endothelial cells and the integrin and selectin profile of their membranes can also support platelet tethering and activation.[5]

With activation, the platelet changes from a smooth discoid shape into a more ameboid shape with filopodia.[5] Cytoskeletal reorganization associated with the shape change also results in the release of the contents of the α-granules and dense granules, which contain substances that recruit and activate additional platelets to the forming clot. The α-granules contain adhesion molecules (e.g., P selectin, vWF, thrombospondin, GPIIb/IIIa [integrin $\alpha_{IIb}\beta_3$]) and coagulation factors (e.g., factors V and VIII and fibrinogen). The dense granules contain smaller ions and nucleotides (e.g., Ca^{2+}, adenosine diphosphate [ADP], adenosine triphosphate, serotonin, histamine).[5] The final change that occurs with platelet activation is a change in the platelet membrane; rearrangement of the membrane phospholipids provides a surface that supports the formation of the complexes that activate factor X (the tenase complex) and factor II (the prothrombinase complex).[5] This final alteration closely links platelet activation to the initiation of secondary hemostasis and clot formation.

Receptors are present on the platelet surface for agonist substances that promote activation (Figure 167-1). The majority of receptors are seven-transmembrane G protein–coupled receptors (GPCRs). There are GPCRs for ADP ($P2Y_1$, $P2Y_{12}$), thrombin (PAR1, PAR4), thromboxane (TP), serotonin ($5\text{-}HT_{2A}$), and epinephrine (β_2-adrenergic) among other agonists. Integrin receptors are linked to cytoskeletal elements and recognize collagen ($\alpha_2\beta_1$) and fibrinogen ($\alpha_{IIb}\beta_3$, also known as the *GPIIb/IIIa receptor*). GPVI is also activated by collagen. The GPIb/IX/V complex, which binds vWF, P selectin, and collagen, is a member of the leucine-rich receptor class. The full host of platelet surface receptors and their actions has been reviewed recently.[5]

Drugs used for antiplatelet therapy primarily have effects on the interactions of various agonists with their specific receptors or on the production of the agonists themselves (Figure 167-2). Although most drugs do not completely inhibit activation of platelets (because there are many redundant activation pathways via the other receptors), they result in a significant decrease of in vitro and in vivo platelet aggregation and have proven benefits for humans with cardiovascular disease. Other drugs eliminate platelet aggregation entirely by inhibiting the ability of the platelet to bind fibrinogen, which is the final common pathway of all platelet agonists.

ANTIPLATELET DRUGS

Adenosine Diphosphate Receptor Antagonists

There are two ADP receptors on the platelet, the $P2Y_1$ receptor and the $P2Y_{12}$ receptor. ADP is released from the α-granules of activated platelets, and so interaction with these platelet surface receptors helps to amplify the platelet aggregation response. Interaction of ADP with both receptors is necessary for full ADP-induced platelet aggregation, but each receptor contributes slightly different platelet effects, which may also differ among species. Agonism at the $P2Y_1$ receptor is associated with platelet shape change and mild, reversible aggregation,[6] whereas agonism at the $P2Y_{12}$ receptor is associated with integrin activation and platelet granule secretion. ADP agonism at $P2Y_{12}$ also

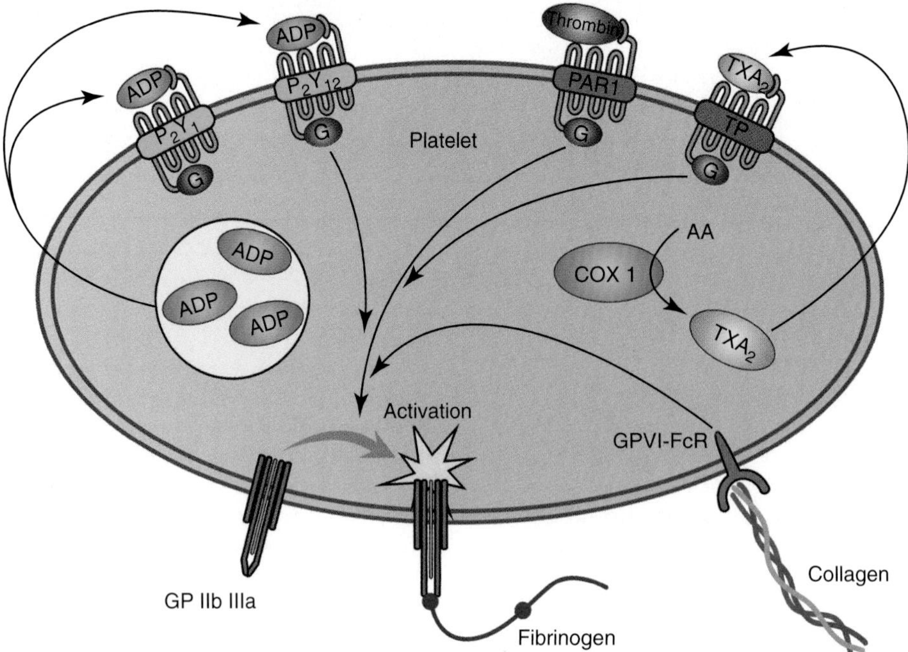

FIGURE 167-1 Schematic of pathways for platelet activation. Many G protein–coupled receptors activate the fibrinogen receptor glycoprotein IIb/IIIa (GPIIb/IIIa) after interaction with specific agonists, including thrombin, adenosine diphosphate (ADP), and thromboxane A_2 (TXA_2). ADP is released from platelet α-granules, and TXA_2 is produced by cyclooxygenase (COX) transformation of membrane-derived arachidonic acid (AA). Collagen also activates the platelet via the GPVI receptor.

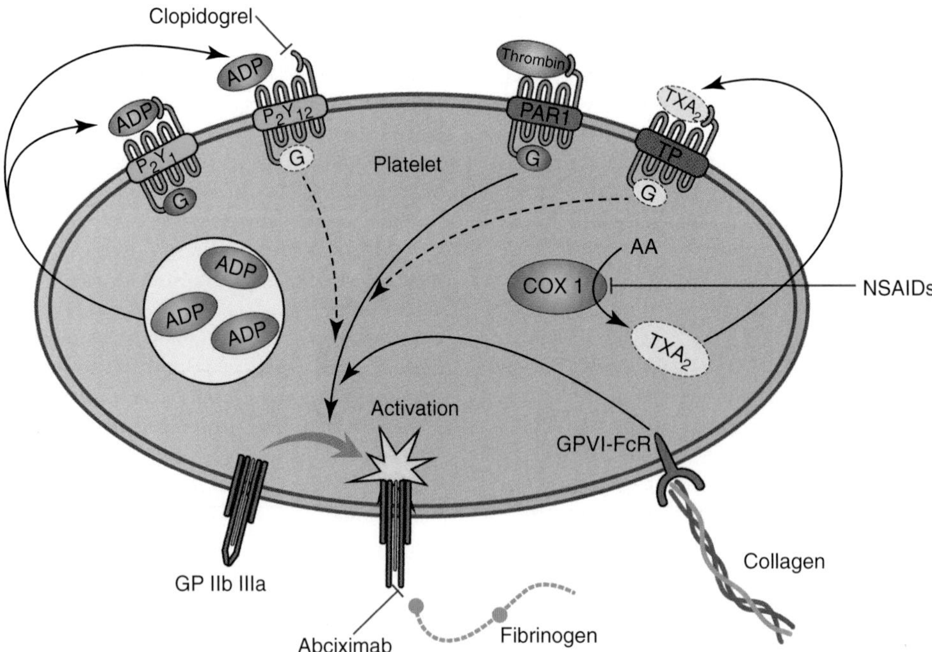

FIGURE 167-2 Same schematic as in Figure 167-1 showing the target receptors of the major antiplatelet medications. Clopidogrel interferes with adenosine diphosphate (ADP) binding at the $P2Y_{12}$ receptor, whereas nonsteroidal antiinflammatory drugs (NSAIDs) interfere with the production of thromboxane A_2 (TXA_2) by platelet cyclooxygenase-1 (COX-1). Abciximab interferes with the binding of fibrinogen to the activated glycoprotein IIb/IIIa (GPIIb/IIIa) receptor.

plays a role in ADP-induced thromboxane A_2 (TXA_2) production.[7] A recent paper described significant postsurgical hemorrhage in a Greater Swiss Mountain Dog with a mutation in the $P2Y_{12}$ receptor.[8] This dog did not show any abnormal bleeding before surgical trauma.

Thienopyridines

The thienopyridines are a class of drugs designed to interfere with ADP-induced platelet aggregation through irreversible binding to the platelet $P2Y_{12}$ receptor. Thienopyridines available for clinical use include clopidogrel (Plavix), ticlopidine (Ticlid, discontinued in the United States), and prasugrel (Effient). All of these agents are pro-drugs requiring hepatic biotransformation into active components via hepatic P-450 enzymes. Alterations of this enzyme system (e.g., through upregulation) may result in altered thienopyridine pharmacokinetics.[9] In human medicine, ticlopidine has been supplanted by clopidogrel or prasugrel due to concerns over drug-induced thrombotic thrombocytopenic purpura (TTP).[9] TTP is also a possible adverse effect of clopidogrel therapy in humans but occurs with a lower incidence. TTP as reported in humans has not been described in the veterinary literature.

Experimental studies of ticlopidine use in cats demonstrated an antiplatelet effect (decreased ADP-induced platelet aggregation, prolonged oral mucosal bleeding time), but the drug resulted in unacceptable toxicity, including anorexia and vomiting, at the dosage at which a consistent antiaggregatory effect was seen (250 mg orally [PO] q12h).[10] Similar effects on platelet aggregation were noted in dogs treated with ticlopidine (62 mg/kg PO q24h).[11] Higher dosages were necessary to achieve the same antiplatelet effects in dogs infected with heartworms *(Dirofilaria immitis)*.[12] Prasugrel is a third-generation thienopyridine and has been evaluated under experimental conditions in dogs; the active metabolite is formed rapidly,[13] and a dose-dependent inhibition of ADP-induced platelet aggregation ensues, with a strong effect seen when the drug was administered at 0.1 mg/kg PO q24h.[14]

Clopidogrel is the most commonly used thienopyridine in veterinary medicine in the United States. Dosages of 18.75 mg per cat PO q24h decreased ADP- and collagen-induced platelet aggregation and platelet serotonin release (an indicator of dense granule secretion).[15] Clopidogrel is thus effective in decreasing the release of the procoagulant molecules from platelet granules and so may slow in vivo thrombus growth by delaying additional platelet activation. Clopidogrel has been studied in experimental[16] and client-owned[17] dogs and effectively decreased ADP-induced platelet aggregation at a dosage of 1 mg/kg PO q24h (Table 167-1).[16] One study showed significant decreases in ADP-induced platelet aggregation as soon as 3 hours following a single oral dose of clopidogrel in dogs,[16] but other studies have used a loading dose of up to 10 mg/kg, followed by a higher maintenance dose.[17] The use of a clopidogrel loading dose (up to 600 mg per person, followed by a maintenance dose of 75 to 150 mg/day) has been advocated in humans undergoing percutaneous coronary intervention for acute coronary syndrome (ACS) to speed platelet inhibition.[18] Variation in the speed and efficacy of platelet inhibition by clopidogrel has been described in humans, which may be a result of polymorphisms in hepatic P-450 enzymes and the speed of generation of the active metabolite.[19] In human medicine, patients who do not experience platelet inhibition (or experience inadequate platelet inhibition or recurrent thrombotic events) while being treated with traditional doses of clopidogrel have been identified and are generally described as having clopidogrel resistance.[20] Although clopidogrel resistance has not been reported in veterinary medicine, it seems likely that variability in P-450 enzyme activity is present in dogs and cats as well, and platelet function testing is recommended in patients who do not respond as expected to clopidogrel therapy.

Table 167-1 Reported Dosing Regimens for Antiplatelet Agents in Dogs and Cats

Drug	Species	Dosage	Comments
Aspirin	Dog	5 mg/kg PO q24h[30]	Analgesic dose higher
	Cat	81 mg/cat PO q48-72h[51] 5 mg/kg PO q48h[41]	Questionable efficacy at either dose
Clopidogrel	Dog Cat	1 mg/kg PO q24h[16] 18.75 mg/cat PO q24h[15]	Rapid onset of action

PO, Per os.

Nucleoside analogs

Nucleoside analogs are also designed to inhibit the effects of ADP on platelet aggregation. Unlike the thienopyridines, these drugs do not require hepatic metabolism for effect and result in a reversible inhibition of the $P2Y_{12}$ receptor. Cangrelor and ticagrelor are currently in use or close to approval for use in humans, with specific indications for platelet inhibition in people with ACS. Ticangrelor is designed for oral use, whereas cangrelor is administered intravenously. Both drugs noncompetitively inhibit ADP binding to the $P2Y_{12}$ receptor through a specific binding site.[21] The nucleoside analogs provide rapid, reversible platelet inhibition; after cessation of ticagrelor therapy in humans, platelet activity returns to normal within 12 hours.[22] Cangrelor results in significant platelet inhibition by 15 minutes after the start of an intravenous infusion, with a return to normal function 1 hour after cessation of the infusion.[22] Although these drugs have been assayed in experimental dogs,[23,24] no evidence is available regarding their use in clinical veterinary patients.

Cyclooxygenase Inhibitors

TXA_2 is a potent vasoconstrictor and platelet agonist. It is produced by activated platelets via a cyclooxygenase (COX) enzyme in the platelet cytosol. Arachidonic acid from the platelet membrane is used to produce TXA_2. At least two isoforms of the COX enzyme have been identified, denoted as *COX-1* and *COX-2*. In general, platelets are thought to contain only the COX-1 isoform, but recent data from humans suggest that COX 2 may be present in the platelets of a subset of people.[25] There is some evidence that a similar phenomenon occurs in dogs as well.[26] Because TXA_2 plays an important role in the recruitment and activation of platelets to the site of vascular injury, drugs that block COX can result in a decreased rate and degree of platelet aggregation.

The archetypical COX inhibitor is acetylsalicylic acid (ASA, aspirin). ASA results in irreversible blockade of platelet COX-1, resulting in long-lasting platelet inhibition.[27] It is generally thought that platelets cannot manufacture additional copies of COX (they lack a cell nucleus), and so blockade by ASA is permanent for the life of the platelet (6.0 ± 1.1 days in dogs,[28] a similar period in cats[29]). This property is the reason for the success of "ultralow-dose" protocols; a small amount of ASA given daily will gradually result in blockade of all platelet COX in the body. Other nonsteroidal antiinflammatory drugs (NSAIDs) can cause reversible blockade of platelet COX and do not result in such profound decreases in platelet activity.[30] Because platelet COX is thought to be primarily COX-1, drugs with a high degree of specificity for the COX-2 isoform (e.g., the coxibs) are thought to have minimal to no effect on platelet reactivity.[30]

In dogs, the effect of ASA and other NSAIDs on platelet function has been extensively described. A dose of 5 mg/kg of ASA given PO q12h for 10 days resulted in significant decreases in platelet aggregation induced by ADP and collagen (see Table 167-1).[30] Carprofen administration (4 mg/kg PO q24h for 10 days) resulted in a lesser degree of inhibition.[30] These studies evaluated platelet aggregation using a low-shear system (aggregometry), which is notable considering that a more recent study in dogs treated with ASA at a dosage of 10 mg/kg PO q12h for 7 days failed to show an inhibition of platelet aggregation as measured using a high-shear system (the PFA-100 platelet function analyzer).[31] Another recent study investigating PFA-100 closure times in mixed breed dogs treated with ASA at 1 mg/kg PO q24h for 10 days showed reliably prolonged closure times in only 8 of 24 treated dogs.[32]

TXA_2 complements the second wave of aggregation; although TXA_2 has a specific receptor on the platelet (the TP receptor), TXA_2 production generally requires platelet activation. The COX activity of platelets can be assayed by using arachidonic acid alone as an aggregating agent. Although many dogs are presumed to have platelets that will aggregate when exposed to TXA_2, there are populations of dogs whose platelets do not show aggregation responses when exposed to arachidonic acid or TXA_2.[33-35] These dogs would presumably be insensitive to the platelet effects of ASA or other NSAIDs. The incidence of this trait among dogs is unknown, but it may reflect a phenomenon similar to the "aspirin resistance" described in humans who do not achieve expected degrees of platelet inhibition from ASA therapy.[20] Of 32 mixed breed dogs evaluated in one study, 50% did not show arachidonic acid–induced aggregation.[33] This is consistent with the above cited study investigating lower-dose ASA (1 mg/kg PO q24h for 10 days) that described variable ASA responses in mixed breed dogs.[32] A study of platelet deposition on polytetrafluoroethylene grafts placed in canine femoral and carotid arteries also showed that dogs who were unresponsive to arachidonic acid–induced aggregation had significantly lower platelet deposition on the graft than responders, and treating the arachidonic acid responders with ASA resulted in similar platelet deposition rates.[34]

Recent studies have evaluated the use of "ultralow-dose aspirin" protocols (usually 0.5 mg/kg PO q24h), as some authors have described this dosage, to decrease platelet aggregation, particularly in animals concurrently treated with glucocorticoids.[36,37] Unfortunately, one canine study that used thromboelastography to assess the ability of ultralow-dose ASA to mitigate the hypercoagulability induced by prednisone therapy failed to show an effect of ASA treatment, although platelet function was not independently evaluated.[36]

Cats in general have reactive platelets and may not benefit from ASA therapy due to the sensitivity of platelets to other agonists that minimize the contribution of TXA_2 to secondary aggregation. Studies evaluating ADP- and collagen-induced platelet aggregation in cats treated with ASA have not shown consistent evidence that ASA is an effective antiplatelet agent in cats, although most studies have evaluated small populations of cats, and whether there is variability in TXA_2 responsiveness (or unresponsiveness) in the general feline population as seen in dogs is unknown.

High-dose ASA in cats (approximately 15 mg/kg PO q48h) decreased collagen-induced platelet aggregation, although ADP-induced aggregation remained unchanged.[38] Better collateral circulation in cats with experimental aortic thromboembolism was achieved following an oral ASA dose of approximately 130 mg/kg PO given 1 hour before thrombosis, and ADP-induced platelet aggregation was decreased in this group.[39] Another study found that feline platelet aggregation in response to collagen, ADP, and thrombin was inhibited by ASA in vitro but was not consistently inhibited in cats treated with single doses of oral or intravenous ASA.[40] These findings are consistent with those of a more recent study that evaluated platelet aggregation and oral mucosal bleeding time in six cats following administration of ASA 5 mg/kg PO q48h for 8 days. In this study, no effects attributable to platelet inhibition were seen, although concentrations of TXB_2 (a stable metabolite of TXA_2) were significantly decreased.[41] ASA did decrease arachidonic acid–induced platelet aggregation in cats treated with 21 mg/kg ASA PO q72h for three doses[42] but did not affect platelet aggregation induced by ADP or collagen. Another study documented decreased arachidonic acid–induced aggregation following a single oral ASA dose of 25 mg/kg, and this decrease persisted for 3 to 5 days.[43] Lower single doses of ASA in this study (5 and 10 mg/kg) did not result in reliable decreases of arachidonic acid–induced aggregation.[43] Although these studies indicate that ASA decreases TXA_2 production by feline platelets, the actual effect on feline platelet reactivity or activation is still unknown.[41] It seems that higher doses of ASA inhibit feline platelet aggregation, but there is no current evidence for or against reliable efficacy for thromboprophylaxis or for clinical inhibition of platelet function.

Fibrinogen Receptor Antagonists

Fibrinogen receptor antagonists are focused on the final common pathway of platelet activation: the expression of an active GPIIb/IIIa fibrinogen receptor. Because therapy is directed at the fibrinogen receptor itself, any variability in platelet response to agonists is minimized because all activated platelets are inhibited from contributing to clot formation. Abciximab (ReoPro) was the first commercially available drug in this class; newer drugs are eptifibatide (Integrilin) and tirofiban (Aggrastat). All of these drugs are available in intravenous formulation only.

Abciximab is a chimeric Fab-fragment molecule and is a noncompetitive inhibitor of GPIIb/IIIa. Eptifibatide and tirofiban are smaller compounds that competitively block the fibrinogen binding site of GPIIb/IIIa and are more specific for this receptor than abciximab.[44] In addition, due to the competitive nature of the receptor blockade by the smaller-molecule drugs, a recovery of platelet function occurs within 4 hours of cessation of infusion of these drugs, whereas up to 48 hours may be required for restoration of platelet function after administration of abciximab.[44] Primary indications for this class of drugs in humans are percutaneous coronary intervention in the treatment of ACS and myocardial infarctions in high-risk patients. In these uses, GPIIb/IIIa inhibitors are frequently combined with other platelet inhibitors and systemic anticoagulants such as heparin.[44] The ability of these drugs to interfere with or displace platelet-fibrinogen binding has resulted in their use to prevent downstream microthrombi following percutaneous coronary intervention and may make them useful as an adjunct to thrombolysis.[44]

Little information is available concerning the use of GPIIb/IIIa inhibitors in small animal medicine. A model of induced carotid thrombus formation in cats investigated treatment with ASA (25 mg/kg PO) or with ASA plus abciximab (administered as a 0.25-mg/kg intravenous [IV] bolus followed by a constant-rate IV infusion of 0.125 mcg/kg/min). This study showed prolongation of mucosal bleeding times and a decrease in thrombus weight with an increase in carotid blood flow in the cats treated with abciximab.[45] In dogs, the in vitro addition of abciximab to whole blood prolonged PFA-100 closure time but did not affect thromboelastography variables.[46] The opportunities for future veterinary application of the GPIIb/IIIa inhibitors, especially in the context of thrombolysis, cardiopulmonary bypass,[47] and high thrombotic risk, merit further study, but their use may be limited because of the availability other, more convenient antiplatelet therapies.

Given the importance of platelets in the pathogenesis of thrombosis and thromboembolism, platelet inhibition remains an important target for novel drug therapies. Current research is directed toward the development of antagonists for the platelet thrombin receptor (PAR1),[48] the vWF receptor (GPIb),[49] and the platelet thromboxane receptor (TP).[50] In addition, new drugs may be directed against elements of the intracellular signaling pathways that support platelet activation and granule release.

REFERENCES

1. Mackman N: Triggers, targets and treatments for thrombosis, Nature 451:914-918, 2008.
2. Moake JL: Von Willebrand factor, ADAMTS-13, and thrombotic thrombocytopenic purpura, Semin Hematol 41:4-14, 2004.
3. Tsai HM, Sussman II, Nagel RL: Shear stress enhances the proteolysis of von Willebrand factor in normal plasma, Blood 83:2171-2179, 1994.
4. Lopez JA, Berndt MC: The GPIb-IX-V complex. In Michelson AD, editor: Platelets, San Diego, 2002, Academic Press/Elsevier Science, pp 85-104.
5. Goggs R, Poole AW: Platelet signaling—a primer, J Vet Emerg Crit Care (San Antonio) 22:5-29, 2012.
6. Hechler B, Eckly A, Ohlmann P, et al: The P2Y1 receptor, necessary but not sufficient to support full ADP-induced platelet aggregation, is not the target of the drug clopidogrel, Br J Haematol 103:858-866, 1998.
7. Garcia A, Kim S, Bhavaraju K, et al: Role of phosphoinositide 3-kinase beta in platelet aggregation and thromboxane A_2 generation mediated by G_i signalling pathways, Biochem J 429:369-377, 2010.
8. Boudreaux MK, Martin M: P2Y12 receptor gene mutation associated with postoperative hemorrhage in a Greater Swiss Mountain dog, Vet Clin Pathol 40:202-206, 2011.
9. Fareed J, Jeske W, Thethi I: Metabolic differences of current thienopyridine antiplatelet agents, Expert Opin Drug Metab Toxicol 9(3):307-317, 2013.
10. Hogan DF, Andrews DA, Talbott KK, et al: Evaluation of antiplatelet effects of ticlopidine in cats, Am J Vet Res 65:327-332, 2004.
11. Boudreaux MK, Zerbe CA: The effect of ticlopidine on canine platelet number, mean platelet volume, and megakaryocyte size, Vet Clin Pathol 20:56-59, 1991.
12. Boudreaux MK, Dillon AR, Sartin EA, et al: Effects of treatment with ticlopidine in heartworm-negative, heartworm-infected, and embolized heartworm-infected dogs, Am J Vet Res 52:2000-2006, 1991.
13. Smith RL, Gillespie TA, Rash TJ, et al: Disposition and metabolic fate of prasugrel in mice, rats, and dogs, Xenobiotica 37:884-901, 2007.
14. Niitsu Y, Sugidachi A, Ogawa T, et al: Repeat oral dosing of prasugrel, a novel P2Y12 receptor inhibitor, results in cumulative and potent antiplatelet and antithrombotic activity in several animal species, Eur J Pharmacol 579:276-282, 2008.
15. Hogan DF, Andrews DA, Green HW, et al: Antiplatelet effects and pharmacodynamics of clopidogrel in cats, J Am Vet Med Assoc 225:1406-1411, 2004.
16. Brainard BM, Kleine SA, Papich MG, et al: Pharmacodynamic and pharmacokinetic evaluation of clopidogrel and the carboxylic acid metabolite SR 26334 in healthy dogs, Am J Vet Res 71:822-830, 2010.
17. Mellett AM, Nakamura RK, Bianco D: A prospective study of clopidogrel therapy in dogs with primary immune-mediated hemolytic anemia, J Vet Intern Med 25:71-75, 2011.
18. Dobesh PP, Beavers CJ, Herring HR, et al: Key articles and guidelines in the management of acute coronary syndrome and in percutaneous coronary intervention: 2012 update, Pharmacotherapy 32:e348-386, 2012.
19. Camilleri E, Jacquin L, Paganelli F, et al: Personalized antiplatelet therapy: review of the latest clinical evidence, Curr Cardiol Rep 13:296-302, 2011.
20. Vadasz D, Sztriha LK, Sas K, et al: Aspirin and clopidogrel resistance: possible mechanisms and clinical relevance. Part I: Concept of resistance, Ideggyogy Sz 65:377-385, 2012.
21. Wallentin L: $P2Y_{12}$ inhibitors: differences in properties and mechanisms of action and potential consequences for clinical use, Eur Heart J 30:1964-1977, 2009.
22. Bernlochner I, Sibbing D: Thienopyridines and other ADP-receptor antagonists, Handb Exp Pharmacol (210):165-198, 2012.
23. van Giezen JJ, Berntsson P, Zachrisson H, et al: Comparison of ticagrelor and thienopyridine $P2Y_{12}$ binding characteristics and antithrombotic and bleeding effects in rat and dog models of thrombosis/hemostasis, Thromb Res 124:565-571, 2009.
24. Ravnefjord A, Weilitz J, Emanuelsson BM, et al: Evaluation of ticagrelor pharmacodynamic interactions with reversibly binding or non-reversibly binding $P2Y_{12}$ antagonists in an ex-vivo canine model, Thromb Res 130:622-628, 2012.
25. Weber AA, Przytulski B, Schumacher M, et al: Flow cytometry analysis of platelet cyclooxygenase-2 expression: induction of platelet cyclooxygenase-2 in patients undergoing coronary artery bypass grafting, Br J Haematol 117:424-426, 2002.
26. Thomason J, Lunsford K, Mullins K, et al: Platelet cyclooxygenase expression in normal dogs, J Vet Intern Med 25:1106-1112, 2011.
27. Jimenez AH, Stubbs ME, Tofler GH, et al: Rapidity and duration of platelet suppression by enteric-coated aspirin in healthy young men, Am J Cardiol 69:258-262, 1992.
28. Heilmann E, Friese P, Anderson S, et al: Biotinylated platelets: a new approach to the measurement of platelet life span, Br J Haematol 85:729-735, 1993.
29. Jacobs RM, Boyce JT, Kociba GJ: Flow cytometric and radioisotopic determinations of platelet survival time in normal cats and feline leukemia virus-infected cats, Cytometry 7:64-69, 1986.
30. Brainard BM, Meredith CP, Callan MB, et al: Changes in platelet function, hemostasis, and prostaglandin expression after treatment with nonsteroidal anti-inflammatory drugs with various cyclooxygenase selectivities in dogs, Am J Vet Res 68:251-257, 2007.
31. Blois SL, Allen DG, Wood RD, et al: Effects of aspirin, carprofen, deracoxib, and meloxicam on platelet function and systemic prostaglandin concentrations in healthy dogs, Am J Vet Res 71:349-358, 2010.
32. Flint SK, Abrams-Ogg AC, Kruth SA, et al: Independent and combined effects of prednisone and acetylsalicylic acid on thromboelastography variables in healthy dogs, Am J Vet Res 72:1325-1332, 2011.
33. Johnson GJ, Leis LA, Dunlop PC: Thromboxane-insensitive dog platelets have impaired activation of phospholipase C due to receptor-linked G protein dysfunction, J Clin Invest 92:2469-2479, 1993.
34. Freeman MB, Sicard GA, Valentin LI, et al: The association of in vitro arachidonic acid responsiveness and plasma thromboxane levels with early platelet deposition on the luminal surface of small-diameter grafts, J Vasc Surg 7:554-561, 1988.
35. Clemmons RM, Meyers KM: Acquisition and aggregation of canine blood platelets: basic mechanisms of function and differences because of breed origin, Am J Vet Res 45:137-144, 1984.
36. Dudley A, Thomason J, Fritz S, et al: Cyclooxygenase expression and platelet function in healthy dogs receiving low-dose aspirin, J Vet Intern Med 27:141-149, 2013.
37. Weinkle TK, Center SA, Randolph JF, et al: Evaluation of prognostic factors, survival rates, and treatment protocols for immune-mediated hemolytic anemia in dogs: 151 cases (1993-2002), J Am Vet Med Assoc 226:1869-1880, 2005.
38. Allen DG, Johnstone IB, Crane S: Effects of aspirin and propranolol alone and in combination on hemostatic determinants in the healthy cat, Am J Vet Res 46:660-663, 1985.
39. Schaub RG, Gates KA, Roberts RE: Effect of aspirin on collateral blood flow after experimental thrombosis of the feline aorta, Am J Vet Res 43:1647-1650, 1982.
40. Hart S, Deniz A, Sommer B, et al: [Effect of acetylsalicylic acid on platelet aggregation and capillary bleeding in healthy cats], Dtsch Tierarztl Wochenschr 102:476-480, 1995.
41. Cathcart CJ, Brainard BM, Reynolds LR, et al: Lack of inhibitory effect of acetylsalicylic acid and meloxicam on whole blood platelet aggregation in cats, J Vet Emerg Crit Care (San Antonio) 22:99-106, 2012.
42. Behrend EN, Grauer GF, Greco DS, et al: Comparison of the effects of diltiazem and aspirin on platelet aggregation in cats, J Am Anim Hosp Assoc 32:11-18, 1996.
43. Greene CE: Effects of aspirin and propranolol on feline platelet aggregation, Am J Vet Res 46:1820-1823, 1985.
44. Kristensen SD, Wurtz M, Grove EL, et al: Contemporary use of glycoprotein IIb/IIIa inhibitors, Thromb Haemost 107:215-224, 2012.
45. Bright JM, Dowers K, Powers BE: Effects of the glycoprotein IIb/IIIa antagonist abciximab on thrombus formation and platelet function in cats with arterial injury, Vet Ther 4:35-46, 2003.
46. Brainard BM, Abed JM, Koenig A: The effects of cytochalasin D and abciximab on hemostasis in canine whole blood assessed by

thromboelastography and the PFA-100® platelet function analyzer system, J Vet Diagn Invest 23:698-703, 2011.
47. Uthoff K, Zehr KJ, Geerling R, et al: Inhibition of platelet adhesion during cardiopulmonary bypass reduces postoperative bleeding, Circulation 90:II269-274, 1994.
48. Leonardi S, Becker RC: PAR-1 inhibitors: a novel class of antiplatelet agents for the treatment of patients with atherothrombosis, Handb Exp Pharmacol 210:239-260, 2012.
49. Bae ON: Targeting von Willebrand factor as a novel anti-platelet therapy; application of ARC1779, an Anti-vWF aptamer, against thrombotic risk, Arch Pharm Res 35:1693-1699, 2012.
50. Davi G, Santilli F, Vazzana N: Thromboxane receptors antagonists and/or synthase inhibitors, Handb Exp Pharmacol 210:261-286, 2012.
51. Smith SA, Tobias AH, Jacob KA, et al: Arterial thromboembolism in cats: acute crisis in 127 cases (1992-2001) and long-term management with low-dose aspirin in 24 cases, J Vet Intern Med 17:73-83, 2003.

CHAPTER 168
ANTICOAGULANTS

Amy Dixon-Jimenez, DVM • Benjamin M. Brainard, VMD, DACVAA, DACVECC

KEY POINTS

- Animals may be predisposed to a hypercoagulable state secondary to cardiac, metabolic, infectious, genetic, and inflammatory diseases.
- Hemostasis is a tightly regulated interplay among various plasma proteins, cellular factors, and the vascular endothelium.
- Anticoagulants act to slow or inhibit different steps within the coagulation pathway and ultimately result in the inhibition of fibrin formation.
- Unfractionated heparin acts with antithrombin to inhibit the activity of factors IIa and Xa, whereas low-molecular-weight heparins primarily impair the activity of factor Xa.
- Vitamin K antagonists (coumarin derivatives) impair the production of coagulation factors II, VII, IX, and X.
- Newer anticoagulants that directly inhibit thrombin or factor Xa activity show promise for anticoagulation of veterinary patients.

Hemostasis is a tightly regulated and precisely balanced interaction between various plasma proteins, cellular factors, and the vascular endothelium. This regulation allows localized coagulation at sites of vascular injury while preventing systemic thrombosis. When regulation of coagulation is disturbed, excessive bleeding or abnormal thrombus formation may result. The diagnosis and management of thrombotic disease is important in human and veterinary medicine due to the associated morbidity and mortality. There are up to 600,000 diagnosed cases of human venous thromboembolism each year, primarily manifested as deep vein thrombosis and pulmonary thromboembolism.[1] People considered at risk of thrombosis include those with inherited disorders (e.g., protein C deficiency or the factor V Leiden mutation), trauma, cancer, heart disease, atrial fibrillation, or prolonged immobilization as well as those receiving certain drugs (e.g., oral contraceptives).[1,2] In veterinary medicine, disorders of hemostasis are frequently encountered in small animal practice and in the critical care setting. Animals are generally thought to be predisposed to a hypercoagulable state secondary to cardiac, metabolic, infectious, genetic, and inflammatory diseases.[3] This chapter discusses the major anticoagulant drug classes; Chapter 167 covers antiplatelet drugs.

PATHOGENESIS

In health, an intact vascular endothelium prevents thrombosis from occurring through several key mechanisms. The endothelial cell surface is itself antithrombotic and inhibits platelet attachment through its negatively charged surface. Tissue factor pathway inhibitor (TFPI) is localized to the endothelial cell surface, where it decreases the procoagulant interaction of tissue factor (TF) with factor VIIa (FVIIa), an important initiator of in vivo clot formation. In addition, endothelial cells actively secrete vasodilators and substances that decrease or inhibit platelet activation. These substances include prostacyclin (prostaglandin I_2), ecto-adenosine diphosphatase, and nitric oxide.[4] The glycocalyx is contained within the extracellular milieu that coats the surface of vascular endothelial cells. In addition to selectins and other signaling molecules, the glycocalyx anchors heparan sulfate, a glycosaminoglycan, which promotes the anticoagulant activity of antithrombin (AT).[2] The presence of heparan sulfate markedly enhances AT inhibition of thrombin, factor Xa (FXa), and factor IXa (FIXa).[2,5] Protein C is also an endogenous inhibitor of coagulation. Activated protein C is generated when thrombin binds thrombomodulin on the endothelial surface. Activated protein C, along with the cofactor protein S, inactivates coagulation factors Va (FVa) and VIIIa (FVIIIa) and also binds thrombin, thereby decreasing fibrin formation.[6] Vascular endothelial cells also create a physical barrier that prevent prothrombotic substances such as von Willebrand factor (vWF), collagen, fibroblasts, and TF from coming into contact with the cellular and plasma proteins within the circulation.[2]

Plasma proteins that participate in coagulation must be activated from their inactive circulating form. Most of the soluble coagulation factors are serine proteases that become sequentially activated, which eventually results in the formation of thrombin from prothrombin. Traditionally, the plasma coagulation components have been described by the cascade model, which defines a series of progressive factor activation steps divided into the extrinsic, intrinsic, and common pathways (Figure 168-1). The extrinsic (or TF) pathway

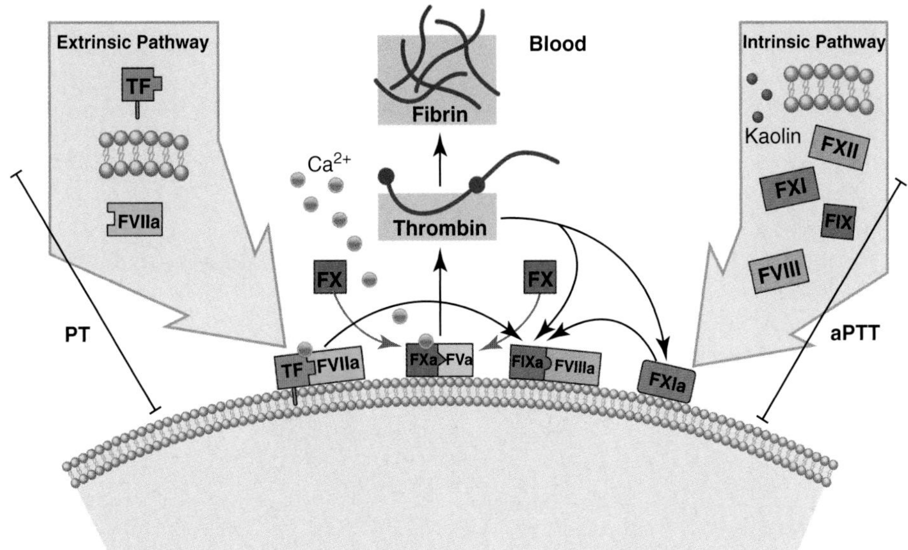

FIGURE 168-1 Prothrombin time (PT) measurement is initiated by the addition of tissue factor (TF), phospholipid, and calcium to citrated plasma. These substances interact with factor VIIa (FVIIa) and a complex is formed of TF, FVIIa, and calcium, which activates factor X (FX) to factor Xa (FXa); FXa combines with activated factor V (FVa), which then forms thrombin and subsequently fibrin; this represents the end of the test. Measurement of activated partial thromboplastin time (aPTT) is initiated by the addition of calcium, a contact activator (e.g., kaolin, ellagic acid), and phospholipid to initiate coagulation via the contact activation pathway. Activation of factor XII results in subsequent activation of factor XI, and then factor IX with its cofactor VIII. Factors IXa and VIIIa with calcium form the tenase complex, activating FX; the process progresses as described previously to result in the formation of thrombin and then fibrin, which is the endpoint of the assay.

initiates coagulation though the interaction of TF and FVIIa.[7] Clinically, the prothrombin time (PT) is used to evaluate the factors that make up the extrinsic pathway and the common (shared) pathway (see Figure 168-1). The intrinsic pathway (also known as the *contact activation pathway*) initiates coagulation through interaction with negatively charged surfaces (such as might be found on indwelling venous catheters) causing activation of factor XII (FXII) within the vascular system and the sequential activation of factors XI, IX, and VIII (to FXIa, FIXa, FVIIIa). This pathway also requires the zymogen prekallikrein and the cofactor high-molecular-weight kininogen, which has a crucial binding site for charged surfaces.[7] The intrinsic and extrinsic pathways converge onto the common pathway, consisting of sequential activation of FXa and FVa, which together promote formation of thrombin from prothrombin (factor II [FII]) and, ultimately, fibrin from fibrinogen (factor I).[8] The activated partial thromboplastin time (aPTT) is the screening test used clinically to evaluate the components of the intrinsic pathway and the common (shared) pathway (see Figure 168-1).

Despite the convenience of the cascade model, recent evidence suggests that the majority of in vivo coagulation is initiated via the extrinsic pathway.[9] The cell-based model of coagulation integrates current understanding of the interaction between the extrinsic, intrinsic, and common pathways and describes three stages of clot formation: initiation, amplification, and propagation. This model emphasizes the role of TF for the initiation of coagulation and of the need for a procoagulant surface for support of clot formation (Figure 168-2). The activated platelet surface frequently provides this procoagulant surface. Cells that express TF are typically located in extravascular locations; however, circulating cells (monocytes, neoplastic cells, and microparticles released from endothelial cells, platelets, or monocytes) can also express TF and activate coagulation in the intravascular space. A small percentage of FVII freely circulates in the vascular space in its active form and, once exposed to a TF-bearing cell, quickly forms the TF-FVIIa complex. This complex catalyzes the conversion of more FVII to FVIIa, which is then available to bind more exposed TF. Complexed FVIIa-TF supports the generation of small amounts of FVa, FIXa, and FXa.[8] Small amounts of thrombin are then formed through the action of the FXa-FVa complex (the "prothrombinase complex"). Thrombin and FIXa can then diffuse from the surface of the TF-bearing cell to nearby platelets, where the amplification stage begins.

The binding of thrombin to receptors on the platelet surface causes the surface to become procoagulant, leads to a change in platelet shape, and triggers the release of platelet granules, which contain numerous procoagulant factors.[8] Thrombin also serves to promote the production of more FXIa and FVa. Importantly, thrombin also helps to separate the components of the circulating vWF-FVIII complex so both are free to participate in coagulation. vWF is critical for platelet localization, adhesion, and aggregation at sites of vascular injury, and FVIII acts as a cofactor for FIX for the activation of FX in the tenase complex.[8]

Propagation of coagulation occurs directly on the platelet surface. FVIIIa complexed with FIXa form the tenase complex, which produces large amounts of FXa.[8] FXa then interacts with FVa to produce thrombin through the cleavage of prothrombin. If not inactivated, thrombin promotes formation of fibrin from fibrinogen and also feeds back to provide an additional positive stimulus for the formation of FXIa and tenase complexes. Fibrin molecules are then cross-linked by FXIIIa and form a matrix to seal over the site of injury.

Thrombus formation is promoted when there is endothelial damage, systemic hypercoagulability, and/or alterations of blood flow (including stasis). These determinants were first described by Virchow in 1856 and represent alterations that can occur within the arterial or venous system.[10] Readers are directed to Chapter 104 for

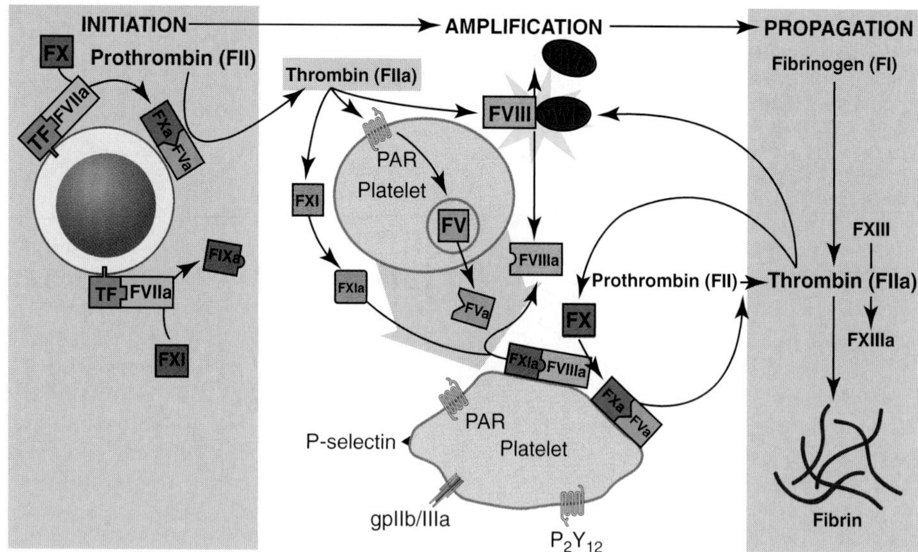

FIGURE 168-2 Diagrammatic representation of the cell-based model of coagulation. Coagulation is initiated by exposure of flowing blood to a tissue factor (TF)–bearing cell or cell particle. The combination of tissue factor with activated factor VII (FVIIa) results in activation of factor X (FXa); FXa, in combination with activated factor V (FVa) from circulation, forms the prothrombinase complex, which activates prothrombin (factor II) to thrombin (factor IIa). The small amount of thrombin formed by this initiating step triggers the amplification step. To amplify coagulation, thrombin activates circulating platelets via interactions with the protease-activated receptor (PAR). In addition, the thrombin releases von Willebrand factor (vWF) from factor VIII (FVIII), which results in activated FVIII (FVIIIa). Thrombin also promotes the activation of factor XI (FXI), which activates factor IX (FIX); the latter combines with FVIIIa to make the tenase complex on the surface of the activated platelet. The tenase complex activates FX, which combines with FVa to produce additional thrombin; this starts the propagation step. The activated platelet also promotes clot propagation; activation of the fibrinogen receptor (glycoprotein IIa/IIIb [GPIIa/IIIb]) allows binding of fibrin, fibrinogen, and vWF, which helps to anchor other platelets at the site of injury and provides additional phospholipid membranes for assembly of the tenase and prothrombinase compounds. Once fibrin strands have formed, activated factor XIII (FXIIIa; also activated by thrombin) forms cross-links between the strands to strengthen the clot.

further discussion of this topic. The amount of platelets and fibrin contained within a thrombus or thromboembolus varies based on its origin in the vasculature. Arterial clots are generally formed under conditions of high shear and include platelets held together by fibrin strands (also known as *white clots*).[11] Clots formed within the venous system and under low-shear conditions consist mostly of fibrin and red blood cells (red clots).[11] Because of these distinctions, therapies to prevent arterial thrombus formation have traditionally included medications that decrease platelet function (see Chapter 167). Anticoagulant medications directly impact the plasma coagulation system and are classically used to inhibit or prevent growth of venous thrombi in human patients. To target clotting in both venous and arterial locations, combination therapy consisting of anticoagulant and antiplatelet drugs may be used.

INDICATIONS FOR ANTICOAGULANT USE

Anticoagulant use is indicated for prevention of thrombosis in diseases that predispose to hypercoagulability. The diagnosis of hypercoagulability is difficult to make in the small animal patient and, once the condition is diagnosed, there is a paucity of information on the appropriate drugs, dosages, and monitoring for these patients. Traditional coagulation testing, such as PT and aPTT, is not optimized to detect hypercoagulability, and there is no evidence that decreased (e.g., shorter) values are indicative of hypercoagulability. Other diagnostic tests such as AT levels and fibrinogen concentration can show loss of endogenous inhibitors of coagulation or increased substrate for clot formation, whereas measurements of fibrin degradation products and D-dimers can detect excessive fibrinolysis. These tests, in general, are insensitive indicators of hypercoagulability in dogs and cats.[11] Thromboelastography (TEG) is a method that describes the changes in whole blood during clot formation and allows evaluation of global hemostasis in a patient. TEG has been used to identify hypocoagulability and hypercoagulability in dogs with immune-mediated hemolytic anemia, neoplasia, and disseminated intravascular coagulation (DIC).[12-14] Diseases in small animal patients that are associated with thrombus formation and may be indications for anticoagulant therapy include pulmonary thromboembolism, portal vein thrombosis, splenic vein thrombosis, vena cava thrombosis, aortic thromboembolism, neoplasia, immune-mediated hemolytic anemia, systemic inflammatory states, sepsis, DIC, protein-losing enteropathies, protein-losing nephropathies, hepatic disease, hyperadrenocorticism, and iatrogenic conditions (see Chapter 104).[15]

ANTICOAGULANTS

Anticoagulants act to slow or inhibit different aspects of the coagulation pathway. They ultimately result in the inhibition of fibrin formation. Importantly, they do not cause lysis or speed breakdown of existing clots. Although anticoagulant medications may prevent the extension of a preexisting clot, clots are typically broken down by the body's fibrinolytic system or through medical or surgical management using local or systemic administration of thrombolytic drugs. The most common anticoagulants used for thromboprophylaxis in people and small animals are the heparins and the vitamin K antagonists (coumarin derivatives).[2,3]

VITAMIN K ANTAGONISTS

Warfarin (coumarin, Coumadin, Panwarfin) has been used in humans for prevention of venous and arterial thrombosis for many years and is the most commonly used oral anticoagulant in people.[3,9] Warfarin administered orally to people is well absorbed, is highly protein bound, and has a long circulating half-life (37 hours), which makes it an attractive drug for long-term management of humans with myocardial infarction, venous thromboembolism, atrial fibrillation, and prosthetic heart valves.[9] There is little veterinary information on the optimal dose of warfarin and the specific diseases for which warfarin is indicated in small animal patients.

Warfarin inhibits the activity of vitamin K epoxide reductase in the liver. FII, FVII, FIX, and FX are produced in the liver as inactive zymogens that must be modified by carboxylation in the presence of vitamin K so that they are able to bind calcium and participate in coagulation.[16] During this process, vitamin K is converted to vitamin K epoxide. Vitamin K epoxide reductase is required to reduce vitamin K epoxide back to the active form necessary for coagulation factor formation. In the presence of warfarin, vitamin K cannot be recycled, which causes a rapid depletion of vitamin K and the dependent coagulation factors (see Figure 111-1). FVII has the shortest half-life, 6.2 hours, so that the first clinical sign of warfarin activity is a prolonged PT.[16] Vitamin K is also required to produce proteins C and S. Because proteins C and S function as anticoagulants, warfarin may have both an anticoagulant and procoagulant effect. In people there is a rapid reduction in protein C and S activity following initiation of warfarin therapy, resulting in a transient procoagulant state.[11] Parenteral heparins (unfractionated or low molecular weight) are used in people when warfarin therapy is initiated to prevent thrombus formation during this transient procoagulant state.

Warfarin dosing in dogs is usually initiated at 0.22 mg/kg by mouth (PO) q12 hr (Table 168-1).[17] In cats, the recommended starting dosage ranges from 0.06 to 0.09 mg/kg PO q24hr (see Table 168-1).[18,19] Among cats with arterial thromboembolic disease due to various causes (primarily cardiomyopathies),[20] those treated with warfarin had median survival times that were similar to or shorter than the median survival times of cats that were given no anticoagulant medications. In addition, the incidence of adverse bleeding events in these cats was high and included fatal hemorrhage.[20] Dogs with arterial thromboembolic disease secondary to hypercoagulability or hypofibrinolysis were administered oral warfarin adjusted to provide an international normalized ratio (INR) of 2.0 to 3.0.[6] In these dogs, warfarin therapy led to improved ambulatory function and was considered an effective treatment.

Adverse Effects

The most common adverse event associated with warfarin administration is hemorrhage, which may be severe. Bleeding can occur in the gastrointestinal and/or urinary tract but can also occur intracranially or in the pulmonary parenchyma. All of these conditions may rapidly become life threatening.

Monitoring

Warfarin requires frequent (initially weekly) monitoring by either PT measurement or determination of the INR. The INR is calculated from the PT of the patient, the laboratory reference mean PT, and the relative strength of the thromboplastin reagent (represented by the international sensitivity index [ISI])[6] as follows:

$$INR = [PT_{patient}/PT_{reference}]^{ISI}$$

The calculation of the INR corrects for intralaboratory and interlaboratory variability as well as for the use of thromboplastin reagents of varying strength. INR values can be compared across laboratories. INR values between 2.0 and 4.0 are considered therapeutic in humans, and dosing is altered based on the INR results.[2] The use of the INR has not been validated for veterinary patients, although its application has been reported for maintenance of dogs receiving warfarin therapy.[6] The intensive monitoring required in humans and small animal patients receiving warfarin may limit the number of animals in whom this drug may be safely used.

HEPARINS

Heparin is the anticoagulant chosen most frequently in veterinary medicine for prevention of thrombus growth and thromboprophylaxis.[21,22] The heparins are inexpensive and can be given intravenously or subcutaneously. They also have the advantage that their action can be readily reversed, if necessary, with protamine sulfate, which binds heparins in a 1:1 ratio. There are many veterinary studies in small and large animals that have assessed the pharmacodynamics of heparins, but direct outcome-based information on the optimal dose of heparins for specific diseases is more limited.

Unfractionated Heparins

Unfractionated heparin (UFH) is a heterogeneous mixture of glycosaminoglycans with molecular weights ranging from 5000 to 30,000 Da.[11] About one third of UFH molecules contain a pentasaccharide sequence that is necessary to bind AT. The fractions of higher-molecular-weight heparin form a large ternary complex that

Table 168-1 Reported Dosages for Anticoagulant Drugs in Dogs and Cats[17-20,28,31-33,35-40,42]

Drug	Species	Dosage	Comments
Warfarin	Dog	0.22 mg/kg PO q12-24h	Adjust using PT or INR
	Cat	0.06-0.09 mg/kg PO q24h	Monitor PT
Unfractionated heparin	Dog	150-300 U/kg SC q8h 30-50 U/kg/hr IV CRI 500 U/kg SC q8-12h	Adjust to target aPTT or anti-Xa level
	Cat	50-300 U/kg SC q6-8h 250 U/kg SC q6h	IV loading doses may be given before starting SC therapy
Low-molecular-weight heparin	Dog	Dalteparin 100-175 U/kg SC q12h Enoxaparin 0.8 mg/kg SC q6h	Optimal dosing interval unknown
	Cat	Dalteparin 100-200 U/kg SC q6-8h Enoxaparin 1.5 mg/kg SC q6-12h	

aPTT, Activated partial thromboplastin time; *CRI*, constant rate infusion; *INR*, international normalized ratio; *IV*, intravenously; *PO*, per os; *PT*, prothrombin time; *SC*, subcutaneously.

inactivates FIIa and FXa, with a ratio of 1:1 for anti-Xa to anti-IIa activity. The lower-molecular-weight heparin molecules are not long enough to bind FIIa but still have affinity for FXa and have a 4:1 ratio of anti-Xa to anti-IIa activity.[2,11] Once bound to AT, UFH inhibits FIXa, FXa, FXIa, FXIIa, and FIIa, with its most profound effects on FIIa and FXa. Heparin is considered an indirect anticoagulant since it works by enhancing the preexisting properties of AT. Heparin also has a direct anticoagulant effect by causing release of TFPI from the endothelial cell surface. The importance of this mechanism in disease states is not known at this time.[23]

UFH is highly protein-bound and also binds to the surface of endothelial cells, macrophages, and platelets.[11] Binding of UFH to endothelial cells and macrophages causes alterations in bioavailability. The activity of UFH is also lower in conditions in which AT activity is decreased. In humans, low AT levels are associated with congenital AT deficiency, acquired AT deficiency, pregnancy, severe burns, hepatic disease, nephrotic syndrome, sepsis, estrogen use, and use of certain chemotherapy agents.[2] Low AT levels have been reported in dogs with nephrotic syndrome and septic peritonitis.[24,25] The effect of AT activity on UFH bioavailability has not been studied in veterinary medicine but may contribute to the observed unpredictable anticoagulant effect of UFH in veterinary patients.

Low-Molecular-Weight Heparins

Low-molecular-weight heparins (LMWHs) contain only glycosaminoglycans with average molecular weights near 5000 Da, but have a heterogeneous distribution in this smaller size range. Between 25% and 30% of the molecules in LMWH preparations contain the pentasaccharide that can bind both AT and FIIa.[9] Due to their size, they exert their primary effect on FXa, and their use in human patients is associated with fewer major bleeding events than with the use of UFH.[2] Unlike UFH, the LMWHs are not highly protein bound and do not bind readily to endothelial cells. This makes the bioavailability of LMWH more predictable (approaching 100% in people following subcutaneous injection).[11] Due to a longer elimination half-life (3 to 6 hours), LMWHs require administration only every 12 to 24 hours in humans, which makes them more convenient than the UFHs.[2,11] Care must be taken in people with impaired renal function since LMWH is excreted mainly by the kidneys. Protamine sulfate can reverse only some of the anticoagulant action of the LMWHs because anti-Xa activity is not completely neutralized.[3] The most frequently used LMWHs in veterinary medicine are dalteparin (Fragmin) and enoxaparin (Lovenox).

Heparin Dosage

The effects of various dosages of UFH on coagulation have been studied in healthy dogs and cats.[3] Heparin is usually administered and dose-adjusted by monitoring aPTT, with the goal of obtaining a value 1.5 to 2.0 times the normal or baseline value.[26] This goal has been extrapolated from human medicine[27] and has not been extensively studied in veterinary patients. A recent study suggests a more conservative target of 1.2 to 1.5 times the baseline aPTT for therapeutic effects in dogs (based on anti-Xa activity).[28] The relationship of the aPTT value to the anti-Xa activity of heparins in vivo is not straightforward, however, and is likely affected by route of administration, inherent patient variation, and the methodology of the clinical laboratory reporting the test results.[21,29] The amount of active circulating heparin is most accurately monitored by measuring anti-Xa activity levels in plasma.[30] Human recommendations for dosing of UFH are based on anti-Xa values and target a therapeutic anti-Xa range between 0.35 and 0.7 U/ml.[27] Guidelines for dosing LMWHs in people for therapy or prophylaxis are also tied to anti-Xa activity levels. The proposed range for prophylactic use (i.e., for patients without existing thrombosis who are undergoing a procedure that may predispose them to thrombus formation) is between 0.1 and 0.3 U/ml.[27] In people with documented thrombosis or evidence of microthrombi (e.g., as manifest by ischemic skin lesions), the target therapeutic LMWH range is 0.5 to 1.0 U/ml.[27] Anti-Xa activity is generally measured 4 to 6 hours after administration. The efficacy of these drugs and the ideal anti-Xa activity levels for thromboprophylaxis or therapy in specific disease conditions have not been extensively studied in veterinary medicine, although evidence suggests that higher overall doses of UFH might be necessary for anticoagulation in patients with a hypercoagulable disease.[11]

Given the unpredictable bioavailability of UFH, empirical dosing recommendations for thromboprophylaxis in dogs vary from 150 to 300 U/kg subcutaneously [SC] q8h (see Table 168-1).[31,32] In healthy dogs given UFH at 250 to 500 U/kg, target anti-Xa activity levels were achieved at all studied doses.[11] However, when UFH was given to dogs at a dosage of 500 U/kg SC q8h, hematoma formation occurred in some dogs.[33] Dogs with immune-mediated hemolytic anemia may require higher doses of UFH (>300 U/kg SC) and/or more frequent dosing (q6h) to obtain target anti-Xa levels.[11] In one study of 18 dogs with immune-mediated hemolytic anemia, administration of UFH at 300 U/kg SC q6h resulted in presumed therapeutic anti-Xa levels (≥0.35 U/ml) in 44% of dogs after the first 40 hours of therapy.[34] Higher doses of UFH may also be necessary in animals with acute inflammation because of the tendency of UFH to bind to other acute-phase proteins.[26] High-dose UFH (900 U/kg/day intravenous constant rate infusion [CRI]) in dogs considered to be at risk of venous thrombosis resulted in hemorrhage in four of six dogs, whereas a lower dosage (300 U/kg/day CRI) did not result in target anti-Xa activity levels.[35] The study of UFH use in cats has been limited. Cats with cardiac disease are at risk of arterial thromboembolism, but there are no studies evaluating the effects of any UFH protocol for cats with this disease. Empirical dosing of UFH ranges from 50 to 300 U/kg SC q6-8h.[20,36] In healthy cats, a UFH dosage of 250 U/kg SC q6h for 5 days resulted in anti-Xa values in the therapeutic range (0.35 to 0.7 U/ml) in most cats for the majority of the study (see Table 168-1).[37]

LMWHs have been studied in dogs and cats. The expense of these drugs is still a large consideration when they are used in the clinical setting. The optimal dose and dosing interval for LMWH is not yet known in veterinary species. In dogs with TF-induced DIC, dalteparin was given as an intravenous CRI to produce anti-Xa activity levels between 0.6 and 0.9 U/ml. Achieving the target anti-Xa levels in this model was associated with less severe hematologic changes.[38] In a study of dogs in an intensive care unit, treatment with dalteparin at 100 U/kg SC q12h failed to achieve plasma anti-Xa levels greater than 0.5 U/ml.[35] Another study investigating dalteparin in dogs used a dosage of 175 U/kg SC q12h and documented mean plasma anti-Xa levels between 0.5 and 1.0 U/mL at 2 and 4 hours after administration, but suggested that a lower dose at more frequent intervals would better maintain therapeutic concentrations for the entire dosing interval without excessive anticoagulation.[39] Dogs given enoxaparin at a dosage of 0.8 mg/kg SC q6h showed consistent anti-Xa levels within the range of 0.5 to 2.0 U/ml for the length of the study period (36 hours) (see Table 168-1).[40]

In cats dalteparin and enoxaparin have rapid absorption and elimination, which results in the need for frequent injections. The bioavailability of dalteparin in cats after subcutaneous injection is approximately 100%.[41] Dalteparin given to cats at 100 U/kg SC q12h did not reliably produce target anti-Xa values (0.3 to 0.6 U/ml).[42] Results from another study confirmed that in cats LMWH needs to be dosed frequently to maintain anti-Xa levels within the therapeutic range. In this study, dalteparin given at 150 U/kg SC q4h and enoxaparin given at 1.5 mg/kg SC q6h provided more reliable achievement of target anti-Xa levels in healthy cats (see Table 168-1).[37] Dalteparin is well tolerated in cats but has not been shown to prevent the occurrence, reduce the severity, or decrease the frequency of arterial thromboembolic disease in cats.[43]

DIRECT THROMBIN INHIBITORS

Direct thrombin inhibitors are small molecules that bind to thrombin at one of two sites[44] and are indicated for prevention of arterial or venous thrombosis in humans, primarily in patients who have experienced heparin-induced thrombocytopenia or other heparin-related complications. This class of drugs includes argatroban (licensed under no trade name), dabigatran (Pradaxa), lepirudin (Refludan), bivalirudin (Angiomax), and ximelagatran (Exanta). The direct thrombin inhibitors have activity against fibrin-bound thrombin and also circulating thrombin. They also do not require AT as a cofactor for this inhibition.[44] They are attractive alternatives for thromboprophylaxis because they do not have as many drug interactions as warfarin and they do not require intensive monitoring with INR determinations.[45] Dabigatran has been shown to be noninferior to warfarin for prevention of thromboembolism and stroke in people with atrial fibrillation, but the cost of this drug has remained prohibitive.[46] Argatroban is available for intravenous administration and has been studied in an experimental dog model of cardiopulmonary bypass. This study found that argatroban was safe and decreased coagulation system activation while dogs were on cardiopulmonary bypass circuits.[47] There are no published clinical studies of the use of direct thrombin inhibitors in veterinary species.

FACTOR Xa INHIBITORS

Oral FXa inhibitors are novel anticoagulants that have been recently approved for use in people for the prevention of venous thromboembolism after total hip replacement and prevention of stroke in patients with atrial fibrillation.[48-52] Unlike UFH and LMWH, these drugs do not require AT for FXa-inhibitory activity. Rivaroxaban (Xarelto) is a direct inhibitor of factor Xa with approximately 80% bioavailability in people after oral administration.[53] The ROCKET AF study in humans compared rivaroxaban with warfarin in patients with atrial fibrillation and found rivaroxaban to be noninferior to warfarin for the prevention of stroke and systemic thromboembolism.[54] In addition, treatment with rivaroxaban was associated with less risk of intracranial hemorrhage and fatal bleeding episodes.[54] In vitro studies of the anticoagulant effect of rivaroxaban on canine and feline blood indicate that these drugs have anticoagulant effects similar to those seen in humans.[55,56] In vivo studies are ongoing and are a necessary step to determine whether veterinary species may benefit from this drug. Apixaban (Eliquis) is another oral FXa inhibitor that appears safe and has an acceptable adverse event profile in humans. An in vitro human model showed that apixaban can also inhibit platelet aggregation through the prevention of thrombin generation via the TF coagulation pathway.[57] Studies in people who have deep vein thrombosis or who require thromboprophylaxis for potential systemic thromboembolism after knee replacement surgery have shown apixaban to be as effective as or superior to currently used anticoagulants.[58,59] Apixaban has not yet been evaluated in veterinary species. Although the anti-Xa drugs can provide an attractive and safe means of oral anticoagulation in veterinary species, prospective studies are necessary to further define the indications for their use.

CONCLUSION

Coagulation abnormalities are commonly encountered in small animal practice. Diseases associated with hypercoagulability and thrombosis include immune-mediated hemolytic anemia, protein-losing enteropathies, protein-losing nephropathies, neoplasia, systemic inflammation, hyperadrenocorticism, and cardiac disease. The most effective anticoagulant and dose regimen for these diseases has yet to be elucidated through controlled, prospective studies. In addition, the tests of choice for monitoring of anticoagulant therapy and the ideal target values for aPTT, anti-Xa activity, and TEG have yet to be discovered. With new anticoagulant drugs on the horizon, the treatment and prophylaxis of thrombosis may become more tailored to the veterinary species.

REFERENCES

1. Srinivasan D, Watzak B: Anticoagulant use in real time, J Pharm Pract 25:1, 2012.
2. Tanaka KA, Key NS, Levy JH: Blood coagulation: hemostasis and thrombin regulation, Anesth Analg 108:1433, 2009.
3. Smith SA: Antithrombotic therapy, Top Companion Anim Med 27:88, 2012.
4. Couto CG: Disorders of hemostasis. In Nelson RW, Couto CG, editors: Essentials of small animal internal medicine, St Louis, 2004, Mosby.
5. Desai UR: New antithrombin-based anticoagulants, Med Res Rev 24(2):151, 2004.
6. Winter RL, Sedacca CD, Adams A, et al: Aortic thrombosis in dogs: presentation, therapy, and outcome in 26 cases, J Vet Cardiol 14(2):333, 2012.
7. Smith SA: Overview of hemostasis. In Feldman BF, Zinkl JG, Jain NC, editors: Schalm's veterinary hematology, Philadelphia, 2000, Lippincott Williams & Wilkins.
8. Smith SA: The cell based model of coagulation, J Vet Emerg Crit Care 19(1):3, 2009.
9. White HD, Gersh BJ, Opie LH: Antithrombotic agents: platelet inhibitors, anticoagulants and fibrinolytics. In Opie LH, Gersh BJ, editors: Drugs for the heart, Philadelphia, 2005, Saunders.
10. Virchow RLK: Gesammelte Abhandlungen zur Wissenschaftlichen Medizin [Frankfurt, 1856, Meidinger Sohn & Co.]. In Thrombosis and emboli (1846-1856), Canton, Mass, 1998, Science History Publications (translated by Matzdorff AC, Bell WR).
11. Dunn M, Brooks MB: Antiplatelet and anticoagulant therapy. In Bonagura JD, Twedt DC, editors: Kirk's current veterinary therapy IX, ed 14, St Louis, 2009, Saunders.
12. Wiinberg B, Jensen AL, Johansson PI, et al: Thromboelastographic evaluation of hemostatic function in dogs with disseminated intravascular coagulation, J Vet Intern Med 22:357, 2008.
13. Kristensen AT, Wiinberg B, Jessen LR, et al: Evaluation of human recombinant tissue factor-activated thromboelastography in 49 dogs with neoplasia, J Vet Intern Med 22:140, 2008.
14. Sinnott VB, Otto CM: Use of thromboelastography in dogs with immune-mediated hemolytic anemia: 39 cases (2000-2008), J Vet Emerg Crit Care (San Antonio) 19:484, 2009.
15. de Laforcade A: Diseases associated with thrombosis, Top Companion Anim Med 27:59, 2012.
16. Prater MR: Acquired coagulopathy I: Avitaminosis K. In Feldman BF, Zinkl JG, Jain NC, editors: Schalm's veterinary hematology, Philadelphia, 2000, Lippincott Williams & Wilkins.
17. Neff-Davis CA, Davis LE, Gillette EL: Warfarin in the dog: pharmacokinetics as related to clinical response, J Vet Pharmacol Ther 4:135, 1981.
18. Smith SA, Kraft SL, Lewis DC, et al: Plasma pharmacokinetics of warfarin enantiomers in cats, J Vet Pharmacol Ther 23:329, 2000.
19. Smith SA, Kraft SL, Lewis DC, et al: Pharmacodynamics of warfarin in cats, J Vet Pharmacol Ther 23:339, 2000.
20. Smith SA, Tobias AH, Jacob KA, et al: Arterial thromboembolism in cats: acute crisis in 127 cases (1992-2001) and long-term management with low-dose aspirin in 24 cases, J Vet Intern Med 17:73, 2003.
21. Pittman JR, Koenig A, Brainard BM: The effect of unfractionated heparin on thromboelastographic analysis in healthy dogs, J Vet Emerg Crit Care (San Antonio) 20(2):216, 2010.
22. Ralph AG, Brainard BM: Update on disseminated intravascular coagulation: when to expect it, when to treat it, Top Companion Anim Med 27:65, 2012.

23. Abildgaard U: Heparin/low molecular weight heparin and tissue factor pathway inhibitor, Haemostasis 23(Suppl 1):103, 1993.
24. Bentley AM, Mayhew PD, Culp WT, et al: Alterations in the hemostatic profiles of dogs with naturally occurring septic peritonitis, J Vet Emerg Crit Care (San Antonio) 23(1):14, 2013.
25. Donahue SM, Brooks M, Otto CM: Examination of hemostatic parameters to detect hypercoagulability in dogs with severe protein-losing nephropathy, J Vet Emerg Crit Care (San Antonio) 21(4):346, 2011.
26. Breuhl EL, Moore G, Brooks MB, et al: A prospective study of unfractionated heparin therapy in dogs with primary immune mediated hemolytic anemia, J Am Anim Hosp Assoc 45:125, 2009.
27. Hirsh J, Bauer KA, Donati MB, et al: Parenteral anticoagulants: American College of Chest Physicians Evidence-Based Clinical Practice Guidelines (8th edition), Chest 133:141S, 2008.
28. Babski DM, Brainard BM, Ralph AG, et al: Sonoclot evaluation of single and multiple dose unfractionated heparin therapy in healthy adult dogs, J Vet Intern Med 26(3):631, 2012.
29. Spinler SA, Wittkowsky AK, Nutescu EA, et al: Anticoagulation monitoring part 2: unfractionated heparin and low molecular weight heparin, Ann Pharmacother 39:1275, 2005.
30. Brooks MB: Evaluation of a chromogenic assay to measure the factor Xa inhibitory activity of unfractionated heparin in canine plasma, Vet Clin Pathol 33:208, 2004.
31. Brooks M: Coagulopathies and thrombosis. In Ettinger SJ, editor: Textbook of veterinary internal medicine, Philadelphia, 2000, Saunders.
32. Couto CG: Disseminated intravascular coagulation in dogs and cats, Vet Med 94:547, 1999.
33. Mischke RH, Schuttert C, Grebe SI: Anticoagulant effects of repeated subcutaneous injections of high doses of unfractionated heparin in healthy dogs, Am J Vet Res 62:1887, 2001.
34. Breuhl EL, Moore G, Brooks MB, et al: A prospective study of unfractionated heparin therapy in dogs with primary immune-mediated hemolytic anemia, J Am Anim Hosp Assoc 45:125, 2009.
35. Scott KC, Hansen BD, DeFrancesco TC: Coagulation effects of low molecular weight heparin compared with heparin in dogs considered to be at risk for clinically significant venous thrombosis, J Vet Emerg Crit Care (San Antonio) 19:74, 2009.
36. Schoeman JF: Feline distal aortic thromboembolism: a review of 44 cases (1990-1998), J Feline Med Surg 1:221, 1999.
37. Alwood AJ, Downend AB, Brooks MB, et al: Anticoagulant effects of low-molecular weight heparins in healthy cats, J Vet Intern Med 21:378, 2007.
38. Mischke R, Fehr M, Nolte I: Efficacy of low molecular weight heparin in a canine model of thromboplastin-induced acute disseminated intravascular coagulation, Res Vet Sci 79:69, 2005.
39. Brainard BM, Koenig A, Babski DM, et al: Viscoelastic pharmacodynamics after dalteparin administration to healthy dogs, Am J Vet Res 73:1577, 2012.
40. Lunsford KV, Mackin AJ, Langston VC, et al: Pharmacokinetics of subcutaneous low molecular weight heparin (enoxaparin) in dogs, J Am Anim Hosp Assoc 45:261, 2009.
41. Mischke R, Schmitt J, Wolken S, et al: Pharmacokinetics of low molecular weight heparin dalteparin in cats, Vet J 192(3):299, 2012.
42. Vargo CL, Taylor SM, Carr A, et al: The effect of a low molecular weight heparin on coagulation parameters in healthy cats, Can J Vet Res 73:132, 2009.
43. Smith CE, Rozanski EA, Freeman LM, et al: Use of low molecular weight heparin in cats: 57 cases (1999-2003), J Vet Med Assoc 225(8):1237, 2004.
44. Siller-Matula JM, Schwameis M, Blann A, et al: Thrombin as a multi-functional enzyme: focus on in vitro and in vivo effects, Thromb Haemost 106:1020, 2011.
45. Garcia D, Libby E, Crowther MA: The new oral anticoagulants, Blood 115(1):15, 2010.
46. Connolly SJ, Ezekowitz MD, Yusuf S, et al: Dabigatran versus warfarin in patients with atrial fibrillation, N Engl J Med 361(12):1139, 2009.
47. Sakai M, Ohteki H, Narita Y, et al: Argatroban as a potential anticoagulant in cardiopulmonary bypass studies in a dog model, Cardiovasc Surg 7:187, 1999.
48. Eriksson BI, Borris L, Dahl OE, et al: Oral, direct Factor Xa inhibition with BAY 59-7939 for the prevention of venous thromboembolism after total hip replacement, J Thromb Haemost 4:121, 2006.
49. Eriksson BI, Borris LC, Dahl OE, et al: Dose-escalation study of rivaroxaban (BAY 59-7939)—an oral, direct Factor Xa inhibitor—for the prevention of venous thromboembolism in patients undergoing total hip replacement, Thromb Res 120:685, 2007.
50. Turpie AG, Fisher WD, Bauer KA, et al: BAY 59-7939: an oral, direct factor Xa inhibitor for the prevention of venous thromboembolism in patients after total knee replacement. A phase II dose-ranging study, J Thromb Haemost 3:2479, 2005.
51. Abdulsattar Y, Bhambri R, Nogid A: Rivaroxaban (Xarelto) for the prevention of thromboembolic disease: an inside look at the oral direct factor Xa inhibitor, P T 34:238, 2009.
52. Wittkowsky AK: New oral anticoagulants: a practical guide for clinicians, J Thromb Thrombolysis 29(2):182, 2010.
53. Kubitza D, Becka M, Voith B, et al: Safety, pharmacodynamics, and pharmacokinetics of single doses of BAY 59-7939, an oral, direct factor Xa inhibitor, Clin Pharmacol Ther 78:412, 2005.
54. Patel MR, Mahaffey KW, Garg J, et al: Rivaroxaban versus warfarin in nonvalvular atrial fibrillation, N Engl J Med 365(10):883, 2011.
55. Conversy B, Blais M-C, Gara-Boivin C, et al: In vitro evaluation of the effect of rivaroxaban on coagulation parameters in healthy dogs, J Vet Intern Med 26:776, 2012 (abstract).
56. Brainard BM, Cathcart CJ, Dixon AC, et al: In vitro effects of rivaroxaban on feline coagulation indices, J Vet Intern Med 25:687, 2011 (abstract).
57. Wong PC, Pinto DJP, Zhang D: Preclinical discovery of apixaban, a direct and orally bioavailable factor Xa inhibitor, J Thromb Thrombolysis 31(4):478, 2011.
58. Lassen MR, Raskob GE, Gallus A, et al: Apixaban or enoxaparin for thromboprophylaxis after knee replacement, N Engl J Med 361(6):594, 2009.
59. Buller H, Deitchman D, Prins M, et al: Efficacy and safety of the oral direct factor Xa inhibitor apixaban for symptomatic deep vein thrombosis. The Botticelli DVT dose-ranging study, J Thromb Haemost 6(8):1313, 2008.

CHAPTER 169

THROMBOLYTIC AGENTS

Daniel F. Hogan, DVM, DACVIM (Cardiology)

KEY POINTS

- Thrombolytic agents are used to return patency to obstructed blood vessels and improve blood flow to infarcted organs.
- The thrombolytic process occurs primarily on recently formed thrombi because older thrombi have extensive fibrin polymerization that makes them more resistant to thrombolysis. Therefore the use of thrombolytic agents carries the greatest chance of success if they are administered as soon as possible following identification of a thrombus.
- Thrombolytic agents are used frequently in emergent patients and are commonly associated with complications such as bleeding and reperfusion injury.
- The thrombolytic agents most commonly used in veterinary medicine are tissue plasminogen activator, streptokinase, and urokinase.
- There is very little clinical experience with the use of these agents in small animals. Additionally, these drugs are quite expensive, which may limit their clinical usefulness in veterinary medicine.

Thrombolysis is the dissolution of thrombi within the cardiovascular system through the enzymatic breakdown of fibrin (fibrinolysis) by the serine protease plasmin. Endogenous thrombolysis is mediated by tissue plasminogen activator (t-PA), synthesized in the vascular endothelial cells, which facilitates the conversion of plasminogen to active plasmin. Plasmin formation takes place in an intimate association among t-PA, plasminogen, and fibrin. Endogenous thrombolysis via t-PA is modulated by multiple substances, of which plasminogen activator inhibitor and thrombin-activatable fibrinolysis inhibitor are the most notable.

Therapeutic thrombolysis is used for conditions including venous thrombosis, pulmonary embolism, systemic arterial occlusive disease, ischemic stroke, and acute myocardial infarction (Box 169-1). Supraphysiologic levels of exogenous plasminogen activators are administered intravenously to cause thrombus dissolution. The thrombolytic process works primarily on recently formed clots; older thrombi have extensive fibrin polymerization that makes them more resistant to thrombolysis. Therefore the use of thrombolytic agents carries the greatest chance for success if they are administered as early as possible following identification of a thrombus (see Box 169-1).

Multiple agents have been approved for use in people to manage pathologic thromboses, including streptokinase, urokinase, anisoylated plasminogen streptokinase, t-PA, and modified forms of t-PA (reteplase and tenecteplase). These agents vary with respect to pharmacokinetics, fibrin specificity, thrombolytic activity, and clinical response. However, there is not a tremendous amount of experience with the use of these agents in veterinary medicine, and scientific reports are limited to examination of streptokinase, urokinase, and t-PA.

SPECIFIC THROMBOLYTIC AGENTS

Streptokinase

Streptokinase combines with plasminogen to form an activator complex that converts plasminogen to the proteolytic enzyme plasmin. Plasmin degrades fibrin, fibrinogen, plasminogen, coagulation factors, and streptokinase. The streptokinase-plasminogen complex converts circulating and fibrin-bound plasminogen and is therefore considered a nonspecific activator of plasmin. This results in a systemic proteolytic state that may predispose to bleeding from loss of coagulation factors and fibrinogen, and an increase in fibrin degradation products. Although the half-life of streptokinase is relatively short (30 minutes), fibrinogenemia can persist for 24 hours.[1]

Streptokinase is produced by streptococci, which can lead to antigenic stimulation in the patient, especially with repeated administrations. Anisoylated purified streptokinase activator complex is a complex of streptokinase and plasminogen that does not require free circulating plasminogen to be effective. Although it does have many theoretic benefits over streptokinase, antigenic stimulation may still

BOX 169-1 *Recommendations for Thrombolytic Therapy in Small Animals*

Clinical Scenarios in Which Thrombolytic Therapy Should Be Considered*

Infarction of organs causing life-threatening consequences
- Cerebral infarction
- Complete bilateral renal infarction
- Complete splanchnic infarction
- Symptomatic and progressive pulmonary embolism

Infarction that may cause irreversible organ dysfunction
- Severe bilateral infarction of the pelvic limbs
- Complete unilateral renal infarction
- Severe unilateral infarction of a thoracic or pelvic limb

Infarction with severe clinical consequences that causes owner to consider euthanasia

Clinical Scenarios in Which Thrombolytic Therapy Could Be Considered

Incomplete infarction of pelvic or thoracic limbs
Symptomatic but static (nonprogressive) pulmonary embolism

Clinical Scenarios in Which Thrombolytic Therapy Should Not Be Considered

Suspected or proven coagulopathies, thrombocytopenia
Evidence of active bleeding
Infective endocarditis
Intracavitary (cardiac) thrombi
Vascularly invasive neoplastic processes

*Some thrombotic states may require surgical intervention instead of thrombolytic therapy.

occur. Use of this product has not been investigated in clinical veterinary patients.

Streptokinase typically is administered by giving 90,000 IU intravenously over 1 hour followed by an infusion of 45,000 IU/hr for up to 12 hours (dogs and cats). Unfortunately, streptokinase is no longer commercially available.

Urokinase

The renal tubular epithelium, not the endothelium, appears to be the primary in vivo source of the proteolytic enzyme urokinase or urokinase plasminogen activator (u-PA). Urokinase is similar in activity to streptokinase but is considered more fibrin specific because of the physical characteristics of the compound. Commercial preparations, derived from human fetal cell cultures, consist of both high-molecular-weight (HMW) and low-molecular-weight (LMW) fractions. Although the HMW fraction predominates, it is converted quickly and continuously within the circulation to the LMW form, which exhibits greater binding to the lysine-plasminogen form of plasminogen.[2,3]

Lysine-plasminogen, in contrast with the glutamate-plasminogen form, differentially accumulates within thrombi and thereby confers fibrin specificity to the u-PA. In addition, glutamate-plasminogen is converted to lysine-plasminogen during thrombolysis, so that the binding of u-PA to plasminogen within the thrombus is increased. It is interesting to note that for u-PA to interact with many cell types, including epithelial cells, the high-affinity u-PA receptor (u-PAR) is required.[4,5] HMW u-PA, but not LMW u-PA, binds to u-PAR, and u-PA associated with the u-PAR is susceptible to the physiologic inhibitor plasminogen activator inhibitor, which suggests a possible clearance mechanism.[6,7]

It also appears that u-PA associated with u-PAR is involved mostly in nonproteolytic activities such as cellular adhesion and migration.[8] Prourokinase, a relatively inactive precursor that must be converted to urokinase before it becomes active in vivo, is under investigation in humans. It is inactive in plasma and does not bind to or consume circulating inhibitors. As with t-PA, prourokinase is somewhat thrombus specific because the presence of fibrin enhances the conversion of prourokinase to active urokinase by an unknown mechanism. Use of this fibrinolytic agent in clinical veterinary patients has not yet been studied.

Urokinase is typically administered as a loading dose of 4400 IU/kg given over 10 minutes, followed by 4400 IU/kg/hr for 12 hours.[9,10] Urokinase is not currently available in the United States, but it may become available again in the near future.

Tissue Plasminogen Activator

The serine protease t-PA is the primary activator of plasmin in vivo; however, it does not readily bind circulating plasminogen and therefore does not induce a systemic proteolytic state at physiologic levels. Plasminogen and t-PA both have a high affinity for fibrin and thereby form an intimate relationship within thrombi, which results in a relatively fibrin-specific conversion of plasminogen to plasmin. However, the fibrin specificity is relative, and when t-PA is given at the recommended high clinical dosages, a systemic proteolytic state and bleeding can be seen.[11] Although the half-life of t-PA is very short (2 to 3 minutes), a sustained fibrinolytic state may persist as a result of protection from the physiologic inhibitors of fibrinolysis (plasminogen activator inhibitor, thrombin-activatable fibrinolysis inhibitor).[12]

The recommended dosing protocol for human recombinant t-PA (Activase) in cats is an intravenous constant rate infusion of 0.25 to 1 mg/kg/hr for a total dose of 1 to 10 mg/kg.[13] Although the clinical experience in dogs is very limited, one dog received multiple 1-mg/kg intravenous boluses every 60 minutes and another received one dose of 1 mg/kg administered intravenously over 60 minutes.[14,15] It would appear reasonable to parallel the cat treatment protocol of 0.25 to 1 mg/kg/hr intravenously for a total dosage of 1 to 10 mg/kg.

Activase is supplied in 50-mg and 100-mg bottles with an estimated cost of $1500 and $3000, respectively. Smaller amounts of t-PA can be purchased (Cathflo Activase) for approximately $100 per 2 mg. This formulation may be more cost effective for small cats or dogs and may also enable owners with budget constraints to afford treatment at the low end of the dosage range. For example, a typical cat weighing 4.5 kg could receive 2.2 mg/kg for about $500. An average-sized dog (15 kg) would require from 15 mg to 150 mg at an approximate cost of $800 to $4500.

The concentration of t-PA is 1 mg/ml when reconstituted, and the preparation is good for up to 8 hours when stored at 2° to 8° C (35.6° to 46.4° F). t-PA has been frozen in a regular freezer (−20° C [−4° F]) for up to 6 months without losing thrombolytic activity in an in vitro feline whole blood thrombus model.[16] This may allow unused portions of the drug to be stored and administered to other animals later. This has been done routinely by ophthalmologists to remove fibrin from within the anterior chamber of the eye. However, there are no preservatives in the final solution, so sterility cannot be guaranteed.

ADVERSE EFFECTS OF THROMBOLYTIC THERAPY

The most common and predictable complication of thrombolytic therapy in humans is bleeding, which may be secondary to thrombocytopenia, platelet dysfunction, hypofibrinogenemia, systemic lytic state, dissolution of hemostatic plugs, or disruption of altered vascular sites.[1,17-20] Fibrin specificity does not appear to have a large clinical effect based on human trials, in which the incidence of bleeding was similar for streptokinase and t-PA.[20] Intracranial hemorrhage, which is the bleeding complication causing most concern, is seen more commonly in patients treated with high levels of t-PA.[19] The reasons for this are not known, but the presence of abnormal vascular sites is suspected based on an increased risk in patients of advanced age.[20]

Reperfusion injury can be seen when metabolic waste and electrolytes are released from infarcted tissues. This most commonly occurs in people who develop arrhythmias after receiving thrombolytic therapy for acute myocardial infarction. The severity of reperfusion injury is proportional to the amount of infarcted tissue, and the more clinically relevant comparison with veterinary medicine may be Leriche syndrome, in which there is infarction of the distal aorta causing ischemia of the pelvic limb musculature. Thrombolytic therapy in these patients results in severe metabolic acidosis and hyperkalemia that often requires aggressive therapy, including hemofiltration or hemodialysis. Similar complications are seen with thrombolytic therapy in cats with distal aortic infarction from cardiogenic embolism (e.g., aortic thromboembolism or saddle thrombus).[9,13,21,22]

THROMBOLYTIC THERAPY IN DOGS

Streptokinase

There is very little reported experience with this thrombolytic agent in dogs. Ramsey et al described a case series of four dogs with thromboembolic disease (one pulmonary, three distal aorta) treated with streptokinase.[23] Partial resolution of the thrombus was noted in one dog, and the other three had complete resolution after one to three doses of streptokinase. All animals experienced partial or complete resolution of clinical signs, with only minor bleeding seen in three that resolved with discontinuation of streptokinase infusion. There was no evidence of reperfusion injury in this study.

Urokinase

Whelan et al[10] described u-PA use in four dogs. Distal aortic infarction was identified by abdominal ultrasonography in three of the dogs, and pulmonary embolism was diagnosed by echocardiography in one dog. The three dogs with aortic infarction had femoral arterial pulses and voluntary motor function before u-PA administration, and there was no identifiable difference after u-PA therapy. Additionally, there was persistence of the thrombi on abdominal ultrasonography. Even though there was no beneficial effect from u-PA therapy in these three dogs, one dog did develop hyperkalemia and metabolic acidosis suggestive of reperfusion injury. All three dogs with aortic thromboembolism were euthanized or died during hospitalization. The dog with pulmonary embolism was reported to have improved clinically with improved echocardiographic indexes, which suggested partial resolution of the pulmonary embolism following u-PA therapy.

Tissue Plasminogen Activator

There are two reports of t-PA therapy for aortic infarction in dogs in the literature. In one report[14] a dog showed a return of femoral arterial pulses after receiving ten 1-mg/kg bolus injections given at 1-hour intervals. However, pulses were again absent 6 days after therapy. Pulses returned after an additional two doses of t-PA, and pulse quality improved after two more doses were given within 24 hours. Short-term follow-up revealed persistence of femoral arterial pulses, normal pelvic limb gait, and resolution of the thrombus on abdominal ultrasonography.

The second report examined the use of t-PA after distal aortic infarction in six dogs.[15] All six dogs failed to improve with the administration of 1 mg/kg of t-PA over a 60-minute period with concurrent heparin therapy.

THROMBOLYTIC THERAPY IN CATS

Many more clinical data are available for cats because of the higher frequency of cardioembolic disease in this species. The incidence of hyperkalemia and reperfusion injury following embolus dissolution with thrombolytic therapy ranges from 40% to 70%.[13,21,22] Reperfusion injury represents the most common cause of death in cats receiving thrombolytic agents, with survival rates ranging from 0% to 43%.[9,13,21,22] Cats that have more complete infarction, such as bilateral paralysis, appear more likely to develop hyperkalemia and metabolic acidosis, probably because of the larger area of ischemia.[13,21]

Streptokinase

There are two retrospective studies evaluating streptokinase therapy for aortic infarction in cats. The first study evaluated eight cats, and all experienced respiratory distress and died suddenly during the maintenance phase of streptokinase therapy.[22] However, two of these cats did have intracavitary thrombi within the left atrium, generally considered a contraindication for thrombolytic therapy. One of these cats was diagnosed as having a right coronary arterial infarction on necropsy that may have resulted from fragmentation of the left atrial thrombus induced by the thrombolytic therapy.

The second study evaluated 46 cats treated for cardioembolic disease.[21] In this study approximately 50% had a return of femoral pulses within 24 hours of initiation of streptokinase therapy. Motor function returned in 30% of the cats, while 80% of those cats regained motor function within 24 hours. Cats with single limb infarction did dramatically better, with 100% regaining pulses and 80% regaining motor function. Of those cats that had infarction of both limbs, only about 50% regained pulses and approximately 25% regained motor function. Adverse effects were seen in 65% of cats that developed abnormal coagulation values after beginning streptokinase therapy. However, some of these cats were also receiving heparin.

Spontaneous bleeding from oral, rectal, or catheter sites was seen in 24% of cats, including 36% of those with abnormal coagulation parameters. Bleeding was severe enough to require transfusions in 27%, with only 18% of these cats surviving streptokinase therapy. Increased respiratory rates were seen in 30% of cats, although this was found to be caused by worsening of congestive heart failure in 21% of the small number of cats in which the underlying cause was pursued (14 of 46). Hyperkalemia developed in approximately 40% of cats and was more likely to be seen with longer infusion periods, which may be related to more complete or severe obstruction. There was an overall survival rate of 33% during hospitalization. However, about 50% of the cats that did survive the hospital stay were euthanized because of complications of therapy or poor prognosis.

Urokinase

There is one retrospective study in 12 cats reporting on the use of u-PA for the treatment of cardioembolic disease.[9] Bilateral aortic infarction was present in 10 of 12 cats (83%), with no palpable pulse in the affected limb(s) in 10 of 12 (83%) and no motor function in 9 of 12 (75%). Urokinase infusion resulted in the return of pulses in 3 of 10 (30%) and return of motor function in 5 of 9 (56%). It is interesting to note that more cats regained motor function than had return of pulses, which suggests that collateral circulation and not thrombolysis resulted in the return of function in at least some cats. Hyperkalemia developed in 3 of 12 cats (25%), including 3 of 7 (43%) that did not have return of pulses or function (which again possibly suggests a role for collateral circulation). There was no evidence of clinical bleeding. Five out of 12 cats survived (42%) and all nonsurvivors were euthanized.

There is also a case report of intraarterial infusion of urokinase in a cat, delivered after intravenous administration of urokinase as well as conservative anticoagulant and antiplatelet therapy failed to result in thrombolysis.[24] A catheter was inserted into the carotid artery and advanced to a location just distal to the renal arteries in the abdominal aorta. Urokinase (60,000 IU) was administered through the intraarterial catheter over 5 minutes and during the third urokinase administration patency of the femoral arteries was noted. Arterial flow to the pelvic limbs was considered partial, so intravenous infusion of urokinase once a day was continued for an additional 6 days with arterial flow considered normal on day 4. The cat did not exhibit any adverse clinical effects from the urokinase therapy, which may be due to the collateral circulation documented on angiography before the intraarterial administration.

Tissue Plasminogen Activator

There have been two clinical trials of t-PA therapy in cats with cardioembolic disease.[13,25] The first study reported a short-term survival rate of 50%, with deaths attributable to reperfusion injury and cardiogenic shock. Of the cats that survived, 100% had bilateral pelvic limb infarction. Perfusion was restored within 36 hours and motor function returned within 48 hours in 100% of surviving cats. Complications included minor hemorrhage from catheter sites (50%), fever (33%), and reperfusion injury (33%).[13] A more recent study of t-PA therapy in cats with arterial thromboembolism reported a 64% survival rate at 24 hours, but only 27% survived to discharge; 91% of the cats had bilateral pelvic limb infarction.[25] In the cats that survived, 50% of infarcted limbs had a palpable pulse at 4 hours after beginning therapy, and 62% had a palpable pulse at 24 hours. Complications were reported in 100% of cats and included azotemia, neurologic signs (45%), arrhythmias (45%), hyperkalemia (36%), acidosis (18%), and sudden death (9%). The study was ended early due to the high incidence of complications.

CONCLUSION

The use of rheolytic thrombectomy machines (e.g., AngioJet system) for rapid removal of pathologic thrombi is under investigation in veterinary medicine. Only one study has been published thus far and described the use of this technology in cats with aortic thromboembolism; successful thrombus dissolution was achieved in five of six cats, and three survived to discharge.[26] Surgical thrombectomy may also be indicated in some animals, especially those with organ infarction (e.g., splenic infarction). Prevention of further thrombus formation in animals with thrombotic disease, regardless of the species or cause, remains a challenging subject in veterinary medicine (see Chapter 168).

REFERENCES

1. Rao AK, Pratt C, Berke A, et al: Thrombolysis in myocardial infarction (TIMI) trial phase I: hemorrhagic manifestations and changes in plasma fibrinogen and the fibrinolytic system in patients treated with recombinant tissue plasminogen activator and streptokinase, J Am Coll Cardiol 11:1, 1988.
2. Gulba DC, Bode C, Runge MS, et al: Thrombolytic agents: an overview, Ann Hematol 73:S9, 1996.
3. Comerota AJ, Cohen GS: Thrombolytic therapy in peripheral arterial occlusive disease: mechanisms of action and drugs available, Can J Surg 36:342, 1993.
4. Blasi F, Conese M, Moller LB, et al: The urokinase receptor: structure, regulation and inhibitor-mediated internalization, Fibrinolysis 8:182, 1994.
5. Barnathan E, Kuo A, Rosenfeld L, et al: Interaction of single-chain urokinase-type plasminogen activator with human endothelial cells, J Biol Chem 265:2865, 1990.
6. Cubellis MV, Andreasson P, Ragno P, et al: Accessibility of receptor-bound urokinase to type-1 plasminogen activator inhibitor, Proc Natl Acad Sci U S A 86:4828, 1989.
7. Ellis V, Wun TC, Behrendt N, et al: Inhibition of receptor-bound urokinase by plasminogen activator inhibitor, J Biol Chem 265:9904, 1990.
8. Blasi F, Carmeliet P: uPAR: a versatile signaling orchestrator, Nat Rev Mol Cell Biol 3:932, 2002.
9. Whelan MF, O'Toole TE, Chan DL, et al: Retrospective evaluation of urokinase use in cats with arterial thromboembolism, J Vet Emerg Crit Care (San Antonio) 15:S8, 2005 (abstract).
10. Whelan MF, O'Toole TE, Chan DL, et al: Retrospective evaluation of urokinase use in dogs with thromboembolism (four cases: 2003-2004), J Vet Emerg Crit Care (San Antonio) 15:S8, 2005 (abstract).
11. Agnelli G: Rationale for bolus t-PA therapy to improve efficacy and safety, Chest 97:161S, 1990.
12. Eisenberg PR, Sherman LA, Tiefenbrunn AJ, et al: Sustained fibrinolysis after administration of t-PA despite its short half-life in the circulation, Thromb Haemost 57:35, 1987.
13. Pion PD, Kittleson MD: Therapy for feline aortic thromboembolism. In Kirk RW, editor: Current veterinary therapy X, ed 10, Philadelphia, 1989, Saunders.
14. Clare A, Kraje BJ: Use of recombinant tissue-plasminogen activator for aortic thrombolysis in a hypoproteinemic dog, J Am Vet Med Assoc 212:539, 1998.
15. Boswood A, Lamb CR, White RN: Aortic and iliac thrombosis in six dogs, J Small Anim Pract 41:109, 2000.
16. Hogan DF: Unpublished data.
17. Gore JM, Sloan M, Price TR, et al: Intracerebral hemorrhage, cerebral infarction, and subdural hematoma after acute myocardial infarction and thrombolytic therapy in the Thrombolysis in Myocardial Infarction Study. Thrombolysis in Myocardial Infarction, Phase II pilot and clinical trial, Circulation 83:448, 1991.
18. Stump DC, Califf RM, Topol EJ, et al: Pharmacodynamics of thrombolysis with recombinant tissue-type plasminogen activator. Correlation with characteristics of and clinical outcomes in patients with acute myocardial infarction, Circulation 80:1222, 1989.
19. Carlson SE, Aldrich MS, Greenberg HS, et al: Intracerebral hemorrhage complicating intravenous tissue plasminogen activator treatment, Arch Neurol 45:1070, 1988.
20. Berkowitz SD, Granger CB, Pieper KS, et al: Incidence and predictors of bleeding after contemporary thrombolytic therapy for myocardial infarction. The Global Utilization of Streptokinase and Tissue Plasminogen Activator for Occluded Coronary Arteries (GUSTO) I Investigators, Circulation 95:2508, 1997.
21. Moore KE, Morris N, Dhupa N, et al: Retrospective study of streptokinase administration in 46 cats with arterial thromboembolism, J Vet Emerg Crit Care 10:245, 2000.
22. Ramsey CC, Riepe RD, Macintire DK, et al: Streptokinase: a practical clot-buster? In Proceedings of the 5th International Veterinary Emergency and Critical Care Symposium, San Antonio, Texas, September 16-20, 1996.
23. Ramsey CC, Burney DP, Macintire DK, et al: Use of streptokinase in four dogs with thrombosis, J Am Vet Med Assoc 209:780, 1996.
24. Koyama H, Matsumoto H, Fukushima R, et al: Local intra-arterial administration of urokinase in the treatment of a feline distal aortic thromboembolism, J Vet Med Sci 72:1209, 2010.
25. Welch KM, Rozanski EA, Freeman LM, et al: Prospective evaluation of tissue plasminogen activator in 11 cats with arterial thromboembolism, J Feline Med Surg 12:122, 2010.
26. Reimer S, Kittleson MD, Kyles AE: Use of rheolytic thrombectomy in the treatment of feline distal aortic thromboembolism, J Vet Intern Med 20:290, 2006.

CHAPTER 170

HEMOSTATIC DRUGS

Angela Borchers, DVM, DACVIM, DACVECC

KEY POINTS

- Coagulopathies may arise from defects in primary hemostasis, secondary hemostasis, or the fibrinolytic system or may be of multifactorial origin.
- In situations in which transfusional therapy is not effective, is not available, or should be avoided altogether, the administration of hemostatic drugs may be considered.
- Several hemostatic agents are currently being used as blood-saving agents in the bleeding human and veterinary patient. However, they cannot replace good medical therapy and surgical technique.

Coagulopathies may arise from defects in primary hemostasis, secondary hemostasis, or the fibrinolytic system, or maybe of multifactorial origin. Although specific defects in primary or secondary hemostasis are often treated with blood products to replenish deficiencies, patients with multiple coagulation abnormalities, severe single coagulation defects, hyperfibrinolysis, or unclassified coagulopathies may not respond adequately to blood product administration. In these cases, administration of nontransfusional hemostatic drugs may be considered as alternative treatment.

Clinical disorders in small animals that may benefit from nontransfusional hemostatic drugs include von Willebrand disease (vWD), hemophilia A and B, and other hereditary coagulation factor deficiencies; hereditary thrombopathies such as Glanzmann's thrombasthenia; acquired thrombopathies; and enhanced hyperfibrinolytic states after surgery or trauma.

Briefly, according to our current understanding, the hemostatic system involves a delicate balance between procoagulation pathways, anticoagulant pathways, and fibrinolysis.

Primary hemostasis initiates the formation of a platelet plug in response to injury to a blood vessel. This process is mediated by von Willebrand factor (vWF), which triggers the adhesion and activation of platelets in response to exposed subendothelium and the formation of the primary platelet plug. *Secondary hemostasis* leads to thrombin generation, which mediates the production of a fibrin fiber meshwork that stabilizes the platelet plug. This process is initiated by the exposure of perivascular tissue factor (TF) to factor VII in blood, which leads to the activation of both the extrinsic and intrinsic coagulation pathways, cumulating in thrombin production (see Chapter 104).

Anticoagulant pathways include antithrombin-mediated factor inactivation, protein C activation via the thrombin-thrombomodulin complex, and TF pathway inhibitor (TFPI).

Fibrinolysis is initiated as tissue plasminogen activator and/or urokinase, which cleave plasminogen into plasmin, are released from the endothelium following injury, ischemia, or exposure to thrombin. Plasmin degrades fibrin into soluble fibrin degradation products.[1-5]

ANTIFIBRINOLYTIC DRUGS

The antifibrinolytic agents most commonly used in human and veterinary medicine are the synthetic lysine analogs ε-aminocaproic acid (6-aminohexanoic acid; EACA) and tranexamic acid (trans-4-aminomethyl cyclohexane carboxylic acid; TXA).[2,6-11]

Aprotinin was previously used widely in human medicine for both its antifibrinolytic and its antiinflammatory properties. The drug was removed from the world markets in May 2008 due to patient safety concerns, including sudden death, thrombotic complications, kidney failure, and myocardial infarction.[8,12]

Plasminogen acts as a fibrinolytic substance by binding to fibrin at a lysine-binding site. Plasminogen is then converted into plasmin, its activated form, which breaks down fibrin into fibrin degradation products. Both, EACA and TXA reversibly block the lysine-binding site on plasminogen, which is essential for binding to fibrin. This step consequently blocks the activation of plasminogen on the surface of fibrinogen and thereby prevents the breakdown of fibrin, although plasmin generation does occur.[6-8]

Indications

In human medicine antifibrinolytic drug therapy has been used extensively for the treatment of intraoperative hemorrhage, particularly in cardiac surgery, liver transplantation, spinal surgery, and orthopedic surgery. Other indications include gastrointestinal bleeding, urinary tract and uterine hemorrhage (both the urinary tract and the endometrium are rich in plasminogen activators),[2,6] and hyperfibrinolytic states, often seen after traumatic events with hypoperfusion or extensive tissue injury.[3,4] A recent comprehensive Cochrane review reported a significant reduction in blood loss and need for blood transfusions after the use of in EACA in patients undergoing major surgery.[13] A similar finding was reported for TXA in a meta-analysis of bleeding surgical patients.[14] Antifibrinolytic drugs have also been used to reduce hemorrhage associated with thrombocytopenia.[15]

Contraindications

Use of antifibrinolytic drugs may be contraindicated in patients with prothrombotic disease processes because there is a concern of promoting thrombus formation. In veterinary medicine these include patients with disseminated intravascular coagulation, aortic thromboembolism, immune-mediated hemolytic anemia, and hyperadrenocorticism.[5] A few case reports have described diffuse thrombotic events and pulmonary embolism in association with antifibrinolytic drug therapy, but a recent comprehensive Cochrane review did not find any supporting evidence for an increased incidence of thrombotic events with the use of EACA or TXA.[2,6,13] Use of antifibrinolytic drugs for treatment of upper urinary tract hemorrhage should be avoided because urinary tract obstruction can occur with thrombus formation.

Table 170-1 **Suggested Drug Dosages for Commonly Used Hemostatic Drugs**

Drug	Dosage	Special Considerations
ε-aminocaproic acid	50-100 mg/kg IV loading dose (over 1 hr) followed by 15 mg/kg/hr CRI or q8h until bleeding is controlled[5,*] 15-40 mg/kg IV bolus followed by 500-1000 mg PO q8h[10]	Dilute in 0.9% saline, LRS, or D5W to 20-25 mg/ml
Tranexamic acid	10-15 mg/kg SC, IM, or slow IV followed by 1 mg/kg/hr CRI for 5-8 hr[5,*]	10 mg/kg q12-24h in renal disease
Desmopressin	Intranasal product: 1-3 mcg/kg SC[5] Parenteral product: 0.3-1 mcg/kg SC, IV (slow)[5,28-30,35,38] Parenteral product: 0.3 mcg/kg IV, SC q12-24h[41]*	Give slowly IV Tachyphylaxis after repeat administration Dilute: 10 ml (<10 kg BW) or 50 ml (>10 kg BW) 0.9% saline for IV administration
Protamine	1 mg for every 1 mg (100 U) heparin slowly IV Decrease dose by 50% for every 30 min elapsed since heparin administration[5,45,*]	May cause severe anaphylaxis, hypotension, and pulmonary hypertension
Conjugated estrogens	0.6 mg/kg IV q24h for 4-5 days[47,*] 50 mg PO q24h for 7 days[46,*] 0.02 mg/kg PO q24h for 5-7 days, then every 2-4 days[60†]	Doses of 1-2 mg/kg may cause myelotoxicity
Recombinant factor VIIa	90 mcg/kg bolus q2h until hemostasis is achieved[49]*	
Yunnan Paiyao	Dogs: <15 kg—1 capsule PO q12h 15-30 kg—2 capsules PO q12h >30 kg—2 capsules PO q8h[61‡] Cats: 1/2 capsule PO q12h[61‡]	Capsules can also be opened and sprinkled on wound

CRI, Constant rate infusion; *D5W*, 5% dextrose in water, *IM*, intramuscularly; *IV*, intravenously; *LRS*, lactated Ringer's solution; *PO*, per os; *SC*, subcutaneous.
*Dosage extrapolated from human literature.
†Dosage extrapolated from veterinary literature for the treatment of urinary incontinence.
‡Dosage based on anecdotal evidence.

Use of Antifibrinolytic Drugs in Cats

Little information is available to date on the use of antifibrinolytic drugs in cats. The few reports of the use of antifibrinolytic drugs in cats in experimental studies report adverse effects, including seizures and myocardial injury.[16,17] It is important to note, however, that the dosing of antifibrinolytic drugs in these studies may not mimic clinical use, and it is difficult to determine if the adverse effects were due to the inhibition of fibrinolysis or were a direct effect of the drug itself. For this reason, the author recommends caution in the use of these drugs in feline patients until more information regarding safety is available.

ε-Aminocaproic acid

EACA competitively inhibits plasminogen activation and at higher doses may also directly inhibit plasmin. The elimination half-life of EACA is 1 to 2 hours in adult human patients. The majority of the drug is eliminated unchanged by renal excretion (65%); about 30% to 35% undergoes hepatic metabolism to adipic acid, which is also excreted in the urine.[6-11,18]

Reported adverse effects in human patients are dose dependent and include hypotension, which is usually associated with rapid intravenous administration, as well as nausea, vomiting, diarrhea, generalized weakness, myonecrosis with myoglobinuria, and rhabdomyolysis.

Limited data are available on the use of EACA in veterinary medicine. In two separate studies, postoperative administration of EACA significantly decreased the prevalence of postoperative bleeding in greyhounds undergoing gonadectomy or limb amputation due to appendicular bone tumors. Neither study reported clinical adverse effects or thrombotic events.[9,10]

EACA can be administered intravenously or orally. The dosages used in veterinary patients are largely extrapolated from human medicine (Table 170-1). Reported dosages in dogs are in the range of 15 to 40 mg/kg intravenously over 30 minutes (rapid administration can cause hypotension and vomiting) and/or 500 to 1000 mg orally per greyhound dog q8h for 5 days, beginning the night of surgery.[9,10] In human medicine EACA is given as a loading dose in an amount on the order of 50 to 100 mg/kg over the first hour, followed by a constant rate infusion of 15 mg/kg/hr thereafter.[19]

Tranexamic Acid

TXA is also a competitive inhibitor of plasminogen activation and at high concentrations is a noncompetitive inhibitor of plasmin. Additionally, TXA competitively inhibits the activation of trypsinogen by enterokinases and noncompetitively inhibits trypsin and thrombin, hence prolonging activated thrombin time at high doses. TXA is about 6 to 10 times more potent in vitro than EACA, with higher and more sustained antifibrinolytic activity,[7,20] and was shown to increase thrombus formation in animal models in a dose-dependent manner.[21] Similar to EACA, TXA is predominantly excreted unchanged via the kidneys (95%). TXA has a terminal half-life of 2 to 3 hours.

Clinical indications are comparable to those for EACA, and a recent randomized multicenter human trial (Clinical Randomisation of an Antifibrinolytic in Significant Haemorrhage 2 [CRASH-2]) found that TXA safely reduced mortality in trauma patients with or at risk of significant bleeding if given early (within 3 hours). TXA given after 3 hours seemed to increase the risk of death due to bleeding.[22,23]

Adverse effects are similar to those reported for EACA in human patients and include hypotension after rapid administration and clinical signs associated with the gastrointestinal tract (nausea, vomiting, diarrhea, abdominal cramps). Concerns regarding thromboembolic complications were not supported by a recent Cochrane review,[8] but care should be taken in patients with renal disease.[24] Convulsive seizures have been reported postoperatively after high doses of TXA were given during cardiac surgery. A potential mechanism for seizures is the structural similarity of TXA with γ-aminobutyric acid.[7]

Limited data are available on the use of TXA in veterinary medicine. An abstract presentation of a retrospective study evaluating 68 dogs with bleeding disorders severe enough to necessitate blood transfusions reported no apparent difference in the total number of blood products used in the group given TXA compared with a control group. TXA was administered intravenously at a mean dose of 8 mg/kg; adverse effects reported were vomiting in two dogs.[25] The human dose used in the CRASH trials was a loading dose of 1 g (~15 mg/kg for a 70-kg person) over 10 minutes followed by 1 g infused over the following 8 hours (~1.8 mg/kg/hr for a 70-kg person).[22] See Table 170-1 for more details regarding dosing.

Topical Antifibrinolytic Therapy

There is a growing interest in human medicine in the efficacy of topical EACA and TXA in major surgical procedures associated with significant blood loss.[26] In addition, antifibrinolytic mouthwashes can be beneficial in controlling bleeding associated with dental procedures in patients who have hemophilia or are taking anticoagulant medications.[27]

DESMOPRESSIN

Desmopressin acetate (1-desamino-8-D-arginine vasopressin, or DDAVP) is a synthetic vasopressin analog. DDAVP is pharmacologically altered from vasopressin by substitution of D-arginine for L-arginine, which virtually eliminates the vasopressor activity (via V_1 receptors) and significantly enhances antidiuretic activity and the stimulation of endothelial release of factor VIII and vWF (via V_2 receptors).[6,18,28] The terminal half-life of DDAVP after intravenous administration is 2.5 to 4.4 hours.[6] The bioavailability of orally administered DDAVP is not reliable because DDAVP is destroyed in the gastrointestinal tract; hence, oral administration of DDAVP is not recommended in the acutely bleeding patient. Plasma concentrations of factor VIII and vWF approximately double to quadruple 30 to 60 minutes after intravenous administration and 60 to 90 minutes after subcutaneous or intranasal administration.[2] For this reason, patients with hemophilia A (congenital deficiency of factor VIII) or type I vWD (low circulating amount of vWF) who are bleeding spontaneously or are scheduled to have surgery benefit from the administration of DDAVP, often in conjunction with blood products.

Administration of DDAVP does not shorten the bleeding times in patients with type II vWD (deficiency of high-molecular-weight vWF multimers) or severe type III vWD (absence of vWF).[2,5]

DDAVP enhances platelet function in uremic thrombocytopathia and other congenital defects of platelet function and also appears to be effective in bleeding disorders caused by chronic liver disease, even though these patients often have normal plasma concentrations of vWF and factor VIII. Patients with prolonged bleeding times due to antiplatelet drugs such as aspirin, ticlopidine, and clopidogrel may also benefit from DDAVP administration. The mechanism of action of DDAVP in human patients is not well understood and may be associated with the induction of supranormal plasma concentrations of vWF, greater concentrations of large multimers of vWF, or high plasma concentrations of factor VIII.[2]

In Doberman Pinschers with type 1 vWD disease, DDAVP administration increased both the quantity of vWF and its functional activity, and there was also a proportional increase in vWF multimer of all sizes in plasma; these results indicate that the primary effect of DDAVP on hemostasis cannot be explained solely by a preferential increase in large vWF multimers, as postulated in humans.[29,30] In addition, the quantitative increase in vWF appears much less pronounced, with an approximately 25% to 70% increase above baseline; in comparison, in humans increases of twofold to fivefold were reported.[30,31]

The effect of DDAVP on factor VIII is dose dependent, and increases ranged from 37% to 140% above baseline in dogs with vWD and in healthy dogs, whereas German Shepherds with hemophilia A did not show substantial increases in plasma factor VIII activity after DDAVP administration.[32-34] Administration of DDAVP improved hemostatic function in Doberman Pinschers with type 1 vWD.[29,35]

DDAVP is often used in human patients who undergo cardiac surgery and other nonurgent elective surgical procedures that are associated with relatively large blood losses, but the true benefit is questionable in patients who do not have an underlying congenital bleeding disorder. A recent Cochrane review did not find any convincing evidence that DDAVP reduces the need for blood transfusions in patients who do not have congenital bleeding disorders.[36]

Adverse effects of DDAVP administration include water retention and hyponatremia due to its antidiuretic actions. Hypotension has been reported after rapid intravenous administration in human patients. The therapeutic effectiveness of DDAVP tends to vary, and tachyphylaxis has been reported after repeat administration within 48 hours, probably because all available factor VIII and vWF has been mobilized from the endothelium.[6,18] Thrombotic events have been reported in individual studies in human patients but did not reach statistical significance in a multicenter review.[36] DDAVP administration may induce transient thrombocytopenia due to excess platelet aggregation in type II vWD.[37] German Shorthaired and Wirehaired Pointers are the only dog breeds reported to be affected with type II vWD; hence, care should be taken when administering DDAVP to these breeds of dogs.

In veterinary medicine, DDAVP has been used for the treatment of diabetes insipidus and congenital bleeding disorders as well as perioperatively in dogs undergoing removal of mammary gland tumors to minimize spread of metastasis and survival of residual cancer cells.[38] DDAVP also proved to be effective in shortening bleeding times in dogs with canine monocytic ehrlichiosis, aspirin-induced platelet dysfunction, and chronic liver disease.[39,40] DDAVP is available for oral, parenteral, and nasal administration. For hemostatic purposes the oral form is not recommended. Parenteral DDAVP is ideal but its use maybe limited due to cost. The human dose for intravenous desmopressin is 0.3 mcg/kg infused over 15 to 30 minutes.[41] In veterinary patients it is common to use the nasal product and inject it subcutaneously at doses of 1 to 2 mcg/kg (see Table 170-1). The dose can be repeated every 6 hours for three to four consecutive doses, after which the therapy should be discontinued for 24 to 48 hours due to concerns of tachyphylaxis.

PROTAMINE

Protamine is a strongly positively charged, alkaline, low-molecular-weight, polycationic amine derived from the sperm of salmon. Approximately 67% of the amino acid composition in protamine is arginine, which contributes to its strong alkalinity. Protamine is routinely used in human medicine after cardiopulmonary bypass to reverse the anticoagulant effects of heparin but is also indicated for the treatment or prevention of bleeding due to administration of either unfractionated or low-molecular-weight heparin.[18,42]

The positively charged, polycationic protamine combines with the negatively charged, polyanionic heparin, forming a protamine-heparin complex that is devoid of anticoagulant activity. Excess protamine is required to neutralize heparin because protamine competes with antithrombin III for binding with heparin.[18,42]

Adverse reactions due to protamine administration in people are often divided into three categories: (1) *systemic hypotension,* which is thought to be the result of histamine release by mast cells after rapid administration of protamine and the involvement of the nitric oxide pathway[42,43]; (2) *anaphylactic reactions,* including antibody-mediated and antibody-antigen complex–mediated anaphylaxis, which is often a problem after repeat administration of protamine in diabetic patients who take protamine-containing insulin daily; and (3) severe *pulmonary hypertension,* which is thought to be due to protamine-heparin complex–induced complement activation and generation of thromboxane A_2 and release of endothelin-1.[42,44]

Other reported adverse effects include delayed, noncardiogenic pulmonary edema and paradoxic bleeding due to thrombocytopenia, thrombocytopathia, and altered thrombin activity after administration of high doses of protamine. The "heparin-rebound effect" is thought to be due to protein-bound heparin that is incompletely bound by protamine. After the protamine-heparin complexes are cleared from the circulation, remaining protein-bound heparin dissociates slowly and binds to antithrombin III to produce an anticoagulant effect. Other causes may include liberation of excess heparin from extravascular spaces or intravascular surfaces, or excess breakdown of protamine by protaminases. Both excess doses of protamine and the heparin-rebound effect can lead to excess bleeding after protamine administration, and the two conditions may be difficult to distinguish from each other and could be misinterpreted as residual heparin anticoagulation.[18,42]

Little is known about the use of protamine in veterinary medicine, but in experimental research it appears to be effective in stopping bleeding in animals that received unfractionated or low-molecular-weight heparin. Adverse effects such as pulmonary hypertension, anaphylactoid reactions, and bleeding after protamine administration have been experimentally induced in dogs.[18,42-44]

The protamine dose is based on the original heparin dose given; each milligram of protamine neutralizes 100 U or more of unfractionated heparin.[45] Given the short half-life of heparin, the dose of protamine should be reduced in accordance with the time elapsed since the original heparin administration. A general guideline is to halve the protamine dose for every 30 minutes that has elapsed (see Table 170-1).[45] Protamine should be given by slow injection over 10 minutes in an effort to avoid hypotension or anaphylactoid reactions.

CONJUGATED ESTROGENS

Conjugated estrogens shorten prolonged bleeding times and stop hemorrhage in patients with uremia. They can be given orally or intravenously and have reportedly shortened the bleeding time by 50% for at least 2 weeks in uremic patients.[6,46] The effect of conjugated estrogens on bleeding times is longer lasting (10 to 15 days) than that of DDAVP (6 to 8 hours); hence, their use should be considered when prolonged hemostasis is desired. Accordingly, conjugated estrogens should be administered for at least 4 to 5 days before an event such as elective surgery to prevent bleeding in patients with renal disease.[6,18,47]

The mechanism of action of conjugated estrogens on bleeding time is unknown, but there is evidence that they increase the levels of vWF and factors VII and XII.[5,6] However, administration of recombinant erythropoietin has become a routine treatment in the management of uremic patients with chronic renal disease because it helps to increase the hematocrit, shortens bleeding times, and improves platelet adhesion. Hence, it appears that administration of conjugated estrogens is rarely required in this subset of patients, and they should be reserved for patients with acute and subacute renal failure and used in combination with DDAVP.[48]

There is limited information about the usefulness of conjugated estrogens for perioperative hemostasis in human and veterinary patients. A few small human studies reported beneficial effects, and conjugated estrogens were well tolerated with negligible adverse effects.[5,6,18] See Table 170-1 for dosing information.

RECOMBINANT FACTOR VIIa

Recombinant factor VIIa (rFVIIa) was developed for the treatment of hemophilia A and B patients with antibodies against factor VIII and IX, respectively. Factor VIIa is a vitamin K–dependent glycoprotein consisting of up to 406 amino acid residues that is originally produced in baby hamster kidney cells and proteolytically converted via chromographic purification into the active two-chain form of rFVIIa.[6,49]

Even though hemophilia A and B are primarily deficiencies of factor VIII and IX, respectively, the extrinsic pathway involving TF and factor VII may also be impaired in hemophilia A patients.[50] The rFVIIa is believed to act in two ways: through the formation of a TF–factor VIIa complex at the site of endothelial damage, which initiates coagulation, production of thrombin, and clot formation; and through a TF-independent mechanism in which rFVIIa at supraphysiologic doses binds directly to the phospholipid membrane of activated platelets, activating factor X and leading to a massive rise in thrombin generation at the platelet surface.[6] Hence, high doses of rFVIIa (up to 10 times higher than physiologic concentrations of factor VII) can compensate for a lack of factor VIII or IX in hemophilia A and B patients. This is called the *bypass effect* and may also explain the effectiveness of rFVIIa in patients with platelet function disorders.[6,49]

rFVIIa has been used successfully in human patients with bleeding problems caused by hemophilia A and B, quantitative and qualitative platelet disorders, vWD, uremia, liver disease, trauma, and surgical procedures, and it may also be administered to patients without preexisting hemostatic defects.[6] The half-life of rFVIIa is short (2.7 hours), and it therefore needs to be administered frequently (every 2 hours) or as a continuous infusion.

Adverse effects are rare, and reports of thromboembolic complications have been limited to a few case studies in human patients.[51] In experimental dog models, rFVIIa administration resulted in a type 1 hypersensitivity reaction.[50]

rFVIIa has been used experimentally in dogs with hemophilia A and B and vWD; it was effective in stopping nail cuticle bleeding in dogs with hemophilia A and B but not in dogs with vWD.[50] The reported half-life in dogs was 2.8 hours, which is very similar to that in humans. It is unclear if rFVIIa will find its way into veterinary medicine. Clinical indications would be comparable to those in human patients, but current cost and the occurrence of hypersensitivity reactions in dog models may limit its future use.

YUNNAN PAIYAO

Yunnan Paiyao (or Yunnan Baiyao) is a Chinese herb mixture that is commonly used to stop bleeding but is also employed for pain relief, reduction of inflammation, and promotion of wound healing. The herbal mixture was developed in the Yunnan province of China in the early 1900s and was historically carried by foreign soldiers as a hemostatic agent for trauma. The exact ingredients of this herbal formula are kept secret, but the main active ingredient is thought to be a pseudoginseng root called *Panax notoginseng*. Biochemical analysis also revealed high concentrations of polysaccharides (94% starch), calcium, and phosphorus.[52-54]

Yunnan Paiyao markedly shortened bleeding and clotting times after experimental oral and topical administration in rabbits, rats, and humans.[53,55] Other mechanisms of action include dose-dependent platelet activation.[56] No adverse effects have been reported after oral and topical administration, but in general, quality control and manufacturing regulations may be lacking for Chinese herbal products, and there is concern about contamination with mycotoxins, heavy metals, microbial agents, and pesticides.[57] Yunnan Paiyao is currently not approved by the U.S. Food and Drug Administration.

Yunnan Paiyao has been widely used in human and veterinary medicine, but evidence supporting the clinical use of Yunnan Paiyao is scarce. One randomized controlled trial evaluating the effect of Yunnan Paiyao on the severity of exercise-induced pulmonary hemorrhage (EIPH) in horses showed no effect of the drug on EIPH severity and other coagulation variables,[58] but Yunnan Paiyao significantly decreased blood loss in a group of human patients undergoing maxillary surgery.[59] See Table 170-1 for dosing information.

REFERENCES

1. Guyton AC, Hall JE: Hemostasis and blood coagulation. In Textbook of medical physiology, 10th ed, Philadelphia, 2000, Saunders, pp 419-429.
2. Mannucci PM: Hemostatic drugs, N Engl J Med 339:245-253, 1998.
3. Brohi K, Cohen MJ, Davenport RA: Acute coagulopathy of trauma: mechanism, identification and effect, Curr Opin Crit Care 13:680-685, 2007.
4. Brohi K, Cohen MJ, Ganter MT, et al: Acute coagulopathy of trauma: hypoperfusion induces systemic anticoagulation and hyperfibrinolysis, J Trauma 64:1211-1217, 2008.
5. Hopper K: Hemostatic agents. In Proceedings of the 6th International Veterinary Emergency and Critical Care Symposium, San Antonio, Texas, 2006.
6. Mahdi AM, Webster NR: Perioperative systemic haemostatic agents, Br J Anaesth 93:842-857, 2004.
7. McCormack PL: Tranexamic acid, Drugs 72:585-617, 2012.
8. Roberts I, Shakur H, Ker K: Antifibrinolytic drugs for acute traumatic injury, Cochrane Database Syst Rev (1):1-20, 2011.
9. Marin LM, Iazbik MC, Zaldivar-Lopez S: Epsilon aminocaproic acid for prevention of delayed postoperative bleeding in retired racing greyhounds undergoing gonadectomy, Vet Surg 41:594-603, 2012.
10. Marin LM, Iazbik MC, Zaldivar-Lopez S: Retrospective evaluation of the effectiveness of epsilon aminocaproic acid for the prevention of postamputation bleeding in retired racing Greyhounds with appendicular bone tumors: 46 cases (2003-2008), J Vet Emerg Crit Care 22:332-340, 2012.
11. Heidmann P, Tornquist SJ, Qu A: Laboratory measures of hemostasis and fibrinolysis after intravenous administration of epsilon aminocaproic acid in clinically normal horses and ponies, Am J Vet Res 66:313-318, 2005.
12. Manufacturer removes remaining stocks of trasylol. Access limited to investigational use. US Food and Drug Administration: Press release, May 14, 2008. Available at http://www.fda.gov/NewsEvents/Newsroom/PressAnnouncements/2008/ucm116895.htm Accessed 11/12/2012.
13. Henry DA, Carless PA, Moxey AJ, et al: Anti-fibrinolytic use for minimizing perioperative allogenic blood transfusion (review), Cochrane Database Syst Rev (3):1-427, 2011.
14. Ker K, Edwards P, Perel P, et al: Effect of tranexamic acid on surgical bleeding: systematic review and cumulative meta-analysis, BMJ 17:344, 2012.
15. Kalmadi S, Tiu R, Lowe C, et al: Epsilon aminocaproic acid reduces transfusion requirements in patients with thrombocytopenic hemorrhage, Cancer 107:136, 2006.
16. Pellegrini A, Giaretta D, Chemello R, et al: Feline generalized epilepsy induced by tranexamic acid (AMCA), Epilepsia 23:35-45, 1982.
17. Hosgor I, Yarat A, Yilmazer S, et al: Collagen deposition in myocardium after inhibition fibrinolytic activity, Blood Coagul Fibrinolysis 16:25-30, 2005.
18. Franck M, Sladen RN: Drugs to prevent and reverse anticoagulation, Anesthesiol Clin North Am 17:799-811, 1999.
19. Aminocaproic acid injection, solution. Available at: http://dailymed.nlm.nih.gov/dailymed/lookup.cfm?setid=1c5bc1dd-e9ec-44c1-9281-67ad482315d9. Accessed 11/12/2012.
20. Verstraete M: Clinical application of inhibitors of fibrinolysis, Drugs 29:236-261, 1985.
21. Sperzel M, Huetter J: Evaluation of aprotinin and tranexamic acid in different in vitro and in vivo models of fibrinolysis, coagulation and thrombus formation, J Thromb Haemost 5:2113-2118, 2007.
22. CRASH-2 Trial Collaborators: Effect of tranexamic acid on death, vascular occlusive events and blood transfusion in trauma patients with significant hemorrhage (CRASH-2): a randomized, placebo controlled trial, Lancet 376:23-32, 2010.
23. CRASH-2 Trial Collaborators: The importance of early treatment with tranexamic acid in bleeding trauma patients: an exploratory analysis of the CRASH-2 randomised trial, Lancet 377:1096-1101, 2011.
24. Martin K, Wiesner G, Breuer T, et al: The risks of aprotinin and tranexamic acid in cardiac surgery: a one-year follow-up of 1188 consecutive patients, Anesth Analg 107:1783-1790, 2008.
25. Kelmer E, Marer Y, Bruchim S, et al: Retrospective evaluation of the safety and efficacy of tranexamic acid (Hexacapron®) for the treatment of bleeding disorders in dogs. In Proceedings of the 11th International Veterinary Emergency and Critical Care Symposium, San Antonio, Texas, 2011.
26. Ipema HJ, Tanzi MG: Use of topical tranexamic acid or aminocaproic acid to prevent bleeding after major surgical procedures, Ann Pharmacother 46:97, 2012.
27. Patatanian E, Fugate SE: Hemostatic mouthwashes in anticoagulated patients undergoing dental extraction, Ann Pharmacother 40:2205, 2006.
28. Kraus KH, Turrentine MA, Jergens AE, et al: Effect of desmopressin acetate on bleeding times and plasma von Willebrand factor in Doberman Pinscher Dogs with von Willebrand's disease, Vet Surg 18:103-109, 1989.
29. Callahan MB, Giger U, Catalfamo JL: Effect of desmopressin on von Willebrand factor multimers in Doberman Pinschers with type 1 von Willebrand disease, Am J Vet Res 66:861-867, 2005.
30. Johnstone IB: Desmopressin enhances the binding of plasma von Willebrand factor to collagen in plasmas from normal dogs and dogs with type I von Willebrand's disease, Can Vet J 40:645-648, 1999.
31. Mannucci PM: Desmopressin (DDAVP) in the treatment of bleeding disorder: the first twenty years, Haemophilia 6:60-67, 2000.
32. Mansell PD, Parry BW: Changes in factor VIII: coagulant activity and von Willebrand factor antigen concentration after subcutaneous injection of desmopressin in dogs with mild hemophilia A, J Vet Intern Med 5:191-194, 1991.
33. Meyers KM, Wardrop KJ, Dodds WJ, et al: Effect of exercise, DDAVP, and epinephrine on the factor VIIIC/von Willebrand factor complex in normal dogs and von Willebrand factor deficient Doberman pinscher dogs, Thromb Res 57:97-108, 1990.
34. Johnstone IB, Crane S: The effect of desmopressin on plasma factor VIII/von Willebrand factor activity in dogs with von Willebrand's disease, Can J Vet Res 2:189-193, 1987.
35. Callahan MB, Giger U: Effect of desmopressin acetate administration on primary hemostasis in Doberman Pinschers with type-1 von Willebrand disease as assessed by a point-of-care instrument, Am J Vet Res 63:1700-1706, 2002.
36. Carless PA, Stokes BJ, Moxey AJ, et al: Desmopressin use for minimizing perioperative allogeneic blood transfusion, Cochrane Database Syst Rev (4):1-52, 2008.
37. Frederici AB, Mannucci PM: Advances in the genetics and treatment of von Willebrand disease, Curr Opin Pediatr 14:23-33, 2002.
38. Hermo GA, Turic E, Angelico D, et al: Effect of adjuvant perioperative desmopressin in locally advanced canine mammary carcinoma and its relation to histologic grade, J Am Anim Hosp Assoc 47:21-27, 2011.
39. Giudice E, Giannetto C, Gianesella M: Effect of desmopressin on immune-mediated haemorrhagic disorders due to canine monocytic ehrlichiosis: a preliminary study, J Vet Pharmacol Ther 33:610-614, 2010.
40. Sakai M, Watari T, Miura T, et al: Effects of DDAVP administration subcutaneously in dogs with aspirin-induced platelet dysfunction and hemostatic impairment due to chronic liver diseases, J Vet Med Sci 65:83-86, 2003.

41. Desmopressin acetate injection. Daily Med website. Available at. http://www.dailymed.nlm.nih.gov/dailymed/lookup.cfm?setid=5fe83452-1670-487d-feb4-27d4bd75a147. Accessed 11/12/2012.
42. Carr JA, Silverman N: The heparin-protamine interaction. A review, J Cardiovasc Surg 40:659-666, 1999.
43. Oguchi T, Doyrsout MF, Kashimoto S, et al: Role of heparin and nitric oxide in the cardiac and regional hemodynamic properties of protamine in conscious chronically instrumented dogs, Anesthesiology 94:1016-1025, 2001.
44. Freitas CF, Faro R, Dragosavac D, et al: Role of endothelin-1 and thromboxane A_2 in the pulmonary hypertension induced by heparin-protamine interaction in anesthetized dogs, J Cardiovasc Pharmacol 43:106-112, 2004.
45. Protamine sulfate injection, solution. Daily Med website. Available at http://dailymed.nlm.nih.gov/dailymed/lookup.cfm?setid=e1964129-33f4-4e4e-86e3-8e6a4e65bd83. Accessed 11/12/2012
46. Shemin D, Elnour M, Amarantes B, et al: Oral estrogens decrease bleeding time and improve clinical bleeding in patients with renal failure, Am J Med 89:436-440, 1990.
47. Livio M, Mannucci PM, Vigano G, et al: Conjugated estrogens for the management of bleeding associated with renal failure, N Engl J Med 315:731-735, 1986.
48. Moia M, Mannucci PM, Vizzotto L, et al: Improvement in the haemostatic defect of uremia after treatment with recombinant human erythropoietin, Lancet 2:1227-1229, 1987.
49. Kristensen AT, Edwards ML, Devey J: Potential uses of recombinant human factor VIIa in veterinary medicine, Vet Clin Small Anim 33:1437-1451, 2003.
50. Brinkhous KM, Hedner U, Garris JB, et al: Effect of recombinant factor VIIa on the hemostatic defect in dogs with hemophilia A, hemophilia B, and von Willebrand disease, Proc Natl Acad Sci U S A 86:1382-1386, 1989.
51. Roberts HR: Clinical experience with activated factor VII: focus on safety aspects, Blood Coagul Fibrinolysis 9(Suppl):S115-S118, 1998.
52. Polesuk J, Amodeo JM, Ma TS: Microchemical investigation of medicinal plants. X. Analysis of the Chinese herbal drug Yunnan Bai Yao, Mikrochim Acta 61:507-517, 1973.
53. Ogle CW, Dai S, Ma JC: The haemostatic effects of the Chinese herbal drug Yunnan Bai Yao: a pilot study, Am J Chin Med 4:147-152, 1976.
54. Shmalberg J, Hill RC, Scott KC: Nutrient and metal analyses of Chinese herbal products marketed for veterinary use, J Anim Physiol Anim Nutr (Berl) 97(2):305-314, 2013. Epub January 31, 2012.
55. Ogle CW, Dai S, Cho CH: The hemostatic effects of orally administered Yunnan Bai Yao in rats and rabbits, Comp Med East West 5:155-160, 1977.
56. Chew EC: Effects of Yunnan Bai Yao on blood platelets: an ultrastructural study, Comp Med East West 5:169-175, 1977.
57. Leung KS-Y, Chan K, Chan C-L, et al: Systematic evaluation of organochlorine pesticide residues in Chinese material medica, Phytother Res 19:514-518, 2005.
58. Epp TS, McDonough P, Padilla DJ, et al: The effect of herbal supplementation on the severity of exercise-induced pulmonary hemorrhage, Equine Comp Exerc Physiol 1:17-25, 2004.
59. Tang Z-L, Wang X, Yi B, et al: Effects of the preoperative administration of Yunnan Baiyao capsules on intraoperative blood loss in bimaxillary orthognathic surgery: a prospective, randomized, double blind, placebo-controlled study, Int J Oral Maxillofac Surg 38:261-268, 2009.
60. Lane IF: Managing refractory urinary incontinence in dogs. In Proceedings of the 84th Annual Western Veterinary Conference, Las Vegas, 2012.
61. Graham L: Everything you need to know about Yunnan Baiyao: a simple and effective herbal therapeutic. In Proceedings of the Wild West Veterinary Conference, Reno, Nevada, 2008.

CHAPTER 171

ANTIARRHYTHMIC AGENTS

Kathy N. Wright, DVM, DACVIM (Cardiology)

KEY POINTS

- Antiarrhythmic agents are useful for managing various tachyarrhythmias, but the clinician must have knowledge of the patient and the arrhythmia, as well as the indications for and adverse effects of each medication.
- Drugs that prolong atrioventricular (AV) nodal refractoriness are useful for AV nodal–dependent and atrial tachyarrhythmias, whereas drugs that prolong myocardial refractoriness are used in atrial, accessory pathway, and ventricular tachyarrhythmias.
- Most antiarrhythmic agents have multiple channel effects, not simply those of their Vaughan Williams class. This must be considered in predicting their potential beneficial and adverse effects.
- Disappointing results regarding the ability of antiarrhythmic agents to prevent sudden death have emerged from several large-scale human studies, and this goal now is pursued largely through device- or catheter-based therapy. Antiarrhythmic agents can be useful in limiting clinical signs related to tachyarrhythmias and thus potentially can prevent euthanasia of veterinary patients.

Antiarrhythmic agents have undergone critical reevaluation during the past two decades with publication of the results of large-scale human studies that have brought to light some of the risks and shortcomings of drug therapy for arrhythmias.[1,2] Once more cavalier in their use of these agents, veterinarians and physicians alike are having to analyze carefully the potential benefits and risks (including proarrhythmic effects) in each patient. Basically, there are two reasons to treat arrhythmias: (1) to alleviate significant clinical signs such as weakness, syncope, or precipitation or exacerbation of congestive heart failure by an arrhythmia, and (2) to prolong survival. Antiarrhythmic drugs, in general, have not been shown to do the latter, although they may in veterinary patients by controlling clinical signs and avoiding an owner decision for euthanasia. Antiarrhythmic devices and procedures are used in human medicine (and increasingly in veterinary cases) to prolong survival. Drugs can be very useful, however, in alleviating clinical signs in individual patients.

CLASSIFICATION SCHEMES

No completely satisfactory or intuitive classification scheme for antiarrhythmic agents has been developed. The most commonly used is the Vaughan Williams classification system, which attempts to group drugs according to their major ion channel or receptor effects. The limitations of this system have been well documented, including the fact that most antiarrhythmic drugs act on multiple channels or receptors, and one must know that when predicting their beneficial and adverse effects. The actions of antiarrhythmic drugs are actually very complex and vary by species (important to veterinarians because much of the data are from humans), age, tissue drug concentration, acid-base and electrolyte balance, presence or absence of myocardial damage, and indirect hemodynamic or autonomic actions.[3]

In spite of its shortcomings, the Vaughan Williams system remains the most widely used to date. An attempt to improve on this system led electrophysiologists to develop the Sicilian Gambit in 1991.[4] This approach attempted to identify the vulnerable parameter for various arrhythmias and did account for the multiple channel and receptor actions of each antiarrhythmic agent, but it was too unwieldy for widespread general use.

Grouping antiarrhythmic agents according to their main use (i.e., supraventricular arrhythmias or ventricular arrhythmias) would seem logical (Box 171-1), but many agents are used to treat multiple types of arrhythmias, so overlap would be inevitable. Despite its inherent limitations, the Vaughan Williams classification is used as the framework for this chapter. Agents that are commonly used in small animal cardiology are discussed.

CLASS I ANTIARRHYTHMIC AGENTS

Class I agents act primarily by inhibiting the fast sodium channel and decreasing the slope of phase 0 of the action potential. The relative potency of their sodium channel effects, whether blockade of the activated or inactivated channel occurs, and their effects on other channels and receptors determine their subclassification.

Class Ia Antiarrhythmic Agents

Class Ia agents have powerful, fast sodium channel–blocking effects and also exhibit moderate blockade of the rapid component of the delayed rectifier potassium current (I_{Kr}). This I_{Kr} blockade results in action potential prolongation and can account for the proarrhythmic effects associated with these drugs in some genetically predisposed individuals.[5] In addition, potent depression of conduction velocity can predispose to intramyocardial reentry. Quinidine, procainamide, and disopyramide are class Ia drugs.

Procainamide is the prototypical agent of this class used in small animal cardiology. It depresses conduction velocity and prolongs the effective refractory period in a wide variety of tissues, including the atrial and ventricular myocardium, accessory atrioventricular (AV) pathways, and retrograde fast AV nodal pathways.[5] Procainamide can thus be effective in a wide variety of arrhythmias, either as a single agent or combined with other agents. It can be administered parenterally for acute termination of severe ventricular or supraventricular tachyarrhythmias. It must be administered slowly intravenously (over 5 to 10 minutes) to prevent hypotension. Procainamide is more effective than lidocaine for acutely terminating ventricular tachyarrhythmias in human patients.[6]

Agents that prolong AV nodal conduction time are given first for acute treatment of atrial tachyarrhythmias, because procainamide can enhance AV nodal conduction and thus worsen the ventricular response rate. Parenteral procainamide is administered in doses of 6 to 8 mg/kg intravenously (IV) over 5 to 10 minutes or 6 to 20 mg/kg intramuscularly (IM) in dogs. A constant rate infusion (CRI) of 20 to 40 mcg/kg/min can be used once a therapeutic response is obtained with slow bolus administration. In cats parenteral procainamide is used cautiously at doses of 1 to 2 mg/kg IV or 3 to 8 mg/kg IM and a CRI of 10 to 20 mcg/kg/min. Sustained-release oral procainamide is not commercially available anymore; however, certain compounding pharmacies offer compounded and presumably sustained-release procainamide. The dosage in dogs is 10 to 30 mg/kg orally (PO) q8h.

Adverse effects commonly are associated with procainamide use but appear to be more frequent in humans and cats than in dogs. Gastrointestinal adverse effects such as anorexia, nausea, and vomiting are seen most commonly in dogs. Adverse effects reported in humans soon after oral procainamide therapy is instituted include rash and fever. Later adverse effects include arthralgia, myalgia, and agranulocytosis. The development of systemic lupus erythematosus is identified rarely in veterinary patients but is reported in one third of human patents who take procainamide for longer than 6 months.[7] A four-way trial of antiarrhythmic drugs in Boxer dogs with ventricular tachyarrhythmias showed that sustained-release procainamide administered at 20 to 26 mg/kg PO q8h reduced the frequency of ventricular ectopy but did not alter the frequency of syncope.[8]

Class Ib Antiarrhythmic Agents

Class Ib antiarrhythmic agents inhibit the fast sodium channel, primarily in the open state with rapid onset-offset kinetics. The window sodium current is also inhibited, which results in the shortening of action potential duration in normal myocardial tissue. This window current is considered to be the steady-state component of the fast sodium current (I_{Na}) resulting from the crossover of the activation and inactivation curves, which govern the opening of the sodium channel. Computer modeling studies support a role for this current in the dispersion of action potential duration across the ventricular wall. Their rapid kinetics explain why class Ib agents have minimal effects on the shorter atrial action potential. The ability of lidocaine and its congeners to block I_{Na} is enhanced in the presence of acidosis, increased extracellular potassium concentrations, and partially depolarized cells. Thus these drugs selectively suppress automaticity and slow conduction velocity in ischemic and diseased ventricular myocardium.

Lidocaine is an intravenous antiarrhythmic agent and typically is the first drug used in the acute treatment of serious ventricular tachyarrhythmias in dogs. It has the benefit of minimal hemodynamic, sinoatrial, and AV nodal effects at standard dosages. A bolus

BOX 171-1 *Antiarrhythmic Agents: General Uses*

Drugs Used to Manage Ventricular Tachyarrhythmias

Class Ia: procainamide, quinidine
Class Ib: lidocaine, mexiletine
Class Ic: flecainide, propafenone
Class II: β-blockers—atenolol, propranolol, metoprolol
Class III: d,l-sotalol, amiodarone

Drugs Used to Manage Supraventricular Tachyarrhythmias

Drugs used to slow atrioventricular nodal conduction

Class II: β-blockers—atenolol, propranolol
Class IV: calcium channel blockers
Other: digoxin

Drugs used to inhibit intramyocardial conduction or prolong myocardial repolarization

Class Ia: procainamide
Class Ic: flecainide, propafenone
Class III: d,l-sotalol, amiodarone

dose of 2 to 4 mg/kg is administered IV over 2 minutes. The bolus can be repeated to a maximum of 8 mg/kg within a 10-minute period, provided adverse effects do not occur. If the lidocaine bolus is successful in converting the ventricular tachycardia to sinus rhythm, it can be followed by a CRI of 25 to 75 mcg/kg/min.

Hepatic clearance of lidocaine determines its serum concentration, and this is directly related to hepatic blood flow. Heart failure, hypotension, and severe hepatic disease can therefore result in decreased lidocaine metabolism and predispose the patient to lidocaine toxicity. The incidence of adverse effects is much higher in cats, with earlier reports of bradyarrhythmias and sudden death. For this reason, caution is recommended in this species. Lower doses of 0.25 to 0.75 mg/kg are administered slowly IV, followed by infusion at rates of 10 to 20 mcg/kg/min.

The most common adverse effects of lidocaine include nausea, vomiting, lethargy, tremors, and seizure activity. These typically resolve quickly with cessation of the infusion. Diazepam may be administered to treat lidocaine-induced seizures.

Mexiletine is the most commonly used oral class Ib agent in dogs. It is highly protein bound and eliminated by renal excretion. Its use and adverse effect profile mirror those of lidocaine. It has been used in dogs in which ventricular tachyarrhythmias are acutely responsive to lidocaine and can be combined with class Ia, II, or III agents. Typical dosing in dogs is 4 to 8 mg/kg PO q8h. There are no data on its use in cats. Tocainide, another lidocaine congener, rarely is used in small animals because of the high incidence of serious adverse effects, including renal failure and corneal dystrophy.[9,10]

Class Ic Antiarrhythmic Agents

Potent blockade of the fast sodium channel with greater effects as the depolarization rate increases (use dependence) highlights class Ic antiarrhythmic drugs.[11] Limited data are available on the use of these agents in clinical veterinary patients. Flecainide and propafenone have been used by veterinary cardiologists to treat certain supraventricular or ventricular tachyarrhythmias in canine patients. Their expense, propensity for proarrhythmia in humans with structural heart disease, and negative inotropic properties, however, have impeded their widespread use in veterinary patients.

CLASS II ANTIARRHYTHMIC AGENTS

β-Adrenergic antagonists, or β-blockers, are some of the most universally useful cardiovascular drugs. β-Blockers have even found their way into the management of dilated cardiomyopathy, a disease for which they were once thought strictly contraindicated. In human patients with stable controlled heart failure, β-blockers reduce all-cause, cardiovascular, and sudden death mortality rates.[12-15] The clinician must be ever cognizant of the animal's underlying heart disease when prescribing β-blockers, however, because this will determine how well the animal tolerates the drug and how slowly it must be introduced. As antiarrhythmics, class II agents (1) inhibit the current I_f, an important pacemaker current that also promotes proarrhythmic depolarization in damaged cardiomyocytes, and (2) inhibit the inward calcium current, I_{Ca-L}, indirectly by decreasing tissue cyclic adenosine monophosphate levels. The magnitude of their antiarrhythmic effect depends on the prevailing sympathetic tone, with the effect increased in higher adrenergic states.

β-Adrenergic antagonists are used to slow AV nodal conduction in supraventricular tachyarrhythmias, slow sinus nodal discharge rate in inappropriate sinus tachycardia (such as that associated with pheochromocytomas), and suppress ventricular tachyarrhythmias thought to be caused, at least in part, by increased sympathetic tone. Their ability to slow AV nodal conduction in dogs appears to be inferior to that of the calcium channel blockers or class IV agents.[16] β-Blockers are often used as first-line antiarrhythmic agents in cats with ventricular or supraventricular tachyarrhythmias. They are often combined with class I or class III agents in dogs with severe ventricular tachyarrhythmias.

β-Blockers are contraindicated in patients that have evidence of sinus nodal dysfunction (sinus arrest, sinoatrial block, persistent sinus bradycardia), AV nodal conduction disturbances, pulmonary disease (particularly true for nonspecific β-blockers or high-dose β_1-selective blockers), or overt congestive heart failure.[5] Fluid retention must be frequently evaluated in patients with congestive heart failure and their condition must be stabilized before β-blockade is instituted. Extremely low dosages must be used in patients with systolic myocardial dysfunction and a course of very slow up-titration followed. Thus, in this subclass of patients, β-blockers are not the choice for acute antiarrhythmic therapy because the amounts required are not generally tolerated.

The drug used can vary according to the situation and the clinician's preference. Esmolol is the intravenous class II agent of choice in small animal cardiology because of its short half-life. A comparison of intravenous negative dromotropic agents in healthy dogs showed that esmolol was a significantly less effective negative dromotrope than diltiazem and caused a severe drop in left ventricular contractility measurements at dosages required to prolong AV nodal conduction.[16] Esmolol is given as an intravenous bolus over 1 to 2 minutes at 0.5 mg/kg. This can be followed by a CRI of 50 to 200 mcg/kg/min. Continuous careful monitoring of the electrocardiogram and blood pressure must be performed during administration of this drug.

The most commonly used oral β-blockers in small animals are atenolol and metoprolol, given their relative β_1 selectivity and long half-life compared with those of propranolol. Heart rate monitoring is useful to determine the appropriate dosage of β-blocker for an individual animal. Atenolol is water soluble and eliminated by the kidney, whereas metoprolol undergoes hepatic metabolism and elimination. These pharmacokinetic differences should be remembered in choosing a β-blocker and dosage for a particular patient.

CLASS III ANTIARRHYTHMIC AGENTS

Class III antiarrhythmic drugs block the repolarizing I_K, which results in prolongation of action potential duration and effective refractory period. Although this effect is beneficial if it occurs at tachyarrhythmia rates, the intrinsic problem is that most class III agents block the rapid component of I_K (I_{Kr}) rather than the slow component (I_{Ks}); thus their effects are accentuated at slower heart rates. This puts the patient at risk of early afterdepolarization and accounts for the proarrhythmic effect of class III antiarrhythmic drugs. This risk is increased with concurrent hypokalemia, bradycardia, intact status in females, increasing age, macrolide antibiotic therapy, and a number of other drugs.[17] Amiodarone, with its blockade of both I_{Ks} and I_{Kr}, makes the action potential pattern more uniform throughout the myocardium and has the least reported proarrhythmic activity of any of the class III agents.

The two class III agents used in small animal cardiology are sotalol and amiodarone, both of which have multiple channel and receptor effects. d,l-Sotalol combines nonselective β-blockade with I_{Kr} inhibition. It is an effective antiarrhythmic agent in both supraventricular and ventricular tachyarrhythmias. Its class II effects predominate at lower dosages and include sinus and AV nodal depression. Its class III effects, seen at higher dosages (>160 mg q24h in humans) are prolongation of the atrial and ventricular myocardial action potential, prolongation of the atrial and ventricular refractory periods, and inhibition of bidirectional conduction along any bypass tract. Prolongation of the action potential duration can result in enhanced calcium entry during the action potential plateau and may explain why the negative inotropic effect of sotalol is far less than expected. Sotalol is hydrophilic, non–protein bound, and excreted solely by the kidneys. The same absolute and relative contraindications apply to sotalol as to β-blockers in general, although, as mentioned earlier, it is better tolerated in animals with significant myocardial dysfunction than other β-blockers.

Two studies of Boxer dogs with familial ventricular arrhythmias compared d,l-sotalol with other antiarrhythmic agents. In the first study, dogs were grouped into asymptomatic, syncopal, and heart failure groups. The dosage of sotalol administered to these dogs was 0.97 to 6.1 mg/kg PO q24h, divided q12h, titrated to effect. Syncopal signs diminished with sotalol therapy, and dogs with systolic dysfunction did not appear to experience untoward drug effects.[18] The second study compared four antiarrhythmic drug regimens for treatment of familial ventricular arrhythmias in Boxers. Sotalol 1.47 to 3.5 mg/kg PO q12h significantly reduced the maximum and minimum heart rates, number of premature ventricular contractions, and ventricular arrhythmia grade. No significant change in the occurrence of syncope, however, was found for sotalol or for any of the other three treatments studied.[8] Finally, a study in German shepherd dogs with inherited ventricular arrhythmias concluded that a sotalol-mexiletine combination was superior to either agent alone.[19] Sotalol typically is administered at 1 to 3 mg/kg PO q12h in dogs and cats.

Amiodarone is the antiarrhythmic agent with the broadest spectrum, exhibiting properties of all four antiarrhythmic classes. It opposes electrophysiologic heterogeneity, which underlies some severe ventricular arrhythmias. The efficacy of amiodarone exceeds that of other antiarrhythmic compounds, including sotalol, in human patients. Furthermore, the incidence of torsades de pointes with amiodarone is much lower than expected from its class III effects. A retrospective study of dogs with severe ventricular or supraventricular tachyarrhythmias concluded that amiodarone resulted in an improvement in the severity of the tachyarrhythmia and clinical signs in 26 of 28 dogs.[20] A major drawback is that amiodarone is associated with a host of multisystemic, potentially serious adverse effects that do not occur with sotalol. A retrospective evaluation of the use of amiodarone in Doberman Pinschers with severe ventricular tachyarrhythmias documented adverse effects in 30% of the 20 patients studied.[21] These adverse effects included vomiting, anorexia, hepatopathies, and thrombocytopenia, and were more common with higher maintenance dosages. Amiodarone typically is reserved for life-threatening ventricular or supraventricular tachyarrhythmias that are not responding to other therapy. Published amiodarone dosages in dogs vary and typically include a loading period.[22] The author usually administers 15 mg/kg PO q24h for 7 to 10 days, then 10 mg/kg PO q24h for 7 to 10 days, then 5 to 8 mg/kg PO q24h long term. Serum amiodarone levels can be measured but may not correlate with tissue concentrations. Amiodarone has not been used in cats. The most common intravenous formulation of amiodarone (Cordarone IV) can result in severe hypotension. This effect has been attributed to the vasoactive solvents of the formulation, polysorbate 80 and benzyl alcohol, both known to exhibit negative inotropic and hypotensive effect. An aqueous formulation of intravenous amiodarone (Amio-Aqueous) does not contain vasoactive excipients and has been shown to be less toxic and cause less hypotension than Cordarone IV.[23] The cost of Amio-Aqueous is significantly more than that of Cordarone IV, however.

CLASS IV ANTIARRHYTHMIC AGENTS

Class IV antiarrhythmics comprise the group of calcium channel–blocking drugs. Nondihydropyridine calcium channel blockers slow AV nodal conduction and prolong the effective refractory period of nodal tissue. This effect is most notable at faster stimulation rates (use dependence) and in depolarized fibers (voltage dependence).[3] These drugs are effective in slowing the ventricular response rate to atrial tachyarrhythmias and can prolong the AV nodal effective refractory period to the point that an AV node–dependent tachyarrhythmia is terminated. They are generally contraindicated in wide-complex tachyarrhythmias.

Diltiazem has gained preference over verapamil because of its more favorable hemodynamic profile (i.e., minimal negative inotropic effect) at effective antiarrhythmic dosages. Intravenous diltiazem (0.125 to 0.35 mg/kg slowly IV over 2 minutes) has been used in dogs to immediately terminate a severe AV nodal–dependent tachyarrhythmia or slow the ventricular response rate to an atrial tachyarrhythmia. A comparison of the electrophysiologic and hemodynamic responses to intravenous diltiazem, esmolol, and adenosine in healthy dogs demonstrated the superior efficacy of diltiazem in slowing AV nodal conduction while maintaining a favorable hemodynamic profile.[16] Nonetheless, adverse effects can be seen, including hypotension and bradyarrhythmias.

Standard oral diltiazem is administered three times daily, which can be difficult, particularly for cat owners. Sustained-release preparations appear to have more variable absorption in companion animals but have been used successfully in dogs with certain supraventricular tachyarrhythmias. A higher incidence of adverse effects of these preparations has been reported in cats, including vomiting, inappetence, and hepatopathies.[24]

OTHER ANTIARRHYTHMIC AGENTS

Digoxin

The electrophysiologic effects of digoxin primarily occur indirectly through the autonomic nervous system by enhancing central and peripheral vagal tone. This results in slowing of the sinus nodal discharge rate, prolongation of AV nodal refractoriness, and shortening of atrial refractoriness. Digoxin is used orally as an antiarrhythmic agent to slow AV nodal conduction in dogs, particularly those with impaired left ventricular systolic function. The ventricular rate is almost never slowed adequately when digoxin is used as a single agent, however, and other drugs must be added. The dosage is 0.005 to 0.01 mg/kg PO q12h in a normokalemic dog with normal renal function and 0.0312 mg PO q24-48h in a normokalemic cat with normal renal function.

Digoxin has a low therapeutic index; owners must be educated about the signs of toxicity. Renal dysfunction, hypokalemia, advancing age, chronic lung disease, and hypothyroidism all predispose to digoxin toxicity and should be corrected (if possible) or the dosage adjusted downward. Serum digoxin concentrations should be monitored to determine the appropriate dosage for an individual animal. The trend in human medicine is toward lower dosages, which appear to be safer and confer benefit with less risk of toxicity. The ideal blood levels remain unknown, but a goal of about 0.5 to 1 ng/ml or 0.6 to 1.2 nmol/L (much lower than before) seems reasonable.[25]

Magnesium Sulfate

Magnesium sulfate intravenous injection is the first-line antiarrhythmic treatment for torsades de pointes and has been used with variable success to treat drug-refractory ventricular tachyarrhythmias or arrhythmias in patients with known hypomagnesemia.[26] It is administered slowly IV at 30 mg/kg (equivalent to 0.243 mEq/kg) over 5 to 10 minutes. Adverse effects include central nervous system depression, weakness, bradycardia, hypotension, hypocalcemia, and QT prolongation.

Adenosine

Adenosine is used widely in the emergency department in human patients to terminate AV node–dependent tachyarrhythmias. A study performed by the author showed that adenosine, even at doses of 2 mg/kg, was ineffective in slowing canine AV nodal conduction.[16] The same result has been found with electrophysiologic study of numerous dogs with orthodromic AV reciprocating tachycardia. A similar study has not been performed in cats.

ANTIARRHYTHMIC DEVICES AND PROCEDURES

Certain supraventricular tachyarrhythmias in dogs can be cured, rather than simply controlled, with transvenous radiofrequency catheter ablation.[27-30] The tachyarrhythmia circuit is first mapped with numerous multielectrode catheters. Once detailed mapping has identified a site in the reentrant circuit or an automatic focus for ablation, a larger-tipped electrode catheter is coupled to a cardiac-specific radiofrequency ablation unit. Radiofrequency energy is delivered to the tip electrode causing thermal desiccation of a small volume of tissue to permanently interrupt the tachycardia circuit. This technique has been used by this author and others in a large number of canine cases.

Permanent pacemaker implantation is a necessary component of the management of certain bradyarrhythmias, such as persistent high-grade AV nodal block and sick sinus syndrome. Rate responsiveness and dual-chamber pacing are all options that are being used or explored by veterinary cardiologists in an attempt to improve patient quality of life and decrease pacing-related complications. Implantable cardioverter-defibrillators have revolutionized treatment for humans with life-threatening ventricular tachyarrhythmias, playing a crucial role in the prevention of sudden cardiac death related to ventricular tachycardia and fibrillation. These devices have been used experimentally in dogs, and their application has been described in one clinical report.[31] For further information on pacing the reader is directed to Chapter 203.

REFERENCES

1. Echt DS, Liebson PR, Mitchell LB, et al: Mortality and morbidity in patients receiving encainide, flecainide, or placebo. The Cardiac Arrhythmia Suppression Trial, N Engl J Med 324:781, 1991.
2. Kuck K, Cappato R, Siebels J, et al: Randomized comparison of antiarrhythmic drug therapy with implantable defibrillators in patients resuscitated from cardiac arrest, Circulation 102:748, 2000.
3. Miller JM, Zipes DP: Therapy of cardiac arrhythmias. In Braunwald E, Zipes DP, Libby P, et al, editors: Braunwald's heart disease: a textbook of cardiovascular medicine, ed 7, Philadelphia, 2005, Saunders.
4. Task Force of the Working Group on Arrhythmias of the European Society of Cardiology: The Sicilian gambit. A new approach to the classification of antiarrhythmic drugs based on their actions on arrhythmogenic mechanisms, Circulation 84:1831, 1991.
5. Opie LH, DiMarco JP, Gersch BJ: Antiarrhythmic drugs and strategies. In Opie LH, Gersch BJ, editors: Drugs for the heart, ed 7, Philadelphia, 2009, Elsevier.
6. Gorgels AP, van den Dool A, Hofs A, et al: Comparison of lidocaine and procainamide in terminating sustained monomorphic ventricular tachycardia, Am J Cardiol 78:43, 1996.
7. Kosowsky BD, Taylor J, Lown B, et al: Long-term use of procaine amide following acute myocardial infarction, Circulation 47:1204, 1973.
8. Meurs KM, Spier AW, Wright NA, et al: Comparison of the effects of four antiarrhythmic treatments for familial ventricular arrhythmias in Boxers, J Am Vet Med Assoc 221:522, 2002.
9. Calvert CA, Pickus CW, Jacobs GJ: Efficacy and toxicity of tocainide for the treatment of tachyarrhythmias in Doberman Pinschers with occult cardiomyopathy, J Vet Intern Med 10:235, 1996.
10. Jacobs G: Tocainide in ventricular arrhythmias. In Proceedings of the 13th American College of Veterinary Internal Medicine Forum, Orlando, Florida, May 18-21, 1995.
11. Ramos E, O'Leary ME: State-dependent trapping of flecainide in the cardiac sodium channel, J Physiol 560(Pt 1):37, 2004.
12. Dargie HJ: β-Blockers in heart failure, Lancet 362:2, 2003.
13. MERIT-HF Study Group: Effect of metoprolol CR/XL in chronic heart failure: metoprolol CR/XL Randomized Trial in Congestive Heart Failure (MERIT-HF), Lancet 353:2001, 1999.
14. The Cardiac Insufficiency Bisoprolol Study II (CIBIS-II): a randomised trial, Lancet 353:9, 1999.
15. Fonarow GC, Albert NM, Curtis AB, et al: Incremental reduction in risk of death associated with guideline-recommended therapies in patients with heart failure: a nested, case-control analysis of IMPROVE HF, J Am Heart Assoc 1:16, 2012.
16. Wright KN, Schwartz DS, Hamlin R: Electrophysiologic and hemodynamic responses to adenosine, diltiazem, and esmolol in dogs, J Vet Intern Med 12:201, 1998.
17. Benoit SR, Mendelsohn AB, Nourjah P, et al: Risk factors for prolonged QTc among US adults: Third National Health and Nutrition Examination Survey, Eur J Cardiovasc Prev Rehabil 12:363, 2005.
18. Meurs KM, Brown WA: Update on Boxer cardiomyopathy. In Proceedings of the 16th American College of Veterinary Internal Medicine Forum, San Diego, May 23-25, 1998.
19. Gelzer AR, Krause MS, Rishniw M, et al: Combination therapy with mexiletine and sotalol suppresses inherited ventricular arrhythmias in German shepherd dogs better than mexiletine or sotalol monotherapy, J Vet Cardiol 12:93, 2010.
20. Pedro P, Lopex-Alvarex J, Fonfara S, et al: Retrospective evaluation of the use of amiodarone in dogs with arrhythmias (from 2003 to 2010), J Small Anim Pract 53:19, 2012.
21. Kraus MS, Ridge LG, Gelzer ARM, et al: Toxicity in Doberman Pinscher dogs with ventricular arrhythmias treated with amiodarone. In Proceedings of the 23rd American College of Veterinary Internal Medicine Forum, Baltimore, June 1-4, 2005.
22. Côté E: Electrocardiography and cardiac arrhythmias. In Ettinger S, Feldman B, editors: Textbook of veterinary medicine, ed 7, St Louis, 2010, Elsevier.
23. Somberg JS, Cao W, Cvetanovic I, et al: Pharmacology and toxicology of a new intravenous amiodarone (Amio-Aqueous) as compared with Cordarone IV, Am J Ther 12:9, 2005.
24. Wall M, Calvert CA, Sanderson SL, et al: Evaluation of extended-release diltiazem once daily for cats with hypertrophic cardiomyopathy, J Am Anim Hosp Assoc 41:98, 2005.
25. Poole-Wilson PA, Opie LH: Digitalis, acute inotropes, and inodilators: acute and chronic heart failure. In Opie LH, Gersch BJ, editors: Drugs for the heart, ed 7, Philadelphia, 2009, Saunders.
26. Keren A, Tzivoni D: Magnesium therapy in ventricular arrhythmias, Pacing Clin Electrophysiol 13:937-945, 1990.
27. Wright KN: Interventional catheterization for tachyarrhythmias, Vet Clin North Am Small Anim Pract 34(5):1171-1185, 2004.
28. Wright KN, Knilans TK, Irvin HM: When, why, and how to perform radiofrequency catheter ablation, J Vet Cardiol 8:95-107, 2006.
29. Santilli RA, Spadacini G, Moretti P, et al: Anatomic distribution and electrophysiologic properties of accessory pathways in dogs, J Am Vet Med Assoc 231:393-398, 2007.
30. Santilli RA, Perego M, Perini A, et al: Radiofrequency catheter ablation of the cavotricuspid isthmus as treatment of atrial flutter in two dogs, J Vet Cardiol 12:59-66, 2010.
31. Nelson OL: Implantable cardioverter defibrillators: a viable option for veterinary patients? In Proceedings of the 22nd American College of Veterinary Internal Medicine Forum, Minneapolis, June 9-12, 2004.

CHAPTER 172

INHALED MEDICATIONS

Carrie J. Miller, DVM, DACVIM (Internal Medicine)

KEY POINTS

- The use of inhaled aerosol medications has stemmed primarily from the need to manage a variety of respiratory diseases in dogs and cats effectively and with minimal adverse effects.
- Aerosol therapy (also known as *nebulization*) is the production of a liquid particulate suspension within a carrier gas (the aerosol) that is inhaled by the patient. Many factors determine whether an inhaled medication will have the desired effect in its desired location.
- Medicinal aerosolized particles are generally described by their mass median diameter (MMD), defined as the average particle diameter by mass.
- The MMD of a particle must be less than 5 μm to reach the small bronchioles and alveoli.
- Three types of systems have been used in veterinary medicine: jet nebulizers, ultrasonic nebulizers, and metered dose inhalers.
- Inhaled bronchodilators and glucocorticoids have been investigated for the treatment of feline bronchopulmonary disease and canine allergic airway disease.
- Inhaled antibiotics have been investigated for the treatment of canine infectious tracheobronchitis and bacterial pneumonia.
- Although nebulized particles are known to reach the lower airways in cats (and presumably in dogs), whether a sufficient number of drug particles are deposited in the lower airways of clinical patients at the recommended drug dosages is unknown.

INTRODUCTION

Administration of medications via inhalation has been commonplace in human medicine for decades.[1] Only recently has inhalant therapy begun to emerge in veterinary medicine, and its use remains primarily empiric. Although few published peer-reviewed studies exist for dogs and cats, clinical use of inhalant medications is clearly on the rise. This chapter summarizes the principles behind aerosol therapy, describes the various delivery systems, and discusses the common respiratory diseases in dogs and cats for which inhalant therapy is prescribed.

PRINCIPLES OF AEROSOL DEPOSITION IN THE LUNGS

The use of aerosol medication has stemmed mainly from the need to manage a variety of respiratory diseases in dogs and cats effectively and with minimal adverse effects. Many of the more common respiratory diseases require glucocorticoids and bronchodilators, which can have severe and costly adverse effects when given systemically.[2,3] In addition, many owners have difficulty administering medications to their cats or dogs, which results in poor owner compliance and inappropriate dosing. Aerosolization may also allow the clinician to effectively manage a disease that may be difficult to treat with systemic medications (e.g., *Bordetella bronchiseptica* infection).[4]

Aerosol therapy (also known as *nebulization*) is the production of a liquid particulate suspension within a carrier gas (the aerosol). Many factors determine whether an inhaled medication will have the desired effect in the correct location. The particles must be small enough in size to travel to the lower airways. Aerosolized particles generally are described by their aerodynamic equivalent diameter (AED). AED is defined as the diameter of a sphere with a standard density of 1 g/cm^3 that falls in air at the same rate as the particle in question.[5] For a particle to be deposited in the small bronchioles and alveoli, it must have an AED of 0.5 to 5 μm. Particles larger than 10 μm usually are deposited in the larynx and nasal turbinates (Table 172-1). The AED is a concept that applies only to aerosols in which the particles are homogenous in size, which is not typical of most therapeutic aerosols. Because therapeutic aerosols contain a range of particle sizes (termed *heterodisperse* aerosols), the unit that is more widely used is mass median diameter (MMD). MMD is defined as the average particle diameter by mass.[6]

Other important factors that affect the deposition of aerosolized particles in the airways are the rate of gravitational fall (gravitational sedimentation), the tendency of the particles to resist change in airflow speed and direction (inertial impaction), and the inherent random motion of particles created by collision with gas molecules (Brownian diffusion). Inertial impaction occurs when there is a sudden change in the direction of gas flow. This is most common in the nasal turbinates and bronchial bifurcations, so it tends to have the most impact in the upper airways for large particles that are larger than 5 μm AED. Gravitational sedimentation has a greater impact in the lower airways where smaller particles travel. Brownian diffusion is thought to affect only particles smaller than 0.1 μm and is probably not clinically relevant.[1,5,6] It is important to remember that the degree of particle deposition by these mechanisms also depends on patient variables such as inspiratory air velocity, tidal volume, and ventilatory pattern.[5]

DELIVERY SYSTEMS

Jet Nebulizers

Compressor (jet) and ultrasonic nebulizers (also called *atomizers*) are commonplace in human medicine, and they are becoming more

Table 172-1 Site of Aerosolized Particle Deposition in the Respiratory Tree

Site of Deposition	Aerodynamic Diameter (μm)
Nasopharynx	>20
Trachea	10-30
Bronchi	5-25
Peripheral airways	0.5-5

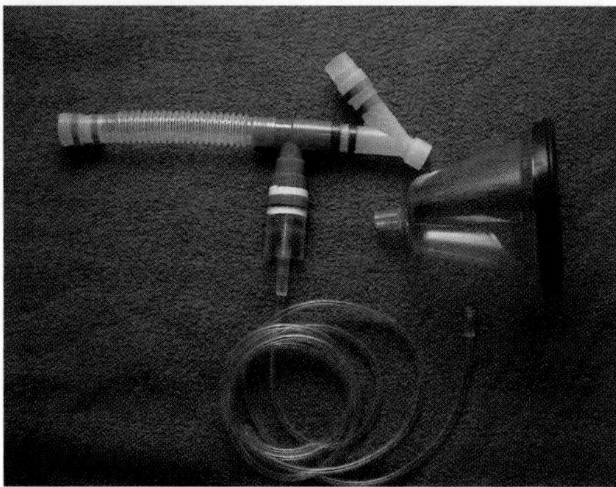

FIGURE 172-1 Example of a jet nebulizer. The tubing delivers the high-velocity gas that comminutes the solution in the nebulizer compartment into a mist. The mist then travels through the tubing and face mask, which will be attached to the patient.

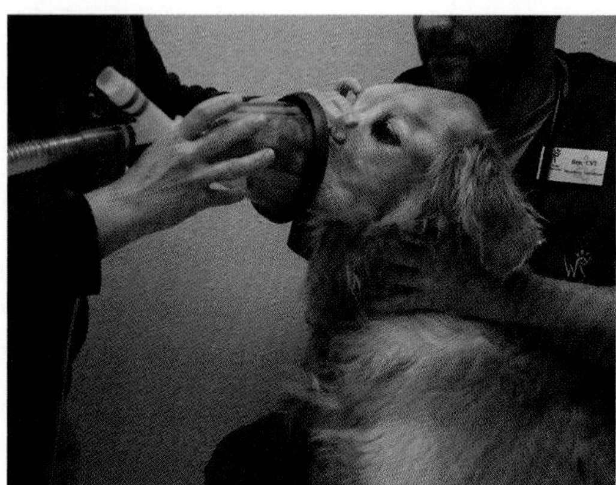

FIGURE 172-2 A patient receiving a nebulization treatment with gentamicin solution. A tight-fitting face mask with minimal dead space should be used.

popular for use in dogs and cats as well. The jet nebulizer uses a narrow, high-velocity stream of gas (typically oxygen) that travels through the designated medicated solution to comminute the liquid into an aerosol mist.[7] The mist is then delivered to the patient through a spacer and face mask (Figures 172-1 and 172-2). Most nebulizers of this type are capable of producing 50 μl of usable aerosol per liter of carrier gas, with an MMD of 3 to 6 μm.[6] This allows a significant portion of the respirable particles to travel to the bronchioles and alveoli, so that they settle principally by gravitational sedimentation in the lower airways.

Certain guidelines must be followed for effective nebulization. The nebulizer and face mask should be kept in an upright position to maximize the effect of nebulization. To enhance particle deposition in the lower airways, it is recommended that a high-output compressor (20 to 30 psi, 8 to 10 L/min) be used. This flow rate will minimize the effects of inertial impaction in the upper airways, and this compressor pressure will ensure adequate particle size as well as decrease the time needed for nebulization. Because inertial impaction can also be affected by the face mask and tubing properties, a shorter tube length, which decreases dead space within the nebulizing system, is recommended. Exhalation into the nebulized mist of medication decreases the proper delivery of the drug, so a one-way inspiratory valve is preferred to maximize drug delivery to the lungs.[5]

Because nebulizers can quickly become contaminated with bacteria and fungi, all parts must be properly disinfected after each use.

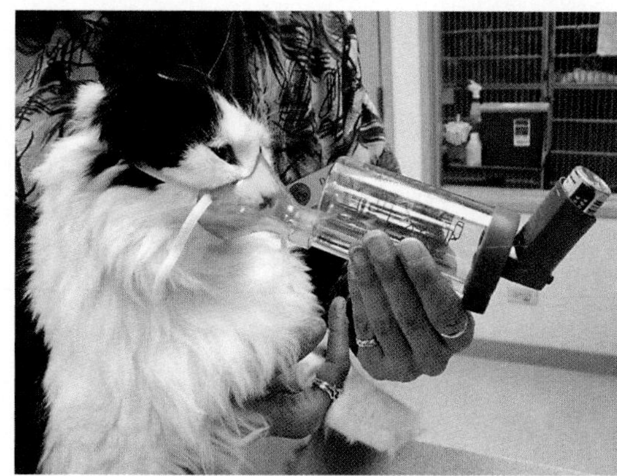

FIGURE 172-3 A patient using a metered dose inhaler attached to a feline spacer and face mask.

Use of disposable nebulizers is not recommended because their efficacy tends to decrease significantly after each use.[5] It is typically recommended that jet nebulizations occur over 5 to 10 minutes.

Ultrasonic Nebulizers

Ultrasonic nebulizers are very similar to jet nebulizers. The source of particle generation, however, is a piezoelectric transducer crystal that converts electrical energy into ultra-high-frequency oscillations that create aerosol particles from the surface of the liquid. There is no need for a compressor gas setup, so these nebulizers are more portable and are even sold for home use. Although the MMD particle size is similar in the two types of nebulizers (3 to 7 μm for ultrasonic nebulizers), the ultrasonic nebulizers can create a denser mist, with aerosols up to 200 μl/L.[6] It is typically recommended that ultrasonic nebulizations occur over 5 to 10 minutes.

Metered Dose Inhalers

Metered dose inhalers (MDIs) have been used in human medicine since 1956.[7] They have made it possible for complete outpatient portable inhalation devices to be used conveniently in human medicine. During the last 20 years, veterinarians have been experimenting with MDIs, and material has been published on how best to use these devices in cats and dogs.[2,8] MDIs consist of a plastic mouthpiece and a holder attached to a sealed aerosol canister, with a metered valve that releases a precisely measured dose of medication when the canister is pressed into the actuator (Figure 172-3). Once the device is actuated, the medication is propelled through the nozzle at a high velocity to form a spray.[7]

Because of the high velocity of the spray and the large MMD, holding chambers have been developed to decrease the velocity and particle size produced by MDI devices. This aids in decreasing the amount of inertial impaction in the upper airways and allows the patient to breathe independently of the actuation of the device. These chambers are termed *spacers* and should be attached to a form-fitting, low-dead-space face mask for veterinary patients. Not only do the spacers provide the aforementioned benefit of decreasing inertial impaction, but they also allow the mist to be sprayed into the chamber before the face mask is applied to the animal patient, which decreases the likelihood that the MDI device will scare the animal. Aerosols are delivered rapidly over 1 to 2 minutes, with an average of 7 to 10 breaths suggested. There are veterinary spacers and face masks manufactured specifically for dogs and cats (AeroKat and AeroDawg, Trudell Medical International, London, Ontario, Canada). Another option is to use a human pediatric spacer and face mask or a veterinary anesthesia face mask.

CLINICAL APPLICATIONS

Feline Bronchopulmonary Disease

Feline bronchopulmonary disease (FBPD) is a syndrome that encompasses a group of common, although incompletely understood, respiratory diseases. Clinical signs are similar to those seen in dogs with chronic bronchitis. The mainstay of treatment for these inflammatory and allergic respiratory diseases is glucocorticoids and bronchodilators (see Chapter 20).[2,3,9] As stated earlier, these medications often have detrimental side effects: glucocorticoids commonly are associated with polyphagia and subsequent weight gain, polydipsia, polyuria, changes in personality, ulceration of the gastrointestinal tract, immunosuppression, hypercoagulability, and diabetes mellitus (with long-term use). Some of the xanthine derivatives (theophylline, aminophylline) can cause vomiting, diarrhea, and inappetence, and all bronchodilators can cause excessive central nervous system stimulation and cardiac arrhythmias.[10] Use of inhaled medications may allow the clinician to control the respiratory disease more effectively without causing undesirable systemic side effects.

Inhaled bronchodilators

Inhaled β_2-adrenergic receptor agonists (albuterol, salmeterol) commonly are used to manage bronchoconstriction secondary to inflammatory lower airway disease. Stimulation of the β_2-receptor causes an increase in intracellular levels of adenylate cyclase, which decreases intracellular calcium levels and subsequently causes smooth muscle relaxation of the bronchial wall.[11,12] β_2-Adrenergic receptor agonists have been administered by nebulization experimentally to dogs at high doses and have had minimal systemic effects. In rats, ulcerated mucosal lesions may develop in the rostral aspect of the nasal cavity, but this was not reported in dogs.[13]

Minimal clinical studies have been published in the small animal veterinary literature evaluating the use of inhaled β_2-agonists for the management of bronchopulmonary disease in veterinary patients. One study showed improvement in lung function following the use of an albuterol inhaler in cats with FBPD.[14] Additional investigators have recommended use of an albuterol inhaler (88 mcg/dose, two puffs with 7 to 10 breaths q12h) for cats with moderate to severe signs of FBPD.[2,8] There is recent research demonstrating that the *R*-albuterol MDI (levalbuterol [Xopenex HFA]) is ideally recommended for cats and dogs; the racemic mixture that includes *S*-albuterol in an MDI (albuterol [ProAir HFA or Ventolin HFA]) may cause an increase in lower airway inflammation due to the proinflammatory effects of the *S*-enantiomer.[15]

Inhaled glucocorticoids

Inhaled glucocorticoids have been studied extensively in laboratory dogs as a model for human asthma, but very few controlled, randomized studies have evaluated the use of inhalant glucocorticoids in the veterinary clinical setting. Interestingly, there are studies showing that the administration of systemic glucocorticoids for at least 48 hours before administration of inhaled bronchodilators causes a significantly greater sensitivity to subsequent β_2-agonist administration. It is thought that glucocorticoids upregulate β_2-adrenergic receptors on bronchial smooth muscle.[16,17] The newer inhaled glucocorticoids tend to have very low systemic absorption and a longer duration of action due to increased lipophilicity.[5]

Inhaled glucocorticoids (e.g., fluticasone propionate [Flovent]) have been suggested for management of FBPD. Use of either a 220, 110, or 44 mcg/dose MDI for fluticasone propionate has been suggested.[2,18,19] Recent studies in cats with experimentally induced asthma indicate that use of the 44 mcg/dose MDI significantly decreases airway eosinophilia. The recommended dosage is two puffs with 7 to 10 breaths q12h in cats with bronchopulmonary disease.[20,21]

Table 172-2 Published Dosages for Inhaled Medications Commonly Used in the Management of Feline Bronchopulmonary Disease

Generic Name	Trade Name	Activity	Dosage
Albuterol	Proventil HFA, ProAir HFA	β_2 Agonist	88 mcg/dose, 2 puffs q12h
Albuterol	Xopenex HFA	β_2 Agonist	44 mcg/dose, no published dosage
Salbutamol	Ventolin HFA	β_2 Agonist	100 mcg/dose, 2 puffs q12h
Salmeterol	Serevent HFA	β_2 Agonist	50 mcg/dose, no published dosage
Fluticasone	Flovent HFA	Glucocorticoid	220 mcg/dose or 110 mcg/dose, 2 puffs q12h
Flunisolide	AeroBid HFA	Glucocorticoid	250 mcg/dose, 2 puffs q12h

Because it takes approximately 2 weeks to obtain steady-state concentrations with fluticasone propionate, oral glucocorticoids should be administered for at least 2 weeks after inhalant therapy is started.[2] At that time, if the cat appears clinically normal, the oral steroids should be tapered slowly. The suggested dosages of inhaled glucocorticoids and bronchodilators commonly used in small animal veterinary medicine are listed in Table 172-2.

Other inhaled medications

Ipratropium bromide is an acetylcholine antagonist that helps to relax smooth muscle. It has minimal systemic absorption and minor inhibitory effects on salivation. It has been used in human medicine in the treatment of patients with bronchitis, although its use for this indication has not been evaluated in veterinary medicine. Additionally, there are some studies in cats with experimentally induced with asthma that show a decrease in airway resistance after long-term treatment with nebulized lidocaine.[22]

Canine Infectious Tracheobronchitis and Pneumonia

The most common bacterial agent in infectious tracheobronchitis is *Bordetella bronchiseptica*. This gram-negative bacterium is predominantly extracellular and has several characteristics that allow the organism to attach to the tracheal cilia. This makes it difficult to decrease *Bordetella* numbers with systemic antimicrobial therapy.[4] Bemis and Appel have shown that parenteral antibiotics do not significantly decrease tracheal numbers of *Bordetella* organisms. They were able to show, however, that aerosolized gentamicin did significantly decrease *Bordetella* numbers in experimentally infected dogs.[23] Animals with symptomatic infectious tracheobronchitis that are treated with aerosolized gentamicin may show significant clinical improvement compared with other patients that are managed with commonly used oral medications.[24] Systemic absorption of aerosolized gentamicin is minimal (<3%) and does not affect renal parameters.[25] The dosage of gentamicin suggested is 6 to 7 mg/kg diluted 1:3 with sterile saline and nebulized for a treatment period of 5 to 10 minutes q8-12h for a minimum of 3 days.[22,24,26]

Medications for Use with Bronchoscopy

One of the more detrimental complications associated with bronchoscopy is bronchospasm, which can result from irritation caused by the bronchoscope itself or can occur during and after bronchoalveolar lavage. Bronchospasm can be particularly life threatening in patients with preexisting bronchoconstriction. Preventive use of bronchodilators has been evaluated in human medicine as well as in one study in cats undergoing bronchoscopy.[20] The study in cats showed that ipratropium bromide administered in combination with salbutamol lowered the incidence of bronchoalveolar lavage–induced bronchoconstriction and may be recommended as a preventive treatment for cats with presumptive FBPD undergoing bronchoscopy. This study used MDIs for delivery of both ipratropium bromide (20 mcg/puff, two puffs) and salbutamol (100 mcg/puff, two puffs) to the cats before sedation or anesthesia.

CONCLUSION

Although nebulized particles are known to reach the lower airways in cats (and presumably in dogs), whether a sufficient number of drug particles are deposited in the lower airways at the recommended drug dosages remains unknown.[27] However, various clinical studies have suggested that inhaled medications do cause an improvement in clinical signs of respiratory disease in dogs and cats. Perhaps as more controlled prospective studies are performed, the veterinary use of inhalant therapy will become more evidence based than empirically based.

REFERENCES

1. Newhouse MT, Ruffin RE: Deposition and fate of aerosolized drugs, Chest 73:936, 1978.
2. Padrid P: Feline asthma diagnosis and treatment, Vet Clin North Am Small Anim Pract 30:1279, 2000.
3. McKiernan BC: Diagnosis and treatment of canine chronic bronchitis, Vet Clin North Am Small Anim Pract 30:1267, 2000.
4. Ford RB: Canine infectious tracheobronchitis. In Greene CE, editor: Infectious diseases of the dog and cat, St Louis, 2006, Elsevier.
5. Hoffman AM: Inhaled medications and bronchodilator usage in the horse, Vet Clin North Am Small Anim Pract 13:519, 1997.
6. Court MH, Dodman NH, Seeler DC: Inhalation therapy, oxygen administration, humidification, and aerosol therapy, Vet Clin North Am Small Anim Pract 15:1041, 1985.
7. Grossman J: The evolution of inhaler technology, J Asthma 31:55, 1994.
8. Padrid P: Use of inhaled medications to treat respiratory diseases in dogs and cats, J Am Anim Hosp Assoc 42:165, 2006.
9. McKiernan BC, Miller CJ: Allergic airway disease. In Wingfield WE, Raffe MR, editors: The veterinary ICU book, Jackson Hole, Wyo, 2002, Teton NewMedia.
10. Boothe DM: Drugs affecting the respiratory system. In Boothe DM, editor: Small animal clinical pharmacology and therapeutics, ed 1, St Louis, 2001, Saunders.
11. Tabachnick IA: A summary of the pharmacology and toxicology of albuterol (Proventil), Ann Allergy 47:379, 1981.
12. Zimmerman I, Walkenhorst W, Ulmer WT: The site of action of bronchodilating drugs (β_2-stimulators) on antigen-induced bronchoconstriction, Respiration 38:65, 1979.
13. Dudley RE, Patterson SE, Machotka SV, et al: One-month inhalation toxicity study of tulobuterol hydrochloride in rats and dogs, Fundam Appl Toxicol 13:694, 1989.
14. Rozanski EA: Lung function and inhaled albuterol in cats with asthma, Proc J Vet Intern Med 13:132, 1999 (abstract).
15. Reinero CR, Delgado C, Spinka C, et al: Enantiomer-specific effects of albuterol on airway inflammation in healthy and asthmatic cats, Int Arch Allergy Immunol 150(1):43-50, 2009.
16. Sauder RA, Tobias JD, Hirshman CA: Methylprednisolone restores sensitivity to β-adrenergic agonists in Basenji-Greyhound dogs, J Appl Physiol 72:694, 1992.
17. Sauder RA, Lenox WC, Tobias JD, et al: Methylprednisolone increases sensitivity to β-adrenergic agonists within 48 hours in Basenji Greyhounds, Anesthesiology 79:1278, 1993.
18. Miller CJ: Rhinitis and sinusitis. In Tilley LP, Smith FWK, Johnson LR, editors: The 5-minute veterinary consult, canine and feline, Baltimore, 2004, Lippincott Williams & Wilkins.
19. Kirschvink N, Leemans J, Delvaux F, et al: Inhaled fluticasone reduces bronchial responsiveness and airway inflammation in cats with mild bronchitis, J Feline Med Surg 8(1):45-54, 2006.
20. Kirschvink N, Leemans J, Delvaux F, et al: Bronchodilators in bronchoscopy-induced airflow limitation in allergen-sensitized cats, J Vet Intern Med 19:161, 2005.
21. Cohn LA, DeClue AE, Cohen RL, et al: Effects of fluticasone propionate dosage in an experimental model of feline asthma, J Feline Med Surg 12(2):91-96, 2010.
22. Nafe LA, Guntur VP, Dodam JR, et al: Nebulized lidocaine blunts airway hyper-responsiveness in experimental feline asthma, J Feline Med Surg 15(8):712-716, 2013.
23. Bemis DA, Appel MJG: Aerosol, parenteral, and oral antibiotic treatment of *Bordetella bronchiseptica* infections in dogs, J Am Vet Med Assoc 170:1082, 1977.
24. Miller CJ: Gentamicin aerosolization for treatment of infectious tracheobronchitis, Proc J Vet Intern Med 17:27, 2003 (abstract).
25. Riviere JE, Silver GR, Coppoc GL, et al: Gentamicin aerosol therapy in 18 dogs: failure to induce detectable serum concentrations of the drug, J Am Vet Med Assoc 179:166, 1981.
26. Greene CE, Watson DJ: Antibacterial chemotherapy. In Greene CE, editor: Infectious diseases of the dog and cat, ed 3, St Louis, 2006, Saunders.
27. Schulman RL, Crochik SS, Kneller SK, et al: Investigation of pulmonary deposition of a nebulized radiopharmaceutical agent in awake cats, Am J Vet Res 65:806, 2004.

CHAPTER 173

COMPLICATIONS OF CHEMOTHERAPY AGENTS

Victoria S. Larson, BSc, DVM, MS, DACVIM (Oncology) • Valerie Madden, DVM

KEY POINTS

- Chemotherapy is one mode of management of cancer in dogs and cats.
- Recent advances in chemotherapy have resulted in increased remission rates and survival times for patients with cancer.
- Complications of chemotherapy occur, and innocent bystanders are also harmed.
- It is imperative that the clinical staff be aware of the toxicities of each chemotherapeutic agent so that complications can be identified.
- Complications should be treated rapidly and thoroughly with supportive measures.

Cancer is a major cause of disease-related death in dogs and cats. Various studies during the last 30 years show that about half of all dogs and one third of all cats will die of cancer. The prevalence of cancer in small animals is increasing, along with an increased awareness of and an expansion of knowledge about diagnosis, treatment options, and prognosis.[1]

As clinicians strive for higher remission rates and longer survival times, treatment protocols are rapidly approaching the cutting edge. The consequence of these advances is that chemotherapy complications have become a reality of practice.

Preparation for, recognition of, and early intervention for such complications are critical for a successful outcome in patients receiving chemotherapy. This chapter focuses on the complications of chemotherapy in dogs and cats.

PRINCIPLES OF CHEMOTHERAPY

Chemotherapy literally means "the management of illness by chemical means."[2]

Simply stated, chemotherapy drugs work by killing cells. Categories of chemotherapy drugs include alkylating agents, antibiotics, antimetabolites, enzymes, hormones, nonsteroidal antiinflammatory drugs (NSAIDs), platinum products, and vinca alkaloids. Each of these effects cell death by various mechanisms of action and all can cause toxicoses because normal cells, as well as cancer cells, are arbitrarily killed in various body systems.

TESTING FOR CHEMOTHERAPY DRUG SENSITIVITY

Many herding dogs have a mutation in the multidrug resistance (MDR1) gene that results in an increased sensitivity to certain drugs, including chemotherapy drugs[3] (Table 173-1). It is currently recognized that dogs such as collies, Shetland Sheepdogs (Shelties), Australian Shepherds, Old English Sheepdogs, English Shepherds, German Shepherds, Long-Haired Whippets, Silken Windhounds, and a variety of mixed breed dogs carry the mutation. Because of this, the authors currently offer testing to all potential chemotherapy patients and recommend that pets of these breeds be tested. The test can be performed in the clinic, with results typically available within 1 week. Dose adjustments or selection of alternative chemotherapy agents may be made pending receipt of results. Further information can be obtained from the Washington State University website (http://www.vetmed.wsu.edu/depts-vcpl).

CHEMOTHERAPY DRUGS

Alkylating agents include cyclophosphamide, chlorambucil, CCNU (1-[2-chloroethyl]-3 cyclohexyl-1-nitrosourea [lomustine]), BCNU (1,3-bis-[2-chloroethyl]-1-nitrosourea [carmustine]), and melphalan. Antibiotic chemotherapy drugs include doxorubicin, actinomycin, epirubicin, bleomycin, and mitoxantrone. Antimetabolites are methotrexate and cytosine arabinoside. L-Asparaginase is an enzyme used in chemotherapy. NSAIDs that commonly are used include piroxicam, meloxicam (Metacam), deracoxib (Deramaxx), etodolac (EtoGesic), and carprofen (Rimadyl). Prednisone is the hormone most commonly used as a chemotherapeutic agent. Platinum products include cisplatin and carboplatin. The vinca alkaloids include vincristine, vinblastine, and vinorelbine.[4-6] Newer chemotherapy drugs include tyrosine kinase inhibitors such as toceranib phosphate and masitinib.[7,8]

Chemotherapy drugs and their potential toxicoses are listed in Table 173-1.

TOXICITIES AND TREATMENT OF CHEMOTHERAPY-RELATED EMERGENCIES

Acute Tumor Lysis Syndrome

Acute tumor lysis syndrome (ATLS) is a rare complication of chemotherapy believed to occur most commonly in patients who have chemotherapy- or radiation-responsive tumors. Risk factors include large tumor burdens, chemotherapy-responsive tumor type, preexisting renal disease, and dehydration.[9,10] This condition results from destruction of tumor cells, which can then lead to release of intracellular electrolytes (potassium, phosphate) as well as the toxic byproducts of cell necrosis into the circulation.[11]

Nucleic acids released from cellular necrosis include purines, which are metabolized to uric acid. Increased levels of uric acid exacerbate metabolic acidosis and renal impairment or failure.[12] Deposition of calcium phosphate salts in the renal tubules in addition to the aforementioned biochemical alterations, intraluminal tubular obstruction, intravascular volume depletion, and release of malignancy-associated nephrotoxins can result in oliguric renal failure.[9]

Biochemical abnormalities include hyperkalemia, hyperphosphatemia, hypocalcemia (as a sequela of elevated phosphate levels), and metabolic acidosis. Azotemia may also be present.[9]

Clinical presentation of ATLS can occur hours to days after therapy has been administered. Characteristically, a patient that has

Table 173-1 **Chemotherapy Drugs and Potential Toxicoses**[4,5,7,8]

Chemotherapeutic Agent	Reported Toxicosis	Specific Toxicities
Alkylating agents	Alopecia Bone marrow suppression Gastrointestinal toxicity Nausea Inappetence Vomiting Diarrhea	CCNU: Cumulative dose–related risk of hepatotoxicity Chlorambucil: neurotoxicity Cyclophosphamide: sterile hemorrhagic cystitis
Antibiotics	Alopecia Bone marrow suppression Gastrointestinal toxicity Nausea Inappetence Vomiting Diarrhea Necrosis, ischemia, and severe soft tissue reaction if given perivascularly	Doxorubicin: Cumulative dose–related risk of dilated cardiomyopathy in dogs, possible renal toxicity in cats, allergic reactions in both species, hemorrhagic colitis
Antimetabolites	Alopecia Bone marrow suppression Gastrointestinal toxicity Nausea Inappetence Vomiting Diarrhea	
Enzymes	Anaphylaxis	L-Asparaginase: Pain on injection, pancreatitis, insulin resistance
Hormones	Iatrogenic excessive hormonal effects	Prednisone/prednisolone: Hypercortisolism, gastrointestinal ulceration, renotoxicity
Nonsteroidal antiinflammatory drugs	Gastrointestinal ulceration Renal toxicity	Carprofen: Liver toxicity
Platinum products	Bone marrow suppression Gastrointestinal toxicity Inappetence Nausea Vomiting Diarrhea	Cisplatin: Pulmonary edema and death in cats, nephrotoxicity in dogs
Protein tyrosine kinase inhibitors (toceranib phosphate, masitinib)	Bone marrow suppression Gastrointestinal toxicity Inappetence Nausea Vomiting Diarrhea	
Vinca alkaloids	Alopecia Bone marrow suppression Gastrointestinal toxicity Ileus Peripheral neuropathies	

CCNU, 1-(2-Chloroethyl)-3 cyclohexyl-1-nitrosourea (lomustine).

ostensibly responded to therapy shows symptoms such as lethargy, vomiting, diarrhea, bradycardia, cardiovascular collapse, and ultimately shock.[10,13]

Workup includes a thorough physical examination, full blood work, and urinalysis. Because the clinical signs of ATLS may mimic other pathologic conditions, additional diagnostic tests such as determination of a coagulation profile, diagnostic imaging, and blood and urine cultures may be indicated.[9,10]

Therapy is directed at cardiovascular support with administration of intravenous fluids and consideration of correction of electrolyte abnormalities and renal parameters. Administration of normal saline is a reasonable choice in patients with hyperkalemia and hyperphosphatemia until such time as the electrolyte abnormalities are corrected, and then a balanced electrolyte solution may be used.[9,10] Please see Chapters 5, 51, and 60 for more detailed recommendations on treatment of shock, fluid therapy, and management of hyperkalemia-associated arrhythmias.

Calcium can be administered parenterally in patients displaying clinical symptoms of hypocalcemia. Due to variability in the production and significance of metabolites, therapies such as urinary alkalinization, administration of allopurinol, and administration of urate oxidases are not currently recommended in veterinary patients.[9]

Allergic Reactions

Acute type I hypersensitivity reactions have been reported upon administration of L-asparaginase. Polysorbate 80, the carrier found in etoposide, can also trigger a type I reaction. Doxorubicin administration can directly stimulate mast cell degranulation, causing an anaphylactoid reaction. This is in contrast to true hypersensitivity reactions, in which mast cell degranulation is activated via immunoglobulin E.

Clinical signs in dogs usually appear within minutes but can occur several hours after administration and can include head shaking, generalized urticaria, erythema, agitation, vomiting, and hypotension leading to collapse. For the most part, dogs tend to manifest allergic reactions in the skin and gastrointestinal (GI) tract. Hypersensitivity reactions are rare in cats and tend to manifest as respiratory signs such as tachypnea, dyspnea, and wheezing.[14]

Hypersensitivity reactions may be prevented by pretreatment with histamine-1 (H_1) and H_2 receptor antagonists. In the emergency setting, therapy should consist of discontinuing the drug, instituting fluid therapy, and administering an H_2 receptor blocker (e.g., diphenhydramine) and glucocorticoids (dexamethasone). Epinephrine can be given in severe and refractory cases.[14]

Bone Marrow Toxicity

Myelosuppression can occur in the oncology patient for a number of reasons, such as secondary to the neoplastic process or as a result of treatment. This chapter addresses bone marrow toxicity resulting from the cytotoxic effects of chemotherapy.

Anemia

Anemia is a common hematologic abnormality in patients with cancer and is most often due to a syndrome of anemia of chronic disease, blood loss, or a paraneoplastic syndrome of immune-mediated hemolytic anemia. Anemia is rarely encountered secondary to chemotherapy because of the longer life span of red blood cells.[14] Although it is uncommon, anemia can occur secondary to bleeding into the GI tract caused by GI ulceration (e.g., from mast cell degranulation and release of vasoactive amines), medications (NSAIDs, glucocorticoids), or chemotherapy. When an animal is bleeding into the GI tract from an ulcer and the underlying cause is a tumor, treatment addresses this underlying cause (resection of the mass, chemotherapy) and supportive care is provided for the gastric ulceration with a proton pump inhibitor (e.g., omeprazole), H_1 receptor antagonist (such as famotidine or ranitidine), and sucralfate. If the ulceration is due to long-term antiinflammatory drug use and this medication is critical to the treatment protocol, the antiinflammatory drugs may be temporarily discontinued, treatment initiated as described earlier, and then antiinflammatory drug therapy reinstituted with the use of a prostaglandin inhibitor. If the bleeding is due to chemotherapy, as in the case of hemorrhagic colitis secondary to doxorubicin chemotherapy, it is usually short term and rarely causes anemia. Supportive care with GI protectants and antidiarrheal medications can be instituted for comfort. The authors prefer the use of sulfasalazine because of its mechanism of action in the large bowel; the diazo bond is cleaved by colonic bacteria to release sulfapyridine and 5-acetylsalicylic acid, which exerts both a local antibiotic and an antiinflammatory action.[15] Anemia secondary to recurrent marrow suppression and exhaustion of the marrow usually is seen after months of therapy and is related to repeated insults to the bone marrow; it is considered irreversible.

Thrombocytopenia

Thrombocytopenia can result from platelet consumption, destruction, decreased production, or loss. For thrombocytopenia resulting from loss into the GI tract, ulcer therapy with antacids and GI protectants, and discontinuation of antiinflammatory drugs is recommended. Thrombocytopenia that results from chemotherapy is rarely of clinical significance and may be treated by delaying the next dose of chemotherapy for 3 to 5 days. Thrombocytosis can be seen in patients after chemotherapy due to bone marrow rebound in response to chemotherapy-induced thrombocytopenia.[14]

Neutropenia

Neutropenia most often is associated with cytotoxic chemotherapy agents. This type of myelosuppression occurs at the nadir, which is defined as the time when the white blood cell count is at its lowest after administration of chemotherapy. The nadir is different for each drug. The nadir for doxorubicin and cyclophosphamide is 7 to 10 days; the nadir for cisplatin is 7 and 16 days; and the nadir for carboplatin is 11 and possibly 21 days after administration. In many instances, treatment is not required for neutropenia because the patient is asymptomatic and the cell counts likely will return to the normal range within a week.

Neutropenia in an oncology patient, even one without a fever, should prompt the veterinary staff to recommend careful monitoring of vital signs (temperature, pulse, and respiratory rate), appetite, and attitude. Neutrophil counts below 1000 cells/mcl warrant prophylactic therapy with broad-spectrum antibiotics for a week. If at any time the patient develops a fever or the clinical condition deteriorates (inappetence, lethargy, depression, vomiting, and diarrhea), aggressive intervention is required to prevent a septic crisis. This should begin with a complete physical examination with an emphasis on auscultation of the lungs, basic blood work and urinalysis, and administration of fluid therapy, in addition to four-quadrant protection with antibiotics (gram-negative, gram-positive, aerobic, and anaerobic coverage). Strict aseptic technique should be used at all times. Serial thoracic radiography should be performed in a neutropenic febrile patient to identify pneumonia early in the course of disease. Additional supportive therapies should be administered as indicated (see Chapter 90).

Neutropenia that is profound or persists for longer than 1 week necessitates therapy with granulocyte colony-stimulating factor. This may be instituted in the hospital and continued for up to 5 days.

Sepsis

Sepsis and septic shock are not uncommon in patients with cancer. Sepsis can be a result of the disease itself or a complication of management (see Chapter 91).

Cardiotoxicity

See Chapter 42.

Dermatologic Toxicity

Dermatologic complications can occur secondary to chemotherapy but rarely require emergency or critical care attention and therefore are not discussed in this chapter.

Extravasation

Extravasation of vesicant chemotherapeutic agents can cause severe local tissue reactions leading to necrosis. Doxorubicin is the chemotherapeutic agent most commonly responsible and arguably results in the most severe reactions, but this may be due to the volume that is extravasated. Other chemotherapeutic agents such as the vinca alkaloids and other anthracyclines can also be locally irritating if delivered outside the vein. Clinical signs of pain, pruritus, erythema, moist dermatitis, and necrosis can occur within 7 to 10 days with doxorubicin and within a week if a vinca alkaloid has extravasated.[16]

If doxorubicin is given accidentally outside the vein, the following recommendations apply:

1. Discontinue administration of the drug immediately.
2. Withdraw as much drug as possible from the catheter.
3. Administer dexrazoxane at 10 times the extravasated dose intravenously within 3 hours of the event and then q24h for 3 days.

4. Monitor the site every other day for 10 days for local tissue reaction.
5. Treat any local reaction symptomatically with topical preparations (antibiotics, steroids), bandaging, Elizabethan collar, and surgical debridement if severe.

If a vinca alkaloid is delivered outside the vein, the following recommendations apply:

1. Discontinue administration of the drug immediately.
2. Withdraw as much drug as possible from the catheter.
3. Some oncologists infiltrate the area with sterile saline or with sterile saline and 8.4% sodium bicarbonate and 4 mg dexamethasone sodium phosphate.
4. Apply warm compress.
5. Treat any local reaction symptomatically with topical preparations (antibiotics, steroids), bandaging, Elizabethan collar, and surgical debridement if severe.

Gastrointestinal Toxicity

Some of the common ongoing health complaints of the oncology patient are cancer cachexia, anorexia, vomiting, and diarrhea.

Cachexia and anorexia

Cachexia and anorexia are common conditions in pets with cancer.[17] Cachexia and sarcopenia are considered emerging phenomena in veterinary patients, and new therapies and management strategies can ameliorate symptoms; however, they are not considered common adverse effects of chemotherapy.[18]

Anorexia, on the other hand, is a significant medical condition in pets receiving chemotherapy, secondary either to the underlying primary condition or to chemotherapy. If it is caused by chemotherapy, management strategies such as dose adjustments, prophylactic therapy with antinausea medications, or symptomatic therapy with antinausea medications, appetite stimulants, and, if not contraindicated by the patient's diagnosis, glucocorticoids may be useful. Placement of a feeding tube in patients that are anorexic is indicated early in the course of disease. The authors recommend placement of a feeding tube when more than 10% of body weight is lost due to therapy. A nasoesophageal tube may be used short term, although this method of feeding typically does not allow for administration of a patient's total daily energy requirement unless feeding is by constant rate infusion, which makes this method useful in hospitalized patients only. An esophageal feeding tube is preferable if the esophagus is functional because it uses esophageal function and is generally well tolerated in dogs and cats.

Vomiting

Vomiting is a common consequence of chemotherapy. Although it is usually self-limiting and stops within 2 to 3 days after it starts, routine supportive care can improve the patient's comfort and shorten the duration of this adverse effect. The authors typically send the patient home with a 5-day course of maropitant citrate (Cerenia) to be administered at the first sign of inappetence or nausea. If the patient does not respond to therapy or continues to vomit for longer than 24 hours, or is vomiting unrelentingly, more aggressive treatment is recommended. This could include admission to the hospital for intravenous fluid therapy, injectable antiemetics (maropitant citrate, ondansetron, or dolasetron, and/or metoclopramide), and GI protectants such as a slurry of sucralfate and an injectable H_2 receptor antagonist (e.g., ranitidine). When a patient has experienced significant vomiting after treatment with a chemotherapy drug, subsequent treatments with the same medication may be reduced in dose by 10% to 25% and ancillary prophylactic medication administered for several days after therapy.

Diarrhea

In oncology patients that are stressed by their treatment or hospitalization, clostridial colitis can result. This condition is characterized by passage of a small volume of loose stool that may or may not have frank blood and mucus in it. Historically, it has been diagnosed by identification of clostridial endospores on a fecal smear in conjunction with clinical signs. An enzyme-linked immunosorbent assay kit is available for detection of *Clostridium perfringens* endospores in fecal specimens. The recommended antimicrobial therapy for clostridial diarrhea is based on sulfasalazine, metronidazole, ampicillin, or tylosin. Dietary management by increasing fiber content in the food through the addition of canned pumpkin or psyllium hydrophilic mucilloid fiber (Metamucil) may also be useful. In mild cases of diarrhea, treatment with bismuth subsalicylate (Pepto-Bismol) often results in resolution of signs within a day or so.

Hemorrhagic colitis is a unique toxicity of doxorubicin (Adriamycin). This form of large bowel diarrhea usually responds to sulfasalazine or metronidazole. If the diarrhea is moderate to severe, persists for longer than 2 to 3 days, or if the patient is exhibiting signs of lethargy, depression, fever, vomiting, or general malaise, more aggressive intervention with hospitalization, resting of the GI tract, fluid therapy, and antibiotics is recommended.

Neurologic Toxicity

Peripheral neuropathies have been reported after administration of the vinca alkaloids, particularly vincristine. Hind limb weakness, partial paralysis, and ileus leading to abdominal pain and constipation have been reported in dogs and cats.[14] Therapy includes supportive care and alleviation of the discomfort of ileus with metoclopramide. Discontinuation of the drug, administering it at a reduced dosage, or substituting vincristine with vinblastine or vinorelbine may be effective.

Cisplatin has resulted in cortical blindness according to a case report of two dogs.[14] 5-Fluorouracil is extremely neurotoxic in cats and should never be administered; it results in a fatal reaction that may include excitability, blindness, tremors, dysmetria, and death. In dogs, it can also result in excitation, seizures, and ataxia.[14]

Urologic Toxicity

Cyclophosphamide has been associated with sterile hemorrhagic cystitis characterized by clinical signs including pollakiuria, hematuria, and dysuria. Diagnosis is made by demonstration of plentiful red blood cells, white blood cells, and the absence of bacteria in urine. Ultrasonography of the bladder reveals a diffusely thickened bladder wall. Therapy consists of discontinuation of the drug, prevention of infection with antibiotics, diuresis, and administration of antiinflammatory medications. Most cases resolve within days to a week after discontinuance of the medication and institution of the supportive measures indicated. Additional therapies reported to be effective in refractory cases are intravesicular administration of a 1% formalin solution and dimethyl sulfoxide (DMSO).[14] It is important to note that cyclophosphamide therapy will likely continue to cause cystitis if it is reinstituted, so substituting chlorambucil for cyclophosphamide may be reasonable. Some cases of sterile hemorrhagic cystitis are reported to be refractory to treatment; however, this has not been the authors' experience. Administration of cyclophosphamide has been associated with the development of transitional cell carcinoma in the bladder later in life.

Nephrotoxicity secondary to cisplatin use has been reported in dogs, and renal failure has been reported in cats after administration of doxorubicin.[14]

Drugs used to treat reactions to chemotherapy are listed in Table 173-2.

Table 173-2 **Drugs Commonly Used to Treat Adverse Effects or Complications of Chemotherapy**[12,14]

Medication	Drug Class	Dose	Frequency	Route	Indications
Amoxicillin or ampicillin	Extended-spectrum penicillin antibiotic	11-22 mg/kg	q8-12h	PO (amoxicillin) or IV, IM (ampicillin)	Infection
Dexrazoxane	Antidote	10 times extravasated dose	Once within 3 hr of event, then q24h for 3 days	IV	Doxorubicin extravasation
Diphenhydramine	H_1 receptor antagonist Antihistamine	1 mg/kg 2-4 mg/kg (not to exceed 40 mg)	q8-12h q8-12h	IV PO	Allergic reaction
Enrofloxacin	Fluoroquinolone antibiotic	5-20 mg/kg (not to exceed 5 mg/kg in cats)	q24h (or divided q12h)	PO or IV	Infection
Famotidine	H_2 receptor antagonist	0.1-0.2 mg/kg	q12h	PO, IV, IM	GI ulcer management *Note:* Anecdotal reports of intravascular hemolysis in cats
Granulocyte colony-stimulating factor	Cytokine hematopoietic agent	5 mcg/kg	q24h until neutrophil count exceeds 3000/mcl for 2 days	SC	Neutropenia
Omeprazole	Proton pump inhibitor	0.5-1.5 mg/kg (0.7 mg/kg for adjunctive therapy)	q24h	PO	GI ulcer management, prevention
Ondansetron	5-HT_3 receptor antagonist	0.5-1 mg/kg	Can be given 0.1-0.5 mg/kg IV over 15 min q8h or 30 min before chemotherapy)	PO	Chemotherapy-related vomiting
Oxybutynin	Genitourinary smooth muscle relaxant	1.25-5 mg total dose (dogs) 0.5-1 mg total dose (cats)	q8-12h	PO	Sterile hemorrhagic cystitis
Maropitant citrate	Antiemetic Neurokinin-1 receptor antagonist	1-2 mg/kg (can give 0.5-1 mg/kg in cats)	1 hr before emetogenic event and then q24h for up to 5 days	PO (2 mg/kg) or SC (1 mg/kg)	Inappetence, nausea or vomiting
Metoclopramide	Central dopaminergic antagonist, peripheral 5-HT_3 receptor antagonist and 5-HT_4 receptor agonist	0.2-0.4 mg/kg	q6h or may be given at 1-2 mg/kg/24 h IV CRI	PO, SC, IM	Vomiting
Metronidazole	Antibiotic	15-25 mg/kg	q12-24h	PO	Diarrhea
Misoprostol	Prostaglandin E_1 analog	2-5 mcg/kg	q6-12h or may be given at 3 mcg/kg q8-24h for prevention of ulcers in pets receiving NSAIDs	PO	Treatment or prevention of GI ulcers
Pantoprazole	Proton pump inhibitor	0.7-1 mg/kg	q24h	IV	GI ulcer management, prevention
Ranitidine	H_2 receptor antagonist	0.5-2 mg/kg (dogs) 1-2 mg/kg (cats)	q12h	PO, IV, IM	GI ulcer treatment, prophylaxis
Sucralfate	Aluminum salt, binds proteinaceous exudate	0.5-1 g (dogs) 0.25-0.5 g (cats)	q8h	PO	GI ulcer management
Sulfasalazine	Sulfonamide, salicylate antibacterial, immunosuppressive	20-40 mg/kg (dogs) 10-20 mg/kg (cats) *Note:* Use caution in cats due to salicylate	q8h q24h	PO PO	Hemorrhagic colitis

5-HT_3, 5-HT_4, 5-Hydroxytriptamine 3 and 4; *CRI,* constant rate infusion; *GI,* gastrointestinal; *H_1, H_2,* histamine 1 and 2; *IM,* intramuscularly; *IV,* intravenously; *NSAIDs,* nonsteroidal antiinflammatory drugs; *PO,* per os; *SC,* subcutaneously.

REFERENCES

1. Withrow SJ: Why worry about cancer in pets? In Withrow SJ, Vail DM, editors: Withrow and MacEwen's small animal clinical oncology, ed 4, St Louis, 2007, Saunders.
2. Blood DC, Studdert VP, Gay CC: Saunders comprehensive veterinary dictionary, ed 3, London, 2007, Elsevier.
3. Mealey KL: Therapeutic implications of the MDR-1 gene, J Vet Pharmacol Ther 27(5):257-264, 2004.
4. Chun R, Garrett L, Vail DM: Cancer chemotherapy. In Withrow SJ, Vail DM, editors: Withrow and MacEwen's small animal clinical oncology, ed 4, St Louis, 2007, Saunders.
5. Kaufman D, Chabner BA: Clinical strategies for cancer treatment: the role of drugs. In Chabner BA, Longo DL, editors: Cancer chemotherapy and biotherapy, principles and practice, ed 2, Philadelphia, 1996, Lippincott-Raven.
6. Ogilvie GK, Moore AS: Chemotherapy: properties, uses, and patient management. In Ogilvie GK, Moore AS, editors: Feline oncology, Trenton, NJ, 2001, Veterinary Learning Systems.
7. London CA, Hannah AL, Zadovoskaya R, et al: Phase 1 dose-escalating study of SU11654, a small molecule receptor tyrosine kinase inhibitor, in dogs with spontaneous malignancies, Clin Cancer Res 9(7):2755-2768, 2003.
8. Hahn KA, Ogilvie G, Rusk T, et al: Masitinib is safe and effective for treatment of canine mast cell tumors, J Vet Intern Med 22(6):1301-1309, 2008.
9. Bergman PJ: Tumor lysis syndrome. In Silverstein D, Hopper K, editors: Small animal critical care medicine, ed 1, St Louis, 2009, Saunders.
10. Mathews K: Oncologic emergencies. In Mathews K: Veterinary emergency and critical care manual, ed 2, Guelph, Canada, 2009, Lifelearn.
11. McCurdy MT, Shanholtz CB: Oncologic emergencies, J Crit Care Med 40(7):2212-2222, 2012.
12. Kosmidis PA, Schrijvers D, André F: ESMO handbook of oncological emergencies, Lugano, Switzerland, 2005, European Society for Medical Oncology.
13. Whol JS, Cotter S: Approach to complications of anti-cancer therapy in emergency practice, J Vet Emerg Crit Care 5(1):61-76, 1995.
14. Couto GC: Management of complications cancer chemotherapy, Vet Clin North Am Small Anim Pract 20:879, 1990.
15. Ramsey I, editor: BSAVA small animal formulary, ed 6, Quedgeley, UK, 2008, British Small Animal Veterinary Association.
16. Langer SW, Sehested M, Jensen PB: Treatment of anthracycline extravasation with dexrazoxane, Clin Cancer Res 6:3680, 2000.
17. Ogilvie GK, Moore AS: Nutritional support. In Ogilvie GK, Moore AS, editors: Feline oncology, Trenton, NJ, 2001, Veterinary Learning Systems.
18. Freeman LM: Cachexia and sarcopenia: emerging syndromes of importance in dogs and cats, J Vet Intern Med 26(1):3-17, 2012.

CHAPTER 174
ANTITOXINS AND ANTIVENOMS

Robert A. Armentano, DVM, DACVIM • Michael Schaer, DVM, DACVIM (Internal Medicine), DACVECC

KEY POINTS

- The main antitoxins used in small animal medicine (tetanus and tick) will vary according to geographic locale.
- Antivenoms are most commonly used to treat poisonous snake bites.

This chapter describes the indications for and use of antivenoms and antitoxins that are available for use against certain toxins and animal venoms. Antivenoms and antitoxins are neutralizing antibodies that are derived from a hyperimmunized donor. In the critically ill dog and cat, there are several conditions that benefit from administration of these antibodies. Tetanus antitoxin and the poisonous snake antivenoms are the products most commonly used in dogs and cats. This section describes each toxin only briefly; the emphasis is on the available products and their applications in treating various conditions.

Antitoxins are antibodies that are used to protect the body by the process of passive immunization. The antibodies are produced in a donor animal by active immunization, and after a period of several weeks to months, the donor's blood is collected and the immunoglobulins are separated into specific components that can be used to provide immunity to the recipient. The donors are commonly horses that undergo a series of immunizations with the organism or toxin against which antibodies need to be produced. These toxins are first treated with formaldehyde to denature the protein and thus render it nontoxic. These denatured proteins are called *toxoids,* and it is the toxoids that are repeatedly injected into a horse or some other host that will produce the desired antitoxin or antibody. The responses of the horses are monitored, and once their antibodies levels are sufficiently elevated, serum is collected.[1] Subsequent injections can be performed using purified toxin. Plasma is separated from the horse blood, and the globulin fraction that contains the antibodies is concentrated, titrated, and dispensed. Antitoxin potency is tested using an international biologic standard.

TETANUS ANTITOXIN

Two tetanus antitoxin preparations are available for veterinary patients: Tetanus Antitoxin Behring produced by Intervet UK (Milton Keynes, U.K.) and Tetanus Antitoxin produced by Fort Dodge Animal Health (Fort Dodge, IA) in the United States. There are also tetanus antitoxin products produced for humans (human tetanus immune globulin) that have been used off label in dogs and cats.[2,3] The reader is referred to the product drug insert for details describing composition, storage, and preparation for injection. The Fort Dodge product is labeled for use in horses, goats, sheep, and swine, but it has been used in dogs and cats.[4] The Intervet tetanus antitoxin is made for use in dogs; it is not recommended for use in cats because of the phenol

BOX 174-1 *Emergency Treatment of Anaphylaxis Due to Antitoxin or Antivenom Administration*

- Slow or stop infusion of antitoxin or antivenom.
- For severe signs:
  - *Epinephrine* 0.01 mg/kg IM; can repeat q15-20min, if necessary.
  - *Diphenhydramine* 3-4 mg/kg IV or IM; can repeat q12h.
  - *Ranitidine* 0.5-1.0 mg/kg IV or famotidine 0.5-1.0 mg/kg IV q12h.

  Note: Glucocorticoids are of no benefit in the emergency setting.
- Other therapeutic measures that might be needed in severe anaphylaxis:
  - Shock fluid resuscitation
  - Vasopressors
  - Bronchodilators
  - Oxygen

IM, Intramuscularly; *IV,* intravenously.

ingredient, which has a high potential for causing anaphylaxis in this species.

Tetanus antitoxin is intended for therapeutic use to enhance recovery rates in animals showing clinical signs of tetanus. It should be combined with other treatments such as antibiotics, muscle relaxants, and general supportive care with fluid therapy and wound care. Tetanus antitoxin binds and neutralizes any free toxin that is circulating in the bloodstream, but it is not effective against toxin that has already bound to nerve tissue.

Anaphylaxis is an anticipated adverse drug reaction to administered tetanus antitoxin. Box 174-1 outlines the emergency treatment protocol. Chapter 152 discusses the management of anaphylaxis in more detail. Results of intradermal skin testing to try to identify animals at greater risk of hypersensitivity are not always dependable for antitoxins and antivenoms because both false-negative and false-positive reactions can occur.[5] In Adamantos and Boag's description of nine dogs that received tetanus antitoxin, only one dog had a mild hypersensitivity reaction after receiving a partial dose.[6] In another report of 16 dogs that received tetanus antitoxin, no signs of hypersensitivity were noted,[4] whereas Burkitt et al reported that 4 of 29 dogs receiving tetanus antitoxin intravenously developed signs of hypersensitivity.[7]

The recommended dose range for tetanus antitoxin is 100 to 1000 U/kg. In various reports the doses of tetanus antitoxin used in dogs ranged from 10 to 1900 U/kg given intravenously.[4,6,7] A case report of tetanus in a cat described the use of a 100-U/kg dose of human tetanus antitoxin administered intramuscularly.[2]

TICK ANTITOXIN

Tick paralysis is a common disorder in dogs and cats in Australia, whereas the syndrome that occurs in the United States affects only dogs. The Australian vector is *Ixodes holocyclus,* whereas the vector in the United States is *Dermacentor* ticks. The syndrome is characterized by a rapidly progressive lower motor neuron neuropathy (see Chapter 85). Treatment entails supportive therapy and removal of the tick. In Australia, treatment also includes the administration of tick antitoxin. There is no tick antitoxin available in the United States.

Until recently antitick serum was produced by the Australian company Commonwealth Serum Laboratories, but it has stopped making this product. Currently tick antitoxin is still available through the Australian Veterinary Serum Company (Lismore, New South Wales, Australia) and Summerland Serums (Alstonville, New South Wales, Australia). The antiserum is prepared from dogs that are hyperimmunized against the venom of *I. holocyclus.* Before its withdrawal from the container, the contents of the bottle should be allowed to reach room temperature. Dosages vary depending on the particular product. Anaphylaxis is the main adverse reaction (see Box 174-1).

There is limited evidence to date to support a benefit, or lack thereof, for tick antitoxin serum therapy in the treatment of tick paralysis in Australia. One major study by Atwell et al[8] involved a prospective survey of tick paralysis in dogs. The population consisted of 577 dogs treated by clinics located along the eastern coast of Australia. The information gathered included signalment, clinical signs, tick-host relationship, treatment, disease progression and recovery, and preventative measures. The mean tick antiserum dose was 0.99 ml/kg for those dogs that did not recover and 1.02 ml/kg for those dogs that did recover, so there was no significant difference in dose. There was no correlation between the severity of the clinical condition and the chosen dose of antitoxin. Any dose between 0.1 ml/kg and 8 ml/kg gave similar results with regard to mortality, time to clinical recovery, and hospitalization time; however, the majority of animals included in this study received an approximately 1-ml/kg dose, which limits the value of these results. Without studies to define the pharmacodynamic and pharmacokinetic properties of tick antitoxin in addition to well-designed prospective trials examining treatment benefit, the exact role of tick antitoxin in the treatment of tick paralysis in Australia cannot be clearly defined. At this time administration of tick antitoxin to animals with tick paralysis in Australia is considered standard of care. Tick antitoxin is generally administered intravenously (IV) in dogs and intramuscularly or intraperitoneally in cats. One suggested administration protocol for IV use in dogs is to dilute the dose 1:1 with 0.9% saline and infuse the total volume over an hour, with appropriate patient monitoring during the administration period.

In another study by Atwell and Campbell,[9] the reactions to tick antitoxin serum and the role of atropine in the treatment of dogs and cats with tick paralysis caused by *I. holocyclus* were described. Data from this pilot survey indicated that more cats than dogs have adverse systemic reactions to tick antitoxin serum and that the majority of the reactions could be related to the Bezold-Jarisch reflex, which involves a variety of cardiovascular and neurologic processes that cause hypopnea and bradycardia. The study concluded that atropine significantly reduced the numbers of adverse reactions.

BOTULISM ANTITOXIN

Dogs can become infected with *Clostridium botulinum* and acquire botulism caused by the type C and D exotoxins. The syndrome is potentially life-threatening because of the severe lower neuron neuropathy that can occur (see Chapter 85). The most severe types involve the muscles of respiration, and ventilator support is required until the effects of the toxin diminish. Unfortunately no type C antitoxin is available, and the type produced for human use is effective only against types A, B, and E. Treatment therefore must be supportive.[10]

BLACK WIDOW SPIDER ANTIVENOM

The reported incidence of black widow spider bites in cats is very low, and there have been no reported black widow bites in dogs. This is probably because cats are very sensitive to black widow venom, whereas dogs are less sensitive to the neurotoxin than cats or humans.[11] The main clinical sign is severe pain, which rapidly follows an almost painless bite. Death can occur in the most severe envenomations. The venom contains five or six biologically active proteins. This includes a very potent α-latrotoxin that induces the release of neurotransmitters from nerve terminals. Other toxic components include acetylcholine, noradrenalin, dopamine, glutamate, and enkephalin. Although calcium gluconate administration has been reported to lessen the intensity of the clinical signs, a commercially available antivenom made for use in humans has been shown to be very effective in a cat.[12] One of the authors of this chapter (M.S.) has also used it in a cat, and it produced a very impressive rapid reversal of clinical signs and a return to normal within a few hours after its administration. Other supportive therapies include morphine, barbiturates, and glucocorticoids.

According to the product description provided by the manufacturer, Merck and Company (Whitehouse Station, NJ), Antivenin (Latrodectus mactans), or black widow spider antivenin, is a sterile nonpyrogenic preparation derived by drying a frozen solution of specific venom-neutralizing globulins obtained from the blood serum of healthy horses immunized against the venom of black widow spiders. It is standardized by a biologic assay in mice. Each vial contains not less than 6000 antivenom units. Twedt et al[12] described the use of the product to treat black widow spider envenomation in a cat. The full amount of the antivenom desiccant was reconstituted with the accompanying diluents and placed in a 50-ml syringe containing 50 ml of 0.9% sodium chloride solution for intravenous injection. The solution was administered over 15 minutes and positive results were evident 2 hours afterward. Intradermal testing before administration has all the limitations described earlier and is of limited benefit.

SCORPION ANTIVENOM

Scorpions are arachnids. The one species causing public health concern in the United States is the bark scorpion *(Centruroides exilicauda)*. It contains an appendage attached at the caudal abdomen known as the *telson* that contains two venom glands and a stinger. The venom can cause systemic envenomation in humans, especially children, and in dogs and cats. The venom blocks voltage-gated potassium and sodium channels in nervous tissue. The clinical signs in humans range from localized pain to severe uncoordinated neuromuscular hyperactivity, oculomotor and visual abnormalities, and respiratory compromise.[13] Dogs and cats are particularly susceptible to clinical signs resulting from the sting. Although there is minimal local inflammation resulting from the sting, the systemic effects are serious and consist of nystagmus, paresthesias, referred pain, and myoclonus. Other signs include excessive salivation, tachycardia, fever, hypertension, and increased respiratory secretions.[14] Rhabdomyolysis has been reported in humans.[15]

Until recently, symptomatic humans were hospitalized in the intensive care unit and received high dosages of benzodiazepines and opioids. Those with respiratory compromise required ventilatory support, sometimes for several days, until the effects of the venom dissipated. An antivenom is now available for use in humans that effectively resolves the signs within 1 to 4 hours after treatment.[13] It was released in August 2011 and consists of a F(ab′)^2 anti-*Centruroides* antivenom marketed as *Centruroides* (Scorpion) Immune F(ab′)^2 (Equine) Injection, or Anascorp (Instituto Bioclon, Mexico City; distributed by Accredo Health Group, Memphis Tenn.). It currently costs approximately $3780 per dose, which will make it difficult for many pet owners to afford. Anascorp is made from the plasma of horses immunized with scorpion venom. The F(ab′)^2 fragments of immunoglobulin bind and neutralize venom toxins, which facilitates redistribution away from target tissues and elimination from the body. The antivenom is composed of venom from *Centruroides noxius, Centruroides limpidus limpidus, Centruroides limpidus tecomanus,* and *Centruroides suffusus suffusus.* The F(ab′)^2 content is not less than 85%. Each vial is reconstituted with 5.0 ml of 0.9% sodium chloride and contains not more than 24 mg/ml of protein and not less than 150 mouse LD_{50} neutralizing units (where LD_{50} is the amount of venom that would be lethal in 50% of mice).

There is no veterinary literature that describes the use of Anascorp in dogs and cats. The high cost is probably a major deterrent to its use in animals. In humans, the initial treatment calls for (1) reconstituting three vials in 5 ml of the accompanying normal saline diluent, (2) combining with and further diluting with normal saline to a total of 50 ml, and (3) infusing IV over 10 minutes. Patients are closely observed for hypersensitivity reactions, which in humans have been reported as vomiting, fever, rash, nausea, headache, rhinorrhea, myalgia, fatigue, cough, diarrhea, and lethargy. The hypersensitivity reaction can be as extreme as anaphylaxis, which requires emergency treatment (see Box 174-1). Serum sickness has also occurred in humans as a rare delayed reaction.

SNAKE ANTIVENOM

Production of Poisonous Snake Antivenom

The production of antivenom is a costly and extensive process. The information that follows is abstracted from Jean-Phillipe Chippaux's textbook *Snake Venoms and Envenomations.*[16] One of the first steps in antivenom production is to detoxify the venom before it is inoculated into the host that is to be hyperimmunized. This can be done by combining the venom with an aldehyde and then adding an adjuvant either before or after the detoxification process. The adjuvant is thought to slow down the resorption of the venom and to maximize the immune reaction.

The immunization protocol depends on the toxicity and the immunogenicity of the venom, the species of animal to be immunized, and the quality of response of the hyperimmunized animal. The horse is commonly used in producing the whole immunoglobulin and F(ab′)^2 snake antivenoms, whereas the sheep is the host for production of the Fab antivenom. The quantity of the injected venom must be adjusted continuously by repeated controls to obtain a sufficient antibody titer. Ten to fifty injections are spread over a period of 3 to 15 months for optimum antibody production. Once this point is reached, blood is collected into anticoagulant (sodium citrate) and the blood product is purified, treated, and then conditioned for sale in liquid or lyophilized forms. Before a new antivenom is marketed, in vivo testing is performed in laboratory animals to evaluate the effect of the antivenom on the lethality of the venom or on a particular biologic activity. In vitro tests are also done to allow evaluation of a particular activity of the venom and its neutralization after the venom is mixed with the antivenom.

Cross reactions between polyvalent antivenoms and several different pit viper venoms have been demonstrated by immunodiffusion and enzyme-linked immunosorbent assay. Cross reactions are frequently seen between related species. However, the cross-precipitation reaction does not necessarily mean cross protection, and it is essential to know which snake venoms are effectively counteracted by each specific product. This information is given in Box 174-2.

Pit Viper Antivenom

The use of polyvalent crotalid antivenom is the mainstay of therapy for moderate to severe pit viper envenomation in the United States. Its use is dictated by affordability and availability. Antivenom administration limits the spread of swelling, reverses coagulopathy, and halts the progression of neuropathy when adequate doses are administered in a timely manner.[17] Although early administration is indicated to reverse hematologic and neurologic abnormalities,

BOX 174-2 *Various Pit Viper Antivenom Products*

Crotalidae Polyvalent Immune Fab (Ovine) (CroFab) (United States)
Antivenom derived from:

Crotalus atrox (western diamondback rattlesnake)
Crotalus adamanteus (eastern diamondback rattlesnake)
Crotalus scutulatus (Mojave rattlesnake)
Agkistrodon piscivorus (cottonmouth or water moccasin)

Also has cross reactivity with:

Crotalus horridus (timber rattlesnake)
Crotalus viridis helleri (Southern Pacific rattlesnake)
Crotalus molossus molossus (blacktail rattlesnake)
Crotalus horridus atricaudatus (canebrake rattlesnake)
Agkistrodon contortrix contortrix (southern copperhead)
Sistrurus miliarius barbouri (southeastern [dusky] pygmy rattlesnake)

Fort Dodge (Equine) (United States)
Antivenom derived from:

Crotalus adamanteus (eastern diamondback rattlesnake)
Crotalus atrox (western diamondback rattlesnake)
Crotalus durissus terrificus (tropical rattlesnake, cascabel)
Bothrops atrox (fer-de-lance)

Additional cross reactivity

Crotalus and *Sisrurus* (rattlesnakes)
Agkistrodon (copperheads and cottonmouths)
Agkistrodon halys of Korea and Japan
Bothrops and subspecies
Crotalus durissus and subspecies
Agkistrodon bilineatus (cantil)
Lachesis mutus (bushmaster of South and Central America)

Antivipmyn Polivalent Anti-snake Fabotherapic (Mexico)
Antivenom derived from:

Crotalus durissus durissus (Central American rattlesnake)
Bothrops asper (fer-de-lance)

Cross reactivity

Crotalus basiliscus (Mexican West Coast rattlesnake)
Crotalus durissus terrificus (South American rattlesnake)
Crotalus simus (shunu or Middle American rattlesnake)
Crotalus polystictus (hocico de puerco, twin spotted rattlesnake)
Crotalus scutulatus (Mojave rattlesnake)
Agkistrodon bilineatus (common cantil)
Agkistrodon bilineatus taylori (Taylor's cantil)
Agkistrodon contortrix contortrix (southern copperhead)
Agkistrodon contortrix laticinctus (broad-banded copperhead)
Agkistrodon contortrix mokeson (northern copperhead)
Agkistrodon contortrix phaeogaster (Osage copperhead)
Agkistrodon contortrix pictigaster (Trans-Pecos copperhead)
Agkistrodon piscivorus piscivorus (eastern cottonmouth)
Agkistrodon piscivorus conanti (Florida cottonmouth)
Agkistrodon piscivorus leucostoma (western cottonmouth)
Sistrurus miliarius ravus (cascabel de neve placas [Mexican])
Sistrurus catenatus catenatus (eastern massasauga)
Sistrurus catenatus edwardsii (desert massasauga)
Sistrurus catenatus tergeminus (western massasauga)
Sistrurus miliarius miliarius (Carolina pigmy rattlesnake)
Sistrurus miliarius barbouri (southeastern [dusky] pygmy rattlesnake)
Sistrurus miliarius strekeri (western pygmy rattlesnake)

PoliVet-ICP (Costa Rica)
Antivenom derived from:

Bothrops asper (fer-de-lance)
Crotalus durissus (neotropical rattlesnake)

Cross reactivity

According to the manufacturer's drug insert it is effective against the venom of most Central American pit vipers but ineffective against the venom of South American pit vipers.

Data from Miami-Dade Fire Rescue Venom Response Program: Antivenom: species covered. Available at http://www.miamidade.gov/fire/library/antivenom-species-covered.pdf.

antivenom does not reverse local tissue necrosis because of the immediate necrotoxic effect of the venom on the tissues.[18]

In moderately to severely affected humans, early intravenous antivenom administration is essential, and the same applies to all vulnerable animal victims.[19] Antivenom is optimally given within 4 hours after the snakebite, although it can still be effective up to 24 hours or longer after envenomation.[19] If the bite results in the injection of a large quantity of venom deep into well-vascularized soft tissues or directly into an artery or vein, death can occur within the first few hours despite vigorous antivenom treatment.

Two currently approved antivenom products are available in the United States: Antivenin (Crotalidae) Polyvalent (ACP) (Boehringer Ingelheim Vetmedica, St. Joseph, Mo.) for dogs, and CroFab (Crotalidae Polyvalent Immune Fab [Ovine], Therapeutic Antibodies, Nashville, Tenn.) for humans. ACP consists of a whole immunoglobulin G (IgG) and horse serum albumin and is the only licensed veterinary antivenom product in the United States. There are also two foreign antivenom products that are effective against North American snakebite envenomation. The first is a $F(ab')^2$ antibody fragment polyvalent product manufactured in Mexico (Antivipmyn [Polivalent Anti-snake Fabotherapic], Instituto Bioclon, Mexico City). The second is a polyspecific IgG product of equine origin from Costa Rica (PoliVet-ICP, Instituto Clodomiro Picado, San José). Obtaining these antivenom products in the United States requires a special importer's permit issued by the U.S. Department of Agriculture (USDA) and the approval of the state veterinarian. All four of these products are clinically effective for venom neutralization in dogs; however, only CroFab and Antivipmyn are effective against Mojave rattlesnake venom.

The ACP product has been used to treat snakebites in humans for over 40 years and is composed of complete immunoglobulin (150 kDa) and albumin from immunized horses.[20] Because the ammonium sulfate precipitation process currently used to prepare this antivenom is inefficient, the serum contains unwanted contaminants in the form of extraneous heterologous proteins such as albumin, α- and β-globulins, and IgM, in addition to the venom-specific IgG. These contaminants are largely responsible for the allergenic properties of this antivenom.[21] Recommended dosing of ACP in dogs varies from 1 to 10 vials depending on the severity of the envenomation, the owner's financial limitations, and the judgment of the clinician. Dosing schedules for dogs have been empirically adopted from human protocols based on severity classification charts and experimental studies, and human doses are extrapolated from the results of in vivo experiments in mice. Since the clinician cannot know the exact amount of venom that was injected into the victim or its subsequent absorption from the tissues, empirical treatment with antivenom is used. Clinical experience is therefore very helpful when managing these cases.

The ACP label recommends the administration of one to five vials intravenously depending on the severity of signs, the time elapsed since the bite, and the size of the snake and size of the victim, with additional doses given every 2 hours as indicated (Antivenin [Crotalidae] Polyvalent [ACP], Boehringer Ingelheim Vetmedica, Inc., St. Joseph, MO). The average amount of ACP used in human patients is 12 vials.[22] It is difficult to determine dosing for dogs based on many of these studies due to the variability in patient size and envenomation dose. The ACP product is sold as a desiccant that must be reconstituted with isotonic saline. The desiccant can take as long as 90 minutes to dissolve, but the process can be speeded by adding the diluent and then gently rolling the bottle under warm flowing tap water. This brings the desiccant into solution within 20 minutes, an important feature when rapid treatment of a severely envenomated patient is vital.[23,24]

PoliVet-ICP is a whole IgG product that is available in Costa Rica. It differs from ACP in that it has no excess proteins.[25] Although the snake species used for immunization for this product *(Bothrops asper, Crotalus durissus)* are not North American snakes, this does not impair its effectiveness against the venom of common North American pit vipers. Its full benefits and risks are unknown.[26] Each milliliter neutralizes not less than 2.5 mg of *B. asper* venom and 2.0 mg of *C. durissus* venom. The manufacturer's recommended dose (as found in the drug insert) for small animals is not less than 4 vials for mild cases, 8 vials for moderate cases, and 16 vials for severe cases.

The newer Fab antivenoms (CroFab [Fab_1], and Antivipmyn [$F(ab')^2$]) are mixed, monospecific, polyvalent products produced by ovine and equine immunization, respectively.[27] The Fab molecules are cleaved from the immunoglobulin, which makes it smaller (50 kDa) and less antigenic.[22] Albumin is also removed. The disadvantage of the smaller molecules is that they are cleared from the bloodstream more rapidly and thus repeated administration is required. One human study recommended that Fab antivenom (CroFab) be readministered every 6 hours for three doses or as clinically indicated based on the progression of swelling and coagulation abnormalities.[28] The reconstitution time for CroFab using hand agitation is rapid, with a median time of 3 to 6.8 minutes. One study showed that the dissolution time can be reduced to a range of 0.9 to 1.1 minutes.[29] Dosing recommendations for dogs are mostly anecdotal and vary from one to several vials. A main disadvantage of CroFab is the cost, but because CroFab has 5.2 times the potency of the ACP product, fewer vials can be used, which possibly narrows the cost differential.[30]

A recent abstract by Bush et al[31] described their experience in using Fab antivenom as a constant rate infusion. The rates of infusion varied from 2 to 4 vials per 24 hours (mean = 3.3 ± 1.0 vials per day) for control or reversal of hematologic abnormalities. The duration of Fab infusion was between 4 and 8 days from the time of envenomation (mean = 6 ± 2 days), after which hematologic values had normalized or were normalizing and continued to do so. The study concluded that the constant rate infusion method may be safer, more efficacious, and more cost effective than observation without Fab treatment or as-needed dosing in high-risk patients.

Antivipmyn, a $F(ab')^2$ antibody fragment antivenom, is cleared from the body faster than IgG but slower than the $F(ab)_1$ antibody fragment.[25] Antivipmyn has been found to be effective in dogs at an initial dose of one to two vials followed by another one to two vials 2 to 4 hours later. A prospective clinical trial is currently being conducted to determine its efficacy in treating North American snakebites.[32]

Anaphylaxis is a rare but potentially life-threatening complication of antivenom treatment because of the equine or ovine origin of the product. Early signs of anaphylaxis such as vomiting, salivation, restlessness, urticaria, and facial pruritus should be treated immediately (see Box 174-1). The optimal rate of antivenom infusion is unknown; however, as long as the patient tolerates any of the products, the entire dose can be administered relatively quickly over 1 hour. A more infrequent complication of antivenom treatment in humans is a type III hypersensitivity reaction (serum sickness), which is a delayed immune complex hypersensitivity response characterized by fever, malaise, nausea, diarrhea, lymph node enlargement, and dermatopathy that can occur over a period spanning 3 days to 2 weeks after antivenom administration.[33] There is an 80% risk of serum sickness in humans who receive ACP, and the incidence is proportional to the dose administered.[34] Unlike in humans, serum sickness has been reported only rarely in dogs, and this may be due to the lower dose administered or a lack of recognition by the patient's immune system.[35]

Coral Snake Antivenom

The IgG coral snake antivenom product that was once available through Wyeth Pharmaceuticals is no longer used in veterinary medicine because there is a limited supply with a Food and Drug Administration extended expiration date and it is available only for human patients. In general, coral snake antivenom is hard to procure because of the difficulty in finding enough coral snakes from which to extract venom, the small amount of venom per snake, and the difficulty in maintaining good health in captive coral snakes.[36]

The product Coralmyn (Polivalent Anti-coral Fabotherapic), marketed by Instituto Bioclon in Mexico City, has been obtainable in the United States after applying for a USDA importer's permit and getting the approval of the state veterinarian. Coralmyn is available in a lyophilized form that requires reconstitution with diluent.

Coralmyn is a polyclonal antivenom $F(ab')^2$ fragment with an equine origin produced using the venom from *Micrurus nigrocinctus nigrocinctus* (black-banded coral snake), which is indigenous to Mexico, Central America, and Columbia. The venom has a strong neurotoxic effect and thus has the same medical significance as venom from the coral snake species found in the southern United States (*Micrurus fulvius fulvius,* or Eastern Coral Snake, and *Micrurus tener tener,* or Texas Coral Snake). Studies in mice have established the efficacy of Coralmyn for neutralizing the venom produced by both *M. fulvius* and *M. tener.*[37,38] Coralmyn is an IgG glycoprotein that has had the Fc fraction removed by enzymatic action, leaving the two Fab fragments, which will neutralize the venom. The $F(ab')^2$ configuration is a lighter-weight product than the whole IgG, which allows it to distribute better in both the vascular and extravascular spaces. The maximum concentration is reached in 1 hour in superficial tissues (in 6 hours in deeper tissues). The $F(ab')^2$ fragment does not activate complement and induces virtually no generation of anti-IgG and anti-IgE antibodies (according to the Coralmyn drug insert). Although Coralmyn has less extraneous protein than an entire IgG product, allergic reactions can still occur, although they are rare. The route of elimination of the antigen-antibody complex is not fully identified, but the reticuloendothelial tissue is apparently involved in the catabolism of the complex $F(ab')^2$ venom.

The authors have used Coralmyn on four dogs and two cats and have found the results to be beneficial as assessed by avoidance of the need for ventilator support and patient survival.[39] These results are observational and there were no paired matched controls, which might have shown that ventilator support can also be avoided in dogs not treated with antivenom. In light of this, the authors' experience with this product has been favorable. Although the manufacturer recommends that the reconstituted product be diluted in 250 ml of 0.9% saline and administered over 4 hours, the authors have injected the reconstituted 10-ml volume over 30 to 45 minutes by using an automatic injection syringe. This technique has been shown to be safe with no adverse effects in this limited population. Although the recommended number of vials for humans ranges from two to nine in the drug insert, the financial restrictions ($750 per vial in 2012) have caused the authors to restrict their doses to one to two vials per patient. Administration of this limited dose might help reduce the number of patients requiring ventilator support, but this outcome is unpredictable. The favorable result observed might also be due to the fact that these particular animals did not receive enough venom to cause respiratory paralysis. Both treated and untreated dogs may progress to require ventilator support, but there is still a chance that the antivenom will help spare them a protracted hospitalization and much greater expense. There have been no blinded studies comparing treatment and nontreatment in dogs to show antivenom efficacy at various dosages.

The Instituto Clodomiro Picado at the University of Costa Rica also produces coral snake antivenom. It is made from purified equine immunoglobulins and contains 0.25% phenol as a preservative. It has proved effective against the Eastern Coral Snake. It is available in both liquid and freeze-dried forms. The shelf life of the freeze-dried antivenom is 5 years; the liquid form can be stored for 3 years at 2° to 8° C.

REFERENCES

1. Tizard IR: Vaccines and their production. In Veterinary immunology—an introduction, ed 7, Philadelphia, 2004, Saunders, p 247.
2. DeRisio L, Gelati A: Tetanus in a cat—an unusual presentation, J Feline Med Surg 5:237, 2003.
3. Green CE: Tetanus. In Greene CE, editor: Infectious diseases in the dog and cat, ed 3, St Louis, 2006, Saunders, p 395.
4. Bandt C, Rozanski EA, Steinberg T, et al: Retrospective study of tetanus in 20 dogs, J Am Anim Hosp Assoc 43:143, 2007.
5. Jurkovich GJ, Luterman A, McCullar K, et al: Complications of Crotalidae antivenin therapy, J Trauma 28(7):1032, 1988.
6. Adamantos S, Boag A: Thirteen cases of tetanus in dogs, Vet Rec 161:298, 2007.
7. Burkitt JM, Sturges BK, Jandrey KE, et al: Risk factors associated with outcome in dogs with tetanus: 38 cases (1987-2005), J Am Vet Assoc 230:76, 2007.
8. Atwell RB, Campbell FE, Evans EA: Prospective survey of tick paralysis in dogs, Aust Vet J 79(6):412, 2001.
9. Atwell RB, Campbell FE: Reactions to tick antitoxin serum and the role of atropine in treatment of dogs and cats with tick paralysis caused by *Ixodes holocyclus:* a pilot survey, Aust Vet J 79(6):394, 2001.
10. Barsanti JA: Botulism. In Greene CE, editor: Infectious diseases in the dog and cat, ed 3, St Louis, 2006, Saunders, p 389.
11. Fowler ME: Veterinary zootoxicology, Boca Raton, Fla, 1993, CRC Press, pp 73-79.
12. Twedt DC, Cuddon PA, Horn TW: Black widow spider envenomation in a cat, J Vet Intern Med 13:613, 1999.
13. Boyer LV, Theodorou AA, Berg RA, et al: Antivenom for critically ill children with neurotoxicity from scorpion stings, N Engl J Med 360:2090, 2009.
14. Brutlag A: Snakes, spiders, and scorpions, oh my! or, managing envenomations. In Proceedings of the 82nd Western Veterinary Conference, February 14-18, 2010, Las Vegas, Nevada, v316.
15. O'Connor A, Ruha AM: Clinical course of bark scorpion envenomation managed without antivenom, J Med Toxicol 8(3):258-262, 2012. Epub May 5, 2012.
16. Chippaux JP: Snake venoms and envenomations, Malabar Fla, 2006, Krieger Publishing Company.
17. Holstege CP, Miller MB, Wermuth M, et al: Crotalid snake envenomation, Crit Care Clin 13(4):889, 1997.
18. Dart RC, Seifert SA, Boyer LV, et al: A randomized multicenter trial of Crotalinae polyvalent immune Fab (ovine) antivenom for the treatment for crotaline snakebite in the United States, Arch Intern Med 161(16):2030, 2001.
19. Juckett G, Hancox JG: Venomous snakebites in the United States: management review and update, Am Fam Physician 65(7):1367, 2002.
20. Dart RC, McNally J: Efficacy, safety, and use of snake antivenoms in the United States, Ann Emerg Med 37(2):181, 2001.
21. Pizon AF, Riley BD, Ruha AM, et al: Antidotes in depth. In Flowmenbaum NE, Goldfrank LR, et al, editors: Goldfrank's toxicologic emergencies, ed 8, New York, 2006, McGraw-Hill, p 1657.
22. Peterson ME: Snakebite: pit vipers, Clin Tech Small Anim Pract 21(4):174, 2006.
23. Norris R: Venom poisoning by North American Reptiles. In Campbell JA, Lamar WW editors: The venomous reptiles of the Western Hemisphere, Ithaca, NY, 2004, Comstock Publishing Associates, p 683.
24. Hill RE, Bogdan GM, Dart RC: Time to reconstitution: purified Fab antivenom vs. unpurified IgG antivenom, Toxicon 39:729, 2001.
25. Chippaux JP, Goyffon M: Venoms, antivenoms and immunotherapy, Toxicon 36(6):823, 1998.
26. Arce V, Rojas E, Ownby CL, et al: Preclinical assessment of the ability of polyvalent (Crotalinae) and anticoral (Elapidae) antivenoms produced in Costa Rica to neutralize the venoms of North American snakes, Toxicon 41(7):851, 2003.
27. Gold BS, Dart RC, Barish RA: Bites of venomous snakes, N Engl J Med 347(5):347, 2002.
28. Dart RC, Seifert SA, Boyer LV, et al: A randomized multicenter trial of Crotalinae polyvalent immune Fab (ovine) antivenom for the treatment for crotaline snakebite in the United States, Arch Intern Med 161(16):2030, 2001.
29. Quan AN, Quan D, Curry SC: Improving Crotalidae polyvalent immune Fab reconstitution times, Am J Emerg Med 28:593, 2010.
30. Consroe P, Egen NB, Russell FE, et al: Comparison of a new ovine antigen binding fragment (Fab) antivenin for United States Crotalidae with the commercial antivenin for protection against venom-induced lethality in mice, Am J Trop Med Hyg 53(5):507, 1995.
31. Bush SP, Seifert SA, Smith SD, et al: Continuous Crotalidae polyvalent Fab (ovine) (FabAV) for selected snakebite patients, Toxicon 60:220, 2012.
32. Peterson ME: What's up with all those antivenoms? In Proceedings of the IVECCS, San Antonio, Texas, 2010, p 355.
33. Waddell LS: Systemic anaphylaxis. In Ettinger SJ, Feldman EC, editors: Textbook of veterinary internal medicine, St Louis, 2010, Saunders, p 531.
34. Berdoulay P, Schaer M, Starr J: Serum sickness in a dog associated with antivenin therapy for snake bite caused by *Crotalus adamanteus*, J Vet Emerg Crit Care 15(3):206, 2005.
35. Holstege CP, Miller MB, Wermuth M, et al: Crotalid snake envenomation, Crit Care Clin 13(4):889, 1997.
36. Najman L, Seshadri R: Rattlesnake envenomation, Compend Contin Educ Vet 29(3):166, 2007.
37. Roodt AR, Paniagua-Solis JF, Dolab JA, et al: Effectiveness of two common antivenoms for North, Central, and South American *Micrurus* envenomations, Clin Toxicol 42:(2)171, 2004.
38. Sanchez EE, Lopez-Johnston JC, Rodriquez-Acosta A: Neutralization of two North American coral snake venoms with United States and Mexican antivenoms, Toxicon 51:297, 2008.
39. Pérez M, Fox K, Schaer M: A retrospective review of coral snake envenomation in the dog and cat: 20 cases (1996 to 2011), J Vet Emerg Crit Care (San Antonio) 22(6):682-689, 2012.

CHAPTER 175

ANTIMICROBIAL USE IN THE CRITICAL CARE PATIENT

Dawn Merton Boothe, DVM, PhD, DACVIM (Internal Medicine), DACVCP

KEY POINTS

- *Staphylococcus, Enterococcus, Escherichia coli,* and *Clostridium* are examples of microbes for which emergent multidrug resistance is limiting therapeutic options.
- Factors that increase the risk of infection with a multidrug-resistant microbe include previous antimicrobial exposure, invasive procedures, longer duration of hospital stay, and inappropriate dosing regimens.
- A number of techniques or policies can be implemented in the critical care environment to improve antimicrobial stewardship and thus reduce antimicrobial resistance.
- Emergence of resistant microbes can be reduced by timely initiation of appropriate antimicrobials at a dosing regimen designed to target the most resistant colonies in an infecting inoculum.

Antimicrobials are among the most common and important drugs prescribed for the critical care patient (CCP).[1] Timely, effective antimicrobial therapy is a crucial determinant of outcome in the CCP[2]; however, the advent of antimicrobial resistance has profoundly altered the use of these agents. The goal of antimicrobial therapy is to eradicate infection safely while minimizing the advent of resistance. The CCP is particularly at risk of developing infections. Cardiovascular, renal, and hepatic dysfunction, as well as altered drug disposition, increase the risk of either adverse drug events or therapeutic failure. Polypharmacy, or the use of multiple medications in an individual patient, increases the risk of adverse drug events and drug interactions. Finally, the sense of urgency accompanying therapeutic decision making in the CCP generally leads to empiric antimicrobial use, which may be based on incorrect assumptions regarding antimicrobial efficacy.[3]

The principles guiding antimicrobial therapy are regularly reviewed.[4] This chapter summarizes those principles, with a focus on their relevance to the CCP. The Infectious Diseases Society of America (http://www.idsociety.org) offers guidelines for the use of antimicrobial agents, many of which are specific to conditions characterized as critical. These guidelines are reassessed and modified on a cyclical basis. The International Society for Companion Animal Infectious Disease (http://www.iscaid.org) also has promulgated guidelines for the treatment of certain infections. However, although they are veterinary specific, they do not focus on critically ill patients.

ANTIMICROBIAL RESISTANCE

The CCP is particularly at risk of developing infection with antimicrobial-resistant bacteria. Risk factors include treatment with antimicrobial therapy within the previous 3 months, hospitalization for longer than 5 days, an environment (community, hospital, or hospital unit) characterized by a high frequency of antimicrobial-resistant organisms, immunosuppressive disease or therapy, and (in human patients) evidence that the infection (pneumonia) is related to health care.[2,4] Other risk factors include the potential for bacterial translocation from the gastrointestinal tract, performance of invasive procedures, and interventions associated with the placement of foreign materials with surfaces conducive to bacterial colonization (e.g., indwelling catheters).

Advent of Resistance

Previous antimicrobial exposure is among the factors most predictive of the development of antimicrobial resistance. The diverse commensal gastrointestinal flora include *Escherichia coli* as the major gram-negative and *Enterococcus* spp as the major gram-positive facultative aerobes; however, the often-underestimated anaerobic flora predominate and are susceptible to unintended effects of antimicrobial therapy. Each microbe maintains an ecologic niche by competing for nutrients and actively suppressing surrounding growth through secretion of antibiotics. Self-destruction does not occur because genes encoding antibiotic secretion generally accompany genes that impart resistance. Constant exposure to antimicrobials also causes surrounding commensal organisms to be primed for resistance. Rapid microbial turnover ensures frequent DNA replication and thus the potential for mutation. Genes imparting resistance are shared among organisms via integrins, plasmids, and transposons that facilitate rapid transfer of multidrug resistance.[4] Resistance to any antimicrobial drug should be anticipated when the population of bacteria reaches or exceeds 10^6 to 10^8 colony-forming units, whether the population is a commensal resident or an infecting pathogen.[5]

The use of broad-spectrum antimicrobial drugs facilitates selection of resistant organisms,[6] although the potential for resistance differs among organisms and the magnitude of resistance varies among drugs. More problematic organisms have emerged since the 1990s including, in order of appearance, methicillin-resistant *Staphylococcus aureus* (MRSA), vancomycin-resistant *Enterococcus* (VRE), fluoroquinolone-resistant *Pseudomonas* (FQRP) and *E. coli,* and, most recently, vancomycin-resistant *S. aureus* (VRSA) and fluoroquinolone-resistant *Clostridium difficile.* Each has developed multidrug resistance, defined as resistance to three or more antimicrobial drugs to which the organism is generally considered susceptible. *E. coli* is also emerging as a multidrug-resistant (MDR) organism, with resistance correlated with fluoroquinolone treatment.[2] Administration of even a single dose of a fluoroquinolone has been associated with changes in the resistance pattern of commensal coliforms in humans.[7] Fluoroquinolone-resistant *E. coli* has been documented in the urinary tract of dogs and in other tissues[8] and has been associated with nosocomial infections in a veterinary teaching hospital.[9] The author has demonstrated that administration of multiple oral doses of either amoxicillin (10 mg/kg q12h) or enrofloxacin (5 mg/kg q24h) in normal dogs is associated with expression of resistance to the treatment drug by fecal *E. coli* within 3 to 5 days of therapy initiation. For each drug, resistance was high level; for enrofloxacin, resistance was multidrug.[10]

Nosocomial Infections

Nosocomial infections occur as a result of medical treatment, usually in a hospital or clinic setting. Nosocomial infections are formally defined as infections arising more than 48 hours after hospital admission. Nosocomial organisms are generally opportunists. The most important source probably is the environment, although transfer from caregivers or other patients is possible. The risk of nosocomial infection is 5- to 10-fold higher in the human critical care ward than in the hospital population at large.[1] Further details regarding nosocomial infections can be found in Chapter 89.

Reducing Microbial Resistance

Wise antimicrobial drug-prescribing behaviors are the most significant mechanism by which bacterial resistance is likely to be reduced in the critical care environment.[11] The Centers for Disease Control and Prevention (CDC) define four primary drivers that reduce the incidence of *C. difficile* infections and the advent of antimicrobial resistance in health care environments (http://www.cdc.gov/getsmart/healthcare/pdfs/Antibiotic_Stewardship_Driver_Diagram_10_30_12.pdf). These include (1) timely and appropriate initiation of antibiotics; (2) appropriate administration and deescalation of antibiotics; (3) data monitoring, transparency, and stewardship infrastructure; and (4) availability of expertise at the point of care.

Notably, one measure that is not effective in reducing antimicrobial resistance is the promulgation of restrictive formularies. As reviewed by Deresinski in 2007,[2] use of such formularies may actually increase problems associated with antimicrobial resistance. The importance of working with a health care team to manage the use of antimicrobials in the CCP cannot be overemphasized. Therapeutic success is more likely to be realized when clinician decisions are supported by the expertise of a veterinary clinical microbiologist and veterinary clinical pharmacologist.

ANTIMICROBIAL SELECTION AND TREATMENT

The following approach is recommended whenever antimicrobial therapy is being considered in the CCP.

Timely Assessment of Need for and Initiation of Antimicrobial Therapy

Perhaps more so than in other patients, the need for antimicrobial prophylaxis or treatment is a consideration generally encountered in the CCP. The sense of urgency and the need for broad-spectrum coverage in the face of an unclear diagnosis lend themselves to the use of empiric antimicrobial therapy. Many hospitals also have standards of care that include routine use of drugs. Yet deescalation of antimicrobial use, including unnecessary use, is a tenet of antimicrobial stewardship. As recognized by the CDC in the Get Smart for Healthcare program (Figure 175-1), up to 53% of hospitalized humans patients receive antibiotics,[6] with such therapy deemed unnecessary in between 14% and 43% of cases.[12] Such statistics are not available for veterinary patients but probably are similar if not worse. Black et al found that use of antimicrobials before bacteriologic culture submission was appropriate in only 30% of critically ill canine patients; the number increased to 75% after culture results were reported (but before minimum inhibitory concentrations [MICs] were available).[13]

The conundrum facing the veterinary critical care specialist is that little information exists to help confirm the presence of infection, yet empiric use of antimicrobials is likely to contribute to resistance. Eventually, molecular diagnostic techniques will catch up with diagnostic needs and provide evidence of infection for the discerning clinician. Until such time, additional consideration should be given to clinical parameters that indicate, but do not necessarily confirm, infection. The development of a fever should not always be assumed to reflect infection. Guidelines have been offered by the Infectious Diseases Society of America (Table 175-1). An exception might be patients with neutropenia in which fever cannot otherwise be explained.[14] Blood cultures (three to four in the first 24 hr) are recommended. Culture results do not necessarily confirm infection because they may not discriminate between normal commensal flora and opportunistic agents (commensals that become pathogenic) or other pathogens (causing harm to the patient). Vibrant and pure growth provides support, but does not confirm, that a cultured organism is the infecting isolate.

Among the approaches used to determine the need for antimicrobial therapy in humans is measurement of biomarkers of inflammation.[15] Kibe et al[16] and Póvoa and Salluh[17] provide excellent systematic reviews of the use of biomarkers to guide antimicrobial therapy in humans. A Cochrane review[18] of the use of procalcitonin as a guide for treatment of acute respiratory infections in humans (encompassing 14 randomized clinical trials not conducted in the United States) found no increased risk of mortality or treatment failure and did find a consistent reduction in antimicrobial use, both in the initial prescribing of antimicrobials and in the duration of therapy. However, the applicability of these findings to dogs and cats and the role of biomarker-based guidance of antimicrobial use requires further research.

Time taken to carefully assess the need for antimicrobial therapy must be balanced against the need for rapid, effective treatment of the CCP. Multiple studies have demonstrated the profound importance of rapid initiation of appropriate therapy. As reviewed by Deresinski,[2] in human patients with septic shock, the survival rate declined by 7.6% for each hour's delay in the administration of appropriate antimicrobial therapy after the onset of hypotension. However, only 50% of patients received appropriate antimicrobial therapy within the first 6 hours. In a cohort study,[19] Gaieski found that mortality was generally decreased from 38.5% to 19% if antimicrobial therapy was initiated within 1 hour of triage. In humans with sterile-site hospital-acquired MRSA infections (also reviewed by Deresinski[2]), survival was higher if appropriate antimicrobial therapy was initiated within 24 hours of collection of culture-positive specimens than if patients did not receive antimicrobials. Notably, therapy was more likely to be inappropriate if the onset of infection occurred within 48 hours of hospital admission, despite the fact that most of these patients had risk factors for hospital-acquired infections.

Identification of the Target and Its Susceptibility

Increasingly, the first mistake in empiric antimicrobial selection is failure to identify the infecting pathogen correctly. Initial empiric therapy should be accompanied by proper collection of culture samples; the drug and dosing regimen is then based on susceptibility testing.[3] The complex nature of nosocomial organisms mandates that they also be cultured.[20] The use of broad-spectrum drugs increases the risk of resistance. Although, by its nature, empiric drug selection is broad, an attempt should be made to narrow the spectrum of the chosen drug. Incorrect empiric choices have been documented in treating close to 50% of patients in shock. Limitations of historical data regarding microbial infections in the various body systems can be profound. Earlier and even current collected data fail (indeed, may not be able) to discriminate commensal from pathogenic isolates. Further, it is only in selected, uncomplicated infections (e.g., urinary tract or skin) that the infecting isolate or its susceptibility to drugs can be predicted with any accuracy. In critically ill patients, organisms generally represent the normal flora of the alimentary canal or nosocomial organisms. The source of infection may help narrow the spectrum of empiric therapy if selected organisms are more likely to

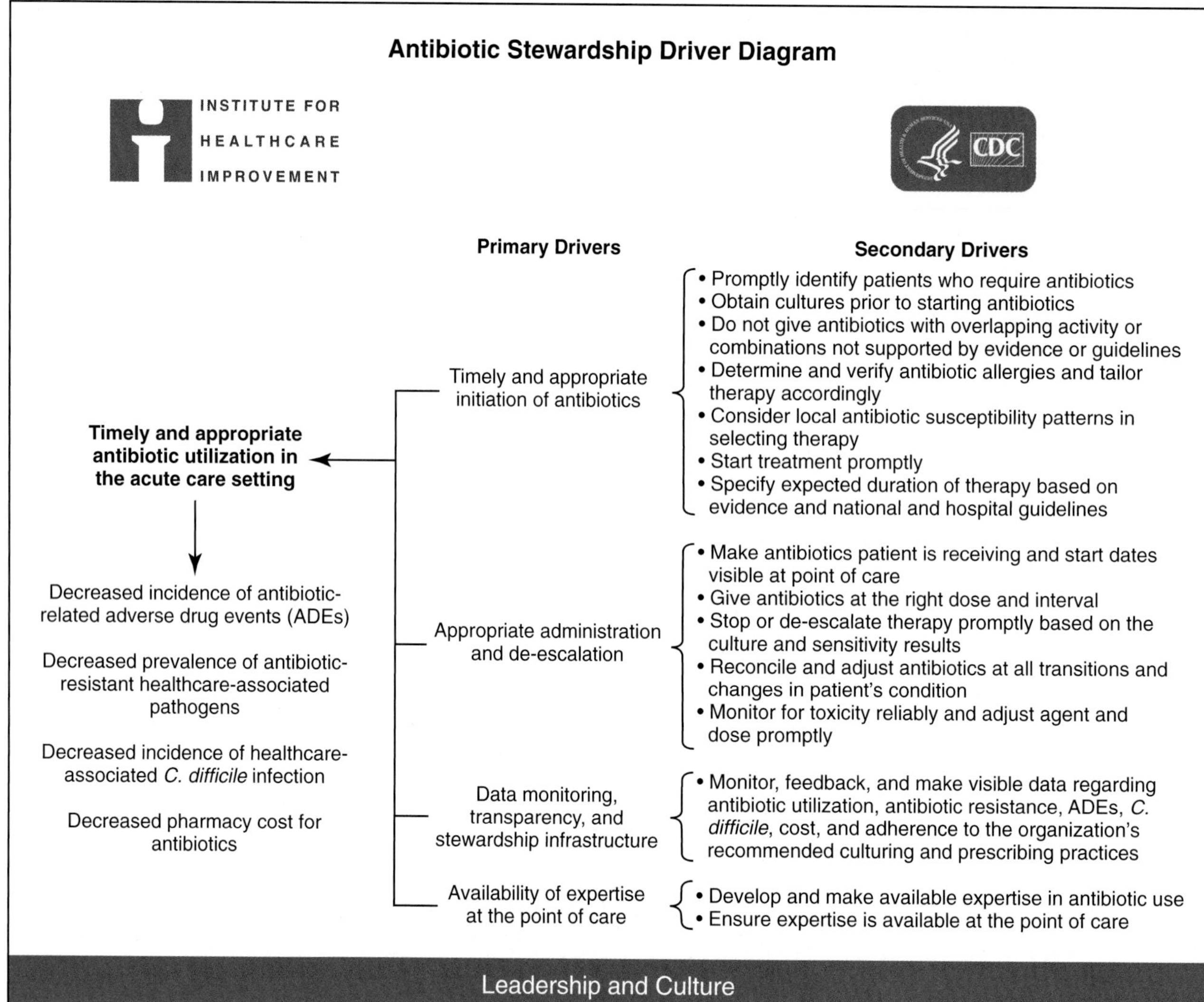

FIGURE 175-1 Through improvement of antimicrobial stewardship in a hospital setting, all patients, and particularly critical care patients, will benefit from reduced antimicrobial resistance. The Centers for Disease Control and Prevention offer an antibiotic stewardship package (http://www.cdc.gov/getsmart/healthcare) that is intended to increase the effectiveness of antimicrobial stewardship in a health care setting. The driver diagram presented here is supported by a framework (not shown) that delineates specific, measurable outcomes upon which the success of a health care stewardship program is based. *(From Centers for Disease Control and Prevention: Implementing and improving stewardship efforts, November 2010. Available at* http://www.cdc.gov/getsmart/healthcare/improve-efforts/driver-diagram/introduction.html. *Accessed April 2013.)*

infect some body systems than others. For example, genitourinary tracts often are infected with gram-negative aerobes, whereas abdominal infections generally are caused by gram-negative aerobes initially, followed by anaerobes. Anaerobic coverage should also be considered in selected infections (e.g., osteomyelitis) and in those involving deep, isolated areas; those affecting hollow organs; and those associated with a foul smell and marked inflammation (i.e., abscess). Granulocytopenic or otherwise immunocompromised patients are more likely to be infected by aerobic gram-negative organisms. Gram staining of cytologic samples with evidence of phagocytized organisms is an often forgotten, but potentially pivotal, method of obtaining guidance for initial selection of antimicrobial therapy. Empiric selection of antimicrobials in the CCP might appropriately be directed initially toward any potential infecting pathogen, including nosocomial organisms with complex patterns of antimicrobial resistance. In a study of 74 canine intensive care unit (ICU) patients for which culture specimens were collected before implementation of antimicrobial therapy, Black et al[13] reported that empiric selection was appropriate, based on susceptibility testing, 75% of the time. The single drug to which isolates were most commonly susceptible was imipenem (79%), and that to which they were least susceptible was ampicillin sulbactam (29%). The combination of imipenem and gentamicin increased susceptibility to 89%.

Even if an organism is correctly identified, prediction of susceptibility patterns may be limited. A history of previous antimicrobial use (the author recommends considering this to be use within the past 3 months, which is supported by human guidelines)[4] indicates selection for resistant organisms. Although the use of β-lactams is likely to have resulted in resistance to other β-lactams, use of fluorinated quinolones is more likely to be associated with MDR bacteria, including MDR methicillin resistance in staphylococci.[21] In their study, Black et al found that 62% of patients had received antimicrobials before submission of culture specimens, and 44% of these cultures were positive for growth.[13] Although 27% of bacteria cultured

Table 175-1 Selected Recommendations for Empiric Antimicrobial Therapy as Indicated for Human Medicine by the Infectious Diseases Society of America[47]

System/Location	Syndrome/Disease	Antibacterial Choices	Reference
Skin, soft tissue Duration: 7-14 days unless slow-growing organisms (*Nocardia:* 3-12 mo, atypical mycobacterium: 3-6 wk)	Impetigo: *Staphylococcus, Streptococcus*	Amoxicillin-clavulanic acid, dicloxacillin, cephalexin, erythromycin, mupirocin topical	48
	MSSA infection	Cefazolin, clindamycin, dicloxacillin, cephalexin, doxycycline/minocycline, TMP-SDZ	48
	MRSA infection	Clindamycin, doxycycline/minocycline, linezolid, vancomycin, TMP-SDZ including combinations	48
Surgical site	Intestinal or genital site infection	Monotherapy: cefoxitin, ceftizoxime, penicillin with β-lactamase inhibitor, imipenem/cilastin, meropenem Combination therapy: fluoroquinolone or third-generation cephalosporin or aztreonam or aminoglycoside with (for anaerobes) clindamycin, metronidazole, chloramphenicol, or penicillin with β-lactamase inhibitor	48
	Nonintestinal site infection	First-generation cephalosporin; if axillary or perineal: cefoxitin, penicillin with β-lactamase inhibitor, or single agents listed earlier for intestinal infection	48
	Necrotizing infection	Streptococci: penicillin plus clindamycin *Staphylococcus aureus:* nafcillin, oxacillin, cefazolin, clindamycin or (if resistant) vancomycin Mixed infection: penicillin with β-lactamase inhibitor with clindamycin or ciprofloxacin; imipenem or meropenem; cefotaxime with metronidazole or clindamycin	48
Hematologic	Neutropenia	Monotherapy with antipseudomonal β-lactam or combination therapy with aminoglycosides as indicated; granulocyte colony-stimulating factors (see also entry for sepsis); fluoroquinolones for prophylaxis	48, 49
Intraabdominal	Extrabiliary, community-acquired infection	Monotherapy: cefoxitin, imipenem/meropenem, moxifloxacin (pradofloxacin), ticarcillin–clavulanic acid or piperacillin-tazobactam Combination therapy: amikacin or gentamicin, cefazolin, ceftriaxone, cefotaxime, ciprofloxacin or levofloxacin with metronidazole	50
	Hospital-acquired infection	*Pseudomonas* or ESBL-producing Enterobacteriaceae: therapy should include aminoglycoside MRSA: therapy should include vancomycin	50
*Urinary	Acute uncomplicated cystitis and pyelonephritis	Nitrofurantoin (5 days), TMP-SDZ (3 days), fosfomycin (single dose); fluoroquinolones (3 days); β-lactams other than amoxicillin or ampicillin (3-7 days) are less effective and thus reserved for cases in which other agents cannot be used	51
	Catheter-associated infection	Insufficient evidence to support routine implementation of prophylactic therapy, methenamine salts, cranberry juice extracts, catheter irrigation with antimicrobials or saline, or addition of antimicrobials or antiseptics in drainage back or treatment of asymptomatic bacteriuria Culture-based therapy for catheter-associated infection (clinical signs) or asymptomatic bacteriuria that persists for 48 hr after catheter removal Duration: 7 days for rapid responders, 10-14 days for delayed responders	51
	Asymptomatic bacteriuria	Culture-based therapy; indications: pregnancy, prostatic surgery (discontinue after surgery), urologic procedure involving mucosal bleeding, persistence for 48 hr after catheter removal	52
Circulatory	Severe sepsis and septic shock	Therapy targeting all potential infecting pathogens that penetrate in adequate concentrations those tissues presumed to be the source of sepsis; combination therapy with two different classes of antimicrobials (β-lactam with macrolide, fluoroquinolone or aminoglycoside) recommended for severely ill, septic patients at high risk of death Duration: 7-10 days, with daily assessment for potential to deescalate	4

Continued

Table 175-1 **Selected Recommendations for Empiric Antimicrobial Therapy as Indicated for Human Medicine by the Infectious Diseases Society of America—cont'd**

System/Location	Syndrome/Disease	Antibacterial Choices	Reference
Oral cavity	Oral decontamination for prevention of sepsis in at-risk patients	For patients receiving assisted ventilation, oral decontamination (chlorhexidine gluconate for oropharyngeal decontamination) and selective oral decontamination	4
Cardiac	Endocarditis	Streptococci (highly susceptible): aqueous penicillin G or ceftriaxone ± aminoglycoside (gentamicin) or vancomycin Staphylococci: nafcillin or oxacillin or cefazolin ± gentamicin; if MRSA, vancomycin ± rifampin and/or gentamicin Enterococci: ampicillin or aqueous penicillin plus gentamicin; vancomycin plus gentamicin; if β-lactamase producer: ampicillin-sulbactam or vancomycin plus gentamicin; if penicillin resistant, aminoglycosides and vancomycin: linezolid for *Enterococcus faecium* and imipenem or ceftriaxone and ampicillin for *Enterococcus faecalis*	53
Respiratory	Community-acquired pneumonia	No antimicrobials within 3 mo: macrolide Comorbidities: fluoroquinolone, or β-lactam with macrolide Intensive care unit patients: β-lactam plus azithromycin or fluoroquinolone *Pseudomonas:* antipseudomonal β-lactam and fluoroquinolone, or aminoglycoside with azithromycin or aminoglycoside with fluorinated quinolone MRSA: vancomycin or linezolid	54

ESBL, Extended-spectrum β-lactamase; *MRSA,* methicillin-resistant *Staphylococcus aureus; MSSA,* methicillin-susceptible *Staphylococcus aureus; TMP-SDZ,* trimethoprim sulfadiazine (or TMP-SMX, sulfamethoxazole, the human FDA-approved formulation; see Chapter 181 for further details).
*Guidelines for the use of antimicrobials for treatment of urinary tract infections in dogs and cats are now available at http://www.hindawi.com/journals/vmi/2011/263768/; accessed January 29, 2014.

from canine ICU patients expressed multidrug resistance, the relationship between previous antimicrobial therapy and multidrug resistance was not explored.

Rational combination antimicrobial therapy can be a powerful tool for enhancing effectiveness while reducing resistance in the CCP. Combination therapy should be routinely considered for treatment of organisms often associated with multidrug resistance (e.g., *Pseudomonas aeruginosa, Enterococcus* spp, and MRSA). The advantage of combination therapy is that a population size of 10^{14} or more colony-forming units must be reached before spontaneous mutations cause resistance to two drugs. In a review of 50 clinical trials involving combination antimicrobial therapy in humans with sepsis or septic shock, combination antimicrobial therapy was associated with increased effectiveness when implemented in the most critically ill patients.[22] However, an increased risk of death was found in low-risk patients, which led the authors to conclude that combination antimicrobial therapy improves survival and clinical response in high-risk, life-threatening infections, particularly septic shock, but may be detrimental in low-risk infections.

Drugs chosen for combination therapy should be selected rationally, based on mechanism of action and target organisms. Mechanisms of action should complement, rather than antagonize, one another.[22] In general, "bacteriostatic" drugs that inhibit ribosomes and thus microbial growth (e.g., chloramphenicol, tetracyclines, and erythromycin) should be avoided in the critically ill patient, particularly in the face of multidrug resistance. If these drugs are used in combination with drugs whose mechanism of action depends on protein synthesis, such as growth of the organism (e.g., β-lactams) or formation of a target protein, the effectiveness of the latter drug will be reduced. For example, the bactericidal activity of β-lactams and fluoroquinolones depends on continued synthesis of bacterial proteins. Antagonistic effects have been well documented between β-lactam antimicrobials and inhibitors of ribosomal activity.[22]

Rather than showing antagonism, drugs that have the same mechanism of action may act in an additive or synergistic fashion. The prototypical example of synergism is the combination of β-lactams and aminoglycosides; aminoglycoside penetration into bacteria is facilitated by penicillin-induced cell wall failure.[22] Indeed, aminoglycoside activity against *Enterococcus* spp and *Staphylococcus* spp should be supported by an agent that acts synergistically with a cell wall–active antibiotic, such as a β-lactam or vancomycin.[23] Synergism has also been demonstrated against some strains of Enterobacteriaceae, *P. aeruginosa,* staphylococci (including MRSA), and other microorganisms. Enhanced movement into the bacteria may occur with other drugs (e.g., potentiated sulfonamides, fluoroquinolones) when combined with a β-lactam. Combination therapy might be considered even with two drugs characterized by low-level resistance (such as might be demonstrated using the epsilon, or Etest [bioMérieux, Durham, N.C.], susceptibility system).

Combination antimicrobial therapy may be selected for treatment of a polymicrobial infection. Aminoglycosides or fluoroquinolones are often combined with β-lactams, metronidazole, or clindamycin to target both aerobic gram-positive and gram-negative infections, and aerobic infections caused by both aerobes and anaerobes. The combined use of selected antibiotics may result in effective therapy against a given microbe even when either drug alone would be ineffective. In humans, broadening the antimicrobial spectrum by combining at least two antimicrobials is recommended in patients with pneumonia. Recommended choices include an aminoglycoside or antipseudomonal fluoroquinolone combined with an antipseudomonal β-lactam (carbapenem if the organism is an extended-spectrum β-lactamase producer) plus vancomycin or linezolid if MRSA is suspected (humans only).[2] The addition of aminoglycosides for treatment of persistent staphylococcal infections (used only in combination with other drugs) is controversial; evidence of enhanced success is mixed in human patients with bacteremia.[24] Further studies are indicated to identify the risk factors or infections for which combination therapy provides the most benefit.

Design of the Dosing Regimen

The timely implementation of a well-designed dosing regimen is second only to selection of the appropriate antimicrobial when striving for therapeutic success and avoidance of resistance in the CCP. Dosing regimens should be designed to reach appropriate pharmacokinetic-pharmacodynamic targets.[2] Three major considerations should influence the design of the dosing regimen: the MIC of the infecting microbe and its relationship to plasma and tissue drug concentrations achieved at the site of infection, and the impact of microbial and host factors that impact active drug concentrations achieved at the site of infection.

Role of the minimum inhibitory concentration in the dosing regimen

Proper identification of the target microbe is not enough. The second major opportunity for error in antimicrobial use in the CCP is in assessing the susceptibility of the infecting isolate to the drug of interest. McKenzie[25] reviewed the principles that guide the design of dosing regimens in CCPs. The risk of antimicrobial resistance is associated with both dose and duration of therapy. Basing drug selection on culture and susceptibility information, with accompanying MIC data, is critical both to identify current bacterial resistance in patients at risk and to design an individual patient dosing regimen.[3,4]

Organisms that might once have been predictably susceptible to a drug may be characterized by an increasing MIC over time, and the MIC may become high enough to render the isolate no longer susceptible to the drug of choice. For example, the percentage of *E. coli* isolates (n = 3000) collected from dogs or cats with spontaneous disease that are resistant to ampicillin (and thus amoxicillin), amoxicillin–clavulanic acid (and thus ampicillin-sulbactam), cephalothin (and thus cephalexin), and doxycycline approximates 50%, 40%, 99%, and 99%, respectively (personal data, September 2013). Further, based on the MIC distributions of these isolates, even isolates considered susceptible by the Clinical and Laboratory Standards Institute are characterized by MICs that are very close to the susceptible breakpoint, which indicates that some level of resistance already has begun to emerge in isolates classified as susceptible.

The importance of hospital-based or regional antibiograms cannot be overemphasized. In treatment of the CCP, an awareness of local susceptibility patterns should weigh into the empiric selection of antimicrobials. Ideally, antimicrobial susceptibility statistics (e.g., antibiograms; Figure 175-2) are generated on an annual basis for each hospital. An important consideration when designing dosing regimens is the relationship between the MIC and the magnitude and time course of the plasma drug concentration (PDC). Based on this relationship, drugs can be categorized as either time dependent or concentration dependent (sometimes referred to as *dosage dependent*). The time-versus-concentration dependency of a drug determines the pharmacokinetic-pharmacodynamic principle to be targeted, which in turn influences dosing regimens.

Time-dependent drugs often act reversibly and thus must be present during most of the dosing interval. Time dependency is exemplified by β-lactams, whose presence is necessary as long as the organism is building new cell walls. The efficacy of β-lactams is best predicted by the percentage of time (T) that the PDC is above the MIC (or T > MIC). Additional time-dependent drugs include other cell wall inhibitors, folic acid inhibitors, and drugs considered to be bacteriostatic. The duration of T > MIC varies with the drug: for first-tier aminopenicillins, T > MIC ideally is 100% of the dosing interval, whereas for third- or fourth-tier carbapenems, the duration should be at least 25% of the dosing interval.[24,26] For time-dependent drugs with very short half-lives (e.g., aminopenicillins), dosing intervals must be shortened. Indeed, for such drugs, constant rate infusions[27] might be ideal, as was demonstrated in an in vitro model of the use of a ceftazidime constant rate infusion for treatment of *P. aeruginosa* infection.[28] The use of slow-release formulations might be more effective than intermittent administration as long as the target maximum concentration (C_{max}) is reached.[29] The impact of drugs with very long half-lives (e.g., cefovecin) on emergent antimicrobial resistance is not clear, but in general their use complicates attempts at deescalation of antimicrobial use by virtue of their prolonged presence in the patient. Administration of a loading dose might be indicated for drugs with a long half-life (e.g., azithromycin).

In contrast to time-dependent drugs, concentration-dependent drugs tend to bind their target irreversibly. These drugs are best represented by the fluoroquinolones and aminoglycosides (both of which result in irreversible inhibition of their targets). Their effectiveness depends on achieving a sufficient concentration of drug molecules at the site so that all target microbial molecules are bound. Their effectiveness is predicted by comparing the C_{max} with the MIC of the infecting organism.[3,24,26] Concentration-dependent drugs often exhibit an excellent postantibiotic effect; that is, effectiveness is maintained even after brief exposure to the drug. A long postantibiotic effect allows a longer dosing interval than might be expected based on the elimination half-life.[30] For such drugs, the magnitude of C_{max}:MIC generally should be a minimum of 10 to 12 and should be higher for more difficult infections (e.g., *P. aeruginosa* infections or those caused by multiple organisms).[31,32] More recently, the effectiveness of concentration-dependent drugs has been best predicted by the area under the inhibitory curve (AUIC), the ratio of the AUC (area under the curve for 24 hours, which is influenced by both dose and interval) to the MIC. An AUIC of over 100 to 125 is generally associated with bacterial killing and decreased resistance.[2] Thus, for treatment of some infections, the dosing regimen might be designed to maximize both the C_{max}:MIC and the AUC:MIC (i.e., a higher dosage, targeting a higher C_{max}:MIC, and a shorter dosing interval, targeting a higher AUC:MIC). For example, if the target C_{max}:MIC of a fluoroquinolone cannot be achieved with a single dose, the addition of a second dose in a 24-hour period may enhance effectiveness by increasing the AUC:MIC. Concentration-dependent drugs, and especially the fluorinated quinolones, demonstrate the importance of going beyond MIC when designing dosing regimens. Dosing regimens that reach the mutant-prevention concentration rather than the MIC at the site of infection are most likely to be effective.[5]

Site of Infection

Among the most important host factors influencing drug concentrations at the location of infection is drug penetrability at the infection site and host response to the infection. Three levels of drug penetration exist in normal tissues. Sinusoidal capillaries, found primarily in the adrenal cortex, pituitary gland, liver, and spleen, present essentially no barrier to bound or unbound drug movement. Fenestrated capillaries such as those located in kidneys and endocrine glands contain pores that do not present a barrier to unbound drug, and movement is thus facilitated between the plasma and interstitium.[33] However, culture and susceptibility testing may be based on an MIC determined in vitro in the absence of protein. Therefore, for those drugs characterized by a high percentage of binding to plasma proteins (e.g., doxycycline), the MIC may underestimate the total plasma concentration of drug necessary for effectiveness. Continuous (nonfenestrated) capillaries, such as those found delivering drug to the brain, cerebrospinal fluid, testes, prostate, muscle, and adipose tissue, present a barrier of endothelial cells with tight junctions that preclude drug movement. For infections in such tissues, the dosing regimen of water-soluble drugs (e.g., β-lactams and aminoglycosides,

Cumulative Antimicrobial Susceptibility Report
Canine Isolates from 1/ 1/ 07 to1/ 1/ 10

PERCENT SUSCEPTIBLE
(No. ISOLATES TESTED) [a]

	No. of Isolates	Amikacin	Amoxicillin/CA	Ampicillin	Cefazolin	Cefpodoxime	Ceftiofur	Cephalothin [b]	Chloramphenicol	Clindamycin	Enrofloxacin	Erythromycin	Gentamicin	Marbofloxacin	Oxacillin + 2% NaCl	Penicillin	Rifampin	Tetracycline	Ticarcillin	Ticarcillin/CA	Trimethoprim/Sulfa
Enterococcus faecalis	128		98	96					84		52	17 (127)		54 (110)		96	54	46 (116)			
Enterococcus faecium	52		31	27					96		6	12		13 (46)		27	54	25 (48)			
Escherichia coli	486	98	68	53	71	70	75 (444)	57 (442)	85		69		85	71				69 (439)	55	68	73
Klebsiella pneumoniae	100	67	60	0	58	61	57 (87)	58 (93)	70		63		64	64				59 (93)	0	61	71
Proteus mirabilis	136	99	95	91	90	96	98 (117)	91 (129)	90		95		92	98				0 (129)	94	100	90
Pseudomonas aeruginosa	250	98							6 (246)		56		89	80 (223)					94	96	
Staphylococcus aureus	30	97	37	17	37	33	21 (28)	37	100	37	50	37	90	50	37	20	93	87			93
Staphylococcus intermedius [b]	480	94	77	20	76	69	72 (411)	78 (441)	98	49 (477)	63	49	90	67	78	18	98 (476)	53 (430)			65
Group G Beta Streptococci	20	45	100	100	100	65	100 (12)	100 (19)	70	95	60	0	65	65		100	100	47 (19)			100

a. Numbers in parentheses represent actual number tested if different from total.
b. Cephalothin acts as a class drug representing cephalothin, cephapirin, cephalexin, cephradine, cefaclor, and cefadroxil.
c. Represents what is presently known as S. *intermedius* group.

FIGURE 175-2 Example of a hospital-based antibiogram, which demonstrates susceptibility patterns. Each cell indicates the percentage of isolates of the organism (delineated by row) susceptible to the drug against which the isolate was tested (delineated by column). If not all isolates were tested against that drug, the number in the cell is in parenthesis. For example, during the data collection period, 68% of *Escherichia coli* isolates collected from dogs during 2007 through 2010 were considered susceptible (based on guidelines promulgated by the Clinical and Laboratory Standards Institute) to amoxicillin–clavulanic acid, which is the model drug for ampicillin-sulbactam. This represents an improvement over the previous years (2003 to 2005) during which only 46% of isolates were susceptible. Cells lacking data represent drugs to which isolates are inherently resistant or for which in vitro data do not predict patient response.

selected sulfonamides, and selected tetracyclines) should be adjusted for potentially poor drug distribution to the site of infection. Indeed, dosages of β-lactams are often adjusted up to 10-fold in treating human central nervous system infections. The bronchus-blood barrier presents an example. Based on studies in human medicine, only 2% to 30% of β-lactams or aminoglycosides in plasma reach bronchial secretions, compared with 30% to 80% of lipid-soluble drugs. For azithromycin, concentrations in bronchial secretions are 17-fold higher than plasma concentrations (as reviewed by Boothe[3]). The effectiveness of some drugs is enhanced because of accumulation of the active (unbound) form in tissues (e.g., macrolides[34]) or phagocytes; such drugs may be of particular efficacy in the presence of marked inflammatory debris.

Culture and susceptibility testing underestimates the effectiveness of drugs that accumulate in tissues or can be applied topically at the site of infection. Note, however, that accumulated drug is not necessarily active drug. Further, drugs excreted in the urine may not concentrate there in the face of altered renal function and may not be able to penetrate uroepithelial cells or biofilm protecting organisms causing cystitis. For topically accessed sites, a level of several thousandfold the MIC may be reached. Although topical application of antimicrobial drugs in the CCP is not common, selected indications should be considered. An example is drug aerosolization for treatment of infections of the respiratory tract, but limited aerosol penetrability and potential adverse effects of aerosolized particles preclude aerosolization as the sole method of drug administration for respiratory tract infections (see Chapter 172). Topical wound management (with or without antimicrobials) may be preferred to systemic antimicrobial therapy.

Disease or other factors can influence drug movement to the site of infection. Pathophysiologic changes associated with the critical nature of a patient's illness have an impact on each drug's disposition, including absorption, distribution, metabolism, and excretion (see Chapter 182). Changes in absorption associated with subcutaneous or intramuscular drug administration can be circumvented by using intravenous administration in critically ill patients. However, distribution may also be impacted by changes in tissue perfusion. The patient in cardiovascular shock may be particularly predisposed to adverse events affecting the cardiovascular and central nervous systems because these organs receive preferential blood flow. Volume replacement may correct some of these changes.

Changes in plasma drug concentration are influenced by changes in the volume to which the drug is distributed.[24] An increase in the volume of distribution decreases plasma drug concentration and vice versa. However, the clinical impact differs with the lipophilicity of the drug. For water-soluble drugs (aminoglycosides, β-lactams, and glycopeptides), distribution is limited to interstitial and other extracellular fluids. Because of this, the volume of distribution can be increased by the accumulation of fluids in peripheral tissues, including the pleural space and peritoneal cavity.[1] Septic shock and trauma are the two most common causes of expansion of volume of distribution in the CCP.[1] Aggressive fluid therapy may also decrease drug concentrations. In each of the foregoing examples, tissue antimicrobial exposure is decreased. Several studies have associated therapeutic failure of aminoglycosides with decreased plasma drug concentrations in septic patients.[1] Dosages should be increased proportionately in these situations. Monitoring of drug concentrations might be considered for patients receiving aminoglycosides to ensure that therapeutic concentrations are achieved at the chosen dosage. Both a peak serum sample collected 1 to 2 hours after administration and a second sample obtained 4 to 6 hours later ideally are collected so that both peak concentration (important for efficacy) and trough concentration (important for safety) can be predicted.

Interestingly, hypoalbuminemia also contributes to decreased antimicrobial exposure, even for drugs that traditionally are not significantly protein bound, probably due to peripheral fluid retention and increased volume of distribution. In general, dosage increases of 1.5-fold to 2-fold are indicated in such cases.[1] Although volume contraction associated with dehydration may cause the opposite effect (higher plasma drug concentrations), volume repletion rather than dosage modification should be implemented. For lipid-soluble drugs, dosage is calculated on a milligram-per-kilogram basis. In addition to affecting plasma drug concentrations, volume of distribution influences drug elimination, expressed as changes in elimination half-life. Elimination half-life is affected by both volume of distribution (directly proportional) and clearance (inversely proportional). For this reason, both may change profoundly (e.g., both volume of distribution and clearance decrease), yet half-life will not be impacted. In general, critical illness decreases drug clearance, although an exception is the hyperdynamic state of septic shock, which is frequently associated with increased clearance. The impact on clearance, like that on volume of distribution, also varies with lipophilicity by virtue of its impact on the site of drug excretion. Water-soluble drugs are generally excreted renally, and their clearance changes proportionately with glomerular filtration. In contrast, lipophilic drugs generally are passively resorbed in the tubules and must be metabolized before clearance. Excretion of these drugs may be decreased in animals with profound hepatic disease (i.e., altered albumin concentration).

Predicting the proper dosing regimen is complicated by the complex pathophysiology of critical diseases. For example, the increased clearance associated with the hyperdynamic state of septic shock may be balanced by decreased renal function; fluid therapy may increase the volume of distribution and thus decrease plasma drug concentrations.

Host Immune Response

On the one hand, immunocompromise increases the risk of infection or therapeutic failure, mandating the need for achievement of bactericidal concentrations of drug at the site of infection. Bactericidal concentrations are paramount to therapeutic success in immunocompromised hosts (e.g., patients with viral infections, patients with granulopoiesis, those receiving immunoinhibiting drugs) or at immunocompromised sites (septicemia, meningitis, valvular endocarditis, and osteomyelitis). However, classification of bactericidal versus bacteriostatic actions is based on in vitro methods, and dosages should be designed to ensure that the minimum bactericidal concentration is achieved at the site of infection in the patient. Nevertheless, for some bacteriostatic drugs, bactericidal concentrations can be achieved in some tissues (e.g., if the drug accumulates at the site of infection).

Although an adequate host immune response facilitates therapeutic success, the host inflammatory response can also profoundly alter drug efficacy. Acute inflammation may initially increase drug delivery to the site of infection. However, marked or chronic inflammation may preclude drug movement and efficacy. Reduced oxygen tension decreases the efficacy of some drugs. Aminoglycosides in particular require active transport into the microbe and may be ineffective in an anaerobic environment, even against facultative anaerobes such as *E. coli.*

Impact of Microbial Factors

In addition to developing resistance, microbes can negatively affect antimicrobial therapy in other ways. Materials released from microbes facilitate invasion, impair cellular phagocytosis, and damage host tissues. The "inoculum effect" increases the risk of failure for several reasons. Larger inocula present more bacterial targets and thus require more drug molecules (higher doses). Moreover, larger inocula present a greater risk of spontaneous mutations resulting in resistance and also produce greater concentrations of destructive enzymes. For example, production of extended-spectrum β-lactamases more often results in cephalosporin resistance with a larger (10^7) than with smaller (10^5) inoculum.

Infection in epithelial tissues (e.g., uroepithelium and respiratory epithelium) is facilitated by bacterial adherence. Materials secreted by organisms often contribute to the marked inflammatory host response and clinical signs of infection. Soluble mediators released by organisms (hemolysin, epidermolytic toxin, leukocidin) may damage host tissues or alter host response. Among the more problematic microbial factors are glycocalyx or biofilm, a virulence factor that facilitates microbe adaptation to new environments. A biofilm is a community that effectively allows a single-cell microbe to become a multicell organism. It consists of microcolonies of both pathogenic and host microbes embedded in a polysaccharide produced by microbes adhering to flat surfaces. These include foreign bodies, wound surfaces, or other tissues.[35] Symbiosis and survival are supported through sophisticated communication and complex patterns of antimicrobial resistance as well as an ability to avoid host immune response. Organisms within the community are often quiescent and thus nonresponsive to antimicrobial therapy. Translocation of the biofilm microflora to sterile tissues may ultimately cause infection, as was demonstrated in dogs undergoing experimental catheterization of the portal vein.[36] However, organism growth in catheters does not necessarily lead to infection, and isolates cultured from urinary catheter tips are not necessarily those causing urinary tract infection.[37]

Adverse Drug Events

Because host (patient) cells are eukaryotic whereas bacterial targets are prokaryotic, antimicrobial drugs generally are safe as a class. Exceptions include those drugs that target shared structures, such as cell membranes (e.g., colistin and polymyxin). Aminoglycosides are predictably nephrotoxic, with toxicity related to the duration of exposure. Toxicity is minimized by dosing once daily so that trough plasma drug concentration (and subsequently urine drug concentration) drops below a threshold (<1 to 2 mg/ml)[38]; ensuring hydration, which may include treatment with sodium-containing fluids[39]; administering in the morning (in diurnal animals); and avoiding nephroactive drugs. In cases of nephrotoxicity, treatment with *N*-acetylcysteine may decrease damage.[40] Fluoroquinolone-induced retinal degeneration in cats reflects the absence of a retinal efflux pump.[41,42] Marbofloxacin, orbifloxacin, and pradofloxacin appear not to cause retinal toxicity, even when administered at dosages exceeding the recommended dosages by severalfold (see also drug package inserts).[42] The use of fluoroquinolones to treat *Staphylococcus pyogenes* infections in humans and *Streptococcus canis* infections in animals has been associated with streptococcal toxic shock syndrome and necrotizing fasciitis.[43,44] The relevance of fluoroquinolone- or macrolide-associated cardiotoxicity (torsades de pointes) to dogs and cats is not clear.[45]

Antimicrobial Deescalation

Deescalation is among the more rational paradigms for empiric antimicrobial use in hospitalized patients with serious bacterial infections.[11,46] The advantages of deescalation include the following: cost minimization, reduction in adverse events, reduced risk of antimicrobial resistance, and a decrease in the incidence of infections related to antimicrobial use, such as *C. difficile* diarrhea or superinfection with MDR isolates of *Candida* species.[2]

The goal of antimicrobial deescalation is to prescribe an initial antibacterial regimen that will cover the most likely bacterial pathogens associated with infection, so that the need for appropriate therapy is addressed and the risk of emerging antibacterial resistance is minimized.[11] Once the decision is made that antimicrobial therapy is indicated, a three-pronged approach to deescalation includes narrowing the antibacterial regimen through culture, assessing the susceptibility for dosage determination, and choosing the shortest course of therapy clinically acceptable.

Although preapproval of selected drug use (e.g., by a committee) and antimicrobial restriction practices may be useful, recommended and more reasonable deescalation procedures include rotating the use of antimicrobial drugs on a regular schedule and designing the dosing regimen so that therapeutic success is maximized at the same time that the lowest-tier drug is used. This enables resistance to be minimized and duration of therapy to be reduced.[46] The use of deescalation procedures in humans has been associated with a return to susceptibility to ceftazidime, piperacillin, imipenem, and fluoroquinolones. The concept of deescalation is most effective when it is implemented under conditions that provide for systematic approaches to antimicrobial therapy.

Deescalation also influences design of the dosing regimen by virtue of its impact on the duration of therapy. In humans, discontinuing unnecessary antimicrobial therapy has been associated with a decrease in hospital stay, cost, antimicrobial resistance, and suprainfection.[6,46] Short courses (i.e., 3 to 5 days) of intensive therapy are increasingly accepted in lieu of the traditional 7 to 10 days of therapy.

An approach to deescalation is offered by Derensinski.[2] Once a culture specimen is collected and empiric therapy is implemented, the first major assessment (both clinical assessment and assessment of relevant microbiologic data) occurs at 48 to 72 hours. If the patient has not shown clinical improvement by that time, microbiologic data should be critically assessed and therapy reexamined. One should be warned that the relevance of antimicrobial data collected before the implementation of antimicrobial therapy which subsequently fails is not clear. It is possible that even though therapy failed, the impact of the antimicrobial on the infecting inoculum may have altered the infecting population or its susceptibility patterns. If the patient has experienced clinical improvement despite microbial data that indicate an inappropriate antimicrobial choice, the clinician may choose to stay the course and monitor or, in a patient at risk, consider the addition of a second antimicrobial supported by the data. However, if the patient has shown clinical improvement and the data indicate that the choice is appropriate, deescalation to a drug with a narrower spectrum or total discontinuation should be considered.

REFERENCES

1. Pea F, Viale P, Furlanut M: Antimicrobial therapy in critically ill patients: a review of pathophysiological conditions responsible for altered disposition and pharmacokinetic variability, Clin Pharmacokinet 44:1009, 2005.
2. Deresinski S: Principles of antibiotic therapy in severe infections: optimizing the therapeutic approach by use of laboratory and clinical data, Clin Infect Dis 45(Suppl 3):S177-183, 2007.
3. Boothe DM: Principles of antimicrobial therapy. In Small animal clinical pharmacology and therapeutics, ed 2, St Louis, 2011, Elsevier, pp 128-188.
4. Dellinger RP, Levy MM, Rhodes A, et al: Surviving Sepsis Campaign: international guidelines for management of severe sepsis and septic shock, 2012, Intensive Care Med 39(2):165-228, 2013.
5. Drlica K, Zhao X: Mutant selection window hypothesis updated, Clin Infect Dis 44(5):681-688, 2007.
6. Salgado CD, O'Grady N, Farr BM: Prevention and control of antimicrobial-resistant infections in intensive care patients, Crit Care Med 33:2373, 2005.
7. Wagenlehner F, Stöwer-Hoffmann J, Schneider-Brachert W, et al: Influence of a prophylactic single dose of ciprofloxacin on the level of resistance of *Escherichia coli* to fluoroquinolones in urology, Int J Antimicrob Agents 15:207, 2000.
8. Smarick SD, Haskins SC, Aldrich J, et al: Incidence of catheter-associated urinary tract infection among dogs in a small animal intensive care unit, J Am Vet Med Assoc 224:1936, 2004.
9. Sanchez S, Stevenson MAM, Hudson CR, et al: Characterization of multidrug resistant *Escherichia coli* isolates associated with nosocomial infections in dogs, J Clin Microbiol 40:3586, 2002.
10. Aly SA, Debavalya N, Suh SJ, et al: Molecular mechanisms of antimicrobial resistance in fecal *Escherichia coli* of healthy dogs after enrofloxacin or amoxicillin administration, Can J Microbiol 58(11):1288-1294, 2012.
11. Kollef M: Appropriate empirical antibacterial therapy for nosocomial infections: getting it right the first time, Drugs 63:2157, 2003.
12. Heckler MT, Aaron DC, Patel NP, et al: Unnecessary use of antimicrobials in hospitalized patients: current patterns of misuse with an emphasis on the antianaerobic spectrum of activity, Arch Intern Med 163:972, 2003.
13. Black DM, Rankin SC, King LG: Antimicrobial therapy and aerobic bacteriologic culture patterns in canine intensive care unit patients: 74 dogs (January-June 2006), J Vet Emerg Crit Care (San Antonio) 19:489, 2009.
14. O'Grady NP, Barie PS, Bartlett JG, et al: Guidelines for evaluation of new fever in critically ill adult patients: 2008 update from the American College of Critical Care Medicine and the Infectious Diseases Society of America, Crit Care Med 36(4):1330-1349, 2008.
15. Jensen JU, Hein L, Lundgren B, et al: Procalcitonin-guided interventions against infections to increase early appropriate antibiotics and improve survival in the intensive care unit: a randomized trial, Crit Care Med 39(9):2048-2058, 2011.
16. Kibe S, Adams K, Barlow G: Diagnostic and prognostic biomarkers of sepsis in critical care, J Antimicrob Chemother 66(Suppl 2):ii33-ii40, 2011.
17. Póvoa P, Salluh JI: Biomarker-guided antibiotic therapy in adult critically ill patients: a critical review, Ann Intensive Care 2(1):32, 2012.
18. Schuetz P, Müller B, Christ-Crain M, et al: Procalcitonin to initiate or discontinue antibiotics in acute respiratory tract infections, Cochrane Database Syst Rev (9):CD007498, 2012.
19. Gaieski DF, Mikkelsen ME, Band RA, et al: Impact of time to antibiotics on survival in patients with severe sepsis or septic shock in whom early goal-directed therapy was initiated in the emergency department, Crit Care Med 38(4):1045-1053, 2010.
20. Schwaber M, Cosgrove SE, Gold H, et al: Fluoroquinolones protective against cephalosporin resistance in gram-negative nosocomial pathogens, Emerg Infect Dis 10:94, 2004.

21. Weese JS, van Duijkeren E: Methicillin-resistant *Staphylococcus aureus* and *Staphylococcus pseudintermedius* in veterinary medicine, Vet Microbiol 140(3-4):418-429, 2010.
22. Kumar A, Zarychanski R, Light B, et al: Early combination antibiotic therapy yields improved survival compared with monotherapy in septic shock: a propensity-matched analysis, Crit Care Med 38(9):1773-1785, 2010.
23. Eliopoulos GM, Moellering RC: Antimicrobial combinations. In Lorian V, editor: Antibiotics in laboratory medicine, Baltimore, 1996, Williams & Wilkins.
24. Lemonovich TL, Haynes K, Lautenbach E, et al: Combination therapy with an aminoglycoside for *Staphylococcus aureus* endocarditis and/or persistent bacteremia is associated with a decreased rate of recurrent bacteremia: a cohort study, Infection 39(6):549-554, 2011.
25. McKenzie C: Antibiotic dosing in critical illness, J Antimicrob Chemother 66(Suppl 2):ii25-ii31, 2011.
26. Mouton JW, Dudley MN, Cars O, et al: Standardization of pharmacokinetic/pharmacodynamic (PK/PD) terminology for antiinfective drugs: an update, J Antimicrob Chemother 55:601, 2005.
27. MacGowan AP, Bowker KE: Continuous infusion of β-lactam antibiotics, Clin Pharmacokinet 35:391, 1998.
28. Alou L, Aguilar L, Sevillano D, et al: Is there a pharmacodynamic need for the use of continuous versus intermittent infusion with ceftazidime against *Pseudomonas aeruginosa?* An in vitro pharmacodynamic model, J Antimicrob Chemother 55:209, 2005.
29. Hoffman A, Danenberg HD, Katzhendler I, et al: Pharmacodynamic and pharmacokinetic rationales for the development of an oral controlled release amoxicillin dosage form, J Control Release 54:29, 1998.
30. Craig WA, Gudmundsson S: Postantibiotic effect. In Lorian V, editor: Antibiotics in laboratory medicine, Baltimore, 1996, Williams & Wilkins.
31. Toutain PL, del Castillo JR, Bousquet-Melou A: The pharmacokinetic-pharmacodynamic approach to a rational dosage regimen for antibiotics, Res Vet Sci 73:105, 2002.
32. Li RC, Zhu ZY: The integration of four major determinants of antibiotic action: bactericidal activity, postantibiotic effect, susceptibility, and pharmacokinetics, J Chemother 14:579, 2002.
33. Barza M: Tissue directed antibiotic therapy: antibiotic dynamics in cells and tissues, Clin Infect Dis 19:910, 1994.
34. Bishai W: Comparative effectiveness of different macrolides: clarithromycin, azithromycin, and erythromycin, Johns Hopkins Division of Infectious Diseases Antibiotic Guide, 2003. Available at http://www.hopkins-abxguide.org.
35. Jacques M, Aragon V, Tremblay YD: Biofilm formation in bacterial pathogens of veterinary importance, Anim Health Res Rev 11(2):97-121, 2010.
36. Howe LM, Boothe DM, Boothe HW: Detection of portal and systemic bacteremia in dogs with severe hepatic disease and multiple portosystemic shunts, Am J Vet Res 60:181, 1999.
37. Smarick SD, Haskins SC, Aldrich J, et al: Incidence of catheter-associated urinary tract infection among dogs in a small animal intensive care unit, J Am Vet Med Assoc 224:1936, 2004.
38. Maller R, Ahrne H, Holmen C, et al: Once-versus twice-daily amikacin regimen: efficacy and safety in systemic gram-negative infections, J Antimicrob Chemother 31:939, 1993.
39. Barclay ML, Begg EJ: Aminoglycoside adaptive resistance: importance for effective dosage regimens, Drugs 61:713, 2001.
40. Kaynar K, Gul S, Ersoz S, et al: Amikacin-induced nephropathy: is there any protective way? Ren Fail 29(1):23-27, 2007.
41. Ramirez CJ, Minch JD, Gay JM, et al: Molecular genetic basis for fluoroquinolone-induced retinal degeneration in cats, Pharmacogenet Genomics 21(2):66-75, 2011.
42. Weibe V, Hamilton P: Fluoroquinolone-induced retinal degeneration in cats, J Am Vet Med Assoc 221:1568, 2002.
43. Ingrey KT, Ren J, Prescott JF: Fluoroquinolone induces a novel mitogen-encoding bacteriophage in *Streptococcus canis*, Infect Immun 71:3028, 2003.
44. Miller CW, Prescott JF, Mathews KA, et al: Streptococcal toxic shock syndrome in dogs, J Am Vet Med Assoc 209:1421, 1996.
45. Briasoulis A, Agarwal V, Pierce WJ: QT prolongation and torsade de pointes induced by fluoroquinolones: infrequent side effects from commonly used medications, Cardiology 120(2):103-110, 2011.
46. Masterson RG: Antibiotic de-escalation, Crit Care Clin 27(1):149-162, 2011.
47. Infectious Diseases Society of America: IDSA practice guidelines, Antimicrobial Stewardship 2013. Available at http://www.idsociety.org/IDSA_Practice_Guidelines. Accessed April 2013.
48. Stevens DL, Bisno AL, Chambers HF, et al: Infectious Diseases Society of America. Practice guidelines for the diagnosis and management of skin and soft-tissue infections, Clin Infect Dis 41(10):1373-1406, 2005.
49. Friedfield AG, Bow EJ, Sepkowitz KA, et al: 2010 Guidelines for the use of antimicrobial agents in neutropenic patients with cancer, Clin Infect Dis 52:e56, 2014; http://www.uphs.upenn.edu/bugdrug/antibiotic_manual/idsaneutropenicfever2010.pdf Accessed Jan 29, 2014.
50. Solomkin JS, Mazuski JE, Bradley, et al: Diagnosis and management of complicated intra-abdominal infection in adults and children: guidelines by the Surgical Infection Society and the Infectious Diseases Society of America, Surg Infect (Larchmt) 11(1):79-109, 2010.
51. Gupta K, Hooton TM, Naber KG, et al: International clinical practice guidelines for the treatment of acute uncomplicated cystitis and pyelonephritis in women: A 2010 update by the Infectious Diseases Society of America and the European Society for Microbiology and Infectious Diseases, Clin Infect Dis 52(5):e103-e120, 2011.
52. Nicolle LE, Bradley S, Colgan R, et al: Infectious Diseases Society of America guidelines for the diagnosis and treatment of asymptomatic bacteriuria in adults, Clin Infect Dis 40(5):643-654, 2005.
53. Baddour LM, Wilson WR, Bayer AS, et al: Infective endocarditis: diagnosis, antimicrobial therapy, and management of complications: a statement for healthcare professionals from the Committee on Rheumatic Fever, Endocarditis, and Kawasaki Disease, Council on Cardiovascular Disease in the Young, and the Councils on Clinical Cardiology, Stroke, and Cardiovascular Surgery and Anesthesia, American Heart Association: endorsed by the Infectious Diseases Society of America, Circulation 111(23):e394-e434, 2005.
54. Mandell LA, Wunderink RG, Anzueto MD, et al: Infectious Diseases Society of America/American Thoracic Society Consensus Guidelines on the Management of Community-Acquired Pneumonia in Adults, Clin Infect Disease 44:S27-S72, 2007.

CHAPTER 176
β-LACTAM ANTIMICROBIALS

Scott P. Shaw, DVM, DACVECC

KEY POINTS

- Penicillins, cephalosporins, and carbapenems are all β-lactam antimicrobials.
- The spectrum of activity of individual β-lactam drugs varies widely.
- Bacteria can produce β-lactamases, cephalosporinases, and carbapenemases that can inactivate these drugs if they are not combined with an appropriate β-lactamase inhibitor. The prevalence of β-lactamase production in bacteria has increased substantially over time.
- Methicillin-resistant *Staphylococcus* spp are resistant to all commonly available β-lactam antimicrobials.

Fleming's observation in 1929 that colonies of staphylococci lysed on a Petri dish contaminated with *Penicillium* mold ushered in the era of modern antimicrobial therapy. His initial efforts to extract the bactericidal substance failed, and it was 11 years before Chain and Florey succeeded in purifying large quantities of the first penicillin from *Penicillium notatum.* By the end of the decade penicillin G was in widespread clinical use. Limitations to penicillin G's efficacy were noticed almost immediately. These included poor bioavailability after oral administration, rapid development of resistance due to the presence of β-lactamase, and poor activity against gram-negative organisms. Development of cephalosporins overcame many of these limitations.[1]

The penicillins, cephalosporins, and carbapenems are referred to as *β-lactam antimicrobials.* All members of this class share a basic structure, the presence of a β-lactam ring. The β-lactam ring is essential for the biologic activity of these drugs. Substitutions can be made on the β-lactam ring for specific purposes such as increasing β-lactamase resistance, enhancing efficacy against specific pathogens, and altering pharmacokinetic properties.[1,2]

MECHANISM OF ACTION

All β-lactam antimicrobials work by interfering with bacterial cell wall synthesis. They do this by binding to and inhibiting the transpeptidases and peptidoglycan-active enzymes, collectively referred to as *penicillin-binding proteins* (PBPs), that catalyze the cross-linking of the glycopeptides which form the bacterial cell wall. β-Lactams are bactericidal, but they do require that the cells be actively growing to be efficacious.[2]

The difference in susceptibility of gram-positive and gram-negative organisms depends on the number and type of drug receptors, the amount of peptidoglycan present (gram-positive organisms have a much thicker cell wall), and the amount of lipid in the cell wall.

PHARMACOLOGY

When administered intravenously, β-lactams are distributed widely in body fluids and tissues. They are lipid insoluble and do not enter living cells well. After oral administration bioavailability varies greatly among drugs depending on their acid stability and protein binding. Ampicillin in particular has poor availability when administered orally; however, the structurally related compound amoxicillin has good bioavailability. Cefovecin is a cephalosporin with an extended half-life so that its dosing interval is markedly longer.[1,3]

Despite their large volume of distribution in interstitial fluid, most of the β-lactams do a poor job of crossing biologic membranes, and their concentration in the eyes, testes, brain, and prostate may be only one tenth of the serum concentration. However, penicillins and cephalosporins are indicated for certain infections within the central nervous system (CNS) because bactericidal levels of drug can be found in the CNS, particularly when there is inflammation of the meninges and a decrease in the blood-brain barrier. Most β-lactams are excreted actively by the kidney into the urine. As a result, urine levels can be severalfold higher than those seen in serum.[1,3]

Classically, cephalosporins were divided into three generations but more recently have been categorized into five. As a general rule, cephalosporins become more gram-negative specific with increasing generation among the first three generations. However, the advent of newer third-generation drugs such as ceftiofur and cefpodoxime, which have a spectrum of action similar to that of first-generation drugs, makes this classification scheme confusing. The fourth-generation cephalosporin drugs generally have both a good gram-positive and good gram-negative spectrum, greater resistance to β-lactamases, and antipseudomonal activity. In recent times fifth-generation cephalosporin drugs have been developed that are effective against methicillin-resistant staphylococci.[1,2] It should be noted that this classification scheme for cephalosporins is not universally accepted.

RESISTANCE

Production of β-Lactamase

Some bacteria such as staphylococci and most gram-negative rods can produce a β-lactamase enzyme that inactivates β-lactams by cleaving the β-lactam ring. More than 60 β-lactamase enzymes have been described; these include penicillinases, cephalosporinases, and carbapenemases. The genes for many of these enzymes are found on plasmids, which allows for transmission of resistance both within and between bacterial species. As a result the prevalence of β-lactamase production and the variety of β-lactamase enzymes have increased substantially over time.[4] Of particular concern is the growing incidence of extended-spectrum β-lactamase (ESBL) production by gram-negative organisms; these enzymes can hydrolyze penicillins, cephalosporins, and aztreonam to variable extents. It should be noted that ESBL production does not confer resistance to the carbapenems.[5] ESBL-producing organisms have been identified in clinical veterinary patients and have been found in the feces of healthy cats and dogs in the community.[6,7] The risk of fecal carriage of ESBL-producing organisms was increased in animals that had received antimicrobials in the 3-month period before testing.[6] See Chapter 103. Novel β-lactam antimicrobial drugs as well as novel β-lactamase inhibitors are currently in development and may be beneficial in the future in the management of multidrug-resistant organisms.[5]

Changes in Cell Wall Permeability

Some bacteria can become resistant to β-lactam antimicrobials by altering their PBPs. The PBPs can still cross-link glycopeptides but prevent the binding of β-lactam antimicrobials. The most important instance if this type of mutation is the acquisition by *Staphylococcus* spp of a gene known as *mecA* that codes for PBP-2a. As a result of this alteration in PBPs, staphylococci become resistant to all commonly available β-lactam antimicrobials (with the exception of fifth-generation drugs) and are known as *methicillin-resistant staphylococci.*[2,8]

SELECTED PENICILLINS AND CEPHALOSPORINS

Penicillin G

In general, penicillin G has a good spectrum of action against gram-positive and anaerobic organisms, with the exception of some *Staphylococcus* spp. Penicillin G is synergistic with aminoglycosides, and this combination may be effective against staphylococci. Penicillin G is the drug of choice for treatment of streptococcal infections (e.g., necrotizing fasciitis), clostridial infection, and actinomycosis.[1]

Extended-Spectrum Penicillins

Both amoxicillin and ampicillin have similar spectrums of action. As a general rule, ampicillin should be given parenterally when treating an infection. The extended-spectrum penicillins are less active against gram-positive and anaerobic organisms than penicillin G, but they have much greater efficacy against gram-negative species. Unfortunately, resistance is a growing problem, and therapeutic failures are becoming common.

Both ampicillin and amoxicillin are available combined with a β-lactamase inhibitor, sulbactam and clavulanic acid, respectively. The addition of a β-lactamase inhibitor results in much greater efficacy against gram-negative organisms as well as some β-lactamase–producing gram-positive and anaerobic organisms.[1-3]

Antipseudomonal Penicillins

The antipseudomonal penicillins (ticarcillin, piperacillin) exhibit greater activity against *Pseudomonas* spp and *Proteus* spp than in seen with other penicillins. It should be noted the antipseudomonal penicillins exhibit variable activity against some gram-negative bacteria such as *Acinetobacter* spp. The combination of ticarcillin and clavulanic acid does provide greater coverage against organisms that produce β-lactamases.[1]

First-Generation Cephalosporins

First-generation cephalosporins (e.g., cefazolin, cephalothin, cephalexin) have increased activity against some β-lactamase–producing organisms such as staphylococci. In general, they display a high level of activity against gram-positive organisms, moderate activity against gram-negative organisms, and minimal activity against anaerobes. Members of this group are used commonly as initial empiric and perioperative therapy because of their spectrum of action and safety profile.[1,2]

Second-Generation Cephalosporins

Because of their stability against β-lactamase, second-generation cephalosporins (cefaclor, cefoxitin, cefotetan, cefuroxime) have a broad spectrum of activity. In general, they are moderately efficacious against gram-positive organisms and have a greater spectrum of activity against gram-negative organisms than the first-generation cephalosporins.[1,3]

Third-Generation Cephalosporins

The third-generation cephalosporins (cefotaxime, ceftriaxone, ceftiofur, cefixime, ceftazidime, cefpodoxime, cefovecin) vary greatly in their spectrum of action, and efficacy of one drug in the class against an organism does not guarantee efficacy if another member of the class is employed. The classic third-generation cephalosporins—cefotaxime, ceftriaxone, cefixime, and ceftazidime—have a high degree of specificity for and efficacy against gram-negative organisms. These drugs are considered the treatment of choice for empiric therapy for infections located within the CNS.[1,3]

Carbapenems

The carbapenems (imipenem, meropenem, and ertapenem) are the only class of antimicrobials that is truly broad spectrum when used as the sole agent. It should be noted that, as with all β-lactam antimicrobials, methicillin-resistant staphylococci are resistant to treatment with carbapenems.[1,3]

Imipenem is administered with cilastatin to decrease renal tubular metabolism. Cilastatin does not affect the antibacterial activity. Imipenem has become a valuable antimicrobial because it has a broad spectrum that includes many bacteria resistant to other drugs. The high activity of imipenem is attributed to its stability against most of the β-lactamases (including ESBL) and its ability to penetrate porin channels that usually exclude other drugs. The carbapenems are more rapidly bactericidal than the cephalosporins and less likely to induce release of endotoxin in gram-negative sepsis in an animal. Resistance to carbapenems has been extremely rare in veterinary medicine.

Meropenem, one of the newer drugs of the carbapenem class, has antibacterial activity approximately equal to or greater than that of imipenem. Other characteristics are similar to those of imipenem. Its advantage over imipenem is that it is more soluble and can be administered in less fluid volume, can be administered more rapidly, and is not as nephrotoxic.

REFERENCES

1. Giguère S, Prescott JF, Dowling PM: Antimicrobial therapy in veterinary medicine, ed 5, Ames, Ia, 2013, Wiley-Blackwell.
2. Katzung B: Basic and clinical pharmacology, ed 12, New York, 2011, McGraw-Hill.
3. Boothe D: Small animal clinical pharmacology and therapeutics, ed 2, Philadelphia, 2012, Saunders.
4. Knapp CW, Dolfing J, Ehlert PA, et al: Evidence of increasing antimicrobial resistance gene abundances in archived soils since 1940, Environ Sci Technol 44:580-587, 2010.
5. Bush K, Macielag MJ: New β-lactam antimicrobials and β-lactamase inhibitors, Expert Opin Ther Pat 20(10):1277-1293, 2010.
6. Gandolfi-Decristophoris P, Petrini O, Ruggeri-Bernardi N, et al: Extended-spectrum β-lactamase-producing Enterobacteriaceae in healthy companion animals living in nursing homes and in the community, Am J Infect Control 41(9):831-835, 2013.
7. Hordijk J, Schoormans A, Kwakernaak M, et al: High prevalence of fecal carriage of extended spectrum β-lactamase/AmpC-producing Enterobacteriaceae in cats and dogs, Front Microbiol 4:242, 2013.
8. Cohn LA, Middleton JR: A veterinary perspective on methicillin-resistant staphylococci, J Vet Emerg Crit Care (San Antonio) 20(1):31-45, 2010.

CHAPTER 177

AMINOGLYCOSIDES

Reid P. Groman, DVM, DACVIM (Internal Medicine), DACVECC

KEY POINTS

- Despite advances in the development of antimicrobial drugs, aminoglycosides still have a place in the treatment of critically ill patients with infections caused by aerobic gram-negative and select gram-positive microorganisms.
- Aminoglycosides exhibit synergistic bactericidal effects when administered in combination with β-lactam antibiotics.
- Aminoglycosides exhibit concentration-dependent killing; that is, bacterial killing is more rapid and effective when they are present in higher concentrations at the site of infection. This distinguishes the aminoglycosides from β-lactams and other commonly used antimicrobials that kill bacteria in a time-dependent fashion.
- Nephrotoxicity is the most serious adverse effect of aminoglycosides.
- Concentration-dependent bacterial killing, adaptive resistance, and the postantibiotic effect all favor the administration of aminoglycosides as a single daily dose.
- The role of therapeutic drug monitoring with single daily dosing is not well defined in small animal medicine.

Aminoglycoside antimicrobial drugs, notably gentamicin and amikacin, are among the best choices for treatment of severe gram-negative infections. Compared with other antimicrobial agents that allow rapid selection of resistant mutants (e.g., β-lactams and fluoroquinolones), the aminoglycosides are predictably effective against many aerobic gram-negative pathogens.[1-3] One of the primary reasons for limiting clinical use of the aminoglycosides is the nephrotoxicity observed with conventional multiple daily dosing.[1,4] Over the past decade, much has been learned about the efficacy and toxicities of the aminoglycosides, and a new pharmacologic strategy has emerged using single daily dosing (SDD).[3-6] Veterinarians are encouraged to reevaluate the role of aminoglycosides in the modern antimicrobial arsenal.

MECHANISM OF ACTION

The aminoglycosides are bactericidal agents.[1,4,7] They penetrate the bacterial cell wall and membrane, and impair protein synthesis by binding to components of the prokaryotic 30s ribosomal subunit.[5,6,8] This binding leads to bacterial misreading of messenger ribonucleic acid (mRNA), with subsequent production of nonfunctional proteins, detachment of ribosomes from mRNA, and cell death.[5]

SPECTRUM OF ACTIVITY

Aminoglycosides are effective against most community-acquired gram-negative aerobes and select gram-positive pathogens. Organisms commonly susceptible to these drugs include *Klebsiella, Citrobacter, Enterobacter, Serratia,* and most *Acinetobacter* spp.[1,5,6] Some isolates of *Stenotrophomonas maltophilia* exhibit endogenous resistance to the aminoglycosides but retain susceptibility to other antibiotic classes.[9] Aminoglycosides are frequently, although not uniformly, effective against multidrug-resistant *Pseudomonas aeruginosa* and *Escherichia coli.*[1,2] Aminoglycosides are not active against anaerobes because their uptake across bacterial cell membranes depends on energy derived from aerobic metabolism.[1,5,7] Consequently, they have markedly reduced activity in areas of low pH and oxygen tension (e.g., abscesses).[1] The aminoglycosides, particularly gentamicin, are active against many *Staphylococcus* spp.[10] Other gram-positive organisms, such as *Streptococcus* spp and many enterococci, are relatively resistant.

Studies of bacteria in cell culture have shown that combining an aminoglycoside with an antibiotic that interferes with cell wall synthesis (e.g., β-lactam agent) results in bacterial killing that is superior to the simple added activity of each drug antimicrobial. This phenomenon is termed *synergy* or *synergism*, and many antibiotic combinations proven to be synergistic in vitro are associated with a better in vivo response.[1,5] The efficacy of the aminoglycosides is enhanced by increased cell permeability induced by the β-lactam antibiotic, which accelerates the uptake of the aminoglycoside into certain bacteria.[7] Specifically, gentamicin synergy is reported by many commercial laboratories for ampicillin-susceptible isolates of *Enterococcus faecium* and *Enterococcus faecalis.* Although specific "synergy" testing is not routinely performed by microbiology laboratories for gram-negative pathogens, clinicians more commonly take advantage of antimicrobial synergy when managing patients with life-threatening gram-negative infections, including those caused by *P. aeruginosa* and many *Enterobacteriaeace.*[1,7,11] Synergy is particularly important when there is low-level resistance to gentamicin or when low tissue pH and low oxygen tension (e.g., abscesses or tissue hypoxia) decrease aminoglycoside transport into bacteria.[1] The aminoglycosides are active against some mycobacteria as well as less common pathogens such as *Yersinia pestis, Brucella* spp, and *Francisella tularensis.*[1,3]

Amikacin and gentamicin are used in similar circumstances, often interchangeably.[1] Amikacin, however, is not degraded by the common enzymes that degrade gentamicin and often shows broader antimicrobial spectrum than gentamicin.[1] Amikacin is thus the preferred agent when refractory or nosocomial infections caused by resistant strains of *Klebsiella* spp and *P. aeruginosa* are encountered.[7] Arbekacin, a newer semisynthetic aminoglycoside licensed in Asia for the treatment of human patients infected with methicillin-resistant *Staphylococcus* spp, has not been evaluated for use in dogs and cats.[6]

INDICATIONS

The introduction of carbapenems, extended-spectrum β-lactam antibiotics, and fluoroquinolones, all of which have a better safety profile than the aminoglycosides, has necessitated a reappraisal of the indications for aminoglycoside therapy. The aminoglycosides are used for short-term treatment (≤ 7 days) of infections caused by susceptible strains of gram-negative microorganisms that are resistant to less toxic antibiotics.[6-8] Empiric treatment is justified for treating life-threatening infections in patients that have recently been hospitalized or received antibiotics. Aminoglycosides are useful for the treatment of severe infections of the abdomen, urinary tract, pulmonary parenchyma, endocardial valves, bloodstream, and surgical wounds.

Monotherapy with an aminoglycoside is seldom appropriate in critically ill patients. Although aminoglycosides may show in vitro activity against some staphylococci and enterococci, their clinical effectiveness as single agents for treating infections caused by these organisms in animals is not reported. Aminoglycosides are traditionally administered in combination with another antimicrobial agent to enhance bactericidal activity and minimize resistance.[1,5,12] More specifically, in patients with life-threatening infections in which mixed organisms are suspected, aminoglycosides are appropriately administered with a β-lactam, β-lactam/β-lactamase inhibitor, or a carbapenem antibiotic.[5,7] This approach provides not only synergistic bacterial activity but also antibacterial coverage during the aminoglycoside-free interval when SDD is used.[1,12]

Metronidazole or clindamycin may be prescribed in combination with an aminoglycoside when coinfection with strict anaerobic pathogens is suspected.

Aerosolized gentamicin may be administered to patients with susceptible pulmonary infections with limited risk of systemic absorption and toxicity (see Chapter 172).[1,5,11] The effectiveness of inhalational therapy with aminoglycosides has not been studied critically in dogs and cats, although aerosolized gentamicin appears to decrease the clinical signs associated with *Bordetella bronchiseptica* infection in dogs.[13]

PHARMACOLOGY AND DOSING

Aminoglycosides are poorly absorbed following oral administration but may act within the gastrointestinal tract, which largely prevents systemic toxicity. Oral neomycin is prescribed to suppress bacterial growth in the large bowel, and paromomycin is effective for enteric salmonellosis and protozoal enteritis in companion animals.[1,14] Although serum levels of neomycin and paromomycin are generally negligible in healthy animals following oral administration, significant systemic absorption and toxicity are possible when the intestinal epithelial barrier is diseased or compromised.[1,14]

Patients receiving parenteral aminoglycosides should be well hydrated, have stable renal function, and have an inactive urine sediment.[1,4] The aminoglycosides are highly water soluble and do not readily cross biologic membranes.[1,7] For this reason, they are largely confined to the extracellular fluid and have a correspondingly small volume of distribution (Vd).[1,8] The aminoglycosides are mainly eliminated unchanged in the urine. They are excreted predominately by glomerular filtration, with a small fraction (<5%) undergoing tubular reabsorption.[4,7] Penetration into cerebrospinal fluid, prostate, and vitreous humor is minimal, and their effectiveness is not reliable in these tissues.[4,7] Therapeutic concentrations are generally achieved in nonexudative pleural and peritoneal effusions, bones, and synovial fluid. Following parenteral administration, adequate tissue levels are generally achieved in the pulmonary parenchyma but not in bronchial secretions. They are usually ineffective for treatment of intracellular pathogens.

The rate and extent to which an aminoglycoside achieves bacterial killing is a function of its concentration.[1,4,6,8,15] For many years, the aminoglycosides were administered in multiple daily doses. However, many in vitro and in vivo studies suggest that administration in an SDD regimen is as effective as or more effective than conventional regimens and reduces the associated toxicities.[6-8,15] SDD implies that the total daily dose is administered as a single dose approximately every 24 hours, rather than in multiple divided doses. Because aminoglycosides possess concentration-dependent activity, the rate and extent of bacterial killing increase when higher aminoglycoside concentrations are achieved with SDD. In addition, outcomes are more favorable and fewer resistant organisms arise.[1,4,10,13]

Aminoglycosides provide a postantibiotic effect (PAE), which means that bacterial replication is impeded even after serum drug concentrations have fallen below the minimum inhibitory concentration (MIC) of the organism in question (Figure 177-1).[1,3,4,8] This

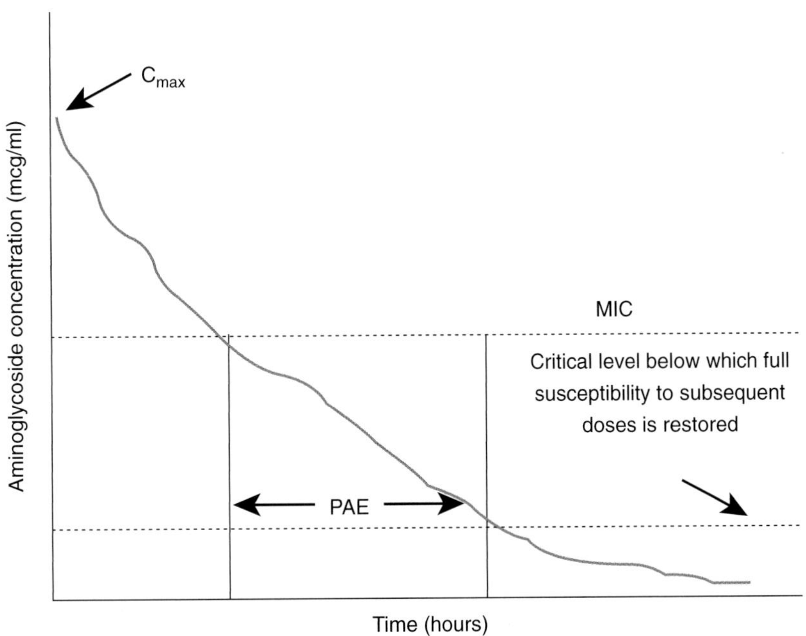

FIGURE 177-1 Graph of hypothetical serum drug concentration versus time following bolus intravenous administration of an aminoglycoside illustrating peak serum concentration (C_{MAX}), minimum inhibitory concentration (MIC), postantibiotic effect, and adaptive resistance. See the section of this chapter on pharmacology and dosing for details.

permits longer dosing intervals. The PAE tends to be longer in vivo than in vitro. Aminoglycosides have a PAE that is linked to (1) the species of bacteria, (2) the MIC of the bacterial strain, and (3) the concentration of drug achieved at the site of infection.[4,8] The PAE of the aminoglycosides permits extended drug-free intervals, without compromising patient outcome; it may be enhanced by the use of higher doses and concurrent administration of a cell wall–active antibiotic such as a β-lactam.[6] Aminoglycosides are associated with a first-exposure effect called *adaptive resistance,* which is most relevant for gram-negative organisms, including *P. aeruginosa.*[1,7] This phenomenon is manifested after the first dose by downregulation of aminoglycoside uptake by bacteria following subsequent doses (see Figure 177-1).[6] When this occurs, there is less bacterial killing with later doses as well as shorter PAEs. Adaptive resistance is most likely to occur with first doses that provide low peak serum concentrations (C_{MAX}). Once the first exposure occurs, the downregulation can last for hours. SDD provides the high serum concentrations necessary to prevent induction of a first-exposure effect, extends the interval between doses to overcome the onset of adaptive resistance, and decreases the incidence of nephrotoxicity.[6,8,12]

The therapeutic effectiveness of the aminoglycosides is correlated with the C_{MAX}, and adverse effects correlate with trough concentrations.[1,3,15] Concentration-dependent bactericidal activity is optimized by attaining a C_{MAX} that exceeds the MIC by a factor of 8 to 10.[6,8,15] The C_{MAX}/MIC ratio is sometimes referred to as the *inhibitory quotient.* The goal of SDD is to obtain a high C_{MAX} while maintaining a drug-free interval of at least 2 to 4 hours (see Figure 177-1). Because of interpatient variability in Vd and renal function, therapeutic drug monitoring (TDM) has been the standard of care in patients treated with traditional multiple daily dosing regimens to ensure adequacy of peak concentrations and prevent toxicity.[1,5,8,15] Rapid turnaround time for test results is crucial if changes are to be made in the regimen before the next scheduled dose. Very few veterinary centers have the benefit of same-day results for drug levels, which effectively precludes the use of TDM in most critically ill companion animals. TDM is not uniformly recommended with SDD unless treatment for longer than 5 to 7 days is anticipated or patients are at high risk of toxicity (e.g., those receiving other nephrotoxic drugs or those with known or suspected preexisting renal impairment).[15] TDM recommendations for SDD include obtaining a peak-level blood sample 20 to 30 minutes after intravenous infusion of the drug and at least two additional samples during the elimination phase of the drug (at 2 and 4 hours after infusion), when feasible.[8] From this information, the drug's Vd, clearance, and half-life may be calculated to determine the most appropriate dosing regimen for a given patient. This monitoring regimen is often impractical, and values can vary significantly on a day-to-day basis in critically ill patients.[3,4,8,12] An acceptable simplified strategy is to obtain a peak-level serum sample 20 to 30 minutes after intravenous administration and a trough-level sample 2 to 4 hours before the next dose to ensure adequate renal clearance that provides a sufficient drug-free period. Trough serum drug concentrations correlate with nephrotoxicity and should be below the limit of detection for most commercial assays. A trough of 1 mcg/ml or more for gentamicin or 2.5 mcg/ml or more for amikacin is indicative (and not a cause) of renal dysfunction and should prompt the clinician to discontinue the aminoglycoside and pursue treatment with a drug of another class.[3,4] In rare instances in which aminoglycoside therapy is the only option, modification of the dosing interval may be considered, but only with frequent monitoring of renal function and intravenous fluid therapy to maintain normal renal blood flow.

A high inhibitory quotient must be achieved with aminoglycoside therapy to reliably kill the offending organism. Pharmacokinetic studies of gentamicin administered using SDD have been completed in healthy dogs and have revealed peak serum levels sufficient for the elimination of most pathogens.[15] However, the initial dose of gentamicin or amikacin necessary to provide adequate peak concentrations in critically ill dogs and cats using SDD has not been evaluated. Measurement of C_{MAX} is useful only if the result is compared with the MIC of the pathogen in question. For example, if an organism has an MIC of 2 mcg/ml, a C_{MAX} of 20 mcg/ml is expected to provide an appropriate inhibitory quotient of 10. This is almost invariably achieved using SDD, but exceptions occur, particularly in critically ill patients, in which a drug's Vd is unpredictable.

Vascular leak syndromes, edematous states, and hypoalbuminemia often are associated with critical illness and an increase in Vd.[1,6,12] Other causes of alterations in Vd include hyperdynamic states in patients with a systemic inflammatory response syndrome (e.g., sepsis, pancreatitis), mechanical ventilation, extensive burn injuries, and severe trauma.[3,6] Aggressive intravenous fluid therapy and parenteral nutrition further contribute to expansion of extracellular water and essentially dilute aminoglycosides in the extracellular compartment of many critically ill patients.[3,6] More specifically, an enlarged Vd associated with any of the aforementioned conditions may result in subtherapeutic aminoglycoside serum levels in patients with systemic inflammatory response syndrome or sepsis (see Chapters 6 and 91).[3,6,12]

TDM may be used to guide proper drug dosing in such cases (Table 177-1). Evaluation of a random sample obtained 8 to 12 hours following administration may be helpful to prevent a prolonged drug-free period. Anticipated trough levels should not be reached by this time in patients with normal renal function.[3,7] However, if serum levels exceed 8 mcg/ml for amikacin or 3 mcg/ml for gentamicin, impaired renal clearance should be suspected and should prompt modification of the dosing regimen or discontinuation of the aminoglycoside.[3] For all patients receiving aminoglycosides, most human hospitals employ specific nomograms based on an individual's serum drug level(s), creatinine clearance, lean body weight, body surface area, gender, and other variables.[4,5,8] Similar formulas have not been developed for companion animals; moreover, the nomograms are not suitable for septic patients.

Although SDD may obviate the need for TDM in many human patients, this has yet to be confirmed by clinical studies in dogs and cats.[4,5,8] Veterinarians are encouraged to incorporate TDM into their practice, even on an intermittent basis, because goal-oriented dosing

Table 177-1 **Aminoglycoside Monitoring Guidelines***

Drug	Dose	Interval	Peak Concentration	Trough Concentration‡
Amikacin	10-15 mg/kg	q24h	30-40 mcg/ml†	≤2.5 mcg/ml or undetectable‡
Gentamicin	6-10 mg/kg	q24h	15-20 mcg/ml†	≤1 mcg/ml or undetectable‡

*Extrapolated from Clinical and Laboratory Standards Institute guidelines, assuming a susceptibility breakpoint concentration of ≤8 mcg/ml for amikacin and ≤2 mcg/ml for gentamicin.
†Obtain sample 30 min after intravenous injection or 60 min after intramuscular injection.
‡Obtain sample 2 to 4 hr before next dose is to be administered.

of aminoglycosides is expected to result in enhanced antibiotic effectiveness and reduced incidence of toxicity.

Gentamicin and amikacin are the most frequently used parenteral aminoglycosides in veterinary medicine. Netilmicin, streptomycin, and tobramycin have been evaluated in companion animals but are seldom used. Gentamicin and amikacin are commonly administered intravenously over 20 minutes, although bolus administration has been described and is well tolerated.[3] The recommended starting dosage for gentamicin is 6 to 10 mg/kg q24h. Amikacin is administered initially at 10 to 15 mg/kg q24h. These dosages are appropriate for intravenous, subcutaneous, and intramuscular routes. The lower end of the published dose is generally recommended for cats. The dosage for obese animals should be based on lean body weight.[1]

The intravenous route is the preferred method of aminoglycoside drug administration in critically ill patients. Patients should be simultaneously receiving sodium-replete intravenous fluids, particularly if there is any question regarding hydration or intravascular volume status. Amikacin and gentamicin are well absorbed following intramuscular and subcutaneous administration in well-hydrated and well-perfused animals.[1] However, these routes of administration are associated with discomfort at the injection site, and absorption is less predictable compared with the intravenous route.[1,15]

Aerosolized antimicrobial therapy for lower respiratory tract infections in animals remains largely unproven (see Chapter 172). This mode of delivery is particularly intriguing for the aminoglycosides because of their limited penetration into respiratory secretions when administered systemically. Limited data support the use of aerosolized gentamicin for inhalation as adjunctive therapy in canine patients infected by *B. bronchiseptica*.[1,13] Injectable gentamicin (6 to 7 mg/kg) diluted 1:2 with sterile saline is placed in the chamber of a jet nebulizer, with each treatment lasting approximately 10 minutes q8-12h.[1,13] Injectable gentamicin is not viscous and can be nebulized using handheld ultrasonic nebulizers as well, although no studies in dogs with naturally occurring respiratory infections are reported using this technology. Systemic absorption is generally negligible. Use of aerosolized aminoglycosides may be reserved for select patients with pulmonary infections that are highly resistant or unresponsive to aggressive conventional therapies, recognizing that it is not known how well or to what extent nebulized agents are distributed to affected pulmonary tissues. Additionally, topical delivery is never adequate alone, and systemic antimicrobials must be administered simultaneously. It remains to be seen if there is a place for administration of nebulized aminoglycosides to dogs and cats with mild to moderately severe lower respiratory tract infections or to intubated patients with severe or ventilator-associated pneumonia.

ADVERSE EFFECTS

Toxic effects of the aminoglycosides generally involve the neuromuscular junction, inner ear apparatus, and, most significantly, renal proximal convoluted tubules.[1,6,7,8]

Reversible neuromuscular paralysis is uncommon and thought to result from interference with the release and uptake of acetylcholine at the neuromuscular junction.[1,4] The aminoglycosides may also inhibit calcium movement into the nerve terminal during depolarization; calcium is required for subsequent release of acetylcholine. Weakness may be produced at dosages just slightly higher than those recommended but is likely to be of clinical consequence only in patients with neuromuscular disorders such as myasthenia gravis or those receiving neuromuscular blocking agents.[1,4-6] Injectable calcium reverses the neuromuscular paralysis produced by aminoglycosides. A cholinesterase inhibitor such as neostigmine also has an antidotal effect.[5]

Aminoglycosides can cause both cochlear and vestibular toxicity by accumulating in the affected tissue and destroying sensory hair cells.[6,7,9,16] Numerous animal studies in which aminoglycosides were administered by a variety of routes for prolonged periods or at very high dosages, or both, reveal that both dogs and cats are susceptible to irreversible aminoglycoside-induced ototoxicity. There appear to be no established standards for assessing, measuring, or defining aminoglycoside-related ototoxicity in companion animals.[10] Moreover, there are scant reports in the literature of drug-induced vestibulocochlear damage in dogs or cats receiving recommended therapeutic dosages of amikacin or gentamicin.[14] In the human literature, the incidence of ototoxicity has not been shown to be significantly different with SDD. Rather, the risk of ototoxicity seems to be related to the duration of treatment with aminoglycosides.[8]

Nephrotoxicity as evidenced by nonoliguric renal insufficiency is a well-known consequence of aminoglycoside administration.[4,6,17,18] Aminoglycosides damage the cells of the proximal renal tubules and reach maximal tubular toxicity around day 9 of therapy.[16] The cationic state of the aminoglycosides facilitates binding to tubular epithelial cells.[4] Intracellular transport results in high concentrations of the aminoglycoside within lysosomes. Lysosomes eventually destabilize and rupture, which disrupts normal cell structure and function. The resulting decline in glomerular filtration is likely multifactorial in origin and involves both tubular and nontubular mechanisms.[4,17]

Results from animal studies suggest that gentamicin is more nephrotoxic than amikacin. However, it is not clear if any real difference exists between the toxicities of the two drugs in the clinical setting, and both have the potential to cause tubular damage.[4,5,8] The physiologic manifestations of nephrotoxicity are varied and often clinically undetectable until extensive injury has occurred.[4,16] Clinically, nephrotoxicity generally manifests as polyuric renal failure, with varying degrees of renal dysfunction.[4,16-18] Glomerular filtration rate decreases as a relatively late event, usually at least 5 to 7 days after initiating therapy. SDD is associated with a lower incidence of nephrotoxicity than administration of the same amount of medication in multiple doses.[1,8,10] Why this regimen is less nephrotoxic is not completely understood, but the cause is believed to be due to less uptake of the drug by renal cortical tissue. Less frequent administration may limit drug accumulation in the renal cortex because the uptake of aminoglycosides appears to be a saturable process.

An area of interest related to aminoglycoside toxicity is the correlation with circadian variation in glomerular filtration.[6,19] Temporal variations in renal toxicity of the aminoglycosides are reported for animals and humans. In diurnal mammals, glomerular filtration rate is slower at rest (at night).[7] An increased incidence of renal toxicity is observed when the drug is injected during the rest period, and lower toxicity is observed when the aminoglycoside is administered during periods of activity (i.e., during the day).[7,19] Moreover, administering gentamicin during the day appears to be more effective. Further investigations are necessary to understand and confirm this phenomenon in dogs and cats with naturally occurring illness.

Evaluating for elevations in blood urea nitrogen and creatinine concentrations is not appropriate to screen for early renal damage.[4,7,16] By the time azotemia is evident, significant intrinsic renal injury already exists and, by definition, the patient is in renal failure.[8,17] Critically ill patients are invariably receiving intravenous fluids, and thus evaluation of urine concentrating ability is of limited utility in assessing for drug-induced renal damage. Enzymuria, the appearance of brush border–derived enzymes such as *N*-acetyl-β-D-glucosaminidase and γ-glutamyl transpeptidase, is one of the earliest signs of aminoglycoside-induced renal damage, but routine measurement is impractical.[1,4,16]

Examination of the urine sediment for granular or cellular casts on a daily basis is recommended.[1,8,14] Ideally, the sediment is examined within 1 or 2 hours of obtaining a urine sample because casts very often dissolve. Urine should also be evaluated with reagent strips because glucosuria and tubular proteinuria may be seen with aminoglycoside-induced renal injury.[4,15] Although some reports describe an inexorable progression of aminoglycoside-induced renal injury and an associated poor prognosis, it is felt that tubular lesions are often reversible and renal function recovers if tubular injury is detected early and therapy discontinued promptly.[6]

Advanced age, duration of therapy, fever, volume depletion, and dehydration increase the risk of aminoglycoside-induced nephrotoxicity.[4,5,16] Other risk factors include concomitant administration of nephroactive drugs (e.g., cisplatin, nonsteroidal antiinflammatory drugs, diuretics such as furosemide, angiotensin-converting enzyme inhibitors), preexisting renal disease, and potassium and magnesium depletion. Penicillins should not be mixed in the same syringe with an aminoglycoside because this inactivates the aminoglycoside.[1] Aminoglycosides should not be administered intravenously with solutions containing calcium, sodium bicarbonate, or heparin.

REFERENCES

1. Greene CE, Boothe DM: Antimicrobial chemotherapy. In Greene CE, editor: Infectious diseases of the dog and cat, St Louis, 2012, Saunders, pp 291-300.
2. Lin D, Foley SL, Qi Y, et al: Characterization of antimicrobial resistance of *Pseudomonas aeruginosa* isolated from canine infections, J Appl Microbiol 113(1):16-23, 2012.
3. Hansen M, Christrup LL, Jarlov JO, et al: Gentamicin dosing in critically ill patients, Acta Anaesthesiol Scand 45:734-740, 2001.
4. Swan SK: Aminoglycoside nephrotoxicity, Semin Nephrol 17:27-33, 1997.
5. Edson RS, Terrell CL: The aminoglycosides, Mayo Clin Proc 74:519-528, 1999.
6. Pagkalis S, Mantadakis E, Mavros MN, et al: Pharmacological considerations for the proper clinical use of aminoglycosides, Drugs 71:2277-2294, 2011.
7. Gonzalez LS 3rd, Spencer JP: Aminoglycosides: a practical review, Am Fam Physician 58:1811-1820, 1998.
8. Avent ML, Rogers BA, Cheng AC, et al: Current use of aminoglycosides: indications, pharmacokinetics and monitoring for toxicity, Intern Med J 41:441-449, 2011.
9. Kralova-Kovarikova S, Husnik R, Honzak D, et al: *Stenotrophomonas maltophilia* urinary tract infections in three dogs: a case report, Vet Med (Praha) 57:380-383, 2012.
10. Papich MG: Selection of antibiotics for methicillin-resistant *Staphylococcus pseudintermedius:* time to revisit some old drugs? Vet Dermatol 23:352-e64, 2012.
11. Reference deleted in pages.
12. Boyd N, Nailor MD: Combination antibiotic therapy for empiric and definitive treatment of gram-negative infections: insights from the society of infectious diseases pharmacists, Pharmacotherapy 31:1073-1084, 2011.
13. Miller CJM, McKiernan BC, Hauser C: Gentamicin aerosolization for the treatment of infectious tracheobronchitis. In Proceedings of the 21st Annual ACVIM Forum, 2003.
14. Gookin JL, Riviere JE, Gilger BC, et al: Acute renal failure in four cats treated with paromomycin, J Am Vet Med Assoc 215:1821, 1999.
15. Albarellos G, Montoya L, Ambros L, et al: Multiple once-daily dose pharmacokinetics and renal safety of gentamicin in dogs, J Vet Pharmacol Ther 27:21-25, 2004.
16. Taber SS, Mueller BA: Drug-associated renal dysfunction, Crit Care Clin 22:357-374, viii, 2006.
17. Rubin SI, Papich MG: Acute renal failure in dogs; a case of gentamicin nephrotoxicity, Comp Cont Educ Small Animal Pract 9:510, 1987.
18. Brown SA, Barsanti JA, Crowell WA: Gentamicin-associated acute renal failure in the dog, J Am Vet Med Assoc 186:686-690, 1985.
19. Widerhon N, Díaz D, Picco E, et al: Chronopharmacokinetic study of gentamicin in dogs, Chronobiol Int 22:731-739, 2005.

CHAPTER 178
FLUOROQUINOLONES

Meredith L. Daly, VMD, DACVECC • Deborah C. Silverstein, DVM, DACVECC

KEY POINTS

- Fluoroquinolone antibiotics exhibit bactericidal properties through their inhibition of deoxyribonucleic acid gyrase and topoisomerase IV.
- Fluoroquinolones are extremely bioavailable and demonstrate a high degree of efficacy at relatively low tissue concentrations.
- They are useful for treating gram-negative and staphylococcal bacterial infections. They have variable efficacy against *Streptococcus* spp and intracellular pathogens.
- Fluoroquinolones have excellent tissue penetration, particularly in the urinary tract, prostate, lung, bile, and inflammatory cells.
- Bacteria are developing resistance to fluoroquinolones.
- Adverse effects of fluoroquinolone antimicrobials include primarily vomiting, diarrhea, nausea, abdominal pain, and cartilage defects. Blindness has occurred in cats.

The fluoroquinolone antimicrobial drugs were introduced into clinical medicine approximately 25 years ago. These agents were regarded initially as model antimicrobial agents because of their broad spectrum of activity, favorable pharmacokinetics, and low incidence of toxicity. The fluoroquinolone antimicrobials are entirely synthetic; all possess a common structure containing a 4-quinolone nucleus. Although the more rarely used first-generation fluoroquinolones (nalidixic acid, flumequine) possess have a limited spectrum of activity, structural modification of the quinolone nucleus has resulted in an increase in potency and a diversification of spectrum in subsequent generations.

As a class, the fluoroquinolones are well absorbed after oral and parenteral administration, have a large volume of distribution, and have extended elimination half-lives, which allows for longer dosing intervals. Fluoroquinolones are bactericidal antibiotics at relatively low tissue concentrations and have a favorable margin of safety. Adverse effects in veterinary medicine are related most frequently to the gastrointestinal (GI) system; however, these agents have been associated with orthopedic, ophthalmologic, neurologic, renal, hepatic, and cardiac toxicity. This chapter reviews chemical, microbiologic, pharmacokinetic, pharmacodynamic, and clinical aspects of these drugs as well as toxicity associated with fluoroquinolone use.

STRUCTURE AND PHYSICAL PROPERTIES

Fluoroquinolones are weak organic acids. They have amphoteric properties as a result of having an acidic group (carboxylic acid) and a basic group (tertiary amine); they are soluble in both alkaline and acidic solutions. All quinolone derivatives in clinical use have a dual-ring structure with a nitrogen at position 1, a carbonyl group at position 4, and a carboxyl group attached to the carbon at the 3 position of the first ring (Figure 178-1).[1] Earlier fluoroquinolones, such as nalidixic acid, did not achieve systemic antibacterial levels. As a result, these agents had limited clinical utility and were suitable only for treating lower urinary tract disease. Fortunately, several structural modifications to the original dual ring have resulted in increased potency, extended spectrum, and enhanced bioavailability.

For example, the addition of a fluorine at position 6 leads to enhanced drug penetration into the bacterial cell as well as increased efficacy against gram-negative bacteria. Addition of a piperazine at position 7 leads to increased antipseudomonal activity, whereas addition of a pyrrolidine group at the same location improves activity against gram-positive organisms.[1,2] At position 8, addition of a halide, fluorine, or methoxy group may increase the drug's half-life, absorption, and efficacy against anaerobic bacteria (see Figure 178-1).[1,2] A more extensive discussion of the relationships between structure and activity of drugs in the quinolone class is beyond the scope of this chapter.

With the increasing use of fluoroquinolone antimicrobials and the structural modifications that have occurred over time, a four-generation classification system has been devised to account for the differences in pharmacokinetic properties and the expanded antimicrobial spectrum of the newer fluoroquinolones. First-generation drugs (e.g., nalidixic acid) achieve minimal serum levels. Second-generation quinolones (e.g., enrofloxacin, difloxacin, marbofloxacin, and ciprofloxacin) have increased gram-negative and systemic activity. Within this class, important differences exist in the rate and extent of biotransformation, rate of elimination, and method of excretion. For example, approximately 40% of enrofloxacin is metabolized to ciprofloxacin; difloxacin is metabolized extensively and excreted as a glucuronide conjugate in bile, with no detectable urine concentrations; and approximately 40% of marbofloxacin is excreted unchanged by the kidney.[3-5] Third-generation drugs (e.g., pradofloxacin) have expanded activity against gram-positive bacteria, atypical pathogens, and some anaerobes. Fourth-generation fluoroquinolones possess significant activity against gram-positive organisms and anaerobes.

Several fluoroquinolones are currently labeled for veterinary use. Enrofloxacin was the first fluoroquinolone approved for use in dogs and cats, followed by orbifloxacin, difloxacin, and marbofloxacin. Pradofloxacin is a newer, third-generation fluoroquinolone that exhibits enhanced bactericidal activity against pathogens that have reduced susceptibility to earlier fluoroquinolones and is now labeled for use in cats in the United States. Ciprofloxacin, though not currently labeled for veterinary use, is commonly used off label in dogs and cats.

MECHANISM OF ACTION

Fluoroquinolone antibiotics exert their antimicrobial effect by inhibiting two enzymes of the topoisomerase class: DNA gyrase (formerly called *topoisomerase II*), and topoisomerase IV. For bacterial replication to proceed, individual strands of bacterial DNA must be separated. This results in "supercoiling," or excessive positive coiling, of DNA strands in front of the replication fork. DNA gyrase is a tetramer composed of two A and two B subunits, encoded by the genes *gyrA* and *gyrB*, that must function together for supercoiling to

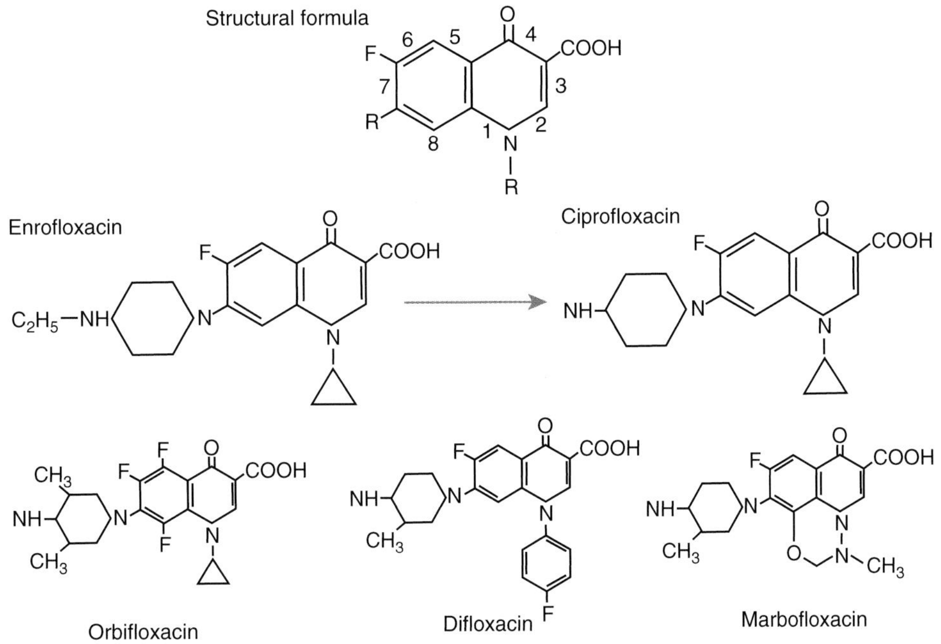

Structural formula

Enrofloxacin

Ciprofloxacin

Orbifloxacin

Difloxacin

Marbofloxacin

FIGURE 178-1 All quinolone derivatives in clinical use have a dual-ring structure with a nitrogen at position 1, a carbonyl group at position 4, and a carboxyl group attached to the carbon at the 3 position of the first ring. The structural modifications to the original dual ring to create many of the available quinolone antibiotics are shown in this figure.

proceed. DNA gyrase is responsible for inducing continuous negative supercoils in the bacterial DNA strand as well as removing positive superhelical twists that accumulate ahead of the DNA replication fork. It accomplishes this via the breakage of both strands of duplex DNA, passage of another segment of DNA through the break, and resealing of the break.[1] Both of these actions serve to relieve the topologic stress of DNA replication.

Quinolones also inhibit the activity of topoisomerase IV. Topoisomerase IV possesses two C and two E subunits, encoded by the genes *parC* and *parE.* Like DNA gyrase, topoisomerase IV is capable of removing positive and negative DNA supercoils, but it is primarily responsible for decatenation, or removing the interlinking of daughter chromosomes, which allows segregation into two daughter cells at the end of a round of replication.[1]

Fluoroquinolones interact with the enzyme-bound DNA complex (i.e., DNA gyrase with bacterial DNA or topoisomerase IV with bacterial DNA) to create conformational changes that result in the inhibition of normal enzyme activity. As a result, the new drug-enzyme-DNA complex blocks progression of the replication fork, thereby inhibiting normal bacterial DNA synthesis and ultimately resulting in rapid bacterial cell death.[2] The comparable mammalian enzyme is not susceptible to the concentrations of quinolones used in clinical practice. Although some degree of overlap may exist, inhibition of topoisomerase IV is responsible for the bactericidal effect of the quinolones on gram-positive bacteria, and DNA gyrase tends to be the primary target for fluoroquinolones in gram-negative organisms.

BACTERIAL SPECTRUM

Although the fluoroquinolone antibiotics all possess the same basic chemical structure, agents within the class exhibit variability in their spectrum and potency (Table 178-1). These antibiotics differ from other antibiotics such as penicillins, tetracyclines, and macrolides in that they exhibit a high degree of efficacy at relatively low serum concentrations. In addition, minimal bactericidal concentrations of quinolones are usually within twofold to fourfold of the minimum inhibitory concentration (MIC) for many of their target organisms.

As a class, the fluoroquinolones are highly effective against aerobic gram-negative bacteria, including most members of the Enterobacteriaceae family *(Escherichia coli, Klebsiella), Pasteurella* spp, *Haemophilus somnus, Bordetella,* and *Campylobacter,* among others.[6] Different fluoroquinolones exhibit variable activity against *Pseudomonas* spp, with ciprofloxacin and levofloxacin being the only quinolones with sufficient potency for use against susceptible strains of *Pseudomonas aeruginosa* in human medicine.[2] Some of the newer fluoroquinolones are active against gram-positive bacteria, including *Staphylococcus aureus, Staphylococcus epidermidis,* and *Neisseria.*[6] Activity against *Streptococcus* spp is limited to a small subset of quinolones, although some newer agents are addressing this deficiency. In general, fluoroquinolones currently available for veterinary use have limited activity against gram-positive and anaerobic organisms. However, pradofloxacin has demonstrated efficacy against *Prevotella* and *Porphyromonas* spp in small animals. Because of their ability to penetrate phagocytic cells, fluoroquinolones have activity against many intracellular pathogens, including *Mycoplasma, Mycobacteria, Chlamydia,* and *Brucella.*[7]

PHARMACOKINETICS AND PHARMACODYNAMICS

As a rule, fluoroquinolones are highly bioavailable after both oral and parenteral administration and exhibit excellent tissue distribution. They are absorbed rapidly after oral administration, with peak serum levels attainable within 0.5 to 2 hours.[4] Quinolone bioavailability may vary between 35% and 100%, depending on the drug and species in question. Table 178-2 summarizes dosing recommendations and peak serum concentrations for commercially available fluoroquinolones labeled for use in small animal patients. Administration of oral antacids containing polyvalent cations (magnesium, aluminum, calcium, iron, and zinc) decreases absorption of quinolone antimicrobial drugs. Food intake does not tend to decrease total serum concentrations of fluoroquinolones, but it may lengthen the time to peak serum concentrations.[1]

Following administration, the quinolones exhibit rapid and extensive tissue distribution. Concentration of quinolone antimicrobials in urine, kidney, lung, prostatic tissue, stool, bile, macrophages,

Table 178-1 Relative Activity of Veterinary Quinolones Against Bacteria Isolated from Animals, as determined by MIC_{90}*

	Concentration (mcg/ml)				
Organism	**Difloxacin**	**Enrofloxacin**	**Marbofloxacin**	**Orbifloxacin**	**Pradofloxacin**
Gram Negative					
Escherichia coli	0.25-16	0.06-20	0.06-20	0.5-4	0.03-02
Klebsiella pneumoniae	0.5	0.12-0.25	0.01-0.06	0.25	0.06-0.25
Proteus spp	1	0.25-0.5	0.125	1	0.25-4
Pasteurella multocida	—	0.016-0.03	<0.008-0.5	ND	0.015
Salmonella spp	0.125	0.03-0.25	0.03	0.25	0.015
Bordetella bronchiseptica	4	0.5	0.5	2	0.25
Pseudomonas aeruginosa	4-8	1-8	0.06-4	4-16	0.5-2
Gram Positive					
Staphylococcus intermedius	1	0.12-0.5	0.25	0.5	0.12
Staphylococcus aureus	1	0.12	0.25-0.5	0.5	
Enterococcus spp	ND	1-2	1-4	16-32	
β-Hemolytic *Streptococcus*	ND	ND	2	1-2	

From Greene CE, Watson ADJ, Greene CE, editors: Infectious diseases of the dog and cat, ed 3, St Louis, 2006, Saunders.
MIC_{90}, Minimum concentration that inhibits the growth of 90% of organisms; *ND,* no data available.
*Lower concentration indicates greater susceptibility. This table should be used as a guide to efficacy. Isolates of the same bacterial species can differ in their antimicrobial resistance depending on differences in time, geography, laboratory methodology, and prior exposure to antimicrobial drugs.

Table 178-2 Peak Serum Concentrations of Quinolones in Dogs and Cats

Drug	Species	Route	Dose (mg/kg)	Peak Serum Concentration (mcg/ml)
Difloxacin	Dogs	PO	5	1.1-1.8
			10	3.6
Enrofloxacin	Dogs	PO	2.75	0.7
			5	1.2-1.41
			5.5	1.4
			7.5	1.9
		SC	20	4.4-5.2
			5	1.3
		IV*	5	1.827
			20	161
Marbofloxaçin	Dogs	PO	1	0.8
			2	1.4-1.47
			2.5	2
			2.75	2
			4	2.9
			5	4.2
			5.5	4.2
Orbifloxacin	Dogs (cats)	PO	2.5	1.37-2.3 (1.6-2.1)
			7.5	6-6.9 (5)
Pradofloxacin	Cats	PO	7.5	1-2.1†
Ibafloxacin	Dogs	PO	7.5	3.72
			15	6.04
			30	12.15
Ciprofloxacin*	Dogs	IV	10	7.8

From Greene CE, editor: Infectious diseases of the dog and cat, ed 3, St Louis, 2006, Saunders.
IV, Intravenously; *PO,* per os; *SC,* subcutaneously.
*Off-label use.
†Based on dose of 5 mg/kg.

and neutrophils often exceeds that in serum.[1,4] For example, quinolone concentrations achieved in bile and urine are often 10 to 20 times greater than those in serum. Because these agents are concentrated in phagocytic cells, they reach higher concentrations at inflammatory sites.[7] Concentrations of quinolones in saliva, prostatic fluid, bone, and cerebrospinal fluid are usually lower than drug concentrations in serum, although they are often adequate for killing susceptible organisms, particularly in the presence of inflammation.[1] Fluoroquinolones are partially metabolized by the liver, and they are excreted in bile or urine unchanged or as metabolites. Most fluoroquinolones are eliminated primarily via the kidney. Depending on the chief mode of excretion, dosage reductions should be considered in animals with renal or hepatic disease.[6]

Fluoroquinolone antibiotics exhibit concentration-dependent bacterial killing; high peak tissue concentrations and persistence of antibiotic concentration above the MIC value for a given organism determines in vivo efficacy. The pharmacodynamic parameters that most closely correlate with the success of these agents include the ratio of the peak serum concentration to the MIC (C_{MAX}/MIC) and the area under the serum concentration curve to the MIC (AUC/MIC). Certain organisms require lower AUC/MIC ratios for prompt eradication by fluoroquinolones. *Streptococcus pneumoniae* and most other gram-positive bacteria are rapidly killed by quinolones at a 24-hour AUC/MIC (AUC/MIC_{24hr}) ratio of 30 to 40 or higher, whereas others, like *P. aeruginosa* and most other aerobic gram-negative bacteria, require much greater exposure over time to quinolones (AUC/MIC_{24hr} ratios of ≥100 to 125).[8,9] Once these target AUC/MIC ratios are achieved, however, there is no evidence to suggest that higher ratios result in more rapid killing or less emergence of bacterial resistance. Pathogen- or species-specific AUC/MIC targets for fluoroquinolones in veterinary patients, although established, are rarely applied to clinical patients.[10,11]

Fluoroquinolones marketed for veterinary use have relatively long half-lives. They are administered once daily to achieve appropriate serum concentrations, which allows higher peak levels and maximal bacterial killing. Fluoroquinolones exhibit a marked postantibiotic effect (PAE) in which they continue to inhibit bacterial growth for up to 8 hours after elimination from the body.[6] A *PAE* is defined as the period of time after serum drug concentration falls below the MIC that bacterial growth continues to be inhibited. Several factors influence the presence and duration of the PAE, including the type of organism, type of antimicrobial, concentration of antimicrobial, duration of antimicrobial exposure, and antimicrobial combinations (synergy). Antimicrobials that induce long PAEs may be administered at longer dosing intervals than indicated by their pharmacokinetic properties such as terminal half-life, which allows fewer daily drug administrations without reducing effectiveness.

The quinolone antibiotics exhibit synergy with other classes of antibiotics; however, their synergistic effects vary in different bacterial infections. Typically they are synergistic with antipseudomonal penicillins, ceftazidime, imipenem, and occasionally rifampin and the aminoglycosides.

RESISTANCE

The effectiveness and consequent widespread use of fluoroquinolones has led to a steady increase in bacterial resistance, particularly among *Staphylococcus, Pseudomonas,* and *E. coli* organisms. There are several known mechanisms of quinolone resistance that work discretely or in combination to confer varying degrees of resistance, ranging from reduced susceptibility to clinically relevant resistance.[12]

Chromosomal point mutations in the genes encoding DNA gyrase and topoisomerase IV are major mechanisms of quinolone resistance. In gram-negative bacteria, the primary target of quinolones is the *gyrA* subunit of DNA gyrase, and in gram-positive organisms the primary target is the *parC* subunit of topoisomerase IV. Resistance tends to occur in a stepwise fashion; the primary target enzyme for an organism is generally the first affected by the mutation, with additional mutations conferring a higher level of resistance. In the genes for both enzymes, point mutations are observed within a site known as the *quinolone resistance–determining region,* which leads to resistance via decreased drug affinity for the altered enzyme-DNA complex.[2,12] Point mutations in the topoisomerase IV subunit genes *parC* and *parE* are also present in gram-negative bacteria, but at a significantly lower frequency than *gyrA* mutations. Likewise, mutations in *gyrA* are seen in gram-positive bacteria with higher levels of fluoroquinolone resistance. Later-generation fluoroquinolone compounds with equal activity against DNA gyrase and topoisomerase IV would require simultaneous mutations in the bacteria at both sites to be rendered ineffective. Double mutants occur rarely; therefore use of these compounds may restrict the development of resistance.

Bacteria are able to increase the expression of energy-dependent efflux systems that prevent the accumulation of effective intracellular concentrations of quinolones via active pumping of drug across the cell membrane.[2,13] The multidrug efflux system AcrA-AcrB-TolC has been shown to be a critical mediator of quinolone efflux in *E. coli* bacteria and may be the primary mechanism of fluoroquinolone resistance in *Salmonella* organisms.[2,11] Gram-negative bacteria can also regulate membrane permeability by altering the levels of outer membrane porins that form the channels responsible for passive diffusion. Loss of, or reduction in, outer membrane porin 1a (OmpF) has been shown to confer antimicrobial resistance by reducing the accumulation of drug within the cytoplasm.[8] It was previously thought that the alterations in efflux systems were capable of producing only low-level resistance to quinolones, becoming clinically relevant only when combined with mutations in target enzymes or membrane alterations.[2,13] However, overexpression of the AcrAB efflux pump, even in the absence of concurrent mechanisms of resistance, has been shown to cause resistance to enrofloxacin and multidrug resistance in *E. coli* bacteria from veterinary patients.[12] This highlights the importance of a continued reappraisal of bacterial resistance mechanisms in small animals and the ways in which resistance may impact therapeutic decisions.

Recently the emergence of plasmid-mediated fluoroquinolone resistance has been reported. Plasmids are extrachromosomal DNA molecules capable of autonomous replication that can confer resistance to the major classes of antimicrobials, including β-lactams, aminoglycosides, tetracyclines, chloramphenicol, sulfonamides, trimethoprim, macrolides, and quinolones.[13] Plasmid-mediated mechanisms typically confer low levels of resistance to fluoroquinolones, but importantly, they favor the selection of bacteria possessing additional chromosome-encoded resistance mechanisms. This could unfortunately select for proliferation of specific, drug-resistant mutant populations and lead to the rapid development of fluoroquinolone and multidrug resistance. A retrospective study evaluating resistance among canine urinary tract isolates from 1992 to 2001 showed a significant increase in resistance in *Proteus* spp, *Staphylococcus intermedius,* and *E. coli* to either enrofloxacin or ciprofloxacin.[14] Similarly, fluoroquinolone use has been correlated with the development of high-level resistance in gram-negative organisms in several human studies.[15,16]

To minimize the development of resistance, fluoroquinolone antibiotics should not be used as first-line agents for infections with organisms that will likely be susceptible to other, less aggressive antimicrobial agents. In addition, adherence to pharmacokinetic and pharmacodynamic parameters of specific antibiotics is important in preventing the selection and spread of resistant strains of bacteria.

CLINICAL USES

Because fluoroquinolone antimicrobial agents exhibit low protein binding, high lipid solubility, and low ionization they have large volumes of distribution with excellent penetration into most tissue beds. They are highly bioavailable and have favorable pharmacokinetic properties allowing for once-daily dosing in most patients. In veterinary medicine, they are used most frequently to treat infections of the urinary tract, respiratory tract, skin, GI tract, and bone. At therapeutic dosages, quinolones are relatively safe, and there are few reported adverse effects.

The bacteria most commonly associated with infections of the urinary tract in the dog include *E. coli, Staphylococcus, Streptococcus, Klebsiella, Proteus,* and *Pseudomonas.* Infections with all of these bacteria have been treated successfully with fluoroquinolone antibiotics. Because fluoroquinolones are concentrated in the urine, several agents within this class are effective for treatment of bacterial cystitis in both the dog and the cat.[14] A recent study evaluated the efficacy of high-dose, short-duration (HDSD) enrofloxacin (18 to 20 mg/kg orally q24h for 3 days) for the treatment of uncomplicated urinary tract infection in dogs and found HDSD enrofloxacin to be noninferior to a 14-day course of amoxicillin-clavulanate, likely as a result of the high urinary concentration achieved by enrofloxacin.[17] Enrofloxacin reaches higher concentrations in prostatic tissue than in serum and is therefore very effective against susceptible organisms causing bacterial prostatitis in the dog.[18]

Fluoroquinolone antibiotics accumulate in lung tissue to levels greater than those found in serum in most domestic animal species. Several fluoroquinolone antibiotics are effective against respiratory pathogens such as *Pasteurella, E. coli,* and *Bordetella* in the dog and cat. In humans, the primary limitation to using fluoroquinolone antibiotics for treatment of community-acquired pneumonia is the limited in vitro susceptibility of *S. pneumoniae* and anaerobic bacteria to ciprofloxacin, ofloxacin, and norfloxacin. However, some of the newer fluoroquinolones, such as gatifloxacin and levofloxacin, have enhanced gram-positive and anaerobic spectra and thus may be more effective for treating pneumonia in humans.[2] Further studies are needed to delineate whether these fluoroquinolones are safe and effective for use in veterinary patients.

Fluoroquinolone antibiotics have been used for the treatment of GI infections, particularly those caused by bacteria resistant to other drugs.[19] The quinolones may also be used in combination therapy in animals with serious systemic gram-negative infections and mixed intraabdominal infections.[6] Fluoroquinolones are used as systemic therapy for treatment of deep pyoderma, other soft tissue infections, and bacterial osteomyelitis.[20,21] Although fluoroquinolones have some efficacy against intracellular pathogens, a study evaluating enrofloxacin for treatment of *Mycoplasma haemofelis* found that a therapeutic effect was achieved only at levels associated with retinal toxicity. Enrofloxacin was not effective in treating *Ehrlichia* infections in experimentally infected dogs.[22,23] However, pradofloxacin, recently approved for use in small cats in the United States (and used in cats and dogs in other countries), possesses activity against *Mycoplasma* species as well as intracellular organisms such as *Rickettsia* spp and *Mycobacteria* spp.[24]

ADMINISTRATION AND DRUG INTERACTIONS

Dosing recommendations for fluoroquinolone antibiotics in dogs and cats can be found in Table 178-2. When given intravenously (*note:* labeled only for intramuscular use in dogs), fluoroquinolone antibiotics should be diluted and administered slowly (i.e., over 30 to 60 minutes). Adverse effects of rapid intravenous administration may include seizures and neurologic sequelae. In addition, intravenous administration of these drugs may cause local tissue reactions or thrombophlebitis. Concurrent administration of antacids decreases GI absorption; oral fluoroquinolones should be given 2 hours before or 6 hours after sucralfate and oral antacids containing polyvalent cations. In addition, some fluoroquinolones inhibit P-450 metabolism and may slow down the metabolism of theophylline and aminophylline, leading to toxicity from elevated levels of methylxanthines. Fluoroquinolone antibiotics may decrease the effectiveness of concurrently administered phenytoin. The use of fluoroquinolones and warfarin concomitantly may result in excessive anticoagulation.[25]

ADVERSE EFFECTS

Fluoroquinolone antibiotics are generally well tolerated. The predominant adverse effects include vomiting, diarrhea, nausea, and abdominal discomfort. These effects are typically mild and dosage related. Discontinuation of the drug or dose reduction often results in relief of clinical signs.

Seizures, tremors, and abnormal electroencephalographic findings have been reported in dogs and cats after administration of fluoroquinolones.[1] Fluoroquinolones directly inhibit γ-aminobutyric acid receptors and stimulate *N*-methyl-d-aspartate receptors in the central nervous system. These effects appear to be exacerbated in the presence of nonsteroidal antiinflammatory medications, theophylline, and other drugs that interfere with the metabolism of fluoroquinolones through the P-450 enzyme system.[26] Occasionally animals may exhibit increases in hepatic transaminase levels or liver function test values.[27] Therefore these antibiotics should be used with caution when administered to animals receiving other hepatotoxic medications or animals with hepatic disease. Renal lesions resulting from precipitation of crystals in the tubular lumens of animals and humans receiving high or supratherapeutic doses of fluoroquinolones have been seen in rare instances.[28]

Fluoroquinolone use has been associated with cartilaginous defects in juvenile animals and humans.[29] The pathogenesis of quinolone-induced cartilage damage is multifactorial. Proposed mechanisms include inhibition of proteoglycan synthesis, chelation of magnesium, and inhibition of mitochondrial dehydrogenase activity. In humans, the damage appears to be reversible with discontinuation of therapy. In one veterinary study, cartilage defects in young dogs were exacerbated by exercise and prevented by exercise restriction.[29] Use of fluoroquinolone antibiotics is contraindicated in young, growing dogs between the ages of 2 and 8 months and up to 18 months in large breed dogs.[6]

Rapid intravenous injection of fluoroquinolones was found to cause dose-related elevations in plasma histamine level in anesthetized dogs. Another study evaluating cardiovascular variables in anesthetized dogs receiving marbofloxacin found that higher than recommended cumulative doses (12 mg/kg, given as a 2 mg/kg bolus followed by a constant rate infusion) resulted in arterial hypotension, decrease in heart rate, and prolongation of the QT interval.[30] A prolonged QT interval and predisposition to torsades des pointes has been reported in human medicine.

Reversible blindness associated with fluoroquinolone use was first reported in human medicine in the early 1990s. Since 1992, several documented cases of blindness have been associated with fluoroquinolone use in cats. Most cats received dosages at the upper limit or above the labeled daily dosage of 5 mg/kg q24h, which suggests that this toxicity is dosage related rather than idiosyncratic.[31] On histopathologic analysis, these cats have evidence of retinal degeneration, with cell death most prominent in the photoreceptor and outer nuclear cell layers. Most cats have irreversible vision loss. This complication is most commonly associated with administration of enrofloxacin but also has been reported with orbifloxacin and marbofloxacin.[23] Reports of fetal toxicity and photosensitization in veterinary medicine are infrequent. Other adverse effects of fluoroquinolone use in humans, such as abnormalities in glycemic control, have not yet been investigated in veterinary medicine.

REFERENCES

1. Spoo JW, Riviere JE: Chloramphenicol, macrolides, lincosamides, fluoroquinolones, and miscellaneous antibiotics. In Adams HR, editor: Veterinary pharmacology and therapeutics, ed 7, Ames, Ia, 1995, Iowa State University Press.
2. Bolon MK: The newer fluoroquinolones, Infect Dis Clin North Am 23:1027, 2009.
3. Boothe DM, Boeckh A, Boothe HW, et al: Tissue concentrations of enrofloxacin and ciprofloxacin in anesthetized dogs following single intravenous administration, Vet Ther 2(2):120, 2001.
4. Frazier DL, Thompson L, Trettien A, et al: Comparison of fluoroquinolone pharmacokinetic parameters after treatment with marbofloxacin, enrofloxacin, and difloxacin in dogs, J Vet Pharmacol Ther 23:293, 2000.
5. Schneider M, Thomas V, Boisrame B, et al: Pharmacokinetics of marbofloxacin after oral and parenteral administration, J Vet Pharmacol Ther 19(1):56, 1996.
6. Greene CE, Watson ADJ: Antibacterial chemotherapy. In Greene CE, editor: Infectious diseases of the dog and cat, ed 3, St Louis, 2006, Saunders.
7. Mandell GM, Coleman E: Uptake, transport, and delivery of antimicrobial agents by human polymorphonuclear neutrophils, Antimicrob Agents Chemother 45(6):1794, 2001.
8. Dudley MN: Pharmacodynamics and pharmacokinetics of antibiotics with special reference to the fluoroquinolones, Am J Med 91:45S, 1991.
9. Zhanel GG, Walters M, Laing N, et al: In vitro pharmacodynamic modeling simulating free serum concentrations of fluoroquinolones against multidrug-resistant *Streptococcus pneumoniae*, J Antimicrob Chemother 47:435, 2001.
10. AliAbadi FS, Lees P: Antibiotic treatment for animals: effect on bacterial population and dosage regimen optimization, Int J Antimicrob Agents 14:307, 2000.
11. Andes D, Craig WA: Animal model pharmacokinetics and pharmacodynamics: a critical review, Int J Antimicrob Agents 19:261, 2002.
12. Shaheen BW, Boothe DM, Oyarzabai OA, et al: Evaluation of the contribution of *gyrA* mutation and efflux pumps to fluoroquinolone and multidrug resistance in pathogenic *Escherichia coli* isolates from dogs and cats, Am J Vet Res 72:25, 2011.
13. Carattoli: Resistance plasmid families in Enterobacteriaceae, Antimicrob Agents Chemother 53:2227, 2009.
14. Cohn LA, Gary AT, Fales WH, et al: Trends in fluoroquinolone resistance of bacteria isolated from canine urinary tracts, J Vet Diagn Invest 15:338, 2003.
15. Ho PL: Increasing resistance of *Streptococcus pneumoniae* to FQ: results of a Hong Kong multicentre study in 2000, J Antimicrob Chemother 48(5):659, 2001.
16. Gagliotti C: Emergence of ciprofloxacin resistance in *E. coli* in isolates from outpatient urine samples, Clin Microbiol Infect 13(3):328, 2007.
17. Westropp JL: Evaluation of the efficacy and safety of high dose short duration enrofloxacin treatment regimen for uncomplicated urinary tract infections in dogs, J Vet Intern Med 26:506, 2012.
18. Dorfman M, Barsanti J, Budsberg SC: Enrofloxacin concentrations in dogs with normal prostate and dogs with chronic bacterial prostatitis, Am J Vet Res 56:386, 1995.
19. Chambers HF: Sulfonamides, trimethoprim, and quinolones. In Katzung BG, editor: Basic and clinical pharmacology, ed 9, New York, 2004, McGraw-Hill.
20. Meunier D, Acar JF, Martel JL, et al: A seven year survey of susceptibility to marbofloxacin of pathogenic strains isolated from pets, Int J Antimicrob Agents 24:592, 2004.
21. Ihrke PJ, Papich MG, Demanuelle TC: The use of fluoroquinolones in veterinary dermatology, Vet Dermatol 10:193, 1999.
22. Dowers KL, Oliver C, Radecki SV, et al: Use of enrofloxacin for treatment of large-form *Haemobartonella felis* in experimentally infected cats, J Am Vet Med Assoc 221:250, 2002.
23. Neer TM, Eddlestone SM, Gaunt SD, et al: Efficacy of enrofloxacin for the treatment of experimentally induced *Ehrlichia canis* infection, J Vet Intern Med 13:501, 1999.
24. Lees P: Pharmacokinetics, pharmacodynamics and therapeutics of pradofloxacin in the dog and cat, J Vet Pharmacol Ther 36:209, 2013.
25. Carroll DN, Carroll DG: Interactions between warfarin and three commonly prescribed fluoroquinolones, Ann Pharmacother 42(5):680, 2008.
26. Petri WA: Sulfonamides, trimethoprim-sulfamethoxazole, quinolones, and agents for urinary tract infections. In Brunton LL, Lazo JS, Parker KL, editors: Goodman and Gillman's the pharmacologic basis of therapeutics, ed 11, New York, 2006, McGraw-Hill.
27. Pallo-Zimmernan LM, Byron JK, Graves TK: Fluoroquinolones: then and now, Compend Contin Educ Vet 32(7):E1, 2010.
28. Vancutsem PM, Babish JG, Schwark WS: The fluoroquinolone antimicrobials: structure, antimicrobial activity, pharmacokinetics, clinical use in domestic animals and toxicity, Cornell Vet 80:173, 1990.
29. Burkhardt JE, Hill MA, Carlton WW, et al: Histologic and histochemical changes in articular cartilages of immature beagle dogs dosed with difloxacin, a fluoroquinolone, Vet Pathol 27(3):162, 1990.
30. Chanoit GP, Schneider M, Woehrlé F, et al: Effect of marbofloxacin on cardiovascular variables in healthy isoflurane-anesthetized dogs, Am J Vet Res 66:2090, 2005.
31. Wiebe C, Pharm D, Hamilton P: Fluoroquinolone-induced retinal degeneration in cats, J Am Vet Med Assoc 221(11):1568, 2002.

CHAPTER 179
MACROLIDES

Scott P. Shaw, DVM, DACVECC

KEY POINTS

- Macrolides are concentrated in macrophages, which results in high drug levels at the site of infection.
- Macrolides exhibit high levels of efficacy against gram-positive organisms and moderate efficacy against anaerobic organisms.

Macrolides represent a large group of similar compounds that are all products of *Streptomyces* spp. Biochemically they are characterized by a macrocyclic lactone ring attached to one or more sugar moieties. Macrolides with the greatest clinical efficacy generally are derived from erythromycin. It should be noted that azithromycin is not technically a macrolide but rather an azalide. It generally is grouped with the macrolides because it shares most of their properties.

MECHANISM OF ACTION

All macrolides work by reversibly binding the 50s ribosome. This results in suppression of ribonucleic acid–dependent protein synthesis. Macrolides are bacteriostatic at clinical concentrations. They are particularly effective against gram-positive organisms and *Mycoplasma* spp. In addition, they have fair efficacy against anaerobic organisms. Many macrolides are actively concentrated in macrophages. This can result in very high drug concentrations at the site of infection.[1]

PHARMACOLOGY

In general, macrolides are characterized by low serum concentrations and large volumes of distribution. They are concentrated in tissues including the lung, heart, and macrophages. Newer macrolides such as azithromycin have high oral bioavailability (40% to 60%) and long half-lives. The main route of excretion is through bile and the intestinal tract.[2]

RESISTANCE

Resistance to macrolides can develop rather quickly. This can occur through a one-step mutation that confers high levels of resistance. This type of resistance can be unstable, but it can develop during treatment. Most low-level resistance is caused by an efflux pump that actively excretes the drug out of the cell. Widespread resistance typically occurs when a gene coding for the methylation of the drug's target site is transferred via a plasmid.[3]

SELECTED MACROLIDES

Erythromycin

Erythromycin is available for both enteral and parenteral administration. When given orally it is subject to rapid degradation by gastric acid. As a result, tablets and capsules typically are protected by an enteric coating. It is important that tablets not be crushed or divided because this can result in inactivation of the drug before it is absorbed.[2]

Dosage-related gastrointestinal (GI) adverse effects are encountered frequently. These are believed to be secondary to the drug's effects on smooth muscle. The parenteral form can cause tissue irritation at the site of injection.[1]

Erythromycin is the drug of choice for treatment of *Campylobacter jejuni* infections. It can also be used as an alternative to penicillin in penicillin-sensitive animals. In small animals, it is employed most commonly in those with liver failure for its prokinetic effects on GI smooth muscle and its ability to limit overgrowth of ammonia-producing organisms within the GI tract.[2] See Chapter 118 for further discussion of the use of erythromycin as a prokinetic agent.

Azithromycin

Azithromycin has greater activity against gram-negative organisms than the other members of the macrolide family. It is effective against *Bartonella, Borrelia, Campylobacter, Chlamydia, Leptospira,* and *Mycoplasma.* It is more stable in acid and as a result has a high oral bioavailability. Azithromycin appears to be taken up rapidly by tissues, then released slowly. Tissue concentrations are generally 10 to 100 times those achieved in serum, and the drug can be concentrated 200 to 500 times in macrophages. This high level of drug in macrophages may not always be advantageous because it can suppress phagocytic activity. Azithromycin does not exhibit any effect on GI smooth muscle. As a result GI adverse effects are uncommon.[1]

Azithromycin commonly is employed by veterinarians to treat severe respiratory infections. It can be highly effective in resolving chronic, refractory cases of pneumonia, particularly those secondary to *Bordetella* infection. Care should be taken when using azithromycin as the sole agent because of the limitations in its gram-negative spectrum and because resistance is a growing problem. In general, azithromycin should be reserved for use as a second-line or third-line agent.

REFERENCES

1. Katzung B: Basic and clinical pharmacology, ed 6, Norwalk, Conn, 1995, Appleton & Lange.
2. Prescott J, Baggot J, Walker R: Antimicrobial therapy in veterinary medicine, ed 3, Ames, Ia, 2000, Iowa State University Press.
3. Boothe DM: Small animal clinical pharmacology and therapeutics, ed 2, St Louis, 2011, Saunders.

CHAPTER 180
ANTIFUNGAL THERAPY

Marie E. Kerl, DVM, MPH, DACVIM, DACVECC

KEY POINTS

- Antifungal drug therapy for systemic fungal infections requires administration for months to resolve disease.
- Amphotericin antifungal drugs must be administered by systemic injection and cause significant nephrotoxicity.
- Azole-type antifungals are administered orally and cause varying degrees of hepatotoxicity.

INTRODUCTION

Limited classes of drugs are available to treat fungal infections. Antifungal drugs used to treat systemic fungal infections include polyene antibiotics and azole derivatives. Antifungal drugs are costly, require long-term administration, and have relatively high toxicity rates. In immunodeficient animals, definitive cure with any therapy is difficult or impossible. This chapter reviews commonly available drugs and provides dosing information to treat various systemic fungal infections in dogs and cats (see Chapter 95).

CLASSES OF ANTIFUNGAL DRUGS

Polyene Antibiotics

Polyene antibiotics used to treat systemic mycoses include amphotericin B (AMB) and lipid-complexed AMB. AMB is produced by the microorganism *Streptomyces nodosus* and is considered the gold standard for antifungal therapy.[1,2] Parenteral administration is required because gastrointestinal (GI) absorption is poor. Following intravenous administration, AMB is protein bound and then redistributes from the blood to the tissues. Metabolic pathways of AMB are poorly understood. Biphasic elimination occurs, with an initial half-life of 2 to 4 days and a terminal half-life of 15 days.[3] Only a small amount undergoes renal and biliary elimination, and central nervous system (CNS) penetration is poor. AMB binds to ergosterol in fungal cell membranes, increasing membrane permeability to cause cell death. There is also affinity for cholesterol found in mammalian cell membranes, which explains its toxic effects. The main toxicity associated with AMB is nephrotoxicity, which is the dose-limiting event with this drug. The drug binds to cholesterol in the proximal tubular cells causing renal vasoconstriction and renal tubular acidosis.[4] Parenteral administration might make AMB a more desirable treatment than oral drugs in animals with severe GI fungal disease because they may absorb oral drugs poorly.

Dosing protocols for AMB include intermittent administration until a cumulative dosage has been achieved, with interruption of therapy in the event of azotemia. Cats typically receive lower intermittent and cumulative dosages than dogs (Table 180-1). To reduce nephrotoxicity, AMB usually is infused in 5% dextrose and administered intravenously over 1 to 5 hours. Blood urea nitrogen concentration should be measured and urine sediment evaluation performed before each dose. Identification of tubular casts in urine sediment is an earlier indicator of ongoing renal tubular damage than serum biochemical test results, and the treatment regimen should be altered if casts are identified. If blood urea nitrogen level exceeds 50 mg/dl, the drug should be discontinued until azotemia resolves.[5] Administration of 0.9% saline intravenously before giving AMB decreases the incidence of nephrotoxicity in humans.[6] Medications with known nephrotoxicity should not be given concurrently with AMB.

Lipid-complexed AMB drugs are newer preparations and have the advantage of being less nephrotoxic than AMB, even when administered at higher cumulative dosages. Formulations that are approved for use in humans include AMB lipid complex (Abelcet), AMB colloidal dispersion (Amphotec), and liposome-encapsulated AMB (AmBisome).[2] All of these compounds require parenteral administration. Few head-to-head comparisons of these drug preparations have been performed, which makes comparisons of efficacy difficult. AMB lipid complex has been used successfully to treat blastomycosis in dogs.[7] The main disadvantage of these drugs is their significantly greater expense compared with AMB.

Azole Antifungals

The azole antifungal drugs inhibit the fungal P-450 enzyme necessary for development of ergosterol in fungal cell walls.[1,8] Broad classifications of this group of drugs include triazoles (e.g., itraconazole, fluconazole, voriconazole, posaconazole) and imidazoles (e.g., ketoconazole, clotrimazole, enilconazole, miconazole).[4] In general, the triazoles have less effect on mammal sterol synthesis and longer elimination times, and the imidazoles have more endocrine adverse effects and greater effects on mammal sterol synthesis.[4] These drugs are administered orally, with peak plasma concentrations occurring within 6 to 14 days. Ketoconazole and itraconazole are weak bases, lipophilic, and protein bound. Administration with food is typically recommended to improve uptake. Absorption is improved in an acid environment, and uptake may be impaired with concurrent use of antacids or histamine-2 receptor antagonists. Distribution occurs through most tissues except the CNS and urine. Fluconazole is minimally protein bound, highly water soluble, and crosses the blood-brain, blood-eye, and blood-prostate barriers.[2] Drugs that are metabolized by the hepatic P-450 enzyme system (especially histamine-2 receptor antagonists) may delay metabolism of azole antifungals, especially ketoconazole, and thereby lead to higher plasma drug concentrations.[3]

Ketoconazole has been effective as a sole agent for treatment of systemic mycoses, but it is less effective than AMB. In serious systemic fungal infections, combination therapy with AMB and ketoconazole may allow reduced dosage and toxicity while maintaining efficacy. Adverse effects of ketoconazole therapy include GI upset, which may be reduced by administering with meals and dividing the dosage into multiple smaller doses daily. Of the commonly used azole antibiotics, ketoconazole is the most likely to induce mammalian P-450 enzymes to cause elevations in hepatic transaminases and alkaline phosphatase. Clinical hepatitis, which may be fatal, has been recognized.[2,3]

Table 180-1 Drug Dosages to Treat Common Systemic Fungal Infections in Dogs and Cats

Infection	Species	AMB*	Liposomal AMB	Ketoconazole†	Itraconazole	Fluconazole
Blastomycosis	Dog	0.5 mg/kg IV 3×/wk Cumulative dose: 4-6 mg/kg	1 mg/kg IV 3×/wk Cumulative dose: 12 mg/kg	5-15 mg/kg PO q12h for at least 3 mo, with AMB initially	5 mg/kg PO q12h for first 5 days, then q24h for 60-90 days, or 30 days beyond resolution	5 mg/kg PO q12h for at least 60 days, or 30 days beyond resolution
	Cat	0.25 mg/kg IV 3×/wk Cumulative dose: 4 mg/kg	—	10 mg/kg PO q12h for at least 3 mo, with AMB initially	5 mg/kg PO q12h for 60-90 days, or 30 days beyond resolution	—
Histoplasmosis	Dog	0.25-0.5 mg/kg IV 3×/wk Cumulative dose: 5-10 mg/kg	—	10 mg/kg PO q12-24h for at least 3 mo, or 30 days beyond resolution	5 mg/kg PO q12h for 4-6 mo, or 60 days beyond resolution	2.5-5 mg/kg PO q12-24h for 4-6 mo, or 30 days beyond resolution
	Cat	0.25-0.5 mg/kg IV 3×/wk Cumulative dose: 4-8 mg/kg	—	See canine recommendations	See canine recommendations	See canine recommendations
Cryptococcosis	Dog	0.25-0.5 mg/kg IV 3×/wk Cumulative dose: 4-10 mg/kg	1 mg/kg IV 3×/wk Cumulative dose: 8-12 mg/kg	10 mg/kg q12-24h, for 4-6 mo	—	5-15 mg/kg PO q12-24h for 6-10 mo, or 30 days beyond resolution
	Cat	0.1-0.5 mg/kg IV or 0.5-0.8 mg/kg SC 3×/wk Cumulative dose: 4-10 mg/kg	—	See canine recommendations	5-10 mg/kg PO q12h, or 20 mg/kg q24h for 6-10 mo, or 30 days beyond resolution	25-50 mg per cat PO q12-24h for 6-18 mo, or until antigen test result is negative
Coccidioidomycosis	Dog	0.4-0.5 mg/kg IV 3×/wk Cumulative dose: 8-11 mg/kg	—	5-10 mg/kg PO q12h for 8-12 mo	5 mg/kg PO q12h up to 12 mo	5 mg/kg PO q12h up to 12 mo
	Cat	—	—	50 mg per cat PO q12-24h up to 12 mo	25-50 mg per cat PO q12-24h up to 12 mo	25-50 mg per cat PO q12-24h up to 12 mo

AMB, Amphotericin B; *IV,* intravenously; *PO,* per os; *SC,* subcutaneously.
*Monitor for nephrotoxicity.
†Administer with food.
Data from Foy DS, Trepanier LA: Antifungal treatment of small animal veterinary patients, Vet Clin North Am Small Anim Pract 40:1171, 2010; Sykes JE, Malik R: Cryptococcosis. In Greene CE, editor: Infectious diseases of the dog and cat, ed 4, St Louis, 2012, Saunders; and Kerl ME: Update on canine and feline fungal diseases, Vet Clin North Am Small Anim Pract 33:721, 2003.

Itraconazole has been effective as a sole agent in blastomycosis, histoplasmosis, coccidioidomycosis, and cryptococcosis. Absorption is most consistent when it is administered with a meal. Itraconazole more selectively inhibits fungal P-450 enzymes than mammalian P-450 enzymes, which limits hepatotoxicity. Mild hepatic transaminase elevation can still occur.[1,9,10]

Cutaneous reactions consisting of localized ulcerative dermatitis and vasculitis occur in a small percentage of dogs receiving itraconazole; dermal lesions resolve following discontinuation of therapy. Itraconazole is available from many veterinary formulating pharmacies at a reduced cost compared with the brand name pharmaceutical preparation (Sporanox); however, efficacy of generic preparations has not been proven. The commercially available liquid form may be better absorbed orally, especially in cats.[9]

Fluconazole is now used instead of ketoconazole for many indications since it is more potent and more soluble, and there is less risk of negative metabolic consequences.[1,4] Increased solubility allows for greater passage through the blood-brain barrier and more consistent oral absorption on an empty stomach. Feeding or compounding into different formulations does not seem to affect absorption.[4] It is indicated for CNS involvement in systemic mycoses and for anorexic animals. Fluconazole has been used successfully to treat cryptococcosis in cats.[11] Fluconazole is metabolized minimally and is excreted mostly in an intact form in the urine. The dosage of fluconazole should be reduced in animals with decreased glomerular filtration rates. Since fluconazole is off patent, it has become a more affordable treatment option for veterinary use.

Voriconazole is a synthetic derivative of fluconazole that has been approved by the U.S. Food and Drug Administration (FDA) and is available to veterinarians. It is licensed for use in humans to treat invasive aspergillosis and oropharyngeal candidiasis in immunocompromised patients. There are minimal data available on clinical therapeutic use of this antifungal agent in dogs and cats. Voriconazole has been associated with adverse neurologic effects in a small case series of cats.[12]

Posaconazole is one of the newer antifungal agents that has been FDA approved for use in people. This drug is similar to itraconazole in structure; however, the major difference is that posaconazole has efficacy against Zygomycetes. No dose ranges have been established for animals.[4]

RECOMMENDATIONS FOR SPECIFIC FUNGAL INFECTIONS

Blastomycosis

Azole antifungals are the treatment of choice for blastomycosis because of efficacy, safety, and convenience of administration.[13] In a study of 112 dogs comparing itraconazole treatment with AMB therapy in historical controls, response and recurrence rates were similar in all groups.[14] A retrospective case series comparing itraconazole treatment with fluconazole therapy in dogs with blastomycosis found that treatment responses and relapse rates were not significantly different in the two groups and that cost of treatment was less for dogs treated with fluconazole than for those given itraconazole.[15] Other treatment options include ketoconazole, AMB, and lipid-complexed AMB. AMB has been used successfully for treatment of blastomycosis. Drawbacks of AMB include the need for parenteral administration and the risk of nephrotoxicity. Lipid-complexed AMB is effective for blastomycosis in dogs, with less risk of nephrotoxicity than conventional AMB.[7] Combinations of AMB and itraconazole or ketoconazole may be used in cases of severe respiratory infection. Refer to Table 180-1 for dosage recommendations.

Histoplasmosis

Azole antifungals are the drugs of choice to treat histoplasmosis. Itraconazole is the most widely studied drug in canine and feline histoplasmosis; however, GI drug absorption of itraconazole can be variable in healthy cats.[9,16] GI drug absorption has not been predicted accurately in animals with GI or disseminated histoplasmosis. Recently, a retrospective case series identified similar recovery and recrudescence rates in cats treated with fluconazole compared with those given itraconazole.[17] Fluconazole has not been studied specifically in dogs. Absorption characteristics of fluconazole make it a more attractive option in animals with CNS involvement or in cases refractory to AMB and itraconazole. In cases of severe GI or disseminated disease, parenteral AMB combined with itraconazole, or high-dose itraconazole, has been recommended for more rapid control of fungal disease.[9]

Treatment should be continued for at least 60 days, or until 1 month following resolution of clinical signs. Complete resolution of GI or disseminated histoplasmosis is challenging to determine, and serologic antibody testing cannot help to identify response to therapy. Animals that experience relapse after discontinuation of therapy should resume antifungal drug treatment. Refer to Table 180-1 for dosage recommendations.

Coccidioidomycosis

Coccidioidomycosis is difficult to cure compared with other fungal infections, with some cases requiring lifelong therapy. Commonly recommended treatments for dogs and cats include azole antibiotics and AMB; however, controlled therapeutic trials are lacking. Respiratory infection can be cleared spontaneously by the host immune response; therefore debate exists over the criteria that must be met to initiate prolonged therapy with expensive and potentially toxic medication.[5] Early initiation of therapy in primary respiratory coccidioidomycosis may be appropriate because dissemination is possible. Generally, treatment should continue for 3 to 6 months beyond resolution of clinical signs.[5]

No specific azole antifungal has been documented as the best therapy for coccidiomycosis in dogs and cats. Ketoconazole, itraconazole, and fluconazole have been reported as treatments for coccidioidomycosis. Given that generic formulations of itraconazole and fluconazole have made these more affordable treatment options with fewer adverse effects, they are typically chosen for first-line therapy.[5] Serologic testing should be repeated within 4 to 6 weeks of initiation of therapy; however, the decision to terminate treatment should not be based on serologic results alone. If the titer is increasing or clinical signs are deteriorating, alternative therapy should be chosen. Prolonged treatment (8 to 12 months) may be needed.[5] AMB is indicated in animals that experience significant adverse effects with azole drugs. Liposome-encapsulated AMB formulations may have fewer adverse effects while retaining efficacy but have not been studied for treatment of this disease.[5] Relapse is common after discontinuation of therapy, particularly in cats.[18] Recommended duration of therapy is generally months. Refer to Table 180-1 for dosage recommendations.

Cryptococcosis

A variety of protocols and regimens have been developed for cryptococcosis in dogs and cats; choice of therapy depends on available drugs, location of infection, and adverse effects. Fluconazole has become the drug of choice for cryptococcosis in cats because of its combination of efficacy and safety compared with other treatment regimens. This drug has better penetration of the CNS, eye, and urinary tract than other azoles.[19] Fluconazole resistance has been reported with some strains of *Cryptococcus gattii* in North America.[19] Itraconazole is a reasonable treatment choice for infections that are not in the eye, CNS, or urinary system. Ketoconazole has been shown to cure infection; however, adverse effects occur more frequently with ketoconazole than with itraconazole.[19]

Subcutaneous or intravenous AMB has been used in combination with other antifungals in serious CNS or disseminated feline and canine cryptococcosis.[2,10] Azole antifungal agents typically are administered for 8 to 10 months, but longer therapy can be required in certain individuals. Recommendations to discontinue therapy 1 month after resolution of clinical signs and a decrease in antigen titer by two orders of magnitude or until results are negative have been proposed for cats.[10] Refer to Table 180-1 for dosage recommendations.

REFERENCES

1. Foy DS, Trepanier LA: Antifungal treatment of small animal veterinary patients, Vet Clin North Am Small Anim Pract 40:1171, 2010.
2. Greene CE: Antifungal chemotherapy. In Greene CE, editor: Infectious diseases of the dog and cat, ed 4, St Louis, 2012, Saunders.
3. Boothe D: Treatment of fungal infections. In Small animal clinical pharmacology and therapeutics, ed 1, Philadelphia, 2001, Saunders.
4. Davis JL, Papich MG, Heit MC: Antifungal and antiviral drugs. In Riviere JE, Papich MG, editors: Veterinary pharmacology and therapeutics, ed 9, Ames, Ia, 2009, Wiley-Blackwell.
5. Greene RT: Coccidiomycosis and paracoccidioidomycosis. In Greene CE, editor: Infectious diseases of the dog and cat, ed 4, St Louis, 2012, Saunders.
6. Branch RA: Prevention of amphotericin B-induced renal impairment. A review on the use of sodium supplementation, Arch Intern Med 148:2389, 1988.
7. Krawiec DR, McKiernan BC, Twardock AR, et al: Use of an amphotericin B lipid complex for treatment of blastomycosis in dogs, J Am Vet Med Assoc 209:2073, 1996.
8. Lu I, Dodds E, Perfect J: New antifungal agents, Semin Resp Infect 17:140, 2002.
9. Brömel C, Greene CE: Histoplasmosis. In Greene CE, editor: Infectious diseases of the dog and cat, ed 4, St Louis, 2012, Saunders.
10. Hodges RD, Legendre AM, Adams LG, et al: Itraconazole for the treatment of histoplasmosis in cats, J Vet Intern Med 8:409, 1994.
11. Malik R, Wigney DI, Muir DB, et al: Cryptococcosis in cats clinical and mycological assessment of 29 cases and evaluation of treatment using orally administered fluconazole, J Med Vet Mycol 30:133, 1992.

12. Quimby JM, Hoffman SB, Duke J, et al: Adverse neurologic events associated with voriconazole use in 3 cats, J Vet Intern Med 24:647, 2010.
13. Legendre AM: Blastomycosis. In Greene CE, editor: Infectious diseases of the dog and cat, ed 4, St Louis, 2012, Saunders.
14. Legendre AM, Rohrbach BW, Toal RL, et al: Treatment of blastomycosis with itraconazole in 112 dogs, J Vet Intern Med 10:365, 1996.
15. Mazepa AS, Trepanier LA, Foy DS: Retrospective comparison of the efficacy of fluconazole or itraconazole for the treatment of systemic blastomycosis in dogs, J Vet Intern Med 25:440, 2011.
16. Boothe D, Herring I, Calvin J, et al: Itraconazole disposition after single oral and intravenous and multiple oral dosing in healthy cats, Am J Vet Res 58:872, 1997.
17. Reinhart JM, KuKanich KS, Jackson T, et al: Feline histoplasmosis: fluconazole therapy and identification of potential sources of *Histoplasma* species exposure, J Feline Med Surg 14:841, 2012.
18. Greene RT, Troy GC: Coccidioidomycosis in 48 cats: a retrospective study (1984-1993), J Vet Intern Med 9:86, 1995.
19. Sykes JE, Malik R: Cryptococcosis. In Greene CE, editor: Infectious diseases of the dog and cat, ed 4, St Louis, 2012, Saunders.

CHAPTER 181
MISCELLANEOUS ANTIBIOTICS

Reid P. Groman, DVM, DACVIM (Internal Medicine), DACVECC

KEY POINTS

- With the emergence of resistant microorganisms and competition from newer antimicrobial agents, it is especially important to revisit and pursue rational approaches to the use of older antimicrobials in small animals.
- Metronidazole, chloramphenicol (CHPC), tetracyclines, potentiated sulfonamides, rifampin, vancomycin, polymyxins, clindamycin, and more recently developed antimicrobials may prove useful in the treatment of various infections in small animal veterinary medicine.
- Metronidazole is predictably effective against obligate anaerobes. Self-limiting neurotoxicity is associated with high dosages or long-term use.
- CHPC is a time-honored broad-spectrum antibiotic with additional activity against spirochetes, rickettsiae, chlamydiae, and *Mycoplasma* spp. Rare complications from human exposure to this drug have limited its use in animals.
- Doxycycline is more lipophilic and has better tissue penetration than tetracycline. It remains the drug of choice for Lyme disease and many rickettsial infections.
- Potentiated sulfonamides are useful agents for a variety of bacterial and protozoal infections, although concerns about adverse events often limit their use.
- Rifampin is the most active antibiotic against staphylococci. Resistance readily develops with monotherapy.
- Vancomycin is presently the last line of defense against multidrug-resistant gram-positive cocci in dogs and cats.
- Polymyxin E (colistin) may prove useful in the treatment of multidrug-resistant gram-negative infections in companion animals.
- Clindamycin is active against most anaerobic pathogens and is the drug of choice for treating toxoplasmosis in dogs and cats.
- Proper use of all antimicrobials, including novel agents such as the streptogramins, oxazolidinones, tigecycline, and the cyclic lipopeptides, is increasingly important to curtail the evolution of antimicrobial resistance.

One of the greatest accomplishments of modern medicine has been the development of antimicrobials for the treatment of potentially fatal infections. However, this has inevitably been followed by the acquisition of resistance toward their antibacterial activity.[1,2] Unfortunately, the past two decades have seen a marked decline in the discovery and development of novel antimicrobials and a remarkable increase in resistance to those in use. In particular, there is substantial worldwide concern with the mounting prevalence of infections caused by multidrug-resistant (MDR) gram-positive and gram-negative bacteria. Veterinary clinicians and microbiologists have been forced to reappraise the value of both relatively older antimicrobials and some more novel agents for the treatment of serious bacterial infections. A concise list of drug doses for the antimicrobial agents discussed in this chapter can be found in Table 181-1.

METRONIDAZOLE

Metronidazole has clinical activity against anaerobic gram-negative bacilli (e.g., *Bacteroides* spp), anaerobic gram-positive bacilli (e.g.,

Table 181-1 Miscellaneous Antimicrobials and Recommended Doses in Small Animals

Drug	Recommended Dose
Chloramphenicol	Dogs: 25-50 mg/kg q8h PO/IV/SC/IM Cats: 12.5-20 mg/kg q12h PO/IV/SC/IM
Metronidazole	Dogs & cats: 10-15 mg/kg q12h PO/IV
Rifampin	Dogs & cats: 5-10 mg/kg q12-24h PO/IV
Minocycline	Dogs & cats: 5-10 mg/kg q12h PO
Clindamycin	Dogs & cats: 10 mg/kg q12h IV/PO
Doxycycline	Dogs & cats: 5-10 mg/kg q12h IV/PO
Trimethoprim/sulfonamide	Dogs & cats: 15-25 mg/kg q12h PO/IV/SC
Vancomycin	Dogs: 15 mg/kg q8h IV

Clostridium spp) anaerobic gram-positive cocci (e.g., *Peptostreptococcus* spp), and some protozoa (e.g., *Giardia*). It does not possess any clinically relevant activity against facultative anaerobes or obligate aerobes. In polymicrobic, or mixed aerobic and anaerobic infections, an antibiotic with activity against aerobic gram-negative enteric pathogens should be used in addition to metronidazole. Although metronidazole's mechanism of action is not entirely clear, the parent drug's nitro group is reduced by electron transport proteins (e.g., nitroreductases) in anaerobic bacteria. The reduction products appear to be responsible for the antimicrobial effects of metronidazole, which include disruption of DNA and inhibition of nucleic acid synthesis. Mammalian cells are unharmed because they lack enzymes to reduce the nitro group of these agents.

Metronidazole diffuses well into tissues and body fluids, including cerebrospinal fluid, bile, and abscesses. Effective tissue penetration and consistent bactericidal activity make metronidazole useful for severe anaerobic infections, including intraabdominal sepsis, pancreatic or hepatic abscesses, and osteomyelitis. The beneficial effects of metronidazole are often attributed to its antiinflammatory properties, in addition to its antibacterial activity. Notably, the immunomodulatory effects of metronidazole may be partly responsible for amelioration of clinical signs in companion animals with inflammatory enteropathies and gingivostomatitis. Until relatively recently, metronidazole for intravenous infusion had to be carefully reconstituted. The pH of the reconstituted solution is very low, thus requiring the addition of sodium bicarbonate to raise the pH before infusion. Currently, ready-to-use (RTU) formulations are widely used in dogs and cats.

Seizures, cerebellar dysfunction, and other neuropathies have been reported with high dosages or long-term use of metronidazole. Although these untoward effects are generally self-limiting, complete recovery may take days to weeks. In general, the dosage should not exceed 20 to 30 mg/kg q24h for dogs and cats, generally divided into twice-a-day dosing. Metronidazole should be used with particular caution in patients with underlying neurologic disorders. Intravenous diazepam administration may lessen the duration and severity of neurologic signs in affected dogs. Patients with severe hepatic disease metabolize metronidazole slowly; therefore 15 to 20 mg/kg q24h is administered in such circumstances.

CHLORAMPHENICOL

Chloramphenicol (CHPC) was the first truly broad-spectrum antibiotic discovered. After initial widespread use, the agent was largely abandoned in developed countries because of concerns over toxicity and the availability of new antimicrobial drugs that appeared safer and similar in spectrum.[2] The rise in antimicrobial resistance to many agents in the 1990s has prompted a reevaluation of CHPC use in human and veterinary medicine.[1-3]

CHPC inhibits protein synthesis in bacteria. It acts primarily on the 50s ribosomal subunit and suppresses the activity of peptidyl transferase, an enzyme that catalyzes peptide bond formation.[1] Depending on the pathogen, the effect of CHPC may be bactericidal or bacteriostatic.[4] CHPC is active against gram-positive and gram-negative aerobic and anaerobic bacteria, as well as spirochetes, rickettsiae, chlamydiae, *Bordetella,* and *Mycoplasma* spp.[1,4] It is often effective for treating *Salmonella* and *Escherichia* infections in the gastrointestinal (GI) tract. Its spectrum of activity generally does not include *Pseudomonas aeruginosa.*[1] CHPC is not predictably active against most *Ehrlichia* spp. Although its lipid solubility permits it to cross the blood-brain barrier, its effectiveness for treating central nervous system (CNS) infections is unpredictable.[1]

The intravenous form, CHPC sodium succinate, is a prodrug hydrolyzed to active CHPC, producing serum levels 70% of those obtained with oral dosing in humans. Metabolism takes place mainly in the liver, and inactive conjugated CHPC is excreted by the kidneys. CHPC should be used with caution in patients with liver disease. Although only a small fraction of active CHPC appears unchanged in the urine, adequate concentrations are achieved to treat many urinary tract infections (in the absence of advanced renal disease).[1]

Reversible bone marrow suppression and GI upset are observed occasionally in small animals, particularly with high dosages or prolonged treatment.[1,2] Cats may be particularly susceptible, although routine blood monitoring is not recommended unless anorexia is observed or when therapy extends beyond 4 weeks.[1,2] The most frequent adverse effects noted in dogs are gastrointestinal signs and weight loss. Inappetence is encountered frequently with oral administration in dogs. Hind limb weakness and tremors associated with CHPC administration are reported in large breed dogs. Ataxia, paresis, and pelvic limb dysfunction are seen in some dogs and reportedly resolve with drug discontinuation or dose reduction.[3] The pathogenesis is not known, although drug-associated distal axonopathies have been reported in human patients receiving CHPC.[3]

Owners should be advised that exposure to CHPC may pose a health risk and to wear gloves when handling medication. Although it is extremely rare, CHPC exposure through aerosolization or oral intake is associated with fatal bone marrow aplasia in humans.[3,4] Contact with mucosal surfaces is required for this severe reaction. Administration of film-coated formulations or capsules may reduce the possibility of contact with active drug.[1] These uncommon reactions are thus essentially avoidable for informed caregivers. CHPC is a cytochrome P-450 inhibitor and thus may decrease the clearance of other drugs that are metabolized by the same enzymes. CHPC may inhibit the metabolism of drugs such as opiates, barbiturates, and propofol. Caution should be exercised when administering other drugs, particularly anesthetics, concurrently with CHPC.[1,2]

Until recently, parenteral administration of CHPC had been all but abandoned in human medicine. Its use had diminished in dogs and cats as well. However, problematic organisms, notably MDR enterococci, methicillin-resistant *Staphylococcus aureus* (MRSA), and methicillin-resistant *Staphylococcus pseudintermedius* (MRSP), often retain in vitro susceptibility to CHPC. Thus it may serve as a viable treatment option for infections with these organisms.[1-3] CHPC is frequently selected as initial treatment of pneumonia in juvenile dogs. It is often effective in these patients, although no prospective studies comparing CHPC with other antimicrobials used to manage lower airway infections have been published. CHPC is rarely administered empirically to cats or dogs. It may be appropriately prescribed for treating select infections when the pathogen is shown to be resistant to safer antibiotics.

Injectable florfenicol is used in cattle and pigs, but elimination in dogs is too rapid for practical clinical use. There is no oral formulation of florfenicol, and effective doses in dogs have not been established.[1,2]

TETRACYCLINES

The tetracyclines are used to treat a variety of infections, including pneumonia and soft tissue and urinary tract infections. This drug class includes tetracycline, oxytetracycline, doxycycline, and minocycline. The tetracyclines are generally considered bacteriostatic. They bind primarily to the 30s subunits of bacterial ribosomes and inhibit protein synthesis.[1,2,4,5] Of the drugs in this group, doxycycline is used more frequently in companion animals, particularly for treating tick-borne diseases or when parenteral therapy is warranted. Doxycycline is the only tetracycline recommended for intravenous use in companion animals. Doxycycline is highly lipophilic, has excellent tissue penetration, and has a broad spectrum of activity against many gram-positive, gram-negative, aerobic, and anaerobic bacteria, including *Mycoplasma* spp, chlamydiae, rickettsiae, spirochetes, and select mycobacteria.[1,5] Doxycycline is occasionally used to treat filarial nematode infections and some protozoal infections in people. It not a first-line treatment for most protozoal infections in dogs or cats. It is the drug of choice for treating Lyme disease, brucellosis, and most *Ehrlichia* infections in dogs. [1,5] Doxycycline is very effective against many strains of *Bordetella bronchiseptica.* Hemotropic mycoplasmosis and infections with *Bartonella* spp may be treated with high-dosage doxycycline. Doxycycline is often a first-line treatment for respiratory infections, especially those caused by *Bordetella bronchiseptica*. Intravenous doxycycline is used for life-threatening infections with *Borrelia burgdorferi* and *Leptospira* spp. Doxycycline is effective for both active bacteremia and the elimination of leptospires from tissues.

Unlike conventional tetracyclines, doxycycline is eliminated largely by nonrenal mechanisms and is considered safe for patients with renal failure.[1,5] Moreover, the half-life and serum levels of doxycycline are not altered in patients with renal failure.[5] Doxycycline has excellent tissue penetration, including the prostate, bile, lung, and bronchial secretions. Drug concentrations measured in most tissues are generally higher than those in serum.[5] As with other tetracyclines, doxycycline possesses a number of nonantibacterial effects including antiinflammation, immunomodulation, inhibition of collagenase activity, and wound healing.[1]

Most adverse effects are associated with oral administration and include GI upset and pill-induced esophageal erosion, particularly in cats.[1,2] The incidence of esophageal damage may be decreased by using coated or liquid forms of the drug and providing at least 10 ml of water or gruel to the patient immediately after administration of the tablet or capsule while maintaining the patient in an upright position to ensure that the medication passes into the stomach.[1-3] There is limited evidence that doxycycline causes tooth discoloration or inhibits bone growth in juvenile patients. Although these effects are well documented with tetracycline (which is known to chelate divalent cations such as calcium), it has not been substantiated for doxycycline.[2] Rapid intravenous administration should be avoided. Drugs in the tetracycline family should never be administered after the medication's expiration date. Ingredients used in the manufacture of these medicines break down over time to form toxins that are particularly damaging to the kidneys.

Although tetracycline susceptibility predicts susceptibility to doxycycline and minocycline, isolates of *S. pseudintermedius* resistant to both tetracycline and doxycycline may remain susceptible to minocycline.[3,6] There has been much less clinical experience with minocycline, although the pharmacokinetics of minocycline are similar to those of doxycycline, and dosing regimens are similar.[2,6]

POTENTIATED SULFONAMIDES

The sulfonamides, known widely as *sulfa drugs,* were the first antibacterial agents and paved the way for the antimicrobial revolution in medicine.[7] Sulfonamide antibiotics such as sulfamethoxazole (SMX), sulfadiazine (SDZ), and sulfadimethoxine (SDM), potentiated by combination with either trimethoprim (TMP) or ormetoprim (OMP), inhibit two consecutive steps in bacterial folic acid synthesis.[1] Folate is necessary for cells to synthesize nucleic acids, and in its absence cells are unable to divide. Folate is not synthesized in mammalian cells but is instead a dietary requirement.[1] This explains the selective toxicity of these agents to bacterial cells.[7]

The potentiated sulfonamides have a broad spectrum of activity that includes urinary, prostate, GI, CNS, bone, joint, skin, soft tissue, and respiratory pathogens.[1,7] They are considered bactericidal against facultative gram-negative bacteria and staphylococci.[7] They have unpredictable activity against streptococci and no activity against enterococci or obligate anaerobes.[1,7] Many strains of *S. aureus, Escherichia coli, Proteus mirabilis, Enterobacter* spp, and *Salmonella enterica* are inhibited by the parenteral combination of TMP-SMX.[1,7] Oral preparations include TMP-SDZ, TMP-SMX, and OMP-SDM. There are no published reports of differences in effectiveness or adverse events between TMP-SDZ and TMP-SMX-TMP. The combination retains variable activity against opportunistic gram-negative pathogens, including *Aeromonas* spp, *Burkholderia cepacia,* and *Acinetobacter* spp. However, *P. aeruginosa* is uniformly resistant.[1]

TMP-SMX is considered a first-line agent for nocardial infections. TMP-SMX, alone or in combination with pyrimethamine, is an alternative treatment for toxoplasmosis in veterinary medicine.[1] Other protozoan and opportunistic mycobacterial infections are susceptible to the potentiated sulfonamides.[7] TMP-SMX is among the treatments of choice for *Pneumocystis* pneumonia in dogs and humans. In vitro, TMP-SMX retains activity against many staphylococcal isolates.[8] However, most isolates of MRSP are resistant.[2] TMP-SMX is generally not effective for *Bacteroides, Serratia, Klebsiella,* or *Enterococcus* spp. Some enterococcal strains may appear to be susceptible to TMP-SMX in vitro using standard growth media. However, enterococci can incorporate exogenously produced folates. Thus all enterococci should be inferred to be resistant to TMP-SMX. When necessary, TMP-SMX can be safely administered intravenously to critically ill dogs and cats. Formulations for subcutaneous administration are available, although their role in the critical care setting is not clear.

Dose-dependent adverse reactions associated with sulfonamide administration include anemia, proteinuria, crystalluria, and hematuria, as well as inhibition of thyroid hormone synthesis.[8,9] Effects on thyroid hormone function are most likely to manifest after 2 to 3 weeks of therapy and are reversible. Idiosyncratic reactions, or sulfonamide hypersensitivity, may be seen after just 5 days of therapy at standard dosages.[9] Sulfonamide hypersensitivities may be observed after a standard course of therapy has been completed. Signs in dogs can include fever, polyarthropathy, hepatotoxicity, skin eruptions, thrombocytopenia, and neutropenia.[9] Coombs-positive hemolytic anemia is observed less commonly than thrombocytopenia or neutropenia.

Idiosyncratic reactions are uncommon events and appear to be much less frequent in cats than in dogs. Larger dogs appear to be predisposed to sulfonamide-associated polyarthropathy. Sulfonamide-induced keratoconjunctivitis sicca is distinct from other adverse events in that the time to onset of signs is often months to years, rather than days to weeks.[9] Thus it is not clear if sulfonamide-induced keratoconjunctivitis sicca is idiosyncratic rather than dosage dependent. Because the incidence is estimated to be 15%, and signs may be reversible if detected quickly, veterinarians are encouraged to evaluate Schirmer tear test results before and during therapy in dogs. Dogs of Doberman Pinscher lineage appear to have a predilection to immune-mediated sulfonamide reactions.[1] Sulfonamides should not be prescribed to dogs with underlying hepatic disease. Cats are more likely than dogs to develop anorexia and vomiting with short-term sulfonamide use. Cats are also more likely to develop azotemia with long-term use. Acetylated sulfonamide metabolites do not accumulate in dogs, which reduces the nephrotoxicity compared with cats.

VANCOMYCIN

Vancomycin, a glycopeptide bactericidal antibiotic, has been used in human medicine for over 40 years. It works by binding to peptide precursors in the bacterial cell wall, preventing cross-linking of peptidoglycan side chains and thereby inhibiting cell wall synthesis.[1] Its spectrum of activity is limited to most aerobic and anaerobic gram-positive organisms, including most isolates resistant to β-lactams. Although vancomycin has been considered the last defense against MDR gram-positive pathogens in humans, the late 1980s saw a rise in vancomycin-resistant bacteria, including vancomycin-resistant enterococci (VRE) and resistant strains of *S. aureus.*[1,2]

Vancomycin is not absorbed across the intestinal wall, and its use is therefore limited to parenteral administration for all infections other than *Clostridium difficile*–associated diarrhea.[2,3] Clinically useful concentrations are achieved in heart, lung, kidney, synovium, and the peritoneal cavity.[1] Vancomycin may not reach therapeutic levels in pleural fluid and bile, although it has been used for treating bacterial cholangiohepatitis in cats. Vancomycin is eliminated almost exclusively by the kidney, and dosage is adjusted in human patients with renal dysfunction. Vancomycin-associated renal impairment is reported, although it is infrequent and generally mild.[1,2] However, vancomycin may potentiate aminoglycoside nephrotoxicity.[10] Rapid infusion of vancomycin can lead to histamine release, and most adverse events (hypotension, tachycardia) can be obviated by slow administration or by preadministration of an antihistamine. For most systemic infections in dogs and cats, vancomycin is given by slow infusion three times daily. Optimal dosing regimens and the need for therapeutic drug monitoring both remain unresolved in human (and veterinary) medicine.[2,10]

Vancomycin use has increased significantly over the past 30 years, and it remains the workhorse agent for β-lactam–resistant staphylococcal and enterococcal infections in most human hospitals. It is a drug of last resort in veterinary medicine, with no published reports of the effective use of vancomycin in small animals. Because reports of vancomycin-resistant gram-positive pathogens in veterinary medicine are rare, this drug is kept in reserve and only prescribed when no other options exist. The only indication for vancomycin use in veterinary medicine is serious infection with methicillin-resistant staphylococci. However, there are almost always other, and usually superior, options for treating dogs and cats.

Other glycopeptides that have been introduced include teicoplanin and telavancin. Teicoplanin, like vancomycin, is widely used to treat MRSA infections outside the United States. Compared with vancomycin, teicoplanin generally has greater potency against streptococci and enterococci. Telavancin was recently approved by the U.S. Food and Drug Administration for the treatment of skin infections caused by susceptible gram-positive pathogens, including MRSA.[8] Neither of these drugs has been studied in companion animals.

POLYMYXINS

Polymyxins B and E have a broad spectrum of activity that includes many gram-negative bacteria. The mechanism of action of polymyxins is not clear. They are cationic detergents that interact with the phospholipids of bacterial cell membranes, which leads to increased cell wall permeability and cell death.[11] In addition to their bactericidal properties, polymyxins can bind and neutralize lipopolysaccharide and prevent the pathophysiologic effects of endotoxin in circulation. Although polymyxin B is still used as a component of topical preparations, parenterally administered polymyxin E (colistin) has been used little since the early 1980s because of the perceived high incidence of drug-related neurotoxicity and nephrotoxicity. However, the mounting prevalence of nosocomial infections caused by highly resistant strains of certain gram-negative bacteria has prompted clinicians and microbiologists to reappraise the clinical value of colistin.[11] Colistin shows bactericidal activity against most strains of *Enterobacter aerogenes*, *Escherichia coli*, *Pseudomonas aeruginosa*, and *Klebsiella pneumoniae*. It has no activity against *Proteus* spp, *Serratia* spp, gram-positive cocci, or anaerobes. In the last decade it has been used intravenously as salvage therapy for infections caused by MDR gram-negative bacteria, or by the inhalational route in select patients with pneumonia due to panresistant strains of *Pseudomonas aeruginosa*. Subcutaneous administration is also reported.

Colistin is not used for routine automated testing and reporting by microbiology laboratories. It is used in some human hospitals on a case-by-case basis, and with the approval of an infectious disease specialist. Nephrotoxicity is dose dependent and reversible following discontinuation of colistin. Long-term use without adverse events is described in human intensive care unit settings, suggesting that colistin use is associated with less severe nephrotoxicity than was once reported.[10,11] Because colistin was introduced over 50 years ago, large pharmacokinetic studies are lacking, and optimal dosing for many infections is not known. Some data suggest that colistin may be used safely and effectively in dogs.[12]

CLINDAMYCIN

The only lincosamide available in the United States is clindamycin. Clindamycin binds to the 50s ribosomal subunit and inhibits protein synthesis in susceptible bacteria.[1] Clindamycin is lipophilic and achieves wide distribution throughout the body. It shares the gram-positive coccal spectrum of erythromycin but is more active (in some cases showing bactericidal activity) against susceptible staphylococci, including some methicillin-resistant isolates, as well as *Toxoplasma gondii*, *Neospora caninum*, *Hepatozoon*, and *Babesia* spp. Clindamycin is the treatment of choice for toxoplasmosis in dogs and cats. Given the protean manifestations of toxoplasmosis in domestic cats, clindamycin is appropriate empirical therapy when *Toxoplasma* infection is suspected. Because it has no clinically significant activity against facultative gram-negative enteric bacteria, clindamycin is appropriately prescribed with an antimicrobial with enhanced gram-negative coverage when treating polymicrobic infections.

Despite increasing resistance, clindamycin remains one of the drugs of choice for most anaerobic infections. It may be preferred over CHPC and metronidazole because of less toxicity. Clindamycin is not useful for enterococci, and it is ineffective for most aerobic gram-negative bacteria.[1] Strains of methicillin-resistant *Staphylococcus pseudintermedius* (MRSP) are variably susceptible. A concern regarding the use of clindamycin for staphylococcal infections is the possible presence of inducible resistance to clindamycin (ICR). ICR is a phenomenon in which the gene for resistance to clindamycin is not expressed until exposure to the antibiotic. Strains with constitutive resistance can be detected readily by standard automated instruments. However, strains with ICR are generally not identified with standard microdilution testing. There is potential for clinical failure when patients infected with strains of staphylococci with ICR are treated with clindamycin. ICR is found worldwide in strains and MRSA and coagulase-negative *Staphylococcus*. Although not common, it is now being recognized with MRSP.[3] Although it is not difficulty to assay for the presence of ICR, most commercial veterinary laboratories do not screen organisms for this phenotype. However, ICR may be suspected when the organism demonstrates in vitro resistance to erythromycin and susceptibility to clindamycin.[3]

Clindamycin is recommended for use in a variety of skin, soft tissue, and respiratory infections. It is widely used for postsurgical orthopedic infections. Clindamycin is widely distributed in body tissues and fluids, including bile, prostatic fluid, and bone.[1] Importantly, clindamycin accumulates in walled-off abscesses, surpassing concentrations of CHPC and penicillins. Although clindamycin achieves very high concentrations in phagocytic leukocytes, it does not have enhanced activity against obligate intracellular pathogens; this is likely because the subcellular location of the antibiotic does not match that of the organism. When clindamycin is administered at recommended dosages, adverse events are infrequent in dogs and cats.[1] Clindamycin may cause anorexia, vomiting, and diarrhea with higher doses.

RIFAMPIN

Rifampin is a bactericidal antibiotic that acts by blocking RNA polymerase. It is active against many gram-negative and most gram-positive bacteria. Rifampin is the most active antibiotic against staphylococci, and veterinarians are familiarizing themselves with this drug because it increasingly appears on susceptibility reports for methicillin-resistant *Staphylococcus* spp. It is active against most strains of MRSP.[2,3] Resistance develops rapidly with rifampin monotherapy, It is generally believed that emergence of resistance is limited by combining rifampin with another antibiotic to which the organism is susceptible.[3] However, a recent study showed rapid appearance of rifampin resistance in MRSP, even when prescribed in combination with other antibiotics.[3] Rifampin is potentially hepatotoxic. Mild elevations in serum alkaline phosphatase levels are common and generally do not warrant concern. Increases in other liver enzymes should prompt cessation of therapy, as hepatotoxicity and acute hepatitis are occasionally reported. Anorexia and vomiting may also occur.[1,2] Hemolytic anemia and thrombocytopenia are rarely observed. Rifampin may produce reversible discoloration (orange tint) of urine, tears, and saliva. To reduce the risk of adverse effects, notably hepatotoxicity, it is recommended that the dosage not exceed 10 mg/kg q24h.[2,3] Rifampin is generally given orally, which may be impractical in the critical care setting. Although injectable rifampin is available and considered safe, use of this formulation is not described in dogs or cats with naturally occurring infections.

NEWER AGENTS ACTIVE AGAINST MULTIDRUG-RESISTANT GRAM-POSITIVE COCCI

The incidence of serious gram-positive infections is increasing at an accelerated rate.[10,13] Resistant strains of *Enterococcus* spp and *Staphylococcus* spp are responsible for a substantial part of this disturbing trend (see Chapter 93). Resistance to β-lactams and other agents has resulted in the increasing use of glycopeptides, such as vancomycin, for treatment of such infections in human medicine. Although vancomycin-resistant enterococci and staphylococci are rare causes of infection in veterinary patients, they are identified frequently in human hospitals. In response to this challenge, a number of new antibiotics have been introduced, including the streptogramins (quinupristin-dalfopristin), the oxazolidinones (linezolid), tigecycline, and the cyclic lipopeptides (daptomycin).[1,8,10,13] Inclusion of these agents here is warranted because they are now part of the pharmacologic armamentarium in human hospitals.[2,8]

The evidence that antimicrobial prescribing is the main driver of antimicrobial resistance is overwhelming, and avoiding unnecessary antimicrobial use is a plausible and easy-to-implement strategy to forestall the emergence of resistance in small animal veterinary patients. None of the following agents has been evaluated adequately in companion animals with naturally occurring infections. Compelling indications for prescribing these agents to dogs and cats do not yet exist.

Daptomycin

Daptomycin, a novel parenterally administered lipopeptide antibiotic, is bactericidal against a range of gram-positive isolates.[8,14] Its exact mechanism of action is not completely understood. It is thought to disrupt plasma membrane function, which leads to the release of intracellular ions, specifically potassium, and results in cell death.[14] It exhibits rapid, concentration-dependent bactericidal activity against susceptible isolates, including MRSA and vancomycin-resistant *Enterococcus faecium* (VREF).[2,14] It is used primarily for skin and soft tissue infections caused by gram-positive bacteria but is also used for complicated urinary tract infections. It is inactivated by surfactant and is not useful for treating pneumonia. It is a relatively safe drug with very few reported adverse effects. Daptomycin has limited hepatic metabolism and is eliminated primarily by the kidneys; dosage adjustments may therefore be necessary in patients with renal dysfunction. There are no reports of its use in veterinary medicine.[2]

Tigecycline

Tigecycline is a member of the glycylcyclines, novel tetracyclines with gram-positive and gram-negative activity. Tigecycline's mechanism of action is similar to that of tetracycline, but it has improved ability to circumvent resistance.[2,8,10] It is one of the newest approved agents with activity against MDR gram-positive pathogens.[14] Tigecycline is used to treat complicated soft tissue and intraabdominal infections in humans. It is active against some resistant *Enterococcus* strains and MRSA, as well as certain β-lactamase–producing Enterobacteriaceae and anaerobes. It is available only for parenteral administration. There are no reports of its use in veterinary medicine to date.[2]

Quinupristin-Dalfopristin

Quinupristin-dalfopristin is a combination of two semisynthetic streptogramin drugs.[2,14] Both have antibacterial capability individually, but they demonstrate synergistic activity when used in combination.[14] Both enter bacterial cells by diffusion and bind to different sites on ribosomes, which results in irreversible inhibition of bacterial protein synthesis.[14] The drug is eliminated through the bile into feces. Quinupristin-dalfopristin is active against a broad spectrum of gram-positive bacteria, including MRSA, VREF, and many streptococci. Quinupristin-dalfopristin also has shown synergy with other antibiotics. Quinupristin-dalfopristin is synergistic in vitro with rifampin against MRSA and with doxycycline against VREF.

Quinupristin-dalfopristin is indicated for the treatment of serious infections caused by MDR organisms, VREF, and MRSA, including soft tissue infections, pneumonia, and bacteremia.[14] It is administered intravenously. Adverse events are reported infrequently but include myalgia, discomfort or thrombophlebitis at the site of injection, nausea, and increases in hepatic transaminase activity.[14] Although uncommon, resistance to quinupristin-dalfopristin has been encountered among VREF and MRSA in the United States. Its use in animals has not been reported.

Linezolid

Linezolid is thought to inhibit the initiation phase of translation and thus interfere with protein synthesis.[13,14] In vitro studies have shown linezolid to be effective against many antibiotic-resistant gram-positive organisms, including MRSA and VRE. In addition, it is effective against gram-negative anaerobes, including *Bacteroides fragilis* and some mycobacteria.[1,13,14] Linezolid has been approved in humans for the treatment of various gram-positive infections, including pneumonia, skin infections, and soft tissue infections.[14] This drug has not been used clinically in veterinary medicine. Linezolid is available for intravenous injection and oral administration. Resistance has been documented in both enterococci and staphylococci, which may limit the use of this drug in the near future.[13] Human patients uncommonly experience adverse events such as nausea and self-limiting thrombocytopenia. Less common, but more serious adverse effects include severe lactic acidosis and a disabling polyneuropathy.[13]

REFERENCES

1. Greene CE, Boothe DM: Antibacterial chemotherapy In Green CE, editor: Infectious diseases of the dog and cat, St Louis, 2012, Saunders, pp 291-302.
2. Papich MG: Selection of antibiotics for methicillin-resistant *Staphylococcus pseudintermedius:* time to revisit some old drugs? Vet Dermatol 23:352-e64, 2012.
3. Frank LA, Loeffler A: Methicillin-resistant *Staphylococcus pseudintermedius:* clinical challenge and treatment options, Vet Dermatol 23:283-e56, 2012.
4. Wareham DW, Wilson P: Chloramphenicol in the 21st century, Br J Hosp Med 63:157-161, 2002.
5. Joshi N, Miller DQ: Doxycycline revisited, Arch Intern Med 157:1421, 1997.
6. Weese JS, Sweetman K, Edson H, et al: Evaluation of minocycline susceptibility of methicillin-resistant *Staphylococcus pseudintermedius,* Vet Microbiol 162:968-971, 2013.
7. Masters PA, O'Bryan TA, Zurlo J, et al: Trimethoprim-sulfamethoxazole revisited, Arch Intern Med 163:402, 2003.
8. Gould IM, David MZ, Esposito S, et al: New insights into methicillin-resistant *Staphylococcus aureus* (MRSA) pathogenesis, treatment and resistance, Int J Antimicrob Agents 39:96-104, 2012.
9. Trepanier LA: Idiosyncratic toxicity associated with potentiated sulfonamides in the dog, J Vet Pharmacol Ther 27:129-138, 2004.
10. Roberts JA, Lipman J: Pharmacokinetic issues for antibiotics in the critically ill patient, Crit Care Med 37:840-851, 2009.
11. Nation RL, Li J: Colistin in the 21st century, Curr Opin Infect Dis 22:535, 2009.
12. Şentürk S: Evaluation of the anti-endotoxic effects of polymyxin E (colistin) in dogs with naturally occurred endotoxic shock, J Vet Pharmacol Ther 28:57-63, 2005.
13. Ager S, Gould K: Clinical update on linezolid in the treatment of Gram-positive bacterial infections, Infect Drug Resist 5:87-102, 2012.
14. Paterson DL: Clinical experience with recently approved antibiotics, Curr Opin Pharmacol 6:486, 2006.

CHAPTER 182

STRATEGIES FOR TREATING INFECTIONS IN CRITICALLY ILL PATIENTS

Mark G. Papich, DVM, MS, DACVCP

KEY POINTS

- Infections in critical care patients should be treated aggressively and promptly.
- Patients may have to be treated empirically initially because there is no time to wait for results of culture and susceptibility testing. Use of empirical selection guidelines for optimum choice of agents is recommended.
- The duration of antimicrobial treatment should be kept as short as possible.
- If patients do not respond to initial treatment, the presence of complicating factors and the possibility of a resistant infection should be considered.

Treatment of infections in critically ill patients is one of the most challenging forms of antimicrobial therapy. These patients are often infected with highly pathogenic, virulent, and sometimes resistant organisms. They usually have comorbidities that produce immunosuppression or confound our ability to treat the infection successfully. Fortunately, there are many advances in our understanding of the use and appropriate administration of antibiotic therapy. A large number of effective drugs are available for small animal veterinary clinicians; some are approved specifically for veterinary use and some are taken from human medicine and used off label. We now have more pharmacokinetic and pharmacodynamic information to guide dosing and make accurate predictions of outcomes. Improved techniques for bacterial identification and susceptibility testing—including revision of breakpoints—have helped to provide information for the most appropriate drug selection. These advances are most important for critical care patients, for it is these patients that often must be treated the most aggressively and promptly with appropriate antimicrobials in situations that can be life threatening. This chapter reviews the current concepts that guide antibiotic therapy in veterinary medicine and provides important strategies for effective dosing.

BACTERIAL SUSCEPTIBILITY

Most bacteria that cause infections in critical care patients are opportunistic, and the infection is often (if not most often) secondary to another primary disease. Regardless of the underlying primary problem, the infection must be treated appropriately for a successful outcome. The bacteria encountered in these patients most often come from the following list: *Staphylococcus pseudintermedius* (formerly called *Staphylococcus intermedius*) and occasionally other staphylococci, *Escherichia coli, Klebsiella pneumoniae, Pasteurella multocida,* β-hemolytic streptococci, *Pseudomonas aeruginosa, Proteus mirabilis* (and occasionally indole-positive *Proteus*), *Enterobacter* spp, and *Enterococcus* spp.

Table 182-1 **Suggested Empirical Treatment Based on Tissue Site***

Infection Site	First-Choice Drugs	Alternate-Choice Drugs
Skin: pyoderma or other skin infection	Amoxicillin-clavulanate Cephalosporin[†]	Trimethoprim-sulfonamide Fluoroquinolone Clindamycin
Urinary tract	Cephalosporin[†] Amoxicillin/ampicillin Amoxicillin-clavulanate	Trimethoprim-sulfonamide Fluoroquinolone[‡] Doxycycline
Respiratory tract	Amoxicillin-clavulanate Fluoroquinolone[‡] Cephalosporin[†]	Macrolide (azithromycin) Aminoglycoside (amikacin, gentamicin) Chloramphenicol Trimethoprim-sulfonamide (for some organisms) Extended-spectrum cephalosporin[§]
Septicemia (blood stream infection)	Amoxicillin-clavulanate Cephalosporin[†] Fluoroquinolone[‡]	Aminoglycoside Extended-spectrum cephalosporin[§]
Bone and joint	Cephalosporin Amoxicillin-clavulanate	Trimethoprim-sulfonamide Clindamycin Extended-spectrum cephalosporin[§] Fluoroquinolone[‡]

*This list includes some (but not all) possible choices for common infections encountered in veterinary medicine. In this list the first-choice drugs are agents with a high likelihood of success, low expense, and few risks. If the first choice has not been effective, or if patient factors (e.g., allergy or adverse effects) preclude using the first choice, the alternate choice should be considered.

[†]Cephalosporin = cefazolin, cephalexin, cefpodoxime, cefadroxil (and in some situations cefovecin).

[‡]Fluoroquinolone = enrofloxacin, marbofloxacin, pradofloxacin, or orbifloxacin.

[§]Extended-spectrum cephalosporin = third-generation drugs (e.g., cefotaxime, cefpodoxime, ceftazidime).

HOW TO PROCEED WITH EMPIRICAL TREATMENT

In critical care situations, the veterinarian may not have the benefit of culture and susceptibility test results to guide initial treatment. These findings are not usually available until at least 24 to 48 hours (or longer) after the specimen is sent to the laboratory. Therefore it is appropriate to institute empirical treatment based on a presumptive diagnosis and a prediction of what is likely to be the most active antimicrobial for each situation (Table 182-1).

If it is possible to perform cytologic analysis of a specimen isolated from a wound, the respiratory tract, or a lesion, it may be possible to narrow the choices down to a gram-positive coccus or gram-negative bacillus (rod). It is not always necessary to perform gram staining. Most cocci are gram positive and most important bacilli are gram negative. If these results are available, then a clinician should assume the most likely pathogen for the site of infection: if the organism is a gram-positive coccus, one should assume that it is a streptococci or *Staphylococcus,* most likely *S. pseudintermedius.* If it is a gram-negative bacillus, one should assume that it is *E. coli.* Even if it turns out to be *K. pneumoniae,* the susceptibility pattern will likely be similar. The only common isolate that has greater likelihood of resistance is *P. aeruginosa,* which is rarely isolated from septic patients or from the airways but can be a cause of urinary tract infections or chronic wound infections. Sometimes the odor or other wound characteristics (e.g., moist environment) are a clue that the pathogen may be *Pseudomonas.* When this approach is used, empirical treatment for the critical care patient can be initiated by following the recommendations in Table 182-2.

Modifications of the treatment regimen can be made after laboratory results are obtained. In the meantime, if the bacteria can be presumptively identified, antibiotic selection is simplified because the susceptibility pattern of many organisms is predicable. For example, if the bacteria are likely to be *Pasteurella, Streptococcus,* or *Actinomyces,* susceptibility is expected to penicillin or an aminopenicillin such as ampicillin, amoxicillin, or amoxicillin–clavulanic acid (Clavamox). Staphylococcus isolated from small animals is most likely to be *S. pseudintermedius* rather than *S. aureus.* Although methicillin resistance is a growing concern, it should initially be assumed that this is a wild-type strain and susceptible to antistaphylococcal agents. These staphylococci usually have predictable susceptibility to β-lactamase-resistant β-lactam antibiotics, such as amoxicillin combined with the β-lactamase inhibitor clavulanic acid (oral), or ampicillin combined with the inhibitor sulbactam (Unasyn, injectable). Cephalosporins active against wild-type strains of *Staphylococcus* include first-generation cephalosporins such as cephalexin (oral) or cefazolin (injectable), or the third-generation cephalosporin cefpodoxime proxetil (Simplicef). Cefovecin (Convenia) is also an appropriate antistaphylococcal agent, but it is not recommended for critical care situations.

Gram-negative bacilli can be less predicable in their susceptibility. For cases in which enteric gram-negative bacilli from the Enterobacteriaceae family are suspected, injectable antibiotics for initial treatment include aminoglycosides (amikacin or gentamicin) or cephalosporins (cefazolin, cefotaxime, or ceftazidime). Of the cephalosporins, cefazolin has less activity than cefotaxime or ceftazidime but may be suitable for initial treatment. Other injectable antibiotics that can be considered for initial treatment include ticarcillin-clavulanate and ampicillin-sulbactam. Any of these injectable antibiotics can be injected by the direct intravenous route (slowly), intramuscular route, or subcutaneous route. Intramuscular or subcutaneous injections can often cause temporary discomfort, but many injectable antibiotics can be reconstituted with lidocaine to decrease this response. The package insert should be checked for determination of compatibility and instructions for reconstituting with lidocaine. The β-lactam antibiotics (penicillin derivatives, cephalosporins, and carbapenems) can also be added to an intravenous infusion. If they are added to an intravenous infusion, the package insert should be consulted for compatibility and stability information. Administration via constant-rate infusion (CRI) ensures a long time-dependent effect for these drugs. A rationale for regimens using time-dependent β-lactam antibiotics is presented later. If an oral

Table 182-2 Empirical Antibiotic Selection for Critical Care Small Animal Patients

Cytologic Characteristics	Presumptive Pathogen	Initial Empirical Treatment by Injection	Initial Empirical Treatment with Oral Medications
Gram-negative bacilli	*Escherichia coli, Klebsiella pneumoniae*	Aminoglycoside (gentamicin, amikacin), ampicillin-sulbactam, cefazolin	Fluoroquinolone (enrofloxacin, marbofloxacin, orbifloxacin), amoxicillin-clavulanate, cefpodoxime proxetil
Gram-negative bacilli	*Pseudomonas aeruginosa*	Amikacin, ciprofloxacin	Fluoroquinolone (enrofloxacin, marbofloxacin)
Gram-positive cocci	*Staphylococcus* spp (usually *Staphylococcus pseudintermedius*)	Cefazolin, ampicillin-sulbactam	Cephalexin, cefpodoxime proxetil, amoxicillin-clavulanate, clindamycin
Mixed population with cellular debris	Anaerobic bacteria	Ampicillin-sulbactam, cefoxitin	Clindamycin, metronidazole, amoxicillin-clavulanate, pradofloxacin (cats)
Gram-negative coccobacillus	*Pasteurella multocida*	Ampicillin, ampicillin-sulbactam, cefazolin	Amoxicillin-clavulanate, cephalexin, cefpodoxime proxetil
Evidence from blood smear or complete blood count of blood-borne pathogen.	*Hemoplasma* spp, *Rickettsia* spp, *Ehrlichia canis*	Doxycycline	Doxycycline, fluoroquinolone (enrofloxacin, marbofloxacin, orbifloxacin, pradofloxacin), chloramphenicol

antibiotic is selected for initial treatment, cefpodoxime proxetil, amoxicillin-clavulanate, or a fluoroquinolone (enrofloxacin, marbofloxacin, orbifloxacin, or pradofloxacin) can be administered.

If a blood-borne pathogen is suspected (e.g., *Hemoplasma* spp, *Rickettsia* spp, or *Ehrlichia canis*), initial treatment almost always consists of doxycycline. Either doxycycline hyclate or doxycycline monohydrate can be used. It may be administered orally or intravenously. Minocycline hydrochloride can be considered as a substitute. For some infections, a fluoroquinolone can be considered as an alternative.

Assessing Initial Response

In critically ill patients, a reasonably rapid response to treatment is expected if the diagnosis is correct and a bacterial infection is producing or contributing to the clinical signs. Response to treatment can be assessed by clinical judgment of improvement; reduction in fever; improvement in complete blood count results, especially white blood cell count; and improvement in other measures of acute infection.

It is important to initiate treatment aggressively with appropriate antibiotics in critically ill patients. The early stages of treatment are a critical time during which appropriate antibiotic therapy is most important. A recent article by Papich and others emphasized the importance of appropriate early intervention and rapid attainment of the pharmacokinetic-pharmacodynamic target.[1] The expression used in the article was "Hit hard and hit fast, for a short duration" to emphasize the need for aggressive treatment, provided early but for a short duration. It was stressed that to increase the likelihood of therapeutic success, for many infections in which the inoculum is large enough to include resistant strains it is important to consider aggressive early treatment with high drug exposure.

If there is initial evidence of treatment success, the duration of treatment should be as short as possible. As discussed more extensively in the previously cited article, there is ample evidence that the duration of dosing should be tempered by the potential for amplification of resistant strains that can occur with prolonged therapies and the risk of inducing the development of chronic infection. When possible, reduction of the number of days of treatment (e.g., to 3 to 5 days, depending on the drug, pathogen, and site of infection) should be considered. However, in some cases (e.g., when the host immune system may be compromised or when there may other complications that may compromise the response to the antimicrobial intervention), clinical judgment should be exercised in deciding whether a longer duration of therapy is necessary.

To Escalate or De-escalate?

As discussed previously, early aggressive treatment is important in critical care patients with infections that can be life threatening. If there is a positive early response, one should continue antibiotics only for as long as necessary—keeping in mind that reducing the number of days of treatment will help decrease the opportunity for emergence of resistance.[2] After treatment has been initiated and culture and susceptibility results have become available, treatment may be modified. Often, if a highly susceptible organism is identified, the regimen can be de-escalated to more common and less expensive agents (sometimes called *first-tier* agents). It is always easier to *de-escalate* after treatment is begun than to *escalate* to more active agents when the first attempts have failed. Although the de-escalation, or step-down, of therapy is often recommended as an important principle of antibiotic stewardship, the true impact of this measure on the control of resistance has yet to be determined. Nevertheless, if the alternative is an escalation protocol after treatment failure with less active agents, problems can be foreseen. By the time that escalation of the regimen is contemplated, the patient may have deteriorated and resistant bacteria may already have had a opportunity to amplify in the patient.[2,3]

WHAT TO DO IF THE INITIAL EMPIRICAL TREATMENT FAILS

If the initial treatment suggested in Table 182-1 or 182-2 is unsuccessful, or if resistant strains of bacteria are either strongly suspected or confirmed with susceptibility testing, treatment should be started with drugs listed in Table 182-3. If the organism is *P. aeruginosa*, *Enterobacter* sp, *K. pneumoniae*, or *E. coli*, resistance against many common antibiotics is possible. A follow-up susceptibility test should be used to confirm the presence of resistance mechanisms. For example, a high percentage of nonenteric *E. coli* strains are resistant to commonly used first-generation cephalosporins and ampicillin. Resistance to fluoroquinolones has been documented in clinical

Table 182-3 Antibiotic Selection for Critical Care Small Animal Patients When Resistance Is Suspected or Initial Treatment (Table 182-1) Has Failed

Presumptive Pathogen	Second Choice (When First Choice Has Failed)	Comments
Escherichia coli, Klebsiella pneumoniae	Cefotaxime, ceftazidime, carbapenem (meropenem), amikacin	Before using amikacin, ensure adequate kidney function.
Pseudomonas aeruginosa	Ceftazidime, carbapenem (meropenem), amikacin	If initial treatment has failed, oral treatment with fluoroquinolones is usually not possible because of resistance.
Staphylococcus spp, (usually *S. pseudintermedius*)	Rifampin, chloramphenicol, aminoglycoside (amikacin, gentamicin), vancomycin	If initial treatment has failed, presumptive methicillin-resistant strain is suspected. Treatment is best guided by susceptibility test results.
Anaerobic bacteria	Metronidazole, carbapenem (meropenem)	Susceptibility tests are rarely performed on anaerobic bacteria. Metronidazole is associated with a low incidence of resistance among anaerobes.

isolates. In one study, 13% to 23% of isolates were intermediate in sensitivity or resistant to fluoroquinolones.[4] In urinary tract infections[5] half of the *E. coli* organisms were resistant to cephalexin and only 22% were sensitive to enrofloxacin. There was a high incidence of resistance in *E. coli* isolates collected from different geographic regions.[6] The multidrug-resistant isolates comprised 56% of the resistant isolates, and over half of these were resistant to amoxicillin, amoxicillin-clavulanate, and enrofloxacin. Based on these data as well as findings of other studies, for initial therapy the gram-negative enteric bacteria are usually expected to be susceptible to aminoglycosides (amikacin and gentamicin) and third-generation cephalosporins. Fluoroquinolones may also be considered, but their activity may be unpredictable if the patient has previously been treated with this class of agents. Previous exposure to fluoroquinolones may select for resistant strains of *E. coli* in dogs that can persist long after drug treatment has been discontinued.[7]

If the organism is suspected to be *P. aeruginosa,* inherent resistance to many drugs is anticipated, but it may be susceptible to fluoroquinolones, aminoglycosides, or an extended-spectrum penicillin such as ticarcillin or piperacillin. The extended-spectrum cephalosporins (third-generation cephalosporins) usually are active against enteric gram-negative bacteria but are not active against *P. aeruginosa* (with the exception of ceftazidime). As with the enteric gram-negative bacilli, if the patient has previously been exposed to these agents, particularly the fluoroquinolones, resistance is more likely.

When a fluoroquinolone is used to treat *P. aeruginosa* infection, administration at the high end of the dosage range is suggested. Of the currently available fluoroquinolones (human or veterinary drugs), ciprofloxacin is the most active in vitro against *P. aeruginosa,* followed by marbofloxacin, enrofloxacin, difloxacin, and orbifloxacin.[8]

If the treatment of *S. pseudintermedius* and other staphylococci fails, methicillin resistance is likely. These organisms are referred to as *methicillin-resistant S. pseudintermedius* (MRSP). They are resistant to all β-lactam antibiotics (penicillins, cephalosporins, and carbapenems) and most are also resistant to other drugs listed previously for treating *Staphylococcus* infection. In these situations, a susceptibility test is strongly recommended and it may be necessary to administer chloramphenicol, rifampin, aminoglycosides, or a tetracycline. A full review of the use of these agents has been provided elsewhere.[9] Similar drugs are considered for treating resistant strains of *Enterococcus* spp. Readers are directed to Chapter 103 for further information.

PENETRATION TO THE SITE OF INFECTION

For most tissues, antibiotic drug concentrations in the serum or plasma approximate the drug concentration in the extracellular space (interstitial fluid). This is because there is no barrier that impedes drug diffusion from the vascular compartment to extracellular tissue fluid.[10] There is really no such thing as "good penetration" and "poor penetration" when referring to most drugs in most tissues. Pores (fenestrations) or microchannels in the endothelium of capillaries are large enough to allow drug molecules to pass through unless the drug is restricted by protein binding in the blood. In tissues lacking pores or channels penetration of some drugs may be inhibited (discussed later).

Diffusion into Tissues

Diffusion of most antibiotics from plasma to tissues is limited by tissue blood flow, rather than drug lipid solubility. This has been called *perfusion rate–limited* drug diffusion. If adequate drug concentrations can be achieved in plasma, it is unlikely that a barrier in the tissue will prevent drug diffusion to the site of infection as long as the tissue has an adequate blood supply. In critical care patients, poor perfusion of tissues owing to compromised hemodynamic function could negatively affect this property. Normally, rapid equilibration between extracellular fluid and plasma is possible because of a high ratio of surface area to volume. That is, the surface area of the capillaries is high relative to the volume into which the drug diffuses. Drug diffusion into an abscess or granulation tissue is sometimes a problem because in these conditions drug penetration relies on simple diffusion and the site of infection lacks adequate blood supply. In an abscess, there may not be a physical barrier to diffusion—that is, there is no impenetrable membrane—but low drug concentrations are attained in the abscess or drug is slow to accumulate because in a cavitated lesion there is low ratio of surface area to volume.

In some tissues a lipid membrane (e.g., tight junctions on capillaries) presents a barrier to drug diffusion. This has been called *permeability rate–limited* drug diffusion. In these instances, a drug must be sufficiently lipid soluble or be actively carried across the membrane to reach effective concentrations in tissues. These tissues include the central nervous system, eye, and prostate. A functional membrane pump (P-glycoprotein) also contributes to the barrier. There also is a barrier between plasma and bronchial epithelium (called the *blood-bronchus* or *blood-alveolar* barrier). This limits concentrations of some drugs in the bronchial secretions and epithelial fluid of the airways. Lipophilic drugs may be more likely to diffuse through the blood-bronchus barrier and reach effective drug concentrations in bronchial secretions.

Urinary Tract

High antibiotic concentrations achieved in renal tubules and the urine after routine therapy with modest doses of antibiotics is often sufficient to cure lower urinary tract infections, even those that are caused by organisms identified on a susceptibility test as "intermediate" in sensitivity.[11,12] Urine concentrations of antibiotics may be at least 100 times the corresponding plasma concentrations because of the tubular concentration. When the infection is confined to the lower urinary tract, these high concentrations are an advantage.[13] Cures of uncomplicated urinary tract infections are possible, even when the antibiotic levels do not attain concentrations high enough to eliminate a systemic infection. However, clinicians should be aware that if the concentrating ability of the kidneys is compromised, antibiotic concentrations in the urine may be low. Patients may have dilute urine because of kidney disease or treatment with corticosteroids, fluid therapy, or diuretics. This is particularly likely in critical care patients. In these situations the clinician should administer doses high enough to ensure that adequate plasma concentrations are attained, which should reach equilibrium with urinary tract tissues.

When the renal tissue is involved, high urine drug concentrations offer no advantage. Drug concentrations in renal tissue—which are equivalent to the renal lymph concentrations—are correlated with plasma drug concentrations, not with the drug concentrations in the urine. An example of an infection in which this applies is pyelonephritis in a critical care patient. Therefore consideration must be given to drugs that attain high concentrations in the renal tissue and that can be administered at doses and intervals that are optimum to achieve the pharmacokinetic-pharmacodynamic relationships required for a clinical cure.

Intracellular Infections

Most bacterial infections are located extracellularly, and a cure can be achieved with adequate drug concentrations in the extracellular (interstitial) space rather than intracellular space. Intracellular infections present another problem. For drugs to reach intracellular sites, they must be carried into the cell or diffuse passively. Generally, lipid-soluble drugs are best able to diffuse through the cell membrane to treat intracellular infections. Examples of drugs that accumulate in leukocytes, fibroblasts, macrophages, and other cells are fluoroquinolones, lincosamides (clindamycin, lincomycin), tetracyclines (doxycycline, minocycline), macrolides (erythromycin, clarithromycin), and the azalides (azithromycin).[14] β-Lactam antibiotics and aminoglycosides do not reach effective concentrations within cells. Organisms such as *Brucella, Chlamydia, Rickettsia, Bartonella,* and *Mycobacteria* are examples of intracellular pathogens. Staphylococci may in some cases become resistant to treatment because of intracellular survival. Fluoroquinolones and tetracyclines such as doxycycline are frequently administered to treat *Rickettsia* and *Ehrlichia* infections. There is good evidence for the efficacy of doxycycline or fluoroquinolones (enrofloxacin has been the only one tested) in treating *Rickettsia* infections, but only doxycycline should be considered because of its efficacy in treating canine ehrlichiosis.

LOCAL FACTORS THAT AFFECT ANTIBIOTIC EFFECTIVENESS

Local tissue factors may decrease antimicrobial effectiveness. For example, pus and necrotic debris may bind and inactivate vancomycin or aminoglycoside antibiotics (gentamicin or amikacin), causing them to be ineffective. Cellular material also can decrease the activity of topical agents such as polymyxin B. Foreign material in a wound (such as surgically implanted material) can protect bacteria from antibiotics and phagocytosis by allowing them to form a biofilm (glycocalyx) at the site of infection.[15,16] Cellular debris and infected tissue can inhibit the action of trimethoprim-sulfonamide combinations through the secretion of thymidine and *p*-aminobenzoic acid, both known to be inhibitors of the action of these drugs. This may explain why trimethoprim-sulfonamide combinations have not been effective in some infected tissues. Cations can adversely affect the activity of antimicrobials at the site of infection. Two important drug groups diminished in activity by cations such as Mg^{2+}, Al^{+3}, Fe^{+3}, and Ca^{2+} are fluoroquinolones and aminoglycosides. (Cations such as Mg^{2+}, Fe^{+3}, and Al^{+3} also can inhibit oral absorption of fluoroquinolones.)

An acidic environment of infected tissue may decrease the effectiveness of clindamycin, macrolides (e.g., erythromycin, azithromycin), fluoroquinolones, and aminoglycosides. Penicillin and tetracycline activity is not affected as much by tissue pH, but hemoglobin at the site of infection decreases the activity of these drugs. An anaerobic environment decreases the effectiveness of aminoglycosides because oxygen is necessary for drug penetration into bacteria.

As mentioned previously, an adequate blood flow is necessary to deliver an antibiotic to the site of infection. Effective antibacterial drug concentrations may not be attained in tissues that are poorly vascularized (e.g., extremities during shock, sequestered bone fragments, and endocardial valves).

PHARMACOKINETIC-PHARMACODYNAMIC OPTIMIZATION OF DOSES

To achieve a cure, the drug concentration in plasma, serum, or tissue fluid should be maintained above the minimum inhibitory concentration (MIC), or some multiple of the MIC, for at least a portion of the dose interval. Antibacterial dosage regimens are based on this assumption, but drugs vary with respect to the peak concentration and the time above the MIC that is needed for a clinical cure. Pharmacokinetic-pharmacodynamic relationships of antibiotics have been examined to explain how these factors can correlate with clinical outcome.[17,18] Shown in Figure 182-1 are some terms used to describe the shape of the plasma concentration versus time profile. C_{MAX} is the maximum plasma concentration attained during a dosing interval. C_{MAX} is related to the MIC by the C_{MAX}:MIC ratio. *AUC* is the total area under the curve. The AUC for a 24-hour period is related to the MIC value by the AUC:MIC ratio. Also shown in Figure 182-1 is the relationship of time to MIC (i.e., time spent above the MIC, or T > MIC), usually expressed as percent of time during the dosing interval that the concentration is above the MIC.

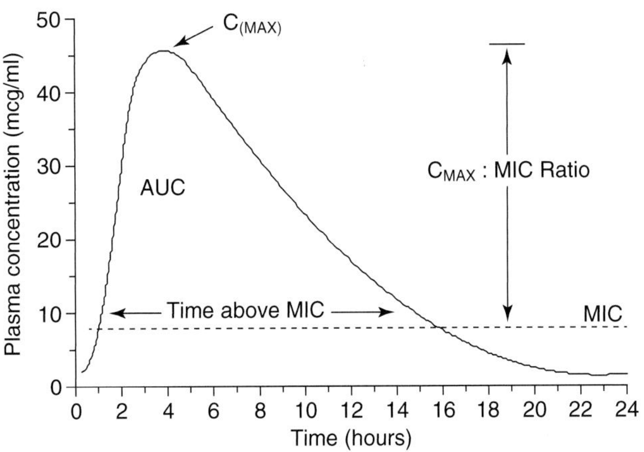

FIGURE 182-1 Pharmacokinetic/pharmacodynamic relationships for antimicrobials. Drug concentrations in relation to the minimum inhibitory concentration (MIC) are shown as time above MIC (T > MIC), ratio of peak concentration to MIC (C_{MAX}:MIC), and ratio of area under the curve to MIC (AUC:MIC).

Antibiotics have been classified as being either bactericidal or bacteriostatic, depending on their in vitro action on the bacteria. However, the clinical distinction between bactericidal and bacteriostatic has become more blurred in recent years.[19] Drugs traditionally considered bactericidal can be bacteriostatic if the concentrations are low. Alternatively, drugs traditionally considered bacteriostatic can be bactericidal against some bacteria and under optimum conditions. Rather than being categorized as bacteriostatic or bactericidal, drugs are now more frequently grouped as either concentration dependent or time dependent in their action. If the drug is concentration dependent, a high enough dose should be administered to maximize the C_{MAX}:MIC ratio or AUC:MIC ratio. If the drug is time dependent, the drug should be administered frequently enough to maximize the T > MIC. For some of the long-acting time-dependent drugs with postantibiotic effects, the AUC:MIC also predicts clinical success. Examples of how these relationships affect drug regimens are provided in the following sections.

Aminoglycosides

Aminoglycosides (e.g., gentamicin, amikacin) are concentration-dependent bactericidal drugs; therefore the higher the drug concentration, the greater the bactericidal effect. An optimal bactericidal effect occurs if a high enough dose is administered to produce a peak of 8 to 10 times the MIC. This can be accomplished by administering a single dose once daily. This regimen is at least as effective, and perhaps less nephrotoxic, than administration of lower doses more frequently.[20] Current regimens for small animals employ this strategy. The single daily dose is based on the drug's volume of distribution (typically in the range of 0.2 to 0.25 L/kg for aminoglycosides in animals). A dosage for gentamicin is 5 to 8 mg/kg q24h for cats and 10 to 14 mg/kg q24h for dogs. An appropriate dosage for amikacin is 10 to 15 mg/kg q24h for cats and 15 to 30 mg/kg q24h for dogs. The efficacy of these regimens has not been tested for conditions encountered in veterinary medicine, but the relationships are supported by experimental evidence. These regimens assume some competency of the immune system. If the animal is immunocompromised, a more frequent interval of administration may be considered. In animals with decreased renal function, longer intervals may be considered, or aminoglycosides should be avoided altogether.

Fluoroquinolones

For the fluoroquinolone antimicrobials, as reviewed by Drusano et al,[21] Papich and Riviere,[22] and Wright et al,[23] investigators have shown that either the peak plasma concentration above bacterial MIC (also known as the *C_{MAX}:MIC ratio*) or the total AUC above the MIC (also known as the *AUC:MIC ratio*) may predict clinical cure in studies of laboratory animals and in a limited number human clinical studies. The optimum value for these surrogate markers has not been determined for treatment of infections in dogs or cats. However, based on other studies, a C_{MAX}:MIC of 8 to 10 or an AUC:MIC of more than 125 has been associated with a cure. As reviewed by Wright et al,[23] in some clinical situations AUC:MIC ratios as low as 30 to 55 have been associated with a clinical cure.

For susceptible bacteria isolated from small animals, the MIC for fluoroquinolones is expected to be low enough that administration of the lowest label dose of any of the currently available fluoroquinolones usually meets the goal of a C_{MAX}:MIC ratio or an AUC:MIC ratio in the range cited earlier. For organisms with MIC values that are slightly higher but still in the susceptible range a higher dose may be required. To take advantage of the wide range of safe doses for fluoroquinolones, low doses have been administered to treat susceptible organisms with low MICs, such as *E. coli* or *Pasteurella.* But for bacteria with higher MICs (e.g., gram-positive cocci) a slightly higher dose is recommended. To achieve the necessary peak concentration for a bacteria such as *P. aeruginosa,* which usually has the highest MIC among susceptible bacteria, use of the highest dose within a safe range is recommended. Bacteria such as streptococci and anaerobes are more resistant, and even at high doses, a sufficient peak concentration or AUC:MIC ratio will be difficult to achieve. An exception to these guidelines is the new fluoroquinolone pradofloxacin, which has an extended spectrum of activity that includes gram-positive cocci and anaerobes.

β-Lactam Antibiotics

β-Lactam antibiotics such as penicillins, potentiated aminopenicillins, and cephalosporins are slowly bactericidal. Their concentrations should be kept above the MIC throughout most of the dosing interval (long T > MIC) for the optimal bactericidal effect.[24] Dosage regimens for the β-lactam antibiotics should consider these pharmacodynamic relationships. Therefore for treating a gram-negative infection, especially a serious one, some regimens for penicillins and cephalosporins require administration three or four times per day. Some long-acting formulations have been developed to prolong plasma concentrations. Some of the third-generation cephalosporins have long half-lives, and less frequent dosing regimens have been used for some of these drugs (e.g., cefpodoxime proxetil). (The long half-life for ceftriaxone seen in people does not occur in animals because of differences in drug protein binding.) Gram-positive organisms are more susceptible to the β-lactams than are gram-negative bacteria, and lower doses and longer intervals are possible when treating infections caused by these bacteria. Additionally, because antibacterial effects occur at concentrations below the MIC (postantibiotic effect) for *Staphylococcus,* longer dose intervals may be possible for staphylococcal infections. For example, cephalexin or amoxicillin-clavulanate has been used successfully to treat staphylococcal infections when administered only once daily (although twice-daily administration is recommended to obtain maximum response). Cefpodoxime proxetil is effective with once-daily administration because of both its high activity (low MIC values) and longer half-life compared with other cephalosporins.

In critical care patients, for optimum treatment β-lactam antibiotics may be administered via CRI to ensure a long T > MIC. Rates of infusion are readily calculated using available parameters for volume of distribution and systemic clearance (Table 182-4). The amount of drug administered over 24 hours is much less with a CRI than with intermittent bolus injections.

Other Time-Dependent Drugs

Drugs such as tetracyclines, macrolides (azithromycin), lincosamides (clindamycin), and chloramphenicol act in a time-dependent manner

Table 182-4 Suggested Loading Doses and Constant-Rate Infusion (CRI) Rates for Selected Antibiotics Used In Critical Care*

Drug	Intravenous Loading Dose (mg/kg)	Intravenous CRI (mg/kg/hr)
Cefazolin	1.3	1.21
Ceftazidime	1.2	1.56
Cefotaxime	3.2	5.04
Ceftriaxone	1.9	1.9
Cefepime	1.4	1.04

*Clinicians should verify the compatibility of each drug with the fluid administered and the stability of the drug for the duration of infusion by consulting the package insert before administration.

against most bacteria, but because they can have long-acting, or postantibiotic, effects the total drug exposure, measured as AUC : MIC, has been used to predict clinical success.

The time-dependent activity of these drugs is demonstrated by studies showing that effectiveness is highest when drug concentrations are maintained above the MIC throughout the dosing interval. Drugs in this group should be administered frequently to achieve this goal. However, a property of some is that they persistent in tissues for a prolonged time, which allows long dosing intervals. The macrolide derivative azithromycin (Zithromax) has shown a tissue half-life as long as 70 to 90 hours in cats and dogs, which permits infrequent dosing. Tissue concentrations of trimethoprim-sulfonamides persist long enough to allow once-daily dosing for many infections. Most published dosing regimens are designed to take the pharmacokinetic properties of these drugs into account.

REFERENCES

1. Martinez MN, Papich MG, Drusano GL: Dosing regimen matters: the importance of early intervention and rapid attainment of the pharmacokinetic/pharmacodynamic target, Antimicrob Agents Chemother 56(6):2795-2805, 2012.
2. Mouton JW, Ambrose PG, Canton R, et al: Conserving antibiotics for the future: new ways to use old and new drugs from a pharmacokinetic and pharmacodynamic perspective, Drug Resist Updat 14:107-117, 2011.
3. Drusano GL, Louie A, Deziel M, et al: The crisis of resistance: identifying drug exposures to suppress amplification of resistant mutant subpopulations, Clin Infect Dis 42:525-532, 2006.
4. Oluoch AO, Kim C-H, Weisiger RM, et al: Nonenteric *Escherichia coli* isolates from dogs: 674 cases (1990-1998), J Am Vet Med Assoc 218:381-384, 2001.
5. Torres SM, Diaz SF, Nogueira SA, et al: Frequency of urinary tract infection among dogs with pruritic disorders receiving long-term glucocorticoid treatment, J Am Vet Med Assoc 227:239-243, 2005.
6. Shaheen BW, Boothe DM, Oyarzabal OA, et al: Antimicrobial resistance profiles and clonal relatedness of canine and feline *Escherichia coli* pathogens expressing multidrug resistance in the United States, J Vet Intern Med 24:323-330, 2010.
7. Boothe DM, Debavalya N: Impact of Routine Antimicrobial Therapy On Canine Fecal *Escherichia coli* antimicrobial resistance: a pilot study, Int J Appl Res Vet Med 9(4):396-406, 2011.
8. Rubin J, Walker RD, Blickenstaff K, et al: Antimicrobial resistance and genetic characterization of fluoroquinolone resistance of *Pseudomonas aeruginosa* isolated from canine infections, Vet Microbiol 131(1-2):164-172, 2008.
9. Papich MG: Selection of antibiotics for methicillin-resistant *Staphylococcus pseudintermedius:* time to revisit some old drugs? Vet Dermatol 23(4):352-360, 2012.
10. Nix DE, Goodwin SD, Peloquin CA, et al: Antibiotic tissue penetration and its relevance: impact of tissue penetration on infection response, Antimicrob Agents Chemother 35:1953-1959, 1991.
11. Lees GE, Rogers KS: Treatment of urinary tract infections in dogs and cats. J Am Vet Med Assoc 189:648-652, 1986.
12. Clinical and Laboratory Standards Institute: Performance standards for antimicrobial disk and dilution susceptibility tests for bacteria isolated from animals; approved standard—third edition, CLSI document M31-A3, Wayne, Pa, 2008, Clinical and Laboratory Standards Institute.
13. Stamey TA, Fair WR, Timothy MM, et al: Serum versus urinary antimicrobial concentrations in cure of urinary-tract infections, N Engl J Med 291:1159-1163, 1974.
14. Pascual A: Uptake and intracellular activity of antimicrobial agents in phagocytic cells, Rev Med Microbiol 6:228-235, 1995.
15. Habash M, Reid G: Microbial biofilms: their development and significance for medical device-related infections, J Clin Pharmacol 39:887-898, 1999.
16. Smith AW: Biofilms and antibiotic therapy: is there a role for combating resistance by the use of novel drug delivery systems? Adv Drug Deliv Rev 57:1539-1550, 2005.
17. Hyatt JM, McKinnon PS, Zimmer GS, et al: The importance of pharmacokinetic/pharmacodynamic surrogate markers to outcome, Clin Pharmacokinet 28:143-160, 1995.
18. Nicolau DP, Quintiliani R, Nightingale CH: Antibiotic kinetics and dynamics for the clinician, Med Clinics North Am 79:477-495, 1995.
19. Pankey GA, Sabath LD: Clinical relevance of bacteriostatic versus bactericidal mechanisms of action in the treatment of gram-positive bacterial infections, Clin Infect Dis 38:864-870, 2004.
20. Freeman CD, Nicolau DP, Belliveau PP, et al: Once-daily dosing of aminoglycosides: review and recommendations for clinical practice, J Antimicrob Chemother 39:677, 1997.
21. Drusano G, Labro M-T, Cars O, et al: Pharmacokinetics and pharmacodynamics of fluoroquinolones, Clin Microbiol Infect 4(Suppl 2):2S27-2S41, 1998.
22. Papich MG, Riviere JE: Fluoroquinolone antimicrobial drugs. In Riviere JE, Papich MG, editors: Veterinary pharmacology and therapeutics, ed 9, Ames, Ia, 2009, Wiley-Blackwell, chap 38.
23. Wright DH, Brown GH, Peterson ML, et al: Application of fluoroquinolone pharmacodynamics, J Antimicrob Chemother 46:669-683, 2000.
24. Turnidge JD: The pharmacodynamics of β-lactams, Clin Infect Dis 27:10-22, 1998.

CHAPTER 183

HEMODYNAMIC MONITORING

Lori S. Waddell, DVM, DACVECC • Andrew J. Brown, MA, VetMB, MRCVS, DACVECC

KEY POINTS

- Hemodynamic monitoring is essential in the treatment of many critically ill patients because it is important in guiding fluid and pharmacologic therapy to optimize cardiovascular function.
- Assessment of hemodynamic status is typically based on physical examination parameters and monitoring of any of the following: continuous electrocardiogram, arterial blood pressure, central venous pressure, mixed venous and central venous oxygen saturation, pulmonary artery pressure, lactate and base deficit, and cardiac output measurements.
- Continuous electrocardiogram monitoring enables the clinician to detect intermittent arrhythmias, determine whether treatment is indicated, and monitor therapeutic effectiveness.
- Direct blood pressure monitoring is the gold standard for blood pressure measurement, but indirect blood pressure monitoring is more readily available and better tolerated by most patients.
- Central venous pressure is relatively easy to monitor and can guide fluid therapy, particularly in patients that are hypovolemic or have septic shock, heart disease, or renal disease.

Hemodynamic monitoring includes monitoring of basic physical examination parameters, continuous electrocardiogram (ECG) and blood pressure, central venous pressure (CVP), central venous oxygen saturation ($ScvO_2$), and lactate clearance and base deficit, as well as the most advanced forms including pulmonary artery pressure (PAP) monitoring, mixed venous oxygen saturation (SvO_2) monitoring, and other technologies to measure cardiac output, cardiac index, systemic vascular resistance, oxygen delivery, and oxygen uptake. See Chapters 184 and 202 for further information on these procedures. The type of monitoring chosen depends on the severity of illness, equipment availability, and the clinician's comfort with the various modalities.

CONTINUOUS ELECTROCARDIOGRAM MONITORING

Continuous ECG monitoring can be very useful in critically ill patients; it provides continuous, hands-off access to the heart rate and rhythm. It allows the clinician to catch arrhythmias that may be intermittent and infrequent, and monitor the need for treatment based on the rate and rhythm. Both standard and telemetric systems are available, with the telemetric models allowing for easier patient movement and less tangling and disconnection of the leads compared with standard systems.

BLOOD PRESSURE MONITORING

Arterial blood pressure monitoring is extremely useful in critical cases and is commonly employed to permit fluid therapy to be tailored to the patient's needs, especially when combined with monitoring of physical examination parameters, urine output, and CVP. It is essential in guiding the use of inotropic agents and vasopressors; these therapies should not be used unless blood pressure can and will be measured frequently. Normal arterial blood pressure values for dogs are as follows: systolic pressure, 150 ± 20 mm Hg; mean pressure, 105 ± 10 mm Hg; and diastolic pressure, 85 ± 10 mm Hg. For cats, normal ranges are 125 ± 10 mm Hg for systolic, 105 ± 10 mm Hg for mean, and 90 ± 10 mm Hg for diastolic.[1] Mean arterial blood pressure can be calculated from these measured values as follows:

$$\text{Mean arterial blood pressure} = \text{diastolic} + \frac{\text{systolic} - \text{diastolic}}{3}$$

Hypotension is defined as a systolic blood pressure of less than 90 mm Hg or a mean arterial pressure of less than 60 mm Hg in either species. Causes of hypotension include decreased cardiac output secondary to reduced circulating volume, myocardial failure, severe bradyarrhythmia or tachyarrhythmia, or decreased systemic vascular resistance due to peripheral vasodilation secondary to sepsis or systemic inflammatory response syndrome. Treatment of hypotension should always be aimed at correcting the underlying problem (see Chapter 8).

Hypertension can be primary (essential hypertension), which is rare in both cats and dogs, or secondary to another disease process that alters renal or neurohormonal function. Kidney injury or failure, whether acute or chronic, is the most frequent cause of secondary hypertension, but hyperthyroidism, diabetes mellitus, hyperadrenocorticism, pheochromocytoma, and various medications (glucocorticoids, cyclosporine A, phenylpropanolamine, and erythropoietin) have also been associated with hypertension.

Blood pressure monitoring can be divided into two main categories, noninvasive and invasive methods. The noninvasive oscillometric or Doppler methods are used most commonly in veterinary patients, although photoplethysmography is also available. Invasive blood pressure monitoring provides direct arterial pressure measurement and is the most accurate method available.

Noninvasive Blood Pressure Monitoring

Noninvasive blood pressure monitoring is based on inflation of a cuff to occlude arterial flow, followed by measurement of the pressure at which flow returns. These methods are technically easy to use and require relatively inexpensive equipment but are prone to error, usually due to selection of an inappropriate cuff size. The guideline for the cuff width is approximately 40% of the circumference of the limb for dogs and 30% of the circumference of the limb for cats. If the cuff is too small, a falsely high pressure will be obtained; if the cuff is too large, a falsely low reading will result.[2] The cuff should be at the level of the right atrium while measurements are being obtained. Keeping the patient motionless in lateral recumbency is ideal for obtaining accurate indirect blood pressure measurements.

The Doppler method is used most commonly in smaller animals such as cats, very small dogs, and exotic species. It is also useful in patients with hypotension or those that have arrhythmias because the oscillometric methods are commonly inaccurate or do not give any readings at all in these circumstances. The Doppler method uses a 10-MHz ultrasound probe to detect blood flow in an artery. The probe is placed over an artery distal to the cuff. Doppler sounds become audible when pressure in the cuff is less than the pressure in the artery. Although the Doppler method typically is regarded as measuring the systolic pressure, one study that compared Doppler readings with direct blood pressure monitoring in anesthetized cats found that the Doppler reading consistently underestimated systolic pressures by 10 to 15 mm Hg and was more closely correlated with mean arterial pressure. This study was performed only in anesthetized healthy cats, so limitations are present.[3]

The oscillometric method of blood pressure determination is commonly used in veterinary medicine. There are a number of different veterinary systems available. The cuff is alternately inflated and deflated, and during deflation alterations in cuff pressure due to pulse pressure changes are sensed by the transducer. The peak amplitude of oscillations equals the mean arterial pressure. Systolic pressure equals the pressure at which oscillations are first detected, and diastolic pressure equals the pressure at which oscillations decrease rapidly.

Oscillometric machines calculate systolic and diastolic blood pressure from the mean arterial pressure using built-in algorithms, so that the mean arterial pressure is the most accurate value. The heart rate is measured as the number of oscillations occurring per minute and should always be compared with the patient's heart rate as determined manually or by ECG. Many of the oscillometric units have been used in studies comparing systolic, mean, and diastolic pressures in anesthetized and awake dogs and cats with variable results, some of which showed acceptable correlation between values obtained with these units and direct arterial blood pressure measurements.[4-9] Later-generation units claim to be more accurate in smaller dogs and cats, but these claims have not held up in more recent studies. Poor agreement was seen using one oscillometric unit in anesthetized dogs compared with direct arterial blood pressure measurements.[10] Readings obtained using three different units were compared with direct arterial blood pressure measurements in anesthetized cats and had poor correlation.[11] Another study showed that pressures measured in awake, ill dogs using the Doppler method and two oscillometric units also were not well correlated with values obtained via direct arterial blood pressure monitoring.[12] Although none of the units currently available would meet validation criteria for humans, these units are readily available, are simpler to use and are associated with fewer potential complications than direct arterial blood pressure monitoring. The American College of Internal Medicine recently drafted a consensus statement on hypertension and proposed new validation recommendations for veterinary devices.[1]

High-definition oscillometry (HDO) is a newer modality for blood pressure monitoring in veterinary medicine. HDO devices are purported to have advantages over standard oscillometric monitors because HDO performs real-time analysis of arterial wall oscillations to obtain pressure-wave amplitudes, so systolic and diastolic pressures are measured instead of calculated. Other reported benefits include accurate readings of values from 5 to 300 mm Hg and high-speed analysis that allows for measurements at heart rates of up to 500 beats/min and during arrhythmias. However, recent studies have not shown good correlation with other blood pressure monitoring methods, although none compared HDO with direct arterial blood pressure monitoring.[13,14] More studies are needed to evaluate HDO, including studies comparing HDO results with values obtained via direct arterial blood pressure monitoring.

Photoplethysmography

Originally designed for use on the human finger, photoplethysmography is based on the "volume clamp" principle. The blood volume in an extremity varies in a cyclic pattern with each cardiac cycle. The variation is detected by a photoplethysmograph attached to a finger (or to the foot or tail in veterinary patients). If the cuff is inflated and deflated fast enough to maintain a constant volume in the finger (or distal extremity), the cuff pressure will equal intraarterial pressure. This allows for a constant, real-time display of cuff pressure, and therefore intraarterial pressure, and measurement of systolic and diastolic pressures.[15] Photoplethysmography has been evaluated in dogs and cats and found to be accurate, but has not come into common use.[3,8]

Invasive Blood Pressure Monitoring

Invasive or direct arterial blood pressure monitoring is considered the gold standard for blood pressure measurement in both veterinary and human patients, both awake and anesthetized. It is usually performed after inserting an arterial catheter that is connected to a pressure transducer and monitor, which allows for continuous monitoring of systolic, diastolic, and mean pressures. Techniques for direct arterial puncture and single-pressure measurement have also been described. See Chapter 201 for further details on placement of these catheters.

When a display monitor is employed, continuous direct arterial pressure monitoring allows for observation of pressure changes and trends (Figure 183-1). Another advantage of placing an arterial catheter is that it can be used to obtain blood samples for arterial blood gas analysis and laboratory testing. Despite its many advantages, direct monitoring should be limited to critically ill patients that will benefit from having blood pressure measured continuously over a defined period (e.g., during anesthesia in a patient with a high anesthetic risk or while hospitalized in an intensive care unit).

Direct arterial blood pressure monitoring in patients with hypovolemic or septic shock is extremely helpful in guiding volume replacement and the use of pressors to maintain an acceptable systemic blood pressure. By evaluating the pressure waveform with various arrhythmias, the clinician can distinguish which ones are causing poor pressures or even pulse deficits, and this can influence the decision to initiate treatment. Direct arterial blood pressure monitoring is not indicated in active, relatively healthy patients because of possible morbidity from arterial catheter placement and the risk of hemorrhage due to disconnection of the arterial line or premature removal by the patient. Animals with arterial catheters must be strictly supervised at all times.

Once an arterial catheter is placed, it is connected to semirigid tubing that has been primed with heparinized saline from a bag of 0.9% sodium chloride with 1 unit of heparin per milliliter of saline. The fluid bag is pressurized to 300 mm Hg to prevent backward flow of arterial blood into the tubing.[16] The tubing from the catheter is attached to a pressure transducer that is connected to a cable and mounted on a board placed at the level of the patient's heart. The pressure transducer converts the pressure changes into an electrical signal that is carried to the monitor by the transducer cable, and then the signal is amplified and displayed on a monitor as a pressure

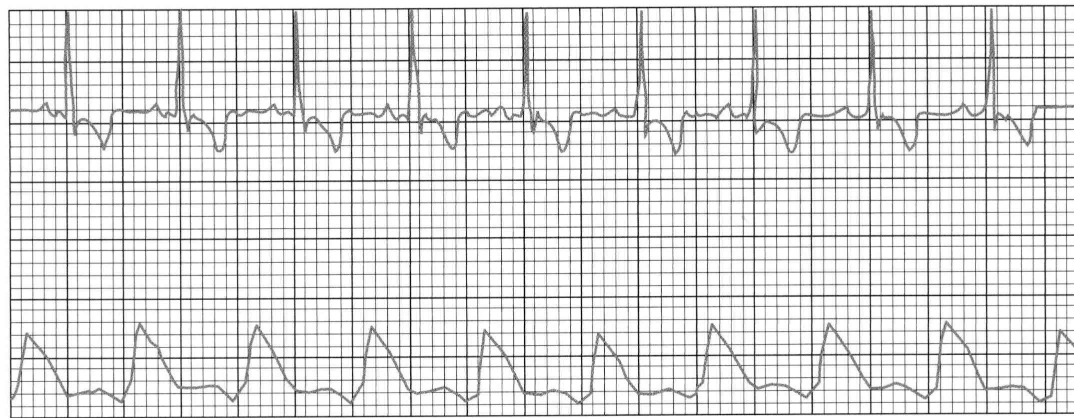

FIGURE 183-1 Direct arterial blood pressure waveform and continuous electrocardiogram. Note that one arterial pressure waveform is seen just after completion of each cardiac complex.

waveform showing the peak systolic pressure, dicrotic notch (which is created by closure of the aortic valve), and diastolic pressure. Monitors can also display numeric values for the systolic, diastolic, and mean arterial pressures.

Although direct arterial monitoring is considered the gold standard for blood pressure monitoring, it can give erroneous results if compliant tubing is used, the catheter is lodged up against the arterial wall, a clot forms at the tip of the catheter, air bubbles are present in the catheter or tubing, or the catheter or tubing becomes kinked. All of these problems can result in the waveform becoming damped, which gives falsely low systolic and falsely high diastolic values. Direct arterial blood pressure monitoring is associated with higher morbidity than noninvasive methods, including hematoma formation at the site of arterial puncture, infection, thrombosis of the artery, or necrosis of the tissues distal to the catheter (particularly in cats that have an indwelling catheter for longer than 6 to 12 hours). Keeping the arterial line patent requires heparinization of the line and catheter, which can be of concern in very small patients. Fortunately, all of the complications other than hematoma formation are quite rare.

Telemetric Blood Pressure Monitoring

Telemetric units are available for implantation into dogs and potentially cats (Data Sciences International, St. Paul, Minn.). These require surgical implantation of a transmitting device that sends digital information to a receiver; this information can then be either collected by a computer and evaluated later or converted into an analog signal for recording on a strip chart.

The device is placed subcutaneously and has a polyurethane catheter with an antithrombogenic coating and a biocompatible gel at the end that is fed into the femoral artery. This technology has been used in laboratory settings for a number of years and is currently used experimentally in both feline and canine patients. These devices allow for free patient movement and prevent the stress of handling and restraint from affecting the blood pressure measurements obtained. These devices are not used commonly in clinical patients but may be a viable option in the future for those that require long-term hospitalization or repeated blood pressure monitoring.

CENTRAL VENOUS PRESSURE MONITORING

CVP is the hydrostatic pressure in the intrathoracic vena cava and, in the absence of a vascular obstruction, is approximately equal to right atrial pressure. When the tricuspid valve is open, right atrial pressure equals right ventricular end-diastolic pressure. This pressure is used to estimate right ventricular end-diastolic volume and the relationship between blood volume and blood volume capacity. It also gives a measure of the relative ability of the heart to pump the volume of blood that is returned to it. Patients that most commonly benefit from CVP monitoring include those that are hypovolemic or have septic shock, heart disease, or renal disease (especially oliguric or anuric kidney injury).

CVP monitoring typically requires a central venous catheter, usually a 16-gauge or 19-gauge jugular catheter, but a femoral vein catheter that extends into the abdominal vena cava has been shown to measure CVP accurately in cats without significant intraabdominal disease[17] and in puppies.[18] The size of the catheter has no effect on measurement of CVP.[19] A study evaluating the correlation between peripheral venous pressure and CVP in awake dogs and cats found that peripheral venous pressure could not be used to approximate CVP.[20]

The tip of the catheter should be positioned in the cranial or caudal vena cava just outside of the right atrium. The catheter is then connected to a three-way stopcock via noncompliant tubing and to a manometer containing heparinized saline or to a pressure transducer as described earlier for direct arterial blood pressure monitoring. The central catheter can be used for CVP monitoring as well as fluid administration or intermittent blood sampling. However, if the CVP is to be monitored continuously and the patient requires additional venous access, a multilumen venous catheter should be placed so that the other ports remain available for fluid therapy, infusions, and blood sampling. Double-lumen and triple-lumen catheters are available in a variety of sizes and lengths (see Chapter 195).

When the central venous catheter is connected to the system, the zero reference point for the bottom of the manometer or the pressure transducer should be the manubrium for a patient in lateral recumbency or the point of the shoulder for a patient in sternal recumbency. Normal ranges for mean CVP are 0 to 5 cm H_2O, but they can vary in individual animals.[21] This makes trends in the CVP much more significant than individual readings. Values can be affected by patient position, so a consistent position should be used when comparing values. Catheter position also affects readings and can be confirmed by radiography or fluoroscopy.

A recent study evaluated the use of ultrasonographically measured hepatic vein diameter, caudal vena cava diameter, and hepatic venous flow velocities, which are multiphasic and correlate with changes in the cardiac cycle in Foxhounds. The investigators found that CVP could be predicted by a multiple linear regression equation using a combination of caudal vena cava diameter, hepatic vein diameter, and the velocity of the *v* wave (the small retrograde wave that occurs during right atrial overfilling near the end of the T wave of the ECG complex—see the later discussion of CVP waveform analysis).[22] This study was limited to Foxhounds that did not have a lot of variation in size; therefore it is difficult to know if this technique would be useful in other breeds or sizes of dogs.

The CVP varies throughout the respiratory and cardiac cycles because CVP reflects right atrial pressure. During inspiration, intrathoracic pressure decreases and the CVP falls. The reverse occurs during exhalation. If a patient has an upper airway obstruction and has difficulty inspiring, these changes will be exaggerated. Positive pressure ventilation will reverse this pattern.

The complexity of the CVP waveform can be seen when it is displayed on a monitor, and the variations that occur during the cardiac cycle can be observed (Figure 183-2, *A* and *B*). Three positive waves are seen, *a*, *c*, and *v* waves, and two negative depressions are seen, x and y descents. The *a* wave represents the increase in the CVP caused by right atrial contraction. The *c* wave is caused by bulging of the tricuspid valve into the right atrium, which increases right atrial pressure and CVP as the right ventricle contracts. The *x* descent is caused by the decrease in atrial pressure during ventricular ejection. The *v* wave is caused by increasing pressure from blood flowing into the right atrium before the tricuspid valve opens. The *y* descent represents rapid emptying of the right atrium as the tricuspid valve opens, allowing blood to flow into the right ventricle. Careful evaluation of the waveform allows abnormalities in each part of the cycle to be detected and differential diagnoses to be considered; for example, large *c* waves are often associated with tricuspid regurgitation.[23,24]

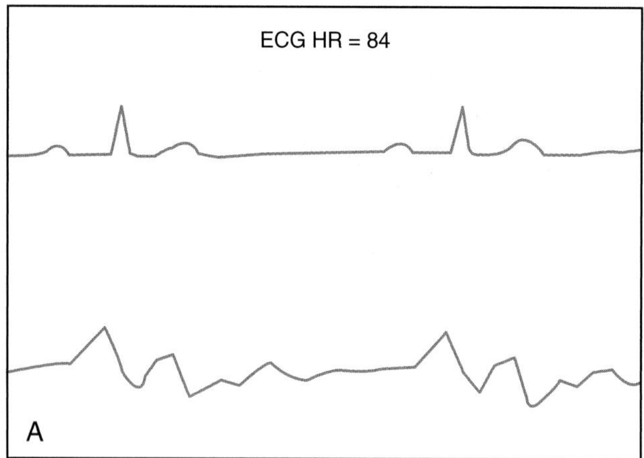

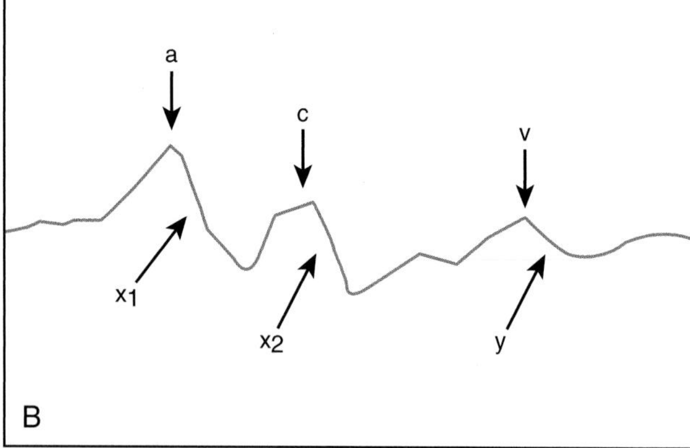

FIGURE 183-2 A, Central venous pressure (CVP) waveform and continuous electrocardiogram. Each phase of the cardiac cycle is reflected in the CVP waveform. **B,** CVP waveform with waves and depressions labeled. *a, a* wave, which represents the increase in the CVP caused by right atrial contraction; *c, c* wave, caused by bulging of the tricuspid valve into the right atrium; *v, v* wave, caused by increasing pressure from blood flowing into the right atrium before the tricuspid valve opens; x_I, x_I descent; x_2, x_2 descent, caused by decreased atrial pressure during ventricular ejection; *y, y* descent, which represents rapid emptying of the right atrium as the tricuspid valve opens.

A low CVP (<0 cm H_2O) indicates hypovolemia due to fluid loss or vasodilation secondary to decreased peripheral venous resistance. A high CVP (>10 cm H_2O) may indicate volume overload, right-sided heart failure, or significant pleural effusion.[25,26] CVP readings of higher than 16 cm H_2O often lead to edema formation or body cavity effusions. Some causes of right-sided cardiac dysfunction are right-sided myocardial failure, pericardial effusion and tamponade, restrictive pericarditis, and volume overload from excessive intravenous fluid administration.

If a CVP reading is questionable, a small test bolus of 10 to 15 ml/kg of an isotonic crystalloid or 5 ml/kg of a synthetic colloid may be given over 5 minutes or less (see Chapter 58). The vascular bed is a very compliant system, able to accommodate changes in volume with minimal changes in pressure. If the patient has a low CVP due to hypovolemia, the CVP will either show no change or will have a transient rise toward normal, then rapidly decrease again. The mean arterial pressure may also increase with the test bolus, then return toward prebolus measurements. A small increase of 2 to 4 cm H_2O with a return to baseline within 15 minutes is usually seen in euvolemic patients. A large increase (>4 cm H_2O) and slow return to baseline (>30 minutes) is seen in hypervolemic animals or those with reduced cardiac compliance.[26]

Contraindications for CVP measurement are few and relate to central venous catheter placement. These include coagulopathies that would make puncture of the jugular or femoral vein an unacceptable risk; high risk of thromboembolic disease, such as in animals with protein-losing nephropathy, hyperadrenocorticism, or immune-mediated disease; and suspicion of increased intracranial pressure, such as in patients with head trauma, seizures, or intracranial disease.

The biggest limitation of CVP monitoring is that it measures the pressures on the right side of the heart instead of the left side because it is the left side that supplies the systemic circulation and drains the pulmonary circulation. Pressures in the left side are more accurate in guiding fluid therapy, but their measurement requires use of a pulmonary artery catheter, which is much more expensive, risky, time consuming, and technically challenging. This makes CVP more readily available and acceptable as an alternative to PAP and pulmonary artery occlusion pressure (PAOP) monitoring.

PULMONARY ARTERY PRESSURE MONITORING

PAP monitoring requires that a catheter be placed in the jugular vein, through the right atrium and ventricle, and into the pulmonary artery. A pulmonary artery catheter allows for measurement of the systolic, diastolic, and mean PAP (see Chapter 202). If the catheter is equipped with a balloon, PAOP (also called the *pulmonary wedge pressure*) can be measured when the balloon at the end of the catheter is inflated in a distal branch of the pulmonary artery. Inflation of the balloon eliminates PAP created by blood flow, and the measured pressure reflects the left atrial filling pressure as it equilibrates across the pulmonary capillary bed.

When the mitral valve is open, left atrial pressure equals left ventricular end-diastolic pressure. This pressure provides the best measure of left ventricular preload and is the best predictor of pulmonary edema secondary to fluid overload. Preload is the amount of stretch in the ventricle at the end of diastole and is an important determinant of cardiac output.

Like CVP, PAP and PAOP can be used for (and are more accurate at) determining the fluid volume status of a patient. Normal PAOP in dogs is 5 to 12 mm Hg.[23] Low PAOP usually signals volume depletion and the need for fluid administration, whereas increased PAOP is indicative of volume overload or cardiac dysfunction so that additional fluid is contraindicated.

Additional parameters that can be monitored with a Swan-Ganz type of catheter are right atrial pressures (used in place of CVP), which are measured via the proximal port of the catheter, and cardiac output, which is determined using the thermodilution technique (thermodilution cardiac output). A known quantity of solution (either saline or 5% dextrose) at a known temperature is injected rapidly into the proximal port of the catheter. The cooler solution mixes and cools the surrounding blood, and the temperature difference is sensed by a thermistor at the distal tip of the catheter. The change in temperature is plotted on a time-temperature curve. The area under the curve is inversely proportional to the cardiac output, which is calculated by a cardiac output monitor. Normal values for cardiac output are 125 to 200 ml/kg/min for dogs and 120 ml/kg/min for cats.[27,28]

Other values that can be calculated include cardiac index (cardiac output ÷ body surface area in square meters), stroke volume (cardiac output ÷ heart rate), stroke volume index (stroke volume ÷ body surface area), systemic vascular resistance ([mean arterial pressure − right atrial pressure] ÷ cardiac index), and pulmonary vascular resistance ([mean PAP − PAOP] ÷ cardiac index).[28] Some catheters are also equipped with an oximeter that will measure central venous hemoglobin saturation (SvO_2). This information, combined with the arterial oxygen saturation (SaO_2), allows for determination of the oxygen content of both arterial and mixed venous blood, oxygen delivery, oxygen consumption, and oxygen extraction (see Chapters 184, 186, and 202).

Placement of these catheters is not without risk because arrhythmias, damage to the tricuspid and pulmonic valves, rupture of a pulmonary artery, and pulmonary thromboembolism have all been reported in humans undergoing the procedure.[29]

MIXED VENOUS AND CENTRAL VENOUS OXYGEN SATURATION

Measurement of SvO_2 (mixed venous oxygen saturation) and $ScvO_2$ (central venous oxygen saturation) is also useful for cardiovascular monitoring. SvO_2 is measured from the pulmonary artery, as mentioned earlier in the section on PAP monitoring, and therefore requires the placement of a catheter in the pulmonary artery. $ScvO_2$, which can be measured from a catheter in the vena cava or the right atrium, is much more accessible. Samples of blood can be removed via these catheters and analyzed with a co-oximeter or a fiberoptic fiber can be embedded in a centrally placed catheter and attached to a monitor for real-time measurements. The normal SvO_2 is greater than 75% and $ScvO_2$ is normally greater than 65%. Typically there is a very strong correlation between the two values, although they can differ by up to 18% in severe shock states.[30,31]

Tissue hypoxia causes increased extraction of oxygen from venous blood, which results in a decrease in both SvO_2 and $ScvO_2$. Increased venous oxygen extraction and resulting venous desaturation is one of the major compensatory responses to help maintain delivery of oxygen to the peripheral tissues in low flow states. Measurements of SvO_2 and $ScvO_2$ reflect systemic oxygen balance and cumulative oxygen debt.

The importance of measurement and optimization of $ScvO_2$ was highlighted in the Rivers et al study in 2001.[32] In this study, patients with severe sepsis or septic shock were treated according to an early goal-directed therapy (EGDT) protocol. One of the endpoints of resuscitation was a $ScvO_2$ of greater than 70%. The goals were to be met within the first 6 hours of therapy. The $ScvO_2$ was increased through the use of vasoactive agents, red blood cell transfusions, and inotropes, in addition to standard therapy. The EGDT group had a significantly lower mortality rate than the conventionally treated group.[32] The EGDT group also had reduced organ dysfunction and injury severity scores, as well as lower lactate concentrations and base deficits, additional values that can be useful in monitoring the cardiovascular status of critically ill patients (see later in chapter for details).

A recent veterinary study evaluated the use of tissue perfusion parameters as predictors of outcome in dogs with severe sepsis or septic shock. $ScvO_2$ and base deficit (see next section) were found to be the best discriminators between survivors and nonsurvivors.[33]

There are some limitations to the measurement of SvO_2 and $ScvO_2$. Both hemoglobin concentration and SaO_2 influence these variables. $ScvO_2$ is much easier to measure, but there can be a loss of correlation between $ScvO_2$ and SvO_2 in very-low-flow states. And finally, if there is an underlying defect in oxygen extraction, as often occurs in patients with severe sepsis, the SvO_2 and $ScvO_2$ values can be normal or even high despite significant oxygen debt.[30]

LACTATE AND BASE DEFICIT

Lactate is produced primarily in periods of insufficient oxygen delivery to the tissues, during anaerobic glycolysis. It is produced from pyruvate by lactate dehydrogenase in the cytosol of cells. When oxygen balance at the cellular level is restored, the process is reversed; and the lactate is used for regeneration of pyruvate, and aerobic metabolism within the mitochondria is resumed. Normally, the liver (and to lesser degree, the kidneys) clears any lactate that is produced, but blood levels increase when production exceeds clearance (see Chapter 56).

Lactate levels at presentation as well as lactate clearance after treatment have been evaluated for prognostic value extensively in humans and to a lesser degree in veterinary patients.[30] Response to therapy, particularly fluid resuscitation, has been shown to have predictive value in humans with trauma and severe sepsis or septic shock. The base deficit has also been evaluated as a marker of anaerobic metabolism. In human studies, patients with persistently high base deficit have higher rates of multiple organ failure and death compared with patients whose base deficit normalizes. The use of lactate and base deficit together may be most helpful in assessing a patient's need for fluid resuscitation and response to fluid therapy. A recent study found that a lower base deficit at presentation was associated with greater survival in dogs with sepsis or septic shock secondary to pyometra.[33] As noted earlier, $ScvO_2$ and base deficit were found to be the best discriminators between survivors and nonsurvivors; lactate level was measured but did not prove useful in this study.[33] Additional studies are needed to prospectively evaluate the outcome prediction utility of lactate and base deficit response to volume resuscitation in dogs and cats.

REFERENCES

1. Brown S, Atkins C, Bagley R, et al: Guidelines for the identification, evaluation, and management of systemic hypertension in dogs and cats, J Vet Intern Med 21:542, 2007.
2. Valtonen MH, Eriksson LM: The effect of cuff width on accuracy of indirect measurement of blood pressure in dogs, Res Vet Sci 11:358, 1970.
3. Caulkett NA, Cantwell SL, Houston DM: A comparison of indirect blood pressure monitoring techniques in the anesthetized cat, Vet Surg 27:370, 1998.
4. Bodey AR, Young LE, Diamond MJ, et al: A comparison of direct and indirect (oscillometric) measurements of arterial blood pressure in anaesthetized dogs, using tail and limb cuffs, Res Vet Sci 57:265, 1994.
5. Bodey AR, Michell AR, Bovee KC, et al: Comparison of direct and indirect (oscillometric) measurements of arterial blood pressure in conscious dogs, Res Vet Sci 61:17, 1996.

6. Stepien RL, Rapoport GS: Clinical comparison of three methods to measure clinical blood pressure in nonsedated dogs, J Am Vet Med Assoc 215:1623, 1999.
7. Meurs KM, Miller MW, Slater MR: Comparison of the indirect oscillometric and direct arterial methods for blood pressure measurements in anesthetized dogs, J Am Anim Hosp Assoc 32:471, 1996.
8. Binns SH, Sisson DD, Buoscio DA, et al: Doppler ultrasonographic, oscillometric sphygmomanometric, and photoplethysmographic techniques for noninvasive blood pressure measurement in anesthetized cats, J Vet Intern Med 9:405, 1995.
9. Pedersen KM, Butler MA, Ersboll AK, et al: Evaluation of an oscillometric blood pressure monitor for use in anesthetized cats, J Am Vet Med Assoc 221:646, 2002.
10. Acierno MJ, Fauth E, Mitchell MA, et al: Measuring the level of agreement between directly measured blood pressure and pressure readings obtained with a veterinary-specific oscillometric unit in anesthetized dogs, J Vet Emerg Crit Care 23:37, 2013.
11. Acierno MJ, Seaton D, Mitchell MA, et al: Agreement between directly measured blood pressure and pressures obtained with three veterinary-specific oscillometric units in cats, J Am Vet Med Assoc 237:402, 2010.
12. Bosiack AP, Mann FA, Dodson JE, et al: Comparison of ultrasonic Doppler flow monitor, oscillometric and direct arterial blood pressure measurements in ill dogs, J Vet Emerg Crit Care 20:207, 2010.
13. Petric AD, Petra Z, Jerneja S, et al: Comparison of high definition oscillometric and Doppler ultrasonic devices for measuring blood pressure in anaesthetised cats, J Feline Med Surg 12:731, 2010.
14. Chetboul V, Tissier R, Gouni V, et al: Comparison of Doppler ultrasonography and high-definition oscillometry for blood pressure measurements in healthy awake dogs, Am J Vet Res 71:766, 2010.
15. Farquhar IK: Continuous direct and indirect blood pressure measurement (Finapres) in the critically ill, Anaesthesia 46:1050, 1991.
16. Burkitt Greedon JM, Raffe MR: Fluid-filled hemodynamic monitoring systems. In Burkitt Creedon JM, Davis H, editors: Advanced monitoring and procedures for small animal emergency and critical care, Ames, Ia, 2012, Wiley-Blackwell.
17. Machon RG, Raffe MR, Robinson EP: Central venous pressure measurements in the caudal vena cava of sedated cats, J Vet Emerg Crit Care 5:121, 1995.
18. Berg RA, Lloyd TR, Donnerstein RL: Accuracy of central venous pressure monitoring in the intraabdominal inferior vena cava: a canine study, J Pediatr 120:67, 1992.
19. Oakley RE, Olivier B, Eyster GE, et al: Experimental evaluation of central venous pressure monitoring in the dog, J Am Anim Hosp Assoc 33:77, 1997.
20. Chow RS, Kass PH, Haskins SC: Evaluation of peripheral and central venous pressure in awake dogs and cats, Am J Vet Res 67:1987, 2006.
21. Jennings PB, Anderson RW, Martin AM: Central venous pressure monitoring: a guide to blood volume replacement in the dog, J Am Vet Med Assoc 151:1283, 1967.
22. Nelson NC, Drost WT, Lerche P, et al: Noninvasive estimation of central venous pressure in anesthetized dogs by measurement of hepatic venous blood flow velocity and abdominal venous diameter, Vet Radiol Ultrasound 51:313, 2010.
23. De Laforcade AM, Rozanski EA: Central venous pressure and arterial blood pressure measurements, Vet Clin North Am Small Anim Pract 31:1163, 2001.
24. Ahrens TS, Taylor LA: Hemodynamic waveform analysis, Philadelphia, 1992, Saunders.
25. Gookin JL, Atkins CE: Evaluation of the effect of pleural effusion on central venous pressure in cats, J Vet Intern Med 13:561, 1999.
26. Hansen B: Technical aspects of fluid therapy. In DiBartola SP, editor: Fluid, electrolyte, and acid-base disorders in small animal practice, ed 4, St Louis, 2012, Saunders.
27. Haskins S, Pascoe PJ, Ilkiw JE, et al: Reference cardiopulmonary values in normal dogs, Comp Med 55:156, 2005.
28. Mellema M: Cardiac output, wedge pressure, and oxygen delivery, Vet Clin North Am Small Anim Pract 31:1175, 2001.
29. Headley JM: Invasive hemodynamic monitoring: physiological principles and clinical applications, Irvine, Calif, 2002, Edwards Scientific.
30. Prittie J: Optimal endpoints of resuscitation and early goal-directed therapy, J Vet Emerg Crit Care 16:329, 2006.
31. Reinhart K, Kuhn HJ, Hartog C, et al: Continuous central venous and pulmonary artery oxygen saturation monitoring in the critically ill, Intensive Care Med 30:1572, 2004.
32. Rivers E, Nguyen B, Havstad S, et al: Early goal-directed therapy in the treatment of severe sepsis and septic shock, N Engl J Med 19:1368, 2001.
33. Conti-Patara A, de Araújo Caldeira J, de Mattos-Junior E, et al: Changes in tissue perfusion parameters in dogs with severe sepsis/septic shock in response to goal-directed hemodynamic optimization at admission to ICU and the relation to outcome, J Vet Emerg Crit Care 22:409, 2012.

CHAPTER 184
CARDIAC OUTPUT MONITORING

Matthew S. Mellema, DVM, PhD, DACVECC • Robin L. McIntyre, DVM

KEY POINTS

- Cardiac output is the volume of blood transferred by the heart to the systemic circulation over time.
- It is a key determinant of oxygen delivery and an early indicator of hemodynamic instability.
- Cardiac output should be measured in any patient for which appropriate clinical decisions cannot be made without this information.
- Both invasive and minimally invasive methods of cardiac output measurement are available for clinical use in dogs and cats.
- Disease states can have a profound and complex impact on cardiac output.
- Complications of pulmonary artery catheters are rare, but placement should be done either by, or under the supervision of, experienced personnel.

Delivery of oxygen to the body and the removal of cellular metabolic waste are the fundamental roles of the cardiovascular and pulmonary systems. To accomplish these vital functions the pulmonary and cardiovascular systems must work in concert in a complex yet deeply integrated fashion. Each system relies on a pumping mechanism to accomplish the transport of blood or respiratory gases to the sites where the exchange of substrates and waste occurs.

In the case of the cardiovascular system, the heart provides the pumping force and the blood vessels serve to conduct and distribute the pumped blood to the tissues. The elastic properties of the vascular tree allow the force generated by the heart to be stored and applied to the column of flowing blood throughout the cardiac cycle. The volume of blood transferred to the systemic circulation over time is termed *cardiac output.* Cardiac output in humans is typically measured in liters per minute (L/min). Veterinary patients come in a broad range of shapes and sizes, and for this reason, cardiac output is often referenced in terms of milliliters of blood per kilogram of body weight per minute (ml/kg/min). Technically, this is a form of cardiac index because the values are being normalized (or indexed) to body mass; however, the term *cardiac output* is more generally applied to this parameter. Normal values for dogs and cats typically range from 120 to 200 ml/kg/min.[1,2] A related measure is formally called *cardiac index* and relates the volume of blood pumped over time to the animal's body surface area rather than body mass because the former is thought to correlate with metabolic rate (a principal determinant of cardiac output). The cardiac index is expressed in liters per minute per square meters (L/min/m^2).[2] The term *combined cardiac output* is used to describe the total volume of blood ejected into the systemic circulation over time when both the right and left ventricles can directly transfer blood to the arterial tree (e.g., fetal circulation, right-to-left patent ductus arteriosus).

Cardiac output is an important measure of cardiovascular function. It provides insights into bulk blood delivery to the body as a whole. When taken together with measurements of the oxygen content of blood, it allows for the determination of whole body oxygen delivery.[1,2] If one knows the patient's heart rate, then knowledge of cardiac output allows the clinician to determine stroke volume. Cardiac output measurements also make it possible for the caregiver to determine important physiologic indicators such as intrapulmonary shunt, systemic and pulmonary vascular resistance, and oxygen consumption. This large array of additional parameters that can be derived once cardiac output is known allow the clinician to potentially make better informed decisions about the need for, or adequacy of, therapeutic interventions and provides a more detailed picture of the patient's cardiovascular status.

INDICATIONS FOR CARDIAC OUTPUT MEASUREMENT

When performed by an experienced and attentive clinician, physical examination of the patient can reveal a great deal about the adequacy of oxygen delivery and cardiac output. Many of the findings of the physical examination relate directly to regional or organ-specific blood flow (e.g., capillary refill time, pulse pressure, mentation). Although these physical examination parameters are invaluable in the repeated assessment of patients and require little more equipment than a wristwatch, some are subjective measures and correlate poorly with an individual patient's actual cardiovascular status.[3] However, it must be noted that although an individual value for capillary refill time, for example, may correlate poorly with more direct measures of cardiac output, the trends in serial physical examination findings in an individual patient typically provide the best and most reliable measure of alterations in that patient's cardiovascular status. Unfortunately, the converse is not true: a patient whose physical examination findings are not changing may be experiencing a decline in cardiac performance that will not be detectable until compensatory mechanisms are exhausted or overcome.

The findings of a thorough physical examination, particularly when complemented with hemodynamic monitoring (see Chapter 183), are sufficient to guide the clinician in directing the care of most patients. However, there exists a subset of critically ill veterinary patients in which more direct assessment of cardiac output (and its derived parameters) is essential for proper case management. Patients with sepsis, septic shock, systemic inflammatory response syndrome, and multiple organ dysfunction syndrome make up the bulk of veterinary patients for which more invasive measures of cardiac output are likely to be required. In patients with severe compromise of the pulmonary or cardiovascular system cardiac output monitoring may also be required to optimize their care. It is in the care of these patients that clinicians may find themselves unable to make appropriate decisions regarding management without the additional information provided via cardiac output monitoring.

In patients with complex disease states such as those mentioned earlier, the individual's cardiovascular and pulmonary systems may be compromised to such an extent that the typical measures of cardiovascular status and performance give contradictory information and suggest therapies that have opposing mechanisms of action (e.g., expanding or depleting extracellular fluid volume). An all-too-common example is a septic patient that has developed capillary leak syndrome (enhanced permeability of systemic capillaries and venules, promoting tissue edema). This patient typically has a low central venous or mean arterial pressure, or both (which suggests that additional intravenous fluid therapy might be of benefit), while at the same time exhibiting marked peripheral edema (which might lead the clinician to want to be less aggressive with fluid administration). The treatment of such a patient would be enhanced by knowledge of cardiac output and oxygen delivery, which are always of primary importance and can mandate a course of action in the face of conflicting findings. Cardiac output can also be a much earlier indicator of deteriorating cardiovascular status because compensatory mechanisms such as reflex vasoconstriction can maintain other indicators like mean arterial pressure near normal levels in the face of worsening cardiac performance.

MEASUREMENT OF CARDIAC OUTPUT

Invasive Methods of Determining Cardiac Output

Nearly all invasive techniques for measuring cardiac output rely on one of two methods: the Fick oxygen consumption method or the indicator dilution method. The commonly used thermodilution method is, in principle, a modification of the indicator dilution method using thermal energy as the indicator. Both methods are discussed here.[4]

Fick oxygen consumption method

The Fick oxygen consumption method is considered the gold standard and is the oldest method of measuring cardiac output. This technique relies on the Fick principle, which states that the total uptake (or release) of a substance by the peripheral tissues is equal to the product of the blood flow to the peripheral tissues and the arteriovenous concentration difference (gradient) of the substance. For a substance that is taken up by the tissues (such as oxygen), the Fick principle says in effect that "what went in minus what came out must equal what was left behind." The Fick principle when applied to cardiac output and oxygen uptake can be expressed as follows:

$$\text{Cardiac output} = \frac{\text{Oxygen consumption}}{\text{Arteriovenous oxygen content difference}}$$

When one uses the original Fick method to determine cardiac output, oxygen consumption is determined by measuring the oxygen concentration difference in the inhaled air and the exhaled air collected from the patient over time (typically 3 minutes). Alternatively, the arteriovenous oxygen content difference can be determined by measuring the oxygen content of both an arterial and a mixed venous blood sample. Although oxygen content analyzers are available, it is more typical for the clinician to measure the oxygen partial pressure (PO_2), hemoglobin saturation (SO_2), and hemoglobin concentration ([Hb]) with a blood gas analyzer and manually calculate oxygen content using the following formula:

$$\text{Oxygen content} = ([\text{Hb}] \times 1.36 \times SO_2) + (0.003 \times PO_2)$$

The principal drawbacks to this approach in veterinary medicine are that it is not a continuous real-time measure of cardiac output and that reliable collection of respiratory gases requires that the patient be intubated. In addition, use of the Fick method relies on the patient's remaining in a stable hemodynamic and metabolic state throughout the period of gas or blood collection; thus the less stable the patient's condition, the less reliable this method becomes. Lastly, results obtained by the Fick method are largely invalid in the presence of significant intracardiac or intrapulmonary shunting of blood.

Carbon dioxide rebreathing methods

The Fick equation can be used to determine cardiac output using carbon dioxide production rather than oxygen uptake. There are two methods, the complete rebreathing technique and the partial rebreathing technique. The following equation is used to calculate cardiac output using the complete rebreathing technique:

$$\text{Cardiac output} = \frac{CO_2 \text{ elimination by the lungs}}{\text{Arteriovenous } CO_2 \text{ difference}}$$

This technique requires breathholding and does not provide continuous measurements.

A monitor has been developed for the partial rebreathing technique (NICO). The partial rebreathing technique combines measurements obtained during a nonrebreathing period with values obtained during a rebreathing period. The following equation is used:

$$\text{Cardiac output} = \frac{\text{Difference in } CO_2 \text{ elimination and end-tidal } CO_2}{\text{Difference in arterial } CO_2 \text{ between baseline and rebreathing phase}}$$

The monitor is connected to a flow and carbon dioxide sensor and an adjustable dead-space breathing loop in the circuit between the patient and the Y piece. The monitor controls a valve that diverts gas flow through the breathing loop during the rebreathing phase. Values for cardiac output are determined every 3 minutes. This method measures only the pulmonary capillary blood flow that participates in gas exchange and calculates the shunt fraction. Values obtained using the NICO monitor have been shown to compare well with those obtained using the lithium dilution method in dogs; however, lower tidal volumes such as those used in lung-protective ventilation strategies have been shown to promote underestimation of cardiac output by partial rebreathing methods compared with the thermodilution technique.[1] The NICO monitor may not provide an accurate determination of cardiac output in smaller dogs.[2] The size of the rebreathing circuit also limits the use of the device in dogs and cats.

Indicator dilution method (including thermodilution)

In actuality, the indicator dilution method is simply an adaptation of the Fick method using indicators that are more easily collected and measured than elemental oxygen. The basis still lies in the Fick principle and conservation of matter (or thermal energy).

In this method an exogenous indicator is injected into the patient's mixed venous blood via a pulmonary artery catheter[5] (see Chapter 202), and the dilution of the indicator is followed continuously until both the original concentration peak associated with injection and a secondary peak due to recirculation are observed. By plotting the concentration of the indicator against time, one can obtain the area under the curve of the concentration versus time plot. Cardiac output is determined by taking the known amount of indicator and dividing it by the area under the curve. Typically this process is an integrated function of the software packages included with modern cardiac monitoring equipment. In the laboratory setting the indicator maybe a dye such as indocyanine green; however, this method is seldom used in clinical patients.

The indicator of choice is often thermal energy. Modern pulmonary artery catheters can be equipped with a sensitive thermocouple that can give highly accurate continuous measurements of blood temperature. This type of pulmonary artery catheter has been termed a *Swan-Ganz catheter* after the physicians who developed it and introduced it into clinical practice in human medicine.

Although the technology has advanced, the technique still relies on the Fick principle. By injecting a known volume of saline at a known temperature (typically room temperature; chilling is no longer needed with modern catheters) into the right-sided circulation, one can use the thermocouple to follow the dilution of this cool sample in the larger, warmer blood volume of the patient. Integration of this temperature signal can provide the clinician with a reliable measure of cardiac output. Recorded values are usually the average of three measurements taken in a short time, one after another. Good agreement is considered to be values that do not vary by more than 10%.

In thermodilution, the indicator is injected into the right atrium and dilution is measured in the pulmonary artery. Dye dilution is performed by injecting dye into the pulmonary artery and measuring the dilution at an arterial site. Transpulmonary thermodilution uses a central venous catheter and a thermistor that is inserted into the femoral artery. This method is potentially as accurate as using a pulmonary artery catheter, and studies in human patients have shown good agreement between the two in the values obtained.[3]

Advances in ion-specific electrode technology have led to novel means of applying indicator dilution principles to determine cardiac output in humans and animals. One such advance is the development of an electrode for lithium ions that can be placed in communication with the patient's arterial bloodstream via an indwelling arterial catheter. Such an electrode can be used to record the dilution of small doses of lithium chloride injected into the venous circulation at either a peripheral or central site. Cardiac output determination by this method has been studied in both dogs and cats, and agreement with cardiac output values obtained via thermodilution methods has generally been good.[6,7] Although the lithium dilution method for determining cardiac output can be termed *minimally invasive,* it is not truly noninvasive because it requires placement of both venous and arterial catheters.

Placement of pulmonary arterial catheters is not a benign procedure, and indications for pulmonary artery catheterization in human patients are controversial. In a large population of critically ill patients, pulmonary artery catheterization was associated with increased 30-day mortality, increased cost of health care, and a longer hospital stay.[4] Another large study found no benefit to therapy directed by pulmonary artery catheter data over standard care.[5] A Cochrane Database systematic review of pulmonary artery catheterization found no difference in mortality or length of stay in critically ill or surgical patients, but it did find increased health care costs associated with pulmonary artery catheterization.[6]

Noninvasive or Minimally Invasive Methods of Determining Cardiac Output

No consensus for pulmonary artery catheter use exists in veterinary medicine. Noninvasive or minimally invasive methods of measuring cardiac output have been developed due to concerns about complications and reliability of pulmonary artery catheterization. Techniques include transesophageal echocardiography, pulse contour analysis, and thoracic bioimpedance.

Transesophageal echocardiography has been used in humans and a number of animal species as a minimally invasive means of tracking changes in cardiac output and performance. Measurement of blood velocity (using Doppler frequency shifts) and aortic diameter (using echocardiography) allow estimates of stroke volume to be made. To obtain truly reliable and quantifiable measurements of cardiac output, one should initially (and periodically) calibrate transesophageal echocardiography measurements against measurements obtained by one of the more invasive methods discussed earlier. In studies involving anesthetized dogs, results using this method are mixed compared with results using thermodilution.[2,7] The utility of this method is also somewhat limited in small animal practice because of equipment limitations, the time required to obtain acceptable studies, patient tolerance of the probe, and the need for highly trained personnel to be on hand to make the measurements. However, it does hold promise in limited applications (e.g., evaluation and monitoring of anesthetized patients).

Measurement of thoracic electrical bioimpedance is a noninvasive method of evaluating changes in the conductivity of the thorax resulting from the pulsatile flow of blood within the thoracic cavity. Sets of electrodes similar to electrocardiograph electrodes are located superficially on the thorax. Although electrocardiograph electrodes simply measure voltage changes resulting from the intrinsic electrical activity of the heart, the electrodes used in the thoracic electrical bioimpedance method both measure and apply voltage. The principle behind the method is Ohm's law, according to which the conductivity (and impedance) of the thorax to the flow of current can be determined by applying a small known voltage to the patient's thorax and then measuring what portion of that initial voltage reaches a distant sensing electrode. Changes in thoracic blood volume (blood and tissue are good conductors, air-filled lungs are not) can be detected, and estimates of stroke volume and cardiac output can be made using computer algorithms. Although this method holds promise in humans, in whom the size and shape of the thorax are somewhat uniform, the variety of species and breeds seen by the small animal clinician may make any single algorithm of limited utility, and estimates may need to be compared with some frequency with results obtained using invasive methods.

Analysis of the arterial pressure waveform, or pulse contour analysis, is an additional form of algorithm-dependent monitoring and can allow real-time determination of cardiac output. Some computers using this technology require calibration before use (PiCCO and PiCCO *plus*) and some do not (FloTrac). Transpulmonary thermodilution (PiCCO, PiCCO *plus*) or lithium dilution (PulsCO/LidCO) is used for the initial calibration, and the PulsCO/LidCO system requires calibration every 8 hours. Determination of cardiac output by transpulmonary thermodilution requires a central venous catheter in addition to an arterial catheter. Once the system has been calibrated, heart rate, area under the curve, aortic compliance, and shape of the pressure curve are used to calculate cardiac output for each pulse waveform. There was good correlation between PiCCO *plus* determinations and cardiac output as assessed by an aortic flow probe in a canine model of hemorrhagic shock.[1] In dogs that have anesthesia-induced hypotension or have rapid changes in cardiac output, the PulsCO system does not accurately predict cardiac output compared with the lithium dilution method.[8,9] A potential disadvantage of the pulse contour analysis approach is that the manufacturers of these monitoring devices often advise that central arterial (aortic) waveforms be monitored rather than peripheral arterial waveforms. In a small animal patient this would generally be achieved by advancing a long catheter into the aorta from a femoral artery insertion site. Any device that requires this more labor-intensive form of achieving arterial access is likely to be used less frequently than those for which peripheral arterial access is known to be sufficient for accurate readings.

NORMAL VALUES

The normal values for cardiac output (and related and derived indexes) for dogs and cats are presented in Table 184-1. Values other than cardiac output and cardiac index are given for the reader's consideration but are discussed in greater detail elsewhere (see Chapters 183 and and 202). The normal values listed in Table 184-1 represent composite values obtained from the literature and measurements made on clinical patients and research animals at the School of Veterinary Medicine at the University of California, Davis.[2] These composites include values from animals that were sedated as well as lightly anesthetized animals. Values for fully awake animals might be considered true "normal" values but would not represent normal values for the setting in which clinical measurements are generally obtained.

POTENTIAL CAUSES OF ERROR

Any form of measurement of any parameter carries an intrinsic degree of error. It is the responsibility of the clinician and the nursing staff to avoid compounding this form of uncertainty by introducing additional sources of error (Table 184-2). To this end, clinicians seeking to measure cardiac output using any of the techniques discussed earlier should ensure that they have been trained by

Table 184-1 **Normal Cardiopulmonary Values for Dogs and Cats**

Parameter (Unit)	Dog	Cat
Heart rate (beats/min)	100-140	110-140
Mean arterial pressure (mm Hg)	80-120	100-150
Cardiac output (ml/kg/min)	125-200	120
Cardiac index (L/min/m^2)	3.5-5.5	—
Stroke volume (ml/beat/kg)	40-60	—
Systemic vascular resistance (mm Hg/ml/kg/min)	0.5-0.8	—
Mean pulmonary artery pressure (mm Hg)	10-20	—
Pulmonary vascular resistance (mm Hg/ml/kg/min)	0.04-0.06	—
Central venous pressure (cm H_2O)	0-10	—
Pulmonary artery wedge pressure (mm Hg)	5-12	—
Oxygen delivery (ml/kg/min)	20-35	—
Oxygen consumption (ml/kg/min)	4-11	3-8
Oxygen extraction (%)	20-30	—

Table 184-2 Sources of Error in Cardiac Output Measurement (Thermodilution Method)

Error Source	Brief Description	Adjustments
Respiratory cycle	Pulmonary artery blood cools during inspiration. Venous return varies with intrathoracic pressure.	Make measurements at end expiration.
Arrhythmias	Arrhythmias cause rapid and marked variations in stroke volume.	Treat arrhythmias as indicated.
Altered intracardiac flow	Shunting and regurgitation can cause some of the injectate to bypass the thermistor or delay arrival of some of the bolus volume.	Thermodilution technique may be invalid in patients with significant flow abnormalities.
Low cardiac output	Slow ejection causes warming of the injectate before it reaches the thermistor.	Further therapeutic interventions will be required to increase cardiac output before values will be valid or repeatable.
Injectate factors	Injectate may be the wrong solution, wrong volume, wrong temperature.	Triple-check all aspects of the bolus before injecting.
Thermistor factors	Thrombus may form on the catheter tip. Catheter may migrate. Catheter may be defective.	Check position and reposition or replace catheter as needed.
Additional infusions	Simultaneous infusion of large volumes of crystalloid or colloid solutions can interfere with thermistor detection of the bolus.	Either interrupt the fluid bolus or postpone cardiac output measurements as dictated by patient's needs.

experienced personnel and have suitable hands-on experience with the method before using it in clinical decision making. Misuse of data from Swan-Ganz catheters by insufficiently trained personnel has on occasion led to iatrogenic injury and poor outcomes, and subsequently the devices have fallen out of favor in some segments of human medicine.

All of the methods for measuring cardiac output that have been discussed rely on the patient's having stable hemodynamics throughout the study period (typically several minutes). In the case of the Fick method, reliable measurements also require that the patient have only small fluctuations in metabolic rate during the study period. With each of the methods discussed, the serial evaluation of measurements is of greater use than any single determination.

DISEASE STATES AND CARDIAC OUTPUT MEASUREMENT

Cardiac output is the product of stroke volume and heart rate. Disease processes that alter either of these factors may alter cardiac output (unless the disease affects both in opposite directions and to equal degrees). Decreasing heart rates may either improve or worsen cardiac output depending on the individual patient. Patients with stiff, noncompliant ventricles or tachyarrhythmias, for example, may benefit from a reduction in heart rate because of greater filling during diastole. Alternatively, a patient with advanced atrioventricular node disease may have reduced cardiac output due to low (ventricular) heart rate. The relationship between heart rate and stroke volume is complex. Moderate increases in heart rate can increase stroke volume via the "staircase effect," whereas greater increases in heart rate may instead reduce stroke volume via impairment of diastolic filling.

Generally, any condition that reduces stroke volume reduces cardiac output if heart rate changes are minimal. Stroke volume is determined by preload, afterload, and contractility. Preload is determined largely by cardiac compliance and filling pressures. Any disease state that reduces filling pressures (e.g., hemorrhage, dehydration) or ventricular compliance (e.g., pericardial tamponade) can reduce preload and cardiac output. Afterload is a complex determinant of stroke volume and is largely dependent on the tone of the vasculature (particularly arterioles) and compliance of the aorta, but in some patients it is influenced by physical abnormalities in the cardiovascular system (e.g., aortic stenosis, arteriovenous fistulas) or the rheology of the blood itself (e.g., hyperviscosity syndromes).

Any process that increases afterload may reduce cardiac output (e.g., α-adrenergic stimulation), and processes that reduce afterload (e.g., reduced blood viscosity, arteriolar dilation) may increase cardiac output. Contractility is a measure of the myocardium's intrinsic ability to generate force and eject blood independent of loading conditions. Contractility may, for example, be depressed by circulating mediators (e.g., sepsis, pancreatitis) or enhanced by β-adrenergic stimulation. Any alteration in a patient's cardiac output should prompt a careful consideration of how disease states may be altering heart rate, preload, afterload, and contractility. Factors known to adversely affect these determinants of cardiac output should be addressed whenever possible.

POTENTIAL COMPLICATIONS

The vast majority of patients in which cardiac output measurements are made experience no direct complications due to the instrumentation or procedures required. However, many complications can occur when hemodynamic data are misinterpreted, and this issue has been discussed earlier in the chapter. A small subset of patients in which Swan-Ganz or other pulmonary artery catheters are placed will experience complications related to the placement, presence, or maintenance of the catheter.[8] These complications include, but are not limited to, the following: catheter-related sepsis, pulmonary artery rupture, damage to cardiac structures, catheter knotting (possibly requiring thoracotomy), hemorrhage, and embolization. For these reasons and others, it is stressed that pulmonary artery catheter placement is not a technique to be learned without the guidance of experienced personnel.

Complications from lithium chloride injection have not been reported in dogs or cats. The other methods of cardiac output determination discussed earlier also are considered to have a very large margin of safety.

REFERENCES

1. Brown AJ: Cardiac output monitoring, MDR notes. Proceedings of the International Veterinary Emergency and Critical Care Symposium, 2008, Phoenix, AZ.

2. Yamashita K, Miyoshi K, Igarashi R, et al: Minimally invasive determination of cardiac output by transthoracic bioimpedance, partial carbon dioxide rebreathing, and transesophageal Doppler echocardiography in beagle dogs, J Vet Med Sci 69(1):43-47, 2007.
3. Busse L, Davison DL, Junker C, et al: Hemodynamic monitoring in the critical care environment, Adv Chronic Kidney Dis 20(1):21-29, 2013.
4. Connors AF Jr, Speroff T, Dawson NG, et al: The effectiveness of right heart catheterization in the initial care of critically ill patients. SUPPORT investigators, JAMA 276:889-897, 1996.
5. Sandham JD, Hull RD, Brant RF, et al: A randomized, controlled trial of the use of pulmonary-artery catheters in high-risk surgical patients, N Engl J Med 348:5-14, 2003.
6. Harvey S, Young D, Brampton W, et al: Pulmonary artery catheters for adult patients in intensive care, Cochrane Database Syst Rev (3):CD003408, 2006.
7. Scansen BA, Bonagura JD, Schober KE, et al: Evaluation of a commercial ultrasonographic hemodynamic recording system for the measurement of cardiac output in dogs, Am J Vet Res 70(7):862-868, 2009.
8. Cooper ES, Muir WW: Continuous cardiac output monitoring via arterial pressure waveform analysis following severe hemorrhagic shock in dogs, Crit Care Med 35(7):1724-1729, 2007.
9. Cheng HC, Sinclair MD, Dyson DH, et al: Comparison of arterial pressure waveform analysis with the lithium dilution technique to monitor cardiac output in anesthetized dogs, Am J Vet Res 66:1430-1436, 2005.

CHAPTER 185
ELECTROCARDIOGRAM EVALUATION

Matthew S. Mellema, DVM, PhD, DACVECC

KEY POINTS

- The electrocardiogram (ECG) is an extremely useful and cost-effective monitoring tool.
- ECG monitoring is indicated for nearly all critically ill patients.
- Rather than a limited study of multiple leads, continuous monitoring of a single lead is the basis of most ECG monitoring in the critically ill patient.
- Interpretation of the ECG should be systematic and thorough to gain the most benefit from its use.
- Trends in ECG alterations may alert the clinician to changes in the patient's condition even when the absolute values of the parameters still fall within the normal ranges.
- Electrolyte abnormalities, hypoxemia, effusions, and pain may cause acute detectable ECG changes without necessarily altering the underlying rhythm.

Disorders of cardiac rhythm and conduction are encountered frequently in critically ill veterinary patients. Arrhythmias may be encountered in patients with primary cardiac disease or may be one manifestation of systemic illness. The severity of rhythm and conduction disturbances can range from inconsequential to acutely life threatening and can progress rapidly from one extreme to the other in some patients.

The electrocardiogram (ECG) is the diagnostic and monitoring tool used to confirm, detect, and define cardiac conduction and rhythm disturbances. In addition, the ECG provides the clinician with continuous real-time data regarding the patient's heart rate and rhythm, which can be informative even in the absence of gross abnormalities. Moreover, the ECG provides clinicians with real-time, continuous information regarding the balance between adrenergic and cholinergic efferent inputs to the heart, and thus insights into the status of the autonomic nervous system can be gained as well. This chapter focuses on the use of the ECG as a monitoring tool. For details on the recognition and treatment of specific cardiac rhythm disorders the reader is referred to other sections of this book (see Chapters 46 to 48).

INDICATIONS

The ECG is an extraordinarily cost effective and useful monitoring tool. In veterinary intensive care the ECG may be second only to serial, well-performed physical examinations in terms of its usefulness in overall patient monitoring. Although a brief multiple-lead evaluation of a patient's ECG is an important part of any diagnostic workup for suspected intrathoracic disease, in the intensive care setting continuous monitoring of cardiac rate and rhythm (typically one or a few leads at a time) is of greatest utility.

Some might argue that all critically ill animals warrant continuous ECG monitoring, and such a statement may be true. However, some patients may have conditions that preclude continuous ECG monitoring and mandate that intermittent evaluations be performed instead. One example of such a patient is a dog with central nervous system disease that is exhibiting circling. In this case, ECG lead wires may present a significant tangling, tripping, or choking hazard to the patient. Also, patients with diffuse dermatologic disease or surface burns may not tolerate typical lead placement. With such exceptions in mind, one can state that most critically ill patients may benefit from continuous ECG monitoring. In particular, any patient with an irregular rhythm, increased heart rate, or decreased heart rate detected on physical examination should undergo ECG monitoring.

ELECTROCARDIOGRAPHIC PRINCIPLES

During depolarization and repolarization of the myocardium, the heart generates an electrical field that can be detected at the surface of the body by ECG leads. The electrocardiographic system used in clinical practice consists of a series of positive and negative leads that when placed around the heart (roughly in the frontal plane either on the trunk or the limbs) will record complexes associated with the various phases of the cardiac electrical cycle. The ECG records the sum of all the electrical impulses generated by the individual myocytes during each cycle. When a positive deflection is seen on the ECG tracing it signifies that the sum of the heart's electrical impulses was moving toward the positive electrode of that lead. A negative deflection signifies that the sum of the impulses was moving away from the positive electrode at that time. Impulses traveling perpendicular to an electrode do not cause a deflection in the tracing. When these deflections are plotted over time, a series of waveforms (P, QRS, and T) are revealed.[1]

The standard leads used in veterinary practice include the three bipolar leads (I, II, and III) and the augmented leads (aVR, aVL, and aVF). Each lead can produce a tracing of the heart's electrical activity from a different orientation. In combination, the information obtained from multiple leads can aid in the diagnosis of rhythm and conduction disturbances. When measurements are made of the P-QRS-T waveforms, these measurements should be taken using a lead II tracing.

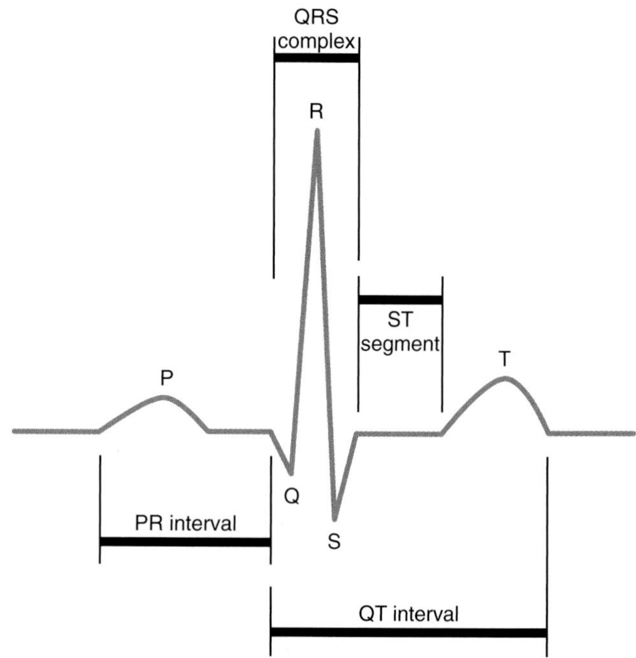

FIGURE 185-1 Component waveforms, segments, and intervals of the normal electrocardiogram.

TECHNIQUE

Many electrode attachment systems are available. When a system is selected, it is important to bear in mind that high-quality ECG recordings require good contact between the electrodes and the patient's skin. If commercially available self-adhesive electrode pads are to be used, then it is advised that the hair be clipped and the skin cleaned and dried before application. Generally, two electrode pads placed over the lateral thorax on each side and a third pad placed in the left inguinal region are sufficient to obtain good-quality tracings. Use of alligator clips is not advised for continuous monitoring because their prolonged use can damage the patient's skin and cause discomfort. Once the electrode pads are placed and clips or wires attached, it is often helpful to place a mesh stockinette shirt around the patient's trunk so that all wires can be collected into a single "stalk" exiting the mesh shirt dorsally. This can enhance patient comfort, prevent lead detachment, and reduce obstacles to patient repositioning.

Leads are created by comparing the voltage signals from one or more electrodes with a reference (e.g., ground or another electrode). When selecting a lead to display during continuous ECG monitoring one should choose the lead that the caregiver believes provides the most easily recognizable waveforms. Lead II is used for rhythm evaluation in cardiac examinations because in most patients this lead lies well within the mean electrical axis of the heart and produces easily recognizable waveforms. However, in the critically ill patient the caregiver may need to evaluate several leads to find the one that gives the most robust signal.

If one is relying on the monitor to calculate heart rates automatically, one will often get more accurate readings if a lead is picked in which the QRS amplitude is markedly different from that of the P and T waves (otherwise, double or triple counting may occur, giving erroneously high heart rate readings). It should always be noted in the patient's record which lead is being monitored. It is essential that the clinician and nursing staff bear in mind that the reference values for canine and feline ECGs are obtained from still animals in right lateral recumbency. During continuous monitoring patients are seldom, if ever, in the ideal position, and changes in waveform amplitude are to be expected relative to normal values. The utility of the continuous ECG is predominantly in monitoring heart rate and rhythm; however, it can also indicate to the clinician whether a standardized recording of all six leads and a rhythm strip should be obtained.

ELECTROCARDIOGRAM WAVEFORMS

Figure 185-1 shows a normal canine lead II P-QRS-T complex with the waveforms, intervals, and ST segment identified. The P wave is a reflection of the depolarization of the atria. Its duration and amplitude should be noted. The PR interval is measured from the beginning of the P wave to the start of the QRS complex and is a measure of the time it took for the electrical impulse to travel from the sinoatrial node to the ventricular myocardium (including the normal delay that occurs as the impulse travels through the atrioventricular node). The QRS complex is a reflection of ventricular depolarization. As with the P wave, the duration and amplitude of the QRS complex should be evaluated. The ST segment is measured from the end of the QRS complex to the beginning of the T wave. Disease states can cause the ST segment to be shifted upward or downward from the baseline, and any such shifts should be noted. The T wave is the result of ventricular repolarization. Although the shape and amplitude of the T wave can be extremely variable in normal dogs, progressive or acute changes in the conformation of the T wave in an individual patient can be a marker of important disease states such as hypoxemia. The QT interval is an indicator of the time required for both ventricular depolarization and repolarization to occur. This interval is measured from the start of the QRS complex to the end of the T wave. The duration of the QT interval can be an important indicator of electrolyte abnormalities but also is strongly dependent on heart rate and must be interpreted in light of this parameter.[1-3]

ELECTROCARDIOGRAM INTERPRETATION

The most important principle in ECG interpretation is that each ECG should be evaluated in the same systematic way. Any thorough evaluation should include the following[1,2]:

1. Calculation of heart rate
2. Determination of the rhythm

Table 185-1 Normal Canine and Feline Lead II Electrocardiogram Values[5]

	Canine	Feline
Heart rate	Puppy: 70-220 beats/min Toy breeds: 70-180 beats/min Standard: 70-160 beats/min Giant breeds: 60-140 beats/min	120-240 beats/min
Rhythm	Sinus rhythm Sinus arrhythmia Wandering pacemaker	Sinus rhythm
P Wave		
Amplitude	Maximum: 0.4 mV	Maximum: 0.02 mV
Duration	Maximum: 0.04 sec (giant breeds, 0.05 sec)	Maximum: 0.04 sec
PR interval	0.06-0.13 sec	0.05-0.09 sec
QRS		
Amplitude	Small breeds: 2.5 mV Large breeds: 3 mV	Maximum: 0.9 mV
Duration	Small breeds: 0.05 sec maximum Large breeds: 0.06 sec maximum	Maximum: 0.04 sec
ST segment		
Depression	No more than 0.2 mV	None
Elevation	No more than 0.15 mV	None
QT interval	0.15-0.25 sec at normal heart rate	0.12-0.18 sec at normal heart rate
T wave	May be positive, negative, or biphasic Not more than one fourth of R-wave amplitude	Usually positive

3. Identification of the waveforms (P-QRS-T) with particular attention paid to changes relative to previous ECG results for this same patient
4. Evaluation of the PR and QT intervals
5. Inspection of the ST segment for elevation or depression

Each of these parameters should be compared with normal values (Table 185-1) and with previous measurements made for the same patient. Serial evaluation can provide important early indications of changes in the patient's condition, even when values fall within the normal range. For example, progressive elongation of the QT interval or QRS duration may signal worsening hyperkalemia in a patient long before the absolute values of these measurements exceed the accepted normal range. Care must be taken when evaluating the amplitude or orientation of the waveforms relative to normal values if they were not obtained from a still animal in right lateral recumbency (as the normal values were). Changes in the durations of the intervals and waveforms seldom are affected by patient position, whereas the orientation and amplitude of the waveforms can vary markedly.

EFFECTS OF DISEASE STATES ON THE ELECTROCARDIOGRAM

Specific arrhythmias and their management are discussed elsewhere in this book (see Chapters 46 to 48). However, many disease states can produce detectable changes in the ECG before they become so severe that they alter the rhythm or shift the heart rate outside the normal range.

Electrolyte Abnormalities

The normal action potentials generated by both contractile and noncontractile cardiac cells are dependent on the sequential opening of a multitude of ion channels and the flow of ionized sodium, potassium, and calcium through these channels across the cell membranes. Further, other electrolytes such as magnesium serve as important cofactors in cellular actions relying on adenosine triphosphate, such as the function of cellular pumps that reestablish resting membrane potential after a depolarization. Magnesium is unusual in that it has a double shell of hydrating water molecules that require a large amount of free energy to be shed. Magnesium must shed this hydration shell before entering divalent cation channels. Thus magnesium is thought to act as an endogenous calcium channel blocker. It is not surprising, therefore, that alterations in electrolyte concentrations can cause alterations in cardiac electrical and mechanical functions.[1-5]

Hyperkalemia

Although most critically ill patients are faced with large ongoing potassium losses or translocation of extracellular potassium to the intracellular compartment, a subset of animals may arrive with (or develop) elevated extracellular potassium levels. Such hyperkalemia may occur as a result of the underlying disease process (e.g., Addison's disease), as a result of treatment (e.g., lysis of a saddle thrombus with subsequent reperfusion), or because of inadvertent administration of excess parenteral potassium ions (e.g., poorly mixed fluids supplemented with potassium chloride). Regardless of the cause, the ECG can serve as an invaluable tool in the detection of hyperkalemia. As serum potassium levels rise above 5.5 mEq/L, the ECG may begin to show tall, peaked T waves. As potassium levels rise to 8 to 9 mEq/L, QRS duration may become prolonged and P-wave amplitude may diminish. With further increases in potassium, the QRS waves may take on a sinusoidal appearance, P waves may no longer be apparent, and ST-segment elevation or depression may be noted. ECG changes are not entirely consistent with varied levels of hyperkalemia. Other factors such as serum ionized calcium concentrations factor into whether ECG changes will manifest at a given serum potassium level.

Hypokalemia

Low serum potassium levels are a common finding in the critically ill patient and frequently need to be addressed when a fluid plan is formulated. When hypokalemia develops it may result in nonspecific ECG changes such as prolongation of the QT interval, reduced T-wave amplitude, and ST-segment depression. Severe hypokalemia may lead to both atrial and ventricular tachyarrhythmias.

Hypercalcemia

Just as they have difficulty in regulating potassium levels, many sick and injured animals struggle to maintain a normal serum ionized calcium level. However, hypercalcemia may occur, resulting from either a primary disease state or administration of intravenous calcium preparations, or both; the elevation in the levels of this ion may be reflected by changes in the ECG. The most notable of these changes is QT-interval shortening, and this finding can be an important signal to the clinician to measure both total and ionized calcium levels.

Hypocalcemia

As one might expect, the effects of hypocalcemia on the ECG are in direct contrast to those caused by hypercalcemia. Prolongation of the QT interval may be an indication of reduced serum calcium concentrations. Nonspecific changes in the shape of the T wave may be noted as well.

Magnesium level

In humans, hypermagnesemia may cause prolonged PR intervals and QRS durations. Little is known about elevated magnesium levels in critically ill dogs and cats, although hypomagnesemia is a recognized condition occurring in a significant number of critically ill veterinary patients. Low magnesium levels cause ECG changes quite similar to those noted for hypokalemia.

Hypoxemia

Low partial pressure of arterial oxygen has a profound effect on cardiac function, sympathetic nervous system activation, and, not surprisingly, the ECG. Severe or prolonged hypoxemia can produce both tachyarrhythmias and bradyarrhythmias and may lead to cardiac arrhythmias. However, in many patients the ECG can also provide early warning signs of worsening tissue oxygenation. Myocardial hypoxia may be reflected by elevation or depression of the ST segment. The sudden appearance of large T waves can herald hypoxemia; thus any abrupt change in T-wave appearance warrants an evaluation of the patient's blood gases.[6]

Intrathoracic Effusions

The accumulation of effusions (or tissues, as may be seen with diaphragmatic hernias) within the pericardial or pleural spaces can result in damping of the ECG waveforms. Diminished or variable amplitude of the QRS complex should prompt the clinician to pursue further diagnostic measures to rule out intracavitary effusions.[3]

Pain

Patient discomfort can lead to nonspecific alterations in the ECG. A progressively increasing heart rate with or without changes in T-wave conformation can be a sign of increasing sympathetic nervous system output. When these changes are seen in a patient exhibiting other signs of discomfort, alleviation of pain may lead to normalization of the ECG parameters.

REFERENCES

1. Tilley LP: Essentials of canine and feline electrocardiography, ed 3, Philadelphia, 1992, Lea & Febiger.
2. Tilley LP, Miller MS, Smith FW Jr: Canine and feline arrhythmias: self-assessment, Philadelphia, 1993, Lea & Febiger.
3. Bonow RO, Mann DL, Zipes DP, et al: Braunwald's heart disease: a textbook of cardiovascular medicine, ed 9, Philadelphia, 2011, Saunders.
4. Darke P, Bonagura JD, Kelly DF: Color atlas of veterinary cardiology, London, 1996, Mosby-Wolfe.
5. Tilley LP, Goodwin J, editors: Manual of canine and feline cardiology, ed 3, St Louis, 2001, Saunders.
6. Channer K, Morris F: ABC of clinical electrocardiography: myocardial ischemia, BMJ 324(7344):1023-1026, 2002.

CHAPTER 186
BLOOD GAS AND OXIMETRY MONITORING

Laurie Sorrell-Raschi, DVM, DACVAA, RRT

KEY POINTS

- Interpretation of blood gas values requires an understanding of acid-base and respiratory physiology.
- There are six basic steps to follow when analyzing arterial blood gas values.
- Pulse oximetry provides a noninvasive means of monitoring oxygenation.
- The final step in blood gas analysis is to evaluate the significance of the findings as they relate to the patient.

> The interpretation of blood gas analysis may be very difficult because it requires an understanding of not only the physiology of acids and bases, but also the physiology of ventilation and gas exchange, the dynamics of electrolyte and water movement, plasma composition, and the renal mechanisms of hydrogen ion, electrolyte and water excretion.[1]
>
> *Rawlston and Qunlan*

Blood gas analysis is an invaluable tool for assessing the physiologic status of critically ill patients. It is necessary, therefore, to develop a method of efficiently and effectively evaluating this information to treat the patient appropriately Although a thorough description of acid-base regulation and blood gas analysis is beyond the scope of this chapter (the reader is directed to Chapters 54 and 55, as well as several additional references[2-11] for a more detailed description of these subjects), what follows is a brief overview of acid-base physiology and a practical method of interpreting blood gas measurements.

HYDROGEN IONS

The proton is one of the basic chemical units of matter. The term *proton* has become synonymous with the term *hydrogen ion* or H^+ in medical physiology. This electrolyte is the end product of many metabolic processes within the body, and the normal H^+ concentration ($[H^+]$) in the extracellular fluid is maintained at around 40 nEq/L. Comparatively, the normal concentrations of most physiologically important electrolytes (e.g., Na^+, K^+, Ca^{2+}, Mg^{2+}, Cl^-,

HCO_3^-) are present in the body in the range of milliequivalents per liter.

Although [H^+] is one millionth the concentration of other electrolytes in the body, its regulation is of paramount importance to normal homeostasis. Hydrogen ions are highly reactive and therefore readily interact with dissociable moieties on proteins. Because proteins play a major role in all biologic functions, alterations in protein structure or function as a result of changes in [H^+] within the body can have catastrophic effects on biologic homeostasis.

BUFFERS

Changes in [H^+] are opposed by buffer systems within the body. These systems consist of an acid (H^+ donator) and its conjugate base (H^+ acceptor) as follows:

$$\underset{acid}{HA} \leftrightarrow H^+ + \underset{base}{A^-}$$

The law of mass action states that the velocity of a reaction is proportional to the concentration of reactants on either side of the equation and their dissociation constants (k):

$$\frac{k_1}{k_2} = K_a = \frac{[H^+][A^-]}{[HA]}$$

Weak acids and their conjugate bases constitute the most effective buffer pairs in the body since they are more capable of accepting or donating H^+ in the presence of changes in H^+ load than are strong acids, which are highly dissociated in many biologic fluids.

HENDERSON-HASSELBALCH EQUATION

In the early 1900s, L.J. Henderson revolutionized the study of acid-base physiology by noting that CO_2 (a primary end product of cellular metabolism) combines with H_2O in the presence of carbonic anhydrase to form H_2CO_3 (carbonic acid). This acid further dissociates into its conjugate base, bicarbonate (HCO_3^-), and H^+:

$$CO_2 + H_2O \xleftrightarrow{\text{carbonic anhydrase}} H_2CO_3 \leftrightarrow HCO_3^- + H^+$$

By applying the laws of mass action and because H_2CO_3 exists in equilibrium with dissolved CO_2, Henderson substituted the value of dissolved CO_2 in his equation. Thus

$$[H^+] = K_a\left(\frac{[CO_2]}{HCO_3^-}\right)$$

This equation had major implications because it not only described one of the first known buffer pairs (H_2CO_3 and HCO_3^-) but also illuminated a process by which the body could buffer changes in H^+ load; namely, ventilation. Later K.A. Hasselbalch would add further utility to the equation by substituting the partial pressure of CO_2 in blood (PCO_2) for dissolved CO_2 and expressing the equation as a logarithm of [H^+], or pH:

$$pH = pK_a + \log\left(\frac{HCO_3^-}{PCO_2 \times SC}\right)$$

where pK_a = the logarithm of the ionization constant K_a for H_2CO_3, and SC = the solubility coefficient of CO_2 in blood (or 0.03).

This is the classic Henderson-Hasselbalch equation.

Regulation of pH

On a daily basis, pH changes within the body are opposed by multiple complex processes that, for the sake of simplicity, can be presented as (1) the actions of intracellular and extracellular buffering systems (chemical buffering), (2) modulation of ventilation (physiologic buffering of the volatile acid CO_2), and (3) renal clearance of titratable (nonvolatile) acid. The three primary chemical buffering systems within the body are proteins (primarily intracellular buffers) and PO_4^- and HCO_3^- (predominately extracellular buffers). Although HCO_3^- comprises only 20% of the total body buffer capacity, its role in [H+] regulation cannot be overemphasized. The reasons are twofold. Not only is the HCO_3^- buffering system capable of responding to an acute change in [H^+], its role in the HCO_3^--H_2CO_3-CO_2 equilibrium equation allows changes in pH to be further modulated by changes in ventilation. The ventilatory arc of the system is capable of reacting within minutes of an acid or alkali load, and this "open system" greatly enhances the buffering capacity of the HCO_3^- system. Finally, the kidneys play a major role in maintaining pH by increasing or decreasing acid elimination in the urine. This system takes hours to days to reach completion but is the most capable of all the processes for returning the body's pH to normal.

BLOOD GAS ANALYSIS: GETTING STARTED

Although blood gas analysis may be performed on venous blood (see Venous Blood Gases later in this chapter), arterial blood gas analysis yields information about oxygenation as well as ventilation and acid-base disorders and is preferentially performed, when possible. There are several potential sites for arterial puncture (e.g., the dorsopedal artery, the digital artery in the front paw, the auricular artery, the lingual artery, the femoral artery). However, the dorsopedal artery is chosen most often due to its size, superficial location, and ease of ensuring adequate hemostasis.

A small amount of local anesthetic such as 0.05 to 0.1 ml of 2% lidocaine injected subdermally 2 to 3 minutes before sampling may aid in restraint. Placement of an arterial catheter may allow for repeated blood gas sampling with less stress for the patient (see Chapter 201). Blood should be drawn into a syringe coated with sodium or lithium heparin (1000 IU/ml) to coat the inside of the syringe. Excess should be discarded since heparin is acidic and excessive amounts in the syringe may alter blood gas values.[12] Any air bubbles should be expelled from the sample, and the sample should be corked or attached to a stopper to prevent further exposure to room air, which could decrease the sample's PCO_2 to zero and the sample's partial pressure of oxygen (PO_2) to that of room air (150 mm Hg at sea level).[12] The sample should be analyzed immediately or held in an ice-water bath at 4° C (39.2° F) (for up to 2 hours) to minimize the effects of cellular metabolism on sample pH, PCO_2, and PO_2.[13]

Temperature Correction

Whether or not to correct blood gas values for temperature remains a controversial subject in both human and veterinary medicine. The issue centers around the hypothesis that as temperature changes, blood gas solubility also changes, and blood gas values may be altered as well. The pH-stat strategy suggests that blood gas values be corrected for patient temperature and the corrected values be maintained within accepted norms for pH and PCO_2. The α-stat strategy assumes that hemoglobin's buffering capacity, which is related to the ionization of the imidazole group of histidine residues, is not affected by temperature changes. Under these circumstances there would be no need to temperature-correct blood gas values.

According to the literature, most attempts at critically applying one strategy versus the other have been made in the context of achieving improved neurologic outcomes in human patients after coronary artery bypass surgery and have shown differing and confounding results.[14,15] There is no clear indication that routine temperature correction in the clinical setting is necessary. It is up to the clinician, therefore, to decide which strategy seems most reasonable and to apply that strategy consistently to serial sampling.

Table 186-1 Normal Arterial Blood Gas Values for Dogs and Cats[16,17]

Parameter	Value (Dogs)	Value (Cats)
pH	7.39 ± 0.03	7.39 ± 0.08
$PaCO_2$ (mm Hg)	37 ± 3	31 ± 6
PaO_2 (mm Hg)	102 ± 7	107 ± 12
HCO_3^- (mEq/L)	21 ± 2	18 ± 4
Base excess (mEq/L)	−2 ± 2	−2 ± 2

HCO_3^-, Bicarbonate; *$PaCO_2$*, partial pressure of arterial carbon dioxide; *PaO_2*, partial pressure of arterial oxygen.

Table 186-2 Acid-Base Disturbances

Acid-base Disturbance	pH	Primary Disorder	Compensation
Respiratory acidosis	Decreased	Increased PCO_2	Increased HCO_3^-
Respiratory alkalosis	Increased	Decreased PCO_2	Decreased HCO_3^-
Metabolic acidosis	Decreased	Decreased HCO_3^-	Decreased PCO_2
Metabolic alkalosis	Increased	Increased HCO_3^-	Increased PCO_2

HCO_3^-, Bicarbonate concentration measured in mEq/L or mmol/L; *PCO_2*, partial pressure of carbon dioxide measured in mm Hg.

Table 186-3 Expected Compensatory Changes to Primary Acid-Base Disorders

Primary Disorder	Expected Compensation
Metabolic acidosis	↓ PCO_2 of 0.7 mm Hg per 1 mEq/L decrease in $[HCO_3^-]$ ±3
Metabolic alkalosis	↑ PCO_2 of 0.7 mm Hg per 1 mEq/L decrease in $[HCO_3^-]$ ±3
Respiratory acidosis—acute	↑ $[HCO_3^-]$ of 0.15 mEq/L per 1 mm Hg ↑ PCO_2 ±2
Respiratory acidosis—chronic	↑ $[HCO_3^-]$ of 0.35 mEq/L per 1 mm Hg ↑ PCO_2 ±2
Respiratory alkalosis—acute	↓ $[HCO_3^-]$ of 0.25 mEq/L per 1 mm Hg ↓ PCO_2 ±2
Respiratory alkalosis—chronic	↓ $[HCO_3^-]$ of 0.55 mEq/L per 1 mm Hg ↓ PCO_2 ±2

$[HCO_3^-]$, Bicarbonate concentration measured in mEq/L; *PCO_2*, partial pressure of carbon dioxide measured in mm Hg, ↑ increased; ↓, decreased.

Step-by-Step Acid-Base Analysis

Number 1: Evaluate the pH

Table 186-1 shows normal arterial blood gas values in dogs and cats.[16,17] Because pH varies inversely with $[H^+]$, any process that increases H^+ load will decrease pH and produce acidosis. Conversely, any process that decreases $[H^+]$ will tend to increase pH and produce alkalosis. The terms *alkalemia* and *acidemia* imply that blood pH is outside the normal range, which may or may not be true depending on the nature of the acid-base disorder and the effectiveness of the organism's compensatory mechanisms (see Chapter 54).

According to the Henderson-Hasselbalch equation, the pH has two components: a ventilatory component (PCO_2) and a metabolic component (HCO_3^-). The pH varies directly with changes in the metabolic component and inversely with changes in the respiratory component. It would follow that pH changes produced by one component may be opposed by opposite changes in the other component. For instance, to compensate for a respiratory acidosis the organism will attempt to increase the concentration of HCO_3^- in the blood. The compensation may be strong, but rarely is it complete, and overcompensation does not normally occur.[4]

Number 2: Evaluate PCO_2 (see also Chapter 16)

Control of ventilation arises from respiratory centers within the brainstem that are sensitive to CO_2-induced changes in cerebral pH.[18] Arterial CO_2 levels are held steady by balancing minute ventilation with metabolic production of CO_2; however, normal ventilatory response to changes in PCO_2 are so sensitive that a 1-mm Hg change in PCO_2 can quadruple minute ventilation. Although ventilation may exceed the production of CO_2, it is unlikely that CO_2 production exceeds ventilatory capacity in healthy animals.

Respiratory acidosis therefore is almost always caused by some aspect of ventilatory failure.[18] Table 186-2, Table 186-3, and Box 186-1 show the most common causes of respiratory acidosis and alkalosis in dogs and cats and the expected acid-base changes that subsequently occur.[6,19-24] It is important to note that although dogs and cats respond similarly to acute respiratory acidosis, there is some question as to whether cats adjust as well to chronic respiratory acidosis as do dogs. This may be because cats lack the adaptive process of urinary ammoniagenesis that allows dogs to bring their pH very close to normal in longstanding chronic respiratory acidosis (>30 days).[21]

Also of note is that the normal renal response to respiratory acidosis and alkalosis (namely, HCO_3^- retention and excretion, respectively) takes several hours to days to correct after correction of the primary respiratory acid-base disorder. The patient may require treatment of the electrolyte changes (in chloride in particular) that accompany the renal response to respiratory acid-base disorders before full correction to baseline HCO_3^- values can be achieved.[6,9]

BOX 186-1 *Causes of Respiratory-Induced Acid-Base Disorders*

Causes of Respiratory Acidosis

Pulmonary and small airway disease
Respiratory center depression
Neuromuscular disease
Restrictive extrapulmonary disorders
Large airway obstruction
Marked obesity
Ineffective mechanical ventilation

Causes of Respiratory Alkalosis

Iatrogenic (mechanical ventilation)
Hypoxemia
Pulmonary disease without hypoxemia
Centrally mediated hyperventilation
Pain, anxiety, fear

Number 3: Evaluate the metabolic indices

Metabolic acid-base disturbances are among the most common acid-base disorders described in veterinary medicine. In the classic approach for characterizing acid-base balance, the Henderson-Hasselbalch equation, pH is described as being proportional to log

BOX 186-2 *Causes of Metabolically Induced Acid-Base Disorders Based on the Base Excess Approach*

Causes of Metabolic Acidosis	Causes of Metabolic Alkalosis
Normochloremic causes	*Chloride-responsive causes*
Lactic acidosis	Vomiting
Ketoacidosis	Diuretic therapy
Toxins	Correction of respiratory acidosis
Renal failure	
Hyperchloremic causes	*Chloride-resistant causes*
Gastrointestinal losses	Primary hyperaldosteronism
Renal failure	Hyperadrenocorticism
Renal tubular acidosis	Overadministration of alkaline fluids
Other	Other

($[HCO_3^-]/PCO_2$). HCO_3^- was used to determine the metabolic component of the body's acid-base status. However, unlike PCO_2, which is an independent variable that the body senses and manipulates to control $[H^+]$, HCO_3^- levels within the body are dependent on many factors (with CO_2 levels being only one of them). Consequently, many attempts were made to find an index that would better reflect whole body buffering capacity.

Base excess/base deficit (BE/BD) is derived from the whole blood buffer curve developed by Siggaard-Anderson in the 1950s and is defined as the amount of acid or base necessary to titrate 1 L of blood to a pH of 7.4 if PCO_2 is held constant at 40 mm Hg.[25,26] Because PCO_2 is held constant, the BE is reflective of the nonrespiratory component of the organism's buffer system. Tables 186-2 and 186-3 and Box 186-2 show the most common causes of metabolic acidosis and alkalosis, as well as relevant acid-base responses. The question remains as to whether cats typically have the expected ventilatory response to metabolic acidoses. There is experimental evidence to suggest that they do not.[7]

Number 4: Determine if there is one problem or many

One of the biggest challenges when analyzing a blood gas measurement is to determine the primary disorder. A good rule of thumb is that the pH of the sample reflects the primary disorder. This sounds simple, but it becomes more and more complicated as compensation and multiple disturbances occur. Various acid-base disturbances may be present simultaneously, except for respiratory alkalosis and acidosis, which are mutually exclusive. Multiple primary disorders that change the pH in the same direction are readily apparent (see Table 186-2). Multiple primary disorders that change the pH in different directions may be distinguished from a single primary disorder with compensation by determining the expected compensation in PCO_2, HCO_3^-, or pH and comparing it with the observed compensation (see Table 186-3). If the two are not equal, there are most likely multiple primary disorders.[3,7-9]

Anion gap

Although BE has been used in human medicine for many years as a bedside index of acid-base analysis it has several short comings. Chiefly, the buffer base nomogram from which the BE equation is derived was created by examining the behavior of blood in vitro; this tends to underestimate whole body buffering capacity. Secondly, this index is fairly insensitive for the detection of complex mixed acid-base disturbances; therefore concurrent but opposing disturbances such as metabolic acidosis and alkalosis may actually be overlooked when this index is used.[27]

In the 1970s the anion gap approach for acid-base analysis was developed to address some of these concerns.[28] As previously mentioned, $[H^+]$ in solution is provided by the dissociation of water into H^+ and OH^-, and the concentration of these two is determined by the concentration of all the other charged ions in the solution. By the law of electroneutrality, the concentration of positively charged ions *(cations)* in solution such as plasma is equal to the concentration of negatively charged ions *(anions)*. The anion gap (AG) is calculated as the difference between all the major cations and anions:

$$AG = ([Na^+]+[K^+]) - ([Cl^-]+[HCO_3^-])$$

However, by the law of electroneutrality there should be no AG. It follows, therefore, that any apparent calculated AG must come from a difference in *unmeasured* cations and anions. Because changes in unmeasured cations of the magnitude necessary to increase the AG are incompatible with life,[28] the AG is generally used as an index to estimate changes in the concentration of unmeasured anions.

In healthy dogs and cats the AGs are approximately *12 to 24 mEq/L* and *13 to 27 mEq/L*, respectively,[7] with the bulk of the unmeasured anions represented by plasma proteins (chiefly albumin), phosphate, and sulfate. Because increases in the AG are much more common than decreases, the AG is most commonly used as an aid in the differentiation of causes of metabolic acidoses.

With organic acidosis (lactic acidosis, ketoacidosis, etc.), HCO_3^- is titrated from H^+ ions of the fixed acids. Consequently, the $[HCO_3^-]$ of the extracellular fluid should decrease, causing an increase in the AG. This is referred to as a *normochloremic metabolic acidosis*. In contrast, when HCO_3^- is lost, as with gastrointestinal loss or renal tubular acidosis, there is a concomitant Cl^- retention; therefore the AG does not change. These types of metabolic acidoses are classified as *normal AG* or *hyperchloremic metabolic acidoses*. Box 186-3 shows causes of metabolic acidosis based on the AG approach.

It is important to keep in mind, however, that because the bulk of the AG is comprised of the negative charge on plasma proteins and phosphates, changes in either of these parameters may have a significant impact on the calculated AG. In fact, the only clinically

BOX 186-3 *Causes of Metabolic Acidosis in Dogs and Cats Based on the Anion Gap (AG) Approach*[7,29,30]

Normal AG (Hyperchloremic)

Diarrhea
Dilutional acidosis (fluid administration with 0.9% NaCl)
Renal tubular acidosis
Carbonic anhydrase inhibitors
Hypoadrenocorticism
Ammonium chloride administration
Cationic amino acid administration

Increased AG (Normochloremic)

Lactic acidosis
Diabetic ketoacidosis
Uremic acidosis
Hyperphosphatemia
Intoxication
- Ethylene glycol
- Metaldehyde
- Salicylates

BOX 186-4 *Anion Gap (AG) Correction for Albumin and Phosphorus*[7,29]

$AG_{Alb\ adj} = AG + 4.2(3.77 - [\text{albumin measured in g/dl}])$
$AG_{Phos\ adj} = AG + 4.2(3.77 - [\text{albumin measured in g/dl}]) + (2.52 - 0.58\ [\text{phosphorus measured in mg/dl}])$

$AG_{Alb\ adj}$, Anion gap adjusted for effect of abnormal serum albumin concentration; *$AG_{Phos\ adj}$* anion gap adjusted for effect of abnormal serum phosphorus concentration.

relevant cause of a decrease in the AG is hypoalbuminemia.[7] It is advisable to adjust the AG as shown in Box 186-4 any time either or both of these values lie outside the normal reference range.[29]

The Stewart approach (see Chapter 55)

In 1983 the mathematician-biophysicist Peter Stewart changed the face of modern acid-base assessment by asserting that, to determine the $[H^+]$ of extracellular fluid, it is necessary to ascertain the dissociation equilibriums for all fully dissociated and partially dissociated ionic compounds and apply three simple rules: (1) *Electroneutrality:* in aqueous solutions, the sum of all of the positively charged ions must equal the sum of all of the negatively charged ions. (2) *Dissociation equilibrium:* the dissociation equilibriums of all incompletely dissociated substances, as derived from the law of mass action, must be satisfied at all times. (3) *Mass conservation:* the amount of a substance remains constant unless it is added, removed, generated, or destroyed. Through a series of mathematically elegant although cumbersome equations, Stewart found that three independent variables fit these criteria: (1) strong ion difference; (2) the concentration of partially dissociated ions, weak acids, or buffer ions (A_{total}); and (3) PCO_2.

In the Stewart approach, PCO_2 also determines the respiratory component of acid-base abnormalities (as in the traditional Henderson-Hasselbalch approach); however, metabolic derangements are defined by changes in SID and $A_{total.}$

Strong Ion Difference. By definition, a strong ion is any substance that is fully dissociated in plasma at body pH. In plasma the most important strong ions are Na^+, K^+, Cl^-, Mg^{2+}, Ca^{2+}, lactate, β-hydroxybutyrate, acetoacetate, and sulfate. The strong ion difference (SID) is defined as the difference between strong cations and anions as follows:

$$SID = ([Na^+]+[K^+]+[Mg^{2+}]+[Ca^{2+}])-([Cl^-]+[A^-])$$

where $[A^-]$ is the concentration of unmeasured strong anions.

This equation is considered the SID apparent (SID_{app}). Under normal conditions the SID_{app} of plasma is approximately 40 to 44 mEq/L. By the law of electroneutrality this charge is balanced by the net negative charge of weak acids, predominately HCO_3^- and A_{total}, which consists of albumin, globulin, and phosphate.[8] This is the SID effective (SID_{eff}).

Changes in SID occur by three basic mechanisms: (1) changes in free water content of plasma, (2) changes in $[Cl^-]$, and (3) changes in unmeasured strong anions $[A^-]^-$). Because Na^+ and Cl^- are quantitatively the most important strong ions clinically it is often acceptable to simplify the SID_{app} as follows:

$$SID_{app} = [Na^+]-[Cl^-]$$

When SID is evaluated, chloride abnormalities must always be considered in relation to free water changes; therefore it is necessary to use corrected Cl values as follows:

$$[CL^-]_{corrected} = [Cl^-]\times([Na^+]_{normal}/[Na^+]_{measured})$$

Box 186-5 depicts the most common causes of changes in SID. An increase in SID correlates with metabolic alkalosis and a decrease in SID correlates with metabolic acidosis.[7,30]

Strong Ion Gap. Although Stewart's equations provide a very sound mechanistic explanation for plasma pH changes, they are too cumbersome (as previously mentioned) to be seen as clinically useful. Consequently, in the 1990s Figge et al developed a modification to the Stewart approach called the *strong ion gap* (SIG).[7] Figge proposed that unmeasured strong ions could be determined by subtracting weak acids (buffer ions) from strong ions, or

$$\begin{aligned} SID_{app} - SID_{eff} &= [Na^+]+[K^+]+[Ca^{2+}]+[Mg^{2+}]-[Cl^-]-[A^-] \\ &\quad -([HCO_3^-]-[\text{albumin}]-[\text{phosphate}]) \\ &= SIG \end{aligned}$$

The advantage that this approach has over the AG is that it should not be affected by changes in albumin and phosphate concentration because both variables are considered in the calculation.

Unfortunately, this formula is equally cumbersome and is not easily applicable to dogs and cats. However, through the work of Constable and McCullough[31,32] and others a simplified SIG (SIG_{simpl}) was developed for dogs at a plasma pH of 7.4 and for cats at plasma pH of 7.35 as follows:

$$\text{For dogs: } SIG_{simpl} = [\text{albumin measured in g/dl}]\times 4.9 - AG$$
$$\text{For cats: } SIG_{simpl} = [\text{albumin measured in g/dl}]\times 7.4 - AG$$

As with the AG, hypophosphatemia may falsely elevate the SIG_{simpl}; therefore the AG should always be corrected for phosphate before calculating the SIG_{simpl}.

The range of normal values for SIG_{simpl} is ±5 mEq/L. An increase in unmeasured strong anions or metabolic acidosis is indicated by a decrease in SIG_{simpl}. Clinically, an increase in SIG_{simpl} is rare but would be indicative of the presence of unmeasured strong cations and thus would produce a metabolic alkalosis. At this time, controlled studies in dogs and cats evaluating the SIG_{simpl} have yet to be published; however, studies in humans are very suggestive that SIG_{simpl} may be a valuable tool for evaluating acid-base balance in the critical care setting.[33]

Base Excess Modification. Despite the pragmatism of Stewart's mechanistic approach to acid-base physiology the practical application of strong ion equations to clinical situation continues to be debated, largely due to the fact that traditional indices of acid-base analysis such as standard base excess (SBE) have been available, are intuitively easy to understand, and, except for very ill patients, show good agreement with indices like the AG. In an effort to try to tackle these issues Fencl, Jabel, et al focused on the concept of improving upon SBE/BD by applying a series of corrective equations to the measured SBE/BD to account for some effects considered in Stewart approach, as shown in Table 55-1.[34] Although base excess gap has not been validated for the dog and cat it is a simple, reasonable way to consider various metabolic components that may be contributing to a patient's overall acid-base status.

Number 5: Determine how well the patient is oxygenating (see also Chapter 15)

Oxygen is necessary for aerobic metabolism. Hypoxia occurs whenever oxygen levels in the blood are low enough to cause abnormal organ function. Hypoxemia occurs when oxygen levels in the blood are too low to meet metabolic demands.[16] PaO_2 is the partial pressure of oxygen dissolved in the arterial blood (plasma). It is the most common blood gas parameter used to monitor the progress of patients with respiratory disorders. Normal PaO_2 values for dogs and cats breathing room air (21% O_2) are shown in Table 186-1. A PaO_2 of less than 80 mm Hg is considered hypoxemia.[16] Although PaO_2 is

BOX 186-5 ***Causes of Metabolically Induced Acid-Base Disorders Based on the Stewart Approach***

SID Acidosis (Decreased SID)

Dilutional acidosis (decreased Na^+)

- With hypovolemia
  - Vomiting
  - Diarrhea
  - Hypoadrenocorticism
  - Third-space loss
  - Diuretic administration
- With normovolemia
  - Psychogenic polydipsia
  - Hypotonic fluid infusion
- With hypervolemia
  - Severe liver disease
  - Congestive heart failure
  - Nephrotic syndrome

Hyperchloremic acidosis (increased Cl^-_{corr})

- Loss of Na^+ relative to Cl^-
  - Diarrhea
- Gain of Cl^- relative to Na^+
  - Fluid therapy (0.9% NaCl, 7.2% NaCl, KCl-supplementation)
- Cl^- retention
  - Renal failure
  - Hypoadrenocorticism

Organic acidosis (increased unmeasured strong ions)

- Uremic acidosis, ketoacidosis, or lactic acidosis
- Toxicities
  - Ethylene glycol
  - Salicylate

SID Alkalosis (Increased SID)

Concentration alkalosis (increased Na^+)

- Pure water loss
  - Water deprivation
  - Diabetes insipidus
- Hypotonic fluid loss
  - Vomiting
  - Nonoliguric renal failure
  - Postobstructive diuresis

Hypochloremic alkalosis (decreased Cl^-_{corr})

- Gain of Na^+ relative to Cl^-
  - Isotonic or hypertonic $NaHCO_3$ administration
- Loss of Cl^- relative to Na^+
  - Vomiting of stomach contents
  - Use of thiazide or loop diuretics

A_{total} Acidosis (Increased A_{total})

Hyperalbuminemia

- Water deprivation

Hyperphosphatemia

- Translocation
  - Tumor cell lysis
  - Tissue trauma or rhabdomyolysis
- Increased intake
  - Use of phosphate-containing enemas
  - Intravenous phosphate administration
- Decreased loss
  - Renal failure
  - Urethral obstruction
  - Uroabdomen

A_{total} Alkalosis (Decreased A_{total})

Hypoalbuminemia

- Decreased production
  - Chronic liver disease
  - Malnutrition or starvation
  - Acute response to inflammation
- Extracorporeal loss
  - Protein-losing nephropathy
  - Protein-losing enteropathy
- Sequestration
  - Inflammatory effusions
  - Vasculitis

A_{total}, Concentration of partially dissociated ions, weak acids, and buffer ions; *Cl^-_{corr}*, corrected Cl^- concentration based on changes in sodium (see text for details); *SID*, strong ion difference.

very useful and reliable, it is dependent on the alveolar partial pressure of oxygen (PAO_2) according to the alveolar gas equation:

$$PAO_2 = (P_B - PH_2O)FiO_2 - \frac{PaCO_2}{R}$$

where P_B = the atmospheric pressure, PH_2O = the partial pressure of water vapor in the air at a given atmospheric pressure, FiO_2 = the fractional inspired concentration of oxygen, and R = the respiratory quotient that is the ratio of oxygen consumption to CO_2 production (0.78 to 0.92 in dogs).[35]

In normal healthy lungs, oxygen diffuses readily from the lungs to the arterial circulation. The PaO_2 should be within 10 mm Hg of the PAO_2 in animals breathing room air and up to 100 mm Hg when the FiO_2 is 100%. It is possible for healthy dogs living at high altitudes to have a PaO_2 of 60 mm Hg (PAO_2 and PaO_2 are decreased at low atmospheric pressure). Similarly, a PaO_2 reading of 100 mm Hg is not acceptable if a dog is anesthetized and breathing 100% oxygen (the PaO_2 should be 500 mm Hg).

The alveolar-arterial (A-a) gradient is calculated as a way to quantify the efficiency of gas exchange. At FiO_2 concentrations of 21%, the A-a gradient is expected to be less than 10 mm Hg; however, at O_2 concentrations of 100% the A-a gradient can normally be up to 100 mm Hg.[35,36] Consequently, the patient's FiO_2 must always be considered when evaluating the A-a gradient.

The ratio of PaO_2 to FiO_2 is another index of oxygenation. Normal values for the PaO_2:FiO_2 (PF) ratio are greater than 400 mm Hg. Values below 300 mm Hg indicate severe defects of gas exchange. Values less than 200 mm Hg may indicate acute respiratory distress syndrome (ARDS; see Chapters 7 and 24).[37] The PF ratio demonstrates some dependency on $PaCO_2$, but this diminishes at an FiO_2 above 50%, which is the point at which this ratio is most likely to be employed.

The oxygen content in milliliters per deciliter (CaO_2) is a calculated value that is included with many blood gas measurements. It is an assessment of the total amount of oxygen carried in the blood. It includes the oxygen dissolved in the plasma and bound to hemoglobin and is an important measure of the oxygen-carrying capacity of the blood, as follows:

$$CaO_2 = (PaO_2 \times 0.003) + (1.34 \times Hb \times SaO_2)$$

where 0.003 = the solubility of oxygen in plasma, 1.34 = the amount of oxygen in milliliters that each gram of hemoglobin (Hb) can hold if it is 100% saturated with O_2, and SaO_2 = oxygen saturation. Normal CaO_2 is 20 ml of O_2 per deciliter of blood.

SaO_2 is a measure of the percentage of the heme groups in an arterial blood sample that are occupied by oxygen molecules as measured using a co-oximeter. The relationship between SaO_2 and PaO_2 is sigmoidal, with maximum saturation seen above a PaO_2 of 100 mm Hg. Most blood gas analyzers do not measure SaO_2 and instead calculate it using a nomogram derived from the oxygen dissociation curve. Under normal circumstances this has few drawbacks; however, if dysfunctional hemoglobin species (such as carboxyhemoglobin, methemoglobin, sulfhemoglobin, or carboxy sulfhemoglobin) or fetal hemoglobin are in circulation, it is important to measure oxygen saturation with a co-oximeter. These devices use four wavelengths of light passed through a blood sample to distinguish between oxygenated hemoglobin and the other types of hemoglobin that are not carrying oxygen or unable to contribute to gas exchange.[3]

Pulse oximetry

Pulse oximeters are bedside monitors that noninvasively measure the SpO_2 rather than the SaO_2 and take advantage of the simple principle used by co-oximeters: blood that is oxygenated is a different color than blood that is not well oxygenated. When light is transcutaneously passed through a tissue bed it is possible to determine the oxygen saturation within that tissue. Deoxygenated hemoglobin absorbs more red light, and oxygenated blood absorbs more infrared light. By using two wavelengths (940 and 660 nm), a high light transmittance speed, fast sample rate, and microprocessor that filters any nonpulsatile data as nonarterial blood flow, it is possible to build a pulse oximeter capable of providing a noninvasive measure of oxygenation.[38]

Pulse oximetry is useful for several reasons. It provides an inexpensive, noninvasive means of monitoring oxygenation that is well tolerated and reliable in dogs and cats when more invasive monitoring is either unwarranted, undesirable, impossible to perform, or some combination thereof.[39-41] The machines are small, quiet, and portable and can be used for extended periods, and their readings may be used as an indirect measure of perfusion.

Recently several studies have been published in human pediatrics as well as adult critical care medicine demonstrating the utility of the SpO_2:FiO_2 ratio (SF) as a reliable noninvasive surrogate marker for the PF ratio. In human medicine the SF ratio has been shown to be a valid diagnostic indicator for ARDS and acute lung injury (ALI); it is especially useful in evaluating the severity of the illness and predicting outcome. A recent pilot study in veterinary medicine suggested that in spontaneously breathing dogs that are not receiving supplemental oxygen, the SF and PF ratios show good correlation. The potential exists, therefore, that pulse oximetry may provide a noninvasive means of monitoring veterinary species that have ARDS/ALI and other forms of respiratory failure.[42] This concept requires further investigation.

As with most screening equipment, there are drawbacks. Pulse oximetry probes typically perform well on the tongue, but this location can be difficult to use in a conscious patient. In cats in particular it may be difficult to obtain accurate readings.[43] The probe may be placed on the shaved skin of the lip, pinna, toe web, flank, or tail, but many conscious patients will not readily tolerate it. Additionally, pulse oximetry readings can be affected by movement, bright overhead lights, vasoconstriction, dark skin pigment, hypothermia, and hypoperfusion. Abnormal hemoglobin also causes the machine to read inaccurately. Carboxyhemoglobin absorbs infrared light similarly to oxygenated hemoglobin and produces falsely high SpO_2 readings. Methemoglobin, on the other hand, absorbs both wavelengths of light equally well. In the presence of this hemoglobin species the pulse oximeter defaults to a value of 85%, reading high or low depending on the patient's actual saturation level.[44] Most importantly, pulse oximetry gives little information about the efficiency of gas exchange. An SpO_2 of 100% in a patient breathing pure oxygen (FiO_2 of 100%) does not evaluate whether the patient's PaO_2 is 500 mm Hg or 100 mm Hg. It is more appropriate to perform arterial blood gas analysis anytime that precise information is needed regarding the patient's oxygenation status.

Number 6: Look at the whole picture

The final step in blood gas analysis is to fit the analysis to the patient. The clinician should make sure the conclusions fit the clinical picture. Regardless of the evaluation methods employed, the clinician must be sure that the conclusions drawn make sense. It is easy to become confused when one is learning acid-base physiology and acid-base analysis; several methods of analysis are possible. The main principles to keep in mind are the following: (1) Everything begins with the patient. (2) The clinician must begin an acid-base analysis with the method with which he or she is most familiar to determine the primary problem. (3) If the answer fits the clinical picture, it is most likely correct. (4) If the answer does not fit, or the therapy is unsuccessful, the clinician should look again using another method (see Chapters 54 and 55).

Venous Blood Gas Values

Venous blood gas samples are often more simple to obtain than arterial blood gas samples. The PCO_2 of venous blood is usually 4 to 6 mm Hg higher and the pH is usually 0.02 to 0.05 units lower than those of arterial blood. Venous blood gas samples are adequate for the clinical assessment of acid-base disorders in patients that are hemodynamically stable.[15,45] Peripheral venous PO_2 values are not representative of arterial oxygen values; however, the blood from veins in the tongue or the claw may be "arterialized" under certain conditions and used for this purpose.[15,46-48] A venous PO_2 of less than 30 mm Hg may suggest poor tissue oxygenation and should be investigated further.

REFERENCES

1. Rawson RE, Quinlan KM: Evaluation of a computer-based approach to teaching acid/base physiology, Adv Physiol Educ 26:85-97, 2002.
2. Muir WW, deMorais HSA: Acid-base balance: traditional and modified approaches. In Thurmon JC, Tranquilli WJ, Benson GJ, editors: Lumb and Jones' veterinary anesthesia, ed 3, Baltimore, 1996, Williams & Wilkins.
3. Martin L: All you really need to know to interpret arterial blood gases, ed 2, Philadelphia, 1992, Williams & Wilkins.
4. DiBartola SP: Introduction to acid-base disorders. In DiBartola SP, editor: Fluid, electrolyte, and acid-base disorders in small animal practice, ed 4, St Louis, 2012, Saunders.
5. DiBartola SP: Metabolic acid-base disorders. In DiBartola SP, editor: Fluid, electrolyte, and acid-base disorders in small animal practice, ed 4, St Louis, 2012, Saunders.
6. Johnson RA, deMorais HA: Respiratory acid-base disorders. In DiBartola SP, editor: Fluid, electrolyte and acid-base disorders in small animal practice, ed 4, St Louis, 2012, Saunders.
7. deMorais HA, Leisewitz AL: Mixed acid-base disorders. In DiBartola SP, editor: Fluid, electrolyte, and acid-base disorders in small animal practice, ed 4, St Louis, 2012, Saunders.
8. deMorais HA, Constable PD: Strong ion approach to acid-base disorders. In DiBartola SP, editor: Fluid, electrolyte, and acid-base disorders in small animal practice, ed 4, St Louis, 2012, Saunders.
9. Rose BD, Post TW: Clinical physiology of acid-base and electrolytes disorders, ed 5, New York, 2001, McGraw-Hill.
10. Corey HE: Stewart and beyond: new models of acid-base balance, Kidney Int 64:777-787, 2003.
11. Matousek S, Handy J, Rees SE: Acid-base chemistry of plasma: consolidation of traditional and modern approaches from a mathematical and clinical perspective, J Clin Monit Comput 25:57-70, 2011.

12. Siggaard-Andersen O: Sampling and storing of blood for determination of acid-base status, Scand J Clin Lab Invest 13:196-204, 1961.
13. Haskins SC: Sampling and storage of blood for pH and blood gas analysis, J Am Vet Med Assoc 170:429-433, 1977.
14. Murkin JM, Martzke JS, Buchan AM, et al: A randomized study of the influence of the perfusion technique and pH management strategy in the 316 patients undergoing coronary artery bypass surgery. II: Neurologic and cognitive outcomes, J Thorac Cardiovasc Surg 110(2):349-362, 1995.
15. Plessis AJ, Jonas RA, Wypij D, et al: Perioperative effects if alpha-stat versus pH-stat strategies for deep hypothermic cardiopulmonary bypass in infants, J Thorac Cardiovasc Surg 114(6):991-1000, 1997.
16. Haskins SC: Blood gases and acid-base balance: clinical interpretation and therapeutic implications. In Kirk RW, editor: Current veterinary therapy VIII, ed 8, Philadelphia, 1983, Saunders.
17. Ilkiw JE, Rose RJ, Martin ICE: A comparison of simultaneously collected arterial, mixed venous, jugular venous, and cephalic venous blood samples in the assessment of blood gas and acid-base status in dogs, J Vet Intern Med 5:294, 1991.
18. Guyton AC, Hall JE: Respiration. In Guyton AC, Hall JE, editors: Textbook of medical physiology, ed 9, Philadelphia, 1996, Harcourt Brace.
19. Jennings DB, Davidson JS: Acid-base and ventilatory adaptation in conscious dogs during chronic hypercapnia, Respir Physiol 58:377-393, 1984.
20. Szlyk PC, Jennings BD: Effects of hypercapnia on variability of normal respiratory behavior in awake cats, Am J Physiol 252:R538-R547, 1987.
21. Lemieux G, Lemieux C, Duplessis S, et al: Metabolic characteristics of cat kidney: failure to adapt to metabolic acidosis, Am J Physiol 259:R277-R281, 1990.
22. deMorais HA, DiBartola SP: Ventilatory and metabolic compensation in dogs with acid-base disturbances, J Vet Emerg Crit Care 1:39-49, 1991.
23. Adrogue HJ, Brensilver J, Cohen J, et al: Influence of steady-state alterations in acid-base equilibrium on the fate of administered bicarbonate in the dog, J Clin Invest 71:867, 1983.
24. Cornlius LM, Rawlings CA: Arterial blood gas and acid base values in dogs with various diseases and signs of disease, J Am Vet Med Assoc 178:992, 1981.
25. Astrup P, Jorgensen K, Siggaard-Andersen O, et al: Acid-base metabolism: new approach, Lancet 1:1035, 1960.
26. Astrup P: New approach to acid-base metabolism, Clin Chem 7:1, 1961.
27. Muir WW, de Morais HAS: Acid-base and fluid therapy. In Grimm KA, Tranquilli WJ, Lamont LA, editors: Essentials of small animal anesthesia and analgesia, ed 2, West Sussex, UK, 2011, Wiley-Blackwell.
28. Oh MS, Carroll HJ: Current concept. The anion gap, N Engl J Med 297:814-817, 1977.
29. Figge J, Jabor T, Kazda A, et al: Anion gap and hypoalbuminemia, Crit Care Med 26(11):1807-1810, 1998.
30. Whitehair KJ, Haskins SC, Whitehair JG, et al: Clinical applications of quantitative acid-base chemistry, J Vet Intern Med 9:1-11, 1995.
31. McCullough SM, Constable PD: Calculation of the total plasma concentration of nonvolatile weak acids and the effective dissociation constant of nonvolatile buffers in plasma for use in the strong ion approach to acid-base balance in cats, Am J Vet Res 64:1047-1051, 2003.
32. Constable PD, Stampfli HR: Experimental determination of net protein charge and A(tot) and K(a) of nonvolatile buffers in canine plasma, J Vet Intern Med 19:507-514, 2005.
33. Funk GC, Doberer D, Sterz F, et al: The strong ion gap and outcome after cardiac arrest in patients treated with therapeutic hypothermia: a retrospective study, Intensive Care Med 35:232-239, 2009.
34. Fencl V, Jabor A, Kazda A, et al: Diagnosis of metabolic acid-base disturbances in critically ill patients, Am J Respir Crit Care Med 162:2246-2251, 2000.
35. Muggenburg BA, Mauderly JL: Cardiopulmonary function of awake, sedated, and anesthetized beagle dogs, J Appl Physiol 37(2):152-157, 1974.
36. Haskins SC: Interpretation of blood gas measurements. In King LG, editor: Textbook of respiratory disease in dogs and cats, ed 1, St Louis, 2004, Saunders.
37. Schuurmans Stekhoven JH, Kreuzer F: Alveolar-arterial O_2 and CO_2 pressure differences in the anesthetized, artificially ventilated dog, Respir Physiol 3:177-191, 1967.
38. Van Pelt DR, Wingfield WE, Wheeler SL, et al: Oxygen-tension based indices as predictors of survival in critically ill dogs: clinical observations and review, J Vet Emerg Crit Care 1(1):19-25, 1991.
39. Dorsch JA, Dorsch SE: Understanding anesthesia equipment, ed 4, Baltimore, 1999, Williams & Wilkins.
40. Fairman NB: Evaluation of pulse oximetry as a continuous monitoring technique in critically ill dogs in the small animal intensive care unit, J Vet Emerg Crit Care 2(2):50-55, 1992.
41. Hendricks JC, King LG: Practicality, usefulness, and limits of pulse oximetry in critical small animal patients, J Vet Emerg Crit Care 3(1):5-12, 1993.
42. Calabro JM, Prittie JE, Palma DA: Preliminary evaluation of the utility of comparing SpO_2/FiO_2 and PaO_2/FiO_2 ratios in dogs, J Vet Emerg Crit Care (San Antonio) 23(3):280-285, 2013.
43. Jacobson JD, Miller MW, Mathews NS, et al: Evaluation of accuracy of pulse oximetry in dogs, Am J Vet Res 53(4):537-540, 1992.
44. Barker SJ, Tremper KK, Hyatt J: Effects of methemoglobinemia on pulse oximetry and mixed venous oximetry, Anesthesiology 70:112-117, 1989.
45. Wingfield WE, Van Pelt DR, Hackett TB, et al: Usefulness of venous blood in estimating acid-base status in the seriously ill dog, J Vet Emerg Crit Care 4:23, 1994.
46. Solter PF, Haskins SC, Patz JD: Comparison of PO_2, PCO_2, and pH in blood collected from the femoral artery and a cut claw of cats, Am J Vet Res 49(11):1882-1883, 1988.
47. Quandt JE, Raffe MR, Polzin D, et al: Evaluation of toenail blood samples for blood gas analysis in the dog, Vet Surg 20(5):357-361, 1991.
48. Wagner AE, Muir WW: A comparison of arterial and lingual and venous blood gases in anesthetized dogs, J Vet Emerg Crit Care 1(1):14-18, 1991.

CHAPTER 187

COLLOID OSMOTIC PRESSURE AND OSMOLALITY MONITORING

Lori S. Waddell, DVM, DACVECC

KEY POINTS

- Determination of colloid osmotic pressure (COP) can guide artificial colloid therapy in veterinary patients.
- Estimation of COP via equations using the patient's albumin and globulin concentrations are unreliable, particularly in critically ill patients that may have altered albumin/globulin ratios.
- Direct measurement via a colloid osmometer is the only reliable way to monitor COP.
- Maintenance of a goal COP of at least 15 mm Hg in whole blood for both dogs and cats reduces the risk of edema formation and secondary organ dysfunction associated with edema.
- Plasma osmolality can be estimated from an equation or measured directly via a freezing point depression osmometer.
- Diagnosis of an osmolal gap (measured plasma osmolality – estimated plasma osmolality) of more than 10 mOsm/kg indicates the presence of an unmeasured osmole(s), such as ethanol or ethylene glycol and its metabolites, and may be clinically useful in diagnosing these toxicities.

Colloid osmotic pressure (COP) is the physiochemical phenomenon that occurs when two solutions with different colloid concentrations are separated by a semipermeable membrane. Oncotic pressure is defined as the osmotic pressure exerted by colloids in solution, so the terms *colloid osmotic pressure* and *oncotic pressure* can be used interchangeably; *colloid oncotic pressure,* a commonly used misnomer, is redundant.

The particles contributing to COP (and the particles that they may hold with them because of their electrical charge) do not pass readily through the semipermeable membrane. This is in contrast to small crystalloid particles such as electrolytes, glucose, and other metabolites, which do pass readily through the membrane. COP is determined using a patient's blood sample and is referenced to normal saline rather than pure water because normal saline is more representative of the fluid in the interstitial space. COP should be thought of as the osmotic pressure exerted by plasma proteins and their associated electrolytes because the electrolytes contribute significantly to the COP. Albumin and its associated cations provide approximately 60% to 70% of the plasma oncotic pressure and globulins provide the remaining 30% to 40%.

Osmolality is the concentration of osmotically active particles (solute) per kilogram of solution. The size and charge of the particles does not matter when determining the osmolality; only the number of particles in solution is relevant.

COLLOID OSMOTIC PRESSURE

Starling's Hypothesis

Starling's hypothesis states that fluid flux at the capillary level is controlled by a balance between hydrostatic pressure and osmotic pressure gradients between the capillaries and interstitial space.

$$J_v = K_{fc}([P_c - P_i] - \sigma[\pi_p - \pi_i])$$

where J_v = the net rate of capillary filtration; K_{fc} = the capillary filtration coefficient; P_c = capillary hydrostatic pressure; P_i = interstitial hydrostatic pressure; σ = the osmotic reflection coefficient; π_p = plasma oncotic pressure; and π_i = interstitial oncotic pressure.

This equation shows the importance of plasma COP in maintaining a normal fluid balance between the intravascular space and the interstitial space (Figure 187-1). If the COP in the capillaries drops lower than the COP in the interstitium, fluid will move out of the vessels and edema formation will be favored. It is important to note that recent evidence has challenged the classic Starling-Landis principle and led to a revised Starling principle that uses the COP of the subglycocalyx space, rather than the COP of the interstitium, to describe fluid movement across some microvascular beds. The colloid osmotic pressure of the fluid in the subglycocalyx space can be substantially lower than that of the free interstitial fluid because of the combined effects of protein sieving by the endothelial glycocalyx and the convective flow of filtered fluid through the endothelial clefts. In addition, this space below the glycocalyx limits fluid reabsorption by the microvasculature.[1]

Of all the variables included in the equation above, only the COP and the capillary hydrostatic pressure can be manipulated clinically. Increasing capillary hydrostatic pressure by administering intravenous fluids tends to increase edema formation. By measuring a patient's COP and using colloid fluid therapy to help maintain normal COP, one can reduce transvascular fluid efflux and the clinical problems associated with it, including interstitial edema and cavitary effusions (see Chapter 11).

Calculated versus Measured Values

Equations have been developed to try to predict COP. In humans, the Landis-Pappenheimer equation can be used:

$$COP = 2.1P + 0.16P^2 + 0.009P^3$$

where P = plasma protein.

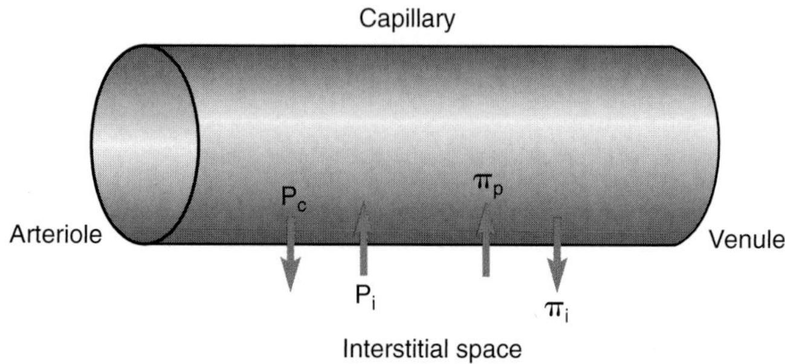

FIGURE 187-1 Starling's hypothesis of fluid flux across the capillary membrane. P_c, Capillary hydrostatic pressure; P_i, interstitial hydrostatic pressure; π_p, plasma oncotic pressure; π_i, interstitial oncotic pressure.

This equation is unreliable in other species, including cats, dogs, cattle, and horses, because they have different albumin/globulin ratios. Species-specific equations have been derived[1a] but are not reliable in critically ill patients, in which protein concentrations (specifically the albumin/globulin ratio) may be altered.[2]

Unfortunately, these equations do not provide an alternative for direct measurement of COP because of the changes associated with illness. Although total solids certainly give an indication of hypoproteinemia and therefore a low COP, refractometry cannot accurately predict COP. Furthermore, once artificial colloids have been administered, the measurement of total solids via refractometry will be inaccurate. The artificial starches available in the United States have a refractometry reading of 4 to 4.2 mg/dl, so the patient's total solids level will appear to approach this range, even if it is actually lower. The only way to predict COP accurately, particularly in critically ill patients and those receiving artificial colloids, is direct measurement via a colloid osmometer (Model 4420, Wescor, Logan, Utah).

Normal Colloid Osmotic Pressure Values

Normal values for COP are species, sample, and laboratory dependent. Published normal values for plasma are 23 to 25 mm Hg for cats and 21 to 25 mm Hg for dogs.[3] For whole blood, normal values are 24.7 ± 3.7 mm Hg for cats and 19.95 ± 2.1 for dogs.[4] A recent study showed a significant difference between COP measured on whole blood and that measured on plasma in healthy dogs.[5] The COP was slightly higher in whole blood (mean magnitude of 0.5 mm Hg) due to the presence of red blood cells, which make a minor contribution to the COP. However, the individual values obtained were all within the expected reference intervals, so either sample may be used clinically. It is recommended that clinicians use the same sample type for comparison in an individual patient.[5] When whole blood is used for COP measurement, samples should be collected with lyophilized heparin, which is commonly available in green-top tubes. Slight variability does occur from one laboratory to another, so normal values should be established for each setting.

Samples of plasma or serum that cannot be processed immediately may be frozen and later thawed for determination of COP with little effect on the accuracy of the values obtained. This practice was evaluated in the study mentioned earlier, which showed changes in frozen samples stored up to 7 days that were minor and would not affect clinical decision making.[5] Whole blood samples can also be refrigerated and processed within 24 hours without any significant effect on the COP. Care should be taken to prevent hemolysis of the sample because free hemoglobin can increase COP. Dilution of the COP due to anticoagulants in the collection tube or syringe can occur; thus lyophilized heparin is preferred. It is provided in a dry form, has a high molecular weight, and is used in a very low concentration so it will have a minimal effect on COP.

Colloid Osmotic Pressure in Critically Ill Patients

COP has been measured in whole blood in 124 critically ill cats and dogs. Mean values obtained were 13.9 ± 3.1 mm Hg (range, 7.6 to 23.8).[6] The normal values for this laboratory were as listed earlier for whole blood. Critically ill cats and dogs can have substantial decreases in their COP values and may benefit greatly from COP monitoring and therapy aimed at correcting a low COP.

How Colloid Osmotic Pressure Is Measured

The colloid osmometer determines the COP of a solution using a semipermeable membrane. The membrane has a uniform pore size that allows only molecules with a molecular weight of 30,000 Da or less to pass through, simulating the capillary endothelium in veterinary patients. This membrane separates two chambers, a reference chamber filled with 0.9% saline and a test chamber into which the patient sample is injected. The sample tested can be serum, plasma, or whole blood (normal ranges vary slightly depending on which is used, as described earlier).

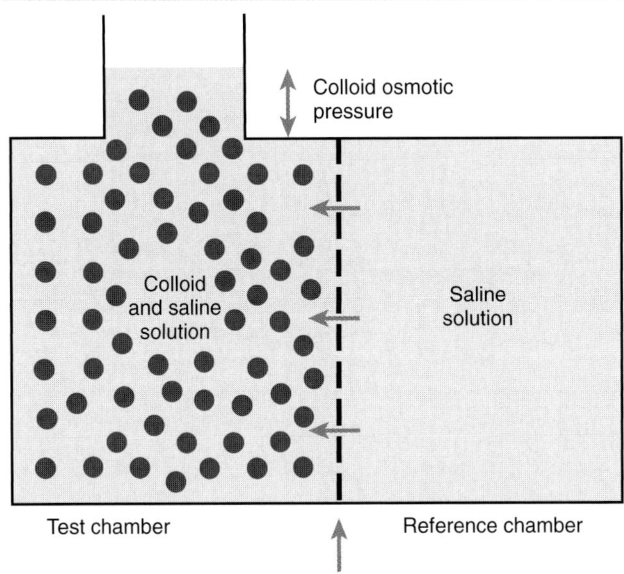

FIGURE 187-2 Measurement of colloid osmotic pressure in a colloid osmometer across a semipermeable membrane. The colloid in the patient's blood sample, placed in the test chamber, cannot move across the semipermeable membrane. Water is therefore drawn across the membrane from the reference chamber. The difference in pressure is measured as the colloid osmotic pressure.

The membrane is relatively impermeable to the proteins because of their large size. Water migrates from the reference chamber into the test chamber as a result of differences in the colloid concentration and COP (Figure 187-2). The COP as determined by the membrane depends not only on the colloid concentration but also on the Gibbs-Donnan effect, which takes into account the negative charge of the proteins. Electroneutrality must be maintained on each side of the membrane. The negative charge of the proteins causes retention of positively charged ions, primarily Na^+, which increases the concentration of these normally diffusible ions in the test chamber.

Because osmotic pressure is proportional to the number of molecules present, not the size of the molecules, the cations contribute significantly to the COP. The actual contribution of these ions to the COP can be determined by the square of the electrical charge carried by the colloid component. Because the total measured COP is determined by both the colloid and the associated positive ions, the COP is related nonlinearly to the colloid concentration. The charge of the proteins in a sample depends on the pH of the sample and the electrophoretic pattern of the proteins. These may be very abnormal in critically ill patients, which makes direct measurement of the COP all the more essential.

After equilibrium has been established between the two chambers (within 30 to 90 seconds), a negative pressure gradient exists in the reference chamber. A sensing diaphragm next to the fluid in the reference chamber is attached to a pressure transducer. Minute pressure changes in the reference chamber are converted into alterations in electrical impedance, which is measured, amplified, then converted into a display on the osmometer that is reported in mm Hg.

Indications for Colloid Osmotic Pressure Measurement

COP measurement should be part of routine monitoring in any patient receiving artificial colloids, in patients with edema, and in patients that are treated with aggressive crystalloid therapy or have low serum albumin concentration. Critically ill patients may have hypoalbuminemia and a decreased COP due to dilution from crystalloid therapy, decreased albumin production caused by anorexia and a shift to production of acute-phase proteins, and increased loss via blood loss, loss into effusions, or loss into the interstitium associated with increased vascular permeability. Monitoring of COP may help prevent edema formation in these patients by allowing the clinician to direct therapy toward correcting a low COP. Fortunately, COP measurement requires a very small sample of blood or serum (less than 0.5 ml). COP can change rapidly in patients receiving large amounts of crystalloid or colloid fluid therapy; therefore daily or twice-daily measurement often is indicated. In a recent study, healthy isoflurane-anesthetized dogs received lactated Ringer's solution at a rate of 0, 10, 20, or 30 ml/kg/hr for 1 hour. In those given the solution at rates of 20 or 30 ml/kg/hr significant decreases in COP were measured at 30 and 60 minutes compared with baseline.[7] Whether this information translates into predictable clinical sequelae is not well studied and most likely depends on other Starling's forces.

Edema of organs such as the heart (which causes increased ventricular stiffness and decreased end-diastolic volume, stroke volume, and cardiac output) and of the lungs (which causes interstitial edema and increased work of breathing) can lead to multiple organ dysfunction long before clinically appreciable peripheral edema is present. By correcting low COP in critically ill patients, some of these secondary problems that contribute to patient morbidity and mortality may be prevented.

A low COP in a critically ill patient can and should be managed with administration of plasma, human or canine albumin solutions, or artificial colloids (e.g., hydroxyethyl starch solutions). In human patients, a lower COP has been associated with decreased survival, particularly before the use of artificial colloids became commonplace.[8] In a later study, COP was not significantly different between survivors and nonsurvivors in patients with a critical illness of at least 7 days' duration. In this study, however, artificial colloids could be used as directed by the patients' physicians, and mean COP in all patients was 16.1 mm Hg.[9] This maintained the COP value above the cutoff that had previously been associated with increased mortality. Further research may find that through management of a patient's low COP with artificial colloids and albumin, this risk factor is eliminated in critically ill patients, and therefore the overall chance of survival is improved.

OSMOLALITY

Definition

Osmolality is the number of particles of solute per kilogram of solvent, and osmolarity is the number of particles of solute per liter of solvent. Both are purely dependent on the number of particles in solution; the particle size, shape, density, or electrical charge has no relevance. In body fluids, they are almost exactly equal because the solvent is primarily water, and 1 kg of water is equal to 1 L of water. Normal values for osmolality are 290 to 310 mOsm/kg in dogs and 290 to 330 mOsm/kg in cats.[10]

Determination of Osmolality

Plasma osmolality can be estimated by using the following equation:

$$\text{Calculated plasma osmolality} = 2(\text{Na}^+) + (\text{BUN} \div 2.8) + (\text{glucose} \div 18)$$

where BUN = blood urea nitrogen and Na^+ = sodium concentration.[11-13]

The sodium concentration is multiplied by a factor of 2 to include the chloride and bicarbonate ions that are present to maintain electroneutrality. Concentrations of urea and glucose are measured in milligrams per deciliter and must be converted to millimoles per liter by the conversion factor of 2.8 for BUN and 18 for glucose. Common causes of increased calculated plasma osmolality include hypernatremia, hyperglycemia secondary to diabetes mellitus, and azotemia (Box 187-1; see later section on effective osmolality). The most common cause of decreased calculated plasma osmolality is hyponatremia (see Chapters 50).

BOX 187-1 *Common Causes of Hyperosmolality in Small Animals*

Effective Osmoles	Ineffective Osmoles
Sodium	Blood urea nitrogen
Glucose	Ethylene glycol and metabolites
Mannitol	Ethanol and methanol
Ketoacids	Acetylsalicylic acid
Lactic acid	Isopropyl alcohol
Phosphates and sulfates (with renal failure)	
Radiopaque contrast solutions	

Serum osmolality can be determined indirectly by using a freezing point depression osmometer or determining the vapor point depression of the solution.[10,12] Freezing point depression is the more common and accurate method because it measures volatile substances in solution (e.g., alcohol) that would be missed using the other method.[11] For every 1 mol of nondissociating molecules dissolved in 1 kg (or 1 L) of water, the freezing point depression is decreased by 1.86°C. The osmolality of this solution would be 1 Osm/kg or 1000 mOsm/kg.[10]

Osmolal Gap

The difference between the measured and calculated serum osmolality is referred to as the *osmolal gap*. Recent evidence has shown a nearly zero osmolal gap in dogs and cats (−5 to 2 with a median of −2 in dogs and −3 to 6 with a median of 2 in cats).[12,13] A measured value that is more than 10 mOsm/kg higher than the calculated plasma value[10] indicates that an unmeasured solute is present in a large amount in the plasma. This could be any solute that is not accounted for in the equation and can include lactic acid, sulfates, phosphates, acetylsalicylic acid, mannitol, ethylene glycol and its metabolites, ethanol, isopropyl alcohol, methanol, radiographic contrast solution, paraldehyde, sorbitol, glycerol, propylene glycol, or acetone (see Box 187-1).[10,14]

It has been reported that commercially available activated charcoal suspensions which contain propylene glycol or glycerol can cause increased serum osmolality in healthy dogs.[15] This may result in difficulty in interpreting serum osmolality when evaluating for some toxins (e.g., ethylene glycol) if activated charcoal is administered before blood samples are obtained for measurement of serum osmolality. An increased osmolal gap can also occur with pseudohyponatremia secondary to hyperlipidemia, marked hyperglycemia, or hyperproteinemia.[10,16] Newer methods of measuring plasma electrolytes with ion-selective electrodes have helped to circumvent this problem.

Effective Osmolality

Because some molecules such as urea are freely diffusible across cell membranes, changes in their concentrations do not cause fluid shifts between the intracellular and extracellular compartments. Other molecules—most importantly sodium, but also glucose, chloride, and others—do not readily cross cell membranes and therefore cause water movement. Effective osmolality, also known as *tonicity,* can be estimated as follows:

$$\text{Calculated effective osmolality} = 2(\text{Na}^+) + (\text{glucose} \div 18)$$

This is the same as the previous equation for calculated plasma osmolality without BUN, which is an ineffective osmole. Tonicity is an important concept when comparing solutions. A solution is hypertonic if it contains a higher concentration of impermeant solutes than a reference solution and hypotonic if it contains a lower concentration of impermeant solutes. Solutions are isotonic if they have equal numbers of impermeant solutes.

Effective osmolality is especially relevant when evaluating azotemic patients. With a very elevated BUN level, the calculated osmolality will be increased, but the effective osmolality or tonicity may be normal or even decreased. The calculated osmolality needs to be used to evaluate these patients; direct measurement of osmolality using the freezing point depression method cannot distinguish between effective and ineffective osmoles.[10]

Evaluation of osmolality, both calculated and measured, can be important for recognition and treatment of several clinical conditions, including sodium disorders, hyperglycemia, and certain toxicities (see Box 187-1). Therapy should be aimed at preventing rapid changes in osmolality because adverse reactions, especially neurologic, may result if the serum osmolality is changed abruptly (see Chapter 50 for more details).

Urine Osmolality

Urine osmolality is the number of molecules (unaffected by the size of the molecules) per kilogram of water and must be measured by an osmometer. It is used to assess the concentrating ability of the kidney and should be interpreted along with the hydration and volume status of the patient. Urine specific gravity (USG) is more commonly used to assess renal concentrating ability because it is easier to measure (through the use of a hand-held refractometer). Specific gravity is a ratio of the density of a substance compared to water, so it is affected by the number of molecules and their molecular weights. Normally, the urine osmolality and USG are linearly correlated. If many high-molecular-weight molecules are present in the urine, USG will overestimate the urine solute concentration, whereas the urine osmolality remains accurate. Some of the molecules that can interfere with USG include albumin, synthetic colloids, and iohexal.[17] Interpretation of urine osmolality requires knowledge of the hydration and intravascular volume status of the patient. This allows for differentiation of an appropriate versus an abnormal physiologic response of the kidneys. The urine osmolality is useful for differentiating sodium disorders, identifying the syndrome of inappropriate antidiuretic hormone (see Chapter 68), differentiating prerenal from renal causes of azotemia, and diagnosing diabetes insipidus.

REFERENCES

1. Levick JR, Michel CC: Microvascular fluid exchange and the revised Starling principle, Cardiovasc Res 87:198, 2010.
1a. Brown SA, Dusza K, Boehmer J: Comparison of measured and calculated values for colloid osmotic pressure in hospitalized animals, Am J Vet Res 55:910, 1994.
2. Thomas LA, Brown SA: Relationship between colloid osmotic pressure and plasma protein concentration in cattle, horses, dogs, and cats, Am J Vet Res 53:2241, 1992.
3. Rudloff E, Kirby R: Colloid osmometry, Clin Tech Small Anim Pract 15:119, 2000.
4. Culp AM, Clay ME, Baylor IA, et al: Colloid osmotic pressure (COP) and total solid (TS) measurement in normal dogs and cats, Proceedings of the IVECCS, San Antonio, September 7-11, 1994 (abstract).
5. Odunayo A, Kerl ME: Comparison of whole blood and plasma colloid osmotic pressure in healthy dogs, J Vet Emerg Crit Care 21:236-241, 2011.
6. King LG, Culp AM, Clay ME, et al: Measurement of colloid osmotic pressure (COP) in a small animal intensive care unit, Proceedings of the IVECCS, San Antonio, September 7-11, 1994 (abstract).
7. Muir WW, Kijtawornrat A, Ueyama Y, et al: Effects of intravenous administration of lactated Ringer's solution on hematologic, serum biochemical, rheological, hemodynamic, and renal measurements in healthy isoflurane-anesthetized dogs, J Am Vet Med Assoc 239:630, 2011.
8. Weil MH, Henning RJ, Puri VK: Colloid oncotic pressure: clinical significance, Crit Care Med 7:113, 1979.
9. Blunt MC, Nicholson JP, Park GR: Serum albumin and colloid osmotic pressure in survivors and nonsurvivors of prolonged critical illness, Anaesthesia 53:755, 1998.
10. DiBartola SP: Disorders of sodium and water: hypernatremia and hyponatremia. In DiBartola SP, editor: Fluid, electrolyte and acid-base disorders in small animal practice, ed 4, St Louis, 2012, Saunders.
11. Barr JW, Pesillo-Crosby SA: Use of the advanced micro-osmometer model 3300 for determination of a normal osmolality and evaluation of different formulas for calculated osmolarity and osmole gap in adult dogs, J Vet Emerg Crit Care 18:270, 2008.
12. Dugger DT, Mellema MS, Hopper K, et al: Estimated osmolality of canine serum: a comparison of the clinical utility of several published formulae, J Vet Emerg Crit Care (in press).
13. Dugger DT, Epstein SE, Hopper K, et al: Comparative accuracy of several published formulae for the estimation of serum osmolality in cats, J Small Anim Pract 54(4):184-189, 2013.
14. Feldman BF, Rosenberg DP: Clinical use of anion gap and osmolal gap in veterinary medicine, J Am Vet Med Assoc 178:396, 1981.
15. Burkitt JM, Haskins SC, Aldrich J, et al: Effects of oral administration of a commercial activated charcoal suspension on serum osmolality and lactate concentration in the dog, J Vet Intern Med 19:683, 2005.
16. Wellman ML, DiBartola SP, Kohn CW: Applied physiology of body fluids in dogs and cats. In DiBartola SP, editor: Fluid, electrolyte and acid-base disorders in small animal practice, ed 4, St Louis, 2012, Saunders.
17. Smart L, Hopper K, Aldrich J, et al: The effect of hetastarch (670/0.75) on urine specific gravity and osmolality in the dog, J Vet Intern Med 23:388, 2009.

CHAPTER 188

INTRAABDOMINAL PRESSURE MONITORING

Guillaume L. Hoareau, DrVet, DACVECC • Matthew S. Mellema, DVM, PhD, DACVECC

KEY POINTS

- Abdominal perfusion pressure, the difference between the mean arterial pressure and the intraabdominal pressure (IAP), can be compromised with IAP elevations.
- Intraabdominal hypertension predisposes patients to developing multiple organ dysfunction and failure.
- Intraabdominal pressure can be dangerously elevated even in disease states that do not primarily involve the abdomen.
- Measurement of IAP can be performed using simple, minimally invasive methods.
- Trends are more useful than a single measurement in helping to assess organ perfusion and can assist in decision making.

Intraabdominal pressure (IAP) and intraabdominal hypertension (IAH) have been recognized in animals and humans for over 150 years.[1,2] A discussion of IAP in pregnancy was published in 1913, and the effects of IAH on renal function in humans was described in 1947.[3,4] One of the first published studies was undertaken simply to determine whether IAP was typically positive or negative in value and involved a series of varied procedures in different species.[1] Original research into the physiologic effects of IAH was performed in several species once the normal IAP was established.[2] These studies used inconsistent protocols, the findings were rarely confirmed independently, and the techniques used would be found unacceptable for technical and humane reasons today. Scientists believed it was important to establish the parameters at that time, though, because surgery and interventional medicine were evolving.

DEFINITIONS AND INCIDENCE

Intraabdominal pressure refers simply to the pressure within the abdominal cavity, regardless of the actual reading. *Intraabdominal hypertension* is defined as a sustained or repeated pathologic elevation of IAP of more than 12 mm Hg.[5,6] An IAH grading system has been proposed with severity graded on the basis of the magnitude of IAP elevation (Table 188-1). *Abdominal compartment syndrome* (ACS) is defined as a sustained increase in IAP of more than 20 mm Hg (with or without an APP < 60 mm Hg) that is associated with new organ dysfunction or failure.[5,6] ACS is considered primary if the site of trauma or disease lies within the abdominal cavity (e.g., fractured liver or spleen, penetrating foreign body, peritonitis, neoplasia, hepatic abscess, pancreatitis) and secondary if the inciting disease is extraperitoneal in origin (e.g., burns or thoracic trauma, usually followed by massive fluid resuscitation or high-pressure mechanical ventilation).

Prevalence studies have reported that approximately 32% to 51% of human intensive care patients experience IAH at some point during their intensive care unit stay. Approximately 14% of these patients have IAP elevations severe enough to be diagnosed with ACS.[7,8] Conzemius et al reported that in a series of 20 dogs with gross abdominal distention and gastric dilation/volvulus, pyometra, acute ascites, or diaphragmatic hernia the period prevalence of IAH was quite high if one applies the human diagnostic criteria (IAP > 12 mm Hg).[9] All of the patients in this study had an IAP of 15 cm H_20 (~11 mm Hg) or more. The prevalence of IAH and ACS in critically ill veterinary patients otherwise remains unknown.

RISK FACTORS

Certain conditions have been associated with an increased risk of IAH in human patients. They are classified by the World Society of the Abdominal Compartment Syndrome as diseases that can lead to the following: (1) diminished abdominal wall compliance, (2) increased intraluminal content, (3) increased abdominal content, or (4) capillary leak syndrome.[10] These same risk factors have been investigated in a series of canine patients.[11] Those patients in which a known risk factor was identified had significantly higher IAP than dogs in the no-risk group, which suggests that these same risks factors are relevant to veterinary as well as human patients. Also, evidence from human studies suggest that physical examination is not always

Table 188-1 Interpretation of Intraabdominal Pressure (IAP) and Recommendations for Therapy

Grade	IAP (cm H_2O)	IAP (mm Hg)	Recommended Action
I	16-20	12-15	Normovolemia should be ensured and the underlying disease should be pursued.
II	21-27	16-20	Volume resuscitation may be necessary, diagnostics to identify the cause should be instituted, and decompression might be considered.
III	28-34	21-25	Volume resuscitation may be necessary, diagnostics to identify the cause should be instituted, and decompression should be considered.
IV	>34	>25	Decompression is necessary to reverse organ damage and prevent further deterioration. Either paracentesis or surgical exploration is strongly recommended.

a reliable tool to evaluate IAP.[12] Clinicians are therefore encouraged to measure and monitor IAP in patients affected by diseases known to predispose to IAH, with or without evidence of IAH on physical examination.

PATHOPHYSIOLOGY

Both primary and secondary ACS are associated with multiple organ dysfunction and a worsened prognosis.[8,13-15] This is an important association because it is highly recommended that IAP be monitored in critically ill patients that do not have intraperitoneal disease. Resolution of the ACS can significantly improve outcome in patients without primary abdominal disease that develop multiple organ dysfunction.[16,17]

The effects of elevated IAP on organ function are well documented.[18-21] Visceral perfusion, abdominal blood flow, central venous pressure (CVP), pulmonary pressures, cardiac output, and renal function are all adversely affected by an increasing IAP, and early changes can be seen when levels exceed 10 cm H_2O. Much of the research documenting the systemic effects of ACS has been performed in dogs.[21-27] Little clinical work in veterinary medicine has documented the effects of ACS in hospitalized patients; however, the disease processes in which it is recognized in humans exist in small animal patients, and the technology for monitoring and responding to changes are the same. Several comprehensive reviews of the subject have been published in the human medical literature.[28-33]

IAH has been documented in human patients with ruptured abdominal aortic aneurysm, abdominal hemorrhage from trauma, occluded mesenteric artery, ruptured or necrotic bowel, bile peritonitis,[20] blunt trauma to any of the abdominal organs, gastric perforation, bladder rupture,[31] and large abdominal mass.[34] In many of these cases, there was a previous surgical procedure and the IAH mandated a reexploration of the abdomen. Fluid infusions and effusions in dogs,[21] morbid obesity,[35] the use of antishock trousers,[36] and pregnancy in humans[3] are also conditions that have been documented to increase IAP.

METHODS OF INTRAABDOMINAL PRESSURE MEASUREMENT

IAP has been measured via catheters placed in the inferior vena cava, stomach,[37,38] urinary bladder, and peritoneal cavity.[39] The urinary bladder method is currently considered the gold standard by the World Society of the Abdominal Compartment Syndrome.[10] Excluding gas in the intestinal tract, the abdominal contents are noncompressible, and thus the pressure at one point is equal to the pressures at all others in the steady state. Therefore bladder pressure measurements reflect the pressure in the abdomen as a whole. Such measurements are relatively simple to obtain in small animal patients and provide consistent, accurate measurements.[39] A urethral catheter is inserted aseptically so that the tip is just inside the trigone of the urinary bladder. A Foley catheter is preferred to ensure that the fenestrations lie just inside the bladder. A sterile urine collection system is attached in the usual way, but two three-way stopcocks are placed in the system (Figure 188-1). A water manometer is attached to the upright stopcock port. A 35-ml to 60-ml syringe of 0.9% sodium chloride or a bag of 0.9% sodium chloride and an intravenous administration set are attached to the distal stopcock port for filling the manometer and infusing the bladder. The bladder is emptied and 0.5 to 1 ml/kg (maximum of 25 ml per patient) of sterile 0.9% sodium chloride is instilled to fill it slightly. This lessens the likelihood that the bladder wall will obstruct the catheter fenestrations.

The system is zeroed to the patient's midline at the symphysis pubis and the manometer is filled with isotonic saline. The stopcock is closed to the fluid source, so that the meniscus in the manometer can drop and equilibrate with the pressure in the urinary bladder. The difference between the reading at the meniscus and the zero point is the IAP. The patient should be laterally recumbent when measurements are obtained. Patient position affects measurement[40] and should therefore be the same at each measurement. End-expiratory readings are standard. Use of appropriate aseptic technique for placement and handling of the urethral catheter and the

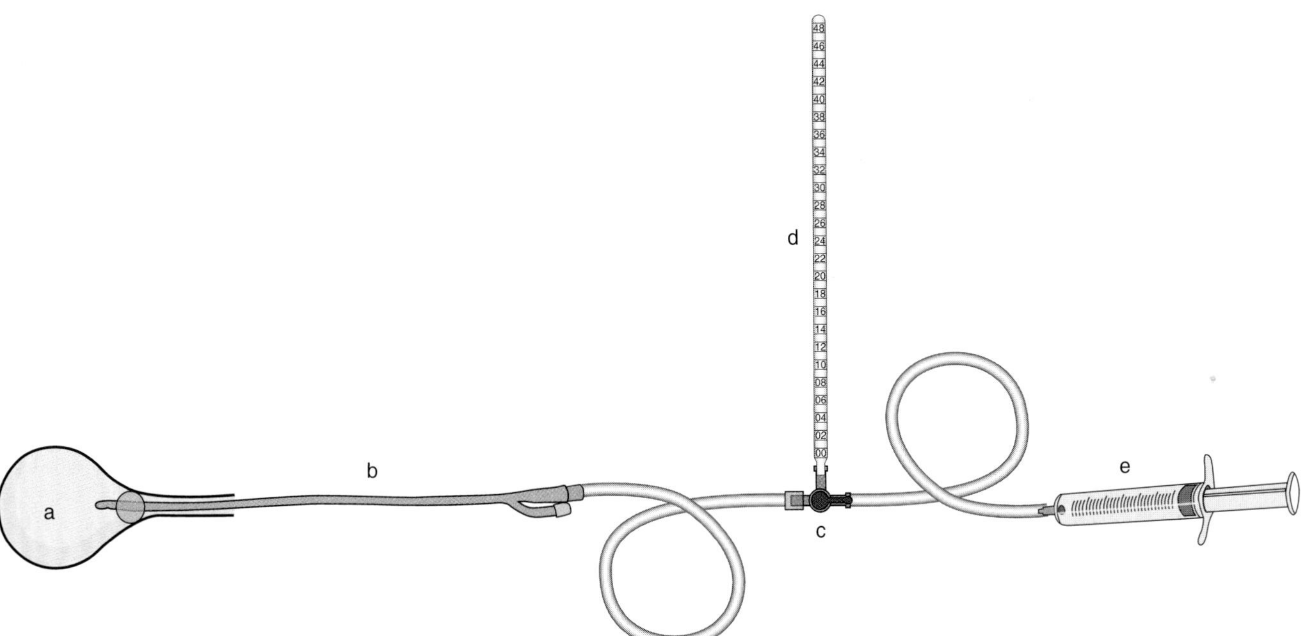

FIGURE 188-1 Setup for measurement of intraabdominal pressure via a urethral catheter. *a,* Urinary bladder; *b,* Foley catheter; *c,* three-way stopcock; *d,* water manometer; *e,* syringe filled with 0.9% NaCl. *(Image courtesy John Doval.)*

BOX 188-1 ***Factors Influencing Intraabdominal Pressure Readings***

- Body positioning
- Body condition
- Pregnancy
- Increased abdominal wall tone
  - Pain
  - Anxiety
- External abdominal pressure application
  - Belly bandages
- Volume of infusate

measurement system prevents a urinary tract infection in an otherwise healthy dog.[9]

Normal IAP in dogs is 0 to 5 cm H_2O. Healthy dogs undergoing elective abdominal surgery (ovariohysterectomy) had a postoperative IAP ranging from 0 to 15 cm H_2O. No problems associated with IAH were observed.[9] Normal IAP ranges from 4 to 8 cm H_2O in sedated cats and 6 to 11 cm H_2O in awake cats.[41] Many factors can impact the measured value of IAP, and following a set protocol minimizes the potential for error. Factors influencing IAP are presented in Box 188-1. In patients at risk of (or suffering from) IAH, IAP should be monitored every 2 to 8 hours. IAP can be monitored more frequently if clinically indicated. In patients for which indwelling bladder catheter placement is not feasible or desirable, measurements made from a catheter tip located in the intraabdominal vena cava may be substituted. Acceptable agreement has been found between intravesicular and caudal vena cava pressures in at least one canine model.[42] Vena cava access may be obtained by advancing a long catheter centrally from a pelvic limb peripheral vein (e.g., lateral saphenous) insertion site (see Chapter 195).

PHYSIOLOGIC EFFECTS OF INTRAABDOMINAL HYPERTENSION

Hemodynamic Effects

Abdominal perfusion pressure (APP) better estimates perfusion pressure to visceral organs than mean arterial pressure (MAP) alone. It is defined as MAP minus IAP. In humans, maintaining APP at or above 60 mm Hg has been associated with improved outcome in patients with IAH and ACS. APP has therefore been proposed as a resuscitation endpoint.[5,6,43]

Increases in IAP lead to elevations in CVP, pulmonary artery pressure, right atrial pressure, pulmonary capillary wedge pressure, MAP, and systemic vascular resistance.[21,44,45] These changes are believed to develop in part because of catecholamine release and a subsequent shift of abdominal vascular volume into the thorax.[44]

Cardiac output may increase transiently with the initial increase in preload resulting from the vascular volume shift. Cardiac output then declines because venous return from the caudal part of the body is reduced and systemic vascular resistance is increased as a result of compression of the abdominal vasculature.[25,26] In a porcine model, an IAP of 30 mm Hg for 4 hours was associated with a significant decrease in cardiac output.[46]

Interestingly, the elevation in IAP may be transmitted to the thoracic cavity and falsely elevate CVP measurements, providing the clinician with a false assessment of the patient's intravascular status.[47] In cases of IAH or ACS, CVP must therefore be interpreted with caution. Other advanced hemodynamic parameters (i.e., pulse pressure variation and global end-diastolic volume) proved more useful than CVP in predicting fluid responsiveness in a porcine model of IAH.[48]

BOX 188-2 ***Abdominal Perfusion Pressure and Filtration Gradient Formulas***

- Abdominal perfusion pressure = mean arterial pressure (MAP) – intraabdominal pressure (IAP)
- Filtration gradient = glomerular filtration pressure – proximal tubule pressure = MAP – IAP – IAP = MAP – 2IAP

When graded increases in IAP were tested in dogs and pigs, urine output decreased,[4,27] and arterial and venous lactate levels increased.[24] These effects are largely due to the reduction in cardiac output. Increasing vascular volume with intravenous fluid infusions improved the reduced cardiac output associated with IAH. Surgical decompression improved oxygenation, cardiac output, and atrial filling pressures within 15 minutes in human patients.[19,49]

Renal Effects

Glomerular filtration rate and urine output were reduced in dogs with an IAP of 10 to 20 cm H_2O. Oliguria and anuria developed in these dogs with moderate to severe IAH of 25 cm H_2O or higher. The evidence suggests that this occurs because of reduced cardiac output and compression of the renal vasculature and parenchyma rather than a postrenal effect of pressure on the ureters.[27] Urine production initially depends on the glomerular filtration gradient (Box 188-2). For the same change in IAP, urine production is reduced beyond the decrease due solely to reduction in APP.[5,50] Porcine models of IAH demonstrated alteration in renal cortical blood flow[51] and anuria at an IAP higher than 30 mm Hg.[46] Azotemia develops secondary to decreased blood urea nitrogen and creatinine excretion. Patients with ACS consistently experience improved urine output and a reduction in azotemia very quickly after surgical decompression.[4,9,19,27,52]

Pulmonary and Thoracic Effects

Pulmonary compliance is reduced with IAH.[40,53] Greater pressure on the peritoneal side of the diaphragm impairs its ability to contract and generate adequate subatmospheric intrathoracic pressure.[44] A small study in human patients with acute lung injury[54] reported that a rise in IAP was associated with a decrease in the overall respiratory system compliance. Partition analysis showed that this was mostly the result of a decrease in chest wall compliance because pulmonary mechanics were unaltered. In mechanically ventilated pigs the negative hemodynamic effects of positive end-expiratory pressure combined with IAH led to a significant increase in blood lactate levels as well as markedly increased CVP, pulmonary capillary wedge pressure, and pulmonary artery pressure.[24,55,56] IAP monitoring is a valuable tool in assessing the numerous factors contributing to changes in pulmonary and hemodynamic function. Patients undergoing mechanical ventilation that have concurrent abdominal disease may benefit from measurement of IAP. To allow the decrease in respiratory compliance to be taken into consideration, volume-controlled mechanical ventilation may be preferred in cases of IAH.[56] Approximately 60% to 70% of the IAP is transmitted to the thoracic cavity as evidenced by a rise in esophageal pressure.[57,58] Thus, when a lung-protective ventilator strategy is being considered, it has been suggested to use ΔP_{Plat}, the difference between the plateau pressure (P_{Plat}) and the IAP.[59]

Even with surgical decompression, human burn patients with ACS experienced more severe lung injury during the 3 days following the burn than those without ACS. This underscores the potential for IAH to trigger pulmonary damage.[60] When pulmonary or cardiovascular parameters deteriorate, if IAH can be ruled out as a cause, the clinician's focus can be better directed to the true cause of deterioration. It has been suggested that elevated positive end-expiratory and peak inspiratory pressures may be the cause, rather than effect, of ACS. Regardless, both should improve with timely intervention when IAP exceeds 25 to 35 cm H_2O.[17]

Central Nervous System Effects

Intracranial pressure is increased with IAH.[35,55,61] Pressure is transmitted from the abdomen to the thorax. Increased thoracic pressures and blood volume in the more compliant compartments reduce venous blood flow in the jugular system and, therefore, drainage from the head.[62] This process has been implicated in the central nervous system abnormalities associated with morbid obesity as well as with iatrogenic pneumoperitoneum during laparoscopic procedures.[63] Patients with IAH should be monitored carefully for signs of increasing intracranial pressure. These include obtundation, changes in and loss of cranial nerve reflexes, vomiting, and seizures.

Visceral Effects

Hepatic, portal, intestinal, and gastric blood flow declined with an associated tissue acidosis in pigs with IAH.[46,64-66] Bowel tissue oxygenation is reduced as measured at the terminal ileum.[67] Laser Doppler microcirculation analysis in a pig model of IAP[51] demonstrated a significant decrease in blood flow to the gastric mucosa, seromuscular layer of the small and large intestine, and renal cortex. Intestinal mucosal blood flow was less affected than blood flow to other layers. Decreased lymphatic drainage[68] and venous return promotes interstitial edema in the viscera, which further promotes IAH. Bacterial translocation across the intestinal wall in association with reduced blood flow in ACS at pressures above 20 mm Hg has been documented in rats.[69,70] In a rabbit model of IAH, an IAP above 20 mm Hg was associated with increased intestinal permeability to fluorescent probes as well as bacterial endotoxin. Translocation of bacteria to the mesenteric lymph nodes and liver was concurrently documented.[71] Although bacterial translocation may predispose the patient to sepsis and its sequelae (i.e., systemic inflammatory response syndrome and multiple organ dysfunction syndrome),[72] it is important to remember that it is also a physiologic process.[73] Additionally, a porcine model showed that pigs subjected to hemorrhagic shock followed by fluid resuscitation and an IAP of 30 mm Hg did not demonstrate a higher rate of bacterial translocation than controls when polymerase chain reaction testing and culture were used to detect bacterial translocation.[74] The link between IAH, ACS, and bacteremia and its association with the development of systemic inflammatory response syndrome and sepsis remains unclear.

Systemic Effects

Several hormonal changes have been documented with IAH. An increase in plasma antidiuretic hormone levels occurred in dogs with externally applied abdominal pressures of 80 mm Hg. This increase was prevented by a prior intravenous infusion of 6% dextran at 8 to 10 ml/kg.[23] Pigs had elevated plasma renin activity and aldosterone levels in response to IAH of 34 cm H_2O.[44] Decompression reversed the hormonal changes. In a pneumoperitoneum model, pigs had elevated levels of epinephrine and norepinephrine at an IAP of 27.2 cm H_2O but not at an IAP of 13.6 cm H_2O.[75] This study did not measure hormone levels after decompression. These changes probably relate to reduced renal perfusion and the baroreceptor and renin-angiotensin responses to a perceived reduction in blood pressure or volume.

Evidence regarding the involvement of IAH and systemic inflammation is growing. Studies in rats[76] and pigs[77] demonstrated a rise in levels of interleukin 1β, interleukin 6, and tumor necrosis factor α as well as lung injury following experimentally induced IAH. This demonstrates the potential for IAH and ACS to injure extraabdominal organs and initiate multiple organ dysfunction syndrome. IAH promotes intraabdominal venous stasis, which is known to encourage thrombosis. The potential for thromboembolism at the time of decompression has been mentioned.[59] To the authors' knowledge there is no consensus guideline regarding anticoagulant therapy in patients with IAH or ACS. Blood flow to the rectus sheath muscles is reduced with IAH, and this may impair wound healing.[78] Thus in postceliotomy patients both systemic and local effects of IAH may promote wound dehiscence and postsurgical complications.

GENERAL CONSIDERATIONS

As a general rule, the following pressure guidelines may be used to assist in clinical decision making in response to elevations in IAP (see Table 188-1):

- If IAP is 10 to 20 cm H_2O, normovolemia should be ensured and the underlying cause should be pursued.
- If IAP is 20 to 35 cm H_2O, volume resuscitation may be necessary, diagnostic modalities to identify the cause should be instituted, and decompression should be considered.
- If IAP is higher than 35 cm H_2O, decompression either by paracentesis or surgical exploration is strongly recommended. Consideration should be given to managing the patient as an open abdomen.

Obviously the breadth of physiologic changes associated with IAH makes the condition a concern in any patient with multisystem disease. Patients with traumatic damage to more than one body cavity often have significant muscle and organ trauma. These patients would benefit from IAP monitoring because bowel ileus, organ ischemia, progressive abdominal hemorrhage, or other problems that are not readily apparent clinically may develop. Dogs with acute, severe pancreatitis can develop effusions and infections that could cause IAH and a rapid deterioration of their clinical status.

IAP measurement provides another objective parameter to use in deciding if and when to perform a surgical exploration. Patients who have had major abdominal surgery may benefit from IAP measurement as a means of early identification of the need for follow-up procedures. For instance, increasing IAP in postoperative patients may indicate dehiscence of surgery sites or peritonitis from any source. If IAP is increasing and urine output is decreasing in spite of adequate fluid therapy, surgical intervention or paracentesis is indicated.[18,19,79] IAP changes can aid in the assessment of the need for paracentesis in patients with severe ascites. Procedures such as therapeutic or diagnostic peritoneal lavage and peritoneal dialysis may be better managed if IAP is monitored in conjunction with monitoring of urine output and patient comfort.

Other situations that can lead to IAH, ACS, and organ dysfunction include intraperitoneal therapies and diagnostic tests. Iatrogenic IAH is generated during diagnostic peritoneal lavage, intracavitary infusion of drugs such as analgesics and antineoplastic agents, and peritoneal dialysis. Patient discomfort and negative effects can be linked to the increased IAP associated with these procedures.[80-82] The long-term effects are unknown, and there is some speculation that the length of time IAH is present can influence the degree of impairment and improvement with decompression.[17] Short-term effects from iatrogenic IAH are more directly associated with patient comfort and quality of life.[80]

IAP is a valuable parameter to monitor in critically ill patients. Regardless of whether primary abdominal disease is present, IAP may rise in response to interventions and treatments and can ultimately result in multiple organ dysfunction and death. Controlled studies still need to be performed in the veterinary clinical setting to better assess which patients will benefit most from measurement of IAP and to establish more specific guidelines for action.

ACKNOWLEDGMENT

In the first edition of this text, this chapter was written by Dr. Sharon Drellich. Dr. Drellich was a highly skilled and well-respected veterinary criticalist who was taken from us at too young an age. She was also a cherished friend and resident-mate of one of the authors (MM). Although the current authors have agreed to update the chapter, the conceptual framework and starting point for this chapter were Sharon's. The authors have elected to continue to have Sharon's name listed as an author posthumously in honor of her memory and many contributions to the field.

REFERENCES

1. Emerson H: Intraabdominal pressures, Arch Intern Med 7:754, 1911.
2. Coombs H: The mechanism of the regulation of intraabdominal pressure, Am J Physiol 61:159, 1922.
3. Paramore RH: The intra-abdominal pressure in pregnancy, Proc R Soc Med 6:291-334, 1913.
4. Bradley SE, Bradley GP: The effect of increased intra-abdominal pressure on renal function in man, J Clin Invest 26:1010-1022, 1947.
5. Malbrain ML, Cheatham ML, Kirkpatrick A, et al: Results from the International Conference of Experts on Intra-abdominal Hypertension and Abdominal Compartment Syndrome. I. Definitions, Intensive Care Med 32:1722-1732, 2006.
6. Cheatham ML, Malbrain ML, Kirkpatrick A, et al: Results from the International Conference of Experts on Intra-abdominal Hypertension and Abdominal Compartment Syndrome. II. Recommendations, Intensive Care Med 33:951-962, 2007.
7. Malbrain MNG, Chiumello D, Pelosi P, et al: Prevalence of intra-abdominal hypertension in critically ill patients: a multicentre epidemiological study, Intensive Care Med 30:822-829, 2004.
8. Malbrain ML, Chiumello D, Pelosi P, et al: Incidence and prognosis of intraabdominal hypertension in a mixed population of critically ill patients: a multiple-center epidemiological study, Crit Care Med 33:315-322, 2005.
9. Conzemius MG, Sammarco JL, Holt DE, et al: Clinical determination of preoperative and postoperative intra-abdominal pressures in dogs, Vet Surg 24:195-201, 1995.
10. Kirkpatrick AW, Roberts DJ, De Waele J, et al: Intra-abdominal hypertension and the abdominal compartment syndrome: updated consensus definitions and clinical practice guidelines from the World Society of the Abdominal Compartment Syndrome, Intensive Care Med 39:1190-1206, 2013.
11. Fetner M, Prittie J: Evaluation of transvesical intra-abdominal pressure measurement in hospitalized dogs, J Vet Emerg Crit Care 22:230-238, 2012.
12. Sugrue M, Bauman A, Jones F, et al: Clinical examination is an inaccurate predictor of intraabdominal pressure, World J Surg 26:1428-1431, 2002.
13. Regueira T, Bruhn A, Hasbun P, et al: Intra-abdominal hypertension: incidence and association with organ dysfunction during early septic shock, J Crit Care 23:461-467, 2008.
14. Vidal MG, Ruiz Weisser J, Gonzalez F, et al: Incidence and clinical effects of intra-abdominal hypertension in critically ill patients, Crit Care Med 36:1823-1831, 2008.
15. Balogh Z, McKinley BA, Holcomb JB, et al: Both primary and secondary abdominal compartment syndrome can be predicted early and are harbingers of multiple organ failure, J Trauma 54:848-859, 2003; discussion 859-861.
16. Hobson KG, Young KM, Ciraulo A, et al: Release of abdominal compartment syndrome improves survival in patients with burn injury, J Trauma 53:1129-1133, 2002; discussion 1133-1124.
17. Kopelman T, Harris C, Miller R, et al: Abdominal compartment syndrome in patients with isolated extraperitoneal injuries, J Trauma 49:744-747, 2000; discussion 747-749.
18. Chang MC, Miller PR, D'Agostino R Jr, et al: Effects of abdominal decompression on cardiopulmonary function and visceral perfusion in patients with intra-abdominal hypertension, J Trauma 44:440-445, 1998.
19. Cullen DJ, Coyle JP, Teplick R, et al: Cardiovascular, pulmonary, and renal effects of massively increased intra-abdominal pressure in critically ill patients, Crit Care Med 17:118-121, 1989.
20. Williams M, Simms HH: Abdominal compartment syndrome: case reports and implications for management in critically ill patients, Am Surg 63:555-558, 1997.
21. Barnes GE, Laine GA, Giam PY, et al: Cardiovascular responses to elevation of intra-abdominal hydrostatic pressure, Am J Physiol 248:R208-213, 1985.
22. Robotham JL, Wise RA, Bromberger-Barnea B: Effects of changes in abdominal pressure on left ventricular performance and regional blood flow, Crit Care Med 13:803-809, 1985.
23. Le Roith D, Bark H, Nyska M, et al: The effect of abdominal pressure on plasma antidiuretic hormone levels in the dog, J Surg Res 32:65-69, 1982.
24. Burchard KW, Ciombor DM, McLeod MK, et al: Positive end expiratory pressure with increased intra-abdominal pressure, Surg Gynecol Obstet 161:313-318, 1985.
25. Kashtan J, Green JF, Parsons EQ, et al: Hemodynamic effect of increased abdominal pressure, J Surg Res 30:249-255, 1981.
26. Ivankovich AD, Miletich DJ, Albrecht RF, et al: Cardiovascular effects of intraperitoneal insufflation with carbon dioxide and nitrous oxide in the dog, Anesthesiology 42:281-287, 1975.
27. Harman PK, Kron IL, McLachlan HD, et al: Elevated intra-abdominal pressure and renal function, Ann Surg 196:594-597, 1982.
28. Watson RA, Howdieshell TR: Abdominal compartment syndrome, South Med J 91:326-332, 1998.
29. Carr JA: Abdominal compartment syndrome: a decade of progress, J Am Coll Surg 216:135-146, 2013.
30. Malbrain ML, Cheatham ML: Definitions and pathophysiological implications of intra-abdominal hypertension and abdominal compartment syndrome, Am Surg 77(Suppl 1):S6-11, 2011.
31. Meldrum DR, Moore FA, Moore EE, et al: Prospective characterization and selective management of the abdominal compartment syndrome, Am J Surg 174:667-672, 1997; discussion 672-663.
32. Nathens AB, Brenneman FD, Boulanger BR: The abdominal compartment syndrome, Can J Surg 40:254-258, 1997.
33. Saggi BH, Sugerman HJ, Ivatury RR, et al: Abdominal compartment syndrome, J Trauma 45:597-609, 1998.
34. Celoria G, Steingrub J, Dawson JA, et al: Oliguria from high intra-abdominal pressure secondary to ovarian mass, Crit Care Med 15:78-79, 1987.
35. Sugerman HJ, DeMaria EJ, Felton WL 3rd, et al: Increased intra-abdominal pressure and cardiac filling pressures in obesity-associated pseudotumor cerebri, Neurology 49:507-511, 1997.
36. Gaffney FA, Thal ER, Taylor WF, et al: Hemodynamic effects of Medical Anti-Shock Trousers (MAST garment), J Trauma 21:931-937, 1981.
37. Collee GG, Lomax DM, Ferguson C, et al: Bedside measurement of intra-abdominal pressure (IAP) via an indwelling naso-gastric tube: clinical validation of the technique, Intensive Care Med 19:478-480, 1993.
38. Sugrue M, Buist MD, Lee A, et al: Intra-abdominal pressure measurement using a modified nasogastric tube: description and validation of a new technique, Intensive Care Med 20:588-590, 1994.
39. Iberti TJ, Kelly KM, Gentili DR, et al: A simple technique to accurately determine intra-abdominal pressure, Crit Care Med 15:1140-1142, 1987.
40. Obeid F, Saba A, Fath J, et al: Increases in intra-abdominal pressure affect pulmonary compliance, Arch Surg 130:544-547, 1995; discussion 547-548.
41. Rader RA, Johnson JA: Determination of normal intra-abdominal pressure using urinary bladder catheterization in clinically healthy cats, J Vet Emerg Crit Care 20:386-392, 2010.
42. Lacey SR, Bruce J, Brooks SP, et al: The relative merits of various methods of indirect measurement of intraabdominal pressure as a guide to closure of abdominal wall defects, J Pediatr Surg 22:1207-1211, 1987.
43. Cheatham ML, White MW, Sagraves SG, et al: Abdominal perfusion pressure: a superior parameter in the assessment of intra-abdominal hypertension, J Trauma 49:621-626, 2000; discussion 626-627.
44. Bloomfield GL, Blocher CR, Fakhry IF, et al: Elevated intra-abdominal pressure increases plasma renin activity and aldosterone levels, J Trauma 42:997-1004, 1997; discussion 1004-1005.

45. Moffa SM, Quinn JV, Slotman GJ: Hemodynamic effects of carbon dioxide pneumoperitoneum during mechanical ventilation and positive end-expiratory pressure, J Trauma 35:613-617, 1993; discussion 617-618.
46. Toens C, Schachtrupp A, Hoer J, et al: A porcine model of the abdominal compartment syndrome, Shock 18:316-321, 2002.
47. Schachtrupp A, Graf J, Tons C, et al: Intravascular volume depletion in a 24-hour porcine model of intra-abdominal hypertension, J Trauma 55:734-740, 2003.
48. Renner J, Gruenewald M, Quaden R, et al: Influence of increased intra-abdominal pressure on fluid responsiveness predicted by pulse pressure variation and stroke volume variation in a porcine model, Crit Care Med 37:650-658, 2009.
49. Peng ZY, Critchley LA, Joynt GM, et al: Effects of norepinephrine during intra-abdominal hypertension on renal blood flow in bacteremic dogs, Crit Care Med 36:834-841, 2008.
50. Sugrue M, Jones F, Deane SA, et al: Intra-abdominal hypertension is an independent cause of postoperative renal impairment, Arch Surg 134:1082-1085, 1999.
51. Olofsson PH, Berg S, Ahn HC, et al: Gastrointestinal microcirculation and cardiopulmonary function during experimentally increased intra-abdominal pressure, Crit Care Med 37:230-239, 2009.
52. Jacques T, Lee R: Improvement of renal function after relief of raised intra-abdominal pressure due to traumatic retroperitoneal haematoma, Anaesth Intensive Care 16:478-482, 1988.
53. Mutoh T, Lamm WJ, Embree LJ, et al: Abdominal distension alters regional pleural pressures and chest wall mechanics in pigs in vivo, J Appl Physiol 70:2611-2618, 1991.
54. Malbrain ML, Deeren DH, Nieuwendijk R, et al: Partitioning of respiratory mechanics in intra-abdominal hypertension, Intensive Care Med 29(Suppl 1):S1-213, 2003.
55. Bloomfield GL, Ridings PC, Blocher CR, et al: Effects of increased intra-abdominal pressure upon intracranial and cerebral perfusion pressure before and after volume expansion, J Trauma 40:936-941, 1996.
56. Wauters J, Claus P, Brosens N, et al: Relationship between abdominal pressure, pulmonary compliance, and cardiac preload in a porcine model, Crit Care Res Pract 2012:763181, 2012.
57. Malbrain M: Effect of intra-abdominal pressure on pleural and filling pressures, Intensive Care Med 29:S73, 2003.
58. Quintel M, Pelosi P, Caironi P, et al: An increase of abdominal pressure increases pulmonary edema in oleic acid-induced lung injury, Am J Respir Crit Care Med 169:534-541, 2004.
59. Malbrain ML: Is it wise not to think about intraabdominal hypertension in the ICU? Curr Opin Crit Care 10:132-145, 2004.
60. Oda J, Yamashita K, Inoue T, et al: Acute lung injury and multiple organ dysfunction syndrome secondary to intra-abdominal hypertension and abdominal decompression in extensively burned patients, J Trauma 62:1365-1369, 2007.
61. Citerio G, Vascotto E, Villa F, et al: Induced abdominal compartment syndrome increases intracranial pressure in neurotrauma patients: a prospective study, Crit Care Med 29:1466-1471, 2001.
62. Bloomfield GL, Ridings PC, Blocher CR, et al: A proposed relationship between increased intra-abdominal, intrathoracic, and intracranial pressure, Crit Care Med 25:496-503, 1997.
63. Josephs LG, Este-McDonald JR, Birkett DH, et al: Diagnostic laparoscopy increases intracranial pressure, J Trauma 36:815-818, 1994.
64. Rasmussen IB, Berggren U, Arvidsson D, et al: Effects of pneumoperitoneum on splanchnic hemodynamics: an experimental study in pigs, Eur J Surg 161:819-826, 1995.
65. Diebel LN, Dulchavsky SA, Wilson RF: Effect of increased intra-abdominal pressure on mesenteric arterial and intestinal mucosal blood flow, J Trauma 33:45-48, 1992; discussion 48-49.
66. Diebel LN, Wilson RF, Dulchavsky SA, et al: Effect of increased intra-abdominal pressure on hepatic arterial, portal venous, and hepatic microcirculatory blood flow, J Trauma 33:279-282, 1992; discussion 282-273.
67. Bongard F, Pianim N, Dubecz S, et al: Adverse consequences of increased intra-abdominal pressure on bowel tissue oxygen, J Trauma 39:519-524, 1995; discussion 524-515.
68. Moore-Olufemi SD, Xue H, Allen SJ, et al: Effects of primary and secondary intra-abdominal hypertension on mesenteric lymph flow: implications for the abdominal compartment syndrome, Shock 23:571-575, 2005.
69. Diebel LN, Dulchavsky SA, Brown WJ: Splanchnic ischemia and bacterial translocation in the abdominal compartment syndrome, J Trauma 43:852-855, 1997.
70. Polat C, Aktepe OC, Akbulut G, et al: The effects of increased intra-abdominal pressure on bacterial translocation, Yonsei Med J 44:259-264, 2003.
71. Cheng JT, Xiao GX, Xia PY, et al: Influence of intra-abdominal hypertension on the intestinal permeability and endotoxin/bacteria translocation in rabbits, Zhonghua Shao Shang Za Zhi 19:229-232, 2003.
72. Deitch EA, Rutan R, Waymack JP: Trauma, shock, and gut translocation, New Horiz 4:289-299, 1996.
73. MacFie J: Current status of bacterial translocation as a cause of surgical sepsis, Br Med Bull 71:1-11, 2004.
74. Doty JM, Oda J, Ivatury RR, et al: The effects of hemodynamic shock and increased intra-abdominal pressure on bacterial translocation, J Trauma 52:13-17, 2002.
75. Mikami O, Fujise K, Matsumoto S, et al: High intra-abdominal pressure increases plasma catecholamine concentrations during pneumoperitoneum for laparoscopic procedures, Arch Surg 133:39-43, 1998.
76. Rezende-Neto JB, Moore EE, Melo de Andrade MV, et al: Systemic inflammatory response secondary to abdominal compartment syndrome: stage for multiple organ failure, J Trauma 53:1121-1128, 2002.
77. Oda J, Ivatury RR, Blocher CR, et al: Amplified cytokine response and lung injury by sequential hemorrhagic shock and abdominal compartment syndrome in a laboratory model of ischemia-reperfusion, J Trauma 52:625-631, 2002.
78. Diebel L, Saxe J, Dulchavsky S: Effect of intra-abdominal pressure on abdominal wall blood flow, Am Surg 58:573-575, 1992.
79. Kron IL, Harman PK, Nolan SP: The measurement of intra-abdominal pressure as a criterion for abdominal re-exploration, Ann Surg 199:28-30, 1984.
80. Mahale AS, Katyal A, Khanna R: Complications of peritoneal dialysis related to increased intra-abdominal pressure, Adv Perit Dial 19:130-135, 2003.
81. Enoch C, Aslam N, Piraino B: Intra-abdominal pressure, peritoneal dialysis exchange volume, and tolerance in APD, Semin Dial 15:403-406, 2002.
82. Morris KP, Butt WW, Karl TR: Effect of peritoneal dialysis on intra-abdominal pressure and cardio-respiratory function in infants following cardiac surgery, Cardiol Young 14:293-298, 2004.

CHAPTER 189
AFAST AND TFAST IN THE INTENSIVE CARE UNIT

Søren R. Boysen, DVM, DACVECC

KEY POINTS

- The focused assessment with sonography for trauma (FAST) scan is not an extensive evaluation of all organs of the abdomen.
- The objective of the FAST scan is to detect free fluid in less than 5 minutes.
- Not all trauma-induced abdominal injury produces free fluid.
- The ultrasound probe should be moved and fanned at each FAST site to increase the sensitivity for detecting smaller localized pockets of free fluid.
- Serial FAST examinations may detect delayed fluid accumulations and can be used to monitor progression or resolution of free fluid accumulations over time.
- Positive findings on FAST scan in trauma patients typically indicate blood; however, ascites, urine, bile, and other forms of peritonitis cannot be ruled out.
- The FAST scan can be used to detect free fluid in nontrauma patients.
- The FAST scan can be extended to include views of the pleural and pericardial space, termed *thoracic focused assessment with sonography for trauma* (TFAST).
- TFAST is used to detect pericardial effusions, pleural effusions, and pneumothorax.
- Pneumothorax can be sonographically detected only when pleural air is located directly beneath the ultrasound probe.
- The glide sign may be difficult to detect in patients that are panting or have rapid shallow respirations.

In contrast to traditional extensive formal ultrasound examinations performed by radiologists and cardiologists, focused assessment with sonography for trauma (FAST) examinations are focused and limited studies performed as a point-of-care emergency procedure to answer specific clinical questions or to facilitate specific procedures (i.e., fluid collection). FAST examinations have become the standard of care in many emergency department and intensive care unit (ICU) settings because they are safe, noninvasive, rapid, repeatable, and portable, and can be performed at the time of initial triage during patient resuscitation.[1,2]

To date, veterinary FAST examinations have involved ultrasound evaluation of the pericardial, pleural, and abdominal spaces for the presence of free fluid, and evaluation of the pleural space for pneumothorax, particularly in patients with cardiovascular instability and those with trauma.[1-3] When the sonographic examination is focused to answer specific questions, ultrasound can be rapidly and effectively used to diagnose and manage patients in the ICU with minimal formal training in the technology.[1-3]

TERMINOLOGY

The terminology for focused emergency ultrasound examinations differs between human and veterinary medicine. As in the original canine veterinary study, human studies use the term *FAST* when referring to emergency ultrasound examinations of the abdomen and *extended* or *E-FAST* when referring to a FAST examination that includes the thorax.[1,4] To differentiate abdominal from thoracic FAST examinations in dogs and cats, the two are also referred to as *abdominal focused assessment with sonography for trauma* (AFAST) and *thoracic focused assessment with sonography for trauma* (TFAST), respectively.[2,3] The AFAST examination in dogs is analogous to the FAST examination in humans, and the two terms are often used interchangeably in veterinary medicine. The TFAST examination in dogs is analogous to the E-FAST examination in humans. This chapter uses the terms *AFAST* and *TFAST* when referring to veterinary studies and *FAST* and *E-FAST* when referring to human studies.

OBJECTIVE OF FOCUSED ASSESSMENT WITH SONOGRAPHY FOR TRAUMA

The objective of FAST examinations is to obtain an immediate answer to a clinically urgent question. FAST examinations are typically performed when obtaining immediate results can help guide resuscitative efforts or delaying the diagnosis can result in deterioration of the patient. Classical situations in which FAST examinations have clinical utility include the patient with cardiovascular instability or the patient in respiratory distress when the underlying cause is uncertain. The chance of ruling in or ruling out a specific pathologic condition is typically maximized by using the FAST examination to answer simple binary (yes-no) questions such as "Is fluid present in the abdomen?" or "Is air present in the pleural space?" It is important to stress that focused emergency ultrasound assessments are not intended to replace more extensive formal ultrasound examinations. AFAST and TFAST examinations should be considered complimentary diagnostic tests performed in the critically ill or unstable patient to provide timely diagnostic information and to help facilitate the use of emergency techniques.

ABDOMINAL FOCUSED ASSESSMENT WITH SONOGRAPHY FOR TRAUMA

There are three applications of focused emergency ultrasound scanning that have been studied in dogs experiencing abdominal trauma: AFAST, serial AFAST, and abdominal fluid scoring.[1,2]

AFAST is a rapid and focused examination of four sites in the abdomen designed to quickly rule in or rule out the presence of free abdominal fluid (typically indicative of hemorrhage). It is not an extensive examination of all the internal abdominal organs and should easily be accomplished within 5 minutes.[1,2] AFAST may be used as an extension of the initial triage examination in patients that have experienced trauma and in patients with cardiovascular instability in which the cause of shock is unknown. Although the use of AFAST is relatively novel in veterinary medicine, preliminary studies in dogs and cats show it to have clinical utility in diagnosing and managing trauma-induced intraabdominal injury.[1,2] Although not specifically studied in veterinary medicine, application of the AFAST

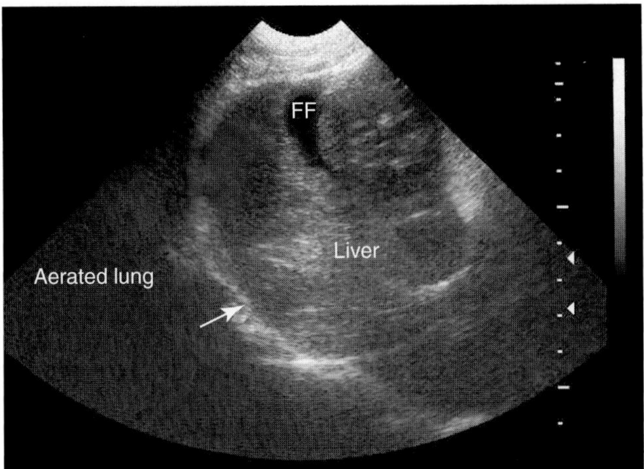

FIGURE 189-1 Subxiphoid view. The subxiphoid view detects free fluid *(FF)* between the liver lobes and between the liver and the diaphragm *(white arrow)*. In this image free fluid appears as an anechoic triangle between liver lobes. The liver and lungs are separated from each other by the diaphragm. This view can also be used to image the pleural and pericardial spaces (see Figure 189.6).

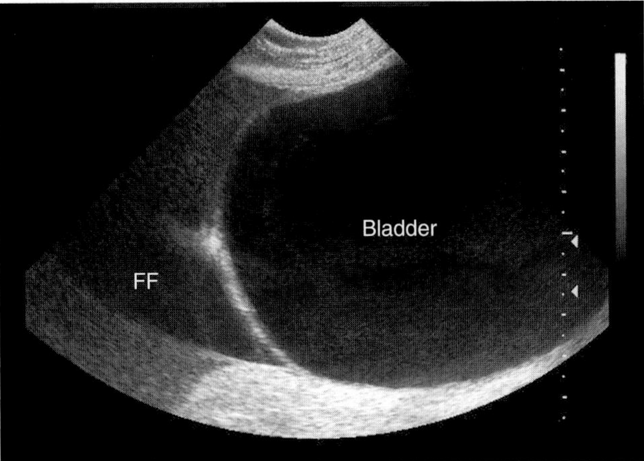

FIGURE 189-2 Bladder view. The midline view over the bladder detects fluid against the external wall of the urinary bladder. In this view free fluid *(FF)* appears as an anechoic triangular shape abutting the urinary bladder wall in the near and far fields of the image.

examination to nontrauma patients for the detection of free fluid due to uroabdomen, nontraumatic hemoabdomen, hollow viscus perforation, and other forms of peritonitis seems reasonable.

The use of serial AFAST examinations has been studied in dogs experiencing blunt abdominal injury and was found to detect changes in the quantity of fluid present in the abdomen over time, especially when combined with determination of abdominal fluid score (AFS).[2] In addition, some dogs with negative results on the initial AFAST examination had positive findings on serial AFAST examinations, which suggests that AFAST has improved sensitivity and specificity for detecting free fluid after blunt trauma when performed serially—similar to what has been shown in people.[2,5] This is particularly true for hollow organ injuries and injuries resulting in only small amounts of free fluid, which are easily missed on the initial AFAST examination.[5] Recommendations regarding when the FAST examination should be repeated vary; however, most studies suggest repeating the FAST examination every 2 to 4 hours, or as needed when the patient's condition is difficult to stabilize or deteriorates following initial stabilization.[2,5]

The AFS is a semiquantitative evaluation of the degree of free fluid (typically hemorrhage) present in the abdomen and is performed by recording the number of sites among the four standard views (see the later section on technique) in which free fluid is detected in the abdomen.[2] It has been suggested that by serially tracking and recording the progression or resolution of intraabdominal hemorrhage, the AFS may help direct therapeutic clinical decisions when considered along with other clinical examination findings.[2] Although the AFS has shown initial promise in the management of dogs experiencing blunt abdominal injury, a study in cats failed to demonstrate such findings.[6] Further studies are needed to assess the value of AFS as an endpoint of resuscitation and its utility in directing fluid therapy or surgical intervention in dogs and cats.

AFAST Technique

The AFAST examination involves visualizing the diaphragm, liver, gallbladder, spleen, kidneys, intestinal loops, and urinary bladder at four sites of the abdomen for the detection of free fluid. Free fluid tends to accumulate in the most dependent areas of the abdomen as anechoic triangles surrounded by organs (Figures 189-1 through 189-4).[1] The examination can be completed without clipping the fur and

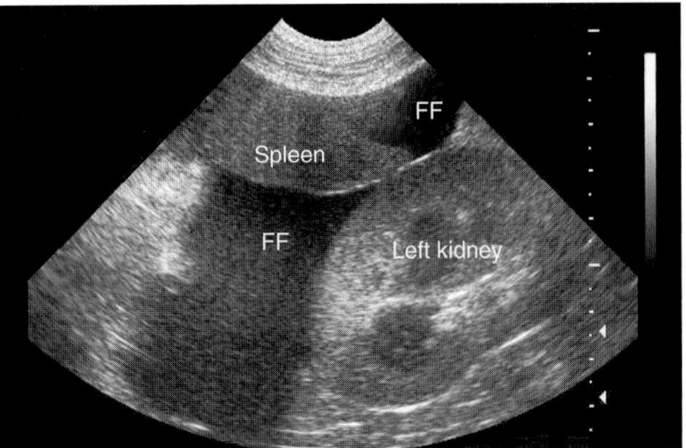

FIGURE 189-3 Left flank view. The left flank view evaluates the splenorenal region. In this image free fluid *(FF)* is seen between the spleen and the left kidney, outlining the borders of both organs.

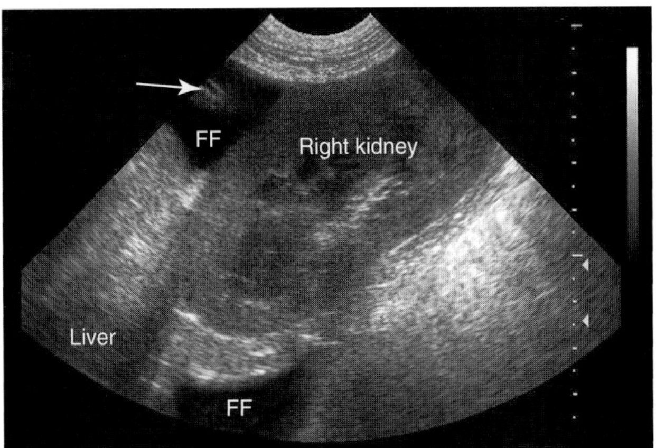

FIGURE 189-4 Right flank view. The right flank view is used to assess the hepatorenal region. In the near field of this image free fluid *(FF)* is seen between the body wall, right kidney, and liver. A loop of intestine *(white arrow)* can be seen "floating" within the free fluid. In the far field free fluid is noted outlining the cranial pole of the right kidney.

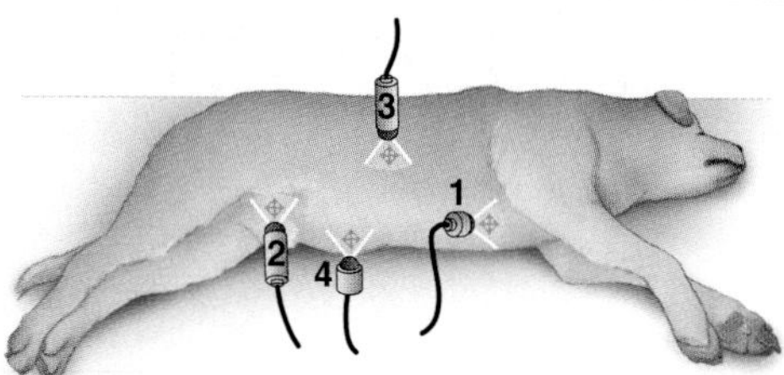

FIGURE 189-5 Transducer placement for the abdominal focused assessment with sonography for trauma examination. The patient can be placed in left or right lateral recumbency. In this figure the patient is shown in left lateral recumbency. The transducer is centered at one of four locations and then moved at least 4 cm and fanned through at least 45 degrees in a cranial, caudal, left, and right direction *(arrows)*. Longitudinal views should be used at each site, and if results are equivocal then a transverse view should also be used. The four sites are (1) the subxiphoid site with the head of the transducer tilted cranially and placed just caudal to the xiphoid process (the transducer often has to be applied with some force to obtain good images, particularly in large breed dogs and when the pleural and pericardial spaces are included); (2) the midline site with the transducer placed over the bladder; (3) the right flank site with the transducer placed over the hepatorenal region; and (4) the left flank site with the transducer placed over the splenorenal region.

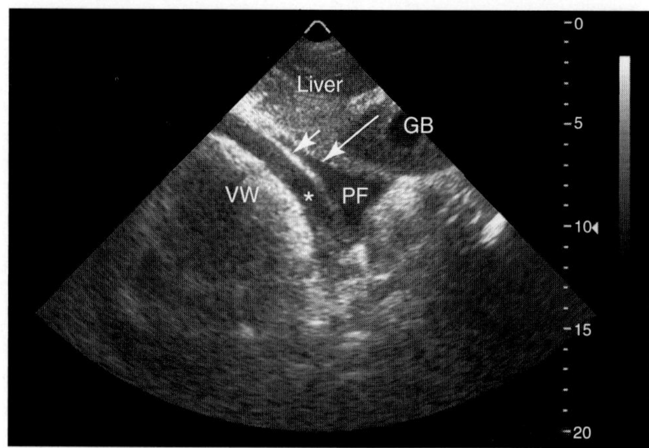

FIGURE 189-6 Subxiphoid view of the thoracic focused assessment with sonography for trauma examination. The subxiphoid view provides an excellent acoustic window into the thorax via the liver, gallbladder *(GB)*, and diaphragm *(large white arrow)*. When the image depth is increased, the subxiphoid view can be used to evaluate the pleural and pericardial spaces. In this image pleural fluid *(PF)* is detected as an anechoic, roughly triangular accumulation located between the diaphragm, pericardial sac *(short white arrow)*, and lung lobes. Pericardial effusion *(*)* is also seen as an anechoic arciform band between the pericardial sac and the ventricular wall of the heart *(VW)*.

with the application of alcohol at the probe-skin interface, although some clinicians prefer to shave a small 2 × 2-inch area of fur at each site and apply ultrasound gel at the probe-skin interface.[1,2]

The AFAST examination can be performed with the patient in right or left lateral recumbency depending on the preference of the sonographer, patient stability, and the position of the patient at presentation (animals brought in left lateral recumbency can be scanned in this position to minimize stress to the patient from movement or manipulation).[1,2] If the animal is in sternal recumbency or is ambulatory, the examiner may choose right lateral recumbency if the volume status of the patient is to be evaluated echographically (e.g., using an echocardiography table) or if the left retroperitoneal space is to be evaluated in detail. Left lateral recumbency may be preferred if the right retroperitoneal space is to be evaluated. Concurrent traumatic injuries including flail chest, fractures, or spinal cord injury may also dictate the AFAST examination position. Dorsal recumbency *is typically avoided* because blunt trauma commonly causes thoracic injury, and pulmonary function may deteriorate when patients with significant thoracic injury are placed in dorsal recumbency.

The four standard views of the AFAST examination are (1) the subxiphoid or diaphragmaticohepatic view to evaluate the hepatodiaphragmatic interface, gallbladder region, pericardial sac, and pleural spaces; (2) the left flank or splenorenal view to assess the splenorenal interface and areas between the spleen and body wall; (3) a midline bladder or cystocolic view to assess the apex of the bladder; and (4) the right flank or hepatorenal view to assess the hepatorenal interface and areas between the intestinal loops, right kidney, and body wall (Figure 189-5).[1,2] The examination can be accomplished using only the longitudinal view at each site, although adding the transverse view is helpful if results of the longitudinal view are equivocal.[1,2] The ultrasound probe should be moved a few inches in several directions at each site and fanned through an angle of 45 degrees until target organs are identified to allow a greater area to be evaluated for the presence of free fluid.[1] The time to complete the examination in dogs is 3 to 6 minutes.[1,2]

The order in which elements of the examination are performed is unlikely to affect the examiner's ability to detect free fluid, but all four sites of the abdomen should be included in the examination, particularly if the AFS is to be determined. The subxiphoid or diaphragmaticohepatic site is often the first site examined because it allows identification of the gallbladder, which can then be used to adjust the ultrasound settings.[1,2] Visualization of the gallbladder is accomplished by tilting and fanning the probe to the right of midline and adjusting the gain until the fluid-filled gallbladder appears anechoic.

Increasing the ultrasound depth at the subxiphoid location allows the examiner to evaluate the thoracic cavity distal to the diaphragm as far as the level of the heart (Figure 189-6). This view of the thorax is part of the TFAST examination and may allow free fluid to be detected in the pleural and pericardial spaces (see the section on TFAST). The sensitivity and specificity for detecting free fluid in the pleural and pericardial spaces via the subxiphoid view has not been reported in dogs or cats. Evaluating the pleural and pericardial spaces via the subxiphoid view may add to the length of time needed to perform the AFAST examination.

Abdominal Fluid Score Technique

Determining the AFS involves recording the number of sites (among the four standard views) in which free abdominal fluid is detected with the animal in lateral recumbency. Animals with an AFS of 0, 1, 2, 3, and 4 would show negative findings at all sites, positive results at one site, positive findings at any two sites, positive results at any three sites, and positive findings at all four sites, respectively.[2] Serial AFAST examinations should be performed every 2 to 4 hours, or more frequently as dictated by clinical findings (e.g., difficulty stabilizing the patient's condition or a deterioration in hemodynamic status).[2,7] Studies evaluating AFS in dogs and cats examined patients in both right and left lateral recumbency; however, it is unknown if patient position with respect to organ injury affects the AFS score. Further studies investigating patient position in relation to AFS score in dogs and cats are warranted.

AFAST for Blunt Abdominal Trauma

FAST examinations are very sensitive and specific for the detection of free abdominal fluid, even when performed by nonradiologists.[8-10] When present, free fluid detected by AFAST in trauma patients is usually indicative of hemorrhage.[1,2] However, trauma-induced abdominal free fluid may be caused by different intraabdominal injuries, including urinary tract rupture, biliary tract rupture, and hollow viscus rupture, so abdominocentesis with fluid analysis (including cytologic examination) is recommended to confirm the diagnosis.[1]

AFAST for Penetrating Abdominal Trauma

FAST examinations are less sensitive at detecting intraabdominal injury following penetrating trauma than following blunt trauma.[11-13] FAST examinations omit large portions of the abdomen and do not reliably exclude localized organ injury. Penetrating trauma often results in localized injury, which may not result in sonographically detectable fluid accumulation, particularly when bowel injury occurs. However, if FAST examination results are positive following penetrating abdominal injury, patients are usually referred for emergency exploratory laparotomy.[11-13] Therefore a positive result on FAST examination can help guide clinical decision making in patients with penetrating abdominal injury, but a negative finding on FAST examination does not rule out intraabdominal injury.[11,13] The sensitivity for detecting free fluid caused by penetrating trauma is improved when serial FAST examinations are performed 12 to 24 hours after the initial insult.[5]

AFAST for Determining the Cause of Intraabdominal Injury

Despite having excellent sensitivity for the detection of free abdominal fluid, FAST is not as sensitive at localizing the site of injury responsible for free abdominal fluid accumulations. Human studies demonstrate that FAST has a limited role in the detection of solid organ injury, which requires greater expertise to detect and adds significantly to the time needed to perform a FAST examination.[14-16] In human studies, the sensitivity for sonographic detection of hepatic and splenic injury (the two most common causes of intraperitoneal hemorrhage in small animals following blunt trauma)[17,18] varies from 41% to 80% depending on the organ affected, the location of the lesion, organ size, and the presence of overlying bowel and gastrointestinal gas.[14-16] The sensitivity and specificity of ultrasound for detecting solid organ injury in human trauma patients is much higher (96.4% and 98%, respectively) when contrast-enhanced ultrasound is used.[19]

Blunt trauma–induced retroperitoneal injury is also difficult to diagnose consistently during FAST examinations in people, with low sensitivity demonstrated in several studies.[20,21] Although the sensitivity for detecting retroperitoneal injury is increased when FAST examinations are performed serially, missed injuries are still frequent. In human trauma cases with negative findings on FAST examination in which retroperitoneal or solid organ injury is still suspected, further testing including computed tomographic scanning is recommended.[20-22] The ability of AFAST to detect trauma-induced retroperitoneal and solid organ injury in veterinary medicine, with or without contrast enhancement, has not yet been investigated.

THORACIC FOCUSED ASSESSMENT WITH SONOGRAPHY FOR TRAUMA

TFAST is a rapid focused evaluation of the thorax.[3] The objective of the TFAST examination is to rule in or out the presence of air or fluid in the pleural space, and to rule in or out the presence of fluid in the pericardial space.[3] In a prospective study of dogs experiencing blunt and penetrating thoracic trauma, the TFAST examination was found to have a sensitivity and specificity for detecting pneumothorax of 78% and 93%, respectively, compared with thoracic radiographs.[3] It should be noted that there were considerable differences in sensitivity when the examinations were performed by an experienced sonographer (95% sensitivity with >70 scans) compared with a novice sonographer (45% sensitivity with <15 scans), which suggests that there is a steep learning curve for the sonographic detection of pneumothorax.[3,23] Despite variation in sensitivity and specificity between experienced and less experienced sonographers, and among published human studies, the negative predicative value of the TFAST examination is high, which indicates that the presence of the glide sign essentially rules out pneumothorax at the site of the transducer.[4,24] However, failure to detect a glide sign may result from conditions other than pneumothorax, including acute respiratory distress syndrome, pulmonary fibrosis, large consolidations, pleural adhesions, atelectasis, right mainstem intubation, and phrenic nerve paralysis.[4,24] Although the sensitivity and specificity of TFAST for detection of trauma-induced pleural and pericardial fluid has not been investigated in veterinary medicine, pericardial and pleural effusions have been diagnosed with TFAST in dogs experiencing trauma.[3] In humans, E-FAST is very sensitive for the detection of trauma-induced pericardial and pleural effusion, and ultrasound has greater sensitivity and specificity for detection of pleural and pericardial effusions than thoracic radiographs, which makes it an ideal modality for diagnosing these conditions.[25]

TFAST Technique

The TFAST examination involves five views of the thorax (Figure 189-7): one on each side of the thorax between the seventh and ninth intercostal spaces (termed the *chest tube site [CTS] view*), one on each side of the chest between the fifth and sixth intercostal spaces over the heart (termed the *pericardial chest site [PCS] view*), and the subxiphoid view of the AFAST examination with the depth of the ultrasound signal adjusted to allow visualization of the pleural and pericardial spaces beyond the diaphragm (see Figure 189-6).[3,26,27] As with AFAST, the animal does not need to be clipped for the TFAST examination to be performed.[3]

The TFAST examination can be performed with the patient in left, right, or sternal recumbency.[3] Since the TFAST examination is often performed concurrently with the AFAST evaluation, the first three views of the TFAST examination (subxiphoid view, CTS and PCS views from the nondependent side of the thorax) are often performed with the patient in lateral recumbency as required for the

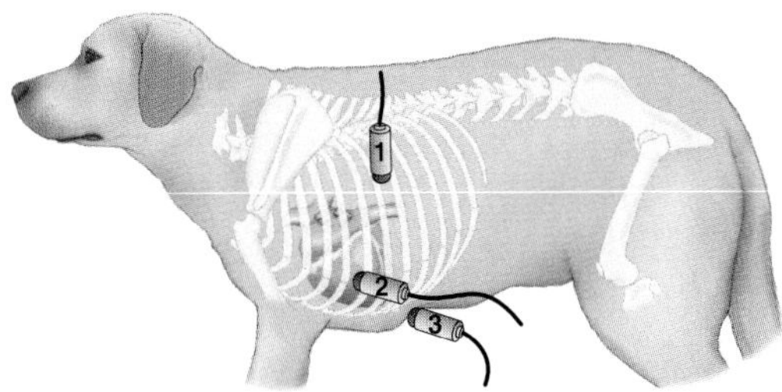

FIGURE 189-7 Transducer placement for the thoracic focused assessment with sonography for trauma (TFAST) examination. The TFAST examination involves bilateral placement of the transducer at the chest tube site *(1)* in the longitudinal plane perpendicular to the ribs at the seventh to ninth intercostal spaces. Scanning at this site is used to rule in or rule out pneumothorax. Pneumothorax is ruled out if the real-time dynamic glide sign and/or B-lines are present. It is important to note that the sonographer must keep the transducer immobile on the chest wall to maximize the chance of detecting the glide sign. Bilateral placement of the transducer at the pericardial site *(2)* in the longitudinal and transverse planes with movement and fanning of the transducer is used to maximize the chances of detecting pleural and pericardial effusions. The fifth view is the subxiphoid view *(3)* of the abdominal focused assessment with sonography for trauma examination with the depth set to allow the pleural and pericardial spaces to be evaluated via the acoustic window through the liver, gallbladder, and diaphragm.

AFAST examination (see earlier). After completion of the AFAST examination, the final two views of the TFAST examination (CTS and PCS on the contralateral side of the thorax) can be completed after the patient is gently rolled into sternal recumbency. In cases in which AFAST is not performed due to severe respiratory compromise, the TFAST examination can be completed with the patient in sternal recumbency.

Chest Tube Site Views

Pleural line and the bat sign

When pneumothorax is present, air within the pleural space will rise to the least dependent area of the chest.[4,24] The least dependent area tends to be the widest part of the chest when the animal is in lateral recumbency and the more dorsal parts of the chest when the animal is in sternal recumbency. Based on this information, the CTS views are used to confirm or rule out pneumothorax.[3] CTS views involve recognition of adjacent ribs and their acoustic shadowing, and identification of the pleural line between adjacent ribs. In healthy animals, the pleural line is composed of the parietal pleura (lining the thorax) and the visceral pleura (lining the lungs). A single plane is evaluated by placing the probe perpendicular to the long axis of the ribs between two adjacent ribs at the seventh and eighth or eighth and ninth intercostal spaces in the dorsal third of the thorax (widest point of the chest with the animal in lateral recumbency).[3] However, the scan must be performed with the probe held motionless to allow movement of the lungs during respiration to be detected.[23] The ribs are identified as hyperechoic (white) arciform structures with distal black shadowing (Figure 189-8). Once the ribs with their acoustic shadowing have been identified, the pleural line is identified. The pleural line is the roughly horizontal white line running between the two ribs and is usually visible just distal to the ribs (the exception being in subcutaneous emphysema, which may prevent the ribs and pleural line from being localized).[3] The image obtained is referred to as the *bat sign*, where the white arciform outline of the ribs represents the wings of a bat and the white hypoechoic pleural line represents the body of the bat (see Figure 189-7).[4] To-and-fro motion of the pleural line as the parietal and visceral pleura slide over one another during inspiration and expiration is known as the *glide sign* (or *lung sliding*).[3,23] The glide sign is the key finding indicating that the parietal and pleural linings are in contact in healthy aerated lung.[4] The glide sign is a dynamic finding and is identified as horizontal movement or shimmering along the pleural line.[23] It may be intermittent with low respiratory rates or apnea because it requires the pleural linings to slide over one another during respirations.[24] It should be noted that the previous technique refers to the TFAST technique described in veterinary patients and that variations, including placement of the probe parallel to the ribs, have been described in humans and veterinary patients.[25,28,29]

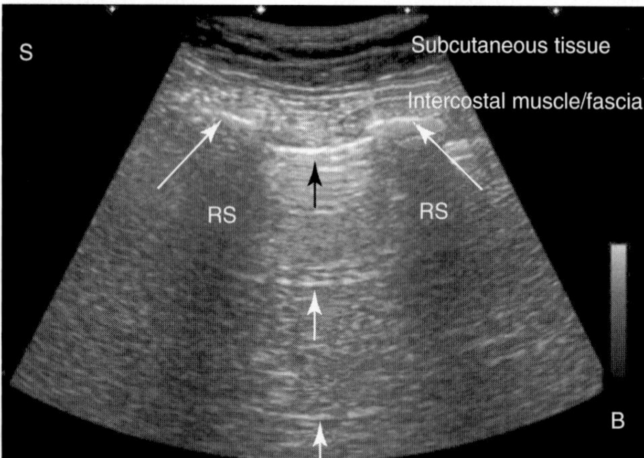

FIGURE 189-8 Longitudinal chest tube site view. The ribs *(long white arrows)* are recognized by their hyperechoic arciform shape with distal acoustic shadowing *(RS)*. The pleural line *(black arrow)* is identified as a hyperechoic horizontal line below the ribs (0.25 cm below the ribs in this image). The pleural line indicates the parietal and visceral pleura with presence of a glide sign in healthy patients. The distinct horizontal white lines seen distal to the pleural line are repetitions of the pleural line, called *A-lines (short white arrows),* which are located equidistant from each other as determined by the distance between the skin and the pleural line. It should be noted that this static image can be seen in patients with and without a pneumothorax. It is the dynamic movement of the parietal and visceral pleura as they slide over each other (which is not possible to see on a static image) that creates the glide sign and rules out pneumothorax.

A-lines

A-lines are horizontal lines of decreasing echogenicity visible in the far field of the image, similar to and equidistant from the pleural line (see Figure 189-8).[23] A-lines should not be confused with the pleural line. A-lines are a result of reverberation artifact as the ultrasound waves reflect off the soft tissue–air interface at the level of the pleural line (which causes the pleural line to be replicated in the sonographic far field).[23,30] The distance between subsequent A-lines corresponds to the same distance between the skin surface and the parietal pleura.[30] A-lines may be seen in patients with and without pneumothorax.[30]

B-lines

In addition to detecting the glide sign, the CTS views often show B-lines (ring-down artifacts), which are a type of comet tail artifact (note that there are multiple types of comet tail artifact).[23,29,30] B-lines are reverberation artifacts originating from the visceral pleura (Figure 189-9).[30] B-lines appear as hyperechoic vertical lines extending from the pleural line to the edge of the far field image, passing through A-lines without fading.[4,23] B-lines move in a to-and-fro fashion with inspiration and expiration, and the movement of B-lines is synchronous with the glide sign.[4,23] An occasional B-line is considered

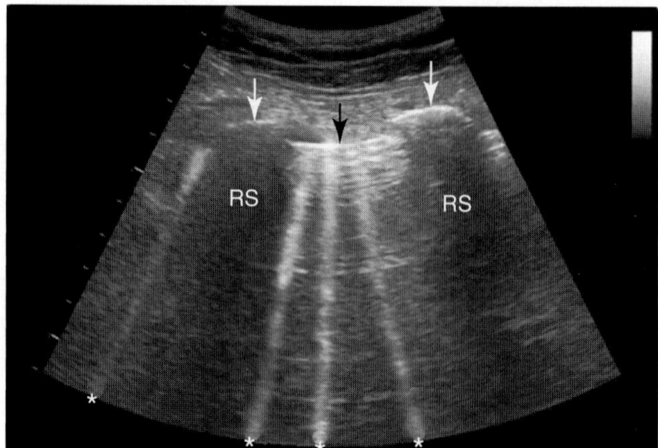

FIGURE 189-9 B-lines. B-lines *(*)* are reverberation artifacts originating from the visceral pleura of the pleural line *(black arrow)*. B-lines appear as hyperechoic vertical lines extending from the pleural line to the edge of the far field image, passing through A-lines without fading. B-lines move in a to-and-fro fashion with inspiration and expiration, and the movement of B-lines is synchronous with the glide sign (only visible in real time). An occasional B-line is considered normal; however, excessive B-lines or B-lines occurring closely together, as seen in this image, suggest interstitial-alveolar lung abnormality. Ribs *(white arrows)* and rib shadowing *(RS)* are visible in this image.

normal; however, excessive B-lines or B-lines occurring closely together (<7 mm apart in humans) are indicative of interstitial-alveolar lung abnormality.[4,23,29] In the case of trauma, numerous B-lines or close proximity of B-lines should be considered diagnostic of pulmonary contusions until proven otherwise.[3,23] When B-lines are numerous they create what is called a *B-pattern,* which is indicative of interstitial-alveolar disease (note that multiple B-lines have also been referred to as *ultrasound lung rockets,* which is synonymous with B-pattern).[23]

Lung curtain

Lung curtain is a term that refers to the lung artifact created by movement of the lungs at the costophrenic angles.[24] Movement of the lung into and out of the ultrasound image at the costophrenic angles creates a vertical sliding artifact similar to the opening and closing of a theater curtain, which should not be confused with the glide sign.[24] The ultrasound probe should be moved cranially if the curtain sign is noted because the curtain sign has not been used for diagnosis of thoracic abnormalities in veterinary patients.

Sonographic signs of pneumothorax

Absence of glide sign and B-lines

With pneumothorax, air separates the visceral pleura from the parietal pleura, which obliterates the glide sign.[23] It is important to emphasize that it is the absence of the glide sign that confirms the presence of pneumothorax and not the presence or absence of the pleural line. The pleural line is visible in both healthy patients (in which it is comprised of both the parietal and pleural linings sliding over one another in a to-and-fro manner) *and* in patients that have pneumothorax (in which it is comprised of only the stationary parietal lining since the visceral lining is separated from the parietal lining by air).[3,23] Pneumothorax will also obliterate the presence of any B-lines because they originate from the visceral pleura.[23] The visceral pleura is not visible (it is displaced distally [to the far field]) when pneumothorax is present.

The severity of pneumothorax can be evaluated by moving the probe in a dorsal to ventral direction and noting when air is no longer present between the lung and chest wall (return of the glide sign).[3,23] The point at which the glide sign returns is known as the *lung point.*[3,23] A linear array probe placed parallel to and between the ribs may help in identifying the lung point. This is a very specific finding and confirms the presence of pneumothorax when seen.[23,24] In the case of massive pneumothorax a lung point will not be detected.[23] Some authors question the ability of the lung point to provide accurate information regarding the size of the pneumothorax and do not use this information in making clinical decisions regarding therapy for pneumothorax.[25] Further studies are required to determine the accuracy of the lung point in determining the size of pneumothorax in veterinary patients.

In summary, pneumothorax is ruled out if a glide sign and/or B-lines are detected, strongly suspected when the glide sign and B-lines are absent, and definitively confirmed if the lung point is identified.

Pericardial Chest Site and Subxiphoid Site Views

The PCS and subxiphoid site views are used to detect the presence of pericardial and pleural effusions (Figure 189-10).[3] Scanning in the PCS views should be performed in transverse and longitudinal planes.[3] The probe should be moved several centimeters or between adjacent rib spaces at each PCS to increase the chances of detecting pericardial and pleural fluid. Increasing the depth (zooming out) allows visualization of the entire heart and its structures, which helps to differentiate pericardial from pleural effusion. Using the subxiphoid view also helps to differentiate pericardial from pleural

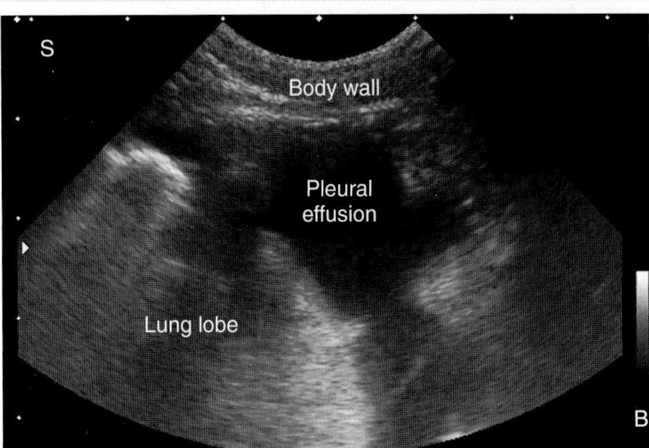

FIGURE 189-10 Pericardial site view. In this image anechoic pleural effusion is visible between the body wall and the lung lobes.

effusion because it provides a good acoustic window into the thoracic cavity (see Figure 189-6).[28]

EMERGENCY LUNG ULTRASOUND TO DETECT INTERSTITIAL-ALVEOLAR LUNG INJURY

The application of focused emergency ultrasound for detection of traumatic and nontraumatic lung injury has recently been investigated in human medicine.[24,30,31] A bedside lung evaluation (BLUE) scan has been used in people to accurately detect the presence of pulmonary contusions, cardiogenic and noncardiogenic pulmonary edema, pneumonia, pulmonary thromboembolism, and other pathologic interstitial-alveolar lung conditions.[31,32] The key concept in this setting is the detection of B-lines that originate from the pleural line. The proximity and number or density of B-lines correlate with extravascular lung water, and the anatomic location of B-lines with respect to lung anatomy correlates with different pathologic lung conditions.[30-32] In veterinary medicine there are preliminary reports of the use of ultrasound to detect similar pathologic processes, including pulmonary alveolar-interstitial edema, through identification of B-lines originating at the pleural-parietal interface of the thorax and lung.[28,29] Emergency lung ultrasound may find a particular niche in differentiating underlying causes of respiratory distress in the severely dyspneic patient that is in too unstable a condition to allow thoracic radiography (e.g., differentiating cardiogenic from noncardiogenic causes of marked respiratory distress in cats and dogs). Emergency point-of-care lung ultrasound protocols similar to human BLUE protocols, such as the Vet Blue protocol, have been proposed in veterinary medicine, although results using these protocols have yet to be published.[26]

REFERENCES

1. Boysen SR, Rozanski EA, Tidwell AS, et al: Evaluation of a focused assessment with sonography for trauma protocol to detect free abdominal fluid in dogs involved in motor vehicle accidents, J Am Vet Med Assoc 225(8):1198-1204, 2004.
2. Lisciandro GR, Lagutchik MS, Mann KA, et al: Evaluation of an abdominal fluid scoring system determined using abdominal focused assessment with sonography for trauma in 101 dogs with motor vehicle trauma, J Vet Emerg Crit Care 19(5):426-437, 2009.
3. Lisciandro GR, Lagutchik SM, Mann KA, et al: Evaluation of a thoracic focused assessment with sonography for trauma (TFAST) protocol to detect pneumothorax and concurrent thoracic injury in 145 traumatized dogs, J Vet Emerg Crit Care 18(3):258-269, 2008.
4. Husain LF, Hagopian L, Wayman D, et al: Sonographic diagnosis of pneumothorax, J Emerg Trauma Shock 5:76-81, 2012.

5. Mohammadi A, Ghasemi-Rad M: Evaluation of gastrointestinal injury in blunt abdominal trauma "FAST is not reliable": the role of repeated ultrasonography, World J Emerg Surg 7(1):2, 2012.
6. Lisciandro G: Evaluation of initial and serial combination focused assessment with sonography for trauma (CFAST) examination of the thorax (TFAST) and abdomen (AFAST) with the application of an abdominal fluid scoring system in 49 traumatized cats, J Vet Emerg Crit Care 22(2):S11, 2012.
7. Pathan A: Role of ultrasound in the evaluation of blunt abdominal trauma, J Liaquat Univ Med Health Sci 4(1):23-28, 2005.
8. Richards JR, McGahan JP, Pali MJ, et al: Sonographic detection of blunt hepatic trauma: hemoperitoneum and parenchymal patterns of injury, J Trauma 17:117-120, 1999.
9. Ma OJ, Kefer MP, Mateer JR, et al: Evaluation of hemoperitoneum using a single- versus multiple-view ultrasonographic examination, Acad Emerg Med 2:581-586, 1995.
10. Shackford SR, Rogers FB, Osler TM, et al: Focused abdominal sonogram for trauma: the learning curve of nonradiologist clinicians in detecting hemoperitoneum, J Trauma 46:553-564, 1999.
11. Boulanger BR, Kearney PA, Tsuei B, et al: The routine use of sonography in penetrating torso injury is beneficial, J Trauma 51:320-325, 2001.
12. Udobi KF, Rodriguez A, Chiu WC, et al: Role of ultrasonography in penetrating abdominal trauma: a prospective clinical study, J Trauma 50:475-479, 2001.
13. Kirkpatrick AW, Sirois M, Ball C, et al: The hand-held ultrasound examination for penetrating abdominal trauma, Am J Surg 187:660-665, 2004.
14. Rothlin MA, Naf R, Amgwerd M, et al: Ultrasound in blunt abdominal and thoracic trauma, J Trauma 34:488-495, 1993.
15. Korner M, Krotz MM, Degenhart C, et al: Current role of emergency US in patients with major trauma, Radiographics 28:225-242, 2008.
16. Cokkinos D, Anypa E, Stefanidis P, et al: Contrast-enhanced ultrasound for imaging blunt abdominal trauma—indications, description of the technique and imaging review, Ultrashall Med 33:60-67, 2012.
17. Kolata RJ, Dudley EJ: Motor vehicle accidents in urban dogs: a study of 600 cases, J Am Vet Med Assoc 167:938-941, 1975.
18. Mongil CM, Drobatz KJ, Hendricks JC: Traumatic hemoperitoneum in 28 cases: a retrospective review, J Am Anim Hosp Assoc 31:217-222, 1995.
19. Valentino M, Ansaloni L, Catena F, et al: Contrast-enhanced ultrasonography in blunt abdominal trauma: considerations after 5 years of experience, Radiol Med 114:1080-1093, 2009.
20. Miller M, Pasquale M, Bromberg W, et al: Not so FAST, J Trauma 54(1):52-59, 2003.
21. Poletti PA, Kinkel K, Vermeulen B, et al: Blunt abdominal trauma: should US be used to detect both free fluid and organ injuries? Radiology 227:95-103, 2003.
22. Shanmurganathan K, Mirvis SE, Sherbourne CD, et al: Hemoperitoneum as the sole indicator of abdominal visceral injuries: a potential limitation of screening abdominal US for trauma, Radiology 212:423-430, 1999.
23. Volpicelli G, Elbarbary M, Blaivas M, et al: International evidence-based recommendations for point-of-care lung ultrasound, Intensive Care Med 38:577-591, 2012.
24. Chandra S, Narasimhan M: Pleural ultrasonography, Open Crit Care Med J 3:26-32, 2010.
25. Hew M, Heinze S: Chest ultrasound in practice: a review of utility in the clinical setting, Internal Med J 42:856-865, 2012.
26. Lisciandro GR: Abdominal and thoracic focused assessment with sonography for trauma, triage, and monitoring in small animals, J Vet Emerg Crit Care 21(2):104-122, 2011.
27. Mantis P: Use of ultrasonography by veterinary surgeons in small animal clinical emergencies, Ultrasound 20:77-81, 2012.
28. Moon Larson M: Ultrasound of the thorax (noncardiac), Vet Clin North Am Small Anim Pract 39:733-745, 2009.
29. Louvet A, Bourgeois JM: Lung down artefact as a sign of pulmonary alveolar-interstitial disease, J Vet Radiol Ultrasound 49(4):374-377, 2008.
30. Nalos M, Kot M, McLean AS, et al: Bedside lung ultrasound in the care of the critically ill, Curr Respir Med Rev 6:271-278, 2010.
31. Gargani L: Lung ultrasound: a new tool for the cardiologist, Cardiovasc Ultrasound 9:6, 2011.
32. Soldati G, Guinta V, Sher S, et al: "Synthetic" comets: a new look at lung sonography, Ultrasound Med Biol 37(11):1762-1770, 2011.

CHAPTER 190
CAPNOGRAPHY

Bruno H. Pypendop, DrMedVet, DrVetSci, DACVAA

KEY POINTS

- Capnography allows the continuous, noninvasive assessment of partial pressure of arterial carbon dioxide.
- The normal gradient between end-tidal and arterial partial pressure of carbon dioxide (PCO_2) is less than 5 mm Hg in small animal species.
- An abrupt decrease in end-tidal PCO_2 to zero or near-zero values may indicate disconnection of the capnograph from the patient or cardiac arrest and should be considered a medical emergency.
- An increased end-tidal to arterial PCO_2 gradient indicates increased alveolar dead-space ventilation.
- Careful examination of a capnogram allows the detection of various abnormalities related to the ventilation equipment or the patient.
- Although capnography can be used in awake, nonintubated patients, results are more accurate in anesthetized and intubated patients.

Capnometry is defined as the measurement and display of carbon dioxide concentration in the respiratory gases on a monitor. Maximum inspired and expired carbon dioxide concentrations during a respiratory cycle are displayed. *Capnography* is defined as a graphic display or recording of carbon dioxide concentration versus time or expired volume during a respiratory cycle (carbon dioxide waveform or capnogram). Time capnograms are most common and are the only ones discussed here; volume capnograms can be used to measure the dead-space volume. A capnograph thus provides more information than does a capnometer; the interpretation of waveforms gives indications on the status of the patient and, in some cases, of the ventilation equipment.

Capnography can be used to confirm endotracheal tube placement, to assess ventilation and carbon dioxide elimination in a noninvasive manner, and (in combination with blood gas analysis) to estimate alveolar dead-space ventilation. Capnography has also been used to monitor the efficacy of cardiopulmonary resuscitation.

NONDIVERTING AND DIVERTING MONITORS

Two types of capnographs are available: nondiverting (mainstream) and diverting (sidestream).[1] As the names indicate, a nondiverting capnograph measures carbon dioxide concentration directly in the breathing system, whereas a diverting device samples gas from the breathing system and measures the carbon dioxide concentration in that gas in the main unit. In nondiverting monitors, the patient's respiratory gas passes through a chamber with two windows. The sensor (light source and detector) fits over that chamber. The sensor also contains a heater to prevent water condensation on the windows. Advantages of mainstream devices include fast response time, no requirement for scavenging gas, ease of calibration (with a sealed chamber containing gas of known carbon dioxide concentration), and use of few disposable items. Disadvantages include the need to place the sensor near the patient (usually at the endotracheal tube connection); increase in apparatus dead space; potential for leaks, disconnection, or obstructions; potential for the sensor to become dislodged from the chamber; exposure of the sensor to damage; and measurement of carbon dioxide only.

In diverting monitors, the sensor is located in the main unit, remote from the breathing system. A pump samples respiratory gas at a constant flow via sampling tubing. Advantages include minimal added dead space, lightweight patient interface, potential for the measurement of multiple gases, and possibility of use in places where the monitor needs to be remote from the patient. Disadvantages include the potential for sampling problems, delayed response (especially with long sampling tubing), removal of gas at a given rate from the circuit, necessity to scavenge gas, potential for change in gas composition (depending on the technology used), need for calibration gas, and potential for gas mixing in the sampling tubing (especially if the tubing is long).

TECHNOLOGY

Various techniques can be used to measure the concentration of carbon dioxide in the expired gas. These include infrared absorption, mass spectrometry, and Raman scattering.[1]

Infrared absorption is the most widely used technique. This technique is based on the concept that gases that have two or more dissimilar atoms in the molecule have unique and specific absorption spectra of infrared light. Infrared absorption can therefore be used to measure not only carbon dioxide but also nitrous oxide and the halogenated anesthetics.

Infrared monitors have a short warm-up time and a quick response time, which allows them to measure inspired and expired concentrations. There is, however, some overlap between the absorption of carbon dioxide and nitrous oxide, and older devices need manual compensatory adjustment when nitrous oxide is used. Water vapor must be removed from the expired gas (e.g., using Nafion tubing, water traps) because it absorbs infrared light at many wavelengths. Infrared absorption is the only technique available in nondiverting (mainstream) devices. It is also available in many diverting units.

Mass spectrometry is not commonly used to measure carbon dioxide concentration in respiratory gases. The mass spectrometer spreads gases and vapors of different molecular weights into a spectrum, according to their mass/charge ratios. When the device is designed properly, it is then possible to direct these different gases and vapors toward targets that can count the number of molecules. The mass spectrometer can be used to measure not only carbon dioxide but also oxygen, nitrogen, nitrous oxide, and the halogenated anesthetics. Depending on the type of mass spectrometer, measurement of a new agent may require hardware or software adaptation. Mass spectrometry can be used to measure gas concentration from one or several locations (up to 31). The device measures gases as concentrations (unlike infrared analyzers and Raman spectrometers, which measure partial pressures) and therefore assumes that the sum of the gases it measures equals 100%. This may result in errors if a gas that is not measured is present in significant concentrations.

The basis of Raman spectrometry is that when laser light interacts with a gas molecule which has interatomic bonds, some of its energy is converted into vibrational and rotational modes, and a fraction of that energy is reemitted at various wavelengths characteristic of the molecule. Venkata Raman won the Nobel Prize in physics in 1930 for the discovery of this phenomenon. Raman scattering was used in one clinical monitor, the Rascal II, which is no longer supported. This device measured oxygen, nitrogen, carbon dioxide, nitrous oxide, and up to five anesthetic agents. It had a fast response time and a very fast startup time. It required little maintenance and was very accurate.

PHYSIOLOGY

A normal time capnogram can be divided into five phases (Figure 190-1).[1,2] Phase 0 corresponds to inspiration, and no carbon dioxide should be measured during that phase. Phase IV is the early part of inspiration, when carbon dioxide–free gas starts entering the airway.

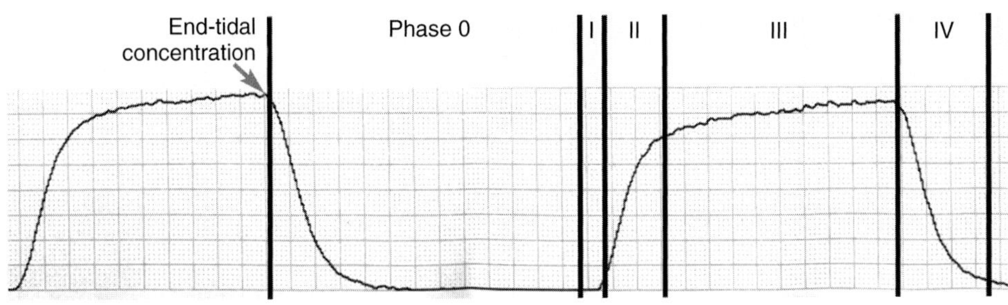

FIGURE 190-1 Normal capnogram.

Some authors include phase IV in phase 0 or in phase III. Expiration is divided into the three remaining phases: I is early expiration, corresponding to the emptying of the anatomic dead space (no carbon dioxide should be measured); II is a rapidly changing mixture of alveolar and dead-space gas, resulting in a steep increase in measured carbon dioxide concentration; and III is the alveolar plateau, during which alveolar concentration of carbon dioxide is measured. The plateau usually has a slight increasing slope. The maximal concentration reached at the end of the plateau is the end-tidal concentration and is assumed to best represent alveolar carbon dioxide concentration (because gas sampled at that time is almost pure alveolar gas). In turn, alveolar partial pressure of carbon dioxide in normal patients is only slightly lower than the arterial partial pressure of carbon dioxide ($PaCO_2$). Therefore, assuming that no significant respiratory or cardiovascular abnormality is present and that accurate end-tidal measurements are made, capnography allows continuous, noninvasive assessment of $PaCO_2$.[2]

$PaCO_2$, and therefore end-tidal PCO_2, result from the balance between carbon dioxide production and carbon dioxide elimination (i.e., alveolar ventilation). Therefore changes in PCO_2 occur only if either production or elimination changes without associated changes in the other component. Because carbon dioxide is the main factor controlling breathing, in a normal, awake animal any change in carbon dioxide production induces a proportional change in alveolar ventilation, so that PCO_2 remains constant. However, in anesthetized animals, or in animals with respiratory, muscular, or neurologic disease, this response to changes in carbon dioxide production may be lost to a variable extent, so that changes in carbon dioxide production may not result in compensatory changes in carbon dioxide elimination; the result is changes in PCO_2. Anesthesia and disease may also alter the normal response to carbon dioxide, so that alveolar ventilation may change (usually decrease) in the absence of changes in carbon dioxide production, which results in changes (usually increases) in PCO_2.[2]

The main information contained in a time capnogram is the inspired carbon dioxide concentration, the respiratory rate, and the end-tidal carbon dioxide concentration, which in most cases is representative of $PaCO_2$. Abnormalities in the shape of a capnogram can provide additional information.[2,3]

As mentioned earlier, the gradient between end-tidal PCO_2 and $PaCO_2$ is normally small (<5 mm Hg in small animal species). Increased dead-space ventilation (i.e., ventilation of alveoli that are not perfused) increases this gradient. Increased dead-space ventilation is commonly related to decreased pulmonary blood flow (e.g., pulmonary thromboembolism, low cardiac output); ventilation-perfusion scattering has a similar effect. In these situations, a larger gradient between end-tidal and $PaCO_2$ may exist, so that end-tidal PCO_2 cannot be used to estimate $PaCO_2$ (but changes in end-tidal PCO_2 usually still correlate with changes in $PaCO_2$).

CAPNOGRAM INTERPRETATION

Even though capnography can be used during spontaneous ventilation in awake or anesthetized patients, it is most useful during mechanical ventilation. Indeed, it provides a breath-by-breath monitoring of the adequacy of ventilation, and it allows the assessment of the response to changes in ventilator settings without having to sample arterial blood. Although arterial blood gas analysis remains the gold standard to assess ventilation, capnography has two major advantages: it provides continuous versus intermittent monitoring, and it is not invasive. It is the only tool used clinically in animals that gives a continuous estimate of $PaCO_2$. Besides noninvasive assessment of $PaCO_2$, capnography allows the detection of various abnormalities pertaining to the breathing equipment or the patient.

Equipment

Increased apparatus dead space, rebreathing with a circle system (e.g., faulty unidirectional valve, exhausted carbon dioxide absorbent), and rebreathing with a nonrebreathing system (inadequate fresh gas flow, leak or disconnection of the inner tubing of a Bain circuit) all result in an elevated baseline, increased inspired PCO_2 and, if ventilation does not change, increased end-tidal PCO_2 (Figure 190-2, *A*). The end-tidal to $PaCO_2$ gradient will be normal or decreased. The slope of phase IV usually is decreased.

Obstruction to expiration is detected by a decrease in the slope of phase II, an increase in the slope of phase III, and sometimes a decrease in end-tidal PCO_2 (if inspiration starts before expiration is complete).

Inadequate sealing around the endotracheal tube usually results in low, nonzero end-tidal readings (see Figure 190-2, *B*).

Patient

Changes in carbon dioxide production without associated changes in alveolar ventilation result in changes in end-tidal PCO_2, with a normal waveform, no inspired carbon dioxide, and a normal end-tidal to $PaCO_2$ gradient. Common causes of increased carbon dioxide production (and increased end-tidal PCO_2) include pain, anxiety, shivering, seizures, hyperthermia, administration of sodium bicarbonate, and carbon dioxide absorption from the peritoneal cavity during laparoscopy.

Apnea obviously results in the absence of a waveform. Hyperventilation leads to a decrease in end-tidal PCO_2, with an otherwise normal waveform, no inspired carbon dioxide, and a normal end-tidal to arterial gradient. Hypoventilation leads to opposite changes. Upper airway obstruction results in changes similar to those described for equipment obstruction.

Decreased transport of carbon dioxide to the lungs (e.g., decreased cardiac output, pulmonary thromboembolism) results in decreased end-tidal PCO_2, a normal capnogram, no inspired carbon dioxide, and an increased end-tidal to $PaCO_2$ gradient. Cardiac arrest results in a sudden decrease of end-tidal PCO_2 to zero or near-zero values. Capnography can be used to monitor the efficiency of cardiopulmonary resuscitation by observing the return of carbon dioxide in the expired gas (related to the return of pulmonary blood flow). End-tidal carbon dioxide values during cardiopulmonary resuscitation have been reported to correlate with resuscitation success (the higher the values, the better the chances of successful resuscitation).

Many types of lung disease result in a scattering of time constants in different areas of the lung. In turn, this results in sequential emptying of "faster" and "slower" alveoli. This manifests on the capnogram by an increase in the slope of phase III. Bronchoconstriction (asthma, bronchospasm) is a typical cause of prolonged expiration (phases II and III) and a decreased slope of phase II and increased slope of phase III.

Cardiogenic oscillations sometimes can be seen on a capnogram. These are small oscillations in phase IV. The slope of this downstroke is also decreased. The frequency of these oscillations corresponds to heart rate. Cardiogenic oscillations are due to gas movement in the airway caused by the heart beat (see Figure 190-2, *C*).

A "curare cleft" is a decrease in carbon dioxide concentration during the alveolar plateau. This is due to a spontaneous inspiratory effort in mechanically ventilated patients (Figure 190-2, *D*).

Graphic examples of normal and abnormal capnograms can be found at http://www.capnography.com.

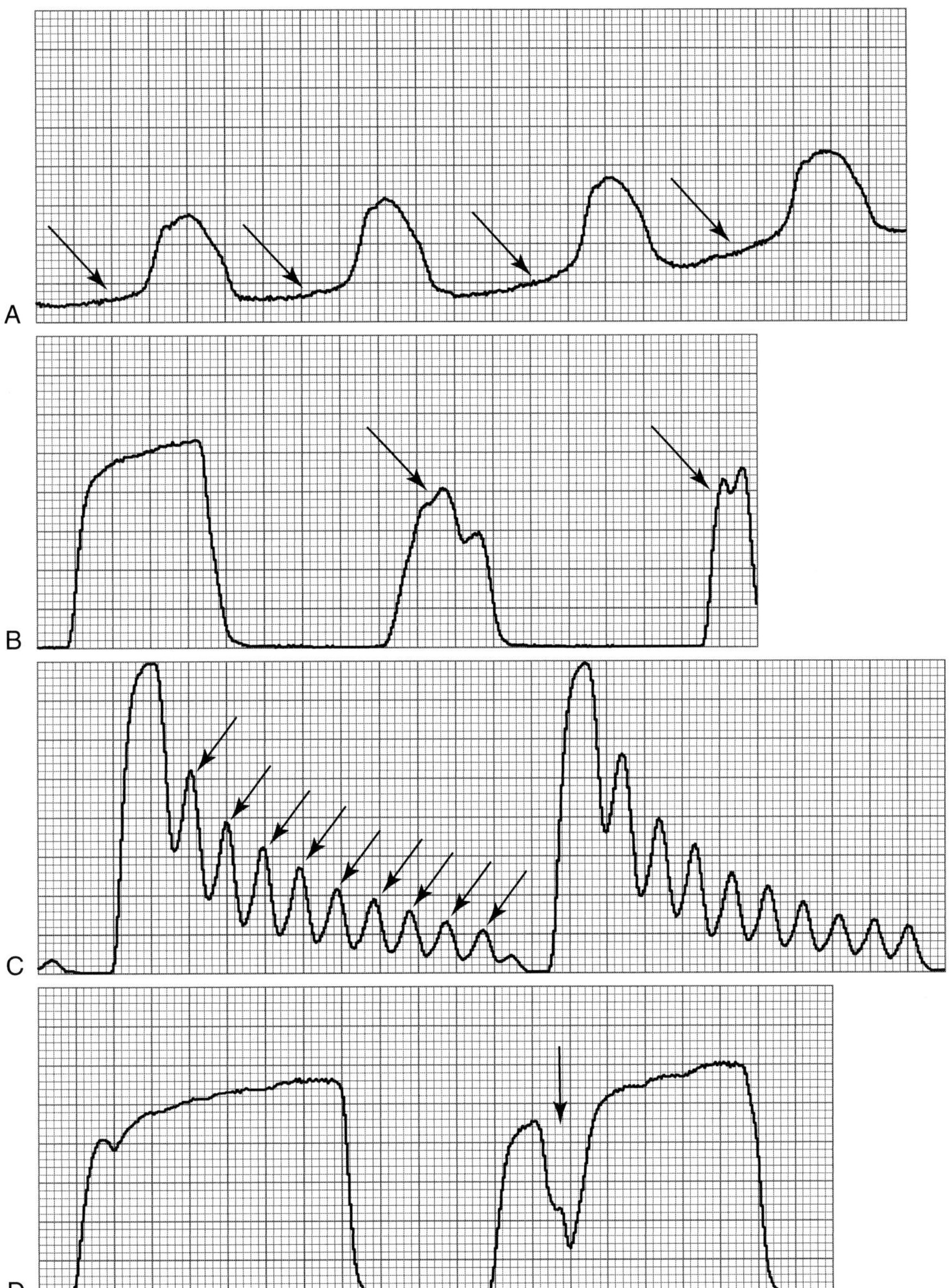

FIGURE 190-2 A, Rebreathing. Note how during expiration, carbon dioxide partial pressure does not return to zero *(arrows)*. **B,** Leak. The first waveform is normal; note how it is altered in subsequent breaths *(arrows)*. **C,** Cardiogenic oscillations. Note that there is a short phase III plateau followed by small oscillations caused by the heartbeat *(arrows)*. **D,** Curare cleft. The first waveform is normal; note the depression during phase III (curare cleft) on the second waveform *(arrow)*.

REFERENCES

1. Dorsh JA, Dorsh SE: Gas monitoring. In Dorsh JA, Dorsh SE, editors: Understanding anesthesia equipment, ed 4, Baltimore, 1998, Williams & Wilkins.
2. Lumb AB: Nunn's applied respiratory physiology, ed 6, Boston, 2005, Butterworth-Heinemann.
3. Thompson JE, Jaffe MB: Capnographic waveforms in the mechanically ventilated patient, Respir Care 50:100, 2005.

CHAPTER 191

INTRACRANIAL PRESSURE MONITORING

Beverly K. Sturges, DVM, MS, DACVIM (Neurology)

KEY POINTS

- Maintaining adequate cerebral perfusion pressure (CPP) is considered the cornerstone of successful treatment of acquired brain injury.
- By monitoring intracranial pressure (ICP) and mean arterial blood pressure (MAP), the clinician can quantitatively assess CPP, as expressed by the formula CPP = MAP − ICP.
- Normal ICP varies between 5 and 10 mm Hg above atmospheric pressure in dogs and cats.
- Catheter tip ICP transducers (fiberoptic or miniature strain gauge) have been used with ease and accuracy in dogs and cats when placed subdurally or intraparenchymally in the brain.
- Monitoring ICP is most important in patients with intracranial hypertension from severe brain disease or head injury and in animals that are anesthetized or comatose.

Acquired brain injury is a common neurologic emergency typically caused by head trauma, brain disease (tumors, meningoencephalitis, hypoxic injury), metabolic derangements, prolonged seizures, or surgical trauma. Increased intracranial pressure (ICP) often is associated with these processes and may affect outcome seriously. Because the intracranial contents (blood, cerebrospinal fluid [CSF], and brain parenchyma) are encased in a rigid container, limited space is available for expansion of the contents. As volume increases in the cranial vault from any cause (edema, hemorrhage, mass), there must be a reciprocal decrease in the other volumes for ICP not to increase beyond limits compatible with life.[1,2]

When compensatory mechanisms in the brain are exhausted, ICP increases and cerebral blood flow is compromised, which results in secondary injury. Secondary injury is a complex sequence of events that leads to further elevations in ICP, reduced cerebral blood flow, tissue hypoxia, and ischemia. This ultimately perpetuates neuronal death and may result in brain herniation.[1,2] Thus secondary injury is a major contributor to the mortality of animals with acquired brain injury. The primary goal in the treatment of these animals is to minimize the impact of the secondary injury by appropriate and timely treatment to maintain adequate cerebral blood flow. In the clinical setting, cerebral blood flow is reflected most accurately by cerebral perfusion pressure (CPP). CPP is dependent on the mean arterial pressure (MAP) and the ICP, and this relationship is expressed by the formula CPP = MAP − ICP.[1,2] By measuring the ICP, the clinician is able to assess whether CPP is maintained adequately in a patient with severe brain disease or injury.[3,4]

Although a growing number of studies in humans have suggested decreased mortality rates and improved long-term outcome with ICP-guided therapy, no randomized clinical trial has been performed showing that ICP monitoring improves outcome. "Guidelines for the Management of Severe Traumatic Brain Injury" (published in 1995 and revised in 2007) outlines the evidence-based recommendations for using ICP monitoring to improve treatment and outcome in severe brain injury.[4] Similar guidelines and recommendations were published in 2004 for the management of severe brain injury in infants and children. As yet, no specific guidelines have been established in veterinary medicine for treating severe brain injury. The standard of care has been primarily that of repeated and careful assessments of an animal's neurologic status in an attempt to detect increases in ICP. Unfortunately, most clinical signs indicating life-threatening intracranial hypertension (ICH) occur as a result of damage to brain tissue, and therapies administered at this point often are ineffective. There are potential benefits gained by monitoring ICP, especially when one expects prolonged and/or life-threatening ICH (Box 191-1).[4,5]

DETERMINATION OF INTRACRANIAL PRESSURE

Intracranial Pressure

Intracranial pressure refers to the pressure exerted by the tissues and fluids against an inelastic cranial vault. The total pressure recorded when ICP is monitored actually consists of several components[1,2]:

1. *Atmospheric pressure* results from the weight of the atmosphere on the brain; for example, a higher altitude results in a higher absolute ICP. Because ICP is always reported relative to the atmospheric pressure, this component is usually not taken into consideration.
2. *Hydrostatic pressure* is influenced by the orientation of the neuraxis relative to gravity (e.g., consider a giraffe vs. a rat).
3. *Filling pressure* refers to the volume of fluid within the cranial vault and affects the compliance or "give" of the brain tissues.

Locations for Monitoring Intracranial Pressure in the Brain

ICP monitoring commonly is done through a burr hole in the skull or a craniectomy site. ICP can be measured directly or reflected through measurement of CSF pressure or brain tissue pressure.[2,3]

BOX 191-1 ***Benefits of Intracranial Pressure (ICP) Monitoring***

1. Allows assessment of actual ICP as well as fluctuations and overall trends in ICP
2. Allows optimization of cerebral perfusion pressure–guided therapy
3. Allows for early intervention
4. Reduces indiscriminate treatment of ICH
5. Allows assessment of the effects of treatment of ICH
6. Allows assessment when clinical monitoring is not possible (anesthetized or comatose animals)
7. Provides assessment of brain death (cerebral perfusion ceases once ICP exceeds diastolic blood pressure)

ICH, Intracranial hypertension.

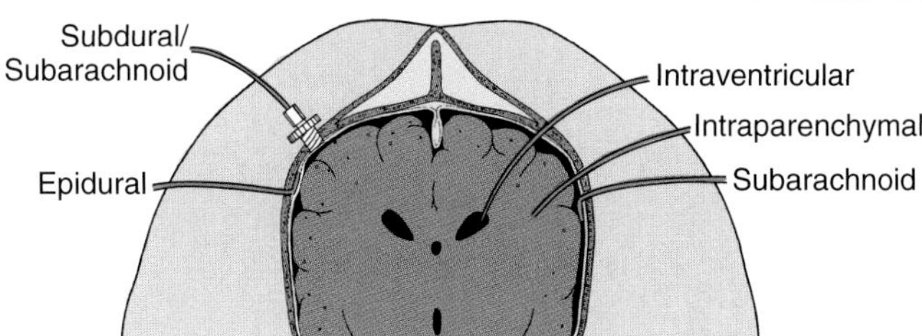

FIGURE 191-1 Intracranial pressure monitoring locations.

CSF pressure measurements can be taken from the lateral ventricles or the cerebral subarachnoid space; brain tissue pressure measurements are taken intraparenchymally from within a cerebral hemisphere. Measurements of ICP from the brain's surface may be taken epidurally or subdurally over a cerebral convexity[1,2,4] (Figure 191-1).

Although there are very few data in veterinary medicine with respect to the role of ICP monitoring in patients with brain disease, several studies in animals have shown that ICP can be monitored accurately. Historically, CSF pressure was measured using a manometer and needle puncture of the cisterna magna. This method requires that the patient undergo general anesthesia and does not allow for the ongoing ICP measurements needed to guide the clinician in treatment decisions. In addition, CSF pressures measured at the cisterna magna may not accurately reflect more compartmentalized elevations in ICP. In animals with global ICH, there is the added risk of brain herniation through the foramen magnum with this method.

Types of Intracranial Pressure Monitoring Devices

Pressure transducers convert ICP into a graded electrical signal that is recorded and displayed. They can be situated either intracranially or extracranially depending on the system used. Extracranial strain gauge–type transducers communicate with the intracranial compartment via fluid-filled tubing and require that ICP measurements be taken at fixed reference points. Pressure transducers situated intracranially are incorporated into the tip of a catheter and implanted into one of several compartments of the brain. Some of the important considerations in choosing a transducer are listed in Box 191-2.[2-4]

BOX 191-2 ***Considerations for Choosing an Intracranial Pressure Transducer***

External Pressure Transducer

Pros

Accurate
May be recalibrated after insertion
Minimal zero drift
Less expensive

Cons

Fluid couple may obstruct and give false readings
Measurements must be taken at fixed reference points
Allows little movement in awake animals
Leakage may occur in the system

Internal Pressure Transducer

Pros

Allows freedom of movement
Accurate
Technically easy to place

Cons

Cannot be rezeroed after insertion
Some zero drift over time
More expensive

Intracranial Pressure Monitoring Systems

Ventriculostomy catheter with external transducer

A ventriculostomy catheter is a fluid-filled hollow tube that is inserted into the lateral ventricle, usually through a burr hole craniotomy. The catheter is connected to an external strain gauge transducer via fluid-filled pressure-resistant tubing. The transducer is leveled or zeroed at an external reference point that represents the level of the foramen of Monro in the brain. Strain gauge transducers convert mechanical pressure (or strain) into a graded electrical signal.[2-4] Changes in ICP cause changes in the pressure exerted on the diaphragm and hence strain on the sensor element. The electrical resistance that is generated is recorded and displayed.

Ventriculostomy catheters provide the most accurate reflection of ICP and have become the gold standard, or reference standard, for monitoring ICP. Not only can ICP measurements be taken from the ventricle, but CSF can be withdrawn as needed for treatment of elevated ICP. Because of this advantage, this method is commonly used in humans. The external landmarks defining the trajectory for accurate placement of a ventriculostomy catheter are easily identified in humans, and the location of the lateral ventricle is reliably predicted most of the time. In dogs and cats, however, several anatomic characteristics impede the feasibility of using this system clinically. These include the marked variation in skull size and shape among breeds of dogs; variation in the size, shape, and location of the lateral ventricles in the brain; and the presence of substantial musculature overlying the cranial vault and obscuring identifying bony landmarks. In addition, when there is distortion of the lateral ventricles caused by intracranial pathologic processes, ventricular catheter placement becomes even more difficult.

Transducer-tipped catheters

Transducer-tipped catheters are a newer class of ICP monitoring devices. The primary pressure transducer is mounted on the distal tip of the implanted catheter. Because the transducer is intracranial, these devices do not require leveling. Both fiberoptic and electrical sensors (miniature strain gauge type) are used in these monitoring systems.[4]

Fiberoptic pressure-sensing methods include intensity modulation and interferometry. A mechanical diaphragm moves with changes in pressure in both methods, and a monitor displays the corresponding ICP value. In the case of intensity modulation, the position of the diaphragm alters the intensity of the light reflected from its rear surface; with the interferometer, the position of the diaphragm is sensed by measuring the ratio of returned light intensities in two spectral bandwidths. This ratio is a function of spectral interference, which varies with the position of the diaphragm. Fiberoptic transducers can record pressures from the intraventricular, intraparenchymal, subarachnoid, and/or subdural compartments of the brain.[2,3]

Fiberoptic ICP monitoring systems, developed for use in humans, have been effective in dogs and cats.[5] ICP can be measured from the CSF or brain parenchyma, and the method is effective in monitoring changes in ICP with the patient under anesthesia and during intracranial surgery.[5]

Catheter tip strain gauge pressure-sensing devices use a miniaturized silicon transducer enclosed in a titanium case and implanted in the tip of a flexible nylon catheter.[6] Changes in the position of the diaphragm cause changes in the electrical resistance, which is recorded and displayed by interface with a control unit for continuous monitoring of ICP. The control unit may then be interfaced with a wide variety of standard patient monitoring systems for ICP values, waveform display, or consolidation of data with other physiologic parameters being monitored. Catheter tip ICP sensors are versatile and may be placed in a ventricle, in brain parenchyma, or in the subarachnoid, subdural, and/or epidural spaces. This system has been used experimentally in awake and anesthetized normal dogs.[6] It has also been used successfully in anesthetized dogs during craniotomy procedures with continued monitoring in awake dogs for 2 to 5 days postoperatively. Placement of the sensor is technically easy, and the system allows complete freedom of movement in awake animals.

Subarachnoid bolt

A subarachnoid bolt is a metal tube or screw secured to the calvaria through a burr hole placed over a cerebral convexity. The tube, which opens into the subarachnoid space, allows for measurement of ICP via fluid coupling to an external pressure transducer or a sensor placed intracranially into the subarachnoid space.[2,3]

Fluid-filled catheter

Epidural or subdural placement of a sensor or a simple fluid-filled catheter connected to an arterial pressure monitoring system is cost effective and adequately serves the purpose of monitoring. Although the accuracy of this system may be questionable, fluctuations and trends in ICP are generally indicated reliably. Dewey et al reported the use of such a system in normal cats and found that it was a reliable alternative to the fiberoptic intraparenchymal monitoring system.[7]

Transcranial Doppler ultrasonography is a noninvasive method of assessing the state of the intracranial circulation and can indirectly predict ICP. It may be useful occasionally in young puppies or hydrocephalic dogs with fontanelles for measuring changes in cerebral vascular resistance.

EVALUATION OF INTRACRANIAL PRESSURE

Normal Intracranial Pressure

Normal ICP values reported in the dog and cat vary from 5 to 12 mm Hg above atmospheric pressure.[5,6] ICP is not a static state, but one that is influenced by several factors. When ICP is recorded, two types of phasic changes can normally be seen in the pressure tracing.[1,2] These fluctuations in ICP are the result of cyclic changes in cerebral blood volume caused by the cardiac and respiratory cycles.

- The CSF fluid pulse pressure wave is caused by contraction of the left ventricle of the heart with resulting distention of the arterioles. The ICP tracing is similar to that of the peripheral arterial blood pressure tracing, with a systolic rise followed by a diastolic fall and a dicrotic notch.
- The pulse pressure waves exhibit characteristic waveforms at faster graphing speed. Changes in the amplitude and shape of this waveform often provide an early indication of changes in ICP and brain compliance[1,2] (Figure 191-2).
- The ICP respiratory waves are slower pressure oscillations that fall with inspiration and rise with expiration. They are produced by fluctuations in both arterial blood pressure and cerebral venous outflow that cause an overall fluctuation in cerebral blood volume and consequently ICP (see Figure 191-2).

Various physiologic phenomena such as coughing, sneezing, straining, or a low head position can raise pressure dramatically in the brain secondary to increased central venous pressure and the resulting retrograde transmission to the CSF.[2,6] In a normal animal, the intracranial tissues are compliant, and such intermittent elevations in ICP are transient and go unnoticed clinically. In animals with intracranial abnormalities and preexisting ICH, ICP may increase precipitously and may remain elevated. Similarly, ICP can be affected by maneuvers such as compression of the jugular veins, suctioning of the back of the throat, and regurgitation.

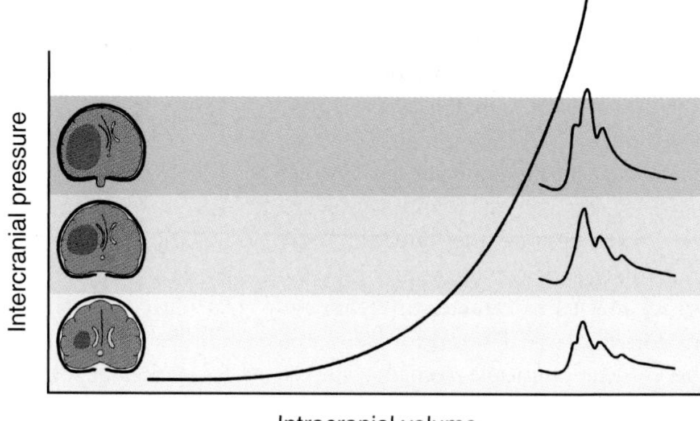

FIGURE 191-2 Intracranial pressure tracings of the pulse pressure waves are shown on the right. Alterations in the amplitude and shape of the waveforms that occur with changes in intracranial pressure and compliance of the neural tissues are shown on the left. This may be used to estimate where a patient's condition falls on the pressure-volume curve.

An absolute level at which ICP is considered pathologically elevated has not been established in humans or animals. Treatment of ICH generally is recommended in humans when ICP measurements are higher than 15 to 20 mm Hg. Because adequate CPP is more important than ICP per se, giving an exact value at which treatment should be initiated in an animal is not possible until studies are done in larger numbers of animals with similar disease processes using similar monitoring systems. General trends in ICP, as well as significant, sustained changes in CPP, may be as useful in guiding therapy and indicating prognosis as the specific ICP measurement recorded. In patients that have not been anesthetized, ICP monitoring is used in combination with meticulous and ongoing visual assessment of the patient to guide treatment decisions for animals with ICH. ICPs of 25 to 40 mm Hg with adequately maintained CPPs are seen routinely in severely brain-injured animals that subsequently fully recover.[5,6] In anesthetized or comatose patients, treatment of ICH should be considered when ICP values are 15 to 20 mm Hg and slowly increasing, when ICP values are lower than 15 mm Hg but rapidly increasing, and when CPP is not being maintained adequately.

Accuracy of Intracranial Pressure Monitoring Systems

In human medicine, with defined limits for treatment of ICH (i.e., 15 to 20 mm Hg), there is considerable discussion regarding the accuracy of ICP monitoring technology; clinicians worry that ICP may be underestimated or overestimated and therefore that they may either incorrectly treat or not treat patients. Although treatment standards have not been as well defined in veterinary medicine, the user must have an understanding of the limitations of the device being employed. In addition, compartmentalization within the cranium, zero drift (with catheter tip transducers), and the need for leveling to obtain accurate measurements (with external transducers) must be taken into account.[4] In particular, fluid-filled systems may have inaccuracies from leakage in stopcocks, improper positioning in the CSF space, and occlusion with debris.[3,7]

Although ventricular pressure measurement is still considered the gold standard for accuracy in monitoring ICP, catheter tip pressure transducers have a similar accuracy. Many studies have looked at the phenomenon of compartmentalization in the brain. ICP can vary within and between the intracranial compartments: brain and CSF, supratentorial and infratentorial locations, and the two hemispheres.[3]

In addition, because the contents are not homogeneous due to variation in tissue and capillary density, pressures may vary throughout the brain even in the absence of a pathologic condition.

In human studies, ICP is assessed most accurately by monitoring the cerebral hemisphere ipsilateral to the lesion.[3] Surface ICP monitors, such as epidural and subdural catheters and bolts, generally are considered less accurate than ventricular catheters or intraparenchymal devices because they are not necessarily reflective of events occurring deep within the brain.[2] In a study monitoring ICP in seven normal dogs using catheter tip strain gauge transducers, no significant difference in ICP was recorded within or between cerebral hemispheres when multiple recordings were taken simultaneously in anesthetized and awake dogs.[6]

Complications of Intracranial Pressure Monitoring

Complications of ICP monitoring are rare overall and should not deter the clinician from deciding to use an ICP monitor if it is indicated.[4] The most common complications reported in humans are infection, hemorrhage, and device malfunction, obstruction, and malposition.[2-4] Infection and hemorrhage are associated more commonly with intraventricular catheter placement, and malfunction (obstruction, breakage) may be more common with catheter-tipped devices.

Indications for Intracranial Pressure Monitoring in Dogs and Cats

The correlation between elevated ICP and a poorer outcome in patients with severe brain injury has been shown in many human studies. Lowering elevated ICP ensures adequate CPP, reduces the risk of herniation, and optimizes recovery. Because placement of an ICP monitor is associated with a small risk of complications as well as added cost, it is reasonable to limit its use to patients that are at most risk of herniation from ICH. ICP monitoring of brain-injured animals is likely to be most useful in the following groups:

1. Animals that are anesthetized or comatose, including animals undergoing and/or recovering from intracranial surgery
2. Animals with severe, progressive neurologic deterioration associated with a disease such as intracranial infection or inflammatory brain disease that may respond to a specific therapy with time
3. Animals with severe and traumatic head injury
4. Research animals

REFERENCES

1. Marmarou AM, Beaumont A: Physiology of the cerebrospinal fluid and intracranial pressure. In Winn HR, Youmans JR, editors: Youmans neurological surgery, ed 5, Philadelphia, 2004, Saunders.
2. Lee KR, Hoff JT: Intracranial pressure. In Youmans JR, editor: Neurological surgery, ed 4, Philadelphia, 1996, Saunders.
3. March K: Intracranial pressure monitoring. Why monitor? AACN Clin Issues 16:456, 2000.
4. Bullock MR, Povlishock JT, editors: Guidelines for the management of severe traumatic brain injury, J Neurotrauma 24:1, 2007.
5. Bagley RS: Options for diagnostic testing in animals with neurologic disease. In Bagley RS, editor: Fundamentals of veterinary clinical neurology, ed 1, Oxford, 2005, Blackwell.
6. Sturges BK, LeCouteur RA, Tripp LD: Intracranial pressure monitoring in clinically normal dogs using the Codman ICP Express and Codman Microsensor ICP transducer, Proceedings of the 18th American College of Veterinary Internal Medicine Forum, Seattle, May 25-28, 2000.
7. Dewey CW, Bailey CS, Haskins SC, et al: Evaluation of an epidural intracranial pressure monitoring system in cats, J Vet Emerg Crit Care 1:20, 1997.

CHAPTER 192
URINE OUTPUT

Sean Smarick, VMD, DACVECC • Terry C. Hallowell, DVM, DACVECC

KEY POINTS

- Measuring urine output assists the clinician in the assessment of perfusion, renal function, and fluid balance.
- Placement of an indwelling urinary catheter is justified for the accurate determination of urine output in critically ill patients.
- Normal urine output is approximately 1 to 2 ml/kg of body weight per hour; however, interpretation of the urine output must be based on the individual patient and clinical situation because urine outputs may vary.
- Oliguric and polyuric states require consideration of prerenal, postrenal, and renal causes, with meticulous attention to fluid therapy.
- Once perfusion and hydration are assessed as normal, urine output can guide fluid administration rates to balance fluid input and urinary output.

URINE OUTPUT AS A MONITORING TOOL

Urine output depends on a number of upstream physiologic processes. For there to be normal urine output, the patient must have adequate tissue perfusion, fluid balance, and renal function.[1] A normal urine output supports the clinical picture of a patient in stable condition; therefore patient fluid input and urine output should be monitored. Abnormal values are of clinical concern and alert the clinician to search for the cause and adjust the patient's therapy. Urine output can reflect a patient's effective circulating blood volume as well as be an indicator of tissue perfusion.[2] Urine output has even been referred to as the "poor man's cardiac output."[1] In human medicine, during the early phases of trauma resuscitation urinary catheters are routinely placed.[3] Novel electric continuous urine collection and measurement systems (e.g., URINFO 2000) are now available that can even provide minute-to-minute information on urine output, and recent studies have shown that low urine output can be an early and reliable indicator of hypovolemia.[2,4]

Once the patient's perfusion and hydration are stabilized, urine output can help guide fluid therapy to maintain fluid balance by matching input with output.[1] A number of conditions often encountered in emergent or critically ill patients warrant monitoring of urine output on some level.

A common condition seen in critically ill patients is acute kidney injury (AKI). AKI is associated with an increase in morbidity, mortality, and length of hospital stay.[5] The RIFLE classification has been validated and is a consensus-based classification system for diagnosing and staging AKI.[5] It further characterizes AKI based on the risk, injury, failure, loss, and end-stage renal disease (RIFLE). AKI is diagnosed on the basis of laboratory findings, such as increases in creatinine concentration or decrease in urine output.[5] The urine output criteria are frequently and arguably incorrectly discarded, and a recent study found a significant difference when the RIFLE system was applied with and without the use of urine output. Omission of the RIFLE urine output criteria for AKI diagnosis led to underestimation of the incidence of AKI and delay in its diagnosis and was also associated with higher mortality.[6] This validates the importance of monitoring urine output in critically ill patients at risk of AKI.

MEASUREMENT OF URINE OUTPUT

Urine output is measured most accurately and easily by collecting urine via an indwelling urinary catheter. The catheter collects urine as it is produced and is indicated for monitoring perfusion and renal function in critically ill patients. The risk of a catheter-associated urinary tract infection can be minimized by following placement and maintenance protocols that include using aseptic technique and leaving the catheter in place for only as long as necessary[7] (see Chapter 208). Graduated cylinders or beakers should be used to measure urine volume because collection bag graduations are inaccurate.

When intensive or precise monitoring of urine output is not necessary, "free catch" methods of collecting urine can be used. These include metabolic cages, collection pans, and absorbent pads. Metabolic cages are rarely used in the clinical setting. Collection pans provide an option for the ambulatory patient. Absorbent pads can be very effective as long as the patient voids the entire urine volume on the pad. Recumbent patients are good candidates for this method because they are forced to urinate in a given position. The absorbent pads are preweighed and then weighed again immediately after the patient urinates. Output is estimated by the change in weight with the assumption that 1 ml of urine weighs 1 g.

In all hospitalized patients, especially those receiving fluid therapy, screening urine output by obtaining a gross estimation of urine volume is indicated as part of ongoing patient assessment. Gross estimation may be adequate for basic monitoring of initial resuscitation, ongoing fluid therapy, and surveillance for obstruction in patients in stable condition. However, more accurate measurement should be performed if the patient remains or becomes critically ill or if the adequacy of urine output is questioned.

DETERMINANTS OF URINE OUTPUT

Urine output depends on the glomerular filtration rate, tubular reabsorption of solutes and water, and patency of the urinary tract. Ultrafiltration of plasma at the glomerulus is the first step in urine production, and any decrease in glomerular filtration rate results in decreased urine output. The ultrafiltrate travels through the nephron, and tubular reabsorption generally leaves less than 1% of the original volume to be excreted as urine. If there is a physiologic or pathologic decrease in these reabsorptive processes, an increase in urine production results, whereas an increase in tubular reabsorption of solutes and water leads to a decrease in urine output. Lastly, urine output depends on an unobstructed path from the kidney to the urethral opening.

Glomerular Filtration Rate

Glomerular filtration rate (GFR) is the volume of fluid filtered from the kidney's glomerular capillaries into Bowman's capsule per unit time.[8] It is determined by the balance of hydrostatic and colloid osmotic forces across the glomerular membrane in addition to the permeability and surface area of this membrane. Between mean arterial blood pressures of 80 and 180 mm Hg, autoregulation maintains renal blood flow, and therefore GFR, constant. Patients with a mean arterial blood pressure below 80 mm Hg will have decreased renal blood flow, GFR, and urine output. Furthermore, decreased baroreceptor stimulation, as occurs in response to hypotension and hypovolemia, increases sympathetic input to the kidneys and circulating catecholamine and angiotensin production. These mediators cause renal arteriolar constriction, which further decreases renal blood flow and GFR in an effort to conserve blood volume.

Tubular Reabsorption of Water and Solutes

Although large volumes of plasma are filtered by the glomerulus, over 99% of the ultrafiltrate normally is reabsorbed by active and passive mechanisms throughout the nephron. This assumes a critical mass of functioning nephrons. The amount of ultrafiltrate that is excreted as urine is fine-tuned by a number of systems that regulate extracellular fluid volume and water balance.

Stretch receptors (baroreceptors) throughout the body are the primary regulators of effective circulating volume. Hypotension and hypovolemia cause decreased stretch, which reduces the activity of these receptors and results in activation of the sympathetic nervous system and renin-angiotensin-aldosterone system. This response increases reabsorption of solutes and water in an effort to maintain the effective circulating volume, which results in decreased urine output. The converse is also true. Increased vascular volume leads to decreased renal reabsorption of solutes and water and increased urine output through activation of atrial natriuretic peptide and decreased stimulation of the renin-angiotensin-aldosterone system.

Antidiuretic hormone (ADH) also influences urine output. It is released primarily in response to increased extracellular osmolality, but it is also released in response to significant decreases in effective circulating volume. ADH increases the amount of water being reabsorbed in the distal nephron and thereby decreases urine output.

Dysfunction of nephrons, pharmacologic interference with the absorptive mechanisms, or abnormalities of the fine-tuning systems can therefore affect urine output.

Impedance to Flow

As the ultrafiltrate leaves the collecting ducts as urine, it flows through the renal pelvis, into the ureter and then the bladder, and finally out the urethra. Obstructions prevent urine flow as well as transmit back pressure to the kidneys, which results in decreased GFR and dysfunction of the affected kidneys.[1,9]

NORMAL URINE OUTPUT

Normal values for urine output have been reported for both adult dogs and cats and are generally accepted as 1 to 2 ml/kg/hr.[1] Urine serves to excrete metabolic waste, and if a patient is anorexic, deprived of food, caged, or in a sedentary state, output may be 0.5 ml/kg/hr or even lower. Conversely, neonates that lack effective urine concentrating abilities and patients receiving fluid therapy at rates exceeding those needed to replenish deficits and meet maintenance requirements may have urine output in excess of 2 ml/kg/hr. Interpretation of urine output depends on the individual patient and clinical situation.[1,9]

ABNORMAL URINE OUTPUT

Abnormal urine output alerts the clinician to consider prerenal, renal, and postrenal causes for the oliguric or polyuric state. As a downstream parameter, abnormal urine output is not specific for any one cause, and abnormal values warrant consideration of a complete rule-out list. For example, although decreased urine output may indicate inadequate resuscitation in a trauma patient in severe shock, it must be considered that oliguria can have other causes such as urinary tract trauma (e.g., ureteral avulsion, bladder rupture). Hence, other indicators of perfusion and urinary tract trauma must be assessed to develop an accurate clinical picture.

Oliguria

A decrease in urine output below what is expected (the lowest normal value in dogs is reported as 0.27 ml/kg/hr) is referred to as *oliguria,* and the total lack of urine production is called *anuria.*[1] In a hydrated and well-perfused patient, urine outputs of less than 1 ml/kg/hr can be considered as an *absolute oliguria.*[1] Although within the normal range for urine production, a urine output of between 1 and 2 ml/kg/hr can be considered a *relative oliguria* in a patient receiving intravenous fluid therapy.[1] Oliguria warrants immediate attention and should prompt the clinician to differentiate between prerenal, renal, and postrenal causes. Prerenal and postrenal causes are ruled out first, followed by evaluation of intrinsic renal abnormalities. Fluid therapy may need to be increased or decreased depending on the cause, and other therapies may be indicated.

Prerenal oliguria

Renal perfusion is necessary to maintain normal urine output. Inadequate renal perfusion decreases GFR and increases tubular resorptive mechanisms as described earlier. Reduced cardiac output or hypotension causes decreased renal perfusion. Common disease processes associated with these changes include severe dehydration, hypovolemia, hemorrhage, cardiac failure, and systemic inflammatory response syndrome and sepsis.

Restoring adequate circulating volume, cardiac function, and vascular tone should restore urine output to normal if poor perfusion is the sole cause of the oliguria.

Urine sodium concentration can also be measured to support the assessment of poor renal perfusion. A urine sodium level of less than 20 mEq/L is consistent with the action of aldosterone and supports the presence of inadequate renal perfusion (in the absence of diuretic administration or intrinsic renal disease).[10]

Postrenal oliguria

A decrease in urine output always warrants an assessment of the patency of the urinary tract, including evaluation of the urinary catheter and closed collection system if one is in place. Obstruction or disruption of the urethra, bladder, or ureters generally leads to oliguria or anuria. A large, inexpressible bladder on palpation warrants evaluation for a lower urinary tract obstruction due to a calculus, tumor, clot, or foreign body. Increased bladder sphincter tone due to upper motor neuron disease or pharmacologic effects of drugs such as opioids should also be considered.

Radiography, abdominal ultrasonography, urinary catheterization with or without retrohydropulsion, or contrast cystourethrography may be warranted to characterize the lesion.

Urethrocystoscopy can also be considered for the evaluation of urethral disease. Unilateral ureteral (or renal pelvic) obstruction or disruption may not result in decreased urine output because the other kidney may compensate. In these patients, urine output depends on the function of the remaining kidney, including the patency of its renal pelvis and ureter. Ureteral obstructions may be challenging to diagnose because "big kidney–little kidney" radiographs are not specific for the condition, and effective imaging with ultrasonography and contrast studies (e.g., iohexol) may require advanced training and equipment. If urinary tract obstruction cannot be relieved readily, fluid therapy must be adjusted to prevent volume overload.

Renal oliguria

A critical mass of functioning nephrons is required to produce an adequate amount of urine. Intrinsic acute renal failure or end-stage chronic renal failure is characterized by a lack of functioning nephrons that simply does not allow enough urine to be made. Renal causes of oliguria are suspected when prerenal and postrenal causes have been ruled out. The history and other diagnostic tests, such as abdominal ultrasonography, may further support this diagnosis. When intrinsic renal disease is being managed, fluid therapy must be adjusted to prevent volume overload. Persistent oliguria or anuria is a poor prognostic indicator in veterinary medicine, especially in the absence of renal replacement therapy.[1]

The syndrome of inappropriate ADH is a potential cause of oliguria in critically ill patients. Causes include recent surgery, administration of μ-agonist narcotics, and the use of positive pressure ventilation. These animals have oliguria despite adequate renal perfusion and do not have evidence of renal or postrenal compromise. Serum hyponatremia is usually evident, and if urine electrolyte levels are measured concurrently, a urine sodium level of more than 40 mEq/L supports the diagnosis. Administration of low-dose loop diuretics such as furosemide usually maintains sufficient urine output until the stimulus is no longer present[1,9,10] (see Chapter 68).

Polyuria

Urine excretion of more than 1 to 2 ml/kg/hr represents polyuria. As with oliguria, prerenal, postrenal, and renal causes should be considered and therapy adjusted accordingly.

Prerenal polyuria

Overhydration caused by administering fluids in excess of what is needed is a common cause of polyuria in the hospitalized patient. Fluid therapy may also result in medullary washout, which leaves the kidney unable to concentrate urine. Primary hormonal alterations, electrolyte abnormalities, osmotic loads, and drugs can also affect the kidney's ability to absorb solute and water (Box 192-1). Careful attention to fluid therapy is required in the polyuric patient to prevent significant abnormalities in hydration. When polyuria occurs in response to excess fluid administration, it is an appropriate response that does not require additional fluid therapy.

Postrenal polyuria

Postobstructive diuresis is a common cause of polyuria often encountered in small animal patients after relief of a urinary tract obstruction. Proximal tubule dysfunction, altered ADH responsiveness, and osmotic diuresis contribute. Aggressive fluid administration is warranted to maintain fluid balance until renal function and solute load return to normal.[1,10]

Renal polyuria

Chronic renal failure usually is characterized in small animals by a progressive loss of nephrons. As a result, the kidney can no longer

BOX 192-1 *Prerenal Causes of Polyuria*

Increased intake Polydipsia (psychogenic) Fluid administration Drugs Diuretics α_2-Agonist sedatives κ-Agonist narcotics Alcohols Glucocorticoids Anticonvulsants Hormonal conditions Hyperadrenocorticism Hypoadrenocorticism Diabetes insipidus Hyperthyroidism	Cerebral salt-wasting syndrome (posttraumatic brain injury) Electrolyte abnormalities Hypokalemia Hypercalcemia Osmotic conditions Diabetes mellitus Salt ingestion or administration Glycols *Escherichia coli* endotoxin Liver disease

fully reabsorb the filtered load of sodium and water and a polyuric state results. In polyuric renal failure, monitoring of urine output assists in balancing fluid administration, and the clinician can quickly recognize deterioration into oliguric renal failure.[1] Conversely, patients recovering from acute renal failure often progress from an oliguric state to one of polyuria.

FLUID BALANCE

Measuring urine output is a valuable tool in balancing fluid therapy in oliguric and polyuric states, or in patients that are critically ill and need tight control over their extracellular fluid volume. In homeostasis, there is no net loss or gain of water and solutes; the excretion is equal to intake. The more one knows about the output part of the equation, the better the fluid plan one can develop. When a patient's fluid output is calculated, both sensible and insensible losses must be considered. Sensible losses are those that can be measured, such as urine, whereas insensible losses are those that cannot be measured, such as from evaporation. Evaporative losses are less than 20 ml/kg/day in sedentary, quiet dogs and cats; however, panting, active dogs can lose as much as 70 ml/kg/day.[1] Drooled saliva and feces can be measured by weighing as described previously, but they often are considered insensible and negligible if normal in amount.

In patients with a normal hydration status, a fluid plan based on matching intake and output is simple and effective. Essentially this fluid plan aims to measure all of the output over a specified period, such as 4 hours, and this volume is then used to determine the new fluid administration rate. This approach can be particularly beneficial in the polyuric patient because excessive fluid loss can occur rapidly.[1,10]

Body weight, physical examination findings, hydration parameters (moistness of mucous membranes, skin turgor, eye position), perfusion parameters (mentation, mucous membrane color, capillary refill time, pulse quality, heart rate, and extremity temperature), packed cell volume, serum total protein level, urine specific gravity, blood pressure, central venous pressure, and lactate levels are parameters that can help assess the hydration and perfusion status of the patient for both initial and ongoing fluid therapy.

CASE EXAMPLE

A 5-kg cat that underwent a procedure to relieve a lower urinary tract obstruction and placement of an indwelling urinary catheter has had a urine output of 120 ml over the previous 4 hours. A 50-ml fluid bolus was given initially and the patient received 2 ml/kg/hr (10 ml/hr) of an isotonic intravenous fluid for the 4-hour period. The patient's intake over the last 4 hours was 90 ml (50-ml bolus + [4 hr × 5 kg × 2 ml/kg/hr]) and the patient's output was 120 ml, a deficit of 30 ml. After it is determined that the patient currently is appropriately perfused and hydrated, the diagnosis of postobstructive diuresis is made. To balance the intake and output, the fluid rate will be increased to replace the 30-ml deficit over the next 4 hours (to a total of 17.5 ml/hr). Once the fluid rate is approximately equal to the urine output, it will be decreased gradually to a maintenance rate; the urine output should follow.

If this same patient generated only 4 ml of urine during the first 4 hours (0.2 ml/kg/hr), inadequate resuscitation, catheter or urinary tract obstruction, or acute renal failure should be considered. If there are signs of inadequate perfusion or dehydration, additional fluids should be administered as appropriate. Integrity and patency of the urinary tract should be assessed by palpating the bladder and flushing the catheter, and if there is still any question regarding the intactness of the lower urinary tract, imaging studies should be performed. Lastly, if no evidence to support prerenal or postrenal causes of oliguria is found, then AKI should be considered.

REFERENCES

1. DiBartola SP, editor: Fluid, electrolyte, and acid-base disorders in small animal practice, ed 4, St Louis, 2012, Saunders.
2. Shamir MY, Kaplan L, Marans RS, et al: Urine flow is a novel hemodynamic monitoring tool for the detection of hypovolemia, Anesth Analg 112:593-596, 2011.
3. Shock. In American College of Surgeons Committee on Trauma: Advanced trauma life support for doctors, ed 6, Chicago, 1997, American College of Surgeons, pp 101-107.
4. Hersch M, Einav S, Izbicki G: Accuracy and ease of use of a novel electronic urine output monitoring device compared with standard manual urinometer in the intensive care unit, J Crit Care 24:629-633, 2009.
5. Singbartl K, Kellum JA: AKI in the ICU: definition, epidemiology, risk stratification, and outcomes, Kidney Int 18:819-825, 2012.
6. Wlodzimirow KA, Abu-Hanna A, Slabbekoorn M, et al: A comparison of RIFLE with and without urine output criteria for acute kidney injury in critically ill patients, Critical Care 16:R200, 2012.
7. Smarick SD, Haskins SC, Aldrich J, et al: Incidence of catheter-associated urinary tract infection among dogs in a small animal intensive care unit, J Am Vet Med Assoc 224:1936, 2004.
8. Legrand M, Payen D: Understanding urine output in critically ill patients, Ann Intensive Care 1:13, 2011.
9. Koeppen BM, Stanton BA: Renal physiology, ed 4, Philadelphia, 2007, Mosby.
10. Rose BD, Post TW: Clinical physiology of acid-base and electrolyte disorders, ed 5, New York, 2001, McGraw-Hill.

CHAPTER 193
PERIPHERAL VENOUS CATHETERIZATION

Harold Davis, BA, RVT, VTS (Emergency/Critical Care; Anesthesia)

KEY POINTS

- There are four primary catheter types: winged, over the needle, through the needle, and multilumen.
- Catheter insertion site selection depends on several factors, including vessel availability and the intended purpose of catheterization.
- Proper vessel immobilization facilitates catheter placement.
- There are several catheter-related complications—phlebitis, thrombosis, catheter embolus, subcutaneous fluid infiltration, and infection—all of which can be minimized by appropriate attention to detail.

Peripheral venous access is a cornerstone of the treatment of the emergent or critically ill patient. Patients often require temporary venous access for administration of medications, fluid and electrolyte replacement, or transfusion of blood products. Medications and fluids with osmolalities of 600 mOsm or less may be administered safely via a peripheral vein.[1] Infusion of more hyperosmolar solutions can cause phlebitis. Site selection depends on the available vessels, condition of the vessels and the patient, expense, and urgency of the situation. Vascular access traditionally involves the insertion of a catheter into the cephalic, saphenous, or auricular vein; however, any visible vessel is a potential candidate for catheterization. Various techniques are used to insert catheters, including percutaneous placement, facilitative relief holes, and venous cutdowns.

CATHETER TYPES

A variety of catheters are commercially available (Figure 193-1). The length and gauge (diameter) of the catheter to be used depend on the species and size of the patient, the veins available and their condition, and the needs of the patient.

Both the radius and the length of the catheter determine the maximum flow rate. A large-gauge, short catheter is needed if fluids are to be administered rapidly, such as in a severely hypovolemic patient. If a slow infusion is acceptable, then a small-gauge catheter might be appropriate. A smaller catheter/vein ratio is considered more "vein friendly."

There are four general categories of intravenous access devices. They include the winged needle and over-the-needle, through-the-needle, and multilumen catheters.

Winged or Butterfly Needle

The winged needle (butterfly) is for short-term use when there is minimal patient movement. Applications include blood collection and administration of nonirritating medications. Common needle sizes range from 25 to 19 gauge. The needles have plastic wings on the shaft to facilitate placement or taping in place. Plastic tubing of various lengths extends from the needle to the syringe connector port. These catheters are easy to place but difficult to maintain because of the ease with which the indwelling sharp needle punctures the vessel wall, which allows subcutaneous infiltration of fluids or medications.

Over-the-Needle Catheter

The over-the-needle catheter is the most commonly used type. It is inexpensive and easy to place. The needle point extends a millimeter or so beyond the catheter tip. Over-the-needle catheters are available in a variety of lengths and gauges and are made of various materials (polytetrafluoroethylene [Teflon], polypropylene, polyvinyl chloride, and polyurethane).

Through-the-Needle Catheter

Catheters passed through the needle are called *through-the-needle* or *inside-the-needle catheters.* Through-the-needle catheters are usually longer (8 to 12 inches) than over-the-needle catheters and come in a variety of diameters. These catheters are used primarily in the jugular vein but can be used peripherally in the medial or lateral saphenous vein. If of appropriate length for the size of the patient, these catheters can be used as peripherally inserted central catheters (PICC lines). They can also be inserted into the cephalic vein but are often difficult to pass beyond the axilla into the larger anterior vena cava. A plastic sleeve prevents catheter contamination during insertion. Once the catheter is placed, the needle is withdrawn from the skin puncture site and either removed completely or covered with a needle guard to prevent the needle from shearing the catheter.

Multilumen Catheter

Arrow International (Reading, Pa.) produces a double-lumen over-the-needle catheter called a *TwinCath.* The TwinCath is more expensive than regular single-lumen catheters, but it allows simultaneous infusion of otherwise incompatible fluids via one catheter. Catheter placement is identical to that of any single-lumen over-the-needle catheter.

Short multilumen catheters placed via the Seldinger technique can also be used for peripheral venous access, usually in a medial or lateral saphenous vein. See Chapter 195 for a description of this technique.

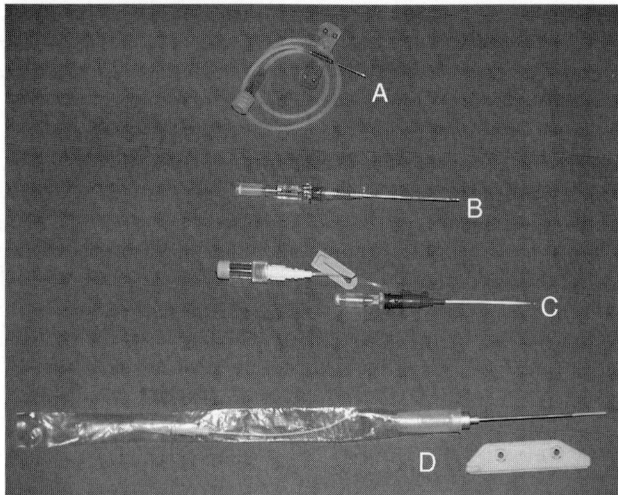

FIGURE 193-1 Example of various types of catheters. **A,** Winged needle or butterfly, **B,** Over-the-needle catheter, **C,** TwinCath double-lumen catheter. **D,** Through-the-needle catheter with needle guard.

ADVANTAGES OF PERIPHERAL VENOUS CATHETERIZATION

- Peripheral catheters tend to be relatively inexpensive, technically simple to place, and well tolerated by most patients.
- Peripheral veins are easily accessible for quick catheterization such as in cardiac arrest or seizures. Placement of two peripheral catheters may be indicated if rapid fluid resuscitation is required.
- Peripheral catheter placement generally requires minimal restraint. Patients experiencing respiratory distress do not tolerate the stress of restraint (e.g., as would be required for central venous catheterization).
- Peripheral venous catheterization is generally associated with fewer significant complications such as hemorrhage, infection, or thrombosis compared with central venous access.

CATHETER INSERTION SITE

Peripheral venous insertion sites include the cephalic, lateral and medial saphenous, pedal, and auricular veins.

Cephalic Vein

The cephalic vein is located on the anterior antebrachium. It crosses from the medial aspect of the leg an inch or so proximal to the carpus to join the brachial vein proximal to the elbow, which ultimately joins the external jugular vein. An accessory cephalic vein on the anterior aspect of the metacarpus passes over the carpus and joins the cephalic vein.[2] If possible, it is best to avoid the insertion of the catheter over the carpus because it will be difficult to secure.

Saphenous Vein

The cranial branch of the lateral saphenous vein obliquely crosses the lateral aspect of the distal tibia.[2] The lateral saphenous is larger than the medial saphenous in the dog, whereas the medial saphenous is larger than the lateral and is more commonly catheterized in the cat.

Pedal Veins

There are several veins crossing the dorsal aspect of all four paws. In large and giant breed dogs these veins can be readily catheterized and may be an option when other more commonly used catheter sites are no longer available.

Auricular Vein

The auricular veins are prominent in some breeds of dogs (Basset, Dachshund, and Bloodhound) and are fairly easy to catheterize. Catheters in these vessels are easily dislodged with motion, which makes them more suitable for anesthetized or largely immobile patients.

INSERTION TECHNIQUE

Percutaneous Placement

The area of the insertion site is generously shaved. Surgical preparation is performed with antiseptic scrub and solution. Aseptic technique is important to prevent indwelling catheter–related infection.[3] Proper aseptic technique may be bypassed in emergency situations, but these catheters should be removed once the crisis has passed.

Following skin preparation, the vein is occluded upstream of the insertion site by a tourniquet or an assistant. The distal portion of the leg is grasped in the palm of the operator's hand and the leg is extended to tense and immobilize the vein. The thumb should not be used to stabilize the vein because this compresses and collapses the vein. Flexion of the carpus will increase the stretch on the vessel and improve vessel immobilization in achondroplastic breeds. With the bevel up, the catheter is inserted through the skin at approximately a 15-degree angle. The catheter is advanced into the vessel; when blood appears in the flash chamber (hub), the needle (stylet) and catheter are advanced as a unit for an additional 1 to 4 mm. This ensures that the end of the catheter is entirely inside the lumen of the vessel. While the stylet is held steady and the longitudinal tension on the leg is maintained, the catheter is then advanced off of the stylet and into the vessel lumen. The catheter is capped with an injection cap or T-set and flushed with heparinized saline.

The technique for percutaneous catheterization of the auricular vein is similar to that for catheterization of any peripheral vein. It may be useful to place roll gauze on the underside of the pinna to stabilize the ear.

Not all procedures are associated with spontaneous bleed back into the hub. If the operator thinks that the needle is in the vessel but does not see a flashback, one option is to attach a syringe filled with heparinized saline and aspirate. Sometimes the flashback occurs, but following catheter insertion blood cannot be aspirated. There are two possibilities: (1) the catheter is in the vein but the vein collapsed around the end of the catheter, or (2) the catheter is not in the vein.

1. Excessive pressure to aspirate may collapse the vein; very gentle aspiration should be attempted.
   - The appearance of any amount of blood in the hub suggests proper placement; the operator should not expect free-flowing blood samples because it is difficult to aspirate from many peripheral catheters.
   - The catheter tip may be occluded by a kink in the vein such as at the flexed elbow for a cephalic catheter; the leg should be extended.
   - The catheter may be large for the vein, obstructing blood flow past it; the vein should be occluded proximally and the foot squeezed to milk more blood into the vein.
   - If the catheter position still cannot be confirmed, the operator should inject a volume of saline into the catheter while watching for a subcutaneous bleb. If a large volume of saline can be injected without forming a subcutaneous bleb, the catheter must be in the vein.
2. The catheter may not be in the vein even though a flashback of blood was observed initially, and this can be attributed to several common technical missteps.

- After the flashback, the tension on the leg and skin was relaxed, which allowed the vein to retract off the end of the needle; the tension must be maintained until after the catheter is inserted.
- The flashback was associated with the needle tip's being in the vein, but the catheter tip was not wholly within the lumen of the vein; when the catheter was introduced it pushed the vein off the needle.
- The needle-and-catheter unit must be inserted a short distance beyond initial vein entry. Sometimes when the needle-and-catheter unit is advanced, it passes through the deep wall of the vein; the catheter will be pushed through the vein. If this is suspected, the needle-and-catheter unit is carefully withdrawn until backflow is evident ("catching the lumen on the way out"). Then re-advance of the catheter into the vessel in the routine manner can be tried.

Facilitative Incision or Relief Hole

Failed catheterization attempts may also be caused by catheter flaring. Flaring of the tip of the catheter may occur when the tip is torn or peeled back during its insertion through the skin. After a failed attempt, the catheter tip should be inspected for such flaring before reuse. Creating a facilitative incision or relief hole reduces the skin tension and friction against the catheter, minimizing catheter flaring, and is an especially important procedure in severely dehydrated patients or those with tough skin. A facilitative incision may be made with a No. 11 scalpel blade or a 20-gauge needle. A 0.5-mm incision is made directly over the vessel, extending through the dermis and with care taken to avoid lacerating the underlying vessel. Local anesthetic blocks are rarely needed; intradermal or subcutaneous lidocaine stings. Following the facilitative procedure, the catheter is inserted as discussed previously.

Venous Cutdown

A venous cutdown is indicated when the veins are small (a small patient or a patient that is severely hypovolemic) or when the veins are obscured (e.g., due to obesity, subcutaneous edema, or hematoma). Following aseptic skin preparation awake animals will require local anesthesia of the region, which should be done with care so as not to inject any agent intravenously. A 1- to 2-cm incision is then made through the skin parallel to the vessel, with care exercised to avoid lacerating the vein. The vessel is dissected free of the surrounding tissue. An encircling suture (absorbable) is placed around the vein proximal and distal to the intended venotomy site. The catheter can be inserted directly through the superficial vessel wall or, if a catheter is to be used without a needle stylet, an incision can be made into the vein while traction is applied on the preplaced sutures. If an incision is made, then once the catheter is inserted, both sutures are tied proximally to prevent bleeding (Figure 193-2). The skin is closed and the catheter site is bandaged.

Peripherally Inserted Central Venous Catheters

Central venous catheterization can be achieved by passing a long catheter from a peripheral insertion site to a central vessel. This can allow easy aspiration of samples, administration of hypertonic fluids, and long-term catheter maintenance (see Chapter 195).

COMPLICATIONS ASSOCIATED WITH CATHETERIZATION

Phlebitis

Phlebitis is inflammation of the vessel wall occurring as a result of damage to the endothelial lining. Phlebitis is characterized by

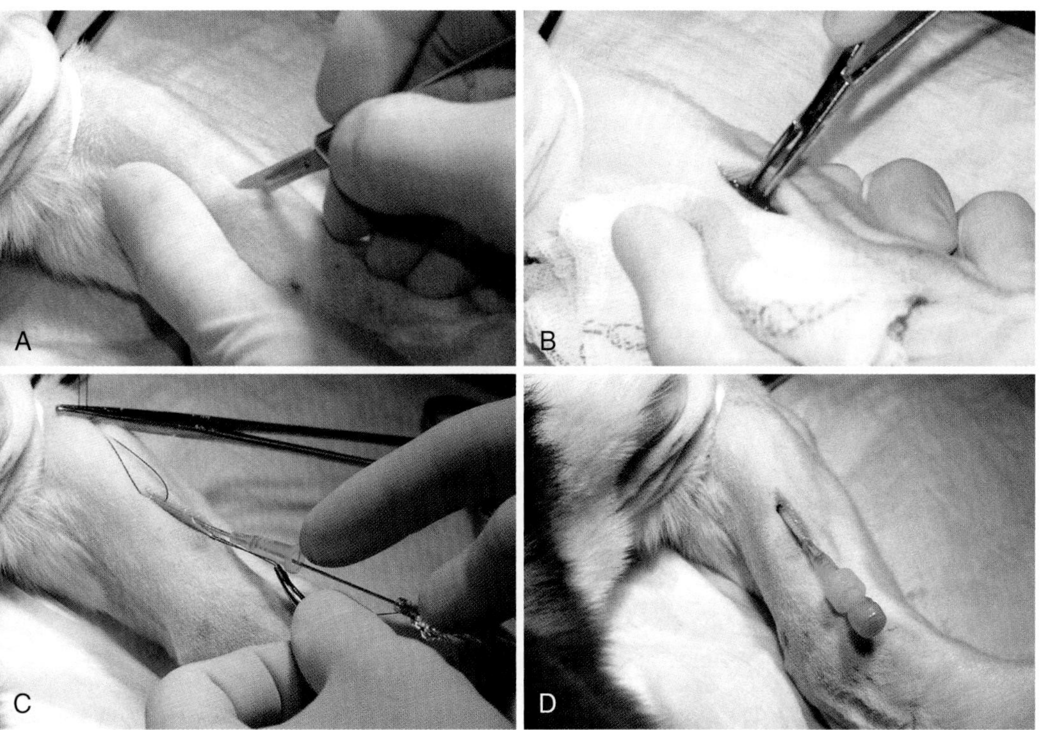

FIGURE 193-2 When the cutdown is performed, drapes are used to facilitate asepsis. Drapes were omitted here for photographic purposes. **A,** A skin incision is made over the cephalic vein. **B,** The vein is isolated using mosquito forceps and blunt dissection. **C,** One encircling suture is placed proximally and another distally to help evaluate the vein. The vein is immobilized while the catheter is inserted. **D,** The proximal suture is tied to help secure the catheter. The skin is closed and the site is bandaged.

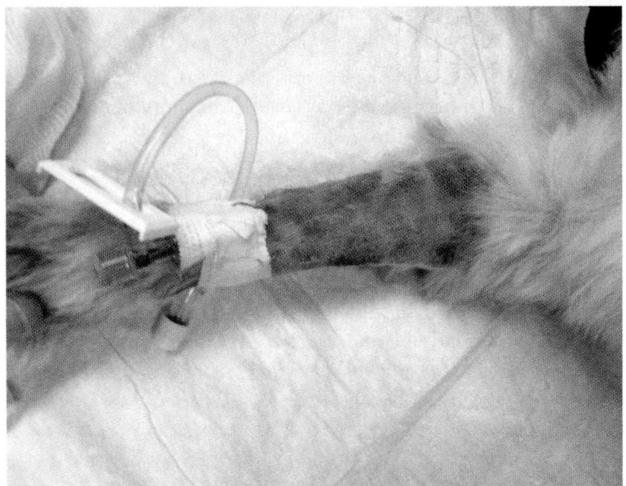

FIGURE 193-3 Patient with phlebitis associated with a cephalic catheter; the catheter insertion site and surrounding tissue are erythematous and painful. The vein feels thickened on palpation.

swelling, tenderness on palpation, and erythema of the skin over the vessel (Figure 193-3). Phlebitis may be caused by the following[4]:

1. Mechanical damage to the vessel by movement of the catheter, so the catheter should be well stabilized.
2. Administration of hyperosmotic fluids or medications; the osmolality of peripherally administered fluids should not exceed 600 mOsm.
3. Infection; aseptic technique should be maintained at all times if possible.

Some patients seem prone to catheter phlebitis for no apparent reason despite the use of good technique.

Thrombosis

Thrombosis is the formation of a thrombus on the catheter or vessel wall (as a consequence of phlebitis). Thrombosis commonly occurs in combination or association with phlebitis (thrombophlebitis). Thrombosis can result from endothelial trauma or an inflammatory reaction to the catheter material. A vein that "stands up" without being held off and feels thick and cordlike characterizes thrombosis.

Catheter Embolism

Catheter embolism occurs when a fragment of the catheter breaks off and enters the circulation. The fragment may be severed when an inside-the-needle catheter is withdrawn. It can also occur if the catheter is cut during bandage change or the patient disturbs the bandage.

Subcutaneous Fluid Infiltration

Infiltration of fluids into the tissues surrounding the vein may occur in the following circumstances:

1. The catheter was never in the vein in the first place.
2. The catheter is displaced out of the vein by excessive skin movement.
3. Upstream vein occlusion by thrombosis has occurred.

Signs of infiltration are swelling and tenderness around the insertion site.

Infection

An indwelling catheter is an excellent pathway for microorganisms to enter the tissues and the venous system. Infection may be heralded by phlebitis and cellulitis (manifesting as a purulent discharge from the insertion site). Use of aseptic technique in catheter placement and maintenance helps to decrease the risk of infection. Fever of unknown origin in a critically ill patient should prompt consideration of replacement of all indwelling catheters.

CATHETER MAINTENANCE

Intravenous catheter care should be performed every 48 hours or on an as-needed basis if the site becomes soiled. The catheter dressing should be removed and the site inspected. The site should be examined for clinical signs of phlebitis, infection, and thrombosis, and, if any is present, the catheter should be removed. While the catheter is flushed with saline or heparinized saline, the insertion site should be observed for fluid leakage or pain during injection. If either is observed, the catheter should be removed.

If any portion of the catheter is exposed, this should be recorded in the medical record and the catheter should not be reinserted. If the catheter site looks good, the site should be cleaned with chlorhexidine solution. When the catheter site is dry, a sterile 2 × 2-inch gauze pad should be placed over it and the bandage reapplied. It is no longer recommended that antibiotic ointment be applied at catheter insertion sites.

Peripheral venous catheters should be replaced when clinically indicated, and routine replacement every 72 to 96 hours is not necessary.[4] It has been the author's experience that as long as routine catheter care is performed and the catheter is removed when problems are first noticed, one can often exceed the 72-hour rule. A study looking at peripheral and jugular venous catheter contamination in dogs and cats supports this experience.[5]

Intravenous catheters should be observed several times a day. If the catheter bandage is wet, the reason should be identified and the bandage should be changed. Swelling distal to the catheter may be indicative of an excessively tight bandage or tape. Swelling proximal to the catheter may be due to infiltration.

REFERENCES

1. Kuwahara T, Asanami S, Kubo S: Experimental infusion phlebitis: tolerance osmolality of peripheral venous endothelial cell, Nutrition 14:496-501, 1988.
2. Evans HE, editor: Miller's anatomy of the dog, ed 3, Philadelphia, 1993, Saunders.
3. Burrows C: Inadequate skin preparation as a cause of intravenous catheter-related infection in the dog, J Am Vet Med Assoc 180:747, 1982.
4. Webster J, Osborne S, Rickard CM, et al: Clinically-indicated replacement versus routine replacement of peripheral venous catheters, Cochrane Database Syst Rev (4):CD007798, 2013.
5. Mathews KA, Brooks MJ, Valliant AE: A prospective study of intravenous catheter contamination, J Vet Emerg Crit Care 6:33, 1996.

CHAPTER 194

INTRAOSSEOUS CATHETERIZATION

Massimo Giunti, DVM, PhD • Cynthia M. Otto, DVM, PhD, DACVECC

KEY POINTS

- Intraosseous catheterization is an emergency procedure that allows rapid access to the central circulation comparable to that achieved with a central venous line.
- Intraosseous catheterization is indicated when emergency vascular access is required and intravenous access cannot be obtained in a timely manner.
- Intraosseous catheterization is an easy, fast, and inexpensive technique that can be performed effectively in various species.
- Intraosseous infusion is contraindicated in recently fractured bones, those in which catheterization has been previously attempted, and the pneumatic bones of birds.
- The rate of complications for intraosseous infusion is extremely low, and osteomyelitis is the primary risk.
- Blood samples obtained from intraosseous catheters can be analyzed for some hematologic, biochemical, and blood gas parameters in steady-state, low-flow conditions and during the early phase of cardiopulmonary resuscitation.

Rapid establishment of vascular access is crucial in critically ill patients, particularly those with life-threatening conditions. Peripheral vessels often constrict or collapse and may grossly disappear in animals with hemodynamic failure. Finding and cannulating vessels is particularly challenging in small and neonatal patients. Attempts to catheterize a peripheral vein can be frustrating, time consuming, and unsuccessful even for the most skilled personnel. In human pediatric prehospital and emergency department settings, peripheral intravenous access could not be obtained in 6% of patients and required over 10 minutes to achieve in 24%, with significantly prolonged times in children younger than 2 years of age.[1]

Compared with percutaneous peripheral venous catheterization, both surgical cutdown and central venous line placement increase the likelihood of successful circulatory access, but they require greater expertise and more time.[1,2] Peripheral venous catheterization within 90 seconds is successful in only 18% of cases. The success rate increases to 37% with subsequent percutaneous femoral vein catheterization.[2]

There are limited alternative routes for drug delivery in animals that require cardiovascular support but lack venous access. The endotracheal route is a last-resort option recommended by the American Heart Association for some resuscitation drugs during cardiac arrest in both adult and pediatric patients.[3,4] This route obviously cannot provide for fluid resuscitation, and even for commonly recommended drugs such as epinephrine the clinical effect is less predictable than when intravenous administration is used.[5] Additionally, the dosage of intratracheal epinephrine has to be increased up to tenfold.[6] Despite this dosage increase, lower circulating epinephrine concentration due to unpredictable absorption from the tracheal mucosa can result in counterproductive β_2-adrenergic stimulation, leading to peripheral vasodilation, low diastolic aortic pressure, and decreased myocardial perfusion pressure.[6]

Two proposed but inadvisable routes of drug administration are the sublingual and intracardiac routes.[7] Intracardiac injections are associated with risks (e.g., lung laceration, hemopericardium, coronary artery perforation, myocardial ischemia, arrhythmias) that exceed the benefits. Alternatives to intravenous access are reported,[7] but they are indicated mainly for volume replacement in states of dehydration (e.g., subcutaneous or intraperitoneal infusion) and are not effective for rapid treatment of hypovolemic patients.

Curiously, an unusual type of emergency vascular access, via the corpus cavernosum, was demonstrated to be fast and feasible for fluid resuscitation in dogs with severe hypovolemia, offering new therapeutic perspectives, even if limited to male dogs.[8] In pediatric and adult patients, intraosseous access is now recommended as the first choice if intravenous access is unavailable.[3,4] The intraosseous route is safe, practical, and reliable for fluid resuscitation, drug administration, and even blood sampling for analysis. This chapter focuses on what makes the intraosseous route suitable for fluid infusion and drug administration. The main indications, contraindications, complications, procedures, and future perspectives for intraosseous access in veterinary patients are presented based on veterinary reports, human studies, and experimental animal models.

HISTORICAL PERSPECTIVES

The possibility of perfusing the tibia of the dog was demonstrated in 1922 by Drinker et al, who were studying the vascular physiology of the bone marrow.[9] With this scientific observation as a starting point, the potential use of the intraosseous route for parenteral infusion of drugs and fluids was addressed by several studies in Europe and North America during the 1930s and 1940s.[10-12] In rabbits, intraosseous infusions of whole blood and hypertonic glucose solutions rapidly corrected anemia and hypoglycemia, respectively.[10] In dogs, intramedullary injection of citrated blood into the sternum effectively restored blood volume.[11] Moreover, an injection of epinephrine into the marrow of the tibia resulted in a clinical response similar to that achieved by injection into the femoral vein.[11]

Intraosseous infusion was established as a reliable and safe technique for rapid, short-term delivery of drugs and fluids into the central circulation in adults and children whose veins were inaccessible (e.g., because of peripheral circulatory failure, burns, or very young age).[11,12] However, with the introduction of plastic catheters for peripheral venous access during the late 1950s, intraosseous infusions fell into disuse.[1,13] A renewed interest in the intraosseous procedure appeared during the 1980s because of its utility in hypotensive patients and efficacy for the administration of lifesaving drugs.[14] The intraosseous route was recommended as an alternative for emergency access in pediatric advanced life support for children younger than 6 years of age, and more recently, resuscitation guidelines extended its use to children of any age and even to adults.[3,4]

PHYSIOLOGY

The bone marrow is a semifluid blood-forming tissue enclosed in a nonexpandable bony case. This protective osseous coating prevents bone marrow vessels from collapsing during peripheral circulatory failure. A rich capillary network drives substances injected into the marrow to the large medullary venous channels and quickly through the nutrient and emissary veins to the central circulation.[9-11]

Several types of fluids (blood and blood components, colloids, crystalloids)[11] and several drugs[15] reach the central circulation with equal effectiveness whether administered through an intraosseous, a central, or a peripheral intravenous line and whether delivered under normotensive, hypotensive, or arrest conditions.[14-16] Particularly during hemodynamic failure, intraosseous infusion of resuscitative fluids (e.g., hydroxyethyl starch solutions) and drugs (e.g., sodium bicarbonate) seems to guarantee a higher magnitude of peak effect and even a prolonged duration of action compared with peripheral venous administration.

Although intraosseously administered drugs reach peak effect more slowly[14,15] because of a reduction in blood flow and an increase in vascular resistance in the bone marrow during systemic hypotension, this effect can be partially overcome by using pressurized infusion, especially when viscous fluids likes colloids are given, or by administering a fluid bolus following the injection of a drug into the intraosseous space.[15] Mean intraosseous infusion flow rates of crystalloid solutions delivered under pressure (300 mm Hg) are limited to approximately 29 ml/min through a 20-gauge needle[17] and 47 ml/min through a 14-gauge needle. Thus rapid delivery of fluids (90 ml/kg within 30 minutes) during severe hypovolemia may not be possible in dogs that weigh more than 15 kg, even when a 14-gauge needle is used. However, intraosseous infusion of hyperoncotic, hypertonic, and even crystalloid solutions effectively reversed hypotension in several animal models of hemorrhagic shock (see Chapter 60).[18-21]

INDICATIONS

There are no studies documenting the incidence or impact of intraosseous catheterization in veterinary clinical practice. Most of the indications have been extrapolated from human experience and experimental animal models.[7,12,17] The information obtained from pediatric patients, in whom the time required to complete an intraosseous catheterization can be less than 1 minute with over 70% to 80% success, may be particularly relevant to small and neonatal animals.[18,19]

Early implementation of the intraosseous route as an alternative to failed intravenous access is now widely accepted and is included in the guidelines for management of cardiac arrest in pediatric and adult human patients. These recommendations are applicable to veterinary patients as well, particularly small and neonatal animals whose veins can be difficult to visualize in health and tend to grossly disappear in shock states.[22] Fluid resuscitation through an intraosseous catheter can usually restore vascular volume sufficiently to allow subsequent catheterization of a peripheral vein.

Conditions such as peripheral vascular thrombosis, peripheral edema, status epilepticus, obesity, and burns may be additional indications for obtaining intraosseous access.[13,18,19] Another advantage of intraosseous catheterization during emergency situations is the potential for blood sampling. Initial assessment of hematologic, biochemical, and acid-base status and subsequent monitoring of the therapeutic response are essential in critically ill patients. Blood sampling can be challenging, however, during cardiovascular collapse.

The reliability of laboratory results obtained on blood collected from intraosseous lines has been investigated in both steady-state conditions and circulatory failure. In normal animals, hemoglobin level, hematocrit, some biochemical parameters (levels of blood urea nitrogen, creatinine, total solids, albumin, bilirubin, sodium, chloride, calcium, phosphorus), and blood gases concentration are sufficiently comparable to those of peripheral or central venous blood to be of clinical value. Values obtained for potassium and glucose, however, need to be interpreted with caution.[23,24] Acid-base values obtained from intraosseous samples in cardiopulmonary resuscitation (CPR) models reflect the mixed venous blood acid-base balance during the first 15 minutes of CPR, but beyond that time values can be influenced by local acidosis.[20,21] In one CPR study, intraosseous and central venous blood biochemical and hemoglobin values remained similar for the first 30 minutes if the intraosseous site was not used for drug infusions.[25]

CONTRAINDICATIONS

The only absolute contraindication to intraosseous catheterization is a fracture in the bone to be used. In cases of failed intraosseous catheter placement in which the cortex has been penetrated, the risk of fluid or drug extravasation is increased.[13,19] To minimize risk, a second cannula of larger diameter should be placed through the same entry site or preferably a different bone should be used. Intraosseous infusions into pneumatic bones of birds are also contraindicated. Clearly, intraosseous catheters should not be placed through infected tissues. Sepsis and septic shock have been suggested as contraindications to the use of intraosseous lines; however, reported complication rates in septic children were low.[1]

METHODS

The increased use of intraosseous catheterization during the last 15 to 20 years[1,19] has been accompanied by the development of new medical equipment. Intraosseous catheters range from traditional manually placed hypodermic needles to dedicated catheters with automated delivery systems.[19,25] The main requirements for any intraosseous delivery system are ease of handling, ability to reload, low expense, and adaptability to most conditions. The supplies necessary for an intraosseous catheterization kit are described in Box 194-1.

Commercial disposable intraosseous infusion needles with a central stylet (Cook Critical Care, Bloomington, Ind.; Cardinal Health, McGaw Park, Ill.) are designed to penetrate the bony cortex, prevent occlusion of the cannula lumen, and establish rapid access to the marrow sinusoids and vascular system (Figure 194-1).[19] However, an 18- to 30-gauge hypodermic needle is useful in neonates with soft cortical bone; an 18- to 22-gauge spinal needle is excellent in cats, small dogs, and birds; and a bone marrow or intraosseous infusion needle is essential in mature dogs.[18]

A bone injection gun is a spring-loaded, impact-driven intraosseous device developed for use in pediatric and adult humans. It propels the intraosseous cannula at high speed through skin, subcutaneous tissues, and bone cortex to a fixed depth. This automatic device was significantly faster than a standard Jamshidi bone marrow needle in obtaining intraosseous access in the proximal tibia of dogs.[25] The high speed of insertion helps to minimize pain; however, local anesthesia is recommended in conscious patients.[25]

Other devices such as a drill for intraosseous access (EZ-IO, Vidacare, San Antonio, Tex.) (Figures 194-2 and 194-3) and a sternal intraosseous device (FAST1, Pyng Medical, Richmond, Canada) are now available.[19] A feline cadaver study found that the EZ-IO system was faster and more likely to be successful than the bone injection gun and manual intraosseous needle placement, regardless of whether the tibia or humerus was used.[26]

BOX 194-1 ***Supplies Necessary for an Intraosseous Catheter Kit***

- Topical antiseptic for skin preparation
- Sterile gloves
- Local anesthetic for the skin and periosteum
- Scalpel blade for making a stab incision through the skin
- Needles
  - Hypodermic (18 to 30 gauge)
  - Spinal (18 to 22 gauge)
  - Bone marrow or intraosseous infusion needles (Jamshidi/Illinois, Cardinal Health, or Cook Critical Care) (see Figure 194-1)
- EZ-IO device (Vidacare): recommended for more rapid access to the intraosseous space (see Figures 194-2 and 194-3)
- Syringe for aspiration of bone marrow to confirm correct placement and potentially collect samples for hematologic or biochemical analysis
- Heparinized saline solution (preservative free)
- Fluid with administration set or catheter cap and pressure bag
- Mechanism to secure the catheter:
  - Tape butterfly and suture material
  - Cyanoacrylates to secure suture directly to hub of needle
  - Commercial intraosseous catheter with flange
  - Bandaging material
- Triple antibiotic ointment or appropriate antiseptic ointment or cream

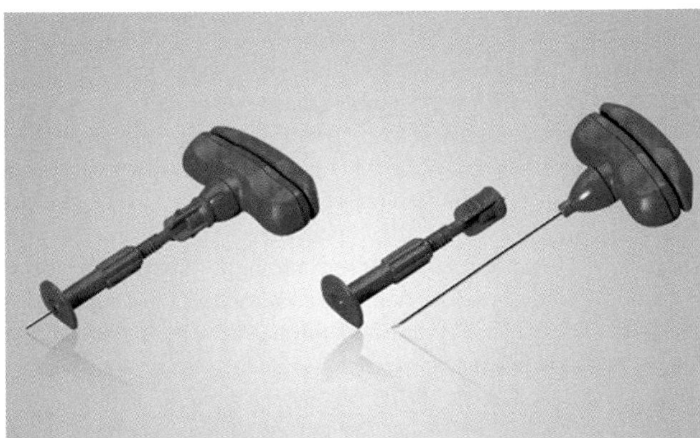

FIGURE 194-1 Intraosseous infusion needle. *(Courtesy Cardinal Health.)*

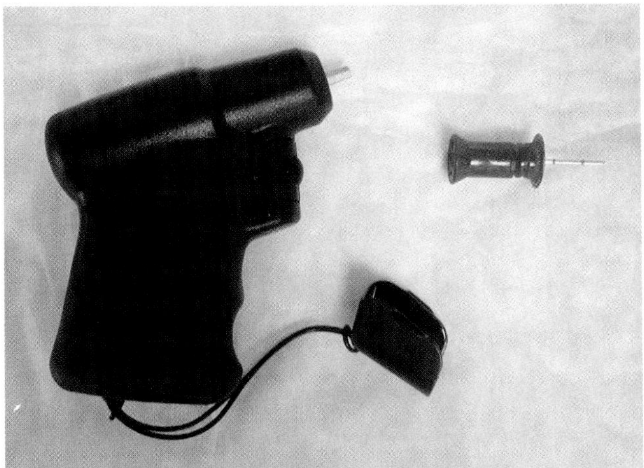

FIGURE 194-2 EZ-IO battery-operated driver with intraosseous needle and stylet.

The access site should be easily accessible and should not interfere with ongoing procedures such as CPR. The most commonly used sites are the flat medial surface of the proximal tibia (1 to 2 cm distal to the tibial tuberosity), the tibial tuberosity itself, and the trochanteric fossa of the femur (Figures 194-4 and 194-5). Alternative approachable points can be considered such as the wing of the ilium, the ischium, and the greater tubercle of the humerus.[18,27] However, no studies in animal patients suggest any one site to be superior. Finally, the choice of a particular site depends on the experience and preference of the clinician, the anticipated duration of use, and the mobility of the patient. Placement in the trochanteric fossa of the femur seems to be well tolerated, allows mobility, and is generally

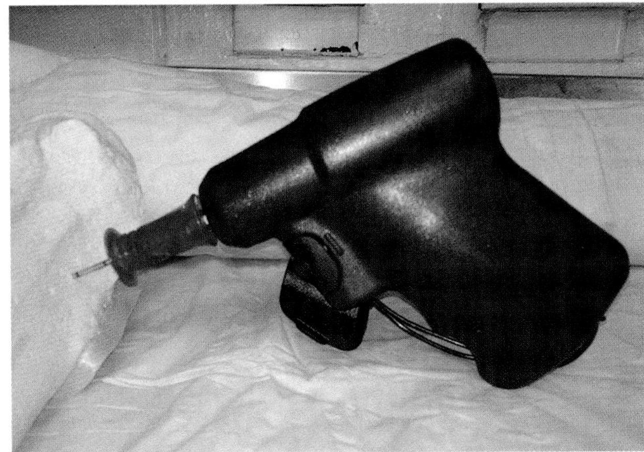

FIGURE 194-3 Insertion of EZ-IO needle into a bone.

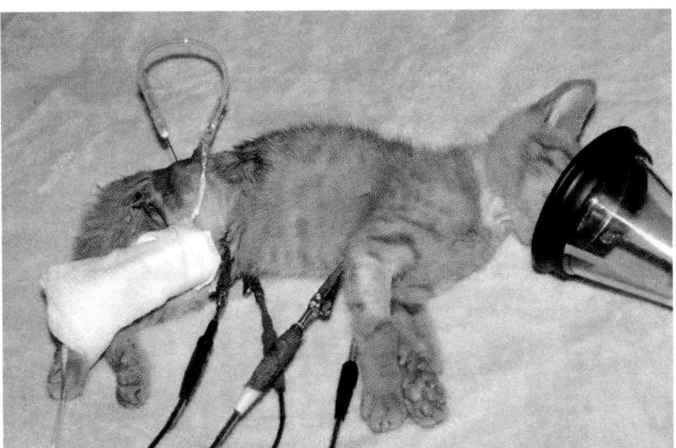

FIGURE 194-4 Intraosseous needle placed in the trochanteric fossa of a sick kitten for fluid resuscitation.

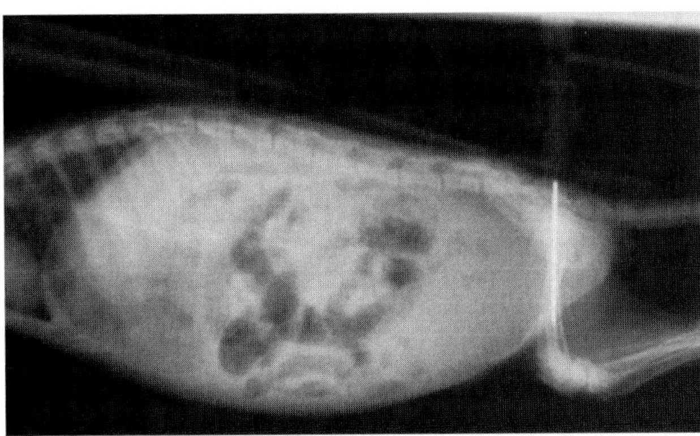

FIGURE 194-5 Radiograph of an intraosseous needle placed through the trochanteric fossa into the shaft of the femur in a ferret.

easy to perform.[18] In obese or very edematous animals or those in status epilepticus, the tibia is probably more accessible.[18]

In humans, alternative sites include the sternum, radius, ulna, and calcaneus.[19] Aseptic preparation of the site is required. The periosteum is highly innervated; therefore when the patient is alert or in stable condition, local infiltration with an anesthetic (e.g., 1% lidocaine) is recommended. A preemptive skin stab incision over the site of penetration of the catheter may prolong the life of the needle.

For placement in the medial tibia, the needle must be directed into the bone slightly distally and away from the proximal growth plate. To prevent sciatic nerve injury during placement in the femur, the needle should be walked off the medial aspect of the greater trochanter into the trochanteric fossa, with the hip joint in a neutral and internally rotated position. Once the desired orientation of the needle is reached, firm pressure should be applied in clockwise and then counterclockwise rotation. This procedure normally generates a small depression that seats the needle in the bone; the pressure is then increased while the same rotation pattern is maintained, and the needle should proceed through the near cortex. A sudden loss of resistance indicates that the needle has penetrated the cortex.

Before fluids or drugs are administered through an intraosseous catheter, verification of correct placement is required. One of the most frequently reported causes of failure of intraosseous catheterization is an error in identifying landmarks. A well-positioned catheter should be firmly seated in the bone and should move with the limb without being dislodged. Gentle aspiration should bring bone marrow into the syringe, although in older animals this may not always be possible. A bolus of heparinized saline solution should flow easily, and there should be no palpable accumulation of fluid in the subcutaneous tissue.

If resistance is encountered, the needle can be rotated 90 to 180 degrees to move the beveled edge away from the inner cortex. The subcutaneous tissue must be observed for fluid extravasation. If extravasation is detected, the needle should be removed to prevent further complications and an alternative bone should be chosen for catheter placement. Once correct placement of the needle is verified, administration of fluids or drugs can be started by syringe or by use of a standard intravenous administration set. To maintain patency during intermittent usage, a catheter plug can be applied and the catheter flushed with heparinized saline solution.

Initial infusion of fluids under pressure causes pain, lasting approximately 1 to 2 minutes, in conscious human patients. In humans, recommendations to minimize pain include withdrawal of a small volume of bone marrow and slow injection of 1% lidocaine over 60 seconds before the infusion is initiated. The intraosseous injection of lidocaine can be toxic, especially to cats. Neither the safety nor the efficacy of intraosseous lidocaine infusions to decrease the pain response to pressurized intraosseous infusions in small animals has been evaluated. To secure the needle properly, a tape butterfly can be wrapped around the hub and sutured to the skin or the periosteum. The suture may also be fixed to the hub of the needle with cyanoacrylate glue. Some intraosseous needles come with permanent butterflies for suturing.

Covering of the area with antiseptic or antibiotic ointment is suggested, and when possible, application of a protective bandage can prevent damage to the needle. Intraosseous catheters require the same nursing care as intravenous catheters. In most cases, the intraosseous catheter is considered a temporary access line that should be replaced by an intravenous catheter as soon as possible. When prolonged intraosseous infusion is required, guidelines for intravenous catheter care should be followed. Although there are limited data, the risk of catheter-related complications is thought to be minimal for up to 72 hours with proper maintenance.[18,26]

COMPLICATIONS

The documented complication rate associated with intraosseous infusions in humans and animals is low. The types of complications include infection, fat embolism, extravasation of fluids, nerve injury, compartment syndrome, and bone fractures.[13,19] One of the most common concerns when performing intraosseous infusion is osteomyelitis. Use of proper sterile technique during placement reduces the risk of infection to 0.6% of cases, with potentially lower risk if the catheter is removed as soon as intravenous access is established or within 72 hours.[1]

Several studies have demonstrated that administration of fluids and drugs via the intraosseous route does not impair bone growth.[28] Fat embolism can occur during intraosseous infusion; however, evidence for clinical significance is lacking. Although extravasation of fluids and compartment syndrome are unlikely with proper technique, they can be associated with major morbidity in humans. Improper catheter placement combined with the use of irritating or hypertonic fluids, high fluid rates, pressure infusion, and large infusion volumes can all predispose to extravasation of fluids and compartment syndrome.[13,19] The latter does not appear to be a major issue in animals; however, if any infiltration is detected, the intraosseous infusion should be discontinued immediately. Also, it is imperative that no additional catheter be placed in the same bone.

Generally intraosseous infusion of hypertonic solutions is considered effective and apparently safe. However, in one laboratory study of combined dehydration and hemorrhagic shock, piglets developed compartment syndrome and associated soft tissue and bone marrow necrosis 48 hours after intraosseous resuscitation with 7.5% hypertonic saline.[29] Compartment syndrome has also been reported after 0.9% saline intraosseous resuscitation of a boy following cardiac arrest.[30] The risk of compartment syndrome associated with intraosseous infusions is reported to be less than 1% in humans and is unknown in veterinary patients[30]; however, one study in dogs did demonstrate an increase in extravasation and tissue pressure associated with infusion of more than 350 ml (~23 ml/kg) of hypertonic contrast dye (Urografin 76; ~2000 mOsm/kg).[31] Finally, appropriate insertion technique, asepsis, frequent monitoring of the intraosseous access site, and prompt removal of the needle once an intravenous line has been established help to reduce risk factors and complication rates.

REFERENCES

1. Rossetti VA, Thompson BM, Miller J, et al: Intraosseous infusion: an alternative route of pediatric intravascular access, Ann Emerg Med 14:885, 1985.
2. Kanter RK, Zimmerman JJ, Strauss RH, et al: Pediatric emergency intravenous access. Evaluation of a protocol, Am J Dis Child 140:132, 1986.
3. 2010 American Heart Association Guidelines for Cardiopulmonary Resuscitation and Emergency Cardiovascular Care Science. Part 14: pediatric advanced life support, Circulation 112(Suppl 3):S876-908, 2010.
4. 2010 American Heart Association Guidelines for Cardiopulmonary Resuscitation and Emergency Cardiovascular Care Science. Part 8: adult advanced cardiovascular life support, Circulation 122(Suppl 3):S729-767, 2010.
5. Niemann JT, Stratton SJ, Cruz B, et al: Endotracheal drug administration during out-of-hospital resuscitation: where are the survivors? Resuscitation 53:153, 2002.
6. Manisterski Y, Vaknin Z, Ben-Abraham R, et al: Endotracheal epinephrine: a call for larger doses, Anesth Analg 95:1037, 2002.
7. Orlowski JP: Emergency alternatives to intravenous access. Intraosseous, intratracheal, sublingual, and other-site drug administration, Pediatr Clin North Am 41:1183, 1994.
8. Stein M, Gray R: Corpus cavernosum as an emergency vascular access in dogs, Acad Radiol 2:1073, 1995.

9. Drinker CK, Drinker KR, Lund CC: The circulation in the mammal bone marrow, Am J Physiol 62:1, 1922.
10. Tocantins LM: Rapid absorption of substances injected into the bone marrow, Proc Soc Exp Biol Med 45:292, 1940.
11. Tocantins LM, O'Neill JF, Jones HW: Infusions of blood and other fluids via the bone marrow: application in pediatrics, JAMA 117:1229, 1941.
12. Heinild S, Sondergaard T, Tudvad F: Bone marrow infusion in childhood: experiences from a thousand infusions, J Pediatr 30:400, 1947.
13. LaRocco BG, Wang HE: Intraosseous infusion, Prehosp Emerg Care 7:280, 2003.
14. Spivey WH, Lathers CM, Malone DR, et al: Comparison of intraosseous, central, and peripheral routes of sodium bicarbonate administration during CPR in pigs, Ann Emerg Med 14:1135, 1985.
15. Orlowski JP, Porembka DT, Gallagher JM, et al: Comparison study of intraosseous, central intravenous, and peripheral intravenous infusions of emergency drugs, Am J Dis Child 144:112, 1990.
16. Warren DW, Kissoon N, Mattar A, et al: Pharmacokinetics from multiple intraosseous and peripheral intravenous site injections in normovolemic and hypovolemic pigs, Crit Care Med 22:838, 1994.
17. Hodge D III, Delgado-Paredes C, Fleisher G: Intraosseous infusion flow rates in hypovolemic "pediatric" dogs, Ann Emerg Med 16:305, 1987.
18. Otto CM, Kaufman MG, Crowe DT: Intraosseous infusion of fluids and therapeutics, Compend Contin Educ Pract Vet 11:42, 1989.
19. Weiser G, Hoffmann Y, Galbraith R, et al: Current advances in intraosseous infusion—a systematic review, Resuscitation 83:20-26, 2012.
20. Kissoon N, Idris A, Wenzel V, et al: Intraosseous and central venous blood acid-base relationship during cardiopulmonary resuscitation, Pediatr Emerg Care 13:250, 1997.
21. Johnson L, Kissoon N, Fiallos M, et al: Use of intraosseous blood to assess blood chemistries and hemoglobin during cardiopulmonary resuscitation with drug infusions, Crit Care Med 27:1147, 1999.
22. Aeschbacher G, Webb AI: Intraosseous injection during cardiopulmonary resuscitation in dogs, J Small Anim Pract 31:629, 1993.
23. Orlowski JP, Porembka DT, Gallagher JM, et al: The bone marrow as a source of laboratory studies, Ann Emerg Med 18:1348, 1989.
24. Dhein CR, Barbee DD: Use of bone marrow serum for biochemical analysis in healthy cats, J Am Vet Med Assoc 206:487, 1995.
25. Olsen D, Packer BE, Perrett J, et al: Evaluation of the bone injection gun as a method for intraosseous cannula placement for fluid therapy in adult dogs, Vet Surg 31:533, 2002.
26. Bukoski A, Winter M, Bandt C, et al: Comparison of three intraosseous access techniques in cats, J Vet Emerg Crit Care 20(4): 393-397, 2010.
27. Hughes D, Beal MW: Emergency vascular access, Vet Clin North Am Small Anim Pract 30:491, 2000.
28. Claudet I, Baunin C, Laporte-Turpin E, et al: Long-term effects on tibial growth after intraosseous infusion: a prospective, radiographic analysis, Pediatr Emerg Care 19:397, 2003.
29. Alam HB, Punzalan CM, Koustova E, et al: Hypertonic saline: intraosseous infusion causes myonecrosis in a dehydrated swine model of uncontrolled hemorrhagic shock, J Trauma 52:18, 2002.
30. Khan LAK, Anakwe RE, Murray A, et al: A severe complication following intraosseous infusion used during resuscitation of a child, Injury Extra 42(10):173-177, 2011.
31. Günal I, Köse N, Gürer D: Compartment syndrome after intraosseous infusion: An experimental study in dogs, J Pediatr Surg 31(11):1491-1493, 1996.

CHAPTER 195

CENTRAL VENOUS CATHETERIZATION

Harold Davis, BA, RVT, VTS (Emergency/Critical Care; Anesthesia)

KEY POINTS

- Central venous catheters are used for hemodynamic monitoring, drug administration, and serial blood sampling.
- Saphenous veins can be used as access points to the central venous circulation.
- Fluids or medications with osmolalities of more than 600 mOsm/L should be administered via a central vein.
- Use of multilumen catheters minimizes the number of veins that need to be catheterized.
- Adherence to aseptic technique for placement is essential to minimize the risk of catheter-related bloodstream infection.

Central venous access is the placement of a catheter in such a way that the catheter is inserted into a venous great vessel.[1] Central venous catheters terminate in the cranial or caudal vena cava. These catheters may be inserted directly into a large central vein such as the jugular vein or inserted via a peripheral vein (peripherally inserted central catheter, or PICC). Placement of a central venous catheter is indicated when hemodynamic monitoring, drug administration, and/or serial blood sampling is needed.[2] Central venous catheters often can be left in place for longer periods than peripheral catheters, which makes them very useful in critically ill patients. A central catheter may be preferable to a peripheral venous catheter for the following purposes:

- To administer multiple types of fluids and drugs that are not compatible with each other, which necessitates the use of multiple catheter lumens
- To administer fluids with an osmolality of more than 600 mOsm/L and constant rate infusions of drugs known to cause phlebitis, such as diazepam, pentobarbital, and mannitol
- To measure central venous pressure
- To monitor central venous blood saturation
- To perform frequent aspiration of blood samples
- To provide total parenteral nutrition
- To maintain venous access for long periods

- To provide access when peripheral catheters are at risk of contamination from vomiting, polyuria, diarrhea, or vaginal discharge because a jugular catheter site may be easier to keep clean
- To facilitate renal replacement therapy or transvenous pacing

GENERAL CONCEPTS

Because introduction of foreign material or infectious agents into the central circulation can have far more serious consequences than peripheral vessel contamination, maintenance of aseptic technique when placing and using central venous catheters is of utmost importance (see Chapter 102). General recommendations for central venous catheter maintenance are to wipe all injection ports with alcohol before needle puncture, keep insertion sites bandaged, prevent catheter hubs from dragging on the ground, and respond immediately to witnessed catheter contamination. This may require cleaning and changing injection ports and fluid lines, or it may necessitate catheter removal. Inadvertent disconnection of fluid lines from a central venous catheter or animal-induced damage to the catheter can lead to significant hemorrhage. Leaving ports of a central venous catheter open to the atmosphere places the patient at risk of air embolism. For this reason the catheter should be occluded by a catheter lock or manual kinking whenever the catheter hub is open to the atmosphere (e.g., when connecting and disconnecting syringes for blood aspiration).

CATHETER TYPES

Through-the-needle catheters, long over-the-needle catheters, long single-lumen catheters, multilumen catheters, and catheter introducers can all be used to access central veins (Figure 195-1).[2-4]

Through-the-Needle Catheter

Through-the-needle catheters were discussed in Chapter 193. They commonly are used to catheterize jugular veins.

Over-the-Needle Catheter

Over-the-needle catheters were discussed in Chapter 193. When used for jugular catheterization, they must be of a length appropriate for the patient's size. The subcutaneous tissues in the region of the jugular vein are very loose, which results in a lot of skin movement. Even when the catheter is well secured to the skin, short catheters can be pulled out of the vein easily.

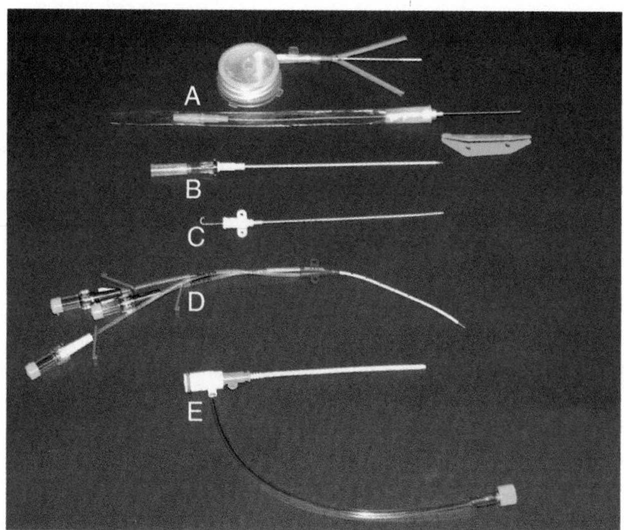

FIGURE 195-1 Examples of catheters used for central venous catheterization. **A,** Two through-the-needle catheters; the top is a Drum-Cartridge catheter and the bottom is an Intracath catheter. **B,** Long over-the-needle-catheter. **C,** Single-lumen central venous catheter. **D,** Triple-lumen catheter. **E,** Catheter sheath introducer.

Long Single-Lumen Catheter

A long single-lumen catheter is inserted using the Seldinger guidewire technique or a peel-off sheathed needle technique.[3] These catheters come in a variety of sizes and lengths. Mila International (Florence, Ky.) and Arrow International (Reading, Pa.) make central venous catheters that are 14 or 16 gauge by 6 or 8 inches (15 or 20 cm). Arrow also makes a 20-gauge by 5-inch (12-cm) and a 22-gauge by 4-inch (10-cm) single-lumen catheter. Smiths Medical SurgiVet (Waukesha, Wis.) makes 5, 6, 7, and 8 Fr central venous catheters; the 5 Fr is 6 inches (15 cm) in length and all others are 10 inches (25 cm).

Single-lumen catheters maybe suitable when there is only one purpose for the central venous catheter, such as serial blood draws or central venous pressure monitoring. Single-lumen catheters can be useful as PICC lines placed in saphenous vessels of small patients.

Multilumen Catheter

Multilumen catheters are placed using the Seldinger guidewire technique or a peel-off sheathed needle technique. Mila International and Arrow International make multilumen catheters. The catheters may be double, triple, or quadruple lumen. They are available in sizes ranging from 4 to 8.5 Fr and 2 to 24 inches (5 to 60 cm) in length.

Multilumen catheters are extremely useful in the critical care setting; they reduce the number of catheters that need to be placed in the critically ill patient. Fluids and drugs that are incompatible can be administered simultaneously. The catheters can be purchased individually or as a kit that contains all the components necessary for insertion. In addition to the catheter and dilators, the kits may include local anesthetic, scalpel, syringe, and so on. Multilumen catheters are more expensive than the commonly used single-lumen catheters.

Percutaneous Sheath Catheter Introducer

Percutaneous sheath introducer systems are large-bore (typically 6 to 8 Fr), relatively short (4 inches) catheters that have a hemostasis valve located in the hub. They also have a short T-extension port for the fluid administration. A central venous catheter, pulmonary artery catheter, or transvenous pacing lead can be passed through the hemostasis valve into the vessel. The hemostasis valve acts as a seal to prevent entry of air into the circulation as well as to prevent blood or fluid loss around the catheter. The introducer is placed using the Seldinger guidewire technique.

CATHETER INSERTION SITE

Central venous insertion sites include the jugular vein and the lateral and medial saphenous veins (see Chapter 193). Long catheters theoretically can be inserted in the cephalic vein and passed up to the level of the cranial vena cava, but they frequently will not pass beyond the elbow. For this reason the cephalic vein rarely is used for PICC lines. In human patients it is recommended to avoid catheter insertion in the femoral region if possible because it is associated with a higher risk of catheter-related bloodstream infection.[4] There are similar concerns in veterinary patients, and the risk of infection is likely to be even greater in patients with diarrhea or urinary incontinence. Catheters insertion sites should not be in close proximity to areas of dermatitis, cellulitis, or abscessation.

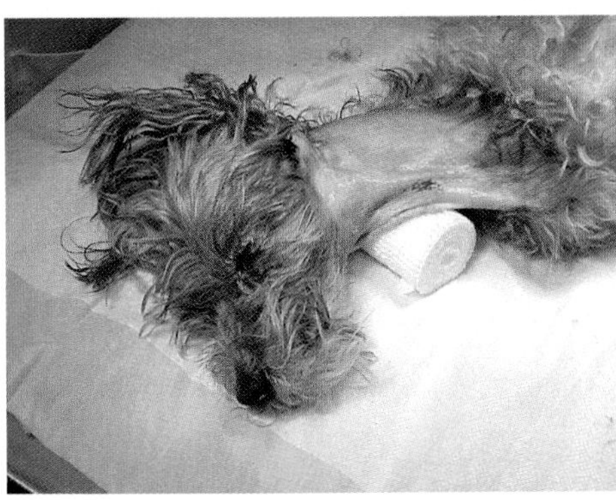

FIGURE 195-2 Placement of roll gauze underneath the patient's neck to provide better exposure to the vessel.

Saphenous Vein

To achieve central venous catheterization via the saphenous vein, long catheters must be used; they are threaded so that they lie in the caudal vena cava. In dogs the lateral saphenous vein is used most commonly, but the medial saphenous vein can also be catheterized. In cats the medial saphenous vein tends to be larger and more easily stabilized for catheterization.

Jugular Vein

The jugular vein is catheterized directly in the cervical region. It lies along a line drawn between the angle of the mandible and the thoracic inlet. Jugular vein catheterization is feasible in both dogs and cats, and the vein may be visible in patients in hemodynamically unstable condition when peripheral venous access is challenging.

The key to jugular catheter insertion is patient positioning and vessel immobilization. If the patient is not positioned properly, it can be difficult to visualize and immobilize the vein. Jugular catheters are placed antegrade, with the tip of the catheter always directed toward the heart. Placement of the jugular catheter is best done with the patient in lateral or dorsal recumbency. The patient's head is extended and its forelimbs positioned caudally by an assistant. Sedation of uncooperative patients is recommended. Placing a bag of fluid, a sandbag, or rolled towels under the neck may be helpful (Figure 195-2). This flexes the neck and helps to make the vessel more accessible. The assistant should hold off the vein by pressing into the thoracic inlet; this should cause the vein to engorge and "stand up." The other end of the vein is immobilized by extending the head.

In some cases venous cutdown may be needed to facilitate placement of a central catheter (see Chapter 193).

CATHETER INSERTION

Strict aseptic technique is followed for all central venous catheterizations. Sterile gloves should be worn and the insertion site draped if the Seldinger technique is used or if the catheter is to be used for total parenteral nutrition. A cap, mask, and gown are worn routinely for central venous catheterization in human patients; this would be ideal in an effort to maximize aseptic technique in veterinary patients, but it has yet to become standard of care.[4,5]

Through-the-Needle Catheter Insertion

When a through-the-needle catheter is used the catheter needle is introduced subcutaneously. The needle tip is positioned over the vein and aligned as closely as possible with the longitudinal axis of the vein. The needle tip is then inserted into the vein; it maybe necessary to angle the needle somewhat to pick up the superficial vein wall. Once it is estimated that the entire needle tip is within the lumen of the vein, the needle is stabilized and the catheter is threaded into the vein. Once the catheter is fully advanced into the vein, pressure is applied over the venous puncture site and the needle is backed out. Once the bleeding has stopped, the needle guard is secured around the needle. The catheter is aspirated to confirm proper placement and to clear it of air. It is then flushed with heparinized saline. The catheter should be capped with an injection cap or T-port and flushed again with heparinized saline. The catheter is sutured or stapled close to the insertion site. The insertion site is then covered with a sterile 2 × 2-inch gauze pad and the catheter site is bandaged.

An alternative method of inserting a through-the-needle catheter is to remove the long single-lumen catheter from the insertion needle provided and thread it through a short over-the-needle catheter instead. Appropriate aseptic technique is maintained. This method is particularly useful for placing PICC lines in saphenous vessels of small patients. The large needle provided with these catheters is commonly too large for effective venipuncture of a peripheral vessel. Using an over-the-needle catheter as an introducer makes initial venipuncture relatively simple, and a through-the-needle catheter maybe more affordable than a multilumen catheter.

In this situation, a common approach is first to insert a short over-the-needle catheter into the medial or lateral saphenous vein (Figure 195-3, *A*). A through-the-needle catheter (with the needle removed) is advanced into the preplaced catheter (see Figure 195-3, *B*). The two catheter hubs are joined tightly together (see Figure 195-3, *C*). Butterfly wing tape is used at the catheter hub juncture to prevent accidental dislodgement. The tape is sutured to the catheter (to prevent the tape from slipping) and the tape wings are sutured to the skin proximally to pull the catheter back toward the insertion site (see Figure 195-3, *D*).

Seldinger Technique

The Seldinger technique uses a smaller introducing catheter or trochar and a guidewire to gain access to vessels or hollow organs. It avoids the requirement of initially puncturing the vessel with a large-bore catheter or trochar.[6] It maybe used to place single-lumen catheters, multilumen catheters, or percutaneous catheter introducer systems. It can also be used to replace an existing catheter in the same location. The Seldinger technique for introduction of a multilumen catheter is described here. The basic concept of this technique is the same for any type of catheter placement in any vessel.[6]

Before the procedure is begun, the required distance for catheter insertion is premeasured. The aim for a jugular catheter is to have the tip lying within the thoracic cavity, just cranial to the right atrium. This distance commonly is estimated by measuring the distance from the intended insertion site to the caudal edge of the triceps muscle or first rib. For PICC lines the distance from the insertion site to the vena cava is measured. These measurements then aid in choosing the most appropriate catheter for that patient.

The insertion site is clipped widely and surgically prepared in a routine manner.[2] Infiltration of the intended insertion site with local anesthetic is recommended in conscious animals. The catheter kit, sterile gauze, scalpel blade, suture material, and instruments are opened on a sterile field. The operator wears sterile gloves; in some circumstances the use of a hat, mask, and sterile gown may also be appropriate, and an assistant can be helpful in challenging cases. The distal port of the multilumen catheter is identified. This is the port that terminates at the very tip of the catheter and is the one through which the guidewire is passed. All ports of the multilumen catheter are flushed with heparinized saline, and all ports, with the exception of the distal port, are capped. The insertion site is draped; this is important because the guidewire is long and flimsy, and the risk of contamination is high if draping is not sufficient.

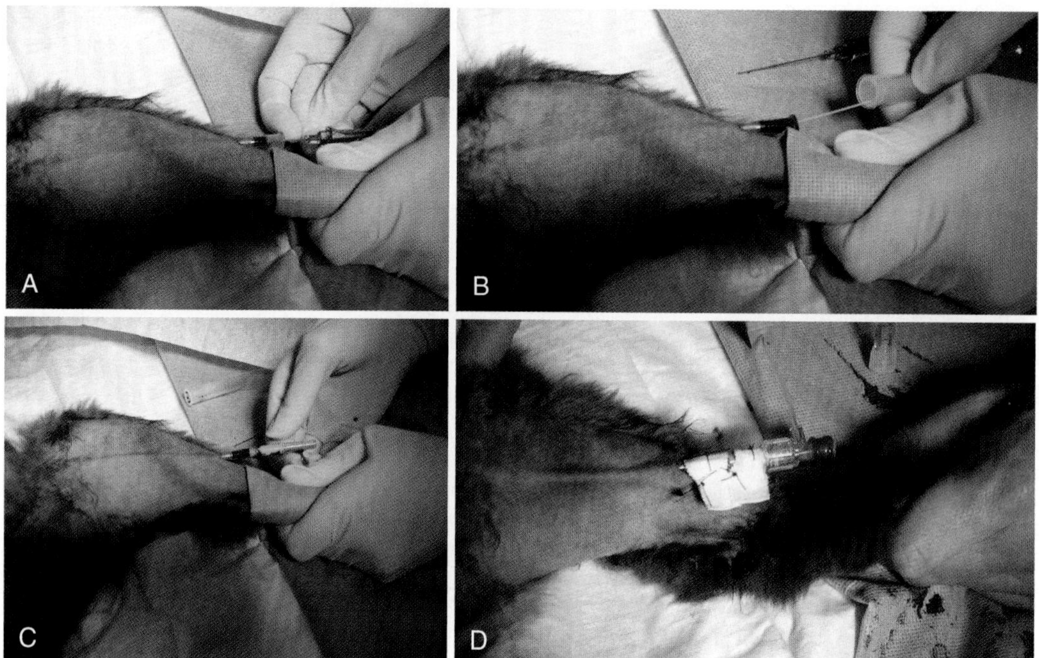

FIGURE 195-3 Placement of a through-the-needle catheter using a short over-the-needle introducer catheter. **A,** The peripheral vein is first catheterized routinely with a short over-the-needle catheter. **B,** The through-the-needle catheter is removed from its accompanying needle and threaded through the peripheral catheter while maintaining aseptic technique. **C,** The two catheter hubs are securely attached to each other. **D,** The catheter is secured to the skin using butterfly tape and sutures.

A small relief incision is made through the dermis with a scalpel blade at the site of intended insertion. The introducing needle or short over-the-needle catheter (Figure 195-4, *A*) enters the skin through the relief incision and is inserted into the underlying vessel. The guidewire is threaded through the inserting needle or catheter into the vein (see Figure 195-4, *B*). The distal end of the wire has a flexible J-tip to prevent puncturing of the vessel wall. It also reduces the likelihood of the wire passing into smaller vessel branches. In some instances when it is difficult to pass the J-tip along the vessel, it maybe advantageous to use the straight end of the guidewire instead. It is important to recognize that this will be more traumatic to the vessel and that gentle technique should be maintained at all times. To prevent embolism of the guidewire, the operator should keep hold of it at all times.

Once the guidewire is inserted, approximately two thirds to three fourths of its length is fed into the vessel. It is held in place while the introducing needle or catheter is removed and a vessel dilator is threaded over the wire. The skin entry site may need to be enlarged with a No. 11 scalpel blade to accommodate the dilator. The dilator is grasped near the distal tip and, with a forward twisting motion, is advanced into the vessel (see Figure 195-4, *C*). To minimize blood loss, pressure is applied over the insertion site with sterile gauze pads as the dilator is removed, with the guidewire left in place.

In the case of a sheath introducer, the dilator is incorporated into the sheath and is removed once the sheath is in place. The multilumen catheter is threaded over the guidewire until the proximal end (the end closest to the operator, not the animal) of the guidewire protrudes from the hub of the catheter. If the guidewire was advanced too far into the vessel, it will be necessary to back it out of the vessel to achieve this. Finally, while the proximal end of the guidewire is held, the catheter is advanced into the vessel the desired distance as determined by previous measurement (see Figure 195-4, *D*). The wire is removed and the port immediately occluded to prevent air embolism occurring.

All ports are then aspirated to remove any air and to ensure that blood is easily drawn through the catheter. If necessary the catheter may be repositioned to allow aspiration of blood. Aseptic technique must be maintained throughout. All ports are flushed with heparinized saline. The catheter is then sutured in place; the insertion site is covered with sterile gauze and bandaged appropriately.

Rewiring of Seldinger Catheters

An exchange technique is employed if an existing catheter has become problematic or it is desirable to replace the catheter with a different type; for example, a lateral saphenous over-the-needle-catheter is to be replaced with a multilumen catheter. Catheters should be rewired only if there is no evidence of catheter-related infection and the insertion site is clean and does not appear inflamed. The Seldinger technique may be used to rewire or exchange a catheter through the existing insertion site. In brief, the wire is passed through the existing catheter and the old catheter is removed; the replacement catheter is then threaded over the wire and into the vein. The advantage of rewiring catheters is that the patient need not undergo an additional venipuncture and the use of other vessels is minimized, which is especially helpful if options are limited.

The procedure is essentially the same as the initial placement of a catheter using the Seldinger technique. Intravenous fluids are disconnected from the intravenous catheter and an injection cap is attached. Any sutures holding the catheter in place are cut and removed, along with all catheter clamps and fasteners. Aseptic technique (use of surgical preparation, gloves, and barrier drape, ± cap and mask) must be followed throughout the procedure. All surfaces of the existing catheter and insertion site are prepped with an antiseptic scrub and solution. A barrier drape is placed. Being careful not to pull out the catheter, an assistant may use sterile mosquito forceps to hold the catheter hub in place. While wearing sterile gloves, the operator exchanging the catheter uses a sterile gauze pad to remove the injection cap. (Some operators double-glove and take off the

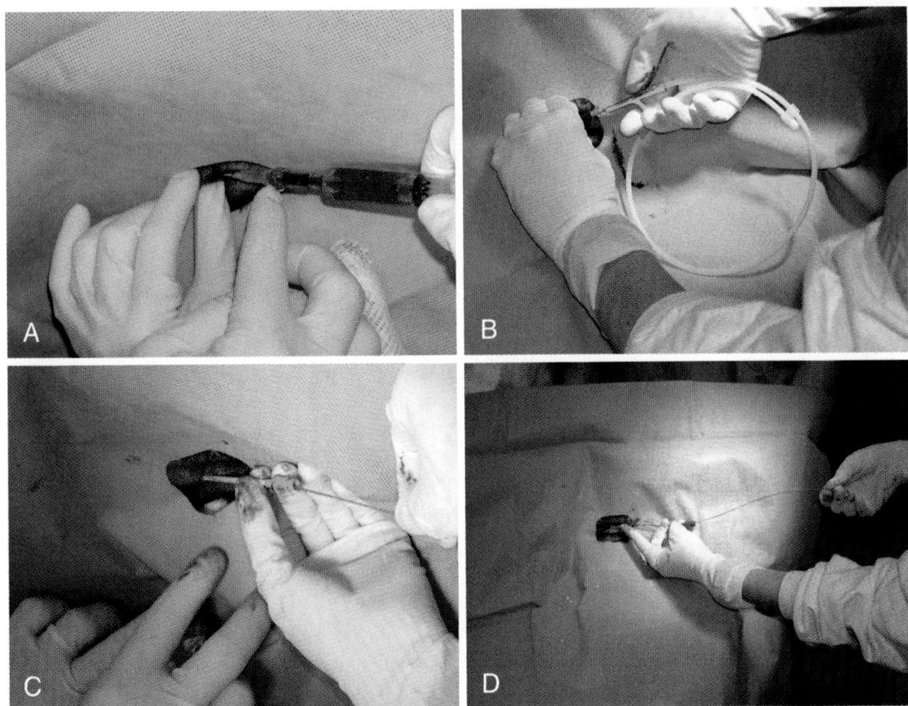

FIGURE 195-4 Seldinger technique for placement of a multilumen catheter. **A,** Initial venipuncture is performed with an over-the-needle catheter. **B,** The guidewire is threaded. **C,** The skin and vessel are dilated. **D,** The catheter is threaded over the guidewire.

outer gloves once the old catheter is removed.) Once the injection cap is removed the exchange wire is threaded through the existing catheter to the desired level. The existing catheter is removed and the exchange wire is left in place. The remainder of the procedure is carried out as previously described for the Seldinger guidewire insertion.

Peel-Off Sheathed Needle Technique

The peel-off sheathed needle (Mila International and Smiths Medical SurgiVet) is similar to an over-the-needle catheter. The sheath has two tabs on the proximal end near the hub of the needle; when the tabs are pulled the sheath splits or peels away. The peel-off sheath technique can be used to place long single-lumen and multilumen catheters.

Peel-off sheath placement is similar to the over-the-needle catheter technique. Once needle and sheath placement is confirmed by bleeding, the needle is removed leaving the sheath in the vessel. The catheter is threaded down the sheath. The sheath is then peeled apart by grasping the tabs and pulling outward and upward. Once the sheath is completely separated, the catheter is positioned and secured.

COMPLICATIONS AND CATHETER MAINTENANCE

The same complications and catheter maintenance described for peripheral venous catheters in Chapter 193 apply to central venous catheters (see also Chapter 102 on catheter-related infections).

Heparinized Saline

Although there is no confirmatory evidence in the veterinary literature, the human literature suggests that normal saline (nonheparinized) may be as effective as heparinized saline in the maintenance of catheter patency.[7,8] All unused ports on central venous catheters should be flushed regularly with saline or heparinized saline. The author uses 4 U/ml of heparinized saline (1000 U/250 ml normal saline) q4h. Bags of heparinized saline should be discarded every 12 to 24 hours to minimize the risk of contamination. If a catheter port will not be used for a prolonged period, an alternative is to implement a heparin lock. The dead space of the catheter is filled with 100 U/ml heparin, replaced q12h. Ideally the concentrated heparin solution is not flushed into the patient; instead, it is aspirated before administering medications or before replacing the heparin lock. Clear labeling of such ports to avoid inadvertent flushing of the concentrated heparin into the patient is important.

REFERENCES

1. American Society of Anesthesiologists Task Force on Central Venous Access; Rupp SM, Apfelbaum JL, Blitt C, et al: Practice guidelines for central venous access: a report by the American Society of Anesthesiologists Task Force on Central Venous Access, Anesthesiology 116:539-573, 2012.
2. Hansen B: Technical aspects of fluid therapy. In DiBartola SP, editor: Fluid, electrolyte and acid-base disorders in small animal practice, St Louis, 2006, Saunders.
3. White RN: Emergency techniques. In King L, Hammond R, editors: Manual of canine and feline emergency and critical care, Cheltenham, UK, 1999, British Small Animal Veterinary Association.
4. Pronovost P, Needham D, Berenholtz S, et al: An intervention to decrease catheter-related bloodstream infections in the ICU, N Engl J Med 355(26):2725-2732, 2006. Erratum in: N Engl J Med 356(25):2660, 2007.
5. How-to guide: prevent central line-associated bloodstream infections (CLABSI), Cambridge, Mass, 2012, Institute for Healthcare Improvement. Available at http://www.ihi.org.
6. Beal MW: Placement of central venous catheters: Seldinger technique, Clinician's Brief, Oct 7, 2005.
7. Arnts IJ, Heijnen JA, Wilbers HT, et al: Effectiveness of heparin solution versus normal saline in maintaining patency of intravenous locks in neonates: a double blind randomized controlled study, J Adv Nurs 67(12):2677-2685, 2011.
8. Wang R, Luo O, He L, et al: Preservative-free 0.9% sodium chloride for flushing and locking peripheral intravenous access device: a prospective controlled trial, J Evid Based Med 5(4):205-208, 2012.

CHAPTER 196

BLOOD FILM EVALUATION

Alan H. Rebar, DVM, PhD, DACVP

KEY POINTS

- Blood film evaluation provides both general information regarding the health status of emergent and critically ill patients and specific diagnostic information in animals with true hematologic emergencies. It is therefore an essential component of the workup for all emergent and critical care patients.
- Blood film evaluation requires a systematic approach. The various cellular elements of the blood (leukocytes, erythrocytes, platelets) should be examined in the same order and manner on every blood film.
- Leukocyte morphology is used to recognize and characterize inflammatory disease. Signposts of inflammation are a neutrophilic left shift, monocytosis, and a persistent eosinophilia. Regenerative left shifts (high neutrophil count, increase in bands) indicate that the bone marrow response is keeping pace with tissue demand; degenerative left shifts (low or normal neutrophil count, increase in bands) indicate that tissue demand is overwhelming the bone marrow (guarded prognosis).
- Neutrophil toxicity indicates either the presence of circulating toxins interfering with neutrophil development in bone marrow or accelerated neutrophil production. Neutrophil toxicity is most commonly (but not exclusively) associated with bacterial infection.
- Lymphocyte patterns and morphology are also important in critically ill patients. Low lymphocyte numbers are generally a reflection of stress (high circulating levels of corticosteroids). Reactive lymphocytes indicate antigenic stimulation.
- The critical step in evaluating anemias is classifying them as regenerative or nonregenerative based on the presence (regenerative) or absence (nonregenerative) of increased numbers of polychromatophils on the blood film. Regenerative anemias are due to blood loss or hemolysis, whereas nonregenerative anemias have a broader range of causes.
- In highly regenerative anemias, red blood cell morphology is extremely important because it may indicate a specific cause for the hemolytic disease. Immune-mediated hemolytic anemia, Heinz body hemolytic anemia, mycoplasmosis, and babesiosis, among others, are all hemolytic diseases that can be diagnosed largely on the basis of red blood cell morphology.
- Thrombocytopenia is the most common primary cause of bleeding disorders in dogs and cats. Thrombocytopenia can result from sequestration of platelets in an enlarged spleen (rare), peripheral utilization in severe inflammation (clinical or subclinical disseminated intravascular coagulation), immune-mediated peripheral destruction (immune-mediated thrombocytopenia), or lack of production in the bone marrow.
- Myeloid and lymphoid leukemias can be recognized in various stages of disease, so peripheral blood findings vary from patient to patient. Severe nonregenerative anemia is the most consistent finding. White blood cell findings are highly variable.

Hematologic abnormalities are among the most common findings in emergent and critically ill patients. Regardless of whether these abnormalities represent primary diseases affecting the hematopoietic system or secondary manifestations of underlying disease in a different organ system, they can usually be recognized through blood film evaluation. Blood film evaluation is therefore an essential component of the clinical workup of all emergent and critically ill patients. This chapter presents a systematic approach to blood film preparation and examination, and highlights the more important hematologic abnormalities seen in the critically ill dog or cat.

BLOOD FILM PREPARATION

To obtain blood films of consistent quality, one must use the same technique every time. A drop of well-mixed blood (blood collected in ethylenediaminetetraacetic acid [EDTA] is often preferred) is placed near the frosted end of the first slide. A second slide (the spreader slide) is placed at about a 30-degree angle to the first and drawn back until it touches the drop of blood. The drop is allowed to spread along the entire edge of the spreader slide by capillary action. At this point the spreader slide is moved quickly and smoothly across the full length of the first slide. The finished blood film is allowed to air dry before staining using a standard Romanowsky technique (Wright stain or a modified quick stain). A well-prepared blood film is flame shaped.[1]

BLOOD FILM EVALUATION

A systematic approach to blood film evaluation is critical to obtaining accurate and complete results. Blood films should first be scanned at low magnification (10× to 20×). All three areas of the blood film (the body of the film near the drop, the monolayer where red blood cells are seen as individual cells and may touch but do not overlap, and the feather edge, which is most distant from the drop) should be examined. The slide should be scanned for clumping of cells (platelets, white blood cells, or red blood cells), rouleaux (orderly stacking of red blood cells), and agglutination (three-dimensional clumping of red blood cells). Any atypical cells or organisms (parasites) should be noted.[1]

Cell morphology is assessed in the monolayer. Even at scanning magnification, one can estimate total white blood cell count and differential. The typical appearance of each leukocyte cell line (neutrophil, eosinophil, monocyte, and lymphocyte) can be assessed. Individual red blood cells can be evaluated for evidence of anisocytosis, polychromasia, and poikilocytosis.

After the slide has been scanned, the entire process should be repeated at oil immersion magnification (100×). Again, most of the evaluation is done in the monolayer. Leukocytes are evaluated for morphologic detail. The presence of neutrophil toxicity, reactive lymphocytes, and inclusions in neutrophils and monocytes are noted. A left shift, which can be recognized at scanning magnifications, is confirmed at oil immersion magnification.

Red blood cell changes suspected at scanning magnification (anisocytosis, polychromasia) also can be confirmed. Poikilocytosis is best assessed at oil immersion magnification. The various types of poikilocytes (spherocytes, schizocytes, acanthocytes, dacryocytes) can all be recognized. Red blood cell inclusions, such as Heinz bodies,

Table 196-1 **General Patterns of Leukocyte Responses**[1]

Condition	WBC	Seg	Band	Lymph	Mono	Eos
Acute inflammation	Increased	Increased	Increased	Decreased or no change	Variable	Variable
Chronic inflammation	Increased or no change	Increased or no change	Increased or no change	Increased or no change	Increased	Variable
Overwhelming inflammation	Decreased or no change	Decreased or no change	Increased	Decreased or no change	Variable	Variable
Excitement leukocytosis	Increased	Increased in dogs; increased or no change in cats	No change	No change in dogs; increased in cats	No change	No change
Stress leukogram	Increased	Increased	No change	Decreased	Increased or no change	Decreased or no change

Eos, Eosinophils; *Mono,* monocytes; *Seg,* segmented neutrophils; *WBC,* white blood cells.

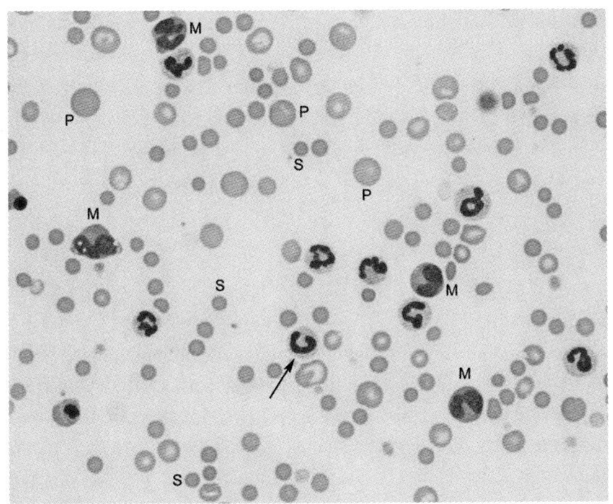

FIGURE 196-1 Blood film from a dog with immune-mediated hemolytic anemia. There is a leukocytosis characterized by neutrophilia with a left shift (band indicated by *arrow*) and monocytosis *(M).* Red blood cell changes include spherocytosis *(S)* and polychromasia *(P).* (Wright stain; original magnification, ×40.)

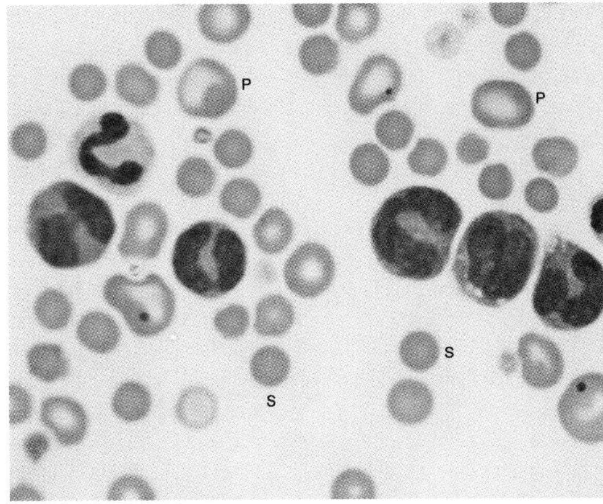

FIGURE 196-2 Higher magnification of the blood film in Figure 196-1 from a dog with immune-mediated hemolytic anemia. The five large leukocytes in a row across the center of the image are monocytes. Also note the spherocytic red blood cells and polychromatophils. (Wright stain; original magnification, ×100.)

and red blood cell parasites, such as *Mycoplasma* and *Babesia,* can be observed (see Chapter 110 for further details).

Oil immersion magnification is best for evaluating platelet numbers. In general, in the monolayer there should be 8 to 15 platelets per (100×) field (see Chapter 106 for further details). This number can be reduced significantly, despite a normal platelet count, if platelet clumps are present.

WHITE BLOOD CELL RESPONSES[1,2]

White blood cell responses are among the best laboratory indicators of the general health status of critically ill patients. Many emergent and critically ill patients have inflammatory diseases. Inflammation is usually indicated by the leukogram. Signs of inflammation include a left shift, monocytosis, or persistent eosinophilia. General patterns of leukocyte responses are presented in Table 196-1.

Left shifts (increased numbers of immature neutrophils in the blood) can be further classified as regenerative or degenerative, depending on whether total neutrophil counts are increased or decreased. Increased numbers of mature neutrophils in conjunction with a left shift is a regenerative left shift (Figure 196-1). Regenerative left shifts indicate that bone marrow production of neutrophils is keeping pace with tissue demand, which is associated with a favorable prognosis for the patient. In contrast, degenerative left shifts are those with normal or decreased numbers of mature neutrophils, which indicates that marrow production is not keeping pace with tissue demand. This in turn signals a guarded prognosis for the patient. A special form of degenerative left shift occurs when total neutrophil counts are increased but over 50% of the neutrophils are immature.

Monocytosis (see Figures 196-1 and 196-2) not only indicates inflammation but is also an indicator of tissue necrosis or a demand for phagocytes. Monocytosis can occur acutely or chronically depending on the inciting cause of the inflammation. Acute systemic diseases such as histoplasmosis and toxoplasmosis can cause monocytosis in as little as 8 to 12 hours after infection. A mild increase in circulating monocytes may also occur as part of a stress leukogram, particularly in dogs.

Persistent eosinophilia usually indicates a systemic hypersensitivity reaction (see Chapter 152). Causes include systemic parasitic infections (e.g., heartworm infections, migrating parasitic larvae), systemic mastocytosis, allergic reactions, feline asthma, and allergic gastroenteritis. In addition to mastocytosis, some other neoplastic diseases, most notably lymphoproliferative disorders, may be associated with systemic hypersensitivity reactions and persistent eosinophilia.

A persistent eosinophilia and lymphocytosis occur in 10% to 15% of canine cases of hypoadrenocorticism (Addison's disease). Patients with Addison's disease may arrive at the hospital in a state of cardiovascular collapse or severe weakness and depression. In these instances, a complete blood count is always warranted.

Other lymphocyte responses can also be quite informative in patients with inflammatory disease. Mild to moderate lymphopenia (counts of 750 to 1500 cells/μl) is usually the result of high circulating levels of corticosteroids (stress response). Marked lymphopenia may be caused by stress alone, but other causes of lymphopenia should also be considered. These include any disease state that interferes with the normal circulatory pattern of lymphocytes (lymph to blood to tissues to lymph). Possibilities include lymphoma, chylous effusions, lymphangiectasia, and lymphedema. Chylous effusions and lymphedema are generally characterized by low plasma and serum protein levels.

White blood cell morphology can be as informative in patients with inflammatory conditions as white blood cell numbers.[1-3] Neutrophils should be assessed for toxicity. The most common feature of toxicity in neutrophils is foamy basophilia of the cytoplasm (Figure 196-3). Döhle bodies, or intracytoplasmic basophilic precipitates of ribonucleic acid (RNA) (Figure 196-4), also represent toxic change. The presence of Döhle bodies indicates significant toxicity in dogs but is far less important in cats, in which they can be seen even in healthy animals. Other features of toxicity include the presence of giant neutrophils and aberrant nuclear shapes such as ring forms.

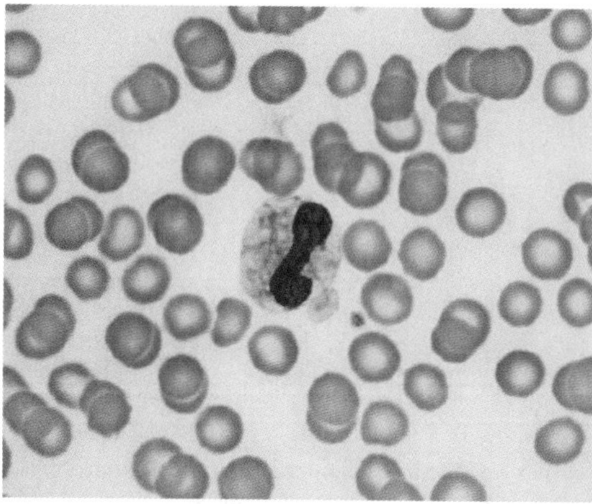

FIGURE 196-3 Blood film from a dog. The central band neutrophil is toxic with foamy basophilic cytoplasm. (Wright stain; original magnification, ×100.)

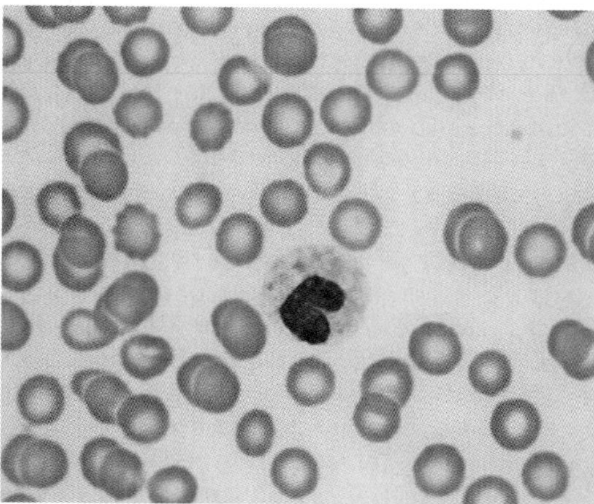

FIGURE 196-4 Toxic band containing several distinct Döhle bodies. (Wright stain; original magnification, ×100.)

Neutrophil toxicity indicates that circulating toxins are interfering with neutrophil development in the bone marrow or that neutrophil production has been accelerated in the bone marrow as a result of increased peripheral demand. Toxicity is most commonly associated with bacterial infections but can be observed in other inflammatory diseases as well. For example, toxicity can be seen following extensive tissue necrosis (e.g., severe trauma).

Following the appearance and disappearance of neutrophil toxicity can be important in the treatment of critically ill patients. The appearance of toxicity may indicate that the patient's condition is worsening. Resolution of toxicity is often an indicator of improvement. However, the assessment of toxicity may be prone to subjective evaluation unless the same person reviews the slide daily, which makes interpretation of changes over time more challenging.

The presence of reactive lymphocytes should also be noted. Reactive lymphocytes are generally larger than normal, with increased amounts of basophilic cytoplasm and large nuclei containing finely granular chromatin. Reactive lymphocytes are antigen stimulated, and their presence indicates that the immune system has been engaged.[1-3]

Monocytes and neutrophils should be examined closely for inclusions. A variety of infectious disease agents, including *Ehrlichia, Histoplasma, Hepatozoon,* and *Leishmania,* can sometimes be observed in circulating phagocytes. Erythrophagocytosis is sometimes seen with certain red blood cell disorders such as immune-mediated hemolytic anemia (IMHA).

RED BLOOD CELL RESPONSES

Anemia is a common problem in emergent and critically ill patients and may be the sole reason the animal is brought to the veterinarian (see Chapter 108). The anemia may be either a primary disease or a secondary accompaniment to some other condition. Blood film evaluation is a critical first step in determining which circumstance exists. The approach to evaluating blood films in anemic animals is summarized in Figure 196-5 and explained in greater detail in the paragraphs that follow.[1-3]

Increased numbers of polychromatophils (large, immature red blood cells that are bluish) on the blood film indicate that the anemia is regenerative and the result of either blood loss or hemolysis (see Figures 196-1 and 196-2). Anemia due to blood loss usually can be easily ruled in or ruled out based on clinical findings, history, and the total protein concentration (decreased with blood loss).

If there is no indication of blood loss and large numbers of polychromatophils are present, then hemolysis should be considered. Careful evaluation of red blood cell morphology may lead to a specific diagnosis in many cases of hemolysis.

For example, spherocytes are red blood cells that are small, stain intensely, and lack central pallor.[1-3] When large numbers of spherocytes are seen in cats or dogs (see Figures 196-1 and 196-2), IMHA is the likely diagnosis. Heinz body hemolytic anemia is diagnosed based on identification of Heinz bodies, which are single to multiple noselike projections from the red blood cell surface that stain like hemoglobin (Figure 196-6).[1-3] In patients with fragmentation hemolytic anemias, large numbers of schizocytes (red blood cell fragments) are usually found on the blood film (Figure 196-7).[1-3] In many cases of infectious hemolytic anemia, the causative disease agent can be observed in affected red blood cells. *Mycoplasma* infections are characterized by the presence of small (1-mcm) basophilic bodies arranged singly or in chains on the red blood cell surface (Figure 196-8).[1,3] In dogs with babesiosis, parasitized red blood cells containing teardrop-shaped *Babesia* (2 to 4 mcm) can often be found.[1,3]

When polychromasia is absent, the anemia is nonregenerative. It is important to remember that in the very acute phase (first 3 days),

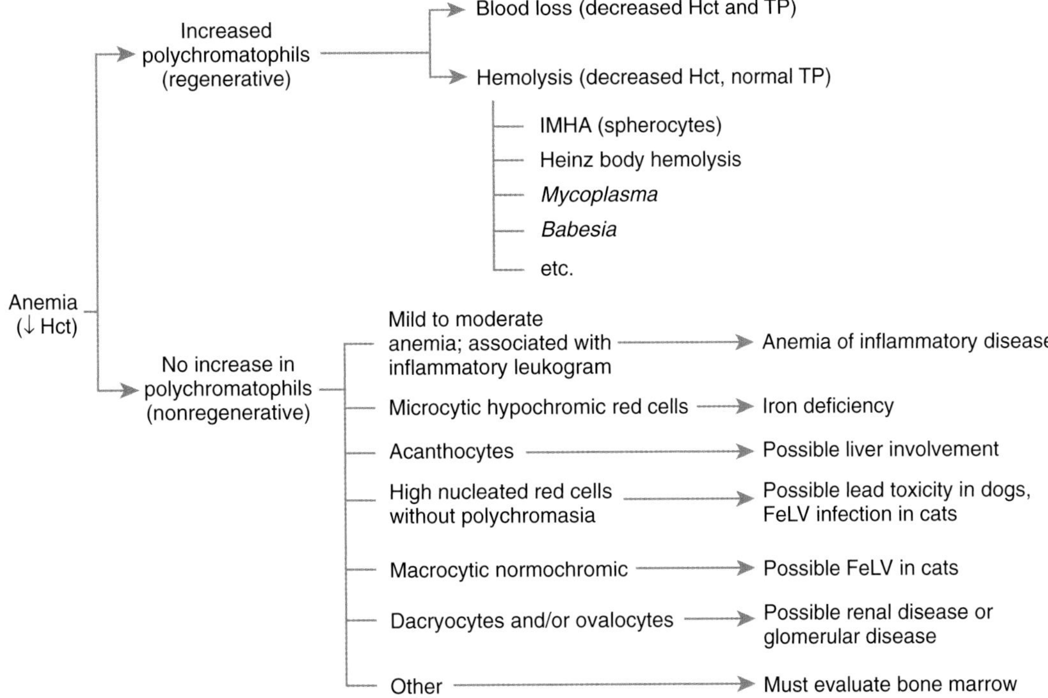

FIGURE 196-5 Evaluation of blood films in anemic patients. *FeLV,* Feline leukemia virus; *Hct,* hematocrit; *IMHA,* immune-mediated hemolytic anemia; *TP,* total protein.

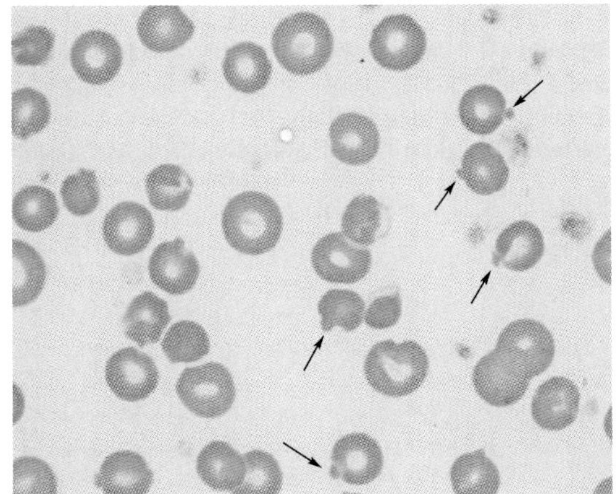

FIGURE 196-6 Heinz body hemolytic anemia. Numerous Heinz bodies *(arrows)* are seen. (Wright stain; original magnification, ×100.)

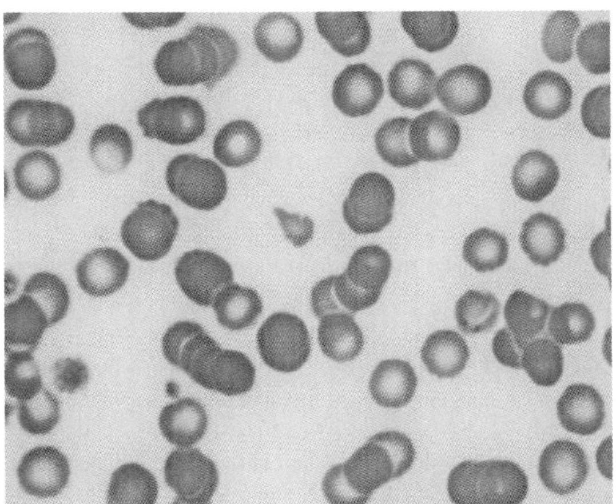

FIGURE 196-7 Blood film from a dog. A triangular schizocyte is seen centrally. (Wright stain; original magnification, ×100.)

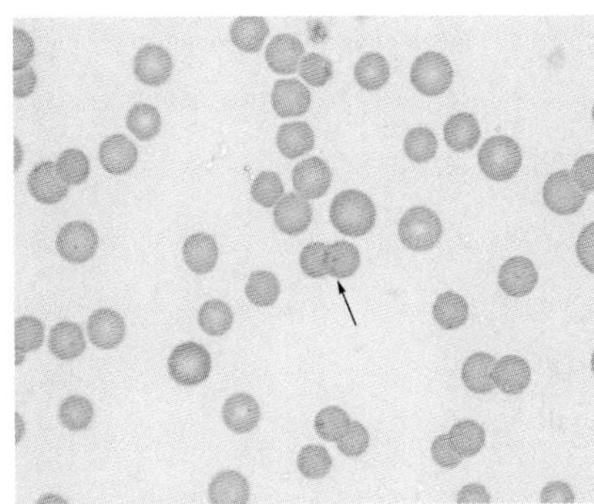

FIGURE 196-8 Hemotrophic mycoplasmosis in a cat. The central red blood cell *(arrow)* contains four organisms. Also note the presence of polychromatophils. (Wright stain; original magnification, ×100.)

even regenerative anemias (blood loss and hemolytic anemias) show very little polychromasia on the blood film and therefore appear nonregenerative. Although most types of nonregenerative anemias require bone marrow evaluation for specific diagnosis, some assumptions can be made based on blood film evaluation. When mild to moderate, normocytic, normochromic nonregenerative anemias (down to hematocrits of 30% in dogs and 25% in cats) occur in conjunction with an inflammatory leukogram, the anemia is almost certainly an anemia of inflammatory disease. The nonregenerative anemia of iron deficiency (severe blood loss) is characterized by small red blood cells with increased areas of central pallor (Figure 196-9).[1-3] Iron-deficient red blood cells are also more fragile than normal, and consequently there are usually more red blood cell fragments (schizocytes). Nonregenerative anemias that have acanthocytes (red blood cells with 2 to 10 elongated, blunt, fingerlike surface projections) on the blood film are suggestive of liver disease.[1-3] Cases of nonregenerative anemia that lack polychromasia but have increased numbers of nucleated red blood cells (>10 per 100 white blood cells counted) most likely result from marrow stromal damage. In dogs this is probably the result of lead poisoning, whereas in cats feline leukemia virus infection should be considered (Figure 196-10). In cats, nonregenerative anemias with macrocytic normochromic red blood cells also are suggestive of feline leukemia virus infection. Some of these patients may even have megaloblasts (giant, fully hemoglobinized red blood cells containing relatively immature, stippled nuclei) on the blood film. Finally, nonregenerative anemias with dacryocytes (teardrop-shaped erythrocytes) or ovalocytes, or both, raise the possibility of myelofibrosis or renal disease (glomerulonephritis) (Figure 196-11).

PLATELET RESPONSES

Platelet numbers should be monitored closely in emergent and critically ill patients[1] (see Chapter 106). Thrombocytopenia is the most common cause of primary bleeding disorders in dogs and cats. Platelet counts can be estimated rapidly by evaluating the blood film.

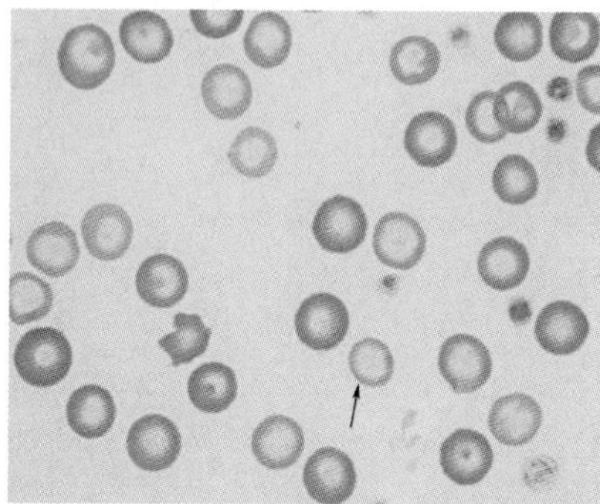

FIGURE 196-9 Blood film from a dog with iron deficiency. Note the small red blood cells with increased areas of central pallor *(arrow)*. (Wright stain; original magnification, ×100.)

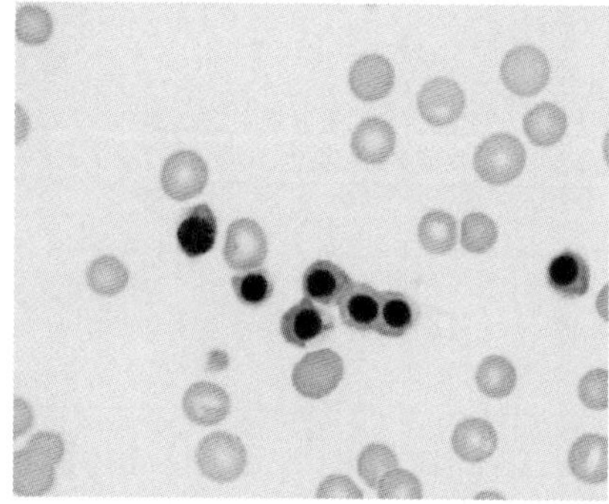

FIGURE 196-10 Blood film from a cat infected with feline leukemia virus. Note the increased number of nucleated red blood cells in the absence of significant polychromasia (inappropriate nucleated red blood cell response). (Wright stain; original magnification, ×100.)

Normally, there are 8 to 15 platelets per 100× oil immersion monolayer field. This correlates with circulating platelet numbers between 200,000 and 800,000 cells/µl. Certain breeds (e.g., Cavalier King Charles Spaniel and Greyhound) may have lower platelet counts normally.

Thrombocytopenia can be a life-threatening event, especially when platelet counts drop below 20,000 to 50,000 cells/µl. Affected animals may have petechiae, ecchymoses, mucosal bleeding, and anemia.

Thrombocytopenia occurs via four mechanisms: sequestration, consumption (utilization), destruction, and hypoproliferation (lack of production) (Table 196-2). Sequestration thrombocytopenia occurs in association with splenomegaly and is extremely rare in animals. Consumption thrombocytopenia is associated with severe inflammation and leads to disseminated intravascular coagulation (DIC). Whenever inflammation is indicated by the leukogram and platelet numbers are even marginally reduced, the possibility of DIC should be considered. In dogs, schizocytes may also be present on the blood film with DIC.

Immune-mediated thrombocytopenia (ITP) occurs as the result of antibody-mediated destruction of circulating platelets. Platelet counts may be extremely low, and as a result platelets often are seen quite rarely on blood films. Bone marrow evaluation reveals increased numbers of platelet precursors (megakaryocytes).

Destruction thrombocytopenia may occur in conjunction with IMHA, so blood films in suspect cases should be evaluated carefully for evidence of spherocytosis. If spherocytosis is seen, a direct antiglobulin test (Coombs' test) is warranted. Patients with combined IMHA and ITP have a more guarded prognosis and are more difficult to treat than those with either IMHA or ITP alone (see Chapters 106 and 110).

Hypoproliferative thrombocytopenia occurs when the marrow's ability to produce platelets is impaired. As in ITP, platelet counts can

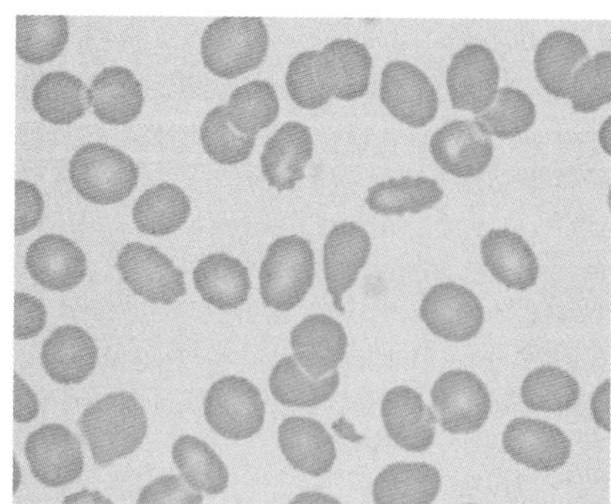

FIGURE 196-11 Blood film from a dog with glomerulonephritis. A dacryocyte is seen centrally. Also note the oval red blood cells. (Wright stain; original magnification, ×100.)

Table 196-2 Causes of Thrombocytopenia[1]

Type	Disorder	Cause
Platelet production defect	Aplasia, hypoplasia Marrow infiltration (myelophthisis) Ineffective megakaryocytopoiesis	Cytotoxic drugs, idiopathic Drugs, infection including viral infections Myelodysplastic syndrome
Accelerated platelet destruction	Immune destruction	Autoantibodies Antibodies to drugs, infection
Peripheral platelet utilization	Nonimmunologic removal	Disseminated intravascular coagulation, vasculitis, severe bleeding, neoplasia, infection
Platelet sequestration	Hypersplenism	Enlarged spleen from numerous causes

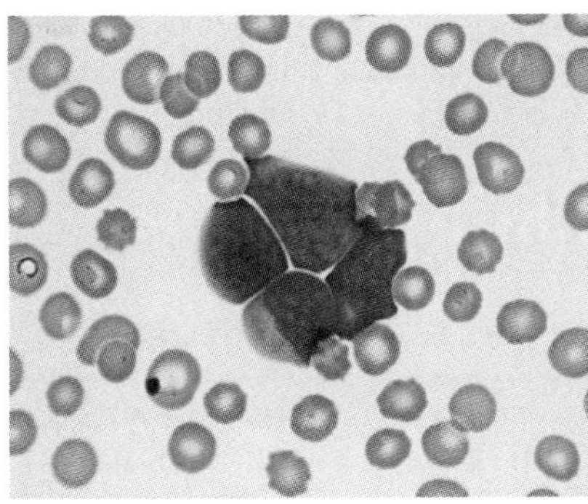

FIGURE 196-12 Lymphoid leukemia in a dog. Four larger-than-normal malignant lymphocytes are seen centrally. Nucleolar whorls can be seen on close inspection. (Wright stain; original magnification, ×100.)

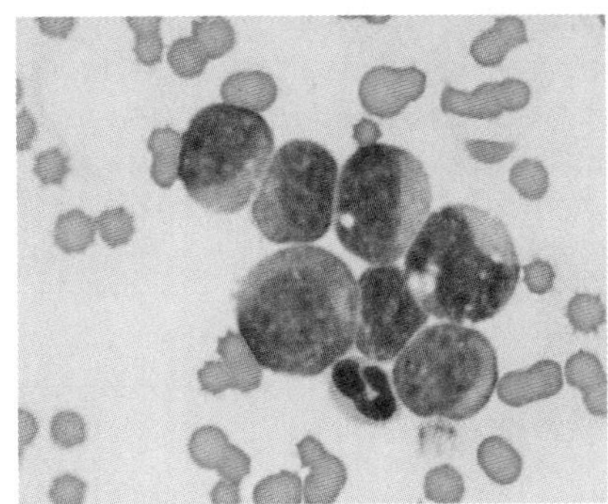

FIGURE 196-13 Acute myelogenous leukemia. Most of the cells are poorly differentiated myeloid precursors. (Wright stain; original magnification, ×100.)

be extremely low. Marrow evaluation reveals a marked reduction in megakaryocytes.

Hypoproliferative thrombocytopenia may occur alone or in conjunction with other cytopenias (e.g., neutropenia, anemia). Although the specific cause of this syndrome is often obscure, hypoproliferative thrombocytopenia may be due to certain infections (viral infections, ehrlichiosis) or toxins. It may also be the result of immune-mediated bone marrow disease (antibodies directed against platelet precursors). It is likely that the hypoproliferative thrombocytopenia seen in some infections is at least partially the result of an immune-mediated reaction.

LEUKEMIA (MYELOID AND LYMPHOID)

Patients with myeloid or lymphoid leukemias are often presented for treatment of emergent conditions that require close monitoring and intensive care. Blood film examination is a critical first step in the diagnosis and evaluation of these conditions. Because patients are presented in various stages of their disease, hematologic findings can vary greatly from case to case.[2]

Perhaps the most consistent finding is a marked nonregenerative anemia. This anemia develops because bone marrow space has been infiltrated by a proliferating neoplastic cell population that is crowding out and interfering with normal red blood cell precursor production. The number of normal circulating leukocytes and platelets is also often decreased.

White blood cell counts may be markedly elevated, normal, or decreased. When white blood cell counts are markedly elevated, it is usually as a result of large numbers of circulating neoplastic cells. In the case of lymphoid leukemias, these cells are typically malignant lymphoblasts, larger-than-normal lymphoid cells with increased amounts of basophilic cytoplasm and large round nuclei containing loose granular chromatin and nucleolar whorls (Figure 196-12). Rarely, blood films from patients with lymphoid leukemia have massively increased numbers of neoplastic, but normal-appearing, small lymphocytes. In the case of myelogenous leukemias, the increase in circulating numbers may be due to the predominance of blasts and progranulocytes (acute leukemia; Figure 196-13) or to the presence of more differentiated, but still abnormal, myelocytes, bands, and segmented cells (chronic leukemia). Special stains may be needed to differentiate acute myelogenous leukemia from lymphoblastic leukemia.

When white blood cell counts are normal, neoplastic cells may or may not be seen on the blood film. If present, they are usually seen only in low numbers. Leukemias with only rare malignant cells in circulation are sometimes called *subleukemic leukemias.* Cases with this clinical presentation require bone marrow evaluation for definitive diagnosis. Bone marrow aspirates generally reveal replacement of normal marrow cellular elements by a relatively monotonous population of malignant cells.

When white blood cell counts are low, there is usually no left shift (unless a secondary infection is present), and red blood cell counts are also almost always extremely low with no evidence of regeneration. Platelet counts are less predictable. The presence of one or more unexplained cytopenias suggests bone marrow disease and is an indication for bone marrow evaluation. Bone marrow aspirates once again reveal replacement of bone marrow elements by a monotonous population of malignant cells, more than 20% of which are blasts. Leukemias in this stage are termed *myelophthisic syndromes* or *aleukemic leukemias.*

REFERENCES

1. Rebar AH, MacWilliams PS, Feldman BF, et al: A guide to hematology in dogs and cats, Jackson Hole, Wy, 2002, Teton NewMedia.
2. Rebar AH: Hemogram interpretation for dogs and cats, Ralston Purina Handbook Series, Wilmington, Del, 1998, The Gloyd Group.
3. Harvey JW: Atlas of veterinary hematology, blood and bone marrow of domestic animals, Philadelphia, 2001, Saunders.

CHAPTER 197

ENDOTRACHEAL INTUBATION AND TRACHEOSTOMY

Mack Fudge, DVM, MPVM, DACVECC

KEY POINTS

- Careful airway assessment is an imperative first step in managing the emergent and/or critically ill patient.
- Prior planning and preparation are key steps to successful endotracheal intubation.
- Knowledge of multiple techniques and adjuncts for airway access improve the odds for successful patient outcomes.
- Effective patient oxygenation should be ensured throughout the intubation process.
- Continuous patient monitoring and intensive nursing care should be provided to ensure successful tracheostomy tube management and patient comfort.
- Care should be taken to prevent damage to the left recurrent laryngeal nerve, major vessels, and esophagus when performing a tracheotomy.
- Long stay sutures should be placed around cartilage rings next to the tracheotomy site to facilitate routine tube replacement and help secure the airway if the tube becomes occluded or dislodged.

Assuring a patent airway is the usual first step in managing emergent and critically ill patients. Airway management in the critically ill is often more challenging because these patients tend to have less physiologic reserve. Complications are more common, both during the initial airway intervention and later once the airway is secured.[1] In patients requiring intervention to secure the airway, endotracheal intubation is perhaps the preferred and most commonly used method. When endotracheal intubation fails, the trachea is typically accessed and secured directly using some form of tracheotomy.

ENDOTRACHEAL INTUBATION

Endotracheal intubation is the procedure of inserting a tube into the lumen of the trachea. The three main reasons for tracheal intubation are (1) provision of a patent airway in a patient with upper airway obstruction, (2) protection against aspiration in a patient without normal airway protective reflexes, and (3) administration of oxygen, gaseous anesthetics, or positive pressure ventilation.[2,3] Intubation is frequently performed and often a lifesaving procedure in critically ill patients. Recognizing the need to intubate and understanding procedures to aid in difficult intubation are essential skills for critical care veterinarians.

Airway Assessment

Airway assessment is the first step in the evaluation of a critically ill or emergent patient. Both airway patency and airway protection must be ascertained. When upper airway disease is severe, rapid induction of anesthesia and tracheal intubation is indicated. Any patient lacking an adequate gag reflex, as may occur with neurologic disease, sedative or anesthetic drug administration, or cardiopulmonary arrest, likewise requires immediate intubation for airway protection, oxygen therapy, and/or positive pressure ventilation as needed.

If orotracheal intubation is unsuccessful, securing a patent airway by another method is required. A temporary tracheostomy is likely the method to be used.

Routine Intubation

Intubation of animals with normal upper airway anatomy is commonly performed using laryngeal visualization and direct insertion of an appropriate-sized, cuffed endotracheal tube. An adequate level of anesthesia is necessary to implement this technique. After correct placement is confirmed, the tube is secured by tying it around the maxilla or mandible caudal to the canine teeth. Alternatively, a tube can be tied around the back of the head. The tube usually is connected to an oxygen source such as a Bain circuit or an anesthetic machine circuit. Finally, the cuff is inflated until it gently occludes the airway exterior to the tube. To determine how much cuff inflation is required, the operator delivers a manual breath while simultaneously inflating the cuff and listening for resolution of the air leak around the endotracheal tube.[3] Alternatively, cuff pressure can be measured with a commercially available cuff pressure monitor or with an aneroid manometer. Ideal tracheal cuff pressures for veterinary patients have not been defined and may vary with the material the tracheal tube is made of. Values of 19 to 24 mm Hg have been targeted in a recent veterinary study.[4]

Dogs

For routine intubation of dogs, a laryngoscope with a blade long enough to allow adequate visualization of the larynx should be used. Intubation is commonly performed with the patient in sternal recumbency. An assistant grasps either side of the maxilla with one hand, keeping the head raised and extended. Either the assistant or the operator opens the mouth by pulling the tongue out and down, and the endotracheal tube is passed between the arytenoids.[3] Alternatively, many dogs can be intubated in lateral or dorsal recumbency without the aid of an assistant.

Cats

Routine intubation of cats is performed in a manner similar to that used for dogs, except that a topical anesthetic such as lidocaine is applied to the larynx before intubation is attempted in an effort to prevent laryngospasm. Some operators favor the use of a stylet to stiffen the endotracheal tube for feline intubation.[3]

Difficult Intubation

The possibility of a difficult intubation should be considered in animals with evidence of upper airway obstruction, trauma, or abnormal anatomy (e.g., brachycephalic breeds). Prior planning for intubation in cases such as these is essential to maximize the likelihood of success.

Preoxygenation

Any delay in intubation of a patient places the animal at risk of hypoxemia. When the patient is breathing room air, complete upper airway obstruction or apnea will lead to hypoxemia within a few minutes. Preoxygenation of the patient by administration of 100% oxygen via a tight-fitting facemask can potentially prevent hypoxemia for up to 10 minutes of airway obstruction or apnea. Although a study in human patients found preoxygenation to be less effective than previously thought, it still is recommended before attempting intubation of any critically ill patient or any patient at risk of a difficult intubation or apnea.[5,6]

Equipment setup

If a difficult intubation is anticipated, all equipment that may be required should be set up before the procedure is started. Endotracheal tubes of the size appropriate for the patient, in addition to several smaller sizes, should be selected. Stylets or guide tubes, such as a polyethylene urinary catheter, should also be available. Large-bore catheters for transtracheal gas insufflation and a surgical kit for an emergent tracheotomy should be included in case intubation is unsuccessful.

Approach

Routine intubation should be attempted initially. Any fluid accumulation in the oropharynx should be removed by suction or with gauze swabs. If routine intubation is unsuccessful, intubation with a smaller endotracheal tube may be possible. If an endotracheal tube cannot be passed, intubation with a guide tube is often possible. An endotracheal tube (routine size or smaller) with lubricant applied can then be passed over the stylet and introduced blindly into the trachea.[3] The stylet is then removed.

Alternative Techniques and Adjuncts

Needle cricothyroidotomy

If nasal or oral intubation is technically difficult and not successful, securing an airway by another route or method may be indicated. In cases of severe respiratory distress there may be insufficient time or inadequate preparation to perform a tracheostomy. Using a needle cricothyroidotomy, oxygen can be provided via a large-gauge needle or catheter inserted through the cricothyroid membrane or through the tracheal wall. This technique is only a temporary measure used for minutes because ventilation will not be effective.[7] However, this technique can buy time until a better prepared, planned surgical procedure can be performed. This percutaneous tracheotomy technique is perhaps quicker and easier to perform than a surgical tracheotomy.[8]

Cricothyroidotomy

In individual animals with prominent cricothyroid membranes, a cricothyroidotomy can be used to secure the airway in patients with severe facial trauma or those requiring an emergent tracheal intubation in which oral or nasal intubation was unsuccessful. Compared with a tracheotomy, cricothyroidotomy is probably less time consuming, easier to perform, associated with fewer complications, and more likely to result in a dependable airway. It may be converted to a tracheostomy later under more controlled conditions. Use of commercially available, prepackaged cricothyroidotomy kits may save time during resuscitation.[2] The potential problem with these kits is that they require the user to be familiar with the contents, and equipment sizes may not be appropriate for a smaller veterinary patient.

Fiberoptic-assisted intubation

Fiberoptic-guided intubation via the oral route may be useful in some patients. The fiberoptic scope is introduced into the caudal oropharynx, which permits glottic visualization and endotracheal intubation. Various specialized fiberoptic laryngoscopes may be used for this purpose.[2] Note that fiberoptic intubations, especially those using the nasal route, may result in more severe pressor and tachycardiac responses than are observed with direct laryngoscopic intubations.[9]

Digital palpation

In certain cases, digitally directed blind intubation may be a prudent and useful technique to perform. Identifying key anatomic structures by palpation may facilitate a gentle insertion of the tip of the endotracheal tube into the airway. It is essential always to verify correct placement of the tube when this technique is used.

Nasal intubation

Intubation using a nasopharyngeal airway can be a useful adjunct method in some patients. This technique is performed commonly in human patients in whom a larger nasal cavity may accommodate a tube large enough for a definitive airway. Nasal tubes used in veterinary patients usually do not permit an airtight seal of the trachea but do provide a good route for oxygen administration. This technique may be contraindicated in trauma patients with basilar skull fracture or disruption of the cribriform plate. In these cases, the airway tube could potentially traverse the fractured cribriform plate and injure the brain.[2]

Retrograde intubation

Retrograde intubation is another method for securing the airway in certain conditions. This technique requires retrograde placement of a guidewire or catheter via the cricothyroid membrane into the trachea and rostrally into the oropharynx. An endotracheal tube (or fiberoptic bronchoscope via the suction port, or a tube changer followed by an endotracheal tube) is then threaded over the guidewire and into the trachea.[2]

Cricoid pressure

Cricoid pressure may be a useful adjunct to tracheal intubation. Firm pressure, directed dorsally over the cricoid cartilage, collapses the esophagus. This tends to prevent passively regurgitated gastric fluid from reaching the hypopharynx and may help direct the endotracheal tube into the trachea. Recent literature brings into question the efficacy of cricoid pressure. Nonetheless, this technique is still used commonly in human patients, especially those with a high likelihood of vomiting or regurgitation.[6,10,11]

Placement Verification

Verification of correct placement of the endotracheal tube is a necessary and critical step. It is not uncommon, especially in hurried or difficult intubations, for the tube to be advanced inadvertently down the esophagus. The simplest and most obvious way to ensure correct placement is through direct visualization of tube placement. Seeing the tube pass through the larynx and into the trachea should ensure correct placement. Measurement of exhaled carbon dioxide can provide an additional level of assurance of correct tube placement. This technique is not recommended for intubations made during cardiac arrest. Other methods such as watching for fogging of the inside of the endotracheal tube during exhalation, observing vapor on shiny surfaces placed at the end of the tube, or noting fluttering of valves on connected anesthesia machines are often misleading and supportive at best.

Complications

Tracheal intubation can be associated with equipment-related or patient-related complications. Some studies report the occurrence of complications related to tracheal intubation in up to 40% of critically ill human patients.[12] Soft or particularly small endotracheal tubes can crimp because of the acute angle created as the tube passes from the oropharynx toward the larynx, which reduces the airflow through the tube. This can lead to hypoventilation and subsequent hypercapnia and hypoxemia. Bending can also create additional pressure at the end of the tube that can damage the dorsal larynx or tracheal mucosa.

Pressure-induced tracheal necrosis is possible when the endotracheal tube cuff is overinflated or the tube is too large for the patient. If the intubation is expected to be prolonged, care should be taken to pad oral soft tissues that come into contact with the endotracheal tube. Prolonged contact of the tube with lips, gingiva, and tongue can cause multiple small areas of pressure necrosis. In rare cases of more extreme damage caused to the trachea by endotracheal tubes, subcutaneous emphysema or even pneumothorax is possible.

Endotracheal tubes may be unintentionally advanced too far and end in a mainstem bronchus, usually the right. This may lead to inadvertent overinflation of the intubated lung and impaired gas exchange. Premeasurement of endotracheal tubes before placement, bilateral thoracic auscultation, radiography, and ultrasound observation may help to avoid inadvertent endobronchial intubation.

Endotracheal intubation can cause increased intracranial pressure and even increased intraocular pressure. It can also cause significant increases in blood pressure and heart rate.[13]Rapid, smooth intubation is important.

TRACHEOSTOMY

Tracheostomy may be indicated for potentially life-threatening upper airway obstruction, oral or pharyngeal surgery, or long-term ventilator support in critically ill patients. Access to the trachea proximal to the nose, mouth, pharynx, and larynx provided by the tracheostomy allows air to enter proximal to obstructions and reduces damage to the oral cavity from prolonged intubation[14]

Tracheostomy Tube Selection

Numerous tracheostomy tubes are commercially available. They can be cuffed or uncuffed and may or may not have an inner cannula. The requirement for a tube cuff depends on individual patient factors. In most cases a cuff is not required, and using an uncuffed tube or keeping the tube cuff deflated may reduce the likelihood of tracheal injury. A cuff may be desirable in patients requiring positive pressure ventilation, although use of this mode may also be feasible with uncuffed tubes. The presence of a tube cuff may make it necessary to use a slightly smaller tracheostomy tube than would be possible without the cuff.

A removable inner cannula allows for easy and effective tube maintenance and is considered desirable. The inner cannula can be removed briefly for cleaning without disrupting airway integrity. Unfortunately, smaller tubes cannot be made with an inner cannula. In the absence of an inner cannula, the entire tracheostomy tube should be replaced every 24 hours (more often if indicated) to prevent occlusion with accumulated secretions.

The size of the tracheostomy tube chosen is based on the diameter of the patient's airway. The largest tube that can be readily accommodated by the trachea is selected. Note that the sizes of tracheostomy tubes do not correspond with the scale used to size endotracheal tubes. An estimate of the appropriate tracheostomy tube size usually can be made by evaluation of the inner lumen diameter of the trachea on a lateral cervical radiograph.

Tracheostomy tubes can also be fenestrated. A fenestration is an opening in the tube that allows airflow through to the upper airway if the external opening is occluded. In human patients this feature is used to enable speech. The utility of a fenestrated tube in veterinary patients is questionable. A fenestrated tube cannot be used with positive pressure ventilation.

If a tracheostomy tube is not immediately available, an endotracheal tube can be shortened and used effectively as an interim substitute.

Percutaneous Tracheostomy

For years the standard technique for tracheostomy was an open surgical approach. Not long after Seldinger described needle replacement over a guidewire, percutaneous tracheostomy techniques were developed. Over the past 20 years, the use of percutaneous dilatational tracheostomy has gained popularity. At present, percutaneous tracheostomy is a common procedure in human intensive care units, with several different techniques and commercially made kits readily available. This method of tracheostomy can be done rapidly, in less than 20 minutes, which makes it a good technique for emergent patients as well. Results are similar to, if not better than, those with a standard surgical technique.[15-21]

A small transverse relief incision is made at the desired location for tube insertion. A small-gauge needle is inserted into the lumen of the trachea. A guidewire is introduced via the needle into the lumen. Next a dilator is passed over the guidewire to make a path for the tracheostomy tube. The tracheostomy tube is then introduced along the dilator over the guidewire. The guidewire and dilator are removed and the tube is secured in place. There are minor variations of this procedure with each technique and kit. Knowledge of the anatomy and experience with the insertion technique and equipment used is essential to achieve success and avoid complications.[22]

SURGICAL TRACHEOSTOMY

Temporary tracheostomy is best performed in a controlled manner with the patient under general anesthesia and an orotracheal tube in place. The animal is placed in dorsal recumbency with the neck carefully extended for exposure of the surgical site. The neck can be elevated from the table by placing it on a cushion. Routine surgical preparation of the ventral cervical region is performed.

A 2- to 5-cm ventral cervical midline skin incision is made extending from the cricoid cartilage toward the sternum. The sternohyoid muscles are separated along their midline with blunt dissection and retracted laterally. The peritracheal connective tissue is removed from the region of the tracheotomy site. Throughout the procedure care must be taken to avoid dissection lateral to the trachea to prevent injury to the left recurrent laryngeal nerve or disruption of tracheal blood supply. The two common surgical approaches for temporary tracheotomy are transverse and vertical incisions.

Transverse incision

In the transverse approach the annular ligament between the third and fourth or fourth and fifth tracheal rings is incised; the incision should extend for no more than 50% of the tracheal circumference. Extreme care must be taken to avoid the left recurrent laryngeal nerve. A small ellipse of cartilage from each tracheal cartilage adjacent to the tracheotomy incision can be made to help reduce tracheal irritation and inflammation. Long loops of suture are placed around the tracheal rings adjacent to the incision to facilitate retraction of the trachea and future replacement of the tube after cleaning (Figure 197-1).[14]

Vertical incision

In the vertical approach a ventral midline vertical incision is made through two to four tracheal rings. Long stay sutures may be placed encircling the cartilage rings lateral to the incision to aid in continued manipulation of the trachea and future tube replacement (Figure 197-2). Segmental lateral tracheal collapse may be a long-term complication of this procedure.[14]

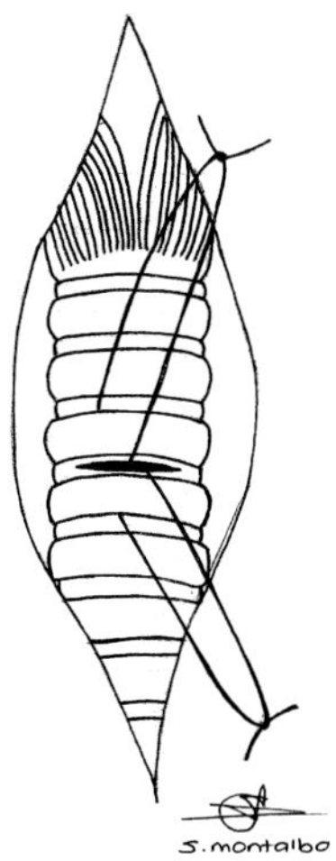

FIGURE 197-1 Transverse incision tracheostomy.

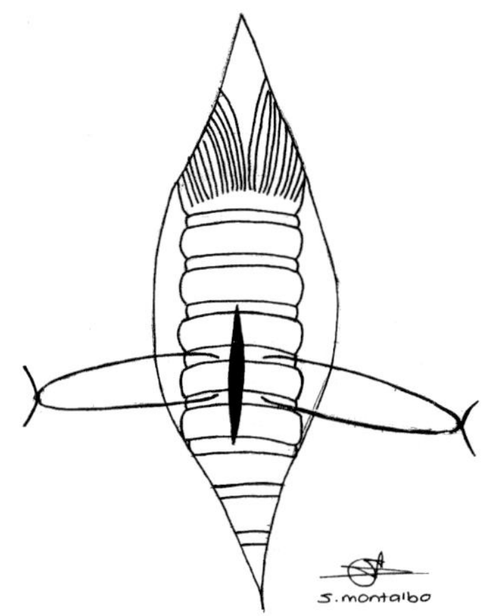

FIGURE 197-2 Vertical incision tracheostomy.

Securing the tracheostomy tube

Following tube placement via either technique the muscles and skin can be closed routinely, but space should be left around the tracheostomy tube so that air can escape easily to prevent subcutaneous emphysema.

The tracheostomy tube can be secured with sutures or with umbilical tape tied around the neck. Commercially made Velcro-fastening tracheostomy tube ties are also available. Tying the tube in place should be considered to facilitate later regular tube replacement and reduce patient discomfort. Tube ties need to be evaluated frequently to prevent inadvertent tube dislodgment.

Tracheostomy Tube Management

Tracheostomy tubes are associated with a high complication rate but a good outcome in most patients. Effective management requires continuous intensive monitoring. When this level of care is unavailable, elective tracheostomy perhaps should not be done. When a tracheostomy is unavoidable, the patient should be transferred to a suitable facility for ongoing care as soon as possible.[14,23]

The major aims of tracheostomy tube management are to prevent tube obstruction, to facilitate removal of airway secretions, and to minimize the risk of airway trauma or nosocomial pneumonia. It is important to recognize that tube occlusion or dislodgment can occur without warning despite ideal tube management, and staff should be prepared for rapid tube replacement (or inner cannula removal) should acute complications develop.[24,25] The placement of stay sutures around tracheal rings adjacent to the tracheotomy site at the time of surgery is essential to allow successful tube replacement. Tape tabs may be placed on the end of each stay suture and labeled "cranial" and "caudal" or "left" and "right" as appropriate. With the use of stay sutures most animals tolerate tube replacement while awake, without sedation.

Patient positioning either in sternal recumbency with the neck extended or in dorsal recumbency with the neck extended is extremely important to facilitate this procedure. Gradual concretion of airway secretions within the lumen of the tracheostomy tube may occur despite regular suctioning. For this reason, removal and cleaning of inner cannulas should be performed every 4 hours, and tubes without an inner cannula should be replaced every 24 hours routinely, even if there are no obvious problems.

BOX 197-1 *Tracheostomy Tube Care Protocol*

- Remove inner cannula (if present) for cleaning and replace with a temporary cannula for the duration of the procedure.
- Humidify airway for 20 minutes before performing suctioning in patients not receiving mechanical ventilation.
- Preoxygenate with 100% oxygen for 3-5 minutes before suctioning.
- Insert a sterile suction catheter to the level of the carina and apply suction as the catheter is removed with a circular motion (taking no longer than 10 seconds).
- Perform suctioning two to four times depending on the amount of exudate and the patient's toleration of the procedure.
- Administer 100% oxygen for 3-5 minutes after each suctioning episode.
- Replace the cleaned inner cannula.
- Clean the incision site surrounding the tracheostomy tube and make sure that the tube is still secured in place appropriately.

Suctioning

Suctioning should be performed frequently to remove secretions from the airway and reduce the likelihood of tube occlusion. See Box 197-1 for a suggested protocol for tracheostomy tube management. Aseptic technique should be used at all times. The suction catheter must be sterile as well as soft and flexible to minimize airway trauma. Human oxygen administration catheters work well for suctioning animal airways.

Sterile physiologic saline solution (1 to 2 ml) can be injected into the trachea through the tracheostomy tube to help loosen exudates before suctioning. The airway should be well humidified, and preoxygenation with 100% oxygen is recommended. The catheter is inserted down the airway several centimeters beyond the length of the tube and suction is applied as the catheter is withdrawn using a circular motion. The duration of suctioning should be brief (no longer than 10 seconds) to minimize small airway collapse, and 100% oxygen should be provided for at least 3 minutes immediately after each suctioning episode.

Tracheostomy tube suctioning is performed routinely every 4 hours, although in some patients it may be necessary more frequently. Respiratory distress or vagal stimulation (retching or vomiting) may occur during tracheal suctioning. Patients may become anxious about the procedure over time and with repetition. Consideration may be given to timing the procedure to coincide with maximum drug effect if analgesics, sedatives, tranquilizers, or anxiolytics are otherwise used in the patient.

Tube Removal

The tracheostomy tube is removed when an adequate upper airway is established. Most small animals that have a tracheostomy for upper airway surgery can be extubated within 48 hours after surgery. After the tube has been removed, the tracheostomy site is left open and allowed to heal by granulation and epithelialization.

Complications

Complications following temporary tracheostomy include tube occlusion or dislodgment, subcutaneous emphysema, pneumothorax, aspiration of fluid or foreign bodies, and pneumonia. Arrhythmias and vagally mediated bradycardia and collapse can occur during suctioning or tube manipulation. With careful management and monitoring, most complications can be prevented.

Summary

Airway management is fundamental in the care of critically ill and emergent patients. Complications resulting from difficulties with airway management may include brain injury, myocardial injury, increased intracranial and intraocular pressures, pulmonary aspiration of gastric contents, trauma to the airways, and death. Shock, respiratory distress, full stomach, airway trauma, cervical spine instability, and head injury may make emergent tracheal intubation a challenging procedure in the critically ill patient. Careful use of pharmacologic agents can greatly enhance the ability to safely secure the airway.

REFERENCES

1. Nolan JP, Kelly FE: Airway challenges in critical care, Anaesthesia 66(Suppl 2):81-92, 2011.
2. Jaber S, Amraoui J, Lefrant JY, et al: Clinical practice and risk factors for immediate complications of endotracheal intubation in the intensive care unit: a prospective, multiple-center study, Crit Care Med 34:2355, 2006.
3. Hartsfield SM: Airway management and ventilation. In Tranquilli WJ, Thurmon JC, Grimm KA, editors: Lumb and Jones' veterinary anesthesia and analgesia, ed 4, Oxford, 2007, Wiley-Blackwell.
4. Briganti A, Portela DA, Barsotti G, et al: Evaluation of the endotracheal tube cuff pressure resulting from four different methods of inflation in dogs, Vet Anaesth Analg 39(5):488-494, 2012.
5. Mort TC: Preoxygenation in critically ill patients requiring emergency tracheal intubation, Crit Care Med 33:2672, 2006.
6. Ehrenfeld JM, Cassedy EA, Forbes VE, et al: Modified rapid sequence induction and intubation: a survey of United States current practice, Anesth Analg 115(1):95-101, 2012.
7. Scrase I, Woollard M: Needle vs. surgical cricothyroidotomy: a short cut to effective ventilation, Anaesthesia 61:962, 2006.
8. Silvester W, Goldsmith D, Bellomo R, et al: Percutaneous versus surgical tracheostomy: a randomized controlled study with long-term follow-up, Crit Care Med 34:2145, 2006.
9. Xue FS, Zhang GH, Sun HY, et al: Blood pressure and heart rate changes during intubation: a comparison of direct laryngoscopy and a fiberoptic method, Anesthesia 61:444, 2006.
10. Stanton J: Literature review of safe use of cricoid pressure, J Perioper Pract 16:250, 2006.
11. Boet S, Duttchen K, Chan J, et al: Cricoid pressure provides incomplete esophageal occlusion associated with lateral deviation: a magnetic resonance imaging study, J Emerg Med 42(5):606-611, 2012.
12. Simpson GD, Ross MJ, McKeown DW, et al: Tracheal intubation in the critically ill: a multi-centre national study of practice and complications, Br J Anaesth 108(5):792-799, 2012.
13. Xue FS, Li CW, Liu KP, et al: The circulatory responses to fiberoptic intubation: a comparison of oral and nasal routes, Anesthesia 61:639, 2006.
14. Hedlund CS: Surgery of the upper respiratory system. In Fossum TW, editor: Small animal surgery, ed 4, St Louis, 2012, Mosby.
15. Cabrini L, Monti G, Landoni G, et al: Percutaneous tracheostomy, a systematic review, Acta Anaesthesiol Scand 56(3):270-281, 2012.
16. Hamaekers AE, Henderson JJ: Equipment and strategies for emergency tracheal access in the adult patient, Anaesthesia 66(Suppl 2):65-80, 2011.
17. Susaria SM, Peacock ZS, Alam HB: Percutaneous dilatational tracheostomy: review of technique and evidence for its use, J Oral Maxillofac Surg 70(1):74-82, 2012.
18. Groves DS, Durbin CG Jr: Tracheostomy in the critically ill: indications, timing and techniques, Curr Opinion Crit Care 13(1):90-97, 2007.
19. Delaney A, Bagshaw SM, Nalos M: Percutaneous dilatational tracheostomy versus surgical tracheostomy in critically ill patients: a systematic review and meta-analysis, Crit Care 10(2):R55, 2006.
20. Al-Ansari MA, Hijazi MH: Clinical review: percutaneous dilatational tracheostomy, Crit Care 10(1):202, 2006.
21. Sengupta N, Ang KL, Prakash D, et al: Twenty months' routine use of a new percutaneous tracheostomy set using controlled rotating dilation, Anesth Analg 99(1):188-192, 2004.
22. Brietzke SE: Percutaneous tracheostomy treatment and management, Medscape Reference, Updated: March 16, 2011. Available at http://www.emedicine.medscape.com.
23. Nicholson I, Baines S: Complications associated with temporary tracheostomy tubes in 42 dogs (1998 to 2007), J Small Anim Pract 53(2):108-114, 2012.
24. St. John RE, Malen JF: Contemporary issues in adult tracheostomy treatment, Crit Care Nurs Clin North Am 16:413, 2006.
25. Boucher MA, Edelman MA, Edmission KW, et al: Tracheotomy. In Mills EJ, editor: Handbook of medical-surgical nursing, ed 4, Philadelphia, 2006, Lippincott Williams & Wilkins.

CHAPTER 198

THORACOCENTESIS

Nadja E. Sigrist, DrMedVet, FVH, DACVECC

KEY POINTS

- Indications for thoracocentesis are pneumothorax and pleural effusions (chyle, transudate, blood).
- Thoracocentesis is an easily performed diagnostic and therapeutic procedure and is relatively safe if performed by skilled personnel.
- Blind thoracocentesis is performed between the seventh and ninth intercostal spaces.
- Thoracocentesis for fluid removal is best guided by ultrasonography.
- Strict aseptic technique is ideal.
- Possible contraindications to thoracocentesis include severe coagulopathies, thrombocytopenia, and thrombocytopathia.

The removal of fluid or air by puncturing the chest with a hollow needle, catheter, or tube is called *thoracocentesis,* and it can be used as both a diagnostic tool and a therapeutic intervention.[1] Unlike in the emergent patient, pleural effusions are more common than pneumothorax in the critically ill patient.[1,2] In this patient population, pleural effusion may be due to the primary disease process or may have secondary cardiovascular or iatrogenic causes. In humans, pleural effusions commonly accompany edematous states caused by heart failure or volume overload, pneumonia, or acute respiratory distress syndrome.[2] Thoracocentesis is an easy and potentially lifesaving procedure that every emergency and critical care veterinarian should be able to perform. Several techniques are discussed in this chapter.[3,4]

INDICATIONS

Animals with pleural space disease experience respiratory distress and may show an inward abdominal movement during inspiration.[5,6] On auscultation, decreased lung sounds may be heard unilaterally or bilaterally. Lung sounds are generally decreased in the dorsal lung fields in association with pneumothorax and in the ventral regions of the chest in association with pleural effusion. Other clinical signs such as a heart murmur, distended jugular veins, increased lung sounds, coughing, bowel sounds heard during chest auscultation, or the feeling of missing organs on abdominal palpation might help in the differentiation of pleural space diseases. Thoracic radiography, ultrasonography, echocardiography, and measurement of packed cell volume, total protein, and albumin may further help identify the cause of respiratory distress and the need for thoracocentesis. Thoracocentesis can be an important diagnostic and lifesaving therapeutic intervention in the animal with severe respiratory distress and should not be withheld in the absence of a confirmed diagnosis of pleural space disease.

Indications for thoracocentesis are diagnosis or suspicion of pneumothorax, tension pneumothorax, or pleural effusion.[1,3] Pneumothorax can be traumatic or spontaneous. Pleural effusion can arise from heart failure, inflammation associated with pneumonia, pancreatitis, pyothorax or feline infectious peritonitis, chylothorax, neoplasia, bleeding disorders, trauma, or lung lobe torsion.[2,7] Thoracocentesis is indicated when air or fluid accumulation in the pleural space is believed to be causing or contributing to respiratory difficulties. Diagnostic thoracocentesis in critically ill patients is indicated for pleural effusions that cannot be otherwise explained. Treatment of suspected infectious processes such as feline infectious peritonitis and pyothorax usually includes pleural drainage.[2,3]

Relative contraindications are pleural space diseases that cannot be treated by thoracocentesis. These include pneumomediastinum, diaphragmatic hernia without fluid accumulation, and pleural masses. Other possible contraindications are bleeding disorders and large bullae because they may lead to deterioration of the patient's respiratory status.[1]

MATERIALS

If oxygen supplementation has not already been initiated, oxygen should be administered to all patients before any handling or restraint.[3] Supplies for orotracheal intubation, including a functional strong light source, should be prepared and ready for use when dyspneic patients are handled. The required materials for the procedure should be prepared before handling the patient. Equipment needed for thoracocentesis is listed in Box 198-1.

Thoracocentesis is performed with a needle, peripheral catheter, or flexible tube placed within the pleural space.[1] It is generally recommended that the catheter or needle used be of the smallest gauge possible.[1] For example, to aspirate air, a 22-gauge butterfly needle can be used in cats and small dogs, and an 18-gauge butterfly needle may be effective in medium and large dogs. The catheter size is generally increased for the aspiration of pleural effusions.

Performing thoracocentesis requires a minimum of two, and ideally three, people. One person is needed to restrain and limit patient movement, one to place and stabilize the needle, and one to

BOX 198-1 ***Equipment Needed for Thoracocentesis***

- Clippers
- Surgical preparation solution
- Lidocaine (1% to 2%)
- Gloves (sterile)
- Butterfly needle or over-the-needle catheter or hypodermic needle of appropriate size
- Extension set
- Three-way stopcock
- 10- to 60-ml syringe, depending on patient size and expected amount of fluid or air
- Tubes for fluid analysis (ethylenediaminetetraacetic acid tube, heparin tube, sterile tube for bacterial culture)
- Sterile saline (if the needle technique is used)

aspirate and collect the fluid or air. The person operating the syringe and stopcock needs both hands, so if only two people are available, the person performing the tap and holding the needle in place also must restrain the patient.

TECHNIQUES

The time of intervention has to be coordinated with all members of the team to minimize patient stress. The animal should choose its most comfortable position. Thoracocentesis can be done with the animal standing, sitting, or lying on its side.[3] The region of the tap is clipped and aseptically prepared. The only exception to this is an animal in severe respiratory distress in which the clinical signs do not allow time for surgical preparation. The anatomic site for thoracocentesis should be based on auscultation results, the position of the animal, and the nature of the suspected problem. Blind thoracocentesis is performed at the seventh to ninth intercostal spaces (Figure 198-1, *A*). If a pneumothorax is suspected, then the needle is inserted in the mid to upper thorax.[3] Fluid may be best aspirated in the lower third of the chest, and fluid thoracocentesis should be performed under ultrasonographic guidance whenever possible. When ventral thoracocentesis is performed, care must be taken to avoid the internal thoracic arteries, which run along the ventral thorax a few centimeters to either side of the sternum, because laceration of one of these arteries can result in significant hemorrhage.[3]

Before puncture, the subcutaneous tissue and the pleura can be infiltrated with a local anesthetic such as lidocaine (1 to 2 mg/kg).[1,3] The puncture site should be cranial to the rib or in the middle of the intercostal space to minimize damage to vessels and nerves located caudally to every rib.[1,8]

Several techniques for thoracocentesis have been described.[1,3,4,9,10] Whichever procedure is used, once the needle has entered the pleural space, the entire needle should be placed parallel to the body wall with the bevel directed toward the lung to avoid iatrogenic lung laceration or puncture (see Figure 198-1, *C*).[9] It might be necessary to redirect the needle, however, and this must be done with the length of the needle parallel to the thoracic wall. Once negative pressure is achieved or the lung can be felt scratching at the needle, it is important to stop aspiration and to remove the needle in the flat position to decrease the risk of lung laceration.[7] Usually, the thorax is emptied maximally, which might require bilateral thoracocentesis.

Needle Insertion Techniques

Thoracocentesis using a butterfly needle

In thoracocentesis using a butterfly needle, a three-way stopcock and syringe can be attached before the puncture is performed (see Figure 198-1, *A*). The needle is inserted through the skin and slowly advanced into the pleural space while gentle negative pressure is applied with the syringe (see Figure 198-1, *B*).[4,9] The needle is advanced until either it feels like the pleura has been penetrated or air or fluid can be aspirated. Once the pleural space has been entered, the needle is angled so that it is lying flat against the chest wall (directed caudally or ventrally) with the needle bevel directed away from the chest wall (see Figure 198-1, *C*). Aspiration is performed gently and is stopped if negative pressure is obtained or the lung can be felt scratching against the needle.

The author prefers this technique for thoracocentesis because it is fast and relatively safe. The short needle is an advantage in small animals but might be too short in large dogs. In large dogs, a hypodermic needle connected to an extension set and collection system can be used as an alternative.[3]

Thoracocentesis using a hypodermic needle with a saline-filled hub

In thoracocentesis using a hypodermic needle with saline-filled hub, the hub of the needle is filled with sterile saline and then the needle is slowly advanced through the skin. The needle is advanced until the saline is either sucked inward (which indicates entry into the pleural space) or expelled (which indicates a tension pneumothorax). The needle is then directed caudally. The extension tubing and stopcock are connected to the needle, and aspiration is performed as described earlier.[3]

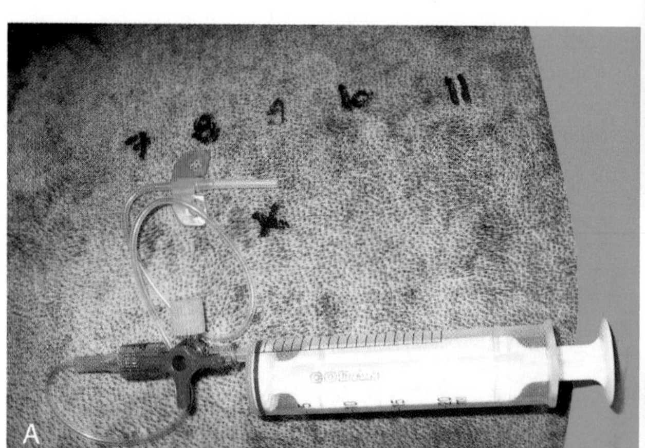

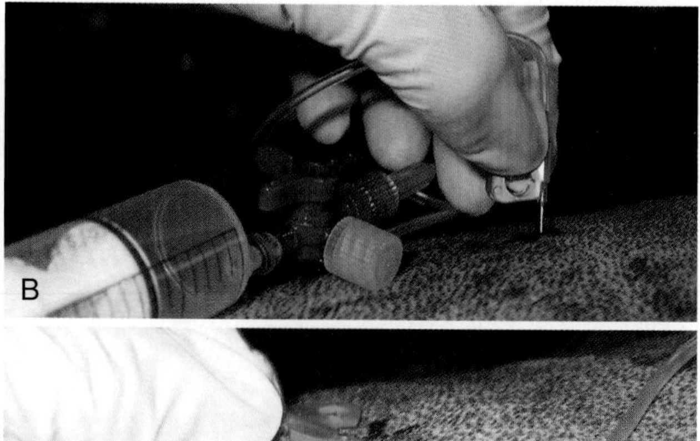

FIGURE 198-1 A, Blind thoracocentesis is performed in the middle or at the caudal border of the seventh, eighth, or ninth intercostal space. The site is clipped and aseptically prepared. A butterfly catheter attached to a three-way stopcock and syringe is pictured. The numbers mark the appropriate rib. **B,** The needle is advanced slowly in a perpendicular fashion. Once the skin is penetrated, 2 to 3 ml of vacuum is applied to the syringe and held constant while the needle is advanced. **C,** Once the pleural space has been entered, air or fluid can be aspirated. At this point, the needle should be angled so that it is lying flat against the chest wall with the bevel directed toward the lung. The needle should be kept parallel to the chest wall during aspiration. Once negative pressure is achieved, the needle is removed in the flat position to decrease risk of lung laceration.

Over-the-Needle Catheter Insertion Technique

Thoracocentesis using an over-the-needle intravenous catheter

Over-the-needle catheters are available in a variety of sizes and lengths and following placement provide a relatively atraumatic option for thoracocentesis. An 18-gauge catheter is recommended for cats and small dogs, a 16-gauge catheter for medium-sized dogs, and a 14-gauge catheter for large dogs. The over-the-needle catheter is advanced through a small relief incision and into the pleural space. Location in the pleural space is confirmed by removal of the stylet and aspiration of fluid or air after connection of the extension tubing and stopcock to the catheter. Alternatively, the extension set can be connected to the stylet and gentle suction applied while the catheter is advanced into the pleural space. When air or fluid is aspirated, which indicates entry into the pleural space, the stylet is retracted a short distance so that the point of the stylet is enclosed within the catheter. The catheter and stylet are then advanced together in a ventral direction as a unit. Once fully inserted, the stylet is removed and the extension set is connected to the catheter.[1] Over-the-needle catheters can be fenestrated with a scalpel blade to improve the ability to aspirate viscous pleural effusions. Care must be taken to make the fenestrations small, evenly spaced, and smooth.

Thoracocentesis using a thoracostomy tube

Commercially available thoracostomy tubes with several holes at the tip can be used for drainage of large amounts of fluid or air. These tubes have a sharp stylet or trochar that can be used to insert the tube into the pleural space. Once the tube enters the pleural cavity, the stylet is held in place and the tube is advanced over the stylet.[2]

Through-the-Needle Catheter Technique

The through-the-needle catheter technique uses a 14- to 18-gauge introducer needle through which a flexible catheter is inserted once the needle enters the pleural space. First the catheter is connected to the extension set, three-way stopcock, and syringe, and then it is set aside. A second syringe is then attached to the empty introducer needle, and gentle suction is applied while the needle is advanced into the pleural space. Once fluid or air can be aspirated, the needle is held in place, the aspiration syringe is detached, and the catheter is inserted quickly through the needle into the pleural space and advanced as far as possible. The needle is then withdrawn from the chest with the catheter left in place.[1]

Seldinger Technique

Use of the Seldinger technique may be indicated to drain large amounts of fluid or air.[11] In this method a guidewire is fed through a needle (similar to the technique described earlier) into the pleural space. The needle is then removed and the guidewire left in place. A flexible catheter with several holes at the tip is then inserted over the guidewire. Once the catheter is inserted into the pleural space the guidewire is removed and the drainage tubing can be connected. This technique can be used for a single thoracocentesis procedure but is more commonly used as a type of indwelling thoracostomy tube.

Diagnostic Evaluation of the Aspirate

The amount of aspirated air or fluid should be measured and diagnostic evaluation of fluid initiated. Measurement of specific gravity, determination of packed cell volume, cell count, total protein measurement, cytologic evaluation, and aerobic and anaerobic culture testing may be indicated.

When there is a negative result on thoracocentesis and strong suspicion of pneumothorax or pleural effusion, it is recommended that the procedure be repeated at another location.

POSTPROCEDURE CARE

Routine thoracic radiographs may not be essential; however, they can be helpful in determining the cause of pleural space disease after fluid or air has been removed. They are also indicated in cases of unsuccessful thoracocentesis. Postprocedure chest radiographs are recommended in human patients who are undergoing mechanical ventilation, and this may be a consideration in veterinary patients as well.[2]

After thoracocentesis, the thorax is auscultated on a regular basis, and respiratory rate and effort are monitored. Thoracocentesis should be repeated whenever the patient's respiratory status deteriorates. If repeat thoracocentesis is necessary, chest tube placement should be considered.

COMPLICATIONS

Thoracocentesis can be associated with a high complication rate in human patients.[2] Pneumothorax and arterial laceration causing hemothorax are the most common complications.[1] The rate of pneumothorax after thoracocentesis has been reported to be as high as 30% in human patients.[2] This rate can be decreased to 0% to 3% by using ultrasonographic guidance when thoracocentesis is performed for pleural effusion.[2] Pneumothorax can occur as a result of laceration of the lung by the needle, introduction of air through the needle or catheter system, puncture of a bulla, or exertion of extreme negative pressure with an nonexpandable lung, leading to pressure-related lung laceration.[1]

Hypotension and reexpansion pulmonary edema may occur if a large volume of fluid or air is evacuated in cases of chronic pleural space disease.[1,2] Vagal reactions have also been reported. Minor complications include formation of a hematoma or seroma at the puncture site. The incidence of complications of thoracocentesis in animals has not been reported.

In the author's opinion, more animals are lost by not doing a thoracocentesis than by performing an unnecessary thoracocentesis, provided appropriate technique is used and asepsis is maintained. Thoracocentesis performed by experienced personnel is a safe, simple, and potentially lifesaving technique.

REFERENCES

1. Blok B, Ibrado A: Thoracocentesis. In Roberts JR, Hedges JR, editors: Clinical procedures in emergency medicine, Philadelphia, 2004, Saunders.
2. Doelken P, Sahn SA: Thoracocentesis. In Fink MP, Abraham E, Vincent JL, et al, editors: Textbook of critical care, Philadelphia, 2006, Saunders.
3. Crowe DT, Devey JJ: Thoracic drainage. In Bojrab MJ, editor: Current techniques in small animal surgery, ed 4, Baltimore, 1998, Williams & Wilkins.
4. Orton C: Pleural drainage. In Orton C, editor: Small animal thoracic surgery, ed 1, Baltimore, 1995, Williams & Wilkins.
5. Sigrist N, Adamik K, Doherr M, et al: Evaluation of respiratory parameters at presentation as clinical indicators of respiratory location in dogs and cats with respiratory distress, J Vet Emerg Crit Care 21:13-23, 2011.
6. Le Boedet K, Arnaud C, Chetboul V, et al: Relationship between paradoxical breathing and pleural diseases in dyspnoeic dogs and cats: 389 cases (2001-2009), J Am Vet Med Assoc 240:1095-1099, 2012.
7. Orton C: Pleural effusion. In Orton C, editor: Small animal thoracic surgery, ed 1, Baltimore, 1995, Williams & Wilkins.
8. Da Rocha RP, Vengjer A, Blanco A, et al: Size of the collateral intercostal artery in adults: anatomical considerations in relation to thoracocentesis and thoracoscopy, Surg Radiol Anat 24:23, 2002.
9. Hansen B: Therapeutic thoracocentesis: butterfly catheter, Atlantic Coast Veterinary Conference, Atlantic City, NJ, October, 2005.
10. Hackett T, Mazzaferro E: Veterinary emergency and critical care procedures, ed 1, Ames, Ia, 2006, Blackwell.
11. Kirsch TD, Mulligan P: Tube thoracostomy. In Roberts JR, Hedges JR, editors: Clinical procedures in emergency medicine, Philadelphia, 2004, Saunders.

CHAPTER 199

THORACOSTOMY TUBE PLACEMENT AND DRAINAGE

Nadja E. Sigrist, DrMedVet, FVH, DACVECC

KEY POINTS

- Chest tubes are used to remove air or fluid from the pleural space.
- The diameter of a chest tube should be similar to the size of the mainstem bronchus. Smaller-diameter tubes can be used for a simple pneumothorax; larger-diameter tubes are used to drain viscous fluid such as purulent exudate.
- Chest tubes are best inserted with the animal anesthetized and intubated. Sedation and local anesthesia may be sufficient in some cases.
- Several tubes and placement techniques exist.
- Thoracic radiography is recommended following tube placement.
- Suction can occur on a continuous or intermittent basis.
- Patients with chest tubes need 24-hour monitoring.
- Strict aseptic placement and management are required.

Therapeutic drainage of the pleural space dates back more than 200 years, and the technique of thoracostomy tube placement for various indications has been adapted and perfected since then.[1] Thoracostomy tubes, also known as *chest tubes* or *thoracic drains,* are used to evacuate air or fluid or both from the pleural space. The reader is also referred to Chapter 198 for a discussion of thoracocentesis. In many cases, tube thoracostomy can be lifesaving. Successful use of the technique, however, requires familiarity with pulmonary and pleural anatomy and physiology. Indications, insertion technique, maintenance, and complications are discussed in this chapter.

INDICATIONS

The purpose of a chest tube is the removal of air or fluid from the pleural space to relieve pulmonary collapse and restore pleural subatmospheric pressure. Pneumothorax and pleural effusion are usually managed initially with thoracocentesis, which can be repeated several times (see Chapter 198). Placement of a thoracostomy tube should be considered if repeated thoracocentesis is required for ongoing air leakage or fluid production, if thoracocentesis is insufficient because of the severity of the disease (e.g., tension pneumothorax), if ongoing fluid production is expected (e.g., chylothorax), if suction as well as lavage is planned (e.g., pyothorax), or if the patient has just undergone thoracic surgery (Box 199-1).[2-6]

In a patient in an unstable condition with ongoing pneumothorax or pleural effusion, there are no absolute contraindications to thoracostomy tube placement. Relative contraindications in patients in stable condition are coagulopathies or pleural adhesions.[2]

THORACOSTOMY TUBE PLACEMENT

Materials

Numerous thoracostomy tubes are commercially available. The tubes come in various sizes and materials. Each has its advantages and disadvantages in terms of material, price, and tissue compatibility.[7]

Thoracostomy tubes are available as single tubes and complete thoracostomy kits. Other tubes can be modified to perform as thoracostomy tubes; however, several criteria must be fulfilled. The tube must be sterile, must elicit minimal tissue reaction in situ, must have multiple fenestrations at the distal end, and must be able to withstand the generation of negative pressure during suctioning without collapsing.[8-10] A radiopaque line along the tube helps identify its position on radiographs. Most commercially available chest tubes come with a stylet to aid insertion into the pleural space and may have an open or closed end.

Adapters such as Christmas tree connectors, tubing with a Luer-Lock fitting, a noncollapsing extension set, and a three-way stopcock are used to connect the tube to the suction device. It is advisable to have a tube thoracostomy set available in the "ready area" of the hospital (Box 199-2).[2]

A key to chest tube size selection is the flow rate of either air or liquid that can be accommodated by the tube.[7] This depends on the diameter and length of the tube and the viscosity and rate of formation of the fluid. In humans, chest tube size is selected based on what type of lung disease is present and whether mechanical ventilation is required. Pleural drainage catheter flow capabilities vary significantly.[7]

Generally chest tube size is chosen with consideration of the nature of the pleural disease and the width of the patient's intercostal space. An unnecessarily large chest tube is likely to be associated

BOX 199-1 ***Indications for Thoracostomy Tube Placement***

- Tension pneumothorax
- Ongoing pneumothorax despite repeated thoracocentesis
- Pyothorax
- Rapidly reoccurring chylothorax
- Penetrating chest injury
- After thoracic surgery
- Performance of pleurodesis

BOX 199-2 ***Tube Thoracostomy Emergency Set***

- Instrument set with hemostat, straight Kelly or Carmalt clamp, forceps, needle holder, scalpel holder, suture scissors, tube clamp
- No. 10 and 15 scalpel blades
- Two 30-cm extension sets
- Two three-way stopcocks
- Christmas tree adapters, two of each size
- 20- and 50-ml syringes, one of each
- Thoracostomy tube of appropriate size
- Sterile gauze
- 3-0 and 1-0 monofilament suture

with increased pain and discomfort. Aspiration of pleural effusion, especially pyothorax, generally is aided by a larger tube diameter to remove clots, cell debris, and fibrin, but thoracostomy tubes for drainage of a pneumothorax do not need to be of maximal diameter.

Anesthesia

Patients requiring chest tube placement should receive supplemental oxygen and should be preoxygenated for anesthesia induction.[2] Analgesia is maintained by infiltration of a local anesthetic at the site of insertion, regional nerve block, or general anesthesia including analgesics.[10] Animals can be sedated; however, the author prefers general anesthesia with the animal intubated to control ventilation and oxygenation. Use of a rapid induction protocol is recommended[10] (see Chapters 142 and 143). If possible, thoracocentesis is performed under local anesthesia before chest tube placement to make the animal a better anesthesia candidate.

Before sedatives or anesthetics are administered, all materials should be ready and the chest wall should be clipped if the animal will tolerate it with minimal stress. Maintaining the animal in sternal recumbency during the procedure may be necessary to avoid respiratory compromise.

Techniques

Thoracostomy tube placement can be classified as either closed or open.[11] The key point in placement is the generation of a subcutaneous tunnel between the skin incision and the point of entry into the pleural space to create an airtight seal around the tube.[8]

Strict aseptic practices are required with all techniques.[1] The lateral thorax is clipped from behind the scapula to the last rib and surgically prepared. The animal ideally is placed in lateral recumbency, provided ventilation and oxygenation are sufficient in this position. Once the area is prepared and appropriate anesthesia or analgesia has been provided, the area is draped. The supplies, including tube, adapter, and suction device as well as a small surgery pack, should already be prepared.

Several techniques exist for closed placement of a chest tube.[2,8,9,11,12] The author prefers the following (Figure 199-1).[8,12] This technique can be used for tubes with trochars and tubes without. The skin over the lateral chest is pulled cranially by an assistant. While the skin is held in this position the appropriate intercostal space is identified, usually the seventh, eighth, or ninth. The length of tube to insert into the thorax is estimated at this time by holding the chest tube alongside the chest with the tip aligned to the second rib, without compromising sterility. A small skin incision, slightly larger than the diameter of the tube, is made overlying the desired intercostal space midway between the dorsal midline and the center of the lateral thorax. The subcutaneous tissue and muscle layers are bluntly dissected with a hemostat. The pleura is then penetrated bluntly using a large hemostat or Carmalt forceps (see Figure 199-1, *A*). During this maneuver, the anesthetist is asked to stop ventilation to minimize injury to the lung.[13] Also, injury to the underlying organs is minimized by holding the hemostat close to the tip with the nondominant hand to avoid overpenetration.

Once the pleura is penetrated, the tips of the hemostat are opened, which creates an opening for the thoracostomy tube (see Figure

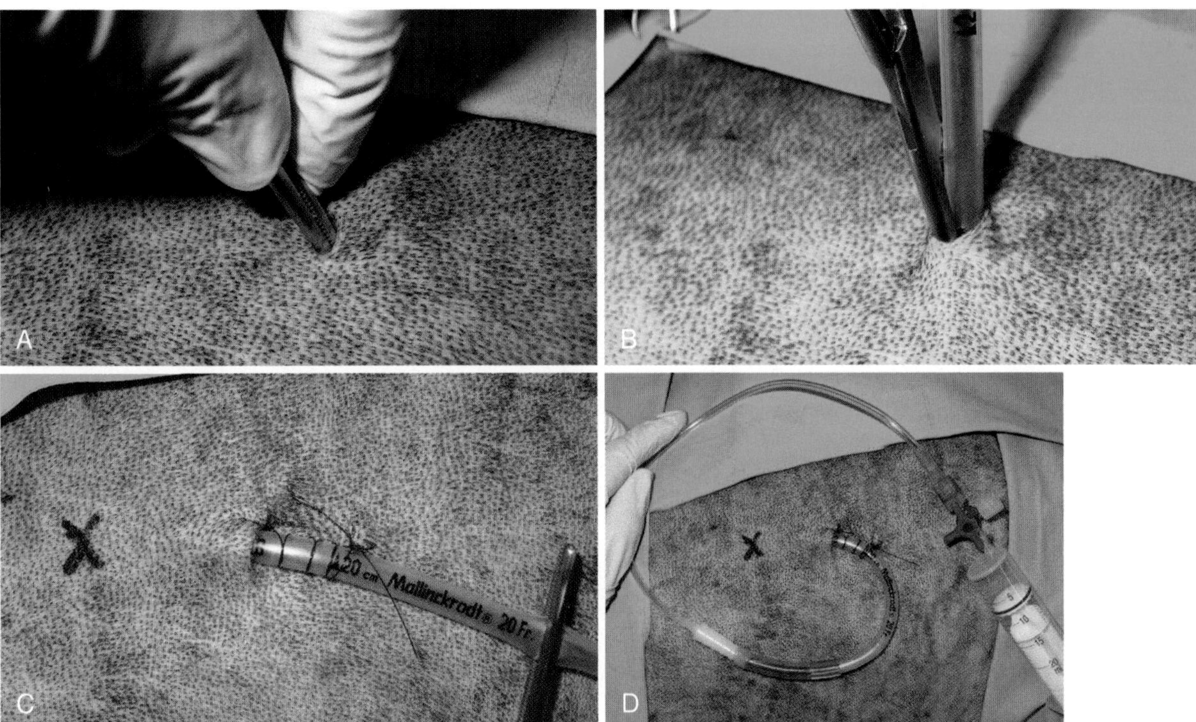

FIGURE 199-1 Thoracostomy tube placement. **A,** While the skin is pulled cranially by an assistant, a skin incision slightly larger than the tube diameter is made, followed by blunt dissection of the subcutaneous tissue and muscles using a hemostat. **B,** To penetrate the pleura, the hemostat or carmalt is held near the tip to prevent overpenetration, and ventilation is stopped. After penetration of the pleura, the tips of the clamp are opened to create an opening for the thoracostomy tube. **C,** The tube is inserted through the opening and advanced toward the uppermost elbow. The stylet can then be removed, and the tube is clamped with a tube clamp. Releasing the skin creates the subcutaneous tunnel (*X* marks the pleural entrance of the tube). The tube is secured to the skin (and the rib periosteum if desired) using a finger-trap suture pattern. **D,** An extension set and three-way stopcock are connected to the thoracostomy tube, and negative pressure is achieved by suctioning with a syringe.

199-1, *B*). Before insertion, the trochar (if present) can be retracted slightly so that the sharp tip is protected by the tube. The tip of the tube is introduced into the thorax and is then advanced toward the uppermost elbow. Once the tip of the tube is well inside the thorax, the hemostat can be removed. The thoracostomy tube should be inserted so that the tip is roughly at the level of the second rib. It is essential that all tube fenestrations be within the thoracic cavity.[2] The stylet is then withdrawn and the tube clamp (Carmalt forceps if a tube clamp not available) can be used to clamp off the tube.

Alternatively, the tube can be connected directly to the suction device. As the skin is released and retracts caudally over the tube, a subcutaneous tunnel is created. The Mac technique can be used to rule out kinking of the tube: the tube is twisted 180 degrees in each direction and then released. If the tube spins back into its position, this is indicative of kinking.[14] Depending on the urgency of pleural evacuation, suction is instituted before or after securing the tube. A purse-string suture is placed around the skin incision if the fit is not firm. The tube is then fixed using a finger-trap suture pattern.[15] A single interrupted suture is placed through the skin at the site of insertion. This suture may pass through the periosteum of the rib (this requires additional local anesthetic) and is tied in a gentle loop, leaving equal and long suture tags. The sutures tags are used to create the finger-trap pattern by placing a single knot on top of the tube, crossing underneath the tube and then placing another single knot on top of the tube, and so on. After four to six finger traps, the tube is once more anchored to the skin, which minimizes the chance of dislocation (see Figure 199-1, *C*). The tube is then connected to the suction system of choice.

The insertion site is covered with sterile gauze, and a bandage is applied to secure the thoracostomy tube to the chest wall and minimize risk of accidental removal.[8]

If no assistant is available to pull the skin forward, the subcutaneous tunnel can be made with a large hemostat or Carmalt forceps. The skin incision is made more caudally (eighth to tenth intercostal space), and the hemostat is tunneled cranially through the subcutaneous tissues by the length of two intercostal spaces to the desired insertion point at the level of the sixth to eighth intercostal space. Then the pleural space is entered and the tube is inserted as described earlier.[2,11]

A thoracostomy tube with a sharp-ended stylet can be placed without the aid of a hemostat[11]; however, the technique of perforating the pleura by punching the distal end of the stylet is not recommended because of increased risk of injury to intrathoracic organs. A combination of blunt dissection through the intercostal space with hemostats and penetration of the pleura with the stylet is preferable.

An alternative for thoracostomy tube placement is the Seldinger technique.[2,16] In this technique the tube is advanced into the thorax with the use of a guidewire that has been inserted through a small needle. After the needle is removed, the guidewire stays in place and the modified tube is advanced over the wire. Once the tube is placed, the guidewire is removed and the tube is secured as described earlier. Care is taken not to compromise the lumen of the catheter with the finger-trap suture. The Seldinger technique has the advantage of requiring a smaller incision using a small-bore tube; it might therefore be less painful and leakage is less likely. Reported complications with small-bore tubes include malpositioning, kinking, and obstruction of the tube.[16]

Open insertion of a thoracostomy tube is performed during thoracotomy, with the advantage that the tube is placed safely under direct visualization. Under certain circumstances, such as when an animal has an open penetrating chest injury, a thoracostomy tube can be inserted directly into the thoracic cavity through the wound. The wound is then sealed with a nonadhesive dressing and the thorax is evacuated immediately. Proper wound débridement and lavage and placement of a new and sterile thoracostomy tube are required as soon as the patient is in stable enough condition for anesthesia.

DRAINAGE

After placement of a thoracostomy tube, negative pressure is generated by manual aspiration or a continuous suction apparatus. The smallest number of connections should be used because they are potential sites for leaks. Cable ties are recommended to secure all connections. Too much negative pressure should be avoided because it can lead to lung tissue trauma and occlusion of the tube by mediastinal or pleural tissue. The normal difference between the pleural pressure and the intraalveolar pressure is 4 to 8 mm Hg, which translates to 5 to 10 ml of vacuum in a syringe.[11]

A thoracic radiography is recommended to confirm proper tube placement, evaluate expansion of the lung, and identify residual pleural fluid or air.[2] Tubes that are kinked or tubes that are not placed between the chest wall and the lung should be partly removed and redirected (only if sterility will not be compromised). Insertion as far as the thoracic inlet might cause extensive pain, and in this case the tube should be pulled back to the level of the second rib.

Further drainage is accomplished using either intermittent or continuous suction. The method used depends on the nature of the pleural space disease and equipment available.[2,8,17,18] In veterinary patients, intermittent manual syringe aspiration every 1 to 6 hours is sufficient in many cases and allows for adequate drainage and maintenance of negative pleural pressure.[11]

Passive Drainage Techniques

Passive drainage of the pleural space relies on the increased intrathoracic pressure generated during exhalation in a spontaneously breathing patient to force air or fluid from the pleural space. Alternatively, in patients undergoing positive pressure ventilation pleural drainage occurs during the inspiratory phase. These techniques generally are not as effective as active drainage and are more suited to mild pleural space disease. Interestingly, in one human study the use of passive drainage following thoracoscopy for spontaneous pneumothorax led to more rapid recovery than the use of active thoracic drainage techniques.[19] Human patients usually are more comfortable with passive drainage than with active drainage. Passive drainage is also enhanced by keeping the patient higher than the drainage apparatus; this may not be possible for larger veterinary patients.

Passive drainage can be achieved with a simple one-bottle water seal (Figure 199-2, *A*) or with a Heimlich valve. Heimlich valves are one-way flutter valves that can be attached to chest tubes to allow pleural air to be expelled during exhalation (if the patient is breathing spontaneously) but prevent entrainment of air into the pleural space during inspiration.[2] They provide a simple and inexpensive option for drainage but are effective only in the management of relatively mild pneumothoraces and are prone to malfunction. The Heimlich valve can be occluded readily by secretions, which may be a life-threatening complication, and constant monitoring is required.

Active Drainage Techniques

In patients with continuous air leaks or severe fluid accumulation, continuous active suction may be necessary. Continuous suction may also allow sustained lung expansion and better healing of leaks by pleural adhesion. Continuous suction requires a water seal between the suction pump and the chest tube; this can be achieved with a two-chamber or three-chamber suction apparatus.[2]

The three-chamber water seal suction apparatus is recommended. These devices are commercially available or can be constructed using three bottles (Figure 199-2, *B*).[2,18] A suction pressure of 10 to 20 cm

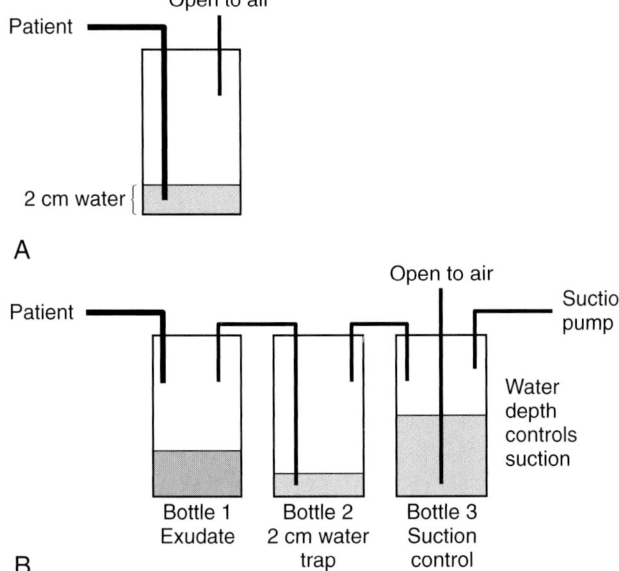

FIGURE 199-2 A, Single-bottle suction apparatus. This single-bottle system acts as both a water seal and a collection chamber so that the depth of liquid may increase with time, which reduces effective drainage. This system is for passive drainage only. Bubbling is evidence of air drainage from the pleural space. **B,** Three-bottle suction apparatus. The three-bottle system has a collection bottle, a water trap, and suction-control bottle. It allows the suction level to be regulated by changing the water depth in bottle 3. There is a water seal so that suction can be turned off without worry that air will leak back into the pleural space. The exudates in bottle 1 can be evaluated and emptied independently. The water trap will bubble if air is evacuated from the pleural space.

H_2O is used.[2,9] This is achieved by filling the third chamber (connected directly to the suction pump) with water to a depth of 10 to 20 cm. The central chamber is the water seal, which is achieved by submerging the tubing entering the second bottle in 2 to 3 cm of water. The first chamber is connected to the chest tube and collects fluid aspirated from the thorax. Pleural effusion can be quantitated by measuring the fluid accumulation in the first chamber. Ongoing air production from a pneumothorax is evidenced by bubbles in the central water seal container. With persistent air leakage, continuous suction may be necessary for several days. If intrapleural air continues to accumulate after more than 2 to 5 days, surgical exploration of the thoracic cavity may be indicated.[2,6,20]

If at any time negative pressure cannot be achieved despite continual aspiration, the tubing should be checked for air leaks, and all adaptors and three-way stopcocks should be checked and replaced in a sequential manner.

MAINTENANCE AND CARE

Strict aseptic care is required. Antibiotic prophylaxis is controversial and depends mostly on the circumstances in which the tube was placed and the animal's underlying disease.[1,21] Prophylactic antibiotics may be indicated in people if thoracostomy tubes are placed because of chest trauma.[22] Thoracostomy tubes increase the risk of nosocomial infections after thoracic surgery in humans.[23]

Bandages should be changed at least daily, and tubing should be wrapped to prevent accidental removal by the animal. A tubing clamp can be placed in addition to the three-way stopcock if the tube is not being aspirated. It is essential that the animal be prevented from damaging the tube, and use of an Elizabethan collar may be required in some cases.

Animals with thoracostomy tubes need 24-hour monitoring. Respiratory rate and effort are checked on a regular basis, and other vital parameters are monitored based on the patient's problem(s). Analgesia is best provided by a combination of intravenous analgesia and administration of local anesthetics through the chest tube (see Chapter 144).

REMOVAL

The decision to remove a chest tube depends on the rate of fluid production or air accumulation in the pleural space. As a general guideline, no air should be retrieved for 24 hours before tube removal. Tube removal can be considered if fluid production falls to less than 2 ml/kg/day.[8] In humans, thoracostomy tubes are removed if daily fluid aspiration is less than 150 to 200 ml.[2,24] Exceptions are patients with septic exudates and those in which the thoracostomy tube is used for lavage. In dogs with spontaneous pneumothorax that require chest tubes, the tubes are left in for an average of 4.5 days (range, 1 to 8 days).[11,25]

Thoracic ultrasound and/or radiography is recommended before tube removal to ensure that the pleural space disease has truly resolved. Tube occlusion or displacement can lead to negative aspiration results despite persistent pleural space disease.[2] Studies in humans recommend routine chest radiography after thoracostomy tube removal only if clinical signs of respiratory distress are present.[26]

For removal, the tube is smoothly withdrawn and a nonadherent pad is pressed firmly over the exit site. A light bandage is applied and the incision is allowed to heal by second intention.

COMPLICATIONS

The most common complication of percutaneous thoracostomy is improper placement.[27] Other complications include hemorrhage, infection, visceral injury, and reexpansion pulmonary edema.[28] In human medicine, the complication rate is between 20% and 30% and depends on the experience of the operator.[29,30]

REFERENCES

1. Watson GA, Harbrecht BG: Chest tube placement, care, and removal. In Fink MP, Abraham E, Vincent JL, et al, editors: Textbook of critical care, Philadelphia, 2006, Saunders.
2. Kirsch TD, Mulligan P: Tube thoracostomy. In Roberts JR, Hedges JR, editors: Clinical procedures in emergency medicine, Philadelphia, 2004, Saunders.
3. Scott JA, Macintire DK: Canine pyothorax: clinical presentation, diagnosis, and treatment, Compend Contin Educ Vet Pract 25:180, 2003.
4. Orton C: Pleural effusion. In Orton C, editor: Small animal thoracic surgery, ed 1, Baltimore, 1995, Williams & Wilkins.
5. Turner W, Breznock E: Continuous suction drainage for treatment of canine pyothorax: a retrospective study, J Am Anim Hosp Assoc 24:485, 1988.
6. Yoshioka M: Treatment of spontaneous pneumothorax in 12 dogs, J Am Anim Hosp Assoc 18:57, 1982.
7. Baumann MH: What size chest tube? What drainage system is ideal? And other chest tube treatment questions, Curr Opin Pulm Med 9:276, 2003.
8. Crowe DT, Devey JJ: Thoracic drainage. In Bojrab MJ, editors: Current techniques in small animals, Baltimore, 1997, Williams & Wilkins.
9. Orton C: Pleural drainage. In Orton C, editor: Small animal thoracic surgery, ed 1, Baltimore, 1995, Williams & Wilkins.
10. Tillson DM: Thoracostomy tubes. Part I. Indications and anesthesia, Compend Contin Educ Vet Pract 19:1258, 1997.
11. Tillson DM: Thoracostomy tubes. Part II. Placement and maintenance, Compend Contin Educ Vet Pract 19:1331, 1997.

12. Hackett TB, Mazzaferro EM: Thoracocentesis and thoracostomy tube placement. In Veterinary emergency and critical care procedures, ed 1, Ames, Ia, 2006, Blackwell.
13. Peek GJ, Firmin RK, Arsiwala S: Chest tube insertion in the ventilated patient, Injury 26:425, 1995.
14. Adame N Jr, Horwood BT, Caruso D, et al: A test to detect chest tube kinking, Acad Emerg Med 13:114, 2006.
15. Smeak D: The Chinese finger-trap suture technique for fastening tubes and catheters, J Am Anim Hosp Assoc 26:215, 1990.
16. Valtolina C, Adamantos S: Evaluation of small-bore wire guided chest drains for management of pleural space disease, J Small Anim Pract 50:290-297, 2009.
17. Cerfolio RJ, Bryant AS, Singh S, et al: The treatment of chest tubes in patients with a pneumothorax and an air leak after pulmonary resection, Chest 128:816, 2005.
18. Fossum TW: Surgery of the lower respiratory system: pleural cavity and diaphragm. In Fossum TW, editor: Small animal surgery, Philadelphia, 2004, Mosby.
19. Ayed AK: Suction versus water seal after thoracoscopy for primary spontaneous pneumothorax: prospective randomized study, Ann Thorac Surg 75:1593, 2003.
20. Boudrieau R, Fossum T, Birchard S: Surgical correction of primary pneumothorax in a dog, J Am Vet Med Assoc 186:75, 1985.
21. Luchette FA, Barrie PS, Oswanski MF, et al: Practice treatment guidelines for prophylactic antibiotic use in tube thoracostomy for traumatic hemopneumothorax: the EAST practice treatment guidelines work group, J Trauma 48:753, 2000.
22. Gonzalez RP, Holevar MR: Role of prophylactic antibiotics for tube thoracostomy in chest trauma, Am Surg 64:617, 1998.
23. El Masri MM, Hammad TA, McLeskey SW, et al: Predictors of nosocomial bloodstream infections among critically ill adult trauma patients, Infect Control Hosp Epidemiol 25:656, 2004.
24. Younes RN, Gross JL, Aguiar S, et al: When to remove a chest tube? A randomized study with subsequent prospective consecutive validation, J Am Coll Surg 195:658, 2002.
25. Valentine A, Smeak D, Allen D, et al: Spontaneous pneumothorax in dogs, Compend Contin Educ Vet Pract 18:53, 1996.
26. Pacharn P, Heller DN, Kammen BF, et al: Are chest radiographs routinely necessary following thoracostomy tube removal? Pediatr Radiol 32:138, 2002.
27. Deneuville M: Morbidity of percutaneous tube thoracostomy in trauma patients, Eur J Cardiothorac Surg 22:673, 2002.
28. Swain FR, Martinez F, Gripp M, et al: Traumatic complications from placement of thoracic catheters and tubes, Emerg Radiol 12:11, 2005.
29. Etoch SW, Bar-Natan MF, Miller FB, et al: Tube thoracostomy. Factors related to complications, Arch Surg 130:521, 1995.
30. Bailey RC: Complications of tube thoracostomy in trauma, J Accid Emerg Med 17:111, 2000.

CHAPTER 200

ABDOMINOCENTESIS AND DIAGNOSTIC PERITONEAL LAVAGE

Karl E. Jandrey, DVM, MAS, DACVECC

KEY POINTS

- The focused assessment with sonography for trauma (FAST) protocol is a rapid and simple technique to detect free abdominal fluid. A needle paracentesis may be successful if directed at these identified areas.
- A blind needle paracentesis may yield peritoneal fluid when a volume of 5.2 to 6.6 ml/kg or more of abdominal fluid is present.
- Complications of abdominocentesis include the introduction or spread of infection, laceration of a viscus, and hemorrhage from a punctured vessel or organ.
- The use of a peritoneal dialysis catheter for abdominocentesis may allow the detection of 1.0 to 4.4 ml/kg of abdominal fluid.
- Significant hemorrhage is present if the packed cell volume of the peritoneal fluid exceeds 5% when the diagnostic peritoneal lavage technique is used.

Abdominal disease can have life-threatening consequences, and in some cases surgical intervention is essential. The clinical challenge is to determine when surgery is indicated because abdominal signs are commonly vague and nonspecific. Serial physical examinations are the most informative portion of the diagnostic evaluation of an emergency or intensive care patient with abdominal disease. Increasing abdominal size and progressive pain can be important clues for intraabdominal injury. Consequently, the abdominal girth at the umbilical level should be measured soon after admission. This baseline measurement can be used to assess subsequent changes. Abdominal rigidity and tenderness are also important clinical signs of peritoneal irritation by blood or intestinal contents. Although physical examination findings can help in the discovery of abdominal disease, they do not further a diagnosis. Samples of peritoneal fluid obtained by abdominocentesis or diagnostic peritoneal lavage, however, may yield the specific diagnosis of an abdominal disease process and lead to directed and specific therapy.

INDICATIONS

Indications for abdominocentesis are (1) radiographic loss of serosal detail; (2) abdominal injury without obvious peritoneal entry wounds; (3) shock, multiple injuries, or signs of abdominal injury after blunt trauma; (4) head or spinal injury precluding reliable abdominal examination; (5) persistent abdominal pain or fluid distention of unknown cause; (6) postoperative complications possibly caused by leakage from an enterotomy or anastomotic site.[1] Periumbilical ecchymosis (Cullen's sign) may indicate hemorrhage in the peritoneum or retroperitoneum. Abdominocentesis may also be performed to relieve abdominal distention and abdominal hypertension due to ascites. Contraindications to abdominocentesis include coagulopathy, organomegaly, or distention of an abdominal viscus. Intestinal or uterine penetration is rare unless the viscus is dilated and adherent to the abdominal wall.[2] Complications include the introduction or spread of infection, laceration of a viscus, and hemorrhage from a punctured vessel. Adhering to the techniques described in this chapter will reduce the risk of complications.

Focused Assessment with Sonography for Trauma

A study that evaluated the use of the focused assessment with sonography for trauma (FAST) protocol in dogs demonstrated that it is a rapid and simple technique for the detection of free abdominal fluid in the emergency department by veterinary clinicians with minimal previous ultrasound experience.[3] In this technique four regions of the abdomen are scanned in longitudinal and transverse planes with the animal in lateral recumbency. These regions are areas where fluid accumulation more commonly occurs: caudal to the xiphoid process, midline over the urinary bladder, and each flank (see Chapter 189).

TECHNIQUE

Abdominocentesis is performed using a single-paracentesis or four-quadrant approach. Single paracentesis can be done using an open- or a closed-needle technique. Use of ultrasound guidance (such as the FAST technique) can highlight a smaller accumulation of fluid and allow for a more directed approach for abdominocentesis.

Preparation of the Patient

Positioning of the patient in left lateral recumbency may be most effective to avoid puncture of the spleen. Restraint may be accomplished manually or with the use of sedatives and analgesics. Before the abdomen is penetrated, a wide surgical clip is performed and the site is prepared using aseptic technique along the ventral midline centered at the umbilicus (Figure 200-1). If abdominal ultrasonography has identified a focal area of peritoneal fluid accumulation, performing a standard aseptic clip and preparation at that location is appropriate.

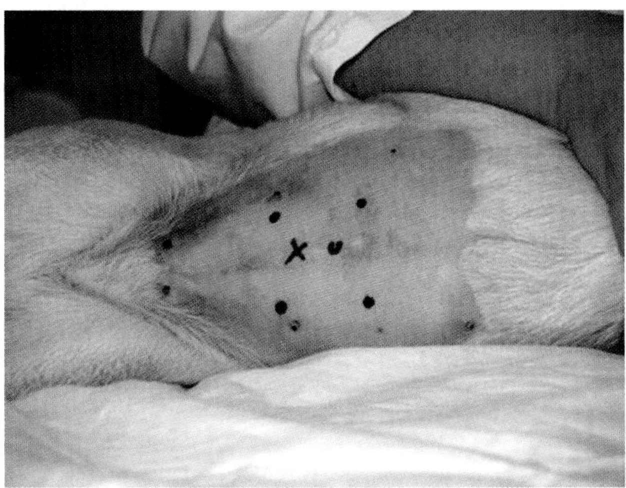

FIGURE 200-1 The patient is placed in left lateral recumbency and is clipped widely centered at the umbilicus *(U).* The X shows the location for a single abdominocentesis or diagnostic peritoneal lavage. The small dots show the sites for a four-quadrant abdominocentesis.

Closed-Needle Abdominocentesis

A closed-needle diagnostic abdominocentesis can be completed using a 20- or 22-gauge needle attached to a syringe or connected to an extension set attached to a 6- or 12-ml syringe. Local anesthetic (2% lidocaine) may be infused at the abdominocentesis site. With the animal in left lateral recumbency, penetration of the abdominal cavity can be completed in the right cranial quadrant caudal to the edges of the liver because peritoneal fluid is gravity dependent and the falciform fat may extend along the midline to the umbilicus. The needle is inserted gently and completely at this site, and further movement of the needle tip should be avoided to prevent laceration of internal structures. Fluid is withdrawn and observed for clots if the fluid is hemorrhagic. Fluid within the abdominal cavity should not clot; hemorrhagic fluid obtained from puncture of the spleen, liver, or any vessel is expected to clot readily. If the fluid sample clots, the needle is removed and abdominocentesis is attempted in another location. Cytologic and biochemical analysis and culture of the abdominal fluid, as indicated, should be completed immediately after fluid removal.

A closed-needle abdominocentesis technique may also be used for therapeutic removal of peritoneal fluid. Instead of a needle, a large-gauge over-the-needle catheter (14 to 18 gauge) can be used, which may allow greater fluid retrieval and lessen the risk of laceration of internal structures. Therapeutic removal of large volumes of fluid may be indicated if the abdominal distention impairs diaphragmatic motion, increases intraabdominal pressure and thus impedes blood flow to the visceral organs, or is painful for the patient. To maintain a closed system, a three-way stopcock can be placed between the syringe and extension set. Another extension set placed on the stopcock can be directed into a bowl or graduated cylinder. Free gas should not be evident on radiographs after a closed-needle abdominocentesis.

Open-Needle Abdominocentesis

An open-needle abdominocentesis is completed in a similar fashion except that the needle alone is inserted into the peritoneal cavity. Fluid from the peritoneum is allowed to flow freely through the needle into a container or a sample submission tube. Rotation of the hub of the needle may facilitate flow. This technique helps prevent occlusion with or aspiration of omentum or intestinal viscera. False-negative results are more likely to occur if suction is applied.[4] The appearance of free abdominal gas on radiographs is possible after this procedure.

Four-Quadrant Abdominocentesis

A modification of the open-needle technique is the four-quadrant abdominocentesis. Instead of one open needle, four open needles are placed simultaneously—one in each quadrant surrounding the umbilicus. Gravity dependency or changes in transabdominal pressure between the needles may increase the likelihood of obtaining fluid. One study in dogs showed that fluid was recovered in 78 of 100 needle paracenteses when 5.2 to 6.6 ml of abdominal fluid per kilogram of body weight was present.[5]

Alternatives to Abdominocentesis

The use of a peritoneal dialysis catheter for abdominocentesis has been shown to detect 1.0 to 4.4 ml of abdominal fluid per kilogram body weight.[6] Its larger diameter and multiple fenestrations make this apparatus more reliable than a standard needle or catheter for detecting smaller volumes of peritoneal fluid. Commercial peritoneal dialysis catheters work well, but over-the-needle catheters can be fenestrated and employed with good results. The use of a 14- or 16-gauge over-the-needle catheter fenestrated manually with a

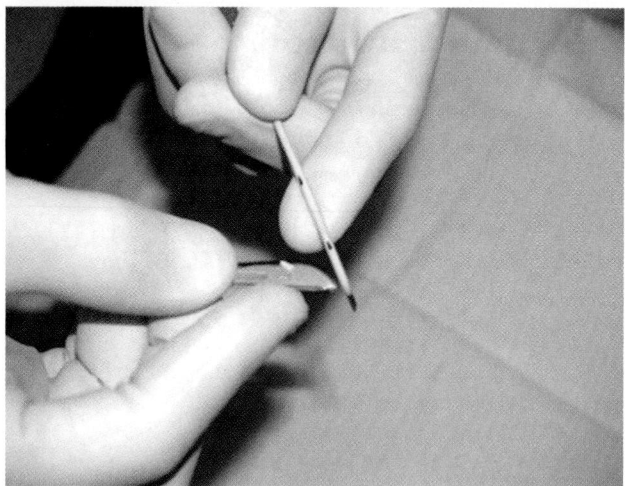

FIGURE 200-2 Use of an over-the-needle catheter with manually created fenestrations increases the surface area for drainage. It is important to make a few small, smooth fenestrations. Fenestrations should not be placed opposite each other on the catheter.

BOX 200-1 ***Supplies Needed for a Diagnostic Peritoneal Lavage***

- Clippers
- Surgical antiseptic scrub
- Peritoneal dialysis catheter *or* 14- to 16-gauge over-the-needle catheter
- No. 11 scalpel blade
- 2% Lidocaine
- Fluid administration set
- 22 ml/kg warm 0.9% saline

No. 10 scalpel blade can increase the surface area for drainage (Figure 200-2). Fenestrations should be small and smooth. Fenestrations should not be too numerous or placed opposite each other on the catheter; this weakens the integrity of the catheter so that a piece of the catheter may break off during removal and remain below the skin or inside the abdomen. The use of a fenestrated catheter increases the likelihood of fluid collection compared with needle abdominocentesis alone.[7]

Diagnostic peritoneal lavage (DPL) is performed when alternative diagnostic methods such as sonography are unavailable or when the patient's condition does not allow other diagnostics or imaging to be performed. Supplies needed to complete a DPL include local anesthetic, scalpel blades, a fluid administration set, and sterile warm 0.9% sodium chloride for infusion (Box 200-1). Patient positioning in left lateral recumbency may be most effective to avoid puncture of the spleen. Administration of sedatives and analgesics increases patient comfort and compliance. Before the abdomen is penetrated, a wide surgical clip is performed and the site is prepared using aseptic technique along the ventral midline centered about the umbilicus. Local anesthetic (2% lidocaine) is infused at the puncture site, either at the umbilicus or 2 to 3 cm lateral to the umbilicus to avoid the falciform fat. A small stab incision is made in the skin with a No. 11 scalpel blade at the site of local anesthetic infusion. A commercial dialysis catheter is introduced through the incision and advanced completely into the abdomen. Slow, gentle rotation of the closed-end dialysis catheter is needed to overcome considerable resistance from fascial planes and the linea alba. If a fenestrated over-the-needle catheter is used, the catheter is advanced completely off the stylet once the tip of the catheter has penetrated the peritoneal cavity. A syringe may be attached to the catheter at this point. If no peritoneal fluid is obtained, saline is infused into the abdomen through the catheter. A volume of 22 ml/kg of warm, sterile 0.9% sodium chloride solution is infused by gravity through a drip set attached to the catheter. The abdomen is gently massaged or the patient is rolled without dislodging the catheter to distribute the saline throughout the abdomen. Either a syringe is attached and fluid is gently aspirated from the catheter or the drip set and fluid bag are allowed to fill by gravity. Large volumes of fluid generally are not obtained due to the wide dispersion of fluid throughout the abdomen. Any amount retrieved should be submitted for biochemical and cytologic evaluation, including culture and susceptibility testing, as appropriate.

Diagnostic peritoneal lavage does not reliably exclude significant injuries to retroperitoneal structures. Kane et al performed computed tomography after diagnostic peritoneal lavage in 44 human blunt trauma patients in hemodynamically stable condition.[8] In 16 patients, computed tomography revealed significant intraabdominal or retroperitoneal injuries not detected by diagnostic peritoneal lavage. Moreover, the findings on computed tomography resulted in a modification to the original treatment plan in 58% of the patients. There are currently no similar studies in veterinary medicine.

ABDOMINAL FLUID ANALYSIS

Packed cell volume (PCV); creatinine, potassium, lactate, and glucose concentrations; and blood urea nitrogen (BUN) level can all be measured in the peritoneal fluid sample. If the PCV of the peritoneal fluid is equal to or exceeds the peripheral PCV, then parenchymal organ laceration or large vascular disruption is suggested. Hemodilution with urine may cause the PCV of abdominal fluid to be decreased in patients with both abdominal hemorrhage and urologic injury. Uroabdomen can be diagnosed by simultaneous measurement of creatinine and potassium levels in both the abdominal fluid and peripheral blood. Higher potassium levels in the abdominal fluid than in peripheral blood (>1.4:1) suggest urologic injury.[8] Because of the high molecular weight of creatinine, a creatinine concentration in the abdominal fluid that is more than twice that in peripheral blood is highly suggestive of free urine in the abdominal cavity.[9] BUN concentration can be assessed rapidly and levels compared in the abdominal fluid and peripheral blood using reagent strip technology. However, BUN concentration can readily equilibrate across the peritoneal lining, and levels are less reliable for the diagnosis of uroabdomen.

Cytologic analysis should be performed on abdominal fluid and abdominal fluid should be submitted for culture and susceptibility testing when septic peritonitis is suspected. Emergent cytologic analysis often assists the clinician in initiating appropriate therapy. In many cases, the correct choice between medical and surgical therapy can be readily apparent before official clinical pathologic analysis is performed. The gross appearance of the fluid should be evaluated. An abdominal fluid sample that is completely clear and colorless makes a diagnosis of peritonitis, severe intraabdominal injury or perforation, or leakage from the gastrointestinal tract less likely.[4] Fluid that appears opaque, cloudy, or flocculent should be examined immediately. A direct smear that has been dried and stained appropriately can be examined at low power for large particulate material such as plant material or crystals. High-power magnification is used to identify bacteria, fungi, and blood cells. Intracellular bacteria (with or without extracellular bacteria) and degenerate neutrophils characterize a septic effusion. One study[10] showed that these features were 100% accurate for the diagnosis of septic peritonitis. Surgical intervention should be considered and undertaken immediately if septic effusion is found, often before confirmation of infection by a reference laboratory. Surgery is not necessarily indicated when only extracellular bacteria are found in the fluid sample. Glucose and lactate levels in peritoneal fluid can also aid in the diagnosis of septic peritonitis. In one prospective analysis, in 18 dogs with septic effusion, peritoneal fluid glucose concentration was always lower than blood glucose concentration.[11] A difference in glucose level between blood and peritoneal fluid of more than 20 mg/dl was 100% sensitive and 100% specific for the diagnosis of septic peritoneal effusion in this study.

Analysis of Diagnostic Peritoneal Lavage Samples

Cytologic characteristics of white cells are more meaningful than absolute cell counts in fluid samples due to the dilutional effects of peritoneal lavage.[2,12] A study comparing preoperative and postoperative DPL samples found that recent surgery can increase the white blood cell counts from normal levels (1000 cells/mcl) to usually less than 10,000 cells/mcl.[13] Elevations in the peritoneal white blood cell count in response to sepsis occur over variable time periods[5] and overlap these normal ranges. Because of dilution the PCV of the DPL fluid cannot be directly compared with the peripheral blood PCV. It has been reported that a DPL fluid PCV of more than 5% is indicative of significant hemorrhage.[12] Serial assessments of the abdominal fluid showing increasing PCV may more clearly define continuing hemorrhage.

Creatinine and potassium elevations in the lavage fluid are more difficult to interpret due to dilutional effects of the 0.9% NaCl. Excretory urography, retrograde contrast cystourethrography, or surgical intervention may be indicated.

With gallbladder or common bile duct injury, appearance of the clinical signs of icterus may be delayed. A dark green to black or dark amber color of peritoneal fluid suggests the presence of bile pigments. Peritoneal fluid can be analyzed for total bilirubin level. If the abdominal fluid bilirubin level is significantly higher than the peripheral bilirubin level, then bile peritonitis is present.

CONCLUSION

Serial physical examinations and diagnostic studies are required to decide whether acute abdominal disease should be surgically explored or treated medically. Blunt abdominal trauma cases present challenging diagnostic problems because the clinical manifestations may be delayed for hours or days. Abdominocentesis is a valuable tool to obtain a sample of peritoneal fluid for laboratory and cytologic analysis in the emergency department or intensive care unit. DPL may be indicated in a patient in which significant abdominal injury has occurred but no fluid accumulation was identified by FAST or obtained by abdominocentesis. Repeated abdominocentesis may also play a role in clinical decision making.

REFERENCES

1. Saxon WD: The acute abdomen, Vet Clin North Am Small Anim Pract 24(6):1207-1224, 1994.
2. Swann H, Hughes D: Diagnosis and management of peritonitis, Vet Clin North Am Small Anim Pract 30(3):603-615, 2000.
3. Boysen SR, Rozanski EA, Tidwell AS, et al: Evaluation of a focused assessment with sonography for trauma protocol to detect free abdominal fluid in dogs involved in motor vehicle accidents, J Am Vet Med Assoc 225(8):1198-1204, 2004.
4. Crowe DT, Crane SW: Diagnostic abdominal paracentesis and lavage in the evaluation of abdominal injuries in dogs and cats: clinical and experimental investigations, J Am Vet Med Assoc 168(8):700-705, 1976.
5. Giacobine J, Siler VE: Evaluation of diagnostic abdominal paracentesis with experimental and clinical studies, Surg Gynecol Obstet 110:676-686, 1960.
6. Kolata RJ: Diagnostic abdominal paracentesis and lavage: experimental and clinical evaluations in the dog, J Am Vet Med Assoc 168(8):697-699, 1976.
7. Glickman LT, Glickman NW, Perez CM, et al: Analysis of risk factors for gastric dilatation and dilatation-volvulus in dogs, J Am Vet Med Assoc 204(9):1465-1471, 1994.
8. Kane NM, Dorfman GS, Cronan JJ: Efficacy of CT following peritoneal lavage in abdominal trauma, J Comput Assist Tomogr 11(6):998-1002, 1987.
9. Schmiedt C, Tobias KM, Otto CM: Evaluation of abdominal fluid:peripheral blood creatinine and potassium ratios for diagnosis of uroperitoneum in dogs, J Vet Emerg Crit Care 11:275-280, 2001.
10. Botte RJ, Rosin E: Cytology of peritoneal effusion following intestinal anastomosis and experimental peritonitis, Vet Surg 12:20, 1983.
11. Bonczynski JJ, Ludwig LL, Barton LJ, et al: Comparison of peritoneal fluid and peripheral blood pH, bicarbonate, glucose, and lactate concentration as a diagnostic tool for septic peritonitis in dogs and cats, Vet Surg 32(2):161-166, 2003.
12. Mann F: Acute abdomen: evaluation and emergency treatment. In: Bonagura JD, editor: Kirk's current veterinary therapy XIII, Philadelphia, 2000, Saunders, pp 160-164.
13. Bjorling DE, Latimer KS, Rawlings CA, et al: Diagnostic peritoneal lavage before and after abdominal surgery in dogs, Am J Vet Res 44(5):816-820, 1983.

CHAPTER 201
ARTERIAL CATHETERIZATION

Elisa M. Mazzaferro, MS, DVM, PhD, DACVECC

KEY POINTS

- Arterial catheters can be placed into the dorsal pedal, radial, femoral, coccygeal, and auricular arteries.
- Arterial catheters can be used for direct blood pressure monitoring and procurement of arterial blood samples for blood gas and other analyses.
- Arterial catheters are generally well tolerated but can easily become dislodged with excessive patient movement.
- Use of arterial catheters should be avoided whenever possible in patients with severe coagulation abnormalities due to the risk of arterial hemorrhage.

The placement of an indwelling arterial catheter is a necessary and useful procedure for many critically ill veterinary patients. Arterial catheters can be used for frequent collection of arterial blood samples when evaluating an animal's arterial oxygenation and ventilation and for direct arterial blood pressure monitoring. To avoid complications associated with hemorrhage or arterial thrombosis, the animal's coagulation status should be considered before placement of a catheter into any artery. If severe thrombocytopenia (<50,000 platelets/µl) or prolonged activated partial thromboplastin time and prothrombin time are present, the patient is at a greater risk of hemorrhage from the site of arterial catheterization.

Arterial catheters are most frequently placed in the dorsal pedal artery.[1] Alternate locations for arterial catheter placement include the auricular artery on the dorsomedial surface of the ear pinna[2] and the femoral, coccygeal, radial, and brachial arteries.[3] With practice, arterial catheterization and maintenance is not technically difficult and can provide information that helps guide lifesaving treatment interventions in the most critically ill veterinary patients.[3]

PATIENT PREPARATION

Although arterial catheters can be placed in an awake patient, placement is generally easier in an anesthetized animal. The dorsal pedal artery is the most suitable site for an awake patient given the restraint necessary.

The site of arterial catheterization should be chosen based on the patient's anatomy and consideration of underlying diseases, such as vomiting, diarrhea, or aural hematomas. For example, placement of a radial artery catheter may be inappropriate in a vomiting patient due to the risk of catheter contamination. Similarly, placement of a femoral, coccygeal, or dorsal pedal artery catheter is inappropriate in a patient with severe diarrhea. Auricular catheters are challenging to maintain in an awake patient and tend to better suited to an anesthetized patient. Because of the increased risks of auricular, femoral, coccygeal, and radial catheter dislodgement in ambulatory patients, dorsal pedal catheters are preferred, whenever possible.[1]

PERCUTANEOUS ARTERIAL CATHETER PLACEMENT

Once the proposed site of arterial catheterization has been chosen, the operator should become familiar with the animal's anatomy, palpating over the artery as it courses along the leg, tail, or ear and feeling carefully for the arterial pulse. The designated site of catheterization should be clipped, then aseptically cleaned with an antimicrobial scrub before catheter placement. The operator should wash his or her hands carefully and ideally wear gloves to maintain aseptic technique during the procedure. Because arterial catheter placement relies largely on palpation of the pulse, it may not always be practical to wear gloves. Careful hand cleaning before catheter placement is recommended if gloves are not worn.

Dorsal Pedal Artery Catheterization

For placement of a catheter in the dorsal pedal artery, the patient should be positioned in lateral recumbency with the leg containing the proposed catheter site located down, adjacent to the table. The fur should be shaved on the anterior portion of the limb from the level of the tarsus distally along the length of the metatarsal bones. The artery is usually palpable just distal to the hock, in between the second and third metatarsal bones.[1] Once the artery has been palpated and the site clipped and aseptically prepared, a 24- to 20-gauge over-the-needle catheter can be placed percutaneously or via a percutaneous facilitation technique.

Percutaneous facilitation refers to the practice of making a small nick in the skin using the bevel of a 20-gauge needle. Care should be taken not to penetrate the artery during this process because arterial spasm is common and can make further attempts at arterial catheterization unsuccessful until a palpable pulse returns. Whether the over-the-needle catheter is placed directly through the skin or through a nick incision created by percutaneous facilitation, the needle and catheter should be inserted through the skin at a 15- to 30-degree angle over the palpable pulse.[1] The needle and catheter should be directed dorsally and laterally to the metatarsals over the site of a palpable pulse in small maneuvers, with careful observation for a flash of blood in the catheter hub. Once a flash of blood is seen in the hub of the catheter, a judgment must be made as to if the catheter itself is within the artery or if a very small advancement is required. The catheter should then be pushed off the stylet into the artery. Pulsatile arterial blood should be observed as soon as the stylet is withdrawn from the catheter if arterial catheterization has been successful.[1] If the catheter snags or does not feed easily, the catheter can be gently pulled over the stylet and another attempt made at catheterization. In some cases, when the original attempt at catheterization has failed, the catheter can be left in its original place and a second attempt made proximally if an arterial pulse is still palpable (Figure 201-1). Leaving the original catheter in place prevents hematoma formation, which may preclude further attempts at arterial catheterization. Should all attempts at arterial catheterization fail, a pressure

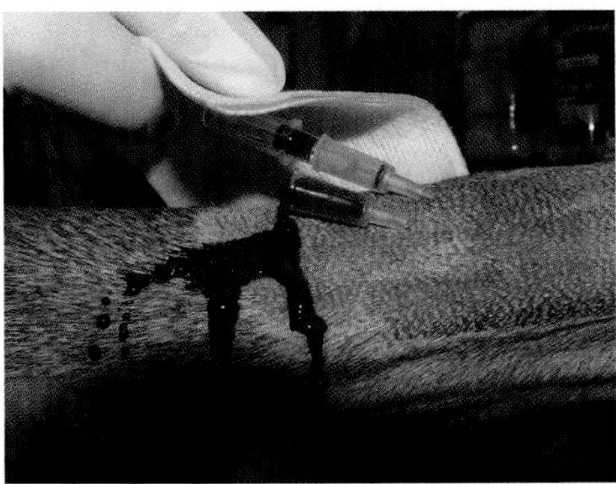

FIGURE 201-1 If percutaneous catheterization is unsuccessful, the original catheter can be left in place and an attempt can be made to place the catheter into the artery more proximally. This technique helps to prevent hematoma formation during catheter placement.

bandage should be placed for a minimum of 15 minutes to prevent hemorrhage and hematoma formation.[1]

Once the dorsal pedal artery catheter is in place, a Luer-Lock T-port or male adapter flushed with heparinized saline should be attached to the catheter hub to prevent further blood loss. The catheter should be flushed with heparinized saline, then secured in place with lengths of ½- and 1-inch white adhesive tape. The catheter hub and adjacent skin and fur should be carefully wiped dry of any blood and other liquids or debris before tape is placed around the catheter hub and distal extremity. The tape should be secured tightly around the catheter hub to prevent dislodgement of the catheter. Additional lengths of 1-inch tape should be secured under the catheter hub and around the distal extremity. Some operators use a combination of surgical glue, suture, and tape to secure the catheter in place,[1] although this is not always necessary. The site of catheter insertion should be covered with bandage material and then labeled "Arterial catheter, not for IV infusion" to prevent inadvertent injection of fluids or drugs into the arterial line.[3]

Femoral Artery Catheterization

Except for anatomic landmarks, percutaneous placement of a femoral artery catheter is similar to placement of a catheter into the dorsal pedal artery. The patient is placed in lateral recumbency, and the medial thigh clipped and aseptically scrubbed from the inguinal region distally to the stifle. The femoral artery pulse is palpable on the medial thigh ventral to the inguinal region and proximal to the stifle. The use of ultrasonography to facilitate identification of the femoral artery has been described and decreases the total time for catheter placement from 10 minutes to 1 minute.[4] The over-the-needle catheter should be placed at a 20- to 30-degree angle through the skin and inserted in a proximal direction, with careful observation for a flash of blood in the catheter hub. Once a flash of blood is seen, the catheter should be advanced off the stylet into the femoral artery. As the stylet is removed from the catheter, pulsatile arterial blood will be visible if the catheter has been placed into the artery. A flushed Luer-Lock T-port or male adapter should be attached to the catheter hub. Once the catheter has been flushed with heparinized saline, a piece of butterfly tape should be placed securely around the catheter hub. The length of butterfly tape can be secured to the patient's skin with sutures on either side of the catheter hub. An additional length of 1-inch white tape should be placed under the catheter and around the limb circumferentially to secure the catheter in place. Bandaging material should be used to cover the catheter. As for all arterial catheters, the bandage should be carefully labeled "Arterial catheter, not for IV Infusion" to prevent inadvertent infusion of drugs or fluids into the arterial line.

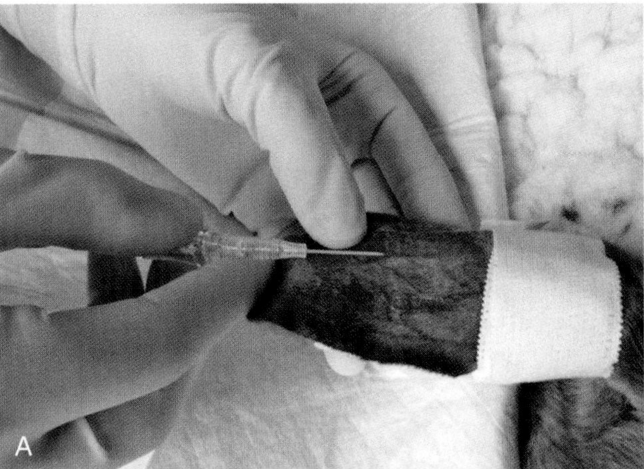

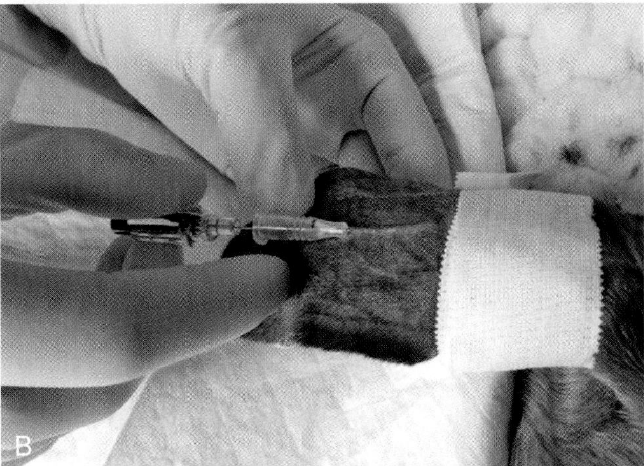

FIGURE 201-2 A, For auricular artery catheterization, the pinna is supported by a roll of gauze held beneath it. The artery is directly visualized, and the catheter is inserted through the skin into the artery. **B,** When a flash of blood is evident in the hub, the catheter is carefully advanced into the artery.

Auricular Artery Catheterization

Catheterization of the auricular artery can be performed in dogs with large ears, such as hounds and hound mixes. The auricular artery is catheterized on the lateral side of the of the ear pinna.[2] This type of catheter is usually placed while the patient is under heavy sedation or general anesthesia. The auricular artery pulse can be palpated on the dorsal aspect of the lateral pinna and the vessel traced toward the ear tip. The fur over the artery should be clipped and the site aseptically scrubbed. With the patient placed in sternal or lateral recumbency, the ear is pulled gently so that the pinna is held perpendicular to the skull. The tip of the ear should be bent ventrally toward the operator with the operator's fingers supporting the pinna from below. The artery is now bent at a perpendicular angle so that it can be traced from the point of a palpable pulse to the ear tip, and the over-the-needle catheter (22 to 24 gauge) can be placed through the skin directly into the artery, with careful observation for a flash of blood in the hub of the catheter (Figure 201-2). Once a flash of blood is seen in the catheter hub, the catheter can be gently fed off of the stylet into the artery. The catheter should be flushed with heparinized saline solution, and a Luer-Lock male adapter or T-port inserted into the catheter hub to prevent further hemorrhage. The skin adjacent to the catheter hub should be dried carefully, and several drops of surgical glue should be placed adjacent to the catheter hub to help secure it to the skin. The catheter can be held in place with lengths of ½-inch tape secured around the catheter hub and under the catheter. The ear can be supported from below with rolled 4 × 4-inch gauze squares or rolls of gauze. Because the weight of the bandage is cumbersome, awake and alert patients may attempt to shake their heads, potentially causing catheter dislodgement. For this reason, the use of an auricular artery catheter is often limited to obtunded, comatose, or anesthetized patients.

Radial Artery Catheterization

Catheterization of a radial artery is technically more difficult than catheter placement in other anatomic locations but can be performed in large dogs. The patient should be placed in lateral recumbency and the palmar aspect of the forelimb clipped just proximal to the large carpal pad and just distal to the accessory carpal pad, where the arterial pulse is palpable. The clipped area should be aseptically scrubbed. The operator should hold the patient's paw in one hand, palpating the arterial pulse with a thumb or forefinger. With the other hand, an over-the-needle catheter should be inserted through the skin at a 15- to 20-degree angle toward the palpable arterial pulse. The operator should watch carefully for a flash of blood in the catheter. As soon as a flash of blood is visible, the catheter should be pushed off of the stylet into the artery. Once in place, the catheter should be flushed with heparinized saline and capped with a Luer-Lock T-port or male adapter. The skin adjacent to the catheter hub should be dried. A length of ½-in white adhesive tape should be secured around the catheter hub and the patient's distal extremity. Additional lengths of 1-inch white adhesive tape should be placed under the catheter hub and then around the patient's limb, with the catheter pushed proximally to secure the catheter in place. The catheter can be bandaged with layers of bandage material. As for all arterial catheters, the bandage should be carefully labeled "Arterial catheter, not for IV infusion" to prevent infusion of drugs and other substances into the artery.

Coccygeal Artery Catheterization

The coccygeal artery pulse is easily palpable on the ventromedial aspect of the tail just distal to the tail base. The fur over the palpable pulse should be clipped, then the site aseptically scrubbed. The patient can be positioned in dorsal or lateral recumbency, depending on operator preference. The arterial pulse should be palpated in between coccygeal vertebrae, and the over-the-needle catheter should be inserted through the skin at a 15-degree angle and pushed cranially toward the tail base until a flash of blood is seen in the catheter (Figure 201-3). Once a flash of arterial blood is visualized, the catheter should be fed off of the stylet and then flushed with heparinized saline. A Luer-Lock T-port or male adapter should be fixed to the catheter hub to prevent hemorrhage. The skin adjacent to the catheter hub should be wiped clean and dry, and a length of ½-inch white adhesive tape should be secured to the catheter hub and around the patient's tail. Additional lengths of 1-inch white adhesive tape should be placed under the catheter hub to push it cranially and secure it in place. The catheter can be wrapped with bandage material to maintain cleanliness. Because coccygeal catheters easily become contaminated with feces during defecation and can become dislodged with patient movement, coccygeal artery catheter use is limited largely to intraoperative procedures.

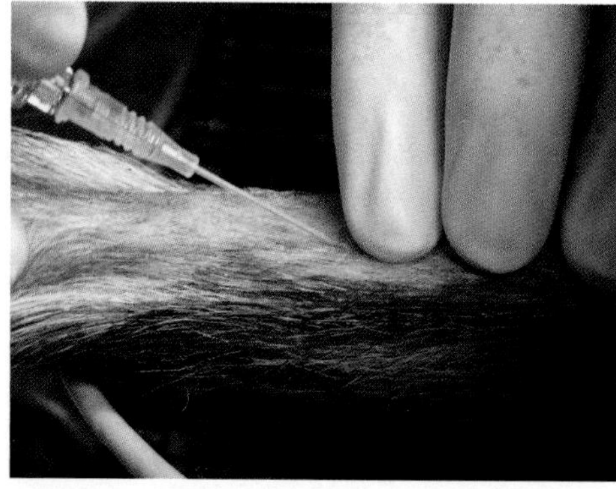

FIGURE 201-3 A coccygeal artery catheter can be placed on the ventral surface of the tail, just caudal to the tail base, in between coccygeal vertebrae.

SURGICAL CUTDOWN FOR ARTERIAL CATHETER PLACEMENT

If percutaneous placement of an arterial catheter is unsuccessful, surgical cutdown can be performed to allow direct visualization and catheterization of the artery. Patient anatomy largely limits surgical cutdown procedures for arterial catheter placement to the dorsal pedal and femoral arteries. Sterile technique should be used at all times. The area over the dorsal pedal or femoral artery should be clipped and aseptically scrubbed, then draped with sterile field towels secured with towel clamps. A small bleb of 2% lidocaine should be inserted in the skin, with care taken to avoid iatrogenic intravenous or arterial administration of the local anesthetic. The skin over the arterial pulse should be incised, with close attention to avoiding laceration of the artery and vein underneath the skin. The artery should be visible directly under the skin, surrounded by perivascular fascia. The dorsal pedal artery is usually visible on top of the metatarsal bones.[3] Several drops of lidocaine should be placed directly over the artery to prevent arterial spasm as the perivascular fascia is bluntly dissected away from the vessel with a curved mosquito hemostat. Once the fascia has been removed from around the artery, a length of suture can be placed around the artery to help lightly elevate it parallel with the skin incision. It is very important to remove every bit of the perivascular fascia before attempting catheter placement.[1] Once the artery has been gently elevated from the incision, the over-the-needle catheter can be inserted directly into the vessel, with care taken to not penetrate through the other side. Excessive traction on the artery can cause arterial spasm, which makes catheterization difficult. A flash of blood will be observed in the hub of the catheter once the catheter has been introduced into the lumen of the artery. The catheter can then be fed off of the stylet, flushed, and capped with a Luer-Lock T-port or male adapter. The suture that was used to elevate the artery can be used to secure the catheter around the catheter hub. The skin over the catheter should be closed with nonabsorbable suture, and the catheter taped in place, bandaged, and labeled as with any other arterial catheter.

MAINTENANCE OF THE ARTERIAL CATHETER

Depending on the mobility of the patient, arterial catheters can be connected to a continuous flushing system with heparinized saline, or intermittently flushed every 1 to 4 hours.[3] In extremely small patients, care needs to be taken to avoid excessive heparinization. Like other vascular catheters, arterial catheters should be examined on a daily basis for signs of erythema or infection. The bandage should be changed daily or more frequently as needed due to soiling. Small volumes of flush solution should be injected to maintain catheter patency. However, other infusions (drugs, fluids, or blood products) should never be administered into an arterial line. Because patient dislodgement of an arterial line can result in significant hemorrhage, it is ideal for patients with indwelling arterial catheters to be under constant supervision. If this is not possible, then measures should be taken to reduce the likelihood of catheter dislodgement, such as application of an Elizabethan collar.

THREE-SYRINGE TECHNIQUE

The three-syringe technique should be employed whenever a blood sample is obtained from an arterial catheter. In this technique, the catheter is first flushed with ½ ml of heparinized saline. The same syringe is then used to withdraw 3 ml of blood from the catheter, and it is saved in an aseptic manner, to be infused back into the patient through a peripheral venous catheter, where possible. The desired volume of arterial blood is then withdrawn into an appropriate syringe. The catheter is then flushed with 2 to 3 ml of heparinized saline and clamped off or reconnected to the continuous flushing system. The arterial blood sample should be analyzed immediately or placed on ice for arterial blood gas analysis.

REFERENCES

1. Hughes D, Beal MW: Emergency vascular access, Vet Clin North Am Small Anim Pract 30(3):491-507, 2000.
2. Waddell LS: Direct blood pressure monitoring, Clin Tech Small Anim Pract 15(3):111-118, 2000.
3. Beal MW, Hughes D: Vascular access: theory and techniques in the small animal emergency patient, Clin Tech Small Anim Pract 15(2):101-109, 2002.
4. Ringold SA, Kelmer E: Freehand ultrasound guided femoral arterial catheterization in dogs, J Vet Emerg Crit Care 18(3):306-311, 2008.

CHAPTER 202

PULMONARY ARTERY CATHETERIZATION

Deborah C. Mandell, VMD, DACVECC

KEY POINTS

- Pulmonary artery catheters (PACs) are placed through the right side of the heart and right ventricular outflow tract into a pulmonary artery (PA).
- PACs may be used to measure cardiac output by thermodilution, calculate systemic vascular resistance, and sample mixed venous blood.
- Information from a PAC may be used to tailor fluid or pressor choices in the anesthetized or critically ill patient.
- A PAC may be placed by following pressure tracings or via fluoroscopic guidance.
- PA catheterization is not a benign procedure and may be associated with significant morbidity; thus a thorough evaluation of the risk/benefit ratio is required.
- Many alternative techniques for measuring cardiac output that do not require placement of a PAC are available for use in veterinary patients.

Pulmonary artery (PA) catheterization is a technique in which a catheter is placed through the right side of the heart and right ventricular (RV) outflow tract into the PA. It is used to measure cardiac output by thermodilution, to calculate systemic vascular resistance, and to sample mixed venous blood. Often, placement is assisted by a latex balloon at the tip of the catheter that allows its course to follow the flow of blood (flow-directed catheter placement).

TYPES OF CATHETERS AND USES

There are many types of pulmonary artery catheters (PACs) designed for angiographic studies or for measuring the blood pressure in the pulmonary arteries. These catheters may be single-lumen or double-lumen catheters.[1] Some catheters have sensors 4 cm distal to the tip of the catheter that allow temperature measurement (e.g., the Swan-Ganz type of catheter). Other catheters may measure blood oxygenation (e.g., the oximetry thermodilution catheter) (Tables 202-1, 202-2, and 202-3). Diameters of thermodilution catheters range from 5 to 7.5 Fr. Angiographic catheters are available in diameters from 4 to 8 Fr. Most Swan-Ganz catheters are made of polyvinyl chloride and are available in lengths of 75 or 110 cm, which are adequate for most small animal species but may not be of sufficient length for horses or other large animals. Other thermodilution catheters are made of polyurethane, which has the characteristic of softening at body temperature.

Table 202-1 **Pulmonary Artery Catheter Types, Sizes, and Manufacturers: Angiographic Catheters**

Name	Company	Diameter (Fr)	Length (cm)
Berman angiographic catheter	Teleflex, Research Triangle Park, NC.	4 5 6 7 8	50 50, 60, 80 60, 90 90, 110 70, 110
Double-lumen pulmonary artery monitoring catheter	Edwards Lifesciences, Irvine, Calif.	5, 6, 7	110
Pulmonary angiography catheter	Edwards Lifesciences	7	110

Table 202-2 **Pulmonary Artery Catheter Types, Sizes, and Manufacturers: Thermodilution Catheters**

Name	Company	Diameter (Fr)	Length (cm)	Notes
Swan-Ganz catheter	Edwards Lifesciences, Irvine, Calif.	5 6, 7, 7.5	75 110	Larger catheters have more lumina (up to six) for infusion
Hands-Off catheter	Teleflex, Research Triangle Park, NC	4 5, 6 6, 7, 7.5	75 80 110	Polyurethane, heparin coated
TDQ continuous cardiac output catheter	ICU Medical, San Clemente, Calif.	8	110	Three-lumen catheters
Criticath thermodilution catheter	Argon Medical Devices, Plano, Tex.	5, 7, 7.5	80 110	Four-lumen or five-lumen catheters, heparin or non–heparin coated

Table 202-3 **Pulmonary Artery Catheter Types, Sizes, and Manufacturers: Other Catheters**

Name	Company	Additional Feature(s)	Diameter (Fr)	Length (cm)
CCO, CCOmbo catheters	Edwards Lifesciences, Irvine, Calif.	Continuous cardiac output monitoring, with or without SvO_2 monitoring	7.5, 8	110
Oximetry thermodilution catheter	Edwards Lifesciences	SvO_2 monitoring (fiberoptic)	4 5.5 7.5	25, 40 75 110
CCOmbo volumetrics catheter	Edwards Lifesciences	Volumetric (RVEDV), with SvO_2 monitoring and continuous cardiac output monitoring	7.5, 8	110
Swan-Ganz pacing catheter, Paceport catheter	Edwards Lifesciences	Pacing ability (or port for introduction of pacing electrodes)	7, 7.5, 8	110
Standard thermodilution catheter	ICU Medical, San Clemente, Calif.	Standard thermodilution catheters, two or three lumens	7, 8	110
OptiQ catheter	ICU Medical	Continuous and intermittent cardiac output monitoring, SvO_2 monitoring	8	110
Criticath pacing catheter	Argon Medical Devices, Plano, Tex.	Additional lumen for temporary ventricular pacing	7.5	110

RVEDV, Right ventricular end-diastolic volume; *SvO_2,* venous oxygen saturation.

Because of the wide diameter, complicated placement, and need to adjust the depth of catheter insertion, it is necessary to place PACs via a catheter introducer sheath. The introducer sheath should be at least one size larger than the catheter itself. For example, a 7 Fr catheter can fit through an 8 or 8.5 Fr introducer sheath, whereas a 6 or 6.5 Fr introducer sheath is adequate for a 5 Fr catheter. For sterility, a plastic sleeve attached to the sheath covers the catheter and keeps the catheter sterile while the PAC is moved into and out of the vessel.

Most commercial catheters designed for thermodilution measurement of cardiac output have multiple ports and lumens (Figure 202-1). The proximal port, or central venous pressure (CVP) port, is used to measure RA or central venous pressure. This port is also used for administration of fluid boluses during cardiac output determination in humans, dogs, and cats. Because the proximal port is located 30 cm from the tip of the catheter where the thermistor is located, a separate catheter must be advanced into the right atrium (RA) in large animals for the purpose of injecting fluid for thermodilution measurements (the proximal port will be located in the RV in the horse).[2] Separate RA catheters have also been used in cats and small dogs, although the proximal port is located outside of the RA.[3] When separate injection catheters are used, it is important that the catheter volume be the same as the injection port on the Swan-Ganz catheter because the *K* constant of the Stewart-Hamilton equation used by cardiac output computers is specific for the catheter type.[4] The *K*

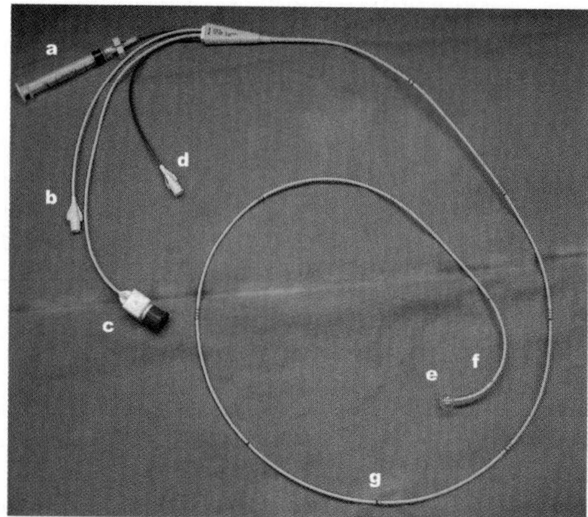

FIGURE 202-1 Swan-Ganz catheter (Edwards Lifesciences, Irvine, Calif.). *a,* Balloon inflation port; *b,* distal infusion port; *c,* connection from the thermistor to the cardiac output computer; *d,* proximal infusion port; *e,* the inflated balloon; *f,* the location of the thermistor; and *g,* the 60-cm distance mark.

constant is a computation constant that is manually entered into the computer. It adjusts for the amount of thermal signal during each measurement, the volume of catheter dead space, and the specific heat, volume, and gravity of the injectate used. The distal port of the catheter is the central lumen and is used to measure both PA pressure and pulmonary capillary wedge pressure (PCWP) also known as *PA occlusion pressure.* Mixed venous blood is also sampled from this port. The balloon port allows for inflation of the balloon tip of the catheter with a small amount of air (usually ≤1.5 ml) for flow-directed catheter placement and measurement of PCWP. The catheter also has an electronic thermistor connection for temperature measurement.

Cardiac Output

A PAC is necessary for evaluation of cardiac output using some thermodilution techniques (see Chapter 184). Briefly, 1.5 ml/kg of saline (or 5% dextrose in water) of a known temperature is injected into the proximal port of the multilumen catheter.[4] In most animals, this proximal port (30 cm proximal to the tip of the catheter) sits either in the RA or in the jugular vein, where it is appropriate to inject the indicator bolus. As mentioned previously, placement of a second injection catheter in the RA may be necessary to perform thermodilution measurements in smaller or larger animals.[2,3] The thermistor probe on the distal end of the catheter measures the change in blood temperature over time and calculates cardiac output based on the area under the temperature curve. Newer Swan-Ganz catheters have thermistor probes near the junction of the proximal port and the catheter to measure the temperature of the injectate more accurately (it may warm significantly during injection). For larger animals such as horses, chilled injectate must be used because subtle changes in blood temperature may not be sensed by the thermistor probe due to the relatively large cardiac output and blood volume in these animals. The indicator bolus must also be administered quickly because slow injection minimizes the change in temperature that is recognized by the thermistor and causes inaccurate readings (if the indicator is injected too slowly, a falsely low cardiac output measurement will be displayed). The use of a power injector pump is recommended for these measurements in large animals, and the bolus should be injected as quickly as possible in small animals.

Pulmonary Capillary Wedge Pressure

Measurement of PCWP via a PAC enables an estimation of left ventricular preload because it can correlate with the left ventricular end-diastolic pressure. This correlation may not be reliable in patients with pulmonary hypertension, mitral regurgitation, or decreased ventricular compliance.[5,6] Airway and intrathoracic pressure can also affect this relationship. The methods for determination of the PCWP are discussed later in the chapter. The PCWP may also be used to derive the pulmonary transcapillary pressure in dogs and cats.[4]

Right Ventricular End-Diastolic Volume

RV end-diastolic volume and index are used increasingly in human medicine to estimate volume status, especially when patients are receiving positive pressure ventilation with positive end-expiratory pressure or in other scenarios in which the PCWP may not accurately indicate left ventricular end-diastolic pressure. These values may be measured via catheters with special rapid-response thermistors that can sense small beat-to-beat changes in temperature induced by an upstream heat filament. These catheters need to be synchronized with the electrocardiogram, and patients must have a regular R-R interval.[7] This same rapid-response thermistor and filament combination is used in catheters that can continuously measure cardiac output without the need for bolus injection (CCO Pulmonary Artery Catheter, CCOmbo Continuous Cardiac Output Catheter, Edwards Lifesciences, Irvine, Calif.).[7]

Selective Pulmonary Angiography

Selective pulmonary angiography via a PAC is sometimes indicated to elucidate complex congenital defects of the cardiopulmonary system in veterinary species.[1] Presurgical right-sided heart catheterization for angiographic purposes is performed commonly in humans before cardiac surgery.[1] In animals, congenital defects such as stenosis of the pulmonic valve may be delineated via angiography and managed with balloon valvuloplasty by inflating a balloon catheter across the stenotic area.[8]

Additional Measurements

Balloon-tipped PACs that measure cardiac output and PCWP can also calculate systemic vascular resistance and pulmonary vascular resistance (see Chapter 184).

INDICATIONS

The indications for placement of a PAC for the purposes of cardiac output measurement or mixed venous blood sampling have received much scrutiny in human medicine because of concerns regarding the risk/benefit ratio. A recent review of randomized controlled trials evaluated the impact of monitoring systems on outcomes in critically ill and perioperative patients undergoing major procedures; the reviewers reported that the majority of studies showed no change in mortality in patients receiving treatment guided by PAC monitoring compared with patients whose therapy was not guided by the PAC data.[9] Interestingly, no monitoring system was associated with a clear-cut improvement in mortality. However, a 1997 consensus conference stated that PACs are useful in the management of hemodynamic instability during and after cardiac surgery and after myocardial infarction.[10] There was uncertain benefit in the use of PAC information to define shock states other than cardiogenic shock. Additionally, there is some evidence that PACs are useful in the treatment of trauma patients as well as in certain pediatric populations.[10,11] A more recent study questioned the usefulness of PACs for management of heart failure, showing no benefit (but no detriment) in the group that received diuretic and afterload reduction therapy based on PAC measurements.[12] A meta-analysis of randomized controlled studies concluded that, although there was no increased morbidity in the group undergoing PAC monitoring, a benefit was not realized from its use.[13,14] Many still believe that PAC monitoring has a role in critically ill patients, and there may be other reasons that no clear benefit has been shown (e.g., inaccurate interpretation of the data, PAC placement that was too late, patient selection criteria, heterogeneity of treatments).[9,15-19]

In veterinary medicine, catheters placed in the PA have been used for thermodilution measurement of cardiac output in many research studies.[20,21] The PAC seems useful for evaluation and treatment of cardiogenic shock. Information such as cardiac output and systemic vascular resistance can be used to guide inotropic and vasodilator therapy. Knowledge of systemic hemodynamics and cardiac output may also be helpful for guiding fluid resuscitation and pressor therapy in the small animal patient with hypovolemic and/or distributive shock. However, studies of the use of PACs in clinical veterinary patients are lacking. Like human medicine, veterinary medicine is also evaluating newer, noninvasive monitoring systems.

Human data have focused on the optimization of oxygen delivery in patients with shock and multiple organ dysfunction syndrome.[22] Although initial studies of this goal-directed therapy have been promising, the overall clinical benefit of this strategy compared with prior techniques has not been ascertained. Swan-Ganz catheters with oximetry probes are available to allow real-time measurement of venous oxygen saturation and optimization of oxygen delivery.

PLACEMENT

Judicious sedation using a benzodiazepine or an opioid may be indicated in some animals during placement of the introducer sheath and PAC (see Chapter 142). In an unanesthetized animal, a local block using lidocaine should be performed because it is often necessary to make a skin incision to facilitate dilation of the vessel and smooth catheter placement. Introducer sheath placement may be performed via cutdown to the external jugular vein, although percutaneous placement via a Seldinger technique is also appropriate and somewhat less complicated.[4] Before the catheter is placed, a wide area of skin should be clipped and prepared aseptically. During placement, sterile drapes should be used to isolate the area, and sterile gown, gloves, and a cap and mask should be worn.

Regardless of technique, it is important to have an idea of the length of catheter required and the distance from cardiac structures before placement. A lateral thoracic radiograph may be helpful for this purpose. Most Swan-Ganz thermodilution catheters are marked with thin black lines every 10 cm and thicker black lines every 50 cm (e.g., 70 cm is represented by one thick line and two thin lines; see Figure 202-1). Placement is accomplished most easily through an introducer sheath placed in the external jugular vein.[5] The introducer catheter has a valve, which allows for ease of catheter placement and subsequent adjustments of catheter position while preventing injection of air or loss of blood from the vessel. The addition of a sterile plastic sleeve allows for preservation of the sterility of the PAC during placement and adjustment. Once the introducer sheath is in place, the neck of the animal should be wrapped to protect the introducer sheath insertion site, as would be done with any jugular catheter.

Before the PAC is fed through the introducer sheath, the integrity of the balloon should be assessed. All ports of the catheter should be flushed with heparinized saline before placement, and the catheter itself may be moistened with saline to allow smooth advancement through the introducer sheath.

Flow-Directed Placement

Classically, PACs are placed by attaching the distal port of the catheter to a calibrated pressure transducer and connecting to a monitor. If continuous monitoring is to be performed, use of a system with a heparinized saline flush is indicated. Monitoring the pressure tracing as the catheter is advanced into the jugular vein (via the preplaced introducer sheath) allows the position of the catheter tip to be deduced by recognition of the different waveforms generated in each area of the heart and vessels (Figure 202-2). After the catheter is inserted into the RA (approximately 20 cm in a medium to large dog), the balloon may be inflated with air (the appropriate volume generally is listed on the port and usually is 1.5 ml) and then advanced further. It may not be necessary to inflate the balloon until the catheter tip is in the RV. The balloon should always be deflated before withdrawal of the catheter to prevent valvular damage and knotting of the catheter, and also after PCWP measurement to avoid unnecessary obstruction of blood flow.

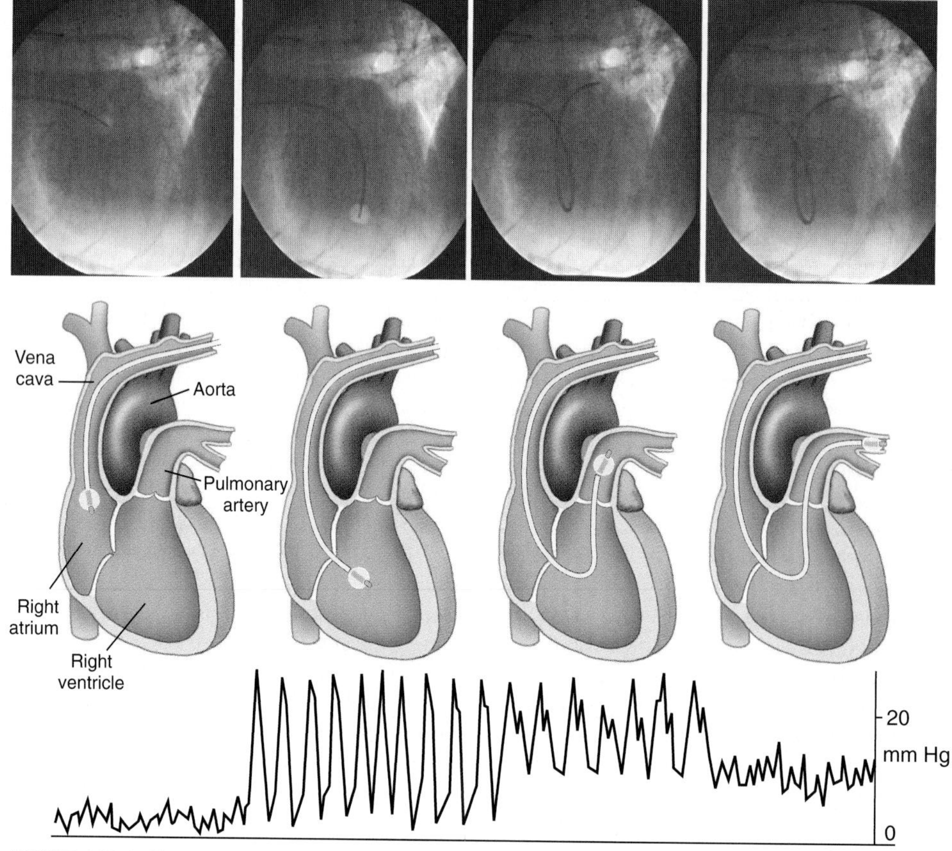

FIGURE 202-2 Characteristic pressure waveforms recognized as the pulmonary artery catheter is fed through (from left to right) the right atrium, the right ventricle, and the pulmonary artery as well as the wedge pressure tracing. A schematic and the fluorographic appearance at each step are shown. In the fluorographic images, the dog is in right lateral recumbency with the dog facing left (Note: The third and fourth images are both in the pulmonary capillary.) *(From Lalli SM: The complete Swan-Ganz, RN 41:64, 1978; and Headley JM: Invasive hemodynamic monitoring: physiological principles and clinical applications, Irvine, Calif, 2002, Edwards Scientific.)*

In humans, the RA is entered at approximately 25 cm, the RV at approximately 30 cm, and the PA at approximately 40 cm; the PCWP can be identified at approximately 45 cm.[18] Thus, if 30 cm of catheter has been introduced but no atrial tracing is yet seen, the catheter tip may have traveled into the azygous vein and should be withdrawn for another attempt. This may be avoided by keeping the tip directed ventrally, combined with slight rotation at the junction of the vena cava and the RA.[1] Once in the RA, the catheter may also become lodged in the coronary sinus or enter the caudal vena cava if it is directed too far caudally or dorsally.[1] If 10 cm of catheter has been introduced after an RA tracing is attained and the tracing has not changed, or reverts to a CVP tracing, inappropriate placement should be suspected. Likewise, once the catheter is in the RV, if the RV waveform persists for a 20-cm advancement after initial appearance, the catheter may be coiling in the RV and should be withdrawn slowly to the RA after deflating the balloon to avoid knotting of the catheter or damage to the tricuspid valve. Ventricular ectopic beats may be observed if the catheter contacts the walls of the RV. After the catheter has been floated into the PA, it should be pulled back 1 to 2 cm to straighten any redundant loops in the RV.

The pressure waveforms have characteristic tracings that allow the operator to identify the position of the catheter tip. The RA tracing is similar to the CVP tracing from the jugular vein. Normal systolic RA pressure ranges from 4 to 6 mm Hg and normal diastolic pressure ranges from 0 to 4 mm Hg in anesthetized cats and dogs, which gives a normal mean RA pressure of 2 to 5 mm Hg. Once the catheter is in the RV, a similar diastolic pressure is measured, but the mean systolic pressure is 15 to 30 mm Hg. The PA tracing is notable because the diastolic pressure no longer decreases to zero due to the pulmonic valve; thus the mean diastolic pressure is 5 to 15 mm Hg (see Figure 202-2). Normal mean PA pressure in dogs is 8 to 20 mm Hg.[1,15]

The characteristic waveform of the PCWP (similar to the RA tracing, but now representing the left atrium) is obtained by advancing the catheter slowly into the PA, with balloon inflated, until a point is reached at which the lumen of the vessel is completely occluded by the balloon (see Figure 202-2). The waveform will change and the mean pressure will be lower than the mean PA pressure on entering the pulmonary capillary (mean PCWP is 5 to 12 mm Hg).[23] The catheter should not remain in a wedged position for longer than 10 to 15 seconds, or two respiratory cycles.[24] Once the PCWP is obtained, the balloon should be deflated, so that once again the PA pressure waveform is displayed. For subsequent readings, because there is a tendency for the catheter to migrate distally as it warms to body temperature and softens, the balloon should be inflated slowly, with constant monitoring of the pressure tracing. PA rupture has been reported secondary to overzealous balloon inflation.[25] In humans, if a PCWP tracing is obtained before the full volume of air is instilled into the balloon (<1.25 ml), it is recommended that the balloon be deflated and the catheter backed out until a PCWP tracing is noted with full inflation with 1.5 ml of air.[23]

When it is in the PA, the balloon should always be inflated slowly over 3 to 5 seconds, not only to avoid overinflation but also because rapid balloon inflation may be associated with spurious results.[23] If the pressure tracing shows a constantly increasing pressure, the tip of the catheter may be covered by the balloon or may be pressed closely on the vessel wall, or it may be in a distal PA branch. This phenomenon, called *overwedging,* may be remedied by deflating the balloon and situating the catheter tip more proximally before reinflating it.

Fluoroscopy

Fluoroscopy provides a way to monitor catheter placement visually. PACs are radiopaque and so may be followed in their path from the jugular vein through the heart via radiography (see Figure 202-2). Fluoroscopy can help to quickly identify misplacement (e.g., into the azygous vein) and may enhance the speed of the procedure. The downside of fluoroscopy is the need for specialized equipment and generation of radiation during the procedure. All participants should wear protective lead aprons. Depending on the condition of the patient, it may not always be prudent to travel to a radiology suite to perform this procedure. Portable (C-arm) fluoroscopy units may simplify this procedure by moving it closer to the bedside.

COMPLICATIONS

Complications of catheter placement reported in the human literature include wire or catheter embolus, cardiac arrhythmias, knotting, cardiac tamponade, carotid artery puncture, tricuspid valve damage, hemothorax, and pneumothorax.[25,26] Many of these complications are related to the initial approach used for vascular access (usually the internal jugular or subclavian veins), which is less of a problem in veterinary species with prominent external jugular veins suitable for placement of the introducer sheath. Insertion of the PAC into the mediastinum or the pleural space has also been reported in humans.[6] More serious complications associated with the use of a PAC include PA rupture from overzealous or erroneous balloon inflation or from direct catheter puncture, although such events are rare (estimated incidence of 0.0031%). Risk factors for PA rupture in humans include advanced age, pulmonary hypertension, and use of improper inflation or positioning techniques.[6] Patients whose blood has been anticoagulated are also at risk. Little veterinary information is available regarding PAC complications; however, one postmortem study in horses that had PACs placed showed evidence of minor endocardial lesions.[27]

During catheter advancement through the heart, cardiac arrhythmias (premature atrial and ventricular contractions) may be seen. In humans, ventricular tachycardia and ventricular fibrillation have been reported, especially in patients with preexisting heart disease. Lidocaine was ineffective in suppressing these arrhythmias in one study, so the most effective way to decrease the incidence of ventricular ectopic beats is expedient passage of the catheter through the RV.[23] Right bundle branch block has also been reported during catheter advancement, which is of concern in patients with preexisting left bundle branch block because complete heart block may result.[6] For this reason, it is recommended that the ability to perform transvenous or transthoracic pacing be available before this procedure is performed in patients with left bundle branch block.[6] Some PACs are also equipped with a separate channel for the placement of pacing leads, and some have electrodes integrated into the catheter. Antiarrhythmic drugs should be available.

Once a PAC is placed, maintenance may be complicated by the formation of thrombi (at the insertion site or at the tip of the catheter), embolic events (from balloon rupture, inadvertent air administration, or thrombi), or distal catheter migration causing pulmonary infarction.[6,23] Infection is also a risk in patients with long-term indwelling PACs.[23] Anticoagulants are not routinely administered after placement of a PAC unless indicated for treatment of the underlying disease process. Anticoagulation in humans may be associated with increased severity of bleeding in the event of a PA rupture.[6] Heparin-coated PACs are available.[28]

ALTERNATIVES

Because of concerns related to the morbidity associated with PACs in critically ill patients, other techniques have been developed to measure cardiac output and systemic oxygenation. Ejection fraction and cardiac output may be measured directly in anesthetized patients using transesophageal echocardiography, a technique that has been investigated in dogs[29] but one which requires some skill in both obtaining and interpreting the images. Another technique for measuring cardiac output is similar to earlier indicator dilution techniques that used indocyanine green dye as a marker of blood flow. Lithium chloride may be used as a "dye," and concentrations measured by an ion-specific electrode may be analyzed and translated into cardiac output via a modified Stewart-Hamilton equation.[30,31] For cardiac output determinations using lithium dilution, the only necessary catheters are an arterial line for sampling and a central venous catheter for injection of the lithium chloride. Peripheral catheters may also be used for injection of the lithium chloride in dogs.[32] This technique has been investigated in dogs, cats, horses, and foals. Lithium ions do not reach toxic levels during routine use of this system.[33,34]

Some systems derive continuous cardiac output measures via analysis of the arterial pressure waveform. The PulseCO system (PulseCO system, LiDCO*plus*, London, U.K.) requires initial calibration with a cardiac output measurement obtained via lithium dilution and only periodic recalibration thereafter.[29] The PulseCO system has been evaluated in dogs and horses.[35,36] Newer systems (e.g., FloTrac, Edwards Lifesciences) do not require calibration to cardiac output.[37] A variation on the Fick principle using partial carbon dioxide rebreathing has also been developed to measure cardiac output. Termed *NICO* (Philips Respironics, Andover, MA), this technique uses a loop of tubing attached to the patient's endotracheal tube to measure the levels of expired carbon dioxide during a brief period of rebreathing.[38-40] An obvious impediment to the use of this technique is the requirement that the patient be intubated. This system has also been evaluated in dogs.[41]

Although a true mixed venous blood sample cannot be obtained without a PAC, alternatives to measuring mixed venous oxygen saturation have been evaluated in human studies. The modification of goal-directed therapy using central venous oximetry has been proposed (see Chapter 5), and central venous catheters with fiberoptic oximetry probes are available for this purpose (PreSep Central Venous Oximetry Catheter, Edwards Lifesciences).[20]

REFERENCES

1. Kittleson MD, Kienle RD: Small animal cardiovascular medicine, ed 1, St Louis, 1998, Mosby.
2. Muir WW, Skarda RT, Milne DW: Estimation of cardiac output in the horse by thermodilution techniques, Am J Vet Res 37:697, 1976.
3. Dyson DH, Allen DG, McDonell WN: Comparison of three methods for cardiac output determination in cats, Am J Vet Res 46:2546, 1985.
4. Mellema M: Cardiac output, wedge pressure, and oxygen delivery, Vet Clin North Am Small Anim Pract 31:1175, 2001.
5. Murphy GS, Nitsun M, Vender JS: Is the pulmonary artery catheter useful? Best Pract Res Clin Anaesthesiol 19:97, 2005.
6. Gomez CMH, Palazzo MGA: Pulmonary artery catheterization in anaesthesia and intensive care, Br J Anaesth 81:945, 1998.
7. Medin DL, Brown DT, Wesley R, et al: Validation of continuous thermodilution cardiac output in critically ill patients with analysis of systematic errors, J Crit Care 13:184, 1998.
8. Sun F, Uson J, Crisostomo V, et al: Interventional cardiovascular techniques in small animal practice—diagnostic angiography and balloon valvuloplasty, J Am Vet Med Assoc 227:394, 2005.
9. Ospina-Tascon GA, Cordioli RL, Vincent J-L: What type of monitoring has been shown to improve outcomes in acutely ill patients? Intensive Care Med 34:800, 2008.
10. Pulmonary Artery Catheter Consensus conference: consensus statement, Crit Care Med 25:910, 1997.
11. Friese RS, Shafi S, Gentilello LM: Pulmonary artery catheter use is associated with reduced mortality in severely injured patients: a National Trauma Data Bank analysis of 53,312 patients, Crit Care Med 34:1597, 2006.
12. Evaluation Study of Congestive Heart Failure and Pulmonary Artery Catheterization Effectiveness: the ESCAPE trial, JAMA 294:1625, 2005.
13. Shah MR, Hasselblad V, Stevenson LW, et al: Impact of the pulmonary artery catheter in critically ill patients: meta-analysis of randomized clinical trials, JAMA 294:1664, 2005.
14. Harvey S, Harrison DA, Singer M, et al: Assessment of the clinical effectiveness of pulmonary artery catheters in management of patients in intensive care (PAC-Man): a randomised controlled trial, Lancet 366:472, 2005.
15. Vincent J-L, Rhodes A, Perel A, et al: Clinical review: update on hemodynamic monitoring—a consensus of 16, Crit Care 15:229, 2011.
16. Vincent J-L, Pinsky MR, Sprung CL, et al: The pulmonary artery catheter: *in medio virtus*, Crit Care Med 36:3093, 2008.
17. Chittock DR, Dhingra VK, Ronco JJ, et al: Severity of illness and risk of death associated with pulmonary artery catheter use, Crit Care Med 32:911, 2004.
18. Iberti TJ, Fischer EP, Leibowitz AB, et al: A multicenter study of physicians' knowledge of the pulmonary artery catheter, JAMA 264:2928, 1990.
19. Hines RL: Pulmonary artery catheters: what's the controversy? J Card Surg 5:237, 1990.
20. Haskins S, Pascoe PJ, Ilkiw JE, et al: Reference cardiopulmonary values in normal dogs, Comp Med 55:156, 2005.
21. Noble WH, Kay JC: Cardiac catheterization in dogs, Can Anaesth Soc J 21:616, 1974.
22. Rivers E, Nguyen B, Havstad S, et al: Early goal-directed therapy in the treatment of severe sepsis and septic shock, N Engl J Med 345:1368, 2001.
23. Headley JM: Invasive hemodynamic monitoring: physiological principles and clinical applications, Irvine, Calif, 2002, Edwards Scientific.
24. Hardy JF, Morissette M, Taillefer J, et al: Pathophysiology of rupture of the pulmonary artery by pulmonary artery balloon-tipped catheters, Anesth Analg 62:925, 1983.
25. Domino KB, Bowdle TA, Posner KL, et al: Injuries and liability related to central vascular catheters, Anesthesiology 100:1411, 2004.
26. Porhomayon J, El-Solh A, Papadakos P, et al: Cardiac output monitoring devices: an analytic review, Intern Emerg Med 7:163, 2012.
27. Schlipf JW, Dunlop CI, Getzy DM, et al: Lesions associated with cardiac catheterization and thermodilution cardiac output determination in horses, Proceedings of the 5th International Congress of Veterinary Anesthesia, Guelph, Canada, August 1994.
28. Randolph AG, Cook DJ, Gonzales CA, et al: Benefit of heparin in central venous and pulmonary artery catheters: a meta-analysis of randomized controlled trials, Chest 113:165, 1998.
29. Lazic T, Riedesel DH, Evans RB: Measurement of cardiac output by transesophageal Doppler ultrasonography in anesthetized dogs: comparison with thermodilution, Vet Anaesth Analg 30:104, 2003.
30. Mason DJ, O'Grady M, Woods JP, et al: Assessment of lithium dilution cardiac output as a technique for measurement of cardiac output in dogs, Am J Vet Res 62:1255, 2001.
31. Mason DJ, O'Grady M, Woods JP, et al: Comparison of a central and a peripheral (cephalic vein) injection site for the measurement of cardiac output using the lithium-dilution cardiac output technique in anesthetized dogs, Can J Vet Res 66:207, 2002.
32. Mason DJ, O'Grady M, Woods JP, et al: Effect of background serum lithium concentrations on the accuracy of lithium dilution cardiac output determination in dogs, Am J Vet Res 63:1048, 2002.
33. McDonell W, Black W: Pharmacokinetics and toxicity of intravenously administered lithium chloride in horses, Vet Anaesth Analg 27:108, 2000.
34. Pittman J, Bar-Yosef S, SumPing J, et al: Continuous cardiac output monitoring with pulse contour analysis: a comparison with lithium indicator dilution cardiac output measurement, Crit Care Med 33:2015, 2005.
35. Chen HC, Sinclair MD, Dyson DH, et al: Comparison of arterial pressure waveform analysis with the lithium dilution technique to monitor cardiac output in anesthetized dogs, Am J Vet Res 66:1430, 2005.
36. Hallowell GD, Corley KT: Use of lithium dilution and pulse contour analysis cardiac output determination in anaesthetised horses: a clinical evaluation, Vet Anaesth Analg 32:201, 2005.
37. Manecke GR: Edwards Flo-Trac sensor and Vigileo monitor: easy, accurate, reliable cardiac output assessment using the arterial pulse wave, Expert Rev Med Devices 2:523, 2005.

38. Jaffe MB: Partial CO_2 rebreathing cardiac output-operating principles of the NICO™ system, J Clin Monit Comput 15:387, 1999.
39. Rocco M, Spadetta G, Morelli A, et al: A comparative evaluation of thermodilution and partial carbon dioxide rebreathing techniques for cardiac output assessment in critically ill patients during assisted ventilation, Intensive Care Med 30:82, 2004.
40. Yamashita K, Igarashi R, Kushiro T, et al: Comparison of noninvasive cardiac output measurements by transthoracic bioimpedance, partial carbon dioxide rebreathing, and transesophageal echocardiography with the thermodilution technique in Beagle dogs, Vet Anaesth Analg 32:13, 2005.
41. Gunkel CI, Valverde A, Morey TE, et al: Comparison of noninvasive cardiac output measurement by partial carbon dioxide rebreathing with the lithium dilution method in anesthetized dogs, J Vet Emerg Crit Care 14:187, 2004.

CHAPTER 203
TEMPORARY CARDIAC PACING

Teresa DeFrancesco, DVM, DACVIM (Cardiology), DACVECC

KEY POINTS

- Temporary cardiac pacing is a minimally invasive or noninvasive modality used to stimulate the heart electrically and increase the heart rate to achieve emergency stabilization in a patient with symptomatic, medically refractory bradycardia, usually as a bridge to permanent cardiac pacing.
- Temporary cardiac pacing is most commonly performed by one of three methods: (1) transvenous, (2) transcutaneous, or (3) transesophageal.
- Temporary transvenous cardiac pacing is achieved by inserting a lead wire into the right ventricle via either the jugular or saphenous vein. A current is generated from a temporary pulse generator that is external to the body.
- Temporary transcutaneous pacing is a noninvasive method in which patch electrodes are placed on the skin of the right and left hemithorax at the cardiac precordium. A current passed between these electrodes stimulates the heart to beat.
- Temporary transesophageal pacing is also noninvasive and is achieved by placing a pacing catheter into the esophagus with the tip positioned just dorsal to the heart. The pacing stimulus delivered consistently paces only the atria and not the ventricles.

Temporary cardiac pacing is a minimally invasive or noninvasive modality used primarily to correct profound medically refractory bradycardia in patients in hemodynamically unstable condition.[1-3] Temporary cardiac pacing is also useful to support heart rate and blood pressure in patients with medically refractory chronotropic insufficiency that are undergoing general anesthesia for permanent pacemaker implantation or another surgery unrelated to the heart such as cataract extraction or cystotomy. Temporary cardiac pacing can be achieved using one of three different techniques—transvenous, transcutaneous, or transesophageal—each having its advantages and disadvantages. Because of the need for specialized equipment and a certain level of expertise, temporary cardiac pacing is usually available only at university or private specialty hospitals in veterinary medicine.

Temporary transvenous cardiac pacing is typically the preferred and most commonly used method in humans.[1,2] In temporary transvenous cardiac pacing a lead wire is inserted via a sheath introducer into either the jugular or saphenous vein and advanced into the right ventricle. A current is generated from a temporary pulse generator that is external to the body. The main advantages of the transvenous system are more consistent capture in patients with either sinus nodal or atrioventricular (AV) nodal disease, improved patient comfort allowing its use in sedated or awake patients, lower cost of equipment, and relative ease of insertion by experienced personnel. The most common complication with transvenous pacing is lead dislodgement and loss of capture, which is most commonly associated with movement of the patient. Other complications include thrombosis, bleeding, infection, ventricular arrhythmias, and cardiac perforation.[4-6]

Noninvasive alternatives to temporary transvenous pacing are transcutaneous pacing and transesophageal pacing. Transcutaneous pacing is preferred over transvenous pacing in life-threatening situations, such as cardiac arrest, because of the shorter time to implementation.[7] Another advantage of transcutaneous pacing is that the patch electrodes have other functions such as cardioversion or defibrillation, which may prove useful if the cardiac rhythm changes to a life-threatening ventricular tachycardia or ventricular fibrillation. The most common complications of transcutaneous pacing are discomfort and musculoskeletal stimulation associated with the pacing stimulus, so that heavy sedation or general anesthesia is required.[8,9] These limit its use to only short-term temporary cardiac pacing. Transesophageal cardiac pacing is also a short-term pacing method because of the requirement for general anesthesia to allow insertion of the pacing catheter into the esophagus.[10,11] The pacing catheter, either a specialized transesophageal pacing lead or a multipurpose electrophysiologic catheter, is inserted into the esophagus just dorsal to the heart. The electrical stimulus usually does not produce any external muscle stimulation unless higher than normal pacing thresholds are used. Another advantage of this system is that it can be implemented more rapidly than transvenous temporary pacing. It is important to recognize that a transesophageal pacing system consistently paces only the atria and not the ventricles. Thus the main disadvantage of transesophageal pacing is that it is useful only in patients with sinus nodal dysfunction and is not useful in patients with AV nodal disease.

INDICATIONS FOR TEMPORARY CARDIAC PACING

The most common application of temporary cardiac pacing is to support heart rate and blood pressure in a patient under general anesthesia for permanent pacemaker implantation. Some cardiologists believe that the use of any type of temporary cardiac pacing is a debatable practice in patients undergoing permanent pacemaker implantation that are in hemodynamically stable condition. However, in patients with erratic ventricular escape rhythms or with extremely low ventricular escape rates (<30 beats/min), temporary pacing does improve cardiac output and blood pressure during anesthesia until the permanent pacing system is in place. Additionally, prophylactic use of temporary pacing during permanent pacemaker implantation ensures rapid rescue if problems such as asystole arise. For this reason, the author uses temporary cardiac pacing in all patients undergoing permanent pacemaker implantation. Arguments against temporary pacing include increased surgical time, likelihood that sedation will be required for placement of the transvenous pacing system, need for specialized equipment for transcutaneous or transesophageal pacing, and lack of evidence for a clear improvement in outcome. In a large retrospective multicenter review of artificial pacemaker practices and outcomes, the use of temporary transvenous pacing in patients undergoing permanent pacemaker implantation varied from 4% to 100%, depending on the institution and personnel performing the procedure.[12] No complications due to temporary transvenous cardiac pacing were reported in this and another similar case cohort.[12,13] Complications of permanent cardiac pacing, in general, were related primarily to the operator's experience level and frequency in placing artificial pacemakers.

In summary, indications for temporary cardiac pacing include the following:

1. Need for heart rate and blood pressure support while patients are under general anesthesia during permanent pacemaker implantation.
2. Need for heart rate and blood pressure support in dogs with clinically silent sinus nodal dysfunction that have experienced an episode of profound and medically refractory bradycardia while undergoing general anesthesia. Typically these dogs were undergoing anesthesia for surgery unrelated to the heart, such as cataract extraction or cystotomy for urolithiasis removal, which was aborted because of the medically refractory and life-threatening bradycardia. If the owner's preference or the dog's clinical status dictates that the surgery be reattempted, these dogs usually require temporary cardiac pacing to tolerate the anesthesia. The author generally does not recommend implantation of permanent pacemakers in dogs with asymptomatic sinus nodal dysfunction.
3. Medically refractory bradycardia in a patient that is in need of a permanent pacemaker but requires hemodynamic stabilization or support before permanent pacing. Some of these patients are being stabilized until permanent pacemaker implantation is possible (e.g., personnel issues). Other patients may have systemic infection or endocarditis so that permanent pacemaker implantation is being postponed until the patient is free of infection or is in more stable condition for general anesthesia. Transvenous pacing is generally selected in such cases because it can be used relatively long term in a sedated or conscious patient.
4. Medically refractory and potentially reversible bradycardia, usually caused by a drug overdose.[14] Drugs that commonly cause medically refractory bradycardias include digoxin, diltiazem, verapamil, and β-blockers. Transvenous pacing is generally chosen in these cases because it can be used long term in a sedated or conscious patient.
5. Cardiac arrest from medically refractory sinus arrest leading to asystole due to drug overdose or natural sinus nodal or AV nodal disease in which a meaningful recovery is possible. Transcutaneous pacing is most useful in these cases because in emergency situations cardiac pacing can be achieved in a shorter time and does not require vascular access. Establishing vascular access, even when the operator is experienced, can cause unacceptable delays in initiation of cardiac pacing.

DESCRIPTION OF THE TEMPORARY PACEMAKER SYSTEMS

All temporary cardiac pacing systems have a pulse generator and a lead wire, catheter, or patch electrodes that deliver the electrical current to stimulate the heart. All of the temporary pulse generators are demand pacemakers that can sense the patient's intrinsic heart rhythm and subsequently suppress the pacing impulse. Each of these systems uses different equipment, and systems vary in how and where the energy is delivered.

Transvenous Pacing System

The equipment needed for temporary transvenous pacing includes a sheath introducer set, a temporary pacing lead wire, and a temporary pacemaker or pulse generator. Additionally, electrocardiography and, ideally, fluoroscopy are used to guide lead wire placement and identify ventricular capture. The sheath introducer set includes a vascular access needle or catheter, placement wire, vessel dilator, and sheath introducer with a one-way hemostatic valve to allow passage of the lead wire. The diameter of the sheath introducer should be big enough to accommodate the pacing wire. The most common catheter size used in dogs is 5 Fr.[3]

The temporary pacing lead is usually a bipolar lead, although quadripolar electrophysiologic catheters are also available. The pacing lead can simply be a semirigid lead wire or can be associated with a balloon-tipped catheter to ease passage across the tricuspid valve. In humans, a new temporary pacing lead wire with active fixation has been described for long-term temporary pacing (days to weeks), such as in a patient with endocarditis.[15] These new active-fixation temporary wires dramatically decrease the rate of dislodgement in long-term temporary pacing. The temporary pulse generator is either a small hand-held battery-operated device or a larger programmer in which heart rate, energy output, and sensitivity can be adjusted to the individual patient.

For the implantation of the temporary transvenous pacing system, the dog is placed in lateral recumbency for central venous access. Whether or not sedation is needed depends on the patient's demeanor and hemodynamic status. Either the jugular or femoral vein is cannulated aseptically with the sheath introducer, using the Seldinger technique. If the temporary transvenous system is being used as a bridge to a permanent transvenous pacing system, the vein used for the temporary system should not be the same one planned for the permanent system. For example, the left jugular vein can be used for the temporary system and the right jugular vein saved for the permanent system. Alternatively, the right saphenous vein can be used for the temporary system and the right jugular vein for the permanent system, which allows the patient to be in the same position during both procedures. The author administers a small subcutaneous infusion of lidocaine for local anesthesia at the catheter insertion site. Once the introducer is in place, it is flushed with heparinized saline and sutured in place.

The pacing lead wire is then inserted via the sheath introducer's hemostatic port, preferably through a plastic contamination guard. The wire is advanced into the right ventricular apex, preferably with fluoroscopic and electrocardiographic guidance, until ventricular capture is noted (Figure 203-1), associated with a smooth coursing of the lead wire into the apex of the right ventricle and ideally seen fluoroscopically or with the aid of transthoracic echocardiography. The pacing lead is connected to the external temporary pacemaker. The temporary pacemaker is usually set for a heart rate between 60 and 100 beats/min. The energy output usually is set at 3 mA initially. At this voltage, the ventricle should be captured with each pacing impulse. One can determine the voltage threshold by gradually turning down the voltage until capture is lost. The pacemaker voltage is then set to at least twice the threshold voltage. The author typically sets the sensitivity at 3 mV for temporary pacing, but this may need to be adjusted to ensure that no oversensing or undersensing of intrinsic beats occurs. Once the pacing wire and external temporary pacemaker settings are made and the lead wire position is deemed adequate, the insertion site is dressed with antimicrobial ointment and the neck is wrapped with a triple-layer bandage to ensure that the wire and external generator are secured and protected.

Transcutaneous Pacing System

A transcutaneous pacing system is an optional feature on some defibrillator/electrocardiogram (ECG) systems. Pacing systems are available from several companies including Phiips (Andover, MA) and Zoll Medical (Chelmsford, MA) both offer devices with optional external cardiac pacing. This pacing system is expensive and is available only at a few veterinary institutions. In addition to the pulse generator, the pacing system requires a good-quality ECG tracing and a pair of disposable transthoracic patch electrodes connected to the pulse generator via pacing leads.[8,9,16,17] Standard ECG leads usually are connected to the dog's footpads to obtain a good-quality recording. The adhesive pacing patch electrodes are then placed on the left and right hemithorax directly over the precordial impulse (Figure 203-2). Proper positioning of the transdermal patch electrodes is critical to the efficacy of temporary pacing.[8,18] The fur is shaved over both the left and right precordia, and a small amount of ECG paste is placed on the electrode patches just before adhesion. One may choose to further secure the patch electrodes with an elastic nonadhesive bandaging material to minimize migration and to improve contact. After the patch electrodes are placed, a good-quality ECG

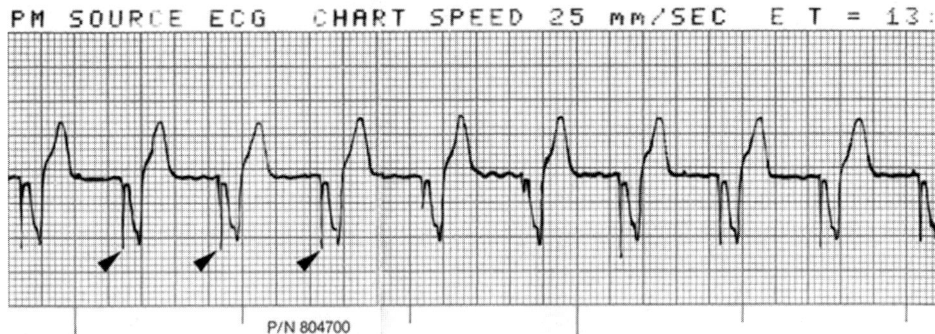

FIGURE 203-1 Electrocardiogram for a dog with a transvenous temporary pacemaker. Note the large pacing spikes *(arrows)* followed by a QRS-T complex, confirming ventricular capture.

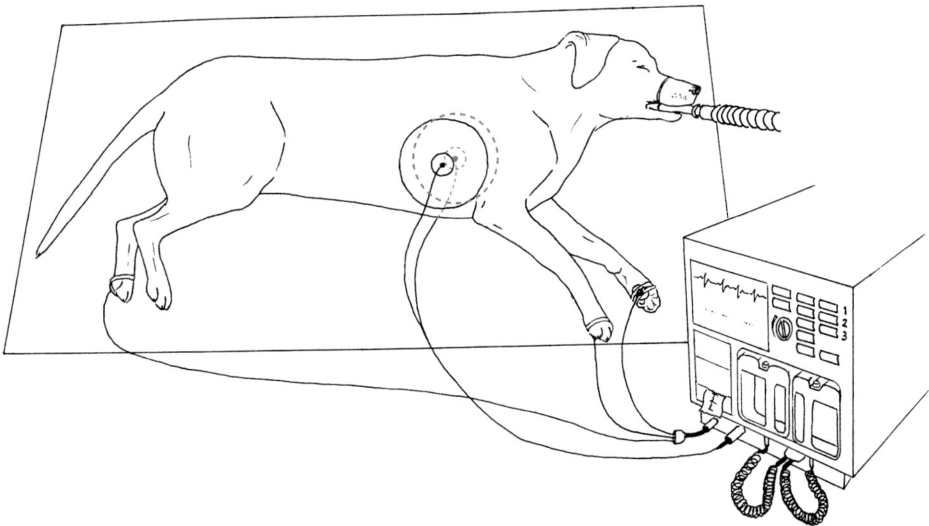

FIGURE 203-2 Schematic illustration of a dog under general anesthesia undergoing noninvasive transthoracic external cardiac pacing. The dog is positioned in lateral recumbency, an electrocardiographic recording is obtained, and after proper sensing of the patient's cardiac rhythm, the pacing stimulus is delivered through the two large patch electrodes placed directly over the precordium on the right and left sides of the thorax. *(From DeFrancesco TC, Hansen BH, Atkins CE: Noninvasive transthoracic temporary cardiac pacing in dogs, J Vet Intern Med 17:663, 2003. Illustration by Petra Guity.)*

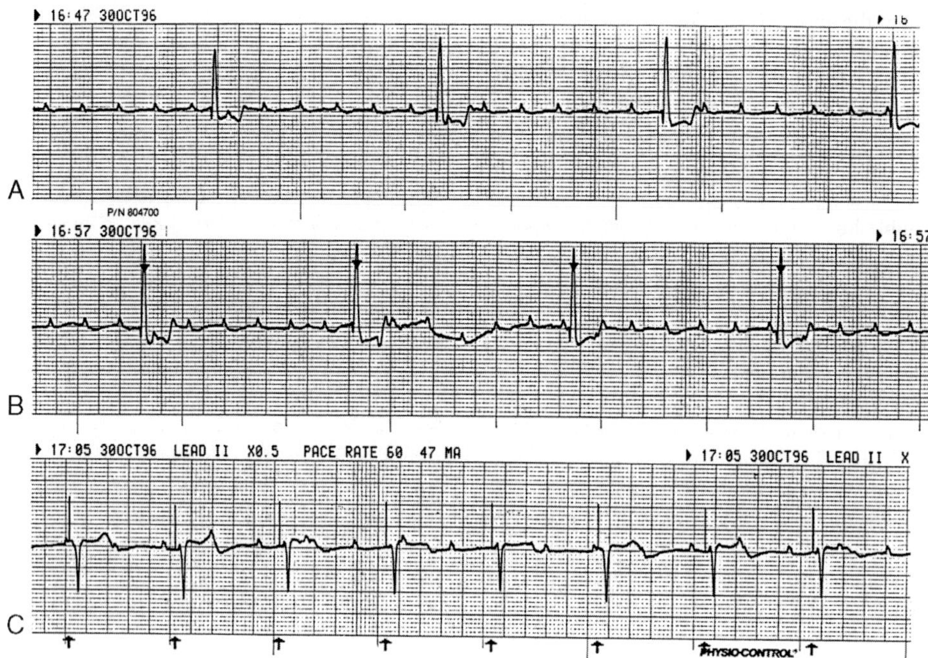

FIGURE 203-3 A, Electrocardiogram for a dog with complete atrioventricular block under general anesthesia for permanent pacemaker implantation. The ventricular rate is 30 beats/min, whereas the atrial rate is 170 beats/min. **B,** Proper sensing of the patient's intrinsic QRS activity is shown with the sensing marker, an inverted triangular symbol on top of the QRS complex. Once accurate sensing is accomplished, the pacemaker is turned on. **C,** Electrical capture of the ventricle by the pacer is shown by a pacing spike followed by a wide QRS-T complex. Each pacing spike is also denoted by an arrow mark just below the paper grid. The ventricular rate is now 70 beats/min (paper speed for all electrocardiographic recordings is 25 mm/sec). *(From DeFrancesco TC, Hansen BH, Atkins CE: Noninvasive transthoracic temporary cardiac pacing in dogs, J Vet Intern Med 17:663, 2003.)*

recording is obtained. Lead selection and ECG gain are optimized to attain accurate sensing of the patient's intrinsic cardiac rhythm by the demand pacing system (Figure 203-3). After accurate QRS sensing is confirmed by the appearance of the sensing marker on the ECG monitor, the desired pacing rate is chosen and the pacing current is increased gradually until ventricular capture is identified on the ECG (see Figure 203-3) and confirmed by palpation of a corresponding arterial pulse. Determination of electrical and mechanical capture can at times be difficult because skeletal muscle is also stimulated, which causes motion ECG and palpation artifact. Ventricular capture is identified by the presence of a wide QRS-T complex after the pacing spike on the ECG monitor. The current output is then maintained just above the capture threshold, usually 10 to 20 mA higher than threshold, for the duration of cardiac pacing. In two clinical canine case series, the current required for pacing ranged from 30 to 160 mA.[8,9] Despite the requirement for general anesthesia, transcutaneous pacing is a good noninvasive alternative to temporary transvenous pacing in many veterinary clinical settings in which short-term temporary pacing is indicated; for example, during permanent pacemaker implantation, replacement, or lead adjustment.

Transesophageal Pacing System

Transesophageal pacing is a relatively newer technique in veterinary medicine. Only a few veterinary centers have this capability, but it offers an attractive noninvasive alternative for heart rate support in animals with sinus nodal dysfunction undergoing general anesthesia.[10,11,19] The equipment needed for transesophageal pacing includes a specialized transesophageal pulse generator, a bipolar pacing catheter, and a semirigid plastic guide (optional). In one study, a disposable esophageal stethoscope with both ends cut was used to insert the pacing catheter.[11] The semirigid tubing is removed once the catheter is in place. The pacing catheter can be a transesophageal pacing lead or a quadripolar electrophysiologic catheter. A recent study in dogs showed lowered pacing thresholds and more consistent pacing with a quadripolar electrophysiologic catheter than with an esophageal pacing catheter.[11] As with all the other pacing systems, electrocardiography (and optionally fluoroscopy) is used to guide pacing catheter placement and identify atrial capture. With the patient in lateral recumbency under general anesthesia, the pacing catheter is inserted transorally into the esophagus, connected to the pulse generator, and advanced to the level of the diaphragm until pacing of the diaphragm is noted. The catheter is then slowly withdrawn until atrial pacing is noted on the ECG. The pacing stimulus is delivered in AAI mode; that is, it paces the atria (A), it senses atrial activity (A), and when atrial activity is sensed it inhibits (I) the pacemaker output. The pacing rate per minute is set to 60 to 100 as needed for support of the patient's heart rate and blood pressure. The pacing amplitude and pulse width are adjusted to ensure capture of the atria and minimize extraneous muscle stimulation. The pulse width is typically initially set between 2 and 10 ms and the pacing amplitude is adjusted between 7 and 30 mA. The initial pacing amplitude is usually set high at 20 to 30 mA and then the amplitude is decreased to an energy level that ensures consistent pacing while minimizing external muscle stimulation. Fluoroscopy can aid in optimal positioning to achieve low pacing thresholds. The lower pacing thresholds are associated with minimal to no external muscle stimulation. Variables such as recumbency, the relationship between the heart and esophagus, breed conformation, catheter shape, and polar surface area can all affect the pacing thresholds.

TROUBLESHOOTING

Common issues with all modalities of temporary pacing are inconsistent pacing and suboptimal sensing of the underlying intrinsic cardiac rhythm. Sensing of the underlying rhythm is more important with sinus nodal dysfunctions than with high-grade AV block. A suboptimal ECG recording resulting in either oversensing or undersensing of the ECG complexes can also result in inconsistent pacing. Changing the lead channel or lead size to ensure that only the QRS complexes are being sensed and not the P or T waves will improve the function of the temporary pacing system. The ECG recording should be pristine. Troubleshooting of inconsistent pacing depends on the type of temporary pacing system used.

Transvenous Pacing System

One potential problem with the initial insertion of the lead wire is that the wire does not advance across the tricuspid valve into the right ventricular apex and continues to loop in the right atrium or goes out the caudal vena cava. Use of balloon-tipped pacing catheters eases the passage across the tricuspid valve into the right ventricle. Additionally, before the wire is inserted, molding 3 to 4 cm of the tip of the wire into a gentle 20- to 30-degree angle may help it slip into the right ventricle. A common problem is inability to capture the ventricle. Pacing spikes are observed, but no QRS complex or capture is seen. This typically results from poor contact of the wire with the ventricular muscle. The position of the wire is checked using fluoroscopy. The ideal placement for the tip of the pacing wire is the apex of the right ventricle. Loss of capture is not uncommon in a conscious patient that is moving. Sedation may help, as may adhering the pacing wire to the sheath introducer to minimize displacement. If no pacing spikes are seen at all, then failure of the battery or pulse generator, or a loose connection is usually at fault. Ideally, a new battery is used for each case.

Transcutaneous Pacing System

Despite the ease and speed of noninvasive transthoracic pacing, especially in arrest situations, the primary disadvantage in human patients is inconsistent pacing success rates.[17] In the author's experience, initial failure to pace in dogs with a transcutaneous pacing system usually results from suboptimal electrode placement and ECG recordings. The patch electrodes should be placed directly over the cardiac impulse beat, but not too close to the sternum, so that the current actually courses across the heart and not along the skin. The author has also noted that the skin and, subsequently, the patch electrodes tend to move with changes in body position, which can cause loss of capture. The position of the patch electrodes should be checked every time the dog is moved. The operator also should be aware that patch electrodes are available in adult and pediatric sizes, and the appropriate electrode size should be used for the dog. Other causes of inconsistent pacing include obesity, barrel-shaped chest conformation, and pleural space or pericardial disease. In dogs with physical reasons for inconsistent pacing, an increase in pacing amplitude, generous use of conducting gel, and wrapping of the chest with a nonadherent bandaging material usually help to achieve capture. In two canine case series, successful pacing was achieved in nearly all dogs, although repositioning of the patch electrodes or optimizing of the ECG recordings was needed in several patients.[8,9]

Transesophageal Pacing System

The author has limited personal experience with transesophageal pacing, but based on the human experience, veterinary case reports, and published canine experimental studies the main problem is inconsistent pacing. The pulse amplitude and pulse width can be increased, in addition to moving the pacing catheter to the optimal position, to achieve cardiac pacing. Fluoroscopy can also be helpful to ensure use of the lowest pacing thresholds and optimal positioning by allowing visualization of the pacing catheter within the esophagus and its relationship to the heart.

COMPLICATIONS

Transvenous Pacing System

Lead dislodgement is the most common complication with temporary transvenous pacing, based on the human literature and the author's experience.[1,2,4-6] Lead dislodgement usually is well tolerated for brief periods but is potentially life threatening in a patient that is entirely pacemaker dependent. Interestingly, there are no reports of complications associated with temporary transvenous pacing in the veterinary literature. Several reports of complications associated with permanent transvenous pacing in dogs[12,13] describe complications similar to those that have been reported in the human literature for temporary transvenous pacing. These include hemorrhage, infection, ventricular arrhythmias, cardiac chamber perforation, and thrombosis. It is important to emphasize that, although the rate of serious complications is probably low for temporary transvenous pacing in dogs, there is the potential for significant and serious sequelae.

Transcutaneous Pacing System

Patient discomfort is a main complication in dogs undergoing transcutaneous pacing, requiring heavy sedation or, more likely, general anesthesia. Although most humans tolerate external cardiac pacing with no or minimal discomfort, conscious dogs do not tolerate transcutaneous pacing. General anesthesia and analgesia are strongly recommended for all dogs in which this technique is employed. In one human case series, the pacing stimulus was described as intolerable by only 10% of patients.[17] These patients described the pacing stimulus as a severe thump or as an intense burning or stinging pain that required termination of pacing. The pain and discomfort associated with noninvasive pacing are increased when pacing current outputs are higher, smaller-diameter patch electrodes are used, and skin abrasions are present at the electrode site.[17] It is unclear whether dogs truly feel pain with transcutaneous pacing or if the element of surprise, combined with the sudden and repetitive nature of the pacing stimuli and skeletal muscle stimulation, make the technique intolerable.

Skeletal muscle stimulation is another complication associated with transcutaneous pacing. This expected side effect is caused by unavoidable electrical stimulation of the skeletal muscles of the thorax and forelegs, which causes the patient to jerk mildly to moderately with each pacing impulse. These movements, although predictable, can increase the difficulty of surgery, especially in smaller dogs, in which the rhythmic motion of the forelegs can be more pronounced. This skeletal muscle jerking can be eliminated with neuromuscular blockade, which then necessitates mechanical ventilation during anesthesia.

Transesophageal Pacing System

Few, mostly minimal complications have been reported with transesophageal pacing. In an experimental animal study, mild focal erosive esophagitis at the site of catheter contact occurred after 24 hours of continuous esophageal pacing.[20] The lesion completely resolved within 7 days. External muscle stimulation is possible at higher pacing thresholds, which may require neuromuscular blockade to suppress. Other complications reported in humans include mild chest pain and irritation associated with catheter placement.

REFERENCES

1. Gammage MD: Temporary cardiac pacing, Heart 83:715, 2000.
2. Kaushik V, Leon AR, Forrester JS Jr: Bradyarrhythmias, temporary and permanent pacing, Crit Care Med 28:N121, 2000.

3. Scansen BA: Interventional cardiology for the criticalist, J Vet Emerg Crit Care (San Antonio) 21:123, 2011.
4. Betts TR: Regional survey of temporary transvenous pacing procedures and complications, Postgrad Med J 79:463, 2003.
5. Murphy JJ: Problems with temporary cardiac pacing, BMJ 323:527, 2001.
6. Hynes JK, Holmes DR, Harrison CE: Five-year experience with temporary pacemaker therapy in the coronary care unit, Mayo Clin Proc 58:122, 1983.
7. White JD, Brown CG: Immediate transthoracic pacing for cardiac asystole in an emergency department setting, Am J Emerg Med 3:125, 1985.
8. DeFrancesco TC, Hansen BH, Atkins CE: Noninvasive transthoracic temporary cardiac pacing in dogs, J Vet Intern Med 17:663, 2003.
9. Noomanová N, Perego M, Perini A, et al: Use of transcutaneous external pacing during transvenous pacemaker implantation in dogs, Vet Rec 167:241, 2010.
10. Sanders RA, Green HW 3rd, Hogan DF, et al: Efficacy of transesophageal and transgastric cardiac pacing in the dog, J Vet Cardiol 12:49, 2010.
11. Chapel EH, Sanders RA: Efficacy of two commercially available cardiac pacing catheters for transesophageal atrial pacing in dogs, J Vet Cardiol 14:409, 2012.
12. Oyama MA, Sisson DD, et al: Practices and outcome of artificial cardiac pacing in 154 dogs, J Vet Intern Med 15:229, 2001.
13. Wess G, Thomas WP, Berger DM, et al: Application, complications and outcomes of transvenous pacemaker implantation in 105 dogs (1997-2002), J Vet Intern Med 20:877, 2006.
14. Syring RS, Costello MF, Poppenga RH: Temporary transvenous cardiac pacing in a dog with diltiazem intoxication, J Vet Emerg Crit Care (San Antonio) 18:75, 2008.
15. de Cock CC, Van Campen CMC, In't Veld JA, et al: Utility and safety of prolonged temporary pacing using an active-fixation lead: comparison with a conventional lead, Pacing Clin Electrophysiol 26:1245, 2003.
16. Zoll PM: Resuscitation of the heart in ventricular standstill by external electrical stimulation, N Engl J Med 13:768, 1952.
17. Zoll PM, Zoll RH, Falk RH: External noninvasive temporary cardiac pacing: clinical trials, Circulation 71:937, 1985.
18. Lee S, Nam SJ, Hyun C: The optimal size and placement of transdermal electrodes are critical for the efficacy of a transcutaneous pacemaker in dogs, Vet J 183:196, 2010.
19. Sanders RA, Green HW 3rd, Hogan DF, et al: Use of transesophageal atrial pacing to provide temporary chronotropic support in a dog undergoing permanent pacemaker implantation, J Vet Cardiol 13:227, 2011.
20. Green HW 3rd, Sanders RA, Ramos-Vara J, et al: Safety of transesophageal pacing for 24 hours in a canine model, Pacing Clin Electrophysiol 32:888, 2009.

CHAPTER 204
CARDIOVERSION AND DEFIBRILLATION

Romain Pariaut, DVM, DACVIM (Cardiology), DECVIM-CA (Cardiology)

KEY POINTS

- Defibrillation is indicated for the treatment of ventricular fibrillation, pulseless ventricular tachycardia and rapid polymorphic ventricular tachycardia.
- Electrical cardioversion is indicated for the treatment of supraventricular and monomorphic ventricular tachyarrhythmias that are nonresponsive to antiarrhythmic drug therapy.
- Shock delivery during cardioversion must be synchronized to the R wave on the electrocardiogram to limit the risk of inducing ventricular fibrillation.
- Hospital personnel should be trained in and aware of the risks of electrical therapies.

DEFINITIONS

Cardioversion and defibrillation are electrical therapies used to terminate tachyarrhythmias and restore sinus rhythm.

Arrhythmias that may respond to cardioversion include supraventricular and ventricular tachycardias, with the exception of ventricular fibrillation and very irregular and rapid polymorphic ventricular tachycardia. Electrical cardioversion is indicated when prompt termination of an arrhythmia causing hemodynamic instability is needed; it is also a treatment option when available antiarrhythmic drugs have failed to restore sinus rhythm.

Defibrillation is indicated for the termination of ventricular fibrillation, a life-threatening emergency characterized by the absence of organized ventricular activity on the surface electrocardiogram. Instead there are rapid and chaotic undulations of varying amplitude. It can also be used for the treatment of rapid polymorphic ventricular tachycardia, whether it is associated with a pulse or not. Ventricular fibrillation, pulseless ventricular tachycardia, asystole, and electromechanical dissociation are three rhythm disturbances that result in cardiac arrest. Therefore defibrillation is always integrated into the advanced life support segment of cardiopulmonary resuscitation (CPR) protocols.

MECHANISM OF CARDIOVERSION AND DEFIBRILLATION

When a shock is delivered to a critical mass of myocardium, most of the ventricular myocyte action potentials experience a coordinated change in voltage (depolarization) and are placed in a refractory state that interrupts further propagation of electrical impulses. This then allows the sinus node to regain control of the cardiac rhythm.

The success of shock in terminating an arrhythmia depends on many factors, including the amount of energy delivered, the path of current relative to the position of the heart, and the transthoracic impedance. Indeed, it appears that as little as 4% of the energy delivered by the defibrillator reaches the myocardium. Importantly, the vector of the shock must travel across at least 70% of the ventricular

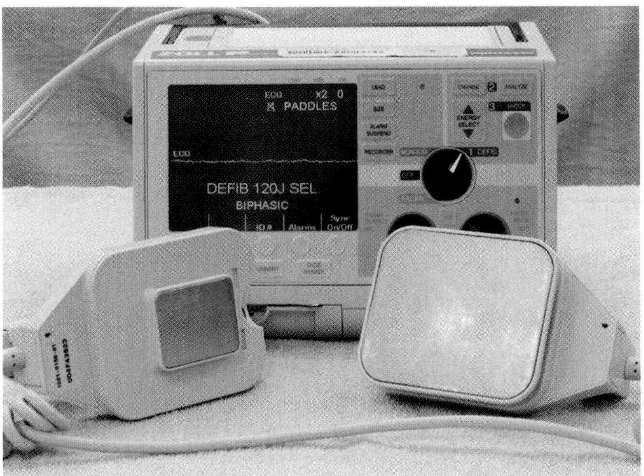

FIGURE 204-1 External biphasic defibrillator-cardioverter. This multifunction device can also be used for external transthoracic pacing. The paddle on the right is adult size. The pediatric-size paddle is on the left.

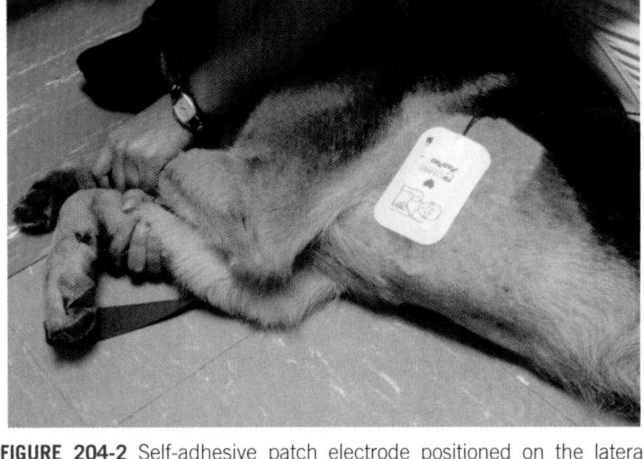

FIGURE 204-2 Self-adhesive patch electrode positioned on the lateral thorax over the palpable cardiac apex beat.

myocardial mass.[1] Finally, high transthoracic impedance decreases the probability of a successful shock. Size and conformation of the chest, water and fat content, pulmonary volume, size and position of the paddles, and force applied to the paddles are factors determining thoracic impedance.[2]

Finally, defibrillation success is a probabilistic event; that is, a shock of the same intensity may succeed or fail on successive attempts.

DEFIBRILLATOR-CARDIOVERTER

A defibrillator is a device designed to quickly deliver a preselected amount of electrical current to the heart. Defibrillation is external when it is performed from the surface of the body; it is termed *internal* when sterile paddles are applied directly to the surface of the heart following a thoracotomy. Defibrillation can also be performed percutaneously via catheters connected to the defibrillator and positioned within the cardiac chambers.

Most defibrillators can be powered from a rechargeable battery, which makes them portable. A transformer converts alternating current (AC) into a direct current (DC) power source because only DC current reliably terminates ventricular fibrillation. The main internal component of the defibrillator is the capacitor, which stores electrical charges supplied by the battery during charging time and then releases them rapidly when the discharge function is triggered. The amount of energy to be delivered is selected by the operator. A set of internal electronic components adjusts the energy, the duration of the shock, and the shock waveform when defibrillation is initiated and charges are released from the capacitor to the paddles.

Most defibrillators are multifunction devices that typically include monitoring and external pacing capabilities. All defibrillators have a display that presents various information, including an electrocardiogram (ECG) tracing obtained from leads directly attached to the patient's limbs or from the "quick-look" defibrillation paddles as well as the preselected amount of energy to be delivered (Figure 204-1). On the front panel, a selector allows the operator to choose between monitoring, pacing, or defibrillation function, and a button is dedicated to switching between synchronous and asynchronous modes. The initiation of a defibrillator's capacitor charging and shock delivery can be triggered from the unit or directly from the paddles. Defibrillators usually produce a continuous sound during charging, which changes in tone when the capacitor is fully charged. Most defibrillators come with a set of adult-size and pediatric-size paddles. Paddles can be replaced by self-adhesive patch electrodes, which are secured on both sides of the chest (Figure 204-2). It is critical that any person who may need to use the defibrillator know precisely how to operate the unit because ventricular fibrillation is an emergency that requires rapid intervention.

Modalities of current delivery to the heart muscle have evolved over the years to increase the probability of first-shock success. An important development has been the transition from monophasic to biphasic shock waveforms. Monophasic defibrillators generate a unidirectional flow of current through the heart. Conversely, biphasic shocks are characterized by an initial positive current flow followed by a negative current flow in the opposite direction. These waveforms have been shown to be more effective than the monophasic configuration in terminating ventricular fibrillation at a lower energy setting, which may also decrease the severity of myocardial damage. Indeed, it appears that the second wave of current eliminates charges from cells that were only partially depolarized by the first phase of the shock and "heals" cell membranes damaged by the first wave of current.[3-5] Finally, biphasic waveforms can take various shapes, with the rectilinear and truncated exponential waveforms being the most common.

Automated external defibrillators have the capability to analyze the rhythm and automatically deliver shocks. They are now widely available in public spaces to be operated by trained bystanders. However, their ability to discriminate between shockable and nonshockable rhythms in dogs is uncertain.

APPROACH TO DEFIBRILLATION

Indications

Defibrillation, which corresponds to the delivery of a shock not synchronized to an R wave, is a critical component of a CPR protocol if ventricular fibrillation or pulseless ventricular tachycardia is the cause of cardiac arrest. Although an attempt to identify the underlying dysrhythmia is important, it should never delay the initiation of basic CPR (attention to airway, breathing, and circulation). Performance of good-quality chest compressions is critical to deliver oxygen and energy substrates to the myocardium before defibrillation (see Chapter 3). Once ventricular fibrillation is confirmed, it is important to initiate defibrillation immediately because the probability of a positive outcome decreases rapidly over time.[6] If ventricular fibrillation is detected within 4 minutes of cardiopulmonary arrest, defibrillation can be performed without an initial cycle of chest compressions.[5] Delivery of an asynchronous shock is also

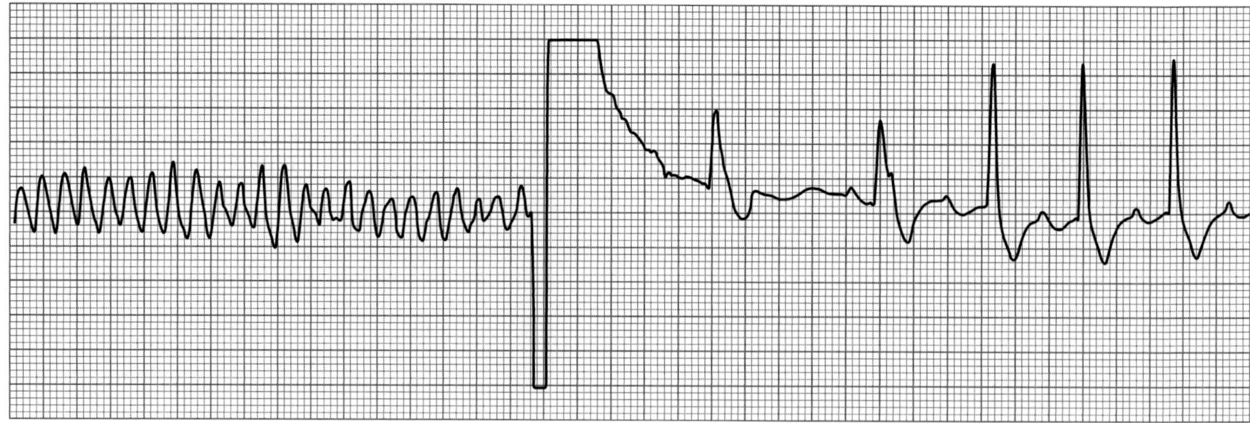

FIGURE 204-3 Termination of ventricular fibrillation and restoration of sinus rhythm via a transthoracic biphasic shock. The two beats with wide QRS complexes following the shock may be ventricular in origin or correspond to sinus beats with aberrant conduction in the ventricles.

indicated for the termination of rapid, irregular polymorphic ventricular tachycardia and pulseless ventricular tachycardia. In fact, when pronounced beat-to-beat changes in QRS morphology are present, synchronization of the shock to the R wave is usually not possible.[6]

Preparation

Although CPR is usually performed with the animal placed in lateral recumbency, it is easier to position the paddles on the chest if the animal is repositioned in dorsal recumbency. It is important to limit the interval between the last chest compression and the delivery of a shock to only a few seconds. The largest paddles or self-adhesive patches that fit on the chest should be used because the large surface of contact with the skin decreases the impedance at the surface of the body. Moreover, good contact between the paddles and the body is paramount. It is improved by applying electrode gel on the paddles and on both side of the chest. Application of gel outside the areas covered by the paddles should be avoided because it can be the cause of short circuits. Ultrasound coupling gel is not a satisfactory alternative since it has poor electrical conductivity. Finally, paddles should not be placed over ECG pads.

Therapy

Selection of paddle size is based on the size of the animal. Pediatric paddles have been recommended for animals weighing less than 15 kg (see Figure 204-1).[7] The paddles are positioned on either side of the lateral thorax over the heart, so that the electrical shock crosses most of the cardiac myocardial mass. Firm manual pressure is then applied to the paddles to literally squeeze the heart between the paddles and decrease the thoracic impedance. Impedance is also influenced by body weight, shape and size of the thorax, lung volume and size, and position of the paddles. As impedance increases, the amount of current that is effectively delivered to the myocardium decreases. However, modern defibrillators can quickly measure thoracic impedance when the paddles are placed on the chest and can automatically adjust the shock waveform characteristics to match the preselected energy to the energy effectively delivered across the chest.[8] Before defibrillation is performed, the person who is responsible for initiating the shock should ascertain that staff are not in contact with the animal and stand clear. The individual holding the paddles should make sure the paddles never come in contact with each other during the procedure to prevent current arcing and sparks. Other safety measures include disconnecting oxygen and anesthetic circuits from the patient to prevent explosions. It is noteworthy that an ECG tracing appears on the monitor of the defibrillator when the paddles are in contact with the chest. This is useful to confirm the rhythm before shock delivery. When it is time to deliver a shock, the operator should loudly say "Clear" and confirm that all personnel are safe before delivering the shock. Delivery of the shock is confirmed by the whole body muscle twitch it triggers.

During ventricular fibrillation, an unsynchronized shock is delivered independently of the cardiac cycle (Figure 204-3). It is believed that monophasic defibrillators usually require higher-energy shock than biphasic defibrillators. The veterinary literature reports values of 2 to 4 J for biphasic shocks.[9] In a research setting the author determined in a few healthy dogs that a biphasic shock with an energy of 4 J/kg consistently terminated ventricular fibrillation, whereas an energy of 3 J/kg was less likely to be successful. Waveform influences the amount of energy that will successfully terminate ventricular fibrillation; it is therefore important to know the device-specific effective waveform dose range provided by the defibrillator manufacturer. It is usually suggested that the operator aim at using the lowest amount of energy possible. However, other reports suggest that higher energies should be selected first to increase the likelihood of a successful first shock. It is also unclear if a fixed-energy protocol should be used when multiple consecutive shocks are necessary to convert ventricular fibrillation or if the energy delivered should be increased on subsequent shocks.[8] With monophasic defibrillators, it was previously recommended to deliver up to three successive shocks if the first one was unsuccessful to decrease transthoracic impedance and therefore increase the amount of energy delivered to the myocardium with the second and the third shocks. This rule does not seem to apply to biphasic defibrillation.[9] Current recommendations are to interpose one 2-minute cycle of chest compressions between each shock.[8]

Open chest cardiac defibrillation is rarely indicated in veterinary patients unless ventricular fibrillation occurs in the operating room. It is performed via sterile internal handles that are connected to the defibrillator to replace the standard paddles. The electrodes at the extremities of the handles consist of 2- to 4-cm metallic disks that are applied directly to the surface of the heart. The electrodes are positioned so that the shock travels across most of the left ventricular mass. Usually, the maximum deliverable energy from internal paddles is limited to 50 J. In dogs, it has been reported that energies of 10 to 30 J can be used to terminate ventricular fibrillation.[10]

Complications

Failure to defibrillate successfully is directly correlated with the duration of ventricular fibrillation.[11] Human studies indicate that the rate of hospital discharge decreases by 10% for every minute of ventricular fibrillation.[12]

The risk of myocardial damage secondary to the delivery of a small number of shocks seems limited except for a transient decrease in cardiac output. In an experimental study in dogs, only a modest increase in cardiac troponin I level was noted after multiple episodes of ventricular fibrillation induction followed by defibrillation.[13]

APPROACH TO SYNCHRONIZED CARDIOVERSION

Indications

There are only a few reports on the use of electrical cardioversion to terminate sustained tachyarrhythmias in an emergency setting.[14] It has been used more extensively, however, as an elective procedure for the management of lone atrial fibrillation. Cardioversion is also indicated for supraventricular tachycardias due to reentry, atrial flutter, and atrial tachycardia. It is more effective at terminating reentrant arrhythmias that are maintained by a self-perpetuating circuit than arrhythmias caused by a rapidly firing ectopic focus. Cardioversion can be used for the treatment of antidromic atrioventricular reentrant tachycardia and preexcited atrial fibrillation that are characterized by rapid activation of the ventricles by an impulse traveling through an accessory pathway. Finally, it is recommended for the treatment monomorphic ventricular tachycardia. Polymorphic ventricular tachycardia is preferably terminated with an asynchronous shock.[6] Short- and long-term maintenance of sinus rhythm following electrical therapy remains the most challenging part of the procedure. Evidence that the use of antiarrhythmic therapy following cardioversion prevents recurrence of tachyarrhythmias is lacking. Dogs without structural cardiac disease or atrial enlargement are more likely to stay in sinus rhythm following cardioversion.[7]

Generally, cardioversion is indicated when standard antiarrhythmic medications have failed to terminate an arrhythmia and the animal's cardiac output is severely compromised.

Preparation

Intravenous access and the ready availability of airway management equipment (including a source of oxygen, endotracheal tubes, and a laryngoscope) are essential before cardioversion is attempted. Antiarrhythmic drugs used to control ventricular tachycardia (lidocaine) and agents to manage unexpected bradycardia (atropine) should also be available. Imbalances in electrolyte levels, including serum magnesium concentration, must be corrected before cardioversion, and adequate oxygenation should be confirmed. An echocardiogram is indicated to evaluate cardiac systolic function, identify the presence of effusions, and determine the most likely substrate for the arrhythmia. The success rate of electrical cardioversion does not seem to improve with the administration of antiarrhythmics before the procedure.[7]

Delivery of a transthoracic shock is a painful and stressful event that requires anesthesia unless the animal is unconscious, which is rarely the case in the presence of tachyarrhythmias, even with heart rates above 300 beats/min. If necessary, opioids with or without a benzodiazepine are commonly used for premedication. Anesthesia induction is obtained via the administration of short-acting intravenous agents such as etomidate or propofol. It is noteworthy that tachyarrhythmias triggered by elevated adrenergic tone may resolve spontaneously after the administration of anesthetics that decrease sympathetic output. Following intubation, anesthesia is maintained with administration of intravenous agents as needed or inhalant anesthetics.

The animal is then placed in dorsal recumbency to facilitate the positioning of the paddles on the chest. It is preferable to cover metallic tables with nonconducting materials. Patches are connected to the animal to provide continuous ECG recording during the procedure. The patches are usually placed above the elbows and stifles to limit the risk of disconnection during the delivery of the shock. It is important to remember that any electrical device connected to the animal during the procedure must be surge protected. Finally, the left and right lateral sides of the thorax are clipped between the third and sixth intercostal spaces.

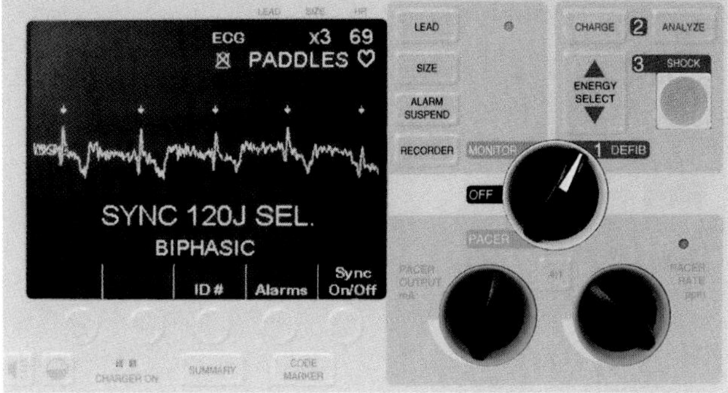

FIGURE 204-4 Synchronized cardioversion. When the defibrillator-cardioverter is in synchronized mode (SYNC), an arrow is visible above each R wave indicating that the cardioversion shock will be timed to the peak of the QRS complex, when the risk of inducing ventricular fibrillation is low.

Therapy

Most of the steps of the procedure are similar to those for defibrillation. It is critical, however, to select the synchronous mode, which times the delivery of a shock to the peak of the R wave; that is, to the absolute refractory period of the myocytes (Figure 204-4). This mode prevents delivery of a shock around the peak of the T wave, which represents the vulnerable period of the ventricles. Delivery of a shock during the vulnerable period increases the risk of initiating ventricular fibrillation because the electrical impulse reaches the ventricles during their repolarization phase, which is characterized by tissue heterogeneity. To use the synchronous mode, ECG cables from the defibrillator are connected to the patient; it is then important to confirm that the defibrillator clearly identifies the R waves, marked by an arrow on the defibrillator-cardioverter display. If the device identifies large T waves rather than R waves, the ECG electrodes should be repositioned or the recording should be switched to a different limb lead. Most defibrillators automatically default back to asynchronous mode after delivery of a synchronous shock. Therefore the "Sync" button must be pressed again and appropriate identification of the QRS complexes by the defibrillator must be confirmed before a second shock is delivered.

Cardioversion generally requires lower energy than defibrillation. The first shock is usually delivered at a level of 1 to 2 J/kg. Subsequent shocks are delivered at higher output until conversion occurs or maximum energy output fails to terminate the arrhythmia. It has been suggested that the presence of structural cardiac disease does not increase significantly the energy required for cardioversion.[7] Although most arrhythmias are stopped with one or two shocks, up to ten shocks may be necessary. Antiarrhythmics may be administered following cardioversion to prevent recurrence of the arrhythmia.

Complications

The main complication of cardioversion is induction of ventricular fibrillation if the shock is not synchronized to the R wave. Ventricular fibrillation should be treated rapidly with a high-energy asynchronous shock. Other complications relate to general anesthesia, skin burns from the external paddles, and thromboembolic events.[2] However, thromboembolism is a rare complication secondary to supraventricular tachycardia or cardioversion in dogs, and anticoagulation is typically not initiated.[15]

REFERENCES

1. Zipes DP, Fischer J, King RM, et al: Termination of ventricular fibrillation in dogs by depolarizing a critical amount of myocardium, Am J Cardiol 36(1):37-44, 1975.
2. Gall NP, Murgatroyd FD: Electrical cardioversion for AF-the state of the art, Pacing Clin Electrophysiol 30(4):554-567, 2007.
3. Murakawa Y, Yamashita T, Kanese Y, et al: Do the effects of antiarrhythmic drugs on defibrillation efficacy vary among different shock waveforms? Pacing Clin Electrophysiol 21(10):1901-1908, 1998.
4. Bright JM, Wright BD: Successful biphasic transthoracic defibrillation of a dog with prolonged, refractory ventricular fibrillation, J Vet Emerg Crit Care (San Antonio) 19(3):275-279, 2009.
5. Rozanski EA, Rush JE, Buckley GJ, et al: RECOVER evidence and knowledge gap analysis on veterinary CPR. Part 4: advanced life support, J Vet Emerg Crit Care (San Antonio) 22(Suppl 1):S44-64, 2012.
6. Link MS, Atkins DL, Passman RS, et al: Part 6: electrical therapies: automated external defibrillators, defibrillation, cardioversion, and pacing: 2010 American Heart Association Guidelines for Cardiopulmonary Resuscitation and Emergency Cardiovascular Care, Circulation 122(18 Suppl 3):S706-719, 2010.
7. Bright JM, Martin JM, Mama K: A retrospective evaluation of transthoracic biphasic electrical cardioversion for atrial fibrillation in dogs, J Vet Cardiol 7(2):85-96, 2005.
8. Deakin CD: Advances in defibrillation, Curr Opin Crit Care 17(3):231-235, 2011.
9. Fletcher DJ, Boller M, Brainard BM, et al: RECOVER evidence and knowledge gap analysis on veterinary CPR. Part 7: Clinical guidelines, J Vet Emerg Crit Care (San Antonio) 22(Suppl 1):S102-131, 2012.
10. Uechi M: Mitral valve repair in dogs, J Vet Cardiol 14(1):185-192, 2012.
11. Strohmenger HU: Predicting defibrillation success, Curr Opin Crit Care 14(3):311-316, 2008.
12. Tabereaux PB, Dosdall DJ, Ideker RE: Mechanisms of VF maintenance: wandering wavelets, mother rotors, or foci, Heart Rhythm 6(3):405-415, 2009.
13. Pariaut R, Saelinger C, Vila J, et al: Evaluation of shock waveform configuration on the defibrillation capacity of implantable cardioverter defibrillators in dogs, J Vet Cardiol 14(3):389-398, 2012.
14. Prosek R: Electrical cardioversion of sustained ventricular tachycardia in three Boxers, J Am Vet Med Assoc 236(5):554-557, 2010.
15. Usechak PJ, Bright JM, Day TK: Thrombotic complications associated with atrial fibrillation in three dogs, J Vet Cardiol 14(3):453-458, 2012.

CHAPTER 205
RENAL REPLACEMENT THERAPIES

Carrie A. Palm, DVM, DACVIM • Kayo Kanakubo, DVM

KEY POINTS

- Renal replacement therapies can provide lifesaving treatments for patients with severe acute kidney injury.
- Life-threatening electrolyte and acid-base derangements nonresponsive to medical management, refractory hyperkalemia, and severe fluid overload are indications for initiation of renal replacement therapy.
- Early initiation of renal replacement therapy should be considered for patients affected with severe acute kidney injury.
- It is critical that clinicians carrying out renal replacement therapies have a solid understanding of the necessary equipment, dialysis prescription, renal physiology, and patient monitoring.

Extracorporeal therapies are modalities in which blood is removed from patient circulation and treated or processed before being returned to the patient. During processing, blood can be cleared of endogenous and exogenous substances, and beneficial substances can also be added to the blood. The most commonly used extracorporeal therapies in veterinary medicine are intermittent hemodialysis (IHD) and, more recently, continuous renal replacement therapy (CRRT). Peritoneal dialysis (PD) is another method for solute and fluid removal that has been applied in veterinary medicine. This method uses the large peritoneal surface area as a natural "dialysis membrane" and is not an extracorporeal therapy because blood is never outside of the patient's body. In veterinary medicine, these modalities are renal replacement therapies (RRTs) that are used primarily for the treatment of acute kidney injury (AKI) but can also be used for fluid removal in congestive heart failure and for treatment of poisonings (see Chapter 75). The availability of IHD and CRRT in veterinary medicine has expanded over the last 10 years, which allows these potentially lifesaving treatments to be used more readily in veterinary patients.

In this chapter the focus is on the use of extracorporeal therapies in the acute critical care setting for the treatment of AKI. Before the intricacies of these modalities are discussed, it is critical to recognize the indications for initiation of RRT in the veterinary AKI patient. In human medicine, several studies have shown that early initiation of RRT improves the prognosis of patients with AKI.[1] Although no studies have proven this in veterinary medicine, it is the author's opinion that a similar phenomenon occurs in animal patients. Many factors must be considered when making the decision to recommend RRT. The presence of significant azotemia is not in and of itself a definitive determinant for initiation of RRT; however, severe azotemia often correlates with increasing patient morbidity. It is the author's experience that the clinical status of most AKI patients is typically unacceptable when blood urea nitrogen (BUN) values are higher than 100 mg/dl and when creatinine values are higher than 10 mg/dl. RRT is indicated in patients with refractory hyperkalemia not responsive to medical management, patients with severe acid-base disturbances, overhydrated patients (especially when anuria or oliguria is present), and patients that are compromised secondary to uremic toxemia and are nonresponsive or minimally responsive to traditional medical management. For the treating clinician, it is important to consider finances when making the decision to recommend initiation of IHD or CRRT. Although significant expense may be associated with IHD and CRRT, early initiation may be cost saving because it may prevent patients from experiencing significant morbidity and may decrease the length of hospital stay.[1]

In veterinary medicine, IHD has been the most commonly used extracorporeal therapy for treatment of AKI. The benefit of this modality is the high maximum removal rate of low molecular weight solutes per unit of time. CRRT is a continuous modality, which most closely mimics endogenous renal function. Once CRRT is started, therapy is continued until the patient's renal function recovers, the goal of the treatment is met (removal of exogenous toxin and/or excessive fluid burden), the patient is transitioned to IHD, or death occurs. CRRT has four distinct modalities: slow continuous ultrafiltration (SCUF), continuous venovenous hemofiltration (CVVH), continuous venovenous hemodialysis (CVVHD), and continuous venovenous hemodiafiltration (CVVHDF). In humans, CRRT is the primary modality prescribed in the intensive care unit (ICU) setting due to its slow removal of toxins, improved removal of higher molecular weight solutes (when hemofiltration is used), ease of use at the bedside, and potential for improved hemodynamic stability compared with IHD. There have been many reports comparing the use of IHD and CRRT in humans, although no clinical benefit has been shown for one modality over the other.[2-4] As is emphasized throughout this chapter, in the hands of an experienced clinician, IHD can be used to obtain the same slow solute removal that can be accomplished with CRRT. Unlike other modalities, PD can be performed without any special equipment or personnel. In veterinary medicine, PD is most often selected when other modalities are not readily available or when patient factors (such as extremely small size) preclude the use of IHD or CRRT.

PRINCIPLES OF DIALYSIS

Dialysis is the movement of solutes between two aqueous solutions separated by a semipermeable membrane. The two major factors that contribute to solute movement are diffusion and convection. Diffusion of solutes depends on the concentration gradient between the two compartments, on solute charge and molecular weight, and on the surface area and permeability of the membrane. Uremic toxins such as BUN (molecular weight, 60 Da) are freely and easily diffusible across the dialysis membrane, whereas a higher molecular weight solute such as albumin (molecular weight, 66,400 Da) does not readily diffuse across.

Convective solute removal occurs when solutes are dragged with plasma water across the dialysis membrane as a result of an osmotic pressure gradient or hydrostatic pressure (solvent drag). The rate of solute removal is dictated by the amount of water movement across the membrane, the membrane pore size, and the membrane surface area. Convection allows for removal of middle (MW 500- to 60,000 Da) and large (MW > 60,000 Da) molecular weight solutes during dialysis.

Solute removal during IHD and the CVVHD mode of CRRT occurs primarily via diffusion, and only a small portion of removal occurs through convection. The countercurrent interactions between the blood and dialysate across the dialyzer semipermeable membrane allow for the most efficient bidirectional movement of solutes from high concentration to low; this means that uremic toxins can be removed from the patient while beneficial substances, such as bicarbonate, can be administered to the patient depending on the dialysis prescription. Due to the properties of diffusive solute removal, a greater portion of uremic toxin clearance (dialysance) occurs at the beginning of the treatment when concentration in the blood is at its maximum.

PD relies on solute removal via diffusive and convective properties when dialysate in the peritoneal cavity equilibrates with the blood compartment through the peritoneal membrane and peritoneal capillaries. The physiologic peritoneal membrane is defined to have three different pore sizes, allowing for movement of both small and larger molecular weight solutes.[5] For maximal clearance of small molecular weight solutes (diffusive property), frequent dialysate exchange is needed so that significant concentration gradients can be maintained. For removal of middle to larger molecular weight solutes (convective property), increased dwell time of dialysate within the peritoneal cavity is needed to permit solute equilibration.

Ultrafiltration is the process of plasma water removal from the intravascular compartment (and ultimately from the interstitial and intracellular spaces as redistribution occurs). In IHD and CRRT, application of negative transmembrane pressure to the dialyzer allows plasma water to shift across the membrane into the dialysate compartment and out of the patient. In SCUF and the CVVH mode of CRRT, in which the treatment modality is purely convective, solute removal occurs only by ultrafiltration. In PD, ultrafiltration is achieved by creating an osmotic pressure gradient between the peritoneal cavity and the peritoneal capillaries, most commonly through the use of dextrose as an osmotic agent.

INDICATIONS

As discussed earlier, the most common application of RRT in small animal medicine is for the treatment of AKI that is nonresponsive to traditional medical management. Iatrogenic overhydration (especially in patients with oliguria and anuria), life-threatening acid-base and electrolyte disturbances such as hyperkalemia, and worsening of blood urea and creatinine values despite medical therapy are occurrences that should signal the clinician to recommend RRT. Despite the known benefits of early initiation of dialysis for human patients, in veterinary medicine initiation of dialysis tends to occur later due to the lack of available dialysis facilities, financial considerations, late diagnosis of disease, and lack of knowledge regarding the benefits of RRT. When owners are readily willing to pursue RRT, initiation of dialysis should not be delayed for affected patients.

Correction of electrolyte abnormalities is achieved by using dialysates with various concentrations of electrolytes. With IHD and CRRT, the dialyzed blood returns directly into the right atrium, which allows for rapid reversal of electrocardiogram abnormalities secondary to severe hyperkalemia, even when total body potassium may still be elevated.

Iatrogenic overhydration in AKI can cause severe morbidity and has been reported to increase mortality rates in humans.[6] In one veterinary study, 55% of dogs diagnosed with AKI secondary to leptospirosis were overhydrated at the time of presentation to a tertiary referral hospital, and 70% of those dogs were oliguric or anuric.[7] Overhydration is a common phenomenon in veterinary patients with AKI, and ultrafiltration via hemodialysis or CRRT is the most effective method for removal of this excessive fluid burden, especially in patients with suboptimal urine output. Removal of fluid may occur readily during the treatment, but the development of hypotension in a compromised patient can make it more difficult to achieve euhydration.

CONTRAINDICATIONS

Potential contraindications for IHD include severe hypotension, severe coagulopathy, and small patient size (due to the required extracorporeal volume). As for human patients, it has been hypothesized that for veterinary patients, CRRT may be safer than IHD in the acute critical care setting due to the slower solute and fluid removal rates. As previously emphasized, experienced clinicians can manipulate the IHD prescription to achieve the same slow solute and fluid removal rates as obtained in CRRT. Financial constraints may preclude treatment; however, it is important to recognize that early initiation of IHD in the appropriate patient can reduce costs by avoiding the need for prolonged ICU and hospital stays. Contraindications for PD in veterinary medicine include peritonitis, recent abdominal surgery, and hypoalbuminemia.

COMPONENTS OF DIALYSIS

Catheters for Intermittent Hemodialysis and Continuous Renal Replacement Therapy

To process (dialyze) large volumes of blood while maintaining rapid blood flows, large-bore catheters are necessary. For extracorporeal RRT, double-lumen temporary dialysis catheters are used most commonly, and are placed in the jugular vein. Catheter size selection is dictated by patient size and vessel diameter. The catheter length is measured so that the tip of the catheter is positioned in the right atrium of the heart, allowing for rapid blood flows. Catheter placement can be performed with the patient under light sedation or under general anesthesia, depending on the patient's clinical condition. The arterial port of the catheter (drawing blood from the patient) communicates with the more proximal side holes, while the venous port (returning blood to the patient) opens on the distal tip of the catheter; this aids to decrease recirculation of blood, which can lead to inefficient treatments. In interdialytic periods, both lumens of the catheter are locked with heparin (typically 100 to 2000 units/ml) to prevent clot formation and maintain catheter patency. Although temporary catheters are constructed to perform efficiently for only a few weeks, they can be successfully maintained for several months, provided that they are managed properly.

Catheters for Peritoneal Dialysis

PD catheters need to allow for adequate inflow and outflow of dialysate so that efficient treatments can be achieved. A majority of PD complications are catheter related. Proper catheter choice, placement technique, and appropriate catheter management are therefore essential for success. There are two main types of PD catheters: acute PD catheters, which are meant for short-term use (<3 days), and chronic PD catheters, which are constructed to function for an extended period of time. To avoid leakage, bacterial infection, and migration, long-term, chronic PD catheters have cuffs to secure the catheter in the subcutaneous exit tract. Long-term catheters are placed via laparotomy or laparoscopy, preferably with partial omentectomy, while acute catheters can be placed percutaneously. In humans, it is recommended to refrain from using a PD catheter for 10 to 14 days after surgical placement to avoid leakage around the catheter site, as immediate use can increase the risk of infection. In veterinary medicine, the need for immediate RRT often requires use of the catheter shortly after placement. To minimize the risk of leaks and other complications when catheters are used immediately after placement, it is recommended that use of large volumes of dialysate be avoided for 24 to 48 hours.

Dialysate

Dialysate is a solution, similar to plasma water, that allows for solute exchange during diffusive dialysis. Bidirectional flow of solute occurs across the semipermeable dialysis membrane via diffusion, depending on the concentration gradient on either side of the membrane. The electrolyte concentration of the dialysate (sodium, potassium, calcium, phosphorus, bicarbonate) is manipulated depending on the patient's blood chemistry. In IHD and the CVVHD and CVVHDF modes of CRRT, the dialysate flows countercurrent to the blood to allow for maximum solute removal. In IHD, dialysate preparation requires a specialized water treatment system, whereas premade dialysate is used for CRRT and PD.

In PD, premade sterile dialysate is infused into the abdomen at defined volumes with defined exchange rates and dwelling times, depending on the treatment goals. Because ultrafiltration in PD is dependent on creation of an osmotic gradient, various osmotic agents with different osmolalities are available. Dextrose-based dialysate is commonly used in veterinary medicine because it is effective and inexpensive. When commercially available PD dialysate is not readily available, lactated Ringer's solution with the addition of dextrose can be used as substitute.[5] Although more concentrated dextrose solutions allow for effective fluid removal from the patient, these concentrates are more likely to lead to secondary peritonitis and dysfunction of the peritoneal membrane.[8]

Dialyzer

Hollow-fiber dialyzers for IHD and CRRT are defined by their membrane characteristics (membrane material, pore size, surface area) and by the blood volume within the hollow fibers. CRRT utilizes both diffusion and convection to achieve solute removal; the pore size and permeability of CRRT dialyzers are therefore larger than that of IHD dialyzers.[9] Improved solute clearance is achieved with bigger dialyzers that have larger pores and surface areas. To ensure that extracorporeal blood volumes are not excessive, dialyzer volume (priming volume) must be considered during dialyzer selection. As discussed previously, the peritoneal cavity and capillaries function as the semipermeable membrane in PD.

Anticoagulation

The extracorporeal circuit and dialyzers are constructed with highly biocompatible materials; however, activation of the coagulation cascade still occurs within minutes of blood contact with the dialyzer.[10] To prevent clotting of blood within the extracorporeal circuit anticoagulation is therefore necessary. Systemic heparinization for IHD and regional citrate anticoagulation for CRRT are most commonly used in veterinary medicine. When heparin-based protocols are used, it is critical to plan all invasive procedures, such as surgery or thoracocentesis, around the hemodialysis associated heparination to minimize the risk of hemorrhage. In addition, comorbidities such as pulmonary or gastrointestinal hemorrhage must be considered when prescribing systemic anticoagulation. When citrate-based protocols are used, although systemic anticoagulation is less likely, hypocalcemia and alkalosis can occur. For patients with thrombocytopenia, coagulopathy, severe gastrointestinal bleeding, or pulmonary hemorrhage, low-dose heparin anticoagulation or no-anticoagulation protocols can be used, but these carry a higher risk of clotting within the extracorporeal circuit. Recently, the use of citrate with IHD has been evaluated for patients at risk of bleeding.[11]

DIALYSIS PRESCRIPTION

The dialysis prescription, including dialysis dose, depends on the treatment goals. In AKI, the fluid balance, degree of uremia, and electrolyte disturbances dictates the dialysis prescription. In IHD, limitations to the rate and amount of ultrafiltration are the dialyzer and the patient's hemodynamic state. Excessive rates of ultrafiltration can induce hypotension, hyperthermia, nausea, and cramping. Degree of overhydration, along with the patient's tolerance of fluid removal (usually <10 ml/kg/hr), in part dictate treatment time.

In severely uremic patients, rapid removal of uremic toxins should be avoided to prevent dialysis disequilibrium syndrome. Rapid removal of osmotically active solutes from the blood compartment creates osmotic pressure gradients between the blood, extravascular, and intracellular compartments. This gradient allows plasma water to shift from the vascular compartment and into the intracellular compartments. When this phenomenon occurs in brain tissue, secondary swelling occurs and this can lead to irreversible neurologic damage or death. To avoid dysequilibrium, when severe uremia is present, initial treatments must be designed to achieve slow solute removal. CRRT was developed to provide slow and safe treatment for patients with severe uremia and for patients in hemodynamically unstable conditions because slow solute and fluid removal can be achieved. As emphasized earlier, in the hands of an experienced clinician, IHD can be used safely to treat patients in critical condition with severely elevated BUN values via manipulation of the prescription. Due to the slow solute clearance rates associated with PD, the risk for dialysis disequilibrium is much lower than in extracorporeal modalities; however, initial prescriptions should still be written with this potential complication in mind.

Careful monitoring of patients, especially during initial treatments, is critical. Patient blood pressure, heart rate, respiratory rate, blood volume change, venous blood saturation, activated clotting time (except for PD), and temperature must be measured frequently. When citrate-based anticoagulation protocols are used, blood calcium level and pH are also measured. Monitoring for nausea, restlessness, hydration status, development of neurologic signs (for early detection of dysequilibrium), and hemorrhage is also necessary. In PD, precise measurements of dialysate inputs and outputs must be recorded to avoid overhydration of the patient. The normal dialysate volume is about 30 to 40 ml/kg per exchange cycle. If fluid balance becomes positive or returning volume decreases to less than 90% of what was administered, the dialysate should be changed to encourage ultrafiltration.[5]

COMPLICATIONS AND OTHER CONSIDERATIONS

Acute complications associated with IHD and CRRT include catheter occlusion, hemorrhage from systemic heparinization, hypocalcemia from regional citrate anticoagulation, hypotension, dialysis disequilibrium syndrome, air embolism, dialyzer membrane reaction, and blood loss through clotting of the extracorporeal circuit.[12,13] The rate of complications with PD is high, although the complications usually are manageable and not life threatening if proper treatments are instituted at an early stage.[14] Common complications are catheter occlusion, catheter site infection, dialysate leakage, septic peritonitis, fluid retention, hypoalbuminemia, dyspnea due to increased abdominal pressure, and hyperglycemia from dialysate with a high glucose concentration.[14-16]

It is a common misconception in veterinary medicine that it is simpler and less expensive to set up a CRRT unit and that it is easier to treat patients with CRRT than with IHD. Some of these misconceptions stem from the fact that CRRT is used at bedside in human ICUs; however, the intensive prolonged treatments required with CRRT and the need to have a dedicated and trained technical staff for the duration of the treatments make it difficult to carry out quality treatments in many veterinary practices. In addition, the cost for premade dialysate can become cost-prohibitive when high dialysate flows were required. In addition, since CRRT is not designed to be a long-term treatment modality, it is necessary to have facilities available to provide longer-term care for patients that remain dependent on RRT. It is critical for any clinician or technical staff member performing extracorporeal RRT to have expertise in renal physiology and extracorporeal medicine to carry out the procedures in a safe manner.

OUTCOME AND PROGNOSIS

There are limited studies in veterinary medicine to compare the efficacy of PD, IHD, and CRRT and no studies to compare the effect of each of these modalities on overall survival and mortality rates. For dogs and cats with AKI, survival rates of 44% and 53%, respectively, have been reported.[17,18] Failure to convert from anuria or oliguria to a nonoliguric state has been associated with a poor prognosis.

In a recent study, 41% of dogs and 44% of cats with AKI of different causes survived with CRRT treatment after failure to improve with medical management.[19] In a retrospective study of 36 dogs with AKI secondary to leptospirosis infection, survival rates were 86% for dogs treated with hemodialysis and 82% for dogs treated conservatively; however, the dogs treated conservatively had less severe disease. The mean initial serum creatinine and BUN concentrations for survivors and nonsurvivors treated conservatively (4.4 and 71 mg/dl, and 8.1 and 156 mg/dl, respectively) were markedly lower than those for dogs treated with IHD (11.4 and 170 mg/dl, and 10 and 176 mg/dl, respectively).[7] In a retrospective study of 22 cats with AKI of different causes treated with PD, 45.5% survived to discharge, and in another study of 6 cats with AKI, 83% of cats recovered kidney function after PD.[14,16]

SUMMARY

The use of RRT has become more and more commonplace in veterinary medicine. When IHD or CRRT is performed, it is critical for the treating clinician to have a solid understanding of renal physiology and dialysis prescription, and a strong technical understanding of the dialysis machine. It is also crucial to recognize the financial and time investments that are necessary to safely and effectively perform dialysis. Once the necessary skills are achieved, RRT can provide a valuable treatment option that can improve patient quality of life and outcome.

REFERENCES

1. Macedo E, Mehta RL: When should renal replacement therapy be initiated for acute kidney injury? Semin Dial 24:132-137, 2011.
2. Marshall MR, Golper TA: Low-efficiency acute renal replacement therapy: role in acute kidney injury, Semin Dial 24:142-148, 2011.
3. Vesconi S, Cruz DN, Fumagalli R, et al: Delivered dose of renal replacement therapy and mortality in critically ill patients with acute kidney injury, Crit Care 13:R57, 2009.
4. Uchino S, Bellomo R, Ronco C: Intermittent versus continuous renal replacement therapy in the ICU: impact on electrolyte and acid-base balance, Intensive Care Med 27:1037-1043, 2001.
5. Cooper RL, Labato MA: Peritoneal dialysis in veterinary medicine, Vet Clin North Am Small Anim Pract 41:91-113, 2011.
6. Mehta RL, Bouchard J: Controversies in acute kidney injury: effects of fluid overload on outcome, Contrib Nephrol 174:200-211, 2011.
7. Adin CA, Cowgill LD: Treatment and outcome of dogs with leptospirosis: 36 cases (1990-1998), J Am Vet Med Assoc 216:371-375, 2000.
8. Ross LA, Labato MA: Peritoneal dialysis. In DiBartola S, editor: Fluid, electrolyte, and acid-base disorders in small animal practice, ed 4, St Louis, 2012, Saunders, pp 665-679.

9. Monaghan KN, Acierno MJ: Extracorporeal removal of drugs and toxins, Vet Clin North Am Small Anim Pract 41:227-238, 2011.
10. Lucchi L, Ligabue G, Marietta M, et al: Activation of coagulation during hemodialysis: effect of blood lines alone and whole extracorporeal circuit, Artif Organs 30:106-110, 2006.
11. Francey T: Regional citrate anticoagulation for extracorporeal blood purification techniques in dogs, Proceedings from the 21st ECVIM-CA Congress, Seville, Spain, September 8-10, 2011.
12. Komeno M, Akimoto A, Fujita T, et al: Role of nitric oxide in hemodialysis-related hypotension in an experimental renal dysfunction dog model, J Vet Med Sci 66:53-57, 2004.
13. Hothi DK, Harvey E: Common complications of haemodialysis. In Warady BA, Alexander SR, editors: Pediatric dialysis, ed 2, New York, 2012, Springer, pp 345-374.
14. Cooper RL, Labato MA: Peritoneal dialysis in cats with acute kidney injury: 22 cases (2001-2006), J Vet Intern Med 25:14-19, 2011.
15. Bersenas AM: A clinical review of peritoneal dialysis, J Vet Emerg Crit Care (San Antonio) 21:605-617, 2011.
16. Dorval P, Boysen SR: Management of acute renal failure in cats using peritoneal dialysis: a retrospective study of six cases (2003-2007), J Feline Med Surg 11:107-115, 2009.
17. Vaden SL, Levine J, Breitschwerdt EB: A retrospective case-control of acute renal failure in 99 dogs, J Vet Intern Med 11:58-64, 1997.
18. Worwag S, Langston CE: Acute intrinsic renal failure in cats: 32 cases (1997-2004), J Am Vet Med Assoc 232:728-732, 2008.
19. Diehl SH, Seshadri R: Use of continuous renal replacement therapy for treatment of dogs and cats with acute or acute-on-chronic renal failure: 33 cases (2002-2006), J Vet Emerg Crit Care 18:370-382, 2008.

CHAPTER 206
APHERESIS

Carrie A. Palm, DVM, DACVIM

KEY POINTS

- Apheresis is an extracorporeal therapy in which the blood is removed from the patient circulation and separated into its components, and one or more of the components is removed or processed before the blood is returned to the patient.
- Therapeutic plasmapheresis or total plasma exchange is an apheresis procedure that involves removal of the plasma component of blood (with concurrent removal of circulating pathologic substances), such as immunoglobulins that may be present in immune-mediated diseases.
- Plasmapheresis has been used successfully to treat veterinary patients with severe and refractory myasthenia gravis and immune-mediated hemolytic anemia.
- Plasmapheresis should be combined with traditional medical management; however, it can be used to supplement treatment when traditional therapies may be contraindicated.

Apheresis is an extracorporeal therapy in which blood is removed from patient circulation, the blood is separated into its components, and one or more of the components is removed or processed before the blood is returned to the patient. Of the extracorporeal therapies, apheresis is the newest form being used more commonly in veterinary patients. Therapeutic plasmapheresis, or therapeutic plasma exchange (TPE), is an apheresis treatment in which the plasma component of blood is removed and replaced with supplemental fluids, or processed before being returned to the patient. Total plasma exchange is the most commonly applied apheresis therapy in veterinary medicine. This chapter focuses on the use of TPE in the critical care setting.

In human medicine, applications for apheresis are vast and are categorized into four groups based on the defined or proven benefit that apheresis provides for each particular disease process or condition. A category I condition, such as myasthenia gravis (MG), is defined as a disease for which apheresis is considered to be a standard of care and is therefore prescribed as a first-line therapy. A category II condition, such as *Amanita* mushroom poisoning, is one in which apheresis is considered to be a supportive therapy, in combination with other therapies. A category III condition, such as acute hepatic failure, is a condition in which controlled trials are limited or their results inconclusive, and a category IV condition is one in which therapy appeared to be ineffective or harmful.[1] Since these therapies have only recently been used more commonly in veterinary medicine, similar categorization is not yet possible; however, the already established human studies can be used as a reference.

EQUIPMENT

Apheresis can be carried out with either centrifugal or filtration methods. In veterinary medicine, both techniques involve the placement of large-bore double-lumen jugular catheters (see Chapter 205 for details). With centrifugation, blood components are separated in order of increasing density (similar to centrifugation for evaluation of packed cell volume) as follows: plasma, platelets, lymphocytes and monocytes, granulocytes, and red blood cells.[2] Once blood components are separated, outlet tubes placed within the apheresis machine allow specific components (i.e., plasma) to be selectively removed from the patient based on the density variation. The other components can be returned to the patient and are mixed with replacement fluids, including colloids and crystalloids, during return. Although not commonly applied in veterinary medicine, removed plasma can also undergo secondary processing, whereby the plasma is run through a secondary column that binds or removes the pathologic substances; the treated plasma is then returned to the patient. To prevent clotting in the extracorporeal circuit, anticoagulation is necessary. For centrifugal apheresis, regional citrate is most commonly used, whereby only the extracorporeal circuit is anticoagulated, without development of systemic anticoagulation. In the United States, centrifugation techniques are most commonly used.

Membrane filtration techniques involve the use of membranes with various pore sizes that can separate out plasma for removal or processing or can remove specific pathologic plasma components, such as immunoglobulins.[3] Membranes may also contain substances such as staphylococcal protein A that can bind plasma components for removal. Filtration techniques cannot be used for removal of specific cell components, whereas centrifugal apheresis can. With filtration apheresis, systemic anticoagulation with heparin is most commonly used.

PRINCIPLES OF APHERESIS

Successful apheresis treatments are based on the principle that the disease being treated is in large part due to pathologic substances within the blood that can be efficiently removed with appropriately prescribed apheresis treatment plans. The ability to remove a substance successfully during TPE depends on the distribution of the substance within the body (the volume of distribution), the rapidity with which the substance equilibrates between body compartments, and the ability to remove adequate amounts of the pathologic substance. As with other extracorporeal therapies, the most successful treatments are achieved with substances that have a small volume of distribution (and are located primarily in the intravascular space), because removal is occurring directly from the intravascular space. As an example, immune-mediated diseases are commonly managed with TPE, which leads to alleviation of or improvement in clinical signs by removing immunoglobulins present in the intravascular space. Immunoglobulin removal has a primary positive effect by decreasing secondary complement fixation and other adverse systemic consequences, and also allows adjuvant medical therapies to be more effective.

With each plasmapheresis treatment, approximately 1 plasma volume is removed and replaced with fluids such as albumin preparations, colloids, and crystalloids. Plasma is not typically used as a replacement fluid in human medicine; rather, a combination of albumin and saline is most commonly used. Due to the potential for complications with repeated human albumin administration in dogs, and given the cost of and lack of experience with canine albumin, albumin has not been used as a replacement fluid by the author. Instead, combinations of saline, hetastarch, and plasma are used. Removal of 1 plasma volume per treatment is based on predicted clearance curves for various substances.[4] For most higher-molecular-weight substances, such as immunoglobulins, the efficiency of pathologic substance removal is not increased when more than 1 or 1.5 plasma volumes are exchanged in a single treatment. If clinical improvement is not seen within three to five apheresis sessions, it is likely that no significant benefit will be gained. Likewise, if clinical remission is achieved after three treatments, there is likely no benefit in performing more treatments at that time. TPE sessions are typically performed every other day. This allows for redistribution of pathologic substance into the intravascular space, which increases efficiency of total body antibody removal with subsequent treatments.

Because case numbers of veterinary patients are small, information regarding complication rate and outcome is limited; however, no significant complications have been encountered. Potential complications include adverse reactions to plasma, hypocalcemia or alkalosis secondary to citrate use, blood loss via clotting of the extracorporeal circuit, hypotension secondary to the large extracorporeal blood volumes (especially in smaller patients with smaller blood volumes), and hypoproteinemia secondary to iatrogenic removal of protein.

INDICATIONS

At the author's institution, apheresis has been used to treat patients with immune-mediated diseases that are severely affected or are refractory or minimally responsive to more traditional therapies. When plasmapheresis is used, traditional medical management is still instituted, with the apheresis techniques serving as an adjuvant therapy to improve patient outcome. It is also important to consider risk/benefit ratio when prescribing apheresis. In the critical care setting, apheresis techniques have been used for the treatment of immune-mediated diseases such as myasthenia gravis and immune-mediated hemolytic anemia. Specifically, TPE has been used for treating these immune diseases. Although case numbers are low, the anecdotal success in these cases is promising. Leukapheresis, or the removal of white blood cells, has also been used to carry out bone marrow transplantation in veterinary patients, and historically, apheresis has been used to treat veterinary patients affected with paraproteinemias, multiple myeloma, acute inflammatory polyradiculoneuritis, and other immune-mediated disease.[5]

MYASTHENIA GRAVIS

MG is an immune-mediated disease characterized by antibody inactivation of the neuromuscular end plate often manifesting as muscle weakness. MG can occur as a focal or generalized disease and can lead to life-threatening complications, such as respiratory depression and aspiration pneumonia secondary to megaesophagus. Traditional medical management involves supportive care and the use of anticholinesterase medications. In cases refractory to medical management or in patients with rapidly progressive disease, apheresis, and specifically TPE, may improve outcome. As noted earlier, MG is a category I condition in human medicine,[6] and given the similarities between human and canine MG, it can be hypothesized that TPE may benefit canine patients. Five dogs with severe generalized and/or rapidly progressive MG have been treated with TPE at the author's institution. Four of the five dogs had resolution of clinical signs after three apheresis treatments. Of those four dogs, two dogs experienced complete remission, one dog redeveloped mild and intermittent regurgitation only (without megaesophagus) approximately 1 month after the final apheresis treatment, and the fourth dog redeveloped significant regurgitation approximately 1 month after discontinuation of therapy. The fifth dog did not show any significant improvement with plasmapheresis treatments. In human medicine, apheresis sessions are used in the acute setting and are often prescribed on a long-term basis if clinical signs recur; however, long-term apheresis is not financially feasible in most veterinary patients. Antibody removal was confirmed for the first three dogs treated at the author's institution via serial measurement of acetylcholine receptor antibody titers during and after apheresis sessions.[7] It is important to note that all patients were treated with concurrent medical therapy in conjunction with TPE. No significant adverse events occurred in any of the treated dogs. Filtration apheresis has been reported for treatment of MG in a canine patient.[7,8]

IMMUNE-MEDIATED HEMOLYTIC ANEMIA

Therapeutic plasma exchange has also been used to treat refractory immune-mediated hemolytic anemia at the author's institution. All patients that were treated with TPE had also received at least 4 days of appropriate immunosuppression before starting apheresis therapy. Use of TPE allowed patients that were previously crossmatch incompatible due to severe agglutination to receive blood transfusions. likely because of a reduction in antibody load. In addition, use of TPE allowed for successful control of disease with the same immunosuppressive protocols that had been previously unsuccessful in those patients.

FUTURE APPLICATIONS

Large-scale studies examining the benefits of apheresis in veterinary medicine are lacking; however, the limited data available suggest that there are likely benefits. With knowledge of the principles of apheresis and use of the human medical experience as a guide, these advanced procedures have the potential to improve outcomes for many veterinary patients. Apheresis techniques may be useful in treating a variety of fulminant immune-mediated diseases, such as immune-mediated thrombocytopenia, polyradiculoneuritis, hyperviscosity syndrome, and *Amanita* mushroom poisoning, among others.[9-13] As more experience is gained in veterinary medicine, apheresis techniques will likely provide therapies for veterinary patients that may lack other viable treatment options.

REFERENCES

1. Szczepiorkowski ZM, Shaz BH, Bandarenko N, et al: The new approach to assignment of ASFA categories—introduction to the fourth special issue: clinical applications of therapeutic apheresis, J Clin Apher 22:96-105, 2007.
2. Burgstaler EA: Current apheresis instrumentation. In McLeod BC, Price TH, Weinstein R, editors: Apheresis: principles and practice, ed 2, Bethesda, Md, 2003, AABB Press, pp 95-130.
3. Gurland HJ, Lysaght MJ, Samtleben W, et al: A comparison of centrifugal and membrane-based apheresis formats, Int J Artif Organs 7:35-38, 1984.
4. Orlin JB, Berkman EM: Partial plasma exchange using albumin replacement: removal and recovery of normal plasma constituents, Blood 56:1055-1059, 1980.
5. Bartges JW: Therapeutic plasmapheresis, Semin Vet Med Surg (Small Anim) 12(3):170-177, 1997.
6. Mantegazza R, Bonanno S, Camera G, et al: Current and emerging therapies for the treatment of myasthenia gravis, Neuropsychiatr Dis Treat 7:151-160, 2011.
7. Palm C, Dickinson P, Sturges B, et al: Plasmapheresis for the treatment of myasthenia gravis in 3 dogs (abstract), American College of Veterinary Internal Medicine Forum, June 15-18, Denver, Colorado, 2011.
8. Bartges JW, Klausner JS, Bostwick EF, et al: Clinical remission following plasmapheresis and corticosteroid treatment in a dog with acquired myasthenia gravis, J Am Vet Med Assoc 196:1276-1278, 1990.
9. Nenov DS, Nenov KS: Therapeutic apheresis in exogenous poisoning and in myeloma, Nephrol Dial Transplant 16:101-102, 2001.
10. Szczepiorkowski ZM, Bandarenko N, Kim HC, et al: Guidelines on the use of therapeutic apheresis in clinical practice—evidence-based approach from the Apheresis Applications Committee of the American Society for Apheresis, J Clin Apher 22:106-175, 2007.
11. Bektas M, Idilman R, Soykan I, et al: Adjuvant therapeutic plasma exchange in liver failure: assessments of clinical and laboratory parameters, J Clin Gastroenterol 42:517-521, 2008.
12. Chhibber V, Weinstein R: Evidence-based review of therapeutic plasma exchange in neurological disorders, Semin Dial 25:132-139, 2012.
13. Stone MJ, Bogen SA: Evidence-based focused review of management of hyperviscosity syndrome, Blood 119:2205-2208, 2012.

CHAPTER 207
CEREBROSPINAL FLUID SAMPLING

Beverly K. Sturges, DVM, MS, DACVIM (Neurology)

KEY POINTS

- Cerebrospinal fluid (CSF) analysis can rapidly provide information that may be useful in making a diagnosis, deciding on a treatment protocol or further diagnostic tests, and monitoring response of central nervous system (CNS) disease to medical treatment.
- The most common indication for CSF analysis in the emergency or intensive care unit setting is suspicion of infectious or inflammatory disease of the CNS.
- In collecting CSF, correct patient positioning and a good understanding of regional anatomy are essential.
- CSF findings uncommonly yield a definitive diagnosis and should be interpreted in light of the patient history, neurologic signs, and other diagnostic results. In addition, they may be normal in spite of significant CNS disease.
- Risks versus benefits of a CSF collection should be considered carefully in patients with elevated intracranial pressure.
- CSF cell counts and cytologic study may be done in house with minimal investment in equipment and give the emergency clinician the most useful information for making a diagnosis.

Cerebrospinal fluid (CSF) collection and analysis may provide rapid information to the clinician investigating a disease affecting the central nervous system (CNS).[1,2] It is particularly useful for confirming the presence of inflammatory and infectious diseases affecting the brain, spinal cord, or nerve roots, especially when the meninges are involved.[1-3] However, CSF analysis should be considered only after an accurate history taking, physical examination, and neurologic assessment has localized a lesion to the CNS and a logical list of differential diagnoses has been considered carefully.[1,2] In most situations, the results of a CSF analysis provide the clinician with a piece of the puzzle that must be used in conjunction with the results of other diagnostic tests, especially magnetic resonance imaging (MRI), to arrive at a correct diagnosis.

CEREBROSPINAL FLUID FORMATION AND FUNCTIONS

The presence of CSF in the subarachnoid space reduces mechanical trauma to the nervous tissue and serves to remove the products of

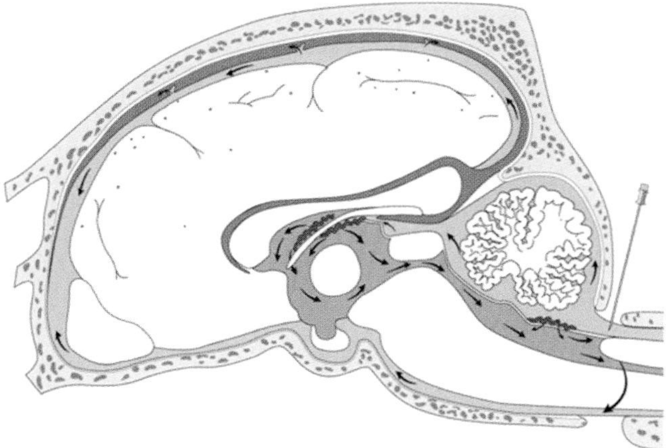

FIGURE 207-1 Cerebrospinal fluid (CSF) pathway and location of cisternal puncture. CSF, secreted by the choroid plexus *(dark blue)*, flows through the ventricular system *(medium blue)* from rostral to caudal: lateral ventricles, third ventricle, mesencephalic aqueduct, and fourth ventricle. From there, most of the CSF exits via the lateral apertures of the fourth ventricle and flows cranially and caudally in the subarachnoid space around the brain and spinal cord *(light blue)*. The remainder of CSF flows caudally down the central canal of the spinal cord. CSF from the cranial subarachnoid space enters the venous system via arachnoid villi. Cisternal puncture is performed by placing a needle in the dorsal subarachnoid space at the craniocervical junction. This space usually becomes accessible when the head is ventroflexed.

brain metabolism (Figure 207-1). It is also an intracerebral transport medium for nutrients, neuroendocrine substances, and neurotransmitters.[4] Most CSF is formed by the choroid plexus in the ventricles via ultrafiltration of plasma and the active transport of selected substances across the blood-brain barrier.[4] The CSF flows caudally through the ventricular system; the majority exits via the fourth ventricle to circulate cranially around the brain and caudally around the spinal cord in the subarachnoid spaces.[4]

Absorption of CSF occurs primarily through the arachnoid villi that penetrate the major dural venous sinuses in the cranium.[4]

INDICATIONS FOR CEREBROSPINAL FLUID COLLECTION AND ANALYSIS

CSF analysis is indicated when a patient has neurologic signs consistent with disease affecting the CNS, including the brain, spinal cord, and nerve roots.[1-3] Performing advanced imaging (e.g., MRI, computed tomography) before CSF collection whenever possible is recommended to help define the underlying neurologic disease.[5] Such imaging gives valuable information relating to the exact location of the lesion and the amount and distribution of associated edema. It also may reveal structural evidence of intracranial hypertension (ICH) such as tentorial or foraminal herniation or blockage of ventricular CSF outflow. Regardless of the findings on advanced imaging, however, animals that are showing rapid neurologic deterioration are most likely to benefit from a diagnostic CSF analysis. Common indications for CSF collection in the emergency or critical care setting include the following:

1. Suspected infectious or inflammatory disease affecting the CNS.[6] Conditions causing meningitis, encephalitis, and myelitis are often moderate to severe by the time animals are showing neurologic signs, and CSF analysis should be done as soon as possible. It is always preferable to collect CSF before treating with medications that may influence the content and, consequently, the interpretation of the findings.
2. Suspected neoplastic disease affecting the CNS.[1,2,6] Except in cases of CNS lymphoma, CSF findings alone are rarely specific for neoplastic disease. However, an analysis is often done to rule out the possibility of inflammatory disease that may also be on the differential list, especially if advanced imaging is not available.
3. Cluster or continuous seizures in animals in which underlying infectious or inflammatory disease or neoplasia is likely.[1]
4. Acute, ascending lower motor neuron signs. Prognosis and treatment vary widely depending on the underlying cause of these signs, and CSF findings may help to differentiate diseases such as acute polyradiculopathy from infectious, inflammatory, or neoplastic disease (e.g., lymphoma).[1]

CSF analysis occasionally may be indicated to monitor short-term response to treatment when an obvious response to therapy is not evident or cannot be monitored. This may be especially applicable to animals that are systemically ill, heavily sedated, or undergoing mechanical ventilation. CSF evaluation, or "the CBC of the CNS,"[1] may be particularly helpful in guiding the clinician in determining further treatment and prognosis in such cases.

CONTRAINDICATIONS AND RISKS

CSF collection requires general anesthesia, the risks of which are inherently higher in animals that might have elevated intracranial pressure (ICP).[3,5] Risks of anesthesia are minimized by the following measures:

1. Using an anesthetic protocol that reduces ICP
2. Treating patients with osmotic diuretics, ventilation, and control of partial pressure of arterial carbon dioxide before anesthetizing if severe ICH is suspected (see Chapter 84)

The emergency clinician should also be aware of the following situations in which the risks of performing CSF collection are likely to outweigh the benefits, and therefore the procedure is not recommended[1,2]:

- Acute traumatic brain injury
- Rodenticide toxicity, aspirin ingestion, serious coagulopathies
- Severe and/or rapidly progressing ICH
- Atlantoaxial luxation or cranial cervical vertebral fracture or luxation

Although CSF analysis is one of the easiest and most direct methods for evaluating the CNS, the proximity of important neural structures to puncture sites makes it possible to penetrate these structures inadvertently during needle placement, especially if there is disease affecting the subarachnoid space.[1]

The most common injury is trauma to the cerebellum, brainstem, or cervical spinal cord. Such injury produces a vestibular syndrome that is apparent when the animal recovers from anesthesia.[1] A rarer, but more serious, consequence is iatrogenic trauma that produces apnea. Immediate treatment with hyperosmolar therapy, mechanical ventilation, and possibly glucocorticoids may save the life of the patient with apnea.[1] Patients with vestibular signs usually recover without treatment in a few days to a couple of weeks. The incidence of these complications is rare when the procedure is performed by a careful, trained individual.

In cases of ICH, herniation of the brain may occur from a rapid reduction of ICP (e.g., pop-off valve effect), producing apnea and unresponsiveness.[1] Usually mydriatic pupils are apparent even while the animal is still anesthetized. Immediate aggressive treatment of ICH is indicated, but these animals have a grave prognosis.

CEREBROSPINAL FLUID COLLECTION TECHNIQUES

Preparation

For CSF collection and examination it is necessary to puncture the subarachnoid space in the cerebellomedullary cistern or in the lower lumbar spine.[1,3,5,6] Small animals must be anesthetized to ensure complete immobility. An infusion of propofol with midazolam or fentanyl, or both, provides excellent anesthesia for performing CSF collection in patients with ICH. The site must be shaved, surgically prepared, and draped with a small, fenestrated, sterile drape. The operator should wear sterile surgical gloves. All equipment should be assembled and ready to use before the patient is positioned. The following items are necessary:

1. Sterile gloves and drape or sterile field
2. Disposable spinal needles with stylets
   - A 22-gauge, 1½-inch spinal needle is used in most cisternal punctures regardless of the size of the dog; it may also be used for cisternal puncture in cats and for lumbar puncture in small dogs and cats.
   - A 22-gauge, 2½-inch spinal needle is occasionally necessary for doing a cisternal puncture in giant breed dogs or in large breed dogs with heavy cervical musculature; it is also commonly used for lumbar punctures in most dogs weighing more than 5 kg.
   - A 22-gauge, 3½-inch spinal needle is used for lumbar punctures in large and giant breed dogs.
   - A 25-gauge, 1-inch spinal needle may be used in small cats and toy breed dogs. These needles are more easily supported by the surrounding tissues in very small animals, and the bevel on the needle is less likely to cause trauma to the brainstem or spinal cord. However, CSF flow is considerably slower through the needle, and this should be remembered when one watches for the flash of CSF in the hub signifying entry into the subarachnoid space.
3. Red-top glass blood collection tubes (Vacutainers)

Collection Sites and Techniques

The site of CSF collection can be the cisterna magna, the lateral ventricle (rarely), or the subarachnoid space in the lumbar region.[1,3,5,6] When focal CNS disease is suspected, CSF findings are more likely to be abnormal and representative of the underlying pathologic condition when CSF is collected caudal to the lesion. In multifocal or diffuse CNS disease, CSF collection at both cisternal and lumbar sites is usually recommended.

Cisternal puncture

Positioning

The subarachnoid space enlarges to form the cerebellomedullary cistern in the dorsal atlantooccipital region (see Figure 207-1).[1,3,5,6] This site is used when the patient's signs suggest brain or cranial cervical spinal cord disease. During cisternal puncture the neck is flexed, and a patent airway must be maintained under anesthesia by use of an endotracheal tube. The animal is placed in lateral recumbency (right lateral is usually easiest for a right-handed operator) and an area from the occipital protuberance to the level of C3 is surgically prepared.

With an assistant standing opposite the person doing the puncture, the patient's neck is flexed moderately (90 to 100 degrees) at the cisternal region while the ears are held out of the way. It is important to make sure that the midline of the neck and the head (from the nose to the occiput) is parallel to the tabletop. If the neck sags, as is common in larger dogs, a small pad can be placed under it. The wings of the atlas are palpated to make sure they are superimposed, which eliminates axial rotation. Positioning is critical in making the puncture exactly on midline.

All landmarks should be palpated before the needle is inserted: external occipital protuberance, spinous process of the C2 vertebra, dorsal arch of the C1 vertebra (this is done by slipping rostrally off of the C2 spine), and the wings of the atlas. Either of the following methods for finding the correct point of insertion may be employed:

1. Using the external occipital protuberance and the spine of C2, the puncture is made on midline halfway between the occiput and the cranial end of the spinous process. If the dorsal arch of C1 can be palpated, the puncture is made on the midline just cranial to it.
2. Using the wings of the atlas, the puncture is made in the center of the triangle formed by the occiput and the wings of the atlas.

With either method, a natural indentation can usually be palpated on midline where the needle is most likely to enter the subarachnoid space.

Needle insertion

The spinal needle is placed perpendicular to the plane of the vertebral column and advanced slowly at a 90-degree angle through the skin and underlying tissues. Extremely tough skin, as in cats, may need to be tented and penetrated before the landmarks are identified for puncture into deeper tissues. Every time a layer of tissue is penetrated, which is detected by a sudden decrease of resistance at the needle tip, the stylet should be removed and the hub of the needle observed for a few seconds for the appearance of CSF. In small dogs and cats, the tissue planes are not as easily ascertained by feel, and the stylet should be removed and checked every 1 to 2 mm. This prevents inadvertent penetration of neural tissue. When the dura is penetrated, resistance decreases and CSF appears in the hub of the needle when the stylet is removed. Occasionally a twitch may be seen or felt when the dura is penetrated, especially if it is inflamed.

Tips for troubleshooting cerebrospinal fluid puncture

1. If pure blood drips from the hub, most likely the needle is slightly off midline and into the vertebral venous plexus, outside of the dura. This poses no harm to the patient, and the needle should be removed and discarded. Landmarks and patient alignment should be rechecked and another puncture attempted.
2. If bloody CSF appears in the hub, most likely the needle has traumatically ruptured vessels in the meninges. The stylet should be replaced for a minute, any blood-tinged CSF allowed to flow out, and CSF collected after it clears. CSF that remains uniformly blood tinged may reflect hemorrhage within the CNS.
3. If the tip of the needle is hitting bone, it is necessary to determine if it is hitting C1 or the occipital bone. Then the needle should be backed out slightly and redirected cranially or caudally along the sagittal plane. If bone is encountered repeatedly, it is best to start over with a new needle after rechecking landmarks and patient positioning.

In cats and small dogs, 1 to 2 ml of CSF can be safely collected by free flow into a sterile glass tube; 6 ml or more may be collected in larger dogs.[1-3] It is best not to aspirate fluid from the hub of the needle because this may collapse the CSF space or initiate hemorrhage.[1] Once enough CSF has been collected, the needle is removed. Historically, the opening pressure of the CSF was measured by attaching a stopcock and manometer to the needle before collecting fluid. However, this practice has largely been abandoned in favor of safer, more accurate ways of measuring CSF pressure and is not recommended.[5]

Precaution. Especially important in the emergency and critical care setting is to exercise caution when collecting CSF from patients with ICH from meningoencephalitis, CNS edema, or an intracranial mass. In these cases it may be dangerous to remove or allow escape of very much CSF. The sudden release of pressure may lead to brain herniation. If CSF flows out of the needle at a high velocity, or if flow is initially very good and then suddenly diminishes, a minimal amount of CSF should be collected. Also in animals with suspected ICH, extreme care should be taken not to flex the animal's head severely or place compression on jugular veins during CSF collection. If there is concern of life-threatening ICH, it may be safer to attempt a lumbar puncture instead of a cisternal puncture.

Lumbar puncture

Positioning

In animals with thoracic, lumbar, or sacral spinal cord disease, CSF should be collected from the lumbar region.[1,6] Additionally, lumbar puncture is usually preferred in animals with ascending lower motor neuron disease or suspected polyradiculopathies. Because of the proximity of the collection site to the diseased cord and the craniocaudal flow of CSF, lumbar fluid is more likely than cisternal fluid to reflect the disease process. In animals that are too ill to undergo general anesthesia or are comatose, a lumbar puncture (and occasionally a cisternal puncture) can be done with a local anesthetic and a tranquilizer if needed.

The technique of lumbar puncture for collection of CSF is the same as that used to place a needle for injection of contrast material into the subarachnoid space for myelography. CSF analysis is usually recommended following advanced imaging (MRI, CT) whenever possible. If myelography is being performed, CSF should be collected and analyzed prior to injecting contrast media to rule out meningomyelitis since injecting a contrast agent in the face of inflammation or infection may further damage an injured spinal cord and possibly disseminate infection. The patient is positioned in lateral recumbency with the right side down (for a right-handed operator). The lumbar spine may be gently flexed to open up the interarcuate space between L4 and L5 (preferred site in large breed dogs), L5 and L6 (preferred site in small breed dogs), or L6 and L7 (preferred site in cats). An area from the midlumbar to the sacral region is clipped and surgically prepared; sterile technique is used as described earlier.

The spinous process is palpated caudal to the desired interarcuate space, and the spinal needle is inserted through the skin at the caudolateral edge of the spinous process. With the needle directed cranially and following the spinous process down, the needle is inserted until the vertebral arch is encountered. Then the needle is "walked" cranially until the interarcuate space is palpated. The needle is advanced gently through the interarcuate ligament and into the vertebral canal until the floor of the canal is encountered. The animal often twitches when the needle penetrates the dura or a nerve root. If spinal fluid is not seen in the hub of the needle within a few seconds, the needle can be rotated and/or retracted slowly until the subarachnoid space is entered and fluid appears. Fluid should be allowed to drip into the collection tube by free flow and should not be aspirated from the needle. If blood is present in the hub, the needle should be withdrawn and discarded and another puncture attempted at a different site.

Note. Although the cauda equina is penetrated in the process of performing the puncture, this usually produces no ill effects.

ANALYSIS OF CEREBROSPINAL FLUID

Many tests can be done on CSF. To perform all possible tests costs money, requires larger volumes of CSF, and rarely gives additional information except in specific situations. For a complete list of these tests and their normal values, the reader is directed to a clinical pathology textbook or the indicated references at the end of this chapter. The following sections describe recommendations for routine analysis of CSF samples.

Specimen Handling and Examination

CSF should be collected in sterile red-top Vacutainer tubes and cytologic analysis performed within 30 to 60 minutes of collection.[1,3,5,6] If it is not possible to evaluate the sample soon after collection, it should be preserved by refrigeration and the addition of 1 drop of fetal calf serum or autologous serum per 0.25 ml of CSF. An aliquot of CSF should be saved in a separate tube for protein measurement.

Table 207-1 Normal Characteristics of Cerebrospinal Fluid (CSF)

Characteristic	Findings in Normal CSF
Color	Colorless
Clarity	Transparent, clear
Refractive index	1.3347 to 1.3350
Protein concentration	*Cisternal:* <25 mg/dl *Lumbar:* <40 mg/dl
Total cell count	*RBCs:* 0/μl *WBCs:* <3/μl cisternal; <5/μl lumbar
WBC differential count	Mononuclear cells *Small mononuclear cells:* 60% to 70% *Large mononuclear cells:* 30% to 40% Polymorphonuclear cells *Neutrophils:* <1% *Eosinophils:* <1% Others *Ependymal lining cells:* rare *Nucleated RBCs:* Rare in lumbar puncture specimens

RBC, Red blood cell; *WBC,* white blood cell.

This portion of the sample may be kept refrigerated or frozen until protein analysis is performed. Most commercial laboratories require a total of about 0.5 ml for routine CSF analysis.

Physical Characteristics

The color and clarity of the CSF should be observed by the clinician at the time of collection (Table 207-1).[1-3,6] Normal CSF is a crystal clear, colorless fluid comparable in appearance to distilled water. Common abnormalities include cloudiness or turbidity, caused by significant pleocytosis, and xanthochromia, a yellow discoloration caused by the breakdown of red blood cells due to recent hemorrhage in the CNS.

Total Cell Count and Differential

Red and white blood cell (RBC and WBC) counts can be performed in private practice using the chamber of a standard hemacytometer (see Table 207-1).[1,3] One to two drops of CSF are placed on each side of the hemacytometer from a standard microhematocrit tube (without anticoagulant) that has first been coated with new methylene blue stain. The nuclei of the nucleated WBCs in the sample will be stained and readily differentiated from the RBCs. The RBCs and WBCs in the nine large squares on each side of the hemacytometer are counted. The mean value of the counts from both sides is multiplied by 1.11 to get the total number of cells per cubic millimeter (microliter) of spinal fluid.

A differential count is done next, with polymorphonuclear cells and mononuclear cells noted. Normal CSF should have fewer than 3 WBCs/μl (slightly higher in lumbar fluid) with no neutrophils, plasma cells, or macrophages. RBCs should not be present in cisternal fluid; however, small numbers are usually considered normal in lumbar fluid. Slight contamination of CSF with blood does not severely affect the counting results.

Higher numbers of RBCs from the peripheral blood may affect the total WBC count, and the following rule of thumb is often used to make a ballpark correction estimate. Because the normal ratio of RBCs to WBCs in blood is about 500 : 1, 1 WBC is subtracted from the total CSF WBC count for every 500 RBCs present in the CSF if the patient's peripheral blood count is in the normal range. For more in-depth discussion on interpreting blood-contaminated CSF, the reader is referred to the reference list.

Cytologic Analysis

Most CSF samples contain low numbers of WBCs, and therefore most samples must be concentrated before morphology is examined microscopically (see Table 207-1).[1,3] Commercial laboratories use a cytocentrifuge to concentrate the cells in a single drop of CSF on a microscope slide. Membrane filtration and sedimentation are alternative methods of cytologic analysis. In-house sedimentation chambers can be constructed easily and used in private practice (see reference list). The slides made using a sedimentation chamber may be examined in house or submitted to a commercial laboratory for morphologic evaluation.

Protein Concentration

Total protein may be measured by several methods, although quantitative protein determinations performed by commercial laboratories are the most accurate (see Table 207-1).[1,3,5,6] Normal values vary by species, laboratory, and site of collection. Most diseases of the CNS cause changes in the CSF protein concentration; elevated protein concentration in the CSF often is used as evidence that neurologic disease is within the CNS. The degree of protein elevation, along with information on the total and differential WBC count, is used to determine the most likely differential diagnoses for the abnormalities seen in the sample. Blood contamination of the CSF (>500 RBCs/μl) may influence protein concentration and should be taken into account. A 1-mg/dl increase in CSF protein level can be estimated for every 1000 RBCs in the sample if the serum protein concentration of the patient is in the normal range. For more in-depth discussion of protein concentration and interpretation, see the reference section.

Other Tests

Many other diagnostic tests may be performed on CSF samples depending on the interpretation of the cytologic findings and protein concentration. These include bacterial culture, antigen-antibody titers, polymerase chain reaction testing, immunocytochemistry, and enzyme, metabolite, and neurotransmitter assays.[1,6]

INTERPRETATION OF COMMON FINDINGS

Although CSF results are usually not specifically diagnostic, certain types of cellular responses can be strongly suggestive of particular diseases.[1-3,5,6] There are many exceptions to the general guidelines presented here, especially when one adds the complexity of evaluating CSF from animals that have chronic disease or have been treated with medications that may affect the cellular content or distribution of cells. It must also be kept in mind that normal CSF findings do not rule out the presence of CNS disease.

1. Mild to moderate predominantly mononuclear pleocytosis typically is seen with inflammatory diseases, especially viral and rickettsial infections (e.g., canine distemper, ehrlichiosis). It may also occur with noninfectious inflammatory brain diseases as well as compressive lesions affecting the spinal cord (intervertebral disk disease [IVDD]).
2. Moderate to marked predominantly neutrophilic pleocytosis most commonly is seen with infectious or inflammatory diseases such as bacterial meningoencephalomyelitis, steroid-responsive meningitis or vasculitis, and feline infectious peritonitis.
3. Moderate to marked predominantly mononuclear pleocytosis classically is seen with granulomatous meningoencephalomyelitis and breed-related forms of necrotizing encephalitis found in Pugs, Maltese, Yorkshire Terriers, Chihuahuas, and others. Lymphoma in the CNS often causes significant mononuclear pleocytosis as well.
4. Marked pleocytosis with a predominance of eosinophils most commonly is caused by eosinophilic meningitis (idiopathic). Other less common conditions, such as migrations of parasites (e.g., *Angiostrongylus*) and protozoal and fungal disease, also should be considered.
5. Mild to marked mixed pleocytosis most often is associated with inflammatory diseases, especially fungal or protozoal meningoencephalomyelitis. Mixed pleocytoses are also commonly seen in infectious or inflammatory disease that is "aging" or being managed with medications that are altering the typical pattern of cells seen. Necrosis of the CNS occurring secondary to vascular infarction, trauma, or neoplasia may also produce a mixed pleocytosis.
6. Albuminocytologic dissociation occurs when the total nucleated cell count is in the normal range (although the distribution of cells may be abnormal) but the protein level is elevated. This finding is very nonspecific and may be seen in virtually any CNS disease, but it is most often indicative of degenerative or demyelinating diseases (degenerative myelopathy), chronically compressive lesions (IVDD, neoplasia, stenoses), and intramedullary pathologic conditions (neoplasia or syringohydromyelia).

REFERENCES

1. Bailey CS, Vernau W: Cerebrospinal fluid. In Kaneko JJ, Harvey JW, Bruss ML, editors: Clinical biochemistry of domestic animals, ed 5, New York, 1997, Academic Press.
2. Chrisman CL: Cerebrospinal fluid analysis, Vet Clin North Am Small Anim Pract 22:781-810, 1992.
3. Wamsley H, Alleman RA: Clinical pathology. In Olby NJ, Platt SR, editors: BSAVA manual of canine and feline neurology, ed 3, Quedgeley, UK, 2000, British Small Animal Veterinary Association.
4. Fishman RA: Cerebrospinal fluid in diseases of the nervous system, ed 2, Philadelphia, 1992, Saunders.
5. Bagley RS: Treatment of important and common diseases involving the intracranial nervous system of dogs and cats. In Bagley RS, editor: Fundamentals of veterinary clinical neurology, ed 1, Oxford, 2005, Blackwell.
6. Tipold A: Cerebrospinal fluid. In Braund KG, editor: Clinical neurology in small animals: localization, diagnosis and treatment, Ithaca, NY, 2003, International Veterinary Information Service. Available at http://www.ivis.org.

CHAPTER 208

URINARY CATHETERIZATION

Sean Smarick, VMD, DACVECC

KEY POINTS

- Urinary catheterization is useful in the critically ill patient to accurately monitor urine output and measure intraabdominal pressure.
- Other purposes include relieving anatomic or functional obstructions, performing radiographic contrast procedures, and supporting selective perioperative patients.
- Catheter-associated urinary tract infection is a potential complication of the procedure but may be limited by following placement and maintenance protocols, restricting the use of indwelling catheters to appropriate patients, and leaving the catheter in place only as long as needed.
- Species, sex, and purpose of catheterization are considerations in choosing a catheter type.
- Indwelling urinary catheters require ongoing care, and their need in individual patients should be reevaluated daily.

Urinary catheterization is performed for diagnostic, treatment, or monitoring purposes and often is indicated in critically ill patients. Sex and species differences may offer anatomic challenges, but these can be overcome with appropriate techniques and practice. Each patient should be evaluated individually to identify a clear indication for the procedure, decide the type of urinary catheter to be used, and determine the duration for which the catheter is to remain in place. Indications for urinary catheter placement can be grouped into those warranting a one-time or intermittent placement and those in which the catheter should be left in place.

INDICATIONS

Intermittent Catheterization

One-time or intermittent urethral catheterization can be used to perform radiographic contrast procedures and relieve an anatomic or functional obstruction leading to urine retention. Urinary contrast imaging procedures, such as contrast urethrocystography, assess the integrity of the lower urinary tract and can help characterize bladder masses, calculi, and urethral obstructions caused by neoplasia, a calculus, or a foreign body. Urethral obstructions may be relieved or bypassed with a urinary catheter. Retrohydropulsion can be used to help dislodge calculi or even retrieve small stones from the bladder. In humans intermittent catheterization has been found to be an alternative to indwelling catheters to address urine retension.[1]

Catheterization can be performed to obtain samples for urinalysis, but it should be considered only if cystocentesis or free-catch samples cannot be obtained. Even a one-time catheterization can introduce bacteria into the lower urinary tract.[2] A urine sample obtained by catheterization can be contaminated by bacterial and red blood cells.[1,3]

Indwelling Catheter

Indwelling urinary catheters allow for continuous urine collection and, based on guidelines for humans issued by the Centers for Disease Control and Prevention, are indicated for critically ill patients or during surgery when accurate urine output determination is required (see Chapter 192), for patients with acute urinary obstruction or retention, for patients whose injuries require immobilization, and for surgical patients undergoing procedures of the genitourinary tract or requiring urine collection during the procedure.[1]

Intraabdominal pressure monitoring can be used in dogs and cats to diagnose intraabdominal hypertension, and the intravesicular pressure in the bladder is the most popular measurement in both people and pets. Continuous monitoring is ideal, followed by frequent intermittent measurement, and the need for either is an indication for placement of an indwelling urinary catheter[4] (see Chapter 188).

Simple recumbency or incontinence and the need for associated nursing care is not a justifiable indication; however, if urine scalding, skin breakdown, or urine contamination of wounds is occurring and other methods have proved ineffective, use of an indwelling catheter can be considered.[1]

These recommendations are generally aimed at preventing complications; namely, catheter-associated urinary tract infection (UTI).

RISKS AND COMPLICATIONS

Infection

Catheter-associated UTIs have been reported in the veterinary literature, and the incidence may exceed 50%. These infections have played a role in nosocomial outbreaks in veterinary intensive care units (ICUs) and have the potential to cause serious morbidity and mortality. Resistant bacteria such as *Klebsiella, Acinetobacter, Enterobacter, Citrobacter, Serratia, Pseudomonas* spp, and *Escherichia coli* may cause veterinary catheter–associated UTI and may serve as a source within the ICU for other nosocomial infections.[5-15] Fungal UTIs have been reported in dogs and cats with lower urinary tract disease, urethrostomies, and indwelling cystotomy tubes but not specifically urinary catheters.[16,17] Catheter-associated fungal UTIs are known to occur in people, but the incidence in dogs and cats is unknown.

Catheter-associated UTIs can occur as a result of introduction of microorganisms into the bladder during catheter insertion. In one study, there was a 20% incidence of UTI following a one-time catheterization in female dogs.[2] Once indwelling, the catheter provides a surface on which bacteria may migrate. This often involves a biofilm, a matrix of microorganisms and their produced glycocalyces, host salts, and proteins. Biofilms allow for the adherence of bacteria to catheter surfaces and provide protection from the host's defenses.[18]

Surveillance for catheter-associated UTIs has not been defined in veterinary medicine. In people, urine obtained aseptically from an indwelling catheter or within 48 hours of removal of a catheter that tests positive for one species of bacteria at a level of 10^5 colony-forming units (CFU)/ml (with no other source of infection) is referred to as *catheter-associated bacteriuria.* Clinical signs of a UTI (e.g., fever) along with a positive finding on urine culture of 10^3 CFU/ml of one species are the criteria for a catheter-associated UTI. Monitoring for asymptomatic bacteriuria in people with an indwelling urinary catheter or after one is removed is not currently recommended.[1,19] The applicability of these guidelines to veterinary patients is unknown. In addition to culturing the urine if there is unexplained fever or other signs of UTI, it would be reasonable to culture the urine more than 2 days after the urinary catheter has been removed.

If there is suspected or confirmed UTI, antibiotics should be administered for 7 to 14 days, guided by results of culture and susceptibility testing. Prophylactic administration of antibiotics to patients with indwelling urinary catheters may offer short-term protection against a UTI, but organisms that are resistant to the antibiotic therapy often emerge. Therefore routine antibiotics prophylaxis for the sole reason of the presence of a urinary catheter are not recommended.[6-9,13,19]

Despite the morbidity and even mortality associated with the use of urinary catheters, appropriate patient selection coupled with adherence to placement and maintenance protocols as described later has allowed achievement of an approximately 10% incidence of catheter-associated UTIs in two veterinary ICUs.[6,8] It should be noted that the patients in these studies had indwelling catheters for an average of 2 days. Increased duration of catheterization has been shown to be a risk factor for the development of catheter-associated UTIs, and for this reason, limiting the time a patient has an indwelling catheter is desirable.

Mechanical Difficulties

During placement, stiff catheters or catheter stylets may cause physical trauma to the urethra or bladder. Appropriate lubrication, judicious use of force, and proper seating of stylets (i.e., stylet contained within the catheter) are indicated to prevent physical trauma. If a soft catheter is advanced too far into the bladder, it may fold back on itself and head back into the urethra. Measuring the required length of catheter before insertion can help prevent this complication. If it is encountered, topical anesthesia and, if needed, sedation usually allow for removal of the catheter with steady traction; however, urethral trauma is a possibility. If this maneuver or manipulation of the catheter with stylets, flushing, and passage of another catheter to force the advancing end back into the bladder are unsuccessful, or the catheter has actually become knotted, surgery is indicated.

CATHETER TYPES

Materials

Urinary catheters are made of a variety of materials that affect stiffness, urethral reactivity, and resistance to bacterial swarming and biofilm formation. Ideally a catheter is soft to promote patient comfort and limit urethral trauma, has minimal reactivity, and has resistance to biofilm formation, which decreases the potential for catheter-associated UTI. The following are available catheter materials, listed in order of decreasing urethral reactivity, increasing biofilm resistance, and hence increasing suitability for long-term indwelling catheter use: plastic, red rubber, latex, siliconized elastomer or Teflon-coated latex, hydrogel-coated latex, and pure silicone. Diffusion from silicone balloons has been reported, resulting in balloon deflation.[20]

In an effort to prevent catheter-associated UTIs, catheters have been coated with antiseptics or antimicrobials. A recent veterinary study in dogs demonstrated reduced formation of biofilm when a chlorhexidine-coated catheter was used.[18] Due to their increased cost, potential to induce reactions, and undetermined efficacy as a primary intervention, the recommendation at this time is that their use in people be limited to patient centers with a high incidence of catheter-associated UTIs where other interventions (e.g., hand-washing compliance, training) have failed.[1,19]

Size

Urinary catheter size is expressed as diameter times length. The diameter is designated using the French (Fr) scale. The scale value, when divided by 3, is the outside diameter of the catheter in millimeters; that is, a 12 Fr catheter has an outside diameter of 4 mm. The appropriate catheter size depends on the patient's size and sex. Cats generally need a 3.5 to 5 Fr, female dogs a 3.5 to 14 Fr, and male dogs a 3.5 to 10 Fr. Males require a longer catheter than females, and some catheters may be too short to reach the bladder in some males. Catheters should be measured before insertion to ensure adequate length in males.

Foley Catheters

Balloon-tipped catheters (with a distal port) are referred to as *Foley catheters,* named after their inventor, Dr. Frederic Foley, who developed them in 1934. Foley catheters are now available in smaller diameters and longer lengths for veterinary patients. They offer the advantage of anchoring the catheter within the bladder when the balloon near the tip is inflated. This eliminates the need to secure the catheter with tape and suture at the vulva or prepuce. They are ideal when an indwelling catheter is needed.

Foley catheters do have the potential for some unique complications related to the balloon. Overfilling the balloon may cause it to occlude the catheter lumen, and overfilling or underfilling the balloon may deviate the tip and result in bladder wall contact. The balloon ideally should be filled with sterile water to prevent contamination in case of permeability or rupture; also, sterile water, unlike saline, will not occlude the small lumen leading to the balloon.[20]

PLACEMENT TECHNIQUE

Before catheter placement, the necessary supplies should be assembled, including a closed collection system if the catheter will be left indwelling (Box 208-1). Universal patient preparation includes placing the patient in lateral recumbency, clipping the hair from the preputial or vulvar area to maintain a hair-free area of at least 3 to 5 cm from the catheter insertion site, and preparing the area with a chlorhexidine scrub and tap water solution. Aseptic technique is maintained by using sterile barrier drapes and sterile gloves, and lubricating the catheter before placement with sterile water–based (lidocaine) lubricating jelly. Before the procedure is started, the catheter is measured from the urethral opening to the bladder, following the path of the urethra (while maintaining sterility). The balloon should be tested before insertion.

Most dogs tolerate the procedure with use of a topical anesthetic, warmed flushing solutions, and appropriate restraint and comforting; however, many cats and some dogs require light sedation. Benzodiazepines, through their action on peripheral skeletal muscle, may induce relaxation of the external urethral sphincter and be of benefit in the sedation cocktail.

Male Dog

In males the penis is held extruded from the prepuce for the entire procedure. After the extruded penis is cleaned of any gross exudate, the prepuce is flushed with 2 to 10 ml of 0.05% chlorhexidine solution five times. With the penis still extruded, the barrier drape is applied and an appropriate-sized urinary catheter is advanced aseptically into the urethral opening and into the bladder.

Female Dog

The vestibule is flushed gently with 2 to 10 ml of a 0.05% chlorhexidine solution five times. Lidocaine jelly or solution (not to exceed 4 mg/kg) may be flushed into the area of the urethral opening a few centimeters into the vulva with a lubricated syringe (without a needle). One hand digitally palpates the urethral papilla while the other hand advances an appropriate-sized catheter under the digit into the urethral opening and into the bladder (Figure 208-1).

Using a stylet or polypropylene catheter to provide some rigidity to a soft catheter may aid in guiding the catheter into the urethral opening. The stylet should be sterile and contained within the catheter to prevent urethral trauma. If this approach is unsuccessful, a disinfected laryngoscope speculum or vaginal speculum with a headlamp or other suitable light source can be used to visualize the urethral opening on the ventral floor of the vestibule-vagina interface (Figure 208-2). The procedure can still be performed with the dog in lateral recumbency, but the individual operator may prefer to place the patient in sternal recumbency with the pelvic limbs over the edge of the table, in standing position, or in dorsal recumbency with the pelvic limbs flexed cranially. Alternatively, an otoscope and attached cone can be used to view the urethral opening. The cone usually will not fit over the distal end of the catheter, which requires that the catheter and closed collection system be modified or that the cone remain attached until the catheter is removed. Small dogs and puppies may require use of a blind technique as described later for female cats.

BOX 208-1 ***Supplies for Urinary Catheter Placement***

General Requirements

Sterile drapes/barrier for work area and patient
Sterile urinary catheter
Gauze sponges
Chlorhexidine surgical scrub and water rinse
Lidocaine or K-Y jelly (single use preferred)
Sterile gloves
Solution of 6.25 ml chlorhexidine 2% in 250 ml sterile water
Syringe for flushing prepuce
Syringe for Foley balloon (3 to 6 ml)

Indwelling but Not a Foley Catheter

Suture (2-0 or 3-0 monofilament nylon)
Needle drivers, scissors, skin forceps
Tape or other securing device

Closed Collection System

Collection bag (appropriate size for animal)
If bag does not have tubing, aspiration port, or male adapter for catheter:
- Male (adapter) connector for urinary catheter
- Extension tubing (1 or 2)
- Three-way Luer-Lok stopcock
- Infusion plug

Cable tie(s) and application gun

Male Cat

The penis is extruded caudally with digital pressure applied to the prepuce craniodorsally. After the extruded penis is cleaned of any gross exudate, the prepuce is flushed with 0.25 to 1 ml of 0.05% chlorhexidine solution five times. With the penis still extruded, an appropriate-sized urinary catheter (usually 3.5 to 5 Fr) is advanced into the urethral opening and into the bladder.

Female Cat

The vestibule is flushed with 0.5 to 2 ml of a 0.05% chlorhexidine solution five times. In larger cats a digital or direct-viewing method as described earlier for female dogs may be attempted, but usually a blind anatomic technique is employed. With the catheter directed along the midline of the ventral floor of the vestibule as it transitions to the vagina, the catheter is advanced blindly into the urethral papilla. Resistance is met at the cervix if the urethral opening is overshot, which necessitates withdrawal and repeating the approach.

Flow of urine from the catheter confirms placement. If the bladder is empty, flushing and aspirating sterile saline from the catheter can provide evidence of proper placement. Imaging (radiography or ultrasonography or both) can be used if placement is still in question. If the catheter is to be indwelling, a sterile closed collection system is connected to the catheter immediately following insertion. One or more cable ties may be used to secure any connections and offer the advantage of visualization over taping of the junctions.

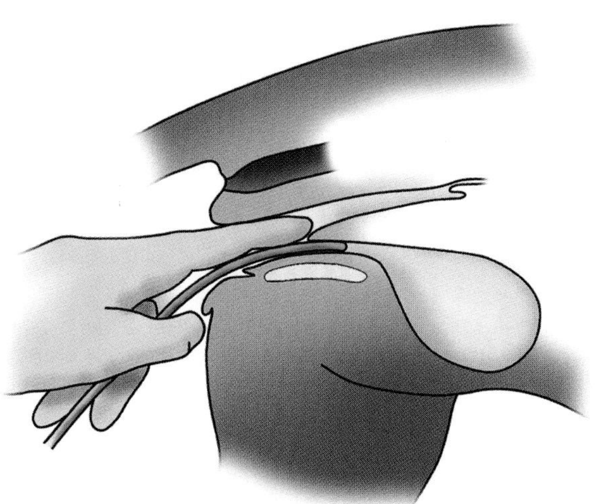

FIGURE 208-1 Urethral catheterization of a female dog. An index finger is placed over the urethral orifice to guide the catheter ventrally into the urethra. *(From Taylor SM: Small animal clinical techniques, St Louis, 2010, Saunders.)*

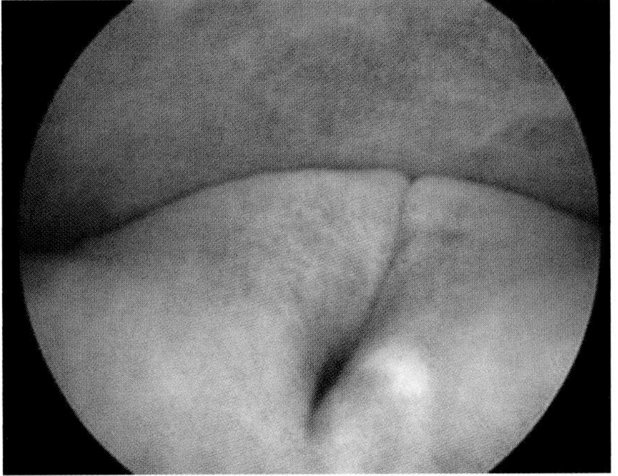

FIGURE 208-2 The canine female urethral opening as viewed through a vaginoscope. The external urethral orifice can be visualized on the ventral floor of the vaginovestibular junction. *(Courtesy Dr. Jodi Westropp, University of California, Davis.)*

Securing the Catheter

To secure a Foley catheter, the catheter is slightly overadvanced into the bladder. The balloon is inflated with sterile water and then the catheter is retracted until resistance is met. For non-Foley catheters, external securing systems must be used. A securing platform may be included that allows the catheter to be sutured to the skin; otherwise, a piece of butterfly tape can be sutured to the vulva or prepuce adjacent to the catheter. The butterfly is an approximately 1-inch piece of 1-inch-wide tape folded upon itself, sandwiching the catheter. The tubing of the sterile collection system is then taped to the patient's tail or leg. Care should be taken to ensure that the collection system is not placing any tension on the urethral catheter or securing site.

Closed Collection System

Use of a sterile closed collection system is the standard of care for all indwelling catheters. Preventing reflux of urine into the bladder is recommended and can be accomplished by ensuring proper operation of the check valve on the urinary collection bag and keeping the bag below the level of the bladder. Contamination of the bag is prevented by avoiding direct contact of the bag especially the spigot, with the floor, other grossly contaminated surfaces, or collection vessels (e.g., graduated cylinders). Ensure that urine is able to flow continuously; if the urinary catheter becomes clogged with debris or blood clots, backflushing with sterile saline may restore flow.[1,19]

If a sterile closed collection system is not available, an empty intravenous fluid bag and sterile fluid administration set may be used. A veterinary study in which such a system was used did not find an increase in catheter-associated UTIs compared with the use of sterile commercial systems; however, a number of caveats must be considered before accepting this as standard operating procedure. The bags used were stored in a cabinet off the ground, were held for no longer than 7 days after original use, were capped with a sterile device while being stored, and did not contain dextrose. Additionally, the average duration of catheterization in the study supporting the use of this system was only 2 days, no catheterization lasted longer than 7 days, and the patient populations were relatively small.[6]

CARE OF AN INDWELLING URINARY CATHETER

When caring for patients with indwelling urinary catheters, hand washing before and after touching each patient is a must, and wearing examination gloves as a universal precaution is good practice.

Every 8 hours or anytime the catheter is visibly soiled, the exposed catheter and external genitalia should be gently cleaned with chlorhexidine scrub and tap water. The prepuce or vestibule should be rinsed and flushed five times with 0.2 to 10 ml (depending on the size of the patient) of diluted chlorhexidine solution (0.05%). Consideration should be given to warming the flush solution for patient comfort, and the solution should do not be introduced into the urethra.[8]

Routine replacement of the catheter or closed collection system is not recommended; however, if the system is thought to be contaminated, a UTI is suspected, or the system is nonfunctional, aseptic replacement is warranted.

Every effort should be made not to break the closed collection system. To obtain urine samples from the closed collection system, the sampling port should be swabbed with alcohol and allowed to dry, then the desired amount should be aspirated with a sterile syringe and 25-gauge needle, and finally the port should be wiped again with alcohol. The infusion plug or closed collection system should be changed only under aseptic conditions and when the integrity of the injection port is compromised.[1,19]

Lastly, as stated earlier, the caregiving team should frequently evaluate whether the benefit of an indwelling catheter outweighs the risks and remove it when it is no longer needed.*

REFERENCES

1. Gould CV, Umscheid CA, Agarwal RK, et al: Guidelines for prevention of catheter-associated urinary tract infections, 2009, Atlanta, 2009, Centers for Disease Control and Prevention. Available at http://www.cdc.gov/hicpac/cauti/001_cauti.html. Accessed February 6, 2014.
2. Biertuempfel PH, Ling GV, Ling GA: Urinary tract infection resulting from catheterization in healthy adult dogs, J Am Vet Med Assoc 178:989, 1981.
3. Comer KM, Ling GV: Results of urinalysis and bacterial culture of canine urine obtained by antepubic cystocentesis, catheterization, and the mid-stream voided methods, J Am Vet Med 179:891, 1981.
4. Smith SE, Sande AA: Measurement of intra-abdominal pressure in dogs and cats, J Vet Emerg Crit Care (San Antonio) 22:530, 2012.
5. Wise LA, Jones RL, Reif JS: Nosocomial canine urinary tract infections in a veterinary teaching hospital, J Am Anim Hosp Assoc 24:627, 1990.
6. Sullivan LA, Campbell V L, Onuma SC: Evaluation of open versus closed urine collection systems and development of nosocomial bacteriuria in dogs, J Am Vet Med Assoc 237:187, 2010.
7. Stiffler KS, McCracken Stevenson MA, Sanchez S, et al: Prevalence and characterization of urinary tract infections in dogs with surgically treated type 1 thoracolumbar intervertebral disc extrusion, Vet Surg 35:330, 2006.
8. Smarick SD, Haskins SC, Aldrich J, et al: Incidence of catheter-associated urinary tract infection among dogs in a small animal intensive care unit, J Am Vet Med Assoc 224:1936, 2004.
9. Ogeer-Gyles J, Mathews K, Weese JS, et al: Evaluation of catheter-associated urinary tract infections and multi-drug-resistant *Escherichia coli* isolates from the urine of dogs with indwelling urinary catheters, J Am Vet Med Assoc 229:1584, 2006.
10. Lippert AC, Fulton RB, Parr AM: Nosocomial infection surveillance in a small animal intensive care unit, J Am Anim Hosp Assoc 24:48, 1988.
11. Glickman LT: Veterinary nosocomial (hospital-acquired) *Klebsiella* infections, J Am Vet Med Assoc 179:1389, 1981.
12. Francey T, Gaschen F, Nicolet J, et al: The role of *Acinetobacter baumannii* as a nosocomial pathogen for dogs and cats in an intensive care unit, J Vet Intern Med 14:177, 2000.
13. Bubenik L, Hosgood G: Urinary tract infection in dogs with thoracolumbar intervertebral disc herniation and urinary bladder dysfunction managed by manual expression, indwelling catheterization or intermittent catheterization, Vet Surg 37:791, 2008.
14. Bubenik LJ, Hosgood GL, Waldron DR, et al: Frequency of urinary tract infection in catheterized dogs and comparison of bacterial culture and susceptibility testing results for catheterized and noncatheterized dogs with urinary tract infections, J Am Vet Med Assoc 231:893, 2007.
15. Barsanti JA, Blue J, Edmunds J: Urinary tract infection due to indwelling bladder catheters in dogs and cats, J Am Vet Med Assoc 187:384, 1985.
16. Jin Y, Lin D: Fungal urinary tract infections in the dog and cat: a retrospective study, J Am Anim Hosp Assoc 41:373, 2005.
17. Pressler BM, Vaden SL, Lane IF, et al: *Candida* spp. urinary tract infections in 13 dogs and seven cats: predisposing factors, treatment, and outcome, J Am Anim Hosp Assoc 39:263, 2003.
18. Segev G, Bankirer T, Steinberg D, et al: Evaluation of urinary catheters coated with sustained-release varnish of chlorhexidine in mitigating biofilm formation on urinary catheters in dogs, J Vet Intern Med 27:39, 2013.
19. Hooton TM, Bradley SF, Cardenas DD, et al: Diagnosis, prevention, and treatment of catheter-associated urinary tract infection in adults: 2009 International Clinical Practice Guidelines from the Infectious Diseases Society of America, Clin Infect Dis 50:625, 2010.
20. Sharpe SJ, Mann FA, Wiedmeyer CE, et al: Optimal filling solution for silicone Foley catheter balloons, Can Vet J 52:1111, 2011.

*References 1, 7-9, 13, 14, 19.

PART XXIII ICU DESIGN AND MANAGEMENT

CHAPTER 209

INTENSIVE CARE UNIT FACILITY DESIGN

Joris H. Robben, DVM, PhD, DECVIM-CA

KEY POINTS

- Intensive care unit (ICU) design should support the staff and organization in their striving to deliver high-quality patient care.
- In human medicine, both patient outcome and staff well-being and performance are improved with better ICU design.
- Inclusion of infection prevention and control measures in ICU design is increasing in importance because of the growing impact of multidrug-resistant bacteria on patient care and outcomes.
- ICU design should offer patients a safe and comfortable environment. The specific needs of veterinary patients, such as cats, deserve special attention during the design process.

The importance of the design of a newly built or renovated intensive care unit (ICU) cannot be overemphasized. The design is often intended to last for a decade or longer and has an impact on a myriad of elements such as staff satisfaction, organizational performance, patient comfort and safety, quality of intensive care, infection prevention and control (IPC), and cost of care delivery.[1] Specific design elements have even been related to improved outcomes for both patients and staff in human hospitals.[2,3]

Although directives in veterinary medicine are limited,[4-6] guidelines in human medicine for the construction of ICUs have become very detailed and are increasingly supported by evidence.[1,3,7-9] Changes in market demand, aging of the population, increased severity of illnesses, rise in hospital-acquired infections, clinical staff shortages, technologic innovations, and environmental concerns—all are shaping the critical care practice in human medicine today.[10] Human guidelines often can be applied to veterinary medicine or can be a valuable source of inspiration despite the fact that the setting is very different.

For the purposes of this chapter, *intensive care* is defined as care for dogs and cats that are in medically unstable or critically ill condition and require constant nursing, continuous monitoring, and intense and sometimes complicated treatment modalities such as continual respiratory support or other intensive interventions. It does not include emergency medicine, but because many ICUs also accommodate intermediate-care patients, the veterinary ICU often services a mix of patients with conditions of varying acuity.

This chapter is not meant to be all encompassing, and the guidelines are intended to indicate desired performance rather than being prescriptive. A *performance guideline* functions to be accommodated, whereas a *prescriptive guideline* provides quantification, such as minimum square footage for a patient cage.[1]

THE DESIGN PROCESS

The type of ICU (intensive versus intermediate/intensive) and the ICU staffing model (open vs. closed) is of primary importance in the choice of ICU design.[11] Therefore unit design begins with an in-depth analysis of the level and volume of patient care, staff resources and workflow patterns, cooperation with support services, and hospital policies. The analysis should lead to the development of a functional (requirements) outline. Development of this outline should predate the actual design process to determine what functions are necessary for the design to support (Table 209-1).[12]

The design process is complex, and the project team should include both clinically oriented and design-based multiprofessional team members. Project team members will likely include hospital administration and hospital service representatives (information technology specialists, caretakers), the clinical multidisciplinary team (including veterinarians, technicians, pet owners, and, if present, infection control specialists, pharmacists, and ancillary staff), the design team (including the architect, engineers, technology planners, and safety hazard officials), and the contractor or construction manager.[1] The program planning and design process involves several steps and should include research of evidence-based recommendations and materials, best practices, design standards, building codes, and other regulatory agency standards.[7,13]

Because design deficiencies are difficult and costly to remedy once the design is in place, it is important to document all decisions.[14] Flawed design that remains uncorrected can result in shortcuts and workarounds that may negatively affect the aspects mentioned earlier, such as IPC.[15] It is of particular importance to include an infection control risk assessment in the design process.[14]

LOCATION IN THE HOSPITAL

An ICU will be situated in a hospital or practice with appropriate departments to ensure that the multidisciplinary needs of intensive care medicine are met.[9] Layout of the ICU should allow easy access to and from the emergency service, the operating theaters, and the recovery room. Connections with the diagnostic imaging department, pharmacy, laboratory, and clinical pathology service have to be considered, especially with limited point-of-care facilities.

A diagram that depicts the relationships between departments and support facilities can help in establishing effective routing for people (staff vs. owners and visitors), patients (gurneys), and equipment and consumables (Figure 209-1). The diagram can contain further detail; for example, by indicating the importance of the

Table 209-1 Factors to Consider in the Design of an Intensive Care Unit

Factor	Related to
Operational considerations	Admission and discharge guidelines Staffing
Unit configuration	Location within the hospital (see Figure 209-1) Size Ground plan (see Table 209-2)
Environmental services	Medical gases, vacuum, and compressed air Electrical power supply Lighting Network and communication Ambient temperature and ventilation Water supply and plumbing Acoustic environment Ceiling finishes Floor and wall surfaces Furnishings and fixtures
Infection prevention and control	See Table 209-3
Safety and security	People safety and security Patient safety and security Backup systems Evacuation planning
Ambiance	Patient comfort (dog versus cat) Owner/visitor Staff
Equipment	Laboratory Monitoring Supportive/care Treatment Crash cart
Communication aspects	Patient record keeping Protocols Bulletin boards

relationships or routing (adjacent, easily accessible, or located within same building) by the thickness of the arrows.[16]

ARRANGEMENT AND SIZE

An ICU should consist of a geographically distinct entity in the hospital with controlled access. The through traffic of patients and provisioning not intended for the ICU should be avoided.

Layout of an ICU is arguably the most important design feature, affecting all aspects of intensive care services including staff working conditions and patient comfort and safety.[17] Overall ICU floor plan and design should be based on patient admission patterns, staff (and visitor) traffic patterns, and the need for support facilities such as a nursing station, storage, clerical space, space for administrative and educational activities, and areas for services that are unique to the individual institution.[12]

The single-patient room, the acuity-adaptable room, and the universal room are new design concepts in human medicine to improve family involvement, infection control, patient safety, comfort, privacy, and confidentiality.[1,18,19] However interesting these concepts may be, staffing, space limitations, and budget constraints will not allow these development to occur in veterinary medicine soon. Nevertheless, creation of complete or partially separated facilities for isolation, infection control, cats, and possibly high-end interventions such as mechanical ventilation and renal replacement therapy deserve consideration.

A human ICU should accommodate a minimum of 6 beds, with 8 to 12 beds considered the optimum.[9] These numbers may also apply to veterinary medicine, although the economic situation as well as the need for the ICU to deal with patients of intermediate- and high-dependency care often results in creation of larger-capacity units. With the increasing availability of intermediate care facilities, diversity in the level of patient care and patient numbers can be reduced in the ICU. Inadequate capacity in an ICU leads to cancellation of planned surgery, transfers of emergency patients, and premature discharge. In human medicine mathematical modeling is available to determine the capacity of a new intensive care unit.[20]

UNIT CONFIGURATION

The floor plan can be divided into three areas: staff work areas, patient care areas, and ancillary services (Table 209-2). Support and ancillary services may be shared with other services.

Staff Work Areas

Because continuous visual (and auditory) surveillance of critically ill patients by the staff is of utmost importance, an unobstructed direct or indirect (e.g., by video monitoring) view of the patient area from the nursing station is mandatory.[1,2,12] The constant visual contact between technician and patient may be achieved by large window openings and glass doors.

The nursing station is foremost an administrative unit and should contain all the necessary equipment to perform this formidable task. The station should support computerized patient charting because it is becoming increasingly popular. These systems provide for "paperless" data management, order entry, and nurse and physician charting. An organizational culture and environment that are supportive of personnel is essential for improving performance and quality of care.[18] Therefore the station should also offer space and comfort to the staff because they spend long hours in the unit.

A staff break room may give the staff an additional opportunity to step back from a physically demanding environment. The presence of a conference or multipurpose room for multidisciplinary patient care conferences may reduce cage-side rounds and thereby limit the amount of staff traffic in the ICU patient area.

Patient Care Areas

The patient areas in current veterinary ICUs are considered open wards, in contrast to the single-patient room designs that are currently drastically changing the patient area layout in human hospitals. This compact design is necessary because a limited number of staff are available to observe and interact with a number of patients with various diseases, procedural histories, and experiences. The increasing amount of bedside equipment, the need for patient and staff comfort, and the requirement for unobstructed movement of persons and equipment are counteracting the striving for compactness. Furthermore, the distance between beds in open ward designs in human medicine plays an important role in IPC.[14] Similar considerations must be kept in mind in companion animal medicine, especially in units that admit very debilitated patients.

A very critical appraisal of storage of consumables and unused equipment in the patient area can minimize unnecessary consumption of room space and help to reduce a crowded, complicated, and confusing visual impression.

Patient modules

A patient module consists of a cage and its direct surroundings. Different frequencies and intensities of care may warrant different types

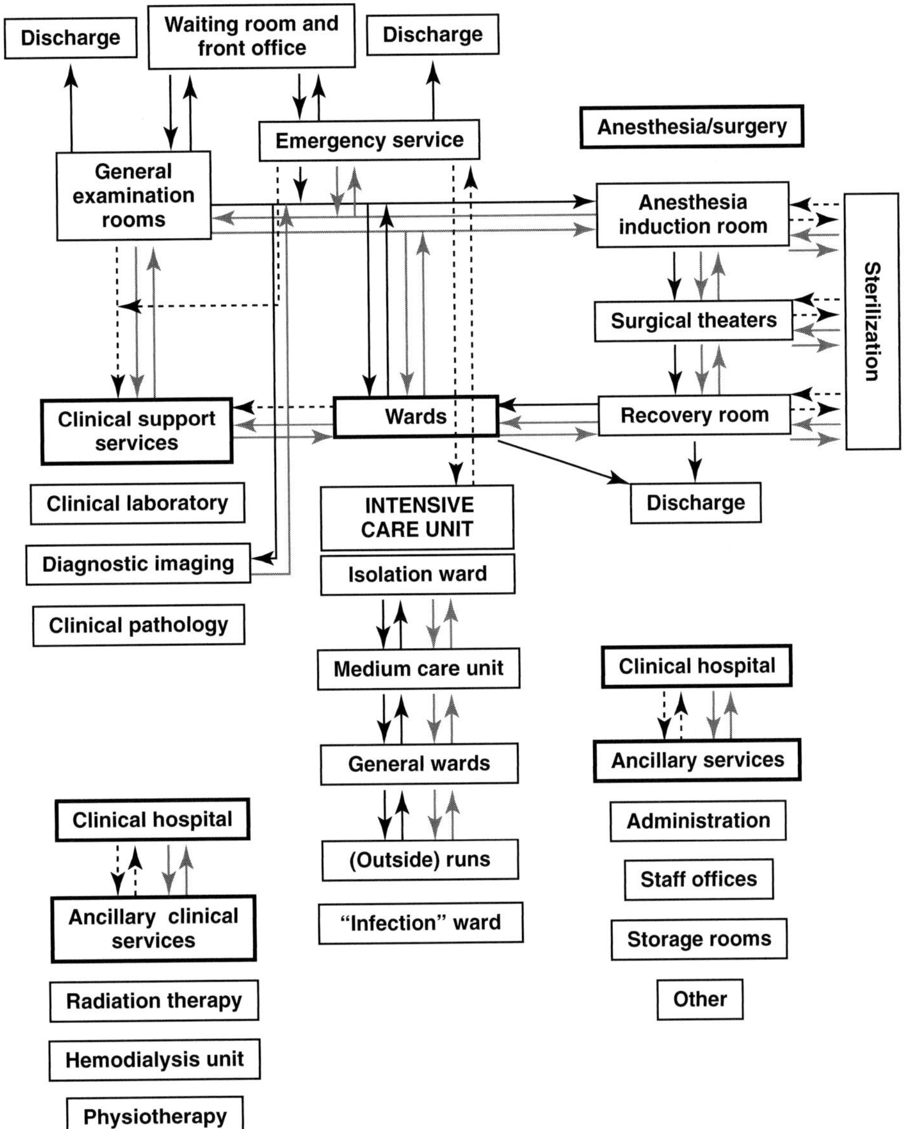

FIGURE 209-1 Schematic portrayal of the hypothetical relationship of the intensive care unit (ICU) to other hospital facilities. The arrows represent possible movement of patients (± owners) *(black)*, staff *(gray)*, and equipment and materials *(black, dotted lines)* between facilities. The construction of such a diagram helps in determining the position and design of the ICU in the hospital or practice. Its incompleteness (here caused by the constraints of the book format) forms a good basis for discussion, improvement, and achievement of consensus.

of patient modules. The presence of a separate intermediate care facility allows a focus on high-end intensive care and patient modules with extended cage-side space.

Provision of sufficient space around the cages is important for comfortable maneuvering of staff and visitors, easy positioning of equipment such as poles with pumps and bags for administering intravenous fluids and medications, and IPC. Essential services such as switches for cage-dedicated light and for medical utility and electrical power outlets can be mounted on a flat wall system, fixed column, suspended column, and boom configuration near the cage.[1] Every cage should have access to at least one outlet for oxygen, vacuum, and compressed air. Modules that are used for mechanical ventilation or continuous renal replacement therapy need access to a higher number of outlets or additional services.[1] Storage for a limited amount of consumables and record keeping facilities also may be necessary in high-end modules.

A wide range of cage types are currently used in veterinary ICUs. Kennels or runs and stacked cages have traditionally been used in many ICU settings. They may be useful for delivering intermediate care but seem inappropriate for high-end intensive care patients. Single cages with enough space around them, such as the "playpen" type, wall-mounted cages, free-standing cages, and oxygen cages, as well as variations on them, give better opportunity to organize and deliver elaborate care to patients (Figure 209-2).[5] When the patient is immobilized, either by anesthesia or neuromuscular disease, use of a table or "bed" increases access to the patient, which provides a more effective, ergonomic working environment (Figure 209-3).

Procedure area and storage

The procedure area is often situated in the patient area itself, with enough room for multiple staff and mobile equipment, such as a mechanical ventilator and a crash cart. It should offer all bedside facilities to allow continued monitoring and treatment of the patient, including light switches, electrical power outlets, and medical outlets. One or two procedure tables can be surrounded on one to three sides by countertops on which disposables and equipment can be arranged

Table 209-2 **Basic Intensive Care Unit Facility Configuration**

Area	Priority	Optional/Shared with Other Services
Staff work areas	Nursing station	
		Staff break room
		Conference/multipurpose room
		Changing room with lockers, shower, toilet
Patient areas	Procedure area	
	Patient modules	
	Equipment/ consumables storage	
	Waste disposal	
		Isolation ward
		Outside runs
Ancillary services	Laboratory facilities	
	Pharmacy	
		Receptionist office with record keeping
		Owner waiting area
		Owner visiting room
		Medical equipment storage
		Consumable supply storage
		Patient grooming room
		Patient food kitchen
		Linen room
		Soiled bedding/waste disposal storage
		Medical offices
		Clinician's overnight room
		Library

and prepared to allow minor medical interventions. Every table should have high-intensity lighting. A hands-free hand-washing and disinfection station should be part of or near to the procedure area. There should be sufficient storage for other equipment and disposable supplies in the procedure area and in the rest of the patient area. A refrigerator, freezer, and fluid incubator may be part of the setup. Provisions should be made for storage and rapid retrieval of one or more crash carts with emergency life-support equipment.

Isolation room

Isolation rooms are equipped with an anteroom for hand washing and protective gowning. The isolation room should be designed and equipped to function as an independent unit. Isolation rooms should have an internal communication system and remote patient monitoring capability with a connection to the nursing station. A dedicated ventilation system is necessary that has the capacity to produce negative or positive air pressure. Provision of a separate circuit for evacuation of contaminated material is recommended.

With the growing incidence of infection with hospital-acquired and multidrug-resistant bacterial strains there may be an increasing demand for infection wards or rooms.

Ancillary Services

All ICUs must have quick and convenient access to 24-hour clinical laboratory services. When these services cannot be provided by the central hospital, a satellite service within or immediately adjacent to the ICU must serve this function. If space is provided in the ICU, it should be adjacent to the patient area, preferably with direct visual contact. The laboratory bench should have sufficient space for centrifuges and laboratory (point-of-care testing) equipment allowing emergency analyses (e.g., packed cell volume, electrolyte levels, blood gas concentrations, glucose level, lactate level) and sufficient electrical and network connections to service this equipment. The laboratory area should have enough room to store administrative records, handbooks, and laboratory consumables. Refrigerators and freezers are necessary for storage of biologic specimens, disposables, and reagents.

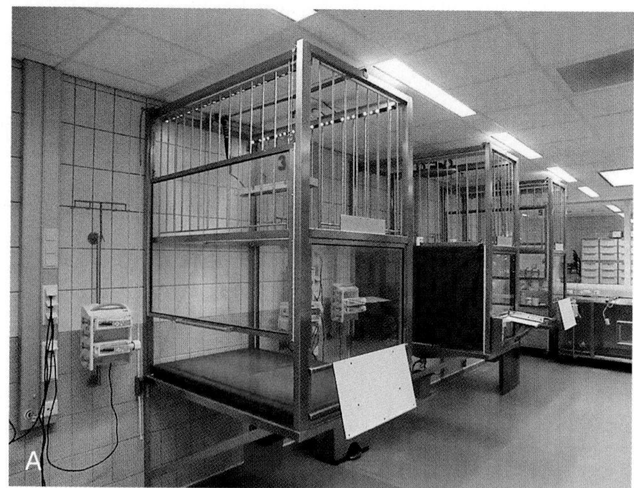

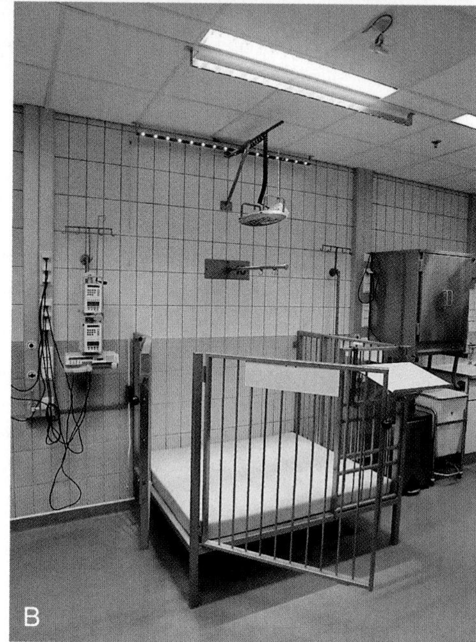

FIGURE 209-2 A, Wall-mounted cage with approach from both sides. When used for cats, direct viewing of dogs can be limited by putting a screen cover over the glass windowpane of the cage. To preserve adequate patient observation, indirect monitoring is maintained over a webcam system (see Figure 209-5). **B,** "Playpen" type of cage for larger dogs. Raising the bottom off the ground improves ergonomics and promotes infection control because the floor cannot be considered a "clean" environment.

The design of the unit must consider the pharmaceutical delivery process. Whether the ICU relies on the hospital pharmacy or a satellite pharmacy within or near the ICU, pharmacy services should be readily accessible, always available, and able to provide all medications needed. A dedicated ICU pharmacy has to abide by local regulations. It should contain temperature-regulated storage for medications

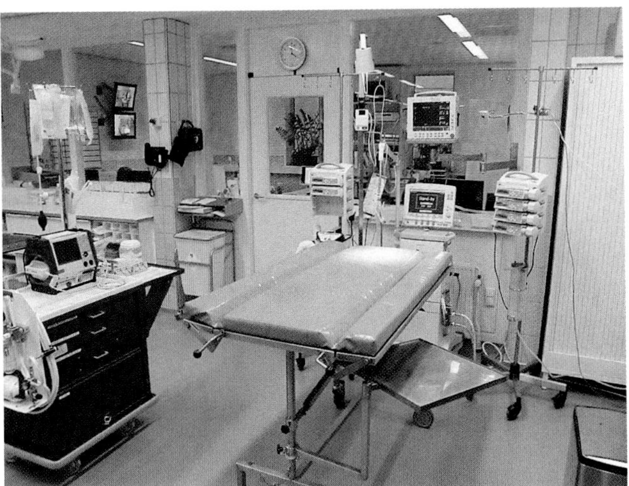

FIGURE 209-3 Mechanical ventilation station. The ventilator, monitoring equipment, airway suction device, and drip poles with infusion pumps are located at the head of the table. The table is a modified surgical table, the top of which is made broader to increase patient comfort. The table can also be tilted.

at room and cooled temperature, storage for intravenous fluids, and a lockable cabinet for controlled substances. Blood products should be stored in a dedicated refrigerator and freezer. A dedicated area to prepare medications is part of the pharmacy.

A special equipment storage room makes it possible to stow unused equipment and relieves the load in the patient area. Adequate grounded electrical outlets for charging and lockable storage for small but valuable items should be available.

The design must consider how supplies will be delivered from central supply processing and bulk stores. A feature of intensive care medicine is that a very large number and variety of specific items (disposables and recyclable equipment) are used in the unit with a high turnover. A three-stage storage system is desirable to reduce the burden of stocking too many supplies in the patient area: central hospital supply facility, clean utility and consumables storage room, and patient area. A limited amount of frequently used items should be stored in the patient area; the majority are stored in the consumables storage room.

Utility storage for soiled items is necessary for controlled and separate removal of waste, soiled bedding, and used recyclable equipment and is an important aspect of the IPC program. This and other support functions and rooms such as a library, patient food and staff kitchen, owner waiting area, patient grooming room, and staff showers, toilets, and lockers are often made available in the rest of the clinic.

UTILITIES

Medical gas (oxygen and compressed air), vacuum and gas evacuation, and electrical outlets should be distributed and arranged in a way to cause minimal interference with nursing care. Local recommendations and regulations often give sufficient guidance for correct technical installation of these services.[8] In human medicine, the choice of system(s) for mounting and organizing electrical, medical gas, and other medical utility outlets has a major impact on patient and staff satisfaction.[1]

Data access points or a wireless intranet may be installed to accommodate computer terminals and mobile computing solutions, such as tablets. Increasing use of technology, but also rapid changes in technology and styles of interfacing, pose formidable design challenges. The design must address workflow, patient confidentiality, future needs, staff preferences, interfaces with the main hospital digital information system, unit-based information technology needs, and other issues, including the fact that members of the care team may need access to data entry and electronic information simultaneously at the patient cage-side and in other areas.

Water supply and plumbing should follow local regulations. Sinks should be strategically placed to support the staff in executing IPC protocols. Each water basin in the ICU should have a dedicated function, either hand-washing and disinfection, disposal of (contaminated) organic liquid materials, or cleaning of equipment. Sinks should enable hands-free operation, and a waste disposal bin should be near. Evidence suggests that the provision of both soap and water and alcohol gel systems is required for maximum performance and hand hygiene adherence.[21]

If the design specifications include the requirement for bedside renal dialysis or continuous renal replacement therapy, appropriately conditioned water and drainage facilities must be provided, with the capacity to deliver deionized water if necessary.[1]

ENVIRONMENTAL ASPECTS

Lighting

Light can be brought into the ICU in the form of either natural or artificial light, and both are used in combination for ambient lighting. Both sources need to be supplied with shading devices and adjustable illumination controls to support observation and movement around the patient at night or whenever the patient requires rest without interruption of its sleep.

Artificial light also serves as independent lighting for specific tasks in limited spaces such as procedure and support areas and patient modules. This flexibility enables the use of brighter and more focused light when necessary. Furthermore, it offers the possibility of maintaining a natural circadian light rhythm in the patient area. Clinical procedures can be supported with specific spotlights with adjustable intensity, field size, and direction.

Air Conditioning

Facilitating the maintenance of good air quality through measures such as effective ventilation, filtration, and appropriate airflow direction and pressure (positive or negative) should be considered thoroughly. A thermoneutral temperature and normal relative humidity should be maintained. System capacity and room air change frequency should take into account the use of water for cleaning the facility.

Acoustic Environment

Of all the environmental factors, lighting conditions and noise have the most impact on people admitted to the hospital. Outside noise should be reduced to a minimum. All sound-producing equipment such as air conditioning systems, refrigerators, and communication systems should be screened for their noise-producing properties. All materials used in the environment (e.g., floors, walls, ceiling, furnishings) should be evaluated for their sound-absorptive properties. Installing high-performance sound-absorbing materials on environmental surfaces becomes even more important in small rooms such as the isolation ward.

Floor and Wall Surfaces, Ceiling Finishes

Easy-to-clean floor, wall, and ceiling coverings should be selected, and proper cleaning and disinfection procedures should be employed. Floor coverings should be seamless and durable, chemically inert, resistant to antiseptics, and sound absorbing. Walls and ceilings should be easy to clean and made of durable materials that are nonabsorbent with low sound transmission. Walls should be fitted with

Table 209-3 **Intensive Care Unit Design Measures for Prevention and Control of Infections**

Feature	Measure
Routing and doors	No through traffic Hands-free door opening
Rooms	Separation of utility rooms for clean and dirty items Isolation and infection room(s)
Ceiling	Easy to clean, including lighting fixtures Prohibits passage of particles from cavity above the ceiling plane
Walls	Easy to clean Smooth with no seams or cracks
Floors	Minimize growth of microorganisms Durable with no seams or cracks Extended a short distance up the wall and coved to form a smooth junction with the wall
Lighting	Proper illumination of support and procedure areas
Room ventilation	Separate systems for isolation/infection wards and storage rooms for dirty items High-pressure or low-pressure rooms Sufficient air exchange rates Effective air filters
Running water	Proper temperature and adequate pressure; stagnation and backflow minimized; dead-end pipes avoided
Patient modules	(Sufficient) separation with open area between cages, effective physical barriers
Hand hygiene	Dedicated and properly designed hand-washing basins, deep and wide enough to prevent splashing, with hands-free operation for taps (strategically positioned) Hand disinfection facilities with alcohol solutions (strategically positioned)
Surfaces of equipment, fixtures, and furnishings	Easy-to-clean surfaces Smooth with no seams or cracks Antimicrobial qualities (?)
Waste receptacles	Hands-free handling
Phones, computer keyboards, and so forth	Easy to clean and disinfect Antimicrobial qualities (?)
Functions	Separation of functions (e.g., purpose-dedicated refrigerators and freezers)

extra protection where there is contact with gurneys, carts, and equipment.

Furnishings

Built-in and freestanding furnishings such as cabinets and carts should be easily cleanable, should have the fewest possible seams, and should be free of fissures or open joints and crevices that retain or permit passage of dirt particles.[18] Furnishings need to be durably constructed to withstand impact with movable equipment without sustaining significant damage.[7]

DETAILS AND COMMON DESIGN ELEMENTS

Infection Prevention and Control

Poor compliance with hand-washing protocols (especially among medical staff) and shortages of nursing staff, together with high-density crowding of patients, promotes horizontal transmission of resistant strains of microorganisms.[22] Although the contribution of the environment to hospital-acquired infection may still be unresolved, few would disagree that hospital design is of paramount importance as a means of preventive medicine. The ICU cannot be rendered sterile, but every effort should be made to reduce the numbers of pathogens and the risk of spread.

The work involved in molding the design of a hospital to infection-control principles is arduous.[23] IPC in the ICU is all about keeping the (multidrug-resistant) bacteria out, preventing cross contamination and spread of microbes, implementing effective and efficient disinfection measures, and using antimicrobial medication appropriately. Numerous aspects of design can help to prevent the introduction and spread of microbes in the ICU (Table 209-3). Of course, design can be effective only in combination with implementation of proper workflows as described in protocols and other directives, appropriate staff behavior, and allowance of sufficient time for staff to comply with hygiene instructions.[15]

Generally speaking, infection transmission occurs via three routes: contact, air, and water. Contact is widely considered the principal or most frequent transmission route. In reality, these three routes may intertwine with each other in the spread of nosocomial infections.[3] Environmental routes of contact-spread infections include direct individual to individual (person or animal) contact and indirect transmission via environmental surfaces.[3]

Because the hands and lower arms of staff play a major role in the spread of microbes, the strategic placement and proper design of hand-washing basins and the strategic positioning of alcohol dispensers is paramount (Figure 209-4).[3,18,25,26] Alcohol-based hand rub dispensers should be installed at the cage-side and in other accessible locations to increase compliance with hand disinfection protocols and reduce contact transmission of infection.

But design measures should also support a reduction in recontamination of clean hands. There is a paucity of scientific evidence

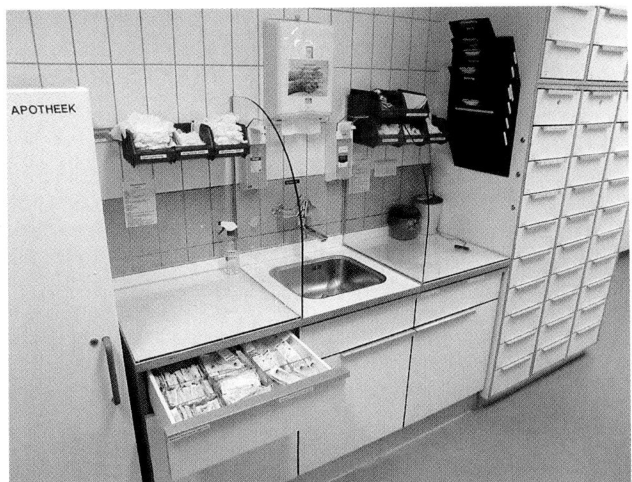

FIGURE 209-4 Hand-washing station. Although proximity of hand-washing stations is essential to support staff compliance, placement too close to procedure areas can be detrimental. Errors in sink placement and design can allow infectious particles from the sink drain to splash onto adjacent areas where sterile disposables and medications are prepared. A cost-effective and minimally invasive solution was found in this example of a hand-washing station in the author's ICU pharmacy by placing glass screens between the sink and preparation area. A recent publication highlighted the issue of flawed positioning and design when a hospital reported an outbreak of infections with a multidrug-resistant organism in the intensive care unit.[24]

identifying which surfaces and furnishings in an ICU are effective in preventing cross transmission and reducing hospital-acquired infection. Current guidelines rely on fundamental principles, such as the epidemiology of infectious diseases, to determine what interventions are most likely to be effective in preventing actual infection.[18] The need to touch surfaces that can easily cause cross contamination such as handles and covers of waste disposal bins should be avoided through the use of automated openers or foot pedals. Items with intensely used surfaces with which contact is unavoidable, such as phones, keyboards, countertops, and carts, should be easy to maintain and clean, and should have a smooth surface without any cracks, seams, or open joints that can retain or permit the passage of dirt. Currently, evidence is lacking regarding the efficacy of applying antimicrobials to, or incorporate them into or onto, the inanimate surfaces of patient care equipment, fixtures, and furnishings, including textiles.[18]

Larger surfaces like walls and ceilings also should be addressed. Floors should be scrubbed regularly but should never be considered "clean": the need to avoid any contact with the floor and isolate the floor should direct the behavior and attitude toward activities, if any, on the floor.

There is a lot of emphasis in human medicine on greater physical separation, isolation, and space per patient, which has currently led to the introduction of single-patient rooms.[3,23,27] That infections increase when the distance between beds is reduced is well recognized in human medicine and has an impact on the positioning of beds.[14] This emphasizes the need for veterinary medicine to use more space and more physical barriers between patients to control infections. If this is not feasible for all cages, then additional space and physical boundaries should at least be considered for the patient modules intended for the high-end patient population, like the mechanical ventilation station or continuous renal replacement therapy module. The provision of a physically separate intermediate care facility can reduce the patient load and allow for more distance between patient cages in the ICU.

Safety and Security

Medical errors are generally triggered by a combination of active failures and latent conditions. Environmental factors that can lead to medical errors include insufficient lighting, noise, lack of space, and other design failures.[3]

Depending on the situation, door and cabinet locks may be necessary to protect staff, patients, and equipment. The ICU design should offer at least two separate exit routes in case of an emergency and an adjoining safe space to which to relocate the patients (e.g., emergency service, recovery room). Emergencies can result from fire, failure of equipment, and biochemical and chemical hazards. The implementation of safety regulations such as the installation of sprinkler systems should be anticipated and introduced early in the design process in consultation with local safety hazard officials.

The basic principles of fire safety are avoidance of fire, limitation of fire, safeguard of life, and reduction of material damage. The hospital should incorporate compartmentalization and local fire control principles into the design. Fire-resistant materials should be applied where necessary.

A set of emergency lights and about 50% of the electrical outlets in the patient area should be identifiable and connected to the facility emergency power system. Control switches (to regulate electrical and gas supply), shut-off valves, and monitoring devices (to monitor pressure in gas pipes) must be located adjacent to the unit where they can be easily operated by the staff in emergency situations.

Patient- and Owner-Centered Care

Human ICU design in the past decade has been driven primarily by a focus on IPC and patient- and family-centered care. In a highly stressful environment like the ICU, the special needs of individual patients, especially cats, deserve more attention.[28] This patient- and owner-centered care will also be driven by higher demands imposed by owners in an ever more competitive veterinary market. Owners are more and more aware of their pets' medical status and feel a need for transparency regarding medical results. The communication among owners and staff is important because it can provide social support to owners, facilitate the owners' involvement in patient care, and also increase owner satisfaction with care. Visiting opportunities may be restricted with limited staffing and space. As a means of addressing the wish of owners to be more involved and to stay connected to their pets while the animals are hospitalized, the author's institution has adopted a system of video streaming of patient images over the Internet that has been applied in neonatal ICUs in the Netherlands to allow parents to see their newborns.[29] The virtual pet visit system (VPVS), called *TelePet,* enables owners to access a website via a password-protected log-in and view the video images produced by a webcam attached to the pet's cage (Figure 209-5). Owner access is maintained and controlled by the staff at all times. The VPVS is not intended to be a replacement of communication but an addition to the owner support measures taken by the staff.

Ambiance

A growing body of literature indicates that management of and climate in the ICU can influence the well-being of health care workers and might even have an impact on patient outcomes.[9] The finding that environmental factors such as distracting nature stimuli and daylight exposure can enhance pain control in human patients indicates the importance of the atmosphere in the ICU.[30]

Hospital design that minimizes environmental stressors (noise) and fosters exposure to stress-reducing or restorative features (nature and art) can help to improve outcomes.[3] Also in veterinary medicine there is an increasing awareness that the ICU is a very hostile

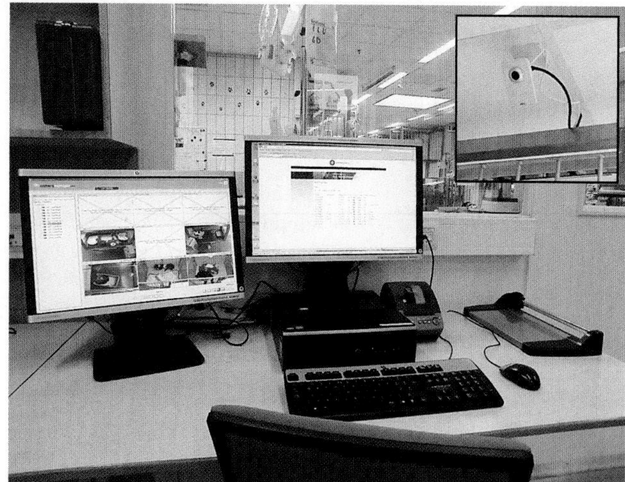

FIGURE 209-5 *TelePet* system used to improve owner satisfaction and involvement. The computer console is used by the staff to control access and set user-specific access codes for the owners. The cameras also offer the staff an alternative view of the patients. *Inset,* Webcam as installed on all cages in the intensive care unit. Mobile webcams are also available; for example, for use at the mechanical ventilation station (see Figure 209-3).

environment, especially for cats.[28] Adjustments can be undertaken such as making the cage a more comfortable patient environment. This is a challenge because many patient-friendly measures decrease the view of the patient (see Figure 209-2, *A*), could interfere with measures for IPC, and may limit the intensity of the care.

Diminished circadian rhythms and sleep deprivation while patients are hospitalized may hinder the healing process and contribute to increased morbidity and mortality in human medicine.[31] The possibility of maintaining a circadian rhythm should be incorporated into the lighting design of the patient area.

Furthermore, some studies have documented the importance of light in modulating circadian rhythms and thereby improving the adjustment to night-shift work among staff.[1]

Communication

Communication among staff is supported by structured patient and multidisciplinary rounds, patient records, protocols, other written directives, and bulletin boards. In the design, patient and staff bulletin boards can be strategically positioned in the ICU to better allow quick and short current communications.

As information technology and medical informatics become more available and both hardware (tablets) and software computer-based order entry systems become more affordable, these emerging technologies could promise a better integration of patient information to caregivers.

REFERENCES

1. Thompson DR, Hamilton DK, Cadenhead CD, et al: Guidelines for intensive care unit design, Crit Care Med 40(5):1586, 2012.
2. Leaf DE, Homel P, Factor PH: Relationship between ICU design and mortality, Chest 137(5):1022, 2010.
3. Ulrich RS, Zimring C, Zhu X, et al: A review of the research literature on evidence-based healthcare design, HERD 1(3):61, 2008.
4. Hardy J: Design and organization of an equine intensive care unit, Vet Clin North Am Equine Pract 20(1):1, 2004.
5. Robben JH, Eveland-Baker JA: ICU design. In Burkitt Creedon JM, Davis H, editors: Advanced monitoring and procedures for small animal emergency and critical care, Chichester, UK, 2012, John Wiley & Sons.
6. Veterinary Emergency and Critical Care Society: Recommendations for veterinary emergency and critical care facilities. Updated August 2013. Available at http://www.veccs.org/index.php?option=com_content&view=article&id=75:recommendations-for-veterinary-emergency-and-critical-care-facilities&catid=38:about-veccs&Itemid=273. Accessed January 17, 2014.
7. Consensus Committee on Recommended Design Standards for Advanced Neonatal Care: Recommended standards for newborn ICU design. In White RD, editor: Report of the eighth consensus conference on newborn ICU design, Clearwater Beach, 2012. Available at http://www.nd.edu/~nicudes/index.html. Accessed January 17, 2014.
8. Facility Guidelines Institute: Guidelines for design and construction of health care facilities, Chicago, 2010, American Society for Healthcare Engineering of the American Hospital Association. Read-only version available at http://www.fgiguidelines.org/guidelines2010.php. Accessed January 17, 2014.
9. Valentin A, Ferdinande P; ESICM Working Group on Quality Improvement: Recommendations on basic requirements for intensive care units: structural and organizational aspects, Intensive Care Med 37(10):1575, 2011.
10. Rashid M: Technology and the future of intensive care unit design, Crit Care Nurs Q 34(4):332, 2011.
11. Gajic O, Afessa B: Physician staffing models and patient safety in the ICU, Chest 135(4):1038, 2009.
12. Guidelines/Practice Parameters Committee of the American College of Critical Care Medicine, Society of Critical Care Medicine: Guidelines for intensive care unit design, Crit Care Med 23(3):582, 1995.
13. White RD: Recommended standards for the newborn ICU, J Perinatol 27(Suppl 2):S4-S19, 2007.
14. Wilson AP, Ridgway GL: Reducing hospital-acquired infection by design: the new University College London hospital, J Hosp Infect 62(3):264, 2006.
15. Anderson J, Gosbee LL, Bessesen M, et al: Using human factors engineering to improve the effectiveness of infection prevention and control, Crit Care Med 38(Suppl 8):S269, 2010.
16. Bennett S: Design, organization and staffing of the intensive care unit, Surgery 30(5):214, 2012.
17. Rashid M: A decade of adult intensive care unit design: a study of the physical design features of the best-practice examples, Crit Care Nurs Q 29(4):282, 2006.
18. Bartley J, Streifel AJ: Design of the environment of care for safety of patients and personnel: does form follow function or vice versa in the intensive care unit? Crit Care Med 38(Suppl 8):S388, 2010.
19. Brown KK, Gallant D: Impacting patient outcomes through design: acuity adaptable care/universal room design, Crit Care Nurs Q 29(4):326, 2006.
20. Costa AX, Ridley SA, Shahani AK, et al: Mathematical modelling and simulation for planning critical care capacity, Anaesthesia 58(4):320, 2003.
21. Provincial Infectious Diseases Advisory Committee: Best practices for hand hygiene in all health care settings, version 2, Ontario, 2010, Ministry of Health and Long-Term Care. Available at http://www.publichealthontario.ca/en/eRepository/2010-12%20BP%20Hand%20Hygiene.pdf. Currently under review. Accessed January 17, 2014.
22. O'Connell NH, Humphreys H: Intensive care unit design and environmental factors in the acquisition of infection, J Hosp Infect 45(4):255, 2000.
23. Levin PD, Golovanevski M, Moses AE, et al: Improved ICU design reduces acquisition of antibiotic-resistant bacteria: a quasi-experimental observational study, Crit Care 15(5):R211, 2011.
24. Hota S, Hirji Z, Stockton K, et al: Outbreak of multidrug-resistant *Pseudomonas aeruginosa* colonization and infection secondary to imperfect intensive care unit room design, Infect Control Hosp Epidemiol 30(1):25, 2009.
25. Boyce JM, Pittet D; Healthcare Infection Control Practices Advisory Committee, HICPAC/SHEA/APIC/IDSA Hand Hygiene Task Force: Guideline for hand hygiene in health-care settings. Recommendations of the Healthcare Infection Control Practices Advisory Committee and the HICPAC/SHEA/APIC/IDSA Hand Hygiene Task Force. Society for Healthcare Epidemiology of America/Association for Professionals in Infection Control/Infectious Diseases Society of America, MMWR Recomm Rep 51(RR-16):1-45, 2002; quiz CE1-4.

26. Tschudin-Sutter S, Pargger H, Widmer AF: Hand hygiene in the intensive care unit, Crit Care Med 38(Suppl 8):S299, 2010.
27. Walsh WF, McCullough KL, White RD: Room for improvement: nurses' perceptions of providing care in a single room newborn intensive care setting, Adv Neonatal Care 6(5):261, 2006.
28. Carney HC, Little S, Brownlee-Tomasso D, et al: AAFP and ISFM feline-friendly nursing care guidelines, J Feline Med Surg 14(5):337, 2012.
29. Spanjers R, Feuth S: Telebaby videostreaming of newborns over internet, Stud Health Technol Inform 90:195, 2002.
30. Malenbaum S, Keefe FJ, Williams AC, et al: Pain in its environmental context: implications for designing environments to enhance pain control, Pain 134(3):241, 2008.
31. Parthasarathy S, Tobin MJ: Sleep in the intensive care unit, Intensive Care Med 30(2):197, 2004.

CHAPTER 210
MANAGEMENT OF THE INTENSIVE CARE UNIT*

Emily Savino, CVT, VTS (ECC) • Lesley G. King, MVB, DACVECC, DACVIM (Internal Medicine)

KEY POINTS

- In the intensive care unit (ICU), a long-term focus (days, possibly weeks) on individual patients blends the immediate need to stabilize and support body systems with the requirement to establish a concrete diagnosis and anticipate and head off predictable complications.
- A cohesive, highly trained, organized, and skilled staff is the foundation for success.
- Specialty certification is available for both clinicians and nurses in the field of emergency and critical care (ECC). An ICU that is staffed with veterinarians who are diplomates of the ACVECC should be expected to function at a state-of-the-art level. To obtain veterinary technician specialty (VTS) certification in ECC, the nurse/technician must have a minimum of 3 years of full-time work experience in ECC medicine, meet rigorous credentialing requirements, and pass the AVECCT examination. Obtaining VTS certification is viewed as demonstrating expertise within a specific field of veterinary medicine.
- The nursing staff must implement most aspects of patient care and should be encouraged to demonstrate initiative and logical, critical thought processes. The specialized skills required to be a successful ICU nurse require additional training, even for those with years of clinical experience in other areas of the hospital. The ideal ratio of technician/nurse to patients is based on several factors, including the seriousness of the patient's condition, the intensity of care required by the patient, and the experience level of the nursing staff.
- The critical care unit is a highly stressful environment where people who come from different backgrounds; possess different goals, values, and expectations; and have different communication styles come together to care for critically ill patients. In this setting, conflict of some sort is inevitable. The more stressful the environment, the more likely that burnout will occur, and the higher the staff turnover rate. Dialogue between staff members and management should be encouraged and various formats can be used, including staff or shift meetings, emails, newsletters, message boards, or communication logs.

*Portions of this chapter were modified with permission from King LG, Carter L: Staffing the intensive care unit. In Wingfield WE, Raffe MR, editors: The veterinary ICU book, ed 1, Jackson, Wyo, 2002, Teton NewMedia, p 1168. The authors would like to acknowledge the contribution of Leslie Carter, MS, RVT, VTS (Emergency and Critical Care), to the original chapter.

Veterinary critical care units provide continual monitoring and specialized care to the highest-risk, most critically ill patient population. The availability of an experienced, well-staffed, well-equipped intensive care unit (ICU) is vital to achieve the most successful patient outcomes.[1] The small animal ICU and its staff should do the following:

- Focus on the sickest patients, predominantly high-risk medical and surgical patients
- Operate 24 hours a day, 7 days a week
- Be equipped to provide state-of-the-art monitoring and therapy
- Be prepared to accept referrals of critically ill patients and new patient admissions at any time, and be prepared for all possible needs of patients in the unit in case of an immediate crisis.

In the ICU, a long-term focus (days, possibly weeks) on individual patients blends the immediate need to stabilize and support body systems with the requirement to establish a concrete diagnosis and anticipate and head off predictable complications.

INTENSIVE CARE UNIT PERSONNEL: STAFF QUALIFICATIONS AND SCHEDULING

An ICU is more than just critically ill patients, advanced monitoring equipment, and a physical location within a hospital—the key component of the ICU is its staff. A cohesive, highly trained, organized, and skilled staff is the foundation for success. When an ICU is being organized, staffing considerations should include scheduling, staff/patient ratios, conflict resolution, and recruitment, training, and retention of staff.

The staff of the ICU consists of a team of physicians and nurses working together side by side. Every ICU team must have a leader who acts as a "point person" for decision making, determination of standards for policy and procedures, and communication both within and outside the unit. In this capacity, the ICU director may be either a veterinarian or a technician. Typically, however, a veterinarian and a technician must work together in a *cohesive partnership* to lead their respective teams for optimal functioning.

Role of the Intensive Care Unit Director

The ICU director is responsible for many key tasks related to the efficient operation of the unit. The following are several of the fundamental responsibilities of the ICU director[2]:

- Administer, direct, and coordinate patient care within the unit and via collaboration with other specialists throughout the hospital
- Evaluate the quality of patient care, review adverse events, develop and enforce plans to avoid medical errors
- Develop and implement policies and procedures within the ICU and throughout the hospital
- Manage personnel: handle scheduling, conduct performance review, manage conflict, assist in career development, advocate for staff, maintain employee morale
- Provide, organize, and facilitate training and education of staff and encourage personal and career development of staff
- Act as a liaison for communication between the ICU staff and patients and their families; clinical staff throughout the hospital; and the hospital administration.
- Perform budgeting: manage costs by reviewing revenue and expenses and implementing policies as needed
- Provide creative thinking: think outside the box, look for innovative solutions to problems

Staffing

Due to the dynamic nature of critical illness and the need for continuous monitoring of affected patients, the ICU should be staffed with qualified personnel on a 24/7 basis. Specialty certification is available for both clinicians and nurses in the field of emergency and critical care (ECC). Achieving specialty certification requires a great deal of commitment and a lot of work but is valuable not only for personal satisfaction but also for quality of patient care and advancement of the field of ECC. Staff may therefore include a combination of board-certified criticalists, non–board-certified veterinarians, ECC residents, interns, veterinary students, nurses, nursing aides, and volunteers.

Veterinarians

The American College of Veterinary Emergency and Critical Care (ACVECC) is a specialty organization that promotes advancement of and high standards of practice for veterinarians involved in veterinary ECC.[3] The organization also establishes requirements for advanced training in the field, monitors residency training programs, and examines and certifies veterinarians as specialists. In addition, the ACVECC exists to encourage research and to promote communication and dissemination of knowledge relating to ECC.

Although individuals can of course practice intensive care medicine without board certification, and many do it well, there is no guarantee as to the quality of training that uncertified individuals have received. In contrast, veterinarians who are board certified by the ACVECC have passed a rigorous training and testing process which ensures that their knowledge base and level of practice reach the highest standards. An ICU that is staffed with diplomates of the ACVECC should be expected to function at a state-of-the-art level.

The need for veterinarians to be physically present in the ICU 24 hours a day varies with the type and number of cases, and the skill and experience of the technical staff. In general, if the veterinarians' shifts do not extend through the full 24-hour period, then a veterinarian must be available at all times to answer questions and respond immediately to changes in the clinical status of patients. Although many questions can be answered over the telephone, it is often necessary for the veterinarian to return to the ICU at once if a change in the patient's condition mandates a physician's attention.

Residents and interns

There is a significant temptation to solve staffing problems by using residents and interns as a means to cover hours. The advantages of this approach are that residents' salaries are often relatively inexpensive compared with those of board-certified specialists, and there is usually a large pool of excellent candidates applying for entry into residency programs. The presence of one or more residents can stimulate discussion, growth, and ongoing learning within a group. Individuals graduating from a residency program can provide a pool from which to hire qualified ICU staff in the future.

Although this solution to the staffing problem seems attractive, there are also some drawbacks. Most importantly, a position in the residency training program is definitively a training position, and a resident requires significant teaching time from the supervising clinician before becoming a staffing asset. The requirements for a residency in the ACVECC program are quite rigidly structured, including significant overlap of clinical duty with the supervising clinician, daily rounds, and weekly didactic sessions.[3] These requirements limit the usefulness of residents for covering hours and can add to the workload of the supervising diplomates.

Thus residents should be used as a means of staffing only if the supervising clinicians are willing to devote a considerable amount of time to teaching and to discussion of cases and the literature.

Nursing staff

It is impossible to overemphasize the importance of a well-trained nursing staff for the smooth running of the unit. The nursing staff must implement most aspects of patient care and should be encouraged to demonstrate initiative and logical, critical thought processes. Effective and timely communication between clinicians and nurses is therefore a vital component of patient care in the ICU. Every effort must be made to include nurses in the decision-making process and to communicate the rationale behind treatment decisions.

The Academy of Veterinary Emergency and Critical Care Technicians (AVECCT) was formed in the mid-1990s and was the first veterinary technician specialty organization to be recognized by the National Association of Veterinary Technicians in America (formerly the North American Veterinary Technicians Association). AVECCT promotes professionalism and excellence in veterinary ECC nursing and is a mechanism for validating the knowledge and skills required for the competent practice of veterinary ECC nursing.[4] To obtain veterinary technician specialty (VTS) certification in ECC, the applicant must have a minimum of 3 years of full-time work experience in ECC medicine, meet rigorous credentialing requirements, and pass the AVECCT examination. Obtaining VTS certification is viewed as demonstrating expertise within a specific field of veterinary medicine.

Because ICU patients are the sickest, the most heavily instrumented, the most dynamic, and at the highest risk of complications or death, it is axiomatic that the ICU must be staffed 24 hours a day with nurses and technicians. These are not patients that can be left unattended overnight. The use of underqualified personnel to fulfill this role—for example, overnight staffing with unsupervised veterinary students—is likely to provide highly variable levels of care and increase the potential for errors. Underqualified staff may provide support during overnight, weekend, and holiday hours. However, if high-quality, state-of-the-art patient care is the expected standard, then these personnel must be supervised by experienced, permanent ICU technical staff on a 24-hour basis.

Scheduling

The number of staff members required to provide patient care depends on the experience level of the staff, the number of patients, the severity of the patient illnesses, and the complexity of patient treatments. An additional scheduling consideration is anticipated variations in caseload. For example, more staffing may be required during the weekday daytime shifts when the caseload is likely to be highest due to increased numbers of hospitalized patients, postoperative patients, and emergency cases.

A minimum of two individuals should be scheduled per shift to ensure that an adequate number of people are available to perform tasks such as placing intravenous catheters or performing cardiopulmonary resuscitation. This staffing model also permits one individual to leave the room (to walk a patient, to take a break) while the second individual remains in the ICU to monitor the patients in the room. Ideally, nurses should be scheduled with some overlap between shifts to communicate patient rounds information, provide additional assistance with patient treatments, and help with organizing the room and restocking supplies between shifts.

When an ICU is staffed, it must be remembered that 1 week represents $7 \times 24 = 168$ hours. Staffing a unit around the clock with just one nurse or one physician at a time, each working 40 hours a week, requires budgeting at least four individuals (160 hours). Ideally, considering vacations and sick days, 4.5 or 5 nurses, working with 4.5 or 5 physicians, are needed to provide one-deep coverage around the clock. Because it is very difficult to fill positions with qualified individuals given current tight budgets and insufficient staff availability, many ICUs have no choice but to compromise staffing numbers at the expense of staff stress and fatigue and a high turnover rate.

Staff/Patient Ratio

The ideal ratio of technician/nurse to patients is based on several factors, including the seriousness of the patient's condition, the intensity of care required by the patient, and the experience level of the nursing staff.[2,3]

In the critical care setting, a very low nurse/patient ratio is required to provide the highest level of patient care. For critical cases such as patients undergoing mechanical ventilation or those that are hemodynamically unstable, a nurse/patient ratio of 1:1 may be needed. In these situations, one nurse should be dedicated to monitoring and treating the patient on a continuous basis in case the patient's status changes quickly and immediate intervention is required. One critically ill patient in very unstable condition may even require the full attention of several staff members, needing care from multiple clinicians and at least one senior nurse simultaneously.

More stable cases may require an average nurse/patient ratio of 1:3. However, patients in more stable condition can sometimes be just as demanding of personnel, although less experienced staff members may be required to care for them. For example, a patient with frequent bouts of diarrhea may require multiple baths, cage cleanings, bedding changes, and catheter rewraps. Even patients in seemingly stable condition can experience a quick change in status, deteriorate, and consequently require more intensive nursing care.

Thus it can be difficult to anticipate ICU staffing needs in advance. Maintaining a well-trained pool of part-time staff that can be called as needed would be an ideal goal to avoid the expenditure of overtime budgets. Currently, a reasonable average ratio of nursing staff to patients in the state-of-the-art small animal ICU is about 1:2 or 1:3, depending on the level of care being provided. This ratio will certainly continue to move more toward 1:1 as the intensity of monitoring and therapeutic protocols continues to increase.

The number of clinicians required per shift varies depending on the patient load and the experience level of the clinicians. Many of the same considerations that apply to the nursing staff apply to physicians: one critically ill patient can consume one clinician to the exclusion of all else. Therefore an ideal goal would be to try to staff the ICU with a minimum of two physicians per shift, at least during the day, to make sure that all of the patients are adequately cared for, even if one patient is demanding the full attention of one physician.

MANAGEMENT OF INTENSIVE CARE UNIT STAFF

Communication

Frequent communication with staff is essential and various formats can be used, including staff or shift meetings, emails, newsletters, message boards, or communication logs. Effective communication between personnel on different shifts is imperative to keep the team unified and focused on common goals. Other equally important aspects of communication include relaying a consistent message and following up with staff and administration regarding past issues. Staff members value managers who respect individual differences and diversity and create an encouraging environment.

It is important for managers to communicate in such a manner that it is not just a one-way conversation. Dialogue between staff members and management should be encouraged. In particular, an open forum must be available for discussion of problem patients or situations and to help resolve misperceptions regarding patient care decisions.

Delegation of Responsibility

It is clear from the list of operational responsibilities for the ICU director that it is unrealistic to expect one person to successfully complete every task. Most successful managers opt to delegate tasks to team members, selecting carefully the tasks they wish to delegate and those they will retain as their own.

Delegation helps to distribute the workload, motivates individuals and the team, creates self-confidence in team members because they have been chosen to carry out an important responsibility, and helps employees feel involved and empowered. It is important that delegation of responsibilities does not leave an employee feeling that he or she has just been given more work with little reward. The employee should be aware that the additional responsibilities also reflect more trust and increased authority and autonomy.

Conflict: Causes, Categories, and Resolution

The critical care unit is a highly stressful environment where people who come from different backgrounds; possess different goals, values, and expectations; and have different communication styles come together to care for critically ill patients. In this setting, conflict of some sort is inevitable. Conflict can play a positive role in the critical care unit by generating new ideas, energizing staff, strengthening relationships, and driving change and evolution. However, unresolved conflicts can decrease efficiency, increase stress, and negatively affect staff morale.

Categories of conflict

Most conflicts fall into one of four distinct categories[2]:

1. **Task/organization:** This type of conflict is caused by a lack or insufficiency of something, such as—lack of inventory, lack of revenue, lack of staff, lack of leadership, and so on. For example, if the unit is short-staffed on a regular basis, the team cannot provide the appropriate level of patient care.
2. **Social/emotional:** These are conflicts that result from interactions between individuals.
3. **Identity/vision:** This type of conflict involves differences of opinion regarding two choices that are mutually exclusive; for

example, end-of-life decisions that involve choosing euthanasia rather than continuing treatment.

4. **Interests/goals/achievements:** Conflicts in this area occur when individuals cannot reach their personal goals, such as obtaining additional training or receiving a salary increase or promotion.

Methods of conflict resolution

Once a conflict has been identified, it is best to work toward resolving the conflict promptly before it escalates and impacts the unit negatively. There are numerous recognized methods of conflict resolution:

1. **Collaboration** does not favor one side over another but instead requires the cooperation of all parties involved to work as a team to reach a creative solution.
2. **Compromise** requires that both sides sacrifice something and both sides get something in return. This approach is often called *meeting halfway.*
3. **Competition** as a means of conflict resolution frequently pits one side against another and ends with a clear winner and a clear loser. This method often produces a very swift conclusion and can result in negative feelings on the side that does not achieve its desired outcome. An example is a decision that is reached based on a popular vote; for instance, staff members vote that the lunch break should be 1 hour rather than the usual 30 minutes.
4. **Accommodation** involves one side's conceding its position and the other side having things its way.

Conflict prevention

Poor communication is a leading cause of conflict in the workplace. Inadequate communication within the critical care team, between the director and the team, and between the director and the administration is problematic.

Skills of effective communicators include the following:

- Assertive communication in which the speaker clearly expresses his or her point in a concise manner but also allows the listener's opinions to be heard.
- Active listening, which involves listening without interrupting and giving the speaker undivided attention. The listener also notes the speaker's nonverbal cues, including hand gestures and facial expressions.
- The use of "I" statements rather than "you" statements, which can be perceived as offensive and blaming.

Recruitment of Intensive Care Unit Nursing Staff

It is challenging to find the ideal nursing staff to work in a critical care unit. Vacancies can be advertised in numerous outlets, including American Veterinary Medical Association–accredited veterinary technician programs, professional veterinary organization websites, relevant listservers, veterinary journals, veterinary conferences, and practice websites. Employers should identify the characteristics that they are seeking in a new employee (e.g., strong medical knowledge base and understanding of disease processes, team approach to patient care, strong communication skills, excellent attention to detail, technical proficiency, good time management skills, and ability to stay calm and focused in a stressful environment).

Hiring officers should recognize that prospective ICU candidates consider many factors when weighing employment options. These may include the facility's reputation, shift requirements, experience requirements, degree of employee turnover, salary, benefits and additional compensation packages, training (paid vs. unpaid, structured vs. unstructured), employer expectations (autonomy of the position, opportunities for career development and advancement), and working conditions (number of staff members per shift, average caseload, employee relationship with management).

Training intensive care unit nurses

The specialized skills required to be a successful ICU nurse require additional training, even for those with years of clinical experience in other areas of the hospital. The training period varies based on each trainee's level of prior clinical experience, self-motivation, and individual learning curve. Senior ICU nurses have advanced technical skills, familiarity with complex monitoring equipment, a good understanding of pathophysiology, and excellent critical thinking abilities. An experienced critical care nurse must competently triage the patients in the room, prioritize patients, and collaborate with the other staff members to assist with delegation of responsibilities to ensure optimal operation of the unit. Knowledgeable ICU nurses have the ability to recognize subtle but significant changes in their patients' status, effectively communicate their concerns to clinicians, and quickly intervene on their patients' behalf.

Nurses who have had limited prior critical care experience benefit from an extensive orientation and training period. Throughout this training period, it is helpful to pair the junior nurse with a senior nurse who is willing to act as a mentor. The mentor's role during training is to provide guidance as the trainee becomes comfortable with the degree of instrumentation and intensity of care required by most critically ill patients. The mentor should provide constructive feedback and help the junior nurse become more at ease in her or his role. During training, the new nurse gains hands-on experience and becomes familiar with the concept of critical thinking. Critical thinking is a difficult skill to develop; most novice nurses have a tendency toward mastering tasks and completing patient treatments rather than thinking critically about cases. It may be necessary to schedule additional experienced nursing staff to ensure that that efficiency of the ICU and the level of patient care are maintained while new staff members are being trained.

During the training period and throughout the nurse's career, it is important to provide feedback on performance at regularly scheduled intervals.. A formal performance review should take place annually.

Retention of Staff: Handling Stress and Burnout

The ICU is frequently an intense, emotionally charged environment. The staff often take their work home with them and experience intense "highs" when they save a patient, balanced by "lows" when all of their best efforts are unsuccessful. Owners are also highly stressed and often distressed or aggressive because they are under intense strain, and this further adds to the difficulties of working with critically ill patients. The more stressful the environment, the more likely that burnout will occur, and the higher the staff turnover rate.

The ongoing demands of critically ill patients around the clock create a high stress level for clinicians in ICUs that are not staffed with qualified physicians 24 hours a day. If qualified staff are not present during overnight hours, ICU clinicians may have a long workday followed by a night of interrupted sleep troubleshooting changes in a patient's condition. Although many ICU clinicians are "adrenaline junkies," this lifestyle inevitably results in burnout. In addition, the absence of a physician in the ICU overnight can add to the stress of overnight nurses, and they may feel guilty if circumstances require frequent calls to the physician during the night.

Staff burnout can lead to decreased employee morale, reduced productivity, and high staff turnover—all of which ultimately have a negative impact on patient care.

There are numerous measures an employer can take to increase employee job satisfaction, reduce burnout, and retain experienced staff:

- **Strive for good working relations.** Foster a collaborative approach to patient care. Include nurses in the decision-making process and offer an explanation for the decisions made.
- **Support the employee's relationship with his or her immediate supervisor.** Ensure that the supervisor is ready available and approachable.
- **Monitor workload.** Ensure that there are enough qualified staff members to provide adequate care to all patients in the ICU. The staff are likely to experience considerable stress if they are too busy to do their best for each animal. Clearly, the unit cannot always be staffed to cope with occasional exceptionally busy times, but efforts should be made to ensure that the unit is adequately staffed to deal with the typical number of patients. The addition of minimally qualified personnel or volunteers, who can keep on top of tasks such as cleaning and stocking, can help to protect the time of the qualified nursing staff. Using on-call or short-notice staff during exceptionally busy times or when regular staff are absent may also ameliorate stress.
- **Include incentives that encourage work-life balance, such as paid time off and flexible schedules.** Flexible scheduling may include allowing employees to work four 10-hour shifts or three 12-hour shifts per week to spend more days per week away from the workplace. It is important to ensure that qualified patient care providers are available to take over when staff members leave. Knowing that the animals are in trusted hands allows staff to leave their patient concerns at work, rather than taking them home.
- **Support staff development and lifelong learning.** Provide a continuing education allowance for employees. Promote career development by encouraging nursing staff to mentor junior staff members, publish, lecture, and obtain specialty certification. Continuing education is of particular importance for the nursing staff to ensure that stress is not resulting from a lack of knowledge about disease processes, protocols, or equipment, or a lack of understanding of management strategies. For example, management of a mechanically ventilated patient can be a very stressful prospect for a nurse who is not comfortable making decisions about ventilator settings, but very satisfying for a well-trained nurse who is comfortable with and challenged by this type of patient. Attending high-quality continuing education sessions also promotes networking with colleagues in the same field who are facing the same challenges.
- **Provide competitive pay and benefits.**

REFERENCES

1. Shortell SM, Zimmerman JE, Rousseau DM, et al: The performance of intensive care units: does good management make a difference? Med Care 32:508-525, 1994.
2. Strack van Schijndel R, Burchardi H: Bench-to-bedside review: leadership and conflict management in the intensive care unit, Critical Care 11:234, 2007.
3. King LG, Carter L: Staffing the intensive care unit. In Wingfield WE, Raffe MR, editors: The veterinary ICU book, ed 1, Jackson, Wyo, 2002, Teton NewMedia, p 1168.
4. Academy of Veterinary Emergency and Critical Care Technicians constitution and bylaws. Available at http://AVECCT.org. http://avecct.org/pdf/constitution.pdf

CHAPTER 211

CLIENT COMMUNICATION AND GRIEF COUNSELING

Michele Pich, MA, MS

KEY POINTS

- Care of a veterinary patient means that the veterinarian has at least two clients: the animal and the human companion(s).
- Taking the time to understand the role that body language, tone of voice, and approach play in effective communication can prevent misunderstandings and unnecessary upset in veterinary clients.
- By knowing what grief resources are available, veterinarians can better help their clients if and when difficult end-of-life decisions have to be made.
- If the client is kept informed of his or her options and the pet's prognosis, the decision-making process can be less adversarial and more like a partnership.

CLIENT COMMUNICATION

Client communication can be difficult when the veterinarian is managing critically ill animals. The veterinarian must explain the relevant medical information and possible diagnostic and therapeutic options in a way that clients can understand. When the individual characteristics of the pet owner are taken into consideration, pet care can be more individualized, and interactions with owners can be more effective and efficient.[1-3]

The Human-Animal Bond

The human-animal bond is a powerful force. It can help us through the most difficult times in our lives.[3] So what happens when there is a rupture in that bond? A break in the human-animal bond can occur for many reasons, the most obvious being death. Other sources of strain and loss can be divorce or separation, or moving (sometimes without being able to take a pet). Members of the armed forces may have periods of time when they are overseas or stationed where their pet cannot be with them. Other stressful times for the human-animal bond include those in which a pet's fate is in jeopardy because of cancer or another chronic illness, an unexpected accident, or behavioral issues such as biting or other concerns of danger. People tend to anthropomorphize and view their animals as a consistent source of social support, which makes the loss even more difficult to bear.[4]

Client Expectations

Clients expect to be given enough information to make an informed decision. The SPIKES six-step model involves paying attention to the setting and the perception, obtaining the invitation of the patient/client, conveying knowledge, expressing empathy, and summarizing the discussion to make sure the client and veterinary staff are partners in the decision-making process.[5] Even when the prognosis is not good, veterinary clients often want a concrete explanation of why one pet responded to a given treatment better than another.[6] The more the veterinarian can discuss the specific factors that make it more or less likely that an animal will experience success with treatment, the better the attending doctor can help a pet owner make an informed decision.[1]

End-of-Life Decisions

Most veterinary professionals understand the importance of and need for compassionate, humane euthanasia of pets that are suffering, but often clients have a more difficult time making this decision. Some clients may be against euthanasia, regardless of the situation, disease process, or prognosis. There are differing opinions about whether it is appropriate to tell clients outright that they need to euthanize their pet. There is often a sense of urgency regarding the need to prevent unnecessary suffering that must be carefully conveyed by a veterinarian, while taking into account the emotional needs of the client.[1] The loss of control associated with losing a pet is many times the most difficult. This is why enlisting the pet owner as much as possible as an informed decision maker in the care and disposition of terminally ill pets can help make the process of grieving progress more smoothly.[5,7]

Compassion Fatigue

Compassion fatigue can be defined as a feeling of not being able to give the best of oneself due to emotional and physical exhaustion from high stress and demanding situations at home or in the workplace, especially when caring for others. Some of the symptoms that can be associated with compassion fatigue are a feeling of numbness or disconnection with the situation, difficulty sleeping or excessive sleeping, isolation, and avoidance.[8,9]

Although anyone caring for an animal can be subject to compassion fatigue, caretakers of pets with stubborn medical problems that require a great deal of care and pets with conditions that result in a high euthanasia rate are especially vulnerable. Pet owners as well as veterinarians and veterinary staff can be especially susceptible.[8,9]

Support for veterinary staff

Veterinarians are often taught that those they work with are the patients or clients in need of care, but it is just as important for veterinarians, veterinary nurses, technicians, and other support staff to seek help as well when situations become too stressful for them. Compassion fatigue is a very real concern for people in any helping profession. Compassion fatigue can be felt by caretakers of humans or animals at home, as well as by those who care for others as a profession. Often the most compassionate individuals are drawn to helping professions, but they are also more susceptible to compassion fatigue and caretaker burnout.[9]

Communicating with Difficult Clients

The Bayer Animal Healthcare Project suggests remembering the acronym *ADOBE* when trying to communicate effectively with veterinary clients. ADOBE stand for acknowledgement of problems, discovering the meaning, opportunities for compassion, boundaries, and extending the system.[10] Nonverbal cues are also an important part of expressing to clients that one cares. A simple phone call, or looking a client in the eye, can make a world of difference to someone and help to prevent miscommunication with clients who are making difficult decisions. Empathizing and summarizing are two ways that a veterinary professional can protect against miscommunication and help build the rapport of a partnership.[10] When the goals and expectations of treatment are clarified in advance and along the way at different stages, better communication with clients can be achieved.[1,2,10] The value of effective communication extends to client satisfaction and even to professional reputation. By communicating clearly and interactively with clients, the veterinary professional can prevent unnecessary complaints, distress, and even lawsuits.[6]

Stages of Grief

Elizabeth Kübler-Ross identified the stages of grief as denial, anger, depression, bargaining, and finally acceptance.[11] Although this literature was initially designed to aid in dealing with human loss, much of it is relevant to the loss of a pet as well. Many people consider their pets to be a part of the family, so it makes sense that they experience many of the same emotions and feelings that people who have lost a human family member or friend experience.

If clients are in denial, they may not fully accept that their pet is terminally ill or even that the pet is deceased. They may continue to talk about their pets in the present tense and avoid people who may orient them to reality.

The anger stage of grieving is sometimes expressed as anger against oneself or anger against the one who gave the person bad news. Unfortunately, veterinarians are often on the receiving end of this anger. Some clients even yell or blame the veterinarian for their pet's death. Although no veterinarian should ever tolerate verbal abuse by clients, it can be helpful to understand that the anger being expressed may actually represent anger about the pet's outcome and displacement of that anger onto the veterinarian.[11]

Depression can be either chronic or acute. Often grieving veterinary clients feel an enormous amount of guilt for the outcome of their pet's care. In most cases, when there is a problem with a client's pet, the client is able to remedy it with actions (e.g., pet is hungry, so feed it; pet is ill, so take it to the vet). In the case of pet death, even if the outcome is that the pet is no longer suffering, the process of consciously accepting this often encounters a few roadblocks.

In the bargaining stage, clients sometimes brood over what they or someone else could have done differently to prevent the ultimate outcome of death.[12] They often focus on the idea that, had a certain thing not been done, the loss would not have occurred. Eventually most clients come to a point of acceptance in which they still miss and love the pet that has died but are able to remember and focus more on the good times with the pet.[11]

TYPES OF GRIEF

Anticipatory Grief

Anticipatory grief occurs when a pet is aging or ill. The pet owner may experience many of the symptoms of grief after loss.[12] Those going through anticipatory grief are often suffering from disenfranchised grief, which is discussed in more depth later in the chapter. Anticipatory grief has been described as "constantly waiting for the other shoe to drop" by several of the grief support clients at the

University of Pennsylvania School of Veterinary Medicine (Penn Vet). When pets or human family members are dying, the people in their lives may begin to disconnect emotionally from the ones dying as a way to prepare emotionally for life without them after they die.[12] This may manifest as a pet owner sounding apathetic or angry at the pet for symptoms or aspects of the pet's illness or condition.

Multiple Losses and "Trigger Grief"

Sometimes the loss of a pet can trigger a more intense grief reaction because the client associates it with the loss of another pet or a person that was important to the individual. Members of veterinary support groups say, for example, that caring for a pet with cancer might make them think about a time when their own parent was terminally ill. By being aware of this potential, veterinarians can better understand that complex emotions are involved in the decision-making and grieving processes. Empathizing with clients can help veterinarians better position themselves to educate clients about their options.[1]

Grief from Expected Loss

When a death is expected, mourning clients may experience many aspects of the grieving process when the pet is still alive through anticipatory grief (explored in more depth earlier in the chapter).[12] They may also have a more difficult time knowing exactly when is the right time to have a pet euthanized since they may have seen the pet make a partial or full recovery from extreme illness previously. There may be additional concerns about feeling the loss of community associated with frequent veterinary visits.

Grief from Unexpected Loss

Veterinarians who work in emergency settings are often charged with helping pet owners understand the severity of a pet's medical condition, while encouraging them to make painful decisions regarding expensive medical treatments that may or may not save the pet.[13] Emergency veterinarians also must deal with telling clients that euthanasia may be the best option for the pet while simultaneously building a rapport with a previously unfamiliar client.[5] By paying attention to the client's words, tone of voice, and body language, the veterinarian can make a better connection with the client in a relatively short period of time, which allows improved decision-making collaboration between physician and client.[10]

Disenfranchised Grief

Feeling alone in one's grieving is a very difficult place to be. Such feelings are common in older individuals and those who move around a lot or do not get out much. Many people feel that they are completely alone once their pet dies.[3] The experience of feeling that one does not have the right to grieve, also known as *disenfranchised grief,* can impede progress through the grieving process.[14] Each society and culture has its own expectations for those who are grieving, and it is important to keep in mind the differences in cultural influence.[15] Differences in religion, country of origin, age, and gender are a few of the things to keep in mind when trying to anticipate whether clients might experience disenfranchised grief.[16] This may even happen when clients try to reach out for help in general (non–animal-specific) bereavement support groups. People might feel that they do not have the right to express their sorrow and difficulty with the loss of their pets when others are grieving the loss of their human family members because they feel that pet loss sounds less important given societal standards.[3] Disenfranchisement of the griever can occur when the relationship was not recognized (e.g., due to attitudes about caring for a pet or failure to acknowledge it), which often happens with employers, friends, and family when a pet dies, or when the grieving person is excluded, either because of physical distance or lack of control or opportunity to grieve.[14,17]

Although the death of a pet is sometimes considered an acceptable form of loss to grieve, grieving for pet loss from other causes is not always recognized by people outside the animal care world.[3] Other forms of loss that are even less accepted by society as valid reasons to grieve, but that still cause a great deal of difficulty for those who experience them, are the loss of a pet through separation or divorce, military or housing displacement, and voluntary surrender of pets that cannot be suitably cared for.[3,14,17] When a pet lover learns of the loss of a pet that was being cared for by an ex-spouse there may be increased feelings of guilt and questions of why the death occurred and whether it could have been prevented if he or she had been present.[3]

COMPLICATING FACTORS

Financial Considerations

Most people do not like to think that money played a role in the treatment of a loved one. However, in reality, finances are often a consideration in deciding whether or not a pet should undergo major surgery or start an expensive treatment protocol, such as chemotherapy or radiation therapy, especially when a client cannot be guaranteed that the treatment will have a successful outcome for the pet.[2] This is why it is important to let clients know when different treatment options are available. Most clients would prefer to do something to help their pets, even if they cannot afford to do everything medically available.[6] Even if the prognosis is worse for a pet that receives a stepped-down level of care, the truth is that providing palliative care and pain management is better than providing no care at all because the owner could not afford it. Discussing money, although uncomfortable, is a necessary part of veterinary care.[2] It is better to discuss expected treatment cost estimates, and to update them as they evolve, to prevent surprises or feelings of unclear motivation. This is important for retention of clients.[2,6]

Mental Health History

Depression and other grief symptoms are not always mutually exclusive. Clients with previous mental health concerns may be more affected by pet loss than those without a history of mental health problems.[12] This history may not always be immediately apparent to the veterinarian. It is important to keep this in mind when working with difficult or seemingly irrational clients. Clients who have a history of depression or anxiety may be more likely to experience these feeling for a prolonged period when grieving significant loss, including loss of a pet. It is especially important to make sure that grieving veterinary clients are connected with sufficient support resources, whether it is a grief counselor, therapist, or, when appropriate, a psychiatrist.[12]

Children and Loss

A child's first experience with death is often the passing of a family pet. Children may not be able to verbalize their feelings when their pet dies. A variety of children's books and workbooks are available to parents who are helping their children cope with the realities and grief associated with pet loss. For example, the book *I'll Always Love You* by Hans Wilhelm[18] and the *My Pet Is Gone Workbook*[19] from the organization Chance's Spot can be quite helpful. Websites such as http://www.veterinarywisdomforpetparents.com have a variety of useful resources for parents as well. Some parents and professionals feel that it is better for the children to be present during a euthanasia experience, whereas others feel that it is better to find other ways for children to be involved in the decision making and memorializing of a pet.[1,3,17] In determining how to talk to a child about pet loss, one must consider the child's age and mental development level. For example, more detail will be given to a 10-year-old than to a

4-year-old. Children who are 3 or 4 years of age do not yet understand that death is permanent, whereas children aged 5 through 8 have a greater understanding of pet loss and will probably ask many more questions. Children aged 9 through 12 may talk most about the experience; teenagers may be more likely to internalize their pain in this loss.[17] The veterinarian may be asked to advise parents on how to talk to their children. Ideally, parents should be as honest as possible with children about the death of their pet because this can prevent backtracking and misunderstandings in the future. They should try to avoid euphemisms such as "put to sleep" or "went away." Otherwise, children may grow to fear sleeping at night or be afraid that if a parent goes away on a business trip he or she may not return either. Also, parents should allow children to ask questions and find individualized ways to express their grief (e.g., through drawings, paintings, poems, collages, songs). In addition, when parents are open about their own grief and sadness, children can learn what it means to grieve in an appropriate way and can realize that they do not need to hide their own feelings of sadness. Parents should also make sure to allow themselves time to grieve without feeling the need to put on a brave face for someone else all of the time.

Pet Loss and Older Adults

Many older adults are on fixed incomes and struggle to provide the best life they can for the pets they love while battling the burden of rising medical bills of their own and the limits of Social Security or pensions in the face of inflation. Older adults are particularly at risk of complications in grieving and disenfranchisement of their grief. Pets are often the only living family members that some senior citizens have, so the care of animal companions of older adults is of particular importance.[3,17] In addition, pets can serve as a form of physical therapy for older adults due to the tactile stimulation of petting and caring for an animal.[17]

VETERINARY RESOURCES

Resources available to veterinarians include the support of a veterinary grief counselor. At Penn Vet, counseling appointments are available for individuals, couples, and families, and there are support groups for those grieving the loss or impending loss of a pet. In addition, a Pet Grief Support Hotline that is staffed by trained veterinary students and overseen by Penn Vet's veterinary grief counselor has recently been launched.

Support Groups

A useful support tool for veterinarians is referral of grieving clients to veterinary support groups. One way for grieving pet owners to combat the loneliness associated with pet loss is to confront the disenfranchised grief by surrounding themselves with others going through something similar.[20] Some support groups focus on helping the pet owner be the best caretaker for a sick or aging pet, such as Cleo's Caregivers Group at Penn Vet. This group addresses issues such as logistical planning, the importance of self-care, available resources, and the need to reach out for support. Other groups focus on helping pet owners deal with all of the emotions and life changes associated with losing a pet. During a 2-year period from April 2010 to March 2012, 104 clients experiencing pet loss attended the Pet Grief Loss Support Group at Penn Vet, not including those who attended only Cleo's Caregivers' Group or participated only in individual counseling. Of those 104 clients, approximately 65% were female. These clients were grieving for 121 different pets; approximately 66% of these pets were dogs, 29% were cats, 2% were birds, 2% were rabbits, and 1% were rats. Group meetings included between 3 and 22 clients, and individual clients attended a mean of 2.74 meetings.

Individual Grief Support Sessions

Some clients experiencing the difficulties of pet loss prefer individual counseling sessions. As with support groups, some clients meet once or twice with the counselor, whereas others meet regularly for a while until they get used to the idea of living their lives without their pet physically by their side each day. The individual's contact with veterinary grief support can take the form of in-person sessions, telephone discussions, or email communications.

Lectures, Seminars, and Workshops

The University of Pennsylvania offers grief support lectures as part of its free Animal Lovers Lecture Series. The topics of these lectures include ruptures in the human-animal bond, grieving, healing, considering a new pet, and reaching out for support. In addition, the grief counselor also provides lectures to veterinary staff at Penn Vet and other veterinary offices on competent client communication, compassion fatigue, and end-of-life decision making, including euthanasia options.

HEALING THROUGH PET LOSS

Finding Meaning

If clients can find meaning in the loss of their pet, it may be easier for them to reach a place of acceptance and healing. Sometimes pet owners can find meaning by having their pet participate in research studies while the pet is alive or by donating the pet's body to support research and learning. Finding meaning when talking with a veterinary client can help prevent miscommunications and can aid in connecting with the client as a partner instead of an adversary.[10] Some clients prefer to use thought journals or become actively involved in causes related to the illness or issues of the pet they are grieving, such as canine cancer research. Others have used online blogging as an avenue of expression and healing from their loss. During the grieving period, clients are likely to call the veterinarian and ask detailed questions about their pet's care. Although this may be alarming or concerning to some veterinarians, it is often part of the healing process for the clients and may help them to make sense of their tragic loss.

Memorializing a Pet

Some veterinary offices offer mementos to clients whose pets have died, such as an ink or clay imprint of the pet's paw. This is a nice way to express to clients that their pet was an individual. Most pet owners prefer to have their pets cremated. Some pet owners select a group cremation in which the pet's ashes are not returned but may be spread at a local pet cemetery with ashes of other pets that have died. Some prefer to have the ashes returned to them, and others choose to take the body home and bury it without cremation. This latter option is not as common in recent years because of sanitary concerns, legal restrictions, and the limited options for relocating remains if the owner moves to another property.[21]

There are many ways of memorializing a pet that veterinarians can suggest to grieving pet owners. Moira Anderson Allen suggests creating a picture book or photo tribute, painting a portrait of the pet, or writing an online tribute.[21]

Many owners find closure in the loss of a pet by donating to a cause related to the pet. The donation may be in the form of money to a pet memorial fund, veterinary research study, or organization, or in the form of supplies to a local animal shelter, and provides a sense of purpose that can help ease the pain of those who struggle with losing a pet. Regardless of whether the donation is a one-time gift or a routine established for holidays, birthdays, or anniversaries, it can help clients find meaning, help others, and create positive feelings regarding their deceased loved one.

REFERENCES

1. Cornell KK, Kopcha M: Client-veterinarian communication: skills for client centered dialogue and shared decision making, Vet Clin North Am Small Anim Pract 37:37-47, 2007.
2. Klingborg DL, Klingborg J: Talking with veterinary clients about money, Vet Clin North Am Small Anim Pract 37:79-93, 2007.
3. Meyers B: Disenfranchised grief and the loss of a companion animal. In Doka KJ, editor: Disenfranchised grief: new directions, challenges, and strategies for practice, Champaign, Ill, 2002, Research Press.
4. Serpell JA: Anthropomorphism and anthropomorphic selection: beyond the "cute response," Soc Anim 10:4, 2002.
5. Shaw JR, Lagoni L: End-of-life communication in veterinary medicine: delivering bad news and euthanasia decision making, Vet Clin North Am Small Anim Pract 37:95-108, 2007.
6. O'Connell D, Bonvicini KA: Addressing disappointment in veterinary practice, Vet Clin North Am Small Anim Pract 37:135-149, 2007.
7. Abood SK: Increasing adherence in practice: making your clients partners in care, Vet Clin North Am Small Anim Pract 37:151-164, 2007.
8. Cohen SP: Compassion fatigue and the veterinary health team, Vet Clin North Am Small Anim Pract 37:123-134, 2007.
9. Stamm BH: Comprehensive bibliography of the effect of caring for those who have experienced extremely stressful events and suffering, 2010. Available at http://www.proqol.org. Accessed June 26, 2012.
10. Morrisey JK, Voiland B: Difficult interactions with veterinary clients: working in the challenge zone, Vet Clin North Am Small Anim Pract 37:65-77, 2007.
11. Kübler-Ross E: On death and dying, London, 1969, Tavistock.
12. Worden JW: Grief counseling and grief therapy, a handbook for the mental health practitioner, ed 4, New York, 2009, Springer.
13. Bateman SW: Communication in the veterinary emergency setting, Vet Clin North Am Small Anim Pract 37:109-121, 2007.
14. Dolka KJ: Introduction. In Doka KJ, editor: Disenfranchised grief: new directions, challenges, and strategies for practice, Champaign, Ill, 2002, Research Press.
15. Sue D, Sue S: Counseling the culturally diverse, ed 6, Hoboken, NJ, 2008, John Wiley & Sons.
16. Dolka JK, Martin TL: How we grieve: culture, class, and gender. In Doka KJ, editor: Disenfranchised grief—new directions, challenges, and strategies for practice, Champaign, Ill, 2002, Research Press.
17. Brandt JC, Grabill CM: Communicating with special populations: children and older adults, Vet Clin North Am Small Anim Pract 37:181-198, 2007.
18. Wilhelm H: I'll always love you, New York, 1985, Crown Publishers.
19. Chance's Spot, Pet Loss and Support Resources: My pet is gone workbook. Available at http://chancesspot.com. Accessed September 12, 2012.
20. McKeon Pesek E: The role of support groups in disenfranchised grief. In Doka KJ, editor: Disenfranchised grief: new directions, challenges, and strategies for practice, Champaign, Ill, 2002, Research Press.
21. Anderson Allen M: Coping with sorrow on the loss of your pet, ed 3, Indianapolis, Ind, 2011, Dog Ear Publishing.

APPENDICES

Appendix 1 Clinical Calculations

Parameter	Formula	Normal Values*
Cardiovascular Parameters		
Arterial oxygen content	CaO_2 (ml/dl) = (Hb [g/dl] × 1.34 × SaO_2) + (PaO_2 [mm Hg] × 0.003)	19-21 ml/dl
Cardiac output	SV (ml/beat/kg) × HR (beats/min)	125-200 ml/kg/min (dog) 200 ml/kg/min (cat)
Cardiac index	CI (ml/kg/min) = CO (ml/min) ÷ BW (kg) CI (L/m^2/min) = CO (L/min) ÷ Body surface area (m^2)	120-200 ml/kg/min 3.5-5.5 L/min/m^2
Oxygen delivery	DO_2 (ml/kg/min) = CI (ml/kg/min) × CaO_2	20-35 ml/kg/min
Oxygen consumption (from Fick equation)	$\dot{V}O_2$ (ml/kg/min) = CO (ml/kg/min) × (CaO_2 − $CmvO_2$)	4-11 ml/kg/min
Oxygen extraction ratio	OER (%) = (CaO_2 − $CmvO_2$) ÷ CaO_2	20%-30%
Systemic vascular resistance	SVR (mm Hg/ml/kg/min) = (MAP − CVP) ÷ CI (ml/kg/min) SVR (dynes · sec/cm^5) = ([MAP − CVP] × 79.9) ÷ CI (L/min/m^2)	0.5-0.8 mm Hg/ml/kg/min 1600-2500 dynes.sec.cm^{-5}
Pulmonary vascular resistance	PVR (mm Hg/ml/kg/min) = (PAP − PAOP) ÷ CI (ml/kg/min) PVR (dynes · sec/cm^5) = ([PAP − PAOP] × 79.9) ÷ CI (L/min/m^2)	0.04-0.06 mm Hg/ml/kg/min 125-250 dynes.sec.cm^{-5}
Stroke volume	SV (ml/beat/kg) = CI (ml/kg/min) ÷ HR SV (ml/beat/m^2) = CI (ml/min/m^2) ÷ HR	1.5-2.5 ml/beat/kg 40-60 ml/beat/m^2
Mean arterial blood pressure	MAP (mm Hg) = ([Systolic BP − Diastolic BP] ÷ 3) + Diastolic BP	Dogs = 80-120 mm Hg Cats = 100-150 mm Hg
Oxygen-Related Parameters		
Alveolar air equation	P_AO_2 (mm Hg) = FiO_2 (P_B − P_{H2O}) − ($PaCO_2$ ÷ RQ)	Depends on FiO_2 and barometric pressure FiO_2 = 0-1 P_{H2O} = 50 mm Hg RQ = 0.8-1
A-a gradient	A-a (mm Hg) = P_AO_2 − PaO_2	Depends on FiO_2 Normal < 15 mm Hg with FiO_2 0.21
PaO_2/FiO_2 ratio	P/F = PaO_2 (mm Hg) ÷ FiO_2 (0–1)	500
Shunt equation	Qs/Qt (%) = (CcO_2 − CaO_2) ÷ (CcO_2 − $CmvO_2$)	<5%
Physiologic dead space	Vd/Vt = ($PaCO_2$ − P_ECO_2) ÷ $PaCO_2$	Normal values (dogs): <40% (spontaneous breathing), <50% (positive pressure ventilation) NOTE: $ETCO_2$ can be used instead of P_ECO_2 for clinical measurements of Vd/Vt, but this may not be accurate in all clinical scenarios (normal dog < 24%)

*Normal values can vary depending on several factors including the laboratory performing the measurements, the method used to obtain the measurements, and the species. Normal values listed here are for dogs (unless noted otherwise) and may differ for feline patients.

Continued

Appendix 1 Clinical Calculations—cont'd

Parameter	Formula	Normal Values*
Fluids and Acid-Base		
Daily maintenance fluid rate	$70 \times BW\ (kg)^{0.75}$ (ml/day) or 2-4 ml/kg/hr	Exponential formula based on body surface area and recommended for use in dogs and cats with body weight <2 kg or >40 kg
Calculated osmolarity	Calculated osmolarity (mOsm/L) = 2(Na) + (BUN [mg/dl] ÷ 2.8) + (Glucose [mg/dl] ÷ 18)	BUN and glucose measured as mg/dl
Osmole gap	Osmole gap (mOsm/L) = measured osmolality − calculated osmolarity	Using the formula given here for calculated osmolarity the expected osmole gap for dogs = 0 to 1 and cats = 2
Anion gap	AG (mmol/L) = (Na + K) − (HCO_3 + Cl)	
Total body water	TBW (L) = 0.6 × BW (kg)	
Free water deficit	Free water deficit (ml) = TBW × ([Na measured ÷ Na normal] − 1)	
Nutrition		
Resting energy requirement	RER (kcal/day) = $70 \times BW\ (kg)^{0.75}$	

A-a, Alveolar-arterial gradient; *AG*, anion gap; *BP*, blood pressure; *BUN*, blood urea nitrogen; *BW*, body weight; *CaO_2*, arterial oxygen content; *CcO_2*, end capillary (pulmonary) oxygen content; *CI*, cardiac index; *CO*, cardiac output; *$CmvO_2$*, mixed venous oxygen content; *CVP*, central venous pressure; *DO_2*, oxygen delivery; $ETCO_2$, end-tidal carbon dioxide; P_ECO_2, mixed exhaled carbon dioxide; *FiO_2*, fraction of inspired oxygen; *Hb*, hemoglobin; *HCO_3*, bicarbonate; *HR*, heart rate; *K*, potassium; *MAP*, mean arterial blood pressure; *Na*, sodium; *O_2*, oxygen; *OER*, oxygen extraction ratio; *$PaCO_2$*, partial pressure of arterial carbon dioxide; *P_AO_2*, partial pressure of alveolar oxygen; *PaO_2*, partial pressure of arterial oxygen; *PAOP*, pulmonary artery occlusion pressure; *PAP*, pulmonary artery pressure; *P_B*, barometric pressure; *P/F*, PaO_2/FiO_2 ratio; *P_{H2O}*, water vapor pressure; *PVR*, pulmonary vascular resistance; *Qs/Qt*, percent of pulmonary arteriovenous shunt; *RER*, resting energy requirement; *RQ*, respiratory quotient; *SaO_2*, arterial oxygen saturation; *SV*, stroke volume; *SVR*, systemic vascular resistance; *TBW*, total body water; *$\dot{V}O_2$*, oxygen consumption.

Appendix 2 Important Physiologic Formulas

Name	Formulas	Comment
Fick equation	$Q = \dot{V}O_2 \div (CaO_2 - CmvO_2)$	
Henderson-Hasselbalch equation for carbonic acid	$pH = 6.1 + Log([HCO_3^-] \div [PCO_2 \times 0.03])$ HCO_3^- measured in mmol/L or mEq/L and PCO_2 measured in mm Hg	
Laplace's law	$P = 2t \div r$	
Modified Bernoulli	$\Delta P = 4V^2$	Used to estimate pulmonary artery pressure on echocardiography
Ohm's law	$Q = \Delta P \div R$	
Poiseuille's law	$Resistance = 8\,\eta l \div 2\pi R^4$	Can combine with Ohm's law to solve for flow (Q)
Reynolds number	$Re = (D \times \rho \times V) \div \eta$	<2000 likely laminar flow >2000 likely turbulent flow
Wall stress	$\sigma \propto (P \times R) \div 2t$	Peak ventricular systolic wall stress is a measure of afterload

CaO_2, arterial oxygen content; *$CmvO_2$*, mixed venous oxygen content; *ΔP*, change in pressure; *D*, diameter; *L*, length; *η*, viscosity; *ρ*, density; *P*, pressure; *Q*, flow (e.g., cardiac output); *r*, radius; *R*, resistance; *t*, wall thickness; *V*, velocity; *$\dot{V}O_2$*, oxygen consumption.

Appendix 3 Ideal Gas Laws

General gas law	$PV = RT$	
Boyle's law	$P_1V_1 = P_2V_2$	
Charles' law	$V_1 \div T_1 = V_2 \div T_2$	
Dalton's law	$P_{total} = P_1 + P_2 + P_3 \ldots\ldots$	NOTE: P here represents gas partial pressure.
Fick's law of diffusion	$J = A/t \times D \times (P_1 - P_2)$	NOTE: P here represents gas partial pressure.

A, Area of tissue gas is diffusing across; *D,* diffusivity measured in length over time; *J,* amount of substance that will diffuse over time; *P,* gas pressure; P_{total}, total pressure of (nonreactive) gas mixture; $P_1+P_2+P_3\ldots\ldots$, partial pressure of individual gases; *R,* gas constant (0.08206 atm·L/mol·K); *t,* thickness of tissue gas is diffusing across; *T,* temperature; *V,* gas volume.

Appendix 4 Surviving Sepsis Campaign 2012 Bundle Recommendations for Humans

To be Completed Within 3 Hours

1. Measure lactate level
2. Obtain blood cultures before administration of antimicrobials
3. Administer broad-spectrum antimicrobials
4. Administer 30 ml/kg isotonic crystalloids intravenously for hypotension or lactate ≥ 4 mmol/L

To be Completed Within 6 Hours

5. Administer vasopressors (for hypotension that does not respond to initial fluid resuscitation) to maintain a mean arterial pressure (MAP) ≥ 65 mm Hg
6. In the event of persistent arterial hypotension despite volume resuscitation (septic shock) or initial lactate ≥ 4 mmol/L (36 mg/dl):
   - Measure central venous pressure (CVP)*
   - Measure central venous oxygen saturation ($S_{CV}O_2$)*
7. Remeasure lactate if initial lactate was elevated*

*Targets for quantitative resuscitation included in the guidelines are CVP of ≥ 8 mm Hg, $S_{CV}O_2$ of ≥70%, and normalization of lactate.

Modified from Dellinger RP, Levy MM, Rhodes A, et al: Surviving Sepsis campaign: international guidelines for management of severe sepsis and septic shock: 2012, *Crit Care Med* 41:580, 2013.

Appendix 5 Constant Rate Infusion Calculations

Micrograms per Kilogram per Minute

$$\frac{\text{Drug dosage rate (mcg/kg/min)} \times \text{Body weight (kg)} \times \text{Volume of fluid (ml)}}{\text{Delivery rate (ml/min)} \times 1000} = \text{Number of mg to add to the volume of fluids}$$

Milligrams per Kilogram per Hour (Using 250 ml bag of fluids)

$$\frac{\text{Drug dosage rate (mg/kg/hr)} \times \text{Body weight (kg)} \times 25\ \text{(hr)}}{\text{Concentration of drug (mg/ml)}} = \text{Volume of drug (ml) to add to a 250-ml bag of fluids and run at 10 ml/hr}$$

Appendix 6 Common Drug Dosages for Constant Rate Infusions

Drug	Intravenous CRI Dosage	Comment
ε-Aminocaproic acid	Loading dose: 50 mg/kg over first hour followed by 15 mg/kg/hr for 5-8 hr	This dose is extrapolated from the human dose for dogs; use in cats is uncertain
Atracurium besylate	Loading dose: 0.2-0.3 mg/kg 4-9 mcg/kg/min	Requires PPV Provides no analgesia
Butorphanol	Loading dose: 0.2-0.4 mg/kg 0.1-0.4 mg/kg/hr	
Calcium gluconate 10%	50-150 mg/kg (0.5-1.5 ml/kg) 5-15 mg/kg/hr (0.05-0.15 ml/kg/hr)	Continuous ECG monitoring recommended
Dexmedetomidine	Loading dose: 0.5-3 mcg/kg 0.5-3 mcg/kg/hr	Can still have adverse cardiovascular effects at these low doses
Diazepam	0.2-1 mg/kg/hr	Administer via central vein; will adsorb to plastic Can see propylene glycol toxicity with prolonged infusions
Diltiazem	Loading dose: 0.15-0.25 mg/kg slowly IV 5-20 mcg/kg/min	
Dobutamine	Dogs: 2-20 mcg/kg/min Cats: 1-5 mcg/kg/min	Continuous ECG monitoring recommended
Dopamine	Low: 1-4 mcg/kg/min Mid: 5-10 mcg/kg/min High: 10-20 mcg/kg/min	Extravasation may cause necrosis Targets dopamine receptors at low doses, β receptors in midrange doses, and α receptors with higher doses
Epinephrine	0.005-1 mcg/kg/min	Potent α and β agonist
Esmolol	Loading dose: 0.05-0.1 mg/kg 50-200 mcg/kg/min	Can cause hypotension
Fentanyl	Loading dose: 1-5 mcg/kg IV Analgesia: 0.05-0.3 mcg/kg/min Anesthesia: Dogs: 0.3-1.5 mcg/kg/min Cats: 0.15-0.7 mcg/kg/min	Use lower loading dose for analgesia May require PPV with higher dosages
Furosemide	Loading dose: 0.5-1 mg/kg 0.1-1 mg/kg/hr	
Glucagon	5 ng/kg/min	Titrate to effect; —treatment for refractory hypoglycemia NOTE: This dose is in nanograms/kg/min
Heparin (unfractionated)	Loading dose: 100 U/kg 25-50 U/kg/hr	Adjust dose to target aPTT or anti-Xa levels
Hydrocortisone	0.25-0.3 mg/kg/day	For pressor refractory septic shock
Hydromorphone	Loading dose: 0.05 mg/kg IV 0.01-0.05 mg/kg/hr	
Regular insulin	2.2 U/kg/day	Monitor blood glucose Will adsorb to plastic, so flush 50 ml of infusion solution through infusion line prior to administration
Isoproterenol	0.04-0.08 mcg/kg/min	May cause hypotension
Ketamine	Loading dose: 1 mg/kg 0.1-1 mg/kg/hr	
Lidocaine	Dog: Loading dose: 2-4 mg/kg slow 25-80 mcg/kg/min Cat: Loading dose: 0.25-0.75 mg/kg slow 10-40 mcg/kg/min	Use with caution in cats
Magnesium sulphate	0.3 to 1 mEq/kg/day	Treatment of hypomagnesemia NOTE: This is not the antiarrhythmic dose
Mannitol	1-2 mg/kg/min Loading dose: 0.25-1 g/kg over 20-30 minutes	Use of in-line filter recommended
Metoclopramide	1-2 mg/kg/24h	Can cause behavior changes (extrapyramidal signs) Higher doses necessary for promotility effects
Midazolam	0.1-0.5 mg/kg/hr	
Milrinone	Loading dose: 30-300 mcg/kg 1-10 mcg/kg/min	

Appendix 6 Common Drug Dosages for Constant Rate Infusions—cont'd

Drug	Intravenous CRI Dosage	Comment
Morphine sulfate	Loading dose: 0.2 mg/kg IM or slow IV Dogs: 0.1-1 mg/kg/hr Cats: 0.1-0.3 mg/kg/hr	IV doses should be given slowly to avoid causing histamine release May require PPV at higher dosages
Nicardipine	0.5-5 mcg/kg/min	
Nitroprusside	0.5-10 mcg/kg/min	Requires constant blood pressure monitoring
Norepinephrine	0.05-3 mcg/kg/min	Primarily α agonist
Pentobarbital	0.2-5 mg/kg/hr	May require PPV
Phentolamine	Loading dose: 0.05-0.1 mcg/kg 5-30 mcg/kg/min	
Phenylephrine	1-3 mcg/kg/min	Pure α agonist
Phosphate	0.01-0.12 mmol/kg/hr	Requires serum phosphorus and calcium monitoring
Procainamide	Loading dose: 6-8 mg/kg IV over 5 minutes titrated until arrhythmia controlled (this dose maybe repeated) 10-40 mcg/kg/min	Dogs only
Propofol	Induction dose: 1-6 mg/kg 0.05-0.4 mg/kg/min	May require PPV
Pyridostigmine	0.01-0.03 mg/kg/hr	
Sufentanil	0.1 mcg/kg/min	Loading dose: 1-2 mcg/kg
Tissue plasminogen activator (tPA)	Cats: 0.25-1 mg/kg/hr IV for a total dosage of 1-10 mg/kg Dogs: 1 mg/kg administered intravenously over 60 minutes	Watch closely for bleeding complications
Tranexamic acid	Loading dose: 10-15 mg/kg slow 1 mg/kg/hr for 5-8 hours	
Vasopressin	1-5 mU/kg/min	For treatment of vasoplegia
Verapamil	0.05-0.15 mg/kg IV 2-10 mcg/kg/min	

aPTT, Activated partial thromboplastin time; *CRI,* constant rate infusion; *ECG,* electrocardiogram; *IM,* intramuscular; *IV,* intravenous; *PPV,* positive pressure ventilation.

NOTE: Many of the drugs and doses included in this table are off-label and require clinician discretion. Owner consent is advised.

INDEX

Page numbers followed by "f" indicate figures, "t" indicate tables, and "b" indicate boxes.

E

F

G

H

Common Conversion Factors

Units Given	Units Wanted	Formula for Conversion
mmol/L	mg/dl	mg/dl = [(mmol/l) × MW] / 10
mg/dl	mmol/L	mmol/L = (mg/dL × 10) / MW
mmol/L	mEq/L	mEq/L = mmol/L × valence
mEq/L	mmol/L	mmol/L = (mEq/L) / valence
%	mg/ml	mg/ml = % × 10
cm	inches	inches = cm × 0.3937
inches	cm	cm = inches × 2.54
°C	°F	°F = °C × (9/5) + 32
°F	°C	°C = (°F − 32) × (5/9)

MW, Molecular weight (mg/mmol) (the sum of the atomic weights of a molecule or compound).

Weight-Unit Conversion Factors

1 lb = 0.4536 kg
1 kg = 2.2046 lb
1 kg = 1000 g
1 kg = 1,000,000 mg
1 g = 1000 mg
1 g = 1,000,000 mcg
1 mg = 1000 mcg
1 oz = 28.35 g
1 g/100 ml = 100%
1 ml water = 1 g

Conversion of Body Weight to Body Surface Area for Cats

kg	m^2
0.50	0.06
1.00	0.10
1.50	0.12
2.00	0.15
2.50	0.17
3.00	0.20
3.50	0.22
4.00	0.24
4.50	0.26
5.00	0.28
5.50	0.29
6.00	0.31
6.50	0.33
7.00	0.34
7.50	0.36
8.00	0.38
8.50	0.39
9.00	0.41
9.50	0.42
10.00	0.44

From Ford RB, Mazzaferro EM: Kirk and Bistner's handbook of veterinary procedures and emergency treatment, ed 8, St Louis, 2006, Saunders Elsevier.

Conversion of Body Weight to Body Surface Area for Dogs

kg	m^2	kg	m^2
0.50	0.06	26.00	0.88
1.00	0.10	27.00	0.90
2.00	0.15	28.00	0.92
3.00	0.20	29.00	0.94
4.00	0.25	30.00	0.96
5.00	0.29	31.00	0.99
6.00	0.33	32.00	1.01
7.00	0.36	33.00	1.03
8.00	0.40	34.00	1.05
9.00	0.43	35.00	1.07
10.00	0.46	36.00	1.09
11.00	0.49	37.00	1.11
12.00	0.52	38.00	1.13
13.00	0.55	39.00	1.15
14.00	0.58	40.00	1.17
15.00	0.60	41.00	1.19
16.00	0.63	42.00	1.21
17.00	0.66	43.00	1.23
18.00	0.69	44.00	1.25
19.00	0.71	45.00	1.26
20.00	0.74	46.00	1.28
21.00	0.76	47.00	1.30
22.00	0.78	48.00	1.32
23.00	0.81	49.00	1.34
24.00	0.83	50.00	1.36
25.00	0.85		

From Ford RB, Mazzaferro EM: Kirk and Bistner's handbook of veterinary procedures and emergency treatment, ed 8, St Louis, 2006, Saunders Elsevier.

Metric Conversions and Abbreviations

Prefix	Number	Weights	Volumes	Lengths
pico	1/1,000,000,000,000	Picogram	Picoliter (pl))	Picometer (pm)
nano	1/1,000,000,000	Nanogram	Nanoliter (nl)	Nanometer (nm)
micro	1/1,000,000	Microgram (mcg)	Microliter (μl)	Micron (μm)
milli	1/1000	Milligram (mg)	Milliliter (ml)	Millimeter (mm)
centi	1/100	Centigram (cg)	Centiliter (cl)	Centimeter (cm)
deci	1/10	Decigram (dg)	Deciliter (dl)	Decimeter (dm)
No prefix	1	Gram (g)	Liter (L)	Meter (m)
kilo	× 1000	Kilogram (kg)	Kiloliter (kl)	Kilometer (km)

Conversion Factors

Metric Unit	US Customary Units
1 milligram	= 1/65 grain
1 gram	= 15.43 grains
1 kilogram	= 2.20 pounds
1 milliliter	= 16.23 minims
1 liter	= 1.06 quarts = 33.80 fluid ounces
1 grain	= 0.065 g
1 dram	= 3.9 g
1 ounce	= 31.1 g
1 minim	= 0.062 ml
1 fluid dram	= 3.7 ml
1 fluid ounce	= 29.57 ml
1 pint	= 473.2 ml
1 quart	= 946.4 ml

Figures in parentheses are commonly employed approximate values.
From Bonagura JD: Kirk's current veterinary therapy XIII: small animal practice, Philadelphia, 2000, Saunders.

Catheter, Wire, and Tubing Size Measurements

Gauge	Approximate External Diameter (mm)	Approximate External Diameter (in)	French Gauge*
30	0.305	0.012	
29	0.330	0.013	1
28	0.356	0.014	
27	0.406	0.016	
26	0.457	0.018	
25	0.508	0.020	
24	0.559	0.222	
23	0.635	0.025	
22	0.711	0.028	2
21	0.813	0.032	
20	0.902	0.035	
19	1.067	0.042	3
18	1.270	0.050	4
17	1.473	0.058	
16	1.651	0.065	5
15	1.829	0.072	
14	2.108	0.083	6
13	2.413	0.095	7
12	2.769	0.109	
11	3.048	0.120	
10	3.404	0.134	

*French Gauge = 3 × external diameter in mm.